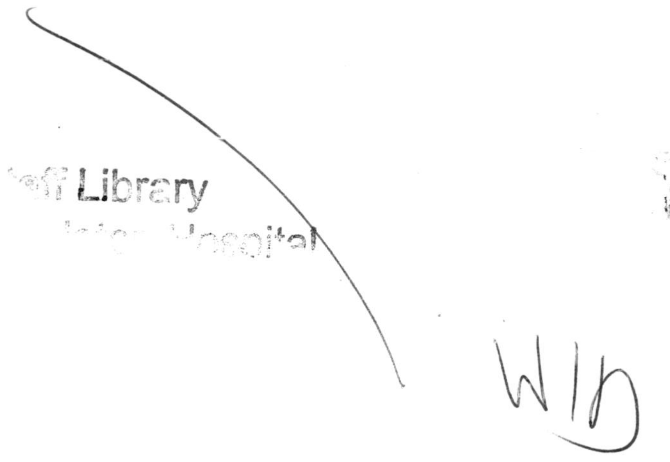
Library

FITZPATRICK'S

DERMATOLOGY IN GENERAL MEDICINE

SIXTH EDITION

IRWIN M. FREEDBERG, MD

George Miller MacKee Professor and Chairman
The Ronald O. Perelman Department of Dermatology
New York University Medical Center
New York, New York

ARTHUR Z. EISEN, MD

The Emma Showman Professor of Dermatology
Program Director, Chief Emeritus
Division of Dermatology
Washington University School of Medicine
St. Louis, Missouri

KLAUS WOLFF, MD, FRCP

Professor and Chairman, Department of Dermatology
University of Vienna Medical School
Vienna General Hospital
Vienna, Austria

K. FRANK AUSTEN, MD

AstraZeneca Professor of Respiratory and Inflammatory Diseases
Department of Medicine
Harvard Medical School
Brigham and Women's Hospital
Boston, Massachusetts

LOWELL A. GOLDSMITH, MD

Professor of Dermatology
University of North Carolina School of Medicine
Chapel Hill, North Carolina
Dean Emeritus
University of Rochester School of Medicine and Dentistry
Rochester, New York

STEPHEN I. KATZ, MD, PhD

Director, National Institute of Arthritis and Musculoskeletal and Skin Diseases
National Institutes of Health
Bethesda, Maryland

FITZPATRICK'S

DERMATOLOGY IN GENERAL MEDICINE

SIXTH EDITION

EDITORS

IRWIN M. FREEDBERG, MD
ARTHUR Z. EISEN, MD
KLAUS WOLFF, MD, FRCP
K. FRANK AUSTEN, MD
LOWELL A. GOLDSMITH, MD
STEPHEN I. KATZ, MD, PhD

VOLUME 1

McGRAW-HILL
Medical Publishing Division

New York Chicago San Francisco Lisbon
London Madrid Mexico City Milan New Delhi
San Juan Seoul Singapore Sydney Toronto

Note: Dr. Stephen Katz's work as editor and author was performed outside the scope of his employment as a U.S. government employee. This work represents his personal and professional views and not necessarily those of the U.S. government.

FITZPATRICK'S DERMATOLOGY IN GENERAL MEDICINE
Sixth Edition

1234567890 KGPKGP 09876543

Set: ISBN 0-07-138076-0
Volume I: ISBN 0-07-138066-3
Volume II: ISBN 0-07-138067-1

This book was set in Times Roman by TechBooks, Inc. The editors were Darlene Cooke, Susan R. Noujaim, Lisa Silverman, and Peter J. Boyle; the production supervisor was Richard Ruzycka; the cover designer was Elizabeth Pisacreta; Barbara Littlewood prepared the index. Quebecor World Kingsport.

This book is printed on acid-free paper.

Library of Congress Cataloging-in-Publication Data
Fitzpatrick's dermatology in general medicine.—6th ed. /
Irwin M. Freedberg . . . [et al.]
p. ; cm.
Includes bibliographical references and index.
ISBN 0-07-138076-0
1. Dermatology. 2. Skin–Diseases. 3. Cutaneous manifestations of general diseases. I. Fitzpatrick, Thomas B. (Thomas Bernard), 1919– II. Freedberg, Irwin M.
[DNLM: 1. Skin Diseases. 2. Skin Manifestations. WR 140 F5593 2003]
RL71.D46 2003
616.5—dc21 2002021932

CONTENTS

PART FOUR

Dermatology and Medicine

SECTION 26 SKIN MANIFESTATIONS OF RHEUMATOLOGIC MULTISYSTEM DISEASES 1677

SECTION 27 SKIN MANIFESTATIONS OF DISEASES IN OTHER ORGAN SYSTEMS 1777

PART FIVE

Diseases Due to Microbial Agents, Infestations, Bites, and Stings

CONTRIBUTORS

Steffen Albrecht, MD, FRCPC

Department of Pathology, The Sir Mortimer B. Davis—Jewish General Hospital and McGill University, Montreal, Quebec, Canada (107)

Honnavara N. Ananthaswamy, PhD

Ashbel Smith Professor and Deputy Chairman, Department of Immunology, The University of Texas M.D. Anderson Cancer Center, Houston, Texas (38)

Karl H. Anders, MD

Chief of Pathology and Director of Laboratories, Department of Pathology, Southern California Permanente Medical Group, Associate Clinical Professor of Pathology and Laboratory Medicine, UCLA School of Medicine, Woodland Hills, California (111)

Richard Rox Anderson, MD

Associate Professor of Dermatology, Harvard Medical School, Massachusetts General Hospital, Boston, Massachusetts (267)

Elliot J. Androphy, MD

Professor and Vice Chair of Research, Barbara and Nathan Greenberg Chair in Biomedical Research, University of Massachusetts Medical School, Worcester, Massachusetts (221, 223)

Grant J. Anhalt, MD

Professor of Dermatology and Pathology, Johns Hopkins Medical Institutions, Baltimore, Maryland (60, 262)

John C. Ansel, MD

Professor and Chairman, Department of Dermatology, Northwestern University Medical School, Chicago, Illinois (20)

Cheryl A. Armstrong, MD

Associate Professor, Department of Dermatology, Northwestern University Medical School, Chicago, Illinois (20)

Kenneth A. Arndt, MD

Professor of Dermatology, Harvard Medical School, Adjunct Professor of Medicine, Dartmouth Medical School, SkinCare Physicians of Chestnut Hill, Chestnut Hill, Massachusetts (271)

Eva Åsbrink, MD, PhD

Associate Professor of Dermatology, Karolinska Institutet at Stockholm Soder Hospital, Stockholm, Sweden (203)

K. Frank Austen, MD

AstraZeneca Professor of Respiratory and Inflammatory Diseases, Department of Medicine, Harvard Medical School, Brigham and Women's Hospital, Boston, Massachusetts (32)

Howard P. Baden, MD

Professor of Dermatology, Department of Dermatology, Cutaneous Biology Research Center, Harvard Medical School, Massachusetts General Hospital, Charlestown, Massachusetts (45, 54, 248)

Lynn A. Baden, MD

Clinical Instructor in Dermatology, Harvard Medical School, Boston, Massachusetts (248)

Philippe Bahadoran, MD

Assistant Professor of Dermatology, Nice University School of Medicine, Nice, France (89, 90)

Maryam Banikazemi, MD

Assistant Professor, Department of Human Genetics, Mount Sinai School of Medicine, New York, New York (151)

Robert Baran, MD

Nail Disease Center, Cannes, France (72, 280)

Raymond L. Barnhill, MD

Chair and Professor of Dermatology and Pathology, Division of Dermatology, The George Washington University School of Medicine, Washington, District of Columbia (93)

Eugene A. Bauer, MD

Department of Dermatology, Stanford University School of Medicine, Stanford, California, (65)

Lisa A. Beck, MD

Assistant Professor of Dermatology and Medicine, Department of Dermatology, Johns Hopkins Medical Institutions; Johns Hopkins Asthma and Allergy Center, Baltimore, Maryland (30)

Michael H. Beck, MD

Honorary Associate Lecturer in Dermatology in the Department of Medicine, University of Manchester School of Medicine, Hope Hospital, Salford, Lancs, England (129)

Ysabel M. Bello, MD

Dermatology Resident, Department of Dermatology and Cutaneous Surgery, University of Miami School of Medicine, Miami, Florida (272)

Donald V. Belsito, MD

Professor and Director, Division of Dermatology, University of Kansas Medical Center, Kansas City, Kansas (120, 121)

Col. Paul M. Benson, MD

Associate Professor, Uniformed Services University of the Health Sciences; Walter Reed Army Medical Center, Washington, District of Columbia (245)

Timothy G. Berger, MD

Professor of Clinical Dermatology, Department of Dermatology, University of California, San Francisco, San Francisco, California (198)

Jeffrey D. Bernhard, MD

Professor of Medicine, Chief, Division of Dermatology, UMass Memorial Medical Center, Worcester, Massachusetts (3)

Arthur P. Bertolino, MD, PhD

Professor and Director, Division of Dermatology, Ohio State University Medical Center, Columbus, Ohio (12)

David R. Bickers, MD

Carl Truman Nelson Professor and Chair, Department of Dermatology, Columbia University, College of Physicians and Surgeons, New York, New York (149)

Michael Bigby, MD

Assistant Professor of Dermatology, Harvard Medical School, Beth Israel Deaconess Medical Center, Boston, Massachusetts (240)

Clifton O. Bingham, III, MD

Assistant Professor of Medicine, New York University School of Medicine, Director, Ambulatory Clinical Research Center, New York, New York (32)

Alf Björnberg, MD

Associate Professor of Dermatology, Department of Dermatology, University of Lund, University Hospital, Lund, Sweden (46)

Andrew Blauvelt, MD

Investigator, Dermatology Branch, Center for Cancer Research, National Cancer Institute, National Institutes of Health, Bethesda, Maryland (119)

Mark Boguniewicz, MD

Division of Pediatric Allergy/Immunology National Jewish Medical and Research Center, Department of Pediatrics, University of Colorado Health Sciences Center, Denver, Colorado (122)

Mark W. Bonner, MD

Staff Dermatologist, Dermatology Clinic, Womack Army Medical Center, Fort Bragg, North Carolina (245)

Irwin M. Braverman, MD

Professor of Dermatology, Yale University School of Medicine, New Haven, Connecticut (183)

Francisco Bravo, MD

Auxiliary Professor of Dermatology and Pathology, Universidad Peruana Cayetano Heredia, Miraflores, Lima, Peru (198)

Stephen Michael Breathnach, MD, PhD, FRCP

Consultant Dermatologist and Senior Lecturer, St. John's Institute of Dermatology, St. Thomas's Hospital, London, United Kingdom (148)

Robert A. Briggaman, MD

Professor and Chair Emeritus, Department of Dermatology, University of North Carolina at Chapel Hill, Chapel Hill, North Carolina (66)

Harold J. Brody, MD

Clinical Professor of Dermatology, Emory University School of Medicine, Atlanta, Georgia (269)

Douglas B. Brown, PhD

Research Scientist, DakDak Photoaging Technologies Division, Charles River Laboratories, Elkins Park, Pennsylvania (247)

June M. Brown, BS

Meningitis and Special Pathogens Branch, Division of Bacterial and Mycotic Diseases, National Center for Infectious Diseases, Centers for Disease Control and Prevention, Atlanta, Georgia (201)

Leena Bruckner-Tuderman, MD

Professor of Dermatology, Department of Dermatology, University Hospital Muenster, Muenster, Germany (16)

Jennifer L. Bub, MD

Dermatology Resident, Division of Dermatology, Department of Medicine, University of Washington School of Medicine, Seattle, Washington (168)

Nigel W. Bunnett, PhD

Professor, Departments of Surgery and Physiology, University of California San Francisco, San Francisco, California (20)

Walter H.C. Burgdorf, MD

Clinical Lecturer, Department of Dermatology, Ludwig Maximilian University, Munich, Tutzing, Germany (97, 99, 105, 106)

Michael J. Camilleri, MD

MRCP, Senior Resident Consultant, Department of Dermatology, Mayo Clinic, Rochester, Minnesota (109)

Ruggero Caputo, MD

Professor and Chairman, Director of the School of Specialization in Dermatology and Venereology, Institute of Dermatological Sciences, Milan, Italy (160, 161)

John A. Carucci, MD, PhD

Assistant Professor of Dermatology, Section of Dermatologic Surgery, Weill Medical College of Cornell University, New York, New York (81)

Christopher T. Cassetty, MD

Fellow, Dermatopharmacology, Department of Dermatology, New York University School of Medicine, New York, New York (256)

Lorenzo Cerroni, MD

Professor of Dermatology, University of Graz, Graz, Austria (83)

K. Andrew Cerveny, Jr., MD

Northeastern Ohio Universities College of Medicine, Wadsworth, Ohio (278)

Mary Wu Chang, MD

Assistant Professor of Dermatology, The Ronald O. Perelman Department of Dermatology, New York University School of Medicine, New York, New York (143)

Mei Chen, MD

Division of Dermatology, LAC and USC Medical Center, Los Angeles, California (66)

Michelle M. Choucair, MD

Assistant Professor, Department of Dermatology, University of Cincinnatti, West Chester, Ohio (272)

Mary-Margaret Chren, MD

Staff Dermatologist, San Francisco VA Medical Center, Associate Professor, UCSF Comprehensive Cancer Care Center, San Francisco, California (2)

Prof. Dr. Enno Christophers

Professor and Chairman of Dermatology, University of Kiel, Kiel, Germany (42, 70)

David H. Chu, MD, PhD

Department of Dermatology, New York University School of Medicine, New York, New York (6)

Mon-Li Chu, PhD

Professor of Dermatology and Cutaneous Biology, Professor of Biochemistry and Molecular Pharmacology, Thomas Jefferson University, Philadelphia, Pennsylvania (14, 15)

Lesley Clark-Loeser, MD

Department of Dermatology, New York University School of Medicine, New York, New York (249)

Jay D. Coffman, MD

Professor of Medicine, Chief, Section of Vascular Medicine, Boston University School of Medicine, Boston Medical Center, Boston, Massachusetts (167)

Jeffrey I. Cohen, MD

Head, Medical Virology Section, Laboratory of Clinical Investigation, National Institutes of Health, Bethesda, Maryland (217)

Philip R. Cohen, MD

Clinical Associate Professor, Department of Dermatology, University of Texas-Houston Medical School, Bellaire, Texas (94)

Suzanne M. Connolly, MD

Associate Professor, Mayo Clinic, Scottsdale, Arizona (87)

Louis Z. Cooper, MD

Professor of Pediatrics, Columbia College of Physicians and Surgeons, New York, New York (210)

Lynn A. Cornelius, MD

Chief, Division of Dermatology, Washington University School of Medicine, St. Louis, Missouri (177)

Melissa I. Costner, MD

Assistant Professor of Dermatology, UT Southwestern Medical Center at Dallas, Dallas, Texas (171, 172)

Thomas G. Cropley, MD

Associate Professor of Medicine, Division of Dermatology, University of Massachusetts Memorial Medical Center, Worcester, Massachusetts (3, 165)

Ponciano D. Cruz, Jr., MD

Professor of Dermatology, University of Texas Southwestern Medical Center, Dallas, Texas (185)

Mark V. Dahl, MD

Professor, Department of Dermatology, Mayo Clinic, Arizona (100)

Jennifer Susan Daly, MD

Associate Professor of Medicine, Clinical Chief, Infectious Disease and Immunology, UMass Memorial Medical Center, Worcester, Massachusetts (237)

Mazen S. Daoud, MD

Fort Myers Dermatopathology, Fort Myers, Florida (48, 49, 50, 77)

Thomas M. DeLauro, DPM

New York College of Podiatric Medicine, Hospital for Joint Diseases-Orthopaedic Institute, Diabetic Foot and Ankle Center, New York, New York (130)

Robert J. Desnick, MD, PhD
Professor and Chairman, Department of Human Genetics, Mount Sinai School of Medicine, New York, New York (151)

A. Damian Dhar, JD, MD
Instructor in Medicine, Chief Resident, Dermatology, Department of Dermatology, Dartmouth-Hitchcock Medical Center, Lebanon, New Hampshire (235)

Charles H. Dicken, MD
Department of Dermatology, Olmstead Medical Center, Rochester, Minnesota (77)

Brian L. Diffey, PhD, DSc
Professor of Photobiology and Medical Physics, Regional Medical Physics Department, Newcastle General Hospital, Newcastle, United Kingdom (247)

John J. DiGiovanna, MD
Director, Division of Dermatopharmacology, Professor, Department of Dermatology, Brown University Medical School, Providence, Rhode Island (51)

Dayna G. Diven, MD
Clinical Associate Professor, University of Texas Medical Branch, Galveston, Texas (220)

Andrzej Dlugosz, MD
Associate Professor, Department of Dermatology and Comprehensive Cancer Center, University of Michigan, Ann Arbor, Michigan (36)

Raphael Dolin, MD
Maxwell Finland Professor of Medicine, Dean for Clinical Programs, Harvard Medical School, Boston, Massachusetts (211, 260)

Jeffrey S. Dover, MD, FRCPC
SkinCare Physicians of Chestnut Hill, Chestnut Hill, Massachusetts (271)

Francesco Drago, MD
Professor of Dermatology, Department of Endocrinology and Metabolic Diseases; Section of Dermatology, University of Genoa, Genova, Italy (216)

Louis Dubertret, MD
Professeur de le Clinique de Maladies Cutania, Universite Paris VII, Paris, France (101)

Karynne O. Duncan, MD
Assistant Professor of Internal Medicine and Dermatology, Department of Dermatology, University of Colorado Health Sciences Center, Denver, Colorado (79)

Madeleine Duvic, MD
Professor, Section Chief, Section of Dermatology, M.D. Anderson Cancer Center, University of Texas Medical School, Houston, Texas (24)

Robert T. Eberhardt, MD
Assistant Professor of Medicine, Director, Vascular Diagnostic Laboratory, Boston University School of Medicine, Boston Medical Center, Boston, Massachusetts (167)

Libby Edwards, MD
Associate Clinical Professor of Dermatology, Wake Forest University School of Medicine, Charlotte, North Carolina (114)

Lawrence F. Eichenfield, MD
Chief of Pediatric and Adolescent Dermatology, Children's Hospital and Health Center, Clinical Professor of Pediatrics and Medicine (Dermatology), UC San Diego School of Medicine, San Diego, California (122)

Alfred R. Eichmann, MD
Associate Professor, Outpatient Clinic of Dermatology and Venereology, Triemli Hospital, Zurich, Switzerland (230, 234)

Arthur Z. Eisen, MD
The Emma Showman Professor of Dermatology, Program Director, Chief Emeritus, Division of Dermatology, Washington University School of Medicine, St. Louis, Missouri (17, 173)

Peter M. Elias, MD
Professor of Dermatology, Department of Dermatology, UC San Francisco, Dermatology Service, Veteran's Affairs Medical Center, San Francisco, California (9, 195)

Dirk M. Elston, MD
Departments of Dermatology and Pathology, Geisinger Medical Center, Danville, Pennsylvania (131)

Patricia G. Engasser, MD
Clinical Professor of Dermatology, University of California, San Francisco School of Medicine and Stanford University School of Medicine, Atherton, California (252)

Ervin H. Epstein, Jr., MD
Research Dermatologist, San Francisco General Hospital, San Francisco, California (5, 82, 110)

Janet A. Fairley, MD
Professor of Dermatology, Medical College of Wisconsin, Milwaukee, Wisconsin (153)

Vincent Falanga, MD
Professor of Dermatology and Biochemistry, Department of Dermatology, Boston University School of Medicine, Roger Williams Medical Center, Providence, Rhode Island (21)

Stella Fatović-Ferenčić, MD, PhD
Institute for the History of Medicine, Croatian Academy of Arts and Sciences, Zagreb, Croatia (1)

David S. Feingold, MD
Professor of Dermatology, Tufts University School of Medicine, Boston, Massachusetts (233)

Kenneth R. Feingold, MD
Professor of Medicine and Dermatology, University of California, San Francisco, Staff Physician, Veterans Affairs Medical Center, San Francisco, California (9)

David E. Fisher, MD, PhD
Associate Professor, Division of Pediatric Hematology/Oncology, Dana Farber Cancer Institute, Harvard Medical School, Boston, Massachusetts (11)

James E. Fitzpatrick, MD
Associate Professor, Department of Dermatology, University of Colorado Health Sciences Center, Aurora, Colorado (139, 246)

Thomas B. Fitzpatrick, MD, PhD, DSc(Hon)
Edward C. Wigglesworth Professor of Dermatology, Emeritus, Chairman Emeritus, Department of Dermatology, Harvard Medical School, Massachusetts General Hospital, Boston, Massachusetts (3, 88, 90, 93, 266)

Raul Fleischmajer, MD
Professor Emeritus, Department of Dermatology, Mount Sinai School of Medicine, New York, New York (186, 187)

Joachim W. Fluhr, MD
Consultant Dermatologist, Head Skin Physiology Laboratory, Dept. of Dermatology and Allergy, Friedrich Schiller University Jena, Jena, Germany (9)

Genoveffa Franchini, MD
Basic Research Laboratory, Division of Basic Sciences, National Cancer Institute, National Institutes of Health, Bethesda, Maryland (224)

Priv.-Doz. Dr. med. Jorge Frank
Dept. of Dermatology and Allergy, University Clinic of the RWTH, Aachen, Germany (149)

Shoshana Frankenburg, PhD
Department of Dermatology and Sharett Institute of Oncology, Hadassah Medical Organization, Jerusalem, Israel (235)

Andrew G. Franks, Jr., MD
Associate Professor of Dermatology, New York University Medical Center, New York, New York (166)

Irwin M. Freedberg, MD
George Miller MacKee Professor and Chairman, The Ronald O. Perelman Department of Dermatology, New York University Medical Center, New York, New York (7, 12, 44)

Peter O. Fritsch, MD

Department of Dermatology and Venereology, University of Innsbruck, Innsbruck, Austria (58, 78)

Vincent A. Fulginiti, MD

Professor Emeritus, University of Arizona Health Sciences Center, Tucson, Arizona (219)

Isabelle Fumal, MD

Department of Dermatopathology, CHU Sart Tilman, University Medical Centre, Liege, Belgium (126)

Richard L. Gallo, MD, PhD

Chief, Dermatology, Associate Professor of Medicine and Pediatrics, VA Medical Center/UCSD, San Diego, California (18)

W. Ray Gammon, MD

Eastern Dermatology, Greenville, North Carolina (66)

Sylvia Garnis-Jones, MSc, MDCM, FRCPC

Clinical Assistant Professor and Director of the Psychodermatology Clinic, Division of Dermatology, Department of Medicine, McMaster University, Oakville, Ontario, Canada (40)

Rachel A. Garton, MD

Department of Dermatology, Wake Forest University School of Medicine, Winston-Salem, North Carolina (192)

Anthony A. Gaspari, MD

Shapiro Professor of Dermatology, University of Maryland, Baltimore, Maryland (255)

Francis P. Gasparro, PhD

Adjunct Research Professor of Dermatology, Thomas Jefferson University, Hamden, Connecticut (247)

Joel M. Gelfand, MD

Department of Dermatology, Hospital of the University of Pennsylvania, Philadelphia, Pennsylvania (132)

Stephen E. Gellis, MD

Assistant Professor of Dermatology (Pediatrics), Harvard Medical School, Boston, Massachusetts (209)

Irma Gigli, MD

The Walter and Mary Mischer Professor in Molecular Medicine, Associate Director, Institute of Molecular Medicine, The University of Texas-Houston, Houston, Texas (117)

Barbara A. Gilchrest, MD

Chief of Dermatology, Boston University School of Medicine, Boston, Massachusetts (33, 144)

Gerald J. Gleich, MD

Professor, Department of Dermatology, University of Utah Health Sciences Center, Salt Lake City, Utah (96)

Richard G. Glogau, MD

Clinical Professor of Dermatology, University of California, San Francisco, San Francisco, California (276)

Mauricio Goihman-Yahr, MD, PhD

Professor of Dermatology, Instituto de Biomedicina, Faculty of Medicine, Central University of Venezuela, Caracas, Venezuela (201)

Lowell A. Goldsmith, MD, MPH

Professor of Dermatology, University of North Carolina School of Medicine, Chapel Hill, North Carolina, Dean Emeritus; University of Rochester School of Medicine and Dentistry, Rochester, New York (5, 8, 45, 54, 76, 145, 147, 150, 189)

Alice B. Gottlieb, MD, PhD

Professor of Medicine, W. H. Conzen Chairman of Clinical Pharmacology, Director, Clinical Research Center, Robert Wood Johnson Medical School, University of Medicine and Dentistry of New Jersey, New Brunswick, New Jersey (263)

Gloria F. Graham, MD

Associate Clinical Professor of Dermatology, Wake Forest University School of Medicine, Winston-Salem, North Carolina (278)

Robin A.C. Graham-Brown, BSc MB FRCP

Consultant Dermatologist, Honorary Senior Lecturer in Dermatology, University of Leicester, The Leicester Royal Infirmary, Leicester, United Kingdom (68, 164)

Richard D. Granstein, MD

George W. Hambrick, Jr. Professor of Dermatology, Chairman, Department of Dermatology, Joan and Sanford I. Weill Medical College of Cornell University, New York, New York (39)

Malcolm W. Greaves, MD, PhD, FRCP

Emeritus Professor of Dermatology, St. Johns Institute of Dermatology, St. Thomas' Hospital, London; Senior Consultant Dermatologist, Singapore General Hospital, Singapore (41)

Justin J. Green, MD

Clinical Instructor of Medicine, Division of Dermatology, UMDNJ, Robert Wood Johnson Medical School at Camden, Marlton, New Jersey (227)

Suzanne Virnelli Grevelink, MD

Department of Dermatology, Children's Hospital Medical Center, Boston, Massachusetts (103)

James M. Grichnik, MD, PhD

Associate Professor, Director Melanocytic Diseases Section, Department of Medicine, Division of Dermatology, Duke University Medical Center, Durham, North Carolina (91)

Douglas Grossman, MD, PhD

Assistant Professor, Departments of Dermatology and Oncological Sciences, Huntsman Cancer Institute, University of Utah, Salt Lake City, Utah (80)

Shireen V. Guide, MD

Stanford University Medical Center, Stanford, California (29)

Anne R. Haake, PhD

Assistant Professor, Information Technology and Bioinformatics, Rochester Institute of Technology, Rochester, New York (6)

Ruth Halaban, PhD

Senior Research Scientist, Department of Dermatology, Yale University School of Medicine, New Haven, Connecticut (11)

Russell P. Hall, III, MD

J. Lamar Callaway Professor of Dermatology, Duke University Medical Center, Durham, North Carolina (63)

Jon M. Hanifin, MD

Professor of Dermatology, Department of Dermatology, Oregon Health and Science University, Portland, Oregon (250)

Rudolf Happle, MD

Professor and Chairman, Department of Dermatology and Allergy, Philipp University of Marburg, Marburg, Germany (188)

Christopher B. Harmon, MD

University of Alabama at Birmingham, Birmingham, Alabama (270)

Conrad Hauser, MD

Associate Professor, Allergy Unit and Department of Dermatology, University Hospital, Geneva, Switzerland (23)

John L.M. Hawk, MD

Professor, Photobiology Unit, St. Thomas' Hospital, London, United Kingdom (134, 135)

Roderick J. Hay, MD

Dean, Faculty of Medicine and Health Sciences, Queens University Belfast, Belfast, Northern Ireland (207)

Harley A. Haynes, MD

Vice Chairman, Department of Dermatology, Brigham and Women's Hospital, Boston, Massachusetts (184)

Peter W. Heald, MD

Professor of Dermatology, Yale School of Medicine, New Haven, Connecticut (157)

Daniel N. Hebert, PhD

Assistant Professor, Department of Biochemistry and Molecular Biology, University of Massachusetts, Amherst, Massachusetts (11)

Peter J. Heenan, MD

Clinical Associate Professor, Department of Pathology, The University of Western Australia, Nedlands, Western Australia (55)

Michael P. Heffernan, MD

Assistant Professor, Division of Dermatology, Washington University School of Medicine, St. Louis, Missouri (170, 205, 206)

G. Scott Herron, MD, PhD

Department of Dermatology, Stanford University School of Medicine, Stanford, California (65)

Warren R. Heymann, MD

Professor of Medicine, Head, Division of Dermatology, UMDNJ-Robert Wood Johnson Medical School at Camden, Marlton, New Jersey (169, 227)

Jan V. Hirschmann, MD

Professor of Medicine, University of Washington School of Medicine, Puget Sound VA Medical Center, Seattle, Washington (259)

Vincent C.Y. Ho, MD

Professor, Skin Care Center, Vancouver, British Columbia, Canada (84)

Gary S. Hoffman, MD

Chair, Department of Rheumatic and Immunologic Disease, The Cleveland Clinic Foundation, Cleveland, Ohio (174)

Rainer Hofmann-Wellenhof, MD

Professor of Dermatology, Department of Dermatology, University of Graz, Graz, Austria (86)

Karen A. Holbrook, PhD

President, Ohio State University, Columbus, Ohio (6)

Steven M. Holland, MD

Senior Clinical Investigator, Laboratory of Host Defenses, NIAID, National Institutes of Health, Bethesda, Maryland (29)

Carlin B. Hollar, MD

Resident, Department of Dermatology, Wake Forest University School of Medicine, Wake Forest University Baptist Medical Center, Winston-Salem, North Carolina (179)

Karl Holubar, MD, FRCP

Professor of Dermatology and Venereology and of the History of Medicine, Chairman, Institute for the History of Medicine, University of Vienna, Vienna, Austria (1, 162)

Herbert Hönigsmann, MD

Professor and Chairman, Division of Special and Environmental Dermatology, Department of Dermatology, University of Vienna Medical School, Vienna, Austria (69, 94, 135, 266)

Yoshiaki Hori, MD (deceased)

Professor and Chairman Emeritus, Department of Dermatology, Yamanashi Medical College, Yamanashi, Japan (90)

Thomas D. Horn, MD

Professor of Dermatology and Pathology, Chair, Department of Dermatology, University of Arkansas for Medical Sciences, Central Arkansas Veterans Healthcare System, Little Rock, Arkansas (118)

Karen R. Houpt, MD

Clinical Associate Professor of Dermatology, Southwestern Medical School, University of Texas Southwestern Medical Center, Dallas, Texas (185)

Anders Hovmark, MD, PhD

Associate Professor of Dermatology, Karolinska Institutet at Stockholm Soder Hospital, Stockholm, Sweden (203)

George J. Hruza, MD

Clinical Associate Professor of Dermatology and Otolaryngology/Head and Neck Surgery, St. Louis University School of Medicine, Town and Country, Missouri (268, 271)

Fred H. Hsieh, MD

Section of Allergy and Immunology, Department of Pulmonary and Critical Care Medicine, Cleveland Clinic Foundation, Cleveland, Ohio (32)

Chung-Hong Hu, MD

Professor of Dermatology and President, Taipei Medical College, Taipei, Japan (47)

Eva A. Hurst, MD

Dermatology Department, Washington University School of Medicine, St. Louis, Missouri (170)

Sam T. Hwang, MD, PhD

Tenure-Track Investigator, Dermatology Branch, Center for Cancer Research, National Cancer Institute, Bethesda, Maryland (27)

William D. James, MD

Vice Chairman and Residency Program Director, Albert M. Kligman Professor, Department of Dermatology, University of Pennsylvania School of Medicine, Philadelphia, Pennsylvania (245)

Prof. Dr. Thomas Jansen

Department of Dermatology and Allergy, Ruhr-University Bochum, Bochum, Germany (74, 124)

Ming H. Jih, MD, PhD

The Ronald O. Perelman Department of Dermatology, New York University Medical Center, New York, New York (7, 44)

Richard Allen Johnson, MDCM

Clinical Associate in Dermatology, Department of Dermatology, Massachusetts General Hospital, Boston, Massachusetts (196, 113, 194, 225)

Graham A. Johnston, MB ChB MRCP

Consultant Dermatologist, Department of Dermatology, The Leicester Royal Infirmary, Leicester, United Kingdom (164)

Joseph L. Jorizzo, MD

Professor and Former (Founding) Chair, Department of Dermatology, Wake Forest University School of Medicine, Wake Forest University Baptist Medical Center, Winston-Salem, North Carolina (179, 192)

Steven Kaddu, MD

Associate Professor, Department of Dermatology, University of Graz, Graz, Austria (85)

Sewon Kang, MD

Associate Professor, Director of Clinical Research Unit, Department of Dermatology, University of Michigan Medical School, Ann Arbor, Michigan (244)

Allen P. Kaplan, MD

Professor of Medicine, Division of Pulmonary, Allergy, and Critical Care; Department of Medicine, Medical University of South Carolina, Charleston, South Carolina (116)

Stephen I. Katz, MD, PhD

Director, National Institute of Arthritis and Musculoskeletal and Skin Diseases, National Institutes of Health, Bethesda, Maryland (64, 67, 95, 178, 254)

David P. Kelsell, MD

Centre for Cutaneous Research, Bart's and The London, Queen Mary's School of Medicine and Dentistry, University of London, London, England (52)

Francisco A. Kerdel, MD

Professor, Department of Dermatology and Cutaneous Surgery, University of Miami School of Medicine, Cedars Medical Center, Miami, Florida (243)

Helmut Kerl, MD

Professor and Chairman, Department of Dermatology, University of Graz, Graz, Austria (83, 85, 86)

A. Ross Kerr, DDS, MSD

Assistant Professor, Department of Oral Medicine, New York University College of Dentistry, New York, New York (112)

Paul A. Khavari, MD, PhD

Department of Dermatology, Stanford University School of Medicine, Stanford, California (65)

Abdul-Ghani Kibbi, MD, FACP

Professor and Chairman, Department of Dermatology, American University of Beirut Medical Center, Beirut, Lebanon (4)

Jenny Kim, MD, PhD

Assistant Clinical Professor of Medicine/Dermatology, Division of Dermatology, UCLA, Geffen School of Medicine, Los Angeles, California (22)

Alexa Boer Kimball, MD, MPH

Assistant Professor, Department of Dermatology, Stanford University School of Medicine, Stanford, California (125)

Arash Kimyai-Asadi, MD

The Ronald O. Perelman Department of Dermatology, New York University Medical Center, New York, New York (7, 44)

Lloyd E. King, Jr., MD, PhD

Professor and Chairman, Division of Dermatology, Department of Medicine, Vanderbilt University Medical Center, Nashville, Tennessee (239)

Richard A. King, MD, PhD

Professor of Medicine and Pediatrics, Institute of Human Genetics, University of Minnesota, Minneapolis, Minnesota (89)

Sidney N. Klaus, MD

Professor of Medicine, Staff Dermatologist, Department of Dermatology, Darmouth Medical School, Dartmouth-Hitchcock Medical Center, Lebanon, New Hampshire (235)

Arnold William Klein, MD

Professor of Medicine/Dermatology, UCLA Geffen School of Medicine, Los Angeles, California (274, 275)

Jeffrey A. Klein, MD

Associate Clinical Professor of Medicine/Dermatology, UCLA Geffen School of Medicine, Los Angeles, California (274)

Alison S. Klenk, MD

Washington University School of Medicine, St. Louis, Missouri (206)

John H. Klippel, MD

Medical Director, Arthritis Foundation, Washington, District of Columbia (181)

Robert Knobler, MD

Associate Professor of Dermatology, Division of Special and Environmental Dermatology, Department of Dermatology, University of Vienna Medical School, Vienna, Austria (266)

John S. Knowland, PhD

Department of Biochemistry, Brasenose College, University of Oxford, Oxford, United Kingdom (247)

Sandra R. Knowles, BScPhm

Lecturer, University of Toronto, Sunnybrook and Women's College Health Sciences Centre, Toronto, Ontario, Canada (138)

Irene E. Kochevar, PhD

Professor, Wellman Laboratories of Photomedicine Department of Dermatology, Massachusetts General Hospital, Harvard Medical School, Boston, Massachusetts (133)

Thomas W. Koenig, MD

Assistant Professor of Psychiatry and Behavioral Sciences, Johns Hopkins Medical Institutions, Baltimore, Maryland (40)

Nellie Konnikov, MD

Professor of Dermatology, Boston University School of Medicine, Boston, Massachusetts (261)

Kenneth H. Kraemer, MD

Chief, DNA Repair Section, Basic Research Laboratory, National Cancer Institute, Bethesda, Maryland (35, 155)

Margaret L. Kripke, PhD

Professor of Immunology, Executive Vice President and Chief Academic Officer, The University of Texas M.D. Anderson Cancer Center, Houston, Texas (38)

James G. Krueger, MD

The Rockefeller University, New York, New York (263)

Jean Krutmann, MD

Professor of Dermatology and Environmental Health, Director, Research Institute for Environmental Health, Heinrich-Heine University, Düsseldorf, Germany (265)

Stephane Kuenzli, MD

Department of Dermatology, Geneva University Medical School, University Hospital, Geneva, Switzerland (257)

Thomas S. Kupper, MD

Chairman, Department of Dermatology, Brigham and Women's Hospital, Boston, Massachusetts (26)

Jeffrey R. LaDuca, PhD, MD

University of Rochester, School of Medicine and Dentistry, Rochester, New York (255)

Nicole LaNatra

Medical Student, New York Medical College, New York, New York (251)

Richard G.B. Langley, MD

Assistant Professor of Dermatology, Dalhousie University, Halifax, Nova Scotia, Canada (93)

Charles M. Lapiere

Emeritus Professor of Dermatology, Universite de Liege, Liege, Belgium (152)

Jo-Ann M. Latkowski, MD

Assistant Professor, Department of Dermatology, New York University School of Medicine, New York, New York (157)

Stephan Lautenschlager, MD

Clinical Lecturer; Staff Physician, Outpatient Clinic of Dermatology and Venereology, Triemli Hospital, Zurich, Switzerland (230, 234)

Robert M. Lavker, PhD

Professor of Dermatology, The Feinberg School of Medicine, Northwestern University, Chicago, Illinois (12)

Thomas J. Lawley, MD

Dean, Professor of Dermatology, Emory University School of Medicine, Atlanta, Georgia (142, 177)

Mark Lebwohl, MD

Professor and Chairman, Department of Dermatology, Mount Sinai School of Medicine, New York, New York (108)

Ken K. Lee, MD

Assistant Professor of Dermatology, Otolaryngology/Head and Neck Surgery, Oregon Health and Science University, Portland, Oregon (279)

Lela A. Lee, MD

Professor of Dermatology and Medicine, University of Colorado School of Medicine, Chief of Dermatology, Denver Health Medical Center, Denver, Colorado (25)

Peter K. Lee, MD

Assistant Professor, Department of Dermatology, University of Minnesota, Minneapolis, Minnesota (194)

David J. Leffell, MD

Professor of Dermatology and Surgery, Department of Dermatology, Yale University School of Medicine, Yale-New Haven Hospital, New Haven, Connecticut (79, 80, 81)

Franz J. Legat, MD

Assistant Professor, Department of Dermatology, Kral-Sranzens-University Graz, School of Medicine, Graz, Austria (20)

Kristin M. Leiferman, MD

Professor, Department of Dermatology, University of Utah Health Sciences Center, Salt Lake City, Utah (96)

Irene M. Leigh, MD, FRCP

Centre for Cutaneous Research, Bart's and The London, Queen Mary's School of Medicine and Dentistry, University of London, London, England (52)

Janie M. Leonhardt, MD

Division of Dermatology, UMDNJ—Robert Wood Johnson Medical School at Camden, Marlton, New Jersey (169)

Donald Y.M. Leung, MD, PhD

Head, Division of Pediatric Allergy/Immunology, National Jewish Medical and Research Center, Professor of Pediatrics, University of Colorado Health Sciences Center, Denver, Colorado (122, 204)

Henry W. Lim, MD

Chairman and C.S. Livingood Chair Department of Dermatology; Director, Academic Programs, Henry Ford Hospital, Detroit, Michigan (136)

Graeme M. Lipper, MD

Research Fellow, Wellman Laboratories of Photomedicine, Department of Dermatology, Massachusetts General Hospital, Boston, Massachusetts (267)

Cynthia A. Loomis, MD, PhD

Assistant Professor, Departments of Cell Biology and Dermatology, New York University School of Medicine, New York, New York (6)

Douglas R. Lowy, MD

Deputy Director, Center for Cancer Research, National Cancer Institute, National Institutes of Health, Bethesda, Maryland (37, 208, 221, 222, 223)

Leslie C. Lucchina, MD

Director of Aesthetic Dermatology, Department of Dermatology, Brigham and Women's Hospital, Boston, Massachusetts (236)

Anne W. Lucky, MD

Department of Pediatrics, Division of Dermatology, Children's Hospital Medical Center of Cincinnati, Cincinnati, Ohio (204)

Thomas A. Luger, MD

Professor and Chairman, Department of Dermatology, University of Munster, Munster, Germany (20)

Calum C. Lyon, MA, MRCP

Clinical Lecturer, Section of Dermatology, University of Manchester/Hope Hospital, Manchester, England (129)

Howard I. Maibach, MD

Professor of Dermatology, Department of Dermatology, University of California, San Francisco School of Medicine, San Francisco, California (252)

Frederick D. Malkinson, MD

Clark W. Finnerud Professor Emeritus, Department of Dermatology, Rush Medical College, Rush-Presbyterian-St. Luke's Medical Center, Chicago, Illinois (128)

Brian F. Mandell, MD, PhD

Clinical Professor of Medicine, Pennsylvania State College of Medicine, Hershey, Pennsylvania (174)

Claire P. Mansur, MD

Assistant Professor of Dermatology, Tufts University School of Medicine, Chair of Dermatology, Tufts-New England Medical Center, Boston, Massachusetts (233)

David J. Margolis, MD, PhD

Associate Professor, Director, Cutaneous Ulcer Center, University of Pennsylvania/ CCEB, Philadelphia, Pennsylvania (132)

M. Peter Marinkovich, MD

Assistant Professor, Director, Bullous Disease Clinic, Department of Dermatology and Program in Epithelial Biology, Stanford University School of Medicine, Stanford, California (65)

Ronald Marks, MD

Emeritus Professor, University of Wales, Cardiff, Penylan, Cardiff, United Kingdom (75)

Adriana R. Marques, MD

Head, Clinical Studies Unit, Laboratory of Clinical Investigation, National Institute of Allergy and Infectious Diseases, National Institutes of Health, Bethesda, Maryland (214)

Ann G. Martin, MD

Assistant Professor of Medicine, Division of Dermatology, Washington University School of Medicine, St. Louis, Missouri (205, 206)

Dieter Maurer, MD

Associate Professor, Director of Immunology, Allergy and Infectious Diseases, Department of Dermatology, University of Vienna Medical School, Vienna, Austria (23)

David I. McLean, MD, FRCP

Professor of Dermatology, Associate Dean, Health Care Systems and Planning, University of British Columbia, Vancouver, British Columbia, Canada (184)

Michael M. McNeil, MD, MPH

Epidemiology and Surveillance Division, National Immunization Program, Centers for Disease Control and Prevention, Atlanta, Georgia (201)

Dean D. Metcalfe, MD

Laboratory of Allergic Diseases, National Institute of Allergy and Infectious Diseases, National Institutes of Health, Bethesda, Maryland (163)

Martin C. Mihm, Jr., MD, FACP

Senior Dermatopathologist, Associate Dermatologist, Pathologist, Clinical Professor of Pathology, Massachusetts General Hospital, Harvard Medical School, Boston, Massachusetts (4, 93)

Robert L. Modlin, MD

Professor of Dermatology and Microbiology and Immunology, Division of Dermatology, David Geffen School of Medicine at UCLA, Los Angeles, California (22, 28, 202)

Akimichi Morita, MD

Associate Professor, Department of Dermatology, Nagoya City University Medical School, Nagoya, Japan (265)

David B. Mosher, MD (deceased)

Department of Dermatology, Harvard Medical School, Massachusetts General Hospital, Boston, Massachusetts (90)

Prof. Dr. Ulrich Mrowietz

Associate Professor of Dermatology, University of Kiel, Kiel, Germany (42, 70)

J. Marcus Muche, MD

Department of Dermatology and Allergy, Humboldt University, Charite Berlin, Berlin, Germany (158)

John Butler Mulliken, MD

Professor of Surgery, Harvard Medical School, Children's Hospital, Boston, Massachusetts (103)

Rhoda S. Narins, MD

Clinical Professor in Dermatology, New York University Medical Center, New York, New York (274)

Kenneth H. Neldner, MD

Professor and Chairman Emeritus, Department of Dermatology, Texas Tech University Health Sciences Center, Lubbock, Texas (146)

Michael M. Nelson, MD

Clinical Research Fellow, Division of Dermatology, Washington University School of Medicine, St. Louis, Missouri (205)

David S. Nieves, MD

Resident in Dermatology, Department of Dermatology, University of Rochester Medical Center, Rochester, New York (145)

Gerhard J. Nohynek, MSc, PhD, DABT

Centre Charles Zviak, L'Oreal Life Sciences Research, Clichy, France (241)

Paul G. Norris, MA, MB

Consultant Dermatologist, Department of Dermatology, Addenbrookes Hospital, Cambridge, United Kingdom (135)

H. Carlos Nousari, MD

Chairman, Department of Dermatology, Cleveland Clinic Florida, Weston, Florida (60, 180, 262)

William S. Oetting, MD

Assistant Professor, Medicine Genetics Office, University of Minnesota, Minneapolis, Minnesota (89)

John E. Olerud, MD

Professor and Chairman, Division of Dermatology, University of Washington Medical School, Seattle, Washington (20, 168)

Elise A. Olsen, MD

Professor of Medicine, Division of Dermatology, Duke University Medical Center, Durham, North Carolina (71)

Seth J. Orlow, MD, PhD

Samuel Weinberg Professor of Dermatology, New York University School of Medicine, New York, New York (143)

Jean-Paul Ortonne, MD

Chief, Department of Dermatology, Hospital Pasteur, Professor of Dermatology, Nice University School of Medicine, Nice, France (88, 89, 90)

Michael N. Oxman, MD

Professor of Medicine and Pathology, University of California at San Diego, Chief, Infectious Diseases and Clinical Virology Sections, VA Medical Center, San Diego, California (215)

Amy S. Paller, MD

Professor of Pediatrics and Dermatology, Northwestern University Medical School, Head, Division of Dermatology, Children's Memorial Hospital, Chicago, Illinois (115, 189, 191)

Johannes Pammer, MD

Associate Professor of Pathology, Clinical Institute for Pathology, University of Vienna Medical School, Vienna, Austria (226)

Renato G. Panizzon, MD

Professor and Chairman, Department of Dermatology, University Hospital CHUV, Lausanne, Switzerland (128)

Madhukar A. Pathak, PhD

Department of Dermatology, Massachusetts General Hospital, Boston, Massachusetts (266)

Alice P. Pentland, MD

Professor and chair, Department of Dermatology, University of Rochester, Rochester, New York (34)

Margot S. Peters, MD

Rochester, Minnesota (96)

Peter Petzelbauer, MD

Department of Dermatology, University of Vienna Medical School, Vienna, Austria (19)

Joan A. Phelan, DDS

Professor and Chair, Department of Oral Pathology, New York University College of Dentistry, New York, New York (112)

Tania J. Phillips, MD

Professor of Dermatology, Boston University School of Medicine, Boston, Massachusetts (272)

Gérald Piérard, MD, PhD

Department of Dermatopathology, CHU Sart Tilman, University Medical Centre, Liege, Belgium (126)

Claudine Piérard-Franchimont, MD, PhD

Department of Dermatopathology, CHU Sart Tilman, University Medical Centre, Liege, Belgium (126)

Warren W. Piette, MD

Professor, Department of Dermatology, University of Iowa College of Medicine, Iowa City, Iowa (156)

Bianca Maria Piraccini, MD, PhD

Department of Dermatology, University of Bologna, Bologna, Italy (13)

Mark R. Pittelkow, MD

Professor, Departments of Dermatology and Biochemistry and Molecular Biology, Mayo Medical School, Rochester, Minnesota (48, 49, 50)

Eniko K. Pivnik, MD

Associate Professor, Department of Pediatrics, University of Tennessee Health Science Center, Memphis, Tennessee (190)

Prof. Dr. Dr. h.c. Gerd Plewig

Department of Dermatology and Allergy, Ludwig-Maximilians-University, Munich, Germany (74, 124)

Jordan S. Pober, MD, PhD

Professor of Pathology, Immunobiology and Dermatology; Director, Interdepartmental Program in Vascular Biology and Transplantation, Boyer Center for Molecular Medicine, Yale University School of Medicine, New Haven, Connecticut (19)

Victor G. Prieto, MD, PhD

Associate Professor of Pathology and Dermatology; Chief of Dermatopathology, Department of Pathology, M.D. Anderson Cancer Center, Houston, Texas (102)

Thomas T. Provost, MD

Distinguished Service Professor, Department of Dermatology, Johns Hopkins Medical Institutions, Baltimore, Maryland (180)

Leena Pulkkinen, PhD

Department of Dermatology and Cutaneous Biology, Thomas Jefferson University, Philadelphia, Pennsylvania (14)

Christopher J. Quirk, MBBS, FACD

Part-time Senior Lecturer, Department of Dermatology, Royal Perth Hospital, Fremantle, Western Australia (55)

Caroline L. Rao, MD

Assistant Professor of Medicine, Duke University Medical Center, Durham, North Carolina (63)

Univ. Prof. Dr. Klemens Rappersberger

Head, Department of Dermatology, Hospital Rudolfstiftung, Vienna, Austria (104)

Helen Raynham, MD

Boston University School of Medicine, Boston, Massachusetts (261)

Thomas H. Rea, MD

Emeritus Professor, Division of Dermatology, LAC/USC Medical Center, Los Angeles, California (202)

Alfredo Rebora, MD

Professor and Director, Department of Endocrinology and Metabolic Diseases, Section of Dermatology, University of Genoa, Genoa, Italy (216)

Thomas E. Redelmeier, PhD

President, Northern Lipids, Inc., Vancouver, British Columbia, Canada (241)

Vivienne Reeve, PhD

Senior Research Fellow, Faculty of Veterinary Science, University of Sydney, New South Wales, Australia (247)

Marvin S. Reitz, Jr., PhD

Institute of Human Virology, University of Maryland Biotechnology Institute, Baltimore, Maryland (224)

Adrienne Rencic, MD, PhD

Department of Dermatology, Johns Hopkins Outpatient Center, Baltimore, Maryland (30, 40)

Steven D. Resnick, MD

Chief, Division of Dermatology, Bassett Healthcare, Cooperstown, New York (195)

Arthur R. Rhodes, MD, MPH

Professor, Department of Dermatology, Rush University, Rush Medical College, Chicago, Illinois (91)

Vincent M. Riccardi, MD

Clinical Professor of Pediatrics (Genetics), The NF Institute, La Crescenta, California (190)

Benjamin E. Rich, PhD

Instructor in Dermatology, Harvard Medical School; Brigham and Women's Hospital, Boston, Massachusetts (26)

June K. Robinson, MD

Director, Division of Dermatology, Loyola University Chicago Stritch School of Medicine, Program Leader of the Skin Cancer Clinical Program, Cardinal Bernardin Cancer Center, Maywood, Illinois (268)

Fred S. Rosen, MD

James L. Gamble Professor of Pediatrics, Center for Blood Research, Harvard Medical School, Boston, Massachusetts (117)

Richard Rothenberg, MD, MPH

Professor, Department of Family and Preventive Medicine, Emory University School of Medicine, Atlanta, Georgia (231, 232)

Adam I. Rubin, MD

Post-Doctoral Residency Fellow, Department of Dermatology, Columbia University College of Physicians and Surgeons; Columbia Presbyterian Medical Center, New York, New York (251)

Ramon Ruiz-Maldonado, MD

Professor, Instituto Nacional de Pediatria, Insurgentes Sur, Mexico City, Mexico (58)

Miguel R. Sanchez, MD

Associate Professor, Ronald O. Perelman Department of Dermatology, New York University School of Medicine, Bellevue Hospital Center, New York, New York (141, 228, 229)

James SanFilippo, MD

Northeastern Ohio Universities College of Medicine, Tallmadge, Ohio (278)

Jean-Hilaire Saurat, MD

Department of Dermatology, Geneva University Medical School, University Hospital, Geneva, Switzerland (257)

Hans Schaefer, PhD

Professor Emeritus, Advisor to the Center of Experimental and Applied Cutaneous Physiology, Department of Dermatology, Charite Hospital, Humboldt-University, Berlin, Germany (241)

Mark Jordan Scharf, MD

Associate Professor, Division of Dermatology, University of Massachusetts Medical School, Worcester, Massachusetts (237)

Jeffrey S. Schechner, MD

Assistant Professor, Department of Dermatology, Yale University School of Medicine, New Haven, Connecticut (19)

Kenneth E. Schmader, MD

Associate Professor of Medicine and Geriatrics, Duke and Durham VA Medical Centers, Durham, North Carolina (215)

Thomas Scholzen, PhD

Department of Dermatology, Ludwig Boltzmann Institute, University Clinical Center of Munster, Munster, Germany (20)

John T. Schroeder, PhD

Assistant Professor of Medicine, Johns Hopkins Asthma and Allergy Center, Baltimore, Maryland (31)

Theresa Schroeder, MD

Assistant Professor, Department of Dermatology, Oregon Health and Science University, Portland, Oregon (176)

Jo L. Seltzer, PhD

Division of Dermatology, Washington University School of Medicine, St. Louis, Missouri (17)

Lori Shapiro, MD, FRCP

Assistant Professor, Departments of Medicine, Dermatology, and Clinical Pharmacology, Sunnybrook and Women's College Health Sciences Centre, Toronto, Ontario, Canada (138)

Christopher R. Shea, MD

Professor of Medicine, Chief, Section of Dermatology, University of Chicago Medical Center, Chicago, Illinois (102)

Neil H. Shear, MD, FRCP

Professor and Chief of Dermatology, University of Toronto, Sunnybrook and Women's Health Sciences Centre, Toronto, Ontario, Canada (138)

Robert L. Sheridan, MD

Assistant Chief of Staff, Shriners Burns Hospital, Boston, Massachusetts (127)

Jonathan A. Ship, DMD

Director, Bluestone Center for Clinical Research, Professor, Department of Oral Medicine, New York University College of Dentistry, New York, New York (112)

Jerome L. Shupack, MD

Professor of Dermatology, The Ronald O. Perelman Department of Dermatology, New York University Medical Center, New York, New York (242, 249, 256)

Robert Sidbury, MD

Assistant Professor, Departments of Pediatrics and Dermatology, University of Washington School of Medicine, Seattle, Washington (250)

Shane G. Silver, MD

The Skin Care Center, University of British Columbia, Vancouver, British Columbia, Canada (84)

David A. Sirois, DMD, PhD

Professor and Chairman, Department of Oral Medicine, New York University College of Dentistry, New York, New York (212)

Michael L. Smith, MD

Assistant Professor of Medicine and Pediatrics, Division of Dermatology, Vanderbilt University Medical Center, Nashville, Tennessee (239)

Renee R. Snyder, MD

Department of Dermatology, University of Texas Medical Branch, Galveston, Texas (220)

Arthur J. Sober, MD

Professor of Dermatology; Associate Chief of Dermatology, Harvard Medical School, Massachusetts General Hospital, Boston, Massachusetts (91, 92, 93)

Richard D. Sontheimer, MD

John S. Strauss Endowed Chair in Dermatology, Professor and Head, Department of Dermatology, University of Iowa College of Medicine/University of Iowa Health Care, Iowa City, Iowa (171, 172)

Apra Sood, MD

Fellow, Contact Dermatitis and Environmental Skin Disease, Department of Dermatology, Cleveland Clinic Foundation, Cleveland, Ohio (137)

Nicholas A. Soter, MD

Professor, The Ronald O. Perelman Department of Dermatology, New York University Medical Center, Tisch Hospital, New York, New York (116, 123, 175, 258)

John R. Stanley, MD

Milton B. Hartzell Professor and Chairman, Department of Dermatology, Hospital of the University of Pennsylvania, Philadelphia, Pennsylvania (59, 61)

Wolfram Sterry, MD

Department of Dermatology and Allergy, Humboldt University, Charite Berlin, Berlin, Germany (158)

Howard P. Stevens, MD

Department of Dermatology, Barnet General Hospital, Barnet, Hertfordshire, United Kingdom (52)

Margaret I. Stewart, MD

Assistant Professor of Medicine, Division of Dermatology, University of Massachusetts Memorial Medical Center, Worcester, Massachusetts (3)

Matthew J. Stiller, MD

Associate Professor of Clinical Dermatology, Director, Clinical Pharmacology Unit, Columbia University College of Physicians and Surgeons; Columbia Presbyterian Medical Center, New York, New York (251)

Georg Stingl, MD

Professor of Dermatology; Head, Division of Immunology, Allergy and Infectious Diseases, Department of Dermatology, University of Vienna Medical School, Vienna, Austria (23, 98, 104)

Stephen P. Stone, MD

Professor of Clinical Medicine, Division of Dermatology, Southern Illinois University School of Medicine, Springfield, Illinois (238)

Stephen E. Straus, MD

Chief, Laboratory of Clinical Investigation, National Institute of Allergy and Infectious Diseases, Director, National Center for Complementary and Alternative Medicine, National Institutes for Health, Bethesda, Maryland (214, 215)

John S. Strauss, MD

Emeritus Professor of Dermatology, University of Iowa College of Medicine/University of Iowa Health Care, Iowa City, Iowa (73)

Bruce E. Strober, MD, PhD

Assistant Professor of Dermatology, The Ronald O. Perelman Department of Dermatology, New York University Medical Center, New York, New York (242)

W.P. Daniel Su, MD

Professor, Department of Dermatology, Mayo Clinic, Rochester, Minnesota (109)

John R. Sullivan, MB, BS, FACD

Director, Centre for Product Testing, Skin and Cancer Foundation, Liverpool and Westmead Hospital, Westmead, New South Wales, Australia (138)

Tung-Tien Sun, PhD

Rudolf A. Baer Professor of Dermatology, Professor of Pharmacology and Urology, New York University School of Medicine, New York, New York (12)

Neil A. Swanson, MD

Professor and Chair of Dermatology, Professor of Otolaryngology/Head and Neck Surgery, Department of Dermatology, Oregon Health and Science University, Portland, Oregon (279)

Morton N. Swartz, MD

Professor of Medicine, Chief, Jackson Firm of Medical Service, Harvard Medical School, Massachusetts General Hospital, Boston, Massachusetts (193, 194, 196, 197, 199)

Susan Sweeney, MD

Chief Resident, Division of Dermatology, University of Massachusetts Medical School, Worcester, Massachusetts (165)

Virginia P. Sybert, MD

Professor, Division of Dermatology, Department of Medicine, University of Washington School of Medicine, Seattle, Washington (53)

Rolf-Markus Szeimies, MD

Assistant Professor, Department of Dermatology, University of Regensburg, Regensburg, Germany (266)

Moyses Szklo, MD, MPH, DrPH

Professor of Chronic Disease Epidemiology, Johns Hopkins University, Bloomberg School of Hygiene and Public Health, Baltimore, Maryland (240)

Gerhard Tappeiner, MD

Associate Professor, Department of Dermatology, University of Vienna Medical School, Vienna, Austria (200, 264)

Francisco A. Tausk, MD

Associate Professor of Dermatology, Johns Hopkins Medical Institutions, Baltimore, Maryland (40)

Charles R. Taylor, MD

Associate Professor of Dermatology, Wellman Laboratories of Photomedicine, Department of Dermatology, Massachusetts General Hospital, Harvard Medical School, Boston, Massachusetts (133)

James S. Taylor, MD

Head, Section of Industrial Dermatology, Department of Dermatology, Cleveland Clinic Foundation, Cleveland, Ohio (137)

Eva Tegner, MD

Associate Professor of Dermatology, University of Lund, University Hospital, Lund, Sweden (46)

Diane M. Thiboutot, MD

Associate Professor of Dermatology, The Pennsylvania State University, The Milton S. Hershey Medical Center, Hershey, Pennsylvania (73)

Antonella Tosti, MD

Associate Professor, Department of Dermatology, University of Bologna, Bologna, Italy (13, 72)

Franz Trautinger, MD

Associate Professor of Dermatology, Division of Special and Environmental Dermatology, Department of Dermatology, University of Vienna Medical School, Vienna, Austria (69)

Janet M. Trowbridge, MD, PhD

Division of Dermatology/Department of Medicine, VA Medical Center/UCSD, San Diego, California (18)

Hensin Tsao, MD

Assistant Professor, Department of Dermatology, Harvard Medical School/ Massachusetts General Hospital, Boston, Massachusetts (92, 196)

Sandy Tsao, MD

Instructor in Dermatology, MGH Dermatology Laser Center, Massachusetts General Hospital, Harvard Medical School, Boston, Massachusetts (218)

Erwin Tschachler, MD

Professor of Dermatology, Ludwig Boltzmann Institute for Venero-Dermatological Infections/Department of Dermatology, University of Vienna Medical School, Vienna, Austria (224, 226)

Maria L. Chanco Turner, MD

Dermatology Branch, National Cancer Institute, Bethesda, Maryland (140)

Jouni Uitto, MD, PhD

Professor and Chairman, Department of Dermatology and Cutaneous Biology, Director, Jefferson Institute of Molecular Medicine, Jefferson Medical College, Philadelphia, Pennsylvania (14, 15)

Robin Unger, MD

New York, New York (277)

Walter Unger, MD

Clinical Professor of Dermatology, Mt. Sinai School of Medicine, New York, New York (277)

Isabel C. Valencia, MD

Dermatology Fellow, Department of Dermatology and Cutaneous Surgery, University of Miami School of Medicine, Miami, Florida (243)

John J. Voorhees, MD

Duncan and Ella Poth Distinguished Professor and Chair, Department of Dermatology, University of Michigan Medical Center, Ann Arbor, Michigan (244)

Susan L. Walker, PhD

Department of Environmental Dermatology, Guy's, King's and St. Thomas' School of Medicine, London, England (134)

John S. Walsh, MD

Assistant Professor of Dermatology, Mayo Clinic Jacksonville, Jacksonville, Florida (153)

Ken Washenik, MD, PhD

Clinical Assistant Professor of Dermatology, Director of Dermatopharmacology, The Ronald O. Perelman Department of Dermatology, New York University Medical Center, New York, New York (242, 249, 256)

Arnold N. Weinberg, MD

Professor of Medicine, Infectious Disease Unit, Massachusetts General Hospital, Boston, Massachusetts (193, 194, 196, 197, 199)

Martin A. Weinstock, MD, PhD

Dermatoepidemiology Unit, VA Medical Center, Providence, Rhode Island (2)

Margaret A. Weiss, MD

Assistant Professor, Department of Dermatology, Johns Hopkins University School of Medicine, Hunt Valley, Maryland (273)

Robert A. Weiss, MD
Assistant Professor, Department of Dermatology, Johns Hopkins University School of Medicine, Hunt Valley, Maryland (273)

C. Bruce Wenger, MD, PhD
Research Pharmacologist, Military Performance Division, US Army Research Institute of Environmental Medicine, Natick, Massachusetts (10)

Richard J. Wenstrup, MD
Professor of Pediatrics, Division of Human Genetics, Cincinnati Children's Hospital Medical Center, Cincinatti, Ohio (154)

Victoria P. Werth, MD
Associate Professor of Dermatology, University of Pennsylvania, Chief, VA Dermatology, Philadelphia, Pennsylvania (166, 253)

Ifor R. Williams, MD, PhD
Assistant Professor of Pathology, Emory University School of Medicine, Atlanta, Georgia (26)

David C. Wilson, MD
Central Virginia Dermatology, Inc., Forest, Virginia (239)

Mary E. Wilson, MD
Chief of Infectious Diseases; Director, Travel Resource Center, Division of Infectious Diseases, Mount Auburn Hospital, Cambridge, Massachusetts (236)

Robert J. Winchester, MD
Director, Division of Autoimmune and Molecular Diseases, Professor of Pediatrics, Medicine and Pathology, Columbia University College of Physicians and Surgeons, New York, New York (43, 182)

Karen Wiss, MD
Associate Professor of Dermatology and Pediatrics, Director, Pediatric Dermatology, University of Massachusetts Memorial Medical Center, Worcester, Massachusetts (213)

Klaus Wolff, MD, FRCP
Professor and Chairman, Department of Dermatology, University of Vienna Medical School, Vienna General Hospital, Vienna, Austria (4, 23, 69, 94, 98, 104, 200, 264, 266)

Elizabeth Ch. Wolff-Schreiner, MD
Associate Professor of Dermatology, University of Vienna, Vienna, Austria (56,57)

Gary S. Wood, MD
Geneva F. and Sture Johnson Professor, Chairman, Department of Dermatology, University of Wisconsin Medical School, Madison, Wisconsin (47, 159)

David T. Woodley, MD
Division of Dermatology, LAC and USC Medical Center, Los Angeles, California (66)

Mina Yaar, MD
Professor of Dermatology, Department of Dermatology, Boston University School of Medicine, Boston, Massachusetts (144)

Kim B. Yancey, MD
Professor and Chair, Department of Dermatology, Medical College of Wisonsin, Milwaukee, Wisconsin (62, 142)

John M. Yarborough, Jr., MD
Tulane University School of Medicine, New Orleans, Louisiana (270)

Antony R. Young, PhD
Department of Environmental Dermatology, Guy's, King's and St. Thomas' School of Medicine, London, England (134)

Benjamin D. Yu, MD
Instructor in Dermatology, Department of Dermatology, University of California San Francisco, San Francisco, California (173)

Stuart H. Yuspa, MD
Chief, Laboratory of Cellular Carcinogenesis and Tumor Promotion, Deputy Director, Center for Cancer Research, National Cancer Institute, Bethesda, Maryland (36)

Huiquan Zhao, MD, PhD
Clinical Geneticist and Pediatrician, Department of Pediatrics, Kaiser Permanente Fontana Medical Center, Fontana, California (154)

Matthew T. Zipoli, MD
Department of Dermatology, University of Minnesota, Minneapolis, Minnesota (194)

PREFACE

The editors and contributors are proud to present to our readers this sixth edition of *Fitzpatrick's Dermatology in General Medicine (DIGM),* a work that has become recognized as a classic medical textbook. Classics often are known by the name of the person most instrumental in their development, and through its past five editions *Fitzpatrick's* (or just *Fitz,* as the text is often called) has become a worldwide resource for physicians, scientists, students, and, in increasing numbers, patients interested in the skin and its diseases. Although the excellence for which *DIGM* is known has come from the input of many clinicians and investigators throughout the world, the driving force for the initial development of the concept and the person who brought *DIGM* to fruition was Thomas B. Fitzpatrick, MD, PhD, Wigglesworth Professor of Dermatology Emeritus at Harvard Medical School. Dr. Fitzpatrick has devoted almost all of his professional energy to bringing dermatology and cutaneous biology into the center of medicine and science throughout the world. He has worked diligently to ensure that the medical and scientific progress made since he first conceived the idea of *DIGM* more than four decades ago was translated rapidly to dermatology. This work remains a testament to his vision.

During the second half of the twentieth century, the period of dermatologic progress covered by the six editions of *DIGM,* great strides have been made in clinical dermatology. It has been our intent to define and document those advances in this sixth edition for our dermatologic colleagues, as well as for the physicians and surgeons of other specialties for whom changes on the skin of their patients are important. Although much has changed over the past decades, the concept for and the purpose of the book remain the same—to provide an all-encompassing, state-of-the-art review of dermatology and to describe the biologic basis for diseases of the skin. Although *DIGM* is truly encyclopedic, it has been edited with the goal of making the entire text easily readable and useful.

The 280 chapters are grouped into 37 sections covering all aspects of the science and clinical care of the skin in health and disease. Fifty new contributors have participated in this edition, many of the chapters are completely new, and a large number of the others have been completely rewritten. Disorders thought to be of only historic importance, such as anthrax and variola, are now central to our twenty-first century world; they are discussed both as dermatologic diseases and as potential agents of mass destruction. Our understanding of disease and pathophysiology has led to novel therapeutic agents such as botulinum toxin, which has proven to be of value in many diverse situations. Thus, the sixth edition of *Dermatology in General Medicine* clearly reflects the complexities and the great potential of our age.

Since complete integration of the basic and clinical sciences is the *DIGM* signature, many new approaches to the biology, structure, and function of the skin are offered in detail. We have introduced a new section on evidence-based dermatology and have expanded the portion of the text dealing with dermatologic changes through the stages of life. Essentially all of the illustrative material is now in full color, and charts and diagrams have been redrawn for ease of interpretation. The therapeutic sections have all been updated to encompass the most recently introduced types of biologic therapy. The progress that has been made in dealing with HIV infection, the scourge of our generation, is clearly described.

We are indebted to the members of our families for their support and for the time with us that they gave up so that *DIGM* could reach all of you. Our thanks to the dedicated staff members at our institutions who helped so much with this edition, to the skilled professionals who participated in the process, including Arlene Stolper Simon, who has assisted in editing the last four editions, and to the McGraw-Hill team, especially Darlene Cooke and Peter Boyle.

Irwin M. Freedberg
Arthur Z. Eisen
Klaus Wolff
K. Frank Austen
Lowell A. Goldsmith
Stephen I. Katz
March 2003

NOTICE

P A R T O N E

Introduction

SECTION 1
GENERAL CONSIDERATIONS

CHAPTER 1

Karl Holubar
Stella Fatović-Ferenčić

Where Have We Come From?

Readily visible alterations of the skin surface have been recognized since the dawn of history. Some were treated; some were not. The equilibrium of the body's humors was considered routinely; the skin was seen as an excretory organ through which bad humors became visible and were drained to the outside world, purifying the body. Skin lesions were believed to have social or even religious significance. Egyptian papyri, Biblical sources, mummies, and classical antiquity attest to this view. *Itching* and changes in *skin color* rank prominently among the abnormalities described. Modern attempts to identify such abnormalities as those representing eczema, leprosy, psoriasis, and similar diseases inevitably fail because the changes represent *inclusive* terms into which half of our latter-day dermatology might well fit. Twenty-five centuries have passed since the apogee of the Hippocratic school, and only very slowly have clinical descriptions improved to the point where they can be identified with disease entities as we know them. Over these many years, medicine and its underlying theories have changed considerably, and yet skin diseases continue to be attributed to divine punishment or personal or ancestral sin.

Little by little, the concepts of *holistic* medicine and *humoral* pathology gave way to organ pathology; the first disease entities were considered, and clinical bedside teaching became a compulsory program in medical school curricula. The enlightenment period eventually brought about the first attempts to systematize and categorize diseases. Clinical observation triumphed, the first therapeutic trials were conducted, scientific periodicals sprang up, and regular exchanges between scientists developed at national and international levels. Balloons lifted humans into the air, ships sailed to the remotest corners of the earth, and good maps became available. The French Revolution was the cogent harbinger of change, and the Napoleonic wars washed away much of the old and opened avenues for medicine as we know it. *Percussion, auscultation,* and local and general *anesthesia* made their appearance, and surgery and "medicine" slowly merged, only to be split up later into the so-called specialty disciplines, dermatology being among the first. It is 200 years since the *first great school of dermatology* became a physical reality and Alibert was entrusted with the directorship of the famous Hôpital Saint-Louis in Paris (1801). The *first textbooks* (Willan's, 1798–1808) and *atlases* (Alibert's, 1806–1814) appeared in print at that time. Skin diseases were described by *individual lesions* (Plenck, 1776), and skin was considered to be an *organ* (Lorry, 1777). Special skin clinics and hospitals were opened.

The *name of the specialty* originated in the form of the (semantically wrong) words *dermologie* (in French, 1764) and, a little later, *dermatologia* (in Latin, 1777). Almost a full century passed before the term *dermatology* was integrated into the various national languages of Europe and was used to identify appointments, departments, and university chairs. Earlier, *diseases of the skin, maladies de la peau, Haut-Krankheiten, malattie della pelle,* and the like were standard. *Dermatopathologia* appeared in 1792 but found its proper use only one century later (Unna's book, 1894). Many journals were founded before the mid-nineteenth century but did not survive. The oldest to continue into our time is the Italian journal, founded in 1866. *Dermatologic societies* began in 1869 (New York Dermatological Society). The American Dermatological Association (ADA) followed in 1876. The first *International Congress of Dermatology* was held in Paris in 1889. The *International League of Dermatological Societies* was formed in Budapest in 1935 and serves as the governing body of world dermatology.

The history of dermatopathology is a century-long story from the early and prophetic thoughts of Henry Seguin Jackson to the first textbook by Unna. The first forays into skin pathology, albeit largely conceptual and semantic, were conducted by Jackson (1792), Gilbert Breschet (1835), and Julius Rosenbaum (1839). Their efforts stalled; both the optical instruments and the cutting and staining techniques were not yet sufficiently developed. Full fruition required several more generations and the hard work and talents of Auspitz, Brocq, Darier, Gans, and Lever.

In the 1930s, two lines of development interacted, one *political*—political on the level of dermatologic organizations and political on the world level—and the other *conceptual*—a shift in emphasis from the purely clinical to investigative dermatology. The interaction, which Rudolf Baer called "revolutionary," began in the United States with three important events that occurred in close succession—the formation of the *American Board of Dermatology* (1932), the foundation of the *Society of Investigative Dermatology* (SID, 1937), and founding of the *American Academy of Dermatology* (AAD, 1938). "Giants" (Baer's word again) like Donald Pillbury, Stephen Rothman, and Marion Sulzberger guaranteed success. On the world scene, and as a consequence of racism, fascism, and Nazism in Europe, Jewish doctors were eliminated—particularly dermatologists, because they constituted the highest percentage in the field and were at the heart and helm of the specialty. Thousands were forced to leave or were killed. This enormous brain drain deprived Europe and dermatology of great strength and enriched the transatlantic regions. The dermatologic center of gravity shifted to America, where this enormous injection of brain power soon made itself felt. Immigrants seldom come with the legal right to practice medicine, a fact that resulted in concentration of the talents of the new arrivals in research areas. American dermatology up to then had concerned itself largely with the clinical, but henceforth the *functional aspect* came to the fore, and *investigative dermatology* was born. From the late 1930s to Stephen Rothman and his classic textbook in 1954 and the contributions of Montagna, the disciplines of histochemistry and cytochemistry were applied to dermatology, and eventually cutaneous immunopathology and molecular biology came into their own.

Meanwhile, Europe took decades to recover. In 1973, the *European Society for Dermatological Research* (ESDR) was founded as a counterpart to the SID, and the *Japanese Society for Investigative Dermatology* (JSID) was founded in 1975. Slowly, a triumverate of research centers emerged—the United States, Europe, and Japan—and regular tricontinental meetings were instituted in support of their dermatologic investigational activities.

The revelation of the function of the Langerhans cell illustrates extremely well the change in the direction of dermatology that took place within the last quarter of the twentieth century. An erstwhile "effete" melanocyte destined to be shed as a useless pensioner within the epidermis, the Langerhans cell moved to the center stage in the research arena with the discovery of its role as the key figure in the elicitation of skin sensitization and immunization. With proper identification of the antigens on "our" cells, dermatology moved to the very center of tissue typing, confirming at last the conviction of Leon Battista Alberti, Donatello, and other humanists of fourteenth and fifteenth century Italy that every individual is singular and special.

Genetics and the human genome, the background for all that we are and stand for, constitute the latest areas of investigation, inseparably linked to the potential capability of altering the preceding singularity, for better or for worse. Many investigators have provided us with discoveries and revelations that are overwhelming. What genetics and genetic engineering have in store for us remains shrouded in the mist of the future.

REFERENCES

The following references are general treatises on the history of dermatology in English, French, German, and Spanish, plus the chapter of the preceding edition of *Dermatology in General Medicine* and the semicentennial issue of the *Journal of Investigative Dermatology* (for the convenience of readers of different ethnic backgrounds and maternal languages). For more specific references and information, we encourage readers to turn to the Web sites of the American History of Dermatology Society (HDS, *http://www.dermato.med.br/hds/*) and the French Society for the History of Dermatology (SFHD, *http://www.bium.univ-paris5.fr/histmed/debut.htm*), which also leads to the European Society for the History of Dermatology and Venereology (ESHDV).

1. Crissey JT, Parish LC: *The Dermatology and Syphilology of the Nineteenth Century.* New York, Praeger, 1981
2. Crissey JT et al: *An Historical Atlas of Dermatology and Dermatologists.* Park Ridge, NJ, Parthenon, 2002
3. Beerman H, Lazarus GS: *The Tradition of Excellence.* Philadelphia, Beerman & Lazarus, 1986
4. Shelly W, Shelley DE: *CMD Congressus Mundi Dermatologiae.* Park Ridge, NJ, Parthenon, 1992
5. Tilles G: *La naissance de la dermatologie (1776–1980).* Paris, éditions Roger Dacosta, 1989 (in French)
6. Scholz A: *Geschichte der Dermatologie in Deutschland.* Berlin, Springer, 1999 (in German)
7. Sierra Valentí X: *Cien años de dermatología 1900–2000.* Madrid, Biblioteca Aula Medica, 2001 (in Spanish)
8. Fifty years of investigative dermatology (semi-centennial issue). *J Invest Dermatol* **92**(suppl):1S–198S, 1989.
9. The Editors: Dermatology in the perspective of general medicine, in *Dermatology in General Medicine,* 5th ed. New York, McGraw-Hill, 1999, pp 3–5
10. Holubar K, Wallach D: History of dermatology: A bicentennial perspective, in *Dermatology in General Medicine,* 5th ed. New York, McGraw-Hill, 1999, pp 5–7

CHAPTER 2

Martin A. Weinstock
Mary-Margaret Chren

The Epidemiology and Burden of Skin Disease

Scientists in health-related fields may focus on different levels. For laboratory scientists, the focus is on phenomena at the molecular, cellular, or organ-system level; for clinical scientists, the focus is on the patient; and for public health practitioners, the focus is on the population. Epidemiology is the basic science of public health.

Epidemiology has many subdivisions and offshoots. Often the *epidemiology of a disease* in a clinical review refers primarily to its frequency and distribution in the population and estimates of the morbidity and mortality of that disease. These data are derived by *descriptive* epidemiology. Case-control, cohort, and cross-sectional studies may seek to identify risk factors and causes of disease and form the core of *analytical* epidemiology. Evaluations of public health interventions (*experimental* epidemiology) constitute the third major branch of *classic epidemiology*. The basic principles of epidemiology have found broad application in many areas, including understanding the public health implications of naturally occurring and synthetic compounds (*molecular epidemiology*), the complex interactions of genetic and environmental factors in disease (*genetic epidemiology*), the formulation of better diagnostic and treatment strategies for patients based on available evidence (*clinical epidemiology*), and the structuring of health care delivery for better outcomes and greater efficiency (*health services research*). The reader is referred to other volumes for a more detailed discussion of dermatoepidemiology.[1,2]

TYPES OF EPIDEMIOLOGIC STUDIES

Three of the many types of epidemiologic studies are mentioned here because of their prominence in epidemiologic research. The randomized, controlled trial is a particularly rigorous type of study appropriate to the evaluation of public health interventions. In general, the intervention is performed on a random sample of the study population, and the entire study population is then observed for the occurrence of the outcome in question. The random assignment of intervention allows the more rigorous application of many statistical techniques and reduces the potential for bias. It is the elimination of many biases that particularly supports the general assumption that these studies more accurately evaluate the efficacy and impact of the intervention than trials that do not assign the intervention condition randomly. Standards have been published[3] and adopted by leading dermatology journals to improve assessment of their validity and their use in subsequent systematic reviews[4] (see Chap. 240).

When evaluating risk factors for disease, it is frequently impossible to assign the risk factor randomly. Hence inference is based on observational studies. In classical cohort studies, a group with exposure to the risk factor and a group without are chosen and observed over time. Occurrences of the study outcome are counted and compared between groups. Although more vulnerable to bias than randomized trials, in cohort studies exposure to the risk factor is known well before the study outcome is knowable, so some potentially serious biases are avoided. In a cohort study, the incidence of the study outcome can be measured directly in each group, and the relative risk can be measured directly as the ratio of the incidence between the two groups.

Cohort studies often are quite expensive to conduct because they require following a large population over time and may be impossible if the outcome being studied is uncommon. Hence observational studies often use the case-control approach, where cases with the outcome being studied and appropriate controls are investigated to determine their past exposure to the risk factor. Relative risks generally can be estimated by this approach, although incidence of the disorder cannot. Readers are referred to standard texts for more detail regarding epidemiologic study designs.[5] Case-control and cohort study methods in dermatology also have been reviewed.[6–8]

BIAS AND CONFOUNDING

The problem with inference from observational studies is that one may be led to draw erroneous conclusions. In particular, an association that is found between an exposure and a disease may be an artifact due to one or more of the many forms of bias or confounding. Proper inference regarding cause and effect requires understanding of these possible artifacts and their potential impacts.[9]

Selection bias occurs when factors that lead to selection of the study population affect the likelihood of the outcomes or exposures evaluated. For example, a case-control study of cutaneous lymphoma may recruit its cases from sources that typically include a high proportion of referred patients. If controls are recruited from a local clinic population, their socioeconomic status and location of residence may be substantially different from those of the cases simply due to the method of recruitment. Under these circumstances, an association of cutaneous lymphoma with occupation may be noted. It then becomes important to note that the observed association may be due not to a carcinogenic chemical in the workplace but rather to the method by which cases and controls were selected. Similarly, if one were conducting a cohort study of the effect of breast feeding on the risk of atopic dermatitis, it would be important to select breast-fed and bottle-fed infants from similar environments.

Information bias occurs when the assessment of exposure or outcome may differ between the groups being compared. People who were exposed to a publicized environmental toxin may be more likely to seek care for minor symptoms or signs (and hence be more likely to be diagnosed and treated) than those who were not so exposed, even if the exposure had no biologic effect. Similarly, people who are diagnosed with a disease may be more likely to recall past exposures than healthy controls.

Confounding occurs when an observed association (or lack thereof) between exposure and disease is due to the influence of a third factor on both the exposure and the disease. For example, people who use sunscreens may be the ones who have the most intense sun exposures, and intense sun exposure is one cause of melanoma. Hence observational studies may mistakenly conclude that sunscreen use is a cause of melanoma when the observed association is due to sunscreen use serving as an indicator of a lifestyle involving intense sun exposure.

CAUSAL INFERENCE

Key issues in the public health arena often must rely on observational data for inferring cause and effect. The criteria for assessment in these circumstances require careful examination of both the validity and generalizability of the individual studies and of the totality of the evidence. The following criteria generally are applied for causal inference when an association is found. Although they are described for inferring causality between an exposure and a disease, they are more generally applicable to epidemiologic causal inference.

Time sequence. The exposure must precede the disease. This is simple and obvious in the abstract but sometimes difficult to establish in practice because the onset of disease may precede the diagnosis of disease by years, and the timing of exposure is often not well defined.

Consistency on replication. Replication of the observed association is key and provides the strongest evidence if the replications are many and diverse and with consistent results. The diversity of the replications refers to varied contexts as well as to study designs with different potential weaknesses and strengths.

Strength of association. True causal relationships may be strong (i.e., high relative risk) or weak, but artifactual associations are unlikely to have a high relative risk. If the association between factors x and y is due to the association of both with confounding variable z, the magnitude of the association between x and y always will be less than the magnitude of the association of either with z.

Graded association. Also described as *biologic gradient,* this criterion refers to an association of the degree of exposure with occurrence of disease, in addition to an overall association of presence of exposure with disease. This dose-response relation may take many forms, since degree of exposure may, for example, refer to intensity, duration, frequency, or latency of exposure.

Coherence. Coherence refers to plausibility based on evidence other than the existence of an association between this exposure and this disease in epidemiologic studies. Coherence with existing epidemiologic knowledge of the disease in question (e.g., other risk factors for the disease and population trends in its occurrence) and other disorders (including but not limited to related disorders) supports inference. Coherence with existing knowledge from other fields, particularly those relevant to pathogenesis, is critically important when those fields are well developed. It may involve direct links, which are preferred, or analogy. Just as observations in the laboratory assume greater significance when their relevance is supported by epidemiologic data, the reverse is equally true.

Experiment. Experimental support is critical when feasible. The strongest inferences derive from results of randomized trials, although other experimental designs and quasi-experimental designs may contribute useful evidence.

More detailed discussions of these issues are available.[10,11]

INVESTIGATION OF DISEASE OUTBREAKS

Although outbreaks of disease vary tremendously, use of a standard framework for investigation is important to address the public health issues efficiently. The Centers for Disease Control and Prevention has described this framework as a series of 10 steps, which are described in more detail elsewhere.[12]

1. *Preparation.* Before initiating fieldwork, background information on the disease must be gathered, and appropriate interinstitutional and interpersonal contacts should be made.
2. *Confirm the outbreak.* Publicity, population changes, or other circumstances may lead to an inaccurate perception that more cases than expected have occurred. Hence local or regional data should be sought to confirm the existence of an increased frequency of disease.
3. *Confirm the diagnosis.* Symptoms and signs of persons affected should be determined and laboratory findings confirmed, perhaps with the assistance of reference laboratories.
4. *Establish a case definition, and find cases.* Careful epidemiologic investigation will involve precise and simple case definitions that can be applied in the field. Efforts to find and count additional cases beyond those reported initially is key to defining the scope of the outbreak.
5. *Establish the descriptive epidemiology.* The cases can now be characterized in terms of *time,* including development of an epidemic curve that describes the changes in magnitude of the outbreak; *place,* including mapping the distribution of cases; and *person,* the demographic and potential exposure characteristics of cases.
6. *Develop hypotheses.* On the basis of the data gathered in steps 1 through 5 and the input of other individuals, plausible hypotheses can be developed for further evaluation.
7. *Conduct analytical epidemiologic investigations.* If the data gathered do not yet clearly prove a hypothesis, cohort and case-control investigations can be conducted to verify or disprove the hypotheses.
8. *Revise hypotheses and obtain additional evidence as needed.* Steps 6 and 7 are repeated, each building on prior iterations, in order to establish the causal chain of events.
9. *Implement control measures.* As soon as the causal chain of events is understood, prevention and control measures are initiated.
10. *Communicate results.* An outbreak investigation is not complete until the results have been appropriately communicated to the relevant communities.

DESCRIPTIONS OF DISEASE IN POPULATIONS: MEASURES OF DISEASE BURDEN

No single number can describe the burden of skin disease because that burden has many dimensions and because the term *skin disease* itself is rather ambiguous. Many disorders with substantial morbidity or mortality, such as melanoma or lupus erythematosus, affect multiple organ systems. The degree of skin involvement may vary widely from patient to patient and within the same patient from time to time. Diseases not typically treated by dermatologists, such as the thermal burns, often are

TABLE 2-1

Skin Disease Deaths, United States, 1998

Cancers	10,740
Melanoma	7,431
Genital	1,040
Lymphoma	122
Other cancers (primarily basal and squamous cell carcinoma)	2,059*
Ulcers	1,813
Bacterial infections	985
Bullous disorders	122
Other causes	420
TOTAL	14,080

*We estimate that approximately half of these are misclassified squamous cell carcinomas arising from mucosal surfaces in the head and neck.[16]

SOURCE: Centers for Disease Control Web site. Available at: www.cdc.gov (verified January 15, 2003).

excluded from estimates of the burden of skin disease even though they primarily involve the skin. In addition, some diseases treated most often by dermatologists may be classified in a different category by funding agencies or others [e.g., melanoma is classified as an oncologic disorder as opposed to dermatologic disorder by the National Institutes of Health and by the *International Classification of Diseases,* 9th revision (ICD-9), even though it almost always arises in the skin]. Organ systems are interrelated, and the overlap is sufficiently great that any definition of skin disease is necessarily arbitrary, and any estimate of the public health burden of these diseases is therefore open to challenge.

Mortality is a critical measure of disease impact. Death certification is universal in the United States, and the ICD code of the underlying cause of each death is recorded. For the year 1998, there were 14,080 deaths reported as due to "skin disease" in the United States, of which most were due to melanoma (Table 2-1). Additional major causes included other skin cancers (primarily keratinocyte carcinomas), infections of the skin, and skin ulcers (primarily decubitus ulcers). Bullous disorders represented about 1 percent of these deaths. The total number of skin disease deaths, of course, depends critically on the definition of skin disease, as noted earlier.

In addition to the total number of deaths, mortality typically is expressed as an age-adjusted rate to facilitate comparisons among populations with different age distributions. Statements of age-adjusted rates of mortality (or anything else that is standardized by age) should be accompanied by an indication of the standard used in the adjustment to avoid potentially misleading inferences. For example, when 1998 melanoma mortality rates are estimated using the 2000 U.S. population standard, the result is 50 percent higher than if the 1940 U.S. standard population is used (1.8 versus 1.2 per 100,000 per year for women and 4.1 versus 2.7 per 100,000 per year for men). Sometimes *years of potential life lost* (YPLL) is also measured, and here again, the reader must be wary of different definitions that may be applied. In one analysis, a decline in mortality from melanoma was noted by one definition that was not observed with another.[13]

Careful analyses of mortality include assessment of the validity of the data. Melanoma mortality statistics appear to be reasonably accurate.[14,15] However, deaths from keratinocyte carcinomas are overestimated by a factor of 2 (mostly due to the erroneous inclusion of mucosal squamous cell carcinomas of the head and neck region),[16] and deaths from cutaneous lymphoma are underestimated by about 40 percent.[14]

Incidence refers to the number of new cases of a disorder. Mortality is low for most skin diseases; hence incidence may be a more useful measure for the assessment of burden of disease. However, many features

TABLE 2-2

New Cases of Selected Reportable Diseases in the United States

	1940	1950	1960	1970	1980	1990	2000
AIDS	—*	—	—	—	—	41,595	40,758
Anthrax	76	49	23	2	1	0	1
Congenital rubella	—	—	—	77	50	11	9
Congenital syphilis	—	—	—	—	—	3,865	529
Diphtheria	15,536	5,796	918	435	3	4	1
Gonorrhea	175,841	286,746	258,933	600,072	1,004,029	690,169	358,995
Hansen's disease	—	44	54	129	223	198	91
Lyme disease	—	—	—	—	—	—	17,730
Measles	291,162	319,124	441,703	47,351	13,506	27,786	86
Plague	1	3	2	13	18	2	6
Rocky mountain spotted fever	457	464	204	380	1.163	651	495
Syphilis (primary and secondary)	—	23,939	16,145	1,982	27,204	50,223	5,979
Toxic shock syndrome	—	—	—	—	—	322	135
Tuberculosis†	102,984‡	121,742‡	55,494	37,137	27,749	25,701	16,377
U.S. population (millions)	132	151	180	204	227	249	273

*Data not available.
†Reporting criteria changed in 1975.
‡Data include newly reported active and inactive cases.
SOURCES: Centers for Disease Control: Annual summary 1984: Reported morbidity and mortality in the United States, *MMWR Morb Mortal Wkly Rep* **33**:124, 1986; Centers for Disease Control and Prevention: Summary of notifiable diseases, United States, 2000, *MMWR Morb Mortal Wkly Rep* **50**:712, 2001; Centers for Disease Control and Prevention: Summary of notifiable diseases, United States, 1990, *MMWR Morb Mortal Wkly Rep* **39**:55, 1991; Eberhardt MS et al: *Urban and Rural Health Chartbook: Health, United States, 2001*, Hyattsville, MD, National Center for Health Statistics, 2001, p 227; adapted with permission from Weinstock MA, Boyle MM: Statistics of interest to the dermatologist, in *The Year Book of Dermatology and Dermatologic Surgery*, edited by BH Theirs, PG Lang, St Louis, Mosby, 2001, p 36.

of skin diseases make their incidence difficult to measure. For example, for many skin disorders there are no diagnostic laboratory tests, and in fact, some disorders may evade physician diagnosis (e.g., allergic reactions). Incidence for reportable communicable diseases in the United States is published periodically based on reports to health departments, although underreporting of skin diseases due to failure to present for medical care or to misdiagnosis is a concern (Table 2-2). Incidences of melanoma and cutaneous lymphoma also have been published based on data from a system of nationwide cancer registries, yet underreporting remains a potential concern with these data.[17,18] Special surveys have been conducted to estimate incidence of other disorders such as keratinocyte carcinomas, although a system of sentinel registries would be required for nationwide assessment.[19] For some diseases unlikely to evade medical detection due to their severity, such as toxic epidermal necrolysis, efforts to estimate incidence have met with considerable success.[20,21] Specific contexts that permit more accurate incidence estimates include the workplace, for example, where occupational skin disease is a prevalent problem.[22]

Cohort patterns of changes in mortality or incidence typically are observed when exposures determined in childhood predict frequency of disease throughout the life span. A classic example is melanoma mortality, for which sun exposure in childhood is an important determinant. A birth cohort is defined as the group of individuals born within a defined (e.g., 10-year) period. Melanoma mortality generally increases as a power function of age within a birth cohort. Until recent decades, each successive birth cohort had higher risk than its predecessor; hence the curves of mortality versus age were shifted upward. Thus the cross-sectional relationship of mortality versus age and the increase in mortality risk during most of the twentieth century followed a cohort pattern. For many countries in the past several decades we have seen a decline in melanoma mortality in the younger age groups despite an increase in older age groups, suggesting a lower baseline in these mortality versus age curves for recent cohorts and hence a likely future decline in overall melanoma mortality.

Prevalence refers to the proportion of the population affected by a disorder. Since many skin diseases are nonlethal yet chronic, prevalence is a particularly important measure of frequency in dermatology. Population-based data on prevalence of skin disease for the United States were obtained in the first Health and Nutrition Examination Survey, which was conducted in the early 1970s.[23] Despite its limitations, this study was notable because the sample was representative of the general U.S. population, the number surveyed was large (over 20,000), and the entire surveyed population was examined by physicians (primarily dermatology residents), so the resulting estimates were not dependent on patients' ability or inclination to seek medical care. Indeed, one of the findings of the survey was that nearly one-third of those examined had one or more skin conditions judged to be significant enough to merit a visit to a physician. The most common conditions and their age- and gender-specific prevalences are indicated in Table 2-3 and Fig. 2-1. A similar survey in the United Kingdom of over 2000 Lodoners

TABLE 2-3

Prevalence of Skin Conditions—United States, 1971–1974*

	Male	Female	Both Sexes
Dermatophytosis	131	34	81
Acne (vulgaris and cystic)	74	66	70
Seborrheic dermatitis	30	26	28
Atopic dermatitis/eczema	20	18	19
Verruca vulgaris	9	6	8
Malignant tumors	6	5	6
Psoriasis	6	5	6
Vitiligo	6	4	5
Herpes simplex	4	5	4

*Cases per 1000 population.
SOURCE: Skin conditions and related need for medical care among persons 1–74 years, United States, 1971–1974, *Vital Health Stat* **11** (212), 1978.

FIGURE 2-1

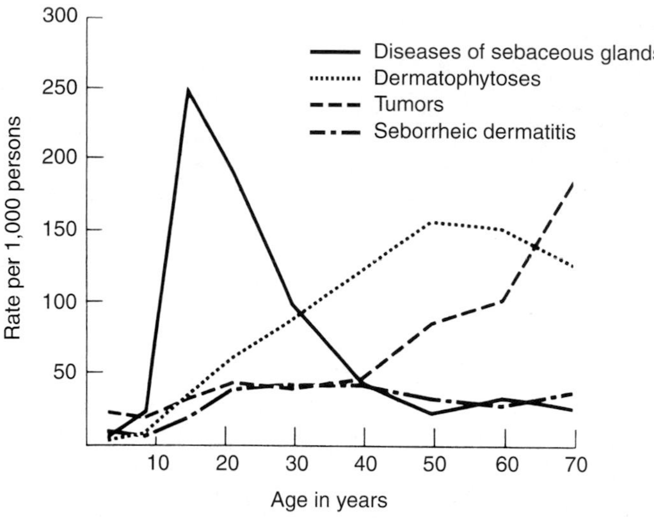

Prevalence rates for the four leading types of significant pathology among persons 1 to 74 years, by age, in the United States, 1971–1974.

in 1975 noted that almost one-quarter of adults had a skin condition serious enough to warrant medical care.[24] Other efforts have focused on obtaining prevalence estimates of specific conditions with special surveys (e.g., see refs. 25 and 26).

Lifetime risks for certain disorders are quoted commonly, although their validity can be questioned. Lifetime risk can be measured only in retrospect, and even then it reflects competing causes of mortality in addition to incidence. It is commonly quoted for disorders such as cutaneous malignancies that are changing substantially in incidence, yet those changes are frequently ignored in its calculation, and in any case, projections of future changes are quite speculative and may be quite misleading.

Number of physician visits for a condition is one practical measure of its frequency that may reflect its incidence, prevalence, and severity, as well as access to health care. Table 2-4 lists frequencies of dermatologist and other physician outpatient visits for some of the most common skin conditions. A feature of using this measure of disease frequency is its direct relation to expenditures for care of the disease.

TABLE 2-4

Visits to Nonfederal Office-Based Physicians in the United States, 1998

	Type of Physician		
Diagnosis	Dermatologist	Other	All Physicians
Acne vulgaris	5,292 (15.8%)	* *	6,035 (0.7%)
Eczematous dermatitis	2,800 (8.4%)	6,586 (0.8%)	9,386 (1.1%)
Warts	1,708 (5.1%)	2,094 (0.3%)	3,801 (0.5%)
Skin cancer	2,289 (6.8%)	1,823 (0.2%)	4,112 (0.5%)
Psoriasis	1,228 (3.7%)	* *	1,439 (0.2%)
Fungal infections	728 (2.2%)	2,388 (0.3%)	3,116 (0.4%)
Hair disorders	788 (2.4%)	* *	1,025 (0.1%)
Actinic keratosis	3,007 (9.0%)	* *	3,289 (0.4%)
Benign neoplasm of the skin	1,925 (5.8%)	1,391 (0.2%)	3,317 (0.4%)
All disorders	33,410 (100%)	795,871 (100%)	829,280 (100%)

*Figure does not meet standard of precision.
NOTE: Estimates in thousands; percentage of total visits is in parentheses.
SOURCES: National Ambulatory Medical Care Survey, National Center for Health Statistics, Centers for Disease Control and Prevention: Personal communication, February 2001; Adapted with permission from Weinstock MA, Boyle MM: Statistics of interest to the dermatologists, in Theirs BH, Lang PG, eds. 2001 The Year Book of Dermatology and Dermatologic Surgery, edited by BH Theirs, PG Lang, St Louis, Mosby, 2001, p 48.

Other Measures of Morbidity: Conceptual Issues

The consequences of skin disease for a population may be difficult to describe because these conditions most often do not affect survival, and the most important gauges of disease status and progression are the physical examination and patients' reports, which are difficult to measure and compile. The World Health Organization has classified the effects on patients of nonfatal diseases into three dimensions.[27] *Impairment* due to disease refers to loss of an anatomic structure or of a physiologic or psychological function. For example, psoriasis can cause thickening and scaling of the palms. *Disability* is restriction on normal performance of an activity due to impairment. Disability from psoriasis may include the loss of ability to use one's hands easily because of skin thickening and scale. Disability may lead to *handicap,* which refers to its consequences for an individual; for example, loss of hand function from psoriasis may render a pianist or dishwasher unable to perform his or her livelihood.

Interpreting and using measures of handicap for groups of persons is complex due to differences in perceptions, expectations, and values. These differences may be related to sociodemographic variables such as age, access to health care, and cultural conceptions of health. For this reason, some have argued that for assessing burden of disease, disability is a more appropriate construct to measure than handicap because it is less prone to cultural differences that might lead to inequities in allocation of resources.[27] A crucial point for skin diseases is that a patient's experiences other than disability are important to a determination of the value patients place on disease effects. For example, experiences such as social stigma and effects of disease on mood may be significant effects of skin diseases that are visible and affect appearance.[28] Thus the measurement and in particular the comparative valuation of nonfatal consequences of disease—and their significance for national policymaking—are controversial. This debate has important implications for dermatology as global health needs, resource allocation, and cost-effectiveness are assessed with single-item metrics that are used for empirical ranking of disease burden.[29,30]

Related to these effects of diseases on patients is the concept of *quality of life,* which refers to the physical, functional, psychological, and social health of the individual.[31] As defined, quality of life includes disability and handicap from a disease and is an important measure of the morbidity of skin conditions, which may cause disfigurement and thus affect patients emotionally as well as physically. Finally, *utility* is a numeric measure of the value a patient attaches to a given health state compared with other health states. This metric is important for the calculation of cost-effectiveness, in which the costs of treatments are compared with the values of the health states they make possible.

Other Measures of Morbidity: Issues in Quantification

Like all assays, measures of the nonfatal consequences of diseases must have certain characteristics of accuracy.[32] For example, they must be *reliable* in that the variability in results among subjects who truly differ should be greater than the variability when a stable subject is examined repeatedly. The measures must have evidence of *validity,* which refers to the extent to which an instrument measures what it is supposed to measure and does not measure something else. Finally, health outcome measures also must demonstrate *responsiveness,* the ability to detect clinical change. In general, the accuracy of measures of disease status and morbidity in dermatology has not been evaluated adequately.[33,34] Furthermore, even when a validated instrument exists, the clinical significance of scores or changes in scores often cannot be judged until the tool is used widely and scores are available for many patients with disease of varying severity. Finally, a significant challenge is developing a consensus among dermatologists about the specific clinical features of an individual disease that are important to include in such measures. For example, criteria for clinically important improvement have been developed for some rheumatologic conditions[35] that, like skin diseases, are chronic and are best assessed using clinical rather than laboratory criteria.

Impairment

The extent to which a specific skin disease disrupts the skin itself is related both to the percentage of body surface area involved and to physical signs of the eruption such as the amount of induration and the degree of scale. Given the pleomorphism of skin eruptions and lesions, most dermatologic severity-of-disease measures are disease-specific. Among the most studied instruments to measure clinical severity of disease are the Psoriasis Area and Severity Index (PASI)[36] and the Severity Scoring of Atopic Dermatitis (SCORAD) index.[37] With the PASI, severity of disease is assessed by judgment of the degree of involvement of four body regions with signs of erythema, induration, and desquamation. The SCORAD index combines an assessment of disease area with six clinical signs of disease intensity (scales to measure pruritus and sleep loss also can be included). These instruments share certain problems; for example, estimates of body surface area are often unreliable,[38] and many investigators (and patients) may not agree that the selected clinical signs represent the important features of disease severity.

Disability

Disease-induced restrictions in the ability of a patient to perform normal activities have been measured for specific skin diseases such as psoriasis. A prototypical instrument is the Psoriasis Disability Index (PDI).[39] The PDI asks patients to rate the effects of their psoriasis on specific aspects of their functioning (e.g., daily activities, work or school, personal relationships, leisure). The PDI has important measurement properties such as validity and responsiveness to change and has been used not only as an outcomes measure in clinical trials but also as a model for measuring disability from other conditions.

Handicap and Quality of Life

Substantial progress has been made in the development and testing of quality-of-life instruments for patients with skin diseases. Several generic instruments exist that are applicable to patients with dermatologic disease of any sort.[40–42] Data continue to be accumulated about the performance of these instruments and the interpretation of their scores. An important conclusion from these studies is that correlations between the quality-of-life effects of skin diseases and their clinical severity as assessed by physicians are modest at best and may in fact be quite low. This finding is also typical of many nondermatologic diseases and implies that a comprehensive assessment of patients with skin disease should include measurement of clinical severity as well as its effects on quality of life.[43]

Utilities

In the measurement of utilities, a variety of procedures are used (such as visual analogue scales and time tradeoff exercises) to assign a numerical value (or utility) to health states. This value reflects patients' preferences for the health states, where 1.0 represents perfect health and 0.0 represents death. With utilities, improvements in morbidity and mortality can be combined into a single weighted metric. Few studies have formally measured utilities of patients with skin diseases, although the approach is feasible[44,45] and has been used for comparing cost-effectiveness of therapies for psoriasis.[46]

Costs

Measurement of costs of skin disease depends on the perspective from which they are measured, since the costs to insurers and patients may be quite different from the overall cost to society. Because most skin diseases are chronic and are cared for in the outpatient setting, estimation of both their monetary and intangible costs is difficult. There are no recent studies of the direct or indirect cost of dermatologic diseases and their care overall. Costs have been estimated, however, for individual diseases. The treatment costs to Medicare of keratinocyte carcinoma (basal cell and squamous cell carcinomas of the skin) in 1995 were estimated to be approximately $285 million, which represented 0.7 percent of the Medicare budget.[47] The direct costs of treating newly diagnosed melanoma in 1997 were estimated at $563 million.[48] The costs of diseases not treated surgically are even more difficult to estimate because valid estimates of drug costs are not widely available. For example, the treatment of acne in the United States generates over 6 million prescriptions annually for oral medications alone, and the total yearly cost of acne likely exceeds $1 billion.[49] Costs also depend on the processes of delivering health care and the technology used. For example, the trend toward increased use of sentinel lymph node biopsies and adjuvant chemotherapy for localized melanoma may increase the costs associated with this disease substantially.

QUALITY OF CARE IN DERMATOLOGY

Health services research uses many of the scientific methods from epidemiology, clinical epidemiology, and the quantitative social sciences to study and improve the quality of health care. From the perspective of health services research, the processes involved in the provision of health care, as well as the particular therapeutic interventions and patient and provider characteristics, are all potentially important determinants of the results (*outcomes* in terms of mortality, morbidity, and cost) of the provision of health care. Dermatologic health services research is still new; much attention has focused on improved outcomes of health care,[50] although the results of well-done clinical trials should inform the process of care as well.[51] Many of the examples cited earlier demonstrate a sharpened focus in dermatology on accurate measurement of the clinical encounter. This capacity to measure the progress of chronic diseases and their care will permit rigorous efforts to evaluate and improve the quality of that care.

REFERENCES

1. Williams HC, Strachan DP, eds: *The Challenge of Dermatoepidemiology.* Boca Raton, FL, CRC Press, 1997
2. Weinstock MA, ed: *Dermatoepidemiology.* Philadelphia, Saunders, 1995

3. Begg C et al: Improving the quality of reporting of randomized controlled trials: The CONSORT statement. *JAMA* **276**:637, 1996
4. Weinstock MA: The JAAD adopts the CONSORT statement. *J Am Acad Dermatol* **41**:1045, 1999
5. Gordis L: *Epidemiology.* Philadelphia, Saunders, 2000
6. Karagas MR: When subjects are not randomly assigned: The cohort approach. *J Cutan Med Surg* **2**:90, 1997
7. Heacock HJ, Rivers JK: Assessing scientific data: The case-control study as it applies to dermatology. Part I. The case-control method. *J Cutan Med Surg* **1**:151, 1997
8. Heacock HJ, Rivers JK: Assessing scientific data: The case-control study as it applies to dermatology. Part 2. Interpreting the results. *J Cutan Med Surg* **2**:35, 1997
9. Sackett DL: Bias in analytic research. *J Chron Dis* **32**:51, 1979
10. Susser M: *Causal Thinking in the Health Sciences: Concepts and Strategies of Epidemiology.* New York, Oxford University Press, 1973
11. Hill AB: Environment and disease: Association or causation? *Proc R Soc Med* **58**:295, 1965
12. Centers for Disease Control Web site. Available at: http://www.cdc.gov/excite/classroom/outbreak_steps.htm#steps. Accessed January 15, 2003
13. Weinstock MA: Epidemiology of melanoma, in *Current Research and Clinical Management of Melanoma,* edited by L Nathanson Boston, Kluwer Academic, 1993, pp 29–56
14. Weinstock MA, Reynes JF: Validation of cause of death certification for outpatient cancers: The contrasting cases of melanoma and mycosis fungoides. *Am J Epidemiol* **148**:1184, 1998
15. Percy C et al: Accuracy of cancer death certificates and its effect on cancer mortality statistics. *Am J Public Health* **71**:242, 1981
16. Weinstock MA et al: Inaccuracies in certification of nonmelanoma skin cancer deaths. *Am J Public Health* **82**:278, 1992
17. Jemal A et al: Recent trends in cutaneous melanoma incidence among whites in the United States. *J Natl Cancer Inst* **93**:678, 2001
18. Weinstock MA, Gardstein BA: Twenty-year trends in the reported incidence of mycosis fungoides and associated mortality. *Am J Public Health* **89**:1240, 1999
19. Weinstock MA: Overview of ultraviolet radiation and cancer: What is the link? How are we doing? *Environ Health Perspect* **103**(suppl 8):251, 1995
20. Roujeau JC et al: Toxic epidemiomal necrolysis (Lyell syndrome): Incidence and drug etiology in France, 1981–1985. *Arch Dermatol* **126**:37, 1990
21. Rzany B et al: Epidemiology of erythema exsudativum multiforme majus, Stevens-Johnson syndrome, and toxic epidermal necrolysis in Germany (1990–1992): Structure and results of a population-based registry. *J Clin Epidemiol* **49**:769, 1996
22. Dickel H et al: Occupational skin diseases in Northern Bavaria between 1990 and 1999: A population-based study. *Br J Dermatol* **145**:453, 2001
23. Johnson M-LT, Roberts J: *Skin Conditions and Related Need for Medical Care Among Persons 1–74 Years, United States, 1971–74* (DHEW Publication No. PHS 79-1660). Hyattsville, MD, National Center for Health Statistics, 1978
24. Rea JN et al: Skin disease in Lambeth: A community study of prevalence and use of medical care. *Br J Prevent Soc Med* **30**:107, 1976
25. Foley P et al: The frequency of common skin conditions in preschool-age children in Australia: Atopic dermatitis. *Arch Dermatol* **137**:293, 2001
26. Brandrup F, Green A: The prevalence of psoriasis in Denmark. *Acta Derm Venereol* **61**:344, 1981
27. Murray CJL: *The Global Burden of Disease: A Comprehensive Assessment of Mortality and Disability from Diseases, Injuries, and Risk Factors in 1990 and Projected to 2020.* Cambridge, MA, Harvard University Press, 1996
28. Ustun TB et al: Multiple-informant ranking of the disabling effects of different health conditions in 14 countries. WHO/NIH Joint Project CAR Study Group. *Lancet* **354**:111, 1999
29. Arnesen T, Nord E: The value of DALY life: Problems with ethics and validity of disability adjusted life years. *Br Med J* **319**:1423, 1999
30. Gross CP et al: The relation between funding by the National Institutes of Health and the burden of disease. *N Engl J Med* **340**:1881, 1999
31. Testa MA, Simonson DC: Assessment of quality-of-life outcomes. *N Engl J Med* **334**:835, 1996
32. Chren MM: Giving "scale" new meaning in dermatology: Measurement matters. *Arch Dermatol* **136**:788, 2000
33. Marks R et al: Assessment of disease progress in psoriasis. *Arch Dermatol* **125**:235, 1989
34. Charman C, Williams H: Outcome measures of disease severity in atopic eczema. *Arch Dermatol* **136**:763, 2000
35. Ward MM: Response criteria and criteria for clinically important improvement: Separate and equal? *Arthritis Rheum* **44**:1728, 2001
36. Fredriksson T, Pettersson U: Severe psoriasis: Oral therapy with a new retinoid. *Dermatologica* **157**:238, 1978
37. Kunz B et al: Clinical validation and guidelines for the SCORAD index: Consensus report of the European Task Force on Atopic Dermatitis. *Dermatology* **195**:10, 1997
38. Tiling-Grosse S, Rees J: Assessment of area of involvement in skin disease: A study using schematic figure outlines. *Br J Dermatol* **128**:69, 1993
39. Finlay AY, Kelley SE: Psoriasis: An index of disability. *Clin Exp Dermatol* **12**:8, 1987
40. Finlay AY, Khan GK: Dermatology life quality index (DLQI): A simple practical measure for routine clinical use. *Clin Exp Dermatol* **19**:210, 1994
41. Chren MM et al: Improved discriminative and evaluative capability of a refined version of Skindex, a quality-of-life instrument for patients with skin diseases. *Arch Dermatol* **133**:1433, 1997
42. Chren MM et al: Measurement properties of Skindex-16: A brief quality-of-life measure for patients with skin diseases. *J Cutan Med Surg* **5**:105, 2001
43. Kirby B et al: Physical and psychologic measures are necessary to assess overall psoriasis severity. *J Am Acad Dermatol* **45**:72, 2001
44. Lundberg L et al: Quality of life, health-state utilities and willingness to pay in patients with psoriasis and atopic eczema. *Br J Dermatol* **141**:1067, 1999
45. Zug KA et al: Assessing the preferences of patients with psoriasis: A quantitative, utility approach. *Arch Dermatol* **131**:561, 1995
46. Chen S et al: Cost-effectiveness and cost-benefit analysis of using methotrexate versus Goeckerman therapy for psoriasis. *Arch Dermatol* **134**:1602, 1998
47. Joseph AK et al: The period prevalence and costs of treating nonmelanoma skin cancers in patients over 65 years of age covered by Medicare. *Dermatol Surg* **27**:955, 2001
48. Tsao H et al: An estimate of the annual direct cost of treating cutaneous melanoma. *J Am Acad Dermatol* **38**:669, 1998
49. Stern RS: Medication and medical service utilization for acne 1995–1998. *J Am Acad Dermatol* **43**:1042, 2000
50. Chren MM: Quality of care in dermatology: The state of (measuring) the art. *Arch Dermatol* **133**:1349, 1997
51. Bigby M: Challenges to the hierarchy of evidence: Does the emperor have no clothes? *Arch Dermatol* **137**:345, 2001

SECTION 2

CLINICAL-PATHOLOGIC CORRELATIONS OF SKIN LESIONS: APPROACH TO DIAGNOSIS

CHAPTER 3

Margaret I. Stewart
Jeffrey D. Bernhard
Thomas G. Cropley
Thomas B. Fitzpatrick

The Structure of Skin Lesions and Fundamentals of Diagnosis

What is most difficult of all? It is what appears most simple: To see with your eyes what lies in front of your eyes.[*]

Goethe

The diagnosis and treatment of diseases that affect the skin rest upon the physician's ability to use the lexicon of dermatology, to recognize the basic and sequential lesions of the skin, and to recognize the various patterns in which they occur in a large variety of diseases and syndromes.[1] The physician who recognizes a malignant melanoma, the rash of Rocky Mountain spotted fever, or the lesions of cutaneous vasculitis will save lives. The physician who fails to perceive cutaneous markers of systemic diseases, or who fails to recognize inconsequential or normal skin lesions for what they are, may fail to make an important diagnosis or subject patients to unwarranted, expensive, and potentially harmful diagnostic procedures.

The visibility and accessibility of the skin are at the root of the challenge and satisfaction of dermatologic diagnosis: there are a myriad of visible lesions and, consequently, a large number of recognizable syndromes and diseases. The general physical examination provides an opportunity to screen for cutaneous markers of systemic disease as well as for skin tumors, and in particular for malignant melanomas at their earliest—and curable—stages.[2,3] Physicians, therefore, must learn to "read" the skin. Certain cutaneous markers, such as the hypomelanotic ash-leaf spot in tuberous sclerosis or necrolytic migratory erythema in glucagonoma syndrome, are signs as sensitive and specific as those seen in an ECG or an x-ray film of the chest.

Individual skin lesions (see Table 3-1 and Figs. 3-1 through 3-16) are analogous to the letters of the alphabet, and groups of lesions can be analogous to words or phrases. Pathologic changes affect various components of the skin (namely, epidermis, dermis, panniculus, and blood vessels). It is helpful to estimate the component of the skin that is *primarily* affected inasmuch as there is a finite number of disorders that produce pathologic changes in the various individual components.

Once the component of the skin affected by a pathologic process is determined to the extent possible by clinical examination, the lesion or lesions should be assessed in terms of their type, shape, arrangement, and distribution. These attributes are discussed fully later in this chapter. Furthermore, as in all other diseases, many skin conditions undergo a characteristic evolution: in many cases, definitive diagnosis may not be possible without the benefit of observation on more than one occasion. Finally, definitive diagnosis may require the information provided by a complete history, physical examination, laboratory tests, and histopathologic analysis.

APPROACH TO THE PATIENT

Dermatologists often prefer to examine the patient *before* obtaining the history and review of systems.[4] This preference is based on three important points. First, that diagnostic accuracy may be higher when visual examination is approached without preconceived ideas.[5,6] This is also true in radiology.[7] Second, that preconceived notions have the power to truncate thinking and to eliminate important considerations from differential diagnosis (the "white bear syndrome": when someone is told not to think about a white bear it is difficult to think about anything else).[8] The third is that some dermatologic lesions and eruptions are so distinctive that a history is not required to make a diagnosis. Some history must always be obtained, however, as misdiagnosis will certainly occur if the opportunity for corroboration of a clinical diagnosis is missed. In many instances, as in the case of a patient with fever and a rash, the complete history is obviously of major importance, but findings from the initial physical examination can be utilized to shape the way the history is obtained. The history, in turn, should provide direction for a subsequent and refined reexamination. In practice, many skilled clinicians obtain much of the history during the clinical examination of the patient.

In patients who present with a skin problem as the chief complaint, the cutaneous process is commonly so readily apparent that the physician's attention is easily diverted from the patient as a whole. This mistake must be avoided; the majority of patients with a "rash" should be approached in the same manner as a patient with a chief complaint of arthralgia or weight loss or dyspnea, when a general medical history is always essential.

The history of a dermatologic illness should include an exact description of the onset, a careful description of the first lesions, and the details of the development and extension of the lesions. In obtaining the history, careful questioning by the examiner is necessary to elucidate

[*]Was ist das Schwerste von allem? Was du das Leichteste dünket: Mit den Augen zu *sehn* was vor den Augen dir liegt.

TABLE 3-1

Types of Skin Lesions

Flat Lesion (Usually in the Plane of the Skin)	Elevated Lesion (Above the Plane of the Skin)	Depressed Lesion (Below the Plane of the Skin
Macule	Papule	Atrophy
Infarct	Plaque	Sclerosis
Sclerosis	Nodule	Erosion
Telangiectasia	Wheal	Excoriation
	Vesicle and bulla	Scar
	Pustule	Ulcer
	Abscess	Sinus
	Cyst	Gangrene
	Exudate (crusts)	
	Scales	
	Scar	
	Lichenification	

the relationship of the onset of the initial eruption or of recurrences to (1) the patient's *occupation;* (2) *treatment* obtained from a previous physician or self-administered; (3) the *diagnosis* such treatment was based on and how it was established; (4) the patient's experience with prescription and nonprescription *drugs;* (5) exposure to *sunlight* and *seasonal variations* (especially in temperate latitudes); (6) the *immediate environment,* including contact with plants, animals, chemicals, metal, and the like; (7) physiologic states such as *menses* or *pregnancy;* and (8) *foods.*

Drugs, given orally or parenterally, are frequent causes of skin eruptions, and therefore the search for a history of drug ingestion or injection must be persistent and detailed (see Chap. 138). The importance of obtaining and recording an accurate medication history cannot be overstated. Drug eruptions usually develop rapidly, so recollection is often not that difficult.

Patients who complain about skin symptoms but who have no visible abnormality of the skin may fall into several categories. Some patients may have genuine organic disease with skin symptoms such as itching or pain.[9] For example, the so-called nonrash of pruritus (itching without visible skin lesions) may be an important sign of an underlying disorder such as thyrotoxicosis.[10] Other "nonrashes," which may range from delusions to dirt accumulated on the skin, have also been described.[11] Cotterill has described the syndrome of dermatologic nondisease, in which patients complain of symptoms such as itching, sweating, burning, excessive hair, or pain in localized areas such as the face, scalp, mouth, or perineum. Some of these patients have deranged body images (dysmorphophobia) and severe, potentially dangerous psychological disturbances.[12,13] Cutaneous artifactual disease is another point at which dermatology and psychiatry intersect.[14] Also in the realm of "invisible dermatoses" are physiologic or pathologic abnormalities of the skin that may not be grossly apparent on clinical examination.[16]

EXAMINATION OF THE SKIN, HAIR, NAILS, AND MUCOUS MEMBRANES

The skin functions as a sensory organ; as an organ of metabolism that has synthesizing, excretory, and absorptive functions; as a protective barrier against the external environment; and as an important factor in temperature regulation. The clinical examination of the skin is partly an appraisal of these particular functions. In addition, however, the skin is synergistic with internal organ systems, and therefore, it reflects pathologic processes that are either primary elsewhere or shared in common with other tissues. The history of medicine suggests that diseases initially characterized as solely cutaneous (e.g., lupus erythematosus, dermatitis herpetiformis, and urticaria pigmentosa) have often subsequently been found to involve several systems.

Inasmuch as visual appreciation of skin lesions is the sine qua non of dermatologic diagnosis, the examiner's eye is undoubtedly the most important instrument at his or her disposal. Yet the standardization of this instrument is a subject that receives scant attention, even though there are surprising variations in physicians' reports of what has been seen. Furthermore, variability persists at every step of the diagnostic process, from description to differential diagnosis. The chances for correct recognition improve, of course, as the examiner gains familiarity with the various disorders of the skin. Even with experience, however, the greatest difficulty in diagnosis is often because of a failure to notice pertinent details from the available evidence.

Feinstein has challenged the tendency to favor laboratory tests that give numerical values as opposed to clinical observations.[17] He wrote that clinicians try to be scientific in the use of inanimate objects but not in the use of their own sensory organs and brain. They often believe that their own human equipment is a hindrance instead of an advantage, an apology rather than an incentive for science in clinical work. Feinstein emphasized the need for more attention to sick people and the human methods of evaluating them, not to inanimate technology. Furthermore, the ability to arrive at a diagnosis through the history and physical examination is probably the most ancient, perhaps defining, and often—from an intellectual point of view—most satisfying attribute of being a physician. Physical diagnosis *is an art, but no less a science because of it,* and nowhere is the *skill* of physical examination more crucial to accurate diagnosis than it is in dermatology.

The examination of the skin should be made in a well-lighted room with natural light, if possible, or a "daylight" type of lamp. When feasible, the patient should be gowned, and examined completely and systematically in sections or quadrants. Articles of clothing are hindrances during the examination and may even be responsible for the inadvertent concealment of large areas of the skin.

The examination should commence with a general assessment of the patient as a whole—a "low-power" scan of the skin surface, during which rapid stock is taken of the skin, nails, and mucous membranes. The survey should include an appreciation of the color, moisture, the turgor, odor and the texture of the skin. Clothing may give clues to the cause of a suspected contact dermatitis or parasitic infestation (e.g., pediculosis).

General Features of the Skin

COLOR Skin color represents an aggregate of the remitted and reflected light, the wavelengths of which depend largely on the presence of four biochromes. Two biochromes are in the epidermis: *melanin* (see discussion in Chap. 11), which is brown and has a broad absorption in the ultraviolet and visible light ranges, and *carotenoids,* which are yellow. Two other biochromes are in the dermis: *oxyhemoglobin,* which is bright red and is found largely in the arterioles and capillaries of the papillary layer, and *reduced hemoglobin,* which is bluish red and is found in the subpapillary venous plexus. The dermal connective tissue may also contribute to the "whiteness" of the skin in lightly pigmented persons. Greater detail on the role of carotenoids in the skin, as well as an in-depth discussion of ceruloderma (blue skin), can be found in Chaps. 145 and 91, respectively.

General Features of the Hair and Nails

The distribution of the body hair, its texture, and amount should be noted as a part of the initial overall survey of the patient's skin, as should examination of the nails. The nails (see Chap. 72) can provide evidence of latent skin disease (psoriasis, lichen planus, alopecia areata, congenital ectodermal defect), as well as suggest the presence of renal or liver disease. Beau's lines (transverse indentations of the nails) and other variations on the theme of transverse white lines across the nails may be associated with a recent febrile or systemic illness, especially a renal or hepatic one. Telangiectasia in the periungual skin is a frequent and important diagnostic finding in systemic lupus erythematosus and dermatomyositis. The hair and nails are discussed in greater detail in Chaps. 71 and 72.

General Features of the Mucous Membranes

(See Chaps. 112 to 114)

The initial general assessment of the patient must also include the oral, genital, and anal regions. The oral mucous membranes indicate the state of hydration and show pigmentary changes that can be racial traits or that may be helpful in the diagnosis of Peutz-Jeghers syndrome and Addison's disease. Among the many skin diseases that have mucous membrane manifestations are lichen planus, pemphigus, pemphigoid, herpes simplex, and erythema multiforme. The tongue may be red and smooth in various states of vitamin B deficiency. Soreness, as well as a beefy-red tongue, may be present as an initial complaint in pernicious anemia. The so-called black hairy tongue may be present as a relatively trivial problem, consisting of darkened, elongate filiform papillae that appear after the use of orally administered antibiotics or without any antecedent cause. The so-called geographic tongue consists of an irregular pattern of areas exhibiting absence of papillae; it may be associated with pustular and other varieties of psoriasis or it may be idiopathic. Lichen planus may be found on the tongue as linear white markings, sometimes in a netlike pattern. Oral thrush (moniliasis) occurs in diseases of altered immunity. Generalized monilial infections involving axillary, oral, periungual, and vaginal areas occur in the syndrome of mucocutaneous candidiasis and the syndrome of Addison's disease with hypoparathyroidism. Oral hairy leukoplakia occurs in HIV infection, often as an early sign.

SKIN LESIONS

Types of Skin Lesions (See Table 3-1)

The basic skin lesions (macules, papules, vesicles, plaques, etc.) are the essential elements upon which clinical diagnosis rests. To read words, one must recognize letters; to read the skin, one must recognize the basic lesions. To understand a paragraph, one must know how words are put together; to arrive at a differential diagnosis, one must know what the basic lesions represent and how they behave, how they are arranged and distributed, when they occur together, and how they evolve. To establish the diagnosis, one must be able to obtain the appropriate history and know when and how to perform appropriate diagnostic tests, such as a biopsy or cytologic preparation.

The lack of standardization of basic terminology has been one of the principal barriers to successful communication among physicians in describing skin lesions. For example, in standard dermatologic texts, the papule is variously described as no greater than 1 cm in size, less than 0.5 cm, smaller than a pea, or ranging from the size of a pinhead to that of a split pea; a nodule is designated as larger than a papule. These are, at best, haphazard standards of measurement, and until there is a more precise system the situation is likely to remain confusing. The International League of Dermatologic Societies has published a glossary of basic lesions that provides a helpful step in this direction.[18] At the very least, the metric ruler must be part of the standard examining apparatus for the skin so that accurate documentation of lesion size will be possible.

Often, identification of the *type* of primary lesion is enough to establish a diagnosis. In many instances, however, it is necessary to observe the evolution of individual lesions or of the eruption as a whole before a diagnostic pattern manifests itself. The evolution of individual lesions results in the formation of *sequential lesions*. Occasionally sequential lesions can be seen at the same time as primary ones. In chickenpox, for example, where new lesions occur in crops, erosions and crusted papules can be seen at the same time as new vesicles: this was helpful in the clinical differentiation of chickenpox from smallpox, in which lesions evolve simultaneously (see Chap. 219). Acral, tender erythematous papules that evolve into purpuric pustules are seen in disseminated gonococcemia. The evolution of an eruption results in a *pattern of spread*. In rubella, the rash involves the entire body within 1 day; in measles (rubeola), the rash takes 3 days to spread from the forehead and behind the ears to the rest of the body. In Rocky Mountain spotted fever, the pattern of spread is from the ankles and wrists, and then to the palms, soles, face, and center of the body surface.

The following *visual glossary* of current descriptive nomenclature is presented with some examples. No attempt has been made to make the examples exhaustive because more comprehensive guides are available.[19,20] Table 3-1 lists the types of lesions to be discussed. A number of infrequently used terms are also defined within this section; others may be found in Leider and Rosenblum.[21]

MACULES (See Fig. 3-1) A *macule* is a circumscribed, flat lesion that differs from the surrounding skin because of its color. Macules may have any size or shape. They may be the result of hyperpigmentation, hypopigmentation, vascular abnormalities, capillary dilatation (*erythema*), or *purpura* (extravasated red blood cells). Some macular lesions are associated with fine scaling. Such scaling may become apparent only after *grattinage*, a combination of light scraping and scratching. We call some such lesions *maculosquamous:* they are not perceptibly raised and therefore cannot be considered plaques (see below).

Telangiectases are permanent dilatations of capillaries that may or may not disappear with application of pressure. They form nonpulsatile, fine, bright red lines or netlike patterns on the skin. Telangiectases are commonly observed on faces of persons chronically exposed to the wind and sun. They are a prominent feature of the erythematous color noted in cutaneous lupus erythematosus. In addition, periungual telangiectases are an important marker for collagen vascular disorders such as lupus erythematosus and dermatomyositis. In hereditary hemorrhagic telangiectasia, the lesions are usually nonpulsatile, dull red, sharply outlined macules or papules, most commonly present on the tongue, lips, face, and fingers. Telangiectases are also a prominent feature of rosacea.

Lesions caused by extravasated red blood cells are included under the term *purpura*. *Petechiae* are small, pinpoint purpuric spots that are often seen in thrombocytopenic states. *Ecchymoses* are larger, bruise-like purpuric lesions. *Suggillations* are swollen "black and blue" marks that are often the consequence of bruising or other injury. The application of pressure with two glass slides or an unbreakable clear lens (*diascopy*) on a red lesion is a simple and reliable method for differentiating redness due to vascular dilatation (erythema) from redness due to extravasated erythrocytes or erythrocyte products (purpura). If the redness remains under the pressure of the slide, the lesion is purpuric.

An *infarct* is an area of cutaneous necrosis resulting from occlusion of blood vessels, as in vasculitis and bacterial embolism. Cutaneous infarcts have a variegated, dusky-red, grayish hue. They are irregularly shaped macules, sometimes depressed slightly below the plane of the skin and often surrounded by a pink zone of hyperemia. They may be tender.

FIGURE 3-1

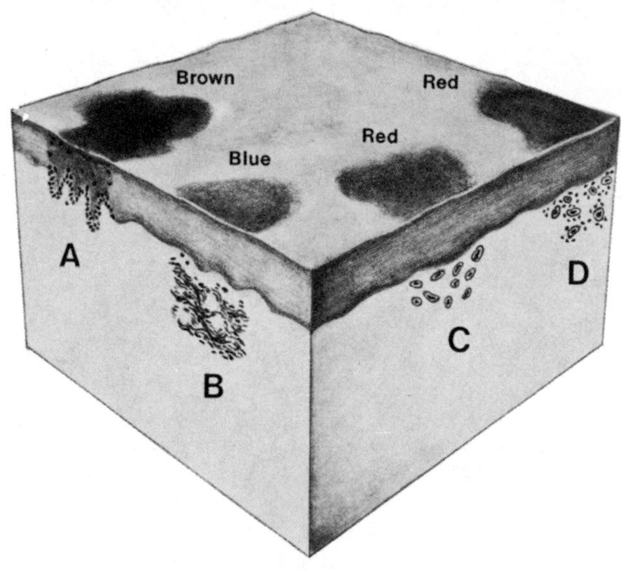

A.

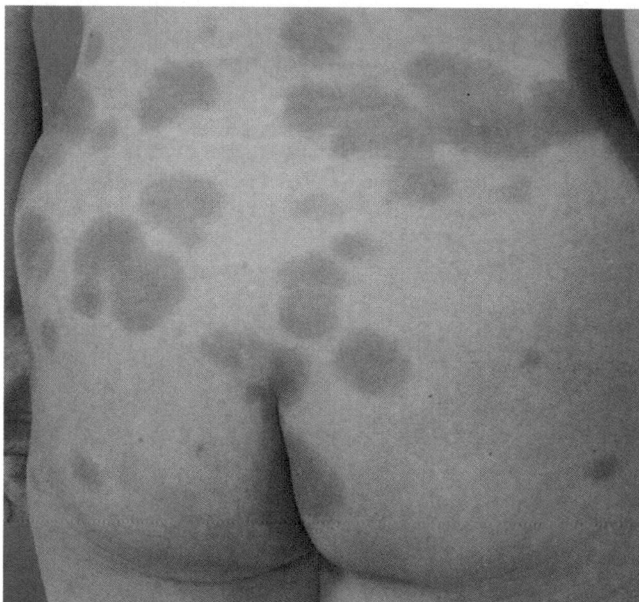

B.

Macule. A macule is a circumscribed, flat lesion that differs from surrounding skin because of its color. Macules may have any size or shape. *A.* They may be the result of hyperpigmentation (A), hypopigmentation, dermal pigmentation (B), vascular abnormalities, capillary dilatation (erythema) (C), or purpura (D). Macules with very-fine scaling are called *maculosquamous,* as in tinea versicolor. *B.* The clinical appearance of an eruption that consists of multiple, well-defined red macules of varying size that blanch upon pressure (diascopy) and are thus due to inflammatory vasodilatation. This eruption represents a drug reaction.

PAPULES A *papule* is a small, solid, elevated lesion (Fig. 3-2) generally smaller than a centimeter or so, and the major portion of a papule projects above the plane of the surrounding skin. *Oblique lighting with a flashlight in a darkened room is often necessary to detect slight elevation.*

Papules may have a variety of shapes. They may be acuminate (pointed), as in miliaria rubra (prickly heat rash); surmounted with scale, as in secondary syphilis; dome-shaped, as in molluscum contagiosum; or flat-topped, as in lichen planus.

Other features, such as color, are also important in the identification of papular lesions. Red papules are seen in psoriasis, often with a superimposed scale that produces bleeding when removed (Auspitz's sign). Papules with scaling are referred to as *papulosquamous lesions.* A copper color is noted in the lesions of secondary syphilis. Flat-topped papules with a violaceous hue are characteristic of lichen planus. The presence of fine, netlike white markings, called Wickham's striae, on the surface of the lesion provides further evidence for the diagnosis of lichen planus. Yellow papules are seen in xanthomatosis. Hemorrhagic or necrotic papules are noted in cutaneous vasculitis and meningococcemia. Purpuric papules—*palpable purpura*—are indicative of vasculitis until proved otherwise. Nevi and melanomas are often characterized by varying shades of red, brown, and black and must be differentiated from pigmented basal cell carcinomas, which often have a somewhat similar appearance. Basal cell carcinomas are waxy-smooth with raised, rolled telangiectatic borders.

Rounded, skin-colored papules may be seen in adenoma sebaceum and amyloidosis. Molluscum contagiosum may be identified as a rounded, translucent papule with a central umbilication; when the papule is punctured, a rounded central "molluscum body" is noted. Pedunculated papules, darker than or the same color as normal skin, occur in neurofibromatosis.

A papule or plaque may consist of multiple, small closely packed, projected elevations that are known as a *vegetation* (Fig. 3-2). Vegetations may be covered with thick dry scales, described as *keratotic* (as in verruca vulgaris), or may be soft and smooth (as in condyloma acuminatum). Seborrheic keratoses are common vegetative lesions, especially in older age groups. They may be yellowish, tan, brown, or black and often have a soft greasy surface. Dry, scaly vegetations occur in actinic keratoses.

All erythematous papules should be examined by diascopy (discussed later in this chapter), inasmuch as a yellow-brown color appears in the papules found in a number of granulomatous disorders, and an erythematous papule that does not blanch on diascopy may be a sign of vasculitis (palpable purpura).

Although certain eruptions may have both macular and papular components, we believe that the abused term *maculopapular* is a non sequitur, or, at best, an oxymoron, and we avoid using it for the sake of clear thinking and communication.[22]

PLAQUES A *plaque* is a mesalike elevation that occupies a relatively large surface area in comparison with its height above skin level (Fig. 3-3). Plaques are often formed by a confluence of papules, as in psoriasis. The typical psoriatic lesion is a raised, erythematous plaque with layers of silvery scale, often described as micaceous.

Repeated rubbing, especially in people with chronic eczema, leads to areas of *lichenification.* Proliferation of keratinocytes and stratum corneum, in combination with changes in the collagen of the underlying dermis, causes lichenified areas of skin to appear as thickened plaques with accentuated skin markings (Fig. 3-3*C*). The lesions may resemble tree bark.

The presence of atrophy, especially in the presence of erythema, scales, pigmentary changes, and follicular plugging, may suggest the diagnosis of cutaneous lupus erythematosus.

"PATCH" According to the *Oxford English Dictionary,* a patch is "a portion of any surface markedly different in appearance or character from what is around it." The *O.E.D.* also states that a patch may be "a small well-defined area of the skin, etc. distinct in color or appearance." Dermatologists have used this term in different ways: some restrict its

FIGURE 3-2

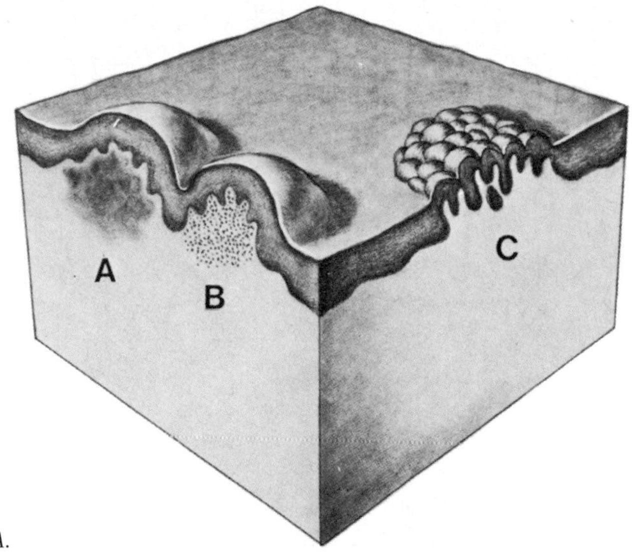

A.

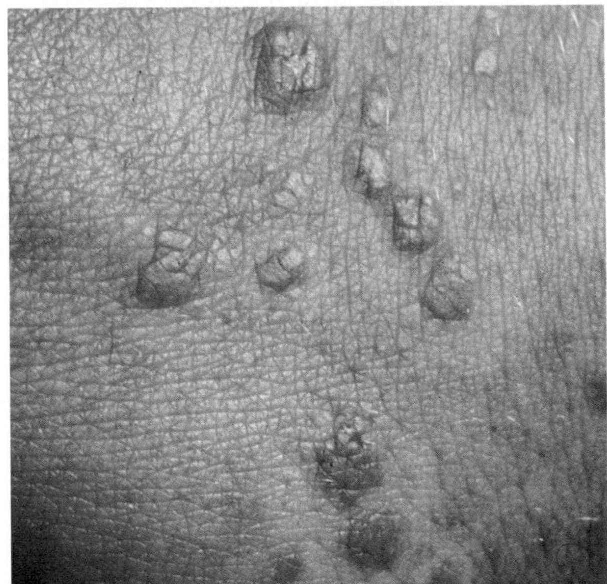

C.

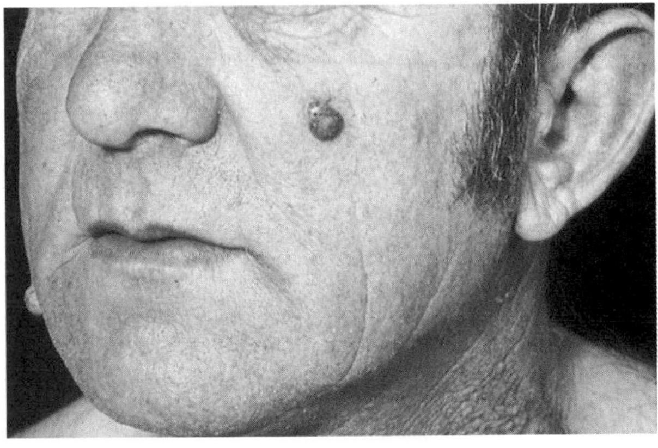

B.

Papule. A papule is a small, solid, elevated lesion. Papules are generally smaller than 1 cm in diameter, and the major portion of a papule projects above the plane of the surrounding skin. *A.* Papules may result, for example, from metabolic deposits in the dermis (A), from localized dermal cellular infiltrates (B), and from localized hyperplasia of cellular elements in the dermis or epidermis (vegetation) (C). Papules with scaling are referred to as *papulosquamous* lesions, as in psoriasis. Clinical examples of papules are shown in: *B.* Two well-defined and dome-shaped papules of firm consistency and brownish color, which are dermal melanocytic nevi; *C.* multiple, well-defined, and coalescing papules of varying size are seen. Their violaceous color, glistening surface, and flat tops are characteristic of lichen planus.

use to the description of very large macules; others use it to refer to relatively thin but large plaques. In general, we feel that accurate description can almost always be better served by more precise terminology, such as large macule, thin and scaling plaque, etc.

NODULES (See Fig. 3-4) A *nodule* is a palpable, solid, round or ellipsoidal lesion. Depth of involvement and/or substantive palpability, rather than diameter, differentiate a nodule from a papule. Depending upon the anatomic component(s) primarily involved, nodules are of five main types: (1) epidermal, (2) epidermal-dermal, (3) dermal, (4) dermal-subdermal, and (5) subcutaneous. Epidermal nodules include, for example, keratoacanthoma, verruca vulgaris, and basal cell carcinoma. Epidermal-dermal nodules include certain compound nevi, malignant melanomas, invasive squamous cell carcinomas, and some lesions of mycosis fungoides. Examples of dermal nodules are lesions of granuloma annulare and dermatofibromas. Erythema nodosum and superficial thrombophlebitis are examples of dermal-subdermal nodules. Lipomas are subcutaneous nodules of adipose tissue.

Nodules in the dermis and subcutis may indicate systemic disease and result from inflammation, neoplasms, or metabolic deposits in the dermis or subcutaneous tissue. For example, late syphilis, tuberculosis, the deep mycoses, xanthomatosis, lymphoma, and metastatic neoplasms all can present as cutaneous nodules. Erythema nodosum presents with tender, subcutaneous nodules on the legs, often as a manifestation of hypersensitivity. Foreign-body reactions, insect bites, and viral and bacterial infections are among other causes of nodular lesions. Because nodules may represent serious systemic disease, unidentified persistent nodules should always be biopsied and cultured.

The terms *tuber* and *phyma* are less often applied and are synonyms for nodule. *Tumor* is a general term for any mass, benign or malignant, and is sometimes used to indicate a large nodule. A *gumma* is, specifically, the granulomatous nodular lesion of tertiary syphilis.

It is always helpful to describe a nodule with measurements and with modifying adjectives such as hard, firm, soft, fleshy, warm, movable, fixed, painless. The surface of a nodule should also be described as, for example, smooth, keratotic, ulcerated, fungating. There has been some semantic confusion in distinguishing nodules from large papules and small tumors. Size is not a major consideration in the definition of nodule. For example, rheumatoid nodules, which are usually located over bony prominences, may be as small as 1 or 2 mm, or as large as several centimeters. In certain instances, more than one term may be satisfactory. In most cases, it is simply best to include measurements and descriptive terms that convey the important features of the lesion in question.

FIGURE 3-3

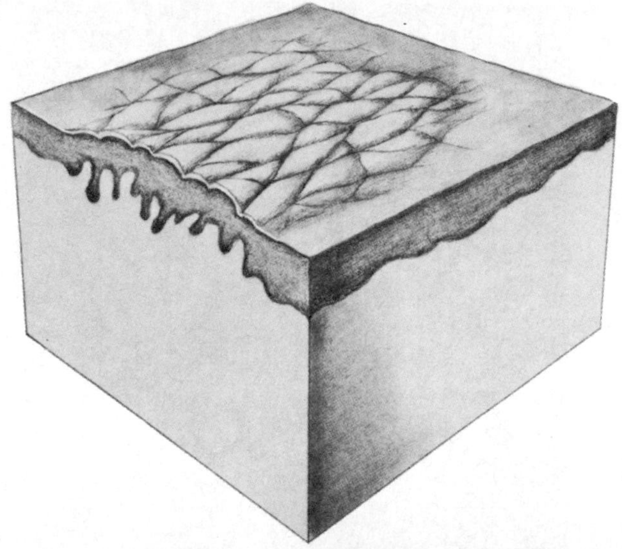

A.

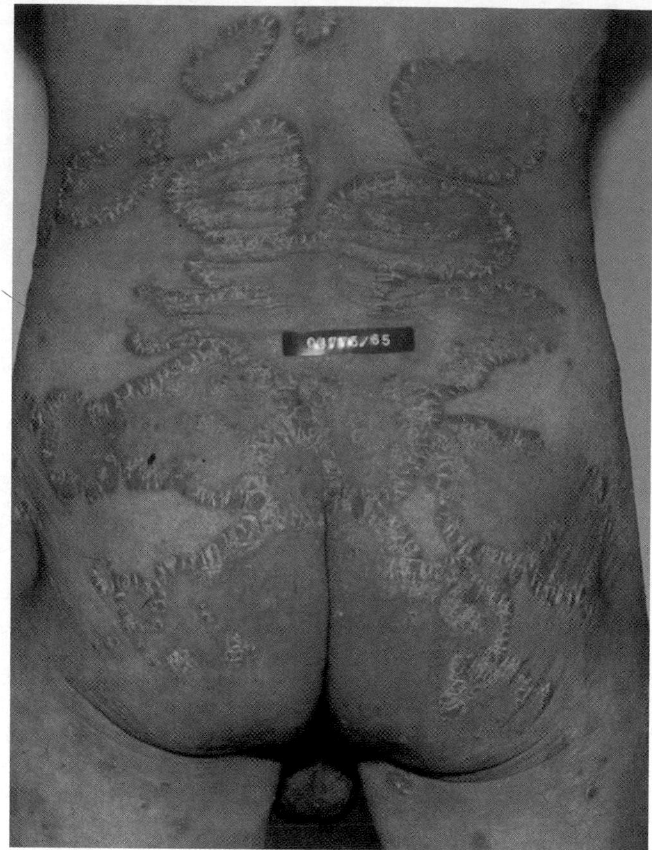

B.

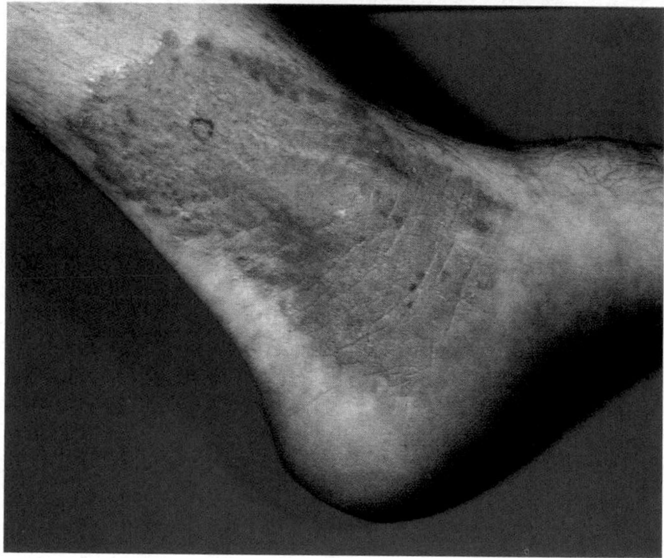

C.

Plaque. A plaque, shown in the drawing (*A*), is a mesa-like elevation that occupies a relatively large surface area in comparison with its height above the skin surface. Well-defined, reddish, scaling plaques that coalesce to cover large areas of the back and buttocks are seen in (*B*). There is some regression in the center, as is typical for psoriasis. *Lichenification* (*C*) represents thickening of skin and accentuation of skin markings. The process results from repeated rubbing and frequently develops in persons with atopy; it can occur in eczematous dermatitis or other conditions associated with pruritus. Lesions of lichenification are not as well defined as most plaques are and often show signs of scratching, such as excoriations and crusts.

WHEALS A *wheal* is a rounded or flat-topped papule or plaque that is characteristically evanescent, disappearing within hours (Fig. 3-5). The epidermis is not affected: there is no scaling. The borders of a wheal, although sharp, are not stable and in fact move from involved to adjacent uninvolved areas over a period of hours. These lesions, also known as hives or urticaria, are the result of edema in the upper portion of the dermis. Wheals are pale red in color, but if the amount of edema is sufficient to compress superficial vessels, they may be white, especially in the center. Wheals may be tiny papules 3 to 4 mm in diameter, as in cholinergic urticaria, or giant erythematous plaques of 10 to 12 cm, as in some cases of urticaria caused by penicillin hypersensitivity. Wheals occur in many shapes: round, oval, serpiginous, annular (ring-shaped).

Wheals can be seen as an allergic response to innumerable initiating agents, such as drugs and insect bites. Wheal-like lesions occur occasionally in dermatitis herpetiformis and bullous pemphigoid. The wheal produced in response to the stroking of a reddish-brown or brownish macule (Darier's sign) is pathognomonic of urticaria pigmentosa (mastocytosis).

Stroking of the skin may produce wheals in some normal persons; this phenomenon is called *dermographism*, classified as one of the physical urticarias. When it is associated with significant itching, it is called *symptomatic* dermographism (see Chap. 116).

Angioedema is a deep, edematous urticarial reaction that occurs in areas with very loose dermis and subcutaneous tissue, such as the lip or scrotum. It may occur on the hands and feet as well, and may cause grotesque deformity. A careful search should be made for laryngeal edema, which may cause airway obstruction (see Chap. 117).

FIGURE 3-4

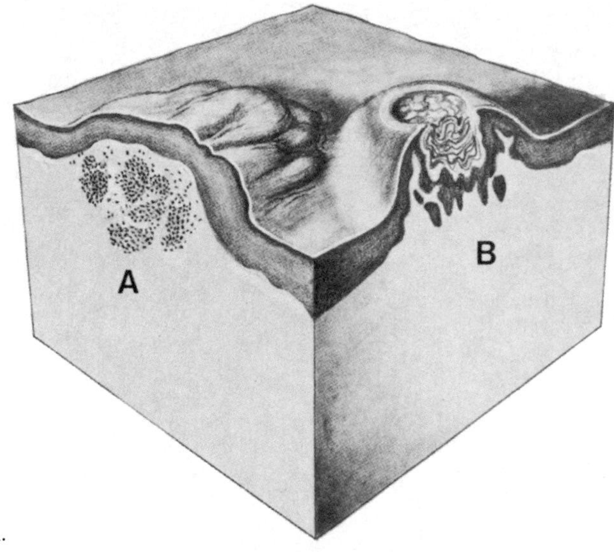

A.

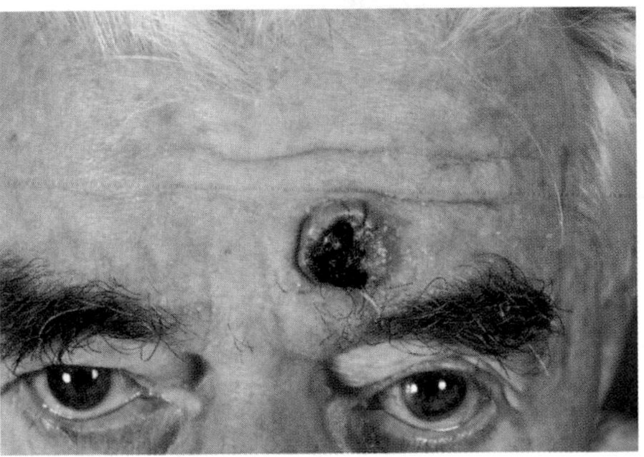

B.

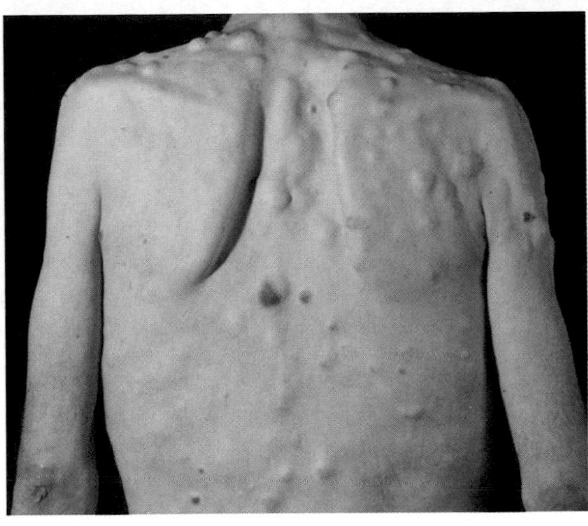

C.

Nodule. A nodule is a palpable, solid, round or ellipsoidal lesion. Depth of involvement and/or substantive palpability rather than diameter differentiate a nodule from a papule. *A.* Nodules may be located in the epidermis (B) or extend into the dermis or subcutaneous tissue (A). *B.* This photograph shows a well-defined, firm nodule with a smooth and glistening surface through which telangiectasia (dilated capillaries) can be seen; there is central crusting indicating tissue breakdown and thus incipient ulceration (nodular basal cell carcinoma). *C.* Multiple nodules of varying size can be seen (melanoma metastases).

VESICLES AND BULLAE A *vesicle* is a circumscribed, elevated lesion that contains fluid (Fig. 3-6). Often the vesicle walls are so thin that they are translucent and the serum, lymph, blood, or extracellular fluid is visible. A vesicle with a diameter greater than 0.5 cm is a *bulla*.

Vesicles and bullae arise from cleavage at various levels of the skin; the cleavage may be within the epidermis (i.e., intraepidermal vesication) (Fig. 3-6), or at or below the dermal-epidermal interface (i.e., subepidermal). Cleavage just beneath the stratum corneum produces a subcorneal vesicle or bulla (A in Fig. 3-6*A*), as in impetigo. Intraepidermal vesication may result from intercellular edema (spongiosis), as characteristically seen in delayed hypersensitivity reactions of the epidermis (e.g., in contact eczematous dermatitis) and in pompholyx. *Spongiotic vesicles* (B in Fig. 3-6*A*) may be detectable microscopically but may not be clinically apparent as vesicles. Loss of intercellular bridges, or desmosomes, is known as *acantholysis,* and this type of intraepidermal vesication (A in Fig. 3-7*A*) is seen in pemphigus vulgaris, where the cleavage is usually just above the basal layer. In pemphigus foliaceus, the cleavage occurs just below the subcorneal layer.

Viruses cause a curious "ballooning degeneration" of epidermal cells (B in Fig. 3-7*A*), as in herpes zoster, herpes simplex, variola, and varicella. Viral bullae often have a depressed ("umbilicated") center. Pathologic changes at the dermal-epidermal junction may lead to subepidermal vesicles and bullae (Fig. 3-8), as are seen in pemphigoid, bullous erythema multiforme, porphyria cutanea tarda, dermatitis herpetiformis, and some forms of epidermolysis bullosa. The thickness of the wall of a bulla may be estimated by its translucency and flaccidity The amount of pressure required to collapse the lesion may help predict whether the bulla is intraepidermal or subepidermal. It has been said that a relatively large, tense bulla suggests pemphigoid, whereas a flaccid bulla suggests pemphigus. There is, however, no reliable means of distinguishing these two diseases except by histologic examination of the lesion and immunofluorescence.

EROSIONS An *erosion* is a moist, circumscribed, usually depressed lesion that results from loss of all or a portion of the viable epidermis (Fig. 3-9). After the rupture of vesicles or bullae, the moist areas remaining at the base are called erosions. Extensive areas of denudation due to erosions may be seen in bullous diseases such as pemphigus. Unless they become secondarily infected, erosions usually do not scar. If inflammation extends into the papillary dermis, an ulcer is present and scarring results, as in vaccinia and variola, and less often in herpes zoster and varicella.

PUSTULES AND OTHER PYODERMATOSES A *pustule* is a circumscribed, raised lesion that contains a purulent exudate (Fig. 3-10). Pus, composed of leukocytes with or without cellular debris, may contain bacteria or may be sterile, as in the lesions of pustular psoriasis. Pustules may vary in size and shape and, depending on the color of

FIGURE 3-5

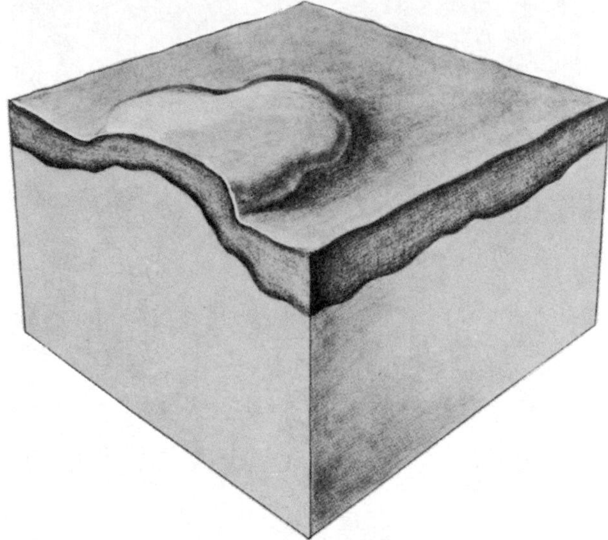

A.

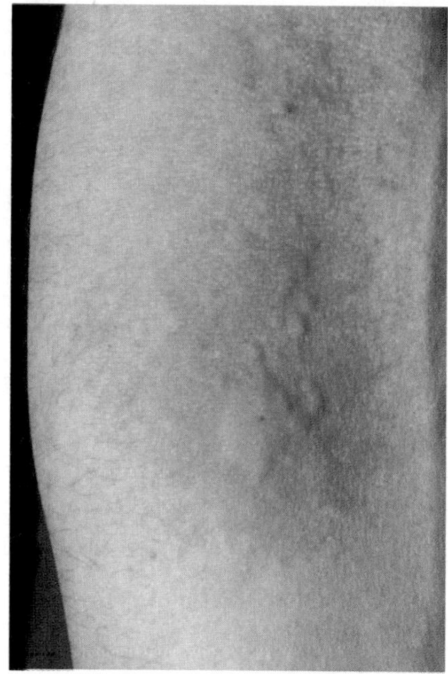

B.

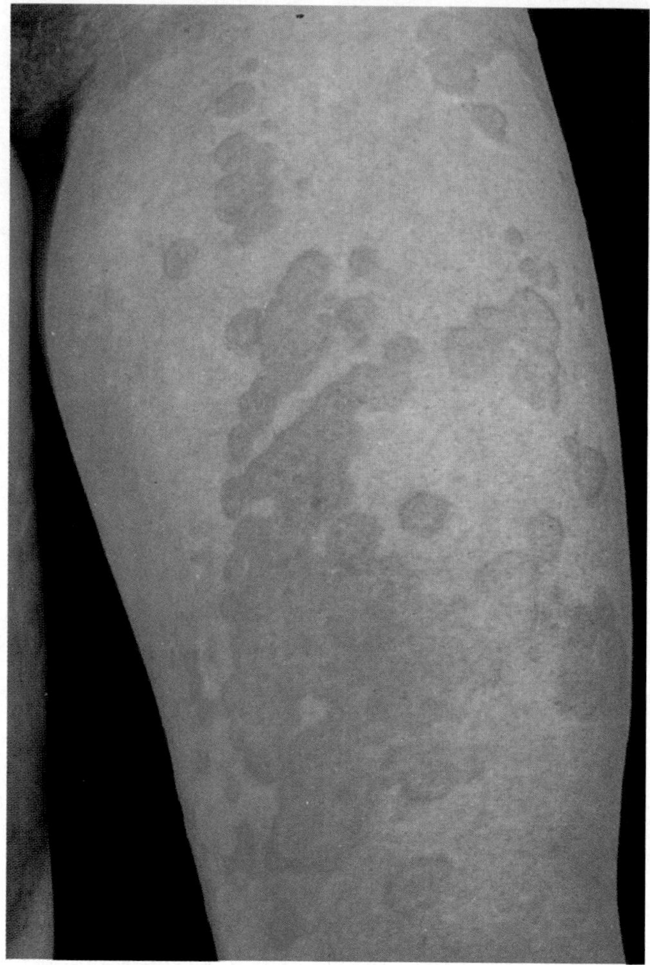

C.

Wheal. A wheal (*A*) is a rounded or flat-topped papule or plaque that is characteristically evanescent, disappearing within hours. Wheals may be tiny papules 3 to 4 mm in diameter, as in cholinergic urticaria [shown in the clinical photograph (*B*)]. They may be large, coalescing plaques, as in allergic reactions to penicillin, other drugs, or alimentary allergens, as shown in (*C*). An eruption consisting of wheals is termed *urticaria* and usually itches.

the exudate, may appear white, yellow, or greenish yellow. Follicular pustules are conical, usually contain a hair in the center, and generally heal without scarring.

Pustules are characteristic of rosacea, pustular psoriasis, Reiter's disease, and some drug eruptions, especially those due to bromide or iodide. Vesicular lesions of some viral diseases (varicella, variola, vaccinia, herpes simplex, and herpes zoster), as well as the lesions of dermatophytosis, may become pustular. A Gram's stain and culture of the exudate from pustules should always be performed.

A *furuncle* is a deep necrotizing form of folliculitis, with pus accumulation. Several furuncles may coalesce to form a *carbuncle*. An *abscess* is a localized accumulation of purulent material so deep in the dermis or subcutaneous tissue that the pus is usually not visible on the surface of the skin. It is red, warm, and tender. An abscess frequently begins as a folliculitis and is commonly a manifestation of cutaneous streptococcal or *Staphylococcus aureus* infection.

A *sinus* is a tract leading from a suppurative cavity to the skin surface or between cystic or abscess cavities. A sinus near the rectum may be seen in rectal abscess, carcinoma of the bowel, or inflammatory bowel disease. Sinuses of the neck suggest actinomycosis, scrofula, branchial pouch, or dental sinus. Deep sinus tracts may occur in hidradenitis suppurativa and acne conglobata.

CYSTS A *cyst* is a sac that contains liquid or semisolid material (fluid, cells, and cell products). A spherical or oval nodule or papule may be suspected of being a cyst if, on palpation, it is resilient; the eyeball, for example, feels like a cyst. The most common cysts are *epidermal (keratinous) cysts* (A in Fig. 3-11*A*), which are lined with squamous epithelium and produce keratinous material. Cysts of pilar (hair follicle) origin that are lined with multilayered epithelium that does not mature through a granular layer are called *pilar cysts* (B in Fig. 3-11*A*).

FIGURE 3-6

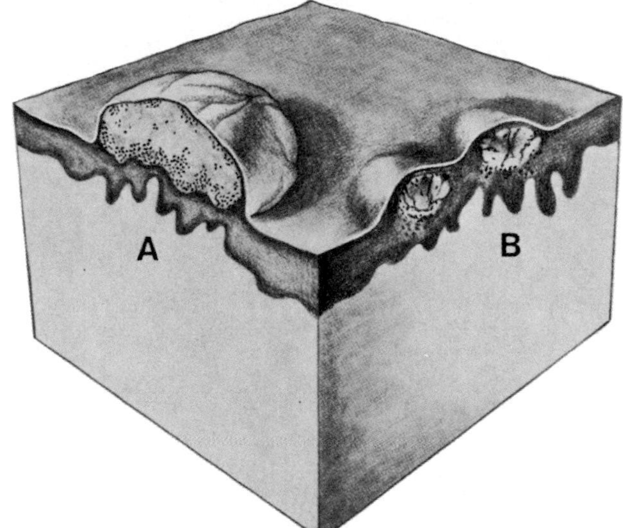

A.

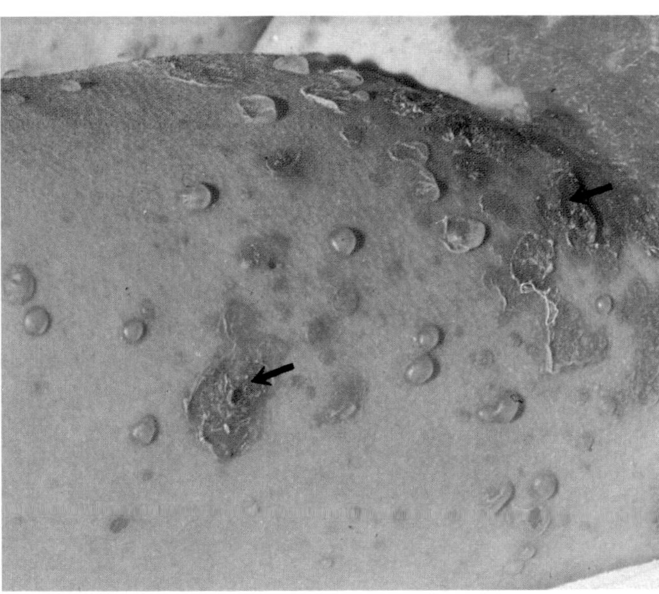

B.

Vesicles and bullae are the technical terms for blisters. A vesicle is a circumscribed lesion that contains fluid. Shown in the drawing (*A*), subcorneal vesicles (A) result from fluid accumulation just below the stratum corneum. Spongiotic vesicles (B) result from intercellular edema. A bulla is a vesicle larger than 0.5 cm. The clinical photograph (*B*) shows multiple translucent subcorneal vesicles that are extremely fragile, collapse easily, and thus lead to crusting (*arrows*). These lesions represent staphylococcal impetigo. Leukocytes present within the vesicles sediment to the lowest portion of the subcorneal cavity when the patient is in an upright position.

ATROPHY *Atrophy* refers to a diminution in the size of a cell, tissue, organ, or part of the body. Epidermal atrophy refers to thinning of the epidermis and is associated with a decrease in the number of epidermal cells (B in Fig. 3-12*A*). Atrophic epidermis may be almost transparent and may or may not retain the normal skin lines. Epidermal atrophy is often associated with alterations in the dermis as well. Senile skin, especially in sun-exposed areas, retains its normal skin lines, exhibits a fine wrinkling, and is somewhat transparent; the deep veins and yellow tendons are easily discernible. Preceding injury or inflammation (e.g., discoid lupus erythematosus) may also cause epidermal atrophy with an "ironed out" appearance and loss of the skin markings.

Dermal atrophy results from a decrease in the papillary or reticular dermal connective tissue and is usually manifested as a depression of the skin (A in Fig. 3-12*A*). Dermal atrophy may follow inflammation or trauma with or without ulceration and is also seen after chronic

FIGURE 3-7

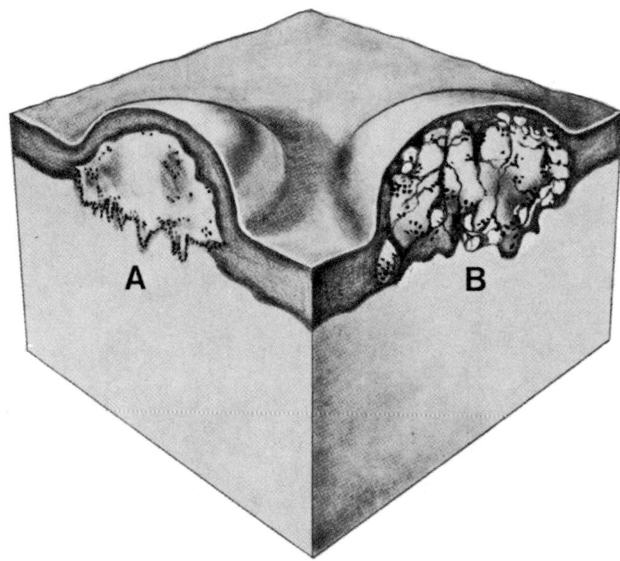

A.

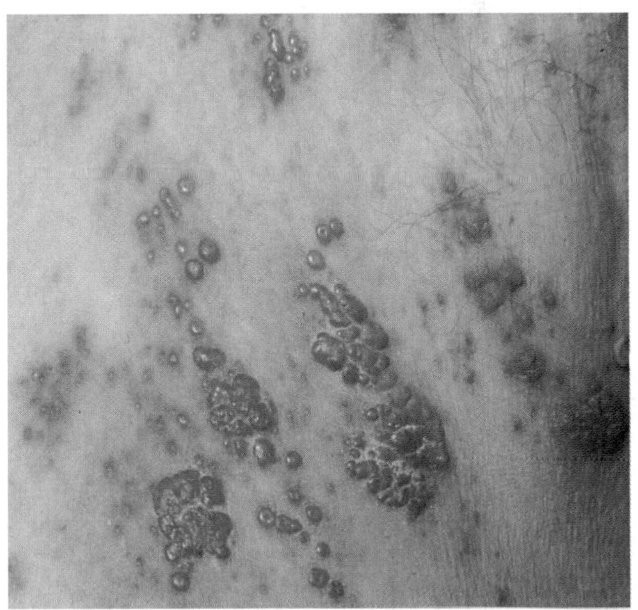

B.

Vesicle. Shown in the drawing (*A*), acantholytic vesicles (A) result from cleavage within the epidermis due to loss of intercellular attachments. Balloon degeneration of epidermal cells leads to the formation of vesicles in certain viral infections (B), such as varicella-zoster. Vesicles characteristic of herpes zoster are shown in (*B*). They appear in crops and are grouped. Central umbilication can be seen in some of them.

FIGURE 3-8

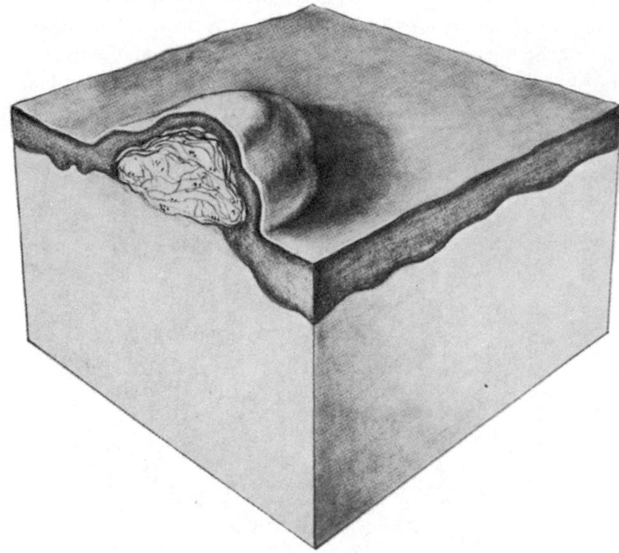

A.

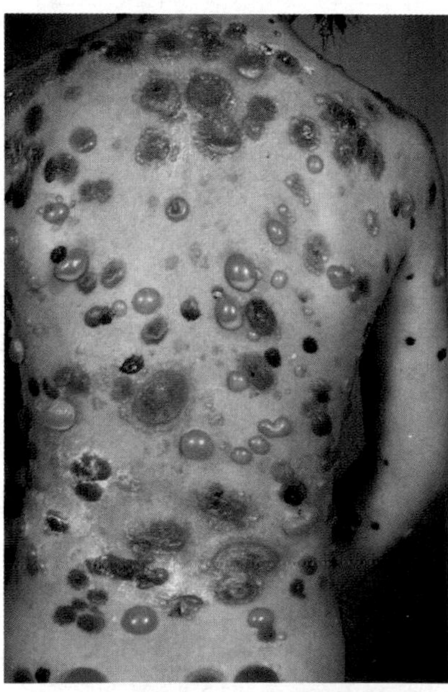

B.

Vesicle. Subepidermal vesicles, as shown in the drawing (*A*), occur as a consequence of pathologic changes in the region of the dermal-epidermal junction. Subepidermal vesicles and bullae are seen in bullous erythema multiforme, porphyria cutanea tarda, epidermolysis bullosa, dermatitis herpetiformis, and bullous pemphigoid. The clinical photograph (*B*) demonstrates bullae in the latter condition. Some of them arise on normal and some on erythematous skin. Most of them are tense and filled with a serous or hemorrhagic fluid; some have collapsed and crusted.

FIGURE 3-9

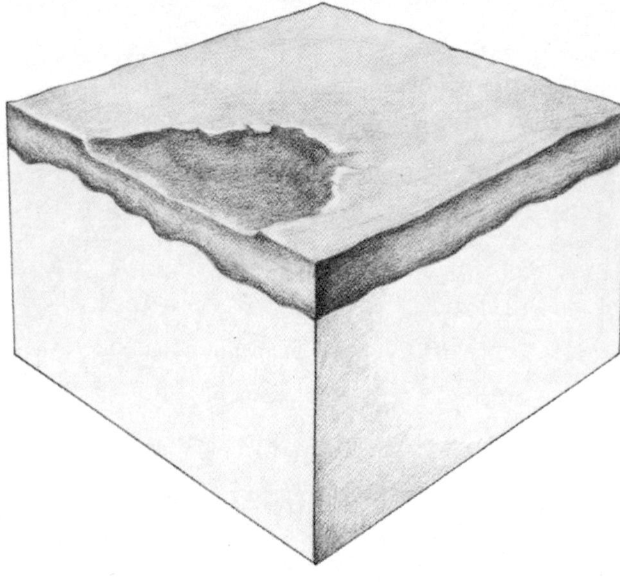

A.

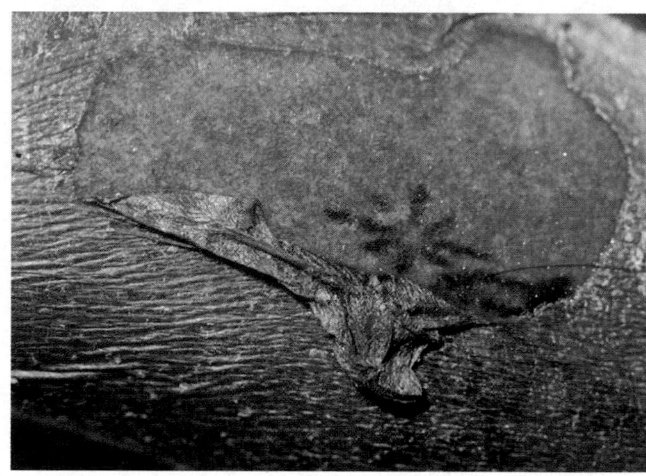

B.

Erosion. An erosion, as shown in the drawing (*A*), is a moist, circumscribed, usually depressed lesion that results from loss of all or a portion of the viable epidermis. Erosions remain after the roofs of vesicles and bullae become detached. Erosions also develop after epidermal necrosis as in toxic epidermal necrolysis, shown in the photograph (*B*). They usually heal without scarring.

application of fluorinated topical steroids. In dermal atrophy occurring without epidermal atrophy, the area of skin is normal in color and markings because the circumscribed depression is produced only by the decrease in dermal tissue. Dermal atrophy may occur with epidermal atrophy, as in the striae of pregnancy, Cushing's disease, or necrobiosis lipoidica; in the latter condition, there are loss of skin markings, increased translucence, and localized depression of the skin. Atrophy is noted in morphea-like basal cell carcinoma, chronic discoid lupus erythematosus, scleroderma, dermatomyositis, and chronic radiodermatitis. If atrophy takes place in the panniculus, depressions of the skin may occur, as in liquefying panniculitis, lipogranulomatosis, progressive lipodystrophy, and poststeroid injections.

ULCERS An *ulcer* is a "hole in the skin" in which there has been destruction of the epidermis and at least the upper (papillary) dermis (Fig. 3-13). Features that are helpful in determining the cause of ulcers and that must be considered in describing them include location, borders, base, discharge, and any associated topographic features of the lesion or surrounding skin, such as nodules, excoriations, varicosities,

FIGURE 3-10

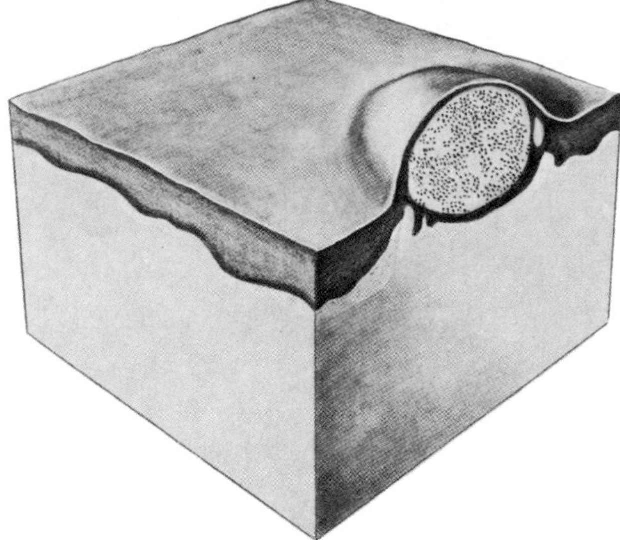

A.

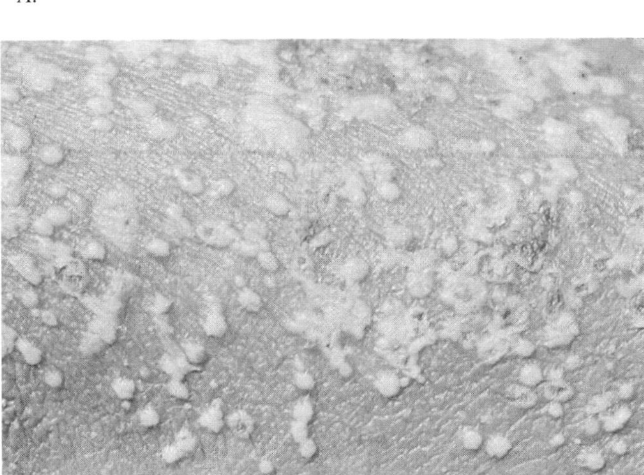

B.

Pustule. A pustule is a papule that contains purulent exudate (*A*). Primary, nonfollicular pustules occur in pustular psoriasis (*B*). These very superficial, subcorneal pustules may coalesce to form lakes of pus.

FIGURE 3-11

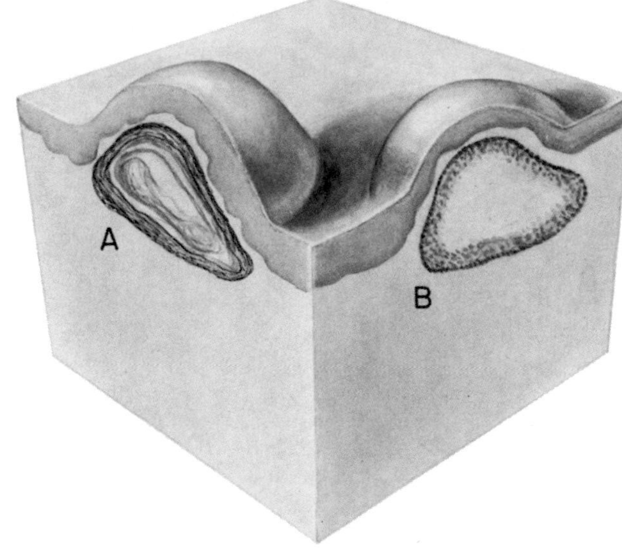

A.

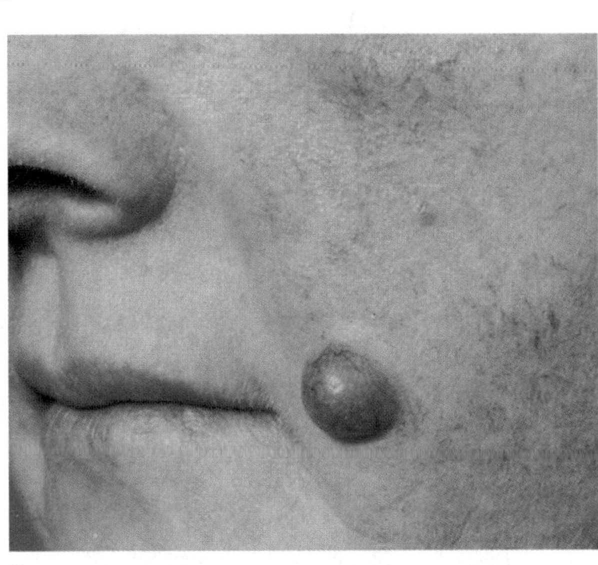

B.

Cyst. A cyst is a sac that contains liquid or semisolid material (fluid, cells, cell products). A spherical or oval nodule or papule may clinically be suspected of being a cyst if, on palpation, it is resilient; the eyeball, for example, feels like a cyst. The most common cysts, shown in the drawing (*A*), are epidermal cysts (A), which are lined with squamous epithelium and produce keratinous material. Cysts of pilar origin that are lined with multilayered epithelium, which does not mature through a granular layer, are pilar cysts (B). The bluish, resilient cyst, shown in (*B*), represents a cystic adnexal tumor (cystic hidradenoma), which is filled with a mucus-like material.

hair distribution, presence or absence of sweating, and adjacent pulses (see Chap. 167). Stasis ulcers are accompanied by pigmentation and, occasionally, by edema or sclerosis. They most commonly begin on the medial aspect of the ankle or lower leg. Hypertensive or ischemic ulcers tend to start on the lateral aspect of the ankle or foot. Factitial ulcerations often have "artificial" shapes, including straight, angular borders. Excoriations that have enlarged into ulcers give a similar appearance but may show the residua of an underlying dermatosis (e.g., eczematous dermatitis associated with chronic venous insufficiency). Pyoderma gangrenosum has purplish, raised, and undermined ragged borders and may be associated with ulcerative colitis or a number of other internal disorders. Decubitus ulcers occur at pressure points.

Ulceration can occur as a result of tissue infarction in areas of large- or small-vessel occlusion or constriction due to various etiologic factors: embolus; thrombosis; ergot poisoning; cryoagglutinins, cryofibrinogenemia, or cryoglobulinemia; polyarteritis; macroglobulinemia; thrombotic thrombocytopenic purpura; polycythemia; generalized Arthus' reaction (purpura fulminans); sepsis; Raynaud's phenomenon; arteriosclerosis obliterans; Wegener's granulomatosis;[23] and calciphylaxis.[24] Ulceration occurs in granulomatous nodules of various types due to deep fungi, tuberculosis, syphilis, and yaws, as well as in a variety of parasitic and bacteriologic disorders. Nodules adjacent to ulcerations suggest granulomatous or neoplastic disease. Neoplasms

FIGURE 3-12

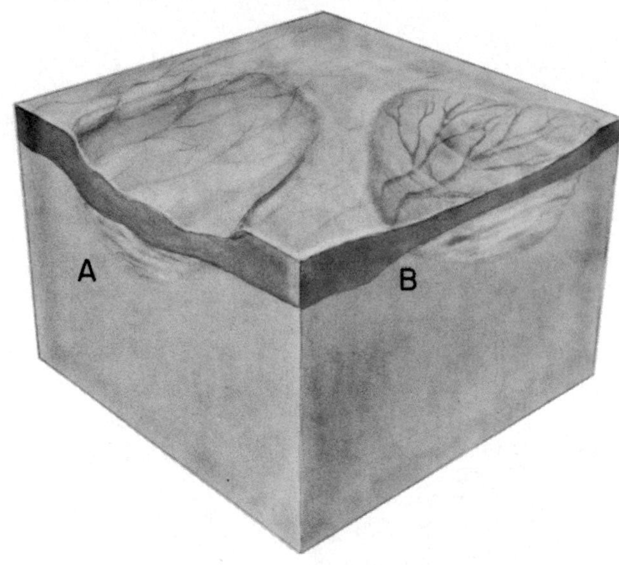

A.

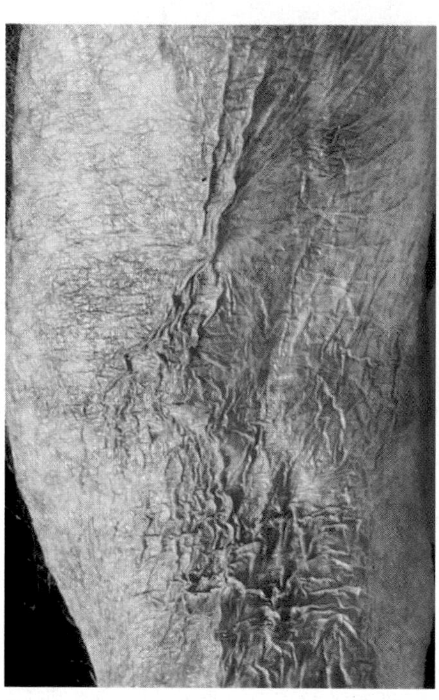

B.

Atrophy. Atrophy refers to a diminution or thinning of the skin. It may be limited to the epidermis or the dermis or may occur simultaneously in both. As shown in the drawing (*A*), epidermal atrophy (B) is manifested by a thin, almost transparent epidermis. Atrophic epidermis may or may not retain the normal skin lines. Dermal atrophy (A) results from a decrease in the papillary or reticular dermal connective tissue and is manifested as a depression in the skin. Atrophy of subcutaneous tissue may also lead to depressions in the skin surface. Marked dermal and epidermal atrophy is shown in the photograph (*B*). Loss of normal skin texture, thinning, and wrinkling are present.

FIGURE 3-13

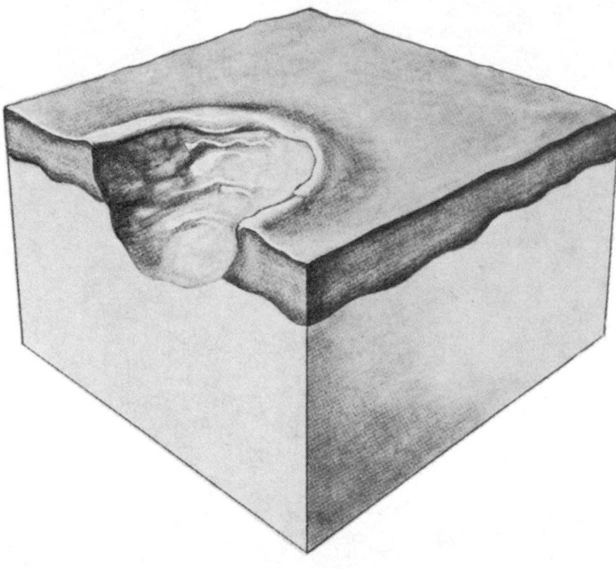

A.

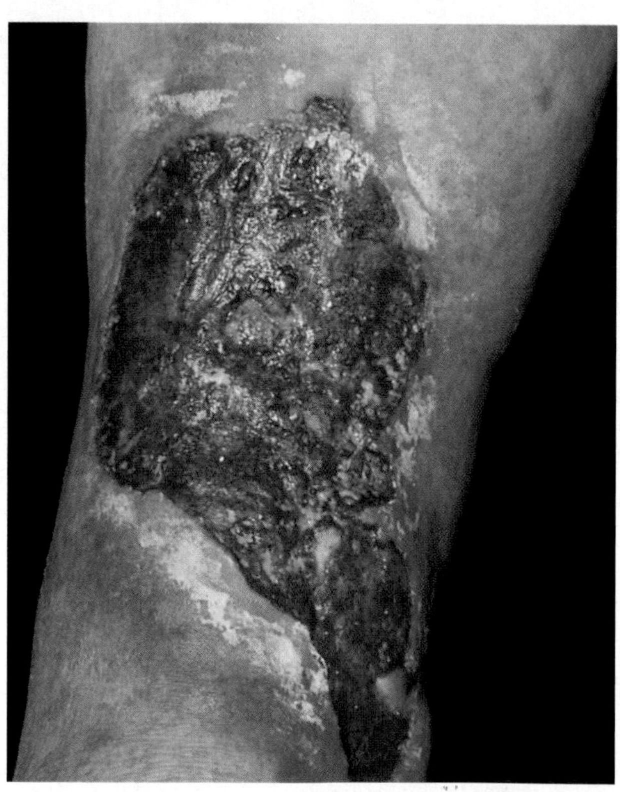

B.

Ulcer. An ulcer, shown in (*A*), is the hole or defect that remains after an area of epidermis and at least part of the dermis have been destroyed or removed. Because the dermis is involved, ulcers heal with scarring. The clinical photograph (*B*) shows a gigantic ulcer with a red, granulating base and well-defined, punched-out borders.

may become necrotic and ulcerated, generally as a result of small-vessel obliteration by the proliferating tumor.

SCAR A *scar* occurs wherever a wound or ulceration has taken place and reflects the pattern of healing in the affected area. Scars may be hypertrophic (A in Fig. 3-14*A*) or atrophic (B in Fig. 3-14*A*). They

FIGURE 3-14

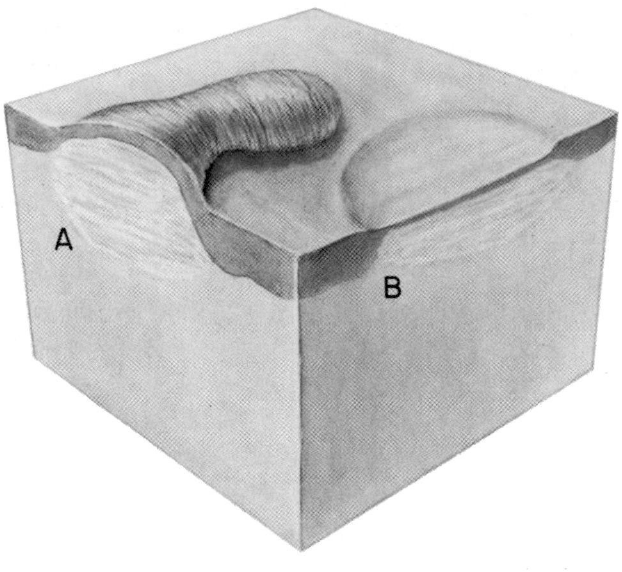

A.

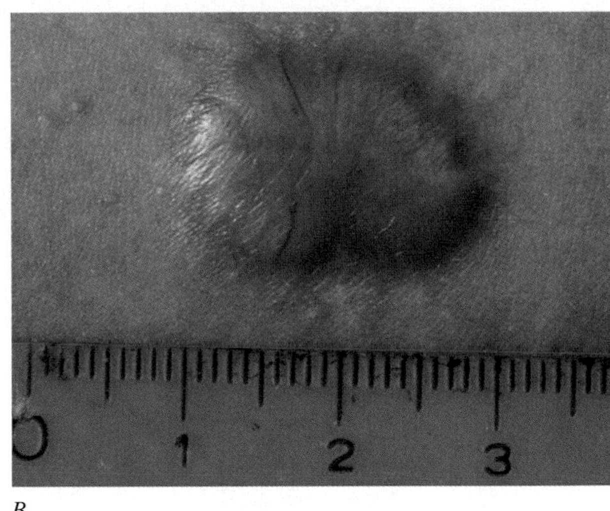

B.

Scar. A scar is the fibrous tissue replacement that develops as a consequence of healing at the site of a prior ulcer or wound. A scar may be hypertrophic (A) or atrophic (B), as shown in the drawing (*A*). A typical clinical example of a hypertrophic scar is shown in the photograph (*B*).

may be sclerotic, or hard, as a consequence of collagen proliferation. The scarred epidermis is thin, generally without normal skin lines and without appendages (B in Fig. 3-14*A*). A depressed scar may resemble a primary atrophic process (see Chap. 105). Scars may occur in the course of acne, some porphyrias, herpes zoster, and varicella. Raynaud's disease, syphilis, tuberculosis (especially on the face), leprosy, or carcinoma may produce *mutilations,* or a loss of tissue that alters major anatomic structures.

SCLEROSIS *Sclerosis* refers to a circumscribed or diffuse hardening or induration in the skin; it is detected more easily by palpation than by inspection. Sclerosis is a component of morphea, linear scleroderma, systemic scleroderma, and porphyria cutanea tarda. It often occurs in chronic stasis dermatitis and chronic lymphedema. Sclerosis may result from dermal or subcutaneous edema, cellular infiltration, or collagen proliferation.

CALCINOSIS *Calcinosis* of the dermis or subcutaneous tissue (e.g., in dermatomyositis and scleroderma) may be felt as *hard* nodules or plaques, with or without visible alteration of the skin surface.

SCALE, DESQUAMATION (SCALING) (See Fig. 3-15) Abnormal shedding or accumulation of stratum corneum in perceptible flakes is called scaling. Under normal circumstances the epidermis is completely replaced approximately every 27 days. The end product of this holocrine process of keratinization is the cornified cell of the outermost layer of the skin—the stratum corneum. The cornified cell is packed with filamentous proteins, normally does not contain a nucleus, and is usually lost imperceptibly. When keratinocyte production occurs at an increased rate, as in psoriasis, immature keratinocytes that retain nuclei reach the skin surface—this is called *parakeratosis.* Parakeratotic cells may pile up and contribute to the formation of *scales*. In psoriasis, scales may appear in thin, mica-like (micaceous) sheets, or accumulate massively, suggesting the appearance of an oyster shell (ostraceous scale). Densely adherent scales that have a gritty feel like sandpaper are typically seen in solar keratosis. Fishlike scale occurs in a group of disorders known as *ichthyoses,* in some of which prolonged retention of the stratum corneum occurs, even though it is produced at a normal rate. Scaling lesions also occur in dermatophyte infections, pityriasis rosea, secondary and tertiary syphilis, and in a large number of conditions in which abnormal keratinization and/or exfoliation of epithelial cells occur.

To the well-trained eye, not all scales are equal, and the expert dermatologist will often obtain diagnostically useful information from close examinations of the type of scale present. Siemens[4] describes the following types of scale: pityriasiform (branny); psoriasiform (brittle platelets of several loose layers); ichthyosiform (like fish scales); cuticular and lamellar (thin, relatively large flakes); membranous or exfoliative (large sheets, peeling); keratotic (composed of horny masses); granular (like small grains); hystrix-like (from the Greek for porcupine); scale formations that appear as little horns; and follicular scale, which may occur as keratotic plugs, spines, filaments, or lichenoid scales. Siemens also points out that scale formation can sometimes be observed only after scratching the lesion, and notes that this phenomenon—latent desquamation—may be found in the early stages of pityriasis rosea as well as in tinea versicolor, parapsoriasis, and psoriasis. Large, heaped-up scale accumulations in psoriasis may be described as ostraceous (oyster-like). Cracklike desquamation can be seen in scabetic burrows and eczema craquelé. Collarettes of scale are seen in pityriasis rosea, superficial mycoses, secondary syphilis, and erythema annulare centrifugum. Seborrheic desquamation refers to the yellow-to-brown, waxy, or greasy scales characteristically seen in seborrheic dermatitis. When exudates such as serum or pus mix with scale, crusts are formed.

Eruptions that consist of scaling papules are referred to as *papulosquamous*. Psoriasis, in which scaling papules coalesce to form plaques, is the classic example of a papulosquamous eruption. *Maculosquamous* refers to flat lesions with fine scaling such as those that can be seen in tinea versicolor and erythrasma. Pityriasis rosea may have papulosquamous, maculosquamous, and even papulovesicular lesions.

FIGURE 3-15

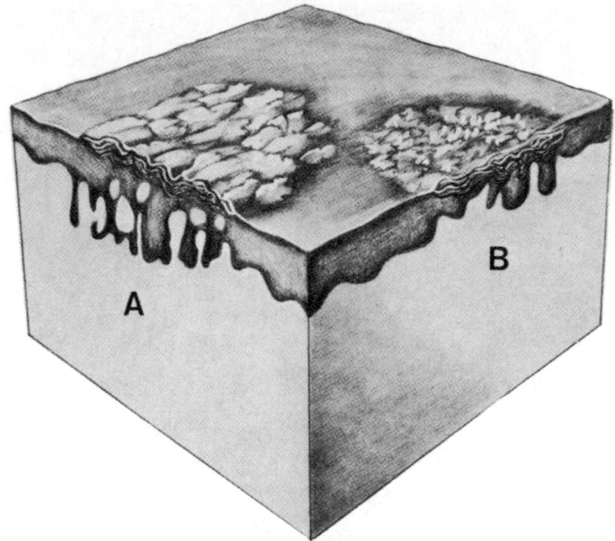

A.

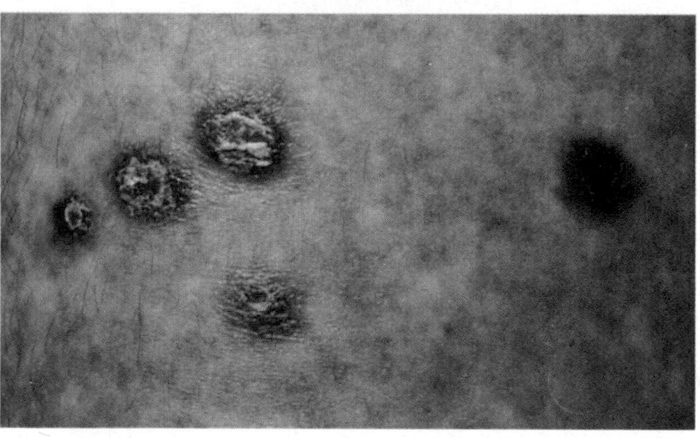
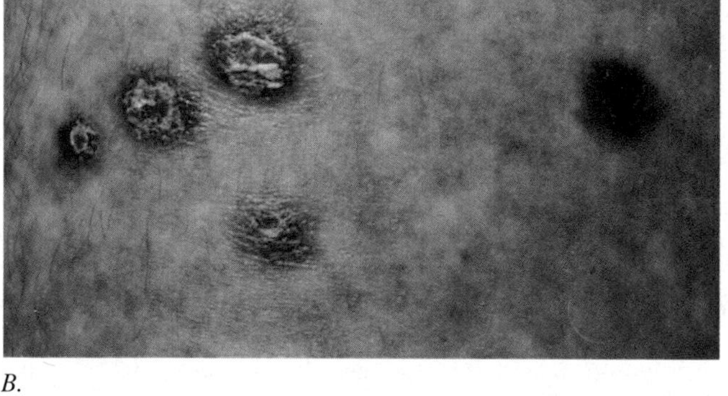

B.

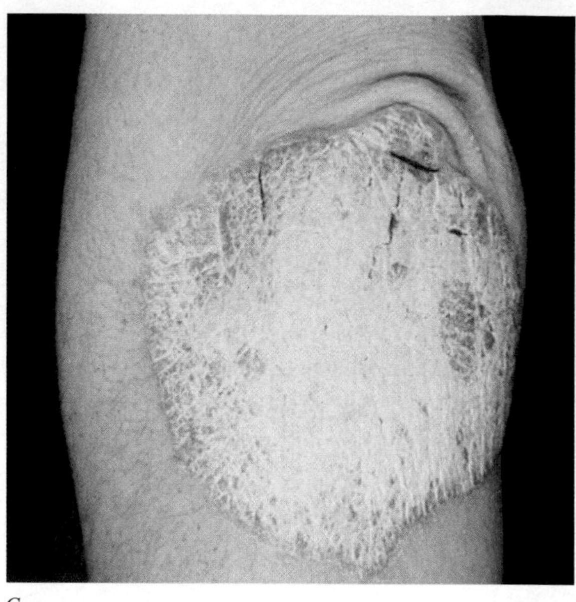

C.

Desquamation. Abnormal shedding or accumulation of stratum corneum in perceptible flakes is called scaling and is shown in the drawing (*A*). Parakeratotic scale (with retained nuclei) may be seen surmounting psoriasiform epidermal hyperplasia (A). Densely adherent scale with a gritty feel from a localized increase in the stratum corneum is seen in actinic keratoses (B). Typical psoriatic scaling is shown in the photograph (*B*). Scales that adhere tightly to the underlying epidermis may build up to form an asbestos-like layer that obscures the underlying lesion, as in the psoriatic plaque shown in (*C*).

CRUSTS (ENCRUSTED EXUDATES) *Crusts* are hardened deposits that result when serum, blood, or purulent exudate dries on the skin surface, and they are characteristic of pyogenic infections. Crusts may be thin, delicate, and friable (A in Fig. 3-16*A*), or thick and adherent (B in Fig. 3-16*A*). Crusts are yellow when formed from dried serum, green or yellow-green when formed from purulent exudate, or when formed from blood. Crusts may be present in acute eczematous dermatitis and impetigo (honey-colored, glistening crusts).

When the exudate or crust involves the entire thickness of the epidermis, the crusts may be thick and adherent; this condition is known as *ecthyma*. A *scutula* is a small, yellowish, cup-shaped crust especially characteristic of superficial fungal infection of the scalp caused by *Trichophyton schoenleinii*.

GANGRENE AND SPHACELUS *Gangrene* refers to a severe necrotizing and sloughing process. Gangrene that results from arterial occlusion is characterized by a sharply demarcated blue-black color. Gangrene from streptococcal or clostridial infection may begin with vesicles that become purplish black followed by rapid necrosis of whole segments of skin.

A *sphacelus* is a densely adherent, dry, necrotic membrane occurring in the floor of an ulcer. It is seen in decubitus ulcers, chronic ulcers due to x-ray damage, diphtheritic or anthrax ulcers, any ischemic ulcer, or factitial dermatosis.

EXCORIATIONS *Excoriations* are superficial excavations of epidermis that may be linear or punctate and result from scratching. They are frequent findings in all types of pruritus and are concomitants of pruritic skin disease, such as atopic eczema, dermatitis herpetiforms, or infestations.

FISSURES *Fissures* are linear cleavages or cracks in the skin and may be painful. They occur particularly in palmar/plantar psoriasis and in chronic eczematous dermatitis of the hands and feet, especially after therapy that has caused excessive drying of the skin. Fissures are frequently noted in perianal psoriasis or at the angles of the mouth (perlèche). Perlèche may be caused by avitaminosis, moniliasis, ill-fitting dentures, or unknown factors.

POIKILODERMA As a morphologic descriptive term, *poikiloderma* refers to the combination of atrophy, telangiectasia, and pigmentary changes (hyper- and hypo-). Poikilodermatous lesions can be seen in radiodermatitis, dermatomyositis, mycosis fungoides, and lupus erythematosus. Because of some confusion stemming from the use of the word poikiloderma in the naming of specific syndromes in the past, it is probably best to restrict it to use as a descriptive, morphologic term and to so indicate when using it.

FIGURE 3-16

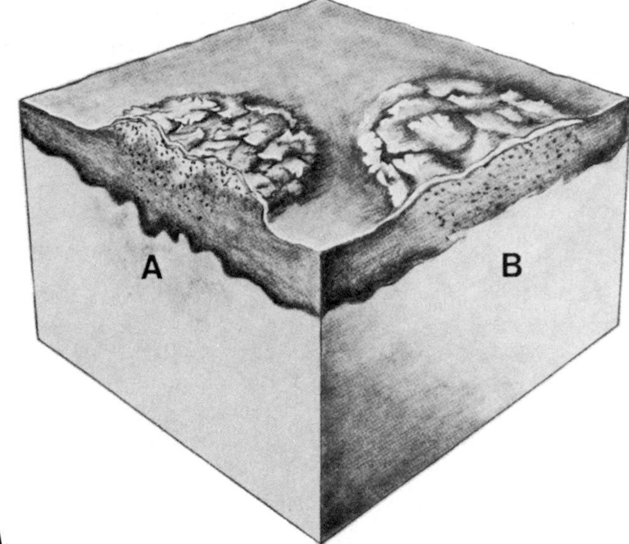

A.

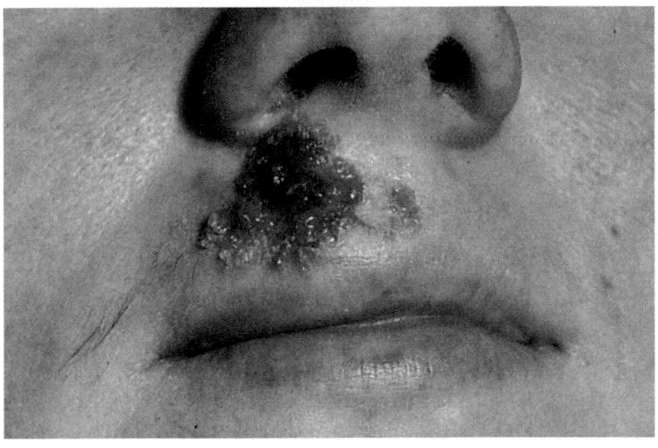

B.

Crusts (encrusted exudates). Crusts result when serum, blood, or purulent exudate dries on the skin surface and are characteristic of injury and pyogenic infections. Crusts may be thin, delicate, and friable (A) or thick and adherent (B), as shown in the drawing (*A*). Crusts are yellow when formed from dried serum, green or yellow-green when formed from purulent exudate, or brown or dark red when formed from blood. Superficial crusts that occur as honey-colored, delicate, glistening particulates on the surface are typical of impetigo and are illustrated in the photograph (*B*).

Shape and Arrangement of Lesions

After the type or types of lesion have been identified, it is necessary to consider their *shape, arrangement* in relation to each other, the pattern of their *distribution*, and their *extent*. The shape, arrangement, and distribution are often helpful and sometimes a key to the diagnosis. The following descriptions of the shape and arrangement of lesions can apply to single or multiple lesions. For example, an annular shape can occur in a single lesion or be derived from the annular arrangement of a number of vesicles, papules, and the like. A single lesion may assume a linear shape, or a number of lesions may be arranged in a linear pattern.

LINEAR LESIONS AND LINEAR ARRANGEMENT Linearity is a simple but important feature of skin lesions because it often indicates an exogenous cause (Fig. 3-17*A*). Vesicles on the leg may convey no

particular meaning until a linear arrangement is observed; this type of arrangement occurs after a vesicant or allergen has been drawn across the skin, as, for example, when there has been contact with *Rhus* leaves. Erythema in linear streaks over an extremity brings to mind the possibility of lymphangitis.

The *Koebner (isomorphic) phenomenon* refers to the fact that in persons with certain skin diseases, especially psoriasis, trauma is followed by new lesions in the traumatized but otherwise normal skin, and these new lesions are identical to those in the diseased skin.[25] The Koebner reaction occurs in traumatized normal skin in vitiligo, psoriasis, and lichen planus, among other conditions. The Koebner phenomenon may occur in recent scars or at pressure points.

Nodules may be linear, inasmuch as they occur along the course of a vein in superficial thrombophlebitis or along an artery in temporal arteritis or polyarteritis nodosa. Deep mycoses (sporotrichosis and coccidioidomycosis) may present as granulomatous nodules along the course of the lymphatics. Vesicles arranged linearly occur in localized herpes zoster (and rarely in herpes simplex) with a distribution that follows a dermatome. Epidermal nevi (nevus unius lateris) may have a striking linear pattern that extends along an entire extremity. Such nevi, as well as a number of other nevoid and acquired skin diseases, may follow the curious *Blaschko's lines,* which do not follow any known vascular or nervous structures in the skin.[26,27] The lesions of factitial dermatosis, which include ulcers, atrophy, scars, or all three, frequently occur in a linear pattern. Linear scleroderma may be recognized by its bands of induration or atrophy that extend along an upper or lower extremity or the midline of the forehead (*coup de sabre*).

ANNULAR AND ARCIFORM LESIONS AND ANNULAR AND ARCIFORM ARRANGEMENTS In most acute erythemas associated with inflammation, the macules are round or oval; Siemens[4] attempted to explain this on the basis of the blood supply, stating that each individual erythematous spot represents the territory of direct blood supply from an individual arteriole. An *annular* (Latin *annulus,* a ring) (Fig. 3-17*B*) lesion may result when the pathologic process in a round lesion spreads peripherally and recedes in the center or when individual lesions occur in a ring-shaped arrangement. A special and important type of annular lesion, the *iris* (Fig. 3-17*C*) or *bull's-eye* lesion, consists of an erythematous annular macule or papule with a purplish or dusky, papular or vesicular center. Iris-type lesions are characteristic of the erythema multiforme syndrome. *Annular* and *round* should not be used interchangeably: annular lesions have clear or contrasting centers, round ones do not. *Nummular* (coin-shaped) and *discoid* (like a disc) are used to describe distinctive round lesions that occur in eczema and cutaneous lupus erythematosus, respectively.

Annular lesions that may be macular or slightly raised occur in erythema marginatum and other figurate erythemas (see Chap. 99), drug eruptions, mycosis fungoides, secondary syphilis, or lupus erythematosus. Annular lesions with scales suggest pityriasis rosea, dermatophytosis, psoriasis, or seborrheic dermatitis. The individual papules of psoriasis often occur in an annular, polycyclic, or arciform arrangement (Fig. 3-17*B*). Lupus vulgaris, sarcoid, granuloma annulare, mycosis fungoides, and tertiary syphilis may exhibit annular or arciform patterns of papules or nodules. As a rule, however, the lesions of tertiary syphilis are arranged in incomplete or broken rings. Secondary syphilis, erythema multiforme, lichen planus, urticaria, lupus erythematosus, dermatophytosis, Lyme borreliosis (erythema migrans), or the figurate erythemas (see Chap. 99) may produce annular papules. A *serpiginous* (snakelike) arrangement of lesions is seen in the wheals of creeping eruptions (larva migrans) and in the papules and nodules of late syphilis and lupus vulgaris.

FIGURE 3-17

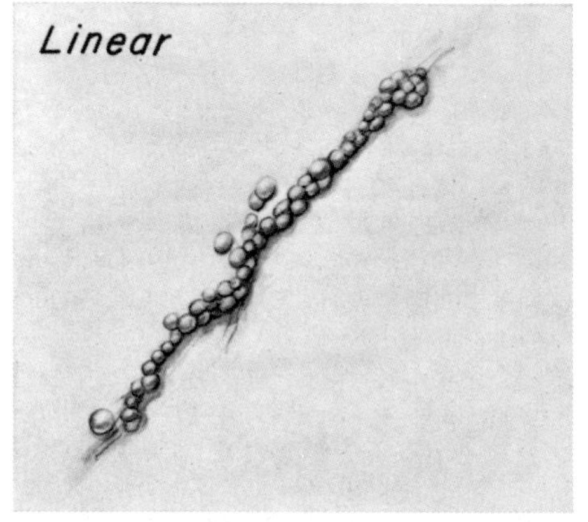

A.

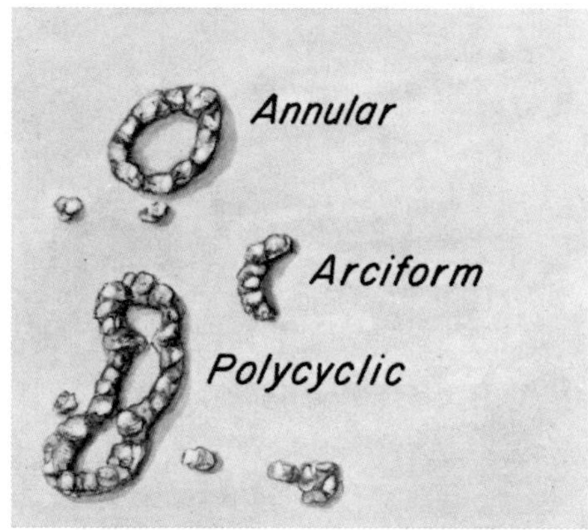

B.

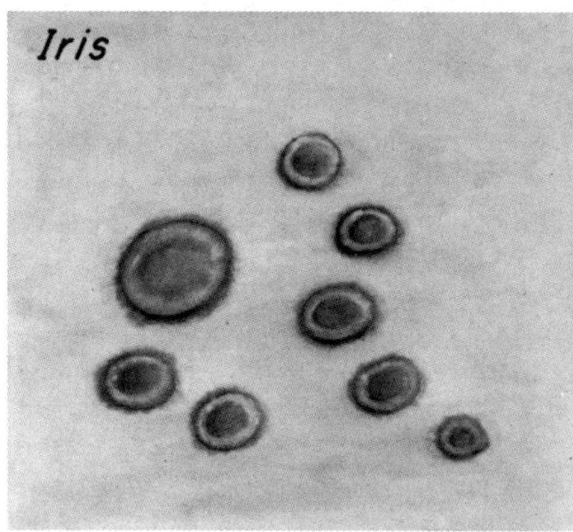

C.

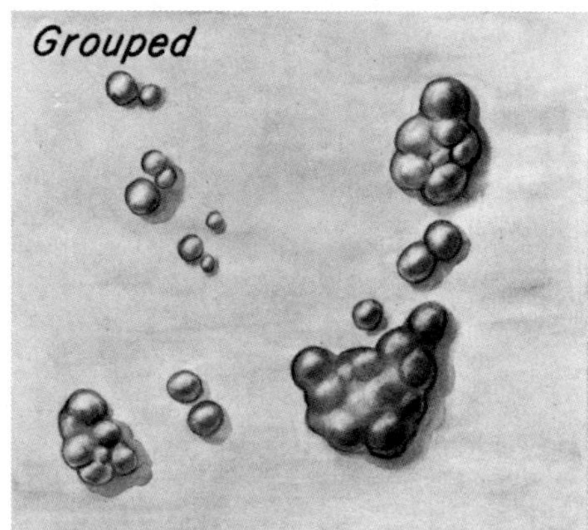

D.

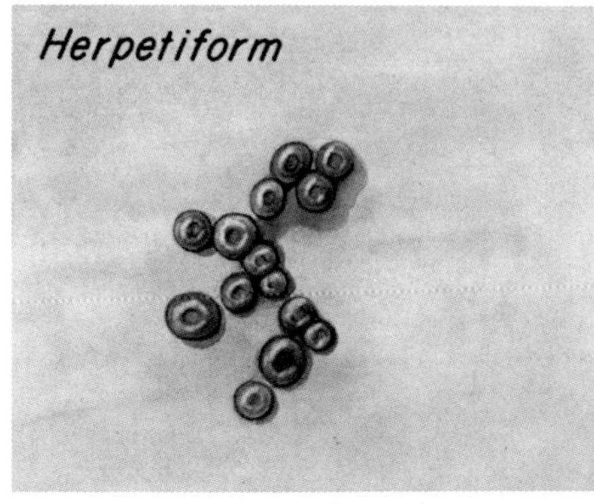

E.

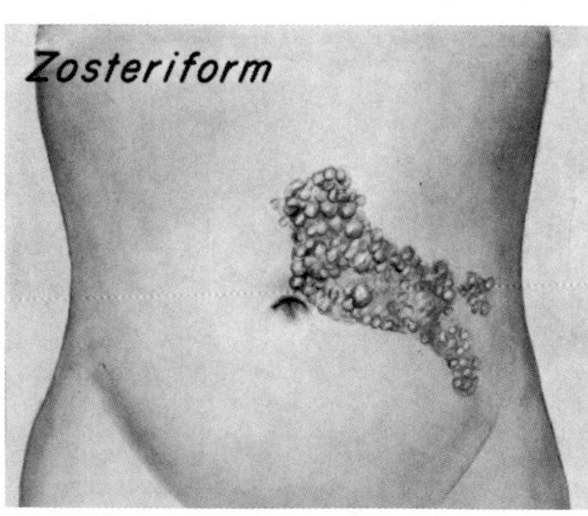

F.

Shape and arrangement of lesions (see text for descriptions).

GROUPED LESIONS Papules, wheals, nodules, and vesicles may occur in groups (Fig. 3-17*D*). These groupings are of little diagnostic value unless they assume a pattern. Clusters or groups of vesicles may occur anywhere on the skin surface, and this arrangement is so characteristic of herpes simplex and herpes zoster that it is termed *herpetiform* (Fig. 3-17*E*). When vesicles or bullae of herpes zoster occur in a bandlike pattern following a dermatome, the arrangement is termed *zosteriform* (Fig. 3-17*F*). A zosteriform or dermatomal arrangement of cutaneous nodules is occasionally observed in metastatic carcinoma of the breast. Nevoid conditions such as melanocytic nevi or epidermal nevi (ichthyosis hystrix) may occur in a zosteriform pattern.

Corymbiform refers to a grouped arrangement that consists of a central cluster of lesions beyond which are scattered individual lesions. The picture is reminiscent of an explosion, or cluster of flowers, and can be seen in verruca vulgaris.

Unpatterned, grouped lesions are noted in verruca plana, lichen planus, urticaria, insect bites (often in groups of three), leiomyoma, and lymphangioma circumscriptum.

RETICULAR ARRANGEMENT A netlike, lacy, or retiform (Latin *reticulum,* "little net") pattern occurs in a number of conditions, the prototype of which is livedo reticularis. Such reticular arrangements also occur in cutis marmorata and erythema ab igne. Individual lesions may also have reticular or lacy components, as, for example, the *Wickham's striae* in lichen planus (see Chap. 49).

Distribution of Skin Lesions

Although it is possible to recognize some skin eruptions by their *patterns of distribution,* the type and shape of the lesion, which have already been discussed, are much more reliable criteria in diagnosis. Inasmuch as the type, shape, and arrangement of lesions and their distribution pattern constitute the important tetrad in dermatologic diagnosis, it is important that the physician be acquainted with some of the more characteristic distribution patterns that are presented in the discussions of individual diseases throughout this book. Skin disorders can be classified as *localized (isolated), regional,* or *generalized;* the term *total (universal)* denotes involvement of the entire skin, the hair, and the nails.

As a first step in the examination of the skin, the physician should view the disrobed patient from a distance. After a survey of the entire skin surface and a close-up inspection of the type and shape of lesions, the distribution pattern can be put in perspective. For example, if eczematous patches are found on the wrist, earlobes, and neck, there is a clue to a metal contact dermatitis from a metal watchband, metal earrings, and a metal necklace.

When an eruption occurs in a bilateral and symmetric distribution, the cause is often endogenous or systemic. This pattern suggests hematogenous dissemination of the pathologic stimulus and is most often indicative of hypersensitivity reactions (e.g., drug sensitization and "allergic" vasculitis), viral exanthems, and certain other skin disorders, such as atopic eczema, dermatitis herpetiformis, etc.

In most cases, the reason for the localization of skin lesions to certain areas is unknown. A few factors, however, account for sites of predilection. Diseases caused or exacerbated by exposure to sunlight are localized to exposed areas such as the dorsa of the hands and arms, the neck, and face, a so-called "photo-distribution." Areas of the face that are usually spared include the skin of the top part of the upper eyelids and the skin of the hair-covered scalp. Cutaneous (discoid) and systemic lupus erythematosus are predominantly localized in exposed areas but may also appear in completely light-shielded areas, such as the skin of the hair-covered scalp, ears, mouth, and feet.

Areas of minor and repeated trauma and areas where skin rubs against skin account for the distribution of lesions of epidermolysis bullosa and some of the lesions in vitiligo and psoriasis. Trauma in combination with light exposure accounts for the skin fragility and bullae localized to the backs of the hands and the face in porphyria cutanea tarda.

Hidradenitis suppurativa consists of abscesses of apocrine sweat glands and is therefore localized to axillae, nipples (in females), and anogenital areas.

Rosacea is usually confined to the "blush" area of the face, and factors that induce blushing are thought to be precipitative; these include alcoholic beverages, certain spicy condiments, hot beverages, and possibly emotional stress.

Candidiasis (moniliasis) is predominantly localized to areas where the skin is warm and moist (axillary, inframammary, and inguinal regions, the intergluteal cleft, the vaginal area, and the mouth). *Candida albicans* is a frequent resident of the gastrointestinal tract and reaches some of these sites by direct contact.

Herpes zoster occurs in a dermatomal pattern because the virus moves along the sensory nerves to the skin.

Lesions may be associated with openings of follicles, as in the follicular keratoses of keratosis pilaris, pityriasis rubra pilaris, and vitamin A deficiency. There is a follicular pattern of involvement in acne, lichen planopilaris, psoriasis, some drug eruptions, fungal infections (particularly *Trichophyton rubrum* and *Trichophyton verrucosum*), various forms of bacterial folliculitis, and some cases of atopic eczema.

During the time taken to survey the distribution pattern of the dermatosis, it is pertinent to review the history, occupation, various forms of exposure (e.g., to light or to airborne and contact allergens), and history of drug ingestion.

PHYSIOLOGIC ABNORMALITIES

Some of the most common disorders in dermatology are basically functional abnormalities of the skin, which include dryness, seborrhea, hyperhidrosis and anhidrosis. These entities are covered in detail in Chap. 76.

PRURITUS

Itching may be a cardinal symptom of general medical significance, the earliest sign of Hodgkin's disease, occult carcinoma, and primary biliary cirrhosis.[10] It is a critical feature of dermatologic disorders such as atopic eczema, dermatitis herpetiformis, and often psoriasis. On the other hand, severe itching can occur as a consequence of mere dryness of the skin. The pathophysiology and clinical aspects of pruritus are discussed in Chap. 41.

INSTRUMENTAL AND LABORATORY PROCEDURES IN DERMATOLOGIC DIAGNOSIS

Aids to Dermatologic Diagnosis: Clinical, Instrumental, and Laboratory

Magnification: To examine the skin surface critically and to detect the fine morphologic detail of skin lesions it is necessary to use a hand lens magnifier (preferably 7×); also, a better image is obtained following application of a drop of mineral oil to the lesion. Magnification is especially helpful in the diagnosis of lupus erythematosus (follicular plugging and atrophy), lichen planus (Wickham's striae), basal cell carcinomas (translucence and delicate telangiectasia), and early malignant melanoma (subtle changes in color, especially gray, slate, or blue). Hand-held magnifying instruments with built-in lighting and a magnification of 10× to 30× have recently become available and these permit better visualization of lesions when used with a drop of oil. Using this small optical instrument or the larger binocular microscope—this technique is called *epiluminescence microscopy*—facilitates the distinction of benign and malignant pigmented neoplasms.[28–30]

Wood's lamp (longwave ultraviolet light, "black" light) is essential for the clinical diagnosis of certain skin and hair diseases and of porphyria. Longwave ultraviolet radiation is obtained by fitting a high-pressure mercury lamp with a specially compounded filter made of nickel oxide and silica (Wood's filter); this filter is opaque to all light except for a band between 320 and 400 nm. When using the Wood's lamp, it is essential for the examiner to become dark-adapted in order to see the contrasts clearly. When the ultraviolet waves emitted by Wood's lamp impinge on the skin, a visible fluorescence occurs. Wood's lamp is particularly useful in the detection of the fluorescence of dermatophytosis (*Microsporum*) in the hair shaft (green) and of erythrasma (coral red) on the skin. Wood's lamp also helps to estimate the variation in the "whiteness" of lesions in relation to the normal skin color, in dark-skinned and especially in fair-skinned persons; for example, the lesions seen in hypomelanotic macules in tuberous sclerosis and in tinea versicolor are not as white as the macules present in vitiligo, which are typically amelanotic. Circumscribed hypermelanosis, such as ephelides and melasma, is much more evident under Wood's lamp, and in lentigo maligna melanoma and acrolentiginous melanoma the Wood's lamp can be used to detect the total extent of the lesion as a guide to total excision. Melanin in the dermis, as in a Mongolian sacral spot, does not become accentuated under Wood's lamp.[31] Therefore, it is possible to localize the site of melanin (epidermal or dermal) by use of the Wood's lamp; this phenomenon is not evident in patients with brown or black skin. The technique is as follows: a grading (minimal, moderate, marked) of the degree of pigmentation is made with visible light and compared with a grading of the degree of color change when examined with Wood's lamp. In epidermal melanin pigmentation the pigment grade increases from minimal to marked, but dermal melanin has the same degree of pigment in both visible light and Wood's lamp illumination.

Diascopy consists of firmly pressing a transparent, hard, flat object (such as a hand lens or *two* microscope slides) over the surface of a skin lesion. The examiner will find this procedure of special value in determining whether the red color of a macule or papule is due to capillary dilatation (erythema) or to extravasation of blood (purpura). Diascopy is also useful for the detection of the hyaline yellowish-brown color of papules or nodules in sarcoidosis, tuberculosis of the skin, lymphoma, and granuloma annulare.

FIGURE 3-18

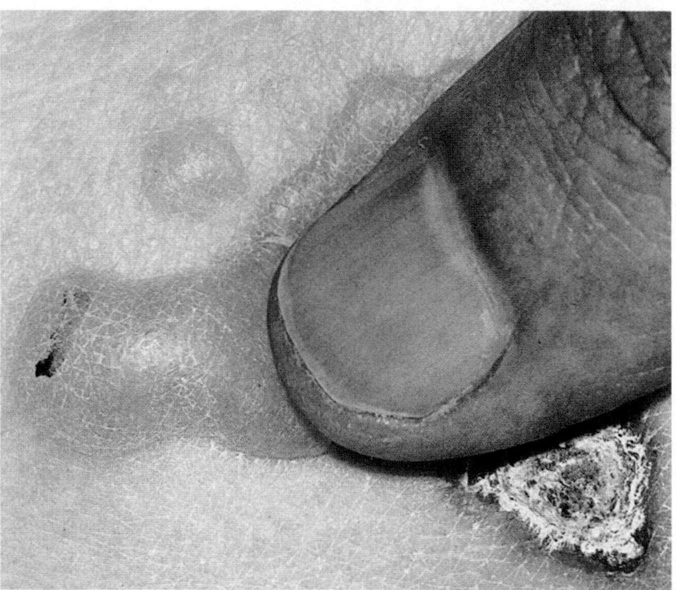

Pemphigus vulgaris. The bulla has been extended by applying pressure with the finger (Nikolsky's sign).

Clinical Signs

The *dimple sign* is a useful maneuver in differentiating dermatofibromas (benign, firm, nodular lesions that are often pigmented) from malignant melanoma. Application of lateral pressure with the thumb and index finger results in the formation of a depression (dimple) in a dermatofibroma, whereas melanoma and melanocytic nevi protrude above their initial plane (become elevated), as does the normal skin when this maneuver is performed.[32]

Nikolsky's sign refers to the sheetlike removal of epidermis (Fig. 3-18) by gentle traction that can be observed in several diseases, the most important of which are pemphigus vulgaris and toxic epidermal necrolysis.[33]

Darier's sign refers to the development of an urticarial wheal in the lesions of urticaria pigmentosa (a brown macule or a slightly elevated papule) after they are rubbed with the rounded end of a pen. The wheal, which is strictly confined to the borders of the lesion, may not appear for 5 to 10 min.

Auspitz's sign refers to the appearance of pinpoint dots of blood at the tops of ruptured capillaries when scale is forcibly removed from psoriatic plaques.[33]

Clinical Tests

Patch testing is used to document and validate a diagnosis of allergic contact sensitization and to identify the causative agent. It may also be of value as a screening procedure in some patients with chronic or bizarre eczematous eruptions (e.g., hand and foot dermatoses). It is a unique means of in vivo reproduction of disease in diminutive proportions, for sensitization affects all the skin and may therefore be elicited at any cutaneous site. The patch test is easier and safer than a "use test" with a questionable allergen, for test items can be applied in low concentrations in small areas of skin for short periods of time. Textbooks on contact dermatitis contain complete lists of antigens used in patch testing.[35]

Photopatch testing is a combination of patch testing and ultraviolet irradiation of the test site and is used to detect photoallergy.

Phototesting is done to determine the patient's sensitivity to various wavelengths of ultraviolet radiation. This is useful in the diagnosis of certain photosensitivities (see Chaps. 135 and 136).

Microscope Examination of Scales, Crusts, Serum, and Hair

Gram's stain and cultures of exudates should be made in lesions suspected of being a bacterial or a yeast (*C. albicans*) infection. Ulcers and nodules require a scalpel biopsy in which a wedge of tissue consisting of all three layers of skin is obtained; the biopsy specimen is minced in a sterile mortar, and the tissue is then cultured for bacteria (including typical and atypical mycobacteria) and fungi.

Microscope examination for mycelia should be made of the roofs of vesicles or of the scales (the advancing borders are preferable) or of the hair and of nails. The tissue is cleared with 10% KOH (20% KOH for nails) and warmed gently. Fungal cultures with Sabouraud's or other appropriate medium should be made. The specifics of dermatophyte and other fungal infections are covered in Chaps. 205 to 207.

Microscope examination of cells obtained from the base of vesicles and bullae (*Tzanck test*) may reveal the presence of giant epithelial cells and multinucleated giant cells (containing 10 to 12 nuclei) in herpes simplex, herpes zoster, and varicella. Material from the base of a vesicle obtained by gentle (do not produce bleeding!) curettage with a scalpel is smeared on a glass slide, stained with Giemsa's (Fig. 3-19) or Wright's stain, and examined for the presence of giant epithelial cells, which are diagnostic. Cultures and rapid immunofluorescent diagnosis for herpes simplex and varicella-zoster are now easily and rapidly available and are more specific than the Tzanck test.

Biopsy of the Skin

Biopsy of the skin is a rewarding diagnostic technique because of the easy accessibility of the skin and the variety of techniques that can be

FIGURE 3-19

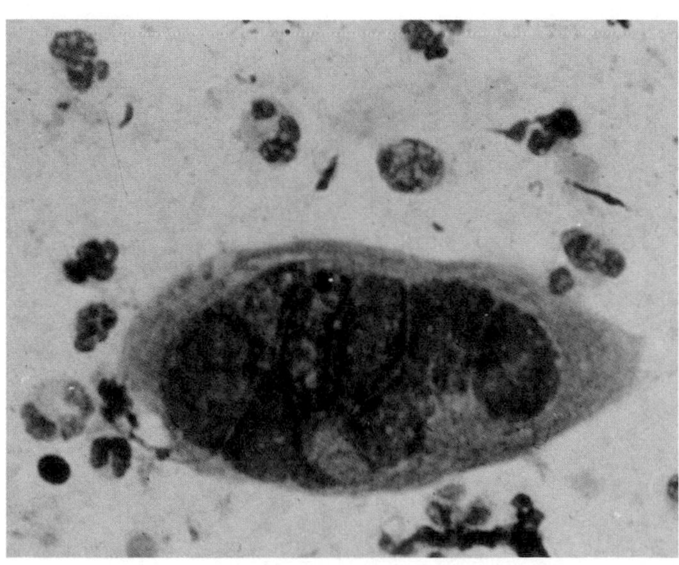

Tzanck preparation showing multinucleate giant epidermal cell (Giemsa's stain). (*Courtesy of Arthur R. Rhodes, M.D.*)

used for the study of the excised specimen, such as immunofluorescence, immunoperoxidase, electron microscopy, and the polymerase chain reaction. In many instances the correlation of the clinical and histologic findings is mandatory, as the histologic diagnosis, especially in noninfectious inflammatory disease, may be nonspecific. A good general rule is that when the histopathology and the clinical findings do not agree, count on the clinical diagnosis, get another biopsy, and see the patient again after a few days or weeks.

The selection of the site of the biopsy is important and is based primarily on the stage of the eruption. Early lesions are usually more typical in vesiculobullous eruptions in which the lesion should be no more than 24 h old. In all other eruptions, older, fully developed lesions are often more characteristic. More than one biopsy may be necessary, especially if the eruption is polymorphous.

A common technique for diagnostic biopsy using local anesthesia is the use of a 4-mm "punch"—a small disposable tubular knife. Immunofluorescence analysis may be done with similar specimens from bullous diseases or lupus erythematosus. For nodules and tumors and, especially, nodules on the leg, a large wedge scalpel biopsy or generous, deep punch biopsy should be obtained including the subcutaneous tissue. Furthermore, all inflammatory nodules suspected of being infectious granulomas should be bisected—one-half for histology, the other half sent in a sterile container for bacterial and mycotic cultures using a tissue mince. Specimens for light microscopy should be fixed immediately in 10% aqueous formalin. A brief but detailed and specific summary of the clinical history and lesions should accompany the specimen. Biopsy is indicated in all suspected neoplasms, in all bullous disorders using immunofluorescence simultaneously, and in all dermatologic disorders in which a specific diagnosis is not possible by clinical examination alone.

More specifics on histology in general and on immunofluorescent and immunoperoxidase techniques in particular, are best described in dermatopathology texts.[36,37]

In summary, dermatologists are physicians who can diagnose a rash! They may also be internists, surgeons, biochemists, or immunologists; but without competency in dermatologic diagnosis they cannot qualify as dermatologists. The sine qua non of the dermatologist is a trained clinical eye for morphologic diagnosis. This diagnostic eye can be acquired only by endlessly repeated encounters in which the physician is forced not only to look at but to observe the rash, while an *experienced mentor points the way.* The most common error in dermatologic diagnosis is to regard the lesions as nonspecific "rashes" rather than as aggregates of specific individual lesions. As in surveying a blood smear, a "general impression" is not enough: the morphologic aspects of each individual cell must be carefully scrutinized and judged to be normal or abnormal. Too often, physicians adopt a speedy, superficial approach to the skin that they would not apply to any other organ that they examine. See Table 3-2.

Lewis Thomas has said that "Medicine is no longer the laying on of hands, it is more like the reading of signals from machines."[37] In dermatology there can be no replacement for the laying on of hands, and the physician is repeatedly gratified by reading signals not from machines, but from people.

TABLE 3-2

Pointers and Pitfalls in Dermatologic Diagnosis

1. Do not remove tissue without sending a portion for histologic examination.
2. If the dermatopathologic findings are at odds with the clinical diagnosis, obtain another biopsy. If disagreement presists, follow the clinical lead (cautiously).
3. Generalized pruritus of more than 1 month's duration and without an obvious cause needs investigation with history, search for lymph nodes (including the supraclavicular nodes), laboratory studies, chest x-ray, and, if indicated, imaging studies.
4. A new or changing mole should be carefully evaluated and excised for diagnosis if it has suspicious features.
5. Examine the entire skin and mucous membranes whenever possible and always in patients presenting with a personal or family history of melanoma or with multiple "moles."
6. Medications can cause almost every type of dermatologic lesion and are always in the list of possible diagnoses. Drug reactions often appear suddenly and are usually symmetric in distribution.
7. A diagnosis of factitial (self-induced) dermatosis can be made only after all other reasonable possibilities are considered. A nervous, strange, or "crazy" affect can be the consequence or the cause of a terrible skin problem.
8. Beware of "snap," "curbside," or "doorway" diagnoses. No other medical specialty engages in this hazardous practice.
9. Be wary of the "atypical" diagnosis. Atypical "this" may be typical "that" to someone who has seen it before.

REFERENCES

1. Jackson R: *Morphological Diagnosis of Skin Disease.* Ontario, Grimsby, 1998
2. Mihm MC Jr et al: Early detection of primary cutaneous malignant melanoma: A color atlas. *N Engl J Med* **289**:989, 1973
3. Boyce JA, Bernhard JD: Total skin examination should be part of routine health maintenance screening. *J Gen Intern Med* **2**:59, 1987
4. Siemens HW: *General Diagnosis and Therapy of Skin Diseases: An Introduction to Dermatology for Students and Physicians* translated by K Wiener. Chicago, Univ of Chicago Press, 1958
5. Haxthausen H: How are dermatological diagnoses made? *Trans St Johns Hosp Dermatol Soc* **30**:3, 1951
6. Jackson R: The importance of being visually literate. *Arch Dermatol* **111**:632, 1975
7. Kundel HL, Wright DJ: The influence of prior knowledge on visual search strategies during the viewing of chest radiographs. *Radiology* **93**:315, 1969
8. Hurst JW: *Notes from a Chairman.* Chicago, Year Book Medical, 1987, p 46
9. Bernhard JD, Haynes HA: Nonrashes 1. The Koebner non-reaction. *Cutis* **29**:158, 1982
10. Bernhard JD (ed): *Itch: Mechanisms and Management of Pruritus.* New York, McGraw-Hill, 1994
11. Brownstein MH: Invisible dermatoses versus nonrashes. *J Am Acad Dermatol* **9**:599, 1983
12. Phillips KA et al: Rate of body dysmorphic disorder in dermatology patients. *J Am Acad Dermatol* **42**:436, 2000
13. Cotterill JA: Clinical features of patients with dermatologic nondisease. *Semin Dermatol* **2**:203, 1983
14. Koblenzer CS: *Psychocutaneous Disease.* Orlando, Grune & Stratton, 1987
15. Gougerot MH: Dermatoses invisibles, leur fréquence, leur intérêt doctrinal et pratique. *Bull Soc Dermatol Syphilol* **47**:361, 1940
16. Requena L, Yus ES: Invisible dermatoses: Additional findings. *Int J Dermatol* **30**:552, 1991
17. Feinstein AR: *Clinical Judgment.* Baltimore, Williams & Wilkins, 1967
18. Winkelmann RK (chairman): The International League of Dermatologic Societies Committee on Nomenclature. Glossary of basic dermatologic lesions. *Acta Derm Venereol Suppl* 130, *(Stockh)*, 1987
19. Fitzpatrick TB, Walker SA: *Dermatologic Differential Diagnosis.* Chicago, Year Book, 1962
20. Goldsmith LA et al: *Adult and Pediatric Dermatology: A Color Guide to Diagnosis and Treatment.* Philadelphia, FA Davis, 1997
21. Leider M, Rosenblum M: *A Dictionary of Dermatological Words, Terms, and Phrases.* New York, McGraw-Hill, 1968, or West Haven, CT, Dome Laboratories, 1976
22. Bernhard JD et al: Maculopapularism. *Am J Dermatopathol* **8**:173, 1986

23. Bernhard JD, Marks EJ: Case records of the Massachusetts General Hospital. Case 17-1986. An 18-year-old man with cutaneous ulcers and bilateral pulmonary infiltrates [Wegener's granulomatosis]. *N Engl J Med* **314**:1170, 1986
24. Oh DH et al: Five cases of calciphylaxis and a review of the literature. *J Am Acad Dermatol* **40**:979, 1999
25. Melski JW et al: The Koebner (isomorphic) response in psoriasis. *Arch Dermatol* **119**:655, 1983
26. Bolognia JL et al: Lines of Blaschko. *J Am Acad Dermatol* **31**:157, 1994
27. Happle R, Assim A: The lines of Blaschko on the head and neck. *J Am Acad Dermatol* **44**:612, 2001
28. Menzies SW et al: *An Atlas of Surface Microscopy of Pigmented Skin Lesions*. New York, McGraw-Hill, 1996
29. Stolz W et al: *Color Atlas of Dermatoscopy*. Germany, Blackwell Science, 1994
30. Kittler H et al: Morphologic changes of pigmented skin lesions: A useful extension of the ABCD rule for dermatoscopy. *J Am Acad Dermatol* **40**:558, 1999
31. Gilchrest BA et al: Localization of melanin pigment on the skin with Wood's lamp. *Br J Dermatol* **96**:245, 1977
32. Fitzpatrick TB, Gilchrest BA: Dimple sign to differentiate benign from malignant pigmented cutaneous lesions. *N Engl J Med* **296**:1518, 1977
33. Goodman H: Nikolsky sign. *Arch Derm Syphilol* **68**:334, 1953
34. Bernhard JD: Auspitz sign is not sensitive or specific for psoriasis. *J Am Acad Dermatol* **22**:1079, 1990
35. Rietschel RL, Fowler JF: *Fisher's Contact Dermatitis*. Philadelphia, Williams & Wilkins, 2001
36. Elder D et al: *Lever's Histopathology of the Skin*. Philadelphia, Lippincott-Raven, 1997
37. Weedon D: *Skin Pathology*. Edinburgh, Churchill Livingstone, 1997
38. Thomas L: *The Youngest Science. Notes of a Medicine-Watcher*. New York, Viking Press, 1983, p 58

CHAPTER 4

Klaus Wolff
Abdul-Ghani Kibbi
Martin C. Mihm

Basic Pathologic Reactions of the Skin

The skin is composed of various tissue compartments that interconnect anatomically and interact functionally. It is difficult to envisage epidermal function without signals from the dermis; in fact, there are only a few pathologic processes that relate solely to the epidermis without involving or being involved by the underlying papillary body or passenger leukocytes traveling to and from the skin. Epidermis, dermis, and subcutaneous tissue by themselves are heterogeneous in nature (see Chap. 6). An analysis of pathologic processes involving the skin should therefore consider both the heterogeneity and the interactions of the individual cutaneous compartments, because only then will it be understood why a few basic reactions lead to a multiplicity of reaction patterns within this tissue.

Pathophysiologically, the skin can be subdivided into three reactive units that extend beyond anatomic boundaries; they overlap and can be divided into different subunits (Table 4-1). These units respond to pathologic stimuli according to their inherent reaction capacities in a coordinated pattern.

The *superficial reactive unit* comprises the epidermis, the subjacent loose connective tissue of the papillary body and its capillary network, and the superficial venular plexus embedded in this connective tissue. The *reticular layer of the dermis* represents another reactive unit and is composed of subunits—hair follicles, glands, and the surrounding connective tissue. The above subunits may respond individually or jointly to pathologic stimuli. Finally, the third reactive unit, the *subcutaneous tissue,* is functionally also heterogeneous; septal and lobular compartments may be involved either alone or together.

SUPERFICIAL REACTIVE UNIT

Epidermis

Keratinocytes, which have the capacity to keratinize, represent the bulk of the epidermis. The epidermis, an ectodermal epithelium, also harbors a number of other cell populations such as melanocytes, Langerhans cells, Merkel cells, and other cellular migrants. The basal cells of the

TABLE 4-1

Reactive Units of the Skin

I Superficial reactive unit
- A Epidermis
- B Junction zone (dermal-epidermal junction)
- C Papillary body
- D Superficial microvascular plexus

II Reticular dermis
- A Connective tissue
- B Appendages (hair follicles, sweat glands, sebaceous glands)
- C Deep vascular plexus

III Subcutis
- A Lobules
- B Septae

epidermis undergo proliferation cycles that provide for the renewal of the epidermis and, as they move toward the surface of the skin, undergo a differentiation process that results in keratinization (Chap. 7). The epidermis is thus a dynamic tissue in which cells are constantly in nonsynchronized motion; the proliferation kinetics and the direction and speed of migration of the individual cell populations differ from each other, so that keratinocytes not only pass each other but also pass melanocytes or Langerhans cells as they move toward the surface of the skin. At the same time they are interconnected through forces of coherence that guarantee the continuity of the epithelium. Stability for this directional cellular flow is provided by the basal membrane complex, which anchors the epidermis to the dermis, and the stratum corneum. It is here that individual cell migration ceases as the keratinizing cells are firmly interconnected by an intercellular cement-like substance (Chap. 9). These forces of cohesion are finally lost at the surface of the epidermis where the individual cornified cells are desquamated. Pathologic changes within the epidermis may therefore relate to the kinetics of epidermal cells or their differentiation and may involve transepidermal migration and intraepidermal cohesion; they also relate to peripatetic leukocytes trafficking to and from the epidermis and adhesion molecules facilitating and directing such cellular movements; and they relate to cytokines and hormones generated by keratinocytes, Langerhans cells, melanocytes, and peripatetic leukocytes. They may affect the entire cell population or individual cells, may be primarily targeted on keratinocytes, or may encompass the other epidermal cell populations. All these processes may occur in an isolated fashion or represent combined phenomena involving all epidermal functions.

DISTURBANCES OF EPIDERMAL CELL KINETICS The mitotic rate of germinative cells, the desquamation rate of corneocytes, and the generation time of epidermal cells determine the homeostasis of the epidermis. Under physiologic conditions, there is a balance among proliferation, differentiation, and desquamation. Enhanced cell proliferation accompanied by an enlargement of the germinative cell pool and increased mitotic rates lead to an increase of the epidermal cell population and thus to a broadening of the epidermis (*acanthosis*) (Fig. 4-1). The causes for acanthosis may reside within the epidermis, as is the case in acanthotic conditions due to epidermotropic viruses, or represent signals that reach the epidermis from the dermis or vasculature. Thus, a shift in the ratio of proliferating to resting cell pools, for example, by a release of the G_1 or G_2 block as in psoriasis (see Chaps. 7 and 42), will lead to both an increase in the turnover of the entire epidermis and to a considerable increase of the volume of germinative cells that have to be accommodated at the dermal-epidermal junction.

The interactions of epidermis and subjacent connective tissue are best illustrated by the process of acanthosis, because thickening of the epidermis and elongation of the rete ridges are usually accompanied by an elongation of the connective tissue papillae, which extend far into the epithelium. This results in an enlargement of the dermal-epidermal interface and, consequently, in an increased area for dermal-epidermal interactions (see Fig. 4-1). A slowing of epidermal cell kinetics results in a reduction of the epidermal cell turnover. This, in turn, leads to a diminution of the germinative cell volume and a flattening of the rete ridges; the epidermis becomes thinner and epidermal *atrophy* results.

Disturbances of epidermal cell kinetics are also reflected in the architecture and composition of the stratum corneum. A simple example is *hyperkeratosis*, where thickening of the stratum corneum may be caused by increased production or a reduced desquamation of corneocytes. In *orthohyperkeratosis*, the stratum corneum may appear qualitatively similar to the normal horny layer, but there may be differences in the packing and cohesion of horny cells. A thickened stratum corneum may

FIGURE 4-1

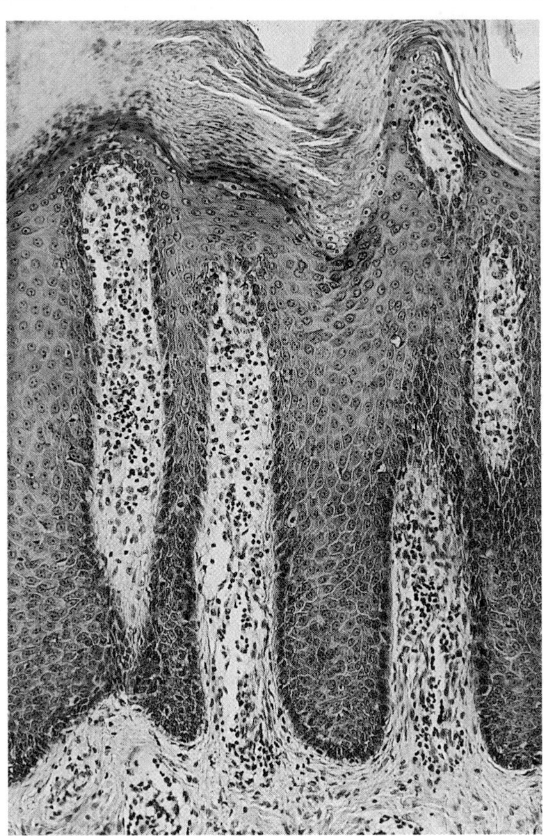

Acanthosis. This sign of increased epidermal kinetics is illustrated in this photomicrograph of psoriasis. Parakeratosis, the retention of nuclei in the horny layer, is evident.

occur in an epidermis exhibiting a rudimentary or a pronounced stratum granulosum.

DISTURBANCES OF EPIDERMAL CELL DIFFERENTIATION A simple example of disturbed epidermal differentiation is parakeratosis, in which faulty and accelerated cornification leads to a retention of pyknotic nuclei of epidermal cells (see Fig. 4-1). In parakeratosis, the stratum granulosum is only rudimentary or may not be present at all, but at the ultrastructural level small keratohyaline granules can be detected. A parakeratotic stratum corneum is not a compact sheet of cornified cells but a loose structure with gaps between cells; these gaps lead to a loss of the barrier function of the epidermis.

Parakeratosis can be the result of incomplete differentiation in postmitotic germinative cells that will become visible morphologically only much later in that layer of the epidermis where keratinization is normally complete, e.g., the stratum corneum. Considering a transit time of 14 days for a postmitotic epidermal cell, a pathologic signal inducing parakeratosis in a cell early in differentiation requires 2 weeks to appear histologically in the stratum corneum. Alternatively, parakeratosis can also be the result of reduced transit time, which does not permit epidermal cells to complete the whole differentiation process. However, "parakeratosis" of cellophane-stripped epidermis becomes microscopically visible as early as 1 h after trauma; here, parakeratosis does not represent disturbed differentiation; rather, it results from

FIGURE 4-2

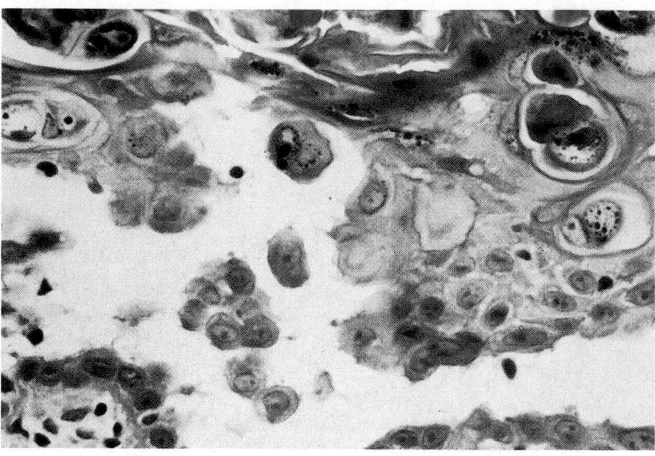

The association of dyskeratosis and acantholysis is seen in this high-power view of Darier's disease, which also demonstrates the intraepidermal cleft formation resulting from these phenomena.

direct cellular injury. Finally, in some skin diseases in which the pathology resides in and around the superficial blood vessels of the dermis, parakeratosis can appear as a secondary epidermal phenomenon 24 h after the eruption. In this case, parakeratosis is the result of a signal delivered to upper epidermal cells already far advanced in differentiation. Therefore, the morphologic term *parakeratosis* signifies both a programmed disturbance of differentiation and maturation and a direct cellular injury.

Dyskeratosis is a term used for premature cornification of individual cells within the viable layers of the epidermis. Dyskeratotic cells have an eosinophilic cytoplasm and a pyknotic nucleus and are packed with keratin filaments arranged in perinuclear aggregates. This leads to a breakdown of the cytoplasmic skeleton of the cell, which loses its ability to adjust its shape and form according to the requirements of adjacent keratinocytes. Such a cell will tend to round up and lose its attachments to the surrounding cells. Dyskeratosis is therefore often associated with acantholysis (see below) but not vice versa (Fig. 4-2).

Dyskeratosis may also signify irreversible cellular damage. In some diseases, it is the expression of a genetically programmed disturbance of keratinization, with keratin filaments detaching from their desmosomal anchoring sites and aggregating in the perinuclear cytoplasm. This is the case in Darier's disease, where keratin filament–desmosome detachments occur in the suprabasal layers, resulting in acantholysis, and only later, as the cell matures, is dyskeratosis apparent. Dyskeratosis may occur in actinic keratosis and squamous cell carcinoma. The morphologic phenomenon of dyskeratosis may also be the result of *apoptosis* (programmed cell death) and may be caused by direct physical and chemical injury. In the sunburn reaction, eosinophilic, apoptotic cells—so-called sunburn cells—are found within the epidermis within the first 24 h after irradiation with UVB (290 to 320 nm), and similar "dyskeratotic," i.e., apoptotic, cells may occur after massive systemic cytotoxic treatment. Individual cell death within the epidermis due to cytotoxic lymphocytes is a regular phenomenon in graft-versus-host reactions of the skin and in erythema multiforme.

DISTURBANCES OF EPIDERMAL COHERENCE Epidermal coherence is the result of a dynamic equilibrium of forming and dissociating intercellular contacts. Epidermal cohesion must permit epidermal cell motion. Both specific intercellular attachment devices (desmosomes) and the intercellular substance are responsible for intercellular cohesion. Desmosomes dissociate and re-form at new sites of intercellular contact as cells migrate through the epidermis, and this requires a functional integrity of epidermal cells. Intercellular cohesion forces are strong enough to guarantee the continuity of the epidermis as an uninterrupted epithelium but, on the other hand, are adaptable enough to permit locomotion, permeability of the intercellular space, and intercellular interactions.

TABLE 4-2

Classification of Intraepidermal Blisters by Anatomic Level with Clinical Examples

Granular layer	Suprabasal
Friction blister	Pemphigus vulgaris
Pemphigus foliaceus	Darier's disease
Subcorneal pustular dermatosis	Basal layer
Staphylococcal scalded-skin syndrome/bullous impetigo	Erythema multiforme
Spinous layer	Lupus erythematosus
Eczematous dermatitis	Lichen planus
Herpesvirus infection	Epidermolysis bullosa simplex
Familial benign pemphigus	

The most common result of disturbed epidermal cohesion is the intraepidermal vesicle, a small cavity filled with fluid. Only rarely, however, is fluid the pathogenetically relevant factor for vesicle formation; loss of cohesion between epidermal cells and the secondary influx of fluid from the dermis is more often responsible for vesiculation. Cell death and lysis of epidermal cells are a third possible cause of the formation of intraepidermal cavities. Despite the multitude of causes and possible pathomechanisms leading to intraepidermal blister formation, distinction can be made on the basis of their anatomic site of origin (see Table 4-2).

Three basic morphologic patterns of intraepidermal vesicle formation are classically recognized. *Spongiosis* is an example of the secondary loss of cohesion between epidermal cells due to the influx of tissue fluid into the epidermis. Serous exudate may extend from the dermis into the intercellular compartment of the epidermis; as it expands, epidermal cells remain in contact with each other only at the sites of desmosomes, acquiring a stellate appearance and giving the epidermis a spongelike morphology (spongiosis). As the intercellular edema increases, individual cells rupture and lyse, and microcavities (*spongiotic vesicles*) result (Fig. 4-3). Confluence of such microcavities leads to larger blisters. Epidermal cells may also be separated by leukocytes, disturbing intraepidermal coherence; thus, the migration of leukocytes into the epidermis and spongiotic edema are often a combined phenomenon. The accumulation of polymorphonuclear leukocytes within the epidermis, the resulting separation of epidermal cells, and their subsequent destruction eventually lead to the formation of a *spongiform pustule*.

Acantholysis is a primary loss of cohesion of epidermal cells. This is initially characterized by a separation of the interdesmosomal regions of the cell membranes of keratinocytes, followed by splitting and a disappearance of desmosomes (see Chap. 59). The cells are intact but are no longer attached; they acquire their smallest possible surface and round up (Figs. 4-2 and 4-4). Intercellular gaps and slits result, and the influx of fluid from the dermis leads to a cavity, which may form in a suprabasal, midepidermal, or even subcorneal location (Fig. 4-5). Keratin filaments within acantholytic cells acquire a perinuclear orientation because they are no longer anchored to desmosomes. However,

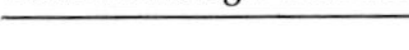

FIGURE 4-3

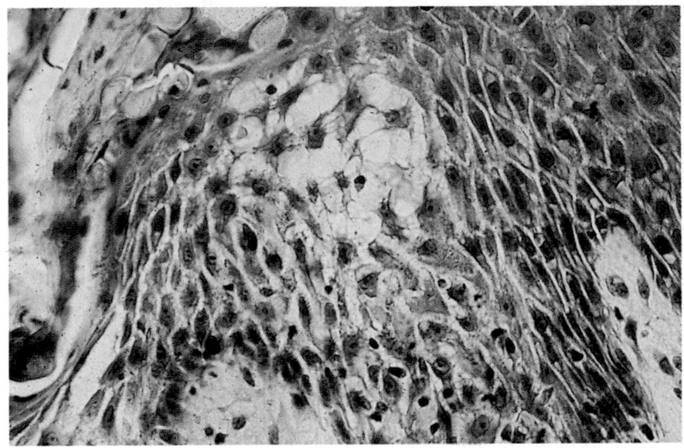

Spongiform vesicle resulting from edematous separation of keratinocytes. These are still partially attached to each other by desmosomes and have thus acquired a stellate appearance.

the cells remain metabolically active (at least for some time) and retain their capacity for DNA synthesis. Degeneration and cell death represent only secondary phenomena. Acantholytic cells can easily be demonstrated in cytologic smears (see Fig. 4-4) and in some conditions have diagnostic significance.

Acantholysis occurs in a number of different pathologic processes that do not have a uniform etiology and pathogenesis. It is important to distinguish between diseases in which acantholysis is the primary event and leads to intraepidermal cavitation (primary acantholysis) and those conditions where epidermal cells are secondarily shed from the walls of established intraepidermal blisters (secondary acantholysis). Primary acantholysis is a pathogenetically relevant event in diseases belonging to the pemphigus group, where it results from the interaction of autoantibodies and antigenic determinants on the keratinocyte membranes (see Fig. 4-5) and is mediated by epidermal proteases (see Chap. 59). This type of acantholysis can also be produced by pemphigus autoantibodies in vitro.

FIGURE 4-4

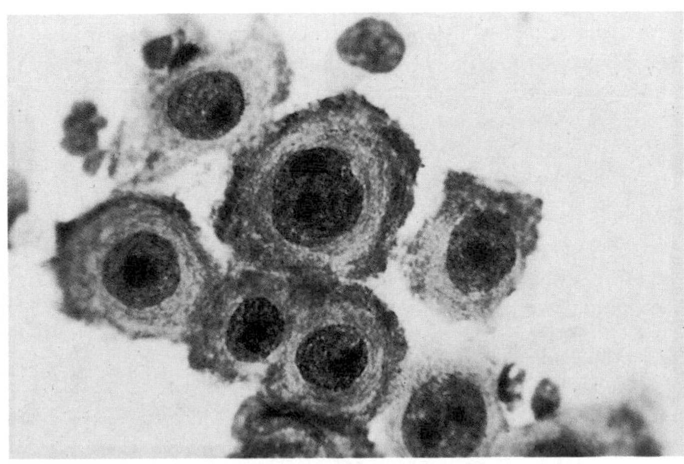

Acantholysis. Single as well as clusters of acantholytic cells are seen. The round shapes result from the loss of intercellular connections. Cytologic smear preparation.

FIGURE 4-5

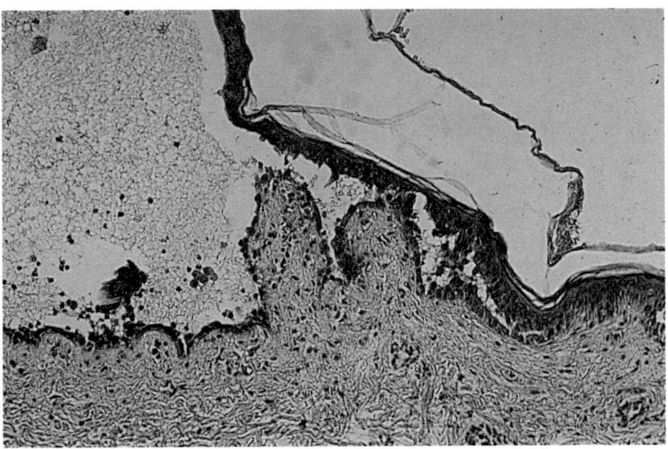

Pemphigus vulgaris. An intraepidermal suprabasal cleft is visible that has resulted from suprabasal acantholysis. It contains acantholytic and inflammatory cells.

Primary acantholysis also occurs in the staphylococcal scalded-skin syndrome, where it is caused by a staphylococcal exotoxin (epidermolysin) that leads to the loss of cohesion of epidermal cells of the subcorneal epidermal layers without impairing cellular integrity (see Chap. 195). Acantholysis in familial benign pemphigus results from the combination of a genetically determined defect of the keratinocyte cell membrane and exogenous factors such as bacterial toxins, trauma, or maceration. In this condition, the loss of intercellular cohesion leads to compensatory development of microvilli on the cell surfaces and an acantholytic separation of cells throughout the whole width of the epidermis (see Chap. 68). A similar phenomenon, albeit more confined to the suprabasal epidermis, occurs in Darier's disease, in which it is combined with dyskeratosis in the upper epidermal layers (see Fig. 4-2) and a compensatory proliferation of basal cells into the papillary body (see Chap. 54). Finally, acantholysis can result from viral infection, but here it is usually combined with other cellular phenomena such as ballooning giant cells and cytolysis (Fig. 4-6) (see Chap. 214).

A loss of epidermal cohesion can result from a dissolution of cells. In the epidermolytic forms of epidermolysis bullosa, basal cells rupture as a result of trauma so that the cleft forms through the basal cell layer independently from preexisting anatomic boundaries (see Chap. 65). Cytolytic phenomena in the stratum granulosum, as are characteristic for epidermolytic hyperkeratosis, result from disturbed differentiation and are the cause of intraepidermal blister formation in bullous congenital ichthyosiform erythroderma, ichthyosis hystrix, and some forms of hereditary palmoplantar hyperkeratosis (see Chaps. 51 and 52).

The Dermal-Epidermal Junction

Epidermis and dermis are interlocked by means of the epidermal rete ridges and the corresponding dermal papillae and footlike cytoplasmic microprocesses of basal cells that extend into corresponding indentations of the dermis. Dermal-epidermal attachment is enforced by hemidesmosomes that anchor basal cells on the basal lamina; this, in turn, is attached to the dermis by means of anchoring filaments and microfibrils (see Chaps. 6, 16, and 65). The basal lamina is not a rigid

FIGURE 4-6

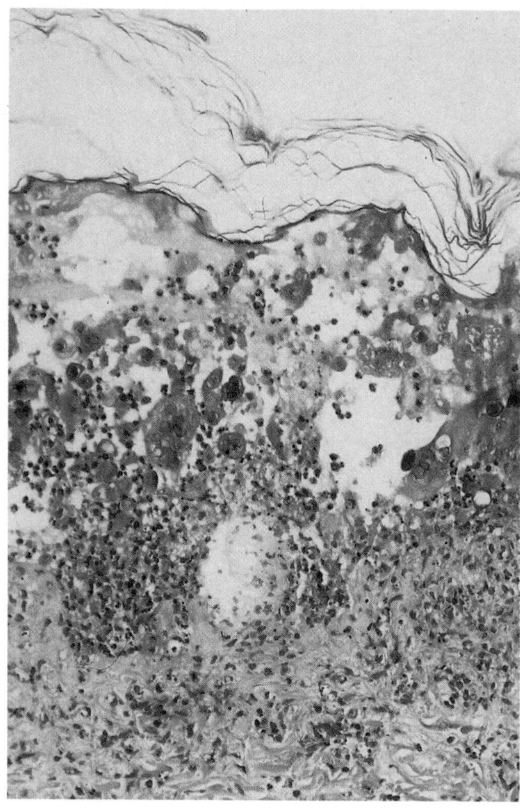

Herpes simplex infection. The epidermis shows marked ballooning degeneration, cytolysis, and intraepidermal vesiculation. Acantholytic and multinucleated epidermal giant cells are a clue to herpetic infection.

structure because leukocytes, Langerhans cells, or other migratory cells pass through it without causing a permanent breach in the junction. After being destroyed by pathologic processes, the basal lamina is reconstituted; this represents an important phenomenon in wound healing and other reparative processes. Functionally, the basal lamina is part of a unit that, by light microscopy, appears as the PAS-positive basal membrane and, in fact, represents the entire junction zone. This consists of the lamina lucida, spanned by anchoring fibrils, and subjacent microfibrils, small collagen fibers, and extracellular matrix (see Chaps. 6, 16, and 65). The junction zone is a functional complex that is primarily affected in a number of pathologic processes.

DISTURBANCES OF DERMAL-EPIDERMAL COHESION The destruction of the junction zone or its components usually manifests as disturbance of dermal-epidermal cohesion and leads to blister formation. These blisters appear to be subepidermal by light microscopy (Fig. 4-7) but in reality may be localized at different levels and result from pathogenetically heterogeneous processes. Subepidermal blister formation can be epidermal (cytolysis of basal cells), as is the case in epidermolysis bullosa simplex (*epidermolytic blistering*) (see Chap. 65). Cytolysis of basal cells can also be the result of a complex inflammatory process that involves the entire junction zone, as is the case in lupus erythematosus, erythema multiforme, or lichen planus; therefore, it may be a phenomenon occurring in a group of etiologically and pathogenetically heterogeneous conditions. In bullous pemphigoid (see Fig. 4-7),

FIGURE 4-7

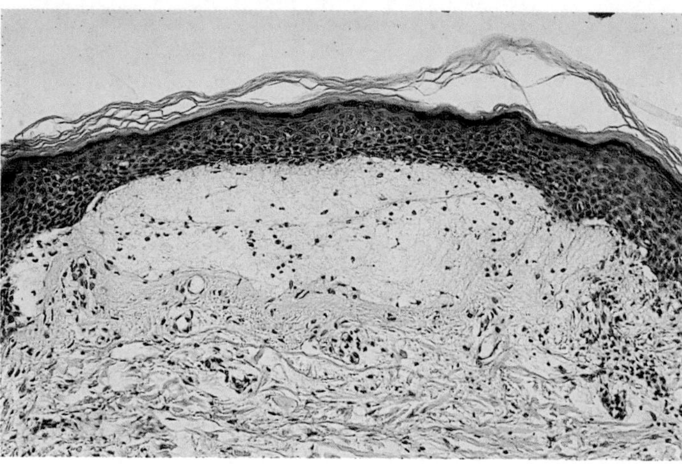

Bullous pemphigoid. Subepidermal (junctional) cleft formation and a perivascular and interstitial lymphoeosinophilic infiltrate are characteristic.

cleft formation runs through the lamina lucida of the basal membrane and is caused by autoantibodies directed against specific antigens on the cytomembrane of basal cells (see Chap. 61). The accompanying inflammation and the hydrodynamic pressure of plasma released from the superficial dermal vessels will eventually lead to a lifting of the basal cells from the basal lamina at the level of injury and thus to blister formation (*junctional blistering*) (see Fig. 4-7). In cicatricial pemphigoid and herpes gestationis, similar mechanisms lead to clefting at the same level, but in the latter there is also destruction of the lamina densa (see Chaps. 62 and 64). Junctional blistering also occurs in the junctional forms of epidermolysis bullosa, but here it is due to the impairment or absence of molecules important for epidermal-dermal cohesion (see Chap. 65) (Table 4-3).

In genuine subepidermal blistering, the target of the pathologic process is below the basal lamina (dermolytic blistering) (see Table 4-3). Reduced anchoring filaments and increased collagenase production result in dermolytic dermal-epidermal separation in recessive epidermolysis bullosa (see Chap. 65); circulating autoantibodies directed against type VII collagen in anchoring fibrils are the cause of dermolytic blistering in acquired epidermolysis bullosa (see Chap. 66). Other immunologically mediated inflammatory mechanisms result in dermolytic blistering in dermatitis herpetiformis (see below and Chap. 67), and physical and chemical changes in the junction zone and papillary body are the cause for a dermolytic cleft formation after trauma in porphyria cutanea tarda (see Chap. 149).

TABLE 4-3

Classification of Blisters at the Dermal-Epidermal Junction by Anatomic Level With Clinical Examples

- Junctional (at the lamina lucida)
  - Junctional epidermolysis bullosa
  - Bullous pemphigoid
- Dermolytic (below basal lamina)
  - Epidermolysis bullosa dystrophicans
  - Epidermolysis bullosa acquisita
  - Porphyria cutanea tarda
  - Dermatitis herpetiformis

Pathologic Reactions of the Entire Superficial Reactive Unit

The papillary body represents a loose connective tissue matrix that supports the epidermis and contains the superficial vascular plexus, the common site of cutaneous inflammatory disease.

As mentioned above, the individual subunits of the superficial reactive unit are only rarely the isolated target of a pathologic process. Examples of isolated reaction patterns are the hyperkeratosis in ichthyosis vulgaris, the hyperproliferative acanthosis, and hyperkeratosis in lamellar ichthyosis. On the other hand, some reaction patterns in the epidermis, such as acantholysis in pemphigus or acantholysis and dyskeratosis in Hailey-Hailey disease, are accompanied by involvement of the superficial papillary dermis. Thus, most pathologic reactions of the superficial skin involve the subunits of the superficial reactive unit jointly. However, the prominence of involvement of one of the components over the other leads to the development of certain clinical pictures. For example, the prominent involvement of the epidermis with hyperplasia leads to psoriatic plaques. Interface dermatitis can result in blister formation as in erythema multiforme. In most cases of bullous diseases dominated by inflammation, different types of inflammatory cells may be characteristic, such as eosinophils in bullous pemphigoid or neutrophils in dermatitis herpetiformis. Interestingly enough, although the transient vasodilatation of urticaria that results in dermal edema and clinical wheal formation affects the dermis predominantly, spongiosis, and even subepidermal blister formation, can occur in severe cases. A few examples of such interactions are detailed below.

CONTACT DERMATITIS (See Chap. 120) In allergic contact dermatitis, there are an inflammatory reaction of the papillary body and superficial microvascular plexus and spongiosis of the epidermis (see Fig. 4-3) with signs of cellular injury and parakeratosis. Lymphocytes infiltrate the epidermis early in the process and aggregate around Langerhans cells, and this is followed by spongiotic vesiculation (Fig. 4-8). Parakeratosis develops as a consequence of epidermal injury, and the inflammation in the papillary body and around the superficial venular plexus stimulates mitotic processes within the epidermis, which, in turn, result in acanthosis and epidermal hyperplasia.

FIGURE 4-8

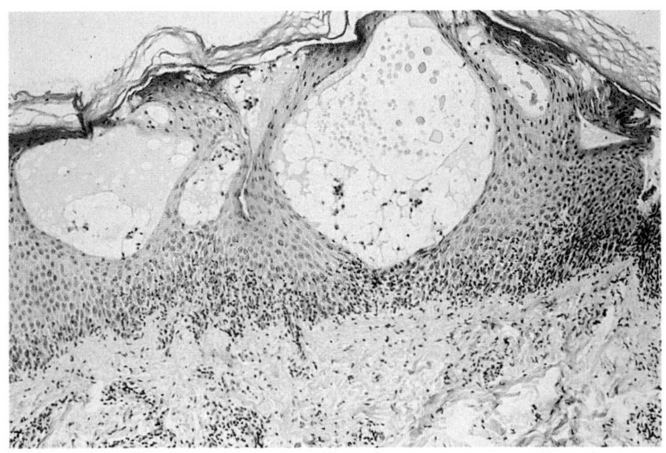

Contact dermatitis. Intraepidermal spongiotic vesicles and pronounced intercellular edema are present in the epidermis. The dermis contains perivascular aggregates of lymphocytes and histiocytes admixed with occasional eosinophils.

PSORIASIS (See Chap. 42) The initial lesion of psoriatic lesions appears to be the perivascular accumulation of lymphocytes and monocytoid elements within the papillary body and superficial venules and focal migration of polymorphonuclear leukocytes into the epidermis. The molecular basis for the sequence of these events is now being clarified. Acanthosis caused by increased epidermal proliferation, papillomatosis, and edema of the elongated dermal papillae together with vasodilatation of the papillary capillary loops and a denser perivascular infiltrate develop almost simultaneously (see Fig. 4-1); the disturbed differentiation of the epidermal cells results in parakeratosis, and neutrophils infiltrating the epithelium from tortuous capillaries (squirting capillaries) lead to spongiform pustules and, in the parakeratotic stratum corneum, to *Munro's abscesses*. It appears that the stimulus for increased epidermal proliferation follows signals released from T cells that are attracted to the epidermis by the expression of adhesion molecules at the keratinocyte surface and are maintained by cytokines released by keratinocytes (see Chap. 42). It is important to note, however, that inflammation of the papillary body and superficial venules, increased epidermal proliferation resulting in acanthosis, disturbance of differentiation leading to parakeratosis, and the infiltration of neutrophils, which, in turn, also disturb the architecture of the epidermis, all result in the composite picture characteristic of psoriasis. The lesion, therefore, results from a combined pathology of the papillary body, superficial venules, the epidermis, and circulating cells.

Psoriasis is a good example of the limited specificity of histopathologic reaction patterns within the skin because psoriasiform histologic features occur in a number of diseases unrelated to psoriasis.

INTERFACE DERMATITIS Inflammation along the dermal-epidermal junction associated with vacuolation characterizes interface dermatitis. This common type of reaction may lead to papules or plaques in some skin diseases and bullae on others.

ERYTHEMA MULTIFORME (See Chap. 58) Two types of reaction occur. In both there is interface dermatitis characterized by lymphocytes scattered along a vacuolated dermal-epidermal junction.

LUPUS ERYTHEMATOSUS (See Chap. 171) Inflammation, edema, and a dense lymphocytic infiltrate in the papillary body and superficial venular plexus, as well as in the deeper layers of the dermis, are a hallmark of this disorder. The main target is the dermal-epidermal junction, where immune complex deposition leads to broadening of the PAS-positive basement membrane zone, accompanied by hydropic degeneration and destruction of basal cells (Fig. 4-9). Scattered inflammatory cells also often appear along the junction. Cytoid bodies result from apoptosis of individual epidermal cells that are infiltrated and coated by immunoglobulins. The changes in the junctional zone reflect on epidermal differentiation resulting in increased orthokeratosis and parakeratosis. Lupus erythematosus readily illustrates the heterogeneity, as well as the lack of specificity, of cutaneous reaction patterns: histologically, it is possible to distinguish between acute and chronic lesions but not between cutaneous and systemic lupus erythematosus. In chronic persisting lesions, the changes in the junctional zone secondarily result in hyperplasia, hyperkeratosis, and an increased interdigitation between epidermis and connective tissue, whereas in acute cases, the destruction of the basal cell layer may lead to subepidermal blistering. Although immune complexes are primarily found within and underneath the basal lamina, blister formation within lupus lesions

FIGURE 4-9

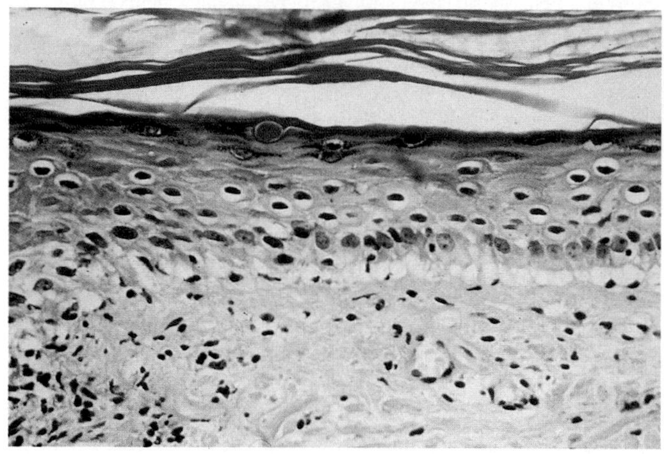

Lupus erythematosus. Hyperkeratosis, thinned epidermis devoid of rete ridges, and vacuolization of the basement membrane zone are present.

occurs above the lamina densa; this is in contrast to the situation in the syndrome of "bullous eruptions in lupus erythematosus" in which blister formation is due to collagen type VII autoantibodies and occurs in the dermis.

LICHEN PLANUS (See Chap. 49) This disease also exhibits a primarily junctional reaction pattern with accumulation of a dense lymphocytic infiltrate in the subepidermal tissue and cytoid bodies at the junction (Fig. 4-10). Lymphocytes encroach upon the epidermis, destroying the basal cells, but they do not infiltrate the suprabasal layers and blister formation only rarely ensues. The destruction of the junctional zone is compensated by a repopulation of the germinative epidermal cell layers through lateral migration from the periphery of the lesion; these alterations are accompanied by changes of epidermal differentiation—there is a widening of the stratum granulosum (*hypergranulosis*) and hyperkeratosis. Identical changes can be seen in graft-versus-host disease (see Chap. 118).

FIGURE 4-10

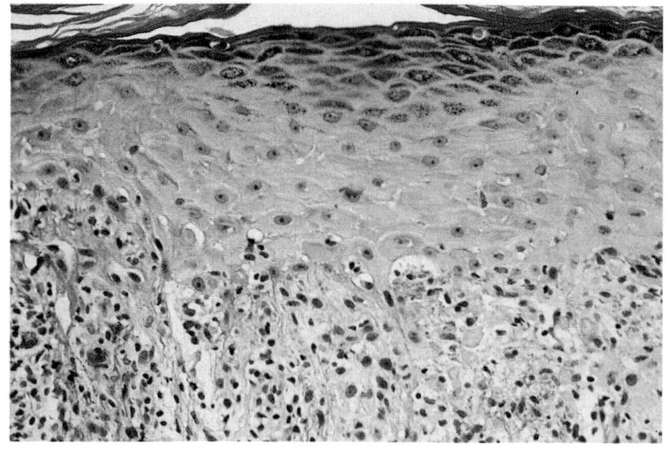

Lichen planus. There is hyperkeratosis, wedge-shaped hypergranulosis, basal cell vacuolization, and a lymphocytic infiltrate at the dermal-epidermal junction. This infiltrate "hugs" the basal cell layer and is associated with many cytoid bodies.

FIGURE 4-11

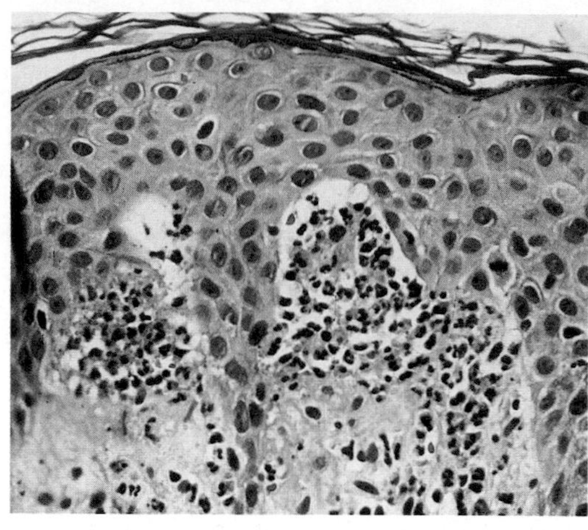

Dermatitis herpetiformis. Two papillae show microabscesses composed of neutrophils. Vacuolization and early cleft formation are evident in both papillae.

DERMATITIS HERPETIFORMIS (See Chap. 67) This condition is usually included among the classic bullous dermatoses; however, it illustrates that the preponderance of one or several pathologic reaction patterns may obscure the true pathogenesis of the condition. The deposition of IgA and complement or fibrillar and nonfibrillar sites within the tips of the dermal papillae represents the primary pathogenic phenomenon. Probably through the activation of the alternative pathway of the complement cascade, there is an influx of leukocytes, which form small abscesses at the tips of the dermal papillae, as well as inflammation and edema (Fig. 4-11). This explains why the primary lesion in dermatitis herpetiformis is urticarial or papular in nature, because only in the case of massive neutrophil infiltration will there be tissue destruction and cleft formation below the lamina densa that results in clinically visible vesiculation.

THE DERMIS

The dermis represents a strong fibroelastic tissue with a network of collagen and elastic fibers embedded in an extracellular matrix with a high water-binding capacity (see Chaps. 6 and 14). In contrast to the tightly interwoven fibrous components of the reticular layer of the dermis, the fibrous texture of the papillary body and the perifollicular and perivascular compartments is loose, and the orientation of the collagen bundles here follows the structures they surround.

The dermis contains vascular networks situated parallel to the skin surface at various levels and connected by vertical communicating vessels. In the upper dermis, they form the superficial plexus that supplies individual vascular districts consisting of several dermal papillae. Superficial and deep networks are connected so intimately that the entire dermal vascular system represents a single three-dimensional unit consisting of vessels of different sizes and dimensions (see Chap. 19). Vascular reaction patterns of the skin should therefore not be viewed too schematically because the vessels are not as regular and geometrically arranged as may appear from schematic drawings. On the other hand, there are profound functional differences between superficial and deep

FIGURE 4-12

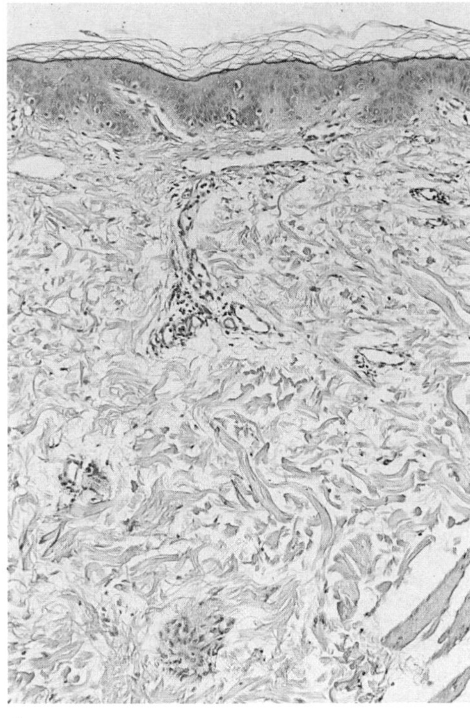

A.

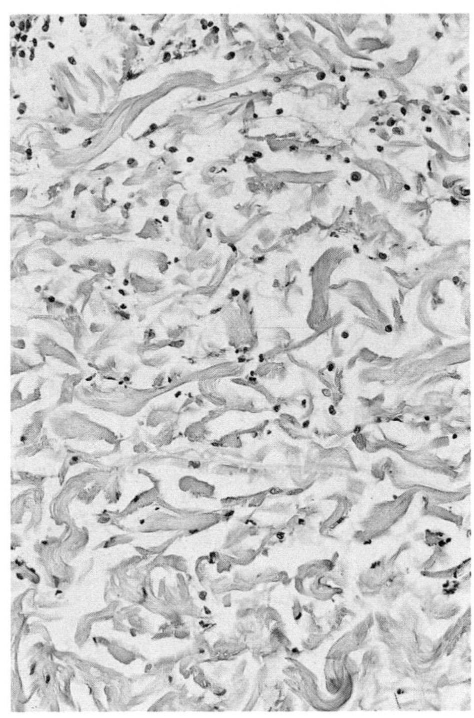

B.

Urticaria. *A.* Characteristic of this reaction is a sparse, perivascular lymphocytic infiltrate with few eosinophils. Note the slight edema in the dermis and around the postcapillary venules. *B.* Higher magnification reveals separation of collagen bundles by edema and sparse interstitial inflammatory infiltrate with eosinophils.

dermal vascular networks, which explains the differences of homing patterns of inflammatory cells to these sites. The architecture of the vascular system is subject to regional modifications because it also depends on the thickness of the subcutaneous fat, which varies from one region to another. Blood vessels and the surrounding loose periadventitial connective tissue represent reaction units embedded three-dimensionally in the connective tissue matrix.

The papillary body with its capillaries and superficial venular plexus represents one functional unit of the dermis. It reacts rather uniformly to a wide spectrum of stimuli, and in a large number of dermatoses it represents the primary target tissue. However, as stated above, the close anatomic and functional relationship to the junctional zone and the epidermis explains why this tissue is affected only rarely in an isolated fashion. Principally, two reaction patterns occur: (1) acute inflammatory processes in which the epidermis and junctional zone are often involved together with the vascular system, and (2) more chronic processes that often remain confined to the perivascular compartment. In this context, it should be noted that the cytologic composition of an inflammatory infiltrate within the skin does not always mirror the acuity of an inflammatory process. Polymorphonuclear leukocytic infiltrates are not always synonymous with an acute process; conversely, chronic processes are not always represented by a lymphohistiocytic infiltrate.

Inflammation confined to the superficial connective tissue–vascular unit is characterized by vascular dilatation, increased permeability, edema, a reduction of intravascular blood flow, and accumulation of red blood cells in the capillary loops. Also, cellular infiltration of the perivascular tissue and an activation of preexisting perivascular histiocytic and connective tissue cells occur. Depending on the degree of vasodilatation, edema, and cellular infiltration, the macroscopic corollary of the histologic changes represents erythematous, urticarial, and infiltrative lesions (wheals, redness, papules). The release of mediators from IgE-laden mast cells in type I immune reactions is histologically manifested primarily as vasodilatation, edema of the papillary body, and a rather sparse infiltrate of leukocytes and histiocytic elements around the superficial venules (Fig. 4-12). These lesions usually resolve relatively rapidly without any residual pathology. The most characteristic example of this type of inflammation is urticaria. More massive reactions, however, lead to a dense perivascular infiltrate (Fig. 4-13*A*), and this may represent a transition to those processes where edema is less pronounced and where dense lymphocytic infiltrates surround the vessels in a sleevelike fashion, as is the case in some cutaneous drug eruptions (Fig. 4-13*B*). More dramatic alterations occur when the vascular system itself is the target of the inflammatory process, which results in a destruction of the vascular channels with all its sequelae, as is the case in necrotizing vasculitis (Fig. 4-14).

Pathologic Reactions of the Dermal Vasculature

Cutaneous necrotizing vasculitis (see Chap. 175) is an inflammatory process that involves vessels of all sizes and, depending on the caliber of vessel and the type of inflammatory reaction, it may lead to clinically and histopathologically different disease patterns. The sequence of pathologic events in vasculitis is best illustrated in necrotizing venulitis of the superficial dermal plexus, where fibrillar and amorphous eosinophilic material is deposited within the vessel wall, which is infiltrated by polymorphonuclear leukocytes and becomes anuclear and necrotic. As leukocytoclasia occurs, nuclear dust is found both within the vessels and in the tissue surrounding the vascular channels. Red blood cells and plasma appear within the perivascular tissue, and these changes give the histologic impression of an "exploded vessel" (see Fig. 4-14). Later, there will also be lymphocytes and histiocytic cells as the tissue damage is repaired. Infiltration of the vascular wall by circulating

FIGURE 4-13

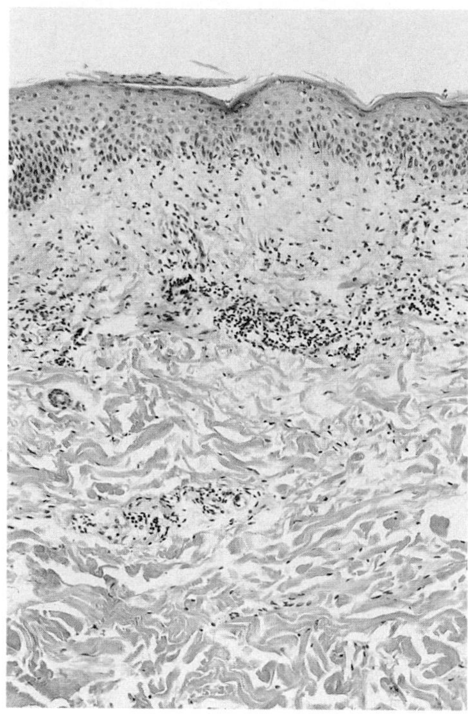

A.

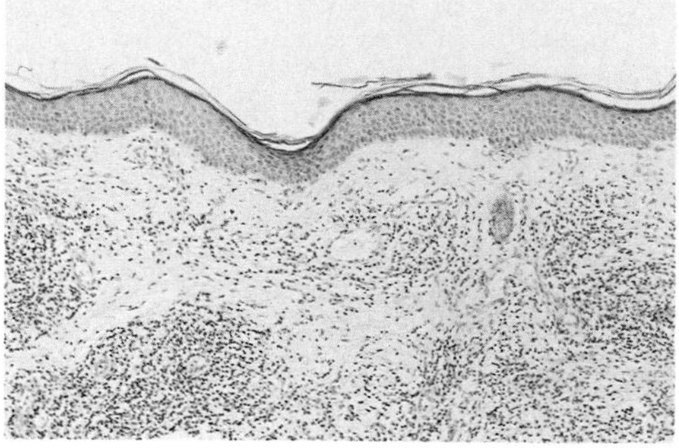

B.

Drug eruption. *A.* Throughout the dermis, perivascular sleeves of mononuclear cells, mainly lymphocytes, are present about superficial and deep venules. There is slight edema in the papillary body and minimal interface dermatitis in this reaction to nifedipine. *B.* More pronounced, even nodular, mononuclear cell infiltrates around vessels in a drug reaction to a beta-blocker.

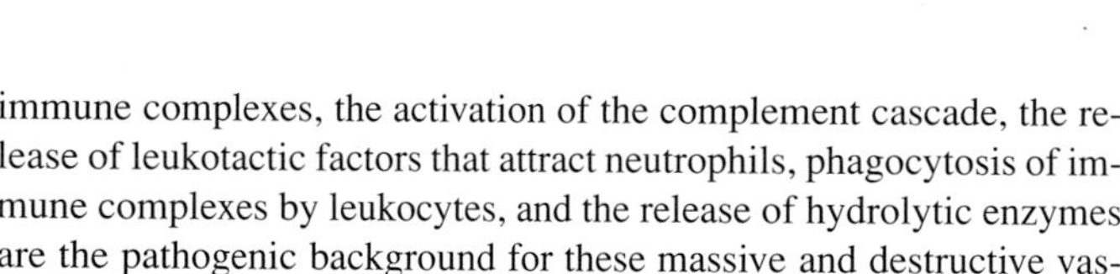

immune complexes, the activation of the complement cascade, the release of leukotactic factors that attract neutrophils, phagocytosis of immune complexes by leukocytes, and the release of hydrolytic enzymes are the pathogenic background for these massive and destructive vascular changes.

Chronic inflammatory reactions of the superficial plexus usually reveal lymphocytic infiltrates in close association with the vascular walls. An example is the superficial erythema occurring with the lymphocytic infiltrates. Also, in purpura simplex (see Chap. 176), damage to the vessel wall is much less evident than in necrotizing vasculitis, but the integrity of the vessels is also impaired as is evidenced by hemorrhage into the tissue. Lymphocytes and, as a secondary reaction, histiocytic elements partly laden with phagocytosed material constitute the inflammatory infiltrate.

FIGURE 4-14

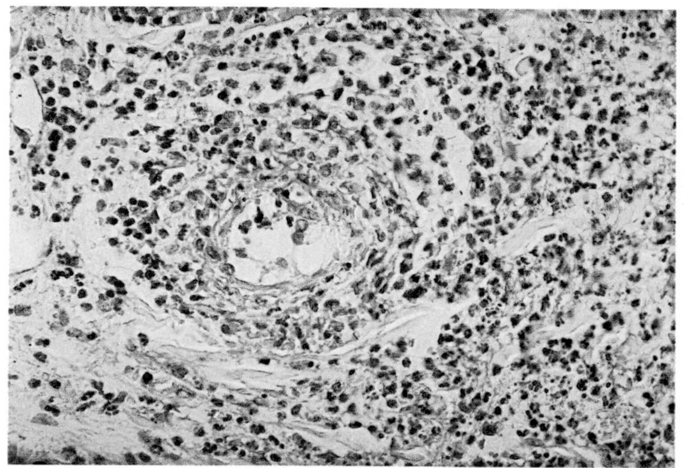

Necrotizing vasculitis. An inflammatory infiltrate composed mostly of neutrophils and nuclear dust is present both around and in the wall of a venule where fibrin is also deposited.

The superficial venules can also be the target of cytolytic processes, with inflammation playing only a secondary role. In erythropoietic protoporphyria (see Chap. 149), endothelial cells are lysed by the phototoxic reaction; plasma, red blood cells, and cellular debris are deposited in the perivascular tissue, causing a massive inflammatory reaction. It is not known whether circulating protoporphyrins sensitize endothelial cells, which are then directly destroyed by a phototoxic reaction, or whether the phototoxic reaction is mediated by the complement system, which has been shown to be activated by porphyrins and light. Regenerating endothelial cells, which use the basal lamina of the destroyed vessel as scaffold, produce new basal lamina material so that after multiple consecutive phototoxic reactions, concentrically arranged basal laminae surround the vascular channels. This basal lamina material and serum proteins that are deposited around the vessels represent the submicroscopic substrate of the massive perivascular hyalinization that is so characteristic of this disease.

The reaction patterns described for the vascular system of the papillary body and the superficial venular plexus also occur in the deep dermis, but there are morphologic and functional differences because here larger vessels are involved. Lymphocytic infiltrates surrounding the vessels in a sleevelike fashion lead to clinical signs only when they are substantial, and then they represent the histopathologic substrate for papular or nodular lesions. This is the case with drug eruptions (see Chap. 138 and Fig. 4-13*B*) and it is also true for deep-seated infiltrates in lupus erythematosus. In the case of necrotizing vasculitis of the medium-sized and larger vessels, there is usually a much more pronounced inflammatory infiltrate, clinically appearing as papular and nodular lesions. Secondary changes due to the interruption of the vascular flow are more pronounced; there may be necrosis and blistering as well as ulceration. Such reactions occur in cutaneous panarteritis nodosa (see Chap. 174), where a total or partial necrosis of the vascular wall is followed by a massive inflammatory reaction, intravascular thrombosis, and hemorrhage. Granulomatous vasculitis also leads to nodular lesions, whereas the hyalinizing vascular changes and vascular occlusion in livedoid vasculitis result in ischemic necrosis (see Chap. 167).

Lymphocytic Infiltrates

Although lymphocytic infiltrates occur in the majority of inflammatory dermatoses, there are a number of pathologic processes in which such infiltrates are the most prominent feature and thus determine the histologic picture. The analysis of these infiltrates is one of the more difficult areas of cutaneous pathology. Lymphocytic infiltrates are formed in inflammatory or proliferative conditions and in the latter may represent a benign or malignant process. They may differ in their cytologic appearance and distribution, may be confined to the periadventitial compartments of the vascular system, or may occur diffusely throughout the collagenous tissue. They may be confined almost exclusively to the reticular dermis and spare the subepidermal compartment or may exhibit pronounced epidermotropism. Because lymphocytes are a heterogeneous population of cells, the analysis of such infiltrates should take into account not only the cytomorphology and distribution pattern but also histochemical properties and immunologic markers. The analysis of round cell infiltrates by monoclonal antibodies (immunophenotyping) and determination of their clonality are at present some of the most important aspects of dermatopathology (see Chaps. 157, 158, and 159).

The distribution pattern of lymphocytic infiltrates can be perivascular, diffuse, or nodular. With superficial localization, secondary involvement of the epidermis may occur and may be of importance: circumscribed parakeratosis occurs, for instance, in the figurate erythemas; pronounced acanthosis often follows inflammatory reactions following insect bites; and massive epidermotropism of lymphocytes occurs in cutaneous T cell lymphoma (see Chap. 157). Vascular involvement, such as hyperplasia of the vessel walls in angiolymphoid hyperplasia (Fig. 4-15), or vasculitis, as in lymphomatoid papulosis, is as important a diagnostic feature as is the involvement of collagen and ground substance by the myxoid changes in lupus erythematosus (Fig. 4-16), lymphocytic infiltration of Jessner-Kanof, and reticular erythematous mucinosis. Extension of the infiltrate into the fat is often a sign of a malignant lymphoma, and the development of lymphoid follicles may either indicate a lymphocytoma or be a sign of centrocytic or centroblastic lymphoma (see Chap. 158). Cytologic examination must include careful determination of whether an infiltrate is monomorphous or polymorphous. In polymorphic infiltrations, the nature of individual cells, such as eosinophils, histiocytes, or other cells, is of importance, as is the consideration of secondary alterations, such as hemorrhage and phagocytosis of cells or cell debris, melanin, or fat, by histiocytic or other mononuclear cells.

FIGURE 4-15

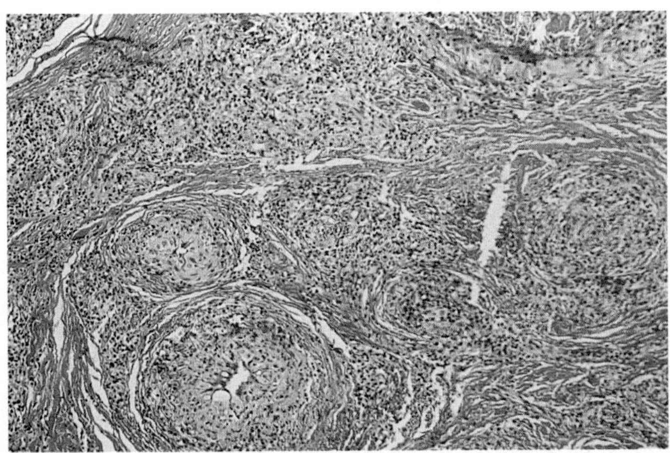

Angiolymphoid hyperplasia. Numerous vascular channels are surrounded by aggregates of inflammatory cells made up of lymphocytes and eosinophils. Note the protrusion of endothelial cells into the lamina of these vessels.

FIGURE 4-16

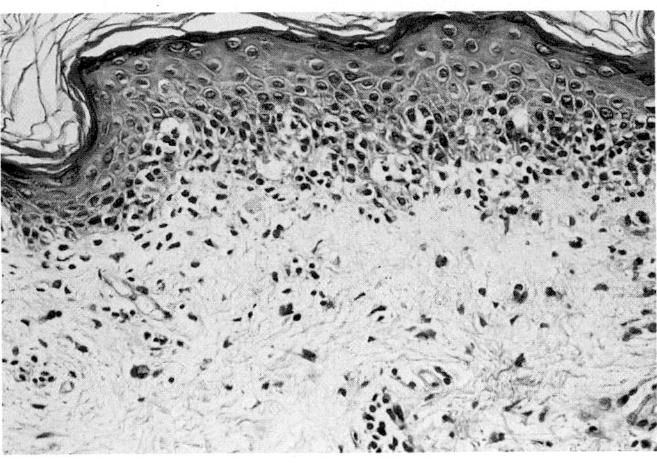

Mucinosis in lupus erythematosus. All the histologic features of lupus erythematosus are illustrated in this photomicrograph (see also Fig. 4-9). Another feature shown is abundant mucin in the superficial dermis, resulting in widely separated collagen bundles.

Among the many possible reaction patterns characterized by lymphocytic infiltrates, several typical patterns can be distinguished.

1. Superficial perivascular infiltrates involve the papillary body and superficial venular plexus and are often accompanied by secondary reactions of the epidermis. Lymphoid cells surround the vascular channels in a sleevelike fashion but often extend diffusely to the epidermis, which may reveal focal parakeratosis in these areas. Clinically, these changes are often characterized as palpable figurate erythemas such as erythema annulare centrifugum, but polymorphic light eruption, drug eruptions (see Fig. 4-13*A*), or insect bites can produce a similar histopathologic picture.

2. Lymphocytic cuffing of venules without involvement of the papillary body and the epidermis may occur in figurate erythemas but also in drug eruptions (see Fig. 4-13*B*). The infiltrates of chronic lymphatic leukemia show a similar distribution pattern but are usually more pronounced.

3. Perivascular lymphocytic infiltrates with a mucinous infiltration of the nonperivascular connective tissue may be found in lymphocytic infiltration of Jessner-Kanof, reticular erythematous mucinosis, or in lupus erythematosus (see Fig. 4-16) and dermatomyositis. In the latter, it may be accompanied by the epidermal changes discussed above and similar alterations in the hair follicles.

4. Nodular lymphocytic infiltrates, which extend throughout the dermis exhibiting focal accumulations of histiocytic cells and thus acquiring the appearance of lymphoid follicles, are typical of lymphocytoma cutis (see Chaps. 159 and 203). Phagocytosed polychrome bodies in histiocytic cells, mitoses in the center of these infiltrates, and an admixture of eosinophils are characteristic features, as is the fact that the papillary body is usually spared so that a conspicuous Grenz zone is found between the infiltrate and the epidermis.

5. Nonfollicular lymphocytic infiltrates sparing the superficial reactive unit may also occur in benign lymphoid hyperplasias, but in these cases, the differentiation from malignant lymphoma is very difficult.

Polymorphic infiltrates showing histiocytes, plasma cells, and occasional eosinophils are usually benign, whereas most malignant non-Hodgkin's lymphomas exhibit a more monomorphous picture.

6. Nodular accumulations of lymphocytes with an admixture of plasma cells and eosinophils accompanied by vascular hyperplasia are characteristic of angiolymphoid hyperplasia (see Fig. 4-15), in which blood vessel walls are thickened and the endothelial cells appear proliferated, swollen, and enlarged. Clinical manifestations also depend on the type and extent of the histopathologic substrate. Involvement of the deep dermis may lead to the inclusion of the subcutaneous tissue into the pathologic process and may thus be manifest clinically as diffuse swelling resembling cellulitis; identical infiltrates and vascular changes confined to the upper dermis clinically lead to well-defined papular and nodular lesions.

7. Atypical lymphocytic infiltrates involving both the superficial and deeper dermis, and cytologically characterized by pronounced pleomorphism of the cellular infiltrate, are characteristic of lymphomatoid papulosis (see Chap. 159). This pseudolymphoma exemplifies the problems that arise when the histopathology of a lesion is used alone to determine whether a process is benign or malignant. Without knowledge of the clinical features and the course of disease, a definite diagnosis is extremely difficult.

Polymorphonuclear Leukocytic Infiltrates

Although neutrophils are the classic inflammatory cells of acute bacterial infections, there are diseases in which neutrophils dominate the histopathology, even in the absence of a bacterial cause. In pyoderma gangrenosum, massive neutrophilic infiltration leads to sterile abscesses, breakdown of the tissue, and ulceration (see Chap. 98). In dermatitis herpetiformis, neutrophils accumulate in the tips of dermal papillae and form papillary abscesses (see Fig. 4-11) that precede the dermolytic blister formation described earlier in this chapter (see also Chap. 67). In erythema elevatum diutinum, neutrophils are the predominant cells centering around superficial and mid-dermal vessels, which exhibit fibrinoid homogenization of their walls (toxic hyalin) and signs of vasculitis (see Chap. 95). The neutrophil is also the predominant cell in the early stages of the more common necrotizing vasculitis (see Fig. 4-14). Neutrophils also represent the majority of the often massive inflammatory infiltrate in acute febrile neutrophilic dermatosis, which is accompanied by pronounced subepidermal edema (see Chap. 94).

Granulomatous Reactions

Skin is an ideal tissue for granuloma formation in which histiocytes play a key role. Although these cells are involved at one time or another in practically all inflammatory processes, it is only the proliferation and focal aggregation of histiocytic cells that may be termed a *granuloma*. When such cells are closely clustered they resemble epithelial tissue, hence the designation *epithelioid cells*. Development of giant cells, storage of phagocytosed material, and the admixture of inflammatory cells such as lymphocytes, plasma cells, and eosinophils may render the histologic picture of a granulomatous reaction more complex. To these have to be added vascular changes and alterations in the fibrous structure of the connective tissue. Granulomas almost always lead to destruction of preexisting tissue, particularly elastic fibers, and in such instances result in atrophy, fibrosis, or scarring. Tissue damage or destruction manifests either as necrobiosis or fibrinoid or caseous necrosis, or it may result from liquefaction and abscess formation or from replacement of preexisting tissue by the histiocytic infiltrate and fibrosis.

Granulomatous reactions of the skin comprise a large spectrum of histopathologic features. Palisading granulomas surround necrobiotic areas of the connective tissue with histiocytes in radial alignment (Fig. 4-17). Granuloma annulare, necrobiosis lipoidica, rheumatoid nodules, and the juxtaarticular nodules of syphilis belong to this group. Necrosis can also develop within the granuloma proper, as is the case for fibrinoid necrosis in sarcoidosis, caseation in tuberculosis, or the necrosis developing in mycotic granulomas.

FIGURE 4-17

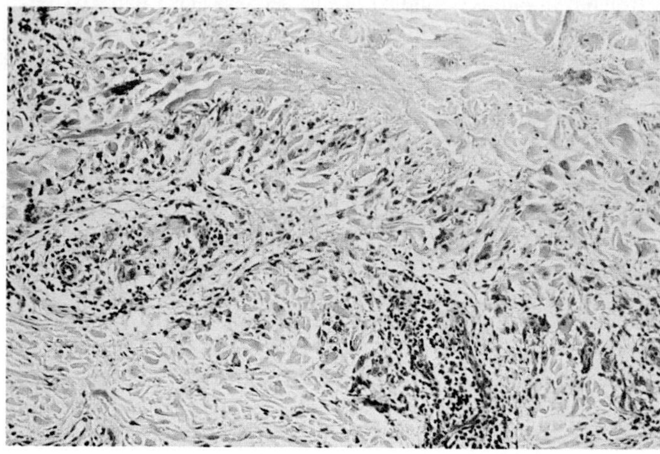

Granuloma annulare. A well-circumscribed palisading granuloma is seen in the dermis. The necrobiotic collagen shown on top is surrounded by histiocytes, lymphocytes, and a few scattered multinucleated giant cells.

Sarcoidal granulomas are typically characterized by naked nodules consisting of epithelioid cells, occasional Langhans' giant cells, and only a small number of lymphocytes (Fig. 4-18). In larger infiltrates, there is often fibrinoid necrosis in the center, the elastic fibers are destroyed, and healing results in atrophy. Silica, zirconium, and beryllium granulomas and a number of foreign-body granulomas may have similar histopathologic features. Consequently, the diagnosis of sarcoidosis should never be made from the histologic appearance of a skin lesion alone; instead, the diagnosis must rely on a combination of the clinical and histopathologic manifestations, the state of cellular immunity, and other symptoms (see Chap. 183). Infectious granulomas with a sarcoidal appearance may occur in tuberculosis, syphilis, leishmaniasis, Hansen's disease, or fungal infections. It is often difficult to classify

FIGURE 4-18

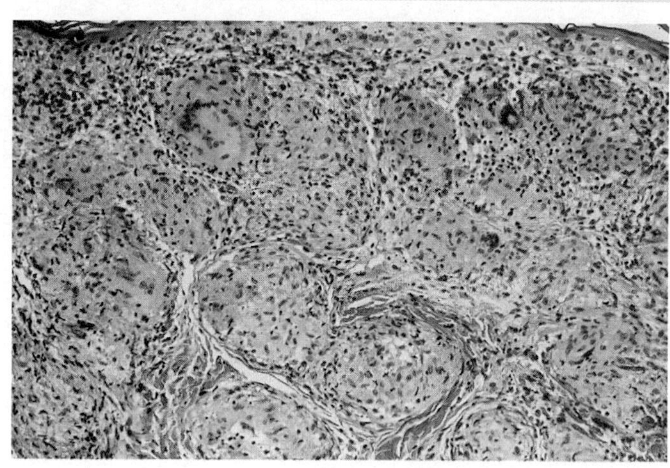

Sarcoidal granuloma. In the dermis numerous "naked" tubercles consisting of epithelioid cells and scant lymphocytes are seen. The overlying epidermis is atrophic.

granulomatous reactions within the skin by the histopathology alone, for even completely different etiologic conditions such as immunopathies and some forms of vasculitis may develop granulomas.

Granulomatous reactions may either extend into the subcutaneous fat or include the superficial reactive unit. In the latter, there is a concomitant reaction of the epidermis, which responds with acanthosis or pseudoepitheliomatous hyperplasia with hyperkeratosis and intraepithelial neutrophilic abscesses, as in bromoderma, or blastomycosis.

A specific form of granulomatous reaction results when the cellular infiltrate consists almost exclusively of the key granuloma cell, the transformed monocyte, commonly referred to as a *histiocyte*. One property of this cell is its capacity to store phagocytosed material. In xanthomatous reaction patterns, histiocytes take up and store fat and are thus transformed into foam cells. They are distributed either diffusely within the dermis with the infiltrate between the collagen bundles, as is the case in diffuse normolipemic xanthomatosis, or as an aggregate infiltrate mimicking a tumor, as is present in the xanthomas occurring in the hyperlipoproteinemias and xanthelasma (see Chap. 150). Less pronounced phagocytosis of fat and giant cells is found in juvenile xanthogranuloma (see Chap. 161); this is mainly located in the upper portions of the reticular dermis and the papillary body and may also acquire a more polymorphous appearance by the admixture of lymphocytes and eosinophils and secondary acanthotic elongations of the rete ridges extending into the granuloma.

An entirely different condition with granulomatous features, in which epidermotropism of histiocytes is a diagnostic sign, is histiocytosis X, or Langerhans cell histiocytosis (see Chap. 160). Depending on the stage and the clinical type, the infiltrate may be predominantly histiocytic or mixed with eosinophils. It may be characterized by phagocytosis of finely dispersed lipid within the histiocytes. Common to all forms is the involvement of the epidermis, into which histiocytic and monocytic cells migrate, which may thus be included in the pathologic process with practically all the reaction patterns it can muster: spongiosis, acanthosis, parakeratosis, spongiotic vesiculation, subepidermal blistering, and necrosis. The identity of histiocytosis X cells with Langerhans cells explains the epidermotropism of the infiltrate in this syndrome.

Reactive proliferative processes of the histiocytic system of the skin include dermatofibroma (Fig. 4-19). There is evidence in some cases that these histiocytic nodules represent a response to insect bites. When dermatofibromas extend into the deep dermis, they may involve the superficial fat by inducing fibrosis; a superficial location involving the papillary body induces a reactive response of the epidermis. Acanthosis, proliferation of the rete ridges, and a pseudobasal cell carcinoma type of epidermal hyperplasia accompany such processes (see Chap. 102).

FIGURE 4-19

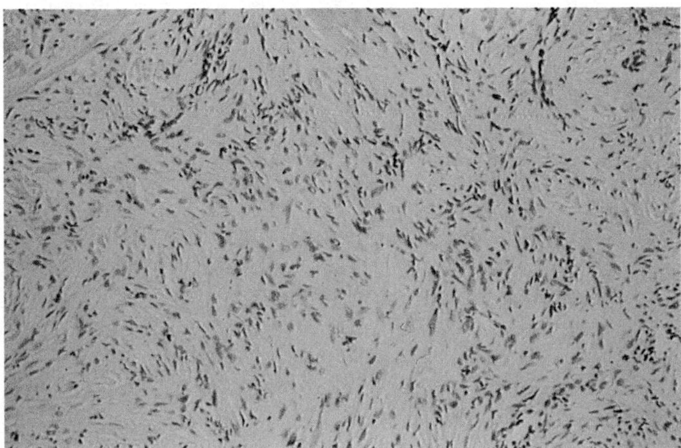

Dermatofibroma. The dermis exhibits spindle cell proliferations that wrap around thickened collagen bundles.

The Fibrous Dermis and Extracellular Matrix

Sclerosing processes of the skin usually reflect dynamic changes of structure and function that involve practically all compartments of this organ. The hallmark of scleroderma (see Chap. 173) is the homogenization and dense packing of the collagen bundles, a narrowing of the interfascicular clefts within the reticular dermis, and the disappearance of the boundary between this portion of the dermis and the papillary body. There is also a diminution of the small papillary and subpapillary vessels, which appear narrowed, and, in the early stages, a perivascular lymphocytic infiltrate and edema of the tissue are constant histopathologic phenomena (Fig. 4-20). The impressive thickening of the dermis not only results from an increase of its fibrous components but is also caused by the fibrosis of the superficial layers of the subcutaneous fat that follows lymphocytic infiltration and a histiocytic reaction.

Sclerodermoid changes may be found in the toxic oil syndrome and L-tryptophan disease, eosinophilic fasciitis (see Chap. 173), and mixed connective tissue disease; they also occur in pachydermoperiostosis, where an increase of fibroblasts and ground substance accompany the sclerotic changes, and in porphyria cutanea tarda, which does not involve the subcutaneous fat and shows typical hyalinization of the papillary vessels. In lichen sclerosus et atrophicus, there is a massive edema of the papillary body and a dense lymphocytic infiltrate that

FIGURE 4-20

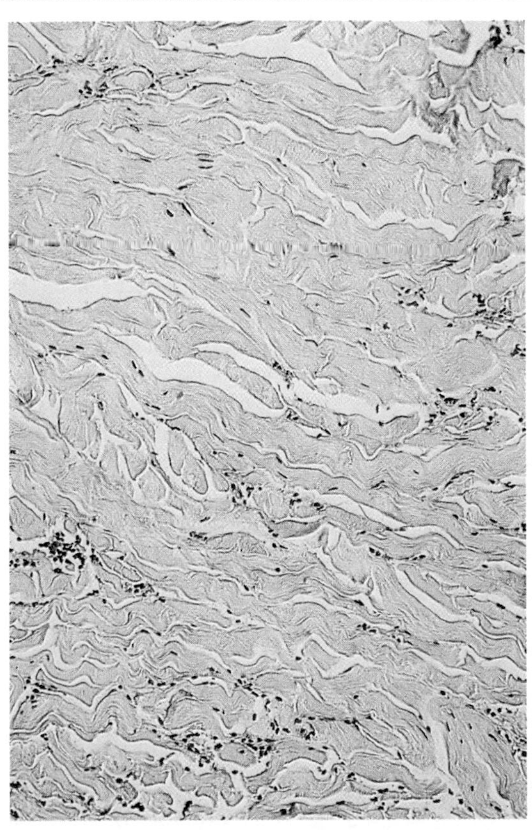

Scleroderma. Extensive homogenization and dense packing of the collagen bundles are seen in the dermis and extending to the subcutis. A sparse inflammatory cell infiltrate is present.

initially hugs the epidermis and later separates the edematous papillary body from the reticular dermis (see Chaps. 113 and 114). As sclerosis sets in, there is also a disappearance of elastic tissue from the papillary body; the concomitant involvement of the epidermis includes hydropic degeneration of basal cells, atrophy, and, at the same time, hyperkeratosis. Changes in the junctional zone in this condition may occasionally lead to a separation of the epidermis from the dermis and thus to blister formation.

Faulty synthesis or cross-linking of collagen results in a number of well-defined diseases or syndromes but leads to relatively few characteristic histopathologic changes. In the different types of the Ehlers-Danlos syndrome (see Chap. 154), the faulty collagen cannot be recognized histopathologically, and only the relative increase of elastic tissue may indicate that something abnormal has occurred in the dermis. On the other hand, pathologic changes of the elastic tissue can be recognized more easily either because elastic fibers have lost their characteristic staining properties or because they appear different with special staining techniques. In generalized elastolysis, a fragmentation of elastic fibers is the histopathologic substrate of the clinical appearance of cutis laxa, and the fragmentation and curled and clumped appearance of elastic fibers are similarly diagnostic in pseudoxanthoma elasticum (see Chap. 154). On the other hand, in actinic elastosis, the histologic substrate of dermatoheliosis, all components of the superficial connective tissue are involved (see Chap. 134). The papillary body, except for a narrow Grenz zone between it and the epidermis, and the superficial layers of the reticular dermis are filled with clumped and curled fibers that progressively become homogenized and basophilic. They are stained by dyes that have an affinity for elastic tissue and thus histochemically behave like elastic fibers; however, there is no doubt that collagen is also involved in this process.

It is not surprising that such profound changes of skin architecture are clinically apparent: the taut and firm connective tissue in scleroderma reflects the sclerotic texture and homogenization of the collagen bundles seen histologically; the loose folds of cutis laxa are a result of the fragmentation of elastic fibers; the cobblestone-like papules in pseudoxanthoma elasticum correspond to the focal aggregation of the pathologically altered elastic material; and the coarseness of skin lines and surface profile in dermatoheliosis are the clinical manifestations of the focal aggregation of elastotic material.

Changes in the extracellular matrix may occur in practically all pathologic processes of an inflammatory or a neoplastic nature. Pronounced accumulation of glycosaminoglycans occurs in inflammatory conditions such as lupus erythematosus, dermatomyositis, or granuloma annulare. In other diseases such as pretibial myxedema and scleredema adultorum (see Chaps. 169 and 186), the accumulation of mucin-like material within the ground substance is the leading alteration. In scleromyxedema (see Chap. 187), similar changes may occur, but a proliferation of fibroblasts may dominate the picture and this is also reflected by the clinical appearance of the skin, which is thickened and hardened.

SUBCUTANEOUS FAT

Inflammatory processes in the subcutaneous adipose tissue take a slightly different course than in the connective tissue of the dermis because of the specific anatomy of the subcutis (see Chaps. 6 and 109). Inflammation of subcutaneous fat reflects either an inflammatory process of the adipose tissue proper or a process arising in the septa; it can involve small venules and capillaries or arise from the larger muscular vessels. The histopathologic manifestations may vary accordingly. Small-vessel pathology is usually manifested locally, involving the neighboring fat lobules, while the destruction or occlusion of a larger vessel will influence the entire tissue segment supplied or drained by this vessel, possibly including even the overlying dermis. Destruction of fat, be it of a traumatic or inflammatory nature, leads to the release of fatty acids that by themselves are strong inflammatory stimuli, attracting neutrophils and scavenger histiocytes and macrophages; phagocytosis of destroyed fat usually results in lipogranuloma formation.

Septal processes that follow inflammatory changes of the trabecular vessels are usually accompanied by massive edema, infiltration of inflammatory cells, and a histiocytic reaction. This is the classic appearance in erythema nodosum (Fig. 4-21); recurring septal inflammation may lead to a broadening of the interlobular septa, fibrosis, and the accumulation of histiocytes and giant cells and may result in vascular proliferation. By contrast, in nodular vasculitis (Fig. 4-22), large-vessel vasculitis in the septal area is accompanied by necrosis of the fat, followed by massive histiocytic reactions and epithelioid cell granulomas within the fat lobules, which often result in a massive fibrotic reaction

FIGURE 4-21

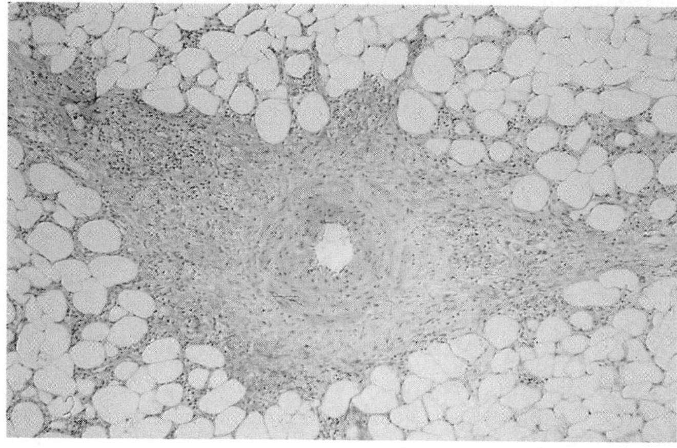

Erythema nodosum. A chronic granulomatous inflammatory infiltrate extends from a septal vessel along the thickened septum into the adjacent fat lobule.

FIGURE 4-22

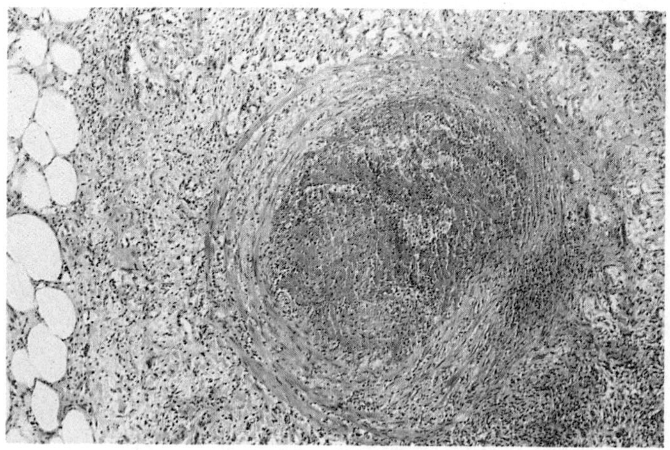

Nodular vasculitis. The characteristic features illustrated are severe vasculitis with necrosis of the large vessel wall and occlusion of the lumen. Necrosis of the fat lobules is present along with an acute and chronic inflammatory cell infiltrate.

FIGURE 4-23

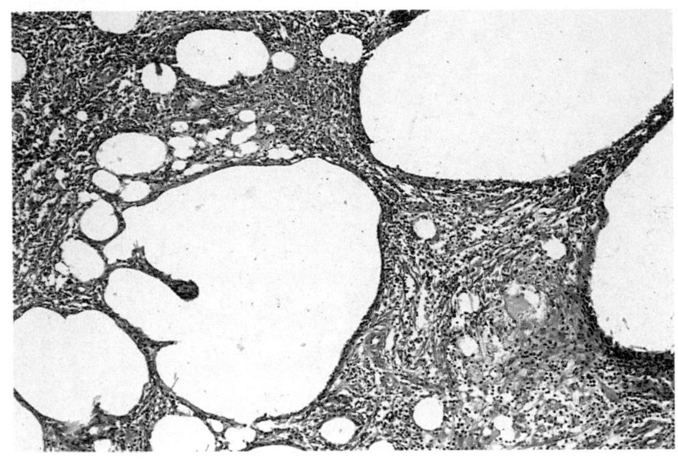

Injection granuloma. The architecture of the panniculus has been obliterated by acute and chronic inflammation in response to fat necrosis with resultant irregular spaces or micropseudocysts.

sclerosing the entire subcutaneous fat layer, Lobular panniculitis, however, results from the necrosis of fat lobules as the primary event, as is the case in idiopathic nodular panniculitis (see Chap. 109), followed by an accumulation of neutrophils and leukocytoclasia. The lipid material derived from necrotic adipocytes contains free and esterified cholesterol, neutral fats, soaps, and free fatty acids, which, in turn, exert an inflammatory stimulus. Histiocytic cells migrate into the inflamed fat, and phagocytosis leads to foam cell formation. Epithelioid granulomas with giant cells may also result, and all types of fibrosis may develop. Fat necrosis is therefore the primary, and inflammation the secondary, event in this type of panniculitis.

The inherent capacity of the adipose tissue to respond characteristically to pathologic stimuli with necrosis, inflammation, and lipogranuloma formation also holds true for disease conditions that affect the subcutaneous tissue only secondarily or result from exogenous factors. Traumatic panniculitis also leads to necrosis of fat lobules and a reactive inflammatory and granulomatous tissue response. After the injection of oils or silicone, large cystic cavities may be formed (Fig. 4-23), whereas after the injection of pentazocine, for instance, fibrosis and sclerosis dominate the histopathologic picture. Oily substances may remain within the adipose tissue for long periods without causing a significant tissue reaction; oil cysts evolve that are surrounded by multiple layers of residual connective tissue, so that the tissue acquires a "Swiss cheese" appearance (Fig. 4-23). Animal or vegetable oils often lead to tuberculoid or lipophagic granulomas with massive histiocytic reactions, foam cells, and secondary fibrosis.

Panniculitis also occurs as a result of infectious agents or specific disease processes. Inflammation, necrosis, and granuloma result from infections by cocci, mycobacteria, and other bacterial organisms and also from mycotic infections where the grade of acuity of the infection and the type of organism determine whether more inflammatory and necrotizing or granulomatous processes result. On the other hand, in sarcoidosis, fat is gradually replaced by epithelioid cell nodules and, in lymphoma, by specific lymphomatous infiltrates. In lupus panniculitis, a dense lymphocytic infiltrate of the septal and lobular tissue determines the histopathologic picture, as does involvement of vessels manifesting as vasculitis. However, destruction of fat, liquefaction, and lipogranuloma may be so pronounced that the vascular component can hardly be recognized, and the histopathologic picture may resemble idiopathic nodular panniculitis.

SUGGESTED READINGS

Ackerman AB et al: *Histologic Diagnosis of Inflammatory Skin Diseases: An Algorithmic Method Based on Pattern Analysis*, 2d ed. Baltimore, Williams & Wilkins, 1997

Ackerman AB: *Resolving Quandaries in Dermatopathology*. New York, Promethean Medical, 1995

Bos JD (ed): *Skin Immune System*, 2d ed. Boca Raton, FL, CRC Press, 1997

Cerroni L et al: An Illustrated Guide to Skin Lymphoma. Oxford, Blackwell Sciences Ltd, 1998

Caputo R et al: *Pediatric Dermatology and Dermatopathology: A Text and Atlas*, vols 1–4. Philadelphia, Lea & Febiger, 1990, 1992, 1997

Crowson A et al: The Melanocytic Proliferations. A Comprehensive Textbook of Pigmented Lesions. Wiley-Liss, Inc, 2001

Elder DE et al: *Lever's Histopathology of the Skin*, 8th ed. Philadelphia, Lippincott, 1997

Farmer ER, Hood AF: *Pathology of the Skin*. 2nd ed, New York, McGraw-Hill Co Inc, 2000

Hood AF et al: A Primer of Dermatopathology, 3rd ed, Norwalk, CT, Appleton & Lange, 2002

Murphy GF et al: Inflammatory Diseases of the Skin, AFIP Fascicle, third series, AFIP September 2002

PART TWO

Biology and Development of Skin

SECTION 3
STRUCTURE AND DEVELOPMENT OF SKIN

CHAPTER 5

Lowell A. Goldsmith
Ervin H. Epstein, Jr.

Genetics in Relation to the Skin

An understanding of genetic principles and methods and the special terminology of genetics is essential for the comprehension of the molecular basis, the familial clustering, and in the not too distant future, the genetic treatment of many skin diseases.[1–5] Important and sometimes confusing terms are defined throughout this chapter. Patients often present with a disease in which the pattern of inheritance (e.g., autosomal dominant) is clear, and penetrance of the gene is high [i.e., those who carry the abnormal gene(s) nearly always have resulting clinical abnormalities, such as X-linked ichthyosis, xeroderma pigmentosum, epidermolysis bullosa simplex]. Individually, these diseases are uncommon; but in aggregate, they comprise a significant fraction of the more severe skin problems.

A second group of patients has diseases with familial clustering (e.g., 25 percent of patients with psoriasis may have an affected first-degree relative), but the pattern of inheritance is uncertain. This group includes very common skin problems—psoriasis, atopic dermatitis, and androgenetic alopecia.

We are now in the midst of an explosion of unprecedented accrual of precise and detailed genetic information about many of the inherited disorders of the skin—partly because of an increased awareness of familial clustering of disease but mostly because of the opportunity to apply knowledge of the sequenced human genome. This precise molecular information will make gene therapy a reality within this decade. Although eventual cures of genetic diseases by gene replacement or modification are as of yet still hoped for, there are now satisfactory treatments aimed at preventing or modifying the deleterious effects of some defective genes. Examples include zinc supplementation to treat acrodermatitis enteropathica, a low-tyrosine and low-phenylalanine diet to treat tyrosinemia II (Richner-Hanhart syndrome), the administration of oral beta-carotene for erythropoietic protoporphyria, and the avoidance of gluten in the treatment of dermatitis herpetiformis.

When the mutant gene in a single dose (or heterozygous state) results in the particular clinical phenotype, the condition is said to be *dominant;* when the mutant gene must be present in double dose (or homozygous state) to produce disease, the resulting disorder is said to be *recessive*. When the mutant gene is on the X chromosome, the condition produced thereby is called *sex-linked* or, more precisely, *X-linked*. X-linked conditions also may be dominant or recessive, depending on whether the heterozygous female does or does not show the phenotype. When the mutant gene is on one of the 22 pairs of autosomes (nonsex chromosomes), the disorder is referred to as *autosomal*.

PEDIGREE PATTERNS

An understanding of the characteristic pedigree patterns of rare, simple inherited (*Mendelizing*) disorders is essential for counseling prospective parents about the risk of having affected children. The three main patterns of inheritance are *autosomal dominant, autosomal recessive,* and *X-linked recessive*.

Autosomal Dominant

Apart from the recipients of new mutations, persons affected with autosomal dominant disorders have one affected parent, and the condition is transmitted from generation to generation. Males and females are affected in approximately equal numbers, and both can transmit the disorder. On average, when an affected person is married to an unaffected person, half the children will have the condition. Figure 5-1 illustrates an idealized autosomal dominant pedigree pattern. Figure 5-2 shows the pedigree of a kindred with monilethrix. It must be emphasized that the exact expected 50:50 ratio probably is found only when many pedigrees (or an exceptionally extensive single pedigree) are available for analysis.

Autosomal Recessive

Typically, rare autosomal recessive disorders occur in siblings, both of whose parents are unaffected. The parents are related to each other more often than the average, and the rarer the condition, the more likely is such parental consanguinity. Provided that affected individuals do not marry a relative, their children are unlikely to manifest the condition. Figure 5-3 shows an idealized pedigree. Figure 5-4 illustrates a kindred with a junctional form of epidermolysis bullosa. Both parents of all the individuals marked as affected could be traced back to one common ancestral couple, one of whom presumably was heterozygous for the mutant gene. This family belonged to the Old Order Amish, where exact pedigree data are available for many generations. This is an example of inbreeding that per se does not alter significantly the frequency of genes in a population. What it does is increase homozygosity and therefore the appearance of undesirable recessive traits. If a person who is homozygous for a particular recessive gene, and therefore affected, does not reproduce because of the grave nature of the hereditary ailment, inbreeding actually may lead to a small decline of the frequency of

FIGURE 5-1

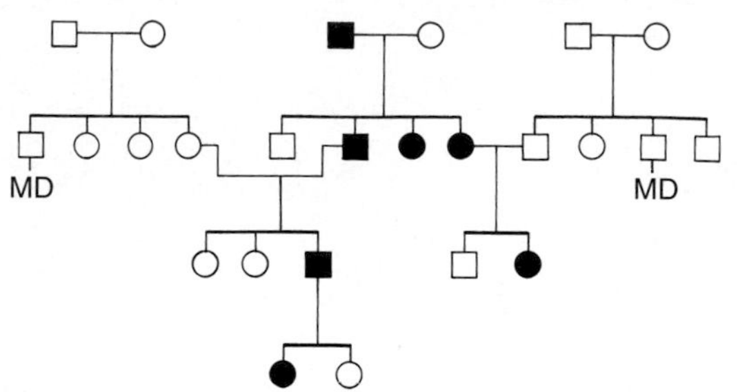

Idealized autosomal dominant pedigree pattern. The condition is transmitted from generation to generation by affected males or females to males or females.

the gene in the given population. Consanguinity plays little part in rare X-linked recessive and/or autosomal dominant disorders. Carriers of a recessive gene are usually clinically normal; a notable exception is that carriers of the gene for Fanconi's anemia have an increased incidence of skin and mucosal malignancies.

X-Linked Recessive

These conditions occur almost exclusively in males, but the gene is transmitted by carrier females, who have the gene only in single dose (heterozygous state). The sons of an affected male all will be normal (since their single X chromosome comes from their clinically unaffected mother). The daughters of an affected male all will be carriers (since all had to have received the single X chromosome that their father had, and that X chromosome carries the mutant copy of the relevant gene). Occasionally, some females show clinical abnormalities as evidence of the carrier state; this phenomenon can be explained by the *Lyon hypothesis.*

Dr. Mary Lyon suggested that (1) early in embryogenesis one X chromosome in each cell of the normal XX female becomes genetically inactive, (2) which X chromosome is inactive is a random matter, and (3) once it had been "decided" whether the X chromosome from the female's mother or that from her father will be the active one in a given cell, all descendants of that cell "abide by the decision." Thus the adult female is a mosaic of two populations of cells, those with the paternal X as the active one and those with the maternal X as the active one. The inactive X chromosome forms the Barr body, or sex chromatin.

The Lyon hypothesis provides an explanation for an intermediate level of gene effect in the heterozygous female and for its rather wide variability. By chance alone, rare individuals may have all cells of a particular type with the mutant X chromosome as the inactive one, in which case no phenotypic abnormality is detectable by even the most sensitive methods. However, in many X-linked conditions, such as anhidrotic ectodermal dysplasia, some carrier females demonstrate abnormal features, suggesting that the X chromosome carrying the mutant gene is active in many cells and that the X chromosome carrying the normal gene is active in relatively few cells. Indeed, patchy abnormalities, such as the Lyon principle would predict, have been observed in females heterozygous for this gene. An idealized pedigree of X-linked inheritance is given in Fig. 5-5, and an example of a family with X-linked ichthyosis is shown in Fig. 5-6. Several individual genes, such as those for steroid sulfatase, abnormalities of which cause X-linked ichthyosis, and those for the Xg^a blood group, do not undergo complete inactivation, but they are the exceptions.

In X-linked dominant inheritance, both males and females are affected, and the pedigree pattern superficially may resemble that of autosomal dominant inheritance. There is, however, one important difference. An affected male transmits the disorder to all his daughters and to none of his sons. X-linked dominant inheritance, lethal in males (Fig. 5-7), has been postulated as a mechanism in incontinentia pigmenti, a condition almost always limited to females. Affected males may be aborted spontaneously or die before implantation.

The term *sex-linked* is used if an autosomal disorder is confined to one sex. Such conditions may be seen in either males or females, and a definite mode of inheritance is not implied by the use of this term. When only males or females in a given family are affected with a condition, this may be an example of *sex limitation,* but it is more likely the result of chance. Sex linkage, better called *X-linkage,* results in a specific pedigree pattern, as described earlier. True sex-limited conditions—that is, disorders that have manifestations in one sex only—are rare. *Sex-influenced* is the term used when an autosomal trait occurs more often but not exclusively in one sex.

A second possible type of sex-linked transmission is that observed with genes

FIGURE 5-2

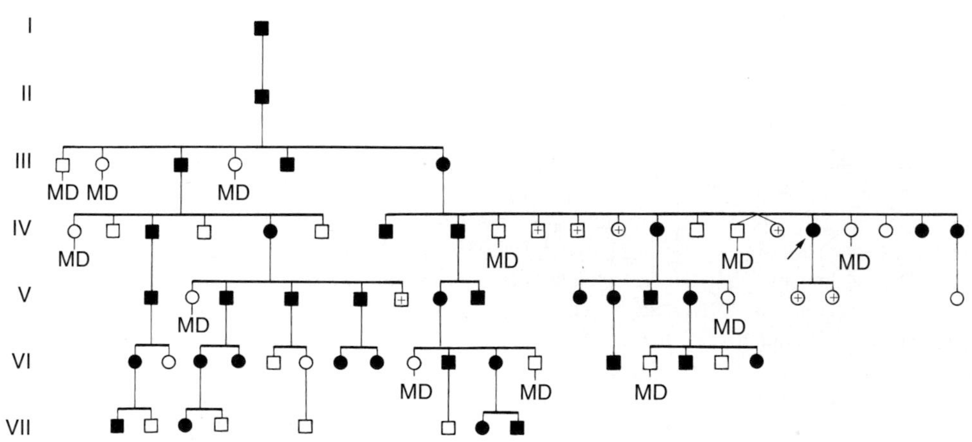

Monilethrix. Although the degree of alopecia was highly variable, all affected persons had an affected parent. (*From McKusick VA:* Medical Genetics 1961–1963: An Annotated Review. *Oxford, England, Pergamon, 1966.*)

FIGURE 5-3

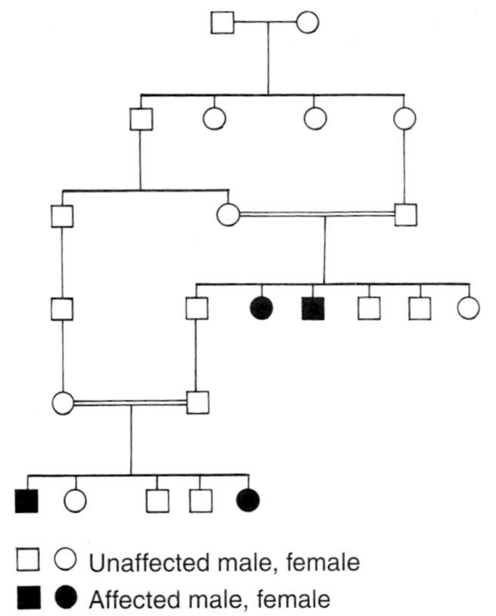

Idealized autosomal recessive pedigree pattern. The parents are unaffected, and consanguinity is common.

carried on the Y chromosome. Since this chromosome determines the maleness of an individual and must be inherited from the father, all the sons and none of the daughters of the affected person will manifest the disorder. There is some evidence that hairy ears (Fig. 5-8), a trait seen more frequently in some areas of India than elsewhere, may be transmitted in this way. An illustrative pedigree is given in Fig. 5-9. The Y chromosome codes for a variety of genes, including genes specifying a testis-specific protein, cytokine receptors, factors whose deficiency leads to azospermia, and other genes. The exact gene causing hairy ears remains to be elucidated.

These disorders are examples of inheritance related to nuclear DNA, but there is also DNA in the mitochondria (mtDNA). Mitochondrial disorders frequently involve the function of the respiratory chain and oxidative metabolism, and the nervous system often is severely affected. The mitochondria in a fertilized ovum are derived from the mother, and the inheritance pattern is maternal. There is no male-to-male transmission (which by itself is characteristic of X-linked inheritance), and *all* the children of an affected woman are affected, although there may be a variation in phenotype. An idealized pedigree of this type of inheritance is illustrated in Fig. 5-10. There often is a mixture of wild-type and mutated mtDNA (defined as *heteroplasmy*) that can lead to random variation in the degree of phenotypic expression. A review of 140 children with mtDNA disease showed that 10 percent of them have skin disorders, including alopecia, pili torti, trichothiodystrophy, hypertrichosis, and hypo- and reticulated hyperpigmentation on sun-exposed areas.[6] Most of these traits are nonspecific but should be looked for in the appropriate clinical setting.

VARIABILITY OF GENETIC DISEASES

The physician must deal with the problem of marked variability in the expression of abnormal genotypes, especially when deciding whether a new mutation has occurred and whether manifestations of a deleterious gene are present in a carrier of that gene who may be asymptomatic. In those cases in which specific quantitative biochemical tests are available, the presence of an abnormal gene, even in a completely asymptomatic carrier, can be determined.

Several terms are used to describe phenotypic (clinically appreciated) variability; their use often is confused, and a brief discussion of these terms is in order. These terms were in use before the molecular bases of the phenomena were established. They can now be reinterpreted through modern insights.

PENETRANCE Penetrance is the presence of any detectable manifestation of an abnormal genotype. If no phenotypic manifestations of a genotype are discernible, the gene is *nonpenetrant*. Thus *penetrance* is an operational term depending on how well one can analyze for evidence of the abnormal genotype. If one can determine detailed DNA sequences of the gene determining the disease, an abnormal genotype always can be detected. If a trait is not penetrant, its expressivity must be none.

EXPRESSIVITY Expressivity defines the degree of expression (severity) of a trait. It is a designation of the qualitative and quantitative manifestations of a specific genotype and is the variability in phenotype produced by a given genotype. Low levels of disease expression may cause familial cases of disease to appear sporadically and complicate genetic analysis.[7]

FIGURE 5-4

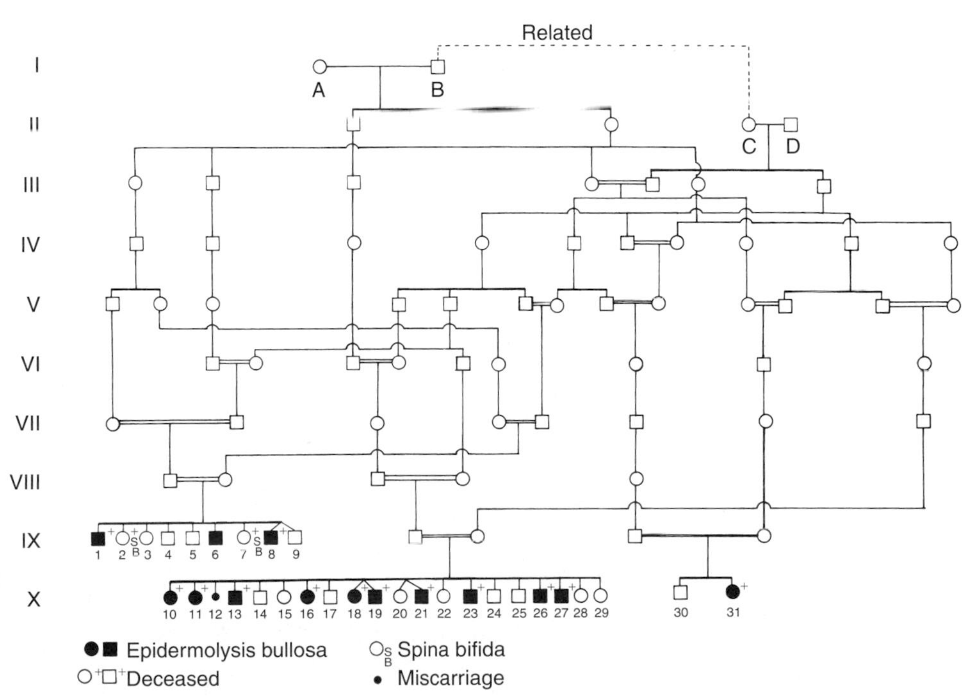

A junctional form of epidermolysis bullosa in a pedigree from the Old Order Amish showing considerable consanguinity.

FIGURE 5-5

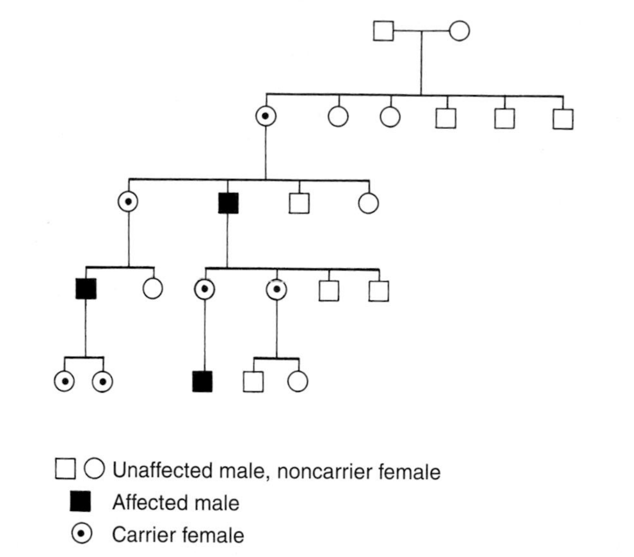

Idealized X-linked recessive pedigree pattern. Only males are affected, and the gene is transmitted by carrier females.

HETEROGENEITY Many diseases called by a single name have greatly disparate phenotypic abnormalities: Patients have heterogeneity in the clinical manifestations of their disease. There are several genetic reasons for such heterogeneity. First, the "disease" actually may be a collection of distinct diseases with only enough similarities to cause them to be lumped together in past classifications. For example, epidermolysis bullosa and ichthyosis today are viewed as groups of clinically distinct diseases, and the genes whose mutations cause these differing diseases themselves are distinct. Thus the gene that is mutant in epidermolysis bullosa simplex causes a defective intracellular protein, and the split is within the basal cells of the epidermis, whereas the clinically quite different junctional epidermolysis bullosa is due to mutations in genes that encode proteins that help to hold the epidermis and dermis together. It is likely that in the future the very definitions of diseases in at least some instances will move from those of a typical constellation of clinical abnormalities to those of a specific mutant gene. This change would mirror the switch of the definition of the clinical entity "consumption" to the definition of the disease tuberculosis, irrespective of whether the disease manifestations are, for example, pulmonary or cutaneous.

Second, even within more narrowly defined diseases, the clinical abnormalities may be caused by mutations in different genes. Such heterogeneity is termed *locus heterogeneity* because the causative mutation may occur at differing genetic loci. This may occur because the differing genes affect independent proteins that function in the same pathway, and it is the abnormality of the pathway that causes the disease manifestations (e.g., the abnormal behavior of basal cell carcinomas may be driven by mutations in either of two interacting proteins in the same pathway—PTCH1 or SMO). Alternatively, the two different genes may encode proteins that actually act together to produce a protein complex (e.g., mutations of either the keratin-5 or the keratin-14 gene may cause epidermolysis bullosa simplex, which is caused by dysfunction of the keratin-5–keratin-14 protein complex).

Third, in most genetic diseases, even those in which there is locus homogeneity—in which the clinical abnormalities are always produced by mutations of the same gene—different patients generally have mutations at different sites of the same gene. These different alleles may produce proteins that are more or less impaired in their functioning and hence may produce clinical abnormalities that are more or less severe. For example, within the spectrum of epidermolysis bullosa simplex, mutations at certain regions of keratin-14 may cause the relatively mild Weber-Cockayne type in which blisters are limited to the hands and feet and appear only with friction, whereas mutations at other sites of the same gene cause the much more severe Dowling-Meara type in which blisters are generalized and appear spontaneously. Thus, different patients have disease of differing clinical severity because they have different versions (alleles) of the gene—there is *allelic heterogeneity.* If the disease is recessive, there is a further opportunity for heterogeneity in that different patients may have different combinations of two mutant alleles—i.e., they are *compound heterozygotes.*

However, patients with the very same mutation (e.g., within a single kindred) still may have disease of differing severity (expressivity). This variation may be due to different external environmental influences (e.g., it is possible to reduce markedly the severity of disease in xeroderma pigmentosum by meticulous avoidance of ultraviolet radiation exposure). In addition, no gene or encoded protein functions in isolation. Rather, they function in the context of an internal environment that varies among patients because they have different versions of other genes (*background-modifying genes*), and these versions may be relatively effective or relatively ineffective at opposing the deleterious effects of the mutant gene. As a mechanistically trivial but heuristically useful example, the development of basal cell carcinomas in patients with the basal cell nevus syndrome may be influenced greatly by skin pigmentation. Patients of African descent and dark skin color have few to no basal cell carcinomas, whereas patients of northern European descent and poor skin melanization have many more of these skin tumors.

FIGURE 5-6

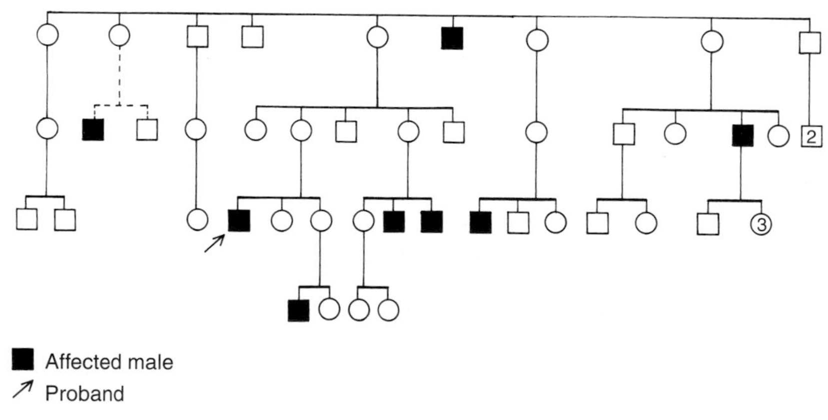

X-linked ichthyosis. No evidence of ichthyosis in the heterozygous females. (Dotted lines are a convention for extramarital relationships.)

Complex Phenotypes

PLEIOTROPY The multiple phenotypic effects due to the primary actions of an abnormal genotype are referred to as *pleiotropy*. Single autosomal genes such as those for Gardner's syndrome, pachyonychia congenita, neurofibromatosis, and basal cell nevus syndrome or the X-linked gene for Menkes' disease cause multiple phenotypic effects in several organ systems. Defining the basic molecular defect in each of these diseases leads to the physiologically based explanation of the complex

FIGURE 5-7

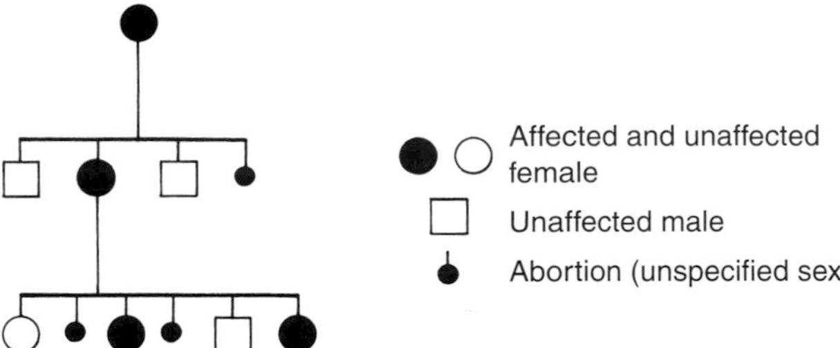

Idealized pedigree pattern of an X-linked dominant trait that is lethal in the male.

phenotype. The expressivity or even the penetrance of these traits may differ in individuals in the same family or between families. The elucidation of the basic defects in these diseases allows understanding of the multiple manifestations of an abnormal genotype. In most cases, pleiotropy is not due to the close linkage of several genes on a chromosome. Those few diseases caused by deletions that remove several adjacent genes on one chromosome are termed *contiguous-gene syndromes*. For example, X-linked ichthyosis in association with Kallman's syndrome is caused by an X-chromosome deletion large enough to delete more than one gene. The Prader-Willi syndrome and the Langer-Giedion syndrome, which may have dermatologic manifestations of hypopigmentation and sparse hair, respectively, often are associated with small chromosomal deletions. In these cases, loss of activity of a portion of a chromosome containing the normal allele of a gene may "uncover" an otherwise silent mutation in a gene on the active chromosome.

Epigenetic phenomena are gene-regulating activities that can persist through one or more generations and *do not* change the basic genetic code.[8,9] Cytosine methylation and histone acetylation or methylation are the basis of imprinting. Over 40 genes are already known to be subject to imprinting. Imprinted genes "remember" the parent of origin and hence may complicate the interpretation of pedigree-derived data. The genes responsible for the Angelman syndrome (maternally derived genes expressed) and the Prader-Willi syndrome (paternally derived genes expressed) are at the same chromosomal location and have hypopigmentation in addition to other phenotypic features.

FIGURE 5-8

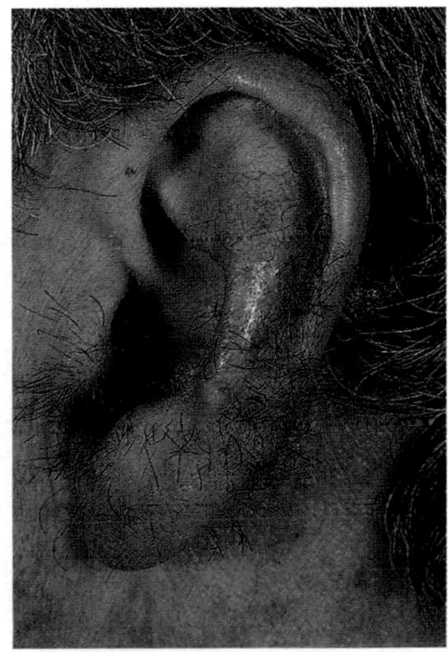

Hairy ear rims in a male.

FIGURE 5-9

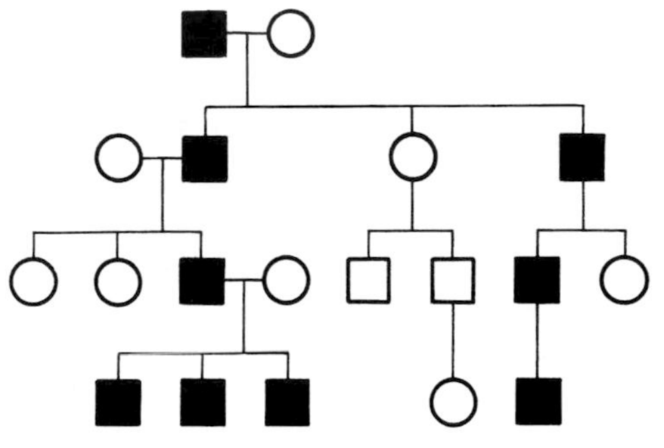

Idealized Y-linked pedigree pattern. All the sons of an affected male must be affected.

Two other terms that are useful in a discussion of some genetic diseases but that often lead to confusion are *phenocopy* and *congenital*.

PHENOCOPY Phenocopy in its broadest sense describes an individual who has the manifestations (phenotype) of a genetic disease but does not have a mutation in the putative gene (e.g., a patient with α-fucosidase deficiency has skin lesions that mimic those of Fabry's disease). Phenocopy is also used to describe those cases in which environmental (nongenetic) causes may mimic inherited diseases. The vascular lesions of the CREST (calcinosis, Raynaud's phenomenon, esophageal motility disorders, sclerodactyly, and telangiectasia) form of systemic sclerosis mimic very closely the telangiectatic lesions of Osler-Rendu-Weber disease. The recognition of phenocopies is of importance for prognosis and counseling for individual patients.

CONGENITAL The words *congenital* ("present at birth") and *familial* do not necessarily imply that a condition is genetically determined. For instance, the developmental abnormalities of newborns due to maternal ingestion of thalidomide during pregnancy are congenital but not, at least as a prime cause, "genetic," and the familial

FIGURE 5-10

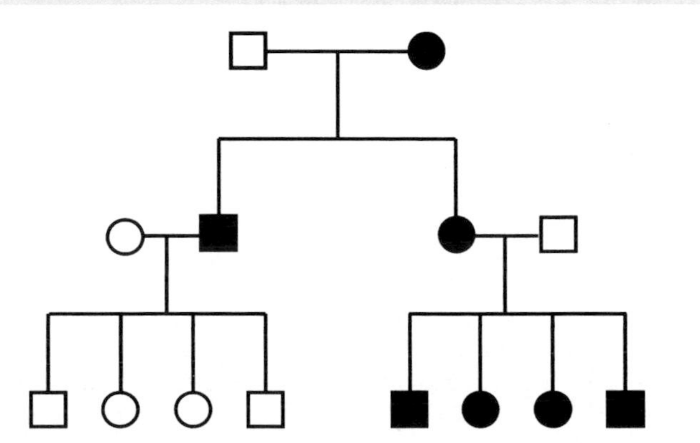

Idealized pedigree demonstrating mitochondrial inheritance. All the children of an affected female are affected, and there is no male-to-male inheritance.

clustering of the ability to use chopsticks or to play basketball with dexterity does not necessarily imply a genetic trait.

MUTATION

A central dogma is that hereditary diseases are caused by abnormalities of DNA sequence, that is, by mutations. DNA in the region of a gene is functionally arranged in alternating blocks of sequences called *exons* and *introns*. All these sequences are transcribed into RNA, and then the introns ("intervening sequences") are spliced out to leave behind the sequences derived from the exons. This process generates the mature messenger RNA (mRNA). The DNA sequences transcribed into mRNA encode the information (three bases per amino acid) that will direct the translation from the nucleic acid "language" to the protein "language" plus regions upstream *(5-prime)* and downstream *(3-prime)* that are important in the metabolism and action of the mRNA. Mutations of a single base pair in an exon may be neutral (may leave unchanged the amino acid that is encoded, may change the amino acid that is incorporated (which may or may not affect the functioning of the encoded protein and may or may not cause phenotypic changes) or may cause premature termination or abnormal elongation of the growing protein chain (which generally abrogates the function of the protein and perhaps even its very presence in the cell). Alternatively, a single base change in an intron, especially if it is at a base adjacent to the start or end of an exon, may cause changes in the splicing—so that an intron is not removed or perhaps an exon is skipped—and thus give rise to a severely abnormal message and hence to a severely abnormal, often truncated protein. Instead of a single base change, mutations may delete or add one or more bases. These commonly lead to premature termination of translation.

TRIPLET REPEATS Several neurologic diseases are caused by expansions of trinucleotide repeats—"runs" of three base pairs that can mutate to form longer and longer such runs. Once some expansion has occurred, further expansion appears to become more likely. Severity of disease often is related to the number of triplets in the expansion. Thus these diseases often show "anticipation," with the onset of clinical disease at progressively younger ages in succeeding generations of a kindred. The mechanisms by which these expanded repeats cause disease are incompletely understood and probably vary in different diseases. Examples of diseases caused by these expansions include Huntington's disease and myotonic dystrophy (which has early-onset androgenetic alopecia).

GENE LOCALIZATION AND IDENTIFICATION

Currently, there are two main strategies for identifying disease-causing mutations. The historical approach was to use knowledge of the manifestations of the disease and of biochemistry and cell biology to hypothesize about what the underlying defect might be. Thus several decades ago Cleaver and colleagues hypothesized that the fundamental defect underlying the extreme sensitivity to ultraviolet (UV) radiation–induced skin cancer in patients with xeroderma pigmentosum might be a failure to repair UV radiation–induced damage to the DNA. Indeed, they were able to demonstrate that repair of DNA was faulty in these patients. Progress in developing this hypothesis is discussed in Chap. 155. Similarly, when enough knowledge was accrued about the mechanisms by which skin pigment is formed normally (when there was clear knowledge of melanocytes, melanosomes, and tyrosinase as the essential enzymatic step), it was not difficult to discover that tyrosinase enzyme activity is lacking in many patients with albinism.

As another example, in the 1970s, groups in Los Angeles and Holland serendipitously found that patients with X-linked ichthyosis lack the enzyme steroid sulfatase. They and others proceeded to isolate that enzyme, to isolate the gene that carries the information for production of steroid sulfatase, to demonstrate that the disease generally arises because of a large deletion of DNA that includes the whole steroid sulfatase gene, and to learn that the failure of normal desulfation of cholesterol sulfate in the stratum corneum underlies the impaired desquamation. Thus, if the correct guess can be made or if by luck a correlation can be detected, the strategies and technologies for investigation are relatively well marked.

However, no one has made such a correct guess or has been the lucky recipient of such serendipitous correlation for most inherited disorders, including psoriasis and atopic dermatitis. For these diseases, a second strategy, that of linkage analysis, is used, and this is the most common approach for disease gene identification today. Linkage analysis has been spectacularly successful during the past 1½ decades in all medical specialties, including dermatology. *Linkage* refers to the occurrence of two loci on one chromosome at sites sufficiently close together that something less than completely independent assortment takes place; that is, they tend to be inherited together. Therefore, conversely, if traits specified by two genes are inherited together all or most of the time, then the two genes probably are located near one another on the same chromosome. This principle underlies the strategy of positional cloning, that is, of identifying a gene whose abnormality causes a disease by finding its chromosomal location rather than by guessing which abnormal biochemical function might cause the disease. Thus the inheritance of the disease is compared with the inheritance of a polymorphic marker at a known chromosomal location (i.e., a "mapped" DNA polymorphism). The raw materials of such an analysis are samples of DNA from multiple members of kindreds in which the disease is inherited and probes that recognize DNA polymorphisms at specific sites. One type of polymorphism commonly studied today is that of different length DNA fragments produced by polymerase chain reaction (PCR) amplification of specific sites with differing numbers of repeated elements, e.g., di- or tetranucleotide repeats. Once the general region of the gene has been identified, careful study of that region can identify sequences that are parts of expressed genes and eventually can identify the actual mutation underlying the disease. This process already has been performed for the whole genome. Such "careful study" has become remarkably easier with the publication of the sequence of the entire human genome—the sequence of nucleic acid bases that comprise the complete genetic information of at least a prototype of our species. Thus, once the candidate chromosomal region has been identified, it no longer is necessary to sequence the region and then identify the genes among these sequences. It is now possible to localize the gene causing the disease, even by a semiautomated genome-wide scan, and then to search the Web to identify candidate genes that can be tested for mutations in the patients. This strategy of positional cloning does not rely at all on knowledge or prescient guessing of the nature of a deranged biochemical pathway. Its power has been amply demonstrated by identification of previously unknown genes, such as those responsible for extracutaneous diseases such as Huntington's disease, Duchenne muscular dystrophy, hereditary retinoblastoma, and cystic fibrosis. These strategies have been applied to heritable Mendelian skin diseases as well, and numerous examples of successful disease gene identification are found in many chapters of this book.

With the great success of identification of genes whose mutations underlie Mendelian diseases, the field is turning now to study of non-Mendelian diseases. These diseases cluster in families, but the clustering fails to follow Mendelian inheritance rules; that is, the relationships among affected individuals cannot be explained by autosomal or X-linked dominant or recessive mechanisms. Such diseases include psoriasis and atopic dermatitis. The risk of psoriasis is markedly increased to 25 percent for those with a first-degree relative from the 2 to 5 percent risk in the general population. Evidence that much of this increase is due to shared genes rather than to shared environment comes from the study of twins. If one twin has psoriasis, the chance of a fraternal twin also having psoriasis is 25 percent, which is about the same as if the siblings were products of separate pregnancies. By contrast, the risk to an identical twin of a sibling with psoriasis is approximately 70 percent. This difference between 25 percent concordance for fraternal twins and 70 percent concordance for identical twins is taken as good evidence that the shared genes are of extreme importance in producing a susceptibility to psoriasis.

The current best-accepted hypothesis to account for this complex inheritance pattern is that susceptibility is controlled by several genes; to be susceptible, individuals must carry susceptibility alleles at more than one gene. It may be that susceptibility alleles at a small number of genes (e.g., three or four) will suffice and that each locus contributes a significant amount to the overall genetic susceptibility. However, it is not formally disproven that susceptibility may be controlled by a much larger number of genes and that susceptibility alleles at each contribute a relatively small amount of the overall genetic susceptibility. If susceptibility to the disease requires susceptibility alleles at more than a few genes, then for diseases that are relatively common (e.g., 2–5 percent for psoriasis in the European population), susceptibility alleles at the relevant genes also must be common. At this writing, the search for loci controlling susceptibility to this group of diseases has been frustratingly unsuccessful. The hope is that it may be possible to identify these genes by looking for polymorphisms at yet smaller intervals. Thus, after the initial sequencing of the genome, there followed immediately the effort to identify single-nucleotide polymorphisms (SNPs). SNPs are specific sites at which alternative bases are found in fairly high incidence (e.g., more than 5–10 percent of the alleles in a given population are the base of minor frequency—the less common allele, and the rest are the more common base—the common allele). SNPs occur as often as every 500 to 1000 bases across the genome, and millions of SNPs have been identified in the hope that they will allow finer-scale mapping of disease-associated genes. Testing of these polymorphisms in thousands of individuals at perhaps hundreds of thousands of sites seems a daunting task and must await the development of cheaper, faster, and more reliable techniques for gathering these data. The importance of these efforts is readily apparent because the diseases of complex inheritance appear to include much of the disease burden, particularly of the populations living in the industrialized parts of the world. However, beyond those diseases such as diabetes, atherosclerosis, asthma, and cancers, it also is hoped that successful unraveling of the genetic bases of complex diseases will lead to significantly improved understanding of diseases in which there is a large environmental component. These diseases include infectious diseases such as tuberculosis or leishmaniasis, in which many are infected, some have clinically apparent disease, and fewer suffer disastrous sequelae. Although environmental factors (e.g., general nutrition) surely help to control these differing responses, currently it is believed that a significant portion of the differential response to infectious diseases is controlled by genetic factors. As examples of genetic influences on the response to infectious disease, the protection afforded against malaria by heterozygosity for sickle hemoglobin has been appreciated for years, whereas the resistance to HIV infection conferred by variant chemokine receptors is a more recent finding. Linkage studies with the HLA locus have determined that

celiac disease is an important model disorder because it has a very specific HLA type. HLA type HLA-DQ2 (A1*0501/B1*0201) and/or HLA-DQ8 (A1*0301/B1*0302) heterodimers are associated with the ability to form a pathogenic immune response to diet-derived gluten and provide an example of how a gene predisposes to an immune reaction to a common environmental antigen.[10] This association, however, does not explain all the susceptibility factors in celiac disease, and other genetic factors seem to be more important than environmental factors except for dietary gluten.

A potential complication in linkage studies is *linkage disequilibrium,* when there is nonrandom association between alleles at different loci. The HLA locus is the classic location that shows linkage disequilibrium, which can complicate gene identification and recombination frequency interpretation. *Haplotypes* are contiguous regions of a chromosome that have a low frequency of recombination and can be used as markers for an adjacent gene of interest. Haplotype analysis can be used to establish ancestral relations between mutant loci that may be in individuals at different geographic locations, as was done for xeroderma pigmentosum loci in families in Turkey and Italy.[11] There are now efforts to apply related strategies to genetically complex skin diseases, and several loci believed to harbor genes important in determining susceptibility (e.g., to psoriasis and atopy) have been found. A distinction is often made between *multifactorial inheritance,*the effect of several genes and the environment, and *multigenic inheritance,* the genetic component of multifactorial inheritance. In such instances, these traits will establish several characteristics: Risk to relatives will be greater than to the general population; the incidence of disease will decrease with increasing distance of genetic relationship; the risk to relatives will increase with the number of affected relatives in the pedigree; and the incidence in first-degree relatives will be greater than the incidence of the disease in the general population. Between typical one-locus (biallelic) inheritance and polygenic inheritance is an example of triallelic recesssive inheritance in the Bardet-Biedl syndrome.[12]

One other technical innovation in the study of hereditary disorders is the insertion into an animal genome of a gene whose abnormality underlies a human disease in order to produce a transgenic animal (e.g., mouse) with the human disease. Such production of a hereditary disease by transferring a mutant gene is analogous to the production of an infectious disease by transferring the causative microbe. Similarly, both approaches allow confirmation of the etiologic role of transferred material, and both offer the possibility of testing experimental therapies in animals instead of humans. For example, insertion of a mutant keratin gene can produce murine epidermolysis bullosa simplex, and insertion of the HLA-B27 gene can produce rat psoriasiform dermatitis and ankylosing spondylitis. Alternatively, mouse DNA sequences coding for specific proteins can be deleted, and these "knockout" mice can be studied as models for human diseases caused by defects in the homologous gene.

For many disorders, it is probably valid to assume genetic equilibrium; the loss of genes from the population, due to failure of the affected individuals to have as many children as the population as a whole, is balanced by the addition of new mutant genes through the process of mutation. The lower the fertility of affected persons, the higher will be the proportion of all cases that are new mutants as opposed to familial cases. For instance, probably about 15 percent of cases of Marfan's syndrome are new mutants. In X-linked recessive conditions such as Duchenne muscular dystrophy or agammaglobulinemia, in which the affected males do not survive to have children, one-third of the cases are new mutants, and two-thirds have a carrier mother and therefore are inherited. In epidermolytic hyperkeratosis, new mutations are common.

TABLE 5-1

Skin Manifestations Associated with Chromosomal Defects (and Frequency of Traits)

Disease	Defect	Skin Manifestations
Turner's syndrome	XO (deficiency of one X chromosome or presence of an abnormal X chromosome XX) (ISO-X)	Congenital and persistent lymphedema Hypoplastic nails Increased number of nevi Redundant skin on neck Low posterior hair line Increased aging of the skin
Klinefelter's syndrome	XXY (XXY mosaics, XXXY, XXYY)	Thirteen percent with leg ulcers
XYY (1:200 males)	Extra Y chromosome	Cystic acne Varicose veins and ulceration
4p—	Deletion of the short arm of chromosome 4	Central scalp defects
Trisomy 8	Extra autosome	Short nails No patella (Important to distinguish trisomy 8 from the nail-patella syndrome)
Inversion 9	Pericentric inversion of chromosome 9	Inversion of 9, usually harmless polymorphism Features of anhidrotic ectodermal dysplasia in obligate females with inversion; obligate females without inversion. One family.
Trisomy 10	Extra autosome	Congenital scalp defect
Isochromosome 12p	Iso 12p mosaicism (Pallister mosaic aneuploid syndrome)	Lymphedema Coarse face Sparse hair—bitemporal Accessory nipples Generalized pigmentary dysplasia with Wood's lamp (marbled with an incontinentia pigmenti pattern)
Trisomy 13 (1:15,000)	Trisomy 13 (D group) Extra autosome	Scalp defects (parietal-occipital) Low posterior hairline Redundant skin on neck Nails narrow and hyperconvex Scrotal-type skin extending to tip of penis
Ring 13	Deletion of portions of 13 associated with ring formation	Epicanthal fold Alopecia and (?) scalp defect Symmetric hypopigmentation (arciform)
Ring 14	Ring of chromosome 14	Epicanthal folds Café au lait macules (some linear) Redundant neck skin Multiple depigmented macules Seizure (myotonic) (Need to consider in differential diagnosis of tuberous sclerosis)
Ring 17	Ring of chromosome 17	Multiple café au lait macules
18p—	Deletion of the short chromosome 18	Congenital alopecia
Trisomy 18 (1:5000)	Extra autosome (E group)	Redundant skin on posterior neck Hypoplastic nails
Trisomy 21, Down's syndrome (1:600)	Trisomy 21 (as an additional autosome or due to a translocation)	Elastosis perforans serpiginosa Vascular instability (acrocyanosis, cutis marmorata) Premature wrinkling of the skin Frequent syringomas Frequent alopecia areata Hyperkeratotic palms, skin, and ichthyosis-like changes Fissured and furrowed skin (xerosis)
Monosomy 21, (mosaic)		EEC syndrome (ectrodactyly, ectodermal dysplasia, cleft lip and palate) Sparse scalp hair
Fragile chromosomal sites	Fragile sites on X chromosome and 7	Primary cutis verticis gyrata

Thus sporadic cases of hereditary disease may represent new-dominant or X-linked mutants. Another frequent mechanism for sporadic cases is the chance occurrence of only one case of a recessive disorder in the family. Human families are small, and a family may have only one child affected by a given recessive disorder. In fact, it can be calculated that of all two-child families with one child affected by a given recessive disorder, the other child will be normal in 86 percent of instances; in three-child families, only one child will be affected in 73 percent of instances; and so on.

TABLE 5-2

Genetic Diseases with Skin Manifestations, Neoplasia, and Chromosomal Instability

Disease	Chromosomal Abnormalities	Associated Neoplastic Diseases
Ataxia-telangiectasia (see Chap. 191)	↑ Chromosome breaks ↑ Endoreduplication	Lymphosarcoma; lymphocytic leukemia Gastric adenocarcinoma
Bloom's syndrome (see Chap. 35)	↑ Chromosome breaks ↑ Chromosome rearrangements ↑ Sister chromatid exchanges Decreased rate of DNA replication ↑ Quadriradial configuration	Leukemia Lymphosarcoma Sigmoid adenocarcinoma Squamous cell carcinoma (oral, esophagus)
Dyskeratosis congenita	↑ Sister chromatid exchanges Normal breaks	Squamous cell carcinoma (tongue, oral, esophagus, nasopharynx, cervix, skin) Mucinous carcinoma Adenocarcinoma (rectum)
Fanconi's aplastic anemia	↑ Breaks ↑ Chromatid exchanges Endoreduplication	Squamous cell carcinoma (anus, vulva, oral) Leukemia, hepatocellular carcinoma Increased skin cancer in carriers
Gardner's syndrome	↑ Tetraploidy in skin fibroblasts	Adenocarcinoma (colon, rectum) Fibrosarcoma, meningioma, leiomyosarcoma
Werner's syndrome	↑ Rearrangements	Osteogenic sarcoma, leukemia Thyroid and liver carcinoma

For the sporadic cases of most autosomal dominant disorders studied from this point of view, it has been possible to demonstrate an effect of paternal age. For example, fathers of children with sporadic cases of achondroplastic dwarfism are, on average, about 7 years older than fathers of children without the disease. By contrast, for new mutations affecting a single gene, maternal age per se probably is not a factor, although a maternal age effect is well known in certain chromosomal aberrations, notably Down's syndrome.

CHROMOSOMES AND CHROMOSOMAL DISORDERS

Genes are arranged and organized in supramolecular groups, the chromosomes. Techniques for the culture of cells and analysis of their chromosomes allowed the definition of the chromosomal basis of several diseases. The use of fluorescent dyes and special staining techniques (banding) has increased the resolution of the cytogenetic techniques possible with the light microscope. Besides a large number of congenital diseases diagnosable by chromosomal analysis, acquired diseases, such as chronic myelogenous leukemia, some T cell lymphomas (mycosis fungoides), and retinoblastoma, also have characteristic chromosomal alterations.

In clinical practice, lymphocytes are stimulated to divide by phytohemagglutinin, and their chromosomes are then studied. The chromosomes of a single such cell are examined with light microscopy at a magnification of about 1800×, and the 46 chromosomes are arranged in what is known as a *karyotype*. The autosomes occur in 22 pairs; the sex chromosomes are X and Y in the male and two X's in the female. Each of the 46 chromosomes consists, at this state of cell division (metaphase), of two chromatids attached at what is called the *centromere*. Each chromatid is destined to form the particular chromosome in one of the two daughter cells.

Abnormalities of chromosome number include trisomy (three of a particular chromosome rather than two), monosomy (absence of an autosome), deletion of a long or a short arm of a chromosome, and the presence of an additional portion of a chromosome (often because of translocation). Since multiple genes will be lost or increased due to a chromosomal aberration, the disorders associated with chromosomes often are serious (or even lethal) and may involve malformations of many organ systems. Skin tumors may lose portions of chromosomes and exhibit *loss of heterozygosity* after one of the two alleles of a gene (the normal allele) is altered or "lost." Such deletion is the "signature" of a nearby tumor-suppressor gene that also is lost along with one allele of the polymorphic marker being assessed.

In certain of the chromosomal disorders, the skin manifestations of the disease are prominent. The prominent skin manifestations are grouped in Table 5-1. The complete phenotypes of many of these syndromes are discussed in other sections of this book.

Several disorders with prominent skin manifestations have evidence of chromosomal instability that is detectable by karyotypic analysis of the cultured cells (Table 5-2). Detailed descriptions of these disorders are given elsewhere in this book. Malignancies of various types are increased in these diseases. In ataxia-telangiectasia and Fanconi's anemia, there is evidence that heterozygotes have an increased incidence of cancer.

GENETIC COUNSELING

Genetic counseling is an integral part of the practice of medicine and usually requires the services of a specialist in medical genetics. Once the diagnosis is established beyond doubt and the mode of inheritance is known, every dermatologist should be able to advise patients correctly and sympathetically. Familiarity with the disease in question allows the dermatologist to discuss with assurance the disease, its various manifestations, and its degree of variability. Genetic counseling must be based on an understanding of genetic principles and on a familiarity with the usual behavior of hereditary and congenital abnormalities not only in terms of mode of inheritance but also in terms of range of severity, social consequences of the disorder, and the availability of therapy.

Counseling should include an explanation of the nature of the defect, the likelihood of recurrence, and what recurrence would entail. Besides being preventive medicine, counseling often relieves parental guilt and can allay rather than increase anxiety. For example, it may not be clear to the person that he or she cannot transmit the given disorder. The unaffected brother of a patient with Fabry's disease or with X-linked ichthyosis need not worry about his children being affected or even carrying the abnormal allele, but he may not know this. The adult unaffected son of a patient with epidermolytic hyperkeratosis (a condition inherited as a dominant) also will not transmit the condition to his children. A person with the recessively inherited form of pseudoxanthoma elasticum (PXE), which leads to serious visual impairment and vascular disease, will have children who will all be clinically normal, provided that he or she does not marry a person who is heterozygous for the PXE gene. In many congenital malformations, such as congenital heart disease and harelip–cleft palate syndrome, and in disorders such as epilepsy, the risk is of the order of a few percent, but the patient often has an exaggerated impression of the risk in future pregnancies.

Generally, unaffected parents who give birth to one child affected with a rare autosomal dominant disorder (e.g., epidermolytic hyperkeratosis) have a negligible chance of having a second affected child. However, such a happy prognosis requires some qualification because the mutation may have occurred not during the development of the sperm or ovum from which the affected child developed but rather during development of the parent so that the parent actually is a mosaic of normal and mutant cells. If the testes or ovaries contain some of the mutant cells, a condition termed *germline mosaicism*, then, for counseling purposes, the clinically unaffected parents must be considered as affected; therefore, as many as half the children also will be affected. Of particular interest to dermatologists are instances in which patients with localized lesions with histology resembling that found in generalized disease (e.g., nevoid, localized Darier's disease, or epidermolytic hyperkeratosis) may be such mosaics who carry the mutation in a small population of skin cells as well as in some germinal cells. Their children then may carry the mutation in all skin cells and have the generalized condition, such as Darier's disease or epidermolytic hyperkeratosis. Hence it is worthwhile (if not necessary) to examine carefully the parents of a child with apparently new mutations causing generalized disease for the presence of localized disease of the same type as that of their child because such a finding would greatly change the estimate of the likelihood of subsequent children being affected.

Special problems that arise during nondirective counseling include the fact that the parents and patients often have a limited knowledge of biology, genetics, and probability. The burden imposed by a disease rather than the strict mathematical risk of recurrence often determines the decision about reproduction. Physicians must be sensitive to cultural and religious beliefs that often determine the attitude of the parents and family to the concept of risk and to the significance

TABLE 5-3

Autosomal Dominant Skin Diseases (Classified According to Major Skin Phenotypic Features)

Blistering
- Epidermolysis bullosa (Cockayne)
- Epidermolysis bullosa dystrophica
- Epidermolysis bullosa simplex
- Pemphigus, benign familial (Hailey-Hailey)

Connective tissue abnormalities
- Cutis laxa
- Ehlers-Danlos syndrome
- Familial pachydermoperiostosis
- Hereditary sclerosing poikiloderma
- Lipoatrophic diabetes
- Marfan's syndrome
- Multiple benign ring-shaped skin creases
- Pseudoxanthoma elasticum
- Sclerotylosis

Gastrointestinal and skin
- Gardner's syndrome
- Keratoderma with esophageal cancer
- Peutz-Jeghers syndrome

Hair abnormalities
- Congenital scalp defect
- Distichiasis and lymphedema
- Hidrotic epidermal dysplasia
- Hypertrichosis universalis
- Marie-Unna hair dystrophy
- Milia and decreased hair density
- Monilethrix
- Pili annulati
- Trichorhinophalangeal syndrome
- Wooly hair

Hyperkeratosis
- Acrokeratosis verruciformis (Hopf)
- Bullous ichthyosiform erythroderma
- Darier's disease
- Erythrokeratoderma variabilis
- Hidrotic ectodermal dysplasia
- Howel-Evans syndrome (with esophageal cancer)
- Ichthyosis hystrix gravior
- Ichthyosis vulgaris (ichthyosis simplex)
- Keratoderma palmaris et plantaris, diffuse, linear punctate
- Naegli's syndrome
- Pachyonychia congenita

Hyperpigmentation
- Alkaptonuria
- Familial lichen amyloidosis
- Familial progressive hyperpigmentation
- Hemochromatosis
- Leopard syndrome (progressive lentiginosis)
- Lipoatrophic diabetes
- Naegli's syndrome
- Peutz-Jeghers syndrome

Hypopigmentation
- Albinism
- Albinism and deafness
- Incontinentia pigmenti achromians

Hypopigmentation (cont'd)
- Piebaldism
- Tuberous sclerosis
- Waardenburg's syndrome

Light sensitivity
- Albinism
- Erythropoietic protoporphyria
- Piebaldism
- Porphyria, variegate (South African)

Nail plate and nail bed defects
- Anonychia ectrodactyly
- Epidermolysis bullosa dystrophica
- Hereditary koilonychia
- Hidrotic ectodermal dysplasia
- Leukonychia totalis
- Nail-patella syndrome
- Pachyonychia congenita
- Pachyonychia congenita with steatocystoma multiplex
- Tuberous sclerosis

Tumors (benign and malignant)
- Basal cell nevus syndrome
- Bushke-Oldendorff syndrome (osteopoikilosis with connective tissue nevus)
- Cowden's syndrome (multiple hamartoma syndrome)
- Epitheliomas, hereditary benign cystic (Brooke-Fordyce)
- Gardner's syndrome
- Malignant melanoma
- Multiple cylindromas (Ancell-Spiegler)
- Multiple leiomyomata
- Multiple lipomatosis
- Neurofibromatosis (von Recklinghausen's)
- Steatocystoma multiplex (multiple sebaceous cysts) with pachyonychia congenita
- Tuberous sclerosis

Urticaria and edema
- Cold hypersensitivity
- Cold hypersensitivity with paramyotonia
- Familial angioedema
- Familial localized heat urticaria
- Lymphedema and distichiasis
- Lymphedema, hereditary (I or Nonne-Milroy type)
- Lymphedema, hereditary (II or Neige type)
- Periodic fever (familial Mediterranean fever)
- Urticaria, deafness, and amyloidosis

Vascular skin lesions
- Blue rubber bleb nevus syndrome
- Glomus tumors
- Hereditary hemorrhagic telangiectasia (Rendu-Weber-Osler)
- Maffuci's syndrome

and burden associated with disease. It must be remembered that if a couple has three children with a given recessive disorder, then the chance of a fourth being affected is still 1:4. "Chance has no memory," and even if the couple has 10 children, the chance with each succeeding pregnancy remains 1:4. Similarly, with autosomal dominant conditions, with one parent affected, the chance of each child having the same condition is 1:2.

The prevailing philosophy in giving genetic counseling is that the counselor states the risk in as precise mathematical terms as possible (with ancillary information on the range of severity that can be expected, the prospects for treatment, and so on) and leaves the decision about the course of action to the prospective parents. Contact information for patient advocacy groups, many of which provide further information for patients and families, is listed in individual chapters and is available online (*http://www.aad.org/patientadvocacy.htlm*).

Prognosis and counseling for those conditions in which the genetic basis is still unclear is more difficult. In such circumstances, empirical data should be used. Persons can be advised, for example, that if both parents have psoriasis, the probability is 60 to 75 percent that a child will have psoriasis; if one parent and a child of that union have psoriasis, then the chance is 30 percent that another child will have psoriasis; and if two normal parents have produced a child with psoriasis, the probability is 15 to 20 percent for another child with psoriasis.

TABLE 5-4

Autosomal Recessive Skin Diseases (Classified According to Major Skin Features)

- Blistering
  - Acrodermatitis enteropathica
  - Congenital erythropoietic porphyria
  - Epidermolysis bullosa dystrophica
  - Epidermolysis bullosa lethalis
  - Tyrosinemia II
- Connective tissue abnormalities
  - Alkaptonuria
  - Cockayne's syndrome
  - Conradi's disease
  - Cutis laxa
  - Ehlers-Danlos syndrome
  - Homocystinuria
  - Lipoid proteinosis
  - Mucopolysaccharidoses
  - Progeria
  - Pseudoxanthoma elasticum
  - Seip-Lawrence syndrome
  - Werner's syndrome
- Hair abnormalities
  - Argininosuccinic aciduria
  - Biotin-responsive carboxylase deficiency
  - Cartilage-hair hypoplasia
  - Chédiak-Higashi disease
  - Cornelia de Lange syndrome
  - Hallermann-Streiff syndrome
  - Homocystinuria
  - Marinesco-Sjögren syndrome
  - Mucopolysaccharidoses
  - Low-sulfur hair syndrome (trichothiodystrophy)
  - Phenylketonuria
  - Vitamin D–resistant rickets (type II) with alopecia
  - Werner's syndrome (premature graying)
- Hyperkeratosis
  - Conradi's syndrome
  - Harlequin fetus
  - Ichthyosiform erythroderma (nonbullous)
  - Ichthyosis, lamellar, of the newborn
  - Keratoderma palmaris et plantaris with corneal dystrophy
  - Keratoderma palmaris et plantaris with periodontopathia (Papillon-Lefèvre syndrome)
- Hyperkeratosis (cont'd)
  - Mal de Meleda
  - Refsum's syndrome
  - Sjögren-Larsson syndrome
  - Tyrosinemia II (Richner-Hanhart syndrome)
- Hyperpigmentation
  - Fanconi's syndrome
  - Gaucher's disease
  - Niemann-Pick disease
  - Wilson's disease
- Hypopigmentation
  - Albinism
  - Chédiak-Higashi syndrome
  - Phenylketonuria
- Light sensitivity
  - Albinism
  - Aspartylglycoaminuria
  - Cockayne's syndrome
  - Congenital erythropoietic porphyria
  - Hartnup's disease
  - Phenylketonuria
  - Xeroderma pigmentosum
- Multiple skin papules
  - Epidermodysplasia verruciformis
  - Farber's lipogranulomatosis
  - Hunter's syndrome
  - Juvenile fibromatosis
  - Lipoid proteinosis
  - Pseudoxanthoma elasticum
- Skin ulcers
  - Prolidase deficiency
  - Werner's syndrome
- Tumors
  - Xeroderma pigmentosum
- Vascular skin lesions
  - Ataxia-telangiectasia
  - Bloom's syndrome
  - Fucosidosis type II
  - Rothmund-Thomson syndrome
  - Sialidosis, juvenile type II

PRENATAL DIAGNOSIS

Molecular diagnoses (identification of specific mutations in individual patients/families) are available for a fee through several laboratories. One company focused on molecular diagnosis of genetic skin diseases is GeneDx (*www.genedx.com/240–453–6285*). In the current absence of effective treatment for many hereditary skin diseases, prenatal diagnosis can provide much appreciated information to couples at risk of having affected children. Three strategies are available.

First, the abnormal genotype may be demonstrable. This soon will become the predominant method of disease detection. Thus identification of the defect of genomic DNA in specific families (e.g., with tyrosinase-negative albinism, most types of epidermolysis bullosa, some severe forms of ichthyosis, and neurofibromatosis) allows analysis of the DNA of noncutaneous fetal cells, generally rapidly and efficiently.

Second, simple karyotyping of fetal cells obtained by chorionic villous sampling or amniocentesis can establish a diagnosis of chromosomal abnormalities and can establish fetal sex, which may indicate the presence of an unaffected fetus should it be a girl and the disease be a recessive X-linked trait.

Third, the phenotype of the disease may be demonstrable. Fetoscopy—direct visualization of the fetus—and skin biopsy in utero allow nearly routinely the prenatal diagnosis of harlequin fetus and some other types of ichthyosis, some forms of epidermolysis bullosa, and albinism. Alternatively, the enzyme deficiency (e.g., steroid sulfatase in kindreds with recessive X-linked ichthyosis) may be demonstrable in noncutaneous fetal cells.

Some dermatologic disorders for which the pattern of inheritance has been established are listed in Tables 5-3 and 5-4. They are separated into groups on the basis of their major phenotypic features. For more detail,[12–17] *McKusick's Catalog of Inherited Diseases*, which is on line (*http://www3.ncbi.nlm.nih.gov/omim/*), has an exhaustive listing of diseases, is continually updated, and is very well referenced.

In summary, for a large number of conditions seen in dermatologic practice, exact information is available about their mode of inheritance, and the basic principles of genetic counseling have been established. With some common disorders such as atopic eczema and psoriasis, the inheritance has, however, not been established beyond doubt, and the etiology is probably multifactorial. In these circumstances, counseling necessarily is more indefinite, but the chance of an affected person having affected children or of unaffected parents with one affected child having other children with the disorder is less than in single-gene conditions and should not be exaggerated.

REFERENCES

1. Genomics Issue. *Arch Dermatol* **137**: 11 (November) [entire issue], 2001
2. Collins F, Guttmacher A: Genetics moves into the medical mainstream. *JAMA* **286**:2322, 2001
3. McKusick V: The anatomy of the human genome: A neo-Vesalian basis for medicine in the 21st century. *JAMA* **286**:2289, 2001
4. Subramanian G et al: Implications of the human genome for understanding human biology and medicine. *JAMA* **286**:2296, 2001
5. Emery A, Rimon D: *Principles and Practice of Medical Genetics,* 3d ed. Edinburgh, Churchill Livingstone, 1996
6. Bodemer C et al: Hair and skin disorders as signs of mitochondrial disease. *Pediatrics* **103**:428, 1999
7. Newman J et al: Mutation in the gene for bone morphogenetic protein receptor II as a cause of primary pulmonary hypertension in a large kindred. *N Engl J Med* **345**:319, 2001
8. Ferguson-Smith A, Surani M: Imprinting and the epigenetic asymmetry between parental genomes. *Science* **293**:1086, 2001
9. Jones P, Takai D: The role of DNA methylation in mammalian epigenetics. *Science* **293**:1068, 2001
10. Papadopoulos G et al: Interplay between genetics and the environment in the development of celiac disease: Perspectives for a healthy life. *J Clin Invest* **108**:1261, 2001
11. Gozukara EM et al: A stop codon in xeroderma pigmentosum group C families in Turkey and Italy: Molecular genetic evidence for a common ancestor. *J Invest Dermatol* **117**:197, 2001
12. Katsanis N et al: Triallelic inheritance in Bardet-Biedl syndrome, a Mendelian recessive disorder. *Science* **293**:2256, 2001
13. Moss C, Savin J: *Dermatology and the New Genetics.* Oxford, Blackwell, 1995
14. Novice F et al: *Handbook of Genetic Skin Disorders.* Philadelphia, Saunders, 1994
15. Scriver CR et al: *The Metabolic and Molecular Bases of Inherited Disease,* 8th ed. New York, McGraw-Hill, 2001
16. Spitz J: *Genodermatosis: A Full-Color Guide to Genetic Skin Disorders.* Baltimore, Williams & Wilkins, 1996
17. Sybert V: *Genetic Skin Disorders.* New York, Oxford University Press, 1997

CHAPTER 6

David H. Chu
Anne R. Haake
Karen Holbrook
Cynthia A. Loomis

The Structure and Development of Skin

Much of the complex structure of skin can be explained in terms of the function of its component cells, cellular organelles, and biochemical composition. This broad image has resulted from the application of immunology, biochemistry, physiology, transgenic models, biophysics, and molecular biology often used in combination with various forms of microscopy, and from alterations in structural and regulatory proteins that are the molecular basis of genodermatoses and skin tumors. This chapter presents a unified concept of structure and function of skin organized according to skin region. These divisions are not independent—they are interdependent, functional units; each region of the skin relies upon and is integrated with the surrounding tissue for regulation and modulation of normal structure and functions at molecular, cellular, and tissue levels of organization.

THE EPIDERMIS

Overview

The epidermis is a continually renewing, stratified, squamous epithelium that keratinizes and gives rise to derivative structures (pilosebaceous units, nails, and sweat glands) called appendages (Figs. 6-1, 6-2, and 6-3). It is approximately 0.4 to 1.5 mm in thickness, as compared to the 1.5- to 4-mm full-thickness skin. The majority of cells in the epidermis are keratinocytes that are organized into four layers named for either their position or a structural property of the cells. Viable cells move outwardly from the basal layer to form layers of progressively more differentiated cells; terminally differentiated (keratinized) keratinocytes are found in the stratum corneum. Intercalated among the keratinocytes at various levels in the epidermis are the immigrant cells—melanocytes and Langerhans cells—and Merkel cells. The melanocytes and Langerhans cells migrate into the epidermis during embryonic development while Merkel cells probably differentiate in situ. Other cells, such as lymphocytes, are transient inhabitants of the epidermis and are extremely sparse in normal skin. The epidermis rests on, and is attached to, a basal lamina that separates epidermis and dermis and mediates their attachment. There are many regional variations in the structure and properties of the epidermis and its appendages; some are apparent grossly, such as thickness (e.g., comparing palm with flexor forearm); other regional differences are microscopic.

The Keratinocyte

The keratinocyte is an ectodermally derived cell that constitutes at least 80 percent of the epidermal cells. All keratinocytes contain cytoplasmic keratin intermediate filaments in their cytoplasm and form desmosomes or modified desmosomal junctions with adjacent cells. Other features of keratinocytes depend upon their location within the epidermis.

Keratin filaments are a hallmark of the keratinocyte and other epithelial cells (reviewed in Refs. 1 and 2). Predominantly, they serve

FIGURE 6-1

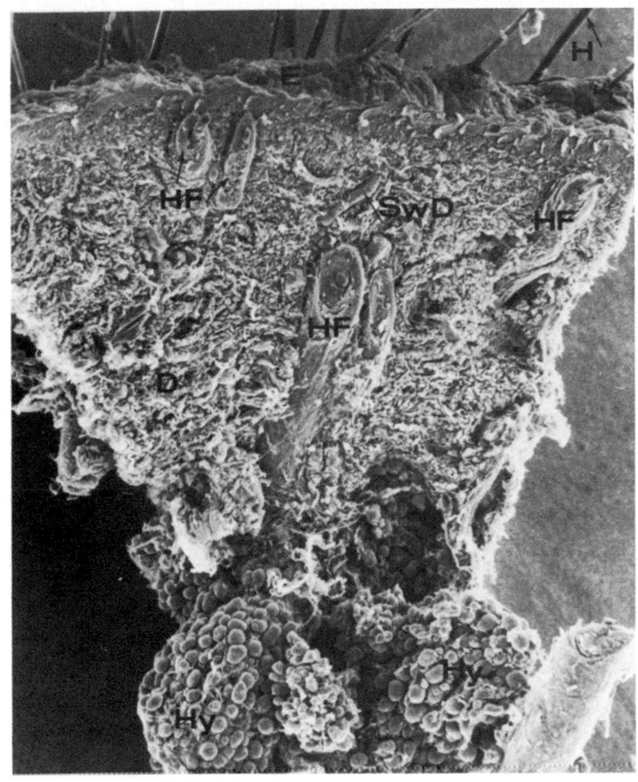

Scanning electron micrograph of full-thickness skin from a newborn infant illustrating all regions of the skin and the appendages. D, dermis; E, epidermis; H, hair; HF, hair follicle; Hy, hypodermis; and SwD, sweat duct. *(From Holbrook KA: An histological comparison of infant and adult skin, in Neonatal Skin Structure and Function, edited by H Maibach, EK Boisits. New York, Marcel Dekker, 1982, p 3, by courtesy of Marcel Dekker.)*

FIGURE 6-2

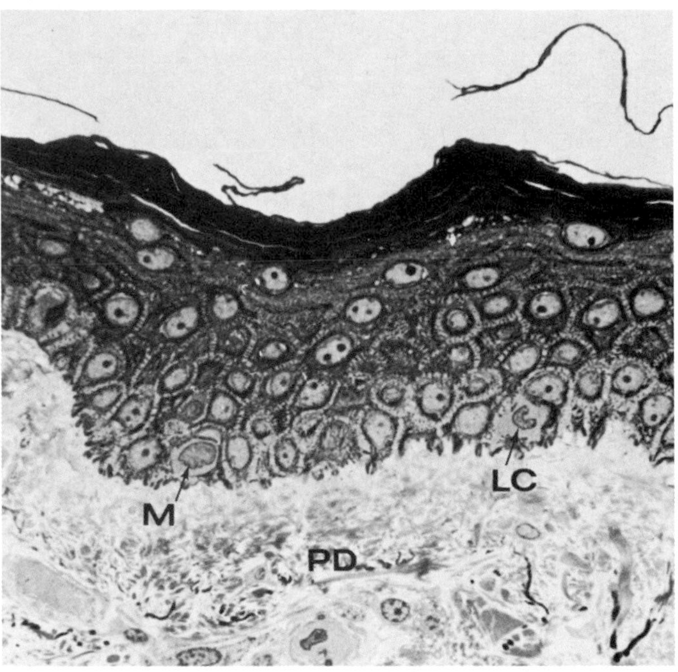

Light micrograph of adult epidermis and papillary dermis (PD). Note the shapes of the cells in each layer. A melanocyte (M) and Langerhans cells (LC) are present among keratinocytes of the basal layer. *(From Holbrook K: Structure and Development of the Skin, in Pathophysiology of Dermatologic Disease, edited by NA Soter, HP Baden. New York, McGraw-Hill, 1991, 2nd edition, p 5, with permission.)*

a structural (cytoskeletal) role in the cells. More than 30 different keratins—approximately 20 epithelial and 10 hair keratins, all within a range of 40- to 70-kDa molecular mass—have been identified in epithelial cells, catalogued, and assigned a number. The keratins are separated into acidic (type I; cytokeratins K10 to K20) and basic-to-neutral (type II; cytokeratins K1 to K9) subfamilies based on their isoelectric points, immunoreactivity, and sequence homologies with type I and type II wool keratins. Keratins assemble into filaments both within cells and when reconstituted in vitro as "obligate heteropolymers," meaning that a member of each family (acidic and basic) must be coexpressed in order to form the filament structure. The coexpression of specific keratin pairs is dependent on cell type, tissue type, developmental stage, differentiation stage, and disease condition. Thus, understanding how keratin expression is regulated provides insight into epidermal differentiation.

Layers of the Epidermis

EPIDERMAL DIFFERENTIATION DEFINES THE CHARACTERISTICS OF THE EPIDERMAL LAYERS The characteristics of each epidermal layer reflect the mitotic and synthetic properties of the keratinocytes and their state of differentiation. Keratinization is a genetically programmed, carefully regulated, complex series of morphologic changes and metabolic events that occur progressively in postmitotic keratinocytes and involve (1) an increase in cell size and flattening of cell shape; (2) the appearance of new cellular organelles and the structural reorganization of those present; (3) change from a generalized cellular metabolism to a more "focused" metabolism associated with the synthesis and modification of molecules (structural proteins and lipids) related to keratinization; (4) alterations in the properties of the plasma membrane, cell surface antigens, and receptors; (5) the eventual degradation of cellular organelles including internucleosomal chromatin fragmentation characteristic of apoptosis; and (6) dehydration. Each stage of differentiation becomes more specialized in cell structure and function. The end point of keratinization is a terminally differentiated, dead keratinocyte (corneocyte) that contains keratin filaments, matrix protein, and a protein-reinforced plasma membrane with surface-associated lipids.

Differentiation is a controlled series of events regulated by both extrinsic (environmental) and intrinsic (systemic and genetic) factors; thus it is vulnerable to alteration at different levels in the keratinization pathway. For many genetic diseases of keratinization, it has been possible to identify a specific defect in an enzyme, the synthesis of a structural protein, or an alteration in lipid metabolism. Understanding this process provides a rational basis for pharmacologic management of some of these disorders.

THE BASAL LAYER The basal layer or stratum germinativum contains mitotically active, columnar-shaped keratinocytes that attach to the basement membrane zone and give rise to cells of the more superficial epidermal layers (Figs. 6-2 and 6-3). Basal cells contain a large nucleus with little marginated heterochromatin and a prominent nucleolus. The typical "housekeeping" organelles, Golgi, rough endoplasmic reticulum, mitochondria, lysosomes, and ribosomes are present in the cytoplasm; in addition, there are membrane-bound vacuoles that contain pigmented melanosomes transferred from melanocytes by phagocytosis (Figs. 6-3 and 6-4).

FIGURE 6-3

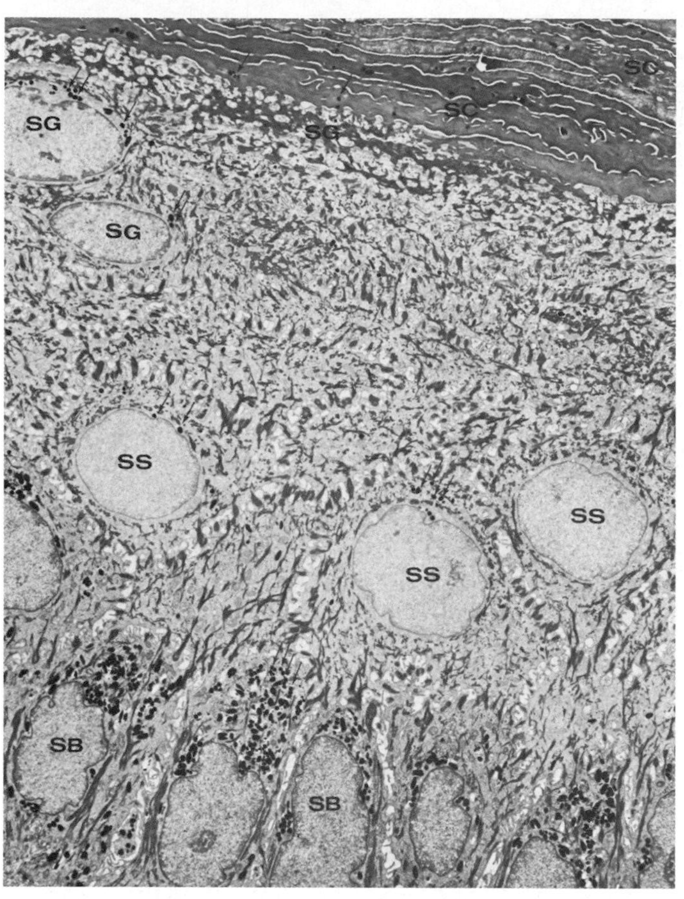

Full-thickness adult epidermis from a black individual. Basal (SB), spinous (SS), granular (SG), and cornified (SC) layers are shown. Melanosomes (*arrows*) are evident in cells of all layers. Note the changes in distribution and organization of keratin filaments. (*From Holbrook K: Structure and Development of the Skin in Pathophysiology of Dermatologic Disease, edited by NA Soter, HP Baden. New York, McGraw-Hill, 1991, 2nd edition, p 4, with permission.*)

The keratin filaments in basal cells are in fine bundles organized around the nucleus, and they insert into desmosomes and hemidesmosomes. The K5 and K14 (approximately 58 kDa/50 kDa) pair of keratins are expressed in the basal layer of the epidermis and other stratifying epithelia. Other keratins are expressed in small subpopulations of basal keratinocytes, including K15 and K19, which are associated with putative stem cells.[3,4] Microfilaments (actin, myosin, and α-actinin) and microtubules are other cytoskeletal elements present in basal cells. Some of the microfilamentous components of the cytoskeleton are also important links with the external environment via their association with the integrin receptors present on basal keratinocytes. Integrins are a large family of cell surface molecules involved in cell-cell and cell-matrix interactions, including adhesion and initiation of terminal differentiation.

The basal layer is the primary location of mitotically active cells of the epidermis. Not all basal cells, however, display equal proliferative potential. Based on cell kinetic studies, three populations coexist within this layer: stem cells, transient amplifying cells, and postmitotic cells. Functional evidence for the existence of long-lived epidermal stem cells comes from both in vivo and in vitro studies.[5,6] Because epidermal cells isolated from small biopsy specimens can be expanded in tissue culture and can be used to reconstitute sufficient epidermis to cover the entire skin surface of burn patients, such a starting population must contain long-lived stem cells with extensive proliferative potential.

The tissue localization of putative epidermal stem cells has been based in part on stem cell characteristics defined in other self-renewing systems, such as bone marrow and fetal liver. Under stable conditions, stem cells cycle slowly; only under conditions requiring more extensive proliferative activity, such as during wound healing or after exposure to exogenous growth factors, do stem cells undergo multiple, rapid cell divisions. A large amount of data supports the existence of multipotent epidermal stem cells within the bulge region of the hair follicle based on these traits. Additional evidence suggests that a subpopulation of surface epidermal basal cells also possesses stem cell characteristics. These basal stem cells appear to be clonogenic, progress rapidly through S-phase of the cell cycle, and divide infrequently during stable self-renewal (retaining ^{3}H-thymidine label over long periods). Additionally, they are capable of cell division in response to exogenous and endogenous agents.

The second type of cell, the transient amplifying cells of the stratum germinativum, arise as a subset of daughter cells produced by the infrequent division of stem cells. These transient amplifying cells provide the bulk of the cell divisions needed for stable self-renewal and are the most common cells in the basal compartment. After undergoing several cell divisions, these cells give rise to the third class of epidermal basal cells, the postmitotic cells. It is the postmitotic cells that undergo terminal differentiation, detaching from the basal lamina and migrating superficially, ultimately differentiating into a corneocyte. In humans, the normal transit time for a basal cell, from the time it detaches from the basal layer to the time it enters the stratum corneum, is at least 14 days. Transit through the stratum corneum and desquamation require another 14 days.

These three functional classes of epidermal basal cells (stem cells, transient amplifying cells and postmitotic cells) are difficult to distinguish in situ based solely on morphology or protein expression. The term *epidermal proliferative unit* has been used to describe vertical columns of progressively differentiating cells in the epidermis (see Chap. 7). Evidence for such columns has come from cell lineage studies and the preferential tracking of a fluorescent dye across gap junctions joining cells within vertical columns rather than laterally within a horizontal plane of cells. Integrin immunolocalization studies, however, suggest that stem cells are largely concentrated in focal areas of the epidermis, such as the deep rete ridges of human palm skin and over the dermal papillae of both scalp and foreskin. The functional significance of these integrin localization patterns is supported by the observations that stem cells can be enriched in culture on the basis of high levels of β_1-integrin expression in vivo and the rapid adhesion of these cells to relevant extracellular matrix proteins. Cells enriched in this manner appear to be clonogenic and suitable for long-term expression of transfected genes.

THE SPINOUS LAYERS The shape, structure, and subcellular properties of spinous cells correlate with their position within the mid-epidermis. They are named for the spine-like appearance of the cell margins in histologic sections (Fig. 6-2). Suprabasal spinous cells are polyhedral in shape and have a rounded nucleus. Cells of the upper spinous layers are larger, more flattened, and contain organelles called "lamellar granules." The cells of all spinous layers contain large and conspicuous bundles of keratin filaments. As in basal cells, the filaments are organized concentrically around the nucleus and insert into desmosomes peripherally.

The K5/K14 keratins present in basal cells are stable and thus remain in the cytoplasm of the spinous cells. In situ hybridization studies show that, except in hyperproliferative disorders where a low level of expression is sustained, the mRNAs for these keratins are not synthesized by suprabasal cells. New synthesis of the K1/K10 (56.5 and 67 kDa) keratin pair occurs in spinous cells. These keratins are characteristic of an epidermal-type pattern of differentiation and thus are referred to as the differentiation- or keratinization-specific keratins. Although this pattern of differentiation is the rule for normal epidermis, the suprabasal keratinocytes in hyperproliferative epidermis (e.g., psoriasis, actinic keratoses, and wound healing) switch to an alternative pathway of differentiation in which the synthesis of K1 and K10 mRNA and protein is downregulated and the synthesis and translation of the messages for K6 and K16 (48- and 56-kDa keratins) are favored. Correlated with this change in keratin expression is a loss of normal phenotypic differentiation in granular and cornified cell layers (see below). The mRNAs for K6 and K16 normally are present in all layers of the epidermis, but the message is translated only when proliferation is stimulated.

FIGURE 6-4

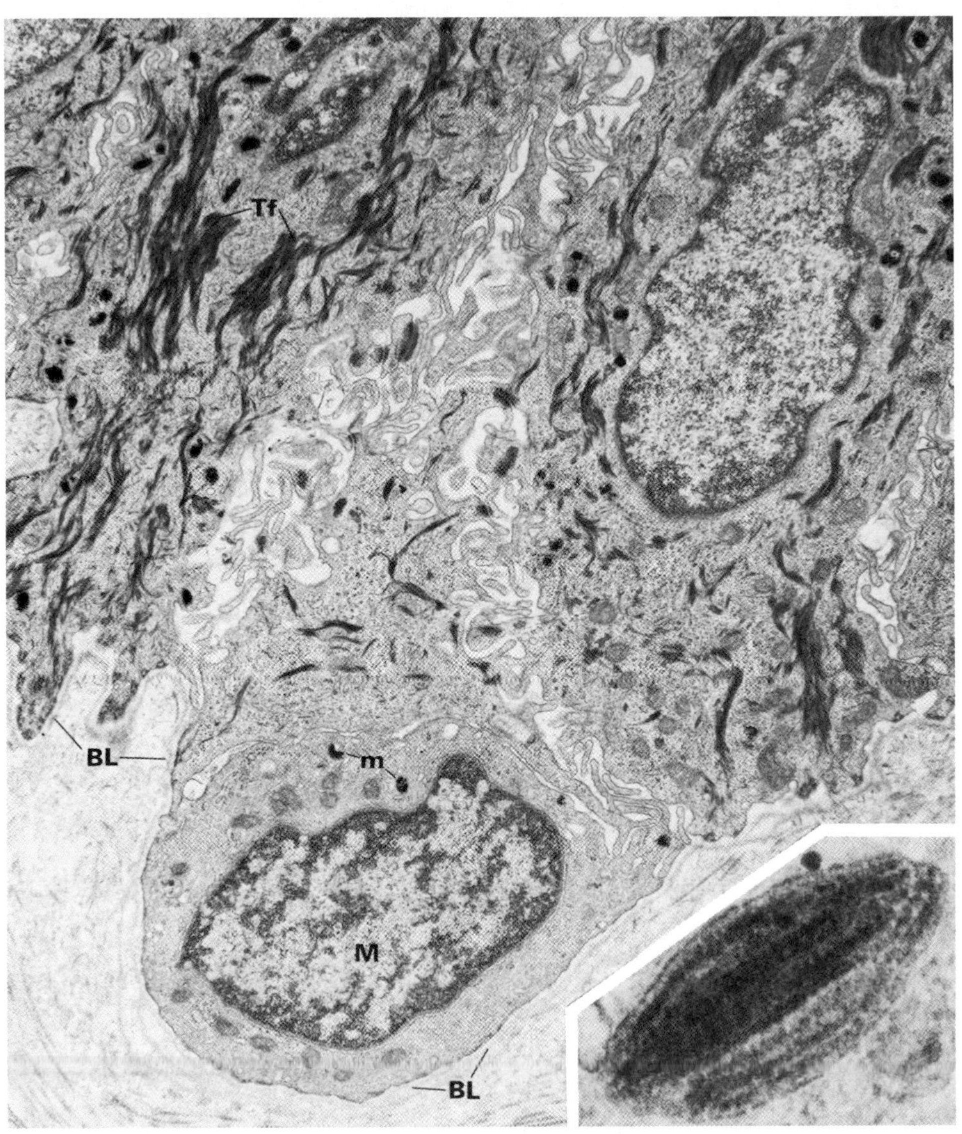

Basal layer of the epidermis. Melanocyte (M) is present at the dermal–epidermal junction protruding into the dermis, still above the basal lamina (BL). It can be distinguished from the keratinocytes by the absence of keratin filaments (Tf) and the presence of melanosomes (m). ×10,000. Inset: Melanosome, ×130,000.

The "spines" of spinous cells are the abundant desmosomes, calcium-dependent cell surface modifications that promote adhesion of epidermal cells and resistance to mechanical stresses (Fig. 6-3). The molecular components of the desmosome have been well characterized.[7] Within each cell there is a desmosomal plaque (Fig. 6-5*A*) associated with the internal surface of the plasma membrane that is composed of six polypeptides: plakoglobin, desmoplakins I and II, keratocalmin, desmoyokin, and band 6 protein (plakophilin). Transmembrane glycoproteins of the cadherin family provide the adhesive properties on the external surface or core of the desmosome. These glycoproteins include desmogleins 1 and 3 and desmocollins I and II. The extracellular domains of these proteins form part of the core. The intracellular domains insert into the plaque, linking them to the intermediate filament (keratin) cytoskeleton. E-cadherins, which are characteristic of adherens junctions, are associated with actin filaments via interaction with catenins,[8] and may regulate the organization of adherens junctions and influence epidermal stratification. The differences in the proteins in the two types of cell attachment structure may be related to specific requirements for the adherens junction–actin relationship as compared with the association of the desmosome proteins and keratin intermediate filaments. A central density/plate bisects the intercellular space between desmosomes (Fig. 6-5*A*).

Abnormal desmosomal structure or disruption of desmosomes causes cells to round, separate (acantholysis), and form blisters and vesicles within the epidermis, and may lead to exfoliation of several epidermal layers. These changes occur in autoimmune diseases such as pemphigus foliaceus and pemphigus vulgaris, in which patients produce antibodies that specifically bind to the extracellular domain of desmogleins 1 and 3, respectively,[9] or in staphylococcal scalded skin syndrome, in which the bacterial exotoxin is a protease that cleaves the extracellular domain of desmoglein 1.[10] In these examples, the desmosomes either disappear entirely or the intercellular association site is destroyed. While desmosomes provide a mechanical coupling between epidermal cells, gap junctions between keratinocytes[11] are sites of physiologic communication (Fig. 6-5*C*). As with desmosomes, gap junctions are more abundant in more differentiated keratinocytes, correlating with the observation that dye is transferred more efficiently among cells of the suprabasal compartment than among basal cells. Communication by means of these junctions is undoubtedly important in the regulation of cell metabolism, growth, and differentiation.

Lamellar granules deliver precursors of stratum corneum lipids into the intercellular space. The granules are first evident in the cytoplasm of the upper spinous cells even though the primary site of their activity is at the granular–cornified layer interface (Fig. 6-6). They are 0.2- to 0.3-μm in diameter, membrane-bound, secretory organelles that contain a series of alternating thick and thin lamellae; these are folded sheets or disk- or liposome-like structures. Lamellar granules contain

FIGURE 6-5

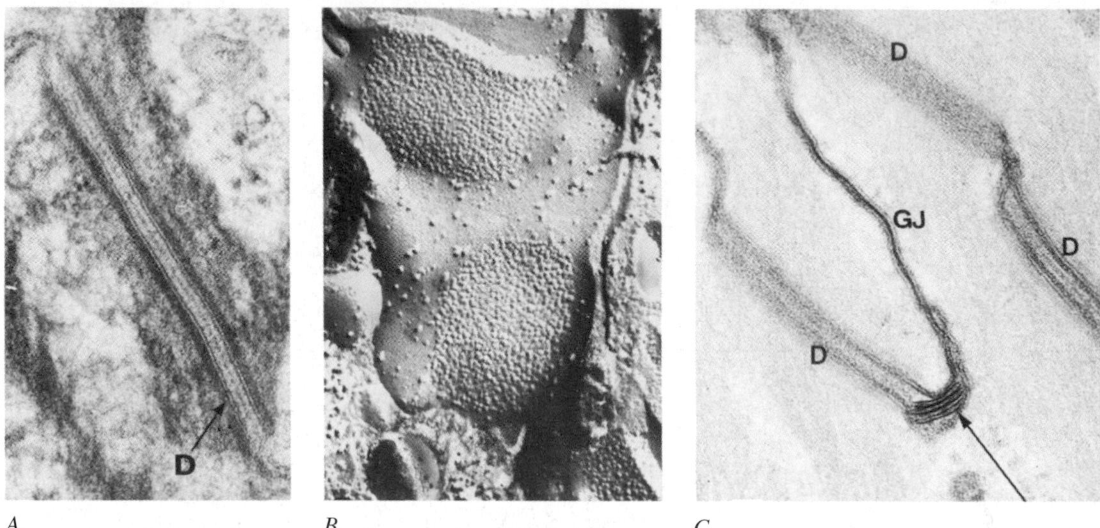

Desmosomes (D) as they appear in skin observed with transmission electron microscopy (*A*) and in the plane of the plasma membrane of tissue prepared by freeze-fracture techniques (*B*). Desmosomes (*arrow*) and a gap junction (GJ) as revealed by aldehyde-potassium ferrocyanide-osmium fixation (*C*). *A Trends in Electron Microscopy of Skin* and *C* ×94,000; *B*×61,700. (*Part C from Wolff K, Wolff-Schreiner EC: J Invest Dermatol 67:39, 1976, with permission.*)

glycoproteins, glycolipids, phospholipids, free sterols, and a number of acid hydrolases, including lipases, proteases, acid phosphatase, and glycosidases. Glucosylceramides, the precursors to ceramides and the dominant component of the stratum corneum lipids, are found in lamellar granules. These enzymes indicate that lamellar granules are a type of lysosome with characteristics of both secretory granules and lysosomes. Roles for the lamellar granule in providing the epidermal lipids responsible for the barrier properties of the stratum corneum, synthesis and storage of cholesterol, and adhesion/desquamation of cornified cells have been hypothesized. These conclusions are based on known defects in structure and composition of lamellar granules and deficits in function of the tissue. Several genodermatoses, including recessive X-linked ichthyosis, involve mutations in genes critical for steroid and lipid metabolism and are characterized by a failure of cornified cells to slough, the result being a retention hyperkeratosis.[12]

FIGURE 6-6

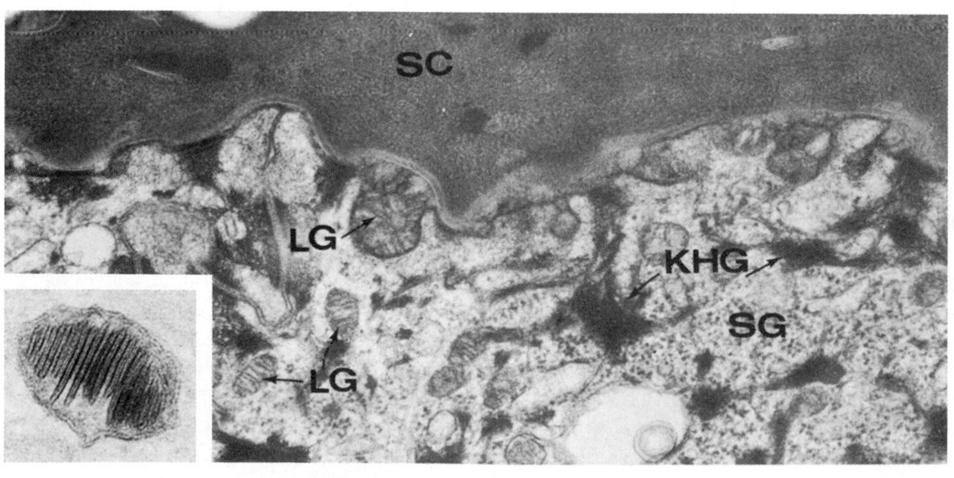

Junction of the stratum granulosum (SG) and stratum corneum (SC). Lamellar granules (LG) are in the intercellular space and cytoplasm of the granular cell. Keratohyalin granules (KHG) are also evident. *Inset:* Lamellar granule, ×28,750. (*From Holbrook K: Structure and Development of the Skin in Pathophysiology of Dermatologic Disease, edited by NA Soter, HP Baden. New York, McGraw-Hill, l991, 2nd edition, p 7, with permission. Inset courtesy of EC Wolff-Schreiner, MD.*)

THE GRANULAR LAYER This layer is characterized by the build-up of components necessary for the process of programmed cell death and formation of a superficial water-impermeable barrier.[13–15] The typical cytoplasmic organelles associated with an active synthetic metabolism are still evident within cells of the stratum granulosum, but the most apparent structures within these cells are the basophilic, keratohyalin granules (Figs. 6-3 and 6-6). Keratohyalin granules are composed primarily of an electron-dense protein, profilaggrin, and keratin intermediate filaments (Fig. 6-6). Loricrin, a protein of the cornified cell envelope (see below), is also found within the keratohyalin granule. Processing of the high-molecular-weight keratins by proteolysis and phosphorylation occurs in the granular layer, thus modifying K1 to K2 (65 kDa) and K10 to K11 (56 kDa).

Profilaggrin is a high molecular mass (>400 kDa), histidine-rich, polyphosphorylated intermediate filament-associated protein made up of tandem repeats of filaggrin monomers joined by small linker peptides. In humans, the 10 to 12 tandem repeats are polymorphic. Although in normal epidermis profilaggrin mRNA is evident only in the granular cell layer and mRNAs for the differentiation-specific keratins are expressed first in the spinous cells, in certain disease states the expression of these two sets of differentiation markers is similarly altered, suggesting some means of coordinate regulation. For example, in some forms of harlequin ichthyosis, there is a low level of expression of K1/K10 and an absence of filaggrin expression. In the restrictive dermopathies, there is similar downregulation of K1/K10 and abnormal structure of the keratohyalin granules.

Conversion of the profilaggrin precursor to oligomeric then monomeric filaggrin subunits occurs stepwise during the transition of a granular cell to a cornified cell by site-specific proteolysis, which involves at least three proteases, and by dephosphorylation. Final proteolysis of filaggrin monomers to free amino acids occurs in the outer layers of the stratum corneum (see below). This is thought to be important for regulation of epidermal osmolarity and flexibility.

The function of filaggrin in the granular cell is uncertain, but in the cornified cell it is thought to serve as the matrix protein that embeds and promotes the aggregation and disulfide bonding of keratin filaments (hence, the name "filaggrin" from *fil*ament *aggr*egation prote*in*) producing the "keratin pattern" structure of the lower cornified cells. The conversion of profilaggrin into its monomeric subunits must be carefully controlled to prevent premature intermediate filament aggregation.

Structural abnormalities in the keratohyalin granule, or the absence of the granules altogether, are histopathologic features of several keratinization disorders; these morphologic changes correlate with abnormalities in filaggrin expression. In many patients with ichthyosis vulgaris there is a marked reduction or an absence of keratohyalin granules, and filaggrin is correspondingly reduced or absent. The effect of this alteration on the organization of the stratum corneum is not substantial, suggesting that even minor amounts of filaggrin can promote keratin filament aggregation.

Other protein markers of keratinization are components of the cornified cell envelope (CE), a 7- to 15-nm thick, dense, protein layer deposited beneath the plasma membrane of cornified cells. Proteins of the CE constitute a significant fraction of the protein in the granular cell and are rendered insoluble by cross-linking via disulfide bonds and N^{ε}-(γ-glutamyl) lysine isopeptide bonds formed by transglutaminases. Involucrin, keratolinin (cystatin-α), loricrin, small proline-rich proteins (cornifin, SPR1, and SPR2), the serine proteinase inhibitor elafin (SKALP), filaggrin linker–segment peptide, and envoplakin have all been found as components of the CE.

Involucrin is an insoluble, 70- to 80-kDa, cysteine-rich protein, first synthesized in the cytoplasm of spinous cells; it becomes cross-linked by transglutaminase(s) in the granular layer into an insoluble cell boundary that is resistant to denaturing and reducing chemicals. Loricrin, a highly insoluble, sulfur- and glycine/serine-rich protein, is a later differentiation product; its mRNA is transcribed only in the uppermost spinous layer and throughout the granular layers. Loricrin is the major CE protein comprising approximately 75 percent of the total CE protein mass. Envoplakin, homologous to desmoplakin, may link the CE to desmosomes and to keratin filaments. The genes encoding loricrin, involucrin, and cornifin have been localized along with profilaggrin and trichohyalin genes to chromosome region 1q21, which may act as a functional cluster of genes. Although the envelope precursors are first synthesized in the spinous and/or granular layers, where they can be recognized biochemically and immunohistochemically, the CE is evident morphologically only in cornified cells. Current models propose that TGase 1 (see below) catalyzes cross-linking of involucrin at the plasma membrane and that less-abundant precursors such as cornifin, elafin, and the SPR proteins are added subsequently. The cytoplasmic surface of the CE is composed primarily of loricrin.

The calcium-requiring transglutaminases are present in all stratified epithelia and in hair follicles. There are three transglutaminases in the epidermis. TGase 1 (keratinocyte TGase) exists in membrane-associated, as well as soluble, full-length proteolytically processed, activated forms. Some TGase 1 activity is present in basal cells, but enzyme activity is especially prevalent in the granular layer of the epidermis. Its membrane-bound, processed form accounts for most of the activity in differentiating keratinocytes. TGase 2 is present in fetal epidermis and in the basal layer of the adult. Soluble TGase 2 appears to

be similar to tissue transglutaminase found in other cells and appears to play a role in apoptosis; it is an autoantigen reacting with dermatitis herpetiformis serum. TGase 3 (epidermal TGase) is expressed after early differentiation markers (e.g., K1 and K10) and coincident with loricrin and profilaggrin. It is less abundant than TGase 1 on the basis of mRNA levels but accounts for a relatively high proportion of epidermal TGase activity. It is clear that the soluble and particulate TGases in the epidermis are distinct, but their independent or coordinated roles in cross-linking the CE have not been fully resolved. How the various components of the CE interact and possibly cross-link with one another is a major area of investigation.

Mutations in the TGM1 gene have been shown to be the genetic basis of some cases of lamellar ichthyosis, an autosomal recessive genodermatosis characterized by large scales and a disruption in the uppermost differentiating layers of the epidermis. These findings underscore the importance of CE formation to the normal process of epidermal keratinization.

As described previously, lamellar granules are first evident in upper spinous layer cells, although their primary site of action is at the interface between the granular and cornified cell layers. In this position they aggregate in clusters, fuse with the plasma membrane, and release their contents into the intercellular space (see Fig. 6-6). The extruded material is stacked into discs, similar to the internal organization of the granule, and is rearranged in various stages, leading to the formation of sheets. The hydrolytic enzymes of the granules are released with the lipids and are involved in their reorganization and subsequent assembly into the intercellular lamellae. The change in morphology corresponds to the remodeling of the "probarrier" lipids (glycolipids, free sterols, and phospholipids) to "barrier" lipids (e.g., sphingolipids that create a hydrophobic seal at the interface between the granular and cornified layers). Epidermis treated with lipid solvents loses its barrier properties. This barrier reduces water loss from the skin and impedes the movement of polar compounds. Animals with an essential fatty acid deficiency have reduced numbers of lamellar granules, lack the barrier lipids, and demonstrate increased water loss from the skin. What triggers exocytosis of the lamellar granules at the granular-cornified interface or what prevents them from discharging their contents within the cell is not understood.

THE TRANSITION FROM A GRANULAR TO A CORNIFIED CELL

The granular cell not only synthesizes, modifies, and/or cross-links new proteins involved in keratinization, it also plays a role in its own programmed destruction. This occurs during the abrupt transition from a granular cell to a terminally differentiated cornified cell. The change involves the loss of the nucleus and virtually all of the cellular contents with the exception of the keratin filaments and filaggrin matrix. DNAse, RNAse, acid hydrolases, esterases, phosphatases, proteases, and plasminogen activator have been identified in the granular cell and implicated in degradation. Morphologic stages of nuclear destruction have been described and occur by an apoptotic mechanism. Individual cells that have characteristics of both granular and cornified cells are identified occasionally within the granular layer. The mechanism for the final dissolution of organelles and disposition of the degraded components is not yet understood, although it is apparent that nucleotides, some amino acids, ions, and trace elements are recovered and reutilized within the epidermis.

THE STRATUM CORNEUM Complete transition from a granular to a cornified cell is accompanied by a 45 to 86 percent loss in dry weight. The layers of resultant cornified, or horny, cells provide mechanical protection to the skin and a barrier to water loss and permeation of soluble substances from the environment (Figs. 6-2, 6-3, and 6-7).[13–16]

FIGURE 6-7

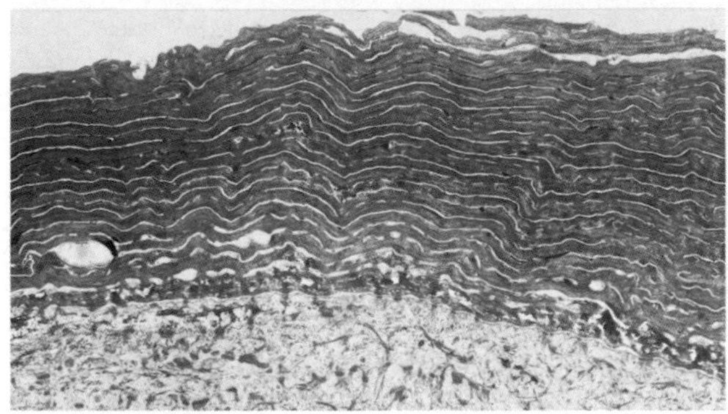

A.

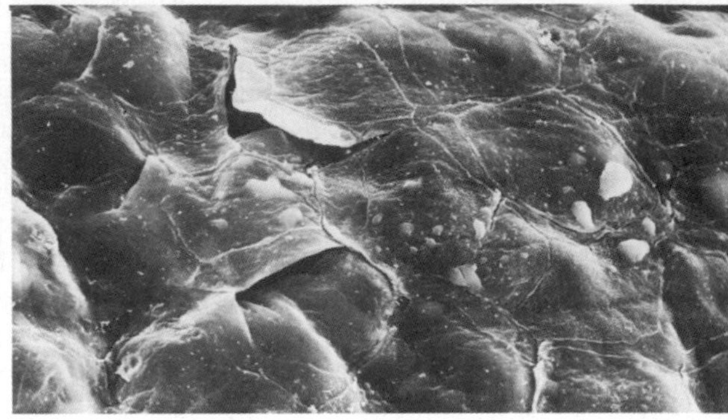

B.

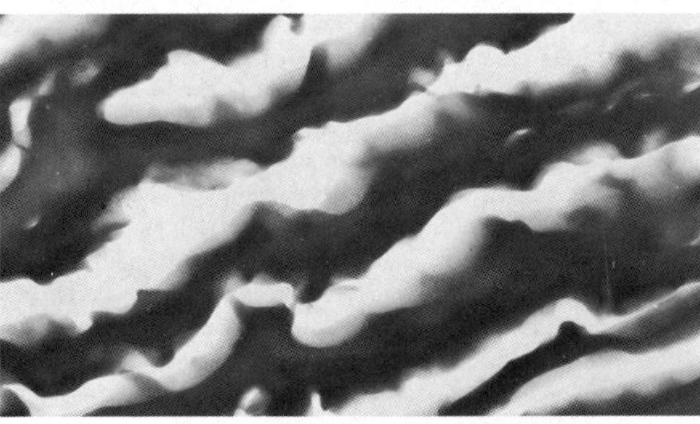

C.

Stratum corneum. Note the closely associated cell layers in the stratum corneum (*A*); the surface markings, thin and flattened shape, and overlapping margins of individual stratum corneum "squames" (*B*); and the interlocking contours of thickly sectioned frozen cornified cells (*C*). *A*, ×5050; *B*, ×450; *C*, ×15,000 in the original magnifications.

The stratum corneum barrier is formed by a two-compartment system of lipid-depleted protein-enriched corneocytes surrounded by a continuous extracellular lipid matrix. The flattened, polyhedral-shaped, horny cell is the largest cell of the epidermis (Fig. 6-7*B*). Its shape and surface features are adapted to maintain the integrity of the stratum corneum yet allow for desquamation (Fig. 6-7). High molecular mass keratins (>60 kDa), stabilized by intermolecular disulfide bonds, account for up to 80 percent of the cornified cell. The remainder of the cell content appears limited to an electron-dense matrix material, probably filaggrin, surrounding the filaments (Fig. 6-7*B*). The nucleus is lost from normal stratum corneum cells but it persists in incompletely keratinized cells (parakeratosis), as seen in psoriasis. Remnants of organelles, especially profiles of membranes and melanin pigment, are occasionally present within the normal cell. Membrane profiles can be particularly abundant in the stratum corneum of patients with excessive numbers of cornified layers, as seen in some of the ichthyoses and in acne. The lipid enrichment results from the deposition of lamellar body contents. Three key lipid types—cholesterol, ceramides, and free fatty acids—form the lamellar bilayers. Lamellar bodies are enriched with glycosphingolipids, phospholipids, cholesterol, and hydrolases. The metabolism and secretion of these contents results in the formation of the lamellar unit structure in the mid-stratum corneum.

Changes in the structure, composition, and function of cornified cells accompany their movement toward the outer surface of the skin. Cells of the deeper layers of the stratum corneum, sometimes called the stratum compactum, are thicker and have more densely packed, organized parallel arrays of keratin filaments, a more fragile cornified CE, and a greater variety of modifications for lateral cell-to-cell attachment [modified desmosomes (Fig. 6-7*A*)], as well as superior–inferior interlocking ridges and villi (Fig. 6-7*B* and *C*), when compared to cells of the outer cornified layers. The latter cell layers are prone to desquamation and thus are referred to as the stratum disjunctum (Fig. 6-7). Cells of the deeper cornified layers have less capacity for water-binding than the mid- and upper regions. Cells in the mid-stratum corneum have the highest concentration of free amino acids and, correspondingly, are able to bind water with greater efficiency. A rigid CE borders the outer stratum corneum cells. The protein composition of the fragile and rigid envelopes is identical; thus differences in the physical properties must reflect maturation of the envelope or perhaps a different association with membrane lipids. The desmosomes undergo proteolytic degradation in the outermost stratum corneum cells, which is one factor that allows individual corneocytes to be shed.

The stratum corneum cell retains some metabolic functions and thus is not the inert covering it has been previously considered. Lipid extraction or metabolic imbalances such as fatty acid deficiency perturb the barrier as well as resulting in epidermal hyperproliferation, scaling, and inflammation. Thus, aberrations in the stratum corneum may initiate skin diseases rather than be the end result of processes in subjacent cell layers.

Regulation of Epidermal Proliferation and Differentiation

Because the epidermis is a continually renewing tissue, its structure and function depend on several processes that must be initiated during development and continue throughout life. These processes include establishment and maintenance of relatively constant cell numbers; interactions between keratinocytes and immigrant cells; adhesion among neighboring keratinocytes, among basal keratinocytes and the basal lamina, among basal lamina and underlying dermis; and keratinocyte terminal differentiation to produce functional corneocytes. Many of the genes and regulatory pathways involved in these processes have been elucidated through tissue culture studies of human and mouse epidermal cells, in vivo studies, and, more recently, transgenic and gene-targeting studies in mice.

The dermis has well-known regulatory influences over epidermal morphogenesis and differentiation.[17] This was determined from studies using tissue recombinants prepared by annealing the epidermis from one source with specific characteristics (e.g., age, species, region) with dermis from another and evaluating the outcome of the recombined skin after it has been grafted to a nude mouse or allowed to differentiate in organ culture. Such experiments, typically performed with embryonic tissues, demonstrate that the thickness, architecture, and pattern of differentiation of the epidermis, and the pattern of the epidermally derived appendages that are formed, conform to the region of the body from which the dermis was obtained. Epidermal–dermal interactions are also critical for the maintenance of postnatal skin structure and function. This can be demonstrated directly and can be observed indirectly in pathologic skin. For example, hyperproliferative keratins are expressed in epidermis that is superficial to a dermal tumor; the extent of K6 and K16 expression correlates with the proximity of the epidermis to the tumor and the degree of tumor cellularity. The products of normal keratinocytes and fibroblasts are also modulated by their interactions. A mutual induction of paracrine growth factor gene expression is induced by coculture of epidermal and dermal cells. The epidermis and dermis also collaborate in the development of the epidermal appendages and in the dermal–epidermal junction (see below).

Integrins

Growth factors, cytokines, and neuropeptides act in concert with cell-cell and extracellular matrix influences to control epidermal homeostasis. An association of matrix molecules with basal keratinocytes through integrin receptors, a family of transmembrane glycoprotein matrix receptors,[18] is important. More than 20 integrin receptors are assembled as heterodimers from one α and one β subunit. The combination of the subunits generally specifies the binding ligand. In keratinocytes, integrins are most evident on basal cells where they are found typically at the sites of focal adhesions and hemidesmosomes. Keratinocytes express several integrins and they have been shown to be involved in a variety of functions important to skin homeostasis.[19,20] The predominant integrins are $\alpha_6\beta_4$, $\alpha_2\beta_1$, and $\alpha_3\beta_1$. The β_1 integrins are found concentrated around the lateral borders between neighboring keratinocytes, whereas $\alpha_6\beta_4$ is found on the basal surface associated with hemidesmosomes. During wound healing, de novo expression of $\alpha_5\beta_1$ and $\alpha_v\beta_6$ integrins, together with a redistribution of β_1 integrins, promotes keratinocyte migration on matrix molecules such as fibronectin. The integrins serve as a physical link and route of communication between matrix molecules, such as collagen, laminin, fibronectin, thrombospondin, and vitronectin, through the plasma membrane to the cytoskeleton of the keratinocyte. What was once thought to be a mechanism for cell anchorage has now been shown to be a route of bidirectional communication that can result in changes, for example, in gene expression, pH, and calcium fluxes. The physical association of basal keratinocytes with the basement membrane is thought to be important in maintaining the phenotype of the cell; separation of the cells from this substrate, the change of cell shape, and relationship to extracellular matrix molecules can induce the onset of terminal differentiation. In culture, it has been demonstrated that differentiating keratinocytes lose adhesiveness to types I and IV collagen, laminin, and fibronectin. Loss of adhesion to fibronectin per se precedes the loss of the integrin receptors for fibronectin. The signal that triggers the decline in ability of an integrin to bind ligand, and hence perhaps an early signal for keratinocyte differentiation, is not yet understood.

Growth Factors

As mentioned above, growth factors regulate epidermal growth and proliferation by autocrine and paracrine mechanisms.[21,22] Much of this evidence comes from studies of transgenic mice that overexpress various factors in the epidermis. Epidermal growth factor (EGF) and transforming growth factor (TGF)-α bind to the same tyrosine kinase activatable receptors on basal and immediately suprabasal epidermal cells to stimulate proliferation.[23] TGF-α is produced by keratinocytes, whereas EGF is synthesized elsewhere in the body. TGF-α is overexpressed in psoriasis and may contribute to the hyperproliferative component of the disease. Targeted overexpression of TGF-α in the mouse epidermis results in a phenotype of hyperplasia, hyperkeratosis, and the formation of spontaneous papillomas, suggesting a potential role of TGF-α in hyperproliferative disorders. Keratinocyte growth factor (KGF), a member of the fibroblast growth factor family, is a potent mitogen for keratinocytes and other epithelia. Although the transcripts for KGF in skin are found only in the dermis, the receptor for KGF is expressed on keratinocytes. Ectopic expression of KGF in the epidermis of transgenic mice results in epidermal thickening as well as regional loss of hair follicles.[24] Other growth factors suppress DNA synthesis and mitosis of keratinocytes and promote differentiation. Among these is TGF-β. The messages for TGF-β_1 and -β_2 are present in low levels in the keratinocytes of the upper epidermal layers but can be upregulated by TGF-β itself and by agents that promote differentiation, such as calcium and phorbol esters. TGF-β requires activation to be effective. Abnormal skin phenotypes in transgenic mice with either increased or decreased levels of functional TGF-β demonstrate that this pathway is part of the endogenous homeostatic regulatory machinery of the epidermis.[25]

Keratinocytes produce other growth factors and cytokines, some of which affect their own proliferation and migration and others of which act on other cells in the epidermis [e.g., basic fibroblast growth factor (bFGF) influences proliferation of melanocytes] and in the dermis [e.g., platelet-derived growth factor (PDGF) produced by keratinocytes is active only on cells in the dermis that bear PDGF receptors]. Dermal cells, in turn, synthesize products that act synergistically with molecules in the epidermis to promote or retard growth.

Cytokines (See Chap. 26)

Keratinocyte-derived cytokines, interleukin (IL)-1α, IL-6, IL-8, and granulocyte-macrophage colony-stimulating factor (GM-CSF) play a role in normal regulation of the epidermis, inflammatory processes, and wound repair in the skin.[26] IL-1α may also promote growth of cultured keratinocytes, an effect that is not implausible because keratinocytes express high affinity IL-1 receptors and thus are a target for autocrine regulation by this molecule.

Retinoids (See Chaps. 244 and 257)

Epidermal homeostasis is dependent on the interaction of several hormones and factors that control the balance between keratinocyte proliferation, differentiation, and apoptosis. One such factor is vitamin A and its derivative compounds and drugs (retinoids).[27] Retinoic acid (RA) can modulate the response of keratinocytes to mitogens and is a pleiotropic regulator of epidermal morphogenesis and differentiation. In the skin, a critical level of RA is necessary for normal morphogenesis and differentiation. The effects of retinoids on the skin in vivo can be appreciated from their use in treating disorders of keratinization and acne.

The diverse cellular effects of retinoids, in the skin and other tissues, result primarily from activation of different sets of responsive genes mediated by specific subtypes of receptors, the retinoic acid receptors (RARs) and retinoid X receptors (RXRs). RA has both positive and negative influences on keratinocyte differentiation that appear to be mediated primarily through the RARγ1 receptor, which is the major RAR subtype of the epidermis. Moreover, the effects of RA on keratinocytes depend on the RA concentration and on the state of the target cell. Micromolar concentrations of RA stimulate slowly growing keratinocytes and act as a mitogen for growth-arrested cells but inhibit proliferation of rapidly proliferating cells in vitro. There is also suppression of genes for differentiation-specific proteins such as K1/K10, filaggrin, and proteins of the cornified envelope when keratinocytes are treated in vitro. Consistent with the finding that the concentration of retinoids in the skin must be tightly controlled, both increased and decreased retinoid signaling can lead to aberrant differentiation in vivo. Long-term RA treatment in vivo results in epidermal hyperproliferation and a modified program of terminal differentiation,[28] whereas formation of an epidermis with compromised barrier function can also result from inactivation of retinoid signaling through expression of a dominant negative receptor.

Vitamin D_3 is another important factor that regulates keratinocyte homeostasis because the skin is both a synthetic and a target organ for vitamin D_3.[27,29] A specific receptor [vitamin D_3 receptor (VDR)], belonging to the same superfamily of nuclear hormone receptors as the retinoid receptors, has been identified in human skin. VDR forms heterodimers with RXR, allowing for crosstalk between these two signaling pathways. The active form of vitamin D_3, 1α,25$(OH)_2D_3$, regulates a decrease in keratinocyte proliferation and an increase in morphologic differentiation of cultured keratinocytes. These effects appear to occur through both changes in gene expression and nongenomic events such as increases in cytosolic calcium. Vitamin D_3 and synthetic analogs are being developed as new clinical tools. Calcipotriene has been studied most extensively and has been shown to be effective in the treatment of psoriasis.

Calcium

The role of calcium in regulating epidermal proliferation and differentiation[29,30] was revealed when it was shown that keratinocytes grown in a low-calcium medium (0.002 to 0.1 mmol Ca^{2+}) failed to stratify and differentiate. There is evidence for a profound effect of calcium on keratinocyte growth and differentiation both in vitro and in vivo. Low calcium stimulates proliferation, which is inhibited by high calcium concentrations in vitro. There is a calcium gradient in native epidermis, increasing from the basal to the upper granular layer. Calcium is required by the epidermis for desmosome formation and activation of enzymes such as transglutaminase. Its effect on differentiation appears to be more related to the block it creates to the establishment of normal tissue architecture than to the regulation of gene expression because a number of differentiation-specific markers are still expressed in cells grown in low-calcium medium. Changes in extracellular calcium levels have a profound and sustained effect on the intracellular calcium levels in normal cultured keratinocytes. The recent discovery that the molecular defects in Hailey-Hailey and Darier diseases are in calcium transporters also suggests that calcium homeostasis plays an important role in maintaining the structural integrity of keratinocytes and the epidermis.[31,32]

The complex interplay of extrinsic and intrinsic factors that regulates the proportion of proliferating and differentiating cells to maintain a constant epidermal thickness as cells desquamate is often perturbed in disease, such as psoriasis or carcinoma. In wound healing, an alteration in the various regulatory factors is essential and advantageous to bringing about enhanced proliferation for epithelial repair.

Apoptosis

Apoptosis, or programmed cell death, is a major cellular homeostatic mechanism in the skin that is affected by the hormones, growth factors, cytokines, and other factors discussed above. Apoptosis is a gene-directed, single-cell death that follows an orderly pattern of morphologic and biochemical changes.[33] Apoptosis functions in the skin in developmental remodeling, regulation of cell numbers, and defense against damaged, virus-infected, or transformed cells. There is evidence that terminal differentiation of the epidermal keratinocyte occurs by a modified apoptotic program that has evolved to adapt the keratinocyte to its specialized functions. As would be predicted for an important homeostatic mechanism, dysregulation of apoptosis has been documented in several diseases of the skin, both immune mediated and genetic, and in skin tumors. Another well-documented occurrence of apoptosis is the formation of the sunburn cell, a typical apoptotic keratinocyte that can be detected in the epidermis following exposure to ultraviolet light. Apoptosis also plays an important role in the hair follicle growth cycle. The mechanism of catagen appears to be related to the onset of apoptosis in the proliferative cells of the hair bulb.

Many studies have focused on the regulatory mechanism of apoptosis because of the obvious significance of the existence of a genetically controlled form of cell death. The skin promises to be one of the primary targets for the generation of new therapeutic strategies to regulate apoptosis because of its widespread occurrence in the skin and the already well-defined pathways controlling epidermal homeostasis.

NONKERATINOCYTES OF THE EPIDERMIS

Melanocytes (See Chap. 11)

The melanocyte is a dendritic, pigment-synthesizing cell derived from neural crest that is confined mainly to the basal layer.[34] In postnatal skin, the cell body of the melanocyte often extends toward the dermis below the level of the basal cell, but always superior to the lamina densa (see Fig. 6-4). Melanocyte processes contact keratinocytes in basal and more superficial layers but do not form junctions with them at any level. Melanocytes are recognized light microscopically by their pale-staining cytoplasm, ovoid nucleus, and the intrinsic color of the pigment-containing melanosomes. Differentiation of the melanocyte correlates with the acquisition of its primary functions: melanogenesis, arborization, and transfer of pigment to keratinocytes.

The melanosome is the distinctive organelle of the melanocyte (Fig. 6-4, inset). It is resolved at the ultrastructural level as an ovoid, membrane-bound structure within which a series of receptor-mediated, hormone-stimulated, enzyme-catalyzed reactions produce melanin. Four different stages (I to IV) of melanosome structure correlate with the degree of melanization. Melanosomes that are involved in the synthesis of brown or black eumelanin are elliptical and have an internal organization of longitudinally-oriented, concentric lamellae; melanosomes that synthesize red or yellow pheomelanin pigments have a spheroidal shape and a microvesicular internal structure. The size of melanosomes is determined genetically; black skin typically contains larger melanosomes than more lightly pigmented skins.

There are important organizational relationships and functional interactions between keratinocytes and melanocytes that the melanocyte depends on for differentiation and function.[35] Approximately 36 basal and suprabasal keratinocytes are thought to coexist functionally with each melanocyte in an epidermal melanin unit, an organizational system that is mimicked in vitro when the two cell types are cocultured. Within this aggregate, melanocytes transfer pigment to associated keratinocytes. As a result, pigment is distributed throughout the basal layer and, to a lesser extent, the more superficial layers where it protects the skin by absorbing and scattering potentially harmful radiation. Once within the keratinocyte, melanosomes exist either individually or in membrane-bound aggregates (melanosome complexes). The distribution of melanosomes within the keratinocyte varies with race (see Chap. 11). Melanosomes within keratinocytes are degraded by lysosomal enzymes as the cells differentiate and move upward. A few melanosomes may still be recognized in the stratum corneum, but these are usually no longer enclosed by a membrane.

The keratinocytes produce soluble factors that regulate melanocyte proliferation, dendricity, and melanization. These phenomena have been observed in cocultures in vitro where undifferentiated and proliferating keratinocytes maintain continuous growth control over melanocytes. Keratinocytes produce growth factors that are mitogenic for melanocytes (e.g., bFGF and TGF-α), but also produce growth inhibitory factors (IL-1, IL-6, TGF-β). Keratinocytes, but not keratinocyte-conditioned medium, induce a dendritic phenotype in melanocytes. The balance between negative and positive regulatory mechanisms involving the keratinocyte requires further investigation. Proliferation of melanocytes and their dendrites, melanogenesis, as well as transfer of pigment also rely on hormonal control (melanocyte-stimulating hormone, agouti signal protein, sex hormones), inflammatory mediators, and vitamin D_3 synthesized within the epidermis.

Merkel Cells

Merkel cells are slow-adapting, type I mechanoreceptors located in sites of high tactile sensitivity. They are present among basal keratinocytes in particular regions of the body[36,37] (Fig. 6-8), and join with them by desmosomal junctions. Merkel cells receive stimuli as keratinocytes are deformed and respond by secretion of chemical transmitters. They are found both in hairy skin and in the glabrous skin of the digits, lips, regions of the oral cavity, and the outer root sheath of the hair follicle. In some of these sites, they are assembled in specialized structures called tactile discs or touch domes. Like other nonkeratinocytes, Merkel cells have a pale-staining cytoplasm. The nucleus is lobulated, and the margins of cells project cytoplasmic "spines" toward keratinocytes. Immunohistochemical markers of the Merkel cell include K18, K8,

FIGURE 6-8

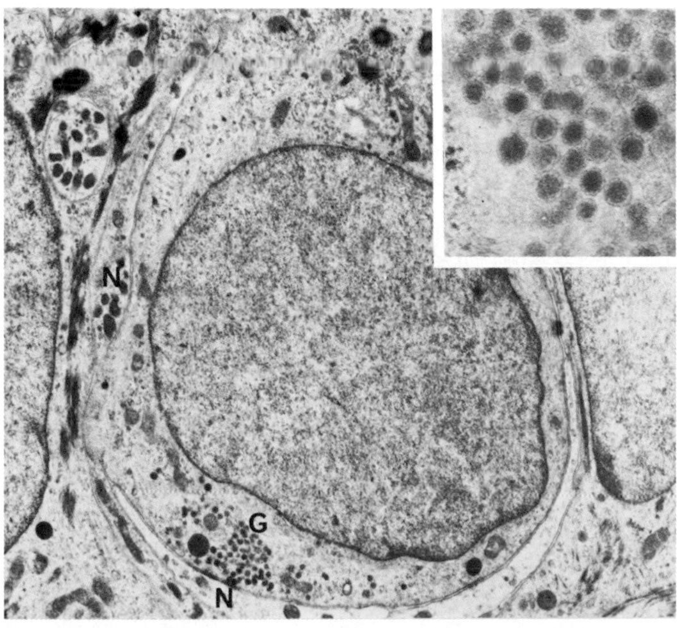

Merkel cell from the finger of a 130-mm CR (crown-rump) 21-week human fetus. Note nerve (N) in direct contact with the lateral and basal of the cell and dense core cytoplasmic granules (G). ×13,925. *Inset:* Merkel cell granules, ×61,450.

K19, and K20 keratin peptides. Keratin 20 is restricted to Merkel cells in the skin and thus may be the most reliable marker.

Merkel cells make synaptic contacts with nerve endings to form the Merkel cell–neurite complex. The cells are easily identified at the ultrastructural level by the 80- to 200-nm diameter, membrane-bounded, dense-core granules that collect opposite the Golgi and proximal to an unmyelinated neurite (Fig. 6-8); the granules are a constant feature of the cell, but the neurite is not always present. The structure of the granule is similar to neurosecretory granules in neurons; they form in the Golgi in the manner of a secretory granule and contain neurotransmitter-like substances and markers of neuroendocrine cells, including metenkephalin, vasoactive intestinal peptide, chromogranin A, acetylcholine, calcitonin gene-related peptide, neuron-specific enolase, and synaptophysin. The granules are also stained positively with the uranaffin reaction, which recognizes amine-storing granules in other neuroendocrine cells, as well as the Merkel cell.

New evidence suggests that Merkel cells are the mechanoreceptors while the nerve terminals transduce the transient phase. The morphology of the contacting membranes of both the Merkel cell and neurite are similar to the pre- and postsynaptic modifications that are characteristic of a synapse. Moreover the presence of neurotransmitter-like substances in the dense core granules suggests that the Merkel cell is the receptor that transmits a stimulus to the neurite via a chemical synapse. Merkel cells may function as targets for the anchorage of nerve endings during embryonic and fetal development, as a stimulus for such fibers to branch or they may participate in induction or alignment of the arrector pili muscles associated with the pilosebaceous unit. Merkel cell neoplasms are discussed in Chap. 86.

The Langerhans Cell: A Nonkeratinocyte Localized in Suprabasal Epidermal Layers (See Chap. 23)

Langerhans cells are bone marrow–derived, antigen-processing and -presenting cells that are involved in a variety of T cell responses.[38] The Langerhans cell is not unique to the epidermis; it is found in other squamous epithelia, including the oral cavity, esophagus, and vagina; in lymphoid organs such as the spleen, thymus, and lymph node; and in the normal dermis.

The life cycle of the Langerhans cells is characterized by two distinct stages. Langerhans cells in the epidermis can ingest and process antigens efficiently but are weak stimulators of unprimed T cells. Activated Langerhans cells that have been induced to migrate after contact with antigen are not phagocytic but are potent stimulators of naïve T cells. They account for 2 to 8 percent of the total epidermal cell population. Like melanocytes, Langerhans cells are dendritic and do not form junctions with any of the cells they appose (Figs. 6-9 and 6-10). They are distributed in the basal, spinous, and granular layers, showing a preference for a suprabasal position. In histologic preparations, Langerhans cells are pale-staining and have convoluted nuclei.

The cytoplasm of the Langerhans cells, as seen by electron microscopy, contains dispersed vimentin intermediate filaments, and small rod- or racket-shaped structures called Langerhans cell granules or Birbeck granules (Fig. 6-10). Serial reconstruction of the Langerhans cell granule shows that it is a cup-shaped disc. The Langerhans cell granule forms when membrane-bound antigen is internalized by endocytosis. Phagolysosomes are common in the cytoplasm of the Langerhans cell. They contain enzymes similar to those of the macrophage and often include particulate material such as melanosomes.

Langerhans cells migrate from the bone marrow to the circulation into the epidermis early in embryonic development and continue to repopulate the epidermis throughout life. A number of the markers expressed by the Langerhans cell are characteristic for other cells of

FIGURE 6-9

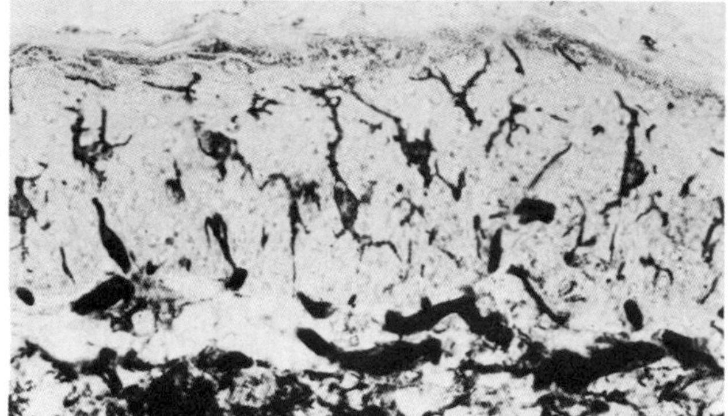

A.

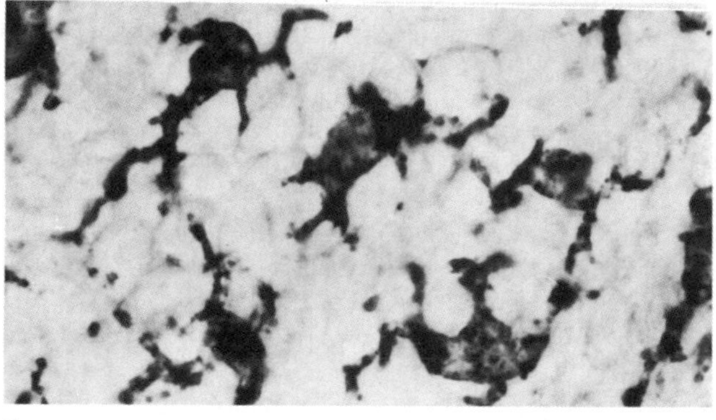

B.

A. Light micrographs of Langerhans cells, as revealed by ATPase staining, in vertical section of epidermis. *B.* Langerhans cells are seen at higher magnification in an isolated epidermal sheet viewed from the dermal side. Note the density and dendritic shape of this nonkeratinocyte population within the epithelium.

the monocyte–macrophage lineage and provide some insight into their function. In vitro studies demonstrate that dendritic cells can differentiate from a number of progenitor cells. Their maturation can be followed by measuring the expression of certain cell-surface molecules, such as cutaneous lymphocyte-associated antigen (CLA), E-cadherin, $\alpha_6\beta_4$ integrin, very-late-activation antigens (VLAs), CD44, integrins of the CD11/CD18 class, as well as intercellular adhesion molecule (ICAM)-1, ICAM-3, and LFA-3. These molecules serve not only as markers of differentiation, but also have a role in Langerhans cell trafficking, adhesion, and costimulation.

Langerhans cells are the primary cells in the epidermis responsible for the recognition, uptake, processing, and presentation of soluble antigen and haptens to sensitized T lymphocytes, and are implicated in the pathologic mechanisms underlying allergic contact dermatitis, cutaneous leishmaniasis, and human immunodeficiency virus infection. They are reduced in the epidermis of patients with certain skin diseases (e.g., psoriasis, sarcoidosis, contact dermatitis) and are impaired functionally by ultraviolet radiation; following UVB irradiation, there is a decrease in the ability of Langerhans cells to present antigen, a decreased production of cytokines (e.g., IL-10 and *cis*-urocanic acid) by keratinocytes, and a depletion in Langerhans cell numbers. Thus, UVB irradiation results in an overall diminished capacity for immune surveillance.

Because of their effectiveness in antigen presentation and lymphocyte stimulation, dendritic cells and Langerhans cells have become prospective vehicles for tumor therapy and tumor vaccines. The principle behind such strategies is to load dendritic cells with tumor-specific antigens, which will then stimulate the host immune response to mount an antigen-specific (and therefore tumor-specific response).

THE DERMAL–EPIDERMAL JUNCTION

(See Chap. 16)

The dermal–epidermal junction (DEJ) is a basement membrane zone that forms the interface between the epidermis and dermis (Fig. 6-11).[39,40] The major function of the DEJ is to attach the epidermis and dermis to each other and to provide resistance against external shearing forces. It serves as a support for the epidermis, determines the polarity of growth, directs the organization of the cytoskeleton in basal cells, provides developmental signals, and serves as a semipenetrable barrier. The structures of the DEJ are almost entirely products of basal keratinocytes, with minor contributions from dermal fibroblasts.

The DEJ can be subdivided into three supramolecular networks: the hemidesmosome–anchoring filament complex, the basement membrane itself, and the anchoring fibrils. The localization of antigens, determination of composition, and the known affinities of some of the matrix molecules present in the basement membrane zone for other matrix molecules (e.g., laminin, entactin/nidogen, and type IV collagen) are the basis for the structural models of this region of the skin and define its function and physical properties. The subdivisions coincide with areas of weakness that can result in dermal–epidermal separation under circumstances of physical stress, genetic disease, an autoimmune process, or trauma.

The hemidesmosome–anchoring filament complex binds basal keratinocytes to the basement membrane. The hemidesmosome has cytoplasmic, membranous, and extracellular components, which have been well characterized. Keratin intermediate filaments insert into the plaque portion (Fig. 6-11), which consists of bullous pemphigoid antigen 230 (BP230; BPAg-1) and plectin. The transmembrane component consists of bullous pemphigoid antigen 180 (BP180; BPAg-2; collagen XVII) and $\alpha_6\beta_4$ integrin. The extracellular domain of BP180 has been localized to the extracellular space beneath the hemidesmosome—the lamina lucida—and has been identified as a type XVII collagen. The intracellular domain of BP180 is localized in the hemidesmosomal plaque. The extracellular matrix components of the hemidesmosome are the subbasal dense plate (Fig. 6-11) and the anchoring filaments. Anchoring filaments originate at hemidesmosomes and insert into the lamina densa. The major component of these filaments is laminin 5 (previously referred to as GB3 antigen, nicein, BM600, kalinin, and epiligrin), which is localized mainly to the lamina densa and the lower lamina lucida and is associated with $\alpha_6\beta_4$ in hemidesmosomes. Laminin-5 consists of three subunits encoded by the genes LAMA3, LAMB3, and LAMC2.

The importance of these structures and molecules in maintaining the integrity of the skin can be surmised from inherited and acquired diseases of the skin in which they are either destroyed, altered, or absent, thereby resulting in dermal–epidermal separation.[41] A similar, although more superficial blistering within the plane of the basal epidermal layer, occurs in patients with the various forms of epidermolysis bullosa simplex caused by mutations in genes that code for the K5 and/or K14 basal cell keratins or other structural proteins specific for this layer (see Chaps. 65 and 66).

The lamina lucida (Fig. 6-11) is the primary location of several noncollagenous glycoproteins: laminins, entactin/nidogen, and fibronectin.[39] Because these molecules self-aggregate (e.g., entactin/nidogen), bind to other matrix molecules (e.g., laminin–entactin/

nidogen, laminin-type IV collagen, and laminin-perlecan) and to cells (e.g., fibronectin, laminin, entactin/nidogen), they are all important in promoting adhesion between the epidermal cell and the lamina densa. Based on structural analysis of the component proteins, a scheme for the supramolecular assembly of the basement membrane has been put forth. This model integrates the role of laminins and their interactions with nidogen, perlecan, and type IV collagen. The lamina lucida appears to be the weakest zone of the DEJ. It separates easily with heat and suction, with treatment with salt solutions and proteolytic enzymes, and in disease.

Type IV collagen is the primary component of the lamina densa. It is a nonbanded, network-forming collagen synthesized by keratinocytes that provides structural support and flexibility to this layer. Type V collagen is codistributed with type IV collagen in the DEJ but not in all basement membranes. Sulfated proteoglycans associated with the lamina densa probably assist in regulating permeability by restricting the passage of cationic macromolecules. Laminin is also within the lamina densa.

The lamina densa functions as a barrier/filter that restricts passage of molecules with a molecular mass ≥40 kDa, but it is penetrated by melanocytes and Langerhans cells during development and, postnatally, by large molecules such as type VII collagen and by neurites associated with Merkel cells; lymphocytes also enter the epidermis in certain inflammatory conditions. It is not clear how penetration occurs in these instances, although cells of invasive carcinomas appear capable of local proteolysis of the lamina densa, in some situations through the production of a type IV collagenase. Repair and remodeling of the DEJ occurs at sites of tissue damage, often in an overly compensated manner recognized ultrastructurally as reduplicated regions of lamina densa. The cause for this excessive synthesis of lamina densa is unclear but probably relates to the stimulatory role of cytokines in promoting synthesis by the epidermis in inflammatory situations.

FIGURE 6-10

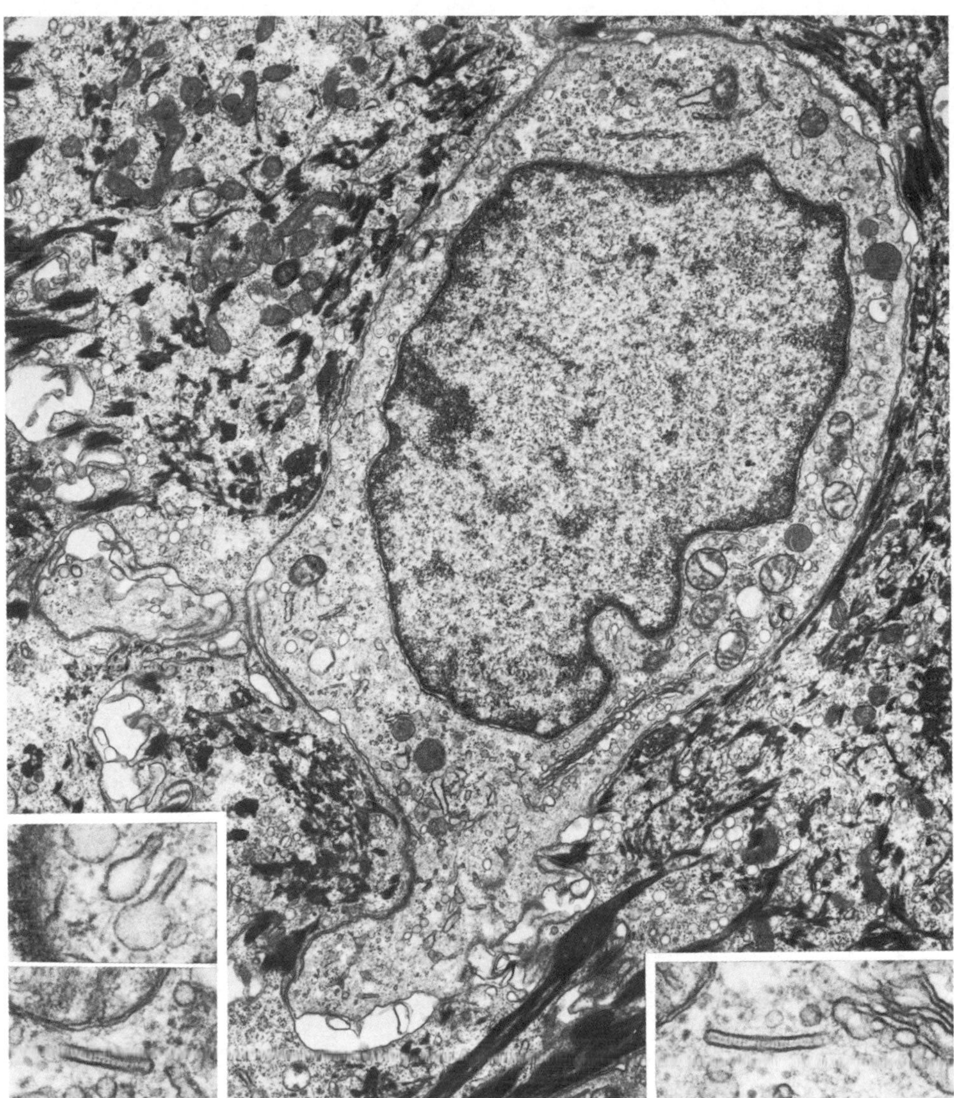

Langerhans cell. Note indented nucleus, rod- and racket-shaped cytoplasmic granules (see also insets), lysosomes, and absence of keratin filaments characteristic of surrounding keratinocytes. ×13,200. *Inset:* Birbeck granules, ×88,000. (*Courtesy of N. Romani, MD.*)

Anchoring fibrils are broad (20 to 60 nm), elongated (200 to 800 nm), flexible, banded, fibrillar structures that originate at the lamina densa and extend into the dermis. The fibrillar portions of anchoring fibrils have the morphologic appearance of collagen fibrils and have been shown to be composed of parallel bundles of end-to-end dimers of type VII collagen molecules, which have the longest helical domains of all collagen molecules and are synthesized primarily by the epidermal keratinocyte.

The anchoring fibrils penetrate into the deepest zone of the DEJ, the sublamina densa region or reticular lamina. Interstitial collagens (types I, III, V, and VI) and procollagens (types I and III) are present in this zone. In addition, the first fibers of the elastic fiber system are organized and probably form part of the complex that anchors the epidermis to the dermis through the basement membrane zone. The oxytalan fibers are bundles of the microfibrillary components of the elastic fibers. They originate from the lamina densa and insert into the planar networks of elaunin elastic fibers organized at the junction between papillary and reticular dermis. Oxytalan fibers are coated with soluble elastin (rather than the cross-linked, insoluble elastin of the mature elastic fibers); they are flexible integrating elements that accommodate deformation of the skin without compromise to structural integrity. The appearance of these fibers in electron micrographs suggests that they can exert tension on the epidermis.

THE DERMIS (See Chaps. 14 and 15)

The dermis is an integrated system of fibrous, filamentous, and amorphous connective tissue that accommodates nerve and vascular networks, epidermally derived appendages, fibroblasts, macrophages, and

FIGURE 6-11

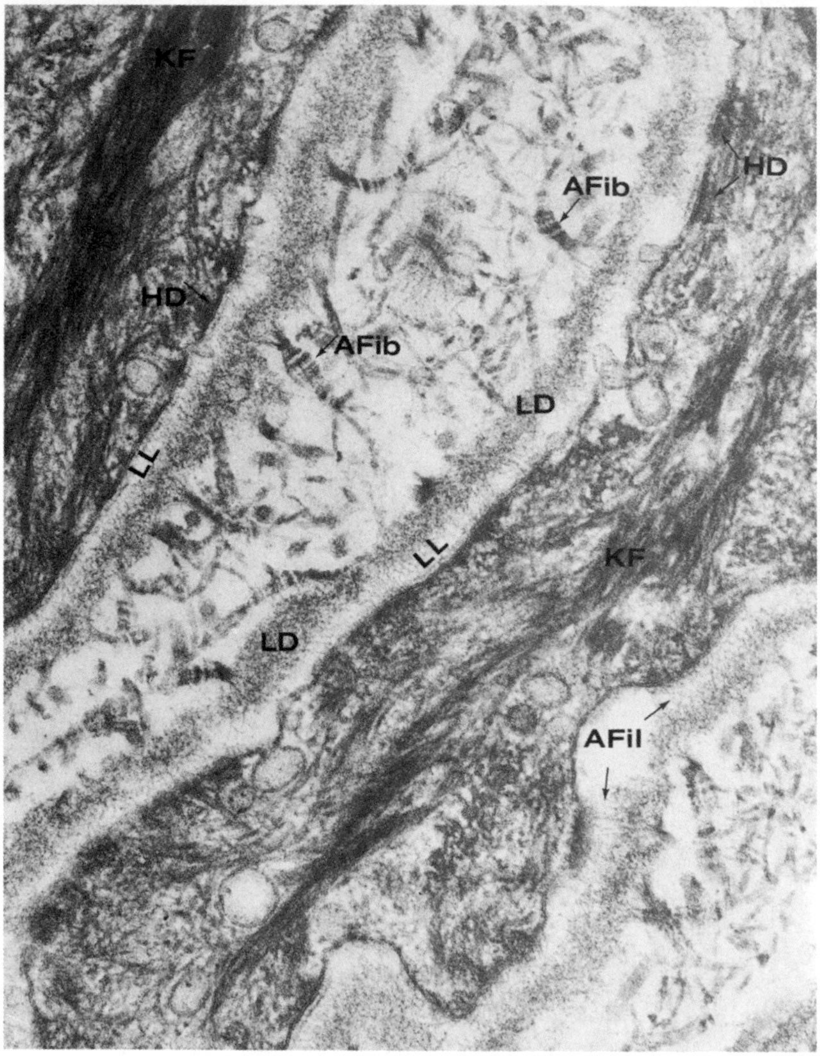

Structure of the dermal-epidermal junction. Tongues of basal keratinocytes contain keratin filaments (KFs). Some of them insert into hemidesmosomes (HD). The lamina lucida (LL) is spanned by anchoring filaments (AFil). Banded anchoring fibrils (AFib) extend into the papillary dermis from the lamina densa (LD). ×71,250 in the original magnification.

mast cells, and other blood-borne cells, including lymphocytes, plasma cells, and other leukocytes, that enter the dermis in response to various stimuli. The dermis makes up the bulk of the skin and provides its pliability, elasticity, and tensile strength. It protects the body from mechanical injury, binds water, aids in thermal regulation, and includes receptors of sensory stimuli. The dermis interacts with the epidermis in maintaining the properties of both tissues,[42] collaborates during development in the morphogenesis of the DEJ and epidermal appendages (teeth, nails, pilosebaceous structures, and sweat glands) and interacts in repairing and remodeling the skin as wounds are healed.

Connective Tissue Matrix of the Dermis

Collagen and elastic connective tissue are the main types of fibrous connective tissue of the dermis (Fig. 6-12). The properties of the matrix molecules themselves and their supramolecular organization into fibrous elements and assembly and integration into an interwoven fabric provide the mechanical properties of the dermis. Other nonfibrous, connective tissue molecules include finely filamentous glycoproteins and the proteoglycans (PGs) and glycosaminoglycans (GAGs) of the "ground substance." The biochemistry of these connective tissue molecules is the topic of subsequent chapters, but each matrix component is introduced in the present chapter in order to reveal the properties and interactions that regulate normal dermal architecture.

COLLAGENOUS CONNECTIVE TISSUE Collagen is the major dermal constituent.[43] It accounts for approximately 75 percent of the dry weight of the skin, and provides both tensile strength and elasticity. The periodically banded, interstitial collagens (types I, III, and V) account for the greatest proportion of the collagen in adult dermis (Fig. 6-12). Approximately 80 to 90 percent of the collagen is type I collagen and 8 to 12 percent is type III collagen. Type V collagen, although less than 5 percent, codistributes and assembles into fibrils with both types I and III collagen in which it is believed to assist in regulating fibril diameter. Type V collagen is polymorphic in structure (granules, filaments) and has been immunolocalized primarily to the papillary dermis and the matrix surrounding basement membranes of vessels, nerves, and epidermal appendages, and at the DEJ. Type VI collagen is abundant throughout the dermis, associated with fibrils and in the interfibrillar spaces, where it can organize into a variety of forms including fine, beaded filaments. Because of its early appearance during development, it is thought to organize the matrix as it is becoming established. Type IV collagen in the skin is confined to the basal lamina of the DEJ, vessels, and epidermal appendages. Type VII collagen forms anchoring fibrils at the DEJ (see above) that interdigitate with the interstitial collagen fibrils in the papillary dermis. Types I and III procollagen molecules and minor collagens, such as $\alpha 1$(I) trimer, are also present in normal dermis.

More than 20 genetically distinct collagens exist in animal tissues. These molecules are composed of three chains that vary according to the collagen type; all chains have a helical domain consisting of (Gly-X-Y)$_n$ repeats, where X and Y are typically proline and hydroxyproline, and globular terminal domains. The chains are glycosylated, assemble into soluble procollagen molecules, and undergo interchain bonding within the rough endoplasmic reticulum. They are then secreted into the extracellular space. Outside of the cell, the amino and carboxyl termini are cleaved proteolytically by collagen metalloproteinases, the molecules align in various patterns (e.g., a staggered array for types I and III collagen molecules, a chicken wire–like network for type IV collagen molecules, and antiparallel dimers for type VII collagen molecules), and are cross-linked. The result is the formation of banded collagen fibrils, filaments, and networks visible by light and electron microscopy. A number of factors such as the physical and chemical properties of the collagen molecules themselves and the interaction in the extracellular space of collagen molecules with proteoglycans and other proteins, including other collagens, influence the assembly of the molecules into fibrils.

ELASTIC CONNECTIVE TISSUE The elastic connective tissue is a complex macromolecular mesh,[44,45] assembled in a continuous network that extends from the lamina densa of the DEJ throughout the dermis and into the connective tissue of the hypodermis. Its organization and

FIGURE 6-12

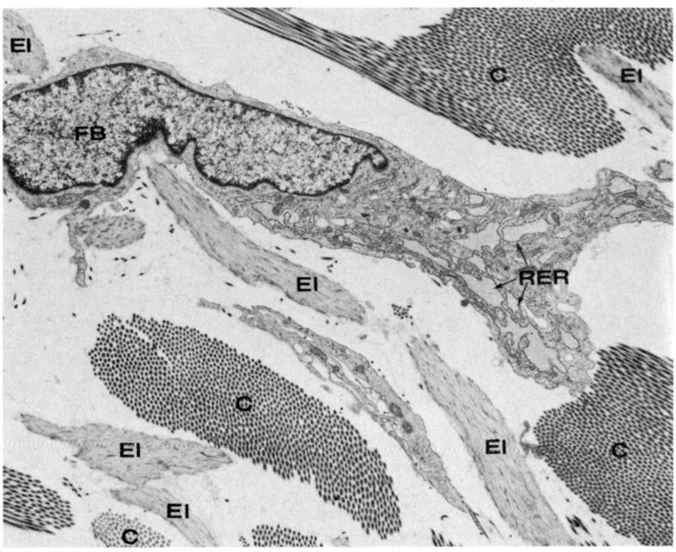

Human dermal fibroblast (FB) and collagen (C) and elastic (El) connective extracellular connective tissue of the extracellular matrix. Note dilation of the rough endoplasmic reticulum (RER). ×5500 in the original magnification. (*From Smith et al., Structure of the dermal matrix during development and in the adult. J. Invest Dermatol 79:93s, 1982, with permission.*)

FIGURE 6-13

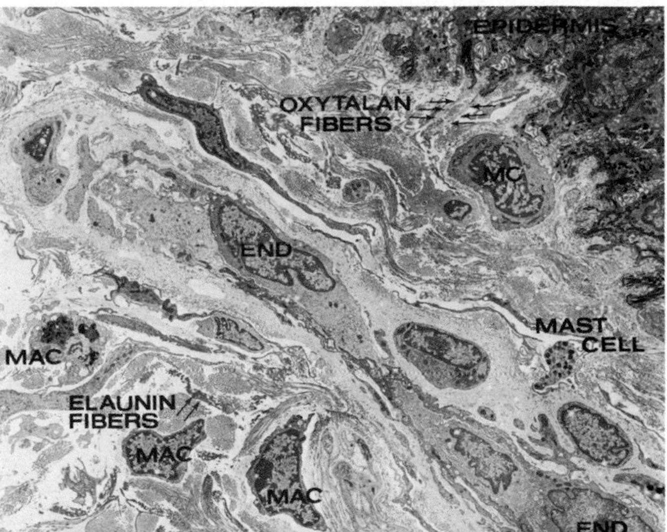

Postcapillary venule of the subpapillary plexus. Note the characteristic rings of basal lamina. Immature elastic fibers (oxytalan and elaunin) are seen above and below the vessel respectively; a melanocyte (MC) bulges down from the epidermis, and a small unmyelinated nerve is subjacent to the vessel. Macrophages (MAC) are seen between the fibrous components. END, endothelial cell. ×3950 in the original magnification.

importance in the dermis is best appreciated when examining samples of skin that have been digested to remove the collagen and other structures of the dermis, but retain the extraordinarily stable elastic fibers. Elastic fibers return the skin to its normal configuration after being stretched or deformed. Elastic fibers are also present in the walls of cutaneous blood vessels and lymphatics and in the sheaths of hair follicles. By dry weight, elastic connective tissue accounts for approximately 4 percent of the dermal matrix protein.

The sequence of elastogenesis is initiated with the synthesis and deposition of microfibrils in a pattern that establishes the position of the elastic fibers. Elastin is then deposited, in variable quantities, on the microfibrillar framework according to the region of the dermis. Mature elastic fibers contain as much as 90 percent elastin; microfibrils are embedded within and collected on the surface of the elastin matrix. Elaunin fibers have an intermediate amount of insoluble, cross-linked elastin (Fig. 6-13). Oxytalan, elaunin, and mature elastic fibers occur in order progressively beginning at the DEJ.

Elastic fibers have microfibrillar and amorphous matrix components (see Fig. 6-12). Several glycoproteins have been identified as constituents of the microfibrils. Among the most characterized of these molecules is fibrillin, a 350-kDa molecule. Mutations in fibrillin have been identified in patients with Marfan's syndrome, an inherited connective-tissue disease in which patients frequently die of an aneurysm in the aorta. Aberrant elastic laminae in the vessel wall may not provide sufficient strength to support the vessel. Elastin, the elastic fiber matrix component, is processed from a secreted, soluble, precursor tropoelastin molecule that is rich in hydrophobic amino acids. Intermolecular, covalent, desmosine cross-links form between four lysyl residues of the tropoelastin molecules to provide exceptional stability and insolubility to the molecule.

The oxytalan fibers extend perpendicularly from the DEJ to the junction between the papillary and reticular dermis, where they merge with the horizontal network of elaunin fibers. Oxytalan fibers are flexible integrating elements that accommodate deformation of the skin without compromise to structural integrity. In turn, the elaunin fibers evolve into the network of mature elastic fibers that extends throughout the reticular dermis. Elastic fibers are positioned between bundles of collagen fibers (Fig. 6-14*C*) except in certain pathologic conditions (e.g., the Buschke-Ollendorff syndrome) where both elastic and collagen fibers are assembled within the same bundle. Cloning and molecular analyses have demonstrated that a variety of well-characterized syndromes involving the skin, as well as cardiovascular, nervous, and/or musculoskeletal systems, result from mutations in genes encoding components of the elastic fiber network. Elastic fibers, which turn over very slowly in the skin, are also damaged by solar radiation and become dysmorphic with aging.[46]

The Diffuse and Filamentous Dermal Matrix

(See Chap. 18)

Several filamentous or amorphous matrix components are present in the dermis between the fibrous matrix elements, associated with the fibers themselves, organized on the surfaces of cells, and in basement membranes. PGs and glycosaminoglycans are the molecules of the "ground substance" that surrounds and embeds the fibrous components.[47,48] They can account for up to 0.2 percent dry weight of the dermis. PGs are unusually large molecules (100 to 2500 kDa) consisting of a core protein that is specific for the molecule and that determines which GAGs will be incorporated into the molecule. Hyaluronic acid (hyaluronan) usually binds to the core protein. The PGs/GAGs can bind up to 1000 times their own volume and thus regulate the water-binding capabilities of the dermis and influence dermal volume and compressibility; they also bind growth factors (e.g., bFGF) and link cells with the fibrillar and filamentous matrix, thereby influencing proliferation, differentiation, tissue repair, and morphogenesis. They are components of basement membranes and are present on surfaces of mesenchymal and epithelial cells.

FIGURE 6-14

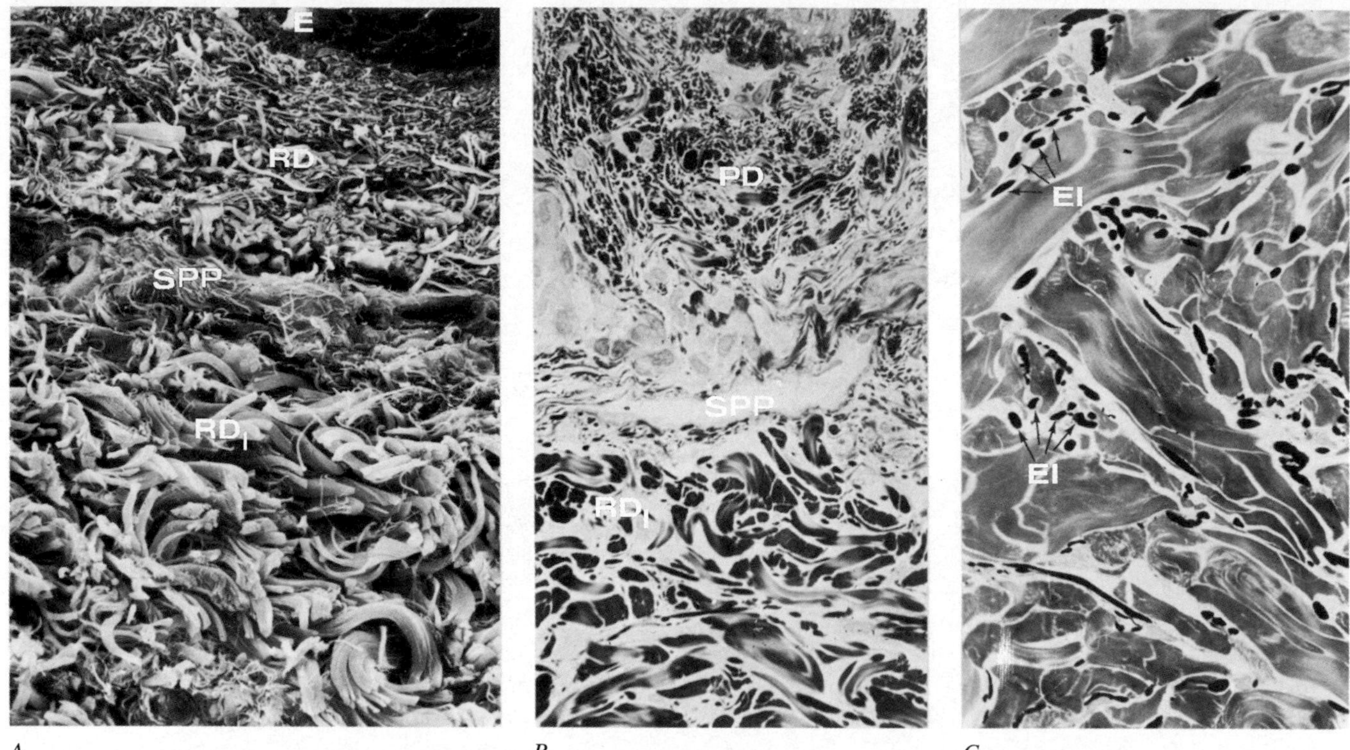

Papillary (PD) and reticular (RD) dermis shown in scanning electron (*A*) and light (*B*, *C*) micrographs. In *A*, the fine PD network is seen beneath the epidermis (E) extending to a vascular boundary created by vessels of the subpapillary plexus (SPP) as shown in *B*. The upper portion of the reticular dermis (RD1) has smaller collagen bundles than the deep reticular dermis. Elastic fibers (E1) border the collagen bundles. *A*, ×525; *B*, ×300; *C*, ×700 in the original magnifications.

The major PGs in the adult dermis are chondroitin sulfates/dermatan sulfate (biglycan, decorin, versican), heparan/heparan sulfate proteoglycans (HSPGs; perlecan, syndecan), and chondroitin-6 sulfate proteoglycans (CSPGs; components of the DEJ). The small dermatan sulfate molecule called PGII, or decorin, is more abundant in the papillary layer of the dermis than the reticular layer. It binds through its core protein to type I collagen where it may influence the lateral growth of fibrils. Versican is a large CSPG found in both papillary and reticular layers of the dermis and is thought to be associated with the microfilaments of the elastic network. HSPGs bind and influence the function of multiple effector molecules (growth factors, cytokines, extracellular matrix, proteases). Syndecan-4, induced in neonatal but not fetal wounds, may be responsible for inflammation and fibrosis.[49] Hyaluronan exists in the dermis as a free GAG and as a component of PGs, although it is much more abundant in fetal dermis where its presence is associated with a more watery, less stable matrix that permits cells to move freely within the tissue. As the dermis matures, the matrix is stabilized by a greater predominance of sulfated GAGs, although rises in hyaluronan are seen in wound healing and other situations analogous to development in which migration of cells is essential to the repair process. Age-related changes in proteoglycan composition of the adult dermis typically occur after age 40 years and involve increases in dermatan sulfate, but decreases in chondroitin-6 sulfate from the basal lamina and native chondroitin sulfate from the dermis.

Fibronectin (in the matrix), laminin (restricted to basement membranes), thrombospondin, vitronectin, and tenascin are glycoproteins found in the dermis and, like the PGs/GAGs, they interact with other matrix components and with cells through specific integrin receptors.[50–54] As a consequence of their binding to other glycoproteins, collagen and elastic fibers, PGs, and to cells, glycoproteins are involved in—in some cases mediate—cell attachment (adhesion), migration, spreading in vitro, morphogenesis (epithelial–mesenchymal interactions, e.g., in follicle development), and differentiation.

Fibronectin is an insoluble, filamentous glycoprotein synthesized in the skin by both epithelial and mesenchymal cells; it ensheathes collagen fiber bundles and the elastic network, is associated with basal laminae, and appears on the surfaces of cells where it is bound to the cell through one of multiple integrin receptors that mediate cell-matrix adhesion. Fibronectin also binds platelets to collagen, is found in fibrin-fibrinogen complexes, and plays a role in organizing the extracellular matrix. Vitronectin is present throughout the dermis in association with the surfaces of all elastic fibers except for oxytalan. Tenascin is a large hexameric extracellular matrix glycoprotein. Minimal quantities of tenascin are present in adult dermis in a distribution restricted to the subepidermal reticular lamina and surrounding smooth muscle of blood vessels, arrector pili muscles, and sweat glands, but expression is strongly upregulated in the papillary dermis in conditions of epidermal hyperproliferation. Epidermal keratinocytes appear to be the primary source. In general, cell adhesion molecules are upregulated during wound healing, in tumors, and during developmental morphogenesis.

Organization of the Dermis: Major Regions of the Dermis[55]

The dermis is organized into papillary and reticular regions (Fig. 6-14); the distinction of the two zones is based largely on their differences in connective tissue organization, cell density, and nerve and vascular patterns. Subdivisions of each of these regions are more or less apparent in mature skin, depending upon the individual. The papillary dermis is proximal to the epidermis, molds to its contours, and is usually no more than twice its thickness. The reticular dermis is the dominant region of the dermis and of the skin as a whole. A horizontal plane of vessels, the subpapillary plexus, marks the boundary between the papillary and reticular dermis. The deep boundary between the dermis and the hypodermis is defined by the transition from fibrous to adipose connective tissue.

PAPILLARY DERMIS The papillary dermis is characterized by small bundles of small-diameter collagen fibrils and oxytalan elastic fibers (Fig. 6-14*A*, 6-14*B*). Mature elastic fibers are usually not found in the normal papillary dermis, but they are common in the skin of patients with certain inherited connective tissue diseases (e.g., dominantly inherited forms of the Ehlers-Danlos syndrome), in aging skin, and in actinically damaged skin. Large, dense, elastic fibers with abnormal structure are the hallmark of sun-damaged skin. The structural characteristics of the matrix in the papillary dermis permit the skin to accommodate to impact. The papillary dermis also has a high density of fibroblastic cells that proliferate more rapidly, have a higher rate of metabolic activity, and synthesize different species of PGs, as compared to those of the reticular dermis. Capillaries extending from the subpapillary plexus project toward the epidermis within the dermal papillae, fingerlike projections of papillary dermis that interdigitate with the rete pegs that project from the epidermis into the dermis (Fig. 6-15).

FIGURE 6-15

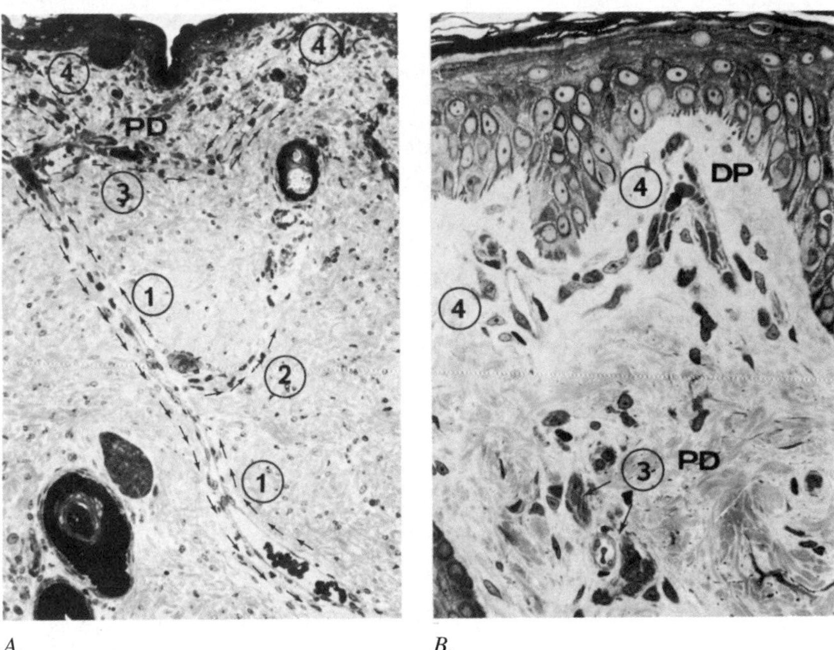

Light micrographs showing the pattern of dermal vasculature seen in the skin of a third trimester fetus (*A*) and an adult (*B*). Ascending/descending vessels pass vertically through the reticular dermis (1) and give off branches to epidermal appendages (2). The ascending vessels terminate at the border between the papillary dermis (PD) and reticular dermis where they form the horizontal subpapillary plexus (3). Capillary loops (4) extend from the plexus into the dermal papillae (*left*). *B*. Enlarged regions of the papillary dermis showing vessels of the subpapillary plexus in cross section (e) and capillary loops in dermal papillae (4) (DP). ×300 in the original magnification. *(Courtesy of LT Smith, PhD.)*

The papillary dermis is generally less involved in pathologic change than the reticular dermis in patients with inherited disorders involving the connective tissue matrix. This suggests that factors other than the connective tissue itself may have a significant role in modulating the structure and function of that tissue. The epidermis and proximal dermis exchange a number of cytokines and growth factors, and matrix components of the dermis are linked to the cytoskeleton of the epidermis through transmembrane receptors; it is possible, therefore, that the organization and composition of the papillary dermis reflect the zone of influence of the epidermis through its soluble and diffusible factors. Connective tissue with the same organization and composition as the papillary dermis ("adventitial dermis") surrounds hair follicles and vessels—situations where matrix also underlies an epithelium.

The sublamina densa region, or reticular lamina, can be identified in some individuals as a subdivision of the papillary dermis. It stains selectively with antibodies to type I procollagen and is characterized by a fine but dense organization of fibrils. Because of this, the structure is sometimes called a *compact zone*. It is a region that is particularly rich in cells that bear receptors for growth factors produced by the epidermis (e.g., PDGF) and it has an abundance of molecules that have adhesive properties (e.g., tenascin). This is also the region containing the ends of anchoring fibrils and related anchoring plaques. This region is more prominent and often thickened in pathologic skin.

RETICULAR DERMIS The reticular dermis is composed primarily of large-diameter collagen fibrils organized into large, interwoven fiber bundles. Mature, bandlike, branching elastic fibers form a superstructure around the collagen fiber bundles (Fig. 6-14*C*). In sectioned specimens of skin, these appear as fine bands at the periphery of the bundles, but scanning electron microscopy provides a more accurate impression of how the two fiber systems are integrated and can interact to provide the dermis with strong and resilient mechanical properties (Fig. 6-14*A*). In normal individuals, the elastic fibers and collagen bundles of the reticular dermis increase in size progressively toward the hypodermis.

Subdivision of the reticular dermis into an upper intermediate zone and a deeper zone is possible because of graded differences in the size and character of the fibrous connective tissue. Intermediate-sized collagen fibrils and fiber bundles and horizontally oriented elaunin elastic fibers characterize the upper zone of the reticular dermis. This zone also has distinct mechanical properties compared with the deeper dermis; it is particularly susceptible to cleavage following trauma, and it may be involved in disease processes (e.g., selective loss of elastic fibers) when other regions are not. Compared to the deeper reticular dermis, the intermediate dermis is also enriched in fibroblastic cells and other connective tissue cells and in inflammatory cells that migrate into the tissue from the subpapillary plexus located in the region.

CELLS OF THE DERMIS Fibroblasts, macrophages, and mast cells are regular residents of the dermis (Figs. 6-12, 6-13, and 6-15 to 6-17). They are found in greatest density in normal skin in the papillary region and surrounding vessels of the subpapillary plexus, but they also occur in the reticular dermis where they are found in the interstices between collagen fiber bundles. Small numbers of lymphocytes collect around blood vessels in normal skin, and, at a site of inflammation, lymphocytes and other leukocytes from the blood are prominent. Pericytes and veil cells ensheathe the walls of blood vessels, and Schwann

FIGURE 6-16

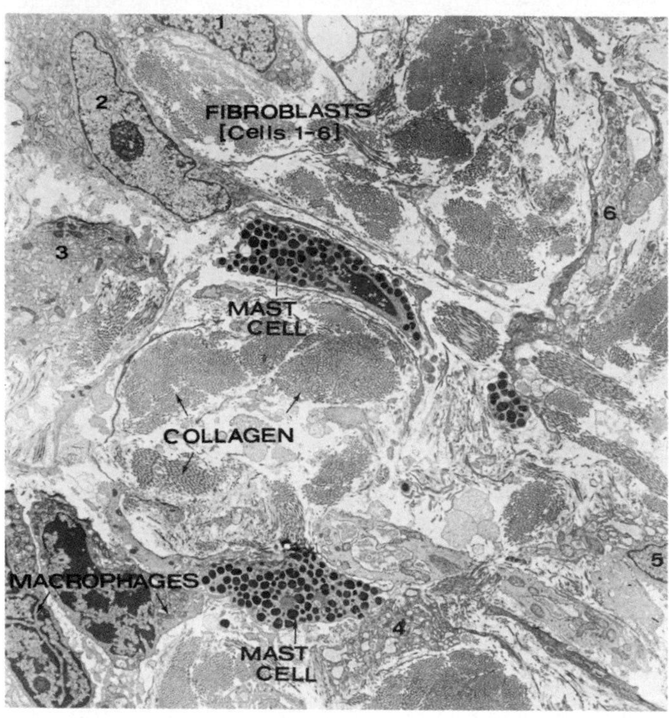

Typical cells of the dermis photographed at the level of the intermediate reticular dermis. ×35,000 in the original magnification. (*Courtesy of SK Anderson.*)

FIGURE 6-17

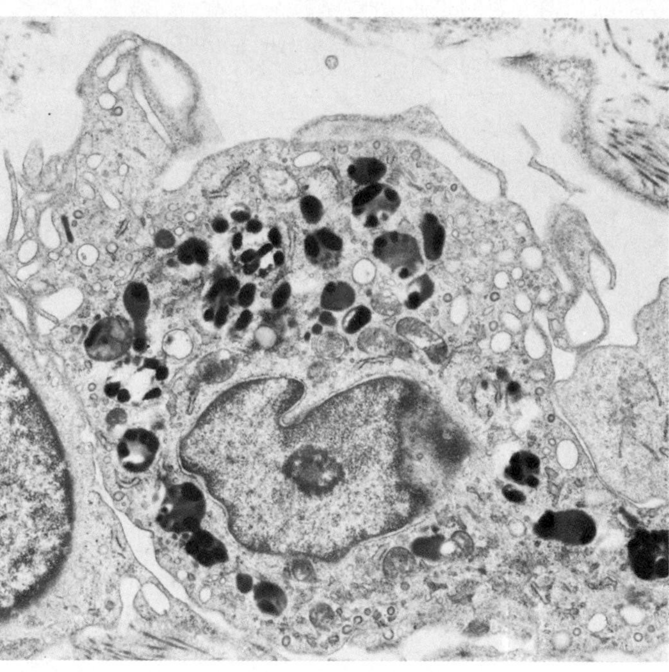

Macrophage. Note melanosomes within the phagosomes. ×15,950.

cells encompass nerve fibers (Figs. 6-13 and 6-15). Once viewed as distinct populations, the separation between fibroblasts, macrophages, and monocytes is no longer clear-cut. Moreover, there is significant heterogeneity among populations of each type based on criteria of structure, function, differentiation, and immunophenotype. Many cells in the dermis previously described as fibroblasts are probably cells with functions different from those of the typical fibroblast.

The *fibroblast* is a mesenchymally derived cell that migrates through the tissue and is responsible for the synthesis and degradation of fibrous and nonfibrous connective tissue matrix proteins and a number of soluble factors (Fig. 6-12). Thus, the function of fibroblasts is to provide a structural extracellular matrix framework as well as to promote interaction between epidermis and dermis by the synthesis of soluble mediators.[42] The same fibroblast is capable of synthesizing more than one type of matrix protein simultaneously. The morphology of the fibroblast often suggests active synthetic activity; the cytoplasm includes multiple profiles of dilated rough endoplasmic reticulum and typically more than one Golgi complex. Focal densities along the plasma membrane are identified as sites where there is communication between the cytoskeleton, transmembrane proteins of the plasma membrane (integrin receptors), and a variety of matrix proteins including laminin, fibronectin, vitronectin, thrombospondin, and collagens. Fibroblasts migrate between and on the surface of fiber bundles in the tissue but rarely do they invade or become trapped within them.

Studies of human fibroblast cell lines indicate that they are a highly diverse population and within a single tissue phenotypically distinct populations exist.[56] There is great interest in fibroblast regulation because of increased proliferative and synthetic activity in wound healing and during formation of hypertrophic scars. Resting and proliferating fibroblasts respond to immune mediators, including IL-1α and IL-1β, by increasing their production of KGF, hepatocyte growth factor (HGF), IL-1α, -1β, and -8. Fibroblasts from hypertrophic scars upregulate and appear abnormally sensitive to TGF-β, whereas interferon (IFN)-1α can decrease their proliferation and collagen production.[57]

Monocytes, macrophages, and dermal dendrocytes The monocytes, macrophages, and dermal dendrocytes are a heterogeneous collection of cells that constitute the mononuclear phagocytic system of cells in the skin. They can be distinguished into the monocyte–macrophage lineage and the dendritic cell lineage on the basis of ultrastructure, histochemistry, and immunocytochemistry. The latter series of cells includes Langerhans cells, indeterminant cells, interdigitating cells, and dermal dendrocytes.

Macrophages[58] are derived from precursor cells of the bone marrow that differentiate into monocytes in the blood, then migrate into the dermis where they differentiate (see Figs. 6-13 and 6-17). Macrophages are difficult to distinguish morphologically from fibroblasts if they do not contain lysosomes and phagocytic vacuoles because both cell types can have well-developed rough endoplasmic reticulum and Golgi, cytoplasmic intermediate filaments, and they occupy similar locations in the tissue.

Several antigenic and enzymatic markers, considered macrophage differentiation antigens, characterize the macrophages and distinguish them from fibroblasts (MAC387, RFD7; KiM8, RFDR); other markers expressed by dermal macrophages are common among tissue macrophages and other cells derived from the monocyte-macrophage lineage. Subsets of macrophages that differ in structure, maturation, function, and position exist in the skin, although all phagocytic skin macrophages appear to coexpress CD11c (KiM1), CD6 (KiM6), and KiM8 antigens.[59]

Macrophages have an expansive list of functions. They are phagocytic; they process and present antigen to immunocompetent lymphoid cells; they are microbicidal (through the production of lysozyme, peroxide, and superoxide), tumoricidal, secretory (growth factors, cytokines, and other immunomodulatory molecules), and hematopoietic; and they are involved in coagulation, atherogenesis, wound healing, and tissue remodeling.

Mast cells (see Chap. 32) are specialized secretory cells distributed in connective tissues throughout the body, typically at sites adjacent to the interface of an organ and the environment.[60] In the skin, mast cells are present in greatest density in the papillary dermis, near the DEJ, in sheaths of epidermal appendages, and around blood vessels and nerves of the subpapillary plexus. They are also common in the subcutaneous fat (see Figs. 6-16 and 6-18). A close association of mast cells with neuropeptide-containing sensory nerves has been found in psoriatic lesional skin. Mast cells are easily identified histologically by a round or oval nucleus and abundant, darkly staining cytoplasmic granules. At the ultrastructural level the granules can be separated into populations of secretory and lysosomal granules. The surface of dermal mast cells is modified by microvilli and, like fibroblasts, they are coated with fibronectin, which probably assists in securing the cells within the connective tissue matrix. The cells are larger in the adult than in the child and contain a greater volume of cytoplasm. Mast cells can become hyperplastic in mastocytosis, a pleomorphic disease that varies with the organ involved.

Mast cells originate in the bone marrow from CD34+ stem cells. Mast cell proliferation depends on the *c-kit* receptor and its ligand, SCF. Mutations in *c-kit* have been documented in patients with mastocytosis.[61] Like basophils, mast cells also contain metachromatic granules and stores of histamine; both cells synthesize eosinophilic chemotactic factor and have IgE antibodies bound to their plasma membranes. Differentiation of the mast cell occurs in the tissue under the influence of factors produced by other cells and extracellular matrix. IL-3 is one of the factors required for this process to occur In rodents, which are frequently used as an animal model system, mast cells can be divided into two distinct subclasses based on their location, content of histamine and T cell responsiveness; this subdivision in humans is far less rigid, however.

Mast cells synthesize an impressive repertoire of mediators. Some of them are preformed and stored in the granules. Histamine, heparin, tryptase, chymase, carboxypeptidase, neutrophil chemotactic factor, and eosinophilic chemotactic factor of anaphylaxis are organized in the predominantly proteoglycan milieu of the granule in a manner that is suggested to retain the enzymes in an inactive state prior to release. The mast cell synthesizes and releases other molecules, without storage, including a number of growth factors, cytokines (IL-1, -3, -4, -5, GM-CSF, and TNF-α), leukotrienes, and platelet-activating factors. Lysosomal granules in the cell contain acid hydrolases that degrade glycosaminoglycans, PGs, and complex glycolipids intracellularly. Several additional enzymes are present in both the lysosomal and the secretory granules. These may be important in initiating the repair of damaged tissue, and/or may help in degrading foreign material.

Various stimuli can trigger release of the contents of the secretory granules. The process of degranulation occurs in the same manner regardless of the type of stimulus. The granules swell and their contents become lucent and disorganized. They fuse with one another and with the plasma membrane, opening channels through which the contents can be released. Release of the mediators into the tissue provokes contraction of vascular smooth muscle and increases vascular permeability, tissue edema, and the recruitment of inflammatory cells into the site. Mast cells are responsible for immediate-type hypersensitivity reactions in the skin and are involved in the production of subacute and chronic inflammatory disease.

The *dermal dendrocyte* is a stellate, dendritic, or sometimes spindle-shaped, highly phagocytic fixed connective tissue cell in the dermis of normal skin. Dermal dendrocytes are not specialized fibroblasts, but rather represent a subset of antigen-presenting macrophages or a distinct lineage that originates in the bone marrow. Similar to many other bone marrow–derived cells, dermal dendrocytes express factor XIIIa and the HLe-1 (CD45) antigen[62] and they lack typical markers of the fibroblastic cell (e.g., Te-7). These cells are particularly abundant in the papillary dermis and upper reticular dermis, frequently in the proximity of vessels of the subpapillary plexus. Dermal dendrocytes are also present around vessels in the reticular dermis and in the subcutaneous

FIGURE 6-18

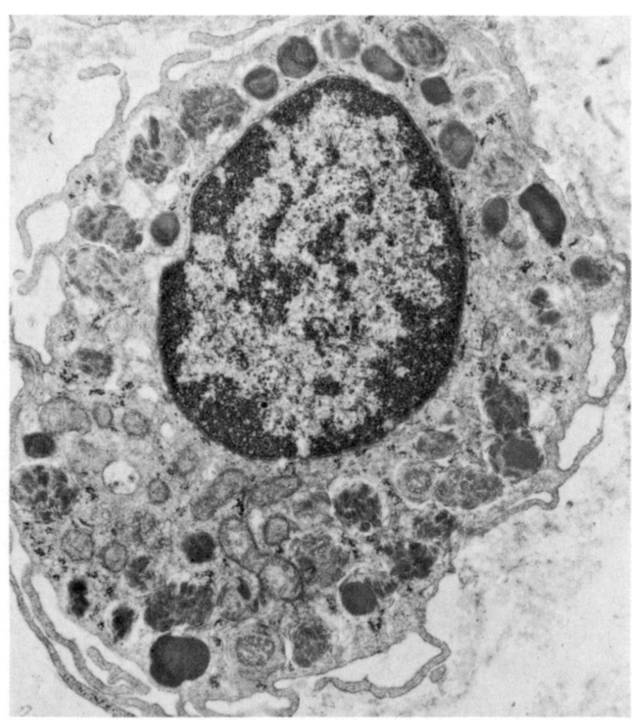

A.

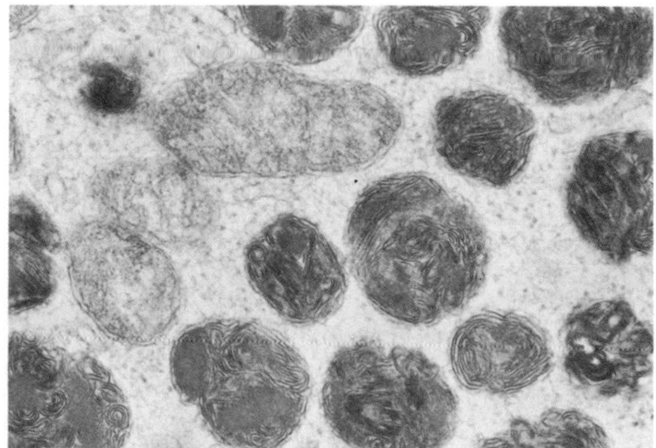

B.

A. Mast cell with cytoplasmic granules and villous projections from the cell surface. ×19,000 in the original magnification. *B.* Secretory granules from another cell. ×43,700 in the original magnification.

fat. The number of dermal dendrocytes is elevated in fetal, infant, photoaged, and certain pathologic adult skin and in association with sites of angiogenesis. Dermal dendrocytes are immunologically competent cells that function as effector cells in the afferent limb of an immune response. They are also highly phagocytic; they can be recognized as melanophages in the dermis or containing other exogenous pigment and iron. They are likely the cell of origin of a number of benign fibrotic proliferative conditions in the skin (e.g., dermatofibromas and fibroxanthomas).

The Cutaneous Vasculature

THE CUTANEOUS BLOOD VESSELS The skin is richly supplied with a vascular network consisting of distributing and collecting channels and horizontal plexuses located at boundaries within the dermis and supplying the epidermal appendages (see Fig. 6-15).[63] The microcirculatory beds in skin include arterioles/terminal arterioles, precapillary sphincters, arterial and venous capillaries, postcapillary venules, and collecting venules. The vessels provide nutrition for the tissues, but for the skin as a whole, the abundance of vessels is more than is needed to meet its metabolic needs. The vasculature is also involved in the regulation of temperature, blood pressure, wound repair, and numerous immunologic events. By comparison with the vasculature of other organs, the vessels of the skin have thick walls supported by connective tissue and smooth muscle cells. This structure is advantageous to an organ that is regularly subjected to shearing forces. All vessels of the cutaneous microcirculation are surrounded by veil cells. These cells are not part of the vessel wall but appear to define a domain for the vessel within the dermis.

The vessels that supply the dermis are small branches from musculocutaneous arteries that penetrate the subcutaneous fat and enter the deep reticular dermis where they are organized into a horizontal, arteriolar plexus. Ascending arterioles extend vertically from the plexus toward the epidermis (see Fig. 6-15). These arterioles have two layers of smooth muscle cells, a discontinuous internal elastic lamina, and pericytes, a second type of contractile cell of the vessel wall. Three-dimensional reconstruction of the smooth muscle reveals an organization of the vessel wall that suggests they are the resistance vessels of the microcirculation. Ascending arterioles may join with one another through vascular arcades. At the junction between the papillary and reticular dermis, terminal arterioles form the subpapillary plexus (see Figs. 6-14, 6-15, and 6-19). The arterioles at this level lack the elastic fibers of the previous segment and have a single layer of smooth muscle cells that is organized in a manner to suggest the vessels' function as precapillary sphincters. Capillary loops extend from the terminal arterioles of the plexus into the papillary dermis, typically one per dermal papilla, but more in areas where the rete ridges are highly developed (see Fig. 6-15). The ascending limb of the loop and all of its intrapapillary portion consist of arterial capillaries that have a continuous endothelium, basal lamina, and a few pericytes that lie external to the subendothelial basal lamina. Pericytes may project through the basal lamina to contact and form tight junctions with endothelial cells. In the thinnest portion of the loop, at its apex, both the endothelium and basal lamina are attenuated, permitting transport of material out of the capillary.

The extrapapillary, descending limb of the loop is a venous capillary. It drains into venous channels of the subpapillary plexus that lie above and below the arteriolar vascular plexus. The venous capillaries and the larger diameter postcapillary venules of the plexus have multiple layers of basal lamina separated by intervening collagen fibrils and a loosely organized sheath of pericytes and veil cells. These elements are more abundant than those of the arterial capillaries. The pericyte–endothelial cell contacts are also enhanced over those that occur in arterial capillaries. The walls of postcapillary venules can become significantly thickened by actinic damage and in metabolic diseases such as diabetes. The postcapillary venules of the subpapillary plexus are physiologically important components of the microcirculation. They respond to mediators such as histamine by developing gaps between adjacent endothelial cells that allow for the extravasation of fluid and escape of cells from the lumen of the vessel and thus are often the site of inflammatory cells in the tissue.

FIGURE 6-19

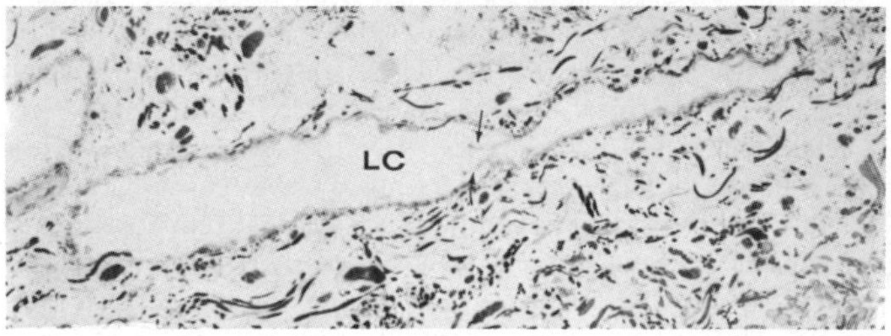

A.

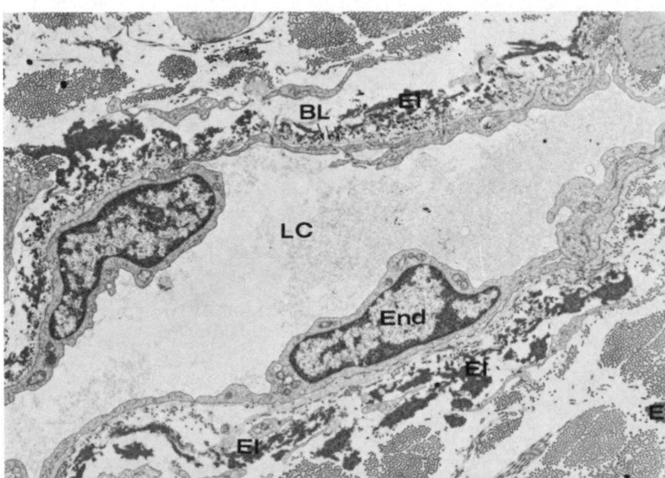

B.

Lymph channels (LC) in adult dermis. Note the valves (*arrows*) (*A*) and that the wall of the channel consists of an endothelium (End), basal lamina (BL), and elastic connective tissue (El). Collagen (C) and elastic fibers of the dermis are also shown (*B*). *A*, ×400; *B*, ×42,000 in the original magnifications.

The postcapillary venules empty into venous channels, parallel to the ascending arterioles, that carry blood to the deep horizontal plexus and then away from the skin. Venules in this location also have the laminated basement membrane structure characteristic of postcapillary venules in the subpapillary plexus. Valves present in the collecting venules exiting the plexus at the junction of the dermis and hypodermis appear to be advantageously placed to insure propulsion of the blood from the skin.

Direct connections exist between arterial and venous circulation in certain regions of the skin (e.g., palms and soles) as alternative bypass routes that shunt blood around congested capillary beds. These sites consist of an ascending arteriole (called a *glomus body*), which is modified by three to six layers of smooth muscle cells and has associated sympathetic nerve fibers and venules. The glomus can close completely when the blood pressure is below a critical level. In the adult, cutaneous vasculature is normally quiescent with the exception of some angiogenesis related to anagen of the hair cycle. This quiescent state is maintained by inhibition of angiogenesis in the normal dermal matrix, by factors such as thrombospondin. Secondary angiogenesis occurs in response to pathogenic stimuli. The major factor stimulated appears to be vascular permeability factor [VPF; vascular endothelial growth factor (VEGF)] secreted by keratinocytes.[64]

THE CUTANEOUS LYMPHATICS The lymph channels of the skin are important in regulating pressure of the interstitial fluid by resorption of fluid released from vessels and in clearing the tissue of cells, proteins, lipids, bacteria, and degraded substances.[65] Lymph flow within the skin depends upon movements of the tissue caused by arterial pulsations and larger-scale muscle contractions and movement of the body. Bicuspid-like valves within the lymphatic vessels may help prevent backflow and stasis of fluid in the vessels.

Dissolved substances, debris, and cells to be removed by lymphatic tissue are collected in blind-ending initial lymphatics (also called lymphatic capillaries, prelymphatic tubules, and terminal or peripheral lymphatics) in the papillary dermis.[65] These vessels are sparse and do not extend as close to the epidermis as the capillary loops. Melanoma cells destroy the endothelial cells of the initial lymphatics to gain entry to the lymph circulation.[66] The lymph capillaries drain into a horizontal plexus of larger lymph vessels located deep to the subpapillary venous plexus. Lymph vessels can be distinguished from blood vessels in the same position by a larger luminal diameter (often difficult to see in their normally collapsed state in the skin) and thinner wall that consists of an endothelium, discontinuous basal lamina, and elastic fibers (Figs. 6-20 and 6-21). Integration of the elastic fibers of the vessel wall with those of the dermal connective tissue matrix has been suggested to serve as a conduit along which fluid can track toward the collecting channels.[65] The endothelial cells are typically flattened and attenuated and either abut one another or overlap; gaps are evident between adjacent endothelial cells in the subpapillary plexus lymphatic vessels in normal and damaged tissue. Gaps are observed less frequently in the vertical lymphatics that carry fluid and debris through the reticular dermis to the deeper collecting plexus at the reticular dermis–hypodermis border. The presence and location of this plexus is more variable in the skin. Smooth muscle cells are present in the walls of lymphatics only at the level of the hypodermis.

Nerves and Receptors of the Skin

OVERVIEW The nerve networks of the skin contain somatic sensory and sympathetic autonomic fibers.[67] The sensory fibers alone (free nerve endings) or in conjunction with specialized structures (corpuscular receptors) function at every point of the body as receptors of touch, pain, temperature, itch, and mechanical stimuli. The density and types of receptors are regionally variable and specific, thus accounting for the variation in acuity at different sites of the body. Receptors are particularly dense in hairless areas such as the areola, labia, and glans penis. Sympathetic motor fibers are codistributed with the sensory nerves in the dermis until they branch to innervate the sweat glands, vascular smooth muscle, the arrector pili muscle of hair follicles, and sebaceous glands.

The skin is innervated by large, myelinated cutaneous branches of musculocutaneous nerves that arise segmentally from spinal nerves (see Fig. 6-20). Small branches that enter the deep dermis are surrounded by an epineurial sheath; perineurial and endoneurial sheaths and Schwann cells envelop fiber bundles and individual fibers, respectively. The pattern of nerve fibers in the skin is similar to the vascular patterns. Nerve fibers form a deep plexus, then ascend to a superficial, subpapillary plexus (see Fig. 6-13). Branches leave both plexuses to supply various regions and structures of the skin. The extent to which fibers retain their sheaths depends upon their terminal distribution.

FIGURE 6-20

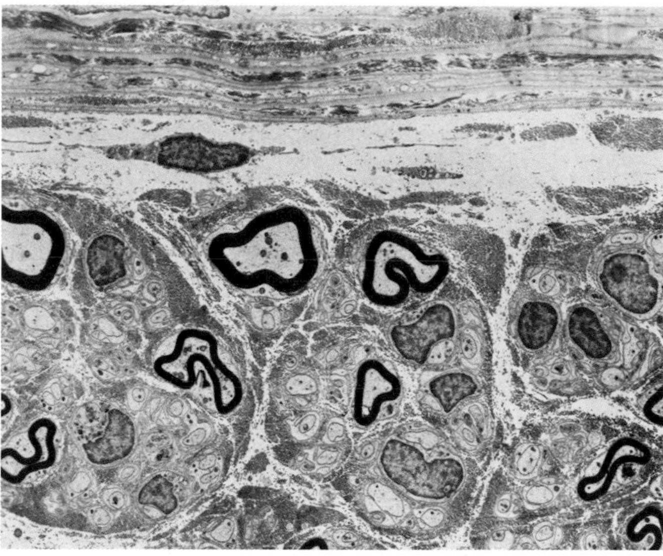

Cutaneous nerve (sural). At the top is the multilayered perineurium consisting of flattened cells interspaced with collagen fibers. This encloses the endoneurial compartment containing bundles of myelinated and unmyelinated axons embedded in collagen. The nuclei seen are those of Schwann cells. ×3350.

ANATOMIC DISTRIBUTION OF NERVES AND RECEPTORS IN THE SKIN The sensory nerves, in general, supply the skin segmentally (dermatomes), but the boundaries are imprecise and there is overlapping innervation to any given area. Autonomic innervation does not follow exactly the same pattern because the postganglionic fibers distributed in the skin originate in sympathetic chain ganglia where preganglionic fibers of several different spinal nerves synapse.

FREE NERVE ENDINGS Free nerve endings are the most widespread and undoubtedly the most important sensory receptors of the body (Figs. 6-21, 6-22). In humans, they are always ensheathed by Schwann cells and a basal lamina. Free nerve endings are particularly common in the papillary dermis just beneath the epidermis (see Figs. 6-13, 6-21, and 6-22); the basal lamina of the fiber may merge with the lamina densa of the basement membrane zone.

The *penicillate fibers* are the primary nerve fibers found subepidermally in hairy skin. Separate, unmyelinated branches from one or more myelinated stem axons are ensheathed collectively by the processes of a single Schwann cell (see Fig. 6–22). The basal lamina of the Schwann cell and longitudinally-oriented collagen fibrils surround each branch to its termination. The penicillate nerve endings are rapidly adapting receptors and function in the perception of touch, temperature, pain, and itch. Discrimination is somewhat generalized (as opposed to punctate) because of the overlapping innervation to any given region. On the other hand, free nerve endings present in nonhairy, ridged skin (palms and soles) have a more precise distribution and project individually and vertically into a dermal papilla without overlapping distribution. These receptors probably function in fine discrimination and are only one of many types of receptors in this tissue, which is richly supplied with encapsulated nerve endings.

Papillary nerve endings are found at the orifice of a follicle. They are branches from nerves that innervate the follicle at a deeper level in the skin. These terminals, in comparison with the penicillate endings, contain more mitochondria and vesicles and are believed to be

FIGURE 6-21

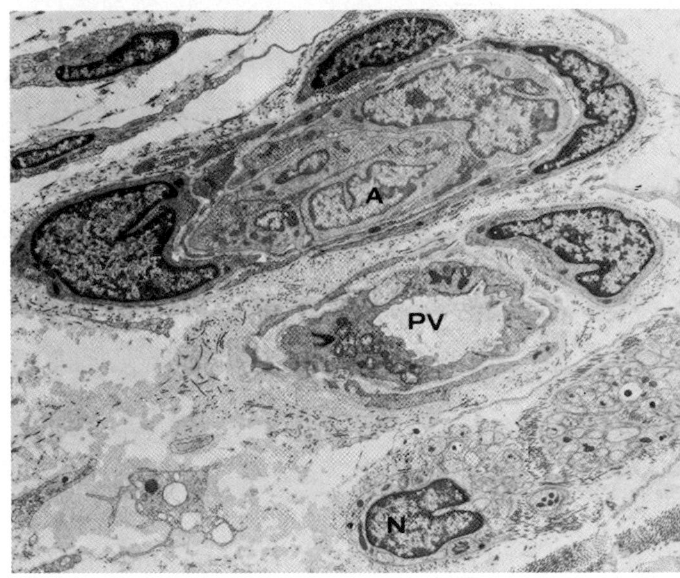

Unmyelinated nerve (N), arteriole (A), and postcapillary venule (PV) of the subpapillary plexus. Note the difference in wall structure of the A and PV. ×4400 in the original magnification.

particularly receptive to cold sensation. Other free nerve endings of the skin are associated with specific structures. Hair follicles, for example, are innervated by fibers that arise from myelinated stem axons in the deep dermal plexus, and they are thought to be slow-adapting receptors that respond to the bending or movement of hairs. Cholinergic sympathetic fibers en route to the eccrine sweat gland and adrenergic and cholinergic fibers to the arrector pili muscle are carried along with the sensory fibers in the hair basket.

Free nerve endings are also associated with individual Merkel cells. As they penetrate the epidermis, they lose all of their sheaths. Complex receptors, described by a number of names (touch domes, Hederiform endings, Iggo's capsule, Pinkus corpuscles, Haarscheibe, etc.), containing as many as 50 Merkel cells, and supplied by a single arborizing nerve, are also present in the skin. In hairy skin, touch domes are associated with certain follicles, particularly those on the neck and dorsal surface of the forearm. In ridged palmar and plantar skin, Merkel cell–neurite assemblies collect at the site where the eccrine sweat duct penetrates a glandular epidermal papilla.

CORPUSCULAR RECEPTORS Corpuscular receptors have a capsule and an inner core and contain both neural and nonneural components. The capsule is a continuation of the perineurium, and the core includes preterminal and terminal portions of the fiber surrounded by lamellated wrappings of Schwann cells. The size of these receptors depends upon their position within the skin (the deeper structures being larger) and, for certain types, upon the age of the individual. Remodeling of the corpuscular receptors occurs throughout life. Corpuscular receptors express neuron-specific enolase, neurofilaments, calbindin D28K and other calcium-binding proteins, S-100, and p75 neurotrophin receptor.

The *Meissner's corpuscle* is an elongated or ovoid mechanoreceptor located in the dermal papillae of digital skin and oriented vertically toward the epidermal surface (Fig. 6-23). One to six myelinated axons enter the base of the corpuscle, lose their myelin coverings, ramify extensively, and terminate in bulboid endings that are surrounded by lamellae.

FIGURE 6-22

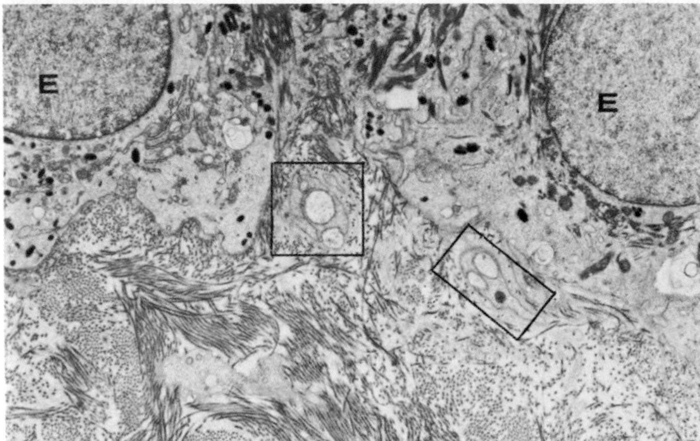

A.

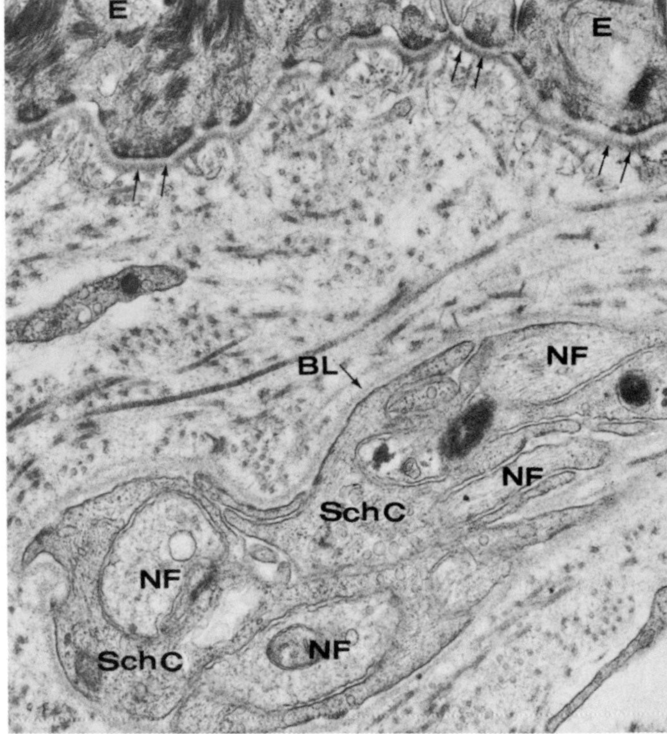

B.

A. Free nerve endings in the papillary dermis. Note the close proximity of these endings (enclosed). E, epidermis. *B.* Nerve fibers (NF) surrounded by a Schwann cell (SchC) are shown in an ending that lies near to the dermal–epidermal junction (*arrows*). *A,* ×6850; *B,* ×20,000 in the original magnifications. (*From Holbrook K: Structure and Development of the Skin. in Pathophysiology of Dermatologic Disease, edited by NA Soter, HP Baden. New York, McGraw-Hill, 1991, 2nd edition, p 15, with permission.*)

The *Pacinian corpuscle* lies in the deep dermis and subcutaneous tissue of skin that covers weight-bearing surfaces of the body (Fig. 6-24). It is distinguished by the structure of its capsule and lamellar wrappings. The perineurium (capsule) is organized into 30 or more concentric layers of cells and fibrous connective tissue. A middle subcapsular zone is composed of collagen and fibroblasts, and the inner core consists of Schwann cell–derived hemilamellae—flattened semicircles that alternate with those of the opposite side. The hemilamellae are packed closely around the nerve fiber and terminals. Pacinian corpuscles serve as rapidly adapting mechanoreceptors responding to vibrational stimuli.

FIGURE 6-23

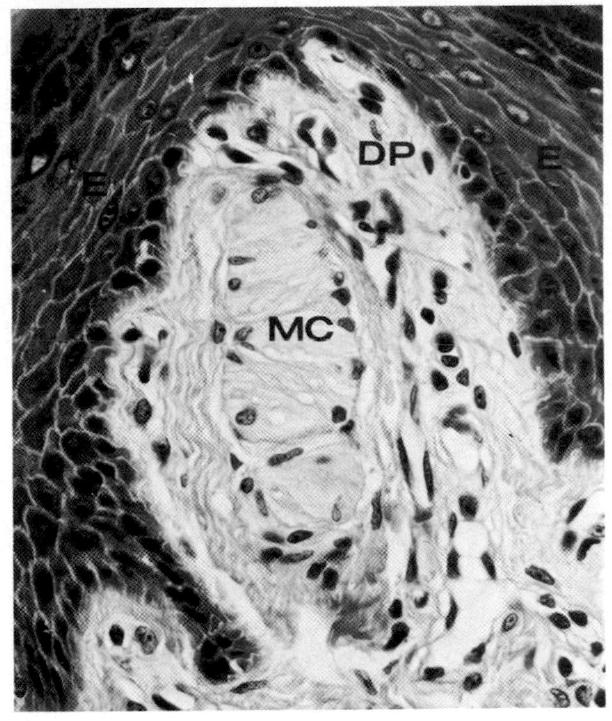

Meissner's corpuscle (MC) within the connective tissue of a dermal papilla (DP) from the sole of the foot. Note the many vessels also in the papilla and the layers of the epidermis (E). ×600.

FUNCTIONAL DISTRIBUTION OF NERVES IN THE SKIN Immunohistochemical staining of nerve fibers in the skin has provided new understanding of the diversity of nerve fibers and complexity of innervation to the skin. The work has demonstrated that nerve fibers have overlapping characteristics. The structures are provided with fibers that release a variety of neurotransmitter substances that may affect their activity. Even though the chemical properties of fibers are recognized, the function of the innervation is not always apparent. Moreover, the distribution of specific types of fibers to zones and structures of the skin from one region of the body may not reflect the innervation for another region of the skin, and the effect of the neurotransmitters may be different among organs.

There are pronounced efferent activities of the cutaneous neurologic system. Neuropeptides released by sensory neurons activate cutaneous target cells to induce inflammatory activities. Neuropeptide receptors and enzymes are expressed by nonneuronal skin cells. Sensory nerve fibers of the skin have been found to synthesize and release calcitonin gene– related peptide, somatostatin, substance P, neurokinin A, vasoactive intestinal peptide (VIP), and melanocyte-stimulating hormone (MSH)-γ or MSH-γ–like peptide.

FIGURE 6-24

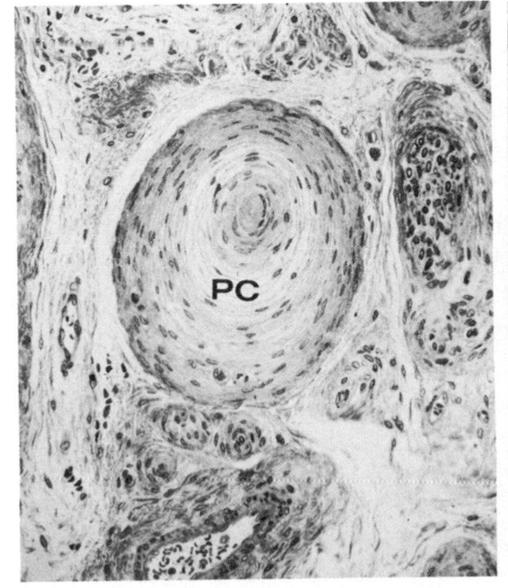

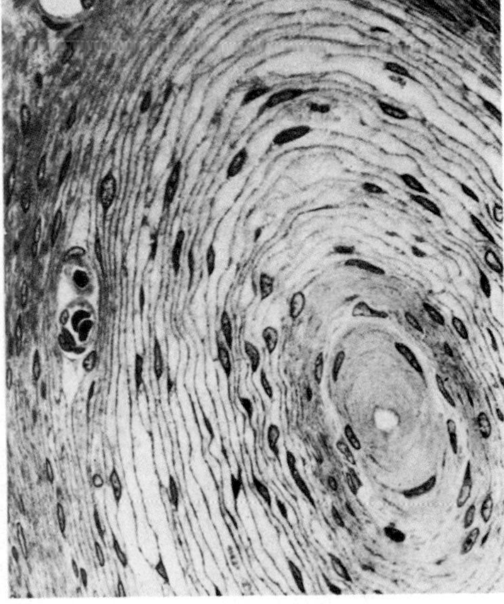

A. *B.*

Pacinian corpuscle (PC) in the subcutaneous plantar tissue. Note the lamellated wrappings and the small vessels interspersed among the layers. A large myelinated nerve is also shown on the right-hand side of *A*. *A*, ×580; *B*, ×1050 in the original magnifications.

Autonomic nerve fibers that supply large vessels and sweat glands in the skin produce the vasoconstrictor neuropeptide Y, tyrosine hydroxylase that is used in the synthesis of catecholamines, VIP, neuron-specific enolase, myelin basic protein, S-100, and possibly somatostatin. Fibers to sweat glands are particularly immunoreactive with antibodies to antinatriuretic peptide, a substance that can function as a diuretic and promote vasodilation, thus possibly assisting the sweat gland in regulating water and electrolyte balance.

THE HYPODERMIS

The boundary between the deep reticular dermis and the hypodermis is an abrupt transition between a predominantly fibrous dermal connective tissue to an adipose tissue–rich subcutaneous region (see Fig. 6-1). Nonetheless, the two regions are structurally and functionally well integrated through nerve and vascular networks and the continuity of epidermal appendages. Actively growing hair follicles extend into the subcutaneous fat, and the apocrine and eccrine sweat glands are normally confined to this depth of the skin.

Mesenchymally derived adipocytes are the primary cells in the hypodermis. They are organized into lobules defined by septa of fibrous connective tissue. Nerves, vessels, and lymphatics are located within the septa and richly supply the region. Subcutaneous fat deposits begin to form in the midtrimester fetus and are already well developed in the newborn infant. The synthesis and storage of fat continues throughout life by enhanced accumulation of lipid within fat cells, proliferation of existing adipocytes, or by recruitment of new cells from undifferentiated mesenchyme.[68,69] The hormone leptin, secreted by adipocytes, appears to provide a long-term feedback signal regulating fat mass. Leptin levels are higher in subcutaneous than omental adipose, suggesting a role for leptin in control of adipose distribution as well. The tissue of the hypodermis insulates the body, serves as a reserve energy supply, cushions and protects the skin, and allows for its mobility over underlying structures. It has a cosmetic effect in molding body contours. The importance of the subcutaneous tissue is apparent in patients with Werner's syndrome, in which subcutaneous fat is absent in lesional areas over bone, or with scleroderma where the subcutaneous fat is replaced with dense fibrous connective tissue. Such regions in Werner's patients ulcerate and heal poorly. The skin of patients with scleroderma is taut and painful. In the hereditary and acquired lipodystrophies, loss of subcutaneous fat is of concern not only cosmetically, but in terms of glucose, triglyceride, and cholesterol regulation as well.

DEVELOPMENT OF SKIN

Overview

Significant advances in the understanding of the molecular processes responsible for the development of the skin have been made over the last several years. Such advances increase the understanding of clinicopathologic correlation among some inherited disorders of the skin, and allow for the early diagnosis of such diseases.[70,71] The developmental progression of various components of the skin is well-documented, and a timeline indicating the events that occur during embryonic and fetal development is provided (Table 6-1).[72,73] Of note, the estimated gestational age (EGA) is used throughout this chapter; this system refers to the age of the fetus, with fertilization occurring on day 1. To avoid confusion, it should be pointed out that obstetricians and most clinicians define day 1 as the first day of the last menstrual period (menstrual age), in which fertilization occurs on approximately day 14. Thus, the two dating systems differ by approximately 2 weeks, such that a woman who is 14 weeks pregnant (menstrual age) is carrying a 12-week-old fetus (EGA).

Conceptually, fetal skin development can be divided into three distinct but temporally overlapping stages, those of specification, morphogenesis, and differentiation. These stages roughly correspond to the embryonic period (0 to 60 days), the early fetal period (2 to 5 months), and the late fetal period (5 to 9 months) of development. The earliest stage, specification, refers to the process by which the ectoderm lateral to the neural plate is committed to become epidermis, and subsets of mesenchymal and neural crest cells are committed to form the dermis. It is at this time that patterning of the future layers and specialized structures of the skin occurs, often via a combination of gradients of proteins and cell-cell signals. The second stage, morphogenesis, is the process by which these committed tissues begin to form their specialized structures, including epidermal stratification, epidermal appendage formation, subdivision between the dermis and subcutis, and vascular formation. The last stage, differentiation, denotes the process by which these newly specialized tissues further develop and assume their mature forms. Table 6-2 integrates specification, morphogenesis, and differentiation with skin morphology and genetic diseases.

For simplification and greater clarity, the stages of development of the epidermis—dermis and hypodermis, dermal–epidermal junction, and epidermal appendages—are presented sequentially.

Epidermis

EMBRYONIC DEVELOPMENT During the third week after fertilization, the human embryo undergoes gastrulation, a complex process of involution and cell redistribution that results in the formation of the three primary embryonic germ layers: ectoderm, mesoderm, and endoderm. Shortly after gastrulation, ectoderm further subdivides into neuroectoderm and presumptive epidermis. The specification of the presumptive epidermis is believed to be mediated by the bone morphogenetic proteins (BMPs). Later during this period, BMPs again appear to play a critical role, along with Engrailed-1 (En1), in specifying the volar versus interfollicular skin.[74–76] By 6 weeks EGA, the ectoderm that covers the body consists of basal cells and superficial periderm cells (Fig. 6-25).

The basal cells of the embryonic epidermis differ from those of later developmental stages. Embryonic basal cells are more columnar than fetal basal cells, and they have not yet formed hemidesmosomes (see below). Although certain integrins (e.g., $\alpha_6\beta_4$) are expressed in these cells, they are not yet localized to the basal pole of the cells. Prior to the formation of hemidesmosomes and desmosomes, intercellular attachment between individual basal cells appears to be medicated by adhesion molecules such as E- and P-cadherin, which have been detected on basal cells as early as 6 weeks EGA. Keratins K5 and K14, proteins restricted to definitive stratified epithelia, are expressed even at these early stages of epidermal formation.

At this stage, periderm cells form a "pavement epithelium." These cells are embryonic epidermal cells that are larger and flatter than the underlying basal cells (Fig. 6-26). Apical surfaces contact the amniotic fluid and are studded with microvilli. Connections between periderm cells are sealed with tight junctions rather than desmosomes. By the end of the second trimester, these cells are sloughed and eventually form part of the vernix caseosa. Like stratified epithelial cells, periderm cells express K5 and K14, but they also express simple epithelial keratins K8, K18, and K19.

Aplasia cutis may reflect focal defects in either epidermal specification or development caused by somatic mosaicism, or mutations that occur postzygotically. The molecular defect for this disorder is not known, however. The fact that few genetic diseases have been described in which epidermal specification or morphogenesis are defective likely reflects the fact that such defects would be incompatible with survival.

EARLY FETAL DEVELOPMENT (MORPHOGENESIS) By the end of 8 weeks' gestation, hematopoiesis has switched from the extraembryonic yolk sac to the bone marrow, the classical division between embryonic and fetal development. By this time, the epidermis begins its stratification and formation of an intermediate layer between the two preexisting cell layers. The cells in this new layer are similar to the cells of the spinous layer in mature epidermis. Like spinous cells, they express keratins K1/K10 and the desmosomal protein desmoglein-3 (pemphigus vulgaris antigen). The cells are still highly proliferative, and during this period of development they evolve into a multilayer structure that will eventually replace the degenerating periderm.

Expression of the p63 gene plays a critical role in the proliferation and maintenance of the basal layer cells. Epidermal stratification does not occur in mice deficient for p63.[77,78] In humans, although no null mutations have been isolated, partial loss of p63 function mutations have been identified in ankyloblepharon, ectodermal dysplasia, and cleft lip/palate syndrome (AEC, Hay-Wells syndrome) as well as ectrodactyly, ectodermal dysplasia, and cleft lip/palate syndrome (EEC).[79–81] The preexisting basal cell layer also undergoes morphologic changes at this time, becoming more cuboidal and expressing new keratin genes, K6, K8, K19, and K6/K16, that are usually expressed in hyperproliferative tissues. The basal layer also begins to elaborate proteins that will ultimately anchor them to the developing basal lamina (see below), including hemidesmosomal proteins bullous pemphigoid antigen 1 (BPAG1), BPAG2, and collagens V and VII.

LATE FETAL DEVELOPMENT (DIFFERENTIATION) Late fetal development reveals the further specialization and differentiation of

TABLE 6-1

Timing of the Major Events in the Embryogenesis of Human Skin*

	First Trimester			Second Trimester			Third Trimester		
	1	2	3	4	5	6	7	8	9
Epidermis									
Appearance of epidermal cell layers									
Stratum basale	X								
Periderm	X								
Stratum intermedium		X							
Stratum granulosum						X			
Stratum corneum						X			
Periderm disappearance						X			
Epidermal cell junctions									
Desmosomes without associated keratin filaments	X								
Desmosomes with associated keratin filaments		X							
Tight junctions	X								
Hemidesmosomes			X						
Antigens									
Pemphigus and pemphigoid antigen			X						
A, B, H blood group antigens			X						
Immigrant cells									
Present, but type uncertain		X							
Melanocyte									
With premelanosomes		X							
With melanosomes that synthesize melanin				X					
Transfer of melanosomes to keratinocytes						X			
Langerhans cells			X						
Merkel cells				X					
Epidermal appendages									
Pilosebaceous apparatus									
Hair follicle development begins			X						
Hair exposed on skin surface and patterns established on the scalp			X						
Sebaceous gland primordium				X					
Sebaceous gland function				X					
Apocrine gland primordium						X			
Apocrine gland function							X		
Eccrine sweat glands (trunk)									
Duct and gland patent and functioning						X			
Nails									
Nail fold and establishment of matrix primordium			X						
Nail plate forms				X					
Keratinization of epidermis and appendages									
Dorsal ridge of presumptive nail			X						
Nail plate				X					
Palmar/plantar surface of digits				X					
Hair cone				X					
Hair tract				X					
Hair shaft					X				
Sebaceous duct					X				
Eccrine sweat gland duct (intraepidermal)						X			
Apocrine duct						X			
Dermis									
Structural organization									
Papillary and reticular regions established				X					
Dermal papillae established					X				
Dermal-subcutaneous boundary		X							
Panniculus adiposus established				X					
Connective tissue matrix proteins									
Collagen present by ultrastructural observation		X							
Collagen present by biochemical analysis									
Type I	?	X							
Type III	?	X							
Elastic microfibrils	?	X							
Elastic matrix				X					
Elastic fibrous networks						X			

*Data are representative of the trunk unless stated otherwise.

TABLE 6-2

Proteins Involved in Cutaneous Development and Differentiation

	Epidermis	Dermis/Subcutaneous	DEJ	Appendages
Specification	**Bone morphogenetic proteins (BMPs)** **Engrailed-1** (Aplasia cutis)	**Lmx-1B** (Nail-patella syndrome) **Engrailed-1** **Wnt 7a**	Not Known	**Lmx-1B** **Wnt 7a** **NGFR**
Morphogenesis	**p63** **Dlx-3** (Tricho-dento-osseous syndrome)	(Restrictive dermopathy) (Focal dermal hypoplasia/Goltz's syndrome) (Proteus syndrome)	**Laminin 1** **Collagen IV** **Heparan sulfate** **Proteoglycans**	**Ectodysplasin A (EDA)** (X-linked hypohidrotic ectodermal dysplasia) **Connexin 30** (autosomal hypohidrotic ectodermal dysplasia, type 2) **EDA receptor** (autosomal hypohidrotic ectodermal dysplasia, type 3) **MSX1** (Witkop syndrome/tooth and nail syndrome) ***c-kit*** (piebaldism) **PAX-3** (Waardenburg's type 1) **p63** (Hay-Wells/AEC, EEC) **β-catenin** (pilomatricomas) **Shh** **Wnt** **BMPs** **FGF5** **LEF1** **Dlx-3**
Differentiation	*Structural proteins* **K5, K14** (EB simplex) **Plectin** (EB with MD) **BPAG2** (GABEB) **$\alpha_6\beta_4$ integrin** (EB with PA) **K1, K10** (BCIE) **K1, K9** (Vorner, Unna-Thost, Greither) **Loricrin** (NBCIE, Vohwinkel's) *Posttranslational modifiers* **LEKTI** (Netherton's) **Transglutaminase 1** (Lamellar ichthyosis; NCIE) **Phytanoyl CoA hydroxylase** (Refsum) **Fatty aldehyde dehydrogenase** (Sjögren-Larsson) **Steroid sulfatase/arylsulfatase C** (X-linked ichthyosis)	(Ehler's-Danlos syndrome) **Collagen VII** (Dystrophic EB) **Fibrillin** (Marfan syndrome) **Elastin** (Cutis laxa) **Type I collagen, a_1 or a_2** (Osteogenesis imperfecta) **MRP6** (PXE) **TIE2** (inherited venous malformations) **Endoglin, activin receptor-like kinase 1** (HHT/Osler-Weber-Rendu) **VEGFR-3** (hereditary lymphedema) **LYVE-1** **Prox-1**	**BPAG2** **Collagen VII** **$\alpha_6\beta_4$ integrin** **Laminin 5** (Junctional EB)	*Hair* **BMPs** **Hoxc13** **Foxn1** **Plakoglobin** (Naxos disease) **Plakophilin/desmosomal band 6** (ectodermal dysplasia, skin fragility syndrome) **Hairless** (papular atrichia) *Nail* **K6a, K16** (pacyhonychia congenita type I) **K6b, K17** (pachyonychia congenita type II, steatocystoma multiplex) Plakophilin *Sebaceous gland* **K6b, K17**

Protein names are indicated in boldface. Associated diseases/genodermatoses are listed in parentheses. Multiple names for the same protein or syndrome are separated by /. Genes and associated diseases can be found online at http://www.ncbi.nlm.nih.gov/omim/ (Online Mendelian Inheritance in Man/OMIM).[70] Abbreviations: AEC, ankyloblepharon-ectodermal dysplasia-clefting; BCIE, bullous congenital ichthyosiform erythroderma; BPAG, bullous pemphigoid antigen; DEJ, dermal-epidermal junction; EB, epidermolysis bullosa; EEC, ectrodactyly-ectodermal dysplasia-clefting; GABEB, generalized atrophic benign epidermolysis bullosa; HHT, hereditary hemorrhagic telangiectasia; K, keratin; MD, multiple dystrophy; NBCIE, nonbullous congenital ichthyosiform erythroderma; NGFR, nerve growth factor receptor; PA, pyloric atresia; PXE, pseudoxanthoma elasticum.

keratinocytes in the epidermis. It is at this time that the granular and stratum corneal layers are formed, and the rudimentary periderm is sloughed (see Figs. 6-25 and 6-26). Keratinization of the surface epidermis is a process of keratinocyte terminal differentiation which begins at 15 weeks EGA. The granular layer becomes prominent, and important structural proteins are elaborated in the basal layer cells. The hemidesmosomal proteins plectin and $\alpha_6\beta_4$ integrin are expressed and correctly localized at this time. Mutations in these genes result in various bullous genodermatoses (reviewed in more detail in Chap. 65). The more superficial cells undergo further terminal differentiation, and the keratin-aggregating protein filaggrin is expressed at this time.

The formation of the cornified envelope is a late feature of differentiating keratinocytes, and it relies on a number of different modifications to create an impermeable barrier. Enzymes such as transglutaminase, LEKTI (encoded by the gene SPINK-5), phytanoyl CoA reductase, fatty aldehyde dehydrogenase, and steroid sulfatase are all important in the elaboration of the cornified envelope and mature lipid barrier, and defects in these enzymes can lead to abnormal epidermal barrier formation (see Table 6-2).

SPECIALIZED CELLS WITHIN THE EPIDERMIS The three major nonepidermal cell types—melanocytes, Langerhans cells, and Merkel

FIGURE 6-25

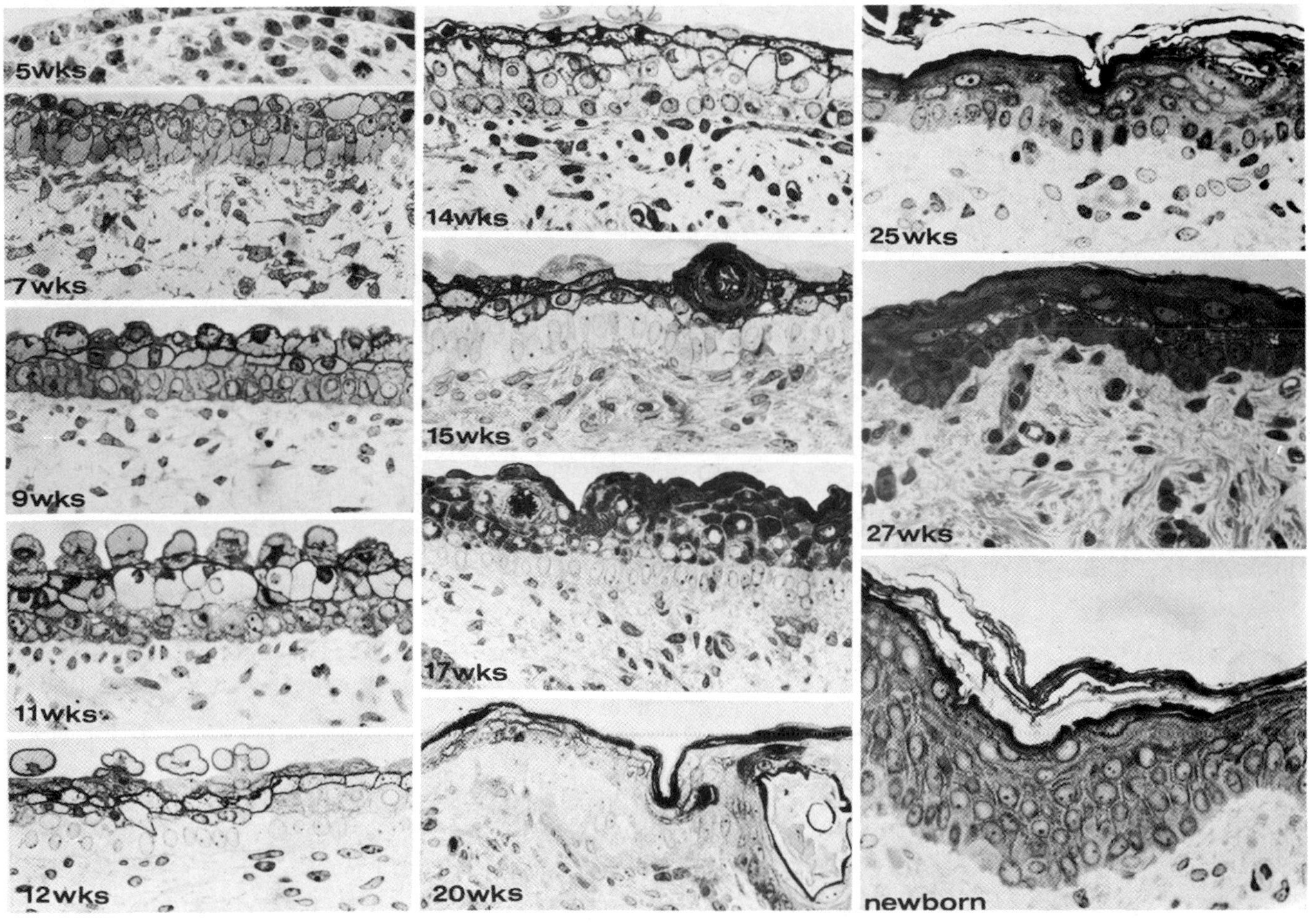

Epidermis and papillary dermis of human embryonic and fetal skin at progressive stages of development. Left column, first trimester; middle column, second trimester; right column, third trimester and newborn. ×120 in the original magnification.

cells—can be detected within the epidermis by the end of the embryonic period. Melanocytes are derived from the neural crest, a subset of neuroectoderm cells. The migratory paths of melanoblast clones are revealed as "Blaschko's lines" in banded pigmentary dyscrasias such as hypomelanosis of Ito and linear and whorled hypermelanosis. The founders of each melanoblast clone originate at distinct points along the dorsal midline, traversing ventrally and distally to take up residence in the epidermis.

Melanocytes are first seen within the epidermis at 50 days EGA. Melanocytes express integrin receptors in vivo and in vitro and may use these to migrate to the epidermis during embryonic development. Migration, colonization, proliferation, and survival of melanocytes in developing skin depend on the cell surface tyrosine kinase receptor, *c-kit*, and its ligand, stem cell factor.[82] Melanin becomes detectable between 3 and 4 months EGA, and by 5 months, melanosomes begin to transfer pigment to keratinocytes. Many genetic disorders of pigmentation have been characterized and are presented in detail in Chaps. 89 and 90.

Langerhans' cells, another immigrant population, are detectable by 40 days EGA. They begin to express CD1 on their surface and to produce their characteristic Birbeck granules by the embryonic–fetal transition. By the third trimester, most of the adult numbers of Langerhans' cells will have been produced.

Merkel cells, as described earlier in the chapter, reside in the epidermis. They are first detectable in the volar epidermis of the 11- to 12-week EGA human fetus. The embryonic derivation of this population of cells is controversial. The strongest evidence thus far for in situ differentiation of Merkel cells from epidermal ectoderm versus immigration of Merkel cells, perhaps from neural crest, comes from studies in which 8- and 11-week EGA fetal volar skin that lacked Merkel cells was transplanted to the nude mouse. Tissue harvested 8 weeks later contained an abundance of human K18-positive Merkel cells within the epidermis, suggesting that the cells differentiated within the grafted tissue.[83] Recent studies show that Merkel cells do not proliferate in the epidermis. This can be interpreted as further evidence that Merkel cells arise from an epidermal stem cell.[84]

DERMAL AND SUBCUTICULAR DEVELOPMENT The origin of the dermis and subcutaneous tissue is more diverse than that of the epidermis, which is exclusively ectodermally derived. The embryonic tissue that forms the dermis depends on the specific body site.[85,86] Dermal mesenchyme of the face and anterior scalp is derived from neural crest ectoderm. The limb and ventral body wall mesenchyme is derived from the lateral plate mesoderm. The dorsal body wall mesenchyme derives from the dermomyotomes of the embryonic somite. Lmx-1B and Wnt7a are important in the specification of the dorsal limb.[87–89] En-1 and BMPs, on the other hand, specify the volar (ventral) limb mesenchyme (see Table 6-2).[78,89]

The embryonic dermis, in contrast to the mature dermis, is cellular and amorphous, with few organized fibers. The mature dermis contains

FIGURE 6-26

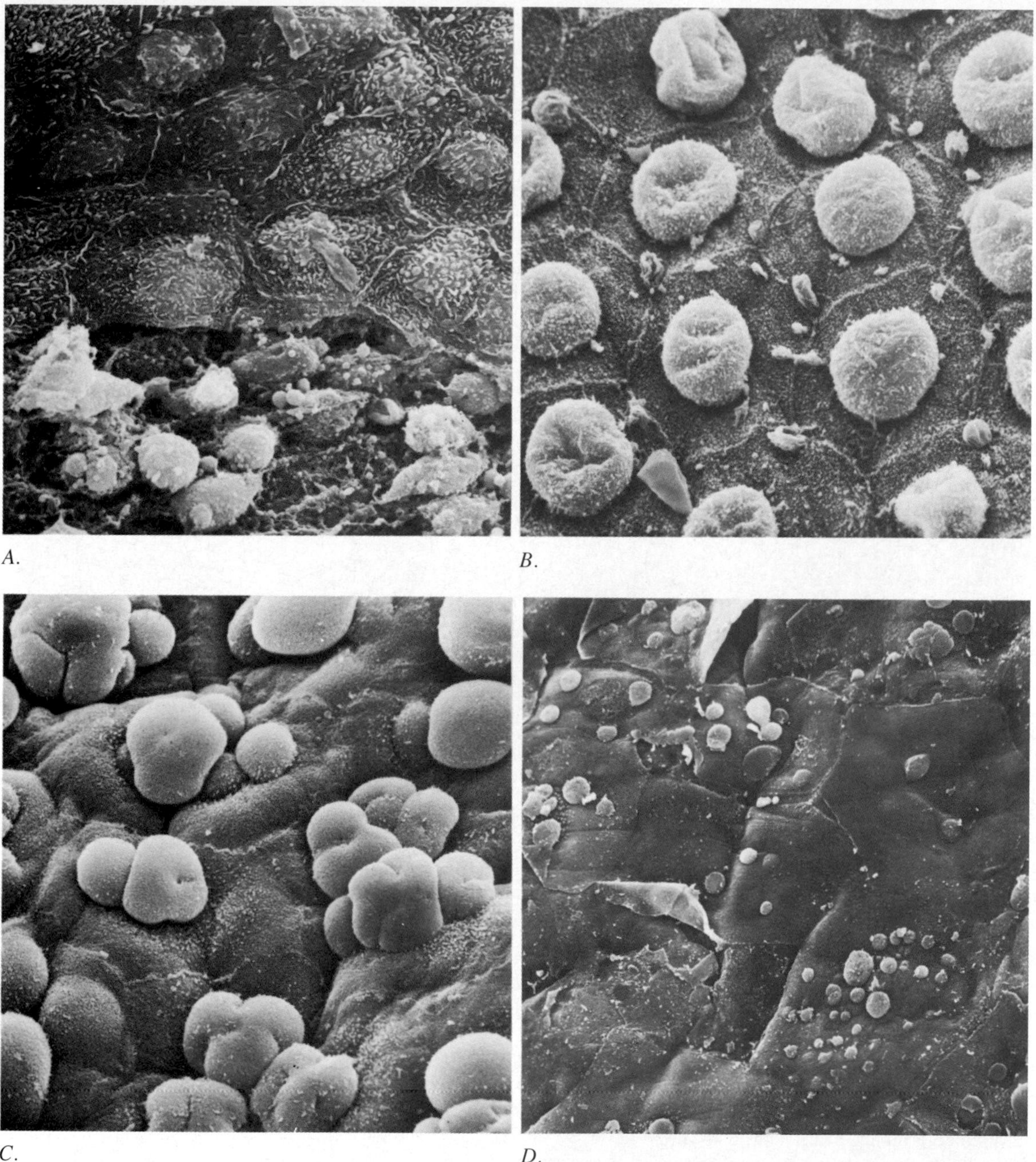

Scanning electron micrographs of the periderm (epidermal surface) of embryonic and fetal skin at progressive stages of development. Cells of the basal layer are revealed where the periderm is torn (*A*). *A*, ×1885; *B* and *C*, ×1450; *D*, ×400.

a complex mesh of collagen and elastic fibers embedded in a matrix of proteoglycans, whereas the embryonic mesenchyme contains a large variety of pluripotent cells in a hydrated gel that is rich in hyaluronic acid. These mesenchymal cells are thought to be the progenitors of cartilage-producing cells, adipose tissue, dermal fibroblasts, and intramembranous bone. Dermal fibers exist as fine filaments, but not thick fibers. The protein components of the future elastin and collagen fibers are synthesized during this period but not assembled. At this point, there is no obvious separation between cells that will become musculoskeletal elements and those that will give rise to the skin dermis.

Although there is no known inherited disorder of dermal development, certain conditions such as restrictive dermopathy, focal dermal hypoplasia (Goltz's syndrome), and Proteus syndrome exhibit focal defects, probably a result of genetic mosaicism affecting genes important in this process. Mutations causing a global defect in this process would likely be incompatible with life.

The superficial mesenchyme becomes distinct from the underlying tissue by the embryonic–fetal transition (about 60 days EGA). By 12 to 15 weeks, the reticular dermis begins to take on its characteristic fibrillar appearance in contrast to the papillary dermis, which is more finely woven. Large collagen fibers continue to accumulate in the reticular dermis, as well as elastin fibers, beginning around mid-gestation and continuing until birth. By the end of the second trimester, the dermis has changed from a nonscarring tissue to a scarring one. As the dermis matures, it also becomes thicker and well-organized, such that at birth, it resembles the dermis of the adult, although it is still more cellular.

Many well-known clinical syndromes and molecules have been discovered that affect this final stage of dermal differentiation. These diseases include dystrophic epidermolysis bullosa (EB) (a collagen VII defect), Marfan syndrome (a defect in fibrillin), Ehlers-Danlos syndrome, cutis laxa (elastin), pseudoxanthoma elasticum (PXE), hereditary hemorrhagic telangiectasia (HHT, or Osler-Weber-Rendu syndrome), and osteogenesis imperfecta (OI) (see Table 6-2). In many of these cases, the specific genetic defect helps to define the many different manifestations of these diseases, although in certain cases (e.g. PXE), the identity of the gene does not readily explain the mechanism of disease.

Specialized Components of the Dermis

BLOOD VESSELS AND NERVES Cutaneous nerves and vessels begin to form early during gestation, but they do not evolve into those of the adult until a few months after birth. The process of vasculogenesis requires the in situ differentiation of the endothelial cells at the endoderm–mesoderm interface. Originally, horizontal plexuses are formed within the subpapillary and deep reticular dermis, which are interconnected by groups of vertical vessels. This lattice of vessels is in place by 45 to 50 days EGA.

At 9 weeks EGA, blood vessels are seen at the dermal–hypodermal junction. By 3 months, the distinct networks of horizontal and vertical vessels have formed. By the fifth month, further changes in the vasculature derive from budding and migration of endothelium from preexisting vessels, the process of angiogenesis. Depending on the body region, gestational age, presence of hair follicles and glands, this pattern can vary with blood supply requirements.

Defects in vascular development have been described, as in the Klippel-Trenaunay and Sturge-Weber syndromes (see Chap. 103). In the Klippel-Trenaunay syndrome, unilateral cutaneous vascular malformations develop, with associated venous varicosities, edema, and hypertrophy of associated soft tissue and bone. In Sturge-Weber syndrome, many cutaneous capillary malformations are seen in the lips, tongue, nasal, and buccal mucosae. Some familial defects in vascular formation result from mutations in the gene encoding TIE2 receptor tyrosine kinase. Capillary malformations seen in hereditary hemorrhagic telangiectasia have been linked to mutations in TGF-β binding proteins, endoglin and activin receptor-like kinase 1.

LYMPHATICS Accumulating evidence suggests that lymphatics originate from endothelial cells that bud off from veins. The pattern of embryonic lymphatic vessel development parallels that of blood vessels. Detailed molecular studies into the development of lymphatics during embryogenesis and fetal development have long been hampered by the lack of lymphatic-specific markers. However, recent studies have identified new genes that appear to be specific for some of the earliest lymphatic precursors. LYVE-1 and Prox-1 are genes considered to be critical for earliest lymphatic specification, whereas VEGF-R3 and SLC may be important in later lymphatic differentiation. Supporting the assertion that VEGF-3 is a critical component of lymphatic formation, some patients with hereditary lymphedema have been found to have defects in the VEGF-3 gene.[90]

NERVES The development of cutaneous nerves parallels that of the vascular system in terms of patterning, maturation, and organization. Nerves of the skin consist of somatic sensory and sympathetic autonomic fibers, which are predominantly small and unmyelinated. As these nerves develop, they become myelinated, with associated decrease in the number of axons. This process may continue as long as puberty.

SUBCUTIS

As mentioned above, by 50 to 60 days EGA, the hypodermis is separated from the overlying dermis by a plane of thin-walled vessels. Toward the end of the first trimester, the matrix of the hypodermis can be distinguished from the more fibrous matrix of the dermis. By the second trimester, adipocyte precursors begin to differentiate and accumulate lipids. By the third trimester, fat lobules and fibrous septae are found to separate the mature adipocytes. The molecular pathways that define this process are currently an area of intense investigation. Although few regulators important in embryonic adipose specification and development have identified, several factors critical for preadipocyte differentiation have been demonstrated, including leptin, a hormone important in fat regulation, and the PPAR family of transcription factors.[69,91]

DERMAL–EPIDERMAL JUNCTION

The dermal–epidermal junction is an interface where many inductive interactions occur that result in the specification or differentiation of the characteristics of the dermis and epidermis. This zone includes specialized basement membrane, basal cell extracellular matrix, the basal-most portion of the basal cells, and the superficial-most fibrillar structures of the papillary dermis. Both the epidermis and dermis contribute to this region.

As early as 8 weeks EGA, a simple basement membrane separates the dermis from the epidermis and contains many of the major protein elements common to all basement membranes, including laminin 1, collagen IV, heparin sulfate, and proteoglycans. Components specific to the cutaneous basement membrane zone, such as proteins of the hemidesmosome and anchoring filaments, are first detected at the embryonic–fetal transition. By the end of the first trimester, or around the time of late embryonic development, all basement membrane proteins are in place. The α_6 and β_4 integrin subunits are expressed earlier than most of the other basement membrane components. However, they are not localized to the basal surface until 9.5 weeks EGA, coincident with the time that the hemidesmosomal proteins are expressed and hemidesmosomes are first observed. At the same time, anchoring filaments (laminin 5) and anchoring fibrils (collagen VII) begin to be assembled. The actual synthesis of collagen VII can be detected slightly earlier, at 8 weeks EGA.

Many congenital blistering disorders have been demonstrated to be a result of defects in proteins of the DEJ (for details, see Chap. 65). The severity of the disease, plane of tissue separation, and involvement of nonskin tissues depend on the proteins involved and the specific mutations. These genes are important candidates for prenatal testing.

DEVELOPMENT OF SKIN APPENDAGES

Skin appendages, which include hair, nails, sweat and mammary glands, are composed of two distinct components: an epidermal portion, which produces the differentiated product, and the dermal component, which regulates differentiation of the appendage. During embryonic development, dermal–epidermal interactions are critical for the induction and differentiation of these structures. Disruption of these signals often has profound influences on development of skin appendages. Our discussion focuses on hair differentiation as a paradigm for appendageal development, because it is the appendage that has been studied most intensely.[92]

Hair

Dermal signals are initially responsible for instructing the basal cells of the epidermis to begin to crowd at regularly spaced intervals, starting between days 75 and 80 on the scalp. This initial grouping is known as the follicular placode or anlage. Based on molecular localization of β-catenin, it has been implicated as a candidate for one of the effectors of this "dermal signal."

From the scalp, follicular placode formation spreads ventrally and caudally, eventually covering the skin. The placodes then signal back to the underlying dermis to form a "dermal condensate," which occurs at 12 to 14 weeks EGA. This process is thought to be a balance of placode promoters and placode inhibitors.[92] Wnt family signaling molecules are proposed to mediate placode promoting effects via the molecules LEF and β-catenin, as well as FGF, TGF-β_2, Msx1 and 2, ectodysplasin A (EDA), and EDAR (EDA receptor). BMP family molecules, on the other hand, act as inhibitors of follicle formation. In model systems, ectopic expression of this family of molecules tends to suppress the formation of follicles. In mice, EDAR and β-catenin expression are required for expression of BMP4 and Sonic hedgehog (Shh), implicating these molecules in early follicular morphogenesis. Furthermore, EDAR may be important for lateral inhibition of cells surrounding the follicles.

Formation of the dermal papilla is thought to be initiated by the "first epithelial signal" that gets transmitted from the follicle epithelium to the underlying mesenchyme. Molecules proposed to be involved in this signaling process include PDGF-A and Shh. After the follicular differentiation process begins, the dermis sends another signal to the epithelial placode cells to proliferate and invade the dermis. The dermal cells associated with the follicle then develop into the dermal papilla. The epithelial cells go on to form the inner root sheath and hair shaft of the mature hair follicle.

In addition to the widened bulge at the base, two other bulges form along the length of the developing follicle, termed the *bulbous hair peg*. The uppermost bulge is the presumptive sebaceous gland, whereas the middle bulge serves as the site for insertion of the arrector pili muscle. This middle bulge is also the location of the multipotent hair stem cells, which are capable of differentiating into any of the cells of the hair follicle, and also have the potential to replenish the entire epidermis, as has seen in cases of extensive surface wounds or burns.

By 19 to 21 weeks EGA, the hair canal has completely formed and the hairs on the scalp are visible above the surface of the fetal epidermis. They continue to lengthen until 24 to 28 weeks, at which time they shift from the active growth (anagen) phase to the degenerative phase (catagen), then to the resting phase (telogen). This completes the first hair cycle. With subsequent hair cycles, hairs increase in diameter and coarseness. During adolescence, vellus hairs of androgen-sensitive areas mature to terminal-type hair follicles.

Sebaceous Glands

Sebaceous glands mature during the course of follicular differentiation. This process begins between 13 and 16 weeks EGA, at which point the presumptive sebaceous gland is first visible as the most superficial bulge of the maturing hair follicle. The outer proliferative cells of the gland give rise to the differentiated cells that accumulate lipid and sebum. After they terminally differentiate, these cells disintegrate and release their products into the upper portion of the hair canal. Sebum production is accelerated in the second and third trimesters, during which time maternal steroids cause stimulation of the sebaceous glands. Hormonal activity is once again thought to influence the production of increased sebum during adolescence, resulting in the increased incidence in acne at this age.

Nail Development

Presumptive nail structures begin to appear on the dorsal digit tip at 8 to 10 weeks EGA, slightly earlier than the initiation of hair follicle development. The first sign is the delineation of the flat surface of the future nail bed. A portion of ectoderm buds inward at the proximal boundary of the early nail field, and gives rise to the proximal nail fold. The presumptive nail matrix cells, which differentiate to become the nail plate, are present on the ventral side of the proximal invagination. At 11 weeks, the dorsal nail bed surface begins to keratinize. By the fourth month of gestation, the nail plate grows out from the proximal nail fold, completely covering the nail bed by the fifth month. Mutations in p63 affect nail development in syndromes such as AEC, as well as EEC. Functional p63 is required for the formation and maintenance of the apical ectodermal ridge, an embryonic signaling center essential for limb outgrowth and hand plate formation. Wnt 7a is thought to be important for dorsal limb patterning, and thus nail formation. In contrast to follicular development, Shh is not required for nail plate formation. Also similar to follicular differentiation, LMX1b and MSX1 are important for nail specification; LMX1b & MSX1 are mutated in nail-patella syndrome and Witkop syndrome respectively.[93–95] Hoxc13 appears to be an important homeodomain-containing gene for both follicular and nail appendages, at least in murine models.[96]

Eccrine and Apocrine Sweat Gland Development

Eccrine glands begin to develop on the volar surfaces of the hands and feet, beginning as mesenchymal pads between 55 and 65 days EGA. By 12 to 14 weeks EGA, parallel ectodermal ridges are induced, which overly these pads. The eccrine glands arise from the ectodermal ridge. By 16 weeks EGA, the secretory portion of the gland becomes detectable. The dermal duct begins around week 16, but the epidermal portion of the duct and opening are not complete until 2 weeks EGA.

Interfollicular eccrine and apocrine glands, in contrast, do not begin to bud until the fifth month of gestation. Apocrine sweat glands usually bud from the upper portion of the hair follicle. By 7 months EGA, the cells of the apocrine glands become distinguishable.

Although not much is known with regard to the molecular signals responsible for the differentiation of these structures, the EDA, EDAR, En1, and Wnt10b genes have been implicated.

PRENATAL TESTING OF CONGENITAL SKIN DISORDERS

The identification of the genes involved in early cutaneous differentiation and development, as well as some of their associated mutations in disease, have made it possible for prenatal testing to diagnose fetuses with life-threatening or debilitating disorders.[97] Candidates for prenatal testing include those fetuses with an affected sibling or family member. A number of techniques have been developed for evaluation of involved genes. For example, chorionic villous sampling (CVS) can be undertaken at 8 to 10 weeks EGA or amniocentesis at 16 to 18 weeks EGA (see Table 6-2). These techniques are associated with less morbidity and mortality to the fetus than the only previously available method, fetal skin biopsy, performed between 19 and 22 weeks EGA. Although these recent advances in prenatal diagnosis allow for the early detection of many severe genodermatoses, certain syndromes, such as harlequin fetus, still require fetal biopsy for diagnosis. Resources for health care providers, including currently available laboratory tests, as well as reviews regarding some of these congenital disorders, can be found at GeneTest (http://www.genetests.org).

REFERENCES

1. Fuchs E: Keratins and the skin. *Annu Rev Cell Dev Biol* **11**:123, 1995
2. Freedberg IM et al: Keratins and the keratinocyte activation cycle. *J Invest Dermatol* **116**:633, 2001
3. Michel M et al: Keratin 19 as a biochemical marker of skin stem cells in vivo and in vitro: Keratin 19 expressing cells are differentially localized in function of anatomic sites, and their number varies with donor age and culture stage. *J Cell Sci* **109**:1017, 1996
4. Lyle S et al: The C8/144B monoclonal antibody recognizes cytokeratin 15 and defines the location of human hair follicle stem cells. *J Cell Sci* **111**:3179, 1998
5. Watt FM: Stem cell fate and patterning in mammalian epidermis. *Curr Opin Genet Dev* **11**:410, 2001
6. Fuchs E et al: At the roots of a never-ending cycle. *Dev Cell* **1**:13, 2001
7. Kowalczyk AP et al: Desmosomes: Intercellular adhesive junctions specialized for attachment of intermediate filaments. *Int Rev Cytol* **185**:237, 1999
8. Yap AS et al: Molecular and functional analysis of cadherin-based adherens junctions. *Annu Rev Cell Dev Biol* **13**:119, 1997
9. Lin MS et al: The desmosome and hemidesmosome in cutaneous autoimmunity. *Clin Exp Immunol* **107**(Suppl 1):9, 1997
10. Hanakawa Y et al: Molecular mechanisms of blister formation in bullous impetigo and staphylococcal scalded skin syndrome. *J Clin Invest* **110**:53, 2002
11. Richard G: Connexins: A connection with the skin. *Exp Dermatol* **9**:77, 2000
12. Herman GE: X-Linked dominant disorders of cholesterol biosynthesis in man and mouse. *Biochim Biophys Acta* **1529**:357, 2000
13. Holbrook KA: Biologic structure and function: Perspectives on morphologic approaches to the study of the granular layer keratinocyte. *J Invest Dermatol* **92**:84S, 1989
14. Nemes Z, Steinert PM: Bricks and mortar of the epidermal barrier. *Exp Mol Med* **31**:5, 1999
15. Presland RB, Dale BA: Epithelial structural proteins of the skin and oral cavity: Function in health and disease. *Crit Rev Oral Biol Med* **11**:383, 2000
16. Elias PM, Feingold KR: Coordinate regulation of epidermal differentiation and barrier homeostasis. *Skin Pharmacol Appl Skin Physiol* **14**(Suppl 1):28, 2001
17. Sengel P: Epidermal–dermal interaction, in *Biology of the Integument*, vol. 2, *Vertebrates*, edited by J Bereiter-Hahn, AG Matoltsy, KS Richards. Berlin, Springer-Verlag, 1986, p 374
18. Hynes RO: Cell adhesion: Old and new questions. *Trends Cell Biol* **9**:M33, 1999
19. Tennenbaum T et al: Differential regulation of integrins and extracellular matrix binding in epidermal differentiation and squamous tumor progression. *J Investig Dermatol Symp Proc* **1**:157, 1996
20. Fuchs E et al: Integrators of epidermal growth and differentiation: Distinct functions for beta 1 and beta 4 integrins. *Curr Opin Genet Dev* **7**:672, 1997
21. Tomic-Canic M et al: Epidermal signal transduction and transcription factor activation in activated keratinocytes. *J Dermatol Sci* **17**:167, 1998
22. Fuchs E, Byrne C: The epidermis: Rising to the surface. *Curr Opin Genet Dev* **4**:725, 1994
23. Jost M et al: The EGF receptor—An essential regulator of multiple epidermal functions. *Eur J Dermatol* **10**:505, 2000
24. Beer HD et al: Expression and function of keratinocyte growth factor and activin in skin morphogenesis and cutaneous wound repair. *J Investig Dermatol Symp Proc* **5**:34, 2000
25. Ito Y et al: Overexpression of Smad2 reveals its concerted action with Smad4 in regulating TGF-beta-mediated epidermal homeostasis. *Dev Biol* **236**:181, 2001
26. Steinhoff M et al: Keratinocytes in epidermal immune responses. *Curr Opin Allergy Clin Immunol* **1**:469, 2001
27. Kang S et al: Pharmacology and molecular action of retinoids and vitamin D in skin. *J Investig Dermatol Symp Proc* **1**:15, 1996
28. Eichner R et al: Effects of long-term retinoic acid treatment on epidermal differentiation in vivo: specific modifications in the programme of terminal differentiation. *Br J Dermatol* **135**:687, 1996
29. Bikle DD et al: Calcium- and vitamin D-regulated keratinocyte differentiation. *Mol Cell Endocrinol* **177**:161, 2001
30. Missiaen L et al: Abnormal intracellular Ca(2+) homeostasis and disease. *Cell Calcium* **28**:1, 2000
31. Sakuntabhai A et al: Spectrum of novel ATP2A2 mutations in patients with Darier's disease. *Hum Mol Genet* **8**:1611, 1999
32. Hu Z et al: Mutations in ATP2C1, encoding a calcium pump, cause Hailey-Hailey disease. *Nat Genet* **24**:61, 2000
33. Nickoloff BJ, Denning M: Life and death signaling in epidermis: Following a planned cell death pathway involving a trail that does not lead to skin cancer. *J Invest Dermatol* **117**:1, 2001
34. Vancoillie G et al: Melanocyte biology and its implications for the clinician. *Eur J Dermatol* **9**:241, 1999
35. Seiberg M: Keratinocyte-melanocyte interactions during melanosome transfer. *Pigment Cell Res* **14**:236, 2001
36. Ogawa H: The Merkel cell as a possible mechanoreceptor cell. *Prog Neurobiol* **49**:317, 1996
37. Johnson KO: The roles and functions of cutaneous mechanoreceptors. *Curr Opin Neurobiol* **11**:455, 2001
38. Jakob T, Udey MC: Epidermal Langerhans cells: From neurons to nature's adjuvants. *Adv Dermatol* **14**:209, 1999
39. Ghohestani RF et al: Molecular organization of the cutaneous basement membrane zone. *Clin Dermatol* **19**:551, 2001
40. Burgeson RE, Christiano AM: The dermal–epidermal junction. *Curr Opin Cell Biol* **9**:651, 1997
41. Uitto J, Pulkkinen L: Molecular genetics of heritable blistering disorders. *Arch Dermatol* **137**:1458, 2001
42. Werner S, Smola H: Paracrine regulation of keratinocyte proliferation and differentiation. *Trends Cell Biol* **11**:143, 2001
43. Burgeson RE, Nimni ME: Collagen types. Molecular structure and tissue distribution. *Clin Orthop* **282**:250, 1992
44. Christiano AM, Uitto J: Molecular pathology of the elastic fibers. *J Invest Dermatol* **103**:53S, 1994
45. Kielty CM, Shuttleworth CA: Microfibrillar elements of the dermal matrix. *Microsc Res Tech* **38**:413, 1997
46. Uitto J, Bernstein EF: Molecular mechanisms of cutaneous aging: Connective tissue alterations in the dermis. *J Investig Dermatol Symp Proc* **3**:41, 1998
47. Iozzo RV: Matrix proteoglycans: From molecular design to cellular function. *Annu Rev Biochem* **67**:609, 1998
48. Scott JE: Supramolecular organization of extracellular matrix glycosaminoglycans in vitro and in the tissues. *FASEB J* **6**:2639, 1992
49. Gallo R et al: Syndecans-1 and -4 are induced during wound repair of neonatal but not fetal skin. *J Invest Dermatol* **107**:676, 1996
50. Schwarzbauer JE, Sechler JL: Fibronectin fibrillogenesis: A paradigm for extracellular matrix assembly. *Curr Opin Cell Biol* **11**:622, 1999
51. Aumailley M, Rousselle P: Laminins of the dermo-epidermal junction. *Matrix Biol* **18**:19, 1999
52. Adams JC: Thrombospondins: Multifunctional regulators of cell interactions. *Annu Rev Cell Dev Biol* **17**:25, 2001
53. Schvartz I et al: Vitronectin. *Int J Biochem Cell Biol* **31**:539, 1999
54. Jones FS, Jones PL: The tenascin family of ECM glycoproteins: Structure, function, and regulation during embryonic development and tissue remodeling. *Dev Dyn* **218**:235, 2000
55. Holbrook KA, Byers PH: Diseases of the extracellular matrix: Structural alterations of collagen fibrils in skin, in *Connective Tissue Disease: Molecular Pathology of the Extracellular Matrix*, edited by J Uitto and A Perejda. New York, Marcel Dekker, 1987, p 10
56. Falanga V et al: Human dermal fibroblast clones derived from single cells are heterogeneous in the production of mRNAs for alpha 1(I) procollagen and transforming growth factor-beta 1. *J Invest Dermatol* **105**:27, 1995
57. Wang R et al: Hypertrophic scar tissues and fibroblasts produce more transforming growth factor-beta1 mRNA and protein than normal skin and cells. *Wound Repair Regen* **8**:128, 2000
58. Cline MJ: Monocytes, macrophages, and their diseases in man. *J Invest Dermatol* **71**:56, 1978
59. Weber-Matthiesen K, Sterry W: Organization of the monocyte/macrophage system of normal human skin. *J Invest Dermatol* **95**:83, 1990
60. Church MK, Clough GF: Human skin mast cells: in vitro and in vivo studies. *Ann Allergy Asthma Immunol* **83**:471, 1999
61. Nagata H et al: *c-Kit* mutation in a population of patients with mastocytosis. *Int Arch Allergy Immunol* **113**:184, 1997
62. Nemes Z et al: Identification of histiocytic reticulum cells by the immunohistochemical demonstration of factor XIII (F-XIIIa) in human lymph nodes. *J Pathol* **149**:121, 1986
63. Braverman IM: The cutaneous microcirculation. *J Investig Dermatol Symp Proc* **5**:3, 2000
64. Detmar M: Molecular regulation of angiogenesis in the skin. *J Invest Dermatol* **106**:207, 1996
65. Ryan TJ: Structure and function of lymphatics. *J Invest Dermatol* **93**:18S, 1989
66. Deutsch A et al: Ultrastructural studies on the invasion of melanomas in initial lymphatics of human skin. *J Invest Dermatol* **98**:64, 1992

67. Johansson O: The innervation of the human epidermis. *J Neurol Sci* **130**:228, 1995
68. Holst D, Grimaldi PA: New factors in the regulation of adipose differentiation and metabolism. *Curr Opin Lipidol* **13**:241, 2002
69. Koutnikova H, Auwerx J: Regulation of adipocyte differentiation. *Ann Med* **33**:556, 2001
70. Online Mendelian Inheritance in Man, OMIM. http://www.ncbi.nlm.nih.gov/omim/. 2001.
71. Novice FM, Collison DW, Burgdorf WHC, Esterly NB. *Handbook of Genetic Skin Disorders*. Philadelphia, W.B. Saunders, 1994.
72. Holbrook KA: Structure and function of the developing human skin, in *Physiology, Biochemistry, and Molecular Biology of the Skin,* edited by LA Goldsmith. New York, Oxford Press, 1991, p 63
73. Loomis CA: Development and morphogenesis of the skin. *Adv Dermatol* **17**:183, 2001
74. Loomis CA et al: The mouse Engrailed-1 gene and ventral limb patterning. *Nature* **382**:360, 1996
75. Ahn K et al: BMPR-IA signaling is required for the formation of the apical ectodermal ridge and dorsal-ventral patterning of the limb. *Development* **128**:4449, 2001
76. Pizette S, Niswander L: Early steps in limb patterning and chondrogenesis. *Novartis Found Symp* **232**:23, 2001
77. Yang A et al: p63 is essential for regenerative proliferation in limb, craniofacial and epithelial development. *Nature* **398**:714, 1999
78. Mills A et al: p63 is a p53 homologue required for limb and epidermal morphogenesis. *Nature* **398**:708, 1999
79. Celli J et al: Heterozygous germline mutations in the p53 homolog p63 are the cause of EEC syndrome. *Cell* **99**:143, 1999
80. McGrath JA et al: Hay-Wells syndrome is caused by heterozygous missense mutations in the SAM domain of p63. *Hum Mol Genet* **10**:221, 2001
81. Wessagowit V et al: Heterozygous germline missense mutation in the p63 gene underlying EEC syndrome. *Clin Exp Dermatol* **25**:441, 2000
82. Okura M et al: Effects of monoclonal anti–*c-kit* antibody (ACK2) on melanocytes in newborn mice. *J Invest Dermatol* **105**:322, 1995
83. Moll I et al: Intraepidermal formation of Merkel cells in xenografts of human fetal skin. *J Invest Dermatol* **94**:359, 1990
84. Moll I et al: Proliferative Merkel cells were not detected in human skin. *Arch Dermatol Res* **288**:184, 1996
85. Christ B et al: Differentiating abilities of avian somatopleural mesoderm. *Experientia* **35**:1376, 1979
86. Noden DM: Vertebrate craniofacial development: Novel approaches and new dilemmas. *Curr Opin Genet Dev* **2**:576, 1992
87. Parr BA, McMahon AP: Dorsalizing signal Wnt-7a required for normal polarity of D-V and A-P axes of mouse limb. *Nature* **374**:350, 1995
88. Cygan JA et al: Novel regulatory interactions revealed by studies of murine limb pattern in Wnt-7a and En-1 mutants. *Development* **124**:5021, 1997
89. Loomis CA et al: Analysis of the genetic pathway leading to formation of ectopic apical ectodermal ridges in mouse Engrailed-1 mutant limbs. *Development* **125**:1137, 1998
90. Oliver G, Detmar M: The rediscovery of the lymphatic system: Old and new insights into the development and biological function of the lymphatic vasculature. *Genes Dev* **16**:773, 2002
91. Rosen ED, Spiegelman BM: Molecular regulation of adipogenesis. *Annu Rev Cell Dev Biol* **16**:145, 2000
92. Millar SE: Molecular mechanisms regulating hair follicle development. *J Invest Dermatol* **118**:216, 2002
93. Dreyer SD, et al: Mutations in LMX1B cause abnormal skeletal patterning and renal dysplasia in nail patella syndrome. *Nature Genet* **19**:47,1998
94. Vollrath D, et al: Loss-of-function mutations in the LIM-homeodomain gene, LMX1B, in nail-patella syndrome. *Hum Mol Genet* **7**:1091, 1998
95. Jumlongras D et al: A nonsense mutation in MSX1 causes Witkop syndrome. *Am J Hum Genet* **69**:67, 2001
96. Godwin AR, Capecchi MR: Hoxc13 mutant mice lack external hair. *Genes Dev* **12**:11, 1998
97. Ashton GH et al: Prenatal diagnosis for inherited skin diseases. *Clin Dermatol* **18**:643, 2000

SECTION 4

BIOLOGY AND FUNCTION OF EPIDERMIS AND APPENDAGES

CHAPTER 7

Arash Kimyai-Asadi
Ming H. Jih
Irwin M. Freedberg

Epidermal Cell Kinetics, Epidermal Differentiation, and Keratinization

The epidermis is the prototype of keratinizing squamous epithelia, also present in the esophagus, vagina, and oral mucosa. The stratified squamous epidermis is composed of a proliferative basal layer containing the self-sustaining stem cell component and spinous and granular cells that express a tightly regulated set of proteins and lipids that are eventually woven into the cornified cell envelope of the corneocyte, providing the skin with its mechanical and chemical barrier. The ability to culture keratinocytes in vitro has provided the opportunity to study many aspects of epidermal proliferation and differentiation. Moreover, a variety of techniques can be used to isolate and characterize the structural and functional proteins of the epidermis and to identify and clone many of the genes responsible for normal epidermal function and for an increasing number of hereditary skin disorders (Tables 7-1 and 7-2). Information about other cells in the epidermis, including melanocytes and Langerhans cells, is found in Chapters 11 and 23, respectively. Hair follicles are considered in Chapter 12, nails in Chapter 13, and sweat glands in Chapter 8. The epidermal barrier is discussed in Chapter 9, and skin structure and development are analyzed in Chapter 6.

EPIDERMAL CELL KINETICS

From a cell kinetic viewpoint, tissues can be divided into three types: (1) static tissues, such as the adult CNS, in which cells do not divide, (2) normally nonproliferative tissues, such as the liver, which retain the ability to divide in response to injury, and (3) constantly renewing tissues, such as the epidermis and gastrointestinal mucosa.

The cell cycle itself is divided into four stages (Fig. 7-1). Mitosis (M) is followed by a resting stage called *gap 1* (G_1). This stage is both the longest and most variable in duration. From G_1, in response to signals that have not been completely defined, cells enter the stage of DNA replication, which is called the *synthesis* (S) stage. The duration of the S phase is relatively constant in mammalian tissues and lasts approximately 7 to 16 h in dividing keratinocytes. During this phase, duplication of the DNA content occurs in anticipation of cell division. During the second gap phase (G_2), which lasts 6 to 8 h, cells complete final preparation for cell division. During the mitotic phase (M), which is the shortest segment of cell division (1–2 h), two daughter cells are produced. There is an additional stage, termed G_0, that some cells may enter during G_1 or possibly G_2. During G_0, cells do not progress through the cell cycle, although they retain the potential to return to the active cell cycle in response to appropriate signals. Progression of the cell through G_1 is controlled by cyclin-dependent kinases, and increases in their inhibitors play a role in the induction of irreversible growth arrest, which is an early and integral step in keratinocyte differentiation.[1]

Measurements related to the cell cycle were of particular focus in the past but today have little direct in vivo physiologic or pathologic significance. The cell cycle time is the time it takes a cell to move from any given point in one cycle to the corresponding point in the next cycle, and in proliferating keratinocytes, it is between 60 and 450 h. The growth fraction is the ratio of proliferating to nonproliferating cells in a given tissue. The mitotic index is the percentage of cells that are in the M phase of the cell cycle. This value is approximately 5 percent in the basal layer and can be determined histologically. The flash-labeling index determines the fraction of cells that take up tritiated thymidine and represents cells in the S phase when thymidine is incorporated into elongating DNA molecules. Thymidine analogues such as bromodeoxyuridine, which can be detected immunologically, as well as fluorescent dyes, which bind stoichiometrically to DNA or other molecules, also can be used to label cells in S phase. Both the mitotic index and the flash-labeling index should include only the proliferative compartment as the denominator and generally are determined as a fraction of the population of basal layer cells. The turnover time is the time required to replace the number of cells of a given tissue compartment, and the transit time is the time between a cell entering and leaving a given tissue compartment. Distinguishing these latter two values from the cell cycle time in the basal layer has been difficult. Moreover, these two values are conceptually identical in the spinous cells and stratum corneum and last approximately 14 days for each.[2] The decreased cell cycle time and increased growth fraction in psoriatic epidermis result in a shorter transit time (see Chap. 42).

TABLE 7-1

Hereditary Diseases Associated with Abnormalities in Epidermal Proteins

FUNCTION	PROTEIN	GENE LOCATION	INHERITANCE	HEREDITARY DISEASE
Intracellular structural	Loricrin	1q21	AD	Vohwinkel syndrome (ichthyotic variant) Progressive symmetric erythrokeratoderma
Desmosomal	Desmoplakin	6p24	AD AR	Striated PPK, PPK, woolly hair, left-sided cardiomyopathy
	Desmoglein 1	18q12.1–q12.2	AD	Striated PPK
	Plakoglobin	17q21	AD	Naxos syndrome
	Plakophilin	1q32	AR	Ectodermal dysplasia/skin fragility syndrome
	β-Catenin	3p22-21.3	AD	Multiple pilomatricomas with muscular dystrophy
Hemidesmosomal	Plectin	8q24	AR	Epidermolysis bullosa simplex with muscular dystrophy
	α_6 β_4 integrin	2 (α_6), 17q11-qter (β_4)	AR	Junctional epidermolysis bullosa with pyloric atresia
	Collagen XVII	10q24.3	AR	Junctional epidermolysis bullosa
	Laminin 5	18q11.2 (α_3), 1q32 (β_3), 1q25–31 (γ_2)	AR	Junctional epidermolysis bullosa
Gap junction	Connexin 26	13q11–q12	AD	Vohwinkel syndrome (classic variant)
	Connexin 30	13q12	AD	Hidrotic ectodermal dysplasia
	Connexin 30.3	1p35.1	AD	Erythrokeratodermia variabilis
	Connexin 31	1p35.1	AD	Erythrokeratodermia variabilis
Calcium ATPases	Ca^{2+} ATPase 2C1	3q21–24	AD	Hailey-Hailey disease
	Ca^{2+} ATPase 2A2	12q23–24.1	AD	Darier-White disease
Enzymes	Transglutaminase 1	14q11.2	AR	Lamellar ichthyosis Congenital nonbullous ichthyosiform erythroderma

NOTE: AD, autosomal dominant; AR, autosomal recessive; for keratin-associated diseases see Table 7-2.

THE CONCEPTS OF STEM CELLS, TRANSIENT AMPLIFYING CELLS, AND DIFFERENTIATED CELLS IN THE EPIDERMIS

In the adult epidermis, cell division is necessary to replace the cells lost through apoptosis or injury in order to maintain cell numbers at a relatively constant level. In stratified epithelia, differentiated cells have a relatively short lifespan. Therefore, throughout adult life, a population of cells is required that is capable of both self-renewal and the formation of cells destined for terminal differentiation. These are the stem cells. In normal skin, two populations of stem cells have been described: those which contribute epidermal keratinocytes destined to become cornified cells and those which contribute cells to the hair follicle and are destined to become the hair shaft. Recent studies have shown that the bulge cells of the hair follicle are at least bipotential, possessing the ability to give rise to both a stratum corneum and a hair shaft[3] (see Chap. 12). Although follicular stem cells are recruited during epidermal wound repair, long-term maintenance of the interfollicular keratinocyte population in adults is thought to be independent of follicular stem cells.[4]

Evidence for the existence of slow-cycling epidermal stem cells initially came from several sources. First, the fact that cultured basal keratinocytes from non-hair-bearing skin can last many years on burn patients suggested a source of self-renewing keratinocytes.[5] In addition, the presence of radio-resistant epidermal cells capable of repopulating the epidermis suggested the presence of a population of cells with prolonged cell cycle times.[6] This has been confirmed by tritiated thymidine labeling of keratinocytes, demonstrating a subpopulation of basal cells with retention of the label for up to 14 months.[7] These stem cells tend to be concentrated in the bulge region of the hair follicle, above the dermal papillae in nonacral skin, and at the deep portion of epidermal rete ridges on acral skin. The bulge is located below the opening of the sebaceous duct and is at the anchoring site of the arrector pili muscle; it is also the deepest part of the permanent portion of the hair follicle.[8] Whereas the bulge is histologically visible in rodent and human fetal hair follicles, it is difficult to visualize in adult hair follicles. Stem cells are relatively small, undifferentiated cells with few organelles and with strong attachments to the basement membrane zone.[8]

Whereas stem cells have an indefinite capacity for self-renewal, transient amplifying cells are defined as proliferating keratinocytes that have limited capacity for self-renewal and will, after a few rounds of mitosis, terminally differentiate.[9] Both stem cells and transient amplifying cells are located within the basal layer, although a third of the latter may be found in the lower spinous layer. That transient amplifying cells divide rapidly is reflected in their avid uptake but short retention of tritiated thymidine, since the marker is diluted with each round of cell division. This is in contrast to prolonged retention of tritiated thymidine by stem cells, reflecting their slow rate of cell division, which serves to protect them from the acquisition of genetic mutations.

Keratinocyte cell cultures, when seeded at low density, demonstrate that some colonies will contain several thousand cells by 2 weeks, whereas others will consist of a small number of terminally differentiated cells.[10] The cells forming the large colonies have the ability to both self-renew and generate daughter cells capable of terminal differentiation and are believed to represent stem cells. The smaller colonies are formed by cells that undergo only a few rounds of mitosis, representing transient amplifying cells. Terminally differentiated keratinocytes lack the ability to divide and thus will not yield clonal colonies in culture, although individual keratinocytes often reassociate in culture, forming colonies composed of a few cells. Thus, each stem cell gives rise to a number of transient amplifying cells that, after a few rounds of mitosis, become terminally differentiated, nonmitotic keratinocytes (Fig. 7-2). Each stem cell and all its progeny have been referred to as the *epidermal proliferative unit.* The histologic correlate of the epidermal proliferative unit can been seen in murine epidermis and occasionally in thin human epidermis, where columns of differentiating cells in the stratum spinosum overlie a cluster of approximately 10 basal cells. These basal cells are arranged with an average ratio of one centrally placed stem cell to nine peripheral transient amplifying cells.[11]

The isolation of stem cells has been hampered by difficulties in finding specific and sensitive markers, such as those present in hematopoietic stem cells. Keratin-19 initially was thought to be such a marker[12] but also was found in many non-label-retaining cells. Moreover, since telomerase activity is necessary for indefinite cell proliferation, it was thought that only stem cells would have high telomerase activity. However, both hematologic and epidermal evidence suggests that telomerase activity is greater in rapidly dividing cells (i.e., transient amplifying cells) than in stem cells.[13,14] Other postulated stem cell markers have included keratin-15, c-Myc, a non-cadherin-associated β-catenin, p63, the antigens recognized by monoclonal antibodies 10G7 and C8/144B, low expression of E-cadherin, and the high expression of delta 1.[15]

TABLE 7-2

Keratin Expression Patterns and Keratin-Associated Diseases

Type II	Type I	Physiologic Location of Expression	Hereditary Diseases
1	10	Suprabasal keratinocytes	Bullous congenital ichthyosiform erythroderma
1	9	Palmoplantar suprabasilar keratinocytes	Epidermolytic PPK Diffuse nonepidermolytic PPK Epidermolytic PPK with polycyclic psoriasiform plaques
2e	10	Upper spinous and granular layer	Ichthyosis bullosa of Siemens
3	12	Cornea	Meesmann's corneal dystrophy
4	13	Mucosal epithelium	White sponge nevus
5	14	Basal keratinocytes	Epidermolysis bullosa simplex
6a	16	Outer root sheath, hyperproliferative keratinocytes, palmoplantar keratinocytes	Pachyonychia congenita type I Focal nonepidermolytic PPK
6b	17	Nail bed, epidermal appendages	Pachyonychia congenita type II Steatocystoma multiplex
8	18	Simple epithelium	Cryptogenic cirrhosis
	19	Embryonic	
Hb 1, 3, 5, 6	Ha1, 2, 3a, 3b, 4–8	Hair follicle	Monilethrix (Hb1 and 6)

FIGURE 7-1

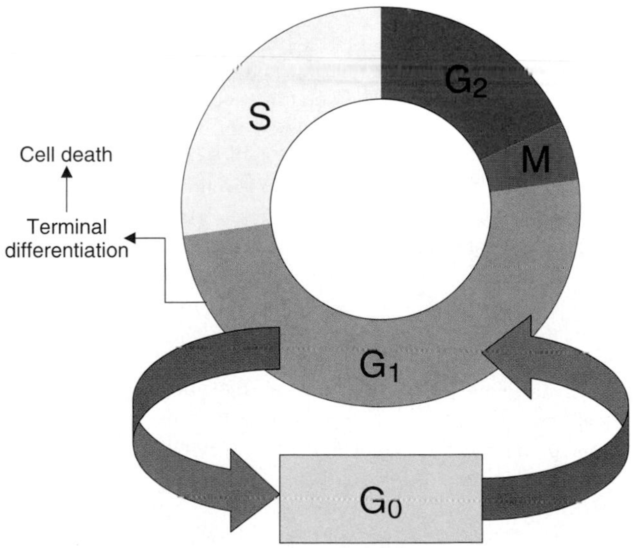

A diagram of the cell cycle. The cycling component starts with cells in the G_1 phase, the most variable part of the cycle. Cells then move into the S phase, during which the DNA content of the cell is doubled. Subsequently, cells enter the second gap phase (G_2), which leads to mitosis and the production of two daughter cells. The daughter cells may proceed through another replicative cycle, enter the differentiation pathway, or enter a resting phase (G_0).

Recently, several lines of evidence have suggested that integrins, the cell adhesion molecules that mediate attachment of basal keratinocytes to collagens, laminins, fibronectin, and vitronectin present in the extracellular matrix, may serve as markers for epidermal stem cells. In the epidermis, integrins are selectively expressed on basal keratinocytes, and the absence of a bound ligand in vitro results in irreversible inhibition of proliferation accompanied by expression of markers of terminal differentiation within a few hours.[16] Of note, β_1 integrin–rich keratinocytes are not distributed at random. Rather, they are concentrated at the tips of dermal papillae in interfollicular skin and at the deep part of the rete ridges in acral skin.[17] These integrin-rich areas have been shown to contain the cells with increased proliferative capacity.[18] Moreover, a number of experiments have shown that keratinocytes with high colony-forming efficiency in vitro can be isolated based on high surface levels of β_1 integrin and rapid adhesion to collagen IV, which is an integrin substrate.[10] The expression of a dominant-negative β_1 integrin mutation in proliferative keratinocytes results in an increased proportion of colonies attributable to transient amplifying cells.[19] However, since many transient amplifying cells and cells of the outer root sheath are also integrin-rich, it is apparent that integrins are not specific markers for epidermal stem cells.

Attempts to isolate epidermal stem cells have significant implications, particularly in the field of gene therapy. Several experiments have shown adequate initial expression of transduced recombinant genes in keratinocytes, with loss of expression after 2 to 6 weeks. This is likely due to terminal differentiation of all transfected cells. Of importance, DNA integration is more efficient in actively dividing cells, requiring selective enrichment and targeting of stem cells in order to gain long-term expression of transduced genes.[20] Enriching stem cells by

FIGURE 7-2

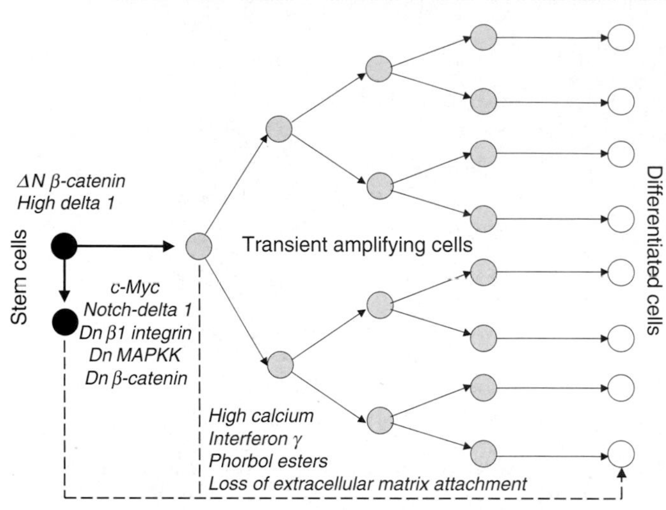

Stem cells, transient amplifying cells, and differentiated keratinocytes. A single stem cell gives rise to a stem cell and a transient amplifying cell, which goes through several rounds of mitosis prior to becoming a nonmitotic cell committed to terminal differentiation. Stabilized amino-terminally deleted β-catenin and high levels of delta 1 promote maintenance of a stem cell compartment, whereas c-Myc and stimulation of Notch by delta 1 on adjacent keratinocytes promote the transformation of stem cells into transient amplifying cells. Expression of dominant negative β_1 integrin, mitogen-activated protein kinase kinase, and β-catenin in keratinocytes also promotes the transformation of stem cells into transient amplifying cells. High concentrations of calcium, interferon-γ, and phorbol esters also promote terminal differentiation, as does loss of contact with the extracellular matrix. Dn, dominant negative. (*Adapted from Bickenbach et al.*[9] *and Watt*[23])

selecting integrin-rich cells with rapid attachment to collagen IV has enabled persistent expression of retrovirally transfected β-galactosidase in vitro for at least 12 weeks.[21] More recently, a sorting method, similar to methods used for the isolation of hematopoietic stem cells, was used to isolate epidermal stem cells from transient amplifying cells.[22] The basal keratinocytes were found to be composed of 90 percent transient amplifying cells, 6.5 percent differentiated cells, and 3.5 percent stem cells. Only stem cells formed large, maintainable, undifferentiated colonies in cell culture. Whereas the transient amplifying cells completely differentiated by 2 months, thereby losing expression of retrovirally transduced genes, persistent gene expression lasting over 6 months was seen in the stem cell population. The maintenance of stem cells appears to depend on β_1 integrin signaling through the mitogen-activated protein kinase (MAPK) pathway as well as by the expression of non-cadherin-associated β-catenin[23,24] (see Fig. 7-2). Catenins are proteins that generally bind cytoskeletal elements such as keratin and actin to cadherins in desmosomal plaques and adherens junctions.

EPIDERMAL DIFFERENTIATION (See Fig. 7-3)

Basal Cell Layer

As discussed earlier, the basal cell layer is composed predominantly of transient amplifying cells that undergo several rounds of mitosis before becoming nonmitotic keratinocytes destined to differentiate into corneocytes. In the basal cell layer, keratinocytes are small and polar,

FIGURE 7-3

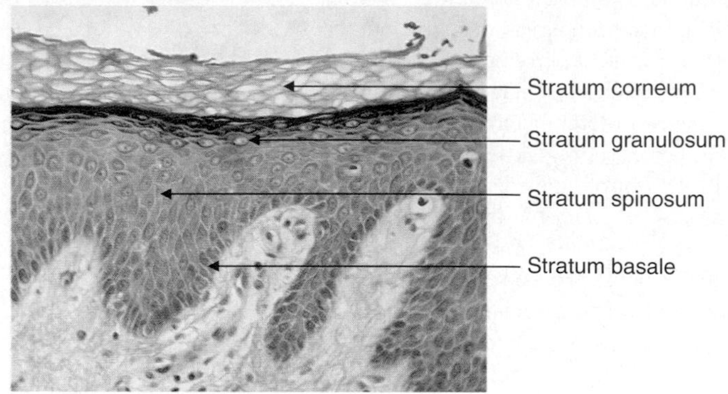

The normal epidermis. The four major steps in epidermal differentiation are represented by (1) an innermost stratum basale composed of mitotically active proliferative cells, (2) a three- to six-cell-layer-thick stratum spinosum containing cells that are still transcriptionally active but are no longer dividing (these cells can devote most of their translational machinery to expressing keratins), (3) a one- to three-cell-layer-thick stratum granulosum with cells that are transcriptionally active, depositing a cornified cell envelope composed of cross-linked proteins and lipids beneath the plasma membrane, and (4) a five- to twenty-cell-layer-thick stratum corneum, which consists of metabolically inert, anucleate squames that are sloughed from the skin surface. The squames sloughed from the skin surface are merely dead sacs surrounded by the cornified cell envelope and full of keratin macrofibrils. Basal cells express keratins 5 and 14, but as they commit to terminal differentiation, they switch off the expression of keratins 5 and 14 and begin expressing keratins 1 and 10. As epidermal cells move up through the spinous layer, they also express keratin 2e, which, like keratin 1, pairs with keratin 10.

expressing keratins 5 and 14. A major function of the basal layer is to provide a mechanical attachment to the underlying basement membrane zone and dermis through hemidesmosomal attachments.

Keratins 5 and 14 are the predominant intermediate filament proteins of basal keratinocytes. The hemidesmosomal and desmosomal plaques anchor cytoplasmic keratins to the plasma membrane and mediate cell attachment to the basement membrane zone and plasma membranes of adjacent cells, respectively (Fig. 7-4). It appears that laminin-5 in the extracellular matrix triggers recruitment of $\alpha_6\beta_4$ integrin heterodimers, keratins, and keratin-associated proteins to the cell surface, initiating hemidesmosomal assembly. The intracellular portion of the hemidesmosome is composed of bullous pemphigoid antigen 1 and plectin, two members of the "plakin" group of proteins that serve to bind the intracellular keratin network to the plasma membrane. This binding is more stable than that seen with intermediate filaments of nonstratified epithelia, providing greater stability to the epidermal keratin filament architecture. The transmembrane portion of the hemidesmosome includes bullous pemphigoid antigen 2, which binds to collagen IV in the lamina densa, and integrins, which bind laminins, fibronectin, and collagens in the basement membrane zone. In addition, extracellular laminin-5 induces phosphorylation and dephosphorylation of $\alpha_6\beta_4$ integrin subunits, thereby allowing the extracellular matrix to modulate cell proliferation, differentiation, apoptosis, migration, and tissue morphogenesis[25] (see Chap. 16).

Spinous Cell Layer

As keratinocytes leave the basal layer, they become nonmitotic and commence terminal differentiation. The suprabasal cells are more metabolically active and larger than those in the basal layer, with most of their protein synthesis devoted to the production of keratins 1 and 10. Concomitantly, the synthesis of the basal layer keratins (5 and 14) is downregulated.

The spinous layer is so named because of the prominent "spines" visible on light microscopy, which represent cytoplasmic attachments via desmosomes, structures that mechanically couple adjacent keratinocytes (Fig. 7-4). The desmosomal plaque is composed of several intracellular plakin proteins, including desmoplakins I and II, envoplakin, periplakin, and plakophilin.[26] Desmoplakins I and II, alternate splicing products of the identical desmoplakin gene, form the major intracellular portion of the desmosomal plaque.[27] The transmembrane portion of the desmosomal plaque includes desmogleins and desmocollins, which are calcium-dependent adhesion molecules (cadherins).[28] Moreover, desmocalmin, a calmodulin-binding protein, promotes calcium-dependent assembly and function of desmosomes. Hereditary and acquired diseases of the desmosomes and hemidesmosomes generally result in abnormal cell-cell and cell-matrix adhesion, respectively, causing blistering disorders, such as pemphigus, pemphigoid, and hereditary epidermolysis bullosa. However, since desmosomes play a significant role in epidermal differentiation and are part of the cornified cell envelope (see below), mutations in desmosomal components also can cause ichthyosiform and palmoplantar dermatoses, such as striated palmoplantar keratoderma, Naxos syndrome, and ectodermal dysplasia/skin fragility syndrome.[29,30] Envoplakin and periplakin, which form homo- and heterodimers in a network radiating from desmosomes and aggregate with keratin intermediate filaments, were identified initially as parts of the cornified cell envelope and are thought to provide the scaffold onto which the cornified cell envelope is later assembled[31] (see below).

FIGURE 7-4

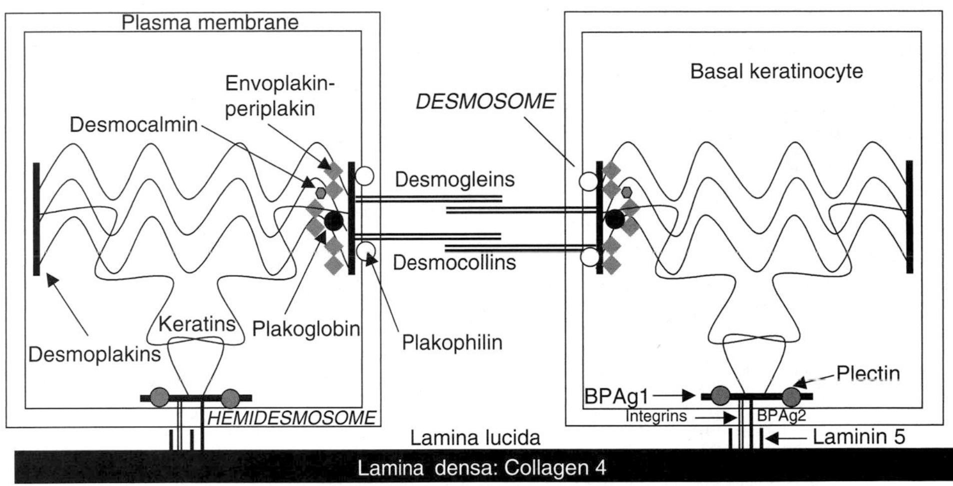

Desmosomal and hemidesmosomal structure. Desmoplakins mediate cell adhesion between adjacent keratinocytes, whereas hemidesmosomes attach keratinocytes to the basement membrane. The intracellular portions of these structures are composed of plakin proteins, which bind keratin to the plasma membrane. The plakins include desmoplakins I and II, periplakin, and envoplakin in the desmosomes and bullous pemphigoid antigen 1 and plectin in the hemidesmosomes. Plakoglobin and plakophilin are also components of the intracellular desmosomal plaque. The transmembrane portions are composed of desmogleins and desmocollins in the desmosomes and bullous pemphigoid antigen 1 and integrins in the hemidesmosomes.

As cells progress through the spinous layer, they accumulate increasing amounts of proteins involved in terminal differentiation. Many of these proteins are encoded by a gene cluster on chromosome 1q21 known as the *epidermal differentiation complex.* This gene complex encodes loricrin, involucrin, profilaggrin, a number of small proline-rich peptides, trichohyalin (a hair follicle protein), and S100A calcium-binding proteins.[32]

Most of the processes of terminal keratinocyte differentiation are controlled by the intracellular calcium concentration[33] (Table 7-3). A low-calcium culture medium maintains keratinocytes in a high-proliferation but low-differentiation state, whereas a high-calcium medium promotes the terminal differentiation of keratinocytes. Similarly, protein kinase C, a regulator of intracellular calcium release, promotes the transition from spinous to granular layer cells. The effects of protein kinase C on protein expression are mediated by AP1 transcription factors, including Jun and Fra.[34] Other transcription factors, such as AP2, SP1, and ETS, also enhance the expression of suprabasal keratins, proteins of the epidermal differentiation complex, and transglutaminases (see below). Inhibition of keratinocyte differentiation is mediated by retinoids and transcription factors such as POU domain proteins and CCAAT enhancer binding proteins.[35]

Electrochemical coupling between cells is mediated by gap junctions, which are formed by the alignment of two connexons on adjacent cell membranes. Each connexon is a hemichannel formed by oligomerization of six homotypic or heterotypic connexin subunits. During epidermal differentiation, there is a progressive change in connexin expression. Connexin 43 in proliferative basal cells is replaced by connexin 26 in nonproliferative spinous keratinocytes.[36,37] Subsequently, connexin 26 is replaced by connexins 31 and 31.1 during terminal differentiation of keratinocytes into corneocytes. These changes in connexin expression cause alterations in intercellular ionic signaling and affect calcium homeostasis via changes in the intercellular flow of both calcium and second messengers that mediate calcium release. Mutations in connexins have been found to underlie three genodermatoses: classic Vohwinkel syndrome, erythrokeratodermia variabilis, and hidrotic ectodermal dysplasia (Clouston syndrome).[38] Moreover, mutations in calcium ATPases that sequester calcium into organelles result in Darier-White disease and Hailey-Hailey disease. The phenotypes seen in these conditions may result from dysregulation of ionic signaling resulting in abnormal keratinocyte differentiation.

TABLE 7-3

Terminal Epidermal Differentiation Processes that are Calcium-Dependent

Differentiation Process	Calcium-Dependent Components
Intercellular structure formation	Desmosome assembly and function Gap junction assembly and function
Protein expression	Involucrin Keratins 1, 2e, 9, and 10 Loricrin Profilaggrin Small proline-rich peptides Transglutaminase
Release of keratohyaline granule contents	Release of loricrin and profilaggrin
Enzyme function	Cleavage of profilaggrin to filaggrin Transglutaminase activity

Granular Cell Layer

As cells reach the granular layer, their appearance changes dramatically with the synthesis of intracellular keratohyaline granules that are visible on light microscopy. The keratohyaline granules contain profilaggrin, a large, highly phosphorylated, calcium-binding precursor protein that consists of several filaggrin repeats separated by short hydrophobic linker sequences, as well as amino- and carboxy-terminal domains. Loricrin, another granule component, is released near the plasma membrane, where it initially binds desmosomal plaque proteins[39] (see below).

The amino-terminal domain of profilaggrin contains functional calcium-binding regions that are believed to be important in its processing to filaggrin.[40] As the keratohyaline granule contents are released into the cytoplasm, profilaggrin is dephosphorylated and cleaved proteolytically into individual filaggrin domains in a calcium-dependent process. Filaggrin is a histidine-rich cationic protein that aggregates keratin, forming macrofilaments.[41] Subsequently, filaggrin is degraded into molecules including urocanic acid and pyrrolidone carboxylic acid, which filter ultraviolet radiation and hydrate the stratum corneum.[41,43]

The lamellar granules of the granular layer, also known as *membrane-coating granules, Odland bodies,* or *keratinosomes,* are dual-function granules that contain both the lipids that provide the permeability barrier of the epidermis and a number of lysosomal enzymes. These granules are first identifiable in the upper spinous layer and become more abundant in the granular layer. The lamellar granule glucosylceramides, the precursors of the stratum corneum ceramides, are formed in the Golgi apparatus by ceramide glucosyltransferase, which is induced during keratinocyte differentiation coincident with the appearance of lamellar granules.[44] Conversely, elevated concentrations of intracellular ceramides inhibit cell proliferation and induce cell differentiation and apoptosis.[45] In the upper granular layer, the lamellar granules orient themselves with the apical surface of the keratinocytes, where they fuse with the plasma membrane and secrete their contents, stacks of membranous lipid-laden disks, into the intercellular space. The lipid-rich lamellae form broad sheets between the keratinocytes and subsequently become part of the cornified cell envelope.

Stratum Corneum and the Cornified Cell Envelope

Drastic remodeling of keratinocytes occurs in the transition to the stratum corneum, where corneocytes devoid of nuclei and other organelles provide a protective barrier. This barrier includes the cornified cell envelope, an extremely durable protein-lipid polymer with a 10-nm insoluble layer of protein covalently linked to the plasma membrane of the keratinocytes and overlaid by a 5-nm lipid envelope. The insoluble protein component of the cornified envelope comprises approximately 90 percent of its total mass, with the lipid component making up the rest. The cornified cell envelope is first formed interior to the cytoplasmic membrane of differentiating keratinocytes but eventually resides on the exterior of cornified cells.[46]

The formation of the cornified cell envelope is a multistep process. Initially, envoplakin and periplakin are expressed at the desmosomal plaques. Subsequently, involucrin, a highly polymorphous, highly soluble, acidic, glutamine-rich protein found in many types of stratified squamous epithelia, localizes to the cytoplasmic membrane. Transglutaminases are also expressed early in differentiation and cross-link involucrin residues to one another and to envoplakin. Transglutaminases (1 and 3) catalyze the formation of isodipeptide bonds between ε-amino groups of lysine and γ-carboxyl groups of glutamine residues. As discussed earlier, after the release of keratohyaline granule contents, loricrin initially accumulates on desmosomes at the cytoplasmic membrane, whereas filaggrin aggregates with keratin intermediate filaments in the cytoplasm.[47] Subsequently, epidermal transglutaminases catalyze the binding of loricrin, keratin macrofilaments, desmosomal peptides, involucrin, small proline-rich peptides, elafin, cystatin A, S100 peptides, cornifins, annexin I, calgizzarin, plasminogen activator inhibitor type 2, and other peptides to the cell membrane in a calcium-dependent fashion, forming the highly insoluble proteinaceous component of the cornified cell envelope at the inner leaflet of the plasma membrane.[1]

It appears that transglutaminase 3, a cytoplasmic enzyme, initially cross-links loricrin and small proline-rich peptides together to form small interchain oligomers, which are then permanently affixed to the developing cornified cell envelope via further cross-linking by transglutaminase 1, a cell membrane–bound and keratinocyte-specific enzyme.[48] Of note, transglutaminase 1 also attaches ω-hydroxyceramide lipids to involucrin glutamine residues, explaining the preferential localization of involucrin to the outer portion of the cornified cell envelope, as opposed to loricrin, which predominates in the inner portions.[49,50] Other studies indicate that desmosomal envoplakin and periplakin also serve as substrates for the attachment of ceramides.[51] Failure to cross-link epidermal proteins and lipids by transglutaminase 1 may explain the phenotypes of lamellar ichthyosis and nonbullous congenital ichthyosiform erythroderma, which can be caused by mutations in the transglutaminase 1 gene.[52]

The exact role of each protein component of the cornified cell envelope is not fully understood, and significant functional overlap exists. Loricrin, as discussed previously, is the major protein component of the cornified cell envelope, comprising over 70 percent of its mass. Loricrin-deficient mice demonstrate congenital erythroderma with a shiny, translucent skin, reduced stratum corneum stability, and easy fragmentation of the cornified cell envelope by mechanical stress. Surprisingly, the skin phenotype disappears 4 to 5 days after birth, concomitant with upregulation of small proline-rich peptides and S100 peptides, which compensate for cornified cell envelope formation.[53] However, transgenic mice expressing a carboxy-terminal truncated form of loricrin demonstrate a phenotype resembling Vohwinkel syndrome.[54] Similarly, involucrin knockout mice appear normal, whereas mice expressing involucrin transgenes demonstrate abnormalities in hair follicle and cornified cell envelope structure.[55,56] These experiments suggest that whereas functional overlap can overcome deficiencies in structural proteins of the cornified cell envelope, expression of an abnormal protein can interfere with cornified cell envelope assembly through dominant-negative effects.

The small proline-rich peptides are members of the epidermal differentiation complex that cross-link with one another and with loricrin in the cornified cell envelope.[57] These peptides are encoded by two *SPRR1,* eight *SPRR2,* and one *SPRR3* genes that are differentially regulated. The peptides share homology with loricrin and involucrin and can be upregulated in the absence of functional loricrin. Whereas loricrin is the major component of the epidermal cornified cell envelope, the small proline-rich peptides, particularly SPRR1a and b, form 70 percent of the cornified cell envelope in the oral mucosa.[58] The exact functional roles of other cornified cell envelope components such as cystatin A, S100 peptides, and cornifin are less well understood.

Corneocyte Shedding

When the final products of this differentiation process, the squames, finally reach the outermost edge of the epidermis, they are mummified cell remnants composed of a cornified envelope surrounded by stacks of lipids and packed with compact keratin macrofilaments. The squames are then shed, only to be replaced by others derived from keratinocytes that have migrated from the basal layer and followed the differentiation pathway described earlier.

To maintain a constant stratum corneum thickness, the process of corneocyte shedding has to be precisely regulated to match the rate of new corneocyte formation. Corneocytes are held together by corneodesmosomes, modified desmosomal structures that appear as homogeneous electron-dense plugs on electron microscopy. In the upper spinous and granular layers, corneodesmosin, a glycine- and serine-rich glycoprotein, is expressed and stored in the lamellar bodies. After transport and release into the extracellular space, corneodesmosin becomes associated with desmosomal desmogleins and desmocollins. Cleavage of corneodesmosin by the stratum corneum tryptic and chymotryptic enzymes causes separation of adjacent corneocytes with resulting cell shedding.[59] Cathepsin D, a lysosomal aspartate proteinase present in the stratum corneum, which is expressed consequent to the calcium concentration change that accompanies terminal epidermal differentiation, also plays a part in the degradation process.[60] The lamellar bodies are known to store many lysosomal enzymes, and the acidic pH (~4.5) of the stratum corneum promotes the enzymatic activities of these proteases.

INTERMEDIATE FILAMENT PROTEINS

In all eukaryotic cells, the cytoskeleton is central to cell structure, function, and differentiation. The cytoskeleton is composed of an elaborate network of structural proteins, including actin microfilaments, microtubules, and intermediate filaments. Named after their assembled diameter (10 nm), intermediate between the thin actin microfilaments (6 nm) and the thick microtubules (25 nm), intermediate filaments are the most heterogeneous of the cytoskeleton proteins and have been divided into six types based on their amino acid sequence and tissue specificity (see Table 7-3).

Keratins

Keratins are the most complex family of intermediate filament proteins, and they provide structural integrity to all epithelial cells. Their relative charges, molecular weights, and antigenic specificity were used by Moll et al.[61] to assign numbered designations to each keratin protein in 1982. Keratin filaments are obligate heterodimers composed of one type I and one type II keratin. Each heterodimer is tissue- and differentiation-specific (Table 7-4). The type I keratins, encoded by a gene cluster on 17q12-q21, are acidic ($pK_i = 4.5$ to 5.5) and relatively smaller in size (~40 to 56.5 kDa), consisting of keratins 9 to 20 in the epidermis and keratins Ha1 to Ha8 in the hair follicle. The type II keratins, encoded by a gene cluster on 12q11–13, are basic or neutral (pKi = 5.5–7.5) and relatively larger in size (~52–67 kDa), consisting of keratins 1 to 8 in the epidermis and Hb1 to Hb6 in the hair follicle. More than one allele exists for several of the keratins, including keratins 1, 2, 4, 5, and 6, but the significance of this is unclear.

TABLE 7-4

Intermediate Filament Types and Tissue Expression Patterns of Intermediate Filament Proteins

TYPE	PROTEIN	TISSUE EXPRESSION
I	Acidic keratin	Epithelia
II	Basic keratin	Epithelia
III	Vimentin	Mesenchymal cells
	Desmin	Muscle
	Peripherin	Peripheral nervous system
	Glial fibrillary acidic protein	Glial cells and astrocytes
IV	α-Internexin	Neurofilaments
V	Lamins	Nucleus
VI	Nestin	Stem cells of central nervous system and skeletal muscle

KERATIN STRUCTURE Keratins share a homologous basic structure with all intermediate filament proteins (Fig. 7-5). The genes for each of the epidermal keratins have been cloned, and their protein structures have been determined. The central α-helical rod domain, composed of 310 to 315 amino acids, is responsible for dimerization and higher-order polymerization and is composed of four highly conserved domains (1A, 1B, 2A, and 2B). The α helix consists of heptad amino acid repeats in which the first and fourth residues are hydrophobic, residing close together on the surface of the helix and enabling two adjacent polypeptides to create a coiled coil. There is a stutter sequence in the helix 2B domain that is associated with reversal of the direction of the α-helix. Mutations that lead to shortening of the rod domain yield keratins that are not only unable to assemble into filaments but also interfere with preexisting keratin filament networks, since keratins are highly dynamic with reversible assembly and disassembly.[62] There is a mutational hotspot in one arginine position of the highly conserved coil 1A region of keratins 9, 10, and 14 that underlies most cases of epidermolytic palmoplantar keratoderma, bullous congenital ichthyosiform erythroderma, and epidermolysis bullosa simplex. This shows that structure and charge are critical elements for keratin assembly and stability.

The four highly conserved α-helical domains are separated by nonhelical linker domains (L1, L12, L2). Since L1 and L12 are rich in both glycine and proline, they disrupt the α helix more effectively than glycine-rich L2. Mutations in keratins 5 and 14 underlying epidermolysis bullosa simplex are clustered in the helix boundary peptides and in the L12 linker domain (see Chap. 65). These linker domain mutations disrupt the β-sheet structure of the L12 domain and prevent proper filament assembly between keratins 5 and 14.[63]

The helix boundary peptides that flank the α-helical rod domain show remarkable evolutionary conservation. Single or few amino acid substitutions and deletions in the most conserved positions of this sequence can result in profound effects on filament assembly in vitro.[64] In addition, there is evidence that the consensus sequence plays an important role in lateral alignment that could affect higher-order interactions in intermediate filaments.[65] All cases of monilethrix and some cases of epidermolysis bullosa simplex are caused by mutations in these helix boundary peptides. Keratin 14 mutants missing the nonhelical carboxy- and amino-terminal domains and small portions of the carboxy end of the rod domain integrate into endogenous keratin filament networks and also form 10-nm filaments with keratin 5. In contrast, small truncations in the amino-terminal end of the rod domain more severely disrupt the filament assembly process and in particular restrict elongation.[66] This demonstrates that the helix boundary peptides are critical for higher-order assembly of keratin filaments.

Finally, the amino-terminal head and carboxy-terminal tail regions, which confer antigenic specificity to individual keratins, consist of the two highly homologous (H) subdomains, two variable (V) subdomains, and two highly charged end (E) subdomains. In hair keratins, these domains are cysteine-rich, permitting the formation of disulfide bonds that confer additional stability to the hair shaft. The end regions of keratins are important for a variety of protein interactions. Mutations affecting the tail domain of keratin 1 cause failure of keratin bundling, retraction of the cytoskeleton from the nucleus, and failed translocation of loricrin to the desmosomal plaques.[67] The glycine loops in the V and E subdomains are thought to form hydrophobic bonds with keratin-associated proteins such as loricrin in the cornified cell envelope. Keratin 5 and 14 truncation experiments have shown that the tails of keratins 5 and 14 are required for filament stabilization, that the head of keratin 5 is required for filament elongation and lateral alignment, and that the highly conserved carboxy R/KLLEGE domain is required for lateral alignment.[68] Interestingly, the ability of keratin 19 (a tail-less keratin) to form filaments demonstrates that this domain is not absolutely necessary for filament formation.

keratin genes are sequentially activated with initial expression of HB5, followed by HB1 and 3, and finally HB6.

The tightly regulated changes in keratin expression are controlled by transcription factors, which are DNA-binding proteins that promote or inhibit expression of nearby genes. Most regulatory sites are found in the promoter region upstream of the structural genes, although introns or downstream sequences also may contain regulatory elements. All keratin promoters have a canonical TATA box or a variant thereof, and basal transcription requires the presence of the TATA box and adjacent initiator sequence. Transcription factor TFIID that binds the TATA box is the only transcription factor common to all keratin genes, although binding sites for AP2 transcription factors are also present in most keratin genes. Other transcription factors that affect keratin gene expression include Sp1, NF1 half sites, retinoic acid–responsive elements, steroid hormone–responsive elements, AP1, NFκB, and a number of other factors.[73]

Many of these transcription factors are activated by extracellular signals[74] (Fig. 7-7). Binding of interferons and several interleukins (3–6, 12) to cell surface receptors activate specific JAK kinases that in turn phosphorylate tyrosines on signal transducing activators of transcription (STATs). STATs subsequently translocate to the nucleus, bind specific DNA sites, and promote gene transcription. A number of peptides (e.g., epidermal growth factor, transforming growth factor α, amphiregulin, and heregulin) bind the epidermal growth factor receptor and cause receptor dimerization, thereby activating a series of proteins including Ras, a MAPK kinase kinase named Raf1, MEKs, and finally ERKs, which also translocate to the nucleus and activate transcription factors such as SAP1 and Elk1.

FIGURE 7-5

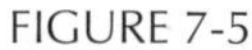

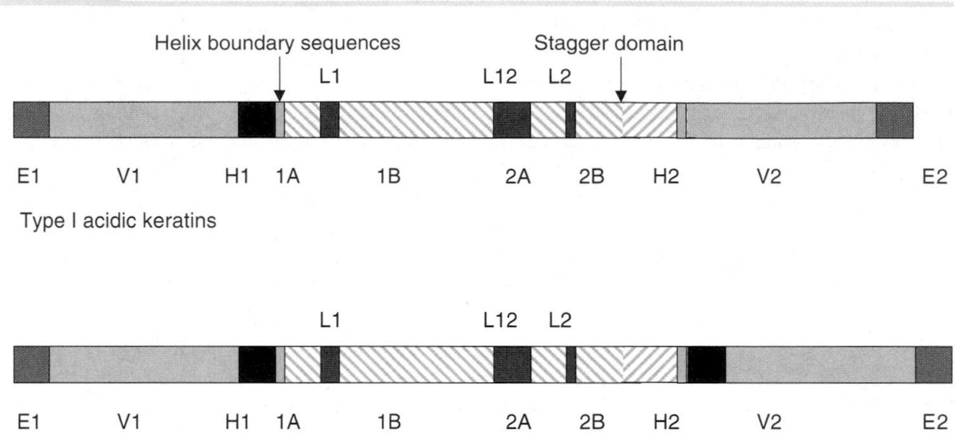

Keratin protein structure. E1 and E2 represent the highly-charged end regions, V1 and V2 represent variable regions, and H1 and H2 represent homologous regions of the end domain. The α-helical rod domain is composed of four α-helical domains (1A, 1B, 2A, 2B), which are separated by nonhelical linker domains (L1, L12, L2) and flanked by the helix boundary peptides. There is a stagger domain in the 2B rod domain in which the direction of the α-helix reverses. Type I (acidic) keratins lack an H2 domain.

KERATIN POLYMERIZATION Whereas other intermediate filaments form homodimers, keratin polypeptides assemble into coiled-coil heterodimers consisting of one type I keratin and one type II keratin. Type I and type II keratins are coexpressed in epithelial cells and form heterodimers spontaneously without the assistance of other proteins or factors. Nonpaired keratins are rapidly degraded ensuring equimolar amounts of the components of each pair.[69] Keratin heterodimers are arranged in a parallel configuration and are aligned axially (Fig. 7-6). The formation of the heterodimers is initiated by highly conserved trigger motifs that have been characterized in the 1B and 2B rod domains.[70] Although keratin pairs not seen in nature can be created in vitro, the resulting keratin filaments are less stable. For instance, the absence of keratin 10 in knockout mice results in increased expression of keratins 6 and 16, which bind keratin 1 but do not fully compensate for the absence of normal keratin 1/10 dimers.[71]

Two keratin heterodimers are arranged in an an antiparallel and staggered configuration to form tetramers (double-coiled coils). Antiparallel alignment of keratin pairs is stabilized by specific amino acid residues in the 1A and 2A rod domains and the L2 linker domain.[72] Tetramers then assemble end-to-end into protofilaments (2–3 nm wide), two of which further assemble into protofibrils (4.5 nm wide), and four protofibrils finally assemble into intermediate filaments (10 nm wide). Within this model of filament formation lie two fundamental interactions: lateral interaction between staggered coiled coils and head-to-tail interactions between the same type keratin. This process of keratin filament formation is dynamic, with coiled-coil subunits constantly being added to and deleted from the structures.

CONTROL OF GENE TRANSCRIPTION IN KERATINOCYTES Keratins account for approximately 30 percent of the total protein of basal keratinocytes, and they comprise 85 percent of the cytoplasmic protein of terminally differentiated keratinocytes. The keratin peptides are expressed in a tissue- and differentiation-specific manner. In the skin, the expression of keratins 5 and 14 in the basal layer gives way to keratins 1 and 10 in the spinous layer and subsequently keratins 2e and 10 in the upper spinous and granular layers. In the hair follicle, type II

FIGURE 7-6

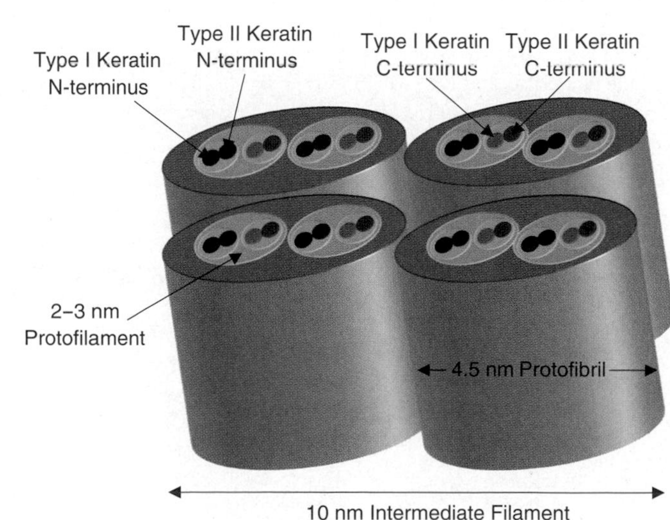

Keratin intermediate filament structure. Each protofilament is composed of two pairs of staggered, antiparallel keratin dimers. Two protofilaments comprise a protofibril, four of which assemble to make the 10-nm keratin intermediate filament.

FIGURE 7-7

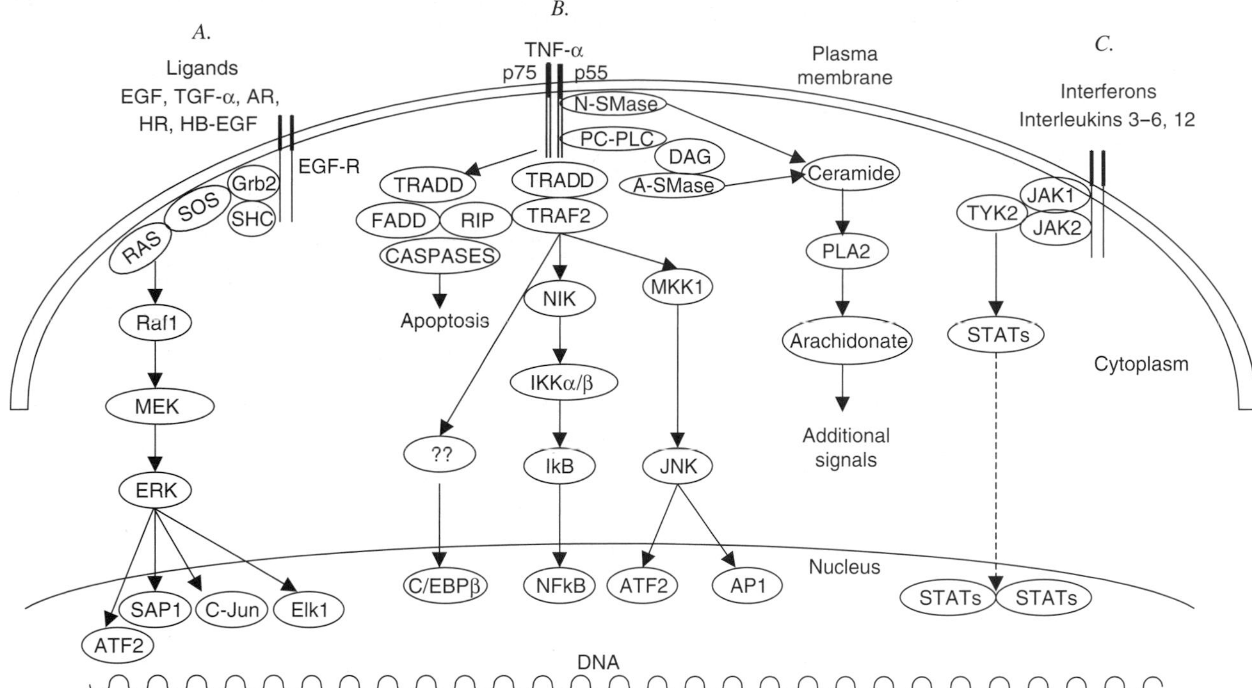

Transcription factor signaling pathways in keratinocytes. *A.* Transforming growth factor *α* (TGF-*α*) and related growth factors bind to the epidermal growth factor receptor (EGF-R) causing dimerization and activation of tyrosine kinase, which lead SHC, Grb2, and SOS to activate RAS that causes downstream activation of several nuclear transcription factors. *B.* There are three principal TNF-*α* signal-transduction pathways: (1) the apoptosis pathway mediated by caspases, (2) the ceramide pathway, and (3) the TRAF2 pathway. TRAF2 causes downstream degradation of I*κ*B, resulting in activation of nuclear NF*κ*B. Other transcription factors induced by TRAF2 include C/EBP*β*, ATF2, and AP1. *C.* The interferon-*γ* (IFN-*γ*) and interleukin (IL) pathways. Binding of ligands to receptors causes association with JAK/TYK kinases that phosphorylate STATS, causing dimerization and translocation to the nucleus and subsequent transcriptional activation. (*Adapted from Freedberg et al.*[73])

Tumor necrosis factor *α* has complex intracellular effects that result in the activation of caspases, resulting in apoptosis, as well as the activation of NFkB, ATF2, and AP1 transcription factors. Although these transcription factor cascades are present in many cell types, there are some keratinocyte-specific transcription factors. These include basonuclin, a zinc finger protein that is found exclusively in the nucleus of the basal and first suprabasal layers, apparently playing a specific role in the control of transcription in the basal layer.[75]

KERATINS IN DISEASE (See Chaps. 51 and 52) Targeted disruption of keratin genes has allowed further delineation of the function of specific epidermal keratins, and keratin gene mutations have been found to underlie a number of hereditary human diseases (see Table 7-4). The effects of keratin mutations on skin physiology can be partially deduced from the phenotypes seen in keratinopathies. Mutations in keratins 1, 2e, 5, 10, and 14 result in keratinocyte ballooning and degeneration, suggesting that the keratin filament network within keratinocytes provides mechanical strength, cellular structure, and assistance in adhesion molecule attachment.

REFERENCES

1. Jetten AM, Harvat BL: Epidermal differentiation and squamous metaplasia: From stem cell to cell death. *J Dermatol* **24**:711, 1997
2. Wright N: Cell population kinetics in human epidermis. *Int J Dermatol* **16**:449, 1977
3. Lenoir MC et al: Outer root sheath cells of human hair follicle are able to regenerate a fully differentiated epidermis in vitro. *Dev Biol* **130**:610, 1988
4. Ghazizadeh S, Taichman LB: Multiple classes of stem cells in cutaneous epithelium: A lineage analysis of adult mouse skin. *EMBO J* **20**:1215, 2001
5. Rheinwald JG, Green H: Serial cultivation of strains of human epidermal keratinocytes: The formation of keratinizing colonies from single cells. *Cell* **6**:331, 1975
6. Withers HR: Recovery and repopulation in vivo by mouse skin epithelial cells during fractionated irradiation. *Radiat Res* **32**:227, 1967
7. Morris RJ, Potten CS: Highly persistent label-retaining cells in the hair follicles of mice and their fate following induction of anagen. *J Invest Dermatol* **112**:470, 1999
8. Akiyama M et al: Characterization of hair follicle bulge in human fetal skin: The human fetal bulge is a pool of undifferentiated keratinocytes. *J Invest Dermatol* **105**:844, 1995
9. Bickenbach JR, Dunnwalk M: Epidermal stem cells: Characteristics and use in tissue engineering and gene therapy. *Adv Dermatol* **16**:159, 2000
10. Jones PH, Watt FM: Separation of human epidermal stem cells from transit amplifying cells on the basis of differences in integrin function and expression. *Cell* **73**:713, 1993
11. Potten CS: Cell replacement in epidermis (keratopoiesis) via discrete units of proliferation. *Int Rev Cytol* **69**:271, 1981
12. Michel M et al: Keratin 19 as a biochemical marker of skin stem cells in vivo and in vitro: keratin 19 expressing cells are differentially localized in function of anatomic sites, and their number varies with donor age and culture stage. *J Cell Sci* **109**:1017, 1996
13. Bickenbach JR et al: Telomerase is not an epidermal stem cell marker and is downregulated by calcium. *J Invest Dermatol* **111**:1045, 1998
14. Chiu CP et al: Differential expression of telomerase activity in hematopoietic progenitors from adult human bone marrow. *Stem Cells* **14**:239, 1996
15. Watt FM: Epidermal stem cells: Markers, patterning and the control of stem cell fate. *Philos Trans R Soc Lond B Biol Sci* **353**:831, 1998
16. Adams JC, Watt FM: Fibronectin inhibits the terminal differentiation of human keratinocytes. *Nature* **340**:307, 1989
17. Jones PH et al: Stem cell patterning and fate in human epidermis. *Cell* **80**:83, 1995
18. Potten CS, Morris RJ: Epithelial stem cells in vivo. *J Cell Sci Suppl* **10**:45, 1988

19. Zhu AJ et al: Signaling via β_1 integrins and mitogen-activated protein kinase determines human epidermal stem cell fate in vitro. *Proc Natl Acad Sci USA* **96**:6728, 1999
20. Miller DG et al: Gene transfer by retrovirus vectors occurs only in cells that are actively replicating at the time of infection. *Mol Cell Biol* **10**:4239, 1990
21. Bickenbach JR, Roop DR: Transduction of a preselected population of human epidermal stem cells: Consequences for gene therapy. *Proc Assoc Am Physicians* **111**:184, 1999
22. Dunnwald M et al: Isolating a pure population of epidermal stem cells for use in tissue engineering. *Exp Dermatol* **10**:45, 2001
23. Watt FM: Epidermal stem cells as targets for gene transfer. *Hum Gene Ther* **11**:2261, 2000
24. Zhu AJ, Watt FM: Beta-catenin signalling modulates proliferative potential of human epidermal keratinocytes independently of intercellular adhesion. *Development* **126**:2285, 1999
25. Jones JC et al: Structure and assembly of hemidesmosomes. *Bioessays* **20**:488, 1998
26. Robinson NA et al: S100A11, S100A10, annexin I, desmosomal proteins, small proline-rich proteins, plasminogen activator inhibitor-2, and involucrin are components of the cornified envelope of cultured human epidermal keratinocytes. *J Biol Chem* **272**:12035, 1997
27. Green KJ et al: Structure of the human desmoplakins: Implications for function in the desmosomal plaque. *J Biol Chem* 265:2603, 1990
28. Cserhalmi-Friedman PB et al: Structural analysis reflects the evolutionary relationship between the human desmocollin gene family members. *Exp Dermatol* **10**:95, 2001
29. Allen E et al: Mice expressing a mutant desmosomal cadherin exhibit abnormalities in desmosomes, proliferation, and epidermal differentiation. *J Cell Biol* **133**:1367, 1996
30. Haftek M et al: Immunocytochemical evidence for a possible role of cross-linked keratinocyte envelopes in stratum corneum cohesion. *J Histochem Cytochem* **39**:1531, 1991
31. DiColandrea T et al: Subcellular distribution of envoplakin and periplakin: insights into their role as precursors of the epidermal cornified envelope. *J Cell Biol* **151**:573, 2000
32. Mischke D et al: Genes encoding structural proteins of epidermal cornification and S100 calcium-binding proteins form a gene complex ("epidermal differentiation complex") on human chromosome 1q21. *J Invest Dermatol* **106**:989, 1996
33. Bikle DD, Pillai S: Vitamin D, calcium, and epidermal differentiation. *Endocr Rev* **14**:3, 1993
34. Rutberg SE et al: Differentiation of mouse keratinocytes is accompanied by PKC-dependent changes in AP-1 proteins. *Oncogene* **13**:167, 1996
35. Eckert RL et al: The epidermis: Genes on—genes off. *J Invest Dermatol* **109**:501, 1997
36. Kamibayashi Y et al: Expression of gap junction proteins connexin 26 and 43 is modulated during differentiation of keratinocytes in newborn mouse epidermis. *J Invest Dermatol* **101**:773, 1993
37. Brissette JL et al. Switch in gap junction protein expression is associated with selective changes in junctional permeability during keratinocyte differentiation. *Proc Natl Acad Sci USA* **91**:6453, 1994
38. Willecke K et al: Biological functions of connexin genes revealed by human genetic defects, dominant negative approaches and targeted deletions in the mouse. *Novartis Found Symp* **219**:76, 1999
39. Hohl D et al: Transcription of the human loricrin gene in vitro is induced by calcium and cell density and suppressed by retinoic acid. *J Invest Dermatol* **96**:414, 1991
40. Presland RB et al: Characterization of two distinct calcium-binding sites in the amino-terminus of human profilaggrin. *J Invest Dermatol* **104**:218, 1995
41. Ishida-Yamamoto A et al: Programmed cell death in normal epidermis and loricrin keratoderma: Multiple functions of profilaggrin in keratinization. *J Invest Dermatol Symp Proc* **4**:145, 1999
42. Scott IR, Harding CR: Filaggrin breakdown to water binding compounds during development of the rat stratum corneum is controlled by the water activity of the environment. *Dev Biol* **115**:84, 1986
43. Morrison H: Photochemistry and photobiology of urocanic acid. *Photodermatology* **2**:158, 1985
44. Madison KC et al: Lamellar granule biogenesis: A role for ceramide glucosyltransferase, lysosomal enzyme transport, and the Golgi. *J Investig Dermatol Symp Proc* **3**:80, 1998
45. Geilen CC et al: Ceramide signaling: Regulatory role in cell proliferation, differentiation and apoptosis in human epidermis. *Arch Dermatol Res* **289**:559, 1997
46. Nemes Z, Steinert PM: Bricks and mortar of the epidermal barrier. *Exp Mol Med* **31**:5, 1999
47. Ishida-Yamamoto A et al: Antigen retrieval of loricrin epitopes at desmosomal areas of cornified cell envelopes: An immunoelectron microscopic analysis. *Exp Dermatol* **8**:402, 1999
48. Candi E et al: Transglutaminase cross-linking properties of the small proline-rich 1 family of cornified cell envelope proteins: Integration with loricrin. *J Biol Chem* **274**:7226, 1999
49. Nemes Z et al: A novel function for transglutaminase 1: Attachment of long-chain omega-hydroxyceramides to involucrin by ester bond formation. *Proc Natl Acad Sci USA* **96**:8402, 1999
50. Steinert PM, Marekov LN: The proteins elafin, filaggrin, keratin intermediate filaments, loricrin, and small proline-rich proteins 1 and 2 are isodipeptide cross-linked components of the human epidermal cornified cell envelope. *J Biol Chem* **270**:17702, 1995
51. Marekov LN, Steinert PM: Ceramides are bound to structural proteins of the human foreskin epidermal cornified cell envelope. *J Biol Chem* **273**:17763, 1998
52. Candi E et al: Biochemical, structural, and transglutaminase substrate properties of human loricrin, the major epidermal cornified cell envelope protein. *J Biol Chem* **270**:26382, 1995
53. Koch PJ et al: Lessons from loricrin-deficient mice: Compensatory mechanisms maintaining skin barrier function in the absence of a major cornified envelope protein. *J Cell Biol* **151**:389, 2000
54. Suga Y et al: Transgenic mice expressing a mutant form of loricrin reveal the molecular basis of the skin diseases, Vohwinkel syndrome and progressive symmetric erythrokeratoderma. *J Cell Biol* **151**:401, 2000
55. Djian P et al: Targeted ablation of the murine involucrin gene. *J Cell Biol* **151**:381, 2000
56. Crish JF et al: Tissue-specific and differentiation-appropriate expression of the human involucrin gene in transgenic mice: an abnormal epidermal phenotype. *Differentiation* **53**:191, 1993
57. Steinert PM et al: Small proline-rich proteins are cross-bridging proteins in the cornified cell envelopes of stratified squamous epithelia. *J Struct Biol* **122**:76, 1998
58. Lee CH, et al: Small proline-rich protein 1 is the major component of the cell envelope of normal human oral keratinocytes. *FEBS Lett* **477**:268, 2000
59. Simon M et al: Refined characterization of corneodesmosin proteolysis during terminal differentiation of human epidermis and its relationship to desquamation. *J Biol Chem* **276**:20292, 2001.
60. Horikoshi T et al: Role of endogenous cathepsin D–like and chymotrypsin-like proteolysis in human epidermal desquamation. *Br J Dermatol* **141**:453, 1999
61. Moll R et al: The catalog of human cytokeratins: Patterns of expression in normal epithelia, tumors and cultured cells. *Cell* **31**:11, 1982
62. Albers K, Fuchs E: Expression of mutant keratin cDNAs in epithelial cells reveals possible mechanisms for initiation and assembly of intermediate filaments. *J Cell Biol* **108**:1477, 1989
63. Galligan P et al: A novel mutation in the L12 domain of keratin 5 in the Kobner variant of epidermolysis bullosa simplex. *J Invest Dermatol* **111**:524, 1998
64. Hatzfeld M, Weber K: Modulation of keratin intermediate filament assembly by single amino acid exchanges in the consensus sequence at the C-terminal end of the rod domain. *J Cell Sci* **99**:351, 1991
65. Hatzfeld M, Weber K: A synthetic peptide representing the consensus sequence motif at the carboxy-terminal end of the rod domain inhibits intermediate filament assembly and disassembles preformed filaments. *J Cell Biol* **116**:157, 1992
66. Coulombe PA, et al: Deletions in epidermal keratins leading to alterations in filament organization in vivo and in intermediate filament assembly in vitro. *J Cell Biol* **111**:3049, 1990
67. Sprecher E et al: Evidence for novel functions of the keratin tail emerging from a mutation causing ichthyosis hystrix. *J Invest Dermatol* **116**:511, 2001
68. Wilson AK et al: The roles of K5 and K14 head, tail, and R/K L L E G E domains in keratin filament assembly in vitro. *J Cell Biol* **119**:401, 1992
69. Kulesh DA, et al: Posttranslational regulation of keratins: Degradation of mouse and human keratins 18 and 8. *Mol Cell Biol* **9**:1553, 1989
70. Wu KC et al: Coiled-coil trigger motifs in the 1B and 2B rod domain segments are required for the stability of keratin intermediate filaments. *Mol Biol Cell* **11**:10, 2000
71. Reichelt J et al: Out of balance: consequences of a partial keratin knockout. *J Cell Sci* **110**:2175, 1997
72. Mehrani T et al: Residues in the 1A rod domain segment and the linker L2 are required for stabilizing the A11 molecular alignment mode in keratin intermediate filaments. *J Biol Chem* **276**:2088, 2001
73. Freedberg IM et al: Keratins and the keratinocyte activation cycle. *J Invest Dermatol* **116**:633, 2001
74. Tomic-Canic M et al: Epidermal signal transduction and transcription factor activation in activated keratinocytes. *J Dermatol Sci* **17**:167, 1998
75. Iuchi S, Green H: Basonuclin, a zinc finger protein of keratinocytes and reproductive germ cells, binds to the rRNA gene promoter. *Proc Natl Acad Sci USA* **96**:9628, 1999

CHAPTER 8

Lowell A. Goldsmith

Biology of Eccrine and Apocrine Sweat Glands

Generalized eccrine sweating is the physiologic response to an increased body temperature during physical exercise or thermal stress and is the most effective means by which humans regulate their body temperature through evaporative heat loss. Failure of this mechanism can lead to heat exhaustion, heat stroke, hyperthermia, and death. Exaggerated local or systemic sweating responses (hyperhidrosis) are a nuisance that may impair social and occupational activities.

Humans have 2 to 4 million eccrine sweat glands distributed over nearly the entire body surface.[1,2] Although each gland weighs only 30 to 40 μg, the total mass of the eccrine sweat glands roughly equals that of one kidney, i.e., 100 g. A well-acclimatized person can perspire as much as several liters per hour and 10 L/day, a secretory rate far greater than that of other exocrine glands. The secretory activity of the human eccrine sweat gland has two major functions: (1) secretion of an ultrafiltrate of a plasma-like precursor fluid by the secretory coil in response to acetylcholine (ACh), which is released from the sympathetic nerve endings, and (2) reabsorption of sodium in excess of water by the duct, producing hypotonic skin surface sweat. Under extreme conditions, where the amount of perspiration reaches several liters a day, the ductal reabsorptive function assumes a vital role in conserving electrolytes. In addition to the secretion of water and electrolytes, the sweat gland excretes heavy metals, organic compounds, and macromolecules.

ANATOMY OF ECCRINE SWEAT GLANDS

In the adult, sweat glands are most numerous on the sole of the foot ($620/cm^2$) and least abundant on the back ($64/cm^2$).[3] Glands first appear in the 3½-month-old fetus on the volar surfaces of the hands and feet.[4] Early in the fifth fetal month, anlagen of the eccrine sweat glands appear in the axillary skin and, a few weeks later, elsewhere on the body. The anlage of the eccrine sweat gland develops from the epidermal ridge as a cord of epithelial cells growing downward; the apocrine gland derives from the upper portion of the hair follicle as a solid epithelial bud. The anlage of the eccrine sweat gland is double-layered, and the lumen is formed between the middle of the fourth and the eighth fetal months. During the eighth fetal month the lumen broadens, and the secretory cells resemble those of the adult gland. The myoepithelial cells are not recognizable until at least the ninth month and are of uncertain origin.[4]

The eccrine sweat gland consists of two segments, a secretory coil and a duct. The secretory coil is composed of three distinct cell types: clear (secretory), dark (mucoid), and myoepithelial. The clear and dark cells occur in approximately equal numbers (Fig. 8-1). The dark cells border nearly all the apical (luminal) surfaces of the secretory tubules. The clear cells rest either directly on the basement membrane or on the myoepithelial cells. Where two or more clear cells abut, intercellular canaliculi are formed. The canaliculi emerge immediately above the basement membrane or the myoepithelial cells and open directly into the lumen of the gland. The only membrane of the clear cell directly exposed to the lumen is that part of the membrane facing the intercellular canaliculus (Fig. 8-2), which is a pouch extending from the luminal space. Spindle-shaped myoepithelial cells, with masses of myofilaments, lie on the basement membrane and abut the clear cells.

The eccrine sweat duct consists of an outer ring of peripheral or basal cells and an inner ring of luminal or cuticular cells. It seems that the proximal (coiled) duct is functionally more active than the distal straight portion because Na^+, K^+-ATPase activity and the number of mitochondria are higher in the proximal portion.[4–6] The luminal cytoplasm of the ductal cells forms a cuticular border consisting of a dense layer of tonofilaments. The basal cells rest on the basement membrane, which is continued from the secretory coil. Their cytoplasmic space contains many mitochondria, suggesting an active role in ductal Na reabsorption. In the epidermis, the duct spirals tightly upon itself.

CELL BIOLOGY AND FUNCTION OF DIFFERENT CELL TYPES

The clear cell contains abundant mitochondria and an autofluorescent body, called a lipofuscin granule, in the cytoplasm. Its cell membrane is rich in villi. In contrast, the dark cell has a relatively smooth cell membrane and contains abundant dark cell granules. The clear cell is most likely responsible for secretion of water and electrolytes. This is suggested by the abundance of membrane villi, membrane infoldings, and mitochondria. Furthermore, when dissociated clear cells are stimulated in vitro by cholinergic agents, they show a dramatic cell shrinkage due to activation of K and Cl channels in the membrane with subsequent net loss of KCl from the cell.[6–8]

In addition, cytoplasmic concentrations of Na, K, and Cl decrease during cholinergic stimulation, concomitant with an increase in intracellular Ca concentration. The abundance of the catalytic subunit of Na^+, K^+-ATPase in the basolateral membrane infoldings of the clear cell further supports the above thesis.[9] 15-Lipoxygenase-2 is in secretory cells but its function is unknown.[10]

The function of dark cells is unknown (Fig. 8-3). Because the dark cells represent the only cell type that stains for PAS, it was assumed that the PAS-positive glycoproteins in sweat might be derived from the dark cells.

The myoepithelial cell is a contractile cell with smooth muscle–like functional characteristics.[9,11] Its cytoplasm is filled with dense myofilaments that react to anti-actin antibodies.[12] The myofilaments also react to antikeratin monoclonal antibodies, suggesting an epidermal origin. Eccrine myoepithelium responds only to cholinergic stimulation, not to α- or β-adrenergic agents.

The duct is composed of two layers of cells, the basal and luminal ductal cells. The basal (or peripheral) cells are morphologically and functionally distinct from the luminal cells. The basal ductal cells are replete with mitochondria, and the circumferences of their cell membranes are rich in ATPase (Fig. 8-4),[9] suggesting that the entire cell membrane is involved in Na pumping for ductal Na absorption. In contrast, the luminal ductal cells have fewer mitochondria, much less ATPase activity, and a dense layer of tonofilaments near the luminal membrane, which is often referred to as the *cuticular border*. The cuticular border provides structural resilience to the ductal lumen, which may dilate whenever ductal flow of sweat is blocked. The entire structural organization of the duct is well designed for the most efficient Na absorptive function; the luminal membrane serves as the absorptive surface by accommodating both Na and Cl channels, and the basal ductal cells serve in Na pumping by providing maximally expanded Na pump sites and efficient energy metabolism. The lumen and the duct contain β-defensin, an antimicrobial, cysteine-rich, low molecular weight peptide.[13]

FIGURE 8-1

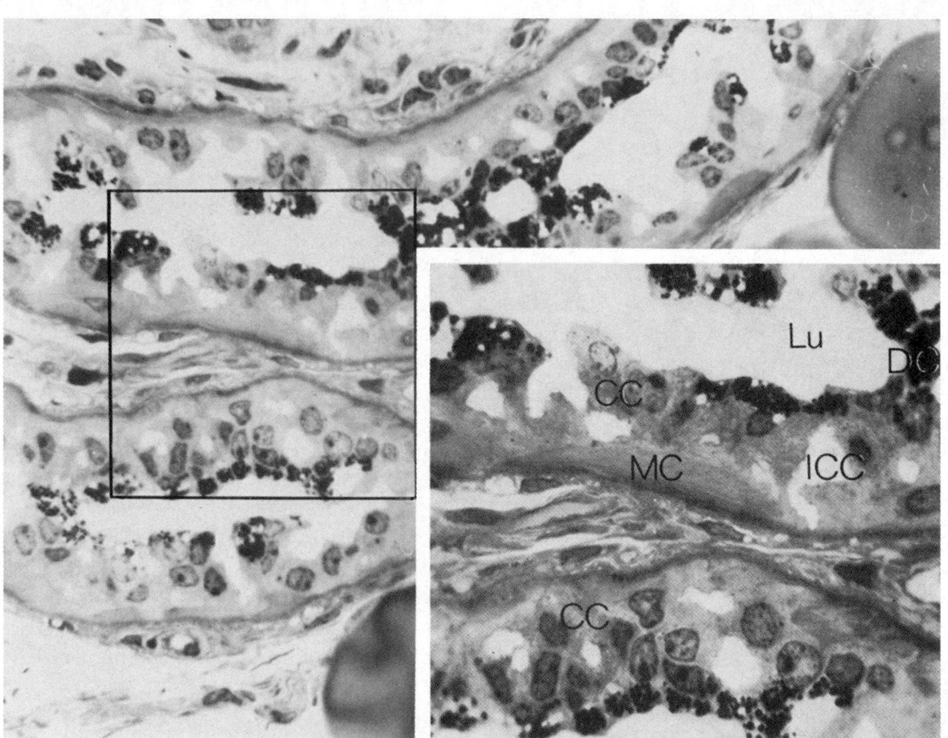

Light photomicrograph of the secretory coil of an acetylcholine-stimulated monkey-palm eccrine sweat gland. A 1-μm thick section was cut from an Epon-embedded specimen and stained with methylene blue. *Inset:* A higher-power view of the area marked by the square. CC, clear cell; DC, dark cell; ICC, intercellular canaliculi; Lu, lumen; MC, myoepithelial cell.

Nervous Control of Eccrine Sweating

Regulation of internal body temperature is among the most fundamental functions of the body. The preoptic hypothalamic area plays an essential role in regulating body temperature: local heating of the preoptic hypothalamic tissue activates generalized sweating, vasodilatation, and rapid breathing, whereas local cooling of the preoptic area causes generalized vasoconstriction and shivering. The elevation of hypothalamic temperature associated with an increase in body temperature provides the strongest stimulus for thermoregulatory sweating responses. Cutaneous temperature influences the rate of sweating. For example, an intense heat stimulus applied to one leg can elicit generalized sweating within 60 s before the tympanic membrane temperature (a measure of hypothalamic temperature) begins to rise, suggesting that neuronal stimuli arising from the heated leg via the cutaneous C fibers activate the hypothalamic sweat center and trigger sweating. Likewise, generalized sweating increases in correlation with an increasing mean skin temperature before core (internal) temperature begins to increase. Nadel et al.[14] quantified various factors involved in determining the rate of local sweating. At a given mean skin and core temperature, an increase in local skin temperature of 10°C triples the local sweating rate until the sweat rate plateaus. On a degree-to-degree basis, an increase in internal temperature is about nine times more efficient than an increase in mean skin temperature in stimulating the sweat center. The local temperature effect is speculated to be due to increased release of periglandular neurotransmitters.

FIGURE 8-2

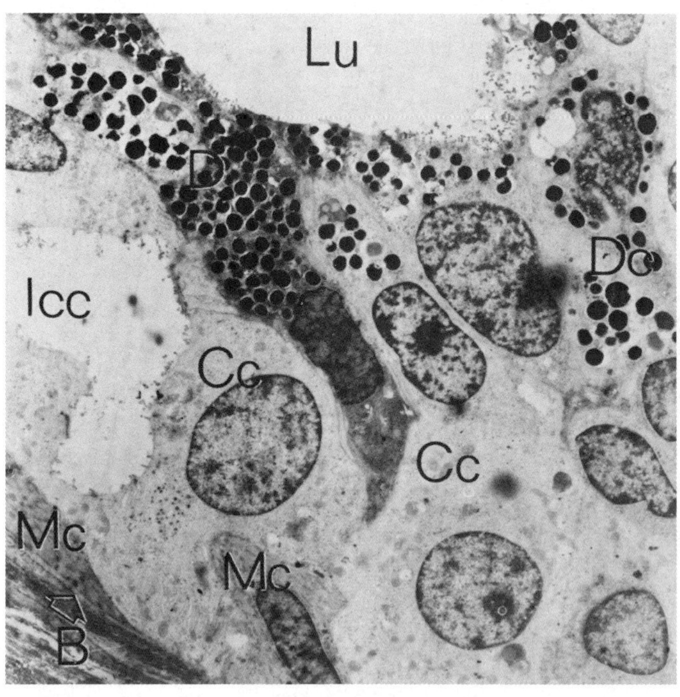

An electron micrograph of the secretory coil of human eccrine sweat gland. Symbols are the same as in Fig. 8-1. B with *arrow,* basal lamina.

INNERVATION Efferent nerve fibers originating from the hypothalamic preoptic sweat center descend through the ipsilateral brainstem and medulla and synapse in the intermediolateral cell columns of the spinal cord without crossing (although sympathetic vasomotor fibers may partially cross).[15] The myelinated axons rising from the intermediolateral horn of the spinal cord (preganglionic fibers) pass out in the anterior roots to reach (through white ramus communicans) the sympathetic chain and synapse. Unmyelinated postganglionic sympathetic class C fibers arising from sympathetic ganglia join the major peripheral nerves and end around the sweat gland. The supply to the skin of the upper limb is commonly from T2 to T8. The face and the eyelids are supplied by T1 to T4, so that resection of T2 for the treatment of palmar hyperhidrosis is likely to cause Horner's syndrome. The trunk

FIGURE 8-3

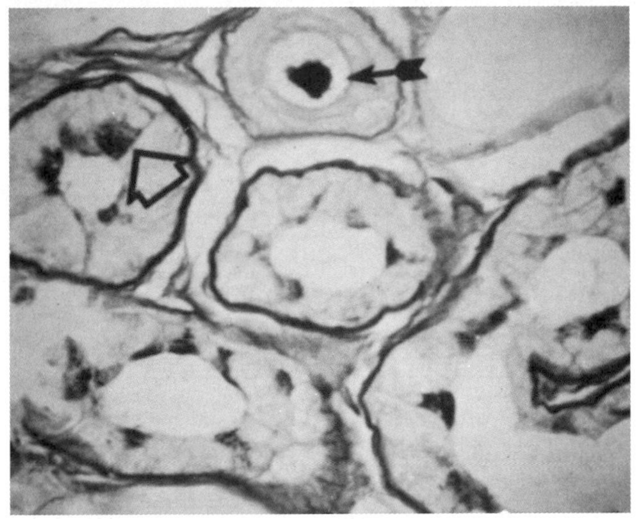

Presence of PAS-positive, diastase-resistant materials in the dark cells (*open arrow*) as well as in the ductal lumen (*solid arrow*).

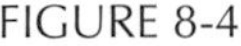

FIGURE 8-4

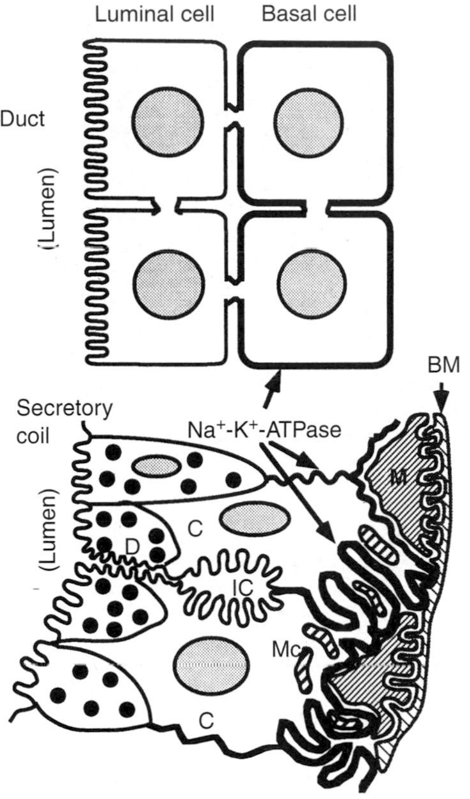

Illustration of the ultrastructures of the eccrine duct and secretory coil and the localization of Na^+, K^+-ATPase. BM, basement membrane; C, clear cell; D, dark cells; M, myoepithelial cell; Mc, mitochondria. The thick lines indicate the localization of Na^+, K^+-ATPase.

is supplied by T4 to T12 and the lower limbs by T10 to L2. Unlike the sensory innervation, a significant overlap of innervation occurs in the sympathetic dermatome because a single preganglionic fiber can synapse with several postganglionic fibers.

The major neurotransmitter released from the periglandular nerve endings is acetylcholine, an exception to the general rule of sympathetic innervation, in which noradrenaline is the peripheral neurotransmitter. In addition to acetylcholine, adenosine triphosphate (ATP), catecholamine, vasoactive intestinal peptide (VIP), atrial natriuretic peptide (ANP), calcitonin gene–related peptide (CGRP), and galanin have been localized in the periglandular nerves. The significance of these peptides or neurotransmitters in relation to sweat gland function is not fully understood.

Botulinum toxin interferes with acetylcholine release. Its heavy chain binds the neurotoxin selectively to the cholinergic terminal and the light chain acts within the cells to prevent acetylcholine release. Type A toxin cleaves sensory nerve action potential (SNAP)-25, a 25-kDa synaptosomal-associated protein; the type B light chain cleaves VAMP (vesicle-associated membrane protein, also named synaptobrevin). The use of the Botulinum toxins are discussed in chapters (Chaps. 76 and 276).

DENERVATION Postdenervation hypersensitivity (of postganglionic fibers) of the eccrine sweat gland remains to be explained. In humans, the sweating response to intradermal injection of nicotine or acetylcholine disappears within a few weeks after denervation of the postganglionic fibers.[16] (Note that the sweating response to thermal sweating should stop immediately after resection of the nerves.) For this reason, the human sweat gland was regarded as being the only exception to Cannon's law—the development of supersensitivity after postganglionic denervation. However, in the cat and monkey, the eccrine sweat gland becomes hypersensitive to adrenaline, nicotine, and methacholine for several weeks after postganglionic denervation and/or the effect of these drugs lasts longer than normal. In contrast, after denervation of preganglionic fibers (by spinal cord injuries or neuropathies), pharmacologic responsiveness of the sweat glands is maintained from several months to 2 years, even though their thermally induced sweating is no longer present.[17]

Emotional Sweating

Sweating induced by emotional stress (emotional sweating) can occur over the whole skin surface in some individuals, but it is usually confined to the palms, soles, axillae, and, in some instances, the forehead. Emotional sweating on the palms and soles ceases during sleep, whereas thermal sweating occurs even during sleep if the body temperature rises. Because both types of sweating can be inhibited by atropine, emotional sweating is cholinergic in nature.

Pharmacology of the Eccrine Sweat Gland and Sweating Rate

Sweat glands respond to cholinergic agents, α- and β-adrenergic stimulants, and other periglandular neurotransmitters, such as VIP and ATP. Periglandular acetylcholine is the major stimulant of sweat secretion, and its periglandular concentration determines the sweat rate in humans. A striking individual difference exists in the degree of sweating response to a given thermal or physical stress. In general, males perspire more profusely than females.[18,19] The sweat rate in a given area of the skin is determined by the number of active glands and the average sweat rate per gland. The maximal sweat rate per gland varies from 2 to 20 nL/min per gland.[3,18] Sweat rate increases during acclimatization, but the morphologic and pharmacologic bases of the individual and regional differences in sweating rate during acclimatization are still poorly understood (Fig. 8-5). In thermally induced sweating, the sweat rate can be mathematically related to the body and skin temperatures in a given subject only at the low sweat rate range. Cholinergic stimulation yields a 5 to 10 times higher sweating rate than does β-adrenergic stimulation. α-Adrenergic stimulation (by phenylephrine) is no more potent than isoproterenol (ISO) (a β-adrenergic agonist) in humans in vivo.[18] Whereas cholinergic sweating begins immediately

FIGURE 8-5

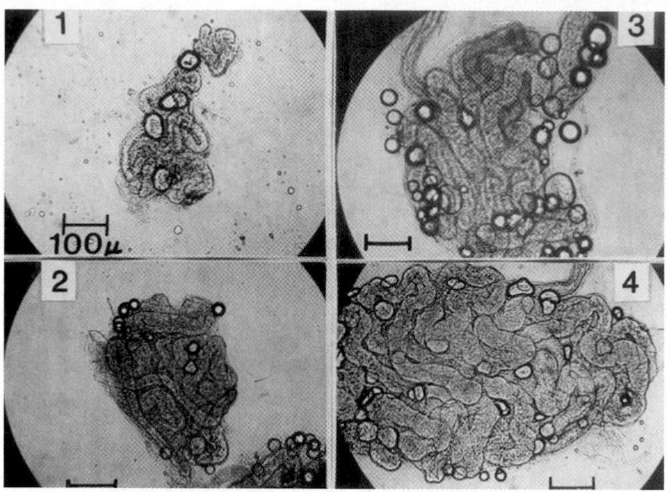

Individual variation in the size of the sweat gland in four male adults, ages 22 to 28. Sweat glands were isolated from biopsy skin specimens obtained from the upper back behind the axilla. Subject 1 is a sedentary man who does not exercise regularly, whereas subject 4 is a well-acclimatized athletic individual.

FIGURE 8-6

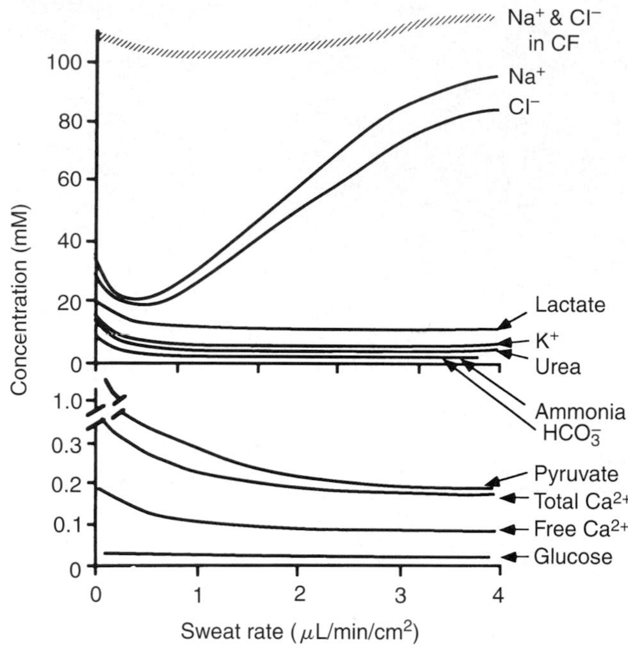

An illustrative relationship between the concentration of sweat ingredients and the sweat rate in thermally induced human sweat. CF, cystic fibrosis.

upon intradermal injection, β-adrenergic sweating requires a latent period of from 1 to 2 min, suggesting that the intracellular mechanism of sweat induction may be different between methacholine (MCh) and ISO. Because the sweat rate by adrenergic agents is rather low, it may be reasonable to surmise that catecholamine in periglandular nerves may be involved in regulation of sweat gland function but not as a stimulant of sweat secretion. One consequence of dual cholinergic and adrenergic innervation is to maximize tissue accumulation of cyclic adenosine monophosphate (cAMP), which may be instrumental in stimulating the synthesis and glandular hypertrophy of the sweat gland. The possibility that periglandular catecholamine is directly involved in emotional sweating or sweating associated with pheochromocytoma[20] may be ruled out because these sweating responses can be blocked by anticholinergic agents.

Pharmacology and Function of Eccrine Myoepithelium

The periodicity of sweat secretion in vivo is caused by the periodicity of central nerve impulse discharges, which occurs synchronously with vasomotor tonus waves. Sweat secretion induced by intradermal injection of pharmacologic agents is steady and does not show such a periodicity.[21] Myoepithelial contraction occurs with cholinergic stimulation, but neither α- nor β-adrenergic agents induce tubular contraction.[22] The myoepithelial cell responds only to cholinergic stimulation: (1) myoepithelial contraction is not a prerequisite for inducing or maintaining sweat secretion by the secretory coil and (2) the amount of so-called preformed sweat is so small, due to the narrow lumen, before stimulation that the initial myoepithelial contraction does not expel a significant amount of preformed sweat. The principal function of the myoepithelium may therefore be to provide structural support for the secretory epithelium, especially under conditions where stagnation of sweat flow (due to ductal blockade) results in an increase in luminal hydrostatic pressure.[11]

Energy Metabolism

Sweat secretion is mediated by the energy (i.e., ATP)-dependent active transport of ions, so a continuous supply of metabolic energy is mandatory for sustained sweat secretion. Endogenous glycogen stored in the clear cells can sustain sweat secretion for less than 10 min; thus the sweat gland must depend exclusively on exogenous substrates for its energy metabolism. Mannose, lactate, and pyruvate are nearly as readily utilized as glucose; other hexoses, fatty acids, ketone bodies, intermediates of the tricarboxylic acid (TCA) cycle, and amino acids are either very poorly utilized or not utilized as substrates. The physiologic significance of lactate or pyruvate utilization by the sweat gland is not yet clear. However, because the plasma level of glucose (5.5 mM) is much higher than that of lactate (1 to 2 mM) or pyruvate (<1 mM), glucose may play a major role in sweat secretion. Oxidative metabolism of glucose is favored as the major route of ATP formation for secretory activity.[22]

Composition of Human Eccrine Sweat

INORGANIC IONS Sweat is formed in two steps: (1) secretion of a primary fluid containing nearly isotonic NaCl concentrations by the secretory coil and (2) reabsorption of NaCl from the primary fluid by the duct. Although a number of factors influence ductal NaCl absorption, the sweat rate (and thus the transit time of sweat) is the most important factor influencing final NaCl concentration—namely, sweat concentration is low at the low sweat rate range but increases with the increasing sweat rate to plateau at around 100 mM (Fig. 8-6). Potassium (K^+) concentration in sweat is relatively constant. It ranges from 5 to 10 mM, which is slightly higher than plasma K^+ concentration. HCO_3^- concentration in the primary sweat fluid is about 10 mM, but that of final sweat is <1 mM, indicating that HCO_3^- is reabsorbed by the duct, presumably coupled by ductal acidification.[23] Sweat NaCl concentration is increased in cystic fibrosis (CF) sweat.

LACTATE The concentration of lactate in sweat usually depends on the sweat rate. At low sweat rates, lactate concentration is as high as 30 to 40 mM, but it rapidly drops to a plateau at around 10 to 15 mM as the sweat rate increases. Acclimatization is known to lower sweat lactate concentrations, whereas arterial occlusion rapidly raises sweat NaCl and lactate concentrations and reduces the sweat rate.[22] Because serum lactate concentration is 1 to 2 mM and an isolated sweat gland produces lactate in vitro,[24] sweat lactate is probably produced by glycolysis of glucose by the secretory cells.

UREA Urea in sweat is derived mostly from serum urea.[25] Sweat urea content is usually expressed as a sweat/plasma ratio (S/P urea). S/P urea is high (=2 to 4) at a low sweat rate range but approaches a plateau at 1.2 to 1.5 as the sweat rate increases.

AMMONIA AND AMINO ACIDS Ammonia concentration in sweat is 0.5 to 8 mM,[26] which is 20 to 50 times higher than the plasma ammonia level. The concentration of sweat ammonia is inversely related to the sweat rate and sweat pH. Free amino acids are in human sweat.[27] Because of the possibility of contamination by the large amounts of amino acids in epidermis, most published data must be reviewed critically.

PROTEINS AND PROTEASES Proteins are present in human sweat. The concentration of sweat protein in the least contaminated, thermally induced sweat is about 20 mg/dL, with the major portion being low molecular weight proteins (i.e., of weight <10,000). Because sweat samples collected by simple scraping, and even those collected with a plastic bag, can be massively contaminated with plasma or epidermal proteins, previous reports on the presence of α- and γ-globulins, transferrin, ceruloplasmin, orosomucoid, and albumin[28,29] and IgE must be carefully reexamined. The sweat samples collected over an oil barrier placed on the skin (the least-contaminated sweat) contain no or trace γ-globulin and a very small amount of albumin. Yokozeki et al.[30] reported the presence of cysteine proteinases and their endogenous inhibitors (CPI) in sweat and the sweat gland. Because epidermal growth factor (EGF) receptors are prominent in the human sweat duct,[33] and because EGF is also present in human eccrine sweat, it is tempting to speculate that the predominance of CPI in the sweat duct could be related, at least in part, to its role in the regulation of EGF receptors in the sweat duct.

Other organic compounds reported to be present in sweat include histamine,[31] prostaglandin,[32] vitamin K–like substances,[33] and amphetamine-like compounds.[34] Sweat also contains traces of pyruvate and glucose. Sweat glucose increases concurrently with a rise in plasma glucose (Fig. 8-7). Some orally ingested drugs,[22] including griseofulvin[35] and ketoconazole,[36] are secreted in sweat.

Mechanism of Sweat Secretion

The current model for sweat secretion is derived from the Na-K-2Cl cotransport model.[37,38] The unique additional features of membrane transport in eccrine clear cells required modification of the original Na-K-2Cl cotransport model—for example, the addition of initial events such as cell shrinkage—and parallel exchangers as shown in Fig. 8-8.[38] The eccrine clear cell is unique in that cholinergic stimulation is followed by dynamic cellular events (as summarized in Table 8-1)—namely, ACh, released from periglandular cholinergic nerve endings in response to nerve impulses, binds to cholinergic receptors, presumably present in the basolateral membrane of the clear cell. The activation of cholinergic receptors somehow stimulates an influx of extracellular Ca into the cytoplasm. The increased cytosolic [Ca] subsequently stimulates Cl channels in the luminal membrane and K channels in the basolateral membrane (see cell 1 in Fig. 8-8), causing a net efflux of KCl from the cell. Consequently, cell volume decreases because water follows the solutes to maintain isoosmolarity. Because the cell cytoplasm also contains osmotically active anions, including amino acids and phosphates (which do not leave the cell so readily), cytoplasmic K and Cl preferentially leave the cell through their respective ion channels, causing a significant decrease in cytoplasmic [K] and [Cl], despite the fact that the cytosolic water remains isoosmotic to the extracellular fluid during cell shrinkage. The decrease in [K] and [Cl] provides a favorable chemical potential gradient (i.e., the driving force) for Na-K-2Cl cotransporters located in the basolateral membrane. The cotransporters carry Na^+, K^+, and $2Cl^-$ into the cell in an electrically neutral fashion (i.e., two cations and two anions cancel out net charges). Because Na channels are absent in the clear cell membrane, Na-K-2Cl cotransporters are the only means by which Na enters the cells. The increase in cytoplasmic [Na] is well known to stimulate Na pumps, which extrude cytoplasmic Na in exchange for extracellular K, but because the Na-K-2Cl cotransporters are continuously operating, [Na] remains higher than the prestimulation level. One of the interesting features of the Na-K-2Cl cotransport model is that in the steady state (i.e., during the sustained sweat secretion, see cell 2 in Fig. 8-8), K and Na recycle across the basolateral membrane without further loss. The movement of Cl across the apical (luminal) membrane, which is down the electrochemical gradient, depolarizes the apical membrane and generates the negative luminal potential (with respect to the bath). The luminal negative potential then attracts Na into the lumen across the Na-conductive intercellular junction (i.e., paracellular pathway).[38] Thus the Na and Cl that enter the lumen across the cell join in the lumen to form NaCl in the isotonic primary fluid. Although the cotransport model may be the major ionic mechanism for sweat secretion, further modifications of the model have become necessary.

FIGURE 8-7

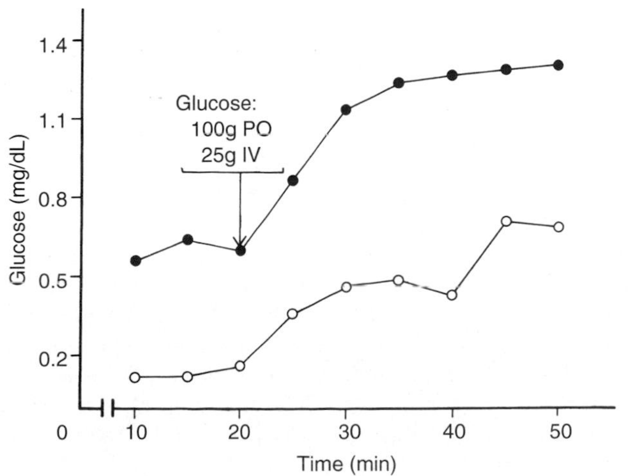

Sweat glucose concentration before and after glucose bolus in two human subjects. Serum glucose was increased from 85 to 360 mg/dL after glucose bolus, indicated by the *arrow*.

Stimulus-Secretion Coupling in Eccrine Sweat Secretion

Douglas and Rubin[39] originally proposed the concept of *stimulus-secretion coupling* to indicate that a cytoplasmic mediator (such as Ca or cAMP) serves as a link between pharmacologic stimulation and the final secretory processes. In the eccrine cell, Ca may serve as such a link by directly stimulating membrane K and Cl channels, thereby stimulating the cotransport system. The role of cAMP has been established as an intracellular mediator of hormones and β-adrenergic agonists in a variety of tissues. The data are consistent with the thesis that cAMP may be an intracellular mediator of β-adrenergic stimulation. Nevertheless, the role of intracellular Ca in cAMP-mediated stimulus secretion coupling is the subject of controversy.

One of the remaining puzzles is whether or not these transporters and channels are completely idle in the resting state.

Mechanism of Ductal Na Reabsorption

The principal function of the sweat duct is absorption of NaCl and HCO_3 from the primary fluid in order to conserve these vital electrolytes for the body. Because Na^+, K^+-ATPase is localized in the entire basal cell membrane[9] and the two cell layers are most likely coupled (and act like a syncytium), the duct functions as though it were made up of a

FIGURE 8-8

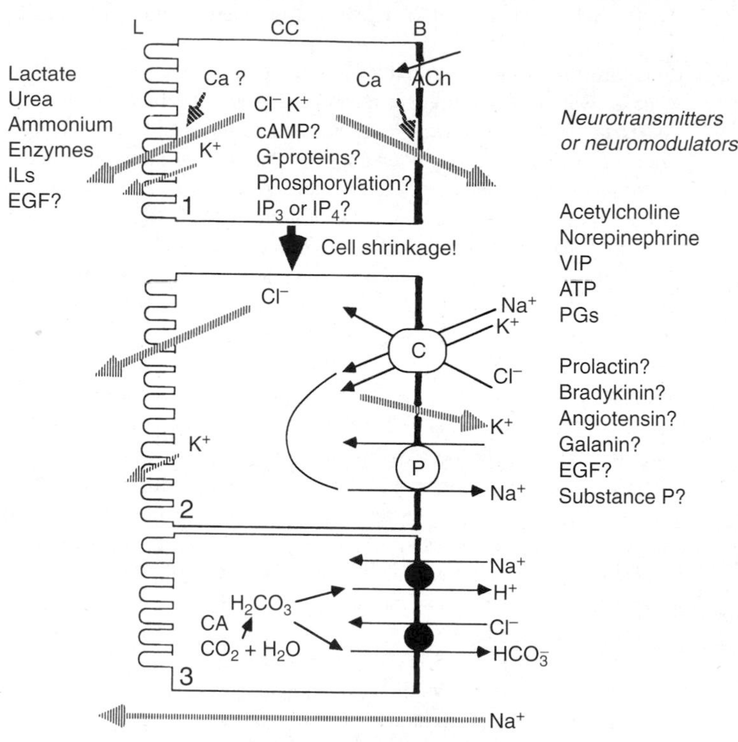

Modified Na-K-2Cl cotransport model for the ionic mechanism of cholinergic eccrine sweat secretion. Cell 2 is similar to the original cotransport model except that a small K conductance was placed across the luminal (apical) membrane.[51] Periglandular neurotransmitters and possible modulators of cellular function are listed on the basal side of the cell. ACh, acetylcholine; B, basolateral membrane; C, Na-K-2Cl cotransporter; Ca, calcium ion; CA in cell 3, carbonic anhydrase; CC, clear cell; EGF, epidermal growth factor; ILs, interleukins; IP_3 and IP_4, inositol triphosphate and inositol tetrakisphosphate, respectively; L, luminal or apical membrane; P, Na^+, K^+-ATPase-dependent Na pump; and shaded thick arrows, conductive flux of ions through ionic channels. Some of the potentially important ingredients are listed in the luminal side of the cell. Na movement across the cell junction is indicated with a shaded arrow at the bottom of the figure. The initial events are summarized in cell 1.

TABLE 8-1

Simplified Sequence of Events During Stimulation of Eccrine Clear Cells with Sustained Sweat Secretion (See Text for Detailed Discussion)

1. Release of acetylcholine (ACh) from the periglandular nerves.
2. Stimulation of Ca influx by ACh.
3. Increase in cytoplasmic [Ca].
4. Activation of K (basolateral) and Cl (apical) channels by Ca.
5. Influx of Cl into the lumen and efflux of K into the basal interstitium.
6. Loss of cytoplasmic KCl, causing cell shrinkage and a decrease in [K] and [Cl].
7. Activation of Na-K-2Cl cotransporters by an increase in gradients.
8. Na influx, causing an increase in cellular [Na].
9. Activation of Na pump by an increase in [Na].
10. From (5): Cl movement into the lumen, generating luminal negative potential.
11. Luminal negative potential, attracting Na into the lumen across cell junctions to form NaCl for the primary sweat.
12. Recycling of K across the basal membrane.
13. Recycling of Na across the basal membrane.
14. Continuation of (2) through (13) as long as ACh is present.

single cell layer, like a nephron (Fig. 8-9). The absorption of NaCl by the duct is due to the active transport of Na ions by the Na pump located in the basal ductal cell membrane. Three homologous sodium epithelial channel subunits have been cloned.[39] Ductal Na reabsorption is ouabain-sensitive[40] and amiloride-sensitive.[41]

Na must be transported against an electrochemical potential gradient as much as 60 to 70 mV. Chloride is also transported against the chemical gradient of 50 mV (against the gradient of from 20 m*M* in the lumen to 130 m*M* in the dermis), but down a favorable electrical gradient of 10 to 20 mV. Thus, Cl must still overcome the electrochemical potential gradient of 30 to 40 mV. It is widely held that the transport mechanism of the sweat duct largely conforms to Ussing's leak pump model.[42] For example, the presence of Cl channels as well as amiloride-sensitive Na channels has been demonstrated in the luminal membrane.[43] As predicted from the model, Na^+, K^+-ATPase and Cl channels are localized in the basal membrane.[43] The presence of ductal acidification or HCO_3 absorption suggests that additional transport processes such as Na-H exchangers or H pumps may also be involved (see Fig. 8-9). In cystic fibrosis, Cl channels in the luminal membrane are defective and those of the basal membrane are significantly decreased,[44] yet sweat ductal acidification is normal and sweat Na absorption is not totally impaired (i.e., sweat Na concentration never reaches 150 m*M* in cystic fibrosis despite the fact that in the primary fluid Na concentration is 150 m*M*, indicating that limited ductal Na absorption is present). Mutations in the transmembrane conductance regulator (CFTR) are the primary defects in cystic fibrosis. The permeability of chloride but not that of sodium is reduced in cystic fibrosis. A current hypothesis is that CFTR is a downregulator of the epithelial sodium channels and that the cystic fibrosis mutation impairs this regulation and results in increased sodium absorption. This further suggests the partial involvement of Cl-HCO_3 or Cl-OH and Na-H exchangers in the sweat duct. Several drugs are known to modify ductal NaCl reabsorption. When aldosterone is injected systemically or locally, the Na/K ratio in sweat begins to decrease within 6 h, reaching a nadir at 24 h and returning to the preinjection level in 48 to 72 h.[45] The effect of aldosterone on the sweat gland, unlike its effect on kidney tubules, is not accompanied by the so-called escape phenomenon.[46] Na deprivation stimulates both renin and aldosterone secretion, but high thermal stress per se [a single 1-h exposure of humans to a temperature of 40°C (104°F)] is a potent stimulator of renin and aldosterone secretion in either the presence or absence of sodium deprivation. Nevertheless, direct evidence is lacking that enhancement of sweat gland function is mediated solely by aldosterone. It appears that ISO (a β-adrenergic agonist) may also enhance ductal NaCl reabsorption.[22] In an in vitro sweat gland preparation, neither acetazolamide (a carbonic anhydrase inhibitor) nor antidiuretic hormone changes ductal or secretory function.

APOECCRINE SWEAT GLAND

The apoeccrine sweat gland, an additional member of the family of sweat glands, was discovered during isolation of human axillary sweat from a patient with axillary hyperhidrosis.[40,47] Although apoeccrine glands (AEG) are readily distinguished from classic eccrine and apocrine glands, the diversity of the gross and fine anatomy of the apoeccrine glands isolated even in the same individual has puzzled investigators (Table 8-2). The AEG develops during puberty from eccrine-like precursor glands and is consistently present in the adult axillae. Its relative frequency varies widely in different adults. However, in patients with axillary hyperhidrosis, as many as 50 percent of all the axillary glands are of the apoeccrine type, whereas in some individuals with no history of axillary hyperhidrosis, the incidence of the apoeccrine glands is

FIGURE 8-9

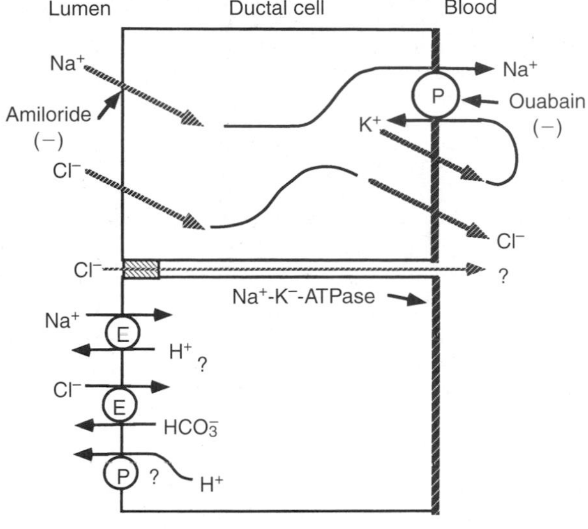

Illustration of ion transport in the sweat duct. The upper cell is similar to Ussing's classical leak-pump model. The lower cell illustrates parallel exchangers and an H pump, which explain ductal acidification of sweat and partial NaCl absorption in the cystic fibrosis duct where the luminal Cl channels are defective. E, exchanger; P, pump. Shaded arrows indicate conductive permeability down the gradient.

much lower. Like the eccrine glands, the AEG has a long duct, which opens directly onto the skin surface (unlike apocrine glands, which open directly into hair follicles). Basically, its secretory tubule consists of a segment of small diameter (as in the eccrine secretory tubule—i.e., less than 80 μm in diameter) and a segment of uniform or irregular dilatation to as much as 500 μm in diameter. These are functionally connected to each other, as was shown by a micropuncture study. The fine morphology of the thick segment is very similar to that of the apocrine gland except that some of the columnar secretory cells contain a large number of mitochondria. The thin segment is indistinguishable from that of the eccrine secretory coil. Like the eccrine gland, the AEG is both cholinergic and adrenergic and its secretory rate is as much as

TABLE 8-2

Some Characteristics of the Apoeccrine Sweat Gland

Appearance	At puberty, develops most likely from an eccrine gland or an eccrine-like precursor.
Size	Variable but larger than eccrine and smaller than apocrine.
Ductal opening	Opens to the nonfollicular skin surface like eccrine.
Duct	Made up of coiled portion and straight portion. Like eccrine duct but tends to have a larger diameter.
Secretory coil	Diameter extremely irregular. Coil is made up of dilated portion and undilated portion. In some coils, the entire secretory coil is irregularly dilated.
Secretory cell type	Very similar to eccrine clear cells in undilated segment, but resembles apocrine cells in dilated portion except that there are some columnar cells. Dilated portion contains rich mitochondria, as in eccrine clear cells.
Intercellular canaliculi	Present in undilated or partially dilated tubules.
Pharmacology	Cholinergic but also responds avidly to epinephrine and isoproterenol and very slighty to phenylephrine.
Sweat secretion	Persistent secretion of clear fluid (as in eccrine) in the presence of acetylcholine.
Sweat rate	Variable but as much as tenfold higher than that of the eccrine glands.

10 times that of the eccrine gland, mainly because of its large glandular size,[5] suggesting that the AEG may play a role in axillary hyperhidrosis. It is interesting that the AEG responds to epinephrine as avidly as to methacholine. The AEG may be basically an eccrine gland that has undergone "apocrinization" due to local growth factor(s). If so, similar apocrinization could occur elsewhere in the body where similar local growth factors are present.

APOCRINE SWEAT GLAND

In addition to the eccrine and apoeccrine sweat glands, described above, apocrine sweat glands are found in humans largely confined to the regions of the axillae and perineum.[48] They do not become functional until just before puberty; thus, it is assumed that their development is associated with the hormonal changes at puberty, although the exact hormones have not been identified. Gonadectomy of mature individuals does not affect the function of the apocrine sweat glands, so that if they are to be considered among the secondary sex characteristics, it should be recognized that it is their development and not the maintenance of their functional activity that is dependent on sex hormones.

Functions

A number of functions have been attributed to the apocrine glands, including odoriferous roles as sexual attractants, territorial markers, and warning signals, a role in increasing frictional resistance and tactile sensibility, as well as a role in increasing evaporative heat loss in some species. The production of pheromones by the apocrine glands of many species is well established.[49]

Because the apocrine glands of humans do not begin to function until puberty and are odor-producing, it is attractive to speculate that they have some sexual function, which may now be vestigial. There are high levels of 15-lipoxygenase-2 in the secretory cells of the apocrine gland. Its product 15-HETE, a ligand for the nuclear receptor peroxisome proliferator-activated receptor-γ, may function as a signaling molecule and function in secretion or differentiation.[10] For nonhuman primates, apocrine glands may have had an odoriferous function, which furred animals then developed for purposes of thermoregulation.

Composition of Secretion

The apocrine sweat of humans has been described as milky and viscid, without odor when it is first secreted. Subsequent bacterial action is necessary for odor production. Little is known of the chemical composition of apocrine secretion in humans, largely because of the difficulties in collecting secretion that has not been contaminated with that of eccrine glands. Furthermore, the presence of a secretory opening in common with that of the sebaceous glands means that apocrine sweat gland secretion will be mixed with sebum. This could account for the milky appearance of the secretion collected by cannulation of the sudosebaceous duct.

Mode of Secretion

Cannulation of the duct of the human apocrine sweat gland has shown that secretion is pulsatile, and it is assumed that contractions of the myoepithelial cells surrounding the secretory cells are responsible for these pulsations.

Control of Secretion

The apocrine sweat glands of humans respond to emotive stimuli only after puberty. They can be stimulated by either epinephrine or norepinephrine given locally or systemically. Denervation does not abolish the response to emotive stimuli,[50] which suggests that the glands can be stimulated humorally either by circulating epinephrine or norepinephrine. Studies on other species have shown that the apocrine glands are controlled by adrenergic nerves; this is in marked contrast to the eccrine glands, which are under cholinergic control.

Denervation experiments on species other than humans have verified that an intact nerve supply is a functional requirement, but the fact that the glands are usually more sensitive to epinephrine than norepinephrine has led to speculation that elevation of circulating levels of epinephrine may supplement the neural stimulus. It is not known whether apocrine glands of all species have both neural and humoral modes of control, although studies on goats have shown that exercise does not stimulate sympathetically denervated glands.

Although an intact nerve supply is a functional requirement of apocrine sweating, the demonstration of nerve endings or varicosities in close proximity to the glands has been difficult.[48] Local capillary circulation may assist in conveying transmitter substance to the sweat gland cells, a form of neurohumoral transmission.

As would be expected, drugs that affect adrenergic systems also have an effect on apocrine sweat glands. Adrenergic neuron–blocking agents inhibit sweating, as do drugs that deplete the stores of transmitter substance in adrenergic neurons. Specific adrenergic receptor–blocking drugs also inhibit sweating, but the types of receptors differ in various species. The type of receptor that mediates the response of the apocrine glands of humans has not been elucidated.

REFERENCES

1. KunoY: *Human Perspiration*. Springfield, IL, CC Thomas, 1956
2. Szabo G: The number of eccrine sweat glands in human skin, in *Advances in Biology of Skin,* vol 3, edited by W Montagna, R Ellis, A Silver. New York, Pergamon, 1962, p 1
3. Sato K, Dobson RL: Regional and individual variations in the function of the human eccrine sweat gland. *J Invest Dermatol* **54**:443, 1970
4. Ellis R: Eccrine sweat glands: Electron microscopy, cytochemistry and anatomy, in *Handbuch der Haut und Geshlechtskrankheiten, vol 1, Normale and pathologische Anatomie der Haut,* 1st ed, edited by J Jadassohn. Berlin, Springer-Verlag, 1967, p 223
5. Hashimoto K, Gross BG, Lever WF: The ultrastructure of the skin of human embryos. I. The intraepidermal eccrine sweat duct. *J Invest Dermatol* **45**:139, 1965
6. Sato K, Dobson RL, Mali JW: Enzymatic basis for the active transport of sodium in the eccrine sweat gland. Localization and characterization of Na-K-adenosine triphosphatase. *J Invest Dermatol* **57**:10, 1971
7. Takemura T, Sato F, Saga K et al: Intracellular ion concentrations and cell volume during cholinergic stimulation of eccrine secretory coil cells. *J Membr Biol* **119**:211, 1991
8. Suzuki Y, Ohtsuyama M, Samman G et al: Ionic basis of methacholine-induced shrinkage of dissociated eccrine clear cells. *J Membr Biol* **123**:33, 1991
9. Saga K, Sato K: Ultrastructural localization of ouabain-sensitive, K-dependent p-nitrophenyl phosphatase activity in monkey eccrine sweat gland. *J Histochem Cytochem* **36**:1023, 1988
10. Shappell S, Keeney D, Zhang J et al: 15-Lipoxygenase-2 expression in benign and neoplastic sebaceous glands and other cutaneous adnexa. *J Invest Dermatol* **117**:36, 2001
11. Sato K, Nishiyama A, Kobayashi M: Mechanical properties and functions of the myoepithelium in the eccrine sweat gland. *Am J Physiol* **237**:C177, 1979
12. Maiorana A, Nigrisoli E, Papotti M: Immunohistochemical markers of sweat gland tumors. *J Cutan Pathol* **13**:187, 1986
13. Ali R, Falconer A, Ikram M et al: Expression of the peptide antibiotics human beta defensin-1 and human beta defensin-2 in normal human skin. *J Invest Dermatol* **117**:106, 2001
14. Nadel ER, Bullard RW, Stolwijk JA: Importance of skin temperature in the regulation of sweating. *J Appl Physiol* **31**:80, 1971
15. Johnson R Spalding J: *Disorders of the Autonomic Nervous System.* Philadelphia, Davis, 1974
16. Coon J, Rothman S: The sweat response to drugs with nicotine-like action. *J Pharmacol Exp Ther* **23**:1, 1941
17. Faden AI, Chan P, Mendoza E: Progressive isolated segmental anhidrosis. *Arch Neurol* **39**:172, 1982
18. Sato K, Sato F: Defective beta adrenergic response of cystic fibrosis sweat glands in vivo and in vitro. *J Clin Invest* **73**:1763, 1984
19. Buceta JM, Bradshaw CM, Szabadi E: Hyper-responsiveness of eccrine sweat glands to carbachol in anxiety neurosis: Comparison of male and female patients. *Br J Clin Pharmacol* **19**:817, 1985
20. Prout BJ, Wardell WM: Sweating and peripheral blood flow in patients with phaeochromocytoma. *Clin Sci* **36**:109, 1969
21. Foster KG, Haspineall JR, Mollel CL: Effects of propranolol on the response of human eccrine sweat glands to acetylcholine. *Br J Dermatol* **85**:363, 1971
22. Sato K: The physiology, pharmacology, and biochemistry of the eccrine sweat gland. *Rev Physiol Biochem Pharmacol* **79**:51, 1977
23. Sato K, Sato F: Na^+, K^+, H^+, Cl^-, and Ca^{2+} concentrations in cystic fibrosis eccrine sweat in vivo and in vitro. *J Lab Clin Med* **115**:504, 1990
24. Sato K, Dobson RL: Glucose metabolism of the isolated eccrine sweat gland. II. The relation between glucose metabolism and sodium transport. *J Clin Invest* **52**:2166, 1973
25. Brusilow SW, Gordes EH: The permeability of the sweat gland to nonelectrolytes. *Am J Dis Child* **112**:328, 1966
26. Brusilow SW, Gordes EH: Ammonia secretion in sweat. *Am J Physiol* **214**:513, 1968
27. Gitlitz PH, Sunderman FWJ, Hohnadel DC: Ion-exchange chromatography of amino acids in sweat collected from healthy subjects during sauna bathing. *Clin Chem* **20**:1305, 1974
28. Page COJ, Remington JS: Immunologic studies in normal human sweat. *J Lab Clin Med* **69**:634, 1967
29. Jirka M, Blanicky P: Micro-isoelectric focusing of proteins in pilocarpine-induced sweat. *Clin Chim Acta* **31**:329, 1971
30. Yokozeki H, Hibino T, Takemura T et al: Cysteine proteinase inhibitor in eccrine sweat is derived from sweat gland. *Am J Physiol* **260**:R314, 1991
31. Garden JW: Plasma and sweat histamine concentrations after heat exposure and physical exercise. *J Appl Physiol* **21**:631, 1966
32. Forstrom L, Goldyne ME, Winkelmann RK: Prostaglandin activity in human eccrine sweat. *Prostaglandins* **7**:459, 1974
33. Seutter E, Sutorius AH: The vitamin K derivatives of some skin-mucins. 3. A route of oxygen transfer. *Int J Vit Nutr Res* **41**:529, 1971
34. Vree TB, Muskens AT, Van R: Excretion of amphetamines in human sweat. *Arch Int Pharmacodyn Ther* **199**:311, 1972
35. Shah VP, Epstein WL, Riegelman S: Role of sweat in accumulation of orally administered griseofulvin in skin. *J Clin Invest* **53**:1673, 1974
36. Harris R, Jones HE, Artis WM: Orally administered ketoconazole: Route of delivery to the human stratum corneum. *Antimicrob Agents Chemother* **24**:876, 1983
37. Sato K, Sato F: Cyclic AMP accumulation in the beta adrenergic mechanism of eccrine sweat secretion. *Pflugers Arch* **390**:49, 1981
38. Sato K: The physiology and pharmacology of the eccrine sweat gland, in *Biochemistry and Physiology of the Skin,* edited by LA Goldsmith. Oxford, Oxford University Press, 1983, p 596
39. Douglas W, Rubin R: The mechanism of catecholamine release from the adrenal medulla and the role of calcium stimulus-secretion coupling. *J Physiol* **167**:288, 1963
40. Sato K, Sato F: Sweat secretion by human axillary apoeccrine sweat gland in vitro. *Am J Physiol* **252**:R181, 1987
41. Garty H, Palmer LG: Epithelial sodium channels: function, structure, and regulation. *Physiol Rev* **77**:359, 1997
42. Ussing HH: Transport of electrolytes and water across epithelia. *Harvey Lect* **59**:1, 1965
43. Sato K et al: Membrane transport and intracellular events in control and cystic fibrosis eccrine sweat glands, in *Cellular and Molecular Basis of Cystic Fibrosis,* edited by G Mastelia, PM Quinton. San Francisco, San Francisco Press, 1988, p 171
44. Sato K, Taylor JR, Dobson RL: The effect of ouabain on eccrine sweat gland function. *J Invest Dermatol* **53**:275, 1969
45. Sato K, Dobson RL: The effect of intracutaneous D-aldosterone and hydrocortisone on human eccrine sweat gland function. *J Invest Dermatol* **54**:450, 1970
46. Conn J et al: The electrolyte content of thermal sweat as an index of adrenal cortical function. *J Clin Invest* **27**:529, 1948
47. Sato K, Leidal R, Sato F: Morphology and development of an apoeccrine sweat gland in human axillae. *Am J Physiol* **252**:R166, 1987
48. Robertshaw D: Apocrine sweat glands, in *Physiology, Biochemistry and Molecular Biology of the Skin,* 2nd ed, edited by LA Goldsmith. Oxford, England, Oxford University Press, 1991, p 763
49. Mykytowycz R: The behavioural role of the mammalian skin glands. *Naturwissenschaften* **59**:133, 1972
50. Shelley W: Apocrine sweat. *J Invest Dermatol* **17**:255, 1951
51. Sato K, Sato F: Nonisotonicity of simian eccrine primary sweat induced in vitro. *Am J Physiol* **252**:R1099, 1987

CHAPTER 9

Peter M. Elias
Kenneth R. Feingold
Joachim W. Fluhr

Skin As an Organ of Protection

Life on dry land exists because plants, arthropods, reptiles, birds, and mammals have developed an outer sheath that protects their aqueous interior from water loss into a relatively desiccated environment. The outer sheath of mammalian skin, the stratum corneum, not only protects against excess water loss but also defends against the entry of microorganisms, as well as natural and synthetic toxins. Finally, the stratum corneum and deeper layers of the skin protect from damage by ultraviolet irradiation, mechanical forces, extreme environmental temperatures, and low-voltage electric current.

FIGURE 9-1

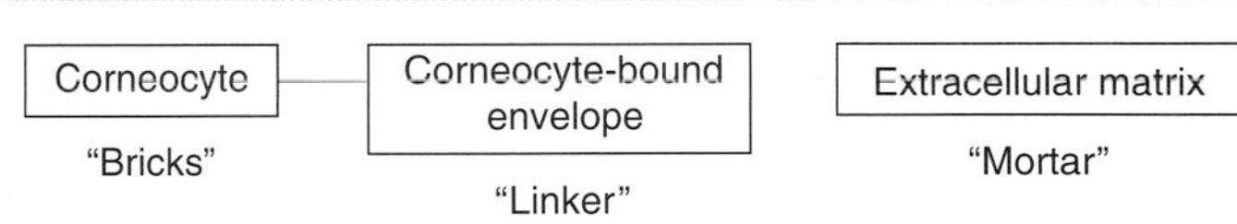

The two-compartment "bricks and mortar" model. The "bricks and mortar" model is shown, with lipids restricted to the stratum corneum interstices. In addition, the corneocyte-bound lipid envelope (CLE) is shown as the potential link between the corneocyte and extracellular matrix compartments.

OVERVIEW OF PROTECTIVE FUNCTIONS OF THE SKIN (See Table 9-1 and Fig. 9-1)

The innermost region of human skin is the *subcutaneous fat layer*. This layer insulates, reduces heat movement into or out of the body, absorbs energy from blunt mechanical trauma, and is active in general energy metabolism. Superficial to the fat layer lies the *dermis,* composed of collagen-glycosaminoglycan complexes, which also protects the body from blunt mechanical trauma. Overlying the dermis is the *epidermis,* which consists of several stratifying layers of nucleated *keratinocytes* and the stratum corneum, which is the major focus of this chapter. *Eccrine sweat glands* and *blood vessels* of the skin aid in the regulation of body temperature. *Sebaceous glands* provide rapid transport of proteins, lipids, and glycerol to the surface of the skin, where the latter is an important determinant of stratum corneum hydration. Afferent and efferent *nerve fibers,* which are chemosensitive, mechanosensitive, and heat sensitive, act as a rapid warning system for potential external trauma.

The *stratum corneum* (SC) is a very resilient tissue, despite its lack of bulk. This resiliency results from these factors: (1) the cornified envelope of individual corneocytes, is highly resistant to both physical and chemical assault; (2) the interdigitation of adjacent corneocytes; (3) the riveting of adjacent corneocytes via specialized desmosomes (corneodesmosomes), which are present and functional in the stratum compactum; and (4) the elasticity (deformability) of the stratum corneum,[1] a property of both its protein and lipid constituents.[2]

TABLE 9-1

Evolving Concepts of Stratum Corneum

1. Unimportant, desquamation: "basket weave" (up to 1960)
↓
2. Tough, resilient, impermeable: "plastic wrap" (up to 1975)
↓
3. Structural, biochemical heterogeneity: "bricks and mortar" (current)
↓
4. Persistent metabolic activity: "living" (current)
↓
5. Interactive with underlying tissues (current)
   a. Metabolic responses to external insults
   b. Pathophysiology—signal cascades
   c. Biosensor—response to shifts in humidity

An interconnected network of structural proteins disperses the force of external physical insults laterally throughout the tissue. Stratum corneum elasticity is also influenced by (1) the extent of hydration of corneocyte cytosolic proteins, a variable that is regulated by the hygroscopic breakdown products of filaggrin;[3] (2) sebaceous gland-derived glycerol, resulting from high rates of triglyceride turnover; and (3) by changes in external humidity.[4,5] Stratum corneum proteins, lipids (especially ceramides), glycerol, and low molecular weight byproducts of keratohyalin (filaggrin) catabolism, known as natural moisturizing factors, bind and retain water in the stratum corneum, thereby maintaining its elasticity.[2]

Because of its loosely organized appearance in skin samples subjected to routine fixation, dehydration, and embedding, the SC was initially not considered functionally important[6] (Table 9-1). Yet, when the SC is frozen-sectioned, and the cornified envelopes of corneocytes are either swollen at alkaline pH or stained with fluorescent, lipophilic dyes, it appears as a compact structure with geometric, polyhedral squames arranged in vertical columns that interdigitate at their lateral margins. Moreover, isolated SC sheets possess both unusually great tensile strength,[1] and very low rates of water permeability.[6] Hence, until the mid-1970s, the SC came to be viewed as a homogeneous film, that is, the "plastic wrap" concept.[6] In the 1970s, the SC was recognized to comprise a structurally-heterogeneous, two-compartment system,[7] with lipid-depleted corneocytes embedded in a lipid-enriched, membranous extracellular matrix (Fig. 9-1). More recently, the SC has come to be appreciated as a tissue with limited types of metabolic activity.[8–12] Most importantly, the SC forms an interface that interacts dynamically with underlying epidermal layers.[13] These recent concepts provide new insights into the mechanisms of permeability barrier homeostasis and into the role of external perturbations in initiating cutaneous pathology.[14] In addition to mechanical integrity, hydration, and barrier function, the outer layers of the epidermis

TABLE 9-2

Protective Mechanisms of the Epidermis

Inflammatory mediators such as prostaglandins, eicosanoids, leukotrienes, histamine, cytokines
Antioxidants including glutathione, oxidases, catalase, cytochrome P_{450} system, vitamins C and E
Heat-shock proteins
UV-absorbing molecules such as melanin, *trans*-urocanic acid, vitamin D, vitamin C metabolites
Water-retaining molecules ("natural moisturizing factors")
Xenobiotic-metabolizing enzymes such as glucuronidation, sulfation, hydroxylation mechanisms
Antimicrobial systems such as surface lipids, surface acidification, ironbinding proteins, complement, antimicrobial peptides

also mediate other critical, protective functions, including water repellence, integrity/cohesion/desquamation, resistance to xenobiotics, antimicrobial defense, UV filtration, and antioxidant defense (Table 9-2). Table 9-3 summarizes current concepts about the structural and biochemical bases for most of these functions.

Defense Against Oxidative Stress

The stratum corneum, as the interface with the ambient environment, is uniquely exposed to several forms of oxidative stress including ozone, ultraviolet (UV) irradiation, air pollution, pathologic microorganisms, and chemical oxidants, as well as topically applied drugs.[15] To prevent epidermal proteins, lipids, and DNA from damage by oxidative stress, the epidermis contains different enzymatic and nonenzymatic antioxidant systems.[16] The lipid-soluble antioxidant alpha-tocopherol is an important antioxidant in extracutaneous tissues[17] and in stratum corneum.[18] Both ozone and UV irradiation deplete the epidermis of vitamin E and induce lipid peroxidation.[19] Moreover, the water-soluble antioxidants vitamin C, uric acid, and glutathione, which recycle vitamin E, are also depleted by UV radiation and/or ozone.[20]

The role of antioxidant enzymes in epidermis is less clear. Patients with vitiligo display low catalase levels in their involved and uninvolved epidermis in association with high levels of hydrogen peroxide.[21] Repigmentation can be induced in vitiligo by topically applied pseudocatalase.[22] Although, levels of superoxide dismutase decline with age, catalase and glutathione reductase activity increase in photoaged, as well as in naturally aged, epidermis, while alpha-tocopherol and ascorbic acid decrease.[23] Acute UV radiation progressively deletes the catalase activity, while UV irradiation over a lifetime increases the catalase activity in the epidermis and dermis.[24] Finally, topically applied antioxidants appear to prevent UV-induced oxidative damage to antioxidative networks, and to SC lipids and proteins.[25] Thus, the epidermis appears to deploy a rich complement of antioxidant mechanisms against various forms of oxidative stress.

Protective, pH-Regulated Functions of the Stratum Corneum

Several of the functions listed in Table 9-3 are potentially regulated by the pH of the SC. These include not only permeability barrier function and inflammation, as discussed above, but also the related functions of SC integrity, cohesion, and desquamation[11] and anti-inflammatory activity, as well as antimicrobial defense.[26] Normal SC demonstrates a markedly acidic pH ("acid mantle").[27] While the origins of the acidic pH of the SC are incompletely understood, exogenous influences, such as lactic acid in sweat,[28] microbial metabolites, and free fatty acids from sebum,[29] have long been considered the most-likely sources. But recent studies point, instead, to three unrelated, endogenous pathways that contribute to SC acidification (Fig. 9-2). The first acidifying mechanism results from the deamination of filaggrin-derived histidine to *trans*-urocanic acid (tUCA) by the enzyme, histidine ammonia-lyase (histidase). This key metabolite, in turn, could impact several pH- and non-pH–related functions[30] (Fig. 9-3). With regard to non-pH–dependent, defensive cutaneous functions, tUCA is an effective UV-filter, but as it absorbs incident UVB, it isomerizes to *cis*-UCA, a potent immunosuppressive molecule that is hypothesized to favor development of UVB- and UVA-induced skin cancers.[31] tUCA, with other filaggrin metabolites, is also a potent endogenous humectant (Fig. 9-3); that is, an important source of SC hydration,[30] which not only regulates skin flexibility (see above), but also regulates downstream effects on epidermal proliferation.[4,32] The second pathway, phospholipid hydrolysis by lamellar body-derived, secretory phospholipase A_2 ($sPLA_2$), generates a pool of free fatty acids (FFA) that contributes to SC acidification, as well as to SC integrity and cohesion[11] (Fig. 9-2). Third, a sodium-proton membrane antiporter, NHE1, is expressed in the outer nucleated layers of the epidermis, where it acidifies localized membrane domains at the SG-SC interface, with a lesser contribution to the bulk pH of the SC[33] (Fig. 9-2).

How does the pH of the SC modulate these many functions? With regard to permeability barrier function, the barrier recovers more slowly after acute insults when exposed to neutral versus acidic buffers.[34] This delay in recovery can be explained by the pH optima of certain key lipid-processing enzymes in the SC interstices (Fig. 9-4). Although $sPLA_2$ displays a neutral pH optimum, two other key lipid-processing

TABLE 9-3

Protective Functions of the Stratum Corneum

Functions	Structural Basis	Biochemical Mechanisms
Mechanical integrity/resilience	Cornified envelope, cytosolic filaments	Cross-linked peptides; e.g., loricrin, keratin filaments
Xenobiotic defense	Lamellar bilayers	Lipid solubility; P_{450} system (outer epidermis)
Antimicrobial defense	Lamellar bilayers; extracellular matrix	Acidic pH; free fatty acids; antimicrobial peptides
Antioxidant defense	Corneocytes and extracellular matrix	Kerations; sebaceous gland-derived vitamin E and other antioxidants
Cytokine signaling	Corneocyte cytosol	Storage and release of pro-IL-1α/β; serine proteases
Permeability barrier	Lamellar bilayers	Hydrophobic lipids
Hydration	Lamellar bilayers; corneocyte cytosolic matrix	Sebaceous gland-derived glycerol; filaggrin break-down products; natural moisturizing factors (NMFs)
Waterproofing/repellence	Lamellar bilayers	Keratinocyte and sebum-derived lipids
Cohesion/desquamation	Corneodesmosomes	Acidic pH; serine proteases
UV protection	Corneocyte cytosol	Structural proteins; *trans*-urocanic acid (tUCA)

enzymes, β-glucocerebrosidase (β-GlcCer'ase) and acidic sphingomyelinase (aSMase), are activated at an acidic pH.[35] Hence, phospholipid catabolism yields locally acidifying products[11] (i.e., FFA), which, in turn, appear to activate β-GlcCer'ase and aSMase, generating ceramides, one of the three key SC barrier lipids, from their polar precursors (Fig. 9-4). Acidification also regulates SC integrity/cohesion, thereby restricting premature desquamation.[11] The basis for this activity relates to corneodesmosome degradation within the SC interstices, a process that requires two serine proteases, the SC chymotryptic and tryptic enzymes, which exhibit neutral-to-alkaline pH optima.[36] Thus, at an acidic pH, low protease activity presumably restricts corneocyte detachment to the low rates that accompany normal desquamation. Furthermore, the release and activation of interleukin (IL)-1α and IL-1β from their preformed precursor pools in the SC also requires serine protease activity, including the SC chymotryptic enzyme. Thus, the earliest, cutaneous proinflammatory events may be triggered by loss of normal SC acidification. Finally, the defensive antimicrobial function of the skin appears to be dependent upon SC acidification (Fig. 9-2).[37] Whereas normal flora, such as micrococci and corynebacteria, grow better at an acidic pH, pathogenic organisms, such as staphylococci, streptococci, and candida, proliferate more avidly at a neutral pH.[37] Thus, SC pH appears to regulate several of the SC's key defensive functions.

FIGURE 9-2

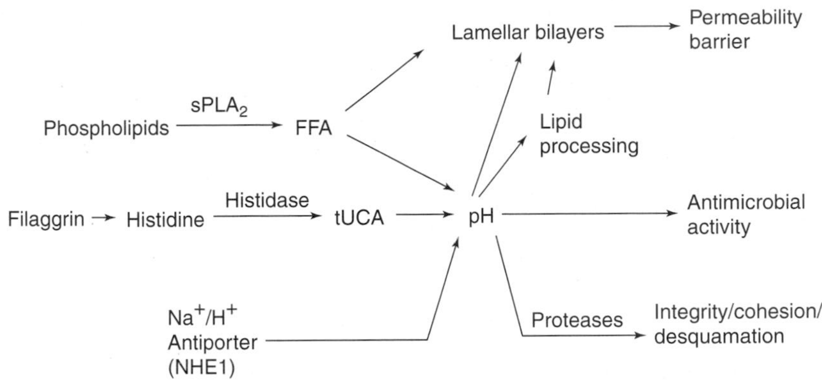

Endogenous pathways for SC acidification. Three endogenous pathways affect SC acidification, thereby regulating one or more of the key SC functions.

FIGURE 9-3

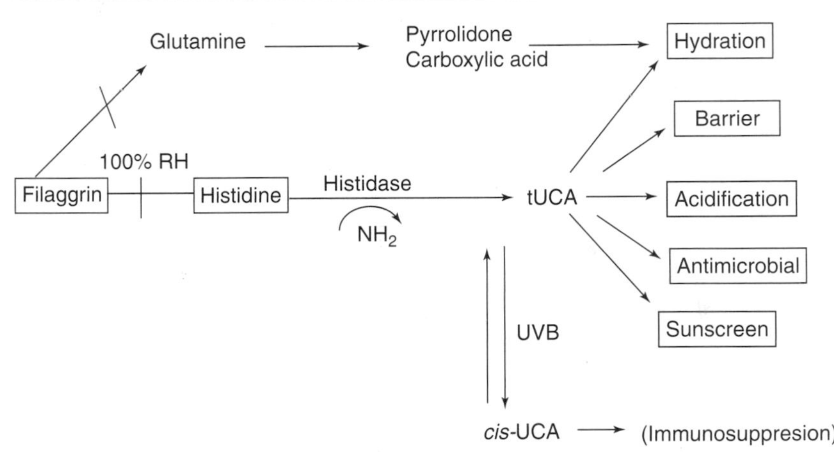

Filaggrin-histidine-urocanic acid pathway—metabolite functions in the SC.

THE TWO-COMPARTMENT MODEL OF THE STRATUM CORNEUM

Evidence for Intercellular Lipid Sequestration

Stratum corneum structure is similar in all keratinizing epithelia, comprising protein-enriched corneocytes embedded in a continuous, lipid-enriched, intercellular matrix in the "bricks-and-mortar" model (see Fig. 9-1).[7,12,38–40] The evidence for such protein-lipid sequestration is based upon freeze-fracture replication; histochemical, biochemical, and cell fractionation; cell separation; and physical–chemical studies.[41] Both freeze-fracture and ruthenium tetroxide postfixation reveal stacks of intercellular bilayers in the intercellular spaces, whereas routine electron microscopy reveals only empty spaces.[42] The two-compartment model also explains both the remarkable capacity of corneocytes to take up water[43] [i.e., the lipid-enriched lamellar bilayers act as semipermeable membranes, while osmotically active molecules (see above) trap water within the cytosol]. However, the two-compartment model must be updated based upon recent evidence both for microheterogeneity (i.e., the presence of extracellular proteins, such as desmosomal components, and abundant hydrolytic enzyme activity within extracellular domains), and for signaling networks that link the stratum corneum to underlying layers (Table 9-1).

FIGURE 9-4

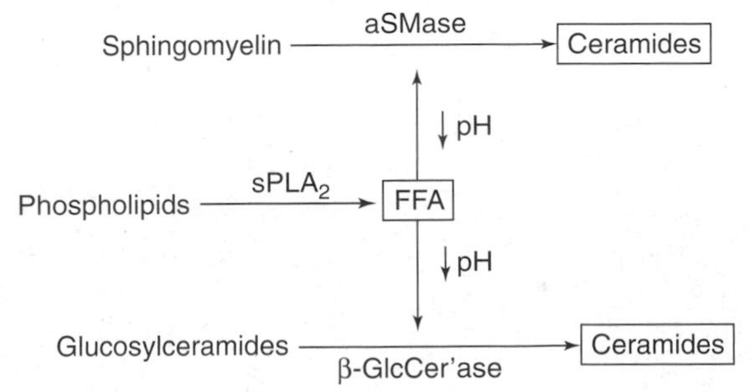

Generation of free fatty acids (FFA) from phospholipids regulates SC pH and, subsequently, the activities of at least two other key SC enzymes.

The Role of Lipids in the Permeability Barrier and Clinical Implications

The importance of stratum corneum lipids for barrier integrity has been known since it was shown that topical applications of organic solvents produce profound alterations in barrier function.[44] Table 9-4 summarizes the key mechanisms by which SC lipids mediate barrier

TABLE 9-4

How Lipids Mediate Permeability Barrier Function

Intercellular localization
Amount of lipid (lipid wt%)
Tortuous pathway
Lamellar organization
Hydrophobic composition
Correct molar ratio
Unique molecular structures

function. More recently, the importance of bulk SC lipids for the barrier was demonstrated by (1) the inverse relationship between the permeability of the stratum corneum to water and water-soluble molecules at different skin sites (e.g., abdomen versus palms and soles) and the lipid content of that site;[45] (2) the observation that organic solvent-induced perturbations in barrier function occur in direct proportion to the quantities of lipid removed;[44] (3) the finding that SC lipid content is defective in pathologic states that are accompanied by compromised barrier function, such as essential fatty acid deficiency;[46] (4) the observation that replenishment of endogenous SC lipids, following lipid removal by solvents or detergents, parallels the recovery of barrier function;[47] and (5) the finding that topically applied SC lipids normalize or accelerate barrier recovery when applied to solvent-treated, tape-stripped, or surfactant-treated skin.[48,49]

These regional differences in SC lipid content have important clinical implications. First, they correlate with susceptibility to the development of contact dermatitis to lipophilic versus hydrophilic antigens at specific skin sites. Whereas allergy to lipophilic antigens, such as poison ivy (urushiol), is more likely to occur on lipid-replete sites, allergy to water-soluble antigens, such as those in metals, foods, flowers, and vegetables, occurs more commonly on lipid-depleted sites such as the palms. Second, persons with atopic dermatitis who display a paucity of SC lipids[10,50–52] are less-readily sensitized to lipid-soluble antigens,[53] but more readily sensitized to hydrophilic antigens, such as nickel.[54] Of course, immunologic abnormalities in atopic individuals could also contribute to differences in sensitization thresholds.[55] Third, percutaneous delivery of topical, lipid-soluble drugs, such as topical steroids and retinoids, occurs more readily on lipid-replete sites, such as the face, axillae, and groin.[56] Hence, the higher propensity to develop cutaneous side effects, such as atrophy from topical glucocorticoids, in these sites. Similarly, lipophilic drugs, such as estradiol, nitroglycerin, scopolamine, clonidine, and fentanyl, are delivered transdermally for systemic therapeutic purposes with relative ease over lipid-replete sites.[57] Finally, the low lipid content of palms and soles explains the increased susceptibility of these sites to the development of soap- or surfactant- and hot water-induced dermatitis;[58] that is, these sites have an intrinsic barrier defect, associated with reduced lipids, and additional lipid removal superimposes a further insult.

Cellular Basis for Lipid-Protein Sequestration (Fig. 9-5)

Since its earliest descriptions, hypotheses have abounded about the function of the epidermal lamellar body.[59] These ellipsoidal organelles, measuring about $0.3 \times 0.5\ \mu$m, appear initially in the first suprabasal cell layer, the stratum spinosum, and continue to accumulate in the stratum granulosum, accounting for about 10 percent of the volume of the granular cell cytosol. The lamellar body contents comprise a plastic sheet, which appears like parallel membrane stacks, enclosed by a limiting trilaminar membrane, in cross-section.[60,61] In the outer granular layer, lamellar bodies move toward the highly invaginated apical surface, where they are poised to undergo rapid exocytosis.[12,59–62] Tracer perfusion studies demonstrate the role of the lamellar body secretory process in barrier formation: The outward egress of water-soluble tracers through the epidermis is blocked at sites where secreted lamellar body contents have been deposited. Membrane specializations, such as tight junctions, are present in these locations, but they are insufficient to account for barrier formation.

The factors that regulate lamellar body secretion were recently elucidated. Low rates of secretion, sufficient to sustain basal barrier function, occur under basal conditions, while both organellogenesis and secretion accelerate under stimulated conditions. For example, acute perturbations of the permeability barrier result in an immediate secretion

FIGURE 9-5

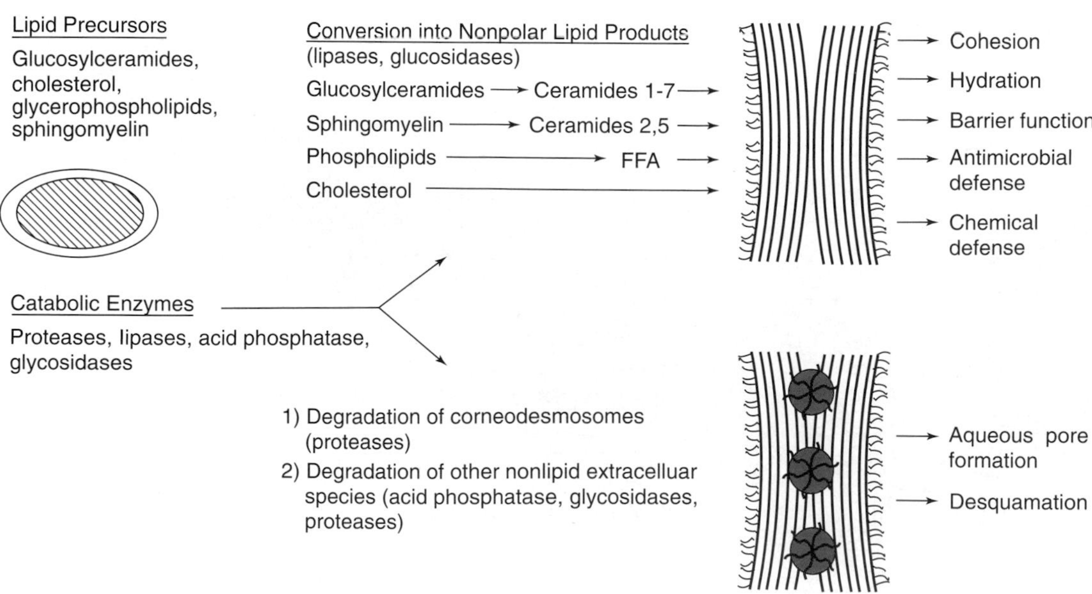

Lamellar body products and functional consequences. Lamellar bodies deliver both lipids and enzymes, which impact barrier-related functions and degradation processes, such as desquamation.

of most lamellar bodies from outermost granular cells, accompanied by a striking reduction in the numbers of these organelles in the cytosol.[61] Changes in the epidermal calcium gradient regulate these differences in secretion.[63] Depletion of extracellular calcium, which accompanies barrier disruption, stimulates lamellar body secretion. As the gradient is reestablished, lamellar bodies reaccumulate in these cells.

Because lamellar bodies are enriched in sugars and lipids, their contents were thought to be important for epidermal cohesion and waterproofing.[12,59,62] Biochemical studies further support a role for this organelle's contents in barrier formation.[60,64–66] Partially purified lamellar body preparations are enriched in glucosylceramides, free sterols, and phospholipids (Fig. 9-5), precursors of the species that account for almost all of the SC intercellular lipids.

In addition to lipids, the lamellar body is enriched in selected hydrolytic catabolic enzymes (Fig. 9-5), including acid phosphatase, certain proteases, a family of lipases, and a family of glycosidases.[12,65,67] As a result of its enzyme contents, the lamellar body has been considered a type of lysosome, but evidence for this concept is lacking. For example, lamellar bodies lack certain acid hydrolases characteristic of lysosomes, such as arylsulfatases A and B, as well as β-glucuronidase.[65] Instead, the lamellar body appears to be a specialized secretory vesicle, analogous to the lamellar body of alveolar type 2 cells. The same enzymes that are concentrated in lamellar bodies occur in highly specific activity in whole stratum corneum, and they are further localized to intercellular domains.[12] These enzymes appear to fulfill dual roles: some play a role in barrier formation and others in desquamation[11,12,36] (Fig. 9-5). The colocalization of the various lipases (phospholipase A_2, sphingomyelinase, steroid sulfatase, acid lipase, and β- glucocerebrosidase) to the same tissue compartment as "probarrier" lipids results in formation of lamellar membrane structures (Table 9-5).[12] Lamellar body-derived serine proteases appear to regulate corneodesmosomal degradation, leading to desquamation[42,68] (Fig. 9-5). Indeed, two of these serine proteases, SC chymotryptic and tryptic enzymes, have been extensively characterized and shown to regulate corneodesmosome degradation.[36,69,70] Finally, recent information suggests that steroid sulfatase, the microsomal enzyme responsible for desulfation of cholesterol sulfate, also reaches SC membrane domains by the lamellar body secretory pathway.[66,71] In summary, a variety of barrier- and nonbarrier-related enzymatic activities persist in the SC. These enzymatic activities can be further localized to either the cytosol, the cornified envelope, or the interstices of the SC. Because of these large amounts of persistent metabolic activity, the SC clearly can no longer be viewed as "dead" or "inert".

TABLE 9-5

Precursors and Products of Stratum Corneum Lipid Processing Enzymes

LIPID PRECURSOR	EXTRACELLULAR HYDROLASE	MATURE SC MEMBRANES
Phospholipids	Secretory phospholipases (group 1 and ? others)	Nonessential free fatty acids
Sphingomyelin	Acid sphongomyelinase	Ceramides 2 and 5+
Cholesterol sulfate	Steroid sulfatase	Cholesterol*
Glucosylceramides	β-Glucocerebrosidase	Ceramides 1, 3, 6, 7+

*Most cholesterol is derived unchanged from lamellar body contents.
+Can be further metabolized to sphingoid base plus free fatty acids by acid ceramidase.

EXTRACELLULAR LIPID PROCESSING

Cosequestration of lipids and selected hydrolytic enzymes within the intercellular spaces of the stratum corneum results from the secretion of the lipid-enriched contents of lamellar bodies from the outermost granular cell. As noted above, barrier formation requires the transformation of the initially secreted lipids (predominantly glucosylceramides, cholesterol, and phospholipids) into a more nonpolar mixture, enriched in ceramides, cholesterol, and free fatty acids, a process that may require acidification of the extracellular domains[9,11,49,60] (see Fig. 9-6). Such an acidic milieu may be required for optimal activation of certain of the key hydrolases, for example, β-glucocerebrosidase, acid lipase, and acid sphingomyelinase. In contrast, secretory phospholipase A_2 and steroid sulfatase, with their neutral pH optima, may be activated at the higher pHs present in the lower SC. Together, these enzymes generate the requisite nonpolar lipid mixture that forms the hydrophobic, intercellular lamellar membrane system (Table 9-5).

Proof of the key role of extracellular β-glucocerebrosidase in this process came from both inhibitor studies (conduritols) and a transgenic murine model.[35,72–74] In both of these models, lack of enzyme activity leads to a barrier abnormality, which appears to be attributable to both accumulation of glucosylceramides and depletion of ceramides. This biochemical change is accompanied by the persistence throughout the SC interstices of immature membrane structures. Such incompletely processed membrane structures also appear in a subgroup of patients with Gaucher's disease (type II), which is characterized by drastically reduced enzyme levels and ichthyosiform skin lesions.[72] Although inadequate to meet the demands of terrestrial life, these immature, glycosylated membrane structures nevertheless appear to suffice in mucosal

FIGURE 9-6

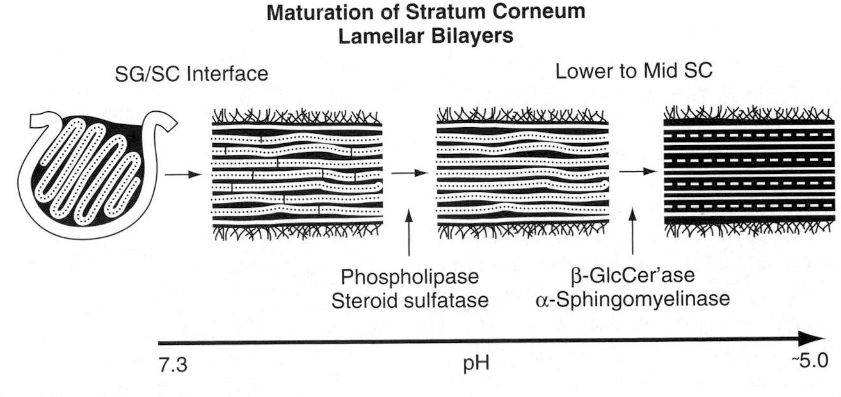

Maturation of stratum corneum lamellar bilayers. Lamellar body lipids are delivered as pleated sheets at the SC/SG (stratum granulosum) interface and subsequently mature into bilayers along a pH gradient.

epithelia.[75] Pertinently, endogenous β-glucosidase levels are reduced in oral mucosa.[76] Thus, the persistence of glucosylceramides could indicate either less stringent barrier requirements and/or additional functions of glucosylceramides unique to these tissues.

Extracellular processing of phospholipids is also required for barrier homeostasis.[77] As with β-glucocerebrosidase, pharmacologic inhibitors of phospholipase A_2 both delay barrier recovery after prior disruption and induce a barrier abnormality in intact murine epidermis.[77] The biochemical abnormality responsible for the barrier defect is product depletion: that is, coapplications of palmitic acid (but not linoleic acid) along with the inhibitors, normalize barrier function. Thus, generation of nonessential FFA by phospholipase-mediated degradation of phospholipids is required for barrier homeostasis. We recently showed the importance of secretory phospholipase A_2-derived FFA for SC acidification, and defined the role of protons derived from this pathway in mediating SC integrity/cohesion.[11]

Recent studies also demonstrate the importance of regulation of acid sphingomyelinase (aSMase) for homeostasis.[9] aSMase is required for the generation of two of the seven ceramides that form the lamellar bilayers.[78] Finally, steroid sulfatase (SSase), which desulfates cholesterol sulfate, is also required for barrier homeostasis.[79] However, rather than supplying cholesterol for the barrier, the principal importance of SSase is removal of excess cholesterol sulfate, which, when present, in excess, provokes excess scale. In summary, four SC extracellular enzymes are required for permeability barrier homeostasis.

EXTRACELLULAR LAMELLAR MEMBRANE GENERATION AND MATURATION

As noted above, lamellar body exocytosis delivers the precursors of the extracellular lamellar membranes to the stratum granulosum–stratum corneum interface (Figs. 9-5 and 9-6).[12] Lamellar body-derived membrane sheets then unfurl, fuse, and transform into broad, uninterrupted membrane sheets, which then metamorphose into lamellar membrane unit structures.[12,42,61,80] This sequence normally occurs in its entirety within the lower two to three cell layers of the SC, correlating with changes in lipid composition, that is, from the polar lipid-enriched mixture of glucosylceramides, phospholipids (including sphingomyelin), and free sterols present in lamellar bodies, to the more nonpolar mixture, enriched in ceramides, free sterols, and free fatty acids, present in the SC. As noted above, these structural changes appear to be completely or partially mediated by a family of lipid hydrolases (Table 9-5),[12] delivered to the SC interstices by lamellar body secretion.

The elucidation of lamellar membrane structure in mammalian SC has been impeded by the extensive extraction artifacts produced during processing for light and electron microscopy.[12] Following the application of freeze-fracture replication to the epidermis, the SC interstices were first shown to be replete with a multilamellar system of broad membrane structures. Further detailed information about intercellular lamellar membrane structures resulted from the application of ruthenium tetroxide postfixation to the study of stratum corneum membrane structures.[42,80,81] With ruthenium tetroxide postfixation, the electron-lucent lamellae appear as pairs of continuous leaflets, alternating with a single fenestrated lamella. Each electron-lucent lamella is separated by an electron-dense structure of comparable width. The entire multilamellar complex lies external to a hydrophobic envelope, containing covalently-bound ceramides. The lamellar spacing or repeat distance of 12.9 ± 0.2 nm of ruthenium tetroxide-fixed lamellae, analyzed by optical diffraction, correlates extremely well with independent measurements of these domains by x-ray diffraction.[80] Because the repeat distance is more than twice the thickness of typical lipid bilayers, each lamellar repeat unit appears to consist of two apposed bilayers.[80] Multiples of these units (up to three) occur frequently in the SC interstices,[80] and simplifications of the basic unit structure, with deletion of one or more lamellae, occur at the lateral surfaces of corneocytes, that is, at three-cell junctures.[80] Electron-dense dilatations of the electron-dense lamellae correspond to comeodesmosomes in the lower SC, and in higher layers, to sites of comeodesmosome hydrolysis.[42,80] It has been proposed that these sites correspond to the aqueous "pore pathway" for water, as well as the route for percutaneous drug and xenobiotic movement (Fig. 9-5).[82]

The membrane complex immediately exterior to the cornified envelope, the covalently-bound lipid envelope replaces the true plasma membrane during terminal differentiation.[3] Although a portion of this trilaminar structure survives exhaustive solvent extraction, it is destroyed by saponification.[83] Lipid extracts of saponified fractions yield long chain, ω-hydroxyacid-containing ceramides that are believed to be covalently attached to glutamine residues in the cornified envelope.[76] Because this envelope persists after prior solvent extraction has rendered the SC porous, it does not itself provide a barrier. However, it is required for normal barrier function,[84] perhaps functioning as a scaffold for the deposition and organization of lamellar body-derived, intercellular bilayers. Although, the origin of the covalently bound envelope remains unknown, it does not appear to originate from the pool of lipids deposited during lamellar body secretion, but rather from fusion of the limiting membrane of lamellar bodies with the plasma membrane, immediately prior to cornification.[71]

MAINTENANCE OF NORMAL STRATUM CORNEUM FUNCTION

Epidermal Lipid Synthesis under Basal Conditions

Studies of cutaneous lipid synthesis demonstrate that[85,86] (1) the skin is a major site of cholesterol synthesis, accounting for 20 to 25 percent of total body synthesis;[87] (2) the skin generates a broad range of lipid species;[88] and (3) most cutaneous sterol and fatty acid synthesis localizes to the dermis—the epidermis is an extremely active site of lipid synthesis, with about 60 to 70 percent of total lipid synthesis occurring in the basal layer.[86,89] However, considerable epidermal lipid synthesis continues in all of the nucleated layers of the epidermis.[89]

It is now clear that systemic factors influence cutaneous lipid synthesis minimally. Whereas hormonal changes, particularly in thyroid, testosterone, or estrogen status, can alter epidermal lipid synthesis, these hormones appear to have little impact on cutaneous lipid synthesis under day-to-day conditions.[86] In addition, changes in circulating sterols from either diet or drugs do not alter epidermal cholesterol synthesis, presumably because of the paucity of low-density lipoprotein receptors on epidermal cells.[86,90] The independence of these layers from circulating influences may have evolutionary significance, because it ensures that the differentiating layers are attuned to their own special functional requirements, that is, barrier homeostasis. Yet, despite its relative autonomy, the epidermis incorporates some circulating lipids such as plant sterols, essential fatty acids, polyunsaturated fatty acids, and arachidonic acid (the epidermis lacks the $^{6}\Delta$-desaturase).[85] Although these lipids are indicators of the capacity of the epidermis to take up exogenous lipids, the quantitative contribution of extracutaneous lipids to the epidermal pool appears to be small in comparison to de novo synthesis.[86]

Metabolic Responses to Barrier Disruption

Despite both its relative autonomy and high basal rates of lipid synthesis, the epidermis responds with a further lipid biosynthetic burst when the permeability barrier is disrupted by topical treatment with either organic solvents, tape stripping, or detergents.[13,86] Regardless of

FIGURE 9-7

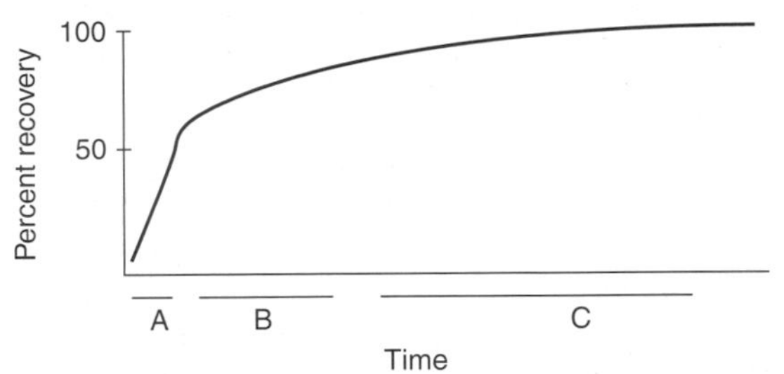

Three phases of barrier recovery after acute perturbations: Regulated metabolic activities in relation to kinetics of recovery.

the manner of barrier disruption, an initial, rapid repair response leads to about 50 percent restoration of normal barrier function in about 12 h in humans, with a slower, late phase leading to complete recovery in 72 to 96 h[91] (Fig. 9-7). These acute forms of barrier perturbation can be analogized to administering a "treadmill" examination to the skin. This assay has been used for several purposes, including the linkage of specific metabolic responses to barrier homeostasis. For example, different metabolic events are associated with the rapid versus slow recovery phase (Fig. 9-7). Immediately after barrier disruption, all of the lamellar bodies in the outermost granular cell are secreted,[61] and an increase occurs in both cholesterol and fatty acid synthesis. In contrast, the late phase of barrier recovery is associated with an increase in ceramide synthesis,[92] as well as a stimulation of epidermal β-glucocerebrosidase[72] and DNA synthesis.[93] That all of these alterations can be attributed to the barrier abnormality is shown by (1) the localization of the increase in synthesis to the underlying epidermis—dermal cholesterol and fatty acid synthetic rates remain unaffected after acute barrier disruption; (2) the extent of the increase in lipid and DNA synthesis is proportional to the degree of the barrier abnormality;[94] (3) the increase in lipid synthesis is prevented when the barrier is artificially restored by application of water vapor-impermeable (but not vapor-permeable) membranes, while the increase in DNA synthesis is partially blocked;[93] and (4) in a sustained model of barrier dysfunction (i.e., rodent essential fatty acid deficiency), lipid synthesis is stimulated, and the increase is normalized when the barrier is restored by either linoleic acid replenishment or occlusion.[94] These results indicate that alterations in barrier function stimulate epidermal lipid synthesis, and suggest further that transcutaneous water loss might be a direct or indirect regulatory factor.

The epidermal activities of the rate-limiting enzymes of the three most abundant lipid species, cholesterol, ceramides, and free fatty acids, are high (Fig. 9-8). These include 3-hydroxy-3-methylglutaryl coenzyme A (HMG-CoA) reductase, serine palmitoyltransferase (SPT), acetyl-CoA carboxylase (ACC), and fatty acid synthase (FAS).[92] Moreover, the activities of all these enzymes increase when the barrier is disrupted under both acute and sustained conditions. Yet, the increase in activities of all these enzymes is blocked when the barrier is restored artificially by occlusion with a vapor-impermeable membrane, indicating that the increase is linked to restoration of normal barrier function.[44] Finally, the changes in enzyme activity are preceded by changes in the mRNA for HMG-CoA synthase, HMG-CoA reductase, squalene synthase, ACC, FAS, and SPT,[95,96] changes that are blocked by occlusion. Transcription of several of these enzymes is, in turn, regulated by one or more transcription factors, sterol regulatory element binding proteins (SREBPs),[97] which modulate cholesterol and fatty acid synthesis in response to changes in the cellular content of these lipids. Thus, acute changes in the barrier initiate a sequence of events, including rapid lamellar body secretion and increased lipid synthesis, which will lead ultimately to barrier restoration. Additional evidence for regulation of lipid synthesis and for an absolute requirement for each of the three key lipids is described below.

SIGNALS OF PERMEABILITY BARRIER HOMEOSTASIS

Ionic Modulations

The ability of occlusion to block the lipid and DNA synthetic response to barrier disruption suggests that transepidermal water loss is a regulatory signal for barrier homeostasis. Yet, a perturbed barrier recovers normally when exposed to isotonic, hypertonic, or hypotonic external solutions, unless calcium, and, to a lesser extent, potassium, are present in the bathing solution.[98] Moreover, calcium and potassium together appear to be synergistic in inhibiting barrier recovery.[98] Because these

FIGURE 9-8

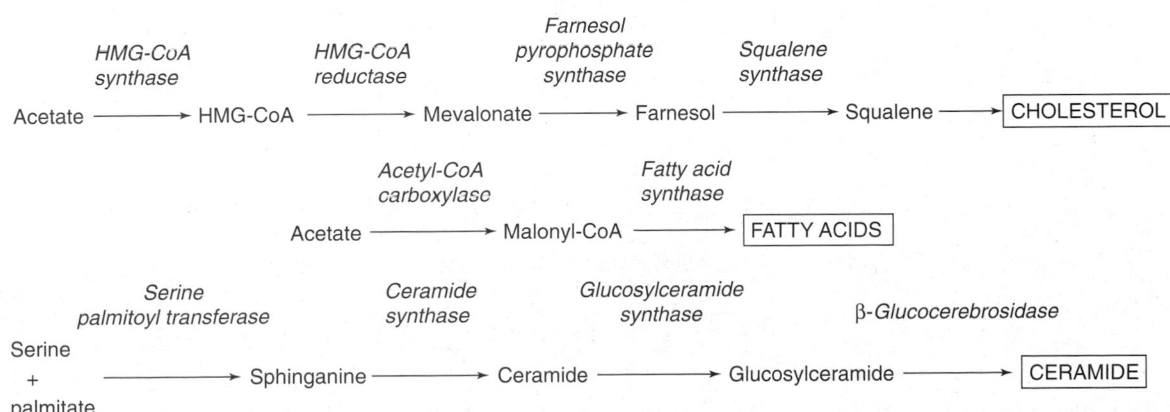

Synthetic pathways and key enzymes for the three key stratum corneum lipids.

FIGURE 9-9

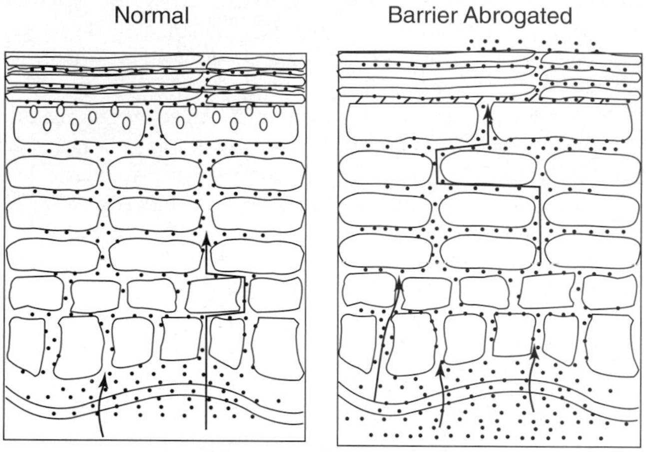

Normal

Barrier Abrogated

Changes in calcium gradient after barrier disruption and during repair regulate lamellar body secretion.

inhibitory influences are reversed by blockade with inhibitors of both L-type calcium channels and calmodulin, translocation of extracellular calcium into the cytosol appears to be required.[98] The mechanism for the negative ionic signal seems to relate to the presence of a calcium gradient in the epidermis (Fig. 9-9). Barrier disruption, regardless of method, results in passive outward displacement of the inhibitory ions into the stratum corneum. It is this depletion of calcium that regulates lamellar body exocytosis[99] (Fig. 9-9). These findings may be clinically relevant, because the incidence of dermatitis, particularly hand eczema, is higher where water supplies contain a high mineral content;[100] i.e., elevated ions in tap water could interfere with barrier recovery in individuals with a damaged skin barrier (e.g., patients with atopic dermatitis). Finally, in contrast to the inverse regulation of lamellar body secretion, changes in the calcium gradient directly regulate mRNA levels of corneocyte-specific proteins. Such upregulation of protein synthesis, leading to optimal differentiation, contributes to basal barrier function, which, itself, regulates the integrity of the calcium gradient[63] (Fig. 9-10).

FIGURE 9-10

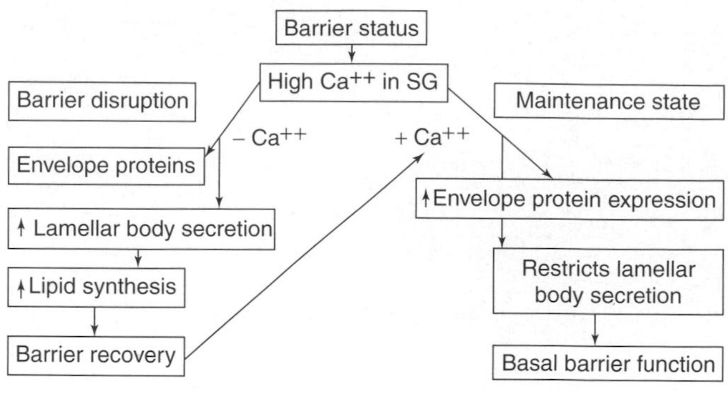

Barrier-impaired changes in calcium gradient regulates epidermal terminal differentiation—the unifying hypothesis.

Cytokine Signaling and Disease Pathogenesis

Whereas the epidermis generates a large number of biologic response modifiers (BRM),[101] the cytokines IL-1α and IL-1β appear to be among the few that are present in the SC under basal conditions.[102] In response to all forms of acute barrier disruption, the preformed pool of IL-1α is released, independent of new cytokine formation.[103] In addition, a rapid increase occurs in the mRNA levels and protein content of several downstream cytokines.[99] Likewise, with sustained barrier disruption, as in essential fatty acid deficiency and in a variety of chronic dermatoses, such as psoriasis and atopic dermatitis, both the mRNA and protein content of several cytokines are increased.[104]

Changes in cytokine expression represent part of the physiologic response to barrier disruption. IL-1α, tumor necrosis factor (TNF)-α, and several other epidermis-derived cytokines are potent mitogens,[101] and both IL-1α and TNF-α regulate lipid synthesis in extracutaneous tissues. Moreover, barrier recovery is delayed in IL-1/TNF receptor knockout mice; conversely, exogenous IL-1α and TNF-α enhance barrier recovery.[8] Hence, it appears that these cytokine responses are homeostatic; that is, they signal metabolic responses leading to barrier recovery. Activation of IL-1α and TNF-α (primary cytokinesis) clearly result in a cytokine cascade that can initiate or sustain inflammation.[103] Yet occlusion with a vapor-impermeable membrane does not block the increase in either mRNA or protein expression for most cytokines (except amphiregulin and nerve growth factor),[105] after acute barrier abrogations.[103,104] Hence, cytokines, via a downstream cascade, operate as physiologic (homeostatic) and pathophysiologic signals. (Figs. 9-11 and 9-12).

Pertinently, barrier disruption is followed by increased migration of mitotically active Langerhans cells into the epidermis.[106] This view represents an *outside* → *inside* concept, as opposed to the dominant *inside* → *outside* view, of the pathogenesis of inflammatory skin diseases (Fig. 9-12).[107] In reality, the "outside–inside" paradigm is not new; rather, it provides an explanation for the isomorphic (Koebner) phenomenon. When downstream activation is sustained and excessive, it can

FIGURE 9-11

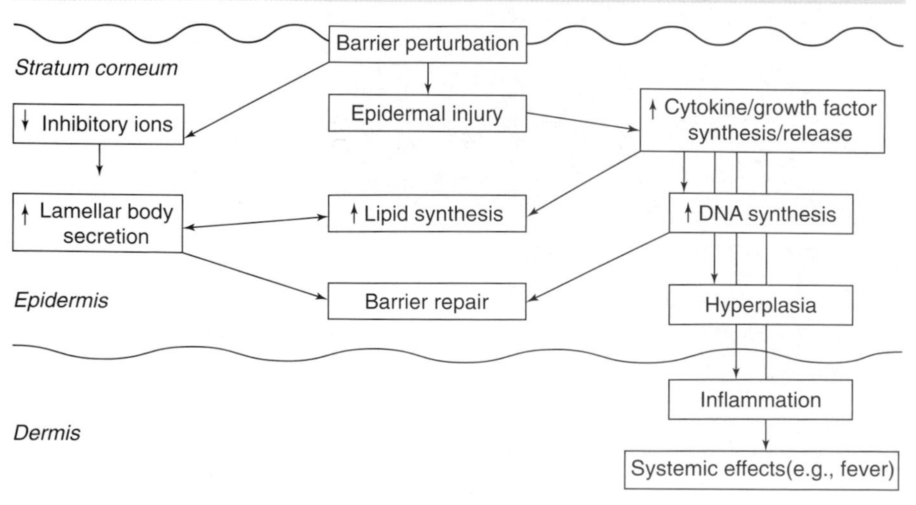

Parallel signaling mechanisms regulate epidermal homeostasis, but simultaneously may induce disease.

FIGURE 9-12

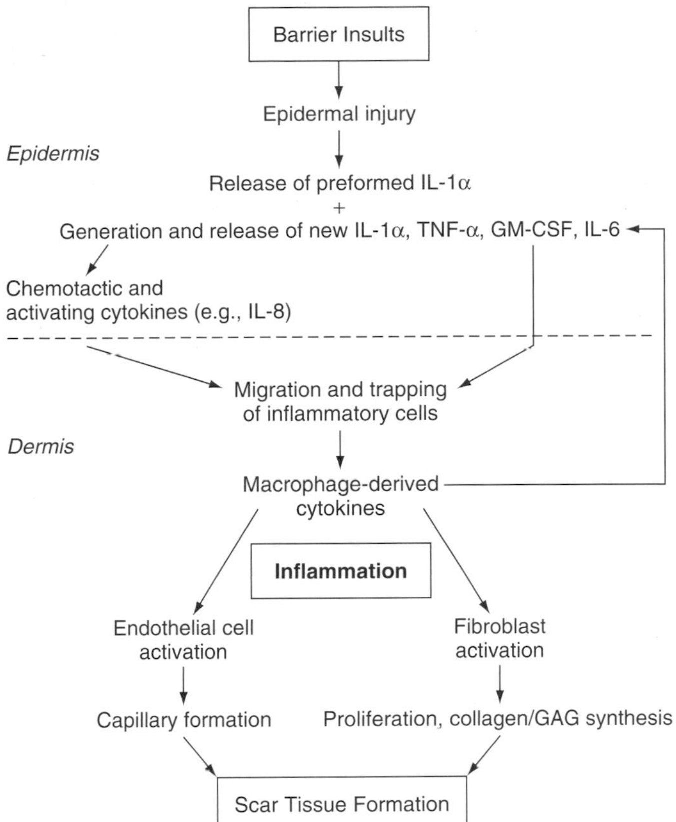

Physiologic and pathophysiologic consequences of barrier disruption. Related downstream mechanisms mediate homeostatic (repair) and pathologic sequences in the skin. The cytokine cascade, resulting from barrier perturbation, can lead to inflammation, as well as to hypertrophic scar and keloids.

FIGURE 9-13

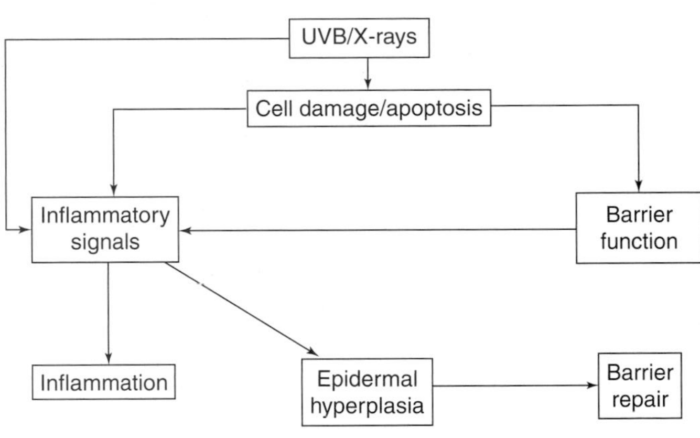

UVB/X-irradiation lead to cell injury with downstream consequences on inflammatory signaling and barrier function.

explain several important dermatoses, such as chronic plaque-type psoriasis, hypertrophic scars/keloids, and a variety of eczemas (Fig. 9-12). Finally, the cytokine cascade, initiated during wound healing, can even lead to fibrosis and endothelial cell proliferation, resulting in hypertrophic scars and keloids (Fig. 9-14).[107]

As noted above, these observations provide an explanation for the pathogenesis of a wide variety of common skin diseases, such as irritant contact dermatitis, psoriasis, and atopic dermatitis, which typically are associated with abnormal barrier function. In Table 9-6, skin diseases are classified as (1) diseases in which a *primary barrier abnormality* exists, that is, under basal conditions or in clinically uninvolved skin; (2) *immunologic abnormalities triggered by* epidermal/*barrier insults*; (3) *disorders sustained* by an *ongoing barrier abnormality,* where occlusion often reverses the pathology; and (4) processes in which a barrier disorder occurs as a result of a *prior immunologic* or *physical disturbance* (true "inside–outside" disorders), where the epidermis is altered secondarily. Examples of disorders with an inside-to-outside pathogen are the delayed barrier abnormalities that follow UVB exposure[108] and X-irradiation[109] (Fig. 9-13).

All of these disorders, unearthed by the cutaneous treadmill examination, can further aggravate the cytokine cascade, and further increase the risk of disease (Fig. 9-14). Awareness of the potential relationship of all of these disorders to the barrier should lead to more rational deployment of barrier repair therapies (see below) and other preventive strategies.[71]

TABLE 9-6

Potential Role of Cutaneous Barrier in Pathophysiology of Skin Disorders

A. Barrier Abnormality Represents Primary or Intrinsic Process
1. Chronological aging (epidermis)
2. Photoaging (epidermis)
3. Atopic dermatitis
4. Premature infants' skin
5. Cheilitis
6. RXLI, Gaucher's (II); Niemann-Pick (1)
7. Burns
8. Ulcers (ischemic, vascular, diabetic)
9. Blisters/bullous disorders (friction, keratin abnormalities)

B. Barrier Abnormality Triggers Immunologic Abnormality
1. Psoriasis (plaque type)
2. Irritant contact dermatitis (acute)
3. Occupational dermatitis (acute)
4. Diaper dermatitis
5. Allergic contact dermatitis

C. Barrier Abnormality Sustains Pathophysiology
1. Atopic dermatitis
2. Irritant contact dermatitis
3. Occupational dermatitis (chronic)
4. Psoriasis
5. Hypertrophic scars and keloids
6. Cheilitis
7. Lamellar ichthyoses
8. Epidermolytic hyperkeratosis

D. Immunologic Abnormality Triggers Barrier Abnormality
1. UVB and X-irradiation
2. Bullous allergic reactions
3. Erythrodermic, pustular, and guttate psoriasis
4. Allergic contact dermatitis

FIGURE 9-14

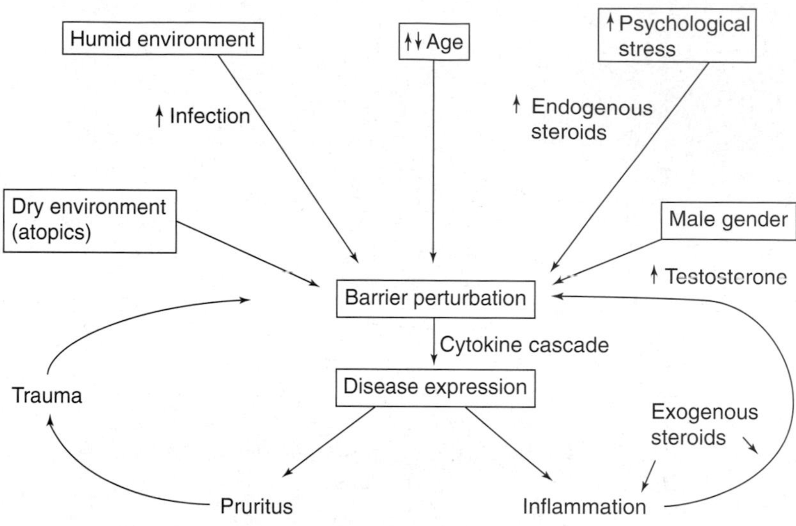

Additional factors that alter barrier homeostasis further amplify cytokine cascade and disease expression.

REQUIREMENTS FOR SPECIFIC LIPIDS VERSUS LIPID MIXTURES FOR BARRIER FUNCTION

Although metabolic studies clearly show that epidermal cholesterol, fatty acid, and ceramide synthesis are modulated by alterations in barrier function, proof that each of these lipids is required for the barrier requires assessment of function after selective deletion of each of these species individually. By using pharmacologic inhibitors of their rate-limiting enzymes (Fig. 9-8), each of the three key lipids is required for barrier homeostasis,[86] that is, deletion of any leads to abnormal barrier recovery and/or abnormal barrier homeostasis in intact skin.

FIGURE 9-15

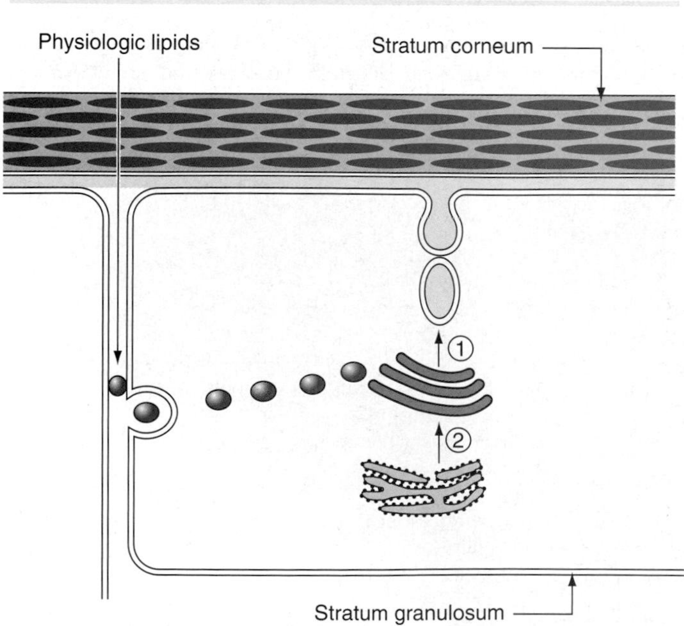

Topical physiologic lipids traverse the stratum corneum and enter the nucleated cell layers. Within the granular cell, they traffic to sites of the lamellar body formation, bypassing the Golgi apparatus. In the trans-Golgi network they mix with newly synthesized lipids, generated in the endoplasmatic reticulum and delivered to the Golgi apparatus. In contrast, nonphysiologic lipids, such as petrolatum, remain restricted to the stratum corneum.

Having shown that each lipid is required individually, the next issue is whether they function cooperatively; that is, when provided topically, must they be supplied in proportions comparable to those present in SC? Indeed, when cholesterol, free fatty acids, ceramides, or even acylceramides are applied alone, they aggravate rather than improve the barrier. Likewise, any two-component system of the three key stratum corneum lipids is deleterious. In contrast, three-component mixtures of the key lipids, or two-component mixtures of acylceramides and cholesterol, allow normal barrier recovery and can even accelerate barrier recovery at optimized proportions of the three key lipids.[77] The mechanism for the aggravation and amelioration of barrier function by the physiologic lipids is the same: after topical applications they are quickly absorbed into the nucleated cell layers,[48] and incorporated into nascent lamellar bodies (Fig. 9-15). Whereas incomplete mixtures yield abnormal lamellar body contents and disordered intercellular lamellae, complete mixtures result in normal lamellar bodies and compact extracellular membrane unit structures.[110] In contrast, inert lipids such as petrolatum provide an immediate barrier by addition of hydrophobic material, which remains restricted to the SC.[111] Physiologic lipid mixtures alone, at equimolar or optimal molar ratios, or in concert with traditional inert ingredients, provide forms of topical therapy that can be deployed strategically for appropriate indications.[71]

The Cutaneous Stress Test

Whereas the above studies demonstrate how stress to the barrier can provoke a cytokine-initiated pathogenesis cascade, the cutaneous stress test can be employed to unmask clinically important skin pathology, analogous to stress tests of any organ system. Table 9-6 lists examples of pathology, revealed by assessment of changes in the kinetics of barrier recovery, after the imposition of acute stress to the barrier, which are inapparent under basal conditions.

REFERENCES

1. Leveque JL et al: Are corneocytes elastic? *Dermatologica* **176**:65, 1988
2. Jokura Y et al: Molecular analysis of elastic properties of the stratum corneum by solid-state ^{13}C-nuclear magnetic resonance spectroscopy. *J Invest Dermatol* **104**:806, 1995
3. Engelke M et al: Effects of xerosis and ageing on epidermal proliferation and differentiation. *Br J Dermatol* **137**:219, 1997
4. Denda M et al: Low humidity stimulates epidermal DNA synthesis and amplifies the hyperproliferative response to barrier disruption: Implication for seasonal exacerbations of inflammatory dermatoses. *J Invest Dermatol* **111**:873, 1998
5. Sato J et al: Water content and thickness of the stratum corneum contribute to skin surface morphology. *Arch Dermatol Res* **292**:412, 2000
6. Scheuplein RJ, Blank IH: Permeability of the skin. *Physiol Rev* **51**:702, 1971
7. Elias PM: Epidermal lipids, barrier function, and desquamation. *J Invest Dermatol* **80**(suppl):44s, 1983
8. Jensen JM et al: Roles for tumor necrosis factor receptor p55 and sphingomyelinase in repairing the cutaneous permeability barrier. *J Clin Invest* **104**:1761, 1999
9. Schmuth M et al: Permeability barrier disorder in Niemann-Pick disease: Sphingomyelin-ceramide processing required for normal barrier homeostasis. *J Invest Dermatol* **115**:459, 2000
10. Hara J et al: High-expression of sphingomyelin deacylase is an important determinant of ceramide deficiency leading to barrier disruption in atopic dermatitis. *J Invest Dermatol* **115**:406, 2000

11. Fluhr JW et al: Generation of free fatty acids from phospholipids regulates stratum corneum acidification and integrity. *J Invest Dermatol* **117**:44, 2001
12. Elias PM, Menon GK: Structural and lipid biochemical correlates of the epidermal permeability barrier. *Adv Lipid Res* **24**:1, 1991
13. Elias PM, Feingold KR: Lipids and the epidermal water barrier: Metabolism, regulation, and pathophysiology. *Semin Dermatol* **11**:176, 1992
14. Elias PM, Feingold KR: Does the tail wag the dog? Role of the barrier in the pathogenesis of inflammatory dermatoses and therapeutic implications. *Arch Dermatol* **137**:1079, 2001
15. Thiele JJ: Oxidative targets in the stratum corneum. A new basis for antioxidative strategies. *Skin Pharmacol Appl Skin Physiol* **1**(14 suppl):87, 2001
16. Thiele JJ et al: The antioxidant network of the stratum corneum. *Curr Probl Dermatol* **29**:26, 2001
17. Traber MG, Sies H: Vitamin E in humans: Demand and delivery. *Annu Rev Nutr* **16**:321, 1996
18. Thiele JJV: Depletion of human stratum corneum vitamin E: An early and sensitive in vivo marker of UV induced photo-oxidation. *J Invest Dermatol* **110**:756, 1998
19. Thiele JJ et al: In vivo exposure to ozone depletes vitamins C and E and induces lipid peroxidation in epidermal layers of murine skin. *Free Radic Biol Med* **23**:385, 1997
20. Weber SU et al: Vitamin C, uric acid, and glutathione gradients in murine stratum corneum and their susceptibility to ozone exposure. *J Invest Dermatol* **113**:1128, 1999
21. Schallreuter KU: Successful treatment of oxidative stress in vitiligo. *Skin Pharmacol Appl Skin Physiol* **12**:132, 1999
22. Schallreuter KU et al: In vivo and in vitro evidence for hydrogen peroxide (H_2O_2) accumulation in the epidermis of patients with vitiligo and its successful removal by a UVB-activated pseudocatalase. *J Investig Dermatol Symp Proc* **4**:91, 1999
23. Rhie G et al: Aging- and photoaging-dependent changes of enzymic and nonenzymic antioxidants in the epidermis and dermis of human skin in vivo. *J Invest Dermatol* **117**:1212, 2001
24. Fuchs J et al: Impairment of enzymic and nonenzymic antioxidants in skin by UVB irradiation. *J Invest Dermatol* **93**:769, 1989
25. Pelle E et al: Protection against endogenous and UVB-induced oxidative damage in stratum corneum lipids by an antioxidant-containing cosmetic formulation. *Photodermatol Photoimmunol Photomed* **15**:115, 1999
26. Bibel DJ et al: Antimicrobial activity of stratum corneum lipids from normal and essential fatty acid-deficient mice. *J Invest Dermatol* **92**:632, 1989
27. Ohman H, Vahlquist A: In vivo studies concerning a pH gradient in human stratum corneum and upper epidermis. *Acta Derm Venereol* **74**:375, 1994
28. Patterson MJ, Galloway SD, Nimmo MA: Variations in regional sweat composition in normal human males. *Exp Physiol* **85**:869, 2000
29. Kearney JN et al: Correlations between human skin bacteria and skin lipids. *Br J Dermatol* **110**:593, 1984
30. Baden HP, Pathak MA: The metabolism and function of urocanic acid in skin. *J Invest Dermatol* **48**:11, 1967
31. Reeve VE et al: Topical urocanic acid enhances UV-induced tumour yield and malignancy in the hairless mouse. *Photochem Photobiol* **49**:459, 1989
32. Denda M et al: Exposure to a dry environment enhances epidermal permeability barrier function. *J Invest Dermatol* **111**:858, 1998
33. Behne MJ et al: NHE1 regulates the stratum corneum permeability homeostasis. *J Biol Chem* **277**:47399, 2002
34. Mauro T et al: Barrier recovery is impeded at neutral pH, independent of ionic effects: Implications for extracellular lipid processing. *Arch Dermatol Res* **290**:215, 1998
35. Holleran WM et al: Beta-glucocerebrosidase activity in murine epidermis: Characterization and localization in relation to differentiation. *J Lipid Res* **33**:1201, 1992
36. Egelrud T et al: Proteolytic degradation of desmosomes in plantar stratum corneum leads to cell dissociation in vitro. *Acta Derm Venereol* **68**:93, 1988
37. Korting HC et al: Differences in the skin surface pH and bacterial microflora due to the long-term application of synthetic detergent preparations of pH 5.5 and pH 7.0. Results of a crossover trial in healthy volunteers. *Acta Derm Venereol* **70**:429, 1990
38. Elias PM et al: Membrane alterations during cornification of mammalian squamous epithelia: A freeze-fracture, tracer, and thin-section study. *Anat Rec* **189**:577, 1977
39. Pilgram GS et al: Cryo-electron diffraction as a tool to study local variations in the lipid organization of human stratum corneum. *J Microsc* **189**:71, 1998
40. Sheu HM et al: Human skin surface lipid film: An ultrastructural study and interaction with corneocytes and intercellular lipid lamellae of the stratum corneum. *Br J Dermatol* **140**:385, 1999
41. Pilgram GS et al: Electron diffraction provides new information on human stratum corneum lipid organization studied in relation to depth and temperature. *J Invest Dermatol* **113**:403, 1999
42. Fartasch M et al: Structural relationship between epidermal lipid lamellae, lamellar bodies, and desmosomes in human epidermis: An ultrastructural study. *Br J Dermatol* **128**:1, 1993
43. Van Hal DA et al: Structure of fully hydrated human stratum corneum: A freeze-fracture electron microscopy study. *J Invest Dermatol* **106**:89, 1996
44. Grubauer G et al: Lipid content and lipid type as determinants of the epidermal permeability barrier. *J Lipid Res* **30**:89, 1989
45. Lampe MA et al: Human stratum corneum lipids: Characterization and regional variations. *J Lipid Res* **24**:120, 1983
46. Grubauer G et al: Relationship of epidermal lipogenesis to cutaneous barrier function. *J Lipid Res* **28**:746, 1987
47. Ahn SK et al: Functional and structural changes of the epidermal barrier induced by various types of insults in hairless mice. *Arch Dermatol Res* **293**:308, 2001
48. Man MM et al: Optimization of physiological lipid mixtures for barrier repair. *J Invest Dermatol* **106**:1096, 1996
49. Mao-Qiang M et al: Extracellular processing of phospholipids is required for permeability barrier homeostasis. *J Lipid Res* **36**:1925, 1995
50. Murata Y et al: Abnormal expression of sphingomyelin acylase in atopic dermatitis: An etiologic factor for ceramide deficiency? *J Invest Dermatol* **106**:1242, 1996
51. Fartasch M, Diepgen TL: The barrier function in atopic dry skin. Disturbance of membrane-coating granule exocytosis and formation of epidermal lipids? *Acta Derm Venereol Suppl (Stockh)* **176**:26, 1992
52. Di Nardo A et al: Ceramide and cholesterol composition of the skin of patients with atopic dermatitis. *Acta Derm Venereol* **78**:27, 1998
53. Rees J et al: Contact sensitivity to dinitrochlorobenzene is impaired in atopic subjects. Controversy revisited. *Arch Dermatol* **126**:1173, 1990
54. Lammintausta K et al: Patch test reactions in atopic patients. *Contact Dermatitis* **26**:234, 1992
55. Bos JD et al: Immune dysregulation in atopic eczema. *Arch Dermatol* **128**:1509, 1992
56. Feldmann RJ, Maibach HI: Regional variation in percutaneous penetration of ^{14}C cortisol in man. *J Invest Dermatol* **48**:181, 1967
57. Shaw JE et al: Testing of controlled-release transdermal dosage forms. Product development and clinical trials. *Arch Dermatol* **123**:1548, 1987
58. Berardesca E et al: Effects of water temperature on surfactant-induced skin irritation. *Contact Dermatitis* **32**:83, 1995
59. Odland GF, Holbrook K: The lamellar granules of epidermis. *Curr Probl Dermatol* **9**:29, 1981
60. Rassner U et al: Coordinate assembly of lipids and enzyme proteins into epidermal lamellar bodies. *Tissue Cell* **31**:489, 1999
61. Menon GK et al: Lamellar body secretory response to barrier disruption. *J Invest Dermatol* **98**:279, 1992
62. Landmann L: The epidermal permeability barrier. *Anat Embryol (Berl)* **178**:1, 1988
63. Mao-Qiang M et al: Calcium and potassium inhibit barrier recovery after disruption, independent of the type of insult in hairless mice. *Exp Dermatol* **6**:36, 1997
64. Wertz PW et al: Sphingolipids of the stratum corneum and lamellar granules of fetal rat epidermis. *J Invest Dermatol* **83**:193, 1984
65. Grayson S et al: Lamellar body-enriched fractions from neonatal mice: Preparative techniques and partial characterization. *J Invest Dermatol* **85**:289, 1985
66. Elias PM et al: Stratum corneum lipids in disorders of cornification. Steroid sulfatase and cholesterol sulfate in normal desquamation and the pathogenesis of recessive X-linked ichthyosis. *J Clin Invest* **74**:1414, 1984
67. Freinkel RK, Traczyk TN: Acid hydrolases of the epidermis: Subcellular localization and relationship to cornification. *J Invest Dermatol* **80**:441, 1983
68. Watkinson A: Stratum corneum thiol protease (SCTP): A novel cysteine protease of late epidermal differentiation. *Arch Dermatol Res* **291**:260, 1999
69. Ekholm IE et al: Stratum corneum tryptic enzyme in normal epidermis: A missing link in the desquamation process? *J Invest Dermatol* **114**:56, 2000

70. Simon M et al: Refined characterization of corneodesmosin proteolysis during terminal differentiation of human epidermis and its relationship to desquamation. *J Biol Chem* **276**:20292, 2001
71. Elias PM, Feingold KR: Coordinate regulation of epidermal differentiation and barrier homeostasis. *Skin Pharmacol Appl Skin Physiol* **1** (14 suppl):28, 2001
72. Holleran WM et al: Permeability barrier requirements regulate epidermal beta-glucocerebrosidase. *J Lipid Res* **35**:905, 1994
73. Holleran WM et al: Consequences of beta-glucocerebrosidase deficiency in epidermis. Ultrastructure and permeability barrier alterations in Gaucher disease. *J Clin Invest* **93**:1756, 1994
74. Takagi Y et al: Beta-glucocerebrosidase activity in mammalian stratum corneum. *J Lipid Res* **40**:861, 1999
75. Wertz PW et al: Comparison of lipids from epidermal and palatal stratum corneum. *J Invest Dermatol* **98**:375, 1992
76. Chang F et al: Covalently bound lipids in keratinizing epithelia. *Biochim Biophys Acta* **1150**:98, 1993
77. Mao-Qiang M et al: Secretory phospholipase A_2 activity is required for permeability barrier homeostasis. *J Invest Dermatol* **106**:57, 1996
78. Uchida Y et al: Vitamin C stimulates sphingolipid production and markers of barrier formation in submerged human keratinocyte cultures. *J Invest Dermatol* **117**:1307, 2001
79. Zettersten E et al: Recessive X-linked ichthyosis: Role of cholesterol-sulfate accumulation in the barrier abnormality. *J Invest Dermatol* **111**:784, 1998
80. Hou SY et al: Membrane structures in normal and essential fatty acid-deficient stratum corneum: Characterization by ruthenium tetroxide staining and x-ray diffraction. *J Invest Dermatol* **96**:215, 1991
81. Madison KC et al: Presence of intact intercellular lipid lamellae in the upper layers of the stratum corneum. *J Invest Dermatol* **88**:714, 1987
82. Menon GK, Elias PM: Morphologic basis for a pore-pathway in mammalian stratum corneum. *Skin Pharmacol* **10**:235, 1997
83. Swartzendruber DC et al: Evidence that the corneocyte has a chemically bound lipid envelope. *J Invest Dermatol* **88**:709, 1987
84. Behne M et al: Omega-hydroxyceramides are required for corneocyte lipid envelope (CLE) formation and normal epidermal permeability barrier function. *J Invest Dermatol* **114**:185, 2000
85. Ziboh VA, Chapkin RS: Metabolism and function of skin lipids. *Prog Lipid Res* **27**:81, 1988
86. Feingold KR: The regulation and role of epidermal lipid synthesis. *Adv Lipid Res* **24**:57, 1991
87. Feingold KR et al: De novo sterologenesis in intact primates. *J Lab Clin Med* **100**:405, 1982
88. Nicolaides N: Skin lipids: Their biochemical uniqueness. *Science* **186**:19, 1974
89. Monger DJ et al: Localization of sites of lipid biosynthesis in mammalian epidermis. *J Lipid Res* **29**:603, 1988
90. Williams ML et al: Free sterol metabolism and low density lipoprotein receptor expression as differentiation markers of cultured human keratinocytes. *J Cell Physiol* **132**:428, 1987
91. Ghadially R et al: The aged epidermal permeability barrier. Structural, functional, and lipid biochemical abnormalities in humans and a senescent murine model. *J Clin Invest* **95**:2281, 1995
92. Holleran WM et al: Regulation of epidermal sphingolipid synthesis by permeability barrier function. *J Lipid Res* **32**:1151, 1991
93. Proksch E et al: Barrier function regulates epidermal DNA synthesis. *J Clin Invest* **87**:1668, 1991
94. Feingold KR et al: Effect of essential fatty acid deficiency on cutaneous sterol synthesis. *J Invest Dermatol* **87**:588, 1986
95. Proksch E et al: Epidermal HMG CoA reductase activity in essential fatty acid deficiency: Barrier requirements rather than eicosanoid generation regulate cholesterol synthesis. *J Invest Dermatol* **99**:216, 1992
96. Harris IR et al: Expression and regulation of mRNA for putative fatty acid transport related proteins and fatty acyl CoA synthase in murine epidermis and cultured human keratinocytes. *J Invest Dermatol* **111**:722, 1998
97. Harris IR et al: Parallel regulation of sterol regulatory element binding protein-2 and the enzymes of cholesterol and fatty acid synthesis but not ceramide synthesis in cultured human keratinocytes and murine epidermis. *J Lipid Res* **39**:412, 1998
98. Lee SH et al: Calcium and potassium are important regulators of barrier homeostasis in murine epidermis. *J Clin Invest* **89**:530, 1992
99. Menon GK et al: Selective obliteration of the epidermal calcium gradient leads to enhanced lamellar body secretion. *J Invest Dermatol* **102**:789, 1994
100. Warren R et al: The influence of hard water (calcium) and surfactants on irritant contact dermatitis. *Contact Dermatitis* **35**:337, 1996
101. Kupper TS: Immune and inflammatory processes in cutaneous tissues. Mechanisms and speculations. *J Clin Invest* **86**:1783, 1990
102. Hauser C et al: Interleukin 1 is present in normal human epidermis. *J Immunol* **136**:3317, 1986
103. Wood LC et al: Barrier disruption stimulates interleukin-1 alpha expression and release from a pre-formed pool in murine epidermis. *J Invest Dermatol* **106**:397, 1996
104. Wood LC et al: Occlusion lowers cytokine mRNA levels in essential fatty acid-deficient and normal mouse epidermis, but not after acute barrier disruption. *J Invest Dermatol* **103**:834, 1994
105. Liou A et al: Amphiregulin and nerve growth factor expression are regulated by barrier status in murine epidermis. *J Invest Dermatol* **108**:73, 1997
106. Proksch E, Brasch J: Influence of epidermal permeability barrier disruption and Langerhans' cell density on allergic contact dermatitis. *Acta Derm Venereol* **77**:102, 1997
107. Elias PM et al: Signaling networks in barrier homeostasis. The mystery widens. *Arch Dermatol* **132**:1505, 1996
108. Haratake A et al: UVB-induced alterations in permeability barrier function: Roles for epidermal hyperproliferation and thymocyte-mediated response. *J Invest Dermatol* **108**:769, 1997
109. Schmuth M et al: Permeability barrier function of skin exposed to ionizing radiation. *Arch Dermatol* **137**:1019, 2001
110. Mao-Qiang M et al: Fatty acids are required for epidermal permeability barrier function. *J Clin Invest* **92**:791, 1993
111. Ghadially R et al: Effects of petrolatum on stratum corneum structure and function. *J Am Acad Dermatol* **26**:387, 1992

CHAPTER 10

C. Bruce Wenger

Thermoregulation

Lying at the boundary between the body and the environment, the skin plays an important role in thermoregulation and serves as both a source of thermal information and an effector organ for controlling heat loss from the body. Living tissue is directly injured if it is heated to temperatures higher than about 45°C (113°F),[1] the level at which heating the skin causes pain, or if it is cooled so that ice crystals form in the cells. Because of its exposed location, the skin is particularly vulnerable to injury by extremes of temperature in the immediate environment, and, in addition to its thermoregulatory responses, local vasodilator responses are elicited when tissue temperature rises toward 40°C (104°F) or falls toward 10°C (50°F); these help to protect the skin against extremes of temperature.

Human beings, like other homeotherms, spend substantial physiologic resources maintaining their internal body temperatures near 37°C (98.6°F) (Fig. 10-1). What biologic advantage is gained by regulating body temperature within such a narrow band? Temperature is a fundamental physicochemical variable that profoundly affects many biologic processes, both through configurational changes affecting the biologic activities of protein molecules—e.g., enzymes, receptors, and membrane channels—and through a general effect on chemical reaction rates. Most reaction rates vary approximately as an exponential function of temperature (T) within the physiologic range, and raising T by 10°C (18°F) increases the reaction rate by a factor of 2 to 3. A familiar clinical example of the effect of body temperature on metabolic processes is the rule that each 1°C (1.8°F) of fever increases a patient's fluid and calorie needs 13 percent.[2]

BODY TEMPERATURES AND HEAT TRANSFER IN THE BODY

The body is divided into a warm internal *core* and an outer *shell*[3] (Fig. 10-2). It is the temperature of the core, which includes the vital organs in the head and trunk, that is regulated within narrow limits. Although normal body temperature is conventionally taken to be 37°C (98.6°F), individual variation and such factors[4,5] as time of day, phase of the menstrual cycle,[6,7] and acclimatization to heat account for differences of up to about 1°C (1.8°F) in core temperatures of healthy subjects at rest. In addition, core temperature may increase several degrees with heavy exercise or fever (Fig. 10-1). Temperature-sensitive neurons and nerve endings at various core sites, including the spinal cord and especially the brain,[8,9] provide the thermoregulatory system with information about the level of core temperature. Shell temperature by contrast is not tightly regulated and is strongly influenced by the environment. Nevertheless, thermoregulatory responses greatly affect the temperature of the shell and especially its outermost layer, the skin. The shell's thickness depends on the environment and the need to conserve body heat. In a warm subject, the shell may be less than 1 cm thick; but in a subject conserving heat in a cold environment, it may extend several centimeters below the skin.

The body loses heat only from tissues in contact with the environment, chiefly the skin. Since heat flows from warmer regions to cooler regions, the greatest heat flows within the body are those from major sites of heat production to the rest of the body and from core to skin. Heat is transported within the body by two means: *conduction* through the tissues; and *convection* by the blood, the process by which flowing blood carries heat from warmer tissues to cooler tissues. Heat flow by conduction is proportional to the change of temperature with distance

FIGURE 10-1

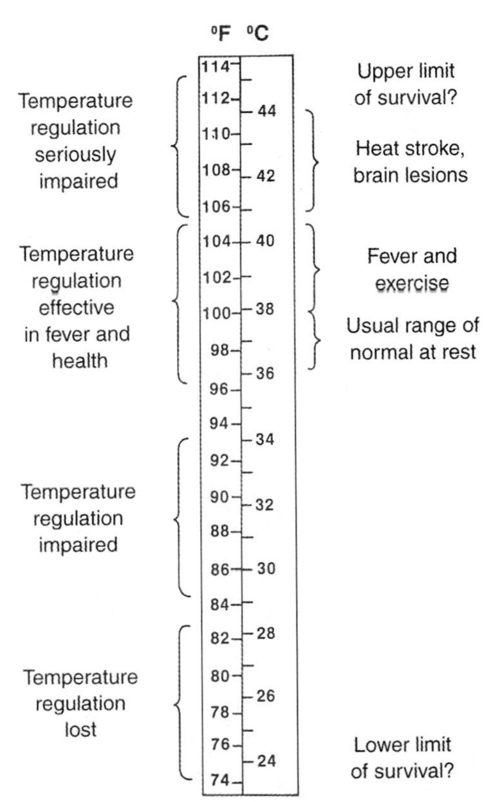

Ranges of rectal temperature found in healthy persons, patients with fever, and persons with impairment or failure of thermoregulation. (*From Wenger CB, Hardy JD: Temperature regulation and exposure to heat and cold, in Therapeutic Heat and Cold, edited by JF Lehman. Baltimore, Williams & Wilkins, 1990, pp 150–178, with permission. Modified from DuBois.*[2])

The views, opinions, and findings in this chapter are those of the author and should not be construed as an official Department of the Army position, policy, or decision unless so designated by other official documentation. Approved for public release, distribution is unlimited.

FIGURE 10-2

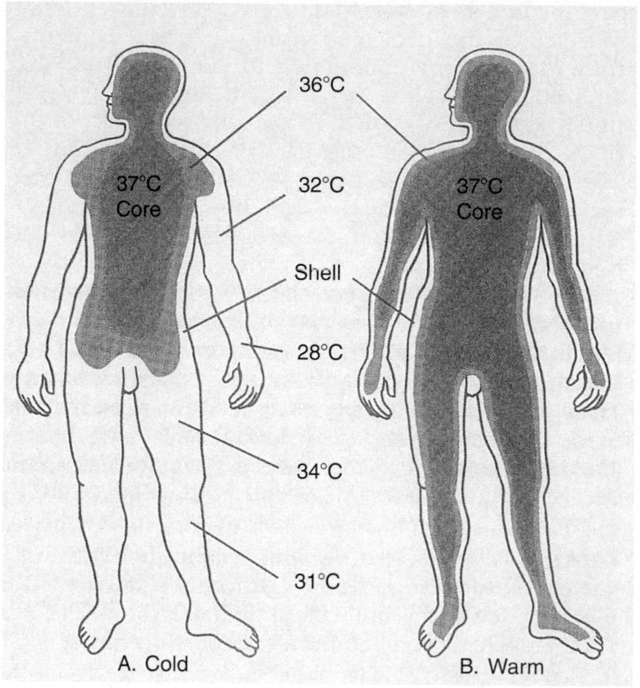

Distribution of temperatures within the body and division of the body into core and shell during exposure to (*A*) cold and (*B*) warm environments. The temperatures of the surface and the thickness of the shell depend on the environmental temperature, so that the shell is thicker in the cold and thinner in the heat. (*From Wenger CB: The regulation of body temperature, in Medical Physiology, edited by RA Rhoades, GA Tanner. Boston, Little, Brown, 1995, pp 587–613, with permission. Based on Aschoff and Wever.*[3])

in the direction of heat flow, and the thermal conductivity of the tissues. As Table 10-1 shows, tissues are rather poor heat conductors. Heat flow by convection depends on the rate of blood flow and the temperature difference between the tissue and the blood supplying the tissue.

Since the shell lies between the core and the environment, all heat leaving the body via the skin must first pass through the shell. Thus, the shell insulates the core from the environment. In a cool subject, skin blood flow is low, so that core-to-skin heat transfer is dominated by conduction; the subcutaneous fat layer adds to the insulation value of the shell, because it increases the thickness of the shell and has a conductivity only about 0.4 times that of dermis or muscle (Table 10-1). In a warm subject, however, the shell is relatively thin and provides little insulation. Furthermore, a warm subject's skin blood flow is high, so that heat flow from the core to the skin is dominated by convection. In these circumstances, the subcutaneous fat layer—which affects conduction but not convection—has little effect on heat flow.

TABLE 10-1

Thermal Conductivities and Rates of Heat Flow through Slabs of Different Materials*

	Conductivity, kcal/(s·m·°C)	Rate of Heat Flow	
		kcal/h	watts
Copper	0.092	33,120	38,474
Epidermis	0.00005	18	21
Dermis	0.00009	32	38
Fat	0.00004	14	17
Muscle	0.00011	40	46
Water	0.00014	51	59
Oak (across grain)	0.00004	14	17
Dry air	0.000006	2.2	2.5
Glass fiber insulation	0.00001	3.6	4.2

*1 m² in area and 1 cm thick, with a 1°C (1.8°F) temperature difference between the two faces of the slab.

Skin temperature is important both in heat exchange and in thermoregulatory control. Skin temperature is affected by thermoregulatory responses such as skin blood flow and sweat secretion and by heat exchange with underlying tissues and the environment. Skin temperature, in turn, is one of the major factors determining heat exchange with the environment. For these reasons, skin temperature provides the thermoregulatory system with important information about the need to conserve or lose body heat. Many bare nerve endings just under the skin are very sensitive to temperature. Depending on the relation of discharge rate to temperature, they are classified as either warm or cold receptors.[8,10] In addition to their responses when skin temperature is stable, these receptors have transient responses during temperature changes. With heating of the skin, warm receptors respond with a transient burst of activity, while cold receptors respond with a transient suppression; the reverse happens with cooling. Because skin temperature is not usually uniform over the body surface, a mean skin temperature ($\bar{T}_{sk}$) is frequently calculated from temperature measurements at several sites. $\bar{T}_{sk}$ is used both to summarize the input from skin temperature into the thermoregulatory system and, along with core temperature, to calculate a mean body temperature to represent the body's thermal state.

BALANCE BETWEEN HEAT PRODUCTION AND HEAT LOSS

Although the body exchanges some energy with the environment in the form of mechanical work, most is exchanged as heat, by conduction, convection, and radiation; and as latent heat through evaporation or (rarely) condensation of water (Fig. 10-3). If the sum of energy production and energy gain from the environment does not equal energy loss, the extra heat is "stored" in or lost from the body. This is summarized in the heat balance equation:

$$M = E + R + C + K + W + S \qquad (10.1)$$

where M is metabolic rate; E is rate of heat loss by evaporation; R and C are rates of heat loss by radiation and convection, respectively; K is the rate of heat loss by conduction (only to solid objects in practice, as explained later); W is rate of energy loss as mechanical work; and S is rate of heat storage in the body,[11,12] which is positive when mean body temperature is increasing.

Metabolic Rate and Sites of Heat Production at Rest

Heat exchange with the environment can be measured by *direct calorimetry* in an insulated chamber specially constructed so that all heat and water vapor leaving the chamber can be captured and measured. From these measurements one can determine the subject's heat loss, which, at steady state, is equal to metabolic rate. More frequently, metabolic rate is estimated *indirect calorimetry*[13] based on measurements of O_2 consumption, because virtually all energy available to the body depends ultimately on reactions that consume O_2. The heat production associated with consumption of 1 L of O_2 varies somewhat with the fuel—carbohydrate, fat, or protein—that is oxidized. For metabolism of a mixed diet, an average value of 20.2 kJ (4.83 kcal) per liter of O_2 is often used. Since the ratio of CO_2 produced to O_2 consumed

FIGURE 10-3

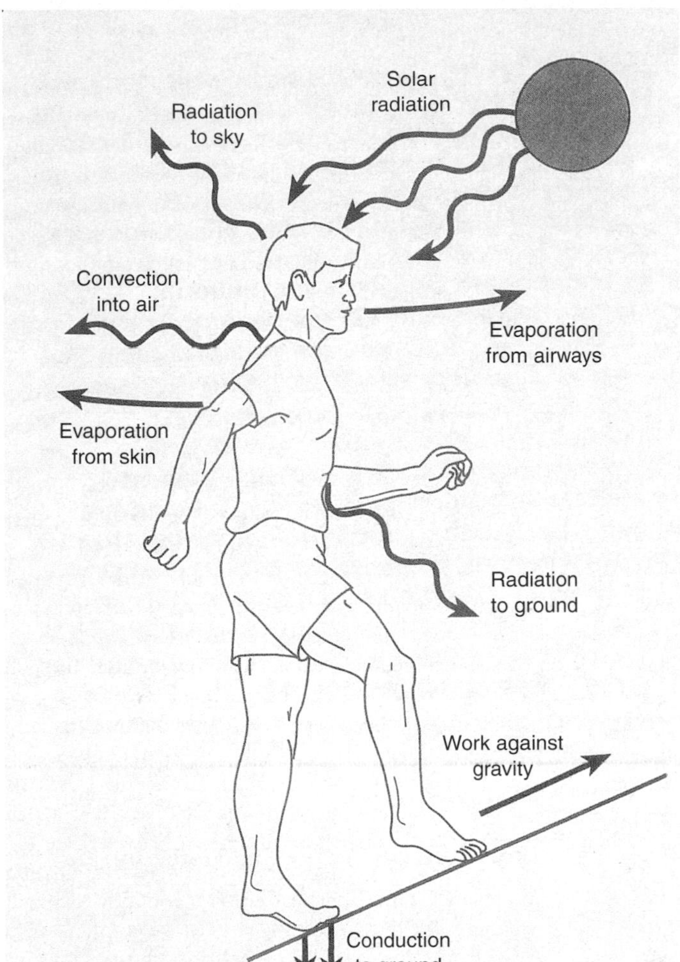

Exchange of energy with the environment. This hiker gains heat from the sun by radiation; he loses heat by conduction to the ground through the soles of his feet, by convection into the air, by radiation to the ground and sky, and by evaporation of water from his skin and respiratory passages. In addition, some of the energy released by his metabolic processes is converted into mechanical work, rather than heat, because he is walking uphill. *(From Wenger CB: The regulation of body temperature, in Medical Physiology, edited by RA Rhoades, GA Tanner. Boston, Little, Brown, 1995, pp. 587–613, with permission.)*

in the tissues is 1.0 for oxidation of carbohydrate, 0.71 for fat, and 0.80 for protein, the accuracy of indirect calorimetry can be improved by also measuring CO_2 production and either estimating the amount of protein oxidized or calculating it from urinary nitrogen excretion.

Metabolic rate at rest is approximately proportional to body surface area. In a fasting young man it is about 45 W/m^2 (81 W or 70 kcal/h for 1.8 m^2 body surface area, corresponding to an O_2 consumption of about 240 mL/min). At rest, the trunk viscera and brain account for about 70 percent of energy production, even though they comprise only about 36 percent of the body mass (Table 10-2). Even during very mild exercise, however, the muscles are the chief source of metabolic energy production; during heavy exercise, they may account for up to 90 percent (Table 10-2). A healthy but sedentary young man performing moderate exercise may reach a metabolic rate of 600 W; and a trained athlete performing intense exercise, 1400 W or more. The overall mechanical efficiency of exercise varies enormously, depending on the activity; at best, no more than one-quarter of the metabolic energy is converted into

TABLE 10-2

Relative Masses and Rates of Metabolic Heat Production of Various Body Compartments During Rest and Severe Exercise

	Percent of Body Mass	Percent of Heat Production	
		Rest	Exercise
Brain	2	16	1
Trunk viscera	34	56	8
Muscle and skin	56	18	90
Other	8	10	1

SOURCE: Modified from Wenger CB, Hardy JD: Temperature regulation and exposure to heat and cold, in *Therapeutic Heat and Cold*, edited by JF Lehman Baltimore, Williams & Wilkins, 1990, pp 150–178.

mechanical work outside the body, and the remaining three-quarters or more is converted into heat within the body.[14] Since exercising muscles produce so much heat, they may be nearly 1°C (1.8°F) warmer than the core. They warm the blood that perfuses them; this blood, returning to the core, warms the rest of the body.

Heat Exchange with the Environment

Radiation, convection, and evaporation are the dominant means of heat exchange with the environment. In humans, respiration usually accounts for only a minor fraction of total heat exchange and is not predominantly under thermoregulatory control, although hyperthermic subjects may hyperventilate. Humans therefore exchange most heat with the environment through the skin.

Every surface emits energy as electromagnetic radiation with a power output that depends on its area, its temperature, and its *emissivity* (identical to its *absorptivity*), a number between 0 and 1 that depends on the nature of the surface and the wavelength of the emitted (or absorbed) radiation. Such *thermal radiation* has a characteristic distribution of power as a function of wavelength, which depends on the temperature of the surface. At ordinary tissue and environmental temperatures, virtually all of the emitted energy is in the infrared part of the spectrum, in a region where most surfaces have emissivities near 1, and thus both emit and absorb at nearly the theoretical maximum efficiency. However, bodies like the sun, which are hot enough to glow, emit large amounts of radiation in the near infrared and visible range, in which light surfaces have lower absorptivities than dark ones. Radiative heat exchange (R) between the skin and the environment is proportional to the difference between the fourth powers of the surfaces' absolute temperatures, but if the difference between $\bar{T}_{sk}$ and the temperature of the radiant environment (T_r) is much smaller than the absolute temperature of the skin, R is nearly proportional to ($\bar{T}_{sk} - T_r$). Some parts of the body surface (e.g., inner surfaces of the thighs and arms) exchange heat by radiation with other parts of the body surface, so that heat exchange between the body and the environment is determined by an *effective radiating surface area* (A_r), which is smaller than the actual surface area. A_r depends on the posture, being closest to the actual surface area in a "spread-eagle" posture and least in someone curled up. The relationship of R to emissivity, temperature, and A_r can be represented by Eq. (10-2) in Table 10-3.

Convection is transfer of heat due to movement of a fluid, either liquid or gas. In thermal physiology, the fluid is usually air or water in the environment, or blood inside the body, as discussed earlier. Fluids conduct heat in the same way as solids do, and a perfectly still fluid

TABLE 10-3

Equations Describing Heat Transfer Between the Skin and the Environment and Between Core and Skin

$$R = h_r e_{sk} A_r(\bar{T}_{sk} - T_r) \qquad (10\text{-}2)$$

where h_r is the radiant heat transfer coefficient, 6.43 W/(m^2·°C) at 28°C; and e_{sk} is the emissivity of the skin.

$$C = h_c \cdot A \cdot (\bar{T}_{sk} - T_a) \qquad (10\text{-}3)$$

where A is the body surface area, $\bar{T}_{sk}$ and T_a are mean skin and ambient temperatures, and h_c is the convective heat transfer coefficient. h_c includes the effects of all the factors besides temperature and surface area that affect convective heat exchange. For the whole body, the most important of these factors is air movement, and convective heat exchange (and, thus, h_c) varies approximately as the square root of the air speed except when air movement is very slight.

$$E = h_e A(P_{sk} - P_a) \qquad (10\text{-}4)$$

where P_{sk} is the water vapor pressure at the skin surface, P_a is the ambient water vapor pressure, and h_e is the evaporative heat transfer coefficient.

$$C = HF_{sk}/(T_c - \bar{T}_{sk}) \qquad (10\text{-}5)$$

where C is shell conductance; HF_{sk} = heat loss through the skin, i.e., total heat loss less heat loss through the respiratory tract; and T_c = core temperature.

transfers heat only by conduction. Because air and water are not good conductors of heat (Table 10-1), perfectly still air or water is not very effective in heat transfer. Fluids, however, are rarely perfectly still, and even nearly imperceptible movement produces enough convection to have a large effect on heat transfer. Thus, although conduction plays a role in heat transfer by a fluid, convection so dominates the overall heat transfer that we refer to the entire process as *convection*. The conduction term (K) in Eq. (10-1) is therefore, in practice, restricted to heat flow between the body and other solid objects and usually represents only a small part of the total heat exchange with the environment. Convective heat exchange between the skin and the environment is proportional to the skin surface area and the difference between skin and ambient air temperatures, as expressed by Eq. (10-3) in Table 10-3. Convective heat exchange depends on air movement; and h_c, the proportionality constant in Eq. (10-3), depends on air speed and on geometric factors that affect heat exchange with moving air.

A gram of water that is converted into vapor at 30°C (86°F) absorbs 2425 J (0.58 kcal), the *latent heat of evaporation,* in the process. In subjects who are not sweating, evaporative water loss is typically about 13 to 15 g/(m^2·h), corresponding to a heat loss of 16 to 18 W for a surface area of 1.8 m^2. About half of this amount is lost through breathing and half as *insensible perspiration,*[10,13] i.e., evaporation of water that diffuses through the skin. Insensible perspiration occurs independently of the sweat glands and is not under thermoregulatory control. Water loss through these routes, however, is quite small compared to what can be achieved by evaporation of sweat. Evaporative heat loss from the skin is proportional to skin surface area and the difference between the water vapor pressure at the skin surface and in the ambient air, as summarized in Eq. (10-4) in Table 10-3. Since water vapor, like heat, is carried away by moving air, air movement and other factors affect E and h_e in just the same way that they affect C and h_c. The water vapor pressure at the skin surface depends on the degree of wetness of the skin surface, and thus on the balance between sweating and evaporation; it is equal to the saturation vapor pressure of water at skin temperature if the skin surface is completely wet. The saturation vapor pressure of water increases substantially over the physiological range of skin temperatures: e.g., from 28.3 torr at 28°C (82.4°F) to 44.6 torr at 36°C (96.8°F). Ambient water vapor pressure, which directly affects evaporation from the skin, is proportional to the actual moisture content in the air. Because the skin is warmed by heat from the body, evaporation from the skin is related only indirectly to relative humidity, which is the ratio between the actual moisture content in the air and the maximum moisture content that is possible at the temperature of the air. This is an important distinction since, for example, sweat can easily evaporate from the skin in cool air even if relative humidity is 100 percent.

HEAT DISSIPATION

Heat produced within the body must be delivered to the skin surface to be eliminated. Heat flows through the shell by two parallel modes: physical conduction through the tissues of the shell and convection by blood perfusing the shell. Since heat flow by each of these parallel modes depends on the temperature difference between core and skin, the power of the shell to transfer heat is expressed as the *conductance* of the shell, and it is calculated by dividing heat flow through the shell by the difference between core and mean skin temperatures, as shown in Eq. (10-5) in Table 10-3. When skin blood flow is minimal [usually at ambient temperatures below about 28°C (82.4°F) in nude resting subjects], the conductance of the shell is determined chiefly by the thickness of the subcutaneous fat layer and is about 16 W/°C in a lean man. Under these conditions a temperature difference between core and skin of 5°C (9°F) will allow a typical resting metabolic heat production of 80 W to be conducted to the skin surface. In a cool environment, $\bar{T}_{sk}$ may be low enough for this to occur easily. However, in a warm environment or, especially, during exercise, shell conductance must increase substantially to allow all the heat produced to be conducted to the skin without at the same time causing core temperature to rise to dangerous or lethal levels. Fortunately, under such circumstances, increases in skin blood flow occur that can raise shell conductance tenfold or more. Thus a crucial thermoregulatory function of skin blood flow is to control the conductance of the shell and the ease by which heat travels from core to skin. A closely related function is to control $\bar{T}_{sk}$: in a person who is not sweating, an increase in skin blood flow tends to bring $\bar{T}_{sk}$ toward T_c, and a decrease allows $\bar{T}_{sk}$ to approach ambient temperature. Since convective and radiative heat exchange ($R + C$) depend directly on skin temperature [Eqs. (10-2) and (10-3)], the body can control heat exchange with the environment by adjusting skin blood flow. The *thermoneutral* zone[11] is the range of conditions of metabolic rate and environment within which adjustments in skin blood flow by themselves are sufficient to allow the body to maintain heat balance. If the heat stress is so great that increasing $R + C$ through increasing skin blood flow is not enough to maintain heat balance, the body secretes sweat to increase evaporative heat loss. Once sweating begins, skin blood flow continues to increase as the person becomes warmer, but now the tendency of an increase in skin blood flow to warm the skin is approximately balanced by the tendency of an increase in sweating to cool the skin. Therefore, after sweating has begun, further increases in skin blood flow usually cause little change in skin temperature or dry heat exchange ($R + C$). The increases in skin blood flow that accompany sweating are important to thermoregulation nevertheless, because they deliver to the skin the heat that is being removed by evaporation of sweat, and facilitate evaporation by keeping the skin warm. Skin blood flow and sweating thus work in tandem to dissipate heat that is produced in the body.

Sympathetic Control of Skin Circulation

Blood vessels in human skin are under dual vasomotor control, involving separate nervous signals for vasoconstriction and for vasodilation.[9,16,17] Reflex vasoconstriction, occurring in response to cold and also as part of certain nonthermal reflexes such as baroreflexes, is mediated primarily through adrenergic sympathetic fibers distributed widely over most of the skin.[18] Reducing the flow of impulses in these nerve fibers allows the blood vessels to dilate. In the so-called acral regions—lips, ears, nose, and palmar/plantar surfaces of the hands and feet[17,18]—and in the superficial veins,[17] vasoconstrictor fibers are the predominant vasomotor innervation, and the vasodilation occurring during heat exposure is largely a result of the withdrawal of vasoconstrictor activity.[19] Blood flow in these skin regions is sensitive to small temperature changes in the thermoneutral range and may be responsible for "fine-tuning" heat loss to maintain heat balance in this range.

In most of the skin, the vasodilation occurring during heat exposure depends on sympathetic nervous signals that cause the blood vessels to dilate, and is prevented or reversed by regional nerve block.[20] Since it depends on the action of nervous signals, such vasodilation is sometimes referred to as *active vasodilation*. It occurs in almost all the skin outside the acral regions[19] and also on the dorsal surfaces of the hands[21] and (presumably) feet. In skin areas where active vasodilation occurs, vasoconstrictor activity is minimal at thermoneutral temperatures; as the body is warmed, active vasodilation does not begin until near the onset of sweating.[17,22] Thus reflex control of skin blood flow in these areas is insensitive to small temperature changes within the thermoneutral range.[19] The neurotransmitter [or other vasoactive substance(s)] responsible for active vasodilation in human skin is not known.[18] However, because sweating and vasodilation operate in tandem in the heat, there has been considerable speculation that the mechanism for active vasodilation is somehow linked to the action of sweat glands.[17,23] Active vasodilation does not occur in the skin of patients with anhidrotic ectodermal dysplasia,[24] even though their vasoconstrictor responses are intact, implying that active vasodilation either is linked to an action of sweat glands or is mediated through nerves that are absent or nonfunctional in anhidrotic ectodermal dysplasia. An early hypothesis,[25] that bradykinin released by sweat glands accounts for active vasodilation, now seems unlikely.[17] The author evaluated thermoregulatory function of a patient with acquired anhidrosis and heat intolerance of 6 months duration who failed to sweat in response to iontophoresis of pilocarpine or injection of acetylcholine (ACh). During 20 min of cycle exercise, sweating was observed only in the popliteal fossae, but forearm blood flow (a widely used index of skin blood flow) increased normally as his core temperature rose to 39°C (102.2°F), even though sensitive dewpoint hygrometry measurements on the same forearm showed no evidence of sweating. Therefore, if active vasodilation does depend on some action of sweat glands, it must be an action that can occur even without sweat secretion.

The finding of nerve endings that contain both vasoactive intestinal peptide (VIP) and ACh near eccrine sweat glands in human skin[26] suggested that active vasodilation may be mediated by release of a vasoactive *cotransmitter* from the cholinergic endings of sudomotor nerves.[27] This notion is supported by a recent study showing that active vasodilation in human skin is blocked by botulinum toxin, a presynaptic inhibitor of ACh release, even though active vasodilation was shown not to be elicited by either a muscarinic or nonmuscarinic action of ACh.[28] However, VIP is unlikely to be the sole mediator of active vasodilation in human skin, because the skin of patients with cystic fibrosis shows normal active vasodilation, even though their sudomotor nerves are deficient in VIP.[29] It may be that control of active vasodilation inludes several branches operating in parallel. For example, some evidence suggests that release of ACh participates in the development of active vasodilation, even though ACh is not necessary to sustain it (see Ref. 30 for a discussion). In addition, nitric oxide appears to contribute to the development of active vasodilation, even though active vasodilation can be elicited when nitric oxide synthesis is blocked.[30,31]

Sweating

Humans can dissipate large amounts of heat by secretion and evaporation of sweat; when the environment is warmer than the skin—usually when the environment is hotter than 36°C (96.8°F), evaporation is the only way to lose heat. Humans possess both *apocrine* sweat glands, which have only a limited regional distribution,[32] and *eccrine* sweat glands, which are widely distributed and are by far the more important type in human thermoregulation. Human sweat glands are controlled through postganglionic sympathetic nerves, which release ACh[33] rather than norepinephrine. Functionally active eccrine glands number about 2 to 3 million.[33] Although this number is fixed before the age of 3,[33] the secretory capacity of the individual glands can change, especially with endurance exercise training and heat acclimatization; a fit man well acclimatized to heat can achieve a peak sweating rate greater than 2.5 L/h.[34,35] (Such rates cannot be maintained, however, and the maximum daily sweat output is probably about 15 L.[36]) Eccrine sweat is essentially a dilute electrolyte solution, though apocrine sweat also contains fatty material. Sweat glands reabsorb Na^+ from the duct by active transport, so that [Na^+] of sweat ranges from less than 5 to 60 meq/L.[37]

THERMOREGULATORY CONTROL

Human thermoregulation includes two distinct subsystems: behavioral thermoregulation and physiologic thermoregulation. Behavioral thermoregulation, through the use of shelter, space heating, and clothing, enables humans to live in the most extreme climates on earth, but it does not provide fine control of body heat balance. Physiologic thermoregulation, on the other hand, is capable of fairly precise adjustments of heat balance but is effective only within a relatively narrow range of environmental temperatures.

Both behavioral and physiologic thermoregulation depend on sensory information about body temperatures. Behavioral thermoregulation is governed by thermal sensation and comfort, and depends largely on conscious actions that reduce discomfort. Warmth and cold on the skin are felt as either comfortable or uncomfortable, depending on whether they decrease or increase the physiologic strain.[38] Thus, a shower temperature that feels pleasant after strenuous exercise may be uncomfortably cold on a chilly morning. Because of the relation between discomfort and physiologic strain, behavioral thermoregulation, by reducing discomfort, also minimizes the physiologic burden imposed by a stressful thermal environment. Thermal sensation and comfort respond to changes in the environment much more quickly than do either core temperature or physiologic thermoregulatory responses.[39,40] Behavioral responses thus appear to anticipate changes in the body's thermal state, presumably reducing the need for frequent small behavioral adjustments.

Physiologic thermoregulation operates through graded control of heat-production and heat-loss responses. Familiar nonliving control systems, such as heating and air-conditioning systems, usually operate at only two levels, because they act by turning a device on or off. In contrast, most physiologic control systems produce a response that is graded according to the disturbance in the regulated variable. In many physiologic systems, including those that control the heat-dissipating responses, changes in the effector responses are proportional to displacements of the regulated variable from some threshold value,[10] and such control systems are called *proportional control* systems (Fig. 10-4). Each response in Fig. 10-4 has a core-temperature threshold, a temperature at which the response starts to increase, and these thresholds depend on mean skin temperature. Thus at any given skin temperature, the change in each response is proportional to the change in core temperature; increasing the skin temperature lowers the threshold level of core temperature and increases the response at any given core temperature.

FIGURE 10-4

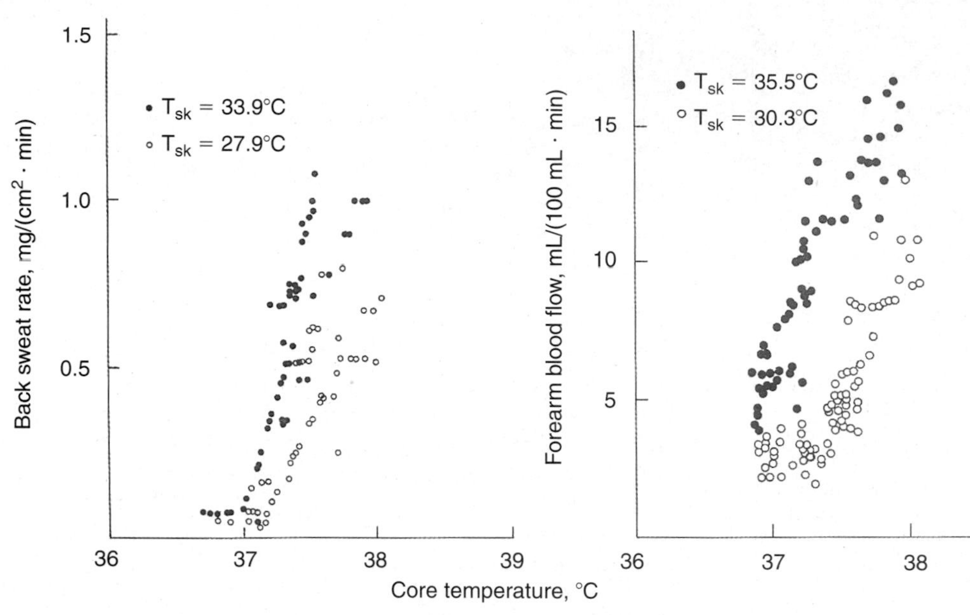

The relations of back (scapular) sweat rate (*left*) and forearm blood flow (*right*) to core temperature and mean skin temperature (T_{sk}). In the experiments shown, core temperature was increased by exercise. (*Left panel drawn from data of Sawka MN et al: Heat exchange during upper- and lower-body exercise. J Appl Physiol 57:1050, 1984. Right panel modified from Wenger CB, et al: Forearm blood flow during body temperature transients produced by leg exercise. J Appl Physiol 38:58, 1975, with permission.*)

FIGURE 10-5

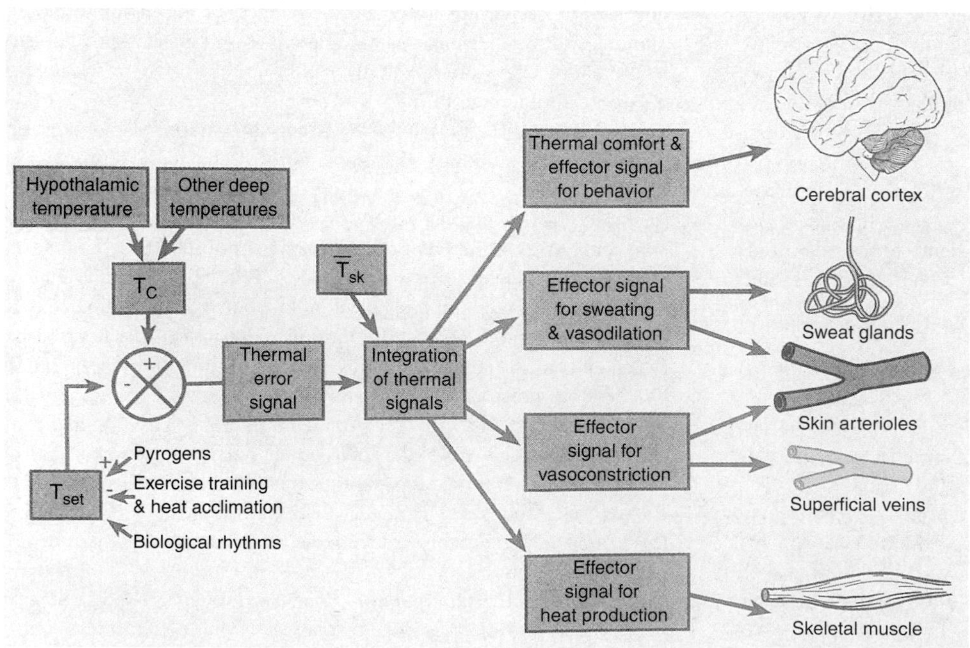

Control of human thermoregulatory responses. The signs by the inputs to T_{set} indicate that pyrogens raise the set point, and heat acclimation lowers it. Core temperature, T_C, is compared with the set point, T_{set}, to generate an error signal, which is integrated with thermal input from the skin to produce effector signals for the thermoregulatory responses. (*From Wenger CB: The regulation of body temperature, in Medical Physiology, edited by RA Rhoades, GA Tanner. Boston, Little, Brown, 1995, pp 587–613, with permission.*)

Integration of Thermal Information

Temperature receptors in the body core and the skin transmit information about their temperatures through afferent nerves to the brainstem, and especially the hypothalamus, where much of the integration of temperature information occurs.[41] The sensitivity of the thermoregulatory responses to core temperature allows the thermoregulatory system to adjust heat production and heat loss to resist disturbances in core temperature. Their sensitivity to skin temperature allows the system to respond appropriately to mild heat or cold exposure with little change in body core temperature, so that environmentally induced changes in body heat content occur almost entirely in the peripheral tissues. For example, the skin temperature of someone who enters a hot environment rises and may elicit sweating even if there is no change in core temperature. On the other hand, an increase in heat production due to exercise elicits the appropriate heat-dissipating responses through a rise in core temperature. Although temperature receptors in other core sites, including the spinal cord and medulla, participate in the control of thermoregulatory responses,[42] the core temperature receptors involved in thermoregulatory control are concentrated especially in the hypothalamus;[42] temperature changes of only a few tenths of 1°C in the anterior preoptic area of the hypothalamus elicit changes in the thermoregulatory effector responses of experimental mammals.

We may represent the central thermoregulatory integrator (Fig. 10-5) as generating thermal command signals for the control of the effector responses. These signals are based on the information about core and skin temperatures that the integrator receives, and on the thermoregulatory *set point*,[4] a reference point which determines the thresholds of all the thermoregulatory responses. We may think of the set point as the setting of the body's "thermostat," and changes in the set point are accompanied by corresponding changes in core temperature at rest. The set point is elevated during fever and lowered slightly by heat acclimatization, as discussed below; it changes in a cyclical fashion with time of day and phase of the menstrual cycle.[4,6,7] The set point reaches a minimum in the early morning, several hours before awaking, and a maximum—which is 0.5 to 1°C (0.9 to 1.8°F) higher—in the late afternoon or evening. During the menstrual cycle the set point is at its lowest point just before ovulation; over the next few days it rises 0.5 to 1°C (0.9 to 1.8°F) and remains elevated for most of the luteal phase.

Peripheral Modification of Skin Vascular and Sweat Gland Responses

Skin temperature affects heat loss responses not only through the reflex actions described above but also through direct actions on the effectors themselves. Local temperature acts on skin blood vessels in two ways. First, local cooling potentiates the constriction of blood vessels in response to nervous signals and vasoconstrictor substances.[18] Second, in skin regions where active vasodilation occurs, local heating dilates the blood vessels (and local cooling constricts them) through a direct action that is independent of nervous signals.[42,44] This direct effect is especially strong at skin temperatures above 35°C (95°F);[44] and when the skin is warmer than the blood, increased blood flow helps to cool the skin and protect it from heat injury. The effects of local temperature on sweat glands parallel those on blood vessels, so that local heating magnifies (and local cooling reduces) the sweating response to reflex stimulation or to ACh,[23] and intense local heating provokes sweating directly, even in sympathectomized skin.[45] During prolonged (several hours) heat exposure with high sweat output, sweat rates gradually diminish and the sweat glands' response to locally applied cholinergic drugs is reduced also. The reduction of sweat gland responsiveness is sometimes called sweat gland "fatigue." Wetting the skin makes the stratum corneum swell, mechanically obstructing the sweat duct and causing a reduction in sweat secretion, an effect called *hidromeiosis*.[46] The glands' responsiveness can be at least partly restored if the skin is allowed to dry (e.g., by increasing air movement[47]), but prolonged sweating also causes histologic changes in the sweat glands.[48]

Thermoregulatory responses may be affected by other inputs besides body temperatures and factors that affect the thermoregulatory set point. Nonthermal factors may produce a burst of sweating at the beginning of exercise,[49,50] and the involvement of sweating and skin blood flow in emotional responses is quite familiar. During exercise and heat stress, skin blood flow is more affected than sweating by nonthermal factors because of its involvement in reflexes that function to maintain cardiac output, blood pressure, and tissue O_2 delivery.

THERMOREGULATORY RESPONSES DURING EXERCISE

At the start of exercise, metabolic heat production increases rapidly, but there is little change in heat loss initially, so heat is stored in the body and core temperature rises. The increase in core temperature, in turn, elicits heat-loss responses, but core temperature continues to rise until heat loss has increased enough to match heat production, so that heat balance is restored and core temperature and the heat-loss responses reach new steady-state levels. The rise in core temperature that elicits heat-dissipating responses sufficient to reestablish thermal balance during exercise is an example of a *load error*,[10] which occurs when any proportional control system resists the effect of some imposed disturbance or "load." Although the elevated T_c of exercise superficially resembles the elevated T_c of fever, there are some crucial differences. First, although heat production may increase substantially (through shivering) at the beginning of a fever, it does not need to stay high to maintain the fever but, in fact, returns nearly to prefebrile levels once the fever is established; during exercise, however, an increase in heat production not only causes the elevation in core temperature but is necessary to sustain it. Second, while core temperature is rising during fever, rate of heat loss is, if anything, lower than before the fever began; during exercise, however, the heat-dissipating responses and the rate of heat loss start to increase early and continue increasing as core temperature rises.

RESPONSE TO COLD

The body's first response to maintain core temperature in the cold is to minimize heat loss by constricting blood vessels in the shell, especially in the skin. Constriction of arterioles reduces heat transfer to the skin by reducing blood flow, and constriction of superficial limb veins further improves heat conservation by diverting venous blood to the deep limb veins, which lie close to the major arteries of the limbs. (This diversion is made possible by the many penetrating veins that connect the superficial and deep veins.) In the deep veins, cool venous blood returning to the core can take up heat from the warm blood in the adjacent deep limb arteries. Thus, some of the heat contained in the arterial blood as it enters the limbs takes a "short circuit" back to the core, and when the arterial blood reaches the skin, it is already cooler than the core and so loses less heat to the skin than it otherwise would. This mechanism can cool the blood in the radial artery of a cool but comfortable subject to as low as 30°C (86°F) by the time it reaches the wrist.[51] Although furred or hairy animals can increase the thickness of their coats by *piloerection,* this response makes a negligible contribution to heat conservation in humans, although it persists as "gooseflesh." If the heat-conserving responses are insufficient to reestablish heat balance, metabolic heat production increases—in adults, almost entirely in skeletal muscles, as a result first of increased tone, and later of frank shivering. Shivering may increase metabolism at rest by more than fourfold acutely, but only about half that amount can be sustained after several hours.

In addition, as the skin is cooled below about 15°C (59°F), its blood flow begins to increase somewhat, a response called *cold-induced vasodilation* (*CIVD*). CIVD is elicited most easily in comfortably warm subjects and is most pronounced in regions rich in arteriovenous anastomoses—i.e., in the hands and feet. The mechanism is uncertain but may involve a direct inhibitory effect of cold on contraction of vascular smooth muscle or on neuromuscular transmission. Although this response increases heat loss from the core somewhat, it keeps the extremities warmer and more functional, and probably protects them from cold injury.

FACTORS THAT ALTER TOLERANCE TO HEAT AND COLD

Prolonged or repeated heat stress, especially when combined with exercise, elicits *acclimatization* to heat, an ensemble of physiologic changes that reduce the physiologic strain that heat stress produces. The classic signs of heat acclimatization are reductions in the levels of core [as much as 1°C (1.8°F)] and skin [1°C (1.8°F) or more] temperatures and heart rate (as much as 30 to 40 beats per minute) reached during exercise in the heat, and increases in sweat production. These changes approach their full development within a week. Heat acclimatization produces other changes[52] as well, including an improved ability to sustain high rates of sweat production; an aldosterone-mediated reduction of sweat sodium concentration (to levels as low as 5 mEq/L), which minimizes salt depletion; an increase in the fraction of sweat secreted on the limbs; and perhaps changes that help protect against heat illness in other ways. The effect of heat acclimatization on performance can be quite dramatic, so that acclimatized subjects can easily complete exercise in the heat that previously was difficult or impossible (see Ref. 53). The mechanisms that produce these changes are not fully understood but include a modest [$\sim$0.4°C (0.72°F)] lowering of the thermoregulatory set point (reducing the thresholds for sweating and cutaneous vasodilation), increased sensitivity of the sweat glands to cholinergic stimulation,[54,55] and a decrease in the sweat glands' susceptibility to hidromeiosis and fatigue. Heat acclimatization disappears in a few weeks if not maintained by repeated heat exposure.

In contrast to heat acclimatization, the changes that occur with cold acclimatization in humans are quite variable and appear to depend on the nature of the acclimatizing cold exposure; they confer only a modest thermoregulatory advantage. For these reasons, it was long questioned whether humans acclimatize to cold. An important adaptive response to cold—although not strictly an example of acclimatization—is enhancement of CIVD. CIVD is rudimentary in hands or feet unaccustomed to cold exposure, but after repeated cold exposure, it begins earlier during cold exposure, produces higher levels of blood flow, and takes on a rhythmical pattern of alternating vasodilation and vasoconstriction, sometimes called the *Lewis hunting response*. This response is often well developed in workers whose hands are exposed to cold, such as fishermen who work with nets in cold water.

Several acute and chronic skin disorders impair thermoregulation through effects on sweating and skin blood flow. Ichthyosis and anhidrotic ectodermal dysplasia are often cited as examples of skin disorders that impair sweating and can profoundly affect thermoregulation in the heat. Since active vasodilation is impaired or absent in anhidrotic ectodermal dysplasia, artificially wetting the skin can only partially correct the thermoregulatory deficit during exercise (when large amounts of body heat need to be carried to the skin) and is likely to be most effective in an environment that is dry enough that evaporation can produce a cool skin. Heat rash (miliaria rubra) also impairs sweating and can reduce exercise tolerance, and its effects may persist after the appearance of the skin has returned to normal.[56] Sunburn also impairs sweating[57] and, in addition, impairs vasoconstriction and heat conservation during cold exposure.[58]

REFERENCES

1. Moritz AR, Henriques FC Jr: Studies of thermal injury: II. The relative importance of time and surface temperature in the causation of cutaneous burns. *Am J Pathol* **23**:695, 1947
2. Du Bois EF: *Fever and the Regulation of Body Temperature.* Springfield, IL, CC Thomas, 1948
3. Aschoff J, Wever R: Kern und Schale im Wärmehaushalt des Menschen. *Naturwissenschaften* **45**:477, 1958
4. Gisolfi CV, Wenger CB: Temperature regulation during exercise: Old concepts, new ideas. *Exerc Sport Sci Rev* **12**:339, 1984
5. Mackowiak PA et al: A critical appraisal of 98.6°F, the upper limit of normal body temperature, and other legacies of Carl Reinhold August Wunderlich. *JAMA* **268**:1578, 1992
6. Hessemer V, Brück K: Influence of menstrual cycle on shivering, skin blood flow, and sweating responses measured at night. *J Appl Physiol* **59**:1902, 1985
7. Kolka MA: Temperature regulation in women. *Med Exerc Nutr Health* **1**:201, 1992
8. Hensel H: Neural processes in thermoregulation. *Physiol Rev* **53**:948, 1973
9. Sawka MN, Wenger CB: Physiological responses to acute exercise-heat stress, in *Human Performance Physiology and Environmental Medicine at Terrestrial Extremes,* edited by KB Pandolf, MN Sawka, RR Gonzalez. Indianapolis, IN, Benchmark Press,1988, pp 97–151
10. Hardy JD: Physiology of temperature regulation. *Physiol Rev* **41**:521, 1961
11. Bligh J, Johnson KG: Glossary of terms for thermal physiology. *J Appl Physiol* **35**:941, 1973
12. Gagge AP, Hardly JD, Rapp GM: Proposed standard system of symbols for thermal physiology. *J Appl Physiol* **27**:439, 1969
13. Ferrannini E: Equations and assumptions of indirect calorimetry: some special problems, in *Energy Metabolism: Tissue Determinants aand cellular Carollaries,* edited by JM Kinney, HN Tucker. New York, Raven, 1992, pp 1–17
14. Åstrand P-O, Rodahl K: *Textbook of Work Physiology.* New York, McGraw-Hill, 1977, pp 523–576
15. Kuno Y: *Human Perspiration.* Springfield, IL, CC Thomas, 1956, pp 3–41
16. Fox RH, Edholm OG: Nervous control of the cutaneous circulation. *Br Med Bull* **19**:110, 1963
17. Rowell LB: Cardiovascular adjustments to thermal stress, in *Handbook of Physiology. Sec 2: The Cardiovascular System. Vol 3: Peripheral Circulation and Organ Blood Flow,* edited by JT Shepherd, FM Abboud. Bethesda, MD, American Physiological Society, 1983, pp 967–1023
18. Johnson JM, Proppe DW: Cardiovascular adjustments to heat stress, in *Handbook of Physiology. Sec 4: Environmental Physiology,* edited by MJ Fregly, CM Blatteis. New York, Oxford University Press for the American Physiological Society, 1996, pp 215–243
19. Roddie IC: Circulation to skin and adipose tissue, in *Handbook of Physiology. Sec 2: The Cardiovascular System. Vol 3: Peripheral Circulation and Organ Blood Flow,* edited by JT Shepherd, FM Abboud. Bethesda, MD, American Physiological Society, 1983, pp 285–317
20. Rowell LB: Active neurogenic vasodilation in man, in *vasodilation,* edited by PM Vanheutte, I Leusen. New York, Raven, 1981, pp 1–17
21. Johnson JM et al: Skin of the dorsal aspect of human hands and fingers possesses an active vasodilator system. *J Appl Physiol* **78**:948, 1995
22. Love AHG, Shanks RG: The relationship between the onset of sweating and vasodilation in the forearm during body heating. *J Physiol (Lond)* **162**:121, 1962
23. Sawka MN et al: Thermoregulatory responses to acute exercise-heat stress and heat acclimation, in *Handbook of Physiology. Sec 4: Environmental Physiology,* edited by MJ Fregly, CM Blatteis. New York, Oxford University Press for the American Physiological Society, 1996, pp 157–185
24. Brengelmann GL et al: Absence of active cutaneous vasodilation associated with congenital absence of sweat glands in humans. *Am J Physiol* **240**:H571, 1981
25. Fox RH, Hilton SM: Bradykinin formulation in human skin as a factor in heat vasodilation. *Physiol (Lond)* **142**:219, 1958
26. Vaalasti A et al: Vasoactive intestinal polypeptide (VIP)-like immunoreactivity in the nerves of human axillary sweat glands. *J Invest Dermatol* **85**:246, 1985
27. Hökfelt T, Johansson O, Ljungdahl Å et al: Peptidergic neurones. *Nature* **284**:515, 1980
28. Kellogg DL Jr et al: Cutaneous active vasodilation in humans is mediated by cholinergic nerve cotransmission. *Circ Res* **77**:1222, 1995
29. Savage MV et al: Cystic fibrosis, vasoactive intestinal polypeptide, and active cutaneous vasodilation. *J Appl Physiol.* **69**:2149, 1990
30. Shastry S, Minson CT, Wilson SA, et al: Effects of atropine and L-NAME on cutaneous blood flow during body heating in humans. *J Appl. Physiol.* **88**:467, 2000
31. Kellogg DL, Jr., Crandall CG, Liu Y et al: Nitric oxide and cutaneous active vasodilation during heat stress in humans. *J Appl. Physiol.* **85**:824, 1998
32. Hurley HJ, Shelley WB: The anatomy of the apocrine sweat gland, in *The Human Apocrine Sweat Gland in Health and Disease,* edited by HJ Hurley, WB Shelley. Springfield, IL, CC Thomas, 1960, pp 6–26
33. Kuno Y: *Human Perspiration.* Springfield, IL, CC Thomas, 1956, pp 42–97
34. Eichna LW et al: The upper limits of environmental heat and humidity tolerated by acclimatized men working in hot environments. *J Indust Hyg Toxicol* **27**:59, 1945
35. Ladell WSS: Thermal sweating. *Br Med Bull* **3**:175, 1945
36. Kuno Y: *Human Perspiration.* Springfield, IL, CC Thomas, 1956, pp 251–276
37. Robinson S, Robinson AH: Chemical composition of sweat. *Physiol Rev* **34**:202, 1954
38. Cabanac M: Physiological role of pleasure. *Science* **173**:1103, 1971

39. Hardy JD: Thermal comfort: skin temperature and physiological thermoregulation, in *Physiological and Behavioral Temperature Regulation,* edited by JD Hardy, AP Gagge, JAJ Stolwijk. Springfield, IL, CC Thomas, 1970, pp 856–873
40. Cunningham DJ et al: Comparative thermoregulatory responses of resting men and women. *J Appl Physiol* **45**:908, 1978
41. Boulant JA: Hypothalamic neurons regulating body temperature, in *Handbook of Physiology. Sec 4: Environmental Physiology,* edited by MJ Fregly, CM Blatteis. New York, Oxford University Press for the American Physiological Society; 1996, pp 105–126
42. Jessen C: Interaction of body temperatures in control of thermoregulatory effector mechanisms, in *Handbook of Physiology. Sec 4: Environmental Physiology,* edited by MJ Fregly, CM Blatteis. New York, Oxford University Press for the American Physiological Society, 1996, pp 127–138
43. Crockford GW et al: Thermal vasomotor responses in human skin mediated by local mechanisms. *J Physiol (Lond)* **161**:10, 1962
44. Wenger CB et al: Effect of nerve block on response of forearm blood flow to local temperature. *J Appl Physiol* **61**:227, 1986
45. Kuno Y: *Human Perspiration.* Springfield, IL, CC Thomas, 1956, pp 277–317
46. Brown WK, Sargent F II: Hidromeiosis. *Arch Environ Health* **11**:442, 1965
47. Nadel ER, Stolwijk JAJ: Effect of skin wettedness on sweat gland response. *J Appl Physiol* **35**:689, 1973
48. Dobson RL et al: Some histochemical observations on the human eccrine sweat glands: III. The effect of profuse sweating. *J Invest Dermatol* **31**:147, 1958
49. Stolwijk JAJ, Nadel ER: Thermoregulation during positive and negative work exercise. *Fed Proc* **32**:1607, 1973
50. Van Beaumont W, Bullard RW: Sweating: its rapid response to muscular work. *Science* **141**:643, 1963
51. Bazett HC et al: Temperature changes in blood flowing in arteries and veins in man. *J Appl Physiol* **1**:3, 1948
52. Wenger CB: Human heat acclimatization, in *Human Performance Physiology and Environmental Medicine at Terrestrial Extremes,* edited by KB Pandolf, MN Sawka, RR Gonzalez. Indianapolis, IN, Benchmark Press, 1988, pp 153–197
53. Pandolf KB, Young AJ: Environmental extremes and endurance performance, in *Endurance in Sport,* edited by RJ Shephard, PO Åstrand. Oxford, England, Blackwell, 1992, pp 270–282
54. Collins KJ et al: The local training effect of secretory activity on the response of eccrine sweat glands. *J Physiol (Lond)* **184**:203, 1966
55. Kraning KK et al: A non-invasive dose-response assay of sweat gland function and its application in studies of gender comparison, heat acclimation and anticholinergic potency, in *Thermal Physiology 1989,* edited by JB Mercer. Amsterdam, Elsevier, 1989, pp 301–307
56. Pandolf KB et al: Persistence of impaired heat tolerance from artificially induced miliaria rubra. *Am J Physiol* **239**:R226, 1980
57. Pandolf KB et al: Human thermoregulatory responses during cold-water immersion after artificially induced sunburn. *Am J Physiol* **262**:R617, 1992
58. Pandolf KB, Gange RW, Latzka WA, et al: Human thermoregulatory responses during cold-water immersion after artificially induced sunburn. *Am J Physiol* **262**:R617, 1992

CHAPTER 11

Biology of Melanocytes

Ruth Halaban
Daniel N. Hebert
David E. Fisher

PIGMENT CELLS

Melanocytes are cells dedicated to the production of melanin (Fig. 11-1). They exert significant biological effects ranging from behavioral consequences of cosmetic importance to the most devastating skin cancer, melanoma. Moreover, additional functions of melanocytes may impact on discrete organ systems, such as hearing and vision, thereby broadening the clinical importance of understanding these cells. Significant progress has been made in unraveling the developmental and mechanistic features of melanocyte biology. Much of this information is derived from molecular studies aimed at probing the basis of inherited conditions and disease syndromes in humans.

Melanin determines skin, hair, and eye pigmentation. The process of melanin production and transfer is highly regulated at the cellular, subcellular, biochemical and genetic levels. The natural display of multiple human skin types, and aberrant pigmentation due to genetic disorders or malignant transformation are a testimony to the complexity of pigmentation. Mutations in more than 90 distinct genes that cause pigmentation defects in animals and insects have led to the identification of crucial molecules that have direct or indirect roles in pigment cell function. Consequently, melanocytes have become a model system for molecular, genetic and developmental processes.

The major events that govern melanocyte distribution and function include:

1. Migration of early melanocyte progenitors, i.e., melanoblasts, from the neural crest, proliferation and localization in the skin and other tissues;
2. Activation of specific cell surface receptors that transmit environmental signals for survival, proliferation and pigmentation;
3. The expression of key enzymes and structural proteins responsible for melanin synthesis;
4. Maintenance of a proper ionic environment within the secretory system conducive to the maturation and activity of key enzymes, as well as to melanosomal organization; and
5. Transport of melanosomes to dendrites and their transfer to epidermal keratinocytes.

Elimination or dysfunction of any of these events by genetic or environmental processes leads to hypo- or hyperpigmentation (see Chap. 90). This chapter summarizes the main aspects of each of these processes. Further information is available from review articles cited for each topic.

FIGURE 11-1

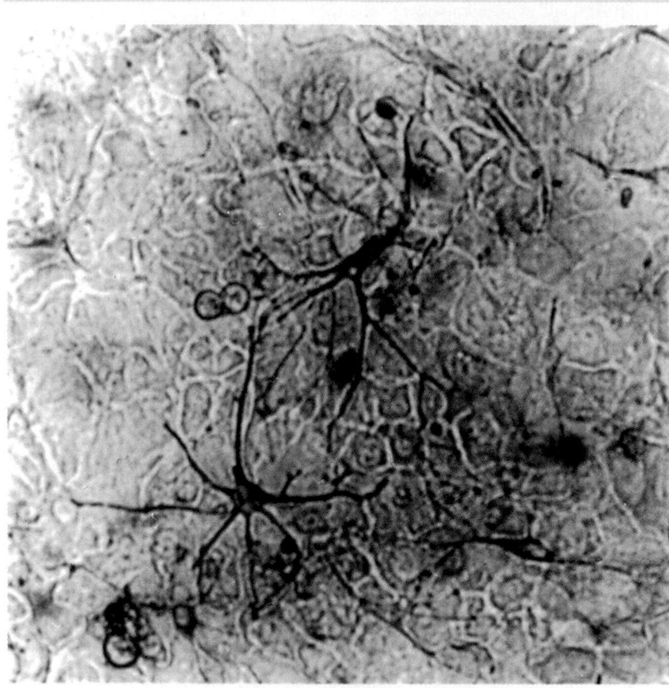

Melanocytes cultured on keratinocytes. Light micrograph showing dendritic melanocytes from a Black donor loaded with melanin and adjacent pigmented keratinocytes due to transfer of melanosomes. (*From Halaban R et al: bFGF as an autocrine growth factor for human melanomas.* Oncogene Res *3:177–186, 1988, with permission.*)

FIGURE 11-2

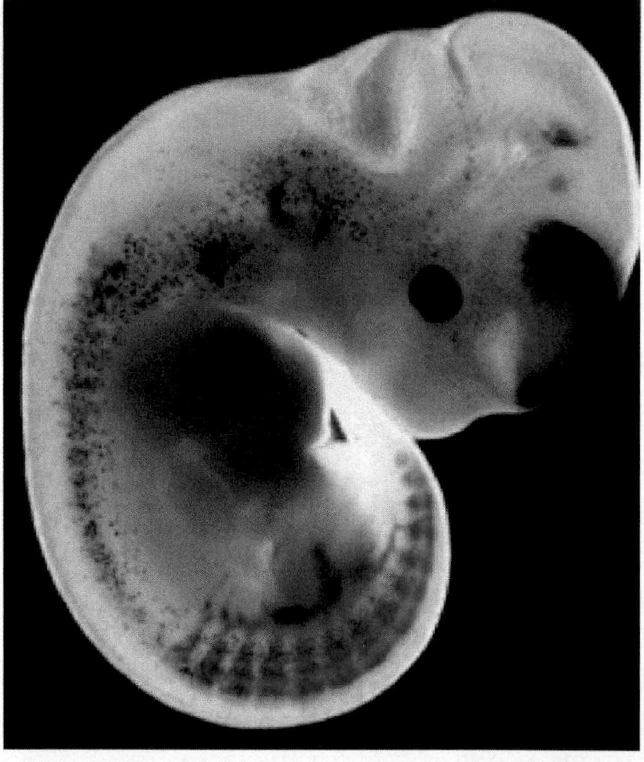

Migration of melanoblast precursors. Migrating melanoblasts in an E11.5 transgenic mouse embryo expressing the Lac Z reporter gene under the control of the melanocyte-specific Dct (DOPAchrome tautomerase) promoter. The melanoblasts are visualized by staining for β-galactosidase. (*Courtesy of Ian Jackson and Alison Wilkie, Medical Research Council, Human Genetics Unit, Western General Hospital, Edinburgh, Scotland.*)

MELANOCYTES DURING DEVELOPMENT

Melanocyte progenitors originate from the neural crest, a transient population of cells localized in the dorsal portion of the closing neural tube. The neural crest cells are pluripotent, capable of giving rise to other lineages including glial cells, neurons, and smooth muscle, as well as bony and cartilaginous components of the head. The neural crest cells destined to become melanocytes migrate, proliferate and differentiate along a dorsolateral pathway, and populate the skin, inner ear, choroid, and part of the iris (Fig. 11-2). They reach their destination via a specific route, guided by discrete diffusable signals produced by the immediate neighboring cells that enhance or suppress their proliferation and/or differentiation. The early signals that induce formation of the neural crest include members of the Wnt, fibroblast growth factor (FGF), and bone morphogenetic protein (BMP) families, as well as Noelin-1 (reviewed in Ref. 1). Some of these signals also help establish the melanocytic lineage by acting as negative or positive activators of melanocyte-specific gene expression. For example, BMP signaling suppresses,[2] whereas Wnt enhances[3] the induction of melanoblasts (early melanocyte progenitors). The positive diffusable factors activate specific cell surface receptors, initiating intracellular signaling cascades that impact on lineage specific gene expression. Deficiencies in these signaling molecules and/or the intracellular cascades that they trigger result in dramatic depigmentation of skin, hair and other sites. The positive signals emanating from the Wnt/β-catenin, the receptor tyrosine kinases Kit and Met, the G-protein linked multiple-membrane spanning receptor endothelin B, and the cell surface adhesion molecules cadherins are described below.

Wnt/β-Catenin

Wnts are secreted glycoproteins that play a critical role in melanocyte determination decisions by activating the Frizzled receptor family. Signaling by Wnt has been genetically implicated in melanocyte development by the severe impact on pigmentation of genetically engineered mice in which Wnt 1 and 3a were eliminated (reviewed in Ref. 1). Wnt controls β-catenin via its influence on the Ser/Thr kinase activity of the key enzyme *glycogen synthase kinase 3β* (GSK3β). In the absence of Wnt, the active GSK3β, in protein complex with APC (adenomatous polyposis coli) and axin, phosphorylates β-catenin on serine residues, facilitating its ubiquitination and proteasome-mediated degradation (Fig. 11-3). Activation of the Frizzled receptor by Wnt, triggers the binding of two inhibitors to GSK3β, Disheveled (Dvl) and Frat 1, suppressing its kinase activity. As a consequence, the levels of β-catenin increase, allowing its translocation to the nucleus, which facilitates the activation of genes by Tcf/Lef transcription factors (T-cell transcription factor/lymphoid enhancer factor) (reviewed in Ref. 4). Lef/β-catenin complexes then upregulate transcription of specific genes. A key target for Tcf /Lef/β-catenin in early melanocyte precursors is *MITF*, encoding a critical regulator of melanocyte specific genes. Mitf thus participates in lineage determination for melanocytes, in agreement with the consequences of mutations that cause Mitf disruption in multiple species including man (reviewed in Refs. 5 and 6)

(Mitf is discussed below under "Regulators of Melanocyte Specific Gene Expression").

Receptor Tyrosine Kinases

STEEL/*C*-KIT The cytokine Steel factor (also known as mast/stem cell factor, M/SCF), and its receptor, *c*-kit, are essential for the development of early melanocyte precursors. Heterozygous loss-of-function mutations in the cytokine or its receptor result in failure of melanocytes to populate broad cutaneous zones, often involving the abdomen or other surfaces. The ventral surface is frequently affected by mutations that disable neural crest cell migration because it represents the area of greatest distance for the dorsal-to-ventral migration of melanocytic precursors (Fig. 11-2). Homozygous loss of Steel Factor or *c*-kit results in complete absence of melanocytes (as well as defects in hematopoietic and germ-cell lineages). Mutations in these genes cause human piebaldism, a condition manifested as broad unpigmented patches reflecting failure of melanocytes to reach the skin (see Chap. 90 and published review[7]).

The *c*-kit receptor is a tyrosine kinase belonging to the PDGF (platelet-derived growth factor) receptor family. Its activation results in stimulation of multiple intracellular signaling cascades, which modulate survival and proliferation (see below, "Melanocyte Growth Factors and Signal Transduction"). Although receptor tyrosine kinases in this family are known to signal to the phosphatidylinositol-3-kinase (PI3K) survival pathway, selective disruption of PI3K signaling does not affect pigmentation, suggesting that the survival effects of *c*-kit stimulation are mediated by different intracellular targets (reviewed in Ref. 8). The presence of Steel factor in keratinocytes contributes to melanocyte localization in the epidermis. First, Steel is expressed by human keratinocytes and activation mutations in *c*-kit further stimulate the melanocytes in the skin and are the cause of hyperpigmentation in mastocytosis.[7,9] Second, in mouse skin, melanocytes are restricted to the hair follicle, except for the ears and tail, controlled by local production of Steel factor.[10] Transgenic mice engineered to express Steel in epidermal keratinocytes, possess increased number of melanocytes in the epidermis, resulting in "humanized" skin.[11]

FIGURE 11-3

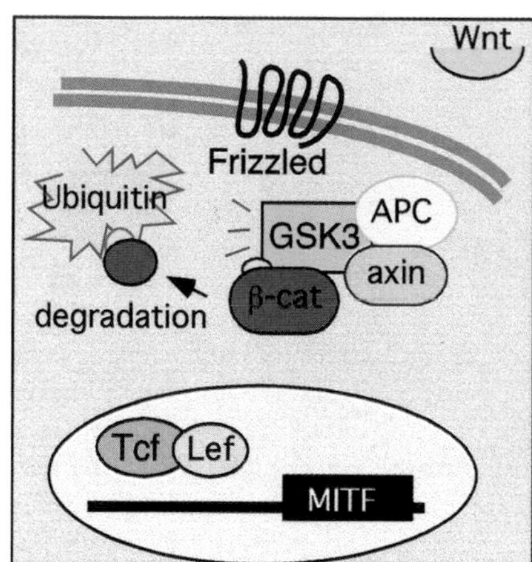

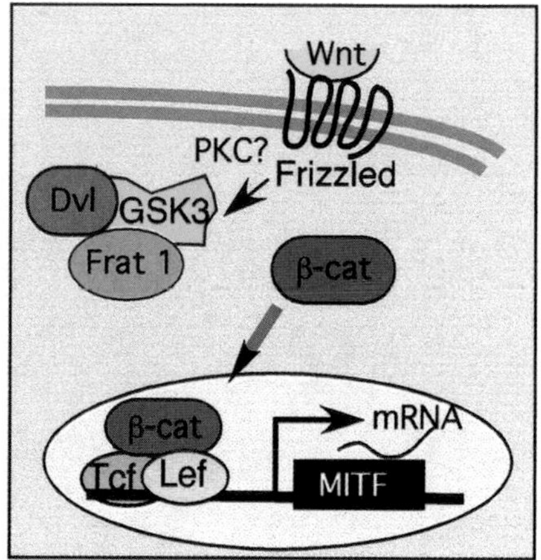

Regulation of Mitf expression by Wnt signaling. Frizzled (Fzl) is a G-protein–linked seven-membrane–spanning domain receptor.[115] It controls β-catenin by modulating GSK3β kinase activity. In the absence of Wnt, GSK3β is in a tetrameric complex with APC (adenomatous polyposis coli), axin and β-catenin. This complex destabilizes β-catenin by enhancing its phosphorylation and proteasome-mediated degradation (*left*). Activation of Frizzled by Wnt (*right*) results in activation of Disheveled (Dvl), which recruits the inhibitory Frat 1 to the protein complex, inhibiting GSK3β kinase activity and blocking β-catenin phosphorylation. Consequently, β-catenin accumulates and translocates to the nucleus where it initiates transcription of Tcf/Lef target genes involved in early development.

HGF/MET Activation of Met by its ligand the hepatocyte growth factor (HGF, also known as Scatter factor, SF) is also required for melanocyte viability and proliferation during development. Targeted ablation of the Met gene in mice (Met –/–) caused a complete loss of melanoblasts, beginning at late stages of neural crest migration (embryonic stage 12).[12] In contrast, overexpression of HGF in various tissues (mtHGF transgenic mice), or specifically in keratinocytes (K14-HGF transgenic mice), enhanced ectopic localization of melanoblasts, and increased the melanocyte population in the dermis and other sites of adult tissues, or only in the dermis, respectively.[12,13] Although Met inactivation has not yet been identified in any human inherited depigmentation syndromes, this receptor system is a good candidate to explore in certain conditions for which no mutations in established target genes have been discovered.

ENDOTHELINS/ENDOTHELIN RECEPTOR B Another cytokine-receptor pair that is implicated in melanocyte development is the endothelin and endothelin receptor family. Endothelins are growth factors (originally identified in endothelial cells) whose mutation produces significant neural crest defects, including melanocyte deficiency. There are three endothelin proteins (ET1, ET2, and ET3) and two receptors (EdnrA and EdnrB). ET3 binds to EdnrB and mutations in either ET3 or EdnrB produce substantial melanocyte loss in humans and mice. ET3 is unlikely to be the only endothelin involved in melanocyte development because the depigmented phenotype of mice null for ET3 is not as severe as in mice with null EdnrB mutation, and even the latter are not always completely devoid of pigment (reviewed in Ref. 14).

Altogether, it is apparent that melanocyte viability, division, and possibly migration, as well as expression of differentiated functions, are severely affected during embryogenesis by inactivating mutations in several receptors or their cognate ligands. The requirement for multiple receptor activities cannot be explained by marked differences in intracellular signaling cascades activated by each receptor. More likely, each receptor/ligand system is critical at specific developmental stages, determined by the timing of receptor expression at the cell surface and the presence of the respective ligand in the adjacent tissue. For example, in vitro studies demonstrate partial rescue of mouse neural crest-derived melanocyte precursors deficient in *c*-kit when grown in the presence of ET3.[15] Judging by the developmental stage at which melanoblasts express a specific receptor, or disappear when a pathway is ablated, it is likely that the Wnt/β-catenin signaling pathway is the first to be activated, followed by *kit*, ET3/endothelin B, and then HGF/Met. It is also possible that simultaneous activation of multiple receptors is required as the melanocyte precursors become more and more differentiated in order to achieve the levels and duration of intracellular signal intermediates and activation of transcription factors essential for proliferation and differentiation (see below, in "Melanocyte Growth Factors and Signal Transduction").

FIGURE 11-4

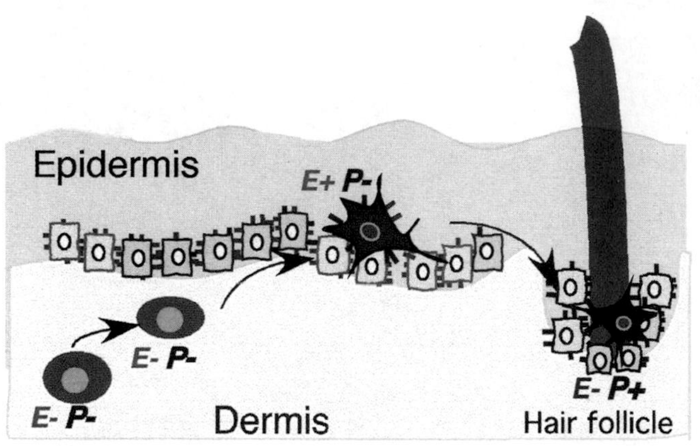

Expression of cadherins in melanocytes and their early precursor. The migrating cadherin–nonexpressing melanoblasts (round orange cells marked E–, P–), start expressing E-cadherin (green bars on dendritic brown cells) as they enter the epidermis and settle among E-cadherin–positive keratinocytes. E-cadherin is suppressed and P-cadherin is upregulated as the melanocytes enter the hair follicle (brown bars on dark brown dendritic cells) settling among similarly P-cadherin–expressing follicular cells. *(Adapted from Nakagawa S and Takeichi*[16] *and Nishimura et al.*[17])

Cadherins and Migration to the Skin

The cadherins are calcium-dependent surface receptors that mediate cell adhesion, homing, and invasion into different layers. The expression of cadherins dynamically changes as neural crest cells emerge from the neural tube. Experiments with chicken embryos show that overexpression of the neuroepithelial cadherin (*N*-cadherin) or a crest cadherin (cad7) suppresses migration of melanocyte precursors from the neural crest, causing their accumulation within the neural tube.[16] Similarly, quantitative studies in mouse embryos reveal that early migrating melanocyte precursors do not express E-cadherin or P-cadherin during their transit into the dermis[17] (Fig. 11-4). However, E-cadherin expression is temporarily upregulated by 200-fold just prior to entering the epidermis, only to be suppressed again as migration continues out of the epidermis into hair follicles. At this transition point, P-cadherin is increased. These patterns of cadherin expression match those of surrounding cells in the same microenvironment.[17,18]

Interestingly, in the "humanized" transgenic mouse skin model in which Steel factor is overexpressed in epidermal keratinocytes, the retained epidermal melanocytes continue to express high levels of E-cadherin.[17] In the K-14-HGF transgenic mice in which melanocytes were restricted to the dermis, there was also downregulation of E-cadherin expression.[13] This is consistent with a role for these homotypic interactions in epidermal homing and invasion. The cadherins are also potential regulators of invasion or metastatic behavior in melanocytic neoplasms.[19]

LOCALIZATION AND FUNCTION OF MELANOCYTES

Melanocytes exist in various tissues in the body. They are localized in the skin at the dermal-epidermal interface, in the hair matrix, the eye in the retinal pigment epithelium and uveal tract, the ear in the stria vascularis and the vestibular region of the inner ear, the leptomeninges and mucous membranes. Although the most visible role of melanocytes is in the production of melanin in the skin for protection against harmful solar radiation, they have important functions in other tissues that may not relate to pigment production.

Melanocytes in the Skin

Melanocytes are located in the epidermal basal layer and project their dendrites into the epidermis where they transfer melanosomes to keratinocytes (Fig. 11-5*A*). These dendritic contacts produce interfaces with multiple keratinocytes, thought to number approximately 36 per melanocyte, giving rise to the "epidermal melanin unit."[20] Melanocytes transfer melanin, packaged within the membrane-bound organelles termed melanosomcs, through these dendritic contacts to adjacent keratinocytes, which, in turn, contain the majority of cutaneous pigment (Fig. 11-5*B*). As keratinocytes mature and differentiate, their most superficial derivatives in the stratum corneum slough off, thus requiring continued synthesis and intercellular transport of melanin for maintaining pigmentation.

The density of epidermal melanocytes varies at different sites in the body. There are about 2000 epidermal melanocytes per square millimeter on the skin of the head and forearm and about 1000 on the rest of the body. This tight regulation of the number of melanocytes in the epidermis is likely to be mediated by keratinocytes that provide growth and survival factors such as fibroblast growth factor 2 (FGF2), also known as basic FGF, to the melanocytes (Fig. 11-5*C*). The density of melanocytes in the skin is the same regardless of racial backgrounds (see Chap. 88). Normal human skin color is thus determined primarily by the melanogenic activity within the melanocytes, the synthesis of melanin, the production of melanosomes, their size, shape, type, and color, the mode in which they are transferred to the keratinocytes, and their distribution in the keratinocytes. In Caucasians, three to eight melanosomes are clustered into membrane-bound groups within keratinocytes, whereas melanosomes of dark-skinned individuals are larger than those of Caucasians and exist within the keratinocytes, predominantly as individual organelles distributed throughout the cytoplasm[21] (Fig. 11-5*D* and *E*). Mislocalization of melanocytes in the dermis is usually associated with pigmented lesions such as nevi and melanomas.

There are apparent changes in the coloration of an individual during life. Almost all infants, including blacks, are lighter at birth and become darker during the first week of postnatal life. Freckles, originally apparent only after sun exposure, become more permanent in the first or second decade of life. The dorsal skin of the hand becomes mottled in color in old age related to an age-induced decline in the number of epidermal melanocytes. In areas not exposed to sun, except for genital sites, there is approximately an 8 to 10 percent reduction in the density of melanocytes per decade of life, whereas the changes in the forehead and cheek are less drastic. The persistence of melanocytes in the genital sites suggests an influence of sex hormones that maintains their constant number.

Melanocytes in the Hair

Melanocytes in the hair follicle provide the melanin for hair shaft pigmentation (Fig. 11-6*A*). The hair bulb melanin unit resides in the proximal anagen bulb, consisting of one melanocyte to five keratinocytes in the hair bulb as a whole, and one melanocyte to one keratinocyte in the basal layer of the hair bulb matrix (Fig. 11-6*B*).[22] Follicular melanogenesis is not a continuous process as in the epidermis, but is rather tightly coupled to the hair growth cycle (see Chap. 12). This cycle involves melanocyte proliferation during the early period of hair shaft production (anagen), maturation during mid to late anagen, and death via apoptosis during the early regression phase in which the lower two-thirds of the hair follicle is resorbed (catagen) (Fig. 11-6*C*). The hair

FIGURE 11-5

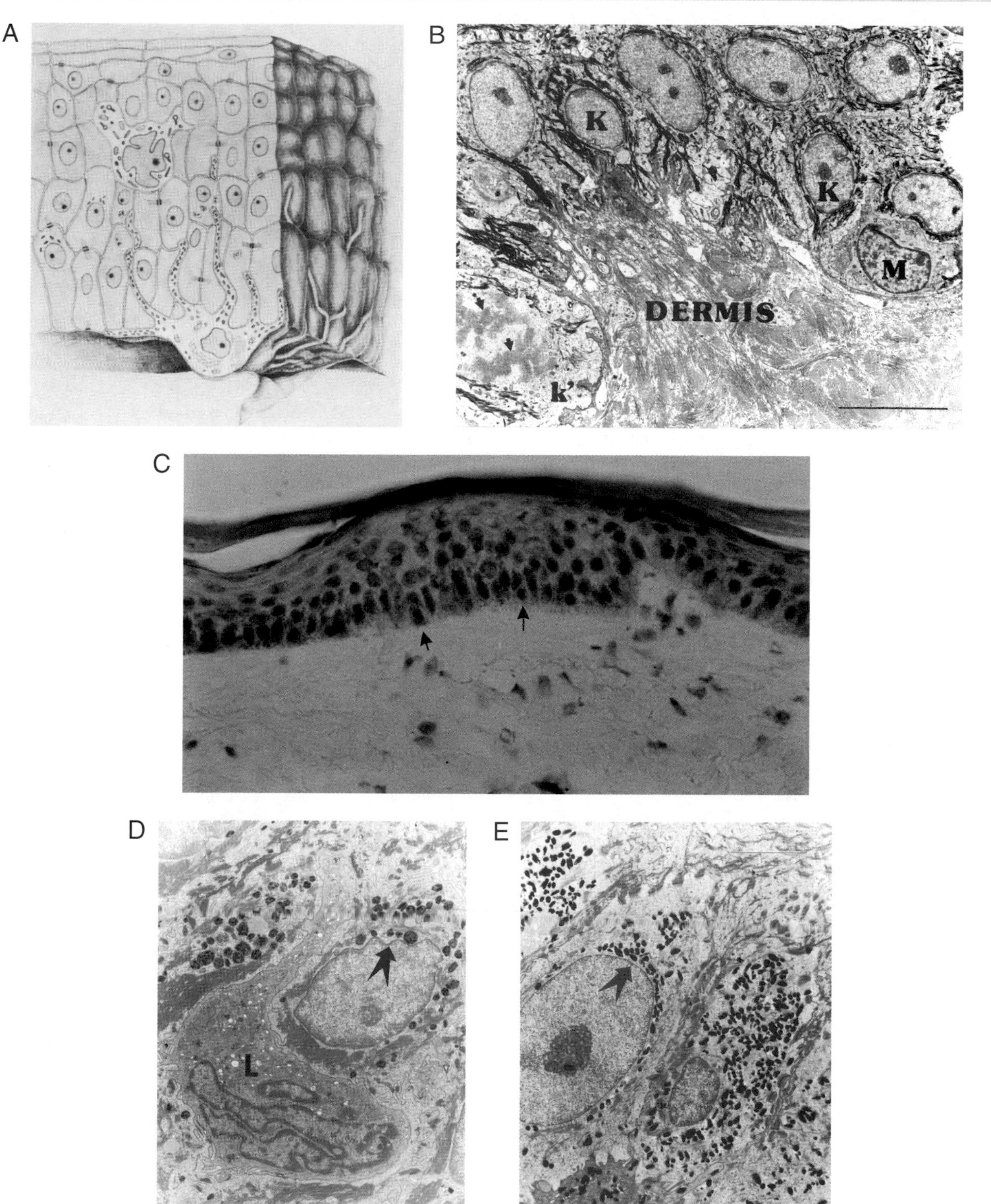

The epidermal melanin unit. *A*. Representation showing the relationship between basal melanocytes, keratinocytes, and Langerhans cells, shown at the upper layer of the epidermis. *(From Quevedo WC Jr. The control of color in mammals.* Am Zoology *9:531, 1969, with permission.) B*. Electron micrograph of the epidermal-dermal junction of human skin showing a dendritic melanocyte (M) among the basal keratinocytes (K). K′ represents a basal keratinocyte undergoing mitosis with condensed chromatin (*arrows*). Bar = $10.0\ \mu m$. *(Illustration courtesy of Raymond E. Boissy, Department of Dermatology, University of Cincinnati, Cincinnati, Ohio.) C*. Human epidermis immunostained for FGF2. The figure shows basal keratinocytes with peroxidase reaction indicating the presence of immunoreactive FGF2. *Arrows* point to melanocytes. *(Courtesy of Glynis Scott, M.D., Department of Dermatology, University of Rochester School of Medicine and Dentistry, Rochester, NY.) D* and *E*. Distribution of melanosomes within keratinocytes in lightly pigmented Caucasian and darkly pigmented African American skin. Melanosomes in lightly pigmented Caucasian skin *(D)* are distributed in membrane-bound clusters. In contrast, in darkly pigmented African American skin *(E)* the melanosomes are individually distributed throughout the cytoplasm of epidermal keratinocytes. Melanosomes in both skin types are frequently concentrated over the apical pole of the nucleus (*arrows*). L, Langerhans ccell. Bar = $3.0\ \mu m$. *(From Minwalla L et al.*[21])

ing a function to melanocytes by comparing pigmented to gray hair, however, suffers from drawbacks due to age-related differences that accompany the process of pigment loss.

FIGURE 11-6

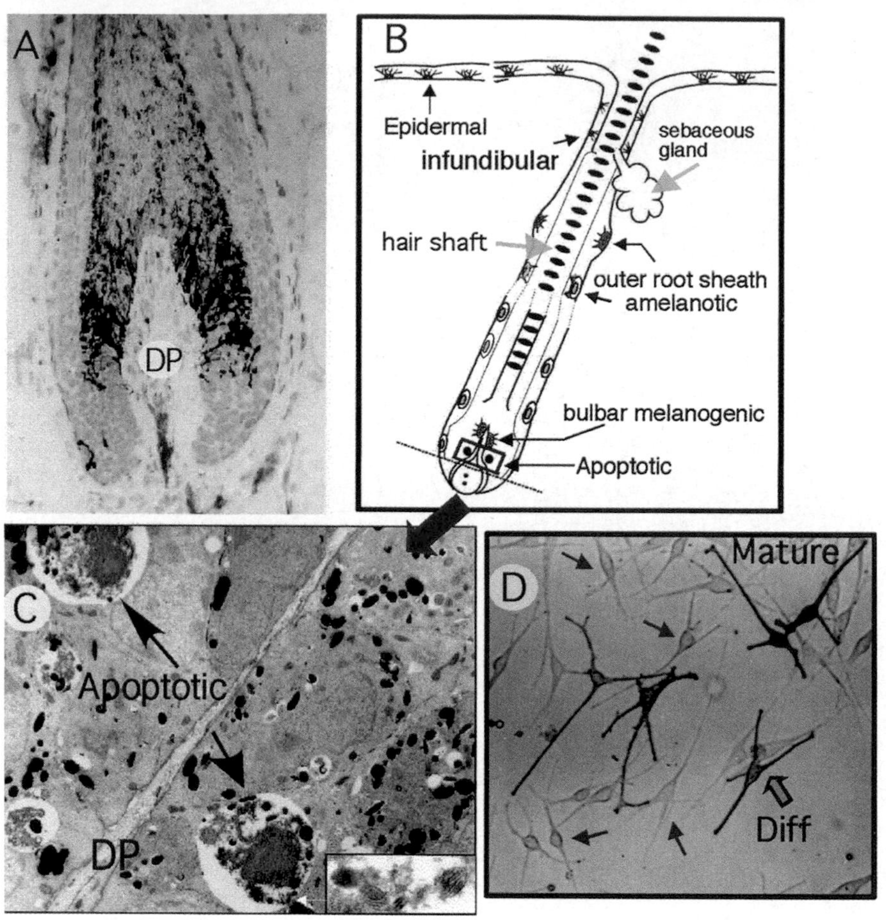

Melanocytes in the hair. *A.* Pigmented human scalp hair follicle in full anagen with high levels of hair bulb melanogenesis. Mature melanin granules are transferred into cortical keratinocyte. DP, dermal papilla. *B.* Hair scalp bulb. Representation of early catagen hair follicle showing loss of some bulbar melanotic melanocytes via apoptosis. *Arrows* point at melanocytes located in epidermal, infundibular, and outer root sheath regions. *C.* Transmission electron micrograph of section of an early catagen hair bulb showing apoptosis of melanotic melanocytes. Inset, high-power view of premelanosomes. DP, dermal papilla. *D.* Primary culture of human scalp hair follicle melanocytes. Mature, fully differentiated (Diff; large arrow), and less differentiated (*small arrows*) are indicated. (*From Tobin DJ and Paus R,*[22] *with permission.*)

follicle contains melanocyte precursors, or possibly melanoblasts, that can even migrate out and populate the interfollicular epidermis upon stimulation[22] (Fig. 11-6*D*). This is particularly visible in patients with vitiligo undergoing repigmentation by PUVA photochemotherapy (psoralen plus ultraviolet light of A wave length) (see Chap. 266). Vitiligo is an inherited or acquired loss of melanocytes in the skin and other sites due to self-destruction, resulting in patches of white skin. In response to PUVA treatment, pigmented spots frequently develop around hair follicles in the vitiliginous skin, apparently due to the outward migration of residual reservoir of melanocytes in the hair follicle. Graying is caused by the gradual decline in the number of melanocytes in the hair follicles in a fashion determined by age and genetic background.

It is not clear whether melanocytes have functions in the hair follicle other than to provide pigment to the hair. They do not serve to protect from UV light, which does not reach the hair follicle. Functions such as restraining keratinocyte proliferation, calcium homeostasis, and protection against reactive oxygen species during rapid cell proliferation and differentiation, have been suggested (reviewed in Ref. 22). Assigning a function to melanocytes by comparing pigmented to gray hair, however, suffers from drawbacks due to age-related differences that accompany the process of pigment loss.

Melanocytes in the Ear

Melanocytes in the ear are critical for proper hearing. Individuals who carry mutations in genes that cause suppression of melanocyte development, such as Waardenburg syndrome (see Chap. 90), suffer from hypopigmentation and impaired hearing (reviewed in Ref. 6). Melanin production, by itself, is not essential, because albinos have normal hearing despite absence of melanin within viable melanocytes (reviewed in Ref. 23). However, because pigmentation confers protection from trauma, albino individuals may suffer from earlier onset of hearing loss due to noise or exposure to toxic drugs (reviewed in Refs. 23 and 24).

Melanocytes in the stria vascularis (known as intermediate cells) are crucial for normal cochlear development and maintenance of endolymphatic potential[24] (Fig 11–7). In their absence, the endolymphatic potential is extremely low and can cause deafness.[25] Endolymphatic fluid in the cochlea is one of the few extracellular fluids which is normally high in K^+. Absence of cochlear melanocytes is associated with significantly diminished endolymphatic K^+, suggesting that melanocytes are either directly or indirectly essential for its maintenance. The melanocytes may perform spatial buffering by transporting K^+ from regions of high to low K^+. This function is carried out by plasma membrane ionic channels, collectively known as inwardly rectifying K^+ channels and voltage-dependent outwardly rectifying K^+ channels. The inwardly rectifying K^+ channel, Kir4.1, was identified in the stria intermediate cells (melanocytes) and is considered to play a central role in stria function and normal hearing.[26]

Loss of melanocytes even after birth can impair endocochlear potential, as shown by mice carrying the dominant B^{lt} mutation at the brown locus. The mutation affects melanocytes specifically because it alters the yet undetermined function of Tyrp1, a melanocyte-specific protein (discussed below in "Melanin Synthesis" and "The Biosynthesis, Distribution, and Transport of Melanosomes"). The B^{lt} mutation causes a progressive loss of melanocytes with age due to self-destruction by oxidation products derived from the tyrosinase reaction.[27] This is true also for humans. Vitiligo (see Chap. 90), a condition manifested as progressive destruction of melanocytes with age, seems to contribute to susceptibility to hearing loss, particularly in males. Another uncommon autoimmune disease, Vogt-Koyanagi-Harada (VKH), that targets melanocyte-specific proteins, causes vitiligo in the skin and other parts of the body including the inner ear.[28] The autoimmunity is manifested as T cell–mediated inflammation around melanocytes and is associated with a high incidence of hearing impairment (reviewed in Refs. 24 and 28; see also Chap. 90).

Melanocytes in the Eye

Melanin-containing pigment cells are present in the choroid and retinal pigment epithelium (RPE) layers of the eye (Fig. 11-8). The choroid is populated by neural crest–derived melanocytes, whereas pigment cells in the RPE originate from the neural ectoderm. RPE cells appear to arise through transdifferentiation from the neuroretina in a fashion largely mediated by Mitf. In the absence of Mitf, RPE cells revert to express neuronal markers and proliferate so as to duplicate neuroretinal structures.[29] However, Mitf expression in RPE melanocytes is not stable and is turned off later in development. Therefore, these cells become rapidly nonpigmented when cultured in vitro in the absence of melanocyte mitogens. In contrast, dividing choroidal melanocytes express melanocytic markers persistently in a fashion similar to that of epidermal melanocytes.

Melanocytes are important for normal development and function of the eye and optic nerves, as manifested by abnormalities in individuals with all forms of albinism regardless of the gene affected, including OCA1 and ocular albinism type 1 (OA1)[30,31] (see Chap. 90). One of the most fascinating functions of melanocytes whose nature still remains unsolved, is in proper routing of the optic nerves at the chiasm during early development of the optic cup. Highly intermixed axons destined to project ipsilaterally and contralaterally to the brain enter the chiasm region and then selectively grow into the correct pathway. Melanin at this crossroad is likely to provide specific guidance cues. In the absence of pigment, the sorting out of intermixed ipsilaterally and contralaterally projecting retinal axons into the appropriate optic tracts is altered, thereby disrupting the gross topographic relationship of fibers in the nerve.

FIGURE 11-7

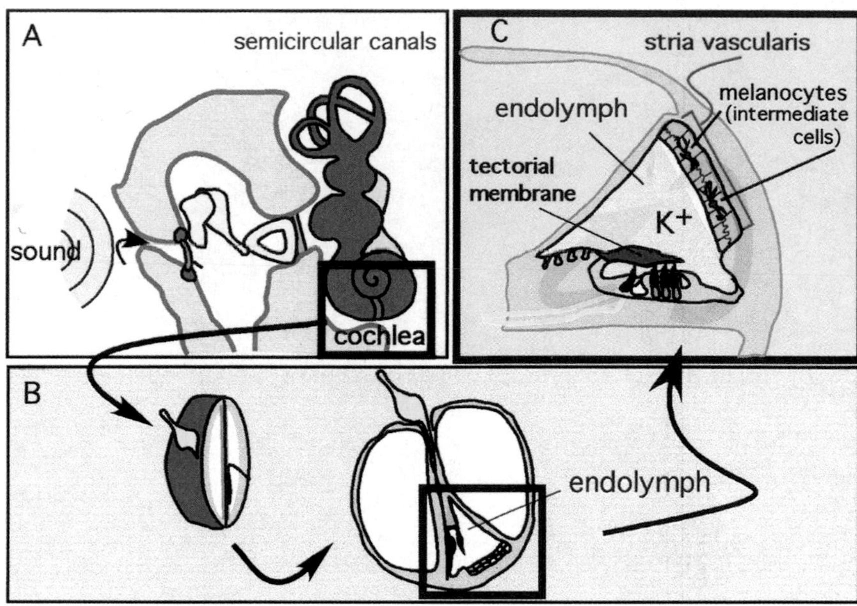

Melanocytes in the ear. *A*. Anatomy of the ear. Sound moves through the pinna, external canal, tympanic membrane, ossicles, and into the endolymphatic fluid contained within the cochlea (inner ear). Transduced vibrations of the appropriate amplitude bend particular sized cilia on hair cells causing a physical opening of ion channels and movement of potassium ions into the hair cells, triggering neuronal firings. *B*. A cross-section of the cochlea reveals three sections. *C*. The potassium-rich endolymph-filled chamber is conditioned by the stria vascularis, made up of intermediate cells (neural crest–derived melanocytes) sandwiched between marginal and basal cells. One wall of this chamber is lined by the motion-sensing hair cells. (*From Price ER and Fisher DE,*[6] *with permission.*)

MELANIN SYNTHESIS

Melanin is the major product of melanocytes and is the main determinant of differences in skin color. Melanin is synthesized in two main forms: the dark-colored brown-black, insoluble eumelanin, and the light-colored red-yellow, alkali-soluble, sulfur-containing pheomelanin. The rate-limiting catalytic activity in the production of both types of melanin is the oxidation of tyrosine by tyrosinase, known as the Raper-Mason pathway[32] (Fig. 11-9). Tyrosinase (monophenol, L-dopa: oxygen oxidoreductase, EC 1.14.18.1) is a melanocyte-specific copper-binding enzyme with homology to polyphenol oxidases and some hemocyanins. It catalyzes the oxidation of monohydric and dihydric phenols (catechols) to their corresponding quinones.[33,34] In vivo, tyrosinase converts tyrosine to DOPAquinone (3,4-dihydroxy- phenylalanine quinone), with the intermediate production of DOPA that remains bound to the active site (Fig. 11-9*A*). DOPA is required for tyrosinase activity (Fig. 11-9*B* and *C*) because it allows the binding of oxygen to the active site of tyrosinase. This process involves the catalytic oxidation of DOPA to DOPAquinone by the *met*-form of the enzyme (Cu II state without bound dioxygen). This step enables the transition to the oxygen-bound form by reducing the copper atoms in the active site. This oxygen-bound form of tyrosinase is now able to use tyrosine and DOPA as substrates.[34]

DOPA is required continuously for tyrosinase activity and is likely to regenerate from the reduction of DOPAquinone. One possible mechanism is the spontaneous endocyclization of DOPAquinone to cyclodopa, which is then converted to DOPAchrome by redox exchange with DOPAquinone.[34] Another alternative is that DOPAquinone is reduced to DOPA through the oxidation of critical sulfhydryl groups on tyrosinase, forming the final disulfide bond(s) required to stabilize the protein in its native/active form. This regeneration step may explain the lag period in tyrosine oxidation by mammalian tyrosinase in vitro in the absence of added DOPA (Fig. 11-9*B*), and the suppression of any enzymatic activity at low pH in which DOPA remains protonated (Fig. 11-9*B* and *C*).

Tyrosinase is the sole supplier of DOPA in melanocytes. Tyrosine hydroxylase, the other DOPA-generating enzyme in dopaminergic neurons, is not expressed in normal melanocytes, and forced expression of a constitutively active form of tyrosine hydroxylase could not substitute for tyrosinase in generating DOPA for the tyrosinase reaction.[35] Interestingly, the structural change induced by DOPA also promotes the maturation of tyrosinase by inducing its transport from the endoplasmic reticulum (ER) to the Golgi[35] (tyrosinase maturation is discussed below, in "Endoplasmic Reticulum Modification and Transport to the Golgi").

Additional steps in the pathway participate in the production of melanin in vivo. These include the oxidation of 5,6-dihydroxyindole (DHI) to indole-5,6-quinone by tyrosinase (reviewed in Ref. 36), the isomerization of DOPAchrome to 5,6-dihydroxyindole-2-carboxylic acid (DHICA) by DOPAchrome tautomerase (DCT) and possibly Tyrp1, and the oxidation of DHICA to carboxylated indole-quinone (Fig. 11-9*A*). Mouse Tyrp1 was also suggested to perform this latter enzymatic activity, but the inability of human Tyrp1 to catalyze the same

FIGURE 11-8

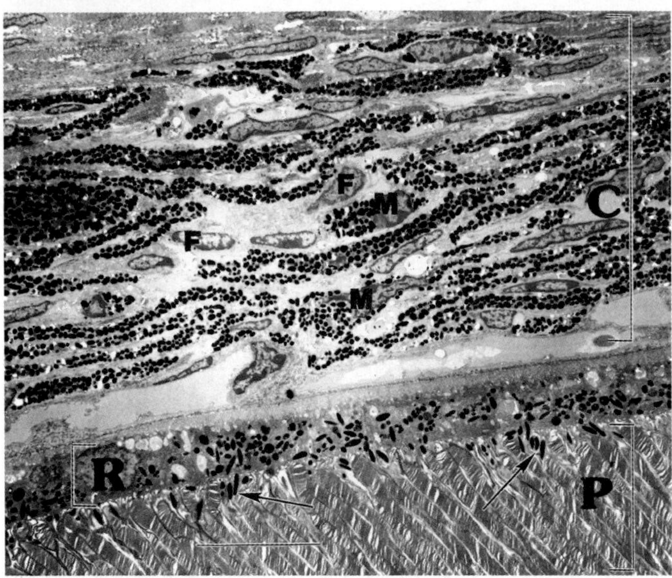

Ocular tissue demonstrating the choroid (C), the retinal pigment epithelium (R), and the photoreceptor cells of the retina (P). The connective tissue of the choroid contains numerous fibroblasts (F) and dendritic melanocytes (M) with cytoplasm filled with mature melanosomes. The retinal pigment epithelium is a single layer of polarized cuboidal melanocytes containing relatively elongated mature melanosomes both within the cell body of the RPE cells and in the numerous slender apical processed (*arrows*) that interdigitate between the rod and cone photoreceptor cells. Bar = 10.0 μm. (*Illustration courtesy of Raymond E. Boissy, Department of Dermatology, University of Cincinnati, Cincinnati, Ohio.*)

FIGURE 11-9

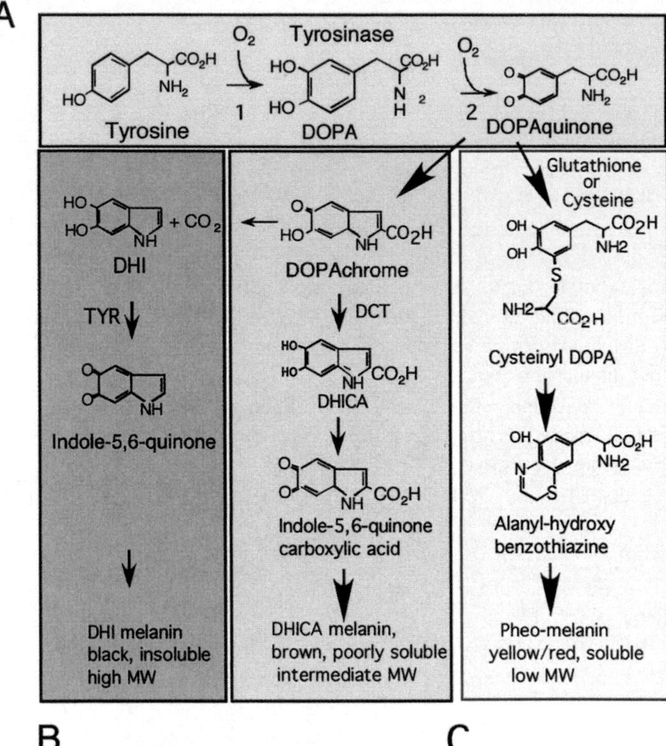

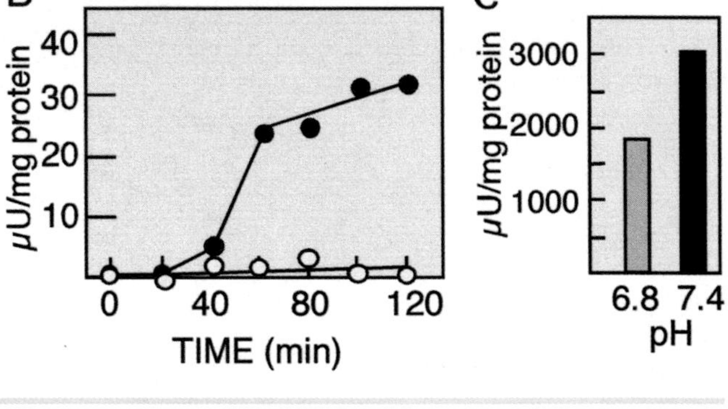

Pathway for melanin biosynthesis. *A.* The intermediates in the oxidation of tyrosine by tyrosinase as described by the Raper Mason pathway[32] and modified by recent studies (reviewed in Ref. 36). Tyrosinase catalyzed the two initial steps (1, 2) as well as the conversion of DHI to indole-5,6-quinone. Some of the intermediates are made by spontaneous conversion and others are formed by enzymatic conversion mediated by newly isolated enzymes. DOPAchrome is converted to 5,6-dihydroxyindole-2-carboxylic acid (DHICA) by DCT (DOPAchrome tautomerase). The identity of the enzyme that converts DHICA to indole-5,6-quinone may not be clear because two proteins, Tyrp1 and Silver, have been suggested to perform this function. *B.* Autocatalytic activation of tyrosinase by DOPA and its suppression at acidic pH. Tyrosinase activity was tested in vitro using extracts from normal human melanocytes in the absence of DOPA at pH 6.8 (*open circles*), or pH 7.4 (*solid circles*). Activity is detected only after 40 min of incubation at an alkaline pH but not at an acidic pH. *C.* Tyrosinase activity in the presence of DOPA. Notice that total activity is about 100-fold higher in the presence compared to the absence of DOPA. The fully activated tyrosinase is still more functional at alkaline compared to acidic pH.

function, in spite of high homology between mouse and human proteins (95 percent identity in the putative catalytic domain and 87 percent total identity), casts doubt on the function of Tyrp1 in this reaction.

The oxidation products of DHICA and DHI provide the building blocks for the brown-black, poorly soluble and insoluble eumelanins, respectively (Fig. 11-9*A*). Pheomelanin is produced from cysteinyldopa and benzothiazine metabolites when DOPAquinone combines with cysteine or glutathione (Fig. 11-9*A*). Melanin is a mixture of pheomelanic and eumelanic monomers and the ratio between the two determines the final color of the skin and hair.[37] The reduction in eumelanin and the predominant presence of pheomelanin, such as in red hair, is regulated in large part by the melanocortin receptor (see below, in "Pigmentation Control by Melanocortins and the Melanocortin Receptor (MCR)").

The main characteristic of melanin is its ability to absorb and scatter UV radiation (280 to 400 nm) and protect against DNA damage.[38] However, the intermediates in melanin biosynthesis and melanin itself can also be harmful. The quinones produced by the tyrosinase reaction are cytotoxic and mediate cell death when they accumulate at high levels. Furthermore, melanin-related molecules enhance UVA radiation (320 to 400 nm)-induced DNA breakage.[39] Melanin reacts avidly with DNA, is photoreactive, and capable of producing damaging reactive oxygen species in response to UVA.[40] Increased levels of pheomelanin and or melanin intermediates induce higher levels of single-strand breaks in UVA-irradiated cultured human melanocytes derived from light-skin individuals as compared to melanocytes from dark-skin individuals.[41] These results suggest that the higher incidence of light-induced melanomas in red-haired and light-skin individuals is due not only to lack of natural protection, but also to enhanced mutagenesis by pheomelanin and/or melanin intermediates. These side effects of melanin may explain the evolutionary pressure to confine its production and localization to the melanosomes.

THE BIOSYNTHESIS, DISTRIBUTION AND TRANSPORT OF MELANOSOMES

Melanosomes are membrane-bound granules of approximately 200 × 900 nm. They are related to lysosomes because both organelles contain similar marker proteins and are positioned after the Golgi in the secretory pathway (reviewed in Refs. 42 and 43). The melanosomes are composed of a distinct set of proteins performing a variety of functions that include building and maintaining the granules, melanin synthesis, and trafficking to the dendritic tips (Table 11–1). The targeting of each of these proteins into the melanosomes is highly regulated, initiating at the site of synthesis on ER-bound ribosomes. The maturation process of melanosomal proteins includes their cotranslational glycosylation and proper folding in the ER, transport to the Golgi where complex carbohydrates are acquired, and vesicular transport to the melanosomes (Fig. 11-10*A*). The specific events governing each step are described in detail for tyrosinase as a model system for other melanocyte-specific proteins.

Tyrosinase is a type I membrane glycoprotein of 529 amino acids, with a signal peptide, and catalytic regions composed of two copper-binding domains coordinated by histidine residues (Fig. 11-10*B*). Tyrosinase also contains 17 cysteine (Cys) residues, one each located in the signal sequence and the cytoplasmic tail, leaving 15 Cys available to form multiple disulfide bonds in the large ectodomain of the protein. While these Cys residues are grouped largely into two Cys-rich domains, their disulfide pairing remains unknown. Tyrosinase has an overall identity of 40 percent with two other cDNAs encoding melanocyte-specific proteins termed tyrosinase-related protein 1 (Tyrp1, also known as TRP1/b-locus/gp75), and DCT (also known as TRP2 or *slaty* locus protein). The homology between these three different proteins is particularly striking in the putative glycosylation sites, the clusters of Cys residues and the two copper-binding sites (Fig. 11-10*B*). However, among these three, only tyrosinase possesses the catalytic activity of converting tyrosine and DOPA to DOPAquinone, and in its absence (and the presence of normal Tyrp1 and DCT), melanocytes remain devoid of any pigment. This is clearly demonstrated by the albino phenotype of melanocytes expressing null mutant tyrosinase and normal Tyrp1 or DCT, and by the pigmented phenotype of melanocytes with normal tyrosinase but with null mutant Tyrp1 protein. Furthermore, only tyrosinase can induce melanin biosynthesis when expressed in heterologous cellular systems, even in the absence of any other melanocyte specific proteins.

Endoplasmic Reticulum Modification and Transport to the Golgi

The *N*-terminal signal sequence of tyrosinase targets the mRNA-ribosome-tyrosinase complex to the ER, the site of entry to the secretory pathway. Upon emergence of the polypeptide chain into the ER, the 18-amino acid *N*-terminal signal sequence is cleaved and human tyrosinase receives six or seven *N*-linked glycosylations cotranslationally, and disulfide bond formation commences. The *N*-linked glycans are attached as a core 14-unit oligosaccharide (glucose$_3$-mannose$_9$-*N*-acetylglucosamine$_2$) by the oligosaccharyl transferase complex on asparagine (Asn) residues that reside in the sequence Asn-X-Thr/Ser (Fig. 11-11*A*).

The newly synthesized tyrosinase polypeptide is subjected to the quality control system in the ER that monitors protein maturation to ensure that defective proteins are not transported throughout the cell (reviewed in Ref. 44). The system includes resident proteins such as calnexin, calreticulin, and the glucosyl transferase that recognize incorrectly folded and misassembled proteins, and target them for ER

TABLE 11-1

Melanocyte Proteins Involved in Organelle Biogenesis, Melanin Synthesis, and Transport of Melanosomes

SITE OF ACTION	PROTEIN	FUNCTION	HUMAN GENETIC DEFECT
Melanosomes	Tyrosinase	Melanin biosynthesis	OCA1
	Tyrp1	Tyrosinase stabilization	OCA3
	DCT	Melanin biosynthesis	Unknown
	Silver/Pmel17/gp100	Melanosomal matrix (DHICA)-converting activity	Unknown
	P-protein	Unknown	OCA2
	OA1	Maintenance of melanosome size/intracellular G- protein–coupled receptor (GPCR)	Ocular albinism 1 (OA1)
	AIM-1/MATP	Maintenance of melanosome size/transporter?	OCA4
Cytosol associated with membranes	CHS	Organelle biogenesis; fusion/fission events in melanosomes and lysosomes; proteins transport	Chédiak-Higashi syndrome
	HPS1	Organelle biogenesis	Hermansky-Pudlak syndrome 1 (HPS1)
Cytosolic surface of transport vesicles or melanosomes	AP-3	Trafficking of integral membrane proteins and sorting to the melanosomes	Hermansky-Pudlak syndrome 2 (HPS2)
	Rab3a	Vesicle trafficking?	Unknown
Cytosol of dendrites	Myosin Va	Melanosome motor that traps melanosomes at the dendritic tips on actin filaments	Griscelli syndrome
	Rab27a	Adaptor protein, vesicle trafficking	Griscelli syndrome
	Mlph	Adaptor protein	Unknown

FIGURE 11-10

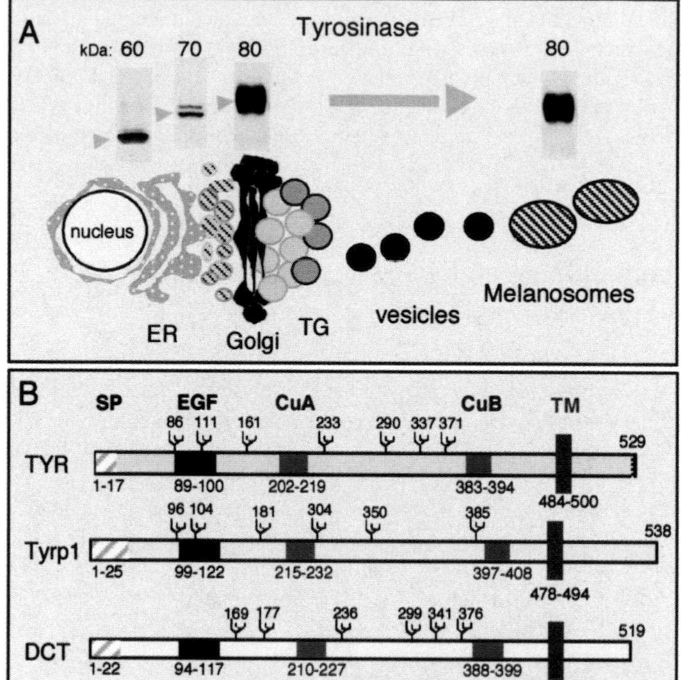

A. Representation of tyrosinase transit through the secretory pathway. Tyrosinase is synthesized on ER-bound ribosomes as the ~58 kDa polypeptide, and cotranslation transfer of six or seven *N*-linked oligosaccharide chains increases tyrosinase's molecular weight to ~70 kDa. The complex sugar modifications in the Golgi apparatus cause a further increase to ~80 kDa, the size of the mature wild-type isoform that is then translocated to the melanosomes. The protein bands of the various tyrosinase forms are Western blots of human tyrosinase from normal melanocytes. *B*. Representation of tyrosinase and two homologous proteins Tyrp1 and Dct. The long horizontal rectangles represent tyrosinase (TYR), Tyrp1, and DCT peptides. The hatched *N*-terminus boxes indicate the signal peptide; the blue areas indicate the EGF-like domain; the green areas indicate the Cu binding sites A and B; and the dark vertical bars indicate the hydrophobic core transmembrane domain (TM). Tyrosinase also possesses an SHL microbodies C-terminal targeting signal represented by the narrow bar at the C-terminus. The range of amino acid for each of these domains is given on the bottom of each bar. The positions of *N*-linked oligosaccharides are represented by the branched structures above the bar, with numbers indicating the position of Asn.

FIGURE 11-11

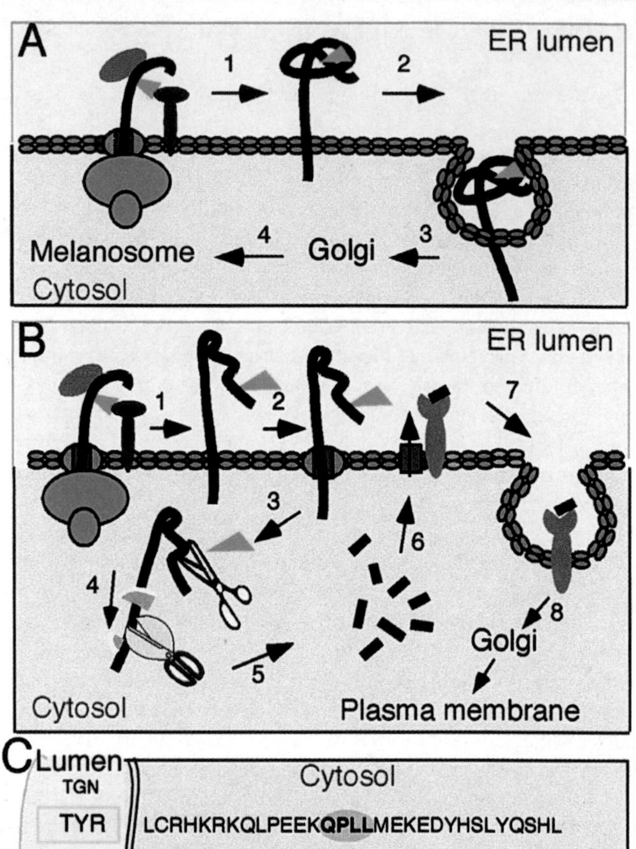

Maturation and degradation of tyrosinase. *A*. Maturation of correctly folded tyrosinase. Tyrosinase is translated by ER-targeted ribosomes (blue spheres). The protein is cotranslationally translocated through the ER membrane (*blue chain*) and *N*-linked glycosylated (*green triangle*). It interacts with the chaperones, calnexin (*red*) and calreticulin (*orange*), in the ER lumen. The fully folded protein emerges from the chaperone complex (1), and is sorted (2) to transport vesicles that bud from the ER membrane (3) for transit to the Golgi then to the melanosomes (4). *B*. Degradation of misfolded tyrosinase. Tyrosinase misfolds (1) in the ER due to mutations or hostile microenvironment and is targeted for retranslocation to the cytosol (2) where its *N*-linked glycans are removed by a cytosolic *N*-glycanase (3). The soluble and unglycosylated tyrosinase is modified by polyubiquitin (4) that sorts the protein to the 26S proteasome for destruction (5). The polypeptides can then be transported back into the ER lumen through the TAP transporter in the ER membrane (6) for binding to MHC class I heavy chain. The peptide-MHC class I heavy chain complex is transported through the secretory pathway to the cell membrane for antigen presentation. *C*. Amino acid sequences of the cytosolic tails of tyrosinase (TYR) and Tyrp1 indicating the di-leucine domain, the recognition site for binding of AP-3 adapter-protein complex (*purple*) that directs intracellular localization to the melanosome.

retention. Calnexin and calreticulin are lectin chaperones that bind specifically to glycoproteins containing monoglucosylated glycans (reviewed in Ref. 44). The monoglucosylated protein is created by the sequential actions of ER glucosidases I and II. The immature, misfolded tyrosinase remains bound to calnexin and calreticulin.[45–47] Chaperone binding may enhance the maturation of wild-type tyrosinase, because the expression of tyrosinase in a heterologous nonmelanogenic cell system (COS7 cells) with overexpressed calnexin permitted an approximately twofold enhancement in the appearance of tyrosinase activity.[48]

Inactivating mutations in tyrosinase, or in other melanocyte-specific proteins such as Tyrp1 and OA1 (the latter a seven-membrane–span G-protein–coupled receptor), can lead to their misfolding and retention in the ER[31,46,49,50] (Fig. 11-11*B*). In the case of OCA1 (see Chap. 89), the consequent disruption in pigmentation is due to inactivation of tyrosinase and the failure of the protein to reach the site of melanin production, the melanosome. These findings have initiated the hypothesis that only functional tyrosinase passes the quality control test performed by resident ER proteins that permit proteins to be transported out of the ER to the Golgi.[35] This quality control test may involve the production of the tyrosinase cofactor DOPA by the oxidation of the tyrosinase substrate, tyrosine. DOPA can then bind to and stabilize nascent tyrosinase, making it competent for transport.

Other proteins, such as Tyrp1 and DCT, can stabilize tyrosinase in the ER. In cells lacking melanosomes, melanosomal proteins are delivered to the lysosomes and both Tyrp1 and DCT are found to stabilize tyrosinase and to increase its activity.[51] This suggested the presence of a melanogenic complex that might not only be important for enzymatic optimization but also for the trafficking of the proteins out of the ER. A high molecular weight complex containing tyrosinase, Tyrp1, and DCT has been identified,[52,53] but understanding the significance of this complex requires further studies.

ER Retention and Production of Antigenic Peptides

Similar to albino melanocytes, melanoma cells are frequently rendered amelanotic due to retention of tyrosinase in the early secretory pathway. In these cells, the wild-type protein is inactivated and misfolded due to a hostile environment within the malignant cells.[45] The ER-retained protein is subsequently retranslocated to the cytosol where it is degraded by the 26S proteasome (Fig. 11-11*B*). These newly generated tyrosinase peptides can become antigenic and elicit an immune response by reentering the ER through TAP (transporter associated with antigen processing) and being presented by the major histocompatibility complex (MHC).[54] Recognition of tyrosinase peptides by tumor-infiltrating lymphocytes in a MHC class I and II restricted manner has been described in patients with melanomas.[55,56]

The destruction of wild-type tyrosinase in melanoma cells is likely to be due to suppression of the oxidoreductive activity of the enzyme by tumor-induced metabolic changes that cause acidification of the extracellular milieu. Melanoma cells, like other solid tumors grown under hypoxic conditions, acidify their extracellular environment because of increased rates of glycolysis and the accumulation of lactic acid, a process known as the *Warburg effect*.[57]

Transport from Golgi to Melanosomes

After tyrosinase is properly folded, stabilized, and possibly oligomerized, it is no longer recognized and retained by the ER quality control machinery. The protein is then packaged into COPII-coated transport vesicles that bud from the smooth ER. The vesicles traffic through the ER-Golgi-intermediate compartment (ERGIC) to the Golgi where complex sugars are added to the high mannose *N*-linked glycans causing an increase in molecular mass of tyrosinase from ~70 kDa to ~80 kDa (Fig. 11-10*A*).

The sorting of tyrosinase and other melanocyte-specific proteins from the Golgi to melanosomes is determined by recognition signals in the cytoplasmic segment (Fig. 11-11*C*). Mutations that cause deletion of tyrosinase's cytoplasmic tail mistarget the protein to the cell surface and generate an OCA1 phenotype.[58] Intracellular localization to the melanosomes is directed by a di-leucine motif present in the tail of tyrosinase, Tyrp1, silver (also known as Pmel17 and gp100), and P-protein[59,60] (Fig. 11-11*C*), by binding to the adapter-like protein complex, AP-3.[61] AP-3, like other adapter complexes, is comprised of four subunits termed $\beta3$-, δ-, $\mu3$, and $\delta3$-adaptin. This heterotetrameric complex is located in the cytosol until it is recruited to the TGN (*trans*-Golgi network) by an ARF-GTPase. Vesicles containing melanocyte-specific proteins are then transported to the lysosome or lysosome-related organelles.

Mutations in AP-3 produce a variety of classical pigmentation and multi-organellar defects in humans, mice, and Drosophila (reviewed in Refs. 14 and 62). Hermansky-Pudlak syndrome (HPS) (see Chap. 90) is a human disease that is characterized by altered storage granules and pigmentation. HPS patients experience excessive bleeding, as well as immunologic and pigmentation deficiencies. The mutation that leads to HPS type 2 (HPS2) has been mapped to the $\beta3$A subunit of the AP-3 adapter. This defect results in the enhanced degradation of the $\beta3$A subunit and the reduction in the overall level of the AP-3 complex. Subsequently, proteins possessing di-leucine–based sorting signals, including melanosomal and lysosomal proteins, are mislocalized to the

plasma membrane (reviewed in Ref. 42). That a mutation in AP-3 affects both pigmentation and blood clotting is indicative of the importance of AP-3 in the trafficking of protein to both melanosomes and platelet-dense granules. However, other determinants must also be involved to direct proteins to the individual compartment.

Melanosome Maturation

Melanosomes develop through a series of morphologically defined stages from an unpigmented (stage I) to a striated organelle enriched in melanin (stage IV) (Fig. 11-12*A*). Stage I melanosomes have an irregular structure and contain internal membranous vesicles that are formed by the invagination of the outer limiting membrane. They likely correspond to the late coated endosomal multivesicular bodies found in nonmelanogenic cells. At stage II, the melanosomes become elongated and form ordered striations. These striations act as templates for melanin polymerization that commences in stage III melanosomes, which possess the functional oxidoreductases and therefore begin to darken. However, stage I melanosomes also possess functional tyrosinase because incubation with DOPA produces melanin within these organelles (Fig. 11-12*B*). Silver is a type I membrane glycoprotein that appears to play a structural role in the formation of these striations because silver expression in nonmelanogenic cells supports the formation of striations within multivesicular bodies.[43]

The assembly of melanosomal enzymes and structural proteins into a membrane-limited granule is not sufficient to produce a functional melanosome. Melanin biosynthesis is dependent on proper pH homeostasis, osmotic pressure, transport of substrate into the melanosome lumen, and other yet uncharacterized activities such as that controlled by the OA1 protein.[63] Proper pH and osmotic pressure are likely to require the activity of multiple spanning membrane transport proteins. Two such candidates are the pink-eyed dilution protein (P-protein) and AIM-1/MATP (for antigen in melanoma-1/membrane-associated transporter protein).[64–68] These two integral membrane melanosomal proteins each possess 12 putative transmembrane domains. Their homology to transport proteins in lower organisms is supportive of a role in ionic regulation in the melanosomes and possibly even in the ER and the Golgi. The P-protein possesses homology to *E. coli* Na^+/H^+ antiporter and MATP to the sucrose/proton transporters in plants, although sucrose transporters have not been previously identified in mammals. Mutations in the human P and MATP genes are the cause of tyrosinase-positive forms of albinism, OCA2 and OCA4, respectively. In the absence of normal P-protein, there is a disruption in melanosomal structure, and misrouting of tyrosinase and Tyrp1 to other sites, including the cell membrane.[65,69] The misrouting of melanosomal proteins in p-null melanocytes suggests a role for the P-protein in trafficking or sorting of melanocyte-specific proteins as they leave the Golgi en route to premelanosomes. The effect of the MATP mutation on transport of melanocyte specific proteins is not yet known. Melanosomes in mouse melanocytes with null MATP (underwhite, or uw) are small, irregularly shaped, and less- or nonpigmented when compared with the round or ovoid pigmented melanosomes in wild-type pigment cells. Further experimentation is required to determine the point at which these transporter proteins enter the melanosomes and their role in melanogenesis.

Melanosome Transport to Dendritic Tips

Once melanosomes become enriched with pigment in the cell body (stage IV), they travel to the dendritic tip in a centrifugal manner for transfer to neighboring keratinocytes in the epidermis. The intracellular transport of organelles requires protein motors, cytoskeletal tracks, and

FIGURE 11-12

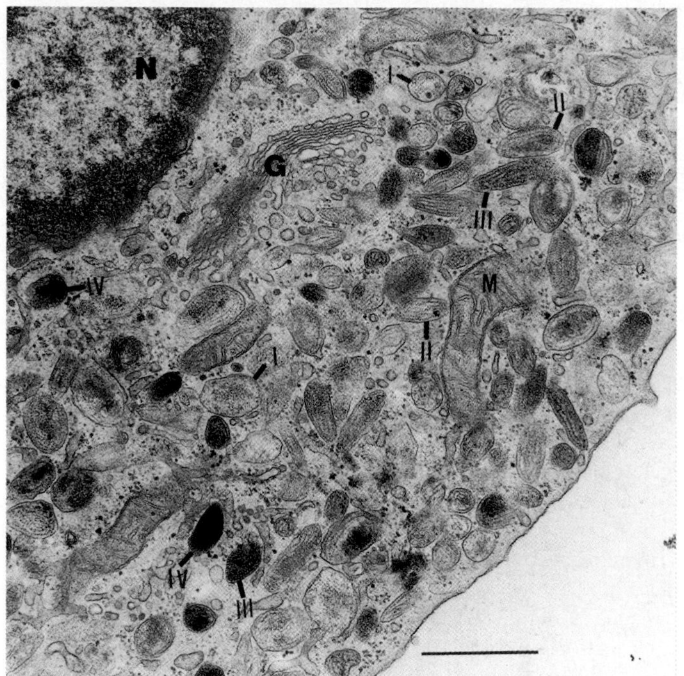

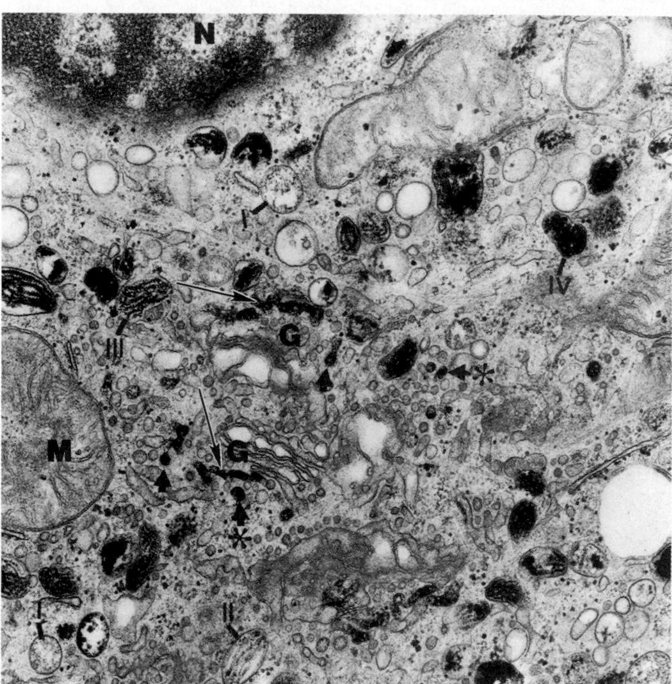

Perinuclear area of normal human melanocytes from a lightly pigmented Caucasian skin demonstrating melanosomes in various stages of maturation. *A.* Melanosomes in the vicinity of the Golgi apparatus (G) exist as stage I premelanosomes (I) that are more oval in shape containing floccular material and short irregular melanofilaments, stage II melanosomes (II) that are more elongated containing an organized, scaffold-like matrix of melanofilaments, stage III melanosomes (III) with melanin being sequentially deposited on the melanofilament matrix, and stage IV melanosomes (IV) with melanin completely filling the organelle and obscuring the matrix. This melanocyte is from a lightly pigmented Caucasian individual and consists of stages II and III melanosomes predominantly, with relatively few stage IV melanosomes. *B.* DOPA reaction products indicating cellular sites of catalytically functional tyrosinase appear in the trans Golgi network (G) including the *trans*-most cisternae (*arrows*), coated vesicles budding from these cisternae (*arrowheads*), and vesicles migrating from the Golgi apparatus (*arrowheads with asterisk*). Reaction products exist in some stage I premelanosomes (I), indicating incorporation of tyrosinase into these organelles. After DOPA histochemistry, this lightly pigmented, white melanocyte consists of stage IV melanosomes predominantly with relatively few stage II and III melanosomes. M, mitochondria; N, nucleus. Bar = 1.0 μm. (*Illustration courtesy of Raymond E. Boissy, Department of Dermatology, University of Cincinnati, Cincinnati, Ohio.*)

adapters/effectors that attach the organelles to the motors. Melanosomes move in a bi-directional manner on microtubules in the dendrites until they are captured at the dendritic tips (Fig. 11-13*A*).

The motor involved in the centrifugal movement of melanosomes to the microtubules and then to the cell periphery remains to be identified. However, genetic analyses of pigmentation mutants that result in the clustering of melanosomes in the cell body or perinuclear region implicate the interplay among several proteins including myosin Va, rab27a, and melanophilin (Mlph).

Myosin V family members such as myosin Va operate in concert with actin filaments that line the cell periphery to move granules to dendritic tips. In the absence of functional myosin Va, the bi-directional movement of melanosomes on microtubules is normal, but the melanosomes fail to accumulate at the dendritic tips. Mutations in Rab27a and Mlph produce a similar phenotype suggesting that these two proteins play a role in the cargo selection by myosin Va. Rab proteins are adapter proteins that are involved in the regulation of intracellular vesicular transport partnered with effector molecules. Together, they provide specificity to steps in the trafficking of intracellular vesicles by promoting the binding and fusion of vesicles destined for specific locations within the cell (reviewed in Ref. 43).

Griscelli syndrome, a rare autosomal recessive disorder, has recently been shown to involve a mutation in *rab27a* and *Myo Va*. While all Griscelli syndrome patients have pigmentation defects, some also possess neurologic or immunologic abnormalities due to defective exocytosis of secretory vesicles from neurons and lytic granules from cytotoxic T lymphocytes, respectively. Griscelli syndrome patients with immune defects have a mutation in rab27a,[70] while patients with neurologic abnormalities have mutations in myosin Va.[71] As expected, defects in these genes cause the accumulation of melanosomes in the cell body[72] (Fig. 11-13*B*), and are likely to have a similar effect on the dispersion of lytic granules in T lymphocytes and secretory vesicles of neurons. The identification and characterization of the melanocyte proteins involved in the transport of melanosomes has helped to provide a more complete diagnosis for patients with Griscelli syndrome.

Melanosome Transfer to Keratinocytes

Melanosomes enriched in pigment at the dendritic tips are translocated to adjacent keratinocytes where the melanin forms a photoprotective cap over the keratinocyte nuclei. Three methods of transfer have been proposed, although the exact mechanism by which this transfer occurs remains unknown (reviewed in Ref. 73).

The first mechanism involves the secretion of the melanosomal contents into the intercellular space by the melanocyte that is then endocytosed by the keratinocyte. This model is supported by the similarities between melanosome and lysosome-related organelles such as secretory lysosomes involved in regulated secretion in hemopoietic cells. This model predicts that the melanosomal proteins could be recycled back to the cell body where they can be used again for melanin production.

The second model proposes the direct fusion of melanocyte and keratinocyte plasma membranes supporting the transfer of melanosomes from one cell to the other. This mechanism predicts the presence of cognate SNARE proteins on the plasma membranes of the melanocyte-keratinocyte that initiate the fusion of the two outer membranes. Model three proposes that the dendritic tips of the melanocyte are phagocytosed by the keratinocyte. Keratinocytes have been observed engulfing dendritic tips and latex beads, exhibiting their phagocytic abilities. This theory further predicts the presence of a keratinocyte receptor because phagocytosis is a receptor-mediated process. Recent studies have identified protease-activated receptor-2 (PAR-2) as a protein that controls melanosome ingestion by keratinocytes after UVB irradiation (see below in "Tanning in Response to UV Light").

FIGURE 11-13

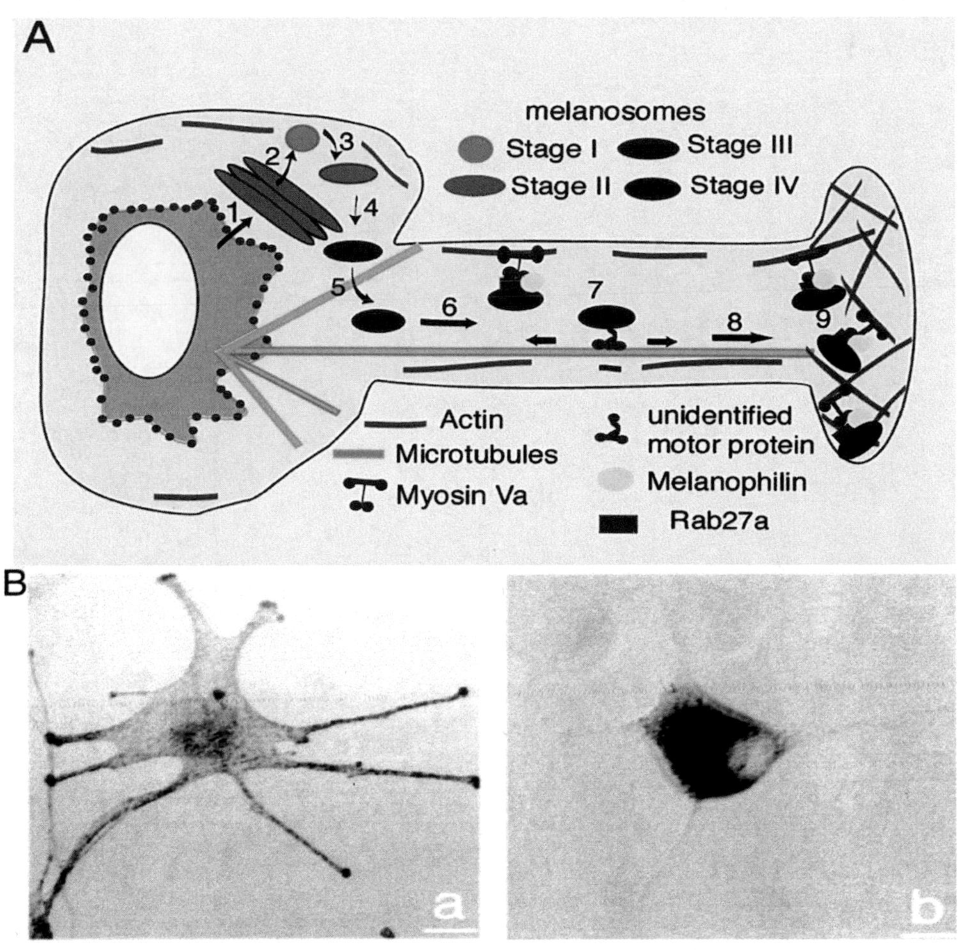

The trafficking of melanosomes and melanosomal-proteins in melanocytes. *A*. Melanosomal proteins are synthesized by cytosolic ribosomes (*blue balls*) that are targeted to the ER (1) where the proteins fold, and receive *N*-linked glycosylations and disulfide bonds. Correctly matured protein is transported through the Golgi cisternae (2) to melanosomes that mature from stage I to stage IV (3 to 5) in the cell body that surrounds the nuclear region. The melanosomes are centrifugally transported to the dendritic tips on microtubules where they are captured by myosin Va-Rab27a-melanophilin complexes associated with actin filaments. This permits the concentration of melanosomes at the cell tip for transfer to neighboring keratinocytes. *B*. Melanosome in melanocytes from a patient with Griscelli syndrome (b) remain restricted to the perinuclear and fail to distribute to the dendrites as seen in normal melanocytes (a). (*From Bahadoran P et al*[72]*, with permission.*)

PIGMENTATION CONTROL BY MELANOCORTINS AND THE MELANOCORTIN RECEPTOR

The Melanocortins and Their Receptors

The melanocortin receptor (MCR) has a central role in constitutive skin color and hair pigmentation and in the ability to tan in response to sunlight. Most red-haired light-skin individuals carry inactive variants of the MCR (see below in "Regulation and Function of MCR Activity"). Our present understanding of the diverse physiologic roles of the MCRs dates back to the first published report by Fuchs, who, in 1912, described an activity in extract from bovine pituitary that caused darkening of frog skin (reviewed in Ref. 74). This easy assay for the detection of biologic activity of what was termed melanocyte-stimulating hormone, or MSH, was instrumental in identifying the ligand and receptor.

The melanocortins (or MSHs) are a group of peptides derived from a common precursor proopiomelanocortin (POMC) produced in the intermediate lobe of the pituitary, as well as in other tissues, such as the skin. POMC encodes several peptides, γ-MSH, α-MSH, ACTH, β-MSH γ-lipotropin, and β-endorphin, with diverse biological functions (reviewed in Refs. 75 and 76) (Table 11–2 and Fig. 11-14*A*). The various peptides are produced by endoproteolytic cleavage mediated by two prohormone convertases (PC1 and PC2) that recognize in each region a paired basic amino acid residue (Arg and Lys) (Fig. 11-14*A*). The hyperpigmentation induced in sun-exposed areas in individuals injected with the superpotent MSH,[77] or the darkening of the skin in patients with Addison's disease that causes hypersecretion of ACTH, indicate that stimulation of the MCR receptor in vivo enhances eumelanin synthesis in human melanocytes. Under normal conditions, the likely source of POMC for melanocytes is skin keratinocytes and not the pituitary, because patients who suffer loss of pituitary function due to tumor growth or other causes have normal pigmentation.

The melanogenic peptides share a tetrapeptide core indispensable for the recognition and activation of the MCR (Fig. 11-14*A*). Each of the processed peptides also undergoes posttranslational modifications, such as amidation, acetylation, and glycosylation that stabilize the protein and/or enhance its biological activity. Although α-MSH is the most potent of the peptides for melanogenic activity, a synthetic peptide in which methionine is replaced with norleucine and L-phenylalanine with D-phenylalanine has a further enhanced activity.[77]

The melanocortins bind to and activate their cognate melanocortin receptor (MC1-R) (Fig. 11-14*B*), a member of a family of receptors for MSH and ACTH peptides, each with a distinct distribution and distinct physiologic roles (Table 11–2). Five genes encoding receptors for melanocortin peptides have been identified, and all belong to

TABLE 11-2

Distribution, Function, and Localization of the Melanocortin Receptor (MCR)

RECEPTOR	LIGAND	FUNCTION	CHROMOSOMAL LOCALIZATION
MC1-R	α-MSH ACTH	Melanocyte pigmentation	16q2
MC2-R	ACTH	Adrenal function	18p11.2
MC3-R	α-MSH γ-MSH ACTH	Cardiovascular regulation	20q13.2
MC4-R	α-MSH ACTH	Energy homeostasis	18q22
MC5-R	α-MSH ACTH	Exocrine secretion	18p11

Among the POMS peptides, the role of β-MSH has not yet been determined, thus its cognate receptor in vivo is not identified. In vitro, β-MSH can bind the MC1-R and induce melanogenesis.

the superfamily of G-protein–coupled seven-membrane–spanning receptors. In addition to pigmentation, they participate in other physiologic functions such as obesity, inflammation, thermoregulation, energy homeostasis, and exocrine gland secretion (reviewed in Refs. 74 to 76).

Regulation and Function of Melanocortin Receptor Activity

MCR activity is mediated through activation or inhibition of adenylyl cyclase that induce changes in intracellular cAMP [cyclic adenosine monophosphate (reviewed in Ref. 74)]. Melanocortins activate, whereas agouti and agouti-related protein (AGRP) block, the stimulation of adenylyl cyclase[78] (Fig. 11-15*A*). The changes in intracellular levels of cAMP modulate the expression of several melanocyte specific genes, including tyrosinase and Tyrp1 (Fig. 11-15*B*, *C*), likely by regulating the activity and expression of the transcription factor Mitf (see below about Mitf in "Regulators of Melanocyte-Specific Gene Expression"). Agouti is a competitive antagonist of the MCR, with high affinities for MC1-R in the skin and MC4-R in the brain (reviewed in Refs. 75 and 79): In mouse skin, agouti is secreted by dermal papillae cells, adjacent to melanocytes. Blockade in melanocortin action at the MC1-R by agouti induces melanocytes to produce the red-yellow color pheomelanin instead of the dark-brown eumelanin (reviewed in Refs. 74 and 79). However, agouti's role in human pigmentation has not yet been established. No polymorphisms in the coding region of *agouti* were found in individuals with different racial backgrounds expressing different levels and kinds of skin and hair coloration, indicating that the human agouti is unlikely to function in normal human pigmentation.[80]

Genetic analysis provides the strongest evidence for the MC1-R receptor function on pigment cells in human skin and hair. The common phenotype of individuals with inactive MC1-R is red hair and pale skin resulting from a low eumelanin-to-pheomelanin ratio. These individuals have normal density of melanocytes in the skin and other sites. Sequencing the MC1-R receptor revealed variation in the coding regions that were more common in red-haired light-skin individuals as compared with dark-haired easy-to-tan individuals (reviewed in Ref. 81). In particular, the red-haired population is homozygous for Arg151Cys, Arg160Trp, or Asp294His, and, in rarer cases, for Arg142His (Fig. 11-14*B*). The presence of one allele carried a sixfold risk ratio of red hair (i.e., heterozygote individuals) and the presence of two alleles carried a twentyfold risk ratio of red hair (i.e., compound heterozygote). Each of these alleles inactivate the MC1-R receptor, suppressing the production of cAMP by adenylate cyclase. An inactivating mutation in POMC is also associated with red hair in addition to a more complicated endocrine phenotype.[76] Therefore, the presence of inactive MC1-R is a major determinant for sun-sensitivity and increased risk to develop melanomas.[81,82] It should be noted, however, that there is a rare red-haired population that do not carry the common inactivating MC1-R variants, nor mutations in POMC, and there are dark-haired individuals carrying MC1-R inactivating variants, indicating that other genes may determine the red hair phenotype (reviewed in Ref. 81).

FIGURE 11-14

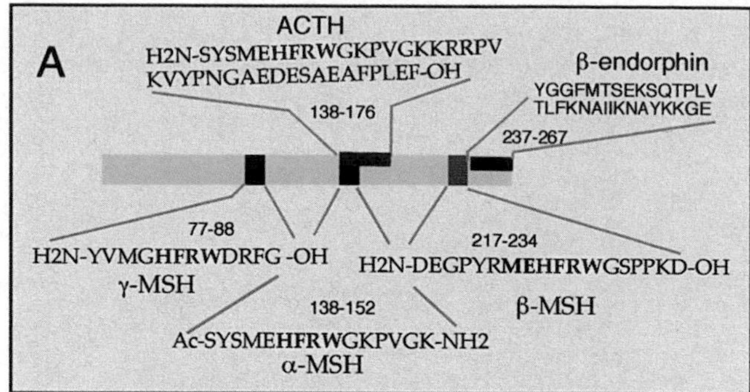

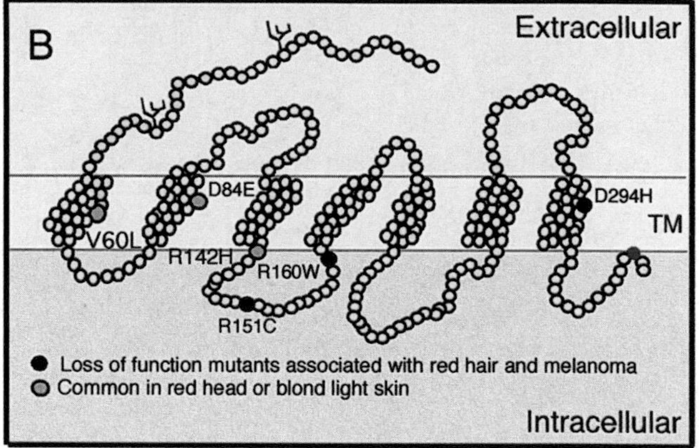

The MCR and its ligands. *A*. Structure of the proopiomelanocortin precursor. Standard abbreviations for amino acids are used. The synthetic superactive α-MSH analogue NDP-α-MSH is modified by the exchange of methionine (M) with norleucine and L-phenylalanine (F) with D-phenylalanine. Ac, acetylated; NH_2, amidated. In red are critical amino acids required for binding to the MCR. *B*. Schematic representation of the human MC1-R receptor. Each of the 318 amino acid residues in the polypeptide chain of the receptor is represented by an empty circle. Branched structures represent *N*-linked glycosylation sites. Reduced function mutants (*red circles*), variants common in red- or blond-haired and fair skin individuals (*orange circles*), and the conserved *C*-terminal cysteine (*green circle*), the possible site for fatty acid acylation and anchoring to the plasma membrane, are indicated. TM, transmembrane domain.

TANNING IN RESPONSE TO UV LIGHT

Sun-exposed tanning is one of the most visible manifestations of pigment cell activity in the skin and is the natural defense against the deleterious effect of UV radiation. The solar radiation that activates melanocytes is in the nonvisible range of ultraviolet (UV) light (290 to 400 nm). UV light acts as a mutagen and a tumor promoter. It induces cellular damage, including oncogenic mutations and promotes melanocyte proliferation. Excessive exposure to UV light early in life can be manifested later on as malignant transformation of melanocytes, i.e., melanomas due to the proliferation of DNA-damaged neonatal melanocyte progenitors[83,84] (see also Chaps. 38 and 134).

Immediate Pigment Darkening

Tanning develops in two phases, the early (transitory) and late (stable) response. The immediate transitory darkening in response to long-wave ultraviolet radiation (UVA, 340 to 400 nm) is known as *immediate pigment darkening* (IPD). Its physiologic role is not clear because it provides very little protection against harmful solar radiation. The principal mechanism is photo-oxidation of preexisting melanin, melanin precursors, and/or melanin metabolites.[85,86] The effect of UVA on melanocytes is direct, as the presence of keratinocytes does not modulate the response.[87] Other proposed changes, such as in cytoskeletal distribution, movement of melanosomes to melanocyte dendrites, increased melanosome transfer, and changes in the pattern of melanosome distribution within keratinocytes, remain controversial[86] (see also Chap. 88).

FIGURE 11-15

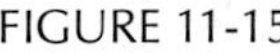

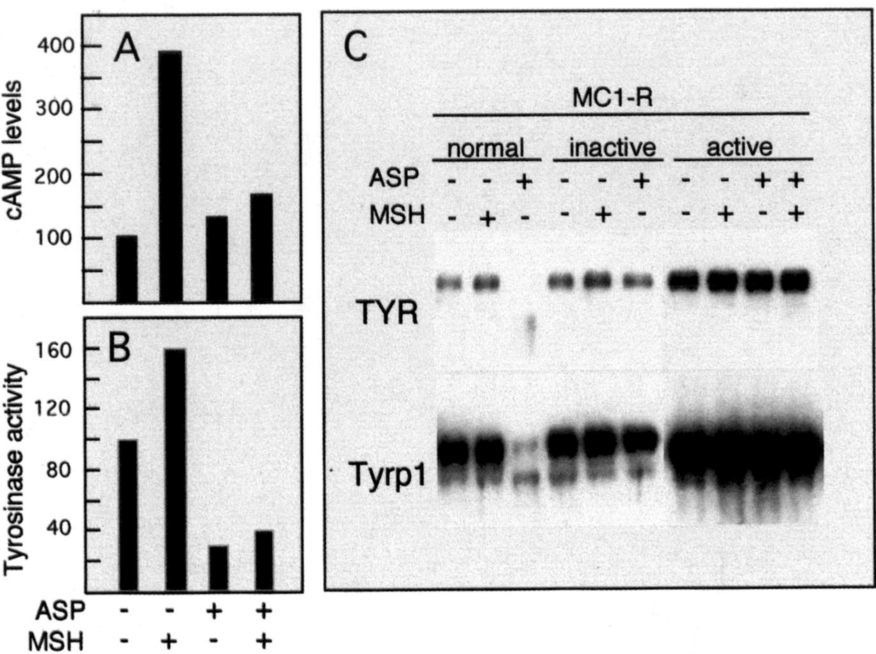

Physiologic evidence that α-MSH and agouti (ASP) act on MC1-R. Mouse melanocytes were incubated in medium with no addition (−), 1 nM α-MSH, 10 nM ASP, or with both (+). *A.* Intracellular levels of cAMP in wild-type mouse melanocytes at the end of 40-min incubation. *B.* Tyrosinase enzymatic activity in wild-type mouse melanocytes at the end of 6-day incubation. Values are expressed as a percent of control (no addition). *C.* Ligand modulation of tyrosinase and Tyrp1 is contingent on the presence of normal, wild-type MC1-R. Mouse melanocytes expressing normal wild-type (E^+/E^+), inactive mutant (e/e), or constitutively active (E^{so}/E^{so}) MC1-R were treated as indicated above each lane. Cell extracts were collected at the end of 6-day incubation and subjected to Western blot analysis for tyrosinase (TYR) and Tyrp1 as indicated.

The Stable Response: Indirect Effects of Ultraviolet on Melanocytes

The long-term effect on pigmentation in response to UV irradiation is due to both direct and indirect effects on melanocytes. UV light activates melanocyte proliferation, the production of melanin and the transfer of melanosomes to keratinocytes. The most convincing evidence for the indirect effect of UV light is the observation that the number of dividing melanocytes increases not only in the exposed skin but also in shielded areas[88] (reviewed in Ref. 89). The major components that mediate the indirect activation are epidermal keratinocytes and probably fibroblasts in the stroma. UVB activates keratinocytes and fibroblasts to produce factors that stimulate melanocytes. These factors include bFGF, HGF/SF, MGF (Steel factor), ET1, POMC, nitric oxide, and proinflammatory cytokines. Some of these factors, such as bFGF, HGF/SF, and ET1, are potent melanocyte mitogens that act in synergy.[90] ET1, in addition, increases dendricity, and MGF/Steel and POMC are particularly efficient at upregulation of pigmentation. UVB activation of POMC expression in keratinocytes in vivo precedes the activation of melanocyte specific genes involved in pigment synthesis such as tyrosinase, Tyrp1, DCT, and gp100/Pmel17, suggesting a cause and effect[91] (Fig. 11-16). The increase in POMC production in response to UVB may also serve to amplify the signal because MSH increases the levels of cell surface receptors in melanocytes.[92] UV enhances the availability of growth factors by regulating the levels of the respective mRNAs for POMC and for various cytokines,[93] or by activation of the plasminogen activator-plasmin system that induces the release of latent stores in the extracellular matrix.[94,95]

Tanning in response to UVB irradiation is further amplified by the enhanced keratinocyte uptake of melanosomes. This process is mediated at least in part by PAR-2.[73,96] PAR-2 is a seven-transmembrane G-protein–coupled receptor that is related to, but distinct from, the thrombin receptors.[73] Cleavage of the extracellular domain of PARs by serine proteases exposes new N-termini, which then act as tethered ligands (Fig. 11-17*A*). This activation process can be mimicked by the synthetic peptide SLIGKV that corresponds to the newly created N-termini, and is inhibited by trypsin inhibitors. A role for PAR-2 in melanosomal uptake was demonstrated by increased melanosome uptake by keratinocytes in response to SLIGKV. Furthermore, UVB irradiation induces secretion of protease in keratinocytes, which cleaves a peptide comprising the PAR-2 cleavage site in a dose-dependent manner. In an experimental skin model, UVB-induced tanning was inhibited by trypsin inhibitor. Similarly, PAR-2 distribution in the human epidermis that is skin-type-dependent is upregulated following UV irradiation (Fig. 11-17*B*), and topical treatments with trypsin inhibitors prevent UV-induced tanning,[96] demonstrating its role in melanosome transfer and the tanning response.

Direct Effect of Ultraviolet B on Melanocytes

UVB induces a transient increase in DNA synthesis and upregulation of melanocyte specific genes in pure cultures of melanocytes, indicating a direct effect not mediated by keratinocytes. This stimulatory activity is likely to be mediated by UV-induced activation of growth factor receptors, as shown for the epidermal growth factor receptor and the insulin receptor.[97,98] Receptor activation leads to signaling through several intermediates, including Grb-2, phospholipase C-γ, and Shc, to the Ras-MAPK cascade (see below, "Melanocyte Growth Factors and Signal Transduction"). This ligand-independent receptor activation is mediated by partial inactivation of receptor-directed tyrosine phosphatases (PTP), such as SHP-1, RPTPα, RPTPσ, and DEP-1, that

FIGURE 11-16

Upregulation of melanocyte-specific genes in human skin in vivo in response to UVB radiation. The expression of POMC in keratinocytes and a panel of melanocyte specific genes (as indicated) in melanocytes is detected by in situ hybridization with gene-specific probes. *A*. POMC expression after 2 days of UVB treatment (equivalent to 2 MED). Very small changes were detected in mRNA levels of melanocyte-specific genes in melanocytes (not shown). *B*. Expression of mRNA after 5 days of UV treatment. Skin sections from control non-irradiated and UVB-irradiated areas stained with the indicated probes are presented. POMC, precursor proopiomelanocortin; TYR, tyrosinase; DCT, DOPAchrome tautomerase. (*From Suzuki I et al,*[91] *with permission.*)

downregulate receptor autophosphorylation.[98] Consequently, receptor activation by UV is likely to involve mostly receptors that are overexpressed at the cell membrane and that undergo spontaneous dimerization and *trans*-phosphorylation/activation.[99] Suppression of PTP by UV could be caused by oxidation of the active center cysteine through an

FIGURE 11-17

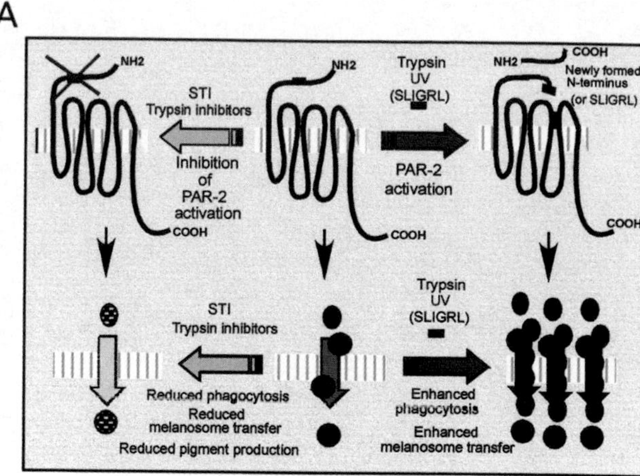

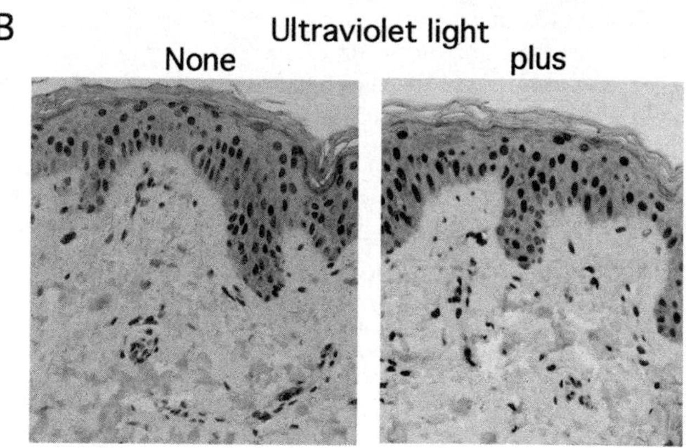

PAR-2 activation and melanosomal transfer in response to UVB irradiation. *A*. Representation of PAR-2 activation and inhibition and the effects on keratinocyte phagocytosis and melanosome transfer. STI, soybean trypsin inhibitor. *(From Seiberg M,*[73] *with permission.)* *B*. UVB upregulates PAR-2 expression in type I human skin. Representative samples of control and 24-h UVR-treated skin sections stained for PAR-2. Control shows predominantly basal distribution of PAR-2, whereas immunoreactivity of PAR-2 in postirradiated skin is throughout the epidermis. (*From Scott GA et al,*[96] *with permission.*)

oxidative intermediate because it was prevented and partially reversed by the thiol-protecting agent *N*-acetylcysteine (NAC).[98]

An alternative pathway, which may contribute to tyrosinase upregulation, involves UVB-induced phosphorylation of the transcription factor USF-1 by the stress kinase p38.[100] In this scenario, constitutive expression of tyrosinase is dependent on Mitf, but activation above basal levels is contingent on USF-1 activation. The p38-signaling cascade plays a major role in the cellular response to stress or proinflammatory cytokines. Therefore, activation of p38 may also be induced indirectly by the proinflammatory cytokines produced by UV-irradiated keratinocytes.[93]

REGULATORS OF MELANOCYTE-SPECIFIC GENE EXPRESSION

Melanocyte-specific genes are induced as neural crest cells destined to become melanocytes migrate out and reach their site of residency. The precise timing of each melanocytic marker is not clear. However, Mitf appear first, followed by DCT, Tyrp1, and tyrosinase.

The among the proteins that have been studied, it is apparent that Kit and observations that Mitf/Kit/DCT/ Tyrp1-positive amelanotic melanocytes are present in the hair follicle, and possibly also in the skin, are consistent with the notion that tyrosinase expression and/or activity are among the last to be established. Therefore, the definitions of a melanoblast and a melanocyte-precursor will be more precise once the panel of melanocyte-specific genes expressed by these cells is determined.

Numerous transcription factors play critical roles in regulating gene expression within developing melanocytes and their precursors. Mitf is most notable among the transcription factors whose mutations specifically affect melanocyte development. Mitf is a transcription factor in the basic/helix-loop-helix/leucine-zipper family, which includes the closely related factors TFE3, TFEC, and TFEB, and the less-closely related Myc proto-oncogene and USF families with which it shares nearly identical DNA binding (and possibly target gene) specificity. Mitf first plays a role in promoting the transition of precursor cells to melanoblasts and, subsequently, in melanoblast survival by influencing Kit expression.[101] Mitf expression is maintained during early and late stages of melanocyte development from the neural crest and later on in the normal adult epidermal melanocytes. Although the precise identity of Mitf's target genes remains incomplete, the consensus DNA sequence recognized by Mitf is found (and highly conserved) in many of the major pigmentation genes including tyrosinase, Tyrp1, DCT, and AIM-1/MATP (reviewed in Refs. 68 and 102). This observation, coupled to Mitf's ability to stimulate artificial promoters derived from these genes, as well as Mitf's regulation by the melanocortin signaling pathway (see below, in "Transcriptional Regulation of Mitf Expression" and "Post-Translational Regulation of Mitf"), suggest that Mitf plays a central role in regulating the pigmentation response in melanocytes.

FIGURE 11-18

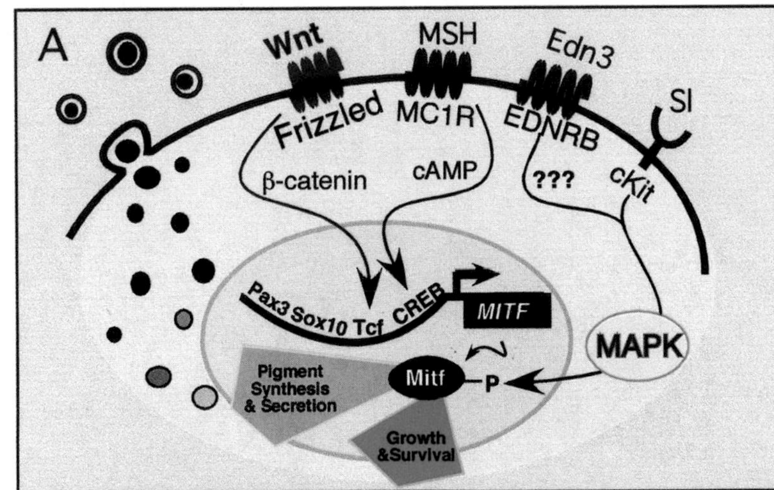

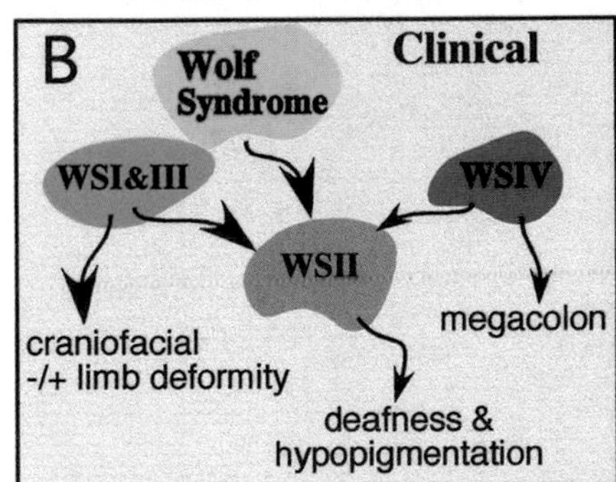

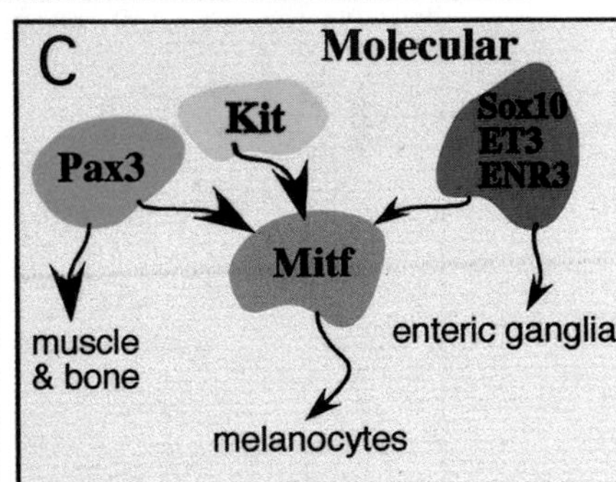

Regulation of Mitf in response to extracellular signals. *A*. Activation of a cell surface receptor induces *MITF* expression via the β-catenin and cAMP pathway (induced by Frizzled and the MCR receptors) that impacts on activation of Tcf/Lef and CREB transcription factors, or via phosphorylation induced by MAPK activation (denoted by P). *B* and *C*. Representation of human syndromic deafness conditions associated with hypopigmentation. *B*. Clinical overlaps and divergences. *C*. Molecular relationships of genes implicated in each syndrome. (*From Price ER, Fisher DE*[6], *with permission.*)

Other transcription factors that exert major effect on melanocytes are Sox10 and Pax3, members of transcription factor families heavily implicated in developmental regulation for multiple organ systems. Both are expressed early in melanocyte development, and both are likely to remain active at later stages as well. As neural crest cells arrive at the dorsolateral surface, there is some evidence that they retain the capacity to differentiate into either glial cells or melanocytes. This dual lineage choice matches the expression pattern for Sox10, which is seen in both glial tumors and melanomas. In fact, these cancer types share a number of biological features, which, for the most part, connote poor prognosis, and it is plausible that Sox10 expression may underlie some of the shared characteristics.[6,103,104]

Transcriptional Regulation of Mitf Expression

The Mitf gene has multiple promoters, each of which contributes alternative initial exons via splicing to a common downstream body of the gene. The major transactivation, DNA binding, and dimerization motifs are all located within the common region of Mitf, so that alternative promoter/first exon usage may be more important for tissue specific expression than for varied protein functions. One of the promoters is thought to be only active in melanocytes and insights into the regulation of this element have provided a remarkable mechanistic linkage for multiple disease genes and factors vital to melanocyte development[5,102,105] (Fig. 11-18*A*, *B*). For example, this melanocyte-restricted Mitf promoter contains a perfect consensus binding sequence for the Tcf/Lef family, which recruits β-catenin as part of the Wnt signaling pathway critical to early neural crest–melanocyte differentiation (Fig. 11-18*C*). Another sequence element, located ~50 base pairs downstream of the TCF/Lef site, is a consensus for the CREB/ATF transcription factor family. CREB becomes activated by phosphorylation after MSH stimulation and is responsible for activating Mitf expression in that context (reviewed in Refs. 5 and 6). Approximately 50 base pairs upstream of the TCF/Lef, site two additional DNA sequence elements are found, one which is recognized by Sox10 and one by Pax3 (Fig. 11-18*C*). Each of these Mitf promoter elements is conserved across species between human and mouse and appears to place the transcriptional regulation of Mitf in the center of multiple signaling and transcriptional pathways, which are vital to melanocyte development.

Posttranslational Regulation of Mitf

Several growth factors receptor systems impact Mitf activity and expression in melanocytes (Fig. 11-18*C*). Activation of Kit by Steel results in MAP kinase-mediated phosphorylation of Mitf at a serine residue

FIGURE 11-19

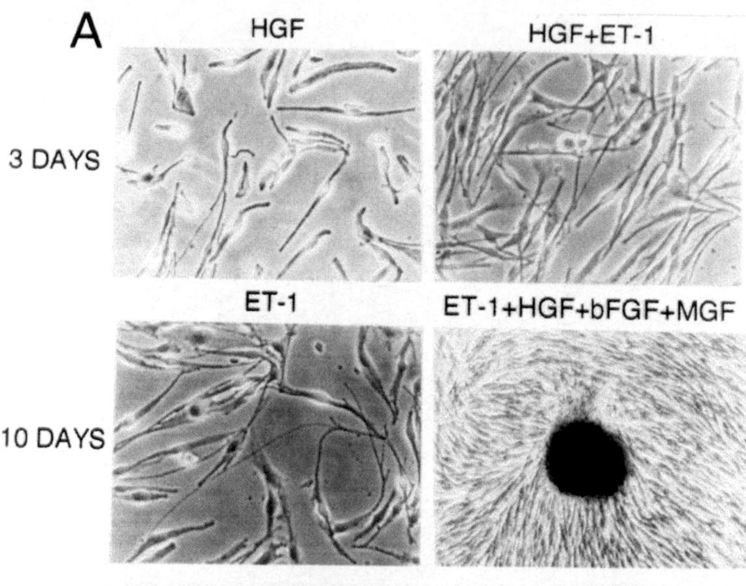

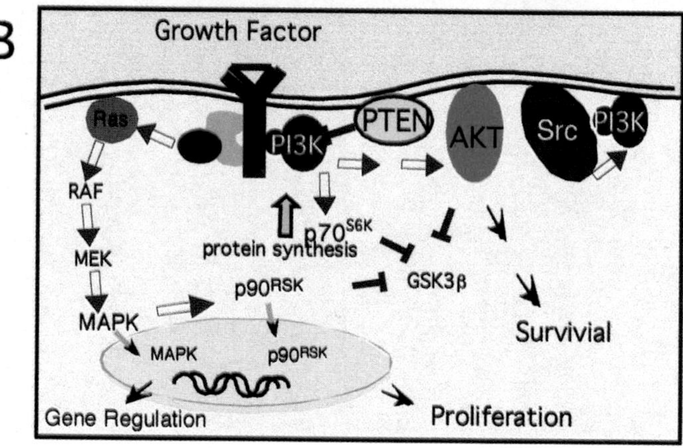

Proliferation and signal transduction in normal human melanocytes. *A.* Proliferative synergism among selected peptide growth factors. Normal neonatal human melanocytes were incubated in chemically defined medium in the presence of specific peptide growth factors. The photomicrographs show morbid melanocytes cultured for 3 days in the presence of HGF/SF alone (*top left*), proliferating melanocytes in HGF/SF plus ET1 (*top right*), surviving cells with ET1 alone for 10 days (*bottom left*), and highly proliferating cells in presence of four growth factors as indicated (*bottom right*). (*From Böhm M et al*[91], *with permission.*) *B.* The critical intermediates in growth factor–mediated signal transduction. The phosphorylated tyrosine residues on the activated receptor create docking sites for several preformed complexes of proteins that induce Ras activation by exchanging GDP (guanine diphosphate) with GTP (guanine triphosphate). Ras, in turn, activates a series of tyrosine and serine/threonine kinases known as the MAPK and the PI3K cascades (*orange arrows*). The message emanating from the cell surface is then delivered to the transcriptional machinery in the nucleus by the translocation of phosphorylated forms of several intermediates including MAPK and $p90^{RSK}$ (*arrows*). In addition, the activated Ser/Thr kinases phosphorylate GSK3β and inactivate its kinase activity (*red bars*). Consequently, factors regulating growth as well as differentiation are induced. Constitutive activation of some members in this pathway, such as aberrant production of growth factors that constantly activate their receptor, overexpression and/or mutational activation of a receptor, and Ras activation (by mutations or by receptor activation), can lead to perpetual mode of proliferation and cellular transformation. *C.* Control of cell-cycle progression by pocket proteins pRb-regulated E2F transcription factors. The model depicts the accepted hypothesis by which mitogenic signals upregulate CDK activity and phosphorylate/inactivate proteins from the retinoblastoma tumor suppressor family (pRb, p107, and p130) (*green arrow*), allowing the production of free E2F transcription factor and the progression from quiescence (G_0/G_1 phase) to DNA synthesis (S phase). Key molecules in CDK regulation are the positive activators cyclins, and the negative regulators, such as $p16^{INK4}$ (*brown arrow*).

(S73), which is highly conserved between species. In addition, MAP kinase activates a second kinase, $p90^{RSK}$, to phosphorylate Mitf at another serine residue (S409). These phosphorylations have the dual effect of enhancing binding by coactivators of the p300 family (thus enhancing gene expression), and targeting Mitf for rapid degradation by the ubiquitin-proteasome pathway, a common end-result for activated transcription factors.[106] Rsk activation is also important because one of its known targets is CREB, through which it is likely to upregulate the Mitf promoter in melanocytes. Other ligand/receptor systems also activate MAP kinase, such as HGF/Met, ET3/EdnrB, and α-MSH/melanocortin, suggesting that Mitf is a common target for extracellular signals (reviewed in Ref. 5).

Mitf and Inherited Human Pigmentation Disorders

Mitf's role as a factor upon which multiple melanocyte developmental pathways converge is highlighted by the phenotypic and molecular defects seen in a group of related human pigmentation disorders. These disorders most prominently affect melanocyte viability (rather than melanin production per se) and therefore exhibit associated clinical features such as deafness, due to deficiencies of inner ear melanocytes. Waardenburg syndrome (WS) encompasses many of these disorders (see also Chap. 90). It is an autosomal dominant disorder (therefore affecting heterozygotes) characterized by a white forelock and sensorineural deafness. The syndrome is subdivided into four subtypes on the basis of presence or absence of additional discrete clinical features. Type II WS exhibits a "core" melanocyte phenotype, while types I and III exhibit, in addition, craniofacial and skeletal deformities and type IV exhibits megacolon due to defective neural crest–derived enteric ganglia. Additional highly related clinical conditions are Wolf syndrome and Tietz-Smith syndrome, both of which exhibit the core melanocyte defects, though of variable severity.

Molecular lesions have been defined for most of these clinical entities and provide a remarkable linkage to the mechanistic pathways outlined above. WSII patients contain either mutations within Mitf itself or another gene yet to be identified. WSI and III patients harbor mutations within Pax3, and WSIV patients contain mutations in Sox10, ET3, or EdnrB.[6] In addition, Tietz-Smith syndrome patients contain Mitf mutations and Wolf syndrome patients contain inactivating mutations in *c*-kit. Thus a picture emerges wherein the phenotypic consequences of specific molecular lesions reflect the developmental requirements for specific factors in melanocytes and sometimes nonmelanocytes. The melanocyte phenotypes for all these mutants might arise through their common targeting of Mitf, while the nonmelanocyte phenotypes are particular to the other lineages in which the factor(s) are expressed (such as enteric ganglia precursors for Sox10). These molecular-phenotypic connections have enlightened the understanding of the pathways through which environmental cues transmit discrete signals to the nucleus, and the resulting transcriptional programs of importance to the developing melanocyte. Because Mitf is such a key transcriptional regulator in melanocytes, it will be of considerable interest to identify its target genes. This point is particularly pertinent because of the evidence implicating Mitf in both proliferation/survival and pigmentation/differentiation pathways.

MELANOCYTE GROWTH FACTORS AND SIGNAL TRANSDUCTION

FIGURE 11-19 (*Continued*)

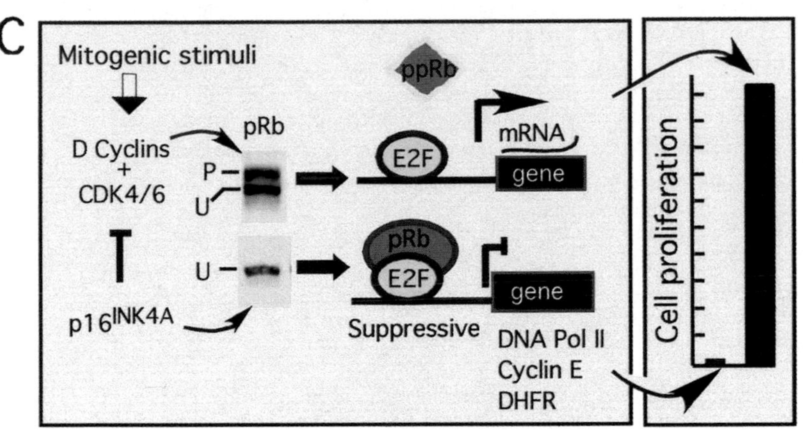

For a long time, the study of melanocyte proliferation in vitro was restricted to the use of melanoma cells (especially the murine melanoma B16 and Cloudman S91 cell lines), because attempts to establish normal melanocytes in culture using the standard, serum-supplemented medium, failed. As it turned out, this particular feature of normal melanocytes is the key for understanding their growth controls, as well as phenotypic changes during malignant transformation. Studies by several investigators have shown that, in addition to common mammalian growth factors such as insulin and transferrin, melanocytes require at least two stimulators that act in synergy (reviewed in Ref. 89) (Fig. 11-19*A*). The list of synergistic peptide mitogens for human melanocytes in vitro, mirrors that required for melanocyte development during embryogenesis. They include HGF, Steel factor, ET1, and FGF2). So far, FGF2 is the only growth factor without a parallel inherited depigmentation defect. One possible reason is the numerous peptide growth factors in this family with overlapping activity (22 all together).

Signal Transduction: Immediate Events

Stimulation by growth factors activates the cognate receptors and triggers within seconds, the activation of key regulators of cell growth, such as Ras, which, in turn, activates multiple effector pathways including the Raf/Mek/MAPK cascade (for short, the MAPK pathway, mitogen-activated protein kinase, known also as extracellular-signal regulated kinase or ERK) and PI3K (reviewed in Ref. 107) (Fig. 11-19*B*). Each of the melanocyte growth factors described above can activate Ras effectors to various degrees, such as the downstream targets MAPK, p90^{RSK}, and p70 S6 kinase.[90,108] The phosphorylation of some of the intermediates, such as MAPK and p90^{RSK}, serves to transport them to the nucleus, where they phosphorylate nuclear factors (such as Mitf and CREB) and change their transcriptional activity via the recruitment of critical elements such as CBP (CREB binding protein). However, proliferation requires high levels and prolonged duration of the phosphorylated/activated state of the signal transduction intermediates, induced only by synergistic growth factors[90] (Fig. 11-19*B*). The stringent requirement for synergistic growth factors may explain the relatively quiescent nature of melanocytes in the skin. Although keratinocytes produce FGF2 continuously, other growth factors, such as ET1 may be induced only in response to UVB irradiation. Interestingly, as melanocytes become senescent and stop proliferating, they also lose their ability to activate the MAPK cascade (reviewed in Ref. 109), in agreement with the pivotal role of this pathway in cell division.

Signal Transduction: The RB/E2F Pathway

The growth factor–activated MAPK pathway mediates transit of quiescent cells into DNA synthesis (G_1- to S-phase of the cell cycle). This occurs, in large part, by activating a group of cyclin-dependent kinases (CDK2, CDK4, and CDK6) responsible for the sequential phosphorylation and inactivation of the pRb (retinoblastoma) family of tumor suppressor proteins (pRb, p107, and p130).[110] The pRb proteins are regarded as master regulators of the cell cycle governing the restriction (R) point, i.e., the point of commitment from quiescence (G_0/G_1) to DNA synthesis (S), by regulating the activity of transcription factors from the E2F family (reviewed in Ref. 111).

The activity of CDKs is coordinated by association with the positive cyclin partners (cyclin D, cyclin A, and cyclin E), and the negative regulators cyclin-dependent kinase inhibitors, termed CKI, belonging to the INK or CIP/KIP families of inhibitors, as well as by site-specific phosphorylations or dephosphorylations carried out by the cyclin activating kinase (CAK) and Cdc25 phosphatase, respectively. Hyperphosphorylation of pRb and family members releases their suppressive association with E2F transcription factors (E2F1 to E2F5). This leads to the accumulation of E2F transcriptional activity and activation of genes responsible for cell-cycle progression (cyclin A, cyclin D1, cyclin E, cdc2, p107, and p21^{CIP1}), DNA synthesis (dihydrofolate reductase and DNA polymerase α), and transcription factors c-MYC, c-MYB, B-MYB, as well as E2F1 and E2F2, that participate in induction of early and late response genes (Fig. 11-19*C*).

Dysregulation of the Rb/E2F pathway is considered a major pathogenic event in cancer cells, including melanomas. Decreased p16^{INK4A} CDK-inhibitory activity, which results from gene deletion, transcriptional silencing, or mutation is common in melanomas (reviewed in Ref. 112). Ablation of p16^{IKN4A} in mice leads to the development of several tumors, including melanoma, a process enhanced by treatments with a carcinogen.[113] However, elimination of the negative regulators of CDKs is not sufficient to cause an immediate change in the growth properties of melanocytes. Individuals homozygous for null p16^{IKN4A} mutations do not always develop melanomas, and mouse melanocytes with homozygous disruption of p16^{INK4A}, p21^{CIP1}, or p27^{KIP1} are dependent on, and respond normally to, mitogenic stimuli. Furthermore, although p21^{CIP1} and p27^{KIP1} were originally described as a CDK inhibitors when artificially expressed at high levels, more recent studies demonstrated that these two proteins have a positive role in proliferation by facilitating multicomplex formation between cyclins, CDK, and associated proteins.

E2F Transcription Factors

Exposure to synergistic growth factors, such as FGF2 in combination with HGF/SF, or ET1, or all three factors, is required for maximum stimulation of cyclin levels (cyclin D1 and cyclin A), phosphorylation of the three pRb family of proteins (pRb, p107, and p130), and the accumulation of free E2F-DNA binding activity[114] (Fig. 11-19*C*). Interestingly, E2F-DNA binding analysis revealed that among the five E2F family members, E2F2 and E2F4 contribute to the major E2F-binding activity in proliferating melanocytes. In growth factor–starved melanocytes, free (and active) E2F-DNA binding activity is drastically reduced, and transcriptional suppressive activity composed of E2F4 in complex with p130, and to a lesser extent pRb, accumulates.[114] In melanoma cells, in contrast, E2F-DNA binding activity is constitutively high, even in the absence of melanocyte growth factors, due mostly to inactivation of pRb by persistent CDK activity and upregulation of the E2F dimerization partner DP1.[114] Inhibition of CDK activity in melanoma cells reconstitutes pRb growth suppressive activity, suggesting a mechanism to control this tumor in patients.

FUTURE PERSPECTIVES

Enormous strides have been made in our understanding of the molecular, cellular, and genetic makeup of pigment cells, since their original description 100 years ago. Indeed, melanocyte biology has emerged as a paradigm for the understanding of tissue-restricted development and homeostasis, based largely upon the rich resource of human and animal genetic mutations whose altered pigmentation minimally affects survival of the host. The future promises increasing opportunities to connect these genetic lesions to the mechanistic pathways they modulate. With the arrival of the postgenomic era, it is increasingly feasible to surmise transcriptional regulatory networks that will connect the effectors of pigmentation to the networks that regulate them. Proteomics promises to provide a new dimension to this analysis, because much of melanocyte biology is regulated at the posttranslational level. Melanocytes represent a novel cell population with the unique mission of protecting and even embellishing the host through pigmentation. Unfortunately, melanocytes also participate in some of the worst human diseases such as melanoma, which will, hopefully, be more effectively treated as the inner workings of this cell are revealed.

REFERENCES

1. Christiansen JH, Coles EG, Wilkinson DG: Molecular control of neural crest formation, migration and differentiation. *Curr Opin Cell Biol* **12**:719, 2000
2. Jin EJ et al: Wnt and BMP signaling govern lineage segregation of melanocytes in the avian embryo. *Dev Biol* **233**:22, 2001
3. Dunn KJ et al: Neural crest-directed gene transfer demonstrates Wnt1 role in melanocyte expansion and differentiation during mouse development. *Proc Natl Acad Sci U S A* **97**:10050, 2000
4. Grimes CA, Jope RS: The multifaceted roles of glycogen synthase kinase 3beta in cellular signaling. *Prog Neurobiol* **65**:391, 2001
5. Goding CR: MITF from neural crest to melanoma: Signal transduction and transcription in the melanocyte lineage. *Genes Dev* **14**:1712, 2000
6. Price ER, Fisher DE: Sensorineural deafness and pigmentation genes: Melanocytes and the Mitf transcriptional network. *Neuron* **30**:15, 2001
7. Vliagoftis H, Worobec AS, Metcalfe DD: The protooncogene *c-kit* and *c-kit* ligand in human disease. *J Allergy Clin Immunol* **100**:435, 1997
8. Blume-Jensen P, Hunter T: Oncogenic kinase signaling. *Nature* **411**:355, 2001
9. Longley BJ Jr et al: Activating and dominant inactivating *c-kit* catalytic domain mutations in distinct clinical forms of human mastocytosis. *Proc Natl Acad Sci U S A* **96**:1609, 1999
10. Ito M et al: Removal of stem cell factor or addition of monoclonal anti-*c-kit* antibody induces apoptosis in murine melanocyte precursors. *J Invest Dermatol* **112**:796, 1999
11. Kunisada T et al: Murine cutaneous mastocytosis and epidermal melanocytosis induced by keratinocyte expression of transgenic stem cell factor. *J Exp Med* **187**:1565, 1998
12. Kos L et al: Met-HGF signaling is critical for melanocyte development: Implications for Waardenburg syndrome Type II. *Pigment Cell Res* **10**:107, 1997
13. Kunisada T et al: Keratinocyte expression of transgenic hepatocyte growth factor affects melanocyte development, leading to dermal melanocytosis. *Mech Dev* **94**:67, 2000
14. Jackson IJ: Homologous pigmentation mutations in human, mouse and other model organisms. *Hum Mol Genet* **6**:1613, 1997
15. Hou L, Panthier JJ, Arnheiter H: Signaling and transcriptional regulation in the neural crest-derived melanocyte lineage: Interactions between KIT and MITF. *Development* **127**:5379, 2000
16. Nakagawa S, Takeichi M: Neural crest emigration from the neural tube depends on regulated cadherin expression. *Development* **125**:2963, 1998
17. Nishimura EK et al: Regulation of E- and P-cadherin expression correlated with melanocyte migration and diversification. *Dev Biol* **215**:155, 1999
18. Jouneau A et al: Plasticity of cadherin-catenin expression in the melanocyte lineage. *Pigment Cell Res* **13**:260, 2000
19. Herlyn M et al: Lessons from melanocyte development for understanding the biological events in naevus and melanoma formation. *Melanoma Res* **10**:303, 2000
20. Fitzpatrick TB, Breathnach AS: Das epidermale Melanin-Einheitsystem. *Dermatol Wochenschr* **147**:481, 1963
21. Minwalla L et al: Keratinocytes play a role in regulating distribution patterns of recipient melanosomes in vitro. *J Invest Dermatol* **117**:341, 2001
22. Tobin DJ, Paus R: Graying: Gerontobiology of the hair follicle pigmentary unit. *Exp Gerontol* **36**:29, 2001
23. King RA: Albinism, in *The Pigmentary System Physiology and Pathophysiology,* edited by JJ Nordlund, R Boissy, VJ Hearing, RA King, J-P Ortonne. New York, Oxford University Press, 1998, p 553
24. Tachibana M: Sound needs sound melanocytes to be heard. *Pigment Cell Res* **12**:344, 1999
25. Holme RH, Steel KP: Genes involved in deafness. *Curr Opin Genet Dev* **9**:309, 1999
26. Ando M, Takeuchi S: Immunological identification of an inward rectifier K+ channel (Kir4.1) in the intermediate cell (melanocyte) of the cochlear stria vascularis of gerbils and rats. *Cell Tissue Res* **298**:179, 1999
27. Cable J, Jackson IJ, Steel KP: Light (Blt), a mutation that causes melanocyte death, affects stria vascularis function in the mouse inner ear. *Pigment Cell Res* **6**:215, 1993
28. Read RW, Rao NA, Cunningham ET: Vogt-Koyanagi-Harada disease. *Curr Opin Ophthalmol* **11**:437, 2000
29. Nguyen M, Arnheiter H: Signaling and transcriptional regulation in early mammalian eye development: A link between FGF and MITF. *Development* **127**:3581, 2000
30. Incerti B et al: OA1 knock-out: New insights on the pathogenesis of ocular albinism type 1. *Hum Mol Genet* **9**:2781, 2000
31. d'Addio M et al: Defective intracellular transport and processing of OA1 is a major cause of ocular albinism type 1. *Hum Mol Genet* **9**:3011, 2000
32. Raper HS: The aerobic oxidases. *Physiol Rev* **8**:245, 1928
33. Lerner AB et al: Mammalian tyrosinase: Preparation and properties. *J Biol Chem* **178**:185, 1949
34. Riley PA: The great DOPA mystery: The source and significance of DOPA in phase I melanogenesis. *Cell Mol Biol* **45**:951, 1999
35. Halaban R et al: Proper folding and ER to Golgi transport of tyrosinase are induced by its substrates, DOPA and tyrosine. *J Biol Chem* **276**:11933, 2001
36. Pawelek JM, Chakraborty AK: The enzymology of melanogenesis, in *The Pigmentary System Physiology and Pathophysiology,* edited by JJ Nordlund, R Boissy, VJ Hearing, RA King, JP Ortonne. New York, Oxford University Press, 1998, p 391
37. Prota G, D'Ischia M, Napolitano A: The chemistry of melanin and related compounds, in *The Pigmentary System Physiology and Pathophysiology,* edited by JJ Nordlund, R Boissy, VJ Hearing, RA King, JP Ortonne. New York, Oxford University Press, 1998, p 307
38. De Leeuw SM et al: Melanin content of cultured human melanocytes and UV-induced cytotoxicity. *J Photochem Photobiol B* **61**:106, 2001
39. Marrot L et al: The human melanocyte as a particular target for UVA radiation and an endpoint for photoprotection assessment. *Photochem Photobiol* **69**:686, 1999
40. Hill HZ, Hill GJ: UVA, pheomelanin and the carcinogenesis of melanoma. *Pigment Cell Res* **8**:140, 2000
41. Wenczl E et al: (Pheo)melanin photosensitizes UVA-induced DNA damage in cultured human melanocytes. *J Invest Dermatol* **111**:678, 1998
42. Dell'Angelica EC et al: Lysosome-related organelles. *FASEB J* **14**:1265, 2000
43. Marks MS, Seabra MC: The melanosome: Membrane dynamics in black and white. *Nat Rev Mol Cell Biol* **2**:738, 2001
44. Helenius A, Aebi M: Intracellular functions of *N*-linked glycans. *Science* **291**:2364, 2001

45. Halaban R et al: Aberrant retention of tyrosinase in the endoplasmic reticulum mediates accelerated degradation of the enzyme and contributes to the dedifferentiated phenotype of amelanotic melanoma cells. *Proc Natl Acad Sci U S A* **94**:6210, 1997
46. Halaban R et al: Endoplasmic reticulum retention is a common defect associated with tyrosinase-negative albinism. *Proc Natl Acad Sci U S A* **97**:5889, 2000
47. Toyofuku K et al: The molecular basis of oculocutaneous albinism type 1 (OCA1): Sorting failure and degradation of mutant tyrosinases results in a lack of pigmentation. *Biochem J* **355**:259, 2001
48. Toyofuku K et al: Promotion of tyrosinase folding in Cos 7 cells by calnexin. *J Biochem* **125**:82, 1999
49. Berson JF et al: A common temperature-sensitive allelic form of human tyrosinase is retained in the endoplasmic reticulum at the nonpermissive temperature. *J Biol Chem* **275**:12281, 2000
50. Toyofuku K et al: Oculocutaneous albinism types 1 and 3 are ER retention diseases: Mutation of tyrosinase or Tyrp1 can affect the processing of both mutant and wild-type proteins. *FASEB J* **15**:2149, 2001
51. Manga P et al: Mutational analysis of the modulation of tyrosinase by tyrosinase-related proteins 1 and 2 in vitro. *Pigment Cell Res* **13**:364, 2000
52. Orlow SJ et al: High-molecular-weight forms of tyrosinase and the tyrosinase-related proteins: Evidence for a melanogenic complex. *J Invest Dermatol* **103**:196, 1994
53. Jimenez-Cervantes C et al: Molecular interactions within the melanogenic complex: Formation of heterodimers of tyrosinase and TRP1 from B16 mouse melanoma. *Biochem Biophys Res Commun* **253**:761, 1998
54. Mosse CA et al: The class I antigen-processing pathway for the membrane protein tyrosinase involves translation in the endoplasmic reticulum and processing in the cytosol. *J Exp Med* **187**:37, 1998
55. Kang XQ et al: Identification of a tyrosinase epitope recognized by HLA-A24-restricted, tumor-infiltrating lymphocytes. *J Immunol* **155**:1343, 1995
56. Topalian SL et al: Human CD4+ T cells specifically recognize a shared melanoma-associated antigen encoded by the tyrosinase gene. *Proc Natl Acad Sci U S A* **91**:9461, 1994
57. Warburg O: On the origin of cancer cells. *Science* **123**:309, 1956
58. Beermann F et al: Misrouting of tyrosinase with a truncated cytoplasmic tail as a result of the murine platinum (c^p) mutation. *Exp Eye Res* **61**:599, 1995
59. Vijayasaradhi S et al: Intracellular sorting and targeting of melanosomal membrane proteins—identification of signals for sorting of the human brown locus protein, gp75. *J Cell Biol* **130**:807, 1995
60. Calvo PA et al: A cytoplasmic sequence in human tyrosinase defines a second class of di-leucine–based sorting signals for late endosomal and lysosomal delivery. *J Biol Chem* **274**:12780, 1999
61. Honing S, Sandoval IV, von Figura K: A di-leucine–based motif in the cytoplasmic tail of LIMP-II and tyrosinase mediates selective binding of AP-3. *EMBO J* **17**:1304, 1998
62. Spritz RA: Multi-organellar disorders of pigmentation: Tied up in traffic. *Clin Genet* **55**:309, 1999
63. Schiaffino MV et al: The ocular albinism type 1 gene product is a membrane glycoprotein localized to melanosomes. *Proc Natl Acad Sci U S A* **93**:9055, 1996
64. Brilliant M, Gardner J: Melanosomal pH, pink locus protein and their roles in melanogenesis. *J Invest Dermatol* **117**:386, 2001
65. Brilliant MH: The mouse p (pink-eyed dilution) and human P genes, oculocutaneous albinism type 2 (OCA2), and melanosomal pH. *Pigment Cell Res* **14**:86, 2001
66. Newton JM et al: Mutations in the human orthologue of the mouse underwhite gene (uw) underlie a new form of oculocutaneous albinism, OCA4. *Am J Hum Genet* **69**:981, 2001
67. Fukamachi S, Shimada A, Shima A: Mutations in the gene encoding B, a novel transporter protein, reduce melanin content in medaka. *Nat Genet* **28**:381, 2001
68. Du J, Fisher DE: Identification of Aim-1 as the underwhite mutant and its transcriptional regulation by MITF. *J Biol Chem* **7**:7, 2001
69. Potterf SB et al: Normal tyrosine transport and abnormal tyrosinase routing in pink-eyed dilution melanocytes. *Exp Cell Res* **244**:319, 1998
70. Menasche G et al: Mutations in RAB27A cause Griscelli syndrome associated with haemophagocytic syndrome. *Nat Genet* **25**:173, 2000
71. Pastural E et al: Two genes are responsible for Griscelli syndrome at the same 15q21 locus. *Genomics* **63**:299, 2000
72. Bahadoran P et al: Rab27a: A key to melanosome transport in human melanocytes. *J Cell Biol* **152**:843, 2001
73. Seiberg M: Keratinocyte-melanocyte interactions during melanosome transfer. *Pigment Cell Res* **14**:236, 2001
74. Lu D, Chen W, Cone RD: Regulation of melanogenesis by MSH, in *The Pigmentary System Physiology and Pathophysiology,* edited by JJ Nordlund, R Boissy, VJ Hearing, RA King, JP Ortonne. New York, Oxford University Press, 1998, p 183
75. Wikberg JE et al: New aspects on the melanocortins and their receptors. *Pharmacol Res* **42**:393, 2000
76. Krude H, Gruters A: Implications of proopiomelanocortin (POMC) mutations in humans: The POMC deficiency syndrome. *Trends Endocrinol Metab* **11**:15, 2000
77. Hadley ME et al: Discovery and development of novel melanogenic drugs. Melanotan-I and-II. *Pharm Biotechnol* **11**:575, 1998
78. Barsh GS et al: Molecular pharmacology of Agouti protein in vitro and in vivo. *Ann N Y Acad Sci* **885**:143, 1999
79. Dinulescu DM, Cone RD: Agouti and agouti-related protein: Analogies and contrasts. *J Biol Chem* **275**:6695, 2000
80. Voisey J, Box NF, van Daal A: A polymorphism study of the human Agouti gene and its association with MC1R. *Pigment Cell Res* **14**:264, 2001
81. Rees JL: The melanocortin 1 receptor (MC1R): More than just red hair. *Pigment Cell Res* **13**:135, 2000
82. Palmer JS et al: Melanocortin-1 receptor polymorphisms and risk of melanoma: Is the association explained solely by pigmentation phenotype? *Am J Hum Genet* **66**:176, 2000
83. Whiteman DC, Whiteman CA, Green AC: Childhood sun exposure as a risk factor for melanoma: A systematic review of epidemiologic studies. *Cancer Causes Control* **12**:69, 2001
84. Noonan FP et al: Neonatal sunburn and melanoma in mice. *Nature* **413**:271, 2001
85. Honigsmann H et al: Immediate pigment darkening phenomenon. A reevaluation of its mechanisms. *J Invest Dermatol* **87**:648, 1986
86. Routaboul C, Denis A, Vinche A: Immediate pigment darkening: Description, kinetic and biological function. *Eur J Dermatol* **9**:95, 1999
87. Duval C, Regnier M, Schmidt R: Distinct melanogenic response of human melanocytes in mono-culture, in co-culture with keratinocytes and in reconstructed epidermis, to UV exposure. *Pigment Cell Res* **14**:348, 2001
88. Stierner U et al: UVB irradiation induces melanocyte increase in both exposed and shielded human skin. *J Invest Dermatol* **92**:561, 1989
89. Halaban R: The regulation of normal melanocyte proliferation. *Pigment Cell Res* **13**:4, 2000
90. Böhm M et al: Identification of $p90^{RSK}$ as the probable CREB-Ser^{133} kinase in human melanocytes. *Cell Growth Diff* **6**:291, 1995
91. Suzuki I et al: Increase of POMC mRNA prior to tyrosinase, TYRP1, DCT, Pmel-17, and P-protein mRNAs in human skin after UVB. *J Invest Dermatol* **118**:73, 2002
92. Chakraborty AK et al: UV light and MSH receptors. *Ann N Y Acad Sci* **885**:100, 1999
93. Li D et al: Rays and arrays: The transcriptional program in the response of human epidermal keratinocytes to UVB illumination. *FASEB J* **15**:2533, 2001
94. DeClerck YA: Interactions between tumour cells and stromal cells and proteolytic modification of the extracellular matrix by metalloproteinases in cancer. *Eur J Cancer* **36**:1258, 2000
95. Fujiwara J et al: Identification of the UV-responsive sequence in the human tissue plasminogen activator gene. *Biosci Biotechnol Biochem* **64**:1084, 2000
96. Scott GA et al: Protease-activated receptor-2 (PAR-2), a receptor involved in melanosome transfer, is upregulated in human skin by ultraviolet irradiation. *J Invest Dermatol* **117**:1414, 2001
97. Coffer PJ et al: UV activation of receptor tyrosine kinase activity. *Oncogene* **11**:561, 1995
98. Gross S et al: Inactivation of protein-tyrosine phosphatases as mechanism of UV-induced signal transduction. *J Biol Chem* **274**:26378, 1999
99. Schlessinger J: Cell signaling by receptor tyrosine kinases. *Cell* **103**:211, 2000
100. Galibert MD, Carreira S, Goding CR: The Usf-1 transcription factor is a novel target for the stress-responsive p38 kinase and mediates UV-induced tyrosinase expression. *EMBO J* **20**:5022, 2001
101. Opdecamp K et al: Melanocyte development in vivo and in neural crest cell cultures: Crucial dependence on the MITF basic-helix-loop-helix-zipper transcription factor. *Development* **124**:2377, 1997
102. Shibahara S et al: Regulation of pigment cell-specific gene expression by MITF. *Pigment Cell Res* **8**:98, 2000
103. Potterf SB et al: Transcription factor hierarchy in Waardenburg syndrome: Regulation of MITF expression by SOX10 and PAX3. *Hum Genet* **107**: 1, 2000

104. Potterf SB et al: Analysis of SOX10 function in neural crest-derived melanocyte development: SOX10-dependent transcriptional control of DOPAchrome tautomerase. *Dev Biol* **237**:245, 2001
105. Fisher DE: Microphthalmia: A signal responsive transcriptional regulator in development. *Pigment Cell Res* **8**:145, 2000
106. Wu M et al: *c-Kit* triggers dual phosphorylations, which couple activation and degradation of the essential melanocyte factor Mi. *Genes Dev* **14**:301, 2000
107. Cobb MH: MAP kinase pathways. *Prog Biophys Mol Biol* **71**:479, 1999
108. Imokawa G, Yada Y, Kimura M: Signaling mechanisms of endothelin-induced mitogenesis and melanogenesis in human melanocytes. *Biochem J* **314**:305, 1996
109. Bandyopadhyay D et al: The human melanocyte: A model system to study the complexity of cellular aging and transformation in non-fibroblastic cells. *Exp Gerontol* **36**:1265, 2001
110. Ewen ME: Where the cell cycle and histones meet. *Genes Dev* **14**:2265, 2000
111. Nevins JR: The Rb/E2F pathway and cancer. *Hum Mol Genet* **10**:699, 2001
112. Ruas M, Peters G: The p16INK4a/CDKN2A tumor suppressor and its relatives. *Biochim Biophys Acta* **1378**:F115, 1998
113. Sharpless NE et al: Loss of p16Ink4a with retention of p19Arf predisposes mice to tumorigenesis. *Nature* **413**:86, 2001
114. Halaban R et al: Deregulated E2F transcriptional activity in autonomously growing melanoma cells. *J Exp Med* **191**:1005, 2000
115. Liu T et al: G protein signaling from activated rat frizzled-1 to the beta-catenin-Lef-Tcf pathway. *Science* **292**:1718, 2001

CHAPTER 12

Robert M. Lavker
Arthur P. Bertolino
Tung-Tien Sun

Biology of Hair Follicles

Hair requires many complex cellular and molecular interactions for its proper formation. Despite its apparent lack of a vital function, for humans the psychological importance of hair is significant. Hair loss can lead to depression, low self-confidence, and humiliation in men and women of all ages. In parallel, growth of facial and body hair in excess of what is deemed culturally acceptable can be just as distressing as hair loss.

From an evolutionary perspective, hairs initially may have served to protect the organism from heat loss and to afford the underlying epidermis a "first line of defense" from abrasion and penetration of noxious chemical agents. The movement of our early ancestors from the shaded tropical rain forests to the exposed savannah may have been accompanied by a gradual loss of dependence on hair as an insulator so that hair on contemporary humans is largely vestigial. While human body hair has little protective value, specialized hairs, such as eyelashes and eyebrows and hairs inside the nostrils and external ears, do afford some protection from the environment. Furthermore, a thick growth of scalp hair provides excellent protection from actinic damage.

Another function of human hair is its role as a "touch organ" involved in sensory reception.[1] All hair follicles have multiple sensory nerve endings that respond to pressure on the hair shaft, thereby providing nearly all the modalities of tactile sensibility. Animals additionally have specialized sinus hairs in the skin of the upper and lower lips, the snout, and above the eyebrows. These tactile hairs (vibrissae), encircled by a blood-filled sinus and with more than 2000 sensory nerve endings, aid nocturnal animals in orientation and function as another set of "eyes." Hair also acts as a conduit in the delivery of scents secreted by the sebaceous and apocrine glands. Finally, hair is an important component of the body image, conveying a vast array of sexual and social messages through its color and the style in which it is worn.

While the hair fiber itself may not have major functional significance, the cyclic nature of the hair follicle has made this epidermal derivative an excellent model system for studying a number of important biologic problems, including morphogenesis, growth regulation, cell differention, pattern formation, and cyclic control. Since many of these processes are influenced by the mesenchyme, the hair follicle is also an ideal system for investigating mesenchymal-epithelial interactions. In addition, the follicle is believed to play a role in maintaining the epidermis, as well as participating in wound healing and skin tumorigenesis (see below). The recent explosion of data in areas of cellular and molecular biology has helped refine concepts concerning the mechanisms, molecules, and genes that control hair follicle formation, growth, disease, and death.

EMBRYOLOGY AND ANATOMY

In human fetuses, the first primordial hair follicles form at approximately 9 weeks' gestation and are distributed mainly in the areas of the eyebrows, upper lip, and chin. The bulk of the remaining follicles begin to develop at approximately 4 to 5 months' gestation in a cephalad to caudad direction. During fetal life, production of follicles occurs in several interspersed waves. Primary and secondary follicles are formed as the skin expands. The secondary follicle develops on each side of the primary follicle, producing typical groupings of three hairs. It is generally assumed that adult skin cannot develop new follicles under normal circumstances.

Follicular morphogenesis begins with inductive events that involve the exchange of signals between epithelial and mesenchymal cells and proceeds through stages of follicular initiation, elongation, and cellular differentiation. The first signal directing hair follicle formation arises in the mesenchyme, inducing a thickening of the overlying epidermis to form a placode. Epithelial cells within the placode become more elongated than adjacent nonplacode cells. Signals from the placode then induce clustering of the underlying dermal cells to form a dermal condensate, and a "second dermal signal" from the condensate then induces the proliferation and downward movement of a column of epithelial cells into the dermis, forming the hair germ[2] (Fig. 12-1*A*). Much progress has been made in identifying the molecules that regulate follicle development. Members of several families of signaling molecules including the Wnt, fibroblast growth factor (FGF), and tumor necrosis factor (TNF) families are potential inducers of epithelial appendages. Wnt signaling appears to be needed for the initial downgrowth of the follicle (placode formation),[3] whereas bone morphogeneic proteins (BMPs) appear to repress placode formation in adjacent skin and thus control the spacing between appendages.[4,5] Recently, follicular papilla cells have been shown to express members of the sonic hedgehog (SHH) and Wnt signaling cascades.[6] It therefore seems likely that the Wnt and SHH signaling pathways are involved in the crosstalk between the ectoderm and mesenchymal condensates leading to the development of the hair germ.

Even the earliest follicular germ cells acquire features that set them apart from the interfollicular epidermal keratinocytes. For example, the follicular cells express neuronal intercellular adhesion molecules (such as N-CAM and I-CAM), which are not expressed by interfollicular keratinocytes. Similarly, mesenchymal cells of the dermal condensate selectively express tenascin, which has been suggested to promote mesenchymal cell aggregation and epithelial cell growth, and p75, a neurotrophin receptor involved in anagen-to-catagen transformation.[7]

The next stage in follicular neogenesis is known as the *follicular peg*, an elongated follicle germ consisting of a column of keratinocytes extending into the dermis roughly perpendicular to the skin surface (see Fig. 12-1*B*). Mesenchymal cells surrounding the epidermal cord become specialized, eventually forming the follicular sheath (also known as the *connective tissue* sheath) whereas mesenchymal cells concentrated at the tip form the follicular papilla. The tip of the epithelial cord is flattened and becomes the matrix portion of the bulb. As the follicle continues to elongate, it becomes the bulbous hair peg (see Fig. 12-1*C*), characterized by the formation of two pouches of outgrowth extending from the outer root sheath cells on the posterior aspect of the follicle. The upper outgrowth gives rise to the sebaceous gland, whereas the lower one gives rise to the bulge, which later becomes the insertion site of the arrector pili muscle. The bulge plays a key role in hair growth because it contains the hair follicular epithelial stem cells (see below).[8]

The deepest portion of the bulbous hair peg forms an invagination encasing the bulk of the follicle-associated and by now highly specialized dermal cells, which develop into the follicular papilla (*dermal papilla*). The matrix keratinocytes of the precortical region ultimately give rise to the hair shaft and inner root sheath. Signaling molecules such as Notch, BMP, and members of the Wnt family are involved in the differentiation of inner root sheath and hair shaft.[5,9] The melanocytes responsible for pigmentation of the hair fiber reside in the proximal bulb of the anagen follicle, situated among the basal keratinocytes of the matrix. The outer root sheath, comprising the most peripheral epithelial cell layers of the follicle, is contiguous with the epidermis and is most likely derived from the cells of the bulge (see below).[10,11] As the follicle begins to produce a hair, the central cells of the rudimentary follicle column degenerate, forming a tunnel through which the newly formed hair fiber can emerge.

A useful way to conceptualize the internal organization of the hair follicle is to view it as a series of concentric epithelial rings bounded by an acellular basement membrane, the so-called glassy membrane (Fig. 12-2). Immediately above the bulb, the outer root sheath consists of a single layer, but higher up the follicle it is composed of multilayers

FIGURE 12-1

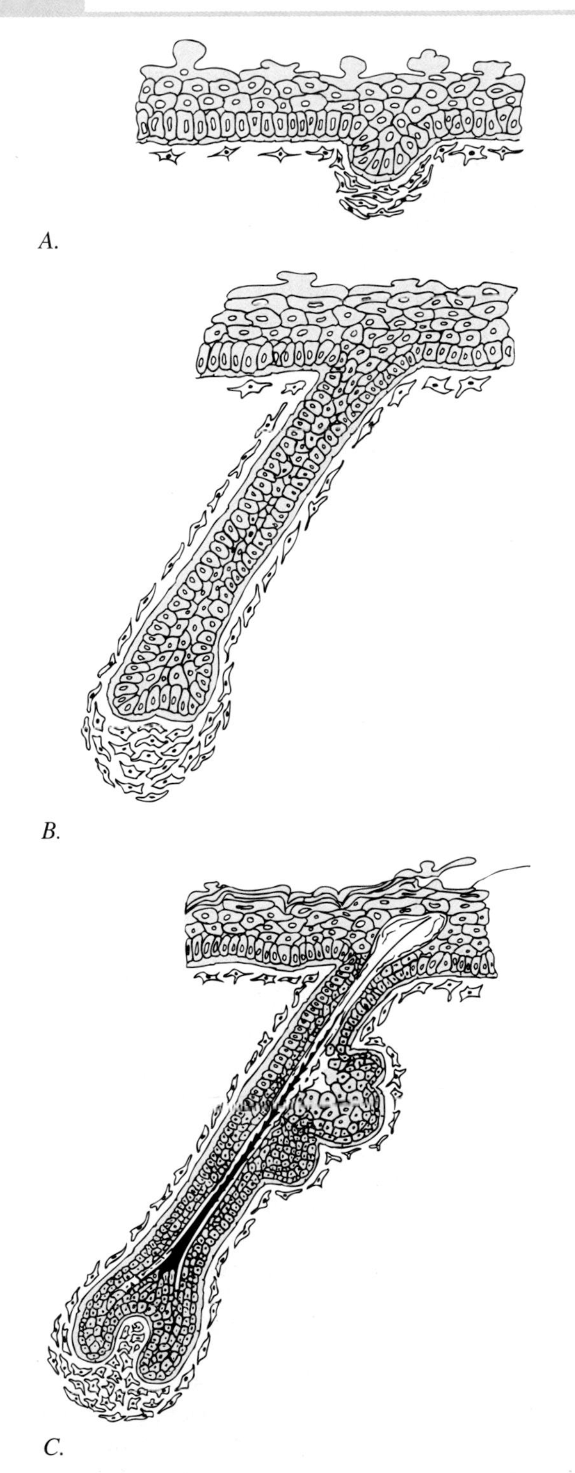

Diagrammatic representation of the major stages of follicular neogenesis. *A.* Follicular germ stage, depicting a condensation of mesenchymal cells just beneath the slight downgrowth or "bud" of fetal basal keratinocytes. *B.* Follicular peg stage, depicting the organization of keratinocytes in the follicle and the mesenchyme of the follicular sheath and follicular papilla located at the tip of the follicle. *C.* Bulbous hair peg stage, depicting regions of the differentiated follicle. Two prominent bulge outgrowths are noted; the uppermost will become the sebaceous gland, and the lowermost is the insertion site of the arrector pili muscle as well as the presumptive site of the hair follicle stem cells. (*From Holbrook et al.*[7] *with permission.*)

FIGURE 12-2

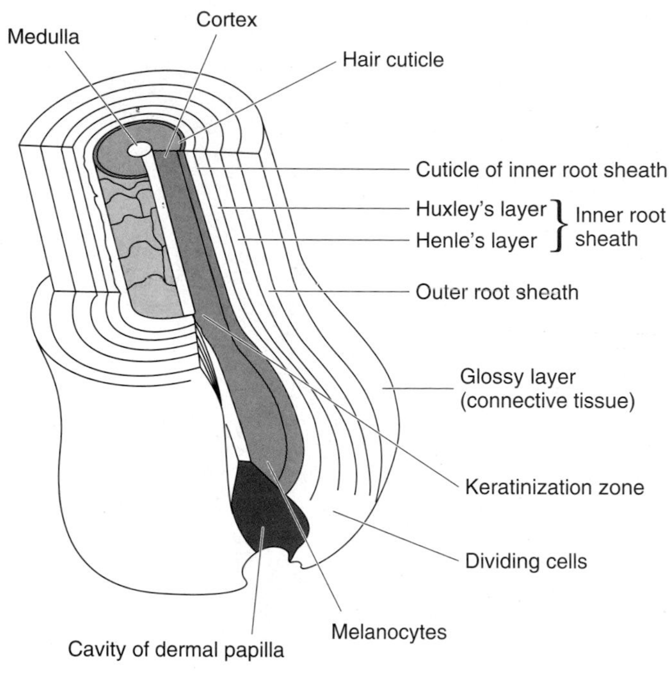

Diagrammatic representation of a cross section of the hair follicle and hair shaft. Both the follicle and hair shaft are organized as a series of concentric compartments. (*Reproduced from Dawber R: Diseases of the Hair and Scalp, Oxford, Blackwell Scientific Publications, with permission.*)

FIGURE 12-3

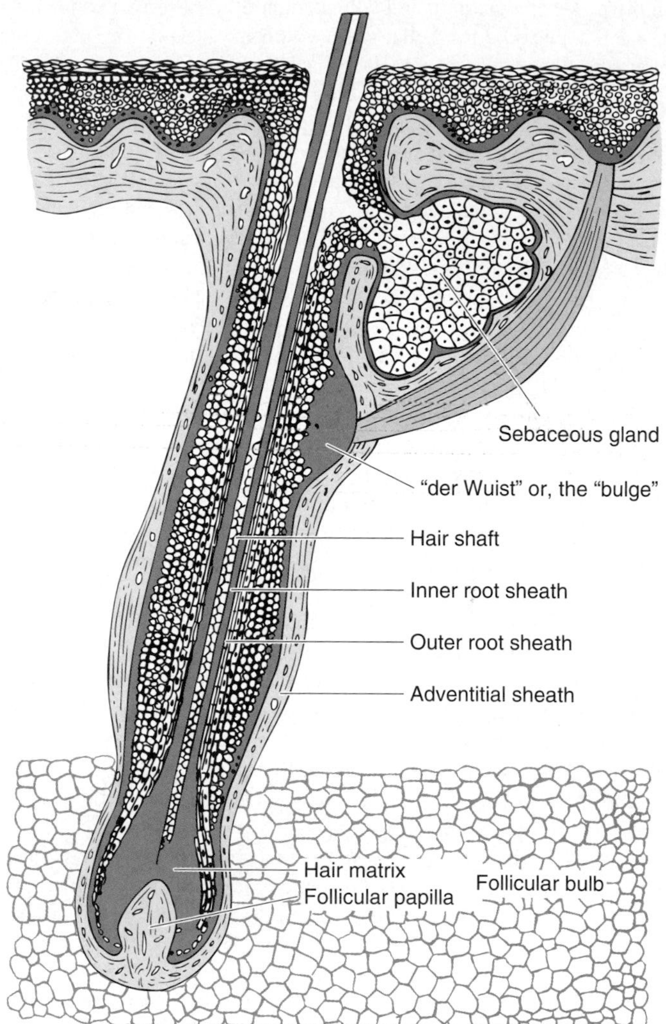

Diagrammatic representation of the adult human hair follicle. The follicle, an invagination of the surface epidermis, is characterized by an infundibulum that communicates directly with the epidermis and extends to the opening of the sebaceous gland. The portion directly beneath the sebaceous gland and terminating at the bulge is the isthmus. The lowermost portion of the hair follicle is the transient region, which begins just beneath the bulge and terminates at the lowermost part of the follicle. The follicular bulb, the lowermost part of the follicle, consists of matrix keratinocytes and specialized mesenchymal cells known as the follicular papilla. The follicular papilla is contiguous with the adventitial sheath, which lines the entire follicle.(*Courtesy of Michael Joffreda, M.D.*)

of cuboidal cells. At the level of the sebaceous gland and above, the outer root sheath is structurally similar to the epidermis. Adjacent to the outer root sheath is the companion layer, which is in contact with the (outermost) Henle's layer of the inner root sheath.[12] In the prekeratogenous regions of the follicle, the companion layer consists of a single row of flattened cells arranged end to end. In the precortical zone, as Henle's layer becomes keratinized, the companion cells become cuboidal with prominent nuclei. Farther up the follicle, where the inner root sheath is degenerating, the companion cells take on irregular shapes and become keratinized. The companion cells contain a unique keratin (K6hf) and express plasminogen activator inhibitor type 2 (PAI-2), which has been postulated to prevent premature cell destruction.[12] Adjacent to the companion layer is the inner root sheath (IRS), composed of three compartments: the outermost Henle's layer, which is the first to keratinize; the intermediate Huxley's layer, which is the major IRS component; and the innermost cuticle layer of the IRS, which is adjacent to the hair shaft. The inner root sheath is thought to mold and hold the hair shaft. The hair shaft also has three compartments: an outermost cuticle layer that interlocks with the cuticle of the IRS, a cortex that forms the bulk of the hair shaft, and a variable medulla.

The longitudinal organization of the follicle can be divided roughly into seven regions with distinct anatomic boundaries (Fig. 12-3): (1) the *hair canal region* extending from the skin surface to the level of the epidermal-dermal junction (its lower part later becomes the intraepidermal "infundibular unit"), (2) the *infundibulum,* which extends down to the opening of the (3) *sebaceous gland,* (4) the *isthmus,* which begins at the sebaceous duct and ends at (5) the *area of the bulge,* the site of insertion of the arrector pili muscle and a region enriched in follicular epithelial stem cells [8,10] (the transient portion of the follicle, located below the bulge/arrector pili muscle complex, extends to the deepest levels of the follicle), (6) the *lower follicle,* which includes the keratogenous zone and extends from the area of the bulge to the top of the hair bulb, and (7) the *hair bulb,* which is the deepest portion of the follicular structure and envelops the follicular papilla. The *critical line of Auber* is at the widest diameter of the bulb and is of significance in that the bulk of the mitotic activity that gives rise to the hair shaft and inner root sheath occurs below this level.

Another important anatomic feature of the follicle is that it lies at an angle relative to the skin surface. The side of the follicle that forms an acute angle with the skin surface is its anterior aspect. When the arrector pili muscle contracts, as in response to cold external temperature, it pulls on the posterior side of the follicle. The temporary alteration in local skin architecture gives rise to what has been described in lay terms as "goose bumps." The associated hair becomes more vertically oriented and therefore provides a greater thermal barrier because the relative thickness of the insulating medium is increased.

THE HAIR CYCLE

While it is well known that hair follicles undergo cycles of growth, involution, and rest (Fig. 12-4), it is important to realize that many other changes occur in the skin as a function of the hair cycle. Investigators have demonstrated that in rats and mice the entire skin changes during the hair cycle, with a generalized thickening of the skin during anagen (the growing phase) and a thinning during telogen (the resting phase).[13] The skin vasculature also undergoes hair cycle–related changes. In murine skin, a greater than fourfold increase in perifollicular vessel size occurs during the anagen phase, followed by a rapid reduction in vessel size during catagen and telogen, suggesting that the growing hair follicle can induce its own blood supply to support its metabolic needs.[14] Finally, it has been demonstrated that anagen follicles have the largest numbers of intrafollicular Langerhans cells, lymphocytes, and perifollicular macrophages.[15] It also has been reported that there is an anagen-associated suppression of contact hypersensitivity as well as photocontact allergy.[15] Such observations have led to the suggestion that anagen phase is associated with an immunosuppressive activity resulting in the formation of a large perifollicular "immune privileged" zone.[15] Taken together, these findings suggest that during the hair cycle the follicle can influence the physiology of many cutaneous structures, such as the sebaceous gland, vasculature, subcutaneous fat, and even immunological activity.

Anagen

Anagen can be subdivided into six substages (I to VI), the first five of which are collectively called *proanagen*. The sixth stage, *metanagen,* is defined by the emergence of the hair shaft above the skin surface. At this stage, the anagen follicle penetrates deeply into the subcutaneous fat.

The length of anagen is known to vary markedly depending on body site and species. The anagen of human hair follicles has been estimated to last 2 to 6 years on the scalp (mosaic pattern), 19 to 26 weeks on the leg, 6 to 12 weeks on the arm, and 4 to 14 weeks on the upper lip (mustache).[16] Interestingly, the hair follicles of the merino sheep are thought to be in a permanent state of anagen lasting the animal's entire lifetime.

Catagen

At the end of anagen, the follicle enters into catagen, which shows morphologic and molecular changes that are characteristic of programmed cell death and apoptosis.[17] At the onset of catagen, the scalp hairs show a gradual thinning and decrease of the pigment at the base of the hair shaft. Melanocytes in the matrix portion of the bulb cease producing melanin, resorb their dendrites, and undergo apoptosis.[15] Matrix keratinocytes abruptly cease proliferating and undergo terminal differentiation so that the lower follicle involutes and regresses. The follicular papillary cells round up and remain within the connective tissue sheath, which contracts, pulling the condensed follicular papilla toward the bottom of the epithelial portion of the regressing follicle. The connective tissue sheath also becomes quite thickened during catagen.[16] At the

FIGURE 12-4

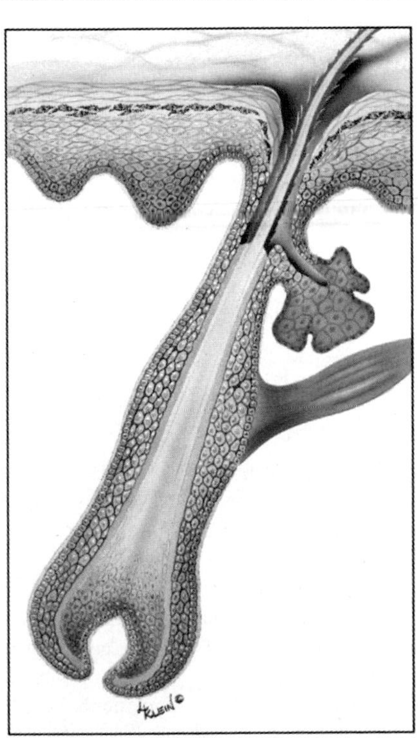

A.

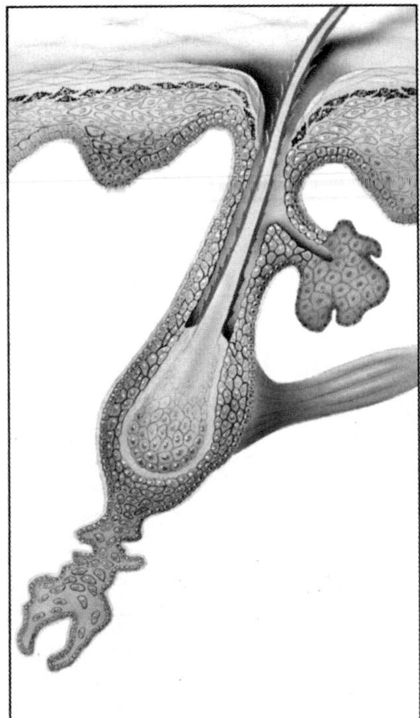

B.

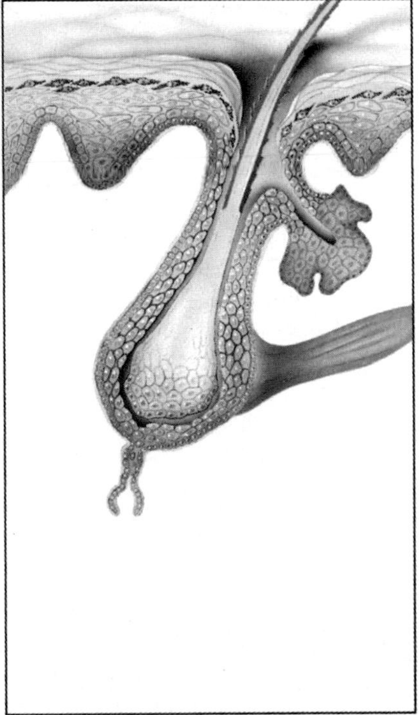

C.

Diagrammatic representation of the changes that occur to the follicle and hair shaft during the hair growth cycle:*(A)* anagen (growth stage), *(B)* catogen (degenerative stage), *(C)* telogen (resting stage). (*Courtesy of Lynn M.Klein, M.D.*)

end of catagen, the follicular papilla comes to rest at the bottom of the permanent portion of the hair follicle.

The molecular signals that trigger catagen are presently unknown. In the catagen follicle there is a decline in an antiapoptotic protein, Bcl-2, and an increase in a proapoptotic protein, Bax.[18] At the onset of catagen, various apoptotic-associated receptors (Fas/Apo, p55TNFR, p75NTR) are observed in the lower portion of the follicular epithelium, and in late catagen, all three receptors are noted in the regressing outer root sheath epithelium.[18] Finally, several transcription factors including c-Myc, and c-Myb, and c-Jun, which have been associated with anagen induction, change immediately before or during catagen.[17] For example, c-Myc decreases in late anagen and catagen, whereas c-Myb and c-Jun only decrease in catagen. Another molecule implicated in the control of the anagen-catagen transition is FGF5.[19] Mice deficient in this factor have a prolonged anagen with a long-haired (angora) phenotype. However, it should be noted that in these mice the follicle still enters catagen, indicating that other signaling molecules are involved in the transition from anagen to catagen. Because insulin-like growth factor, keratinocyte growth factor (KGF), and hepatocyte growth factor (HGF) are downregulated at the initiation of catagen, whereas transforming growth factor beta (TGF-β1) and several neurotrophins are upregulated at the same time, the changes in concentration of these molecules have been suggested to play a role in anagen-catagen transition.[15]

Telogen

The telogen hair has a club-shaped proximal end within the hair follicle, and it is typically shed from the follicle during telogen or the subsequent anagen. The new hair produced from the subsequent anagen does not "push out" the hair from the previous cycle and may on occasion be found adjacent to a so-called retained club hair within a follicle. The inner root sheath, which normally disintegrates in the anagen follicle at the level of the sebaceous duct opening, is absent from the telogen follicle. Eventually, a new growing phase occurs, and the cycle is repeated.

On human scalp, the anagen period is generally quite long; however, catagen lasts only about 2 weeks and telogen 1 to 3 months.[16]

Exogen

Recently, attention has been directed to studying the mechanism of hair shedding, and the term *exogen* has been coined to denote the hair shedding phase.[20] This term describes the relationship between the hair shaft and the base of the telogen follicle rather than the cycling activity of the underlying follicle.[15] Since hairs can be retained for more than one cycle, the shedding phase is most likely independent of anagen and telogen. While little is known about what controls exogen, proteolytic pathways have been implicated in club hair formation and removal.[15]

Although the cyclic nature of hair growth just described is similar in humans and in animals, the pattern of growth and rest and the rate of growth vary depending on species and body site. For example, hair growth can occur either in a wave, where all follicles are relatively synchronized, or in a mosaic pattern, where the activity of each follicle is independent of its neighbors.[21] Even though it has been stated dogmatically that sometimes hair growth in mice, rats, hamsters, and rabbits occurs in wave patterns, this is true only for the first two hair cycles. Subsequent cycles in these species become less synchronized and eventually assume a mosaic pattern. Guinea pigs, cats, dogs, subhuman primates, and humans exhibit a mosaic pattern of hair cycling.[22] Although humans initially display a wave pattern of hair growth in utero and during the early postnatal period, this synchronization is later lost. At 26 to 28 weeks' gestation, most human scalp hair follicles make the transition to telogen in a wave pattern that spreads from the frontal to parietal regions, marking the last stage of the first hair cycle.[23] Many of these primary hairs are shed in utero,[24] although this may be delayed in some individuals, resulting in abundant hair at birth.[23] It is also typical for a bandlike area of occipital hair follicles to enter the first telogen near birth and for these hairs to shed synchronously 2 to 3 months later.[23,25] Waves of hair growth occur before the establishement of the mosaic pattern, which is usually present by the end of the first postnatal year.

At any one time, about 85 to 90 percent of human scalp hair follicles are in anagen, about 13 percent are in telogen, and less than 1 percent are in catagen.[16] It is believed that each follicle goes through the hair cycle 10 to 20 times in a lifetime. However, the assumption that all human follicles traverse regularly through the hair growth cycles is unsubstantiated. Investigations of murine hair follicles suggest that follicles remain in telogen for progressively longer periods of time. This makes good biologic sense considering the tremendous amount of energy required to sustain a hair follicle in anagen for several years. The idea that the cycle for human hair follicles also may be discontinuous and/or heterogeneous should be given serious consideration.

DISTRIBUTION OF HAIR

Hair follicles are distributed throughout the integument with the exception of the palms, soles, and portions of the genitalia (so-called glabrous skin). The highest density of follicles is on the scalp, where it has been reported as 1135/cm^2 at birth, diminishing to 795 by the end of the first year and 615 by the third decade, commensurate with an increase in scalp skin surface area.[26] Headington[27] used transverse skin sectioning (histologic) techniques to examine scalp skin and found normal adult follicular density to be in the range of 310 to 500/cm^2. Pecoraro et al.[28] reported average scalp hair shaft densities ranging from 170 to 250/cm^2 in prepuberal children. By carefully examining the growth of hairs from hair transplant grafts in adults, Unger[29] observed emergent hairs in the range of about 100 to 200/cm^2. It should be noted that the follicular densities obtained by counting emergent hair shafts are significantly less that the number observed in tissue sections due to the fact that very small hairs as well as unpigmented hairs may be missed in clinical counting. The total number of hair follicles in the scalp is approximately 100,000 in people with brown-black hair. It is about 10 percent greater in blondes and 10 percent less in redheads.

HAIR AS A BIOLOGIC FIBER

Mature hair shafts are nonliving biologic fibers. Their integrity and physical properties are due to the accumulation of several groups of highly specialized hair-differentiation products, including the hair ("hard") keratins, and to the strong intercellular attachments between the various cells of the hair fiber. An important biochemical feature that contributes to the physical properties of the fiber is disulfide bonding between various structural proteins. Such links between the keratins and the high-sulfur proteins produce a sturdy, dense network that largely fills the keratinocytes. These disulfide bonds also help maintain the texture and shape of the fibers; they are chemically broken during the first stage of hair styling with permanents or during straightening and are re-formed after the desired change has been accomplished so that the new form is maintained. Mutations in hair proteins can lead to certain hair diseases.[30]

Outer Root Sheath and Companion Layer

Outer root sheath cells contain several epithelial ("soft") keratin intermediate filament proteins, including the K5/K14 pair characteristic of basal epidermal cells[31] and the K6/K16 pair characteristic of hyperproliferative keratinocytes.[31] K19 also has been detected in the outer root sheath cells of the adult human hair follicle, with the greatest concentration observed in the bulge region.[32,33] K17 has been detected in the outer root sheath in a distinct cluster of matrix keratinocytes and in the medulla of murine hair.[34] In human hair extracts, K17 was found in eyebrow and facial hair but not in hairs from other body sites. Based on its polarized location in the matrix and presence in the medulla, K17 has been proposed to play a role in determining hair shape and orientation.[34] Finally, K6hf, a novel human cell type II keratin, has been demonstrated to be exclusively expressed in the companion layer of the hair follicle.[35]

Cortex

The cortex is the major part of the human hair fiber, and it contains the bulk of the hair ("hard") keratins. The hair keratin filaments are built on the same molecular plan as the epidermal intermediate filaments, in which the 400 to 500 amino acid residues of individual chains are arranged in sequences containing many heptad repeats. Consequently, they can pair together to form coils. Recent work focused on characterizing human hair keratin genes has shown that in the human hair follicle there are nine functional type I (acidic) hair keratin genes located on chromosome 17q12–21 and six functional type II (basic) hair keratin genes located on chromosome 12q13.[36,37] The type I hair keratins were sorted into three groups on the basis of structure: group A (hHa1, hHa3-I, hHa3-II, and hHa4) and group B (hHa7 and hHa8), each containing highly related hair keratins, and group C (hHa2, hHa5, and hHa6), which contains structurally unrelated hair keratins. The type II hair keratins were sorted into two groups: group A (hHb1, hHb3, and hHb6), containing the highly related hair keratins, and group C (hHb2, hHb4, and hHb5), containing the less related hair keratins.

Other major proteins found in the cortex, known as keratin-associated proteins, can be divided into two groups: (1) the high-sulfur proteins, rich in cysteine (9–25 kDa), which form a biologic "glue" between the keratin filaments of the cortex, and (2) a less prominent group of high-glycine/tyrosine-containing proteins (6–9 kDa).[38] Sequence analysis of one of these glycine/tyrosine-containing proteins has revealed its capacity to form glycine loops, which could interact with similar glycine loops of the hair keratin filaments. This type of interaction would produce a tightly packed structure for the cortex keratin.[38]

With respect to expression patterns within the anagen hair follicle, hHa5 and hHb5 are detected in the nonproliferating matrix keratinocytes and the precortical cells, sites of early hair follicle differentiation. Somewhat later expression was noted for the type I keratins hHa1, hHa3-I/II, and hHa4 that were expressed sequentially in the cortex. Type II keratins hHb1, hHb3, and hHb6 also were seen in the cortex. The high-sulfur proteins are the last to be produced in the cortex.[38,39]

Medulla

In the medulla, which is morphologically distinct from the cortex, there are the citrulline-containing ϵ-(γ-glutamyl)lysine cross-linked proteins. These medullary proteins, along with trichohyalin, an intermediate filament–associated protein, are also found in the inner root sheath.[40]

Cuticle

The cuticle of the hair shaft is also very important in maintaining the integrity of the fiber. It may be likened to a layer of armor that resembles reptilian scales and protects the cortex. With respect to expression patterns of the hair keratins, the hHa5/hHa2 and hHb5/hHb2 keratins are coexpressed throughout the cuticular cells. As was the case for the cortex, the high-sulfur proteins are the last to be produced in the cuticle.[38] When the cuticle is damaged from physical or chemical exposures, the fiber is more likely to break. When this happens along the shaft (e.g., trichorrhexis nodosa), the fiber is likely to become severed with minor subsequent manipulation; when this happens at the distal end of the shaft, the fiber is likely to fracture longitudinally, producing trichoptilosis ("split ends").

There are variations in the cross-sectional features of hair fibers. Typical diameters of scalp hairs range from 40 to 120 μm,[41] with hair from whites and blacks generally having narrower diameters than hair from Asians. There are also tendencies for scalp hairs from different races to have specific characteristics: The hair of whites is usually oval in cross section and somewhat curly; the hair of blacks is usually oval and sometimes flattened in cross section and twisted; and the hair of Asians is round in cross section and straight.[42] These relationships do not apply to hairs from other body sites—e.g., eyelashes, beard hairs, and pubic hairs—which tend to share similar features in all races.

HAIR PIGMENTATION

The basic color of the hair is determined by the melanocytes. Hair is actively pigmented only when it grows because the melanogenic activity of follicular melanocytes is coupled to the anagen stage of the hair cycle. In catagen and telogen, melanin formation is switched off. Melanocytes located in the matrix area of the anagen follicle, in the region above the follicular papilla, produce the pigment. Pigment-laden dendritic processes from these melanocytes course among the differentiating hair keratinocytes, which engulf portions of the pigmented dendrites. Although a follicle usually produces only one type of pigment at any given time, two types of pigment can be produced. Eumelanin is the pigment in brown-black hairs, and pheomelanin is the pigment in red-blond hairs. The pigment is predominantly located in the cortex of the hair shaft. Typically, it is not found in the hair shaft during the early stages of new hair formation, and so new hair tips do not usually contain pigment. Similarly, pigment typically is not found in the portion of the hair shaft produced just before the follicle enters the resting phase of the hair cycle, so the proximal portion of normally shed ("club," or telogen) hair also lacks pigment. One of the more perplexing issues that remains to be solved is what happens to the melanocytes during the catagen/telogen phase of the hair growth cycle. Current belief is that melanocyte loss during catagen is replenished from an undifferentiated melanocyte pool in the "permanent portion" of the hair or from another, as yet unidentified precursor pool.[43]

Variations in the spectrum of hair color shades are relatively simple, yet the factors that produce subtle variations are more complex. The intensity of color is generally proportional to the amount of pigment in the fiber. In the extreme, absence of pigment produces white hair, whereas markedly diminished pigment produces gray hair. Lighter shades of a given color result when less pigment is incorporated in the hair shaft. Subtle variations in hue depend on the refraction and reflection of incident light at the various internal interfaces of the hair shaft as well as the interfaces with the external environment and/or materials that may coat the fiber.

Work in mice has provided insights into the mechanisms of patterning in the hair coat as well as potential genes involved in the control of hair pigmentation. Follicular papillary cells have been found to express the *agouti* gene, which encodes a signaling molecule that causes hair follicle melanocytes to synthesize yellow instead of black pigment.[44] Expression of this gene was shown to be under the control of two different promoters. One is active at the midpoint of anagen, thus controlling the anagen-specific production of pigment. The other remains active throughout the hair cycle but only on the ventral surface, causing mice to have black dorsal hairs and yellow ventral hairs.[45] Another gene, *bcl-2,* that encodes a protooncogene involved in blocking apoptosis, was expressed in the follicular papillae of cycling murine and human hair follicles during the entire cycle. Interestingly, genetic ablation of this gene in mice resulted in the formation of gray hair during the second hair cycle because of a reduced number of follicular melanocytes, suggesting that expression of *bcl-2* might be essential for melanocyte survival. Other molecules implicated in hair pigmentation are stem cell factor (SCF) and its receptor, c-Kit. Evidence for this comes from observations that (1) c-Kit is required for postnatal melanocyte activation, (2) melanocytes in newborn mice are c-Kit–dependent, (3) melanocytes undergo apoptosis when c-Kit receptors are blocked, and (4) proliferating, differentiating, and melanin-producing melanocytes express c-Kit, whereas the putative melanocyte precursors do not.[46] Furthermore, studies in normal and SCF-overexpressing mice reveal that SCF/c-Kit is required for the formation and trafficking of functional melanocytes during each new hair cycle, whereas the putative melanocyte precursor cells are not dependent on SCF/c-Kit.[47] Since cultured human follicular papillary cells can secrete SCF as well as *agouti* gene product, these cells may play an active role in regulating the pigmentation of hair follicles.[48]

TYPES OF HAIR

Hairs can be classified according to their texture and length; this is species-dependent, since humans and mice have rather different hair types. Thus humans have lanugo hair, vellus hair, intermediate hair, and terminal hair. Lanugo hair is the soft, fine hair that covers much of the fetus and usually is shed before birth. The other terms have most relevance to scalp hair, although the basic principles convey some meaning for other hair sites. The classification is not exact and basically relates to the final length of the hairs: Vellus scalp hairs achieve lengths less than 1 cm, indeterminate scalp hairs are approximately 1 cm in length, and terminal scalp hairs grow longer than 1 cm. The prominence of various hair-shaft features, in general, increases with progression through this series (e.g., amount of pigment, hair-shaft diameter, and extent of medulla formation).

Although the types of hairs are not clearly defined in terms of fiber length for other body sites, the general relationships cited above are conveyed when such terminology is used. Eyebrow or eyelash hairs are typically less than 1 cm in length but are considered terminal hairs. Yet the usual lengths (several millimeters) of beard hairs along with their associated features in normal women would best be described as vellus hair. Using the phrase *terminal beard hair growth* with regard to a woman would indicate that there is a departure from the norm, with the presence of the longer, coarser hairs typical of hirsutism or hypertrichosis.

REGULATION OF THE HAIR GROWTH CYCLE

Much of the recent excitement in the hair field has focused on elucidating the location and biology of the follicular epithelial stem cells, characterizing the follicular papillary cells and their products, identifying the molecular mechanisms involved in the epithelial/mesenchymal regulation of the hair growth cycle, and defining further the hormonal aspects of hair growth regulation.

Follicular Epithelial Stem Cells

A knowledge of follicular epithelial stem cells is essential because these cells play a central role in long-term maintenance of the hair follicle, regulation of the hair growth cycle, and skin tumor initiation.[10,49] It has been shown that the bulge region of the outer root sheath is a major site of follicular epithelial stem cells because epithelial cells within this region exhibit several important stem cell features.[49] For example, the bulge cells are slow cycling; they can be induced to proliferate in response to various growth stimuli; they are relatively undifferentiated, as evidenced by a primitive-appearing cytoplasm; they have a greater proliferative capacity than epithelial cells from other regions of the hair follicle; and being located at the lowermost part of the permanent portion of the follicle, they are spared from the cellular destruction that occurs during every catagen. The identification of hair follicle stem cells in the bulge region provided a mechanistical model to explain some important features of the hair cycle[8] (the *bulge-activation hypothesis*) (Fig. 12-5). According to this hypothesis, the bulge epithelial stem cells, on receiving mesenchymal signals from the abutting dermal papilla, undergo transient proliferation during early anagen, giving rise to a population of rapidly proliferating, transit amplifying (TA)

FIGURE 12-5

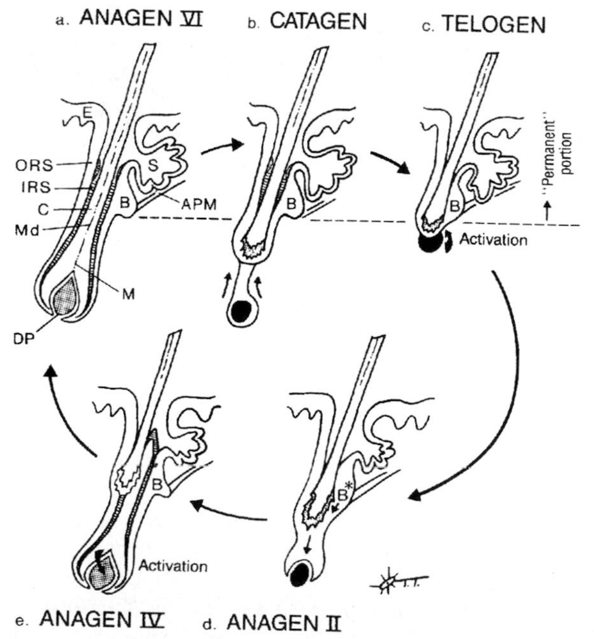

Hair cycle: the bulge activation hypothesis. Illustrated are the sequential phases of the hair cycle. Abbreviations include epidermis (E), sebaceous glands (S), bulge (B), arrector pili muscle (APM), outer root sheath (ORS), inner root sheath (IRS), hair cortex (C), hair medulla (Md), matrix (M), and follicular (dermal) papilla (DP). Structures above the dashed line constitute the permanent portion of the hair follicle; keratinocytes below this line degenerate during catagen and telogen and therefore are dispensable. Four important tenets of the bulge activation hypothesis include (1) upward movement of the follicular papilla during catagen that will lead to its close proximity to the bulge during telogen,(2) activation of the bulge cells by the adjacent follicular papilla,(3) downward movement of the follicular papilla as anagen begins, followed shortly thereafter by a "turning off" of the now proliferating (B*) bulge cells, and (4) activation of the follicular papilla by the new matrix. This hypothesis predicts that a hair cycle will have a duration based on the finite proliferative potential of the matrix TA cells. (*Adapted from Cotsarelis et al.*[8] *with permission.*)

cells that form an epithelial column growing downward, pushing away the dermal papilla cells. Once the dermal papilla signals are removed, the bulge stem cells resume their slow-cycling state. Since the matrix keratinocytes are TA cells, they have a limited proliferative capacity, and once this growth potential is exhausted, they undergo terminal differentiation/apoptosis—a key event of catagen.

Recent data have provided strong support to the bulge stem cell theory. For example, using a double-labeling technique, Taylor et al.[10] showed that the progeny of the bulge stem cells can migrate downward toward the hair matrix and can give rise to several hair cell types, including the cortex and medulla. Oshima et al.[11] showed by microdissection experiments that the bulge cells of mouse vibrissa can give rise to all cell types of the follicle as well as the sebaceous gland. Taken together, these data strongly support the concept that bulge stem cells can give rise not only to all the cell types of the hair follicle but also to some of the hair-related structures such as the sebaceous gland.

The Hair Follicle as a Guardian of the Epidermis

It has long been appreciated that the follicle may play a role in epidermal wound repair. It is well known, for example, that when the murine epidermis is removed experimentally using a felt wheel, some keratinocytes emigrate out from the follicles, contributing to regeneration of the interfollicular epidermis.[10] A similar follicular origin for repairing keratinocytes was reported in the reepithelialization of human skin following a severe burn. Using a double-labeling method that selectively tagged the progeny (TA) cells of the bulge stem cells, Taylor et al.[10] showed that these bulge-derived TA cells not only can move downward to form the outer root sheath, the matrix, and the hair shaft of the hair follicle but also can move upward to populate the basal layer of the epidermis. Emigration of upper follicular epithelial cells into the epidermis was observed in normal neonatal mouse skin, as well as in adult skin in response to a full-thickness skin wound. Such an upward emigration of follicular epithelial TA cells into even normal epidermis suggests a much closer relationship between the follicle and normal epidermis than was appreciated previously and supports the idea that bulge-derived keratinocytes may be involved in long-term maintenance of the epidermis.[8,10,50] The upward migration of the bulge stem cell–derived progeny cells into normal epidermis, combined with the downward migration of the stem cell progeny to form the hair shaft, suggests that the bulge stem cells are at least bipotent[10,49] (Fig. 12-6). Microdissection studies by Oshima et al.[11] also showed that the β-galactosidase–tagged bulge cells of mouse vibrissae follicles can give rise not only to the entire follicle but also to the epidermis. Taken together, these studies provide strong evidence that multipotent epithelial stem cells are located within the bulge and that these cells are capable of maintaining the epidermis, the hair follicle, and the sebaceous gland.

Involvement of the Hair Follicle in Skin Cancer

Since stem cells are known to represent a key target of tumor initiation,[10,50] it is important to know whether some skin cancers originate from hair follicular stem cells. Several lines of evidence suggest that this is the case. First, many basal cell carcinomas (BCCs) exhibit histologic and biologic features of the hair follicle, including their accumulation of cytoplasmic glycogen similar to that of the outer root sheath and their occasional resemblence to the matrix keratinocytes and to trichoepitheliomas.[50] Second, although ionizing radiation targeting the superficial rat epidermis produces few, if any, skin tumors, deeper radiation causing follicular damage can effectively induce skin tumor formation. Third, skin chemical carcinogenesis studies revealed that topical application of a carcinogen to mice at the onset of anagen (when bulge cells are proliferating) produced greater numbers of tumors than telogen application (when bulge cells are quiescent), suggesting that follicular stem cells can give rise to experimentally induced skin cancers.[51] Fourth, papilloma formation in a *v-Ha-ras* transgenic mouse line showed that the upper follicle is the origin of the tumor.[52] Fifth, studies on papilloma formation using domestic rabbits that have been infected with cottontail rabbit papilloma virus showed that the virus infects primarily the follicle cells that have the highest keratinocyte colony-forming ability (derived from stem cell–enriched regions of the hair follicle).[53] Sixth, a puzzling feature of many of the experimentally induced skin tumors is that they are associated with the infundibulum of the upper follicle rather than the bulge.[52,55] This observation may be explained by the fact that the upper hair follicle contains a population of early (young) TA (progenitor) cells that still have a high growth potential. These upper follicle TA cells are highly proliferative, making them particularly susceptible to DNA damage and possibly to tumor initiation.[10] Taken together, these findings support the idea that the hair follicle is the origin of at least some skin tumors and that both the bulge region and the upper follicle may be involved in neoplastic transformation.

FIGURE 12-6

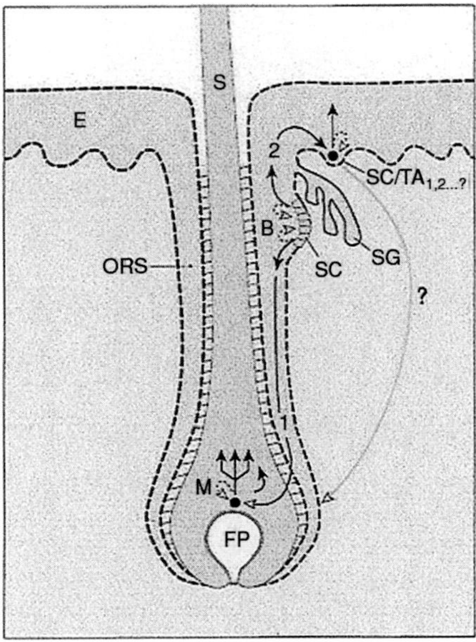

A schematic diagram of an epidermopilosebaceous unit in hair-bearing skin. The unit consists of the epidermis and the hair follicle with its associated sebaceous gland. The bulge contains a population of putative keratinocyte stem cells that can give rise to (pathway 1) a population of pluripotent and rapidly dividing progenitor (TA) cells in the matrix that yields the hair shaft. Alternatively, the bulge stem cells can give rise to the stem/progenitor cells of the epidermis (pathway 2). It is hypothesized here that the epidermal stem cell represents a form of bulge-derived, young TA cell ($SC/TA_{1,2...}?$). The long, curved arrow denotes the demonstrated capability of adult epidermal cells to form a new hair follicle in response to appropriate mesenchymal stimuli. (B, bulge; E, epidermis; FP, follicular or dermal papilla; M, matrix keratinocytes; ORS, outer root sheath; S, hair shaft; SC, stem cells; SG, sebaceous gland; TA, transit amplifying cells.) (*Reproduced from Lavker and Sun*[49] *with permission.*)

Molecular Control of Hair Follicle Development, Differentiation, and Cycling

As mentioned previously, a large number of genes have been implicated in hair follicle development as well as the hair growth cycle. These genes may act on the stem cell population, the matrix keratinocytes, and the follicular papilla.[56,58] These molecules include members of the Wnt, Notch and SHH signaling pathways, as well as EGF/TGF-α,

TGF-β, BMP, and the FGF families. Ectodysplasin and its receptor (EDA/EDAR) and PGDF-A also have been implicated in follicle development.

Wnt SIGNALING Members of the Wnt signaling pathway have been implicated in regulating hair follicle development and growth. Extracellular Wnt ligands bind to Frizzled receptors, thus inactivating a complex of proteins that normally target β-catenin for degradation. Thus activation of Wnt signaling causes β-catenin to accumulate, translocate to the nucleus, bind transcription factors of the TCF/LEF family, and regulate the expression of target genes.[58] β-Catenin mRNA is upregulated in placodes, and LEF-1 is also expressed in both the ectodermal placodes and the dermal condensates. A reporter gene sensitive to the activity of the LEF–β-catenin complex is expressed in the placodes and dermal condensates of developing follicles, suggesting that Wnt signaling is important for the crosstalk between epithelium and mesenchyme.[5] Consistent with this hypothesis, mice lacking LEF-1 or β-catenin have reduced numbers of hair follicles.[3] Conversely, ectopic expression of LEF-1 or stablized forms of β-catenin in the epidermis mimic an activated Wnt signaling pathway and result in precocious hair follicle formation and, in the presence of β-catenin, hair follicle tumorigenesis. Stabilizing mutations in the β-catenin gene are implicated in the etiology of human pilomaticoma, a tumor of hair follicle matrix cells.[58]

Members of the Wnt pathway also may play a role in regulating hair shaft formation. The β-catenin–LEF-1 complex is active in the more differentiated matrix cells (precursors of the hair shaft) of the fully formed hair follicle.[58] Furthermore, Wnt3 and a Wnt effector gene, *Disheveled2,* are expressed in the precortical zone, and the ectopic expression of Wnt3 in the outer root sheath alters hair shaft differentiation, resulting in a shortened hair phenotype.[59] Similar stunted hair growth was observed in mice overexpressing the β-catenin–related protein plakoglobin.[60] The plakoglobin-induced short hair phenotype was due to a significant decrease in the length of anagen, an early onset of apoptosis, and a reduction in the proliferative rate of the follicular keratinocytes. Thus Wnt family members may provide key signals to the cells that differentiate into various components of the hair shaft.

The Wnt pathway also may be involved in activating the normally quiescent hair follicle stem cells during early anagen of the hair cycle. TCF3 protein, a repressor of the Wnt signaling pathway, is expressed in the bulge region of the hair follicle. In mice carrying a reporter gene responsive to the β-catenin–LEF complexes, the reporter gene was found to undergo transient expression in bulge cells at the start of anagen.[58] Overexpression of TCF3 leads to suppression of epidermal differentiation and promotion of outer root sheath differentiation. In addition, TCF3 was found to function in the maintenance of the stem cell phenotype, suggesting that the repression of Wnt target genes is required to maintain the stem cells in an undifferentiated state. Lifting of this repression and activation of the Wnt signaling pathway thus may be necessary for the conversion of stem cells to TA cells at anagen onset.[58] Further evidence of the potential involvement of Wnt signaling in the determination of hair follicle stem cell fate comes from the observation that in the absence of epithelial β-catenin, keratinocytes can only adopt an epidermal phenotype, whereas in the presence of β-catenin, follicular epithelial stem cells can differentiate into follicular or epidermal lineages.[3]

SHH SIGNALING SHH can be produced by one cell to affect the developmental process of its neighboring target cell.[61] SHH interacts with and blocks the function of a cell surface receptor called patched-1 (Ptc1) that normally inhibits a third protein called Smoothened (Smo). Inhibition of Smo activates the expression of genes encoding Ptc1 itself, as well as the transcription factor Gli1. The SHH signaling pathway plays a critical role in regulating hair follicle development. In SHH-deficient mice, hair development is arrested, and the expression of Gli1 and Ptc1, downstream effector molecules in the SHH pathway, is greatly reduced in both epithelial and mesenchymal components, suggesting that SHH signals to both the epithelial and mesenchymal cells of the developing hair follicle.[62] However, mesenchymal condensates do develop in SHH-null mice, suggesting that SHH may act later than Wnt signaling in regulating hair follicle development.

Recent results suggest that SHH plays an important role in regulating early anagen. For example, inactivation of SHH protein does not prevent anagen onset but blocks progression of follicles through anagen.[63] Consistent with this, intradermal overexpression of SHH in mouse skin with an adenoviral vector caused telogen follicles to enter anagen.[64] As in morphogenesis, SHH may act downstream of Wnt signaling in early anagen, since anagen onset does not occur in mice lacking epithelial β-catenin.[3]

The hair follicle exhibits several histologic and biologic features of BCCs.[50] In humans, BCCs are known to develop from both follicular and interfollicular epidermis. Given the fact that SHH is required for hair follicle morphogenesis, it is not surprising that SHH signaling also may play a role in BCC formation (see Chaps. 81 and 82). For example, recent data indicate that BCC in humans results from inappropriate activation of the SHH pathway in the epidermis and is often associated with mutations in *Ptc.*[65,66] It also has been demonstrated that skin tumors arise in mice following overexpression of SHH and the effectors of the SHH pathway (Gli1, and Gli2) and that many of these tumors resemble BCCs and other hair follicle–derived neoplasias such as trichoepitheliomas and trichoblastomas.[67,69] Given the fact that the follicular epithelial stem cells are the likely source of many skin tumors, it is possible that the levels of SHH and/or the Gli transcription factors could alter the growth regulation of these stem cells, resulting in BCC development.

NOTCH SIGNALING Notch is a transmembrane receptor that, on ligand binding, undergoes proteolytic release of the Notch intracellular domain (NICD). NICD translocates to the nucleus, where it acts as a part of the transcription complex with CBF1/Su(H)/Lag1 (CSL) proteins. Ligands for Notch include Delta, Jagged-1, and Jagged-2 in vertebrates.[9] Within the hair follicle, the Notch1 receptor colocalizes with its ligand Jagged-1 in the precortical cells. Thus the Notch–Jagged-2 pair may be involved in the transition of matrix cells into the more differentiated components of the hair shaft.[70] Recently it was found that the ectopic expression of Notch1 in the cortex resulted in the abnormal development of the medulla and cuticle, supporting the idea that Notch expression in one cell type may direct the differentiation of adjacent cell types.[9]

ADDITIONAL INTERCELLULAR SIGNALING MOLECULES The formation of placode seems to be promoted by EDA, a protein related to tumor necrosis factor, and its receptor (*ectodermal dysplasia receptor-EDAR*). The *EDA* gene is mutated in human X-linked anhidrotic ectodermal dysplasia and in the *Tabby* mouse, in both cases causing a reduction in the number of hair follicles.[71] Conversely, members of the BMP family appear to inhibit follicle formation.[71] With respect to hair follicle differentiation, transgenic mice ectopically expressing Noggin (an inhibitor of BMP) in the hair matrix cells and precortical cells were found to have cycling cells present in the precortex and hair shaft. This indicates that BMP signaling suppresses matrix cell proliferation and is required to induce the terminal differentiation of the hair shaft progenitors located in the precortical cells.[4] Another molecule implicated in the conversion of the dermal condensate into the dermal papilla is PDGF-A. Mice lacking PDGF-A have small dermal papilla and correspondingly thin hair when compared with wild-type mice.[72]

The Follicular Papilla

As mentioned earlier, the follicular papilla is a group of specialized mesenchymal cells that plays a central role in follicular development and hair cycle control. For example, the diameter and length of the hair fiber are directly related to the volume of the follicular papilla.[73] A recent study showed that the number of follicular papilla cells and the volume of their associated extracellular matrix were positively correlated with the size of the hair cortex.[73] The hairless phenotype of the *hr/hr* mutant mouse was shown to be due to a failure of the follicular papilla to ascend during the first catagen phase.[74] Perhaps the most striking demonstration of the significance of the follicular papilla in hair growth came from the demonstration that isolated follicular papillae from rat vibrissae, when combined with an interfollicular epidermis, can induce new hair formation.[75] More recently, papillary cells derived from pelage follicles were found to induce pelage-type follicles, whereas cells from the vibrissae induced large vibrissae-type follicles.[76] The hair-inducing ability of follicular papilla cells was further demonstrated when cultured keratinocytes were mixed with either fibroblasts or follicular papilla cells and grafted to a nude mouse.[77] Hair follicles formed if follicular papilla cells were present; however, no hair follicles were formed in the presence of dermal fibroblasts. It is also apparent that the specialized cells located within the connective tissue sheath that surrounds the follicle have the capacity to form a follicular papilla and to induce hair growth.[78] Taken together, these findings clearly demonstrate that follicular papillary cells and dermal sheath cells are distinct from the regular dermal fibroblasts because they can send out signals that can induce hair formation.

Follicular papillary cells produce several growth factors, cytokines, and transcription factors that play a role in regulating the hair cycle. For example, KGF has a stimulatory effect on hair follicle growth in vivo.[79] mRNAs for insulin-like growth factor–binding proteins are localized to the follicular papilla and connective tissue sheath of anagen follicles, suggesting a possible role in modulating insulin-like growth factor during the hair cycle.[80] mRNA for the protease nexin-1, a potent serine protease inhibitor, also has been localized in the follicular papillae of human and rat anagen follicles but not in those of catagen or telogen.[12] Recently, mRNA for osteopontin, a secreted glycosylated phosphoprotein known to play diverse roles in mediating cell-matrix interactions, growth regulation, and various aspects of the inflammation/tissue repair cascade, has been localized to the follicular papillae of catagen follicles but not those in anagen or telogen.[81] This last observation is of particular interest in that it shows that specific genes are turned on during catagen, which is therefore not simply a passive "degenerative" phase. While the functional role of osteopontin in catagen is unclear, it may promote the formation of a tightly aggregated follicular papilla and/or protect the follicular papilla cells from apoptosis induced by cytokines or hypoxia during catagen.[81] In another study, freshly isolated mouse follicular papilla cells were shown to express Ptch and Gli1, molecules in the SHH signaling cascade, as well as Wnt5a, Frizzled 7, Disheveled 2, GSK, β-catenin, and LEF-1, all components of the Wnt signal transduction cascade.[6] Thus the follicular papillary cells elaborate proteases and their inhibitors, extracellular matrix molecules, growth factors, receptors, and signal-transduction molecules that are involved in the regulation of the hair cycle.

Hormones as Regulators of the Hair Cycle

Systemic factors such as androgens, estrogens, glucocorticoids, thyroid hormones, and growth hormones all can modulate hair growth.[82] Hamilton[83] was the first to recognize the importance of androgens in human hair growth when he noted that men castrated before the age of puberty neither became bald nor grew beards unless they were treated with testosterone. Castration of older men prevented balding. Androgens are known to upregulate the pubic hair, axillary hair, and beard hair but to downregulate genetically predisposed scalp hair follicles in androgenetic alopecia (common baldness).[84] The fact that only select populations of hairs demonstrate such responses exemplifies the diverse responses of hair follicles to similar stimuli. The follicular papilla appears to be the target for androgen effects because these cells have been demonstrated to express androgen receptors and androgen-metabolizing enzymes (such as 5α-reductase, types I and II.)[85] Follicular papillae in the balding scalp have been demonstrated to have higher levels of androgen receptors than those from nonbalding skin.[86]

Some insight into androgen action has been gained from common forms of androgen insensitivity resulting from defects in the androgen receptor or 5α-reductase (the enzyme that converts testosterone to the more potent dihydrotestosterone).[82] Testosterone can have a species-dependent stimulatory or inhibitory effect on cultured dermal papilla cells. For example, in vitro studies employing cultured dermal papillary cells from human beard and scalp follicles have shown that when beard cells are incubated with testosterone, they secrete mitogenic factors that stimulate the growth of other dermal papillary cells and outer root sheath cells.[87] Conversely, in studies using dermal papilla cells from the macaque, testosterone stimulates cells from androgen-sensitive follicles to synthesize inhibitory factors that dampen the growth of follicular epithelial cells in culture.[88] Beard-derived follicular papillary cells express greater amounts of insulin-like growth factor I (IGF-1) in response to testosterone, suggesting that IGF-1 may be a regulatory molecule in hair growth.[89] While a unified mechanism for hormonal control of hair growth is presently lacking, further studies using the preceding approaches should yield a better understanding of the differential actions of androgens on hair.

REFERENCES

1. Halata Z: Sensory innervation of the hairy skin (light- and electronmicroscopic study). *J Invest Dermatol* **101**:75s, 1993
2. Hardy MH: The secret life of the hair follicle. *Trends Genet* **8**:159, 1992
3. Huelsken J et al: β-Catenin controls hair follicle morphogenesis and stem cell differentiation in the skin. *Cell* **105**:533, 2001
4. Kulessa H et al: Inhibition of BMP signaling affects growth and differentiation in the anagen hair follicle. *EMBO J* **24**:6664, 2000
5. Reddy S et al: Characterization of *Wnt* gene expression in developing and postnatal hair follicles and identification of *Wnt5a* as a target of sonic hedgehog in hair follicle morphogenesis. *Mech Dev* **107**:69, 2001
6. Kishimoto J et al: Wnt signaling maintains the hair-inducing activity of the dermal papilla. *Gene Dev* **14**:1181, 2000
7. Holbrook KA et al: Expression of morphogens during human follicle development in vivo and a model for studying follicle morphogenesis in vivo. *J Invest Dermatol* **101**:39S, 1993
8. Cotsarelis G et al: Label-retaining cells reside in the bulge of the pilosebaceous unit: Implications for follicular stem cells, hair cycle, and skin carcinogenesis. *Cell* **61**:1329, 1990
9. Lin M-H et al: Activation of the *Notch* pathway in the hair cortex leads to aberrant differentiation of the adjacent hair-shaft layers. *Development* **127**:2421, 2000
10. Taylor G et al: Involvement of follicular stem cells in forming not only the follicle but also the epidermis. *Cell* **102**:451, 2000
11. Oshima H et al: Morphogenesis and renewal of hair follicles from adult multipotent stem cells. *Cell* **104**:233, 2001
12. Jensen PJ et al: Serpins in the human hair follicle. *J Invest Dermatol* **114**:917, 2000
13. Muller-Rover S et al: A comprehensive guide for the accurate classification of murine hair follicles in distinct hair cycle stages. *J Invest Dermatol* **117**:3, 2001
14. Yano K et al: Control of hair growth and follicle size by VEGF-mediated angiogenesis. *J Clin Invest* **107**:409, 2001

15. Stenn KS, Paus R: Controls of hair follicle cycling. *Physiol Rev* **81**:449, 2001
16. Kligman AM: The human hair cycles. *J Invest Dermatol* **33**:307, 1959
17. Seiberg M et al: Changes in expression of apoptosis-associated genes in skin mark early catagen. *J Invest Dermatol* **104**:78, 1995
18. Linder G et al: Analysis of apoptosis during hair follicle regression (catagen). *Am J Pathol* **151**:1601, 1997
19. Hebert JM et al: FGF5 as a regulator of the hair growth cycle: Evidence from targeted and spontaneous mutations. *Cell* **78**:1017, 1994
20. Stenn KS et al: Growth of the hair follicle: A cycling and regenerating biological system, in *Molecular Basis of Epithelial Appendage Morphogenesis,* edited by C-M Chuong. Austin, Landes, 1998
21. Chase HB et al: Critical stages of hair development and growth in the mouse. *Physiol Zool* **24**:1, 1951
22. Takashima I, Kawagishi I: Comparative study of hair growths in mammals, with special reference to hair grouping and hair cycle, and hair growth rate in the juvenile stumptailed macaque, in *Biology and Disease of Hair,* edited by T Kobori, W Montagna. Baltimore, University Park Press, 1976
23. Barman JM et al: The first stage in the natural history of the human scalp hair cycle. *J Invest Dermatol* **48**:138, 1967
24. Kligman AM: Pathologic dynamics of human hair loss. *Arch Dermatol* **83**:175, 1961
25. Saadat M et al: Measurement of hair in normal newborns. *Pediatrics* **57**:960, 1976
26. Giacometti L: The anatomy of the human scalp, in *Advances in Biology of the Skin,* edited by W Montagna. Oxford, Pergamon Press, 1964
27. Headington JT: Transverse microscopic anatomy of the human scalp: A basis for a morphometric approach to disorders of the hair follicle. *Arch Dermatol* **120**:449, 1984
28. Pecoraro V et al: The normal trichogram in the child before puberty. *J Invest Dermatol* **42**:427, 1964
29. Unger WP: *Hair Transplantation*. New York, Decker, 1979
30. Jones LN, Steinert PM: Hair keratinization in health and disease. *Dermatol Clin* **14**:633, 1996
31. Sun T-T et al: Classification, expression and possible mechanisms of evolution of mammalian epithelial 2 keratins: A unifying model, in *Cancer Cells,* edited by A Levine, W Toop, G Vande Woude, J D Watson. Cold Spring Harbor, Cold Spring Harbor Laboratory, 1984, vol I, p169.
32. Stasiak PC et al: Keratin 19: Predicted amino acid sequence and broad tissue distribution suggest it evolved from keratinocyte keratins. *J Invest Dermatol* **92**:707, 1989
33. Michel M et al: Keratin 19 as a biochemical marker of skin stem cells in vivo and in vitro: Keratin 19 expressing cells are differentially localized in function of anatomic sites, and their number varies with donor age and culture stage. *J Cell Sci* **109**:1017, 1996
34. Mcgowin KM, Coulombe PA: Keratin 17 expression in the hard epithelial context of the hair and nail, and its relevance for the pachyonychia congenita phenotype. *J Invest Dermatol* **114**:1101, 2000
35. Winter H et al: A novel human type II cytokeratin, K6hf, specifically expressed in the companion layer of the hair follicle. *J Invest Dermatol* **111**:955, 1998
36. Langbein L et al: The catalog of human hair keratins: I. Expression of the nine type I members in the hair follicle. *J Biol Chem* **274**:19874, 1999
37. Langbein L et al: The catalog of human hair keratins: II. Expression of the six type II members in the hair follicle and the combined catalog of human type I and II keratins. *J Biol Chem* **276**:35123, 2001
38. Rogers GE, Powell BC: Hair follicle keratins, in *Handbook of Mouse Mutations with Skin and Hair Abnormalities*, edited by JP Sundberg. Boca Raton, CRC Press, 1994
39. Lynch MH et al: Acidic andbasic hair/nail ("hard") keratins: in Their colocalization in upper cortical and cuticle cells of the human hair follicle and their relationship to "soft" keratins. *J Cell Biol* **103**:2593, 1986
40. Fietz MJ et al: Analysis of the sheep trichohyalin gene: Potential structural and calcium-binding roles of trichohyalin in the hair follicle. *J Cell Biol* **121**:855, 1993
41. Hayashi A et al: Trichogram. *J Invest Dermatol* **60**:70, 1975
42. Lindelof B et al: Human hair form. *Arch Dermatol* **124**:1359, 1988
43. Tobin DJ et al: The fate of hair cycle melanocytes during the hair growth cycle. *J Invest Dermatol* **4**:323, 1999
44. Miller MW et al: Cloning of the mouse *agouti* gene predicts a secreted protein ubiquitously expressed in mice carrying the *Lethal-Yellow* mutation. *Gene Dev* **7**:454, 1993
45. Vrieling H et al: Differences in dorsal and ventral pigmentation result from regional expression of the mouse agouti gene. *Proc Natl Acad Sci USA* **91**:5667, 1994
46. Okura M et al: Effects of monoclonal anti-c-Kit antibody (ACK2) on melanocytes in newborn mice. *J Invest Dermatol* **105**:322, 1995
47. Botchkareva NV et al: SCF/c-Kit signaling is required for cyclic regeneration of the hair pigmentation unit. *FASEB J* **15**:645, 2001
48. Hibberts NA et al: Dermal papilla cells derived from beard hair follicles secrete more stem cell factor (SCF) in culture than scalp cells or dermal fibroblasts. *Biochem Biophys Res Commun* **222**:401, 1996
49. Lavker RM, Sun T-T: Epidermal stem cells: Properties, markers, and location. *Proc Natl Acad Sci USA* **97**:13473, 2000
50. Lavker RM et al: Hair follicle stem cells: Their location, role in hair cycle, and involvement in skin tumor formation. *J Invest Dermatol* **101**:16S, 1993
51. Miller SJ et al: Mouse skin is particularly susceptible to tumor initiation during early anagen of the hair cycle: possible involvement of hair follicle stem cells. *J Invest Dermatol* **101**:591, 1993
52. Hansen LA, Tennant RW: Follicular origin of epidermal papillomas in *v-Ha-ras* transgenic TG.AC mouse skin. *Proc Natl Acad Sci USA* **91**:7822, 1994
53. Schmitt A et al: The primary target cells of the high-risk cottontail rabbit papillomavirus colocalize with hair follicle stem cells. *J Virol* **70**:1912, 1996
54. Binder RL et al: Squamous cell hyperplastic foci: Precursors of cutaneous papillomas induced in SENCAR mice by two-stage carcinogenesis regimen. *Cancer Res* **58**:4314, 1998
55. Morris RJ et al: Evidence that the epidermal targets of carcinogen action are found in the interfollicular epidermis or infundibulum as well as in the hair follicles. *Cancer Res* **60**:226, 2000
56. Millar SE: The role of patterning genes in epidermal differentiation, in *Cytoskeletal-Membrane Interactions and Signal Transduction,* edited by P Cowin, M Klymkowsky. Austin, Landes Bioscience, 1997 p 87
57. Oro AE, Scott MP: Splitting hairs: Dissecting roles of signaling systems in epidermal development. *Cell* **95**:575, 1998
58. Fuchs E et al: At the roots of a never ending cycle. *Dev Cell* **1**:13, 2001
59. Millar SE et al: Wnt signaling in the control of hair growth and structure. *Dev Biol* **207**:133, 1999
60. Charpentier E et al: Plakoglobin suppresses epithelial proliferation and hair growth in vivo. *J Cell Biol* **149**:503, 2000
61. Dlugosz A: The hedgehog and the hair follicle: a growing relationship. *J Clin Invest* **104**:851, 1999
62. Chiang C et al: Essential role for sonic hedgehog during hair follicle morphogenesis. *Dev Biol* **205**:1, 1999
63. Wang LC et al: Conditional disruption of hedgehog signaling pathway defines its critical role in hair development and regeneration. *J Invest Dermatol* **114**:901, 2000
64. Sato N et al: Induction of the hair growth phase in postnatal mice by localized transient expression of sonic hedgehog. *J Clin Invest* **104**:855, 1999
65. Hahn H et al: Mutations of the human homolog of *Drosophila patched* in the nevoid basal cell carcinoma syndrome. *Cell* **85**:841, 1996
66. Johnson RL et al: Human homolog of *patched*, a candidate gene for the basal cell nevus syndrome. *Science* **272**:1668, 1996
67. Oro AE et al: Basal cell carcinomas in mice overexpressing sonic hedgehog. *Science* **276**:817, 1997
68. Nilsson M et al: Induction of basal cell carcinomas and trichoepitheliomas in mice overexpressing Gli-1. *Proc Natl Acad Sci USA* **97**:3438, 2000
69. Grachtchouk M et al: Basal cell carcinomas in mice overexpressing Gli2 in skin. *Nature Genet* **24**:216, 2000
70. Powell BC et al: The *Notch* signaling pathway in hair growth. *Mech Dev* **78**:189, 1998
71. Barsh GS: Of ancient tales and hairless tails. *Nature Genet* **22**:315, 1999
72. Karlsson L et al: Roles for PGDF-A and sonic hedgehog in development of mesenchymal components of the hair follicle. *Development* **126**:2611, 1999
73. Elliott K et al: Differences in hair follicle dermal papilla volume are due to extracellular matrix volume and cell number: Implications for the control of hair follicle size and androgen responses. *J Invest Dermatol* **113**:873, 1999
74. Montagna W et al: Skin of hairless mice: I. Formation of cysts and the distribution of lipids. *J Invest Dermatol* **19**:83, 1952
75. Oliver RF: The experimental induction of whisker growth in the hooded rat by implantation of the dermal papilla. *J Embryol Exp Morphel* **18**:43, 1967

76. Jahoda CA, Reynolds AJ: Dermal-epidermal interactions: Follicle-derived cell populations in the study of hair-growth mechanisms. *J Invest Dermatol* **101**:335, 1993
77. Kamimura J et al: Primary mouse keratinocyte cultures contain hair follicle progenitor cells with multiple differentiation potential. *J Invest Dermatol* **109**:534, 1997
78. Robinson M et al: In vivo induction of hair growth by dermal cells isolated from hair follicles after extended organ culture. *J Invest Dermatol* **117**:596, 2001
79. Danilenko DM et al: Keratinocyte growth factor is an important endogenous mediator of hair follicle growth, development, and differentiation. *Am J Pathol* **147**:145, 1995
80. Batch JA et al: Identification and localization of insulin-like growth factor-binidng protein (IGFBP) messenger RNAs in human hair follicle dermal papilla. *J Invest Dermatol* **106**:471, 1996
81. Yu D-W et al: Osteopontin gene is expressed in the dermal papilla of pelage hair follicles in a hair cycle–dependent manner. *J Invest Dermatol* **117**:1554, 2001
82. Paus R, Cotsarelis G: The biology of hair follicles. *New Engl J Med* **341**:491, 1999
83. Hamilton JB: Male hormone stimulation is a prerequisite and an incidant in common baldness. *Am J Anat* **71**:451, 1942

84. Randall VA: Androgens are the main regulator of human hair growth, in *Hair and Its Disorders: Biology, Pathology, and Management,* edited by F Camacho, VA Randall, V Price. London, Martin Dunitz, 2000, p 69
85. Randall VA et al: Androgen action in cultured dermal papilla cells from human hair follicles. *Skin Pharmacol* **7**:20, 1994
86. Hibberts NA et al: Balding hair follicle dermal papilla cells contain higher levels of androgen receptors than those from non-balding scalp. *J Endocrinol* **156**:59, 1998
87. Randall VA et al: Mechanism of androgen action in cultured dermal papilla cells derived from human hair follicles with varying responses to androgens in vivo. *J Invest Dermatol* **98**:86S, 1992
88. Obana N et al: Inhibition of hair growth by testosterone in the presence of dermal papilla cells from the frontal bald scalp of the postpubertal stumptailed macaque. *Endocrinology* **138**:356, 1997
89. Randall VA: The use of dermal papilla cells in studies of normal and abnormal hair follicle biology, in *Dermatologic Clinics,* edited by DA Whiting. Philadelphia, Saunders, 1996, vol 14

CHAPTER 13

Antonella Tosti
Bianca Maria Piraccini

Biology of Nails

The nail apparatus consists of a horny "dead" product, the nail plate, and four specialized epithelia: the proximal nail fold, the nail matrix, the nail bed, and the hyponychium (Fig. 13-1).

The nail apparatus develops during the ninth embryonic week from the epidermis of the dorsal tip of the digit as a rectangular area, the nail field, which is delineated by a continuous groove.[1] The proximal border of the nail field extends downward and proximally into the dermis to form the nail matrix primordium. By the fifteenth week, the nail matrix is completely developed and starts to produce the nail plate, which will continue to growth until death.

FIGURE 13-1

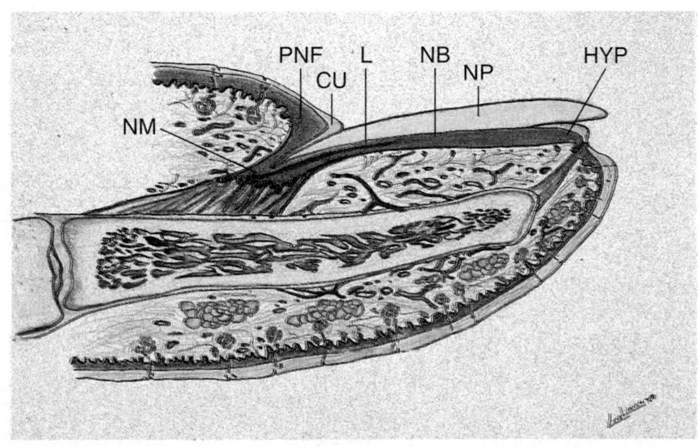

Drawing of a normal nail. CU, cuticle; HYP, hyponychium; L, lunula region; NB, nail bed; NM, nail matrix; NP, nail plate; PNF, proximal nail fold.

The nail apparatus lies immediately above the periosteum of the distal phalanx. The intimate anatomic relationship between the nail and the bone is responsible for the common occurrence of bone alterations in nail disorders and vice versa. The shape of the distal phalangeal bone also determines the shape and the transverse curvature of the nail.

Fingernails usually present a longitudinal major axis and toenails a transverse major axis. The ratio between length and width is important for the esthetical appearance of the nails. The size of the nails varies in the different digits, the biggest nail being that of the first toe, which covers about 50 percent of the dorsum of the digit.

The nails have numerous functions. Fingernails not only contribute to the esthetic of the hands, but are very important in protecting the distal phalanges, and in enhancing tactile discrimination and the capacity to pick up small objects. They are also widely used for scratching and grooming, and are an efficient natural weapon. Toenails protect the distal toes and contribute to pedal biomechanics.

NAIL PLATE

The nail plate is a fully keratinized structure that is continuously produced throughout life. It results from maturation and keratinization of the nail matrix epithelium and it is firmly attached to the nail bed, which partially contributes to its formation. Proximally and laterally the nail plate is surrounded by the nail folds that cover its proximal and lateral margins. At the tip of the digit, the nail plate separates from the underlying tissues at the hyponychium. The nail plate is rectangular in shape, translucent, and transparent. It is curved in both the longitudinal and transverse axes, especially in the toes. The nail plate surface is smooth, but frequently shows mild longitudinal ridges that increase with aging. The pattern of these ridges can be used for forensic identification. The bottom of the nail plate shows longitudinal ridges that correspond to the rete ridges of the nail bed. The nail plate is homogeneously pink in color, except for its free edge that is white. The pink color of the nail plate is due to the nail bed blood vessels. The proximal part of the fingernails, especially of the thumbs, shows a whitish, opaque, half-moon–shaped area, the lunula, which is the visible portion of the nail matrix. In this area, the nail plate attachment to the underlying epithelium is loose. More than 90 percent of fingernails show a thin distal transverse white band, the onychocorneal band, which marks to the most distal portion of firm attachment of the nail plate to the nail bed.[2] This area represents an important anatomic barrier against environmental hazards and its disruption produces nail plate detachment with onycholysis. The onychocorneal band is separated from the nail plate white free edge by a 1- to 1.5-mm pink band called the *onychodermal band.*

In transverse sections, the nail plate consists of three portions: dorsal nail plate, intermediate nail plate, and ventral nail plate.[3] The dorsal and the intermediate portions of the nail plate are produced by the nail matrix, whereas its ventral portion is produced by the nail bed. Above the lunula, the nail plate is thinner and consists only of the dorsal and intermediate portions. There is a natural line of cleavage between the dorsal and the intermediate nail plate.

The nail plate progressively thickens from its emergence to its distal margin, the mean toenail thickness at the distal margin being 1.65 ± 0.43 mm in men and 1.38 ± 0.20 mm in women. Fingernails are thinner, their mean thickness being 0.6 mm in men and 0.5 mm in women. There is an increase in nail thickness with age, particularly in the first two decades. Nail thickness depends on the length of the nail matrix and nail bed.[4] Thinning of the nails is usually a sign of nail matrix disorders, whereas nail thickening is most commonly a consequence of nail bed disorders.

PROXIMAL NAIL FOLD

The proximal nail fold is a skin fold that consists of a dorsal and a ventral portion (Fig. 13-2). The dorsal portion is anatomically similar to the skin of the dorsum of the digit but thinner and devoid of pilosebaceous units. The ventral portion, which cannot be seen from the exterior, and which proximally is in continuity with the germinative matrix, covers approximately one-fourth of the nail plate. It closely adheres to the nail plate surface and keratinizes with a granular layer. The limit between the proximal nail fold and the nail matrix can be established histologically at the site of disappearance of the granular layer.

The horny layer of the proximal nail fold forms the cuticle, which is firmly attached to the superficial nail plate and prevents the separation of the plate from the nail fold. The integrity of the cuticle is essential for maintaining homeostasis of this region. The dermis of the proximal nail fold contains numerous capillaries that run parallel to the surface of the skin. Capillary microscopy permits the observation of both the arterial and the venous limbs of the capillaries, which are arranged in parallel rows and appear as fine regular loops with a small space between the afferent and efferent limbs. The morphology of proximal nail fold capillaries is typically altered in connective tissue diseases.

FIGURE 13-2

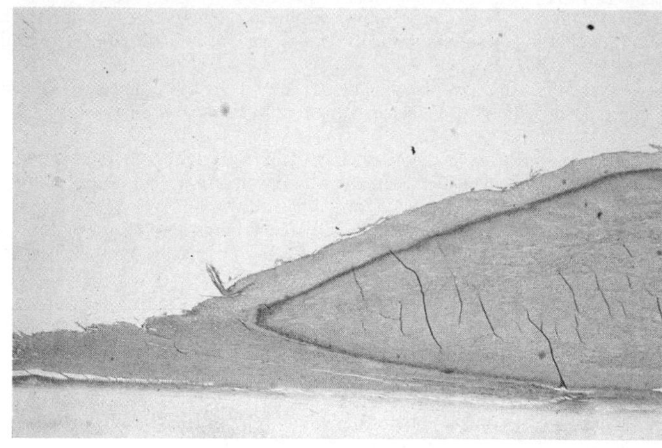

Histologic section showing the dorsal and the ventral portions of the proximal nail fold. The cuticle provides adhesion between the ventral nail fold and the nail plate.

NAIL MATRIX

The nail matrix is a specialized epithelial structure that lies above the mid-portion of the distal phalanx. After elevation of the proximal nail fold, the matrix appears as a distally convex crescent with its lateral horns extending proximally and laterally.

In longitudinal sections, the matrix has a wedge-shaped appearance and consists of a proximal (dorsal) and a distal (ventral) portion (Fig. 13-3). Nail matrix keratinocytes divide in the basal cell layer and keratinize in the absence of a granular zone. Cornified onychocytes are composed mainly of keratin filaments, high-sulfur matrix proteins, and the marginal band, which consists of precipitated proteins on the cytoplasmic side of the cell membrane. The site of keratinization

FIGURE 13-3

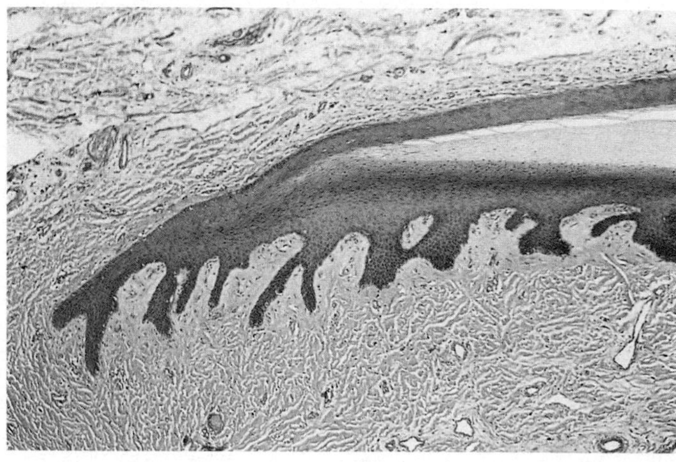

Histologic section of the proximal nail matrix. (*Courtesy of C. Misciali, M.D.*)

(keratogenous zone) of nail matrix onychocytes can be clearly distinguished in histologic sections as an eosinophilic area in which cells show fragmentation of their nuclei and condensation of their cytoplasm.[1] In this area, nuclear fragments are destroyed by DNAase and RNAase enzymes. In some conditions, nuclear fragments may persist within the intermediate nail plate, producing leukonychial spots. These, however, frequently disappear before reaching the nail free edge, due to persistence of active DNA and RNA lytic enzymes within the horny nail plate.

Maturation and differentiation of nail matrix keratinocytes do not follow a vertical axis, as in the epidermis, but occur along a diagonal axis that is distally oriented. For this reason, keratinization of the proximal nail matrix cells produces the dorsal nail plate and keratinization of the distal nail matrix cells produces the intermediate nail plate.

In some fingers, the distal matrix is not completely covered by the proximal nail fold, but is visible through the nail plate as a white half-moon-shaped area, the lunula. The white color of the lunula results from two main anatomic factors: (1) the keratogenous zone of the distal matrix contains nuclear fragments that cause light diffraction; and (2) the nail matrix capillaries are less visible than nail bed capillaries due to the relative thickness of the nail matrix epithelium.[5]

Nail Matrix Keratinocytes

The nail matrix cells are able to synthesize both "soft" or skin-type and "hard" or hair-type keratins. According to Kitahara and Ogawa the dorsal nail matrix keratinocytes in vivo produce soft keratins, while the ventral nail matrix keratinocytes produce hard keratins. Results from in vitro studies, however, indicate that all cells are able to change their course of differentiation and express multiple keratins.[6] When cultured in a chemically defined medium, nail matrix cells are considerably larger than epidermal keratinocytes and show a low nucleus/cytoplasm and a high euchromatin/heterochromatin ratio. The growth rate of cultured nail matrix cells is higher than that of epidermal keratinocytes.[7] When cultured in serum-containing medium, the nail matrix cells show spontaneous migration and stratified growth in a semilunar area, which resembles the architecture of the nail matrix.

Melanocytes

Nail matrix melanocytes are usually quiescent and therefore not detectable in pathologic sections. By using immunohistochemical techniques, two different populations of melanocytes have been recognized in the nail: (1) DOPA-negative, dormant melanocytes localized in the proximal and distal matrix and in the nail bed; and (2) DOPA-positive, activatable melanocytes localized in the distal matrix.[8] DOPA-positive melanocytes possess the key enzymes that are necessary for melanin production and may become activated by a large number of physiologic and pathologic conditions. Nail matrix melanocyte activation produces diffuse or banded nail pigmentation and is more common in blacks and Japanese than in Caucasians.

Nail matrix melanocytes are frequently arranged in small clusters among the suprabasal layers of the nail matrix epithelium.[9] Suprabasal location of nail matrix melanocytes may be a consequence of the distribution of the adhesion molecules in the nail epithelium, where $\alpha_3\beta_1$ integrin, which possibly regulates melanocyte-keratinocyte adhesion, is expressed in basal and suprabasal locations.[10]

Electron microscopically, nail matrix melanocytes of Caucasians do not contain mature melanosomes, which are normally found in nail matrices of Japanese and blacks.[11]

Langerhans Cells

Langerhans cells are more numerous in the proximal than in the distal nail matrix. As in normal epidermis, Langerhans cells are predominantly found in the suprabasal layers. They may, however, occasionally be seen within the basal layer of the nail matrix epithelium.

Merkel Cells

The presence of Merkel cells has been demonstrated in the nail matrix. By using antibodies against CK8 and CK20 cytokeratins, we detected more than 20 Merkel cells per nail matrix section in adults.[12]

NAIL BED

The nail bed, which contains sparse DOPA-negative melanocytes,[8] extends from the distal margin of the lunula to the onychodermal band and is completely visible through the nail plate. The nail bed epithelium is so adherent to the nail plate that it remains attached to the undersurface of the nail when a nail is avulsed. The nail bed epithelium is thin and consists of two to five cell layers. Its rete ridges, which are longitudinally oriented, interdigitate with the underlying dermal ridges in a tongue-in-groove–like fashion.

Nail bed keratinization produces a thin horny layer that forms the ventral nail plate, and in toto, the nail bed contribution to nail plate formation corresponds to about one-fifth of the terminal nail thickness and mass.[13] In histologic sections, the ventral nail plate is easily distinguishable because of its light eosinophilic appearance. Nail bed keratinization is not associated with the formation of a granular layer. A granular layer may, however, appear when the nail bed becomes exposed after nail avulsion.[1]

HYPONYCHIUM

The hyponychium marks the anatomic area between the nail bed and the distal groove, where the nail plate detaches from the dorsal digit. Its anatomic structure is similar to that of plantar and volar skin, and keratinization occurs through the formation of a granular layer. The horny layer of the hyponychium partially accumulates under the nail plate free margin.

The hyponychium is normally covered by the distal nail plate, but it may become visible in nail biters.

BASEMENT MEMBRANE ZONE

The antigenic structure of the basement membrane zone of the nail is identical to that of the epidermis and there are no differences in the antigenic composition of the basement membrane zone between the different portions of the nail apparatus.[14] This may explain the involvement of the nails in conditions characterized by mutations of basement membrane-associated genes, as well as in autoimmune skin diseases involving the basement membrane zone antigens.[15]

THE DERMIS

The nail apparatus is devoid of subcutaneous tissue, and its dermis does not contain pilosebaceous units. The arrangement of the rete ridges varies in the different portions of the nail apparatus. The dermis beneath the proximal nail matrix consists of condensed connective tissue that forms a tendon-like structure connecting the matrix to the periosteum of the proximal phalangeal bone (posterior ligament) (Fig. 13-1). A small amount of subdermal fat tissue is present close to the periosteum of the base of the phalanx.[16] The close connection between the lateral horns and the periosteum is possibly responsible for the nail plate's lateral convexity. The rete ridges of the dermis underneath the nail matrix are characteristically long and root-like–shaped, running from lunula to hyponychium.[1] The dermis under the distal matrix consists of a loose network of connective tissue containing numerous blood vessels and rare glomus bodies. The longitudinal orientation of the capillary vessels within the nail bed grooves explains the linear pattern of the nail bed hemorrhages (splinter hemorrhages). The nail bed dermis contains numerous glomus bodies and connective tissue bundles radiating to the phalangeal periosteum.

BLOOD AND NERVE SUPPLY

The nail apparatus has an abundant blood supply provided by the lateral digital arteries. These run along the sides of the digits and produce branches that supply both the matrix and the proximal nail fold and arches that supply the matrix and the nail bed. The matrix therefore has two different sources of blood supply.

The nail bed is richly supplied (10 to 20/cm^2) by encapsulated neurovascular structures containing one to four arteriovenous anastomoses and nerve endings. These glomus bodies are possibly involved in the regulation of the blood supply to the digits in cold weather.

The cutaneous sensory nerves, which originate from the dorsal branches of the paired digital nerves, run parallel to the digital vessels.

CHEMICAL PROPERTIES

The nail plate, like hair, consists mainly of low-sulfur filamentous proteins (keratins) embedded in an amorphous matrix composed of high-sulfur proteins rich in cystine. Other nail constituents include water, lipids, and trace elements. Nail keratins consist of 80 to 90 percent hard "hair-type" keratins and 10 to 20 percent soft "skin-type" keratins. Hard keratins have been identified as the acidic 44K/46K and basic 56K to 60K keratins. Soft keratins have been identified as the 50K/58K and 48K/56K keratin pairs[17] (see Chap. 7).

In normal conditions, the water content of the nail plate is 18 percent, most of it being in the intermediate nail plate.[18] This may, however, significantly vary due to the high porosity of the nail plate, which can be rapidly hydrated and dehydrated. Dehydration is faster when the nails are kept long. When the water content decreases below 18 percent, the nail becomes brittle; when it increases above 30 percent, it becomes opaque and soft.

The nail contains less than 5 percent lipids, mainly cholesterol. Lipid composition of the nail plate varies with age and sex under the influence of sex hormones.[19] The nail also contains traces of several inorganic elements including iron, zinc, and calcium. These, however, do not contribute to nail hardness. Permeability of the nail plate to drugs and water is considerably different from that of the skin (Table 13-1).

TABLE 13-1

Differences Between Nail Plate and Epidermal Horny Layer

	NAIL PLATE	HORNY LAYER
Thickness	500–1000 μm	10–40 μm
S-S bonds	10.6%	1.2%
Maximal swelling (in water)	25%	200–300%
Lipid content	1–5%	10–20%
Permeability behavior	Hydrophilic membrane	Lipophilic membrane

The nail, in fact, behaves like a hydrophilic gel membrane that is easily penetrated by small hydrophilic molecules.[20]

PHYSICAL PROPERTIES

The nail plate is hard, strong, and flexible. Hardness and strength are due to the nail plate's high content of hard keratins and cystine-rich, high-sulfur proteins, while its flexibility depends on its water content and increases with nail plate hydration.[21] The double curvature of the nail plate along its longitudinal and transverse axes enhances nail plate resistance to mechanical stress.[22]

The strength of fingernails is similar to that of wool and human hair, with a maximum elastic stress varying from 420 to 880 kg/cm^2.[23]

The physical properties of the nail also depend on the arrangement and adhesion of onychocytes in the different portions of the nail plate, as well as on the orientation of the keratin filaments within the nail plate onychocytes.[22] The dorsal and ventral nail plate contain keratin filaments oriented parallel and perpendicular to the nail growth axis, whereas the intermediate nail plate contains keratin filaments oriented perpendicular to the nail growth axis.[24] This explains why the nail plate is more susceptible to transverse than to longitudinal fractures.

At an ultrastructural level, the corneocytes of the dorsal nail plate are flat, with their shorter diameter perpendicular to the nail plate surface. The average sizes of these cells are 34 μm in length, 64 μm in width, and 2.2 μm in height.[25] Cell adhesion is strong and this portion of the nail is responsible for nail plate hardness and sharpness. The onychocytes of the intermediate nail plate show multiple interdigitations of their cell membranes. The average dimensions of these cells are 40 μm in length, 53 μm in width, and 5.5 μm in height. Cell adhesion is provided by desmosomes and complex interdigitations. This part of the nail plate is responsible for nail pliability and elasticity. The ventral nail plate is thin and consists of soft keratins. It provides adhesion to the underlying nail bed.

NAIL GROWTH

The nail plate grows continuously during life. Fingernails grow faster than toenails, mean growth being 3 mm per month for fingernails and 1 mm per month for toenails. Complete replacement of a fingernail requires about 100 to 180 days (6 months). When the nail plate is avulsed, it takes approximately 40 days before the new fingernail will first emerge from the proximal nail fold. After a further 120 days, it will reach the fingertip. The total regeneration time for a toenail is 12 to 18 months. As a consequence of the slow nail growth rate, diseases of the nail matrix become evident with a considerable delay with respect to their onset and require a long time to disappear after treatment.

Nail growth rate varies among different individuals and among the different digits of the same individual. It depends on the turnover rate of the nail matrix cells and is influenced by several physiologic and pathologic conditions. Nail growth rate is slow at birth, slightly increases during childhood, usually reaches its maximum between the second and the third decades of life, and then sharply decreases after the age of 50 years.[26] Conditions that are associated with a slow growth rate include systemic illness, malnutrition, peripheral vascular or neurologic diseases, and treatment with antimitotic drugs. Nails affected by onychomycosis frequently exhibit a slow growth rate. An arrest of nail growth is a typical feature of the yellow-nail syndrome (see Chap. 72). A reduction in the longitudinal nail growth is usually associated with nail thickening. Accelerate nail growth may cause nail thinning and/or longitudinal ridging of the nail plate (nail beading).

Due to their slow growth rate, the nails may provide information on pathologic conditions that have occurred up to several months before the time of observation. Because drugs and toxic substances are stored within the nail, nail clippings can be used to detect previous exposure to drugs or chemicals. The nail of the big toe is the best site for investigation because of its size and slow growth rate.

In some metabolic diseases, nail plate analysis can be used for diagnostic and therapeutic purposes. Nail clippings may also be used for genetic analysis and determination of blood groups. DNA can, in fact, be extracted easily from fingernail clippings and used for enzymatic amplification and genotypic or individual identification.

REFERENCES

1. Zaias N: Fundamentals and techniques, in *The Nail in Health and Disease,* 2d ed, edited by N Zaias. Norwalk, CT, Appleton & Lange, 1990, p. 3
2. Sonnex TS et al: The nature and significance of the transverse white band of human nail. *Semin Dermatol* **10**:12, 1991
3. Dawber RPR: The ultrastructure and growth of human nails. *Arch Dermatol Res* **269**:197, 1980
4. Johnson M et al: Determination of nail thickness and length. *Br J Dermatol* **130**:195, 1994
5. Cohen PR: The lunula. *J Am Acad Dermatol* **34**:943, 1996
6. Kitahara T et al: Cellular features of differentiation in the nail. *Microsc Res Tech* **38**:436, 1997
7. Picardo M et al: Characterization of cultured nail matrix cells. *J Am Acad Dermatol* **30**:434, 1994
8. Perrin CH et al: Anatomic distribution of melanocytes in normal nail unit. *Am J Dermatopathol* **19**:462, 1997
9. Tosti A et al: Characterization of nail matrix melanocytes using anti-PEP1, anti-PEP8, TMH-1 and HMB-45 antibodies. *J Am Acad Dermatol* **31**:193, 1994
10. Cameli N et al: Expression of integrins in human nail matrix. *Br J Dermatol* **130**:583, 1994
11. Hashimoto K: Ultrastructure of the human toenail. *J Invest Dermatol* **56**:235, 1971
12. Cameli N et al: Distribution of Merkel cells in adult human nail matrix. *Br J Dermatol* **139**:541, 1998
13. Johnson M et al: Nail is produced by the normal nail bed: A controversy resolved. *Br J Dermatol* **125**:27, 1991
14. Sinclair RD et al: The basement membrane zone of the nail. *Br J Dermatol* **131**:499, 1994
15. Cameli N et al: Characterization of the nail matrix basement membrane zone: An immunohistochemical study of normal nails and of the nails in Herlitz junctional epidermolysis bullosa. *Br J Dermatol* **134**:178, 1996
16. Drape J-L et al: The lunula: A magnetic resonance imaging approach to the subnail matrix area. *J Invest Dermatol* **106**:1081, 1996
17. Lynch MH et al: Acid and basic hair/nail ("hard") keratins: Their localization in upper cortical and cuticle cells of the human hair follicle and their relationship to "soft" keratins. *J Cell Biol* **103**:2593, 1986
18. Jemec GBE et al: Ultrasound structure of the human nail plate. *Arch Dermatol* **125**:643, 1989
19. Helmdach M et al: Age and sex variation in lipid composition of human fingernail plates. *Skin Pharmacol Appl Skin Physiol* **13**:111, 2000
20. Kobayashi et al: Drug permeation through the three layers of the human nail plate. *J Pharm Pharmacol* **51**:271, 1999
21. Finlay AY et al: An assessment of factors influencing flexibility of human fingernails. *Br J Dermatol* **10**:103, 1980
22. Forslind B: Biophysical studies of the normal nail. *Acta Derm Venereol* **50**:161, 1970
23. Young RW et al: Strength of fingernails. *J Invest Dermatol* **44**:35, 1965
24. Garson JC et al: Histological structure of human nail as studied by synchrotron x-ray microdiffraction. *Cell Mol Biol* **46**:1025, 2000
25. Achten G et al: Nails in light and electron microscopy. *Semin Dermatol* **10**:54, 1991
26. Bean WB: Nail growth: 30 years of observation. *Arch Intern Med* **134**:497, 1974

SECTION 5

BIOLOGY OF EXTRACELLULAR MATRIX, BLOOD VESSELS, AND NERVES

CHAPTER 14

Collagen

Jouni Uitto
Leena Pulkkinen
Mon-Li Chu

STRUCTURE

The closely related proteins of the collagen family are the main fibrillar components of the connective tissues and the major extracellular proteins of the human body.[1–4] The physiologic role of collagen fibers in the skin is to provide the tensile properties that allow the skin to serve as a protective organ against external trauma. In human skin, collagen fibers form the bulk of the extracellular matrix and comprise more than 70 percent of the dry weight of the dermis. The bulk of collagen in dermis is deposited as large bundles of regularly oriented fibers composed of fibrils and microfibrils. The fibrils are aligned in a parallel manner, resulting in a pattern of cross-striations that can be visualized by electron microscopy (Fig. 14-1). The most prominent cross-striations appear as repeating bands spaced approximately 70 nm apart.

The prototype of the collagens is type I collagen, the most abundant collagen in the dermis and in other connective tissues (Fig. 14-2). The type I collagen molecule has an approximate molecular mass of 290 kDa and is composed of three polypeptide chains, each having a molecular mass of about 94 kDa. These three polypeptides, known as α chains, are coiled around each other much like strands of rope, so that the collagen molecule has a triple-helical structure. This conformation gives the molecule a rigid, rodlike shape with approximate dimensions of 1.5×300 nm (Fig. 14-2).

The special structure of the collagen triple helix is largely explainable by the unusual amino acid composition of the α chains. Each α chain of type I collagen has approximately 1000 amino acids, and glycine, the smallest amino acid, accounts for approximately one-third of the total number of amino acids, evenly distributed in the collagenous portion of the polypeptide. Consequently, the polypeptide chains of collagen can be considered to be repeating triplets represented as $(Gly\text{-}X\text{-}Y)_{333}$ (Fig. 14-2). The X and Y positions of the repeating sequence can be occupied by a variety of amino acids, but the X position is often occupied by proline and the Y position is occupied by hydroxyproline. These two amino acids account for about 22 percent of the total amino acid composition of type I collagen. The relatively high contents of these amino acids and the characteristic distribution of glycine in every third position are necessary for the triple-helical conformation of the collagen molecule, and hydroxyproline plays a critical role in stabilizing the triple helix at body temperature (see below). The triple-helical conformation gives collagen many of its unique properties and is essential for normal fibrillogenesis. Mutations that affect the formation of the stable triple helix prevent collagen from forming fibers, resulting in serious defects of connective tissue function.[3,5]

FIGURE 14-1

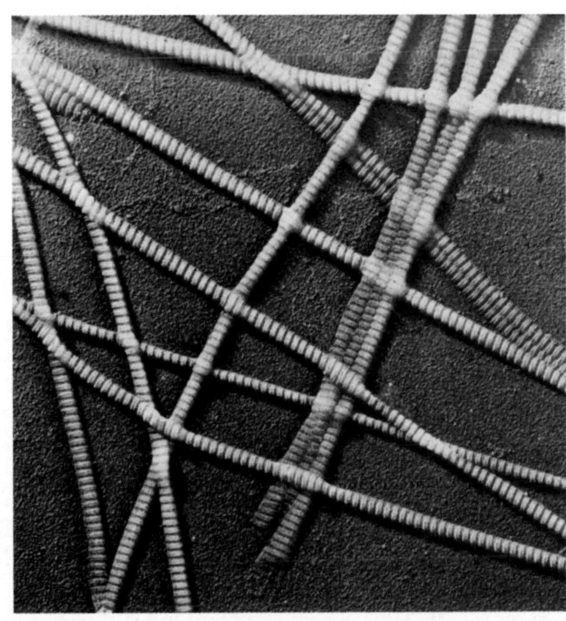

Electron micrograph of collagen fibers from a preparation of human dermis demonstrating the regular banding pattern at approximately 70-nm intervals. × 45,000.

FIGURE 14-2

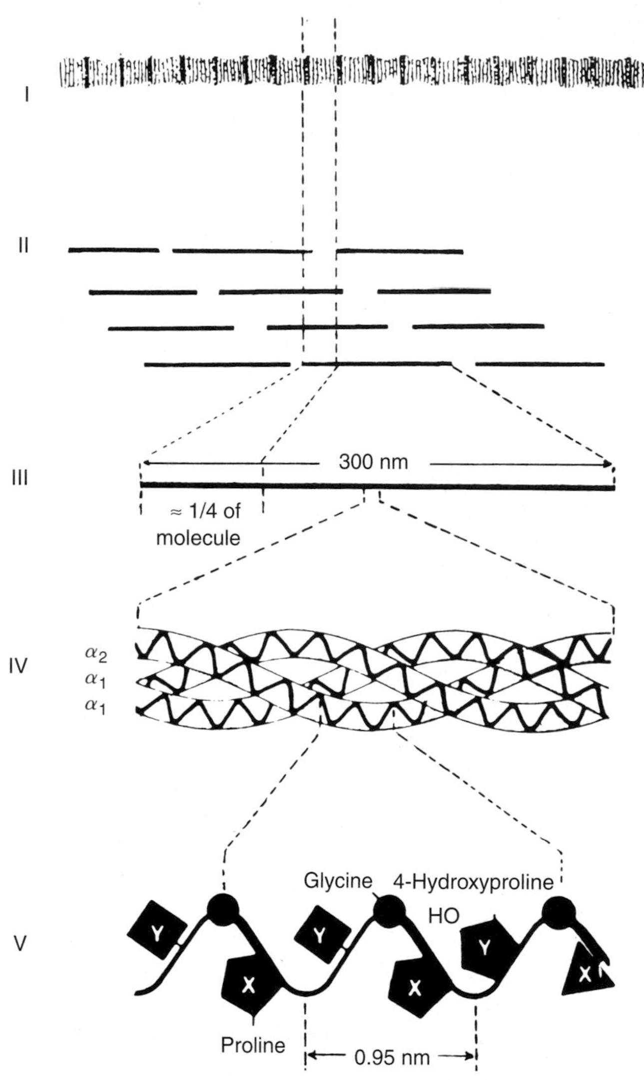

Representation of the structure of type I collagen. The collagen fibers (I), which on electron microscopy demonstrate a repeating periodicity (see Fig. 14-1), are composed of individual collagen molecules aligned in a quarter-stagger arrangement (II). Each type I collagen molecule is an approximately 300-nm-long rodlike structure (III) consisting of three individual polypeptides, known as α chains, that are twisted around each other in a right-handed triple helix (IV). Each chain is composed of amino acids in a repeating Gly-X-Y sequence (V); as indicated, the X position is frequently occupied by a prolyl residue, and the Y position is frequently occupied by a 4-hydroxyprolyl residue. The individual α chains have a left-handed helical secondary structure with a pitch of 0.95 nm. (*From Uitto J et al: Collagen structure, function, and pathology, In* Progress in Diseases of the Skin, *vol 1, edited by R Fleischmajer. New York, Grune & Stratton, 1981, p 103, with permission.*)

GENETIC HETEROGENEITY

Collagen comprises a family of closely related yet genetically distinct proteins. In the human genome there are as many as 36 different genes encoding α chains with variable amino acid sequences; these α chains correspond to at least 21 different types of collagen, which have been assigned Roman numerals I to XXI (Table 14-1). Furthermore, several additional collagenous proteins have been identified, largely through recombinant DNA technology or search of the genome database, but the lack of precise information about the structure and the α-chain composition of these collagens precludes assignment of a Roman numeral at this time. In addition to well-characterized collagens, short, triple-helical collagenous segments are present in other proteins, including acetylcholinesterase, the C1q component of the complement system, pulmonary surfactant proteins, macrophage scavenger receptors, and ectodysplasin A, a product of the gene mutated in X-linked anhidrotic ectodermal dysplasia.[6,7] However, these proteins are not included in the collagen family because the collagenous domains are not a predominant part of the molecules, and the proteins do not function primarily as structural components of the extracellular matrix of connective tissue.

The genetically distinct collagens can be separated on the basis of their physicochemical properties. Also, peptide mapping with limited enzymatic digestion or chemical reagents, such as cyanogen bromide, which cleaves the polypeptides at each methionyl residue, greatly facilitates the early identification of different genetic forms of collagens. More recently, molecular cloning approaches and near completion of the human genome database have enabled identification of additional collagen genes with precise knowledge of their chromosomal locations (Table 14-2).

On the basis of the fiber architecture in tissues, the genetically distinct collagens can be divided into different classes (Table 14-1). Collagen types I, II, III, V, and XI align into relatively large fibrils and are therefore designated *fibril-forming collagens.* Type IV is arranged in an interlacing network within the basement membranes, whereas type VI is a distinct microfibril-forming collagen and type VII collagen forms anchoring fibrils. A recently described group, *FACIT* (fibril-associated collagens with interrupted triple helices) collagens,[8] includes types IX, XII, XIV, XIX, XX, and XXI. Many of these collagens are associated with larger collagen fibers and may serve as molecular bridges important for the organization and stability of the extracellular matrices. Type XIII and XVII collagens are transmembrane proteins. An overview of the collagens potentially contributing to skin physiology and pathology is presented below (see Table 14-2). Other collagen types (including II, IX, X, XI, XIX, XX, and XXI) are not discussed in detail because they are apparently not present in the skin in significant quantities.

Type I collagen, the most widely distributed and most extensively characterized form of collagen, is found predominantly in bone and tendon and it accounts for approximately 80 percent of the total collagen of adult human dermis. The type I collagen molecule contains two identical α chains, designated α1(I), and a third chain, called α2(I), clearly different in its amino acid composition. Thus, the chain composition of type I collagen is $[\alpha1(I)]_2\alpha2(I)$. Collagen molecules that consist of three identical α1(I) chains have also been detected, but these so-called α1(I) trimer molecules with chain composition of $[\alpha1(I)]_3$ appear to represent a minor fraction of collagen in connective tissues, such as the skin.[9] Collagen types I and III form the relatively broad extracellular fibers that are primarily responsible for the tensile strength of the human dermis. Mutations in the type I and III collagen genes can result in connective tissue abnormalities in the skin and joints, among other tissues, in different forms of the Ehlers-Danlos syndrome and fragility of bones in osteogenesis imperfecta.[3,5]

Type III collagen, another genetically distinct form of collagen, predominates in gastrointestinal and vascular connective tissues, but it also represents approximately 10 percent of the total collagen in the adult human dermis.[10] Type III collagen was initially designated *fetal collagen,* as it predominates in human skin during embryonic life. However, the synthesis of type I collagen accelerates during the early postnatal period until the ratio of type I to type III collagen in adult human skin is ~8:1.[10] Type III collagen is composed of three identical α chains, α1(III), distinguished from the chains of type I collagen by a relatively high content of hydroxyproline and glycine and the presence of a cysteine residue. Mutations in the type III collagen gene cause the vascular type of Ehlers-Danlos syndrome (see below).

Type IV collagen is abundantly present in basement membranes.[11] In the skin, type IV collagen is found in the basement membrane at the dermal–epidermal junction, primarily within the lamina densa, where it forms a lattice rather than the fibers characteristic of dermal collagens.[12]

The type IV collagen present in human skin is predominantly a heterotrimer, $[\alpha1(IV)]_2\alpha2(IV)$, although, occasionally, the homopolymers $[\alpha1(IV)]_3$ and $[\alpha2(IV)]_3$ may be assembled. The molecular masses of the $\alpha1(IV)$ and $\alpha2(IV)$ chains are 185 and 175 kDa, respectively. The type IV collagen molecule is characterized by the presence of noncollagenous interruptions within the triple-helical domain, thus conferring flexibility to the molecule. More recently, four additional α chains—$\alpha3(IV)$, $\alpha4(IV)$, $\alpha5(IV)$, and $\alpha6(IV)$—have been identified.[13] The type IV collagen molecules containing these subunit polypeptides appear to be expressed primarily in glomerular basement membranes and their importance for renal physiology is attested by the fact that mutations in the gene encoding the $\alpha5(IV)$ polypeptide result in Alport's syndrome,[14] an X-linked renal disease. Furthermore, autoantibodies recognizing the $\alpha3(IV)$ chains underlie Goodpasture's syndrome.[15] Finally, the $\alpha5$ chain of type IV collagen has been shown to be a target of circulating IgG autoantibodies in a novel autoimmune disease with sub-epidermal blisters and renal insufficiency.[16]

TABLE 14-1

Genetic Heterogeneity of Collagen

Collagen Type	Chain Composition*	Molecular Characteristics/ Supramolecular Assembly	Tissue Distribution/ Cell Source†
I	$[\alpha1(I)]_2\ \alpha2(I)$	Fibrillar	Skin, bone, tendon
I-trimer	$[\alpha1(I)]_3$	Fibrillar	Tumors, skin
II	$[\alpha1(II)]_3$	Fibrillar	Cartilage
III	$[\alpha1(III)]_3$	Fibrillar	Fetal skin, blood vessels, gastrointestinal tract
IV	$[\alpha1(IV)]_2\alpha2(IV)^‡$	Basement membrane	Ubiquitous
V	$[\alpha1(V)]_2\alpha2(V)$; $[\alpha1(V)]_3{}^‡$	Fibrillar	Ubiquitous
VI	$\alpha1(VI)\alpha2(VI)\alpha3(VI)$	Microfibril	Ubiquitous
VII	$[\alpha1(VII)]_3$	Anchoring fibril	Papillary dermis of the skin and other epithelial tissues (gastrointestinal tract, trachea, esophagus)
VIII	$[\alpha1(VIII)]_3$	Network forming	Endothelial cells
IX	$\alpha1(IX)\alpha2(IX)\alpha3(IX)$	FACIT	Cartilage
X	$[\alpha1(X)]_3$	Network forming	Hypertrophic cartilage
XI	$\alpha1(XI)\alpha2(XI)\alpha3(XI)$	Fibrillar	Cartilage
XII	$[\alpha1(XII)]_3$	FACIT	Tendons, ligaments, perichondrium, periosteum, cornea
XIII	$[\alpha1(XIII)]_3$	Transmembrane	Ubiquitous including epidermis (17 splice combinations known)
XIV	$[\alpha1(XIV)]_3$	FACIT	Skin, tendons, cornea
XV	Unknown	Basement membrane	Ubiquitous
XVI	$[\alpha1(XVI)]_3$	FACIT	Skin, internal organs, cartilage
XVII	$[\alpha1(XVII)]_3$	Transmembrane	Hemidesmosomes of basal keratinocytes in dermal-epidermal junction of the skin
XVIII	Unknown	Basement membrane	Ubiquitous
XIX	Unknown	FACIT	Basement membrane
XX	Unknown	FACIT	Corneal epithelia, embryonic skin, sternal cartilage, tendon, lung
XXI	Unknown	FACIT	Smooth muscle cell in blood vessel walls, developing heart

*The precise chain composition of some of the recently described collagens is not known.
†The predominant tissue distribution is indicated; lesser amounts may be present in other tissues.
‡Additional α chains exist (see text).

Type V collagen consists of a subfamily of similar interrelated collagens that contain four different types of α chains. The predominant form in the skin is $[\alpha1(V)]_2\alpha2(V)$. Type V collagen is present in most connective tissues, and in the skin type V collagen represents less than 5 percent of the total collagen. The importance of type V collagen has been demonstrated by discovery of mutations in the type V collagen genes in patients with classical, autosomal dominant forms (types I and II) of the Ehlers-Danlos syndrome (EDS).[17,18] It is of interest that a clinically similar, classic type of EDS, can be derived from absence of tenascin-X expression, leading to an autosomal recessive form of the disease.[19] Tenascin-X is developmentally associated with collagen fibrillogenesis and its absence could explain defective collagen fibers similar to those in patients with mutations in the type V collagen genes. The pathoetiologic role of tenascin-X was confirmed by development of TNX null mice, which exhibit progressive hyperextensibility and reduced tensile strength of their skin.[20]

Type VI collagen was initially thought to be a minor collagen in tissues such as the dermis. However, improved biochemical isolation procedures demonstrate that type VI collagen may be a relatively abundant component in a variety of tissues, including skin.[21] The type VI collagen molecules consist of three distinct α chains—$\alpha1(VI)$, $\alpha2(VI)$, and $\alpha3(VI)$—which fold into a triple-helical domain of about 100 nm in length, with globular domains at both ends of the molecule.[22] Type VI collagen assembles into relatively thin microfibrils that form a network independent of the previously mentioned broad collagen fibers, which consist primarily of types I and III collagens.[23] The microfibrillar network may perform an anchoring function by stabilizing the assembly of the broad collagen fibers as well as basement membranes. Recent studies demonstrate that mutations in each of the three type VI collagen genes can lead to different forms of congenital muscular dystrophy, with no apparent phenotype in the skin but with limited joint hypermobility.[24,25]

Type VII collagen, the major component of the anchoring fibrils at the dermal–epidermal basement membrane zone was originally designated as long-chain (LC) collagen because it has an unusually

TABLE 14-2

Molecular Genetics of Collagens Present in Human Skin

Collagen Type	Constituent Polypeptide	Gene Designation	Chromosomal* Location of the Gene
I	α1(I)	COL1A1	17q21-q22
	α2(I)	COL1A2	7q21-q22
III	α1(III)	COL3A1	2q24-q33
IV	α1(IV)	COL4A1	13q33-q34
	α2(IV)	COL4A2	13q33-q34
	α3(IV)	COL4A3	2q36-q37
	α4(IV)	COL4A4	2q36-q37
	α5(IV)	COL4A5	Xq22
	α6(IV)	COL4A6	Xq22
V	α1(V)	COL5A1	9q34.2-34.3
	α2(V)	COL5A2	2q24-q32
	α3(V)	COL5A3	19p13.2
	α4(V)	COL5A4	ND
VI	α1(VI)	COL6A1	21q22.3
	α2(VI)	COL6A2	21q22.3
	α3(VI)	COL6A3	2q37
VII	α1(VII)	COL7A1	3p21
VIII	α1(VIII)	COL8A1	3q11.1-13.2
	α2(VIII)	COL8A2	1p32.3-34.3
XII	α1(XII)	COL12A1	6q12-13
XIII	α1(XIII)	COL13A1	10q22
XIV	α1(XIV)	COL14A1	8q23
XV	α1(XV)	COL15A1	9q21-22
XVI	α1(XVI)	COL16A1	1p34-35
XVII	α1(XVII)	COL17A1	10q24.3
XVIII	α1(XVIII)	COL18A1	21q22.3
XIX	α1(XIX)	COL19A1	6q12-q13
XXI	α1(XXI)	COL21A1	6p11-12

*ND, not determined.

long triple-helical region of about 450 nm.[26] It has only one type of α chain, α1(VII), and the triple-helical domain contains interchain disulfide bonds and a pepsin-sensitive, nonhelical site close to the center of the molecule.[27] The triple-helical collagenous domain is flanked by a large, nonhelical domain (NC-1) at the amino terminus and a shorter carboxyl terminal nonhelical domain (NC-2). Type VII collagen is a major constituent of the anchoring fibrils that extend from the dermal–epidermal junction to the papillary dermis. Type VII collagen molecules become organized into anchoring fibrils through the formation of antiparallel dimers linked through their carboxyl terminal ends.[26] The large amino-terminal, noncollagenous domains of type VII collagen are thought to interact at one end with type IV collagen and/or laminin 5 components of the dermal–epidermal basement membrane and at the other end with basement membrane–like structures, known as anchoring plaques, found in the papillary dermis.[26,28] These types of structural organizations of the anchoring fibrils could stabilize the attachment of the dermal–epidermal basement membrane to the underlying dermis. Alternatively, it has been suggested that most anchoring fibrils form U-shaped loops that entrap larger fibers consisting of type I and III collagens.[29] Thus, alterations in the expression, structure, or molecular interactions of type VII with other basement membrane components could result in skin fragility. Such a situation is exemplified by *dystrophic epidermolysis bullosa (DEB),* a group of heritable mechanobullous diseases characterized by blistering of the skin as a result of minor trauma[30–32] (see Chap. 65). A scarcity of type VII collagen and abnormalities in the anchoring fibrils have been demonstrated in the dominant dystrophic form of epidermolysis bullosa (EB), and anchoring fibrils and type VII collagen are absent in some cases of severe recessive dystrophic EB. Distinct mutations in different forms of DEB have been demonstrated in more than 300 families, and none of the families with DEB studied so far has revealed mutations in genes other than that encoding the α1(VII) polypeptide of type VII collagen.[31,32] Furthermore, type VII collagen serves as the autoantigen in the acquired form of EB[33] (see Chap. 66).

Type VIII collagen refers to a molecule initially isolated from cultures of endothelial cells and other cell types.[34] It consists of two separate polypeptides, α1(VIII) and α2(VIII), and forms the hexagonal lattices in Descemet's membrane of corneas. These observations explain the finding that mutations in the type VIII collagen gene (COL8A2) result in a form of corneal dystrophy.[35]

Type XII collagen belongs to the group of *FACIT* collagens that contain more than one triple-helical domain separated by noncollagenous segments. They do not undergo proteolytic processing from a larger proform, and therefore are not secreted as procollagens. The FACIT collagens form fibers only in association with fibrillar collagens. For example, type XII collagen, consisting of three identical α1(XII) chains, is localized in dense connective tissues in association with type I collagen. However, skin shows relatively little reactivity with the type XII collagen-specific antibodies, and the precise quantitation and the physiologic role of type XII collagen in the skin remain to be elucidated. However, it has been suggested that type XII collagen mediates interactions between banded collagen fibers and modulates extracellular matrix deformability.[36]

Type XIII collagen, a transmembrane protein, is ubiquitously distributed in small amounts in most tissues, and in particular, the expression of this collagen has been detected in normal human skin and cultured keratinocytes.[37] Immunolabeling studies localized type XIII collagen epitopes in the epidermis to cell-cell contact sites as well as in dermal–epidermal junctions. More refined localization suggested that this collagen may, in fact, be a component of the adherens junctions.[37] An unusual observation is that type XIII collagen mRNAs are present in as many as 17 splice variants, which display differential tissue expression patterns.[38] However, the functional differences of the proteins derived from these splice variants of mRNA are currently unknown.

Type XIV collagen belongs to the FACIT group and has a high structural homology with type XII collagen. By analogy with type IX collagen, a well-characterized component of the cartilaginous matrices, type XIV collagen may be oriented parallel to the surface of large collagen fibers composed of collagen types I and III. Type XIV collagen, like other FACIT collagens, may be involved in determining the interaction of collagen fibrils with each other and with other components of the extracellular matrix.

Type XVII collagen was initially identified as the 180-kDa bullous pemphigoid antigen *(BPAG2),* which was recognized by circulating autoantibodies in the sera of some patients with bullous pemphigoid or herpes gestationis.[39] This antigen, which is synthesized by basal keratinocytes, was localized by immunoelectron microscopy to the hemidesmosomes at the dermal–epidermal basement membrane zone of human skin. Type XVII collagen is a transmembrane protein in type 2 topography; that is, the amino-terminal end is intracellular while the carboxy-terminal ectodomain is in the extracellular space.[40] The ectodomain consists of 15 collagenous domains with the characteristic repeating Gly-X-Y sequences that form triple helices.[41] These collagenous domains are separated by noncollagenous segments of variable sizes, and consequently, type XVII collagen is a protein characterized by alternating collagenous and non-collagenous segments.[40] The type XVII collagen gene was mapped to the long arm of human chromosome 10. This location is distinct from any previously mapped collagens and also distinguishes BPAG2 from BPAG1, the 230-kDa bullous pemphigoid antigen, which has been mapped to the short arm of chromosome 6.[42] The importance of the type XVII collagen was also shown by mutations in the corresponding gene *(COL17A1)* that underlie a nonlethal variant of junctional EB, generalized atrophic benign epidermolysis bullosa *(GABEB)*.[40,43] These patients have protracted, lifelong blistering of the skin, atrophic scarring, alopecia, and nail dystrophy.

Collagens of types XV, XVI, XVIII, XIX, XX, and XXI were recently discovered by cDNA cloning or by examination of the genome database, and their complete primary structures are established.[44–51] These all contain multiple triple-helical domains separated by short noncollagenous regions. In addition, they possess a large globular domain at the amino terminus, which shares sequence similarity with the N-termini of minor fibrillar collagens, FACIT collagens, and thrombospondin. These collagens are further divided into two subgroups. Types XV and XVIII collagens contain a large, homologous C-globular domain and both are expressed in basement membranes. Interestingly, C-terminal fragments of type XV and XVIII collagens have been identified as endostatin, an inhibitor of angiogenesis and tumor growth.[52] Types XVI, XIX, XX, and XXI collagens share the characteristic C-terminal features of the FACIT collagens, but it is not known whether they are associated with fibrillar collagen. Type XVI collagen has been localized to the upper papillary dermis at the cutaneous basement membrane zone, in close vicinity to type VII collagen. Furthermore, type XVI collagen colocalizes with fibrillin-1 at the dermal–epidermal junction, but not in deeper layers of the dermis. These observations suggest that type XVI collagen may contribute to the stability of the cutaneous basement membrane zone.[53]

COLLAGEN GENE STRUCTURE

The collagen genes, like most eukaryotic genes, are large, multiexon genes interrupted at several points by noncoding DNA sequences of unknown function called *introns*.[54] Thus, the eukaryotic gene coding for a protein is much larger than would be predicted from the amino acid sequences of the final protein. An example of the complexity of collagen genes is the intron–exon organization of the type VII collagen gene *(COL7A1)* (see Fig. 14-3), which consists of 118 exons, the largest number in any published gene.[55]

During the early stages of gene expression, the entire gene is transcribed into a high-molecular-weight precursor mRNA, which is a complementary copy of the coding strand of the double-helical DNA. The precursor mRNA undergoes posttranscriptional modifications, such as capping and polyadenylation, and the introns are removed by splicing to yield a linear, uninterrupted coding sequence with 5′ and 3′ untranslated flanking regions. The mature mRNA is then transported into the cytoplasm and translated in cells, such as dermal fibroblasts.

Complementary and genomic DNA clones corresponding to the α chains of various collagen molecules have been described in different laboratories. These clones have been extensively characterized and hybridized with the corresponding mRNA molecules to examine the temporal and topographic expression of these genes by Northern blot and in situ hybridization techniques, respectively. In addition, their nucleotide sequence homology with the corresponding amino acid sequences in the collagen α chains in various animal species has been determined, thus allowing estimates of the evolutionary conservation of certain segments within the collagens.[56] A high degree of conservation implies a region of functional importance within a protein molecule.

Recombinant DNA technology has also facilitated determination of the precise chromosomal location of the different collagen genes within the human genome (Table 14-2). With few exceptions, the collagen genes are widely scattered throughout the human genome. For example, the genes coding for the two constituent polypeptide chains of type I collagen, $\alpha 1$(I) and $\alpha 2$(I), are located on separate chromosomes, 17 and 7, respectively. Knowledge of the precise chromosomal location of the genes coding for collagens in human skin will allow development of polymorphic markers within the genes and in the flanking DNA for use in genetic linkage studies. In addition, sophisticated mutation detection strategies, based on scanning of the genes, have led to identification of a large number of mutations in different collagen genes with characteristic phenotypic consequences (see, e.g., Refs. 3 to 5, 31, 32, and 57).

TRANSLATION OF COLLAGEN POLYPEPTIDES

Under physiologic conditions, collagen molecules spontaneously assemble into insoluble fibers. This observation presented a logistic problem because it was difficult to visualize how a collagen molecule could be synthesized inside the cell and then secreted into the extracellular space without premature assembly of the molecules into insoluble fibers. This problem was solved by the demonstration that collagen is initially synthesized as a larger precursor molecule, procollagen, which is soluble under physiologic conditions.

The precursor polypeptides of procollagen, so-called prepro-α chains, are synthesized on the ribosomes of the rough endoplasmic reticulum in fibroblasts and related cells (Fig. 14-4). This initial translation product, the prepro-α chain, contains an amino-terminal signal (or leader) sequence. The signal sequence, a characteristic feature of many secreted proteins, is rich in hydrophobic amino acids and probably serves as a signal for attachment of the ribosomes to the membranes of the rough endoplasmic reticulum and vectorial release of the nascent polypeptides into the cisternae of the rough endoplasmic reticulum. During the transmembrane transport of the polypeptides, the signal sequence is enzymatically removed in a reaction catalyzed by signal peptidase (Table 14-3). The polypeptides released inside the lumen of the rough endoplasmic reticulum are termed *pro-α chains* and are larger than collagen α chains because they contain additional peptide sequences at both ends of the molecule. Various studies show that these noncollagenous extension peptides are different from the collagenous portion of the molecule in that they do not have glycine in every third position, they are relatively poor in proline and hydroxyproline, and they are relatively rich in acidic amino acids. These extension peptides also contain cysteine and tryptophan, which are not present, for example, in type I and II collagens. These noncollagenous domains often contain motifs homologous with sequences found as building blocks in other extracellular matrix proteins, such as the fibronectin III domain, von Willebrand factor A domain, and thrombospondin N-terminal domain sequences. It should be noted that, in spite of their homology, these domains do not have the functional characteristics of the original proteins.

POSTTRANSLATIONAL MODIFICATIONS OF POLYPEPTIDE CHAINS

After the assembly of amino acids into prepro-α chains on the ribosomes, the polypeptides undergo several modifications before the completed collagen molecules are deposited into extracellular fibers (Fig. 14-4). Most of these modification reactions are catalyzed by specific enzymes, and many of the modifications are characteristic of the biosynthesis of collagen (Tables 14-3 and 14-4). These events are often termed *posttranslational modifications* to emphasize that these reactions are not directly controlled by the information in the mRNA but occur in the polypeptide chains after the amino acids have been linked together by peptide bonds. The posttranslational modification reactions of

FIGURE 14-3

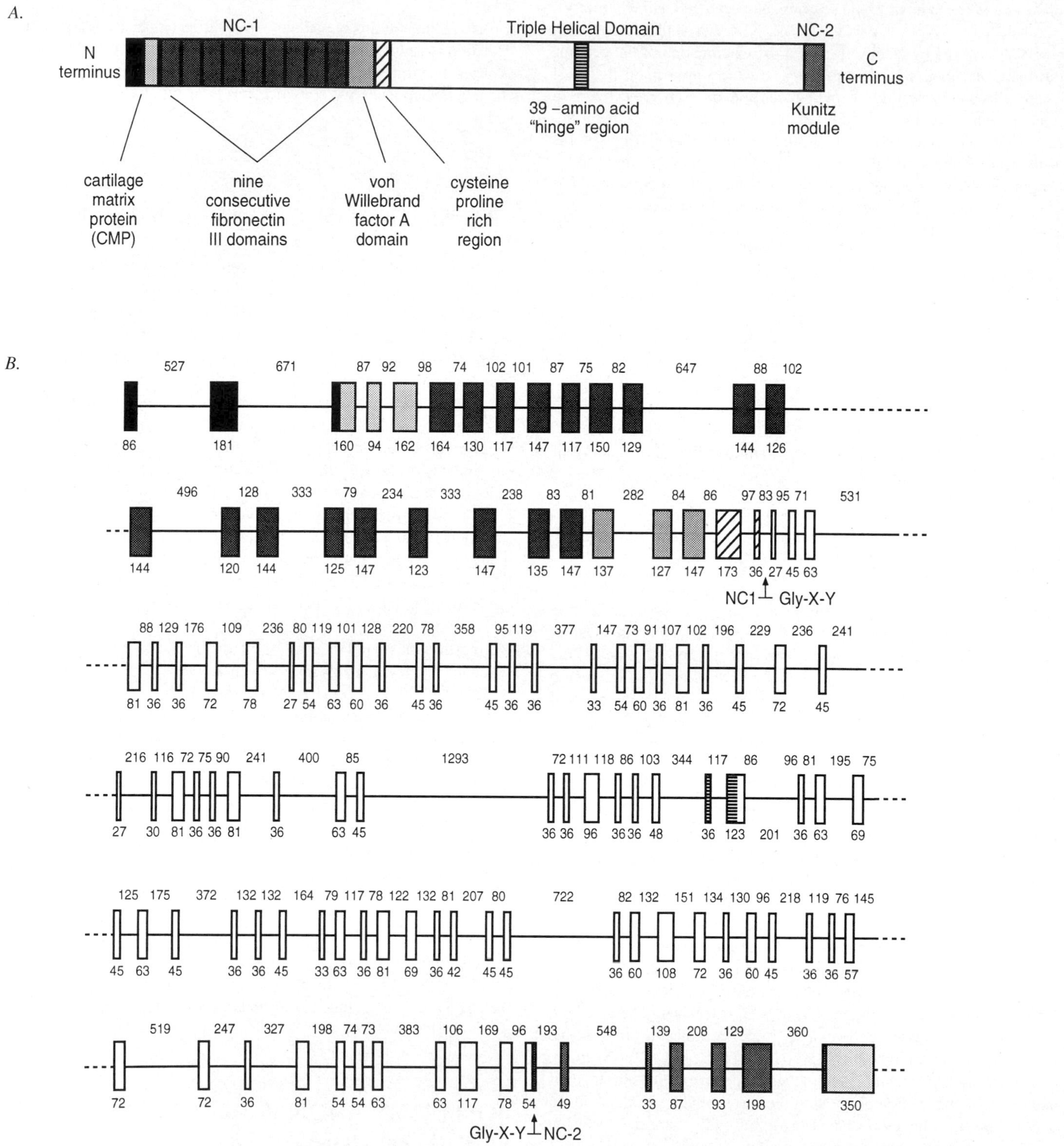

A.
NC-1
Triple Helical Domain
NC-2
N terminus
C terminus
39 -amino acid "hinge" region
Kunitz module
cartilage matrix protein (CMP)
nine consecutive fibronectin III domains
von Willebrand factor A domain
cysteine proline rich region
B.
527 671 87 92 98 74 102 101 87 75 82 647 88 102
86 181 160 94 162 164 130 117 147 117 150 129 144 126
496 128 333 79 234 333 238 83 81 282 84 86 97 83 95 71 531
144 120 144 125 147 123 147 135 147 137 127 147 173 36 27 45 63
NC1 Gly-X-Y
88 129 176 109 236 80 119 101 128 220 78 358 95 119 377 147 73 91 107 102 196 229 236 241
81 36 36 72 78 27 54 63 60 36 45 36 45 36 36 33 54 60 36 81 36 45 72 45
216 116 72 75 90 241 400 85 1293 72 111 118 86 103 344 117 86 96 81 195 75
27 30 81 36 36 81 36 63 45 36 36 96 36 36 48 36 123 201 36 63 69
125 175 372 132 132 164 79 117 78 122 132 81 207 80 722 82 132 151 134 130 96 218 119 76 145
45 63 45 36 36 45 33 63 36 81 69 36 42 45 45 36 60 108 72 36 60 45 36 36 57
519 247 327 198 74 73 383 106 169 96 193 548 139 208 129 360
72 72 36 81 54 54 63 63 117 78 54 49 33 87 93 198 350
Gly-X-Y NC-2

Structural organization of the type VII collagen polypeptide, the $\alpha 1$(VII) chain, as deduced from molecular cloning, and the intron-exon organization of the corresponding gene, *COL7A1*. *A*. The $\alpha 1$ (VII) polypeptide consists of a triple-helical domain that contains imperfections or interruptions in the Gly-X-Y repeat sequence, including a 39–amino acid "hinge" region. The central collagenous domain is flanked by noncollagenous segments, the amino-terminal NC-1 domain and the carboxyl-terminal NC-2 domain. The NC-1 domain consists of submodules with homology to known adhesive proteins, as indicated below the molecule. The NC-2 domain has a segment of homology with the Kunitz proteinase inhibitor molecule. *B*. The type VII collagen gene consists of a total of 118 exons *(vertical blocks)*, which are separated from each other by intervening noncoding intronic sequences *(horizontal lines)*. The sizes (in base pairs) of the introns *(above the lines)* and the exons *(below the blocks)* are indicated. (*Modified from Christiano et al.,*[58] *with permission.*)

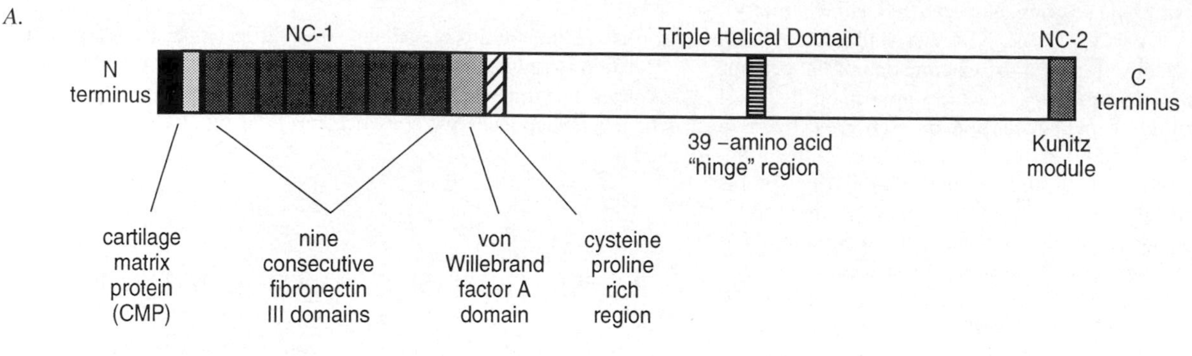

FIGURE 14-4

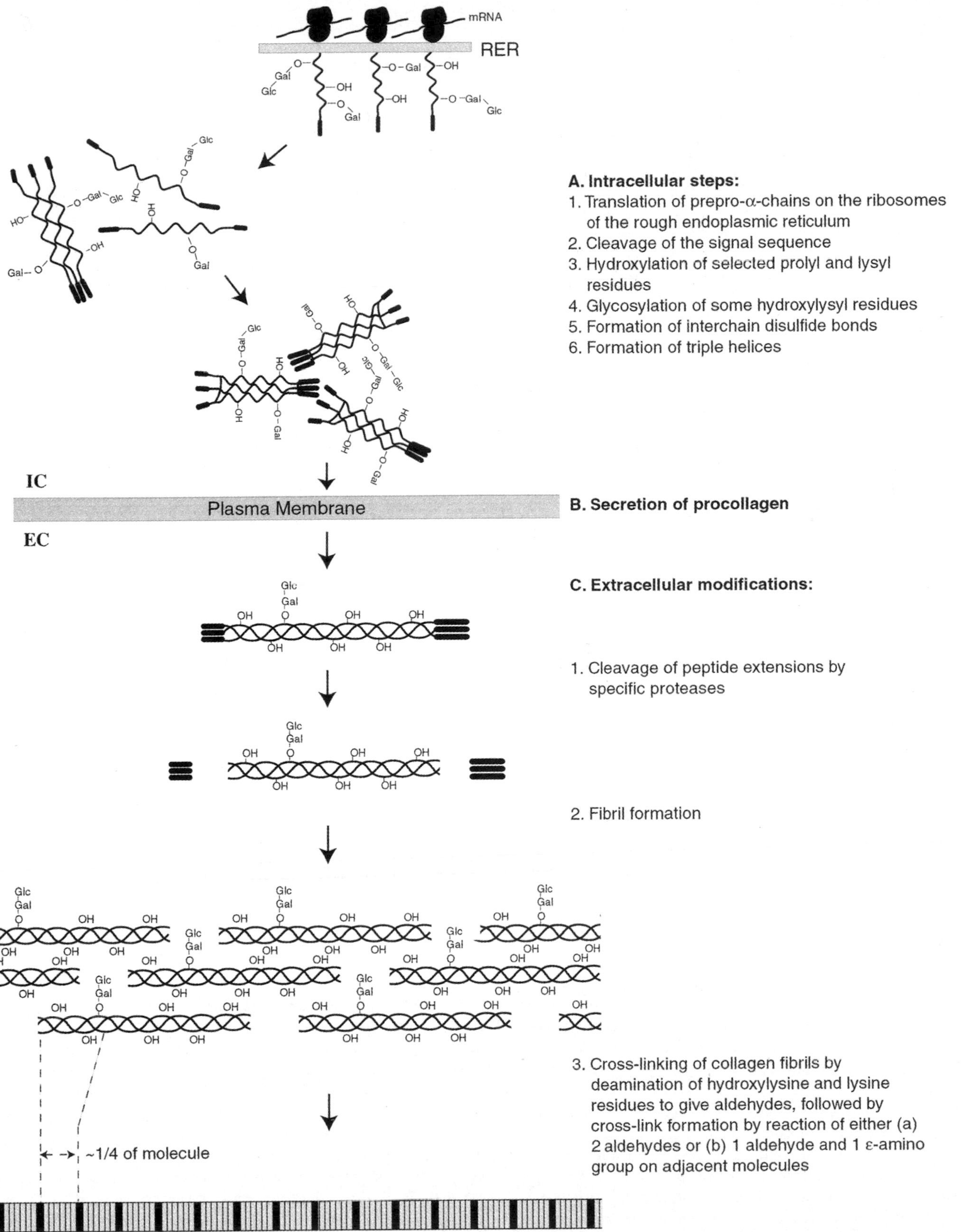

Biosynthesis of procollagen and the assembly of collagen molecules into the extracellular fibers. Glc-Gal, glucosylgalactose attached to a hydroxylysyl residue; mRNA, messenger RNA; –OH, hydroxyl group of hydroxyproline or hydroxylysine; RER, rough endoplasmic reticulum.

TABLE 14-3

Characteristics of Enzymes Participating in the Biosynthesis of Collagen

Enzyme*	Substrate	Product	Cofactors and Cosubstrates
Signal peptidase	Nascent prepro-α chains	Pro-α chains	None known
Prolyl-4-hydroxylase	Prolyl residue in x-pro-gly sequence in pro-α chains†	4-Hydroxyproline	O_2, Fe^{2+}, α-ketoglutarate, ascorbic acid
Prolyl-3-hydroxylase	Prolyl resisdue in pro-hyp-gly sequence in pro-α chains†	3-Hydroxyproline	O_2, Fe^{2+}, α-ketoglutarate, ascorbic acid
Lysyl hydroxylase	Lysyl residue in lys-gly, lys-ser, or lys-ala sequence in pro-α chains†	Hydroxylysine	O_2, Fe^{2+}, α-ketoglutarate, ascorbic acid
Collagen galactosyl transferase	Hydroxylysine in pro-α chains†	Gal-*O*-hydroxylysine	Mn^{2+}, UDP-galactose
Collagen glucosyl transferase	Galactosyl-*O*-hydroxylysine in pro-α chains†	Glc-gal-*O*-hydroxylysine	Mn^{2+}, UDP-glucose
Protein disulfide isomerase‡	Cysteine residues in the extensions of pro-α chains	S-S bonds stabilizing the correct protein conformation	Thiols
Procollagen N-proteinase (ADAMTS-2)	Procollagen or p_n-collagen	P_c-collagen or collagen§	Ca^{2+}
Procollagen C-proteinase	Procollagen p_c-collagen	P_n-collagen or collagen§	Ca^{2+}
Lysyl oxidases	Lysyl or hydroxylysyl residue in fibrillar collagen	Aldehyde derivatives of lysine or hydroxylysine	Cu^{2+}, O_2

*The action of these enzymes (with the exception of signal peptidase) is relatively specific to collagen; the complete sequences of procollagen synthesis and collagen degradation involve additional, less-specific enzymes, such as those of transcription and translation.
†These reactions are terminated when the pro-α chains fold into the triple-helical conformation.
‡It has not been established whether the formation of interchain disulfides in procollagen involves enzymatic catalysis, as occurs in some other proteins, or whether their synthesis takes place spontaneously.
§If intact procollagen is used as a substrate, partially modified products are formed; however, if the partially cleaved proteins serve as substrates, collagen is produced. P_n-collagen refers to collagen molecule with N-terminal propeptide still attached while C-propeptide is cleaved off; P_c-collagen has the C-terminal propeptide still attached while the N-propeptide has been removed.

collagen include (1) synthesis of hydroxyproline by hydroxylation of selected prolyl residues; (2) synthesis of hydroxylysine by hydroxylation of selected lysyl residues; (3) attachment of carbohydrates, galactose or glucosylgalactose, onto certain hydroxylysyl residues; (4) chain association, disulfide bonding and triple-helix formation; (5) proteolytic conversion of procollagen to collagen; and (6) fiber formation and cross-linking. Current evidence indicates that modification reactions (1) to (4) are intracellular events, whereas proteolytic conversion, fiber formation, and cross-linking probably take place extracellularly (Fig. 14-4).

Synthesis of Hydroxyproline

A characteristic feature of collagen is the presence of relatively large amounts of hydroxyproline (Fig. 14-5). Small amounts of hydroxyproline are also found in elastin (see Chap. 15), as well as in some proteins in which the collagenous domains are a minor portion of the molecule, such as acetylcholinesterase, the C1q component of the complement system, the macrophage scavenger proteins, and ectodysplasin A (see Refs. 6 and 7). The hydroxyproline in collagen is found in two isomeric forms. *Trans*-4-hydroxy-L-proline accounts for more than 95 percent of the total hydroxyproline in type I and type III collagens. The minor form is *trans*-3-hydroxy-L-proline, which is found in greater amounts in type IV collagen.[58]

The functional role of hydroxyproline in collagen is well established. A critical amount of *trans*-4-hydroxy-L-proline is required for the folding of α chains into the triple helix, the conformation required for the normal secretion of procollagen molecules out of the cells (Fig. 14-6). Thus, in the absence of hydroxyproline, collagen polypeptides would not form the critical triple-helical structure under physiologic conditions, and no functional collagen fibers would appear in the extracellular space.

Although hydroxyproline accounts for about 10 percent of the total amino acids in type I collagen, free hydroxyproline is not incorporated into newly synthesized collagen polypeptides. The hydroxyprolines are synthesized by hydroxylation of certain prolyl residues that are already in peptide linkages (Fig. 14-5). The formation of *trans*-4- and *trans*-3-hydroxyproline is catalyzed by two separate enzymes—prolyl-4-hydroxylase and prolyl-3-hydroxylase—which have been purified and extensively characterized from various vertebrate tissues, including human skin. The prolyl-4-hydroxylase recognizes only prolyl residues in the Y position of the repeating triplet sequence Gly-X-Y of collagen. In contrast, prolyl-3-hydroxylase only hydroxylates prolyl residues in the X position when the Y position is already occupied by a *trans*-4-hydroxyproline. Thus, 3-hydroxyproline is typically found in collagen in a glycine-(3-hydroxyproline)-(4-hydroxyproline)-glycine sequence. The prolyl hydroxylases require molecular oxygen, ferrous iron, α-ketoglutarate, and a reducing agent such as ascorbate as cosubstrates or cofactors for the reactions (Fig. 14-5 and Table 14-3).

The hydroxylation of appropriate prolyl residues begins while the pro-α chains are growing on the ribosomes, and the hydroxylation is completed soon after the release of full-length polypeptide chains from the ribosomes.[58] The enzyme prolyl-4-hydroxylase has been localized to the rough endoplasmic reticulum (Fig. 14-6). Prolyl hydroxylases do not hydroxylate prolyl residues if the collagen substrate is in a triple-helical conformation. Because triple-helix formation takes place in the cisternae of the rough endoplasmic reticulum (see below), hydroxyproline formation must be completed before the procollagen molecules leave this cellular compartment.

As noted above, prolyl hydroxylase requires a reducing agent, such as ascorbate, for its activity. Therefore, ascorbic acid deficiency leads to a decreased formation of collagen fibers, explaining some of the clinical manifestations in scurvy, such as poor wound healing and decreased tensile strength of the connective tissues.[59] An analogous situation may exist in tissues with relative anoxia, because molecular oxygen is a specific requirement for the formation of hydroxyl groups in hydroxyproline. Studies with animal models demonstrate that wound healing is relatively poor under hypobaric conditions, and in such situations the low O_2 levels may limit the synthesis of hydroxyproline.[60] This observation may also explain the decreased healing tendency of wounds and ulcers in peripheral tissues that are anoxic due to relatively poor blood supply.

Synthesis of Hydroxylysine

Hydroxylysine is another amino acid characteristic of collagen (Fig. 14-7). During the intracellular synthesis of procollagen, hydroxylysine serves as an attachment site for the sugar residues and is critical to the formation of cross-links that stabilize the extracellular collagen matrix. Free hydroxylysine is not incorporated into nascent polypeptide chains, but certain lysyl residues in peptide linkages are converted to hydroxylysine. The hydroxylation reaction is catalyzed by an enzyme, lysyl hydroxylase, which, like the prolyl hydroxylases, requires O_2, Fe^{2+}, α-ketoglutarate, and ascorbate as cofactors and cosubstrates. Despite certain similarities, the prolyl and lysyl hydroxylases are different enzyme proteins and products of different genes. Lysyl hydroxylase, like prolyl-4-hydroxylase, hydroxylates only lysyl residues in the Y position of the repeating Gly-X-Y sequence. Even though hydroxylation of lysyl residues in collagen is initiated while the polypeptides are still assembled on the ribosomes, the formation of hydroxylysine continues for some time after the release of peptides from the ribosomes.

The extent to which lysyl residues in the Y position of the Gly-X-Y sequence are hydroxylated varies greatly among the collagens from different sources. In particular, type I and type III collagens are frequently hydroxylated to a lesser degree, so that these collagens normally contain approximately four to eight hydroxylysine residues per 1000 amino acids, whereas type II collagen has approximately four to five times as many hydroxylysine residues. In type IV collagen, most of the lysyl residues are converted to hydroxylysine. This variation can be explained in part by differences in the actual number of lysyl residues that are available for maximal hydroxylation in the pro-α chains. The variation in the hydroxylation of lysyl residues can also be explained by the fact that the nature of the amino acids in the X position and in the adjacent triplets influences the rate at which lysyl residues in Gly-X-Lys sequences are hydroxylated. In addition, lysyl hydroxylase does not hydroxylate a collagen substrate that is in the triple-helical conformation.[58] Therefore, folding of the pro-α chains into a triple helix terminates the intracellular formation of hydroxylysyl residues. The rate at which pro-α chains of different genetic types fold into the triple helix varies, and, in particular, the rate of triple-helix formation is considerably slower during the synthesis of type II procollagen than of type I procollagen. Thus, folding of the procollagen polypeptides into their triple-helical conformation can regulate the amount of hydroxylysyl residues in newly synthesized collagen molecules.

TABLE 14-4

Major Steps in the Biogenesis and Degradation of Collagen and Their Functional Significance

STEP*	FUNCTIONAL SIGNIFICANCE
I. Expression of genes coding for collagen polypeptides	
a. Gene selection	Determines the collagen isotype to be synthesized
b. Transcription	Formation of mRNA precursor
c. Processing of mRNA precursor	Formation of functional mRNA
d. Translation	Assembly of polypeptide chains
e. Control of the rate of transcription, mRNA processing or translation	Determines the amount of polypeptide synthesized
II. Intracellular cotranslational and posttranslational modifications.	
a. Removal of the signal sequence	May be necessary for secretion
b. Synthesis of 4-hydroxyproline	Stabilization of triple helix
c. Synthesis of 3-hydroxyproline	Unknown
d. Synthesis of hydroxylysine	Stabilization of covalent cross-links; attachment site for glycosylation
e. Synthesis of hydroxylysine-*O*-glycosides	May influence cross-link formation and determine the morphology and stability of the fibers
f. Glycosylation of the extension peptides	Unknown
g. Degradation of nonhelical chains	Removal of defective polypeptides and modulation of collagen production
h. Chain association and disulfide bonding	Facilitation of triple-helix formation
i. Triple-helix formation	Prerequisite for proper secretion
III. Secretion	Transport of procollagen through Golgi apparatus to the extracellular space
IV. Extracellular modifications	
a. Removal of the extension peptides from procollagen	Necessary for fiber formation
b. Deamination of certain lysine and hydroxylysine residues	Necessary for cross-link formation
c. Nonenzymatic glycosylation	May interfere with fiber formation
V. Fiber formation	
a. Alignment of the molecules	Formation of microfibrils
b. Formation of cross-links	Stabilization of the fiber structures
c. Supramolecular assembly	Architectural organization of collagen in tissues
d. Interactions with other extracellular macromolecules	Determines the physiologic properties of tissues
VI. Extracellular degradation	
a. Cleavage by specific collagenases	Rate-limiting step in degradation
b. Further degradation by peptidases and enzymes metabolizing free amino acids	Removal of degradation products

*These are the major steps in the sequence in the order in which they are likely to occur under physiologic conditions in vivo; some of the reactions can, however, occur simultaneously or in reverse order.

The critical importance of lysyl hydroxylation of collagen is attested to by the deficiency of lysyl hydroxylase in patients with the scoliotic (type VI) form of EDS, characterized by hyperextensible skin, loose-jointedness, severe kyphoscoliosis, and ocular fragility.[61]

Glycosylation

Collagen is a glycoprotein that contains galactosyl and glucosylgalactosyl residues attached to the molecule. The sugar residues are attached to collagen polypeptides during intracellular biosynthesis in a sequential manner, so that a galactosyl residue is first added to the molecule and

FIGURE 14-5

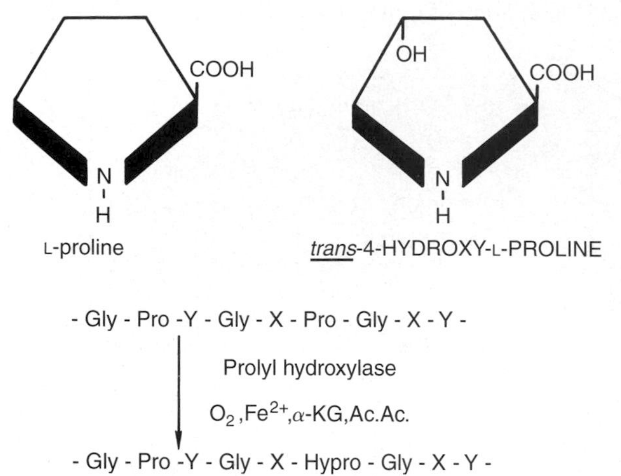

Structures of proline and hydroxyproline, and schematic representation of the enzymatic hydroxylation of prolyl residues in the Y position of the repeating Gly-X-Y sequence of collagen polypeptides. (*From Uitto J, Prockop DJ: Inhibition of collagen accumulation by proline analogues:* The mechanism of their action, in Collagen Metabolism in the Liver, *edited by H. Popper, K Becker. New York, Stratton intercontinental, 1975, p 139, with permission.*)

then a glucose moiety is attached to some of the galactosyl residues[61] (Figs. 14-4 and 14-5). The link between the carbohydrate unit and the polypeptide is an *O*-glycosidic bond through the hydroxyl group of hydroxylysine. Therefore, the synthesis of hydroxylysine is a prerequisite for the glycosylation of collagen. The two glycosylation reactions are catalyzed by separate, specific enzymes called collagen galactosyl-transferase and collagen glucosyl-transferase (Table 14-3). These enzymes have been extensively purified from a variety of sources; both of them use uridine diphosphate (UDP)-sugars as a source of the carbohydrate and require Mn^{2+} as a cofactor.

The relative number of sugar residues in genetically distinct forms of collagen shows considerable variation. In particular, types II and IV collagens are relatively rich in carbohydrates, whereas collagens of types I and III contain only a few sugar residues. The glycosylation of pro-α chains begins on nascent polypeptides after the synthesis of hydroxylysyl residues. The glycosylation reactions are terminated when the polypeptides fold into a triple-helical conformation, because the transferase enzymes do not glycosylate collagen substrates in a triple-helical form. It appears that the addition of galactose and glucose is accomplished in the cisternae of the rough endoplasmic reticulum and that the rate at which the procollagen polypeptides fold into the triple-helical conformation may partly explain the variability in the number of sugars in various types of collagens. In addition to sugars attached to the hydroxylysyl residues in the triple-helical portion of the molecule, the nonhelical extension peptides contain complex carbohydrates, consisting mainly of mannose. The function of the sugar residues in collagen and also in the extension peptides is not known.

FIGURE 14-6

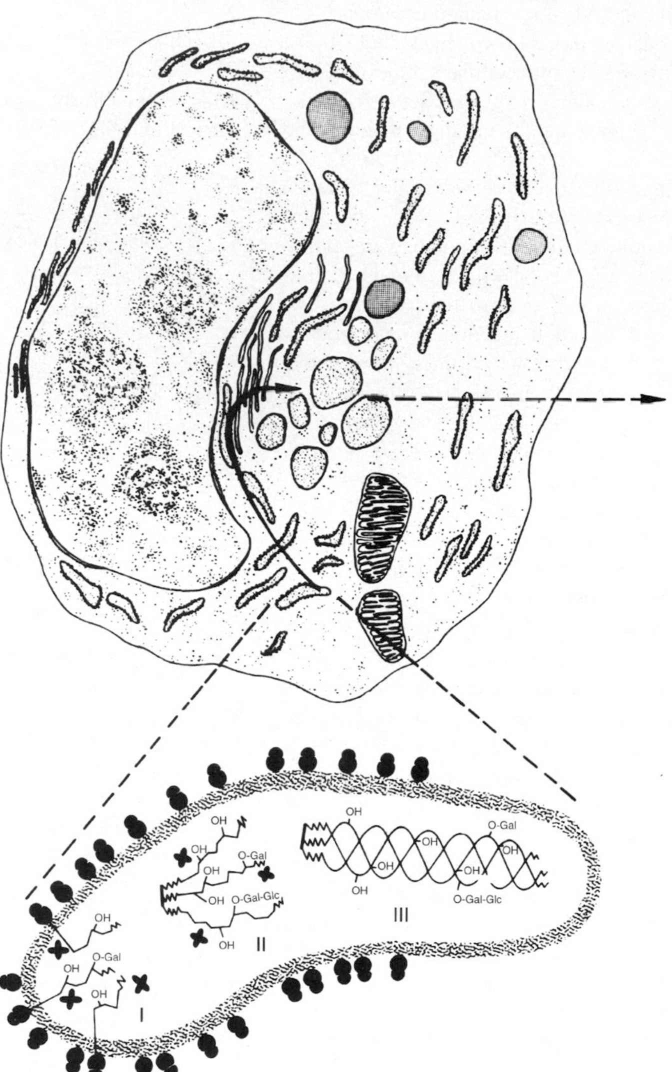

Representation of the synthesis and secretion of procollagen by a fibroblast. The enlarged area demonstrates events taking place in the rough endoplasmic reticulum of the cells during the synthesis of procollagen. In the first stage (I), the polypeptide chains of procollagen are synthesized on the membrane-bound ribosomes, and the nascent chains are fed into the cisternae of the rough endoplasmic reticulum. Hydroxylation of prolyl and lysyl residues and glycosylation of hydroxylysyl residues are initiated on the growing polypeptide chains. These reactions are completed soon after release of full-size chains from ribosomes (II). Three pro-α chains are linked together by the formation of interchain disulfide bonds, and the collagenous portions of the polypeptides assume a triple-helical conformation (III). The procollagen molecules are then transferred from the rough endoplasmic reticulum to Golgi vesicles, and are secreted from these vesicles into the extracellular milieu. –OH, hydroxyl groups of hydroxyproline and hydroxylysine; –Gal, galactosyl residue attached to hydroxylysine; –Gal Glc, glucosylgalactosyl residue attached to hydroxylysine; the cloverleaf-like structures signify the hydroxylating and glycosylating enzymes. (*After Prockop DJ et al: Intracellular steps in the biosynthesis of collagen, in* Biochemistry of Collagen, *edited by GN Ramachandran, AH Reddi. New York, Plenum, 1976, p 163, with permission.*)

CHAIN ASSOCIATION, DISULFIDE BONDING, AND TRIPLE-HELIX FORMATION

A critical step in the intracellular biosynthesis of procollagen is the association of three pro-α chains and subsequent folding of the collagen portion of the polypeptides into a triple helix (Fig. 14-6). The noncollagenous peptide extensions on the individual pro-α chains assume globular conformations soon after their translation and this conformation contains the specific information that directs the correct

FIGURE 14-7

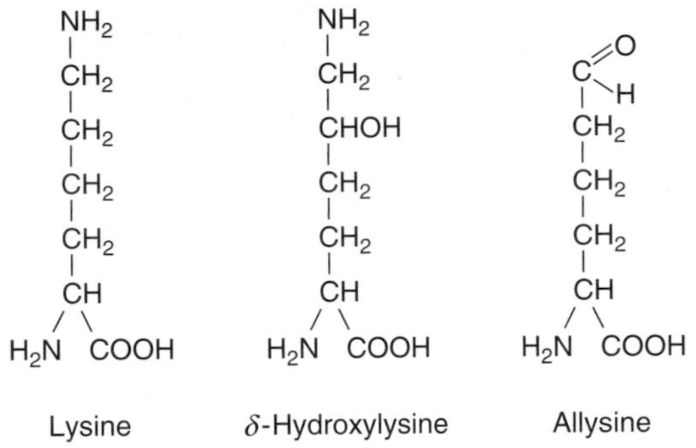

Lysine	δ-Hydroxylysine	Allysine
NH_2	NH_2	$C(=O)H$
CH_2	CH_2	CH_2
CH_2	CHOH	CH_2
CH_2	CH_2	CH_2
CH_2	CH_2	CH
CH	CH	H_2N COOH
H_2N COOH	H_2N COOH	

Structures of lysine, hydroxylysine, and allysine, the aldehyde derivative of lysine. (*From Uitto J, Lichtenstein JR: Defects in the biochemistry of collagen in diseases of connective tissue.* J Invest Dermatol *66:59, 1976, with permission.*)

association of the three pro-α chains. Such a mechanism might explain the association of pro-α1 and pro-α2 chains in a proper 2:1 ratio during the synthesis of type I procollagen. It would also explain the rapid and efficient association of the pro-α chains and folding of the molecule into the triple helix. The latter point is emphasized by the observation that fully processed collagen α chains isolated from tissues renature into a triple helix very slowly, and 24 h or more are required for about 50 percent of the molecules to become helical. In contrast, newly synthesized pro-α chains of type I procollagen, which contain intact nonhelical amino- and carboxyl terminal extensions, associate and fold into the triple-helical conformation within 5 to 10 min from the time they are synthesized on the ribosomes. The association of the extensions at the carboxyl terminal ends of the polypeptide chains appears to facilitate folding of the molecules into the triple helix, perhaps by providing a nucleation site from which the formation of the triple helix is propagated throughout the collagenous portion of the molecule.

During the process of chain association, the cysteine residues on the extension peptides of the pro-α chains form interchain disulfide bonds linking three pro-α chains together (Fig. 14-6). The interchain disulfide bonds of types I and II procollagens are located in the carboxyl terminal ends of the molecules. Experiments with freshly isolated connective tissue cells have demonstrated that the synthesis of interchain disulfide bonds closely parallels the rate at which the procollagen molecules fold into the triple-helical conformation (Fig. 14-6). On the basis of this observation and other experimental evidence, it appears that the formation of the interchain disulfide bonds may play a role in helix formation during the biosynthesis of procollagen. In addition, it has been shown that the rate at which the pro-α chains fold into the triple helix varies during the intracellular synthesis of genetically different types of procollagens. In particular, studies with isolated matrix-free cells have shown that triple-helix formation by type II procollagen is considerably slower than that by type I procollagen, and the triple-helix formation by type IV procollagen is even slower. As discussed earlier, triple-helix formation limits some of the post-translational modification reactions, such as hydroxylation of certain lysyl residues and subsequent glycosylation of hydroxylysines. Consequently, the differences in the rate of helix formation may, at least in part, explain the variations in the content of hydroxylysine and glycosylated hydroxylysine, in that type II and type IV collagens, both of which demonstrate relatively slow rates of triple-helix formation, also have the highest hydroxylysine and glycosylated hydroxylysine contents.

SECRETION OF PROCOLLAGEN

Pro-α chains, the precursor polypeptides of procollagen, are assembled on the membrane-bound ribosomes, and the newly synthesized polypeptides are translocated into the cisternae of the rough endoplasmic reticulum. In this cellular compartment, three pro-α chains, which have been hydroxylated and glycosylated, fold into a triple helix, and the triple-helical procollagen molecules are then transported into the extracellular space (Fig. 14-6). Procollagen is secreted in Golgi vacuoles or in vesicles of the cells' smooth endoplasmic reticulum. (Fig. 14-6) The intracellular translocation also involves microtubules, because colchicine and other microtubule-disrupting agents delay the secretion of procollagen, and the procollagen molecules then accumulate in the Golgi vesicles. The rate of procollagen secretion also varies among different types of collagens, as measured in matrix-free cell systems derived from different embryonic tissues. The secretion of type I procollagen by matrix-free tendon cells takes about 15 to 20 min whereas the secretion of type II procollagen by cartilage cells requires 30 to 35 min. The secretion of type IV procollagen is even slower and the secretion of procollagen synthesized by matrix-free lens cells requires approximately 60 min. The reasons for these differences are not completely understood. However, slower secretion of type II and type IV procollagen may be explained, in part, by delayed triple-helix formation, because triple-helical conformation is required for the secretion of procollagen molecules at an optimal rate.

CONVERSION OF PROCOLLAGEN TO COLLAGEN

After secretion into the extracellular space, procollagen molecules are converted to collagen by limited proteolysis, which removes the extension peptides on the molecule.[62] The conversion of type I procollagen to collagen is catalyzed by two specific enzymes, procollagen N-proteinase and procollagen C-proteinase, that separately remove the amino-terminal and carboxyl terminal extensions, respectively (Table 14-3). Furthermore, the N-proteinase catalyzing the conversion of type III procollagen to collagen is a separate, specific enzyme.[63]

The N-proteinase capable of cleaving type I procollagen belongs to the ADAMTS (a disintegrin and metalloprotease with thrombospondin motifs) family of extracellular proteases, and is specifically ADAMTS-2.[64] The activity of this enzyme is dependent on the native conformation of the amino-terminal propeptides in procollagen, as they do not catalyze the removal of the extension peptides from isolated pro-α chains. Furthermore, the partially purified N-proteinase is inhibited by metal chelators, suggesting a requirement for divalent cations.[63,65]

C-proteinase is required for removal of the carboxyl-terminal extension from types I, II, III, and V procollagens, allowing the fully processed molecules to form functional fibers.[62] Cloning of the type I procollagen C-proteinase revealed that it is identical with *bone morphogenic protein-1 (BMP-1)*, a metalloprotease implicated in pattern formation during development of diverse organisms and also capable of inducing ectopic bone formation.[65,66] The activity of the C-proteinase/BMP-1 is stimulated by procollagen C-proteinase enhancers, glycoproteins that bind to the C-terminal propeptide of type I procollagen.[67,68] Thus, the conversion of procollagen to collagen is a complex, carefully controlled process, and lack of removal of either the amino- or the carboxyl terminal extensions results in impaired tensile strength of collagen fibers in the skin. Specifically, deficiency in the removal of the amino-terminal propeptide of type I collagen in vivo causes dermatosparaxis, a disease of fragile skin, originally recognized in various animal species, and more recently recognized in humans.[69,70] Specifically, the human counterpart is the dermatosparaxis type of EDS (type VIIc), caused by deficiency in N-proteinase activity.[69] It should be noted that a phenotypically similar disease, the arthrochalasia type EDS (types VIIa and b), can be caused by mutations in the type I collagen genes (COL1A1 or COL1A2, respectively) at the cleavage site for the N-proteinase.[71]

FIBER FORMATION AND CROSS-LINKING

After removal of the extension peptides in the extracellular space, the collagen molecules spontaneously align to form fibers. These fibers, however, do not attain the necessary tensile strength until the molecules are linked together by specific covalent bonds known as *cross-links*.[72] The most common forms of cross-links in collagen are derived from lysine or hydroxylysine. The first step in the cross-linking of collagen is the enzymatic synthesis of aldehyde derivatives by removal of the ε-amino groups of some of the lysyl and hydroxylysyl residues (Figs. 14-4 and 14-6). The aldehydes then form cross-links by two kinds of reactions. One reaction involves condensation of an aldehyde with an ε-amino group, still present in unmodified lysine or hydroxylysine, to form a Schiff base type of covalent cross-link (Fig. 14-8). The second type of reaction is an aldol condensation between two aldehydes. In addition to these cross-links, collagen contains several more complex cross-links that also involve lysyl or hydroxylysyl residues. The lysine- and hydroxylysine-derived cross-links can be either intramolecular, occurring between two adjacent α chains in the same collagen molecule, or intermolecular, stabilizing the alignment of neighboring collagen molecules along the microfibril.

The first step in collagen cross-linking, the oxidative deamination of certain lysyl and hydroxylysyl residues, is catalyzed by lysyl oxidase. This enzyme requires copper as a cofactor, and its activity is readily inhibited by nitriles, such as β-amino-propionitrile, which produce lathyrism in animals. Lysyl oxidase functions in the extracellular space, and it has much greater activity with collagen that has been precipitated as native fibrils as compared with denatured collagen or isolated α chains. It should be noted that several additional lysyl oxidase-like (LOXL) proteins have been identified by molecular cloning. Thus, lysyl oxidase is a family of copper-dependent enzymes although the precise functions of the LOXL proteins is currently unknown.[73] The in vivo formation of aldehydes appears to occur primarily after the onset of fibril formation. Because the cross-links of collagen provide the tensile strength required in certain tissues, a defect in the formation of these covalent bonds could lead to a disturbance in connective tissue function. An example is the occipital horn syndrome (previously known as the Ehlers-Danlos syndrome type IX), which results from reduced lysyl oxidase activity. The primary defect resides in perturbed copper metabolism caused by mutations in a copper transport enzyme protein, an ATPase encoded by the gene MNK-1 that is also involved in Menkes' syndrome.[74,75] As a result, serum copper levels are reduced, leading to reduced lysyl oxidase activity.

FIGURE 14-8

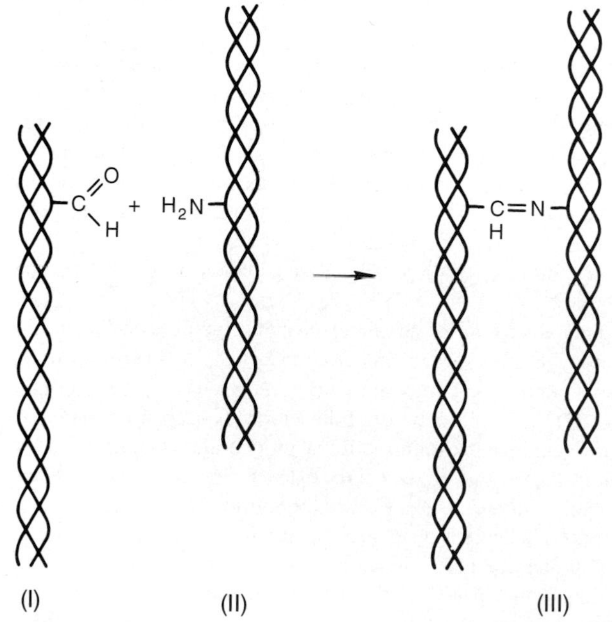

Representation of the formation of intermolecular cross-links of collagen. The cross-linking is initiated by oxidative deamination of either a lysyl or hydroxylysyl residue to form a corresponding aldehyde derivative (I). The aldehyde then reacts with an ε-amino group on an unmodified lysyl or hydroxylysyl residue in an adjacent collagen molecule (II), and they form a Schiff-base-type covalent cross-link. (*From Uitto J, Lichtenstein JR: Defects in the biochemistry of collagen in diseases of connective tissue.* J Invest Dermatol *66:59, 1976, with permission.*)

CONTROL OF COLLAGEN PRODUCTION

A major question in collagen biology concerns the mechanisms that control the deposition of collagen in tissues. Such control must exist in vivo, because the consequences of uncontrolled collagen accumulation are demonstrated by diseases such as progressive systemic sclerosis and various other fibrotic conditions.[76]

On the basis of theoretical considerations, the accumulation of collagen in tissues can be controlled at several different levels of biosynthesis and degradation. The possible sites of control include (1) transcriptional and posttranscriptional control of the formation of functional procollagen mRNA molecules; (2) control of the rate of polypeptide assembly through translation of mRNA; (3) posttranslational control of the triple-helix formation, secretion, and conversion of the precursor forms to collagen; and (4) degradation of newly synthesized pro-α chains and removal of extracellular collagen fibers.

Several observations suggest that an important control mechanism acts at the level of mRNA formation through regulation of the transcriptional activity of gene expression.[54,77] In fact, there is a good correlation between collagen biosynthesis and the level of procollagen mRNAs in several in vitro models by using cultured cells, such as skin fibroblasts. At least in these models, the production of procollagen is primarily regulated at the transcriptional level.

The transcriptional regulation of collagen gene expression involves both *cis*-acting elements and *trans*-acting factors. The *cis*-acting elements are nucleotide sequences in the promoter region of the gene that serve as binding sites for *trans*-acting cellular proteins, which can up or downregulate the transcriptional promoter activity. Some of the *trans*-acting factors are nuclear receptors, such as the retinoic acid receptors (RAR and RXR)[78] that form a complex with the ligand (a retinoid) and then bind to the retinoic acid-responsive elements (RARE) in the target gene. Retinoids, such as all-*trans*-retinoic acid, modulate type I collagen gene expression both in vitro and in vivo. In particular, quiescent nonproliferating cells can be stimulated by retinoic acid to activate collagen gene expression. This may have relevance to the elevated collagen synthesis observed in photodamaged dermis after topical application of all-*trans*-retinoic acid.[79]

One of the most powerful modulators of connective tissue gene expression is transforming growth factor β (TGF-β), a member of a family of growth factors that upregulate the expression of several extracellular matrix protein genes, including those encoding collagen types I, III, IV, V, VI, and VII.[80] In the case of these collagens, the elevated mRNA levels result primarily from the enhanced transcription of the collagen promoter, as determined in transient cell transfections with corresponding collagen promoter/reporter gene constructs.[81] Contributing to the elevation of collagen mRNA levels in fibroblast cultures incubated with TGF-β_1 is the increased stability of type I collagen mRNAs. Thus, the elevated collagen mRNA levels observed in cells incubated with TGF-β could result from a combination of enhanced transcriptional activity and reduced turnover of the mRNA.

PHARMACOLOGIC PERSPECTIVE

In addition to transcriptional modulators of collagen gene expression, such as retinoids, the multiplicity of posttranscriptional reactions can serve as a source of regulation during procollagen production and may provide opportunities for pharmacologic manipulation of collagen production.[82] Of particular interest is the role of prolyl hydroxylation in limiting the formation of triple-helical collagen. As indicated earlier, the presence of *trans*-4-hydroxyproline is necessary for the formation of the triple helix at physiologic temperatures. The triple helix is required, in turn, for normal secretion of procollagen and subsequent collagen fiber formation. Thus, if formation of 4-hydroxyproline is inhibited, the production of collagen decreases. In several experimental systems designed to limit the synthesis of *trans*-4-hydroxyproline, the production of triple-helical procollagens is decreased concomitantly.[82] These observations suggest that the formation of *trans*-4-hydroxyproline could be rate-limiting in procollagen production in vivo. In support of this suggestion, it has been found that the activity of prolyl hydroxylase in tissues correlates with the rate of procollagen synthesis in various clinical and experimental conditions. From these data it is clear that prolyl hydroxylase activity has the capacity to limit collagen production, but it has not been demonstrated thus far that such activity would be rate-limiting under physiologic conditions.

Another control mechanism that determines the amount of extracellular collagen involves degradation of the molecules. Some newly synthesized pro-α chains are degraded intracellularly before secretion,[83] although there are technical difficulties in determining the exact fraction of pro-α chains degraded by this pathway. It has been suggested that this mechanism removes defective pro-α chains that are not able to fold into a triple helix. In addition to the intracellular degradation, continuous removal of extracellular collagen fibers by specific collagenases regulates the amount of tissue collagen (see Chap. 17).

The manner by which hormones regulate collagen gene expression has not been defined in all cases, but a number of endocrinologic disorders dramatically affect the amounts of collagen found in connective tissues.[84] Of special interest is the effect of various glucocorticoids on collagen in the dermis and other connective tissues. The biosynthesis of collagen is inhibited by hydrocortisone and various fluorinated glucocorticoids used in clinical dermatology.[85] The inhibition is much more pronounced with fluorinated steroids as compared with hydrocortisone. In lower concentrations, the glucocorticoids affect collagen gene expression primarily by inhibiting the rate of transcription, thus resulting in reduced levels of procollagen mRNA. In higher concentrations, glucocorticoids also reduce the activity of prolyl hydroxylase, leading to deficient hydroxylation of collagen polypeptides. As a result, the amount of newly synthesized collagen decreases, possibly explaining connective tissue side effects, such as atrophy of the dermis, often observed after intralesional or prolonged topical application of high potency glucocorticoids.[86]

COLLAGEN DISEASES

The term *collagen disease* implies that a clinical condition involves an abnormality in the structure, synthesis, or degradation of collagen. This term is frequently used to characterize a clinically heterogeneous group of diseases, including lupus erythematosus, scleroderma, and dermatomyositis. In the classic sense, the use of the term in these diseases was based on morphologic changes, known as *fibrinoid degeneration,* that have been interpreted to represent changes in collagen fibers. However, there is currently no conclusive evidence that fibrinoid degeneration of collagen fibers is indicative of a defect in collagen. On the basis of available biochemical evidence, scleroderma is the only clinical condition among the classical collagen diseases that involves any detectable abnormality in the structure or metabolism of collagen (see also Chap. 173).

As discussed above, collagen is an unusual protein in many respects, and its structure and metabolism involve a number of special features that are critical for deposition of normal collagen fibers. Based on our understanding of the biochemistry of normal collagen, it is now possible to identify discrete points at which defects could be introduced into collagen molecules or mature fibers. A defect at any one of these levels could produce a "true" collagen disease.[84] Based on these considerations, the term *collagen disease* should be reserved for conditions in which a defect in collagen can be demonstrated clearly at the molecular level. In a primary collagen disease, such a defect could be an inherited abnormality in the structure of the collagen or procollagen or in the enzymes participating in the biosynthesis and degradation of collagen. In a secondary, acquired type of collagen disease, changes in collagen may be a consequence of initially unrelated metabolic changes. According to these definitions, several clinical disorders that are true collagen diseases are currently known (Table 14-5).

Recently, progress in understanding the basic principles of collagen biology in normal tissues has created a foundation for exploration of collagen abnormalities in a variety of diseases affecting the connective tissues. Indeed, there are many diseases in which a basic biochemical defect in collagen has been described, and several heritable connective tissue diseases with cutaneous involvement are now known to result from specific molecular defects in collagen (Table 14-5). Many of these diseases involve insertions, deletions, or single-base substitutions in the collagen genes, which alter the primary structure of the protein. In several acquired diseases, the regulation of collagen gene expression is disturbed, leading to altered deposition of collagen in tissues. The diversity of collagen pathology is exemplified by the Ehlers-Danlos syndrome and fibrotic skin diseases (see Chaps. 154 and 173). The Ehlers-Danlos syndrome comprises a group of phenotypically similar conditions that frequently result from abnormalities in the structure of collagen.[87] In contrast, the fibrotic skin diseases exemplify conditions with altered regulation of collagen gene expression that leads to excessive accumulation of collagen in tissues.

TABLE 14-5

Heritable Connective Tissue Diseases with Cutaneous Involvement

DISEASE	INHERITANCE*	MUTATED GENES‡	AFFECTED PROTEIN
Ehlers-Danlos syndrome	AD, AR	COL1A1, COL1A2, COL3A1, COL5A1, COL5A2	α Chains of types I, III, and V collagens
		PLOD	Procollagen-lysine 2-oxoglutarate 5-dioxygenase (lysylhydroxylase),
		ADAMTS-2	Procollagen N-peptidase
		TNX	Tenascin-X
		B4GALT-7	Xylosylprotein 4-beta-galactosyl-transferase
Osteogenesis imperfecta	AD, AR,	COL1A1, COL1A2	α_1 and α_2 Chains of type I collagen
Cutis laxa	AD, AR, XR†	ELN	Elastin
		MNK-1 (ATP7A)	ATP-dependent copper transporter
Homocystinuria	AR	CBS	Cystathionine β-synthase
Menkes' syndrome	XR	MNK-1 (ATP7A)	ATP-dependent copper transporter
Focal dermal hypoplasia	XD	ND	
Tuberous sclerosis (shagreen patches)	AD	TSK-1	Hamartin 1
Familial cutaneous collagenoma	AD	ND	
Epidermolysis bullosa	AD, AR	COL7A1 COL17A1	α1 Chains of types VII and XVII collagens

*AD, autosomal dominant; AR, autosomal recessive; XD, X-linked dominant; XR, X-linked recessive; ND, not determined.
†Most cases involve abnormalities in the elastic fibers, and in some cases, mutations in the elastin gene (ELN) have been disclosed. Occipital horn syndrome, a copper deficiency syndrome, allelic to the Menkes' syndrome gene (MNK-1), was previously known as x-linked cutis laxa and also Ehlers-Danlos syndrome IX (see Chap. 154).
‡For detailed discussion on these genes, see Refs. 4 and 87.

REFERENCES

1. Prockop DJ, Kivirikko KI: Collagens: Molecular biology, diseases, and potentials for therapy. *Annu Rev Biochem* **64**:403, 1995 etc
2. Brown JC, Timpl R: The collagen superfamily. *Int Arch Allergy Immunol* **107**:484, 1995
3. Myllyharju J, Kivirikko KI: Collagens and collagen-related diseases. *Ann Med* **33**:7, 2001
4. Pulkkinen L et al: Progress in heritable skin diseases: Molecular bases and clinical implications. *J Am Acad Dermatol* **47**:91, 2002
5. Kuivaniemi H et al: Mutations in fibrillar collagens (types I, II, III, and XI), fibril-associated collagen (type IX), and network-forming collagen (type X) cause a spectrum of diseases of bone, cartilage, and blood vessels. *Hum Mutat* **9**:300, 1997
6. Elomaa O et al: Cloning of a novel bacteria-binding receptor structurally related to scavenger receptors and expressed in a subset of macrophages. *Cell* **80**:603, 1995
7. Kere J et al: X-linked anhidrotic (hypohidrotic) ectodermal dysplasia is caused by mutation in a novel transmembrane protein. *Nat Genet* **13**:409, 1996
8. Shaw LM, Olsen BR: FACIT collagens: Diverse molecular bridges in extracellular matrices. *Trends Biochem Sci* **16**:191, 1991
9. Uitto J: Collagen polymorphism: Isolation and partial characterization of α1(I)-trimer molecules in normal human skin. *Arch Biochem Biophys* **192**:371, 1979
10. Epstein EH Jr: [α1(III)]$_3$ Human skin collagen, release by pepsin digestion and preponderance in fetal life. *J Biol Chem* **249**:3225, 1974
11. Heikkilä P, Soininen R: The type IV collagen gene family. *Contrib Nephrol* **117**:105, 1996
12. Timpl R et al: A network model for the organization of type IV collagen molecules in basement membranes. *Eur J Biochem* **120**:203, 1981
13. Lohi J et al: Expression of type IV collagen α1(IV)–α6(IV) polypeptides in normal and developing human kidney and in renal cell carcinomas and oncocytomas. *Int J Cancer* **72**:43, 1997
14. Tryggvason K: Mutations in type IV collagen genes and Alport phenotypes. *Contrib Nephrol* **117**:154, 1996
15. Merkel F et al: Autoreactive T-cells in Goodpasture's syndrome recognize the N-terminal NC1 domain on α3 type IV collagen. *Kidney Int* **49**:1127, 1996
16. Ghohestani RF et al: The α5 chain of type IV collagen is the target of IgG autoantibodies in a novel autoimmune disease with subepidermal blisters and renal insufficiency. *J Biol Chem* **275**:16002, 2000
17. Schwarze U et al: Null alleles of the COL5A1 gene of type V collagen are a cause of the classical forms of Ehlers-Danlos syndrome (types I and II). *Am J Hum Genet* **66**:1757, 2000
18. Michalickova K et al: Mutations of the α2(V) chain of type V collagen impair matrix assembly and produce Ehlers-Danlos syndrome type I. *Hum Mol Genet* **3**:249, 1998
19. Schalkwijk J et al: A recessive form of Ehlers-Danlos syndrome caused by tenascin-X deficiency. *N Engl J Med* **345**:1167, 2001
20. Matsumoto K et al: Tumour invasion and metastasis are promoted in mice deficient in tenascin-X. *Genes Cells* **6**:1101, 2001
21. Olsen DR et al: Collagen gene expression by cultured human skin fibroblasts: Abundant steady-state levels of type VI procollagen mRNAs. *J Clin Invest* **83**:791, 1989
22. Timpl R, Chu M-L: Microfibrillar collagen type VI, in *Extracellular Matrix Assembly and Structure,* PD Yurchenko, DE Birk, RP Mecham, eds. Academic Press, San Diego, 1994, p 207
23. Keene DR et al: Ultrastructure of type VI collagen in human skin and cartilage suggests an anchoring function for this filamentous network. *J Cell Biol* **107**:1995, 1988
24. Scacheri PC et al: Novel mutations in collagen VI genes: Expansion of the Bethlem myopathy phenotype. *Neurology* **58**:593, 2002
25. Camacho-Vanegas O et al: Ullrich scleroatonic muscular dystrophy is caused by recessive mutations in collagen type VI. *Proc Natl Acad Sci U S A* **98**:7516, 2001
26. Burgeson RE: Type VII collagen, anchoring fibrils, and epidermolysis bullosa. *J Invest Dermatol* **101**:252, 1993
27. Christiano AM et al: Cloning of human type VII collagen: Complete primary sequence of the α1(VII) chain and identification of intragenic polymorphisms. *J Biol Chem* **269**:20256, 1994
28. Rousselle P et al: Laminin 5 binds the NC-1 domain of type VII collagen. *J Cell Biol* **138**:719, 1997
29. Shimizu H et al: Most anchoring fibrils in human skin originate and terminate in the lamina densa. *Lab Invest* **76**:753, 1997
30. Fine J-D et al: Revised classification system for inherited epidermolysis bullosa: Report of the Second International Consensus Meeting on diagnosis and classification of epidermolysis bullosa. *J Am Acad Dermatol* **42**:1051, 2000
31. Pulkkinen L, Uitto J: Mutation analysis and molecular genetics of epidermolysis bullosa. *Matrix Biol* **18**:29, 1999
32. Uitto J et al: The molecular basis of the dystrophic forms of epidermolysis bullosa, in *Epidermolysis Bullosa: Clinical, Epidemiologic and Laboratory Advances, and the Findings of the National Epidermolysis Bullosa Registry,* edited by J-D Fine, EA Baner, J McGuire, AN Moshell. Baltimore, The Johns Hopkins University Press, 1999, p 326
33. Lapiere JC et al: Epitope mapping of type VII collagen: Identification of discrete peptide sequences recognized by sera from patients with acquired epidermolysis bullosa. *J Clin Invest* **92**:1831, 1993
34. Levy SG et al: The composition of wide-spaced collagen in normal and diseased Descemet's membrane. *Curr Eye Res* **15**:45, 1996
35. Munier BS et al: Missense mutations in COL8A2, the gene encoding the α2 chain of type VIII collagen, cause two forms of corneal endothelial dystrophy. *Hum Mol Genet* **10**:2415, 2001

36. Nishiyama T et al: Type XII and XIV collagens mediate interactions between banded collagen fibers in vitro and may modulate extracellular matrix deformability. *J Biol Chem* **269**:28193, 1994
37. Peltonen S et al: A novel component of epidermal cell-matrix and cell-cell contacts: Transmembrane protein type XIII collagen. *J Invest Dermatol* **113**:635, 1999
38. Peltonen S et al: Alternative splicing of mouse α1(XIII) collagen RNAs results in at least 17 different transcripts, predicting α1(XIII) collagen chains with length varying between 651 and 710 amino acid residues. *DNA Cell Biol* **16**:227, 1997
39. Li K et al: Cloning of type XVII collagen. Complementary and genomic DNA sequences of mouse 180-kilodalton bullous pemphigoid antigen (BPAG2) predict an interrupted collagenous domain, a transmembrane segment, and unusual features in the 5′-end of the gene and the 3′-untranslated region of the mRNA. *J Biol Chem* **268**:8825, 1993
40. Gatalica B et al: Cloning of the human type XVII collagen gene (COL17A1), and detection of novel mutations in generalized atrophic benign epidermolysis bullosa. *Am J Hum Genet* **60**:352, 1997
41. Areida SK et al: Properties of the collagen type XVII ectodomain. Evidence for N- to C-terminal triple helix folding. *J Biol Chem* **276**:1594, 2001
42. Sawamura D et al: Bullous pemphigoid antigen: cDNA cloning and mapping of the gene to the short arm of human chromosome 6. *Genomics* **8**:722, 1990
43. McGrath JA et al: Mutations in the 180-kD bullous pemphigoid antigen (BPAG2), a transmembrane hemidesmosomal collagen (COL17A1), in generalized atrophic benign epidermolysis bullosa. *Nat Genet* **11**:83, 1995
44. Kivirikko S et al: Distribution of type XV collagen transcripts in human tissue and their production by muscle cells and fibroblasts. *Am J Pathol* **147**:1500, 1995
45. Pan TC et al: Cloning and chromosomal location of humanα1(XVI) collagen. *Proc Natl Acad Sci U S A* **89**:6565, 1992
46. Oh SP et al: Cloning of cDNA and genomic DNA encoding human type XVIII collagen and localization of the α1(XVIII) collagen to mouse chromosome 10 and human chromosome 21. *Genomics* **19**:494, 1994
47. Sumiyoshi H et al: Ubiquitous expression of the α1(XIX) collagen gene (COL19A1) during mouse embryogenesis becomes restricted to a few tissues in the adult organism. *J Biol Chem* **272**:17104, 1997
48. Koch M et al: α1(XX) Collagen, a new member of the collagen subfamily, fibril-associated collagens with interrupted triple helices. *J Biol Chem* **276**:23120, 2001
49. Fitzgerald J et al: A new FACIT of the collagen family: COL21A1. *FEBS Lett* **505**:275, 2001
50. Chou M-Y, Li H-C: Genomic organization and characterization of the human type XXI collagen (COL21A1) gene. *Genomics* **79**:395, 2002
51. Tuckwell D: Identification and analysis of collagen α1(XXI), a novel member of the FACIT collagen family. *Matrix Biol* **21**:63, 2002
52. O'Reilly MS et al: Endostatin: An endogenous inhibitor of angiogenesis and tumor growth. *Cell* **88**:277, 1997
53. Grassel S et al: Collagen XVI is expressed by human dermal fibroblasts and keratinocytes and is associated with the microfibrillar apparatus in the upper papillary dermis. *Matrix Biol* **18**:309, 1999
54. Chu M-L, Prockop DJ: Collagen: Gene structure, *in Connective Tissue and Its Heritable Disorders:* Molecular, Genetic and Medical Aspects, 2nd ed, edited by PM Royce, B Steinmann. New York, Wiley-Liss, 2002, p 223
55. Christiano AM et al: Structural organization of the human type VII collagen gene (COL7A1), composed of more exons than any previously characterized gene. *Genomics* **21**:169, 1994
56. Blumberg B et al: Basement membrane procollagen IV and its specialized carboxyl domain are conserved in Drosophila, mouse and human. *J Biol Chem* **262**:5947, 1987
57. Christiano AM et al: A strategy for identification of sequence variants in COL7A1 and a novel 2-bp deletion mutation in recessive dystrophic epidermolysis bullosa. *Hum Mutat* **10**:408, 1997
58. Berg RA: Determination of 3- and 4-hydroxyproline. *Methods Enzymol* **82**:372, 1982
59. Davidson JM et al: Ascorbate differentially regulates elastin and collagen biosynthesis in vascular smooth muscle cells and skin fibroblasts by pretranslational mechanisms. *J Biol Chem* **272**:345, 1997
60. Uitto J, Prockop DJ: Synthesis and secretion of underhydroxylated procollagen at various temperatures by cells subject to temporary anoxia. *Biochem Biophys Res Commun* **60**:313, 1974
61. Burrows NP: The Ehlers-Danlos syndrome: On beyond collagens. *J Clin Invest* **24**:99, 1999
62. Prockop DJ et al: Procollagen N-proteinase and procollagen C-proteinase. Two unusual metalloproteinases that are essential for procollagen processing probably have important roles in development and cell signaling. *Matrix Biol* **16**:399, 1998
63. Colige A et al: cDNA cloning and expression of bovine procollagen I N-proteinase: A new member of the superfamily of zinc-metalloproteinases with binding sites for cells and other matrix components. *Proc Natl Acad Sci U S A* **94**:2374, 1997
64. Tang BL: ADAMTS: A novel family of extracellular matrix proteases. *Int J Biochem Cell Biol* **33**:33, 2001
65. Kessler E et al: Bone morphogenetic protein-1: The type I procollagen C-proteinase. *Science* **271**:360, 1996
66. Li SW et al: The C-proteinase that processes procollagens to fibrillar collagens is identical to the protein previously identified as bone morphogenic protein-1. *Proc Natl Acad Sci U S A* **93**:5127, 1996
67. Takahara K et al: Type I procollagen COOH-terminal proteinase enhancer protein: Identification, primary structure, and chromosomal localization of the cognate human gene (PCOLCE). *J Biol Chem* **269**:26280, 1994
68. Scott IC et al: Structural organization and expression patterns of the human and mouse genes for the type I procollagen COOH-terminal proteinase enhancer protein. *Genomics* **55**:229, 1999
69. Nusgens BV et al: Evidence for a relationship between Ehlers-Danlos type VII in humans and bovine dermatosparaxis. *Nat Genet* **1**:214, 1992
70. Colige A et al: Human Ehlers-Danlos syndrome type VII C and bovine dermatosparaxis are caused by mutations in the procollagen I N-proteinase gene. *Am J Hum Genet* **65**:308, 1999
71. Byers PH et al: Ehlers-Danlos syndrome type VIIA and VIIB result from splice-junction mutations or genomic deletions that involve exon 6 in the COL1A1 and COL1A2 genes of type I collagen. *Am J Med Genet* **72**:94, 1997
72. Rucker RB, Murray J: Cross-linking amino acids in collagen and elastin. *Am J Clin Nutr* **31**:1221, 1978
73. Mäki JM et al: Cloning and characterization of a fifth human lysyl oxidase isoenzyme: The third member of the lysyl oxidase-related subfamily with four scavenger receptor cysteine-rich domains. *Matrix Biol* **20**:493, 2001
74. Kaler SG et al: Occipital horn syndrome and a mild Menkes phenotype associated with splice site mutations at the MNK locus. *Nat Genet* **8**:195, 1994
75. Das S et al: Diverse mutations in patients with Menkes disease often lead to exon skipping. *Am J Hum Genet* **55**:883, 1994
76. Uitto J, Kouba DJ: Cytokine modulation of extracellular matrix gene expression: Relevance to fibrotic skin diseases. *J Dermatol Sci* **24**:S60, 2000
77. Karsenty G, Park RW: Regulation of type I collagen genes expression. *Int Rev Immunol* **12**:177, 1995
78. de Thé H et al: Identification of a retinoic acid responsive element in the retinoic acid receptor β gene. *Nature* **343**:177, 1990
79. Griffiths CEM et al: Restoration of collagen formation in photodamaged human skin by tretinoin (retinoic acid). *N Engl J Med* **329**:530, 1993
80. Roberts AB: The ever-increasing complexity of TGF-β signaling. *Cytokine Growth Factor Rev* **13**:3, 2002
81. Mauviel A, Uitto J: The extracellular matrix in wound healing: Role of the cytokine network. *Wounds* **5**:137, 1993
82. Uitto J et al: Pharmacological inhibition of excessive collagen deposition in fibrotic diseases. *Fed Proc* **43**:2815, 1984
83. Rennard SI et al: Intracellular degradation of newly synthesized collagen. *J Invest Dermatol* **79**(suppl 1):77s, 1982
84. Uitto J, Prockop DJ: Molecular defects in collagen and the definition of "collagen disease," in *Molecular Pathology,* edited by RA Good, SB Day, JJ Yunis. Springfield, IL, Charles C. Thomas, 1975, p 670
85. Oikarinen AI, Uitto J: Molecular mechanisms of glucocorticosteroid action on connective tissue metabolism, in *Diseases of Connective Tissue: The Molecular Pathology of the Extracellular Matrix,* edited by J Uitto, AJ Perejda, in series: *The Biochemistry of Disease: A Molecular Approach to Cell Pathology,* series editors E Farber, HC Pitot. New York, Marcel Dekker, 1987, p 385
86. Booth BA et al: Steroid-induced dermal atrophy: Effects of glucocorticosteroids on collagen metabolism in human skin fibroblast cultures. *Int J Dermatol* **21**:333, 1982
87. Uitto J et al: Heritable disorders of connective tissue—Ehlers-Danlos syndrome, pseudoxanthoma elasticum and cutis laxa, in *Dermatology,* edited by Bologna JL, Jorizzo JL, Rapini RP. London, Harcourt Publishers (in press)

CHAPTER 15

Jouni Uitto
Mon-Li Chu

Elastic Fibers

STRUCTURE AND DEVELOPMENT OF THE ELASTIC FIBERS

Elastic fibers of the connective tissue form a network responsible for the resilient properties of various organs.[1–3] The distribution of elastic fibers is variable in different tissues. Their relative concentration is highest in the aorta and arterial blood vessels, but they are also abundant in the lungs (Table 15-1). Elastic fibers are also present in the skin, although they are only a minor component (Fig. 15-1). Specifically, in sun-protected human skin, the elastin content is about 1 to 2 percent of the total dry weight of dermis[4] (Table 15-1). In the papillary dermis, elastic fibers are present either as bundles of microfibrils (oxytalan fibers) or with small amounts of cross-linked elastin (elaunin fibers). In the reticular dermis, the elastic fibers, which consist primarily of elastin, are oriented horizontally in a network with vertical extensions to the papillary dermis in the form of oxytalan fibers.

Examination of elastic connective tissues by transmission electron microscopy has demonstrated that mature elastic fibers consist of two distinct components (Fig. 15-2). The major component is composed of a well-characterized connective tissue protein, elastin, that shows no distinct periodic banding pattern. This amorphous, electron-lucent elastin component, when visualized by transmission electron microscopy, is surrounded by distinct microfibrillar structures that have a regular diameter of 10 to 12 nm (Fig. 15-2). The microfibrillar component is composed of a variety of recently characterized proteins.[3]

Fetal Development

Elastin and the microfibrils exist in close association in various connective tissues. However, the relative proportions of these components vary during embryonic development. The first elements of elastic fibers that form during human fetal development consist of bundles of microfibrils that can be visualized by electron microscopy early in the first trimester of gestation. During the second trimester, the elastic fibers remain relatively immature in structure and composition, but with increasing fetal age and maturation of the fibers, the amorphous elastin component becomes more prominent. Fully developed elastic fibers consist of a central amorphous core surrounded by an envelope of microfibrils, although some microfibrils are also dispersed within the amorphous component. Electron microscopic estimations of the fully matured elastic fibers suggest that the elastin protein represents well over 90 percent of the total content of such fibers.[5] It should be noted, however, that skin as well as other tissues, contain microfibrils devoid of elastin.

TABLE 15-1

Relative Concentrations of Elastin and Collagen in Various Tissues*

Tissue	Percentage of Dry Weight	
	Elastin	Collagen
Skin	0.6–2.1	71.9
Lung	3–7	10
Aorta	28–32	12–24
Ligamentum nuchae	74.8	17
Achilles tendon	4.4	86.0
Liver	0.16–0.30	3.9

*The values represent determinations from different animal species.

The biochemical characterization of elastin and the microfibrils was hampered for many years by the relative insolubility of these structures, and early information about the structural features of these fibers was gained through electron microscopic observations. However, several recent innovations and improvements in biochemical technology, including the techniques of molecular biology, have greatly facilitated the characterization of these proteins, so that features of their basic structures and several aspects of their biosynthesis are now well understood. Interest in the biochemistry of the elastic connective tissues has increased with the realization that marked changes in the structure of these proteins are observed in various disease processes, many of them affecting the skin.

BIOLOGY OF THE ELASTIC FIBERS

Elastin

PROTEIN STRUCTURE The fibers composed of elastin, when visualized by transmission or scanning electron microscopy, appear as amorphous, branching structures forming continuous sheets in some connective tissues (Figs. 15-2 and 15-3). The isolation and characterization of the basic polypeptide unit of elastin was hindered for a long time by the extreme insolubility of elastin in mature animal tissues. It was discovered, however, that this insolubility is attributable to the presence of complex covalent cross-links, known as desmosines (see below), whose formation can be prevented by maintaining the animals on a copper-deficient diet or by feeding them lathyrogens, such as β-aminopropionitrile, which inhibit elastin and collagen cross-linking. Once the formation of the cross-links is prevented, a large fraction of newly synthesized elastin can be extracted from the tissues. By these methods, large quantities of soluble elastin were initially purified from porcine aorta, and short peptide fragments were sequenced.[6] The precise amino acid sequence of human elastin has been deduced from cloned complementary DNAs (cDNAs).[7,8]

The basic molecular unit of elastin is a linear polypeptide, known as tropoelastin, that consists of approximately 800 amino acids with a molecular mass of about 70 kDa. Elastin is relatively rich in hydrophobic residues—such as valine and alanine—and its amino acid composition is similar to that of collagen in that about one-third of the total number of amino acid residues consist of glycine. However, glycine is not evenly distributed in elastin, as it is in a typical collagen sequence. Instead, the glycine residues are grouped in valine and proline-rich regions, which are interspersed with alanine-rich sequences. Elastin also contains some hydroxyproline, but the relative content of this amino acid is considerably lower than that in collagen, and the values for hydroxyproline are variable. Elastin does not contain hydroxylysine or carbohydrate moieties covalently linked to the polypeptide chain.

Several models for the molecular structure of elastin have been proposed to account for the special resilient nature of the fibers. The various aspects considered in these models include the prevalence of random-coil conformation, the presence of α helices in the monomeric unit, the frequency and distribution of stabilizing cross-links, and the degree of hydration of the protein.[9,10] One of the earlier theories described elastin as a rubber-like elastomer with an amorphous network structure.[10] According to this theory, the covalent cross-links, which are randomly distributed, link up to four tropoelastin polypeptides, but there are no specific interactions between the individual chains. According to another theory, elastin is described as an "oiled-coil" that is interrupted by regularly repeating cross-link and α-helical regions.[9] In this model, each desmosine or isodesmosine cross-link connects two individual polypeptides. The oiled-coil regions consist of repeating sequences relatively rich in hydrophobic amino acids. Based on these considerations, one could speculate that during stretching of the fiber network, the hydrophobic groups are exposed to the surrounding aqueous milieu, and the energy for contraction of the fiber is derived from the return of these groups to a nonpolar environment.

FIGURE 15-1

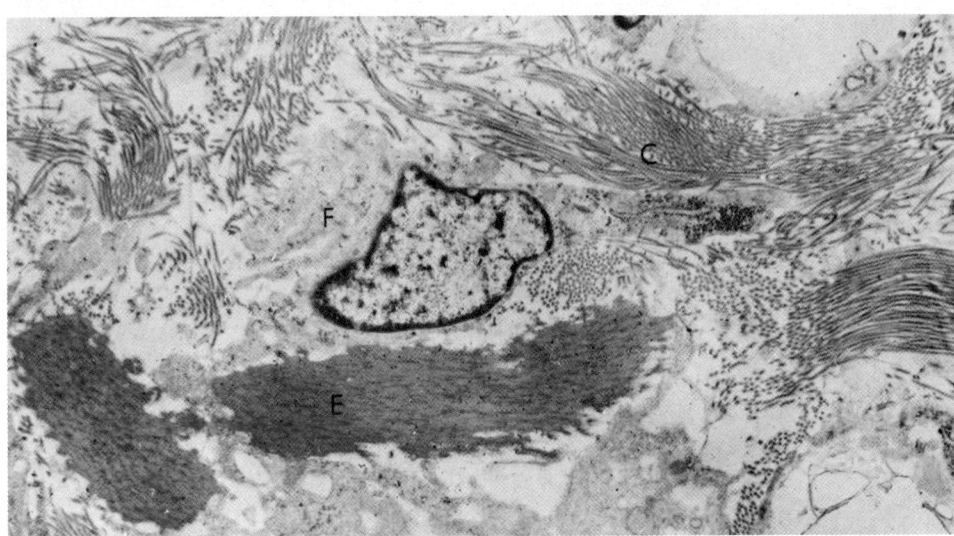

Transmission electron microscopy of human skin demonstrating a fibroblast (F) surrounded by elastic structures (E) and collagen fibers (C).

FIGURE 15-2

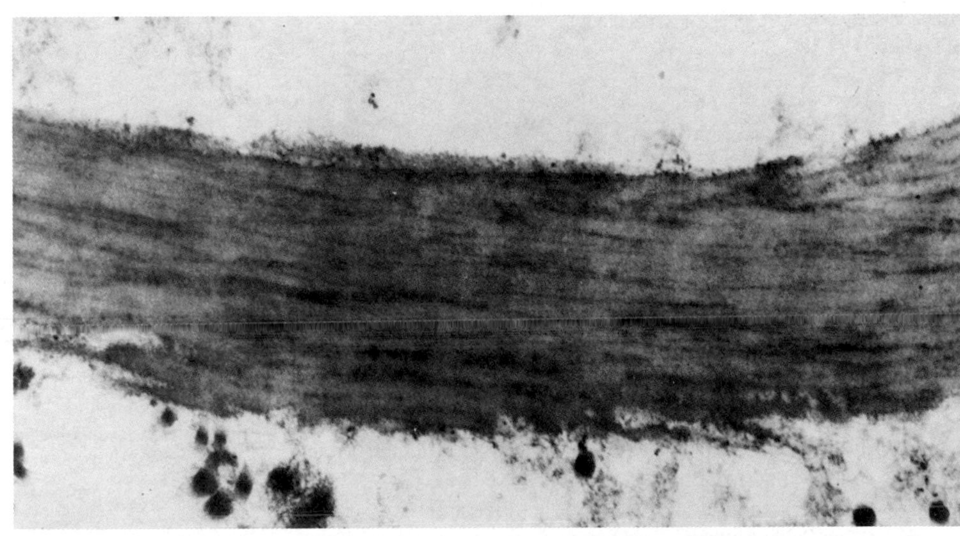

Transmission electron microscopy of the elastic fibers in normal human skin. Elastin, the electron-lucent core of the fiber, is surrounded by thin, electron-dense microfibrils. Original magnification ×16,000.

One characteristic feature of elastic fibers is the presence of cross-links that covalently bind elastin polypeptide chains into a fiber network. The two major cross-link compounds, desmosine and its isomer, isodesmosine, are structures that appear to be unique to elastin[11] (Fig. 15-4). The content of desmosines in various elastin preparations has been shown to be fairly constant, approximately 1.5 residues per 1000 amino acids. Consequently, assay of desmosine and isodesmosine can provide a quantitative measure of the elastin content in tissues.[12]

GENE STRUCTURE Cloning of cDNAs corresponding to the human elastin messenger RNA (mRNA), approximately 3.5 kb in size, has allowed elucidation of the entire primary sequence of tropoelastin[8] (Fig. 15-5). The deduced amino acid sequence depicts alternating segments of cross-link domains, characterized by the presence of lysyl residues separated by two or three alanine residues, and hydrophobic domains. The cross-link domains and the hydrophobic regions are encoded by separate exons[13] (Fig. 15-5). The human elastin gene consists of 34 separate exons spanning a total of 45 kb of genomic DNA[13] (Fig. 15-5). The elastin gene has been mapped to the long arm of chromosome 7 (Fig. 15-6).[14]

CONSTITUTIVE AND ALTERNATIVE SPLICING The information stored in the DNA sequence of the elastin gene is transcribed in the nucleus of the cells to a large mRNA precursor, which undergoes several

FIGURE 15-3

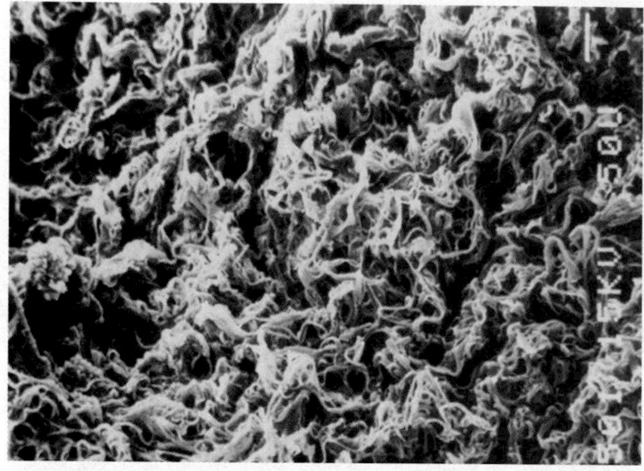

A.

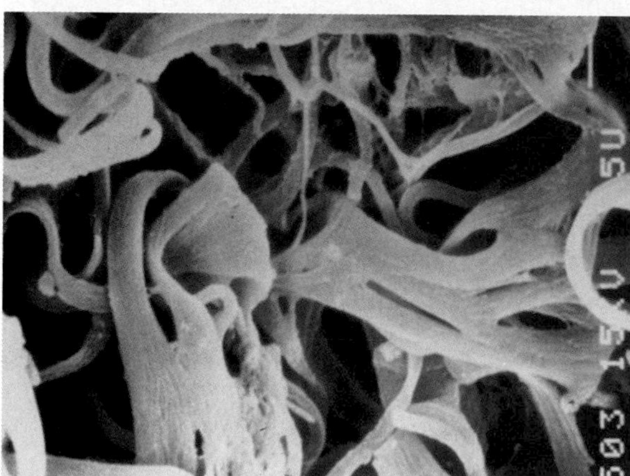

B.

Scanning electron microscopy of the elastic fibers in human skin. Original magnifications: *A.* ×2000; *B.* ×5000.

posttranscriptional modifications, including splicing and polyadenylation. The processed molecules are then transported to the cytoplasm, where the functional mRNAs serve as templates for the synthesis of elastin polypeptides during translation. Several lines of evidence suggest that the rate of elastin biosynthesis is largely regulated by the abundance of the functional mRNA.

An early observation during the isolation of human elastin cDNAs was that several overlapping clones were identical, with the exception of short sequences that were absent in some clones but present in others.[7,8,15] Comparison of these sequences in the cDNAs with the corresponding genomic DNA segments indicated that the differences were due to alternative splicing of certain exons during posttranscriptional processing of the elastin pre-mRNA. In fact, as many as six exons in the human gene are reported to be subject to alternative splicing, and several of the variant mRNAs are translated into protein. This mechanism can provide significant variation in the amino acid composition of individual elastin polypeptides and presumably in the function of the elastic fibers in tissues. However, the developmental significance and tissue specificity of alternative splicing has not been elucidated in detail.

REGULATION OF ELASTIN GENE EXPRESSION Expression of genes at the transcriptional level is regulated by the activity of the

FIGURE 15-4

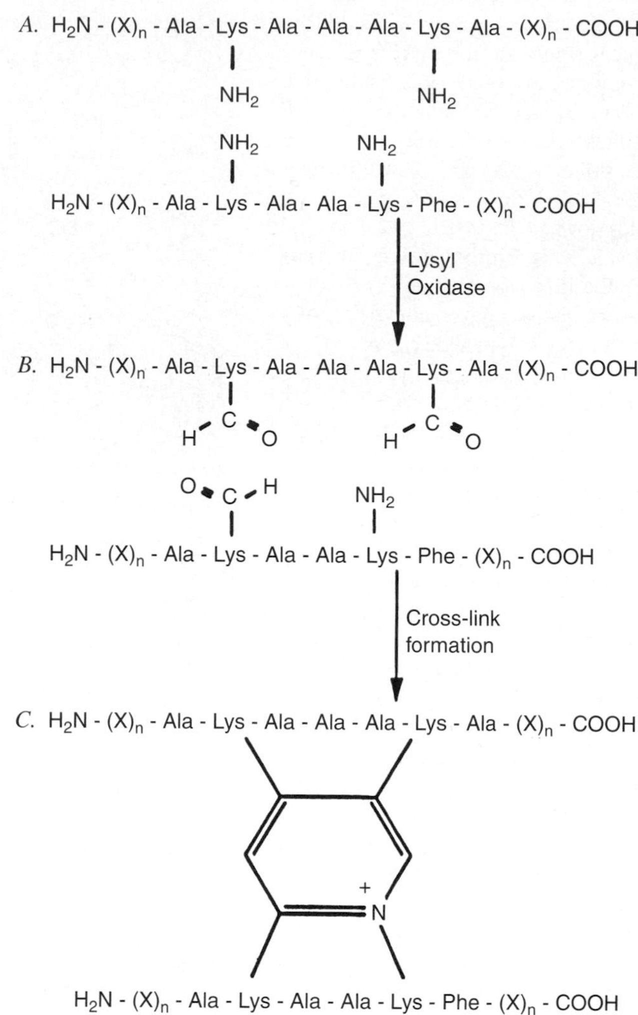

Formation of intermolecular cross-links, desmosine and isodesmosine, between two tropoelastin polypeptides. *A.* Amino acid sequences of a potential cross-link region within the tropoelastin polypeptides. Note the ε-amino group (NH_2) of the four contributing lysyl residues. *B.* Three of the lysyl residues undergo oxidative deamination catalyzed by lysyl oxidase to yield corresponding aldehyde derivatives, allysines. *C.* Three of the allysines and the fourth unmodified lysyl residue, still containing an ε-amino group, fuse into a stable desmosine cross-link. (*From Uitto et al.,*[74] *with permission.*)

promoter region upstream from the 5′ end of the coding region. The elastin promoter contains a remarkable constellation of potential binding sites for transcriptional regulatory factors indicative of complex transcriptional regulation. These include multiple Sp1 and AP2 binding sites, putative glucocorticoid-responsive elements, and TPA- and cAMP-responsive elements (CRE). The absence of a TATA box in the promoter region suggests that there may be multiple sites of transcriptional initiation, and various molecular tests, including S1 protection and primer extension analyses, confirm this fact.[13] Functional analyses of the human elastin promoter segment have been carried out by constructing a panel of promoter-reporter gene [chloramphenicol acetyl transferase (CAT)] constructs.[16] These constructs have been used in transient transfections with a variety of cultured cells, including human skin fibroblasts. These studies indicate that the core promoter necessary for basal expression of the gene is contained within the region −128 to −1 (in reference to translation initiation site −1, +1), and the upstream sequences contain several up- and down-regulatory elements. The positive regulatory and core promoter activities may be explained, at least in part, by the presence of multiple Sp1 and AP2 binding sites within these regions, which may act as general enhancer elements; DNAase footprinting experiments indicate that Sp1 and AP2 sites indeed interact with their respective *trans*-acting factors. This is supported by the observation that deletion of the segment −134 to −87, containing three putative Sp-1 binding sites, reduced the activity to less than 20 percent of the reference construct −475 to −1. Development of transgenic mice expressing the human elastin promoter has revealed that 5.2 kb of DNA flanking the human elastin gene contains the elements necessary for tissue-specific expression.[17] In addition to the 5′ upstream sequences, the first introns of both the bovine and human elastin genes contain regions of extremely strong sequence homology. Because it has been demonstrated that the first intron of three different collagen genes contains segments that act as enhancer elements of the promoter activity,[18] the strong conservation within intron 1 of the elastin gene suggests the possible presence of an enhancer in this gene as well. However, functional testing of the homologous segments has thus far not provided conclusive support for this possibility.

FIGURE 15-5

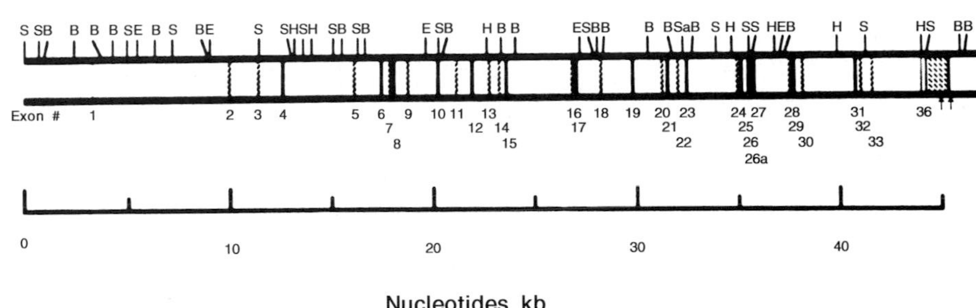

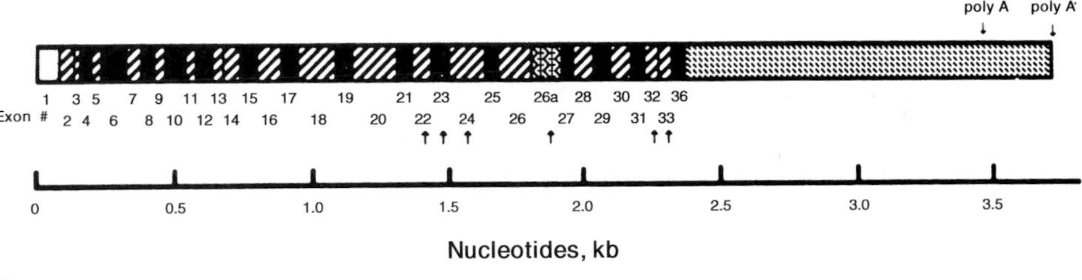

Representation of the human elastin gene (*A*) and the corresponding cDNA (*B*). *A*. The exons have been numbered starting from the 5′ end of the gene and correspond to those shown in the cDNA (see *B*). The presence of restriction endonuclease cleavage sites: *BamHI* (B), *EcoRI* (E), *HindIII* (H); kb = kilobases. *B*. The cDNA, about 3.5 kb in size, is divided into separate exons that are numbered from 1 to 36 and drawn to scale. Note that the human elastin gene contains only 34 exons. However, to maintain a consistent numbering system between the bovine and human elastin genes, the last exon is designated as number 36; thus, the human gene is missing the counterparts of bovine exons 34 and 35. The arrows indicate the exons that have been shown to be subject to alternative splicing. (*From Uitto et al.,*[74] *with permission.*)

CYTOKINE AND HORMONAL REGULATION The presence of multiple *cis*-acting elements in the elastin promoter region suggests that elastin gene expression is subject to modulation at the transcriptional level by *trans*-acting factors. For example, previous studies have indicated that tumor necrosis factor (TNF)-α decreases elastin mRNA abundance primarily by suppressing promoter activity.[19] In other studies, transforming growth factor (TGF)-β has been shown to upregulate the abundance of human elastin mRNA by up to about 30-fold,[20] but evidence from transient transfection assays suggests that this upregulation is, at least in part, posttranscriptional.[20] In fact, assay of elastin mRNA half-life suggests that TGF-β stabilizes the elastin mRNA, leading to elevated steady-state levels. At the same time, subcutaneous injection of TGF-β in transgenic mice expressing the human elastin promoter enhanced the promoter activity in a time-dependent manner up to 10-fold.[21] The latter results suggested that the 5.2-kb upstream segment of the human elastin gene contains *cis*-elements responsive to TGF-β. Regardless of the mechanism, however, these observations collectively suggest that mediators released from inflammatory cells can modulate elastin gene expression, and such modulation may play a role in diseases characterized by altered accumulation of elastic fibers in tissues.

Vitamin D_3 also modulates elastin gene expression. Specifically, incubation of fibroblasts with vitamin D_3 results in an 80 to 90 percent decrease in total accumulation of tropoelastin accompanied by a parallel decrease in steady-state levels of the corresponding mRNA.[22] At the same time, insulin-like growth factor (IGF)-1 enhances elastin gene expression at the transcriptional level.[23] Although there is preliminary evidence for modulation of elastin gene expression by selective growth factors and hormone-like substances, the precise details are largely unknown.

ELASTIN BIOSYNTHESIS Elastin biosynthesis involves several specific steps necessary for the assembly of elastic fibers (Table 15-2). Several studies show that smooth muscle cells in culture synthesize relatively large quantities of elastin, suggesting that they may be the major source of elastin in tissues rich in elastic fibers, such as vascular connective tissue.[24] In addition to smooth muscle cells, human dermal fibroblasts in culture also express the elastin gene, and elastin production by cultured fibroblasts has been demonstrated by immunoblotting using anti-elastin antibodies and by molecular hybridization of mRNA with elastin-specific DNA probes.[15,25] The amount of elastin synthesized by cultured human skin fibroblasts is relatively small; nonetheless, fibroblasts may be the primary source of elastin in the dermis. Elastin gene expression has also been suggested to occur in cultured epidermal keratinocytes, although the level of expression in keratinocytes is extremely low in comparison to dermal fibroblasts.[26] The biologic significance of elastin gene expression in keratinocytes is unclear.

After the completion of translation, newly synthesized polypeptides are translocated into the cisternae of the rough endoplasmic reticulum, in a manner similar to that occurring during the biosynthesis of collagen

FIGURE 15-6

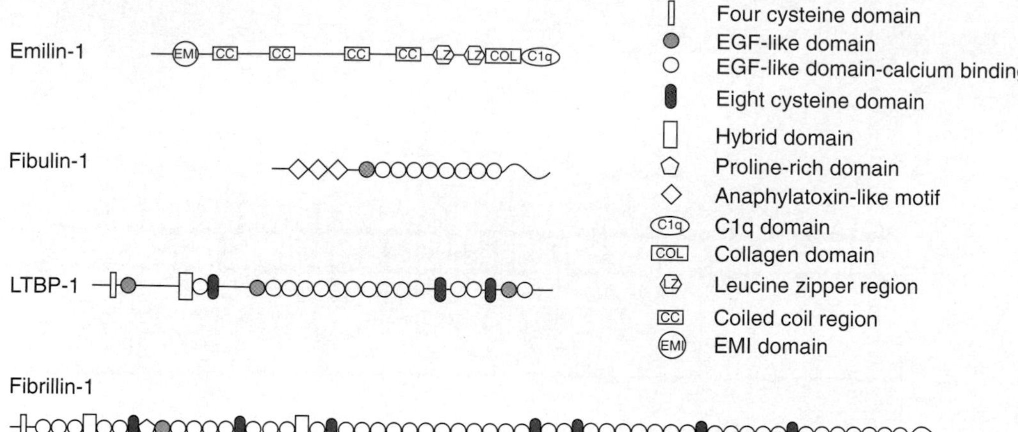

Modular domain structures of selected elastin associated microfibrillar proteins, including fibrillin (FBN), latent TGF-β–binding protein (LTBP), fibulin (FBLN), and emilin. The first member of each gene family is represented. The FBN, LTBP, and FBLN families are related because they share common protein motifs. (Adapted from references 3, 59, and 68).

and other proteins destined for export from the cell. The polypeptides are then transferred from the rough endoplasmic reticulum into the extracellular space by transport mechanisms whose functioning in the case of elastin is not completely understood. It has been demonstrated, however, that incubation of cells synthesizing elastin with colchicine decreases the rate of elastin secretion and that the polypeptides accumulate intracellularly.[27,28] This observation suggests that the secretion of elastin polypeptides is a process that involves the microtubules of the cells, and that the molecules may be transferred out of the cells packaged in Golgi vacuoles or related vesicles.

An interesting feature of elastin is the presence of 4-hydroxyproline. However, the relative hydroxyproline concentration in various elastin preparations is considerably lower than in collagen. Amino acid analyses of elastin isolated from various sources indicate that the hydroxyproline content of the protein can vary from 7 to 25 residues per 1000 amino acids, and that hydroxyproline accounts for about 10 to 20 percent of the total imino acid (proline plus hydroxyproline) content of the molecule.[27,29] Previous studies clearly demonstrated that hydroxyproline plays an important functional role in the synthesis and secretion of collagen. In contrast, the presence of hydroxyproline is not required for the synthesis and secretion of elastin. This conclusion is based on studies in which cells synthesizing both elastin and procollagen are incubated with α,α'-dipyridyl, an inhibitor of prolyl hydroxylase, which prevents the formation of hydroxyproline. Under such conditions, the cells continue to synthesize and secrete tropoelastin at the normal rate, whereas no intact triple-helical procollagen is recovered in the medium.[27,29] The hydroxyproline found in elastin, therefore, appears to be a coincidental feature of the molecule in terms of synthesis and secretion of this protein. It has been suggested that, in fact, hydroxyproline may be present in elastin serendipitously, as the elastin polypeptides are synthesized in the same region of the rough endoplasmic reticulum as is procollagen.[27] Thus, prolyl hydroxylase, which is

TABLE 15-2

Steps at Various Levels of Biosynthesis and Degradation of Elastin and the Functional Significance of These Steps*

Step	Functional Significance
1. Expression of the gene encoding for elastin polypeptides	
a. Transcription	Formation of mRNA precursor
b. Constitutive and alternative splicing of the mRNA precursor	Formation of functional mRNAs
c. Translation	Synthesis of polypeptides
d. Control of the rate of transcription and translation	Determines the quantity of polypeptide synthesis
2. Intracellular cotranslational and posttranslational modifications	
a. Removal of the signal sequence*	Necessary for secretion
b. Formation of 4-hydroxyproline	Unknown
c. Intracellular degradation of some of the polypeptides*	Removal of defective polypeptides and modulation of elastin production
3. Secretion	Transport through Golgi apparatus to the extracellular space
4. Extracellular posttranslational modifications	
a. Oxidative deamination of some lysyl residues by lysyl oxidase	Necessary for cross-link formation
5. Fiber formation	
a. Assembly with the microfibrillar proteins	Formation of elastic fibers
b. Formation of covalent cross-links	Stabilization of the fibers
c. Interactions with other extracellular macromolecules and cells	Determines the physical properties of tissues
6. Extracellular degradation	
a. Cleavage by specific elastases and other proteolytic enzymes	Turnover of the extracellular fibers

*These are the major steps in the sequences in which they are likely to occur in vivo.
The steps marked by an asterisk have not been explored in detail in the case of elastin, but by analogy with other proteins, they are likely to occur.

located in this cellular compartment, hydroxylates some of the prolyl residues occurring in Pro-Gly sequences of the elastin polypeptides. Because the activity of prolyl hydroxylase in the cells can be variable, depending on several factors, including the concentration of cofactors and cosubstrates, this suggestion explains the variability in the hydroxyproline content encountered in elastin isolated from different tissues.

As discussed elsewhere (see Chap. 14), during the intracellular biosynthesis of procollagen, in addition to hydroxylation of prolyl residues, several other posttranslational modifications occur; these include hydroxylation of certain lysyl residues, subsequent glycosylation of certain hydroxylysyl residues, and glycosylation of the precursor-specific extension peptides using the lipid-carrier mechanism. In the case of elastin, none of these modifications has been demonstrated. In particular, amino acid analyses have failed to disclose the presence of hydroxylysine,[6] and earlier chemical analyses have not detected any carbohydrates in elastin.[30]

FIBRILLOGENESIS AND CROSS-LINKING The formation of desmosines occurs in the extracellular space, where the first step is the oxidative deamination of lysyl residues to corresponding aldehydes, known as allysines. This conversion is catalyzed by a copper-requiring enzyme, lysyl oxidase.[31] The desmosines are formed by the fusion of three allysines and a fourth unmodified lysyl residue in two adjacent tropoelastin chains. Thus, the desmosines link the individual elastin polypeptides into an insoluble network (see Fig. 15-4).

The oxidative deamination of lysyl residues in elastin is catalyzed by lysyl oxidase, an enzyme that requires copper and molecular oxygen as cofactors. It has been shown that in copper-deficient animals the production of functional enzyme is reduced and that the newly synthesized elastic fibers are not stabilized by the formation of desmosines.[32] Consequently, the individual tropoelastin polypeptides remain soluble and the elastin-rich tissues are fragile. Because lysyl oxidase is synthesized and secreted by human skin fibroblasts in culture,[33] these cells are presumably one source of the enzyme in vivo.

Lysyl oxidase contains at least three possible copper-binding domains.[31] The human lysyl oxidase (LOX) gene was originally mapped to chromosomal locus 5q23.[34] This enzyme is also identical to a tumor suppressor gene, rrg, whose expression is reduced in transformed cells.[35] Therefore, lysyl oxidase may have a broader spectrum of biologic activity than previously anticipated. More recently, additional genes have been identified encoding proteins with homology to lysyl oxidase.[36] These lysyl oxidase-like (LOXL) genes have been mapped to different chromosomal regions, and the total number of lysyl oxidase genes is currently five (LOX and LOXL1 to 4). Although the enzymatic activity of the LOXL gene products has not been demonstrated, lysyl oxidases seem to form a family of multifunctional amine oxidases.[36]

DEGRADATION AND REMODELING Although the metabolic turnover of elastin is very slow when compared to proteins in general, a portion of the body's elastin is continuously degraded and may partly be replaced by newly synthesized fibers.[37] In addition, degradation of elastin is markedly increased in a variety of pathologic conditions.[38] Thus, the tissues containing elastin must contain proteolytic enzymes that are capable of degrading elastic fibers.

Evidence for elastase, a specific elastolytic enzyme, was first obtained from study of the pancreas, and, subsequently, elastolytic enzymes have been detected in several other tissues, as well as in a variety of cell types, including polymorphonuclear leukocytes, monocyte/macrophages, and platelets.[39,40]

The classic elastases are serine proteases that degrade insoluble elastic fibers at neutral or slightly alkaline pH. The activity of these enzymes is inhibited by serum factors, such as α_1-antitrypsin and α_2-macroglobulin. Assay of the amino-terminal amino acids of elastin degradation products demonstrates that these enzymes preferentially cleave the polypeptide at bonds involving glycine, alanine, and valine. However, elastases from different sources (pancreas versus polymorphonuclear leukocytes) have different cleavage specificities, as shown by peptide mapping of degradation products.[41]

In addition to the classic elastases, which are serine proteases, others were recently shown to be metalloenzymes requiring calcium for their activity. One such enzyme is secreted by macrophages isolated from human alveolar macrophages exudates.[42] This metalloenzyme is different from leukocyte or pancreatic elastases (see Chap. 17).

Elastin-like small molecular weight synthetic substrates, such as succinyl-L-(alanyl)$_3$-paranitroanilide (SAPNA), are often used to detect elastase activity. A convenient feature of these substrates is their degradation even in the presence of inhibitors, such as α_2-macroglobulin, which interfere only with the degradation of large protein substrates by the elastases. By using SAPNA as substrate, an elastase-like enzyme activity has been detected in human serum.[43] This enzyme is clearly inhibited by metal chelators, such as ethylenediaminetetraacetic acid (EDTA), but not by serine protease inhibitors, suggesting that its activity depends on calcium or another divalent cation. Values elevated up to 100-fold over normal have been demonstrated in the serum of a patient with autosomal recessive cutis laxa with histologically demonstrable fragmentation of elastic fibers in the skin.[43]

Of particular dermatologic interest is the demonstration of elastase activity in the blister fluid from lesions of dermatitis herpetiformis and bullous pemphigoid.[44,45] The elastase activity in the lesions of dermatitis herpetiformis is due to a serine protease and probably originates from polymorphonuclear leukocytes abundantly present in the lesions. The activity in the bullous pemphigoid lesions is caused by a metalloenzyme of unknown cellular origin. Regardless of the origin of the elastase activity, these enzymes could play a role in the development of the blisters by degrading the elastic fibers and other structures in the dermal–epidermal junction.

The Microfibrillar Proteins

Microfibrils consist of apparently tubular structures about 10 to 12 nm in diameter. Their staining properties and susceptibilities to enzymatic digestion differ from those of the amorphous elastin. At high resolution, the microfibrils appear in cross-section as an outer electron-dense shell surrounding an inner lucid core and in longitudinal section as a beaded chain, suggesting that they may be composed of more than one protein. Apparently similar microfibrils are present in many tissues, including those containing abundant elastin and those in which there is no visible or immunoreactive elastin, such as the ocular ciliary zonule and the periodontal ligament. In the dermis, the microfibrillary bundles that connect the deep dermal elastic plexus with the dermal–epidermal junction region consist of microfibrils indistinguishable from those associated with elastic fibers. In their superficial distribution, no immunoreactive elastin is associated with them; but as they traverse the dermis, they are associated with an increasing amount of amorphous elastin.

Because of their insolubility and apparent complexity, chemical characterization of the microfibrils progressed slowly until recently. The problem of identifying these structurally important components was compounded by the observation that small amounts of several proteins, including amyloid P and decay-accelerating factor, have been localized to the elastic microfibrils by immunoelectron microscopy. While they may have some functional role, it is unlikely that any one of the latter is a major structural component of the microfibrils. Progress, however, has been made in the identification of a number of proteins as structural components of the elastic microfibrils.

These structural proteins can be divided into several groups based upon their molecular characteristics. Table 15-3 lists these proteins and provides some distinguishing features, including their human

TABLE 15-3

Microfibrillar Component Proteins

MICROFIBRILLAR PROTEIN	CHARACTERISTIC FEATURES	HUMAN CHROMOSOMAL LOCUS
Fibrillins	350 kDa	
FBN1	Contain EGF and TGF-β–binding protein motifs	15q15–q21
FBN2		5q23–q31
Latent TGF-β binding proteins (LTBPs)	125 to 310 kDa	
LTBP 1	Contain EGF and TGF-β–binding protein motifs	2p22–24
LTBP2	Secreted as a complex with latent TGF-β but also found as a free protein	14q22–q33
LTBP3		11q12
LTBP4		19q13.1–13.2
Fibulins	60 to 240 kDa	
FBLN1	Contain EGF and anaphylatoxin motifs	22q13.3
FBLN2		3p24–p25
FBLN3		2p16
FBLN4		11q13
FBLN5	Mutations in cutis laxa	14q32.1
Microfibril-associated glycoproteins (MAGPs)		
MAGP1 (MFAP2)	31 kDa; widely distributed in microfibrils	1p36.1–p35
MAGP2 (MP25)	25 kDa	12p12.3–p13.1
Microfibril-associated proteins		
MFAP1	Very acidic	15q15–q21
MFAP2		1p36.1–p35
MFAP3		5q32–q33.2
MFAP4	Frequently deleted in Smith-Magenis syndrome	17p11.2
βig-h3		5q31
Lysyl oxidase	Probably not a structural component	5q23–q31
Emilin-1 (gp115)		2p23
Emilin-2		18p11.3

chromosomal localizations. These groups include several gene families that share protein domain motifs and are discussed below.

FIBRILLINS The largest of the microfibrillar proteins and, quantitatively, perhaps the most important ones, are the fibrillins, 350-kDa glycoproteins that form an integral part of the microfibril structure.[46,47] Electron microscopic images of human monomeric fibrillin synthesized by fibroblasts in culture show an extended flexible molecule approximately 148 nm long and 2.2 nm wide. Multiple fibrillin molecules align in a parallel head-to-tail fashion to form microfibrils. Molecular cloning studies have so far identified two distinct homologous human genes encoding fibrillins: fibrillin-1 (FBN1) located on chromosome 15q15-21 and fibrillin-2 (FBN2) on chromosome 5q23-q31.[48,49] Analysis of the fibrillin amino acid sequences, deduced from cloned cDNAs, showed that these proteins contain multiple repeats of a sequence motif previously observed in epidermal growth factor precursor molecule, each motif having six conserved cysteines.[47] Many of these repeats contain consensus sequences that have been associated with calcium binding. A second motif containing eight cysteines, originally found in latent TGF-β–binding proteins (LTBPs)[50] has also been identified in the fibrillins (see Fig. 15-6 for comparison of structures of the FBNs and LTBPs). Of interest is the report of a protein in jellyfish having extensive homology to mammalian fibrillin, thus identifying fibrillin as a very ancient protein that evolved well before elastin.[51]

LATENT TGF-β–BINDING PROTEINS Several members of the LTBP family have been cloned and shown to contain repeating domains similar to those found in FBN1 and FBN2 (Fig. 15-6). TGF-β is always secreted as a latent complex, and in some cases, this complex is bound to a LTBP.[50,52] To date, four distinct LTBPs (LTBP1 to 4) have been cloned and characterized, ranging in size from 125 to 310 kDa.[53] The function of LTBPs remains to be determined, but it is clear that they are not necessary to maintain TGF-β in an inactive form and they do not appear to bind mature TGF-β. Although LTBPs may facilitate the secretion of TGF-β or binding of the inactive complex to the cell surface where activation takes place, they are also found as free proteins associated with components of the extracellular matrix. Recent development of an LTBP3 knockout mouse has revealed craniofacial malformations, perturbed ossification, and development of osteosclerosis and osteoarthritis.[54] These observations were interpreted to mean that LTBP3 is important for the control of TGF-β action and, specifically, that LTBPs may modulate TGF-β bioavailability.

Immunohistologic studies have localized both LTBP1 and LTBP2 to microfibrils in elastic fibers, strongly suggesting that one or more of the LTBPs may be a component of these fibrils.[55,56] Furthermore, levels of LTBP1 are altered in a number of pathologic conditions, including solar elastosis and actinic keratosis.[57]

FIBULINS The fibulins (FBLNs) are a family of extracellular matrix glycoproteins that contain tandem epidermal growth factor (EGF)-like repeats similar to fibrillins and LTBPs.[58,59] Molecular cloning has identified as many as five distinct fibulin genes[58–62] (Table 15-3). The deduced amino acid sequences reveal that the molecules are modular, having the EGF-like repeats and a common carboxyl terminal globular domain (Fig. 15-6). FBLN1 and FBLN2 contain an anaphylatoxin-like domain (Fig. 15-6). FBLN1 is alternatively spliced and four variants have been identified differing from one another at their carboxyl termini. Fibulin proteins are widely distributed in connective tissues, including the skin, and enriched in developing elastin-containing tissues. Fibulins

TABLE 15-4

Clinical Features, Histopathology, Inheritance, Associated Biochemical Findings, and Predisposing Clinical Conditions in Cutaneous Diseases with Elastic Fiber Abnormalities*

Disease	Inheritance†	Clinical Manifestations	Histopathology of Skin	Biochemical Findings‡ Related to Elastic Fibers and Predisposing Clinical Conditions
Pseudoxanthoma elasticum	AR, sporadic§	Yellowish papules coalescing into plaques Inelastic skin Cardiovascular and ocular abnormalities	Accumulation of pleiomorphic and calcified elastic fibers in the mid-dermis	Deposition of calcium apatite crystals, excessive accumulation of glycosaminoglycans on elastic fibers; D-penicillamine treatment; mutations in the *ABCC6* gene
Buschke-Ollendorf syndrome	AD	Dermatofibrosis lenticularis disseminata and osteopoikilosis	Accumulation of interlacing elastic fibers in the dermis	Increased desmosine content in the skin
Cutis laxa	AR, AD, or NH	Loose, sagging, inelastic skin Pulmonary emphysema Tortuosity of aorta Urinary and gastrointestinal tract diverticuli	Fragmentation and loss of elastic fibers	Decreased desmosine content and reduced elastin mRNA levels; increased elastase activity in some cases; D-Penicillamine treatment, inflammatory and urticarial skin lesions (e.g., drug reaction); mutations in the *ELN* or *FBLN5* gene in limited cases
DeBarsy syndrome	AR	Cutis laxa-like skin changes Mental retardation Dwarfism	Rudimentary, fragmented elastic fibers	Reduced elastin mRNA levels
Wrinkly skin syndrome	AR	Decreased elastic recoil of the skin Increased number of palmar and plantar creases	Decreased number and length of elastic fibers	
Mid-dermal elastolysis	NH	Fine wrinkling of the skin, primarily in exposed areas	Fragmentation and loss of elastin in the mid-dermis	Inflammatory; sun exposure
Anetoderma	NH	Localized areas of atrophic, saclike lesions	Loss and fragmentation of elastic fibers in the dermis	Reduced desmosine content in the lesions; often secondary to inflammatory lesions
Elastosis perforans serpiginosa	NH	Hyperkeratotic papules, commonly on the face and neck	Accumulation and transepidermal elimination of elastic fibers	D-Penicillamine–induced abnormalities in elastin cross-linking
Elastoderma	Unknown	Loose and sagging skin with loss of recoil	Accumulation of pleiomorphic elastotic material without calcification in the mid- and lower dermis and the subcutaneous tissue	
Isolated elastomas	NH	Dermal papules or nodules	Accumulation of thick elastic fibers in the dermis	
Elastofibroma dorsi	NH	Deep subcutaneous tumor, usually on subscapular area	Accumulation of globular elastic structures encased in collagenous meshwork	Trauma on the lesional area
Actinic elastosis	NH	Thickening and furrowing of the skin	Accumulation of irregularly thickened elastic fibers in upper dermis	Chronic sun exposure
Marfan's syndrome	AD	Skeletal, ocular, and cardiovascular abnormalities, hyperextensible skin; striae distensae	Fragmentation of the elastic structures in the aorta	Mutations in the FBN1 gene

(continued)

TABLE 15-4 (*Continued*)

Clinical Features, Histopathology, Inheritance, Associated Biochemical Findings, and Predisposing Clinical Conditions in Cutaneous Diseases with Elastic Fiber Abnormalities*

Disease	Inheritance†	Clinical Manifestations	Histopathology of Skin	Biochemical Findings‡ Related Elastic Fibers to Predisposing and Clinical Conditions
Congenital contractural arachnodactyly	AD	Camptodactyly and joint contractures		Mutations in the *FBN2* gene
Williams syndrome	AD	Supravalvular aortic stenosis; velvety skin; dysmorphic facies	Disruption of smooth muscle and matrix relationship affecting blood vessels	Allelic deletion of the *ELN* gene; contiguous gene deletion syndrome

*Most of these conditions represent a group of diseases with clinical, genetic, and biochemical heterogeneity.
†AD, autosomal dominant; AR, autosomal recessive; NH, not a heritable disease.
‡The biochemical abnormalities have been demonstrated in only a limited number of patients in each group, and it is not known whether the biochemical changes are the same in each patient with any given disease.
§Rare cases with a distinct acquired form of pseudoxanthoma elasticum have been described.

1, 2, and 5 are located within the elastic fibers but in somewhat different distribution. Specifically, FBLN1 was found to reside within the elastin core in the skin,[63] while FBLN2 is located at the interface between the fibrillin-1 microfibrils and the elastic core.[64] FBLN5 binds both smooth muscle cells and elastin, thus facilitating the cell-matrix interactions. Particularly interesting is the clinical phenotype of FBLN-5 knockout mice, which show progressive laxity of skin associated with vascular abnormalities and emphysematous lung changes;[61,62] these changes are reminiscent of those noted in patients with congenital cutis laxa.[38] In fact, mutations in the FBLN5 gene have been recently documented in some cases with cutis laxa.[65]

OTHER MICROFIBRILLAR PROTEINS A number of other proteins, unrelated to the FBNs, LTBPs, and FBLNs, are constituents of the microfibrils. When bovine nuchal ligament, a tissue rich in microfibrils, was extracted with saline under reducing conditions, five major bands having apparent molecular weights of 340, 78, 70, 31, and 25 kDa were identified upon gel electrophoresis.[56] Molecular cloning of the 25- and 31-kDa components, designated microfibril-associated glycoproteins (MAGPs), shows that these two proteins share limited regions of homology.[66,67] The observation that these proteins can be extracted from tissues by solvents containing a strong reducing agent suggests that intermolecular disulfide bonding is an important feature of the association of the polypeptide chains in the fibrils.

Other candidate microfibril components include the lysyl oxidases,[31] interface proteins called *emilins*,[68] and several proteins designated microfibril-associated proteins (MFAPs) (see Table 15-3).[69–71] Among the latter, MFAP1 is remarkable in that it is extremely acidic, with glutamic acid comprising 23 percent and aspartic acid 6 percent of the residues. The extremely acidic nature of the protein suggests that it may have an important function in the assembly of the very basic tropoelastin molecules.

Despite characterization and cloning of several microfibrillar proteins, a number of questions regarding microfibril structure and function remain unresolved. A completely satisfactory molecular model of the microfibrils has yet to be developed, and the precise relationships between the fibrillins and other proposed components of the microfibrils remain obscure. Moreover, while apparently identical microfibrils have been identified ultrastructurally both with and without associated elastin, it has yet to be determined whether structural or compositional differences exist between these two groups or among microfibrils in different tissues.

PATHOLOGY OF THE ELASTIC FIBERS IN CUTANEOUS DISEASES

Several heritable and acquired connective tissue diseases have been shown to affect the elastic fibers, including pseudoxanthoma elasticum (PXE), cutis laxa, and Buschke-Ollendorf syndrome (Table 15-4). In addition, clinically distinct entities with phenotypes closely resembling PXE (e.g., elastoderma) or cutis laxa (e.g., wrinkly skin syndrome) can be recognized. The clinical, genetic and molecular features of these disorders are detailed in recent reviews.[38,72–74]

REFERENCES

1. Kielty C et al: Elastic fibers. *J Cell Sci* **115**:2817, 2002
2. Midwood KS, Schwarzbauer JE: Elastic fibers: Building bridges between cells and their matrix. *Curr Biol* **12**:R279, 2002
3. Rosenbloom J, Abrams WR: Elastin and the microfibrillar apparatus, in *Connective Tissue and Its Heritable Disorders*, 2nd ed, edited by RM Royce, B Steinmann. New York, Wiley-Liss, 2002, pp 249–269
4. Uitto J et al: Elastic fibers in human skin: Quantitation of elastic fibers by computerized digital image analyses and determination of elastin by radioimmunoassay of desmosine. *Lab Invest* **49**:499, 1983
5. Ross R et al: The morphogenesis of elastic fibers. *Adv Exp Biol Med* **79**:7, 1977
6. Sandberg LB, Davidson JM: Elastin and its gene. *Pept Prot Rev* **3**:169, 1984
7. Indik Z et al: Alternative splicing of human elastin mRNA demonstrated by sequence analysis of cloned genomic and complementary DNA. *Proc Natl Acad Sci U S A* **84**:5680, 1987
8. Fazio MJ et al: Cloning of full-length elastin cDNAs from a human skin fibroblast recombinant cDNA library: Further elucidation of alternative splicing utilizing exon-specific oligonucleotides. *J Invest Dermatol* **91**:458, 1988
9. Gray WR et al: Molecular model for elastin structure and function. *Nature* **246**:461, 1973
10. Hoeve CAJ: The elasticity in the presence of diluents. *Adv Exp Med Biol* **79**:607, 1977
11. Akagawa M, Suyama K: Mechanism of formation of elastin crosslinks. *Connect Tissue Res* **41**:131, 2000
12. Starcher BC: Determination of the elastin content of tissues by measuring desmosine and isodesmosine. *Anal Biochem* **79**:11, 1977
13. Bashir M et al: Characterization of the complete human elastin gene. *J Biol Chem* **264**:8887, 1989
14. Fazio MJ et al: Human elastin gene: New evidence for localization to the long arm of chromosome 7. *Am J Hum Genet* **48**:696, 1991

15. Fazio MJ et al: Isolation and characterization of human elastin cDNAs, and age-associated variation in elastin gene expression in cultured skin fibroblasts. *Lab Invest* **58**:270, 1988
16. Kähäri V-M et al: Deletion analyses of 5′-flanking region of the human elastin gene. *J Biol Chem* **265**:9485, 1990
17. Hsu-Wong S et al: Tissue-specific and developmentally regulated expression of human elastin promoter activity in transgenic mice. *J Biol Chem* **269**:18072, 1994
18. Hormuzdi SG et al: A gene-targeting approach identifies a function for the first intron in expression of the α1(I) collagen gene. *Mol Cell Biol* **18**:3368, 1998
19. Kähäri V-M et al: Tumor necrosis factor-α down-regulates human elastin gene expression. *J Biol Chem* **267**:26134, 1992
20. Kähäri V-M et al: Transforming growth factor-β upregulates elastin gene expression in human skin fibroblasts. *Lab Invest* **66**:580, 1992
21. Katchman SD et al: Transforming growth factor-β up-regulates human elastin promoter activity in transgenic mice. *Biochem Biophys Res Commun* **203**:485, 1994
22. Pierce RA et al: 1,25-dihydroxyvitamin D_3 repress tropoelastin expression by a posttranscriptional mechanism. *J Biol Chem* **267**:11593, 1992
23. Wolfe BL et al: Insulin-like growth factor-1 regulates transcription of the elastin gene. *J Biol Chem* **268**:12418, 1993
24. Giro MG et al: Quantitation of elastin production in cultured vascular smooth muscle cells by a sensitive and specific enzyme-linked immunoassay. *Collagen Rel Res* **4**:21, 1984
25. Sephel GC et al: Heterogeneity of elastin expression in cutis laxa fibroblast strains. *J Invest Dermatol* **93**:147, 1989
26. Kajiya H et al: Cultured human keratinocytes express tropoelastin. *J Invest Dermatol* **109**:641, 1997
27. Uitto J et al: Synthesis of elastin and procollagen by cells from embryonic aorta: Differences in the role of hydroxyproline and the effects of proline analogs on the secretion of the two proteins. *Arch Biochem Biophys* **173**:187, 1976
28. Rosenbloom J, Cywinski A: Biosynthesis and secretion of tropoelastin by chick aorta cells. *Biochem Biophys Res Commun* **69**:613, 1976
29. Rosenbloom J, Cywinski A: Inhibition of proline hydroxylation does not inhibit secretion of tropoelastin by chick aorta cells. *FEBS Lett* **65**:246, 1976
30. Grant ME et al: Carbohydrate content of insoluble elastins prepared from adult bovine and calf ligamentum nuchae and tropoelastin isolated from copper deficient porcine aorta. *Biochem J* **121**:197, 1971
31. Smith-Mungo LI, Kagan HM: Lysyl oxidase: properties, regulation and multiple functions in biology. *Matrix Biol* **16**:387, 1998
32. Rucker RB: Isolation of soluble elastin from copper-deficient chick aorta. *Methods Enzymol* **82A**:559, 1982
33. Kuivaniemi H et al: Abnormal copper metabolism and deficient lysyl oxidase activity in a heritable connective tissue disorder. *J Clin Invest* **69**:710, 1983
34. Hämäläinen ER et al: Molecular cloning of human lysyl oxidase and assignment of the gene to chromosome 5q23.3-31.2. *Genomics* **11**:508, 1991
35. Kenyon K et al: Lysyl oxidase and rrg messenger RNA. *Science* **253**:802, 1991
36. Csiszar K: Lysyl oxidases: A novel multifunctional amine oxidase family. *Prog Nucleic Acid Res Mol Biol* **70**:1, 2001
37. Goldstein RA, Starcher BC: Urinary excretion of elastin peptides containing desmosine after intratracheal injection of elastase in hamsters. *J Clin Invest* **61**:1286, 1978
38. Uitto J, Pulkkinen L: Heritable diseases affecting the elastic tissues: Cutis laxa, pseudoxanthoma elasticum and related disorders, in *Emery & Rimoin's Principles and Practice of Medical Genetics*, 4th ed, edited by DL Rimoin, JM Connor, R Pyeritz, BR Korf. New York, Churchill Livingstone, 2002, p 4044
39. Bieth J: Elastases: Structure, function and pathological role. *Front Matrix Biol* **6**:1, 1978
40. Werb Z et al: Proteinases and matrix degradation, in *Textbook of Rheumatology*, 3d ed, edited by WN Kelley, ED Harris Jr, S Ruddy, CB Sledge. Philadelphia, Saunders, 1989, p 300
41. Senior RM et al: Comparison of the elastolytic effects of human leukocyte elastase and porcine pancreatic elastase. *Adv Exp Med Biol* **79**:249, 1977
42. Shapiro SD et al: Elastase of U-937 monocyte-like cells: Cloning and characterization of a unique elastolytic metalloproteinase produced by human alveolar macrophages. *J Biol Chem* **268**:23824, 1993
43. Anderson LL et al: Characterization and partial purification of a neutral protease from the serum of a patient with autosomal recessive pulmonary emphysema and cutis laxa. *J Lab Clin Med* **105**:537, 1985
44. Oikarinen AI et al: Demonstration of collagenase and elastase activities in the blister fluids from bullous skin diseases: Comparison between dermatitis herpetiformis and bullous pemphigoid. *J Invest Dermatol* **81**:261, 1983
45. Oikarinen AI et al: Proteolytic enzymes in blister fluids from patients with dermatitis herpetiformis. *Br J Dermatol* **114**:295, 1986
46. Sakai LY et al: Fibrillin, a new 350-kDa glycoprotein, is a component of extracellular microfibrils. *J Cell Biol* **103**:2499, 1986
47. Handford PA et al: Fibrillin: From domain structure to supramolecular assembly. *Matrix Biol* **19**:457, 2000
48. Lee B et al: Linkage of Marfan syndrome and a phenotypically related disorder to two different fibrillin genes. *Nature* **352**:330, 1991
49. Maslen CL et al. Partial sequence of a candidate gene for the Marfan syndrome. *Nature* **352**:334, 1991
50. Kanzaki T et al: TGF-β_1 binding protein: A component of the large latent complex of TGF-β_1 with multiple repeat sequences. *Cell* **61**:1051, 1990
51. Reber-Muller S et al: An extracellular matrix protein of jellyfish homologous to mammalian fibrillin forms different fibrils depending on the life stage of the animal. *Dev Biol* **169**:662, 1995
52. Bashir MM et al: Analysis of the human gene encoding latent transforming growth factor-β–binding protein-2. *Int J Biochem Cell Biol* **28**:531, 1996
53. Oklu R, Hesketh R: The latent transforming growth factor-beta–binding protein (LTBP) family. *Biochem J* **352**:601, 2000
54. Dabovic B et al: Bone abnormalities in latent TGF-[beta]–binding protein (Ltbp)-3-null mice indicate a role for Ltbp-3 in modulating TGF-[beta] bioavailability. *J Cell Biol* **156**:227, 2002
55. Taipale J et al: Latent transforming growth factor-β_1 associates to fibroblast extracellular matrix via latent TGF-β–binding protein. *J Cell Biol* **124**:171, 1994
56. Gibson MA et al: Bovine latent TGF-β_1–binding protein-1: Molecular cloning, identification of tissue isoforms and immunolocalization to the elastin-associated microfibrils. *Mol Cell Biol* **15**:6932, 1995
57. Karonen T et al: Transforming growth factor beta 1 and its latent form binding protein-1 associate with elastic fibres in human dermis: Accumulation in actinic damage and absence in anetoderma. *Br J Dermatol* **137**:51, 1997
58. Argraves WS: Fibulin is an extracellular matrix and plasma glycoprotein with repeated domain structure. *J Cell Biol* **111**:3155, 1990
59. Pan T-C et al: Structure and expression of fibulin-2, a novel extracellular matrix protein with multiple EGF-like repeats and consensus motifs for calcium binding. *J Cell Biol* **123**:1269, 1993
60. Giltay R et al: Sequence, recombinant expression and tissue localization of two novel extracellular matrix proteins, fibulin-3 and fibulin-4. *Matrix Biol* **18**:469, 1999
61. Nakamura T et al: Fibulin-5/DANCE is essential for elastogenesis in vivo. *Nature* **415**:171, 2002
62. Yanagisawa H et al: Fibulin-5 is an elastin-binding protein essential for elastic fibre development in vivo. *Nature* **415**:168, 2002
63. Roark EF et al: The association of human fibulin-1 with elastic fibers: An immunohistological, ultrastructural, and RNA study. *J Histochem Cytochem* **43**:401, 1995
64. Reinhardt DP et al: Fibrillin-1 and fibulin-2 interact and are colocalized in some tissues. *J Biol Chem* **271**:19489, 1996
65. Loeys B et al: Homozygosity for a missense mutation in fibulin (FBLN5) results in a severe form of cutis laxa. *Human Mol Genet* **11**:2113, 2002
66. Gibson MA et al: Further characterization of proteins associated with elastic fiber microfibrils including the molecular cloning of MAGP-2 (MP25). *J Biol Chem* **271**:1096, 1996
67. Faraco J et al: Characterization of the human gene for microfibril-associated glycoprotein (MFAP2), assignment to chromosome 1p36.1-p35, and linkage to D1S170. *Genomics* **25**:630, 1995
68. Colombatti A et al: The EMILIN protein family. *Matrix Biol* **19**:289, 2000
69. Yeh H et al: Structure of the human gene encoding the associated microfibrillar protein (MFAP1) and localization to chromosome 15q15-q21. *Genomics* **23**:443, 1994
70. Abrams WR et al: Molecular cloning of the microfibrillar protein MFAGP3 and assignment of the gene to human chromosome 5q32-q33.2. *Genomics* **26**:47, 1995
71. Lausen M, et al: Microfibril-associated protein 4 is present in lung washings and binds to the collagen region of lung surfactant protein D. *J Biol Chem* **274**:32234, 1999
72. Milewicz DM et al: Genetic disorders of the elastic fiber system. *Matrix Biol J* **19**:471, 2000
73. Uitto J, Bernstein EF: Molecular mechanisms of cutaneous aging: Connective tissue alterations in the dermis. *J Invest Dermatol Symp Proc* **3**:41, 1998
74. Uitto J et al: Elastic fibers of the connective tissue, in *Biochemistry and Physiology of Skin*, 2d ed, edited by L Goldsmith. New York, Oxford University Press, 1991, p 530

CHAPTER 16

Leena Bruckner-Tuderman

Basement Membranes

Basement membranes underlie epithelial and endothelial cells and separate them from each other or from the adjacent stroma. Another form of basement membrane surrounds smooth muscle or nerve cells. The physiologic functions of basement membranes are diverse. As early as the gastrula stage of development, extracellular macromolecules form scaffolds for cell attachment and migration, and serve as boundaries between cells of different destinies. The resulting compartmentalization is determined and maintained throughout life. As the various organ systems mature, basement membranes continue to serve as substrates and provide support for differentiated cells, maintain tissue architecture during remodeling and repair, and, in some cases, acquire specialized functions, including the ability to serve as selective permeability barriers, e.g., the glomerular basement membrane or the basement membrane of the blood-brain barrier, or acquire strong adhesive properties, like the basement membrane surrounding smooth muscle cells, or that at the dermal-epidermal junction, which provide the tissues resistance against shearing forces.

Ultrastructurally, basement membranes most often appear as trilaminar structures, consisting of a central electron-dense region, known as the *lamina densa,* adjacent on either side to an apparently less-dense area, known as the *lamina lucida* or *lamina rara*. The lamina lucida directly abuts the plasma membranes of the adherent cells. Where basement membranes separate cells from a stromal matrix, the electron-translucent region immediately adjacent to the plasma membrane is defined as the *lamina lucida interna,* whereas the opposite side of the basal lamina is referred to as the *subbasal lamina*. The relative size of each of these regions varies between basement membranes of different tissues, between the basement membranes of the same tissue at different ages, and as a consequence of diseases. For example, the trilaminar glomerular basement membrane in humans varies from 240 to 340 nm in width, whereas the bilaminar basement membrane of the dermal-epidermal junction measures 50 to 90 nm.

Different basement membranes contain both common and unique components. All share a basic network structure to which specific macromolecules have been appended. These molecules are responsible for the specialized structures and functions of different basement membranes. Studies using recombinant proteins and transgenic and knockout mouse technologies have provided a wealth of new information on these aspects (discussed below). Also the recent availability of the complete genomic sequences of humans, *Drosophila melanogaster,* and *Caenorhabditis elegans* makes it possible to compare the genomes and address questions about basement membrane composition and functions with much more confidence than before.[1] Cell adhesion to basement membranes appears ancient and exquisitely conserved. Coelenterates have basement membranes, as do all more complex animals. The basic constituents of these structures are collagen IV, laminin, nidogen/entactin, and proteoglycans of the perlecan type, which all are highly conserved. Comparative analysis demonstrated that the four molecules formed the basis of an early basement membrane that has been preserved in molecular detail. The number of the polypeptide subunits and their individual structures vary between species, but many interesting features, e.g., the organization of collagen IV genes in an antiparallel head-to-head arrangement with a common promoter, can be found in both vertebrates and in Drosophila, suggesting important functional characteristics.

ULTRASTRUCTURE OF THE DERMAL-EPIDERMAL JUNCTION

The dermal-epidermal junction is an example of a highly complex form of basement membrane,[2,3] which underlies the basal cells and extends into the upper layers of the dermis (Fig. 16-1*A*). This basement membrane is continuous along the epidermis and skin appendages, including sweat glands, hair shafts, and sebaceous glands. In the upper regions of the dermis, different basement membranes surround capillaries and nerves, but these are excluded from the present discussion. The dermal-epidermal junction can be divided into three distinct zones. The first zone contains the keratin filament-hemidesmosome complex of the basal cells and extends through the lamina lucida to the lamina densa. The plasma membranes of the basal cells in this region contain numerous electron-dense plates known as hemidesmosomes. The intracellular architecture and organization of the basal cells are maintained by keratin intermediate filaments, 7 to 10 nm in diameter, also known as tonofilaments, that course through the basal cells and insert into the desmosomes and hemidesmosomes. External to the plasma membrane is a 25- to 50-nm–wide lamina lucida that contains anchoring filaments, 2 to 8 nm in diameter, originating in the plasma membrane and inserting into the lamina densa. The anchoring filaments can be seen throughout the lamina lucida but they are concentrated in the regions of the hemidesmosomes. Ultrastructurally, the anchoring filaments appear to secure the epithelial cells to the lamina densa.

The existence of the lamina lucida in vivo has been questioned. When the ultrastructure of the basement membrane is evaluated following high-pressure preservation techniques, the lamina densa appears intimately associated with the epithelial cell surface.[2,4] When the dermal-epidermal junction is similarly prepared, no distinct lamina lucida is seen (Fig. 16-1*B*). This suggests that the lamina lucida may result from shrinkage of the cell surface away from the lamina densa due to dehydration. The appearance of anchoring filaments spanning the lamina lucida may then result from the firm attachment of constituents of the lamina densa at the hemidesmosome that is subsequently pulled from the lamina densa by shrinkage. Other components that are also tightly fixed to the keratinocyte plasma membrane, either at the hemidesmosomes or at other sites along the membrane between the hemidesmosomes, may similarly become displaced into the shrinkage space. This may account for the localization of laminins to both the lamina lucida and the lamina densa, because laminins are bound to the cells by specific integrins

FIGURE 16-1

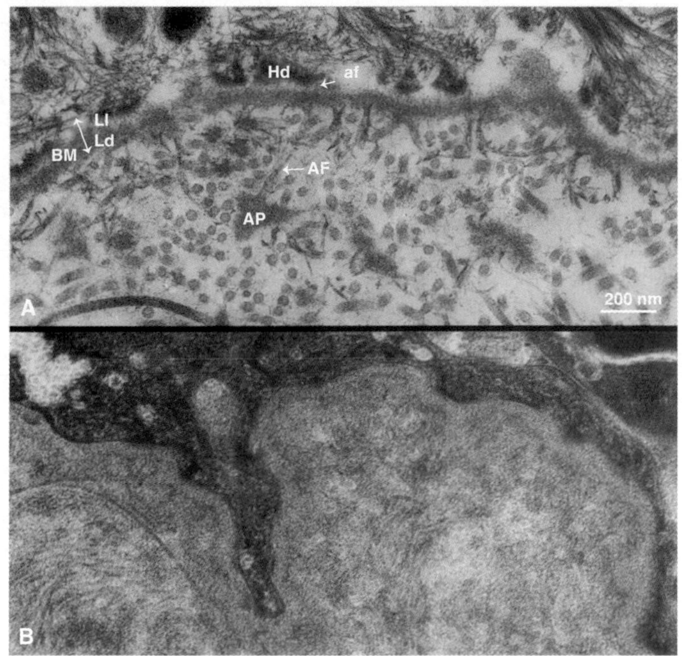

A. Ultrastructure of the human dermal-epidermal junction as visualized by transmission electron microscopy following standard fixation and embedding protocols. af, Anchoring filament; AF, anchoring fibril; AP, anchoring plaque; BM, basement membrane; Hd, hemidesmosome; Ll, lamina lucida; Ls, lamina densa. Bar = 200 nm. *B.* Ultrastructure of the human dermal-epidermal junction by transmission electron microscopy following protocols using high-pressure fixation and embedding techniques. Note the dense character of both the basement membrane and the subjacent papillary dermis. Anchoring filaments, anchoring fibrils, and anchoring plaques are not distinguishable. (*Both photos courtesy of Douglas R. Keene, MD, Shriners Hospital, Portland, Oregon.*)

(discussed below). Regardless of its actual occurrence in vivo, the evaluation of the lamina lucida by standard electron microscopy techniques has allowed identification of specific structures that would otherwise have been difficult to detect.

The second zone, the lamina densa, appears as an electron-dense amorphous structure 20 to 50 nm in width. The dermal-epidermal lamina densa is similar in appearance to analogous structures in other organs. At high magnification, it has a granular-fibrous appearance.[2] The major molecular components of the lamina densa are collagen IV, nidogen/entactin, perlecan, and laminins which all can polymerize to networks of variable thickness (Fig. 16-2).[5]

The subbasal lamina contains microfibrillar structures. Two of these are readily distinguishable. The first structure, known as *anchoring fibrils,* appears as condensed fibrous aggregates 20 to 75 nm in diameter.[6] At high resolution, they appear to have a nonperiodic cross-striated banding pattern (Fig. 16-1*A*). The length of the anchoring fibril is difficult to measure because of its random orientation in relation to the plane of the section. In toad skin, these structures have lengths of approximately 800 nm. The anchoring fibrils in human skin appear to be somewhat shorter. The ends of the anchoring fibrils appear to be less-tightly packed, giving a somewhat frayed appearance. The proximal end inserts into the basal lamina, and the distal end is integrated into the fibrous network of the dermis.[7] Many of the anchoring fibrils originating at the lamina densa loop back into the lamina densa in a horse shoe-like manner;[8] others insert their opposite ends into amorphous-appearing structures, termed *anchoring plaques.*[9] These structures are believed to be independent "islands" of electron-dense material, although some controversy exists in the literature.[8] Anchoring fibrils are primarily aggregates of collagen VII.[9]

Tubular fibrillin-containing *microfibrils,* 10 to 12 nm in diameter, are also localized in the sublamina densa region. On the basis of classic histochemical staining procedures, these have been identified as elastic-related fibers.[10] Elastic components of the dermis are formed from microfibrillar and amorphous components.[11] The microfibrillar component in the absence of amorphous component was previously named the oxytalan fibers; the microfibrillar component in the presence of small amounts of amorphous component were designated as the elaunin fibers; and the microfibrillar component in the presence of abundant amorphous component is known as the *elastic fiber.* In the papillary dermis, the microfibrils insert into the basal lamina perpendicular to the basement membrane and extend into the dermis, where they gradually merge with the elastic fibers to form a plexus parallel to the dermal-epidermal junction. These two elastic components appear to be continuous with the elastic fibers present deep within the reticular dermis.[11] The gradient of an increasing amorphous component from the basal lamina into the reticular dermis may represent a system of increasingly mature elastic fibers.

In summary, the ultrastructure of the dermal-epidermal junction strongly suggests that the lamina densa functions as a structural scaffold for the attachment of the epidermal cells at one surface, secured by anchoring filaments extending from the lamina densa to the hemidesmosomes. The latter also serve as insertion points for intracellular keratin filaments that provide an internal cytoskeleton for the basal cells. On the opposite surface, the extracellular matrix suprastructures of the dermis are firmly attached to the lamina densa. The interaction of different dermal fibers with the basal lamina appears to be mediated by the anchoring fibrils. The elastic system of the dermis inserts directly into the basal lamina via the microfibrils. Thus, the dermal-epidermal junction provides a continuous series of attachments between the reticular dermis and the internal cytoskeleton of the basal cells. These observations suggest three major functions for the epidermal basement membrane: It provides (1) a structural foundation for the secure attachment and polarity of the epidermal basal cells; (2) a barrier function, separating the components of the epidermis and the dermis; and (3) firm attachment of the dermis to the epidermis through a continuous system of structural elements. Biologic and molecular analyses indicate that the basement membranes also modify cellular functions, such as organization of the cytoskeleton and rescue from apoptotic signaling.[12]

BIOCHEMICAL CHARACTERIZATION OF THE BASEMENT MEMBRANE

Basement membranes contain collagenous and noncollagenous glycoproteins, and proteoglycans. The unusual amino acids hydroxyproline and hydroxylysine are found almost exclusively in collagens, and their presence is considered a marker for this family of proteins (for review, see Ref. 13). The hydroxyproline content suggests that collagen accounts for 40 to 65 percent of the total basement membrane protein. All basement membranes contain collagen IV as the major collagen and the heparan sulfate proteoglycan perlecan, irrespective of tissue source. In addition, many other glycoproteins have been found in basement membranes, including several laminins, nidogen/entactin, fibulins, and fibronectin.[14,15]

In contrast to the ubiquitous components within all basement membranes, some molecules demonstrate a restricted distribution. Certain collagen IV isoforms, collagens VII and XVII, or several laminins,

FIGURE 16-2

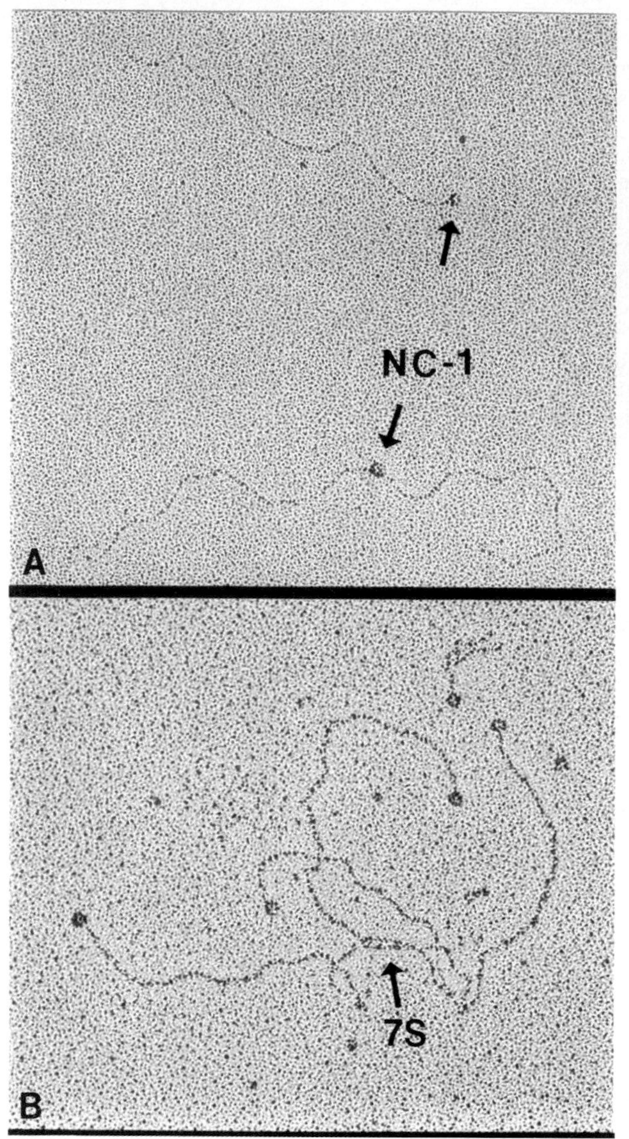

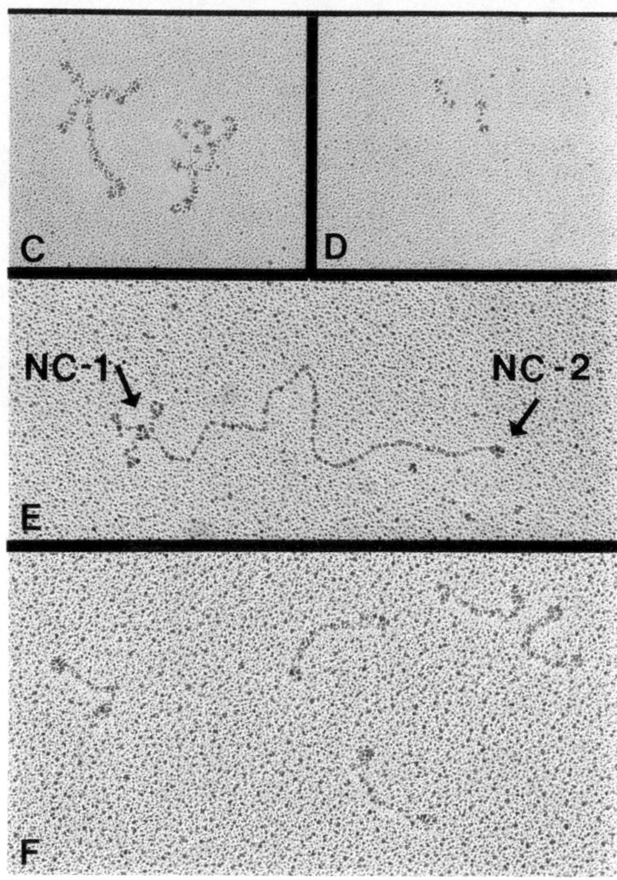

Images of basement membrane molecules visualized by rotary shadowing. *A*. Collagen IV monomer and a dimer resulting from aggregation of C-terminal NC-1 domains. *B*. Collagen IV tetramer ("spider") demonstrating the 7-S domain with the four protruding molecules and their large terminal NC-1 domains. *C*. Laminin 1 molecules. *D*. Nidogen molecules. *E*. Procollagen VII. The NC-1 and NC-2 regions are indicated. *F*. Laminin five molecules. (*All micrographs were provided by Douglas R. Keene, MD, Shriners Hospital, Portland, Oregon.*)

are not ubiquitous. For example, the $\alpha 3$ chain of collagen IV is localized in the basement membrane of the kidney and lung, but not in those of the skin and blood vessels and, vice versa, collagens VII and XVII are associated with the squamous epithelia of skin but are not found in glomerular and alveolar basement membranes.[14,15] Differences in macromolecular composition are responsible for morphologic and functional variance of basement membranes. Some of these differences reflect tissue-specific accessory structures, while others result from differences in the constituents of the lamina densa itself (discussed below).

Ubiquitous Components of Basement Membranes

COLLAGEN IV Advances in our knowledge of collagen IV structure have substantially contributed to our understanding of basement membrane architecture.[16] In addition to its unique primary structure, the chain composition and supramolecular organization of collagen IV is different from the classical interstitial collagens (for review, see Refs. 17 and 18).

Collagen IV has a structure closely related to the procollagen form, typical of many collagens (see Chap. 14). A collagen IV α-chain contains three distinct domains (Fig. 16-2*A*), the N-terminal cysteine-rich (7-S) domain, a central triple-helical domain, and a C-terminal globular domain (NC-l). The chain composition is determined by the NC-l domains, and the α chains are linked to each other by covalent interactions through these domains.[16] The triple helix of collagen IV measures 330 nm, which is longer than that of interstitial collagens. It is not helical throughout its length, but it does contain several sites at which glycine is not present in every third position.[15] These minor discontinuities result in increased flexibility in the collagen IV helix, but also render it susceptible to a variety of proteases.[15]

The characteristic fibril structure of the interstitial collagens results from aggregation of molecules in a staggered array, producing a cross-banding pattern in electron microscope after appropriate staining. In contrast, the ultrastructure of the lamina densa indicates no periodic cross-striations, strongly suggesting that the aggregates of collagen IV are different. The suprastructure of collagen IV has been partially elucidated by rotary shadowing electron microscopy that indicated that the major interactions among collagen IV molecules occur at their amino- and carboxyl-terminal domains, and by lateral association of their triple helices (Fig. 16-2*A*).[15] Covalent interactions among 7-S regions of different molecules are the basis for the specialized network characteristic of basement membranes (Fig. 16-2*B*).[15] The individual 7-S regions overlap in both the parallel and antiparallel directions, producing a characteristic four-legged "spider" form. The NC-l domains at the end of each leg of the spider interact with the NC-l domain of the adjacent aggregates (Fig. 16-2*B*). Association is stabilized by covalent bonds. These end-to-end interactions result in an extended two-dimensional network that is the basis of basement membrane organization.

The high flexibility of the basement membrane network structure makes the possibility of interactions with other collagens or noncollagenous molecules very attractive. An open meshwork of collagen IV with, for example, laminins or perlecan, can be easily visualized.[17] The implied porosity of this structure would then be limited by the size of the pores in the collagen network and by structural elements associated with it. This model of the basement membrane structure allows considerable mechanical stability while retaining physiologic flexibility. These properties of strength and elasticity would be expected for a dynamic surface, such as that seen in the epidermal-dermal junction and surrounding blood vessels.

Collagen IV molecules in different basement membranes contain genetically distinct but structurally homologous α chains. Six different α chains have been identified. The $\alpha 1$ and $\alpha 2$ chains are ubiquitous, but the $\alpha 3 \alpha 4$, $\alpha 5$, and $\alpha 6$ chains show restricted distribution among tissues.[18] Recent studies have elucidated the chain organization and the discriminatory interactions that govern network assembly in the basement membranes of the glomerulus and smooth muscle. The existence of two networks, namely $\alpha 1/\alpha 2$-containing and $\alpha 3/\alpha 4/\alpha 5$-containing networks, was established in the glomerular basement membrane. The chains are linked to each other by covalent interactions through the NC-l domain, indicating that these domains contain recognition sequences for selection of chains that are sufficient to direct the assembly of the $\alpha 1/\alpha 2$-containing or $\alpha 3/\alpha 4/\alpha 5$-containing networks.[16] Smooth muscle basement membranes have an $\alpha 1/\alpha 2/\alpha 5/\alpha 6$-containing network in addition to the classical $\alpha 1/\alpha 2$-network.[19] The $\alpha 1/\alpha 2/\alpha 5/\alpha 6$-network represents a new arrangement in which a triple-helical molecule containing the $\alpha 5$ and $\alpha 6$ chains is linked to an adjoining molecule composed of the $\alpha 1$ and $\alpha 2$ chains. Together, the six chains of collagen IV are distributed in three major networks, $\alpha 1/\alpha 2$, $\alpha 3/\alpha 4/\alpha 5$, and $\alpha 1/\alpha 2/\alpha 5/\alpha 6$, whose chain composition is determined by the NC-l domains. In the skin, the $\alpha 1/\alpha 2$-containing collagen IV network dominates within the dermal-epidermal junction, but $\alpha 1/\alpha 2/\alpha 5/\alpha 6$-containing network is also likely to be present.[20]

The $\alpha 3$(IV) chain is the antigen recognized by the circulating autoantibodies in the Goodpasture syndrome,[21] and autoantibodies directed against the NC-l domain of the $\alpha 5$(IV) collagen chain were found in a novel autoimmune disease characterized by subepidermal bullous eruptions and renal insufficiency.[22] Structural aberrations in the genes encoding the $\alpha 3$, $\alpha 4$, $\alpha 5$, and $\alpha 6$ chains cause different forms Alport syndrome, a genetic disease characterized by nephritis and deafness.[18,23]

LAMININS Laminins are members of a family of very large glycoproteins (600 to 950 kDa) with semirigid and extended structures (for review, see Refs. 24 and 25). Three types of subunit chains have been designated α (200 to 400 kDa), β (220 kDa), and γ (155 to 200 kDa) chains. The molecular structure of all laminins is a trimeric aggregate of one of each, α, β, and γ chains. With rotary shadowing electron microscopy the molecules were shown to have an asymmetric cross-like structure (Fig. 16-2*C*). The long arm of the cross is approximately 125 nm in length; the short arms are variable, but the largest measure approximately 80 nm. The laminin molecule is divided into globular and rodlike sections. The four extremities of the crosslike structure contain globular domains, and the three short arms of the cross contain globular domains approximately 20 nm from their free ends. The globular and rodlike domains of laminin have been individually implicated in various functions, including cell attachment and spreading, aggregation with itself and with other components of the lamina densa (Fig. 16-3), with neurite outgrowth, and with cellular differentiation.

Laminins are present in all basement membranes[24,25] and ultrastructural studies indicate that they are localized to the lamina lucida/lamina densa. Exceptions may form the $\gamma 3$ chain-containing laminins 14 and 15 that can be found in tissues without classical basement membranes, such as the central nervous system.[26] By interacting with integrins and other cell surface components laminins can control cellular activities such as adhesion, migration, proliferation, and polarity, or promote neurite outgrowth.[25] The integrins bind to the LG domain of the α chain, at the foot of the long arm of the laminin cross.[27]

To date, 15 laminin isoforms have been identified (for review, see Refs. 24 to 27). The $\alpha 1$ chain containing laminin 1 ($\alpha 1 \beta 1 \gamma 1$) is the "prototype" laminin. The $\alpha 2$ chain containing laminins 2 and 4 are present primarily within the basement membranes of the muscle fibers, nerves, neuromuscular junction, and glomerulus. Mutations in the laminin $\alpha 2$ chain cause progressive muscular dystrophy and a significant decrease in the amount of basement membrane accumulated surrounding muscle cells.[28] The absence of the muscle basement membrane leads to progressive degeneration of the muscle due to cell death. Therefore, the prediction is that laminins, and basement membranes in general, are required to prevent apoptosis by the cell types they surround.[14] Three additional laminin α chain variants—$\alpha 3$, $\alpha 4$, and $\alpha 5$—are known. The $\alpha 3$ chain is involved in epithelial adhesion[29] (see below), and the $\alpha 4$ and $\alpha 5$ chains are found in a variety of tissues including endothelia, mature epithelia, neuromuscular junction, and glomerulus as components of laminins 8 to 11.[30] Three β-chain variants are known: $\beta 1$, $\beta 2$, and $\beta 3$. The distribution of the $\beta 2$ chain is largely restricted to the neuromuscular junction, but it is also found in nonmuscle tissues such as the glomerular basement membrane of kidney and the capillary basal lamina.[24,25] Targeted ablation of the $\beta 2$ gene leads to muscular dystrophy and renal failure in mice, due to a loss of the neuromuscular folds and the ingrowth of the glial cells within the neuromuscular junction and to fusion of the glomerular podocyte foot processes, respectively. The $\beta 3$ chain is involved in epithelial adhesion (see below). At the present time, three γ chain variants—$\gamma 1$, $\gamma 2$, and $\gamma 3$—are known. The $\gamma 2$ chain is found only in laminin 5 (see below), and the $\gamma 3$ chain is found only in laminins 14 ($\alpha 4$, $\beta 2$, and $\gamma 3$), and 15 ($\alpha 5$, $\beta 2$, and $\gamma 3$), which may play roles in the central nervous system, e.g., in retinal photoreceptor production, stability, and synaptic organization.[31]

NIDOGEN/ENTACTIN Laminin is strongly associated with another lamina densa glycoprotein nidogen/entactin. Rotary shadowing of nidogen indicates a dumbbell shape (Fig. 16-2*D*). Nidogen binds laminin at a specific site within the $\gamma 1$ chain in a calcium-dependent manner.[32] Nidogen also binds collagen IV, perlecan, and fibulins.[33] Because isolated laminin will self-assemble in the presence of calcium, these observations support the concept of basement membrane structure where separate networks of collagen IV, perlecan, and laminin are linked by nidogen. Recently, a second nidogen, nidogen 2, was identified.[34] In light of the central role of nidogen as a basement membrane linker, it was surprising that no pathologic phenotype was observed in mice with targeted ablation of the nidogen 1 gene.[35] This led to the prediction that nidogen 2 compensates functionally for the lack of nidogen 1 in the tissues and, therefore, more information on the functions of these

FIGURE 16-3

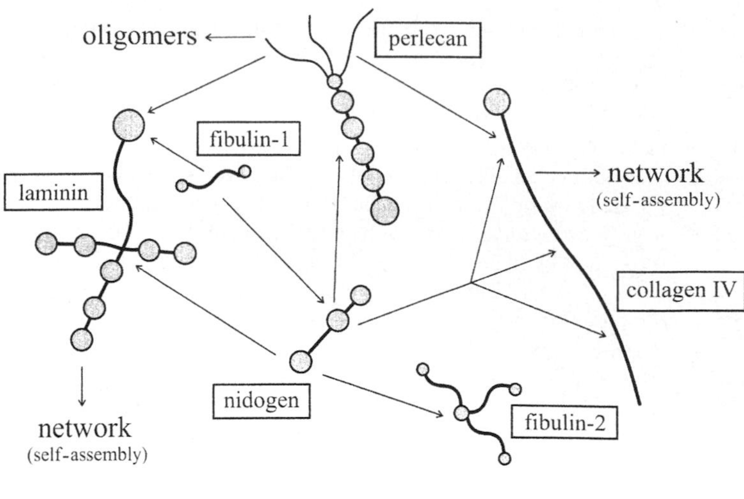

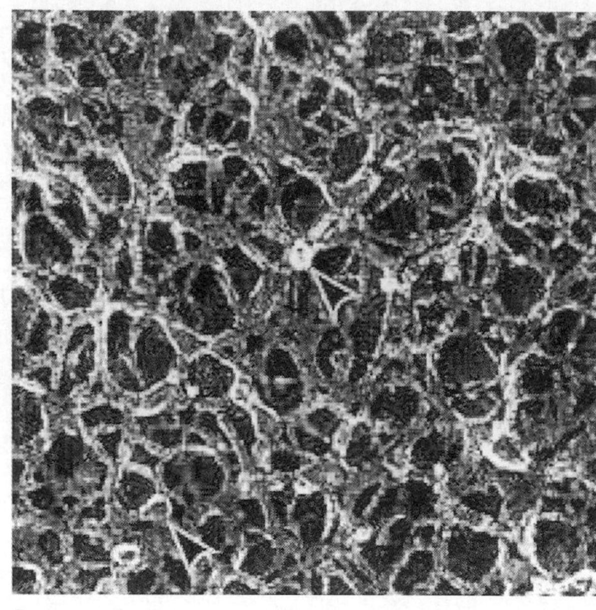

A. *B.*

A. Representation of the networks formed by the ubiquitous components of the basement membranes. Monomeric collagen IV self-assembles into dimers and tetramers that further aggregate into a complex lattice. Laminins self-polymerize into networks. Perlecan can oligomerize in vitro, and the glycosaminoglycan side chains interact with the collagen IV framework. Nidogen/entactin is thought to bind components of all three networks and also fibulins. Nidogen therefore plays a central role as a stabilizer of the lamina densa framework. Individual molecules are not drawn to scale. (*Drawing courtesy of Ulrike Mayer, PhD, Wellcome Trust Centre for Cell-Matrix Research, Manchester, UK.*) *B*. Rotary shadowing image of a quick-freeze, deep-etch replica of collagen IV polymers. The replica shows an extensive, branching and anastomosing network with occasional globular structures (*arrowhead*), which can be visualized as a model for the structure of the lamina densa. (*Photo kindly provided by Toshihiko Hayashi, PhD, University of Tokyo, Japan. See also Ref.*[94])

ubiquitous basement membrane components can be expected from future double knockout mice lacking both nidogen 1 and 2.

FIBULINS Fibulins are a newly identified family of highly conserved, calcium-binding extracellular matrix proteins, with at least six members. They are located in vessel walls, basement membranes, and microfibrillar structures.[36] Fibulin-2 binds fibrinogen, fibronectin, nidogen, and several other basement membrane molecules, such as the proteoglycans aggrecan and versican.[37] Therefore, fibulins are likely to contribute to the structural networks of different basement membranes and their ligands.

HEPARAN SULFATE PROTEOGLYCANS Another class of ubiquitous integral basement membrane constituents are the proteoglycans.[38] Three proteoglycans are characteristically present in vascular and epithelial basement membranes: perlecan, agrin, and bamacan. They consist of a core protein of various lengths, and the first two carry primarily heparan sulfate side chains, whereas the latter carries primarily chondroitin sulfate. The name *perlecan* is derived from its rotary shadowing appearance reminiscent of a string of pearls. Perlecan represents a complex multidomain proteoglycan with enormous dimensions and a number of posttranslational modifications.[39] Knockout mice lacking perlecan exhibited abnormalities in many tissues, including basement membranes, and embryonic lethality.[40] The morphology of the basement membranes was not altered but the membranes deteriorated in regions under increased mechanical stress, such as myocardium or skin, resulting in lethal cardiac abnormalities and skin blistering. *Agrin* is a major heparan sulfate proteoglycan of neuromuscular junctions and renal tubular basement membranes. *Bamacan* is likely to be the chondroitin sulphate proteoglycan previously identified in many basement membranes. The proteoglycans are capable of interactions with several other basement membrane components and are believed to contribute to the overall architecture of the basement membrane as well as provide tissue-specific functions (see Fig. 16-3). The high sulfate content of the proteoglycans makes them highly negatively charged and hydrophilic. The charge density of these molecules is responsible for providing the selective permeability of the glomerular basement membrane.

Syndecans are transmembrane heparan sulfate proteoglycans that are present on most cell types, including basal keratinocytes of the epidermis. They regulate a variety of biologic processes, ranging from growth factor signaling, cell adhesion to ECM and subsequent cytoskeletal organization, to infection of cells with microorganisms.[41]

EPITHELIAL-SPECIFIC BASEMENT MEMBRANE COMPONENTS

The dermal-epidermal junction of skin is an excellent example of specific divergence in basement membrane structure. The structural components of hemidesmosomes, anchoring filaments, and anchoring fibrils in the basement membrane zone have been identified and characterized (for review, see Refs. 2, 3, 12, and 14). A cartoon depicting the relative locations of the proteins found at the dermal-epidermal junction is shown in Fig. 16-4. These proteins are listed in Table 16-1 and discussed below.

The Hemidesmosomes

Ultrastructurally, the hemidesmosome closely resembles one-half of the desmosome at cell-cell junctions in the epidermis. However, the components of these two structures are distinct.[42] Characterization of the hemidesmosomal proteins was initially aided by the use of autoantibodies in serum of patients with bullous pemphigoid. The antigens recognized by the sera ranged in mass from 120 to 230 kDa, with a considerable variability between individual serum samples.[43–46] Monoclonal antibodies and cloning of the cDNAs for the proteins helped identify three distinct proteins: 230 kDa, 180 kDa, and 120 kDa.[45,46] The 230-kDa protein, *BPAg-1* (bullous pemphigoid antigen-1, or BP230), is a coiled-coil dimeric proteins with homology to plakins, which are able to bind intermediate filaments.[45] BPAg-1 is the major component of the hemidesmosomal inner dense plaque. In a transgenic mouse model, deletions in BPAg-1 caused epidermolysis bullosa simplex (see Chap. 65). The 180-kDa protein, previously called BPAg-2 or BP180, is a transmembrane collagen now known as *collagen XVII,* where the collagenous domain is extracellular.[46–48] Mutations in collagen XVII cause junctional epidermolysis bullosa (see Chap. 65), indicating that it directly or indirectly stabilizes interactions of the epithelial cells with the basement membrane. Its intracellular ligands are plectin, BPAg-1 and $\beta 4$ integrin.[42] The extracellular ligands are $\alpha 6$ integrin and laminin 5.[49] The 120-kDa protein is the shed ectodomain of collagen XVII.[44,47,48]

Plectin, another dimeric plakin homologue, is also a component of the hemidesmosome. However, its tissue distribution is not limited to hemidesmosome-containing basement membranes. Mutations causing the loss of plectin result in epidermolysis bullosa simplex and progressive muscular dystrophy (see Chap. 65), indicating a role for this molecule in the stability of cell-basement membrane adhesion in a variety of tissues.

One key component of the hemidesmosome is the *integrin* $\alpha 6\beta 4$. Integrins are a large class of transmembrane extracellular matrix binding proteins that provide cell attachment and subsequent signal transduction. Integrin $\alpha 6\beta 4$ has a high affinity for laminin 5,[42] and therefore is essential to integration of the hemidesmosome with the underlying basement membrane and stroma. Mutations in either the $\alpha 6$ or $\beta 4$ chains result in dermal-epidermal instability. In mice, null mutations cause severe junctional epidermolysis bullosa.[50,51] In humans, different mutations in the $\alpha 6$ or $\beta 4$ chains are associated with variably severe skin blistering associated with pyloric atresia.[52,53]

Recently, a member of the cell surface transmembrane proteins of the tetraspan superfamily, *CD151,* was identified as a component of the hemidesmosome.[54] It colocalizes with $\alpha 3\beta 1$ and $\alpha 6\beta 4$ integrins at the basolateral surface of basal keratinocytes and its recruitment into the hemidesmosomes seems to be regulated by $\alpha 6\beta 4$ integrin. It was suggested that CD151 plays a role in the formation and stability of hemidesmosomes by providing a framework for the spatial organization of the different components.[54]

FIGURE 16-4

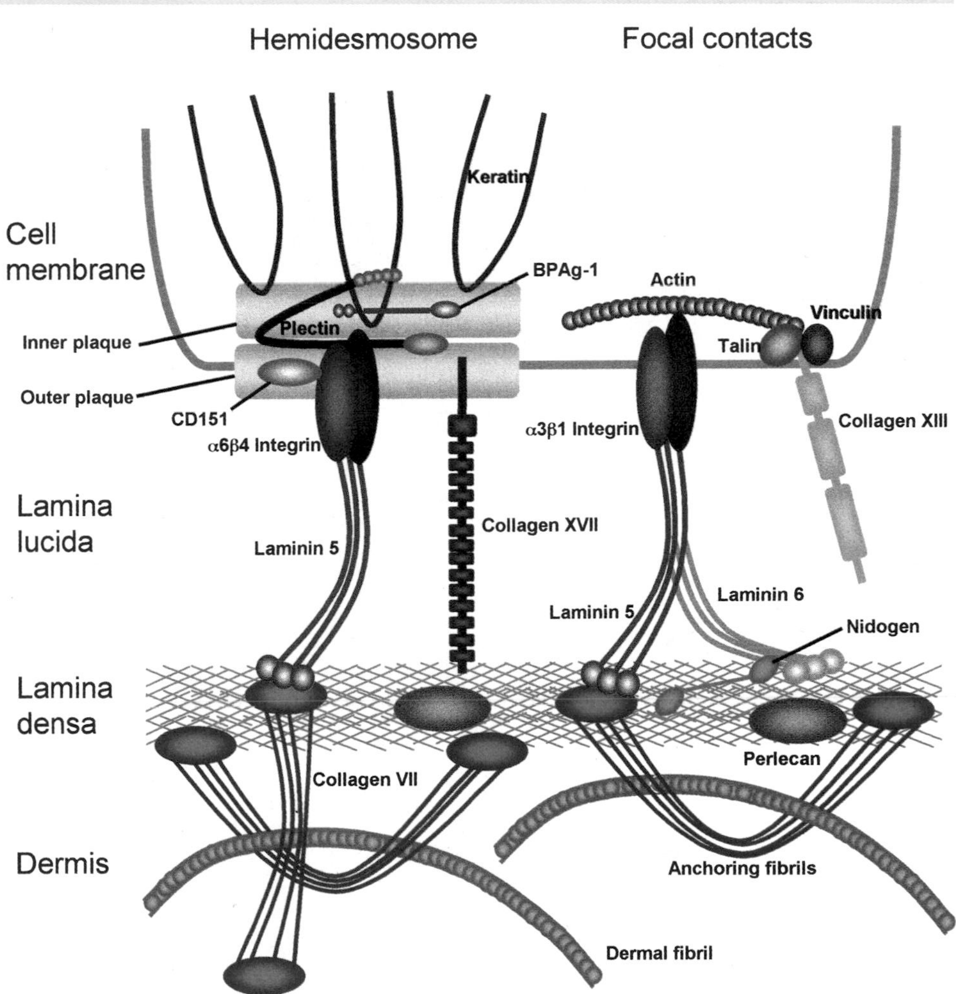

Model of the hypothetical relationships of molecules within the dermal-epidermal junction basement membrane. The illustration depicts monomeric laminin 5 as the bridge between the transmembrane hemidesmosomal integrin $\alpha 6\beta 4$ and the collagen VII NC-1 domain. The tight binding of laminin 5 to $\alpha 6\beta 4$ and to collagen VII provides the primary resistance to frictional forces. The transmembrane collagen XVII also participates in this stabilization, because its extracellular domain also binds laminin 5. Within the epithelial cell, the transmembrane elements bind the proteins of the hemidesmosomal dense plaque, BPAg-1 and plectin, which then associate with the keratins. Experimental evidence suggests that collagen XVII binds BPAg-1, integrin $\alpha 6\beta 4$, and plectin, and that integrin $\alpha 6\beta 4$ binds plectin. The laminin 5–6 complex is shown within the basement membrane between hemidesmosomes, bound by integrin $\alpha 3\beta 1$ where it potentially functions to maintain basement membrane assembly or stability. In vitro, integrin $\alpha 3\beta 1$ and another transmembrane collagen, type XIII, are localized to the focal contacts. In these structures, they may function, together with vinculin and talin, as the link between the basement membrane and the epithelial cortical actin network. In the lamina densa, collagen IV and perlecan networks are stabilized by nidogen. Anchoring fibrils are secured to the lamina densa by the implanted NC-1 domain of collagen VII. The fibrils project into the dermis and either terminate in anchoring plaques or loop back to the lamina densa. The anchoring fibril network entraps dermal fibrils, thus securing the adhesion of the lamina densa to the papillary dermis. None of the molecules is drawn to scale.

Anchoring Filaments

Several proteins are candidates for the anchoring filament component(s). *Laminin 5* has been localized to the anchoring

TABLE 16-1

Molecular Components of the Dermal-Epidermal Junction

Molecule	Special Features	Gene(s)	Genetic Abnormalities
Hemidesmosome components			
BPAg-1	Cytoskeleton linker, isoforms	BPAG1	EB simplex in mice; no human mutations found so far
Plectin	Cytoskeleton linker, isoforms	PLEC1	EB simplex with muscular dystrophy
$\alpha6\beta4$ Integrin	Transmembrane component	ITGA6, ITGB4	Junctional EB with pyloric atresia
Collagen XVII	Transmembrane component, shed ectodomain	COL17A1	Junctional EB non-Herlitz
$\alpha3\beta1$ Integrin	Transmembrane component, between hemidesmosomes	ITGA3, ITGB1	Disruption of $\alpha3$ in mice: minor skin blistering, kidney failure
Lamina lucida/lamina densa components			
Laminin 5 ($\alpha3\beta3\gamma2$)	In anchoring filaments, central role in dermal-epidermal adhesion	LAMA3 LAMB3 LAMC2	Junctional EB, Herlitz and non-Herlitz forms
Laminin 6 ($\alpha3\beta1\gamma1$)	Binds covalently to laminin 5, between hemidesmosomes	LAMA3 LAMB1 LAMC1	LAMA3 defects; junctional EB Herlitz, others not known
Laminin 10 ($\alpha5\beta1\gamma1$)	Function in basement membrane development?	LAMA5 LAMB1 LAMC1	Disruption of $\alpha5$ in mice: embryonic lethal
Laminin 2 ($\alpha2\beta1\gamma1$)	Functions at the dermal-epidermal junction unknown	LAMA2 LAMB1 LAMC1	Congenital muscular dystrophies, no obvious skin abnormalities
Collagen IV $\alpha1$(IV)/$\alpha2$(IV) $\alpha3$(IV)/$\alpha4$(IV) $\alpha5$(IV)/$\alpha6$(IV)	Basic basement membrane scaffold; tissue-specific isoform networks; at the dermal-epidermal junction $\alpha1$(IV)/$\alpha2$(IV) and $\alpha5$(IV)/$\alpha6$(IV) chain-containing networks	COL4A1 COL4A2 COL4A3 COL4A4 COL4A5 COL4A6	Disruption of $\alpha1$ and $\alpha2$ in mice; embryonic lethal; in man, X-linked and autosomal Alport syndrome, diffuse leiomyomatosis
Nidogen 1 and 2	Multiple ligands, network connectors	NID1 NID2	Disruption of nidogen-1 in mice: no obvious phenotype
Perlecan	Heparan sulfate proteoglycan	HSPG2	Disruption of perlecan in mice: abnormalities in many tissues including basement membranes, embryonic lethal
Anchoring fibril components			
Collagen VII	Proteolytically processed, dimers polymerize to fibrils	COL7A1	Dystrophic EB, all forms

EB, epidermolysis bullosa.

filaments.[12,24,25,28,55] It is a disulfide-bonded complex of $\alpha3$, $\beta3$, and $\gamma2$ chains. Rotary shadowing imaging indicates that laminin 5 has a rod-like structure terminating in the globular regions (see Fig. 16-2*F*). The component chains are considerably truncated relative to other laminin chains, and this truncation is reflected in the loss of the structures equivalent to the short arms of other laminins. Additionally, the $\alpha3$ and $\gamma2$ chains of laminin 5 are proteolytically processed after secretion from the keratinocyte, further shortening the short arm structures.[56,57] The shape of the molecule is consistent with its potential to be the anchoring filament protein. Laminin 5 has high affinity for $\alpha6\beta4$ integrin,[42] and it forms covalent complexes with laminin 6 ($\alpha3\beta1\gamma1$),[58] binds to the NC-1 domain of collagen VII, the anchoring fibril protein[59,60] and to the distal ectodomain of collagen XVII.[49] Genetic evidence suggests that laminin 5 is essential in keratinocyte adhesion, as null mutations in any of its component $\alpha3$, $\beta3$, or $\gamma2$ chains result in severe Herlitz' junctional epidermolysis bullosa (see Chap. 65). Targeted disruption of the LAMA3 gene in mice prevented the synthesis of both laminin 5 and 6 molecules (both contain the laminin $\alpha3$ chain) and resulted in abnormal hemidesmosomes, lack of survival of mutant epithelial cells, severe junctional blistering, and perinatal lethality.[29] Therefore, the severity of the laminin 5 null phenotype reflects the loss of its ability to bridge the hemidesmosomes and the anchoring fibrils, resulting in a separation within the lamina lucida. The mouse model also demonstrated that defects in the epithelial basement membrane can cause abnormalities of ameloblast differentiation in developing teeth, thus suggesting a role for laminin 5 in enamel formation.[29]

The extracellular domain of *collagen XVII* localizes to the region of the anchoring filament.[61] This protein exists in two forms, as a transmembrane protein, and as a soluble shed ectodomain.[47,48,62] It is now known that the 120-kDa and 97-kDa antigens recognized by antisera from patients with linear IgA dermatosis, which have been localized to the lamina lucida/anchoring filament region, represent derivatives of collagen XVII.[63–67] The 120-kDa antigen is the intact shed ectodomain, and the 97-kDa antigen is a partially degraded fragment.[44] Proteins implicated as anchoring filament components have also included LAD-1,[64] which several lines of evidence suggest is identical with the shed ectodomain of collagen XVII.[44,65,67] Yet another antigen, recognized by monoclonal antibody 19-DEJ-1, localizes to the region of the lamina lucida beneath hemidesmosomes.[68] This antigen appears to be sulfated and may be a proteoglycan. Its identity has so far remained elusive.

The Epithelial Lamina Densa

The basement membrane beneath and between the hemidesmosomes contains the $\alpha1/\alpha2$-containing collagen IV network, probably some

$\alpha 1/\alpha 2/\alpha 5/\alpha 6$-containing *collagen IV* network, as well as nidogen, perlecan, and laminin $\alpha 3$-containing molecules.[14,20,55] The laminin $\alpha 3$ chain is also contained in laminin 6, which has the unique property of forming disulfide-bonded dimers with laminin 5.[58] It is probable that the major $\alpha 3$-containing laminin in the lamina densa between hemidesmosomes is the laminin 5-6 complex.[55,58] As the laminin $\alpha 3$-chain is a ligand for integrin $\alpha 3\beta 1$ present between hemidesmosomes, it is expected that binding of laminin 5 to 6 to the intracellular actin cytoskeleton is mediated by integrin $\alpha 3\beta 1$. This is consistent with studies in mice in which targeted ablation of the integrin $\alpha 3$-chain causes loss of the basement membrane between hemidesmosomes but not beneath them.[69] The laminin 5–6 complex contains a $\gamma 1$ chain and can therefore bind nidogen and the collagen IV network.[32] There are additional laminins within the dermal-epidermal basement membrane, one of which was assumed to be laminin 1. However, it is now believed that laminin 1 is a relatively minor component, if present at all, and that laminin 10 ($\alpha 5\beta 1\gamma 1$) is more abundant.[24,25,70] Laminin 2 may also exist at the dermal-epidermal basement membrane.[71]

Anchoring Fibrils

Collagen VII is the major component of the anchoring fibrils.[7–9,72] The collagen VII molecule is distinguished from other collagens in that it has a triple-helical domain that is 450 nm in length. Globular domains exist at both ends of the triple helix, the N-terminal domain NC-1 is very large and trident-like (see Fig. 16-2*E*). Collagen VII is synthesized and secreted mainly by keratinocytes as a monomeric procollagen.[72] This is processed by BMP-1, a proteinase that removes the C-terminal propeptide,[73] to yield a mature collagen VII that rapidly dimerizes through disulfide crosslinks at the carboxy terminus. The C-propeptides are believed to facilitate the formation of the centrosymmetric dimers.[74] The dimers then aggregate laterally to form the anchoring fibrils.[7,8,72] The fibrils are stabilized by the enzyme tissue transglutaminase which catalyzes the formation of covalent γ-glutamyl-ε-lysine cross-links.[75]

The NC-1 domain binds to laminin 5 and collagen IV within the lamina densa (Fig. 16-3).[59,60] The triple helical domains of an antiparallel collagen VII dimer make the length of the anchoring fibril. It extends perpendicularly from the lamina densa and either loops back into the lamina densa, or inserts into the anchoring plaques.[7–9,72] The anchoring plaques are electron-dense structures that contain collagen IV and laminin 5, and perhaps other basement membrane components, but which are believed to be independent of the lamina densa itself.[7] They are distributed randomly in the papillary dermis below the lamina densa and are interrelated by additional anchoring fibrils. The anchoring fibril network forms a scaffold that entraps large numbers of dermal fibrils, securing the lamina densa to the subjacent dermis.[7–9,72] Correspondingly, null mutations in COL7A1, the gene encoding collagen VII, result in severe, generalized dystrophic epidermolysis bullosa (see Chap. 65). To date, more than 300 COL7A1 mutations have been found in both recessive and dominant forms of dystrophic epidermolysis bullosa,[72,76] and the spectrum of biologic and clinical phenotypes is much broader than anticipated.[72,77] Collagen VII–deficient mice recapitulated the clinical and morphologic characteristics of severe recessive dystrophic epidermolysis bullosa in humans.[78]

Recent gene transfer experiments have indicated that an ex vivo gene therapy approach is promising for treatment of dystrophic epidermolysis bullosa. Transfection with a PAC vector carrying the entire COL7A1 gene increased collagen VII production in a keratinocyte line[79] and reverted the collagen VII–deficient phenotype of keratinocytes derived from the skin of a patient with severe dystrophic epidermolysis bullosa.[80] In another approach, a cosmid containing the entire human COL7A1 gene was used to generate transgenic mice.[81] The cosmid was capable of directing stable expression of human collagen VII in the skin of the transgenic mice for at least 19 months.[81]

In the acquired form of epidermolysis bullosa, epidermolysis bullosa acquisita, and in bullous systemic lupus erythematosus, autoantibodies target the NC-1 domain,[82,83] although epitopes in other domains of collagen VII have also been identified.[74,84]

THE ORIGIN OF THE BASEMENT MEMBRANES

The basement membrane constituents are products of both epithelial and mesenchymal cells. Models of rodent intestinal development suggested that both laminin and collagen IV were synthesized by mesenchymal cells.[85] In vitro modeling of basement membrane formation clearly shows that, under at least some conditions, the dermal-epidermal junction basement membrane is contributed to by both tissue compartments, and it has been proposed that differentiated fibroblasts exist adjacent to epithelial tissues in vivo, which produce basement membrane components and assist in basement membrane assembly.[86,87] Of the known basement membrane components, only laminins 5 and 6 are exclusively produced by the epidermis. Epithelial cells also manufacture most of collagen VII, whereas mainly mesenchymal cells synthesize collagen IV, nidogen, perlecan, and the laminin $\alpha 2$ chain.[88] In skin equivalent cultures,[86,87] and developing mouse organs,[88,89] fibroblasts are the only source of nidogen at the epithelial-mesenchymal interface. Because the mesenchymal products are translocated to the basolateral epithelial surface where they condense, that surface must provide the localization cues. Integrins $\alpha 6\beta 4$ and $\alpha 3\beta 1$, and perhaps collagen XVII, provide this function, suggesting that the laminins initiate basement membrane polymerization. As nidogen is thought to be required for stabilization of the basement membrane, and because it is a mesenchymal product, it is likely that the dermis is essential to development of basement membranes.[20,24,25,86] An interesting regulatory step to basement membrane formation may be added by dermal enzymes, e.g., BMP-1, which process epithelial cell products, such as laminin 5 and procollagen VII, to mature basement membrane molecules.[56,73]

THE FUNCTION OF BASEMENT MEMBRANES

Basement membranes have five major functions: (1) they serve as a scaffold for tissue organization and as a template for tissue repair; (2) the renal basement membranes serve as selective permeability barriers for the ultrafiltration of serum, and other basement membranes also demonstrate selective filtration; (3) they are physical barriers between different types of cells or between cells and their underlying extracellular matrix; (4) they firmly link an epithelium to its underlying matrix or to another cell layer; and (5) they regulate cellular functions. All of these characteristics of basement membranes are used during development and differentiation of multicellular organisms.

Their ultrastructure demonstrates that basement membranes serve as substrates for the attachment of differentiated cells and fix their polarity. Their continuity throughout the various organ systems stabilizes the established tissue orientations and provides a template for orderly repair after traumatic injury.[90] In the dermal-epidermal junction, the basement membrane mediates the connections of the basal cells with the connective tissue in the dermis. Tissue healing in adults depends on the presence of both the correct cell types and an intact basement membrane. Major disruptions in the basement membrane result in the formation of scar tissue and the loss of function in that area.

The selective permeability in the kidney is due to the renal basement membranes. Molecules with diameters >7 nm, i.e., larger than serum albumin, infrequently cross the basement membrane.[91] However, size is not the only criterion for membrane permeability; the transmembrane passage of negatively charged molecules is retarded in relation to neutral molecules of equivalent diameter, and the passage of positively charged molecules is facilitated. The components of basement membrane function as molecular sieves and as electrostatic barriers. The strong negative charge of heparan sulfate proteoglycans is believed to be directly responsible for the ion selectivity. The nearly ubiquitous distribution of heparan sulfate proteoglycans in all basement membranes suggests that these serve as selective permeability barriers in multiple locations, including the blood-brain barrier.[92] Ultrafiltration may be especially important during development and morphogenesis of all tissues.

Basement membranes also provide physical separation between different germ layers and between stratified epithelia and their underlying extracellular matrices. This barrier is especially important in the containment of tumors. With the exception of certain cells of the immune system, nonmalignant cells seldom cross a basement membrane. Benign tumor cells, when placed upon isolated amniotic basement membranes, are unable to cross this barrier in vitro. In contrast, malignant cells bind the basement membrane, regionally disrupt its structure at the site of the attachment, and migrate through the rupture. Laminins mediate the tumor-cell binding, and the basement membrane dissolution is catalyzed by metalloproteases produced by the tumor cell (see Chap. 17). The absence of distinguishable basement membranes in tumor biopsies has been an indicator of malignancy, and there appears to be a high correlation between metastasis and basement membrane degradation.[93] These observations underline the importance of the basal lamina as an obstacle to cell migration.

Several mouse models with deficiency of extracellular matrix components have proved the importance of the basement membranes in morphogenesis. The deposition of the basement membrane components between the different germ layers is one of the first manifestations of embryologic compartmentalization of tissues with distinctive developmental roles. These specialized matrices provide a substrate for organized cellular migration leading to morphogenesis. It is likely that basement membranes function in the selective exchange of molecules involved in early tissue-inductive interactions.

By binding biologically active signaling molecules basement membranes can regulate a multitude of biologic events, such as cell adhesion and migration, cytoskeleton and cell form, cell division, differentiation and polarization, and apoptosis. For example, basement membrane proteoglycans can bind growth factors that can be released from the complexes by various matrix-degrading proteinases from fibroblasts or inflammatory cells. The growth factors, including transforming growth factor-β or fibroblast growth factors, are potent regulators of cell growth, and extracellular matrix formation, in addition to their immunomodulatory and regulatory roles.

REFERENCES

1. Rubin GM et al: Comparative genomics of the eukaryotes. *Science* **287**:2204, 2000
2. Keene DR et al: Immunodissection of the connective tissue matrix in human skin. *Microsc Res Tech* **38**:394, 1997
3. Eady RA et al: Ultrastructural clues to genetic disorders of skin: The dermal-epidermal junction. *J Invest Dermatol* **103**:13S, 1994
4. Goldberg M, Escaig-Haye F: Is the lamina lucida of the basement membrane a fixation artifact? *Eur J Cell Biol* **42**:365, 1986
5. Erickson AC, Couchman JR: Still more complexity in mammalian basement membranes. *J Histochem Cytochem* **48**:1291, 2000
6. Palade GE, Farquhar MG: A special fibril of the dermis. *J Cell Biol* **27**:215, 1966
7. Keene DR et al: Collagen VII forms an extended network of anchoring fibrils. *J Cell Biol* **104**:611, 1987
8. Shimizu H et al: Most anchoring fibrils in human skin originate and terminate in the lamina densa. *Lab Invest* **76**:753, 1997
9. Sakai LY et al: Collagen VII is a major structural component of anchoring fibrils. *J Cell Biol* **103**:1577, 1986
10. Handford PA et al: Fibrillin: From domain structure to supramolecular assembly. *Matrix Biol* **19**:457, 2000
11. Ramirez F: Pathophysiology of the microfibril/elastic fiber system. *Matrix Biol* **19**:455, 2000
12. Ryan MC et al: The functions of laminins: Lessons from in vivo studies. *Matrix Biol* **15**:369, 1996
13. Myllyharju J, Kivirikko KI: Collagens and collagen-related diseases. *Ann Med* **33**:7, 2001
14. Burgeson RE, Christiano AM: The dermal-epidermal junction. *Curr Opin Cell Biol* **9**:651, 1997
15. Yurchenco PD, Schittny JC: Molecular architecture of basement membranes. *FASEB J* **4**:1577, 1990
16. Boutaud A et al. Type IV collagen of the glomerular basement membrane. Evidence that the chain specificity of network assembly is encoded by the noncollagenous NC1 domains. *J Biol Chem* **275**:30716, 2000
17. Colognato H, Winkelmann DA, Yurchenco PD: Laminin polymerization induces a receptor-cytoskeleton network. *J Cell Biol* **145**:619, 1999
18. Hudson BG, Reeders ST, Tryggvason K: Type IV collagen: structure, gene organization, and role in human diseases. Molecular basis of Goodpasture and Alport syndromes and diffuse leiomyomatosis. *J Biol Chem* **268**:26033, 1993
19. Borza DB et al. The NC1 domain of collagen IV encodes a novel network composed of the alpha 1, alpha 2, alpha 5, and alpha 6 chains in smooth muscle basement membranes. *J Biol Chem* **276**:28532, 2001
20. Fleischmajer R et al: There is temporal and spatial expression of alpha1 (IV), alpha2 (IV), alpha5 (IV), alpha6 (IV) collagen chains and beta1 integrins during the development of the basal lamina in an in vitro skin model. *J Invest Dermatol* **109**:527, 1997
21. Netzer KO et al. The Goodpasture autoantigen. Mapping the major conformational epitope(s) of alpha3(IV) collagen to residues 17–31 and 127–141 of the NC1 domain. *J Biol Chem* **274**:11267, 1999
22. Ghohestani RF et al: The alpha 5 chain of type IV collagen is the target of IgG autoantibodies in a novel autoimmune disease with subepidermal blisters and renal insufficiency. *J Biol Chem* **275**:16002, 2000
23. Jais JP: X-linked Alport syndrome: natural history in 195 families and genotype-phenotype correlations in males. *J Am Soc Nephrol* **11**:649, 2000
24. Ekblom M et al: Laminin isoforms and epithelial development. *Ann N Y Acad Sci* **857**:194, 1998
25. Aumailley M, Smyth N: The role of laminins in basement membrane function. *J Anat* **193**:1, 1998
26. Koch M et al: Characterization and expression of the laminin gamma3 chain: A novel, non-basement membrane-associated, laminin chain. *J Cell Biol* **145**:605, 1998
27. Timpl R et al: Structure and function of laminin LG modules. *Matrix Biol* **19**:309, 2000
28. Helbling-Leclerc A et al: Mutations in the laminin alpha-2-chain gene (LAMA2) cause merosin-deficient congenital muscular dystrophy. *Nat Genet* **11**:216, 1995
29. Ryan MC et al: Targeted disruption of the LAMA3 gene in mice reveals abnormalities in survival and late stage differentiation of epithelial cells. *J Cell Biol* **145**:1309, 1999
30. Sixt M et al: Endothelial cell laminin isoforms, laminins 8 and 10, play decisive roles in T cell recruitment across the blood-brain barrier in experimental autoimmune encephalomyelitis. *J Cell Biol* **153**:933, 2001
31. Libby RT et al: Laminin expression in adult and developing retinae: Evidence of two novel CNS laminins. *J Neurosci* **20**:6517, 2000
32. Mayer U, Kohfeldt E, Timpl R: Structural and genetic analysis of laminin-nidogen interaction. *Ann N Y Acad Sci* **857**:130, 1998
33. Ries A et al: Recombinant domains of mouse nidogen-1 and their binding to basement membrane proteins and monoclonal antibodies. *Eur J Biochem* **268**:5119, 2001
34. Kohfeldt E et al: Nidogen-2: A new basement membrane protein with diverse binding properties. *J Mol Biol* **282**:99, 1998
35. Murshed M et al: The absence of nidogen 1 does not affect murine basement membrane formation. *Mol Cell Biol* **20**:7007, 2000
36. Zhang H et al: Fibulin-1 and fibulin-2 expression during organogenesis in the developing mouse embryo. *Dev Dyn* **205**:348, 1996
37. Olin AI et al: The proteoglycans aggrecan and versican form networks with fibulin-2 through their lectin domain binding. *J Biol Chem* **276**:1253, 2001

38. Iozzo RV: Heparan sulfate proteoglycans: intricate molecules with intriguing functions. *J Clin Invest* **108**:165, 2001
39. Hopf M et al: Mapping of binding sites for nidogens, fibulin-2, fibronectin and heparin to different IG modules of perlecan. *J Mol Biol* **311**:529, 2001
40. Costell M et al: Perlecan maintains the integrity of cartilage and some basement membranes. *J Cell Biol* **147**:1109, 1999
41. Woods A: Syndecans: Transmembrane modulators of adhesion and matrix assembly. *J Clin Invest* **107**:935, 2001
42. Nievers MG et al: Biology and function of hemidesmosomes. *Matrix Biol* **18**:5, 1999
43. Stanley JR: Autoantibodies against adhesion molecules and structures in blistering skin diseases. *J Exp Med* **181**:1, 1995
44. Schumann H et al: The shed ectodomain of collagen XVII/BP180 is targeted by autoantibodies in different blistering skin diseases. *Am J Pathol* **156**:685, 2000
45. Tamai K et al: The human 230-kD bullous pemphigoid antigen gene (BPAG1). Exon-intron organization and identification of regulatory tissue specific elements in the promoter region. *J Clin Invest* **92**:814, 1993
46. Giudice GJ, Emery DJ, Diaz LA: Cloning and primary structural analysis of the bullous pemphigoid autoantigen BP180. *J Invest Dermatol* **99**:243, 1992
47. Schäcke H et al: Two forms of collagen XVII in keratinocytes. A full-length transmembrane protein and a soluble ectodomain. *J Biol Chem* **273**:25937, 1998
48. Hirako Y et al: Cleavage of BP180, a 180-kDa bullous pemphigoid antigen, yields a 120-kDa collagenous extracellular polypeptide. *J Biol Chem* **273**:9711, 1998
49. Tasanen K et al. The ectodomain of collagen XVII organises and stabilises the anchorage of basal keratinocytes to the basement membrane. *Submitted for publication*
50. Georges-Labouesse E et al: Absence of integrin alpha 6 leads to epidermolysis bullosa and neonatal death in mice. *Nat Genet* **13**:370, 1996
51. van der Neut R et al: Epithelial detachment due to absence of hemidesmosomes in integrin beta 4 null mice. *Nat Genet* **13**:366, 1996
52. Ruzzi L et al. A homozygous mutation in the integrin alpha6 gene in junctional epidermolysis bullosa with pyloric atresia. *J Clin Invest* **99**:2826, 1997
53. Vidal F et al: Integrin beta 4 mutations associated with junctional epidermolysis bullosa with pyloric atresia. *Nat Genet* **10**:229, 1995
54. Sterk LM et al. The tetraspan molecule CD151, a novel constituent of hemidesmosomes, associates with the integrin alpha6beta4 and may regulate the spatial organization of hemidesmosomes. *J Cell Biol* **149**:969, 2000
55. Nishiyama T et al: The importance of laminin 5 in the dermal-epidermal basement membrane. *J Dermatol Sci* **1**:(suppl S51), 2000
56. Amano S et al: Bone morphogenetic protein 1 is an extracellular processing enzyme of the laminin 5 gamma 2 chain. *J Biol Chem* **275**:22728, 2000
57. Gagnoux-Palacios L et al: The short arm of the laminin gamma2 chain plays a pivotal role in the incorporation of laminin 5 into the extracellular matrix and in cell adhesion. *J Cell Biol* **153**:835, 2001
58. Champliaud MF et al: Human amnion contains a novel laminin variant, laminin 7, which, like laminin 6, covalently associates with laminin 5 to promote stable epithelial-stromal attachment. *J Cell Biol* **132**:1189, 1996
59. Rousselle P et al: Laminin 5 binds the NC-1 domain of collagen VII. *J Cell Biol* **138**:719, 1997
60. Chen M et al: Development and characterization of a recombinant truncated type VII collagen "minigene". Implication for gene therapy of dystrophic epidermolysis bullosa. *J Biol Chem* **275**:24429, 2000
61. Nonaka S et al: The extracellular domain of BPAG2 has a loop structure in the carboxy terminal flexible tail in vivo. *J Invest Dermatol* **115**:889, 2000
62. Franzke C-W et al: Transmembrane collagen XVII, an epithelial adhesion protein, is shed from the cell surface by ADAMs. *Submitted for publication*
63. Zone JJ et al. Identification of the cutaneous basement membrane zone antigen and isolation of antibody in linear immunoglobulin A bullous dermatosis. *J Clin Invest* **85**:812, 1990
64. Marinkovich MP et al: LAD-1, the linear IgA bullous dermatosis autoantigen, is a novel 120-kDa anchoring filament protein synthesized by epidermal cells. *J Invest Dermatol* **106**:734, 1996
65. Zone JJ et al: The 97-kDa linear IgA bullous disease antigen is identical to a portion of the extracellular domain of the 180-kDa bullous pemphigoid antigen, BPAg2. *J Invest Dermatol* **110**:207, 1998
66. Egan CA et al: Bullous pemphigoid sera that contain antibodies to BPAg2 also contain antibodies to LABD97 that recognize epitopes distal to the NC16A domain. *J Invest Dermatol* **112**:148, 1999
67. Kromminga A et al: Patients with bullous pemphigoid and linear IgA disease show a dual IgA and IgG autoimmune response to BP180. *J Autoimmun* **15**:293, 2000
68. Fine JD et al: Detection and partial characterization of a midlamina lucida–hemidesmosome associated antigen (19-DEJ-1) present within human skin. *J Invest Dermatol* **92**:825, 1989
69. DiPersio CM et al: Defects in matrix organization and keratinocyte adhesion in the epidermis of mice deficient in alpha3beta1 integrin. *J Cell Biol* **137**:729, 1997
70. Sorokin LM et al: Developmental regulation of the laminin alpha5 chain suggests a role in epithelial and endothelial cell maturation. *Dev Biol* **189**:285, 1997
71. Sewry CA et al: Diagnosis of merosin (laminin-2)-deficient congenital muscular dystrophy by skin biopsy. *Lancet* **347**:582, 1996
72. Bruckner-Tuderman L et al: Biology of anchoring fibrils: Lessons from dystrophic epidermolysis bullosa. *Matrix Biol* **18**:43, 1999
73. Rattenholl A et al: BMP-1 and mTLL-1 process procollagen VII to mature collagen VII. *J Biol Chem*, in press
74. Chen M et al: The carboxyl terminus of type VII collagen mediates antiparallel dimer formation and constitutes a new antigenic epitope for epidermolysis bullosa acquisita autoantibodies. *J Biol Chem* **276**:21649, 2001
75. Raghunath M et al: Cross-linking of the dermo-epidermal junction of skin regenerating from keratinocyte autografts. Anchoring fibrils are a target for tissue transglutaminase. *J Clin Invest* **98**:1174, 1996
76. Whittock NV et al: Comparative mutation detection screening of the type VII collagen gene (COL7A1) using the protein truncation test, fluorescent chemical cleavage of mismatch, and conformation sensitive gel electrophoresis. *J Invest Dermatol* **113**:673, 1999
77. Zimmer P et al: Dysphagia and esophageal stenosis: An extracutaneous form of dystrophic epidermolysis bullosa due to mutations in the collagen VII gene. *Gastroenterology* **122**:220, 2002
78. Heinonen S et al. Targeted inactivation of the type VII collagen gene (Col7a1) in mice results in severe blistering phenotype: A model for recessive dystrophic epidermolysis bullosa. *J Cell Sci* **112**:3641, 1999
79. Compton SH et al: Stable integration of large (>100 kb) PAC constructs in HaCaT keratinocytes using an integrin-targeting peptide delivery system. *Gene Ther* **7**:1600, 2000
80. Mecklenbeck S et al: Microinjection of the COL7A1 gene into collagen VII-deficient epidermolysis bullosa keratinocytes leads to synthesis and secretion of normal procollagen VII. *Human Gene Ther,* in press
81. Sat E et al: Tissue-specific expression and long-term deposition of human collagen VII in the skin of transgenic mice: implications for gene therapy. *Gene Ther* **7**:1631, 2000
82. Hallel-Halevy D et al: Epidermolysis bullosa acquisita: Update and review. *Clin Dermatol* **19**:712, 2001
83. Shirahama S et al: Bullous systemic lupus erythematosus. Detection of antibodies against noncollagenous domain of type VII collagen. *J Am Acad Dermatol* **38**:844, 1998
84. Tanaka H et al: A novel variant of acquired epidermolysis bullosa with autoantibodies against the central triple-helical domain of type VII collagen. *Lab Invest* **77**:623, 1997
85. Simon-Assmann P, Kedinger M: Tissue recombinants to study extracellular matrix targeting to basement membranes. *Methods Mol Biol* **139**:311, 2000
86. Fleischmajer R et al: Skin fibroblasts are the only source of nidogen during early basal lamina formation in vitro. *J Invest Dermatol* **105**:597, 1995
87. Marinkovich MP et al: Cellular origin of the dermal-epidermal basement membrane. *Dev Dyn* **197**:255, 1993
88. Salmivirta K, Sorokin LM, Ekblom P: Differential expression of laminin alpha chains during murine tooth development. *Dev Dyn* **210**:206, 1997
89. Ekblom P et al: Role of mesenchymal nidogen for epithelial morphogenesis in vitro. *Development* **120**:2003, 1994
90. Nguyen BP et al: Deposition of laminin 5 in epidermal wounds regulates integrin signaling and adhesion. *Curr Opin Cell Biol* **12**:554, 2000
91. Deen W'M, Lazzara MJ, Myers BD: Structural determinants of glomerular permeability. *Am J Physiol Renal Physiol* **281**:F579, 2001
92. Pardridge WM: Blood-brain barrier biology and methodology. *J Neurovirol* **5**:556, 1999
93. Liotta LA, Kohn EC: The microenvironment of the tumour-host interface. *Nature* **411**:375, 2001
94. Nakazato K et al: Gelation of the lens capsule type IV collagen solution at a neutral pH. *J Biochem* **120**:889, 1996

CHAPTER 17

Jo L. Seltzer
Arthur Z. Eisen

The Role of Extracellular Matrix Metalloproteinases in Connective Tissue Remodeling

Maintenance of the normal tissue architecture of human skin and other tissues requires the deposition, assembly, and turnover of extracellular matrix (ECM) macromolecules, including the collagens, elastin, glucosaminoglycans, and glycoproteins. The ability of resident cells to organize and remodel the surrounding ECM is essential for morphogenesis, angiogenesis, and wound healing. In a great number of pathologic situations, including tumor invasion/metastasis, the arthritides, fibrotic diseases, and inflammatory processes, there is derangement of the dynamic balance between ECM breakdown and synthesis. ECM remodeling in general is a cooperative multistep process involving localized degradation of the existing ECM, cytoskeletal rearrangement, cell translocation, and the deposition of new ECM components. Although each of these steps is controlled by a variety of molecular mechanisms, the initial step may depend on the presence of proteinases capable of initiating the degradation of ECM macromolecules. These enzymes comprise the matrix metalloproteinase (MMP) gene family,[1–3] which includes the collagenases, the gelatinases, the stromelysins, the matrilysins, metalloelastase, enamelysin, and the membrane-type MMPs (Fig. 17-1 and Table 17-1). The MMPs have been given historically based numerical designations (see Table 17-1), but the descriptive names will be used in this chapter.

GENERAL DESCRIPTION OF THE MATRIX METALLOPROTEINASES

The MMP family is distinguished by several common characteristics. All contain zinc at the active site, complexed to the conserved sequence HEXXHXXGXXHXXXXXXXM. All analyzed thus far by crystallography contain an additional structural zinc.[3] All require octahedral binding of calcium ions to maintain structural integrity. The propeptide portions contain an absolutely conserved PRCVPD sequence immediately upstream of the amino terminus of the active enzyme, important in zymogen activation. Finally, all are inhibited by the tissue inhibitor of metalloproteinases (TIMP) family of proteins.

Analysis of the primary structures of these enzymes allows the identification of structural domains shown in Fig. 17-1. The propeptide domain is immediately amino-terminal to the catalytic domain, containing the zinc binding site. In the collagenases, stromelysins, metalloelastases, and membrane-type MMPs (MT-MMPs), the catalytic domain is attached by a short "hinge" to the carboxyl-terminal pexin-like domain. The pexin-like domain consists of four hemopexin repeats shown by crystallographic analysis to be arranged in a propellar-like structure. A fibronectin-like domain is present only in gelatinases A and B (MMP-1 and -9) and consists of three 58-residue head-to-tail repeats homologous to the type II motif of the collagen-binding domain of fibronectin. This domain is amino-terminal to the catalytic zinc within the catalytic domain. Gelatinase B contains a unique 54-amino-acid-long proline-rich domain, homologous to the $\alpha 2$ chain of type V collagen, also inserted into the catalytic domain, carboxyl-terminal to the zinc. In the MT-MMPs, a short hydrophobic membrane-spanning domain is inserted in the fourth pexin repeat. Crystal structures have been obtained for several complete MMPs, as well as some additional active-site domains.[3]

The structures of a number of the metalloproteinase genes have been determined, and the similarities suggest a common precursor. For example, interstitial collagenase (human and rabbit) and stromelysin (human and rat) consist of 10 exons virtually identical in length. A cluster of MMP genes—*collagenase-1, -2,* and *-3, stromelysin-1* and *-2, matrilysin-1, metalloelastase,* and *enamelysin*—has been mapped

FIGURE 17-1

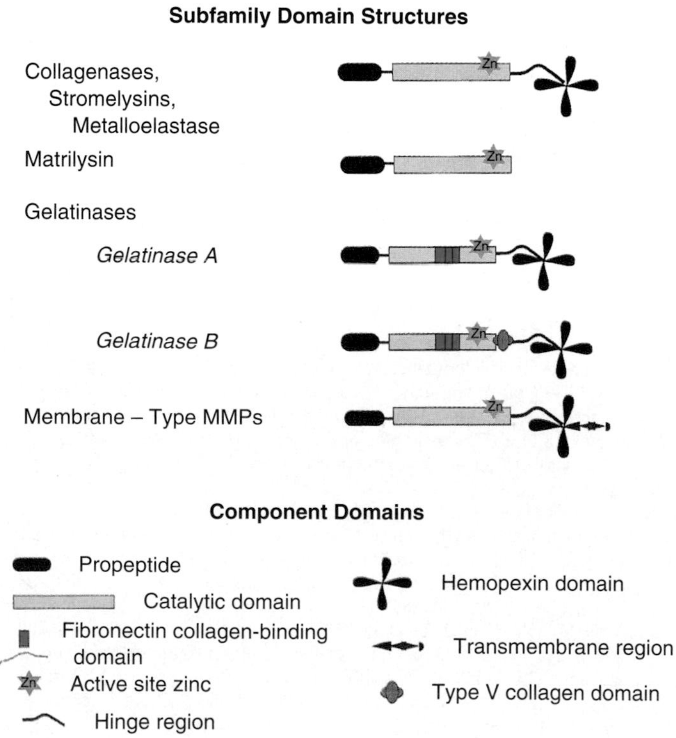

Domain structure of matrix metalloproteinases.

TABLE 17-1

Matrix Metalloproteinases

Enzyme	MMP Number	Alternate Name	Proenzyme Mol. Wt.	Known Matrix Substrates
Interstitial collagenase	MMP-1	Type I collagenase	52,000	Collagens I, II, III, VII, VIII, X, entactin, tenascin, aggrecan, denatured collagens, IL-1β, myelin basic protein, L-selectin
Neutrophil collagenase	MMP-8		75,000	Collagens I, II, III, V, VII, VIII, X, gelatin, aggrecan, fibronectin
Collagenase-3	MMP-13		52,000	Collagens I, II, IV, IX, X, XIV, aggrecan
Gelatinase A	MMP-2	72-kDa type IV collagenase	72,000	Denatured collagens, collagens IV, V, VII, X, XI, XIV, collagen 1, species-dependent, elastin, fibronectin, laminin, aggrecan, myelin basic protein
Gelatinase B	MMP-9	92-kDa type IV collagenase	92,000	Denatured collagens, collagens IV, V, VII, X, XIV, elastin, entacin, aggrecan, fibronectin, osteonectin, IL-1β, plasminogen, myelin basic protein
Stromeylsin-1	MMP-3	Proteoglycanase	57,000	Proteoglycan core protein, laminin, fibronectin collagens I, IV, V, IX, X, XI, gelatin, elastin, tenascin, aggrecan, myelin basic protein, entactin, decorin, osteonectin
Stromelysin-2	MMP-10	Transin-2	55,000	Proteoglycan core protein, collagens III, IV, V, laminin, fibronection, elastin, aggrecan
Stromelysin-3	MMP-11		61,000	Alpha$_1$ proteinase inhibitor
Martrilysin	MMP-7	PUMP Matrilysin-1	28,000	Collagen IV, denatured collagens, laminin, fibronectin, elastin, aggrecan, tenascin, myelin basic protein
Matrilsyin-2	MMP-26	Endometase	28,000	Gelatin, alpha$_1$ proteinase inhibitor
Membrane type matrix metalloproteinase-1	MMP-14	MTI-MMP	63,000	Progelatinase A, denatured collagen, fibronectin, laminin, vitronectin, entactin, proteoglycans
Membrane type matrix metalloproteinase-2	MMP-15	MT2-MMP	72,000	Progelatinase A
Membrane type matrix metalloproteinase-3	MMP-16	MT3-MMP	64,000	Progelatinase A
Membrane type matrix metalloproteinase-4	MMP-17	MT4-MMP	70,000	Unknown
Membrane type matrix metalloproteinase-5	MMP-24	MT5-MMP	73,000	Progelatinase A
Membrane type matrix metalloproteinase-6	MMP-25	MT6-MMP	63,000	Unknown
Metalloelastase	MMP-12		54,000	Elastin, collagen IV, vitronectin, plasminogen, laminin, entactin, fibrinogen, fibrin, fibronectin
Enamelysin	MMP-20		54,000	Amelogenin, aggrecan
MMP-19	MMP-19	RASI-1	57,000	Gelatin, aggrecan, fibronectin
MMP-21	MMP-21		Unknown	Unknown
MMP-22	MMP-22		Unknown	Unknown
MMP-23	MMP-23		44,000	Unknown
Epilysin	MMP-28		56,000	Unknown

to the long arm of human chromosome 11. *Matrilysin 2* [4] is on the short arm of chromosome 11. The *gelatinase A* and *B* genes have three additional exons coding for each of the three fibronectin-like repeats, suggesting that exon shuffling resulted in recruitment of the functional domain from fibronectin to the enzyme protein. The *gelatinase A* and *B* genes have been colocalized on chromosome 16.[5] Chromosomal locations of other MMPs are diverse.

GENERAL DESCRIPTIONS OF INDIVIDUAL MMPs

The MMPs show a great deal of overlapping substrate specificities (see Table 17-1). The identity of the particular enzymes involved in various instances of remodeling and tissue destruction depends to a large degree on tissue specificity and regulation by agents such as cytokines and growth factors. Specific enzymologic differences in members of the same subclass of MMPs, such as collagenases, are subtle but are most likely physiologically meaningful.

Interstitial Collagenases

Interstitial collagenase (MMP-1) was the first enzyme of the MMP family to be discovered. Triple-helical collagen was resistant to all known vertebrate proteinases until Gross and Lapiere[6] demonstrated collagenolytic activity in the medium of cultured tadpole tail skin explants. Human skin collagenase was then isolated in active form from culture medium of skin explants[7] and subsequently as a proenzyme from monolayer fibroblast cultures.[8] Many other cell types, including keratinocytes, synovial cells, and monocytes-macrophages, express an identical enzyme. Interstitial collagenase, like the other MMPs, contains intrinsic zinc in the active site and requires calcium for activity and thermostabilization.

Fibroblasts synthesize collagenase as a preproenzyme and secrete the enzyme as two proenzyme forms with molecular masses of 57 and 52 kDa (see Table 17-1). The minor 57-kDa proenzyme form is the result of posttranslational addition of N-linked complex oligosaccharides to a fraction of the 52-kDa proenzyme. Both potential N-glycosylation sites are contained within the active form of the enzyme.[9] Newly synthesized procollagenase, secreted rapidly after biosynthesis with negligible intracellular storage, is converted extracellularly to the 42- or 47-kDa active enzyme by removal of an 81-amino-acid peptide from the amino-terminal end of the molecule.

Interstitial collagenase degrades collagen types I, II, and III at physiologic pH and temperature by catalyzing a single cleavage three-quarters of the distance from the amino terminus in each of the three polypeptide chains comprising the helical native collagen molecule. Collagenase specifically cleaves the $\alpha1$(I) chains at a Gly-Ile bond (residues 775 and 776), and the $\alpha2$(I) chain at a Gly-Leu bond in the homologous region. Ten other Gly-Ile or Gly-Leu bonds within the triple-helical domain of the interstitial collagens are not cleaved, suggesting that the local conformation of the collagenase cleavage site is a major factor in determining substrate specificity. This region is more hydrophobic than other parts of the collagen molecule and lacks hydroxyproline residues that stabilize the triple helix. Indeed, human fibroblast collagenase catalyzes multiple cleavages in the denatured chains of all collagen types at Gly-Ile and Gly-Leu bonds. Thus it appears that the triple helix of native collagen can drastically after the ability of human fibroblast collagenase to catalyze cleavages that would be permissible from primary sequence cosideration alone. Moreover, even under optimal conditions of cleavage, collagen degradation by human fibroblast collagenase proceeds slowly for an enzymatic process, with a turnover number of approximately 25 molecules of fibrillar collagen degraded per molecule of collagenase per hour. This catalytic rate k_{cat} is the lowest of any mammalian enzyme described to date.

In addition to cleaving interstitial collagen types I, II, and III, fibroblast collagenase also cleaves type VII collagen (anchoring fibrils)[10] and type X collagen but does not degrade collagen types IV and V. Interstitial collagenase produces limited specific cleavages in a variety of noncollagenous substrates such as the plasma antiproteinases: α_2-macroglobulin, α_1-trypsin inhibitor, and α_1-antichymotrypsin. The cleavage sites are often different from those identified in the interstitial collagens. A bulky hydrophobic residue usually occurs on the amino-terminal side of the cleaved bond, similar to the substrate specificity of the bacterial metalloproteinase thermolysin.

Human neutrophil interstitial collagenase (MMP-8) attacks collagens at the same site as does fibroblast collagenase to produce the characteristic three-quarters/one-quarter collagen fragments. The cloned enzyme is highly homologous to fibroblast collagenase but has a molecular mass of 75 kDa due to a high degree of glycosylation. It is not immediately secreted but is stored in granules. Although both collagenases have similar affinities (K_m) for types I and III collagen, fibroblast collagenase degrades soluble type III collagen with a higher turnover rate,[9] whereas neutrophil collagenase degrades soluble type I collagen more rapidly.[8] For both enzymes, the differences in specificity against monomeric collagens are largely abolished when the substrates are reconstituted into the insoluble fibrillar forms found in tissues.

Collagenase-3 (MMP-13), first cloned from breast carcinoma, is homologous to rodent collagenase. The purified recombinant enzyme cleaves helical collagens, giving the characteristic three-quarters/one-quarter fragments. Unlike interstitial and neutrophil collagenases, however, collagenase-3 acts 5 to 10 times more rapidly on soluble type II collagen than on types I and III. Because of its preferential cleavage of type II collagen, and because it is made by both normal and osteoarthritic chondrocytes, collagenase-3 is thought to play an important role in osteoarthritis. Collagenase-3, unlike the other collagenases, can be activated by MT1-MMP.

At physiologic temperature, the products of collagen cleavage become soluble, are thermally unstable, and denature spontaneously, forming gelatins. These denatured gelatins are susceptible to attack by other proteinases. Thus the interstitial collagenases stand at a key point in connective tissue metabolism; they initiate the proteolytic events resulting in the complete degradation of collagen.

Stromelysins

Prostromelysin-1 is constitutively secreted by fibroblasts as a major 57-kDa form and a minor glycosylated 60-kDa form.[12] As with interstitial collagenase, a single mRNA species codes for both secreted proenzyme forms. Stromelysin has a broad substrate specificity, degrading proteoglycans, type IV collagen (principally in its nonhelical region), laminin, and fibronectin. It displays low activity against gelatin and casein (see Table 17-1) Stromelysin does not cleave type I collagen, but it degrades types III and IX collagens and acts as a telopeptidase by cutting intact types II and XI collagens at sites between the cross-linking hydroxylysine residue and the start of the triple helix.[13] It is not known whether stromelysin ever acts in concert with type IV collagenase to degrade basement membrane collagens.

Stromelysin-2 appears to have much the same substrate specificity as stromelysin-1 (see Table 17-1) but differs in tissue distribution. For example, stromelysin-1, but not stromelysin-2, is found in rheumatoid synovia. Both stromelysin-1 and stromelysin-2 are present during bone development, but at different locales; e.g., osteoclasts contain only stromelysin-2.[14] In keratinocytes, stromelysin-2 is induced by cytokines, whereas stromelysin-1 is not. A temporal progression of stromelysin-1 and stromelysin-2 expression is seen in keratinocytes during wound healing (see below).[15]

Stromelysin-3, first cloned from breast carcinoma,[16] differs substantially from the other members of its family. When the full-length enzyme was expressed in a mammalian system, it was found not to cleave the extracellular matrix components normally considered as stromelysin substrates but to cleave α_1-trypsin inhibitor in a specific manner.[17] In order to render the enzyme active against normal stromelysin substrates, the carboxyl-terminal domain had to be deleted and a mutation made in Asp-235.[18]

Unlike most other secreted MMPs, stromelysin-3 cannot be activated by organomercurial compounds. The presumably active enzyme is found in the extracellular space with the propeptide already removed. Interestingly, a stretch of 10 amino acids between the propeptide and catalytic domain is suitable for cleavage by the Golgi proteinase furin.

Cotransfection of furin and prostromelysin-3 into COS-7 cells resulted in a fully processed proteinase. Furin inhibitors and brefeldin A have been used to confirm that maturation of stromelysin-3 occurs in the trans-Golgi apparatus, followed by secretion.

Because proteolytic activity of stromelysin-3 seems to be limited, its physiologic role is uncertain, although it is found ubiquitiously in stroma surrounding tumors of epithelial origin. It has been suggested[17] that its function is to inactivate serine proteinase inhibitors (serpins) and thus allow enzymes such as plasmin to play a role in the degradation of matrix proteins.

Gelatinases (Type IV Collagenases)

The major component in all basement membranes is type IV collagen, accounting for 40 to 65 percent of the total protein. Interstitial collagenases do not cleave type IV collagen, whereas stromelysins cleave only the globular portions of the molecule. An MMP that could cleave the helical portion of type IV collagen into the prototypical three quarters/one-quarter fragment was first described by Salo et al.[20] from mouse melanoma cell culture. The human enzyme was cloned subsequently as a 72-kDa proenzyme[21] and found to be identical to gelatinase A from fibroblasts and human skin explants.[22] Gelatinase A (MMP-2) has a marked preference for protein substrates with a collagenous primary structure and was hypothesized to be the enzyme responsible for completing the degradation of collagen after cleavage by interstitial collagenase. Gelatinase A digests gelatin more than 100 times faster than does interstitial collagenase and rapidly cleaves collagenous peptides as small as six amino acid residues.[23]

Normal human macrophages, granulocytes, keratinocytes, and other cell types, including many transformed cells, secrete the related MMP gelatinase B (MMP-9). The primary structure of this enzyme contains all the elements of gelatinase A with an additional unique 54-amino-acid proline-rich domain, homologous to the $\alpha 2$ chain of type V collagen, inserted next to the zinc-binding active center domain [24] (see Fig. 17-1). Gelatinase B is a glycoprotein; the role of glycosylation in secreted metalloproteinases is not understood.

As shown in Fig. 17-1, in addition to the three domains also present in interstitial collagenase and stromelysin, both gelatinases A and B contain an insertion of three contiguous copies of fibronectin type II homology units immediately in front of the conserved zinc-binding site. Experiments investigating the functional role of this domain showed it to be responsible for the binding of progelatinases to gelatin,[25] although there is some question whether gelatin binding mediated by this domain is the rate-limiting step in gelatin hydrolysis. Recent studies by Collier et al.,[26] applying fractal kinetics to the digestion of gelatin in a three-dimensional matrix, have shown that the carboxyl-terminal hemopexin-like domain plays a role in allowing the gelatinase molecule to move laterally to new binding sites in the solid substrate.

The actual cleavage sites catalyzed by gelatinase A proteolysis were determined in cyanogen bromide peptides of type I gelatin. In addition to the expected cleavages between glycine and hydrophobic residues (Leu, Ile, Ala, Phe), unexpected cleavages were found between glycine and nonhydrophobic residues, specifically Glu, Asn, and Ser. Hexapeptides containing these unexpected cleavages sites were cleaved readily by gelatinase A. Of particular significance with regard to the enzyme's preference for gelatin as a protein substrate was the finding that hydroxyproline brackets the cleavage site at the P5 and P5′ positions. A kinetic investigation using synthetic substrates in which hydoxyprolines at these positions were systematically varied showed that the hydroxyprolines increased affinity (lowered K_m) for the substrates.[23] Although gelatinase B digests a similar profile of matrix proteins as gelatinase A (see Table 17-1), careful enzymatic analysis showed major differences in their specificity. Gelatinase A is twice as active against type I gelatin as gelatinase B, whereas gelatinase B digests type IV collagen two to three times faster than gelatinase A. Furthermore, substrates designed to give optimal turnover numbers for gelatinase A were digested at least an order of magnitude slower by gelatinase B.[23]

A unique feature of the gelatinase subclass is that portions of both proenzymes are secreted complexed to a specific MMP protein inhibitor. Some secreted progelatinase B molecules are noncovalently complexed at the carboxyl terminus with the tissue inhibitor of metalloproteinases, TIMP-1.[24] Progelatinase A is complexed in a similar fashion with a related but distinct tissue inhibitor of metalloproteinases, TIMP-2.[27] Nonetheless, both enzymes can be activated by organomercurials; the propeptide domain from the amino terminus is autocatalytically cleaved and removed as with MMPs not complexed to an inhibitor.

Matrilysin

Matrilysin-1 (MMP-7) is the smallest of the MMPs with a proenzyme of only 28 kDa. The only member of this family encoded without a hemopexin-like domain,[28] it contains only the pre, pro, and catalytic domains. Matrilysin displays broad substrate specificity degrading many extracellular matrix proteins including type IV collagen, fibronectin, entactin, elastin, and aggrecan (see Table 17-1). It also cleaves $\beta 4$ integrin. Because matrilysin lacks the carboxyl-terminal hemopexin-like domain, it is inhibited by the TIMPs approximately three orders of magnitude less strongly than other secreted MMPs.

The most distinguishing characteristic of matrilysin aside from its size is its tissue distribution. It is found almost exclusively in epithelium of glandular structures and in monocyte-derived marcrophages.[28,29] It is found in the germinative basal cell layer of fetal epidermis, appendageal buds, and developing hair follicles and sweat glands. In the adult, it is present in the secretory cells of the sweat glands[30] and is produced by other exocrine glands such as mammary and parotid glands, pancreas, liver, prostate, and peribronchial glands of the lung. In many ductal structures it appears to be secreted into the lumen, leading to a suggestion that one of its main functions is to prevent clogging of the ducts.

Matrilysin is found in most carcinomas examined, often in the early stages. In situ hybridization experiments show it to be localized to the tumor islands, in contrast to many other MMPs, which are made by the surrounding stroma.[31]

A new matrix metalloprotienase lacking a carboxy-terminal domain was cloned recently (MMP-26). At first termed *endometase*[32] because it is normally expressed only in endometrium, it also was found in placenta and in tumors of diverse origins and renamed *matrilysin-2*.[4,33] Like matrilysin, it has a broad substrate specificity, including activation of gelatinase B. In amino acid sequence, matrilysin-2 is most analogous to metalloelastase (MMP-12).

Membrane-Type Matrix Metalloproteinases

Membrane-type matrix metalloproteinases (MT-MMPs) are bound to the cell membrane, in contrast to all other MMPs, which are secreted extracellularly as proenzymes.[34] With six known MT-MMPs (see Table 17-1), this group is the newest and now largest division of this enzyme family. Widely distributed in both normal and neoplastic tissues, each MT-MMP has a characteristic tissue specificity.

MT-MMPs resemble other MMPs structurally (see Fig. 17-1), with a prodomain, catalytic domain, hinge region, and hemopexin-like domain. In addition, there are three conserved sequence insertions. An extension of the carboxyl terminus is rich in hydrophobic residues, allowing anchoring in the plasma membrane. All except MT4-MMP and M6-MMP have a short cytoplasmic tail.[35] A short (11 amino acid) furin recognition site in the prodomain of all MT-MMPs enables intracellular activation of the zymogen, probably in the trans-Golgi region. Stromelysin-3 also contains this site. MT-MMPs 1, 2, 3, and 5 contain a unique eight-residue insertion in the catalytic domain, possibly related to substrate specificity.[36]

All MT-MMPs, except MT4-MMP, are able to activate progelatinase A (MMP-2) (see below). They are potent proteinases with a broad range of substrates, including collagens, fibronectin, and proteoglycans.[37] The tissue location varies. Synthesis of MT1-MMP as defined by in situ hybridization is mainly confined to fibroblastic cells adjacent to the tumor islands.[38] Immunohistologic staining in some cases has shown the enzyme to be present on the plasma membranes of carcinoma cells. Furthermore, reminiscent of gelatinase A, carcinoma cells in culture can produce MT-MMP. At the cellular level, MT1-MMP is localized to specialized structures descriptively called *invadopodia.* The cytoplasmic tail of the enzyme contains potential phosphorylation sites that might have a role in localizing MT1-MMP at such specific cellular sites. Clustered $\beta 1$ integrins form another locus associated with MT1-MMP, which could have a role in cell-matrix interactions.[37]

Miscellaneous Matrix Metalloproteinases

Several members of the growing MMP family do not fit clearly into any of the subfamilies described earlier. Whereas much information is available on metalloelastase, others are simply chromosomal DNA sequences (MMP-21and -22). Since technology increasingly has allowed for the discovery of enzymes by structure rather than by catalytic activitiy, finding even more miscellaneous MMPs can be expected.

MACROPHAGE METALLOELASTASE Macrophage metalloelastase (MMP-12) was discovered as a cDNA clone from a human alveolar macrophage library.[39] It is relatively potent as an elastase with a turnover rate comparable with that of matrilysin and gelatinase B, i.e., approximately 30 percent the rate of human leukocyte elastase.[39] In the lung, metalloelastase accounts for most of the pathologic destruction of elastin; mice lacking the enzyme do not develop emphysema when made to smoke cigarettes.[40] It is also the most potent MMP in generating angiostatin by cleavage of plasminogen. Angiostatin inhibits endothelial cell proliferation and thus is an inhibitor of angiogenesis.

The cDNA of macrophage metalloelastase shows a domain structure similar to that of the interstitial collagenases and stromelysins. However, while medium harvested from alveolar macrophage cultures contains metalloelastase proenzyme, manipulation of the medium during purification produces a mature proteinase of 22 kDa. Activation of the proenzyme in vitro involves removal of the propeptide as well as rapid removal of the carboxyl-terminal domain. It is not known in what form metalloelastase is found in vivo.

Metalloelastase is made at the end stage of monocyte differentiation into alveolar macrophages. Peripheral blood monocytes do not make this enzyme, although they do secrete matrilysin, which is an efficient elastase.

OTHER NEWLY FOUND MMPs: MMP-19, -20, -23, AND -28 MMP-19, -20, and -28 all contain the same basic domain structure as collagenase and stromelysin. Enamelysin (MMP-20) is restricted to dental tissues and can degrade amelogenin, the major protein component of the enamel matrix.[41] MMP-19[42] and -28[43,44] have broad tissue distributions and are closely related to each other. Because the catalytic domain of MMP-19 is able to hydrolyze a number of basement membrane proteins, and because of relatively strong expression in normal tissues, it is suggested that these enzymes may play a role in normal tissue turnover.

MMP-23, expressed predominantly in ovary, testis, and prostate, shows homologies to other MMPs in the catalytic domain but significant differences in the other domains. It lacks a signal sequence. The putative activating sequence in the prodomain contains an unpaired cyteine but is ALCLLPA instead of the conserved PRCGVPD and is followed by a furin activation sequence. The carboxyl-terminal domain is short and has no similarity to hemopexin. The recombinant enzyme has been shown to cleave peptide substrates.[45]

Adamalysins

Adamalysins are a growing family of cell surface metalloproteinases containing both a metalloproteinase and a disintegrin domain. The best characterized is TACE, the TNF-α converting enzyme. A discussion of these enzymes is beyond the scope of this chapter.

REGULATION OF MMP ACTIVITY

ECM metalloproteinase activity is modulated by gene expression, by the activation of the latent proenzymes, and by interaction with inhibitors.

Regulation of Gene Expression

Cells secrete ECM metalloproteinases in a complex pattern of response to multiple growth factors and oncogenes, indicating a corresponding complexity of gene regulation. Responses to inducers and inhibitors tend to be cell-type specific. For example, transforming growth factor beta (TGF-β) inhibits production of collagenase (MMP-1) in fibroblasts but stimulates its production in keratinocytes[15]; interferon-1 induces responses similar to TGF-β.

The genes of all the secreted MMPs, with the exception of gelatinase A, contain in their promoter regions a TATA box for binding transcription initiation factors. Enhancer elements have been identified in the 5′ untranslated portions of most MMP genes, including *PEA3, AP1, AP2,* and *SP2.* The best characterized and most universal enhancer is the 8-bp sequence TGAGTCAC, called the *activator protein-1* (AP-1) site, that binds transcription factors Fos and Jun as a heterodimer.[46] Agents such as interleukin 1 (IL-1), epidermal growth factor (EGF), platelet-derived growth factor (PDGF), tumor necrosis factor alpha (TNF-α), and the chemical tumor promoter TPA upregulate Fos and Jun proteins that in turn bind to the AP-1 sites, resulting in increased expression of MMPs. Ultraviolet light exposure upregulates collagenase in fibroblasts through an autocrine loop, generating IL-1α and basic fibroblast growth factor (bFGF), which in turn upregulates the production of Fos and Jun. Fos and Jun then bind to the AP-1 site.[46]

The AP-1 site is also crucial to glucocorticoid downregulation of MMP synthesis in fibroblasts, as shown by deletion experiments.[46] Glucocorticoids bind to receptors in the cytoplasm. The receptor-ligand complex is then transported to the nucleus, where it can act on glucocorticoid response elements in the genes. In the case of MMP repression, the receptor-ligand complex interacts with Jun, inducing a conformational change. The ability of the Jun-Fos heterodimer to bind to the AP-1 site is greatly reduced, resulting in a suppression of MMP gene transcription. Inhibition of MMP synthesis by retinoids, which have specific receptors in the nucleus, likewise appears to occur via protein interactions that ultimately decrease the binding of the Fos-Jun heterodimer to the AP-1 site.

The structure of the gelatinase A (MMP-2) promoter is completely different from that of the other secreted MMPs. It lacks a conventional TATA box, AP-1 sites, or indeed any sites common to the other MMP 5′ untranslated regions. Enhancer and silencer elements have been reported,[46] but reports of actual responses to such agents as cytokines have been inconclusive. Production of gelatinase A by fibroblasts is inhibited by glucocorticoids and retinoids, but due to the lack of an AP-1 site, the mechanism of repression is of necessity different from that of other MMPs.

The immunoglobulin superfamily is involved in MMP regulation through the extracellular matrix metalloproteinase inducer (EMMPRIN). This highly glycosylated transmembrane protein, identical to CD147 or basigin, is enriched on the surface of tumor cells. In cocultures, it stimulates fibroblasts to produce elevated levels of interstititial collagenase, gelatinase A, stromelysin-1, MT1-MMP, and MT2-MMP.[47]

The MMPs also may respond to alterations in the matrix proteins themselves via integrin and other receptors. Production of several MMPs is increased or induced by culturing cells on type I collagen,[48] although enzyme levels are further modulated by cytoskeletal alterations in the fibroblasts[15]; it has been shown that production of interstitial collagenase and stromelysin-1 is increased through the fibronectin integrin receptor.[31]

Proenzyme Activation

MMPs are synthesized as inactive proenzymes. The extent of proenzyme activation thus becomes an important element in the ultimate regulation of connective tissue turnover. In vitro activation of interstitial collagenase has been studied extensively and can be considered the model for most of the secreted MMPs. Either limited proteolysis or treatment with an organomercurial compound such as aminophenyl mercuric acetate sets up a chain of events causing conversion to the fully active form by complete removal of the propeptide.

The serine proteinase trypsin rapidly converts the latent 52-kDa procollagenase to an active 42-kDa enzyme form. The initial cleavage is made between Arg-55 and Asn-56 in the propeptide, generating a 46-kDa conversion intermediate. Further processing of this intermediate is independent of the presence of trypsin and leads to the formation of the stable 42-kDa active collagenase with Val-101 at the amino terminus.[49] The second cleavage is blocked by inhibitors of metalloproteinase activity such as EDTA and 1,10-phenanthroline, as well as the specific tissue inhibitors of metalloproteinases (TIMPs), indicating autoproteolysis.[49] Treatment with organomercurials activates the proenzyme with no initial loss in molecular mass, followed by cleavage to a 44-kDa intermediate, then finally to the 42-kDa active enzyme form, identical to the one obtained with trypsin treatment.

A satisfactory explanation for both pathways of proenzyme activation is the cysteine switch model.[50] The highly conserved propeptide sequence PRCGVPDV immediately upstream from the amino terminus of the active enzyme contains the only unpaired cysteine in the proenzyme molecule. In the latent enzyme this cysteine forms a coordination bond with the zinc atom in the active center, thus effectively chelating the metal necessary for activity. Treatment with an organomercurial compound forms a mercaptide with the cysteine residue, allowing the active center zinc to be exposed with a water molecule substituted in the coordination complex. The release of the cysteine coordination thus creates an active proteinase. Likewise, limited proteolytic cleavage within the propeptide domain allows the cysteine in this conserved PRCGVPDV sequence to be uncoordinated from the active center zinc. Again, the exposed zinc catalyzes autoproteolytic removal of the remainder of the propeptide. The transition from inactive zymogen to the enzymatically active species always involves removal of the amino-terminal propeptide. In addition, interstitial collagenase can be superactivated by proteolytic treatment with stromelysin-1 (MMP-3).[51]

With the exception of gelatinase A, all secreted MMP proenzymes can be similarly activated by serine proteinases or organomercurials. Gelatinase A (MMP-2) cannot be easily activated by serine proteinases, although the propeptide is effectively removed by the cysteine switch mechanism with organomercurials. The cell-associated MT-MMPs are believed to be the physiologic activators of this enzyme, with MT1-MMP (MMP-14) being the best understood. MT1-MMP is anchored in the plasma membrane with a short cytoplasmic tail and the active site domain oriented extracellularly.[34] It acts both as a receptor for gelatinase A (MMP-2)[52] and as a proteolytic activator. As a receptor, MT1-MMP binds the amino terminus of the inhibitor TIMP-2 to its active site. The carboxyl-terminal end of the TIMP-2 can then bind to the carboxyl terminus of progelatinase A. A neighboring MT1-MMP molecule, free of TIMP-2, proteolytically cleaves the bound progelatinase A at Asn-37–Leu-38 in the prodomain. The shortened progelatinase A molecule autocatalytically removes the remainder of the prodomain and can be released to the extracellular space.[37] Because active gelatinase A binds to $\alpha_v\beta_3$ integrin in some cells, clustering of MT1-MMP and integrins in invadopodia may cause the gelatinase A to be immediately tethered to the cell membrane.[37,53] Also noteworthy is that this activation mechanism is exquisitely sensitive to TIMP-2 concentration. At moderately low TIMP-2 concentrations, there are enough free MT1-MMP molecules to catalyze gelatinase A activation. As TIMP-2 concentration increases, MT1-MMP active sites become saturated with inhibitor (i.e., are in receptor form), and there are no working molecules to cleave the progelatinase.[52]

The cellular MT-MMPs are also produced as proenzymes. Their mode of activation is not yet fully understood, but these enzymes, as well as stromelysin-3 (MMP-11), contain a sequence susceptible to the Golgi processing enzyme furin in their propeptides.[30] Whether furin or another enzyme in that family is actually responsible for MT-MMP activation is not as yet known.

Regulation of Enzyme Activity by Inhibitors

MACROMOLECULAR INHIBITORS Once proenzymes have been activated, inhibitors can modulate proteolysis. Human serum potently inhibits MMPs; α_2-macroglobulin, a nonspecific antiproteinase, accounts for more than 95 percent of this inhibitory activity. However, because of its large size, the role of α_2-macroglobulin probably is confined to inactivation of proteinases that have gained access to the bloodstream rather than those found within the interstices of organized connective tissue. The tissue inhibitors of metalloproteinases (TIMPs) are considered to be the major tissue inhibitors.[54]

To date, four TIMPs have been described. They are small proteins, and glycosylation accounts for most of the differences in molecular weight; for example, TIMP-1 (~29 kDa) is a glycoprotein with 184 amino acids, whereas TIMP-2 (~21 kDa) is unglycosylated with 194 aminino acids All form tight 1:1 stoichiometric complexes with the active site of MMPs, and most MMPs are inhibited by all TIMPs, with some differences in binding constants. An important exception is that TIMP-1 does not inhibit MT-MMPs. The TIMPs share about 40 percent sequence homology and consist of two domains, each stabilized by three disulfide bonds. The amino-terminal domain is the inhibitory domain, as shown by using truncated molecules. The carboxy-terminal domain is involved in the binding of TIMP-1 to progelatinase B (MMP-9) and TIMP-2 and -4 to progelatinase A (MMP-2).[54,55]

TIMPs are secreted proteins, but TIMP-3 is unique in being tightly bound to the extracellular matrix. A mutation in TIMP-3 that apparently deranges the normal disulfide bonding has been correlated with Sorsby's fundus dystrophy, a rare autosomal dominant eye disease in which the structure of Bruch's membrane is compromised. TIMP-3 also differs in that it specifically inhibits TACE, the TNF-α-converting enzyme.[54]

The balance between proteolytic enzymes and their inhibitors is tightly regulated during tissue remodeling and physiologic processes. The TIMPs, like the MMPs, are regulated by various agents, although TIMP-1 is generally more responsive to cytokines than TIMP-2.[56] The responses are cell- and tissue-specific. In some cases, the regulation is coordinated with that of MMPs. For example, retinoids induce a two- to threefold increase in the production of TIMP-1 in cultured human fibroblasts, accompanied by decreased quantities of interstititial collagenase mRNA. This inverse regulation suggests tissue stabilization.[54,58]

In pathologic processes, however, the situation is not so clear. While it has been shown that overexpression of TIMPs can inhibit tumor growth, metastasis, and angiogenesis in experimental models, high levels of TIMPs in human tumors often are correlated with an adverse prognosis.[56] The paradoxical findings concerning TIMPs in disease states may reflect the fact that they have functions other than inhibitory. When TIMP-1 was first cloned, it was found identical to an erythroid-potentiating factor. Both TIMP-1 and- 2 subsequently have been shown to act as mitogens on a number of cell lines. TIMP-1 suppresses apoptosis in Burkitt's lymphoma cell lines,[59] but overexpression of TIMP-3 induces programmed cell death in some cancer cell lines.[56] These functions are independent of MMP inhibition. Furthermore, the role of TIMP-2 in progelatinase A activation may lead to either tissue destruction or maintenance depending on its level relative to MT-MMP levels (see above). The physiologic function of the progelatinase B–TIMP-1 complex described earlier is not known.

SYNTHETIC MMP INHIBITORS Crystallographic analysis is an important tool for design of specific inhibitors. High-resolution structures have been obtained for the active site domain of several MMPs, including interstitial collagenase, stromelysin-1, and MT1-MMP. All are similar oblate ellipsoids, with the active site cleft notched into the flat ellipsoid surface. All contain a structural zinc and two or three bound calciums.[3] TIMPs also have been mapped, including the TIMP-2 bound to the MT1-MMP active site and TIMP-1 bound to the stromelysin active site.[60] The hemophexin domain of gelatinase A has been crystallized[61] and shows great topologic resemblance to the hemopexin domain of the whole porcine collagenase-1 molecule. This domain consists of four blades arranged in a propeller shape and containing more bound calcium and other ions.

The first group of synthetic molecules to be used as MMP-inhibiting drugs contained a zinc-binding group, such as hydroxamate, bound to structures derived from the Leu-Ala-Gly sequence on the carboxyl-terminal side of the interstitial collagenase collagen cleavage site. Because of promising results in animal models, some molecules such as marimastat, AG3340, and BAY 12-9566 have been tested in human clinical trials against arthritis and cancer. The results generally have been disappointing because of debilitating side effects in some cases and ineffectiveness in others. However, because increased synthesis and activation of MMPs are associated with many pathologies (Table 17-2), the search for MMP-inhibiting drugs remains an active area of pharmaceutical research.

MMP PHYSIOLOGY

Evidence for the involvement of the MMPs in both normal and pathologic events has been accumulating at a logarithmic rate (see Table 17-2). In normal physiology, the appearance and disappearance of the individual enzymes and inhibitors are under rigorous temporal control. In pathologic conditions, tissue destruction that accompanies uncontrolled increase in these proteinases may lead to irreversible damage, as in tumor metastasis and aneurysms. In many cases, the severity of the inflammatory response and resulting tissue destruction may be modulated by anti-inflammatory drugs.

TABLE 17-2

Processes Known to Involve MMPs

NORMAL PHYSIOLOGY	PATHOLOGY
Wound healing	Tumor invasion and metastasis
	Osteoarthritis
Morphogenesis	Rheumatoid arthritis
	Liver fibrosis
Reproductive physiology	Atherosclerosis
	Emphysema
Immune functions	Multiple sclerosis
	Abdominal aneurysms
Angiogenesis	Corneal ulcerations
	Dermatitis herpetiformis
	Sorsby's fundus dystrophy
	Bullous pemphigoid
	Recessive dystrophic epidermolysis bullosa
	Acute lichen planus
	Periodontal disease
	Inflammation
	Restenosis
	Multicentric osteolysis

Normal Functions of MMPs

The discovery of interstitial collagenase in the resorbing tissue of the metamorphosing tadpole established a role for MMPs in development. The rise and fall of specific MMPs and their inhibitors has been documented carefully for invasive and remodeling events ranging from implantation to angiogenesis.[62] For example, in the development of human skin, epidermal cells and appendageal buds express matrilysin during mesenchymal invasion.[30] Later in embryogenesis, matrilysin is concentrated only in cells at the distal portion of invading hair follicles and sweat gland appendageal cords. In adult skin, matrilysin is found only in the sweat glands.[29] Gelatinase A can be localized to the stroma directly under developing appendageal cords and is correlated with loss of type VII collagen from the basement membrane zone.[63] Given the precision of these enzymatic appearances, it is quite puzzling that genetic knockout mice lacking specific MMPs develop nearly normally and are fertile. Only mice lacking MT1-MMP (MMP-14) have severe skeletal defects that lead to death in early adulthood.[64] It is hypothesized that because the secreted MMPs have overlapping specificities, one proteinase can substitute for another.

Although expressed at very low levels in normal adult tissues, MMPs become dramatically increased during connective tissue remodeling. The precise enzymes expressed are regulated in a time-dependent and cell-specific manner. The orchestration of the rise and fall of MMPs and their inhibitors is exemplified by recent investigations of wound healing and of the menstrual cycle. In wound healing, keratinocytes migrating over the wound area acquire mRNA for interstitial collagenase (MMP-1) and stromelysin-2 (MMP-10) when they come in contact with the dermal type I collagen. The migrating keratinocytes do not express TIMP. Stromelysin-1 (MMP-3) is expressed by keratinocytes still in contact with basement membrane in the proliferative area just behind the migrating front. With wound closure, keratinocytes ceases production of these enzymes.[15]

MMPs in the cycling endometrium rise and fall with the menstrual cycle. Gelatinase A and TIMP-1 mRNAs are present at all times. Messenger RNAs for matrilysin (MMP-7) in the epithelium and stromelysin-3 (MMP-11) in the stroma are found in all phases except early secretory. All enzymes investigated—interstitial collagenase; gelatinases A and B; stromelysin-1, -2, and -3; and matrilysin—are produced in the menstrual phase, undoubtedly playing a role in tissue sloughing.[65]

It has long been known that interstitial collagenase (MMP-1) rises dramatically in the postpartum uterus,[13,17] enabling postpartum uterine resorption. In mice, matrilysin (MMP-7), stromelysin-2 (MMP-10), and collagenase-3 (MMP-13) are all elevated in involuting uterus, but matrilysin-deficient mice involute normally. In these mice, other MMPs are elevated during involution, lending substance to the theory that functionally many of these enzymes are interchangeable.[66] Interstitial collagenase, stromelysin-1 (MMP-3), and matrilysin are expressed at high levels in the trophoblast; gelatinase A (MMP-2) and MTI-MMP (MMP-14) appear to be expressed coordinately at the site of implantation.

The immune response involves release of MMPs. Stimulated macrophages release relatively large quantities of interstitial collagenage, stromelysin-1, matrilysin, metalloelastase (MMP-12), and gelatinase B (MMP-9),[67] contributing to connective tissue remodeling. T cells release low levels of the gelatinases, perhaps facilitating their migration through connective tissues. The MMPs released during the inflammatory response are able to cleave TNF-α from its membrane-bound precursor, presumably leading to an augmentation loop of proteolytic activity. MMP inhibitors are able to prevent the release of TNF-α and have a protective effect against septic shock.

MMPs in Disease

TUMOR INVASION AND METASTASIS Both in vitro and in vivo, tumor invasion and metastasis are consistently correlated with increased levels of MMPs. There is great variation in the specific enzymes overexpressed in different tumors, depending on tissue of origin and tumor type. Gelatinases A and B (MMP-2 and -9), matrilysin (MMP-7), stromelysin-3 (MMP-11), and MT1-MMP (MMP-14) have been reported elevated most often, but studies of the more recently discovered MMPs may change this generalization. Within the tumor itself, the MMPs are distributed in a cell-specific manner. For example, in human breast cancer,[68] only matrilysin is produced by epithelial cells, with gelatinase A, stromelysin-3, and MT1-MMP localized to stromal fibroblasts, although having different distribution patterns. Gelatinase B is found only in endothelial and inflammatory cells. Elevated MMP levels are considered prognostic indicators in many instances; expression of interstitial collagenase, for example, is associated with poor prognosis in esophageal and colorectal cancers. In squamous cell carcinomas (SCC), stromelysin-3 is associated with local invasiveness in the head and neck, whereas the level of gelatinase A expression correlates with the prognosis for cervical SCC. Overexpression of collagenase-3 in SCCs of head, neck, and vulva correlates with increased metastasis.

The complexity of the physiologic role of MMPs in tumor invasion and metastasis is just beginning to be understood. Given the ability of these enzymes to digest all components of extracelluar matrix, it has long been felt that their main function is to create spaces for growing tumors and pathways for metastasizing cells. From the first observation that the ability to digest type IV collagen was correlated with metastatic capacity in melanoma cells,[69] experimental data have substantiated the importance of proteolytic activity.[37,70] In melanoma cell lines, active gelatinase A is present only in highly invasive cells lines; the activation is attributed to the expression of MT1-MMP.[71] Conversely, increasing inhibitiory potential by transfection of TIMP-1 into melanoma or *ras*-transformed fibroblasts inhibits invasion and metastasis in vivo.[72] Transfection of a single MMP gene into tumor lines has been shown to affect their invasive and metastatic properties. When a normal mouse mammary epithelial cell line was induced to make stromelysin, the cells became tumorigenic and invasive.[73]

Close examination has revealed that MMPs may affect tumor growth itself. Transfection of a normally matrilysin-negative colon carcinoma cell line with the matrilysin gene increased its tumorigenicity in nude mice; transfection of antisense matrilysin into a matrilysin-positive colon carcinoma cell line reduced its tumorigenicity and subequent metastasis to the liver.[74] Likewise, melanoma cells made to overexpress TIMP-1 were shown to extravasate and form lung colonies when injected into nude mice, but the colonies were extremely small.[70] It is quite possible that MMP effects on tumor growth have to do with release of growth factors stored in the extracelluar matrix. For example, digestion of decorin by stromelysin generates TFG-β, which affects cell proliferation and angiogenesis. MMPs can release insulin-like growth factor (IGF) from inhibitory association with IGF-binding proteins. Angiogenesis, which is necessary for tumor maintenance, seems to require MT-MMP and gelatinase A activity; synthetic MMP inhibitors have been shown to inhibit tumor angiogenesis.

MMPs are able to digest proteins other than ECM structural proteins. Different enzymes have been reported to cleave serpins, E-cadherin, and other MMPs. They can digest integrins and thus disrupt cell-matrix attachments, leading to a promigratory phenotype. Proteolysis of some matrix components is also promigratory. Digestion of laminin-5 by gelatinase A generates a cleavage product that promotes keratinocyte migration.[70]

Knockout and transgenic mice have underscored the importance of MMPs in tumor invasion and metastasis. When a strain of mice with a genetic predisposition to intestinal tumors was made matrilysin null, tumors decreased 58 percent.[74] Gelatinase A–deficient mice show reduced angiogenesis, tumor growth, and metastasis in response to injected Lewis lung carcinoma and B16-BL6 melanoma cells.[75] Gelatinase B knockout mice also show reduced tumor growth, probably due to impaired angiogensis.[62] Mice lacking stromelysin-3 have a lowered tumorigenic response to chemical mutagenesis. Transgenic mice in which stromelysin is overexpressed in mammary glands show increased premalignant changes and malignant conversions.[73]

Although the discovery of new MMPs still progresses at a rapid rate, understanding of their function remains a challenge. For example, a puzzling recent discovery is the existence of a human knockout syndrome, in which three families with inherited multicentric osteolysis were found to be gelatinase A (MMP-2) null. One mutation in the enzyme showed an early stop codon, whereas another was a single base substitution leading to a nonfunctional protein.[76] The osteolytic phenotype seems counterintuitive to lack of proteolytic capacity; it has been suggested that decreased TGF-β processing in the absence of gelatinase A may be responsible for the numerous bone problems seen in these patients.[77]

MMP inhibitors have been shown to reduce tumor growth and metastasis in a number of animals models. For example, batimastat inhibits local invasive growth and spread of human colorectal carcinoma implanted into mice. However, human clinical trials thus far have proved disappointing. Many patients develop dose-limiting side effects from some of the inhibitors. Other potential drugs are less effective than placebo in treating the late-stage cancers against which they have been used. Evidence seems to be accumulating that the most effective use of these drugs will be as an adjuctive therapy in early stages of the disease.

ARTHRITIS The extensive tissue destruction in osteoarthritis and rheumatoid arthritis is accompanied by high levels of both interstitial collagenase (MMP-1) and stromelysin-1 (MMP-3). In cells such as those in proliferating rheumatoid synovial tissue, the mRNAs for these two proteinases may represent as much as 2 percent of the total mRNAs. The mRNA is accompanied by a high concentration of the secreted proteins. Cartilage extracts from patients with these diseases also show high levels of these enzymes, and the level of enzyme activity correlates with the severity of the disease. In addition, synovial fluid from osteoarthritic patients shows higher than normal levels of these enzymes.[78]

Because of its preferential cleavage of type II collagen, it is speculated that collagenase-3 (MMP-13) plays an important role in arthritis. It has been found expressed in the synovial membranes of patients with both osteoarthritis and rheumatoid arthritis.[79] Surprisingly, in cell culture, the enzyme is expressed by chondrocytes but not synoviocytes; it has been detected in articular cartilage from osteoarthritic but not normal patients.[78,80]

OTHER DISEASES Diseases in which MMPs have been implicated are listed in Table 17-2. It is safe to conclude that MMPs are elevated in any conditions in which connective tissue architecture is deranged, from corneal ulcerations to abdominal aortic aneurisms. Wherever inflammatory infiltrates are present, proteolytic enzymes that can destroy ECM are likely to be released. In addition, any situation in which cytokines such as IL-1 or TNF-α are released likely will result in elevated levels of MMPs.

CONCLUSIONS AND FUTURE DIRECTIONS

Although many questions remain unanswered about MMPs and their inhibitors, their involvement in the maintenance and remodeling of connective tissue seems well established. The discovery that MMPs can cleave TNF-α from its membrane-bound precursor and that an MMP inhibitor was able to protect mice from a lethal dose of endotoxin by inhibiting TNF-α processing and release opens up new classes of physiologic processes in which MMPs may be involved. Indeed, the cellular localization of the newest subfamily, the MT-MMPs, and the discovery of intracellular processing of gelatinase A in normal cells[81] raise the possibility of implicating MMPs in cytoskeletal rearrangements and other intracellular events. Finally, the development of specific inhibitors based on crystallographic structures will be an important tool in evaluating the roles of the different MMPs in both physiologic and pathologic processes. These specific inhibitors could lead to new classes of drugs useful in the treatment of the many diseases in which MMPs are involved.

REFERENCES

1. Murphy G et al: Evaluation of some newer matrix metalloproteinases. *Ann NY Acad Sci* **878**:25, 1999
2. Nagase H, Woessner JF Jr: Matrix metalloproteinases. *J Biol Chem* **274**:21491, 1999
3. Bode W et al: Structural properties of matrix metalloproteinases. *Cell Mol Life Sci* **55**:639, 1999
4. Uria JA, Lopez-Otin C: Matrilysin-2, a new matrix metalloproteinase expressed in human tumors and showing the minimal domain organization required for secretion, latency, and activity. *Cancer Res* **60**:4745, 2000
5. Huhtala P et al: Completion of the primary structure of the human type IV collagenase preproenzyme and assignment of the gene (CLG4) to the q21 region of chromosome 16. *Genomics* **6**:554, 1990
6. Gross J, Lapiere CM: Collagenolytic activity in amphibian tissues: A tissue culture assay. *Proc Natl Acad Sci USA* **54**:1197, 1962
7. Eisen AZ et al: Human skin collagenase: Isolation and mechanism of attack on the collagen molecule. *Biochem Biophys Acta* **151**:637, 1968
8. Bauer EA et al: Collagenase production by human skin fibroblasts. *Biochem Biophys Res Commun* **64**:232, 1975
9. Wilhelm SM et al: Human fibroblast collagenase: Glycosylation and tissue-specific levels of enzyme synthesis. *Proc Natl Acad Sci USA* **83**:3756, 1986
10. Seltzer JL et al: Cleavage of type VII collagen by interstitial collagenase and type IV collagenase (gelatinase) derived from human skin. *J Biol Chem* **264**:3822, 1989
11. Freije JM et al: Molecular cloning and expression of collagenase-3, a novel human matrix metalloproteinase produced by breast carcinomas. *J Biol Chem* **269**:16766, 1994
12. Wilhelm SM et al: Human skin fibroblast stromelysin: Structure, glycosylation, substrate specificity, and differential expression in normal and tumorigenic cells. *Proc Natl Acad Sci USA* **84**:6725, 1987
13. Wu JJ et al: Sites of stromelysin cleavage in collagen types II, IX, X, and XI of cartilage. *J Biol Chem* **266**:5625, 1991
14. Bord S et al: Stromelysin-1 (MMP-3) and stromelysin-2 (MMP-10) expression in developing human bone: Potential roles in skeletal development. *Bone* **23**:7, 1998.
15. Parks WC et al: Matrix metalloproteinases in tissue repair, in *Matrix Metalloproteinases,* edited by WC Parks, RW Mecham. San Diego, Academic Press, p 263
16. Basset P et al: A novel metalloproteinase gene specifically expressed in stromal cells of breast carcinomas. *Nature* **348**:699, 1990
17. Pei D et al: Hydrolytic inactivation of a breast carcinoma cell–derived serpin by human stromelysin-3. *J Biol Chem* **269**:25849, 1994
18. Noel A et al: Identification of structural determinants controlling human and mouse stromelysin-3 proteolytic activities. *J Biol Chem* **270**:22866, 1995
19. Pei D, Weiss SJ: Furin-dependent intracellular activation of the human stromelysin-3 zymogen. *Nature* **375**:244, 1995
20. Salo T et al: Purification and characterization of a murine basement membrane collagen-degrading enzyme secreted by metastatic tumor cells. *J Biol Chem* **258**:3058, 1983
21. Collier IE et al: H-*ras* oncogene–transformed human bronchial epithelial cells (TBE-1) secrete a single metalloprotease capable of degrading basement membrane collagen. *J Biol Chem* **263**:6579, 1988
22. Seltzer JL et al: Purification and properties of a gelatin-specific neutral protease from human skin. *J Biol Chem* **256**:4662, 1981
23. Xia T et al: Comparison of cleavage site specificity of gelatinases A and B using collagenous peptides. *Biochem Biophys Acta* **1293**:259, 1996
24. Wilhelm SM et al: SV40-transformed human lung fibroblasts secrete a 92-kDa type IV collagenase which is identical to that secreted by normal human macrophages. *J Biol Chem* **264**:17213, 1989
25. Collier IE et al: Alanine scanning mutagenesis and functional analysis of the fibronectin-like collagen-binding domain from human 92-kDa type IV collagenase. *J Biol Chem* **267**:6776, 1992
26. Collier IE et al: Substrate recognition by gelatinase A: The C-terminal domain facilitates surface diffusion. *Biophys J* **81**:2370, 2001
27. Stetler-Stevenson WG et al: Tissue inhibitor of metalloproteinase (TIMP-2): A new member of the metalloproteinase inhibitor family. *J Biol Chem* **264**:17374, 1989
28. Wilson CL, Matrisian LM: Matrilysin: An epithelial matrix metalloproteinase with potentially novel functions. *Int J Biochem Cell Biol* **28**:123, 1996
29. Parks WC, Sires UI: Matrix metalloproteinases in skin biology and disease. *Curr Opin Dermatol* **3**:240, 1995
30. Karelina TV et al: Matrilysin (PUMP) correlates with dermal invasion during appendageal development and cutaneous neoplasia. *J Invest Dermatol* **103**:482, 1994
31. MacDougall JR, Matrisian LM: Contributions of tumor and stromal matrix metalloproteinases to tumor progression, invasion and metastasis. *Cancer Metastas Rev* **14**:351, 1995
32. Park HI et al: Identification and characterization of human endometase (matrix metalloproteinase-26) from endometrial tumor. *J Biol Chem* **275**:20540, 2000
33. de Coignac AB et al: Cloning of MMP-26: A novel matrilysin-like proteinase. *Eur J Biochem* **267**:3323, 2000
34. Sato H et al: A matrix metalloproteinase expressed on the surface of invasive tumour cells. *Nature* **370**:61, 1994
35. Velasco G et al: Human MT6-matrix metalloproteinase: Identification, progelatinase A activation, and expression in brain tumors. *Cancer Res* **60**:877, 2000
36. Llano E et al: Identification and characterization of human MT5-MMP, a new membrane-bound activator of progelatinase A overexpressed in brain tumors. *Cancer Res* **59**:2570, 1999
37. Ellerbroek SM, Stack MS: Membrane-associated matrix metalloproteinases in metastasis. *Bioessays* **21**:940, 1999
38. Okada A et al: Membrane-type matrix metalloproteinase (MT-MMP) gene is expressed in stromal cells of human colon, breast, and head and neck carcinomas. *Proc Natl Acad Sci USA* **92**:2730, 1995
39. Shapiro SD: Elastolytic metalloproteinases produced by human mononuclear phagocytes: Potential roles in destructive lung disease. *Am J Respir Crit Care Med* **150**:S160, 1994
40. Shapiro SD: Mighty mice: Transgenic technology "knocks out" questions of matrix metalloproteinase function. *Matrix Biol* **15**:527, 1997

41. Llano E et al: Identification and structural and functional characterization of human enamelysin (MMP-20). *Biochemistry* **36**:15101, 1997
42. Stracke JO et al: Biochemical characterization of the catalytic domain of human matrix metalloproteinase 19: Evidence for a role as a potent basement membrane degrading enzyme. *J Biol Chem* **275**:14809, 2000
43. Marchenko GN, Strongin AY: MMP-28, a new human matrix metalloproteinase with an unusual cysteine-switch sequence is widely expressed in tumors. *Gene* **265**:87, 2001
44. Lohi J et al: Epilysin, a novel human matrix metalloproteinase (MMP-28) expressed in testis and keratinocytes and in response to injury. *J Biol Chem* **276**:10134, 2001
45. Velasco G et al: Cloning and characterization of human MMP-23, a new matrix metalloproteinase predominantly expressed in reproductive tissues and lacking conserved domains in other family members. *J Biol Chem* **274**:4570, 1999
46. Fini ME et al: Regulation of matrix metalloproteinase gene expression, in *Matrix Metalloproteinases*, edited by WC Parks, RW Mecham. San Diego, Academic Press, p 299
47. Sameshima T et al: Glioma cell extracellular matrix metalloproteinase inducer (EMMPRIN) (CD147) stimulates production of membrane-type matrix metalloproteinases and activated gelatinase A in co-cultures with brain-derived fibroblasts. *Cancer Lett* **157**:177, 2000
48. Lee AY et al: Intracellular activation of gelatinase A (72-kDa type IV collagenase) by normal fibroblasts. *Proc Natl Acad Sci USA* **94**:4424, 1997
49. Grant GA et al: The activation of human fibroblast procollagenase: Sequence identification of the major conversion products. *J Biochem* **262**:5886, 1986
50. Birkedal-Hansen H: Proteolytic remodeling of extracellular matrix. *Curr Opin Cell Biol* **7**:728, 1995
51. He CS et al: Tissue cooperation in a proteolytic cascade activating human interstitial collagenase. *Proc Natl Acad Sci USA:* **86**:2632, 1989
52. Strongin AY et al: Mechanism of cell surface activation of 72-kDa type IV collagenase: Isolation of the activated form of the membrane metalloprotease. *J Biol Chem* **270**:5331, 1995
53. Murphy G, Gavrilovic J: Proteolysis and cell migration: Creating a path? *Curr Opin Biol* **11**:614, 1999
54. Brew K et al: Tissue inhibitors of metalloproteinases: Evolution, structure and function. *Biochem Biophys Acta* **1477**:267, 2000.
55. Nagase H et al: Engineering of selective TIMPS. *Ann NY Acad Sci* **878:**1, 1999
56. Gomez DE et al: Tissue inhibitors of metalloproteinases: Structure, regulation and biological functions. *Eur J Cell Biol* **74**:111, 1997
57. Clark SD et al: Regulation of the expression of tissue inhibitor of metalloproteinases and collagenase by retinoids and glucocorticoids in human fibroblasts. *J Clin Invest* **80**:1280, 1987
58. Mauviel A, et al: Cell-specific induction of distinct oncogenes of the *jun* family is responsible for differential regulation of collagenase gene expression by transforming growth factor-beta in fibroblasts and keratinocytes. *J Biol Chem* **271**: 10917, 1996
59. Guedez L et al: In vitro suppression of programmed cell death of B cells by tissue inhibitor of metalloproteinases-1. *J Clin Invest* **102**:2002, 1998
60. Bode W, Huber R: Structural basis of the endoproteinase-protein inhibitor interaction. *Biochem Biophys Acta* **1477**:241, 2000
61. Libson AM et al: Crystal structure of the haemopexin-like C-terminal domain of gelatinase A. *Nature Struct Biol* **2**:938, 1995
62. Werb Z et al: Matrix-degrading proteases and angiogenesis during development and tumor formation. *APMIS* **107**: 11, 1999
63. Karelina TV et al: Basement membrane zone remodeling during appendageal development in human fetal skin: The absence of type VII collagen is associated with gelatinase-A (MMP2) activity. *J Invest Dermatol* **114**:371, 2000
64. Holmbeck K et al: MT1-MMP–deficient mice develop dwarfism, osteopenia, arthritis, and connective tissue disease due to inadequate collagen turnover. *Cell* **99**:81, 1999
65. Rodgers WH et al: Patterns of matrix metalloproteinase expression in cycling endometrium imply differential functions and regulation by steroid hormones. *J Clin Invest* **94**:946, 1994
66. Fata JE et al: Cellular turnover and extracellular matrix remodeling in female reproductive tissues: Functions of metalloproteinases and their inhibitors. *Cell Mol Life Sci* **57**:77, 2000
67. Goetzl EJ et al: Matrix metalloproteinases in immunity. *J Immunol* **156**:1, 1996
68. Heppner KJ et al: Expression of most matrix metalloproteinase family members in breast cancer represents a tumor-induced host response. *Am J Pathol* **149**:273, 1996
69. Liotta LA et al: Metastatic potential correlates with enzymatic degradation of basement membrane collagen. *Nature* **284**:67, 1980
70. McCawley LJ, Matrisian LM: Matrix metalloproteinases: Multifunctional contributors to tumor progression. *Mol Med Today* **6**:149, 2000
71. Hofmann UB et al: Matrix metalloproteinases in human melanoma. *J Invest Dermatol* **115**:337, 2000
72. Ray JM, Stetler-Stevenson WG: The role of matrix metalloproteases and their inhibitors in tumour invasion, metastasis and angiogenesis. *Eur Respir J* **7**:2062, 1994
73. Sternlicht MD et al: The stromal proteinase MMP3/stromelysin-1 promotes mammary carcinogenesis. *Cell* **98**:137, 1999
74. Fingleton BM et al: Matrilysin in early stage intestinal tumorigenesis. *APMIS* **107**:102, 1999
75. Westermarck J, Kahari VM: Regulation of matrix metalloproteinase expression in tumor invasion (review). *FASEB J* **13**:781, 1999
76. Martignetti JA et al: Mutation of the matrix metalloproteinase 2 gene (MMP2) causes a multicentric osteolysis and arthritis syndrome. *Nature Genet* **28**:261, 2001
77. Vu TH: Don't mess with the matrix. *Nature Genet* **28**:202, 2001
78. Smith RL: Degradative enzymes in osteoarthritis. *Frontiers Biosci* **4**:D704, 1999
79. Wernicke D et al: Cloning of collagenase 3 from the synovial membrane and its expression in rheumatoid arthritis and osteoarthritis. *J Rheumatol* **23**:590, 1996
80. Reboul P et al: The new collagenase, collagenase-3, is expressed and synthesized by human chondrocytes but not by synoviocytes: A role in osteoarthritis. *J Clin Invest* **97**:2011, 1996
81. Karelina TV et al: Localization of 92-kDa type IV collagenase in human skin tumors: Comparison with normal human fetal and adult skin. *J Invest Dermatol* **100**:159, 1993

CHAPTER 18

Richard L. Gallo
Janet M. Trowbridge

Proteoglycans and Glycosaminoglycans of Skin

Proteoglycans and their glycosaminoglycan components constitute a considerable portion of the cellular membrane and extracellular milieu of the skin. Their ability to bind and alter protein–protein interactions or enzymatic activity has identified them as important determinants of cellular responsiveness in development, homeostasis, and disease. Because proteoglycans are a structurally unique and highly diverse group of macromolecules, it is important to become familiar with their structure and organization to understand their function. The most distinguishing structural characteristic of proteoglycans is that they comprise both a core protein and covalently linked linear carbohydrate chains known as glycosaminoglycans (GAGs). GAGs are highly polyanionic and bear the highest charge density of any vertebrate macromolecule. It has long been recognized that GAGs are a major component of the skin. More recently, it has been appreciated that the content and composition of GAGs in the skin can change during development and a variety of pathologic processes, and that both core protein and GAGs impart a unique set of functions that are critical to a large number of biologic processes.

STRUCTURE AND NOMENCLATURE

In the past, terms such as *ground substance* or *mucopolysaccharide* were used to describe proteoglycans because of their appearance histologically and their thick and mucinous nature when isolated. Because of these physical properties, proteoglycans were difficult to study and poorly understood. Glycobiology has clearly defined proteoglycans as essential regulatory molecules that control many cellular functions. To attain this understanding, important advances have been made in the identification of specific proteoglycan core proteins and the assembly of their GAG side chains.

Proteoglycans are known by specific gene families based on amino acid sequence information derived from their core proteins and carbohydrate compositional analysis of their GAG side chains. The prototypical proteoglycan consists of a single core protein linked to one or more GAGs (Fig. 18-1). Each core protein has the capacity to accept a variety of GAG chains. Therefore, the nomenclature for proteoglycans is complicated in that individual molecules must be defined based on the core protein and the associated GAGs.

THE GAG CHAIN

The GAG chain is defined based on the assembly of essential sugar residues. These sugars are organized as disaccharide pairs that usually consist of an acidic sugar that is either an iduronic acid or glucuronic acid alternating with a hexosamine that is either glucosamine or galactosamine. When assembled as disaccharides, the choice of sugars and the linkage between them is used to assign a name to the GAG chain. Thus, several terms are used to define GAGs (Fig. 18-1*B*), including hyaluronic acid, containing a glucuronic acid alternating with *N*-acetylglucosamine linked β1–3 and β1–4; heparan sulfate, containing iduronic or glucuronic acids alternating with *N*-acetylglucosamine linked β1–4; chondroitin sulfate, containing glucuronic acid alternating with *N*-acetylgalactosamine linked β1–3 and β1–4; and keratan sulfate, containing galactose alternating with *N*-acetylglucosamine linked β1–4 and β1–3 (not shown). A fifth general term used to describe GAGs, and of particular importance to cutaneous biology, is *dermatan sulfate*. This form of GAG (also known as chondroitin sulfate B) is similar to other chondroitin sulfates except that it contains a high proportion of iduronic acids in place of glucuronic acid and has more variable sulfation. Dermatan sulfate shares features of both chondroitin sulfate (*N*-acetyl galactosamine) and heparan sulfate (iduronate) (Fig. 18-1*B*).

The nomenclature described above for GAGs only partly defines the nature of these molecules. The linear chains of linked disaccharide units in a GAG are highly variable in size, ranging from as few as 10 disaccharides to several thousand. Thus, the mass of naturally occurring GAGs typically ranges between 5×10^3 daltons and 10^7 daltons for hyaluronic acid. Further variability is introduced into the GAG chain by epimerization reactions and sulfation reactions. The control of these reactions depends both on the nature of the GAG, the core protein to which it may be attached, the cell type, and the cell environment. For example, the simplest GAG, hyaluronic acid, is never sulfated. Other GAGs can be variably sulfated. Heparan sulfate can be sulfated at the N, C-2, and C-6 positions of *N*-acetylglucosamine and at the C-2 position of iduronic acid. Dermatan sulfate can be sulfated at C-2 of iduronate and at C-4 and C-6 of *N*-acetylgalactosamine. These highly sulfated sugars tend to occur in specific regions of the GAG chain and are interspersed with areas of low sulfation. Such discreet domains of low or high sulfation are believed to determine the interactions between proteoglycans and glycosaminoglycans and their many binding partners.

In heparan sulfate from human dermal fibroblasts, the highly sulfated regions resemble the sulfation found in heparin, which are responsible for the anticoagulant activity of heparin. However, heparin lacks the regions of low sulfation found in heparan sulfate. Thus, it is important to distinguish heparin from heparan sulfate for both functional and structural considerations.

The size, disaccharide composition, and sulfation are of utmost importance in understanding GAGs. These parameters influence function and are the mechanism by which instructions are defined within the molecule. Thus, the linear GAG should be considered as a molecule containing information similar to the way information is encoded in a protein. GAG synthesis (with the exception of hyaluronan) occurs in the Golgi apparatus. Sequence information is determined by the activity and location of multiple specific enzymes along this pathway. Today, many of the synthetic enzymes that control heparan sulfate synthesis and those enzymes responsible for postsynthetic modifications have been identified and characterized.[1] The sulfated GAGs are all synthesized on core proteins. The tetrasaccharide xylose, galactose, galactose, glucuronic acid is first assembled on the core protein by beginning with a xylosyltransferase forming a linkage between xylose and a serine residue in the core protein. Subsequent elongation reactions that occur in the Golgi apparatus define the nature of the GAG chain. It is appreciated that part of the information necessary to direct synthesis of the GAG is encoded within the core protein sequence itself. The final product, core protein with attached GAG, defines the proteoglycan (see Fig. 18-1*A*). Hyaluronan, the only GAG produced without attachment to a core protein, is synthesized by an enzyme complex at the plasma membrane and then extruded into the extracellular space.

FIGURE 18-1

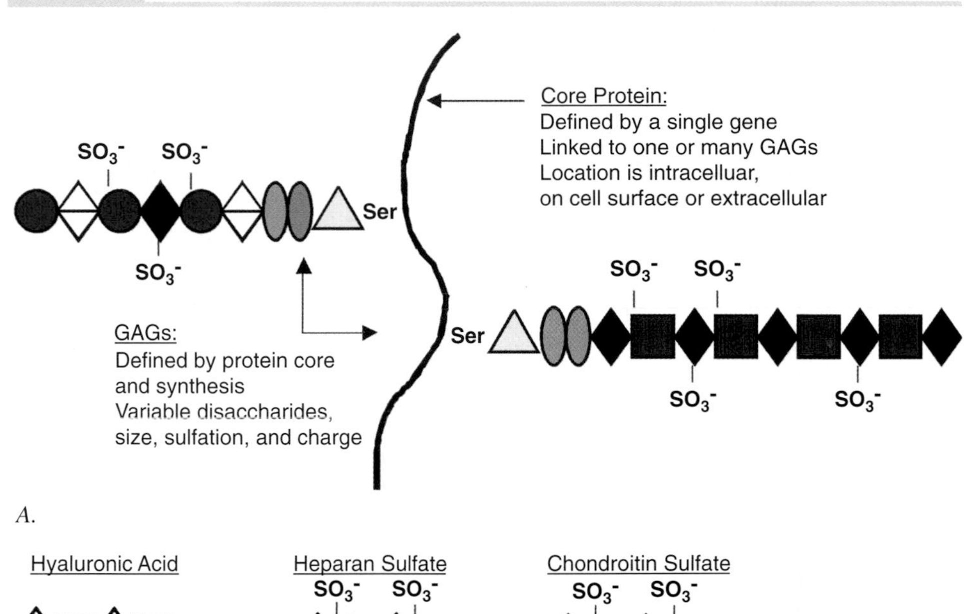

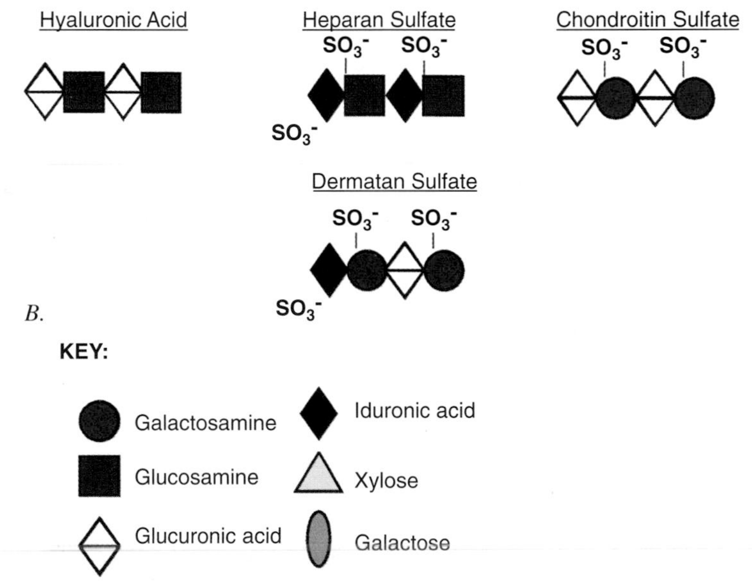

A. Prototype of proteoglycan structure. Core proteins may contain from 1 to 100 glycosaminoglycan (GAG) chains, depending on the core protein sequence. Two different GAG chains are shown: dermatan sulfate (*top left*) and heparan sulfate (*bottom right*). Sites of potential sulfation are indicated. Ser represents a serine amino acid residue in the core protein to which GAGs are attached. *B*. Disaccharide repeating units of glycosaminoglycans shown as tetrasaccharides. Structures of heparan sulfate, dermatan sulfate, chondroitin sulfate A/C, and hyaluronan are shown. Sulfation can vary in heparan sulfate and dermatan sulfate. Chondroitin sulfate A is chondroitin 4-sulfate. Chondroitin sulfate C is chondroitin 6-sulfate.

THE CORE PROTEIN

Our understanding of proteoglycans has advanced dramatically as a result of increased information about their core proteins and the subsequent use of molecular tools to study the expression and function of both the protein core and GAG components. Many specific proteoglycans can now be defined and studied based on their core protein sequence. For purposes of organization, it is useful to group proteoglycans based on their site of expression by the cell. Specific proteoglycan core proteins have been identified within the cell, attached to the cell surface, bound within the extracellular matrix, and released in soluble form (Table 18-1).

Serglycin is the best known intracellular proteoglycan and is found within the secretory granules of hematopoietic cells including mast cells, leukocytes, and eosinophils. This core protein is processed further to contain either heparan sulfate or chondroitin sulfate GAG. The heparan sulfate form is found in serosal mast cells and is a major source from which heparin is pharmacologically derived. The serglycin peptide core is composed primarily of tandem serine-glycine repeats and has an estimated mass of 16 to 18 kDa before GAG addition and 60 to 750 kDa after the addition of multiple heterogenous GAG chains.[2] Thus, serglycin is a unique proteoglycan because of its distinctive core protein sequence and intracellular localization. In the skin, serglycin is found whenever mast cells or eosinophils enter the dermal stroma. Upon release, serglycin becomes a major source for delivery of highly sulfated heparan sulfate GAG.

Several cell surface proteoglycans have been identified and are the subject of much recent interest because of their ability to function at the interface between the plasma membrane and the extracellular environment. These cell proteoglycans can be found attached to the cell surface either by a phospholipid anchor (e.g., glypican family) or as membrane-spanning core proteins (e.g., syndecan family). The mammalian glypican family is currently known to consist of six distinct proteins: glypican, cerebroglycan, OCI-5, K-glypican, glypican-5, and glypican-6.[3] This family of core proteins shares the glycophosphatidyl inositol (GPI) anchorage mechanism and a unique cysteine motif that is likely to impart a compact tertiary structure to the proteoglycans. Consequently, glypicans can be visualized as a compact protein presenting GAG chains in close proximity to the outer surface of the plasma membrane. Individual members of the glypican family have been identified in a variety of cells and tissues, including lung, kidney, brain, and intestine.[4,5]

TABLE 18-1

Core Proteins of Proteoglycans

CORE PROTEIN	LOCATION	USUAL GAG COMPONENT
Intracellular		
Serglycin	Mast cells, basophils	HS CS
Cell Surface		
Syndecan-1	Keratinocytes, other epithelia	HS CS
Syndecan-2	Fibroblasts, endothelia, bone	HS
Syndecan-3	Neural cells, limbs	HS
Syndecan-4	Ubiquitous, lymphoid	HS CS
NG-2	Neural, melanoma	CS
Glypican (GPC-1)	Brain, vascular endothelia	HS
Cerebroglycan (GPC-2)	Brain only	HS
OCI-5 (GPC-3)	Intestine and mesenchymal	HS
K-glypican (GPC-4)	Kidney, brain	HS
Glypican-5 (GPC-5)	Brain, kidney, bone	HS
Glypican-6 (GPC-6)	Intestine, kidney, lung	HS
Epican	Keratinocytes	HS CS KS
Betaglycan	Fibroblasts, epithelia	HS
Endocan	Endothelia	DS
Thrombomodulin	Endothelia	DS
Extracellular Matrix		
Aggracan	Cartilage	KS CS
Versican	Fibroblasts	CS DS
Brevican	Brain	CS
Neurocan	Brain	CS
Phosphocan	Brain	CS KS
Decorin	Fibroblasts, others	DS
Biglycan	Bone	DS
Epiphycan	Cartilage	DS
OIF	Cartilage	
Fibromodulin	Fibroblasts	KS
Lumican	Cornea	KS
Agrin	Brain	HS
Perlecan	Basement membranes	HS
Bamacan	Basement membranes	CS

CS, chondroitin sulfate; HS, heparan sulfate; KS, keratan sulfate.

The surface of most cells contains another important family of proteoglycans known as the syndecans. Syndecans, like glypicans, are found in a wide variety of cells and tissues. The structure of these cell surface proteoglycans differs from that of the glypicans. Syndecan core proteins consist of a short C-terminal cytoplasmic region, a transmembrane domain, and an extracellular region containing attachment sites for GAG chains. Unlike glypicans, syndecans span the plasma membrane and extend beyond the surface of the cell. In this way, syndecans are in a unique position to connect extracellular GAG to structures within the cytoplasmic space. The cytoplasmic domain imparts the ability of syndecans to participate in intracellular signal transduction via the protein kinase C pathway. Expression of syndecans is abundant in skin. Syndecan transcripts and proteins are expressed in distinct patterns during development[6] and in mature tissues.[7] Syndecan-1 is particularly abundant on keratinocytes and can vary the nature of attached GAG chains as keratinocytes differentiate.[8] During wound repair, syndecans-1 and -4 are greatly induced in the dermis and granulation tissue.[9] Deletion of syndecan-4 from mice greatly decreases the rate of wound repair.[10] During malignant transformation, syndecan-1 expression decreases in the epidermis[11] and expression can alter malignant behavior in select cell types.[12] Thus, syndecans have received particular attention as proteoglycans that modify cell function. Because syndecans and other proteoglycans can contain more than one GAG species either simultaneously or under different cellular circumstances, GAG expression in addition to protein expression provides an additional mechanism of regulation.

Two other cell surface proteoglycans are worth special mention. Epican and betaglycan are examples of cell surface proteins that are "part-time" proteoglycans. Epican, a splice variant of the cell surface molecule CD44 that can exist as a heparan, chondroitin, or keratin sulfate proteoglycan, mediates cell–cell adhesion, growth, and differentiation.[13] Betaglycan is also known as the transforming growth factor-beta (TGF-β) type III receptor. Both betaglycan and epican exist as variants without GAG chains and may exert their function at the cell surface with or without GAG addition.

The extracellular matrix contains multiple proteoglycans that have now been identified and studied. As has been discussed for proteoglycans at the cell surface, the extracellular matrix proteoglycans have a variety of distinct structural characteristics. Aggrecan, a large proteoglycan found in cartilage, has been studied extensively. This core protein contains a region with over 100 Ser-Gly dipeptides that serve as attachment sites for chondroitin sulfate GAG. The ~230 kDa core protein can be modified to contain up to 130 GAG chains and have a final mass of ~2200 kDa.[14] This densely packed multiple GAG configuration has been described as a "bottle-brush" to illustrate the predicted structure. The aggrecan core protein also contains sites for keratan sulfate attachment and a domain for noncovalent binding to hyaluronic acid. As many as 100 aggrecan molecules can bind to a single hyaluronic acid molecule. Thus, the overall proteoglycan aggregate (from which the name *aggrecan* is derived) can have a mass near 200,000 kDa.

In the skin, fibroblasts produce large aggregating proteoglycans similar to aggrecan. The best known of these large proteoglycans is called *versican*. The core protein of versican contains attachment sites for 12 to 15 GAG chains, which are primarily chondroitin sulfate or dermatan sulfate. Versican, like aggrecan, also binds hyaluronic acid, enabling it to form large aggregates. In skin, versican has been identified in the dermis (fibroblasts) and epidermis (keratinocytes) and demonstrates selective upregulation in response to TGF-β.[15] Thus, the size, distribution, and abundance of versican in the skin suggest that this is an important molecule in the regulation of the behavior of the skin.

In contrast to the large aggregating extracellular matrix proteoglycans represented by aggrecan and versican, several genes encoding smaller proteoglycans have been identified in the extracellular matrix. One family of the proteoglycans is characterized by a leucine-rich repeat motif. The prototype of this family is decorin, an approximately 36-kDa secreted proteoglycan. Decorin is in abundance in skin and cartilage and is thought to be a ubiquitous component of connective tissue. The relatively small decorin core protein has a single dermatan sulfate chain covalently bound to a serine residue at amino acid position 4 and, like many other proteoglycans, also has N-linked oligosaccharides. Thus, after GAG addition and glycosylation, decorin can have a mass of 80 kDa. Decorin received its name from observations that this molecule closely associates with collagen fibrils and can be seen to "decorate" the fibrils in vivo. This interaction is attributed to the ability of the decorin core protein to directly bind to collagen type I.[16] Decorin's single GAG chain binds to tenascin-X, another extracellular matrix protein that colocalizes with collagen fibrils in connective tissues.[17] These binding interactions contribute to collagen fibril formation and influence function. Interestingly, similar phenotypes (see below) showing abnormal collagen morphology are seen in a patient deficient in tenascin-X and in the murine decorin knockout model.[18,19]

FUNCTION

To understand how proteoglycans function in the skin it is essential to recall the basics of their organization, as previously discussed: (1) Proteoglycans are part protein and part GAG; (2) GAGs are heterogeneous but encode specific information; (3) proteoglycan core proteins are expressed in different cellular compartments; and (4) proteoglycan expression and GAG composition vary according to cellular context. These characteristics are important because the fundamental influence dictating proteoglycan function is the ability to bind to other molecules in its environment. Therefore, the sequences (both amino acid sequence and disaccharide sequence) of the core protein and GAG control proteoglycan function by influencing binding.

Similar GAGs can be found on multiple core proteins. This ability to interchange GAGs among cores adds complexity in studying proteoglycan function. Therefore, in many cases, proteoglycan function is discussed purely in terms of the function of GAG chains. This implies that a number of genes encoding core proteins containing these GAGs may have a similar function. Figure 18-2 illustrates some of the functions attributed to proteoglycans containing heparan sulfate and dermatan sulfate. The functions proposed for proteoglycans containing these GAGs derive from the ability of these molecules to bind to other components of the extracellular environment and mediate assembly of larger molecular complexes.

The list of molecules to which the major skin proteoglycans heparan sulfate and dermatan sulfate bind is quite extensive (Table 18-2). Therefore, several functions for proteoglycans have been proposed that include the particular biologic system in which the ligand is involved. Some of the most compelling experimental evidence for functions of heparan and dermatan sulfate proteoglycans includes the ability to bind several growth factors, cytokines, and components of the extracellular matrix.[20] Numerous laboratories have shown that heparan sulfate is required for the function of several growth factors including several members of the fibroblast growth factor family,[21,22] hepatocyte growth factor/scatter factor,[23] and vascular endothelial growth factor.[24] In this model, the heparan sulfate proteoglycan can be found either at the cell surface or in a soluble form. The molecules then assemble to form a ternary complex at the cell surface between the growth factor, its specific high-affinity signaling receptor, and the proteoglycan (Fig. 18-2*A*).[25] Only after this ternary complex is formed does the cell receive the growth factor's signal to begin to proliferate, differentiate, or migrate. Dermatan sulfate's ability to participate in these interactions was only recently demonstrated.[26,27] The significance of this assembly to skin biology is illustrated during wound repair. Heparan sulfate-dependent growth factors, such as members of the fibroblast growth factor family, are induced in a healing wound[28] and influence the wound repair process through the stimulation of keratinocyte proliferation, fibroblast growth, and angiogenesis. Heparan sulfate proteoglycans such as syndecan-1 and -4 are also induced at these sites[29] and enable activity of the growth factor. Because dermatan sulfate is the predominant GAG in wound fluid and because it can bind a variety of growth factors, cytokines, and extracellular matrix proteins, the further study of this GAG and the proteoglycans it comprises promises to be a very exciting subject for future investigation.

The influence of the proteoglycan core protein on cell behavior is thought to relate to the ability of the core protein to influence the amount and localization of GAG expression. In the example of wound repair, heparan and dermatan sulfate expression is influenced by the expression of the syndecan core proteins to which the GAGs are covalently

FIGURE 18-2

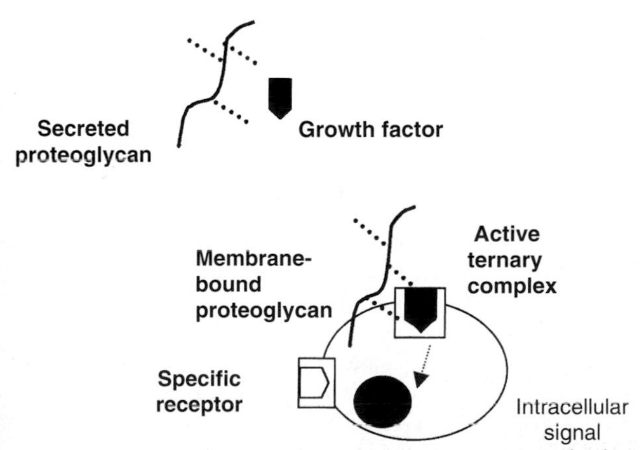

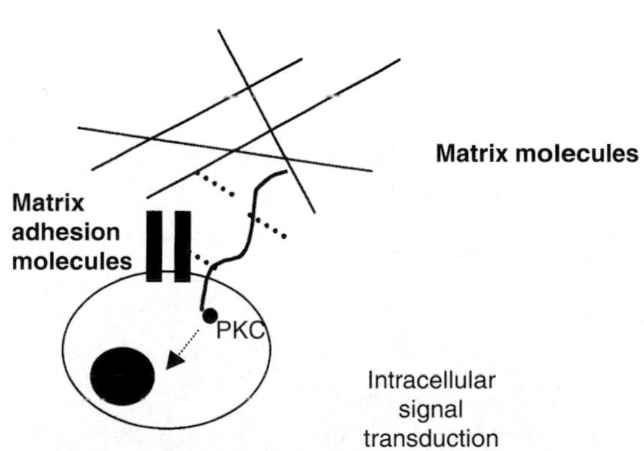

Theoretical models for proteoglycan function. *A*. Proteoglycans as coreceptors for growth factors. Proteoglycan, growth factor, and specific receptor must all assemble at the cell surface before growth factor can activate the cell. Secreted extracellular proteoglycans may sequester and stabilize growth factors. *B*. Proteoglycans as extracellular matrix receptors. Proteoglycan can assemble with other matrix adhesion receptors (e.g., integrins) to aid in cell adherence. The proteoglycan syndecan-4 also interacts and signals through protein kinase C (PKC) to enable cell activation by matrix adhesion.

TABLE 18-2

Binding Interactions of Heparan Sulfate, Dermatan Sulfate, and Heparin

CATEGORY	LIGAND
Extracellular matrix components	Collagen types I, III, IV, V Fibronectin Laminin Pleiotropin Tenascin-X Thrombospondin Vitronectin wnt-I wnt-induced secretory protein
Growth factors (GF)	Fibroblast GF family Hepatocyte GF/scatter factor Heparin-binding epidermal GF Platelet-derived GF Schwannoma-derived GF Vascular endothelial GF
Growth factor binding proteins (BP)	Follistatin Insulin-like growth factor BP-3 TGF-β BP
Cytokines	TGF-β Interleukin 8 Interferon-γ inducible protein-10 Interferon-γ Macrophage inhibitory protein-1α
Cell adhesion molecules (CAM)	CD45 L-Selectin Mac-1 Neural cell adhesion molecule Platelet/endothelial CAM
Proteases/Antiproteases	Elastase Thrombin Tissue plasminogen activator Antithrombin III Heparin cofactor II Leuserpin Plasminogen activator inhibitor-I Protein C inhibitor Protease nexin I
Pathogens	gC and gB of herpes simplex virus gC-11 of cytomegalovirus gp 120 of HIV *Staphylococcus aureus* surface proteins Penetrin of *Trypanosoma cruzi* *Streptococcus mutans* surface proteins *Neisseria gonorrhoeae* surface proteins Mycobacterial surface proteins Adhesin proteins of *Borrelia burgdorferi*

attached. Other molecules, such as the syndecan-inducer PR-39,[29] the syndecan-inhibitor tumor necrosis factor–α,[30] and TGF-β, can have significant influence on the wound repair process by controlling GAG and proteoglycan expression.[31]

Recently, further study of the expression of proteoglycans has expanded the direct evidence for a function for these molecules. In addition to growth factor binding, heparan sulfate proteoglycans are important molecules involved in adhesion to the extracellular matrix. In this model, cell surface proteoglycan helps the cell adhere to the extracellular matrix in conjunction with other matrix-binding molecules such as the integrins (Fig. 18-2*B*). Syndecan-4 is selectively enriched in dermal fibroblasts at sites consistent with this function. Furthermore, the formation of these focal adhesions requires heparan sulfate and the subsequent activation of protein kinase C by a domain in the syndecan-4 core protein cytoplasmic tail.[32] In this example, both the extracellular GAG and intracellular core protein of the proteoglycan have demonstrable function.

Other proteoglycans also interact with matrix molecules. Chondroitin sulfate and dermatan sulfate bind fibronectin and laminin.[33] As mentioned above, decorin, to which dermatan sulfate is typically attached, is known to associate primarily with type I collagen via its core protein.[16] In mice, selective disruption of the decorin gene leads to mice with abnormal collagen morphology and increased skin fragility.[18] Thus, through targeted disruption in the mouse, the function of decorin as a stabilizer of collagen fibrils has been directly confirmed.

The function of the large extracellular matrix proteoglycans in skin is thought to reside primarily in physical properties inherent in their large mass and charge density. Hyaluronan has been studied extensively from this perspective because of its extreme hydrophilicity and viscosity in dilute solution. As discussed earlier, hyaluronic acid is pure GAG and is synthesized extracellularly without a core protein. The genes for human hyaluronan synthase have been cloned and identified.[34] The expression of hyaluronan is developmentally regulated in skin[35] and changes during wound repair. It has been proposed that the physicochemical properties of hyaluronan serve to expand the matrix and thus aid cell movements. Other physical properties attributed to GAG and large proteoglycan complexes, such as those formed with versican or basement membrane proteoglycans, include their ability to act as anionic filters and elastic cushions and their function in salt and water balance. In fetal skin, the high relative content of hyaluronan has been associated with the ability of fetal skin to heal without scar.

Clues to the functions of proteoglycans and GAGs have been gathered from numerous reports of abnormal GAG composition associated with human disease. The well-known mucopolysaccharidoses are lysosomal storage disorders caused by a genetic deficiency of enzymes that degrade GAGs. A disorder in the ability to degrade hyaluronic acid has also been described.[36] These disorders reflect the severe pathology that can be caused by an excess of select GAGs.

The clinical manifestations of a deficiency in a specific proteoglycan are seen in the fetal overgrowth syndrome known as the Simpson-Golabi-Behmel syndrome. This X-linked condition is characterized by pre- and postnatal overgrowth with numerous visceral and skeletal abnormalities. The genetic defect for this syndrome in some families was identified as the cell surface proteoglycan OCI-5, also known as glypican-3.[37]

Multiple cutaneous disorders are associated with abnormal proteoglycan synthesis or deposition. A deficiency of decorin core protein has been described as the etiology of a variant form of Ehlers-Danlos syndrome. Affected individuals have skin that is thin and easily bruised with poor healing or chronic ulcers.[38] Rapid changes in select proteoglycans occur in the skin following injury.[39,40] This is consistent with their role as growth factor and matrix receptors. Infectious disease is influenced by proteoglycan expression. For example, decorin-deficient mice are somewhat resistant to infection with *Borrelia burgdorferi*. Presumably this resistance is caused by a partial dependence of the organism on decorin for binding in the dermis.[41] During aging, the composition of GAG in the skin undergoes a marked change.[42,43] It has been proposed that the observed decrease in hyaluronic acid can explain diminished skin turgor in aged skin. Retinoids also effect this response.[44] In keloids, hyaluronic acid synthesis is elevated.[45] Thyroid hormone also has a marked effect on the synthesis of proteoglycans and GAGs. The manifestation of this response is seen in pretibial myxedema, where the mucinous material deposited is predominantly hyaluronic acid and chondroitin sulfate. Other pathologic skin conditions, including pseudoxanthoma elasticum,[46] scleroderma,[47] psoriasis,[48] a variant form of Ehlers-Danlos syndrome,[38] lichen myxedema,[49] and UVB-irradiated skin,[50] have also been reported to have abnormal amounts of proteoglycans. These associations do not imply that abnormal proteoglycan metabolism is responsible for these disorders, yet they suggest that much of the pathophysiology of skin disease can be influenced by the function of cutaneous proteoglycans.

In summary, proteoglycans are best thought of as central regulatory molecules that act to influence a variety of cell behaviors. As more information becomes available regarding the regulation of proteoglycan and GAG synthesis, we have seen that these molecules are essential to cutaneous biology. The time has come to abandon archaic descriptions such as "ground substance" in the dermatology lexicon.

REFERENCES

1. Esko JD, Lindahl U: Molecular diversity of heparan sulfate. *J Clin Invest* **108**:169, 2001
2. Schick BP: Regulation of expression of megakaryocyte and platelet proteoglycans. *Stem Cells* **14**(suppl 1):220, 1996
3. Bernfield M et al: Functions of cell surface heparan sulfate proteoglycans. *Annu Rev Biochem* **68**:729, 1999
4. Litwack E et al: Expression of the heparan sulfate proteoglycan glypican-1 in the developing rodent. *Dev Dyn* **211**:72, 1998
5. Veugelers M et al: Glypican-6, a new member of the glypican family of cell surface heparan sulfate proteoglycans. *J Biol Chem* **274**:26968, 1999
6. Rapraeger AC: Molecular interactions of syndecans during development. *Semin Cell Dev Biol* **12**:107, 2001
7. Kim C et al: Members of the syndecan family of heparan sulfate proteoglycans are expressed in distinct cell-, tissue-, and development specific patterns. *Mol Biol Cell* **5**:797, 1994
8. Sanderson RD et al: Syndecan, a cell surface proteoglycan, changes in size and abundance when keratinocytes stratify. *J Invest Derm* **99**:1, 1992
9. Gallo RL et al: Syndecans-1 and -4 are induced during wound repair of neonatal but not fetal skin. *J Invest Dermatol* **107**:667, 1996
10. Echtermeyer F et al: Delayed wound repair and impaired angiogenesis in mice lacking syndecan-4. *J Clin Invest* **107**:R9, 2001
11. Inki P, Jalkanen M: The role of syndecan-1 in malignancies. *Ann Med* **28**:63, 1996
12. Hirabayashi K et al: Altered proliferative and metastatic potential associated with increased expression of syndecan-1. *Tumour Biol* **19**:454, 1998
13. Zhou J et al: Growth and differentiation regulate CD44 expression on human keratinocytes. *In Vitro Cell Dev Biol Anim* **35**:228, 1999
14. Watanabe H et al: Roles of aggrecan, a large chondroitin sulfate proteoglycan, in cartilage structure and function. *J Biochem (Tokyo)* **124**:687, 1998
15. Tiedemann K et al: Cytokine regulation of proteoglycan production in fibroblasts: Separate and synergistic effects. *Matrix Biol* **15**:469, 1997
16. Keene DR et al: Decorin binds near the C terminus of type I collagen. *J Biol Chem* **275**:21801, 2000
17. Elefteriou F et al: Binding of tenascin-X to decorin. *FEBS Lett* **495**:44, 2001
18. Danielson KG et al: Targeted disruption of decorin leads to abnormal collagen fibril morphology and skin fragility. *J Cell Biol* **136**:729, 1997
19. Burch GH et al: Tenascin-X deficiency is associated with Ehlers-Danlos syndrome. *Nat Genet* **17**:104, 1997
20. Iozzo R: *Proteoglycans: Structure, Biology and Molecular Interactions*. New York, Marcel Dekker, 2000, p 1–4
21. Ornitz DM, Itoh N: Fibroblast growth factors. *Genome Biol* **2**:Reviews 3005.1–3005.12, 2001
22. Loo BM et al: Binding of heparin/heparan sulfate to fibroblast growth factor receptor 4. *J Biol Chem* **276**:16868, 2001
23. Sergeant N et al: Stimulation of DNA synthesis and cell proliferation of human mammary myoepithelial-like cells by hepatocyte growth factor/scatter factor depends on heparan sulfate proteoglycans and sustained phosphorylation of mitogen-activated protein kinases p42/44. *J Biol Chem* **275**:17094, 2000
24. Tessler S et al: Heparin modulates the interaction of VEGF165 with soluble and cell associated flk-1 receptors. *J Biol Chem* **269**:12456, 1994
25. Schlessinger J et al: Crystal structure of a ternary FGF-FGFR-heparin complex reveals a dual role for heparin in FGFR binding and dimerization. *Mol Cell* **6**:743, 2000
26. Penc SF et al: Dermatan sulfate released after injury is a potent promoter of FGF-2 activity. *J Biol Chem* **273**:28116, 1998
27. Lyon M et al: The mode of action of heparan and dermatan sulfates in the regulation of hepatocyte growth factor/scatter factor. *J Biol Chem* **31**:31, 2001
28. Werner S et al: Large induction of keratinocyte growth factor expression in the dermis during wound healing. *Proc Natl Acad Sci USA* **89**:6896, 1992
29. Gallo RL et al: Syndecans, cell surface heparan sulfate proteoglycans, are induced by a proline-rich antimicrobial peptide from wounds. *Proc Natl Acad Sci U S A* **91**:11035, 1994
30. Kainulainen V et al: Suppression of syndecan-1 expression in endothelial cells by tumor necrosis factor-alpha. *J Biol Chem* **271**:18759, 1996
31. Brown CT et al: Characterization of proteoglycans synthesized by cultured corneal fibroblasts in response to transforming growth factor beta and fetal calf serum. *J Biol Chem* **274**:7111, 1999
32. Oh E et al: Syndecan-4 proteoglycan regulates the distribution and activity of protein kinase C. *J Biol Chem* **272**:8133, 1997
33. Ruoslahti E: Structure and biology of proteoglycans. *Ann Rev Cell Biol* **4**:229, 1988
34. Shyjan AM et al: Functional cloning of the cDNA for a human hyaluronan synthase. *J Biol Chem* **271**:23395, 1996
35. Agren UM et al: Developmentally programmed expression of hyaluronan in human skin and its appendages. *J Invest Dermatol* **109**:219, 1997
36. Natowicz MR et al: Clinical and biochemical manifestations of hyaluronidase deficiency. *N Engl J Med* **335**:1029, 1996
37. Pilia G et al: Mutations in GPC3, a glypican gene, cause the Simpson-Golabi-Behmel overgrowth syndrome. *Nat Genet* **12**:241, 1996
38. Wu J et al: Deficiency of the decorin core protein in the variant form of Ehlers-Danlos syndrome with chronic skin ulcer. *J Dermatol Sci* **27**:95, 2001
39. Brown CT et al: Synthesis of stromal glycosaminoglycans in response to injury. *J Cell Biochem* **59**:57, 1995
40. Oksala O et al: Expression of proteoglycans and hyaluronan during wound healing. *J Histochem Cytochem* **43**:125, 1995
41. Brown EL et al: Resistance to Lyme disease in decorin-deficient mice. *J Clin Invest* **107**:845, 2001

42. Carrino DA et al: Age-related changes in the proteoglycans of human skin. *Arch Biochem Biophys* **373**:91, 2000
43. Ghersetich I et al: Hyaluronic acid in cutaneous intrinsic aging. *Int J Dermatol* **33**:119, 1994
44. Lundin A et al: Topical retinoic acid treatment of photoaged skin: Its effects on hyaluronan distribution in epidermis and on hyaluronan and retinoic acid in suction blister fluid. *Acta Derm Venereol* **72**:423, 1992
45. Alaish SM et al: Hyaluronic acid metabolism in keloid fibroblasts. *J Pediatr Surg* **30**:949, 1995
46. Passi A et al: Proteoglycan alterations in skin fibroblast cultures from patients affected with pseudoxanthoma elasticum. *Cell Biochem Funct* **14**:111, 1996
47. Kuroda K, Shinkai H: Decorin and glycosaminoglycan synthesis in skin fibroblasts from patients with systemic sclerosis. *Arch Dermatol Res* **289**:481, 1997
48. Seyger MM et al: Altered distribution of heparan sulfate proteoglycans in psoriasis. *Acta Derm Venereol* **77**:105, 1997
49. Turakainen H et al: Synthesis of glycosaminoglycans and collagen in skin fibroblasts cultured from a patient with lichen myxedematosus. *Arch Dermatol Res* **277**:55, 1985
50. Margelin D et al: Alterations of proteoglycans in ultraviolet-irradiated skin. *Photochem Photobiol* **58**:211, 1993

CHAPTER 19

Peter Petzelbauer
Jeffrey S. Schechner
Jordan S. Pober

Endothelium

The systemic vascular system is formed by a continuous series of hollow tubes that carry blood from the heart to the tissues and back again. Blood exits the heart through the aorta, a large elastic artery, which gives rise to a series of diverging, progressively narrower muscular arteries and arterioles that deliver the blood to all of the organs of the body. The terminal arterioles arborize into an interconnecting network of microvessels, mostly capillaries, which nourish and cleanse the peripheral tissues. The capillary network empties into a series of converging venules and progressively larger veins that ultimately return the blood to the heart. All segments of this vascular system, as well as the heart itself, are lined by a simple, one-cell–thick layer of epithelial-like cells called *endothelium*. All of these endothelial cells share common features and perform common functions, and hence may be collectively described as one cell type. However, endothelia from one segment of the vascular system may differ in significant ways from the endothelia at other anatomic sites. In the first sections of this chapter, we consider both the commonality and diversity of endothelia, beginning with functional properties of endothelium. We then describe the development of the vascular endothelial system, summarize the shared and morphologic features exhibited by diverse endothelia, describe the shared and variable molecular markers of endothelia as they appear in different segments of the vasculature, discuss the role of endothelial cells in inflammation, and conclude with a consideration of the specialized features of skin endothelium.

PROPERTIES OF ENDOTHELIAL CELLS

As the lining of the vasculature, all endothelial cells must perform three important constitutive functions. First, vascular endothelial cells must maintain homeostasis of the blood that consists of about equal volumes of fluid (plasma) and cellular elements (mostly erythrocytes with a lesser mass of leukocytes and platelets). The plasma contains the proteins of the coagulation system that have the capacity to self-assemble into an insoluble matrix of fibrin, i.e., to form an intravascular thrombus or an extravascular clot when placed in contact with tissue cells or extracellular matrix. In addition, both the leukocytes and the platelets have membrane receptors that trigger cellular activation upon contact with the extravascular environment. The endothelial cell lining acts to prevent intravascular activation both of the coagulation system and of these responsive cellular elements, yet it keeps both systems poised to respond to appropriate stimuli, e.g., wounds or infections. In other words, vascular endothelium forms a blood-compatible container that prevents inappropriate activation of the blood without disabling protective responses.

The second function that must be performed by endothelial cells is to form a barrier that separates circulating blood from the tissues. The barrier formed by endothelial cells permits limited passage of fluid and solutes, allowing the blood to nourish the tissues, while displaying "permselectivity" for macromolecules, and a virtually impenetrable barrier for blood cells (except at specialized sites of high permeability and leukocyte trafficking). In other words, vascular endothelium regulates rather than completely prevents interactions between blood and tissues.

The third constitutive function that must be performed by endothelial cells is to regulate the extent of local blood flow. Blood flow may be shunted, within limits, from one organ to another. Perfusion of particular vascular beds is determined by vessel luminal diameter, which, in turn, is regulated by the tension generated by the smooth-muscle cell layer that invests the endothelial lining of the arteries and arterioles, particularly at the "precapillary sphincter" of the terminal arteriole. Although the tension of these investing smooth muscle cells is tonic, i.e., these cells are never completely relaxed, the level of contraction can be varied. The physiologic signals that affect vascular smooth-muscle tone are largely mediated through the endothelial cell lining, which can produce potent vasodilating or vasoconstricting substances. Remarkably, many direct constrictors of isolated vascular smooth-muscle cells (e.g., acetylcholine or bradykinin) are actually physiologic vasodilators because their actions on smooth-muscle cells are overwhelmed by their ability to concomitantly induce endothelial cells to release potent vasodilators such as nitric oxide (NO) or endothelial-derived hyperpolarizing factor (EDHP). In other words, endothelial cells integrate extrinsic signals and set the level of local vascular smooth-muscle cell tone and tissue perfusion.

These three constitutive functions of endothelium are performed, to some extent, by all vascular endothelial cells. However, endothelium is specialized at various anatomic sites, and the capacity to perform constitutive functions may be influenced by these specializations. For example, the ability of endothelial cells to interact with circulating cells and macromolecules varies with vessel type. Arterial endothelia are the major producers of von Willebrand factor, a protein that strengthens platelet adhesion so it may resist strong shear forces, which typically are found only in arteries. Leukocytes preferentially interact with venules where endothelia most intensely express adhesion proteins that bind leukocytes. Arterial and arteriolar endothelium are specialized to regulate vasomotor tone and are the primary producers of NO and EDHP. Capillaries are the major site of nutritive exchange with the peripheral tissues, and capillary endothelial cells maintain a high degree of curvature, narrowing the vessel lumen so as to maximize the ratio of lumenal surface to lumenal volume. Moreover, different capillary beds display widely different degrees of permeability and selectivity, from the high resistance tight junction of brain microvessels to the open spaces between the sinusoidal endothelial cells of liver and, in humans, of spleen. Such functional differences among endothelia lining different vascular segments and in different tissues is important in the skin endothelial cell system. Injury to endothelium can lead to impairment or loss of constitutive functions, producing phenomena collectively referred to as *endothelial cell dysfunction*. The consequences of endothelial cell dysfunction also depend on the anatomic site of endothelial cell injury. Such differences have relevance for the role of endothelium in skin diseases.

In addition to their constitutive functions, endothelial cells respond to various proinflammatory stimuli by altering morphology and phenotype. These changes are part of host defense, i.e., they are functional rather than dysfunctional, and are referred to as *endothelial activation* (see below). Endothelial activation can result in an increased local influx of circulating humoral and cellular elements into the vessel wall and surrounding tissues. Again, features of these inducible functions are shared by all endothelium, but activation responses are also modulated by endothelial differences displayed among different vascular segments or in different organs. For example, although venular endothelial cells have become specialized for recruitment and activation of leukocytes in response to inflammatory stimuli, adhesion molecule expression in the lungs also occurs in the capillaries of the alveolar wall, an alternative site of leukocyte trafficking.

ENDOTHELIAL ORIGIN AND DEVELOPMENT OF THE VASCULAR SYSTEM

The first endothelial cells arise from an embryonic progenitor cell type called the *angioblast*. There are few established markers for angioblasts, and until recently, angioblasts were generally identified only after they had differentiated into endothelial cells. The best current marker for angioblasts may be expression of receptors for vascular endothelial growth factor (VEGF, see below) and platelet endothelial cell adhesion molecule (PECAM)-1 (CD31). Early angioblasts may arise from an even more primitive cell type, the hemangioblast, which also gives rise to hematopoietic progenitor cells.[1] In other words, some vascular endothelia may share a common embryonic origin with circulating blood cells rather than with other with vascular (e.g., smooth muscle) or tissue cells. This is reflected in the fact that many markers originally thought to be restricted to hematopoietic cells (e.g., CD34, CD36, and stem cell factor CD117) are also expressed by endothelia, and many markers originally thought to be unique for endothelia (e.g., PECAM-1, CD31; endoglin, CD105; VEGFR-2; Tie-1 and Tie-2) have been found on circulating blood cells. Hemangioblasts arise from mesodermal cells in the yolk sac and, at slightly later stages, from cells of the dorsal mesoderm, and differentiate to form the "blood islands" at these sites. Angioblasts initially arise from within the blood islands. Some angioblasts further differentiate in situ to form the endothelial cell lining of the blood islands while others migrate to elsewhere in the embryo to form the rudimentary vasculature. Later in development, some angioblasts appear to arise directly from cells of the splanchnic mesoderm without passing through a hemangioblast stage. The distinct embryologic origin of angioblasts is not known to result in functional differences among endothelial cells.

Newly formed angioblasts typically migrate as individual cells, differentiating into endothelial cells within tissues of endodermal origin (e.g., lung, heart, and gut).[2] Upon differentiation from individual angioblasts, endothelial cells spontaneously self-associate to form cords and, ultimately, hollow tubes. These tubes of endothelium are the first blood vessels. Endothelial cell tubes subsequently recruit and induce the differentiation of primitive mesenchymal cells into the investing cells of the vessel wall (e.g., smooth-muscle cells and pericytes).

Vessels that supply tissues of ectodermal and mesodermal origin arise primarily from outgrowth of endothelial cells present within preexisting endodermal vessels rather than differentiating from angioblasts. These differentiated endothelial cells typically migrate as cords, rather than as individual cells. The migrating cords of endothelium spontaneously form hollow tubes that, once again, recruit primitive mesenchymal cells to differentiate into investing vessel wall cells.

The formation of endothelial-lined tubes, i.e., primitive blood vessels, from differentiating angioblasts is called *vasculogenesis,* and the development of new blood vessels from preexisting endothelial-lined blood vessels is called *angiogenesis*. The maturation of a simple endothelial-lined tube into a mature blood vessel invested by stromal supporting cells (e.g., pericytes or vascular smooth muscle cells) is a form of *vascular remodeling*. Vascular remodeling also refers to both the growth of some microvessels into larger structures (i.e., arteries and veins) and the concomitant disappearance of other microvessels, largely by apoptosis, as large vessels are formed. Vasculogenesis, angiogenesis, and vascular remodeling are all required for the normal development of the vasculature. The vasculature is the first organ system to be formed in the embryo, but it continues to change throughout fetal and postnatal development. Vasculogenesis is completed during early embryonic development and angiogenesis is completed slightly later during embryonic development (although physiologic angiogenesis resumes in the adult female ovary during the ovulatory cycle). All subsequent development of the vascular system is through vascular remodeling, which normally continues to occur until adulthood.

In the adult, mature endothelial cells retain the capacity to regenerate and, when tissues are injured, new blood vessels can develop as part of the repair process. These vessels are thought to arise primarily by angiogenesis, initiated by endothelial cells in vessels neighboring the wound site. However, recent studies suggest that bone marrow-derived angioblasts present in adult blood are capable of "seeding" the site of injury to supplement angiogenesis.[3] New vessels formed early in wound healing undergo vascular remodeling as young granulation tissue matures. Vascular remodeling may also occur in mature vessels subjected to various stimuli (e.g., hypertension and increased flow).

Vasculogenesis and angiogenesis in the embryo (and angiogenesis in wound healing) require regulation of endothelial proliferation and migration as well as the coordination between the endothelial and supporting cells. Transgenic and genetic knockout murine models have revealed that the signals that mediate this complex process largely depend on the binding of secreted molecules such as VEGF and angiopoietins, and membrane-bound ephrins that bind to specific receptor tyrosine kinases.[4]

Molecules of the VEGF family are required to initiate the formation of primitive vessels. VEGF was initially identified for its ability to induce vascular permeability and endothelial proliferation, and is now known to also promote migration and inhibit apoptosis. VEGF is a highly specific mitogen for endothelial cells and does not act on vascular smooth muscle, fibroblasts, or epithelial cells. VEGF synthesis by stromal or epithelial cells is increased in settings of hypoxia, and VEGF is largely responsible for angiogenesis that develops in hypoxic tissues. This family of molecules includes five VEGF splice variants (VEGF A–E) and the homologue placental growth factor (PlGF). These molecules variably bind a family of closely related receptor tyrosine kinases named VEGFR-1 (Flt-1), VEGFR-2 (KDR or Flk-1), and VEGFR-3 (Flt-4). VEGFR-2 is the main mediator of VEGF growth and permeability effects on endothelial cells, playing the primary role in driving vascular development and angiogenesis in adults, and binding all VEGF isoforms. The activity of VEGFR-2 can be enhanced by binding of VEGF A to neuropillin-1, which appears to function as a coreceptor. VEGFR-1 binds PlGF and VEGFs A and B, and may have a downregulatory role or act as a decoy receptor. PlGF binding to VEGFR-1 appears to amplify endothelial cell responses to VEGF. Early in embryonic development VEGFR-3 is widely expressed on vascular endothelium, but it later becomes restricted to lymphatic endothelium. VEGFR-3 binds VEGFs C and D, which play a critical role in lymphatic development and post natal lymphangiogenesis.

The importance of tight regulation of VEGF expression during vascular development has been demonstrated in several murine development models. Mice that have undergone the targeted disruption of VEGF or VEGFR-2 genes fail to develop a vasculature. VEGF is so critical for vasculogenesis that even heterozygous knockout animals, which produce 50% as much VEGF as normal animals, show embryonic lethality. Conversely, knockout of the downregulatory VEGFR-1 results in the formation of immature leaky vessels. Similar results are observed when VEGF A is overexpressed. Disruption of VEGFR-3 results in the disorganization of large vessels and lymphatic hypoplasia. A missense mutation in VEGFR-3 occurs in primary human lymphedema. Transgenic overexpression of VEGF C results in lymphatic hyperplasia, indicating the important role of this splice variant in lymphatic development.[4–6]

Fibroblast growth factors 1 and 2 (also called acidic and basic FGF, respectively) have been proposed as participants in vasculogenesis and angiogenesis during embryonic development, but this has not been firmly established. The principal signaling receptor for these molecules is FGFR-I.[7] However, knock out of this receptor in mice produces death in the gastrula stage, i.e., before vasculogenesis begins, so specific evaluation of FGF function in vascular development is not possible in these animals. Both FGF-1 and -2 are potent endothelial cell mitogens, although they are not specific for endothelial cells (i.e., they also act on smooth-muscle cells and fibroblasts), and they are active in the same bioassays of angiogenesis as is VEGF. Interestingly, the FGFs can "synergize" with VEGF in stimulating cultured endothelial cell mitogenesis and in bioassays of angiogenesis, giving greater responses than those seen with either agent alone. In the adult, FGF-1 and -2 are stored in the cytoplasm of a variety of cells, consistent with the fact that these proteins lack signal sequences required for efficient secretion. Stored FGFs are released when cells are injured, acting as "wound hormones" to stimulate local angiogenesis and connective tissue growth.[7]

Other polypeptide factors have also been found to act on endothelial cells in vivo and in vitro, including epidermal growth factor (EGF),[8] heparin-binding EGF-like growth factor,[9] and hepatocyte growth factor/scatter factor.[10] These molecules have some angiogenic potential, but their role in embryonic development is not clear.

Subsequent to the initial vasculogenic actions of VEGFs, another family of receptor tyrosine kinases, Tie-1 and Tie-2 (Tek), are required for vascular remodeling and stabilization. Tie-2 mediates the "dialog" between primitive mesenchymal cells and the endothelium of the immature blood vessel through binding to angiopoietins 1 (Ang-1), 2 (Ang-2), murine angiopoietin 3 (Ang-3), and its human orthologue angiopoietin 4 (Ang-4). Ang-1 binding appears to primarily positively effect vascular stability. Mouse embryos lacking either Ang-1 or Tie-2 develop a normal primary vasculature, but fail to undergo further vascular remodeling. In the heart, there is impaired association between the endocardium and the underlying myocardium. There are defects in the remodeling of vascular beds that appear be due to a similar lack of appropriate association with underlying support cells. Furthermore, venous malformations are found in humans with a Tie-2 mutation, which are typified by enlarged vascular channels with a relative lack of supporting smooth muscle cells. Ang-2 appears to be a competitive inhibitor of Ang-1, and Ang-2 overexpression in transgenic mice results in a phenotype resembling an Ang-1 knockout animal.[11] This suggests that Ang-2 may serve to antagonize Ang-1, perhaps as an early step in angiogenesis and vascular remodeling, i.e., when a preexisting vessel must be destabilized to permit endothelial cell outgrowth and migration. This hypothesis is supported by the impairment of certain forms of postnatal vascular remodeling in Ang-2 knockout mice, and the upregulation of Ang-2 in settings of intense angiogenesis such as in highly angiogenic tumors, and in response to hypoxia and VEGF treatment. Although the ligands for Tie-1 are not known, knockout of this receptor results in similar defects in vascular maturation later in embryonic development.[4,12]

An important role has recently been identified for the eph family of receptor tyrosine kinases and their corresponding ephrin ligands. Both the eph receptors and the ephrin ligands are membrane bound and it appears that they mediate bidirectional cell to cell signaling. Based on membrane attachment characteristics, the ephrins are divided into two classes, the A class (ephrin-A1 to A5) that generally bind the eight ephA receptors (ephA1 to A8), and the B class (ephrin-B1 to B3) that bind the six ephB receptors (ephB1 to B6). Ephrin-A1 has activity during inflammatory angiogenesis induced by tumor necrosis factor (TNF). Ephrin-B1 promotes endothelial capillary assembly in vitro. Recent knockout mouse studies suggest key roles for ephrin-B2 and its ephB4 receptor during vascular development. Mice lacking ephrin-B2 and its ephB4 receptor have lethal defects in early angiogenic remodeling.[13] During vascular development ephrin-B2 marks the endothelial cells of early arterial vessels and ephB4 marks the endothelium of early veins. This distribution supports the proposal that ephrin-B2 and ephB4 are involved in establishing venous versus arteriolar identity. As development proceeds ephrin-B2 continues to mark the arteriolar endothelium, with additional expression on surrounding arteriolar smooth muscle cells and pericytes, and may be involved in regulating endothelial–smooth muscle interactions.[14]

Other endothelial cell-derived signals that act on the mesenchymal cells during vascular remodeling have not been identified with certainty, but two leading candidates are platelet-derived growth factor (PDGF) and transforming growth factor-β (TGF-β).[21] Both PDGF and TGF-β are molecules that are secreted by endothelial cells, acting on mesenchymal cells to promote migration, matrix biosynthesis and differentiation. PDGF is a mesenchymal cell mitogen, whereas TGF-β may promote or inhibit cell growth. Like VEGF and FGF, PDGF acts through receptor protein tyrosine kinase. In contrast, the TGF-β signaling receptor is a protein serine/threonine kinase rather than a protein tyrosine kinase. TGF-β also uses a number of nonsignaling receptors that "present" TGF-β to the signaling receptor. The dimeric nonsignaling endothelial cell TGF-β binding protein, endoglin (CD105), appears to play an important role in vascular development and angiogenesis. A truncation mutation in the endoglin gene causes a hereditary form of vascular malformations (hereditary hemorrhagic telangiectasia type I)[15] Similar multisystemic vascular dysplasia and hemorrhage are seen in mice heterozygous for CD105. Interestingly, endoglin knockout mice die of defective vascular development. A role for at least some isoforms of PDGF in vascular remodeling in the embryo was recently confirmed in knockout animals. Similar confirmation is lacking for TGF-β, but it has been difficult to effectively knock out the function of this molecule because complete absence of TGF-β causes embryonic lethality. In rare, live-born, TGF-β knockout animals, it is likely that TGF-β was provided to the developing fetus by the mother. Such animals die young and cannot be easily bred.

Matrix glycoproteins (e.g., fibronectin and laminin) and receptors for matrix glycoproteins (especially $\beta 1$ and $\beta 3$ integrins) are also believed to play a role in vasculogenesis/angiogenesis.[16] This seems intuitive because neither endothelial cells nor mesenchymal cells can survive unless they interact with matrix proteins via integrin receptors. Knock-out of most of these molecules causes early embryonic lethality, usually prior to development of the vascular system, preventing a direct test of their role in vascular embryology. An exception to this is knock out of B3 integrin, which shows normal development and enhanced tumor angiogenesis. Finally, two other classes of molecules have been implicated in vessel formation, namely coagulation factors and proinflammatory cytokines. One key coagulation factor, tissue factor, is implicated in vasculogenesis by observations of defective vascular development in tissue factor knockout mice.[17] Coagulation factor V knockout mice may also have some vascular defects, but this phenotype is more variable. It was recently suggested that the effects of deficiencies in the coagulation cascade on vascular development may be the indirect result of defective thrombin production, because knockout of the thrombin receptor PAR-1 produces similar phenotypes. Evidence for a role of proinflammatory cytokines in angiogenesis has come largely from in vivo bioassays. It is not clear if these molecules act directly on endothelial cells, or whether they act by causing release of primary vasculogenic/angiogenic factors (e.g., VEGF or FGF) by other cells (e.g., from mesenchymal cells or from recruited leukocytes).[18] Knockout mice lacking inflammatory cytokines do not show defects in vasculogenesis or angiogenesis. Endothelial cell molecules involved in adhesion of leukocytes [e.g., E-selectin or vascular cell adhesion molecule (VCAM)-1] have also been reported to be signals for angiogenesis, but roles for E-selectin or VCAM-1 in vascular development have also not been confirmed in knockout mice.

The specialization of endothelial cell types at different anatomic sites occurs during vascular remodeling. It has been proposed that specialization is induced by signals that vary with anatomic location. In the adult, vascular remodeling is influenced by mechanical signals such as shear stress or stretch. Cultured endothelial cells respond to mechanical forces,[19] and it is likely that this occurs in the embryo as well. Because mechanical forces differ with anatomic position, they are a candidate for inducing endothelial specialization. In general, mechanical forces are most pronounced in the arterial tree. Mechanical forces can act either through force applied directly to the cell (detected by some unknown signal transducer) or indirectly by "tugging" on the integrin-mediated attachments of endothelial cells to underlying *basement membrane,* a specialized region of the extracellular matrix that forms on the ablumenal surface of the endothelial cells.

The basement membrane itself is an even better candidate to determine endothelial specialization than are mechanical forces. The basement membrane varies in macromolecular composition (both glycoprotein and proteoglycan) and in its structural organization with anatomic site or vessel type. In certain vascular beds (e.g., in splenic sinusoids), the basement membrane is not well formed, i.e., there is a absence of matrix condensation as viewed by electron microscopy. However, all endothelial cells are attached to matrix and will undergo apoptosis if they become detached. Both endothelial cells and nonendothelial cells contribute to basement membrane synthesis and maintenance. The contribution of the surrounding nonendothelial cells to basement membrane composition thus provides a means for the local tissue to influence endothelial cell specialization. This hypothesis is supported by the observation that endothelial cells cultured on specialized basement membranes made by nonendothelial cells may acquire specialized features, e.g., the formation of fenestrae on endothelial cells grown on basement membrane made by epithelial cells.[20] However, cultured endothelial cells may retain some tissue-specific differences, regardless of the matrix used for their culture. Endothelial cell specialization may also be influenced directly by other cells either through cell-cell contact or through diffusable signals. For example, astrocytes cocultured with endothelial cells may stimulate formation of high-resistance junctions, which are characteristic of microvessels in the central nervous system.[21]

When angiogenesis and vascular remodeling occur following injury, the endothelial cells lining the new vessels may not display the same characteristics as the original endothelial cells resident at that anatomic site. For example, capillary endothelia in injured liver may be continuous and lose fenestrae. Similar alterations in the endothelial cell phenotype have been observed in certain skin diseases. We refer to this change in the endothelial cell phenotype as *metaplasia,* analogous to the changes observed in reparative epithelial cells as a response to chronic injury. This term does not imply that individual endothelial cells have changed from one type of specialized endothelium to another, but rather that new endothelial cells arising from angiogenic repair processes may have a distinct phenotype.

MORPHOLOGIC FEATURES AND MOLECULAR MARKERS OF ENDOTHELIUM

General Morphologic Features of Endothelial Cells

Endothelial cells are flattened epithelial-like cells, with a thickness typically less than 10 μm, and a surface area covering up to 1000 μm^2. In large vessels, endothelial cells assume an elongated shape with their long axis oriented in the direction of blood flow. Endothelial cells located in regions of turbulent flow, i.e., at branch points of the arterial tree, are often polygonal rather than elongated. Cultured endothelial cells are typically more polygonal, but elongate when flowing medium is passed over them for periods of 24 h or more.[22] These observations have led to the conclusion that shear stress, the force imparted by viscous drag of flowing liquid, is responsible for inducing a cytoskeletal rearrangement and the change of shape from polygonal to elongated. The nucleus is centrally located in both polygonal and elongated cells. Interestingly, the microtubular organizing center of endothelial cells, is always found located near the nucleus, oriented toward the heart (i.e., upstream of flow in arteries and downstream of flow in veins) regardless of the direction of blood flow.[23] The basis for this phenomenon is unknown.

In most vessels, the endothelial cells form a continuous monolayer, in which each endothelial cell forms junctional complexes with all of its neighbors. Endothelial cells are in contact with neighboring endothelial cells through gap junctions, and evidence has been presented that they may additionally form functional gaps with both surrounding vessel wall cells and, on occasion, with bound leukocytes. Endothelial cells are normally polarized, concentrating integrin receptors for matrix macromolecules on the basal surface while displaying adhesion molecules for leukocytes almost exclusively on their apical surface, which faces the lumen of the blood vessel.[24]

Specialized Organelles of Endothelial Cells

Endothelial cells have a number of characteristic organelles, the best described of which are Weibel-Palade bodies (WPB), fenestrae, and the caveolar system. WPB are elongated, membrane-bound organelles that display longitudinal striations by electron microscopy. WPB are distributed randomly throughout the cytoplasm in vascular endothelial cells of most vertebrates, and are found in arteries (most prominently), veins, capillaries, and endocardium, but not of lymphatics. They may or may not be expressed in glomerular endothelial cells or in the sinusoidal endothelial cells of liver or spleen. WPB constitutively contain von Willebrand factor (vWF; also called factor VIII-related antigen), P-selectin (CD62P),[25] lysosomal-membrane–associated glycoprotein 3 (LAMP-3 or CD63),[26] 1, 3-fucosyltransferase VI,[27] and interleukin 8.[28] The longitudinal striations within the WPB are formed by highly polymerized forms of vWF, reaching sizes up to 20 Md, and are responsible for cell surface expression of the integral membrane proteins P-selectin and CD63. Upon release, vWF polymers may attach to the basement membrane and stabilize platelet adhesion to the subendothelial matrix, particularly in high-velocity arterial flow. Although vWF is commonly used as an endothelial cell marker (see below), it is also found in megakaryocytes, which appear to lack a physiologic mechanism of release, synthesizing vWF only for storage within the α granules of their platelet progeny. P-selectin is also found in the membranes of platelet α granules. P-selectin mediates leukocyte adhesion to endothelium (see below). CD63 is a 53-kDa lysosomal membrane glycoprotein belonging to the TM4 superfamily that may interfere with neutrophil adhesion to endothelium.

Because vascular endothelium forms a continuous monolayer, most transendothelial transport takes place in the junctions between cells. One important exception is in the fenestrae of capillaries in lymph nodes, capillaries in the intestinal mucosa, renal glomerular endothelial cells, and in hepatic and bone marrow sinusoids. Fenestrae are 175 nm in diameter, are grouped into structures resembling sieve plates, and occupy 6 to 8 percent of the surface capillaries. They are specialized annular patches of attenuated cytoplasm and membrane characterized by an increased concentration of anionic lipids.[29] Fenestrated capillaries are much more permeable to water and small-molecular-size solutes than those of the continuous type. The anionic charge probably precludes the *trans*-fenestral passage of anionic plasma proteins. Fenestrae are unique to endothelial cells. Various factors such as pressure, alcohol, serotonin, nicotine, and infection change the number and diameter of fenestrae.[29] However, even endothelium of the continuous type may become transiently fenestrated.

A second important transport system is vesicular transport. All endothelial cells appear to contain numerous micropinocytotic vesicles beneath the folded surface, both, luminal and abluminal, indicating a high vesicle transport rate in these cells. Although such structures were originally interpreted as vesicles caught in the process of budding off or fusing to the membrane, upon careful examination most of these vesicles turned out to have narrow tubular connections to the plasma membrane. These flask-shaped caveolae, literally "little caves," are part of the surface membrane, either as single caveola or as more complex racemose invaginations. In fact, free plasmalemmal vesicles are extremely rare in capillary endothelium. Caveolae are maintained by a network of investing protein, called *caveolin*. The lipid composition of the caveolar membranes are enriched for cholesterol and sphingomyelin. It is becoming evident that caveolae serve to harbor signal transducing subcompartments of the plasma membrane, particularly receptor tyrosine kinases associated with growth factor responses (e.g., platelet-derived growth factor receptors), as well as associated proteins such as phosphatidylinositol 3-kinase, Src-like kinases, and phospholipase C. Endothelial nitric oxide synthase is also found associated with caveolin-1. Mice lacking caveolin-1, the main protein component of caveolae, have impaired nitric oxide and calcium signaling in the cardiovascular system, causing aberrations in endothelium-dependent relaxation, contractility, and maintenance of myogenic tone.[30] The caveolar systems are not unique for endothelial cells, but they are particularly well developed in this cell type, especially in brain capillaries.

Endothelial Junctions

Neighboring endothelial cells connect to each other by forming interdigitating protrusions connected by junctions. Junctions possess different degrees of complexity along the vascular tree, reflecting different permeability for proteins and cells. Intercellular tight (occluding) junctions constitute the anatomic basis for the tightly regulated interfaces of the blood-testis and blood-brain barriers.[31] They consist of a continuous belt-like meshwork of six anastomosing junctional strands, which prevent the transport of macromolecules, such as horseradish peroxidase, into the tissue. The transmembrane protein occludin, linked to ZO-1 cytoplasmic proteins, appears to provide the molecular basis of this function. In addition, junctional adhesion molecules, called JAMs, members of the immunoglobulin superfamily, form homophilic adhesion sites in tight junctions and play a role in the generation of cell polarity.[32] Arterial endothelium also possess tight junctions, however they consist of only one to two junctional strands. Tight junctions are virtually absent in postcapillary venules.

Adherens junctions are found in all vascular endothelium. They are multimeric protein structures consisting of two transmembrane proteins, CD144 (also called cadherin 5 or VE-cadherin) and CD31 (also called PECAM-1) that are linked by proteins of the catenin family to the actin-based cytoskeleton.[33] VE-cadherin is strictly localized to endothelial junctions, whereas PECAM-1 is more broadly distributed over the cell surface. Adherens junction proteins appear to be involved in three different cell functions. First, they participate in capillary tube formation. Indirect evidence for the role of the transmembrane molecules PECAM-1 and VE-cadherin in vessel formation came from investigations of malignant endothelial tumors with primitive or abortive vascular (luminal) differentiation, which had little to no VE-cadherin or PECAM-1 expression. Blocking VE-cadherin and PECAM-1 interactions with monoclonal antibodies inhibited vessel formation in normal endothelial cells.[34] VE-cadherin–negative endothelial cells derived by gene targeting failed to organize in vessel-like structures.[35] Second, PECAM-1 and VE-cadherin participate in the regulation of leukocyte transendothelial migration. Third, PECAM-1 and VE-cadherin may indirectly regulate cell growth by regulating the free cytoplasmic pool of β-catenin. Endothelial cells also express a neuronal cadherin, N-cadherin. However, this protein is localized outside the junction and appears to be nonfunctional.

The existence of a third type of junction has been demonstrated by transfer of microinjected small-molecular-weight tracers between adjacent endothelial cells indicating the presence of gap junctional interendothelial communications. In endothelium, the gap junctional proteins are connexins-43, -37, and -40.

A fourth kind of adhering junction ("complexus adherens" or "syndesmos") is particularly abundant in the endothelium-related, stellate cells which form the three-dimensional filter meshwork of the lymph node sinus. They contain cadherin 5, plakoglobin, and desmoplakin, but are negative for vinculin and α-actinin.

Endothelial Cell-Matrix Interactions

In general, continuous as well as fenestrated endothelium rest on a basal lamina. It is thought that fenestrae are partially or completely occluded in all vascular beds by this basal membrane except in hepatic and bone marrow sinusoidal cells. The basal lamina is predominantly formed by both endothelium itself and surrounding cells, and consists of laminin-1, collagens, fibronectin, nidogen (entactin), and heparan sulfate proteoglycans. Surprisingly, immunohistochemical investigations do not reveal qualitative differences between the basal lamina of newly formed capillary sprouts and established vasculature. Interaction with these matrix molecules is essential for maintaining normal endothelial function. For example, the laminin A chain peptide supports endothelial branching and formation of new capillaries.[36] Furthermore, a 20-kDa C-terminal fragment of collagen XVIII specifically inhibits endothelial proliferation and angiogenesis,[37] indicating that collagen XVIII also appears to be a positive regulator of vessel growth. On the other hand, endothelium–collagen V interactions inhibit endothelial attachment and growth. Endothelial cells interact with these components of the basal lamina by numerous transmembrane adhesion molecules. The complexities of these interactions have only been partially characterized. Members of the integrin family are particularly important for this function. For example, $\alpha_6\beta_1$, $\alpha_2\beta_1$, $\alpha_5\beta_1$, and $\alpha_V\beta_3$ receptor complexes are important for endothelial attachment to, and migration on, laminin, collagen, and tenascin therefore serving important roles in angiogenesis. In addition, ligation of integrins by matrix proteins also has a multitude of intracellular effects on the organization of the endothelial actin skeleton and on signaling processes within the cell.[38] Endothelial growth factors have been shown to differentially upregulate the biosynthesis of α_2, α_5, β_1, and β_3 integrins, in order to serve the different needs of endothelium during growth, spreading, and new vessel formation. Moreover, integrins show certain tissue and vessel restricted expression, for example, $\alpha_1\beta_1$is found only in small blood vessels and capillaries, but not in large-vessel endothelium. Matrix proteins such as thrombospondins may also serve as inhibitors of angiogenesis.[39]

Morphologic Specialization of Endothelial Cells

As we noted in the preceding sections, endothelial cells differ along the course of the vasculature with regard to numbers of Weibel-Palade bodies, extent of the development of the caveolar system, the presence or absence of fenestrae, the type of intercellular junction, and the nature of the basement membrane composition and interactions. Additional morphologic specializations also may develop. The best characterized of these occurs in the postcapillary venules of the lymph nodes and mucosal-associated lymphoid tissues. Such endothelial cells loose their characteristic flat morphology of vascular endothelium and acquire a distinct "high" or cuboidal shape. For this reason, these microvessels are called *high endothelial venules* (HEVs). Their endothelial cells display more prominent biosynthetic organelles and synthesize basement membrane highly enriched with sulfated glycosaminoglycans.[40] These features are thought to facilitate transendothelial diapedesis of lymphocytes. Similar morphologic features may be acquired by venular endothelium at sites of chronic inflammation and may represent an adaptation to elevated levels of leukocyte trafficking.[41]

A second specialized type of endothelial cell is the sinusoidal endothelial cell of the spleen. Sinuses in the spleen are not found in all mammals. For example, they are well formed in humans and rats, but are absent in mice. In the spleen, where sinusoids exist, arteries open into splenic parenchyma, and blood is reabsorbed into sinusoids through open spaces at the end, and through interendothelial slits. The spleen sinus traps erythrocytes with denatured hemoglobin (Heinz bodies) by a yet unknown mechanism. The sinusoids drain into the venous system.

Molecular Markers of Endothelial Cells

Endothelial cells display a number of common biochemical/molecular features that have been used to define an antigenic phenotype. The single most widely used marker for vascular endothelium is vWF, which may be detected in WPB or within the biosynthetic organelles (Golgi apparatus or endoplasmic reticulum). vWF is displayed by almost all vascular endothelium, but its level may vary. vWF is essentially undetectable in renal glomerular capillaries. vWF is also found in megakaryocytes and platelets. CD31 (PECAM-1) is shared by endothelium and platelets, but is also found on circulating leukocytes (see below). All endothelium can be recognized by acetylated low-density lipoprotein (acLDL) uptake via the "scavenger cell pathway" of LDL metabolism. There are at least four different types of scavenger receptors.[42] Some of these receptors are shared with or are unique to macrophages, while some are probably unique to endothelium. However, the uptake of fluorescence-tagged acetylated or oxidized LDL has been used as a marker of endothelium, but does not distinguish among receptors, or between endothelial cells and macrophages. Nearly all endothelial cells secrete and then bind CD143 (angiotensin-converting enzyme) to the cell surface. This characteristic is shared with macrophages. Most endothelial cells express the anticoagulant protein CD141 (thrombomodulin). This feature is shared with trophoblast cells of the placenta, which, like endothelium, form a blood-compatible surface that prevents coagulation.

Some endothelial markers are not proteins. Endothelial cells display proteoglycans rich in heparan sulfate glycosaminoglycans that bind and activate antithrombin III, i.e., have anticoagulant properties. Human vascular endothelial cells express blood group H antigens recognized by the lectin ulex europaeus agglutinin-1 (UEA-1). This expression is also shared with erythrocytes and certain specialized epithelia. Endothelial cells of species other than higher primates (including humans) and Old World monkeys lack a particular fucosyltransferase and cannot synthesize blood group H, but have related carbohydrate moieties that instead bind lectins such as Bandeiraea simplicifolia, peanut, and Dolichos biflorus agglutinin.

Combinations of vWF expression, receptor-mediated acLDL uptake, angiotensin-converting enzyme (ACE) expression, thrombomodulin expression, and blood group H expression are used as molecular identifiers of endothelial cells in vitro and in vivo. As we have noted, none of these markers alone is truly endothelial specific. More recently, VEGF receptors 1 and 2 have been used, but these receptors have recently been found on a growing list of other cell types. Tie-1 and Tie-2 have been suggested to be more specific, but these markers have not been adequately examined as to specificity. Although less widely used, intercellular adhesion molecule (ICAM)-2 may be the single best marker for endothelium. It is not generally found on other cell types and transgenic receptor genes expressed using the ICAM-2 promoter appear to be expressed only on endothelial cells.[43] Other helpful markers are P-selectin and, following cytokine treatment (see below), E-selectin (CD62E). E-selectin expression, when present, appears to be absolutely specific for endothelium, but is not inducible on all endothelial cells.

All endothelial cells share numerous surface proteins with various subpopulations of hematopoietic cells such as CD9, CD13, CD31, CD40, CD54, CD58, CD105 (endoglin), complement receptors for C1q and C5a, and complement regulatory proteins such as CD46, CD55, CD59, and Thy-1. This probably reflects the common embryologic origin of the angioblast and the hematopoietic stem cell. Moreover, endothelial cells express proteins broadly found on many cell types, such as CD26, CD44, CD47, and CD146 (MUC18). Endothelial cells also express class I major histocompatibility complex (MHC) molecules and a characteristic array of integrins. Finally, it should be noted that in normal tissues in vivo, endothelial cells investing blood vessels can be differentiated from endothelial cells investing lymphatics, the latter being Prox-1, Lyve-1 (lymphatic vessel endothelial hyaluronan receptor), podoplanin, and VEGF receptor 3 positive.[44]

True blood capillaries consist of tubes formed by a continuous string of elongated endothelial cells, each curved to form a segment of a hollow cylinder. Capillary endothelial cells express a series of microvessel-specific proteins not found on large vessels such as the

PAL-E antigen.[45] Blood capillaries also express CD34, which is also expressed on immature hematopoietic cells. Interestingly, monoclonal antibodies to different CD34 epitopes variably stain hematopoietic cells but uniformly stain endothelial cells.[46] In large mammals, microvascular endothelial cells express class II MHC molecules. CD36 is found on all microvessels with exception of brain endothelial cells and subtypes of skin microvessels,[46,47] which are CD36 negative. Certain molecules are restricted to distinct microvascular beds such as CD32 and CD206 for liver and skin and CD71 for brain.[48–50] Microvascular endothelial cells in certain organs may express unique sialomucins. In the gastrointestinal tract and the breast, they are contained within the 60-kDa core protein MadCAM-1.[51] In the lymph nodes, especially the high endothelial venule, they may be found in the secreted sialomucin GlyCAM-1. Moreover, certain surface proteins of endothelial cells may be decorated with sulfated sialylated and fucosylated carbohydrates, which react with antibody MECA-79, are collectively called peripheral node addressins, and function as L-selectin ligands.[40] They are specifically found in peripheral nodes, but may also be expressed on skin endothelium.[41]

In addition to the constitutively expressed molecules, endothelial cells show a characteristic pattern of inducible markers. At sites of inflammation, endothelial cells may express E-selectin and VCAM-1 (CD106). P-selectin may be increased on the cell surface, as is ICAM-1. Tumor vessels may display ICAM-3.

ENDOTHELIUM IN INFLAMMATION

Innate Immunity

Innate immunity, also called natural or native immunity, comprises the host's defense systems against microbes that are independent of T and B lymphocytes and their receptors for specific antigens. The innate immune system is much older in evolutionary terms than the T- and B-cell–specific immune system, and elements of innate immunity have been found in invertebrates such as sponges and starfish. The principal effector cells of innate immunity in humans are the phagocytic leukocytes, including both neutrophils and mononuclear phagocytes (i.e., blood monocytes and their progeny, tissue macrophages), natural killer (NK) cells, a primordial lymphocyte. Innate immunity has a humoral component, primarily involving the complement system and its alternative pathway of activation. Various acute phase proteins made by the liver cells, macrophages, and vascular endothelium also participate in innate immunity. The cells of the innate immune response, like those of the specific immune response, communicate with each other through release of cytokines. Endothelial cells are both a target and a source of the inflammatory cytokines of innate immunity.

The innate response to microbes is initiated by recognition by the host of the presence of non-self. In general, only a few prototypic foreign structures are recognized and the range of responses of innate immunity are limited. The two key responses are to viruses and bacteria. Cells infected with replicating viruses, but not normal mammalian cells, form double-stranded RNA molecules. Double-stranded RNA signals the presence of non-self by activating certain kinases. The kinases, in turn, trigger the synthesis of interferons α and β (IFN-α/β). IFN-α/β, also called type I IFN, is a cytokine that induces resistance to viral infections in host cells and renders infected cells more susceptible to lysis by host effector cells.[52] IFN-α/β also activates NK cells, which are major effector cells of innate immunity.

Antibacterial responses are initiated against bacterial cell-wall constituents not found in mammalian cells, such as lipopolysaccharide (LPS), which comprises the outer wall of gram-negative bacteria. LPS binds to the LPS-binding protein in plasma and is delivered to the cell surface receptor CD14, expressed on the surface of monocytes/macrophages. This complex can activate the transmembrane signaling receptor toll-like receptor 4 and its accessory protein MD2. LPS stimulation activates several intracellular signaling pathways that include the IκB kinase-NFκB and mitogen-activated protein kinase (MAPK) pathways. These signaling pathways in turn activate a variety of transcription factors that include NFκB (p50/p65) and AP-1 (c-fos/c-jun), which coordinate the induction of many genes encoding inflammatory mediators. Endothelial cells lack CD14 but respond to complexes of LPS with soluble CD14. As in macrophages, endothelial activation occurs through toll-like receptor 4.[53] Endothelial cells also express toll-like receptor 2, which serves as a signaling receptor for gram-positive cell wall components. Certain vascular beds express the macrophage mannose receptor (CD206), a receptor for oligosaccharides on the cell wall of bacteria, yeasts, and parasites. Other receptors of the innate immune system include a variety of lectin-type molecules, such as mannose-binding protein or galactins, that recognize bacterial carbohydrates. Mannose-binding protein may activate the alternative pathway of complement activation.

The cellular response to bacterial products such as LPS involves the secretion of several key cytokines, including TNF (sometimes called TNF-α), interleukin-1β (IL-1β), IL-6, IL-10, IL-12, and IL-15. TNF and IL-1β act on endothelial cells to induce proinflammatory changes that are discussed in detail below. TNF also acts on neutrophils to potentiate their oxidative burst response. IL-6 triggers the liver and other cells to make acute phase proteins. IL-12 acts on NK cells to induce secretion of IFN-γ; IFN-γ, in turn, further activates neutrophils and macrophages, combining with TNF to induce more potent antimicrobial mechanisms such as increased generation of reactive oxygen intermediates and possibly nitric oxide. IL-15 acts as a growth factor for NK cells. Whereas all of the above mentioned cytokines promote inflammation, IL-10 serves to dampen the response, downregulating the synthesis of other cytokines. Knockout mice lacking IL-10 show uncontrolled inflammation, especially in the gut where LPS is abundant.

TNF and IL-1β appear to be central to many different types of inflammatory reactions. In general, endothelial responses to TNF and IL-1 are similar and are considered together. At least five changes in the phenotype of endothelial cells that promote inflammation, collectively called "endothelial activation", have been described.

VASODILATORS TNF- or IL-1β–treated endothelial cells acquire increased capacities to produce vasodilators, such as prostaglandin I_2 (PGI_2) and NO. PGI_2, sometimes called prostacyclin, is synthesized in endothelial cells by a series of three sequential enzyme-catalyzed reactions. First, cytosolic phospholipase A_2 ($cPLA_2$) releases arachidonic acid from the SN-2 position of membrane phosphatidyl choline. Endothelial cells contain an enzyme that can acetylate the now vacant SN-2 hydroxyl group of phosphatidyl choline, generating biologically active platelet-activating factor (PAF); PAF is a potent activator of neutrophils. Second the liberated arachidonic acid is oxidized by O_2 in a two-step reaction catalyzed by prostaglandin H synthase (also called cyclooxygenase) to form prostaglandin H_2(PGH_2). Third, the PGH_2 is converted to PGI_2 by the enzyme prostacyclin synthase. The total reaction sequence is initiated by the activation of $cPLA_2$. $cPLA_2$ is constitutively expressed in endothelial cells, normally in an inactive form.[54] The enzymatic activity of $cPLA_2$ is increased by phosphorylation, catalyzed either by mitogen-activated protein (MAP) kinases such as ERK-1 or ERK-2, or by stress-activated protein (SAP) kinases such as p38. TNF and IL-1β efficiently activate p38 in endothelial cells, contributing to $cPLA_2$ activation, whereas autacoids like histamine probably work through ERK-1 or ERK-2. However, in order for activated $cPLA_2$ to efficiently interact with the cellular membrane, where phosphatidyl choline is sequestered, there must also be a rise in cytosolic free calcium. Neither TNF or IL-1β can cause a rise in cytosolic free calcium in endothelial cells, and this second signal is typically provided by autacoids such as histamine or the complement-derived anaphylatoxin C5a. LPS is an activator of the alternative pathway of complement, which can generate C5a. C5a not only acts on endothelial cells directly, but can also trigger perivascular mast cells to release histamine, which, in turn, acts on endothelial cells.

Endothelial cells express one isoform of prostaglandin H synthase, PGHS-1, also called cyclooxygenase (COX)-1, that is constitutively active. Once $cPLA_2$ is activated to release arachidonic acid, PGHS-1 becomes rate limiting. Treatment of endothelial cells with TNF or IL-1β dramatically increases the level of PGHS activity by inducing de novo expression of a second isoform, PGHS-2, which is also called COX-2. This response markedly increases the capacity of the cell to make PGH_2 from arachidonic acid. It is not known whether prostacyclin synthase activity is limiting or whether it is regulated by cytokines.

NO is synthesized by the oxidative conversion of arginine to citrulline and NO. This reaction is catalyzed by an enzyme called nitric oxide synthase (NOS). Normally, endothelial cells express a single isoform of NOS, called NOS-III or endothelial NOS (e-NOS). This enzyme is activated by rises in cytosolic free calcium that are signaled through the calcium-binding protein calmodulin. As noted earlier, TNF or IL-1β do not directly effect cytosolic calcium levels, but they increase NOS activity by increasing the level of a normally limiting cofactor, tetrahydrobiopterin. (This effect is enhanced by the presence of IFN-γ).

The net result of these TNF and IL-1β actions is to increase the synthesis of the vasodilatory molecules PGI_2 and NO by endothelial cells. PGI_2 or NO both relax smooth-muscle cell tension thereby producing local vasodilation and increasing tissue perfusion and hence delivery of leukocytes to the site of cytokine generation. Pharmacologic reduction in the generation of PGI_2 is thought to contribute to the anti-inflammatory actions of aspirin and nonsteroidal anti-inflammatory drugs (NSAIDs) that inhibit PGHS activity.

LEUKOCYTE ADHESION TNF- or IL-1β–treated endothelial cells exhibit a change in their cell surface that favors the initial tethering, rolling, and, ultimately, firm adhesion of leukocytes. Adhesion is a prelude to extravasation of leukocytes into the tissues. The initial tethering is typically mediated by selectins expressed on the leukocyte or on the endothelial cell.[55] There are three structurally related selectin proteins: L-selectin (CD62L), E-selectin (CD62E), and P-selectin (CD62P). L-selectin is constitutively and exclusively expressed on leukocytes. It binds to certain sialylated and fucosylated carbohydrates that may be attached to several different endothelial plasma membrane proteins, or proteoglycans, including CD34 and MadCAM-1, or on the endothelial cell–secreted proteoglycan, GlyCAM-1. In general, microvessels in peripheral tissues, do not constitutively synthesize L-selectin ligands, even though they express CD34 protein. However, these endothelial cells can change their pattern of glycosaminoglycan synthesis when exposed to TNF or IL-1β so that L-selectin ligands are now synthesized and displayed.

E-selectin, which binds carbohydrate ligands related to sialylated Lewis X or A moieties on leukocytes, is expressed exclusively by endothelial cells. Endothelial cells do not normally synthesize E-selectin, but its transcription and expression are induced by TNF or IL-1β. Studies using cultured endothelial cells suggest that synthesis of E-selectin is transient (onset 30 to 60 min, peak 2 to 4 h) and that the level cell surface expression generally conforms to the level of new synthesis, implying rapid internalization and degradation of expressed protein. However, these processes may be partly dissociated, so that E-selectin expression on the cell surface may persist for hours or even days after mRNA synthesis has been downregulated. The relevant glycan moieties expressed on neutrophils that are recognized by E-selectin are principally attached to two different proteins: E-selectin ligand-1 (ESL-1) and L-selectin. The protein that displays E-selectin ligands on lymphocytes appears to be P-selectin ligand-1 (PSGL-1, see below).[56]

P-selectin is found in the membrane of secretory storage granules in platelets (i.e. α granules) and endothelial cells (i.e., WPB). P-selectin is rapidly translocated to the endothelial cell surface in response to autacoids. In mice, but not humans, TNF or IL-1β may increase P-selectin levels by inducing new synthesis in chronic inflammatory settings. The ligands for P-selectin include glycans similar to those for E-selectin and sulfated sialomucins similar to those for L-selectin, but these are displayed on distinct leukocyte surface glycoproteins, principally PSGL-1.[57]

The initial interaction of a selectin with its ligand results in leukocyte "tethering" to the endothelial surface, a low-affinity attachment. In the presence of flowing blood, the tethered leukocyte is propelled in the direction of blood flow, rapidly breaking and reforming selectin-mediated attachments. This results in rolling of the leukocyte along the endothelial cell surface. It should be noted that the ligands involved in selectin-mediated adhesion that participate in the initial tethering may not be the same as those involved in rolling, e.g., neutrophils may switch from L-selectin to ESL-1 as the principal E-selectin ligand during these two phases of the interaction.[58] Studies using blocking monoclonal antibodies or adhesion molecule knockout mice have confirmed that selectins are required for neutrophil rolling and subsequent recruitment in vivo, although E- and P-selectin functions may be redundant (i.e., both molecules must be knocked out or inhibited for complete loss of rolling). It is not clear whether this redundancy also applies to humans where E- and P-selectin expression is controlled by different signals.

Firm adhesion of leukocytes to endothelium is generally mediated by leukocyte integrins. Leukocytes utilize two different types of integrins to interact with endothelial cells. The first of these are the CD18 or β_2 integrins, including LFA-1 ($\alpha_L\beta_2$ or CD11a/CD18) and Mac-1 ($\alpha_M\beta_2$ or CD11b/CD18). Both of these integrins bind to ICAM-1 (also called CD54), a member of the immunoglobulin superfamily of proteins.[59] ICAM-1 is constitutively expressed at low levels by endothelial cells, although typically at higher levels than on tissue cells. However, ICAM-1 synthesis and expression can be dramatically (twentyfold or more) upregulated by TNF or IL-1β (onset 4 h, plateau at 24 h). IFN-γ causes a limited and gradual increase in endothelial cell expression of ICAM-1 (as compared to its rapid and potent effect on keratinocyte or melanocyte ICAM-1 expression), but IFN-γ can potentiate the effects of TNF in endothelium. Endothelial cells also constitutively express a structurally related molecule, called ICAM-2 (CD102) that can be recognized by LFA-1 but not Mac-1. Despite the constitutive expression of ICAM-2 at levels comparable to that of induced ICAM-1, there is little evidence that ICAM-2 actually mediates firm adhesion of leukocytes to endothelial cells. Antibody blocking experiments suggest that LFA-1 is more important than Mac-1 for the firm adhesion of neutrophils to endothelium, and that Mac-1 may play a more important role in neutrophil activation (especially in phagocytosis, because Mac-1 is also a receptor for complement protein fragment C3bi). However, this hierarchy may depend on the activating signal (see below).

The adhesion mediated by LFA-1 or Mac-1 recognition of ICAM-1 is much stronger than that mediated by selectins so that once these molecules have engaged ICAM-1, leukocytes no longer roll. In the case of neutrophils, integrin engagement results in a gradual slowing of rolling velocity. In contrast, lymphocytes abruptly convert from rolling to firm adhesion. Once adherent, leukocytes spread out and then slowly crawl along the endothelial cell surface until they reach a cell junction where they diapedese through the vessel wall into the tissues. It is likely that LFA-1-mediated attachment, disengagement, and reattachment to ICAM-1 play a role in the spreading, crawling, and diapedesis of leukocytes. Although ICAM-1 is initially (at 4 h) upregulated diffusely on the luminal surface of the endothelial cell, it tends to preferentially localize to the intercellular junctions over the first few days.[24] Studies with blocking antibodies in knockout mice confirm that β_2 integrins and ICAM-1 play a major role in leukocyte adhesion to endothelium and in subsequent recruitment.

The second group of integrins on leukocytes that mediate attachment to endothelium are the $\alpha_4$integrins (CD49d), which may pair with either β_1(CD29) to form VLA-4 or with β_7 to form LPAM-1. Both $\alpha_4\beta_7$ and $\alpha_4\beta_1$ bind to vascular cell adhesion molecule-1 (VCAM-1 or CD106) and to the CS-1 domain of the cell-associated fibronectin isoform. $\alpha_4\beta_7$ can also bind MadCAM-1, recognizing an immunoglobulin-like domain distinct from the sialomucin moiety recognized by L-selectin. $\alpha_4\beta_7$ interactions with MadCAM-1 are thought to mediate lymphocyte homing to mucosal lymphoid tissues and will be discussed later in this chapter when we address homing of T cells to skin. In humans, VLA-4 is not found on circulating neutrophils, being restricted in expression to monocytes, T cells, eosinophils and basophils. In rodents, it is expressed on neutrophils as well.

The principal endothelial cell ligand for VLA-4 is VCAM-1. This immunoglobulin superfamily member is not expressed on resting endothelial cells under normal circumstances, but is upregulated by TNF or IL-1β with a time course similar to that observed for ICAM-1. VCAM-1 may be selectively upregulated by interleukin-4, a cytokine associated typically with certain types of specific rather than innate immunity. Although VCAM-1 expression is not responsive to IFN-γ itself, IFN intensifies TNF-induced VCAM-1 expression.[60] Interestingly, VCAM-1 may support initial tethering and rolling of leukocytes, as well as firm adhesion, depending on whether the affinity/avidity of the leukocyte VLA-4 is increased by leukocyte activation. Both VLA-4 and VCAM-1 knockout mice are embryonic lethal mutations and shed no light on inflammatory processes; antibody-blocking experiments, however, confirm a role for these molecules in leukocyte recruitment in vivo.[61]

LEUKOCYTE ACTIVATION TNF- or IL-1β–treated endothelial cells promote the activation of tethered or rolling leukocytes, triggering the transition from selectin-mediated low-affinity attachment to integrin-mediated firm adhesion and the transition from spherical, immotile leukocytes to spread, migrating forms. In some experiments, engagement of selectins appears to be adequate by itself to trigger some of these changes, but most experiments implicate the requirement for a distinct signal. One candidate activator is the lipid mediator PAF, which can be displayed in the endothelial cell plasma membrane. As noted earlier, PAF synthesis is initiated by $cPLA_2$ activation, i.e., the same reaction that provides arachidonic acid for PGI_2 synthesis. (In endothelial cells, PAF contains acyl lipids rather than the alkyl lipids favored by leukocytes.) It has been reported that IL-1α (but not IL-1β) may promote PAF synthesis in endothelial cells, but most studies emphasize the role of autacoids (e.g. histamine), rather than cytokines, as inducers of PAF synthesis.

The chemokines constitute an important group of TNF- or IL-1β induced leukocyte activators, that are defined by the presence and number of amino acids between two N-terminal cysteine residues (i.e. C-C, C-X-C, etc.). Chemokines induce migration and/or activation of various types of leukocytes through interaction with a group of seven *trans*-membrane G-protein-coupled receptors. The C-X-C chemokines (such as IL-8) are particularly important for neutrophil activation and C-C chemokines (such as MCP-1) are important for monocyte activation. Both IL-8 and MCP-1 are synthesized and secreted by TNF- or IL-1β–treated endothelial cells. Furthermore, endothelial cells can display their secreted chemokines in a complex with cell surface proteoglycans in a manner that renders them bioavailable to tethered or rolling leukocytes. The bound chemokines displayed by endothelial cells could be made by endothelial cells or could be captured and displayed once made by tissue cells or leukocytes. In addition, there is a transmembrane protein form of a chemokine called fractalkine, with its chemokine domain presented at the top of a mucin-like stalk. Fractalkine can be induced in vascular endothelial cells and functions as an adhesion molecule. Accumulating evidence suggests that fractalkine mediates vascular injury during glomerulonephritis, in allograft rejection and atherosclerotic disease.[62,63,64] Chemokines may also play a role in activation and recruitment of specific lymphocyte subsets, as will be discussed later in this chapter.

EXTRAVASATION OF LEUKOCYTES The interaction between TNF- and IL-β–treated endothelial cells and leukocytes results in degradation of cellular and extracellular matrix barriers that normally separate leukocytes from the tissue space. The endothelial junctions contain proteins, such as PECAM-1 (CD31) that appear to contribute to leukocyte transmigration and, as noted above, chronically activated endothelial cells also concentrate adhesive ligands, such as E-selectin, ICAM-1, and VCAM-1, at these same junctions. The details of interaction between leukocytes and endothelial cells during diapedesis in vivo are unknown, although antibody to PECAM-1 does appear to inhibit this process. A PECAM-1 knockout mouse has a surprisingly mild phenotype with only minor effects on leukocyte transmigration. The two junctional proteins, VE-cadherin and JAM-1, are localized at endothelial adherens and tight junctions, respectively. They control paracellular permeability and leukocyte transmigration by a mechanism not yet fully understood.[65] Recent observations have also implicated CD99 as an endothelial cell junctional protein that participates in trans-endothelial cell migration.

TNF- or IL-1β–treated endothelial cells secrete and activate matrix metalloproteinases (MMPs), which degrade the condensed region of connective tissue matrix, i.e., the basement membrane, that underlies the endothelial monolayer. Endothelial cells may also trigger leukocytes to synthesize or release MMPs, and the signals for this release may be cytokine-inducible molecules such as VCAM-1 or chemokines.[66]

VASCULAR LEAKAGE AND PROVISIONAL MATRIX TNF- or IL-1β–treated endothelial cells permit the nonspecific extravasation of fluid and plasma proteins commonly called "vascular leak." The loss of permselectivity and consequent vascular leak is a hallmark of inflammation. The principal purpose of this response is to allow plasma proteins, such as fibronectin and fibrinogen, to deposit in the tissues where they form a provisional matrix that can be used by motile leukocytes. This is important because circulating leukocytes typically lack receptors that allow them to interact with the normal extracellular matrix, composed largely of interstitial collagens.

Collectively, these five TNF- or IL-1β-mediated responses of endothelial cells promote the development of an inflammatory infiltrate initially comprised of neutrophils and, later, of mononuclear phagocytes. The infiltrating leukocytes serve to phagocytose the eliciting microbes (e.g., bacteria) and clean up damaged tissue. Infiltrating phagocytes also can cause tissue damage through the same mediators and enzymes they use to eradicate microbes (e.g., reactive oxygen intermediates, nitric oxide, and matrix degrading enzymes such as elastase and MMPs). These mechanisms can and often do injure local endothelial cells, manifested by endothelial cell retraction and/or denudation and often accompanied by intravascular thrombosis. Intravascular thrombi exacerbate tissue ischemia and injury. Fortunately, TNF-or IL-1β–treated endothelial cells become more resistant to injury through expression of protective gene products such as detoxifying agents for reactive oxygen intermediates, such as manganese-superoxide dismutase and hemoxygenase, protease inhibitors such as plasminogen activator inhibitor-1 and tissue inhibitors of metalloproteinases (TIMPs), and cytoprotective genes such as the zinc finger protein A20 and Bcl-related antiapoptotic genes such as A1. These protective responses allow endothelial cells to survive many inflammatory reactions without triggering thrombosis and consequent tissue infarction.

The acquisition of cytoprotective features has been observed in the endothelial cells of organ grafts that have evaded transplant rejection.[67] However, these protective responses are not always adequate. Moreover, some other TNF- or IL-1β–mediated endothelial responses, for example, induction of procoagulant proteins such as tissue factor coupled with loss of anticoagulant proteins, such as thrombomodulin, may actually exacerbate tissue and vascular injury. This combination of neutrophil recruitment and activation with alterations in the endothelial coagulation system may underlie the tissue injury that can result from LPS in such experimental models as the local Shwartzman reaction or in gram-negative septicemia.

In summary, endothelial cells, through their responses to cytokines, can contribute to host defense reactions mediated by the innate immune system. However, these same effector mechanisms may lead to endothelial injury and exacerbate tissue damage.

To date, the only known function of class I and class II MHC molecules is to present peptides to T cells. Vascular endothelial cells constitutively express class I MHC molecules, as well as the proteins involved in generating peptides and involved in loading these peptides into nascent class I molecules.[68] The expression of class I genes (and the gene encoding the associated β_2-microglobulin molecule), as well as for the proteins involved in peptide generation and class I MHC molecule peptide loading, are all upregulated by cytokines, particularly by interferons (IFN-α, β, and γ), and by TNF.[69] Cultured human endothelial cells do not normally express class II MHC molecules or the proteins responsible for peptide loading of class II molecules; these proteins are all induced by IFN-γ, but these actions of IFN-γ are inhibited by IFN-α/β or TNF. In large mammals, including humans, class II molecules are basally expressed on microvascular cells in vivo.[69,70] It is unclear whether this "constitutive" expression depends upon low levels of circulating IFN-γ or is truly constitutive. Class II molecule expression on microvascular endothelial cells of guinea pigs and mice are readily induced upon IFN-γ exposure; this seems not to occur in rats, although cultured rat endothelial cells do respond to IFN-γ by expressing class II molecules. These species differences could affect the capacities of endothelial cells to present antigens to CD4+ T cells in vivo.

The typical diameter of a capillary lumen is less than 10 μm, i.e., narrower than the diameter of a circulating lymphocyte. Consequently, circulating T cells are forced to encounter antigenic peptides complexed to both class I and class II MHC molecules displayed on the microvascular endothelial surface during the course of normal circulation. A key question is what effect does this encounter have on the T cell? Upon recognition of peptide-MHC molecule complexes, T cells may become activated, may remain unchanged, which is a response called immunologic ignorance, or may become inactivated and unable to respond to future encounters (i.e., enter a state of "anergy"). Moreover, activation is a graded response and need not be all or none.

Studies of the consequences of T cell recognition of antigen presented by endothelial cells have largely used cell culture systems and have been primarily concerned with allogeneic responses, which are a cross-reaction of T cells specific for foreign peptides complexed with self allelic forms of MHC molecules with peptides (self or foreign) complexed to non-self allelic forms of MHC molecules as may be encountered in transplantation.[71] Such in vitro experiments suggest that naïve T cells ignore antigens presented by endothelial cells (or, in some instances, may become anergized), whereas resting memory T cells or recently activated T blasts respond by new cytokine gene expression and a limited degree of proliferation. However, endothelial cells are not particularly effective at promoting T cell differentiation as compared to specialized antigen-presenting cells such as dendritic cells. This limitation may correlate with the observation that human endothelial cells are deficient in expressing certain costimulator molecules, e.g., B7.1 (CD80) and B7.2 (CD86) expressed on dendritic cells, and must costimulate T cells largely with LFA-3 (CD58).[71] Interestingly, in certain other species (e.g., pigs) endothelial cells do express B7.2 and well as LFA-3.

It is our hypothesis that the primary role of human endothelial cell antigen presentation, which occurs in the capillaries, is to boost the adhesion of circulating memory T cells specific for the antigen by increasing the affinity/avidity of LFA-1 for ICAM-1 (and perhaps ICAM-2). This adhesive response would serve to promote T cell attachment to endothelium, most likely in the venules that drain the capillaries where antigen was presented, thus initiating local T cell diapedesis. This mechanism, if true, would serve to contribute to the efficiency of immune surveillance. This is a potentially important function because T cells specific for any one antigen, even among memory T cells expanded by prior encounter with antigen, are rare (fewer than 1 in 10,000 to 100,000) and presentation of antigen by endothelial cells could markedly increase the likelihood that antigen will be recognized in a timely manner.

T cells may differentiate into specialized cytokine-producing subsets. For CD4+ T cells, such responses may become polarized into T_H1 responses, dominated by T cells that produce IFN and lymphotoxin (LT), or into T_H2 responses, dominated by T cells that produce IL-4 and IL-5. The T_H1 subset favors recruitment and activation of mononuclear phagocytes and (in mice, at least) favors production by B cells of antibody isotypes that can efficiently opsonize bacteria for phagocytosis by these cells. The T_H2 subset favors recruitment and activation of eosinophils and favors production of antibody isotypes that target parasites for eosinophil-mediated killing, and trigger mast cells and basophils to release vasoactive mediators and cytokines. It is possible that these same sets of cytokines preferentially alter the adhesion molecule expression pattern of vascular endothelium to favor particular patterns of leukocyte and lymphocyte subset recruitment. For example, IFN-γ may combine with LT to cause prolonged expression of E-selectin, an important ligand for T_H1 T cells. T_H1 cells, but not T_H2 cells, are able to bind to P-selectin and E-selectin. Migration of T_H1 cells into inflamed skin can be blocked by antibodies against P- and E- selectin.[72] PSGL-1 appears to functions as P- and E-selectin ligands for T_H1 cells.[72,73] Although PSGL-1 is expressed on both, T_H1 and T_H2 cells, it only supports binding of T_H1 cells to selectins. The increased expression of the α_3-fucosyltransferases in T_H1 cells correlated with the ability of T_H1, but not T_H2, cells to bind to P-selectin. Thus, the regulation of the binding of effector T_H1 cells to the endothelium, and subsequent trafficking to inflammatory sites, appears to be controlled by the fucosylation state of PSGL-1 mediated by the selective expression of the α_3-fucosyltransferases.

In contrast, IL-4 increases VCAM-1 expression while suppressing E-selectin, a cell surface molecule that may favor eosinophil and perhaps T_H2 cell recruitment. In other words, T cell cytokines, produced by specific subsets, may modify the innate endothelial cell responses, e.g., to TNF, in a way that biases leukocyte recruitment toward recruitment of specific effector cells. Finally, differential expression of chemokine receptors may also account for selective recruitment of T cell subsets; e.g., CCR5 and, to a lesser degree, CXCR3 are preferentially found on T_H1 cells, whereas CCR4, CCR8, and, more controversially, CCR3 and CXCR4 are preferentially found on T_H2 cells.

ENDOTHELIUM OF THE SKIN

Morphology and Molecular Markers

ARCHITECTURE OF THE SKIN VASCULATURE The dermal microvasculature consists of two interconnected systems. The superficial vascular plexus (SVP) is comprised of paired arterioles and venules that form an interconnected network of vessels coursing on a plane parallel to and just beneath the epidermal surface.[74] Capillaries arise from the arterioles, extend upward within the papillary dermis at sites between the epidermal rete ridges, and then loop back down to the venules forming arcade-like structures. In normal skin, most of this capillary loop is invested with a basement membrane that resembles that of the arteriole. The capillaries acquire a venular-like investiture only at the level of the deepest rete just proximal to the anastomosis with the venule of the SVP.[75] The arteriolar portion of the papillary loop has a homogeneous-appearing basement membrane, which becomes multilayered at the venular portion. There are no ultrastructural differences between capillary loops at different sites of the skin. Inflammatory leukocytes extravasate through the venule-like portions of the capillary and through the venule proper, but only rarely infiltrate through the arteriole-like portions of the capillary or the arteriole itself.

The arterioles and venules of the SVP are connected by short, straight vessels to the arterioles and venules of a deeper planar network of anastomosing vessels called the deep vascular plexus (DVP). The plane of the DVP is parallel to that of the SVP and courses above the boundary between the reticular dermis and the underlying subcutis. The DVP is fed through penetrating vessels from the subcutis. The DVP is drained by valve-containing veins into the subcutaneous fat. Valves are at most places where the small vessels join the larger ones and imply a mechanism involved in forward propulsion of blood. The DVP contains arterioles and venules of larger caliber consisting of three layers—an intima, media, and adventitia—whereas those found within the SVP are smaller, and do not possess an internal or external elastic membrane. The vessel wall in the SVP consists of discontinuous layers of elastic fibers and smooth muscles. Capillary networks connecting the arterioles and venules of the DVP provide nourishment for the adnexal structures within the reticular dermis. The venules of the DVP serve as portals of entry for leukocytes associated with inflammation of the adnexa or for inflammation within the reticular dermis itself, as occurs in cellulitis.

Dermal microvessels are surrounded by flat adventitial cells, ultrastructurally most closely resembling a fibroblast, called *veil cells.*[76] Veil cells are external to the wall, demarcating the vessel from the surrounding dermis. These cells are negative for T or B cell markers, are HLA-DR and CD1a negative, and express factor XIIIa, and therefore are also called XIIIa-positive dendrocytes. Interestingly, factor XIIIa-positive dendrocyte rarefaction is found in the classic type of Ehlers-Danlos syndrome, but the significance of this finding is not clear. Unlike veil cells, pericytes are an integral component of the cell wall. They extend long cytoplasmic processes over the surface of the endothelial cells and make interdigitating contacts. The coverage of endothelial cells by pericytes varies considerably between different microvessel types and the location of pericytes on the microvessel is not random but appears to be functionally determined. At points of contact, communicating gap junctions, tight junctions, and adhesion plaques are present. Specifically in the postcapillary venule, there is an intimate interdigitation between pericytes and endothelial cells, one pericyte making contact with two to four endothelial cells. Pericytes are rich in contractile proteins, together with the complex interdigitation with endothelium in postcapillary venules, it can be assumed that they are responsible, at least in part, for gap formation in response to, e.g., histamine or bradykinin (although cultured endothelial cells are capable of contraction in the absence of pericytes). Moreover, interaction between pericytes and endothelium is important for the maturation, remodeling, and maintenance of the vascular system via the secretion of growth factors or modulation of the extracellular matrix. There is also evidence that pericytes are involved in the transport across the blood-brain barrier and the regulation of vascular permeability.

MOLECULAR MARKERS OF SKIN ENDOTHELIUM In addition to molecules expressed on all endothelium, the skin vasculature shows several site-specific characteristics. Postcapillary venules of the SVP are CD36 negative and thus distinct from capillaries of the DVP and from capillaries of other tissues which are CD36 positive.[77] CD36 antigen is a cellular receptor for thrombospondin, collagen, low-density lipoproteins, long-chain fatty acids, and platelet-agglutinating protein p37.[78] Moreover, CD36 functions as one of the receptors that mediates the adhesion of *Plasmodium falciparum*-infected erythrocytes to microvascular endothelium. The functional consequences of the disparate CD36 expression on SVP versus DVP endothelium are unknown. Microvessels express an epitope recognized by antibody PAL-E, which distinguishes them from lymphatic endothelium.

Postcapillary venules of the skin express toll-like receptor family members, CD206 (macrophage mannose receptor, also expressed on lymphatics) and CD32 molecules (FcγRIIa).[48] CD32 binds complexed IgG and is thought to function in the elicitation of type III hypersensitivity (immune complex-mediated) as well as in immune complex clearing. Moreover, skin microvessels in situ constitutively express HLA class II molecules at their luminal surfaces, which, as discussed previously, implies that endothelial cells may directly participate in the elicitation of antigen-driven immune responses. Indeed, skin microvessels in cell culture appear able to process and present antigen in a class II–restricted manner to T cells.[79]

Skin Microvessels in Inflammation and Repair

SKIN MICROVESSELS IN CUTANEOUS INFLAMMATION It is clear that vascular endothelial cells are important participants in the development of inflammatory responses. Recently, it was elucidated that tissue-specific differences in endothelial cells may partly determine the unique patterns of inflammation observed in different organs. One mechanism by which vascular endothelium may contribute to tissue-specific inflammatory patterns is through distinctive patterns of adhesion molecule expression, resulting in selective recruitment and diapedesis of circulating leukocytes bearing the proper ligands. In the skin, E-selectin, VCAM-1, and ICAM-1 may be particularly important in this process, and they have been extensively evaluated in normal and disease states. In noninflamed skin there is no significant microvascular expression of E-selectin and VCAM-1, and low levels of ICAM-1, as opposed to lesions of active dermatitis and psoriasis, where there is a small amount of VCAM-1, and high levels of E-selectin and ICAM-1.[47,77,80] In cutaneous T cell lymphoma (CTCL) there are high levels of VCAM-1.[86]

There appear to be differences in the inducibility of these adhesion molecules by leukocyte derived cytokines in different disease states as well. In normal and nonlesional skin explants, E-selectin is inducible by the inflammatory cytokines IL-1 and TNFα, whereas the inducibility of VCAM-1 varies in different disease states. VCAM-1 may only be inducible in skin that has been inflamed (e.g., spongiotic dermatitis), or in perilesional skin as well (e.g., on postcapillary venules of the superficial vascular plexus in psoriasis),[77] or in both lesional and nonlesional skin in CTCL.[86] The changes in dermal endothelial cells that permit VCAM-1 induction in these settings are unknown, but they cannot be reproduced with cytokines.

The induction of E-selectin appears to be particularly important in cutaneous inflammatory reactions. In addition to being readily inducible by cytokines, and uniformly associated with leukocytic infiltration, it may play a role in the selective recruitment of lymphocytes to cutaneous sites of inflammation through binding to the cutaneous lymphocyte antigen (CLA).[81,82] CLA is a carbohydrate moiety on the surface of T cells closely related to sialylated Lewis-X, which has homology to the core structure of P-selectin glycoprotein-1.[56] By using the identifying monoclonal antibody HECA-452, CLA has been found on 80 to 90 percent of skin infiltrating lymphocytes as compared to 5 to 10 percent at other peripheral sites. CLA is also present on circulating precursor Langerhans cells, and presumably plays a role in their eventual localization to the skin. The expression of E-selectin in cultured dermal microvascular endothelial cells is relatively persistent compared to endothelium derived from other sources. This persistent expression of E-selectin in vivo has been proposed to be responsible for the preferential homing of a CLA positive lymphocytes to the skin. Recent work in a chimeric human mouse model of inflammation suggests that CLA-positive lymphocytes specifically migrate through the superficial, as opposed to the deep, vascular plexus.[83] It is unlikely that E-selectin–CLA interactions alone are sufficient for the homing of lymphocytes to the skin. The transmigration of CLA-positive lymphocytes across activated endothelium is dependent on interactions with VCAM-1 and ICAM-1, in addition to E-selectin.

The induction of E-selectin on cutaneous microvessels also appears to play a role in immediate hypersensitivity reactions in atopic individuals. These reactions are characterized by an IgE-dependent biphasic response. Within minutes after exposure, the relevant antigen crosslinks IgE bound to the high affinity FcRε receptors on the surface of mast cells, resulting in histamine release. Histamine-dependent stimulation of endothelial cells leads to vasodilatation and increased vascular permeability that produces the classic wheal and flare response, typically resolving within 30 to 90 min. This reaction, known as the early phase response, is not accompanied by endothelial E-selectin upregulation or inflammatory cell recruitment. The late phase reaction begins 3 to 4 h after antigen challenge, and is characterized by the infiltration of eosinophils, neutrophils, and mononuclear cells into the inflamed area. Granulocytes are most prominent at 6 to 8 h, and by 24 to 48 h the cellular infiltrate consists largely of mononuclear cells. The expression of E-selectin, indicating endothelial activation, is detectable at the onset of infiltration. Although this E-selectin induction may simply be due to cytokine release from infiltrating inflammatory cells, there is evidence that the necessary mediators are released from skin resident cells. In skin organ culture, the addition of antigen either prior to or during the culture period results in significant E-selectin expression without inflammatory infiltrate.[84]

VCAM-1 may play a role in the specific homing of leukocytes to the skin through binding to the integrin $\alpha_4\beta_7$ on the surface of lymphocytes. This integrin is associated with the specific localization of lymphocytes to the gut through binding to the vascular adhesion molecule MadCAM-1 on the endothelium of intestinal microvessels.[86] Another ligand for $\alpha_4\beta_7$ includes fibronectin. Recently, $\alpha_4\beta_7$ has been found to be expressed on a high percentage of intraepidermal lymphocytes, particularly in CTCL, and, to a lesser degree, in spongiotic dermatitis.[86] Interestingly, in CTCL, the expression of $\alpha_4\beta_7$ strongly correlated with the expression of integrin $\alpha_E\beta_7$. $\alpha_E\beta_7$ is also found on a high percentage of gut (intraepithelial) and intraepidermal lymphocytes.

In chronic inflammatory conditions such as psoriasis and CTCL, the cutaneous microvascular endothelium develops a high endothelial venule morphology similar to that seen in peripheral lymph nodes. This is accompanied by the expression of the peripheral lymph node addressin L-selectin ligands identified by the antibody MECA-79. Interestingly, there was MECA-79 reactivity in the perifollicular vessels in noninflamed skin. This has led to the speculation that peripheral node addressins in chronic T cell–mediated skin diseases are responsible for sustained lymphocyte recruitment. The constitutive expression in normal skin may serve a function in continuous lymphocyte recirculation.[85]

Chemokines may also play a role in the selective homing of T cells to the skin. CCR4 is expressed at high levels by CLA-positive memory T cells. The CCR4 receptor TARC is constitutively expressed on endothelial cells in cutaneous postcapillary venules. In vitro TARC triggers CLA-positive T cells that are rolling on E-selectin to firmly adhere ICAM-1. Another skin-associated chemokine, CCL27 (CTACK), is produced by keratinocytes, and also preferentially attracts CLA-positive memory T cells.[87]

ANGIOGENESIS IN THE SKIN The details of the interactions between endothelial cells and angiogenic factors in physiologic and pathologic states were previously outlined. This section focuses on the role of angiogenesis in wound healing, inflammation, and tumorigenesis in the skin.

Cutaneous wound healing is a complex process that is, in part, dependent on angiogenesis. The revascularization of wounds is regulated by a combination of adhesion molecules and soluble growth factors derived from endothelial cells, keratinocytes, and inflammatory cells. Two soluble peptides that are particularly important are FGF-2 and VEGF. VEGF is produced by the keratinocytes and infiltrating macrophages in healing wounds. The splice variants of VEGF produced by keratinocytes are potent mitogens for dermal microvascular endothelial cells.[88,89] VEGFR-2 is also upregulated on endothelial cells at the site of injury.[90] Hypoxia, which often is present in healing wounds and rapidly growing tumors, induces keratinocytes, dermal fibroblasts, and endothelial cells to produce VEGF in vitro.[89] Angiopoietins 1 and 2 are also upregulated during injury, consistent with the role they are thought to play in the destabilizing, followed by stabilization of the vasculature. This allows a window for VEGF-mediated sprouting and elongation, followed by Ang-1–mediated remodeling.[4] FGF-2 is released in cutaneous wounds derived from endothelial cells and by infiltrating macrophages. When blocking antibodies directed against FGF-2 are used, wound angiogenesis is nearly completely inhibited.[91]

Adhesion molecules are necessary for physiologic angiogenesis in the skin. The expression of integrin $\alpha_v\beta_3$ on the tips of growing capillaries appears to facilitate endothelial migration, and appears to be required for wound healing. In an in vivo model in which human skin placed on immunodeficient mice is wounded, blocking antibodies directed against $\alpha_v\beta_3$ inhibited both angiogenesis and wound healing. In a similar model, blocking of the binding of CD31 and cadherin 5 with filamentous actin also blocked wound vascularization and healing.[34]

Tumor growth is dependent on the growth of nutritive blood vessels. Tumors are known to produce angiogenic factors such as VEGF, FGF-2, EGF, and HGF/SF.[92] Some of theses growth factors play a role in the pathogenesis of both benign and malignant skin tumors. There is a significant vascular component to the growth and metastases of cutaneous melanoma and an increased numbers of vessels in cutaneous melanoma as compared to severely atypical nevi. This vascular proliferative response appears to be in part mediated by FGF-2, which is known to be produced by melanoma cells. Antisense oligonucleotides directed against FGF-2 inhibit the proliferation of both primary and malignant melanoma.[94] HGF/SF and VEGF are also produced by melanoma cells, and may also contribute to their vascularization.

Peptide growth factors also appear to play a role in the pathogenesis of benign and malignant vascular tumors. Human endothelial cells acquire a Kaposi's sarcoma cell-like morphology when cultured in the presence of HGF/SF.[94] The spindle cells of Kaposi's sarcoma also produce large amounts of VEGF. The proliferative phase of hemangiomas contain high levels of FGF-2 and VEGF. There is increased FGF-2 in the involuting phase of these benign vascular tumors as well. VEGF-C–mediated tumor lymphangiogenesis is also associated with breast cancer metastasis.[95] The effective use of several angiogenesis inhibitors in murine tumor models have shown that tumor growth and metastases is dependent on an adequate vascular supply. These data have resulted in the ongoing investigational use of angiogenesis inhibitors as anticancer therapy.

Vascular remodeling appears to play a role in the pathogenesis of some inflammatory skin diseases, notably psoriasis. Psoriatic vessels become tortuous and elongated, and the normally well defined boundary between capillary endothelium resting on an arteriolar-like homogenous basement membrane and endothelial cells on a venular-like laminated basement membrane becomes unclear. The intrapapillary portions of capillaries acquire a venular phenotype,[96] corresponding to direct metaplasia from a arteriolar to a venular phenotype. It should be noted that this elongation of the capillary loops occurs without the formation of new vessels. Light microscopic investigations on eruptive guttate psoriatic lesions demonstrated that vascular alterations are the first ultrastructurally detectable alterations within the dermal compartment. These alterations consist of gap formation within postcapillary venules, endothelial cell hypertrophy (they acquire a cuboidal shape similar to that seen in high endothelial venules), and compression of the vascular lumen, all of which precedes the invasion of inflammatory cells into the tissue.[96] This morphologic alteration is accompanied by altered endothelial function. For example, there is increased blood flow in perilesional psoriatic skin even in the absence of any microscopically detectable changes.[97] The role angiogenic factors play in vascular remodeling in psoriasis has been partly characterized. It has been suggested that these vascular alterations may, in part, be mediated by increased production of VEGF by keratinocytes in the hyperplastic epidermis. There is also increased expression of the VEGFR1 and VEGFR2 on the papillary dermal microvascular endothelial cells.[98] VEGF appears to directly upregulate expression of ICAM-1, VCAM-1, and E-selectin on endothelial cells. The VEGF-mediated vascular leak and adhesion molecule upregulation can be inhibited by concurrent overexpression of Ang-1. The role of angiogenesis in inflammatory processes has been further exemplified by the anti-inflammatory effects of angiogenesis inhibitors.[99]

REFERENCES

1. Pardanaud L et al: Relationship between vasculogenesis, angiogenesis and haemopoiesis during avian ontogeny. *Development* **105**:473, 1989
2. Risau W, Flamme I: Vasculogenesis. *Annu Rev Cell Dev Biol* **11**:3, 1995
3. Asahara T et al: Isolation of putative progenitor endothelial cells for angiogenesis. *Science* **275**:964, 1997
4. Yancopoulos GD et al: Vascular-specific growth factors and blood vessel formation. *Nature* **407**:242, 2000
5. Makinen T et al: Inhibition of lymphangiogenesis with resulting lymphedema in transgenic mice expressing soluble VEGF receptor-3. *Nat Med* **7**:199, 2000
6. Karkkainen MJ et al: A model for gene therapy of human hereditary lymphedema. *Proc Natl Acad Sci U S A* **98**:12677, 2000
7. Fernig DG, Gallagher JT: Fibroblast growth factors and their receptors: An information network controlling tissue growth, morphogenesis and repair. *Prog Growth Factor Res* **5**:353, 1994
8. Gospodarowicz D et al: Control of proliferation of human vascular endothelial cells. Characterization of the response of human umbilical vein endothelial cells to fibroblast growth factor, epidermal growth factor, and thrombin. *J Cell Biol* **77**:774, 1978
9. Ushiro S et al: Heparin-binding epidermal growth factor-like growth factor: p91 activation induction of plasminogen activator/inhibitor, and tubular morphogenesis in human microvascular endothelial cells. *Jpn J Cancer Res* **87**:68, 1996
10. Grant DS et al: Scatter factor induces blood vessel formation in vivo. *Proc Natl Acad Sci U S A* **90**:1937, 1993
11. Maisonpierre PC et al: Angiopoietin-2, a natural antagonist for Tie2 that disrupts in vivo angiogenesis. *Science* **277**:55, 1997
12. Jones N et al: Rescue of the early vascular defects in Tek/Tie2 null mice reveals an essential survival function. *EMBO REP* **2**:438, 2001
13. Adams RH et al: Roles of ephrinB ligands and EphB receptors in cardiovascular development: Demarcation of arterial/venous domains, vascular morphogenesis, and sprouting angiogenesis. *Genes Dev* **13**:295, 2000
14. Gale NW et al: Ephrin-B2 selectively marks arterial vessels and neovascularization sites in the adult, with expression in both endothelial and smooth-muscle cells. *Dev Biol* **230**:151, 2000
15. McAllister KA et al: Endoglin, a TGF-beta binding protein of endothelial cells, is the gene for hereditary haemorrhagic telangiectasia type 1. *Nat Genet* **8**:345, 1994
16. Beck L, D'Amore PA: Vascular development: cellular and molecular regulation. *FASEB J* **11**:365, 1997
17. Carmeliet P et al: Role of tissue factor in embryonic blood vessel development. *Nature* **383**:73, 1996
18. Folkman J: Angiogenesis in cancer, vascular, rheumatoid and other disease. *Nat Med* **1**:27, 1995
19. Resnick N, Gimbrone MA: Hemodynamic forces are complex regulators of endothelial gene expression. *FASEB J* **9**:874, 1995
20. Milici AJ et al: The formation of fenestrations and channels by capillary endothelium in vitro. *Proc Natl Acad Sci U S A* **82**:6181, 1985
21. Janzer RC, Raff MC: Astrocytes induce blood-brain barrier properties in endothelial cells. *Nature* **325**:253, 1987
22. Remuzzi A et al: Orientation of endothelial cells in shear fields in vitro. *Biorheology* **21**:617, 1984
23. Rogers KA, Kalnins VI: Comparison of the cytoskeleton in aortic endothelial cells in situ and in vitro. *Lab Invest* **49**:650, 1983
24. Bradley JR, Pober JS: Prolonged cytokine exposure causes a dynamic redistribution of endothelial cell adhesion molecules to intercellular junctions. *Lab Invest* **75**:463, 1996
25. Bonfanti R et al: PADGEM (GMP140) is a component of Weibel-Palade bodies of human endothelial cells. *Blood* **73**:1109, 1989
26. Vischer UM, Wagner DD: CD63 is a component of Weibel-Palade bodies of human endothelial cells. *Blood* **82**:1184, 1993
27. Schnyder CS et al: Localization of α1,3-fucosyltransferase VI in Weibel-Palade bodies of human endothelial cells. *Proc Natl Acad Sci U S A* **97**:8369, 2000
28. Wolff B et al: Endothelial cell "memory" of inflammatory stimulation: Human venular endothelial cells store interleukin 8 in Weibel-Palade bodies. *J Exp Med* **188**:1757, 2000
29. Wisse E et al: Structure and function of sinusoidal lining cells in the liver. *Toxicol Pathol* **24**:100, 1996
30. Drab M et al: Loss of caveolae, vascular dysfunction, and pulmonary defects in caveolin-1 gene-disrupted mice. *Science* **293**:2449, 2000
31. Shivers RR et al: Isolated rat brain capillaries possess intact, structurally complex, interendothelial tight junctions; freeze-fracture verification of tight junction integrity. *Brain Res* **324**:313, 1984
32. Bazzoni G et al: Interaction of junctional adhesion molecule with the tight junction components ZO-1, cingulin, and occludin. *J Biol Chem* **275**:20520, 2000
33. Petzelbauer P et al: Endothelial adherens junctions. *J Invest Dermatol Symp Proc* **5**:10, 2000
34. Matsumura T et al: Endothelial cell tube formation depends on cadherin 5 and CD31 interactions with filamentous actin. *J Immunol* **158**:3408, 1997
35. Vittet D et al: Targeted null-mutation in the vascular endothelial-cadherin gene impairs the organization of vascular-like structures in embryoid bodies. *Proc Natl Acad Sci U S A* **94**:6273, 1997
36. Grant DS et al: Interaction of endothelial cells with a laminin A chain peptide (SIKVAV) in vitro and induction of angiogenic behavior in vivo. *J Cell Physiol* **153**:614, 1992
37. O'Reilly MS et al: Endostatin: An endogenous inhibitor of angiogenesis and tumor growth. *Cell* **88**:277, 1997
38. Miyamoto S et al: Integrin function: Molecular hierarchies of cytoskeletal and signaling molecules. *J Cell Biol* **131**:791, 1995
39. Detmar M: Tumor angiogenesis. *J Invest Dermatol Symp Proc* **5**:20, 2000
40. Yeh JC et al: Novel sulfated lymphocyte homing receptors and their control by a core1 extension β1,3-*N*-acetylglucosaminyltransferase. *Cell* **105**:957, 2000
41. Lechleitner S et al: Peripheral lymph node addressins are expressed on skin endothelial cells. *J Invest Dermatol* **113**:410, 1999
42. Adachi H et al: Expression cloning of a novel scavenger receptor from human endothelial cells. *J Biol Chem* **272**:31217, 1997
43. Cowan PJ et al: Targeting gene expression to endothelial cells in transgenic mice using the human intercellular adhesion molecule 2 promoter. *Transplantation* **62**:155, 1996
44. Karkkainen MJ et al: Lymphatic endothelium: A new frontier of metastasis research. *Nat Med* **4**:E2, 2002
45. Schlingemann RO et al: Monoclonal antibody PAL-E specific for endothelium. *Lab Invest* **52**:71, 1985
46. Fina L et al: Expression of the CD34 gene in vascular endothelial cells. *Blood* **75**:2417, 1990
47. Petzelbauer P et al: Inducibility and expression of microvascular endothelial adhesion molecules in lesional, perilesional, and uninvolved skin of psoriatic patients. *J Invest Dermatol* **103**:300, 1994
48. Gröger M et al: Dermal microvascular endothelial cells express CD32 receptors in vivo and in vitro. *J Immunol* **156**:1549, 1996
49. Gröger M et al: Dermal microvascular endothelial cells express the 180-kDa macrophage mannose receptor in situ and in vitro. *J Immunol* **165**:5428, 2000
50. Jefferies WA et al: Transferrin receptor on endothelium of brain capillaries. *Nature* **312**:162, 1984

51. Berg EL et al: L-selectin-mediated lymphocyte rolling on MAdCAM-1. *Nature* **366**:695, 1993
52. Gresser I: Wherefore interferon? *J Leukoc Biol* **61**:567, 1997
53. Faure E et al: Bacterial lipopolysaccharide activates NF-6B through toll-like receptor 4 (TLR-4) in cultured human dermal endothelial cells. Differential expression of TLR-4 and TLR-2 in endothelial cells. *J Biol Chem* **275**:11058, 2000
54. Newby AC, Henderson AH: Stimulus-secretion coupling in vascular endothelial cells. *Annu Rev Physiol* **52**:661, 1990
55. Pober JS, Cotran RS: Immunologic interactions of T lymphocytes with vascular endothelium. *Adv Immunol* **50**:261, 1991
56. Fuhlbrigge RC et al: Cutaneous lymphocyte antigen is a specialized form of PSGL-1 expressed on skin-homing T cells. *Nature* **389**:978, 1997
57. Bevilacqua MP: Endothelial-leukocyte adhesion molecules. *Annu Rev Immunol* **11**:767, 1993
58. Lawrence MB et al: Neutrophil tethering to and rolling on E-selectin are separable by requirement for L-selectin. *Immunity* **1**:137, 1994
59. Tonnesen MG et al: Adherence of neutrophils to cultured human microvascular endothelial cells. Stimulation by chemotactic peptides and lipid mediators and dependence upon the Mac-1, LFA-1, p150,95 glycoprotein family. *J Clin Invest* **83**:637, 1989
60. Lechleitner S et al: Interferon enhances tumor necrosis factor-induced vascular cell adhesion molecule 1 (CD106) expression in human endothelial cells by an interferon- related factor 1-dependent pathway. *J Exp Med* **187**:2023, 2000
61. Albelda SM et al: Adhesion molecules and inflammatory injury. *FASEB J* **8**:504, 1994
62. Umehara H et al: Fractalkine and vascular injury. *Trends Immunol* **22**:602, 2000
63. Matsukawa A et al: Chemokines and innate immunity. *Rev Immunogenet* **2**:339, 2000
64. Yoshie O et al: Chemokines in immunity. *Adv Immunol* **78**:57, 2000
65. Dejana E et al: Interendothelial junctions and their role in the control of angiogenesis, vascular permeability and leukocyte transmigration. *Thromb Haemost* **86**:308, 2000
66. Madri JA et al: The roles of adhesion molecules and proteinases in lymphocyte transendothelial migration. *Biochem Cell Biol* **74**:749, 1996
67. Bach FH et al: Accommodation of vascularized xenografts: Expression of "protective genes" by donor endothelial cells in a host Th2 cytokine environment. *Nat Med* **3**:196, 1997
68. Collins T et al: Immune interferon activates multiple class II major histocompatibility complex genes and the associated invariant chain gene in human endothelial cells and dermal fibroblasts. *Proc Natl Acad Sci U S A* **81**:4917, 1984
69. Lapierre LA et al: Three distinct classes of regulatory cytokines control endothelial cell MHC antigen expression. Interactions with immune gamma interferon differentiate the effects of tumor necrosis factor and lymphotoxin from those of leukocyte alpha and fibroblast beta interferons. *J Exp Med* **167**:794, 1988
70. Page C et al: Antigenic heterogeneity of vascular endothelium. *Am J Pathol* **141**:673, 1992
71. Pober JS et al: Can graft endothelial cells initiate a host anti-graft immune response? *Transplantation* **61**:343, 1996
72. Austrup F et al: P- and E-selectin mediate recruitment of T-helper-1 but not T-helper-2 cells into inflamed tissues. *Nature* **385**:81, 1997
73. Hirata T et al: P-selectin glycoprotein ligand 1 (PSGL-1) is a physiological ligand for E-selectin in mediating T helper I lymphocyte migration. *J Exp Med* **192**:1669, 2000
74. Yen A, Braverman IM: Ultrastructure of the human dermal microcirculation: the horizontal plexus of the papillary dermis. *J Invest Dermatol* **66**:131, 1976
75. Braverman IM, Yen A: Ultrastructure of the human dermal microcirculation. II. The capillary loops of the dermal papillae. *J Invest Dermatol* **68**:44, 1977
76. Braverman IM: Ultrastructure and organization of the cutaneous microvasculature in normal and pathologic states. *J Invest Dermatol* **93**:2S, 1989
77. Petzelbauer P et al: Heterogeneity of dermal microvascular endothelial cell antigen expression and cytokine responsiveness in situ and in cell culture. *J Immunol* **151**:5062, 1993
78. Febbraio M et al: CD36: A class B scavenger receptor involved in angiogenesis, atherosclerosis, inflammation, and lipid metabolism. *J Clin Invest* **108**:785, 2000
79. Vora M et al: Antigen presentation by human dermal microvascular endothelial cells. Immunoregulatory effect of IFN-gamma and IL-10. *J Immunol* **152**:5734, 1994
80. Das PK et al: Differential expression of ICAM-1, E-selectin, and VCAM-1 by endothelial cells in psoriasis and content dermatitis. *Acta Derm Vvenerol Suppl* **186**:21, 1994
81. Berg EL et al: The cutaneous lymphocyte antigen is a skin lymphocyte homing receptor for the vascular lectin endothelial cell-leukocyte adhesion molecule 1. *J Exp Med* **174**:1461, 1991
82. Picker LJ et al: A unique phenotype of skin-associated lymphocytes in humans: preferential expression of the HECA-452 epitope by benign and malignant T cells at cutaneous sites. *Am J Pathol* **136**:1053, 2000
83. Kunstfeld R et al: HECA-452+ T cells migrate through superficial vascular plexus but not through deep vascular plexus endothelium. *J Invest Dermatol* **108**:343, 1997
84. Leung DY et al: Expression of endothelial-leukocyte adhesion molecule-1 in elicited late phase allergic reactions. *J Clin Invest* **87**:1805, 1991
85. Hamann A et al: Role of alpha 4-integrins in lymphocyte homing to mucosal tissues in vivo. *J Immunol* **152**:3282, 1994
86. Schechner JS, Edelson RL, McNiff JM, Heald PW, Pober JS: Expression of integrin $\alpha_4\beta_7$ on epidermotropic cutaneous T cells in cutaneous T cell lymphoma and spongiotic dermatitis. Lab Inves¯t **79**:601, 1999
87. Pober JS et al: Human endothelial cell presentation of antigen and the homing of memory/effector T cells to skin. *Ann N Y Acad Sci* **941**:12, 2000
88. Brown LF et al: Expression of vascular permeability factor (vascular endothelial growth factor) by epidermal keratinocytes during wound healing. *J Exp Med* **176**:1375, 1992
89. Detmar M et al: Hypoxia regulates the expression of vascular permeability factor/vascular endothelial growth factor (VPF/VEGF) and its receptors in human skin. *J Invest Dermatol* **108**:263, 1997
90. Detmar M et al: Keratinocyte-derived vascular permeability factor (vascular endothelial growth factor) is a potent mitogen for dermal microvascular endothelial cells. *J Invest Dermatol* **105**:44, 1995
91. Broadley KN et al: Monospecific antibodies implicate basic fibroblast growth factor in normal wound repair. *Lab Invest* **61**:571, 1989
92. Leek RD et al: Cytokine networks in solid human tumors: Regulation of angiogenesis. *J Leukoc Biol* **56**:423, 1994
93. Becker D et al: Proliferation of human malignant melanomas is inhibited by antisense oligodeoxynucleotides targeted against basic fibroblast growth factor. *EMBO J* **8**:3685, 1989
94. Naidu YM et al: Role of scatter factor in the pathogenesis of AIDS-related Kaposi sarcoma. *Proc Natl Acad Sci USA* **91**:5281, 1994
95. Skobe M et al: Induction of tumor lymphangiogenesis by VEGF-C promotes breast cancer metastasis. *Nat Med* **7**:192, 2000
96. Braverman IM, Sibley J: Role of the microcirculation in the treatment and pathogenesis of psoriasis. *J Invest Dermatol* **78**:12, 1982
97. Brody I: Dermal and epidermal involvement in the evolution of acute eruptive guttate psoriasis vulgaris. *J Invest Dermatol* **82**:465, 1984
98. Detmar M et al: Overexpression of vascular permeability factor/vascular endothelial growth factor and its receptors in psoriasis. *J Exp Med* **180**:1141, 1994
99. Lange-Asschenfeldt B et al: Increased and prolonged inflammation and angiogenesis in delayed-type hypersensitivity reactions elicited in the skin of thrombospondin-2-deficient mice. *Blood* **99**:538, 2002

CHAPTER 20

Franz J. Legat
Cheryl A. Armstrong
Thomas Scholzen
John E. Olerud
Nigel W. Bunnett
Thomas A. Luger
John C. Ansel

Neurobiology of the Skin

The skin is innervated by a three-dimensional network of nerve fibers that not only participate in the transmission of sensory impulses but also contribute to neurocutaneous inflammation and wound healing. Neuropeptides that are released by cutaneous sensory nerves in response to a variety of noxious stimuli can also mediate a broad range of biologic effects through the interaction with a variety of target cells in the skin.[1–4] Likewise, neurohormones such as alpha-melanocyte–stimulating hormone (α-MSH), which are capable of modulating a range of cellular activities, can be detected in peripheral nerves and are produced by different cell types in the skin.[5] The biologic activities of these released cutaneous neuropeptides and neurohormones include the modulation of cell proliferation, cytokine production, and cellular adhesion molecule expression in cutaneous target cells such as keratinocytes, microvascular endothelial cells, Langerhans cells, melanocytes, fibroblasts, dermal leukocytes, and mast cells.[1–8] The cutaneous neuroinflammation cascade is regulated by the expression of specific neuropeptide and neurohormone receptors on epidermal and dermal cells, as well as by the activity of proteolytic enzymes in the skin that degrade released neuropeptides, thereby terminating the neuroinflammatory response.[1] Neurocutaneous interactions and responses also depend on the production and activity of neurotrophic factors, such as nerve growth factor (NGF), that can be secreted by skin cells under physiologic and pathophysiologic conditions and can modulate the growth and proliferation of cutaneous nerve fibers.[1,9] This chapter discusses the role of different components of the sensory nervous system in mediating cutaneous inflammation and wound healing. An overview of our current understanding of the key components of neurogenic inflammation in the skin is presented.

NEUROGENIC INFLAMMATION

Background

The cutaneous sensory nervous system is responsible for relaying sensory information from the skin to the central nervous system (CNS). Early in the twentieth century, Bayliss and Bruce noted that patients with defective cutaneous sensory systems were incapable of mounting normal inflammatory responses in the skin to topically applied proinflammatory agents.[10,11] Likewise, for many years, clinicians observed that patients with certain cutaneous sensory disorders, such as congenital analgesia syndromes, postherpes analgesia, and diabetic neuropathy, had defective responses to inflammatory stimuli.[12] Such clinical observations had led investigators to examine the role of the cutaneous neurologic system in modulating cutaneous inflammation.

Hallmarks of Neurogenic Inflammation: Vasodilation and Plasma Leakage

The definition of neurogenic inflammation has expanded as our understanding of the complex network of neuropeptides, target cell receptors, and degradatory enzymes involved in this process has grown. Nicholas Jansco coined the term *neurogenic inflammation* to describe the inflammatory response in the skin by direct electrical stimulation of sensory nerves or by stimulation of these nerves by chemical irritants, such as capsaicin, mustard oil, formalin, xylene, or hypertonic solutions.[13,14] Major consequences of neuroinflammatory responses include vasodilation, increased vascular permeability, and plasma leakage. Jansco first used capsaicin (*trans*-8-methyl-*N*-vanillyl-6-nonenamide), the pungent ingredient in hot chili peppers, as a specific research tool to induce sensory nerve activation and neuroinflammatory responses, when administered in low doses. An increasing number of subsequent studies support the contribution of capsaicin-sensitive nerve fibers and released neuropeptides in mediation of inflammation in the skin.[15] Capsaicin induction of neuropeptide release from sensory nerves triggers a cascade of inflammatory events, such as pain, erythema, and edema in skin and mucosa. The phenomenon of capsaicin-induced *desensitization* that renders nerves in the treated area insensitive to further stimulation by chemical irritants is caused by sensory nerve depletion of neuropeptides, such as substance P and calcitonin gene–related peptide (CGRP), as well as by the destruction of free sensory nerve endings.[15,16] A specific functional capsaicin-sensitive vanilloid receptor has been identified on sensory nerves. This receptor is believed to respond primarily to localized heat and acidic stimuli.[17]

Local Effector Function of Sensory Nerve Endings and Axon Reflex Model

Neurogenic inflammation in response to the application of capsaicin to the skin is not inhibited by local anesthetics and, thus, the release of neuropeptides from cutaneous sensory nerves appears to be independent of the induction of the neuronal action potential.[15] Released cutaneous neuropeptides are capable of diffusing into surrounding tissues to initiate various inflammatory responses. By this mechanism, nerve endings in the skin mediate local effector inflammatory responses and may act as the first component of the innate immune response after cutaneous injury.

There are also mechanisms by which the activation of sensory nerves can spread to branched nerve endings that are not directly stimulated. The application of cutaneous irritants or the injection of histamine into a localized region of the skin causes reddening (erythema) and edema (wheal), as well as an arteriolar vasodilation (flare) that spreads far beyond the site of initial stimulation. The flare component of this so-called triple response in the skin is dependent on an intact sensory innervation of the skin, because it does not take place in denervated skin. This neurosensory phenomenon may be explained by the so-called axon-reflex model of neurogenic inflammation. This model proposes that after injury of tissue innervated by the sensory nervous system, an immediate orthodromic signal, elicited by the sensory nerves to the dorsal root ganglia and the CNS, allows the host to sense and respond to the injury rapidly by a withdrawal and avoidance response. In addition to this orthodromic response to the CNS, other branched components of these afferent nerves pass nerve impulses antidromically in the reverse direction back to the peripheral innervated tissue.[15,18] In this antidromic response, neuropeptides are released into the injured tissue where they can interact with potential target cells located in close proximity to the activated sensory nerve fibers.[15,18]

THE CUTANEOUS SENSORY NERVOUS SYSTEM

Neuroanatomy

The cutaneous sensory nervous system is an important component of the peripheral nervous system. Sensory nerves are derived from dorsal root ganglion neurons and are present in all parts of the skin, representing the initial somatic portion of the afferent sensory pathway.[19] The presence of intraepidermal and dermal nerves has been demonstrated in human skin by using electron microscopy[20] and confocal laser-scanning microscopy[21] and by immunohistochemistry with antibodies directed against neuronal derived proteins (Fig. 20-1). These studies demonstrate that the epidermis is innervated by a three-dimensional network of unmyelinated, fine nerve fibers with free branching endings that converge in the dermis. These afferent sensory neurons in the peripheral nervous system synthesize a heterogeneous group of at least 17 different neuropeptides[18] consisting of 2 to more than 40 amino acids in size. Neuropeptides in the skin are synthesized and released predominantly by a subpopulation of small neurofilament-poor (unmyelinated) afferent neurons (C fibers) designated as *C-polymodal nociceptors,* which represent about 70 percent of all cutaneous C fibers, and, to a far lesser extent, by small myelinated Aδ-fibers (Aδ mechanothermal receptors).[22] Immunohistochemical studies in the skin demonstrate the presence of multiple neuropeptides and neurohormones such as substance P, neurokinin A, CGRP, vasoactive intestinal peptide, and α-MSH[1,22] in sensory nerves. Substance P is often considered to be the prototype of the neuropeptides released from sensory C fibers in the skin that are capable of a range of proinflammatory activities.[1–4]

Although cutaneous nerves are the principal source of neuropeptides in the skin, there is also evidence that neuropeptides or neurohormones may be produced by skin cells such as keratinocytes, microvascular endothelial cells, and fibroblasts.[22] In addition, immune cells that either constitutively reside in the skin or infiltrate the skin under inflammatory conditions both respond to and have been reported to produce certain neuropeptides and neurohormones.[22] Somatostatin, atrial natriuretic peptide, and proopiomelanocortin (POMC) peptides, such as α- and γ-MSH or β-endorphin, have been detected in human skin or skin cells.[5,22] POMC peptides, which were originally discovered as pituitary hormones, have also been detected in cutaneous melanocytes, keratinocytes, microvascular endothelial cells, Langerhans cells, mast cells, and fibroblasts, as well as in immune cells such as monocytes and macrophages.[5] A major regulator of POMC transcription is corticotrophin-releasing hormone (CRH), which was also recently detected in the skin. CRH belongs to the stress-responsive mediators and is likely to play a crucial role in modulating immune–neuroendocrine interactions. Stress-induced CRH may affect POMC

FIGURE 20-1

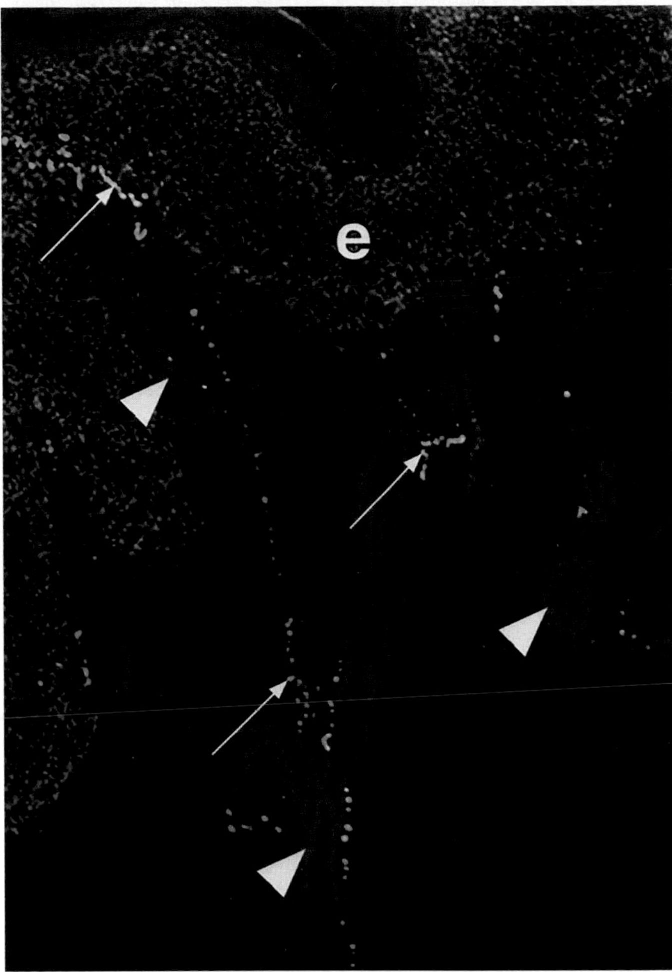

Nerve fibers in the skin. Confocal microscopy demonstrates CGRP immunoreactivity of nerves in the epidermis and dermis (*small arrows, green staining*). The cutaneous nerves are in close proximity to microvascular structures in the dermis, which are demonstrated by CD34 immunoreactivity (*arrowheads, red staining*).

gene transcription not only in the pituitary, but also in peripheral tissues, including the skin. Thus, POMC peptides can function as mediators of immune and inflammatory responses and influence the course of certain skin diseases.[5,23]

Neuropeptide Receptors

Different types of neuropeptide receptors have been identified on neuronal and nonneuronal cells in the skin. Three principal neurokinin (NK) receptors have been described to date—NK-1R, -2R, and -3R—that bind with high affinity to substance P, NK A, and NK B, respectively, although there is considerable cross-reactivity between these different neurokinin peptides and the three NK receptors.[24] NK receptors are seven-transmembrane G protein-coupled peptides.[25] Recent studies indicate that murine keratinocytes predominantly express NK-2R, whereas human keratinocytes and dermal endothelial cells express NK-1R.[26] Thus, these important target cells in the skin that participate in a wide range of cutaneous inflammatory responses express the appropriate receptors for neurokinins released by sensory fibers. Additionally, two subtypes of CGRP receptors have been identified, based on different pharmacologic and biologic responses after activation by various CGRP agonists and antagonists.[28,29] Dermal microvascular endothelial cells and Langerhans cells have been reported to respond specifically to CGRP.[3,22] In contrast POMC peptides exert their effects via a group of five G protein-coupled receptors with seven-transmembrane domains, designated as melanocortin (MC) receptors (MC-1R through MC-5R). Epidermal and dermal cells, as well as inflammatory and immunocompetent cells, almost exclusively express MC-1R, which exhibits the highest affinity for αMSH.[5,23,30]

Neuropeptide-Degrading Enzymes

In addition to released neuropeptides and appropriate target cell neuropeptide receptors, another key determinant of the neurogenic inflammatory response is the expression of neuropeptidases such as neutral endopeptidase (NEP, CD10).[1,22] NEP is a cell membrane-associated protease capable of degrading neurokinins such as substance P and is believed to be an important regulator in terminating neurogenic inflammation. This proteolytic enzyme is often colocated on the cell membrane of the target cells that express NK receptors and thus can effectively diminish the inflammatory effect by degrading excess released neuropeptides.[1,22,31] Recent work indicates that significant NEP expression and bioactivity can be detected in the epidermis and microvascular endothelial cells of the dermis[32] (Fig. 20-2). The spontaneous vascular leakage and cutaneous edema, which occur in the dermis of mice that lack the NEP gene, also indicate the important function of this enzyme in preventing constitutive neurogenic-mediated inflammation in the skin.[33]

The carboxypeptidase angiotensin-converting enzyme (ACE) also appears to have biologic effects similar to those of NEP. Blockade of ACE by inhibitors of this enzyme (e.g., captopril and enalapril) in wild-type mice caused elevated plasma extravasation, which was mediated by diminished degradation of substance P and bradykinin.[34] This may be of clinical consequence to patients who receive these drugs.

FIGURE 20-2

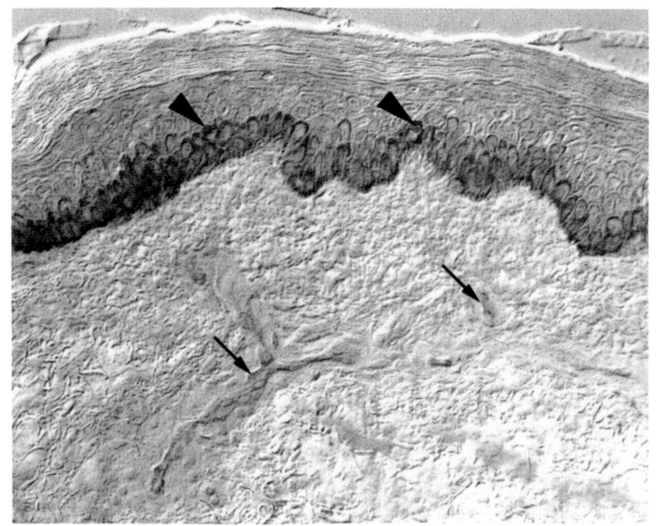

Neutral endopeptidase in the skin. Immunohistochemistry demonstrates significant neutral endopeptidase in the basal layer of the epidermis (*arrowheads*), as well as in microvascular endothelial cells in the dermis (*small arrows*).

To control the production of POMC peptides, the presence of several peptide processing neuropeptidases, named prohormone convertases, are required. These enzymes have recently been detected in the skin and are upregulated by proinflammatory stimuli such as UV light.[5]

These data indicate that the complex process known as neurogenic inflammation depends on a number of biologic factors, including the types and quantities of neuropeptides released, the types of receptors located on target cells, the presence and localization of NEP and other proteases, the activation state of target cells, as well as the presence of other mediators of inflammation such as prostaglandins and cytokines.

Neurotrophins

Neurotrophic growth factors are essential for the growth, proliferation, and maintenance of cutaneous nerves. Neurotrophic factors that may play a role in the skin include nerve growth factor (NGF), brain-derived NGF, neurotrophin-3, and human neurotrophin-4/5.[1,9] NGF is the best characterized member of the neurotrophin family. It was isolated more than 40 years ago as an agent that stimulates neurite growth and development in embryonic sensory cells.[35] In the adult animal, NGF plays a continuous dynamic role in regulating peptide neurotransmitter levels and synthesis in mature neurons.[36] NGF is synthesized in increased quantities in inflamed tissue, and after uptake and retrograde transport by sensory nerves, contributes to increased neurite neuropeptide synthesis.[37] During cutaneous inflammation the nerves innervating the inflamed skin demonstrate increased NGF content and eventually increased neuronal substance P and CGRP levels.[38] This increase of neuropeptide content in sensory nerves was prevented by anti-NGF antibodies indicating that NGF plays an important role in the stimulation of neuropeptide synthesis during cutaneous inflammation.[38]

Murine and human keratinocytes also express, synthesize, and release NGF.[9] NGF synthesis and release from keratinocytes is increased by cutaneous neuropeptides such as substance P and neurokinin A,[39] after UV-irradiation,[9] and in cutaneous wounds.[40] Greater amounts of NGF are secreted by proliferating preconfluent keratinocytes than by more differentiated stratified cells.[9] In addition, NGF stimulates the proliferation of human dermal microvascular endothelial cells (HDMEC).[41] After skin injury, increased amounts of NGF may contribute to wound healing by direct stimulatory effects on keratinocytes, as well as on dermal microvascular endothelial cells,[9,41,42] and by the regeneration of damaged nerves and reinnervation of the damaged skin area.[16]

Recent studies similarly demonstrate neurotrophic activity for the angiogenic factors such as vascular endothelial growth factor (VEGF). VEGF stimulates axonal outgrowth from dorsal root ganglia by the activation of the VEGF receptor flk-1,[43] suggesting cross-talk between the nervous and vascular system.

NEUROPEPTIDE–TARGET CELL INTERACTIONS IN SKIN INFLAMMATION

A key experimental finding that has expanded our understanding of neurogenic inflammation was the observation that various nonneural cells express specific neuropeptide receptors and thus are capable of responding to released neuropeptides.[1] Lymphoid cells, such as T cells, B cells, and monocytic cells, express specific receptors for neurotransmitters[1] so that they can respond to these neuropeptides with the induction of modified cytotoxic activities, antibody secretion, cytokine production, and adhesion molecule expression.[22,44] Thus, in a direct way the neurologic system may be able to modulate immune responses.

It has been established by a number of investigators that neuropeptides are capable of activating mast cells to release mediators of immediate hypersensitivity such as histamine.[45] Mast cells are also capable of secreting mediators of late-phase inflammatory responses such as tumor necrosis factor (TNF)-α. Substance P specifically induces mast cell TNF-α mRNA expression and increases secreted TNF-α activity.[1,4] Additionally, substance P treatment of skin explants causes mast cell degranulation and subsequent TNF-α–mediated induction of E-selectin on postcapillary venular endothelial cells.[1,4] In addition, UVB-induced CGRP release from sensory afferent nerve fibers and the subsequent CGRP-induced release of TNF-α from skin mast cells play an important role in the UVB-induced suppression of the cutaneous hypersensitivity (CHS) reaction to dinitrofluorobenzene (DNFB).[46] Thus, these studies support the role of the neurologic system in directly activating mast cells and modulating immediate and delayed inflammatory responses in the skin.

Recently, a new mechanism of sensory nerve–mast cell interaction was reported in which mast cell-derived tryptase was found to be able to directly stimulate the release of neuropeptides such as substance P and CGRP, by the activation of protease-activated receptor-2 (PAR-2) on sensory afferent nerves.[47] The protease-induced local release of neuropeptides eventually induces localized neurogenic inflammation.[47] In addition, small amounts of PAR-2 agonists, including mast cell tryptase, are able to sensitize sensory afferent neurons and induce thermal and mechanical hyperalgesia.[48] Thus, this new mechanism of protease-induced neurogenic inflammation may contribute to the proinflammatory effects of mast cells in human disease. In normal human skin, PAR-2 receptors are also found on epidermal and dermal cells, with increased expression of PAR-2 receptors noted in keratinocytes and endothelial cells in inflamed atopic and psoriatic skin. In these skin diseases, the number of mast cells was also found to be increased.[49] PAR-2 activation of mast cells may contribute to the pathophysiology of these chronic inflammatory diseases.

It has been noted that cutaneous sensory fibers extend into the epidermis where they come in direct contact with both keratinocytes and Langerhans cells[3,50] (see Fig. 20-1). Neuropeptides released by epidermal nerve fibers may modulate cutaneous inflammation, in part by the induction of keratinocyte cytokine production. Substance P is capable of directly activating both murine and normal human keratinocytes to secrete cytokines such as interleukin-1 (IL-1) in a dose-dependent manner in vitro and in vivo. This effect was inhibited by specific NK receptor antagonists.[1,22] A number of recent studies also have focused on the relationship between Langerhans cells and CGRP, released from cutaneous sensory nerve fibers.[3] It has been proposed that CGRP is capable of suppressing delayed-type hypersensitivity (DTH) reactions and CHS reactions by the reduction of Langerhans cell density and the inhibition of Langerhans cell antigen presentation to T cells.[3,51,52] CGRP was also found to inhibit both proliferation and antigen presentation of peripheral blood mononuclear cells.[53] It has been proposed that CGRP may also impair antigen presentation required for cutaneous CHS and DTH reactions by the induction of anti-inflammatory cytokines, such as IL-10, that may, in turn, suppress T cell functions.[53]

Dermal microvascular endothelial cells are also potentially important targets and modulators of cutaneous neurogenic inflammation. Cutaneous sensory nerve fibers are found in close contact with dermal microvascular endothelial cells[27] (see Fig. 20-1). Cutaneous neuropeptides affect two important inflammatory activities of endothelial cells: cytokine production and cellular adhesion molecule expression. Neuropeptides such as CGRP released by cutaneous sensory nerves induce IL-8 production in normal HDMEC.[1] IL-8 is a principal chemotactic factor for neutrophils and facilitates their vascular transmigration. HDMEC also can be activated directly by substance P to express increased cellular adhesion molecules in a dose-dependent fashion in vitro and in vivo.[1,27] Thus, released cutaneous neuropeptides can directly modulate HDMEC inflammatory activities.

Among the multiple POMC peptides, α-MSH and β-endorphin are regarded as neurohormones with extensive immunomodulatory capacities. β-Endorphin is synthesized in peripheral blood mononuclear cells and has been demonstrated to favor a Th2-type immunoresponse.[54] α-MSH regulates proliferation and differentiation of keratinocytes and melanocytes and modulates fibroblast and endothelial cell cytokine production in vitro.[5,55,56] Locally, as well as systemically, α-MSH impairs immunologic functions and induces anti-inflammatory cytokines such as IL-10.[5,23] Additionally, α-MSH antagonizes the proinflammatory effects of cytokines such as IL-1, IL-6, and TNF-α, and downregulates the production of interferon-γ by T cells, as well as the expression of accessory molecules such as CD86 and CD40, which are required for T cell activation. These observations suggest that this neurohormone may play a crucial role in the downregulation of inflammatory reactions within the skin.[5,23,57]

THE ROLE OF NEUROGENIC INFLAMMATION IN CUTANEOUS DISEASE AND WOUND HEALING

There are a number of human clinical diseases that appear to have a significant neurogenic component, including ophthalmic herpesvirus infections, inflammatory bowel disease, asthma, and inflammatory arthritis.[1] In the skin, there is evidence of a neurogenic component in the pathogenesis of urticaria, psoriasis, atopic dermatitis, and hypersensitivity reactions, and in the physiologic process of wound healing.[1]

As previously indicated, there is a close anatomic association of cutaneous nerves and mast cells in the skin, thus providing a direct physical link for these two systems to interact.[58] The ability of neuropeptides to activate mast cells and induce urticaria has been appreciated for a number of years.[45] Investigators have demonstrated that NKs such as substance P are capable of binding to and directly activating mast cells and triggering the release of immediate hypersensitivity mediators.[45] Neuropeptides may also be responsible for the release of mast cell cytokines, which can mediate late-phase inflammatory responses.[1] In addition, recent reports also revealed the induction of neurogenic inflammation by mast cell tryptase via the activation of PAR-2 on sensory afferent nerves.[47]

A neurogenic component for the pathophysiology of psoriasis is suggested by both clinical and experimental findings.[59–61] Clinically, lesions often have a symmetric distribution and occur in regions that are traumatized. The so-called Koebner phenomenon in psoriasis may be partly initiated by the release of proinflammatory neuropeptides in the traumatized skin.[60] Investigators also report increased levels of neuropeptides and sensory nerves in psoriatic skin lesions, and capsaicin, a chemical that is capable of depleting neuropeptides from nerve endings, is reported to have some therapeutic value in clearing psoriatic lesions.[59,61] In addition, NGF, which plays an important role in synthesis and release of neuropeptides in sensory nerves, is significantly increased in inflamed lesional skin from psoriatic patients when compared to normal healthy skin.[62] Likewise, in atopic dermatitis, increased lesional staining of cutaneous nerves and abnormal cutaneous responses to injected neuropeptides have been reported.[63,64]

The role of POMC peptides in the pathogenesis of atopic dermatitis is supported by the in vitro observation that α-MSH modulates IgE production and the finding of increased levels of POMC peptides in the skin of patients with atopic dermatitis.[65,66] Recently, the POMC-derived neurohormone α-MSH also was shown to induce the release of the potent pruritogen histamine from human skin mast cells and from skin bunch biopsies in a dose-dependent manner.[67]

Neuropeptides appear to play a role in both immediate and DTH reactions in the skin. CGRP and substance P have been demonstrated to participate in or modulate immediate-type skin hypersensitivity reactions. DTH and CHS are delayed T cell–mediated immune reactions occurring in the skin after a first injection (as in DTH) or contact sensitization (as in CHS) with an antigen, followed by a second contact with the hapten (elicitation). Topical application of substance P on mouse ears significantly increases the ear-swelling response to a contact allergen,[68] whereas inhibitors of substance P diminish CHS and DTH responses in mice and humans.[69,70] These experiments suggest a proinflammatory effect of substance P in CHS and DTH. Other neuropeptides appear to have a suppressive effect on hypersensitivity reactions in the skin. CGRP, which is released by sensory neurons during the elicitation phase of CHS,[71] appears to suppress DTH and CHS reactions through interactions with Langerhans cells, as described above.[3,52] Systemic pretreatment of adult mice with capsaicin, which causes the depletion of neuropeptides from sensory nerves, results in an increased CHS to contact allergens as well as increased DTH to alloantigens, suggesting both proinflammatory and immunosuppressive effects of neuropeptides released from cutaneous sensory nerves in CHS and DTH.[71,72]

α-MSH is one of the most powerful neurohormones in terms of its ability to modify CHS reactions. α-MSH inhibits both the sensitization and elicitation phase of CHS and induces hapten-specific tolerance in mice.[73] This is mediated, at least in part, by the inhibition of accessory signals on antigen-presenting cells and the induction of the immunosuppressive cytokine IL-10, which has been shown to inhibit the elicitation phase of CHS and induce tolerance.On the other hand, the effect of α-MSH on the elicitation phase could be explained by its capacity to downregulate the endothelial cell adhesion molecule expression required for adhesion and transmigration of inflammatory cells.[5,23]

Interestingly, many skin diseases in which neuropeptides are proposed to play a role are affected by UV light. Phototherapy of psoriasis, atopic dermatitis, as well as prurigo nodularis is well established, and phototherapy is able to suppress chronic urticaria as well as skin CHS reaction.[74] The release of neuropeptides such as substance P and CGRP from cutaneous sensory nerves by erythemogenic doses of UV-light and the reduction of UV-induced inflammation by receptor antagonists to substance P and CGRP, as well as the increase of UV-induced inflammation in genetically engineered mice deficient for NEP, clearly indicate that neuropeptides are important mediators of UV-induced cutaneous inflammation.[75–77] Furthermore, experimental phototherapy with repeated suberythemogenic doses of UVB significantly increased the content of substance P and CGRP in sensory nerves and augmented the mustard oil-induced cutaneous inflammation.[78]

The involvement of neuropeptides in UV-induced immunosuppression is also well established. CGRP is an important mediator in UVB-induced local and systemic immunosuppression, in part by the interaction with skin mast cells.[46,79–81] The role of CGRP in UV-induced immunosuppression has been confirmed by the ability of the CGRP-antagonist CGRP8-37, applied at cutaneous UV-irradiated sites before sensitization to a contact allergen, to restore the UV-induced suppression of the CHS reaction induced by DNFB.[46,81] The inhibitory effects of CGRP on antigen presentation by Langerhans cells and macrophages was previously discussed.[3] In addition, CGRP applied to rat skin reduced the number of Langerhans cells in the epidermis to that of UV-exposed rat skin.[81] UV light also induces the release of α-MSH from keratinocytes, and upregulates the expression of POMC mRNA. α-MSH, then, is able to exert a variety of antiinflammatory and immunomodulating effects.[82] Taken together these studies suggest that effects of phototherapy on diseases such as psoriasis or atopic dermatitis may, at least in part, be explained by its modulation of the cutaneous sensory nervous system and neurohormones.

There is also increasing evidence that the neurologic system may also play an important role in mediating normal wound healing responses. Released neuropeptides may modulate a number of important aspects of normal wound healing such as cell proliferation, cytokine and growth factor production, and neovascularization.[22] NEP expression appears to be both increased and redistributed in the wound environment during the healing processes.[32] Abnormal wound healing responses in the lower limbs of insulin dependent diabetics is also accompanied by overexpression of cutaneous NEP.[83] Surgical resection of cutaneous nerves results in delayed wound healing in animal models.[84] In addition, patients with cutaneous sensory defects due to lepromatous leprosy, spinal cord injury, or diabetic neuropathy develop ulcers that fail to heal in spite of aggressive wound care and wound protection.[1] Experimental evidence indicates that the neurologic system also appears to have an important trophic effect for tissue integrity and function.[1]

SUMMARY

The neurobiologic system of the skin plays a much wider role than simply the transmission of sensory impulses to the CNS. It is now appreciated that in the skin there are complex interactions between sensory nerve fibers, released neuropeptides, cutaneous target cells bearing neuropeptide receptors, proteases that degrade cutaneous neuropeptides, and neurotrophins that influence innervation. Indeed, the cutaneous neurosensory system may represent an important early component of the innate immune system in the skin. New therapies for inflammatory skin diseases or impaired wound healing, which are mediated by the modulators of neurocutaneous interactions, are likely to result from continued scientific investigations in this field.

REFERENCES

1. Ansel JC et al: Interactions of the skin and nervous system. *J Invest Dermatol Symp Proc* **2**:23, 1997
2. Brain SD: Sensory neuropeptides in the skin, in *Neurogenic Inflammation*, edited by P Geppetti, P Holzer. Boca Raton, FL, CRC Press, 1996, p 229
3. Hosoi J et al: Regulation of Langerhans cell function by nerves containing calcitonin gene-related peptide. *Nature* **363**:159, 1993
4. Lotti T et al: Neuropeptides in skin. *J Am Acad Dermatol* **33**:482, 1995
5. Luger TA et al: Cutaneous immunomodulation and coordination of skin stress responses by α-melanocyte–stimulating hormone. *Ann N Y Acad Sci* **840**:381, 1998
6. Slominski A et al: Corticotropin-releasing hormone and proopiomelanocortin involvement in the cutaneous response to stress. *Physiol Rev* **80**:979, 2000.
7. Toyoda M et al: Calcitonin gene–related peptide upregulates melanogenesis and enhances melanocyte dendricity via induction of keratinocyte-derived melanotrophic factors. *J Invest Dermatol Symp Proc* **4**:116, 1999
8. Slominski A, Wortsman J: Neuroendocrinology of the skin. *Endocr Rev* **21**:457, 2000.
9. Pincelli C, Yaar M: Nerve growth factor: Its significance in cutaneous biology. *J Invest Dermatol Symp Proc* **2**:31, 1997
10. Bayliss W: On the origin from the spinal cord of vasodilator fibers of the hind limb, and on the nature of these fibers. *J Physiol* **26**:173, 1901
11. Bruce AN: Vasodilator axon reflexes. *Q J Exp Physiol* **6**:339, 1913
12. Lewis T, Marvin H: Observations relating to vasodilatation arising from antidromic impulses, to herpes zoster and trophic effects. *Heart* **14**:27, 1927
13. Jancso N: Role of the nerve terminals in the mechanism of inflammatory reactions. *Bull Millard Fillmore Hosp (Buffalo, NY)* **7**:53, 1960
14. Jancso N et al: Direct evidence for neurogenic inflammation and its prevention by denervation and by pretreatment with capsaicin. *Br J Pharmacol Chemother* **31**:138, 1967
15. Holzer P: Capsaicin: Cellular targets, mechanism of action, and selectivity for thin sensory neurons. *Pharmacol Rev* **43**:144, 1991
16. Schicho R, Skofitsch G, Donnerer J: Regenerative effect of human recombinant NGF on capsaicin-lesioned sensory neurons in the adult rat. *Brain Res* **815**:60, 1999

17. Caterina MJ, Julius D: The vanilloid receptor: A molecular gateway to the pain pathway. *Annu Rev Neurosci* **24**:487, 2001
18. Holzer P: Local effector functions of capsaicin-sensitive sensory nerve endings: Involvement of tachykinins, calcitonin gene-related peptide and other neuropeptides. *Neuroscience* **24**:739, 1988
19. Sternini C: Organization of the peripheral nervous system: Autonomic and sensory ganglia. *J Invest Dermatol Symp Proc* **2**:1, 1997
20. Hilliges M et al: Ultrastructural evidence for nerve fibres within all vital layers of the human epidermis. *J Invest Dermatol* **104**:134, 1995
21. Reilly DM et al: The human epidermal nerve fibre network: Characterization of nerve fibres in human skin by confocal microscopy and assessment of racial variations. *Br J Dermatol* **137**:163, 1997
22. Scholzen T et al: Neuropeptides in the skin: Interactions between the neuroendocrine and the skin immune systems. *Exp Dermatol* **7**:81, 1998
23. Luger TA et al: The role of alpha-MSH as a modulator of cutaneous inflammation. *Ann N Y Acad Sci* **917**:232, 2000
24. Hershey A et al: Organization, structure, and expression of a gene encoding the rat substance P receptor. *J Biol Chem* **266**:4366, 1991
25. Krause J et al: Structure, functions, and mechanisms of substance P receptor action. *J Invest Dermatol* **98**:2SA, 1992
26. Song I-S et al: Substance P induction of murine keratinocyte PAM 212 interleukin 1 production is mediated by the neurokinin 2 receptor (NK-2R). *Exp Dermatol* **9**:42, 2000
27. Quinlan KL et al: Neuropeptide regulation of human dermal microvascular endothelial cell ICAM-1 expression and function. *Am J Physiol* **275**:C1580, 1998
28. Aiyar N et al: A cDNA encoding the calcitonin gene-related peptide type 1 receptor. *J Biol Chem* **271**:11325, 1996
29. Dumont Y et al: A potent and selective CGRP2 agonist, [Cys(Et)2,7] hCGRP alpha: Comparison in prototypical CGRP1 and CGRP2 in vitro bioassays. *Can J Physiol Pharmacol* **75**:671, 1997
30. Cone RD et al: The melanocortin receptors: Agonists, antagonists, and the hormonal control of pigmentation. *Recent Prog Horm Res* **51**:287, 1996
31. Okamoto A et al: Interactions between neutral endopeptidase (EC 3.4.24.11) and the substance P (NK1) receptor expressed in mammalian cells. *Biochem J* **299**:683, 1994
32. Olerud JE et al: Neutral endopeptidase (NEP) expression by human keratinocytes: Distribution in skin and wounds. *J Invest Dermatol* **112**:873, 1999
33. Lu B et al: The control of microvascular permeability and blood pressure by neutral endopeptidase. *Nat Med* **3**:904, 1997
34. Grady E et al: Mechanisms attenuating cellular responses to neuropeptides: Extracellular degradation of ligands and desensitization of receptors. *J Invest Dermatol Symp Proc* **2**:69, 1997
35. Levi-Montalcini R: The nerve growth factor: Thirty-five years later. *EMBO J* **6**:1145, 1987
36. Lindsay RM et al: Neuropeptide expression in cultures of adult sensory neurons: Modulation of substance P and calcitonin gene-related peptide levels by nerve growth factor. *Neuroscience* **33**:53, 1989
37. Raivich G et al: NGF receptor mediated reduction in axonal NGF uptake and retrograde transport following sciatic nerve injury and during regeneration. *Neuron* **7**:151, 1991
38. Donnerer J et al: Increased content and transport of substance P and calcitonin gene-related peptide in sensory nerves innervating inflamed tissue: Evidence for a regulatory function of nerve growth factor in vivo. *Neuroscience* **49**:693, 1992
39. Burbach GJ et al: The neurosensory tachykinins substance P and neurokinin A directly induce keratinocyte nerve growth factor. *J Invest Dermatol* **117**:1075, 2001
40. Matsuda H et al: Role of nerve growth factor in cutaneous wound healing: Accelerating effects in normal and healing-impaired diabetic mice. *J Exp Med* **187**:297, 1998
41. Raychaudhuri SK et al: Effect of nerve growth factor on endothelial cell biology: Proliferation and adherence molecule expression on human dermal microvascular endothelial cells. *Arch Dermatol Res* **293**:291, 2001
42. Tuveri M et al: NGF, a useful tool in the treatment of chronic vasculitic ulcers in rheumatoid arthritis. *Lancet* **356**:1739, 2000
43. Sondell et al: Vascular endothelial growth factor is a neurotrophic factor which stimulates axonal outgrowth through the flk-1 receptor. *Eur J Neurosci* **12**:4243, 2000
44. Bhardwaj R et al: Evidence for the differential expression of the functional alpha-melanocyte-stimulating hormone receptor MC-1 on human monocytes. *J Immunol* **158**:3378, 1997
45. Church MK et al: Mast cells, neuropeptides and inflammation. *Agents Actions* **27**:8, 1989
46. Niizeki H et al: Calcitonin gene-related peptide is necessary for ultraviolet B-impaired induction of contact hypersensitivity. *J Immunol* **159**:5183, 1997
47. Steinhoff M et al: Agonists of protease-activated receptor-2 induce inflammation by a neurogenic mechanism. *Nat Med* **6**:151, 2000
48. Vergnolle N et al: Proteinase-activated receptor-2 and hyperalgesia: A novel pain pathway. *Nat Med* **7**:821, 2001
49. Steinhoff M et al: Proteinase-activated receptor-2 in human skin: Tissue distribution and activation of keratinocytes by mast cell tryptase. *Exp Dermatol* **8**:282, 1999
50. Dalsgaard C-J et al: Cutaneous innervation in man visualized with protein gene product 9.5 (PGP 9.5) antibodies. *Histochemistry* **92**:385, 1989
51. Torii H et al: Calcitonin gene-related peptide and Langerhans cell function. *J Invest Dermatol Symp Proc* **2**:82, 1997
52. Asahina A et al: Inhibition of the induction of delayed-type and contact hypersensitivity by calcitonin gene-related peptide. *J Immunol* **154**:3056, 1995
53. Fox FE et al: Calcitonin gene-related peptide inhibits proliferation and antigen presentation by human peripheral blood mononuclear cells: Effects on B7, interleukin 10, and interleukin 12. *J Invest Dermatol* **108**:43, 1997
54. Panerai AE, Sacerdote P: Beta-endorphin in the immune system: A role at last? *Immunol Today* **18**:317, 1997
55. Hartmeyer M et al: Human dermal microvascular endothelial cells express the melanocortin receptor type 1 and produce increased levels of IL-8 upon stimulation with alpha-melanocyte-stimulating hormone. *J Immunol* **159**:1930, 1997
56. Schulte U et al: Evidence for a functional melanocortin receptor on human fibroblasts. *J Invest Dermatol* **110**:479, 1998
57. Taylor AW et al: Alpha-melanocyte stimulating hormone suppresses antigen-stimulated T cell production of gamma-interferon. *Neuroimmunomodulation* **1**:188, 1994
58. Naukkarinen A et al: Immunohistochemical analysis of sensory nerves and neuropeptides, and their contacts with mast cells in developing and mature psoriatic lesions. *Arch Dermatol Res* **285**:341, 1993
59. Bernstein JE et al: Effect of topically applied capsaicin on moderate and severe psoriasis vulgaris. *J Am Acad Dermatol* **15**:504, 1986
60. Farber EM et al: Stress, symmetry and psoriasis: Possible role of neuropeptides. *J Am Acad Dermatol* **14**:305, 1986
61. Naukkarinen A et al: Quantification of cutaneous sensory nerves and their substance P content in psoriasis. *J Invest Dermatol* **92**:126, 1989
62. Fantini F et al: Nerve growth factor is increased in psoriatic skin. *J Invest Dermatol* **105**:854, 1995
63. Giannetti A, Girolomoni G: Skin reactivity to neuropeptides in atopic dermatitis. *Br J Dermatol* **121**:681, 1989
64. Pincelli C et al: Neuropeptides in skin from patients with atopic dermatitis: An immunohistochemical study. *Br J Dermatol* **112**:745, 1990
65. Glinski W et al: Increased concentration of beta-endorphin in the sera of patients with severe atopic dermatitis. *Acta Derm Venereol* **75**:9, 1995
66. Aebischer I et al: Neuropeptides are potent modulators of human in vitro immunoglobulin E synthesis. *Eur J Immunol* **24**:1908, 1994
67. Grutzkau A et al: Alpha-melanocyte stimulating hormone acts as a selective inducer of secretory functions in human mast cells. *Biochem Biophys Res Commun* **278**:14, 2000
68. Gutwald J et al: Neuropeptides enhance irritant and allergic contact dermatitis. *J Invest Dermatol* **96**:695, 1991
69. Wallengren J: Substance P antagonist inhibits immediate and delayed-type cutaneous hypersensitivity reactions. *Br J Dermatol* **124**:324, 1991
70. Scholzen TE et al: Neutral endopeptidase terminates substance P-induced inflammation in allergic contact dermatitis. *J Immunol* **166**:1285, 2001
71. Ek L, Theodorsson E: Tachykinins and calcitonin gene-related peptide in oxazolone-induced allergic contact dermatitis in mice. *J Invest Dermatol* **94**:761, 1990
72. Girolomoni G, Tigelaar RE: Capsaicin-sensitive primary sensory neurons are potent modulators of murine delayed-type hypersensitivity reactions. *J Immunol* **145**:1105, 1990
73. Grabbe S et al: Alpha-melanocyte-stimulating hormone induces hapten-specific tolerance in mice. *J Immunol* **156**:473, 1996
74. Horio T: Indications and action mechanisms of phototherapy. *J Dermatol Sci* **23**:(suppl 1)S17, 2000
75. Benrath J et al: Calcitonin gene-related peptide, substance P and nitric oxide are involved in cutaneous inflammation following ultraviolet irradiation. *Eur J Pharmacol* **293**:87, 1995
76. Scholzen TE et al: Effect of ultraviolet light on the release of neuropeptides and neuroendocrine hormones in the skin: Mediators of photodermatitis and cutaneous inflammation. *J Invest Dermatol Symp Proc* **4**:55, 1999
77. Benrath J et al: Differential time course of skin blood flow and hyperalgesia in the human sunburn reaction following UV irradiation of the skin. *Eur J Pain* **5**:155, 2001

78. Legat FJ et al: UVB irradiation with non-erythematogenic doses increases neuropeptides in the skin of rat ears. *Photochem Photobiol* **69**:55, 1999
79. Garssen J et al: A role for neuropeptides in UVB-induced systemic immunosuppression. *Photochem Photobiol* **68**:205, 1998
80. Hart PH et al: Mast cells in UVB-induced immunosuppression. *J Photochem Photobiol B* **55**:81, 2000
81. Gillardon F et al: Calcitonin gene-related peptide and nitric oxide are involved in ultraviolet radiation-induced immunosuppression. *Eur J Pharmacol* **293**:395, 1995
82. Luger TA et al: Role of epidermal cell-derived alpha-melanocyte stimulating hormone in ultraviolet light mediated local immunosuppression. *Ann N Y Acad Sci* **885**:209, 1999
83. Spenny M et al: Neutral endopeptidase inhibition improves wound repair in diabetic mice. *J Invest Dermatol* **117**:441, 2001
84. Lusthaus S et al: Effect of denervation on incision wound scars in rabbits. *J Ger Dermatol* **1**:11, 1993

CHAPTER 21

Vincent Falanga

Mechanisms of Cutaneous Wound Repair

Wound healing and *wound repair* are terms often used interchangeably, but they actually stand for two quite different sets of events and outcomes. *Wound healing* is a term that technically should be used only in the context of regeneration, when the original architecture and structure of an organ or anatomic part is completely restored to the way it was before injury. More primitive animals, such as small amphibians and reptiles, are still capable of this type of regeneration. However, as animals became larger and more complex, regeneration was no longer possible. In adult humans, with the possible exception of the liver, true regeneration does not occur. Rather, humans and other higher vertebrates heal by a process of repair, whereby the eventual outcome is not anatomic restoration but a functional compromise. Teleologically and from an evolutionary standpoint, the process of repair for higher animals needed to be rapid and to allow for immediate survival of the organism. As noted below, this type of repair is characterized by a substantial amount of scarring and fibrosis. Another consideration is that most of the mechanisms of wound repair that have evolved are aimed at addressing acute tissue injury. From an evolutionary standpoint, humans were not supposed to develop degenerative diseases or live long enough to develop arterial, venous, and pressure ulcers or neuropathic ulcers from diabetes. Therefore, humans are quite unprepared for these types of chronic wounds, and there are no specific mechanisms that have evolved to deal with them in an effective way.

There are three recognized phases that characterize the cutaneous repair process: the inflammatory phase, the proliferative or migratory phase (tissue formation), and the remodeling phase (Fig. 21-1). Each phase will be discussed individually and the main components and events that characterize each will be identified. However, it should be noted that breaking down the overall process of wound repair into these three phases is somewhat artificial because they overlap considerably.[1]

FIGURE 21-1

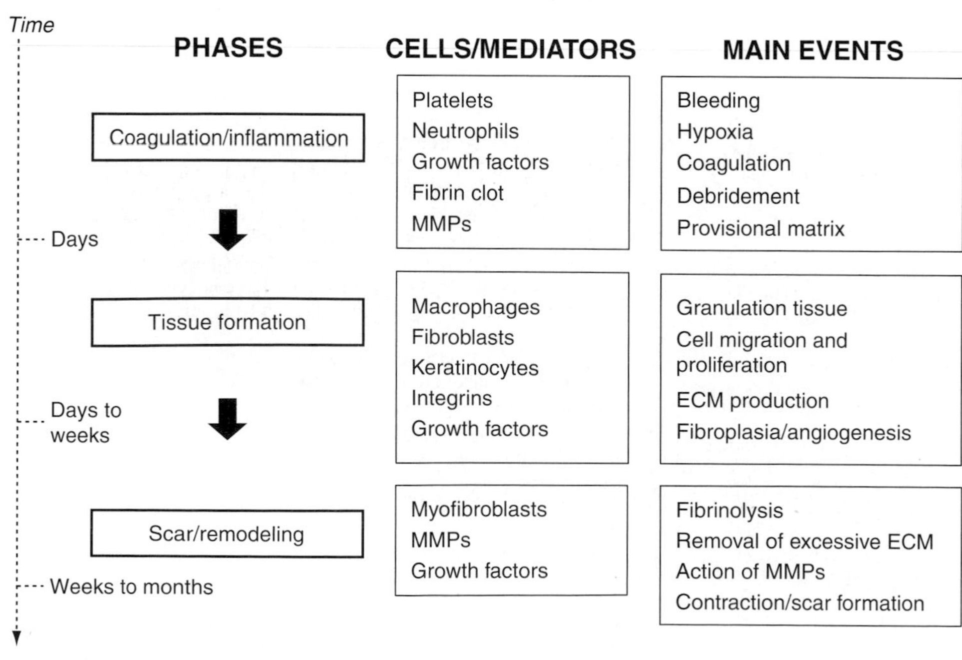

Schematic representation of the different phases of wound repair and the cells and events involved at different time points. ECM, extracellular matrix, MMP, matrix metalloproteinase.

INFLAMMATORY PHASE (PHASE 1)

The first phase, that of inflammation, begins immediately after an acute injury. Disruption of blood vessels leads to local release of blood cells and blood-borne elements resulting in clot formation. While the blood clot within the vessel lumen provides hemostasis, the clot within the injury site acts as a provisional matrix for cell migration.[2] The inflammatory phase is dominated by the platelet, which directs clotting of the fresh wound by the intrinsic and extrinsic coagulation pathways. Platelets also release a number of chemotactic factors that attract other platelets, leukocytes, and fibroblasts to the site of injury. The inflammatory phase continues as leukocytes, specifically neutrophils and macrophages, enter the scene. Their initial role is to debride the wound by phagocytosing and killing bacteria and scavenging cellular debris. However, it should be recognized that neutrophils and macrophages also release growth factors and other important mediators during this period of time.

This first phase of wound repair can be best understood by breaking it down into the following components: (1) platelet release and aggregation, (2) the processes of coagulation and inflammation, and (3) recruitment of leukocytes. Each of these processes will be discussed in turn, again emphasizing that such events are high interrelated.

Platelet Release and Aggregation

Platelets are essential components of the repair process and are critical to successful hemostasis. Tissue injury leads to blood vessel damage, platelet release, and activation of blood coagulation.[3] Platelets first adhere to interstitial connective tissue and then aggregate. Platelets at the wound site are exposed to thrombin and fibrillar collagen, which trigger their activation, adhesion, and aggregation. During aggregation, platelets release many mediators, including adenosine diphosphate, (ADP), and also express several clotting factors on their membrane surface. The process of coagulation is greatly facilitated by these platelet products that, in turn, lead to further platelet activation.

Besides ADP, the mediators released by the alpha granules of activated platelets include several adhesive proteins, such as fibrinogen, fibronectin, thrombospondin, and von Willibrand factor VIII. Fibrinogen, fibronectin, and thrombospondin serve as ligands for platelet aggregation, whereas von Willibrand factor VIII facilitates platelet adhesion to fibrillar collagens.[4] These activities result in the formation of a platelet plug. Thrombin polymerization of fibrinogen leads to fibrin, which amplifies the clot and will form part of the provisional extracellular matrix required for the migration of cells into the wound. It should be emphasized that no cell acts alone at any stages of the wound healing process. For example, in this platelet-dominated phase, endothelial cells produce several factors that limit platelet aggregation and clot formation to the area of injury. Among these activities are inhibition of platelet aggregation(by prostacyclin), inhibition of thrombin activity (by antithrombin III), degradation of coagulation factors V and VIII (by protein C), and initiation of clot lysis by converting plasminogen to plasmin with plasminogen activator.[5]

In addition to these critical roles in clot formation and the inflammatory phase of wound repair, platelets also release a number of growth factors and cytokines. These factors participate in the initial inflammatory phase but, equally important, also serve as signals for the migration of certain critical cells to the site of injury. Among these growth factors are platelet-derived growth factor (PDGF), transforming growth factor $\beta 1$ (TGF-$\beta 1$), platelet factor 4, connective tissue activating peptide (CTAP-III), beta-thromboglobulin, and neutrophil-activating peptide 2 (NAP-2). It should be noted that platelets are the most important storage site for TGF-$\beta 1$, one of three TGF-β isoforms, that plays a critical role in wound repair.[6]

The Process of Coagulation and Inflammation

During the process of coagulation, plasma and other blood elements leak from injured blood vessels and contribute to the formation of a thrombus through the intrinsic and extrinsic pathways. The intrinsic pathway is initiated when blood is exposed to subendothelial tissue, an event that leads to activation of factor X. Conversely, the extrinsic pathway begins when thromboplastin activates factor VII. The intrinsic and extrinsic pathways both lead to the formation of thrombin, which cleaves fibrinopeptides A and B as well as other fragments from fibrinogen and ultimately leads to polymerization of fribrinogen to fibrin.[7,8] However, the stability of fibrin and, indeed, its biologic activity are very much dependent on its cross-linking, which occurs as a result of the action of factor XIII.[9] Blood coagulation ends when the different stimuli for the activation of the coagulation cascade resolve. However, there are also active processes in place to downregulate the coagulation cascade. Among these are the inhibition of platelet aggregation by prostacyclin, inhibition of thrombin activity when this molecule binds to antithrombin III, and the action of protein C, an "anticoagulant" factor that degrades factors V and VIII.

Migration to the site of injury of a number of key cells, such as keratinocytes, fibroblasts, endothelial cells, and monocytes, is aided by their receptors for various components of the thrombus. However, a host of other mediators is produced and plays an important role in the amplification of the inflammatory/coagulation phase. For example, the formation of bradykinin, as well as C3a and C5a, is stimulated by activated Hageman factor.[5,9] The end result of the action of these and other mediators is increased vascular permeability, neutrophil and monocyte recruitment, and release of factors from mast cells. Cleavage of fibronogen, as mentioned, leads to a number of active fragments, such as the fibrinopeptides, that are important in stimulating migration to the wound site of certain cells, including fibroblasts.

Recruitment of Leukocytes

There is a constant cascade of inflammatory molecules and recruitment of inflammatory cells during the early phases of wound healing.[10] Neutrophils and monocytes arrive at the site of injury at about the same time. Initially, neutrophils are present in greater numbers because they constitute a larger fraction of peripheral white cells. Both neutrophils and monocytes are attracted to the wound by such chemotactic factors as kallikrein, fibrinopeptides released from fibrinogen, and fibrin degradation products. However, the list of reactants and chemotactic agents is long. In addition to the growth factors released by the platelets and the fragments resulting from the polymerization and cross-linking of fibrinogen, there are other by-products of proteolysis and other matrix components, as well as formyl methionyl peptides cleaved from bacterial proteins.[11] These and other chemotactic factors also stimulate the expression of CD11/CD18 complex on the surface of neutrophils, thereby enhancing the adherence of neutrophils to blood vessel endothelium and facilitating their diapedesis between adjacent endothelial cells.[12,13] It is important to understand that in order to enter the wound, leukocytes must exit the circulation, a process that is highly regulated by molecular changes on the surface of endothelial cells in blood vessels within and adjacent to the wound. This endothelial-leukocyte interaction provides the means to select the types of leukocytes entering the site of tissue injury. As a response to injury, endothelial cells express selectins, which by their adhesion properties cause the circulating leukocytes to slow down, roll, and be pulled from the blood. Both E and P selectins probably are required for the full recruitment of neutrophils and macrophages.[14] Once these weaker adhesions slow down the leukocytes, tighter interactive adhesions provided by β_2 integrins cause the leukocytes to negotiate the space between endothelial cells and reach the wound.[15]

Neutrophils are important in tissue debridement and in bacterial killing, events that produce further products of complement activation with inflammatory and chemotactic properties. New evidence suggests that neutrophils are also a rich source of cytokines, such as PDGF-like molecules. Connective tissue growth factor (CTGF) is one such peptide.[16,17] The action of neutrophils is enhanced by integrins, cell surface receptors that facilitate cell-matrix interactions.[18–20] However, neutrophils do not appear to be absolutely critical for wound repair, since neutropenia by itself does not interfere with the healing process.[21] Similarly, guinea pigs depleted of neutrophils are able to heal normally.[21]

As the inflammatory process continues, within 24 to 48 h after injury, monocytes replace neutrophils and become the predominant leukocyte. Monocytes are attracted to the injury site by some of the same chemoattractants responsible for recruitment of neutrophils, such as kallikren, fibrinopeptides, and fibrin degradation products.[13] Other, more specific chemoattractants then take over in recruiting monocytes, and they include fragments of collagen, fibronectin, elastin, and TGF-β1. Monocytes undergo a phenotypic change to tissue macrophages and, unlike neutrophils, they are critical for the progression of wound healing. Macrophages phagocytose and kill bacteria and scavenge tissue debris.[22] They also release several growth factors, including PDGF, fibroblast growth factor (FGF), TGF-β, and TGF-α, thereby stimulating migration and proliferation of fibroblasts, as well as production and modulation of extracellular matrix. It has long been stated that the macrophage is the central and critical cell for wound repair. The basis for this assertion is experiments in which animals depleted of macrophages by the use of antimacrophage serum and steroids failed to heal properly.[23] However, it is important to consider that what may delay or impair healing is not so much the presence or absence of inflammation and certain cells but rather an inappropriate inflammatory response. For example, there is evidence that healing may occur in the absence of an inflammatory infiltrate.[24] Conversely, experiments in mice constitutively expressing the chemotactic cytokine IP-10 show that an intense inflammatory infiltrate can impair neovascularization and the formation of appropriate granulation tissue.[25] Therefore, the true role of inflammation in tissue repair remains somewhat controversial from an experimental point of view. From a clinical standpoint, one can make the observation that in certain cutaneous wounds, such as pemphigus or pyoderma gangrenosum, downregulation of inflammation with the use of glucocorticoids is generally helpful. Possibly, modulation and "correction" of the inflammatory response by glucocorticoids may be helpful in these selected clinical entities.

A few days after tissue injury, the remaining neutrophils are phagocytosed by tissue macrophages, and the first phase of wound healing comes to an end, whereas the second phase of proliferation and tissue formation is under way.

PROLIFERATION AND TISSUE FORMATION (PHASE 2)

The first phase of wound repair lays the groundwork for the more formative second phase of proliferation and tissue formation (see Fig. 21-1). The term *tissue formation,* rather than *proliferation,* is clearly more appropriate. In this phase of wound repair, one is dealing with both cellular proliferation and migration, processes that are aided by a number of events, such as hypoxia, as well as specific adhesion proteins and extracellular matrix components. Platelet aggregation and release, the early inflammatory process, and entry into the wound of neutrophils and subsequently monocytes-macrophages have served a number of functions that will now allow and facilitate the proliferation of key resident cells, such as fibroblasts, the migration of endothelial cells and the process of neovascularization, and keratinocyte migration. Keratinocytes undergo a remarkable change in morphology and function. They migrate to the wound bed, release a number of proteins and enzymes that help facilitate their migration and other cellular functions, and ultimately reconstitute the damaged epidermis and basement membrane.[26,27] The later stages of the second phase of wound repair feature formation of granulation tissue and reconstitution of the dermal matrix (fibroplasia) and development of new blood vessels (angiogenesis) (Figs. 21-1 and 21-2). Fibroblasts and endothelial cells undergo activation, phenotypic alteration, and migration much like keratinocytes do. Another critical background component of this phase is hypoxia, which begins immediately after injury and severance of blood vessels but whose effects have a profound impact on the migration and

FIGURE 21-2

Reepithelializing Acute Wound

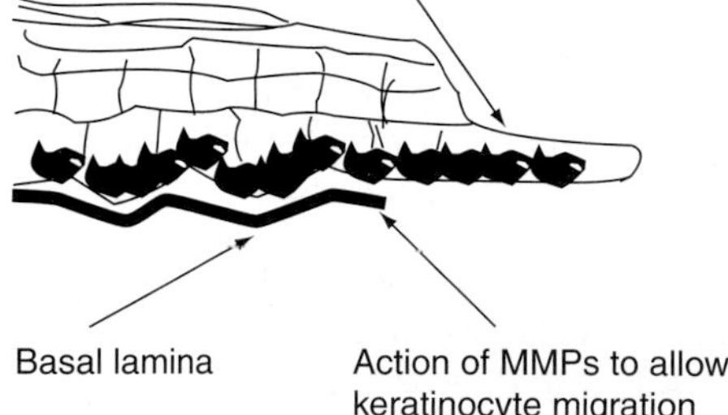

DERMIS

- Formation of a clot and provisional matrix
- Influx of macrophages
- Fibroplasia and angiogenesis
- Formation of granulation tissue

Non-Healing Chronic Wound

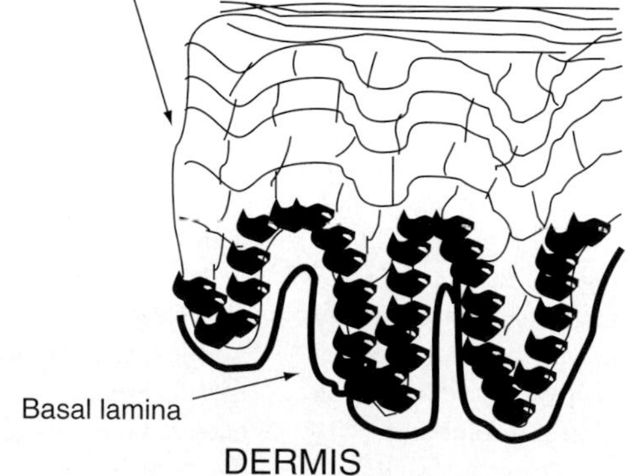

DERMIS

- Inability to move from one phase of wound repair to the next
- Excessive amounts of ECM and faulty fibrinolysis
- Trapping of growth factors
- Abnormal phenotype of resident wound cells

Diagrammatic representation of the epidermal edge of a normally healing wounds (*left*) and of a nonhealing wound (*right*). The healing wound shows separation from the underlying basal lamina and a thick epithelial tongue. The chronic wound edge shows the typical acanthotic epidermis. The bottom portion of the figure shows events presents in the dermis during repair.

proliferation of fibroblasts and endothelial cells as well as, possibly, keratinocyte migration. In the context of this second phase of wound repair, the following components and events will be discussed: (1) hypoxia, (2) fibroplasia, (3) angiogenesis, (4) keratinocyte migration, (5) extracellular matrix production, and (6) the role of integrins.

Hypoxia

Immediately following acute injury, the wound becomes temporarily hypoxic due to severence of blood vessels. There are some common misconceptions about hypoxia and its role in wound repair, possibly for two reasons. The major reason is that one incorrectly equates hypoxia with ischemia. The latter implies that both blood flow and oxygen delivery are impaired. However, hypoxia by itself, without a significant decrease in blood flow, may have different biologic consequences. The second reason for misconceptions about hypoxia is that chronic wounds are often treated with hyperbaric oxygen. Whether this type of treatment is helpful or not is beyond the scope of this discussion. However, the very fact that high oxygen delivery is sought by some clinicians caring for difficult to heal wounds implies that low oxygen tension is always highly undersirable.

However, from a physiologic standpoint, there is evidence that low oxygen tension actually plays an important stimulatory role in the early tissue repair process. Evidence points to low oxygen tension as an important early stimulus for fibroblast (and endothelial cell) activation. Fibroblast replication and longevity are enhanced in hypoxia,[28] and low oxygen tension stimulates clonal expansion of dermal fibroblasts seeded as single cells.[29] Moreover, the synthesis of a number of growth factors is enhanced in hypoxic cells. Macrophages secrete an angiogenic substance only when they are exposed to low oxygen tension. This reversible effect was observed at an oxygen tension of 15 to 20 mmHg.[30] TGF-β1 transcription and peptide synthesis are enhanced in cultures of human dermal fibroblasts exposed to a similar level of hypoxia.[31] In addition, hypoxia upregulates the synthesis of endothelin-1,[32] PDGF B chain, [33] and VEGF in endothelial cells.[34] It appears that, at least in some cases, the effect of hypoxic conditions is mediated by hypoxic inducible factor 1 (HIF-1), a DNA-binding complex shown to contain at least two basic helix-loop-helix PAS-domain proteins.[35,36]

In a totally anaerobic (anoxic) environment, the synthesized procollagen is underhydroxylated and accumulates intracellularly. Thus, in studies where fibroblasts were exposed to temporary (90 min) but absolute anoxia followed by reexposure to atmospheric oxygen at 37°C, the secreted procollagen was found to be about 15 percent underhydroxylated.[37] While hypoxia enhances collagen mRNA levels,[38] reoxygenation may be necessary to the excretion of a final functional product. There is, of course, a high likelihood that periods of reoxygenation are common in wounds. How oxygen radicals formed during reoxygenation affect collagen synthesis is not known.[39,40] These highly reactive oxygen species include the superoxide anion, hydrogen peroxide, and hydroxyl radical. However, it has been shown that interleukin 1α (IL-1α) and IL-6 are increased in endothelial cells exposed to a cycle of hypoxia/reoxygenation. Interestingly, dismutase and glutathione peroxidase prevented these increases in IL-1 and IL-6, suggesting a role for oxygen-derived free radicals in cytokine synthesis.[41]

Fibroplasia

During the process of reepithelialization, the wound is also undergoing fibroplasia and angiogenesis (discussed below). *Fibroplasia* refers to formation of granulation tissue and reconstitution of the dermal matrix. The key cell in this aspect of wound repair is the fibroblast. It is generally accepted that fibroblasts migrate into the wound; produce large amounts of collagens, proteoglycans, elastin, and other matrix proteins; and participate in wound contraction. Fibroblasts, like keratinocytes, undergo phenotypic changes that modify their interactions with the extracellular matrix, allowing them to perform a number of functions.[42] There is evidence for the existence of subpopulations of fibroblasts, with each subpopulation responsible for a different aspect of healing.[43,44] For example, the response of clonal populations of fibroblasts to certain signals, including growth factors, is quite heterogeneous.[43,44] Because fibroblasts and other mesenchymal or epithelial cells do not have easily definable markers, like lymphocytes do, this heterogeneity in fibroblast subpopulations is not understood. However, the next several years are likely to see improvements in the techniques available to identify mesenchymal and epithelial cells of the same lineage.

Soon after injury, the formation of a clot provides an appropriate early matrix for cell migration. Fibrin and fibronectin, components of that clot, act as the provisional matrix for fibroblast migration. The behavior of fibroblasts is highly linked to PDGF, a peptide to which they are exposed immediately after wounding.[45] It should be recognized that fibroblasts in unwounded skin are surrounded by a collagen-rich matrix, are biosynthetically inactive, and express high levels of the collagen integrin receptor α_2. This changes dramatically when the fibroblasts arrive at the provisional matrix and are exposed to a number of highly active peptides, including PDGF. Fibroblasts in the fibrin-fibronectin environment of the provisional matrix that are exposed to PDGF upregulate the integrin subunits α_3 and α_5.[45] Gelsolin, a protein involved in capping and the severing of actin may be critical to subsequent movement related to the actinomyosin cytoskeleton during fibroblast migration.[46] These integrins facilitate fibroblast migration into the wound bed, where fibroblasts may be influenced by other growth factors and cytokines to proliferate or undergo further phenotypic changes. Ultimately, as the wound heals, the new collagen-rich extracellular matrix will cause downregulation of fibroblast integrins α_3 and α_5 while increasing levels of α_2.[45] Other factors are at work in regulating fibroblast migration into the wound.[45,47–51] Gelsolin is a downstream effector of Rac, a GTPase molecule that is activated by PDGF. Just as it attracts monocytes and neutrophils to the wound area, TGF-β1 also has been implicated as an important chemoattractant for fibroblasts.[52] As stated earlier, TGF-β1 upregulates the expression of provisional matrix integrins $\alpha_5\beta_1$ and $\alpha_v\beta_3$.[53,54] However, there are other mechanisms by which TGF-β1 might affect locomotion.[55] It has been shown that production of hyaluronan (HA) and RHAMM, a cell surface receptor for HA, is increased by TGF-β1 and is necessary for locomotion of tumor cells.[56]

Another HA receptor, CD44, has slightly different functions from the RHAMM receptor, but it ultimately mediates movement of fibroblasts on HA substrates.[57–59] Fibroblasts in hypertrophic scar tissue express greater amounts of CD44 and have decreased internalization of CD44 in the presence of HA.[60]

Fibroblasts begin to migrate into the wound 48 h after injury. They move along the fibrin-fibronectin matrix deposited in the initial clot, and they themselves produce fibronectin, which can facilitate their movement. Other extracellular matrix components, such as tenascin, are additional signals for fibroblast adhesion and movement. The Arg-Gly-Asp-Ser (RGDS) tetrapeptide, which is common to these and other extracellular matrix proteins, is important in the binding of these molecules to cell surface integrin receptors.[61,62]

Fibroblasts produce other extracellular matrix components, including type I and III collagen, elastin, glycosaminoglycans, and proteoglycans. Type III collagen, which is present in large quantities in fetal dermis but not in adult dermis, is the predominant collagen type during early wound repair. Synthesis of type III collagen becomes maximal 5 to 7 days after injury. [61,63] TGF-β has been shown to stimulate fibroblast production of types I and III collagen both in vitro and in vivo.[43] There is evidence that fibroblast clones with a greater collagen synthetic phenotype are selected during the early stages of wound repair.[44]

As the new connective tissue is formed, some fibroblasts undergo a further phenotypic change to actin-rich myofibroblasts. These cells display features characteristic of fibroblasts and smooth muscle cells. They contain an extensive network of rough endoplasmic reticulum, presumably needed to produce large amounts of matrix proteins.[64] Myofibroblasts are largely responsible for wound contraction and are prominently present in granulation tissue.[64,65] Unlike other cells involved in the wound healing process, myofibroblasts undergo organized arrangements along the lines of contraction.[66] Exposure to a number of mediators, including angiotensin, prostaglandins, bradykinis, and endothelins, leads to muscle-like contractions of the myofibroblasts. PDGF isoforms AB and BB also play an important role in how myfibroblasts contract the collagen matrix.[1] Understanding myofibroblasts and their function has other implications besides tissue repair. Hypertrophic scars and Dupuytren's contracture are conditions in which myofibroblasts play important roles.[67] The ultimate amount of wound contraction depends to a large extent on the depth of the wound. Skin wounds can be classified as either full or partial thickness. In full-thickness wounds, the injury extends deeper than the adnexa. These wounds heal at least in part by contraction, which results in an approximate 40 percent decrease in wound size.[68] In full-thickness wounds, epithelialization occurs from the wound edge alone. Partial-thickness wounds, in contrast, are not as deep, and parts of the adnexa remain in the wound bed. Partial-thickness wounds display less contraction, and epithelialization occurs from both the wound edge and from the adnexal structures with the wound bed.[69]

Angiogenesis

Antiogenesis describes the process by which new vessel growth, called *neovascularization,* takes place. Angiogenesis occurs at the same time as fibroplasia, and in fact, the two are interdependent. As with other processes of wound repair, new vessel formation occurs in the context of the changing extracellular matrix. The chief cell of angiogenesis is the endothelial cell, which, like the keratinocyte and fibroblast, must undergo specific changes in order to migrate to the wound bed, proliferate, and direct new vessel formation. Migration of endothelial cells into the wound depends on chemotactic signals supplied by the extracellular matrix and neighboring cells. FGF-2, or basic fibroblast growth factor, appears to be critical to these procecces. For example, blocking of this peptide will greatly interfere with angiogenesis (Table 21-1). Some of the effects of FGF-2 may be mediated through vascular endothelial growth factor (VEGF), although this peptide also may be stimulated in the wound by keratinocyte growth factor (KGF) and transforming growth factor α (TGF-α). Receptors for these peptides are upregulated by endothelial cells at the site of injury. Among these are flt-1, a VEGF receptor. VEGF receptor 2 and its coreceptor neuropilin 1 are also upregulated. There is evidence that like reepithelialization, cell migration is a more important component of angiogenesis than proliferation. However, many signals that are involved in endothelial cell migration, such as fibronectin and heparin, also may stimulate proliferation.[1,2,42]

Aside from their role in angiogenesis, endothelial cells play an active role in the inflammatory stage of wound healing. They produce several factors that control propagation of the initial clot, thereby limiting platelet aggregation and clot formation to the area of injury. These mediators include prostacyclin, which inhibits platelet aggregation; antithrombin III, which inhibits thrombin activity; protein C, which degrades coagulation factors V and VIII; and most important, plasminogen activator, which initiates clot lysis by converting plasminogen to plasmin.[5]

Experiments with the avascular cornea have shown that phenotypic alteration of endothelial cells during wound healing includes the development of pseudopodia that project through fragmented basement membranes. The stimulus for this phenotypic change is not as well known as those outlined for keratinocytes and fibroblasts. By the second day following acute injury, endothelial cells at the wound edge begin to migrate into the perivascular space, and those remaining in the blood vessel begin to proliferate.[42]

A number of factors have been implicated in stimulating angiogenesis. As described before, low oxygen tension in the early wound environment appears to potentiate angiogenesis and fibroplasias.[70] Low oxygen tension also may stimulate macrophages to produce and secrete angiogenic factors.[30] Growth factors shown to be angiogenic include TGF-β1 and FGF. Of interest is that TGF-β1 is a potent inhibitor of endothelial cell proliferation, yet it induces a dramatic angiogenic response when injected into the dermis. This is probably so because TGF-β leads to the recruitment of macrophages, which in turn secrete substances that stimulate endothelial cell ingrowth. This example underscores the complexities involved in this phase of wound repair and the difficulty in assigning definite effects to any particular factor or cell. However, it does appear that the FGF family is by far the most important in stimulating angiogenesis. These peptides are released by macrophages and interact with heparin, which enhances their biologic activity. As discussed earlier, macrophages are essential to the wound healing process.

As it does with other phases of wound healing, the extracellular matrix plays a critical role in angiogenesis. One component of the provisional matrix is secreted protein acidic and rich in cysteine (SPARC). Released from fibroblasts and macrophages, SPARC, or its proteolytic fragments, stimulate angiogenesis during formation of granulation tissue.[71] SPARC, tenascin, and thrombospondin are all components of the early provisional matrix and also can be found in tissues where cells are dividing or migrating.[72] They are considered antiadhesive proteins and have been shown to promote cell rounding and partial detachment.[71] In addition to these effects, SPARC also can stimulate the production of collagenase, stromalysin, and gelatinase. Heparin and fibronectin, two other components of the provisional matrix, stimulate endothelial cells to project pseudopodia through basement membrane defects at the site of injury.[42] FGF further stimulates cells to release procollagenase and plasminogen activator (PA).[42] PA converts plasminogen to plasmin and activates collagenase. These enzymes help to break down the basement membrane and facilitate endothelial cell migration into the perivascular space.

TABLE 21-1

Partial List of Growth Factors and Cytokines in the Context of Wound Repair and Their Roles in Some Cellular Functions and Matrix Production

RESPONSES	EGF	FGF	GMCSF	IL-1	PDGF	TGF-β1	VEGF	CTGF
Fibroblast proliferation	+	+		+	++	+		+
Keratinocyte proliferation	+	+		+		−		
Angiogenesis	+	+	+	+	+	+	++	
Matrix formation		+			++	++		++
Inflammatory cell migration chemotaxis			++	+		+		

NOTE: EGF, epidermal growth factor; FGF, fibroblast growth factor; GMCSF, granulocyte-macrophage colony-stimulating factor; HGF, hepatocyte growth factor; IL-1, interleukin 1; IGF-1, insulin growth factor 1; PDGF, platelet-derived growth factor; TGF-β1, transforming growth factor β1; VEGF, vascular endothelial growth factor; CTGF, connective tissue growth factor. Blank cell, no definite response; +, definite but mild response; ++, definite and marked response.

Just as with other stages of wound healing, cell-to-cell and cell-to-matrix interactions play a key role in determining endothelial cell invasion, migration, and proliferation. During wound repair, a number of adhesive proteins are expressed in the basement membrane zone of blood vessels, including vWF, fibronectin, and fibrinogen. Studies have shown that several integrin receptors, especially $\alpha_v\beta_3$, are upregulated on the surface of smooth muscle cells and endothelial cells during angiogenesis.[73] $\alpha_v\beta_3$ is the endothelial cell receptor for vWF, fibrinogen/fibrin, and fibronectin. In one study, $\alpha_v\beta_3$ was found to be expressed in newly formed blood vessels in granulation tissue but not in normal unwounded skin.[73]

Keratinocyte Migration

The process of reepithelialization begins several hours after tissue injury. Keratinocyte migration, rather than proliferation, is actually responsible for most of the resurfacing of the epidermal defect. The process by which reepithelialization occurs in acute wounds is quite different from what one observes in wounds that fail to heal. Figure 21-2 shows a diagrammatic representation of the migrating epithelial tongue in acute wounds, contrasting it with the acanthotic epidermis generally seen in wounds that do not heal. This point will be discussed in more detail below because it is pertinent to understanding the overall mechanisms of wound repair. The events regulating keratinocyte migration are highly heterogenous and yet interrelated. These events have to do with changes in the shape of keratinocytes, in restructuring of their cytoskeleton and keratin expression, and in expression of proteases. Phenotypic alteration of keratinocytes enables them to migrate both from the wound edge and from any adnexal structures remaining in the wound bed. One to two days after the initial injury, epidermal cells at the wound edge and within the wound begin to divide and proliferate, thereby contributing to the population of migrating cells. For small wounds, the proliferative event is minor and probably not as important. However, for large wounds, there is a very dramatic burst of proliferative activity without which proper and timely resurfacting of the wound would not occur. This discrepancy between small and large wounds has created some confusion, and frequently one hears the erroneous statement that proliferation is not important for keratinocyte migration.

Nevertheless, several studies have shown that, in a pure sense, keratinocyte migration and proliferation can be regarded as two independent processes. One way to investigate this is to block keratinocyte proliferation with TGF-β, which is a prominent and potent inhibitor of epithelial cell growth. In one such study,[74] investigators exposed keratinocytes to a matrix of collagen that stimulated marked motility and later to TGF-β, which resulted in marked inhibition of proliferation. Despite this effect, the keratinocytes continued to migrate. In fact, migration was enhanced by TGF-β.[74]

As discussed previously, keratinocytes undergo profound changes in morphology as they migrate or, perhaps stated more properly, as they are empowered to migrate. Basal keratinocytes undergo a morphologic change from their normal cuboidal shape to a flattened cell with extended lamellipodia that project into the wound bed.[75] Hemidesmisomes are retracted from the plasma membrane, and the number of gap junctions increases. Integrin receptor expression changes to facilitate keratinocyte movement on collagens, and keratinocytes begin to synthesize and release types I and IV collagenases.

The expression of new integrins clearly aids keratinocyte migration. For example, the ability of keratinocytes to get hold of and migrate over the provisional matrix is intimately linked to their expression of $\alpha_5\beta_1$ and $\alpha_v\beta_6$ fibronectin/tenascin receptors.[76] Vitronectin and its integrin receptor ($\alpha_v\beta_5$) are also critical components of this migration. Indeed, in a model of bioengineered skin, vitronectin and its integrin counterpart have been found to be essential for the migration of keratinocytes over the surface of the construct (epiboly). Keratinocyte migration begins

and is associated with several morphologic and biochemical changes.[77] The keratinocytes at the edges of the wound upregulate proteases to allow their migration in the context of a fibrin clot. Experimental observations indicate that the process of occlusion greatly aids this migration and that in such circumstances the keratinocyte actually may migrate indiscriminately over a number of surfaces placed within the wound. Thus occlusion may speed up reepithelialization by stimulating keratinocytes to migrate in less specific ways. For keratinoyctes to migrate, they need to detach themselves from the basal lamina to which they are attached through the hemidesmosomes, anchoring contacts linking laminin via $\alpha_6\beta_6$ to the keratinocyte's keratin filament network.[78] The migration of keratinocytes over extracellular matrix as well as the provisional wound matrix is aided by the expression of new integrins, mainly the $\alpha_5\beta_1$ and $\alpha_v\beta_6$ fibronectin/tenascin receptors and the $\alpha_v\beta_5$ vitronectin receptors. Movement over collagen requires the $\alpha_2\beta_1$ integrin.[79–82] Crawling over these surfaces by the keratinocytes is achieved through morphologic changes and lamellopodial movement. The cytoskeleton is critical to these changes and to cell migration. Thus contraction of the actinomyosin filaments inserting into adhesion complexes results in and facilitates cell crawling. It is now thought that crawling and movement are not confined to the basal keratinocytes at the wound edge. Rather, suprabasal keratinocytes seem to "leapfrog" over the basal cells. Strength for keratinocyte locomotion is provided by keratins, which are important in both lamellopodial crawling and in the pursestring-type of closure observed in embryonic wounds. Keratins 6, 16, and 17 are induced in keratinocytes at the wound's edge.[83]

Various cytokines and matrix proteins stimulate keratinocyte migration on the wound bed. Connective tissue promoters of migration include fibronectin and type IV collagen, both of which can be synthesized by keratinocytes,[84] and native denatured type I collagen.[75] Growth factors, such as TGF-β and epidermal growth factor (EGF), stimulate keratinocytes to migrate. TGF-β also increases keratinocyte production of fibronectin. Signal-transduction pathways critical to keratinocyte migration are being elucidated. The p38-MAPK/SAPK pathway is required for the migration of keratinocytes on a collagen substrate.[85]

As in other physiologic processes, stops or brakes are in place to allow an end to the events facilitating keratinocyte migration. One such signal is the reconstitution of laminin, which is a major component of the lamina lucida zone of the basement membrane. In intact unwounded skin this large glycoprotein acts by preventing direct contact between keratinocytes and collagens contained within the basement membrane (types IV and VII) and dermis (types I, III, and VI).[26,75,86] With injury to the skin, the laminin component is disrupted, and this event allows contact of keratinocytes with the underlying collagens, thereby stimulating migration. It has been shown that laminin reappears in the dermal-epidermal junction after keratinocytes have migrated and resurfaced the wound and thus serves as a signal for keratinocytes to stop migrating.[2]

The process of reepithelialization could not occur unimpeded without the appropriate expression and action of enzymes needed to dissolve substrates and matrix materials for keratinocytes to migrate.[87–89] Ultimately, these enzymes also play a fundamental role in tissue remodeling. Migrating keratinocytes upregulate tissue-type plaminogen activator (tPA) and the urokinase-type plaminogen activator (uPA) and its receptor. These enzymes are critical for the movement of keratinocytes through the fibrin clot.[90–92] Other proteases are also important. The matrix metalloproteinases (MMPs) enzyme family comprises more than 20 different members, some of which, during the process of cutaneous repair, are very tightly expressed and regulated. MMPs are zinc-dependent endopeptidases that are activated by other proteinases such as plasmin. Their activity is blocked or downregulated by tissue inhibitors of metalloproteinases. Collagenase-1

(MMP-1), stromelysin-2 (MMP-10), and the 92-kDa gelatinase (MMP-9) are expressed by keratinocytes at the edges of the wound. MMP-1 is needed for keratinocyte migration on type I collagen and is upregulated in keratinocytes at the very edge of the wound, after the cells have freed themselves from the basal lamina, a process that is aided by MMP-9. MMP-10 degrades a number of extracellular matrix proteins other than collagen. Other MMPs are spatially upregulated just proximal to the wound's edge. In this category are stromelysin-2 (MMP-10) and the newly described epilysin (MMP-28), which is associated with keratinocyte proliferation rather than migration during wound repair.[93] There is evidence that keratinocyte migration is blocked by inhibitors of MMPs.[94]

Integrin expression is also regulated by growth factors, including TGF-β, PDGF, and VEGF. The expression of $\alpha_5\beta_1$ and $\alpha_v\beta_3$ in cultured fibroblasts and the β_4 subunit in cultured keratinocytes is increased by TGFβ-1.[95–97] This cytokine also upregulates $\alpha_5\beta_1$ and $\alpha_v\beta_5$ in keratinocytes.[86] The effect of cytokines and growth factors on the regulation of integrin expression must be viewed in context of the matrix surrounding the target cell. It has been shown that PDGF-BB, a prominent component of the early wound environment, upregulates $\alpha_5\beta_1$ and $\alpha_3\beta_1$ expression in fibroblasts grown in fibronectin-rich tissue culture of fibrin.[45] However, fibroblasts grown on collagen gels, thereby approximating the normal dermis or late wound environment, do not show upregulation of these integrins, even in the presence of PDGFF-BB. The vast array of cytokines affecting integrin expression are initially released by aggregating platelets in the early wound.[98] Later they are produced by fibroblasts, keratinocytes, monocytes, and macrophages.[86]

TISSUE REMODELING (PHASE 3)

In the third and final phase of wound repair, the formed tissue is degraded and remodeled, and cells undergo apoptosis and other drastic changes. Typically, this phase can last several months. Although the functional outcome is not ideal, in that tissue regeneration has not occurred, the remodeling process allows the host to develop a stable scar that has approximately 70 percent of the original strength. Closure of the wound is of paramount importance from a survival and evolutionary standpoint, and the outcome of repair reflects this priority and is a compromise between functional and structural needs. In many ways, this phase of wound repair resembles many other unrelated physiologic processes in which the initial outcome is exaggerated. Thus, during the process of wound repair, there is probably an overabundance of cellular migration and proliferation and even excessive deposition of many types of extracellular matrix components. This "exaggeration" of the repair response is important in ensuring a proper inflammatory reaction and clearing of bacteria, wound debridement, and removal of necrotic tissue. Fibroplasia and angiogenesis are critical to the development of the appropriate wound bed required for keratinocyte migration and reepithelialization. However, as stated, the abundance of cells and extracellular matrix material must now be dealt with, and a remodeling process is required for downregulating the response and returning to an approximation of the prewounded state. Apoptotic mechanisms and the enzymatic activity of MMPs and other proteinases will be at work to achieve a balance within the newly reepithelialized wound.

Events of remodeling are closely linked to those which have allowed the deposition of certain extracellular matrix components and migration of cells to the wound site in the first place. The reason for this is that no remodeling can take place unless the primary stimulatory signals are turned off. Therefore, the discussion about what is critical to the formation of tissue is appropriate when viewed in the context of how this formed tissue is now modified. To be sure, this third phase of wound repair is not as well studied as the processes of inflammation and proliferation, and therefore, many more questions remain. It also should be recognized that the remodeling phase does not occur homogeneously within the wound, either in location or in time. In the context of the remodeling phase of wound repair, the following events and key extracellular matrix components will be discussed in turn: (1) fibronectin and associated components, (2) hyaluronic acid and proteoglycans, (3) collagen, and (4) contraction and the emergence of myofibroblasts.

Fibronectin and Associated Components

Fibroblasts produce fibronectin as they enter the wound site, and at least initially, the concentrations of fibronectin are very high. By 4 to 5 days after injury, the fibronectin network is well established.[54] It is important to note that the process by which fibroblasts leave their collagen-rich environment to enter the wound site requires them to modify their behavior and characteristics. Fibroblasts need to become activated and modify their integrin repertoire, which will dictate what they bind to and where they will go. To a certain extent, this is regulated by cytokines. For example, exposure of fibroblasts to PDGF can upregulate the integrin subunits α_3 and α_5, which are considered more adapt at binding to provisional wound matrix components. Conversely, the α_2 integrin subunit is upregulated in fibroblasts in a collagen-rich environment. The production of fibronectin is stimulated by a number of growth factors, but certainly TGF-β, which also upregulates integrin receptors' binding to fibronectin.[45,99] This cytokine is critical in the deposition of extracellular matrix and is often implicated in the pathogenesis of excessive scarring and fibrosis. TGF-β is a chemoattractant for fibroblasts[100] and stimulates their proliferation,[101] as well as causing an overall increase in extracellular matrix formation.[99] There is directionality to the deposition of fibronectin, which is important in the way other extracellular matrix proteins are laid down. For example, collagen deposition will align itself after the fibronectin pattern, which in turn mirrors the axis of alignment of fibroblasts.[54] Ultimately, during remodeling and contraction, myofibroblasts will make use of the fibronectin network to cause wound contraction.

A number of hypotheses have been proposed for the mechanims in addition to fibronectin underlying the adhesion of fibroblasts to extracellular matrix. One hypothesis is proteinase-based, whereby the assembly of the actin cytoskeleton is dictated by the action of proteinases on specific cellular sites.[72] The deposition of ECM-associated molecules, such as tenascin, SPRC, thrombospondin, and dermatan sulfate, is another way of influencing and modifying the overall ECM makeup.[72] For example, SPARC upregulates fibroblast expression of metalloproteinases, especially collagenase, whereas thrombospondin and tenascin have both adhesive and antiadhesive properties.[102] To a large extent, regulation of how SPARC induces collagenase expression is related to which ECM components fibroblasts are exposed to. Thus SPARC leads to collagenase production in fibroblasts grown on collagen types I, II, III, and V and on vitronectin, but not on collagen type IV. Eventually, the fibronectin-rich environment of the initial wound is modified and remodeled by cell and plasma proteases. Over time, fibronectin is replaced by type III collagen and ultimately by type I collagen.

Hyaluronic Acid and Proteoglycans

The glycosaminoglycan (GAG) hyaluronic acid (hyaluronan) is also an abundant component of the provisional matrix and one whose deposition needs to be modified during the remodeling process. High levels of hyaluronic acid are present in the early embryo, where it is thought to offer less resistance to cell migration. Indeed, embryonic wound repair is characterized by a hyaluronic acid–rich environment, thought to be at least in part responsible for the "scarless" healing of embryonic wounds. Fibroblasts from early granulation tissue produce large amounts of hyaluronic acid, and proliferating cells express CD44, which is the receptor for this GAG molecule.[99,103] Besides the issue of offering less resistance to cell movement, hyaluronic acid may stimulate cell motility by altering cell-matrix adhesion. One example of this is that hyaluronic acid weakens the adhesion of heparan sulfate and fibronectin.[104] Perhaps more important from a physical/spatial standpoint is that hyaluronic acid creates a highly hydrated structure leading to tissue swelling and interstitial spaces and thus an environment more conducive to cell movement.[99] The effects of hyaluronic acid are also regulated by growth factors and cytokines. Upregulation of hyaluronic acid expression and its receptors (e.g., RHAAMM) by TGF-$\beta 1$ stimulates fibroblast motility.[105,106]

Eventually, as remodeling occurs, hyaluronic acid is degraded by hyaluronidase and replaced by sulfated proteoglycans, which contribute a stronger structural role in late granulation tissue formation and in scars while being less able to stimulate cellular movement. Two major proteoglycans, chondroitin-4-sulfate and dermatan sulfate, are produced by mature scar fibroblasts.

Collagen

Three main classes of collagens are present normally in connective tissue: fibrillar collagens (types I, III, and V), basement membrane collagen (type IV), and other interstitial collagens (types VI, VII, and VIII). These are merely examples of the many different types of collagen present in skin. Importantly, however, the fibrillar collagens serve as the major structural collagens in all connective tissues.[42,99]

During the initial phases of wound repair, it appears that the wound tends to recapitulate the processes involved in embryogenesis. Thus granulation tissue is initially comprised of large amounts of type III collagen, which is a minor component of adult dermis and indeed is present in larger amounts in fetal wound repair. During the phase of remodeling, over a period of a year or more, type III collagen is gradually replaced by type I collagen. Type I collagen replacement is associated with increased tensile strength of the scar. However, the final tensile strength of a scar is only about 70 percent of that of preinjured skin.[106] The process of converting the collagen content of the dermis from type III to type I collagen is controlled by interactions involving synthesis of new collagen with lysis of old collagen.[43] Key to this process of conversion are metalloproteinases and specifically the collagenases.

Matrix-degrading metalloproteinases (MMP) are proenzymes that need to be activated and are considered to be the physiologic mediators of matrix degradation. The prototypic MMP is interstitial collagenase, but over 20 such enzymes have been described. There are three broad classes of these zinc-dependent enzymes: collagenases, gelatinases, and stromelysins. The collagenases include interstitial collagenase (fibroblast collagenase, MMP-1), which acts on collagens I, II, III, VII, and X. Collagen type II is a particularly good substrate for MMP-1. Another important member of the collagenase class is neutrophil collagenase (MMP-1), which also degrades type II and III collagens but is particularly active against type I collagen. Gelatinases break down denatured collagen (gelatin). Among the most important gelatinases are gelatinase A (MMP-2), which breaks down gelatins, collagen IV, and elastin. Another key gelatinase is gelatinase B (MMP-9), which is produced by many cell types, including macrophages, neutrophils, and keratinocytes. Stromelysins have a relatively broad substrate specificity. Both stromelysin 1 (MMP-3) and 2 (MMP-10) act on proteoglycans, fibronectin, laminin, gelatins, and collagens III, IV, and IX. Another member of the stromelysin family, matrilysin (MMP-7), degrades mainly fibronectin, gelatins, and elastin. One of the newest member of the MMP family is epilysin (MMP-28), which appears to be produced by proliferating keratinocytes distal to the wound edge.[93] It may be needed to restructure the basement membrane.

Stimulation of the production of MMPs and their activation are not only by growth factors and cytokines, such as IL-1, but also by extracellular matrix components and other chemicals. For example, trypsin, organomercurials, plasmin, and SDS can activate MMPs, whereas calcium stabilizes them. As stated, MMPs are dependent on zinc, which is located at the center of the molecule at a conserved sequence known as HEXGH. A number of chelators, including tissue inhibitor of metalloproteinase (TIMP), inhibit several members of the MMP family, whereas α_2-macroglobulin entraps them.[1,87,89]

The remodeling phase is more than a breakdown of excess macromolecules formed during the proliferative phase of wound healing. Cells within the wound are returned to a stable phenotype, extracellular matrix material is altered (i.e., collagen type III to type I), and the granulation tissue that was so exuberant during the early phases of wound healing disappears.

Myofibroblasts and Contraction

During the earlier stages of wound repair, beginning around 4 days after injury, granulation tissue forms.[1] Granulation tissue is so named based on its granule-like appearance, which is rich in vascular structures. In the more mature wound and during remodeling, this granulation tissue has to be modified. One of the primary events is wound contraction. There are different degrees of contraction depending on the host, the location of the wound, and its depth. For example, rodents heal in large part by contraction, which must be kept in mind when extrapolating to humans the results of experimentally induced wounds in mice and rats. The location of the wound is important too; much more contraction appears to occur over rounded surfaces, such as shoulders and the nose. The reasons for these differences due to location are not known. Certainly, more tension may be present in certain locations, and this could modify the type of extracellular matrix laid down, as well as having an effect on fibroblast phenotype and selection. However, of the utmost importance to the development and extent of contraction is wound depth. Partial-thickness wounds, down only to papillary dermis, heal with less scarring and contraction. Full-thickness wounds, which encompass the fat and subcutaneous tissue, tend to heal with much more scarring and rely on contraction for faster repair. Anyhow, the mass of tissue that has formed in the earlier phases of wound repair must now be made smaller, and contraction is an effective and dependable way of doing so. The myofibroblast plays a critical role in the contraction process. One often reads that myofibroblasts are "transformed" wound fibroblasts that express α-smooth muscle actin and are smooth muscle–like cells. The term *transformed* is incorrect, since transformation is used properly only in the context of the path to neoplasia. The mechanisms leading to the myofibroblast phenotype are largely unknown, but certain growth factors, such as TGF-$\beta 1$, can regulate this process. It is also known that myofibroblasts can play a fundamental pathogenic role in certain fibrotic conditions, such as Dupuytren's contracture, and have critical consequences for the clinical expression of certain other conditions. For example, hypertrophic scars are myofibroblast-rich and thus both contract and eventually resolve over time. In contrast, keloids generally lack a significant component of myofibroblasts and therefore neither contract nor resolve easily.[42,64–66]

THE WORLD OF CHRONIC WOUNDS

The preceding discussion has been centered on cutaneous wound repair after acute injury. It must be recognized, however, that the applicability of those events and processes is limited when it comes to chronic wounds, such as in diabetes, in venous and arterial insufficiency, and in a variety of situations complicated by inflammatory processes and faulty response from the host. Acute wounds, such as those created by surgery or trauma, have a predictable time frame for healing and generally heal quite readily. However, chronic wounds display what has been called a "failure to heal." A number of observations have been made with regard to chronic wounds, and hypotheses have been proposed for their failure to heal. The scientific rigor of these hypotheses and possible mechanisms is less than what has been described in the preceding discussion for the general principles of wound repair, for it has been far more difficult to study chronic wounds in humans, and experimental models of chronic injury are few and not ideal. Yet it is useful to briefly describe some of the abnormalities that have been found and thus provide a contrast with the highly regulated principles of the different phases of wound repair.

Perhaps the best example where some progress has been made in understanding a chronic wound and its failure to heal is in ulcers due to venous insufficiency. The underlying abnormality in the development of venous ulcers is venous hypertension, which refers to the inability of venous pressure in the foot to decrease in response to exercise. In this sense, the term *hypertension* is a misnomer, for the pressure is not increased in an absolute sense. Venous "hypertension" is most commonly the result of faulty valves in the lower extremities, with or without blockage of blood flow in the deep veins. However, it should be recognized that the calf muscle pump, responsible for propelling blood back toward the heart, acts as a unit made up of veins and muscles. Thus a decrease in muscle function also could result in venous "hypertension". The first true hypothesis to address the pathophysiology of venous ulceration in a rational way suggested that the loss of tissue integrity and the development of ulceration were the result of venous "hypertension" and the leakage of fibrinogen from the intravascular compartment.[107–110] The fibrinogen quickly polymerized to fibrin around blood vessels ("fibrin cuffs"). It was hypothesized that the fibrin cuffs would prevent the diffusion of oxygen and other nutrients from the blood to the dermis. This "functional ischemia" was proposed to lead to loss of tissue integrity and, ultimately, ulceration. Since the fibrin cuff hypothesis was first proposed, there has been continued reassessment of its validity. While fibrin cuffs have been found in more than 90 percent of biopsies from venous ulcers and surrounding skin, at the same time a strong dynamic relationship between the presence or absence of these cuffs and ulceration has not been detected. Also, it has been realized that polymerized fibrin has gaps within its structure that are large enough for oxygen and large molecules to get through. Still, further reevaluation has determined that given a sluggish blood flow, pericapillary fibrin cuffs could contribute to the pathogenesis by altering or decreasing the exchange of certain substances between blood and dermis. Moreover, there is substantial evidence that patients with venous disease and ulceration have decreased fibrinolytic capacity, which contributes to the development and persistence of fibrin cuffs.[108]

Hypotheses for the development of chronic wounds are not necessarily mutually exclusive. The complexity of chronic wounds is such that a number of pathogenic steps are involved. It has been reported that as a consequence of venous "hypertension", damage to the endothelium occurs and neutrophils adhering to the damaged blood vessels release a number of inflammatory mediators that compound the damage. Another hypothesis has to do with the unavailability of growth factors in chronic wounds.[110] There is evidence that growth factors in chronic wounds are bound to and trapped by macromolecules such as albumin, fibrinogen, α_2-macroglobulin leaking into the dermis. The α_2-macroglobulin molecule is a scavenger for growth factors, including PDGF.[111,112]

The critical importance of MMPs in cutaneous wound repair, particularly in the context of keratinocyte migration has been discussed previously. However, in chronic wounds, MMPs may have a darker side. For example, in venous ulcers and other types of chronic wounds, the wound fluid contains excessive amounts of metalloproteinases, which break down the extracellular matrix and, most likely, cytokines and growth factors.[113–116]

It also should be recognized that tissues around chronic wounds are not normal and that indeed they are altered by the primary pathogenic mechanisms that had to the inability to heal readily. Clinically, the best example of this is the intense fibrosis surrounding venous ulcers, which is termed *lipodermatosclerosis*. Once lipodermatosclerosis becomes established, it can lead to ulcers and becomes the site of ulcer recurrence. Indeed, venous ulcers surrounded by lipodermatosclerosis are much more difficult to heal. The reason for these observations may lie in an increasing body of evidence suggesting that the cellular makeup of wounds that do not heal is altered. Because of the ease with which they are grown and studied in culture, the best evidence comes from wound fibroblasts. We now know that ulcer fibroblasts are senescent[117,118] and are unresponsive to certain selected cytokines and growth factors. For example, it has been shown that venous ulcer fibroblasts are unresponsive to the action of transforming growth factor (TGF-β1)[119] and platelet-derived growth factor (PDGF).[120] The synthetic program of cells in diabetic ulcers also may be altered so that such chronic wounds are said to be "stuck" in a certain phase of the repair process. There is evidence for this in diabetic ulcers.[121] A close relationship has been reported between some of these abnormalities and the inability to heal. For example, a correlation has been found between fibroblast senescence and wounds that do not heal.[117]

CONCLUSION

Characterizing the number of events and the interrelationships that occur after tissue injury represents a rather daunting task. Yet, over the last several decades, the orderly progression from injury to inflammation and coagulation, to the development of a provisional matrix, to the formation of granulation tissue, and to tissue remodeling has been elucidated. Although somewhat artificial, the different phases of wound repair described here are the platform on which more knowledge can be built. Much still needs to be learned, but the framework is there for understanding tissue repair and for developing ways to accelerate it. Indeed, due to breakthroughs in science and technology, progress has been exponential in the last few years. In the long run, one would like to discuss how skin can be regenerated and not simply repaired. For that to occur, we will need an even greater understanding of the science involved. What may look detailed today will turn out to be sketchy tomorrow. It is also possible that lessons learned from failure to heal, as in chronic wounds, will provide valuable lessons for the general principles of wound healing.

REFERENCES

1. Clark RA: Wound repair: overview and general considerations, in *The Molecular and Cellular Biology of Wound Repair,* 2d ed, edited by RAF Clark. New York, Plenum, 1996, p 3
2. Clark RA et al: Fibronectin and fibrin provide a provisional matrix for epidermal cell migration during wound reepithelialization. *J Invest Dermatol* **79**:264, 1982
3. Santoro SA: identification of a 160,000 dalton platelet membrane protein that mediates the initial divalent cation-dependent adhesion of platelets to collagen. *Cell* **46**:913, 1986

4. Moncada S et al; An enzyme isolated from arteries transforms prostaglandin endoperoxides to an unstable substance that inhibits platelet aggregation. *Nature* **263**:663, 1976
5. Loskutoff DJ, Edgington TE: Synthesis of a fibrinolytic activator and inhibitor by endothelial cells. *Proc Natl Acad Sci USA* **74**:3903, 1977
6. Roberts AB: Transforming growth factor-beta, in *The Molecular and Cellular Biology of Wound Repair,* 2d ed, edited by RAF Clark, New York, Plenum, 1996, p 275
7. Furie B: The molecular basis of blood coagulation. *Cell* **53**:505, 1988
8. Weisel JW et al: The sequence of cleavage of fibrinopeptides from fibrinogen is important for protofibril formation and enhancement of lateral aggregation in fibrin clots. *J Mol Biol* **232**:285, 1993
9. Weiss E et al: Un-cross-linked fibrin substrates inhibit keratinocyte spreading and replication: Correction with fibronectin and factor XIII cross-linking. *J Cell Physiol* **174**:58, 1998
10. Dipietro LA et al: Modulation of macrophage recruitment into wounds by monocyte chemoattractant protein-1. *Wound Repair Regen* **9**:28, 2001
11. Riches X: Macrophage involvement in wound repair, remodelling and fibrosis, in *The Molecular and Cellular Biology of Wound Repair,* 2d ed, edited by RAF Clark. New York, Plenum, 1996, P 95
12. Tonnesen MG: Neutrophil-endothelial cell interactions: Mechanisms of neutrophil adherence to vascular endothelium. *J Invest Dermatol* **93**:535, 1989
13. Doherty DE et al: Human monocyte adherence: A primary effect of chemotactic factors on the monocyte to stimulate adherence to human endothelium. *J Immunol* **138**:1762, 1987
14. Subramaniam M et al: Role of endothelial selectins in wound repair. *Am J Pathol* **150**:1701, 1997
15. Springer X: Traffic signals for lymphocyte recirculation and leukocyte emigration: The multistep paradigm. *Cell* **76**:301, 1994
16. Grotendorst GR: Connective tissue growth factor: A mediator of TGF-beta action on fibroblasts. *Cytokine Growth Factor Rev* **8**:171, 1997
17. Hubner G et al: Differential regulation of pro-inflammatory cytokines during wound healing in normal and glucocorticoid-treated mice. *Cytokine* **8**:548, 1996
18. Gresham HD et al: A novel member of the integrin receptor family mediates Arg-Gly-Asp–stimulated neutrophil phagocytosis. *J Cell Bio* **108**:1935, 1989
19. Grinnell F: Wound repair, keratinocyte activation and integrin modulation. *J Cell Sci* **101**:1, 1992
20. Cass DL et al: Epidermal integrin expression is upregulated rapidly in human fetal wound repair. *J Pediatr Surg* **33**:312, 1998
21. Simpson DM, Ross R: The neutrophilic leukocyte in wound repair a study with antineutrophil serum. *J Clin Invest* **51**:2009, 1972
22. Newman SL et al: Phagocytosis of senescent neutrophils by human monocyte-derived macrophages and rabbit inflammatory macrophages. *J Exp Med* **156**:430, 1982
23. Leibovich SJ, Ross R: The role of the macrophage in wound repair: A study with hydrocortisone and antimacrophage serum. *Am J Pathol* **78**:71, 1975
24. Hopkinson-Woolley J et al. Macrophage recruitment during limb development and wound healing in the embryonic and foetal mouse. *J Cell Sci* **107**:1159, 1994
25. Luster AD et al: Delayed wound healing and disorganized neovascularization in transgenic mice expressing the IP-10 chemokine. *Proc Assoc Am Physicians* **110**:183, 1998
26. Kubo M et al: Fibrinogen and fibrin are anti-adhesive for keratinocytes: A mechanism for fibrin eschar slough during wound repair. *J Invest Dermatol* **117**:1369, 2001
27. Hauck CR et al: The focal adhesion kinase: A regulator of cell migration and invasion *IUBMB Life* **53**:115, 2002.
28. Packer L, Fuehr K: Low oxygen concentration extends the lifespan of cultured human diploid cells. *Nature* **267**:423, 1977
29. Falanga V, Kirsner RS: Low oxygen stimulates proliferation of fibroblasts seeded as single cells. *J Cell Physiol* **154**:506, 1993
30. Knighton DR et al: Oxygen tension regulates the expression of angiogenesis factor by macrophages. *Science* **221**:1283, 1983
31. Falanga V et al: Hypoxia upregulates the synthesis of TGF-beta 1 by human dermal fibroblasts. *J Invest Dermatol* **97**:634, 1991
32. Kourembanas S et al: Hypoxia induces endothelin gene expression and secretion in cultured human endothelium. *J Clin Invest* **88**:1054, 1991
33. Kourembanas S et al: Oxygen tension regulates the expression of the platelet-derived growth factor-B chain gene in human endothelial cells. *J Clin Invest* **86**:670, 1990
34. Shweiki D et al: Vascular endothelial growth factor induced by hypoxia may mediate hypoxia-initiated angiogenesis. *Nature* **359**:843, 1992
35. Semenza GL et al: Hypoxia-inducible factor 1: From molecular biology to cardiopulmonary physiology. *Chest* **114**:405, 1998
36. Wang GL et al: Hypoxia-inducible factor 1 is a basic-helix-loop-helix-PAS heterodimer regulated by cellular O_2 tension. *Proc Natl Acad Sci USA* **92**:5510, 1995
37. Uitto J, Prockop DJ: Hydroxylation of peptide-bound proline and lysine before and after chain completion of the polypeptide chains of procollagen. *Arch Biochem Biophys* **164**:210, 1974
38. Falanga V et al: Low oxygen tension increases mRNA levels of alpha 1 (I) procollagen in human dermal fibroblasts. *J Cell Physiol* **157**:408, 1993
39. Faller DV: Endothelial cell responses to hypoxic stress. *Clin Exp Pharmacol Physiol* **26**:74, 1999
40. Stadman X: Protein oxidation and aging. *Science* **267**:1220, 1992
41. Ala Y et al: Hypoxia/reoxygenation stimulates endothelial cells to promote interleukin-1 and interleukin-6 production: Effects of free radical scavengers. *Agents Actions* **37**:134, 1992
42. Singer AJ, Clark RA: Cutaneous wound healing. *New Engl J Med* **341**:738, 1999
43. Yamaguchi Y et al: Lack of co-ordinate expression of the alpha 1 (I) and alpha 1 (III) procollagen genes in fibroblast clonal cultures. *Br J Dermatol* **143**:1149, 2000
44. Falanga V et al: Human dermal fibroblast clones derived from single cells are heterogeneous in the production of mRNAs for alpha 1(I) procollagen and transforming growth factor-beta 1. *J Invest Dermatol* **105**:27, 1995
45. Xu I, Clark RA: Extracellular matrix alters PDGF regulation of fibroblast integrins. *J Cell Biol* **132**:239, 1996
46. Witke W et al: Hemostatic, inflammatory, and fibroblast responses are blunted in mice lacking gelsolin. *Cell* **81**:41, 1995
47. McClain SA et al: Mesenchymal cell activation is the rate-limiting step of granulation tissue induction. *Am J Pathol* **149**:1257, 1996
48. Greiling D, Clark RA: Fibronectin provides a conduit for fibroblast transmigration from collagenous stroma into fibrin clot provisional matrix. *J Cell Sci* **110**:861, 1997
49. Georges-Labouesse EN et al: Mesodermal development in mouse embryos mutant for fibronectin. *Dev Dyn* **207**:145, 1996
50. Ffrench-Constant C et al: Reappearance of an embryonic pattern of fibronectin splicing during wound healing in the adult rat. *J Cell Biol* **109**:903, 1989
51. Brown GL et al: Enhancement of epidermal regeneration by biosynthetic epidermal growth factor. *J Exp Med* **163**:1319, 1986
52. Hartwig JH et al: Thrombin receptor ligation and activated Rac uncap actin filament barbed ends through phosphoinositide synthesis in permeabilized human platelets. *Cell* **82**:643, 1995
53. Eckes B et al: Interactions of fibroblasts with the extracellular matrix: Implications for the understanding of fibrosis. *Springer Semin Immunopathol* **21**:415, 1999
54. Welch MP et al: Temporal relationships of F-actin bundle formation, collagen and fibronectin matrix assembly, and fibronectin receptor expression to wound contraction. *J Cell Biol* **110**:133, 1990
55. Samuel SK et al: TGF-beta 1 stimulation of cell locomotion utilizes the hyaluronan receptor RHAMM and hyaluronan. *J Cell Biol* **123**:749,1993
56. Hardwick C et al: Molecular cloning of a novel hyaluronan receptor that mediates tumor cell motility. *J Cell Biol* **117**:1343, 1992
57. Estes JM et al: Hyaluronate metabolism undergoes an ontogenic transition during fetal development: Implications for scar-free wound healing. *J Pediatr Surg* **28**:1227, 1993
58. Thomas L et al: CD44H regulates tumor cell migration on hyaluronate-coated substrate. *J Cell Biol* **118**:971, 1992
59. Underhill C: CD44: The hyaluronan receptor. *J Cell Sci* **103**:293, 1992
60. Messadi DV, Bertolami CN: CD44 and hyaluronan expression in human cutaneous scar fibroblasts. *Am J Pathol* **142**:1041, 1993
61. Mosher X: Assembly of extracellular matrix. *Curr Opin Cell Biol* **4**:810, 1992
62. Wu C et al: The alpha 5 beta 1 integrin fibronectin receptor, but not the alpha 5 cytoplasmic domain, functions in an early and essential step in fibronectin matrix assembly. *J Biol Chem* **268**:21883, 1993
63. Kurkinen M et al: Sequential appearance of fibronectin and collagen in experimental granulation tissue. *Lab Invest* **43**:47, 1980
64. Majno G et al: Contraction of granulation tissue in vitro: similarity to smooth muscle. *Science* **173**:548, 1971
65. Gabbiani G et al: Granulation tissue as a contractile organ: A study of structure and function. *J Exp Med* **135**:719, 1972
66. Grinnell F: Fibroblasts, myofibroblasts, and wound contraction. *J Cell Biol* **124**:401, 1994
67. Chiu HF, McFarlane RM: Pathogenesis of Dupuytren's contracture: A correlative clinical-pathological study. *J Hand Surg [Am]* **3**:1, 1978

68. Bailey AJ et al: Characterization of the collagen of human hypertrophic and normal scars. *Biochim Biophys Acta* **405**:412, 1975
69. Levenson X: The healing of rat skin wounds. *Ann Surg* **161**:293, 1965
70. Falanga X: Growth factors and wound healing. *Dermatol Clin* **11**:667, 1993
71. Gailit J, Clark RA: Wound repair in the context of extracellular matrix. *Curr Opin Cell Biol* **6**:717, 1994
72. Tremble PM et al: SPARC, a secreted protein associated with morphogenesis and tissue remodeling, induces expression of metalloproteinases in fibroblasts through a novel extracellular matrix-dependent pathway. *J Cell Biol* **121**:1433, 1993
73. Brooks PC et al: Requirement of vascular integrin alpha v beta 3 for angiogenesis. *Science* **264**:569, 1994
74. Sarret Y et al: Human keratinocyte locomotion: The effect of selected cytokines. *J Invest Dermatol* **98**:12, 1992
75. Woodley DT et al: Re-epithelialization: Human keratinocyte locomotion. *Dermatol Clin* **11**:641, 1993
76. Regezi JA et al: Tenascin and beta 6 integrin are overexpressed in floor of mouth in situ carcinomas and invasive squamous cell carcinomas. *Oral Oncol* **38**:332, 2002
77. Gabbiani G et al: Cytoplasmic filaments and gap junctions in epithelial cells and myofibroblasts during wound healing. *J Cell Biol* **76**:561, 1978
78. Krawczyk WS, Wilgram GF: Hemidesmosome and desmosome morphogenesis during epidermal wound healing. *J Ultrastruct Res* **45**:93, 1973
79. Haapasalmi K et al: Keratinocytes in human wounds express alpha v beta 6 integrin. *J Invest Dermatol* **106**:42, 1996
80. Breuss JM et al: Expression of the beta 6 integrin subunit in development, neoplasia and tissue repair suggests a role in epithelial remodeling. *J Cell Sci* **108**:2241, 1995
81. Cavani A et al: Distinctive integrin expression in the newly forming epidermis during wound healing in humans. *J Invest Dermatol* **101**:600, 1993
82. Yamada X: Provisional matrix, *The Molecular and Cellular Biology of Wound Repair,* 2d ed, edited by RAF Clark. New York, Plenum, 1996, p 51
83. Paladini RD et al: Onset of re-epithelialization after skin injury correlates with a reorganization of keratin filaments in wound edge keratinocytes: defining a potential role for keratin 16. *J Cell Biol* **132**:381, 1996
84. O'Keefe EJ et al: Spreading and enhanced motility of human keratinocytes on fibronectin. *J Invest Dermatol* **85**:125, 1985
85. Li W et al: The p38–MAPK/SAPK pathway is required for human keratinocyte migration on dermal collagen. *J Invest Dermatol* **117**:1601, 2001
86. Gailit J et al: TGF-beta 1 stimulates expression of keratinocyte integrins during re-epithelialization of cutaneous wounds. *J Invest Dermatol* **103**:221, 1994
87. Circolo A et al: Differential regulation of the expression of proteinases/antiproteinases in fibroblasts: Effects of interleukin-1 and platelet-derived growth factor. *J Biol Chem* **266**:12283, 1991
88. Laiho M et al: Transforming growth factor-beta induction of type-1 plasminogen activator inhibitor: Pericellular deposition and sensitivity to exogenous urokinase. *J Biol Chem* **262**:17467, 1987
89. Overall CM et al: Independent regulation of collagenase, 72-kDa progelatinase, and metalloendoproteinase inhibitor expression in human fibroblasts by transforming growth factor-beta. *J Biol Chem* **264**:1860, 1989
90. Grondahl-Hansen J et al: Urokinase-and tissue-type plasminogen activators in keratinocytes during wound reepithelialization in vivo. *J Invest Dermatol* **90**:790, 1988
91. Romer J et al: Differential expression of urokinase-type plasminogen activator and its type-1 inhibitor during healing of mouse skin wounds. *J Invest Dermatol* **97**:803, 1991
92. Romer J et al: The receptor for urokinase-type plasminogen activator is expressed by keratinocytes at the leading edge during re-epithelialization of mouse skin wounds. *J Invest Dermatol* **102**:519, 1994
93. Saarialho-Kere U et al: Epilysin (MMP-28) expression is associated with cell proliferation during epithelial repair. *J Invest Dermatol* **119**:14, 2002
94. Nagase H, Brew K: Engineering of tissue inhibitor of metalloproteinases mutants as potential therapeutics. *Arthritis Res* **4**:551, 2002
95. Roberts CJ et al: Transforming growth factor beta stimulates the expression of fibronectin and of both subunits of the human fibronectin receptor by cultured human lung fibroblasts. *J Biol Chem* **263**:4586, 1988
96. Heino J et al: Regulation of cell adhesion receptors by transforming growth factor-beta: Concomitant regulation of integrins that share a common beta 1 subunit. *J Biol Chem* **264**:380, 1989
97. Ignotz RA et al: Regulation of cell adhesion receptors by transforming growth factor-beta: Regulation of vitronectin receptor and LFA-1. *J Biol Chem* **264**:389, 1989
98. Assoian RK et al: Transforming growth factor-beta in human platelets: Identification of a major storage site, purification, and characterization. *J Biol Chem* **258**:7155, 1983
99. Lawrence X: Physiology of the acute wound. *Clin Plast Surg* **25**:321, 1998
100. Postlethwaite AE et al: Stimulation of the chemotactic migration of human fibroblasts by transforming growth factor beta. *J Exp Med* **165**:251, 1987
101. Loef X: Induction of c-six RNA and activity similar to platelet-derived growth factor by transforming growth factor-beta: A proposed model for indirect mitogenesis involving autocrine activity. *Proc Natl Acad Sci USA* **83**:2453, 1986
102. Lawler X: Cell attachment to thrombospondin: The role or ARG-GLY-ASP, calcium and integrin receptors. *J Cell Biol* **107**:2351, 1988
103. Laurent TC, Fraser JR: Hyaluronan. *Faseb J* **6**:2397, 1992
104. Lark MW et al: Close and focal contact adhesions of fibroblasts to a fibronectin-containing matrix. *Fed Proc* **44**:394, 1985
105. Yang B et al: Identification of two hyaluronan-binding domains in the hyaluronan receptor RHAMM. *J Biol Chem* **268**:8617, 1993
106. Abercrombie X: Wound contraction in relation to collagen formation in scorbutic guinea pigs. *J Embryol Exp Morphol* **4**:167, 1956
107. Browse NL, Burnand KG: The cause of venous ulceration. *Lancet* **2**:243, 1982
108. Falanga V et al: Dermal pericapillary fibrin in venous disease and venous ulceration. *Arch Dermatol* **123**:620, 1987
109. Falanga V et al: Heterogeneity in oxygen diffusion around venous ulcers. *J Dermatol Surg Oncol* **17**:336, 1991
110. Coleridge Smith PD: The microcirculation in venous hypertension. *Vasc Med* **2**:203, 1997
111. Higley HR et al: Extravasation of macromolecules and possible trapping of transforming growth factor-beta in venous ulceration. *Br J Dermatol* **132**:79, 1995
112. Falanga V, Eaglstein WH: The "trap" hypothesis of venous ulceration. *Lancet* **341**:1006, 1993
113. Grinnell F et al: Degradation of fibronection and vitronectin in chronic wound fluid: analysis by cell blotting, immunoblotting, and cell adhesion assays. *J Invest Dermatol* **98**:410, 1992
114. Ladwig GP et al: Ratios of activated matrix metalloproteinase-9 to tissue inhibitor of matrix metalloproteinase-1 in wound fluids are inversely correlated with healing of pressure ulcers. *Wound Repair Regen* **10**:26, 2002
115. Wysocki AB, Grinnell F: Fibronectin profiles in normal and chronic wound fluid. *Lab Invest* **63**:825, 1990
116. Wysocki AB et al: Wound fluid from chronic leg ulcers contains elevated levels of metalloproteinases MMP-2 and MMP-9. *J Invest Dermatol* **101**:64, 1993
117. Stanley A, Osler T: Senescence and the healing rates of venous ulcers. *J Vasc Surg* **33**:1206, 2001
118. Stanley AC et al: Reduced growth of dermal fibroblasts from chronic venous ulcers can be stimulated with growth factors (see Discussion). *J Vasc Surg* **26**:994, 1997
119. Hasan A et al: Dermal fibroblasts from venous ulcers are unresponsive to the action of transforming growth factor-beta 1. *J Dermatol Sci* **16**:59,1997
120. Agren MS et al: Proliferation and mitogenic response to PDGF-BB of fibroblasts isolated from chronic venous leg ulcers is ulcer-age dependent. *J Invest Dermatol* **112**:463, 1999
121. Loots MA et al: Differences in cellular infiltrate and extracellular matrix of chronic diabetic and venous ulcers versus acute wounds. *J Invest Dermatol* **111**:850, 1998

SECTION 6

CELLULAR AND MOLECULAR BIOLOGY OF INFLAMMATION, REPAIR, AND CARCINOGENESIS

CHAPTER 22

Jenny Kim
Robert L. Modlin

Innate Immunity and the Skin

Throughout evolution, the immune system has developed complex and intricate mechanisms to defend the host against infection and cancer. The ability of the immune system to distinguish self from non-self is critical in determining when a response will be elicited. The immune system of higher vertebrates uses both rapid (innate) and sustained (adaptive) immune responses, which differ in the way they recognize foreign antigens, and the speed in which they respond (Fig. 22-1). The innate immune system uses germ-line–encoded pattern recognition receptors to respond to biochemical structures commonly shared by a number of different pathogens and elicits a rapid response against encountered pathogens, although no lasting immunity is generated. In contrast, cells of the adaptive immune system recognize molecules specific to particular pathogens, and clonally expand cells bearing antigen-specific receptors. A few of these cells become memory cells when the infection subsides, and thus have the capability of providing long lasting protective immunity. Together, the innate and adaptive immune systems defend the host against infections and disease, making survival possible. This chapter describes the distinct role of the innate immune responses in generating host defense mechanisms in skin.

INNATE IMMUNITY

While adaptive immunity occurs only in vertebrates, the innate immune system exists in all multicellular organisms. Defense mechanisms that are used by the host immediately after encountering a foreign ligand are referred to as innate immunity. These include physical barriers such as the skin and mucosal epithelium, soluble factors such as complement, antimicrobial peptides, chemokines, and cytokines, and cells of the innate immune system including monocytes/macrophages, dendritic cells, and polymorphonuclear leukocytes (PMNs) (Fig. 22-2).

Physical Barrier

Physical structures prevent most pathogens and environmental toxins from harming the host. The skin and the epithelial lining of the respiratory, gastrointestinal, and the genitourinary tract provide physical barriers between the host and the external world. Skin, once thought to be an inert structure, plays a vital role in protecting the individual from the external environment. The epidermis impedes penetration of microbial organisms, chemical irritation, and toxins, absorbs and blocks solar and ionized radiation, and inhibits water loss.

The stratum corneum, the outermost layer of the epidermis that results from the terminal differentiation of the keratinocytes, forms the primary layer of protection from the external environment. This layer of anucleated keratinocytes is composed of highly cross-linked

FIGURE 22-1

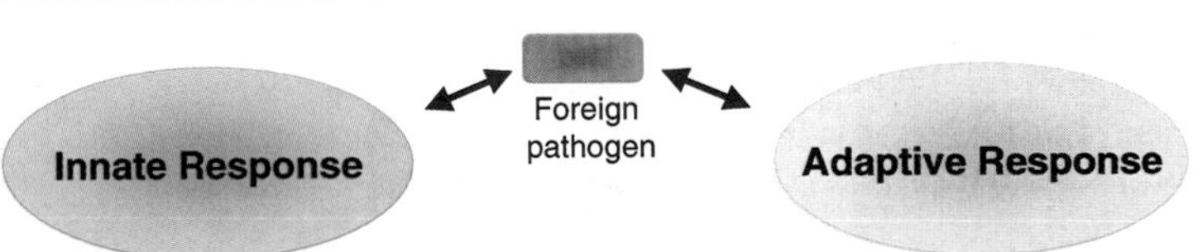

The immune system of higher vertebrates uses both innate and adaptive immune responses. These immune responses differ in the way they recognize foreign antigens, and the speed in which they respond; yet, they complement each other in eradicating foreign pathogens.

FIGURE 22-2

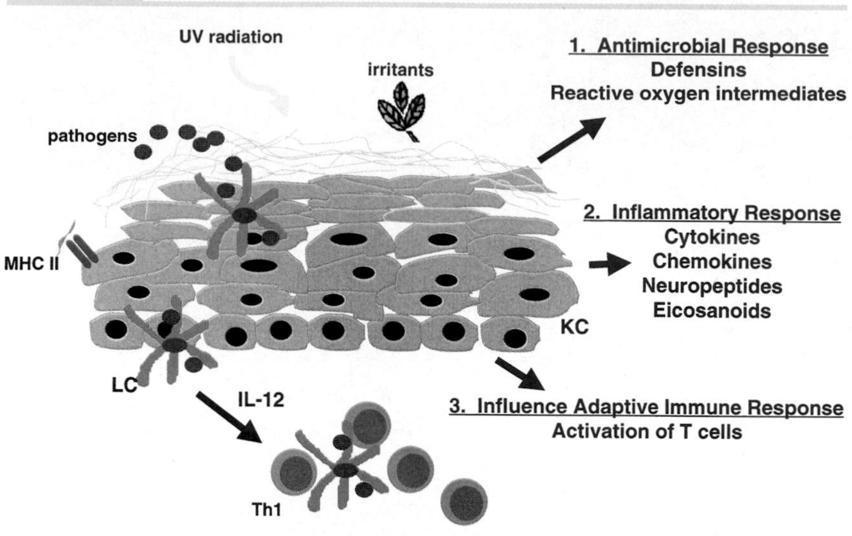

The innate immune response in skin. In response to exogenous factors such as foreign pathogens, UV radiation, and chemical irritants, innate immune cells mount multiple immune responses including (1) release of antimicrobial agents; (2) induction of inflammatory mediators, including cytokines, chemokines, neuropeptides, and eicosanoids; and (3) influencing the type of adaptive immune response. KC, keratinocytes; LC, Langerhans cells; MHC, major histocompatibility complex; SC, stratum corneum.

proteinaceous cellular envelopes with extracellular lipid lamellae consisting of ceramides, free fatty acids, and cholesterol[1] (see Chaps. 7 and 9). The free fatty acids create an acidic environment that inhibits colonization by certain bacteria such as *Staphylococcus aureus,*[2] providing further protection.

The oral mucosa, gastrointestinal, and respiratory linings have special features to protect the body from microbes and other foreign materials. In the mouth and in the upper gastrointestinal tract, chemical substances such as digestive enzymes and acidic secretions inhibit microbial growth. Furthermore, nonpathogenic microbes colonize the epithelium of the gut and prevent invasion by pathogenic microbes. The protective role of the normal flora becomes clear when the use of antibiotics destroys these nonpathogenic bacteria, opening up a window of opportunity for invasion by pathogenic bacteria. Finally, the upper respiratory tract is lined by ciliated columnar epithelium, and the movement of cilia protects inhaled foreign particles from entering the alveolar space. Given these vital functions, it is not surprising that a break in this physical barrier, as often occurs in patients with severe burn or large wounds, results in high morbidity and mortality.

COMPLEMENT COMPONENTS (See Chap. 33)

One of the first innate defense mechanisms awaiting pathogens that overcome the epithelial barrier is the alternative pathway of complement. Unlike the classical complement pathway that requires antibody triggering, the alternative pathway of complement activation can be activated by microbial surfaces in the absence of specific antibody. In this way, the host defense mechanism comes into play immediately after encountering the pathogen without the 5 to 7 days required for antibody production.

Initially, the complement component C3 undergoes spontaneous hydrolysis to give C3(H_2O), which binds to factor B, allowing it to be cleaved by factor D into Ba and Bb. The C3(H_2O)Bb complex, which is a C3 convertase, forms cleaving C3 to C3a and C3b. C3b can attach covalently through its reactive thioester group to the surfaces of host cells or to pathogens. The bound C3b is able to bind factor B, which is then cleaved by factor D to yield Ba and the active protease Bb. If C3bBb forms on the surface of the host cells, it is rapidly inactivated by complement regulatory proteins expressed on the host cell such as CR1 (complement receptor 1), DAF (decay-accelerating factor), factor H, and MCP (membrane cofactor of proteolysis). However, bacterial surfaces do not express complement regulatory proteins, and properidin (factor P) binds and stabilizes the C3bBb complex. C3bBb complex also is a C3 convertase and initiates the cleavage of further molecules of C3 leading to opsonization by C3b and the generation of $C3b_2Bb$, the alternative pathway C5 convertase, leading to activation of the terminal complement components.

Not all microbial surfaces allow for activation of the alternative complement pathway. Although the content of sialic acid (high levels are present on the surfaces of vertebrate cells) has been implicated as one of the factors that determine the ability to trigger the alternative complement pathway, it is not clear exactly what distinguishes surfaces that allow the complement cascade to proceed.

KERATINOCYTES

Once thought to be inert, keratinocytes, the predominant cells in the epidermis, can mount an immune response through secretion of antimicrobial peptides. Human epithelial cells produce β-defensins, cysteine-rich cationic low molecular weight antimicrobial peptides. Antimicrobial peptides are an important evolutionarily conserved innate host-defense mechanism in many organisms. The first human β-defensin, HBD-1, was isolated from human hemofiltrate obtained from a patient with end-stage renal disease.[3] HBD-1 is constitutively expressed in the epidermis, is not transcriptionally regulated by inflammatory agents,[4] and has antimicrobial activity against gram-negative bacteria.[5] In addition, recent findings suggest that HBD-1 plays a role in keratinocyte differentiation.[6] A second human β-defensin, HBD-2, was discovered in extracts of lesions from psoriasis patients.[7] Unlike HBD-1, HBD-2 expression is inducible by microbes including *Pseudomonas aeruginosa, S. aureus,* and *Candida albicans.*[7–9] In addition to stimulation by microbes, proinflammatory cytokines such as tumor necrosis factor (TNF)-α and interleukin (IL)-1 can also induce HBD-2 transcription in keratinocytes.[7–9] When tested for antimicrobial activity, HBD-2 also showed effective activity against gram-negative bacteria such as *Escherichia coli* and *P. aeruginosa,* but not against gram-positive bacteria such as *S. aureus.*[7] Recently, a third β-defensin, HBD-3, was isolated and characterized.[10] Contact with TNF-α and with bacteria were found to induce HBD-3 mRNA expression. In addition, HBD-3 demonstrated potent antimicrobial activity against *S. aureus* and vancomycin-resistant *Enterococcus faecium.* Therefore, HBD-3 is among the first human β-defensins in skin to demonstrate effective antimicrobial activity against a gram-positive bacteria. The localization of human β-defensins to the outer layer of the skin and the fact the β-defensins have antimicrobial activity against a variety of microbes suggest that human β-defensins are essential parts of cutaneous innate immunity.

Furthermore, evidence indicating that human β-defensins attract dendritic cells and memory T cells via the chemokine receptor CCR6,[11] provide a link between the innate and the adaptive immunity is skin.

Other innate antimicrobial peptides, called *cathelicidins,* have also been identified in skin.[12] Animal studies show that these cathelicidins are an important component of innate host defense in mice and protect against necrotic skin infections produced by group A streptococci. These peptides are produced in increasing amounts following skin wounding due to their release by neutrophils and increased synthesis by keratinocytes.[12,13]

Keratinocytes can also mount an immune response through the secretion of inflammatory cytokines. Keratinocytes constitutively release very low levels of cytokines; however, upon injury or stimulation with exogenous factors such as lipopolysaccharides (LPS), silica, poison ivy catechols, *Staphylococcus* toxins, and UV radiation, keratinocytes secrete high levels of IL-1, IL-6, IL-8, IL-10, and TNF-α (see Chap. 26). These cytokines can induce differentiation and growth of keratinocytes and other resident or migrating cells in the epidermis, dermis, and vessels. Furthermore, they are important mediators of both local and systemic inflammatory and immune responses.

In addition to cytokines, keratinocytes secrete other factors such as neuropeptides, eicosanoids, and reactive oxygen species. These mediators have potent inflammatory and immunomodulatory properties and play an important role in the pathogenesis of cutaneous inflammatory and infectious diseases as well as in aging.

PHAGOCYTES

Effective host defense against invading microorganisms requires detection of the foreign pathogens and the rapid deployment of an effective antimicrobial response. This function is imparted to the innate immune system that recognizes the molecular structures of microbial invaders. The microbes are rich with molecular arrays or patterns that are shared among groups of pathogens. Examples include LPS of gram-negative bacteria, lipoteichoic acids of gram-positive bacteria, lipoproteins of bacteria and parasites, glycolipids of mycobacteria, mannans of yeast, bacterial DNA sequences, and double-stranded RNA of viruses. Phagocytes, such as macrophages and PMNs, are the major cellular component of the innate immune system and have the capacity to detect these microbial patterns using complement receptors on their surface.

In the epidermis, there are skin-specific cells known as Langerhans cells. After encountering a pathogen in the epidermis, Langerhans cells take up the pathogen by an endocytotic process and migrate to the draining lymph nodes where they develop into mature dendritic cells. These migrating cells lose the ability to take up and process antigen but they upregulate MHC molecules and costimulatory molecules to activate naïve T cells.

Neutrophils are normally not present in skin; however, during inflammatory processes, these cells migrate to sites of infection and inflammation where they are the earliest phagocytic cells to be recruited. PMNs can phagocytose microbes coated with antibody and with the complement component C3b. In addition, PMNs have specific receptors that recognize pathogens directly.

Phagocytes express pattern recognition receptors that function to recognize pathogen-associated molecular patterns. Examples of pattern recognition receptors include the mannose receptor that recognizes mannan and CD14 that recognizes the lipid A portion of LPS. Pattern recognition receptors are nonclonal receptors that are present on all cells of a class, e.g., macrophages, and do not depend on immunologic memory because they are germ-line encoded. Recently, a new mammalian pattern recognition receptor, the Toll-like receptor, has been identified and important studies are emerging to provide new insights into the mechanisms by which the innate response recognizes and combats microbial invaders.

Pattern Recognition Receptors

How do phagocytes recognize foreign pathogens? One way that pathogens can be recognized and destroyed by the innate immune system is via receptors on phagocytic cells. Unlike adaptive immunity, the innate immune response relies on a relatively small set of germ-line–encoded receptors that recognize conserved molecular patterns found only on microorganisms. The phagocytic cells recognize pathogen-associated molecular patterns that are shared by a large group of pathogens. These pathogen-associated molecular patterns are usually conserved molecular structures required for survival of the microbes and therefore are not subject to selective pressure. In addition, pathogen-associated molecular patterns are specific to microbes and are not expressed in the host system. Consequently, the innate immune system has mastered a clever way of distinguishing between self and non-self and of relaying this message to the adaptive immune system.

Molecules that recognize pathogen-associated molecular patterns are known as pattern-recognition receptors. Pattern-recognition receptors can be divided into several families of proteins by their structure. For example, Toll and CD14 are pattern-recognition receptors that contain leucine-rich repeats, collectins have calcium-dependent lectin domains, and macrophage scavenger receptors contain scavenger-receptor protein domains. These pattern-recognition receptors can also be divided into three different classes by their function: secreted, endocytic, and signaling. Secreted pattern-recognition receptors function as opsonins by binding to microbial cell walls and flagging them for recognition by the classical complement system and phagocytes. The best-characterized receptor of this class is the mannan-binding lectin. The macrophage mannose receptor is an endocytic pattern recognition receptor that functions by recognizing carbohydrates with a large number of mannose residues that are characteristic of microorganisms, and mediating their phagocytosis by macrophages. Signaling receptors recognize pathogen-associated molecular patterns and activate signal transduction pathways that lead to the expression of a number of immune response genes, including cytokine genes. The recently identified family of Toll-like receptors is a pattern-recognition receptor family.

Toll

There is now substantial evidence to support a role for mammalian Toll-like receptors in innate immunity (Fig. 22-3). First, Toll-like receptors are pattern-recognition receptors that recognize pathogen-associated molecular patterns present on a variety of bacteria and fungi. Second, Toll-like receptors are expressed at the interface with the environment where the host must defend against microbial threats. Third, the activation of Toll-like receptors induces expression of costimulatory molecules and the release of cytokines that instruct the adaptive immune response. Fourth, Toll-like receptors directly activate host defense mechanisms that then combat the foreign invader.

Toll was first identified in dorsoventral patterning in the *Drosophila melanogaster* embryo and in antifungal defense in adult flies.[14,15] Since then, at least 10 mammalian Toll homologues, Toll-like receptors, have been identified. The extracellular domain has leucine-rich repeats and recognizes a spectrum of microbial products. Studies suggest that mammalian Toll homologues, Toll-like receptors, mediate responsiveness to specific molecular structures from both gram-positive and gram-negative organisms. For example, LPS activates Toll-like receptor 4; microbial lipoproteins, peptidoglycans, and *S. aureus* lipoteichoic

FIGURE 22-3

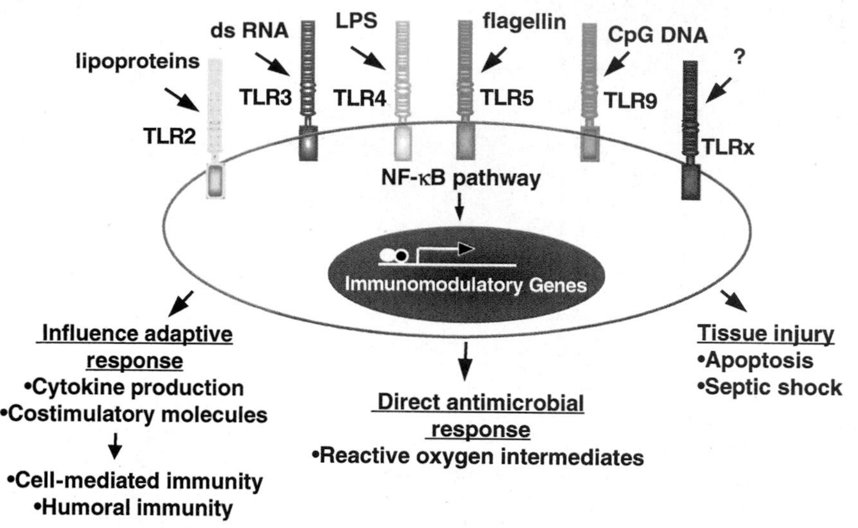

Toll-like receptors mediate innate immune response in host defense. Activation of Toll-like receptors by specific ligands induces (1) cytokine release and costimulatory molecules that instruct the type of adaptive immune response; (2) direct antimicrobial response; and (3) tissue injury.

acid activate Toll-like receptor 2[16–21]; a specific bacterial DNA, an unmethylated cytidine-phosphate-guanosine (CpG) activates Toll-like receptor 9[22]; bacterial flagellin activates Toll-like receptor 5[23]; and double-stranded RNA activates Toll-like receptor 3.[24]

The intracellular domain of Toll-like receptors has homology to the IL-1 receptor and shares common signaling molecules of the Rel/NF-κB pathway.[16,17] Considerable progress has been made toward understanding the cell-signaling events that occur after Toll-like receptor activation with emphasis on the activation of NF-κB, a transcription factor involved in the expression of many proinflammatory cytokines. The Toll-like receptor signaling pathway has been analyzed and found to share features in common with Toll signaling in *Drosophila*.[25,26] LPS activation via Toll-like receptors has been shown to induce an intracellular signaling cascade involving MyD88, IL-1 receptor accessory protein kinase (IRAK), TNF-receptor associated factor (TRAF-6), and NF-κB–inducing kinase (NIK) leading to activation of NF-κB and subsequent immunoregulatory gene transcription.[25–27] Further study of mammalian Toll-like receptor signaling pathways could identify different downstream events according to the nature of the microbial ligand and Toll-like receptor family member that has been activated.

Toll-like receptors were initially found to be expressed in all lymphoid tissue but were most highly expressed in peripheral blood leukocytes.[28] Expression of Toll-like receptor mRNA has been found in monocytes, B cells, T cells, granulocytes, and dendritic cells.[29,30] Protein expression of toll family members has been verified by using monoclonal antibodies for B cells, monocytes, and dendritic cells. Underhill et al. suggest that following phagocytosis, Toll-like receptors are recruited to the pathogen-containing phagosomes and discriminate between gram-positive and gram-negative bacteria,[31] thus surveying the intracellular compartments of the cells for microbial invaders. The expression of Toll-like receptors on cells of the monocyte/macrophage lineage is consistent with the role of Toll-like receptors in modulating inflammatory responses via cytokine release. Because these cells migrate into sites that interface with the environment, lung, skin, and gut, the location of Toll-like receptor expressing cells would be situated to defend against invading microbes. Toll-like receptor expression by adipocytes, intestinal epithelial cells, and dermal endothelial cells supports the notion that Toll-like receptors serve a sentinel role for invading microorganisms. The regulation of Toll-like receptor expression is critical to their role in host defense, yet few factors have been identified that modulate their expression. IL-4 acts to downregulate Toll-like receptor expression,[32] suggesting that T_H2 cell adaptive immune responses might inhibit Toll-like receptor activation.

LPS and lipoproteins have historically been known to be potent inducers of cytokine production. However, not until the identification of Toll-like receptors was a receptor linked to this response. Medzhitov et al. first demonstrated that constitutive activation of Toll-like receptor 4, using a dominant active construct transfected in a human monocytoid line, induced cytokine production and upregulation of costimulatory molecules.[33] Since then, critical proinflammatory and immunomodulatory cytokines, such as IL-1, IL-6, IL-8, IL-10, IL-12, and TNF-α, have been shown to be induced following activation of Toll-like receptors by microbial ligands.[18,28,33,34] Evidence suggests that monocyte-derived dendritic cells produce the proinflammatory IL-12, and not the anti-inflammatory IL-10, upon activation with lipoproteins. Activation of Toll-like receptors on dendritic cells triggers their maturation, in terms of expression of CD83, MHC class II, as well as the costimulatory molecules CD80 and CD86. In this manner, the activation of dendritic cells via Toll-like receptors enhances their ability to present antigen to T cells and generate T_H1 cytokine responses critical for cell-mediated immunity (CMI). Consequently, activation of Toll-like receptors, as part of the innate response, can lead to instruct the nature of the adaptive T cell response.

In *Drosophila, Toll* is critical for host defense. Flies with a mutation in *Toll* are highly susceptible to fungal infection. It is now evident that mammalian Toll-like receptors play a prominent role in directly activating host defense mechanisms. Activation of Toll-like receptor 2 by microbial lipoproteins induces activation of the inducible nitric oxide (iNOS) promoter, which leads to the production of nitric oxide (NO), a known antimicrobial agent. There is strong evidence that Toll-like receptor 2 activation leads to killing of intracellular *Mycobacterium tuberculosis* in both mouse and human macrophages.[35] In mouse macrophages, bacterial lipoprotein activation of Toll-like receptor 2 leads to a nitric oxide–dependent killing of intracellular tubercle bacilli. In human monocytes and alveolar macrophages, bacterial lipoproteins similarly activated Toll-like receptor 2 to kill intracellular *M. tuberculosis;* however, this occurred by an antimicrobial pathway that is nitric oxide independent. These data provide evidence that mammalian Toll-like receptors have retained not only the structural features of *Drosophila* Toll that allow them to respond to microbial ligands, but also the ability directly to activate antimicrobial effector pathways at the site of infection. In *Drosophila,* activation of Toll leads to the NF-κB–dependent induction of a variety of antimicrobial peptides, including metchnikowan, defensins, cecropins, and drosomycin.[14,36,37] The clues from *Drosophila* suggest that exploring the mechanisms of induction of antimicrobial peptides in mammalian cells is warranted. In this regard, it was recently shown that LPS induces β-defensin-2 in tracheobronchial epithelium,[38] suggesting the conservation of the *Drosophila* Toll pathway of antimicrobial peptide induction.

The activation of Toll-like receptors can also be detrimental, leading to tissue injury. The administration of lipopolysaccharides to mice can result in manifestations of septic shock, which is dependent on Toll-like receptor 4.[39] Evidence suggests that Toll-like receptor

2 activation by *Propionibacterium acnes* induces inflammatory responses in acne vulgaris leading to tissue injury (J. Kim and R.L. Modlin, unpublished). Aliprantis et al. demonstrated that microbial lipoproteins induced features of apoptosis via Toll-like receptor 2.[19] Thus, microbial lipoproteins have the ability to induce both Toll-like receptor–dependent activation of host defense and tissue pathology. This dual signaling pathway is similar to TNFR and CD40 signaling, which can induce both NF-κB activation and apoptosis.[40] In this manner, it is possible for the immune system to activate host defense mechanisms, and then, by apoptosis, to downregulate the response to prevent it from causing tissue injury. Activation of Toll-like receptors can lead to the inhibition of MHC class II antigen presentation pathway, which can downregulate immune responses leading to tissue injury but could also contribute to immunosuppression.[41]

The susceptibility of mice with spontaneous mutations in Toll-like receptors to bacterial infection implicates Toll-like receptors as critical receptors in mammalian host defense.[42–44] Toll-like receptor 4 mutations are associated with lipopolysaccharide hyporesponsiveness in humans.[45] By inference, we anticipate that humans with genetic alterations in other Toll-like receptors may have increased susceptibility to certain microbial infections. Furthermore, it should be possible to exploit the pathway of Toll-like receptor activation as a means to adjuvant immune responses in vaccines and treatments for infectious diseases, as well as to abrogate responses detrimental to the host.

Effector Functions of Phagocytes

Activation of phagocytes by pathogens induces several important effector mechanisms. One such mechanism is the triggering of cytokine production. A number of important cytokines are secreted by macrophages in response to microbes, including IL-1, IL-6, TNF-α, IL-8, IL-12, and IL-10. IL-1, IL-6, and TNF-α play critical roles in inducing the acute-phase response in the liver and in inducing fever for effective host defense. TNF-α induces a potent inflammatory response to contain infection; IL-8 is important as a mediator of PMN chemotaxis to the site of infection.

One of the most important cytokines produced by monocytes is IL-12 (see Chap. 26). Both in murine models of infection and in human infectious disease, susceptibility or resistance to infection is often determined by the T_H1 and T_H2 T cell cytokine patterns. It has become increasingly evident that IL-12 is a pivotal regulator of T_H1 responses and hence is essential for promoting CMI against intracellular microbial pathogens. In this manner, the ability of the innate immune system to release IL-12 influences the nature of the adaptive immune response.

Phagocytes also secrete an inhibitory cytokine, IL-10, that has many anti-inflammatory activities. The importance of IL-10 is underscored in both human disease and murine infection models. IL-4 and IL-10 production is associated with the progressive forms of leishmanial, schistosomal, and trypanosomal infections. In leprosy, IL-10 expression in lesions correlates with susceptibility to infection.[46] Thus, IL-10 appears to inhibit aspects of CMI required for the effective elimination of intracellular pathogens.

There is strong evidence that dysregulation of IL-10 is associated with human allergic diseases. In addition, a number of studies have reported the production of IL-10 in association with malignant cell types including carcinomas of skin, breast, colon, kidney, bladder, ovary, and lung. The production of IL-10 by tumors has been implicated as one of the mechanisms that neoplastic cells use to evade the local immune response.[47]

Another important defense mechanism triggered in phagocytes in response to pathogens is the induction of a direct antimicrobial responses. Phagocytic cells such as PMNs and macrophages recognize pathogens, engulf them, and induce antimicrobial effector mechanisms to kill the pathogens. PMNs generate oxygen-dependent or oxygen-independent killing. The release of toxic oxygen radicals, lysosomal enzymes, and antimicrobial peptides such as the human neutrophil defensins, leads to direct killing of the microbial organisms.[48,49] Similarly, activation of Toll-like receptors on macrophages by microbial ligands upregulates iNOS, which results in rapid generation of NO and powerful microbicidal activity. Macrophages use this mechanism to contain some infectious organisms not susceptible to PMN attack, such as mycobacteria, certain fungi, and parasites. In addition, stimulation of monocytes by activated T cells also leads to the generation of NO.

Finally, Langerhans cells, monocytes, and macrophages present antigens to T and B lymphocytes, the adaptive immune cells. Upon pathogen recognition, monocytes are able to discriminate self from non-self molecules and foreign antigens are presented to lymphocytes for initiation of adaptive immune response. This important function of antigen presenting cells is discussed in detail in Chap. 23.

CD40

Phagocytic cells of the innate immune system can also be activated by cells of the adaptive immune system. CD40 is a 50-kDa glycoprotein present on the surface of B cells, monocytes, dendritic cells, and endothelial cells, and its ligand is CD40L. CD40–CD40L interactions play a crucial role in the development of effector functions. CD40–CD40L interactions between T cells and macrophages play a role in maintenance of T_H1 type cellular responses and mediation of inflammatory responses. Other studies have established a role for CD40–CD40L interactions in B cell activation, differentiation, and in Ig class switching.[51] In addition, CD40–CD40L interaction leads to upregulation of B7.1 and B7.2 on B cells. This costimulatory activity induced on B cells then acts to amplify the response of the T cells.[52] These mechanisms underscore the importance of the interplay between the innate and the adaptive immune system in generating an effective host response.

Thus, the innate immune response is a critical first line of defense. It is rapid, allowing for early detection of microbial pathogens and control of infection. Using germ-line–encoded receptors, the innate immune system distinguishes pathogens from self-antigens and activates appropriate effector mechanisms. Furthermore, the innate immune response controls the initiation of the adaptive immune response by regulating costimulatory molecules and releasing effector cytokines. In contrast, the adaptive immune response is delayed in onset, is characterized by highly specific receptors that are distributed clonally on subsets of particular cells, and involves immunologic memory. Not only do the innate and adaptive immune response complement each other, they are interactive in that the innate immune response influences the type of adaptive response and the adaptive immune response influences the function of innate cells.

REFERENCES

1. Elias PM et al: Lipid-related barriers and gradients in the epidermis. *Ann N Y Acad Sci* **548**:4, 1988
2. Fluhr JW et al: Generation of free fatty acids from phospholipids regulates stratum corneum acidification and integrity. *J Invest Dermatol* **117**:44, 2001
3. Bensch KW et al: hBD-1: A novel beta-defensin from human plasma. *FEBS Lett* **368**:331, 1995
4. Valore EV et al: Human beta-defensin-1: An antimicrobial peptide of urogenital tissues. *J Clin Invest* **101**:1633, 1998
5. Goldman MJ et al: Human beta-defensin-1 is a salt-sensitive antibiotic in lung that is inactivated in cystic fibrosis. *Cell* **88**:553, 1997
6. Frye M et al: Expression of human beta-defensin-1 promotes differentiation of keratinocytes. *J Mol Med* **79**:275, 2001
7. Harder J et al: A peptide antibiotic from human skin. *Nature* **387**:861, 1997

8. Singh PK et al: Production of beta-defensins by human airway epithelia. *Proc Natl Acad Sci U S A* **95**:14961, 1998
9. Harder J et al: Mucoid *Pseudomonas aeruginosa,* TNF-alpha, and IL-1beta, but not IL-6, induce human beta-defensin-2 in respiratory epithelia. *Am J Respir Cell Mol Biol* **22**:714, 2000
10. Harder J et al: Isolation and characterization of human beta-defensin-3, a novel human inducible peptide antibiotic. *J Biol Chem* **276**:5707, 2001
11. Yang D et al: Beta-defensins: Linking innate and adaptive immunity through dendritic and T cell CCR6. *Science* **286**:525, 1999
12. Nizet B et al: Innate antimicrobial peptide protects the skin from invasive bacterial infection. *Nature* **22**:414, 2001
13. Dorschner RA et al: Cutaneous injury induces the release of cathelicidin antimicrobial peptides active against group A Streptococcus. *J Invest Dermatol* **117**:91, 2001
14. Lemaitre B et al: The dorsoventral regulatory gene cassette spatzle/Toll/cactus controls the potent antifungal response in Drosophila adults. *Cell* **86**:973, 1996
15. Hashimoto C et al: The Toll gene of Drosophila, required for dorsal-ventral embryonic polarity, appears to encode a transmembrane protein. *Cell* **52**:269, 1988
16. Gay NJ et al: Drosophila Toll and IL-1 receptor. *Nature* **351**:355, 1991
17. Belvin MP et al: A conserved signaling pathway: The Drosophila toll-dorsal pathway. *Annu Rev Cell Dev Biol* **12**:393, 1996
18. Takeuchi O et al: Differential roles of TLR2 and TLR4 in recognition of gram-negative and gram-positive bacterial cell wall components. *Immunity* **11**:443, 1999
19. Aliprantis AO et al: Cell activation and apoptosis by bacterial lipoproteins through Toll-like receptor-2. *Science* **285**:736, 1999
20. Means TK et al: Human Toll-Like receptors mediate cellular activation by *Mycobacterium tuberculosis*. *J Immunol* **163**:3920, 1999
21. Yoshimura A et al: Recognition of gram-positive bacterial cell wall components by the innate immune system occurs via Toll-like receptor 2. *J Immunol* **163**:1, 1999
22. Hemmi H et al: A Toll-like receptor that recognizes bacterial DNA. *Nature* **408**:740, 2000
23. Hayashi F et al: The innate immune response to bacterial flagellin is mediated by Toll-like receptor 5. *Nature* **410**:1099, 2001
24. Alexopoulou L et al: Recognition of double-stranded RNA and activation of NF-kappaB by Toll-like receptor 3. *Nature* **413**:732, 2001
25. Muzio M et al: The human toll signaling pathway: Divergence of nuclear factor and JNK/SAPK activation upstream of tumor necrosis factor receptor-associated factor 6 (TRAF6). *J Exp Med* **187**:2097, 1998
26. Yang RB et al: Signaling events induced by lipopolysaccharide-activated toll-like receptor 2. *J Immunol* **163**:639, 1999
27. Kawai T et al: Unresponsiveness of MyD88-deficient mice to endotoxin. *Immunity* **11**:115, 1999
28. Yang RB et al: Toll-like receptor-2 mediates lipopolysaccharide-induced cellular signalling. *Nature* **395**:284, 1998
29. Akashi S et al: Cutting edge: Cell surface expression and lipopolysaccharide signaling via the toll-like receptor 4-MD-2 complex on mouse peritoneal macrophages. *J Immunol* **164**:3471, 2000
30. Muzio M et al: Differential expression and regulation of toll-like receptors (TLR) in human leukocytes: selective expression of TLR3 in dendritic cells. *J Immunol* **164**:5998, 2000
31. Underhill DM et al: The Toll-like receptor 2 is recruited to macrophage phagosomes and discriminates between pathogens. *Nature* **401**:811, 1999
32. Staege H et al: Human toll-like receptors 2 and 4 are targets for deactivation of mononuclear phagocytes by interleukin-4. *Immunol Lett* **71**:1, 2000
33. Medzhitov R et al: A human homologue of the Drosophila Toll protein signals activation of adaptive immunity. *Nature* **388**:394, 1997
34. Toura I et al: Cutting edge: Inhibition of experimental tumor metastasis by dendritic cells pulsed with alpha-galactosylceramide. *J Immunol* **163**:2387, 1999
35. Thoma-Uszynski S et al: Induction of direct antimicrobial activity through mammalian toll-like receptors. *Science* **291**:1544, 2001
36. Lemaitre B et al: Drosophila host defense: Differential induction of antimicrobial peptide genes after infection by various classes of microorganisms. *Proc Natl Acad Sci U S A* **94**:14614, 1997
37. Hoffmann JA et al: Phylogenetic perspectives in innate immunity. *Science* **284**:1313, 1999
38. Becker MN et al: CD14-dependent LPS-induced beta-defensin-2 expression in human tracheobronchial epithelium. *J Biol Chem* **275**:29731, 2000
39. Poltorak A et al: Defective LPS signaling in C3H/HeJ and C57BL/10ScCr mice: Mutations in Tlr4 gene. *Science* **282**:2085, 1998
40. Aliprantis AO et al: The apoptotic signaling pathway activated by Toll-like receptor-2. *EMBO J* **19**:3325, 2000
41. Noss EH et al: Toll-like receptor 2-dependent inhibition of macrophage class II MHC expression and antigen processing by 19-kDa lipoprotein of *Mycobacterium tuberculosis*. *J Immunol* **167**:910, 2001
42. O'Brien AD et al: Genetic control of susceptibility to *Salmonella typhimurium* in mice: Role of the LPS gene. *J Immunol* **124**:20, 1980
43. Cross A et al: The importance of a lipopolysaccharide-initiated, cytokine-mediated host defense mechanism in mice against extraintestinally invasive *Escherichia coli*. *J Clin Invest* **96**:676, 1995
44. Medina E et al: Resistance ranking of some common inbred mouse strains to *Mycobacterium tuberculosis* and relationship to major histocompatibility complex haplotype and Nramp1 genotype. *Immunology* **93**:270, 1998
45. Arbour NC et al: TLR4 mutations are associated with endotoxin hyporesponsiveness in humans. *Nat Genet* **25**:187, 2000
46. Yamamura M et al: Defining protective responses to pathogens: Cytokine profiles in leprosy lesions. *Science* **254**:277, 1991
47. Kim J et al: IL-10 production in cutaneous basal and squamous cell carcinomas. A mechanism for evading the local T cell immune response. *J Immunol* **155**:2240, 1995
48. Leffell MS et al: Intracellular and extracellular degranulation of human polymorphonuclear azurophil and specific granules induced by immune complexes. *Infect Immun* **10**:1241, 1974
49. Ganz T et al: Defensins. Natural peptide antibiotics of human neutrophils. *J Clin Invest* **76**:1427, 1985
50. Tian L et al: Activated T cells enhance nitric oxide production by murine splenic macrophages through gp39 and LFA-1. *Eur J Immunol* **25**:306, 1995
51. Hollenbaugh D et al: The role of CD40 and its ligand in the regulation of the immune response. *Immunol Rev* **138**:23, 1994
52. Grewal IS et al: Requirement for CD40 ligand in costimulation induction, T cell activation, and experimental allergic encephalomyelitis. *Science* **273**:1864, 1996

CHAPTER 23

Georg Stingl
Dieter Maurer
Conrad Hauser
Klaus Wolff

The Skin: An Immunologic Barrier

Microbial attack poses a major, potentially lethal threat to all higher organisms. Anatomically, the first barrier to microbiologic invasion is the skin, particularly the epidermis. Today we know that the capacity of the skin to protect the integrity of the host not only is based on its physical and structural properties, but also includes an immunologic component of both the innate (e.g., rapid production and release of proinflammatory cytokines and antimicrobial peptides by epidermal cells exposed to microbial pathogens) and the adaptive type. A robust innate reaction is also the major trigger of an adaptive response initiated by dendritic antigen-presenting cells in the epidermis [Langerhans cells (LCs)] and dermis [dermal dendritic cells (DDCs)]. When appropriately stimulated and loaded with antigenic peptides, these cells can leave the skin and migrate to regional lymphoid tissues where they induce lymphocyte activation and expansion at a clonal level.

In the recent past, we began to understand that the immunosurveillance function of the skin is finely tuned and tailored to the needs of the host. Inasmuch as it guarantees the rapid recognition of and response to microbial danger signals, it also prevents the occurrence of such a reaction toward harmless and innocuous substances.

This chapter describes the contributions of the cell populations of skin to the immunologic barrier function of this organ and points to some of the factors that injure and/or restore its function.

ANTIGEN-PRESENTING CELLS: LANGERHANS CELLS AND DERMAL DENDRITIC CELLS

Definition

In 1868, the medical student Paul Langerhans, driven by his interest in the anatomy of skin nerves, identified a population of dendritically shaped cells in the suprabasal regions of the epidermis after impregnating human skin with gold salts.[1] These cells, which later were found in virtually all stratified squamous epithelia of mammals, are now eponymously referred to as *Langerhans cells.* There also exist substantial numbers of dendritic leukocytes in the dermis. Although some of them represent LCs on their way into or out of the epidermis, most of these cells are phenotypically slightly different from LCs and are generally referred to as *dermal dendritic cells*.[2] LCs and DDCs are lineage-negative (Lin–), bone marrow-derived leukocytes endowed with exquisite antigen-presenting properties. Thus, they phenotypically and functionally resemble other dendritic cells (DCs) present in most, if not all, lymphoid and nonlymphoid tissues.[3] As the gatekeepers of the immune system, they control the response to events perturbing tissue homeostasis.

Morphology

LCs/DDCs cannot be readily recognized in routinely fixed and stained paraffin-embedded sections of mammalian skin. Apart from identifying LCs on the basis of their unique ultrastructural markers, that is, the Birbeck granules (see below), LCs/DDCs can be selectively visualized at the light microscopic level with certain histochemical and, more importantly, immunolabeling procedures.

HISTOCHEMICAL METHODS The demonstration of a membrane-bound, formalin-resistant, sulfhydryl-dependent adenosine triphosphatase (ATPase) is an excellent method for the identification of LCs in humans and rodents.[4] Intraepidermal ATPase+ cells are found mainly at a suprabasal position (Fig. 23-1). Their pronounced dendritic shape, as well as their distribution and density, can be even better appreciated by an *en face* view of whole epidermal mounts that have been subjected to this staining procedure (Fig. 23-2).

IMMUNOLABELING PROCEDURES Extensive antibody screening of LCs has led to the identification and characterization of many surface and/or cytoplasmic antigenic determinants on these cells (Table 23-1). Although all these moieties may be important for the functional repertoire of LCs, the only ones that can be used for the identification of intraepidermal LCs are those that are displayed by essentially all LCs, but which are not expressed by other cells in the epidermis.

In human epidermis, markers fulfilling these criteria include (1) CD1a antigens, that is, major histocompatibility antigen (MHC) class I-related restriction elements also found on cortical thymocytes; (2) MHC class II-encoded human leukocyte antigen (HLA)-DR/DQ/DP antigens;

FIGURE 23 1

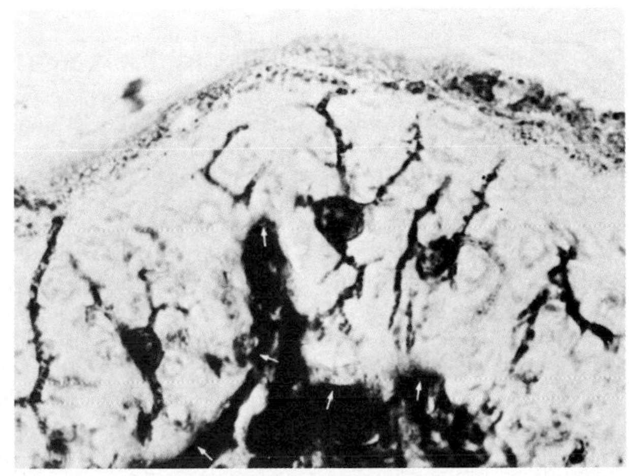

Suprabasal dendritic Langerhans cells in human epidermis as revealed by the ATPase technique. Arrows denote the dermal–epidermal junction. *(From Wolff K: Die Langerhans-Zelle. Ergebnisse neuerer experimenteller Untersuchungen. Arch Klin Exp Dermatol 229:54, 1967, with permission.)*

FIGURE 23-2

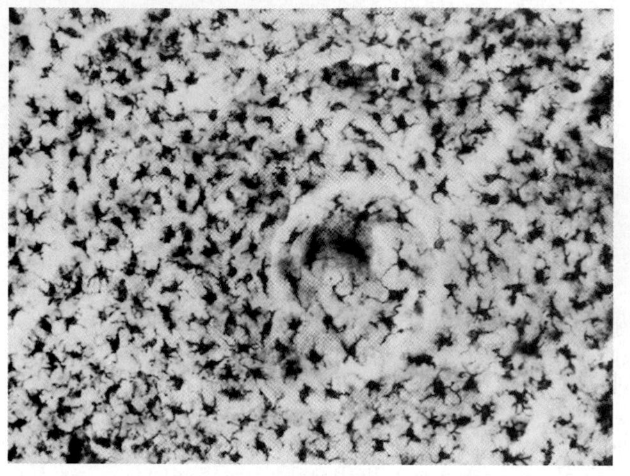

Histochemical (ATPase technique) demonstration of the Langerhans cell population in a sheet preparation of guinea pig epidermis. *(From Wolff K et al: Proceedings of the 13th International Congress of Dermatology, Munich, 1967, vol 2. Berlin, Springer, 1968, p 1502, with permission.)*

(3) a Birbeck granule-associated antigen defined by the monoclonal antibodies (MAb) Lag and DCGM4; and (4) CD39, recently identified as LC ATPase.[5]

Among these markers, the authors consider anti-CD1a immunolabeling the most reliable approach for identifying intraepidermal human LCs. Because of its high expression density on both the surface and in the cytoplasm, even one-step immunolabeling procedures usually suffice for reliable LC labeling. Equally important is that, in the epidermis, CD1a is selectively present on LCs not only in normal skin, but, with few exceptions, also in perturbed/inflamed skin. The situation is quite different for HLA-DR antigens, which, while confined to LCs in normal epidermis, are also expressed by keratinocytes in many inflammatory skin diseases. This makes it often difficult, if not impossible, to recognize HLA-DR–bearing LCs in perturbed skin.

Bone marrow-derived DDCs are somewhat heterogeneous, and the various subtypes cannot always be easily distinguished and differentiated from each other. In addition to LCs migrating in or out of the epidermis, there exists the distinctive population of DDCs that reportedly express MHC class I and II molecules, CD45, CD1c and to a lesser extent CD1a, CD11c, CD40, CD54, CD80, the myeloid markers CD33 and CD36, and subunit A of the clotting proenzyme factor XIII (factor XIIIa). As opposed to classical macrophages, they express only low to negligible amounts of CD14.

ELECTRON MICROSCOPY (Fig. 23-3) In 1961, Birbeck et al.[6] established the criteria that allow the recognition and identification of LCs at any location. These criteria include a clear cytoplasm devoid of tonofilaments, desmosomes, or melanosomes; a lobulated, frequently convoluted nucleus; and the presence of a distinctive, pentilaminar cytoplasmic organelle, termed a *Langerhans cell granule* or *Birbeck granule*. This granule usually appears as a rod-shaped organelle of variable length and position; but, occasionally, the limiting membrane may expand on one of the rod's ends, thus giving the granule a tennis racket-shaped appearance. From the variable images obtained in different planes of section, it can be assumed that the Birbeck granule is usually a flat, platelike, occasionally twisted or cup-shaped structure with a vesicular bleb protruding from one of its ends (reviewed in Ref. 4).

The derivation and function of Birbeck granules have long been a matter of debate. Most investigators now favor the "endocytosis theory," which claims that these organelles originate from the cell membrane and subserve intracellular transport functions. Support for this hypothesis came from studies with the LC-specific MAb DCGM4, which stains both the cell surface and the cytoplasm. By immunoprecipitation, DCGM4 identifies a 40-kDa molecule, termed *Langerin*. It is a type II Ca^{2+}-dependent lectin displaying mannose-binding specificity. While sparing MHC class II+ cytoplasmic compartments, Langerin colocalizes with Birbeck granules. When incubated with freshly isolated LCs, the anti-Langerin MAb is internalized into Birbeck granules. Together with the demonstration of Birbeck granule formation after transfection of Langerin cDNA into fibroblasts, this finding indicates that Langerin is an antigen-capturing molecule that channels the antigen into Birbeck granules and, perhaps, provides access to a nonclassical, non-MHC class II-dependent antigen-processing pathway.[7]

Ultrastructurally, DDCs exhibit a folded nucleus and a highly ruffled, irregular surface. Their cytoplasm is relatively dark and contains the organelles needed for an active cellular metabolism, but it is devoid of Birbeck granules.[2]

Tissue Distribution

Apart from their occasional occurrence at extraepithelial sites (dermis, dermal lymphatics, aortic wall, lymph nodes, thymus), LCs, as defined by the presence of Birbeck granules, are essentially confined to stratified squamous epithelia of mammals.[4] Certain intraepidermal ATPase+ DCs contain very few, or even no Birbeck granules, but are otherwise indistinguishable from classic LCs. Some of these "indeterminate" cells probably represent "activated" LCs (see below), prepared to begin their journey from the epidermis to the regional lymph node.

In the epidermis, the density of the LC population varies regionally. In the mouse, LC densities differ considerably according to strain, sex, age, and body region. LCs are sparse in the tail epidermis because of the structural patterning of this particular region. They are virtually absent from parakeratotic scale regions but are present in orthokeratotic interscale zones. Such observations have prompted speculations about the involvement of LCs in the control of epidermal cell proliferation. The paucity or, even, absence of LCs in the mouse tail, as well as in other areas such as the central cornea, and hamster cheek pouch may contribute to the impaired ability of a contactant to induce sensitization when applied to these sites (see below).

There also exist regional differences in the number of LCs per unit area of human skin. On head, face, neck, trunk, and limb skin, the LC density ranges between 600 and $1000/mm^2$. Comparatively low densities ($\sim 200/mm^2$) are encountered in palms, soles, anogenital and sacrococcygeal skin, as well as the buccal mucosa. The density of human LCs decreases with age, and LC counts in skin with chronic actinic damage are significantly lower than those in skin not exposed to ultraviolet (UV) light.

DDCs are located primarily in the vicinity of the superficial vascular plexus.

Life Cycle (Fig. 23-4)

Although it has been known for a long time that LCs originate from precursors in the bone marrow,[8] individual steps of LC ontogeny were elucidated only recently.

A major breakthrough in the understanding of LC development came from the observation that the exposure of CD34+ hematopoietic progenitor cells (HPCs) to granulocyte-macrophage colony-stimulating factor (GM-CSF) and tumor necrosis factor-α (TNF-α) gives rise to a progeny of CD1a+, E-cadherin+, Birbeck granule-containing cells with immunostimulatory properties strikingly resembling those of LCs isolated from human skin.[9] Subsequent studies have delineated the phenotype of LC progenitors at their various states of

TABLE 23-1

Phenotype of Resident vs. Cytokine-Activated Human Epidermal Langerhans Cells

Property	Resident LC	Cytokine-activated LC	Property	Resident LC	Cytokine-activated LC
Morphology			**Costimulatory molecules/**		
Birbeck granules	+++	+/−	**activation markers**		
Cytoplasmic veils	+	+++	CD24	−	++
Enzyme profiles			CD40	+/−	+
Adenosine triphosphatase/	+++	+/−	CD50 (ICAM-3)	++	++
CD39			CD54 (ICAM-1)	+/−	++
Antigenic profiles			CD58 (LFA-3)	+	++
MHC class I	+	++	CD69	+	−
MHC class II	++	+++	CD80 (B7-1)	−	+
CD1a	+++	+	CD83	−	+
CD1b	−	−	CD86 (B7-2)	+/−	++
CD1c	+	−	CD98	++	+
CD3-TCR	−	−	CD101	?	+
CD4	+	?	B7-H1, B7-H2, B7-H3	?	?
CD8	−	+/−	Dectin-1, Dectin-2	++	?
CD14	−	−	**Cytokine receptors/receptors**		
CD15	−	−	**for chemotactic factors**		
CD19	−	−	GM-CSFRα (CD116)	+	++
CD20	−	−	GM-CSFRβ (CD131)	+/−	++
CD45	++	++	M-CSFR (CD115)	−	−
CD45RA	−	−	TNF-RII (75kD) (CD120b)	+	+/−
CD45RB	−	+	IL-1RI (CD121a)	+	+/−
CD45RO	+	−	IL-1RII (CD121b)	+	++
FcαR (CD89)	−	−	IL-2Rα (CD25)	−	++
FcγRI (CD64)	−	−	IL-2Rβ (CD122)	−	+
FcγRII (CD32)	+	−	IFN-γR (CDw119)	+	+
FcγRIII (CD16)	−	−	CCR1	−	−
FcϵRI	+	−	CCR2	−/+	−
Antigen uptake receptors			CCR3	−	−
DEC-205 (CD205)	+	++	CCR5	−	−
Macrophage mannose	−	−	CCR6	++	−
receptor (CD206)			CCR7	−/+	++
Langerin (CD207)	++	+/−	CXCR1	−	−
DC-Lamp (CD208)	+/−	++	CXCR3	−	−
DC-Sign (CD209)	−	−	CXCR4/Fusin	+/−	+/−
Adhesion molecules			CXCR5	−	−
β_1 integrins	+ or ++	? ($\alpha4\uparrow$, $\alpha6\downarrow$)	C5aR (CD88)	+/−	+
β_2 integrins	+ or +/−	?/++ (CD11c)			
CD44					
pan	+	++			
v7/v8	+	−			
v4 v6, v9	+/−	++			
E-cadherin	++	+/−			
CLA	+	+ or ++			

maturation/differentiation. It is now clear that, already at the CD34+ precursor stage, cells exist that are committed to the LC lineage. A useful marker for the identification of these cells is the cutaneous lymphocyte-associated antigen (CLA), which is detectable on both skin-homing T cells and on LCs in situ. CLA is abundantly expressed by LC precursors rather than by cells giving rise to non-LC DCs. It remains to be determined whether this E- and P-selectin ligand can mediate skin homing of LCs/LC progenitors.

A great deal about the developmental steps of LCs and DDCs was learned from studies by Caux et al.[10] demonstrating the emergence of two distinctive subsets of LC/DC precursor cells in GM-CSF– and TNF-α–supplemented liquid cultures of CD34+ HPCs. Precursor cells in the CD1a+/CD14– subset, when isolated and further cultured in GM-CSF– and TNF-α–supplemented medium for 12 to 14 days, develop into cells displaying all the features of LCs including the expression of E-cadherin and Birbeck granules.[10] Evidence exists that a cell type with phenotypic features indistinguishable from those of in vitro generated CD1a+/CD14– LC precursors exists in the peripheral blood. It starts to express E-cadherin and Langerin and to display Birbeck granules within 1 day of culture in the presence of GM-CSF, interleukin (IL)-4, and transforming growth factor (TGF)-β1.

The second DC precursor subset appearing in GM-CSF– and TNF-α–stimulated HPC cultures displays the CD1a–/CD14+ phenotype.[10] The lineage commitment of these cells is much less restricted than that of the CD1a+ precursors. While they give rise to a monocyte/macrophage progeny when exposed to macrophage colony-stimulating factor (M-CSF), they develop into cells with a DDC phenotype in the presence of GM-CSF and TNF-α as evidenced by their expression of CD1a, CD11b, CD11c, CD36, CD68, and factor XIIIa and by their lack of E-cadherin and Birbeck granules.

With regard to the factors promoting the development of DCs and LCs/DDCs in particular, stem cell factor (SCF) and Flt3 ligand (FL)

FIGURE 23-3

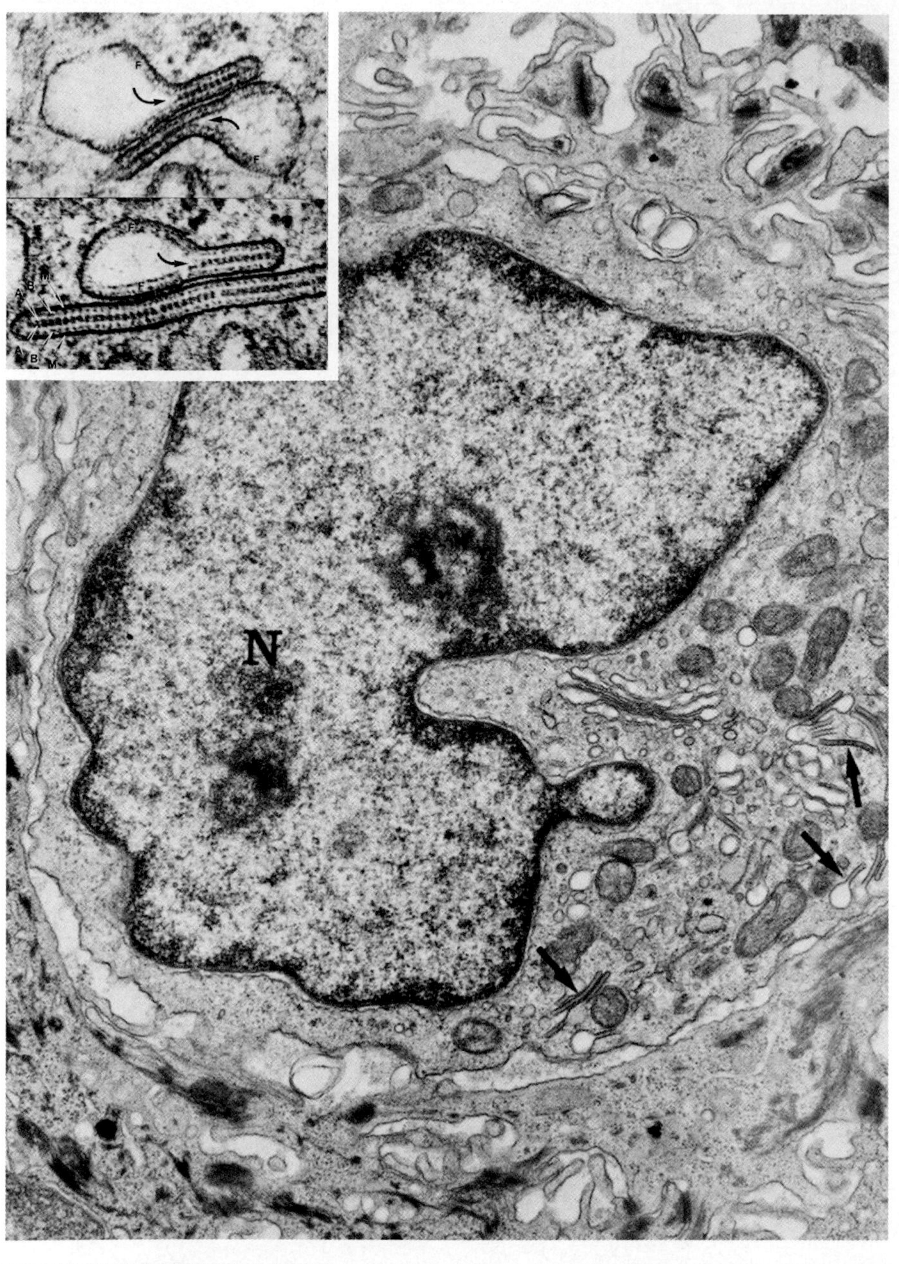

Electron micrograph of a Langerhans cell in human epidermis. Arrows denote Birbeck granules. N, nucleus. (*From Stingl G: New aspects of Langerhans cell functions. Int J Dermatol 19:189, 1980, with permission.*) Inset: High-power electron micrograph of Birbeck granules. The curved arrows indicate the zipper-like fusion of the fuzzy coats (*F*) of the vesicular portion of the granule. The delimiting membrane (*M*) envelops two sheets of particles (*B*) attached to it and a central lamella composed of two linear arrays of particles (*A*). (*From Wolff K: The fine structure of the Langerhans cell granule. J Cell Biol 35:466, 1967, with permission.*)

do apparently amplify the DC differentiation pathway initiated by GM-CSF and TNF-α, but without any selectivity for LCs/DDCs.

The factor most critically needed for the development of LCs/DDCs is TGF-β1. This is evidenced by the lack of LCs in TGF-β1–/– mice, and by the absolute requirement of TGF-β1 for the generation of LCs in GM-CSF– and TNF-α–supplemented serum-free stem cell cultures.[11] In vitro data show that paracrine stimulation with TGF-β1 of CD14+/CD11c+/CD11b– and CD14+/CD11c+/CD11b+ cells developing in GM-CSF– and TNF-α–stimulated HPC cultures results in bona fide LCs and DDCs, respectively.[12] Cells with an identical phenotype exist within normal human dermis, and the generation of true LCs from CD14+/CD11c+ dermal cells was recently demonstrated.[13] There also exist reports on the transformation of peripheral blood monocytes into LCs or DCs with LC features by TGF-β1 and IL-15, respectively. It remains to be seen under which conditions such events would occur in vivo.

The mechanisms responsible for the rather selective homing of LCs/DDCs or their precursors to the skin and of LCs/LC precursors to the epidermis are still not completely understood. Recent evidence points to an important role of macrophage inflammatory protein 3α (MIP-3α)/CCL20 in the recruitment of LCs to the epidermis: (1) on day 6 of GM-CSF– and TNF-α–supplemented HPC cultures, CD1a+ LC precursors express only one CC chemokine receptor, CCR6, in a prominent fashion and migrate to its ligand MIP-3α/CCL20 in a selective manner[14]; and (2) CD14+ LC precursors as well as LCs in situ express CCR6.[13,14] IL-10, and probably also TGF-β1, are mainly responsible for CCR6 induction and upregulation on LCs/LC precursors, whereas IL-4 and interferon (IFN)-γ suppress this event.

However, CCR6 is also expressed on certain non-LC DCs in Peyer's patches, and its ligand MIP-3α/CCL20 is expressed in epithelia other than the epidermis. Thus, the actual significance of this chemokine/chemokine receptor combination in LC recruitment to the epidermis has yet to be resolved. Another chemokine possibly involved in this process is the cutaneous T cell-attracting chemokine (CTACK).[15] It is constitutively produced by keratinocytes, and its ligand, CCR10, is expressed by endothelial cells, fibroblasts, melanocytes, T cells, and LCs, but not by other DCs.[16] The role, if any, of CCR10 and other cytokines in the regulation of LC influx in the epidermis (e.g., TNF-α, IL-6, IL-12) is still unclear.

Within the epidermis, LCs are anchored to surrounding keratinocytes by E-cadherin–mediated homotypic adhesion.[17] This event and the display of TGF-β1 also prevent terminal differentiation and migration (see below), thus securing intraepidermal residence for the cells under homeostatic conditions.

HLA-DR+/ATPase+ DCs can be identified in the human epidermis by 6 to 7 weeks of estimated gestational age. These cells must originate from hemopoietic stem cells in the yolk sac or fetal liver, the primary sites of hemopoiesis during the embryonic period. Until the twelfth week of pregnancy, these cells are CD1a– and lack Birbeck granules. Thereafter, there occurs a dramatic increase in LC CD1a expression, an event that coincides with the initiation of bone marrow function.

The fact that epidermal LCs originate from bone marrow precursors does not mean that every LC that either leaves or is removed from the

FIGURE 23-4

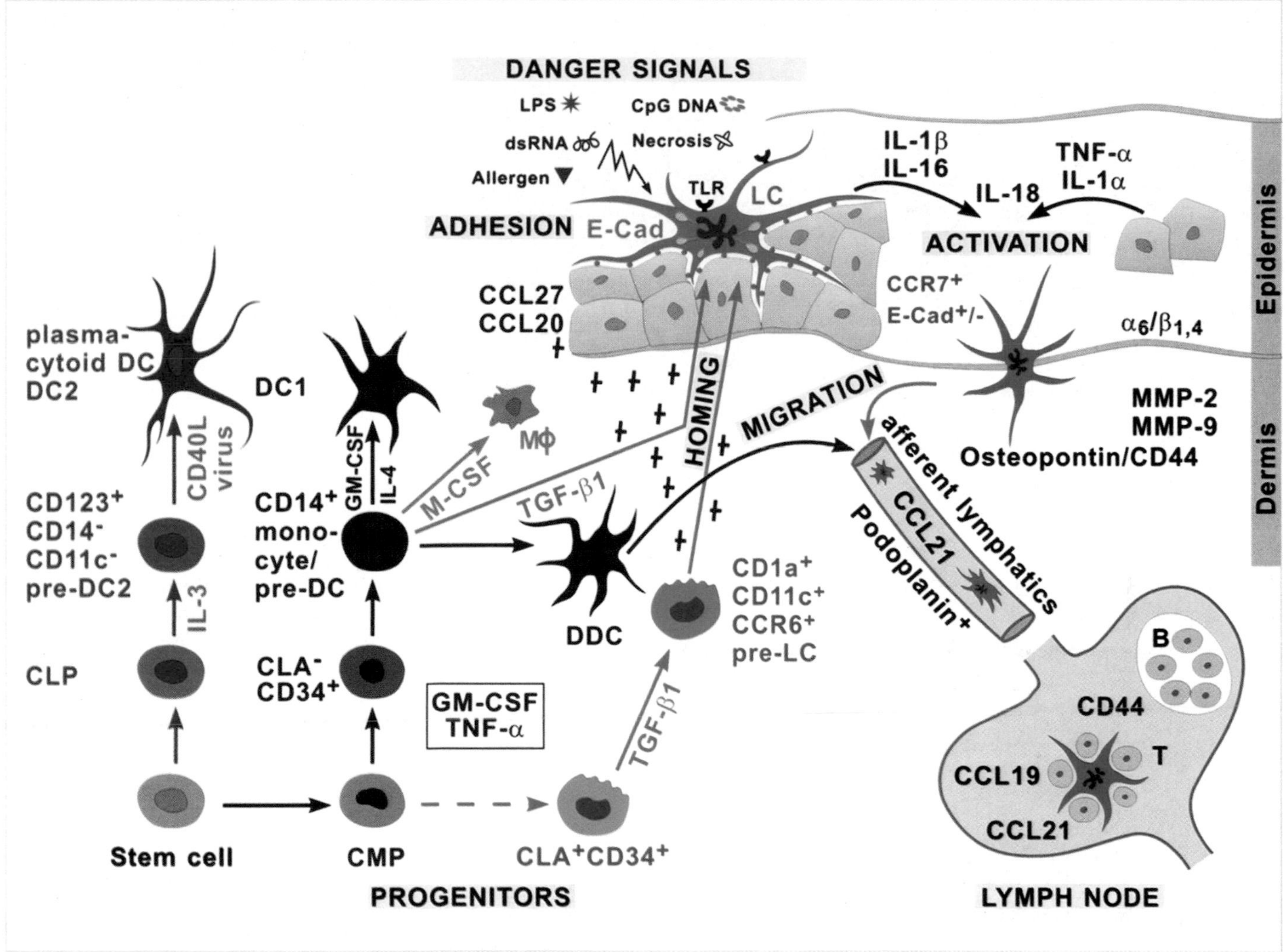

Schematic of ontogeny, migration, and maturation pathways of cutaneous dendritic leukocytes. $\alpha_6/\beta_{1,4}$ integrins; B, B cells; CCL, CC chemokines; CCR, CC chemokine receptor; CD, cluster of differentiation-nomenclature of leukocyte antigens; CLA, cutaneous lymphocyte-associated antigen; CLP, common lymphoid progenitor cell; CMP, common myeloid progenitor cell; CpG DNA, immunostimulatory cytosine- and guanine-rich sequences of deoxyribonucleic acid; DC, dendritic cell; DDC, dermal dendritic cell; dsRNA, double-stranded ribonucleic acid; E-Cad, E-cadherin; GM-CSF, granulocyte/macrophage colony-stimulating factor; IL, interleukin; LC, Langerhans cell; LPS, lipopolysaccharide; Mϕ, macrophage; M-CSF, macrophage colony-stimulating factor; MMP, matrix metalloproteinase; T, T cells; TGF-β1, transforming growth factor beta 1; TLR, toll-like receptor; TNF-α, tumor necrosis factor alpha.

epidermis is replenished by a precursor cell newly immigrating into the skin. Cell division probably also contributes to the maintenance of epidermal LC numbers as evidenced by the demonstration of cycling/mitotic events in these cells,[4] as well as by the finding that the LC population of human skin grafted onto a nude mouse remains rather constant for the life of the graft, despite epidermal proliferation and the absence of circulating cells. The partial depletion of LCs from these grafts by UV radiation, topical glucocorticoids, or tape stripping is followed by their restoration, within a few weeks, to pretreatment levels, and by a substantial increase in dividing LCs.

Finally, there remains the question about the ultimate fate of the epidermal LC population. Major perturbation of the cutaneous microenvironment (danger signal[18]) leads to their activation, resulting either in their elimination via the stratum corneum[4] or, more importantly, in their migration to lymphoid tissues where they initiate type 1 (T_H1/T_c1)-dominated T cell responses (see below). By contrast, what happens in normal skin is unclear. Does LC shedding occur under physiologic (nondanger) conditions? Is there a natural flux of LCs/DDCs to the regional lymph nodes? If so, what are the functional consequences of such an occurrence? Evidence exists that melanin granules captured in the skin accumulate in the regional lymph nodes but not in other tissues. The further observation of only very few melanin granule-containing cells in TGF-β1 –/– mice suggests that, under steady-state conditions, epidermal and/or dermal antigens are carried to the regional lymph nodes by TGF-β1–dependent cells (most likely LCs/DDCs) only. Evidence now exists that T lymphocytes encountering such antigen-presenting cells (APCs) in vivo are rendered unresponsive in an antigen-specific manner.[19] It may therefore be assumed that absence of pathogenic T cell autoimmunity and/or lack of reactivity against innocuous environmental compounds (e.g., aeroallergens) in the periphery is primarily the consequence of an active immune response rather than the result of its nonoccurrence.

FIGURE 23-5

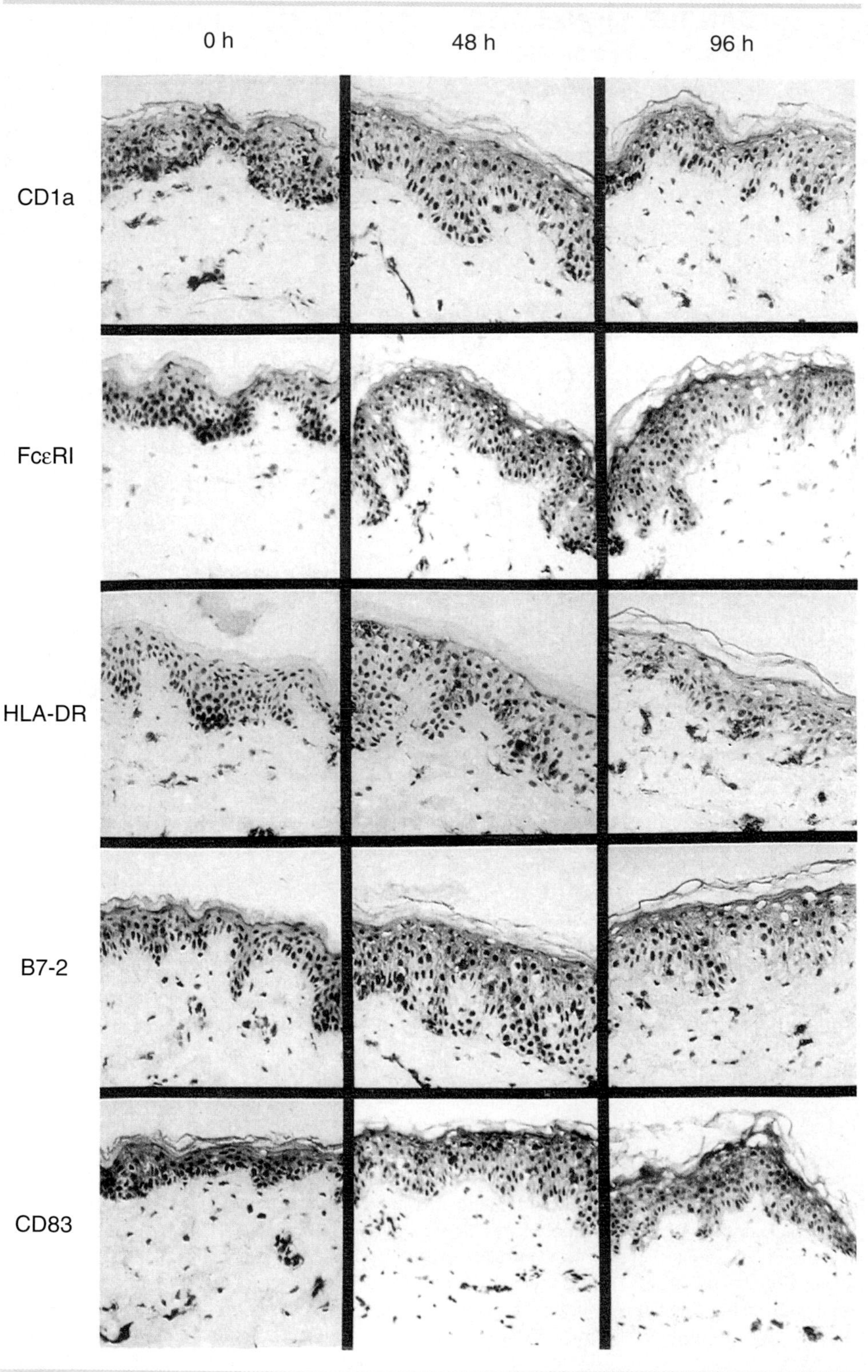

Phenotypic changes and emigration of epidermal Langerhans cells (LCs) after perturbation of the cutaneous microenvironment. Cryostat sections of freshly excised or ex vivo cultured (48 h, 96 h) human split-thickness skin were reacted with antibodies against CD1a, FcεRI, HLA-DR, B7-2, or CD83 and then processed for peroxidase immunolabeling. Before culture, LCs are CD1a+, FcεRI+, CD83– and reside mainly at a suprabasal position within the epidermis. In skin organ culture, LCs progressively lose surface-bound CD1a and FcεRI; upregulate HLA-DR, B7-2, and CD83; and move downward.

Upon receipt of danger signals (e.g., chemical haptens, hypoxia), the situation is quite different. After a few hours, LCs begin to enlarge, to display increased amounts of surface-bound MHC class II molecules, and to migrate downward in the dermis where they enter afferent lymphatics and, finally, reach the T cell zones of draining lymph nodes. During this process, LCs undergo phenotypic changes similar to those that occur in single epidermal cell cultures[20]; that is, downregulation of molecules/structures responsible for antigen uptake and processing as well as for LC attachment to keratinocytes (e.g., Fc receptors, Birbeck granules, E-cadherin) and upregulation of moieties required for active migration and stimulation of robust responses of naive T cells (e.g., CD40, CD80, CD83, CD86) (Table 23-1; Fig. 23-5).

The mechanisms governing LC migration are becoming increasingly clear. TNF-α and IL-1β (in a caspase 1-dependent fashion) are critical promoters of this process, whereas IL-10 inhibits its occurrence. Increased cutaneous production and/or release of the proinflammatory cytokines is probably one of the mechanisms by which certain immunostimulatory compounds applied on or injected in the skin [e.g., imiquimod, unmethylated cytosine-guanosine (CpG) oligonucleotides] accelerate LC/DDC migration. IL-16 induces LC mobilization. This event could perhaps be operative in atopic dermatitis. In this disease, DCs of lesional skin exhibit surface IgE bound to high affinity Fc receptors (FcεRI), and allergen-mediated receptor cross-linking results in enhanced IL-16 production.

An important hurdle for emigrating LCs is the basement membrane. During their downward journey, LCs probably attach to it via α_6-containing integrin receptors and produce proteolytic enzymes such as type IV collagenase (matrix metalloproteinase 9) to penetrate it and to pave their way through the dense dermal network into the lymphatic system. Evidence is accumulating that LC/DDC migration occurs in an active, directed fashion. Osteopontin is a chemotactic protein that is essential in this regard. It initiates LC emigration from the epidermis and attracts LCs/DDCs to draining nodes by interacting with an N-terminal epitope of the CD44 molecule.[21] The entry into and active transport of cutaneous DCs within lymphatic vessels appears to be mediated by macrophage chemotactic proteins (MCPs) binding to CCR2 and by the secondary lymphoid-organ chemokine (SLC)/CCL21 produced by lymphatic endothelial cells of the dermis and binding to CCR7 on maturing LCs.[22]

Besides its presence on mature DCs, CCR7 is expressed by naive T cells and by a small subset of circulating, lymph node-seeking "central memory" T lymphocytes. These expression patterns suggest that the interaction between CCR7 and its ligands SLC/CCL21 and Epstein-Barr virus (EBV)-induced molecule 1 ligand chemokine (ELC)/CCL19 are of central importance in bringing together mature DCs and naive T cells in the T cell zones of the lymph nodes.

The question of where and how the life cycle of an LC ends has not yet been completely resolved, but some evidence exists that DCs, upon cognate interaction with T cells, physically disappear from the lymph nodes.[23] This is largely due to an apoptotic process triggered by ligation of CD40 on mature LCs and is effected by the interaction of CD95/Fas-bearing mature LCs and CD95L/FasL-expressing activated T cells. The biologic significance of this finding is underscored by studies in humans and experimental animals deficient in this or other death receptor/death receptor ligand pairs.[24] Their capacity for clearing antigen-bearing LCs in lymph nodes is significantly delayed. As a consequence, ongoing T cell responses are not sufficiently downregulated or terminated, and signs of autoimmunity may develop.

Functional Properties

Compelling evidence exists that LCs and other skin DCs, as members of the family of "professional" APCs, play a pivotal role in the induction of adaptive immune responses against pathogens and cancer cell-associated neoantigens introduced into and/or generated in the skin (immunosurveillance). The immunogenic potential of DCs is regulated by surface receptors triggered by ligands secreted or presented by other somatic cells or, alternatively, by microbial products (danger or competence signals). Many of the receptor structures that sense such signals are "rented" from the innate immune system where they are used to recognize molecular patterns demarcating infectious nonself, as well as normal and abnormal self (pattern recognition receptors). Thus, and according to Janeway and Medzhitov's theory, innate immunity controls the development and nature of adaptive immunity.[25] Some evidence also exists that DCs that have not received such competence signals are not stimulatory, but actively downregulate or prevent potentially harmful immune responses by tolerizing T cells or by inducing T cells with suppressive properties (regulatory T cells). For a better understanding of the functional properties of skin DCs, the basic principles of antigen uptake, processing, and presentation are briefly reviewed.

GENERAL PRINCIPLES OF ANTIGEN PRESENTATION (Fig. 23-6) Unlike B cells, T cells cannot recognize soluble protein antigen per se; their antigen receptor T cell receptor (TCR) is designed to see antigen-derived peptides bound to MHC locus-encoded molecules expressed by APCs.[26] For the antigen-specific activation of T helper (T_H) cells, exogenous antigen-derived peptides are usually presented in the context of MHC class II molecules.[27] In this situation, peptides are generated in the endocytic, endo-/lysosomal pathway and are bound to MHC class II; the resulting MHC–peptide complex is expressed at the APC surface for encounter by the TCR of CD4+ T_H cells. In contrast, most CD8+ T cells, destined to become cytotoxic T cells, recognize the endogenous antigen in association with MHC class I molecules.[27] Because most nucleated cells transcribe and express MHC class I genes/gene products, it is evident that many cell types can serve as APCs for MHC class I-restricted antigen presentation and/or as targets for MHC class I-dependent attack by T cells. In the MHC class II-dependent antigen-presentation pathway, DCs, including LCs and DDCs (see below), B cells, and monocytes/macrophages are the major APC populations.

MHC CLASS I-RESTRICTED ANTIGEN PRESENTATION[28]

The classic MHC class I presentation pathway Immediately after their biosynthesis, MHC class I heavy and light (β_2-microglobulin) chains are inserted into the membranes of the endoplasmic reticulum. The third subunit of the functional MHC class I complex is the peptide itself. The major sources of peptides for MHC class I loading are cytosolic proteins, which can be targeted for their rapid destruction through the catalytic attachment of ubiquitin. Cytosolic proteinaceous material undergoes enzymatic digestion by the proteasome to yield short peptide chains of 8 to 12 amino acids, an appropriate length for MHC class I binding. In its basic conformation, the proteasome is a constitutively active "factory" for self-peptides. IFN-γ, by replacing or adding certain proteasomal subunits, induces "immunoproteasomes," presumably to fine-tune the degradation activity and specificity to the demands of the immune response. The processed peptides are translocated to the endoplasmic reticulum by the transporter associated with antigen processing (TAP), an MHC-encoded dimeric peptide transporter. With the aid of chaperons (calnexin, calreticulin, tapasin), MHC class I molecules are loaded with peptides, released from the endoplasmic reticulum, and transported to the cell surface. Several infectious antigens with relevance to skin biology have adopted strategies to subvert MHC class I presentation and, thus, the surveillance of cell integrity by interfering with defined molecular targets. Important examples for such an interference are the inhibition of proteasomal function by the Epstein-Barr virus-encoded EBNA-1 protein, the competition for peptide-TAP interactions by a herpes simplex virus protein, and the retention/destruction of MHC class I molecules by adenovirus- and human cytomegalovirus-encoded products.

Alternative MHC class I presentation pathways (cross-presentation) Under certain conditions, exogenous antigen can reach the MHC class I presentation pathway. Significant evidence for this cross-presentation first came from in vivo experiments in mice demonstrating that viral, tumor, and MHC antigens can be transferred from MHC-mismatched donor cells to host bone marrow-derived APCs to elicit antigen-specific cytotoxic T cell responses that are restricted to self MHC molecules.[29] In vitro studies have now defined that exosomes (i.e., small secretory vesicles of about 100 nm in diameter secreted by various cell types including tumor cells), heat shock proteins (hsp), immune complexes, and apoptotic cells (taken up via CD36 and $\alpha v\beta 3$ or $\alpha v\beta 5$ integrins) can all serve as vehicles for the delivery of antigen to DCs in a manner that permits the cross-presentation of antigen. In all in vitro systems in which a direct comparison has been made, DCs, but not monocytes/macrophages, were capable of cross-presentation. Three distinct pathways are currently exploited by which antigen can access MHC class I molecules of DCs: (1) a recycling pathway for MHC class I in which antigen is loaded in the endosome; (2) a pathway by which retrograde transport of the antigen from the endosome to the endoplasmic reticulum facilitates entry into the classic MHC class I antigen presentation pathway; and (3) an endosome to the cytosol transport pathway, again allowing antigen processing via the classic MHC class I antigen presentation pathway.

MHC CLASS II-RESTRICTED ANTIGEN PRESENTATION[30] MHC class II molecules predominantly bind peptides within endo-/lysosomal compartments. Sampling peptides in these subcellular organelles allows class II molecules to associate with a broad array of peptides derived from proteins targeted for degradation after internalization by fluid phase or receptor-mediated endocytosis, macropinocytosis, or phagocytosis. One of the striking structural differences between MHC class I and class II molecules is the conformation of their peptide-binding grooves. Whereas MHC class I molecules have binding pockets to accommodate the charged termini of peptides and, thus, selectively associate with short peptides, the binding sites of MHC class II molecules are open at both ends. Thus, MHC class II molecules bind peptides with preferred lengths of 15 to 22 amino acids but can also associate with longer moieties.

FIGURE 23-6

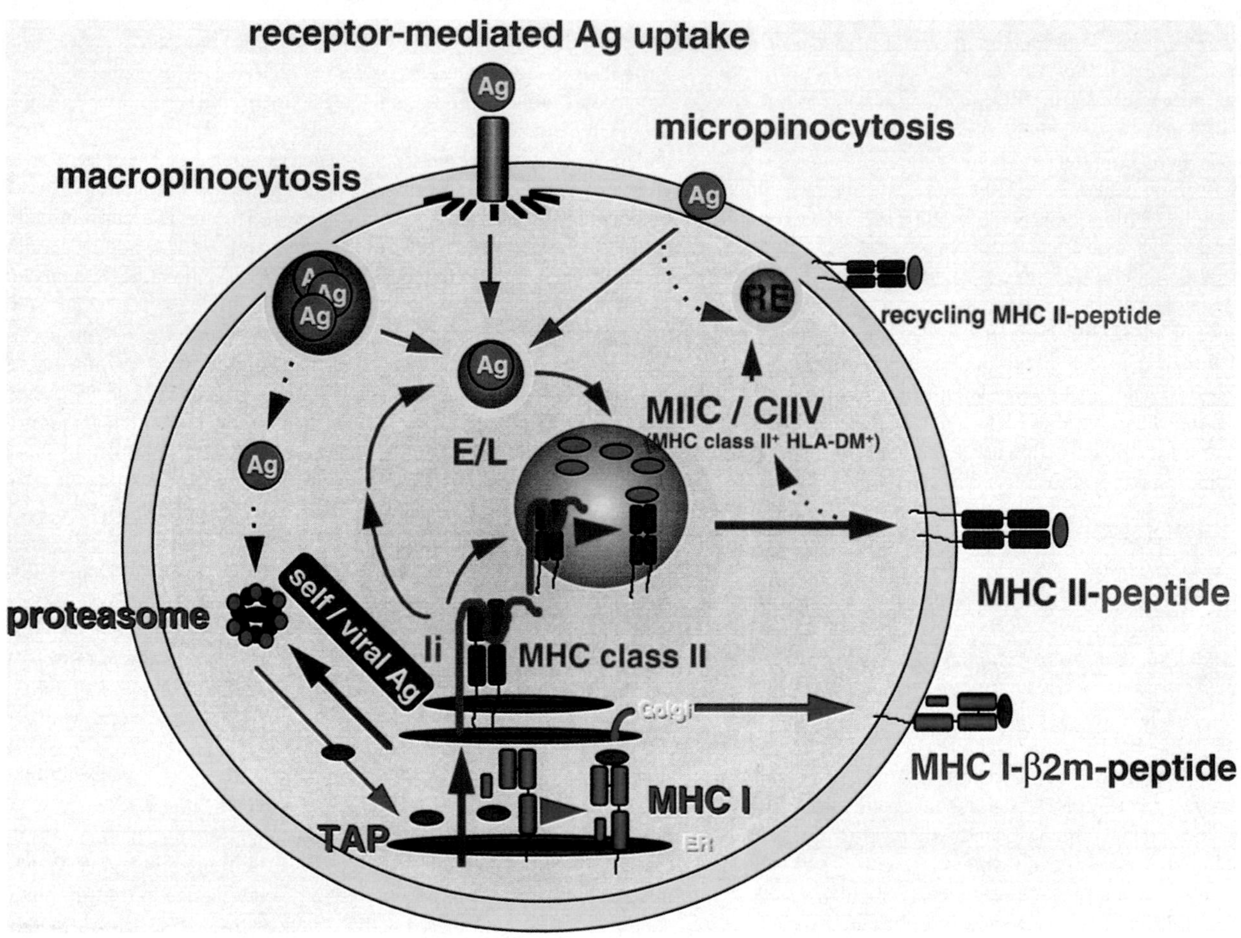

Schematic of MHC class I- and MHC class II-dependent antigen-presentation pathways. *MHC class II presentation (red):* Exogenous antigens (Ag) taken up via fluid phase micro- or macropinocytosis or via receptor-mediated endocytosis enter the endo-/lysosomal (E/L) pathway of protein degradation. Resulting peptides reach subcellular organelles rich in MHC class II and HLA-DM/H2M antigens [MHC class II compartments (MIIC); class II-containing vesicles (CIIV)]. Newly synthesized MHC class II antigens arrive in these compartments because of their physical association with the invariant chain (Ii), which then undergoes proteolysis by the action of cellular enzymes leaving only a small fragment of Ii [class II-associated invariant peptide (CLIP)] in the place of the MHC class II peptide binding groove. Upon removal of CLIP by HLA-DM/H2M, the newly synthesized MHC class II moieties can bind the exogenous Ag-derived peptides generated in the endo-/lysosomal system. As also outlined in this figure, cell surface-bound MHC class II can be internalized into recycling endosomes (*RE*) and, within these compartments, acquire certain peptides derived from exogenous Ag.

MHC class I presentation pathway (green): In the classic form, the proteasome degrades cytosolic Ag synthesized by the cell itself (e.g., self and viral Ag). The resulting peptides are then imported into the endoplasmic reticulum (*ER*) in a TAP-dependent manner, loaded onto MHC class I molecules and, finally, transported to the cell surface in the form of a peptide-MHC class I $\beta 2$ microglobulin ($\beta 2$m) complex en route of the Golgi complex. At least in certain APCs, not only endogenous but also exogenous Ag-derived peptides can get access to the MHC class I presentation pathway (see text). This MHC class I peptide loading can occur either in a TAP-dependent (e.g., following a macropinosome to cytosol transfer of exogenous Ag) or in a TAP-independent fashion (e.g., targeting of MHC class I molecules into MIIC/CIIV followed by their loading with peptides generated in endolysosomes).

Newly synthesized MHC class IIα and β subunits assemble in a stoichiometric complex with trimers of the type II transmembrane glycoprotein invariant chain (Ii). The association with Ii contributes in at least three different ways to the function of class II molecules: (1) Ii assembly promotes the proper folding of class II molecules in the endoplasmic reticulum; (2) the abluminal portion of Ii contains signal sequences that facilitate the export of MHC class II–Ii complexes through the Golgi system to endo-/lysosomes; and (3) Ii prevents class II molecules from premature loading by peptides intended for binding to MHC class I molecules in the endoplasmic reticulum. The segment of Ii functioning as a competitor for peptide binding to class II is termed class II-associated Ii peptide (CLIP; residues 81 to 104 of Ii). Once the nascent MHC class IIα/β–Ii trimers arrive in the endo-/lysosomal system, Ii is subject to proteolysis by acid hydrolases. The last proteolytic step, the generation of CLIP, is catalyzed by cathepsin S in DCs, by cathepsin L in thymic epithelial cells, and by cathepsin F in macrophages. Upon HLA-DM–chaperoned exchange of CLIP for exogenous antigen-derived peptide, fully assembled class II molecules are exported to the cell surface and acquire a stable conformation. Depending on the cell type and the activation status of a cell, the half-life of class II-peptide complexes varies from a few hours to days. It is particularly long (more than 100 h) on DCs that have matured into potent immunostimulatory cells of lymphoid organs upon encounter with an inflammatory stimulus in nonlymphoid tissues. The very long retention of peptide-class II complexes on mature DCs ensures that only those peptides generated at sites of inflammation will be displayed in lymphoid organs for T cell priming.

CD1-DEPENDENT ANTIGEN PRESENTATION[31] Recently, it became clear that, besides peptides, self glycosphingolipids and bacterial lipoglycans may act as T cell stimulatory ligands. Molecules that bind and present these moieties belong to the family of nonpolymorphic, MHC class I- and II-related CD1 proteins. In the skin, members of the CD1 family are expressed mainly by LCs and DDCs (see above). The CD1 isoforms, CD1a, b, c, and d, sample both recycling endosomes of the early endocytic system and late endosomes and lysosomes to which lipid antigens are delivered. In contrast to the MHC class II pathway, antigen loading in the CD1 pathway occurs in a vacuolar acidification-independent fashion. T cells expressing a Vα24-containing canonic TCR, natural killer (NK) T cells, and CD4–/CD8– T cells, include the most prominent subsets of CD1-restricted T cells. CD1-restricted T cells play important roles in host defense against microbial infections. Accordingly, human subjects infected with *M. tuberculosis* showed elevated responses to CD1c-mediated presentation of a microbial lipid antigen, when compared to control subjects, and activation of CD1d-restricted NK T cells with a synthetic glycolipid antigen resulted in improved immune responses to several infectious pathogens. Thus, the CD1 pathway of antigen presentation and glycolipid-specific T cells may provide protection during bacterial and parasite infection, probably by the secretion of proinflammatory cytokines, the direct killing of infected target cells, and B cell help for immunoglobulin production.

DENDRITIC CELLS IN THE CONTEXT OF SKIN IMMUNITY

Induction of protective immunity via the skin Both in vitro and in vivo studies imply that the major function of LCs and of other skin DCs is to provide the sensitizing signal for the occurrence of skin-induced immune responses against a wide variety of antigens, including alloantigens, tumor antigens, microorganisms, and contact allergens. This is best illustrated by the early observations (1) that the epidermal LC density positively correlates with the outcome of the immune response to the contact sensitizers dinitrofluorobenzene (DNFB), trinitrochlorobenzene (TNCB), and oxazolone,[32] and (2) that LC-containing, but not LC-depleted, epidermal cell suspensions pulse-exposed to either soluble protein antigens or haptens elicit a genetically restricted, antigen-specific, proliferative in vitro response in T cells.[33] Murine skin that is either naturally deficient in LCs (tail skin) or experimentally depleted of LCs (by UV light or glucocorticoids) failed to induce contact hypersensitivity (CHS),[32] and skin grafts depleted of LCs by vigorous tape stripping enjoy a prolonged survival on class II-disparate recipients. Similarly, the attempt to sensitize Syrian hamsters via the cheek pouch epithelium, a unique tissue because of its low LC density and virtual absence of lymphatic drainage, is not followed by a productive immune response. This failure to sensitize is frequently not an immunologic "null event" but can also result in a state of specific immunologic unresponsiveness that is associated with and probably caused by the generation of suppressor/regulatory T lymphocytes (see below).

Although these observations clearly show that the LC/DC system is indispensable for the occurrence of antigen-specific skin immunity, it is equally clear that LCs/DCs as they occur in their tissue residence are poorly, if at all, stimulatory for naive T cells. In 1986, Inaba et al.[34] found that freshly isolated murine LCs ("immature" LCs) can present soluble antigen to primed MHC class II-restricted T cells but are only weak stimulators of naive, allogeneic T cells and primary antibody responses. In contrast, LCs purified from epidermal cell suspensions after a culture period of 72 h or LCs purified from freshly isolated murine epidermal cells and cultured for 72 h in the presence of GM-CSF and IL-1 ("mature" LCs) are extremely potent stimulators of primary T cell-proliferative responses to alloantigens,[34] soluble protein antigens,[35] and haptens,[35] and of primary T cell-dependent B cell responses. The strong immunostimulatory potential of mature LCs for resting T cells does not mean that they are superior to freshly isolated, immature LCs in every functional aspect. In fact, immature LCs far excel cytokine-activated LCs in their capacity to take up and process native protein antigens.[36] Accordingly, immature rather than mature LCs/DDCs express antigen uptake receptors/pattern recognition receptors including the mannose-binding receptors Langerin (expressed by LCs only)[7] and macrophage mannose receptor (expressed by DDCs), the C-type lectin receptor DEC-205, the low-affinity IgG receptor CD32/FcγRII, the high-affinity IgE receptor FcεRI, and the thrombospondin receptor CD36 (Table 23-1). Immature LCs present the resulting peptide fragments as effectively as they can present peptides loaded onto the cells from the exterior. Mature LCs, while fully capable of presenting these peptides, have lost their capacity to process and present the native protein.[36] This cytokine-/culture-induced switch from the processing/peptide loading to the presentation mode is a highly regulated LC function attributable to fundamental molecular changes in protein synthesis and vesicle trafficking. LCs in their immature state display MHC class II antigens in lysosomal, HLA-DM–containing, peptide-loading compartments (MIIC) and, to a much lesser extent, on the cell surface. When LCs mature in situ, the degree of class II and HLA-DM colocalization decreases, and MHC class II molecules are transferred to the plasma membrane. Likewise, MHC class I surface expression is upregulated during the process of DC maturation. While MHC class II and invariant chain synthesis is high in the immature state, it is diminished or entirely shut off during the process of LC maturation.

The display of MHC-peptide complexes on the DC surface delivers the "first signal" to T cells; that is, the triggering of the TCR by the APC-bound peptide-MHC complex. However, this signal alone is insufficient for the induction of productive and protective T cell immunity. In fact, certain cell types that express MHC class II molecules in an inducible fashion (keratinocytes, endothelial cells, fibroblasts) or xenogeneic cells that are genetically engineered to express the antigen/MHC complex, when encountered by antigen-specific T cells, induce a state of anergy in these cells.[37] "Second signals" delivered by professional APCs critically determine the occurrence, the magnitude, and the quality of T cell responses. In skin DCs, as well as in DCs from other locations, molecules that deliver second signals are upregulated in a strictly maturation-dependent fashion (Table 23-1). Second signals include membrane-bound costimulators and secreted cytokines. The best-defined costimulators for T cells are the two members of the B7 family, B7.1/CD80 and B7–2/CD86.[38] LCs/DCs in situ do not express or express only minute amounts of these costimulatory molecules, but greatly upregulate these moieties during maturation. The necessity for these costimulatory molecules is best illustrated in experiments showing that when T cells are exposed to an antigen-pulsed APC in the presence of B7 antagonists, or if CD28-deficient T cells encounter an antigen, the cells do not expand but are anergized or undergo apoptosis.[39] Other costimulatory molecules include the intercellular adhesion molecule (ICAM)-1 that binds to lymphocyte function-associated antigen (LFA)-1, and LFA-3, the ligand of T cell-expressed CD2. Further important ligand-receptor pairs mediating APC-T cell interactions include heat-stable antigen (CD24)/CD24 ligand (L), CD40/CD40L, CD27L/CD70, OX40L/OX40 (CD134), and RANKL/RANK.

Although inducible by rather simple manipulations, that is, by culture of explanted skin (Fig. 23-5), LC/DC maturation is a highly regulated process that is initiated by the triggering of surface receptors. Evidence exists that cytokines released as a consequence of physicochemical or infection-associated tissue perturbation (e.g., keratinocyte-derived GM-CSF, TNF-α, IL-1) and/or ligation of CD40 molecules on LCs can provide the critical signals for the induction of LC maturation. Epicutaneously applied contact sensitizers, but not irritants or tolerogens, activate certain protein tyrosine kinases, modify the cellular content and structure of intracytoplasmic organelles (increase in coated pits and vesicles, endo- and lysosomes, and Birbeck granules) and, thus, induce LC maturation directly or indirectly via the release of cytokines from keratinocytes. Of particular importance is that microbes, microbial products, and the consequences of microbial tissue damage can deliver signals that regulate DC maturation and, thus, decisively control whether protective immunity or immunologic paralysis ensues.[40] Maturation signals are delivered to DCs by the uptake of necrotic, but not of apoptotic, cells,[41] virus-derived double-stranded RNA, intact microorganisms (e.g., leishmania major amastigotes, dengue virus), and compounds that trigger members of the family of Toll-like receptors (TLRs). Toll receptors are evolutionary conserved between insects and humans and are regarded as prototype innate defense receptors because of their affinity for pathogens/pathogenic products. Ten members of the TLR family have been classified so far.[42] LC express at least TLR1 to TLR4. Ligands of TLR2 include lipoproteins from *Mycobacterium tuberculosis, Borrelia burgdorferi, Treponema pallidum,* mycobacterial lipoarabinomannan, lipopolysaccharide (LPS), peptidoglycan, zymosan, and glycophosphatidyl inositol anchors from *Treponema pallidum* and *Trypanosoma cruzi* lipoproteins. TLR4 binds hsp60 and is the most important receptor for LPS from gram-negative bacteria. TLR7 recognizes the synthetic substance imiquimod, and CpG-rich DNA triggers TLR9.[42,43] Signals initiated by TLR and by certain other DC receptors result in the maturation-related downregulation of antigen/pathogen uptake receptors. Thus, maturation signals force skin DCs to focus on the presentation of skin-related dangerous antigens and prevent them from taking up irrelevant moieties during the final journey of the cells from the epidermis–dermis to the regional lymph node.

The importance of LC/DC maturation and migration to regional lymph nodes for the induction of adaptive immunity is best evidenced by the findings that (1) LCs disappear from the epidermis and migrate via dermal lymphatics to the regional lymph nodes in response to contact sensitizers[44]; (2) mature, but not immature, DCs, after intracutaneous injection, migrate efficiently to regional nodes; (3) the inhibition of LC migration toward regional nodes by genetic ablation or antibody-mediated inhibition of migration-inducing factors (e.g., IL-1β, osteopontin, CD44, SLC) can prevent the occurrence of sensitization to topically applied contact allergens[21,45,46]; and (4) DCs, isolated from skin-draining nodes after hapten application to the skin, can induce CHS when administered into naive mice, and can stimulate the proliferation of nonsensitized T cells. These and other experiments strongly indicate that hapten-bearing DCs appearing in the regional lymph nodes after epicutaneous application of the contact-sensitizing hapten are derived from the skin. They most likely represent LCs (and DDCs) that had left the skin after epicutaneous sensitization, migrated to the regional lymph node, and, on arrival, initiated allergen-specific T cell activation. The finding that the injection of particulate antigen into the skin converts dermal monocytic cells into fully stimulatory DCs that migrate to the regional nodes, highlights the enormous plasticity of the skin immune system.

The restriction elements presenting hapten/haptenated peptide epitopes include MHC class I and MHC class II. The LC-expressed ATPase CD39/ectonucleotidase triphosphate diphosphohydrolase can also function as a hapten-presenting molecule when high hapten concentrations are applied.[47] In line with a critical role of CD39 in LC function is also the observation that CD39 knockout mice show severely attenuated CHS responses to oxazolon.[5] Surprisingly, these mice have exacerbated skin inflammation to topically applied irritant chemicals as a result of a deficiency in catalyzing keratinocyte-derived extracellular ATP/ADP (adenosine diphosphate). As LCs are the only epidermal cells with ATPase activity, the results point to an unexpected function of LCs in the maintenance of epidermal homeostasis; that is, the scavenging of inflammation-inducing nucleotides.

Once LCs arrive in the lymph nodes, they exert their superior immunostimulatory activity not only by their cell surface molecules but also by their secretory activity. Difficulties in isolating sufficient numbers of LCs and other skin DCs prevented detailed analyses of their secretory repertoire for a considerable time period, but the development of sensitive molecular techniques and in vitro culture systems to expand LCs and DDC-like cells from hematopoietic precursors allowed important accomplishments. Pioneering work in this field demonstrated that, after exposure to contact allergens, LC rapidly upregulates IL-1β mRNA expression[48]; this finding suggests an important role for IL-1β in the initiation of primary immune responses. Subsequently, the expression of TNF-α, IL-6, MIP-1α, MIP-1γ, and IL-12 by isolated LCs has been reported. In vitro-generated LCs and DDCs both produce a broad array of immunologically relevant cytokines.[49] Both LCs and DDCs spontaneously produce mRNA encoding IL-1α, IL-1β, IL-6, IL-7, IL-12 (p35 and p40), IL-15, IL-18, TNF-α, TGF-β, M-CSF, and GM-CSF, but lack expression of IL-2, IL-3, IL-4, IL-5, IL-9, and IFN-γ. IL-12 secretion was maximal after triggering of CD40. LCs, even after activation, fail to express the immunoregulatory cytokine IL-10, whereas the DDC-like cells could secrete this cytokine, even in the absence of stimulatory agents.

A massive body of evidence suggests that the mode of DC activation/maturation determines the quality of T cell responses. On the basis of the type of lymphokines they produce, CD4+ helper T cells can be divided into three major subsets: T_H1, T_H2, and T_H0.[50] T_H1 cells produce IFN-γ and predominantly promote delayed-type hypersensitivity, whereas T_H2 cells, which produce IL-4, IL-5, and IL-13, provide help for certain B cell responses. T cells exhibiting a not (yet) polarized secretion pattern with the production of cytokines typical of both T_H1 and T_H2 exist in both humans and rodents and were designated T_H0 cells. Differentiation toward the T_H1 or T_H2 phenotype is directed by cytokines present at the time of the first APC–T cell encounter. The key factors are IL-4 and the heterodimeric cytokine IL-12. IL-4 promotes T_H2 cell development, whereas IL-12 is a potent inducer of T_H1 cells. Consistent with this concept are the findings that IL-12p40 –/– as well as STAT-4 –/– (signal transducer and activator of transcription, involved in IL-12 receptor signaling) mice are defective in IFN-γ production and almost completely lack the ability to generate a T_H1 response. Conversely, knocking out the IL-4 or STAT-6 (involved in IL-4 receptor signaling) genes resulted in deficient T_H2 responses. Although DCs, including LCs, do not produce IL-4, they can elaborate significant amounts of IL-12 when appropriately stimulated. IL-12-inducing stimuli are signals that are delivered during the T cell–APC interaction (cross-linking of CD40 or HLA-DR on the APC surface, IFN-γ)[49] as well as microorganisms.[40] In fact, ingestion of yeast cells from *Candida albicans* activates DCs for IL-12 production and priming of protective T_H1 cells, whereas ingestion of *Candida albicans* hyphae inhibits IL-12, induces T_H2 cells, and does not lead to protective antifungal immunity.[51] Similarly, IL-10, glucocorticoids, and prostaglandin E_2 render DCs deficient in IL-12 production and promote the development of T_H2 cells.[52] The recently identified new members of the B7 family, B7H/B7RP-1 and B7-H1, ligands of the T cell-expressed activation-induced costimulator ICOS and a yet to be characterized T cell receptor, respectively, induce high-level production of the immunosuppressive cytokine IL-10 and thus a T_H2-like or T regulatory (see below) profile in T cells.[53] In view of their inability to secrete IL-12, B cells may be involved in the elicitation of T_H2 responses only, whereas DCs, depending on their activation state and the milieu surrounding them, may promote either T_H1 or T_H2 differentiation.

LCs are also implicated in the generation of cytotoxic T cell responses. Indeed, it is the current view that LC-dependent activation of CD8+ T cells is the major pathogenic mechanism of allergic contact dermatitis[54] and may be of relevance in several other immune-mediated inflammatory skin diseases (see below). Evidence exists that LCs/DCs induce the generation of MHC class I-restricted allo-, hapten-, and virus-specific cytotoxicity in resting T lymphocytes. Such DC-induced proliferative and cytotoxic responses are MHC class I-restricted and can occur even in the absence of CD4+ T helper cells when DCs have been stimulated via their CD40 surface receptor.[55]

Therapeutic use of the immunostimulatory capacity of DCs to induce protective immunity Driven by the discovery of the superior stimulatory capacity of mature LCs for CD4+ and CD8+ T cells, a solid body of evidence has been compiled suggesting that skin DCs are capable of inducing protective immunity against cancer. Grabbe et al.[56] demonstrated that the repeated subcutaneous injection of GM-CSF–activated LCs that had been loaded with tumor fragments derived from a spindle cell tumor line resulted in host resistance to a subsequent challenge with viable tumor cells. In keeping with this observation is the finding that murine epidermal DCs, pulsed with synthetic ovalbumin (OVA) peptides (e.g., SIINFEKL, amino acids 257 to 264 of OVA) and injected subcutaneously, elicit OVA-specific CD8+ T cells that lyse OVA-expressing target cells in vitro and prevent the growth of OVA-transfected, but not of nontransfected, melanoma cells in vivo. This potent immunostimulatory function is apparently mediated by mature LCs. As long as this advanced maturational stage has not been reached, the exposure of LCs to suppressive factors, for example, IL-10, can abrogate their capacity to induce antitumor immunity, whereas the fully matured cells become resistant to this inhibitory effect. These data support the hypothesis that immune surveillance exists in the epidermis and that LCs are the critical cellular elements of this host defense mechanism.

According to this concept, the development of protein/peptide- and DNA-based immunization strategies to optimize antigen presentation by skin DCs is a rational approach to anticancer vaccine design. Cutaneous genetic immunization with naked DNA results in the transfection and/or uptake of DNA-encoded proteins by skin DCs, which migrate to draining lymph nodes and efficiently elicit antigen-specific, cytotoxic, and helper T cell responses.[57] Other strategies currently being pursued aim at introducing tumor antigen-encoding cDNA under the control of DC-specific promoters, cancer cell-derived RNA, tumor antigen-derived peptides, tumor antigen–hsp complexes, tumor cell-derived exosomes, or even apoptotic or necrotic tumor cells selectively into skin DCs or into ex vivo purified or in vitro-generated DCs for the induction of cytotoxic T cell responses. What has been learned from the human trials reported so far is that administration of DCs is safe and under certain conditions leads to substantial immune responses and to limited clinical responses.[58]

Downregulation of immune responses via the skin Early observations indicated that the application of hapten to LC-deficient skin/mucosa caused hapten-specific T cell tolerance (see above). More recent evidence suggests that both the site onto which the allergen is applied as well as its dose may be critical for whether T cell immunity or tolerance occurs. Steinbrink et al.[59] demonstrated that the painting of minute quantities of hapten onto ears of naive mice results in a state of long-lasting, hapten-specific tolerance, whereas the application of standard immunizing doses to ears of control animals was followed by the regular delayed-type ear swelling response that appears after hapten challenge. Although it is tempting to speculate that DCs with tolerizing potential are present in the skin, it must be remembered that haptens diffuse rapidly from the application site, spread through the circulation, and, thus, may be presented by immature DCs in many organs, or even by nonprofessional or non-APCs. "Low zone" tolerance is associated with a lymphokine secretion pattern suggestive of a T_H2-biased immune reaction. The recently identified "regulatory" T cells, cells with the capacity to antigen specifically or nonspecifically downregulate T cell-mediated immune reactions in vitro and in vivo, display a T_H2-like cytokine secretion profile.[60] Regulatory T cells display the IL-2 receptor α-chain/CD25, the B7 ligand CTLA-4, and secrete IL-10, TGF-β, and, depending on their derivation, IFN-γ. Immature, but not mature, DCs stimulate the induction or, at least, the expansion of regulatory T cells.[61] UV radiation can induce a distinct T regulatory type 1-like T suppressor cell population that may block the activation of T_H1 cell-mediated immune responses.[62] Hapten-reactive CD4+ T regulatory cells that produce high levels of IL-10, low levels of IFN-γ, and no IL-4 have been isolated from the blood and skin of allergic individuals, and these cells express an adhesion molecule and chemokine receptor pattern that supports their skin-homing properties; these findings suggest that, during every immune response induced via the skin, the effector arm (i.e., cytotoxic T cells, CD4+ effector cells) and a downregulatory component are activated.[63] Thus, the balance between the two components in sensitized individuals critically determines whether a given antigen or pathogen that appears in the skin is subject to immune attack or is recognized but ignored by the immune system.

LCs may also directly downregulate ongoing immune reactions. Experimental evidence suggests that they may impose suppressive effects during the elicitation phase of contact hypersensitivity and, when stimulated by CD40 ligation, but not by LPS or IFN-γ, can kill T cells in a FasL-dependent fashion.

Phenotypic and Functional Alterations in Disease

ALLERGIC DISORDERS

Contact hypersensitivity Studies in the late 1970s and early 1980s first claimed a role for LCs in the development of CHS.[32] Today we know that certain haptens but not irritants, when applied to the skin, can induce changes in its cellular constituents, resulting in conditions that promote activation of LCs/DDCs and their migration to the draining lymph nodes where they stimulate the proliferation of nonsensitized T cells in a hapten-specific manner. The likelihood of sensitization depends on the chemical structure of the hapten and on the genetic susceptibility of the individual exposed to it. In vitro studies are in progress to predict the allergenicity of a given chemical on the basis of its capacity to induce maturational events in DCs and to endow them with immunostimulatory properties. As opposed to the earlier view that CHS responses are mediated by CD4+ type 1 T cells, it now appears that CD8+ type 1 T cells are the main effector cells and that the concomitantly generated, hapten-specific CD4+ T cells are downregulating this response.[54]

Notwithstanding the critical role of LCs/DDCs in CHS induction, epidermal LCs are apparently not needed for the challenge reaction to occur. The cell(s) actually responsible for it has (have) yet to be identified.

Atopic dermatitis Lesional skin of patients with atopic dermatitis (AD) contains increased numbers of DCs in both the epidermis and the dermis. In the epidermis, they represent either classical LCs or so-called inflammatory dendritic epidermal cells (IDECs). IDECs can be distinguished from LCs by a limited set of markers including FcεRI^{high}, FcγRII/CD32^{high}, CD1b, and CD36.[64] In patients with AD and hyperimmunoglobulinemia E, IDECs and, to a lesser extent, LCs often express FcεRI-bound surface IgE. Allergen-induced cross-linking of these IgE moieties in vitro facilitates their processing and presentation to T cells[65] and induces transcription and expression of proinflammatory molecules including IL-1, TNF-α, and IL-16.[66] Should these processes also be operative in vivo, they may well be responsible not only for the often severe and rapid outbreaks of eczematous skin lesions after allergen exposure, but also for the maintenance and, thus, chronicity of allergic tissue inflammation.

INFECTIOUS DISEASES Cutaneous DCs play a pivotal role in the host defense against pathogenic microorganisms penetrating or introduced into the skin (see above). As might be expected, microorganisms have found ways and strategies to circumvent immunosurveillance by these cells. Examples of this microbial escape include the downregulation of MHC class II molecules on epidermal LCs in *Lyme* *borreliosis,* the inhibition of LC migration by *Schistosoma mansoni*-derived prostaglandin D_2, and the prevention of LC/DC maturation and differentiation on infection with measles virus. LCs/DDCs are also an important target of HIV infection[67] and, at mucosal sites, could be an important point of virus entry during sexual intercourse. Once infected, LCs can sustain viral replication[68] and supposedly transmit the infection to the lymphoid tissue. Very active HIV-1 replication has been observed in DC–T cell conjugates emigrating from skin explants.[69] The in vivo role, if any, of DC-SIGN in the uptake and presentation of the virus[70] has yet to be determined. Patients with AIDS have reduced LC numbers because of viral cytopathicity and/or immunologic elimination.

SKIN CANCER The outcome of immune responses triggered by LCs/DDCs is critically dependent on the state of cell maturation. While terminally differentiated IL-12–producing LCs/DDCs favor the development of type 1 T cell-dominated responses and, thus, of protective microbial and cancer immunity, cells with a more immature phenotype promote the generation of type 2 T cells, or even regulatory T cells (see above). In the case of cancer, the latter scenario is highly undesirable and may have disastrous consequences for the affected individual. Thus, it is not surprising that the presence of fully matured LCs/DCs within or around the neoplasm is usually associated with tumor regression, whereas progressive cancers are mostly infiltrated with and surrounded by immature DCs. This is best demonstrated in melanoma and Langerhans cell histiocytosis itself. Prevention of DC maturation is caused by the production and release of immunoinhibitory cytokines and, perhaps, certain angiogenetic factors by cancer cells, as well as the direct negative effects of certain carcinogens.[71]

Decreased LC densities have been encountered in lesions of squamous cell and basal cell carcinoma, in Bowen's disease, in actinic keratoses, and in human papillomavirus (HPV)-induced acanthomas. Several factors may be responsible for this phenomenon, including UV- and/or drug-induced immunosuppression of the host, as well as putative adverse effects of HPV on the LC population.

Effects of Physicochemical Agents and Drugs

UVB UVB has many adverse biologic effects, the most severe being the initiation and promotion of skin cancers. Originally, it was thought that UVB promotes the development of cutaneous neoplasia solely by its direct transforming effect on the genome of the host cells. Later, it was recognized that UVB induces a state of immunodeficiency, which is best exemplified by the inability of UVB-irradiated mice to mount a protective immune response against highly immunogenic UVB-induced tumors. These and other observations led to the concept that there exists a link between UVB-induced immune dysfunction and carcinogenesis.[72]

Many investigators set out to probe this concept by using CHS as a read-out system. In one series of experiments, mice were irradiated with very high, nonphysiologic ($>10^5$ J/m^2) doses of UVB and were then exposed to the hapten either at the irradiated site or at a distant, nonirradiated site. In both instances, mice developed a hapten-specific unresponsiveness that could be transferred to naive recipients. Although UVB does not penetrate further than the upper dermis, these high-dose UVB-irradiated animals develop a systemic defect of APC function. In contrast to this high-dose model of UVB-induced immunosuppression, Toews et al.[32] irradiated mice with 100 J/m^2 of UVB on 4 consecutive days and then applied the hapten to either the irradiated or the nonirradiated site. While they succeeded in inducing CHS via the nonirradiated site, application of the hapten to the irradiated site did not result in sensitization. This hapten-specific unresponsiveness could not be reversed by resensitization with the same hapten at a distant skin site, but it could be adoptively transferred by spleen and lymph node cells into immunologically naive syngeneic mice. Although not inducible in all mouse strains, this low-dose model of UVB-induced immunosuppression is certainly biologically more relevant than the high-dose model because it uses fluences of UVB (100 to 300 J/m^2 per single exposure) that are equivalent to one minimal erythema dose in humans. Although evidence exists that hapten sensitization is less likely to occur via UVB-irradiated skin than via non UVB-exposed skin in humans, human epidermal cells appear to be less susceptible to UVB than their murine counterparts. It is important to account for these differences in susceptibility when data on the effects of UVB radiation on the immune system in rodents are extrapolated to humans.

LCs are probably the major targets in the induction of UVB-induced immunosuppression: (1) UVB irradiation of skin leads to their dose-dependent reduction and injury[32]; (2) the injection of purified UVB-irradiated LCs into naive mice not only fails to sensitize, but even tolerizes these animals[73]; and (3) UVB irradiation of single epidermal cells leads to a dose-dependent inhibition of their immunostimulatory properties.[33] This finding is true for type 1 (T_H1, T_c1) T cells but not for type 2 or regulatory T cells.

With respect to the mechanism(s) of UVB-induced immunosuppression, the generation of cyclobutane pyrimidine dimers and, as a consequence, apoptosis appear to be the key events.[74] Indeed, the excision of these dimers by a liposome-incorporated repair enzyme restores the antigen-presenting activity of cutaneous DCs.[75] In this context, it should be mentioned that accelerated excision repair can also be accomplished by IL-12,[76] a cytokine critical for the induction and expansion of type 1 T cells.

In addition to its direct DNA-damaging effect, UVB also triggers the production/release by epidermal cells of substances that downregulate or prevent the occurrence of immune responses dominated by type 1 T cells.

A cytokine that probably plays an essential role in this process is IL-10. This mediator is secreted by UV-irradiated keratinocytes and can be found in skin biopsies and suction blister fluid from UV-exposed human volunteers as well as in the serum of UV-irradiated animals. In addition to its inhibitory action on IFN-γ production by activated type 1 T cell clones, IL-10 profoundly alters the function of APCs by blocking their synthesis and/or upregulation of costimulatory molecules such as IL-1β, CD54, and CD80. Studies from several laboratories convincingly demonstrate that (1) IL-10-treated LCs can tolerize T_H1 cells; (2) in vivo administration of recombinant IL-10 induces tolerance to contact-sensitizing haptens[77]; and (3) IL-10 knockout mice are resistant to the UVB-induced suppression of certain delayed type hypersensitivity reactions. Another molecule implicated in UVB-induced immunosuppression is urocanic acid. It is synthesized normally in skin in the *trans*-isomerized form via deamination of histidine within keratinocytes. After absorption of UVB radiation, *trans*-urocanic acid is converted to the *cis* isomer. Both in vivo and in vitro studies indicate that *cis*-urocanic acid can suppress T cell-mediated responses by interfering with the antigen-presenting function of LCs/DCs.[78]

On the basis of the observation that mice treated with indomethacin become resistant to UVB-induced suppression of CHS, it was suggested that prostaglandins, predominantly PGE_2, are somehow involved in generating immunosuppression. It now appears that PGE_2 exerts its effects by increasing IL-10 secretion and, conversely, by downregulating IL-12 and TNF-α production/secretion.

Although the above data are perfectly consistent with the concept of LCs playing a critical role in UVB-induced immunosuppression, the derivation and nature of the cells(s) delivering tolerizing signals in the lymphoid tissues have not yet been elucidated. Because conflicting data exist about the effect of UVB irradiation on LC migration and LC maturation, several, non-mutually exclusive scenarios are conceivable. First, UVB, while arresting LCs in an immature state, allows them to migrate to T cell zones in the regional lymph nodes. In the absence of costimulatory molecules, LCs would transmit tolerizing signals. Second,

LCs of UVB-irradiated skin undergo apoptosis and are replaced by a population of IL-10-producing, tolerance-inducing APCs.[79] Third, UVB pushes LCs into apoptosis and thus prevents their migration to the lymph nodes. Antigenic material would reach the afferent lymphatics and be transported to the lymph node in unbound form. Uptake of this material by immature DCs residing there would again result in tolerization.

UVA, PUVA UVA can also adversely affect the number, phenotype, and function of LCs,[80] resulting in a state of immunosuppression. Recent data indicate that UVA II acts primarily on epidermal LCs, whereas UVA I leaves LCs apparently unaltered, but induces emigration of DDCs from the skin. The actual epidermal damage seen after UVA (and also UVB) irradiation has been ascribed, in part, to the generation of reactive oxygen intermediates. Reports exist that antioxidants (e.g., vitamin C, vitamin E, flavonoids) can prevent, at least partially, the deleterious effects of UV irradiation on cutaneous immunity.

In both humans and experimental animals, PUVA treatment causes a transitory reduction and a functional impairment of ATPase+/MHC class II+ epidermal cells in a dose-dependent fashion. It remains to be seen whether these effects contribute to PUVA carcinogenicity.

IONIZING RADIATION Both x-radiation and Grenz rays produce significant reductions in the number and/or function of LCs.

HYPERTHERMIA Prolonged exposure of mice to mild whole-body hyperthermia enhances LC migration in the absence of foreign antigen. This finding indicates that increases in local or systemic body temperature, as they occur during infection and inflammation, have per se a regulatory effect on immune function.

IMMUNOSTIMULATORY COMPOUNDS When applied to or injected into the skin, imidazoquinolones such as imiquimod and resiquimod as well as CpG-containing oligonucleotides induce activation and functional maturation of LCs/DDCs. This opens new and exciting avenues for the induction of protective, type 1 T cell-dominated antimicrobial and antitumor immune responses.

IMMUNOSUPPRESSIVE DRUGS Many of the immunoinhibitory and/or anti-inflammatory substances used in dermatology (glucocorticoids, cyclosporine, tacrolimus, methotrexate, azathioprine, and vitamin D_3 analogues) may adversely influence LCs/DDCs at the phenotypic and/or functional level. It is not always clear whether the effects of the respective drugs are a result of their direct or indirect (via their symbionts) actions on cutaneous DCs.

RETINOIDS Controversy exists as to whether or not retinoids can protect LCs from depletion by UVB or tumor-promoting phorbol esters.

KERATINOCYTES

The contention that the regulatory effects of cytokines on the phenotype and function of dendritic APCs in vitro are of great in vivo relevance gains support from immunomorphologic studies documenting a close proximity between dendritic APCs and resident skin cells that produce soluble mediators of the inflammatory and immune response.

DDCs are members of the "dermal microvascular unit" and can conceivably receive signals from the other cellular components of this unit; that is, endothelial cells, pericytes, mast cells, and T cells. In the epidermis, the LC enjoys an even closer association with its symbionts. Evidence exists that nerves containing calcitonin gene–related peptide (CGRP) frequently impinge on LCs of the human epidermis.[81] This

physical interaction is probably of great functional importance because CGRP and the neuropeptide substance P can inhibit the immunostimulatory capacity of LCs.

Although LCs may also have occasional encounters with melanocytes and Merkel cells, their most important epidermal partner is, unquestionably, the keratinocyte.

Keratinocytes not only have structural functions but also participate actively in inflammatory and immunologic processes. This action became evident when it was discovered that these cells produce a wide variety of biologically active molecules, some of which act as mediators of the inflammatory reaction and the immune response, for example, cytokines, neuropeptides, antimicrobial peptides, and eicosanoids.

In addition to their role as immunomodulating cells, keratinocytes can also participate directly in immune reactions as both inducers and targets. As such, they play a pivotal role in the pathogenesis and expression of many skin diseases, including eczema, psoriasis, pemphigus, erythema multiforme, and graft-versus-host-disease (GVHD).

Secretory Functions

CYTOKINES Keratinocytes are capable of producing/secreting a large number of cytokines that may affect neighboring cells (paracrine pattern), modulate their own functional status (autocrine pattern), and, in situations of massive release, reach the circulation and affect the function of cells at distant sites (endocrine pattern). Some of these factors [e.g., IL-1, IL-1 receptor antagonist, IL-6, IL-7, IL-8 and other chemokines, IL-10, IL-12, IL-15, IL-18 (IFN-γ–inducing factor, IGIF), TNF-α, GM-CSF, M-CSF, SCF] are important mediators of the inflammatory and/or immune response, whereas others (e.g., TGF-α and -β, platelet-derived growth factor, basic fibroblast growth factor, keratinocyte growth factor, nerve growth factor, vascular endothelial cell growth factor) regulate the growth of different epithelial and/or mesenchymal cells (Table 23-2). The latter factors are dealt with elsewhere in this volume (see Chap. 26).

TABLE 23-2

Keratinocyte-Derived Cytokines and Cytokine Receptors

Interleukins
- IL-1α (IL-1F1), IL-β (IL-1F2) and homologues (IL-1F5, IL-1F7, IL-1F9, IL-1F10), IL-1RA (IL-1F3), IL-18 (IGIF, IL-1F4)
- IL-6, IL-7, IL-10, IL-12, IL-15
- TNF-α, lymphotoxin-α, LIF, MIF, IFN-α, IFN-β, IFN-κ

Chemokines
- CXC chemokines: Groα (CXCL1), IL-8 (CXCL8), Mig (CXCL9), IP-10 (CXCL10), I-TAC/IP-9 (CXCL11)
- CC chemokines: MCP-1 (CCL2), RANTES (CCL5), TARC (CCL17), MIP-3α/LARC (CCL20), MDC (CCL22), CTACK (CCL27)

Colony-stimulating factors
- GM-CSF, M-CSF, SCF (c-*kit*), flt-3 ligand

Other growth factors
- TGF-α, TGF-β, KGF, PDGF, NGF, bFGF, VEGF

Cytokine receptors
- IL-1R type I (active) and II (decoy receptor)
- TNF-αR type 1 (p55)
- IL-4Rα, IL-6R, IL-10R1, IL-13Rα1, IL-18R, IL-20R1/IL-20R2, IL-22R1/IL-20R2
- IFN-γ receptor, IL-17R (by inference)

Chemokine receptors
- CXCR1, CXCR2, CCR3, CCR6

Keratinocytes of unperturbed skin produce only a few of these mediators, such as IL-1, IL-7, and TGF-β, constitutively. Resident keratinocytes contain large quantities of preformed and biologically active IL-1α, as well as immature IL-1β in their cytoplasm.[82] The likely in vivo role of this stored intracellular IL-1 is that of an immediate initiator of inflammatory and repair processes after epidermal injury; that is, after its release into the extracellular space. IL-7 is an important lymphocyte growth factor that, in the mouse, promotes the proliferation of dendritic epidermal T cells (DETCs) and keeps them alive. The role of this cytokine in the survival and proliferation of the T lymphocytes of human skin is unclarified. Some evidence exists for the IL-7–driven propagation of Sézary lymphoma cells.

TGF-β, in addition to its growth-regulating effects on keratinocytes and fibroblasts, modulates the inflammatory as well as the immune response,[83] and is important for LC development (see above).[11]

Upon delivery of certain noxious, or at least potentially hazardous stimuli (e.g., hypoxia, trauma, nonionizing radiation, haptens and other rapidly reactive chemicals, microbial toxins), the production and/or release of many cytokines is often dramatically enhanced. The biologic consequences of this event are manifold and include the initiation of inflammation (IL-1, TNF-α, IL-6, members of the chemokine family), the modulation of LC phenotype and function (IL-1, GM-CSF, TNF-α, IL-10, IL-15), T cell activation (IL-15, IL-18), T cell inhibition (IL-10, TGF-β), and skewing of the lymphocytic response in the type 1 direction (IL-12).[82,84–87] In some cases, keratinocytes may also play a role in amplifying inflammatory signals in the epidermis originating from numerically minor epidermal cell subsets. One prominent example is the induction of proinflammatory cytokines such as TNF-α in keratinocytes by LC-derived IL-1β in the initiation phase of allergic contact dermatitis.[48]

In the case of a robust stimulus, keratinocyte-derived cytokines may be released into the circulation in quantities that cause systemic effects. During a severe sunburn reaction, for example, serum levels of IL-1, IL-6, and TNF-α are clearly elevated and probably responsible for the systemic manifestations of this reaction, such as fever, leukocytosis, and the production of acute phase proteins.[88] There is also evidence that the UV-inducible cytokines IL-6 and IL-10 can induce the production of autoantibodies and, thus, be involved in the exacerbation of autoimmune diseases such as lupus erythematosus. The fact that secreted products of keratinocytes can reach the circulation could conceivably also be used for therapeutic purposes. The demonstration by Fenjves et al.[89] that grafting of apolipoprotein E (apo-E) gene-transfected human keratinocytes onto mice results in the detection of apo-E in the circulation of the mouse supports the feasibility of such an approach.

Another important function of keratinocytes is the production/secretion of factors governing the influx and efflux of leukocytes into and out of the skin. Two good examples are the chemokines TARC (CCL17) and CTACK (CCL27) that have corresponding receptors selectively expressed on skin-homing T lymphocytes. Blocking of both chemokines drastically inhibited the migration of T cells to the skin in a murine model of CHS.[90] Another more distinct function of a keratinocyte-derived chemokine in the recruitment of leukocyte subpopulations to the epidermis is suggested by the selective expression of the MIP-3α receptor, CCR6, on LCs and LC precursors[14] (see above). Because certain cytokines function as inducers of others, it could often not be decided whether a given cytokine triggered a particular tissue reaction by acting directly or indirectly, that is, via the induction of other mediators, on the relevant target cell(s). Studies with genetically modified animals, that is, animals overexpressing or lacking a particular gene, proved to be valuable tools in this regard. Examples include (1) the appearance of an inflammatory and hyperproliferative skin disease in mice overexpressing IL-1α or IL-1 receptor type I in basal keratinocytes; (2) the inhibition of some aspects of skin inflammation in mice overexpressing the IL-1 receptor type II (decoy receptor); (3) the impaired development of CHS to TNCB in some, but not all, IL-1β–deficient mice; (4) the occurrence of cachexia and GVHD-type skin changes in keratin-14 (K14) promoter-driven TNF-α transgenic mice; (5) the presence of subtle epidermal changes but absence of leukocytic infiltration in K14/IL-6 transgenic mice; (6) the recruitment to skin of LCs and other DCs in mice overexpressing monocyte chemoattractant protein 1 in basal keratinocytes; (7) the occurrence of exaggerated cutaneous inflammatory responses in IL-10–deficient mice; (8) the development of a lymphoproliferative skin disease in K14/IL-7 transgenic mice; and (9) the inhibition of skin development by overexpression of TGF-β1 in the epidermis of transgenic mice.

NEUROPEPTIDES The skin is a rich source of neuropeptides including neurotransmitters (e.g., CGRP, substance P, somatostatin) and neurohormones. The inhibitory effects of CGRP and substance P on LC antigen presentation function already were briefly discussed. The neurohormone proopiomelanocortin (POMC) is produced by the pituitary gland as well as by a number of cell types, including keratinocytes.[91] POMC is synthesized as a large prohormone and is cleaved posttranslationally in active peptide hormones such as α-, β-, and γ- melanocyte-stimulating hormone (MSH), adrenocorticotropin (ACTH), corticotropin-like intermediate lobe peptide, and others. Resident and freshly isolated keratinocytes produce very low amounts of POMC peptides. When stimulated with IL-1, UVB, or tumor promoters, these cells abundantly express POMC transcripts and release bioactive α-MSH. POMC peptides exert their bioactivities by binding to one of the melanocortin receptors, which differ with regard to their cellular expression as well as their binding specificity and avidity. For example, the melanocortin receptor 1, which exclusively binds α-MSH, is expressed on melanocytes, mononuclear phagocytes, and probably also on keratinocytes.

α-MSH profoundly affects the inflammatory and the immune responses. It antagonizes the effects of proinflammatory cytokines. and modulates IgE synthesis in vitro. It appears that the anti-inflammatory properties of this neuropeptide are because of its IL-10–inducing effect, its ability to induce CD25+CD4+ regulatory T cells, or its capacity to interfere with important effector pathways, for example, inhibition of the inducible macrophage isoform of nitric oxide synthase (NOS-II) in macrophages. In the skin, α-MSH can downregulate the differentiation-driven hsp70 expression by keratinocytes and thus appears to regulate the cells' cytoprotective protein equipment. α-MSH reportedly suppresses both the sensitization and elicitation limbs of hapten-induced contact allergy. This hyporesponsiveness probably reflects a state of hapten-specific tolerance mediated by the α-MSH–triggered production of IL-10.[92]

ANTIMICROBIAL PEPTIDES Antimicrobial peptides are increasingly recognized as important players in the innate immune system.[93] Also, keratinocytes produce such peptides including cathelicidins (LL-37)[94] and β-defensins (BD-1, BD-2, BD-3).[95] Their antimicrobial mechanism of action may relate to membrane insertion and pore formation. Adrenomedullin, members of the calcitonin-related peptide superfamily, α-MSH, and secretory leukocyte protease inhibitor (SLPI, ALP, HUSI-I) are among previously identified peptides with antimicrobial activities discovered later. BD-1 is constitutively produced by keratinocytes. Its production and that of others (LL-37, BD-2, and SLPI) is enhanced/induced by bacteria, proinflammatory cytokines,[95] or trauma.[96] Although these natural antibiotics generally have broad and overlapping antimicrobial spectra, it has recently been shown that selective deficiency of LL-37 in mice can aggravate skin infections with group A streptococci.[97] Additional functions of these peptides include the chemotactic attraction of leukocytes, induction of cell proliferation, and alteration of cell metabolism. An example of the close interplay between constituents of innate and adaptive immunity is the capacity of human BD-2 to attract T lymphocytes and DCs through binding to CCR6.[98] Cathelicidins may play a role in skin host defense by attracting neutrophilic granulocytes, and BD-2 and LL-37 by induction of mediator release from mast cells via a G protein-dependent IgE-independent mechanism.

OTHER MEDIATORS Other secreted protein mediators that can be synthesized and released from keratinocytes and that may play a role in host defense are the complement components C3 and factor B. Keratinocytes are among the cells that synthesize eicosanoids, an ensemble of lipid mediators regulating inflammatory and immunologic reactions. They can produce and release the cyclooxygenase product PGE_2 that has both proinflammatory and immunosuppressive properties and, when acting on DCs, promotes the development of type 2 T cells responses.[52] Other keratinocyte-derived eicosanoids include the neutrophil chemoattractant leukotriene $(LT)B_4$, the proinflammatory 12-lipoxygenase product 12(s)-hydroxyeicosatetraenoic acid (12(S)HETE), and 15-HETE, an anti-inflammatory and immunosuppressive metabolite of the 15-lipoxygenase pathway.

Another group of biologic response modifiers originating in keratinocytes and other epidermal cells are free radical molecules, now generally referred to as reactive oxygen species. These include the superoxide radical (O_2), hydrogen peroxide (H_2O_2), the hydroxyl radical (HO), nitric oxide (NO), and others. These radicals are generally viewed as dangerously reactive entities threatening the integrity of many tissues. The skin is particularly at risk because it is exposed to O_2 from both inside and outside, and because of the activation of oxygen by light. Free radicals probably contribute to solar damage and photoaging of the skin. However, certain reactive oxygen species have potent inflammation-inducing (e.g., oxygen free radicals) as well as immunomodulatory (e.g., NO) properties, and thus provide an important host defense mechanism against microbial invasion. For discussion of these molecules, the reader is referred to appropriate reviews.[99,100]

The Keratinocyte as an Immunologic Target Cell

The demonstration of cytokine receptors on and cytokine responsiveness by keratinocytes (Table 23-2) established that the functional properties of these cells can be subject to regulation by cells of the immune system. As a consequence, keratinocytes express or are induced to express immunologically relevant surface moieties that can be targeted by leukocytes for stimulatory or inhibitory signal transduction.

Keratinocytes can synthesize complement and related receptors, including the C3b receptor (CR1, CD35), the Epstein-Barr virus receptor CR2 (C3d receptor, CD21), the C5a receptor (CD88), the membrane cofactor protein (CD46), the decay-accelerating factor (CD55), and complement protectin (CD59). CD59 may protect keratinocytes from attack by complement. Its engagement by CD2 stimulates the secretion of proinflammatory cytokines from keratinocytes. Membrane cofactor (CD46) is reported to be a receptor for M protein of group A streptococci. Its ligation induces proinflammatory cytokines in keratinocytes such as IL-α, IL-6, and GM-CSF.

Cross-linking of CD23 (FcεRII), induced by IFN-γ or IL-4 on cultured keratinocytes, results in the secretion of TNF-α, IL-6, IL-10, and nitric oxygen via inducible NOS. CD40 is very weakly expressed by keratinocytes under steady-state conditions. It is upregulated by IFN-γ, an event probably operative in psoriasis. Engagement of CD40 induces enhanced keratinocyte ICAM-1 and Bcl-x expression, the release of IL-8, and the arrest of the cell cycle followed by keratinocyte differentiation.

In addition to their role in maintaining and securing the structural properties of the epidermis (see Chap. 6), keratinocyte-bound adhesion molecules may also subserve immune functions. A particular role was suspected for the LFA-1 (integrin) ligand ICAM-1 because it is expressed in keratinocytes in a large variety of inflammatory skin conditions. When this adhesion molecule was overexpressed under the control of a K14 promoter, however, no phenotype was found, even under inflammatory conditions. Gluing together keratinocytes is also not the sole function of E-cadherin. Homotypic interactions with LCs anchor these cells in the epidermis,[17] and heterotypic binding to $\alpha_E\ \beta_7$ helps to immobilize murine DETCs as well as CD8+ T lymphocytes in this tissue.

Cytokine action on keratinocytes not only leads to a modulation of the inflammatory and/or immune response but can also result in a change of their proliferation and differentiation program. For example, IFN-γ and IL-1 induce the de novo expression of keratin 17 and keratin 6/16, respectively.[101] MIP-1α reportedly inhibits the proliferation of undifferentiated keratinocytes.

ROLE OF MHC CLASS I ON KERATINOCYTES Attempts to quantitate surface molecules on nonstimulated keratinocytes revealed that MHC class I products are expressed on these cells in even higher density than on nonstimulated LCs. As outlined above, peptides derived from self or foreign (e.g., viral) antigens synthesized in the cytosol associate with MHC class I and are displayed at the cell surface as ligands for antigen receptors of T cells. Because the CD8 molecule binds to nonpolymorphic framework determinants of the MHC class I heavy chain, keratinocytes represent targets for CD8+ cytotoxic T lymphocytes.

Cytotoxic T cells may induce cytolysis either by secretory products (perforin, granzymes; TNF-α, lymphotoxin-α and -β) or through cell-bound ligands (CD95L, TRAIL) of death-domain–carrying receptors on the target cell (e.g., CD95/Fas/Apo-1, TRAMP/DR3/Apo-3, TRAIL receptors 1, 2, 3).[102,103] Although through different receptor/signaling pathways, both mechanisms can result in apoptosis of the target cell (a form of cell death that involves protein synthesis and DNA fragmentation). MHC class I-restricted T cell-mediated keratinocyte lysis is apparently an important event in CHS,[104] and may be involved in herpes simplex virus infection, lichen planus, acute cutaneous GVHD, and other skin disorders exhibiting a lichenoid T cell infiltrate and keratinocyte damage. Keratinocyte apoptosis was recently shown to be involved in spongiosis, a histologic feature of various forms of eczema.

Massive keratinocyte apoptosis occurs in toxic epidermal necrolysis in an MHC-independent fashion. Evidence exists that this event can be halted by the administration of pooled intravenous immunoglobulins through blocking of keratinocyte CD95 interaction with its ligands.[105] In addition to being susceptible to the cytotoxic effects of perforin and granzyme, keratinocytes can produce these very same molecules and, thus, contribute to skin inflammation and host defense. Fas-induced apoptosis is also a consequence of UV irradiation (sunburn cell formation on a histologic level) and involves pathways that are either dependent on or independent of its ligand.

INDUCTION AND FUNCTION OF MHC CLASS II ON KERATINOCYTES Keratinocytes of normal skin fail to display MHC class II molecules, but their expression can be triggered by several factors, particularly IFN-γ. IFN-γ exerts this effect via the induction of transcription factors for MHC class II α- and β-chain genes, among them the class II transactivator, CIITA, and RFX5, a DNA-binding protein of the RFX family. As a consequence, IFN-γ-stimulated keratinocytes start to express not only MHC class II α- and β-chains, but also acquire two other central elements of the MHC class II presentation pathway—the invariant chain of MHC class II and HLA-DM. In many skin disorders, MHC class II expression by keratinocytes has been found in connection with a prominent lymphocytic infiltration and, thus, has been attributed to IFN-γ production by the infiltrating T cells.[106]

MHC class II-bearing keratinocytes are capable of inducing proliferation in allogeneic CD4+ T cell lines but not in resting T cells.[107] Although containing many essential elements of the MHC class II presentation pathway, keratinocytes do not efficiently display peptides from exogenously added protein antigens in their surface-bound MHC class II. It remains to be seen whether this relates to inefficient liberation of immunogenic peptides or to a poor accessibility of MHC class II-containing vesicles for exogenous material in these cells. Nevertheless, keratinocytes present processing-independent, synthetic peptides to T cell hybridomas, indicating that these cells can display functional peptide/class II complexes. In vivo, this presentation pathway may become operative when sufficient regurgitation of peptides from antigen processing-competent cells (i.e., LCs) occurs. Alternatively, it is conceivable that many of the IFN-γ–inducible MHC class II moieties are occupied by peptides derived from cellular proteins.

Studies of the functional consequences of MHC class II presentation to T cells have demonstrated that, at least in T_H1 clones, class II+ keratinocytes can induce antigen-specific nonresponsiveness (tolerance) to subsequent restimulation.[107,108] While primed T cells enter a state of functional anergy on encountering keratinocyte-bound antigen, naive T cells may undergo apoptosis on receipt of the same antigenic stimulus displayed on the epithelial cell surface.[109] Nondelivery of costimulatory signals or production of inhibitory factors (e.g., TGF-β, PGE_2) may be responsible for T cell downregulation. In vivo, the injection of hapten-modified, MHC class II+ keratinocytes into naive mice leads to a specific, yet transient, hyporesponsiveness to subsequent sensitization by hapten.

Class II+ keratinocytes can also be killed by MHC class II-restricted T cells.[107] DCs and class II+ T cell blasts are apparently well suited for the elicitation of CD4+ T cells with cytotoxic potential. Perforin/granzyme B and Fas ligand are the proapoptotic effector molecules used by CD4+ T cells. The antigenic moieties recognized by these cells include minor transplantation and viral antigens. Thus, it is likely that CD4+ cytotoxic T cells critically contribute to the keratinocyte damage in a variety of autoimmune-mediated, allergic, infectious, and other (still idiopathic) skin disorders.

LYMPHOCYTES

Normal skin is the prototype of a nonlymphoid organ, that is, an organ in which primary lymphocyte responses are not initiated. However, normal skin is not entirely devoid of lymphocytes.

In murine epidermis, for instance, there exists a distinctive population of T lymphocytes* that are uniformly dendritic in shape (hence their name dendritic epidermal T cells) and exhibit a very restricted TCR repertoire.[112] In fact, almost all DETCs carry virtually identical TCRs encoded by $V\gamma3/J\gamma1/C\gamma$ and $V1\delta/D\delta2/J\delta1/C\delta$ genes rearranged in the canonical sequence. The same TCR configuration is found on early fetal thymocytes which, in all likelihood, are the natural DETC predecessors.[113]

The (patho)physiologic function(s) of DETCs remain(s) elusive. Several, partly contradictory concepts have received experimental support. One suggests that DETCs represent a broadly acting, first-line defense system that, upon perturbation of the skin (e.g., by stress, carcinogens, microbial assault, and haptens), undergoes activation and expansion to ultimately eliminate the pathogen or restore the integrity of the skin/epidermis. An entirely different concept suggests that DETCs act as regulatory cells suppressing or eliminating T effector cells, thus protecting the epidermis from excessive immunologic injury.

Although T cells represent the vast majority of lymphocytes in human skin and outnumber, by far, NK cells and B cells, a human analogue of the rodent DETC population has not been identified. On the contrary, most T cells of human skin are round to polygonal in shape, reside in the dermis rather than in the epidermis, and predominantly express TCR $\alpha\beta$ rather than TCR $\gamma\delta$.[114,115] Although the ratio of TCR $\alpha\beta$+ and $\gamma\delta$+ T cell subsets in human skin is similar to that in blood,[115] the TCR repertoire of skin-associated T cells is apparently not determined by random sampling of peripheral blood T cells, as evidenced by a restricted usage of $V\alpha$, $V\beta$, and $V\delta/J\delta$ specificities in normal human skin as compared to the blood.

Dermal T cells, which comprise more than 90 percent of the T cell population of the skin, are preferentially clustered around postcapillary venules of the superficial plexus high in the papillary dermis (Fig. 23-7). They are often situated just beneath the dermal–epidermal junction and within, or in close proximity to, adnexal appendages, such as hair follicles and eccrine sweat ducts. Dermal T cells express the classic markers CD2 and CD5 and are primarily single positive for CD4 or CD8 coreceptors, showing either an equal distribution or preference for the CD4+ subset. Most belong to the CD45RO+ memory population and are CD7 negative.

FIGURE 23-7

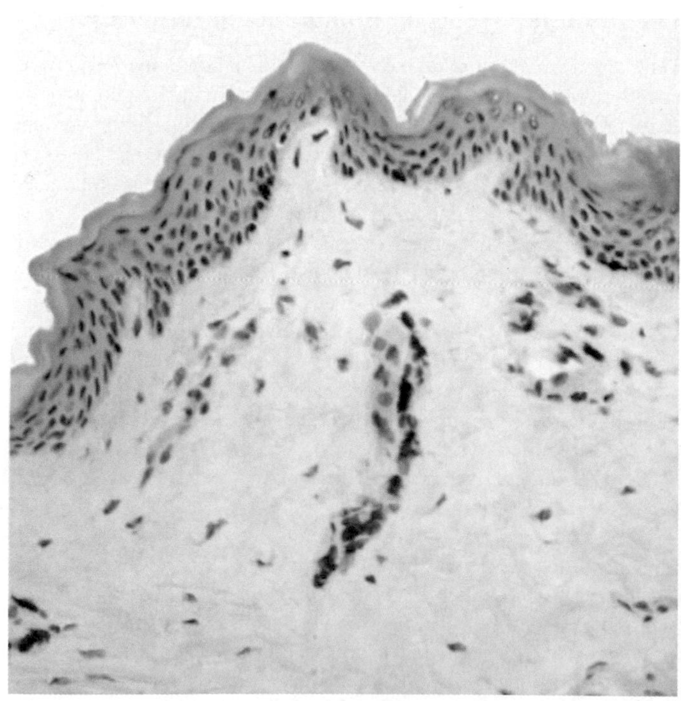

Visualization of T lymphocytes in a cryostat section of normal human skin using a monoclonal anti-CD3 antibody in an indirect immunoperoxidase technique. Stained cells are predominantly located around the superficial vascular plexus in the dermis and, to a much lesser extent, in the basal layer of the epidermis. (*Courtesy of Christine Bangert, MD.*)

*For our purpose, T cells are defined by the surface expression of CD3-associated TCRs. TCR species identified so far include $\alpha\beta$ and $\gamma\delta$ heterodimers.[110] TCRs $\alpha\beta$ are expressed on most peripheral T cells and usually recognize the antigenic fragment in conjunction with MHC,[26] occasionally also together with CD1 antigens.[31] TCRs $\gamma\delta$ are present on early fetal thymocytes, on a minor fraction of adult thymocytes and peripheral T cells, and, at least in the mouse system, on various proportions of lymphocytes populating epithelial tissues. These TCR $\gamma\delta$-bearing cells recognize a heterogeneous array of ligands including classic and nonclassic MHC antigens, bacterial heat shock proteins, and multiple self proteins.[111]

Approximately half of these CD3+ cells express the skin-homing receptor CLA with no obvious difference between the CD4+ and CD8+ subsets.[116]

At perivascular sites, most T cells express HLA-DR and/or CD25, indicating that some of them represent effector cells and others belong to the recently defined subset of regulatory T cells.[117]

Epidermal T cells account for approximately 2 to 3 percent of all CD3+ cells in normal human skin. They reside primarily in the basal and suprabasal layers (Fig. 23-7), often in close apposition to LCs. Most of them bear TCR$\alpha\beta$ dimers and exhibit the single positive (CD4−/CD8+>>CD4+/CD8−) and, occasionally, the double negative[118] (CD4−/CD8−) phenotype. CD4−/CD8+ TCR$\alpha\beta$-bearing epidermal cells express the CD8$\alpha\alpha$ homodimer at frequencies considerably higher than those in paired samples of peripheral blood.

Human epidermal T cells are typically CD2+ and CD5+, often lack the CD7 antigen, and mostly have the memory cell phenotype (CD45RO+/CD45RA−). Various portions express CD25 (IL-2Rα), CD57, and Fas (CD95). Many T cells of the human epidermis react with the MAb HECA-452 and HML-1, which define CLA and the $\alpha_E\beta_7$ integrin (CD103), respectively. A minor population of human epidermal T cells display TCR$\gamma\delta$ heterodimers, and most of these are CD4−/CD8−. In sharp contrast to epidermal T cells of rodents, human epidermal T cells exhibit an irregular distribution, being particularly abundant in volar skin and in the acrosyringeal epithelium of eccrine sweat ducts.

The derivation of intraepidermal memory cells can be explained in two, mutually nonexclusive ways. First, they might be generated by chronic antigenic stimulation of naive T cells residing indigenously in the epidermis. Alternatively, they could enter the skin/epidermis in an already sensitized state. Although the existence of an indigenous T cell population in the human epidermis is still a matter of speculation, one should not forget that some of the T cell subsets in the human epidermis, that is, TCR$\alpha\beta$+CD8+ and CD4−/CD8− T cells, respond to nonpeptide lipid and glycolipid antigens in a CD1-restricted fashion.[31] Because expression of CD1 proteins is a prominent feature of LCs and DDCs, it could be hypothesized that cutaneous immunosurveillance also includes the sensitization of resident epidermal T cells to skin-specific pathogens via skin-associated APCs. Another line of thought postulates that TCR$\alpha\beta$+CD8+ epidermal T cells represent potentially autoreactive cells.[119] In unperturbed skin, they would be kept in a state of anergy towards self-antigens by immature DCs (LCs) and nonprofessional APCs (keratinocytes). After the delivery of danger signals, keratinocytes and LCs would express costimulatory molecules and could conceivably activate these epidermal T cells. Although attractive, this concept still awaits experimental proof.

The theory that the pool of intraepidermal memory cells would derive from and be continuously replenished by primed T cells recruited from the peripheral blood to the skin is mainly based on studies with the MAb HECA-452. This antibody reacts with 10 to 20 percent of peripheral blood T cells exhibiting the memory cell phenotype, with the vast majority of skin-infiltrating T cells in cutaneous sites of chronic inflammation, with more than half of epidermal T cells of normal human skin (see above), but with relatively few T cells in extracutaneous inflammatory sites.[116,120] Cell attachment experiments have shown that memory T cells, but not naive T cells, adhere to E-selectin+ endothelial cells and that the HECA-452+ T cell subset is the predominant E-selectin–binding population among circulating lymphocytes. The further observations that E-selectin is preferentially expressed on endothelial cells of venules in inflammatory skin lesions and that these venules are associated with a predominantly HECA-452+ T cell infiltrate suggest that, in inflamed skin, the interaction between CLA and E-selectin is of critical importance for the adhesion and, finally, transmigration of memory T cells to/through the dermal microvasculature. The question still remains as to which mechanism is operative in T cell homing to clinically normal skin. The possibility exists that, even at sites of only subclinical inflammation, E-selectin expression is induced on dermal microvascular endothelial cells in quantities sufficient for trapping CLA-bearing memory T cells.

Leukocytes and nonleukocytes residing in the skin can produce chemokines with T cell chemotactic properties such as IL-8, GR0 α, IP-10, monokine-induced by interferon-γ (Mig), MCP-1, 2, 3, RANTES (regulated on activation, normal T cell expressed and secreted), MIP-1α, MIP-1β, and lymphotactin. Of particular importance for the homing of CLA+ T cells to the skin, at least under inflamed conditions, appears to be the CC chemokine CCL27/CTACK.[15] It is produced by basal keratinocytes and is also displayed on the surface of dermal endothelial cells. Its expression is upregulated by IL-1β and TNF-α and downregulated by glucocorticoids. The receptor for CCL27, CCR10, is expressed on CLA+ T cells, and in vivo experiments have demonstrated a pivotal role for CCL27–CCR10 interactions in T cell-mediated skin inflammation.[121]

The recruitment of CLA-expressing type 2 (T_H2) T cells into the skin, as apparently happens in atopic dermatitis, can also be mediated by thymus and activation-regulated chemokine (TARC). This CC chemokine is expressed in basal keratinocytes of atopic dermatitis lesions and attracts CLA+ T cells by binding and signaling to CCR4 expressed on those cells.[122]

Adhesion molecule interactions that help to anchor T cells in the epidermis include the attachment of LFA-1 (CD11a)-bearing T cells to ICAM-1 (CD54)+ keratinocytes in inflamed skin and, more physiologically, the $\alpha_E\beta_7$–E-cadherin–mediated binding of T cells to nonactivated keratinocytes.

With regard to the factors responsible for the survival and/or expansion of human epidermal cells, it appears that analogous to the mouse system, IL-7 and IL-15 play important roles in these processes. Both T cell growth factors can be produced by human epidermal cells, and both are overexpressed in the T cell-rich skin lesions of patients with tuberculoid leprosy.

Despite the large preponderance of memory cells, small numbers of CD45 RA+/RO– T cells also exist in normal human skin. Little is known about their functional repertoire and about the mechanisms governing their influx into the skin. The homing of CCR7-expressing naive T cells to secondary lymphoid organs is known to occur via so-called high endothelial venules (HEVs). The attachment of naive T cells to HEV is mediated by the interaction of lymphocyte L-selectin and so-called peripheral node addressins defined by the MAb MECA-79. The actual transmigration and attraction of the cells into the nodes is accomplished by the CCR7 ligands CCL21/SLC and CCL19/MIP-3β/ELC.

MECA-79–reactive endothelial cells have been detected in the perifollicular areas of chronically inflamed skin and, to a much lesser extent, in normal human skin.[123] It is possible, therefore, to speculate that the presence of HEV-like vessels allows for a minor influx of naive T cells into the skin under steady-state conditions and that this process can be amplified when conventional migratory pathways of lymph node-primed T memory cells do not sufficiently eliminate the pathogen.

SYNOPSIS (Fig. 23-8)

Evidence presented in this chapter demonstrates that the skin is both a physical barrier between the host and the environment as well as an immunologic gatekeeper destined to optimally serve the needs of the host.

On recognition of "danger" signals (e.g., microbial invasion) by receptors of the innate immune system, a cascade of cellular and molecular events is initiated that allows dendritic APCs (LCs, DDCs)

FIGURE 23-8

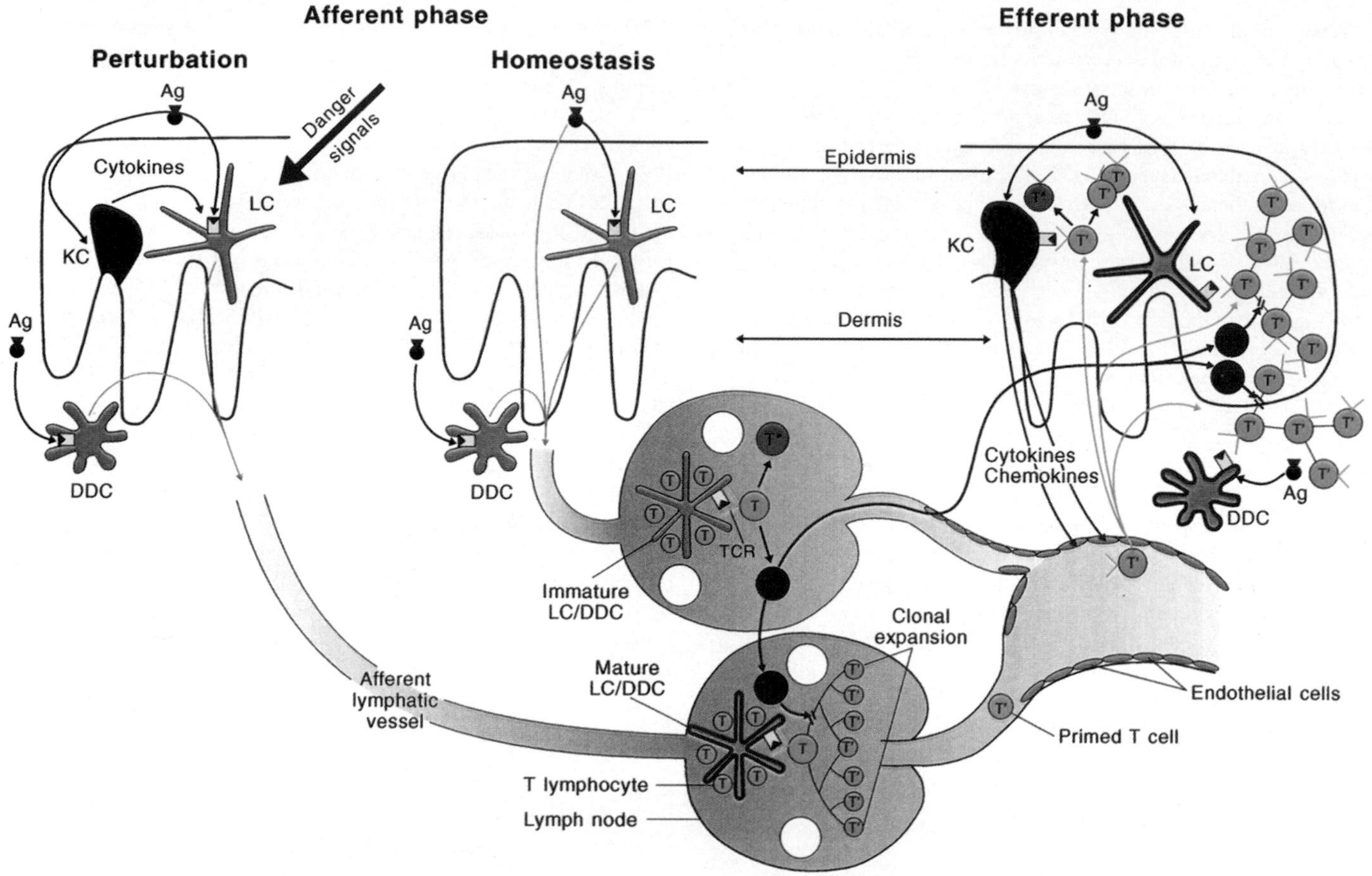

The mechanisms operative in the initiation, expression, and downregulation of cutaneous immune responses.

Induction of productive T cell immunity via the skin: The epi-and/or intracutaneous de novo appearance of antigens (i.e., pathogens such as microorganisms and haptens) results in the elicitation of productive antigen-specific immunity when "danger signals" (i.e., DNA rich in CpG repeats in microbacteria, Toll-like receptor ligands, etc.) are present at the time of antigenic exposure. The receipt of danger signals leads to tissue perturbation as evidenced by the increased secretion of GM-CSF, TNF-α, and IL-1 by KCs and other skin cells. Antigen-presenting cells (LCs, DDCs) that pick up the antigen, process it, and reexpress it as a peptide/MHC complex on the surface are also profoundly affected by danger signals or danger signal-induced cytokines. The alterations of LCs/DDCs include the increased expression of MHC antigens, costimulatory molecules, and cytokines (IL-1β, IL-6, IL-12), as well as the enhanced emigration of these cells from the skin to the paracortical areas of the draining lymph nodes. At this site, the skin-derived dendritic cells provide activation stimuli to naive resting T cells surrounding them. This occurs in an antigen-specific fashion and, thus, results in the expansion of the respective clone(s). These primed T cells begin to express skin homing receptors (e.g., cutaneous lymphocyte-associated antigen) as well as receptors for various chemoattractants that promote their attachment to dermal microvascular endothelial cells of inflamed skin and, ultimately, their entry into this tissue.

Elicitation of T cell-mediated tissue inflammation and pathogen defense: On receipt of a renewed antigenic stimulus by cutaneous antigen-presenting cells (LCs, DDCs), the skin-homing primed T cells expand locally and display the effector functions needed for the elimination or, at least, the attack of the pathogen. Alternatively, primed T cells may encounter the antigen on the surface of nonprofessional antigen-presenting cells (e.g., MHC class II-bearing KCs), a situation that conceivably results in a state of clonal T cell anergy.

Downregulation and prevention of cutaneous T cell immunity: In the absence of danger signals (tissue homeostasis), antigen-loaded LCs/DDCs also leave the cutaneous compartment and migrate towards the draining lymph node. These cells or, alternatively, resident lymph node dendritic cells that had picked up antigenic moieties from afferent lymphatics present this antigen in a nonproductive fashion; that is, induce antigen-specific T cell unresponsiveness or allow the responding T cell(s) to differentiate into immunosuppressive T regulatory cells. The latter may limit antigen-driven clonal T cell expansion during primary immune reactions in lymph nodes and during secondary immune reactions at the level of the peripheral tissue. Such events can result in the downregulation of both desired (antitumor, antimicrobial) and undesired (hapten-specific, autoreactive) immune responses. Ag, antigen; DDC, dermal dendritic cell; KC, keratinocyte; LC, Langerhans cell; T, T cell (naive); T′, primed T cell; T*, anergic T cell; TCR, T cell receptor; Treg, T regulatory cell.

to pick up and process the antigens, to emigrate from the skin, and to terminally (i.e., irreversibly) mature into extremely potent immunostimulatory cells. On arrival in the secondary lymphoid organs, they trigger pathogen-specific protective immune responses in naive, resting lymphocytes. T cell blasts generated in skin-draining peripheral lymph nodes, but not those originating from other lymphoid tissues, begin to express skin-specific homing receptors such as CLA. The interaction with corresponding addressins on cytokine-activated endothelial cells of the dermal microvasculature allows these cells to find their way back to the site harboring the pathogen, which, under optimal circumstances, would then be neutralized or eliminated.

In other situations (steady-state conditions, UV irradiation, application of immunosuppressive compounds), LC/DDC activation fails to occur. Such immunologically immature DCs and perhaps also other, nonprofessional APCs (e.g., keratinocytes, fibroblasts) will deliver signals directly or indirectly to silence T cells.

It thus appears that the components of skin-associated lymphoid tissues[124] (i.e., dendritic APCs, cytokine-producing keratinocytes, and skin-homing T cells originating in skin-draining peripheral lymph nodes) can subserve a dual function. On the one hand, they provide the skin with unique immune surveillance mechanisms for the successful prevention of or combat against cancer and infectious diseases. On the other hand, they secure the homeostasis of the integument by preventing the development of exaggerated, tissue-destructive immune responses against per se innocuous moieties such as autoantigens and allergens.

REFERENCES

1. Langerhans P: Über die Nerven der menschlichen Haut. *Virchows Arch* **44**:325, 1868
2. Cerio R et al: Characterization of factor XIIIa positive dermal dendritic cells in normal and inflamed skin. *Br J Dermatol* **121**:421, 1989
3. Banchereau J, Steinman RM: Dendritic cells and the control of immunity. *Nature* **392**:245, 1998
4. Wolff K: The Langerhans cell, in *Current Problems in Dermatology*, vol IV. Basel, Karger, 1972, p 79. Editor: J.W.H. Mali, Nijmegen, the Netherlands
5. Mizumoto N et al: CD39 is the dominant Langerhans cell-associated ecto-NTPDase: Modulatory roles in inflammation and immune responsiveness. *Nat Med* **8**:358, 2002
6. Birbeck M et al: An electron microscope study of basal melanocytes and high-level clear cells (Langerhans cells) in vitiligo. *J Invest Dermatol* **37**:51, 1961
7. Valladeau J et al: Langerin, a novel C-type lectin specific to Langerhans cells, is an endocytic receptor that induces the formation of Birbeck granules. *Immunity* **12**:71, 2000
8. Katz SI et al: Epidermal Langerhans cells are derived from cells originating in bone marrow. *Nature* **282**:324, 1979
9. Caux C et al: GM-CSF and TNF-α cooperate in the generation of dendritic Langerhans cells. *Nature* **360**:258, 1992
10. Caux C et al: CD34+ hematopoietic progenitors from human cord blood differentiate along two independent dendritic cell pathways in response to GM-CSF + TNF-α. *J Exp Med* **184**:695, 1996
11. Strobl H et al: TGF-β1 promotes in vitro development of dendritic cells from CD34+ hemopoietic progenitors. *J Immunol* **157**:1499, 1996
12. Jaksits S et al: CD34+ cell-derived CD14+ precursor cells develop into Langerhans cells in a transforming growth factor β1-dependent manner. *J Immunol* **163**:4869, 1999
13. Larregina AT et al: Dermal-resident CD14+ cells differentiate into Langerhans cells. *Nat Immunol* **2**:1151, 2001
14. Charbonnier A-S et al: Macrophage inflammatory protein 3α is involved in the constitutive trafficking of epidermal Langerhans cells. *J Exp Med* **190**:1755, 1999
15. Morales J et al: CTACK, a skin-associated chemokine that preferentially attracts skin-homing memory T cells. *Proc Natl Acad Sci U S A* **96**:14470, 1999
16. Homey B et al: Cutting edge: the orphan chemokine receptor G protein-coupled receptor-2 (GPR-2, CCR10) binds the skin-associated chemokine CCL27 (CTACK/ALP/ILC). *J Immunol* **164**:3465, 2000
17. Tang A et al: Adhesion of epidermal Langerhans cells to keratinocytes mediated by E-cadherin. *Nature* **361**:82, 1993
18. Matzinger P: Tolerance, danger, and the extended family. *Annu Rev Immunol* **12**:991, 1994
19. Hawiger D et al: Dendritic cells induce peripheral T cell unresponsiveness under steady state conditions in vivo. *J Exp Med* **194**:769, 2001
20. Schuler G, Steinman RM: Murine epidermal Langerhans cells mature into potent immunostimulatory dendritic cells in vitro. *J Exp Med* **161**:526, 1985
21. Weiss JM et al: Osteopontin is involved in the initiation of cutaneous contact hypersensitivity by inducing Langerhans and dendritic cell migration to lymph nodes. *J Exp Med* **194**:1219, 2001
22. Kriehuber E et al: Isolation and characterization of dermal lymphatic and blood endothelial cells reveal stable and functionally specialized cell lineages. *J Exp Med* **194**:797, 2001
23. Ingulli E et al: In vivo detection of dendritic cell antigen presentation to CD4+ T cells. *J Exp Med* **185**:2133, 1997
24. Wang J et al: Inherited human caspase 10 mutations underlie defective lymphocyte and dendritic cell apoptosis in autoimmune lymphoproliferative syndrome type II. *Cell* **98**:47, 1999
25. Medzhitov R, Janeway CA Jr: Innate immunity: Impact on the adaptive immune response. *Curr Opin Immunol* **9**:4, 1997

26. Davis MM et al: Ligand recognition by $\alpha\beta$ T cell receptors. *Annu Rev Immunol* **16**:523, 1998
27. Germain RN, Margulies DH: The biochemistry and cell biology of antigen processing and presentation. *Annu Rev Immunol* **11**:403, 1993
28. Pamer E, Cresswell P: Mechanisms of MHC class I-restricted antigen processing. *Annu Rev Immunol* **16**:323, 1998
29. Huang AYC et al: Role of bone marrow-derived cells in presenting MHC class I-restricted tumor antigens. *Science* **264**:961, 1994
30. Watts C: Capture and processing of exogenous antigens for presentation on MHC molecules. *Annu Rev Immunol* **15**:821, 1997
31. Porcelli SA, Modlin RL: The CD1 system: Antigen-presenting molecules for T cell recognition of lipids and glycolipids. *Annu Rev Immunol* **17**:297, 1999
32. Toews GB et al: Epidermal Langerhans cell density determines whether contact hypersensitivity or unresponsiveness follows skin painting with DNFB. *J Immunol* **124**:445, 1980
33. Stingl G et al: Antigen presentation by murine epidermal Langerhans cells and its alteration by ultraviolet B light. *J Immunol* **127**:1707, 1981
34. Inaba K et al: Immunologic properties of purified epidermal Langerhans cells. Distinct requirements for stimulation of unprimed and sensitized T lymphocytes. *J Exp Med* **164**:605, 1986
35. Hauser C, Katz SI: Activation and expansion of hapten- and protein-specific T helper cells from nonsensitized mice. *Proc Natl Acad Sci U S A* **85**:5625, 1988
36. Romani N et al: Presentation of exogenous protein antigens by dendritic cells to T cell clones. Intact protein is presented best by immature, epidermal Langerhans cells. *J Exp Med* **169**:1169, 1989
37. Mueller DL et al: Clonal expansion versus functional clonal inactivation: A costimulatory signaling pathway determines the outcome of T cell antigen receptor occupancy. *Annu Rev Immunol* **7**:445, 1989
38. Greenfield EA et al: CD28/B7 costimulation: A review. *Crit Rev Immunol* **18**:389, 1998
39. van Parijs L, Abbas AK : Homeostasis and self-tolerance in the immune system: Turning lymphocytes off. *Science* **280**:243, 1998
40. Rescigno M et al: Coordinated events during bacteria-induced DC maturation. *Immunol Today* **20**:200, 1999
41. Sauter B et al: Consequences of cell death: exposure to necrotic tumor cells, but not primary tissue cells or apoptotic cells, induces the maturation of immunostimulatory dendritic cells. *J Exp Med* **191**:423, 2000
42. Akira S et al: Toll-like receptors: critical proteins linking innate and acquired immunity. *Nat Immunol* **2**:675, 2001
43. Hemmi H et al: Small anti-viral compounds activate immune cells via the TLR7 MyD88-dependent signaling pathway. *Nat Immunol* **3**:196, 2002
44. Silberberg-Sinakin I et al: Antigen-bearing Langerhans cells in skin, dermal lymphatics and in lymph nodes. *Cell Immunol* **25**:137, 1976
45. Weiss JM et al: An essential role for CD44 variant isoforms in epidermal Langerhans cell and blood dendritic cell function. *J Cell Biol* **137**:1137, 1997
46. Engeman TM et al: Inhibition of functional T cell priming and contact hypersensitivity responses by treatment with anti-secondary lymphoid chemokine antibody during hapten sensitization. *J Immunol* **164**:5207, 2000
47. Stoeckl J et al: Monomorphic molecules function as additional recognition structures on haptenated target cells for HLA-A1-restricted, hapten-specific CTL. *J Immunol* **167**:2724, 2001
48. Enk AH, Katz SI: Early molecular events in the induction phase of contact sensitivity. *Proc Natl Acad Sci U S A* **89**:1398, 1992
49. de Saint-Vis B et al: The cytokine profile expressed by human dendritic cells is dependent on cell subtype and mode of activation. *J Immunol* **160**:1666, 1998
50. Abbas AK et al: Functional diversity of helper T lymphocytes. *Nature* **383**:787, 1996
51. Fè d'Ostiani C et al: Dendritic cells discriminate between yeasts and hyphae of the fungus *Candida albicans*. Implications for initiation of T helper cell immunity in vitro and in vivo. *J Exp Med* **191**:1661, 2000
52. Kalinski P et al: Final maturation of dendritic cells is associated with impaired responsiveness to IFN-γ and to bacterial IL-12 inducers: Decreased ability of mature dendritic cells to produce IL-12 during the interaction with Th cells. *J Immunol* **162**:3231, 1999
53. Dong H et al: B7-H1, a third member of the B7 family, costimulates T-cell proliferation and interleukin-10 secretion. *Nat Med* **5**:1365, 1999

54. Xu H et al: T cell populations primed by hapten sensitization in contact sensitivity are distinguished by polarized patterns of cytokine production: interferon γ-producing (Tc1) effector CD8+ T cells and interleukin (IL) 4/IL-10-producing (Th2) negative regulatory CD4+ T cells. *J Exp Med* **183**:1001, 1996
55. Ridge JP et al: A conditioned dendritic cell can be a temporal bridge between a CD4+ T-helper and a T-killer cell. *Nature* **393**:474, 1998
56. Grabbe S et al: Tumor antigen presentation by murine epidermal cells. *J Immunol* **146**:3656, 1991
57. Condon C et al: DNA-based immunization by in vivo transfection of dendritic cells. *Nat Med* **2**:1122, 1996
58. Steinman RM, Dhodapkar M: Active immunization against cancer with dendritic cells: The near future. *Int J Cancer* **94**:459, 2001
59. Steinbrink K et al: Low zone tolerance to contact allergens in mice: A functional role for CD8+ T helper type 2 cells. *J Exp Med* **183**:759, 1996
60. Shevach EM et al: Control of T-cell activation by CD4+ CD25+ suppressor T cells. *Immunol Rev* **182**:58, 2001
61. Jonuleit H et al: Induction of interleukin 10-producing, nonproliferating CD4+ T cells with regulatory properties by repetitive stimulation with allogeneic immature human dendritic cells. *J Exp Med* **192**:1213, 2000
62. Shreedhar VK et al: Origin and characteristics of ultraviolet-B radiation-induced suppressor T lymphocytes. *J Immunol* **161**:1327, 1998
63. Cavani A et al: Effector and regulatory T cells in allergic contact dermatitis. *Trends Immunol* **22**:118, 2001
64. Wollenberg A et al: Langerhans cell phenotyping: a new tool for differential diagnosis of inflammatory skin diseases. *Lancet* **346**:1626, 1995
65. Stingl G, Maurer D: IgE-mediated allergen presentation via FcεRI on antigen-presenting cells. *Int Arch Allergy Immunol* **113**:24, 1997
66. Kraft S, Bieber T: FcεRI-mediated activation of transcription factors in antigen-presenting cells. *Int Arch Allergy Immunol* **125**:9, 2001
67. Tschachler E et al: Epidermal Langerhans cells—A target for HTLV-III/LAV infection. *J Invest Dermatol* **88**:233, 1987
68. Kawamura T et al: Low levels of productive HIV infection in Langerhans cell-like dendritic cells differentiated in the presence of TGF-β1 and increased viral replication with CD40 ligand-induced maturation. *Eur J Immunol* **31**:360, 2001
69. Pope M et al: Conjugates of dendritic cells and memory T lymphocytes from skin facilitate productive infection with HIV-1. *Cell* **78**:389, 1994
70. Geijtenbeek TBH et al: DC-SIGN, a dendritic cell-specific HIV-1-binding protein that enhances *trans*-infection of T cells. *Cell* **100**:587, 2000
71. Woods GM et al: Carcinogen-modified dendritic cells induce immunosuppression by incomplete T-cell activation resulting from impaired antigen uptake and reduced CD86 expression. *Immunology* **99**:16, 2000
72. Kripke ML: Photoimmunology. *Photochem Photobiol* **52**:919, 1990
73. Cruz PD Jr et al: Disparate effects of in vitro low-dose UVB irradiation on intravenous immunization with purified epidermal cell subpopulations for the induction of contact hypersensitivity. *J Invest Dermatol* **92**:160, 1989
74. Kripke ML et al: Pyrimidine dimers in DNA initiate systemic immunosuppression in UV-irradiated mice. *Proc Natl Acad Sci U S A* **89**:7516, 1992
75. Vink AA et al: The inhibition of antigen-presenting activity of dendritic cells resulting from UV irradiation of murine skin is restored by in vitro photorepair of cyclobutane pyrimidine dimers. *Proc Natl Acad Sci U S A* **94**:5255, 1997
76. Schwarz A et al: Interleukin-12 suppresses ultraviolet radiation-induced apoptosis by inducing DNA repair. *Nat Cell Biol* **4**:26, 2002
77. Enk AH et al: Induction of hapten-specific tolerance by interleukin 10 in vivo. *J Exp Med* **179**:1397, 1994
78. Beissert S et al: Regulation of tumor antigen presentation by urocanic acid. *J Immunol* **159**:92, 1997
79. Hammerberg C et al: Active induction of unresponsiveness (tolerance) to DNFB by in vivo ultraviolet-exposed epidermal cells is dependent upon infiltrating class II MHC+ CD11b bright monocytic/macrophagic cells. *J Immunol* **153**:4915, 1994
80. Aberer W et al: Ultraviolet light depletes surface markers of Langerhans cells. *J Invest Dermatol* **76**:202, 1981
81. Hosoi J et al: Regulation of Langerhans cell function by nerves containing calcitonin gene–related peptide. *Nature* **363**:159, 1993
82. Kupper TS, Groves RW: The interleukin-1 axis and cutaneous inflammation. *J Invest Dermatol* **105**:62S, 1995
83. Cerwenka A, Swain SL: TGF-β1: Immunosuppressant and viability factor for T lymphocytes. *Microbes Infect* **1**:1291, 1999
84. Schroeder J-M: Cytokine networks in the skin. *J Invest Dermatol* **105**:20S, 1995
85. Enk AH, Katz SI: Identification and induction of keratinocyte-derived IL-10. *J Immunol* **149**:92, 1992
86. Blauvelt A et al: Interleukin-15 mRNA is expressed by human keratinocytes, Langerhans cells, and blood-derived dendritic cells and is downregulated by ultraviolet B radiation. *J Invest Dermatol* **106**:1047, 1996
87. Stoll S et al: Production of IL-18 (IFN-γ–inducing factor) messenger RNA and functional protein by murine keratinocytes. *J Immunol* **159**:298, 1997
88. Koeck A et al: Human keratinocytes are a source for tumor necrosis factor α: Evidence for synthesis and release upon stimulation with endotoxin or ultraviolet light. *J Exp Med* **172**:1609, 1990
89. Fenjves ES et al: Systemic distribution of apolipoprotein E secreted by grafts of epidermal keratinocytes: implications for epidermal function and gene therapy. *Proc Natl Acad Sci U S A* **86**:8803, 1989
90. Reiss Y et al: CC chemokine receptor (CCR)4 and the CCR10 ligand cutaneous T cell- attracting chemokine (CTACK) in lymphocyte trafficking to inflamed skin. *J Exp Med* **194**:1541, 2001
91. Schauer E et al: Proopiomelanocortin-derived peptides are synthesized and released by human keratinocytes. *J Clin Invest* **93**:2258, 1994
92. Grabbe S et al: α-Melanocyte–stimulating hormone induces hapten-specific tolerance in mice. *J Immunol* **156**:473, 1996
93. Risso A: Leukocyte antimicrobial peptides: Multifunctional effector molecules of innate immunity. *J Leukoc Biol* **68**:785, 2000
94. Frohm M et al: The expression of the gene coding for the antibacterial peptide LL-37 is induced in human keratinocytes during inflammatory disorders. *J Biol Chem* **272**:15258, 1997
95. Harder J et al: Isolation and characterization of human β–defensin-3, a novel human inducible peptide antibiotic. *J Biol Chem* **276**:5707, 2001
96. Dorschner RA et al: Cutaneous injury induces the release of cathelicidin anti-microbial peptides active against group A *Streptococcus*. *J Invest Dermatol* **117**:91, 2001
97. Nizet V et al: Innate antimicrobial peptide protects the skin from invasive bacterial infection. *Nature* **414**:454, 2001
98. Yang D et al: β-Defensins: linking innate and adaptive immunity through dendritic and T cell CCR6. *Science* **286**:525, 1999
99. Darr D, Fridovich I: Free radicals in cutaneous biology. *J Invest Dermatol* **102**:671, 1994
100. Bruch-Gerharz D et al: Nitric oxide in human skin: Current status and future prospects. *J Invest Dermatol* **110**:1, 1998
101. Freedberg IM et al: Keratins and the keratinocyte activation cycle. *J Invest Dermatol* **116**:633, 2001
102. Kaegi D et al: Molecular mechanisms of lymphocyte-mediated cytotoxicity and their role in immunological protection and pathogenesis in vivo. *Annu Rev Immunol* **14**:207, 1996
103. Chan FK-M et al: Signaling by the TNF receptor superfamily and T cell homeostasis. *Immunity* **13**:419, 2000
104. Kehren J et al: Cytotoxicity is mandatory for CD8+ T cell-mediated contact hypersensitivity. *J Exp Med* **189**:779, 1999
105. Viard I et al: Inhibition of toxic epidermal necrolysis by blockade of CD95 with human intravenous immunoglobulin. *Science* **282**:490, 1998
106. Volc-Platzer B et al: Evidence of HLA-DR antigen biosynthesis by human keratinocytes in disease. *J Exp Med* **159**:1784, 1984
107. Gaspari AA, Katz SI: Induction and functional characterization of class II MHC (Ia) antigens on murine keratinocytes. *J Immunol* **140**:2956, 1988
108. Bal V et al: Antigen presentation by keratinocytes induces tolerance in human T cells. *Eur J Immunol* **20**:1893, 1990
109. Marelli-Berg FM et al: Antigen presentation by epithelial cells induces anergic immunoregulatory CD45RO+ T cells and deletion of CD45RA+ T cells. *J Immunol* **159**:5853, 1997
110. Clevers H et al: The T cell receptor/CD3 complex: A dynamic protein ensemble. *Annu Rev Immunol* **6**:629, 1988
111. Hayday AC: $\gamma\delta$ Cells: A right time and a right place for a conserved third way of protection. *Annu Rev Immunol* **18**:975, 2000
112. Stingl G et al: Thy-1+ dendritic epidermal cells express T3 antigen and the T-cell receptor chain. *Proc Natl Acad Sci U S A* **84**:4586, 1987
113. Havran WL, Allison JP: Origin of Thy-1+ dendritic epidermal cells of adult mice from fetal thymic precursors. *Nature* **344**:68, 1990

114. Foster CA et al: Human epidermal T cells predominately belong to the lineage expressing α/β T cell receptor. *J Exp Med* **171**:997, 1990
115. Bos JD et al: T-cell receptor $\gamma\delta$ bearing cells in normal human skin. *J Invest Dermatol* **94**:37, 1990
116. Bos JD et al: Skin-homing T lymphocytes: Detection of cutaneous lymphocyte-associated antigen (CLA) by HECA-452 in normal human skin. *Arch Dermatol Res* **285**:179, 1993
117. Levings MK et al: Human CD25+ CD4+ T regulatory cells suppress naive and memory T cell proliferation and can be expanded in vitro without loss of function. *J Exp Med* **193**:1295, 2001
118. Groh V et al: Double-negative (CD4– CD8–) lymphocytes bearing T-cell receptor α and β chains in normal human skin. *Proc Natl Acad Sci U S A* **86**:5059, 1989
119. Shiohara T, Moriya N: Epidermal T cells: Their functional role and disease relevance for dermatologists. *J Invest Dermatol* **109**:271, 1997

120. Picker LJ et al: A unique phenotype of skin-associated lymphocytes in humans. Preferential expression of the HECA-452 epitope by benign and malignant T cells at cutaneous sites. *Am J Pathol* **136**:1053, 1990
121. Homey B et al: CCL27-CCR10 interactions regulate T cell-mediated skin inflammation. *Nat Med* **8**:157, 2002
122. Vestergaard C et al: A Th2 chemokine, TARC, produced by keratinocytes may recruit CLA+CCR4+ lymphocytes into lesional atopic dermatitis skin. *J Invest Dermatol* **115**:640, 2000
123. Lechleitner S et al: Peripheral lymph node addressins are expressed on skin endothelial cells. *J Invest Dermatol* **113**:410, 1999
124. Streilein JW: Skin-associated lymphoid tissues (SALT): Origins and functions. *J Invest Dermatol* **80**:12S, 1983

CHAPTER 24

Madeleine Duvic

Influence of the HLA System on Disease Susceptibility

ORIGINS AND STRUCTURE OF HLA

In 1948, Gorer and coworkers found that rejection of tissue transplants between two incompatible members of the same species is caused by an immunologic reaction against "histocompatibility" antigens expressed on the surface of cells.[1] In humans, the major histocompatibility complex (MHC) or human leukocyte antigen (HLA) system is highly polymorphic; that is, each gene can have many variations or alleles. Human MHC is found on chromosome 6p21, where it extends over about 4000 kilobases of DNA[2] (Fig. 24-1). Antigens A, B, and C were defined by antibody reactivity from sera of multiparous women, and D was initially defined by lymphocyte cross reactivity. The C locus is located between A and B, and D lies on the other side of B. The genes for the fourth component of complement were localized between those for HLA-B and HLA-D. Class I, II, and III genes are usually inherited as a genetic unit, the haplotype. A haplotype consists of the complete set of A, B, C, and D (-DR, -DQ, and -DP) antigens present on one chromosome, but in approximately 1 percent of the population genetic recombination (crossover) occurs.[2] Each person expresses two antigens (alleles) for each locus (A, B, C, D), and each parent has two haplotypes. The child inherits (according to Mendelian laws) one haplotype from each parent.

Class I HLA antigens (A, B, C) are 43- to 45-kDa cell surface glycoproteins with three external domains that complex with a smaller β_2-microglobulin encoded by a gene on chromosome 19. Class I antigens are expressed on all nucleated cells but not on red blood cells. Several other nonclassical MHC class I–like, or class Ib, genes encode nonpolymorphic molecules: CD1, the neonatal Fc receptor for IgG, HLA-G, HLA-E, the MHC class I chain–related gene A, and Hfe.[3]

Class II genes (D) encode surface B cell alloantigens or Ia antigens expressed only on immunocompetent cells: B lymphocytes, macrophages, dendritic cells, and Langerhans cells. Three major subregions of class II are HLA-DR, -DQ, and -DP. Class II molecules present antigens to the T cell receptors on helper (CD4+) T cells.[4] Both immune response and immune suppression genes are thought to exist in the D region.

The class III region contains complement genes and genes for the tumor necrosis factors. Class III genes encode the C2 and C4 components of the classical complement pathway and factor B (Bf) of the alternate complement pathway.[5] Tumor necrosis factor (alpha and beta) and the steroid hormone 21-hydroxylase are in this region.

FIGURE 24-1

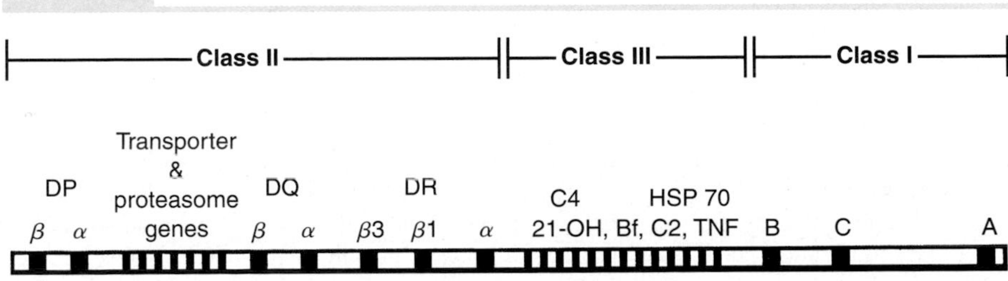

A simplified map of the major histocompatibility complex on the short arm (p) of chromosome 6. Only genes encoding a known protein product are shown, and class I and II genes are given special attention.

The Trimolecular Complex

The trimolecular complex or immunologic synapse is composed of the antigen-presenting cell expressing the HLA molecules, antigen, and the T cell receptor (TCR).[6] Antigen-presenting cells contain proteolytic enzymes that process proteins and transporter-associated proteins (TAPs) to load peptides onto the appropriate class I or class II MHC chain within the endoplasmic reticulum (see Figs. 24-2 and 28-3). Small polypeptides of 8 or 9 amino acids or 12 to 15 amino acids bind to MHC class I or class II molecules and are presented to CD8+ or CD4+ T cells, respectively. TCR is a heterodimer consisting of an α and β chain, each containing a variable and constant region. The presence or absence of costimulatory molecules (B7, CD28) on T cells and antigen-presenting cells is also critical in determining whether a T cell becomes activated or remains quiet (tolerance).[6,7] TCRs occur solely on T cell surfaces and recognize antigen fragments only when they are bound to MHC molecules from an identical source.[7] Thus, T cells are largely responsible for the control of self versus non-self differentiation.

HLA AND DISEASE ASSOCIATIONS

Autoreactive helper T cells are involved in the onset and maintenance of autoimmune disease. Environmental injury (toxin, viral disease, or bacterial pathogen) may trigger autoimmunity by providing antigen that mimics a host protein (molecular mimicry).[8] HLA antigens control which peptides are ultimately seen by T cells and thereby may be a major disease determinant for immunologically mediated diseases. HLA and other genetic factors are termed *susceptibility genes* as they modify the risk of getting a disease but are neither necessary nor sufficient for it to develop. For most autoimmune skin diseases, HLA-DQ genes are the primary susceptibility genes in this region, although other genes may contribute.

In addition to traditional antigen presentation, specific sequences on HLA chains can link superantigens to the TCR, resulting in T cell proliferation.[9] With respect to skin diseases, γ-interferon can induce keratinocytes to express HLA class II molecules, in turn, activating T cells in the presence of superantigens.[10] Several skin diseases, including Kawasaki's disease, atopic dermatitis/eczema, psoriasis, and cutaneous T cell lymphoma (CTCL), are thought to be initiated or exacerbated by streptococcal or staphylococcal bacterial superantigens. Superantigens bypass the need for antigen processing but depend on specific amino acids for binding to HLA class II molecules.

Certain HLA alleles are more common among different ethnic groups, and they are inherited together as a common haplotype. Thus, connections between disease incidence and frequency of HLA alleles often differ by race or ethnicity. In some cases, however, the same epitopes that cause susceptibility may be carried on other haplotypes. In studying HLA frequency in a disease, the control group must be composed of healthy, unrelated persons and must coincide with the disease group for ethnic lineage and geographic area of residence. A quantitative measure of the strength of an association between a given disease and an HLA antigen is called the *relative risk* (RR). The RR represents a measure of the risk of contracting a disease for an individual who possesses the antigen in question, as compared to the risk for an individual lacking that antigen (see footnote to Table 24-1 for calculation of RR).

The first HLA disease associations in humans related to cancer—nasopharyngeal carcinoma and the antigen HLA-Bw46 (formerly Singapore 2). This antigen is found only in those areas of Asia where nasopharyngeal carcinoma is comparatively common. (In antigen designations that include a w, such as Bw46, the w indicates a working status; the antigen has not been completely or officially acknowledged internationally.) In the Japanese and black Africans, in whom B27 is rare, ankylosing spondylitis is also rare, whereas in North American Indians, in whom B27 is common, ankylosing spondylitis is also common.[11]

TABLE 24-1

HLA Alleles and Dermatologic Disease Associations

Disease	Allele	Relative Risk*
Psoriasis	DR406	21.6
	Cw6	7.0
Psoriatic arthritis	B27	
	B39	
	DQw3	
Dermatitis herpetiformis	DQw2	Infinity
	DR3	68.6
Systemic lupus erythematosus	C4A*Q0 with DR2	24.9
	DR2	1.70
	DR3	2.65
	DQA0501	
Systemic sclerosis	DQA2	
	C4A*Q0	
Pemphigus vulgaris	Dw10/DR4	31.9
	DRB1*0402	
	Dw10	26.7
	DR4	14.60
	DRw6 (DR14)	
Pemphigus foliaceus	DRB1*0102	7.3
Alopecia areata	DR4	2.8
	DRB1*1104	16.5
	DQB1*0301	12.0
	DQB1*03	12.14
Lichen planus	DR6 (w/HepC)	4.9
	DR1	3.68
	DR10	8.27
	Bw61/DRw9	6.0
Behçet's syndrome	B51	9.3, 18.2
	B52	2.8
Epidermolysis bullosa acquisita	DR2 (black)	4.8
	DR2 (white)	13.1
Erythema multiforme (herpes-associated)	DQB1*0301	6.5
Mycosis fungoides	DR5 (DRw11)	4.4†
	DQB1*03	2.15†
Sézary syndrome	DQB1*0502	7.75†

*The RR is calculated in the following manner:

$$RR = \frac{\text{(patients antigen-positive)} \times \text{(controls antigen-negative)}}{\text{(patients antigen-negative)} \times \text{(controls antigen-positive)}}$$

The RR represents the measure of risk of developing a disease for an individual who possesses the HLA antigen in question, as compared to the risk for an individual lacking the antigen.
†Odds ratio.

A positive association of a gene with a disease can arise in one of two ways: (1) the associated polymorphism truly does have a pathogenic role in the disease, or (2) it is in linkage disequilibrium with a pathogenic mutation on another gene nearby. An individual's MHC ancestral haplotype is the clearest single determinant of susceptibility to MHC-associated immunopathologic diseases, and it defines the alleles carried at all loci in the MHC. There are 150 to 200 genes in the MHC, but their direct effect in causing disease is difficult to determine because recombination occurs only at defined hot spots.[12]

Because HLA chain variable sequences are critical for peptide binding, there was an expectation that associated peptides could be isolated from the HLA groove and unlock the secret of autoimmune diseases. This has proven to be more difficult than expected. Furthermore, in the case of psoriasis, as noted below, HLA associations appear to result only from linkage disequilibrium with an unknown disease-causing gene. In this case, the polymorphic alleles of the HLA region served as the first genetic markers for finding disease-related genes through association and linkage studies. Table 24-1 outlines some published associations between HLA antigens with selected dermatologic diseases discussed below.

Psoriasis (See Chap. 42)

Psoriasis is a T cell–mediated immune reaction causing increased keratinocyte proliferation. Like type I diabetes, psoriasis is a complex genetic trait with major susceptibility conferred by the HLA locus and an environmental trigger.[13] Psoriasis was first associated with HLA class I alleles and subsequently with the extended HLA haplotype: HLA-DR4, -DR7, -DQw7, -DQw9, -DP15, and -DP18.[14] The RR for Cw6 in all forms of psoriasis is only 7.0, whereas for HLA-DR*406 it is 21.6.[15] The sequences of DR4 subtypes show a unique serine substitution for tyrosine at position 37 in DR406 that may influence the configuration of the HLA groove and peptide binding.[16]

Type I or early onset psoriasis is associated with the HLA-Cw6, allele Cw*0602, found in up to 67 percent of patients with psoriasis. Psoriasis develops in only about 10 percent of HLA-Cw6-positive individuals.[13,14] Guttate psoriasis can be triggered by group A β-hemolytic streptococcus superantigen.[17] All patients with guttate psoriasis have the HLA-Cw*602 allele, in contrast to 20 percent of controls having the allele, suggesting an important and highly significant relationship (odds ratio = infinity; 95 percent confidence limits 25.00-infinity; P corrected < 0.0000002).[18]

Recent studies suggest that Cw6 is not the disease-conferring gene; rather, it is found on a common inherited ancestral haplotype in linkage disequilibrium with a more closely linked putative disease-causing gene PSORS1.[13] The psoriasis gene resides within a 111-kb interval telomeric to HLA-C and centromeric to the corneodesmosin gene.[19] Several genes, including corneodesmosin (S-gene) and HCR, have been excluded, and the OTF3 polymorphism may confer susceptibility independent of HLA-Cw*602.[13,19–22] Psoriasis susceptibility loci have also been mapped to other chromosomes.[14,23,24]

Approximately 5 to 7 percent of patients with psoriasis also have psoriatic arthritis, and genetic heterogeneity is suggested. HLA-B38 and -B39 are increased in those whose peripheral joints are affected, but these antigens are not in linkage with HLA-Cw6. Although the strong association between ankylosing spondylitis and B27 is widely known, HLA-B27 also is found among 50 percent of patients with psoriasis who have arthritis of the spine (sacroiliitis or spondylitis). Antigens B27, B39, and DQw3 have also been shown to be risk factors for (and important predictors of) progression of psoriatic arthritis. Pustular forms of psoriasis also have a strong association with HLA-B27 (56 to 75 percent of patients versus 8 percent of normal control subjects) but not with Cw6, B13, B17, or B37. An increased frequency of HLA-DRB1*0402 is found in psoriasis patients with rheumatoid arthritis (RA)-like arthritis.[25] Thus, these patients differ, clinically and genetically, from those having psoriasis vulgaris limited to the skin.[26]

Vasculitis (See Chaps. 174 and 175)

Vasculitis, a heterogeneous group of disorders, is characterized by vessel type and size and composition of circulating immune complexes. Various genes, including the MHC, gender, and environmental factors may account for differences in clinical presentation.[27] In giant cell arteritis, HLA-DRB1*04 alleles are associated with risk of ominous visual complications. Takayasu's arteritis, involving the aorta and coronary arteries, occurs in Japan in association with the haplotype HLA-Bw52, Dw12, DRB2, and DQw1.[27] In Kawasaki's disease, a polymorphism of the MHC class I chain-related gene (MICA), located near HLA-B, is associated with susceptibility to coronary aneurysm formation.[28]

There are no clear-cut HLA associations to distinguish primary systemic vasculitides involving medium to small vessels: polyarteritis nodosa (PAN), microscopic polyangiitis, Wegener's granulomatosis (WG), and Churg-Strauss syndrome (CSS). WG is associated with HLA-DR1, DR2, and HLA-DQw7.[28] An HLA class I deficiency has been reported in a few patients with destructive granuloma in the respiratory mucosa resembling WG who were found to have defective expression of the TAP-2, an HLA locus gene.[29]

Small vessel vasculitis includes Henoch-Schönlein purpura (HSP), hypersensitivity vasculitis, cutaneous leukocytoclastic angiitis (CLA), and vasculitis secondary to essential mixed cryoglobulinemia. Patients with HSP may have deficiencies in the second and fourth components of complement, including C4 gene deletion. Associations with HLA-B35, HLA-DRB1*01, and DRB1*11 have been described.[30] HLA-DRB1*11 is associated with hepatitis C–associated cryoglobulinemia with vasculitis.[31]

Behçet's Syndrome (See Chap. 192)

Behçet's syndrome is characterized by severe uveitis, aphthae-like lesions of the mouth and genitalia, arthritis, and diffuse vasculitis. The etiology is unknown, but there is a strong association with HLA-B51, which suggests a genetic basis. The disorder is prevalent in males in the Near and Far East. Arber et al. found that HLA-B51 and -B52 were present in 24 of 38 (63 percent) Jews and 8 of 38 (21 percent) Arabs in Israel, as compared with 13 of 151 (9 percent) control subjects (RR = 18.2 and 2.8, respectively).[32] B51 antigen has 21 alleles, B*5101–B*5121.[33] Although HLA-B*5101 and HLA-B*5108 are increased in Italian and Arab patients, HLA-B*5101 is most highly significant in Japanese patients (RR = 9.3).[33,34] In Chinese patients, DQ alleles associated with mucocutaneous disease distinguished Behçet's syndrome from recurrent aphthous stomatitis.[35]

What is the significance of the B51 association? Excessive function of peripheral blood neutrophils in Behçet's syndrome has been related to B51. Behçet's syndrome is found only in B51 suballeles sharing amino acid residues at positions 63 and 67 and positions 77 to 83 for specific peptide binding and natural killer (NK) cell interactions.[34] Finally, a non-HLA gene carried on the HLA-B*5101 haplotype may be responsible for susceptibility to Behçet's syndrome.[36]

Sarcoidosis (See Chap. 183)

Sarcoidosis, a systemic noncascating granulomatous disorder of unknown etiology, affects skin as well as other organs. Sarcoid is associated with HLA-A1, -B8, and -DR3 in European patients. HLA alleles are associated with specific clinical features: HLA-B27 with lung disease, HLA-B13 and -B35 with early onset, and HLA-DR3 with good outcome. HLA may interact with immunoglobulin to influence severity of the disease. One cluster, HLA-DR4, C4BQ0, Gm (1, 3, 17 23 5*, 21, 28), and BfF, is associated with stage II sarcoidosis, and another, HLA-DR3, C4AQ0, κ_m (1) and Gm (3 23 5*), is associated with stage I disease.[37]

In multiplex families, multipoint nonparametric linkage (NPL) analysis showed linkage (NPL score > 2.5; $P < 0.006$) for the entire MHC region with a maximum NPL score of 3.2 ($P = 0.0008$) at marker locus D6S1666 in the class III gene cluster.[38] Lung-restricted expansions of T cells with a specific T cell receptor are associated with HLA-DRB1*0301 (DR17) and -DRB3*0101 alleles, suggesting the presence of a specific antigen triggering sarcoidosis.[39]

Bullous or Blistering Diseases

The bullous diseases have a humoral response to distinct adhesion molecules in epidermis or dermoepidermal basement membrane zone.

Autoreactive T cells play a role in antibody production and are HLA restricted.

PEMPHIGUS VULGARIS AND FOLIACEUS (See Chap. 59) Pemphigus vulgaris (PV) is a potentially fatal autoimmune blistering disease, more common in Jewish persons in the fourth or fifth decades. Susceptibility to PV is associated with HLA-DR4 serologic specificity among Ashkenazi Jews, and with DR4 (DRB1*0402) as well as DR6 (DR14) in linkage disequilibrium with DQB1*0503 in other ethnic groups.[40] Serum from patients with PV has autoantibodies against desmoglein 3 (Dsg3), whereas pemphigus foliaceus (PF) is characterized by more superficial ulcerations and by autoantibodies to desmoglein 1. Nine Japanese patients with PV and five of seven patients with PF carried one or two alleles of HLA-DRB1*04 (*0403, *0406) and HLA-DRB1*14 (*1401, *1405, *1406) subtypes. Sequence analysis of DRB1*04 and DRB1*14 alleles showed conservation of phenylalanine at position 26 and valine at position 86 with the DRB1*0402 allele that reportedly also confers a strong susceptibility to PV in Ashkenazi Jews.[41]

In a study of 87 Italian patients with PV and PF, DRB1*04 and DRB1*14 were increased, while DRB1*07 was decreased in both groups of patients relative to control subjects.[42] A significant association was found between DRB1*1401 and PV ($P < 0.0001$) as well as PF ($P < 0.0001$) in addition to a significant increase of the linked DQB1*0503 (PV $P < 0.0001$; PF $P < 0.0001$). The association between DRB1*0402 and PV ($P < 0.0001$) has been confirmed; and furthermore, PV and PF share DRB1*1401 and DQB1*0503, as susceptible HLA alleles, whereas DRB1*0402 is found to be associated only with PV.

Three groups of Brazilian patients with fogo selvagem (FS) carried DRB1*0404, *1402, or *1406 ($P < 0.005$, RR = 14). These share the same amino acid sequence at positions 67 to 74 on the third hypervariable region of the DRB1 gene, LLEQRRAA, suggesting that inheritance of this epitope is involved in the susceptibility to FS ($P < 0.00001$, RR = 6.4). Because both PV and PF carry the same susceptible HLA alleles, the explanation for differences in the diseases are not yet known and are hypothesized to reside in other genes or in environmental exposure. The HLA alleles associated with drug-triggered pemphigus are identical to those predisposing to idiopathic pemphigus, suggesting that HLA alleles may be true disease susceptibility genes in pemphigus. Of interest, healthy unaffected relatives with the same HLA types as affected patients with pemphigus may also have pemphigus autoantibodies.[43]

Pemphigoid gestationis (see Chap. 64) is a rare autoimmune vesiculobullous disease associated with pregnancy that is closely related to the pemphigoid group of blistering disorders. It is characterized by linear deposition of C3 along the basement membrane zone (BMZ) of perilesional skin. The disease may be triggered by inappropriate expression of HLA on the placenta, presenting antigen that cross-reacts with skin. DR3 and DR4 class II are associated with pemphigoid gestationis.[44]

BULLOUS PEMPHIGOID (See Chap. 61) In mucous membrane pemphigoid (MMP) circulating IgA or IgG antibodies detect BMZ antigens (BP230 and BP180). The HLA-DQB1*0301 allele confers a predisposition to all subgroups of MMP. DQB1*0301 is increased in patients with detectable circulating anti-BMZ IgG compared with those negative for IgG ($P < 0.0096$, P corrected < 0.019) but not for the subgroups with or without BP180 or BP230 target antigens. Haplotype frequencies show an increase in DRB1*04, DQB1*0301 (P corrected < 0.000066) and DRB1*11, DQB1*0301 (P corrected < 0.000002) among patients when compared with controls.[45]

ERYTHEMA MULTIFORME (See Chap. 58) Erythema multiforme (EM) includes EM minor, EM major (Stevens-Johnson syndrome), and toxic epidermal necrolysis (TEN). Autoantibodies against the desmosomal proteins desmoplakin I and II are detected in patients with EM defining clinical subsets. There is an increased frequency of certain HLA antigens reported in association with EM, including HLA-B15(B62), HLA-B35, HLA-A33, HLA-DR53, and, more recently, HLA-DQB1*0301.[46] Recurrent EM in young adults follows recurrent herpes simplex where it is highly associated with the DQB1*0301 allele (RR = 6.5; $P < 0.001$).[47]

Certain HLA-DQB1 alleles may also be related to severity of mucous membrane or ocular involvement. Of 21 patients with herpes-associated EM, 13 had only minor or no involvement of mucous membranes and carried the HLA allele DQB1*0302 (phenotype frequency 61.9 percent versus 18.8 percent in controls, P corrected = 0.0008). All three patients with major involvement of mucous membranes had the rare HLA allele DQB1*0402 (phenotype frequency in controls 6.4 percent, P corrected = 0.017).[47] In another study, HLA-DQB1*0601, but not DQB1*0302, was found in a significantly disproportionate number of white patients with Stevens-Johnson syndrome and ocular complications.[48]

DERMATITIS HERPETIFORMIS (See Chap. 67) Dermatitis herpetiformis (DH), an autoimmune blistering disease in which granular IgA is deposited at the dermal–epidermal junction, is associated with gluten-sensitive enteropathy or celiac disease. HLA-DR3 is expressed in 95 percent and HLA-DQw2 in 100 percent of patients with DH.[49] Both DH and celiac disease are strictly associated with class II HLA alleles A1*0501 and B1*02 encoding the HLA-DQ2 heterodimer.[50] Both are most highly associated with HLA DRB1*0301 (91 percent versus 22 percent of controls), HLA DQB1*02 (100 percent versus 32 percent of controls), and DPB1*0101 (39 percent and 14 percent). All patients with DH are positive for the DQA1*0501/DQB1*02 dimer in *cis* or *trans,* and this is probably responsible for presenting gliadin peptide implicated in the disease process.[50] HLA-DQw2 sequences in patients with DH do not differ from those in normal HLA-DQw2 subjects.

Patients with celiac disease are homozygous for DR2 in contrast to patients with DH (65 percent versus 39 percent). Differences in dosage of HLA class II genotypes between DH and celiac disease may explain the milder gastrointestinal symptoms characteristic of DH.[51] There may be interactions between a specific DQ molecule and one of several different DPB1 alleles that contribute to susceptibility to the intestinal lesion that is common to DH and celiac disease. Sex differences have been found with regard to HLA DQ2 susceptibility in females.[51]

The ancestral haplotype 8.1 (HLA-A1, C7, B8, C4AQ0, C4B1, DR3, DQ2) is carried by most whites with HLA-B8 and contains the tumor necrosis factor allele polymorphism TNF2.[52] This haplotype is also associated with accelerated HIV disease and susceptibility to insulin-dependent diabetes mellitus (IDDM), systemic lupus erythematosus (SLE), common variable immunodeficiency, IgA deficiency, myasthenia gravis, and several other conditions.[17]

EPIDERMOLYSIS BULLOSA (See Chap. 65) Epidermolysis bullosa (EB) has many variations caused by mutations in the components of the anchoring fibrils and BMZ proteins. In a small study, patients with recessive dystrophic EB had higher gene frequencies of haplotypes HLA-Bw62, HLA-DR4, DQw3, and HLA-Bw60, DR4, DQ3 than expected.[53]

EPIDERMOLYSIS BULLOSA ACQUISITA (See Chap. 66) Epidermolysis bullosa acquisita (EBA) and bullous SLE both have circulating IgG autoantibodies that react with type VII collagen molecules in anchoring fibrils.[54] HLA-DR2 is significantly increased in both black and white patients with EBA, and in patients with bullous SLE.[54]

SYSTEMIC LUPUS ERYTHEMATOSUS (See Chap. 171) Susceptibility to SLE is governed by a number of genes in the HLA region.[55] In whites, the association between the haplotype carrying HLA-B8, HLA-DR3, C4A gene deletion and tumor necrosis factor α (TNFα)–308A, the polymorphic variant of TNF-α, is well described.[55,56] In Native Americans, DQ4 and DR8 are associated with SLE; and B7, DR2, and DQ6 are associated with SLE in Asians. In a large study of minority populations with lupus, HLA-DRB1*0301 (DR3), DRB1*1503 (DR2), and DRB1*08 (DR8) alleles were more frequently found in whites, African Americans, and Hispanics, respectively. Hispanics were more likely to have cardiac and renal disease; African Americans were more likely to have neurologic and renal disease. Patients with HLA-DRB1*01 had less renal disease. Disease severity was associated with poor socioeconomic status, suggesting that both genetic and environmental factors govern the presentation of SLE.[56]

As many as 100 other genes may participate in SLE pathogenesis, and the contribution of the MHC is weak with a RR of 2 to 3.[57] Complete deficiency of one of the early complement components is the strongest known genetic risk factor for SLE. When the homozygous C4A null phenotype and HLA-DR2 are both present, the RR for SLE is 24.9. Davies et al.[56] found that the strongest association with SLE was for the combination of DQA*0501 and C4A*QO. Both DQA*0501 ($P =$ 0.02) and C4A*QO ($P = 0.03$) seemed to have significant individual effects on SLE susceptibility, with a significant statistical interaction between the two loci ($P = 0.01$). Distinguishing between the effects of null genes for C4 and HLA-DR3 has been difficult due to marked linkage disequilibrium between DR3 and a null allele of C4A (C4A QO) in white populations.

In patients who were negative for the anti-La antibody, only C4A*QO had a significant individual effect, although a significant statistical interaction between DQA*0501 and C4A*QO was again detected. These results suggest that susceptibility to SLE is related to several genes with different roles; HLA-DQA*0501 may affect autoantibodies, while C4A*QO may be implicated in immune complex clearance.[56]

Autoantibodies to nucleic acids as well as proteins have been reported in the sera of patients with SLE (Table 24-2). The presence of particular autoantibodies or clinical manifestations are more highly correlated with specific HLA alleles in both SLE and systemic sclerosis than is the development of the disease per se.[57]

SYSTEMIC SCLEROSIS (See Chap. 173) Scleroderma [systemic sclerosis (SSc)] is an autoimmune disease with fibrosis of the skin and internal organs. A large study of 202 patients with SSc and with well-defined clinical phenotypes and serologic typing for the presence of disease-specific autoantibodies showed strong associations between the clinical phenotype and the presence of specific autoantibodies.[58] Antitopoisomerase autoantibody (ATA) was associated with pulmonary fibrosis ($P = 0.00002$), the anti-RNA polymerase autoantibody (ARA) with renal involvement ($P = 0.0000006$) and diffuse skin disease ($P = 0.00001$), and the anticentromere autoantibody (ACA) with limited skin involvement ($P = 0.00002$) and protection against pulmonary fibrosis ($P =$ 0.0000003). HLA-DPB1*1301 was significantly associated with the ATA (P corrected $=$ 0.0001). In addition, ATA was associated with HLA-DRB1*11 and the ACA with HLA-DRB1*04, HLA-DRB1*08 ($P = 0.001$) and HLA-DQB1 alleles with a glycine residue at position 26.

HLA-DQB1*0301 is significantly associated with SSc per se in all ethnic groups. Whites were likely to have more ACA and African Americans more anti-U1-ribonucleoprotein (RNP) and anti-U3-RNP (fibrillarin) autoantibodies. HLA-DRB1*11 correlated with the anti-topoisomerase I antibody response, and HLA-DRB1*01, DRB1*04, and DQB1*0501 with ACA.[59] The frequency of antibodies to fibrillin differs among ethnic groups but is not associated with HLA alleles.

TABLE 24-2

HLA-Determined Autoantibody Associations*

Disease	Autoantibody	HLA Alleles
Systemic lupus erythematosus	Anti-Ro (SS-A)	HLA-DQA1,-DQB1
	Anti-La (SS-B)	HLA-DQA1,-DQB1
	Anti-phospholipids	HLA-DQB1
	Anti-Sm	HLA-DQA1*0102, -DQB1*0602
	Anti-nRNP	HLA-DQA1*0101, -DQB1*0501,
	Anti-dsDNA	HLA-DQB1*0201, *0602,0302
	Anti-EBA	HLA-DR2
Systemic sclerosis	Anticentromere	HLA-DQB1*0301, *0501,0402
	Anti-Topo I	HLA-DQB1*0301, *0302,*0602
	Anti-PM-Sci	HLA-DQB1*0201, (linked DR3)
	Anti-U1-RNP	HLA-DR4
	Anti-U3-RNP (fibrillarin)	HLA-DQB1*0602, *0604

*See Fig. 24-2.
SOURCE: SLE: from Arnett and Reveille,[90] with permission; SSc: from Arnett,[88] with permission.

FIGURE 24-2

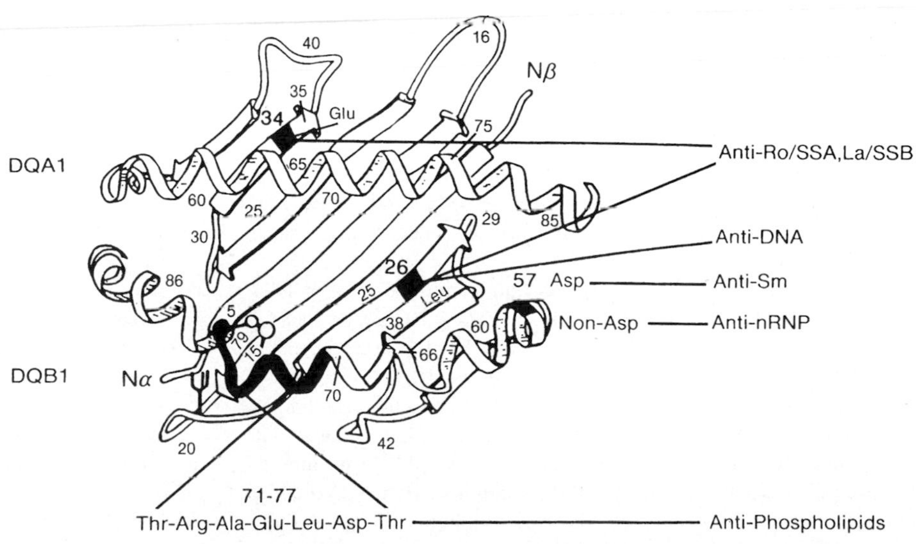

Representation of class II MHC structure for HLA-DQ molecules. Numbers indicate outermost domain amino acid positions encoded by HLA-DQA1 and -DQB1 alleles. Specific amino acid positions showing the strongest associations with selected lupus autoantibodies are highlighted. (*From Arnett and Reveille,*[90] *with permission.*)

Class II antigens may influence the ability of the immune system to generate a response to intracellular autoantigens such as ATA to which it is not tolerized.[59]

Previous studies have shown associations of DRB1 alleles with SSc but have rarely determined DQA1 allele frequencies. The DQA1*0501 allele is significantly increased among men with SSc as compared to healthy men [odds ratio (OR) 2.3, $P = 0.006$, P corrected $= 0.04$]. DQA1*0501 is associated with diffuse SSc in men (OR 3.0, $P = 0.004$, P corrected $= 0.03$) but not with limited SSc in men. DRB1 associations may be due to linkage disequilibrium with DQA1. The contribution of HLA genes to the risk of SSc appears to be greater in men than in parous women.[60]

Lichen sclerosis et atrophicus and morphea are both considered as localized variants of scleroderma with distinct presentations and occasional *Borrelia burgdorferi* infection. In a small case series, five of seven patients with lichen sclerosis and morphea had HLA-DQ7.[61,62]

LICHEN PLANUS (See Chap. 49) Lichen planus (LP) is a T cell–mediated immune response similar to graft-versus-host disease. HLA alleles may vary depending on the cutaneous manifestations and with the presence of hepatitis C virus. Across ethnic groups, there appear to be no uniform HLA associations with LP. In Israeli Jewish patients with oral erosive LP, there was a significant association with HLA-DR2 (RR = 4.7) and a decrease in DR4 (RR = 0.3).[63] Arab patients with cutaneous LP had significant increases in the frequencies of HLA-DR1 (RR = 3.68) and DR10 (RR = 8.27).[64] Among 42 Japanese patients with oral LP, the frequency of DRw9 was significantly increased (RR = 3.3), and when DRw9 was carried on a Bw61/DRw9 haplotype, the RR was increased to 6.0.[65] In white British patients, HLA-Bw57 appeared to predispose a person to oral LP, whereas HLA-DQ1 seemed to be associated with resistance to it.[66]

Patients with exclusive oral LP and hepatitis C virus infection possess the HLA-DR6 allele more frequently than patients with exclusive oral LP without hepatitis C virus infection (52 percent versus 18 percent, respectively; P corrected $= 0.028$, RR = 4.93).[67]

ALOPECIA AREATA (See Chap. 71) Alopecia areata (AA) is an organ-specific autoimmune reaction with T cells targeted to the hair follicle and phenotypic heterogeneity with progression to complete hair loss (alopecia totalis and universalis). In a study of identical twins, there was 55 percent concordancy, similar to psoriasis, which suggests that both genetic and environmental factors play a role.[68]

Class I HLA associations for AA include HLA-B12 (RR = 5.4) for patchy AA, and HLA-B18, -B13, and -B27.[69] In 88 white Americans with AA, HLA-DR4 and -DR5 were increased relative to controls, and DRB3-w52a was significantly reduced ($P = 0.00001$).[70] The DR5 (DRw11) subtype DRB*1104 is significantly associated with persistent AA and juvenile onset.[71]

DR5 associations reflect linkage disequilibrium with DQ alleles. Class II HLA-DQB1*03 alleles (*0301, *0302, or *0303) are found in 80 percent of all white patients with AA (n = 85) and in 92 percent of the subset with alopecia totalis or alopecia universalis (P corrected $=$ 0.00003) (RR = 12).[71] DQB1*03 alleles are thought to participate directly in the pathogenesis of AA by binding peptides that initiate the immune response. These alleles all have a proline at position 55 that may interact in forming salt bridges between HLA-DQ α and β heterodimers and stabilizing the HLA heterodimers.[71]

In a cohort of Turkish patients with AA, the frequencies of HLA-A1, HLA-B62 (B15), HLA-DQ1, and HLA-DQ3 were significantly higher than those in control subjects, while HLA-DR16 was less frequent. Juvenile and severe involvement were related to HLA-Cw6 and HLA-DR1, respectively.[72]

To confirm association studies in unrelated patients with AA, transmission dissociation testing and linkage were performed in AA multiplex families.[73] There is a significant association between AA and alleles of HLA-DQB ($P = 0.009$) and HLA-DR ($P = 0.008$). In particular, DQB1*302 ($P = 0.0002$), DQB1*601 ($P = 0.041$), DQB*603 ($P = 0.027$), HLA-DR4 ($P = 0.005$), and HLA-DR6 ($P = 0.005$) are associated with AA in families. Linkage between AA and class II loci is supported with a maximal logarithm of odds (LOD) score of 2.42 to HLA-DQ at 5 percent recombination and 2.34 to HLA-DR at 0 percent recombination.

VITILIGO (See Chap. 90) Vitiligo is seen in association with other autoimmune diseases and after treatment of melanoma; it is mediated by skin-homing CD8+ lymphocytes. In Italians, HLA-BfS, -C4A3, -C4B1, -DR5, and -DQW3 characterize the early onset form of vitiligo, while HLA-BfS, -C4A3, -C4B1, -DR7, and -DQw2 distinguish the adult form.[74] Vitiligo may have an autosomal dominant pattern of inheritance with linkage to HLA alleles affecting the age of onset.

In a family-based case-control association study, linkage and association of the DRB4*0101 allele were found with vitiligo (P corrected $= 0.0016$, RR = 2.21). Evidence for linkage and association of the DQB1*0303 allele was found ($\chi^2 = 7.36$, $P = 0.006$). The DRB4*0101/0101 genotype carries a 3.58 percent risk of developing vitiligo. Both DRB4*0101 and DQB1*0303 alleles provide significant susceptibility for vitiligo.[75]

Skin Cancer

MALIGNANT MELANOMA (See Chap. 93) Antitumor immune responses to melanoma-associated antigens involves HLA antigen presentation, which is vital for developing vaccines and other immunotherapies. HLA associations in malignant melanoma have been correlated with response to immunotherapy and with disease progression. HLA-A2 class I associations were first reported and correlated with melanoma antigens (MARTs) and with peptides derived from tyrosinase.[76] Melanoma predominantly affects whites, a population in whom expression of HLA-A2 is prevalent. Among HLA-A2 subtypes, HLA-A*0201 is widely expressed; and HLA-A*0201-restricted, tumor-reactive cytotoxic T lymphocyte responses have been studied extensively.[77] Non-HLA-A*0201 subtypes (*0202, *0204, and *0205) may also be found in patients with melanoma who show responses to different peptide antigens. Specific peptides of tyrosinase, Ty 56-70 and Ty 448-462, which are HLA-DRB1*0401 restricted, are recognized by CD4+ T cells. Other tyrosinase antigens are also HLA-A2 restricted and may elicit a CD8+ T cell tumor necrosis factor response.

For all patients, Lee et al. showed that HLA-DQB1*0301 is associated with an increased risk for cutaneous melanoma.[78] HLA-DQ1 was recently associated with clinical response and with prolonged survival in patients treated with interleukin 2 immunotherapy.[79] In Japanese individuals, HLA-B13 is increased in patients with melanoma compared with control subjects and is particularly common in nodular melanoma, whereas HLA-B61 is decreased in patients with melanoma. Almost 50 percent of patients with acral lentiginous melanomas express HLA-B51, which is not found in any patients with nodular melanomas.[80]

The importance of lower expression of HLA-A and HLA-B antigens on melanomas and its mechanisms are controversial.[81] About 15 percent of melanomas studied have deletions in or loss of chromosome 6p and consequently do not express HLA antigens, which could increase their selective survival.[82] Defective TAP could also lead to lower HLA expression on melanomas.[83]

NONMELANOMA SKIN CANCER (See Chaps. 80 and 81) Data for HLA associations with nonmelanoma skin cancers (basal cell and squamous cell carcinomas) are from immunosuppressed and renal transplant patients at increased risk for squamous cell cancer. HLA-DR1 is increased in nonimmunosuppressed patients who are younger than 60 years old and have multiple squamous cancers.[84] Bouwes Bavinck et al. found a significant negative association between HLA-11 and skin cancer (RR = 0.05) in one study and an increased risk (RR = 1.7) in a second study.[85] HLA-B27 is associated with the development of basal cell carcinomas.[86]

CUTANEOUS T CELL LYMPHOMA (See Chap. 157) Mycosis fungoides (MF) and its leukemic variant, Sézary syndrome, are the most common variants of CTCL. HLA-DR5 was initially reported to be associated with MF. HLA-DQB1*03 alleles linked to DR5 are more significantly associated with MF.[87] The strongest association for MF is between DQB1*0502 and Sézary syndrome (odds ratio = 7.75).[87]

SIGNIFICANCE

Histocompatibility antigens play a critical role in determining the type of response a host can raise to a particular peptide antigen, whether self-antigen, viral antigen, or superantigen. HLA chains bind antigen for presentation to T cells, with HLA class I being important for CD8+ activation and HLA class II being important for CD4+ helper T cells. The details of these interactions and epitopes or sequences of the HLA chains and the peptides have yet to be clarified in most skin diseases. T cells are also important in evoking humoral or antibody responses. HLA alleles are significantly associated with specific autoantibody responses rather than with the disease.[88]

The allelic polymorphisms of the HLA antigens are useful markers for other disease susceptibility genes, even when they are not themselves disease enabling. HLA alleles confer susceptibility underlying immune or autoimmune skin reactions, and may influence time of onset, severity, or sex predilection. In the future, knowledge of an individual's HLA type could be invaluable to prevent autoimmune skin diseases, especially when recognized trigger factors or viral infections call for immediate therapeutic intervention. Understanding the immune response at the molecular level offers the possibility of blocking the reaction by anti-idiotypic antibodies, DNA vaccines, or peptides that bind to specific areas of the receptors.[89]

REFERENCES

1. Benacerraf B, Rock KL: The significance of MHC restriction, in *Major Histocompatibility System: The Gorer Symposium,* edited by P Medawar, T Lehner. London, Blackwell Scientific, 1985, p 16
2. Dupont B: The HLA system: An introduction, in *The HLA System: A New Approach,* edited by J Lee. New York, Springer-Verlag, 1990, p 1
3. Blumberg RS et al: The multiple roles of major histocompatibility complex class I-like molecules in mucosal immune function. *Acta Odontol Scand* **59**:139, 2001
4. Kumar V, Sercarz E: An integrative model of regulation centered on recognition of TCR peptide/MHC complexes. *Immunol Rev* **182**:113, 2001
5. Moulds JM: Ethnic diversity of class III genes in autoimmune disease. *Front Biosci* **6**:D986, 2001
6. Bromley SK et al: The immunological synapse and CD28–CD80 interactions. *Nat Immunol* **2**:1159, 2001
7. Rudolph MG et al: Crystal structure of an isolated V(alpha) domain of the 2C T-cell receptor. *J Mol Biol* **314**:1, 2001
8. Mackay IR, Rosen FS: Autoimmune diseases. *N Engl J Med* **345**:345, 2001
9. Janeway CA: Are there cellular superantigens? *Immun Rev* **131**:189, 1993
10. Strange P et al: Interferon gamma treated keratinocytes activate T cells in the presence of superantigens: Involvement of major histocompatibility complex class II molecules. *J Invest Dermatol* **102**:150, 1994
11. Reveille JD et al: HLA-B27 and genetic predisposing factors in spondyloarthropathies. *Curr Opin Rheumatol* **13**:265, 2001
12. Price P et al: The genetic basis for the association of the 8.1 ancestral haplotype (A1, B8, DR3) with multiple immunopathological diseases. *Immunol Rev* **167**:257, 1999
13. Elder JT et al: The genetics of psoriasis 2001: The odyssey continues. *Arch Dermatol* **137**:1447, 2001
14. Barker JN: Genetic aspects of psoriasis. *Clin Exp Dermatol* **26**:321, 2001
15. Harrison P et al: Association of HLA-antigens with psoriasis. *J Invest Dermatol* **98**:557A, 1992
16. Hall JR, Arnett FC: The HLA system and cutaneous diseases, in *Immunologic Diseases of the Skin,* edited by RE Jordon. Norwalk, CT, Appleton & Lange, 1991, p 101
17. Leung DY et al: Evidence for a streptococcal superantigen-driven process in acute guttate psoriasis. *J Clin Invest* **96**:2106, 1995
18. Mallon E et al: HLA-C and guttate psoriasis. *Br J Dermatol* **143**:1177, 2000
19. Oka A et al: Association analysis using refined microsatellite markers localizes a susceptibility locus for psoriasis vulgaris within a 111-kb segment telomeric to the HLA-C gene. *Hum Mol Genet* **8**:2165, 1999
20. O'Brien KP et al: The HCR gene on 6p21 is unlikely to be a psoriasis susceptibility gene. *J Invest Dermatol* **116**:750, 2001
21. Gonzalez S et al: The OTF3 gene polymorphism confers susceptibility to psoriasis independent of the association of HLA-Cw*0602. *J Invest Dermatol* **115**:824, 2000
22. Enerback C et al: Stronger association with HLA-Cw6 than with corneodesmosin (S-gene) polymorphisms in Swedish psoriasis patients. *Arch Dermatol Res* **292**:525, 2000
23. Bowcock AM et al: Insights into psoriasis and other inflammatory diseases from large-scale gene expression studies. *Hum Mol Genet* **10**:1793, 2001
24. Lee YA et al: Genomewide scan in German families reveals evidence for a novel psoriasis-susceptibility locus on chromosome 19p13. *Am J Hum Genet* **67**:1020, 2000
25. Gladman DD et al: HLA-DRB1*04 alleles in psoriatic arthritis: Comparison with rheumatoid arthritis and healthy controls. *Hum Immunol* **62**:1239, 2001
26. Barton AC et al: Genetic studies of psoriatic arthritis: Dissecting joints and skin. *J Rheumatol* **28**:3, 2001
27. Gonzalez-Gay MA, Garcia-Porrua C: Epidemiology of the vasculitides. *Rheum Dis Clin North Am* **27**:1, 2001
28. Huang Y et al: Polymorphism of transmembrane region of MICA gene and Kawasaki disease. *Exp Clin Immunogenet* **17**:130, 2000
29. Hauser C: Granulomatous disease associated with HLA class I deficiency. *Br J Dermatol* **144**:901, 2001
30. Amoli MM et al: HLA-DRB*01 association with Henoch-Schönlein purpura in patients from northwest Spain. *J Rheumatol* **28**:1266, 2001
31. Cacoub P et al: HLA-DR phenotypes influence the risk of hepatitis C virus-associated mixed cryoglobulinemia. *Arthritis Rheum* **43**(suppl):S1911, 2000
32. Arber N et al: Close association of HLA-B51 and B52 in Israeli patients with Behçet's syndrome. *Ann Rheum Dis* **50**:351, 1991
33. Mizuki N et al: HLA-B*51 allele analysis by the PCR-SBT method and a strong association of HLA-B*5101 with Japanese patients with Behçet's disease. *Tissue Antigens* **58**:181, 2001
34. Kotter I et al: Comparative analysis of the association of HLA-B*51 suballeles with Behçet's disease in patients of German and Turkish origin. *Tissue Antigens* **58**:166, 2001
35. Sun A et al: Some specific human leukocyte antigen (HLA)-DR/DQ haplotypes are more important than individual HLA-DR and -DQ phenotypes for the development of mucocutaneous type of Behçet's disease and for disease shift from recurrent aphthous stomatitis to mucocutaneous type of Behçet's disease. *J Oral Pathol Med* **30**:402, 2001
36. Gul A et al: Linkage mapping of a novel susceptibility locus for Behçet's disease to chromosome 6p22-23. *Arthritis Rheum* **44**:2693, 2001
37. Martinetti M et al: HLA-Gm/κm interaction in sarcoidosis. Suggestions for a complex genetic structure. *Eur Respir J* **16**:74, 2000
38. Schurmann M et al: Familial sarcoidosis is linked to the major histocompatibility complex region. *Am J Respir Crit Care Med* **162**:861, 2000
39. Grunewald J et al: Lung T-helper cells expressing T-cell receptor AV2S3 associate with clinical features of pulmonary sarcoidosis. *Am J Respir Crit Care Med* **161**:814, 2000
40. Scharf SJ et al: Specific HLA-DQB and HLA-DRB1 alleles confer susceptibility to pemphigus vulgaris. *Proc Natl Acad Sci U S A* **86**:6215, 1989
41. Miyagawa S et al: HLA-DRB1*04 and DRB1*14 alleles are associated with susceptibility to pemphigus among Japanese. *J Invest Dermatol* **109**:615, 1997

42. Lombardi ML et al: Common human leukocyte antigen alleles in pemphigus vulgaris and pemphigus foliaceus Italian patients. *J Invest Dermatol* **113**:107, 1999
43. Ahmed AR et al: Linkage of pemphigus vulgaris antibody to the major histocompatibility complex in healthy relatives of patients. *J Exp Med* **177**:419, 1993
44. Engineer L et al: Pemphigoid gestationis: A review. *Am J Obstet Gynecol* **183**:483, 2000
45. Setterfield J et al: Mucous membrane pemphigoid: HLA-DQB1*0301 is associated with all clinical sites of involvement and may be linked to antibasement membrane IgG production. *Br J Dermatol* **145**:406, 2001
46. Schofield JK et al: Recurrent erythema multiforme: Tissue typing in a large series of patients. *Br J Dermatol* **131**:532, 1994
47. Malo A et al: Recurrent herpes simplex virus-induced erythema multiforme: Different HLA-DQB1 alleles associate with severe mucous membrane versus skin attacks. *Scand J Immunol* **47**:408, 1998
48. Power WJ et al: HLA typing in patients with ocular manifestations of Stevens-Johnson syndrome. *Ophthalmology* **103**:1406, 1996
49. Hall RP et al: Alterations in HLA-DP and HLA-DQ antigen frequency in patients with dermatitis herpetiformis. *J Invest Dermatol* **93**:501, 1989
50. Spurkland A et al: Dermatitis herpetiformis and celiac disease are both primarily associated with the HLA-DQ (alpha 1*0501, beta 1*02) or the HLA-DQ (alpha 1*03, beta 1*0302) heterodimers. *Tissue Antigens* **49**:29, 1997
51. Holopainen P et al: Candidate gene regions and genetic heterogeneity in gluten sensitivity. *Gut* **48**:696, 2001
52. McManus R et al: TNF2, a polymorphism of the tumor necrosis-alpha gene promoter, is a component of the celiac disease major histocompatibility complex haplotype. *Eur J Immunol* **26**:2113, 1996
53. Vaidya S et al: HLA and epidermolysis bullosa. Association between the HLA complex and recessive dystrophic epidermolysis bullosa. *Arch Dermatol* **127**:1524, 1991
54. Gammon WR et al: Increased frequency of HLA-DR2 in patients with autoantibodies to epidermolysis bullosa acquisita antigen: Evidence that the expression of autoimmunity to type VII collagen is HLA class II allele associated. *J Invest Dermatol* **91**:228, 1988
55. Sullivan KE: Genetics of systemic lupus erythematosus. *Rheum Dis Clin North Am* **26**:229, 2000
56. Davies EJ et al: Relative contributions of HLA-DQA and complement C4A loci in determining susceptibility to systemic lupus erythematosus. *Br J Rheumatol* **34**:221, 1995
57. Tan FK, Arnett FC: The genetics of SLE. *Curr Opin Rheumatol* **10**:399, 1998
58. Gilchrist FC et al: Class II HLA associations with autoantibodies in scleroderma: A highly significant role for HLA-DP. *Genes Immun* **2**:76, 2001
59. Reveille JD et al: Systemic sclerosis in 3 US ethnic groups: A comparison of clinical, sociodemographic, serologic, and immunogenetic determinants. *Semin Arthritis Rheum* **30**:332, 2001
60. Lambert NC et al: HLA-DQA1*0501 is associated with diffuse systemic sclerosis in Caucasian men. *Arthritis Rheum* **43**:2005, 2000
61. Farrell AM et al: Genital lichen sclerosis associated with morphea or systemic sclerosis: Clinical and HLA characteristics. *Br J Dermatol* **143**:598, 2000
62. Azurdia RM et al: Lichen sclerosus in adult men: A study of HLA associations and susceptibility to autoimmune disease. *Br J Dermatol* **140**:79, 1999
63. Roitberg-Tambur et al: Serologic and molecular analysis of the HLA system in Israeli Jewish patients with oral erosive lichen planus. *Tissue Antigens* **43**:219, 1994
64. White AG, Rostom AI: HLA antigens in Arabs with lichen planus. *Clin Exp Dermatol* **19**:236, 1994
65. Watanabe T et al: Analysis of HLA antigens in Japanese with oral lichen planus. *J Oral Pathol Med* **15**:529, 1986
66. Porter K et al: Class I and II HLA antigens in British patients with oral lichen planus. *Oral Surg Oral Med Oral Pathol Oral Radiol Endod* **75**:176, 1993
67. Carrozzo M et al: Increased frequency of HLA-DR6 allele in Italian patients with hepatitis C virus-associated oral lichen planus. *Br J Dermatol* **144**:803, 2001
68. Jackow C et al: Alopecia areata and cytomegalovirus infection in twins: Genes versus environment. *J Am Acad Dermatol* **38**:418, 1998
69. Zhang L et al: HLA associations with alopecia areata. *Tissue Antigens* **38**:89, 1991
70. Duvic M et al: HLA-D locus associations in alopecia areata: DRw52 may confer disease resistance. *Arch Dermatol* **127**:64, 1991
71. Colombe BW et al: HLA class II antigen associations help to define two types of alopecia areata. *J Am Acad Dermatol* **33**:757, 1995
72. Kavak A et al: HLA in alopecia areata. *Int J Dermatol* **39**:589, 2000
73. de Andrade M et al: Alopecia areata in families: Association with the HLA locus. *J Invest Dermatol Symp Proc* **4**:220, 1999
74. Finco O et al: Age of onset in vitiligo: Relationship with HLA supratypes. *Clin Genet* **39**:48, 1991
75. Zamani M et al: Linkage and association of HLA class II genes with vitiligo in a Dutch population. *Br J Dermatol* **145**:90, 2001
76. Rivoltini L et al: Binding and presentation of peptides derived from melanoma antigens MART-1 and glycoprotein-100 by HLA-A2 subtypes: Implications for peptide-based immunotherapy. *J Immunol* **156**:3882, 1996
77. Anichini A et al: Cytotoxic T cells directed to tumor antigens not expressed on normal melanocytes dominate HLA-A2.1–restricted immune repertoire to melanoma. *J Immunol* **156**:208, 1996
78. Lee JE et al: HLA-DQB1*0301 association with increased cutaneous melanoma risk. *Int J Cancer* **59**:510, 1994
79. Brady MS et al: CD4(+) T cells kill HLA-class-II-antigen-positive melanoma cells presenting peptide in vitro. *Cancer Immunol Immunother* **48**:621, 2000
80. Ichimiya M et al: Putative linkage between HLA class I polymorphism and the susceptibility to malignant melanoma. *Australas J Dermatol* **37**(suppl 1):S39, 1996
81. Gasparollo A et al: Unbalanced Expression of HLA-A and -B antigens: A specific feature of cutaneous melanoma and other non-hemopoietic malignancies reverted by gamma interferon. *Int J Cancer* **91**:500, 2001
82. Sette A et al: HLA expression in cancer: Implications for T cell-based immunotherapy. *Immunogenetics* **53**:255, 2001
83. Kamarashev J et al: TAP1 down-regulation in primary melanoma lesions: An independent marker of poor prognosis. *Int J Cancer* **95**:23, 2001
84. Glover MT et al: HLA antigen frequencies in renal transplant recipients and non-immunosuppressed patients with non-melanoma skin cancer. *Eur J Cancer* **29A**:520, 1993
85. Bouwes Bavinck JN et al: The risk of skin cancer in renal transplant recipients in Queensland, Australia: A follow-up study. *Transplantation* **61**:715, 1996
86. Czarnecki D et al: Skin cancers and HLA frequencies in renal transplant recipients. *Dermatology* **185**:9, 1992
87. Jackow CM et al: HLA-DR5 and DQB1*03 class II alleles are associated with cutaneous T-cell lymphoma. *J Invest Dermatol* **107**:373, 1996
88. Arnett FC: HLA and autoimmunity in scleroderma (systemic sclerosis). *Int Rev Immunol* **12**:107, 1995
89. Wang E et al: T-cell-directed cancer vaccines: The melanoma model. *Expert Opin Biol Ther* **1**:277, 2001
90. Arnett FC, Reveille JD: Genetics of systemic lupus erythematosus. *Rheum Clin North Am* **18**:865, 1992

CHAPTER 25

Lela A. Lee

Immunoglobulin Structure and Function

During evolution, jawed vertebrates developed the capacity to respond with exquisite specificity to foreign organisms.[1] Specific immunity is characterized by an enormous diversity of possible responses and by refinement in the immune response with successive exposures to the organism.[2] The cells that can discriminate with fine specificity through their vast repertoire of receptors are lymphocytes. Specific immunity, also called *adaptive immunity* because it develops as an adaptation to infection, can be segregated into humoral immunity, mediated by antibodies produced by B lymphocytes, and cellular immunity, mediated by T lymphocytes. These two forms of specific immunity developed to serve different functions. Humoral immunity is directed primarily toward extracellular antigens, such as circulating bacteria and toxins. Cellular immunity is directed primarily toward antigens that infect or inhabit cells. To combat extracellular pathogens, the defending agent needs to be abundant and widely distributed in the body, particularly at its interfaces with the environment. Antibodies fulfill these characteristics by being capable of being secreted in great quantity from the cells that produce them and by being distributed in blood, mucosa, and interstitial fluid. In addition, antibodies can attach through Fc receptors to the surface of certain other cells of the immune system, such as mast cells, conferring antigen specificity to cells that do not have their own endogenously produced antigen-specific receptors.

ANTIBODY STRUCTURE

Antibodies, or immunoglobulins (Ig), are a family of glycoproteins that share a common structure.[2–4] The antibody molecule has a symmetric Y shape consisting of two identical light chains, each about 24 kDa, that are covalently linked to two identical heavy chains, each about 55 or 70 kDa, that are covalently linked to one another (Fig. 25-1). Within the light and heavy chains are variable and constant regions. The major function of the variable region is to recognize antigens, whereas the constant region mediates effector functions. The light and heavy chains contain a series of repeating, homologous units of about 110 amino acids that assume a globular structure and are called *Ig domains.* The Ig domain motif is found not only in antibody molecules but also in a variety of other molecules of the Ig "superfamily," including the T cell receptor, the major histocompatibility complex (MHC), CD4, CD8, and intercellular adhesion molecule 1 (ICAM-1), among other molecules. The light chains have two major domains, a variable (V_L) and a constant (C_L) domain. The heavy chains have four or five domains, a variable (V_H) and three (in IgA, IgD, and IgG) or four (in IgM and IgE) constant (C_H1–4) domains. In IgA, IgD, and IgG, there is a hinge region between C_H1 and C_H2 that confers additional flexibility to the molecule. The variable domains are at the N terminus. At the C terminus are the constant domains and, in the heavy chains of membrane-bound antibodies, the transmembrane and cytoplasmic domains.

Within the variable regions of the light and heavy chains are three areas of intense variability called *hypervariable regions.* These three regions, which are in proximity to one another in the three-dimensional (3D) structure of the antibody, are the areas most responsible for binding antigen. Because the hypervariable regions form a shape complementary with that of the antigen, the hypervariable regions are also called the *complementarity-determining regions* (CDRs). The unique areas formed by the hypervariable regions are present in too low an amount in the individual to generate self-tolerance. Thus the immune system may not distinguish the unique portion of the antibody as self and may produce antibodies to that region of the antibody. The area

FIGURE 25-1

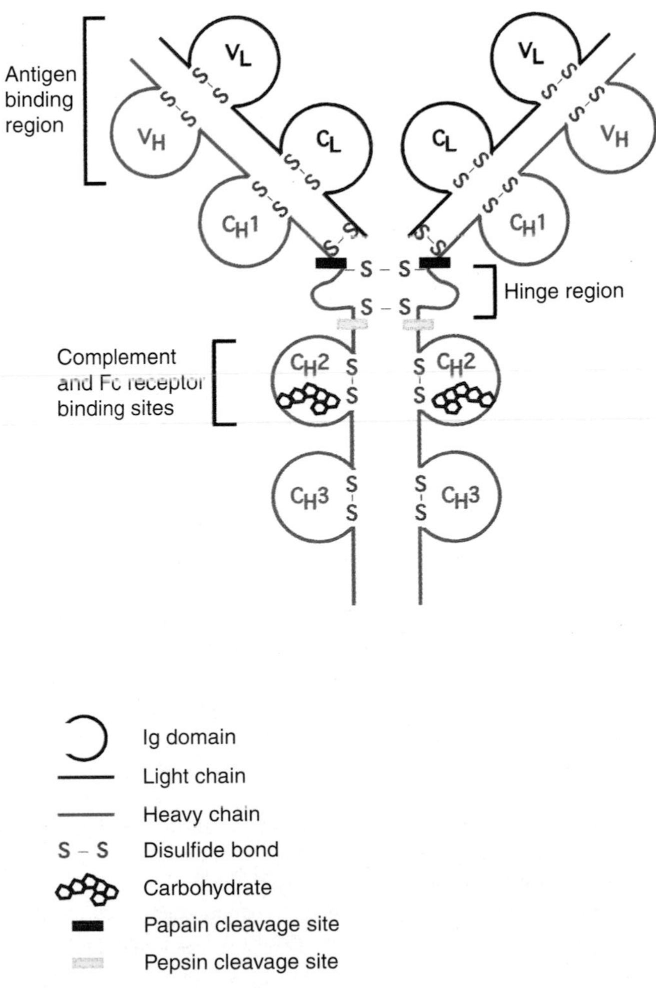

Schematic representation of an IgG molecule.

TABLE 25-1

Immunoglobulin Classes and Their Functions

Class	Subtypes	Secreted Form	Approximate MW of Secreted Form, kDa	Serum Concentration, mg/mL	Serum Half-Life, Days	Functions
IgM	None	Pentamer	970	1.5	5	Primary antibody response; antigen receptor on naive B cells; complement activation
IgD	None	Monomer	180	Trace	3	Antigen receptor on naive B cells
IgA	IgA1, 2	Monomer, polymer (usually dimer)	160 (monomer), 390 (secretory IgA)	3.5	6	Mucosal immunity; neonatal immunity
IgG	IgG1, 2, 3, 4	Monomer	150	13	23	Neonatal immunity; opsonization; complement activation (except IgG4); phagocytosis; ADCC*; feedback inhibition of B cells
IgE	None	Monomer	190	Trace	2	Immediate hypersensitivity; defense against parasites

*Antibody-dependent cell-mediated cytotoxicity.

of the antibody capable of generating an immune response is called an *idiotope,* and antibody responses to idiotopes result in a network of idiotypic–anti-idiotypic interactions that may help regulate the humoral immune response.[5]

There are two types of light chains, κ and λ, each encoded on different chromosomes. Each antibody molecule has either two κ or two λ chains, never one of each. The functional differences, if any, between κ and λ are not known. There are five types of heavy chains, α, δ, ε, γ, and μ, corresponding to the antibody classes IgA, IgD, IgE, IgG, and IgM, respectively. The different heavy chain classes have significantly different functions, as will be discussed below. The IgA and IgG classes contain closely related subclasses, consisting of IgA1 and IgA2 and IgG1, IgG2, IgG3, and IgG4 (Table 25-1).

Enzymatic digestion of IgG molecules by papain results in three cleavage products, two identical Fab fragments consisting of a light chain bound to the V-C_H1 region of the heavy chain and an Fc portion consisting of two C_H2-C_H3 heavy chains bound to each other. Fab was so named for its property of antigen binding, and Fc was so named for its property of crystallizing. When IgG is digested by pepsin, the C-terminal region is digested into small fragments. The remaining product consists of the Fab region along with the hinge region. Fab fragments containing the hinge region are termed Fab′. When the two Fab′ fragments in an antibody molecule remain associated, the fragment is called $F(ab')_2$.

ANTIBODY CLASSES (see Table 25-1)

IgM

IgM is the first Ig molecule to be expressed during B cell development. Its secretory form is a pentamer consisting of five IgM molecules joined at their C termini by tail pieces and stabilized by a molecule called a *joining (J) chain.* The engagement of membrane-bound IgM by antigen results in the activation of naive B cells. Secreted IgM recognizes antigen, usually through low-affinity interactions, and it can activate complement. IgM is the major effector of the primary antibody response. Although IgM interactions typically are low-affinity, IgM can be very effective in responding to a polyvalent antigen (such as a polysaccharide with repeating epitopes) because its pentameric structure allows for multiple low-affinity interactions, resulting in a high-avidity interaction. (*Avidity* refers to the overall strength of attachment, whereas *affinity* refers to the strength of attachment at a single antigen-binding site.)

IgD

The IgD molecule exists primarily in a membrane-bound form and is the second antibody class to be expressed during B cell development. Its function is not completely understood, but in its membrane-bound form it can serve as an antigen receptor for naive B cells.[6]

IgA

IgA is the most abundant Ig in the body, being present in large quantity at mucosal sites. It is responsible for mucosal immunity and is secreted in breast milk, thus contributing to neonatal immunity. In its secreted form, it exists as a monomer, dimer, or trimer, with the multimers being formed by interactions between tail pieces and stabilized by the J chain. For transport across epithelial surfaces, IgA dimers attach to a type of Fc receptor called the *polymeric Ig receptor.*[7] Once the transport process is complete, the IgA dimers remain attached to the extracellular portion of the receptor, called the *secretory component,* that protects the IgA from proteolysis. Cells of the immune system that have receptors for IgA include neutrophils, eosinophils, and monocytes.

IgG

IgG is the most abundant Ig in the circulation. Its secreted form is a monomer. IgG plays an important role in secondary antibody responses, and its interactions with antigen tend to be high-affinity, particularly as the immune response matures. A number of cells have Fc receptors for IgG, including monocytes, neutrophils, eosinophils, natural killer (NK) cells, and B cells. IgG opsonizes (coats) antigen, allowing phagocytosis of the antigen, and activates complement. An exception is IgG4, which does not activate complement. IgG is the only Ig class to cross the placenta, and therefore, it plays an important role in neonatal immunity. The interaction of IgG with the MHC class I–related receptor FcRn is involved in the delivery of IgG across the placenta as well as in prolonging its level in the circulation.[8] The serum half-life of IgG is 23 days, considerably longer than that of the other Ig classes.

IgE

IgE is found in very small amounts in the circulation. High-affinity receptors for the Fc portion of IgE are present on mast cells, basophils, and eosinophils, and low-affinity receptors are present on B cells and Langerhans cells. In mast cells, basophils, and eosinophils, IgE engagement with antigen activates the cells. IgE mediates immediate hypersensitivity, but its principal protective role may be to combat parasites.

MECHANISMS FOR THE GENERATION OF ANTIBODY DIVERSITY

The information encoded by an individual's DNA is limited by the need for the DNA to fit into a package the size of a cell. This space is far too small for sufficient DNA to encode billions of different lymphocyte receptors if the genes were encoded separately. Lymphocytes have adapted to this limitation by special mechanisms that increase by orders of magnitude the number of different possible antigen receptors.[9] Each clone of B cells produces identical antigen receptors (i.e., antibodies) with unique specificities. It is estimated that an individual has about 10^9 different B cell clones, resulting in 10^9 distinct antibodies. A major mechanism for generating this enormous diversity is gene rearrangement, whereby segments of DNA within a lymphocyte undergo somatic recombinations.[10] Light chain genes contain three regions, V (variable), J (joining), and C (constant), and heavy chain genes contain four regions, V, D (diversity), J, and C. Within each region are many gene segments from which to select for the final antibody product, which is comprised of one gene segment from each region. The initial event in antibody formation is the joining of one D and one J segment from a heavy chain gene, with subsequent deletion of the DNA between the two segments. Next, a V segment is selected to join to the DJ segment, and any remaining D segments are deleted. The VDJ complex has attached 3′ to it any remaining J segments plus the C region. The unused J segments are removed during RNA processing. A similar process occurs in light chain loci; because there are no D segments in light chain loci, a VJ rather than a VDJ complex is formed.

The ability to select one segment each from the many segments available in the V, D, and J regions leads to a vast increase in the repertoire of possible antibodies. Additional diversity is generated by the juxtaposition of a rearranged light chain to a rearranged heavy chain and by the addition, deletion, or transposition of nucleotides at the junctions between V and D, D and J, and V and J segments, a phenomenon called *junctional diversity.*

B CELL MATURATION

Bone marrow and fetal liver stem cells that give rise to B cells are initially pluripotent.[2] The stem cells may proceed to develop in the lymphocytic pathway, where they can give rise to B, T, or NK cells. The earliest cell committed to the B cell lineage is called a *pro-B cell.* At the pro-B cell stage, the cell expresses recombinase-activating gene (RAG) and terminal deoxyribonucleotidyl transferase (TdT), which will be needed subsequently for somatic recombination and nucleoside transfers involved in junctional diversity, respectively. At the pro-B cell stage, somatic recombination has not taken place, and therefore, Ig is not yet expressed.

The next stage of B cell maturation is represented by the pre-B cell and is marked by the synthesis of a cytoplasmic μ heavy chain. Since light chains are not yet expressed at this stage, surface Ig is not present. Some of the μ heavy chains associate with invariant molecules called *surrogate light chains* to form complexes called *pre-B cell receptors.* These receptors are then expressed on the pre-B cell surface and provide important signals for the proliferation and maturation of the developing B cell.[11]

The formation of light chains marks the next stage in B cell maturation, the immature B cell. When light chains join with the μ heavy chains, an IgM molecule results and can be expressed on the cell surface. The cytoplasmic tails of IgM molecules are too short to transduce signals. Signal transduction is rather a function of two other molecules, called Igα and Igβ, associated with IgM in a B cell receptor complex on the cell surface. Although the presence of a B cell receptor complex confers the ability to recognize specific antigens, at this stage such recognition does not result in proliferation or differentiation. Rather, the cells may undergo negative selection when antigen is encountered. Immature B cells recognizing self-antigen may be deleted through apoptosis[12] or may undergo receptor editing, a process by which a new, non-self specificity is acquired.[13]

Acquisition of the ability to express IgD as well as IgM is the hallmark of the next stage, the mature B cell. The cell is naive because it has not been activated by antigen, but it is competent to respond to antigen. Mature B cells exit the bone marrow and migrate to blood and lymphoid tissues, where they constitute the majority of B cells in those locations.

The encounter of antigen by mature naive B cells leads to B cell activation, proliferation, and differentiation. A subset of B cells become memory B cells, which are then activated if the antigen is encountered subsequently.[14] Another subset of B cells differentiates into cells that make progressively less membrane-bound Ig and more secreted Ig. These cells can undergo class switching from IgM and IgD to IgA, IgE, or IgG.[15] The terminally differentiated B cells committed to the production of secreted Ig are plasma cells and have abundant rough endoplasmic reticulum, consistent with the function of the cells as antibody factories.

ANTIGENS BOUND BY B CELLS

B cells recognize a variety of macromolecules, including proteins, lipids, and nucleic acids. The portion of the macromolecule recognized by the antibody is called an *epitope* or *determinant.* B cells recognize both linear epitopes (epitopes formed by several adjacent amino acids) and, quite commonly, conformational epitopes (epitopes present as a result of folding of the macromolecule).[16] In contrast to B cells, T cell responses are almost entirely restricted to linear epitopes of peptides.

Macromolecules, particularly large proteins, may contain several different epitopes, and a humoral response to a macromolecule typically is comprised of multiple different antibodies. Although each different antibody is specific for a given epitopic configuration, similarities in epitopes may exist such that an antibody to a given epitope on a given macromolecule also may be able to bind a different epitope on a different macromolecule. This phenomenon is called *cross-reactivity* and may be important in the genesis of autoimmune antibody responses.

Macromolecules that have multiple identical epitopes are classified as being polyvalent or multivalent. Antibodies to these macromolecules or aggregates of macromolecules may form complexes called *immune complexes* with the antigen. At a particular concentration of antibody and antigen, called the *zone of equivalence,* a large network of linked antigens and antibodies forms. At lower or higher concentrations of antibody or antigen, the complexes are much smaller. Immune complexes, formed in the circulation or in tissue, may be responsible for disease through the initiation of an inflammatory response.

B CELL AND ANTIBODY FUNCTION

On engagement of the mature B cell receptor by antigen, clustering of receptors initiates signaling transduced by Igα and Igβ. The resulting signaling cascade eventuates in the expression of genes involved in B cell activation. B cell activation is facilitated by second signals, one of which may be provided by the complement protein C3d.[17]

The subsequent response to an antigen often involves a complex interaction between B cells and T cells, leading to a fine-tuning of the immune response. B cells are capable of functioning as antigen-presenting cells. In response to a protein antigen, B cells take up the antigen, process it, and present peptide–class II MHC complexes to T cells. T cells recognizing the peptide–class II MHC complexes receive a primary signal from the complex and a secondary signal from costimulatory interactions, notably binding of B7-1 and B7-2 on B cells to CD28 on T cells.[18] These T cells are activated, and their activation in turn provides signals to the B cells through the actions of cell surface molecules (in particular, CD40 on B cells and CD40 ligand on T cells) and cytokines [e.g., interleukin 2 (IL-2), IL-4, IL-5, and IL-6].[2] The overall effects on B cells are activation, proliferation, and differentiation. T cell interaction with B cells also results in class switching from IgM to IgA, IgE, or IgG and affinity maturation, whereby the affinity of antibodies for the antigen progressively increases. During affinity maturation, somatic hypermutations in antibody genes result in antibodies with both greater and lesser affinity for the antigen.[19,20] Those antibodies with greater affinity confer a survival advantage on the B cells that produce them. Progressively, the population of B cells evolves in favor of those producing higher-affinity antibodies for the antigen.

As noted earlier, T cell responses are limited almost entirely to peptides. Thus B cell responses to non-protein antigens may not result in T cell help through the mechanisms described earlier.[21] One type of T cell–independent B cell response produces so-called natural antibodies, IgM antibodies that are largely anticarbohydrate antibodies produced without apparent antigen exposure.[22] These natural antibodies are characterized by a limited repertoire and are thought to be produced by B1 peritoneal cells stimulated by bacteria that colonize the gut.

Antigen occupation of antibody-binding sites leads to functional results, called *effector functions.* Many effector functions are mediated through the binding of Ig to Fc receptors (FcRs)[23] FcRs generally are divided into those that trigger cell activation and those that do not. Those that can trigger activation contain one or more motifs called *immunoreceptor tyrosine-based activation motifs* (ITAMs). Of those that do not trigger activation, some can inhibit cell activation and contain a motif called the *immunoreceptor tyrosine-based inhibition motif* (ITIM). FcRs that neither activate nor inhibit cell activation are involved in the transport of Ig through epithelia and the prolongation of the half-life of IgG.

The effector functions of antibodies serve to eliminate the antigen that initiated the immune response and also to downregulate the immune response when activation is not required. Effector functions of antibodies include neutralization of antigen, complement activation, cell activation (of monocytes, neutrophils, eosinophils, and B cells), phagocytosis (by monocytes and neutrophils), and antibody-dependent cell-mediated cytotoxicity (mediated by NK cells). In addition, engagement of IgG by antigen provides a negative signal to B cells, mediated through the binding of the antigen-antibody complex to an Fcγ receptor, FcγIIB, on the B cell.[24]

B CELLS AND ANTIBODIES IN DISEASE

Disorders of B cells or antibodies cause or contribute to many diseases of dermatologic relevance.[25–30] Immunodeficiency diseases may result from abnormalities of B cell development or activation or from abnormalities in effector function pathways. B cell lymphomas may result from failure to regulate proliferation, differentiation, or programmed cell death. Antibodies may initiate an inflammatory response that results in injury, as in IgE-mediated allergic reactions or immune-complex diseases. In some cases, the antigen may not be obviously harmful, but the response to the antigen is. In other cases, the antigen may be pathogenic, but the character or magnitude of the immune response is inappropriate or inadequately controlled. The regulatory systems that protect an organism from attack by its own immune system occasionally fail. In some cases, autoimmunity may be initiated as a result of an immune response to a pathogen. The pathogen may act as a nonspecific activator of the immune system or may activate the immune response specifically, e.g., by containing an epitope or epitopes that are cross-reactive with an autoepitope. These responses may be particularly difficult to control because the major stimulus for the immune response, the antigen, is a normal component of "self" and cannot be eliminated. Thus, through many mechanisms, the normal protective B cell response, which developed as an elegant means to discriminate very finely among various potential pathogens, can be subverted to result in harm to the organism.

REFERENCES

1. Litman GW et al: Evolution of antigen binding receptors. *Annu Rev Immunol* **17**:109, 1999
2. Abbas AK et al: *Cellular and Molecular Immunology,* 4th ed. Philadelphia, Saunders, 2000
3. Alzari PM et al: Three-dimensional structure of antibodies. *Annu Rev Immunol* **6**:555, 1988
4. Davies DR, Metzger H: Structural basis of antibody function. *Annu Rev Immunol* **1**:87, 1983
5. Pan Y et al: Anti-idiotypic antibodies: Biological function and structural studies. *FASEB J* **9**:43, 1995
6. Preud'homme JL et al: Structural and functional properties of membrane and secreted IgD. *Mol Immunol* **37**:871, 2000
7. Mostov KE: Transepithelial transport of immunoglobulins. *Annu Rev Immunol* **12**:63, 1994
8. Ghetie V, Ward ES: Multiple roles for the major histocompatibility complex class I–related receptor FcRn. *Annu Rev Immunol* **18**:739, 2000
9. Honjo T: Immunoglobulin genes. *Annu Rev Immunol* **1**:499, 1983
10. Gellert M: Recent advances in understanding V(D)J recombination. *Adv Immunol* **64**:39, 1997
11. Ghia P et al: B-cell development: A comparison between mouse and man. *Immunol Today* **19**:480, 1998
12. Norvell A et al: Engagement of the antigen-receptor on immature murine B lymphocytes results in death by apoptosis. *J Immunol* **154**:4404, 1995
13. Casellas R et al: Contribution of receptor editing to the antibody repertoire. *Science* **291**:1541, 2001
14. Fearon DT et al: Arrested differentiation, the self-renewing memory lymphocyte, and vaccination. *Science* **293**:248, 2001
15. Stavnezer J: Antibody class switching. *Adv Immunol* **61**:79, 1996
16. Benjamin DC et al: The antigenic structure of proteins: A reappraisal. *Annu Rev Immunol* **2**:67, 1984
17. Mongini PK et al: The affinity threshold for human B cell activation via the antigen receptor complex is reduced upon co-ligation of the antigen receptor with CD21 (CR2). *J Immunol* **159**:3782, 1997
18. Lenschow DJ et al: CD28/B7 system of T cell costimulation. *Annu Rev Immunol* **14**:233, 1996
19. Martin A, Scharff MD: Immunology: Antibody alterations. *Nature* **412**:870, 2001
20. Wagner SD, Neuberger MS: Somatic hypermutation of immunoglobulin genes. *Annu Rev Immunol* **14**:441, 1996
21. Mond JJ et al: T cell-independent antigens type 2. *Annu Rev Immunol* **13**:655, 1995
22. Boes M: Role of natural and immune IgM antibodies in immune responses. *Mol Immunol* **37**:1141, 2000
23. Daeron M: Fc receptor biology. *Annu Rev Immunol* **15**:203, 1997
24. Cambier JC et al: The unexpected complexity of Fc gamma RIIB signal transduction. *Curr Top Microbiol Immunol* **244**:43, 1999
25. Paller AS: Update on selected inherited immunodeficiency syndromes. *Semin Dermatol* **14**:60, 1995
26. Cerroni L, Kerl H: New concepts in cutaneous B-cell lymphomas. *Curr Top Pathol* **94**:79, 2001
27. Kay AB: Allergy and allergic diseases, part 2. *N Engl J Med* **344**:109, 2001
28. Lotti T et al: Cutaneous small-vessel vasculitis. *J Am Acad Dermatol* **39**:667, 1998; quiz 688
29. Lin MS et al: The desmosome and hemidesmosome in cutaneous autoimmunity. *Clin Exp Immunol* **107**(suppl 1):9, 1997
30. Lee LA: Lupus erythematosus, in *Dermatology,* edited by JL Bolognia, JL Jorizzo, RP Rapini. London, Mosby, 2002

CHAPTER 26

Ifor R. Williams
Benjamin E. Rich
Thomas S. Kupper

Cytokines

When cells and tissues in complex organisms communicate over distances greater than one cell diameter, soluble factors are required. A subset of these factors is produced or released transiently under infectious or injurious challenge to orchestrate complex and carefully choreographed responses in the microenvironment of the tissues. Such responses mobilize certain circulating white blood cells to the relevant injured area (but not elsewhere), and guide other leukocytes, particularly T and B cells, involved in host defense to specialized lymphatic tissue remote from the infectious lesion but sufficiently close to contain antigens from the relevant pathogen. After a limited period of time in this setting (i.e., lymph node), antibodies produced by B cells and effector memory T cells can be released into the circulation and localize at the site of infection. Soluble factors produced by resident tissue cells at the site of injury, by leukocytes and platelets that are recruited to the site of injury, and by memory T cells ultimately recruited to the area, all conspire to generate an evolving and effective response to a challenge to host defense. The degree of this response must be appropriate to the challenge, and the duration of response must be transient—that is, long enough to decisively eliminate the pathogen but short enough to minimize damage to healthy host tissues. The cell-to-cell communication involved in the coordination of this response is accomplished by cytokines.

Cytokines (which include the large family of chemokines, discussed in Chap. 27) are soluble polypeptide mediators that play pivotal roles in communication between cells of the hematopoietic system and other cells in the body.[1] Cytokines influence many aspects of leukocyte function including differentiation, growth, activation, and migration. Although many cytokines are substantially upregulated in response to injury to allow a rapid and potent host response, cytokines also play important roles in the development of the immune system and in homeostatic control of the immune system under basal conditions. The growth and differentiation effects of cytokines are not limited to leukocytes, but soluble factors that principally mediate the growth and differentiation of cells other than leukocytes are not discussed in this chapter.

General features of cytokines are their pleiotropism and redundancy. Before the advent of a systematic nomenclature for cytokines, most newly isolated cytokines were named according to the biologic assay being used to isolate and characterize the active molecule (e.g., T cell growth factor for the molecule that was later renamed interleukin-2). Often, independent groups studying quite disparate bioactivities isolated the same molecule, thus revealing the pleiotropic effects of these cytokines. For example, before being termed interleukin-1 (IL-1), this cytokine had been variously known as endogenous pyrogen, lymphocyte-activating factor, and leukocytic endogenous mediator.[2] Many cytokines have a wide range of activities, causing multiple effects in responsive cells and a different set of effects in each type of cell capable of responding. The redundancy of cytokines typically means that in any single bioassay (such as induction of T cell proliferation), multiple cytokines will display activity. In addition, the absence of a single cytokine (such as in mice with targeted mutations in cytokine genes) can often be largely or even completely compensated for by other cytokines with overlapping biologic effects.

HISTORIC PERSPECTIVES

The first cytokines described had distinct and easily recognizable biologic activities, exemplified by IL-1, IL-2, and the interferons (IFNs). The term *cytokine* was first coined in 1975 to describe several such activities released into the supernatant of an epithelial cell line.[3] Before this time, such activities had been thought to be the exclusive domain of lymphocytes (lymphokines) and monocytes (monokines), and were considered a function of the immune system. Keratinocyte cytokines were first discovered in 1981,[4] and the list of cytokines produced by this epithelial cell rivals that of nearly any other cell type in the body.[5] The number of molecules that can be legitimately termed cytokines has exploded in recent years and has brought under the cytokine rubric molecules with a broad range of distinct biologic activities. The progress in genomic approaches has led to identification of novel cytokine genes based on homologies to known cytokine genes. Making sense of this plethora of mediators is a greater challenge than ever, and strategies to simplify the analysis of the cytokine universe are sorely needed.

The concept of "primary" and "secondary" cytokines continues to be extremely useful for discussion of cytokine function.[6] Primary cytokines are those cytokines that can, by themselves, initiate all the events required to bring about leukocyte infiltration in tissues. IL-1 (both α and β forms) and tumor necrosis factor (TNF; includes both TNF-α and TNF-β) function as primary cytokines, as do certain other cytokines that signal through receptors that trigger the nuclear factor κB (NF-κB) pathway (e.g., IL-18). IL-1 and TNF induce cell adhesion molecule expression on endothelial cells [both selectins and immunoglobulin superfamily members such as intercellular adhesion molecule-1 (ICAM-1) and vascular cell adhesion molecule-1 (VCAM-1)], induce a variety of cells to produce a host of additional cytokines, and induce expression of chemokines that provide a chemotactic gradient, allowing the directed migration of specific leukocyte subsets into a site of inflammation (see below). Primary cytokines can be viewed as part of the "innate" immune system, and in fact, share signaling pathways with the so-called Toll-like receptors (TLRs), a recently described family of receptors that recognize molecular patterns characteristically associated with microbial products.[7,8] In spite of sometimes potent inflammatory activity, other cytokines do not duplicate this full repertoire of activities. Many qualify as secondary cytokines, whose production is induced after cell stimulation by IL-1 and/or TNF family molecules. The term "secondary" does not imply that they are less important or less active than primary cytokines; rather, it indicates that their spectrum of activity is more restricted.

Another concept that has withstood the test of time is the assignment of many T cell-derived cytokines into one of two groups on the basis of which of the two helper T cell subsets (T_H1 and T_H2) produce them (see Chap. 28).[9] Commitment to one of these two patterns of cytokine secretion also occurs with CD8 cytotoxic T cells and $\gamma\delta$ T cells, leading to the suggestion that the type 1 and type 2 terminology should not be restricted to CD4+ $\alpha\beta$ T cells, but should be applied instead to all classes of T cells.[10] Dominance of type 1 or type 2 cytokines in a T cell immune response has profound consequences for the outcome of immune responses to certain pathogens and extrinsic proteins capable of serving as allergens.[9,10] A third pattern of T cell cytokine production by CD4 T cells, in which transforming growth factor-β (TGF-β) is the dominant cytokine produced, has also been recognized. These T_H3 cells typically function as regulatory T cells.[11]

Not all useful classifications of cytokines are based solely on analysis of function. Structural biologists, fueled by improved methods of generating homogeneous preparations of proteins and establishment of new analytic methods (e.g., solution magnetic resonance spectroscopy) that complement the classic x-ray crystallography technique, have solved the three-dimensional structure of many cytokines. These efforts led to the identification of groups of cytokines that fold to generate similar three-dimensional structures and bind to groups of cytokine receptors that also share similar structural features. For example, most of the cytokine ligands that bind to receptors of the hematopoietin cytokine receptor family are members of the four-helix bundle group of cytokines.[12] These proteins have a shared tertiary architecture consisting of four antiparallel α-helical stretches separated by short connecting loops. The normal existence of some cytokines as oligomers rather than monomers was discovered in part as the result of structural investigations. For example, IFN-γ is a four-helix bundle cytokine that naturally exists as a noncovalent dimer. The bivalency of the dimer enables this ligand to bind and oligomerize two IFN-γ receptor complexes, thereby facilitating signal transduction.[13] TNF-α and TNF-β are both trimers that are composed almost exclusively of β sheets folded into a "jelly roll" structural motif. Ligand-induced trimerization of receptors in the TNF receptor family is believed to be critical for initiation of signaling by these receptors.[14]

CYTOKINE SIGNAL TRANSDUCTION PATHWAYS

To mediate their effects, cytokines must first bind with specificity and high affinity to receptors on the cell surface of responding cells. Many aspects of the pleiotropism and redundancy manifested by cytokines can be understood through an appreciation of the shared mechanisms of signal transduction mediated by cell surface receptors for cytokines. In the early years of the cytokine biology era, the emphasis of most investigative work was on the purification and eventual cloning of new cytokines and a description of their functional capabilities in vitro and in vivo. In recent years, many of the cytokine receptors have been cloned, and several of the signaling cascades initiated by cytokines have been described in detail. Most cytokine receptors can be classified into a relatively small number of families and superfamilies (Table 26-1), the members of which function in an approximately similar fashion. A major theme of this chapter is that most cytokines send signals to cells through pathways that are very similar to those of other cytokines using the same class of receptors. The fact that individual cytokines often use several downstream pathways of signal transduction accounts in part for the pleiotropic effects of these molecules. Nevertheless, we propose that a few major signaling pathways account for most effects attributable to cytokines. Of particularly central importance are the NF-κB pathway and the Jak-STAT pathway.

NF-κB, IκB, and Primary Cytokines

A major mechanism contributing to the extensive overlap between the biologic activities of the primary cytokines IL-1 and TNF is the shared use of the NF-κB signal transduction pathway. IL-1 and TNF use completely distinct cell surface receptor and proximal signaling pathways, but these pathways converge at the activation of the NF-κB transcription factor. NF-κB is of central importance in immune and inflammatory processes because a large number of genes that elicit or propagate inflammation have NF-κB recognition sites in their promoters. NF-κB regulated genes include cytokines, chemokines, adhesion molecules, nitric oxide (NO) synthase, cyclooxygenases, and phospholipase A_2.[15]

In nonstimulated cells, NF-κB heterodimers formed from p65 and p50 subunits are inactive because they are sequestered in the cytoplasm as a result of tight binding to inhibitor proteins in the IκB family (Fig. 26-1). Signal transduction pathways that activate the NF-κB system do so through the activation of an IκB kinase complex consisting of two kinase subunits (IKKα and IKKβ) and a regulatory subunit (IKKγ). The IKK complex phosphorylates IκBα and IκBβ on specific serine residues, yielding a target for recognition by an E3 ubiquitin ligase complex. The resulting polyubiquitination marks this IκB for rapid degradation by the 26S proteasome complex in the cytoplasm. Once IκB has been degraded, the free NF-κB (which contains a nuclear localization signal) is able to pass into the nucleus and induce expression of NF-κB–sensitive genes.[16] Among the genes regulated by NF-κB are IL-1β and TNF-α; this endows IL-1β and TNF-α with the capacity to establish a positive regulatory loop that favors persistent inflammation.[15] Most cytokines (other than IL-1 and TNF) do not activate the

TABLE 26-1

Major Families of Cytokine Receptors

Receptor Family	Example	Major Signal Transduction Pathways(s) Leading to Biologic Effects
IL-1 receptor family	IL-1R, type I	NF-κB activation via TRAF6
TNF receptor family	TNFR1	NF-κB activation involving TRAF2 and TRAF5 Apoptosis induction via "death domain" proteins
Hematopoietin receptor family (class I receptors)	IL-2R	Activation of Jak-STAT pathway
Interferon/IL-10 receptor family (class II receptors)	IFN-γR	Activation of Jak-STAT pathway
Immunoglobulin superfamily	M-CSFR	Activation of intrinsic tyrosine kinase
TGF-β receptor family	TGF-βR, type I and II	Activation of intrinsic serine/threonine kinase coupled to SMADs
Chemokine receptor family	CCR5	Seven transmembrane receptors coupled to G-proteins

M-CSF, macrophage colony-stimulating factor; SMAD Sma- and Mad-related protein.

NF-κB pathway as part of their signal transduction mechanisms, although the presence of κB recognition sites in the promoters of these same cytokines is very common.

FIGURE 26-1

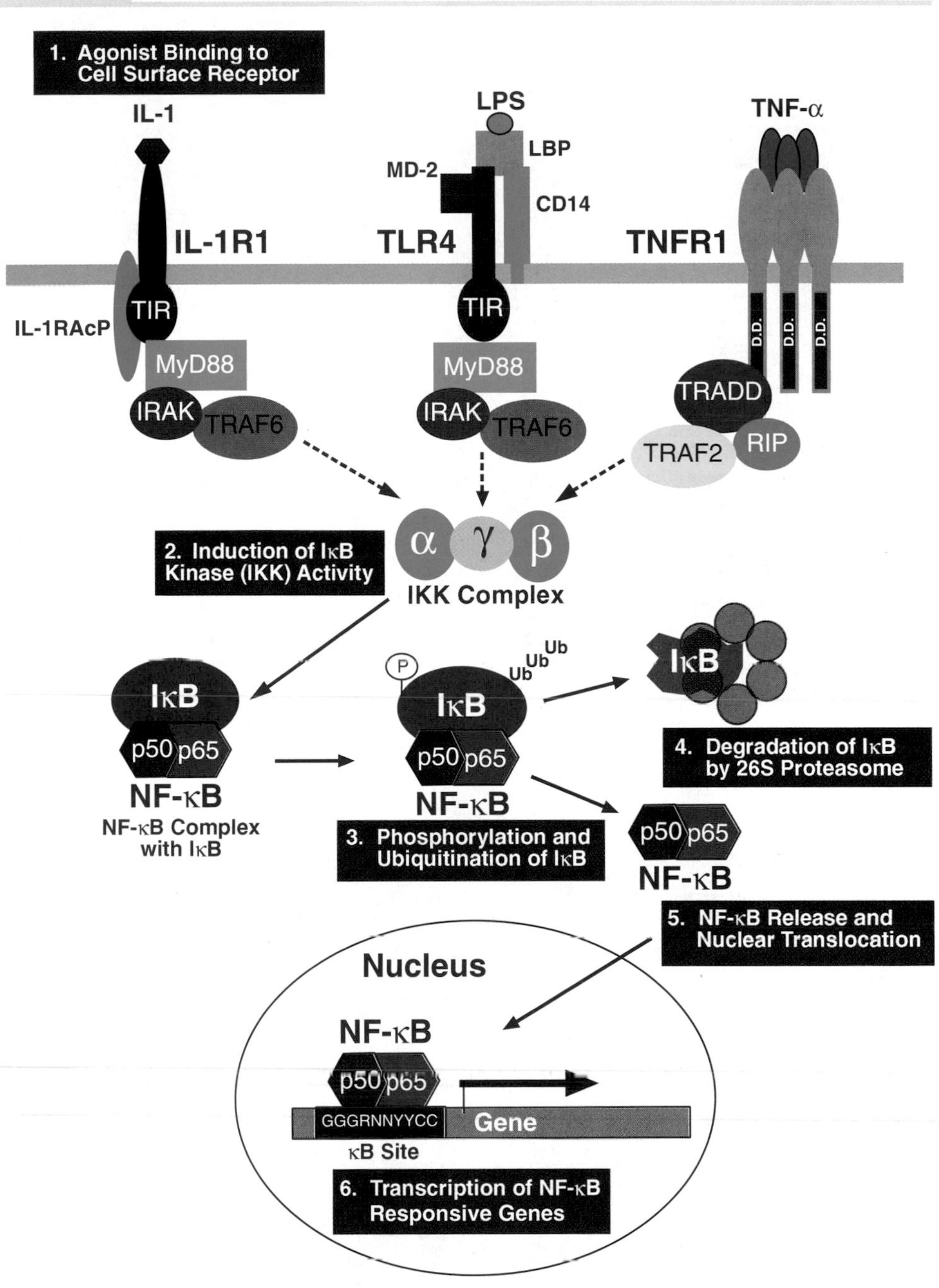

Activation of NF-κB regulated genes after signaling by receptors for primary cytokines or by TLRs engaged by microbial products. Under resting conditions, NF-κB (a heterodimer of p50 and p65 subunits) is tightly bound to an inhibitor called IκB, which sequesters NF-κB in the cytoplasm. Engagement of one of the TLRs or the signal transducing receptors for IL-1 or TNF family members leads to induction of IκB kinase activity that phosphorylates IκB on critical serine residues. Phosphorylated IκB becomes a substrate for ubiquitination, which triggers degradation of IκB by the 26S proteasome. Loss of IκB results in release of NF-κB, permitting it to move to the nucleus and activate transcription of genes whose promoters contain κB recognition sites. DD, death domain; TRADD, TNFR1-associated DD protein; RIP, receptor-interacting protein.

Proinflammatory cytokines are not the only stimuli that can activate the NF-κB pathway. Bacterial products (e.g., lipopolysaccharide), oxidants, activators of protein kinase C (e.g., phorbol esters), viruses, and ultraviolet radiation are other stimuli that can stimulate NF-κB activity.[15] Recently, a cell surface receptor for the complex of lipopolysaccharide (LPS), LPS-binding protein, and CD14 was identified as TLR4.[17] The cytoplasmic domain of TLR4 is similar to that of the IL-1R1 and other IL-1R family members,[18] and is known as the TIR domain (for Toll/IL-1 receptor). When ligand is bound to this TIR domain, an adapter protein called MyD88 is recruited. In turn, MyD88 recruits one or more of the IL-1R–associated kinases (which include IRAK-1, -2, and -M),[19] which then signal through TRAF6, a member of the TNF receptor-associated factors (TRAF) family, to activate the IKK complex. Because most incident solar UV radiation is absorbed by resident cells in the epidermis and dermis, UV radiation effects on the NF-κB pathway are particularly relevant to the biology of skin. The cell surface receptors for IL-1, TNF, and epidermal growth factor (EGF) are rapidly clustered and internalized after exposure to UV radiation, leading to ligand-independent activation of both NF-κB and the c-Jun *N*-terminal kinases (JNKs).[20]

Hench's discovery of the anti-inflammatory effects of glucocorticoids was acknowledged with a Nobel Prize in 1950. Glucocorticoids inhibit as broad a range of proinflammatory effects as primary cytokines induce, and while their pharmacologic use is rife with potential complications, their anti-inflammatory activity is undisputed. A link between glucocorticoids and primary cytokines was made through the discovery that these pharmacologic agents increase the gene expression of IκBα, thus serving to replace IκBα degraded by proteasomes after phosphorylation and ubiquitination, and ultimately to sequester NF-κB dimers in the cytoplasm.[21] Effectively, then, glucocorticoids tip the balance between sequestered and active NF-κB by inducing IκBα synthesis, while primary cytokines promote inflammation by liberating NF-κB from its association with IκB. Thus, glucocorticoids attack the central pathway by which primary cytokines work, and the plethora of effects that they have on inflammation is mirrored by those of genes inducible by NF-κB.

Jak-STAT Signal Transduction Pathway

A major breakthrough in the analysis of cytokine-mediated signal transduction was the identification of a common cell surface to nucleus

cytokine receptors via this interaction. Homodimeric or heterodimeric STAT proteins are phosphorylated by the Jak kinases and subsequently translocate to the nucleus. In the nucleus, they bind recognition sequences in DNA and stimulate transcription of specific genes, often in cooperation with other transcription factors.[24] As shown in Table 26-2, the same STAT molecules can be involved in signaling by multiple different cytokines. The specificity of the response in these instances may depend on the formation of complexes involving STATs and other transcription factors that then selectively act on a specific set of genes.

Further investigation into the regulation of the Jak-STAT signaling has identified at least three general regulatory pathways that dampen the effects of Jak-STAT–mediated cytokine signaling.[25] The actions of tyrosine phosphatases such as SHP-1 attenuate the effects of tyrosine phosphorylation occurring after cytokine receptor activation. Members of the suppressor of cytokine synthesis (SOCS) family are negative regulatory proteins that are induced by cytokines and inhibit cytokine signaling as part of a negative feedback loop. Finally, protein inhibitor of activated STAT (PIAS) family members mediate their inhibition of cytokine signaling by inhibiting the DNA-binding activity of STATs.

FIGURE 26-2

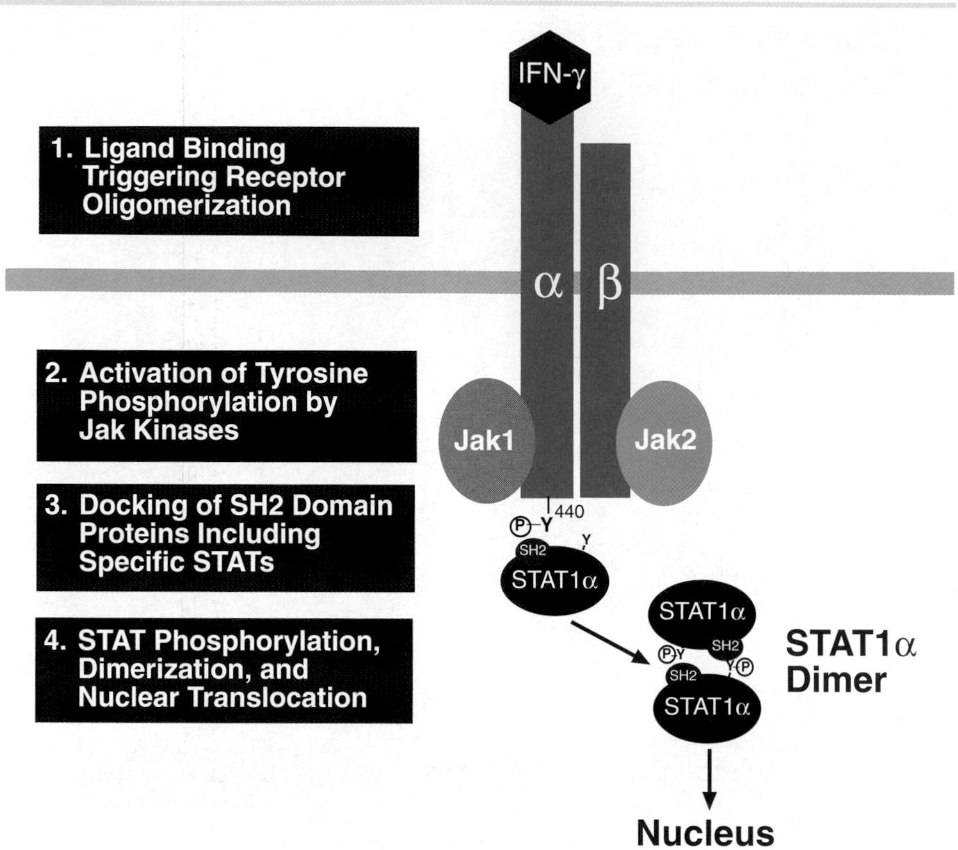

Participation of Jak and STAT proteins in IFN-γ signaling. Binding of human IFN-γ (a dimer) to its receptor brings about oligomerization of receptor complexes composed of α and β chains. The nonreceptor protein tyrosine kinases Jak1 and Jak2 are activated and phosphorylate critical tyrosine residues in the receptor, such as the tyrosine at position 440 of the α chain (Y^{440}). STAT1α molecules are recruited to the IFN-γ receptor based on the affinity of their SH2 domains for the phosphopeptide sequence around Y^{440}. Receptor-associated STAT1α molecules then dimerize through reciprocal SH2-phosphotyrosine interactions. The resulting STAT1α dimers translocate to the nucleus and stimulate transcription of IFN-γ regulated genes.

pathway used by most cytokines. This "Jak-STAT" pathway was first elucidated through careful analysis of signaling initiated by interferon receptors (Fig. 26-2),[22] but was subsequently shown to play a role in signaling by all cytokines that bind to members of the hematopoietin receptor family.[23] The Jak-STAT pathway operates through the sequential action of a family of four nonreceptor tyrosine kinases (the Jaks or *Ja*nus family *k*inases) and a series of latent cytosolic transcription factors known as STATs (*s*ignal *t*ransducers and *a*ctivators of *t*ranscription). The cytoplasmic portions of many cytokine receptor chains (Table 26-2) are noncovalently associated with one of the four Jaks (Jak1, Jak2, Jak3, and Tyk2).

Jak activity is upregulated after stimulation of the cytokine receptor. Ligand binding to the cytokine receptors leads to the association of two or more distinct cytokine receptor subunits and brings the associated Jaks into close proximity with each other. This promotes cross-phosphorylation or autophosphorylation reactions that in turn fully activate the kinases. Tyrosines in the cytoplasmic tail of the cytokine receptor, as well as tyrosines on other associated and newly recruited proteins, are also phosphorylated. A subset of the newly phosphorylated tyrosines can then serve as docking points for attachment of additional signaling proteins bearing src homology 2 (SH2) domains. Cytoplasmic STATs possess SH2 domains and are recruited to the phosphorylated

IL-1 FAMILY OF CYTOKINES (IL-1α, IL-1β, IL-18)

IL-1 is the prototype of a cytokine that has been discovered many times in many different biologic assays.[2] Distinct genes encode the α and β forms of human IL-1, with only 26 percent homology at the amino acid level. Both IL-1s are translated as 31-kDa molecules that lack a signal peptide, and both reside in the cytoplasm. This form of IL-1α is biologically active, but the 31-kDa IL-1β molecule must be cleaved by caspase-1 (initially termed IL-1β–converting enzyme or ICE) to generate an active molecule[26]; this process occurs concurrently with release from the cell through a recently defined pathway of microvesicle shedding.[27] IL-1α can be cleaved by calpain to a 17-kDa form to facilitate its release from cells.[28]

IL-1β appears to be the dominant form of IL-1 produced by monocytes, macrophages, Langerhans cells, and dendritic cells. IL-1α predominates in epithelial cells including keratinocytes, probably because epithelial IL-1α is stored in the cytoplasm of cells that comprise an interface with the external environment. Such cells, when injured, can release biologically active 31-kDa IL-1α and therefore can initiate inflammation.[6] However, if uninjured, these cells will differentiate and effectively release their IL-1 contents into the environment. Leukocytes, including dendritic and Langerhans cells, carry their cargo of IL-1 inside the body, where its unregulated release could cause significant tissue damage. Thus, the release of biologically active IL-1β from cells is controlled at several levels: IL-1β gene transcription, caspase-1 gene transcription, and transcription of the protease that activates caspase-1 to generate mature IL-1β, all of which must occur efficiently for such cells to release IL-1β. The role of IL-1β in the migration of Langerhans cells from the epidermis during the initiation of contact hypersensitivity was explored in several recent studies, leading some to suggest that this event is pivotal in the egress of Langerhans cells from the epidermis and the generation of successful sensitization.[29] Recent studies of mice deficient in IL-1α and IL-1β genes suggest that both molecules are important in contact hypersensitivity, but that IL-1α is more critical.[30]

Active forms of IL-1 bind to the IL-1R1, or type I IL-1 receptor.[18] IL-1R1 is the sole signal transducing receptor for IL-1, and its cytoplasmic domain bears little homology to other cytokine receptors, showing greatest homology with the *Toll* gene product identified in *Drosophila*. A second cell surface protein, the IL-1R associated protein (IL-1RAcP), must associate with the IL-1R1 for signaling to occur. Both IL-1R1 and the IL-1RAcP are essential for IL-1 signaling, as mice deficient in either of these molecules exhibit absent IL-1 signaling.[31] When IL-1 associates with the IL-1R1/IL-1RAcP complex, the MyD88 adapter is recruited, followed by association of one or more of the IRAKs. In turn, these kinases associate with TRAF6.[32] Stepwise activation and recruitment of additional signaling molecules culminates in the induction of IKK activity. The net result is the NF-κB–mediated activation of a series of genes, including adhesion molecules, chemokines, secondary cytokines, nitric oxide synthase, and cyclooxygenases.

TABLE 26-2

Use of Janus Kinases and STAT Proteins in Signal Transduction by Selected Cytokine Receptors

Cytokine	Receptor Chains and CD Designations*	Jak Kinases	STAT Protein(s)
IFN-α, β	α (CD118), β	Jak1, Tyk2	STAT1, STAT2
IFN-γ	α (CD119), β	Jak1, Jak2	STAT1
IL-2	α (CD25), β_c (CD122), γ_c (CD132)	Jak1, Jak3	STAT3, STAT5
IL-3	α (CD123), β_c (CDw131)	Jak1, Jak2	STAT5
IL-4	α (CD124), γ_c (CD132)	Jak1, Jak3	STAT6
IL-4 and IL-13	α (CD124), α1 (CD213a1)	Jak1, Jak2	STAT6
IL-5	α (CDw125), β_c (CDw131)	Jak1, Jak2	STAT1, STAT5
IL-6	α (CD126), gp130 (CD130)	Jak1, Jak2, Tyk2	STAT1, STAT3
IL-7	α (CD127), γ_c (CD132)	Jak1, Jak3	STAT1, STAT3, STAT5
IL-9	α (IL-9Rα), γ_c (CD132)	Jak1	STAT1, STAT3, STAT5
IL-10	α (CDw210), β (IL-10Rβ)	Jak1, Tyk2	STAT1, STAT3
IL-12	β_1 (CD212), β_2	Jak2, Tyk2	STAT1, STAT3, STAT4
IL-15	β_c (CD122), γ_c (CD132)	Jak1, Jak3	STAT5
IL-17	α (CDw217)		STAT2, STAT3
IL-19	α (IL-20Rα), β (IL-20Rβ)		
IL-20	α (IL-20Rα), β (IL-20Rβ) α (IL-22Rα), β (IL-20Rβ)		STAT3
IL-21	α (IL-21R), γ_c (CD132)	Jak1, Jak3	STAT1, STAT3
IL-22	α (IL-22Rα), β (IL-10Rβ)		STAT1, STAT3, STAT5
IL-24	α (IL-22Rα), β (IL-20Rβ) α (IL-20Rα), β (IL-20Rβ)		STAT1, STAT3
GM-CSF	α (CD116), β_c (CDw131)	Jak1, Jak2	STAT5

*CD designations reflect the 2000 update agreed upon at the seventh International Workshop on Human Leukocyte Differentiation Antigens. Several cytokine receptor chains have not yet been sufficiently characterized with monoclonal antibodies to receive a CD designation.

A molecule known as the IL-1 receptor antagonist, or IL-1ra, can bind to the IL-1R1, but does not induce signaling through the receptor.[33] This IL-1ra exists in three alternatively spliced forms, and an isoform produced in monocytes is the only ligand for the IL-1R1 that both contains a signal peptide and is secreted from cells. Two other isoforms of the IL-1ra, both lacking signal peptides, are contained in epithelial cells.[34] The function of the IL-1ra seems to be as a pure antagonist of IL-1 ligand binding to the IL-1R1, and binding of IL-1ra to the IL-1R1 does not induce the mobilization of the IL-1RAcP. Consequently, while both IL-1α/β and the IL-1ra bind with equivalent affinities to the IL-1R1, the association of the IL-1R1 with IL-1RAcP increases the affinity for IL-1α/β manyfold, without affecting the affinity for the IL-1ra. This finding is consistent with the observation that a vast molar excess of IL-1ra is required to fully antagonize the effects of IL-1. The biologic role of IL-1ra is likely to be in the quenching of IL-1–mediated inflammatory responses, and mice deficient in the IL-1ra have exaggerated and persistent inflammatory responses.[35]

A second means of antagonizing IL-1 activity occurs via expression of a second receptor for IL-1, the IL-1R2. This receptor has a short cytoplasmic domain and binds IL-1α/β and IL-1ra. IL-1R2 is a 68-kDa receptor that can be cleaved from the cell surface by an unknown protease and released as a stable soluble 45-kDa molecule that retains avid IL-1α/β binding function, but loses affinity for IL-1ra.[36] By binding the functional ligands for the IL-1R1, the IL-1R2 serves to inhibit IL-1–mediated responses. It is likely that the IL-1R2 inhibits IL-1 activity in another way—by associating with the IL-1RAcP at the cell surface and removing and sequestering it from the pool available to associate with the IL-1R1. Thus, soluble IL-1R2 binds to free IL-1, while cell surface IL-1R2 sequesters IL-1RAcP. Expression of the IL-1R2 can be upregulated by a number of stimuli, including glucocorticoids and IL-4.[37] However, IL-1R2 can also be induced by inflammatory cytokines, including IFN-γ and IL-1, probably as a compensatory signal designed to limit the scale and duration of the inflammatory response.[38] Production of the IL-1R2 serves to make the producing cell and surrounding cells resistant to IL-1–mediated activation. Some of the most efficient IL-1-producing cells are also the best producers of the IL-1R2.

IL-18 was first identified by its capacity to induce IFN-γ.[39] One name initially proposed for this cytokine was IL-1γ, because of its homology to IL-1α and β. Like IL-1β, it is translated as an inactive precursor molecule of 23 kDa, and is cleaved to an active 18-kDa species by caspase-1. It is produced by multiple cell types in skin, including keratinocytes, Langerhans cells, and monocytes.[40] IL-18 induces proliferation, cytotoxicity, and cytokine production by T_H1 and NK cells, mostly synergistically with IL-12.[41] The IL-18 receptor bears striking similarity to the IL-1R1.[18] The binding chain (IL-18R) is an IL-1R1 homologue, originally cloned as IL-1Rrp1. IL-18R alone is a low-affinity receptor that must recruit IL-18RAcP (a homologue of IL-1RAcP). As for IL-1, both chains of the IL-18 receptor are required for signal transduction. Although there is no IL-18 homologue of the IL-1ra, a molecule known as IL-18 binding protein (IL-18BP) binds to soluble mature IL-18 and prevents it from binding to the IL-18R complex.

It is clear that there is a large family of receptors homologous to the IL-1R1 and IL-18R molecules,[18] having in common a TIR motif (see Fig. 26-1). Some of them may be receptors for recently cloned molecules homologous to IL-1α and IL-1ra. All of them share analogous signaling pathways initiated by the MyD88 adapter molecule. Thus, the IL-1R1, the IL-18R, the TLRs, and their ligands, are all best viewed as elements of the innate immune system that signal the presence of danger/injury to the host.

When IL-1 produced by epidermis was originally identified, it was noted that both intact epidermis and stratum corneum contained significant IL-1 activity. This observation led to the concept that epidermis was a shield of sequestered IL-1 surrounding the host, waiting to be released upon injury. More recently, it was observed that high levels of the IL-1ra coexist in keratinocytes[42]; however, repeated experiments show that in virtually all cases, the amount of IL-1 present is sufficient to overcome any potential for inhibition mediated by the IL-1ra. Mechanical stress to keratinocytes promotes the release of large amounts of IL-1 in the absence of cell death.[43] Release of IL-1 induces expression of endothelial adhesion molecules, including E-selectin, ICAM-1, and VCAM-1, as well as chemotactic and activating chemokines. This attracts not only monocytes and granulocytes, but also a specific subpopulation of memory T cells that bear cutaneous lymphocyte antigen (CLA) on their cell surface. CLA+ memory T cells are abundant in inflamed skin, comprising the majority of T cells present. Therefore, any injury to the skin, no matter how trivial, releases IL-1 and attracts this population of memory T cells. If the cells encounter their antigen in this microenvironment, their activation and subsequent cytokine production will amplify the inflammatory response. This process of injury and subsequent cytokine release has been proposed as the basis of the clinical observation known as the Koebner reaction.[43]

TNF: THE OTHER PRIMARY CYTOKINE

TNF-α is the prototype for a family of related signaling molecules that mediate their biologic effects through a family of related receptor molecules. TNF-α was initially cloned on the basis of its ability to mediate two biologic effects: (1) hemorrhagic necrosis of malignant tumors and (2) inflammation-associated cachexia. Although TNF-α exerts many of its biologically important effects as a soluble mediator, newly synthesized TNF-α exists as a transmembrane protein on the cell surface. A specific metalloprotease known as TNF-α–converting enzyme (TACE) is responsible for most TNF-α release by T cells and myeloid cells.[44] Closely related to TNF-α is TNF-β, also known as lymphotoxin α (LT-α). Other related molecules in the TNF family include lymphotoxin β (LT-β), Fas ligand (FasL), TNF-related apoptosis-inducing ligand (TRAIL), TNF-related activation-induced cytokine (TRANCE), and CD40 ligand (CD154).[14] Although some of these other TNF family members have not been traditionally regarded as cytokines, their structure (all are type II membrane proteins with an intracellular N terminus and an extracellular C terminus) and signaling mechanisms are closely related to those of TNF. The soluble forms of TNF-α, LT-α, and FasL are homotrimers; and the predominant form of lymphotoxin-β is a membrane-bound heterotrimer of one LT-α chain and two LT-β chains. Trimerization of TNF receptor family members by their trimeric ligands appears to be required for initiation of signaling and expression of biologic activity.

The initial characterization of TNF receptors led to the discovery of two receptor proteins capable of binding TNF-α with high affinity. The p55 receptor for TNF (TNFR1) is responsible for most biologic activities of TNF, but the p75 TNF receptor (TNFR2) is also capable of transducing signals (unlike the IL-1R2, which acts solely as a biologic sink for IL-1). TNFR1 and TNFR2 have substantial stretches of close homology and are both present on most types of cells. Nevertheless, there are some notable differences between the two TNFRs (see below).

Unlike cytokine receptors from several of the other large families, TNF signaling does not involve the Jak-STAT pathway. TNF-α evokes two types of responses in cells: proinflammatory effects and induction of apoptotic cell death. The proinflammatory effects of TNF-α, which include upregulation of adhesion molecule expression and induction of secondary cytokines and chemokines, stem in large part from activation of NF-κB and can be transduced through both TNFR1 and TNFR2. Induction of apoptosis by signaling through TNFR1 depends on a region known as a "death domain," which is absent in TNFR2, and the association of additional proteins with death domains with the TNFR1 signaling complex. Signaling initiated by ligand binding to TNFR1, Fas, or other death domain-containing receptors in the TNF family eventually leads to activation of caspase-8 or -10 and the nuclear changes and DNA fragmentation characteristic of apoptosis.[14]

At least two TNF receptor family members (TNFR1 and the LT-β receptor) also contribute to the normal anatomic development of the lymphoid system.[45] Mice deficient in TNF-α lack germinal centers and follicular dendritic cells. TNFR1 mutant mice have the same abnormalities plus an absence of Peyer's patches. Mice with null mutations in LT-α or LT-β have further abnormalities in lymphoid organogenesis and fail to develop peripheral lymph nodes.

TNF-α is an important mediator of cutaneous inflammation, and its expression is induced in the course of almost all inflammatory responses in skin. Normal human keratinocytes and keratinocyte cell lines produce substantial amounts of TNF-α after stimulation with LPS or UV light.[46] Cutaneous inflammation stimulated by irritants and contact sensitizers is associated with strong induction of TNF-α production by keratinocytes , a response that is blunted by administration of anti-TNF and in TNF-α–deficient mice.[47,48] Intradermal injection of TNF-α is associated with the migration of Langerhans cells to draining lymph nodes, allowing for sensitization of naive T cells.[49] One molecular mechanism that may contribute to TNF-α–induced migration of Langerhans cells toward lymph nodes is reduced expression of the E-cadherin adhesion molecule after exposure to TNF-α.[50] The predominant TNF receptor expressed by keratinocytes is TNFR1[51]; autocrine signaling loops involving keratinocyte-derived TNF-α and TNFR1 lead to keratinocyte production of a variety of TNF-inducible secondary cytokines.

The central role of TNF-α in inflammatory diseases, including rheumatoid arthritis and psoriasis, has become evident from clinical studies. Two new clinical drugs target the TNF pathway: a humanized anti–TNF-α antibody infliximab (Remicade) and the soluble TNF receptor etanercept (Enbrel). Although larger studies are needed, these drugs appear to have a more profound effect on psoriasis than any other biologic response modifiers.[52,53] Paradoxically, they do not work in all autoimmune diseases—multiple sclerosis appears to worsen slightly after treatment with these reagents.

CLASS I (HEMATOPOIETIN RECEPTOR) FAMILY OF CYTOKINE RECEPTORS AND THEIR LIGANDS

The hematopoietin receptor family (also known as class I cytokine receptor family) is the largest of the cytokine receptor families and comprises a number of structurally related type I membrane-bound glycoproteins. The cytoplasmic domains of these receptors associate with non-receptor tyrosine kinase molecules including Jak and src family kinases. After ligand binding and receptor oligomerization, these associated non-receptor tyrosine kinases phosphorylate intracellular substrates leading to signal transduction. Most of the multiple chain receptors in the hematopoietin receptor family consist of a cytokine-specific α chain subunit paired with one or more shared receptor subunits. Four shared receptor subunits have been described: the common γ chain (γ_c);

the common β chain shared between the IL-2 and IL-15 receptors; a distinct common β chain shared between the granulocyte-macrophage colony-stimulating factor (GM-CSF), IL-3, and IL-5 receptors; and, finally, the gp130 molecule, which participates in signaling by IL-6 and related cytokines.

Cytokines with Receptors That Include the γ_c Chain: IL-2, IL-4, IL-7, IL-9, IL-15, and IL-21

The receptor complexes that use the γ_c chain are the IL-2, IL-4, IL-7, IL-9, IL-15, and IL-21 receptors.[54] Two of these receptors, the IL-2R and the IL-15R, also use the IL-2Rβ_c chain. The γ_c chain is physically associated with Jak3 kinase, and activation of Jak3 kinase is critical to most signaling initiated through this subset of cytokine receptors.[55]

IL-2 AND IL-15 IL-2 and IL-15 can each activate natural killer (NK) cells and stimulate proliferation of activated T cells. IL-2 is a product of activated T cells, and IL-2R is largely restricted to lymphoid cells. The IL-15 gene is expressed by nonlymphoid tissues, and its transcription is induced by UVB light in keratinocytes and fibroblasts and by LPS in monocytes and dendritic cells. Multiple isoforms of IL-15Rα are found in various hematopoietic and non-hematopoietic cells. The IL-2R and IL-15R complexes of lymphocytes incorporate up to three receptor chains, whereas most other cytokine receptor complexes have two. The affinities of IL-2R and IL-15R for their respective ligands can be regulated, and, to some extent, IL-2 and IL-15 compete with each other. The highest affinity receptor complexes for each ligand ($\sim 10^{-11}$ M) consist of the IL-2Rβ_c and γ_c chains, as well as their respective α chains (IL-2Rα, also known as CD25, and IL-15Rα). γ_c and IL-2Rβ_c without the α chains form a functional lower affinity receptor for either ligand (10^{-8} to 10^{-10} M). While both ligands transmit signals through the γ_c chain, those signals elicit overlapping but distinct responses in various cells. Activation of naive CD4 T cells by T cell receptor (TCR) and costimulatory molecules induces expression of IL-2, IL-2Rα, and IL-2Rβ_c, leading to vigorous cell proliferation. Prolonged stimulation of the TCR and IL-2R leads to expression of Fas ligand and activation-induced cell death (AICD). While IL-2 signaling facilitates the death of CD4 T cells in response to sustained exposure to antigen, IL-15 inhibits IL-2 mediated AICD as it stimulates growth. Similarly, IL-15 promotes proliferation of memory CD8 T cells while IL-2 inhibits such proliferation. These contrasting biologic roles are illustrated by mice deficient in IL-2 or IL-2Rα that develop autoimmune disorders and mice deficient in IL-15 or IL-15Rα that have lymphopenia and immune deficiencies. Thus, IL-15 appears to have an important role in promoting effector functions of antigen-specific T cells, whereas IL-2 is involved in controlling autoreactive T cells.[56]

IL-4 AND IL-13 IL-4 and IL-13 are products of activated T_H2 cells that share limited structural homology ($\sim$30 percent) and overlapping but distinct biologic activities. A specific receptor for IL-4, which does not bind IL-13, is found on T cells and NK cells. It consists of IL-4Rα (CD124) and γ_c and transmits signals via Jak1 and Jak3. A second receptor complex that can bind either IL-4 or IL-13 is found on keratinocytes, endothelial cells, and other nonhematopoietic cells.[57] It consists of IL-13Rα1 (CD213a1) and IL-4Rα and transmits signals via Jak1 and Jak2. These receptors are expressed at low levels in resting cells and their expression is increased by various activating signals. Both signal transduction pathways appear to converge with the activation of STAT6, which is both necessary and sufficient to drive T_H2 differentiation, as well as the insulin receptor substrates 1 and 2 (IRS-1 and IRS-2) and Shc. Another cell surface molecule homologous to IL-13Rα1, termed IL-13Rα2 (CD213a2), binds with high affinity to IL-13 but is not known to transmit any signals and may function as a decoy receptor.[58]

The biologic effects of engagement of the IL-4 receptor vary depending on the specific cell type, but most pertain to its principal role as a growth and differentiation factor for T_H2 cells.[59] Exposure of naive T cells to IL-4 stimulates them to proliferate and differentiate into T_H2 cells, which produce more IL-4; this cycle leads to autocrine stimulation that prolongs T_H2 responses. Thus, the expression of IL-4 early in the immune response can initiate a cascade of T_H2 cell development leading to a predominately T_H2 response. The genes encoding IL-4 and IL-13 are located in a cluster with IL-5 that undergoes structural changes during T_H2 differentiation that are associated with increased expression. While naive T cells can make low levels of IL-4 when activated, it is also produced by activated NKT cells. Mast cells and basophils also release preformed IL-4 from secretory granules in response to FcεRI-mediated signals.[60] A prominent activity of IL-4 is the stimulation of class switching of the immunoglobulin genes of B cells. As critical factors in T_H2 differentiation and effector function, IL-4 and IL-13 are mediators of atopic immunity. In addition to controlling the behavior of effector cells, they also act directly on resident tissue cells such as in inflammatory airway reactions.

IL-7 Mutations abrogating the function of IL-7, IL-7Rα (CD127), γ_c, or Jak3 in mice or humans cause profound immunodeficiency as a result of T and NK cell depletion.[55] This is principally due to the indispensable role of IL-7 in promoting the expansion of lymphocytes and regulating the rearrangement of their antigen receptor genes. IL-7 is a potent mitogen and survival factor for immature lymphocytes in the bone marrow and thymus. The second function of IL-7 is as a modifier of effector cell functions in the reactive phase of certain immune responses. IL-7 transmits activating signals to mature T cells and certain activated B cells. Like IL-2, IL-7 stimulates proliferation of cytolytic T cells (CTL) and lymphokine-activated killer (LAK) cells in vitro, and enhances their activities in vivo. Monocytes exposed to IL-7 release IL-6, IL-1α, IL-1β, and TNF-α, and exhibit enhanced tumoricidal activity in vitro. IL-7 is a particularly significant cytokine for lymphocytes in the skin and other epithelial tissues. It is expressed by keratinocytes in a regulated fashion, and this expression is thought to be part of a reciprocal signaling dialogue between dendritic epidermal T cells and keratinocytes in murine skin. Keratinocytes release IL-7 in response to IFN-γ and dendritic epidermal T cells secrete IFN-γ in response to IL-7.[61]

IL-9 AND IL-21 IL-9 is a product of activated T_H2 cells that acts as an autocrine growth factor as well as a mediator of inflammation.[62] It is also produced by mast cells in response to IL-10 or stem cell factor. It stimulates proliferation of T and B cells and promotes expression of IgE by B cells. It also exerts proinflammatory effects on mast cells and eosinophils. Mice deficient in IL-9 have deficits in mast cell and goblet cell differentiation. Thus, IL-9 appears to be a potent effector of allergic inflammatory processes. IL-21 is a recently discovered cytokine that triggers signals through a receptor composed of a specific α chain (IL-21R) and γ_c.[63] IL-21 elicits varied responses from different lymphocytes; most notably it promotes proliferation and maturation of NK cells.

Cytokines with Receptors That Use the IL-3Rβ Chain: IL-3, IL-5, and GM-CSF

The receptors for IL-3, IL-5, and GM-CSF consist of unique cytokine-specific α chains paired with a common β chain known as IL-3Rβ, or β_c (CDw131). Each of these factors acts on subsets of early hematopoietic cells.[64] IL-3, previously known as multilineage colony-stimulating factor, is principally a product of CD4+ T cells and causes proliferation, differentiation, and colony formation of various myeloid cells from bone marrow. IL-5 is a product of T_H2 CD4+ cells, as well as of activated mast cells, that conveys signals to B cells and eosinophils. IL-5 has costimulatory activity on B cells in that it enhances their proliferation and immunoglobulin expression in conjunction with antigen. In conjunction with an eosinophil-attracting chemokine known as eotaxin, IL-5 plays a central role in the accumulation of eosinophils that accompanies parasite infections and some cutaneous inflammatory processes. IL-5 appears to be required to generate a pool of eosinophil precursors in bone marrow that can be rapidly mobilized to the blood, while eotaxin recruits these eosinophils from blood into specific tissue sites.[65] GM-CSF is a growth factor for myeloid progenitors in the bone marrow. It is produced by activated T cells, phagocytes, keratinocytes, fibroblasts, and vascular endothelial cells. In addition to its role in early hematopoiesis, GM-CSF has potent effects on macrophages and dendritic cells. Fresh Langerhans cells cultured in vitro in the presence of GM-CSF are transformed into mature dendritic cells with maximal immunostimulatory potential for naive T cells. The effects of GM-CSF on dendritic cells probably account for the dramatic ability of GM-CSF to evoke therapeutic antitumor immunity when tumor cells are engineered to express it.[66]

IL-6 and Other Cytokines with Receptors That Use GP130

Receptors for a group of cytokines including IL-6, IL-11, leukemia inhibitory factor (LIF), oncostatin M (OSM), ciliary neurotrophic factor (CNTF), and cardiotrophin-1 (CT-1) interact with a hematopoietin receptor family member, gp130 (*g*lyco*p*rotein, *130* kDa), that does not appear to interact with any ligand by itself. gp130 is recruited into signaling complexes with other receptor chains when they engage their cognate ligands; these complexes may result in the formation of gp130 homodimers (as in the case of IL-6 and IL-11 signaling) or heterodimers between gp130 and the cytokine-specific α chain (as occurs with LIF, OSM, CNTF, and CT-1).[67]

IL-6 is the most thoroughly characterized of the cytokines that use gp130 for signaling, and it serves as a paradigm for discussion of the biologic effects of this family of cytokines. IL-6 is yet another example of a highly pleiotropic cytokine with multiple effects. Different names (including interferon-β2, B cell stimulatory factor 2, plasmacytoma growth factor, cytotoxic T cell differentiation factor, and hepatocyte-stimulating factor) were used for IL-6 before it was recognized that a single molecular species could account for all of these activities. IL-6 acts on a wide variety of cells of hematopoietic origin. IL-6 stimulates immunoglobulin secretion by B cells and has mitogenic activity on B lineage cells and plasmacytomas. IL-6 also promotes maturation of megakaryocytes and differentiation of myeloid cells. In addition to its participation in hematopoietic development and reactive immune responses, IL-6 is a central mediator of the systemic acute phase response. Increases in circulating IL-6 levels stimulate hepatocytes to synthesize and release acute phase proteins.

Two distinct signal transduction pathways are triggered by IL-6.[67] The first is mediated through the gp130 molecule, which dimerizes on engagement by the complex of IL-6 and IL-6Rα. Homodimerization of gp130 and its associated Jak kinases (Jak1, Jak2, Tyk2) leads to activation of STAT3. A second pathway of gp130 signal transduction involves Ras and the MAP kinase cascade and results in phosphorylation and activation of a transcription factor originally designated nuclear factor of IL-6 (NF-IL6).

IL-6 is an important cytokine for skin and is subject to dysregulation in several human diseases including some with skin manifestations.[68] IL-6 is produced in a regulated fashion by keratinocytes, fibroblasts, and vascular endothelial cells, as well as by leukocytes infiltrating the skin. IL-6 can stimulate the proliferation of human keratinocytes under some conditions.[69] Psoriasis is one of several inflammatory skin diseases in which the expression of IL-6 is elevated.[69] Human herpesvirus-8 (HHV-8) produces a viral homologue of IL-6 that may be involved in the pathogenesis of HHV-8–associated diseases, including Kaposi's sarcoma and body cavity-based lymphomas.[70]

The other cytokines that use gp130 as a signal transducer have diverse bioactivities. IL-11 inhibits production of inflammatory cytokines and has shown some therapeutic activity in patients with psoriasis.[71] Exogenous IL-11 also stimulates platelet production and has been used to treat thrombocytopenia occurring after chemotherapy.[72] As their names imply, OSM and LIF can suppress growth and metastasis of certain malignant cells; while in other systems, they either promote or inhibit differentiation, tissue repair, and other cellular processes.

IL-12: The Pivotal Cytokine for T_H1 Responses

IL-12 is distinct from most other cytokines in that in its active form it is a heterodimer of two proteins, p35 and p40. IL-12 is principally a product of antigen-presenting cells such as dendritic cells, monocytes, and macrophages, as well as certain B cells in response to bacterial components, GM-CSF, and IFN-γ. Activated keratinocytes are an additional source of IL-12 in skin. Human keratinocytes constitutively make the p35 subunit, and expression of the p40 subunit can be induced by stimuli such as contact allergens, phorbol esters, and UV radiation.[73]

IL-12 is a critical immunoregulatory cytokine that is central to the initiation and maintenance of T_H1 responses.[74] T_H1 responses that depend on IL-12 provide protective immunity to intracellular bacterial pathogens, while IL-12–mediated T_H1 responses are central to several autoimmune diseases. IL-12 also has stimulatory effects on NK cells, promoting their proliferation, cytotoxic function, and the production of cytokines including IFN-γ. IL-12 stimulates protective antitumor immunity in a number of animal models.[66]

Two chains that are part of the cell surface receptor for IL-12 have been cloned. Both are homologous to other β chains in the hematopoietin receptor family and are currently designated β_1 and β_2. The β_1 chain is associated with Tyk2, and the β_2 chain interacts directly with Jak2. The signaling component of the IL-12R is the β_2 chain. The β_2 chain is expressed in T_H1 but not T_H2 cells and appears to be critical for the commitment of T cells to production of type 1 cytokines. IL-12 signaling induces the phosphorylation of STAT1, STAT3, and STAT4, but it is STAT4 that is essential for induction of a T_H1 response.[74]

Recently, a novel cytokine that uses the p40 chain of IL-12 was discovered. IL-23, which is comprised of the IL-12 p40 chain and a distinct p19 chain, has activities that overlap with those of IL-12, but also appears to induce proliferation of memory T cells.[75]

THE CLASS II FAMILY OF CYTOKINE RECEPTORS AND THEIR LIGANDS

A second major class of cytokine receptors with common features includes two types of receptors for interferons, the IL-10R, and the recently discovered receptors for additional IL-10–related cytokines, including IL-19, IL-20, IL-22, and IL-24.

Interferons: Prototypes of Cytokines Signaling through a Jak-STAT Pathway

IFNs were one of the first families of cytokines to be characterized in detail. The IFNs were initially subdivided into three classes: IFN-α

(the leukocyte IFNs), IFN-β (fibroblast IFN), and IFN-γ (immune IFN). The α and β IFNs are collectively called type I IFNs, and all of these molecules signal through the same two-chain receptor (the IFN-$\alpha\beta$ receptor).[76] The second IFN receptor is a distinct two-chain receptor specific for IFN-γ.[13] Both receptors are present on many cell types in skin, as well as in other tissues. Each of the chains comprising the two IFN receptors is associated with one of the Jak kinases (Tyk2 and Jak1 for the IFN-$\alpha\beta$R and Jak1 and Jak2 for the IFN-γR). Only in the presence of both chains and two functional Jak kinases does effective signal transduction occur after IFN binding.

Viruses, double-stranded RNA, and bacterial products are among the stimuli that elicit release of the type I IFNs from cells. Many of the effects of the type I IFNs directly or indirectly increase host resistance to the spread of viral infection. Additional effects mediated through the IFN-$\alpha\beta$R are increased expression of major histocompatibility complex (MHC) class I molecules and stimulation of NK cell activity.[76] In addition to its well-known antiviral effects, IFN-α also can modulate T cell responses by favoring the development of a T_H1 type of T cell response.[77] Finally, the type I IFNs also inhibit the proliferation of a variety of cell types, providing a rationale for their use in the treatment of some types of cancer.[77] Forms of IFN-α are used clinically to treat hairy cell leukemia, various lymphoid and nonlymphoid cutaneous malignancies, and papillomavirus infections.

Production of IFN-γ is restricted to NK cells, CD8 T cells, and the subset of CD4 T cells producing type 1 cytokines (T_H1 cells). T_H1 cells produce IFN-γ after engagement of the T cell receptor, and IL-12 can provide a strong costimulatory signal for T cell IFN-γ production.[74] NK cells produce IFN-γ in response to cytokines released by macrophages including TNF-α, IL-12, and IL-18. IFN-γ has antiviral effects but is a less potent mediator than the type I IFNs for induction of these effects. The major physiologic role of IFN-γ is its capacity to modulate immune responses. IFN-γ induces synthesis of multiple proteins that play essential roles in antigen presentation to T cells, including MHC class I and class II glycoproteins, invariant chain, the Lmp2 and Lmp7 components of the proteasome, and the TAP1 and TAP2 intracellular peptide transporters. These changes increase the efficiency of antigen presentation to CD4 and CD8 T cells. IFN-γ is also required for activation of macrophages to their full antimicrobial potential, permitting them to eliminate microorganisms capable of intracellular growth. Like type I interferons, IFN-γ also has strong antiproliferative effects against some cell types. Finally, IFN-γ is an inducer of selected chemokines (e.g., IP-10 and Mig) and an inducer of endothelial cell adhesion molecules (e.g., ICAM-1 and VCAM-1). Because of the breadth of its activities, IFN-γ comes the closest of the T cell cytokines to behaving as a primary cytokine.

IL-10: An "Anti-inflammatory" Cytokine

IL-10 is one of several cytokines that primarily exert regulatory rather than stimulatory effects on immune responses.[78] IL-10 was first identified as a cytokine produced by T_H2 T cells that inhibited cytokine production after activation of T cells by antigen and antigen-presenting cells. IL-10 acts through a cell surface receptor on macrophages, dendritic cells, neutrophils, B cells, T cells, and NK cells. The ligand binding chain of the receptor is homologous to the receptors for IFN-α/β and IFN-γ, and signaling events mediated through the IL-10 receptor use a Jak-STAT pathway. IL-10 binding to its receptor activates the Jak1 and Tyk2 kinases and leads to the activation of STAT1 and STAT3. Inhibitory effects of IL-10 on antigen-presenting cells such as monocytes, macrophages, and dendritic cells include inhibition of expression of class II MHC and costimulatory molecules (e.g., B7-1, B7-2) and decreased production of T cell-stimulating cytokines (e.g., IL-1, IL-6, and IL-12). At least four viral genomes harbor viral homologues of IL-10 that are biologically active after binding to the IL-10R. There are several cell types for which IL-10 has stimulatory rather than inhibitory effects; IL-10 stimulates B cell synthesis of class II MHC molecules and costimulates the growth of mast cells.

Epidermal keratinocytes are a major source of IL-10 in skin. IL-10 production by keratinocytes is upregulated after cell activation; one of the best characterized activating stimuli for keratinocytes is UV irradiation.[79] UV-induced keratinocyte IL-10 production leads to local and systemic effects on immunity. Some of the well-documented immunosuppressive effects that occur after exposure to UV light exposure are the result of the liberation of keratinocyte-derived IL-10 into the systemic circulation.[80] IL-10 also plays a dampening role in other types of cutaneous immune and inflammatory responses, because the absence of IL-10 predisposes mice to exaggerated irritant and contact sensitivity responses.[81]

Novel IL-10–Related Cytokines: IL-19, IL-20, IL-22, and IL-24

Cytokines related to IL-10 have been identified and shown to engage a number of receptor complexes with shared chains. IL-19, IL-20, and IL-24 transmit signals via a complex consisting of IL-20Rα and IL-20Rβ. Transgenic mice overexpressing IL-20 develop severe cutaneous inflammation and altered epidermal proliferation and differentiation. Expression of the IL-20R chains is strongly induced when they are triggered and they are only detected on keratinocytes, endothelial cells, and certain monocytes in association with inflammatory conditions such as psoriasis.[82] IL-22 activates a receptor consisting of IL-22R and IL-10Rβ, while IL-20 and IL-24 also engage a complex incorporating IL-20Rβ and IL-22R.[83,84] The profound effects of IL-20 expression in transgenic mice and the association of IL-20R expression with psoriasis point toward a central role for these cytokines in the epidermal changes associated with cutaneous inflammation.

THE TGF-β FAMILY AND ITS RECEPTORS

TGF-β1 was first isolated as a secreted product of virally transformed tumor cells capable of inducing normal cells in vitro to show phenotypic characteristics associated with transformation. More than 30 additional members of the TGF-β family have been identified and are grouped into several families: the prototypic TGF-βs (TGF-β_1 to TGF-β_3), the bone morphogenetic proteins (BMPs), the growth/differentiation factors (GDFs), and the activins.[85] The TGF name for this family of molecules is somewhat of a misnomer, because TGF-β has antiproliferative rather than proliferative effects on most cell types. Many of the TGF-β family members play an important role in development, influencing the differentiation of uncommitted cells into specific lineages. TGF-β family members are made as precursor proteins that are biologically inactive until a large pro-domain is cleaved. Monomers of the mature domain of TGF-β family members are disulfide-linked to form dimers that strongly resist denaturation.[86]

Participation of at least two cell surface receptors (type I and type II) with serine/threonine kinase activity is required for biologic effects of TGF-β. Ligand binding by the type II receptor (the true ligand-binding receptor) is associated with the formation of complexes of type I and type II receptors. This allows the type II receptor to phosphorylate and activate the type I receptor, a "transducer" molecule responsible for downstream signal transduction. Downstream signal transmission from the membrane-bound receptors in the TGF-β receptor family to the nucleus is primarily mediated by a family of cytoplasmic Smad proteins that translocate to the nucleus and regulate transcription of target genes.[87]

TGF-β has a profound influence on several types of immune and inflammatory processes. A combination of effects of TGF-β on fibroblast function make it one of the most fibrogenic of all cytokines studied.[88] Fibroblasts treated with TGF-β display enhanced production of collagen and other extracellular matrix molecules. In addition, TGF-β inhibits the production of metalloproteinases by fibroblasts and stimulates the production of tissue inhibitors of the same metalloproteinases (TIMPs). TGF-β effects on fibroblasts may be important in promoting wound healing. An immunoregulatory role for TGF-β_1 was identified in part through analysis of TGF-β_1 knockout mice. These mice develop a wasting disease at 20 days of age that is associated with a mixed inflammatory cell infiltrate involving many internal organs. Development of cells in the dendritic cell lineage is also perturbed in mice deficient in TGF-β_1, as evidenced by an absence of epidermal Langerhans cells and specific subpopulations of lymph node dendritic cells.[89]

CHEMOKINES: SECONDARY CYTOKINES CENTRAL TO LEUKOCYTE MOBILIZATION

Chemokines are a large superfamily of small cytokines that have two major functions. First, they guide leukocytes via chemotactic gradients in tissue. Typically, the purpose is to bring an effector cell to where its activities are required. Second, a subset of chemokines has the capacity to increase the binding of leukocytes via their integrins to ligands at the endothelial cell surface, thus facilitating firm adhesion and extravasation of leukocytes in tissue. The complex activities of this important class of cytokines are discussed in Chap. 27.

THE CYTOKINE NETWORK—THERAPEUTIC IMPLICATIONS AND APPLICATIONS

Although many things may change in the world of cytokines, certain key concepts have stood the test of time. Principal among them is the idea that cytokines are emergency molecules, designed to be released locally and transiently in tissue microenvironments. When cytokines are released persistently, the result typically is chronic disease. One potential way to treat such diseases is with cytokine antagonists or other drugs that target cytokines or cytokine-mediated pathways.

For the clinician, certain key questions have arisen around the therapeutic use of cytokines. Several cytokines have already entered clinical trials, and some, such as type I interferons, have been used for years to treat melanoma and cutaneous lymphomas. With certain notable exceptions, systemic cytokine therapy has been disappointing and is often accompanied by substantial morbidity. In contrast, the local administration of cytokines, including transduction of autologous melanoma cells with factors such as GM-CSF or IL-12, may yield more promising results.[66] This is consistent with the idea that if used locally and transiently, cytokines are powerful biologic response modifiers. The use of GM-CSF and IL-12 as vaccine adjuvants is being extensively tested. Conversely, agents that specifically block cytokine activity are also being developed. The natural antagonist of IL-1 (IL-1ra), antibodies to TNF-α, and a recombinant soluble TNFR1 have already been approved for clinical use. These antagonists of TNF-α activity appear highly effective at inducing durable remissions in patients with psoriasis.[52,53] Specific antagonists of other cytokines are also being developed. Cytokines that have predominantly anti-inflammatory effects, such as IL-10 and IL-11, are being used to treat inflammatory skin diseases such as psoriasis.[71,90] Finally, fusion toxins linked to cytokines, such as DAB_{389}IL-2 (Ontak), exploit the cellular specificity of certain cytokine receptor interactions to kill target cells.[91] Each of these approaches is still new and open to considerable future development. An understanding of cytokines by clinicians of the future is likely to be central to effective patient care.

REFERENCES

1. Oppenheim JJ: Cytokines: Past, present, and future. *Int J Hematol* **74**:3, 2001
2. Dinarello CA: Interleukin-1. *Cytokine Growth Factor Rev* **8**:253, 1997
3. Bigazzi PE et al: Production of lymphokine-like factors (cytokines) by simian virus 40-infected and simian virus 40-transformed cells. *Am J Pathol* **80**:69, 1975
4. Luger TA et al: Epidermal cell (keratinocyte)-derived thymocyte-activating factor (ETAF). *J Immunol* **127**:1493, 1981
5. Kupper TS: The activated keratinocyte: A model for inducible cytokine production by non-bone marrow-derived cells in cutaneous inflammatory and immune responses. *J Invest Dermatol* **94**:146S, 1990
6. Kupper TS: Immune and inflammatory processes in cutaneous tissues. Mechanisms and speculations. *J Clin Invest* **86**:1783, 1990
7. Rock FL et al: A family of human receptors structurally related to *Drosophila* Toll. *Proc Natl Acad Sci U S A* **95**:588, 1998
8. Sieling PA, Modlin RL: Toll-like receptors: mammalian "taste receptors" for a smorgasbord of microbial invaders. *Curr Opin Microbiol* **5**:70, 2002
9. Mosmann TR, Coffman RL: T_H1 and T_H2 cells: Different patterns of lymphokine secretion lead to different functional properties. *Annu Rev Immunol* **7**:145, 1989
10. Mosmann TR, Sad S: The expanding universe of T-cell subsets: T_H1, T_H2 and more. *Immunol Today* **17**:138, 1996
11. Weiner HL: Induction and mechanism of action of transforming growth factor-β–secreting T_H3 regulatory cells. *Immunol Rev* **182**:207, 2001
12. Nicola NA, Hilton DJ: General classes and functions of four-helix bundle cytokines. *Adv Protein Chem* **52**:1, 1998
13. Bach EA et al: The IFNγ receptor: a paradigm for cytokine receptor signaling. *Annu Rev Immunol* **15**:563, 1997
14. Chan KF et al: Signaling by the TNF receptor superfamily and T cell homeostasis. *Immunity* **13**:419, 2000
15. Barnes PJ, Karin M: Nuclear factor-κB: A pivotal transcription factor in chronic inflammatory diseases. *N Engl J Med* **336**:1066, 1997
16. Karin M, Delhase M: The IκB kinase (IKK) and NF-κB: Key elements of proinflammatory signaling. *Semin Immunol* **12**:85, 2000
17. Poltorak A et al: Defective LPS signaling in C3H/HeJ and C57BL/10ScCr mice: Mutations in Tlr4 gene. *Science* **282**:2085, 1998
18. Sims JE: IL-1 and IL-18 receptors, and their extended family. *Curr Opin Immunol* **14**:117, 2002
19. Jensen LE, Whitehead AS: IRAK1b, a novel alternative splice variant of interleukin-1 receptor-associated kinase (IRAK), mediates interleukin-1 signaling and has prolonged stability. *J Biol Chem* **276**:29037, 2001
20. Rosette C, Karin M: Ultraviolet light and osmotic stress: Activation of the JNK cascade through multiple growth factor and cytokine receptors. *Science* **274**:1194, 1996
21. Scheinman RI et al: Role of transcriptional activation of IκBα in mediation of immunosuppression by glucocorticoids. *Science* **270**:283, 1995
22. Darnell JE Jr et al: Jak-STAT pathways and transcriptional activation in response to IFNs and other extracellular signaling proteins. *Science* **264**:1415, 1994
23. Leonard WJ: Role of Jak kinases and STATs in cytokine signal transduction. *Int J Hematol* **73**:271, 2001
24. Takeda K, Akira S: STAT family of transcription factors in cytokine-mediated biological responses. *Cytokine Growth Factor Rev* **11**:199, 2000
25. Greenhalgh CJ, Hilton DJ: Negative regulation of cytokine signaling. *J Leukoc Biol* **70**:348, 2001
26. Thornberry NA et al: A novel heterodimeric cysteine protease is required for interleukin-1β processing in monocytes. *Nature* **356**:768, 1992
27. MacKenzie A et al: Rapid secretion of interleukin-1β by microvesicle shedding. *Immunity* **15**:825, 2001
28. Kobayashi Y et al: Identification of calcium-activated neutral protease as a processing enzyme of human interleukin 1α. *Proc Natl Acad Sci U S A* **87**:5548, 1990
29. Enk AH et al: An essential role for Langerhans cell-derived IL-1β in the initiation of primary immune responses in skin. *J Immunol* **150**:3698, 1993

30. Nakae S et al: IL-1α, but not IL-1β, is required for contact-allergen-specific T cell activation during the sensitization phase in contact hypersensitivity. *Int Immunol* **13**:1471, 2001
31. Cullinan EB et al: IL-1 receptor accessory protein is an essential component of the IL-1 receptor. *J Immunol* **161**:5614, 1998
32. Cao Z et al: TRAF6 is a signal transducer for interleukin-1. *Nature* **383**:443, 1996
33. Hannum CH et al: Interleukin-1 receptor antagonist activity of a human interleukin-1 inhibitor. *Nature* **343**:336, 1990
34. Muzio M et al: Cloning and characterization of a new isoform of the interleukin 1 receptor antagonist. *J Exp Med* **182**:623, 1995
35. Hirsch E et al: Functions of interleukin 1 receptor antagonist in gene knockout and overproducing mice. *Proc Natl Acad Sci U S A* **93**:11008, 1996
36. Symons JA et al: Soluble type II interleukin 1 (IL-1) receptor binds and blocks processing of IL-1β precursor and loses affinity for IL-1 receptor antagonist. *Proc Natl Acad Sci U S A* **92**:1714, 1995
37. Colotta F et al: Interleukin-1 type II receptor: A decoy target for IL-1 that is regulated by IL-4. *Science* **261**:472, 1993
38. Groves RW et al: Inducible expression of type 2 IL-1 receptors by cultured human keratinocytes. Implications for IL-1-mediated processes in epidermis. *J Immunol* **154**:4065, 1995
39. Dinarello CA et al: Overview of interleukin-18: More than an interferon-γ inducing factor. *J Leukoc Biol* **63**:658, 1998
40. McInnes IB et al: Interleukin 18: A pleiotropic participant in chronic inflammation. *Immunol Today* **21**:312, 2000
41. Nakanishi K et al: Interleukin-18 regulates both T_H1 and T_H2 responses. *Annu Rev Immunol* **19**:423, 2001
42. Hammerberg C et al: Interleukin-1 receptor antagonist in normal and psoriatic epidermis. *J Clin Invest* **90**:571, 1992
43. Lee RT et al: Mechanical deformation promotes secretion of IL-1α and IL-1 receptor antagonist. *J Immunol* **159**:5084, 1997
44. Killar L et al: Adamalysins. A family of metzincins including TNF-α converting enzyme (TACE). *Ann N Y Acad Sci* **878**:442, 1999
45. von Boehmer H: Lymphotoxins: from cytotoxicity to lymphoid organogenesis. *Proc Natl Acad Sci U S A* **94**:8926, 1997
46. Kock A et al: Human keratinocytes are a source for tumor necrosis factor α: Evidence for synthesis and release upon stimulation with endotoxin or ultraviolet light. *J Exp Med* **172**:1609, 1990
47. Piguet PF et al: Tumor necrosis factor is a critical mediator in hapten induced irritant and contact hypersensitivity reactions. *J Exp Med* **173**:673, 1991
48. Pasparakis M et al: Immune and inflammatory responses in TNF-α-deficient mice: A critical requirement for TNF-α in the formation of primary B cell follicles, follicular dendritic cell networks and germinal centers, and in the maturation of the humoral immune response. *J Exp Med* **184**:1397, 1996
49. Cumberbatch M et al: Langerhans cell migration. *Clin Exp Dermatol* **25**:413, 2000
50. Schwarzenberger K, Udey MC: Contact allergens and epidermal proinflammatory cytokines modulate Langerhans cell E-cadherin expression in situ. *J Invest Dermatol* **106**:553, 1996
51. Trefzer U et al: The 55-kD tumor necrosis factor receptor on human keratinocytes is regulated by tumor necrosis factor-α and by ultraviolet B radiation. *J Clin Invest* **92**:462, 1993
52. Mease PJ et al: Etanercept in the treatment of psoriatic arthritis and psoriasis: A randomised trial. *Lancet* **356**:385, 2000
53. Chaudhari U et al: Efficacy and safety of infliximab monotherapy for plaque-type psoriasis: A randomised trial. *Lancet* **357**:1842, 2001
54. Taniguchi T: Cytokine signaling through nonreceptor protein tyrosine kinases. *Science* **268**:251, 1995
55. Notarangelo LD et al: Of genes and phenotypes: the immunological and molecular spectrum of combined immune deficiency. Defects of the γ_c-JAK3 signaling pathway as a model. *Immunol Rev* **178**:39, 2000
56. Waldmann TA et al: Contrasting roles of IL-2 and IL-15 in the life and death of lymphocytes: Implications for immunotherapy. *Immunity* **14**:105, 2001
57. Kawakami K et al: The interleukin-13 receptor α2 chain: An essential component for binding and internalization but not for interleukin-13-induced signal transduction through the STAT6 pathway. *Blood* **97**:2673, 2001
58. Bernard J et al: Expression of interleukin 13 receptor in glioma and renal cell carcinoma: IL13Rα2 as a decoy receptor for IL13. *Lab Invest* **81**:1223, 2001
59. Seder RA et al: The presence of interleukin 4 during in vitro priming determines the lymphokine-producing potential of CD4+ T cells from T cell receptor transgenic mice. *J Exp Med* **176**:1091, 1992
60. Plaut M et al: Mast cell lines produce lymphokines in response to cross-linkage of FcεRI or to calcium ionophores. *Nature* **339**:64, 1989
61. Takashima A et al: Interleukin-7-dependent interaction of dendritic epidermal T cells with keratinocytes. *J Invest Dermatol* **105**:50S, 1995
62. Soussi-Gounni A et al: Role of IL-9 in the pathophysiology of allergic diseases. *J Allergy Clin Immunol* **107**:575, 2001
63. Vosshenrich CA, Di Santo JP: Cytokines: IL-21 joins the γ_c-dependent network? *Curr Biol* **11**:R175, 2001
64. Geijsen N et al: Specificity in cytokine signal transduction: lessons learned from the IL-3/IL-5/GM-CSF receptor family. *Cytokine Growth Factor Rev* **12**:19, 2001
65. Collins PD et al: Cooperation between interleukin-5 and the chemokine eotaxin to induce eosinophil accumulation in vivo. *J Exp Med* **182**:1169, 1995
66. Mach N, Dranoff G: Cytokine-secreting tumor cell vaccines. *Curr Opin Immunol* **12**:571, 2000
67. Taga T, Kishimoto T: Gp130 and the interleukin-6 family of cytokines. *Annu Rev Immunol* **15**:797, 1997
68. Paquet P, Pierard GE: Interleukin-6 and the skin. *Int Arch Allergy Immunol* **109**:308, 1996
69. Grossman RM et al: Interleukin 6 is expressed in high levels in psoriatic skin and stimulates proliferation of cultured human keratinocytes. *Proc Natl Acad Sci USA* **86**:6367, 1989
70. Neipel F et al: Human herpesvirus 8 encodes a homolog of interleukin-6. *J Virol* **71**:839, 1997
71. Trepicchio WL et al: Interleukin-11 therapy selectively downregulates type I cytokine proinflammatory pathways in psoriasis lesions. *J Clin Invest* **104**:1527, 1999
72. Schwertschlag US et al: Hematopoietic, immunomodulatory and epithelial effects of interleukin-11. *Leukemia* **13**:1307, 1999
73. Enk CD et al: UVB induces IL-12 transcription in human keratinocytes in vivo and in vitro. *Photochem Photobiol* **63**:854, 1996
74. Sinigaglia F et al: Regulation of the IL-12/IL-12R axis: A critical step in T-helper cell differentiation and effector function. *Immunol Rev* **170**:65, 1999
75. Oppmann B et al: Novel p19 protein engages IL-12p40 to form a cytokine, IL-23, with biological activities similar as well as distinct from IL-12. *Immunity* **13**:715, 2000
76. Bogdan C: The function of type I interferons in antimicrobial immunity. *Curr Opin Immunol* **12**:419, 2000
77. Belardelli F, Gresser I: The neglected role of type I interferon in the T-cell response: Implications for its clinical use. *Immunol Today* **17**:369, 1996
78. Moore KW et al: Interleukin-10 and the interleukin-10 receptor. *Annu Rev Immunol* **19**:683, 2001
79. Enk CD et al: Induction of IL-10 gene expression in human keratinocytes by UVB exposure in vivo and in vitro. *J Immunol* **154**:4851, 1995
80. Shreedhar V et al: A cytokine cascade including prostaglandin E2, IL-4, and IL-10 is responsible for UV-induced systemic immune suppression. *J Immunol* **160**:3783, 1998
81. Berg DJ et al: Interleukin 10 but not interleukin 4 is a natural suppressant of cutaneous inflammatory responses. *J Exp Med* **182**:99, 1995
82. Blumberg H et al: Interleukin 20: Discovery, receptor identification, and role in epidermal function. *Cell* **104**:9, 2001
83. Dumoutier L et al: Cutting edge: STAT activation by IL-19, IL-20 and mda-7 through IL-20 receptor complexes of two types. *J Immunol* **167**:3545, 2001
84. Wang M et al: Interleukin 24 (MDA-7/MOB-5) Signals through two heterodimeric receptors, IL-22R1/IL-20R2 and IL-20R1/IL-20R2. *J Biol Chem* **277**:7341, 2002
85. Kingsley DM: The TGF-β superfamily: New members, new receptors, and new genetic tests of function in different organisms. *Genes Dev* **8**:133, 1994
86. Bonewald LF: Regulation and regulatory activities of transforming growth factor-β. *Crit Rev Eukaryot Gene Expr* **9**:33, 1999
87. Miyazono K et al: TGF-β signaling by Smad proteins. *Adv Immunol* **75**:115, 2000
88. Denton CP, Abraham DJ: Transforming growth factor-β and connective tissue growth factor: Key cytokines in scleroderma pathogenesis. *Curr Opin Rheumatol* **13**:505, 2001
89. Strobl H, Knapp W: TGF-β1 regulation of dendritic cells. *Microbes Infect* **1**:1283, 1999
90. McInnes IB et al: IL-10 improves skin disease and modulates endothelial activation and leukocyte effector function in patients with psoriatic arthritis. *J Immunol* **167**:4075, 2001
91. Gottlieb SL et al: Response of psoriasis to a lymphocyte-selective toxin (DAB389IL-2) suggests a primary immune, but not keratinocyte, pathogenic basis. *Nat Med* **1**:442, 1995

CHAPTER 27

Sam T. Hwang

Chemokines

The skin is an organ in which the migration, influx, and egress of leukocytes occurs in both homeostatic and inflammatory processes. Chemokines and their receptors are accepted as vital mediators of cellular trafficking. Since the discovery of the first *chemo*attractant cyto*kine* or chemokine in 1977, 50 new chemokines and 17 chemokine receptors have been discovered. Most chemokines are small proteins with molecular weights in the 8 to 10 kDa range; they are synthesized constitutively in some cells and can be induced in many cell types by cytokines. Initially associated only with recruitment of leukocyte subsets to different inflammatory sites, it has become quite clear that chemokines play roles in angiogenesis, neural development, cancer metastasis, hematopoiesis, and infectious diseases.[1]

This chapter focuses primarily on the function of chemokines in inflammatory conditions, but it also touches on the role of these molecules in other settings. An overview of the structure of chemokines and chemokine receptors as well as details of the molecular signaling pathways initiated by the binding of a chemokine to its cognate receptor is provided. Expression patterns of chemokine receptors are noted, particularly in light of the many types of immune cells that potentially can be recruited to skin under inflammatory conditions. Individual chemokine receptors are highlighted in regard to observed biologic function, including facilitation of migration of effector T cells into the skin and the egress of antigen-presenting cells out of the skin. Finally, the roles of chemokines and their receptors in disease—atopic dermatitis, psoriasis, cancer, and infectious disease—are described to emphasize the diversity of chemokine functions in skin.

STRUCTURE

Chemokines can be grouped into four subfamilies based on the spacing of amino acids between the first two cysteines. The CXC chemokines (also called α-chemokines) show a C-X-C motif with one non conserved amino acid between the two cysteines. The other major subfamily is termed the CC subfamily (or β-chemokines) because of the lack of the additional amino acid. The two remaining subfamilies contain only one member each: the C subfamily is represented by lymphotactin, and fractalkine is the only member of the CXXXC (or CX3C) subfamily. Chemokines can also be assigned to one of two broad, and perhaps overlapping, functional groups. One type mediates the attraction and recruitment of immune cells to sites of active inflammation [e.g., regulated on activation, normal T cell expressed and secreted (RANTES); macrophage inflammatory protein (MIP)-1α/β; and liver and activation-regulated chemokine (LARC)], while other chemokines [e.g., secondary lymphoid-tissue chemokine (SLC) and stromal-derived factor-1 (SDF-1)] appear to play roles in constitutive or homeostatic migration pathways.[1]

The complexity and redundancy in the nomenclature of chemokines has led to the proposal by Zlotnik and Yoshie[1] for a systematic nomenclature for chemokines based on the type of chemokine (C, CXC, CX3C, or CC) and a number based on the order of discovery. For example, SDF-1, a CXC chemokine, has the systematic name CXCL12. Because this nomenclature is not yet universally used and because the original names (abbreviated in most cases) are commonly found in the literature, an original name with an abbreviation is used throughout this chapter. Table 27-1 provides a list of chemokine receptors that are discussed in this chapter, as well as the major chemokine ligands that bind to them. The systematic names of the chemokines are also shown.

Chemokines are highly conserved and have similar secondary and tertiary structures. On the basis of crystallography studies, a disordered amino terminus followed by three conserved antiparallel β-pleated sheets is a common structural feature of chemokines. Fractalkine is unique in that the chemokine domain sits atop a mucin-like stalk tethered to the plasma membrane via a transmembrane domain and short cytoplasmic tail.[2] Although CXC and CC chemokines form multimeric structures under conditions required for structural studies, these associations may be relevant only when chemokines associate with cell-surface components such as glycosaminoglycans (GAGs) or proteoglycans. Because most chemokines have a net positive charge, these proteins tend to bind to negatively charged carbohydrates present on GAGs. Indeed, the ability of positively charged chemokines to bind to GAGs is thought to enable chemokines to preferentially associate with the lumenal surface of blood vessels despite the presence of shear forces from the blood that would otherwise wash the chemokines away.

CHEMOKINE RECEPTORS AND SIGNAL TRANSDUCTION

Chemokine receptors are seven transmembrane-spanning domain membrane proteins that couple to intracellular heterotrimeric G proteins containing α, β, and γ subunits.[1] They represent a part of a large family of G-protein coupled receptors (GPCR), including rhodopsin, that have critical biologic functions. Leukocytes express three Gα protein subtypes (s, i, and q), while the β and γ subunits have 5 and 11 known subtypes, respectively. This complexity in the formation of the heterotrimeric G-protein may account for specificity in the action of certain chemokine receptors. Normally, G-proteins are inactive when guanosine diphosphate (GDP) is bound, but they are activated when the GDP is exchanged for guanosine triphosphate (GTP) (Fig. 27-1). After binding to ligand, chemokine receptors rapidly associate with G-proteins, which, in turn, increases the exchange of GTP for GDP. Pertussis toxin is a commonly used inhibitor of GPCR that irreversibly adenosine diphosphate (ADP)-ribosylates Gα subunits of the α_i class and subsequently prevents most chemokine receptor-mediated signaling. Activation of G-proteins leads to the dissociation of the G_α and $G_{\beta\gamma}$ subunits (Fig. 27-1). The G_α subunit activates protein tyrosine kinases and mitogen-activated protein kinase, leading to cytoskeletal changes

TABLE 27-1

Chemokine Receptors in Skin Biology

CHEMOKINE RECEPTOR	CHEMOKINE LIGAND	EXPRESSION PATTERN	COMMENTS	REFERENCES
CCR1	MIP-1α (CCL3), RANTES (CCL5), MCP-3 (CCL7)	T, Mo, DC, NK, B	Migration of DC and monocytes; strongly upregulated in T cells by IL-2	(58)
CCR2	MCP-1 (CCL2), -3, -4 (CCL13)	T, Mo	Migration of T cells to inflamed sites	(58)
CCR3	Eotaxin (CCL11) > RANTES, MCP-2 (CCL8), -3, -4	Eo, Ba, T_H2, K	Migration of T_H2 cells and "allergic" immune cells	(21, 41)
CCR4	TARC (CCL17), MDC (CCL22)	T	Expression in $T_H2 > T_H1$ cells; highly expressed on CLA^+ memory T cells; TARC expression by keratinocytes may be important in atopic dermatitis	(8, 20, 36, 37)
CCR5	RANTES MIP-1α, β (CCL3,4)	T, Mo, DC	Marker for T_H1 cells; migration to acutely inflamed sites; may be involved in transmigration of T cells through endothelium; major HIV-1 fusion co-receptor	(12, 58)
CCR6	LARC (CCL20)	T, DC, B	Expressed by memory, not naive, T cells; possibly involved in arrest of memory T cells to activated endothelium and recruitment of T cells to epidermis in psoriasis	(15, 45, 66)
CCR7	SLC (CCL21), ELC (CCL19)	T, DC, B	Critical for migration of naïve T cells and "central memory" T cells to secondary lymphoid organs; required for mature DC to enter lymphatics and localize to lymph nodes	(13, 27, 67, 68)
CCR10	CTACK (CCL27)	T	Preferential response of CLA^+ T cells to CTACK in vitro; may be involved in T cells homing to epidermis, where CTACK is expressed	(7, 26)
CXCR1, 2	IL-8 (CXCL8), MGSA/GRO α (CXCL1), ENA-78 (CXCL5)	N, NK, En	Recruitment of neutrophils (e.g., epidermis in psoriasis); may be involved in angiogenesis	(69, 70)
CXCR3	IP-10 (CXCL10), Mig (CXCL9), I-TAC (CXCL11)	T	Marker for T_H1 cells and may be involved in T cell recruitment to epidermis in CTCL; induces arrest of activated T cells on stimulated endothelium	(17, 25)
CXCR4	SDF-1α, β (CXCL12)	T, DC, En	Major HIV-1 fusion coreceptor; involved in vascular formation	(58)
CX3CR1	Fractalkine (CX3CL1)	T, Mo, MC, NK	May be involved in adhesion of activated T cells, Mo, NK cells to activated endothelium	(2,16)

ABBREVIATIONS: B, B cells; Ba, basophils; CLA, cutaneous lymphocyte-associated antigen; CTACK, cutaneous T cell attracting chemokine. DC, dendritic cells; En, endothelial cells; Eo, eosinophils; GRO, growth-regulated oncogene; HIV, human immunodeficiency virus; IL-8, interleukin-8; I-TAC, interferon-inducible T cell α chemoattractant; LARC, liver and activation-regulated chemokine (also known as MIP-3α); MC, mast cells; MCP, monocyte chemattractant protein; MDC, macrophage-derived chemokine; MGSA, melanoma growth stimulatory activity; Mig, monokine-induced by IFN-γ; MIP, macrophage inflammatory protein; Mo, monocytes; NK, natural killer cells; RANTES, regulated upon activation, normal T expressed and secreted; SDF, stromal-derived factor; SLC, secondary lymphoid-tissue chemokine; T, T cells; TARC, thymus and activation-regulated chemokine; T_H1, 2, T helper 1, 2 cell.

and gene transcription. The G_α subunit retains GTP, which is slowly hydrolyzed by the GTPase activity of this subunit. This GTPase activity is both positively and negatively regulated by GTPase-activating proteins [also known as regulator of G-protein signaling (RGS) proteins]. The $G_{\beta\gamma}$ dimer initiates critical signaling events in regard to chemotaxis and cell adhesion. It activates phospholipase C (PLC),[3] leading to formation of diacylglycerol (DAG) and inositol triphosphate [Ins(1,4,5)P_3]. Ins(1,4,5)P_3 stimulates Ca^{2+} entry into the cytosol, which, along with DAG, activates protein kinase C isoforms. Although the $G_{\beta\gamma}$ subunits are critical for chemotaxis, the $G_{\alpha i}$ subunit has no known role in chemotactic migration. There is also evidence that binding of chemokine receptors results in the activation of other intracellular effectors including Ras, Rho, and phosphatidylinositol-3-kinase (PI3K).[4] RhoA and protein kinase C appear to play a role in integrin affinity changes, whereas PI3K may be critical for changes in the avidity state of leukocyte factor antigen-1 (LFA-1). Other proteins have been found that regulate the synthesis, expression, or degradation of G-protein coupled receptors. For example, receptor–activity-modifying proteins (RAMPS) act as chaperones of seven transmembrane-spanning receptors and regulate surface expression as well as the ligand specificity of chemokine receptors (see Fig. 27-1). After chemokine receptors are exposed to appropriate ligands, they are frequently internalized, leading to an inability of the chemokine receptor to mediate further signaling. This downregulation of chemokine function, which is termed *desensitization,* occurs because of phosphorylation of Ser/Thr residues in the C-terminal tail by proteins termed *GPCR kinases* (GRK) and subsequent internalization of the receptor (see Fig. 27-1). Desensitization may be an important mechanism for regulating the function of chemokine receptors by inhibiting cell migration as leukocytes arrive at the primary site of inflammation.

CHEMOKINES AND CUTANEOUS LEUKOCYTE TRAFFICKING

Generally speaking, chemokines are thought to play at least three different roles in the recruitment of host defense cells, predominantly

FIGURE 27-1

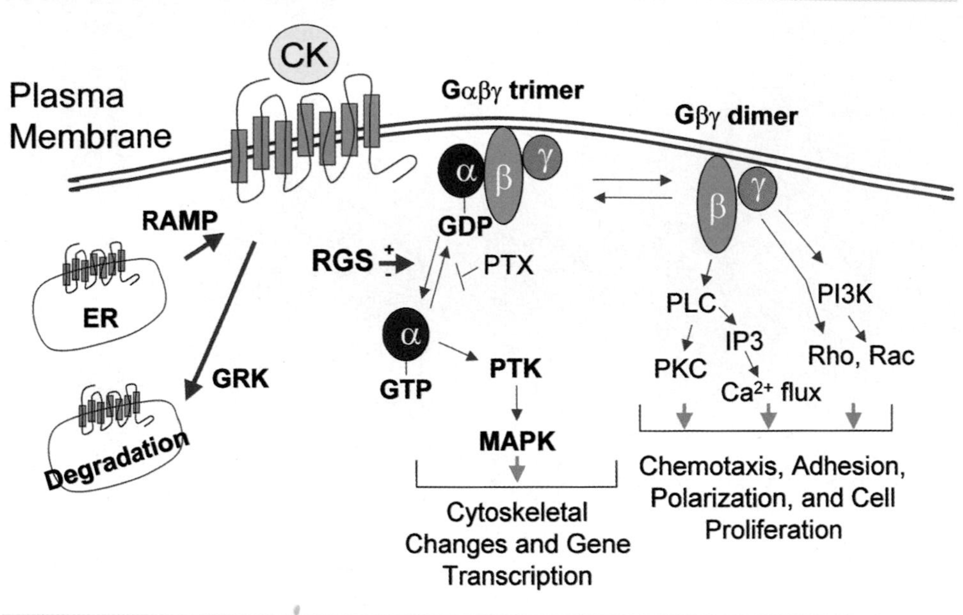

Chemokine receptor-mediated signaling pathways. CK, chemokine; DG, 1,2-diacylglycerol; ER, endoplasmic reticulum; GRK, G-protein coupled receptor kinase; IP3, inositol-1,4,5-triphosphate; MAPK, mitogen-activated protein kinase; PIP2, phosphatidylinositol-4,5-bisphosphate; PKC, protein kinase C; PLC, phospholipase C; PTK, protein tyrosine kinase(s); PTX, pertussis toxin; RAMP, receptor–activity-modifying protein; RGS, regulator of G-protein signaling.

FIGURE 27-2

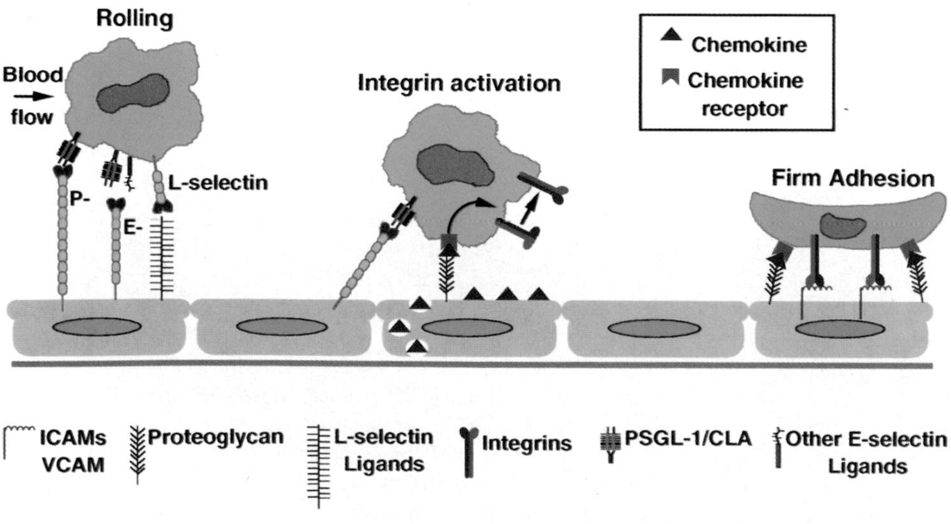

Multistep model of leukocyte recruitment. Leukocytes, pushed by the bloodstream, first transiently bind or "roll" on the surface of activated endothelial cells via rapid interactions with P-, E-, or L-selectin. Chemokines are secreted by endothelial cells and bind to proteoglycans that present the chemokine molecules to chemokine receptors on the surface of the leukocyte. After chemokine receptor ligation, intracellular signaling events lead to a change in the conformation of integrins and changes in their distribution on the plasma membrane resulting in "integrin activation." These changes result in high-affinity/avidity binding of integrins to endothelial cell intercellular adhesion molecules (ICAMs) and vascular cell adhesion molecule (VCAM)-1 in a step termed *firm adhesion,* which is then followed by transmigration of the leukocytes between endothelial cells and into tissue. PSGL-1/CLA, P-selectin glycoprotein ligand-1/cutaneous lymphocyte-associated antigen.

leukocytes, to sites of inflammation. First, they provide the signal or signals required to cause leukocytes to come to a complete stop (i.e., arrest) in blood vessels at inflamed sites such as skin. Second, chemokines have a role in the transmigration of leukocytes from the lumenal side of the blood vessel to the ablumenal side. Third, after transmigration, chemokines likely drive the migration of leukocytes to sites of inflammation either in the dermis or even the epidermis. Keratinocytes are a rich source of chemokines when stimulated by appropriate cytokines. In addition, chemokines and their receptors play critical roles in the emigration of resident skin dendritic cells (DC) (i.e., Langerhans cells and dermal DC) from the skin to draining lymph nodes via afferent lymphatic vessels, a process that is essential for the development of acquired immune responses.

This section is divided into three subsections. The first introduces basic concepts of how all leukocytes arrest in inflamed blood vessels before transmigration by introducing the multistep model of leukocyte recruitment; the second details mechanisms of T cell migration; and the final subsection focuses on the mechanisms by which chemokines mediate the physiologic migration of DC from the skin to regional lymph nodes.

Multistep Model of Leukocyte Recruitment

For leukocytes to adhere and migrate to peripheral tissues, they must overcome the pushing force of the vascular blood stream as they bind to activated endothelial cells at local sites of inflammation. According to the multistep or cascade model of leukocyte recruitment (Fig. 27-2), one set of homologous adhesion molecules termed *selectins* mediates the transient attachment of leukocytes to endothelial cells, while another set of adhesion molecules termed *integrins* and their receptors (*immunoglobulin superfamily members*) mediates stronger binding (i.e., arrest) and transmigration.[5] The selectins (E, L, and P) show great homology and are part of a larger family of carbohydrate-binding proteins termed lectins. E- and P-selectin are expressed by endothelial cells and platelets (P-selectin only), whereas L-selectin is expressed by all classes of leukocytes. The selectins bind their respective carbohydrate ligands with low affinity and rapid on/off kinetics, enabling the behavior noted in the transient binding or "rolling" of leukocytes on endothelial cells.

The major skin-associated vascular selectin is E-selectin. It is upregulated on endothelial cells by inflammatory cytokines such as tumor necrosis factor (TNF)-α and binds to sialyl Lewis x-based carbohydrates. E-selectin ligands are detected on a subset of human memory T cells by a monoclonal antibody (HECA452).[6] Because most T cells at inflamed skin sites express these carbohydrate epitopes, this antigen has been termed the *cutaneous lymphocyte-associated antigen* (CLA). CLA is expressed by 10 to 40 percent of memory T cells and has been suggested as a marker for skin-homing T cells.[6] At least two chemokine receptors (CCR10 and CCR4) show preferential expression in CLA$^+$ memory T cells.[7,8] While E-selectin is likely to be an important component of skin-selective homing, there is evidence to suggest that L-selectin may also be involved in T cell migration to skin.[9,10]

In the second phase of this model, leukocyte integrins such as those of the β_2 family must be "turned on" or activated from their resting state in order to bind to their counterreceptors such as intercellular adhesion molecule-1 (ICAM-1) that are expressed by endothelial cells. A vast array of data suggests that the binding of chemokines to leukocyte chemokine receptors plays a critical role in activating both β_1 and β_2 integrins.[4,11] Activation of chemokine receptors leads to a complex signaling cascade (see Fig. 27-1) that causes a conformational change in individual integrins, which leads to increases in the affinity of individual leukocyte integrins for their ligands. Moreover, chemokine receptor signaling causes clustering of integrins in certain areas on the plasma membrane, prompting an increase in the avidity of these integrins for their ligands (see Fig. 27-2). Furthermore, later steps of migration (i.e., transmigration or diapedesis) are also dependent on chemokines in selective cases.[12] The ability of neutrophils to roll on inflamed blood vessels likely depends on their expression of L-selectin and E-selectin ligands, whereas their arrest on activated endothelia likely depends on their expression of CXCR1 and CXCR2 as described below for wound healing. Integrin activation via chemokine-mediated signals appears to be more complex in T cells, which appear to use multiple chemokine receptors, as described in more detail below.

Chemokine-Mediated Migration of T Cells

Antigen-inexperienced T cells are termed *naive* and can be identified by expression of three cell surface proteins: CD45RA (an isoform of the pan-leukocyte marker), L-selectin, and the chemokine receptor CCR7. These T cells migrate efficiently to secondary lymphoid organs (e.g., lymph nodes), where they may make contact with antigen-bearing DC from the periphery. Once activated by DC presenting antigen, T cells then express CD45RO, are termed *memory* T cells, and appear to express a variety of adhesion molecules and chemokine receptors that facilitate their extravasation from blood vessels to inflamed peripheral tissue. A specific subset of CCR7-negative, L-selectin-negative memory T cells has been proposed to represent an effector memory T cell subset that is ready for rapid deployment at peripheral sites in terms of cytotoxic activity and ability to mobilize cytokines.[13]

Although chemokines are both secreted and soluble, the net positive charge on most chemokines enables them to bind to negatively charged proteoglycans such as heparan sulfate that are present on the lumenal surface of endothelial cells. Thus, chemokines, in effect, are presented to T cells as they roll along the lumenal surface (see Fig. 27-2). After ligand binding, chemokine receptors send intracellular signals that lead to increases in the affinity and avidity of T cell integrins such as LFA-1 and very-late antigen-4 (VLA-4) for their endothelial receptors ICAM-1 and vascular cell adhesion molecule-1 (VCAM-1), respectively. Only a few chemokine receptors (CXCR4, CCR7, CCR4, and CCR6) are expressed at sufficient levels on resting peripheral blood T cells to mediate this transition. With activation and interleukin (IL)-2 stimulation, increased numbers of chemokine receptors (e.g., CXCR3) are expressed on activated T cells, making them more likely to respond to other chemokines. In several different systems, inhibition of specific chemokines produced by endothelial cells dramatically influences T cell arrest in vivo[14] and in vitro.[15]

The possible roles of several chemokines including thymus and activation-regulated chemokine (TARC), eotaxin, LARC, the interferon-inducible protein-10 (IP-10), and fractalkine have been described in relationship to T cell homing and arrest in cutaneous sites. Several of these are discussed separately in the section dealing with chemokines and specific skin diseases. However, all can be expressed by inflamed endothelial cells and induce arrest of T cells in vitro. Potentially, these chemokines could regulate the entry of different T cell subsets to the skin under specific inflammatory conditions.

Fractalkine, the sole member of the CX3C chemokine family, can present itself because its chemokine domain sits atop a relatively rigid mucin-like, protein stalk that is tethered to the membrane surface of endothelial cells. Like LARC, fractalkine is highly upregulated by endothelial cells that are stimulated with TNF-α. Fractalkine may be of particular importance in recruiting natural killer (NK) cells and monocytes, both of which highly express the fractalkine receptor CX3CR1.[16] It may also be involved in recruiting activated T cells, which begin to express CX3CR1 after exposure to IL-2.[16]

CXCR3 serves as a receptor for chemokine ligands monokine-induced by interferon-γ (Mig), IP-10, and interferon-inducible T cell α chemoattractant (I-TAC). These three chemokines are distinguished from other chemokines by being highly upregulated by interferon-γ (IFN-γ). Resting T cells do not express functional levels of CXCR3 but upregulate this receptor with activation and cytokines such as IL-2. Once expressed on T cells, CXCR3 is capable of mediating arrest of memory T cells on activated endothelial cells.[17] The expression of its chemokine ligands is strongly influenced by IFN-γ, which synergistically works with proinflammatory cytokines such as TNF-α to increase expression of these ligands by activated endothelial cells[17] and epithelial cells.

In general, activation of T cells by cytokines such as IL-2 is associated with the enhanced expression of chemokine receptors including CCR1, CCR2, CCR5, and CXCR3. Just as T_H1 and T_H2 (T helper cells 1 and 2) subsets have different functional roles, it might have been predicted that these two subsets of T cells would express different chemokine receptors. Indeed, the chemokine receptors CCR4[18–20] and CCR3[21] are associated with T_H2 cells in vitro, whereas T_H1 cells are associated with other receptors such as CCR5 and CXCR3.[22]

In some instances, chemokine receptors may be regarded as functional markers that identify T_H1- versus T_H2-type lymphocytes, while also promoting their recruitment to inflammatory sites characterized by "allergic" or "cell-mediated" immunity, respectively. In T_H1-predominant disease, many infiltrating T cells express CCR5 and CXCR3.[23] When T cells are activated in vitro in the presence of T_H1-promoting cytokines, the same chemokine receptors—CCR5 and CXCR3—appear to be highly expressed, whereas in the presence of T_H2-promoting cytokines, the receptors CCR4, CCR8, and CCR3 predominate. There is likely to be some overlap as demonstrated under some conditions in which both T_H1- and T_H2-type T cells express CCR4.[19]

After T cells have extravasated from the bloodstream and enter dermal tissue, they likely home to the epidermis via chemokines as well. The epidermis is a particularly rich source of chemokines, including RANTES, MCP-1, IP-10, IL-8, LARC, and TARC. Keratinocytes from patients with distinctive skin diseases appear to express somewhat different chemokine expression profiles. For instance, keratinocytes derived from patients with atopic dermatitis synthesized mRNA for RANTES at considerably earlier time points in response to IL-4 and TNF-α than did keratinocytes derived from normal individuals and patients with psoriasis.[24] Keratinocytes derived from patients with psoriasis synthesized higher levels of IP-10 with cytokine stimulation as well as higher constitutive levels of IL-8,[24] a chemokine that recruits neutrophils. This finding has also been observed in the lesional skin of patients with psoriasis (a T_H1-predominant skin disease) and may explain the large numbers of neutrophils that localize to the suprabasal and cornified layers of the epidermis in this disease. IP-10 may recruit activated T cells of the T_H1 phenotype to the epidermis and has been postulated to have a role in the recruitment of malignant T cells to the skin in cutaneous T cell lymphomas.[25]

A new chemokine, termed *cutaneous T cell attractant chemokine* (CTACK), was recently described and is selectively expressed in the epidermis.[26] Expression is constitutive, although it is upregulated under inflammatory conditions. CTACK has been reported to preferentially attract CLA$^+$ memory T cells in vitro and may play a role in recruiting, and perhaps even in retaining, skin-homing T cells in the epidermis.[26]

Chemokines in the Trafficking of Dendritic Cells from Skin to Regional Lymph Nodes

Antigen-presenting cells, including DC of the skin, are critical initiators of immune responses, and their trafficking patterns are thought to influence immunologic outcomes. Their mission includes taking up antigen at sites of infection or injury and bringing these antigens to regional lymph nodes where they both present antigen and regulate the responses of T and B cells. When activated by inflammatory cytokines, lipopolysaccharide, or injury, DC leave peripheral sites such as the skin, enter afferent lymphatic vessels, and migrate to draining regional lymph nodes, where they encounter both naïve and memory T cells.

Chemokines guide the DC on the journey from the skin to a regional draining lymph node via afferent lymphatic vessels. After a skin DC such as a Langerhans cell is activated by a variety of stimulating molecules including lipopolysaccharide, TNF-α, and IL-1β, it migrates out of the epidermis and enters the dermis. During this process, E-cadherin expression is downregulated (presumably so that Langerhans cells can detach from keratinocytes). At the same time, activated (migrating) DC strongly upregulate synthesis of CCR7, the major receptor for SLC, which is expressed constitutively by lymphatic endothelial cells.[27,28] Presumably, sensing a gradient of SLC, DC then enter dermal lymphatic vessels and flow with the lymph to regional draining lymph nodes (Fig. 27-3).

Secondary lymphoid organs such as lymph nodes strongly express SLC in the paracortical T cell zones and express other chemokines in B cell zones. Presumably, SLC acts as signal to retain maturing DC in T cell–rich areas. DC may also have direct effects on B cells, which localize to B cell areas of secondary lymphoid organs via expression of CXCR5.[29] CXCR5 is expressed by a subset of skin DC and may be involved in targeting some DC to B cell areas that express the CXCR5 ligand, B lymphocyte chemoattractant (BLC).[30] Naïve T cells also strongly express CCR7 and use this receptor to arrest on high endothelial venules.[14] The importance of the CCR7 pathway is demonstrated by Langerhans cells from CCR7 knockout mice that demonstrate poor migration from the skin to regional lymph nodes[31] and by the observation that antibodies to SLC block migration of DC from the periphery to lymph nodes,[27] inhibiting contact hypersensitivity responses.[32] Thus, CCR7 and its ligands facilitate the recruitment of at least two different kinds of cells—naïve T cells and DC—to the lymph nodes through two different routes. The expression of CCR7, however, by naïve T cells appears to be constitutive, whereas the expression of CCR7 is highly regulated by DC and triggered only by activation and maturation.

After DC reach the lymph nodes, they must physically interact with naive and memory T cells. The resulting contact zone between the DC and T cell is termed the *immunologic synapse* and is critical for T cell activation. Activated DC secrete many different chemokines, including RANTES, macrophage-derived chemokine (MDC), and TARC,[33] which would presumably attract T cells to the vicinity of DC. Moreover, skin-derived DC release sufficient MDC into the culture medium to stimulate the chemotaxis of antigen-primed, but not naïve, T cells.[34] Recent data show that chemokine expression by DC leads to the rapid attachment of antigen-primed T cells to DC in a pertussis toxin–sensitive manner.[35] Therefore, chemokines orchestrate a complex series of migration patterns by bringing both DC and T cells to the confines of the lymph nodes, where the expression of chemokines by DC themselves appears to be a direct signal for binding of the T cells.

FIGURE 27-3

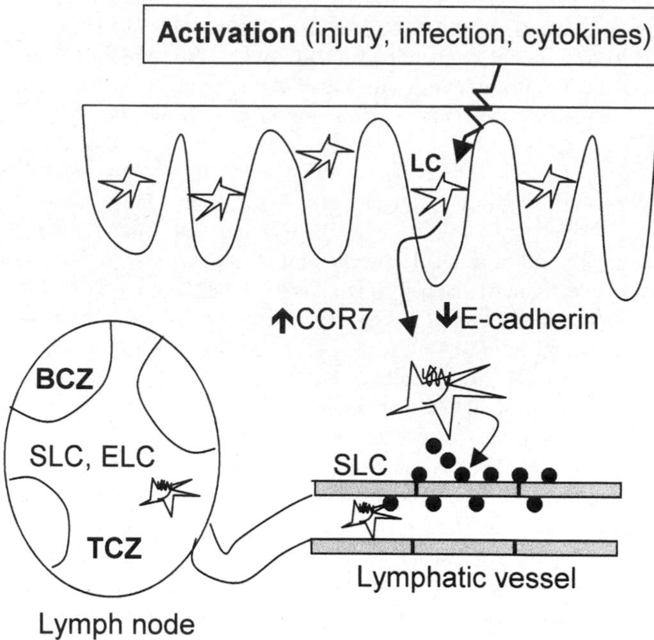

Trafficking of epidermal Langerhans cells to regional lymph nodes. Langerhans cells (LC) are activated by a variety of stimuli including injury, infectious agents, and cytokines such as IL-1β and TNF-α. Having sampled antigens, the activated LC downregulate E-cadherin and strongly upregulate CCR7. Sensing the CCR7-ligand and SLC, that is produced by lymphatic endothelial cells, the LC migrate into lymphatic vessels, passively flow to the lymph nodes, and stop in the T cells zones (TCZ) that are rich in two CCR7 ligands—SLC and Epstein-Barr virus–induced molecule 1 ligand chemokine (ELC). BCZ, B cell zones.

CHEMOKINES IN DISEASE

Atopic Dermatitis (See Chap. 122)

Atopic dermatitis is a T_H2-mediated allergic skin disease. It is manifested by xerotic, red, scaly, and sometimes lichenified patches of skin in characteristic locations, and other systemic "allergic" symptoms. The inflammatory infiltrate in atopic dermatitis usually contains variable numbers of eosinophils, lymphocytes, mast cells, and monocytes/macrophages. The serum IgE level is usually elevated due to enhanced IL-4 production. The pathogenesis of atopic dermatitis is unclear, although its course is often self-limited. Acute or seasonal flare-ups, however, may occur over the lifetime of the patient. Therapy often consists of skin hydration and topical anti-inflammatory medications, including glucocorticoids and tacrolimus.

The mechanism of lymphocyte homing to skin in the setting of atopic dermatitis has been clarified by experimental data showing that the T_H2-associated chemokine receptor, CCR4, in conjunction with its ligand, TARC, may play a role in recruiting T cells to atopic skin. A mouse model of atopic dermatitis (the NC/Nga mouse) has been described, in which skin at 8 weeks of age spontaneously begins to exhibit erosions, dryness, and erythema. Histologically, an infiltrate similar to that of human atopic dermatitis begins at the same time, and IL-4 is abundantly produced in the skin. As in humans, the serum IgE level is strikingly increased. An exogenous pathogen (allergen) is suspected to play a role in the development of the atopic dermatitis-like lesions because lesions do not appear when the animals are raised in an environment that is cleaner than those of conventional mice. Agents (glucocorticoids and tacrolimus) that are effective in the treatment of human atopic dermatitis are also effective in the skin lesions of these mice.

TARC was strongly expressed in the basal cell layer of lesional, but not unaffected, skin of NC/Nga mice.[36] In contrast, TARC expression in the skin was negligible when animals were raised under clean conditions. In humans with atopic dermatitis, CLA^+CCR4^+ lymphocytes were increased in number in the peripheral blood compared to control subjects.[20] Moreover, serum levels of TARC in patients with atopic dermatitis were tenfold higher than concentrations found in unaffected individuals and correlated with disease severity,[37] while patients with psoriasis showed only a minimal elevation of TARC in the serum. Thus, there are strong correlative data in humans to support a role for TARC and CCR4 in the pathogenesis of atopic dermatitis.

Other chemokine receptors may also play a role in atopic dermatitis. The recruitment of eosinophils to skin is a frequent finding in allergic skin diseases, including atopic dermatitis and cutaneous drug reactions. Eotaxin, initially isolated from the bronchoalveolar fluid of guinea pigs after experimental allergic inflammation, binds primarily to CCR3, a receptor expressed by eosinophils,[38] basophils, and T_H2-type T cells.[21] Injection of eotaxin into the skin promotes the recruitment of eosinophils, whereas antieotaxin antibodies delay the dermal recruitment of eosinophils in the late-phase allergic reaction in mouse skin.[39]

CCR3 was recently shown to be expressed by keratinocytes, but it is generally expressed at lower levels than those found in eosinophils.[40,41] Immunoreactivity and mRNA expression of eotaxin and CCR3 were both increased in lesional skin of patients with atopic dermatitis, but not in nonatopic control subjects.[42] Eotaxin increases proliferation of CCR3-expressing keratinocytes in vitro.[40] Serum levels of eotaxin, RANTES, MCP-1, and MIP-1β are elevated in patients with atopic dermatitis.[43] Finally, expression of eotaxin (and RANTES) by dermal endothelial cells correlates with the appearance of eosinophils in the dermis in patients with onchocerciasis who experience allergic reactions after treatment with ivermectin.[44] Thus, the production of eotaxin in the skin may contribute to the recruitment of eosinophils and T_H2 lymphocytes via direct binding to CCR3. In addition, CCR3 expression by keratinocytes may actually play a role in driving keratinocyte proliferation.

Psoriasis (See Chap. 42)

Psoriasis, an inflammatory skin disorder characterized by thickened, pruritic plaques, does not have a clear etiology, although it is considered a T cell–mediated, autoimmune disease. Histologically, there are abundant neutrophils in the epidermis, T cells in the epidermis and dermis, and other immune cells, such as mast cells, which may be present in greater than normal numbers.

Multiple potential trafficking pathways may be mediated by chemokines in psoriasis. Chemokines expressed by vascular endothelial cells likely induce the arrest of effector memory T cells. LARC mediates the arrest of a subset of T cells expressing CCR6 to activated endothelial cells under conditions in vitro that simulate blood flow.[15] Besides endothelial cells, keratinocytes produce LARC, which may be a factor in recruiting T cells and immature DC to the epidermis.[45,46] Indeed, LARC and CCR6 are upregulated in the skin of patients with psoriasis.[45]

TARC is produced by dermal endothelial cells from psoriatic skin lesions.[8] Although its receptor, CCR4, has been associated with T_H2-type T cells,[18] there is evidence suggesting that T_H1-type T cells can also express this receptor.[19] Although TARC is expressed in lesional skin in atopic dermatitis, it is unknown whether or not keratinocytes in psoriatic skin lesions express this chemokine.

Neutrophils in the epidermis of psoriatic skin are likely to be attracted there by high levels of IL-8, which would act via CXCR1 and CXCR2. In addition to attracting neutrophils, IL-8 is an ELR^+ CXC chemokine that is angiogenic and able to attract endothelial cells (see "Cancer" below). This proangiogenic effect may lead to the formation of the long, tortuous capillary blood vessels in the papillary dermis that are characteristic of psoriasis. Moreover, keratinocytes also express CXCR2 and thus may be autoregulated by the expression of CXCR2 ligands in the skin.

Multiple chemokines, including TARC, LARC, RANTES, Mig, and CTACK,[26] are expressed in psoriatic epidermis, but they are also found in a variety of skin diseases, including cutaneous T cell lymphomas (CTCL) and atopic dermatitis.[24] Activated T cells would generally express all the chemokine receptors required to signal through the five chemokines noted above. The necessity of any one of them to the recruitment of T cells to the epidermis is difficult to discern without a specific way of individually blocking their activity. The very redundancy of chemokine expression in psoriasis suggests that blocking any single chemokine pathway may not prove to be effective in the clinical management of this disease. Keratinocytes derived from patients with psoriasis do seem to express more IL-8 and IP-10, whereas claims have been made for greater expression of TARC from keratinocytes of patients with atopic dermatitis.[20] Both RANTES and MCP-1 were produced by stimulated cultured keratinocytes from patients with psoriasis and atopic dermatitis.[24] Whether these patterns of expression may be applied to larger populations of patients with psoriasis and atopic dermatitis is unknown.

Cancer

Chemokines may play a role in tumor formation and immunity in several distinct ways including the control of angiogenesis and the induction of tumor immune responses.[47] CXC chemokines that express a three amino acid motif consisting of Glu-Leu-Arg (ELR) immediately preceding the CXC signature are angiogenic, whereas most non-ELR CXC chemokines, except SDF-1, are angiostatic. It is not clear that ELR^- chemokines actually bind to chemokine receptors to reduce angiogenesis. It has been proposed that they act by displacing growth factors from proteoglycans. In any event, the balance between ELR^+ and ELR^- chemokines is thought to contribute to the complex regulation of angiogenesis at tumor sites. IL-8, a prototypical ELR^+ chemokine, can be secreted by melanoma cells and has been detected in conjunction with metastatic dissemination of this cancer.[48] IL-8 may also act as an autocrine growth factor for melanoma,[49] as well as for several other types of cancer. Although CXCR1 and CXCR2 bind IL-8 in common, several other ELR^+ CXC chemokines, including growth-regulated oncogene α (GRO α) and epithelial-neutrophil–activating peptide-78 (ENA-78), bind primarily to CXCR2. CXCR2 appears, in most instances, to be associated with both the angiogenic and growth regulatory properties of tumors.[50]

Tumors, including melanoma, have long been known to secrete chemokines and are capable of attracting a variety of immune cells. The question arises as to why this behavior is not deleterious to the tumor itself. Breast cancers, for instance, secrete macrophage chemotactic protein-1 (MCP-1), which attracts macrophages through CCR2. Higher tissue levels of MCP-1 correlate with increasing numbers of macrophages in the tissue. An initial hypothesis might be that the attraction of immune cells would contribute to the immunologic clearance of the tumor. Recent data, however, suggest that inflammatory cells such as macrophages may actually play a critical role in tumor invasion and metastasis. First, MCP-1 may increase expression of macrophage IL-4 through an autocrine feedback loop and possibly skew the immune response from a cell-mediated (antitumor) response to one that is humoral. Secondly, there is evidence that certain immune cells, such as macrophages, actually promote tumor invasion and metastasis. Mice that are deficient in colony-stimulating factor-1 (CSF-1), a factor required for the survival and development of macrophages, have a decreased risk for developing invasive/metastatic tumors.[51] Although the precise mechanism by which macrophages delay tumor progression is unknown, growth factors, angiogenic factors, and matrix metalloproteases produced by macrophages could all possibly influence tumor growth and metastasis. Thus, the production of chemokines by tumors and the corresponding recruitment of certain cells, such as macrophages, may be advantageous in terms of increasing vascularity and promoting metastasis.

The antitumor effects of particular chemokines may occur by a variety of mechanisms. ELR^{-} CXCR3 ligands such as IP-10 are potently antiangiogenic and may act as downstream effectors of IL-12–induced, NK cell–dependent angiostasis.[52] Of note, some tumors, such as breast cancer, can synthesize LARC, and these tumors attract immature DC that express CCR6.[53] Experimentally, LARC has been transduced into murine tumors, where it attracts DC in mice and suppresses tumor growth in experimental systems.[54] It is not clear, however, that in humans the ability of tumors to express LARC correlates with a better clinical prognosis.

The production of cytokines and chemokines at tumor sites or by tumors may at first seem to be disadvantageous to the tumor. However, many tumors initially arise from chronically inflamed sites (i.e., chronic wounds in the case of squamous cell carcinoma) or as a result of infection [i.e., Kaposi's sarcoma and human herpesvirus (HHV)-8]. The initial setting of many tumors may indeed be one in which the recruitment of inflammatory cells is advantageous to the organism as a whole. Tumors that arise and survive in such a milieu may be resistant to the usual antitumor effects of immune cells.

Tumor metastasis is the most common source of mortality and morbidity in cancer. With skin cancers such as melanoma, there is a propensity for specific sites such as brain, lung, and liver, as well as distant skin sites. Cancers may also metastasize via afferent lymphatics and eventually reach regional draining lymph nodes. The discovery of nodal metastasis often portends a poor prognosis. In fact, the presence of nodal metastases is the most powerful predictor of poor survival in melanoma.

Chemokines may play an important role in the site-specific metastases of cancers of the breast and of melanoma. Human breast cancer as well as melanoma cell lines express the chemokine receptors CXCR4 and CCR7, whereas normal breast epithelial cells and melanocytes do not appear to express these receptors.[55] Extracts from tissues that are the common sites of breast cancer metastasis (e.g., lung) induce the chemotaxis of breast cancer cell lines in a CXCR4-dependent manner.[55] Furthermore, in a nude mouse system, anti-CXCR4 antibodies blocked metastasis of human breast cancer cell lines.[55] Given the clear demonstration that CCR7 is involved in the migration of DC into afferent lymphatics and draining lymph nodes after activation (see earlier section "Chemokine-Mediated Migration of T Cells"), the acquisition of CCR7 by cancer cells may allow these cells to home to afferent lymphatics and the draining lymph nodes as well. In support of this hypothesis, CCR7-transfected B16 murine melanoma cells were found to metastasize at significantly higher efficiency to regional lymph nodes than parental mock-transfected B16 cells after inoculation into the footpads of mice.[56] Neutralizing anti-SLC antibodies coinjected with the CCR7-expressing melanoma cells prevented the metastasis to the regional lymph nodes,[56] suggesting that therapy directed toward CCR7 ligands (or CCR7 itself) may be of value in reducing nodal metastasis.

Infectious Diseases

Although chemokines and chemokine receptors may have evolved as a host response to infectious agents, recent data suggest that infectious organisms may have co-opted chemokine- or chemokine receptor-like molecules to their own advantage in selected instances. Various microorganisms, including cytomegalovirus and Kaposi's sarcoma herpesvirus (human herpesvirus-8), express chemokine receptor–like proteins once they are integrated within the host cell. In the case of Kaposi's sarcoma herpesvirus GPCR, this receptor is able to promiscuously bind several chemokines. More importantly, it is constitutively active and may work as a growth promoter in Kaposi's sarcoma.[57]

The human immunodeficiency virus (HIV)-1 is an enveloped retrovirus that enters cells via receptor-dependent membrane fusion.[58] CD4 is the primary fusion receptor for all strains of HIV-1 and binds to HIV-1 proteins gp120 and gp41. However, different strains of HIV-1 have emerged that preferentially use CXCR4 (T-tropic), or CCR5 (M-tropic), or either chemokine receptor as a receptor for entry. While other chemokine receptors can potentially serve as coreceptors, most clinical HIV-1 strains are primarily dual-tropic for either CCR5 or CXCR4.[58]

The discovery of a 32-base pair deletion ($\Delta 32$) in CCR5 in some individuals that leads to low levels of CCR5 expression in T cells and DC, and that correlates with a dramatic resistance to HIV-1 infection, demonstrated a clear role for CCR5 in the pathogenesis of HIV-1 infection.[59] The frequency of $\Delta 32$ mutations in humans is surprisingly high, and the complete absence of CCR5 in homozygotes has been associated only with a more clinically severe form of sarcoidosis. Otherwise, these individuals are healthy. In fact, there is an association of less severe autoimmune disease with this mutation.[60]

Langerhans cells reside in large numbers in the genital mucosa and may be one of the first initial targets of HIV-1 infection.[61] Because infected (activated) Langerhans cells likely enter dermal lymphatic vessels (see the earlier section "Chemokines in the Trafficking of Dendritic Cells from Skin to Regional Lymph Nodes") and then localize to regional lymph nodes, the physiologic migratory pathway of Langerhans cells may also coincidentally lead to the transmission of HIV-1 to T cells within secondary lymphoid organs. CCR5 is expressed by immature or resting Langerhans cells in the epidermis, and analogues of RANTES block HIV infection in Langerhans cells.[62] By preventing CCR5 expression on Langerhans cells, the $\Delta 32$ mutation may reduce HIV-1 infection of Langerhans cells as well as of T cells. Thus, CCR5 antagonists may be of therapeutic use in the treatment or prevention of HIV-1 disease.

CXCR4 may also play a role in the transmission of HIV-1 through skin DC. As DC mature, they strongly express CXCR4 along with CCR7. In this setting, they may be able to be infected with dual-tropic viruses or with T-tropic viruses and migrate to draining lymph nodes. The role of CXCR4 clinically is unclear because human polymorphisms in CXCR4 have not been unequivocally associated with either a protective or a deleterious effect in HIV-1 disease. There is a single-nucleotide polymorphism in the $3'$ untranslated region of SDF-1; however, that may be related to delayed progression of HIV-1 disease.[63] Deletion mutants in humans for CXCR4 are unlikely to exist because CXCR4 appears to be essential for the formation of vascular systems in the gut and heart, as demonstrated by neonatal lethality after targeted deletion of CXCR4 in mice.[64]

Inasmuch as chemokines constitute a mechanism to protect higher organisms from microbes, microbes have evolved mechanisms for usurping chemokines and their receptors for their own advantage. Of note, microbes themselves (e.g., molluscum contagiosum virus and HHV-8) produce broad-spectrum chemokine antagonists that may be responsible for the lack of inflammation at the site of infection. Recent work with chemokine antagonists of CCR5 suggests the real possibility that chemokine-based agents will be used to treat or prevent HIV-1 disease and that refinement of chemokine antagonists may lead to the development of effective anti-inflammatory agents.[65]

Signaling pathways are just beginning to be understood, and further work needs to be done to understand the regulation of these receptors, the specificity of their intracellular activities, and the mechanisms by which they work in the face of multiple chemokines present in inflammatory sites.

REFERENCES

1. Zlotnik A,Yoshie O: Chemokines: A new classification system and their role in immunity. *Immunity* **12**:121, 2000
2. Bazan JF et al: A new class of membrane-bound chemokine with a CX3C motif. *Nature* **385**:640, 1997
3. Jiang H et al: Pertussis toxin-sensitive activation of phospholipase C by the C5a and fMet-Leu-Phe receptors. *J Biol Chem* **271**:13430, 1996
4. Constantin G et al: Chemokines trigger immediate $\beta2$ integrin affinity and mobility changes: Differential regulation and roles in lymphocyte arrest under flow. *Immunity* **13**:759, 2000
5. Springer TA: Traffic signals for lymphocyte recirculation and leukocyte emigration: The multistep paradigm. *Cell* **76**:301, 1994
6. Berg EL et al: The cutaneous lymphocyte antigen is a skin lymphocyte homing receptor for the vascular lectin endothelial cell-leukocyte adhesion molecule 1 (ELAM-1). *J Exp Med* **174**:1461, 1991
7. Homey B et al: The orphan chemokine receptor G protein-coupled receptor-2 (GPR-2, CCR10) binds the skin-associated chemokine CCL27 (CTACK/ALP/ILC). *J Immunol* **164**:3465, 2000
8. Campbell JJ et al: The chemokine receptor CCR4 in vascular recognition by cutaneous but not intestinal memory T cells. *Nature* **400**:776, 1999
9. Lechleitner S et al: Peripheral lymph node addressins are expressed on skin endothelial cells. *J Invest Dermatol* **113**:410, 1999
10. Hwang ST, Fitzhugh DJ: Aberrant expression of adhesion molecules by Sézary cells: Functional consequences under physiologic shear stress conditions. *J Invest Dermatol* **116**:466, 2001
11. Campbell JJ et al: Chemokines and the arrest of lymphocytes rolling under flow conditions. *Science* **279**:381, 1998
12. Kawai T et al: Selective diapedesis of Th1 cells induced by endothelial cell RANTES. *J Immunol* **163**:3269, 1999
13. Sallusto F et al: Two subsets of memory T lymphocytes with distinct homing potentials and effector functions. *Nature* **401**:708, 1999
14. Stein JV et al: The CC chemokine thymus-derived chemotactic agent 4 (TCA-4, secondary lymphoid tissue chemokine, 6Ckine, Exodus-2) triggers lymphocyte function-associated antigen 1-mediated arrest of rolling T lymphocytes in peripheral lymph node high endothelial venules. *J Exp Med* **191**:61, 2000
15. Fitzhugh DJ et al: Cutting edge: CC chemokine receptor-6 (CCR6) is essential for arrest of a subset of memory T cells on activated dermal microvascular endothelial cells under physiologic flow conditions in vitro. *J Immunol* **165**:6677, 2000
16. Imai T et al: Identification and molecular characterization of fractalkine receptor CX3CR1, which mediates both leukocyte migration and adhesion. *Cell* **91**:521, 1997
17. Piali L et al: The chemokine receptor CXCR3 mediates rapid and shear-resistant adhesion-induction of effector T lymphocytes by the chemokines IP10 and Mig. *Eur J Immunol* **28**:961, 1998
18. Imai T et al: Selective recruitment of CCR4-bearing Th2 cells toward antigen-presenting cells by the CC chemokines thymus and activation-regulated chemokine and macrophage-derived chemokine. *Int Immunol* **11**:81, 1999
19. Andrew DP et al: C-C chemokine receptor 4 expression defines a major subset of circulating nonintestinal memory T cells of both Th1 and Th2 potential. *J Immunol* **166**:103, 2001
20. Vestergaard C et al: A T_H2 chemokine, TARC, produced by keratinocytes may recruit CLA+CCR4+ lymphocytes into lesional atopic dermatitis skin. *J Invest Dermatol* **115**:640, 2000
21. Sallusto F et al: Selective expression of the eotaxin receptor CCR3 by human T helper 2 cells. *Science* **277**:2005, 1997
22. Bonecchi R et al: Differential expression of chemokine receptors and chemotactic responsiveness of type 1 T helper cells (Th1s) and Th2s. *J Exp Med* **187**:129, 1997
23. Qin S et al: The chemokine receptors CXCR3 and CCR5 mark subsets of T cells associated with certain inflammatory reactions. *J Clin Invest* **101**:746, 1998
24. Giustizieri ML et al: Keratinocytes from patients with atopic dermatitis and psoriasis show a distinct chemokine production profile in response to T cell-derived cytokines. *J Allergy Clin Immunol* **107**:871, 2001
25. Sarris AH et al: Interferon-inducible protein 10 as a possible factor in the pathogenesis of cutaneous T-cell lymphomas. *Clin Cancer Res* **3**:169, 1997
26. Morales J et al: CTACK, a skin-associated chemokine that preferentially attracts skin-homing memory T cells. *Proc Natl Acad Sci U S A* **96**:14470, 1999
27. Saeki H et al: Cutting edge: Secondary lymphoid-tissue chemokine (SLC) and CC chemokine receptor 7 (CCR7) participate in the emigration pathway of mature dendritic cells from the skin to regional lymph nodes. *J Immunol* **162**:2472, 1999
28. Gunn MD et al: A chemokine expressed in lymphoid high endothelial venules promotes the adhesion and chemotaxis of naïve T lymphocytes. *Proc Natl Acad Sci U S A* **95**:258, 1998
29. Förster R et al: A putative chemokine receptor, BLR1, directs B cell migration to defined lymphoid organs and specific anatomic compartments of the spleen. *Cell* **87**:1037, 1996
30. Saeki H et al: A migratory population of skin-derived dendritic cells expresses CXCR5, responds to B lymphocyte chemoattractant in vitro, and colocalizes to B cell zones in lymph nodes in vivo. *Eur J Immunol* **30**:2808, 2000
31. Förster R et al: CCR7 coordinates the primary immune response by establishing functional microenvironments in secondary lymphoid organs. *Cell* **99**:23, 1999
32. Engeman TM et al: Inhibition of functional T cell priming and contact hypersensitivity responses by treatment with anti-secondary lymphoid chemokine antibody during hapten sensitization. *J Immunol* **164**:5207, 2000
33. Sallusto F et al: Distinct patterns and kinetics of chemokine production regulate dendritic cell function. *Eur J Immunol* **29**:1617, 1999
34. Tang HL, Cyster JG: Chemokine upregulation and activated T cell attraction by maturing dendritic cells. *Science* **284**:819, 1999
35. Wu M et al: Cutting edge: CC chemokine receptor-4 (CCR4) mediates antigen-primed T cell binding to activated dendritic cells. *J Immunol* **167**:4791, 2001
36. Vestergaard C et al. Overproduction of TH2 specific chemokines in NC/Nga mice exhibiting atopic dermatitis-like lesions. *J Clin Invest* **104**:1097, 1999
37. Kakinuma T et al: Thymus and activation-regulated chemokine in atopic dermatitis: Serum thymus and activation-regulated chemokine level is closely related with disease activity. *J Allergy Clin Immunol* **107**:535, 2001
38. Combadiere C et al: Cloning and functional expression of a human eosinophil CC chemokine receptor. *J Biol Chem* **271**:11034, 1996
39. Teixeira MM et al: Chemokine-induced eosinophil recruitment. Evidence of a role for endogenous eotaxin in an in vivo allergy model in mouse skin. *J Clin Invest* **100**:1657, 1997
40. Petering H et al: Characterization of the CC chemokine receptor 3 on human keratinocytes. *J Invest Dermatol* **116**:549, 2001
41. Wakugawa M et al: Expression of CC chemokine receptor 3 on human keratinocytes in vivo and in vitro—upregulation by RANTES. *J Dermatol Sci* **25**:229, 2001
42. Yawalkar N et al: Enhanced expression of eotaxin and CCR3 in atopic dermatitis. *J Invest Dermatol* **113**:43, 1999
43. Kaburagi Y et al: Enhanced production of CC-chemokines (RANTES, MCP-1, MIP-1alpha, MIP-1beta, and eotaxin) in patients with atopic dermatitis. *Arch Dermatol Res* **293**:350, 2001
44. Cooper PJ et al: Eotaxin and RANTES expression by the dermal endothelium is associated with eosinophil infiltration after ivermectin treatment of onchocerciasis. *Clin Immunol* **95**:51, 2000
45. Homey B et al: Upregulation of macrophage inflammatory protein-3α/CCL20 and CC chemokine receptor 6 in psoriasis. *J Immunol* **164**:6621, 2000

46. Dieu MC et al: Selective recruitment of immature and mature dendritic cells by distinct chemokines expressed in different anatomic sites. *J Exp Med* **188**:373, 1998
47. Schneider GP et al: The diverse role of chemokines in tumor progression: Prospects for intervention (review). *Int J Mol Med* **8**:235, 2001
48. Singh RK et al: Expression of interleukin 8 correlates with the metastatic potential of human melanoma cells in nude mice. *Cancer Res* **54**:3242, 1994
49. Schadendorf D et al: IL-8 produced by human malignant melanoma cells in vitro is an essential autocrine growth factor. *J Immunol* **151**:2667, 1993
50. Addison CL et al: The CXC chemokine receptor 2, CXCR2, is the putative receptor for ELR+ CXC chemokine-induced angiogenic activity. *J Immunol* **165**:5269, 2000
51. Lin EY et al: Colony-stimulating factor 1 promotes progression of mammary tumors to malignancy. *J Exp Med* **193**:727, 2001
52. Yao L et al: Contribution of natural killer cells to inhibition of angiogenesis by interleukin-12. *Blood* **93**:1612, 1999
53. Bell D et al: In breast carcinoma tissue, immature dendritic cells reside within the tumor, whereas mature dendritic cells are located in peritumoral areas. *J Exp Med* **190**:1417, 1999
54. Fushimi T et al: Macrophage inflammatory protein 3alpha transgene attracts dendritic cells to established murine tumors and suppresses tumor growth. *J Clin Invest* **105**:1383, 2000
55. Müller A et al: Involvement of chemokine receptors in breast cancer metastasis. *Nature* **410**:50, 2001
56. Wiley H et al: Expression of CC chemokine receptor-7 (CCR7) and regional lymph node metastasis of B16 murine melanoma. *J Natl Cancer Inst* **93**:1638, 2001
57. Arvanitakis L et al: Human herpesvirus KSHV encodes a constitutively active G-protein–coupled receptor linked to cell proliferation. *Nature* **385**:347, 1997
58. Locati M, Murphy PM: Chemokines and chemokine receptors: Biology and clinical relevance in inflammation and AIDS. *Annu Rev Med* **50**:425, 1999
59. Liu R et al: Homozygous defect in HIV-1 coreceptor accounts for resistance of some multiply-exposed individuals to HIV-1 infection. *Cell* **86**:367, 1996
60. Gerard C, Rollins BJ: Chemokines and disease. *Nat Immunol* **2**:108, 2001
61. Blauvelt A: The role of skin dendritic cells in the initiation of human immunodeficiency virus infection. *Am J Med* **102**:16, 1997
62. Kawamura T et al: Candidate microbicides block HIV-1 infection of human immature Langerhans cells within epithelial tissue explants. *J Exp Med* **192**:1491, 2000
63. Winkler C et al: Genetic restriction of AIDS pathogenesis by an SDF-1 chemokine gene variant. ALIVE Study, Hemophilia Growth and Development Study (HGDS), Multicenter AIDS Cohort Study (MACS), Multicenter Hemophilia Cohort Study (MHCS), San Francisco City Cohort (SFCC). *Science* **279**:389, 1998
64. Tachibana K et al: The chemokine receptor CXCR4 is essential for vascularization of the gastrointestinal tract. *Nature* **393**:591, 1998
65. Schön MP, Ruzicka T: Psoriasis: The plot thickens. *Nat Immunol* **2**:91, 2001
66. Liao F et al: CC-chemokine receptor 6 is expressed on diverse memory subsets of T cells and determines responsiveness to macrophage inflammatory protein 3α. *J Immunol* **162**:186, 1999
67. Gunn MD et al: Mice lacking expression of secondary lymphoid organ chemokine have defects in lymphocyte homing and dendritic cell localization (see comments). *J Exp Med* **189**:451, 1999
68. Förster R et al: CCR7 coordinates the primary immune response by establishing functional microenvironments in secondary lymphoid organs. *Cell* **99**:23, 1999
69. Kulke R et al: Colocalized overexpression of GRO-alpha and IL-8 mRNA is restricted to the suprapapillary layers of psoriatic lesions. *J Invest Dermatol* **106**:526, 1996
70. Rossi D, Zlotnik A: The biology of chemokines and their receptors. *Annu Rev Immunol* **18**:217, 2000

CHAPTER 28

Robert L. Modlin

Lymphocytes

The unique role of lymphocytes in the immune system is the ability to recognize, with great specificity, the diversity of foreign antigens. All lymphocytes derive from a common bone marrow stem cell. This finding has been exploited in various clinical settings; it is possible to restore the entire lymphocyte pool by bone marrow or stem cell transplantation. There are three kinds of lymphocytes: B cells, natural killer (NK) cells, and T cells.

TYPES OF LYMPHOCYTES

B cells mature in the fetal liver and adult bone marrow. B cells produce antibodies: protein complexes that bind specifically to particular molecules known as antigens. Each B cell produces a different antibody molecule. Some of this antibody is present on the surface of the B cell, conferring the unique ability of that B cell to recognize a specific antigen. Much of the antibody is secreted; the secreted antibody mediates humoral immune responses. In skin, humoral immunity contributes to the immune defense against extracellular pathogens. Antibodies bind to microbial agents and neutralize them or facilitate uptake of the pathogen by phagocytes that destroy them. Antibodies are also responsible for mediating certain pathologic conditions in skin. In particular, antibodies against self-antigens lead to autoimmune disease, typified in the pathogenesis of pemphigus and bullous pemphigoid. Furthermore, IgE antibodies to foreign substances contribute to allergic disease, including atopic dermatitis.

NK are large granular-appearing lymphocytes that survey the body, looking for altered host cells. All nucleated cells express the major histocompatibility complex (MHC) class I molecules. NK cells have receptors, called killer inhibitory receptors, which recognize the self MHC class I molecules.[1,2] Recognition of self MHC class I delivers a negative signal to the NK cell that paralyzes it. However, if a nucleated cell loses expression of its MHC class I molecules, the NK cell, upon encountering it, will become activated and kill it. Because many virus infected cells and tumor cells have reduced expression of MHC class I molecules, NK cells are able to recognize and kill them. In addition, NK cells have activating receptors that bind MHC-like ligands on target cells.

T cells mature in the thymus where they are selected to live or die. Those T cells that will have the capacity to recognize foreign antigens are positively selected and can enter the circulation. Those T cells that react to self are negatively selected and destroyed. If the immune system is envisioned as a bureaucracy, the T cell is the ideal bureaucrat. T cells have the unique ability to direct other cells of the immune system. They do this by releasing cytokines. For example, T cells contribute to cell-mediated immunity, required to eliminate intracellular pathogens, by releasing cytokines that activate macrophages and other T cells. T cells release cytokines that activate NK cells, and also release cytokines that permit the growth, differentiation and activation of B cells.

TRAFFICKING OF LYMPHOCYTES INTO SKIN

Lymphocytes are not prominent in normal human skin; in fact, only a small number can be detected around blood vessels. This contrasts to normal mouse skin, in which a resident population of dendritic T cells have been observed in the epidermis.[3,4] The few T cells present in normal skin are likely on a mission: to survey the skin and detect foreign antigens which pose a threat to the host. No one knows for sure. However, in inflammatory skin conditions, there is a dramatic increase in the number of lymphocytes found in skin. Depending on the condition, lymphocytes may be evident in the epidermis, dermis, and/or the subcutaneous fat. Part of the increase in cell number may be due to the local proliferation of resident lymphocytes. Most of the increase in cell number is due to the rapid influx of lymphocytes. How do lymphocytes get into skin?

The mechanism by which T lymphocytes traffic into skin depends on a chain of molecular interactions between cells (Fig. 28-1). For many inflammatory conditions, the foreign antigen, be it a contact allergen, bacterial molecule, or tumor-associated protein, is initially encountered in the epidermis. The antigen is first taken up by Langerhans cells, dendritic-appearing cells that form a network lattice in the epidermis for detecting and capturing foreign substances. It has been documented clearly that the Langerhans cell with this foreign antigen exits the skin via the lymphatics and travels to draining lymph nodes.

Langerhans cells are part of the family of "dendritic cells"; professional antigen-presenting cells with dendritic morphology and extraordinary antigen-presenting function. The encounter of the Langerhans cell with antigen upregulates its immunostimulating capacity by inducing expression of antigen presenting elements such as major histocompatability molecules; costimulatory molecules, such as B7-1 required for optimal presentation; and cytokines, such as interleukin (IL)-12 required for the generation of cell-mediated immunity (CMI). In the lymph node, these activated Langerhans cells present the antigen to T cells. Next, the T cells become activated and expand. They enter blood vessels and journey towards the skin. The interaction of T cells with antigen and Langerhans cells results in the induction of a cell surface molecule known as cutaneous lymphocyte antigen (CLA).[5] CLA is a glycoprotein that defines a subset of memory T cells that home to skin. CLA is a glycosylated form of P-selectin glycoprotein ligand-1 (PSGL-1), that is expressed constitutively on all human peripheral-blood T cells. The level of CLA on cells is regulated by an enzyme, $\alpha(1,3)$-fucosyl transferase VII, that modifies PSGL-1. In this manner, CLA-positive cells bind to both E-selectin and P-selectin, strengthening the interaction between circulating T cells and cutaneous endothelium, whereas CLA-negative cells bind P-selectin but do not bind E-selectin.[6,7]

In patients with contact dermatitis, the CLA+ subset, but not the CLA– subset, contains the T cells with the capacity to respond to the allergen.[8] Furthermore, greater than 90 percent of T cells in inflammatory skin disease are CLA+. CLA facilitates the entry of T lymphocytes into skin by mediating tethering and rolling of T cells on vascular endothelial cells, through binding to E-selectin. Chemokines released by the endothelial cells activate T cells to express adhesion molecules, leukocyte factor antigen (LFA)-1 and very-late antigen (VLA)-4. T cells firmly adhere to endothelium by the interaction of LFA-1 with intercellular adhesion molecule (ICAM) and VLA-4 with vascular cell adhesion molecule (VCAM). The interaction with the endothelial cells is sufficiently strong to permit transmigration of the T cell into the skin and allow their participation in the inflammatory process.

FIGURE 28-1

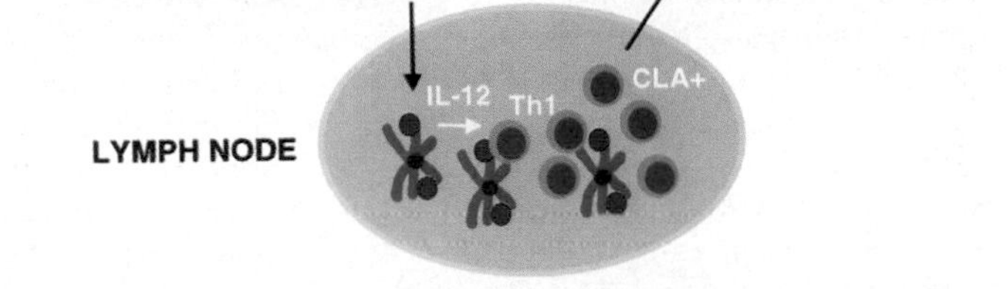

How T cells get into skin. Langerhans cells (LC) pick up antigen in skin and traffic via lymphatics to draining lymph nodes. There, antigen presentation induces expression of cutaneous lymphocyte antigen (CLA), the skin homing receptor, on T cells. These activated T cells traffic via blood vessels to skin, where they can participate in an immune response. Keratinocyte release of interleukin (IL)-10 can downregulate the local T cell response.

T CELL POPULATIONS IN SKIN

The accumulation of T cells in skin is not stochastic. It is abundantly clear that specific populations of T cells, identified by cell surface determinants and their cytokine profile, localize to the skin. Various cell surface determinants on T cells enable us to detect their presence. Initially, functional T cell populations could be delineated in skin according to their expression of the CD4 and CD8 molecules. In the majority of inflammatory conditions studied, including lichen planus, psoriasis, atopic dermatitis and basal cell carcinoma, CD4+ T cells outnumbered CD8+ T cells, in a manner similar to or somewhat greater than that present in the peripheral blood. However, in the study of human leprosy skin lesions, CD4+ T cells were found to be predominant in the tuberculoid form of the disease and CD8+ T cells were found to be predominant in the lepromatous form of the disease.[9] Because all leprosy patients had an excess of CD4+ T cells in their blood, the abundance of CD8+ T cells in lepromatous skin lesions provides clear evidence for the specific accumulation of T cell populations in skin.

A perhaps more relevant marker of T cell populations is the diversity of their T cell receptor (TCR). The TCR is the part of the T cell that

FIGURE 28-2

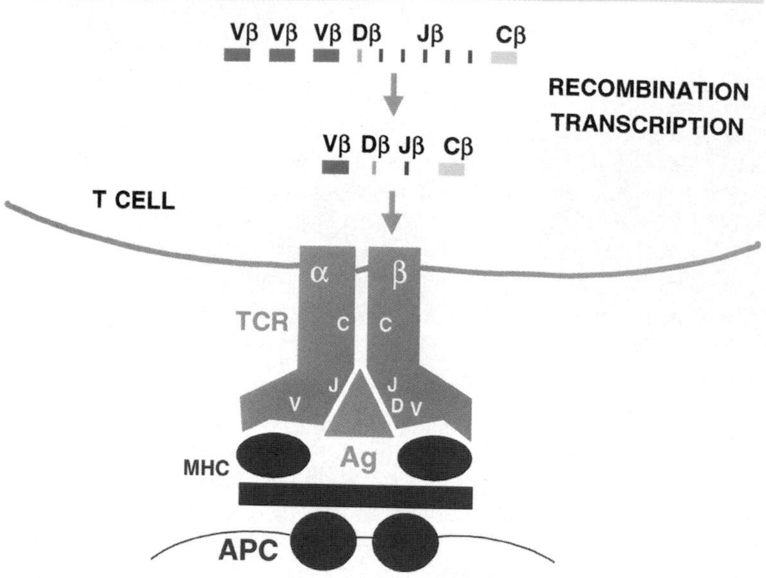

T cell receptor gene rearrangements. This diagram shows how diversity in TCRs is generated by gene rearrangement. In this instance, rearrangement of the β chain is shown. The encoded TCR can then recognize antigen in the context of an appropriate antigen-presenting molecule.

recognizes antigen. The TCR is found to be associated with a set of cell surface proteins known collectively as CD3 that are specific for T cells. One characteristic of CD3 is the presence of a long cytoplasmic tail. When the TCR is triggered by antigen, a signal is delivered through the cytoplasmic tail of CD3 that results in T cell activation.

The majority of T cells have a TCR heterodimer composed of α and β protein chains. A smaller population of peripheral T cells has been identified in which the T cells have a TCR composed of γ and δ protein chains. Most T cells in skin have $\alpha\beta$ TCRs; however, in some conditions, such as human leprosy and leishmaniasis, $\gamma\delta$ T cell accumulations can represent as many as 35 percent of infiltrating cells.[10] The function of these $\gamma\delta$ T cells may be to recognize small nonpeptide pyrophosphate molecules, which are ubiquitous to microbial pathogens and thus form an initial line of defense against infection.[11] $\gamma\delta$ T cells may provide immune surveillance against malignancy, using additional cell surface receptors to kill cancer cells.[12]

The diversity of T cells infiltrating skin can be more precisely assessed by examining the repertoire of TCRs in the infiltrate (Fig. 28-2). The TCR complex is composed of a variable (V), diversity (D), joining (J), and constant region gene segments that define the antigen specificity of the T cell. The accumulation of specific populations of T cells in skin can be inferred by finding a dominant V gene usage in the infiltrate. This is accomplished by using the polymerase chain reaction to amplify small numbers of skin biopsy-derived mRNAs that encode for the TCR proteins. The clearest example is the clonality of the T cell population in cutaneous T cell lymphoma (CTCL), in which a single V gene usage is found to predominate in different skin lesions from the same individual.[13] The dominant expression of several TCR V genes in an infiltrate is thought to indicate that a small number of antigens drive the local inflammatory response. A limited TCR V gene usage has been reported to be present in the skin lesions of leprosy,[14] psoriasis,[15] basal cell carcinoma, and countless other reactions in which T cells are present. However, in no instance has the limited set of antigens been defined and correlated with the TCR usage.

The most direct indication of relevant T cell populations in skin is to determine the number of T cells which recognize the antigen. It has been documented that 1/1000 to 1/10,000 T cells in the peripheral blood recognize a given antigen. However in the skin, approximately 1/50 to 1/100 T cells recognize the antigen causing the disease.[16,17] Thus, there is as much as a 100-fold enrichment of antigen-reactive T cells at the site of cutaneous inflammation.

ANTIGEN PRESENTATION IN SKIN

To carry out its specific mission, the recruited T cell must recognize its antigen in skin so that it can be activated to perform its effector function. In 1972, Doherty and Zinkernagel discovered that T cells recognize antigen in the context of antigen-presenting molecules, a discovery for which they won the Nobel prize in 1996. It has been the paradigm, since the early 1980s, that T cells recognize peptide antigens in association with the MHC encoded structures, which vary from individual to individual (Fig. 28-3) (see Chap. 23). These molecules present small peptides to T cells.[18] Specifically, CD4+ T cells recognize 15-amino-acid peptides bound to MHC class II molecules, such as HLA-DR. CD8+ T cells recognize 8- to 9-amino-acid peptides in the context of MHC class I molecules, such as HLA-A or HLA-B. Many of the HLA associations seen in human skin disease are likely to reflect the ability of that particular MHC molecule to present a disease-relevant peptide to T cells.

Peptide presentation by MHC class I and II molecules is now widely accepted as the basic mechanism underlying specific T cell recognition of viruses, bacteria, multicellular parasites and many types of tumors. These antigen-presenting molecules have different mechanisms by which they encounter antigen[19,20] (Fig. 28-4). Most of the peptides presented by class I molecules are derived from the degradation of proteins in the cytoplasm. This degradation is thought to occur in a multisubunit unit complex of low molecular weight proteins called the *proteasome*. Peptides are transported from the cytoplasm to the ER by TAP, a transporter located in the ER and *cis*-Golgi membranes. Within the ER and *cis*-Golgi, peptides can be loaded into class I molecules by displacing invariant chain peptides and the new peptide–class I complex is exported to the cell membrane. In contrast, most of the peptides presented by the class II pathway are extracellular in origin. Proteins that enter the cells by endocytosis traffic to endosomes, where they are processed into small peptides. Upon acidification of the endosome to pH 5, these peptides can be loaded into MHC class II molecules with the assistance of the loading facilitator, HLA-DM. The stable peptide–MHC class II complex can be exported to the cell surface.

A third pathway of antigen presentation has been identified and this pathway has been demonstrated to contribute to immunologic responses in skin. The human CD1 family is encoded by five genes with an intron/exon structure similar to MHC class I genes. The genes encode polypeptides with a modest but significant level of homology to both MHC class I and II proteins. However, unlike the MHC molecules that are polymorphic, in that they differ from individual to individual, CD1 molecules are nonpolymorphic, in that they are identical in all individuals. At least four human CD1 proteins (the CD1a, -b, -c, and -d isoforms) are expressed on the surface of cells in association with β_2-microglobulin. Human CD1a, -b, and -c proteins are also expressed on a variety of specialized antigen-presenting cells, including dendritic cells in skin. These CD1 molecules can be induced on virtually all circulating human monocytes by exposure to granulocyte-macrophage colony-stimulating factor (GM-CSF) and IL-4, suggesting that they might be upregulated on tissue macrophages in many inflammatory lesions.

FIGURE 28-3

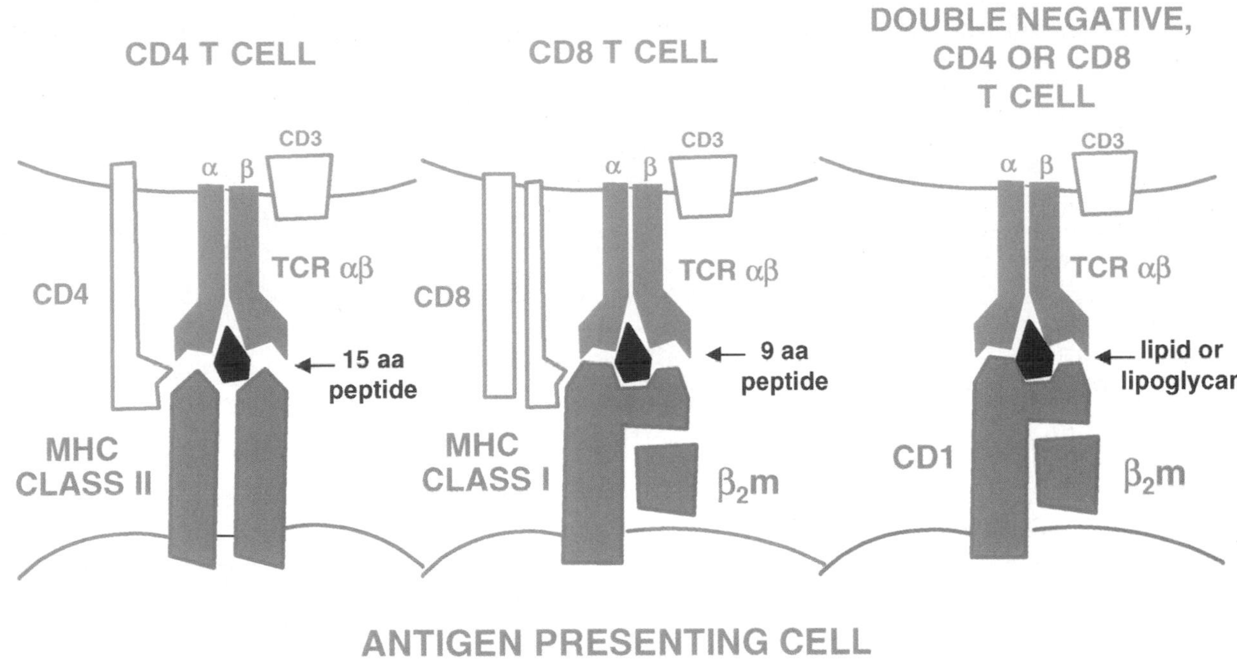

Types of antigen presentation. The molecules that mediate antigen presentation and the types of antigens presented are shown.

The unique feature of the CD1 system is its ability to participate in the presentation of nonpeptide antigens to T cells (see Fig. 28-3). So far, the CD1 antigen presentation pathway has been shown to be involved in the presentation of lipid and glycolipid antigens.[21,22] CD1-restricted T cell responses have been shown to contribute to CMI in the skin lesions of patients with leprosy, by releasing interferon (IFN)-γ and lysing macrophages containing bacteria. Given the expression of the CD1 molecule on Langerhans cells and dermal dendritic cells, it is anticipated that CD1-mediated presentation is involved in other infectious and inflammatory conditions in skin.

FIGURE 28-4

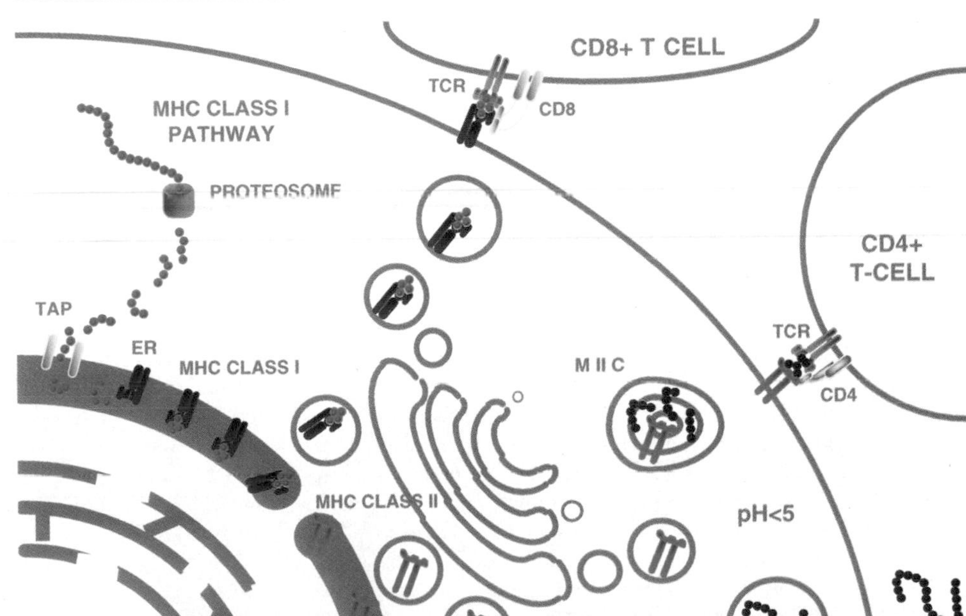

Antigen-processing pathways. The intracellular antigen processing pathways for MHC class I and MHC class II presentation are shown. The MHC class I pathway involves the processing of cytoplasmic proteins; whereas, the MHC class II pathway involves the processing of exogenous proteins.

COSTIMULATORY MOLECULES

Antigen presentation by MHC molecules or MHC-like molecules provides one of two signals required for proper T cell activation. The second signal is delivered by the interaction of cell surface proteins present on the T cell with determinants on the antigen-presenting cell, collectively termed *costimulatory molecules*. One crucial interaction appears to involve CD28 present on the T cell with B7-1 or B7-2 located on the antigen-presenting cell.[23] The engagement of the T cell receptor by the antigen/MHC complex in the absence of costimulation can induce T cell unresponsiveness, a condition known as *anergy*. Of special interest to cutaneous immunity, B7-1 is not normally expressed on Langerhans cells, but upon activation by antigen or other exogenous stimuli, Langerhans cells express B7 molecules. In this manner, it is possible to regulate immunologic reactions in skin through the induction of B7 expression.

CYTOTOXIC T CELLS

In responding to an intracellular pathogen, either a virus, bacteria, or parasite, the T cell must lyse the infected cell. This reduces the reservoir of infected cells, dispersing the pathogen so that activated macrophages can take up and destroy the released microorganisms. The process of targeted T cell lysis is called cytotoxicity. Two distinct subsets for cytotoxic T cells have been identified and can be differentiated by the mechanism by which they kill targets.[24] The end result is the induction of a programmed cell death known as *apoptosis*.[25,26] The first mechanism of cytotoxicity involves the interaction of two cell surface proteins, Fas ligand on the T cells with Fas on the target. Ligation of these molecules delivers a signal through Fas that induces the apoptosis cascade in the target. The second mechanism involves the release of cytoplasmic granules present in such T cells. These granules contain perforin that induces a pore in the target, and granzymes, serine esterases that, when injected into cells, trigger the apoptotic pathway. Such granules also contain *granulysin*, a protein with a broad spectrum of antimicrobial activity against bacteria, fungi, and parasites.[24,27] In this manner, cytotoxic T cells can directly kill microbial invaders. Besides contributing to host defense against infection and tumors, cytotoxic T cells can also contribute to tissue injury. For example, cytotoxic T cells recognize self-antigens of melanocytes and may contribute to the pathogenesis of vitiligo.[28]

THE T_H1/T_H2 PARADIGM

T cells regulate cytotoxic T cell induction, B cell function and macrophage function. They do this by the release of cytokines. How are they able to achieve specificity in the kind of immune response they trigger?

A major paradigm shift in how we think about immunoregulation resulted from the analysis of cytokine patterns produced by murine CD4+ T cell clones[29] (Fig. 28-5). T cells that produce IL-2 and IFN-γ, termed *T_H1 cells*, contribute to cell-mediated immune reactions, whereas T cells that produce IL-4, IL-5, and IL-10, termed *T_H2 cells*, augment humoral responses. In murine models of intracellular infection, resistant versus susceptible immune responses appear to be regulated by these two T cell subpopulations.[30–32] T_H1 cells, primarily by the release of IFN-γ, activate macrophages to kill or inhibit the growth of the pathogen and trigger cytotoxic T cell responses, resulting in mild or self-healing disease. In contrast, T_H2 cells facilitate humoral responses and inhibit some cell-mediated immune responses, resulting in progressive infection. These cytokine patterns are cross-regulatory. The T_H1 cytokine IFN-γ, downregulates T_H2 responses. The T_H2 cytokines, IL-4 and IL-10, downregulate both T_H1 responses and macrophage function. The result is that the host responds in an efficient manner to a given pathogen by making either a T_H1 or T_H2 response. Sometimes the host chooses an inappropriate cytokine pattern, resulting in clinical disease.

The discovery that T_H1/T_H2 responses could contribute to the outcome of human disease caused by a single antigen, was first delineated by the study of leprosy. Because leprosy presents as a spectrum of clinical manifestations that correlate with the immune response to the pathogen, it provides an extraordinary window onto immune regulation in humans: At one end of the spectrum, patients with tuberculoid leprosy typify the resistant response that restricts the growth of the pathogen. The number of lesions is few, although tissue and nerve damage is frequent. At the opposite end of this spectrum, patients with lepromatous leprosy represent extreme susceptibility to *Mycobacterium leprae* infection. In lepromatous leprosy, the skin lesions are numerous and growth of the pathogen is unabated, resulting in many viable bacteria throughout the skin lesions. These clinical presentations correlate with the level of CMI against *M. leprae*. The standard measure of CMI to the pathogen is the Mitsuda reaction. Patients are challenged by intradermal injection of *M. leprae* and induration is measured 3 weeks later. The test is positive in tuberculoid patients and negative in lepromatous patients. It is widely agreed that T cells involved in CMI are pivotal in determining the outcome of infection with *M. leprae*, because skin test and lymphocyte reactivity are positive in tuberculoid patients, but negative in lepromatous patients. Yet, there is an interesting paradox in that CMI and humoral responses exhibit an inverse relationship. Anti-*M. leprae* antibodies are most elevated in patients with the lepromatous form of the disease, and therefore, are not thought to play a role in protection.

FIGURE 28-5

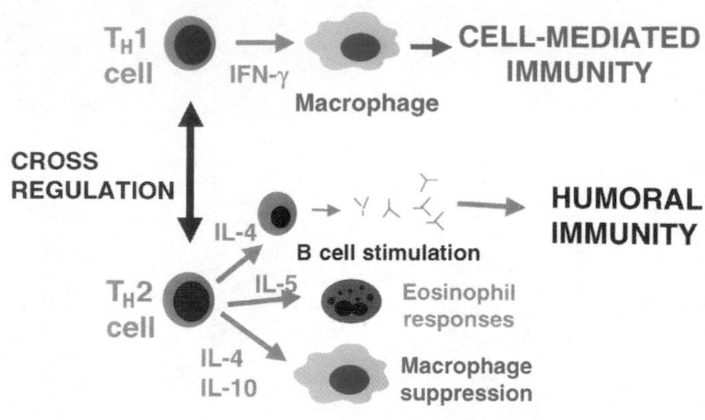

The T_H1/T_H2 paradigm. Two major subsets of T cells can be differentiated according to their cytokine patterns. These two subsets have different functional roles in immunologic responses.

This paradox can best be explained according to the patterns of cytokines in the lesions.[33,34] The T_H1 cytokines, principally IL-2 and IFN-γ, are more strongly expressed in tuberculoid lesions; while the T_H2 cytokines, notably IL-4, IL-5, and IL-10, are characteristic of lepromatous lesions. These cytokine patterns can be assigned to the major T cell subset observed in the lesions: CD4+ T cells predominate in tuberculoid lesions and CD8+ T cells predominate in lepromatous lesions. All of the *M. leprae*-specific CD4+ T cells derived from tuberculoid patients produce IL-2 and IFN-γ and are designated CD4+ "type 1" cells. The CD8+ T cells derived from lepromatous lesions produce high levels of IL-4 and low levels of IFN-γ and are designated CD8+ "type 2" cells.

In terms of the immunopathogenesis of leprosy, the abundance of IL-2 and IFN-γ in tuberculoid lesions is likely to contribute to the resistant state of immunity in these patients. IL-2 may contribute to host defense by inducing the clonal expansion of immune-activated cytokine-producing T cells and augmenting the production of IFN-γ. IFN-γ is well known to enhance production of reactive oxygen and nitrogen intermediates by macrophages and stimulate them to kill or restrict the growth of intracellular pathogens. The cytokines found to be increased in lepromatous lesions might be expected to contribute to the immune unresponsiveness and failure of macrophage activation in these individuals. IL-4 may contribute to the elevated anti-*M. leprae* antibodies in lepromatous patients via its role in differentiation and immunoglobulin class switching of B cells but it also has a negative immunoregulatory effect on CMI, downregulating T cell and macrophage function.

Of particular interest to immunologists is the delineation of factors that influence the T cell cytokine pattern. The innate immune response is one important factor involved in determining the type of T cell cytokine response (Fig. 28-6). Innate immunity pertains to those cells that have been preprogrammed to respond to foreign molecules using pattern recognition receptors that respond to biochemical patterns of foreign ligands (see Chap. 22). Cells of the innate immune response include macrophages, NK cells, and mast cells. Innate immunity can be contrasted to acquired immunity, which involves the selection and expansion of immune cells with the development of memory. The acquired immune response involves T and B cells, with highly specific receptors that are selected by gene rearrangement. Cells of the innate immune response release cytokines that, in turn, bias the cytokine profile of the acquired T cell response.

FIGURE 28-6

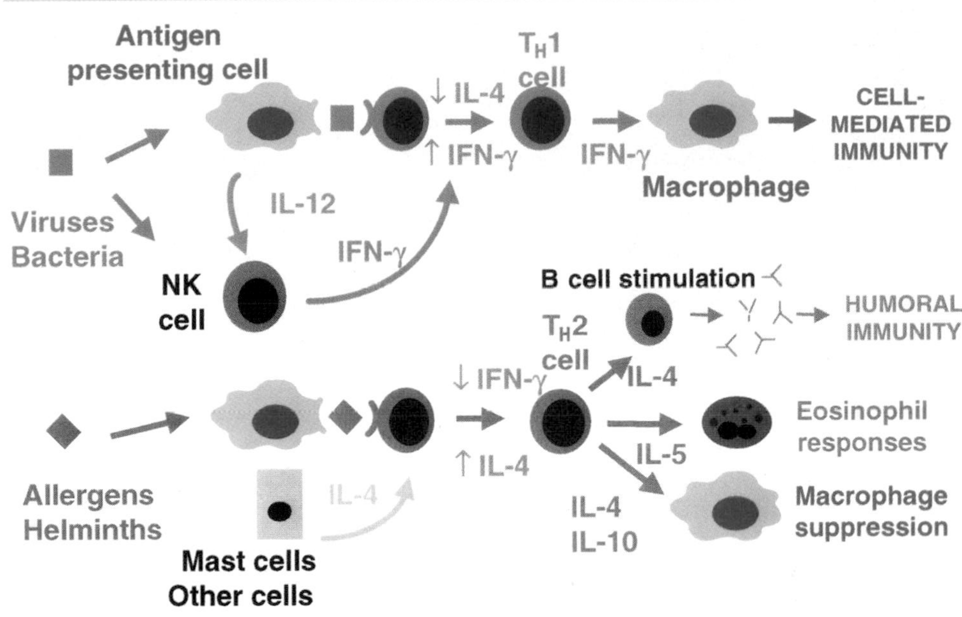

The role of innate immunity in determining the type of cytokine response.

The ability of the innate immune response to induce the development of a T_H1 response is mediated by release of IL-12, a 70-kDa heterodimeric protein.[35–37] For example, in response to an intracellular pathogen, macrophages release IL-12, which acts on NK cells to release IFN-γ. The presence of IL-12, IL-2, and IFN-γ, with the relative lack of IL-4, facilitates T_H1 responses. In contrast, in response to allergens or extracellular pathogen, mast cells or basophils release IL-4, which, in the absence of IFN-γ, leads to differentiation of T cells along the T_H2 pathway. It is intriguing to speculate that keratinocytes may also influence the nature of the T cell cytokine response. Keratinocytes can produce IL-10, particularly after exposure to UVB.[38] The released IL-10 can specifically downregulate T_H1 responses, thus facilitating the development of T_H2 responses.

The T_H1/T_H2 paradigm provides insight into the pathogenesis of many skin diseases in which T cells have an immunologic role. There is ample evidence that the T_H1–T_H2 paradigm is not rigid; there are situations in which a mixture of cytokines is found and examples of T cell clones, known as *T_H0 cells*, that secrete a combination of T_H1 and T_H2 cytokines. However, it has been possible to find a number of dermatologic conditions in which either a T_H1 or T_H2 cytokine pattern predominates. In the realm of cutaneous infection, leishmaniasis is an outstanding example of a disease with a clinical spectrum in which T_H1 and T_H2 cytokines appear to have a pathogenic role. Leishmaniasis, like leprosy, is not a single disease entity, but a set of clinical entities, each with a differing immunopathogenesis. Similar to leprosy, the type 1 cytokine pattern is characteristic of leishmaniasis lesions in which CMI to the parasite is strong and the lesions self-cure; the type 2 pattern typifies lesions in which immunity to the parasite is weak and the cutaneous lesions are progressive.[39,40] Studies in animal models suggest that it may be possible to induce effective CMI by vaccination using a combination of parasite antigens and recombinant IL-12.[41] This immunotherapeutic strategy engenders a T_H1 cytokine response. T_H1 responses are involved in immunologic resistance to *Borrelia burgdorferi*, the causative agent of Lyme disease.[42]

Pathogenic concepts of atopic dermatitis include a central role for allergen-specific T cells that produce T_H2 or "type 2" cytokines, including IL-4 and IL-5. Allergen-specific T cells that produce this cytokine profile have been demonstrated in the peripheral blood and skin lesions of subjects with active disease.[43–45] In addition, the lesions of atopic dermatitis contain abundant IL-10, although the source of this cytokine is likely to be tissue macrophages and keratinocytes.[46] Together the T_H2 pattern of cytokines is thought to induce increased immunoglobulin production, particularly IgE mast cell growth and the infiltration of eosinophils. These cytokines may also downregulate T_H1 responses, accounting for the increased susceptibly to cutaneous bacterial infection. To alter the T_H2 response in atopic dermatitis, clinical trials involving the administration of IFN-γ have shown that treatment with IFN-γ induces significant, but modest, improvement in some patients.[47] Interestingly, moderate clinical improvement occurred in the absence of reduction in the levels of IgE. It is thought, however, that T cells producing T_H2 cytokines help B cells produce autoantibodies in pemphigus vulgaris.[48]

In allergic contact dermatitis, sensitization involves the development of a T_H1 response. T_H1 cytokines predominate in murine T cells sensitized in vitro to haptenated antigen-presenting cells.[49] Likewise, in humans with contact dermatitis, nickel-specific T cells produce a T_H1 cytokine pattern.[50] Induction of contact hypersensitivity involves the production of IL-12; in fact, neutralization of IL-12 leads to tolerance or nonresponsiveness to the allergen.[51] In the examination of the lesions during the elicitation phase of allergic contact dermatitis, a T_H2 response is found, both in animal models and in human reactions.[52,53] The mechanism underlying the switch from a T_H1 to a T_H2 response is unknown. For a long time now, allergic contact dermatitis has been regarded as a delayed-type hypersensitivity response (type IV immune reaction). Yet, in 1938, Sulzberger and Baer suggested that "the contact-type of reaction of the human skin is a form of allergy with special and peculiar characteristics which are not necessarily identical with the cutaneous hypersensitivity. . . ."[54] The presence of a T_H2 cytokine pattern in the elicitation phase of allergic contact dermatitis, as compared to the T_H1 pattern in tuberculin hypersensitivity,[46] points to the existence of distinct immunologic mechanisms underlying these cutaneous reactions. Alternatively, the T_H2 cytokines IL-4 and IL-10 may act to downregulate and shut off the allergic response.

T_H1/T_H2 responses may be involved in antitumor immunity. For example, IL-4 and IL-10 predominate in the lesions of basal cell and squamous cell carcinoma, as compared to the T_H1 response present in benign neoplasms.[55] The source of the IL-10 in these cutaneous carcinomas is the tumor itself, a mechanism by which the cancer can downregulate antitumor T cell responses. Similarly, CTCL represents a T_H1 cytokine response, whereas patients with the more progressive Sézary syndrome exhibit a T_H2 cytokine response.[56] Finally, T_H1 cytokine responses predominate in skin lesions of psoriasis, including uninvolved skin from psoriatic patients.[57,58] These T_H1 cells may be autoimmune, responding to self-antigens in the epidermis.

Whatever the role for the observed cytokine patterns in human skin disease, the T_H1–T_H2 paradigm exposes new targets for therapy. Trials are underway to exploit this knowledge through the use of cytokine agonists and antagonists to shift the balance between the T_H1 and T_H2 patterns for the benefit of the patient. In general, understanding the functional role of lymphocytes in skin, both in terms of normal function and in disease, will enhance our ability to help our patients.

REFERENCES

1. Moretta A et al: Existence of both inhibitory (p58) and activatory (p50) receptors for HLA-C molecules in human natural killer cells. *J Exp Med* **182**:875, 1995
2. Pende D et al: The natural killer cell receptor specific for HLA-A allotypes: A novel member of the p58/p70 family of inhibitory receptors that is characterized by three immunoglobulin-like domains and is expressed as a 140-kD disulfide-linked dimer. *J Exp Med* **184**:505, 1996
3. Caughman SW et al: Culture and characterization of murine dendritic Thy-1+ epidermal cells. *J Invest Dermatol* **86**:615, 1986
4. Tigelaar RE et al: TCR gamma/delta+ dendritic epidermal T cells as constituents of skin-associated lymphoid tissue. *J Invest Dermatol* **94**:58S, 1990
5. Butcher EC, Picker LJ: Lymphocyte homing and homeostasis. *Science* **272**:60, 1996
6. Fuhlbrigge RC et al: Cutaneous lymphocyte antigen is a specialized form of PSGL-1 expressed on skin-homing T cells. *Nature* **389**:978, 1997
7. Robert C et al: Interaction of dendritic cells with skin endothelium: A new perspective on immunosurveillance. *J Exp Med* **189**:627, 1999
8. Santamaria Babi LF et al: Circulating allergen-reactive T cells from patients with atopic dermatitis and allergic contact dermatitis express the skin-selective homing receptor, the cutaneous lymphocyte-associated antigen. *J Exp Med* **181**:1935, 1995
9. Modlin RL et al: T lymphocyte subsets in the skin lesions of patients with leprosy. *J Am Acad Dermatol* **8**:182, 1983
10. Modlin RL et al: Lymphocytes bearing antigen-specific gamma/delta T-cell receptors in human infectious disease lesions. *Nature* **339**:544, 1989
11. Tanaka Y et al: Nonpeptide ligands for human gamma delta T cells. *Proc Natl Acad Sci U S A* **91**:8175, 1994
12. Girardi M et al: Regulation of cutaneous malignancy by gamma delta T cells. *Science* **294**:605, 2001
13. Wood GS et al: Detection of clonal T-cell receptor gamma gene rearrangements in early mycosis fungoides/Sézary syndrome by polymerase chain reaction and denaturing gradient gel electrophoresis (PCR/DGGE). *J Invest Dermatol* **103**:34, 1994
14. Wang X-H et al: Selection of T lymphocytes bearing limited T-cell receptor beta chains in the response to a human pathogen. *Proc Natl Acad Sci U S A* **90**:188, 1993
15. Chang JC et al: CD8+ T cells in psoriatic lesions preferentially use T-cell receptor V beta 3 and/or V beta 13.1 genes. *Proc Natl Acad Sci U S A* **91**:9282, 1994
16. McCluskey RT et al: Studies on the specificity of the cellular infiltrate in delayed hypersensitivity reactions. *J Immunol* **90**:466, 1963
17. Modlin RL et al: Learning from lesions: Patterns of tissue inflammation in leprosy. *Proc Natl Acad Sci U S A* **85**:1213, 1988
18. Engelhard VH: Structure of peptides associated with class I and class II MHC molecules. *Annu Rev Immunol* **12**:181, 1994
19. Germain RN, Margulies DH; The biochemistry and cell biology of antigen processing and presentation. *Annu Rev Immunol* **11**:403, 1993
20. Cresswell P: Assembly, transport, and function of MHC class II molecules. *Annu Rev Immunol* **12**:259, 1994
21. Beckman EM et al: Recognition of a lipid antigen by CD1-restricted $\alpha\beta$+ T cells. *Nature* **372**:691, 1994
22. Sieling PA et al: CD1-restricted T cell recognition of microbial lipoglycans. *Science* **269**:227, 1995
23. Linsley PS, Ledbetter JA: The role of the CD28 receptor during T cell responses to antigen. *Annu Rev Immunol* **11**:191, 1993
24. Stenger S et al: Differential effects of cytolytic T cell subsets on intracellular infection. *Science* **276**:1684, 1997
25. Berke G: The binding and lysis of targeT cells by cytotoxic lymphocytes: Molecular and cellular aspects. *Annu Rev Immunol* **12**:735, 1994
26. Kagi D et al: Cytotoxicity mediated by T cells and natural killer cells is greatly impaired in perforin-deficient mice [see comments]. *Nature* **369**:31, 1994
27. Stenger S et al: An antimicrobial activity of cytolytic T cells mediated by granulysin. *Science* **282**:121, 1998
28. Palermo B et al: Specific cytotoxic T lymphocyte responses against Melan-A/MART1, tyrosinase and gp100 in vitiligo by the use of major histocompatibility complex/peptide tetramers: The role of cellular immunity in the etiopathogenesis of vitiligo. *J Invest Dermatol* **117**:326, 2001
29. Mosmann TR et al: Two types of murine helper T cell clones I. Definition according to profiles of lymphokine activities and secreted proteins. *J Immunol* **136**:2348, 1986
30. Heinzel FP et al: Reciprocal expression of interferon gamma or interleukin 4 during the resolution or progression of murine leishmaniasis. Evidence for expansion of distinct helper T cell subsets. *J Exp Med* **169**:59, 1989
31. Pearce EJ et al: Downregulation of T_H1 cytokine production accompanies induction of T_H2 responses by a parasitic helminth, *Schistosoma mansoni*. *J Exp Med* **173**:159, 1991
32. Pond L et al: Evidence for differential induction of helper T cell subsets during *Trichinella spiralis* infection. *J Immunol* **143**:4232, 1989
33. Yamamura M et al: Defining protective responses to pathogens: Cytokine profiles in leprosy lesions. *Science* **254**:277, 1991
34. Salgame P et al: Differing lymphokine profiles of functional subsets of human CD4 and CD8 T cell clones. *Science* **254**:279, 1991
35. Gately MK et al: Regulation of human lymphocyte proliferation by a heterodimeric cytokine, IL-12 (cytotoxic lymphocyte maturation factor). *J Immunol* **147**:874, 1991
36. Manetti R et al: Natural killer cell stimulatory factor [interleukin 12 (IL-12)] induces T helper type 1 (T_H1)-specific immune responses and inhibits the development of IL-4-producing T_H cells. *J Exp Med* **177**:1199, 1993
37. Trinchieri G: Interleukin-12: A proinflammatory cytokine with immunoregulatory functions that bridge innate resistance and antigen-specific adaptive immunity. *Annu Rev Immunol* **13**:251, 1995
38. Enk AH, Katz SI: Identification and induction of keratinocyte-derived IL-10. *J Immunol* **149**:92, 1992
39. Pirmez C et al: Cytokine patterns in the pathogenesis of human leishmaniasis. *J Clin Invest* **91**:1390, 1993
40. Caceres-Dittmar G et al: Determination of the cytokine profile in American cutaneous leishmaniasis using the polymerase chain reaction. *Clin Exp Immunol* **91**:500, 1993
41. Afonso LC et al: The adjuvant effect of interleukin-12 in a vaccine against Leishmania major. *Science* **263**:235, 1994
42. Yssel H et al: *Borrelia burgdorferi* activates a T helper type 1-like T cell subset in Lyme arthritis. *J Exp Med* **174**:593, 1991
43. Van Reijsen FC et al: Skin-derived aeroallergen-specific T-cell clones of T_H2 phenotype in patients with atopic dermatitis. *J Allergy Clin Immunol* **90**:184, 1992
44. van der Heijden FL et al: High frequency of IL-4-producing CD4+ allergen-specific T lymphocytes in atopic dermatitis lesional skin. *J Invest Dermatol* **97**:389, 1991
45. Hamid Q et al: Differential in situ cytokine gene expression in acute versus chronic atopic dermatitis. *J Clin Invest* **94**:870, 1994
46. Ohmen JD et al: Overexpression of IL-10 in atopic dermatitis: Contrasting cytokine patterns with delayed-type hypersensitivity reactions. *J Immunol* **154**:1956, 1995
47. Hanifin JM et al: Recombinant interferon gamma therapy for atopic dermatitis. *J Am Acad Dermatol* **28**:189, 1993
48. Lin MS et al: Development and characterization of desmoglein-3 specific T cells from patients with pemphigus vulgaris. *J Clin Invest* **99**:31, 1997
49. Hauser C: Cultured epidermal Langerhans cells activate effector T cells for contact sensitivity. *J Invest Dermatol* **95**:436, 1990

50. Kapsenberg ML et al: TH1 lymphokine production profiles of nickel-specific CD4+T- lymphocyte clones from nickel contact allergic and non-allergic individuals. *J Invest Dermatol* **98**:59, 1992
51. Riemann H et al: Neutralization of IL-12 in vivo prevents induction of contact hypersensitivity and induces hapten-specific tolerance. *J Immunol* **156**:1799, 1996
52. Brown MS, Goldstein JL: A receptor-mediated pathway for cholesterol homeostasis. *Science* **232**:34, 1986
53. Gautam SC et al: Anti-inflammatory action of IL-4. Negative regulation of contact sensitivity to trinitrochlorobenzene. *J Immunol* **148**:1411, 1992
54. Sulzberger MB, Baer RL: Sensitization to simple chemicals: III. Relationship between chemical structure and properties, and sensitizing capacities in the production of eczematous sensitivity in man. *J Invest Dermatol* **1**:45, 1938
55. Kim J et al: IL-10 production in cutaneous basal and squamous cell carcinomas. A mechanism for evading the local T cell immune response. *J Immunol* **155**:2240, 1995
56. Saed G et al: Mycosis fungoides exhibits a T_H1-type cell-mediated cytokine profile whereas Sézary syndrome expresses a T_H2-type profile. *J Invest Dermatol* **103**:29, 1994
57. Uyemura K et al: The cytokine network in lesional and lesion-free psoriatic skin is characterized by a T-helper type 1 cell-mediated response. *J Invest Dermatol* **101**:701, 1993
58. Schlaak JF et al: T cells involved in psoriasis vulgaris belong to the T_H1 subset. *J Invest Dermatol* **102**:145, 1994

CHAPTER 29

Shireen V. Guide
Steven M. Holland

Regulation of the Production and Activation of Neutrophils

Human bone marrow commits enormous resources to the creation of neutrophils, producing about 10^{11} daily with a circulating half-life of about 7.5 hours and tissue survival of 1 to 2 days. In contrast, erythropoiesis yields cells that last 120 days, and the products of lymphopoiesis may last a lifetime. Neutrophils are absolutely required for the prevention of infection and are not yet amenable to significant external replacement therapy. The neutrophil not only plays a central role in host defense but also can be responsible for significant tissue damage. Understanding the pathophysiology of the neutrophil indicates pathways that can be exploited to enhance protection from infection. Selective abrogation of those pathways that are injurious in certain settings is also possible. Future clinical studies will focus on enhancement of neutrophil recruitment, adherence, and activation; prevention of these same activities in the setting of myocardial, cerebral, or bowel infarction may reduce injury. Regulation of neutrophil responses in the skin is a major concern. This chapter will present an overview of neutrophil biology and function and use a few well-characterized defects of myeloid function as illustrations.

NEUTROPHIL ONTOGENY AND DEVELOPMENT

Like the other components of the hematopoietic system, the neutrophil is ultimately derived from a pluripotent stem cell. The commitment of a myeloid cell down a developmental pathway is largely determined by ambient cytokines and reflected in its surface markers, morphology, and functional characteristics. The myeloblast is fully committed to the neutrophil lineage and is the first morphologically distinct cell in neutrophil development. All subsequent stages of neutrophil development occur in the setting of granulocyte colony-stimulating factor (G-CSF) and granulocyte-macrophage colony-stimulating factor (GM-CSF). Four to six days are required for maturation through the mitotic phase to the myelocyte and 5 to 7 days more for the myelocyte to develop into a mature neutrophil. Following the myelocyte stage, the maturing neutrophil passes through the metamyelocyte and band stages before acquiring the fully developed neutrophil phenotype. Development of neutrophils through the myelocyte stage occurs exclusively in the bone marrow, which is composed of about 60 percent developing neutrophils. The mature neutrophil measures 10 to 12 μm and has a highly condensed, segmented, multilobulated nucleus, usually with three to five lobes. As noted above, approximately 10^{11} neutrophils are generated daily, but this number can rise tenfold in the setting of infection. The calculated circulating granulocyte pool is 0.3×10^9 cells per kilogram of blood, and the marginated pool is 0.4×10^9 cells per kilogram of blood, comprising only 3 and 4 percent of the total granulocyte pool, respectively.[1] The bone marrow releases 1.5×10^9 cells per kilogram of blood per day to this pool but keeps 8.8×10^9 cells per kilogram of blood in the marrow in reserve. An additional reserve of immature and less competent neutrophils, 2.8×10^9 cells per kilogram of blood, is also available.

Granulocyte colony-stimulating factor (G-CSF) is a glycoprotein that is critically important for neutrophil production. Mice lacking the G-CSF gene show only 20 to 30 percent of normal neutrophil numbers and are unable to upregulate neutrophil numbers in response to infection.[2] Mice heterozygous for the G-CSF deletion show lower levels of neutrophils than wild-type mice, suggesting a gene dosage effect. Exogenously administered human G-CSF was able to significantly elevate circulating neutrophil counts in these animals, similar to the effect seen in human neutropenia.[2] Dong et al.[3] have recognized dominant mutations in the G-CSF receptor that are associated with severe neutropenia and eventual development of leukemia. However, the mutations leading to severe congenital neutropenia and cyclic neutropenia are not in the G-CSF or G-CSF receptor genes but rather in those for neutrophil elastase.[4]

GRANULE CONTENT AND FUNCTION

Neutrophils are characterized by cytoplasmic granules and partially condensed nuclei. Granules are first found at the promyelocyte stage. Primary (azurophilic) granules are the first to arise, measure about 0.8 μm in diameter, and contain numerous antimicrobial products, including lysozyme, myeloperoxidase, and defensins (Table 29-1). All the primary granules that will be available to the mature neutrophil are synthesized at the promyelocyte stage, which leads into the myelocyte, the last cell of the neutrophil lineage with proliferative potential. Therefore, cytokines or agents that increase total neutrophil production must act at or before the myelocyte stage. During the myelocyte stage, the smaller secondary (specific) granules appear. These granules measure about 0.5 μm in diameter and contain lactoferrin, collagenase, gelatinase, vitamin B_{12}–binding protein, and complement receptor 3 (CR3; CD11b/CD18). gp91^{phox} and p22^{phox} comprise the specific granule component cytochrome b_{558}, defects in which cause chronic granulomatous disease (CGD), characterized by infections with particular catalase-producing bacteria. Gelatinase has been shown recently to cleave and potentiate the activity of interleukin 8 (IL-8).[5] Primary granules are synthesized only during the promyelocyte stage and distributed to daughter cells during division, so they are eventually outnumbered by about 3:1 by the specific granules that are produced throughout the myelocyte stage.

Granules fuse in a sequential fashion with incoming phagocytic vacuoles, such as ingested bacteria. Secondary granules fuse to the phagosome within the first 30 s after ingestion and release their enzymes, many of which function best at neutral or alkaline pH.[6] By 3 min after ingestion, the primary granules have fused to the phagolysosome, leading to rapid and marked lowering of the intravacuolar pH. In the presence of foreign objects too large to be ingested or certain stimuli, degranulation to the cell surface occurs, and granule contents are released into the surrounding environment. This can be inferred by detection of lactoferrin levels in blood.

Neutrophil granules and their content are critical to effective neutrophil function.[7] There are two genetic examples of disordered granule biogenesis. Chediak-Higashi syndrome (CHS) is a rare autosomal recessive disorder with a generalized abnormality of primary granule and lysosome formation. Cells of almost all lineages fail to form lysosomes and other intracytoplasmic granules appropriately. Giant azurophilic granules in neutrophils are seen on light microscopy. Abnormal skin and hair pigmentation is due to defective melanin distribution, leading to partial oculocutaneous albinism and silvery hair. Associated findings are photophobia, nystagmus, peripheral neuropathy, and mental retardation. Neutrophil bactericidal activity is reduced, as is natural killer (NK) cell function. Many patients die in childhood from infection, and about half the patients who survive into adolescence develop an aggressive "lymphoproliferative" phase with diffuse organ infiltration and death. In adulthood, an aggressive, severe, debilitating peripheral neuropathy is common. Many mammalian mutants have the autosomal recessive traits of giant lysosomes and pigmentary dilution characteristic of CHS. The *beige* mouse has been used extensively as a model for the neutrophil dysfunction of CHS. The gene responsible for CHS has been cloned and identified as *lyst* (lysosomal transporter). Understanding the function of this gene promises to better inform our knowledge of pigmentation, neuropathy, and immune response.

Neutrophil-specific granule deficiency is a rare autosomal recessive condition clinically characterized by a profound susceptibility to bacterial infections. There is a paucity or absence of neutrophil-specific granules, specific granule proteins (e.g., lactoferrin), and their respective mRNAs and very low levels of the primary granule products defensins and their mRNAs. Specific granule deficiency is due to loss of the transcriptional factor CCAAT/enhancer binding protein ε (C/EBP-ε), which is essential in normal myeloid development.[8] Acquired abnormalities of neutrophil granules are seen in some myeloid leukemias in which

TABLE 29-1

Human Neutrophil Granule Components

Azurophil (Primary) Granules	Specific (Secondary) Granules	Other Granules*
Microbicidal enzymes		
Bactericidal permeability-increasing protein (BPI)		
Defensins	p15s	
Lysozyme	Lysozyme	
Myeloperoxidase		
Elastase		
Cathepsin G		
Proteinase 3	Proteinase 3	
Azurocidin		
Phospholipase A_2 (PLA_2)		
Acid hydrolases		
Cathepsin B	Cathepsin B	Cathepsin B
Cathepsin D	Cathepsin D	Cathepsin D
β-Glycerophosphatase		β-Glycerophosphatase
β-Glucuronidase		β-Glucuronidase†
N-acetyl-β-glucosaminidase		*N*-Acetyl-β-glucosaminidase
α-Mannosidase		α-Mannosidase†
Receptors		
	N-Formyl-methionyl-leucyl-phenylalanine (fMLF)	
	CR3 (Mac-1, CD18-CD11b) (binds to C3bi)	
	Laminin	
	Vitronectin	
Other		
Collagenase	Procollagenase	Metalloproteinases
	Progelatinase	
	Gelatinase	Gelatinase
	Lactoferrin	
	Vitamin B_{12}–binding proteins	
	Cytochrome b_{558}	
	Histaminase	

*Heterogeneous population of organelles including the C-particles, and secretory vesicles.
†Location not entirely certain.
SOURCE: Adapted from Refs. 7 and 54.

primary granule contents may be aberrantly accumulated (e.g., Auer rods in acute myelogenous leukemia). In acute thermal injury, secondary granules degranulate shortly after injury. The discharge of secondary granules may contribute to the neutrophil hypofunction sometimes seen in severe burns.[9]

CHEMOATTRACTANTS AND CHEMOTAXIS

The ability of neutrophils to move toward very slight gradients of chemical signals was noted by Metchnikoff over a century ago. The classic chemoattractants *N*-formyl-methionyl-leucyl-phenylalanine (fMLF), complement factor 5a (C5a), leukotriene B_4 (LTB_4), and platelet-activating factor (PAF) were known to be potent agents for the migration of neutrophils.[10] More recently, chemokines (chemoattractant cytokines), a class of small (<10 kDa), extremely active chemoattractant proteins, have been identified. The chemokines fall into several broad families: CXC chemokines tend to be chemoattractant to neutrophils and T lymphocytes and have a cysteine-X-cysteine motif in the amino-terminal portion of the molecule; CC chemokines tend to be chemoattractant for monocytes and T lymphocytes and have a cysteine-cysteine motif in the amino-terminal portion of the molecule; other classes of chemokines have a C or a CX_3C motif. Among the CXC chemokines, the peptide sequence glutamic acid–leucine–arginine (ELR) immediately proximal to the CXC motif confers potent neutrophil chemoattraction. The CXC chemokine genes are all 25 to 90 percent identical to each other and are physically located on chromosome 4q12-q21. The CC chemokine genes are all 25 to 70 percent identical to each other and located on chromosome 17, suggesting common evolutionary origins for these gene families.

IL-1 activates the release of IL-8 from neutrophils. IL-8 is a potent chemoattractant and neutrophil activator. Blockade of IL-8 by neutralizing anti–IL-8 antibody in rabbit models of pulmonary inflammation was successful in preventing neutrophil accumulation and reperfusion injury, confirming the central role for this chemokine in neutrophil recruitment to sites of inflammation.[11,12] Many different cellular sources for IL-8 have been identified, including neutrophils, monocytes, T cells, B cells, NK cells, basophils, eosinophils, fibroblasts, endothelial cells, keratinocytes, and smooth muscle. Exudative neutrophils are particularly effective at synthesizing IL-8, probably through a calcium-regulated mechanism.[13]

Exuberant neutrophil function is implicated in Sweet's syndrome (acute febrile neutrophilic dermatosis), as shown by the frequent association of the syndrome with hematologic malignancies, dysmyelopoiesis, and sometimes the use of G-CSF.[14]

The classic chemoattractants and chemokines use receptors that have in common seven predicted transmembrane regions and an extracellular amino-terminal domain and transduce their signals through pertussis toxin–sensitive heterotrimeric G-proteins. These are the same type of receptor through which is mediated signal transduction for light, neuropeptides, and neurotransmitters. Chemoattractant receptor binding by a cognate ligand leads to exchange of bound GDP for GTP by the α subunit of the heterotrimeric G protein, which, in turn, leads to the dissociation of the β-γ subunit of the complex, stimulation of phospholipase C, and generation of inositol triphosphate and diacylglycerol from phosphatidylinositol bisphosphate. Inositol triphosphate stimulates the release of calcium from intracellular "calciosomes," whereas diacylglycerol activates protein kinase C. Extracellular calcium also enters the cell, preparing it for subsequent movement, generation of oxidants, and secretion of vesicles (Fig. 29-1).

Ras-related GTPases of the Rho superfamily are other key signaling intermediates involved in actin cytoskeletal regulation and adhesion.[15] Phosphatidylinositol-3-kinase (PI3K) is activated by Rho and Ras and is a pivotal signaling molecule shown recently to be necessary for the neutrophil respiratory burst, adhesion, endothelial transmigration, and chemotaxis.[16] Mitogen-activated protein kinases (MAPKs) are serine-threonine kinases that include p38, Erk1, Erk2, and Jnk and are involved in neutrophil signaling and adhesion. Inhibition of p38 impairs chemotaxis and tumor necrosis factor α (TNF)α mediated superoxide production and adhesion along with impaired release of secondary granules.[17] Erk activation is required for neutrophil homotypic aggregation. Interestingly, salicylate inhibition of neutrophil adhesion has been shown to act through Erk inhibition.[18]

The medical interest in chemokines and their receptors has been vastly augmented by numerous reports that several chemokine receptors function as HIV coreceptors. HIV is unable to penetrate CD4+-expressing T lymphocytes or monocytes in the absence of specific chemokine receptors. The demonstration of a defect in the chemokine receptor CCR5 that is protective against HIV infection has spawned a whole new field of investigation into uses of chemokine receptor blockade to prevent the acquisition or spread of HIV infection.[19]

ADHESION

Neutrophils exist in at least two states in the circulation: free flowing (that which is sampled on blood drawing) and marginated (those cells which are attached to the endothelium or are traversing the lung). Neutrophils rolling along the endothelium recognize sites of activation (e.g., chemokine expression), adhere to those sites, and traverse the endothelium to enter the tissue and fight infection. Leukocyte physical interaction with endothelium and other leukocytes is mediated by three main sets of molecules: integrins, selectins, and members of the immunoglobulin supergene family (intercellular adhesion molecules, ICAMs) (Fig. 29-2).

Elaboration of chemoattractants or display of activation markers on endothelium triggers leukocyte high-affinity binding by β_2 integrins, heterodimeric surface molecules stored in the secondary granules of neutrophils that are displayed on the cell surface on leukocyte activation. There are three β_2 integrin heterodimers comprised of different α chains, CD11a, -b, and -c, and a common β chain, CD18. Each CD11-CD18 complex has separate and overlapping activities. CD11a-CD18 (leukocyte function–associated molecule 1, LFA-1) binds to other leukocytes and mediates tight adhesion to the endothelium through ICAM-1 and ICAM-2. CD11b-CD18 (Mac-1, Mo-1, or complement receptor 3, CR3) binds to the inactivated form of the third component of complement (C3bi) and thereby facilitates complement-mediated phagocytosis. CD11b-CD18 also binds to bacteria directly, to fibrinogen, and to endothelium through ICAM-1. Divalent cations Ca^{2+} and Mg^{2+}/Mn^{2+} also mediate adhesion through β_2 integrin A domains containing a metal ion–dependent adhesion site (MIDAS). CD11b-CD18 is thought to mediate transendothelial migration and may induce the expression of the β_1 integrin VLA-6 (CD49f-CD29), derived from neutrophil granules, to aid in tissue infiltration. The integrin-associated protein (IAP or CD47), expressed on both neutrophils and endothelial cells, is also involved in the transendothelial migration of neutrophils.[20] Metalloproteinases may be involved in cleavage of L-selectin, allowing neutrophil migration through the basement membrane.[21]

Absence of CD18 causes leukocyte adhesion deficiency type 1 (LAD1) and is characterized by a clinical picture that is largely predicted from the molecular defect. Neutrophils lacking CD18 roll normally along the endothelium but are unable to stick to the vessel wall or exit the circulation after chemotactic stimulation.[22] Absence of LFA-1

FIGURE 29-1

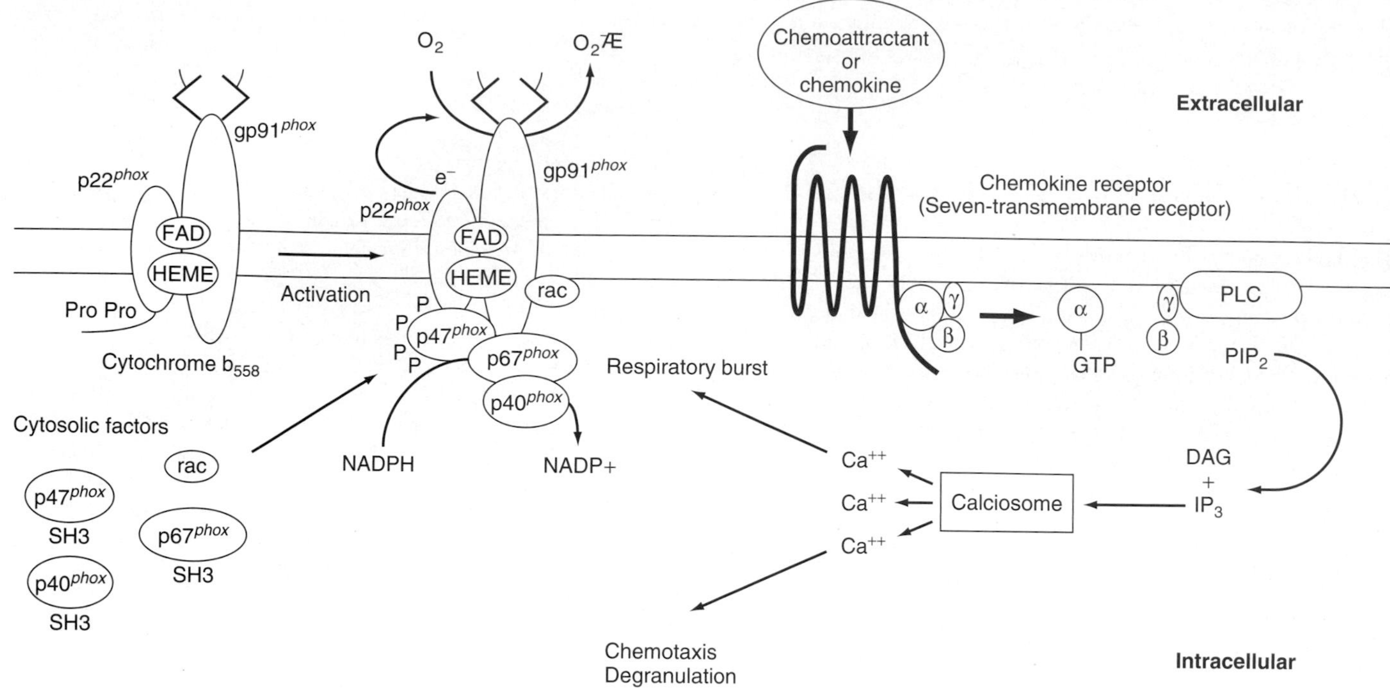

The neutrophil can be activated by interaction of a chemoattractant with its receptor on the cell surface, leading to release of secondary mediators and resulting in an increase in intracellular calcium concentration. Ligation of the seven-transmembrane receptor results in dissociation of the heterotrimeric G protein, leading to activation of phospholipase C (PLC) and generation of phosphatidylinositol bisphosphate (PIP_2), diacylglycerol (DAG), and inositol triphosphate (IP_3). Assembly of the NADPH oxidase following cellular activation is depicted. The cytosolic factors p47^{phox}, p67^{phox}, and p40^{phox} are shown with *src*-homology 3 (SH3) domains. The proline-rich tail of p22^{phox} is schematized (ProPro). Following activation, p47^{phox} is multiply phosphorylated (P) and binds to p67^{phox}. This complex then binds via the p47^{phox} SH3 domain to the p22^{phox} proline tail. An electron is taken from NADPH and transferred to molecular oxygen in the extracellular space or inside a phagolysosome. p40^{phox} appears to serve a regulatory role. Defects in any of the four structural proteins of the NADPH oxidase lead to inability to produce superoxide and cause CGD. FAD, flavin adenine dinucleotide. α, β, and γ are subunits of the heterotrimeric GTP-coupled receptors.

(CD11a-CD18) makes neutrophils unable to bind tightly to and traverse activated endothelium to infected areas. Affected patients have chronic neutrophil leukocytosis, presumably from inability of neutrophils to bind tightly to endothelium and exit the circulation, thus leading to a reduction in the marginated pool and an increase in the circulating pool. Patients have poor neutrophil penetration to sites of bacterial invasion, leading to necrotic ulcers that are characteristically lacking neutrophils on biopsy. Absence of Mac-1 (CD18-CD11b or CR3) leads to inability to perform complement-mediated phagocytosis, although antibody-mediated phagocytosis remains intact.

LAD1 is a rare autosomal recessive disorder that falls into two broad categories depending on the degree of CD18-CD11 deficiency.[23] Severe LAD1 ($<$1.0 percent of normal protein expression) is manifested by delayed umbilical stump separation, umbilical stump infection, persistent leukocytosis in the absence of active infection ($>$15,000/μL), and severe, destructive periodontitis with associated loss of teeth and alveolar bone. Recurrent infections of the skin, upper and lower airways, bowel, and perirectal area and septicemia are common and usually due to *Staphylococcus aureus* or gram-negative rods. Severe LAD1 patients should receive bone marrow transplantation as early as possible. Patients with moderate LAD1 (2.5 to 30 percent of normal protein expression) tend to be diagnosed later in life and less commonly have life-threatening infections. Leukocytosis is still the rule, as are delayed wound healing and periodontal disease. Patients with the moderate form of the disease are less ill and tend to live past childhood. Fluorescent-activated cell sorting (FACS) showing reduction or absence of CD18 and the coexpressed molecules CD11a, CD11b, and CD11c confirms the diagnosis.

The ability of neutrophils to roll along the endothelium is mediated by selectins, surface glycoproteins on the endothelium, and sialyl-Lewis^x (CD15s), a highly fucosylated surface glycoprotein on neutrophils.[24] Endothelial cells express E-selectin (CD62E) and P-selectin (CD62P), whereas leukocytes express L-selectin (CD62L). Although endothelial E-selectin and P-selectin bind to the sialyl-Lewis^x (CD15s) antigen on neutrophils, the neutrophil molecule L-selectin probably binds to distinct antigens on endothelium, including CD34, and is highly sensitive to glycosylation.[24] L-selectin is shed by neutrophils on activation, allowing neutrophil migration into sites of inflammation. Cross-linking of L-selectin on neutrophils results in superoxide generation and may result in upregulation of TNF-α, IL-8, and tyrosine phosphorylation and activation of MAP kinase.[25] Leukocyte adhesion deficiency type 2 (LAD2) occurs in the absence of properly fucosylated CD15s, leading to neutrophilia, recurrent pulmonary, periodontal, and cutaneous infections, and abnormal chemotaxis. The underlying defect is in the inability to fucosylate CD15 as well as other molecules. Three cases of LAD2 have been reported, confirming the critical role of selectins in neutrophil function. Since the enzyme responsible for this defect is a GDP-fucose transporter, this disease is now classified as a congenital disorder of glycosylation (CDG) and known as CDG-IIc.[26] Interestingly, although infections are common early in life, LAD2 (CDG-IIc) patients appear to improve with age.[27] Administration of fucose to patients with LAD2 has been reported to be therapeutic.[28] The patients reported also had mental retardation, short stature, distinctive facies, and the Bombay (*hh*) blood phenotype, indicating the multiple systems in which fucosylation is critical.

FIGURE 29-2

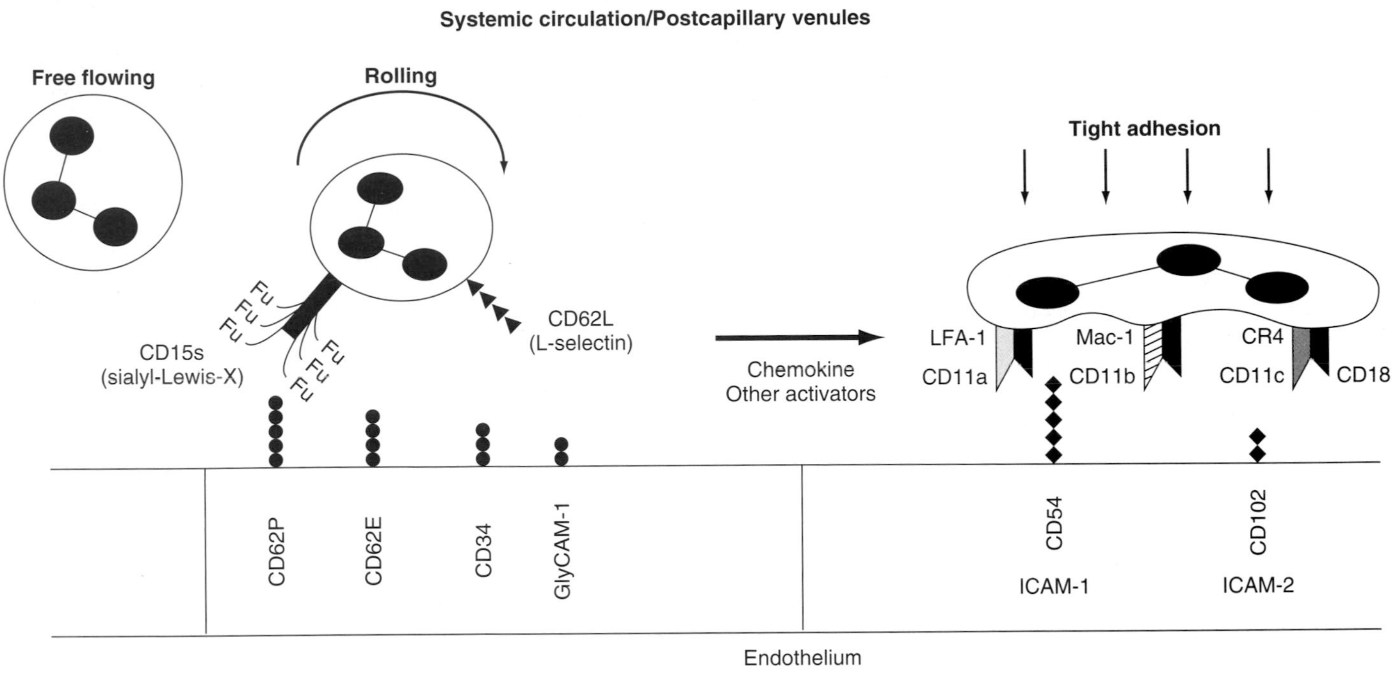

The interaction of selectins and integrins with endothelia is depicted. One population of neutrophils flows freely in the circulation. A substantial number of neutrophils roll gently along the endothelial wall using endothelial and leukocyte selectins and glycoproteins. CD15s interacts with CD62P and CD62E, whereas CD62L interacts with CD34 and GlyCAM-1. Abnormalities in fucosylation of CD15s cause leukocyte adhesion deficiency 2 (congenital defect of glycosylation IIc). Activation of the neutrophils leads to display of higher-affinity leukocyte integrins with common CD18 chains that bind to CD54 and CD102 on the endothelial surface. Defects in CD18 (black) lead to inability to exit the circulation at sites of infection, causing leukocyte adhesion deficiency 1.

Doerschuk and coworkers have recognized that while the CD18-containing integrin pathway is critically important for inflammation in the skin, it is not necessary for accumulation of neutrophils in the lung or peritoneum in mice.[29,30] CD18-deficient mice have normal or above-normal recruitment of neutrophils into pulmonary alveoli and alveolar septa in response to *Streptococcus pneumoniae* or *Escherchia coli* and normal or above-normal recruitment of neutrophils into peritoneum in response to *S. pneumoniae* or the sterile irritant thioglycollate. In contrast, CD18-deficient mice do not recruit neutrophils into skin irritated with croton oil. These findings remain remarkable, since administration of blocking antibody to CD18 in normal mice blocks neutrophil accumulation at most sites of infection.[31] In addition, CD11a-deficient mice show a defect in thioglycollate peritonitis. Overall, these data indicate that while CD18-dependent pathways are critical for cutaneous inflammation, CD18-independent pathways exist for pulmonary inflammation. Further, in the setting of congenital absence of CD18, compensatory pathways exist in the mouse to respond to peritoneal inflammation.

PHAGOCYTOSIS

Recognition, binding, signaling, adherence, cytoskeletal remodeling, engulfment, and membrane fusion are required for the complex process of phagocytosis. Two mechanisms are well characterized, one mediated by immunoglobulin and one mediated by complement.

Receptors for the Fc portions of IgG (FcγR) are present on many components of the cellular immune response, including neutrophils, monocytes, macrophages, eosinophils, and basophils. FcγRI (CD64) is a receptor for IgG_1 and IgG_3 on monocytes, macrophages, and eosinophils and is upregulated on neutrophils after interferon-γ stimulation. FcγRII (CD32) binds IgG with rather low affinity, with the binding of IgG_1 and IgG_3 greater than that of IgG_2 and IgG_4. FcγRIII (CD16) binds IgG_1 and IgG_3 with intermediate affinity.[32] The form of FcγRIII expressed on neutrophils, FcγRIIIB, is bound to the membrane through a glycan phosphatidyl inositol (GPI) linkage, which is largely cleavable by phosphatidyl inositol–specific phospholipase C. Since FcγRIIIB has no cytoplasmic domain, its role in signal transduction requires further clarification. It may function through association with FcγRII.[33] Cross-linking of these receptors by antibody leads to rapid engulfment of targets with release of granule contents and oxygen metabolites into the phagolysosome. In the event that the target is too large for ingestion, degranulation occurs against the antibody-coated surface.[34]

The complement receptors CR1 and CR3 are expressed on the surfaces of neutrophils, eosinophils, and basophils. Complement receptor 1 (CR1) is designated CD35 and is found on many cell types. It binds C3b and enhances its degradation to C3dg by factor I, thereby removing that molecule from further activation of the alternative pathway.[35] Complement receptor 3 (CR3, CD11b-CD18) binds iC3b and fibrinogen, as well as certain bacteria, parasites, and fungi. CR1 and CR3 are not able *per se* to stimulate phagocytosis, but in the presence of a second signal, such as one given through FcγR or by cytokines, phagocytosis proceeds.

MECHANISMS OF KILLING

Neutrophil granules contain enzymes and proteins for killing ingested bacteria and fungi. Some of these bactericidal mechanisms are dependent on the generation of oxygen metabolites for microbicidal activity, but others are not. In addition to mobilizing its own resources, neutrophils produce a multitude of cytokines that stimulate and attract other phagocytes as well as lymphocytes.[36]

Oxygen-Independent Pathways

Bactericidal/permeability-increasing protein (BPI) is a highly potent antibacterial granule protein synthesized at the time of development of the primary granules in which it is stored.[37] BPI is a highly basic (pH > 9.6) protein of 452 amino acids and about 58 kDa.[38] Sequence homology to lipopolysaccharide-binding protein (LBP), a critical endotoxin-binding acute-phase reactant,[39] suggests that it acts by directly binding to LPS. BPI is cytotoxic to gram-negative bacteria at concentrations as low as 10^{-9} M, but it is much less effective against gram-positive organisms. Binding to lipopolysaccharide (LPS) leads to insertion of BPI into the outer membrane of the organism and eventual insertion into the inner membrane. Arrest of bacterial growth occurs by mechanisms not yet characterized but is solely dependent on the N-terminal half of the molecule. The C-terminal fragment serves as an anchor to the membrane.[38] BPI appears to exert its effect within the phagolysosome. Not all gram-negative rods are sensitive to BPI, especially *Burkholderia (Pseudomonas) cepacia* and *Serratia marcescens,* pathogens in patients who lack oxidative killing.

Defensins are small (<4 kDa) cationic proteins found in the primary granules of neutrophils involved in killing ingested gram-positive and gram-negative bacteria.[40] Defensins are synthesized during the promyelocyte-myelocyte stage as prepropeptides, stored predominantly in a dense subset of the primary neutrophil granules as propeptides, and released during neutrophil degranulation.[41] Defensins generally require an actively metabolizing target and are capable of killing transformed mammalian cells as well as prokaryotes and yeasts. Defensins and BPI act synergistically against gram-negative bacteria. As primary granule contents, defensins are present in reduced amounts in the Chediak-Higashi syndrome[42] but are absent in specific granule deficiency, indicating that defensin transcription is controlled by C/EBPε.[43]

Proteinase 3 (PR-3), the antigen against which the cANCA is directed in Wegener's granulomatosis, is found predominantly in primary granules but also in secondary and secretory granules. Synthesis and surface display are upregulated by cytokines such as TNF-α.[44] Elastase is another myeloid serine protease found in primary granules that has remarkable roles in host defense. On the one hand, mice with elastase defects have decreased resistance to gram-negative bacteria.[45] On the other hand, human neutrophil elastase deficiency is the cause of severe congenital neutropenia and cyclic neutropenia.[4] There are many forms of phospholipase A_2 (PLA_2) that are also found in neutrophil granules, where they act both directly and synergistically with BPI to kill intracellular bacteria.[46]

Lactoferrin is an iron-binding protein present in specific granules of neutrophils and in mucosal secretions. When released into the phagolysosome, lactoferrin binds iron and inhibits the growth of phagocytosed bacteria and some fungi. The mechanisms through which lactoferrin exerts its antimicrobial action probably include the depletion of iron from an organism's environment, but iron-binding–independent antimicrobial activities and direct immunomodulatory effects are also reported.[47] Lactoferrin is readily released into the circulation following burns and experimental endotoxemia, presumably from neutrophil degranulation.[48]

Oxygen-Dependent Pathways

An extremely potent microbicidal property of neutrophils is the ability to produce toxic oxygen metabolites through the assembly of the reduced nicotinamide dehydrogenase phosphate (NADPH)–oxidase complex. This enzyme complex catalyses the addition of an electron to molecular oxygen, leading to the formation of superoxide anion, which is converted to hydrogen peroxide by superoxide dismutase (see Fig. 29-1). In the presence of the primary granule component myeloperoxidase, hydrogen peroxide is combined with halogen (chloride in neutrophils) to form hypohalous acid (bleach). The NADPH oxidase is a multiprotein complex that in the basal state exists in separate membrane-bound and cytosolic compartments. On cell activation, the cytosolic components translocate to the membrane, resulting in an active NADPH oxidase (see Fig. 29-1) that yields the respiratory burst.

The genes required for mounting the respiratory burst have been cloned and sequenced and are named as members of the phagocyte oxidase complex (*phox*). Secondary granules contain cytochrome b_{558}, a heme- and flavin-binding protein heterodimer composed of a 91-kDa glycosylated beta chain (gp91^{phox}) and a 22-kDa alpha chain (p22^{phox}). The cytosolic compartment contains three factors, p47^{phox}, p67^{phox}, and the small guanine nucleotide (GTP)–binding protein Rac. Assembly of the NADPH complex is caused by diverse stimuli. p47^{phox} and p67^{phox} contain *src*-homology type 3 domains (SH3 boxes) that bind to proline-rich targets in themselves and other members of the NADPH complex. Stimulation leads to structural changes in p47^{phox} that promote its interaction with p22^{phox} through p47^{phox} SH3 domains and p22^{phox} C-terminal proline-rich sequences (see Fig. 29-1).

Pathologic mutations in the four required components destroy the generation of phagocyte superoxide and cause chronic granulomatous disease (CGD), a disease characterized by recurrent life-threatening infections with bacteria and fungi and exuberant granuloma formation.[49] The reported frequency is 1 in 200,000 persons, but the real frequency is likely higher. About 70 percent of cases are X-linked (gp91^{phox}), and the remainder are autosomal recessive mutations in the other three structural proteins. CGD is quite variable, ranging in time of presentation from infancy to late adulthood, with the majority of patients diagnosed as toddlers and young children.[50] Frequent sites of infection are skin, lung, lymph nodes, liver, bone, perianal region, and gingiva. The most common infectious agents in CGD are S. *aureus, B. cepacia, S. marcescens, Nocardia* sp., and *Aspergillus* sp.[49,50] Granulomata in CGD originate from an improperly regulated inflammatory response to persistent infection or irritation (e.g., sutures, residual bacterial or fungal antigens). The fact that these inflammatory responses are abnormally exuberant in the absence of superoxide production indicates the critical role that superoxide and its metabolites play in resolution of inflammation through degradation of leukotrienes, complement, and other chemotactic factors.[51]

Interferon-γ (IFN-γ) is a potent T lymphocyte cytokine that acts on myeloid cells and enhances host defense activity in patients with CGD through mechanisms as yet unknown but independent of superoxide formation.[52] Homologous recombinant knockout animals have been made for the gp91^{phox} and p47^{phox} genes (reviewed in Ref. 49). These animals display no superoxide production and are highly susceptible to agents similar to those found in human CGD patients. The p47^{phox} knockout has a phenotype like human CGD, with spontaneous infections, granulomatous inflammation, abnormally exuberant inflammatory reactions, and reduction in infections seen with prophylactic IFN-γ.[53]

PHARMACOLOGIC MODULATION

As neutrophils are overrecruited to tissues in neutrophilic dermatoses, they produce reactive oxygen intermediates, activate proteinases, and release chemotactic cytokines, all of which contribute to further tissue injury and inflammation. Therefore, the development of treatments to inhibit neutrophil adhesion and chemotaxis, suppress generation of or damage by reactive oxygen intermediates, and suppress the release of lysosomal enzymes and chemotactic factors is a high priority.

Dapsone is often used for chronic neutrophilic dermatoses such as subcorneal pustular dermatosis or erythema elevatum diutinum. Dapsone is thought to suppress neutrophil adherence and subsequent migration, scavenge reactive oxygen intermediates, and interfere with the myeloperoxidase-halide system. Thalidomide augments CD8+ lymphocyte activity and interferes with the stability of TNF-α mRNA. Colchicine inhibits neutrophil chemotaxis, presumably through the inhibition of microfilament formation that may have effects on the release of lysosomal enzymes, and the production of oxygen intermediates. Antibiotics such as tetracyclines, macrolides, and metronidazole also have putative antioxidant properties and may interfere with neutrophil chemotaxis. Sulfasalazine induces neutrophil apoptosis and enhances adenosine release at sites of inflammation.

REFERENCES

1. Athens JW et al: Leukokinetic studies: IV. The total blood, circulating and the granulocyte turnover rate in normal subjects. *J Clin Invest* **40**:989, 1961
2. Lieschke GJ et al: Mice lacking granulocyte colony-stimulating factor have chronic neutropenia, granulocyte and macrophage progenitor cell deficiency, and impaired neutrophil mobilization. *Blood* **84**:1737, 1994
3. Dong F et al: Mutations in the gene for the granulocyte colony-stimulating factor receptor in patients with acute myeloid leukemia preceded by severe congenital neutropenia. *N Engl J Med* **333**:487, 1995
4. Aprikyan AA, Dale DC: Mutations in the neutrophil elastase gene in cyclic and congenital neutropenia. *Curr Opin Immunol* **13**:535, 2001
5. Van den Steen PE et al: Neutrophil gelatinase B potentiates interleukin-8 tenfold by aminoterminal processing, whereas it degrades CTAP-III, PF-4, and GRO-alpha and leaves RANTES and MCP-2 intact. *Blood* **96**:2673, 2000
6. Bainton DF: Sequential degranulation of the two types of polymorphonuclear leukocyte granules during phagocytosis of microorganisms. *J Cell Biol* **58**:249, 1973
7. Borregaard N, Cowland JB: Granules of the human neutrophilic polymorphonuclear leukocyte. *Blood* **89**:3503, 1997
8. Lekstrom-Himes JA et al: Neutrophil-specific granule deficiency results from a novel mutation with loss of function of the transcription factor CCAAT/enhancer binding protein epsilon. *J. Exp Med* **189**:1847, 1999
9. Davis JM et al: Neutrophil degranulation and abnormal chemotaxis after thermal injury. *J Immunol* **124**:1467, 1980
10. Zigmond SH: Ability of polymorphonuclear leukocytes to orient in gradients of chemotactic factors. *J Cell Biol* **75**:606, 1977
11. Broaddus VC et al: Neutralization of IL-8 inhibits neutrophil influx in a rabbit model of endotoxin-induced pleurisy. *J Immunol* **152**:2960, 1994
12. Sekido N et al: Prevention of lung reperfusion injury in rabbits by a monoclonal antibody against interleukin-8. *Nature* **365**:654, 1993
13. Kuhns DB, Gallin JI: Increased cell-associated IL-8 in human exudative and A23187-treated peripheral blood neutrophils. *J Immunol* **154**:6556, 1995
14. Hensley CD, Caughman SW: Neutrophilic dermatoses associated with hematologic disorders. *Clin Dermatol* **18**:355, 2000
15. Hall A: Rho GTPases and the actin cytoskeleton. *Science* **279**:509, 1998
16. Hirsch E et al: Central role for G protein-coupled phosphoinositide 3-kinase gamma in inflammation. *Science* **287**:1049, 2000
17. Ward RA et al: Priming of the neutrophil respiratory burst involves p38 mitogen-activated protein kinase-dependent exocytosis of flavocytochrome b_{558}–containing granules. *J Biol Chem* **275**:36713, 2000
18. Capodici C et al: Phosphatidylinositol 3-kinase mediates chemoattractant-stimulated, CD11b/CD18-dependent cell-cell adhesion of human neutrophils: Evidence for an ERK-independent pathway. *J Immunol* **160**:1901, 1998
19. Baggiolini M, Moser B: Blocking chemokine receptors. *J Exp Med* **186**: 1189, 1997
20. Cooper D et al: Transendothelial migration of neutrophils involves integrin-associated protein (CD47). *Proc Natl Acad Sci U S A* **92**:3978, 1995
21. Walcheck B et al: Neutrophil rolling altered by inhibition of L-selectin shedding in vitro. *Nature* **380**:720, 1996
22. von Andrian UH et al: In vivo behavior of neutrophils from two patients with distinct inherited leukocyte adhesion deficiency syndromes. *J Clin Invest* **91**:2893, 1993
23. Anderson DC, Springer TA: Leukocyte adhesion deficiency: An inherited defect in the Mac-1, LFA-1, and p150,95 glycoproteins. *Annu Rev Med* **38**:175, 1987
24. McEver RP: Selectins. *Curr Opin Immunol* **6**:75, 1994
25. Frohlich D et al: The Fcγ receptor–mediated respiratory burst of rolling neutrophils to cytokine-activated, immune complex–bearing endothelial cells depends on L-selectin but not on E-selectin. *Blood* **91**:2558, 1998
26. Lubke T et al: Complementation cloning identifies CDG-IIc, a new type of congenital disorders of glycosylation, as a GDP-fucose transporter deficiency. *Nature Genet* **28**:73, 2001
27. Etzioni A, Tonetti M: Leukocyte adhesion deficiency II-from A to almost Z. *Immunol Rev* **178**:138, 2000
28. Etzioni A, Tonetti M: Fucose supplementation in leukocyte adhesion deficiency type II. *Blood* **95**:3641, 2000
29. Hogg JC, Doerschuk CM: Leukocyte traffic in the lung. *Annu Rev Physiol* **57**:97, 1995
30. Mizgerd JP et al: Neutrophil emigration in the skin, lungs, and peritoneum: Different requirements for CD11/CD18 revealed by CD 18-deficient mice. *J Exp Med* **186**:1357, 1997
31. Conlan JW, North RJ: *Listeria monocytogenes,* but not *Salmonella typhimurium,* elicits a CD18-independent mechanism of neutrophil extravasation into the murine peritoneal cavity. *Infect Immun* **62**:2702, 1994
32. Kurlander RJ, Batker J: The binding of human immunoglobulin G_1 monomer and small, covalently cross-linked polymers of immunoglobulin G_1 to human peripheral blood monocytes and polymorphonuclear leukocytes. *J Clin Invest* **69**:1, 1982
33. Boros P et al: IgM anti-FcγR autoantibodies trigger neutrophil degranulation. *J Exp Med* **173**:1473, 1991
34. Johnston RB Jr et al: Generation of superoxide anion and chemiluminescence by human monocytes during phagocytosis and on contact with surface-bound immunoglobulin G. *J Exp Med* **143**:1551, 1976
35. Medof ME et al: Unique role of the complement receptor CR1 in the degradation of C3b associated with immune complexes. *J Exp Med* **156**:1739, 1982
36. Cassatella MA: The production of cytokines by polymorphonuclear neutrophils. *Immunol Today* **16**:21, 1995
37. Elsbach P et al: Integration of antimicrobial host defenses: Role of the bactericidal/permeability-increasing protein. *Trends Microbiol* **2**:324, 1994
38. Ooi CE et al: A 25-kDa NH_2-terminal fragment carries all the antibacterial activities of the human neutrophil 60-kDa bactericidal/permeability-increasing protein. *J Biol Chem* **262**:14891, 1987
39. Schumann RR et al: Structure and function of lipopolysaccharide-binding protein. *Science* **249**:1429, 1990
40. Lehrer RI et al: Defensins: Endogenous antibiotic peptides of animal cells. *Cell* **64**:229, 1991
41. Rice WG et al: Defensin-rich dense granules of human neutrophils. *Blood* **70**:757, 1987
42. Ganz T et al: Microbicidal/cytotoxic proteins of neutrophils are deficient in two disorders: Chediak-Higashi syndrome and "specific" granule deficiency. *J Clin Invest* **82**:552, 1988
43. Gallin JI et al: Human neutrophil-specific granule deficiency: A model to assess the role of neutrophil-specific granules in the evolution of the inflammatory response. *Blood* **59**:1317, 1982
44. Witko-Sarsat V et al: Presence of proteinase 3 in secretory vesicles: Evidence of a novel, highly mobilizable intracellular pool distinct from azurophil granules. *Blood* **94**:2487, 1999
45. Belaaouaj A et al: Mice lacking neutrophil elastase reveal impaired host defense against gram-negative bacterial sepsis. *Nature Med* **4**:615, 1998
46. Degousee N et al: Groups IV, V and X phospholipases A_2 in human neutrophils: Role in eicosanoid production and gram-negative bacterial phospholipid hydrolysis. *J Biol Chem* **6**:6, 2001
47. Brock J: Lactoferrin: A multifunctional immunoregulatory protein? *Immunol Today* **16**:417, 1995
48. Kuhns DB et al: Increased circulating cytokines, cytokine antagonists, and E-selectin after intravenous administration of endotoxin in humans. *J Infect Dis* **171**:145, 1995
49. Segal BH et al: Genetic, biochemical, and clinical features of chronic granulomatous disease. *Medicine* **79**:170, 2000
50. Winkelstein JA et al: Chronic granulomatous disease: Report on a national registry of 368 patients. *Medicine* **79**:155, 2000
51. Segal B et al: Leukotrienes, the NADPH oxidase, and complement are critical regulators of thioglycollate peritonitis in mice. *J Leukocyte Biol* **71**:410, 2002
52. A controlled trial of interferon gamma to prevent infection in chronic granulomatous disease. The international Chronic Granulomatous Disease Cooperative Study Group. *N Engl J Med* **324**:509, 1991
53. Jackson SH et al: IFN-γ is effective in reducing infections in the mouse model of chronic granulomatous disease (CGD). *J Interferon Cytokine Res* **21**:567, 2001
54. Bainton D: Developmental biology of neutrophils and eosinophils. In *Inflammation: Basic Principles and Clinical Correlates,* edited by Gallin JI, Snyderman R, Philadelphia, Lippincott-Raven, 1998.

CHAPTER 30

Adrienne Rencic
Lisa A. Beck

Regulation of the Production and Activation of Eosinophils

Eosinophils are bone marrow-derived cells that normally account for 1 to 3 percent of peripheral blood leukocytes or less than 350 cells per cubic millimeter of blood. As proinflammatory cells, their presence within tissue sites is usually associated with diseased states. In general, the diseased states can be divided into parasitic infections, atopic diseases, reactive eosinophilias, and idiopathic eosinophilic syndromes. This chapter reviews the biologic actions of eosinophils with particular focus on what controls eosinophil production, activation, and tissue trafficking. It ends with a review of the mechanisms of several antieosinophilic treatment strategies with particular attention paid to their theoretical mode of action.

BONE MARROW PRODUCTION AND TISSUE DISTRIBUTION

Eosinophils are derived from a common myeloid progenitor known as the colony-forming unit-granulocyte/erythroid/macrophage/megakaryocyte (CFU-GEMM), which is a pluripotent stem cell that also gives rise to red blood cells, platelets, monocytes, neutrophils, and basophils. It is hypothesized that cytokines generated at sites of inflammation act in a paracrine fashion on stromal cells in the bone marrow microenvironment to differentiate CFU-GEMMs into more cell-specific progenitors. In the case of eosinophil production, this is thought to be the eosinophil/basophil-CFU (Eo/B-CFU). This hybrid cell, which has been found in the circulation of patients with atopic dermatitis, is characterized by granule contents that have features of both cell types as well as by the expression of the interleukin (IL)-5 receptor and the chemokine receptor CCR3.[1] Eo/B-CFUs have been found in inflamed tissues of patients with allergic diseases. Because these tissues also produce many of the hematopoietic cytokines, it has been proposed that some hematopoiesis may occur within sites of inflammation in addition to the bone marrow.[2]

The cytokines important in the development of eosinophilia from these bone marrow progenitors have been extensively studied in mouse models. These studies demonstrate the primary importance of the hematopoietic cytokine, IL-5, and the CCR3 ligand, eotaxin. For example, IL-5 transgenic mice develop peripheral blood and tissue eosinophilia, whereas experiments with neutralizing anti-IL-5 antibodies in wild-type mice lead to a significant reduction in baseline levels of circulating eosinophils and diminished eosinophilia in response to infection with various parasites or challenge with allergen.[3,4] Despite the massive eosinophilia in IL-5 transgenic mice, these mice do not develop the tissue damage observed in eosinophilic diseases, probably because eosinophils must also be activated to degranulate and/or release their inflammatory mediators. The chemokine eotaxin has been thought to act as both a granulocyte-macrophage colony-stimulating factor by increasing myeloid progenitors in general and, more specifically, as a facilitator of emigration of Eo/B-CFU progenitors and mature eosinophils from the bone marrow compartment into the systemic circulation.[5] Mice deficient in both eotaxin and IL-5 have the greatest reduction in tissue eosinophils in experimental models of asthma.[6]

With the development of antibodies specific for eosinophil granule major basic protein (MBP), it has become possible to screen both diseased and normal human tissues for the presence of degranulated eosinophils as well as intact eosinophils. These studies demonstrate that eosinophils are a significant component of the inflammatory infiltrate in several cutaneous diseases such as urticaria and atopic dermatitis (AD), which contains few intact eosinophils but extensive MBP-staining of the dermal collagen fibers. Furthermore, in samples of normal tissue, eosinophils are resident cells in lymph nodes, thymus, and spleen where they are largely intact.[7] This finding supports the notion that eosinophils predominantly reside in the tissues, much like mast cells and basophils. Similarly, eosinophils are present in the lamina propria of the stomach and intestines in healthy individuals, but appreciable degranulation is observed at these sites. It is surmised from this constitutive tissue localization that eosinophils probably play a role in innate immunity.[8]

Eosinophil Ultrastructure and Surface Receptors

ULTRASTRUCTURE The eosinophil is easily identifiable by light microscopy by virtue of its basic granules, which have a high affinity for acidic dyes such as eosin, Giemsa, and fluorescein derivatives such as FITC (fluorescein isothiocyanate), and typically stain with a distinctive tinctorial property (Fig. 30-1*A*).[9] The availability of fluorescent-labeled eosinophil granule-specific antibodies has made it possible to demonstrate degranulated eosinophils as well (Fig. 30-1*B*). Eosinophils typically contain a bilobed nucleus; however, their distinguishing feature is the distinctive cytoplasmic granules. By electron microscopy these so-called specific or secondary granules consist of two compartments, the outer matrix and the inner electron-dense crystalline core (Fig. 30-1*C*). Four highly basic proteins are found within these granules: MBP, eosinophil cationic protein (ECP), eosinophil-derived neurotoxin (EDN), and eosinophil peroxidase (EPO).

MBP is the most abundant of the granule proteins (786 mg/10^6 eosinophils).[10] It is the only one of the four basic proteins located in the core of the secondary granule. ECP is present in the matrix of the granules and is 10 times less abundant than MBP. EDN is also located in the matrix and is much less abundant than either MBP or ECP. EPO is the least abundant of these four proteins and is also located in the matrix. EPO is the granule protein most specific for eosinophils because MBP is found in basophils, neutrophils, and placental X cells; ECP is found in basophils, neutrophils, and monocytes; and EDN is found in neutrophils and basophils. Other proteins found in the secondary granules include enzymes, cytokines, growth factors, and chemokines.

Other cytoplasmic granules are relatively nonspecific and consist of unicompartmental primary granules, lipid bodies, small granules, vesicles, and elongated tubules. The Charcot-Leyden crystal protein

(CLC-P), also known as galectin-10, is found in primary granules. It was first described in the postmortem blood and spleen of a leukemia patient, in 1853, by Charcot and Robin, and later, in 1872, by Leyden in the sputum of patients with asthma. Although its role in eosinophil function is unclear, its distinctive hexagonal bipyramidal crystals tend to be found at sites of eosinophil infiltration and degranulation. It was once thought to possess lysophospholipase activity but has more recently been found to bind to lysophospholipases.[11] Although once considered to be an exclusive marker of eosinophilia, CLC-P has been identified in basophils as well. Lipid bodies and small granules increase in number in response to eosinophil activation. Recent work suggests that lipid bodies may be the site of eicosanoid production and cytokine storage. Small granules are probably analogous to lysosomes in other cell types. Rough endoplasmic reticulum and Golgi structures are present but are not prominent in mature eosinophils.[12]

Surface Receptors

Multiple receptors are present on the surface of eosinophils, but no single surface protein is uniquely expressed. These receptors have been identified either by flow cytometry or by functional assays, and can be grouped as follows: chemotactic factor receptors (chemokine, complement, and others); immunoglobulin and other immunoglobulin supergene family (IgSF) members; cytokine receptors; adhesion molecule receptors; and receptors involved in apoptosis[13] (Table 30-1).

CHEMOTACTIC FACTOR RECEPTORS Chemotactic factors are thought to be important in orchestrating cellular trafficking to sites of inflammation as well as physiologic homing (e.g., gastrointestinal tract). Many chemotactic agents [leukotrienes (LTB_4), platelet-activating factor (PAF), bacterial products (fMLP), and complement components (C5a)] have potent effects on eosinophils but are nonselective. In as much as many eosinophilic diseases are characterized by tissue eosinophilia with little to no neutrophilia, the identification of more selective chemotaxins such as LTD_4, LTE_4, C3a, and C-C chemokines was an important breakthrough.

Specific members of the chemokines or chemotactic cytokines family are thought to be essential for the cellular trafficking of eosinophils. Chemokines are a family of 8- to 15-kDa proteins that can be subdivided into four structural subfamilies based on the number and location of conserved cysteine residues in their primary sequence: CC, CXC, C, and CX3C (see Chap. 27).[14] The biologic effects of chemokines are mediated through specific, high-affinity chemokine receptors, which are typically selective for unique but overlapping subsets of chemokines. The binding of chemokines to their respective receptors on the eosinophil mediates many biologic effects in addition to cell shape change and migration, such as cell activation, receptor internalization, induction of the respiratory burst, and transient activation of integrin adhesiveness (see "Trafficking of Eosinophils into Tissues," below).

The chemokine receptor CCR3 and its major ligands [eotaxin 1–3, monocyte chemoattractant protein (MCP)-4, and regulated on activation, normal T cell expressed and secreted (RANTES)] play a critical role in both the homeostatic and inflammation-induced recruitment of eosinophils to tissue sites.[11] The most highly expressed CCR present on human eosinophils is CCR3, with occasional individuals expressing modest levels of CCR1. Although there appears to be some variability in the expression of the major chemokine receptors CCR3 and CCR1 on eosinophils from different donors, our work and that of others suggest that this finding cannot be explained by in vitro priming, and expression levels of allergic and nonallergic donors do not differ. Under the influence of various stimuli in vitro, eosinophils express other chemokine receptors, such as CXCR2 through 4, and it is implied that they express CCR6 because they migrate in response to its ligand, macrophage inflammatory protein (MIP)-3α.[15,16]

IMMUNOGLOBULIN RECEPTORS AND MEMBERS OF THE IMMUNOGLOBULIN SUPERGENE FAMILY In the immunoglobulin family the receptor most highly expressed on eosinophils is FcγR11 (CD32), which binds aggregated IgG, particularly of the subclasses IgG_3 and IgG_1. The binding of IgG to this receptor can alter eosinophil survival. There is conflicting evidence concerning the presence of the high affinity IgE receptor FcεR1 on the surface of eosinophils.[17] The intracellular α chain may account for the immunohistochemical findings suggesting that eosinophils express FcεR1. FcαRI (CD89), the IgA receptor, is present on the surface of eosinophils.[18] The binding of IgA-opsonized particles to this receptor triggers a variety of immune effector functions. This finding and the fact that there are many eosinophils in the lamina propria of the stomach and intestines suggest that eosinophils play an important role in mucosal immunity.

Members of the IgSF are type I transmembrane molecules that share common structural characteristics of the globular domains in immunoglobulins. Intracellular adhesion molecule (ICAM)-1 (CD54) and ICAM-3 (CD50) are expressed on eosinophils and are thought to be important in leukocyte–leukocyte and leukocyte–tissue cell adhesion using leukocyte function-associated antigen (LFA)-1($\alpha L\beta_2$; CD11a) as its counterligand. CD4 is present at low levels on the surface of eosinophils and binds HIV.[19] Lastly, like all leukocytes, eosinophils express HLA-class I and on activation express HLA-DR (class II).

CYTOKINE RECEPTORS Cytokine receptors are present at low levels on the surface of eosinophils. Receptors for IL-3 (CD123), IL-5 (CD125), and granulocyte-macrophage colony-stimulating factor (GM-CSF) (CD116) are most readily detectable, and all share a common β chain (CD132). Eosinophil activation by a variety of other cytokines has been identified despite the fact that their receptors are not readily detected by flow cytometry. These include stem cell factor (*c-kit* receptor; CD117), interferon (IFN)-γ (CD119), tumor necrosis factor (TNF)-α (CD120), IL-4 (CD124), IL-9 (CD129 and CD132), IL-13β receptor (gp65), IL-2 (CD25), and transforming growth factor (TGF)-β receptors.

ADHESION MOLECULE RECEPTORS Adhesion molecule receptors are expressed on the eosinophil cell surface to mediate trafficking to tissues and within tissues, and for general cell–cell interactions. These receptors fall into three groups: IgSF, selectins and their glycoprotein counterligands, and integrins. L-selectin (CD62L) and P-selectin glycoprotein ligand-1 (PSGL-1, CD162) are expressed at high levels, whereas E-selectin ligands [e.g., sialyl-Lewis X (CD15s)] are expressed at very low levels. P selectin and PSGL-1 are the most important selectin pair in eosinophil migration into tissues.[20]

Eosinophils express a variety of integrins on their surface, which facilitate their adhesion to the extracellular matrix proteins vascular cell adhesion molecule (VCAM)-1 (CD106) on activated endothelium or ICAM-1 on resting or activated epithelium and activated endothelium. Eosinophils express β_1, β_2, and β_7 integrins. Integrins are composed of two subunits that exist as noncovalently associated heterodimers, with an α and a β subunit. The β_1 integrins expressed on eosinophils include $\alpha_4\beta_1$ (VLA-4), which binds to both VCAM-1 on activated endothelium and an alternatively spliced form of fibronectin. Eosinophil adhesion to fibronectin induces the autocrine production of eosinophil survival cytokines (IL-3, IL-5, and GM-CSF). The other β_1 integrin expressed on eosinophils is $\alpha_6\beta_1$, which binds laminin.[21] Four β_2 integrins are found on eosinophils: $\alpha L\beta_2$ (LFA-1), $\alpha M\beta_2$ (Mac-1), $\alpha X\beta_2$, and $\alpha D\beta_2$. These integrins bind to ICAM-1, -2, and -3; VCAM-1; fibrinogen; and the complement fragment C3bi. Lastly, eosinophils also express $\alpha_4\beta_7$, the ligand for the gut mucosal addressin cell adhesion molecule-1 (MAdCAM-1), which is thought to be important in homing

FIGURE 30-1

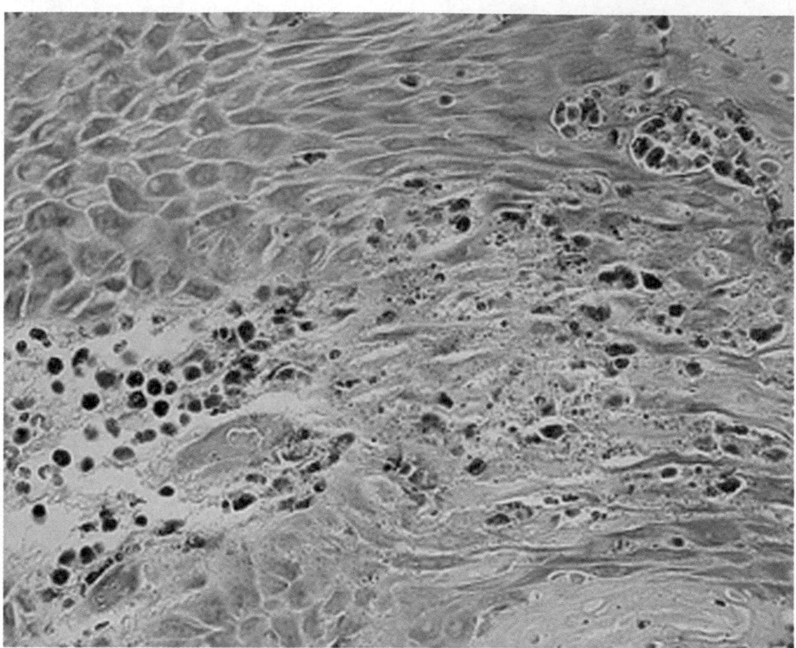

A.

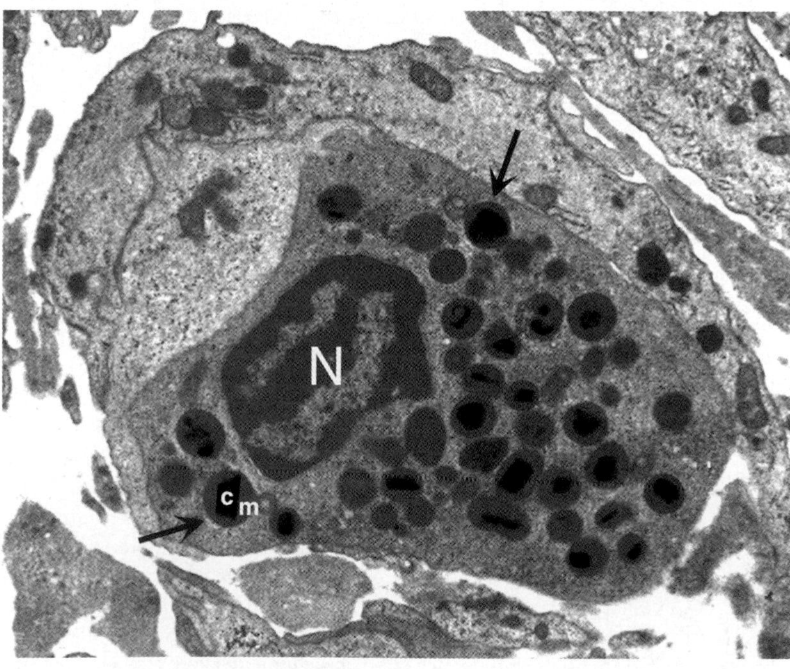

C.

Eosinophil morphology. *A.* Giemsa-stained section of skin from a patient with idiopathic hypereosinophilic syndrome. Eosinophils stain a bright red color. In the reproduction, the color is pink/purple. There are both intact eosinophils and free cytoplasmic granules within the dermis (×400 magnification). *B.* FITC-conjugated anti-MBP staining of a human skin biopsy specimen from a regulated on activation, normal T cell expressed and secreted (RANTES)-challenged site. Both intact and degranulated eosinophils are present. This technique is probably the most sensitive one for identification of tissue eosinophil (×160 magnification). *C.* Representative electron micrograph of a tissue eosinophil illustrating the secondary or specific granules that contain the eosinophil basic proteins: MBP, ECP, EDN, and ECP (*arrows*). In one of the granules, the electron-dense core (c) and lucent matrix (m) are labeled. N, nucleus.

of eosinophils to intestinal mucosa.[11] $\alpha_4\beta_7$ also mediates adhesion to fibronectin and VCAM-1.

RECEPTORS INVOLVED IN APOPTOSIS Apoptosis plays an important role in many biologic processes. Diseases characterized by eosinophilia are thought to result in part from a delayed or defective apoptotic pathway in eosinophils. Eosinophils have at least two cell surface receptors, CD95 (fas) and CD69, that induce apoptosis on activation.[22] In contrast, CD9, and receptors for IL-3, IL-5, GM-CSF, and IFN-γ are involved in eosinophil survival.

ACTIVATION

Various inflammatory mediators, including cytokines (TNF-α, GM-CSF, IL-3, and -5, and IFN-γ), complement components (C3a and C5a), lipid mediators (LTC_4 and PAF), engagement of IgA and IgG Fc receptors, and chemokines, activate eosinophils. Several members of the CC chemokine subfamily (eotaxin, eotaxin-2, RANTES, and MCP-2 to -4) are potent activators of eosinophils as demonstrated by actin polymerization/chemotaxis, respiratory burst, and production of reactive oxygen species.[14] Eosinophils activated in vitro or in vivo develop phenotypic changes that include a reduction in the number of granules, vacuolization, and an expansion of their cytoplasm, leading to a decrease in cell density. They are referred to as hypodense, in contrast to normal-density eosinophils (normodense). The number of hypodense cells has been correlated with allergic disease severity, and it is believed that this finding primarily reflects in vivo exposure to eosinophil survival cytokines (see above). A cell surface marker that can distinguish hypodense from normodense eosinophils has not been identified. There are, however, several surface markers with enhanced expression on in vitro or in vivo activated or hypodense cells: αM integrin (CD11b), αX integrin (CD11c), FcγR111 (CD16), hyaluronic acid receptor (CD44), ICAM-1 (CD54), CD69, and HLA-DR.[23]

INFLAMMATORY MEDIATORS AND POTENTIAL PHYSIOLOGIC EFFECTS

Eosinophils contain many substances that mediate inflammation,[10] including the four cationic granule proteins, arachidonic acid–derived lipids, hydrolytic enzymes, neuropeptides, reactive oxygen species, and cytokines/chemokines. MBP serves a variety of toxic functions. It is an antihelminthic toxin, bactericidal, and cytotoxic. It causes histamine release from basophils and rat mast cells and activates neutrophils to release IL-8.[24] It is thought to have procoagulant activity because it neutralizes heparin, likely through its inactivation of thrombomodulin, and it is a strong platelet agonist.[25] ECP has activities similar to those of MBP. Some of its other functions include potent neurotoxicity, weak RNase activity, and the ability to alter fibrinolysis. EDN is also a potent neurotoxin, with RNase activity and antihelminthic activity. EPO in the presence of hydrogen peroxide and halide kills microorganisms and tumor cells. It causes histamine release and degranulation from rat mast cells. The activities of these granule proteins are likely responsible for some of the signs and symptoms of eosinophilic skin diseases (see Chap. 96).

All four of the cationic granule proteins likely contribute to the edema in many eosinophilic diseases in that they induce the release of histamine from mast cells and basophils. MBP injected into the skin of humans causes a dose-dependent wheal-and-flare response. NERDS (nodules, eosinophilia, rheumatism, dermatitis, and swelling), bullous pemphigoid, herpes gestationis, episodic angioedema with eosinophilia, urticaria, Well's syndrome (eosinophilic cellulitis), and even insect bite reactions have various degrees of edema.[26]

Membrane damage and muscle contraction can be a direct result of toxic granules. The application of MBP, ECP, or EPO to airway epithelium in primates produces ciliostasis, desquamation, and hyperreactivity of respiratory smooth muscle. MBP and ECP damage parasite membranes. In idiopathic hypereosinophilic syndrome (IHES), the damage to the endothelium is thought to be the initiating factor in the cardiomyopathy in these patients. Pulmonary disease in IHES and Churg-Strauss syndrome is initially characterized by airway hyperreactivity.

Thrombosis has been noted in IHES, and several cases of hepatic vein obstruction (Budd-Chiari syndrome) have been reported. The etiology of this thrombosis is not completely clear. It could be the result of direct endothelial damage or of the procoagulant activity of MBP and ECP. MBP and ECP neutralize heparin, and MBP is a strong platelet agonist. PAF is an additional eosinophil-derived inflammatory mediator that could potentiate this effect by inducing platelet aggregation.

The lipid mediators released by eosinophils are primarily arachidonic acid metabolites. LTC_4 is the only leukotriene produced intracellularly by eosinophils. LTC_4 and its metabolites, LTD_4 and LTE_4, are called cysteinyl leukotrienes and were previously referred to as the slow-reacting substances of anaphylaxis (SRS-A). These molecules cause bronchoconstriction, increased airway reactivity, increased mucus secretion, hypotension, and increased vascular permeability. The cysteinyl leukotrienes and PAF are likely major mediators of asthma. The predominant lipid mediator produced in eosinophils via the cyclooxygenase pathway is thromboxane B_2, but this and the other mediators produced through this pathway are minor when compared to those produced by the lipoxygenase pathway.

FIGURE 30-1 (*Continued*)

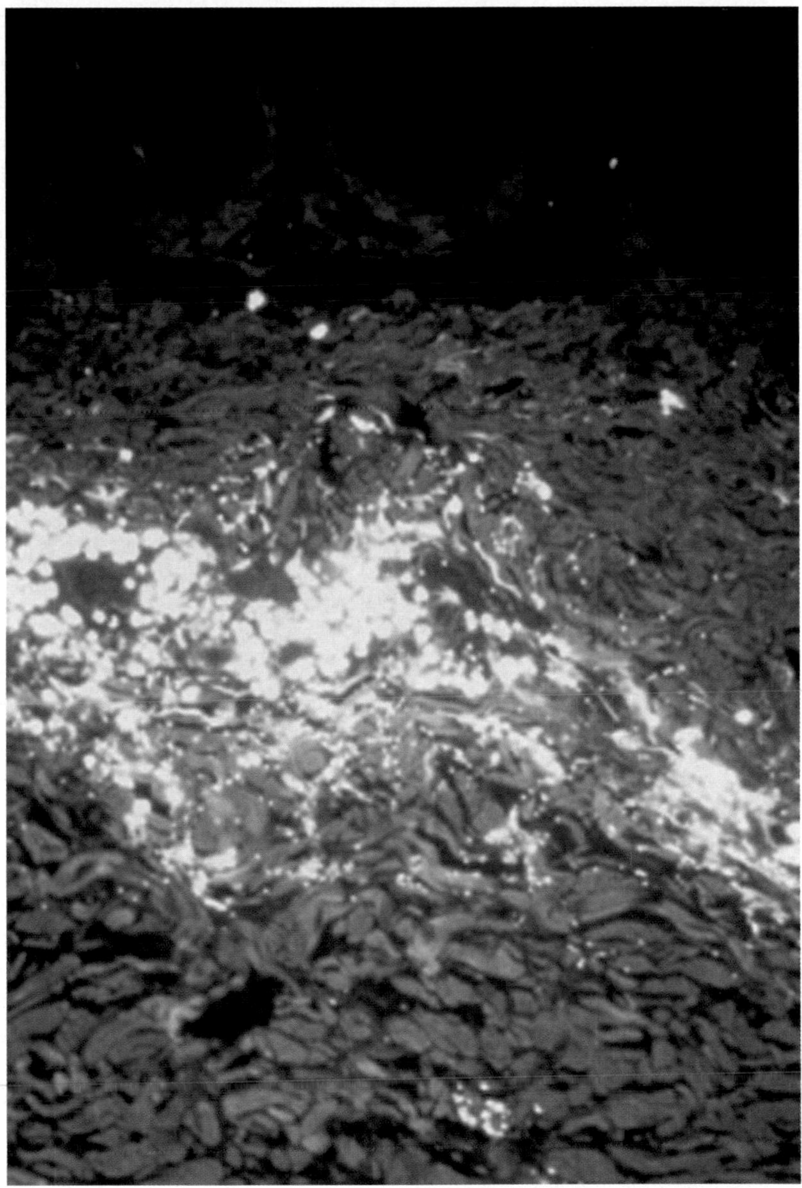

B.

Many hydrolytic enzymes have been identified in human eosinophils, but their role in disease remains largely speculative. Arylsulfatase B, β-glucuronidase, acid phosphatase, catalase, 5-lipoxygenase, phospholipase A_2 (PLA_2), and histaminase are present in eosinophil small granules. Eosinophils stimulated with IL-5 or PAF release matrix metalloproteinase-9, which is thought to be important in migration through the basement membrane.[27] Collagenase, which degrades type I and type III collagen, may play a role in tissue remodeling during wound healing.

The reactive oxygen species that are important in tissue injury and are induced by eosinophils include superoxide and hydrogen peroxide. They are produced by NADPH oxidase during the respiratory burst initiated on eosinophil activation. Hydrogen peroxide can generate cytotoxic hypohalous acids through the action of EPO. Reactive oxygen species can also propagate the inflammatory response by inducing gene expression and T cell proliferation.[28]

Eosinophils from both healthy and diseased individuals produce several neuro-active mediators, including vasoactive intestinal peptide (VIP) and substance P. This fact, and the fact that eosinophils (both intact and degranulated) are often observed in close approximation to nerve endings, suggest some crosstalk. Eosinophil-induced nerve dysfunction is thought to be responsible for the gastric dysmotility that occurs in patients with food allergies or the dysfunction of vagal muscarinic M2 receptors in patients with asthma.[29]

A variety of cytokines and chemokines are produced by eosinophils: TGF-α, TGF-β, nerve growth factor (NGF), platelet-derived growth factor (PDGF)-β, TNF-α, IL-1α, IL-2 thru -6, IL-10, IL-12, IL-16,

TABLE 30-1

Receptors on Eosinophils

CHEMOKINE, CHEMOTACTIC FACTORS, AND COMPLEMENT RECEPTORS	
CD35 (CR1)	LTB_4R
CD88 (C5a)	LTD_4R
C3aR	LTE_4R
PAFR	fMLPR
CXCR2	CCR1
CXCR3	CCR3
CXCR4	CCR6
CYTOKINES	
CD25 (IL-2)	CD124 (IL-4)
CD116 (GM-CSF)	CD 125 (IL-5)
CD117 (c-*kit,* SCF)	CD129
CD119 (IFN-γ)	CD131 (IL-3, IL-5, GM-CSF) (common beta chain)
CD120 (TNF-α)	IL-13R
CD123 (IL-3)	TGF-βR
ADHESION MOLECULES	
CD11a (LFA-1α)	β_7-integrin
CD11b* (Mac-1α, C3biR)	CD29 (β_1-integrin)
CD11c*(p150, 95 α)	CD44* (hyaluronate receptor)
αD integrin	CD49d (VLA-4 a chain)
CD15 (Lewis X)	CD49f (VLA-6 a chain)
CD15s (sialyl-Lewis X)	CD54 (ICAM-1)
CD18 (β_2-integrin)	CD62L (L selectin)
CD162 (PSGL-1)	
IMMUNOGLOBULIN SUPERGENE FAMILY	
CD4	CD66
CD16* (FcγR11)	CD89 (FcαRI)
CD31	CD100
CD32(FcγR11)	
CD47	CD101
CD48	HLA class I
CD50	HLA-DR*
CD54	FcεRI
CD58	Siglec-8
Siglec-8L	
APOPTOSIS, SIGNALING, AND MISCELLANEOUS	
CD9	CD82
CD17 (lactosyl ceramide)	CD92
CD24	CD95 (fas)
CD37	CD97
CD39	CD98
CD43	CD99
CD52 (CAMPATH-1)	CD137
CD53	CD139
CD63 (granulophysin)	CD148
CD65 (ceramide dodecasaccharide)	
CD69*	CD149
CD76	CD151
CD81 (TAPA-1)	CD161
	CD165

*Present on activated eosinophils.
GM-CSF, granulocyte-macrophage colony-stimulating factor; HLA, human leukocyte antigen; ICAM, intercellular adhesion molecule; IL, interleukin; LFA, leukocyte factor antigen; TGF, transforming growth factor; TNF, tumor necrosis factor; VLA, very-late antigen;
SOURCE: Modified from Abu-Ghazaleh RI et al.

GM-CSF, IL-8, MIP-1α, lymphocyte chemoattractant factor (LCF), eotaxin, and RANTES.[30]

The release of TGF-α and TGF-β from eosinophils and the ability of eosinophil mediators to induce platelet release of TGF-β lead to fibroblast proliferation and extracellular matrix production. Other eosinophilic mediators may contribute to altered fibrinolysis including ECP, MMP-9, and collagenase. The clinical correlate to this is the fibrosis in the lungs and the heart of patients with IHES. Additionally, this may contribute to the fibrosis in Schulman's syndrome (eosinophilic fasciitis), eosinophilia myalgia syndrome, and toxic oil syndrome.

Eosinophils have other physiologic functions related to their ability to secrete chemokines and cytokines. Chemoattractants, colony-stimulating factors, and endothelial-activating cytokines released by eosinophils lead to augmentation of cellular infiltrates. Moreover, eosinophils may be able to act as antigen-presenting cells.[31] They express CD4, the IL-2 receptor (CD25), and HLA-DR (MHC class II) on their cell surface.

Eosinophils have been found in a variety of cancers, particularly in lymphomas, leukemias, and colon cancer. They are thought to confer a poor prognosis in several tumors such as nodular sclerosing Hodgkin's disease, Sézary syndrome, and gastric carcinoma.[32] One possible explanation is that the tumor cells produce IL-5, thereby inducing eosinophil production, and such production reflects the tumor burden. Clinical studies have also suggested that tumors associated with tissue and/or peripheral eosinophilia may have a more favorable prognosis.[33] The specific nature of eosinophil-dependent antitumor activity has not been sufficiently explored, but it might include direct cytotoxic effects on tumor cells by eosinophil cationic proteins, antigen presentation, vascular compromise via microthrombi formation (secondary to release of heparinases and PAF), or enhancement/synergism with the antitumor response of other leukocytes (e.g., superoxide and nitric oxide generation).[34,35]

We and others have observed similar eosinophil accumulation and activation in biopsies from postvaccination tumor delayed hypersensitivity responses in humans after autologous GM-CSF gene-transduced renal cell carcinoma and melanoma cell trials.[36,37] One patient undergoing treatment for renal cell carcinoma developed objective evidence of tumor regression as noted by chest CT. At approximately the same time, this patient developed an unusually large area (80 × 80 mm) of erythema and induration at a tumor skin test site, which was characterized by an intense infiltration of eosinophils with prominent degranulation as measured by extracellular MBP staining.[37]

TRAFFICKING OF EOSINOPHILS INTO TISSUES

The selective recruitment of eosinophils into sites of inflammation is largely a function of eosinophil-activating cytokines, endothelial-activating cytokines, and chemokines.

Eosinophil-Activating Cytokines

The eosinophil-activating cytokines (IL-3, IL-5, and GM-CSF) enhance eosinophil survival, maturation, chemotactic responses, and leukotriene production. IL-5 is most specific for eosinophils, whereas the others have similar effects on other leukocytes. For example, eosinophils from patients with atopic dermatitis have increased migratory responses in vitro to several common chemotaxins (N-fMLP, IL-4, and PAF) in comparison to eosinophils from normal individuals, suggesting that they were exposed to one of these activating cytokines in vivo.[38] In fact, IL-5 treatment of eosinophils from normal donors induced the migratory responses seen with eosinophils from patients with atopic dermatitis. Similarly, we have observed that the kinetics of eosinophil recruitment in response to intradermal challenge with RANTES are profoundly faster in allergic individuals.[39] Eosinophils from patients with atopic dermatitis demonstrate prolonged survival ex vivo when compared to eosinophils from normal controls, providing further evidence that they have been primed in vivo by activating cytokines like IL-5.[40] Although eosinophil-activating cytokines can be produced by many cell types (keratinocytes, endothelial cells, monocytes, and T cells), eosinophils themselves may be a major source, and thus there may be an autocrine feedback loop.[40] The local reactions observed in response to GM-CSF administered subcutaneously as an adjunct to chemotherapy demonstrate both intact and degranulated eosinophils, suggesting that eosinophil activation by GM-CSF coupled with cutaneous trauma may be sufficient to induce tissue recruitment.[41]

Endothelial-Activating Cytokines and Chemokines

The regulation of endothelial adhesion molecules important in cell migration is discussed in Chap. 27. The initial step of eosinophil recruitment involves rolling on endothelial selectins (and perhaps the L-selectin counterligand or VCAM-1). This step is followed by a firm adhesion, or "tethering" of the eosinophil. Recent in vitro studies show that tethering or firm adhesion of eosinophils to VCAM-1 or ICAM-1 is a process that is substantially increased by eotaxin, MCP-3, and RANTES.[42] This is thought to be mediated by transient effects of chemokines on β_1 and β_2 integrin avidity. Thus, the transition of an eosinophil from a rolling cell to a firmly adherent one is likely to be facilitated, if not primarily mediated, by chemokines on the endothelial surface. Chemokines produced by structural cells such as fibroblasts, smooth muscle cells, and epithelium are probably important in directing migration and activation of eosinophils in tissues.

THERAPEUTIC STRATEGIES

Although many available therapies (glucocorticoids, myelosuppressive drugs, IFN-α, IFN-γ, leukotriene antagonists, and possibly even antihistamines) inhibit eosinophilic inflammation, none is specific for eosinophils. Glucocorticoids are the most effective. They are thought to affect tissue eosinophil infiltration by three mechanisms: induction of eosinophil apoptosis, reduction of eosinophil production by bone marrow, and inhibition of the cytokines and chemokines important in eosinophil trafficking.[43] Steroids suppress the production of several cytokines important for the induction of adhesion molecules on endothelial cells (IL-1, TNF-α, IL-4, and IL-13) and the release of eosinophil-active chemokines (eotaxin, MCP-3, MCP-4, RANTES). The immediate reduction (<3 h) in circulating eosinophils observed after systemic administration of steroids is thought to occur as a consequence of sequestration into extramedullary organs (liver, spleen, and lymph nodes), as shown in rodents. The mechanism for this action may be that steroids induce the expression of CXCR4 on eosinophils, thereby enabling them to respond to the CXCR4 ligand stromal cell–derived factor-1 (SDF-1) that is produced by stromal cells in extramedullary organs.[15]

Several myelosuppressive drugs (hydroxyurea, interferons, and cyclophilins) are beneficial in eosinophilic disorders alone or as steroid-sparing agents. Interferons are thought to act by inhibiting eosinophil degranulation and inflammatory mediator release.[44] Cyclophilins (cyclosporine, FK506, and ascomycin) are thought to act by inhibiting T cell cytokine release, including cytokines that induce eosinophilic inflammation (IL-4, IL-5, and GM-CSF). Leukotriene antagonists, including 5-lipoxygenase inhibitors (zileuton) and cysLT1 receptor antagonists (zafirlukast and montelukast) decrease tissue eosinophils in allergic individuals and may diminish the biologic actions of eosinophil-derived leukotrienes.[45] Lastly, there have been conflicting reports about the ability of the newer generation antihistamines (cetirizine and fexofenadine) to inhibit eosinophil recruitment in cutaneous and airway allergen challenge models.[46]

With advances in our understanding of eosinophil biology, new, more specific therapeutic strategies have emerged. The approaches that are in preclinical or early clinical development include: anti-IL-5 humanized monoclonal antibodies, small molecular weight antagonists for CCR3 and VLA-4, antisense molecules to VCAM-1 and ICAM-1, and glycomimetics to PSGL-1, the p-selectin ligand on eosinophils.[45]

REFERENCES

1. Sehmi R, Denburg JA: Differentiation of human eosinophils, in *Human Eosinophils: Biological and Clinical Aspects,* edited by G Marone. Basel, Karger, 2000, p 29
2. Kim Y-K et al: Immunolocalization of CD34 in nasal polyposis: Effect of topical corticosteroids. *Am J Respir Cell Mol Biol* **20**:388, 1999
3. Tominaga A et al: Transgenic mice expressing a B-cell growth and differentiation factor gene (interleukin-5) develop eosinophilia and autoantibody production. *J Exp Med* **173**:429, 1991
4. Foster PS et al: Interleukin 5 deficiency abolishes eosinophilia, airways hyperreactivity, and lung damage in a mouse asthma model. *J Exp Med* **183**:195, 1996
5. Peled A et al: The chemotactic cytokine eotaxin acts as a granulocyte-macrophage colony-stimulating factor during lung inflammation. *Blood* **91**:1909, 1998
6. Mould AW et al: The effect of IL-5 and eotaxin expression in the lung on eosinophil trafficking and degranulation and the induction of bronchial hyperreactivity. *J Immunol* **164**:2142, 2000
7. Kato M et al: Eosinophil infiltration and degranulation in normal human tissue. *Anat Rec* **252**:418, 1998
8. Rothenberg ME et al: Gastrointestinal eosinophils. *Immunol Rev* **179**:139, 2001
9. Spry CJF: *Eosinophils: A Comprehensive Review, and Guide to the Scientific and Medical Literature*. Oxford, Oxford University Press, 1988
10. Gleich GJ et al: Eosinophils, in *Inflammation: Basic Principles and Clinical Correlates,* 2nd ed, edited by JI Gallin, IM Goldstein, R Snyderman. New York, Raven, 1992, p 663
11. Ackerman SJ et al: Charcot-Leyden crystal protein (galectin-10) is not a dual-function galactin with lysophospholipase activity, but binds a lysophospholipase inhibitor in a novel structural fashion. *J Biol Chem* **277**:14859, 2002
12. Dvorak AM, Weller PF: Ultrastructural analysis of human eosinophils, in *Human Eosinophils: Biological and Clinical Aspects,* edited by G Marone. Basel, Karger, 2000, p 1
13. Tachimoto H, Bochner BS: The surface phenotype of human eosinophils, in *Human Eosinophils: Biological and Clinical Aspects,* edited by G. Marone. Karger, Basel, 2000, p 45
14. Nickel R et al: Chemokines and allergic disease. *J Allergy Clin Immunol* **104**:723, 1999
15. Nagase H et al: Glucocorticoids preferentially upregulate functional CXCR4 expression in eosinophils. *J Allergy Clin Immunol* **106**:1132, 2000
16. Nagase H et al: Regulation of chemokine receptor expression in eosinophils. *Int Arch Allergy Immunol* **125**:29, 2001
17. Seminario M et al: Intracellular expression and release of Fc epsilon RI alpha by human eosinophils. *J Immunol* **162**:6893, 1999
18. Abu-Ghazaleh RI et al: IgA-induced eosinophil degranulation. *J Immunol* **142**:2393, 1989
19. Weller PF et al: Infection, apoptosis, and killing of mature human eosinophils by human immunodeficiency virus-1. *Am J Respir Cell Mol Biol* **13**:610, 1995
20. Symon FA et al: Functional and structural characterization of the eosinophil P-selectin ligand. *J Immunol* **157**:1711, 1996
21. Georas SN et al: Expression of a functional laminin receptor ($\alpha_6\beta_1$, VLA-6) on human eosinophils. *Blood* **82**:2872, 1993
22. Walsh GM et al: Ligation of CD69 induces apoptosis and cell death in human eosinophils cultured with granulocyte-macrophage colony-stimulating factor. *Blood* **87**:2815, 1996
23. Matsumoto KJ et al: CD44 and CD69 represent different types of cell-surface activation markers for human eosinophils. *Am J Respir Cell Mol Biol* **18**:860, 1998
24. Page S et al: Stimulation of neutrophil IL-8 production by eosinophil granule major basic protein. *Am Respir Cell Mol Biol* **21**:230, 1999
25. Mukai H et al: MBP binding to thrombomodulin potentially contributes to the thrombosis in patients with eosinophilia. *Br J Hematol* **90**:892, 1995

26. Butterfield J et al: Nodules, eosinophilia, rheumatism, dermatitis and swelling (NERDS): A novel eosinophilic disorder. *Clin Exp Allergy* **23**:571, 1993
27. Okada S et al: Migration of eosinophils through basement membrane components in vitro: Role of matrix metalloproteinase-9. *Am J Respir Cell Mol Biol* **17**:519, 1997
28. Pahl H, Baeuerle P: Activation of NF-kappa B by ER stress requires both Ca^{2+} and reactive oxygen intermediates as messengers. *FEBS Lett* **392**:129, 1996
29. Jacoby DB et al: Human eosinophil major basic protein is an endogenous allosteric antagonist at the inhibitory muscarinic M2-receptor. *J Clin Invest* **91**:1314, 1993
30. Lacy P, Moqbel R: Eosinophil cytokines, in *Human Eosinophils: Biological and Clinical Aspects,* edited by G Marone. Basel, Karger, 2000, p 134
31. Shi H et al: Lymph node trafficking and antigen presentation by endobronchial eosinophils. *J Clin Invest* **105**:945, 2000
32. Suchin K et al: Increased interleukin 5 production in eosinophilic Sézary syndrome: Regulation by interferon alfa and interleukin 12. *J Am Acad Dermatol* **44**:28, 2001
33. Goldsmith MM et al: The importance of the eosinophil in head and neck cancer. *Otolaryngol Head Neck Surg* **106**:27, 1992
34. Kubo H et al: Cytotoxin properties of eosinophil granule major basic protein for tumor cells. *Int Arch Allergy Immunol* **118**:426, 1999
35. Hung K et al: The central role of CD4+ T cells in the antitumor immune response. *J Exp Med* **188**:2357, 1998
36. Soiffer R et al: Vaccination with irradiated autologous melanoma cells engineered to secrete human granulocyte-macrophage colony-stimulating factor generates potent antitumor immunity in patients with metastatic melanoma. *Proc Natl Acad Sci U S A* **1998**:13141, 1998
37. Simons JW et al: Bioactivity of autologous irradiated renal cell carcinoma vaccines generated by ex vivo granulocyte-macrophage colony-stimulating factor gene transfer. *Cancer Res* **57**:1537, 1997
38. Dubois GR et al: IL-4 induces chemotaxis of blood eosinophils from atopic dermatitis patients, but not from normal individuals. *J Invest Dermatol* **102**:843, 1994
39. Beck LA et al: Cutaneous injection of RANTES causes eosinophil recruitment: Comparison of nonallergic and allergic subjects. *J Immunol* **159**:2962, 1997
40. Wedi B et al: Delayed eosinophil programmed cell death in vitro: A common feature of inhalant allergy and extrinsic and intrinsic atopic dermatitis. *J Allergy Clin Immunol* **100**:536, 1997
41. Mehregan DR et al: Cutaneous reactions to granulocyte-monocyte colony-stimulating factor. *Arch Dermatol* **128**:1055, 1992
42. Cooper PJ et al: Sequential expression of RANTES and eotaxin by the dermal vascular endothelium is associated with the appearance of eosinophils in the skin after the treatment of onchocerciasis with ivermectin. *Clin Immunol* **95**:51, 2000
43. Schleimer RP et al: Inhibition of inflammatory cell recruitment by glucocorticoids: cytokines as primary targets, in *Topical Glucocorticoids in Asthma: Mechanisms and Clinical Actions,* edited by RP Schleimer, WW Busse, P O'Byrne. New York, Marcel Dekker, 1997, p 203
44. Stevens SR et al: Long-term effectiveness and safety of recombinant human interferon gamma therapy for atopic dermatitis despite unchanged serum IgE levels. *Arch Dermatol* **134**:799, 1998
45. Hansel TT, Barnes PJ: *New Drugs for Asthma, Allergy and COPD*. Basel, Karger, 2001
46. Charlesworth EN et al: Effect of cetirizine on mast cell-mediator release and cellular traffic during the cutaneous late-phase response. *J Allergy Clin Immunol* **83**:905, 1989

CHAPTER 31

John T. Schroeder

Regulation of the Production and Activation of Basophils

The basophil has long been recognized as an effecter cell in allergic inflammation. It secretes histamine and leukotriene (LT) C_4, two of the most potent inflammatory mediators contributing to the acute symptoms associated with diseases such as allergic rhinitis, asthma, and urticaria. Furthermore, there is now firm evidence that basophils are a major source of interleukin (IL)-4 and IL-13, arguably the two most critical proinflammatory cytokines contributing to the pathogenesis of allergic disease. This information, along with new evidence that basophils selectively infiltrate allergic lesions, particularly in the skin, emphasizes the growing belief that these cells play an essential and unique role in the intricate cellular interactions of allergic disease.

HISTORICAL ASPECTS

Although they are easily distinguished from other leukocytes when properly stained (Fig. 31-1), the fact that basophils are rare, representing less than 1 percent of the white blood cells, initially made it difficult for investigators to study their function. It was not until the early 1950s that basophils were identified as the sole source of histamine released in a reaction dependent on IgE among blood leukocytes challenged with specific antigen.[1] The belief that they might be a substitute for studying the hard-to-recover tissue mast cell was supported by evidence that the releasability of a patient's basophils in response to ragweed antigen, in vitro, could predict the clinical responsiveness of the patient to this allergen during ragweed season.[2] The "surrogate" concept, however, was abandoned during the 1980s, with advances in the methods for isolating both cell types. Subsequent studies showed that many functional differences exist between basophils and mast cells. Basophils, in fact, were found to be far more "excitable" than mast cells, releasing histamine after exposure to a diverse assortment of substances and independent of IgE/receptor cross-linking.

The recent movement toward studies of IgE-mediated cytokine generation arose from work published in 1989, showing that IL-3–dependent murine mast cells generated, de novo, IL-4, IL-5, IL-6, and other cytokines that were previously thought to be made only by a subset of activated CD4+ T cells, T helper 2 (T_H2) cells.[3] The basophil, by secreting T_H2 cytokines in addition to histamine and LTC_4, possesses

FIGURE 31-1

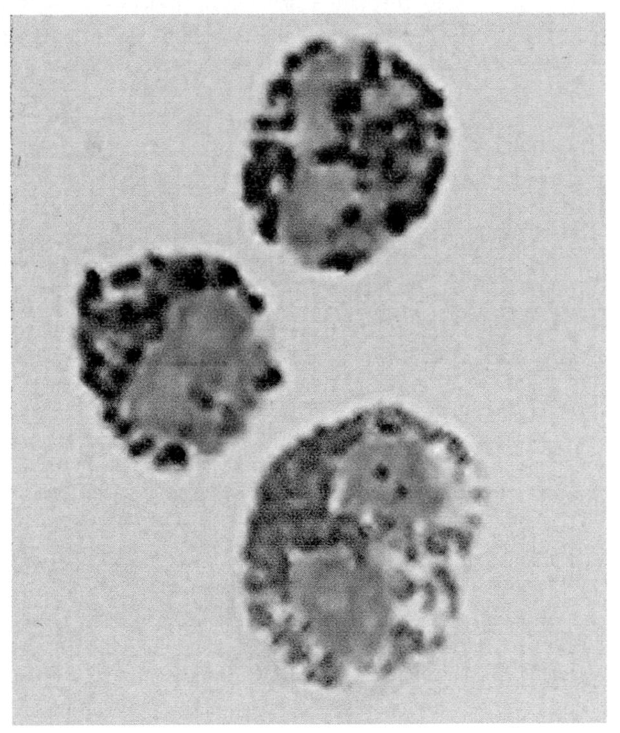

Wright's stain showing two basophils with one eosinophil. Original magnification × 400.

both effector and modulatory functions in allergic lesions. Table 31-1 summarizes the more common characteristics of basophils.

ONTOGENY AND DEVELOPMENT

As with other hematopoietic cells, basophils are ultimately derived from a pluripotent stem cell. However, unlike mast cells, which mature at specific tissue sites in the lung, gut, and skin after the release of a committed progenitor from the bone marrow, basophils are thought to mature in the marrow and to be released as cells with essentially no capacity

TABLE 31-1

Selected Properties of Human Basophils

PROPERTY	FEATURES
Morphology	5–8 μm in size Large and few cytoplasmic granules Lobed nucleus
Natural history	Originates and matures in bone marrow Important growth factor: IL-3 Life span: days (without IL-3)
Major surface receptors	FcεRI (30,000–1,000,000) High IL-3 receptor expression Low c-*kit* expression CD40L
Major inflammatory mediators released	Histamine (1 μg/10^6 cells) Leukotriene C_4 (60 ng/10^6 cells)
Specific cytokines secreted	IL-4 (10–1000 pg/10^6 cells) IL-13 (0–1000 pg/10^6 cells) MIP-1α (0–1500 pg/10^6 cells)

for further development.[4] Evidence shows that basophils are more developmentally related to eosinophils than to mast cells. The number of eosinophil/basophil progenitors is higher in the bone marrow and blood of patients with asthma than in normal subjects,[5,6] and allergen provocation increases the frequency of these cells.[7] Much of the knowledge about the factors involved in the maturation of human basophils has come from studies in which these cells are cultivated in vitro from CD34+ precursor cells found in bone marrow, cord blood, and whole blood. It is currently accepted that IL-3 possesses substantial activity for the development of basophils and is likely the key factor involved.[8] Other cytokines, however, particularly granulocyte-macrophage colony-stimulating factor (GM-CSF), IL-5, and, to a lesser extent, nerve growth factor (NGF), have all been reported to influence basophil development.[9,10] Furthermore, in vivo studies with nonhuman primates show increased numbers of basophils, eosinophils, and their progenitors in the blood of animals infused with either IL-3 or GM-CSF.[11]

PHENOTYPIC MARKERS

Basophils share with other leukocytes, the expression of various adhesion molecules, including members of the selectin, immunoglobulin, and integrin superfamilies, that enable these cells to migrate from the blood across the endothelial barrier and into tissue (reviewed in Refs. 12 and 13). Of particular importance is their expression of $\alpha_4\beta_2$ integrins, which are also found on eosinophils and subclasses of T lymphocytes. These adhesion molecules specifically bind vascular cell adhesion molecule-1 (VCAM-1), and it is this interaction that is most responsible for the selective migration of these cell types into sites of allergic inflammation.[14–16]

Basophils also express receptors that bind various chemokines and cytokines that play a key role in the trafficking and activation of these cells. The eotaxins (I and II) and RANTES (regulated on activation, normal T cell expressed and secreted) are potent chemoattractants for basophils that interact through the highly expressed CCR3 receptor on these cells (see Chap. 27). The CCR1 and CCR2 receptors provide overlapping specificity for the monocyte chemotactic proteins (MCP)-1, -3, and -4, all of which activate basophils. Basophils also express the CXCR4 receptor—a coreceptor important for HIV entry into lymphocytes. The most prominent cytokine receptor expressed on basophils is that for IL-3 (i.e., CD123), which binds this cytokine with high affinity, initiating signals important for both the survival and activation of these cells. Other cytokine receptors on basophils include those for IL-5, GM-CSF, NGF, IL-2, IL-4, and IL-8. Indirect evidence for the expression of receptors for stem cell factor (SCF), interferon-γ (IFN-γ), and tumor necrosis factor α (TNF-α) on basophils comes from studies reporting that these cytokines modulate mediator release.

Basophils and mast cells differ from other immune cells in that they express the high affinity receptor for IgE (FcεRI). The cloned receptor consists of an α, a β, and two γ subunits associated with one another to form an $\alpha\beta\gamma_2$ tetramer. Although monocytes, certain dendritic cells, Langerhans cells, and eosinophils all are reported to express FcεRI, none of these cells appear to have the full tetrameric structure on their cell surface. Like basophils and mast cells, each of these cells also expresses the α-subunit, which confers the high affinity (Ka $<10^{10}$/M) for IgE. However, these cells lack the β subunit, which is thought to play a critical role in amplifying the intracellular signals initiated upon cross-linking of IgE/receptor complexes.[17]

The expression of FcεRI on basophils differs significantly among donors, ranging from 30,000 to 1,000,000 per cell. Studies conducted more than 25 years ago suggested a positive correlation between FcεRI expression on basophils and the levels of total IgE in serum.[18] Credence for this belief has come with the recent development of anti-IgE therapy. For instance, MacGlashan et al. showed that serum IgE levels in patients allergic to dust mites were reduced by more than 90 percent with the infusion of a humanized anti-IgE antibody (E25 or Omalizumab).[19] Subsequently, there was a decrease in the expression of FcεRIα on the basophils of these individuals and a significant loss of reactivity to the antigen. Upon completion of the therapy, both the IgE serum levels and FcεRIα expression returned, as did the responsiveness to dust mite antigen.[20] Basophils also bind IgG through the expression of FcγRII (CD32). Cross-linking antigen-specific IgG bound to this receptor with antigen-specific IgE on FcεRI induces intracellular signals that prevent degranulation and mediator release.[21]

Other activation-linked markers are found on basophils, including the ligand for CD40, CD40L. This molecule, which was previously found on the cell surface of only a few cell types, such as activated T cells, dendritic cells, and endothelial cells, plays a critical role in costimulating B lymphocytes for IgE synthesis. As a result, basophils provide both the soluble factors (IL-4/IL-13) and the cellular interactions (via CD40L) required to induce IgE production by B cells in vitro.[22]

IgE-DEPENDENT ACTIVATION

Release and Function of Preformed Mediators

Cross-linking of IgE/FcεRI complexes on the surface of basophils and mast cells, either by the natural interaction with antigen or by artificial stimulation with anti-IgE, initiates a cascade of intracellular events that leads to the rapid release of preformed and newly generated products. Histamine is a preformed mediator of most interest in the basophil, and its release is essentially complete 20 min after cell stimulation. On average, basophils store approximately 1 pg/cell of histamine in their cytoplasmic granules, as compared to the 3 to 8 pg/cell found in mast cells. As noted above, essentially all of the histamine present in normal human blood is derived from basophils, a fact that has long allowed the use of washed leukocytes in studies of the parameters of IgE-mediated secretion of histamine. The physiologic importance of histamine lies in its ability to contract smooth muscle and to induce vascular leakage by binding to receptor sites in lung tissue, skin, and mucosa. Although tryptase and major basic protein are thought to be mast cell- and eosinophil-specific products, respectively, low amounts of α-tryptase[23] and major basic protein have been identified in human basophils.

Monoclonal antibodies have been developed that identify other granule-specific proteins found only in basophils. The monoclonal antibody 2D7 identifies a 72-kDa protein that is released on cell degranulation.[24] The monoclonal antibody BB1 is specific for a high-molecular-weight complex of $\sim 5 \times 10^6$ Da referred to as basogranulin.[25] As discussed below, these antibodies have greatly facilitated the detection of basophils in tissue.

Newly Generated Mediators and Function

LEUKOTRIENES Through enzymatic activity mediated largely by cytosolic phospholipase A_2 (PLA_2), activated basophils cleave phospholipids (such as phosphatidylinositol and phosphatidylcholine) to release arachidonic acid. The arachidonic acid provides the substrate for LTC_4 synthesis. Unlike mast cells, basophils do not synthesize prostaglandins. The amount of LTC_4 generated by basophils (10 to 100 fg/cell) varies among donors and is much less than the amount of histamine released from these cells. It is, however, far more potent than histamine at inducing smooth-muscle constriction. These cysteinyl leukotrienes are the major mediators involved in the late-phase response (see below). The clinical efficacy of the cysteinyl leukotriene receptor antagonists and 5-lipoxygenase inhibitors supports this belief.[26,27]

CYTOKINES As noted above, the cytokines made by basophils, which include IL-4 and IL-13, are commonly found in allergic lesions and could be critical for IgE synthesis by B cells. In fact, more mRNA and protein for these cytokines are produced by basophils than by any other leukocyte circulating in blood (reviewed in Ref. 28), as evidenced in studies with stimuli that specifically activate basophils and in studies with antigen stimulation, which is capable of also activating T lymphocytes.[29] The explanation for this finding is relatively straightforward: all basophils (i.e., approximately 1 in 200 leukocytes) potentially express antigen-specific IgE, whereas the number of antigen-specific T lymphocytes in blood is estimated at 1 in several thousand.

The biologic activities of both IL-4 and IL-13 suggest that basophils, by producing these cytokines, could play a critical role in orchestrating allergic inflammation (Fig. 31-2). The synthesis of IgE by B cells depends on the ability of these cytokines to induce isotype-switching from IgM to IgE. Both also enhance the expression of major histocompatibility complex (MHC) class II antigens on antigen-presenting cells (APCs) and VCAM-1 on endothelial cells. Individually, IL-4 is currently the only cytokine capable of fostering the development of T_H2 cells from T_H0 lymphocytes, whereas IL-13 has been implicated in mucus production and collagen synthesis.

The parameters important for the production of IL-4 and IL-13 by basophils, resulting from IgE-mediated activation, strongly indicate that signals are initiated for the de novo synthesis of these cytokines. Cycloheximide, an inhibitor of protein synthesis, completely inhibits the secretion of IL-4 and IL-13 by basophils, which suggests that little, if any, protein for these cytokines is stored in the cytoplasmic granules. Unlike histamine and LTC_4, both of which are released minutes after activation, the accumulation of IL-4 mRNA in basophils is first evident at a time (~30 min) when mediator release is essentially over. The secretion of protein for IL-4 peaks 4 to 6 h after activation. The generation of IL-13 appears to be more variable, with much of the current evidence suggesting that its production, while slower to develop, is more protracted than that of IL-4. Protein for IL-13 is first measurable 1 to 2 h after cell stimulation, and its levels peak 18 to 20 h after stimulation (Fig. 31-3). The secretion of both IL-4 and IL-13 is exquisitely dependent on the prolonged changes in cytosolic calcium initiated with concentrations of antigen (or anti-IgE) that are nearly tenfold less than those optimal for mediator release. This finding, combined with pharmacologic evidence that the immunosuppressants FK506 and cyclosporin A (CsA) are potent inhibitors of this response, has implicated a role for the nuclear factor of activated T cells (NFAT) family of transcription factors in the generation of these cytokines.

Of those agents previously shown to inhibit mediator release, including B_2 agonists, H_1 agonists, glucocorticoids, and cyclosporine/FK506, essentially all are relatively more potent against cytokine production.[30–33] However, it remains to be seen whether this ability to inhibit mediator release and cytokine secretion from basophils can be attributed to the clinical efficacy of these drugs.

Activation of Basophils Independent of IgE Cross-Linking

Many substances that activate basophils for mediator release, independently of IgE/FcεRI cross-linking, have essentially no effect on mast cells. Some of the earliest substances described were complement factors (i.e., C5a) and bacterial-derived peptides (i.e., f-met-leu-phe,

FIGURE 31-2

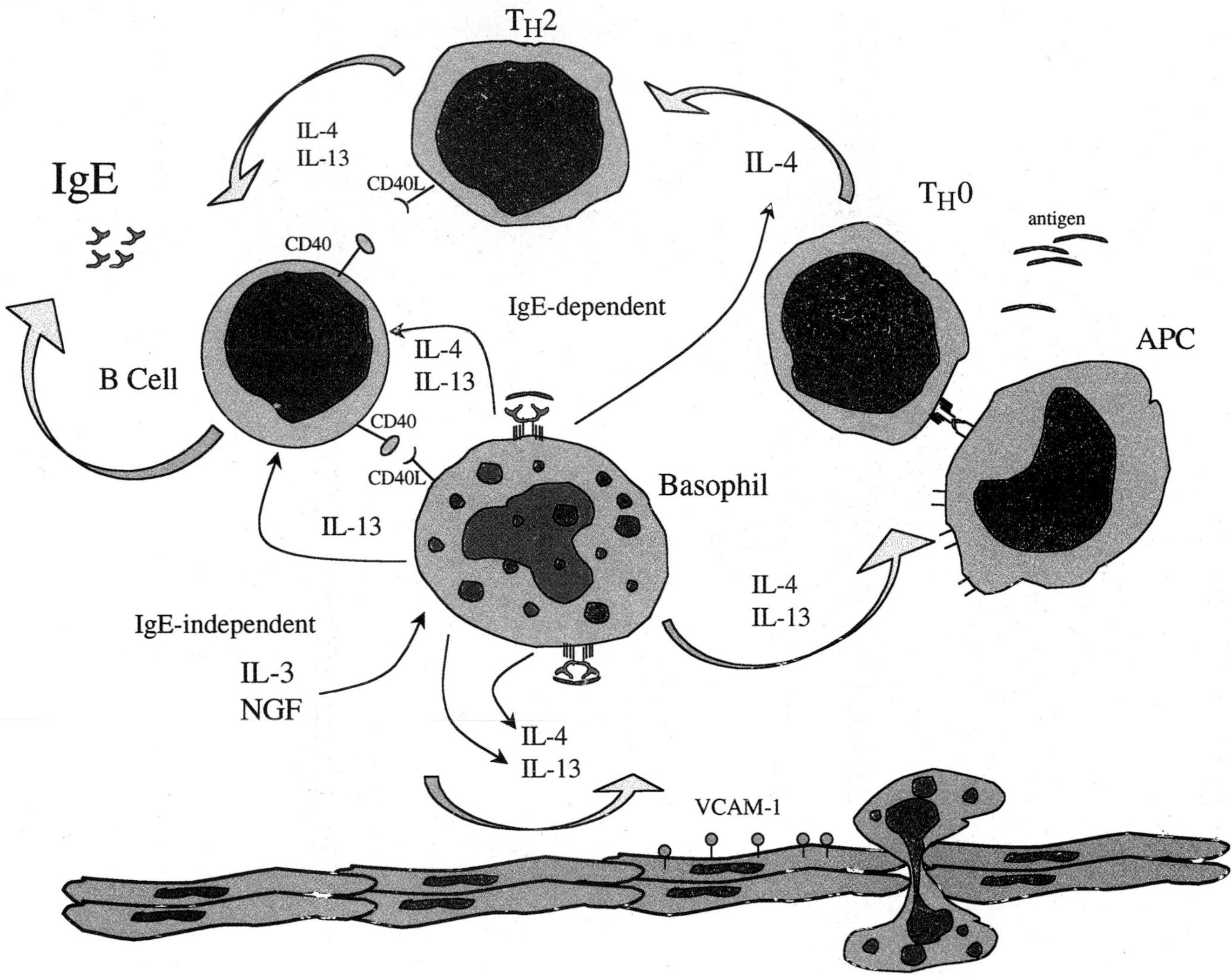

Potential biologic functions for IL-4 and IL-13 secreted by human basophils. Basophils secrete IL-4 and IL-13 in response to IgE-dependent stimuli (i.e., antigen). Substances such as IL-3 and NGF, which act independently of IgE, can also stimulate basophils for IL-13 secretion. These cytokines, along with the costimulatory effects of CD40L (on basophils) interacting with CD40, can induce IgE synthesis in B lymphocytes. Both IL-4 and IL-13 also upregulate VCAM-1 expression on endothelium, thus promoting the migration of eosinophils, basophils, and lymphocytes into lesion sites. By upregulating the expression of major histocompatibility complex class II molecules, these cytokines also facilitate antigen presentation to T cells. Finally, the IL-4 required for the development of T_H2 cells also may be derived from activated basophils.

fMLP). Although they induce mediator release, neither stimulus induces IL-4 or IL-13 secretion sufficiently in the absence of a costimulus, indicating a dissociation between mediator release and cytokine secretion. This characteristic is also seen among the various chemokines that activate basophils. The MCPs (MCP 1, -3, and -4), RANTES, the eotaxins (I and II), and stromal-derived factor-1 (SDF-1) all induce histamine release, albeit primarily from basophils isolated from allergic donors. There are no reports of these chemokines directly inducing either IL-4 or IL-13. Overall, it seems apparent that the chemokines are less effective at inducing cytokine production and mediator release from basophils than they are at promoting cell migration.

In addition to the chemokines listed above, several other cytokines (predominately growth factors) modulate basophil function. In particular, IL-3 modulates several aspects of the basophil response. It plays a critical role in the development and maturation of basophils from precursor cells; exerts antiapoptotic-like activity on mature basophils, facilitating their survival in culture for weeks[34]; and affects both early and late activation responses in basophils. Early effects, which occur within 15 min of exposure, include the ability to "prime" or enhance the secretion of histamine, LTC_4, and cytokines in response to IgE-dependent and -independent activation. In fact, at high concentrations (e.g., 300 n*M*), IL-3 directly induces histamine release from cells of some allergic patients. When used alone, IL-3 also induces relatively late, yet protracted, production of IL-13 from basophils, with secreted protein first detected after 4 hours incubation and continuing for more than 48 hours.[35] Remarkably, this production of IL-13 is not sensitive to FK506, unlike the case with FcεRI-mediated cell activation.[31] Both IL-5 and GM-CSF, which bind to receptors that share a common β-chain with the IL-3 receptor, are also reported to prime basophils for increased histamine release, but these cytokines do not appear to mediate the same late effects, such as IL-13 production, that are seen with IL-3 exposure.[36] However, NGF, which also primes basophils for increased mediator release by binding to the so-called TrkA receptor, was recently shown to activate basophils for IL-13 production, with parameters similar to those seen with IL-3 activation.[37]

FIGURE 31-3

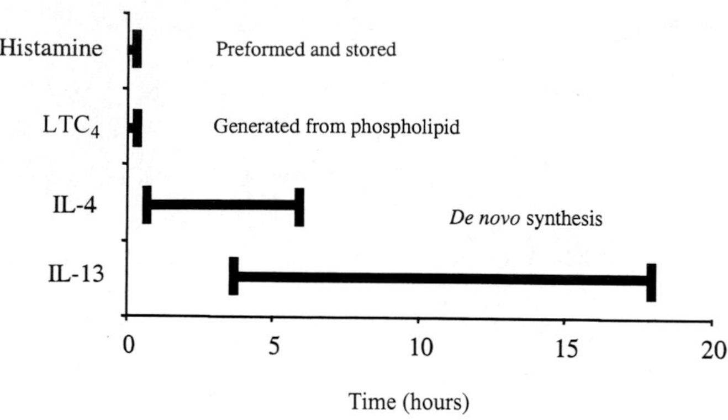

Relative duration of mediator release (histamine and LTC_4) and cytokine secretion (IL-4 and IL-13) resulting from the IgE-dependent activation of basophils in vitro.

Both mediator release and cytokine secretion are enhanced in basophils exposed to recombinant histamine-releasing factor (HRF). Originally referred to as IgE-dependent HRF, this protein is now thought to be a cytokine that binds a specific receptor on basophils, eosinophils, and lymphocytes, rather than IgE.[38,39] HRF directly induces histamine release and IL-4 secretion from the basophils of certain allergic individuals,[40] whereas it primes for IgE-mediated release of histamine, IL-4, and IL-13 from cells of nonallergic individuals.[41] Collectively, HRF and the cytokines noted above, all of which have been identified in allergic lesions, are thought to amplify ongoing allergic responses, in part by enhancing and/or prolonging the responses of basophils and other immune cells.

BASOPHILS IN DISEASE

Under specific pathologic conditions, basophils selectively migrate into tissue sites, accumulating in numbers manyfold those circulating in normal blood. Nowhere has this recruitment been more evident than in the allergic inflammation associated with the so-called late-phase response (LPR) resulting from experimental allergen challenge. These reactions unfold 6 to 12 h after a reduction in symptoms resulting from the early response. LPR lesional sites have long been characterized by a striking influx of eosinophils and mononuclear cells. Nonetheless, basophils have been identified in all models of the LPR, including those of the upper and lower airways and in the skin.[42–44] As a result, some portion of the symptoms associated with the LPR could be basophil-mediated.

A resurgence in studies investigating the role basophils play in allergic lesions has arisen from two developments: the use of monoclonal antibodies allowing their identification in tissues with immunohistochemistry, and the discovery that basophils produce large quantities of IL-4 and IL-13 in vitro. In two independent studies, each using different monoclonal antibodies, basophils were identified in late reactions of the skin 6 to 24 h after experimental allergen challenge.[45,46] The results from both studies were remarkably similar, showing that the percentage of basophils infiltrating these skin lesions approached nearly 50 percent of the infiltrating eosinophils, and thus suggest a far greater presence of these cells than that previously reported. These antibodies have also identified basophils in the lung and nose 6 to 24 h after allergen challenge, albeit at percentages somewhat less than those described in the skin.[46–48]

Recent evidence shows that the basophils infiltrating LPR lesions also secrete IL-4. In one study, the ex vivo production of IL-4 by cells recovered in bronchoalveolar lavage (BAL) samples was seen only in fractions containing basophils.[9] In another study, dual-staining immunohistochemical techniques showed the presence of IL-4 mRNA and protein in cells colabeled with the basophil-specific antibody 2D7.[50] In this study, basophils accounted for nearly 80 percent of the cells expressing IL-4. These findings challenge the long-held belief that T lymphocytes are the major source of IL-4 in allergic reactions. It remains to be seen whether the IL-13 expressed in the LPR[51] is also derived from basophils.

Other studies show the involvement of basophils in natural disease. With the 2D7 monoclonal antibody, large numbers of basophils were found in the lungs of individuals dying from asthma.[52] In the same study, basophils were not found in the lungs of individuals dying from nonasthma–related causes, including those with a history of asthma. Basophils have been identified in skin lesions of patients with atopic dermatitis and urticaria.[53–55] Increasing evidence shows that basophils from patients presenting with these diseases, in particular atopic dermatitis, are reactive to enterotoxins derived from *Staphylococcus aureus* organisms.[56] It seems certain that future studies will address the role of basophils in such lesions now that their detection in tissue can be facilitated with the monoclonal antibodies described.

Finally, it has long been demonstrated that basophils selectively migrate into the so-called cutaneous basophilic hypersensitivity (CBH) reaction, which closely resembles the Jones-Mote reactions originally described in guinea pigs. Unlike LPRs, these reactions are reported to evolve independently of IgE and instead are thought to have a cell-mediated component responsible for modulating the influx of basophils. During the 1970s, the Dvoraks demonstrated CBH in humans after inducing allergic contact dermatitis reactions with rhus toxoid (the active agent in poison ivy) or dinitrochlorobenzene in patch tests.[57,58] They also noted the appearance of basophils in several other conditions involving a cellular component, including tumor and skin allograft rejection,[59,60] bullous pemphigoid,[61] Crohn's disease,[62] and viral hypersensitivity.[63] The active degranulation process (so-called piecemeal degranulation) occurring in the basophils in all of these conditions has suggested a commonality for their activation in these lesions.

REFERENCES

1. Ishizaka T et al: Identification of basophil granulocytes as a site of allergic histamine release. *J Immunol* **108**:1000, 1972
2. Lichtenstein L et al: Clinical and in vitro studies on the role of immunotherapy in ragweed hay fever. *Am J Med* **44**:514, 1968
3. Plaut M et al: Mast cell lines produce lymphokines in response to cross-linkage of Fc epsilon RI or to calcium ionophores. *Nature* **339**:64, 1989
4. Murakami I et al: Studies on the kinetics of human leukocytes in vivo with ^{3}H-thymidine autoradiography. II. Eosinophils and basophils. *Acta Haematol* **32**:384, 1969
5. Denburg J: The origins of basophils and eosinophils in allergic inflammation. *J Allergy Clin Immunol* **102**:S74, 1998
6. Denburg JA et al: Increased numbers of circulating basophil progenitors in atopic patients. *J Allergy Clin Immunol* **76**:466, 1985
7. Wood L et al: Changes in bone marrow inflammatory cell progenitors after inhaled allergen in asthmatic subjects. *Am J Respir Crit Care Med* **157**:99, 1998
8. Kirshenbaum AS et al: IL-3-dependent growth of basophil-like cells and mastlike cells from human bone marrow. *J Immunol* **142**:2424, 1989
9. Tsuda T et al: Synergistic effects of nerve growth factor and granulocyte-macrophage colony-stimulating factor on human basophilic cell differentiation. *Blood* **77**:971, 1991
10. Dvorak AM et al: Ultrastructure of eosinophils and basophils stimulated to develop in cord blood mononuclear cell cultures containing recombinant human interleukin-5 or interleukin-3. *Lab Invest* **61**:116, 1989

11. Dvorak A et al: Ultrastructure of monkey peripheral blood basophils stimulated to develop in vivo by recombinant human interleukin-3. *Lab Invest* **61**:677, 1989
12. Agis H et al: Comparative immunophenotypic analysis of human mast cells, blood basophils, and monocytes. *Immunology* **87**:535, 1996
13. Bochner B: Systemic activation of basophils and eosinophils: Markers and consequences. *J Allergy Clin Immunol* **106**:S292, 2000
14. Schleimer RP et al: IL-4 induces adherence of human eosinophils and basophils but not neutrophils to endothelium. *J Immunol* **148**:1086, 1992
15. Moser R, Fehr J: IL-4 controls the selective endothelium-driven transmigration of eosinophils from allergic individuals. *J Immunol* **149**:1432, 1992
16. Thornhill MA et al: IL-4 increases human endothelial cell adhesiveness for T cells but not for neutrophils. *J Immunol* **144**:3060, 1990
17. Donnadieu E et al: A second amplifier function for the allergy-associated Fc(epsilon)RI- beta subunit. *Immunity* **12**:515, 2000
18. Malveaux FJ et al: IgE receptors on human basophils. Relationship to serum IgE concentration. *J Clin Invest* **62**:176, 1978
19. MacGlashan D Jr et al: Down-regulation of FcεRI expression on human basophils during in vivo treatment of atopic patients with anti-IgE antibody. *J Immunol* **158**:1438, 1997
20. Saini S et al: Down-regulation of human basophil IgE and Fc epsilon RI alpha surface densities and mediator release by anti-IgE-infusions is reversible in vitro and in vivo. *J Immunol* **162**:5624, 1999
21. Kepley C et al: Negative regulation of FcepsilonRI signaling by FcgammaRII costimulation in human blood basophils. *J Allergy Clin Immunol* **106**:337, 2000
22. Gauchat J-F et al: Induction of human IgE synthesis in B cells by mast cells and basophils. *Nature* **365**:340, 1993
23. Xia HZ et al: Quantitation of tryptase, chymase, FcεRIα, and FcεRIγ messenger RNAs in human mast cells and basophils by competitive reverse transcription-polymerase chain reaction. *J Immunol* **154**:5472, 1995
24. Kepley C et al: Identification and partial characterization of a unique marker for human basophils. *J Immunol* **154**:6548, 1995
25. McEuen A et al: Development and characterization of a monoclonal antibody specific for human basophils and the identification of a unique secretory product of basophil activation. *Lab Invest* **79**:27, 1999
26. Calhoun W et al: The effect of Accolate (zafirlukast) on cellular mediators of inflammation: BAL findings after segmental allergen challenge. *Am J Respir Crit Care Med* **157**:1381, 1998
27. Kane GC et al: A controlled trial of the 5-lipoxygenase inhibitor, zileuton, on lung inflammation produced by segmental antigen challenge in human beings. *J Allergy Clin Immunol* **97**:646, 1996
28. Schroeder J, MacGlashan D Jr, Lichtenstein L: Human basophils: Mediator release and cytokine production. *Adv Immunol* **77**:93, 2001
29. Devouassoux G et al: Frequency and characterization of antigen-specific IL-4– and IL-13–producing basophils and T cells in peripheral blood of healthy and asthmatic subjects. *J Allergy Clin Immunol* **104**:811, 1999
30. Gibbs B et al: Inhibition of interleukin-4 and interleukin-13 release from immunologically activated basophils due to the actions of anti-allergic drugs. *Naunyn Schmiedebergs Arch Pharmacol* **357**:573, 1998
31. Redrup A et al: Differential regulation of IL-4 and IL-13 secretion by human basophils. Their relationship to histamine release in mixed leukocyte cultures. *J Immunol* **160**:1957, 1998
32. Schroeder J et al: Inhibition of cytokine generation and mediator release by human basophils treated with desloratadine. *Clin Exp Allergy* **31**:1, 2001
33. Schroeder J et al: Regulation of IgE-dependent IL-4 generation by human basophils treated with glucocorticoids. *J Immunol* **158**:5448, 1997
34. MacGlashan D Jr et al: In vitro regulation of FcεRIα expression on human basophils by IgE antibody. *Blood* **91**:1633, 1998
35. Ochensberger B et al: Human blood basophils produce interleukin-13 in response to IgE-receptor–dependent and –independent activation. *Blood* **88**:3028, 1996
36. Miura K et al: Differences in functional consequences and signal transduction induced by IL-3, IL-5, and nerve growth factor in human basophils. *J Immunol* **167**:2282, 2001
37. Sin A et al: Nerve growth factor or IL-3 induces more IL-13 production from basophils of allergic subjects than from basophils of nonallergic subjects. *J Allergy Clin Immunol* **108**:387, 2001
38. MacDonald S: Human recombinant histamine-releasing factor. *Int Arch Allergy Appl Immunol* **113**:187, 1997
39. Wantke F et al: The human recombinant histamine releasing factor: Functional evidence that it does not bind to the IgE molecule. *J Allergy Clin Immunol* **103**:642, 1999
40. Schroeder J, Lichtenstein L, MacDonald S: An IgE-dependent recombinant histamine-releasing factor induces IL-4 secretion from human basophils. *J Exp Med* **183**:1265, 1996
41. Schroeder J, Lichtenstein L, MacDonald S: Recombinant histamine releasing factor enhances immunoglobulin E-dependent interleukin-4 and -13 secretion by human basophils. *J Immunol* **159**:447, 1997
42. Bascom R et al: The influx of inflammatory cells into nasal washings during the late response to antigen challenge. *Am Rev Respir Dis* **138**:406, 1988
43. Guo C-B et al: Identification of IgE-bearing cells in the late phase response to antigen in the lung as basophils. *Am J Resp Cell Mol Biol* **10**:384, 1993
44. Charlesworth EN et al: Cutaneous late-phase response to allergen. Mediator release and inflammatory cell infiltration. *J Clin Invest* **83**:1519, 1989
45. Irani A-M et al: Immunohistochemical detection of human basophils in late-phase skin reactions *J Allergy Clin Immunol* **101**:354, 1998
46. Macfarlane AJ et al: Basophils, eosinophils, and mast cells in atopic and nonatopic asthma and in late-phase allergic reactions in the lung and skin. *J Allergy Clin Immunol* **105**:99, 1999
47. Gauvreau G et al: Increased numbers of both airway basophils and mast cells in sputum after allergen inhalation challenge of atopic asthmatics. *Am J Respir Crit Care Med* **161**:1473, 2000
48. KleinJan A et al: Basophil and eosinophil accumulation and mast cell degranulation in the nasal mucosa of patients with hay fever after local allergen challenge. *J Allergy Clin Immunol* **106**:677, 2000
49. Schroeder J et al: IL-4 production by human basophils found in the lung following segmental allergen challenge. *J Allergy Clin Immunol* **107**:265, 2001
50. Nouri-Aria K et al: Basophil recruitment and IL-4 production during human allergen-induced late asthma. *J Allergy Clin Immunol* **108**:205, 2001
51. Huang S-K et al: IL-13 expression at the site of allergen challenge in patients with asthma. *J Immunol* **155**:2688, 1995
52. Kepley C et al: Immunohistochemical detection of human basophils in postmortem cases of fatal asthma. *J Allergy Clin Immunol* **107**:A160, 2001
53. Henocq E, Gaillard J: Cutaneous basophil hypersensitivity in atopic dermatitis. *Clin Allergy* **11**:13, 1981
54. Mitchell E et al: Basophils in allergen-induced patch test sites in atopic dermatitis. *Lancet* **1**:127, 1982
55. Mitchell E et al: Cutaneous basophil hypersensitivity to inhalant allergens in atopic dermatitis patients: Elicitation of delayed responses containing basophils following local transfer of immune serum but not IgE antibody. *J Invest Dermatol* **83**:290, 1984
56. Leung D et al: Presence of IgE antibodies to staphylococcal exotoxins on the skin of patients with atopic dermatitis. Evidence for a new group of allergen. *J Clin Invest* **92**:1374, 1993
57. Dvorak HF et al: Cutaneous basophil hypersensitivity. II. A light and electron microscopic description. *J Exp Med* **132**:558, 1970
58. Dvorak HF, Mihm MC Jr: Basophilic leukocytes in allergic contact dermatitis. *J Exp Med* **135**:235, 1972
59. Dvorak HF: Role of basophil leukocytes in allograft reactions. *J Immunol* **106**:279, 1971
60. Dvorak H et al: Rejection of first-set skin allografts in man. The microvasculature is the critical target of the immune response. *J Exp Med* **150**:322, 1979
61. Dvorak AM et al: Bullous pemphigoid, an ultrastructural study of the inflammatory response: Eosinophil, basophil and mast cell granule changes in multiple biopsies from one patient. *J Invest Dermatol* **78**:91, 1982
62. Dvorak AM, Monahan RA: Crohn's disease. Ultrastructural studies showing basophil leukocyte granule changes and lymphocyte parallel tubular arrays in peripheral blood. *Arch Pathol Lab Med* **106**:145, 1982
63. Dvorak HF, Hirsh MS: Role of basophil leukocytes in cellular immunity to vaccinia virus infections. *J Immunol* **107**:1576, 1971

CHAPTER 32

Fred H. Hsieh
Clifton O. Bingham, III
K. Frank Austen

The Molecular and Cellular Biology of the Mast Cell

The mast cell (MC) has long been recognized as a primary effector cell in immediate-type hypersensitivity reactions. Recent studies have focused on its lineage development and tissue heterogeneity and its response to innate and adaptive immunologic stimuli. These insights provide evidence that the MC participates in a broad spectrum of biologic processes ranging from allergic inflammation to innate immune responses against gram-negative bacteria and helminths. Mast cells also may play a physiologic role in wound healing, tissue remodeling, and angiogenesis. The focus of this chapter is on the biology of the human MC with references to rodent systems as necessary for completeness.

DISTRIBUTION AND IDENTIFICATION

Mast cells are dispersed widely throughout the body, although their numbers are highest at mucosal surfaces, where they are exposed to foreign stimuli.[1] The number of MCs increases at inflammatory sites in various disorders, including atopic dermatitis, inflammatory bowel disease, multiple sclerosis, and asthma.[2–5] Dermal MCs often are located in close proximity to blood vessels, nerves, and lymphatics, with an estimated density of 7000 to 20,000 MCs per cubic millimeter of skin.[1]

Mast cells can be identified by numerous granules that undergo red-purple metachromatic staining with the basic dye toluidine blue. These cells exhibit a variable morphology ranging from round to spindle-shaped with sizes up to 25 μm. A unilobed nucleus may be round to oval in shape and typically is positioned eccentrically. Monoclonal antibodies directed against the membrane receptor c-*kit* and the granule proteases tryptase, chymase, and carboxypeptidase A identify MCs in situ. Chloroacetate esterase, which reacts with the granule proteases of MCs, identifies MCs in tissues but also reacts with cathepsin-G in neutrophil granules.

The cytoplasmic granules of human MCs contain macromolecular complexes of proteoglycans and proteases with distinct morphology that are detected by immunocytochemistry and electron microscopy.[1] This characteristic led to an early descriptive classification based on anatomic localization and staining characteristics (Fig. 32-1). Mast cells containing only tryptase (MC_T or reactive MC phenotype) demonstrate scroll-like granules by electron microscopy. They tend to predominate in the intestinal mucosa and lung parenchyma. Mast cells containing tryptase, chymase, and carboxypeptidase A (MC_{TC} or constitutive tissue phenotype) tend to predominate in the skin and submucosa of many tissues. Their granules are scroll-poor with a grating or lattice-like structure with periodicity.[6] Mast cells with granules containing chymase without tryptase (referred to as MC_C) have been identified in the skin, lymph nodes, and intestinal submucosa. Thus there exists every combination of phenotypic heterogeneity for these three proteases.

DEVELOPMENTAL BIOLOGY

Mast cells originate from hematopoietic committed progenitors (PrMC) in the bone marrow that mature and differentiate in the target tissue. The development of tissue MCs in both rodents and humans requires the interaction between the receptor tyrosine kinase c-*kit* (CD117) and its fibroblast- or stromal cell–derived ligand stem cell factor (SCF). It is further modulated by additional factors in the tissues that account for MC functional and immunohistochemical heterogeneity. In particular, a constitutive baseline MC subpopulation resides in perivascular connective tissues and varies in number depending on the anatomic site, whereas an immunohistochemically and functionally distinctive reactive MC subpopulation develops and expands in mucosal surfaces in response to T cell–derived growth factors.[7,8]

The earliest evidence that the interaction between SCF and c-*kit* profoundly influences MC development came from analyses of mice with naturally occurring MC deficiencies. The W/W_v mouse strain lacks MCs due to a mutation of the gene that encodes c-*kit*, whereas the Sl/Sl_d mouse strain also lacks MCs and has a mutation of the gene that encodes for SCF (also known as the *kit* ligand or Steel factor).[7] The MC deficiency of W/W_v mice was corrected by transplantation of bone marrow cells from normal congenic mice, thereby confirming the hematopoietic origin of MCs and indicating that correction of the defect in c-*kit* permitted normal MC development. In several cytokine-independent human and rodent MC lines, a single-amino-acid substitution in the tyrosine kinase domain of the cytoplasmic portion of c-*kit* results in a constitutively phosphorylated and activated receptor.[9,10] Functional mutations of the same type have been found in association with several types of systemic mastocytosis in humans—indolent mastocytosis, systemic mastocytosis with an associated clonal hematologic non-mast cell lineage disease, and mast cell leukemia.[11] Thus decreased signaling through c-*kit* results in MC deficiency, whereas excessive activation of this receptor leads to aberrant MC proliferation.

Human PrMCs were recognized initially as CD34+, c-*kit*+, CD14− mononuclear progenitor cells found in bone marrow[12] and peripheral blood with SCF-dependent culture systems.[13] These observations supported the bone marrow origin of human MCs and suggested that human PrMCs also reach target tissues by the peripheral circulation and differentiate in an SCF-dependent manner. Human MCs can be derived in culture from various sources, including cord blood, using SCF in combination with accessory cytokines such as interleukin 6 (IL-6) and IL-10.[14–16] Whereas SCF and intact c-*kit* are essential and sufficient to support normal numbers of constitutive-tissue MCs, additional factors are necessary for the expansion of MC subpopulations. The importance of IL-3 in reactive intestinal mucosal MC hyperplasia is demonstrated by targeted disruption of the IL-3 gene.[17] Mice lacking the IL-3 gene have a markedly attenuated jejunal intraepithelial MC

FIGURE 32-1

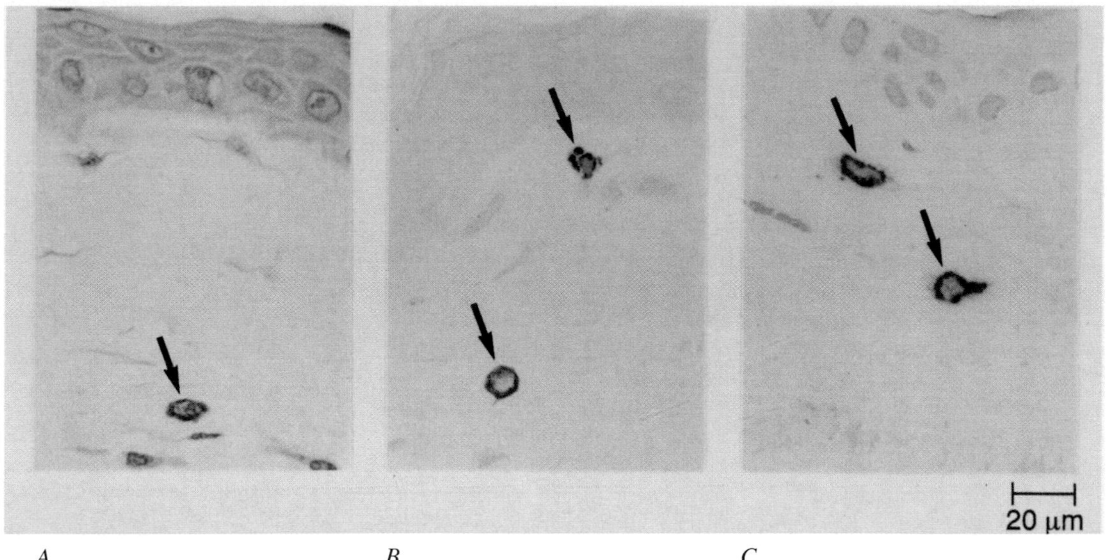

A. B. C.

Human skin MCs (*arrows*) identified by three different staining methods: (*A*) the basic dye toluidine blue; (*B*) immunochemical reaction with chloroacetate esterase; (*C*) immunoalkaline phosphatase staining with monoclonal antibody against tryptase. (*Courtesy of Daniel S. Friend, M.D., Brigham and Women's Hospital.*)

hyperplasia in response to helminth infection even though they have normal numbers of constitutive submucosal MCs. Humans with T cell immunodeficiencies lack MCs in the intestinal mucosa but not in the adjacent submucosa, thereby providing evidence for the existence of a constitutive T cell–independent population of MCs as well as a reactive population dependent on T cells for expansion.[18] Other T cell–derived cytokines, including IL-4, IL-5, IL-6, and IL-9, function synergistically with SCF to amplify the numbers of MCs in human cord blood–derived cultures[16] and at inflamed mucosal sites in mice.[19] Thus important developmental parallels are seen in the mouse and human MC, since both require SCF and its intact receptor *c-kit* to maintain in situ development of constitutive and T cell–modulated populations.

MAST CELL RECEPTORS, LIGANDS, AND CHEMOTAXIS

Mast cell activation occurs through perturbation of the high-affinity IgE receptor FcεRI that is expressed on the surface of not only MCs but also basophils and Langerhans cells.[20] In MCs and basophils, FcεRI is a tetrameric structure consisting of one alpha chain that binds the Fc portion of IgE, one transmembrane β chain, and two disulfide-linked γ chains participating in signal transduction. The two γ chains are disulfide-linked and display significant structural homology to the zeta chain of the T cell receptor with two tandem cytoplasmic immunoregulatory tyrosine activation motifs (ITAMs).[21] Activation through FcεRI occurs when adjacent IgE-bearing receptors are cross-linked by a multivalent antigen or by an immune complex composed of IgE.

Inhibitory receptors that attenuate FcεRI activation have been identified on both human and mouse MCs. Both the low-affinity IgG receptor FcγRIIb1 and gp49B1, a transmembrane receptor member of the immunoglobulin supergene family, contain immunoregulatory tyrosine-based inhibition motifs (ITIMs) in their cytoplasmic domains. Coligation of FcεRI with either FcγRIIb1 or gp49B1 leads to decreased MC degranulation and cysteinyl leukotriene generation.[22,23] Phosphorylation of the ITIM motif of FcγRIIb1 activates polyphosphoinositol 5-phosphatase (SHIP), and phosphorylation of the ITIM motif on gp49B1 activates Src homology protein tyrosine phosphatase 1 (SHP-1).[24,25] Whereas FcεRIIb1 is recruited by the Fc portion of an immune complex during an adaptive immune response, the ligands for gp49B1 are believed to be innate and may include an integrin.[26] The targeted disruption of either FcεRIIb1 or gp49B1 increases the susceptibility of mice to anaphylactic reactions.[27,28]

Chemotactic proteins such as chemokines play an essential role in the selective recruitment and activation of MCs at sites of inflammation (see Chap. 27). Eotaxin and RANTES (regulated on activation, normal T cell expressed and secreted) are members of the beta or CC chemokine family and are chemotactic for cord blood–derived MCs.[29] RANTES binds to the CCR1, CCR3, and CCR5 chemokine receptors, and progenitor cord blood–derived MCs express CCR5; progenitor and mature MCs express CCR3.[16] In situ MCs in the skin and intestinal submucosa express CCR3. Stromal cell–derived factor 1α (SDF-1α), a member of the α or CXC chemokine family, can induce calcium flux and concentration-dependent transendothelial migration in cord blood–derived MCs by binding to CXCR4.[30] IL-8, which binds to the CXCR1 and CXCR2 chemokine receptors, stimulates chemotaxis in cord blood–derived MCs and the immature human MC line HMC-1.[31] SCF also can act as a chemotactic factor for HMC-1, an effect dependent on fibronectin and blocked by antibodies to SCF.[32] Other factors such as the anaphylatoxins C3a and C5a are able to stimulate the laminin-dependent migration of cord blood– or skin-derived MCs.[33]

MAST CELL–DERIVED MEDIATORS

Mast cell–derived mediators can be preformed and stored in secretory granules, newly generated from phospholipid membrane components, or induced by de novo gene expression. This sequence with redundant functions likely allows the MCs to participate in sustained inflammatory responses.

Preformed Secretory Granule Mediators

Histamine is a biogenic amine produced by MCs, basophils, and platelets and is stored in secretory granules.[34] Histamine is exocytosed rapidly in response to immunologic and nonimmunologic stimuli. Histamine acts through the H_1 receptor to mediate increased vascular permeability, bronchial and intestinal smooth muscle contraction, and increased nasal mucus production; it acts through the H_2 receptor to increase vascular permeability, gastric acid secretion, and airway mucus production.[35] H_3 and H_4 receptors have been cloned recently to describe an entire family of G protein–coupled receptors; the precise function of these new receptors is still being addressed.[36]

The metachromatic staining of MC granules is due to sulfated anionic *proteoglycans* composed of a novel peptide core, serglycin, common to all hematopoietic cell secretory granule proteoglycans, and of adducts such as heparin and chondroitin sulfate.[37] Human lung MCs contain both heparin and chondroitin sulfate proteoglycans.[38] Mast cells developed from transgenic mice strains defective in heparin synthesis have altered granule morphology with defects in histamine and MC proteases, suggesting posttranslational control of granule constituents.[39,40]

The tryptase gene family encodes the predominant *proteases* of the human MCs. This serine endopeptidase exhibits trypsin-like substrate specificity and cleaves basic amino acid residues from proteins. Several members of the family have been described, including α, β, γ, and mouse MC protease 7 (mMCP-7)–like tryptases. The tryptase locus resides on chromosome 16p13.3, and sequencing of the locus led to identification of a novel tryptase gene related to mMCP-7. Along with mMCP-6, mMCP-7 has been shown to play a distinct role in inflammation.[41] The γ-tryptases, also on this chromosome, contain a C-terminal hydrophobic domain that may serve as a membrane anchor.[42,43]

The tryptases are stored as a cationic tetramer with heparin.[44] β-Tryptase is stored in the secretory granule and released during exocytosis. Serum levels of β-tryptase rise within 15 min of anaphylactic events and peak at 1 to 2 hours.[45] α-Tryptase is constitutively released from MCs, and levels of both α- and β-tryptase are elevated in patients with mastocytosis due to an increased burden of MCs.[45,46] Tryptase levels are elevated in the bronchoalveolar lavage (BAL) fluid of patients with asthma and in nasal secretions of those with allergic rhinitis.[47,48]

Tryptase inactivates certain neuropeptides, including the bronchodilatory vasoactive intestinal peptide, and also targets matrix metalloproteinases, procoagulant proteins, and proteinase-activated receptor 2.[49,50] In vitro, tryptase stimulates fibroblast proliferation and mRNA synthesis for procollagen and upregulates the expression of IL-8 and intercellular adhesion molecule 1 (ICAM-1) in bronchial epithelial cells.[51,52] Recombinant human β_1-tryptase instilled into the mouse trachea increases the number of neutrophils in the BAL fluid and improves bacterial clearance in the lungs of W/W_v mice; this finding suggests a role for β_1-tryptase in innate immune responses in the lung. α-Tryptase was ineffective in this regard, and thus it appears that relevant functional distinctions exist in vivo.[53]

The MC_{TC} subpopulation of human MCs contains the chymotryptic-like serine endopeptidase *chymase* and/or a second member of this gene family, cathepsin-G.[54] A single human MC chymase gene composed of five exons has been identified on chromosome 14.[55] Chymase also binds to heparin in a macromolecular complex.[34] In vitro, chymase has a 100-fold greater potency than angiotensin-converting enzyme in the conversion of angiotensin I to angiotensin II. It inactivates bradykinin and the neuropeptides vasoactive intestinal peptide and substance P; cleaves laminin, type IV collagen, and fibronectin with attendant basement membrane degradation; and can convert the precursor of IL-1β to an active form, stimulating secretion from airway serous cells.[56]

Mouse MCs contain five separate chymases (mMCP-1, -2, -4, -5, and -9). These chymases have been cloned and immunochemically defined to allow further study of the phenotypic diversity and plasticity of MCs influenced by various cytokines in vitro and in vivo.[57] The mouse chymase genes are located on chromosome 14 and exhibit a similar genomic organization to the human genes, with mMCP-5 being the closest in evolution.[58] Cytokine regulation of the profile of chymase family expression in vitro is based on induction of transcript stability.[59] The diversity of chymase expression during the initiation and resolution of intestinal mastocytosis during helminth infection in the mouse likely reflects such transcript regulation in situ by T cell–secreted cytokines.

Lipid-Derived Mediators of Inflammation

Lipid mediators are newly formed from membrane phospholipids after cell activation. Membrane phospholipids serve as the source of the 20-carbon arachidonic acid substrate used to form the prostaglandins (PGs) and leukotrienes (LTs). Phospholipase (PL) A_2 enzymes release arachidonic acid from the *sn*-2 position of phospholipids to provide substrate for eicosanoid products and platelet-activating factor (PAF). The integral perinuclear membrane PG endoperoxide synthases (PGHS-1 and -2, or cyclooxygenase 1 and 2) metabolize the released arachidonic acid directly to the intermediates PGG_2 and PGH_2 for processing by terminal PG synthases. Mast cells contain hematopoietic cell–type PGD_2 synthase, which converts PGH_2 to PGD_2.[60]

In activated mouse bone marrow–derived mast cells (BMMCs), the two isoforms of PGHS serve different functions. A constitutive phase of PGD_2 generation occurring within minutes after activation of MCs via FcεRI or the c-*kit* receptor is linked to the constitutively expressed PGHS-1. This immediate PGD_2 production is accompanied by the rapid phosphorylation and translocation of cytosolic PLA_2 ($cPLA_2$) to a membrane compartment, an event dependent on the MAP kinase pathway.[61] A delayed phase of PGD_2 generation occurring over several hours in response to SCF and IL-10 plus FcεRI cross-linking requires the de novo induction of PGHS-2 and is linked to heparin-sensitive cell membrane–associated low-molecular-weight PLA_2 and $cPLA_2$.[62]

PGD_2 appears in bronchial and nasal secretions after allergen challenge, and its metabolite, $9\alpha,11\beta$-PGF_2, appears in the urine of patients with systemic mastocytosis and in those with aspirin-induced asthma.[63,64] The intradermal injection of PGD_2 leads to a wheal and flare response due to vasodilation and increased vascular permeability, and the inhalation of PGD_2 causes the bronchoconstriction of airway smooth muscle.[65] Two seven-transmembrane G protein–coupled receptors for PGD_2 have been described: the DP receptor, which is expressed on endothelial and airway smooth muscle cells, and CRTH2, which is selectively expressed on T_H2 cells, eosinophils, and basophils.[66,67] The binding of PGD_2 to CRTH2 may provide a positive-feedback pathway between MCs and T_H2 lymphocytes in allergic inflammation. T_H2 cells would support cytokine-mediated, SCF-dependent coproliferation of mucosal MCs with augmented capacity to generate cysteinyl leukotrienes, whereas PGD_2 would continue to recruit T_H2 cells to the inflammatory focus.

The first enzyme in the leukotriene pathway, 5-lipoxygenase (5-LO), undergoes calcium-dependent translocation to the perinuclear membrane after cell activation. There, arachidonic acid released by $cPLA_2$, in the presence of the integral membrane protein 5-lipoxygenase–activating protein (FLAP), is presented to 5-LO for conversion to the epoxide leukotriene A_4 (LTA_4). LTA_4 is subsequently converted into the cysteinyl leukotriene LTC_4 by LTC_4 synthase, an integral perinuclear membrane protein that conjugates glutathione to LTA_4.[68] The targeted disruption of LTC_4 synthase has demonstrated that this enzyme, and not microsomal or cytosolic glutathione-*S*-transferases, is the major

LTC_4-producing enzyme in vivo. Cysteinyl leukotrienes are the predominant mediators of the permeability changes that accompany IgE-dependent MC activation.[69]

Activated human MCs produce LTC_4, which undergoes carrier-mediated export for conversion to the active metabolites LTD_4 and LTE_4. The three cysteinyl leukotrienes each increase microvascular permeability, are potent inducers of long-lasting wheal and flare responses, and when inhaled, elicit bronchoconstriction, with LTC_4 and LTD_4 providing more than 1000-fold greater potency than histamine.[70] Levels of cysteinyl leukotrienes are elevated in the nasal secretions of patients with allergic rhinitis and in BAL fluid from patients with asthma. The gene for human LTC_4 synthase is localized distal to the gene cluster for the T_H2-type cytokines IL-3, IL-4, IL-5, and IL-13 and granulocyte-macrophage colony-stimulating factor (GM-CSF) on chromosome 5.[71] Two cysteinyl leukotriene receptors have been described, CysLT1 and CysLT2, with CysLT1 having a greater binding affinity for LTD_4 than LTC_4 or LTE_4, and CysLT2 having equal affinities for LTC_4 and LTD_4 and poor affinity for LTE_4.[72,73] IL-4 priming of cord blood–derived human MCs uncovers a response to LTC_4 and to pyrimidinergic ligands that is blocked by CysLT1 receptor inhibitors and is subject to cross-desensitization between these ligands.[74]

Human MCs from different tissues have different capacities to generate eicosanoids. Both total PGD_2 generation and the PGD_2–cysteinyl leukotriene ratio are marked by quantitative and relative tissue-related differences.[8] In mouse BMMCs, upregulation of the intermediate enzymes for prostaglandin or leukotriene generation depends on different cytokines, e.g., SCF for the PGD_2 pathway and IL-3 for the cysteinyl leukotriene pathway.[75] In human MCs derived in vitro from cord blood, IL-4, IL-3, and IL-5 prime for increased cysteinyl leukotriene production, with each cytokine targeting distinct steps in the cysteinyl leukotriene biosynthetic pathway. IL-4 induces the expression of $Fc\varepsilon RI$ and LTC_4 synthase, whereas IL-3 and IL-5 translocate 5-lipoxygenase to the nucleus.[76]

Cytokines and Chemokines: Constitutive and Induced

The MC is increasingly recognized as a source of multifunctional cytokines that may participate in the recruitment and activation of other cells in the inflammatory microenvironment. Mast cells with different secretory granule protease phenotypes exhibit differences in their cytokine profiles, thus indicating further heterogeneity based on tissue localization.[77]

Human tissue MCs demonstrate transcripts and immunoreactive protein for IL-4 in situ, and dispersed human lung MCs release IL-4 and IL-5 after activation with IgE and antigen.[77,78] When mouse BMMCs are stimulated with SCF plus IL-10, the mRNA transcripts for IL-6 are upregulated, but little protein is released. However, when IL-1β is added to the culture, steady state transcripts persist with attendant IL-6 protein release due to the induction of a stabilizing factor that prolongs the half-life of IL-6 mRNA and permits its translation.[79] Cord blood–derived human MCs can release IL-5, IL-13, GM-CSF, and tumor necrosis factor α (TNF-α), as well as the chemokine macrophage inhibitory protein 1α (MIP-1α), after activation through $Fc\varepsilon RI$.[80]

Although TNF-α (cachexin) can be constitutively stored in the granule, most is induced with immunologic activation of mouse MCs.[81] TNF-α also can be released in response to bacterial infection through the interaction of lipopolysaccharide with toll-like receptor 4 or bacterial FimH with CD48.[82,83] Recent studies with MC-deficient W/W_v mice have demonstrated the importance of MC-derived TNF-α in neutrophil recruitment in bacterial peritonitis[83,84] and in protection from endotoxic shock, a response mediated by Janus kinase 3.[85] Mast cell–derived TNF-α also upregulates endothelial leukocyte adhesion molecule 1 (ELAM-1) and ICAM-1 expression on endothelial cells, facilitating

adhesion and ingress of eosinophils and T cells to the inflammatory locus.[86]

Transcripts for transforming growth factor β (TGF-β), a potent fibroblast activator and proliferation factor, are localized in human MCs from fibrotic lung and rheumatoid synovium.[87] Cultured mouse BMMCs activated through $Fc\varepsilon R1$ release bioactive TGF-β, which upregulates α_1 (I) collagen mRNA transcripts in fibroblasts.[88] Rat peritoneal MCs synthesize nerve growth factor (NGF), as determined by both transcript and protein.[89] Mouse MCs contain the chemokines RANTES and members of the MIP family.[90]

The biology of the MC traditionally has been studied in the context of the cell's central pathobiologic role in allergy and allergic inflammation. Recent studies have focused on MC development in the hematopoietic lineage and integrin-selective tissue localization of committed circulating progenitors. Detailed histologic and molecular analysis of the determinants of MC heterogeneity in tissues has led to the concept of constitutive and reactive MC populations developed from a single lineage of committed progenitors. Compelling evidence has been evolving to identify MCs involved in innate host defense against bacteria as those of the constitutive phenotype, whereas MCs involved in the host defense against helminths arise from prelocalized resident progenitors that amplify, mature, and differentiate under the control of T cell signals.

REFERENCES

1. Weidner N, Austen KF: Evidence for morphologic diversity of human mast cells: An ultrastructural study of mast cells from multiple body sites. *Lab Invest* **63**:63, 1990
2. Damsgaard TE et al: Mast cells and atopic dermatitis: Stereological quantification of mast cells in atopic dermatitis and normal human skin. *Arch Dermatol Res* **289**:256, 1997
3. Bischoff SC et al: Quantitative assessment of intestinal eosinophils and mast cells in inflammatory bowel disease. *Histopathology* **28**:1, 1996
4. Ibrahim MZ et al: The mast cells of the multiple sclerosis brain. *J Neuroimmunol* **70**:136, 1996
5. Crimi E et al: Increased numbers of mast cells in bronchial mucosa after the late-phase asthmatic response to allergen. *Am Rev Respir Dis* **144**:1282, 1991
6. Irani AA et al: Two types of human mast cells that have distinct neutral protease compositions. *Proc Natl Acad Sci USA* **83**:4464, 1986
7. Galli SJ et al: The kit ligand, stem cell factor. *Adv Immunol* **55**:1, 1994
8. Austen KF, Boyce JA: Mast cell lineage development and phenotypic regulation. *Leuk Res* **25**:511, 2001
9. Furitsu T et al: Identification of mutations in the coding region of the proto-oncogene c-*kit* in a human mast cell leukemia cell line causing ligand independent activation of c-*kit* product. *J Clin Invest* **92**:1736, 1993
10. Tsujimura T et al: Ligand independent activation of c-*kit* receptor tyrosine kinase in a murine mastocytoma cell line P-815 generated by a point mutation. *Blood* **83**:2619, 1994
11. Valent P et al: Diagnostic criteria and classification of mastocytosis: A consensus proposal. *Leuk Res* **25**:603, 2001
12. Kirshenbaum AS et al: Demonstration of the origin of human mast cells from CD34+ bone marrow progenitor cells. *J Immunol* **146**:1410, 1991
13. Rottem M et al: Mast cells cultured from the peripheral blood of normal donors and patients with mastocytosis originate from a CD34+/FcεR1- population. *Blood* **84**:2489, 1994
14. Furitsu T et al: Development of human mast cells in vitro. *Proc Natl Acad Sci USA* **86**:10039, 1989
15. Mitsui H et al: Development of human mast cells from umbilical cord blood cells by recombinant human and murine c-*kit* ligand. *Proc Natl Acad Sci USA* **90**:735, 1993
16. Ochi H et al: T helper type-2 cytokine-mediated comitogenic responses and CCR3 expression during differentiation of human mast cells in vitro. *J Exp Med* **190**:267, 1999
17. Lantz CS et al: Role for interleukin-3 in mast cell and basophil development and in immunity to parasites. *Nature* **392**:90, 1998
18. Irani AM et al: Deficiency of the tryptase-positive, chymase-negative mast cell type in gastrointestinal mucosa of patients with defective T lymphocyte function. *J Immunol* **138**:4381, 1987

19. Finkelman FD, Urban JF Jr: The other side of the coin: The protective role of TH2 cytokines. *J Allergy Clin Immunol* **107**:772, 2001
20. Bieber T et al: Human epidermal Langerhans cells express the high affinity receptor for immunoglobulin E (FcεRI). *J Exp Med* **175**:1285, 1992
21. Scharenberg AM, Kinet JP: FcεRI and the FcRβ amplifier. *Int Arch Allergy Immunol* **117**:113, 1997
22. Katz HR et al: Mouse mast cell gp49B1 contains two immunoreceptor tyrosine-based inhibition motifs and suppresses mast cell activation when coligated with the high affinity Fc receptor for IgE. *Proc Natl Acad Sci USA* **93**:10809, 1996
23. Daeron M et al: Regulation of high-affinity IgE receptor-mediated mast cell activation by murine low affinity IgG receptors. *J Clin Invest* **95**:577, 1995
24. Ono M et al: Role of the inositol phosphatase SHIP in negative regulation of the immune system by the receptor FcγRIIB. *Nature* **383**:263, 1996
25. Lu-Kuo JM et al: gp49B1 inhibits IgE-mediated mast cell activation through both immunoreceptor tyrosine-based inhibitory motifs, recruitment of the src homology 2 domain-containing phosphatase-1, and suppression of early and late calcium mobilization. *J Biol Chem* **274**:5791, 1999
26. Castells MC et al: gp49B1-alpha v beta 3 interaction inhibits antigen-induced mast cell activation. *Nature Immunol* **2**:436, 2001
27. Ujike A et al: Modulation of immunoglobulin (Ig)E-mediated systemic anaphylaxis by low-affinity Fc receptors for IgG. *J Exp Med* **189**:1573, 1999
28. Daheshia M et al: Increased severity of local and systemic anaphylactic reactions in gp49B1-deficient mice. *J Exp Med* **194**:227, 2001
29. Romagnani P et al: Tryptase-chymase double-positive human mast cells express the eotaxin receptor CCR3 and are attracted by CCR3-binding chemokines. *Am J Pathol* **155**:1195, 1999
30. Lin TJ et al: Human mast cells transmigrate through human umbilical vein endothelial monolayers and selectively produce IL-8 in response to stromal cell–derived factor-1α. *J Immunol* **165**:211, 2000
31. Nilsson G et al: Mast cell migratory response to interleukin-1 is mediated through interaction with chemokine receptor CXCR2/interleukin-8RB. *Blood* **93**:2791, 1999
32. Nilsson G et al: Stem cell factor is a chemotactic factor for human mast cells. *J Immunol* **153**:3717, 1994
33. Hartmann K et al: C3a and C5a stimulate chemotaxis of human mast cells. *Blood* **89**:2863, 1997
34. Schwartz LB et al: Quantitation of histamine, tryptase, and chymase in dispersed human T and TC mast cells. *J Immunol* **138**:2611,1987
35. Falus A, Meretey K: Histamine: An early messenger in inflammatory and immune reactions. *Immunol Today* **13**:154, 1992
36. Hough LB: Genomics meets histamine receptors: New subtypes, new receptors. *Mol Pharmacol* **59**:415, 2001
37. Avraham S et al: Cloning and characterization of the mouse gene that encodes the peptide core of secretory granule proteoglycans and expression of this gene in transfected rat fibroblasts. *J Biol Chem* **264**:16719, 1989
38. Stevens RL et al: Identification of chondroitin sulfate E and heparin proteoglycans in the secretory granules of human lung mast cells. *Proc Natl Acad Sci USA* **85**:2284, 1988
39. Forsberg E et al: Abnormal mast cells in mice deficient in a heparin-synthesizing enzyme. *Nature* **400**:773, 1999
40. Humphries DE et al: Heparin is essential for the storage of specific granule proteases in mast cells. *Nature* **400**:769, 1999
41. Huang C et al: Regulation and function of mast cell proteases in inflammation. *J Clin Immunol* **18**:169, 1998
42. Caughey GH et al: Characterization of human gamma-tryptases, novel members of the chromosome 16p mast cell tryptase and prostasin gene families. *J Immunol* **164**:6566, 2000
43. Wong GW et al: Cloning of the human homolog of mouse transmembrane tryptase. *Int Arch Allergy Immunol* **118**:419, 1999
44. Schwartz LB: Structure and function of human mast cell tryptase, in *Biological and Molecular Aspects of Mast Cell and Basophil Differentiation and Function,* edited by Y Kitamura New York, Raven, 1995
45. Schwartz LB et al: Time course of appearance and disappearance of human mast cell tryptase in the circulation after anaphylaxis. *J Clin Invest* **83**:1551, 1989
46. Schwartz LB et al: The α form of human tryptase is the predominant type present in blood at baseline in normal subjects and is elevated in those with systemic mastocytosis. *J Clin Invest* **96**:2702, 1995
47. Wenzel SE et al: Activation of pulmonary mast cells by broncheoalveolar allergen challenge: In vitro release of histamine and tryptase in atopic subjects with and without asthma. *Am Rev Respir Dis* **137**:1002, 1988
48. Rasp G, Hochstrasser K: Tryptase in nasal fluid is a useful marker of allergic rhinitis. *Allergy* **48**:72, 1993
49. Tam EK, Caughey GH: Degradation of airway neuropeptides by human lung tryptase. *Am J Respir Cell Mol Biol* **3**:27, 1990
50. Corvera CU et al: Mast cell tryptase regulates colonic myocytes through proteinase-activated receptor-2. *J Clin Invest* **100**:1383, 1997
51. Gruber BL et al: Synovial procollagenase activation by human mast cell tryptase: Dependence upon matrix metalloproteinase 3 activation. *J Clin Invest* **84**:1657, 1989
52. Cairns JA, Walls AF: Mast cell tryptase is a mitogen for epithelial cells: Stimulation of IL-8 production and intracellular adhesion molecule-1 expression. *J Immunol* **156**:275, 1996
53. Huang C et al: Evaluation of the substrate specificity of human mast cell tryptase β_1 and demonstration of its importance in bacterial infection of the lung. *J Biol Chem* **276**:26276, 2001
54. Schechter NM et al: Identification of a cathepsin G-like proteinase in the MCTC type of human mast cell. *J Immunol* **145**:2652, 1990
55. Caughey GH et al: Structure, chromosomal assignment, and deduced amino acid sequence of a human gene for mast cell chymase. *J Biol Chem* **266**:12956, 1991
56. Fukami H et al: Chymase: Its pathophysiological roles and inhibitors. *Curr Pharm Des* **4**:439, 1998
57. Gurish MF et al: Tissue-regulated differentiation and maturation of a v-*abl*-immortalized mast cell-committed precursor. *Immunity* **3**:175, 1995
58. Gurish MF et al: A closely linked complex of mouse mast cell specific chymase genes on chromosome 14. *J Biol Chem* **268**:11372, 1993
59. Xia Z et al: Post-transcriptional regulation of chymase expression in mast cells: A cytokine-dependent mechanism for controlling the expression of granule neutral proteases of hematopoietic cells. *J Biol Chem* **271**:8747, 1996
60. Kanaoka Y et al: Cloning and crystal structure of hematopoietic prostaglandin D synthase. *Cell* **96**:449, 1997
61. Murakami M et al: The immediate phase of c-*kit* ligand stimulation of mouse bone marrow-derived mast cells elicits rapid leukotriene C_4 generation through posttranslational activation of cytosolic PLA_2 and 5-lipoxygenase. *J Exp Med* **182**:197, 1995
62. Bingham CO III et al: A heparin-sensitive phospholipase A_2 and prostaglandin endoperoxide synthase are functionally linked in the delayed phase generation of prostaglandin D_2 generation in mouse bone marrow-derived mast cells. *J Biol Chem* **271**:25936, 1996
63. O'Sullivan S et al: Increased urinary excretion of the prostaglandin D_2 metabolite $9\alpha,11\beta$-prostaglandin F_2 after aspirin challenge supports mast cell activation in aspirin-induced airway obstruction. *J Allergy Clin Immunol* **98**:421, 1996
64. Roberts LJ II et al: Increased production of prostaglandin D_2 in patients with systemic mastocytosis. *N Engl J Med* **180**:1400, 1980
65. Hardy CC et al: The bronchoconstrictor effect of inhaled prostaglandin D_2 in normal and asthmatic men. *N Engl J Med* **311**:209, 1984
66. Narumiya S et al: Prostanoid receptors: structures, properties, and functions. *Physiol Rev* **79**:1193, 1999
67. Hirai H et al: Prostaglandin D_2 selectively induces chemotaxis in T helper type 2 cells, eosinophils, and basophils via seven-transmembrane receptor CRTH2. *J Exp Med* **193**:255, 2001
68. Lam BK et al: Leukotriene C_4 synthase. *J Lipid Mediat Cell Signal* **12**:333,1995
69. Kanaoka Y et al: Attenuated zymosan-induced peritoneal vascular permeability and IgE-dependent passive cutaneous anaphylaxis in mice lacking leukotriene C_4 synthase. *J Biol Chem* **276**:22608, 2001
70. Arm JP, Lee TH: Sulphidopeptide leukotrienes in asthma. *Clin Sci (Colc)* **84**:501, 1993
71. Penrose JF et al: Molecular cloning of the gene for human leukotriene C_4 synthase, organization, nucleotide sequence, and chromosomal localization to 5q35. *J Biol Chem* **271**:11356, 1996
72. Lynch KR et al: Characterization of the human cysteinyl leukotriene cysLT1 receptor. *Nature* **399**:789, 1999
73. Heise CE et al: Characterization of the human cysteinyl leukotriene 2 (CysLT2) receptor. *J Biol Chem* **275**:30531, 2000
74. Mellor EA et al: Cysteinyl leukotriene receptor 1 is also a pyrimidinergic receptor and is expressed by human mast cells. *Proc Natl Acad Sci USA* **98**:1964, 2001
75. Murakami M et al: Interleukin 3 regulates development of the 5-lipoxygenase/leukotriene C_4 synthase pathway in mouse mast cells. *J Biol Chem* **270**:22653, 1995
76. Hsieh FH et al: T helper cell type 2 cytokines coordinately regulate IgE-dependent cysteinyl leukotriene production by human cord blood–derived mast cells: Profound induction of leukotriene C_4 synthase expression by IL-4. *J Exp Med* **193**:123, 2001

77. Bradding P et al: Heterogeneity of human mast cells based on cytokine content. *J Immunol* **155**:297, 1995
78. Jaffe JS et al: Human lung mast cell IL-5 gene and protein expression: Temporal analysis of upregulation following IgE mediated activation. *Am J Resp Cell Mol Biol* **13**:665,1995
79. Lu-Kuo JM et al: Post-transcriptional stabilization by interleukin-1β of interleukin-6 mRNA induced by c-*kit* ligand and interleukin 10 in mouse bone marrow-derived mast cells. *J Biol Chem* **271**:22169, 1996
80. Ochi H et al: IL-4 and -5 prime human mast cells for different profiles of IgE-dependent cytokine production. *Proc Natl Acad Sci USA* **97**:10509, 2000
81. Gordon JR, Galli SJ: Release of both preformed and newly synthesized tumor necrosis factor alpha (TNF-α)/cachectin by mouse mast cells stimulated via the FcεRI: A mechanism for the sustained action of mast cell-derived TNF-α during IgE-dependent biological responses. *J Exp Med* **174**:103, 1991
82. Malaviya R et al: The mast cell tumor necrosis factor alpha response to FimH-expressing *Escherichia coli* is mediated by the glycosylphosphatidylinositol-anchored molecule CD48. *Proc Natl Acad Sci USA* **96**:8110, 1999
83. Supajatura V et al: Protective roles of mast cells against enterobacterial infection are mediated by toll-like receptor 4. *J Immunol* **167**:2250, 2001

84. Echtenacher B et al: Critical protective role of mast cells in a model of acute septic peritonitis. *Nature* **381**:75,1996
85. Malaviya R et al: Role of Janus kinase 3 in mast cell-mediated innate immunity against gram-negative bacteria. *Immunity* **18**:313, 2001
86. Klein LM et al: Degranulation of human mast cells induces an endothelial antigen central to leukocyte adhesion. *Proc Natl Acad Sci USA* **86**:8972, 1989
87. Qu Z et al: Mast cells are a major source of basic fibroblast growth factor in chronic inflammation and cutaneous hemangioma. *Am J Pathol* **1147**:564, 1995
88. Gordon JR, Galli SJ: Promotion of mouse fibroblast collagen gene expression by mast cells stimulated via the FcεRI: Role for mast cell-derived transforming growth factor β and tumor necrosis factor α. *J Exp Med* **180**:2027, 1994
89. Leon A et al: Mast cells synthesize, store, and release nerve growth factor. *Proc Natl Acad Sci USA* **91**:3739, 1994
90. Burd PR et al: Interleukin 3-dependent and -independent mast cells stimulated with IgE and antigen express multiple cytokines. *J Exp Med* **170**:245, 1989

CHAPTER 33

Irma Gigli

Human Complement System

The complement system consists of a group of plasma and cell membrane proteins that mediate a number of biologic reactions. Investigations in humans and the development of experimental disease models have demonstrated the participation of complement in inflammation, tissue injury, hemostasis, and antigen-specific immune responsiveness. These diversified tasks are achieved either by complement components alone or by their interaction with other plasma proteins or specific cell membrane receptors (complement receptors).

The components of the classical pathway and the membrane attack sequence are named by the letter C followed by a number: C1, C4, C2, C3, C5, C6, C7, C8, and C9. Some of the earlier components were named before their position in the sequence was known, thus leading to the apparent inconsistency in their order in the nomenclature. C1 consists of three distinct subcomponents, designated C1q, C1r, and C1s. The activation components of the mannan-binding lectin (MBL) pathway are designated by capital letters representing the initials of the proteins involved: MBL and mannan-associated serine proteases (MASPs). The proteins of the alternative pathway are designated by capital letters: B, D, P, H, and I. C3 is an essential protein of all pathways. Because it was originally recognized as a component of the classical pathway, the original nomenclature is retained. Activation fragments and fragments resulting from regulatory cleavage of a component are denoted by lowercase letters, as in C3a, C3b, C3c, C3dg, and C3d; the letter i signifies an inactive product of a component, as in iC3b.[1] Receptors for fragments of complement proteins (CR) are named after their ligand or indicated by an arabic number: CR for C3b/C4b = CR1; CR for C3dg = CR2; and CR for iC3b = CR3.

The activation of the complement system is organized in three pathways (classical, mannan-binding lectin, and alternative) and in a final common event, the assembly of the membrane attack complex (MAC). Activation is controlled by a number of plasma and cell membrane proteins. Complement activation results in the development of active enzymes from their precursors in a series of limited proteolytic processes, in which the product of one reaction is the catalyst for the next. The terminal components in the sequence form a nonenzymatic, self-associating multimolecular complex that binds firmly to target membranes by means of hydrophobic interactions with the membrane lipid bilayer. Extensive structural information that is now available through the cloning and sequencing of DNA coding for complement proteins and receptors reveals homologies among a number of proteins in the system.[2] This information, together with studies on the chromosomal localization of the genes, provides evidence of genetic linkage among complement and noncomplement genes. Polymorphic variants for most complement proteins have been described, a number of which are of clinical relevance.[2]

BIOCHEMISTRY OF THE PROTEINS OF THE COMPLEMENT SYSTEM AND ACTIVATION MECHANISMS

Central to the functions of the complement system is the activation of the third component, C3. This protein is activated by two enzymes termed *C3 convertases,* which are generated during complement activation (Fig. 33-1). Complement activation can be triggered by antigen–antibody complexes (classical pathway) and by bacterial, viral, and surface carbohydrates (MBL pathway), but C3 also has the capability for direct recognition of foreign materials (alternative pathway). The latter two forms of complement activation represent a primitive antibody-independent immune system (native immunity).

Activation of the Classical Pathway (Table 33-1, Fig. 33-1)

The activation of the classical pathway is initiated primarily by antibody complexed with an antigen, which may be a cell surface constituent or a soluble protein.[1] Activation can also be initiated in the absence of antibody by certain oligosaccharides, porins from gram-negative bacteria, ligand-bound C-reactive protein, and a variety of charged substances. Photoactive substances, double-stranded DNA, some oncoviruses, and products of tissue damage, such as mitochondrial cardiolipin, mitochondrial proteins, and nucleic acid, may also activate the classical pathway. These mechanisms of activation most likely differ from that afforded by antigen–antibody complexes and may involve the MBL pathway.[3]

Aggregation of IgG or IgM molecules, either specifically by interaction with an antigen or nonspecifically by heat or by chemical cross-linking, is necessary for the binding and activation of the recognition unit of the classical pathway, C1.[4] At least two IgG molecules are required for C1 activation, whereas only one IgM molecule bound to two or more antigenic sites is sufficient. C1 is a Ca^{2+}-dependent molecular complex composed of three distinct proteins, C1q, C1r, and C1s.[5] C1 reacts with antigen–antibody complexes, and probably with other activators, through the C1q subunit. C1q has an unusual amino acid composition; it contains glycine, hydroxyproline, and hydroxylysine residues, with glycosylgalactosyl residues coupled to them.[6] This composition indicates the presence of a collagen-like structure. C1q is visualized by electron microscopy as a molecule consisting of six peripheral globular units joined by connective strands to a common central fibril-like portion. The globular segments are, in fact, the binding sites for the Fc portion of IgG[7] or for the constant domain of IgM.[8] IgG3 binds C1q most efficiently, followed by IgG1 and IgG2, whereas in most cases, IgG4 does not bind C1q. On binding to the antigen–antibody complexes, C1q is thought to produce an allosteric change in the proenzyme C1r that triggers its autocatalytic activation.[9] Activated C1r hydrolyzes a single peptide bond in precursor C1s and generates a serine esterase active site, activated C1s. C1r and C1s are very similar in size, and the amino acid sequence of the active site has considerable homology with other

FIGURE 33-1

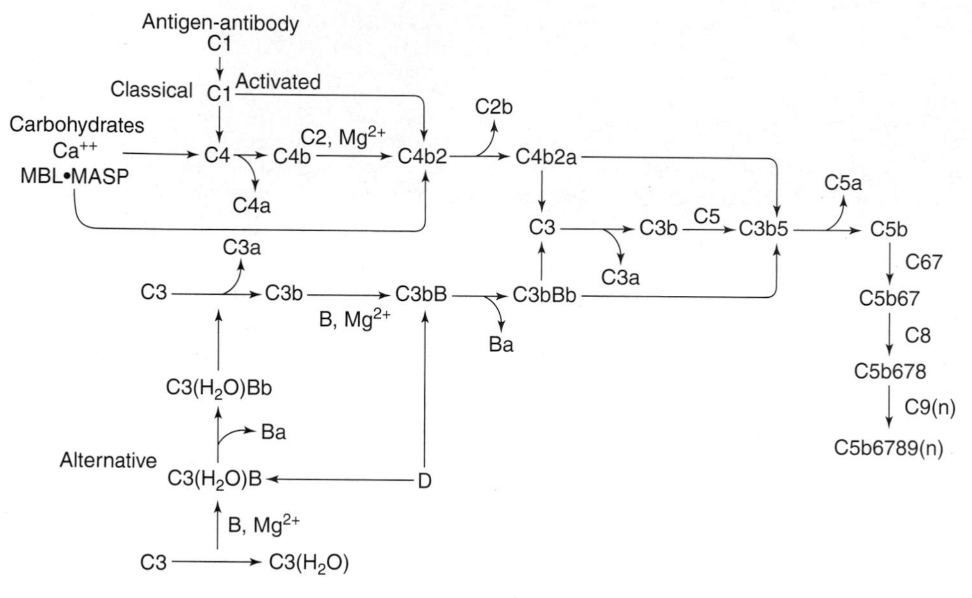

Activation of the classical, mannan-binding lectin (MBL), and alternative pathways, and formation of the membrane attack complex.

TABLE 33-1

Proteins of the Classical and the Mannan-Binding Lectin Pathways

	Molecular Mass (kDa)	Subunit Structure Chains (kDa)	Chromosome Localization	Serum Concentration (μg/mL)
Activation				
C1q	460	A (26 kDa × 6) B (26 kDa × 6) C (24 kDa × 6)	1	80
C1r	83	Single	12	50
C1s	83	Single	12	50
Mannan-binding lectin	~600	Multimer of 32	10	10
Serine proteases:				
MASP1 and 2	85	Single	?	?
C4	209	α (97 kDa) β (75 kDa) γ (35 kDa)	6	600
C2	102	Single	6	30
C3	185	α (110 kDa) β (75 kDa)	19	1400
Regulation				
Plasma				
C1INH	110	Single	11	180
C4bp	500	8 (70 kDa) α subunits β subunit	1	250
Factor I	80	α (50 kDa), β (38 kDa)	4	35
Cell membrane				
CR1/CD35	160–250	Single	1	
DAF/CD55	70	Single	1	

NOTE: DAF, decay accelerating factor; MCP, membrane cofactor protein.

serine esterases, yet their substrate specificity is quite distinct.[9] The only natural substrate of C1r is precursor C1s, whereas C1s will hydrolyze bonds only in the next two components in the sequence, C4 and C2.[1]

C4 is a highly polymorphic protein composed of three disulfide-linked polypeptide chains: α, β, and γ. C4 is synthesized as a single-chain precursor and is posttranslationally cleaved into its three chains.[10] The amino acid sequence of the α chain shows homology with the sequence of C3 and C5, suggesting that these three proteins may have originated by gene duplication.[11]

During complement activation, C1s cleaves the α chain of C4 at the N terminus, releasing C4a, a 9-kDa peptide.[11] C4a is one of three complement-derived peptides with anaphylatoxin activity. The larger fragment, C4b, has a transiently active binding site, provided by an internal thioester.[12] It can react with hydroxyl or amino groups in immune complexes or membranes, resulting in the stable binding of C4b to them. Although most activated C4 molecules remain free in the fluid phase and quickly become inactive (iC4b), the high serum concentration of C4 enables a single C1s molecule to deposit a large number of C4b molecules at the site of an antigen–antibody complex. The cleavage of C4 exposes an acceptor site in the resulting C4b molecule that permits, in the presence of Mg^{2+}, the reversible binding of C2.[13] C2 is a single-chain molecule that is cleaved by C1s to generate the fragments C2a and C2b. C2a (73 kDa) remains attached to C4b in a thermolabile protein-protein enzymatic complex, C4b2a, the classical pathway C3 convertase.[1] C2a contains the catalytic site and activates C3 and C5. The smaller fragment, C2b (34 kDa), is released into the fluid phase, and it has been reported to develop kinin-like activity if cleaved by plasmin.[14]

C3 is a glycoprotein; it is also synthesized as a single-chain precursor and is posttranslationally cleaved into two covalently bonded chains, α and β.[15] C3 is the complement protein present in the highest concentration in plasma and is essential for the classical, MBL, and alternative pathways. The catalytic site within the C4b2a complex hydrolyzes a single peptide bond from the N terminus of the α chain of C3 to generate two fragments, C3a and C3b.[1] The C3a peptide (9 kDa), containing the 77 N-terminal amino acids, is a potent anaphylatoxin.[16] The major fragment, C3b, like C4b, is transiently capable of forming a stable linkage with immune complexes and cell surfaces through an internal thiol ester within the α chain.[12] If an appropriate binding site is not available, the C3b is inactivated in the fluid phase (iC3b).

Activation of the Mannan-Binding Lectin Pathway (Table 33-1, Fig. 33-1)

An antibody- and C1-independent pathway leading to the assembly of the classical C3 convertase, C4b2a, was recently discovered.[3] This pathway uses MBL and calcium to recognize bacterial, viral, and fungal pathogens expressing terminal mannose or *N*-acetylglucosamine on their surfaces. MBL is structurally similar to C1q, consisting of four to six C-lectin domains connected to a central region by triple-helical collagen stems.[17] MBL circulates in blood in a complex with zymogen forms of serine proteases called MASPs, which have modular structures identical to C1r and C1s. Thus, the MBL–MASPs complex is structurally similar to the C1 complex (C1q, C1r, C1s). Binding of MBL to carbohydrate structures on pathogens results in activation of the single-chain zymogen MASP to an active two-chain serine protease, which, in turn, sequentially cleaves C4 and C2, resulting in the formation of pathogen-bound C3 convertase C4bC2a. In addition, human MBL is able to substitute for C1q and interact directly with C1r, and C1s to activate the classical pathway. A potential link between the specific immune response and native immunity has been suggested following the observation that agalactosyl immunoglobulins (Ig-GO) complex with MBL and bind C1r and C1s so that complement activation proceeds. Thus, MBL may be viewed as a molecule of the innate immune system with pluripotent activities.[17]

Activation of the Alternative Pathway

(Table 33-2, Fig. 33-1)

The alternative pathway of complement activation endows the host with a natural humoral defense mechanism against infections.[18] Although antigen–antibody complexes are capable of initiating the alternative pathway,[19] more often activation occurs independent of immunoglobulins. The lack of a requirement for antibodies or the early components of the classical pathway is readily demonstrable with sera from individuals congenitally deficient in gamma globulins or in C4 and C2. The alternative pathway may be activated by bacteria, virus-infected cells, certain viruses, some lymphoblastoid cell lines, and abnormal erythrocytes. The plasma proteins involved in the alternative pathway are C3, factor B, factor D, and the regulatory protein properdin (P). Proteolytic generation of C3b from native C3 is necessary for the alternative pathway to function, and the central enzyme of the pathway that cleaves C3 contains C3b as an essential component.[20] This initial step includes $C3(H_2O)$, a nonenzymatic event that results from the spontaneous hydrolysis of an internal thioester in the C3 molecule upon interaction with H_2O.[21] This C3, modified only at the thioester site, binds factor B in a Mg^{2+}-dependent reaction $[C3(H_2O)B]$ and allows its cleavage by the serine protease factor D.[22] Factor D is present in plasma in active form but cleaves factor B only when it is bound to $C3(H_2O)$ or C3b. In this process, a 33-kDa fragment, Ba, is released, while the major fragment, Bb, remains associated with $C3(H_2O)$ to form $C3(H_2O)Bb$.[21] This is the initial C3 convertase; the catalytic site is located in the Bb

TABLE 33-2

Proteins of the Alternative Pathway

	Molecular Mass (kDa)	Subunit Structure Chains (kDa)	Chromosome Localization	Serum Concentration (μg/mL)
Activation				
C3	185	α (110 kDa) β (75 kDa)	19	1400
Factor B	90	Single	6	210
Factor D	25	Single	9?	2
Regulation				
Plasma				
Properdin	225	4 (55-kDa) subunits	X	26
Factor H	150	Single	1	450
Factor I	80	α (50 kDa), β (38 kDa)	4	35
Cell membrane				
CR1	160–250	Single	1	
DAF	70	Single	1	
MCP	45–70	Single	1	

NOTE: DAF, decay accelerating factor; MCP, membrane cofactor protein.

TABLE 33-3

Proteins of the Membrane Attack Complex

	Molecular Mass (kDa)	Subunit Structure Chains (kDa)	Chromosome Localization	Serum Concentration (μg/mL)
Formation				
C5	190	α (115 kDa) β (74 kDa)	9	70
C6	120	Single	5	65
C7	110	Single	5	55
C8	150	α (64 kDa) β (64 kDa) γ (22 kDa)	1 1 9	55
C9	69	Single	5	60
Regulation				
Plasma				
S-protein (vitronectin)	83	Single	17	500
Cell membrane				
CD59/HRF20	20	Single	11	

subunit, and it hydrolyzes additional C3 molecules at the same site as does C4b2a. Once formed, C3b either is inactivated by regulatory proteins or initiates amplified C3b deposition by forming the alternative pathway C3 convertase (C3bBb). This enzyme amplifies the cleavage of C3 and the deposition of newly generated C3b.[21–23] The C3b-dependent positive feedback is a unique feature of the alternative pathway.

Assembly of the Membrane Attack Complex

(Table 33-3, Fig. 33-1)

The classical and MBL pathway C3 convertase C4b2a, as well as the alternative pathway convertase C3bBb, can function in the cleavage of the next component, C5, provided that additional C3b molecules are available in close proximity.[24] The role of C3b is to transiently bind C5[25] and modify its conformation so that a peptide bond may be cleaved from the N terminus of the α chain to generate C5a and C5b. C5a is released into the fluid phase and functions as the most potent complement-derived anaphylatoxin.[26] The larger fragment, C5b, becomes, without further enzymatic cleavage, the focal point for the assembly of MAC. C5b is composed of the rest of the α chain and the β chain that expresses labile binding sites. One site allows the transient association of C5b with membranes, and a second interacts with C6. C5b6 reacts with the next component, C7, to form a trimolecular complex, C5b67. The binding site in the nascent C5b67 differs from the binding site on C3b in that C5b, despite structural homologies with C3 and C4, lacks the internal thiolester.[12] The complex does not bind to membranes covalently; rather, it attaches firmly to the lipid moiety through hydrophobic groups exposed on the surface of C7.[27] C5b67 interacts with C8, which penetrates the lipid portion of the cell membrane and induces the polymerization of multiple C9 molecules.[28] Polymerized C9 leads to the insertion of MAC into membranes and the formation of transmembrane channels that allow water, ions, and small molecules to enter the cell, thereby causing cell swelling and lysis. Nucleated cells are more resistant to lysis because ion pumps counteract the influx of ions and water through the channel and limit cell swelling. In addition, an active recovery process takes place by removal of MAC from the cell membrane by either endocytosis or exocytosis.[28] Nucleated cells can recover from limited complement damage, but their function may be altered (Table 33-4).

REGULATION MECHANISMS OF COMPLEMENT ACTIVATION AND FUNCTION

The activation process and functions of the complement system are strictly regulated by plasma proteins that prevent spontaneous or abnormal activation in the fluid phase, by plasma proteins that downregulate or upregulate normal activation against target substances, and by membrane proteins that protect host cells from the lytic action of complement.

Regulation of the Classical and the MBL Pathways (Fig. 33-2)

The classical pathway convertase is readily activated in serum by immune complexes, but little activation takes place in their absence. Although C1 may autoactivate by an intramolecular mechanism, autoactivation is controlled by the inhibitor of the first component of complement (C1INH).[29] C1INH prevents the proteolysis of C1r and C1s by interacting with a form of C1 that is in a transitional state, conformationally distinct from native C1 but not yet activated. C1INH also inhibits the enzymatic activities of C1r and C1s by covalently binding to the catalytic site of these proteins, dissociating them from C1q and preventing the cleavage of C4 and C2. Immune complexes activate C1 in serum because the activation rate of the enzyme is faster than its inactivation by C1INH. The interaction of C1INH with C1 has physiologic relevance that is not limited to the regulation of the classical pathway. At the cellular level, the binding site on C1q for the C1q receptor on peripheral blood leukocytes and monocytes becomes available only after C1 interacts with C1INH.[4] Similar to its action on C1r and C1s, the C1INH inhibits activated MASP.[17] Thus, the C1INH may regulate the activation of the MBL pathway in a manner similar to the classical pathway. In addition to its action on C1, C1INH is a point of convergence of the complement system with the clotting and kinin-forming systems, two other effector systems of the inflammatory process[30,31] (see Chap. 117).

The assembly and function of the C3 convertase generated by the classical and MBL pathways are regulated by the inherent instability of the C4b2a enzyme at 37°C (98.6°F) and by two plasma proteins: C4b-binding protein (C4bp), and the enzyme C4b/C3b inactivator (factor I), for which C4bp is a cofactor.[32] C4bp is a multivalent protein that can

TABLE 33-4

Nonlytic Effects of C5b-9 on Human Cells

Cell	Biologic Effects
Neutrophil	Reactive oxygen metabolites and LTB_4 production Vesiculation
Platelet	Prothrombinase activation Vesiculation TXB_2 production
Monocyte–macrophage	Reactive oxygen metabolites, PGE_2, and TXB_2 production
Synovial cells	Reactive oxygen metabolites and PGE_2 production

Note: LT, leukotriene; PG, prostaglandin; TX, thromboxane.

FIGURE 33-2

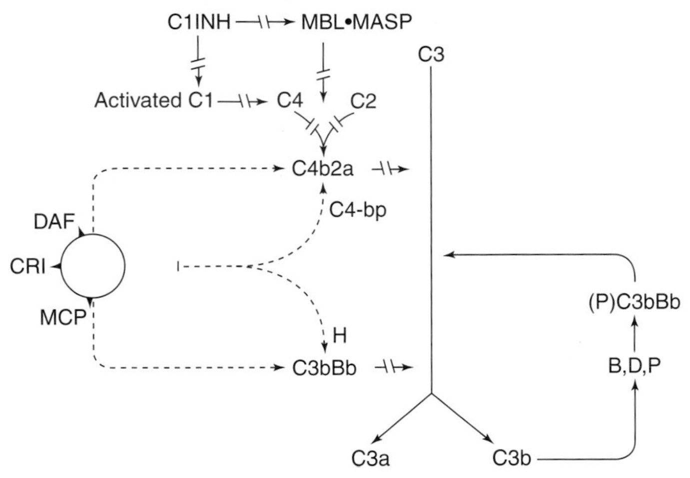

C1INH —⊣⊢→ MBL•MASP

C3

Activated C1 —⊣⊢→ C4 C2

C4b2a ⊣⊢

C4-bp

DAF

CRI

MCP

I

H

C3bBb ⊣⊢

(P)C3bBb

B,D,P

C3a C3b

Regulation of the classical, mannan-binding lectin (MBL), and alternative pathways by plasma and cell membrane proteins. CR1, C3b receptor; DAF, decay accelerating factor; MCP, membrane cofactor protein.

bind to a number of C4b molecules. This interaction mediates three functional changes: (1) it accelerates the dissociation of C2a from the C4b2a enzyme; (2) it prevents the uptake of C2 by C4b; and (3) it facilitates the proteolytic cleavage of C4b by factor I.[33] Factor I cleaves two peptide bonds from the α' chain of C4b, thereby generating three fragments. One fragment, C4d, remains attached to the activating particle; the other two fragments, α_3 and α_4, remain covalently bonded to the β chain, forming C4c, and no longer participate in the activation of the system. Complement activation on cell membranes is controlled by three membrane proteins that act in a similar way to C4bp. The decay accelerating factor (DAF)[34] prevents the binding of C2 to C4b and dissociates the C4b2a complex once it is formed. The C3b receptor (CR1) and the membrane cofactor protein (MCP) also have cofactor activity for factor I.[35]

The fluid phase and membrane cofactor proteins (C4bp, factor H, CR1, DAF, and MCP) share structural features. Each is constructed from a limited number of structural domains with highly conserved cysteine residues (short consensus repeats) present in multiple copies in the molecules.[36]

Regulation of the Alternative Pathway (Fig. 33-2)

The effectiveness of regulatory proteins to either limit or amplify the deposition of C3b-9 molecules on activating substances discriminates between nonactivators and activators of the alternative pathway.[23,37] The presence or absence of sialic acid on the activating surface seems to determine the accessibility of the deposited C3b to plasma regulatory proteins.[38] Substances poor in sialic acid favor activation, whereas those rich in sialic acid do not. Some of the proteins that regulate C4b2a also regulate the alternative pathway. The C3b/C4b inactivator (factor I), CR1, MCP, and DAF are common to both the classical and the alternative pathways, whereas factors H and P function exclusively in the regulation of the alternative pathway (Tables 33-1 and 33-2). Factor H accelerates the temperature-dependent dissociation of Bb from the C3bBb complex,[39] prevents the uptake of factor B by C3b, and impairs the formation of the amplification convertase. It also promotes the cleavage of the α' chain of C3b by factor I. This process results in the generation of an inactive form of the protein (iC3b) that consists of 43- and 68-kDa fragments linked to the intact β chain (Fig. 33-2). The cell membrane proteins CR1, MCP, and DAF have a function similar to that of factor H. They prevent amplification of C3b deposition by accelerating the decay of Bb from the C3bBb complex; however, only CR1 and MCP serve as cofactors for factor I. CR1 is the only cofactor molecule that catalyzes further cleavage of the 68-kDa fragment to generate C3dg and C3c.[40] In contrast to these proteins that downregulate the formation of C3bBb, P upregulates its function. P is recruited from plasma; it binds to C3bBb (C3bBbP), retarding both the temperature- and factor H-dependent dissociation of Bb.[21,37]

Regulation of the Membrane Attack Complex

(Table 33-3)

The final step in the activation of the complement system, the assembly of the C5b-9 complex (MAC), is also strictly regulated, resulting in the protection of cells from lysis. The formation and function of MAC may be prevented by several plasma inhibitors, the most important being the adhesive molecule vitronectin (S-protein). This acidic glycoprotein binds to C5b67 at a site that prevents the formation of a stable, membrane-bound C5b67 complex and polymerization of C9.[41] Binding of nascent C5b67 to membranes is also inhibited nonspecifically by plasma lipoproteins.

A glycolipid-anchored membrane protein has been described that is presumably responsible for protecting the cells of the host from lysis when complement activation takes place (Table 33-3). This ~20-kDa[42,43] protein has been assigned different names—membrane inhibitory protein (MIP), MACIF, HRF 20, and CD59. It acts by binding to C8 and C9 on the cell membrane, successfully preventing C9 polymerization and channel formation.

BIOLOGIC ACTIVITY OF THE PRODUCTS OF COMPLEMENT ACTIVATION

The biologic significance of the complement system is not limited to the completion of the reaction sequence and the role it plays in the death of affected cells. Perhaps of greater importance are the various other biologic effects that are mediated by three kinds of products of complement activation, namely, antigen-bound components, inactive fluid-phase intermediates, and enzyme-cleaved peptides that may serve as ligands to specific receptors on a variety of cells.

Biologic Effects of Complement Activation on Target Particles

EARLY COMPLEMENT COMPONENTS IN VIRUS NEUTRALIZATION[44] The biologic activities that result from the binding and subsequent activation of C1, C4, and C2 are relatively unknown. In vitro C1 and C4 enhance the capacity of specific IgM antibodies to neutralize herpes simplex virus.[45] The neutralization of vesicular stomatitis virus by normal human serum involves the components of the classical pathway through C3 and a nonimmunoglobulin serum factor. The reaction is initiated by the direct attachment of C1 to the external glycoprotein of the virus, which leads to the deposition of complement components on the viral envelope. Complement-mediated neutralization of influenza[46] and Epstein-Barr viruses (EBV)[47] by low levels of specific or cross-reacting antibodies together with C1, C4, C2, and C3, but not with late-acting components, has also been observed. The viruses that cause Newcastle disease and vaccinia are similarly neutralized. These studies indicate that virus neutralization generally requires activation of the classical pathway only through the C3 step. Enveloped viruses are also susceptible to complement-dependent lysis that leads to irreversible loss of viral activity.[48]

COMPLEMENT RECEPTORS AND VIRAL INFECTIONS Some complement receptors serve as fusion proteins for certain viruses. The surface glycoprotein gp 57/67, known to participate in the binding of measles virus to host cells, has been identified as the complement regulatory protein MCP/CD46.[49,50] A second complement receptor involved in the infection of B lymphocytes by EBV is the CR2 receptor. The binding of CR2 to EBV allows the virus to penetrate and infect B lymphocytes.[51,52] Complement also appears to participate in all stages of the HIV life cycle. The mechanism of entry of the virus into the cell, the activation of proviral DNA through signaling via complement receptors, viral budding, and extracellular survival of the virus all involve complement products.[53]

C3B-MEDIATED SOLUBILIZATION OF IMMUNE COMPLEXES In vitro the interaction of antibodies and antigen at high concentrations results in the formation of large aggregates that precipitate. In vivo this precipitation is inhibited by complement proteins, thereby preventing the deposition of insoluble complexes in tissue.[54,55] The binding of C3b to the immune complexes interferes with lattice formation, limits aggregation, and renders the immune complexes more soluble. Although activation of the classical pathway alone may suffice, optimal solubilization of immune aggregates requires participation of both the classical and the alternative pathways. The significance of these processes in disease pathogenesis is demonstrated by the high incidence of immune complex-mediated diseases in patients deficient in C3, C1, C4, or C2.[56]

MEMBRANE ATTACK COMPLEX IN CELL ACTIVATION The terminal complex C5b-9 has been regarded as the lytic event in complement activation. However, the assembly of MAC on the membranes of nucleated cells that are resistant to lysis by homologous complement may result in cell stimulation and the release of proinflammatory molecules.[28] In vitro MAC induces the production and release of reactive oxygen metabolites, eicosanoids, enzymes, and other proinflammatory mediators (see Table 33-4).

Biologic Effects Mediated by the Interaction of Products of Complement Activation with Cell Membrane Receptors

Some of the most important biologic activities of complement known today stem from products of activation and degradation of C3 and C5. The interaction of complement fragments with cells bearing receptors for them may set off a variety of cellular reactions that depend on the cell types carrying the receptors (Table 33-5). At least three distinct reactions may be triggered by receptor–ligand interactions: phagocytosis of immune complexes bearing complement fragments, immune regulation and differentiation of cells, and changes in cellular metabolism.

PHAGOCYTOSIS AND CLEARANCE OF IMMUNE COMPLEXES The rate and amount of phagocytosis of antigen–antibody complexes containing IgG by neutrophils and macrophages are greatly augmented by the presence of C3b and iC3b.[56] This reaction is mediated by the presence of specialized receptors for C3b (CR1) and iC3b (CR3) on the membrane of phagocytic cells[57] (Table 33-5). CR1 has the widest distribution of all complement receptors, but more than 90 percent of CR1 in blood is expressed on erythrocytes. Immune complexes bearing C3b become bound to erythrocytes and are transported to the liver, where they are cleared by fixed macrophages.[58] The binding of immune complexes to erythrocytes is an active process; the C3b on the immune complexes attached to CR1 is cleaved by factor I, and the complex is released. The immune complex is gradually reduced in size and becomes more soluble. Thus, under physiologic conditions, complement and erythrocytes have a synergistic role to facilitate removal and prevent precipitation of immune complexes.

TABLE 33-5

Function and Localization of C3 Receptors

	CR1/CD35	CR2/CD21	CR3/CD11b-CD18
Ligand	C3b and C4b (iC3b)	C3d and C3dg	iC3b
Molecular mass (kDa)	190–250 (single chain)	140 (single chain)	260 (α chain 165) CD11b (β chain 95) CD18
Cell type	Erythrocytes Polymorphonuclear leukocytes Eosinophils Monocytes Macrophages B lymphocytes T lymphocytes Langerhans cells Keratinocytes	B lymphocytes NK cells Follicular dendritic cells Keratinocytes	Polymorphonuclear leukocytes Monocytes/macrophages NK cells Cytotoxic T cells
Function	Regulation of complement activation: acts as cofactor of factor I in the cleavage of bound C3b and C4b Processing of immune complexes: erythrocyte CR1 binds immune complexes bearing C3b and carries them to the liver, where they are apparently cleared by local macrophages Enhancement of phagocytosis and ADCC Enhancement of antibody-independent cellular response	Enhancement of ADCC Binds EBV Cell growth stimulation Antibody response (T cell-dependent)	Enhancement of ADCC through cell–target interaction Enhancement of phagocytosis

NOTE: ADCC, antibody-dependent cellular cytotoxicity; EBV, Epstein-Barr virus; NK, natural killer.

CR3 is present, among other cells, on neutrophils, macrophages, dendritic cells, and lymphocytes involved in antibody-dependent cell cytotoxicity. The primary ligand for CR3 is iC3b.[59] CR3 is composed of two chains, α (CD11b) and β (CD18); the β chain is identical to the β chain of the leukocyte surface protein, leukocyte function-associated–1 antigen (CD11a/CD18).[60] The presence of CR3 on phagocytes is essential for normal clearance of foreign particles; individuals deficient in CR3 experience impaired phagocytosis and repeated bacterial infections.[60] A molecule similar in function to CR3 but distinct in the size of its chain has been named CR4.

COMPLEMENT RECEPTORS AND IMMUNE REGULATION

Cells bearing receptors for complement may carry immune complexes to specific sites where such cells accumulate. The concentration of complexes at such sites may explain the phenomenon of localization of particular antigens in B cell areas of lymphoid organs.[61] The finding that the complexes are released from C3b receptors as a result of the action of factor I, thus acquiring the ability to bind to C3d receptors (CR2),[62] supports the hypothesis that complexes containing C3d are transportable by cells having receptors for them.[63] B lymphocytes, follicular dendritic cells, and natural killer cells express CR2.[64,65] CR2 binds C3dg and C3d as well as the Epstein-Barr virus (EBV), but the EBV-binding site is distinct from the C3 fragment-binding site.[51,52]

Several lines of evidence support the view that the interaction of complement fragments and complement receptors plays a role in the control of antigen-specific immune responsiveness. Animals depleted of complement may be immunocompromised. It has been suggested that the binding of C3b and C3d triggers the proliferation of B lymphocytes.[66] The production of C3b and C3d in serum may account, in the absence of T lymphocytes, for the activation of B lymphocytes with thymus-dependent antigens.[67,68] Complement may also play a role in maintaining immunologic memory. Thymectomized, C3-depleted animals do not produce memory B cells, whereas thymectomized animals with an intact complement system do. Moreover, animals that are depleted of C3 or are genetically deficient in C3 or CR2 do not exhibit a secondary immune response.[63,68–70] The evidence obtained from animal models has not yet been related to humans.

Anaphylatoxins (Table 33-6)

Among the peptides generated by enzyme cleavage during the activation of the complement system are the three anaphylatoxins, C4a, C3a, and C5a (Table 33-6).[26,71] They cause release of histamine from mast cells, degranulation of basophils, contraction of guinea pig ileum in vitro with tachyphylaxis, and a local increase in vascular permeability when injected intracutaneously in humans and guinea pigs. C3a also induces 5-hydroxytryptamine release from platelets and thromboxane release from macrophages, and it mediates the directed chemotaxis of eosinophils but not neutrophils. The injection of C3a and C5a into human skin results in erythema, edema, and pruritus; pretreatment with antihistamines abolishes the reaction to C3a.[72] The significance of C4a in vivo is not clear. The action of the anaphylatoxins C3a and C5a is attributed to their ability to bind to specific G protein-coupled seven transmembrane receptors on a variety of cells.[26,73,74] Most of the chemotactic activity in serum induced by immune complexes, endotoxins, and bacterial products may be ascribed to C5a and C5a des-arg. Moreover, the injection of highly purified C5a into the skin of laboratory animals results in massive accumulation of polymorphonuclear leukocytes followed by the accumulation of macrophages. In vitro C5a is chemotactic for monocytes, macrophages, and eosinophils, as well as for polymorphonuclear leukocytes, and produces neutrophil adhesiveness. It also stimulates neutrophil oxidative metabolism and the production of toxic oxygen species. It induces the release of lysosomal enzymes from a variety of phagocytic cells, the secretion of IL-1, IL-6, IL-8 from macrophages, and the secretion of platelet-activating factor from numerous cell types. The biologic functions of the three anaphylatoxins are modulated by the carboxypeptidase N in serum.[75] This protein cleaves the C-terminal arginine residue (des-arg) of all three anaphylatoxins. C3a and C4a become inactive. C5a des-arg loses its spasmogenic activity, but it retains chemotactic and other neutrophil-stimulating effects at a reduced potency. Evidence for the biologic significance of anaphylatoxins in inflammatory processes has centered on neutrophil adhesiveness and degranulation. In disease processes,

TABLE 33-6

Function of Anaphylatoxins in Human Tissue

	C3a	C5a*†
Mast cells	Secretion of vasoactive amines	Secretion of vasoactive amines Production of leukotrienes Downregulation of adenylate cyclase
Monocytes/macrophages	Secretion of IL-1 Production of prostaglandins	Chemotaxis Production of leukotrienes Enhancement of immune response Secretion of IL-1, IL-6, IL 8
Lymphocytes	Impairment of antibody production	Enhancement of specific primary humoral response
Polymorphonuclear leukocytes	Enzyme release	Chemotaxis Stimulation of cellular metabolism Aggregation
Eosinophils	Chemotaxis ECP release	Chemotaxis ECP release
Smooth muscle	Contraction	Contraction
Skin	Erythema Edema	Erythema Edema
Blood vessels	Capillary permeability changes	Capillary permeability changes
Hepatocytes		Acute phase protein synthesis

*C5 des-arg activity 100 times lower than C5a.
†Receptor for C5a present in epithelial cells in a variety of tissues—neurons, microglia, and astrocytes—but functional significance is not known.
NOTE: ECP, eosinophil cationic protein; IL, interleukin.

anaphylatoxins have been identified as possible mediators in complications of hemodialysis and cardiopulmonary bypass procedures, pulmonary leukostasis, and other inflammatory processes involving blood vessels.

REFERENCES

1. Müller-Eberhard HJ: Molecular organization and function of the complement system. *Annu Rev Biochem* **57**:321, 1988
2. Crawford K, Alper CA. Genetics of the complement system. *Rev Immunogenet* **2**:323, 2000
3. Petersen SV et al: The mannan-binding lectin pathway of complement activation: biology and disease association. *Mol Immunol* **38**:133, 2001
4. Hughes-Jones N: The classical pathway, in *Immunobiology of the Complement System,* edited by GD Ross. New York, Academic Press, 1986, p 21
5. Gigli I et al: Preparation of the unactivated form of the first component of human complement, C1, and investigation of the mechanism of action. *Biochem J* **157**:541, 1976
6. Reid KBM: A collagen-like amino acid sequence in a polypeptide chain of human C1q (subcomponent of the first component of complement). *Biochem J* **141**:189, 1974
7. Burton DR et al: C1q receptor site on immunoglobulin G. *Nature* **288**:338, 1980
8. Wright JF et al: C1 binding by murine IgM. The effect of a Pro-to-Ser exchange at residue 436 of the μ chain. *J Biol Chem* **263**:11221, 1988
9. Arlaud GJ et al: Purified proenzyme C1r. Some characteristics of its activation and subsequent proteolytic cleavage. *Biochim Biophys Acta* **616**:116, 1980
10. Gigli I et al: The isolation and structure of C4, the fourth component of human complement. *Biochem J* **165**:439, 1977
11. Gorski JP et al: C4a: The third anaphylatoxin of the human complement system. *Proc Natl Acad Sci U S A* **76**:5299, 1979
12. Tack BF: The β-Cys-γ-Glu thiol ester bond in human C3, C4, and α_2-macroglobulin. *Springer Semin Immunopathol* **6**:259, 1983
13. Nagasawa S, Stroud RM: Cleavage of C2 by C1s into the antigenically distinct fragments C2a and C2. *Proc Natl Acad Sci U S A* **74**:2998, 1977
14. Strang CJ et al: Angioedema induced by a peptide derived from complement component C2. *J Exp Med* **168**:1685, 1988
15. Brade V et al: Biosynthesis of pro C3, a precursor of the third component of complement. *J Exp Med* **146**:759, 1977
16. Hugli TE: Structure and function of C3a anaphylatoxin. *Curr Topics Microbiol Immunol* **153**:181, 1990
17. Kawasaki T: Structure and biology of mannan-binding protein, MBP, an important component of innate immunity. *Biochim Biophys Acta* **1473**:186, 1999
18. Fearon DT, Austen KF: Current concepts in immunity. The alternative pathway—a system for host resistance to microbial infections. *N Engl J Med* **303**:259, 1980
19. Müller-Eberhard HJ, Schreiber RD: Molecular biology and chemistry of the alternative pathway of complement. *Adv Immunol* **29**:1, 1980
20. Müller-Eberhard HJ, Goetz O: C3 proactivator convertase and its mode of action. *J Exp Med* **135**:1003, 1972
21. Pangburn MK, Müller-Eberhard HJ: The alternative pathway of complement, in *Complement,* edited by HJ Müller-Eberhard, PA Miescher. Berlin, Springer, 1984, p 185
22. Fearon DT et al: Formation of a hemolytically active cellular intermediate by the interaction between properdin factors B and D and the activated third component of complement. *J Exp Med* **138**:1305, 1973
23. Schreiber RD et al: Initiation of the alternative pathway of complement: Recognition of activators by bound C3b and assembly of the entire pathway from six isolated proteins. *Proc Natl Acad Sci U S A* **75**:3948, 1978
24. Müller-Eberhard HJ: The membrane attack complex, in *Complement,* edited by HJ Müller-Eberhard, PA Miescher. Berlin, Springer, 1984, p 22
25. Isenman DE et al: The interaction of C5 with C3b in free solution: A sufficient condition for cleavage by fluid phase C3/C5 convertase. *J Immunol* **124**:326, 1980
26. Ember JA, Hugli TE. Complement factors and their receptors. *Immunopharmacology* **38**:3, 1997
27. Tschopp J et al: The membrane attack complex of complement: C5b-8 complex as C9 receptor and catalyst of C9 polymerization. *J Immunol* **134**:495, 1985
28. Morgan BP: Complement membrane attack on nucleated cells: Resistance, recovery and non-lethal effects. *Biochem J* **264**:1, 1989
29. Ziccardi RJ: The first component of human complement (C1): Activation and control, in *Complement,* edited by Müller-Eberhard, PA Miescher. Berlin, Springer-Verlag, 1985, p 167
30. Schreiber AD et al: Inhibition by C1INH of Hageman factor fragment activation of coagulation, fibrinolysis, and kinin generation. *J Clin Invest* **52**:1402, 1973
31. Gigli I et al: Interaction of plasma kallikrein with the C1 inhibitor. *J Immunol* **104**:574, 1970
32. Gigli I et al: Modulation of the classical pathway C3 convertase by the plasma proteins C4-binding protein and C3b inactivator. *Proc Natl Acad Sci U S A* **76**:6596, 1979
33. Fujita T et al: Human C4-binding protein. II. Role in proteolysis of C4b by C3b-inactivator. *J Exp Med* **148**:1044, 1979
34. Nicholson-Weller A et al: Isolation of a human erythrocyte membrane glycoprotein with decay-accelerating activity for C3 convertases of the complement system. *J Immunol* **129**:184, 1982
35. Liszewski MK et al: Control of the complement system. *Adv Immunol* **61**:201, 1996
36. Hourcade D et al: The regulators of complement activation (RCA) gene cluster. *Adv Immunol* **45**:381, 1989
37. Fearon DT, Austen KF: Activation of the alternative complement pathway due to resistance of zymosan-bound amplification convertase to endogenous regulatory mechanisms. *Proc Natl Acad Sci U S A* **74**:1683, 1977
38. Fearon DT: Relation by membrane sialic acid of β1H-dependent decay-dissociation of amplification C3 convertase of the alternative complement pathway. *Proc Natl Acad Sci U S A* **75**:1971, 1978
39. Pangburn MK et al: Complement C3 convertase: Cell surface restriction of β1H control and generation of restriction on neuraminidase-treated cells. *Proc Natl Acad Sci U S A* **75**:2416, 1978
40. Davis AE et al: Physiologic inactivation of fluid phase C3b: Isolation and structural analysis of C3c, C3dg (α2D) and C3g. *J Immunol* **132**:1960, 1984
41. Podack ER et al: Inhibition of C9 polymerization within SC5b-9 complex of complement by S protein. *Acta Pathol Microbiol Immunol Scand* **92**:89, 1984
42. Sugita Y et al: Molecular cloning and characterization of MACIF, an inhibitor of membrane channel formation of complement. *J Biochem* **106**:555, 1989
43. Okada N et al: A novel membrane glycoprotein capable of inhibiting membrane attack by homologous complement. *Int Immunol* **1**:205, 1989
44. Cooper NR, Nemerow GR: Complement, viruses and virus infected cells, in *Complement,* edited by HJ Müller-Eberhard, PA Miescher. Berlin, Springer, 1984, p 345
45. Daniels CA et al: Neutralization of sensitized virus by purified components of complement. *Proc Natl Acad Sci U S A* **65**:528, 1970
46. Beebe DP et al: Neutralization of influenza virus by normal human sera: Mechanisms involving antibody and complement. *J Immunol* **130**:1317, 1983
47. Nemerow GR et al: Neutralization of Epstein-Barr virus by nonimmune human serum: Role of cross-reacting antibody to herpes simplex virus and complement. *J Clin Invest* **70**:1081, 1982
48. Leddy JP et al: Effect of selective complement deficiency on the rate of neutralization of enveloped viruses by human sera. *J Immunol* **118**:28, 1977
49. Naniche D et al: Human membrane cofactor protein (CD46) acts as a cellular receptor for measles virus. *J Virol* **67**:6025, 1993
50. Manchester M et al: Multiple isoforms of CD46 (membrane cofactor protein) serve as receptors for measles virus. *Proc Natl Acad Sci U S A* **91**:2161, 1994
51. Nemerow GR et al: Identification and characterization of the Epstein-Barr virus receptor on human B lymphocytes and its relationship to the C3d complement receptor (CR2). *J Virol* **55**:347, 1985
52. Fingerroth JD: Epstein-Barr virus receptor of human B lymphocytes is C3d receptor CR2. *Proc Natl Acad Sci U S A* **81**:4510, 1984
53. Stoiber H et al: Role of complement in HIV infection. *Annu Rev Immunol* **15**:649, 1997
54. Schifferle JA, Paccaud JP: Complement and its receptor: A physiological transport system for circulating immune complexes, in *Contributions to Nephrology,* edited by G D'Amico et al. Basel, Karger, 1989, p 1
55. Miller GW, Nussenzweig V: A new complement function: Solubilization of antigen-antibody aggregates. *Proc Natl Acad Sci U S A* **72**:418, 1975
56. Ehlenberger AG, Nussenzweig V: The role of membrane receptors for C3b and C3d in phagocytosis. *J Exp Med* **145**:357, 1977
57. Ahearn JM, Fearon DT: Structure and function of the complement receptors, CR1 (CD35) and CR2 (CD21). *Adv Immunol* **46**:183, 1989
58. Shifferli JA et al: The role of complement and its receptor in the elimination of immune complexes. *N Engl J Med* **315**:488, 1986

59. Ross GD, Rabellino EM: Identification of a neutrophil and monocyte complement receptor (CR3) that is distinct from lymphocyte CR1 and CR2 and specific for a site contained with C3bi (abstr). *Fed Proc* **38**:1467, 1979
60. Arnaout MA et al: Deficiency of a granulocyte-membrane glycoprotein (gp150) in a boy with recurrent bacterial infections. *N Engl J Med* **306**:693, 1982
61. Bianco C et al: Follicular localization of antigen: Possible role of lymphocytes bearing a receptor for antigen-antibody complement complexes, in *Morphological and Functional Aspects of Immunity,* edited by K Lindahl-Kiessling et al. New York, Plenum, 1971, p 251
62. Ross GD et al: Two different complement receptors on human lymphocytes. One specific for C3b and one specific for C3b inactivator-cleaved C3b. *J Exp Med* **138**:798, 1973
63. Croix DA et al: Antibody response to a T-dependent antigen requires B cell expression of complement receptors. *J Exp Med* **183**:1857, 1996
64. Miller GW, Nussenzweig V: Complement as regulator of interactions between immune-complexes and cell membranes. *J Immunol* **113**:464, 1974
65. Wahlin B et al: C3 receptor on human lymphocyte subsets and recruitment of ADCC effector cells by C3 fragments. *J Immunol* **130**:2831, 1983
66. Meuth JL et al: Suppression of T lymphocyte functions by human C3 fragments. I. Inhibition of human T cell proliferative responses by kallikrein cleavage fragment of human iC3b. *J Immunol* **130**:2605, 1983
67. Fearon DT, Carroll MC. Regulation of B lymphocyte responses to foreign and self-antigens by CD19/CD21 complex. *Ann Rev Immunol* **18**:393, 2000
68. Hebell T et al: Suppression of the immune response by soluble complement receptor of B lymphocytes. *Science* **254**:102, 1991
69. Carroll MC: The role of complement in B cell activation and tolerance. *Adv Immunol* **74**:61, 2000
70. Fischer MB et al: Regulation of the B cell response to T-dependent antigens by classical pathway complement. *J Immunol* **157**:549, 1996
71. Bitter-Suermann D: The anaphylatoxins, in *The Complement System,* edited by K Rother, GO Till. Berlin, Springer, 1988, p 367
72. Wuepper KD et al: Cutaneous response to human C3a anaphylatoxin in man. *Clin Exp Immunol* **11**:13, 1972
73. Gerard C, Gerard NP: C5a anaphylatoxin and its seven transmembrane-segment receptor. *Annu Rev Immunol* 12:775, 1994
74. Drouin SM et al: Expression of the complement anaphylatoxin C3a and C5a receptors on bronchial epithelial and smooth muscle cells in models of sepsis and asthma. *J Immunol* **166**:2025, 2001
75. Bokisch VA, Müller-Eberhard HJ: Anaphylatoxin inactivator of human plasma: Its isolation and characterization as a carboxypeptidase. *J Clin Invest* **49**:2427, 1970

CHAPTER 34

Alice P. Pentland

Eicosanoids

Arachidonic acid and its metabolites, termed *eicosanoids,* are ubiquitous bioactive mediators formed from the unsaturated fatty acids present in cell membranes. Eicosanoids function as local hormones, regulating many important physiologic and pathologic processes such as pain, fever, clotting, and parturition.[1,2] Medications that alter their formation are readily available. Biochemically, they are formed by the addition of oxygen to polyunsaturated fatty acids such as arachidonic acid and linoleic acid, which leads to the formation of a large array of biologically active mediators. The fatty acid metabolism of arachidonic acid has been most thoroughly studied, because it is the most common substrate for cyclooxygenase, lipoxygenase, and monooxygenase enzymes. Studies of this class of compounds began in the 1930s with the discovery of prostaglandins.[3,4]

BIOCHEMISTRY

Eicosanoids have potent biologic effects in picomolar amounts. The extreme biologic potency of this class of compounds necessitates careful regulation of their synthesis and degradation. Arachidonic acid is stored in the phospholipids of cell membranes and is released by phospholipases after the specific stimulation of cell surface receptors.[1] In addition to carefully regulated release by receptor stimulation, arachidonic acid is released during membrane dissolution induced by cellular necrosis or apoptosis.[2,5] Once cleaved from the membrane, arachidonic acid is immediately oxygenated to form products that are released from the cell or are reesterified into membrane phospholipids. Because arachidonic acid metabolites are not stored, the synthesis of products of arachidonic acid is synonymous with their release.[1,2]

Eicosanoid synthesis has specific structural requirements. Eicosanoids are derived from the essential omega-6 fatty acids [eicosatetraenoic acid (20:4n-6) and eicosatrienoic acid (20:3n-9)] and their omega-3 derivatives, eicosapentaenoic acid (EPA, 20:5n-3) and docosahexaenoic acid (DHA, 22:6n-3). Among these fatty acids, arachidonic acid, also known as 5,8,11,14-eicosatetraenoic acid (20:4n-6), is the usual substrate for eicosanoid formation and is usually stored in the sn-2 position of phospholipid (Fig. 34-1). The essential role of eicosanoids in physiologic processes is believed to be the reason for the dietary requirement for omega-6 fatty acids. The terminology of the eicosanoids formed from omega-6 and omega-3 fatty acids is dictated by the number of double bonds present in the substrate fatty acid. For example, prostaglandin (PG) E_2 is derived from arachidonic acid and has two double bonds remaining in its side chain, whereas PGE_1 is derived from linoleic acid and has only one double bond remaining.

A specific location of double bonds in the *cis* configuration is required for synthesis of eicosanoid products from fatty acid precursors. The usual location of double bonds in arachidonic acid is shown in Fig. 34-1. Folding of the arachidonic acid molecule to form a prostaglandin requires these specific areas of desaturation to allow the final molecular conformation.

FIGURE 34-1

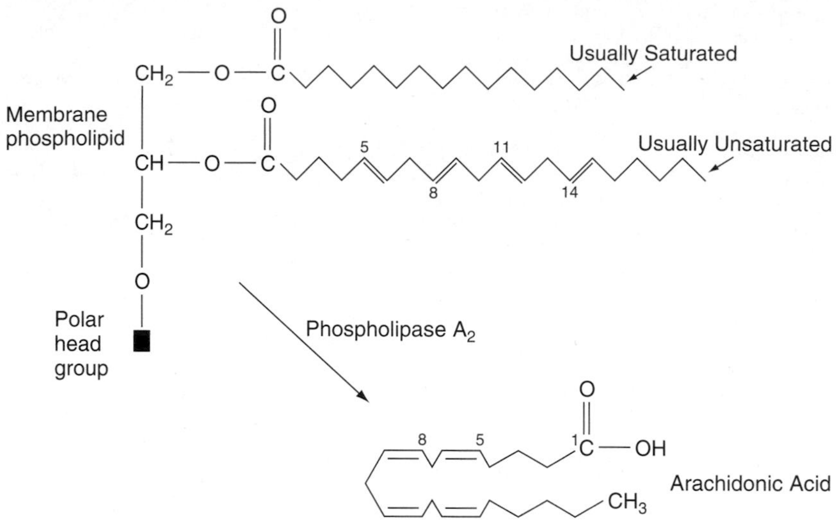

Membrane phospholipid

Usually Saturated

Usually Unsaturated

Polar head group

Phospholipase A_2

Arachidonic Acid

Synthesis of eicosanoids. Unsaturated fatty acids are required as a substrate. These are usually stored in the sn-2 position of membrane phospholipids.

Arachidonic acid and its metabolites act locally to regulate autocrine and paracrine functions. Their metabolism does not affect the function of cells at distant sites.[1,6] These local actions are regulated in several ways. The array of products that can be synthesized from free arachidonic acid are not produced in each cell type; each cell has a unique set of enzymes and receptors that permit rapid, selective, local regulation (Table 34-1).[2,7] Each cell has a characteristic set of enzymes for eicosanoid synthesis, which determines its product profile. The nature of the stimulus also influences the products that are formed by each type of cell (i.e., particulate versus soluble).[7]

In addition to regulating the synthesis of these compounds, cells also tune their responses by regulating the expression of their receptors for detecting prostaglandins and leukotrienes.[8,9] A cell in its resting state may express only a few products, but after cytokine stimulation it may synthesize new enzymes and receptors or may downregulate receptors selectively. The complexity of this regulatory system explains the diverse effects that a single metabolite of arachidonic acid may have between tissues as well as in different species.[7,10]

Phospholipases

Because arachidonic acid is a membrane constituent, its release from membrane phospholipids by phospholipase is a key regulatory event in initiating eicosanoid synthesis.[1,11] Phospholipases have unique substrate interaction characteristics that influence how they can act to release substrate. Because the substrate is present in membranes, the phospholipase enzyme must first bind to the membrane (an equilibrium reaction), after which it "scoots" on the membrane surface to liberate its substrate.[11]

Multiple phospholipases exist that can selectively hydrolyze fatty acid from the phospholipid present in cell membranes. They are named for the location of the bond they attack during substrate hydrolysis. The enzymes attacking these four sites of hydrolysis are named phospholipase A_1 (PLA_1), phospholipase A_2 (PLA_2), phospholipase C (PLC), and phospholipase D (PLD).[12] In addition to the nomenclature based on substrate specificity, mammalian PLA_2s are divided into two major types: secretory and cytosolic.

SECRETORY PHOSPHOLIPASES Secretory phospholipases require calcium for catalysis, are generally of low molecular weight (approximately 14 kDa), and fall into two major groups: pancreatic (type I, digestive) and nonpancreatic (type II, inflammatory). For example, secretory phospholipases play a role in mast cell-mediated inflammation, where mast cell-derived secretory phospholipase releases arachidonic acid for metabolism by adjacent cells (termed *transcellular metabolism*). They show no selectivity in their hydrolysis of fatty acid from the sn-2 position of membrane phospholipid, leaving lysophospholipid and free fatty acid. Secretory phospholipases are thought to be key in the release of arachidonic acid in inflammatory disease states, such as arthritis.[12–15]

CYTOSOLIC PLA_2 In contrast to the secretory phospholipases, cytosolic phospholipases are higher in molecular weight (39 to 100 kDa) and are generally selective in their preference for arachidonic acid over other fatty acid constituents of membrane phospholipid. Some of these enzymes are calcium dependent, while others are not. High-molecular-weight, calcium-dependent, cytosolic phospholipase A_2 ($cPLA_2$) is thought to be responsible for the majority of eicosanoid product formation. Cytosolic phospholipase is a major source of arachidonic acid in skin.[12,13,16,17]

PHOSPHOLIPASE C In some tissues (such as platelets) arachidonic acid is released indirectly by PLC. This enzyme cleaves inositol-containing phospholipids, releasing diacylglycerol. Diacylglycerol is subsequently cleaved by diacylglycerol lipase to generate free arachidonic acid.[18] PLC-mediated release of diacylglycerol is also important because diacylglycerol is a cofactor for protein kinase C activation.[19] Activation of this pathway also results in the simultaneous release of inositol phosphates, which mobilize intracellular calcium.[20] Therefore, after PLC activation, three different mediators are produced: arachidonic acid, inositol phosphates, and diacylglycerol.

Once free arachidonic acid is in the cell cytosol, there are three main pathways of metabolism: cyclooxygenase, lipoxygenase, and monooxygenase. Cyclooxygenase metabolism leads to the synthesis of prostaglandins and thromboxanes, which interact with specific receptors to initiate tissue responses (Fig. 34-2). Lipoxygenase enzymes catalyze the formation of 5-, 12-, or 15-hydroperoxyeicosatetraenoic acid (HPETE) intermediates, which are subsequently reduced, leading to the formation of hydroxyeicosatetraenoic acid (HETE) as shown in Fig. 34-3.[21–23] The 5-lipoxygenase pathway is particularly important among these lipoxygenase reactions because it forms the highly active leukotriene derivatives of arachidonic acid,[24] which interact with specific receptors, and also contributes to lipoxin formation.[25] Lastly, monooxygenases (members of the cytochrome P_{450} family) are also responsible for the formation of arachidonic acid oxygenation products. In addition, these pathways play an important role in both eicosanoid degradation and in the formation of products with biologic activity.[26]

Prostaglandins and Thromboxanes

Arachidonic acid is converted to prostaglandins by the prostaglandin endoperoxide synthase, also known as cyclooxygenase. There are two isoforms of cyclooxygenase known as COX-1 and COX-2. COX-1 is present constitutively in most prostaglandin-producing cells. COX-2 expression is inducible by exposure of cells to agents such as growth factors and cytokines, such as interleukin-1, and in inflammatory states. COX-2 is an endoplasmic reticulum-associated homodimer composed of 72-kDa subunits requiring heme binding and glycosylation for activity.[6,27,28] The PGH_2 produced by prostaglandin endoperoxide synthase serves as a substrate for the formation of PGE_2, PGF_2, PGD_2, thromboxane (TX) A_2, and prostacyclin (PGI_2) through the action of specific isomerases.[29]

In the small vessels of the skin, TXA_2, PGE_2, and PGI_2 are key mediators in regulating peripheral vascular tone and clotting. When appropriately stimulated (as by a breach in the endothelium or the presence of bacteria), blood elements such as platelets, monocytes, and macrophages synthesize TXA_2 through the action of the microsomal cytochrome P_{450} enzyme, thromboxane synthase.[30] TXA_2 is a potent inducer of vasoconstriction and platelet aggregation. TXA_2 has a very short half-life (30 s); it spontaneously hydrolyzes to TXB_2, an inactive degradation product. This short half-life allows modulation of vasoconstriction over very short time periods.

PGD_2 is the primary prostaglandin synthesized in mast cells, and therefore is an important mediator in allergic responses.[31] It also appears to be the predominant prostaglandin formed by Langerhans cells.[32] It is found abundantly in the central nervous system and male genitalia. Two types of enzyme synthesize PGD_2: the lipocalin, or brain type, and the hematopoietic type, which is the predominant form in skin. PGD_2 is a peripheral vasodilator, allergic and inflammatory mediator, mediator of nociceptive responses, and an inhibitor of platelet aggregation. Its effects outside skin include sleep induction and centrally induced hypothermia.[33–35]

To balance the formation of the potent vasoconstrictor TXA_2 by blood elements, vascular endothelium and smooth muscle actively synthesize PGI_2 and PGE_2, which are potent vasodilators, via their respective microsomal cytochrome P_{450} synthases.[36–39] In addition to its vasodilatory properties, PGI_2 is an antiaggregatory agent, making it capable of stopping proliferation of a platelet thrombus. Like TXA_2, it has a very short 10-min half-life, after which it hydrolyzes spontaneously to 6-keto-$PGF_{1\alpha}$. PGE_2 is synthesized in endothelium and causes capillary vascular smooth muscle dilatation and plasma exudation, potentiates histamine- and bradykinin-induced effects on vascular permeability, and enhances the sensation of pain from these mediators.[6,40–42] Its actions are more long-lasting than those of PGI_2. Thus, the balance between the synthesis of vasodilators by

TABLE 34-1

Effects of Arachidonic Acid Metabolites and Their Tissue Source in Skin

COMPOUND	EFFECTS	TISSUE SOURCE
PGE_2	Plasma exudation Stimulates cell proliferation Hyperalgesia Relaxes smooth muscle Antagonizes renal H_2O reabsorption Inhibits gastric secretion Stimulates LHRH release Facilitates blastocyst implantation	Epithelium, fibroblasts, macrophages
$PGF_{2\alpha}$	Bronchoconstriction Vasopressor Stimulates cell proliferation	Keratinocytes
PGD_2	Relaxes smooth muscle Sleep induction Central hypothermia Inhibits platelet aggregation Bronchoconstriction	Mast cells, Langerhans cells
PGI_2	Inhibits platelet aggregation Relaxes smooth muscle Rapidly metabolized to 6-keto $PGF_{1\alpha}$	Endothelium, vascular smooth muscle, fibroblasts, macrophages
TXA_2	Stimulates platelet aggregation Constricts smooth muscle Rapidly broken down into TXB_2	Platelets, macrophages
12-HETE	Enhances endothelial cell invasion Stimulates smooth muscle migration 12-R-HETE inhibits Na^+, K^+-ATPase, increases $\alpha II\beta 3$ integrin expression	Keratinocytes, mast cells, leukocytes
15-HETE	Hyperalgesia Inhibits cyclooxygenase Inhibits mixed lymphocyte reaction Stimulates cytotoxic suppressor T cell formation	Eosinophils, keratinocytes
LTB_4	Induces neutrophil chemotaxis (as potent as C5 or FMLP) Chemokinesis Neutrophil degranulation	Macrophages, neutrophils
LTC_4	Plasma exudation Vasodilation in skin Bronchoconstriction Stimulates mucus secretion	Mast cells
LTD_4	Vasoconstriction in lung Vasodilation in skin Bronchoconstriction Stimulates mucus secretion	Mast cells
Lipoxin A	Bronchoconstriction Arteriolar dilation Antagonizes LTB_4-induced inflammation Inhibits PMN adhesion to endothelial cells	Leukocytes
Lipoxin B	Bronchoconstriction Stimulates monocyte colony formation	Leukocytes
Knockout mouse		
COX-1	Decreased pup survival	
COX-2	Impaired renal function Cardiac myofibrosis Infertility	

ABBREVIATIONS: 12-HETE, 15-HETE, 12- or 15- hydroxyeicosatetraenoic acid; LHRH, luteinizing hormone–releasing hormone; LT, leukotriene; PG, prostaglandin; PGI_2, prostacyclin; PMN, polymorphonuclear leukocyte; TX, thromboxane.

FIGURE 34-2

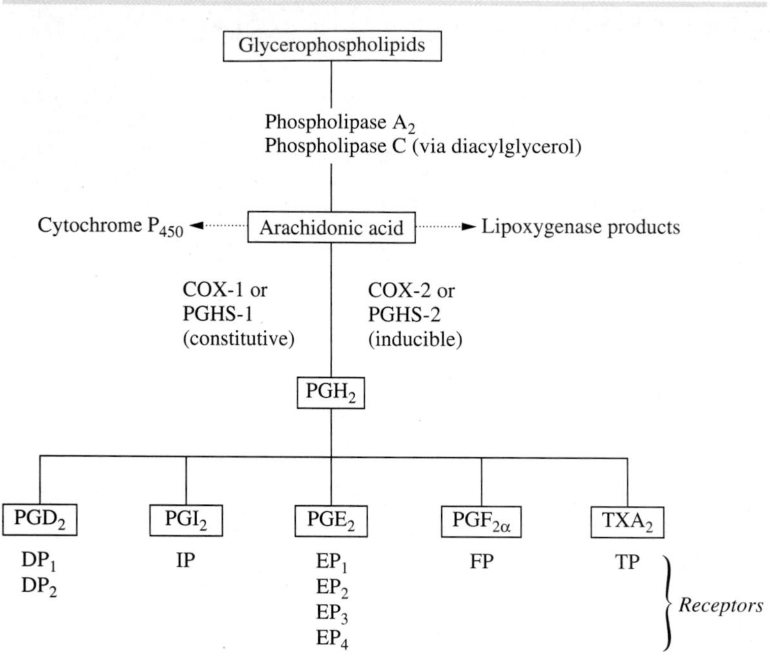

Prostaglandin and thromboxane formation. Prostaglandins are formed by the serial action of phospholipases and cyclooxygenases. Their effects are mediated through specific receptor activation. COX, cyclooxygenase; PGHS, prostaglandin endoperoxide synthase; DP, IP, EP, FP, and TP are receptors for PGD_2, PGI_2, PGE_2, $PGF_{2\alpha}$, and thromboxane, respectively.

vascular cells and vasoconstrictors released from blood cells can determine vascular tone and modulate clot propagation and inflammatory pain.

$PGF_{2\alpha}$ is synthesized by keratinocytes in skin, as well as in a number of other organs, by the action of PGF synthase. It can act as a vasopressor, can stimulate fibroblast proliferation,[2] and is important in labor and delivery.[43] Three separate pathways lead to the formation of $PGF_{2\alpha}$: 9,11-endoperoxide reduction of PGH_2, 11-ketoreduction of PGD_2, and 9-ketoreduction of PGE_2. Conversion of PGH_2 to $PGF_{2\alpha}$ appears to be the predominant pathway. Two different active sites on PGF synthase are responsible for the reduction of both PGD_2 and PGH_2.[44–46] PGD_2 can also be metabolized to a diastereoisomer of $PGF_{2\alpha}$ by an NADPH-dependent mechanism. This compound has the same biologic activities as the $PGF_{2\alpha}$ produced by 9,11-endoperoxide reduction of PGH_2.[47]

Prostaglandins produce their effects through interaction with specific G-protein–linked receptors (see Fig. 34-2). Prostaglandin receptors have a structural motif common to G-protein–coupled rhodopsin-type receptors, with seven putative transmembrane domains, an extracellular amino-terminal domain, and an intracellular carboxyl-terminal domain that specifies G-protein interactions.[8] This carboxyl-terminal domain determines linkage to different intracellular signaling pathways. Specific receptors have been identified for each of the major prostaglandin types: the thromboxane receptor, termed TP; four PGE_2 receptors, designated as EP_1, EP_2, EP_3, and EP_4[48,49]; the $PGF_{2\alpha}$ receptor, FP; the PGI_2 receptor, IP; and two distinct PGD_2 receptors, DP and DP_2.[50,51] Structural analysis of the receptors shows that their overall homology is not high. The TP, EP_2, and EP_3 receptors are on chromosomes 10, 15, and 3, respectively. Their structural homology is restricted to the consensus sequence of the seventh transmembrane domain and the second extracellular loop.[8]

Three major types of signaling pathways may be triggered by prostaglandin binding. Depending upon the structure of the receptor and the G protein associated with it, stimulation of the prostaglandin receptors may trigger a rise in calcium, mediate a rise in intracellular levels of cyclic adenosine monophosphate (cAMP), or inhibit cAMP formation.

FIGURE 34-3

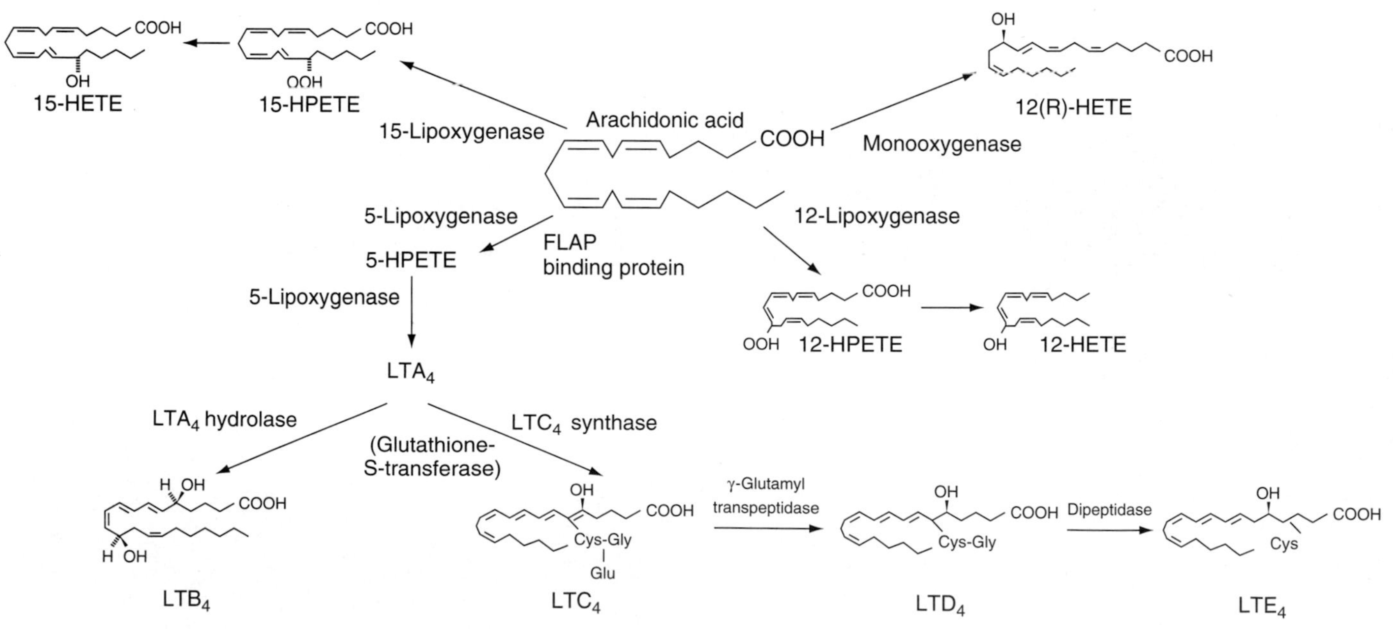

Synthesis of leukotrienes and HETEs.

On the basis of these signaling responses, prostaglandin receptors can be grouped into three general categories. The relaxant receptors (IP, DP_1, EP_2, and EP_4) increase levels of cAMP and induce smooth muscle relaxation. The contractile receptors (TP, FP, DP_2, and EP_1) mediate Ca^{++} mobilization and induce smooth muscle contraction. Lastly, the EP_3 and DP_2 receptors are able to decrease levels of cAMP. The EP_3 receptor inhibits smooth muscle contraction in this way, while DP_2 receptors are present on eosinophils and counteract eosinophil responses mediated through the DP_1 receptor. The balance between the DP receptors may have a role in eosinophil recruitment in asthma. Great potential for the development of useful new therapeutic agents exists as specific agonists and antagonists of prostaglandin receptors are developed.[8,48,49,52]

Lipoxygenases

Lipoxygenases are a family of enzymes in mammalian cells that catalyze the insertion of oxygen into unsaturated fatty acids to produce a hydroperoxy derivative.[2] Three classes of lipoxygenase enzymes insert oxygen into the 5-, 12-, or 15-carbon of arachidonic acid and are designated by their substrate site preference as 5-, 12-, or 15-lipoxygenases (see Fig. 34-3).

The 5-lipoxygenase pathway is particularly important in the regulation of biologic systems, because it is necessary for the formation of leukotrienes.[22,24] Leukotrienes are so named because of their predominant synthesis by leukocytes and their conjugated triene structure. 5-Lipoxygenase translocates to the nuclear membrane in the presence of Ca^{2+}, where it interacts with the 5-lipoxygenase-activating protein (FLAP) to form the leukotriene intermediate, leukotriene (LT) A_4.[53–55] 5-Lipoxygenase is present in neutrophils, macrophages, mast cells, and lung epithelium.[22] LTA_4 hydrolase can act on LTA_4 to form LTB_4. LTA_4 hydrolase is cytosolic and is found in a wide variety of tissues, including leukocytes, lung, heart, and intestine.[54] Some tissues that contain LTA_4 hydrolase do not contain 5-lipoxygenase and therefore depend upon LTA_4 being provided transcellularly for their synthesis of leukotrienes. LTB_4 is one of the most potent chemotactic and chemokinetic substances known, with maximal activities in the 10^{-9} M range. LTB_4 can induce degranulation of polymorphonuclear leukocytes and their adherence to vascular endothelium. LTB_4 is the predominant eicosanoid metabolite of neutrophils and is also produced by macrophages.[54,55] 5-Lipoxygenase activity has been reported in keratinocytes by some investigators,[56] but its presence has since been refuted.[57]

The actions of LTB_4 are mediated by interaction with its receptors.[58] In the neutrophil, LTB_4 receptors are associated with a guanosine triphosphate (GTP)-binding protein that regulates receptor affinity for LTB_4 and transduces the signal. Two receptor populations have been described. The high-affinity binding site dissociation constant is 4 to 5×10^{-10} M, in the range of the minimal effective concentration for chemotaxis. The low-affinity binding site has a molar dissociation constant of 0.6 to 5.0×10^{-7} M, in the concentration range required for secretion of neutrophil granules.[55,58] Thus, chemotaxis of neutrophils is initiated toward a site of inflammation through activation of their high-affinity receptor. Degranulation then occurs when the concentration of LTB_4 surpasses that necessary for activation of the low-affinity receptor, nearer the site of inflammation.

The 5-lipoxygenase pathway also leads to the generation of the cysteinyl leukotrienes, also known as slow-reacting substance of anaphylaxis.[24,55,58] LTC_4 is formed by the action of LTC_4 synthase, which adds glutathione at the 6-carbon position of LTA_4. The removal of glutamic acid from LTC_4 by γ-glutamyl transpeptidase produces LTD_4. Dipeptidase can further metabolize LTD_4 by removal of a glycine residue. Once the leukotrienes have been formed, their release from the cell is mediated by an export carrier system. LTB_4 and LTC_4 have individual carrier systems. The LTC_4 transporter is a 190-kDa glycoprotein, which also can transport related substances out of the cell. Transport is adenosine triphosphate (ATP)-dependent for both LTC_4 and LTB_4.[55,58,59] To eliminate these potent mediators, oxidative inactivation occurs via the combination of hydrogen peroxide produced through the respiratory burst of activated cells and extracellular chloride ion to produce hypochlorous acid, which attacks the sulfur of the cysteinyl adduct. This inactivation is important in the local environment of a site of inflammation. However, in primates LTE_4 is primarily eliminated through urinary excretion.[60,61]

As is the case for the prostaglandin receptors, the leukotriene receptors are highly heterogeneous. Receptors for LTB_4, LTC_4, and LTD_4 have been cloned. Biochemical evidence indicates the LTB_4 receptors are linked via a G-protein to PLC. Cysteinyl leukotrienes also appear to be coupled via a Gq protein to IP3 turnover and increases in intracellular Ca^{2+}.[55,58,60] Two classes of LTC_4 receptors are present, termed cysteinyl leukotriene $(CysLT)_1$ and $CysLT_2$.[62] Leukotriene receptors are expressed in the airway as well as in smooth muscle, microvasculature, blood elements, and skin. Splice variants of the $CysLT_1$ have been identified in the mouse, suggesting the opportunity for specific pharmacology.[62]

Arachidonate 12-lipoxygenase activity is found in platelets, leuko-cytes, mast cells, and epithelial cells, where it is present in abundance.[63–65] 12-S-hydroxyeicosatetraenoic acid has been reported to enhance tumor cell growth, endothelial cell invasion, and $\alpha IIb\beta 3$ integrin expression.[66] The leukocyte isoform is capable of metabolizing linoleic acid to [9Z,11E,(13S)]-13-hydroperoxyoctadecadienoic acid (13-HpODE), which is subsequently reduced to 13-hydroxyoctadecadienoic acid (13-HODE). These compounds are capable of forming DNA adducts, increasing epidermal growth factor-dependent signaling, and stimulating progression of breast carcinoma in a mouse model.[67–69]

The third major lipoxygenase enzyme present in mammalian cells is 15-lipoxygenase. The 15-lipoxygenase metabolic pathway is prominent in eosinophils and human airway epithelial cells. 15-HETE has been reported to induce hyperalgesia. It can also influence the synthesis of lipoxygenase and leukotriene products in mast cells, platelets, neutrophils, and eosinophils and has been implicated in atherogenesis. The 15-lipoxygenase is also capable of forming 13-HODE from linoleic acid.[70,71]

The lipoxins are a family of compounds that can be derived from arachidonic acid by the serial action of 5-, 12-, or 15-lipoxygenase, followed by further lipoxygenase metabolism. Lipoxins A_4 and B_4 contain a conjugated tetraene structure and appear to be generated by transcellular events during cell-cell interactions.[25] Studies in vitro have shown that lipoxin A_4 causes arteriolar dilation, antagonizes LTB_4-induced inflammation, and inhibits polymorphonuclear (PMN) leukocyte adhesion to endothelial cells. Lipoxin B_4 can stimulate monocyte colony formation, and both products are bronchoconstrictors.[2,25,72] The lipoxin receptor has recently been cloned. It is a classic seven transmembrane domain-type receptor, and its mRNA is found in lung, myeloid cell types, and tissues with a high degree of phagocytic infiltrates.[72] Lipoxin A_4 binding on PMNs is G-protein coupled. Lipoxins also act on a pharmacologically defined subclass of LTC_4-LTD_4 receptor; thus their actions may be like those of leukotrienes at these receptor sites.[73]

Cytochrome P_{450} enzymes can also metabolize eicosanoids. In contrast to cyclooxygenases and lipoxygenases, which introduce molecular oxygen (O_2) into their substrates, cytochrome P_{450} monooxygenation reactions introduce one atom of an oxygen molecule while cooxygenating a nearby molecule.[26] The epoxy acids have several significant physiologic functions. They are able to mobilize microsomal calcium and to alter K^+ and Na^+ ion flux. This capacity to regulate ion transfer may make monooxygenase products important in regulating cell water balance. ω-Hydroxylation by cytochrome P_{450} enzymes is also a predominant metabolic pathway for LTB_4.[26,58]

PROSTAGLANDIN ACTIONS IN NORMAL ORGAN FUNCTION

Information about normal function due to specific eicosanoids interacting with their receptors comes from studies of knockout animals and receptor localization studies (Table 34-2). The E series prostaglandins are important modulators of normal cell proliferation and play an important role in wound repair.[6,8] Cyclooxygenase inhibitors decrease epithelial proliferation and migration across a wound bed by 50 percent. Production of collagen fibrils in the dermal matrix is also decreased in the absence of PGE_2. In addition, collagenase activity from stimulated monocytes and macrophages depends upon the concomitant synthesis of PGE_2. In the epidermis and intestine, normal apoptotic sloughing of intestinal epithelium is regulated by COX-2–dependent PGE_2 synthesis. However, in the stomach, mucus secretion is modulated by COX-1–dependent PGE_2 synthesis.[74–77]

Prostaglandins mediate many key functions beyond the skin. PGE_2-mediated regulation of water balance in the kidney occurs due to the selective presence of receptors and the presence of inducible COX-2. EP_3 receptors are expressed in the tubular epithelium of the outer medulla, EP_1 receptor is in the papillary collecting ducts, and EP_4 receptor is in the glomerulus. This distribution pattern matches with known PGE_2-mediated functions in the kidney regulating ion transport, water reabsorption, and glomerular filtration. The contribution of COX-2 to regulation of renal function is demonstrated by selective knockout studies in transgenic mice.[74] The elimination of COX-2 disturbs normal renal tubular water balance because antidiuretic hormone responses in the proximal tubule are mediated by COX-dependent PGE_2 synthesis.[8,78,79]

PGE_2 also modulates fertility, where its absence decreases conception. Luteinizing hormone and follicle-stimulating hormone induce high levels of COX-2 and EP_2 receptor signaling, which act together to enhance cumulus expansion and rupture of the oocyte in the ovary. An important contribution to the oocyte's ability to be fertilized is also made via this signaling pathway; in mice lacking the EP_2 receptor, fertilization is decreased more than tenfold. Implantation is also supported by COX-2–mediated synthesis of PGI_2.[80] At the end of pregnancy, onset of labor is stimulated by the production of $PGF_{2\alpha}$, which is COX-1 dependent. This delayed onset of labor causes decreased pup survival.

TABLE 34-2

Major Phenotypes of Mice Deficient in Prostanoid Receptors*

Disrupted Gene	Major Phenotypes of Knockout Mice
DP	Reduced responses in allergic asthma
EP_1	Reduction in carcinogen-induced colorectal neoplasia
EP_2	Impaired ovulation and fertilization Salt-sensitive hypertension
EP_3	Impaired febrile response to pyrogens Impaired duodenal bicarbonate secretion
EP_4	Patent ductus arteriosus Decreased inflammatory bone resorption
FP	Parturition failure
IP	Thrombotic tendency, decreased inflammatory swelling
TP	Bleeding tendency

*Extensive studies have used knockout mouse strategies to demonstrate the functional role played by prostanoid receptors.[8]

These effects on fertility are observed primarily in knockout animals and are subtle if inhibitors are used.

EP_4 receptor activation is needed for closure of the ductus arteriosus immediately after birth. Knockout animals have a high mortality rate from failure of the ductus to close at birth. The EP_4 receptor is also important in bone remodeling; bone resorption is greatly decreased in EP_4 receptor knockout mice.[8]

EICOSANOID FORMATION AND ACTION IN INFLAMMATION, INJURY, AND DISEASE

Many of the early events in inflammation are extensively influenced by metabolites of arachidonic acid. After the skin is exposed to inflammatory stimuli, mast cells located perivascularly release PGD_2 and LTC_4 (converted to LTD_4 and LTE_4), which promote vasodilation and plasma exudation.[34,55,58,81,82] Mast cell histamine stimulates PGI_2 synthesis by vascular endothelium and PGE_2 synthesis by nearby fibroblasts; these mediators, in turn, potentiate the effects of histamine in the vessels of the dermis. Secretory phospholipase release also allows release of arachidonic acid from nearby cells. This mediator release appears clinically as a wheal-and-flare response.

In mastocytosis, there is a well-documented role for PGD_2 in the vasodilation and syncope that accompany the syndrome. In addition to the release of histamine by mast cells, PGD_2 is important in mediating the symptoms of the disease. Effective treatment of symptoms is often achieved by the simultaneous use of aspirin and antihistamines.[83]

In acute injury, the release of thromboxane by platelets contributes to platelet aggregation and clot formation. Neutrophils release LTB_4 at the injury site, recruiting more neutrophils in the initial phases of inflammation.[55,58] Macrophages arrive somewhat later at the injury site and release more TXA_2, $PGF_{2\alpha}$, PGE_2, LTB_4, and LTC_4, further contributing to the inflammation. Phospholipase activation enhances the inflammation. The synthesis of these inflammatory mediators contributes significantly to the pattern of inflammation observed early in the injury response.[7]

Another common form of injury in which prostaglandin synthesis plays a role is ultraviolet light (UVB) injury. After exposure to three times the minimal erythema dose of UVB, there occurs a prolonged increase in the release of PGE_2, $PGF_{2\alpha}$, and 6-keto-$PGF_{1\alpha}$.[84–86] In the first 24 h after UV exposure, this prostaglandin release contributes substantially to the pain and erythema induced. Early treatment with indomethacin inhibits erythema, demonstrating the role of prostaglandins in the process.[87,88] Increased synthesis of $cPLA_2$ is partially responsible for increased prostaglandin formation in the first 24 h. At later time points, an increase in COX-2 occurs.[17,85,88]

Substantial evidence demonstrates the deranged metabolism of eicosanoids in psoriasis. Increased levels of 12-HETE and free arachidonic acid are reported in lesional skin.[89,90] In addition, increased amounts of the potent chemotactic agent LTB_4 are found, which is likely a result of the presence of neutrophils in psoriatic skin samples.[91] However, evidence for the importance of these metabolites in the pathophysiology of the disease remains circumstantial. Drugs that decrease the synthesis of lipoxygenase products (steroids, anthralin) improve psoriasis,[2,92] whereas inhibitors of prostaglandin synthesis may exacerbate the disease.[93] The exact role of these changes in the pathogenesis of psoriasis remains obscure.

Eicosanoids are very important to pain and fever responses. The first evidence supporting the role of prostaglandins in pain and fever was the discovery that aspirin is an inhibitor of cyclooxygenase.[6,8] Further work with knockout animals has shown that fever is mediated by the EP_3 receptor,[8] while pain perception is modulated by the EP_1 receptor.[94] The role of specific prostaglandins in mediating pain is supported by the location of receptors in neurons of the dorsal root ganglion.

Recent evidence also implicates cyclooxygenase in the pathogenesis of cancer of the colon.[95–97] Studies in individuals with familial polyposis demonstrate that long-term treatment with nonsteroidal anti-inflammatory drugs (NSAIDs, COX inhibitors) decreases the incidence of colon carcinoma by 50 percent. This result appears to be due to the regulation of PGE_2-dependent growth in the intestine, which stops progression of initiated tumor cells. Similar profound inhibition of tumor formation has been demonstrated with UV-induced tumors in mice.[98–100]

Reductions in the risk of myocardial infarction have been demonstrated in patients taking the COX-inhibitor aspirin. Individuals with unstable angina who take low-dose aspirin have a 33 percent decrease in their risk of a cardiovascular event. Similar reductions in the risk of stroke occur, and the risk of death is decreased by one-sixth.[101] Prostaglandins are also important in toxemia of pregnancy, as demonstrated by the decrease of toxemia symptoms in patients treated with low-dose aspirin beginning in the second trimester.[102]

Epidemiologic and clinical studies suggest than NSAIDs can inhibit the progression of Alzheimer's disease. Histochemical stains show that there is an increased level of COX-1 in β-amyloid plaques in the brains of patients with Alzheimer's disease, suggesting that COX-1 activity may be important in patients with this disorder.[103]

In asthma, it is well documented that there is airway hyperresponsiveness, increased airway smooth-muscle contraction, mucus hypersecretion, and increased vascular permeability. When asthma is triggered by a specific antigen, the initial event is antigen-mediated mast cell activation.[58] Similar mechanisms are involved in allergic responses of the skin.[81] In cases of exercise induced asthma, local dehydration is thought to result in hyperosmolarity, resulting in mast cell activation. Mast cells permeate the airways in individuals with asthma. When stimulated, these cells release stored histamine from granules and synthesize PGD_2 and leukotrienes. LTC_4, LTD_4, and LTE_4 control at least three signs of asthma: smooth muscle contraction, mucus secretion, and edema formation. LTE_4 is generally less potent than LTC_4 or LTD_4. In the asthmatic airway, the leukotrienes potentiate the effect of histamine 1000-fold. Leukotrienes are 2000 times more potent as bronchoconstrictors than histamine.[58]

INHIBITORS OF EICOSANOID FORMATION AND ACTION

Despite the extensive knowledge about the physiology of arachidonic acid metabolites and their receptors, most of the drugs presently available to the physician in practice to manipulate eicosanoid formation are not specific. Aspirin and most NSAIDs act through the inhibition of cyclooxygenase activity.[6] Whereas these drugs are relatively specific in their inhibition of the cyclooxygenases, the synthesis of all prostaglandins and thromboxanes occurs via these enzymes. Efforts to produce selective inhibitors of COX-2 have resulted in two new selective agents: rofecoxib (Vioxx) and celecoxib (Celebrex).[104] Drugs of this class permit COX-1–mediated activities, such as clotting and stomach mucus secretion, to occur, while COX-2–mediated prostaglandin synthesis contributing to inflammation is blocked. These drugs are highly efficacious in arthritis and have demonstrated some efficacy as cancer chemopreventive agents.[95–98] Studies are ongoing of their activity as skin cancer chemopreventive agents. This is likely to add to the already observed benefit of NSAIDs in colon carcinoma.

Some prostaglandin analogues are currently available that are used for their specific therapeutic benefit. For example, the PGE_1 analogue misoprostol is used for the prevention of NSAID-induced gastric ulcers,[105] the PGE_2 analogue dinoprostone is used for cervical ripening and reduction of time in labor, and the $PGF_{2\alpha}$ analogue latanoprost is used for glaucoma.[106]

Leukotriene receptor antagonists are now available for treatment of asthma. Because they are receptor blockers, they must bind to the CysLT receptor to prevent agonist-stimulated synthesis of leukotrienes. Several such drugs are now on the market, such as Montelukast (Singulair) and zafirlukast (Accolate). Both these drugs bind to the $CysLT_1$ receptor, leaving an opportunity for better drug development if antagonists to the $CysLT_2$ receptor can also be developed. A second drug interfering with leukotriene synthesis is zileuton (Zyflo), a competitive inhibitor of 5-lipoxygenase.[107,108] Like the leukotriene receptor antagonists, it must be present before the induction of leukotriene synthesis to be effective. These drugs are often combined with prednisone to produce maximum benefit in patients with asthma. Prednisone influences the synthesis of eicosanoids by two methods. First, it decreases the synthesis of $cPLA_2$, thereby decreasing the release of arachidonic acid.[102,109] Second, it blocks the synthesis of COX-2, thereby decreasing the synthesis of prostaglandins.[110] Prednisone also has an important effect on eicosanoid synthesis in mast cells by stabilizing the cell membranes, thereby decreasing cell degranulation in response to antigen or other stimuli.[108]

In summary, the metabolism of eicosanoids by mammalian cells is a ubiquitous process that locally regulates many fundamental cellular functions. Eicosanoids play important roles in the normal inflammatory response and are also involved directly or indirectly in the pathophysiology of many diseases. Clearly, there is a great opportunity for the development of therapeutic agents that modulate eicosanoid action. Effective drugs are available to regulate the synthesis of prostaglandins as a group; and selective agents for inhibiting the release of arachidonic acid, its metabolism into lipoxygenase or monooxygenase products, or interaction of its metabolites with specific receptors are being developed. Steroids suppress the formation of some of these metabolites.

REFERENCES

1. Fitzpatrick FA, Soberman R: Regulated formation of eicosanoids. *J Clin Invest* **107**:1347, 2001
2. Fogh K, Kragballe K: Eicosanoids in inflammatory skin diseases. *Prostaglandins Other Lipid Mediat* **63**:43, 2000
3. Goldblatt MW: Properties of human seminal plasma. *J Physiol* **84**:208, 1935
4. Van Euler US: A depressor substance in the vesicular gland. *J Physiol* **84**:21P, 1935
5. Marnett LJ: Aspirin and the potential role of prostaglandins in colon cancer. *Cancer Res* **52**:5575, 1992
6. Marnett LJ et al: Arachidonic acid oxygenation by COX-1 and COX-2. *J Biol Chem* **274**:22903, 1999
7. Tripp CS et al: Calcium ionophore enables soluble agonists to stimulate macrophage 5-lipoxygenase. *J Biol Chem* **260**:5895, 1985
8. Narumiya S et al: Prostanoid receptors: Structures, peptides and functions. *Phys Rev* **79**:1193, 1999
9. Dahlen SE: Pharmacological characterization of leukotriene receptors. *Am J Respir Crit Care Med* **161**:S41, 2000
10. Marks F, Furstenberger G: Cancer chemoprevention through interruption of multistage carcinogenesis. The lessons learnt by comparing mouse skin carcinogenesis and human large bowel cancer. *Eur J Cancer* **36**:314, 2000
11. Gelb MH et al: Do membrane-bound enzymes access their substrates from the membrane or aqueous phase: Interfacial versus non-interfacial enzymes. *Biochim Biophys Acta* **1488**:20, 2000
12. Hurley JH et al: Floundering about at cell membranes: A structural view of phospholipid signaling. *Curr Opin Struct Biol* **10**:737, 2000
13. Dennis EA: Diversity of group types, regulation, and function of phospholipase A2. *J Biol Chem* **269**:13057, 1994
14. Cho W: Structure, function, and regulation of group V phospholipase A(2). *Biochim Biophys Acta* **1488**:48, 2000

15. Mao-Qiang M et al: Secretory phospholipase A2 activity is required for permeability barrier homeostasis. *J Invest Derm* **106**:57, 1996
16. Pickard RT et al: Identification of essential residues for the catalytic function of 85-kDa cytosolic phospholipase A_2. Probing the role of histidine, aspartic acid, cysteine, and arginine. *J Biol Chem* **271**:19225, 1996
17. Gresham A et al: Increased synthesis of high-molecular-weight $cPLA_2$ mediates UV-induced PGE_2 in human skin. *Am J Physiol* **39**:C1037, 1996
18. Hokin LE: Receptors and phosphoinositide-generated second messengers. *Ann Rev Biochem* **54**:205, 1985
19. Nakamura S et al: Lipid mediators and protein kinase C activation for the intracellular signaling network. *J Biochem* **115**:1029, 1994
20. Exton JH: Regulation of phosphoinositide phospholipases by hormones, neurotransmitters, and other agonists linked to G proteins. *Ann Rev Pharm Toxicol* **36**:481, 1996
21. Yedgar S et al: Inhibition of phospholipase A(2) as a therapeutic target. *Biochim Biophys Acta* **1488**:182, 2000
22. Radmark O: Arachidonate 5-lipoxygenase. *J Lipid Mediat Cell Sig* **12**:171, 1995
23. Kuhn et al: Arachidonate 15-lipoxygenase. *J Lipid Mediat Cell Sig* **12**:157, 1995
24. Henderson WR: The role of leukotrienes in inflammation. *Basic Sci Rev* **121**:684, 1994
25. Serhan CN, Romano M: Lipoxin biosynthesis and actions: role of the human platelet LX-synthase. *J Lipid Mediat Cell Sig* **12**:293, 1995
26. Carroll MA, McGiff JC: A new class of lipid mediators: cytochrome P_{450} arachidonate metabolites. *Thorax* **55**:S13, 2000
27. Morita I et al: Different intracellular locations for prostaglandin endoperoxide H synthase-1 and -2. *J Biol Chem* **270**:10902, 1995
28. Picot D et al: The x-ray crystal structure of the membrane protein prostaglandin H_2 synthase-1. *Nature* **367**:243, 1994
29. Jakobsson PJ et al: Identification of human prostaglandin E synthase; a microsomal, glutathione-dependent, inducible enzyme, constituting a potential novel drug target. *Proc Nat Acad Sci U S A* **96**:7220, 1999
30. Hsu PY et al: Expression, purification and spectroscopic characterization of human thromboxane synthase. *J Biol Chem* **274**:762, 1999
31. Roberts LJ et al: Prostaglandin, thromboxane and 12-hydroxy-5,8,10, 14-eicosatetraenoic acid production by ionophore-stimulated rat serosal mast cells. *Biochim Biophys Acta* **575**:185, 1979
32. Rosenbach I et al: Comparison of eicosanoid generation by highly purified human Langerhans cells and keratinocytes. *J Invest Dermatol* **95**:104, 1990
33. Urade Y, Hayaishi O: Biochemical, structural, genetic, physiological and pathophysical features of lipocalin-type prostaglandin D synthase. *Biochim Biophys Acta* **1482**:259, 2000
34. Matsuoka T et al: Prostaglandin D_2 as a mediator of allergic asthma. *Science* **287**:2013, 2000
35. Satoh S et al: Promotion of sleep induced by prostaglandin D_2 in rats. *Proc Natl Acad Sci U S A* **93**:5980, 1996
36. Tanioka T et al: Molecular identification of cytosolic prostaglandin E_2 synthase that is functionally coupled with cyclooxygenase-1 in immediate prostaglandin E_2 biosynthesis. *J Biol Chem* **275**:32775, 2000
37. Jakobsson PJ et al: Identification of human prostaglandin E synthase: A microsomal, glutathione-dependent, inducible enzyme, constituting a potential novel drug target. *Proc Nat Acad Sci U S A* **96**:7220, 1999
38. Nowak J, Fitzgerald GA: Redirection of prostaglandin endoperoxide metabolism at the platelet-vascular interface in man. *J Clin Invest* **83**:380, 1989
39. Hara S et al: Isolation and molecular cloning of prostacyclin synthase from bovine endothelial cells. *J Biol Chem* **269**:19897, 1994
40. Pentland AP, Needleman PN: Modulation of keratinocyte proliferation in vitro by endogenous prostaglandin synthesis. *J Clin Invest* **77**:246, 1986
41. Rheins LA et al: Suppression of the cutaneous immune response following topical application of the prostaglandin PGE_2. *Cell Immunol* **106**:33, 1987
42. Santoli D et al: Suppression of interleukin-2–dependent human T cell growth in vitro by prostaglandin E (PGE) and their precursor fatty acids. *J Clin Invest* **85**:424, 1990
43. O'Brien WF: The role of prostaglandins in labor and delivery. *Clin Perinatol* **22**:973, 1995
44. Watanabe K et al: Enzymatic formation of prostaglandin $F_{2\alpha}$ from prostaglandin H and D. *J Biol Chem* **260**:7035, 1985
45. Hong Y et al: The role of selenium-dependent and selenium-independent glutathione peroxidases in the formation of prostaglandin $F_{2\alpha}$. *J Biol Chem* **264**:13793, 1989
46. Watanabe K et al: Stereospecific conversion of prostaglandin D_2 to (5Z,13E)-(15S)-9 alpha-11 beta, 15-trihydroxyprosta-5,13-dien-1-oic acid (9 alpha, 11 beta-prostaglandin F_2) and of prostaglandin H_2 to prostaglandin F_2 alpha by bovine lung prostaglandin F synthase. *Proc Natl Acad Sci U S A* **83**:1583, 1986
47. Liston TE, Roberts LJ: Transformation of prostaglandin D_2 to 9 alpha, 11-beta-(15S)-trihydroxyprosta-(5Z, 13E)-dien-1-oic acid (9 alpha, 11 beta-prostaglandin F_2): A unique biologically active prostaglandin produced enzymatically in vivo in humans. *Proc Natl Acad Sci U S A* **82**:6030, 1985
48. Negishi M et al: Prostaglandin E receptors. *J Lipid Mediat Cell Sig* **12**:379, 1995
49. Kotani M et al: Molecular cloning and expression of multiple isoforms of human prostaglandin E receptor EP_3 subtype generated by alternative messenger RNA splicing: Multiple second messenger systems and tissue-specific distributions. *Mol Pharmacol* **48**:869, 1995
50. Monneret G et al: Prostaglandin D_2 is a potent chemoattractant for human eosinophils that acts via a novel DP receptor. *Blood* **98**:1942, 2001
51. Hirai H, et al: Prostaglandin D_2 selectively induces chemotaxis in T helper type 2 cells, eosinophils, and basophils via seven-transmembrane receptor CRTH2. *J Exp Med* **193**:255, 2001
52. Coleman RA et al: International Union of Pharmacology classification of prostanoid receptors: Properties, distribution and structure of the receptors and their subtypes. *Pharmacol Rev* **46**:205, 1994
53. Rouzer CA, Samuelsson B: Reversible, calcium-dependent membrane association of human leukocyte 5-lipoxygenase. *Proc Natl Acad Sci U S A* **84**:7393, 1987
54. Haeggstrom JZ: Structure, function, and regulation of leukotriene A4 hydrolase. *Am J Respir Crit Care Med* **161**:S25, 2000
55. Samuelsson B: The discovery of the leukotrienes. *Am J Respir Crit Care Med* **161**:S2, 2000
56. Grabbe J et al: Production of LTB-like chemotactic arachidonate metabolites from human keratinocytes. *J Invest Dermatol* **85**:527, 1985
57. Breton J et al: Human keratinocytes lack the components to produce leukotriene B4. *J Invest Dermatol* **106**:162, 1996.
58. Devillier P et al: Leukotrienes, leukotriene receptor antagonists and leukotriene synthesis inhibitors in asthma: An update. Part 1: Synthesis, receptors and role of leukotrienes in asthma. *Pharmacol Res* **40**:3, 1999
59. Jakobsson PJ et al: Identification and characterization of a novel human microsomal glutathione S-transferase with leukotriene C4 synthase activity and significant sequence identity to 5-lipoxygenase-activating protein and leukotriene C4 synthase. *J Biol Chem* **271**:22203, 1996
60. Metters KM: Leukotriene receptors. *J Lipid Mediat Cell Sig* **12**:413, 1995
61. Orning L et al: In vivo metabolism of leukotriene C4 in man: Urinary excretion of leukotriene E4. *Biochem Biophys Res Commun* **130**:214, 1985
62. Maekawa A et al: Identification in mice of two isoforms of the cysteinyl leukotriene-1 receptor that result from alternative splicing. *Proc Natl Acad Sci U S A* **98**:2256, 2001
63. Funk CD et al: Molecular cloning, primary structure and expression of the human platelet/erythroleukemia cell 12-lipoxygenase. *Proc Natl Acad Sci U S A* **87**:5638, 1990
64. Yoshimoto T et al: Cloning and sequence analysis of the cDNA for arachidonate 12-lipoxygenase of porcine leukocytes. *Proc Natl Acad Sci U S A* **87**:2142, 1990
65. Holtzman MJ et al: A regiospecific monooxygenase with novel stereo preference is the major pathway for arachidonic acid oxygenation in isolated epidermal cells. *J Clin Invest* **84**:1446, 1989
66. Honn KV et al: 12-lipoxygenases and 12(S)-HETE: Role in cancer metastasis. *Cancer Metastasis Rev* **13**:365, 1994
67. Liehr J et al: Lipid hydroperoxide-induced endogenous DNA adducts in hamsters: Possible mechanism of lipid-hydroperoxide-mediated carcinogenesis. *Arch Biochem Biophys* **316**:38, 1995
68. Wang M, Liehr J: Identification of fatty acid hydroperoxide cofactors in the cytochrome P450-mediated oxidation of estrogens to quinone metabolites. *J Biol Chem* **269**:284, 1994
69. Rose DP et al: Effects of linoleic acid on the growth and metastasis of two human breast cancer cell lines in nude mice and the invasive capacity of these cell lines in vitro. *Cancer Res* **54**:6557, 1994
70. Zhao H et al: Lipoxygenase mRNA in cultured human epidermal and oral keratinocytes. *J Lipid Res* **36**:2444, 1995
71. Yla-Herttuala S et al: Transfer of 15-lipoxygenase gene into rabbit iliac arteries results in the appearance of oxidation-specific lipid-protein

adducts characteristic of oxidized low-density lipoprotein. *J Clin Invest* **95**:2692, 1995
72. Serhan CN, Oliw E: Unorthodox routes to prostanoid formation: New twists in cyclooxygenase-initiated pathways. *J Clin Invest* **107**:1481, 2001
73. Papayianni A et al: Lipoxin A4 and B4 inhibit leukotriene-stimulated interactions of human neutrophils and endothelial cells. *J Immunol* **156**:2264, 1996
74. Morham SG et al: Prostaglandin synthase 2 gene disruption causes severe renal pathology in the mouse. *Cell* **83**:473, 1995
75. Langenbach R: Prostaglandin synthase 1 gene disruption in mice reduces arachidonic acid-induced inflammation and indomethacin-induced gastric ulceration. *Cell* **83**:483, 1995
76. Blumenkrantz N, Sondergaard I: Effects of prostaglandin E_1 and $F_{1\alpha}$ on biosynthesis of collagen. *Nature* **239**:246, 1972
77. Leong L et al: Cyclooxygenases in human and mouse skin and cultured human keratinocytes: Association of COX-2 expression with human keratinocyte differentiation. *Exp Cell Res* **224**:79, 1996
78. Lin L et al: Role of prostanoids in renin-dependent and renin-independent hypertension. *Hypertension* **17**:517, 1991
79. Breyer MD, Breyer RM: Prostaglandin E receptors and the kidney. *Am J Physiol Renal Physiol* **279**:F12, 2000
80. Hizaki H et al: Abortive expansion of the cumulus and impaired fertility in mice lacking the prostaglandin E receptor subtype EP(2). *Proc Nat Acad Sci U S A* **96**:10501, 1999
81. Soter NA et al: Local effects of synthetic leukotrienes (LTC_4, LTD_4, LTE_4, and LTB_4) in human skin. *J Invest Dermatol* **80**:115, 1983
82. Maurice PDL et al: The effect of prostaglandin D_2 on the response of human skin to histamine. *J Invest Dermatol* **89**:245, 1987
83. Roberts LJ et al: Increased production of prostaglandin D_2 in patients with systemic mastocytosis. *N Engl J Med* **303**:1400, 1980
84. Pentland AP et al: Enhanced prostaglandin synthesis after ultraviolet injury is mediated by endogenous histamine stimulation. *J Clin Invest* **86**:566, 1990
85. Black AK et al: Time course changes in levels of arachidonic acid and prostaglandins D_2, E_2, $F_{2\alpha}$ in human skin following ultraviolet B irradiation. *Br J Clin Pharmacol* **10**:453, 1980
86. Hruza LL, Pentland AP: Mechanisms of UV-induced inflammation. *J Invest Dermatol* **100**:35S, 1993
87. Snyder DS, Eaglstein WH: Topical indomethacin and sunburn. *Brit J Dermatol* **90**:91, 1974
88. Grewe M et al: Analysis of the mechanism of ultraviolet (UV) B radiation-induced prostaglandin E_2 synthesis by human epidermoid carcinoma cells. *J Invest Derm* **101**:528, 1993
89. Hammarstrom S et al: Arachidonic acid transformations in normal and psoriatic skin. *J Invest Dermatol* **73**:180, 1979
90. Duell EA et al: Determination of 5-, 12-, and 15-lipoxygenase products in keratomed biopsies of normal and psoriatic skin. *J Invest Dermatol* **91**:446, 1988
91. Bain SD: Psoriasis and leukotriene B_4. *Lancet* **2**:762, 1982
92. Bedford CJ et al: Anthralin inhibition of mouse epidermal arachidonic acid lipoxygenase in vitro. *J Invest Dermatol* **81**:566, 1983

93. Katayama H, Kawada A: Exacerbation of psoriasis induced by indomethacin. *J Dermatol* **8**:323, 1981
94. Stock JL et al: The prostaglandin E_2 EP_1 receptor mediates pain perception and regulates blood pressure. *J Clin Invest* **107**:325, 2001
95. Rao CV et al: Modulation of experimental colon tumorigenesis by types and amounts of dietary fatty acids. *Cancer Res* **61**:1927, 2001
96. Rao C et al: Chemoprevention of colon carcinogenesis by sulindac, and nonsteroidal anti-inflammatory agent. *Cancer Res* **55**:1464, 1995
97. Prescott SM, Fitzpatrick FA: Cyclooxygenase-2 and carcinogenesis. *Biochim Biophys Acta* **1470**:M69, 2000
98. Pentland AP et al: Reduction o UV-induced skin tumors in hairless mice by selective COX-2 inhibition. *Carcinogenesis* **20**:1939, 1999
99. Fisher SM et al: Chemopreventive activity of celecoxib, a specific cyclooxygenase-2 inhibitor, and indomethacin against ultraviolet light-induced skin carcinogenesis. *Mol Carcinog* **25**:231, 1999
100. Giovannucci E et al: Aspirin use and the risk for colorectal cancer and adenoma in male health professionals. *Ann Intern Med* **121**:241, 1994
101. Day L, Barnfield M: Who should be taking aspirin? *Practitioner* **239**:426, 1995
102. Dekker GA, Sundler R: Dexamethasone down-regulates the 85-kDa phospholipase A_2 in mouse macrophages and suppresses its activation. *Biochem J* **307**:499, 1995
103. Yermakova A, O'Banion MK: Cyclooxygenases in the central nervous system: implications for treatment of neurological disorders. *Current Pharm Des* **6**:1755, 2000
104. Crofford LJ et al: Basic biology and clinical application of specific cyclooxygenase-2 inhibitors. *Arthritis Rheum* **43**:4, 2000
105. Moses MF et al: Prevention of acute graft rejection by the PGE_1 analog misoprostol in renal transplant recipients treated with cyclosporine and prednisone. *N Engl J Med* **322**:1183, 1990
106. Rulo AH et al: Reduction of intraocular pressure with treatment of latanoprost once daily in patients with normal-pressure glaucoma. *Ophthalmology* **103**:1276, 1996
107. Barnes NC: Effects of antileukotrienes in the treatment of asthma. *Am J Respir Crit Care Med* **161**:S73, 2000
108. Devillier P et al: Leukotrienes, leukotriene receptor antagonists and leukotriene synthesis inhibitors in asthma: An update. Part II. Clinical studies with leukotriene receptor antagonists and leukotriene synthesis inhibitors in asthma. *Pharmacol Res* **40**:15, 1999
109. Dolan-O'Keefe M et al: Transcriptional regulation and structural organization of the human cytosolic phospholipase A(2) gene. *Am J Physiol Cell Physiol* **278**:L649, 2000
110. Irahara M et al: Glucocorticoid receptor-mediated post-ceramide inhibition of the interleukin-1 beta-dependent induction of ovarian prostaglandin endoperoxide synthase-2 in rats. *Biol Reprod* **60**:946, 1999

CHAPTER 35

Kenneth H. Kraemer

Cellular Hypersensitivity and DNA Repair

A group of heritable diseases with differing clinical features share the common characteristics of in vitro or in vivo cellular hypersensitivity to damage by several physical or chemical agents.[1–3] These diseases include those with ultraviolet hypersensitivity (xeroderma pigmentosum, Cockayne syndrome, trichothiodystrophy, and familial melanoma with dysplastic nevi), those with x-ray hypersensitivity (ataxia-telangiectasia and basal cell nevus syndrome), and those with chromosome instability (Bloom syndrome, Fanconi anemia, and ataxia-telangiectasia). This cellular hypersensitivity may be of diagnostic utility and may suggest measures for therapeutic or prophylactic intervention. Knowledge of the molecular basis of the cellular hypersensitivity is rapidly emerging. In this chapter, the major tests used to assess cellular hypersensitivity and DNA repair are outlined. The clinical features and cellular abnormalities in these disorders are included in Chaps. 82, 93, and 155.

USE OF CULTURED CELLS FOR ASSESSMENT OF HYPERSENSITIVITY

Cells obtained directly from patients and grown in culture medium are termed *primary* cultures. Dermal fibroblasts generally grow easily in culture and can be subcultured. Recent advances in cell-culture techniques have permitted prolonged growth and subculture of keratinocytes and melanocytes. Lymphocytes may be stimulated to divide by means of 'mitogens' such as phytohemagglutinin (PHA), a plant lectin, or interleukin (IL)-2.

Primary cultures of skin dermal fibroblasts can generally be established from a 2- to 4-mm sterile skin punch biopsy. The inner surface of the upper arm has proven to be a suitable site because this area heals easily, the resulting scar is not readily visible, the site is shielded from ultraviolet radiation, and a large proportion of the attempts to establish cultures have been successful. The tissue is placed in sterile culture medium (or sterile saline) with antibiotics and transported to a cell-culture laboratory at room temperature.

Primary cultures have a limited life span. Their growth rate slows dramatically and they cannot be successfully subcultured. To avoid this cellular senescence, techniques have been developed to immortalize cultured cells. Transformation of lymphocytes with Epstein-Barr (EB) virus or fibroblasts with SV40 virus results in cultures of cells that grow indefinitely without senescence. Transformed lymphocytes, termed lymphoblastoid cell lines, resemble immature lymphoid cells. Lymphoblastoid cell lines can generally be established by EB virus treatment of 10 to 20 mL of sterile whole blood [collected in sterile tubes containing acid citrate dextrose (ACD) or heparin].

Established cell cultures may be frozen at liquid nitrogen temperatures and stored indefinitely in a state of suspended animation. When thawed, the cells resume growth in fresh culture medium. Human cell cultures (skin fibroblasts or blood cells) are established, frozen, and made available for research by the Human Genetic Mutant Cell Repository (401 Haddon Ave, Camden, NJ 08103, telephone 800-752-3805; http://locus.umdnj.edu/ccr/).

ASSESSMENT OF CELLULAR HYPERSENSITIVITY

Tests to assess cellular hypersensitivity to physical or chemical agents may be divided into tests of intact cellular function or chromosome integrity (Table 35-1) and tests that measure the mechanism of impairment of cell function such as DNA repair.

Tests of Intact Cell Function

Tests of cellular function measure the capacity of the intact cell to recover from the damage induced. These tests do not provide information as to the specific type of damage resulting in cellular injury or the mechanism of cellular recovery, but they do form the basis for identifying cells as hypersensitive.

TABLE 35-1

Tests of Cellular Sensitivity to Physical or Chemical Agents

Intact cell function
Growth rate
Colony-forming ability
Cell mutagenesis
Host–cell reactivation
Chromosome integrity
Chromosome breakage
Sister chromatid exchanges

GROWTH RATE One of simplest tests of cellular function is the assessment of the growth rate of cells in mass culture following exposure to UV or x-ray. Cells from patients with xeroderma pigmentosum or Cockayne syndrome are hypersensitive to UV and cells from patients with ataxia-telangiectasia are hypersensitive to killing by x-ray.

COLONY-FORMING ABILITY Colony-forming ability assesses the capacity of a single cell to proliferate enough to form a visible colony. Xeroderma pigmentosum fibroblasts from two affected siblings (XP12TA and XP25TA), their father (XPH27TA), unaffected brother (35TA), and normal fibroblasts (96TA and HSTA) were treated with 254-nm ultraviolet radiation (UVC) and colony-forming ability determined (Fig. 35-1). The XPC fibroblast strains from the affected siblings

FIGURE 35-1

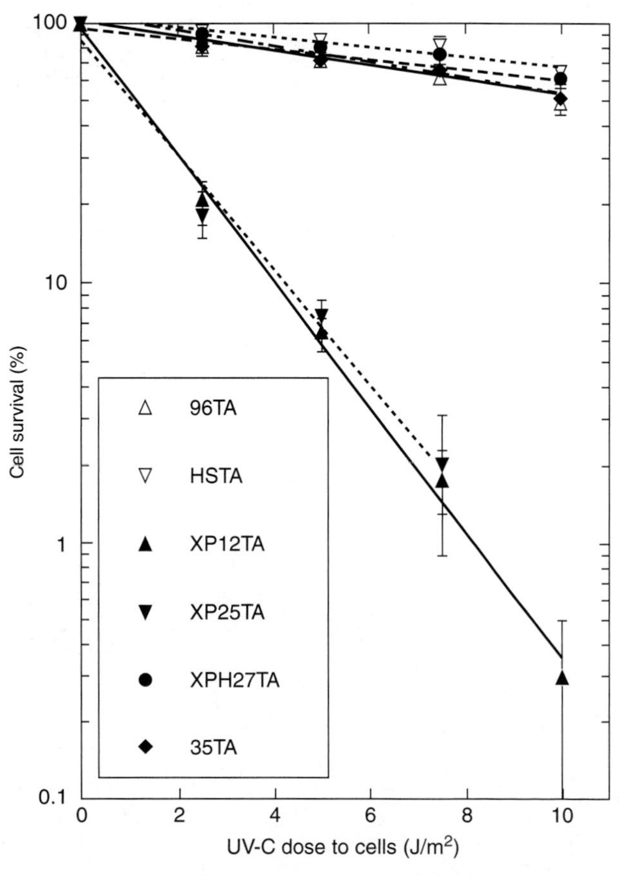

Colony-forming ability assay of cell sensitivity. Ultraviolet sensitivity of XP complementation group C fibroblasts. Colony forming ability of fibroblasts from two affected siblings (XP12TA and XP25TA) following exposure to various doses of UVC was reduced compared to that of the normal controls (96TA and HSTA). Fibroblasts from the clinically normal father (XPH27TA) who is an obligate XPC heterozygote and the unaffected brother (35TA) had normal post-UV colony-forming ability.[4]

were much more sensitive than the normal strains and showed similar post-UV hypersensitivity. Cells from the unaffected brother and the clinically normal father, a heterozygous carrier of the XPC defect, had normal post-UV survival.[4]

MUTAGENESIS Assays of induced mutations measure the frequency of induction of mutated cells following treatment with damaging agents. A limited number of mutated characteristics, such as thioguanine resistance [resulting from loss of activity of the enzyme hypoxanthine guanine phosphoribosyltransferase (HGPRT)] and ouabain resistance [caused by an alteration in membrane adenosine triphosphatase (ATPase)] have been examined in culture. The growing cells can have mutations (alterations in DNA sequence) induced in their DNA by treatment with UV. Such somatic mutations are thought to be related to induction of cancer in vivo. Cells from XP patients are hypermutable after UV exposure.

HOST-CELL REACTIVATION These assays rely on the fact that DNA viruses or plasmids do not have the ability to repair damage to their DNA but depend on cellular repair systems. Thus, damaged viruses or plasmids would be expected to grow better on cells with normal repair capacity than on cells with reduced repair capacity.

Host-cell reactivation assays (Fig. 35-2) have been developed that utilize plasmids, which are small, double-stranded DNA that can replicate independently in bacteria and often carry genes for antibiotic resistance. Molecular biologic techniques have been used to modify plasmids to permit expression of bacterial genes in mammalian cells.

FIGURE 35-2

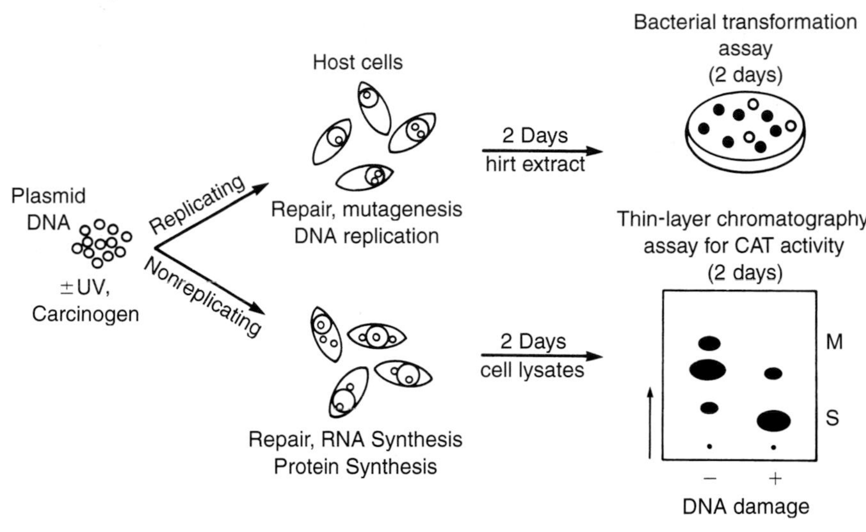

Plasmid host-cell reactivation assays of cell sensitivity. Plasmid DNA is treated in vitro with UV radiation or another carcinogen and then introduced into the human host cells by transfection. A nonreplicating plasmid is used to measure the DNA repairability of the host cell (lower path). A replicating plasmid measures DNA replication and mutagenesis in addition to DNA repair (upper path). See text for further details.

A plasmid DNA repair assay uses a nonreplicating plasmid, pRSV-CAT, which contains a gene for the bacterial enzyme chloramphenicol acetyl transferase (CAT), or for luciferase, which is constructed to permit expression in human cells. The plasmid is damaged by UV radiation and introduced into cultured human cells by a transfection technique. The cells' DNA repair enzymes repair the damage in a similar manner to the repair of cellular DNA. Repaired DNA will then function to transcribe mRNA, which then results in synthesis of the CAT enzyme in the human cell. The amount of CAT activity reflects the efficiency of the cellular DNA repair system. This assay can also be used to determine the complementation group by cotransfecting UV-treated plasmid plus plasmids expressing wild-type XP cDNA.

Figure 35-3 shows the results of plasmid host-cell reactivation experiments and complementation group assignment with DNA excision repair-deficient XP65BE cells. UV treated plasmid showed low expression in the XP65BE cells that was increased only by cotransfection with a plasmid expressing the wild-type *XPG* cDNA. This result indicates that XP65BE cells are in XP complementation group G.

Replicating plasmids can be used to measure mutagenesis in human cells. Xeroderma pigmentosum and Cockayne syndrome cells show post-UV plasmid hypermutability.[5]

Tests of Chromosome Integrity

CHROMOSOME BREAKAGE Chromosome breakage is usually assessed in primary cultures of mitogen-stimulated peripheral blood leukocytes or in long-term cultures of fibroblasts or lymphoblastoid cell lines. Cell-cycle progression is stopped at metaphase by treatment of the cells with a mitotic inhibitor such as colchicine. With this procedure, the 23 pairs of metaphase chromosomes from a single cell are spread over a discrete area of the slide and stained (usually with Giemsa). Chromosome preparations may be analyzed for the number of chromosomes per metaphase, the morphology of the individual chromosomes, and the attachments or rearrangements of chromosomes with each other. Increased spontaneous chromosome breakage is seen in three cancer-prone diseases; Bloom syndrome, ataxia-telangiectasia, and Fanconi anemia. Chromosome breakage may also be assessed after treatment of cells with DNA-damaging agents. Xeroderma pigmentosum cells are hypersensitive to chromosome breakage following ultraviolet radiation. Ataxia-telangiectasia cells are hypersensitive to chromosome breakage following treatment with x-rays or bleomycin.

In another assay, *G2 chromosome breakage,* fibroblasts or lymphocytes are exposed to low-dose x-rays and metaphases are collected beginning 1.3 h later. (Cells in metaphase at that time were in the G2 phase at the time of x-ray exposure.) The frequency of chromatid breaks and gaps is scored at several time intervals. With normal cells, there is a rapid decline in frequency of chromatid breaks and gaps. Cells from XP patients show a normal initial level of breaks and gaps but these persist longer than normal.[6] With obligate XP heterozygotes (parents of XP patients), the initial level of damage was similar, but there was an intermediate level of persistent breaks and gaps.[7] This assay has also been found to be abnormal with other genetic disorders such as ataxia-telangiectasia, familial melanoma with dysplastic nevi, basal cell nevus syndrome, Bloom syndrome, Fanconi anemia, and retinoblastoma.

SISTER CHROMATID EXCHANGE During cell growth, chromatids occasionally exchange positions along the arms of a chromosome. This "sister chromatid exchange" (SCE) may be detected by permitting the cells to grow through two cycles of replication in medium containing the nucleic acid analogue bromodeoxyuridine (BrUdR) (Fig. 35-4). After the first cycle of replication, the DNA of the newly synthesized strand is labeled with BrUdR while the older strand is unlabeled. Such chromosomes appear uniformly dark with Giemsa stain. After a second cycle of replication in BrUdR-containing medium, one arm of a chromosome will contain two labeled chromatids, while the other will contain one labeled and one unlabeled chromatid. The doubly substituted arm will

FIGURE 35-3

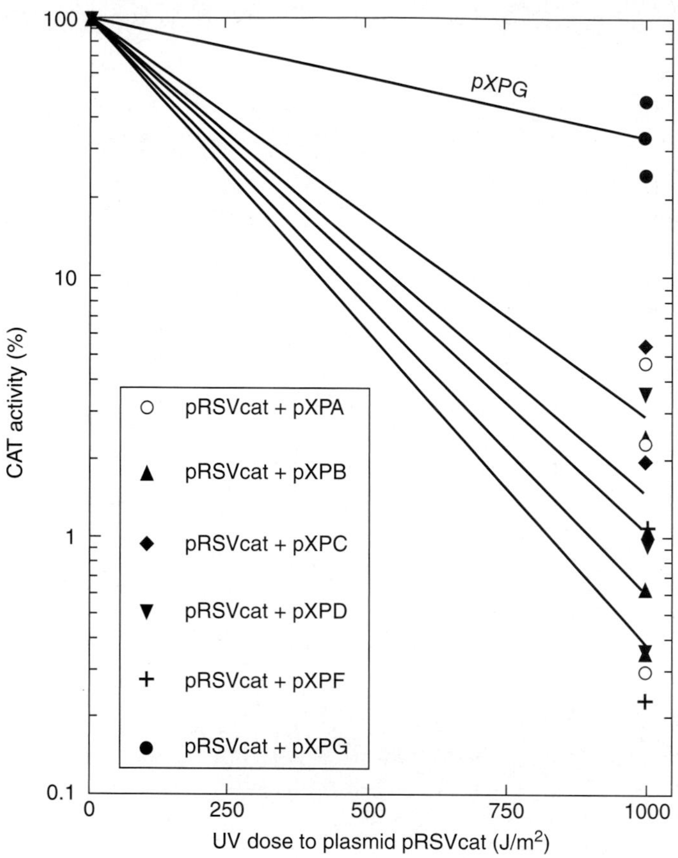

Plasmid host cell reactivation and assignment to XP complementation group G. A 1000 J/m^2 UVC-treated reporter gene plasmid (pRSVcat) was cotransfected with a wild-type XP cDNA containing plasmid [pXPA (*open circle*), pXPB (*triangle*), pXPC (*diamond*), pXPD (*inverted triangle*), pXPF (*cross*), pPXG (*closed circle*)] into triplicate cultures of primary patient fibroblasts (XP65BE). Each symbol represents the relative reporter gene activity in an independent transfection experiment 48 h after transfection compared with the corresponding unirradiated control reporter gene plasmid. The low level of host-cell reactivation typical of XP cells was increased only by adding the plasmid expressing wild-type XPG cDNA, indicating that the XP65BE cell is in XP complementation group G.[15]

FIGURE 35-4

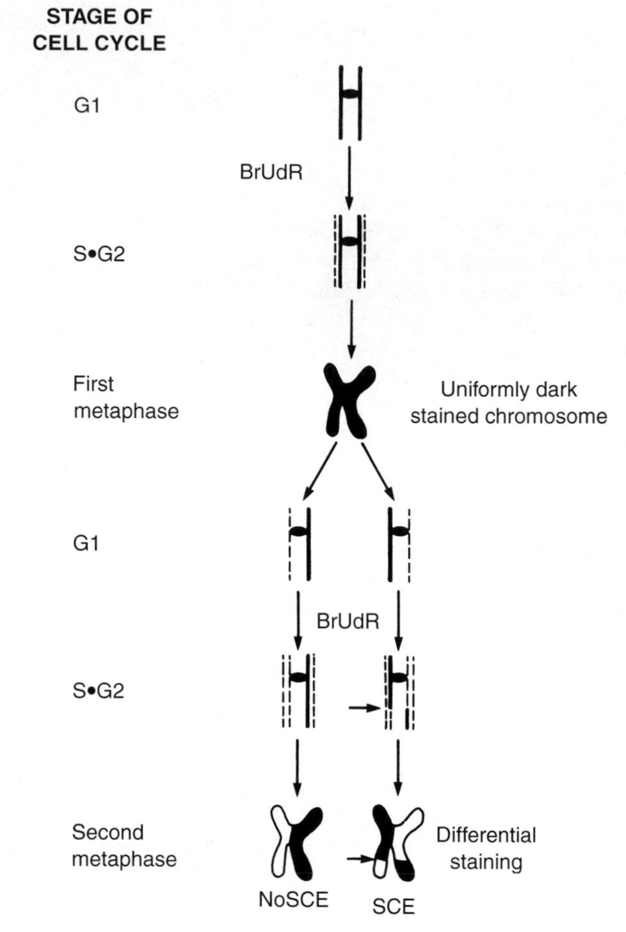

Schematic of sister chromatid exchange (SCE) assay of cell sensitivity. Cultured cells are permitted to go through two cycles of replication in medium containing bromodeoxyuridine. Staining with Giemsa or Hoechst dye number 33258 differentiates singly substituted from doubly substituted chromosomes, thus permitting recognition of SCEs.

stain lightly, while the singly substituted arm will stain darkly. If an SCE occurred during replication, a portion of each chromosome arm would be doubly substituted and the remainder singly substituted with BrUdR. SCEs are thought to be related to DNA damage and repair, although their precise significance is not understood. Figure 35-5 shows the appearance of mitogen-stimulated peripheral blood lymphocytes from a patient with Bloom syndrome that have been treated to reveal the elevated frequency of spontaneous SCEs. Lymphocytes from normal individuals generally have 8 to 10 SCEs per metaphase. The Bloom syndrome metaphase shown has 152 SCEs[8]. Xeroderma pigmentosum cells have an abnormally great increase in SCEs after UV radiation.

DNA REPAIR

Many environmental physical and chemical agents kill cells by damaging the cellular DNA. Table 35-2 lists some of the agents commonly used in laboratory studies on human cells and the type of damage induced. Normal cells contain enzyme systems that repair DNA damage. In bacteria, yeast, and rodent cells, many mutants that are hypersensitive to killing by physical agents (UV, X-ray) or chemicals have defective DNA repair. Some of these same hypersensitivity characteristics have been found in cells from patients who may also have defective DNA repair.

DNA Repair Pathways

The nucleotide excision repair (NER) pathway is known to act on DNA damaged with UV radiation (forming cyclobutane pyrimidine dimers and other photoproducts) or damaged with certain carcinogens (such as benzo-[a]-pyrene) (Table 35-2). In this pathway, the damaged nucleotide is removed and replaced with undamaged DNA. This pathway is defective in most XP patients and is discussed in more detail later in this chapter. Other pathways involve base excision repair, mismatch repair, photoreactivation, and bypass repair. More extensive descriptions of these pathways may be found in references.[1–3]

One of the most commonly used tests of NER is unscheduled DNA synthesis (UDS). This test has been used to measure DNA repair in intact human skin, in cultured epidermal or dermal cells, in blood cells, and for prenatal diagnosis using amniotic fluid cells. UDS measures the combined action of endonuclease, exonuclease, and polymerase in the nucleotide excision repair system. Cells are treated with UV radiation or another DNA-damaging agent and then incubated in medium containing radioactive thymidine. During the process of NER, the damage is removed and the radioactive thymidine is incorporated into the repaired region. The cells are treated with fixative, coated with autoradiographic (photographic) emulsion, kept in the dark for an appropriate interval, and then the emulsion is developed. During the exposure interval, the decay of tritium from the thymidine incorporated into the DNA exposes a small portion of the overlying emulsion. The tritium is revealed as a microscopic, dark grain in the developed emulsion above the cellular location of the incorporated thymidine. UV radiation of normal fibroblasts results in a large increase in the number of grains over all the nuclei. In marked contrast, radiation of the (DNA repair-defective) XP fibroblasts results in very few grains over their nuclei (Figs. 35-6 and 35-7).

FIGURE 35-5

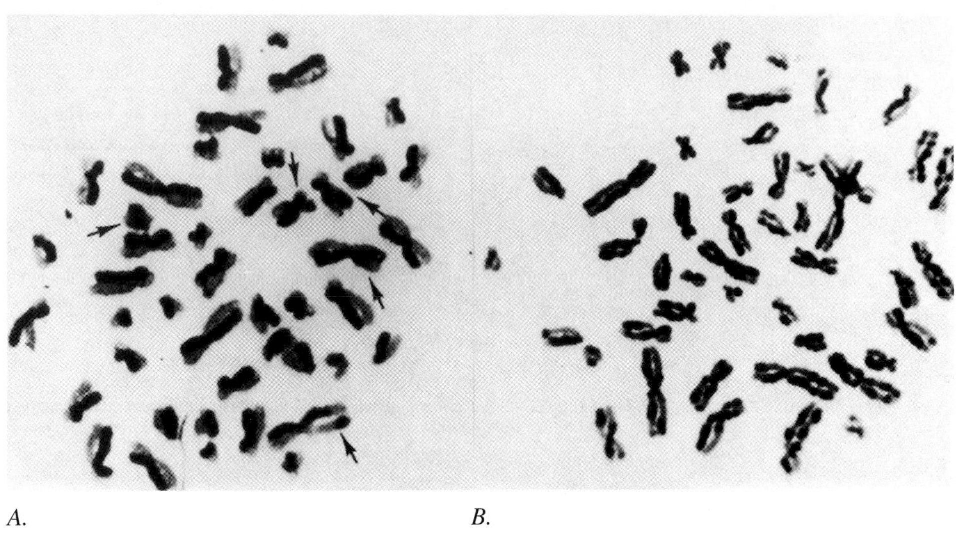

Sister chromatid exchange (SCE) assay of cell sensitivity. *A.* Undamaged normal cultured peripheral blood lymphocytes have about 10 SCEs per metaphase. *B.* Cultured peripheral blood lymphocytes from a patient with Bloom syndrome have a manyfold increase in SCEs. (*From Chaganti et al.,*[14] *with permission.*)

Complementation Groups

Cell fusion studies have been used to determine whether cells have different types of DNA repair defects. Fusion of fibroblasts from two XP patients with different DNA repair defects is followed by UV exposure and autoradiographic determination of unscheduled DNA synthesis (Figs. 35-6 and 35-7). The heterokaryons (from different donors) have a markedly increased amount of unscheduled DNA synthesis in comparison with the homokaryons (from a single donor) or the unfused mononuclear XP cells. This implies that the two fused XP strains had complementary DNA repair defects. Each strain supplied what the other was lacking. Such XP fibroblasts are said to be in different DNA repair complementation groups. Heterokaryons resulting from XP patients with the same DNA repair defect do not show an increase in post-UV unscheduled DNA synthesis. Such cells are said to be in the same complementation group. Seven complementation groups (genes) have been identified with fibroblasts from patients with XP, two from patients with Cockayne syndrome (CS) and three from trichothiodystrophy (TTD) patients (Table 35-3). This implies that each of these clinical disorders can be associated with more than one molecular defect.

TABLE 35-2

Cellular Damage Induced by Physical and Chemical Agents

Agent	Damage
Ultraviolet radiation	DNA: dipyrimidine cyclobutane dimers (TT, TC, CT, or CC), pyrimidine-pyrimidone (6-4) photoproducts (mostly TC), thymine glycols, DNA protein cross-links
X-radiation	DNA strand breaks, altered bases (thymine glycols)
Psoralens plus UVA	DNA–psoralen monoadducts, DNA interstrand cross-links (binds to T at TA sequences), psoralen–protein binding (high dose)
Mitomycin C	DNA interstrand cross-links
Benzo-[a]-pyrene	Binds to guanine in DNA making bulky adducts
Oxidation	Base damage (8-oxo-deoxyguanine)

FIGURE 35-6

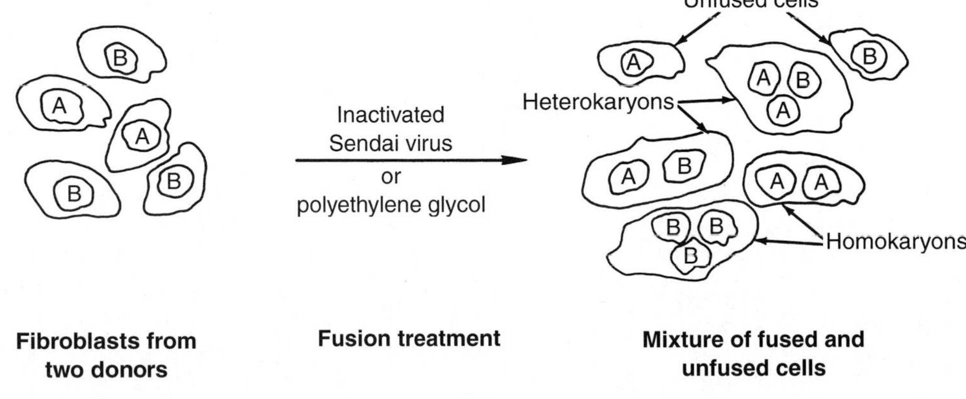

Schematic of cell fusion technique. Cocultured fibroblasts from two donors (A + B) are treated with inactivated Sendai virus or polyethylene glycol to induce cell fusion.

FIGURE 35-7

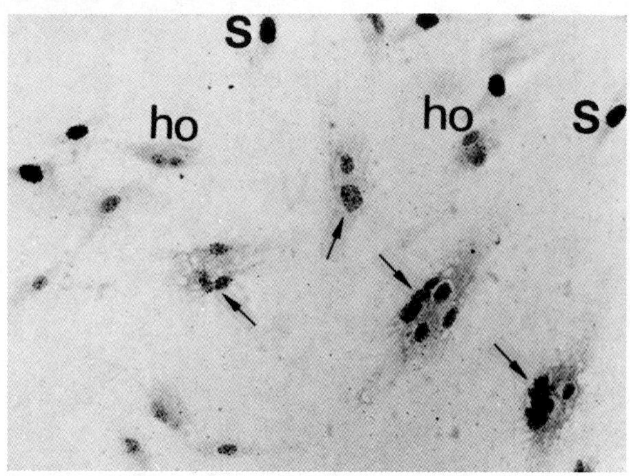

Increased unscheduled DNA synthesis in complementing xeroderma pigmentosum heterokaryons. A mixed culture of fused xeroderma pigmentosum fibroblasts was exposed to UV radiation and unscheduled DNA synthesis was determined. The nuclei of S-phase cells (*S*) are heavily labeled with radioactive thymidine. The unfused mononuclear cells have the same low level of unscheduled DNA synthesis as the fused homokaryons (*ho*). The heterokaryons (*arrows*), containing nuclei from both xeroderma pigmentosum fibroblast strains, have increased unscheduled DNA synthesis, indicating mutual correction of their DNA repair defects.

FIGURE 35-8

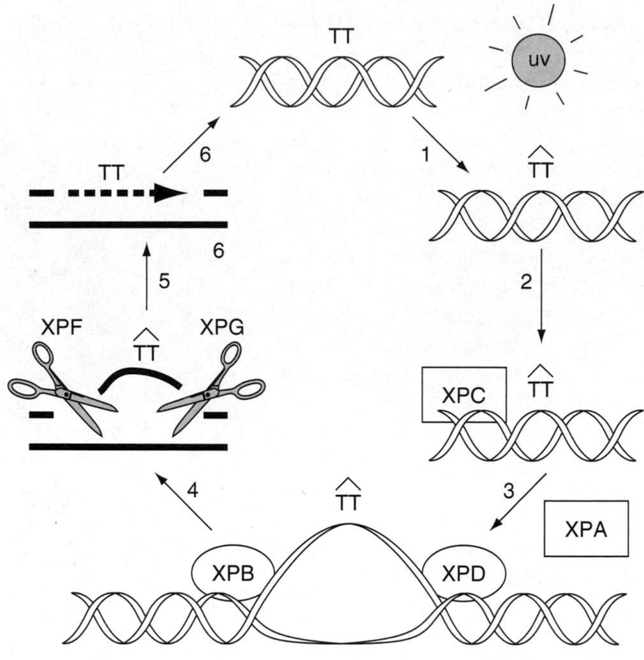

DNA excision repair scheme. Undamaged DNA contains adjacent pyrimidines in one strand (*top*). (1) Exposure to ultraviolet radiation in sunlight results in formation of photoproducts at the adjacent pyrimidines. (2) The XPC protein (in conjunction with other proteins such as XPE) detects the presence of the photoproduct and binds to the DNA, thereby marking the site for further processing. (3) The XPB and XPD proteins (in a complex containing the components of basal transcription factor TFIIH) unwind the DNA helix in the region of the photoproduct. (4) The XPF and XPG proteins (in complex with other proteins) make single-strand cuts 5′ and 3′ to the photoproduct, resulting in a gap of about 30 nucleotides. (5) The gap is filled in by DNA polymerase, which synthesizes new DNA using the other (undamaged) strand as a template. (6) DNA ligase joins the newly synthesized DNA to the older portion of the DNA strand, restoring the original undamaged DNA sequence. Further details are in the text.

HUMAN DNA REPAIR GENES

In recent years, more than 100 DNA repair genes have been identified (www.cgal.icnet.uk/DNA_Repair_Genes.html#NER).[9] Figure 35-8 shows a schematic of the repair of DNA by several of the XP proteins acting in concert.

XP Complementation Group A

The *XPA* gene is located on human chromosome 9 and codes for a messenger RNA of about 1000 bases, corresponding to a protein of 273 amino acids that binds to damaged DNA. Most XP-A patients have XP with neurologic abnormalities. More than 90 percent of Japanese XP-A patients have the same single base substitution mutation in this gene.[10] A diagnostic test for this mutation based on the polymerase chain reaction (PCR) and differences in enzymatic digestion of normal and mutated products and has been developed for rapid diagnosis of XP-A homozygotes and heterozygotes, as well as for prenatal diagnosis.[11]

TABLE 35-3

Cloned DNA Repair Genes Associated with Human Diseases

Gene*	Chromosome Location	Protein Size	Function
XPA	9q22.3	273 aa	Binds damaged DNA
XPB (ERCC3)	2q21	782 aa	DNA helicase, part of TFIIH
XPC	3p25	940 aa	Binds damaged DNA, global genome repair
XPD (ERCC2)	19q13.3	760 aa	DNA helicase, part of TFIIH
XPE (DDB2)	11p12-q11	427 aa	Binds damaged DNA
XPF (ERCC4)	16p13.3-p13.11	916 aa	DNA endonuclease
XPG (ERCC5)	13q22	1186 aa	DNA endonuclease
CSA (ERCC8)	5	396 aa	Transcription-coupled repair
CSB (ERCC6)	10q11	1493 aa	Transcription-coupled repair
XPV (polymerase eta)	6p21.1-p12	713 aa	DNA damage bypass polymerase

*The genes designated XP are defective in the corresponding xeroderma pigmentosum complementation group and those designated CS are defective in the corresponding Cockayne syndrome complementation group. ERCC refers to human excision repair cross-complementing genes that correct defects in cultured hamster cells.

XP Complementation Group B

The *XPB* gene on human chromosome 2 codes for a 2900-base messenger RNA, which corresponds to a protein of 782 amino acids that functions as a 3′ to 5′ DNA helicase in unwinding DNA (Fig. 35-8). Remarkably, this *XPB* gene was also found to be part of the TFIIH complex that is involved in regulation of the basal rate of transcription (RNA synthesis) of active genes. Analysis of the DNA of XP-B cells showed a single-base substitution mutation within the *XPB* (ERCC3) gene.[10] The XP-B phenotype was seen in three patients with the XP/CS complex and one with TTD.

XP Complementation Group C

The *XPC* gene on chromosome 3 codes for a 3500-base messenger RNA that corresponds to a protein of 940 amino acids. The XPC protein is involved with recognition of DNA damage (Fig. 35-8). Single-base substitution and splice mutations have been found in XP-C patients[12]; most XP-C patients have XP without neurologic abnormalities.

XP Complementation Group D

The *XPD* gene on chromosome 19 codes for a 760-amino acid protein that, like the XPB protein, is also a DNA helicase (but unwinds DNA in the 5′ to 3′ direction) and part of basal transcription factor TFIIH (Fig. 35-8). Different base substitution mutations within the *XPD* gene result in the different clinical phenotypes seen: XP, XP with neurologic abnormalities, the XP/CS complex, TTD, and XP/TTD.[13,14]

XP Complementation Group E

The *XPE* gene on chromosome 11 codes for a DNA damage-binding protein of 1140 amino acids. While two XP-E patients had mutations in the *XPE* gene, other XP-E patients did not have mutations.[10] These patients generally have mild skin symptoms without neurologic abnormalities.

XP Complementation Group F

The *XPF* gene on chromosome 16 codes for a 905-amino acid protein that serves as a DNA endonuclease 5′ to the lesion (Fig. 35-8). XP-F patients generally have XP without neurologic abnormalities. Most were described in Japan.[10]

XP Complementation Group G

The *XPG* gene on chromosome 13 codes for a protein of 1186 amino acids that functions as a DNA endonuclease 3′ to the lesion (Fig. 35-8). Mutations resulting in markedly truncated proteins are found in XP-G patients with the XP/CS complex, whereas XP-G patients without neurologic disease have missense mutations that retain some activity.[15]

CS Complementation Group A

The *CSA* gene on chromosome 5 codes for a 396 amino acid protein that is involved with transcription-coupled DNA repair. Mutations have been reported in a few patients.[10]

CS Complementation Group B

The *CSB* gene on human chromosome 10 codes for a protein of 1493 amino acids, which is a DNA helicase involved in transcription-coupled DNA repair. Mutations have been described in 24 patients.[16,17]

XP Variant

The XPV gene (polymerase eta) codes for an error-prone polymerase on chromosome 6 (Table 35-3).[18,19] XP variant patients are clinically identical to other XP patients with cutaneous symptoms without neurologic abnormalities.

ROLE OF DNA REPAIR GENES IN EXCISION REPAIR

The cloning of the human DNA repair genes has permitted study of the role of their encoded proteins in DNA excision repair. Several laboratories have developed cell-free assay systems that partially reconstitute portions of the nucleotide excision repair system using defined proteins.[20,21] A more detailed picture of nucleotide excision repair is emerging. Figure 35-8 shows a schematic version of the functions of XP genes in nucleotide excision repair. Double-stranded DNA contains adjacent pyrimidines. (1) Exposure to UV radiation from sunlight forms cyclobutane dimers or other photoproducts at adjacent pyrimidines, thereby distorting the DNA. (2) The *XPC* or *XPA* gene products bind to the damaged DNA, marking it for further processing. The *XPC* gene product may function in conjunction with the *XPE* gene product in lesion recognition. The *XPA* gene product probably functions in conjunction with replication protein A (RPA), TFIIH, and ERCC1. (3) The *XPB* and *XPD* gene products partially unwind the DNA in the region of the damage, thereby exposing the lesion for further processing. These proteins are part of the TFIIH basal transcription factor and appear to prefer to repair damage to actively transcribing genes before inactive genes. (4) The *XPF* gene product, in a complex with ERCC1, makes a single-strand nick at the 5′ side of the lesion, while the *XPG* gene product makes a similar nick on the 3′ side, resulting in the release of a region of about 30 nucleotides containing the damage. (5) The resulting gap is filled by DNA polymerase using the other (undamaged) strand as a template in a process involving proliferating cell nuclear antigen (PCNA). (6) DNA ligase I seals the region restoring the original undamaged sequence.

Recently, mouse models of DNA repair-deficient disorders have been generated by using recombinant DNA technology to alter embryonal mouse stem cells.[22] This gene targeting may be used to either completely inactivate a DNA repair gene, resulting in a knockout mutant, or to partially inactivate a gene by introducing the same mutations that are found in humans with disease. Like XP patients, these mice are hypersensitive to UV exposure and have an increased post-UV skin cancer susceptibility. Mouse models for CS and TTD have also been produced. These mice have some skin symptoms similar to those of humans but differ with respect to neurologic disease. This area of research is just beginning. Future studies may provide insights into multiple effects of DNA repair genes including immune abnormalities and possible interactions among these genes.

REFERENCES

1. Van Steeg H, Kraemer KH: Xeroderma pigmentosum and the role of UV-induced DNA damage in skin cancer. *Mol Med Today* **5**:86, 1999
2. Bootsma D et al: Nucleotide excision repair syndromes: Xeroderma pigmentosum, Cockayne syndrome, and trichothiodystrophy, in *The Genetic Basis of Human Cancer*, edited by B Vogelstein, KW Kinzler. New York, McGraw-Hill, 1998, p 245
3. Hoeijmakers JH: Genome maintenance mechanisms for preventing cancer. *Nature* **411**:366, 2001
4. Slor H et al: Clinical, cellular, and molecular features of an Israeli xeroderma pigmentosum family with a frameshift mutation in the XPC Gene: Sun protection prolongs life. *J Invest Dermatol* **115**:974, 2000
5. Gözükara EM et al. The human DNA repair gene, ERCC2 (XPD), corrects ultraviolet hypersensitivity and ultraviolet hypermutability of a shuttle vector replicated in xeroderma pigmentosum group D cells. *Cancer Res* **54**:3837, 1994
6. Parshad R et al: Cytogenetic evidence for differences in DNA incision activity in xeroderma pigmentosum group A, C, and D cells after X-irradiation during G2 phase. *Mutat Res* **294**:149, 1993
7. Parshad R et al: Carrier detection in xeroderma pigmentosum. *J Clin Invest* **85**:135, 1990
8. Chaganti RS et al: A manyfold increase in sister chromatid exchanges in Bloom's syndrome lymphocytes. *Proc Natl Acad Sci U S A* **71**:4508, 1974

9. Wood RD et al: Human DNA repair genes. *Science* **291**:1284, 2001
10. Cleaver JE et al: A summary of mutations in the UV-sensitive disorders: Xeroderma pigmentosum, Cockayne syndrome, and trichothiodystrophy. *Hum Mutat* **14**:9, 1999
11. Kore-eda S et al: A case of xeroderma pigmentosum group A diagnosed with a polymerase chain reaction (PCR) technique. Usefulness of PCR in the detection of point mutation in a patient with a hereditary disease. *Arch Dermatol* **128**:971, 1992
12. Chavanne F et al: Mutations in the XPC gene in families with xeroderma pigmentosum and consequences at the cell, protein, and transcript levels. *Cancer Res* **60**:1974, 2000
13. Lehmann AR: The xeroderma pigmentosum group D (XPD) gene: One gene, two functions, three diseases. *Genes Dev* **15**:15, 2001
14. Broughton BC et al: Two individuals with features of both xeroderma pigmentosum and trichothiodystrophy highlight the complexity of the clinical outcomes of mutations in the XPD gene. *Hum Mol Genet* **10**:2539, 2001
15. Emmert S et al: Relationship of neurologic degeneration to genotype in three xeroderma pigmentosum group G patients. *J Invest Dermatol* **118**:972, 2002
16. Mallery DL et al: Molecular analysis of mutations in the CSB (ERCC6) gene in patients with Cockayne syndrome. *Am J Hum Genet* **62**:77, 1998.
17. Colella S et al: Alterations in the CSB gene in three Italian patients with the severe form of Cockayne syndrome (CS) but without clinical photosensitivity. *Hum Mol Genet* **8**:935, 1999
18. Johnson RE et al: hRAD30 mutations in the variant form of xeroderma pigmentosum. *Science* **285**:263, 1999
19. Masutani C et al: The XPV (xeroderma pigmentosum variant) gene encodes human DNA polymerase eta. *Nature* **399**:700, 1999
20. Araujo SJ et al: Nucleotide excision repair of DNA with recombinant human proteins: Definition of the minimal set of factors, active forms of TFIIH, and modulation by CAK. *Genes Dev* **14**:349, 2000
21. Petit C, Sancar A: Nucleotide excision repair: From *E. coli* to man. *Biochimie* **81**:15, 1999
22. Friedberg EC, Meira LB: Database of mouse strains carrying targeted mutations in genes affecting cellular responses to DNA damage. Version 4. *Mutat Res* **459**:243, 2000

CHAPTER 36

Andrzej Dlugosz
Stuart H. Yuspa

Carcinogenesis: Chemical

CUTANEOUS CANCER AND PUBLIC HEALTH

Cutaneous cancers account for more than half of all malignancies in North America, totaling more than 1 million nonmelanoma skin cancers [mainly basal cell carcinomas (BCCs) and squamous cell carcinomas (SCCs)] and 50,000 melanomas in 2001. Death rates from nonmelanoma skin cancers equal those of Hodgkin's disease and uterine cancer, while deaths from melanoma are increasing at an alarming rate. Cutaneous cancers also significantly impact health care costs, and treatment is associated with considerable morbidity and cosmetic defects. For these reasons, understanding the etiology and pathogenesis of cutaneous cancers is a significant public health goal, and development of rational nondeforming therapies to reduce morbidity and mortality is urgently needed. The high prevalence of skin cancer, the external location of the tumors, and well-defined preneoplastic lesions provide an excellent opportunity for studying the factors regulating cutaneous cancer induction in humans. Those qualities that facilitate the study of cutaneous neoplasms in human populations have also been useful in establishing relevant animal models. Advances in molecular genetics, keratinocyte cell culture, and construction of genetically altered mice have greatly facilitated the analysis of basic mechanisms of cutaneous carcinogenesis. This chapter focuses on nonmelanoma skin cancer: the reader is referred to Chap. 93 for further discussion of melanoma.

CHEMICALS ASSOCIATED WITH SKIN CANCER INDUCTION IN HUMANS

The ultraviolet radiation (UVR) in sunlight is the primary etiologic agent for all skin cancers, and thus UVR is the major carcinogen in the human environment. The powerful carcinogenic activity of UVR is attributable to its ability to damage DNA and cause mutations, its capacity to clonally expand incipient neoplastic cells whose altered signaling pathways provide a survival advantage in the face of ultraviolet-induced cytotoxicity, and its activity as an immune suppressant (see Chaps. 38 and 39). The association of UVR with skin cancer is so strongly supported by clinical, epidemiologic, and experimental data that it represents the most clear-cut etiologic factor in human malignancy. Also implicated in the development of human skin cancer are various chemicals, as a result of environmental, occupational, or medicinal exposures (Table 36-1). In 1775, Sir Percivall Pott[1] attributed the increased incidence of scrotal cancer in chimney sweeps to repeated exposure to soot. This report provided the first link between occupational exposure and the development of cancer, as well as the first example of chemical carcinogenesis. In the last 30 years, the mechanisms by which chemicals cause cancer have been unraveled and they reveal striking similarities to the properties responsible for UVR carcinogenicity, namely DNA damage, selective cytotoxicity, and immune suppression.

The carcinogenic potential of coal and petroleum derivatives is now firmly established as a result of experimental animal studies and epidemiologic reports. Petroleum products and grease, as well as insecticides, herbicides, and fungicides, are particularly pathogenic for SCC, whereas fiberglass and dry-cleaning agents increase the incidence of BCC. Recent evidence suggests that cigarette and pipe smokers have an overall twofold increased risk for cutaneous SCC, and the risk increases with the intensity of the tobacco use.[2]

Arsenic exposure is associated with the development of premalignant keratoses, Bowen's disease, SCC, and BCC, as well as a number of internal malignancies.[3] While Fowler's solution (1% potassium arsenite) is no longer used in medical practice, certain herbal medicines are still a source of arsenic exposure. Occupational exposures to arsenic as a component of agricultural pesticides, sheep and cattle dip, mining and smelting, glass manufacturing, and other industries are well-documented. A more insidious source of environmental arsenic exposure is contaminated drinking water or shell fish, and analysis of affected populations shows a dose-dependent increase in skin cancer. Mouse models provide evidence for an interaction of ingested arsenic acting as a cocarcinogen with solar radiation to increase the frequency and size of cutaneous carcinomas and reduce the latency period.[4]

TABLE 36-1

Environmental Agents Associated with the Development of Human Skin Cancer

Agent	Individual at Risk	Route of Exposure	Tumor Types
UV radiation	General population	T	BCC, BD, SCC, M
Cigarette smoke	Smokers	T or S	SCC
Soot	Chimney sweep	T	SCC
Coal tar, pitch	Coker of coal, steel worker	T	SCC
Petroleum oils	Machinist, textile worker	T and S	SCC
Arsenic	Agriculture worker, etc.	S and/or T	BD, SCC, BCC
4,4′-Bipyridyl	Pesticide manufacturer	T	SCC, BD
PCB	Petrochemical worker	T or S	M
Dry-cleaning reagents	Dry cleaner	T or S	BCC
Fiberglass	Insulators	T	BCC
Psoralen (PUVA)	Psoriasis patient	T and S	SCC, BCC, M
Nitrogen mustard	CTCL patient	T	SCC
Immunosuppressants	Transplant recipients, etc.	S	SCC, BCC
Ionizing radiation	Various skin disorders	T	BCC, SCC

ABBREVIATIONS: BCC, basal cell carcinoma; BD, Bowen's disease; CTCL, cutaneous T cell lymphoma; M, melanoma; PCB, polychlorinated biphenyl; S, systemic; SCC, squamous cell carcinoma; T, topical.
SOURCE: Modified from Dlugosz A et al,[19] with permission of Blackwell Publishing, Oxford, UK.

A variety of medications have been associated with the development of skin cancer. Systemic treatment with immunosuppressive agents results in an increased incidence of both benign and malignant skin lesions.[5] Topical nitrogen mustard also increases the risk of developing skin cancer. Despite the clear-cut association between occupational exposure to tars and skin cancer, the use of crude coal tar in the treatment of psoriasis appears to pose a relatively low risk for the development of skin tumors. In contrast, the use of ionizing radiation to treat a variety of skin diseases increases the risk of BCC in all treated patients and SCC in individuals with sun-sensitive skin.[6]

Systemic administration of 8-methoxypsoralen combined with ultraviolet A treatments (PUVA) is associated with a dose-dependent increase in the risk of developing cutaneous SCC that persists following discontinuation of therapy.[7] Patients receiving high-level exposures ($\geq$ 337 PUVA treatments) had more than a 100-fold increase in SCC incidence while those receiving $<$100 treatments had a fivefold higher than expected incidence. Of individuals with PUVA-associated SCC, 3.8 percent developed metastases, and SCCs developed on the male genitalia much more frequently than in the general population. The incidence of BCC and melanoma is also increased in PUVA patients. PUVA is thus a potent stimulus for the induction of epithelial skin cancer in humans and also induces SCC in mice. While this implies that PUVA is a complete carcinogen by virtue of its DNA-damaging properties, the frequent detection of human papilloma virus DNA in PUVA-induced cancers suggests that immunosuppression may also contribute to carcinogenesis in this setting.[8]

THE NATURE OF CHEMICAL CARCINOGENS: CHEMISTRY AND METABOLISM

How can such a diverse group of chemical and physical agents contribute to cutaneous cancer when the great majority of environmental agents to which humans are exposed are not carcinogenic? We now know that carcinogens can be genotoxic, nongenotoxic, or both. Genotoxic carcinogens have high chemical reactivity (such as alkylating agents like nitrogen mustard) or they can be metabolized to reactive intermediates by the host (such as petroleum products). They form covalent adducts with macromolecules and target DNA in the nucleus and mitochondria.[12] Because there is a good correlation between the ability to form covalent DNA adducts and the potency to induce tumors in laboratory animals, DNA is considered the ultimate target for most genotoxic carcinogens. The interaction with DNA is not random, and each class of agents reacts selectively with purine and pyrimidine targets.[9] Furthermore, targeting of carcinogens to particular sites in DNA is determined by nucleotide sequence, by host cell, and by selective DNA repair processes, making some genetic material at risk over others. As expected from this chemistry, genotoxic carcinogens are potent mutagens, particularly adept at causing base mispairing or small deletions, leading to missense or nonsense mutations. Others may cause macrogenetic damage such as chromosome breaks and large deletions. In all cases, mutations detected in tumors represent a combination of the effect of the mutagenic change on the function of the protein product and the effect of the functional alteration on the behavior of the specific host cell type.

A number of chemicals that cause cancers in laboratory rodents and contribute to human skin cancer incidence are not demonstrably genotoxic. Synthetic pesticides and herbicides, dry-cleaning reagents, and arsenic may fall within this group. The mechanism of action by nongenotoxic carcinogens is controversial and may be related in some cases to toxic cell death and regenerative hyperplasia. Induction of endogenous mutagenic mechanisms such as DNA oxyradical damage, depurination of DNA, and deamination of 5-methylcytosine may contribute to carcinogenicity of these agents. Nongenotoxic carcinogens may interfere with host protective mechanisms, as has been suggested for the action of arsenic in suppressing DNA repair or inhibiting the activity of tumor-suppressor genes.[4] Thus, nongenotoxic carcinogens may serve as modifiers in concert with genotoxic agents such as UVR.

A number of metabolic pathways activate or detoxify carcinogens and procarcinogens (chemicals that can be transformed into active carcinogens). These pathways are complex and interactive,[10] and genetic polymorphisms, both in animal models and in humans, contribute to cancer susceptibility. In general, metabolic activation of carcinogens involves oxidation at carbon–carbon double bonds or saturated carbon atoms, or oxidation or reduction at nitrogen moieties yielding reactive intermediates that bind to DNA. Conjugates are also frequent intermediates of metabolism of many carcinogens and can be both activating and detoxifying pathways.[10] Metabolic activation of carcinogens and the polymorphic nature of metabolic activity among individuals provide an approach to estimate individual risk profiles for particular exposures. Furthermore, a number of metabolic pathways are inducible and modified by diet, hormones, and additional exposures, adding further complexity to the process of carcinogenesis.

HEREDITARY CANCER SYNDROMES

If DNA is the target for carcinogens and mutagenesis is the underlying mechanism of cancer pathogenesis, how do we determine the genetic targets that contribute to the phenotype of cutaneous neoplasms? Considerable insight into the genetic basis of sporadic skin cancers has come from the elucidation of specific genes or genetic loci that define hereditary skin tumor syndromes (Table 36-2).[11,12] In particular, the importance of DNA as a target for carcinogenesis was strongly supported by the discovery of defects in DNA repair genes that comprise the complementation groups of skin cancer prone xeroderma pigmentosum (XP) families (see Chap. 35). At least six independent genes, on distinct chromosomal loci, define proteins involved in nucleotide excision repair, a process critical for the protection of DNA against both UVR and chemical carcinogen-induced damage. Among these are proteins that recognize and bind to sites of DNA damage (XPA, XPC), helicases (XPB, XPD), and endonuclease components (XPG, XPF), defects in any of which give a skin cancer–prone phenotype. Potential polymorphisms with functional consequences in these and other DNA repair genes may also contribute to susceptibility states in the general population.[13,14] Examination of SCCs and BCCs from XP patients has also revealed potential target genes for cancer induction because signature mutations in *PTCH1, Ras, p53,* and *INK4a-ARF* (*p16^{INK4a}* and *ARF*) have been found with high frequency.[15,16] Chromosomal mapping studies in the nevoid basal cell carcinoma syndrome (Chap. 82), coupled with genetic and functional studies in *Drosophila,* implicated mutations in the *PTCH1* gene and other defects in the Sonic hedgehog (Shh) signaling pathway in the development of hereditary and many sporadic BCCs.[17] The *INK4a* locus, and specifically mutations in the *p16^{INK4a}* gene, was identified in the etiology of hereditary melanoma[18] through mapping of the inheritance pattern of familial melanoma. Detection of specific mutations in Cowden's syndrome (*PTEN*), Muir-Torre syndrome (*MSH2, MLH1*), pilomatricoma [*CTNNB* (*β-catenin*)], and trichoepithelioma (*PTCH1, p16^{INK4a}*) has illuminated defects associated with the development of adnexal tumors. The delineation of the specific genes mutated in other syndromes where locus mapping is confirmed (see Table 36-2) should provide even more insight into the broader spectrum of skin neoplasms.

ANIMAL MODELS VERIFY THE GENETIC BASIS FOR CUTANEOUS NEOPLASMS

Using human hereditary cancer syndromes as a guide, genetically based animal models have been developed that validate the contribution of individual genes to human cancer susceptibility by prospective experimental analysis.[19] These models have also contributed to the understanding of gene-environment interactions by testing the influence of chemical and physical carcinogens on tumor development in the setting of an altered genetic makeup. The discovery of inactivating *PTCH1* and *SMO* mutations in BCCs (Fig. 36-1) led to the development of several mouse models exploring the role of deregulated Shh signaling in BCC tumorigenesis. Keratinocyte-targeted overexpression of Shh or an

TABLE 36-2

Gene Targets for Mutations in Hereditary and Sporadic Cutaneous Cancers

GENE	FUNCTION	LOCUS	TUMOR TYPE	SYNDROME	SPONTANEOUS
p53	DNA repair, apoptosis, cell cycle regulation	17p13.1	BCC, SCC	Li Fraumeni (but no increase in skin cancers)	Yes
XPA, XPB *XPC, XPD* *XPF, XPG*	DNA repair	3p25, 2q21 9q22.3, 19q13.3 16p13.3-13, 13q22	BCC, SCC, melanoma	Xeroderma pigmentosum	Possible
PTCH1	Sonic hedgehog receptor	9q22.3	BCC, trichoepithelioma	Nevoid basal cell carcinoma	Yes
SMO	Sonic hedgehog effector	7q31-32	BCC	?	Yes
p16^{INK4a}	Cyclin inhibitor	9p21	Melanoma, SCC, trichoepithelioma	Dysplastic nevus	Yes
CTNNB (*β-catenin*)	Cell–cell adhesion, transcription factor	3p22-p21.3	Pilomatricoma	?	Yes
CYLDI	Unknown	16q12-13	Cylindroma	Multiple cylindroma	Yes
PTEN	Phosphatase	10q23.3	Trichilemmoma	Cowden's	Unknown
MSH2 *MLH1*	Mismatch repair	2p22-p21 3p21.3	Sebaceous gland carcinoma	Muir-Torre	Unknown
?	?	9p21	Trichoepithelioma	Multiple trichoepithelioma	Unknown
?	?	Xq24-q27	BCC	Bazex	Unknown
?	?	9q31	Keratoacanthoma	Ferguson-Smith	Unknown

SOURCE: Reprinted from Dlugosz A et al,[19] with permission of Blackwell Publishing, Oxford, UK.

FIGURE 36-1

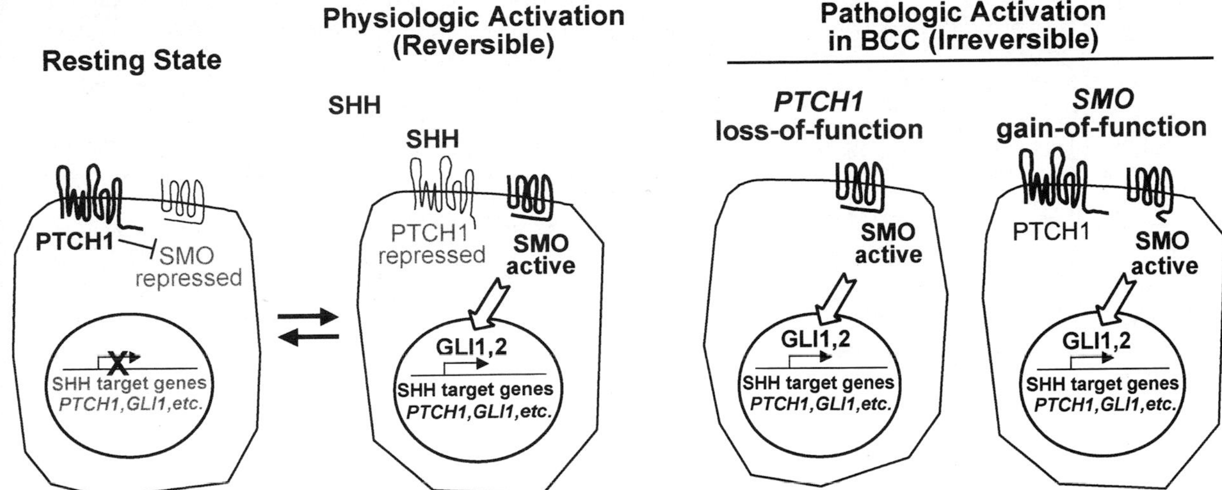

Current model depicting proposed molecular basis of basal cell carcinoma. In contrast to the stepwise evolution of SCC, which affects multiple signaling pathways, clinical and experimental studies suggest that deregulation of the SHH pathway plays a central role in BCC development, and may be sufficient for tumorigenesis. In the absence of SHH in normal cells (resting state), signaling is repressed due to inhibition of the transmembrane protein SMO by PTCH1. During physiologic activation of this pathway, secreted SHH binds and inhibits PTCH1, resulting in SMO-mediated signaling and induction of the SHH target genes *PTCH1, GLI1,* and others, which are likely to influence cellular growth control. GLI1 and GLI2 are candidate nuclear effectors regulating expression of target genes. In contrast to reversible, SHH-dependent signaling under normal conditions, this pathway is constitutively activated in basal cell carcinomas and certain other tumors: *PTCH1* mutations result in functional loss of the inhibitory PTCH1 protein, while *SMO* mutations result in an altered SMO protein that is largely resistant to inhibition by PTCH1. (*Modified from Dlugosz A et al,*[19] *with permission of Blackwell Publishing, Oxford, UK.*)

activated form of the downstream signaling molecule SMO (M2SMO) resulted in the development of basal cell–like proliferations in newborn mouse skin. Overexpression of SHH in human keratinocytes grafted onto severe combined immunodeficiency disease (SCID) mice also resulted in BCC-like lesions. Mice with heterozygous disruption of the *Ptchl* gene have features in common with nevoid basal cell carcinoma syndrome patients, including microscopic hair follicle–derived tumors and various macroscopic skin tumors, including BCCs, after treatment with UVR or ionizing radiation.[20] When Gli1 or Gli2 transcription factors, which are nuclear effectors of Shh signaling, are targeted to mouse keratinocytes, multiple BCCs develop. Interestingly, Gli1 mice displayed a variety of follicle-derived tumors with relatively few BCCs,[21] while Gli2 mice developed BCCs exclusively.[22] Collectively, these findings provide strong evidence that constitutive Shh signaling plays a key role in, and may be sufficient for, BCC development.

The multistage induction of cutaneous SCC (Fig. 36-2) and the absence of a hereditary syndrome that specifically imparts uniquely high susceptibility to this lesion have made the delineation of specific genetic loci involved in SCC induction more complex. Nevertheless, the analysis of genetic defects in human SCCs has focused attention on specific targets such as DNA repair genes, *Ras, p53, p16*^{INK4a}, and the epidermal growth factor receptor (EGFR) pathway (Table 36-3). Mouse models for XPA, XPC, and XPD deficiency have been constructed, and all show sensitivity to UVR and enhanced development of SCC after either UVR or chemical carcinogen exposure.[23] A number of other DNA repair-deficient mutant mice are also being tested for cancer susceptibility and may reveal the mechanistic basis for new clinical syndromes by reverse genetics.[23] Mouse mutants targeting the *ras* gene have revealed important information concerning the contribution of the Ras pathway to particular stages of SCC development. Heterozygous activating *ras* gene mutations are sufficient to induce a benign squamous papilloma, the precursor to SCC, and the yield of chemically induced tumors in mice genetically deleted in the *H-ras* allele is markedly reduced.[24] Homozygosity of a mutant *ras* gene is associated with progression to SCC, suggesting that high penetrance of the Ras pathway can recruit additional changes required for progression. Transgenic targeting of oncogenic *ras* to suprabasal epidermis produces terminally benign tumors while targeting to basal cells or hair follicle outer root sheath cells encourages progression to SCC, indicating that the target cell for early mutations may also determine the tumor phenotype.[25] While heterozygous *p53* inactivation is detected early in human SCC, *p53* deletion in mice enhances malignant progression but does not increase benign tumor formation. This may be analogous to the common loss of heterozygosity (LOH) seen at the *p53* locus later in human SCC development.[26] Of particular interest for human tumor development is the frequent observation that double heterozygotes for *p53* deletion and other cancer-prone phenotypes (such as DNA repair deficiency) further sensitize mouse skin to tumor induction by UVR or chemical carcinogens.[23] Mice with genetically defined defects in the *p16*^{INK4a} locus or its downstream effector CDK4 are sensitive to both squamous tumor and melanoma induction after treatment with carcinogenic chemicals, consistent with defects in this pathway detected in both melanoma and nonmelanoma human skin cancers.[27,28]

TUMOR BIOLOGY AND BIOCHEMISTRY

General Principles

Malignant tumors exhibit fundamental alterations in behavior that distinguish them from the normal tissues in which they arise. These differences include a reduced requirement for growth stimuli, impaired response to growth inhibitory/differentiation signals, alterations in apoptosis, delayed or blocked senescence, prolonged angiogenesis, and the capacity for invasion and metastasis. Although one or more of these abnormalities can be detected at different stages of tumor progression and may thus be seen in premalignant lesions, all are present in advanced

FIGURE 36-2

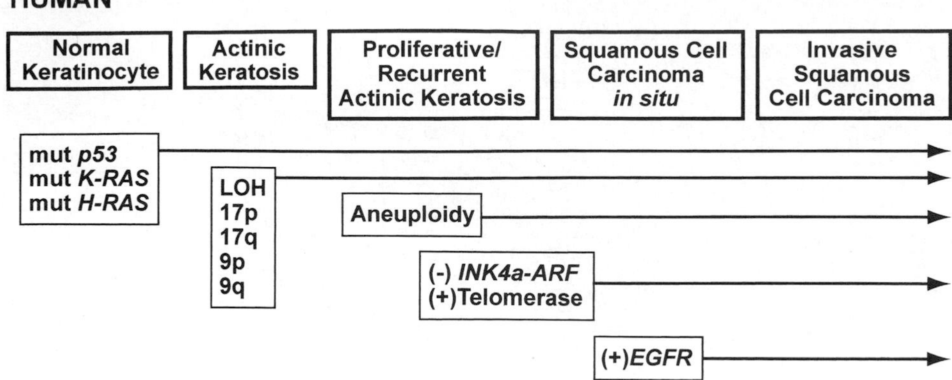

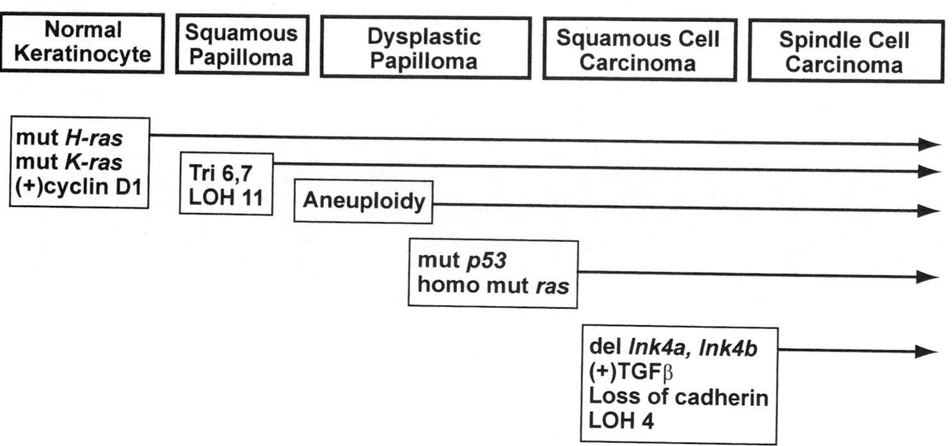

Genetic changes associated with development of cutaneous squamous cell carcinomas. The multistage evolution of invasive squamous cell cancer in humans is depicted schematically with frequently associated genetic changes. Single base mutations in early lesions frequently are characteristic of ultraviolet light-induced damage, while later changes are associated with genomic instability. Increased activity of telomerase (deletion of inhibitor) or epidermal growth factor receptor (EGFR) tyrosine kinase (gene amplification) may also result from epigenetic changes. In chemically induced mouse cutaneous squamous cell carcinoma, the multistage evolution to anaplastic or spindle cell tumors in this model is highly ordered, both temporally and genetically. *Ras* mutations are characteristic of chemical mutagens used to initiate tumor formation. Early upregulation of cyclin D1 and later upregulation of transforming growth factor (TGF)-β_1 occur through epigenetic mechanisms and appear to be important components of carcinogenesis. (*Modified from Dlugosz A et al,[19] with permission of Blackwell Publishing, Oxford, UK. Assistance for the construction of this figure was provided by Luowei Li, M.D.*)

cancers. The driving force behind these changes is genomic instability, which facilitates the accumulation of mutations in both oncogenes and tumor-suppressor genes that contribute to the observed aberrations in cell function.[29] While some of these changes are cell autonomous and can be studied in purified populations of tumor cells, others depend on various additional cell types recruited to participate in the development and progression of cancer in intact organisms. Both the intrinsic alterations in neoplastic keratinocytes and the influence of collaborating cell types in skin tumor biology are being elucidated through the use of experimental models.

From analyses of both human SCC pathogenesis and experimental skin tumor induction by chemical carcinogens, specific premalignant and malignant stages have been identified that have typical phenotypic, genetic and biochemical characteristics (Fig. 36-2). Note that in contrast to SCCs and most other cancers, BCCs do not appear to have precursor lesions or give rise to more aggressive cancers. This is likely related to the observation that the genomic instability that fuels neoplastic progression in other tumor types is largely missing in BCCs, even though a substantial proportion of these tumors harbor *p53* mutations that would be expected to facilitate the accumulation of additional genetic defects. SCC starts as a single or small number of specific mutations in a cell that has the capacity to cycle, a change understood as the "initiation" of carcinogenesis. Upon clonal expansion, initiated cells form a premalignant lesion, such as a squamous papilloma in the mouse or an actinic keratosis in the human. Agents that enhance clonal expansion of initiated cells are called tumor promoters. Tumor promotion may occur as a consequence of exogenous exposures such as UVR, topical chemicals or medications, infections, or wound healing. Promotion may be an endogenous process influenced by diet, smoking, or immune suppression. The acquisition of additional mutations that provide a growth advantage to the incipient cancer cell may also serve as an autonomous promoting stimulus. Premalignant lesions undergo further phenotypic changes, often in a predictable sequence and commonly multifocal within a single lesion.[30] Some foci or lesions progress at a faster rate than others, and these are at highest risk for malignant conversion.[31] Premalignant progression encompasses the majority of the tumor latency period prior to malignant conversion, when the lesion shows invasive properties.

Initiation is usually a low-frequency genetic event and is directly dependent on carcinogen dose. A large variety of carcinogen classes can initiate skin tumors in rodents (Table 36-3). The phenotype of initiated epidermal cells as defined from in vitro analysis includes a defect in maturation, escape from senescence, and an enhanced growth potential, but initiated cells are still responsive to negative regulation, for example by TGF-β. At the molecular level, initiation involves an alteration in signal transduction pathways that regulate cellular responses to extracellular signals, and these are internally regulated by protooncogenes and tumor-suppressor genes.[32] Tumor promotion is generally a nongenotoxic stimulus that results in a disturbance of tissue homeostasis.[30] Multiple classes of agents have promoting properties in experimental skin carcinogenesis (Table 36-3). The mechanisms of tumor promotion include activation of cell surface receptors, activation or inhibition of cytosolic enzymes and nuclear transcription factors, stimulation of proliferation, inhibition of apoptotic cell death, and direct cytotoxicity. Genotoxic carcinogens also can have promoting

TABLE 36-3

Examples of Agents Capable of Inducing Skin Cancer in Rodents

Initiating Agents	Promoting Agents
Polycyclic aromatic hydrocarbons	Phorbol esters
Benzo[a]pyrene*	12-*O*-Tetradecanoylphorbol-13-acetate
7,12-Dimethylbenz[a]anthracene	Croton oil*
3-Methylcholanthrene	Aromatics
Tobacco tar*	Phenol*
Dibenz(a,h)anthracene*	Anthralin*
Aromatic amines	7-Bromomethylbenz[a]anthracene
2-Acetylaminofluorene	Other
Alkylating agents	Dihydroteleocidin (fungal product)*
β-Propiolactone*	Wounding*
4-Nitroquinoline-*N*-oxide	Abrasion*
Bis(chloromethyl)ether*	Cigarette smoke condensate*
Nitrogen mustard*	Benzoyl peroxide*
Cisplatin*	2,3,7,8-Tetrachlorodibenzo-*p*-dioxin*
Nitrosamines and nitrosamides	Diacylglycerols
N,N′-Dimethylnitrosourea*	Ultraviolet radiation*
N-Methyl-*N′*-nitro-*N*-nitrosoguanidine*	Dodecane
Other	Retinoic acid*
Urethane*	
Dinitropyrene*	
Ionizing radiation*	
Ultraviolet radiation*	

*Known human contact.

properties, and repeated exposures to low concentrations of genotoxic carcinogens can induce tumors more effectively than fewer exposures to the same total dose in experimental carcinogenesis. Exogenous tumor promoters can determine the target site for tumor formation, and the promoting action of UVR may, in part, contribute to skin targeting for tumors when germ-line mutations produce an initiated state in multiple cell types. In general, initiated cells respond differently to promoters than normal cells, allowing for clonal selection of an initiated population.[33] Premalignant progression in an initiated cell clone occurs spontaneously but is accelerated by additional exposures to genotoxic agents including some cancer chemotherapeutic drugs.[34] Premalignant progression in chemically induced mouse skin carcinogenesis is associated with nonrandom, sequential chromosomal aberrations including amplifications, duplications, deletions, and loss of heterozygosity, suggesting repeated episodes of cell selection, producing specific chromosomal aberrations that become modally dominant within the progressing focus. Thus, at least one function of the relevant genetic events in premalignant progression must result in a growth advantage for the affected cell. Epigenetic changes are also associated with malignant conversion, and upregulation of AP-1 transcriptional activity, alterations in cell-cycle regulatory genes and secreted proteases, and changes in gene splicing and expression of modified cell surface molecules have all been reported. Together these changes could facilitate migration and invasion that characterize the malignant phenotypes. Alterations in methylation of DNA in tumor cells could also contribute to this stage of carcinogenesis.[35]

The Pathogenesis of Basal Cell Carcinomas

(see Chaps. 81 and 82)

Animal models for induction of skin tumors by chemical and physical agents have been extremely valuable for exploring mechanisms of carcinogenesis in an experimental setting (Table 36-4). Rats exposed to chemical carcinogens [3-methylcholanthrene (MCA), 7,12-dimethylbenzanthracene (DMBA)] or ionizing radiation preferentially develop BCCs that are phenotypically similar to human BCCs. In contrast, mice are resistant to BCC induction in the absence of genetic modification, and even *Ptch1*± mutant mice (modeling patients with nevoid basal cell carcinoma syndrome) develop SCC in addition to BCC when treated with UVR.[20] Interestingly, mice develop BCC when exposed either subcutaneously or topically to dehydroretronecine,[36] an observation that has never been explored mechanistically.

As noted earlier, BCCs represent an intriguing exception to the rule of multistage cancer development. These tumors consist of homogeneous, slowly growing cells that very rarely metastasize, although they can cause extensive local damage. Even those rare BCCs exhibiting cellular atypia generally have a benign course, suggesting that the full complement of factors driving malignant progression in SCCs and other neoplasms is not operating in these tumors. BCC cells exhibit abnormalities in growth control and terminal differentiation, induce clinically apparent angiogenesis, and invade their immediate surroundings. However, transplantation studies using human BCCs or transgenic mouse skin with BCC-like lesions suggest that the tumor cells are critically dependent on adjacent stroma for survival. This property may help explain both the lack of BCC metastases and the difficulty in establishing BCC cell lines.

Studies performed using human and rodent BCCs have identified candidate molecules that may be important in the biology of these tumors. Upregulation of various matrix metalloproteases (MMPs), both in tumor cells and stroma, is likely to be important in the local invasion of BCC, and may impact on growth control and other cellular functions given the emerging role of MMPs in regulating signaling at multiple levels.[37] Expression of several adhesion molecules is downregulated in BCCs, which may account for the characteristic appearance of clefts

TABLE 36-4

Animal Models for Cutaneous Cancer Induction by Exogenous Agents

Experimental Models for Basal Cell Carcinoma		
Agent	**Species**	**Comments**
MCA	Rat	Other skin tumors
DMBA	Rat	SCC > BCC; lower DMBA doses may increase BCC incidence
Ionizing radiation	Rat	Other skin tumors
Dehydroretronecine	Mouse	BCC > SCC, also internal tumors
Experimental Models for Squamous Cell Tumor Induction		
Agent	**Species**	**Comments**
(PAH, NA, AA) + promoter	Mouse, rat	Predominantly papilloma
(PAH, NA, AA) repeated	Mouse, rat	Predominantly SCC
UVB	Mouse	p53 mutations, immune suppression, SCC
UVA	Mouse	Papillomas and SCC

Abbreviations: AA, aromatic amines; DMBA, 7,12-dimethyl-benzanthracene; MCA, 3-methylcholanthrene; NA, nitrosamines; PAH, polycyclic aromatic hydrocarbons.

between tumor cells and stroma in histologic sections, but the functional significance of this finding in BCC biology has not been established. The antiapoptotic molecule Bcl-2 is consistently upregulated in BCCs, but does not appear sufficient to block apoptosis in these tumors as it does in other settings. Indeed, the remarkably slow growth rate of BCCs has been attributed to apoptotic cell loss. Expression studies in human BCCs and experimental models suggest the involvement of growth factor signaling pathways such as platelet-derived growth factor (PDGF).[38] Several lines of evidence point to components of the cell-cycle machinery as potentially critical targets in mitogenic responses to Shh signaling. Keratinocytes overexpressing Shh have enhanced proliferative potential and fail to undergo growth arrest in response to the cell cycle inhibitor p21;[39] in the absence of Shh, Ptch1 interacts with and may sequester Cyclin B1, a component of M-phase promoting factor that is required for mitosis and cell-cycle progression;[40] and Shh can drive proliferation of immature cerebellar cells by causing prolonged induction of Cyclins D1, D2, and E.[41] As additional Shh target molecules are uncovered, their potential involvement in keratinocyte tumor biology can be examined using the recently-developed mouse models of BCC.

The Pathogenesis of Squamous Cell Carcinomas

(see Chaps. 79 and 80)

Both mice and rats are sensitive to SCC induction by a variety of chemical and physical agents (see Table 36-4), and the induction of SCC in mice by UVR closely mimics the pathogenesis of SCC in human skin. In addition, multistage chemical carcinogenesis in mouse skin is a powerful tool for delineating many of the fundamental concepts underlying epithelial carcinogenesis in other organs. Building on the association of deregulated EGFR signaling in human cancer, mouse models suggest that constitutive EGFR activation is an important component of skin tumor formation because transgenic targeting of TGF-α to the epidermis can produce a benign tumor phenotype in the absence of activating *ras* mutations.[42] However, activation of the EGFR by ligand overexpression is not sufficient for autonomous tumor formation because many of these tumors regressed. Nevertheless, small benign skin tumors form upon oncogenic *ras* transformation of *EGFR* null keratinocytes, suggesting that a *ras*-induced compensatory pathway for tumor growth exists in the premalignant tumor.[43] Additional evidence implicating enhanced growth factor signaling in SCC is provided by transgenic studies that use a dominant form of SOS, an adapter molecule involved in transducing growth-stimulatory signals from receptor tyrosine kinases such as EGFR, which result in spontaneous development of papillomas in mouse skin.[44] Overexpression of ErbB2, a receptor tyrosine kinase related to and capable of interacting with EGFR, results in spontaneous skin tumor development in transgenic mice.[45] Insulin-like growth factor-1 (IGF-1), when overexpressed in mouse skin, also triggerled development of squamous papillomas, some of which progressed to carcinomas.[46] While most of these studies invoke an autocrine mechanism for growth stimulation of tumor cells, factors produced by cells in the tumor stroma may also supply mitogenic or angiogenic signals to keratinocytes.[47] Additional studies performed in mice suggest that specific components of the cell-cycle machinery, including E2F1, cyclin D1, and Cdk4, can contribute to SCC development and/or progression.

In addition to deregulated growth control, there is a progressive loss in the capacity for terminal differentiation during SCC progression (see Fig. 36-2), culminating in a tumor with a spindle cell morphology that is indistinguishable from malignancies originating in mesenchymal tissues. Although the mechanisms responsible for defective differentiation at different stages of human skin cancer are not known, there is evidence that deregulation of the protein kinase C (PKC) family of enzymes plays a role in aberrant differentiation of mouse skin keratinocytes expressing the *ras* oncogene.[30] PKCδ, which has been implicated in terminal differentiation of normal epidermal keratinocytes, is rendered inactive as a result of tyrosine-phosphorylation in ras-transformed keratinocytes. Restoring PKCδ to its native, nontyrosine phosphorylated state reversed the block to terminal differentiation in ras-transformed keratinocytes. In addition, overexpression of PKCδ in the skin of transgenic mice inhibits the development of squamous papillomas and carcinomas.[48] In contrast, skin-targeted overexpression of PKCε resulted in less differentiated SCCs that rapidly metastasized to regional lymph nodes.[49] Additional work is needed to better understand the mechanism by which SCC tumor cells evade signals that trigger differentiation of normal keratinocytes.

Prostaglandin metabolism (see Chap. 34) is activated by UV radiation and is constitutively induced in human SCCs, probably due to overexpression of the enzyme cyclooxygenase-2 (COX-2). Although the mechanism by which changes in prostaglandins influence skin cancer is not clear, prostaglandins appear to operate at the tumor promotion stage. Telomerase activity is detected in a substantial proportion of human skin cancers, suggesting that these tumor cells are capable of evading cellular senescence, and telomerase-deficient mice are resistant to chemical carcinogenesis.[50] Additional contributors that are likely to be involved in SCC development and progression include mediators of angiogenesis, MMPs, and integrins, as well as other molecules involved in cellular adhesion and migration.

Spontaneous or carcinogen-induced tumor formation on genetically modified mice has revealed genes and pathways that appear to be important in skin cancer induction but would not have been apparent from hereditary cancer syndromes or analysis of human skin cancers. Suprabasal targeting of c-Myc in transgenic mice permits suprabasal cells to cycle and produces the papilloma phenotype while basal cell targeting of c-Myc is not oncogenic.[51] Deletion of the cyclin/CDK inhibitor p21^{waf1}, a downstream effector of p53, increases the number of benign tumors but not the rate of premalignant progression.[52,53] TGF-β suppresses premalignant progression but is required for progression from SCC to a spindle-cell phenotype.[54] Two AP-1 transcription factors influence distinct stages of skin tumor development, where c-Jun is essential for papilloma and c-Fos is essential for SCC development.[55] Additional molecules now implicated in experimentally induced mouse SCCs are ornithine decarboxylase, p16^{Ink4a}, p15^{Ink4b}, and E-cadherin.[56–58] These pathways are frequently altered in human SCC, but their contribution to pathogenesis remains to be proven by studies that directly transform human keratinocytes and study them in an in vivo setting.

Constitutional Modifiers of Carcinogenesis

Inbred mouse strains differ in susceptibility to particular carcinogenic exposures by several orders of magnitude, and transplantation studies indicate sensitivity resides in the target tissue rather than systemically. Genomic scans of backcrossed mice among sensitive and resistant mouse strains indicate that constitutional determinants are multigenic and distinct for benign tumor formation or progression.[59] Similar studies indicate genetic loci determine the survival potential for tumor-bearing animals.[60] While identifying genes involved in susceptibility and resistance in animal models is likely to reveal determinants important for human skin cancer risk, the classic genetic approaches are difficult and complex because multiple interacting loci are likely to be involved.[61] Genetically modified mouse models have revealed pathways associated with skin tumor susceptibility. Alterations in p53, drug metabolizing enzymes, T cell function, and DNA repair modify risk for experimental skin cancer induction. Remarkably, polymorphisms in drug metabolizing enzymes and DNA repair pathways,[62,63] and variable responses in the p53 tumor-suppressor pathway or in T cell immunity after exposure to skin carcinogens,[64] modify the human risk for skin cancer.

Exogenous Modifiers of Carcinogenesis

In experimental models, antioxidants and agents that alter microsomal metabolism of carcinogens can reduce or prevent tumor initiation by inhibiting the formation of ultimate carcinogens or accelerating their detoxification (Table 36-5). Similar mechanisms may influence ultraviolet light or ionizing radiation mutagenesis through inhibition of mutagenic oxyradicals produced endogenously following exposure. Scavengers prevent reactive mutagens from reaching critical targets. Cell-cycle inhibitors prevent fixation of mutations, allowing for DNA repair while cytotoxic agents kill initiated cells prior to their expansion into a tumor mass.

A number of agents are effective in the postinitiation phase of experimental tumor development, and some are being clinically evaluated. Inhibitors of COX-2 (celecoxib, indomethacin) and ornithine decarboxylase (difluoromethylornithine) prevent both UVR and chemically induced tumors.[65,66] While the mechanism of action of retinoids as modifiers of tumor development is not clear, retinoids are effective inhibitors of benign tumor formation in mouse skin carcinogenesis studies, and show promise as inhibitors of actinic keratoses and cutaneous tumors in human studies (see Chap. 257). Predictable and parallel alterations in retinoid receptors in mouse and human cutaneous SCC indicate that the retinoid pathway must be central to cancer development in epidermis.[67] Considerable interest has developed in dietary factors that modify skin carcinogenesis. Restricted fat/energy diets reduce papilloma incidence in mouse models[68] and decrease the frequency of actinic keratoses in human populations.[69] Diverse dietary or natural factors such as green tea, caffeic acid phenethyl ester from honey bee hives, resveratrol from grapes, silymarin from milk thistle, ginger extract, crocetin, and ursolic acid from the rosemary plant are among natural products shown to be effective inhibitors of skin tumor formation by topical application or systemic exposure.[70] Several of these agents are believed to be antioxidants, but the precise mechanism of inhibition and their effectiveness as chemopreventive agents for human skin cancer remain to be established. Finally, immune response modifiers such as imiquimod may be effective for treating some types of skin cancer by modulating cytokine expression.[71]

TABLE 36-5

Modifiers of Carcinogenesis

INHIBITOR CLASS	EXAMPLES
	INHIBITORS OF INITIATION
Antioxidants, scavengers	Butylated hydroxyanisole; butylated hydroxytoluene; selenium; vitamin C; vitamin E; ellagic acid
Inducers of mixed function oxidase	Polycyclic aromatic hydrocarbons; TCDD; PCB
Inhibitors of mixed function oxidase	α-Naphthoflavone; glucocorticoids
Cytotoxic agent	Sulfur mustard
Suppressor of tumor development	Retinoids
	INHIBITORS OF PROMOTION
Antiproliferative	Anti-inflammatory steroids: dexamethasone, fluocinolone acetonide; inhibitors of arachidonic acid metabolism: indomethacin, celecoxib; inhibitors of polyamine metabolism: α-difluoromethylornithine
Antioxidant	Antioxidants: tert-butylhydroxyanisole, selenium; protease inhibitors: leupeptin, tosyl lysine chloromethylketone; superoxide dismutase; copper (II) 3,5-diisopropylsalicylic acid
Natural products and dietary factors	Retinoic acid; vitamin D; green tea; silymarin; resveratrol; ursolic acid; caffeic acid phenethyl ester; curcumin; 1,25-dihydroxyvitamin D_3

ABBREVIATIONS: PCB, polychlorinated biphenyl; TCDD, 2,3,7,8-tetrachlorodibenzo-*p*-dioxin.

NOVEL MOLECULAR TARGETS BASED ON NEW MECHANISTIC DATA

The substantial progress in our understanding of factors involved in skin tumor pathogenesis holds the promise of new approaches to treatment and prevention. In addition to the identification of new therapeutic targets, improved strategies are being developed for altering gene and protein function in skin with great selectivity. The abundance and unrivaled accessibility of skin cancers and precancers makes them prime targets for rigorous translational studies and clinical trials. Based on the basic research studies outlined above, potential therapeutic targets include p53; COX-2; telomerase; EGFR or other receptor tyrosine kinases, and intracellular signaling elements such as SOS; Ras; ornithine decarboxylase; the DNA repair machinery; MMPs; PKC; molecules involved in cell-cycle progression, such as cyclins D1 and D2, CDK4, $p16^{INK4a}$, and E2F1; retinoid receptors; and c-Fos. In all cases, the potential efficacy of the proposed treatments would need to be carefully evaluated in animal models or human tissues grown in immune-deficient mice. Because the great majority of cutaneous SCCs are effectively treated using surgery or radiation therapy, perhaps the greatest utility of these studies for dermatology patients would be in the identification of agents capable of preventing the appearance of premalignant lesions or blocking neoplastic progression to SCC in predisposed individuals. Along these lines, a recent double-blind study reported a significant reduction in the development of actinic keratoses and BCCs in xeroderma pigmentosum patients treated topically with the DNA repair enzyme T4 endonuclease V, administered over a 1-year period.[72]

In contrast to the multiple genetic and biochemical changes associated with SCC development, the majority of BCCs have mutations in *PTCH1* or *SMO*, and essentially all of these tumors exhibit uncontrolled activation of the Shh pathway. Because several experimental models suggest that deregulated Shh signaling may be sufficient for BCC formation, this pathway is a prime target for mechanism-based drug development. Cyclopamine and related molecules block Shh signaling by inhibiting SMO function and may therefore be useful clinically. However, Shh is a key embryonic signaling molecule whose inhibition causes profound developmental defects, so attempts to treat or prevent human BCCs by modulating this pathway will need to be approached with care. Given the recent advances in our understanding of nonmelanoma skin cancer, it seems likely that new, rationally designed medical approaches for intervention will soon be available for these common neoplasms.

REFERENCES

1. Pott P: Cancer scrotic, in *Chirurgical Observations Relative to the Cataract, the Polypus of the Nose, the Cancer of the Scrotum, the Different Kinds of Ruptures, and the Mortification of the Toes and Feet.* London, Hawes, Clarke, and Collins, 1775, p 63
2. De Hertog S et al: Relation between smoking and skin cancer. *J Clin Oncol* **19**:231, 2001
3. Schwartz RA: Arsenic and the skin. *Int J Dermatol* **36**:241, 1997
4. Rossman TG et al: Arsenite is a cocarcinogen with solar ultraviolet radiation for mouse skin: An animal model for arsenic carcinogenesis. *Toxicol Appl Pharmacol* **176**:64, 2001
5. Penn I: Post-transplant malignancy: The role of immunosuppression. *Drug Saf* **23**:101, 2000
6. Lichter MD et al: Therapeutic ionizing radiation and the incidence of basal cell carcinoma and squamous cell carcinoma. The New Hampshire Skin Cancer Study Group. *Arch Dermatol* **136**:1007, 2000
7. Stern RS et al: Oral psoralen and ultraviolet-A light (PUVA) treatment of psoriasis and persistent risk of nonmelanoma skin cancer. PUVA Follow-up Study. *J Natl Cancer Inst* **90**:1278, 1998
8. Harwood CA et al: Detection of human papillomavirus DNA in PUVA-associated non-melanoma skin cancers. *J Invest Dermatol* **111**:123, 1998
9. Dipple A: DNA adducts of chemical carcinogens. *Carcinogenesis* **16**:437, 1995
10. Yuspa SH, Shields PG: Etiology of Cancer: Chemical Factors, in *Cancer Principles of Oncology,* 5th ed, edited by VT DeVita, S Hellman, SA Rosenberg. Philadelphia, Lippincott-Raven, 1997, p 185
11. Halpern AC, Altman JF: Genetic predisposition to skin cancer. *Curr Opin Oncol* **11**:132, 1999
12. Tsao H: Genetics of nonmelanoma skin cancer. *Arch Dermatol* **137**:1486, 2001
13. Wood RD et al: Human DNA repair genes. *Science* **291**:1284, 2001
14. Winsey SL et al: A variant within the DNA repair gene XRCC3 is associated with the development of melanoma skin cancer. *Cancer Res* **60**:5612, 2000
15. Soufir N et al: Association between INK4a-ARF and p53 mutations in skin carcinomas of xeroderma pigmentosum patients. *J Natl Cancer Inst* **92**:1841, 2000
16. Bodak N et al: High levels of patched gene mutations in basal-cell carcinomas from patients with xeroderma pigmentosum. *Proc Natl Acad Sci U S A* **96**:5117, 1999
17. Bale AE, Yu KP: The hedgehog pathway and basal cell carcinomas. *Hum Mol Genet* **10**:757, 2001
18. Hussussian CJ et al: Germline p16 mutations in familial melanoma. *Nat Genet* **8**:15, 1994
19. Dlugosz A et al: Progress in cutaneous cancer research. *J Invest Dermatol* 2003 (in press)
20. Aszterbaum M et al: Ultraviolet and ionizing radiation enhance the growth of BCCs and trichoblastomas in patched heterozygous knockout mice. *Nat Med* **5**:1285, 1999
21. Nilsson M et al: Induction of basal cell carcinomas and trichoepitheliomas in mice overexpressing GLI-1. *Proc Natl Acad Sci U S A* **97**:3438, 2000
22. Grachtchouk M et al: Basal cell carcinomas in mice overexpressing Gli2 in skin. *Nat Genet* **24**:216, 2000
23. Friedberg EC, Meira LB: Database of mouse strains carrying targeted mutations in genes affecting cellular responses to DNA damage. Version 4. *Mutat Res* **459**:243, 2000
24. Ise K et al: Targeted deletion of the H-ras gene decreases tumor formation in mouse skin carcinogenesis. *Oncogene* **19**:2951, 2000
25. Brown K et al: The malignant capacity of skin tumours induced by expression of a mutant H-ras transgene depends on the cell type targeted. *Curr Biol* **8**:516, 1998
26. Ahmadian A et al: Genetic instability in the 9q22.3 region is a late event in the development of squamous cell carcinoma. *Oncogene* **17**:1837, 1998
27. Krimpenfort P et al: Loss of p16Ink4a confers susceptibility to metastatic melanoma in mice. *Nature* **413**:83, 2001
28. Sotillo R et al: Invasive melanoma in Cdk4-targeted mice. *Proc Natl Acad Sci U S A* **98**:13312, 2001
29. Lengauer C et al: Genetic instabilities in human cancers. *Nature* **396**:643, 1998
30. Yuspa SH: The pathogenesis of squamous cell cancer: Lessons learned from studies of skin carcinogenesis—Thirty-third G.H.A. Clowes Memorial Award Lecture. *Cancer Res* **54**:1178, 1994
31. Hennings H et al: Induction of papillomas with a high probability of conversion to malignancy. *Carcinogenesis* **6**:1607, 1985
32. Blume-Jensen P, Hunter T: Oncogenic kinase signaling. *Nature* **411**:355, 2001
33. Hennings H et al: Development of an in vitro analogue of initiated mouse epidermis to study tumor promoters and antipromoters. *Cancer Res* **50**:4794, 1990
34. Hennings H et al: Enhanced malignant conversion of benign mouse skin tumors by cisplatin. *J Natl Cancer Inst* **82**:836, 1990
35. Robertson KD, Jones PA: DNA methylation: past, present and future directions. *Carcinogenesis* **21**:461, 2000
36. Johnson WD et al: Dehydroretronecine-induced skin tumors in mice. *J Natl Cancer Inst* **61**:85, 1978
37. Sternlicht MD, Werb Z: How matrix metalloproteinases regulate cell behavior. *Annu Rev Cell Dev Biol* **17**:463, 2001
38. Xie J et al: A role of PDGFRalpha in basal cell carcinoma proliferation. *Proc Natl Acad Sci U S A* **98**:9255, 2001
39. Fan H, Khavari PA: Sonic hedgehog opposes epithelial cell cycle arrest. *J Cell Biol* **147**:71, 1999
40. Barnes EA et al: Patched1 interacts with cyclin B1 to regulate cell cycle progression. *EMBO J* **20**:2214, 2001
41. Kenney AM, Rowitch DH: Sonic hedgehog promotes G(1) cyclin expression and sustained cell cycle progression in mammalian neuronal precursors. *Mol Cell Biol* **20**:9055, 2000
42. Dominey AM et al: Targeted overexpression of transforming growth factor α in the epidermis of transgenic mice elicits hyperplasia, hyperkeratosis, and spontaneous squamous papillomas. *Cell Growth Differ* **4**:1071, 1993
43. Hansen LA et al: The epidermal growth factor receptor is required to maintain the proliferative population in the basal compartment of epidermal tumors. *Cancer Res* **60**:3328, 2000
44. Sibilia M et al: The EGF receptor provides an essential survival signal for SOS-dependent skin tumor development. *Cell* **102**:211, 2000
45. Kiguchi K et al: Constitutive expression of erbB2 in epidermis of transgenic mice results in epidermal hyperproliferation and spontaneous skin tumor development. *Oncogene* **19**:4243, 2000
46. DiGiovanni J et al: Constitutive expression of insulin-like growth factor-1 in epidermal basal cells of transgenic mice leads to spontaneous tumor promotion. *Cancer Res* **60**:1561, 2000
47. Skobe M, Fusenig NE: Tumorigenic conversion of immortal human keratinocytes through stromal cell activation. *Proc Natl Acad Sci U S A* **95**:1050, 1998
48. Reddig PJ et al: Transgenic mice overexpressing protein kinase C delta in the epidermis are resistant to skin tumor promotion by 12-*O*-tetradecanoylphorbol-13- acetate. *Cancer Res* **59**:5710, 1999
49. Jansen AP et al: Protein kinase C-epsilon transgenic mice: A unique model for metastatic squamous cell carcinoma. *Cancer Res* **61**:808, 2001
50. Gonzalez-Suarez E et al: Telomerase-deficient mice with short telomeres are resistant to skin tumorigenesis. *Nat Genet* **26**:114, 2000
51. Waikel RL et al: Deregulated expression of c-Myc depletes epidermal stem cells. *Nat Genet* **28**:165, 2001
52. Missero C et al: The absence of $p21^{Cip1/WAF1}$ alters keratinocyte growth and differentiation and promotes *ras*-tumor progression. *Genes Dev* **10**:3065, 1996
53. Weinberg WC et al: Genetic deletion of $p21^{WAF1}$ enhances papilloma formation but not malignant conversion in experimental mouse skin carcinogenesis. *Cancer Res* **59**:2050, 1999
54. Portella G et al: Transforming growth factor β is essential for spindle cell conversion of mouse skin carcinoma in vivo: Implications for tumor invasion. *Cell Growth Differ* **9**:393, 1998
55. Young MR et al: Transgenic mice demonstrate AP-1 (activator protein-1) transactivation is required for tumor promotion. *Proc Natl Acad Sci U S A* **96**:9827, 1999
56. Clifford A et al: Role of ornithine decarboxylase in epidermal tumorigenesis. *Cancer Res* **55**:1680, 1995
57. Linardopoulos S et al: Deletion and altered regulation of $p16^{INK4a}$ and $p15^{INK4b}$ in undifferentiated mouse skin tumors. *Cancer Res* **55**:5168, 1995
58. Navarro P et al: A role for the E-cadherin cell–cell adhesion molecule during tumor progression of mouse epidermal carcinogenesis. *J Cell Biol* **115**:517, 1991
59. Mock BA et al: Multigenic control of skin tumor susceptibility in SENCAR/Pt mice. *Carcinogenesis* **19**:1109, 1998
60. Nagase H et al: A subset of skin tumor modifier loci determines survival time of tumor-bearing mice. *Proc Natl Acad Sci U S A* **96**:15032, 1999
61. Balmain A: Cancer as a complex genetic trait. Tumor susceptibility in humans and mouse models. *Cell* **108**:145, 2002

62. Nelson HH et al: The XRCC1 Arg399Gln polymorphism, sunburn, and non-melanoma skin cancer: Evidence of gene-environment interaction. *Cancer Res* **62**:152, 2002
63. Lear JT et al: Detoxifying enzyme genotypes and susceptibility to cutaneous malignancy. *Br J Dermatol* **142**:8, 2000
64. Ramachandran S et al: Susceptibility and modifier genes in cutaneous basal cell carcinomas and their associations with clinical phenotype. *J Photochem Photobiol B* **63**:1, 2001
65. Fischer SM et al: Chemopreventive activity of celecoxib, a specific cyclooxygenase-2 inhibitor, and indomethacin against ultraviolet light-induced skin carcinogenesis. *Mol Carcinog* **25**:231, 1999
66. Takigawa M et al: Inhibition of mouse skin tumor promotion and of promoter-stimulated epidermal polyamine biosynthesis by difluoromethylornithine. *Cancer Res* **43**:3732, 1983
67. Xu XC et al: Progressive decreases in nuclear retinoid receptors during skin squamous carcinogenesis. *Cancer Res* **61**:4306, 2001

68. Birt DF et al: High-fat diet blocks the inhibition of skin carcinogenesis and reductions in protein kinase C by moderate energy restriction. *Mol Carcinog* **16**:115, 1996
69. Black HS et al: Effect of a low-fat diet on the incidence of actinic keratosis. *N Engl J Med* **330**:1272, 1994
70. Gupta S, Mukhtar H: Chemoprevention of skin cancer through natural agents. *Skin Pharmacol Appl Skin Physiol* **14**:373, 2001
71. Marks R et al: Imiquimod 5% cream in the treatment of superficial basal cell carcinoma: Results of a multicenter 6-week dose-response trial. *J Am Acad Dermatol* **44**:807, 2001
72. Yarosh D et al: Effect of topically applied T4 endonuclease V in liposomes on skin cancer in xeroderma pigmentosum: A randomised study. Xeroderma Pigmentosum Study Group. *Lancet* **357**:926, 2001

CHAPTER 37

Douglas R. Lowy

Oncogenes and Viral Carcinogenesis

The study of carcinogenesis induced by viruses has been influenced by several complementary goals. The cornerstone has been to detect transmissible etiologic agents of naturally occurring human tumors. The principal clinical importance of this goal is that once such viral agents are identified, it may be possible to use this information to intervene prophylactically or therapeutically by focusing attention on the virus. Prophylactic approaches to intervention include interrupting viral transmission through the development of effective prophylactic vaccines and the establishment of appropriate public health measures. Therapeutic approaches include viral-specific therapies via vaccines and drugs that interfere with an important viral function.

In recent years, compelling evidence has been presented for the role of viruses in the pathogenesis of several types of human tumors (Table 37-1).[1–5] Identification of hepatitis B virus as a cause of hepatocellular carcinoma and the development of an effective prophylactic vaccination against this virus demonstrated that the vaccine can reduce the incidence of liver carcinomas in an endemic area.[6]

Another important goal of viral carcinogenesis is to use tumor viruses to develop models for the experimental study of carcinogenesis (Table 37-2).[3,7,8] The ability of certain animal viruses to induce tumors experimentally in animal hosts was first shown in the early part of the twentieth century.[9] Since then, many animal viruses have been found to cause tumors either in their natural host species or in heterologous species. In addition to providing enormous insight into the mechanisms by which animal and human tumor viruses induce tumors, results derived from the analysis of viral carcinogenesis have also had direct implications for the pathogenesis of nonvirally induced tumors. These experimental studies uncovered a group of cellular genes (called *oncogenes* or *transforming genes*) that play an important pathogenetic role in many naturally occurring human tumors, as well as in those induced experimentally by viruses, carcinogens, and ionizing radiation.[7,8,10] Tumor virology has also provided important insights into the function of *tumor-suppressor genes*. This class of cellular genes, which normally inhibit unrestrained cell growth, also plays key roles in the development of many human tumors not associated with viruses.[11,12] Tumor virus systems emphasize the theme that tumors are induced by specific proteins, which can be encoded either by viral or cellular genes, as well as the important contribution of host and environmental factors in determining whether infection will result in a benign or malignant outcome.[11,13,14]

EXPERIMENTAL VIRAL CARCINOGENESIS

Tumor viruses are usually identified by their capacity to induce tumors in animal hosts.[15] Members of several different families of DNA viruses may have oncogenic potential.[1–3] Among the RNA viruses, some retroviruses are clearly tumorigenic.[16] Retroviruses may be considered a form of DNA virus in that their entire genetic information is converted to DNA after infection of the host cell, although their viral genetic information is RNA when these viruses are particles outside the cell. Some hepatocellular carcinomas are attributable to infection with hepatitis C virus, an RNA virus that does not have a DNA form.[17,18] The finding that one member of a given virus family may be oncogenic does not mean that all viruses from the family will share this capacity.

TABLE 37-1

Viruses That Are Tumorigenic in Animals

VIRUS FAMILY*	EXAMPLES: VIRUS (HOST SPECIES†)	BENIGN OR MALIGNANT	TUMORS IN NATURAL HOST
Adenovirus	Many human serotypes (hamsters)	Malignant	No
Papovavirus			
Polyomavirus group	Polyoma, SV40 (hamsters)	Both	No
Papillomavirus group	Bovine papillomavirus (cows, rodents) Rabbit papillomavirus (rabbits)	Both	Yes
Poxvirus	Rabbit fibroma (rabbits)	Benign	Yes
Herpesvirus	Marek's disease (chickens)	Malignant	yes
Hepadnavirus	Woodchuck hepatitis (woodchuck)	Malignant	Yes
Retrovirus	Avian leukosis, Rous sarcoma, murine leukemia, Harvey sarcoma (many host species)	Malignant	Yes

*These are DNA viruses, except for retroviruses. Retroviruses contain their genetic information as RNA in virions; the RNA is converted to DNA in infected host cells.
†The host species in which tumors are induced.

Each tumor virus induces a reproducible spectrum of tumors in a given host. In addition to the virus, tumor formation may depend on host factors as well as on the virus. Consequently, it is not uncommon for a virus to be oncogenic in one host but not in another. In some instances, such as some adenoviruses and polyomaviruses, the virus may induce tumors in heterologous species but not in its natural host species. Only a few animal herpesviruses cause tumors in their natural hosts. Oncogenic retroviruses typically induce malignant disease in their natural hosts, while papillomaviruses and poxviruses usually induce benign tumors. However, a small proportion of the benign tumors induced by certain human papillomaviruses and animal papillomaviruses can progress to frank malignancy. Such viruses clearly have malignant potential, despite the fact that the frequency of benign tumor formation (warts) induced by these viruses far exceeds that of malignant growths.[19,20]

In general, a virus will induce a tumor only after the virus has actually infected the target cell (the cell that will ultimately give rise to the tumor). In most instances, however, infection of a potential target cell by itself may not be sufficient for tumor formation. Tumor formation thus represents the outcome of the interaction between the virus and the infected target cell. Even those viruses that are highly oncogenic will infect many more cells than will ultimately give rise to tumors. For a given virus, the cells that become malignant therefore represent only a small subset of the infected cells. The risk of malignancy is often increased by immunologic impairment of the host, especially in the case of tumors attributable to viral infection.[21] Hormonal factors may also play a role. Exposure to certain environmental agents, such as carcinogens that are active in the target cell, may shorten the latency period to malignancy and increase the frequency with which malignant tumors develop.

TABLE 37-2

Viruses Associated with Human Tumors

VIRUS GROUP	VIRUS	TUMOR
Papillomavirus	Several HPV types (especially 5, 8, 16, 18, 31, 33)	Cutaneous carcinomas in epidermodysplasia verruciformis, urogenital carcinomas
Hepadnavirus	Hepatitis B	Hepatocellular carcinoma
Flavivirus	Hepatitis C	Hepatocellular carcinoma
Herpesvirus	HHV-8/KSHV	Kaposi's sarcoma
Retrovirus	HTLV, HIV	Some T cell lymphomas, AIDS-related malignancies

Virus-induced tumors usually do not produce infectious virus particles even when tumor growth continues to require the expression of some viral genes. This fact should be considered when searching for evidence of participation of a virus in the production of a tumor of unknown etiology. Once the virus particle (virion) gets inside the target cell, the viral genetic information required for tumor formation often does *not* include those viral genes actually encoding the proteins that form new virions; it often does include virus-encoded nonvirion protein(s). The production of virion proteins is presumably selected against in the tumor cell because their presence might be directly toxic to the cell and/or render the cell susceptible to destruction by the immune defenses of the host. In some instances of malignancy attributable to viral infection, nonmalignant cells may continue to produce virus particles. In Marek's disease, a lymphomatosis of chickens induced by a herpesvirus, the lymphoid tumor cells express some viral genes but do not produce virus particles; infectious virus is, however, produced in the otherwise normal skin appendages of the same bird.

Viral-mediated immunosuppression can also lead indirectly to tumor formation. For example, immunosuppression secondary to infection with the human immunodeficiency virus (HIV) is associated with Kaposi's sarcoma and a number of other tumors, but the tumor cells do not appear to contain HIV.[22–24] Instead, the evidence suggests that the immunologic impairment induced by HIV permits other infectious agents to induce the tumors, such as HHV-8/KSHV in Kaposi's sarcoma.[25,26]

MECHANISMS OF TUMORIGENESIS

As described in other chapters, tumors may also be induced experimentally by noninfectious agents, such as chemicals or ultraviolet radiation (see Chaps. 36 and 38). One of the most important conclusions derived from the study of chemically induced tumors (where viruses are not involved) is that the transition of a cell from normal to malignant is typically a multistep (rather than a single-step) process. Most investigators believe that the most important changes in the tumor cell represent alterations in cellular genes.[11]

The cellular mechanisms by which virus infection may give rise to tumors may be usefully considered in the context of the multistage theory of carcinogenesis. If a virus is thought of as a group of foreign genes that have been introduced into the potential target cell by means of the virus particle, tumor induction by viruses may be viewed as occurring by one of three general mechanisms:

1. The genes of a virus may directly specify all the functional changes (one or more viral-encoded proteins) required to convert a normal cell to a malignant one. Such a virus would induce tumors in a single step; the growths would therefore develop after a very short latency period. Because the virus was supplying all the abnormal

functions for the cell, the continued presence of the virus would be required for the malignant properties of the cell to be maintained. Under some circumstances, the high-level expression of a single retroviral oncogene may induce malignant tumors, although combinations of two oncogenes, which are found in some transforming animal retroviruses, are usually required for the direct induction of malignant tumors. Most DNA tumor viruses contain more than one viral oncogene, and each contributes to the oncogenic properties of the virus. In vitro studies show that some oncogenes, whether from retroviruses or from DNA viruses, serve principally to prolong the life span of the cell, while others directly stimulate cell growth and division. Both functions are necessary for tumor formation.[7,27] In the absence of a cooperating immortalizing gene, expression of an oncogene that stimulates abnormal cell growth usually also induces the cell to undergo senescence or apoptosis (programmed cell death), a potent mechanism to protect the organism from cancer.[5,28] Immortalizing genes blunt the apoptotic mechanism, thus accounting for the strong oncogenic activity when an immortalizing and a directly transforming gene are expressed together.

2. A virus may directly specify some, but not all, of the functional changes required for tumor development. In these instances, the virus would help the infected cell on its way to become a tumor cell, but certain additional cellular changes (such as alterations in cellular genes) would be required for the cell to give rise to a tumor. This appears to be by far the most common mechanism by which viruses induce tumors in people. The cellular changes in tumors fall into one of two functional classes. Most frequently, the changes are alterations that complement the viral functions, in which case the presence of viral genetic information would continue to be required. Alternatively, in some experimental tumors the changes have supplanted the viral functions, so that persistence of the virus is no longer necessary (as in some Abelson murine leukemia virus-induced tumors).[29] Tumors that require cellular changes in addition to viral infection typically take considerably longer, months to years, to develop as compared to tumors in which the virus supplies all the abnormal functions required for tumor formation. In well-studied forms of experimental viral carcinogenesis, most tumors require the continued presence of at least a portion of the viral genetic information. The same seems to be true of most virally associated human tumors.
3. Viruses can induce tumors by an even more indirect process. Instead of directly supplying some of the specific abnormal functions associated with tumorigenesis, infection by the virus may simply increase the likelihood that the cellular changes required for tumor formation will occur. Activation of the expression of a cellular proto-oncogene by chromosomal integration of the viral regulatory elements near the proto-oncogene,[30] is a occurs with some retroviruses and the woodchuck hepatitis virus,[31] clear example of this process. Tumor viruses that function by this mechanism typically induce tumors only after a very long latency period.

TUMOR-PROMOTING GENES AND TUMOR-SUPPRESSOR GENES

An important biologic feature of many tumor viruses is that they (or their isolated viral genetic sequences) can induce morphologic transformation of at least some cells in culture.[15] Here, transformation means that the cells are converted toward the tumorigenic phenotype. The capacity of these viruses to transform cells in vitro usually correlates with their ability to induce tumors in animals. These in vitro systems make it possible to define the mechanisms by which these viruses transform cells. Such in vitro studies have shown that the capacity of tumor viruses to directly transform cells is due to the expression of one or more genes encoded by the virus. These genes are called viral oncogenes or transforming genes.

Although most viral genes are not closely related to cellular genes, the oncogenes of retroviruses are actually derived from a class of cellular genes that are highly conserved in evolution.[7,30] These cellular genes are normally present in all species from yeasts to humans (more than 100 such genes have now been found in humans). This group of cellular genes was first identified by their close homology to retroviral oncogenes, so its members have been called proto-oncogenes. Most of them serve important roles in normal growth and development. While the expression and activity of proto-oncogenes are carefully controlled, these genes become constitutively active when they are present in retroviruses. A variation on this activation within the virus occurs during tumorigenesis by retroviruses that lack their own viral oncogene. In many instances, members of this class of retrovirus integrate their viral DNA near a proto-oncogene, leading to the deregulated expression of the proto-oncogene.

Deregulation of one or more proto-oncogenes occurs in a wide variety of human and animal tumors, regardless of etiology.[11,32] As with retroviral oncogenes, such deregulation renders the proto-oncogene constitutively active, which probably serves an important pathogenic role in the tumors. Most of these deregulated proto-oncogenes can induce morphologic transformation of tissue culture cells; the normal forms will be negative, or less active, in the same assay. Viral genes that promote tumorigenesis may also do so by the inhibition of cellular senescence, apoptosis, DNA repair, genetic stability, or immune defense mechanisms. Analogous changes are also found in cancers that lack an infectious etiology.[10,12]

The oncogenes of DNA tumor viruses are not derived directly from cell-encoded proteins. Most of the oncogenic activities of their encoded proteins fall into one of three categories. Some, such as the epidermal growth factor homologues of poxviruses, mimic activities of proteins encoded by cellular proto-oncogenes.[33] Others, such as the middle T antigen of polyoma virus, activate proteins encoded by proto-oncogenes.[34] Still others, such as the E6 and E7 proteins of some papillomaviruses, the large T antigen of SV40 virus, or the E1A and E1B proteins of adenoviruses, bind to and functionally inactivate cellular proteins encoded by tumor-suppressor genes.[15,35–37] Most genes of this class inhibit the growth of the target cell, so that the loss of this inhibitory activity contributes to transformation by these viral oncoproteins. Functional inactivation of tumor-suppressor genes, usually by genetic alteration, has been identified in many nonviral tumors in animals and humans.[11,12]

VIRUSES IN HUMAN TUMORS

In humans, members of several different virus families are associated with the development of malignancy (see Table 37-1). The evidence for believing viruses are involved in these tumors includes the regular association of a specific virus with certain tumors, epidemiologic data that infection with the virus is a risk factor for tumor development, finding viral genetic information in the tumor tissue, increased incidence of the tumor in immunosuppressed individuals, and the observation that similar animal viruses may be oncogenic when inoculated into experimental animals. In addition, Epstein-Barr and hepatitis B viruses are oncogenic for experimental animals, and specific genes of Epstein-Barr virus, HHV-8, and certain papillomaviruses can induce cellular transformation in vitro. These viruses are associated with a long latency period, which implies that cellular changes, in addition to viral infection, are required for malignancy.

The Epstein-Barr virus (EBV),[38,39] which is the etiologic agent of infectious mononucleosis, is implicated in African Burkitt's lymphoma (but not in most American cases), in nasopharyngeal carcinomas in the Far East, in immunoblastic B cell lymphomas in immunosuppressed patients, and in Hodgkin's disease.[40,41] EBV is well known for its capacity to immortalize normal lymphoid cells. African Burkitt's lymphoma seems to exemplify the situation in which virus infection may be necessary, but not sufficient for malignancy. In virtually all cases of EBV-associated Burkitt's lymphoma, there is deregulated expression of the *myc* proto-oncogene, in addition to EBV infection. Because overexpression of *myc* can induce B cell neoplasms in mice, it is reasonable to conclude that the constitutive *myc* expression contributes, in concert with EBV, to the malignant phenotype in these lymphomas.

Certain human papillomaviruses (HPVs) are associated with the development of malignancy.[19,20,42] Only a limited number of the HPV types are associated with malignant potential, and typical cutaneous warts should not be considered premalignant lesions. In epidermodysplasia verruciformis, there is a close relationship between the virus-induced benign papillomas and subsequent cutaneous squamous cell carcinomas. Although the malignant lesions do not contain viral particles, the HPV genetic information is retained in primary tumors and metastatic lesions. Papillomaviruses are also found regularly in bowenoid papulosis and in many noncutaneous urogenital carcinomas. Virtually all cases of cervical carcinomas contain HPV DNA.[43] As with adenovirus and SV40, the oncoproteins of the genital papillomaviruses functionally inactivate proteins of tumor-suppressor genes.[35–37]

A retrovirus that does not contain a cell-derived oncogene [human T cell lymphoma/leukemia virus (HTLV)] is implicated in the pathogenesis of some adult T cell lymphomas/leukemias.[44] This tumor was originally described in certain regions of Japan, but has a worldwide distribution. Tumor cells from many patients have been shown to harbor this virus or portions of its genetic information. HTLV shares many features with feline and bovine leukemia viruses, retroviruses that are causative agents of lymphomas/leukemias in cats and cattle, respectively.

The consistent finding of HHV-8/KHSV in Kaposi's sarcoma, whether associated with AIDS or with the African or classic forms, argues that this virus contributes to the development of the condition.[25,26,45] As with other human tumor viruses, only a subset of infected individuals appear to develop the tumors.

The identification of specific viruses as etiologic agents of human tumors suggests it may be possible to prevent tumors by vaccination. As noted earlier, this has been accomplished with the vaccine against hepatitis B leading to a reduction in liver cancer associated with this virus.[6] Vaccination with the major structural viral protein of papillomavirus has produced excellent protection against experimental animal papillomavirus infection.[46–48] The development of effective therapies against HIV has reduced the incidence of some AIDS-associated malignancies, especially Kaposi's sarcoma.[49]

REFERENCES

1. Minson A, Neil J, McCrae M, editors: *Viruses and Cancer,* vol 51. Cambridge, Cambridge University Press, 1994, p 309
2. Morris JDH et al: Viral infection and cancer. *Lancet* **346**:754, 1995
3. Knipe DM, Howley PM et al, editors: *Fields Virology*. New York, Lippincott Williams & Wilkins, 2001
4. Zur Hausen H: Viruses in human cancers. *Eur J Cancer* **35**:1878, 1999
5. Young LS et al: Viruses and apoptosis. *Br Med Bull* **53**:509, 1997
6. Chang MH: Universal hepatitis B vaccination in Taiwan and the incidence of hepatocellular carcinoma in children. *N Engl J Med* **26**:1855, 1997
7. Cooper GM: *Oncogenes*. Boston, Jones and Barlett, 1995
8. Lowy DR: The causes of cancer, in *Molecular Oncology,* edited by JM Bishop, RA Weinberg. New York, Scientific American, 1996, p 41
9. Rous P: Transmission of a malignant new growth by means of a cell-free filtrate. *JAMA* **56**:198, 1911
10. Kinzler K, Vogelstein B, editors: *The Genetic Basis of Human Cancer*. New York, McGraw-Hill, 1998
11. Weinberg RA, Hanahan D: Molecular pathogenesis of cancer, in *Molecular Oncology,* edited by JM Bishop, RA Weinberg. New York, Scientific American, 1996, p 41
12. Hanahan D, Weinberg R: The hallmarks of cancer. *Cell* **100**:57, 2000
13. Khanna R et al: Immune regulation in Epstein-Barr virus-associated diseases. *Microbiol Rev* **59**:387, 1995
14. Doria G et al: Genetic control of immune responsiveness, aging and tumor incidence. *Mech Ageing Dev* **96**:1, 1997
15. Nevins JR: Cell transformation by viruses, in *Fields Virology*, edited by D Knipe, P Howley, et al. New York, Lippincott Williams & Wilkins, 2001, p 245
16. Coffin JM: *Retroviruses*. Plainview, NY, Cold Spring Harbor Laboratory Press, 1997
17. Monto A, Wright T: The epidemiology and prevention of hepatocellular carcinoma. *Semin Oncol* **28**:441, 2001
18. Bonkovsky H, Mehta S: Hepatitis C: A review and update. *J Am Acad Dermatol* **44**:159, 2001
19. IARC: *Human Papillomaviruses. IARC Monographs on the Evaluation of Carcinogenic Risks to Humans,* vol 64. Geneva, WHO, 1995
20. Lowy D, Howley P: Papillomaviruses, in *Fields Virology,* edited by DM Knipe, PM Howley et al. New York, Lippincott Williams & Wilkins, 2001, p 2231
21. Frisch M et al: Association of cancer with AIDS-related immunosuppression in adults. *JAMA* **285**:1736, 2001
22. Knowles DM: Etiology and pathogenesis of AIDS-related non-Hodgkin's lymphoma. *Hematol Oncol Clin North Am* **10**:1081, 1996
23. Aboulafia DM, Mitsuyasu RT: Lymphomas and other cancers associated with acquired immunodeficiency syndrome, in *AIDS: Biology, Diagnosis, Treatment and Prevention,* edited by VT DeVita, S Hellman, SA Rosenberg. Philadelphia, Lippincott-Raven, 1997, p 319
24. Haller JO: AIDS-related malignancies in pediatrics. *Pediatr Oncol Imaging* **35**:1517, 1997
25. Boshoff C, Chang Y: Kaposi's sarcoma-associated herpesvirus: A new DNA tumor virus. *Annu Rev Med* **52**:453, 2001
26. Herndier B, Ganem D: The biology of Kaposi's sarcoma. *Cancer Treat Res* **104**:89, 2001
27. Hunter T: Cooperation between oncogenes. *Cell* **64**:249, 1991
28. Pan HCY, Van Dyke T: Apoptosis and cancer mechanisms. *Cancer Surv* **29**:305, 1997
29. Gunwald DJ et al: Loss of viral gene expression and retention of tumorigenicity by Abelson lymphoma cells. *J Virol* **43**:92, 1982
30. Varmus H: An historical view of oncogenes, in *Oncogenes and the Molecular Origins of Cancer,* edited by RA Weinberg RA. Cold Spring Harbor, NY, Cold Spring Harbor Laboratory, 1989
31. Buendia MA: Hepatitis B viruses and liver cancer: The woodchuck model, in *Viruses and Cancer,* vol 51, edited by A Minson, J Neil, M McCrae. Cambridge, Cambridge University Press, 1994, p 173
32. Bishop JM: Molecular themes in oncogenesis. *Cell* **64**:235, 1991
33. Buller RML et al: Cell proliferative response to vaccinia virus is mediated by VGF. *Virology* **164**:182, 1988
34. Courtneidge SA. Further characterization of the complex containing middle T antigen and pp60. *Curr Top Microbiol Immunol* **144**:121, 1989
35. Howley P, Lowy D: Papillomavirus replication, in *Fields Virology,* vol 2, edited by D Knipe, P Howley et al. New York, Lippincott Williams & Wilkins, 2001, p 2197
36. Huibregtse JM, Beaudenon SL: Mechanism of HPV E6 proteins in cellular transformation. *Semin Cancer Biol* **7**:317, 1996
37. Jones DL, Munger K: Interactions of the human papillomavirus E7 protein with cell cycle regulators. *Semin Cancer Biol* **7**:327, 1996
38. Rickinson AB, Kieff E: Epstein-Barr virus, *Fields Virology*. New York, Lippincott Williams & Wilkins, 2001, p 2511
39. Farrell PJ et al: Epstein-Barr virus genes and cancer cells. *Biomed Pharmacother* **51**:258, 1997
40. Niedobitek G et al: Epstein-Barr virus infection and human malignancies. *Int J Exp Pathol* **82**:149, 2001
41. Oudejans JJ et al: Epstein-Barr virus in Hodgkin's disease: More than just an innocent bystander. *J Pathol* **181**:353, 1997
42. Zur Hausen H: Papillomavirus infections—A major cause of human cancers. *Biochim Biophys Acta Rev Cancer* **1288**:F55, 1996
43. Walboomers JM et al: Human papillomavirus is a necessary cause of invasive cervical cancer worldwide. *J Pathol* **189**:12, 1999
44. Yoshida M: Multiple viral strategies of HTLV-1 for dysregulation of cell growth control. *Annu Rev Immunol* **19**:475, 2001

45. Gillison ML, Ambinder RF: Human herpesvirus-8. *Curr Opin Oncol* **9**:440, 1997
46. Breitburd F et al: Immunization with virus-like particles from cottontail rabbit papillomavirus (CRPV) can protect against experimental CRPV infection. *J Virol* **69**:3959, 1995
47. Suzich JA et al: Systemic immunization with papillomavirus L1 protein completely prevents the development of viral mucosal papillomas. *Proc Natl Acad Sci U S A* **92**:11553, 1995

48. Harro CD et al: Safety and immunogenicity trial in adult volunteers of a human papillomavirus 16 L1 virus-like particle vaccine. *J Natl Cancer Inst* **93**:284, 2001
49. Rabkin CS. AIDS and cancer in the era of highly active antiretroviral therapy (HAART). *Eur J Cancer* **37**:1316, 2001

CHAPTER 38

Margaret L. Kripke
Honnavara N. Ananthaswamy

Carcinogenesis: Ultraviolet Radiation

Cancer of the skin is the most common type of neoplasm in countries with predominantly Caucasian populations and high levels of ambient solar radiation. The incidence of new cases of skin cancer exceeds 1 million per year in the United States alone.[1] Precise information on the incidence of and mortality from skin cancer is difficult to obtain; with the exception of cutaneous melanoma, skin cancers generally are not reported to cancer registries, and skin cancer as a cause of death probably is underreported. However, the incidence of nonmelanoma skin cancer is thought to have been increasing since the early part of the twentieth century, and special surveys have indicated that it is continuing to climb.[1,2] Most of these nonmelanoma skin cancers are thought to result from chronic exposure of the skin to solar ultraviolet (UV) radiation. This idea originated around the turn of the twentieth century from the astute observations of physicians who noted that skin cancers occurred in the sun-damaged skin of persons who pursued outdoor occupations. Thus sunlight was one of the first agents recognized to be carcinogenic for humans.

The increasing incidence of skin cancers, including melanoma, has been attributed to increasing exposure of the population to sunlight. During the past century, changes in clothing styles, recreational activities, longevity, and other aspects of lifestyle have resulted in increases in exposure to sunlight. Other factors, such as chemicals or viruses, also may be playing a role in the increasing incidence of skin cancer, but at present there is no evidence to support this idea. The wavelengths of solar radiation involved in tumor induction appear to be within the UV region of the spectrum (wavelengths between 200 and 400 nm), especially in the UVB (290–320 nm) range. A relatively small amount of UVB radiation is present in sunlight because wavelengths in this region are strongly absorbed by the layer of ozone present in the upper atmosphere. UV wavelengths below 290 nm (UVC radiation) are completely absorbed by ozone and thus are not present in natural sunlight (see Chap. 133). Experimental evidence suggests that stratospheric ozone may have been decreasing since around 1980 because of the release of chlorofluorocarbon compounds (from human uses) into the atmosphere. This downward trend is expected to continue into the early years of the twenty-first century and then gradually to return to the pre-1980 equilibrium over the next 50 years, assuming that the worldwide phaseout of these chemicals proceeds as expected.[3] Decreases in the concentration of stratospheric ozone are expected to cause a corresponding increase in the amount of UV radiation in sunlight, particularly in the UVB region. The increasing incidence of nonmelanoma skin cancer experienced to date is unlikely to be related to ozone depletion, however. This is so because the estimated decreases in ozone concentration over populated parts of the globe are small and have occurred too recently to have had an impact on skin cancer incidence.[3] On the other hand, the likelihood that the ozone concentration will remain lower than normal for another half-century implies that the incidence of skin cancer has not peaked and will continue to rise in the future.

ULTRAVIOLET CARCINOGENESIS IN HUMANS

Although it is not possible to prove directly that sunlight, particularly the UVB radiation in sunlight, causes skin cancer in humans, the circumstantial evidence for its role is quite convincing. Taken together, epidemiologic studies and experimental studies in laboratory animals indicate that repeated exposure to solar UV radiation is the primary cause of most nonmelanoma skin cancers in light-skinned populations.

Epidemiologic Findings

Evidence supporting the idea that sunlight causes nonmelanoma skin cancers in humans comes from a variety of observations on human subjects.[4] Most compelling is the finding that these skin cancers, especially squamous cell carcinomas, appear on parts of the body that receive maximum exposure to sunlight in sites that exhibit chronic UV damage. The face, head, neck, backs of the hands, and arms are the predominant sites for development of nonmelanoma skin cancers. The incidence of these skin cancers increases with increasing age as well, implying that cumulative lifetime exposure to sunlight is responsible for skin cancer induction.[5]

Persons who spend the most time out of doors, such as those with outdoor occupations, generally have a higher incidence of squamous cell carcinoma than those who work indoors, suggesting that there is a dose-response relationship between sunlight exposure and skin cancer incidence. An interesting illustration of this point comes from a study of Maryland watermen, a relatively stable and homogeneous group of Caucasians who make their living fishing on the Chesapeake Bay. Among this group, the incidence of squamous cell carcinoma, but not basal cell carcinoma, correlated directly with the individual's personal exposure to sunlight. The higher the dose of UVB radiation received, the higher was the probability of developing squamous cell carcinoma.[6]

Geographically, there is a direct association between the amount of environmental solar radiation and the incidence of skin cancer in light-skinned individuals in the population.[4] Thus the incidence of skin cancer in Caucasians increases as one approaches the equator. The latitude gradient is steeper for squamous cell than for basal cell carcinomas.[5] This finding suggests that the incidence of squamous cell carcinoma is more dependent on sunlight exposure than that of basal cell carcinoma and that other factors in addition to sunlight may be involved in the induction of basal cell carcinoma. In fact, epidemiologic studies suggest that the incidence of basal cell carcinoma correlates poorly with cumulative lifetime exposure to sunlight[6,7] and may be more related to intermittent (recreational) exposure and exposure during the childhood years.[7,8]

Pigmentation, which is protective against sunburning, is also protective against skin cancer. The most striking example of this is seen in the high incidence and early occurrence of squamous cell carcinomas in African albinos compared with the extremely low incidence in their pigmented counterparts.[8] In addition to albinism, there are other genetic diseases associated with increased incidence of skin cancers on sun-exposed body sites. Xeroderma pigmentosum is characterized by extreme sun sensitivity, development of multiple skin cancers on sun-exposed parts of the body, and a decreased ability of somatic cells to repair UV-induced lesions in DNA (see Chap. 35). The association between defective DNA repair and skin cancer development constitutes direct evidence in humans that the UV radiation in sunlight is responsible for its carcinogenic effects. Another genetic disease, basal cell nevus or Gorlin's syndrome, is associated with a high incidence of multiple basal cell carcinomas, which occur preferentially on sun-exposed areas or in skin exposed to x-rays (see Chap. 82). These genetic diseases are discussed in further detail below.

Taken together, these findings present compelling evidence that exposure to sunlight is the cause of most nonmelanoma skin cancers. Furthermore, the studies of patients with xeroderma pigmentosum and the Maryland watermen strongly suggest that the carcinogenic wavelengths in sunlight fall mainly within the UVB region of the solar spectrum. This suggestion has been substantiated by many types of experiments in laboratory animals and by recent molecular studies of human and murine skin cancers.

Factors Affecting Carcinogenesis

Clearly, susceptibility to nonmelanoma skin cancer is dictated by a combination of factors, including sun exposure habits, occupation, and the degree of skin pigmentation. In addition to these major factors, other less obvious ones also may contribute to an individual's susceptibility to solar carcinogenesis. For example, persons with erythrodysplasia verruciformis sometimes develop squamous cell carcinomas. When this occurs, the tumors generally appear on sun-exposed body sites.[9] This observation suggests that there may be an interaction between papillomaviruses and sunlight exposure that promotes the development of skin cancer.

Once a person has developed a nonmelanoma skin cancer, the risk of developing a second primary tumor is greatly increased over the risk of persons of comparable skin type developing skin cancer. In one prospective study, one-third of the patients with basal cell carcinoma developed a second cancer within 5 years.[10] Thus, having had skin cancer constitutes a risk factor for the development of subsequent tumors.

One factor that has been clearly associated with an increased risk of nonmelanoma skin cancers is chronic immunosuppression. This observation came from studies of malignancies arising in renal transplant patients, which demonstrated that the risk of developing skin cancer was increased four to sevenfold in areas of low sun exposure and more than twentyfold in areas of high sun exposure.[11] These tumors appear predominantly on sun-exposed body sites and generally occur within a few years of transplantation. Careful examination of the skin of such patients revealed a high incidence of warts as well as carcinoma in situ and squamous cell carcinoma.[12] Human papillomavirus has been associated with the skin cancers as well as with benign warts, suggesting that immune suppression, papillomaviruses, and UV radiation all may interact to produce skin cancer in these individuals. These observations imply that a person's immune status is an important component in the risk of developing skin cancer.

It is also possible that exposure to certain chemicals may enhance the induction of skin cancers by UV radiation. Studies in animal models have demonstrated that there are many possible types of interactions between chemicals and UV radiation that can increase or even decrease tumor formation. For example, repeated application of a chemical tumor-promoting agent such as croton oil to murine skin initiated with UV radiation results in a high incidence of skin cancers, even though treatment with either agent alone produces few or no tumors.[13] In humans, however, such interactions have been documented only in the case of psoralens, which are photosensitizing compounds. The long-term use of 8-methoxypsoralen plus UVA radiation (PUVA) for therapy of psoriasis has been associated with an increased incidence of squamous cell carcinoma in some studies.[14] However, these skin cancers do not occur preferentially on parts of the body that receive the highest solar UV radiation, suggesting that they are related to the therapy alone rather than to an interaction between solar UV radiation and PUVA therapy. Recent molecular studies support the view that PUVA is carcinogenic for humans by itself.

Based on studies of xeroderma pigmentosum, it seems likely that the intrinsic ability of one's cells to repair UV-induced lesions in DNA also influences the risk of developing skin cancer. Because many genes are involved in the repair of DNA damage, one might expect individuals to differ in the ability of their cells to repair DNA damaged by chemicals and radiation and, consequently, to differ in their susceptibility to UV carcinogenesis. Such a correlation was, in fact, noted in a comparison of the ability of skin fibroblasts from patients with basal cell carcinoma and normal control subjects to repair cyclobutylpyrimidine dimers induced in vivo by solar-simulated UV radiation. The occurrence of basal cell carcinoma was associated with decreased excision repair of such lesions in DNA.[15] Molecular epidemiologic studies showed that lymphocytes from basal cell carcinoma patients also exhibited reduced DNA repair capacity and that persons with more than four basal cell cancers had the lowest DNA repair capability.[16] Therefore, DNA repair capacity also may contribute to an individual's risk of developing skin cancer.

EXPERIMENTAL UV CARCINOGENESIS

Much of our information on UV carcinogenesis has come from investigations of the process in animal models, particularly in the mouse. This system is especially convenient for quantitative studies of carcinogenesis because the carcinogen can be delivered in an accurately measured dose. In addition, the carcinogen is present only during the time of application and does not persist in the tissues, and it does not require metabolic activation. Furthermore, the tumors can be identified at an early stage, and their development, progression, or regression can be followed by visual observation without the need for invasive procedures.

Tumor Induction by UV Radiation

Skin cancers have been induced experimentally with UV radiation in a variety of laboratory animals, including mice, rats, guinea pigs, and opossums. The tumor types vary somewhat depending on the species, but in mice they are mainly squamous cell carcinomas, fibrosarcomas, and undifferentiated or spindle cell tumors. Many factors influence the induction of tumors by UV radiation, even within a single species.[17] For example, hairless mice develop primarily squamous cell carcinomas after UV radiation, whereas haired mice tend to develop tumors of spindle cell morphology. Within a single mouse strain, tumor types can be influenced by UV dose. Different strains of mice can differ in their rate of tumor development, the proportions of different histologic types of tumors, and the anatomic sites of tumor development. Other variables influencing carcinogenesis include the amount of pigmentation in the skin, skin thickness, thickness of the keratin layer, and the age of the skin at the time of the first radiation.

Wavelength

The first studies of experimental UV carcinogenesis were carried out by Findlay,[18] who demonstrated that chronic exposure of albino mice to UV radiation from a quartz-mercury vapor lamp produced skin tumors on the ears and depilated dorsal skin. Shortly thereafter, Roffo[19] performed experiments with albino rats using sunlight filtered through window glass to produce skin cancers. These studies demonstrated that UV radiation could be used to produce skin cancers in laboratory rodents and determined that the primary carcinogenic waveband of sunlight fell within the wavelength range between 290 and 320 nm. Since that time, a number of different approaches have been used in an attempt to define more precisely an action spectrum for UV carcinogenesis, which is a plot of relative carcinogenic effectiveness as a function of wavelength. Knowledge of the action spectrum for UV carcinogenesis would be useful for several reasons. First, it could give information about the mechanisms of cancer induction by UV radiation. Second, knowing the important wavelengths for UV carcinogenesis would be helpful for designing sunscreens to prevent cancer induction. Third, knowledge of the action spectrum is essential for estimating the increased risk of skin cancer development resulting from ozone depletion.

Using combinations of light sources and filters, several groups have provided evidence that the action spectrum for carcinogenesis in the albino hairless mouse closely approximates the action spectra for UV-induced erythema in human skin[20] and UV-induced edema in murine skin.[21] Thus the most effective wavelengths for cancer induction in the hairless mouse are between 295 and 305 nm, and the activity decreases sharply with increasing wavelengths above this range (Fig. 38-1). Because of the similarity of this action spectrum to that of the erythema-inducing activity of UV radiation on human skin, and because of similarities in the dose-response relationships between UV carcinogenesis in humans and in mice, this action spectrum is often used as an approximation of the carcinogenic effectiveness of UV radiation for human skin.

Studies on the wavelength dependence of UV carcinogenesis in mice indicate that UVB radiation is around 1000 times more efficient than UVA radiation in producing murine skin cancers. This does not mean, however, that UVA radiation is noncarcinogenic. On the contrary, when given in sufficient doses, UVA radiation also produces skin cancers in mice.[22] Whether UVA radiation contributes to solar carcinogenesis in human skin is not clear, however. Although its carcinogenic effectiveness is much less than that of UVB radiation, it is present in much greater amounts in sunlight. Some experimental studies have suggested that UVA radiation actually potentiates cancer induction by UVB radiation, but whether it does so under natural environmental conditions is uncertain. Molecular analysis of human skin cancers does not support a role for UVA radiation as a mutagenic initiator of carcinogenesis; however, UVA radiation could serve as an important tumor promoter.

FIGURE 38-1

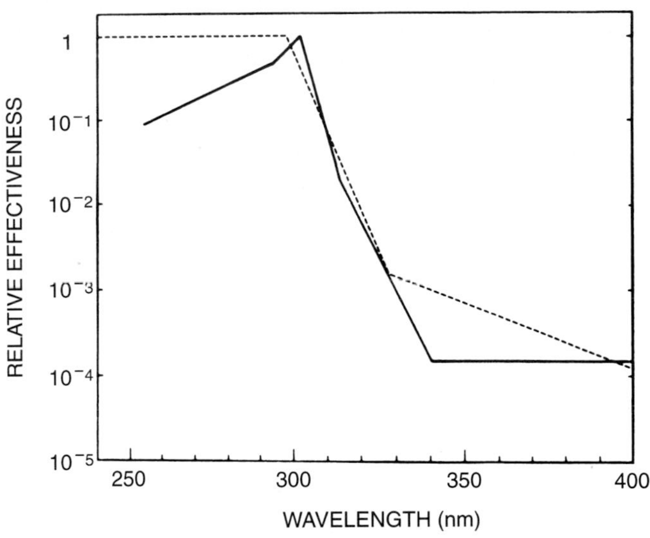

Action spectrum for photocarcinogenesis in the hairless albino mouse (—) and a standardized action spectrum for UV-induced erythema in humans (---). (*Adapted from van der Leun JC et al: Human health, in UN Environment Programme: Environmental Effects Panel Report. New York, United Nations, November 1989, p18, with permission of the authors.*)

Dose Response

Beginning around 1940, Blum[23] and colleagues initiated a monumental series of quantitative studies of tumor formation on the ears of haired albino mice exposed to UV radiation from various sources. These studies, which used large numbers of animals and carefully monitored light sources, addressed the energy requirements and time and dose relationships for tumor induction.

An important finding from this work was that cessation of irradiation before tumors appeared did not inhibit tumor formation. It did, however, reduce the rate of tumor formation dramatically compared with that in animals in which the irradiations were continued until tumors appeared. This finding suggests that limiting sun exposure in persons already exhibiting solar damage may at least retard tumor development. Another interesting feature of this system is that reciprocity of time and dose is observed only within a narrow range of conditions and that, in general, UV radiation given as many small doses is more carcinogenic than the same total dose of UV radiation given in a few very large doses. The basis for this lack of reciprocity is not known; it may be due to greater repair of DNA damage during the longer intervals between treatments with the high doses of UV radiation. Alternatively, the high doses may be killing many cells, thereby removing them from the pool of potential cancer cells. Regardless of the mechanisms involved, these studies indicate that UV carcinogenesis is achieved most efficiently with multiple low doses of UV radiation.

Interactions with Other Agents

One of the conclusions Blum drew from his studies was that UV carcinogenesis was a continuous process in which the effects of the UV radiation accumulated to lead, eventually, to the formation of skin cancers. This interpretation was reevaluated following the proposal by Berenblum[24] that chemical carcinogenesis in mouse skin was a two-stage process involving an irreversible initiation step and a reversible promotion phase. Subsequent studies demonstrated that a single, noncarcinogenic dose of UV radiation followed by repeated applications of a tumor-promoting agent (croton oil) produced tumors in murine skin.[13] This finding demonstrated that UV radiation was an initiator of carcinogenesis, like many of the chemical carcinogens. UV radiation also can serve as a tumor promoter after an initiating dose of a chemical carcinogen. Thus UV radiation may play a variety of roles during cutaneous carcinogenesis.

In addition to its interactions with other initiators and tumor promoters, tumor induction by UV radiation can be influenced by a variety of chemical and physical agents. One of these is retinoic acid, which has been shown both to augment and to reduce UV carcinogenesis under different experimental conditions. Antioxidants, such as butylated hydroxytoluene (BHT) and vitamin C, have been shown to inhibit UV carcinogenesis, suggesting that oxygen-dependent mechanisms are involved in tumor induction by UV radiation, most likely in the promotion phase. Studies in both mice and humans have demonstrated that a low-fat diet can reduce skin cancer induction.[25] The mechanisms involved are not known.

Obviously, any agent that reduces the amount of UV radiation reaching the target cells in the skin by either blocking or absorbing the radiation has the potential to inhibit carcinogenesis. Absorbers of UV radiation commonly used in commercial sunscreen preparations include *para*-aminobenzoic acid, cinnamates, benzophenones, and 2-ethylhexyl-*para*-dimethylaminobenzoate; blocking agents are zinc oxide and titanium dioxide (see Chap. 247).

Physical factors also have been shown to influence UV carcinogenesis. There are suggestions that x-irradiation may act synergistically with UV radiation in the production of skin cancers and that high temperature, wind, and high relative humidity can all increase susceptibility to UV carcinogenesis.

Immunology

Studies of UV carcinogenesis in the mouse demonstrated that there is an important immunologic component to tumor induction in this system. Investigation of the antigenic properties of skin cancers induced in haired, inbred mice demonstrated that these tumors are highly antigenic. When transplanted into normal, genetically identical mice, most of these tumors are rejected by the immune system of the recipient animal, although they will grow progressively in immunosuppressed mice. This finding raised the question of how such highly antigenic tumors were able to persist and grow in the primary host. Transplantation experiments demonstrated that early in the course of chronic UV radiation, before primary tumors were evident, the mice lost their ability to reject UV-induced tumors. Thus UV radiation had a systemic effect on the mice that interfered with tumor rejection.[26] The importance of the systemic effect for tumor induction was shown by experiments in which mice were exposed to UV radiation for a limited period to induce the systemic effect and then exposed to carcinogenic doses of UV radiation at a separate site. Mice that had been preirradiated at a distant site showed an increase in the rate of tumor induction.[27] Similar studies using UV radiation as the initiator and croton oil as the promoter suggested that the systemic effect of UV radiation was exerted during the promotion phase of two-stage carcinogenesis.[28]

The inability of UV-irradiated mice to reject UV-induced tumors could be passively transferred with lymphoid cells, demonstrating that the systemic alternation was immunologic in nature. Subsequent studies demonstrated that T lymphocytes were responsible for this effect and that these T suppressor cells inhibited the rejection of primary UV-induced skin cancers.[26] Recent evidence indicates that the T suppressor cells belong to a specialized subset of cells with features of both natural killer cells and T lymphocytes termed NK-T cells that regulate immune responses to lipid-containing molecules.[29] These studies indicated that exposure of the skin to UV radiation caused profound systemic changes in immune function and, moreover, that the immunosuppressive effects of UV radiation were of critical importance in the process of UV carcinogenesis. Mechanisms of UV-induced immunosuppression are discussed in Chap. 39.

The demonstration of an increased incidence of skin cancers in immunosuppressed human subjects supports the notion that immunologic factors are also important in UV carcinogenesis in humans. Moreover, recent studies have demonstrated that patients with sunlight-associated skin cancers are more sensitive to UV-induced immunosuppression than are normal subjects.[30] This finding implies, in addition, that susceptibility to the immunologic effects of UV radiation may be an important determinant of skin cancer development in humans. UV-induced immune suppression also has been suggested as a possible explanation for the latitude gradient of non-Hodgkin's lymphoma and the increased incidence of this malignancy in persons with nonmelanoma skin cancer. In support of this notion, recent experimental studies showed that UV radiation accelerates that development of lymphoid malignancies in genetically susceptible mice.[31]

GENETICS

Cancers of many types involve mutations in genes that control cellular growth. Some genes facilitate cell growth (cellular oncogenes); others inhibit this process (tumor suppressor genes). A mutation that results in activation or overexpression of an oncogene or production of an altered oncogene product ultimately can lead to cancer formation. Similarly, mutations that inactivate genes or the products of genes involved in negative regulation of cell growth can contribute to cancer induction. In addition, alterations in genes involved in the repair of UV-induced DNA damage can lead to the development of UV-associated cancers. The occurrence of rare hereditary diseases associated with a high incidence of specific types of cancer has led to the identification of several genes involved in skin cancer development. Xeroderma pigmentosum is an autosomal recessive disease caused by the mutation of genes involved in DNA repair. Nine such genes have been identified so far. The disease is characterized by a high incidence of both melanoma and nonmelanoma skin cancers with an early age of onset. The association of skin cancer with defective DNA repair indicates the importance of DNA repair genes as determinants of susceptibility to UV carcinogenesis. As mentioned earlier, DNA repair capacity seems to be a determinant of skin cancer susceptibility in the general population as well as in xeroderma pigmentosum patients.

Patients with Li-Fraumeni syndrome, another hereditary disease, have a high incidence of multiple internal malignancies. These individuals inherit one defective copy of *p53,* a gene involved in regulation of the cell cycle. This tumor suppressor gene is lost or mutated in a variety of cancers, especially in skin and lung carcinomas. In both mice and humans, UV-induced skin cancers exhibit a high frequency (60–100 percent) of mutations in *p53,* and these can be detected in irradiated skin long before skin cancers are apparent.[32] It has been found that *p53* knockout mice with only one copy of the *p53* gene are highly susceptible to UV carcinogenesis.[33] Mice lacking both copies of the *XPA* or *XPC* DNA repair genes also exhibit increased susceptibility to skin cancer induction by UV radiation, and mice lacking both copies of *XPC* and one copy of *p53* are even more susceptible.[34,35]

Studies of patients with Gorlin's syndrome, also known as *nevoid basal cell carcinoma syndrome,* have led to the identification of genes associated with basal cell carcinoma. This syndrome is a rare autosomal dominant disorder characterized by multiple basal cell carcinomas that appear at a young age on sun-exposed areas of the skin. Patients with Gorlin's syndrome were found to have germ-line mutations in the human homologue of the *patched* gene *(ptc)* that is involved in the regulation of development in *Drosophila.*[36] This gene is mutated in tumors from many patients with sporadic basal cell carcinoma as well, suggesting that genetic alterations in the *ptc* gene also may play a role in the development of sporadic basal cell carcinoma. *Ptc* normally functions to inhibit the sonic hedgehog (Shh) signal transduction pathway, and binding of Shh to *ptc* relieves the inhibition, allowing for transduction to continue through a series of additional steps. Mutations in *ptc* result in loss of its function and subsequent overexpression of downstream proteins, leading to uncontrolled cell division. Mutations resulting in overexpression of Shh also can lead to basal cell carcinoma formation[37] (see Chaps. 81 and 82).

The *ras* family of oncogenes is also mutated in a small percentage of murine and human skin cancers (10–40 percent).[38] These genes are also involved in the transduction of signals from the cell membrane to the nucleus. Mutations that activate *ras* genes lead to persistent signal transduction, resulting in a loss of normal cellular growth control. *Ras* mutations are present in other types of solid tumors as well. One other gene that has been implicated in susceptibility to skin cancer in humans is the gene for glutathione *S*-transferase 1 *(GSTM1)*. Alleles of this gene code for enzymes involved in detoxification of electrophilic molecules and reactive oxygen species. Persons homozygous for the null allele, which makes no enzyme, have a slightly elevated risk of developing multiple basal and squamous cell carcinomas.[39] The mechanism by which these isoenzymes protect against skin carcinogenesis is not clear, but they could counteract certain steps in tumor promotion by either UV radiation or chemicals.

MOLECULAR MECHANISMS

From the experimental studies of UV carcinogenesis, it is clear that UV radiation can play a variety of roles in the development of skin cancers. It can serve as a complete carcinogen and induce tumors in animals and in cells in vitro in the absence of any other stimulus. It also can serve as an initiating agent in multistage carcinogenesis, in which tumor promoters are required for tumor development. UV radiation also shares many properties with chemical tumor promoters, such as induction of proliferation, stimulation of the production of enzymes involved in tumor promotion, and induction of inflammation, all of which probably contribute to the carcinogenic process. The immunosuppressive effect of UV radiation also contributes to its carcinogenic activity. In addition, UV radiation may have other effects on the local environment in which the tumors develop—such as increased vascularity and production of growth factors—that could contribute to tumor growth and progression. Finally, any one of these effects of UV radiation may contribute to the induction of skin cancers by other agents such as x-rays, viruses, or chemical carcinogens. Thus UV radiation may serve as a cofactor in other types of cutaneous carcinogenesis in addition to inducing skin cancers directly.

The molecular mechanisms by which UV radiation exerts its varied effects are not completely understood. The carcinogenic process probably involves multiple sequential steps, some, but not all of which involve alterations in DNA structure (mutations). Evidence that UV-induced lesions in DNA are involved in the formation of skin cancer comes from a variety of systems. In humans, the association between defective DNA repair and sunlight-induced skin cancers in xeroderma pigmentosum patients provides strong evidence for the involvement of UV-induced lesions in DNA. Experimental studies using species whose cells contain a light-activated DNA repair enzyme suggest further that cyclobutyl pyrimidine dimers induced by UV radiation between adjacent pyrimidine bases on the same strand of DNA are a critical component of the carcinogenic process. Studies with the Amazon molly (*Poecilia formosa*) demonstrated that the formation of UV-induced cancers of the thyroid tissue could be prevented by exposing the tissue to visible light after UV radiation.[40] The visible light activated an enzyme that specifically repairs pyrimidine dimers in DNA. Studies with the South American opossum (*Monodelphis domestica*) demonstrated similarly that skin cancer induction by chronic UV radiation could be inhibited by exposure of the skin to UVA radiation plus visible light after each UV radiation exposure.[41]

Theoretically, any alteration capable of causing a mutation in specific target genes could contribute to UV carcinogenesis because there is a close correlation between mutation and transformation by UV radiation. Other lesions in DNA produced after UVB radiation include [6–4] photoproducts, purine photoproducts, cytosine photohydrates, single-strand breaks, and sister chromatid exchanges. Furthermore, DNA damage can result from reactive oxgyen species, such as singlet oxygen, superoxide anion, and hydrogen peroxide, that are generated during exposure of mammalian cells to UV radiation. Based on detailed molecular analysis of the mutations in the *p53* gene in both human and murine skin tumors, cyclobutyl pyrimidine dimers and [6–4] photoproducts seem to be the predominant mutagenic lesions contributing to skin cancer induction. Most *p53* mutations are C→T transitions and CC→TT double-tandem mutations at dipyrimidine sites, which result from cyclobutyl pyrimidine dimers and [6–4] photoproducts. These mutations are characteristic of UVB and UVC radiation but not of UVA radiation or chemical carcinogens, implying that UVB radiation is the most important mutagenic agent for the induction of skin cancer by sunlight.[42] Therefore, other molecular alterations must contribute to carcinogenesis by causing mutations in genes other than *p53* or by contributing to nonmutational steps in the carcinogenic process.

Molecular analysis of *p53* mutations in murine skin cancers induced by PUVA revealed that PUVA also induced unique mutations in this gene, different from those induced by UVB radiation. This information prompted a study of *p53* mutations in skin cancers obtained from patients undergoing PUVA therapy to ascertain the etiology of these cancers. Although some were UVB signature mutations, the majority of the *p53* mutations observed in skin cancers from these patients occurred at or adjacent to 5'-TA/5'-TAT sites, which are characteristic of PUVA-induced mutations.[43] Thus this study suggests that PUVA is carcinogenic in humans and that the majority of the skin cancers that occur in patients undergoing PUVA therapy are related to the treatment rather than to sunlight exposure.

UV RADIATION AND MELANOMA

In contrast to the clear relationship between UV exposure and basal cell and squamous cell carcinomas, the role played by UV radiation in the induction and pathogenesis of cutaneous melanoma remains unclear. Only lentigo maligna melanoma exhibits a relationship to sunlight exposure similar to that of the nonmelanoma skin cancers. The other types of melanoma do not occur preferentially on the most heavily exposed body sites, nor does their incidence continue to rise with increasing age. Furthermore, their occurrence does not correlate with occupational or cumulative lifetime exposure to sunlight.[5] On the other hand, there is a latitude gradient for melanoma, although the relationship is not as strong as that for either basal cell or squamous cell carcinoma.

More attention has been focused on this issue in recent years because of concerns about the consequences of ozone depletion and the rapid rise in the incidence of melanoma. Although the evidence remains largely circumstantial, it supports the conclusion that UV radiation is a contributing factor in the development of at least some cutaneous melanomas in addition to being the primary cause of lentigo maligna melanoma. This evidence can be summarized as follows:

1. Case-control studies indicate that a higher risk of melanoma development is associated with intense sun exposure early in life.[44]
2. The increasing incidence of melanoma parallels that of nonmelanoma skin cancer.[2]
3. Pigmentation is inversely correlated with the incidence of cutaneous melanoma.[45]
4. The risk of melanoma development in patients with xeroderma pigmentosum is 2000 times higher than that in the general population. Furthermore, there is evidence that at least some of these melanomas have UV-induced mutations in oncogenes (see Chap. 93).
5. Immigrant studies demonstrate an increased incidence of melanoma among persons who are native to sunny regions or who immigrate to such areas before the age of puberty as compared with persons who immigrate later in life.[46]

In addition, there is evidence from animal models that supports a relationship between exposure to UV radiation and melanoma induction. In addition to other types of skin and ocular tumors, cutaneous melanomas occur in the marsupial *M. domestica* after long-term chronic exposure of adults[47] or after acute exposure of neonates[48] to UV radiation. Furthermore, precancerous melanotic lesions were prevented by treatment with visible light after UV irradiation, suggesting that they may result from UV-induced lesions in DNA.[47] Certain hybrid species of tropical fish are prone to melanoma development following exposure to UV radiation. In this model also photoactivation of an enzyme that repairs thymine dimers reduces the incidence of melanoma.[49] However, an action spectrum for the induction of melanoma in the fish model demonstrated that UVA radiation also induced melanoma.[50] This finding has raised questions about the accuracy of predictions concerning the increased risk of melanoma that would result from ozone depletion (which affects only UVB) and and has generated concern about the effectiveness of UVB sunscreens for preventing skin cancer.

In mice, melanomas can be induced by combinations of UV radiation and tumor promoters and chemical carcinogens and UV radiation.[51] In addition, exposing murine skin to UV radiation has been reported to accelerate the development of both primary[51] and transplantable[52] melanomas within the site of UV radiation. Studies on the mechanism of this effect of UV radiation suggest that both the production of melanoma-specific growth factors from UV-irradiated epidermis and decreased immunologic reactivity of the skin may be involved.

The weight of evidence, though admittedly circumstantial, favors the conclusion that UV radiation contributes in some way to the induction and pathogenesis of cutaneous melanoma. The relationship between exposure to UV radiation and the development of melanoma clearly differs from that of solar UV radiation and the nonmelanoma skin cancers in terms of dose response, age dependence, and perhaps the participation of other carcinogenic factors. Molecular evidence for the involvement of UV radiation as an initiator of melanoma induction is quite limited. In contrast to the high frequency of UV-induced mutations in *p53* in skin carcinomas, *p53* is rarely mutated in melanomas and therefore is unlikely to play a major role in melanoma development. However, genetic abnormalities in $p16^{INK4a}$ and $p14^{ARF}$ genes have been shown to play a role in human melanoma.[53] The *INK4a-ARF* locus on human chromosome 9p21 encodes two proteins, $p16^{INK4a}$ and $p14^{ARF}$ ($p19^{ARF}$ in mice), known to function as tumor suppressors via the retinoblastoma or the p53 pathway.[54] Deletions and mutations in $p16^{INK4a}$ and $p14^{ARF}$ have been reported in familal and sporadic melanoma,[53,55,56] and studies using $p16^{INK4a}$ and $p19^{ARF}$ knockout mice have shown that these mice develop both spontaneous and chemical carcinogen-induced malignant melanoma.[57,58] These studies support the notion that $p16^{INK4a}$ and $p19^{ARF}$ genes play a critical role in the pathogenesis of malignant melanoma. An additional melanoma-associated gene is that coding for hepatocyte growth factor (or scatter factor). A single erythemal UV radiation exposure of neonatal, but not adult, transgenic mice that overexpress hepatocyte growth factor/scatter factor results in the development of cutaneous melanoma.[59] This mouse model may be useful for determining the reasons for the association between childhood sunburn and the subsequent development of melanoma in humans. Aside from its possible function as an initiator, UV radiation probably can play a number of different roles in the induction of melanoma. Also, UV radiation may be only one of several carcinogens involved in the pathogenesis of this tumor. To date, however, other such carcinogens have not been identified.

PREVENTION

For the nonmelanoma skin cancers, the most logical approach to prevention is to limit exposure of the skin to natural and artificial sources of UV radiation. This can be achieved in numerous ways, including the use of sunscreens, the avoidance of outdoor activities during the noon hours when the amount of UV radiation in sunlight is maximal, and the use of protective clothing. Reducing the lifetime dose of UV radiation reduces the risk of skin cancer development in mice and presumably in humans as well. Because the effects of UV radiation in causing nonmelanoma skin cancers are cumulative, we would expect that reducing sunlight exposure at any age would retard the rate of tumor development.

For melanoma and perhaps even for some basal cell carcinomas, it is not clear whether this strategy would be effective because there is not a simple, direct relationship between dose of UV radiation and melanoma induction. For example, if melanoma results from childhood exposure to UV radiation, as has been suggested, reducing sunlight exposure during adult life may not be beneficial in attempting to decrease the incidence of melanoma. Obviously, more information on the dose response, wavelength dependence, and mechanism of action of UV radiation in the induction of melanomas is needed to devise effective strategies for preventing even the melanomas that are sunlight-related.

REFERENCES

1. Rowe DE et al: Prognostic factors for recurrence, metastasis, and survival rates in squamous cell carcinoma of the skin, ear, and lip. *J Am Acad Dermatol* **26**:976, 1992
2. Glass AG, Hoover RN: The emerging epidemic of melanoma and squamous cell skin cancer. *JAMA* **262**:2097, 1989
3. Madronich S et al: Changes in ultraviolet radiation reaching the earth's surface. *Ambio* **24**:143, 1995
4. Urbach F: Geographic pathology of skin cancer, in *The Biologic Effects of Ultraviolet Radiation*, edited by F Urbach. Oxford, England, Pergamon, 1969, p 635

5. Fears TR et al: Mathematical models of age and ultraviolet effects on the incidence of skin cancer among whites in the United States. *Am J Epidemiol* **105**:420, 1977
6. Vitasa BC et al: Association of nonmelanoma skin cancer and actinic keratosis with cumulative solar ultraviolet exposure in Maryland watermen. *Cancer* **65:**2811, 1990
7. Kricker A et al: Does intermittent sun exposure cause basal cell carcinoma? A case-control study in western Australia. *Int J Cancer* **60**:489, 1995
8. Kricker A et al: Sun exposure and non-melanocytic skin cancer. *Cancer Causes Control* **5**:367, 1994
9. Jablonska S et al: Epidermodysplasia verruciformis as a model in studies on the role of papovavirus in oncogenesis. *Cancer Res* **32**:583, 1972
10. Robinson JK: Risk of developing another basal cell carcinoma: A 5-year prospective study. *Cancer* **60**:118, 1987
11. Penn I: Tumors of the immunocompromised patient. *Annu Rev Med* **39**:63, 1988
12. Bouwes-Bavinck JN: Epidemiological aspects of immunosuppression: Role of exposure to sunlight and HPV on the development of skin cancer. *Hum Exp Toxicol* **14**:98, 1994
13. Epstein JH, Roth HL: Experimental ultraviolet light carcinogenesis: A study of croton oil promoting effects. *J Invest Dermatol* **50**:387, 1968
14. Stern RS, Lander EJ: Risk of squamous cell carcinoma in patients treated with oral methoxsalen (psoralen) and UV-A radiation: A meta-analysis. *Arch dermatol* **134:**1582, 1998
15. Alcalay J et al: Excision repair of pyrimidine dimers induced by simulated solar radiation in the skin of patients with basal cell carcinoma. *J Invest Dermatol* **95**:506, 1990
16. Wei Q et al: DNA repair and aging in basal cell carcinoma: A molecular epidemiologic study. *Proc Natl Acad Sci USA* **90**:1614, 1993
17. Ananthaswamy HN, Kripke MK: Experimental skin carcinogenesis by ultraviolet radiation, in *Pathophysiology of Dermatologic Disease,* edited by NA Soter, HP Baden. New York, McGraw-Hill, 1990 p 483.
18. Findlay GM: Ultraviolet light and skin cancer: *Lancet* **215**:1070, 1928
19. Roffo AH: Cancer et soleil: Carcinomes et sarcomes provoques par l'action du soleil in toto. *Bull Assoc France Etude Cancer* **23**:590, 1934
20. Sterenborg HJCM, van der Leun JC: Action spectra for tumorigenesis by ultraviolet radiation, in *Human Exposure to Ultraviolet Radiation: Risks and Regulations*, edited by WF Passichier, BFM Bosnjakovic. Amsterdam, Elsevier, 1987, p 173
21. Cole CA et al: An action spectrum for photocarcinogenesis. *Photochem Photobiol* **4**:275, 1986
22. Sterenborg HJCM, van der Leun JC: Tumorigenesis by a long wavelength UV-A source. *Photochem Photobiol* **51**:325, 1990
23. Blum HF: *Carcinogenesis by Ultraviolet Light*. Princeton, NJ, Princeton University Press, 1959
24. Berenblum I: A speculative review: The probable nature of promoting action and its significance in the understanding of the mechanism of carcinogenesis. *Cancer Res* **14:**471, 1954
25. Black HS et al: Evidence that a low-fat diet reduces the occurrence of non-melanoma skin cancer. *Int J Cancer* **62**:165, 1995
26. Kripke ML: Immunology and photocarcinogenesis: New light on an old problem. *J Am Acad Dermatol* **14**:149, 1986
27. deGruiji F, van der Leun JC: Systemic influence of pre-irradiation of a limited skin area on UV-tumorigenesis. *Photochem Photobiol* **35**:379, 1982
28. Strickland PT et al: Enhancement of two-stage skin carcinogenesis by exposure of distant skin to UV radiation. *J Natl Cancer Inst* **74**:1129, 1985
29. Moodycliff AM et al: Immune suppression and skin cancer development regulation by NKT cells. *Nature Immunol* **1**:521, 2000
30. Yoshikawa T et al: Susceptibility to effects of UVB radiation on induction of contact hypersensitivity as a risk factor for skin cancer in human. *J Invest Dermatol* **95**:530, 1990
31. Jiang W et al: UV irradiation augments lymphoid malignancies in mice with one functional copy of wild-type *p53*. *Proc Natl Acad Sci USA* **98**:9790, 2001
32. Ananthaswamy HN et al: Sunlight and skin cancer: Inhibition of *p53* mutations in UV-irradiated mouse skin by sunscreens. *Nature Med* **3**: 310, 1997
33. Jiang W et al: *p53* protects against skin cancer induction by UV-B radiation. *Oncogene* **18**:4247, 1999
34. Nakane H et al: High incidence of ultraviolet-B–or chemical-carcinogen–induced skin tumours in mice lacking the xeroderma pigmentosum group A gene. *Nature* **377**:165, 1995
35. Cheo DL et al: Synergistic interactions between *XPC* and *p53* mutations in double-mutant mice: Neural tube abnormalities and accelerated UV radiation-induced skin cancer. *Curr Biol* **6**:1691, 1996
36. Johnson RL et al: Human homolog of *patched,* a candidate gene for the basal cell nevus syndrome. *Science*. **272**:1668, 1996
37. Ingham PW: Transducing hedgehog: The story so far. *EMBO J* **17**:3505, 1998.
38. Ananthaswamy HN, Pierceall WE: Molecular mechanisms of ultraviolet radiation carcinogenesis. *Photochem Photobiol* **52**:1119, 1990
39. Heagerty AHM et al: Glutathione *S*-transferase *GSTM1* phenotypes and protection against cutaneous tumours. *Lancet* **343**:366, 1994
40. Hart RW et al: Evidence that pyrimidine dimers in DNA can give rise to tumors. *Proc Natl Acad Sci USA* **74**:5574, 1977
41. Ley RD et al: UVA/visible light suppression of ultraviolet radiation–induced skin and eye tumors of the marsupial *Monodelphis domestica*. *Photochem Photobiol* **47**:45S, 1998
42. Nataraj AJ et al: *p53* gene mutations and photocarcinogenesis. *Photochem Photobiol* **62**:218, 1995
43. Nataraj AJ et al: *p53* mutation in squamous cell carcinomas from psoriasis patients treated with psoralen plus UVA (PUVA). *J Invest Dermatol* **109**:238, 1997
44. Lew RA et al: Sun exposure habits in patients with cutaneous melanoma: A case control study. *J Dermatol Surg Oncol* **9**:981, 1983
45. Crombie IK: Racial differences in melanoma incidence. *Br J Cancer* **40**:185, 1979
46. Holman CDJ, Armstrong BK: Cutaneous malignant melanoma and indicators of total accumlated exposure to the sun: An analysis separating histogenetic types. *J Natl Cancer Inst* **73**:75, 1984
47. Ley RD et al: Ultraviolet radiation-induced malignant melanoma in *Mondelphis domestica. Photochem Photobiol* **50**:1, 1989
48. Robinson ES et al: Malignant melanoma in ultraviolet irradiated laboratory opossums: Initiation in suckling young, metastasis in adults, and xenograft behavior in nude mice. *Cancer Res* **54:**5986, 1994
49. Setlow RB et al: Animal model for ultraviolet radiation–induced melanoma: Platyfish-swordtail hybrid. *Proc Natl Acad Sci USA* **86**:8922, 1989
50. Setlow RB et al: Wavelengths effective in induction of malignant melanoma. *Proc Natl Acad Sci USA* **90**:6666, 1993
51. Romerdahl CA et al: The role of ultraviolet radiation in the induction of melanocytic skin tumors in inbred mice. *Cancer Commun* **4**:209, 1989
52. Romerdahl CA et al: Effect of UV-B radiation on the in vivo growth of murine melanoma cells. *Cancer Res* **48**:4007, 1988
53. Fitzgerald MG et al: Prevalence of germ-line mutations in *p16*, $p19^{ARF}$, and *CDK4* in familial melanoma: Analysis of a clinically-based population. *Proc Natl Acad Sci USA* **93**:8541, 1996
54. Quelle DE et al: Alternative reading frames of the *INK4a* tumor suppressor gene encodes two unrelated proteins capable of inducing cell cycle arrest. *Cell* **83**:993, 1995
55. Pollock PM et al: Evidence for UV induction of *CDKN2* mutations in melanoma cell lines. *Oncogene* **11**:663, 1995
56. Flores JF et al: Loss of $p16^{INK4a}$ and $p15^{INK4b}$ genes, as well as neighboring 9p21 markers, in sporadic melanoma. *Cancer Res* **56**:5023, 1996
57. Chin L et al: Cooperative effects of *INK4a* and *ras* in melanoma susceptibility in vivo. *Genes Dev* **11**:2822, 1997
58. Krimpenfort P et al: Loss of $p16^{INK4a}$ confers susceptibility to metastatic melanoma in mice. *Nature* **413**:83, 2001
59. Noonan FP et al: Neonatal sunburn and melanoma in mice. *Nature* **413**:271, 2001

CHAPTER 39

Richard D. Granstein

Photoimmunology

Photoimmunology is the science that concerns itself with the effects of nonionizing radiation on the immune system. Although some data are available from human studies, most of the information currently available concerns the effects of ultraviolet radiation (UVR) in murine systems. Nonetheless, this work may have great relevance for understanding analogous or similar effects in humans.

SKIN-ASSOCIATED LYMPHOID TISSUES

The protective role of the skin includes collective properties that allow it to be considered as an immune organ. The skin contains antigen-presenting cells [Langerhans cells, (LC)] capable of communicating with T, and probably non-T, lymphocytes. In addition, keratinocytes can produce a number of cytokines that may also participate in immune recognition in the skin (see below). Streilein and his colleagues labeled these cells and the regional draining lymph nodes as *skin-associated lymphoid tissues* (SALT).[1]

Skin can clearly serve as an environment for antigen presentation in both the elicitation phase of an immune response (such as contact dermatitis) and in the induction phase of the immune response. Overwhelming evidence shows that LC are capable of presentation of various antigens to T cells (see below) and much data support the concept that certain T cells preferentially circulate between the skin and its regional lymph nodes.[1] Recently, a specific antigen, known as the *cutaneous lymphocyte antigen* (CLA), has been found to be expressed on memory T cells that traffic to the skin.[2] CLA appears to interact with E-selectin on endothelial cells.[2]

It has long been known that normal epidermis contains lymphocytes. In the mouse, most of these are highly dendritic and bear gamma/delta T cell receptors.[3] In the human, the majority are not dendritic and bear conventional alpha/beta T cell receptors.[4]

As the main barrier between the organism and the environment, the skin encounters viruses, fungi, bacteria, and chemical and physical carcinogens from which the organism must be protected. Presumably, SALT has evolved to meet the antigenic challenges of protecting the organism from infection and, perhaps, from cutaneous carcinogenesis. Immunosuppressed patients have increased rates of skin cancer, suggesting that immunosurveillance against skin cancer exists.[5]

IMMUNOLOGIC ASPECTS OF ULTRAVIOLET CARCINOGENESIS

This topic is covered in detail in Chap. 38; it is dealt with briefly here. Unna is generally credited with first describing the relationship between skin cancer and exposure to sunlight.[6] Early studies, in the 1920s, demonstrated that UVR can cause skin cancer in mice.[7] Midrange UVR (UVB, 280 to 320 nm) is more efficient than short-wave UVR (UVC, 200 to 280 nm) in producing tumors in mice.[8,9] Also, no UVC radiation reaches the earth's surface; it is totally absorbed by the atmospheric ozone layer. Long-wave UVR (UVA, 320 to 400 nm), when added to UVB radiation, may accelerate carcinogenesis.[10] UVA radiation alone, however, appears to be at least 1600 times less carcinogenic than UVB radiation.[10]

DNA Effects

The transformation of cells by UVR is thought to occur, at least in part, as a consequence of changes induced in DNA. The energy required to damage DNA increases greatly for longer wavelengths, with at least four times more energy required at 310 nm than at 254 to 300 nm.[11] Pyrimidine dimer production by UVR (290 to 360 nm) occurs in vivo in human skin.[12] The role of DNA damage in the production of some human carcinomas by UVR is supported by the finding that cells from patients with xeroderma pigmentosum, a condition marked by numerous sunlight-related cutaneous malignancies, are defective in their ability to repair UV-damaged DNA.[13,14]

Evidence that UV-induced pyrimidine dimers in DNA can give rise to tumors comes from studies of a small fish that can be grown in clones, the Amazon molly *Poecilia formosa*.[15] Thyroid tissue irradiated with 254-nm radiation and transplanted into the abdominal cavity of another fish grows into a tumor. However, if the 254-nm radiation is followed by photoreactivating illumination (to activate photoreactivating enzyme, which removes pyrimidine dimers), the percentage of fish yielding tumors is markedly reduced. Additionally, the marsupial *Monodelphis domestica* expresses photoreactivating enzyme. This animal develops both nonmelanoma and melanoma skin tumors after appropriate exposure to UVB radiation.[16] Photoreactivating illumination reduces both nonmelanoma and melanoma tumors.[16] Other evidence suggests that certain other DNA photoproducts are mutagenic and thus may also be involved in carcinogenesis.[17,18]

DNA photochemistry is believed to exert its effects by producing activation of oncogenes and mutations in tumor suppressor genes. Involvement of pyrimidine dimers in activation of the *N-ras* oncogene in vitro has been shown.[19] There are conflicting reports on the rate of mutations within ras oncogenes in human nonmelanoma and melanoma skin cancers.[20] However, there is much evidence for mutations in the tumor suppressor gene *p53* in human nonmelanoma skin cancer.[21] Mutations in the genes of the hedgehog signaling pathway (especially in *patched-1* and *smoothened*) appear central to the development of basal cell carcinoma.[22] This area is covered in detail within chapters dealing specifically with each type of skin cancer (see Chaps. 79 to 82 and 93).

Antigenicity of UVR-Induced Tumors

As early as 1939, it was reported that UVR-induced skin cancers were difficult to transplant, even to isogenic mice. At the time, this

Portions of this chapter were modified from Granstein RD: Ultraviolet radiation effects on immunologic function. *Reg Immunol* 3:112, 1990, © Wiley, Inc, 1990.

was attributed to bacterial contamination.[23] Later, it was found that most UVR (280 to 320 nm)-induced fibrosarcomas and squamous cell carcinomas were highly antigenic, at least in some strains of mice. These tumors regressed when transplanted to syngeneic normal mice but grew in immunosuppressed mice.[24] Furthermore, UV-irradiated nontumor–bearing mice were susceptible to challenge with syngeneic UVR-induced tumors, even when subcarcinogenic doses of UVR were given.[25] Second-set rejection of syngeneic UVR-induced tumors in animals that had been specifically immunized before UVR exposure was normal,[25] implying that a specific step in acquiring immunity is most likely affected by UVR.

FIGURE 39-1

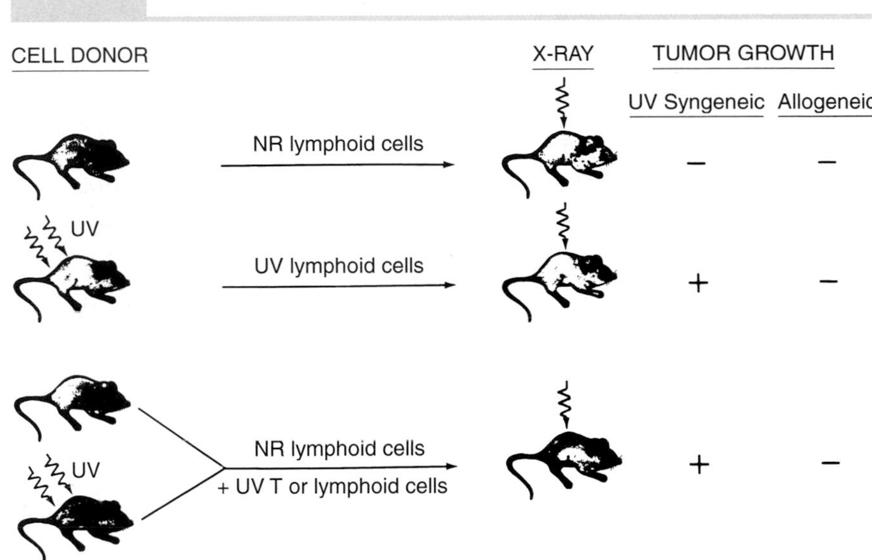

Experimental protocol used to demonstrate the immunologic basis of the UV in radiation-induced systemic alteration. Lymphoid cells from normal or UV-irradiated mice were used to reconstitute the immune system of lethally x-irradiated animals. Susceptibility to the growth of UVR-induced skin cancers was transferred with lymphoid cells taken from UVR-irradiated mice and was specific for UVR-induced syngeneic tumors. Mixing studies demonstrated that the effect was due to T lymphocytes in the lymphoid cell preparation. NR, nonirradiated age-matched controls. (*Reprinted from Kripke ML: Immunology and photocarcinogenesis. New light on an old problem. J Am Acad Dermatol* ***14****:149, 1986, with permission from Mosby-Year Book, Inc.*)

Regulatory T Cells

Normal mice can be rendered susceptible to syngeneic UVR-induced tumors by the adoptive transfer of lymphoid cells from either tumor-bearing or non-tumor-bearing UV-irradiated donors (Fig. 39-1). These cells, which have been shown to be T cells,[26] recognize UVR-induced specificities found on most UVR-induced tumors as their adoptive transfer renders the recipients susceptible to most UV-induced tumors. Lethally x-irradiated mice reconstituted with lymphoid cells from normal donors are resistant to UVR-induced tumor challenge, whereas those receiving lymphoid cells from UV-irradiated donors do not reject tumor. Mice given equal numbers of cells from both categories of donor also do not reject tumor.[27] These findings imply that the T cells involved in inducing susceptibility to tumors are suppressor cells. Experiments demonstrate that CD4+ T cells account for this phenomenon.[28] Because these cells appear to arise in UV-irradiated mice prior to animals developing tumors, UVR tumor-associated antigenic determinants are presumably induced in the skin by UVR even before the overt appearance of a tumor.

There is additional evidence that suppressor T cells (TS) cells are necessary for the development of primary skin cancers.[29] Groups of lethally x-irradiated mice had their lymphoid systems reconstituted with spleen and lymph node cells from syngeneic normal mice, with cells from chronically UV-irradiated mice, or with a mixture of both types of cells. Four weeks later, all three groups of mice received skin grafts from the irradiated areas of mice that had received chronic exposure to UVR. Significantly more tumors arose in the skin grafted to mice reconstituted with lymphoid cells from UVR-treated mice or a mixture of lymphoid cells from UVR-treated and normal mice than in the skin of those that had received only normal cells. In additional experiments, groups of mice were given intravenous injections of T cells from either normal or chronically UVR-irradiated syngeneic mice. These mice, as well as mice that had not received injections, were then exposed to UVR until tumors developed. Recipients of T cells from UVR-treated mice developed more tumors than did uninjected mice or mice that had received normal T cells; they also developed them earlier.[29] These two experiments demonstrate that the TS cells induced in mice by UVR not only inhibit the rejection of tumor transplants but also play an important role in carcinogenesis. This study illustrates the importance of immunologic regulatory mechanisms in the control of cancer growth in the primary host.

Antigen-Presenting Cell Function in UVR-Treated Mice

Studies show that splenic antigen-presenting cells (APC) from UV-irradiated mice do not present antigen effectively for priming UV-irradiated mice for a delayed-type hypersensitivity (DTH) response. This defective antigen presentation not only prevents the induction of a normal DTH response, it also stimulates the production of TS cells that are specific for the "improperly" presented antigen.[30]

Defective antigen presentation may explain the appearance of suppressor cells in UVR-irradiated animals that prevent the rejection of UVR-induced tumors. After UVR exposure, new antigens, related in specificity to tumor antigens, presumably appear in the skin. At the same time, the defect in antigen presentation occurs with inappropriate presentation of certain of these antigens to the lymphoid system, resulting in the formation of TS cells with specificity for certain tumor antigens present in UVR-induced skin cancers. In this regard, LC pulsed in vitro with tumor-associated antigens (TAA) can present TAA for in vivo antitumor immunity[31] when administered subcutaneously to naive mice. Furthermore, a number of cytokines, including granulocyte-macrophage colony-stimulating factor (GM-CSF), interleukin (IL) 10, and tumor necrosis factor (TNF)-α, modulate the ability of LC to present TAA for induction of antitumor immunity.[31] Exposure to GM-CSF is necessary for LC to induce substantial immunity against an experimental tumor. Exposure of LC to IL-10 before, but not after, activation with GM-CSF inhibits the ability of LC to prime naive mice for immunity to a tumor. Conversely, TNF-α exposure inhibits the ability of LC to present TAA when exposure occurs after, but not before, activation with GM-CSF. In addition, in vitro exposure of LC to UVB radiation inhibits LC presentation of TAA. These results highlight the complexity of the interaction of regulatory signals in vivo. The recent finding that the epidermis can serve as a source of both cellular and humoral elements that are capable of downregulation of immunity may be important in this regard. These studies have been performed primarily in contact hypersensitivity and in vitro systems and are discussed in detail below.

Human Studies

Involvement of the immune system in human cutaneous carcinogenesis is suggested by the increased risk of malignancy in patients undergoing immunosuppressive therapies. The frequency of skin cancers including basal cell carcinomas, squamous cell carcinomas and possibly melanoma is increased in immunosuppressed patients.[32,33] The overall increased risk of skin cancer in renal transplant patients is approximately sevenfold, mostly due to squamous cell carcinomas that are increased over 36-fold.[34]

B and T lymphocytes have been isolated from both human basal cell carcinomas and squamous cell carcinomas in numbers comparable to those found in biopsies of DTH reactions.[35] Some patients demonstrate immunologic reactivity against tumor cells by their own serum or peripheral blood lymphocytes.[36] However, patients in another study with large (>3 cm) squamous cell carcinomas were found to have defective cell-mediated immunity as measured by intradermal antigen reactivity and dinitrochlorobenzene (DNCB) sensitization.[37]

These studies suggest that some human skin tumors are antigenic and demonstrate that immunosuppression leads to an increased risk of some skin malignancies. The possibility that factors other than immunosuppression alone may play a role in skin cancer susceptibility in transplant patients comes from the findings that recipients of renal transplants lacking HLA-A11 are resistant to the development of skin cancer[38] and that recipients mismatched for HLA-B antigens (but not HLA-A or HLA-DR) demonstrate an increased risk of cutaneous squamous cell carcinoma but not basal cell carcinoma.[39] This latter study also indicated that there may be a slightly higher risk of squamous cell carcinoma in recipients homozygous for HLA-DR. The reasons for an increased rate of squamous cell carcinoma in HLA-B-mismatched recipients remain unclear, and these patients did not have higher cumulative doses of immunosuppressive drugs.

FIGURE 39-2

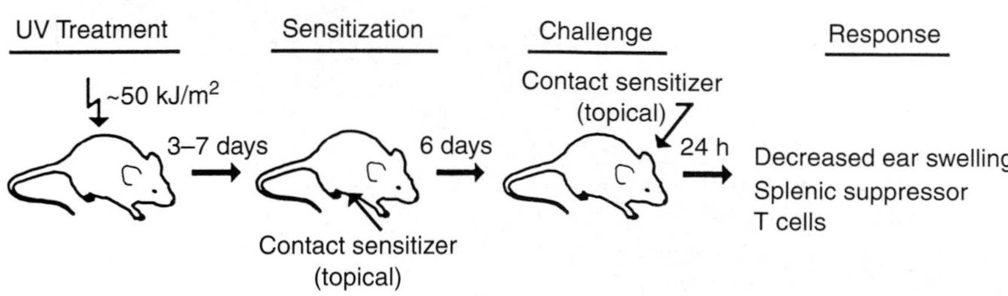

Mice are irradiated on the dorsum, then 3 to 7 days later sensitized on the ventral surface. Upon elicitation of contact hypersensitivity 6 days later, a decreased response is observed compared to nonirradiated controls in association with the development of splenic antigen-specific suppressor T cells. *(Reprinted from Kripke ML: Photoimmunology Photochem Photobiol* ***52***:*919, 1990, with permission from Pergamon Press.)*

Thus, in the murine system, immunologic changes induced in the host by UVR are of great significance in the development and growth of UVR-induced skin tumors. UVR appears to have at least two effects in mice: it both induces transformation of epidermal cells and produces specific immunologic changes that result in the appearance of TS cells with activity for UVR-induced tumors. The development of these cells accompanies or even precedes the development of clinically overt UVR-induced tumors. These cells are demonstrated by adoptive transfer and appear to be responsible for the failure of immune mechanisms to destroy the tumor.[28,29]

The relevance of these findings to human skin cancer is difficult to evaluate directly. The types of experiments described here cannot be performed with human tumors because of ethical considerations and the lack of a syngeneic testing system. Nonetheless, this murine system provides important evidence that immunologic regulatory pathways control the immune response to some types of cancer, even in the primary host. Findings that UVR-treated mice have an increased incidence of leukemia and lymphoma suggest that UV-induced immunologic changes may have significance for cancers in organs other than the skin.[40,41]

EFFECTS OF UVR ON CONTACT AND DELAYED-TYPE HYPERSENSITIVITY

Studies examining UVR effects on contact hypersensitivity (CHS) and DTH in animal models provide clues as to possible mechanisms by which UVR induces the immunologic changes that, at least in part, permit UVR regressor tumors to develop and grow. Two murine models have been extensively studied: one, termed high-dose, employs relatively large doses of short-term UVB radiation that suppresses the ability to induce CHS even at irradiated and nonirradiated sites; the other, termed low-dose, employs doses of UVB radiation that do not induce marked changes in murine skin and lead to the suppression of CHS only after induction at the irradiated sites.

In the high-dose model, mice are given doses of UVR that induce gross changes in their skin within a few days.[42] Mice are immunized by contact sensitization with a hapten at a nonirradiated site. Upon challenge several days later for a CHS response, a reduced response is observed compared to control animals (Fig. 39-2). This suppressed response is associated with the appearance of a population of TS lymphocytes in the spleens of these mice. Evidence suggests that these cells are T helper ($T_{H}1$) cells.[43] Similar irradiation schedules will also suppress the induction of DTH to subcutaneously injected antigens.[44] A causal relationship between the apparent defect in antigen presentation and the suppressed induction of CHS has been hypothesized. The mechanisms by which UVR exposure induces these changes is not well understood. Several hypotheses have been formulated. Cutaneous exposure to UVR may induce release of mediators that circulate and alter immunologic events throughout the animal. In support of this possibility, sera from mice exposed to short-term high-dose UVR downregulate the induction of CHS along with the appearance of transferable TS cells.[45] Furthermore, UVR exposure of keratinocytes in vitro causes the release of factors that suppress the induction of CHS.[46,47] At least one of these factors is IL-10. A large body of work supports the idea that release of IL-10 subsequent to UVR exposure of the skin is responsible for the inhibition of the ability of mice to be sensitized to subcutaneously injected proteins (DTH), while release of TNF-α plays a role in inhibition of sensitization to contact sensitizers[47] (see below). Indeed, IL-10–deficient, gene-targeted mice are not suppressed by UVB radiation for induction for a DTH response but are normally suppressed for induction of CHS.[48]

It has also been suggested that urocanic acid, present in the stratum corneum and epidermis, may play a role. *trans*-Urocanic acid undergoes an isomerization after exposure to UVB radiation to the *cis* form. *cis*-Urocanic acid is immunosuppressive in a number of models.[49] Prostaglandins may also have a role in these effects because indomethacin treatment of irradiated mice prevents immunosuppression.[50] There is substantial evidence that *cis*-urocanic acid suppresses DTH reactions but not CHS, in a manner similar to IL-10.[51] In this regard, *cis*-urocanic acid appears to modulate the rate of IL-10 formation in the epidermis after UVR exposure.[51] There is also a report that *cis*-urocanic acid may produce its effects by inducing mast cell degranulation with release of mediators including IL-10.[52] The exact role of *cis*-urocanic acid remains unclear as other data suggest that there is not a good relationship between *cis*-urocanic acid formation and suppression of the induction of DTH by UVB radiation.[53] In addition to *cis*-urocanic acid, there is also evidence in the literature suggesting that the neuropeptide calcitonin gene–related peptide (CGRP) is a mediator of UVB-induced suppression of contact hypersensitivity in this model.[54] CGRP has also been studied in the low-dose model (see below).

Other hypotheses to explain the effects of high-dose UVB radiation on APC function in this model include the possibility that UVR may reach and alter APC as they circulate through the dermal microvasculature; the suggestion that LC are altered by UVR exposure and then migrate to other anatomic sites where they function as abnormal APC; and the possibility that inflammation produced by UVR exposure alters trafficking of immunocompetent cells with consequences that manifest in an inability to induce CHS in animals at nonirradiated sites. Available evidence does not support these mechanisms as having major responsibility for the effects observed.

In the low-dose model of UVR-induced suppression of the induction of CHS, gross changes are not induced in the skin[55] and immunization with a hapten must be performed at the irradiated site. A suppressed response is observed, accompanied by induction of specific tolerance (inability to be subsequently immunized to the same antigen seen through the UVR-exposed site) and the appearance of splenic hapten-specific TS cells (Fig. 39-3). Recent data suggest that these cells are also T_H1 cells.[56] Susceptibility to this local effect of UVR appears to be genetically determined.[57] As mentioned above, however, data suggest that induction of the release of TNF-α locally by UVR exposure may mediate the suppression of CHS.[57] Thus, the difference between UVR-susceptible and UVR-resistant strains may relate to their ability to produce or respond to TNF-α after exposure to UVR. In this model, application of the sensitizer at a nonirradiated site produces a normal response. The mechanisms by which UVR produces these effects are not entirely clear. Immunosuppressive factors released by keratinocytes, similar to those discussed above, or release of TNF-α may mediate the suppression observed. Also, a direct effect of UVR on LC function in situ may be involved. Certain aspects of LC function, including the ability to present certain antigens, are disturbed by UVR exposure in vitro.[58,59] Other studies have demonstrated that exposure of LC to UVB radiation in vitro prevents normal presentation of antigen by LC to T_H1 cells but spares their ability to present antigens to T_H2 cells.[59] There is also evidence that CGRP plays a role in immune suppression in this model.[60,61] CGRP changes the number and morphology of epidermal LC and the presence of a CGRP inhibitor can block the UVB-induced suppression. In the same report, evidence supporting a role for nitric oxide in UVB-induced immunosuppression was also presented.[60] Some evidence exists that this effect of CGRP may be mediated by induction of mast cell degranulation with release of mediators including TNF-α and IL-10.[61] This hypothesis would, perhaps, unify the data implicating TNF-α with the data supporting a role for CGRP in the low-dose immunosuppression model. Indeed, there is some evidence that while TNF-α plays a role in failure of induction of immunity, IL-10 is important for induction of tolerance in the low-dose model.[62] Alterations in LC antigen processing and presentation by these various mechanisms may then lead to inappropriate presentation of antigen, resulting in predominant induction of downregulation of immunity. In this regard, it is also of interest that cellular elements within the epidermis can induce tolerance and/or suppression when exposed to antigen and injected intravenously without UVR exposure.[63,64] Finally, LC, after exposure to UVR in vitro, will also induce downregulation of immunity in this manner.[63] These observations might suggest that UVR exposure alters LC so that they do not efficiently present antigen for CD4-dependent immunity while preserving or enhancing the ability of epidermal elements to generate signals for immunologic downregulation. With regard to the mechanism(s) by which the induced suppressor cells mediate downregulation of immunity, there is evidence that they function, at least in part, by inducing Fas/Fas ligand-mediated apoptosis in hapten-coupled APC.[65]

Data also suggest a role for pyrimidine dimers (the major DNA photoproduct after UVR exposure) in both the local and systemic models of UVR suppression of CHS.[66] By using the marsupial *Monodelphus domestica* (which expresses photoreactivating enzymes), it was demonstrated that after UVR exposure in both the high- and low-dose models, subsequent exposure to 320- to 500-nm light ("photoreactivating light") prevented suppression of the induction of CHS. Photoreactivating light removed about 85 percent of the dimers. Further support for involvement of DNA comes from experiments utilizing the bacterial enzyme T4 endonuclease V, which accelerates the repair of cyclobutylpyrimidine dimers in mice. Application of this enzyme to murine skin after UVR exposure inhibits suppression of the induction of CHS at a nonirradiated site.[67] This observation supports the involvement of DNA photoproducts in the systemic suppression of CHS by UVR. Use of this enzyme to minimize pyrimidine dimers after UVR exposure, however, only partially inhibited suppression of CHS in the low-dose local model,[68] suggesting involvement of other mechanisms in local suppression.

Given the clear effects of UVR on these immunologic parameters, the question of whether UVR can alter immune responses to

FIGURE 39-3

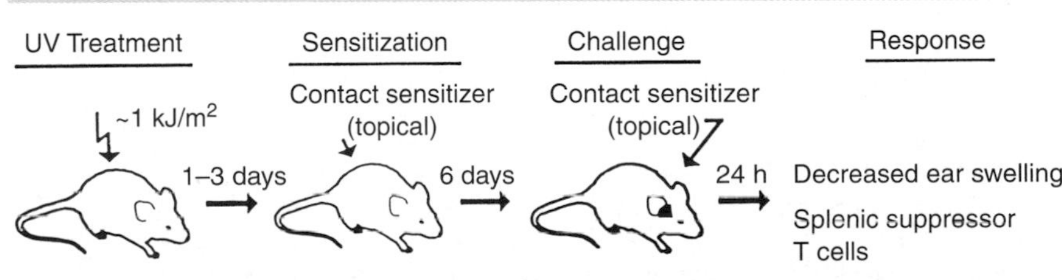

Mice are irradiated on the dorsum. Then, 1 to 3 days later they are sensitized at the irradiated site. Upon elicitation of a contact hypersensitivity response 6 days later, a decreased response is observed in association with the development of antigen-specific splenic suppressor T cells. (*Reprinted from Kripke ML: Photoimmunology. Photochem Photobiol* ***52*** *:919, 1990, with permission from Pergamon Press.)*

infectious organisms has been explored. In mice, exposure of the site of inoculation to UVR 24 h before and every 48 to 72 h after inoculation with *Leishmania major* promastigotes results in inhibition of skin lesion development.[69] Furthermore, this irradiation regimen suppresses the induction of DTH to leishmanial antigens. The number of parasites recovered from injection sites was the same in control and irradiated animals. Thus, the locus of UVR appears to be host reactivity rather than the parasites themselves. Other studies also using a murine model have shown that a single large dose of UVR inhibits DTH to *Candida albicans*. This inhibition is associated with the generation of transferable splenic-suppressor cells if irradiation occurs prior to immunization.[70] However, if irradiation occurs after immunization, DTH is still inhibited, but without the appearance of splenic-suppressor cells.[70] In addition, UVR inhibits the ability of rats to clear *Listeria monocytogenes*.[71] UVR exposure results in more severe primary infection to herpes simplex virus type 1 in mice,[72] and inhibits murine T_H1 immune responses to *Borrelia burgdorferi,* while leaving T_H2 responses intact.[73] Also, it has been shown that local UVR exposure reduces the granulomatous reaction to lepromin in sensitized individuals.[74] However, no effect of UV radiation was observed in a murine model of infection with *Schistosoma mansoni*.[75]

FIGURE 39-4

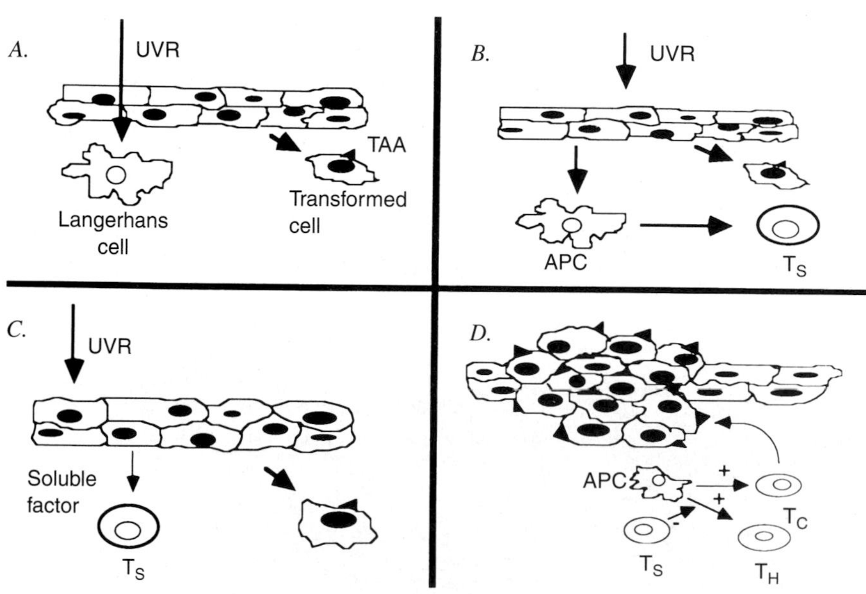

Model of UVR-induced tumorigenesis. Experimental evidence exists to suggest several mechanisms for UVR-induced downregulation of the immune response to UVR-induced tumor-associated antigens (TAA). A. Direct functional derangement or elimination of antigen-presenting cells (APC, presumably Langerhans cells) from the epidermis that are capable of presenting antigen from transformed cells for CD4-dependent responses. B. Selection or preservation of UVR-resistant APC (I-A+; or Thy 1+) that may present TAA for activation of T suppressor (TS) cells. C. UVR-induced release of an epidermal factor(s) resulting in preferential activation of TS cells and immunologic downregulation. D. Clonal proliferation of transforming cell clone expressing TAA. Immune rejection is inhibited by lack of functional APC to induce T helper activity directed against TAA (A), or presence of APC primed for suppression (B), and/or epidermal immunosuppressive factor release (C). (*Reprinted with permission from Gallo RL et al: Physiology and pathology of skin photoimmunology, in* Skin Immune System, *edited by JD Bos. Boca Raton, CRC Press, 1989, p 381. Copyright CRC Press, Inc., Boca Raton, FL.*)

Hypothetical Pathway for UVR-Induced Skin Cancer Formation

Correlation of data from studies examining UVR effects on CHS and the photocarcinogenesis experiments discussed above might suggest the following hypothesis as to the mechanism by which UVR-induced immunologic changes participate in the generation of UVR-induced skin cancers (Fig. 39-4). UVR may produce two effects. Presumably, it induces a transformation of keratinocyte targets to a malignant phenotype with the expression of TAA. Additionally, UVR would produce changes in epidermal antigen-presenting function with alteration of the balance between the induction of immunity and the induction of tolerance/suppression toward downregulation. This may occur through UVR-induced changes in LC, mediated in part by UVR-induced cytokine signals, preventing efficient presentation of antigen for effector immune mechanisms with preservation or enhancement of downregulatory signals. Certain TAA are then presented for the induction of TS cells that prevent immunologic destruction of the incipient tumor. Although not shown directly, this hypothesis is consistent with the available data.

Human Studies

The importance of these observations for humans is difficult to evaluate. Nonetheless, some observations might suggest that similar mechanisms may apply. Relatively modest exposures of UVR have immunologic effects on normal persons.[76,77] Exposure to 1 h of summer sunlight on 12 occasions resulted in significant increases in suppressor/cytotoxic (CD8) lymphocytes and a decrease in helper phenotype (CD4) cells in peripheral blood.[76] These subjects also demonstrated increased nonspecific suppressor cell activity in their peripheral blood mononuclear cell (PBMC) populations. In a similar study, individuals given 30-min exposures in a commercial solarium with an irradiation source emitting 0.04% UVB radiation and 10.6% UVA radiation demonstrated reduced cutaneous responses to DNCB, increased nonspecific suppressor cell activity, decreased natural killer cell activity, and a decrease in the CD4 to CD8 cell ratio compared to controls.[77] A report suggests that humans may vary in their susceptibility to the ability of local UVB radiation to inhibit the induction of CHS.[78] In this study, a dose of UVB radiation that depletes LC from skin was followed by application of DNCB. Sixty percent of individuals became sensitive to DNCB from this protocol (UVB-sensitive), whereas others did not. Skin cancer patients had a higher rate of nonresponse (92 percent), and 45 percent of them became tolerant to DNCB, while no normal subjects became tolerant. The analogy to the situation with inbred strains of mice (discussed above) might suggest a genetic basis for UVB susceptibility in this manner and that the ability to suppress CHS with UVB radiation might be a risk factor for skin cancer susceptibility.[78]

Human epidermal cells obtained after exposure to UVB radiation are capable of activating suppressor-inducer lymphocytes. This activity appears to reside in non-Langerhans CD1-DR+ macrophage-like APC that appear in the epidermis 1 to 3 days after exposure to UVB radiation.[79] Macrophages recruited into skin by UVR exposure are also capable of inducing immunologic downregulation to a hapten.[80] There are data suggesting that the suppressive activity of these cells relates to release of IL-10 and TNF-α after binding of iC3b to these cells.[81] There are also data from mice indicating that similar mechanisms also play a role in UV-induced immunosuppression in mice.[82] These findings suggest mechanisms by which UVR exposure of human skin might enhance suppressor pathways.

In addition to the studies suggesting that exposure to UVR can alter immunologic parameters in humans, there is evidence that human skin cancer development is at least partially under immunologic control. As mentioned above, immunosuppressed persons, suppressed either due to underlying illness or because of immunosuppressive treatment for cancer or for the maintenance of transplanted organs, have greatly increased rates of skin cancer. Squamous cell carcinomas are increased 30- to 40-fold, and smaller increases in the incidence of basal cell carcinomas have been documented.[32,34] The rate of melanoma occurrence in these patients may also be increased.[34] The majority of the nonmelanoma skin cancers in these individuals occur in sun-exposed areas.

LANGERHANS CELLS

Exposure of LC to UVR in vitro alters their ability to present antigen in some situations.[58,59] LC are bone marrow-derived, dendritic, Ia-bearing cells capable of presenting various antigens to T lymphocytes.[31,83,84] When isolated in vitro, these cells mature, at least partly under the influence of GM-CSF, to become much more potent antigen-presenting cells for primary immune responses. They are very similar to dendritic cells found in lymphoid organs.[84,85]

For 40 years LC have been known to be sensitive to UVR.[86] After UVR exposure in vivo, LC density decreases, as determined by Ia antigen expression and ATPase staining;[87] some LC appear to be present in the epidermis when examined by electron microscopy, although with altered morphology. The ability to induce CHS in mice appears to have a relationship to the density of ATPase-positive cells in the epidermis.[88] Furthermore, if LC are UVR-exposed in vitro, coupled to hapten, and transferred to primed mice by subcutaneous administration, immunity fails to develop;[89] instead, a state of specific tolerance occurs associated with the appearance of transferable splenic TS cells. Thus, exposure to UVR alters antigen presentation by a mixed population of epidermal cells. This does not, however, prove that such effects are due to changes in LC.

KERATINOCYTE-DERIVED CYTOKINES

Keratinocytes are able to produce a number of cytokines with immunologic or inflammatory activities, depending on their state of activation. These include IL-1α, IL-1β, IL-3, IL-6, IL-7, IL-8, IL-12, IL-15, granulocyte colony-stimulating factor, macrophage-stimulating factor, GM-CSF, TNF-α, transforming growth factor-α, and transforming growth factor-β, among others[90–94] (see also Chap. 26). IL-1, IL-6, IL-8, IL-10, TNF-α, and GM-CSF expression are reportedly increased in keratinocytes after UVB exposure.[84,90,95,96] IL-7 expression is downregulated by UVB radiation,[91] and controversy exists regarding the effects of UVB radiation on IL-15 expression in keratinocytes.[94,97] Additionally, serum or plasma levels of IL-1 activity increase after total-body exposure to UVR in mice,[98] rabbits,[99] and also humans.[98,100] Similarly, it has been found that exposure of humans to UVR results in increased circulating IL-6 and TNF-α activity.[101,102] Hypothetically, alterations in cytokine production secondary to exposure to UVR may play a role in the immunologic changes observed after exposure of animals to UVR

in vivo. As discussed above, there is evidence that release of IL-10 and TNF-α, subsequent to in vivo UVR exposure, plays a role in UVR-induced immunosuppression. Although not proven, it is thought that production of these cytokines occurs in the skin. Changes in cytokine release by epidermal cells after UVR exposure might also play a role in the exacerbation of certain autoimmune diseases by sunlight exposure.

UVR may also affect the biology of adhesion molecules. Exposure of keratinocytes to UVR inhibits the ability of cytokines to induce intercellular adhesion molecule (ICAM)-1, an important cell surface molecule involved in the adhesion function of certain cells including keratinocytes and endothelial cells.[103,104] This effect might also be involved in the modulation of cutaneous inflammatory activity by UVR. The effect of UVB radiation on expression of the costimulatory molecules B7-1 (CD80) and B7-2 (CD86) has also been examined. Irradiation of LC in vitro inhibited the upregulation of B7-1 and B7-2 that occurs when LC are cultured.[105] However, exposure of human skin in-situ with erythemogenic doses of solar simulating UV radiation resulted in strong up-regulation of B7-1 and B7-2 between 12 and 24 h after exposure.[106] The importance of an understanding of the effect of UVR on expression of these molecules relates to their importance in activation of T cells. Indeed, interactions of CD86 with its receptors appears to be important for UVR-induced immune suppression.[107] Transgenic mice with a functional disruption in B7-mediated stimulation of T cells have reduced UVR-induced skin cancer formation.[108]

EFFECTS OF WHOLE-BODY EXPOSURE TO UVR ON LYMPHOCYTES IN HUMANS

As early as 1928, investigators were interested in the medical effects of nonionizing radiation[109] because of the perception that both sunlight and artificial sources of radiation might be of clinical benefit in some disease states. It was found that acute or chronic exposure to radiation increased the number of PBMC. These studies are difficult to interpret because various radiation sources were used, and both healthy subjects and patients with disease were examined.

This question was later reexamined.[110] Normal subjects were given a single, whole-body exposure to UVB radiation to produce a mild or a marked erythema. Circulating leukocytes in these subjects were monitored over the following 72 h. Shortly after exposure to UVR, the subjects who developed erythema had a decreased proportion of circulating T lymphocytes. This effect was most pronounced at 8 to 12 h after exposure, followed by a return to normal levels by 72 h. The proportion of B cells did not change. This effect was accompanied by a fall in the response of the circulating cells to the T cell mitogen phytohemagglutinin. Subjects who developed only a slight erythema did not show this decrease in reactivity to phytohemagglutinin, suggesting that this effect may be dose-related. Both groups showed an increase in the number of circulating polymorphonuclear leukocytes. Also, as discussed above, Hersey et al. demonstrated that individuals exposed to 1 h of summer sunlight for 12 exposures or to 30-min exposures in a commercial solarium demonstrated a decrease in the ratio of CD4+ to CD8+ lymphocytes in their peripheral blood.[92]

Taken together, it is clear that ultraviolet radiation alters a number of parameters of immunologic function after exposure both in vitro and in vivo. Table 39-1 summarizes the observations that have been made in this regard. These findings, of course, do not speak to the pathways by which UVR alters the immunologic status of an intact organism. A major challenge for the future is to understand the interactions of these various phenomena within a whole animal. These questions are

TABLE 39-1

Ultraviolet Radiation Effects

In vitro
Alters ability of antigen-presenting cells (including Langerhans cells) to present antigen
Alters ability of lymphocytes to respond to mitogens or antigens
Alters cytokine production
Induces the release of immunosuppressive factors
In vivo
Induces skin cancer formation
Alters Langerhans cell morphology and function
Suppresses the induction of contact hypersensitivity
Suppresses the induction of delayed-type hypersensitivity
Alters cell trafficking
Increases circulating levels of certain cytokines
Alters proportions of lymphocyte subtypes in peripheral blood

of importance to medicine. For example, it is of clinical relevance to understand the mechanisms by which nonionizing radiation interacts with the skin to induce exacerbations of autoimmune disease. Also, a further understanding of the role of UVR exposure in infectious and neoplastic conditions may be important in designing new therapeutic modalities.

Perhaps the area in which photoimmunology has received the most attention is photocarcinogenesis (see Chap. 38). Skin cancer induced in animal models by UVR clearly represents a system in which the skin, the immune system, and light interact to produce pathology. Circumstantial evidence indicates that similar mechanisms may be involved in human cutaneous photocarcinogenesis. As discussed above, there is epidemiologic evidence demonstrating increased rates of skin cancer in immunosuppressed individuals, highlighting the role of the immune system in the regulation of these tumors. Also, as discussed above, modest doses of UVR clearly induce changes in immunologic parameters in humans that are at least measurable. The direct relevance of these changes for future disease is, of course, unknown. It would seem clear that avoidance of exposure to prolonged and excessive sunlight is prudent, given the current state of knowledge of the role of sunlight in the development of cutaneous malignancies; it would also prevent sunlight-induced aging of the skin. The possible role of exposure to sunlight in the development of other pathologies, such as infectious disease, remains to be more fully investigated.

REFERENCES

1. Streilein JW, Tigelaar RE: SALT: Skin-associated lymphoid tissues, in *Photoimmunology,* edited by JA Parrish ML Kripke, WL Morison. New York, Plenum, 1983, p 95
2. Santamaria LF et al: Allergen specificity and endothelial transmigration of T cells in allergic contact dermatitis and atopic dermatitis are associated with the cutaneous lymphocyte antigen. *Int Arch Allergy Immunol* **107**:359, 1995
3. Steiner G et al: Characterization of T cell receptors on resident murine dendritic epidermal cells. *Eur J Immunol* **18**:1323, 1988
4. Groh V et al: Human lymphocytes bearing T cell receptor gamma/delta are phenotypically diverse and evenly distributed throughout the lymphoid system. *J Exp Med* **169**:1277, 1989
5. Kinlen LJ et al: Collaborative United Kingdom–Australia study of cancer in patients treated with immunosuppressive drugs. *Br Med J* **2**:1461, 1979
6. Unna PG: *The Histopathology of the Disease of the Skin.* Edinburgh, WF Clay, 1894
7. Findlay GM: Ultra-violet light and skin cancer. *Lancet* **2**:1070, 1928
8. Freeman RG et al: Ultraviolet wavelength factors in solar radiation and skin cancer. *Int J Dermatol* **9**:232, 1970
9. Urbach F et al: Ultraviolet carcinogenesis: Experimental, global, and genetic aspects, in *Sunlight and Man: Normal and Abnormal Photobiologic Responses,* edited by MA Pathak LL Harber, M Seiji, A Kukita; TB Fitzpatrick, consulting editor. Tokyo, University of Tokyo Press, 1974, p 259
10. Appendix F, in *Protection Against Depletion of Stratospheric Ozone by Chlorofluorocarbons*. Washington, DC, National Academy of Sciences, 1979, p 325
11. Tan EM et al: Action spectrum of ultraviolet light-induced damage to nuclear DNA in vitro. *J Invest Dermatol* **55**:439, 1970
12. Sutherland BM et al: Pyrimidine dimer formation and repair in human skin. *Cancer Res* **40**:3181, 1980
13. Cleaver JE: Defective repair replication of DNA in xeroderma pigmentosum. *Nature* **218**:652, 1968
14. Epstein JH et al: Defect in DNA synthesis in skin of patients with xeroderma pigmentosum demonstrated in vivo. *Science* **168**:1477, 1970
15. Hart RW et al: Evidence that pyrimidine dimers in DNA can give rise to tumors. *Proc Natl Acad Sci U S A* **74**:5574, 1977
16. Ley RD, Reeve VE, Kusewitt DF: Photobiology of *Monodelphus domestica*. *Dev Comp Immunol* **24**:503, 2000.
17. Brash DE, Haseltine WA: UV-induced mutation hotspots occur at DNA damage hotspots. *Nature* **298**:189, 1982
18. Brash DE: UV mutagenic photoproducts in *Escherichia coli* and human cells: A molecular genetics perspective on human skin cancer. *Photochem Photobiol* **48**:59, 1988
19. van der Lubbe JLM et al: Activation of *N-ras* induced by ultraviolet light in vitro. *Oncogene Res* **3**:9, 1988
20. Campbell C et al: Codon 12 Harvey-*ras* mutations are rare events in non-melanoma human skin cancer. *Br J Dermatol* **128**:111, 1993
21. Ren ZP et al: Human epidermal cancer and accompanying precursors have identical *p53* mutations different from *p53* mutations in adjacent areas of clonally expanded non-neoplastic keratinocytes. *Oncogene* **12**:765, 1996
22. Bonifas J et al: Activation of expression of hedgehog target genes in basal cell carcinoma. *J Invest Dermatol* **116**:739, 2001
23. Rusch HP, Baumann CA: Tumor production in mice with ultraviolet irradiation. *Am J Cancer* **35**:55, 1939
24. Kripke ML: Antigenicity of murine skin tumors induced by ultraviolet light. *J Natl Cancer Inst* **53**:1333, 1974
25. Kripke ML, Fisher MS: Immunologic parameters of ultraviolet carcinogenesis. *J Natl Cancer Inst* **57**:211, 1976
26. Spellman CW, Daynes RA: Modification of immunological potential by ultraviolet radiation. II. Generation of suppressor cells in short-term UV-irradiated mice. *Transplantation* **24**:120, 1977
27. Fisher MS, Kripke ML: Systemic alteration induced in mice by ultraviolet light irradiation carcinogenesis. *Proc Natl Acad Sci U S A* **74**:1688, 1977
28. Ullrich SE, Kripke ML: Mechanisms in the suppression of tumor rejection produced in mice by repeated UV irradiation. *J Immunol* **133**:2786, 1984
29. Fisher MS, Kripke ML: Suppressor T lymphocytes control the development of primary skin cancers in ultraviolet-irradiated mice. *Science* **216**:1133, 1982
30. Greene MI et al: Impairment of antigen-presenting cell function by ultraviolet radiation. *Proc Natl Acad Sci U S A* **76**:6591, 1979
31. Grabbe S, Granstein RD: Modulation of antigen-presenting cell function as a potential regulatory mechanism in tumor-host reactions. *In Vivo* **7**:265, 1993
32. Hill BHR: Immunosuppressive drug therapy potentiator of skin tumors in five patients with lymphoma. *Aust J Dermatol* **17**:46, 1976
33. Jensen P et al: Skin cancer in kidney and heart transplant recipients and different long-term immunosuppressive therapy regimens. *J Am Acad Dermatol* **40**:177, 1999
34. Hoxtell EO et al: Incidence of skin carcinoma after renal transplantation. *Arch Dermatol* **113**:436, 1977
35. Viac J et al: Characterization of mononuclear cells in the inflammatory infiltrates of cutaneous tumors. *Br J Dermatol* **97**:1, 1977
36. Nairn RC et al: Specific immune response in human skin carcinoma. *Br Med J* **4**:701, 1971
37. Weimar VM et al: Cell-mediated immunity in patients with basal and squamous cell skin cancer. *J Am Acad Dermatol* **2**:143, 1980
38. Bouwes Bavinck JN et al: HLA-A11-associated resistance to skin cancer in renal transplant recipients. *N Engl J Med* **323**:1350, 1990
39. Bouwes Bavinck JN et al: Relation between skin cancer and HLA antigens in renal-transplant recipients. *N Engl J Med* **325**:843, 1991
40. Eaton GJ et al: Effects of ultraviolet light on nude mice: Cutaneous carcinogenesis and possible leukemogenesis. *Cancer* **42**:182, 1978
41. Ebbesen P: Enhanced lymphoma incidence in BALB/c mice after ultraviolet light treatment. *J Natl Cancer Inst* **67**:1077, 1981
42. Noonan FP et al: Suppression of contact hypersensitivity in mice by ultraviolet irradiation is associated with defective antigen presentation. *Immunology* **43**:527, 1981

43. Shreedhar VK et al: Origin and characteristics of ultraviolet-B radiation-induced suppressor T lymphocytes. *J Immunol* **161**:1327, 1998
44. Molendijk A et al: Suppression of delayed-type hypersensitivity to histocompatability antigens by ultraviolet radiation. *Immunology* **62**:299, 1987
45. Schwartz T et al: Inhibition of the induction of contact hypersensitivity by a UV-mediated epidermal cytokine. *J Invest Dermatol* **87**:289, 1986
46. Kim TY et al: Immunosuppression by factors released from UV-irradiated epidermal cells: Selective effects on the generation of contact and delayed hypersensitivity after exposure to UVA or UVB radiation. *J Invest Dermatol* **94**:26, 1990
47. Rivas JM, Ullrich SE: The role of IL-4, IL-10 and TNF-alpha in the immune suppression induced by ultraviolet radiation. *J Leuk Biol* **56**:769, 1994
48. Beissert S et al: Impaired immunosuppressive response to ultraviolet radiation in interleukin-10–deficient mice. *J Invest Dermatol* **107**:553, 1996
49. DeFabo EC, Noonan FP: Mechanism of immune suppression by ultraviolet radiation in vivo. I. Evidence for the existence of a unique photoreceptor in skin and its role in photoimmunology. *J Exp Med* **158**:84, 1983
50. Chung H-T et al: Involvement of prostaglandins in the immune alterations caused by the exposure of mice to ultraviolet radiation. *J Immunol* **137**:2478, 1986
51. Moodycliffe AM et al: Differential effects of a monoclonal antibody to cis-urocanic acid on the suppression of delayed and contact hypersensitivity following ultraviolet irradiation. *J Immunol* **157**:2891, 1996
52. Reeve VE et al: Differential photoimmunoprotection by sunscreen ingredients is unrelated to epidermal cis urocanic acid formation in hairless mice. *J Invest Dermatol* **103**:801, 1994
53. Hart PH et al: A critical role for dermal mast cells in cis-urocanic acid-induced systemic suppression of contact hypersensitivity responses in mice. *Photochem Photobiol* **70**:807, 1999
54. Garssen J, Buckley TL, Van Loveren H: A role for neuropeptides in UVB-induced systemic immunosuppression. *Photochem Photobiol* **68**:205, 1988
55. Elmets CA et al: In vivo low dose UVB irradiation induces suppressor cells to contact sensitizing agents, in *The Effect of Ultraviolet Light on the Immune System,* edited by JA Parrish. Skillman, NJ, Johnson & Johnson Press, 1983, p 317
56. Schwarz A et al: Evidence for functional relevance of CTLA-4 in ultraviolet-radiation-induced tolerance. *J Immunol* **165**:1824, 2000
57. Streilein JW et al: Functional dichotomy between Langerhans cells that present antigen to naive and to memory/effector T lymphocytes. *Immunol Rev* **117**:159, 1990
58. Stingl G et al: Antigen presentation by murine epidermal cells and its alteration by ultraviolet B light. *J Immunol* **127**:1707, 1981
59. Simon JC et al: Low dose ultraviolet B-irradiated Langerhans cells preferentially activate CD4+ cells of the T helper 2 subset. *J Immunol* **145**:2087, 1990
60. Gillardon F et al: Calcitonin gene-related peptide and nitric oxide are involved in ultraviolet radiation-induced immunosuppression. *Eur J Pharmacol* **293**:395, 1995
61. Kitazawa T et al: Hapten-specific tolerance promoted by calcitonin gene–related peptide. *J Invest Dermatol* **115**:942, 2000
62. Niizeki H et al: Hapten-specific tolerance induced by acute, low-dose ultraviolet B radiation of skin is mediated via interleukin-10. *J Invest Dermatol* **109**:25, 1997
63. Tan K-C et al: Epidermal cell presentation of tumor-associated antigens for induction of tolerance. *J Immunol* **153**:760, 1994
64. Sullivan S et al: Induction and regulation of contact hypersensitivity by resident, bone marrow derived, dendritic epidermal cells: Langerhans and Thy-1+ epidermal cells. *J Immunol* **137**:2460, 1986
65. Schwarz T et al: Ultraviolet light-induced immune tolerance is mediated via the Fas/Fas ligand system. *J Immunol* **160**:4262, 1998
66. Applegate LA et al: Identification of the molecular target for the suppression of contact hypersensitivity by ultraviolet radiation. *J Exp Med* **170**:1117, 1989
67. Kripke ML et al: Pyrimidine dimers in DNA initiate systemic immunosuppression in UV-irradiated mice. *Proc Natl Acad Sci U S A* **89**:7516, 1992
68. Wolf P et al: Sunscreens and T4N5 liposomes differ in their ability to protect against ultraviolet-induced sunburn cell formation, alterations of dendritic epidermal cells, and local suppression of contact hypersensitivity. *J Invest Dermatol* **104**:287, 1995
69. Giannini MS: Suppression of pathogenesis in cutaneous leishmaniasis by UV radiation. *Infect Immun* **51**:838, 1986
70. Denkins Y et al: Exposure of mice to UV-B radiation suppresses delayed hypersensitivity to *Candida albicans*. *Photochem Photobiol* **49**:615, 1989
71. Goettsch W et al: Effects of ultraviolet-B exposure on the resistance to *Listeria monocytogenes* in the rat. *Photochem Photobiol* **63**:672, 1996
72. El-Ghorr AA, Norval M: The effect of UV-B irradiation on secondary epidermal infection of mice with herpes simplex virus type 1. *J Gen Virol* **77**:485, 1996
73. Brown EL et al: Modulation of immunity to *Borrelia burgdorferi* by ultraviolet irradiation: Differential effect on Th1 and Th2 immune responses. *Eur J Immunol* **25**:3017, 1995
74. Cestari TF et al: Ultraviolet radiation decreases the granulomatous response to lepromin in humans. *J Invest Dermatol* **105**:8, 1995
75. Noonan FP, Lewis FA: UVB-induced immune suppression and infection with *Schistosoma mansoni*. *Photochem Photobiol* **61**:99, 1995
76. Hersey P et al: Alteration of T cell subsets and induction of suppressor T cell activity in normal subjects after exposure to sunlight. *J Immunol* **131**:171, 1983
77. Hersey P et al: Immunological effects of solarium exposure. *Lancet* **1**:545, 1983
78. Yoshikawa T et al: Susceptibility to effects of UVB radiation on induction of contact hypersensitivity as a risk factor for skin cancer in humans. *J Invest Dermatol* **95**:530, 1990
79. Cooper KD: Cell-mediated immunosuppressive mechanisms induced by UV radiation. *Photochem Photobiol* **63**:400, 1996
80. Hammerberg C et al: Active induction of unresponsiveness (tolerance) to DNFB by in vivo ultraviolet-exposed epidermal cells is dependent upon infiltrating class II MHC+; CD1b bright monocytic/macrophage cells. *J Immunol* **153**:4915, 1994
81. Yoshida Y et al: Monocyte induction of IL-10 and down-regulation of IL-12 by iC3b deposited in ultraviolet-exposed human skin. *J Immunol* **161**:5873, 1998
82. Hammerberg C: Activated complement component 3 (C3) is required for ultraviolet induction of immunosuppression and antigenic tolerance. *J Exp Med* **187**:1133, 1998
83. Katz SI et al: Epidermal Langerhans cells are derived from cells originating in bone marrow. *Nature* **282**:324, 1979
84. Grabbe S et al: Mechanisms of ultraviolet radiation carcinogenogenesis. *Chem Immunol* **58**:291, 1994
85. Schuler G, Steinman RM: Murine epidermal Langerhans cells mature into potent immunostimulatory dendritic cells in vitro. *J Exp Med* **161**:526, 1985
86. Fan J et al: A study of the epidermal clear cells with special reference to their relationship to the cells of Langerhans. *J Invest Dermatol* **32**:445, 1959
87. Aberer W et al: Ultraviolet light depletes surface markers of Langerhans cells. *J Invest Dermatol* **76**:202, 1981
88. Toews GB et al: Epidermal Langerhans cell density determines whether contact hypersensitivity or unresponsiveness follows skin painting with DNFB. *J Immunol* **124**:445, 1980
89. Sauder DN et al: Induction of tolerance to topically applied TNCB using TNP-conjugated ultraviolet light-irradiated epidermal cells. *J Immunol* **127**:261, 1981
90. Luger TA, Schwarz T: Epidermal cell-derived cytokines, in *Skin Immune System,* edited by JD Bos. Boca Raton, FL, CRC Press, 1990, p 257
91. Takashima A et al: Interleukin-7-dependent interaction of dendritic epidermal T cells with keratinocytes. *J Invest Dermatol* **105**:50S, 1995
92. Venner TJ et al: Interleukin-8 and melanoma growth-stimulating activity (GRO) are induced by ultraviolet B radiation in human keratinocyte cells lines. *Exp Dermatol* **4**:138, 1995
93. Yawalkar N et al: Constitutive expression of both subunits of interleukin-12 in human keratinocytes. *J Invest Dermatol* **106**:80, 1996
94. Blauvelt A et al: Interleukin-15 mRNA is expressed by human keratinocytes, Langerhans cells, and blood-derived dendritic cells and is down-regulated by ultraviolet B radiation. *J Invest Dermatol* **106**:1047, 1996
95. Gahring L et al: Effect of ultraviolet radiation on production of epidermal cell thymocyte-activating factor/interleukin 1 in vivo and in vitro. *Proc Natl Acad Sci U S A* **81**:1198, 1984
96. Ansel JC et al: The effect of in vitro and in vivo UV irradiation on the production of ETAF activity by human and murine keratinocytes. *J Invest Dermatol* **81**:519, 1983
97. Mohamadzadeh M et al: Ultraviolet B radiation up-regulates the expression of IL-15 in human skin. *J Immunol* **155**:4492, 1995
98. Granstein RD, Sauder DN: Whole-body exposure to ultraviolet radiation results in increased serum interleukin-1 activity in humans. *Lymphokine Res* **6**:187, 1987

99. Ansel JC et al: Fever and increased serum IL-1 activity as a systemic manifestation of acute phototoxicity in New Zealand White rabbits. *J Invest Dermatol* **89**:32, 1987

100. Konnikov N et al: Elevated plasma interleukin-1 levels in humans following ultraviolet light therapy for psoriasis. *J Invest Dermatol* **92**:235, 1989

101. Urbanski A et al: Ultraviolet light induces increased circulating interleukin-6 in humans. *J Invest Dermatol* **94**:808, 1990

102. Kock A et al: Human keratinocytes are a source for tumor necrosis factor alpha: Evidence for synthesis and release upon stimulation with endotoxin or ultraviolet light. *J Exp Med* **172**:1609, 1990

103. Norris DA et al: Ultraviolet radiation can either suppress or induce expression of intercellular adhesion molecule 1 (ICAM-1) on the surface of cultured human keratinocytes. *J Invest Dermatol* **95**:132, 1990

104. Krutmann J et al: Tumor necrosis factor beta and ultraviolet radiation are potent regulators of human keratinocyte ICAM-1 expression. *J Invest Dermatol* **95**:127, 1990

105. Denfeld RW et al: Further characterization of UVB radiation effects on Langerhans cells: altered expression of the costimulatory molecules B7-1 and B7-2. *Photochem Photobiol* **67**:554, 1998

106. Laihia JK et al: Up-regulation of human epidermal Langerhans' cell B7-1 and B7-2 co-stimulatory molecules in vivo by solar-simulating irradiation. *Eur J Immunol* **27**:984, 1997

107. Ullrich SE et al: Antibodies to the costimulatory molecule CD86 interfere with ultraviolet radiation-induced immune suppression. *Immunology* **94**:417, 1998

108. Beissert S et al: Reduced ultraviolet-induced carcinogenesis in mice with a functional disruption is B7-mediated costimulation. *J Immunol* **163**:6725, 1999

109. Laurens H: The physiological effects of radiation. *Physiol Rev* **8**:1091, 1928

110. Morison WL et al: In vivo effects of UVB on lymphocyte function. *Br J Dermatol* **101**:513, 1979

PART THREE

Disorders Presenting in the Skin and Mucous Membranes

SECTION 7
NONCUTANEOUS MANIFESTATIONS OF SKIN DISEASES

CHAPTER 40

Thomas W. Koenig
Sylvia Garnis-Jones
Adrienne Rencic
Francisco A. Tausk

Psychological Aspects of Skin Diseases

Scientific advances are shedding new light on the understanding and treatment of long-recognized conditions located at the interface of dermatology and psychiatry. Both arising from ectoderm, the skin and the nervous system are connected by more than just their common origins. The skin is one of the major avenues by which we perceive the world, and, in turn, are perceived by it. When these perceptions go awry, great distress may result to the patient, as is the case in delusional parasitosis. When the skin itself is markedly affected by a primary dermatologic condition, psychological sequelae often follow, greatly impacting the patient's self-esteem, confidence, and overall quality of life.

The central nervous system can influence the health (both actual and perceived) of other organ systems including the skin. Psychophysiologic mechanisms for this interaction range from the stress responses mediated by neuroadrenal connections and associated changes in immunologic function, to the systemic and local action of various neuropeptides and neurohormones.[1,2]

ROLE OF THE DERMATOLOGIST IN TREATING PSYCHOCUTANEOUS PATIENTS

Between 20 and 40 percent of patients seeking treatment for skin complaints have some type of psychiatric or psychological problem causing or complicating the presenting symptoms. A large number of these patients lack insight into the possible psychogenic origin of their symptoms and are often reluctant to accept any kind of psychiatric referral. Therefore, in the absence of a psychiatry liaison clinic in the dermatologic setting, the dermatologist must be familiar with the most common of these diagnoses, their clinical manifestations (both psychological and dermatologic), and the basic principles of treatment.

CLASSIFICATION OF PSYCHOCUTANEOUS DISEASES

Following the original description of C. Koblenzer,[3] psychocutaneous diseases can be classified based on their primary etiology as:

- Primary psychiatric disorders, which can present with a variety of symptoms and behaviors, that can lead to perceived or actual dermatologic conditions, or
- Primary dermatologic disorders that can be exacerbated through psychophysiologic mechanisms such as stress or that may cause demoralization, anxiety, and distress through their impact on the patient's physical appearance and well being.

Primary Psychiatric Disorders

MONOSYMPTOMATIC HYPOCHONDRIACAL PSYCHOSIS—DELUSIONAL PARASITOSIS Dermatologic patients will occasionally show evidence of psychosis, characterized by the presence of delusions, hallucinations, or formal thought disorder. Delusions are fixed false beliefs that patients hold with unshakeable conviction not endorsed by the larger cultural, ethnic, or religious community. Hallucinations are sensory perceptions that occur without any external stimulus, and can occur in any of the five sensory modalities. Misinterpretations of existing stimuli (e.g., an inanimate piece of fiber seen as a worm or other parasite) are better understood as illusions or delusional misrepresentations. Formal thought disorder describes the disorganization of thought processes as reflected in the speech of the patient. The most frequent form of this condition seen by dermatologists is *delusional parasitosis* (DP). Because this "monosymptomatic hypochondriasis" is frequently the only overt manifestation of the subject's psychosis, these patients most often present to dermatologists and entomologists rather than to psychiatrists.

Epidemiology This disease predominates in middle aged to elderly females with premorbid social isolation. "Folie a deux" occurs when delusional symptoms have been "induced" in another individual (usually a family member) by a patient.

Clinical characteristics Patients with delusional parasitosis frequently present to the clinician in an anxious, ruminative, overwhelmed state, with a history of visits to multiple prior physicians without satisfaction. In addition to proffering a long and detailed history that includes visual or tactile hallucinations of the organisms, the patient also frequently provides "evidence" of the parasitic infection in the form of lint, fibers, and the like, which are delusionally misinterpreted as entire organisms, body parts, larvae, or ova. Skin manifestations can be quite variable, if [illegible] they reflect unsuccessful attempts at treating the infestation resulting in lesions ranging between mild excoriations to large ulcers,[4] including the damage from "topical" treatments undertaken by the patient in an attempt to free themselves of the perceived infestation.

Differential diagnosis Actual infestation must be ruled out. Subsequently, the differential diagnosis of psychosis must be parsed through, distinguishing between the primary psychiatric conditions that manifest with delusions of infestation. True monosymptomatic hypochondriasis represents a form of delusional disorder characterized by a rather discrete, circumscribed delusional belief with possible associated hallucinations without clear syndromic changes in affect or personality.[5] On the contrary, patients with uni- or bipolar depressive psychosis will describe classic changes in mood, motivations, sleep, and appetite, along with altered self-attitude. Schizophrenic patients often show a deterioration in global functioning, impaired social relatedness, thought disorder, and more bizarre delusions and hallucinations.

Treatment The critical tenet of treatment is to keep the patient engaged. Because these patients will frequently reject psychiatric referrals,[6] various authors have suggested means by which patients can be retained in treatment paving the road leading to the psychiatric referral.[6,7] Targeted therapy is undertaken with antipsychotic medications.[4] Pimozide has been used historically as the drug of choice, although it is now replaced by atypical antipsychotics such as olanzapine and risperidone, which are associated with fewer side effects.

Course and prognosis Although often regarded as chronic, unremitting and difficult to treat, these patients have a good recovery rate following appropriate pharmacologic therapy.

BODY DYSMORPHIC DISORDER *Body dysmorphic disorder* (BDD) is a condition characterized by an excessive preoccupation or concern with a presumed defect in physical appearance despite normal or only minimally objective anomalous findings. Also known as *dysmorphophobia,* this is a psychological experience that also results in functional impairment in various arenas of the patient's life.[5]

The nosological classification of BDD revolves around the intensity with which patients hold on to their abnormal beliefs. Those with unshakeable convictions are currently diagnosed as having a delusional disorder.[5] However, there appears to be a continuum of intensity and insight from preoccupations, through overvalued ideas to clear delusions.[8] There are no differences in the demographics, family history, course of illness, or, perhaps most importantly, response to specific treatments in patients with the psychotic and nonpsychotic forms of this illness. The evidence linking BDD to the obsessive-compulsive spectrum of disorders[9] has significant potential treatment implications.

Epidemiology The prevalence of BDD, is estimated to be from 1 percent in the general population to 12 percent in dermatology clinic patients. Classic presentation is in the mid to late teens without a significant gender prevalence, often in association with mood disorders. A lifetime history of psychotic and obsessive-compulsive disorders is also seen with increased frequency.[10]

Clinical manifestations Patients present with intensely articulated distress about various body parts. Most patients also develop ideas of reference in which they think or are convinced that others notice and comment upon the presumed defect.[10] Frequent, almost compulsive behaviors often accompany the worrisome thoughts, consuming hours each day, including repeated examination in mirrors, covering up the defect and asking others for reassurance. Consultations with other physicians are common and a history of past operations on the perceived defect is seen in a significant proportion of patients. Marked restriction in social and occupational functioning is seen in up to 98 percent of individuals, and 30 percent of patients were described as housebound.[10] Thoughts and attempts of suicide, some occasionally successful, are frequent. Current or past suicidal ideation should thus be routinely assessed by the practitioner.

Treatment As noted before, many patients with body dysmorphic disorder will seek dermatologic, surgical, or other nonpsychiatric treatment over the course of their illness. Evidence suggests that if patients receive such treatment they do not improve, are usually disappointed with the results, and may even experience an exacerbation of their symptoms. Thus, it is strongly recommended that these lines of treatment be avoided.

Pharmacologic trials show a good response to selective serotonin reuptake inhibitors (SSRIs) including fluoxetine, paroxetine, fluvoxamine, sertraline and the tricyclic antidepressant clomipramine. Adequate titration and persistence are important, because these patients require higher doses and longer treatment times than those used in the typical treatment of major depression. Although starting doses are lower, average effective doses are in the range of 40 to 60 mg/day of fluoxetine, 175 mg/day of clomipramine, and 240 mg/day of fluvoxamine with average time to response between 7 and 14 weeks. A significant proportion of patients who fail one adequate SSRI trial respond favorably to a trial with another SSRI, suggesting that serial trials of similarly acting agents should be administered in initially refractory cases. Interestingly, patients with delusional and nondelusional forms of body dysmorphic disorder respond at least equally well to treatment with SSRIs.[10,11] Responses to other treatments are not as promising. Lack of clear success has been noted with other agents such as antipsychotics (including pimozide), tricyclic antidepressants (other than clomipramine), benzodiazepines, and anticonvulsants.[10,11]

Course and prognosis Body dysmorphic disorder is a chronic illness without clear evidence for spontaneous remission without treatment. As seen above, pharmacotherapy with appropriate medications may lead to improvement in a majority of patients. However, the data also suggest that recurrence rates are extremely high with discontinuation of treatment[10] and thus patients may require long-term treatment, which may also include insight oriented psychotherapy.

Self-Inflicted Dermatoses (Factitious Disorders)

TRICHOTILLOMANIA This is a condition currently classified as an impulse control disorder,[5] which is characterized by repetitive pulling of hair resulting in alopecia. Strict criteria also include a build up of tension before hair pulling or when resisting an urge to do so, pleasure or relief after pulling out the hair, and significant functional impairment and distress in the patient.

Epidemiology Prevalence rates are estimated to be between 0.5 and 3.5 percent with a mean age of onset between 10 and 13 years. Despite its current classification, there are marked similarities with obsessive-compulsive disorder, which may have important treatment implications. Comorbid psychiatric disorders are depression, anxiety, and obsessive-compulsive disorder.

Clinical characteristics (Fig. 40-1) Trichotillomania presents clinically with nonscarring alopecia, most commonly with hairs broken at different lengths; occasionally, repeated trauma may ultimately result in some scarring. Body areas involved typically include the scalp, eyelashes, eyebrows, and pubic hair, with a majority of patients pulling hair from more than one site. Rarely, this is followed by the ingestion of the hair, leading to the potentially dangerous complication of trichobezoar. Awareness of the behavior is partial to complete in a vast majority of patients, and frequently occurs while patients are engaged in isolated, sedentary activities. Attempts to resist the behavior and to disguise its cosmetic sequelae are common. Typical histopathologic findings that may be helpful in confirming the diagnosis in questionable cases include catagen hairs, pigment casts, and traumatized hair bulbs without significant inflammation or scarring.

TREATMENT Because of trichotillomania's similarities to obsessive-compulsive disorder, the use of SSRIs and clomipramine has received much attention. Successful monotherapy with paroxetine,

FIGURE 40-1

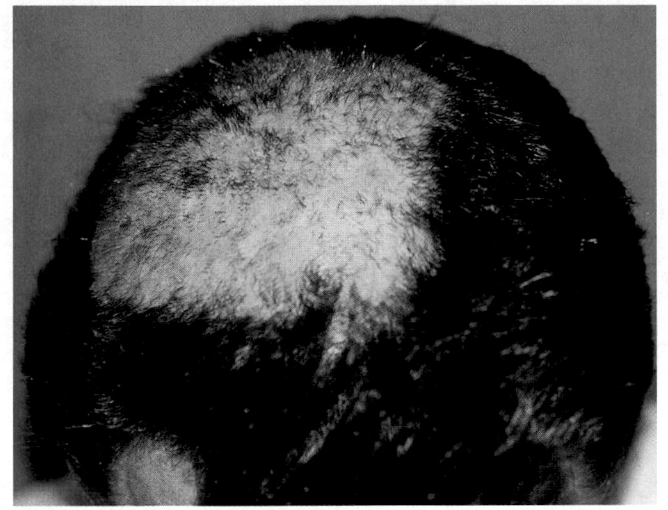

Trichotillomania. Hairs broken at different lengths. (*Courtesy of Ciro Martins, MD.*)

sertraline, venlafaxine, olanzapine, and clomipramine have been reported, as well as the augmentation of serotonin reuptake inhibitors with the addition of olanzapine, risperidone, or pimozide. Low-dose atypical antipsychotic agents in combination with SSRIs appear to have promising results. Nonpharmacologic treatment of trichotillomania relies heavily upon behavioral therapies, especially habit reversal, which entails engaging the patient in a behavior incompatible with hair pulling when the urge appears, such as performing a manual task that occupies both hands. Cognitive-behavioral treatment also has an important role and is even more effective than treatment with clomipramine;[12] hypnotherapy may also be very useful, particularly in the treatment of the pediatric population.[13] Insight-oriented psychotherapy also has good results.

Course and prognosis Trichotillomania is a chronic disorder and data on long-term success of pharmacologic and psychotherapeutic interventions are inconclusive. Although short-term success occurs, sustained improvement has yet to be shown convincingly.

DERMATITIS ARTEFACTA This is a form of factitious disorder in which patients will intentionally feign symptoms and produce signs of disease in an attempt to assume the patient role. Unlike patients with malingering who engage in similar behavior for external or "secondary gain" (such as monetary reward or relief from occupational or other social responsibilities), the factitious patient seeks the "primary gain" of the emotional and psychological benefits that accrue to those who are "ill." Patients with borderline personality disorder may also exhibit self-mutilatory behavior. Occasionally, a psychologically disturbed adult will induce skin lesions in their children, a form of Munchausen syndrome by proxy.

Epidemiology Predominating in females, the age of onset varies significantly with patients in adolescence through the seventh and eighth decades of life. Patients with factitious disorder have often been exposed to (through upbringing) or engaged in some aspect of the health professions. Comorbid depressive and personality disorders may also be seen.

Clinical characteristics (Figs. 40-2 and 40-3) Although it has long been observed that patients with dermatitis artefacta may present with lesions in virtually all areas of the body that can mimic most dermatoses, some common elements may hint at this diagnosis. Lesions are often in areas readily accessible to the patient, and may have geometric patterns or angulated borders surrounded by completely healthy skin. Morphology is often bizarre and does not conform to typical presentations of known dermatoses (Figs. 40-4 and 40-5). Patients are often unable to provide a clear history of the initial appearance or evolution of the process, and typically deny any role in the production of the lesions. Characteristically, the histopathology is unrevealing.

FIGURE 40-2

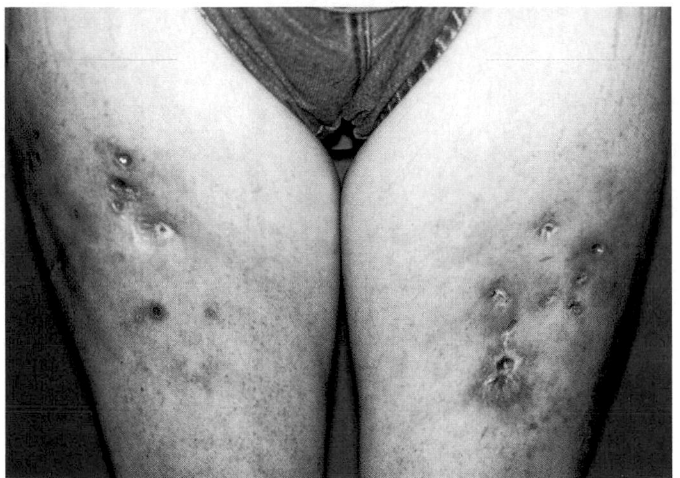

Dermatitis artefacta, secondary to subcutaneous injections of Demerol, and persistent excoriations.

Differential diagnosis As in all cases of factitious disease, the clinician must rule out possible disease entities that are consistent with the history and clinical findings. Unusual presentations of common illnesses and rare conditions must be entertained. However, exhaustive searches for primary skin pathology without supporting clinical evidence may compound the problem and actually perpetuate the patient's factitious behavior. Occlusive dressings (e.g., an Unna boot) or other means of preventing manipulation by the patient lead to healing of the lesions and are often helpful strategies in clarifying the diagnosis.

Treatment A supportive, nonconfrontational, empathic approach to the patient is indicated initially. Immediate confrontation regarding the suspicion that the patient's lesions are self-induced can be counterproductive in that the patient will often flee from treatment at that point. Frequent visits and symptomatic topical treatments are useful in

FIGURE 40-3

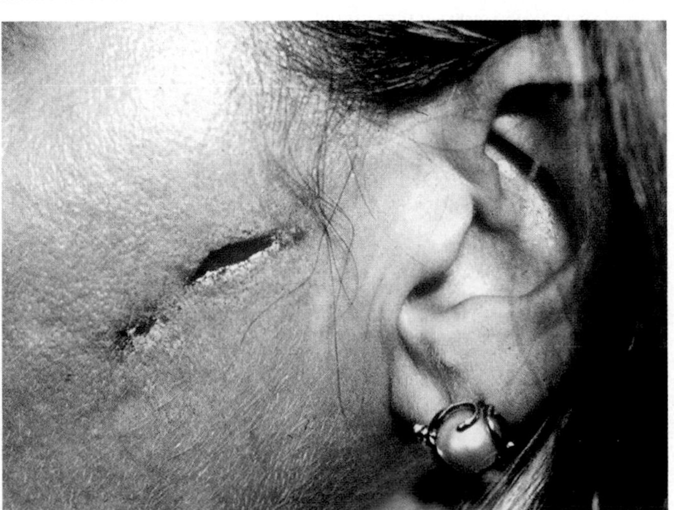

Dermatitis artefacta. Linear sharply bordered ulcer.

FIGURE 40-4

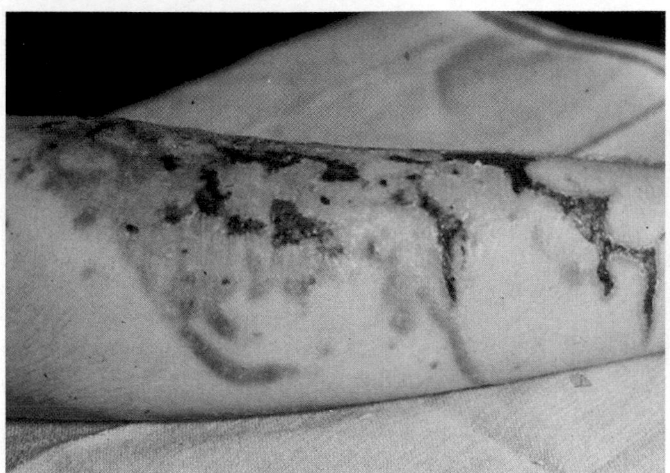

Dermatitis artefacta. Telltale linear streaks from application of caustic solution. (*Courtesy of Hahnemann University Hospital.*)

FIGURE 40-5

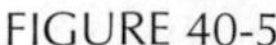

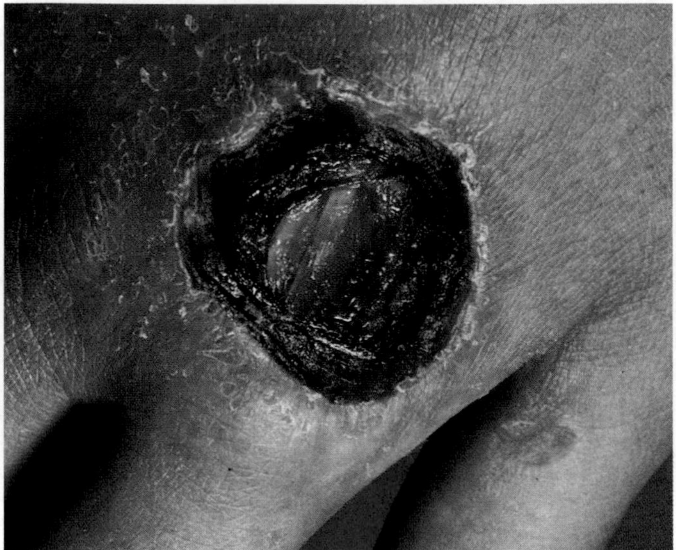

A.

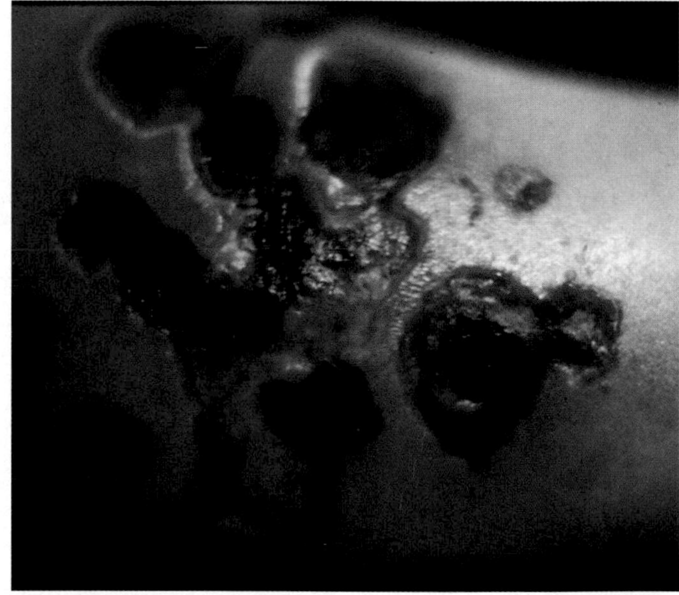

B.

Dermatitis artefacta. *A.* Solitary ulcer on the dorsum of the hand; tendons are visible at the base. *B.* Deeply and sharply punched-out ulcerations with necrotic eschars. (*Courtesy of the Hospital of the University of Pennsylvania.*)

the beginning. However, the clinician must be careful not to collude in the patient's abnormal illness behavior and, ultimately, the recognition of the patient's role in the production of the lesions must be broached. The goal is to establish a trusting and supportive enough relationship with the patient that he or she will accept a psychiatric referral to explore the complex personality and behavioral derangements that often underlie this condition. Antidepressants and low-dose atypical antipsychotics have also been reported to be useful adjunctive therapies.[14,15] In the case of Munchausen syndrome by proxy, in which the lesions are induced in children by parents or caregivers, child protective services or equivalent agencies must be alerted immediately to safeguard the welfare of the child.

Course and prognosis These are fundamentally determined by the underlying psychopathology. In those patients with severely disturbed personalities, the recurrent self-defeating and destructive behaviors are likely to continue.

NEUROTIC EXCORIATIONS This is also a condition in which patients induce skin lesions through repetitive, compulsive excoriation of their skin. However, unlike patients with dermatitis artefacta, these patients admit their role in the production of the lesions. This condition seems to be associated with underlying obsessive-compulsive personality traits and depressive disorders.

Epidemiology Neurotic excoriations have been reported in up to 2 percent of dermatology clinic patients with a predominance in middle-aged females, and is frequently associated with obsessive-compulsive personality and mood disorders.

Clinical characteristics Patients with neurotic excoriation often describe significant itch leading to persistent scratching, which is frequently antedated by considerable psychological stressors. The development of this disorder has also been noted to be associated with the marked limitation in activity seen in illness or senescence.[16] The repeated excoriation can lead to the development of an "itch–scratch cycle," perpetuating the behavior. Patients present with multiple excoriations in various stages of evolution and healing, with postinflammatory hyperpigmentation and frequent scarring (Fig. 40-6). The distribution of the lesions reflects their self-inflicted nature with most being on the extensor surfaces of the extremities, upper back, and face, sparing unreachable areas. Frequently, patients develop neurotic excoriations overlying preexisting dermatosis, such as folliculitis and acne. Prurigo nodularis can be considered an extreme variant of this entity, characterized by severely pruritic nodules that may vary from a few millimeters to 1 to 2 cm in diameter, preferentially located on the lower extremities.

Differential diagnosis The clinician must evaluate the patient for causes of pruritus (see Chap. 41) and rule out possible internal diseases including neoplasms. The differential for the underlying psychiatric disorder, if present, must include depressive and anxiety disorders and, more rarely, excoriations secondary to delusions of parasitosis.

Treatment Treatment should be directed at underlying psychopathology when identifiable. Antidepressants, helpful in the treatment of both depressive and anxiety disorders including obsessive-compulsive disorder, may have some utility. Supportive psychotherapeutic approaches are usually helpful and well-tolerated, and behavioral interventions similar to that used to treat self-injurious behaviors in Tourette's syndrome may be useful.

FIGURE 40-6

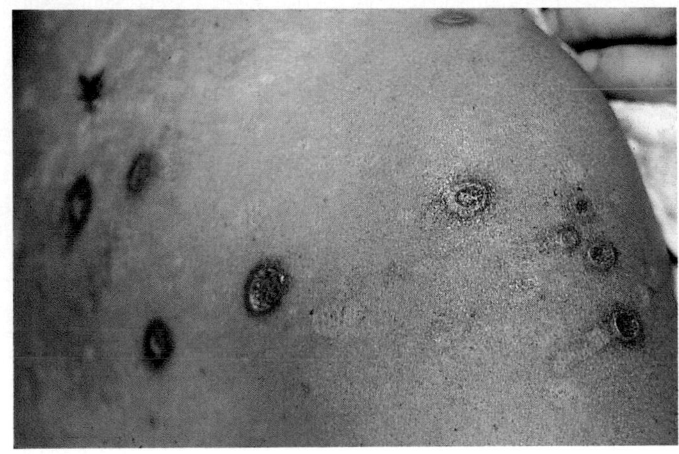

Neurotic excoriations. Lesions present in all stages of evolution.

Course and prognosis This can be a chronic condition whose prognosis depends on the underlying psychiatric illness. With appropriate therapy, patients with affective and anxiety disorders may have excellent outcomes, with a symptom-free, normally functioning state.

ATYPICAL CHRONIC PAIN SYNDROME Occasionally, patients will present to dermatologists with complaints of burning, pain, or dysesthesias in the skin or mucus membranes for which no identifiable pathology can be found. This can be a frustrating situation for patient and clinician alike. A psychiatric approach to these patients may offer a means of understanding the complex factors underlying this syndrome, such as comorbid affective disorders, personality vulnerabilities, behavioral problems, and life circumstances that may perpetuate the pain cycle and maintain the patient in an illness role.

There is a significantly increased rate of depression in patients with chronic pain syndromes and a clear relationship between lifetime depression and the development of medically unexplained symptoms, including pain. Depression not only worsens the experience of pain by psychologically magnifying negative perceptions, but may also interfere with the function of descending monoaminergic neurons that dampen nociceptive transmission. This could explain the role for tricyclic antidepressants in analgesia. Other complicating factors include anxiety, which is also commonly seen in patients with chronic pain. Personality disorders influence all aspects of patients' lives and may make the burden of a chronic condition more challenging to bear. At times, family or social environments may unwittingly play a role in undermining the chronic pain patient's rehabilitation by rewarding illness behaviors with well-meaning, yet oversolicitous, attention. Pain states can further be complicated if the patient develops an inappropriate pattern of using prescribed analgesics. For all of these reasons, the best course of action for patients presenting with poorly explained chronic pain is to refer them to a multidisciplinary pain center where thorough evaluation and treatment can be undertaken.

PSYCHOGENIC PRURITUS Psychogenic pruritus and itch in general are discussed in Chap. 41.

PSYCHOTROPIC MEDICATIONS USED IN DERMATOLOGY

A number of different classes of psychotropic medications are routinely used by those dermatologists who elect to treat psychocutaneous disorders. Knowledge of the drugs and their actions, indications, side effects, therapeutic doses, and potential drug interactions is, therefore, critical.

These drugs are classified according to their clinical utility (e.g., antidepressants or antipsychotics) and further identified by their chemical structure and/or mechanism of action. All of the drugs discussed in this section exert their clinical effects through modulation of neurotransmitter function in the central nervous system by altering presynaptic reuptake of the transmitters, blocking their pre- and/or postsynaptic receptor binding, stimulating those receptors or some combination of the above. The most appropriately used in each of the following three major classes are discussed: antipsychotics, antidepressants, and anxiolytics.

Antipsychotics

These medications have a wide variety of uses in psychiatry, but their primary indication in psychocutaneous medicine is in the symptomatic treatment of disorders characterized by delusions and/or hallucinations. The most common indications in dermatology are delusional parasitosis and, less frequently, for the treatment of self-induced dermatosis.[14,17] The drugs are believed to exert their beneficial effects by the blockade of postsynaptic dopamine receptors in the central nervous system (CNS). Dopaminergic tracts in the mesolimbic and mesocortical systems are felt to be the most important with regard to the production of symptoms of psychotic illness. However, dopamine is found widely throughout the brain and its blockade in the nigrostriatal and tuberoinfundibular pathways can lead to significant side effects.

Antipsychotics are now classified as typical (or conventional) and atypical. The older, typical antipsychotics include pimozide, haloperidol, fluphenazine, and chlorpromazine. These drugs are potent, nonspecific blockers of postsynaptic D_2 dopamine receptors and have varying degrees of inherent anticholinergic activity. The newer atypical antipsychotics have different affinities for dopamine receptors subtypes and serotonergic blocking properties at the 5-HT_2 receptor. This combination allows a continued potent antipsychotic effect but with a much more preferable neurologic side-effect profile because of decreased interference with dopamine transmission in the basal ganglia. Agents in this subclass include olanzapine, risperidone, quetiapine, and ziprasidone.

DOSING Of the typical antipsychotics, pimozide was the most widely used in dermatology, although evidence for its utility from convincing double-blind, placebo-controlled trials is sparse at best. Following appropriate cardiac evaluation and monitoring, a starting dose of 1 mg daily can be gradually increased in 1 mg increments on a weekly to biweekly basis, depending on clinical response and side effects; doses above 6 mg/day have little clinical utility. Because of the important cardiovascular and neurologic side effects associated with this drug, we now tend to use alternatives in the form of atypical antipsychotics (see above). We discuss olanzapine as a prototype of this subclass. A typical starting dose of 1.25 mg (one-half tablet) to 2.5 mg at bedtime may be increased slowly by 2.5 mg increments. Dermatologic patients reportedly respond extremely well to very low doses of this drug, (ranging between 1.25 and 5 mg/day).[14,17] However, because no clear evidence exists yet for established dosage ranges for the treatment of delusional parasitosis, close follow-up with gradual titration is necessary. Doses beyond 20 mg daily are unlikely to yield increasing clinical response although higher doses are used in the treatment of schizophrenia. As with the typical antipsychotics, clinical response may take weeks for full effect, although some results can be seen early. In addition to its antipsychotic action this drug has antihistamine activity (H_1) and anxiolytic properties at low doses (2.5 to 5 mg), making it a valuable addition to the dermatologic armamentarium.

SIDE EFFECTS The most dramatic side effects of the typical antipsychotics, including pimozide, are neurologic. They are divided into acute and delayed. The acute neurologic side effects are a result of dopaminergic blockade in the striatum causing (1) dystonias (acute increases in tone and abnormal posturing, typically involving muscles of the face, neck, tongue, and pharynx), (2) parkinsonism (with tremor, gait disturbance, stiffness, cog wheeling rigidity, marked facies, and general bradykinesia), and (3) akathisia (an experience of marked restlessness in the muscles which should be distinguished from psychic anxiety or agitation). These acute neurologic side effects are best managed by coadministration of an anticholinergic medication such as benztropine 0.5 to 2.0 mg twice daily or diphenhydramine 75 to 100 mg po IM for severe acute dystonia. The most worrisome delayed side effect of antipsychotic treatment is tardive dyskinesia (TD), characterized by repetitive movements that usually involve the lips, tongue, face, and upper extremities. It is rare in patients with fewer than 6 months of treatment. Risk factors for the development of TD may include older age, female gender, and the presence of affective disorder. Treatment of TD includes decrease or discontinuation of the antipsychotic if the underlying psychiatric illness allows, and stopping anticholinergic medications. A majority of patients will have significant, if not total, improvement of the dyskinetic movements.

Nonneurologic side effects include sedation, galactorrhea and the effects on the QT interval. Because of pimozide's effect on the repolarization phase of cardiac conduction, prolongation of the QT interval is possible, which is a potential risk factor for the development of fatal ventricular tachyarrhythmias. Baseline electrocardiograms (ECGs) should be obtained on all patients and after dose changes. In those patients with existing QTc prolongation, or in those patients who develop it during treatment, pimozide should be discontinued. Finally, neuroleptic malignant syndrome (NMS), characterized by fever, autonomic instability, diffuse increase in muscle tone, mental status changes, rhabdomyolysis and renal failure, is, fortunately, a rare but potentially fatal complication of antipsychotic treatment. This can occur at any time during treatment, but is more common during the first few weeks or months, or during rapid dose increases. Patients presenting with such features should be referred for emergent evaluation and subsequent treatment if indicated.

The atypical antipsychotics have a much more favorable neurologic side effect profile secondary to less interference in striatal dopamine transmission. This includes the acute neurologic symptoms as well as a lower risk for developing TD. Serious NMS may also be seen, albeit much less frequently. The most common side effects of treatment with olanzapine are sedation and weight gain (which can be very significant). Patients may develop glucose intolerance, and signs and symptoms of hyperglycemia should be monitored during the treatment. In general, olanzapine and other atypical antipsychotics are fairly well-tolerated by patients, which make them the treatment of choice over the older typical antipsychotics.

Antidepressants

A wide array of antidepressant options currently exist. This section discusses the classes of antidepressants most commonly used by dermatologists: tricyclic antidepressants and SSRIs. In dermatology, these drugs are used to treat affective disorders such as major depression, anxiety disorders, and obsessive-compulsive spectrum disorders such as trichotillomania and body dysmorphic disorder.

TRICYCLIC ANTIDEPRESSANTS The tricyclic antidepressants are agents that block the presynaptic reuptake of monoamines from the synapse in the central nervous system. Thus, norepinephrinergic and serotonergic transmission is potentiated. Most agents in this class block this reuptake rather nonspecifically, although the drug clomipramine acts most prominently on serotonin reuptake, which underlies its special utility in the treatment of some obsessive-compulsive disorders.

The tricyclic doxepin has found frequent use in dermatology (perhaps even more than psychiatry currently) because of its potent antihistaminergic properties in addition to its antidepressant effects. In those patients with anxious depressions in whom pruritus is a significant comorbid dermatologic symptom, this may be the antidepressant of choice.

Dosing Typical dose ranges for the most commonly prescribed tricyclic antidepressants are listed in Table 40-1. In general, low initial dosing with gradual titration to therapeutic levels is advised. As most are sedating, bedtime dosing is recommended. An advantage of this class of antidepressants is that serum levels are readily obtainable and can aid in the choice of appropriate daily doses. Because individual metabolism of these compounds varies radically, objective evidence of actual blood levels is quite helpful. These levels can inform the clinician about patient compliance and subtherapeutic dosing, two major factors that must be considered when the treatment regimen is unsuccessful.

Side effects The tricyclic antidepressants not only affect monoaminergic transmission in the CNS, but also have varying degrees of anticholinergic, antihistaminergic, and peripheral anti–α_1-adrenergic properties that can lead to significant side effects. These side effects include constipation, dry mouth, urinary retention, marked sedation, and orthostatic hypotension. Orthostatic pulse and blood pressure measurements should be documented in the record for all patients receiving tricyclic antidepressants. These drugs can also lead to significant alteration in the repolarization phase of cardiac conduction, increasing the risk for ventricular tachyarrhythmias. A baseline ECG should be obtained in all patients. Tricyclics should not be used in those patients with significant prolongation of the QTc interval, left bundle-branch block, or bifascicular block. They also cause tachycardia as a result of a reflex increase secondary to orthostatic hypotension and

TABLE 40-1

Dose Ranges and Receptor-Mediated Side Effects of Commonly Used Antidepressants

	Dose Range (mg/day)	Anti Cholinergic	Sedation*	Orthostatic Hypotension†
Tricyclics				
Amitriptyline	100–300	+++	+++	+++
Nortriptyline	50–150	++	++	++
Clomipramine	75–250	+++	+++	+++
Doxepin	100–300	+++	++++	+++
SSRIs				
Fluoxetine	10–80	—	—	—
Sertraline	50–200	—	—	—
Paroxetine	10–40	+	+	—
Citalopram	10–60	—	—	—
Fluvoxamine	100–300	—	++	—

*Antihistaminergic effects.
†Anti-α_1-adrenergic effects.
Adapted from Arana GW, Rosenbaum JF: Handbook of Psychiatric Drug Therapy Philadelphia, Lippincott Williams & Wilkins, 2000.

a general decrease in vagal tone to the heart. They may also induce seizures.

Like all antidepressants, the tricyclics have the potential to precipitate an episode of mania or hypomania if used in patients with bipolar affective disorder. These patients should be screened for such a history before initiating therapy and referred to a psychiatrist who can follow the patient closely for signs of an emerging manic episode. Tricyclics are also potentially fatal in overdose; therefore patients who express suicidal ideations are best treated by a psychiatrist.

SELECTIVE SEROTONIN REUPTAKE INHIBITORS As their name implies, SSRIs selectively block the reuptake of serotonin into the presynpatic nerve terminal. Effective antidepressants, they are also very valuable agents in the treatment of anxiety and obsessive-compulsive disorders.

Dosing Table 40-1 lists the usual dose ranges for SSRIs. For obsessive-compulsive spectrum disorders, sometimes higher doses of these agents are required for clinical effect.

Side effects These are generally well-tolerated medications, even in the geriatric population. Unlike tricyclics, most of these drugs are somewhat stimulating and morning dosing is the rule. Decreased appetite, insomnia, akathisia, nausea, and diarrhea (due to serotonin's action on gut motility) are fairly common. These are typically seen upon initiation of therapy or after dose changes, and often disappear with continued treatment. Approximately 30 percent of patients will experience sexual dysfunction, with decreased libido and orgasmic delay or anorgasmia being seen in both sexes. Like the tricyclics, SSRIs can lead to manic episodes in bipolar patients. They may actually be more likely to cause rapid cycling in which the patient experiences several depressive and manic swings in a relatively short period of time.

The SSRIs are relatively safe in overdose. Because of their lack of effect on the myocardium and minimal, if any, impact on seizure threshold, they do not have the same risks as tricyclics. However, because they can be somewhat activating, patients with suicidal ideation treated with SSRIs should be followed extremely closely as energy may return before the dysphoria and suicidal wishes disappear.

These drugs also inhibit subtypes of the cytochrome P_{450} system; therefore, other drugs metabolized by this system are subject to significant alterations in serum levels. Dose adjustment and careful monitoring are important when coadministering such medications.

Anxiolytics

Although antidepressants can be used to treat anxiety disorders, the symptomatic treatment of anxiety occasionally involves the use of other anxiolytics. Benzodiazepines are currently the most widely used class of anxiolytics, supplanting previous use of barbiturates. Buspirone, a nonbenzodiazepine anxiolytic, has also found some limited utility in certain patients.

Benzodiazepines are CNS depressants, exerting their influence through action at the GABA receptor. GABA is the major inhibitory neurotransmitter in the CNS. Thus, in addition to treating anxiety, other effects include sedation, loss of muscle coordination and possible amnesia or blackouts. Buspirone is a partial 5-HT_{1A} receptor agonist without the same liability for dependence and subsequent withdrawal phenomena common to all GABA active agents. Because of the potential for physical and psychological dependence, benzodiazepines should be used with great caution. Potent, short-acting benzodiazepines such as alprazolam and lorazepam may have more of a possibility of inducing dependency. In general, the short-term symptomatic treatment of anxiety symptoms while other more definitive pharmacologic and psychotherapeutic measures are being undertaken remains the main indication for the use of these medications by the nonpsychiatrist.

Buspirone is an anxiolytic medication approved for the treatment of generalized anxiety disorder. It is thought to mediate its effects through serotonergic mechanisms. Unlike benzodiazepines, buspirone must be taken chronically for anxiolytic effects to be seen. It is generally prescribed at 5 mg three times daily with increase to a total daily dose of 30 mg.

NONPHARMACOLOGIC TREATMENTS FOR PSYCHOCUTANEOUS DISORDERS

The dermatologist should request a consultation with a psychiatrist or a liaison clinic during the treatment of patients with psychocutaneous disorders as soon as it is amenable to the patient. Although dermatologists are becoming more comfortable with the use of certain psychotropic medications, they generally do not have the time or the training to use effectively other treatment modalities such as psychotherapy and hypnosis. It is therefore sufficient that the practicing dermatologist be aware that a variety of psychotherapeutic approaches are available, including insight-oriented, cognitive-behavioral, supportive, and, to a lesser extent in current practice, psychodynamic therapy. Certain types of therapies may be more effective for a given condition which underscores a fundamental point: diagnosis should drive choice of therapy and patients should not be formulated based upon rigid therapeutic/theoretical biases.

Primary Dermatologic Diseases

THE ROLE OF STRESS IN SKIN DISEASES The presence of a force that threatens to disrupt the organism's homeostatic balance is perceived as a stressor, and the ensuing reaction reflects the normal response aimed at the preservation of life. Mammalian organisms respond to external (i.e., physical, environmental) or internal provocations (infections, anxiety, or anticipatory stress) by triggering a cascade of events that ultimately activate the hypothalamus-pituitary-adrenal (HPA) axis,[18] allowing the organism to cope with noxious stimuli and mount a successful "fight-flight" reaction. This adaptation to challenges ("stress response"[19]) is critical for survival following an acute provocation; however, its persistence chronically can lead to exhaustion, distress, and, eventually, disease. Whereas short-lived (acute) stressors are known to enhance immunity, chronic stress has an adverse effect on health and life expectancy, alters immunity, and favors the progression of infections as well as an increase in the development of experimentally induced neoplasms.[2] A number of studies provide clear evidence that psychosocial factors, including stress and other emotional states (such as depression), have a deleterious effect on the outcome of numerous human diseases including those of the skin.[2,20]

Although suspected for many years, retrospective and prospective studies have provided the clinical basis to support the notion that stressful events can correlate with the onset or exacerbation of skin diseases. Additional evidence was gleaned from the results of therapeutic trials utilizing psychotherapeutic approaches and stress reducing interventions[21] in the treatment of dermatologic ailments such as atopic eczema, psoriasis, urticaria, herpes simplex infection, alopecia areata, warts, and malignant melanoma, among others.

Atopic eczema More than most other skin diseases, atopic eczema exemplifies the delicate balance between inherited factors, environmental influences and psychosocial issues in the maintenance of health. Up to 70 percent of atopic subjects reported preceding emotional stressors prior to the first episode of dermatitis,[22] while numerous patients with eczema suffer exacerbations of their skin symptoms following episodes of psychological stress. These subjects have increased anxiety, altered coping mechanisms, and a close connection between severity of symptoms and stressful life events. Psychodynamic approaches have emphasized the role played by an abnormal family structure and altered mother-child relationships in this disease, an issue that is highlighted by the improvement in the symptoms of children with atopic eczema when their mothers receive psychological treatment. Other psychosocial interventions found to be effective as sole or adjuvant therapies for pediatric and adult patients[21] include behavioral therapies and biofeedback, stress reduction regimens, psychoanalysis, hypnosis, and relaxation techniques.

Psoriasis Psychosocial issues appear to be closely linked to the well-being of patients with psoriasis. Stressors often precede the initial onset of the disease or subsequent flares. Individual or group psychotherapy, behavioral approaches, and biofeedback, among other techniques, have resulted in improvement of the psoriatic plaques, as well as enhancement of overall well being.[23,24] Recent randomized controlled trials showed that highly suggestible patients treated with hypnosis significantly improved when compared to the control group,[25] and patients who used meditation tapes at the time of phototherapy cleared in half the time when compared to those who did not use them.[26]

Herpes simplex There is strong evidence to support the role of stress in the evolution of herpes simplex virus (HSV) infections. Experimental restraint stress correlates with the reactivation of latent HSV infection in the dorsal root ganglion neuron of rats. Human studies show that persistent, but not single, stressful events are associated with the frequency of recurrences,[27] which is in accordance with findings that chronic but not acute stress correlates with the development of experimental viral infections in normal volunteers.[28] Furthermore, psychosocial interventions decrease the frequency of recurrences of herpes simplex infections.

Urticaria The relationship between stress and some forms of urticaria is supported by numerous anecdotal observations. Patients suffering from adrenergic urticaria report that their symptoms invariably follow acute stressful events. Others, with hereditary angioedema are known to have symptoms frequently triggered by emotional stress. The finding that stress mediates the degranulation of mast cells via corticotropin-releasing factor (CRF)[29] and neuropeptides,[30] supports its putative role in the pathogenesis of urticaria.

Almost all inflammatory skin diseases have been anecdotally reported at one time or another to be associated to stressors. Up to 50 percent of females with acne suffer flares following stress, and patients with seborrheic dermatitis, lichen planus, pemphigus vulgaris, and alopecia areata have been reported to have symptoms triggered or exacerbated by emotional stress.

MECHANISMS OF STRESS IN THE SKIN The underlying mechanisms that could explain how stressful events can modify skin diseases relate to (1) the effect of steroid hormones and catecholamines on immune cells, (2) abnormalities in the HPA axis, and (3) local (tissue) factors such as the secretion of neuropeptides and neurohormones and alterations in the barrier function of the skin.

Effect of stress hormones on immunity The bi-directional communication between immune and endocrine-neural systems is highlighted by the effects that follow a stressful event: CRF from the paraventricular nucleus of the hypothalamus is secreted into the pituitary, stimulating the release of adrenocorticotropic hormone (ACTH) from the pituitary leading to cortisol secretion from the adrenal glands. Simultaneously, cortical and limbic input also act on the locus ceruleus, activating the sympathetic system, mediating the resulting surge in norepinephrine and the release of peripheral neuropeptides.[18] However, the stress response is not only triggered by psychological or physical provocations. For example, infections induce monocyte/macrophage-derived inflammatory cytokines such as interleukin (IL)-1, IL-6, and tumor necrosis factor (TNF)-α, which cross the blood-brain barrier, resulting in CRF release from the hypothalamus. The secretion of cortisol and norepinephrine causes profound effects on the immune system by regulating the differentiation of T cells and macrophages, and by modifying inflammation and immunity.[31] Two distinct populations of T helper (T_H) lymphocytes, which generally oppose each other, regulate immune function through the secretion of stimulatory or suppressive soluble cytokines (see Chap. 26). T_H1 cells mediate cellular immunity through the production of interferon (IFN)-γ and IL-2, and T_H2 induce humoral immunity through IL-4, IL-5, IL-10, and IL-13. The cytokines from one cell type curb the differentiation and proliferation of the other type. Physiologic doses of glucocorticosteroids inhibit the transcription of cytokines and chemokines and act on macrophages leading to a shift towards a T_H2 response,[32] while pharmacologic doses lead to the suppression of both T cell subsets (hence their use in the treatment of T_H1-, as well as T_H2-, driven diseases). Similarly, catecholamines also stimulate differentiation of the T_H2 phenotype through binding to lymphocyte β_2 adrenergic receptors, and the suppression of IFN-γ. These neurotransmitters inhibit macrophage IL-12, which is critical in the induction of T_H1 cells, and induce secretion of macrophage derived IL-10, a potent suppressor of antigen presentation, as well as an inducer of the T_H2 response. Some of these effects that lead to the inhibition of cellular immunity and stimulation of immunoglobulin production are not prevented by hypophysectomy or adrenalectomy, which could be explained by the other pathways such as the direct innervation of immune organs and cells.

This combined effect on the T_H1/T_H2 balance may explain why the activity of some diseases appears to fluctuate during periods of stress or concurrent infections. Autoimmune diseases including pemphigus or systemic lupus erythematosus (SLE), or conditions with T_H2 predominance, such as acute stages[33] of atopic eczema may deteriorate if the immunity is shifted toward the humoral T_H2 response with concomitant increased production of immunoglobulins, particularly IgE. Additionally, atopic patients that are exposed to experimental stress demonstrate alterations in lymphocyte trafficking, cytokine profiles, and distribution of eosinophils and T cells.[34] Similarly, when patients with SLE are confronted with a stressor such as an infection, the T_H1-mediated symptoms could improve, while T_H2-mediated involvement (i.e., immune complex-mediated pathology) may deteriorate. Also, steroidal (among other) hormonal changes during pregnancy may shift the T_H1/T_H2 balance in patients with diseases in which there is T_H1 predominance, such as psoriasis or acne, inducing the transient improvement of symptoms seen in these women.

The nature, timing, and duration of the stressor is critical in determining its effect on the immune system. Short-lived (acute) stress is usually associated with enhancement, whereas chronic stress is linked to suppression of the immune functions.[35]

Abnormalities of the HPA axis Genetic factors can condition the stress response and its influence on inflammation. Indeed, some rat strains have an inherited hypothalamic deficiency that makes them hypo-responsive to stress, succumbing to T_H1-type inflammatory diseases secondary to the inadequate production of corticosterone following exposure to stressors. Interestingly, a similar mechanism has been reported in patients with rheumatoid arthritis,[36] and in children and adult patients with atopic eczema, who were found to have an impaired cortisol response to laboratory stressors or to infused CRF, when compared to healthy controls.[37] These findings may explain why some patients with chronic eczema, who have a T_H1/T_H2combined profile with T_H1 predominance (thus differing from the acute phase), suffer clinical exacerbations during concomitant stressful events due to the inability to maintain appropriate cortisol levels during these adverse events.

Environmental factors have also been found to modify the stress response at the level of the central nervous system. Traits acquired during early life condition responses to stressors in adulthood. For example, women who suffered physical, or sexual abuse during childhood have significant alterations in the HPA axis response to stressors as adults.[38]

Local effect of neuropeptides and neurohormones Cutaneous nerves have a direct effect on inflammation of the skin, either through direct innervation or through the release of neuropeptides and neurohormones (see Chap. 20). During acute stress, leukocytes are mobilized and redistributed to accumulate in peripheral organs, such as the skin, to prepare the organism to confront foreign challenges (e.g., an infection).[39] This type of stress not only enhances overall cellular immunity, but also increases delayed-type hypersensitivity (DTH) in the skin,[39] and induces the degranulation of mast cells, a process involving neurokinins, peripheral nerves and cutaneous production of urocortin and CRH, which promote local inflammation.[29,40,41]

In contrast, chronic stress has opposite effects; it suppresses DTH[39] and significantly impairs wound healing in animals and humans. Some of these effects could be mediated by α–melanocyte-stimulating hormone (MSH), a peptide with local immunosuppressive effects[41] that also suppresses skin DTH when administered to the brain either exogenously, or endogenously, as it occurs under stress.

The effects of emotional stress on the skin are not only restricted to changes in the local immunity, but also induce alterations in skin barrier functions, which can be reversed by glucocorticosteroid receptor antagonists or by the administration of anxiolytics.[2,42] This phenomenon may explain the effect of stress on the evolution of some skin diseases with altered *trans*-epidermal water loss, such as atopic dermatitis and psoriasis.[43]

THE ROLE OF SKIN DISEASES ON PSYCHOSOCIAL WELL-BEING The physical or perceived disfigurement of the integument itself can become a source of significant stress, with a considerable impact on an individual's psychological, social, and physical well being. This is often overlooked or underestimated by the general public, many health insurers, and the medical community, including dermatologists. Although dermatologic conditions are responsible for a significant source of social stigmatization in many human societies and cultures, it is only recently that we have begun to quantitate the effect of skin disease on an individual's quality of life (QOL). Psoriasis, for example, impairs the social life of 40 percent of patients and 64 percent feel that their disease significantly impacts their socioeconomic functioning. The impairment of QOL correlates with disease severity in patients with atopic dermatitis, which is also associated with high levels of anxiety, sleep, and mood disturbances. Urticaria patients suffer QOL impairments similar to that of patients with coronary artery disease waiting for bypass surgery. Children with alopecia areata suffer significant psychiatric impact from their disease, with higher levels of anxiety, depression, decreased concentration, and increased aggression or withdrawal. Acne patients, with fewer symptoms than those with conditions such as psoriasis or eczema, have similar levels of deleterious emotional states.

The Dermatology Life Quality Index (DLQI)[44] and the Skindex-16[45] are simple and practical validated instruments that can be used both in the office setting and for research purposes to quickly evaluate QOL. Specific instruments, are also available for patients with psoriasis, eczema, acne, and urticaria among others. These tests are helpful tools that can assess improvement in both the physical and the psychosocial aspects of a patient's disease.

The sum of observations, studies, and therapeutic interventions suggests that stress plays a significant role in the biology and clinical expression of skin diseases, and supports the notion that therapies that address this issue may have a positive impact on the well being of patients with dermatologic diseases. Adjuvant psychosocial interventions could also mediate an increased adherence to medical treatments, provide social support, decrease stress or alter the response to stress, ameliorate anxiety, aid patients to develop better coping mechanisms,

improve depression, and help with self image or distorted body perception.

REFERENCES

1. Panconesi E, Hautmann G: Psychophysiology of stress in dermatology. The psychobiologic pattern of psychosomatics. *Dermatol Clin* **14**:399, 1996
2. Tausk FA, Nousari H: Stress and the skin. *Arch Dermatol* **137**:78, 2001
3. Koblenzer CS: *Psychocutaneous Disease*. Orlando, FL, Grune and Stratton, 1987
4. Driscoll MS et al: Delusional parasitosis: A dermatologic, psychiatric, and pharmacologic approach. *J Am Acad Dermatol* **29**:1023, 1993
5. American Psychiatric Association:*DSM-IV. Diagnostic and Statistic Manual of Mental Disorders,* 4th ed. Washington, DC, Author, 1994
6. Gould WM, Gragg TM: Delusions of parasitosis. An approach to the problem. *Arch Dermatol* **112**:1745, 1976
7. Koblenzer C: Psychologic aspects of skin diseases, in *Fitzpatrick's Dermatology in General Medicine,* 5th ed, edited by Freedberg IM, Eisen AZ, Wolff K, Austen KF, Goldsmith LA, Katz SI, Fitzpatrick TB, New York, McGraw-Hill, 1999, p 475
8. Hollander E, Phillips K: *Body Image and Experience Disorders*. Washington, DC, American Psychiatric Press, 1993
9. Phillips KA et al: Body dysmorphic disorder: An obsessive-compulsive spectrum disorder, a form of affective spectrum disorder, or both? *J Clin Psychiatry* **56**(suppl 4):41, 1995
10. Phillips KA et al: Body dysmorphic disorder: 30 cases of imagined ugliness. *Am J Psychiatry* **150**:302, 1993
11. McElroy SL et al: Body dysmorphic disorder: Does it have a psychotic subtype? *J Clin Psychiatry* **54**:389, 1993
12. Ninan PT et al: A placebo-controlled trial of cognitive-behavioral therapy and clomipramine in trichotillomania. *J Clin Psychiatry* **61**:47, 2000
13. Cohen HA et al: Hypnotherapy: An effective treatment modality for trichotillomania. *Acta Paediatr* **88**:407, 1999
14. Koblenzer CS: Dermatitis artefacta. Clinical features and approaches to treatment. *Am J Clin Dermatol* **1**:47, 2000
15. Garnis-Jones S et al: Treatment of self-mutilation with olanzapine. *J Cutan Med Surg* **4**:161, 2000
16. Gupta MA et al: Neurotic excoriations: A review and some new perspectives. *Compr Psychiatry* **27**:381, 1986
17. Gupta MA, Gupta AK: Olanzapine is effective in the management of some self-induced dermatoses: Three case reports. *Cutis* **66**:143, 2000
18. Chrousos GP: The hypothalamic-pituitary-adrenal axis and immune-mediated inflammation. *N Engl J Med* **332**:1351, 1995
19. Selye H: The general adaptation syndrome and the disease of adaptation. *J Clin Endocrinol* **6**:117, 1946
20. Kimyai-Asadi A, Usman A: The role of psychological stress in skin disease. *J Cutan Med Surg* **5**:140, 2001
21. Gupta MA, Gupta AK: Psychodermatology: An update. *J Am Acad Dermatol* **34**:1030, 1996
22. Faulstich ME, Williamson DA: An overview of atopic dermatitis: Toward a bio-behavioural integration. *J Psychosom Res* **29**:647, 1985
23. Ginsburg IH: Coping with psoriasis: A guide for counseling patients. *Cutis* **57**:323, 1996
24. Ginsburg IH: Psychological and psychophysiological aspects of psoriasis. *Dermatol Clin* **13**:793, 1995
25. Tausk F, Whitmore SE: A pilot study of hypnosis in the treatment of patients with psoriasis. *Psychother Psychosom* **68**:221, 1999
26. Kabat-Zinn J et al: Influence of a mindfulness meditation-based stress reduction intervention on rates of skin clearing in patients with moderate to severe psoriasis undergoing phototherapy (UVB) and photochemotherapy (PUVA). *Psychosom Med* **60**:625, 1998
27. Cohen F et al: Persistent stress as a predictor of genital herpes recurrence. *Arch Intern Med* **159**:2430, 1999
28. Cohen S et al: Psychological stress and susceptibility to the common cold. *N Engl J Med* **325**:606, 1991
29. Theoharides TC et al: Corticotropin-releasing hormone induces skin mast cell degranulation and increased vascular permeability, a possible explanation for its proinflammatory effects. *Endocrinology* **139**:403, 1998
30. Singh LK et al: Acute immobilization stress triggers skin mast cell degranulation via corticotropin releasing hormone, neurotensin, and substance P: A link to neurogenic skin disorders. *Brain Behav Immun* **13**:225, 1999
31. Chrousos GP: The hypothalamic-pituitary-adrenal axis and immune-mediated inflammation. *N Engl J Med* **332**:1351, 1995

32. Elenkov IJ, Chrousos GP: Stress hormones, Th1/Th2 patterns, pro/anti-inflammatory cytokines and susceptibility to disease. Trends Endocrinol Metabol **10**:359, 2000
33. Grewe M et al: A role for Th1 and Th2 cells in the immunopathogenesis of atopic dermatitis. *Immunol Today* **19**:359, 1998
34. Schmid-Ott G et al: Different expression of cytokine and membrane molecules by circulating lymphocytes on acute mental stress in patients with atopic dermatitis in comparison with healthy controls. *J Allergy Clin Immunol* **108**:455, 2001
35. Kiecolt-Glaser JK et al: Psychoneuroimmunology and psychosomatic medicine: Back to the future. *Psychosom Med* **64**:15, 2002
36. Gudbjornsson B et al: Intact adrenocorticotropic hormone secretion but impaired cortisol response in patients with active rheumatoid arthritis. Effect of glucocorticoids. *J Rheumatol* **23**:596, 1996
37. Buske-Kirschbaum A et al: Psychobiological aspects of atopic dermatitis: An overview. *Psychother Psychosom* **70**:6, 2001
38. Heim C et al: Pituitary-adrenal and autonomic responses to stress in women after sexual and physical abuse in childhood. *JAMA* **284**:592, 2000
39. Dhabhar FS, McEwen BS: Enhancing versus suppressive effects of stress hormones on skin immune function. *Proc Natl Acad Sci USA* **96**:1059, 1999
40. Singh LK et al: Potent mast cell degranulation and vascular permeability triggered by urocortin through activation of corticotropin-releasing hormone receptors. *J Pharmacol Exp Ther* **288**:1349, 1999
41. Slominski A et al: Corticotropin releasing hormone and proopiomelanocortin involvement in the cutaneous response to stress. *Physiol Rev* **80**:979, 2000
42. Garg A et al: Psychological stress perturbs epidermal permeability barrier homeostasis. *Arch Dermatol* **137**:53, 2001
43. Taieb A: Hypothesis: From epidermal barrier dysfunction to atopic disorders. *Contact Dermatitis* **41**:177, 1999
44. Finlay AY, Khan GK: Dermatology Life Quality Index (DLQI)—A simple practical measure for routine clinical use. *Clin Exp Dermatol* **19**:210, 1994
45. Chren MM et al: Measurement properties of Skindex-16: A brief quality-of-life measure for patients with skin diseases. *J Cutan Med Surg* **5**:105, 2001

CHAPTER 41

Malcolm W. Greaves

Pathophysiology and Clinical Aspects of Pruritus

Pruritus (itching) is the predominant symptom of skin disease and can best be defined indirectly as a sensation that leads to a desire to scratch. Pain and itch are separate and distinct sensations, although both modalities follow the same gross neural pathways. Because of the subjective nature of itching, with difficulty in arriving at a precise definition and reproducible methods of measurement, as well as a lack of convincing animal models, progress in this field has been slow. However significant progress has been made in the past few years, mainly as a result of application of new technology, especially the use of microneurography that enables recordings to be made from individual afferent neurons following stimulation in man in vivo. The concept of "central" itch—itch generated in the central nervous system, rather than peripherally, has gained more support and this has led to a new neuropathophysiology-based classification of itch (discussed below). These advances have yet to be translated into new safe and effective antipruritic treatments, but these are round the corner.

CLASSIFICATION AND TYPES OF ITCH

Recently, Twycross et al.[1] proposed classifying itches into pruritoceptive (originates in diseased skin); neurogenic (due to molecular or neurophysiologic dysfunction in the nervous system, e.g., cholestasis, opioid-induced pruritus); neuropathic (due to nervous system pathology, e.g., multiple sclerosis, Creutzfeldt-Jakob disease); and psychiatric (e.g., parasitophobia). This classification system recognizes the important role the central nervous system plays as a source of itch as well as a regulator of itch traffic.

ITCHY SKIN: ALLOKNESIS

That pruritoceptive itch, which is itself heterogeneous, was recognized by Bickford,[2] who described two responses to an itchy stimulus applied to the skin: an itch that is well localized to the site of the stimulus, persisting only briefly after the itch is removed, and a subsequent, diffuse, poorly localized area that does not itch spontaneously but that itches intensely when subjected to light touch or other minor stimulus. Bickford called the former "spontaneous itch" and the latter "itchy skin." We use the term *alloknesis* to describe "itchy skin." Alloknesis is analogous to the better known allodynia (injury to skin results in well-localized, short-lived, intense pricking pain and a surrounding diffuse area of hyperalgesia). Whether spontaneous itch involves different sensory fibers than does alloknesis is unclear. It was originally suggested[3] that these two qualities are served by rapidly conducting (A delta) and slowly conducting (C) fibers, respectively. An alternative, more attractive explanation from Graham et al.[4] states that the more diffuse state of alloknesis is due to activation within sensory relays of the cord of interneuronal facilitating circuits following low-intensity stimulation of pain fibers. Possibly the facilitation may be peripheral, due to local release of pharmacologic activity in the skin as proposed for allodynia by Lewis[5] and more recently by Lynn.[6]

The phenomenon of alloknesis is familiar to the dermatologist. The development of an urticarial wheal is associated with well-defined localized spontaneous itching, as well as with a surrounding area of skin that responds with itching to any mild mechanical stimulus, persisting for hours or even days after the wheal has subsided. The same phenomenon may account, to a greater or lesser degree, for the itchy discomfort of patients with atopic eczema, who frequently experience bouts of intense pruritus due to sweating.

ITCH ORIGINATING FROM NERVES IN THE SKIN

A characteristic of itch is that the only peripheral tissues from which it can be evoked are skin, mucous membranes, and cornea. Itch sensitivity is not evenly distributed; there are itch points in a spotty distribution.[7–9] Shelley and Arthur[9] inserted itch-producing spicules from the plant *Mucuna pruriens* to varying levels below the skin surface and showed maximum itch sensitivity at the basal layer. When itch-producing substances are injected deeply into skin, they produce pain, and when the epidermis is removed, itch can no longer be generated.[9,10] Itch cannot be produced from completely denervated skin as in herpes zoster or leprosy.[10] The C neuron toxin capsaicin, although initially producing intense irritation, abolishes the ability to produce itch after repeated application.[11] Itch persists even when all the large A neurons are blocked by an inflated sphygmomanometer cuff.[1,9] It is evident that C and perhaps A delta neurons are unique in their ability to provoke itch. Although it is widely accepted that there are no specialized structures behaving as "itch receptors" in skin, free nerve endings specifically serving the sensation of itch have not yet been identified. Light and ultrastructural studies have demonstrated the presence of intraepidermal free nerve endings that stain positively for neuropeptides, but it could not be confirmed that these served the sensation of itch.[12]

The Search for Specific Itch Neurons in Human Skin

Classic theory proposes that itch and all other primary sensations are associated with activation of specialized neurons, one for each sensation. Search for a so-called itch fiber has been enabled by the development of human microneurography in which an ultrafine glass microelectrode is inserted percutaneously into peripheral nerves to record active single neurons in conscious individuals. By this method recordings were made from unmyelinated neurons that responded to *Mucuna pruriens* spicules or histamine.[13] By using electrical field stimulation coupled with microneurography in ulnar and peroneal nerves, a subset of ultraslow-conducting C neurons innervating a wide territory of skin was identified by Handwerker and colleagues.[14] These neurons, which represent 10 to 15 percent of the total number of C fibers in the nerve were coresponsive to heat. This finding could explain the well-known observation that the itch threshold is lowered in warmed skin.[15] The same technique can be used to produce microstimulation within a neuron. Occasionally, this stimulation produces a sensation of itch.

The existence of a subset of dedicated itch-transmitting C neurons receives further support from recent studies of spinal cord pathways. Itch-transmitting primary afferent C neurons synapse with secondary transmission neurons that cross over to the contralateral spinothalamic tract and ascend to the thalamus. In the cat, microneurography identified lamina 1 neurons in the lateral spinothalamic tract that selectively responded to histamine, suggesting a central dedicated nerve pathway for itch.[16]

Itch-Producing Mediators in Skin

HISTAMINE Histamine applied in low concentrations at the level of the dermoepidermal junction causes intense itching, but deeper intracutaneous injections cause pain. Histamine is synthesized in the mast cells of the skin and stored in mast cell granules. It is released by these cells in response to a variety of injurious stimuli. Histamine acts to produce itch by way of the H_1 receptor and not via H_2 receptors.[17] Histamine also causes rapid tachyphylaxis with respect to vasodilation and increased vascular permeability.[17] Therefore, it is unlikely to behave as a mediator of sustained inflammation, although it is an important mediator in short-lived wheal-and-flare reactions of the urticarial type. Some itch-producing substances owe their action to release of histamine from mast cells. Prior depletion of histamine from these cells abolishes itch caused by these substances that act by way of mast cells. Therefore, pharmacologic studies to characterize new itch-producing substances should include investigation for their ability to degranulate mast cells.

SEROTONIN (5-HYDROXYTRYPTAMINE) This amine, present in platelets but not in human mast cells, can cause itching in skin through histamine release from dermal mast cells,[18] but probably also has a more important regulatory action on itch via 5-HT_3 receptors within the central nervous system (discussed below).

ENDOPEPTIDASES Endopeptidases such as trypsin or papain (present in the spicules of *Mucuna pruriens*) cause itch. Trypsin is an important component of dermal mast cells, and is secreted upon mast cell activation. Recent studies[19] suggest that mast cell-derived tryptase, by its action on proteinase-activated receptor-2 (PAR-2) contained in adjacent C neuron terminals, evokes release of pruritogenic neuropeptides by the same terminals. This forms an additional pathway for itch, and represents an example of interaction between the immune and nervous systems. Kallikrein is a kinin-forming enzyme, the best known product of which, bradykinin, causes predominantly pain rather than itch, by a peripheral action.

NEUROPEPTIDES Substance P, localized in C neuron terminals, is released from this site by the action of mast cell tryptase on PAR-2 (discussed above) and causes itching both by a direct action, and by release of dermal mast cell histamine via NK-1 receptors.[20] Opioid peptides have both a central and a peripheral itch-producing action. Low doses of intradermal morphine produce itch, and the effect is independent of prostaglandins or mast cell degranulation. One site of action of opioid receptor agonists is on the dorsal root ganglia or spinal cord, because low doses of epidural morphine cause segmental itching. Patients with cholestatic itching obtain relief from the selective μ receptor opioid antagonist naloxone, but it is unknown whether this is a central or peripheral action.[21] However, opioid agonists acting on opioid κ receptors are antipruritic, raising the possibility that some types of itch could be relieved by a combination of opioid μ receptor antagonists and κ receptor agonists.[22]

EICOSANOIDS Arachidonic acid transformation products (prostaglandins, leukotrienes, and other hydroxy fatty acids) possess powerful proinflammatory properties but are not directly pruritic. Prostaglandin E (PGE), although not itself a cause of itching, does enhance itching due to other mediators. Pretreatment of human skin by low concentrations of PGE_1 lowered the threshold of the treated skin to itch produced by subsequent intradermal injection of histamine at the same site.[23] However, aspirin, a cyclooxygenase inhibitor, does not relieve pruritus.[24]

CENTRAL MECHANISMS OF ITCH

Two issues remain to be addressed: Why is itch specific to skin and why does it not affect deep tissues? Why does itch respond (temporarily) to scratching? By comparison with deep tissue, skin is characterized by the ability to localize itch stimuli precisely. This is achieved by the presence in the sensory pathways of effective surround inhibition. This is illustrated by applying a very gentle point stimulus to a sensitive area such as the lip. This causes poorly localized itching. Enlarging the area of application, for example, by applying a weak blunt stimulus, abolishes the itch as a consequence of activating surround inhibition. The punctate stimulus activated a small group of C neurons to cause itching, whereas the blunt stimulus caused inhibition to activation of inhibitory neuronal circuits in the dorsal horn. Scratching and rubbing activate low threshold touch-and-pressure–conducting myelinated A neurons, setting up surround inhibition involving suppression of both pre- and postsynaptic pathways. The practical consequence of this observation was the setting up of *trans*-epidermal nerve stimulation as a treatment for itch.[25] The arrival of volleys in large A fibers inhibits the response of spinal cord cells to C neuron input.

Gate Control

The dorsal horn of the cord receives afferent impulses but is also subject to powerful descending controls from the brain. Histamine-induced discharge of dorsal horn cells is strongly suppressed by stimulation of the midbrain periaqueductal grey. This is one example of many descending inhibitory controls, but there are equally important excitatory controls. All these pathways form the descending limbs of the gate control,[26] which enables higher centers to exert influence on the severity of itch—possibly one reason for the common observation that itching is generally more severe at night.

ITCHING IN PATHOLOGIC STATES

Pruritus associated with underlying internal disease is often multifactorial, involving both systemic and external factors, including ambient temperature and humidity. Itching associated with skin disease may also include central (neurogenic) and pruritogenic components.

Pruritus of Chronic Renal Disease (See also Chap. 165)

Pruritus is one of the most distressing symptoms of chronic renal failure. It affects 20 to 50 percent of patients, especially those on dialysis, although it is recently becoming less prevalent, probably due to more efficient dialysis techniques.[27] Scratching is common and the patient may be heavily excoriated. However, the skin may show nummular eczematous, prurigo nodularis-like, or lichenified appearances. The back is invariably affected, and the arm bearing the arteriovenous fistula is also a common site in dialysis patients. Patients being dialyzed with membranes that are less permeable and biocompatible (cuprophan) are more likely to suffer pruritus than those patients who are using more permeable polysulphone membranes. Patients with uremic pruritus often have a dry skin, but correction of this by emollients usually provides only mild relief. The expanding number of alleged pathogenetic factors bears testimony to the elusiveness of the causes. These include secondary hyperparathyroidism, increased numbers of dermal mast cells, elevated plasma histamine levels, abnormal levels of divalent cations, proliferation of sensory nerve endings in skin, release of pruritogenic cytokines during hemodialysis, and elevated levels of vitamin A.[28–32] Secondary hyperparathyroidism, though common in patients with renal failure, is a rare cause of renal pruritus. The proliferation of nerve endings in skin is most likely a response to incessant scratching and rubbing, rather than a primary cause of pruritus in these patients. Elevation of histamine levels, with or without increased population density of dermal mast cells, is also unlikely to be important because antihistamines are rarely effective. Recent evidence based upon response of patients to naltrexone, a selective opioid antagonist, raises the possibility that opioid peptides may be involved, although this finding has been challenged.[33,34]

Pruritus of Cholestasis (See also Chap. 164)

The highly distressing and persistent pruritus of biliary obstruction often begins with an acral distribution, but later becomes more generalized. Both peripheral and central mechanisms are important. Cholestatic pruritus is associated with high plasma levels of bile salts, but there is little or no evidence of a correlation between concentrations of bile salts and itching, whether the bile salts are measured in the blood or skin itself.[35] However it is evident that bile salts are highly pruritic when applied to blister bases or to scarified skin. Furthermore, administration of an exchange resin, cholestyramine, which lowers bile salt levels, does provide some relief. This finding also probably explains the benefit of plasma perfusion through charcoal beads.

That patients with cholestatic itching also have elevated plasma opioid levels was first demonstrated by Thornton and Losowsky in 1988.[36] They found elevated concentrations of methionine enkephalin and leucine enkephalin, and showed that the pruritus improved after treatment by the opioid antagonist nalmefene. These observations were later developed and extended by Bergasa and Jones.[37] Briefly, their evidence may be stated as follows. Animal models of cholestasis are associated with elevated levels of opioid peptides and scratching, relieved by naloxone[38] and with increased proenkephalin mRNA expression in the adult rat liver.[39] Also, plasma from patients with pruritus of cholestasis, which was relieved by naloxone,[40] causes scratching in monkeys when injected into the dorsal horn. Human-controlled trials of naloxone infusions showed a significant benefit in patients with pruritus of cholestasis.[21,41] In the light of these findings, combination of both bile salt-lowering and opioid antagonist strategies appear reasonable in the management of pruritus of cholestasis.

Pruritus of Endocrine Disease

Generalized intractable itching is a recognized feature of thyrotoxicosis and may be a presenting symptom[42] (see Chap. 169). This is usually due to increased blood flow, which raises the skin temperature, which, in turn, reduces the threshold to itching.[15] The skin is warm, moist, and flushed. However, itching in thyrotoxicosis may be localized to the anogenital area, in which case, it is usually due to mucocutaneous candidosis. Hypothyroidism may also present with widespread pruritus, in this case, due to excessive skin dryness. The skin is cool, dry, slightly scaly, and may be thickened and sallow (myxedema).

Generalized itching is not a feature of diabetes mellitus. Although there was a suggestion in the early literature that widespread pruritus could be a presenting feature, this is not substantiated by more recent studies.[43] However, anogenital itching is common, is often a presenting feature, and is due to mucocutaneous candidosis. Localized itching of the scalp can also be a manifestation of diabetic neuropathy,[44] which may respond to topical capsaicin treatment.[45] Postmenopausal pruritus may be generalized or localized, and, in the latter case, it is usually anogenital and due to candidosis. Generalized pruritus is less common, often episodic, and associated with postmenopausal hot flushes. The presence of elevated plasma levels of pituitary luteinizing hormone and follicular stimulating hormone should support the diagnosis.

Iron Deficiency

The role of iron deficiency in the causation of pruritus is controversial. Several reports have implicated iron deficiency as a cause of pruritus in otherwise normal-looking skin.[46] Pruritus and iron deficiency are sometimes associated in patients with polycythemia vera, the cause of the deficiency usually being venesection. In these patients, correction of iron deficiency is associated with clinical improvement.[47] However, a study of a large series of patients with severe iron deficiency revealed no evidence of pruritus in any of these over a period of 6 months.[48] Although patients with iron deficiency may complain of pruritus, it is unlikely that iron deficiency is responsible and other causes should be sought.

Pruritus in Hematologic Disease (See also Chaps. 157, 158 and 163)

Itch is common in hematologic disorders. In Sézary syndrome (T cell leukemia) it is invariable, intense, and generalized. In polycythemia vera, it occurs in about 50 percent of patients, is often precipitated by contact with water ("bath itch") and is associated with raised blood histamine levels.[49–51] In Hodgkin's disease, it may be a presenting symptom,[52] and may persist after remission. In cutaneous mastocytosis, itching occurs locally following rubbing the skin, although it can be widespread in severely affected patients, when it is usually associated with systemic symptoms. Itching may occur in patients with myeloid and lymphatic leukemia and myelodysplasia.

Pruritus as a Manifestation of Solid Malignant Tumors

Traditionally the onset of pruritus in a middle-aged or elderly patient with an otherwise normal-looking skin prompts a thorough investigation for underlying systemic causes including internal neoplasia, although the latter is an uncommon cause. Although pruritus may occasionally be present years before the tumor becomes clinically detectable, even if resources are available, full investigation for a causative solid tumour is probably not worthwhile.[53,54]

Pruritus of HIV-1 Infection (See also Chap. 225)

Itch is an early symptom of HIV disease and may be associated with skin disease (scabies, pediculosis, seborrheic eczema, xerosis) or a result of systemic causes (hepatic disease, renal disease, lymphoma, adverse drug reaction, systemic and skin infection including *Staphylococcus aureus* and Pityrosporum). However, it may occur as a primary symptom of HIV. Eosinophilic folliculitis is an intensely pruritic eruption characteristically occurring in HIV-positive individuals with a CD4 count less than 300/μL. Clinically, it presents with follicular and nonfollicular urticarial papules and plaques, which may or may not be pustular on the upper trunk, extremities, and face.[55] It may be associated with elevated serum IgE and may flare up on administration of antiretroviral treatment.[56]

Itching in Senescence (See also Chap. 144)

At least 50 percent of persons aged 70 years or older will suffer from prolonged bouts of troublesome pruritus. Pruritic skin diseases such as scabies, lichen planus prebullous pemphigoid, pemphigoid nodularis, or low-grade eczema should be considered, as well as underlying systemic disease, especially cholestasis and renal failure. However, in many instances, no cause is found. In many of these cases, the cause is desiccation of the skin due to a combination of decline in natural moisturizing factors in aging skin and low atmospheric humidity, as in a heated institutional environment. Occasionally, the pruritus may be provoked by water contact, mimicking aquagenic pruritus (discussed below). However, unlike true aquagenic pruritus, water-evoked itching in senescent skin responds well to emollient treatment.

Itching as a Manifestation of Psychiatric Disease

(See also Chap. 40)

Localized pruritus, especially anogenital pruritus, is a common manifestation of chronic anxiety, although candidosis with or without accompanying diabetes mellitus, pinworms, and dermatitis medicamentosa must always be excluded. In cases in which these have been excluded, sympathetic explanation of the cause of the itch, advice regarding local hygiene, change in lifestyle, and prescription of a mild anxiolytic drug such as a beta blocker may be all that is required. If the localized area is persistently rubbed, lichenification may develop (lichen simplex, neurodermatitis). Parasitophobia is a much more serious problem, the patient persisting in claiming skin infestation, although careful inspection reveals no evidence of parasites. The patient will often bring "evidence" in the form of collected fragments, although on examination the material proves to be nonspecific debris. One patient of the author's habitually brought to the outpatient clinic not only debris, but also her own small portable microscope to make sure her "evidence" was fully examined! Such patients have a delusional psychosis and a psychiatric referral is wise.

MISCELLANEOUS ITCHES

Aquagenic Pruritus

Originally described by Shelley[57] and subsequently characterized by Greaves et al.,[58] aquagenic pruritus is a rare but well-recognized and intractable pruritus mainly of the middle-aged and elderly. Characteristically, local itching is provoked by contact with water at any temperature, provoking a bout of itching lasting for 30 to 60 min, with no visible signs in the skin. During attacks patients are usually considerably distressed, but there are no other systemic manifestations. Laboratory investigations are negative, but occasionally patients with aquagenic pruritus and normal blood indices can progress to polycythemia vera.[59] The condition is persistent and most patients present with a history going back several years. Because of the lack of a visible rash, these patients are frequently labeled as "neurotic." However elevated levels of histamine are found in blood and skin.[58] The condition must be distinguished from water-induced itching of the elderly (unlike true aquagenic pruritus, this condition is relieved by emollients) and from the "bath itch" of polycythemia vera. The cause of aquagenic pruritus is unknown, but both acetylcholine and histamine are involved, although antihistamines are usually ineffective in reducing the itching. Increased acetylcholinesterase activity is present in cutaneous nerve fibers in affected skin, and the itch can be relieved by local application of atropine-like drugs.[58] Increased tissue fibrinolytic activity has also been demonstrated in the skin of patients with this condition.[60] Table 41-1 lists case reports of disease associations with aquagenic pruritus. Aquagenic pruritus has been comprehensively reviewed.[61]

Hydroxyethyl Starch-Induced Pruritus

There have been several reports, mainly in European journals, of intense itching, lasting for as long as 1 year, following hydroxyethyl starch intravenous infusion for vascular insufficiency. The pruritus is associated with ultrastructural evidence of deposition of hydroxyethyl starch in the Schwann cells of peripheral nerve fibers, endothelial cells, and macrophages, and is probably an example of a neurogenic itch.[67]

TABLE 41-1

Case Reports of Disease/Drug Associations with Aquagenic Pruritus

Underlying Abnormality	Reference
Hypereosinophilic syndrome	Newton JA et al.[62]
Myelodysplastic syndrome	Mc Grath JA, Greaves MW[63]
Juvenile xanthogranuloma	Handfield-Jones SE et al.[64]
Squamous carcinoma of the cervix	Ferguson JA et al.[65]
Antimalarial drug therapy (for lupus)	Jimenez-Alonso J et al.[66]

Notalgia Paraesthetica

This is a common chronic localized itch, affecting mainly the interscapular area especially the T2–T6 dermatomes, but occasionally with a more widespread distribution, involving the shoulders, back, and upper chest. The sensation perceived by the patient is part itch, part paraesthesia. There are no specific cutaneous signs, apart from those attributed to scratching and rubbing. Amyloid deposition may be found in skin biopsies, but this is a secondary event. The current view on etiology is that it is a neuropathic itch due to entrapment of spinal nerves as they emerge through the epaxial muscles of the back.[68] It may respond to topical capsaicin treatment.

Brachioradial Pruritus

This localized pruritus is becoming increasingly common. Patients, usually fair skinned, affluent, and middle aged, habitually indulge in golf, tennis, sailing, or other leisure outdoor activities in sunny climates.[69] They develop persistent pruritus of the outer surface of the upper arm elbow and forearm, associated with clinical evidence of chronic sun damage and xerosis in the pruritic skin. The itch may gradually become more widespread. Results of phototesting are negative and the problem seems consequent upon straightforward chronic ultraviolet overexposure. It may respond to capsaicin cream.

Pruritus of Anorexia Nervosa

Pruritus has long been a recognized feature of the symptomatology of anorexia nervosa[70] and usually subsides following weight restoration. Possible causes include compulsive washing, impaired renal or hepatic function, and thyroid disease. However, in many patients, no cause is apparent. A recent study of 19 patients suggests that abnormalities of regional blood flow, serotonergic, and opioid tone may underlie this symptom.[71] It is suggested that anorexia nervosa should be considered as a cause in any low-body-weight patient with otherwise unexplained pruritus.

Pruritus of Creutzfeldt-Jakob Disease ("Prion Pruritus")

Three patients have been reported as presenting with intense itching during the prodromal period of the disease. Creutzfeldt-Jakob disease is a spongiform encephalopathy related to scrapie, also a prion disease of animals, regularly associated with itching and scratching.[72] All three of these patients had evidence of brainstem dysfunction and it is proposed that "prion pruritus" is a central (neuropathic) pruritus in patients with no evidence of other systemic or cutaneous causes.

Itching in Atopic Eczema (See also Chap. 122)

This remains a controversial area and the molecular basis of pruritus in atopic eczema remains largely unexplained. Whether the itch precedes the eczema, or the other way round is also an unresolved issue. What is certain is that an itch-scratch vicious cycle exists in atopic patients, in which scratch damage enhances itch. Itching is particularly acute in response to punctate stimuli such as wool fibers; rubbing or scratching elicits surround inhibition (discussed earlier). Alloknesis (discussed earlier) is a prominent feature of the itch of atopic eczema and explains the bouts of intense itching associated with sweating, sudden changes in temperature, dressing, and undressing. That there is a central (neurogenic) component to the itch of atopic eczema is suggested by the poor response to low sedation H_1 antihistamines.[73] This also suggests that histamine is not a major mediator of atopic eczema;[74] alternative candidates include cytokines. Opioid peptides may serve as central mediators because opioid antagonists are effective in some patients. Nocturnal scratching is a major problem in atopic eczema, occurs during sleep stages 1 and 2 (superficial sleep), and occupies 10 to 20 percent of the total sleeping time, leading to tiredness and irritability. Treatment should be directed first at managing dryness and infection—two important and remediable causes of itch. Sedative antihistamines may be useful. Topical steroids allay itching where this is a result of inflamed skin, using the lowest effective concentration. Phototherapy (UVB, photochemotherapy) may be effective in some patients. For selected, severely handicapped, treatment-resistant patients, recourse may be made to oral azathioprine or to cyclosporin. Most recently, tacrolimus, a topically applied macrolide immunosuppressive with an action resembling that of oral cyclosporin, was shown to be effective in relieving the pruritus of atopic eczema.[75]

Prurigo Nodularis

Prurigo nodularis is a chronic papulonodular intensely itchy eruption of unknown cause. It occurs symmetrically, predominantly on the extensor surfaces of the limbs, lower back, and abdomen. The palms, soles, head, and neck are rarely involved. The surrounding skin looks healthy. Histologically, apart from the obvious hyperkeratosis and massive acanthosis, there is also "colossal hyperplasia" of neural fibers (Pautrier's neuroma) although this is the result of chronic scratching or rubbing, and is not diagnostic.[76] Recently, immunoelectron microscope studies demonstrated overexpression of p75 nerve growth factor receptor in Schwann cells and perineurium cells, which may be the immediate cause of the hyperplasia.[77] Topical treatment, including emollients, corticosteroids, and possibly capsaicin, may be beneficial. Systemically, sedative antihistamines may help patients sleep at night. Some authors advocate cyclosporin, but probably the most effective treatment is thalidomide,[78] but it must not be administered to fertile women, and polyneuropathy is a troublesome side effect.

INVESTIGATION OF GENERALIZED PRURITUS WITH NO RASH

Careful history, including a full drug history, and physical examination are the starting points, and the latter should include rectal, and in women, pelvic, examination. The history should take into account the multidimensional nature of itching and should include details of quality, distribution, and timing. Any patient referred with generalized pruritus should be assumed to have scabies until proved otherwise—skin signs may be clinically inapparent, perhaps confined to a few small nodules on the genitalia. Investigations should include full blood count, including a differential count for eosinophilia, urinalysis, stool examination for evidence of parasites, and occult blood. Chest x-ray, thyroid, liver function, and renal function tests should be carried out, together with a search for evidence of infection by hepatitis B or C, HIV, plasma protein electrophoresis, immunoelectrophoresis, and an analysis of serum iron. A CT scan of the abdomen is usually justifiable to help rule out lymphoma. A skin biopsy is useful to exclude clinically inapparent cutaneous mastocytosis.

TREATMENT OF PRURITUS

Treatment of pruritus depends upon identifying and removing the cause whether systemic or cutaneous. False hopes of highly effective treatment for those patients in whom no cause can be found should not be raised; there are no effective selective systemic or topical antipruritic agents with acceptable tolerability. One reason for this is the lack of convincing animal models for itch and the paucity of quantitative statistically analyzable methods for measuring itch; most methods are indirect, involving quantification of scratch or subjective in which a visual analogue scale is used. It is important to elicit from a detailed history—taking the precise quality, timing, and distribution of the itch, so that more focused therapy can be instituted. The "Eppendorf itch questionnaire" is an example of this approach.[79]

General Measures

The sensation of itching is heightened if the skin is warm,[15] therefore measures should be taken to cool the skin down, including tepid showering, light clothes, and air conditioning where appropriate. Cooling lotions, such as calamine or oil-in-water vanishing creams, may help. Aqueous menthol lotion 1% is effective in the treatment of histamine-induced itching.[80] Menthol can also be formulated in an aqueous cream base. Topical steroids are not antipruritic, and are not indicated unless there is evidence of cutaneous inflammation as a cause for the itching. For localized itches, topical capsaicin (8-methyl-*N*-vanillyl-6-nonenamide), the active ingredient of chili pepper, may be effective. Unfortunately, compliance is poor because initial application causes intense irritation because of the release of neuropeptides via an action on C neuron terminals via VR1 receptors.[81] Doxepin is a tricyclic antidepressant with potent anti-H_1-and anti-H_2 histamine-receptor properties. Topical application of a doxepin 5% cream is effective in eczema-associated pruritus, but its usefulness is limited by sedation because of percutaneous absorption. Other strategies for intractable localized pruritus include electrical stimulation treatment by TENS (transepidermal electrical nerve stimulation) and CFS (cutaneous field stimulation).[82,83] These probably work by creating surround inhibition (discussed earlier).[25] Other measures possibly worth trying include paroxetine, a selective serotonin reuptake inhibitor (SSRI; claimed to be effective in relieving the itch of terminal cancer sufferers),[84] 5-HT_3–receptor antagonists such as odansetron,[85] and opiate receptor antagonists administered orally or parenterally.[86]

Chronic Renal Disease

Excessive dryness of the skin should be treated with emollients. Where secondary hyperthyroidism is responsible, this should be dealt with.[28] UVB phototherapy, including narrow band UVB, is effective, and probably the treatment of choice for most patients.[87] Remissions may last for as long as 18 months. This treatment decreases the population density of mast cells by inducing apoptosis, causes nerve dysfunction, and reduces divalent cations in the skin. Naltrexone was shown to be effective in a double-blind randomized crossover trial,[33] although this finding has been challenged,[34] and odansetron may also be of value.[88]

Cholestasis

Cholestyramine is effective in the treatment of cholestatic itch, especially in primary biliary cirrhosis, but it is ineffective in the presence of total biliary obstruction. It chelates intestinal bile acids, therefore reducing the enterohepatic circulation of bile salts. Usually 4 g is administered before and after breakfast, and repeated at midday and evening meals (maintenance, 12 g/day). Unfortunately patient compliance is poor because of nausea; the treatment is unpalatable. Rifampicin is also useful and acts as a hepatic enzyme inducer, in addition to inhibiting hepatocyte uptake of bile salts. The controlled trial evidence of the value of the opioid antagonist naloxone has already been referred to (see above)[21] and oral opioid μ-receptor antagonists (naltrexone, nalmefene) are also available.[89] Development of opioid withdrawal symptoms has been noted in some treated cholestasis patients.[21,36] This can be avoided by giving a slow infusion of naloxone [0.002 μg/kg per min (160 to 200 μg/24h)], doubling the rate of infusion every 3 h if no adverse events occur. Other treatments worth trying include codeine,[90] hydroxyethyl rutosides,[91] ultraviolet phototherapy,[92] ursodcoxycholic acid,[93] charcoal superfusion,[94] and odansetron.[95]

Aquagenic Pruritus and Water-Induced Itching of Polycythemia Vera

Antihistamines are rarely of value, despite the association of elevated histamine levels with this disorder. Although UVB phototherapy is effective in some patients, PUVA is the preferred treatment.[96] At least 50 percent of patients experience sustained improvement, although the treatment may have to be repeated on a 6 month or annual basis.[96] In the case of aquagenic pruritus associated with polycythemia vera, repeated venesection often relieves the pruritus. Aspirin has been advocated by some authors. Other treatments which have been advocated include attenuated androgens and interferon-α2b.[97,98]

Pruritus of HIV

As indicated above, pruritus is an extremely common complaint in HIV sufferers and the causes are legion. Very thorough examination needs to be carried out, both in the skin and systemically, bearing in mind that there may be concurrently more than one cause. Pruritic papular eruptions including eosinophilic folliculitis are often treatment resistant. Phototherapy (UVB)[99] is well worth trying. Other measures include PUVA and pentoxifylline.[100]

REFERENCES

1. Twycross R et al: Itch: More than scratching the surface. *QJM* **96**:7, 2003
2. Bickford RGL: Experiments relating to itch sensation, its peripheral mechanism and central pathways. *Clin Sci* **3**:377, 1938
3. Rothman S: Physiology of itching. *Physiol Rev* **21**:357, 1941
4. Graham DT et al: Neural mechanisms involved in itch, "itchy skin" and tickle sensations. *J Clin Invest* **30**:37, 1951
5. Lewis T: Experiments relating to cutaneous hyperalgesia and its spread through somatic nerves. *Clin Sci* **2**:373, 1936
6. Lynn B: Cutaneous hyperalgesia. *Br Med Bull* **33**:103, 1977
7. Frey M von: Zur physiologie der juckempfinding. *Arch Neerl Physiol* **7**:142 1922
8. Bishop GH: Responses to electrical stimulation of single sensory units of skin. *J Neurophysiol* **6**:361, 1943
9. Shelley WE, Arthur RP: The neurohistology and neurophysiology of the itch sensation in man. *Arch Dermatol* **76**:296, 1957
10. Torok L: Uber das Wesen der Juckempfinding. *Ztschr Psychol* **46**:23, 1907

11. Toth Kasa I et al: Capsaicin prevents histamine-induced itching. *Int J Clin Pharmacol Res* **6**:163, 1986
12. Hillige M, Wang L et al: Ultrastructural evidence for nerve fibers within all vital layers of the human epidermis. *J Invest Dermatol* **104**:134, 1995
13. Torebjork HE: Afferent C units responding to mechanical, thermal and chemical stimuli in human non-glabrous skin. *Acta Physiol Scand* **92**:374, 1974
14. Schmelz M et al: Specific C receptors for itch in human skin. *J Neurosci* **17**:8003, 1997
15. Fruhstorfer H et al: The effect of thermal stimulation on clinical and experimental itch. *Pain* **24**:259, 1986
16. Andrew D, Craig AD: Spinothalamic lamina 1 neurons selectively sensitive to histamine: A central neural pathway for itch. *Nat Neurosci* **4**:72, 2001
17. Davies MG, Greaves MW: Sensory responses of human skin to synthetic histamine analogues and to histamine. *Br J Pharmacol* **9**:255 1967
18. Greaves MW, Shuster S: Responses of skin blood vessels to bradykinin, histamine and 5-hydroxytryptamine. *J Physiol* **193**:255, 1967
19. Steinhoff M et al: Agonists of proteinase-activated receptor 2 induce inflammation by a neurogenic mechanism. *Nature Medicine* **6**:151, 2000
20. Jorrizo JL et al: Vascular responses of human skin to substance P and mechanism of action. *Eur J Pharmacol* **87**:67, 1983
21. Bergasa NV et al: Effects of naloxone infusions in patients with the pruritus of cholestasis. A double blind randomized controlled trial. *Ann Int Med* **123**:161, 1995
22. Kumagai H, Sasamua H, Hayashi M et al: Prospects for a novel opioid κ receptor agonist TRK-820 in uremic pruritus. *Proc Int Workshop on Itch, Singapore,* p 59, 2001
23. Greaves MW, Mc Donald Gibson W: Itch, the role of prostaglandins. *BMJ* **3**:601, 1967
24. Daly, BM, Shuster, S, Effect of aspirin in pruritus. *BMJ* **293**:907, 1986
25. Wall PD, Sweet WH: Temporary abolition of pain in man. *Science* **155**:108, 1967
26. Melzack R, Wall PD: Pain mechanisms: A new theory. *Science* **150**:971, 1965
27. Szepietowski JC, Schwartz RA: Uremic pruritus. *Int J Dermatol* **37**:247, 1998
28. Hampers CL et al: Disappearance of "uremic" itching after subtotal parathyroidectomy. *N Engl J Med* **279**:695, 1968
29. Cawley EP: Presidential address: A surfeit of mast cells in the skin of patients with uremia. *Arch Dermatol* **111**:1663, 1663
30. Carmichael AJ et al: Serological markers of renal itch in patients receiving long-term haemodialysis. *BMJ* **296**:1575, 1988
31. Pereira, BJG Dinarello, CA, Production of cytokines and cytokine inhibitory proteins in patients on dialysis. *Nephrol Dial Transplant* **9**(suppl 2):60, 1994
32. Berne B et al: UV treatment of uraemic pruritus reduces the vitamin A content of the skin. *Eur J Clin Invest* **14**:203, 1968
33. Peer G et al: Randomised crossover trial of naltrexone in renal pruritus. *Lancet* **348**:1552, 1996
34. Pauli-Magnus C, Mikus G, Alscher DM et al: Naltrexone does not relieve uremic pruritus: Results of a randomised, placebo-controlled crossover study. *J Am Soc Nephrol* **11**:514, 2000
35. Ghent CN et al: Elevations in skin tissue levels of bile acids in human cholestasis: Relation to serum levels and to pruritus. *Gastroenterology* **73**:1125, 1977
36. Thornton JR, Losowsky MS: Opioid peptides and primary biliary cirrhosis. *BMJ* **297**:1501, 1988
37. Bergasa NV, Jones EA: The pruritus of cholestasis: Potential pathogenic and therapeutic implications of opioids. *Gastroenterology* **108**:1582, 1995
38. Bergasa NV et al: Cholestasis in the male rat is associated with naloxone-reversible antinociception. *J Hepatol* **20**:85, 1994
39. Bergasa NV et al: Cholestasis is associated with proenkephalin mRNA expression in the adult rat liver. *Am J Physiol* **268**:G346, 1995
40. Bergasa NV et al: Plasma from patients with pruritus of cholestasis induces opioid receptor-mediated scratching in monkeys. *Life Sci* **53**:1253, 1993
41. Bergasa NV et al: A controlled trial of naloxone infusions for the pruritus of chronic cholestasis. *Gastroenterology* **102**:544, 1992
42. Caravati CM Jr et al: Cutaneous manifestations of hyperthyroidism. *South Med J* **62**:1127, 1969
43. Neilly JB et al: Pruritus in diabetes mellitus: Investigation of prevalence and correlation with diabetes control. *Diabetes Care* **9**:273, 1986
44. Scribner M: Diabetes and pruritus of the scalp. *JAMA* **237**:1559, 1977
45. Ross DR, Varipapa RJ: Treatment of painful diabetic neuropathy with topical capsaicin. *N Engl J Med* **321**:474, 1989
46. Lewiecki EM, Rahman F: Pruritus: A manifestation of iron deficiency. *JAMA* **236**:2319, 1976
47. Salem HH et al: Pruritus and severe iron deficiency in polycythaemia vera. *BMJ* **285**:91, 1982
48. Tucker WFG et al: Absence of pruritus in iron deficiency following venesection. *Clin Exp Dermatol* **9**:186, 1984
49. Berlin, NI: Diagnosis and classification of polycythaemias. *Semin Hematol* **12**:339, 1975
50. Gilbert HS et al: A study of histamine in myeloproliferative disease. *Blood* **78**:795, 1966
51. Archer CB et al: Polycythaemia vera can present with aquagenic pruritus. *Lancet* **1**:1451, 1988
52. Botero F: Pruritus as a manifestation of systemic disorders. *Cutis* **21**:873, 1978
53. Kantor GR, Lookingbill DP: Generalised pruritus and systemic disease. *J Am Acad Dermatol* **9**:375, 1983
54. Paul R et al: Itch and malignancy prognosis in generalized pruritus: A 6-year follow up of 125 patients. *J Am Acad Dermatol* **16**:1179, 1987
55. Rosenthal D et al: Human immunodeficiency virus-associated eosinophilic folliculitis: A unique dermatosis associated with advanced human immunodeficiency virus infection. *Arch Dermatol* **127**:206, 1991
56. Rodwell GEL, Berger TG: Pruritus and cutaneous inflammatory conditions in HIV disease. *Clin Dermatol* **18**:479, 2000
57. Shelley WB: Questions and answers: Post-wetness (aquagenic) pruritus. *JAMA* **212**:1385, 1970
58. Greaves MW et al: Aquagenic pruritus. *BMJ* **282**:2008, 1981
59. Archer, CB et al: Polycythaemia vera can present with aquagenic pruritus. *Lancet* **1**:1451, 1988
60. Steinman HK et al: Polycythaemia rubra vera and water induced pruritus: Blood histamine levels and cutaneous fibrinolytic activity before and after water challenge. *Br J Dermatol* **116**:329, 1987
61. Menage HduP, Greaves MW: Aquagenic pruritus. *Semin Dermatol* **14**:313, 1995
62. Newton JA et al: Aquagenic pruritus associated with the idiopathic hypereosinophilic syndrome. *Br J Dermatol* **122**:103, 1990
63. Mc Grath JA, Greaves MW: Aquagenic pruritus and the myelodysplastic syndrome. *Br J Dermatol* **123**:414, 1990
64. Handfield-Jones SE et al: Aquagenic pruritus associated with juvenile xanthogranuloma. *Clin Exp Dermatol* **18**:253, 1993
65. Ferguson JA et al: Aquagenic pruritus associated with metastatic squamous cell carcinoma of the cervix. *Clin Exp Dermatol* **19**:257, 1994
66. Jimenez-Alonso J et al: Antimalarial drug-induced aquagenic-type pruritus in patients with lupus. *Arthritis Rheum* **41**:744, 1998
67. Metze D et al: Persistent pruritus after hydroxyethyl starch infusion therapy: A result of long-term storage in cutaneous nerves. *Br J Dermatol* **136**:553, 1997
68. Eisenberg E et al: Notalgia paraesthetica associated with nerve root impingement. *J Am Acad Dermatol* **37**:998, 1997
69. Walcyk PJ, Elpern DJ: Brachioradial pruritus: A tropical dermopathy. *Br J Dermatol* **115**:177, 1986
70. Taniguchi S et al: Generalised pruritus in anorexia nervosa. *Br J Dermatol* **134**:510, 1996
71. Morgan JF, Lacey JH: Scratching and fasting: A study of pruritus and anorexia nervosa. *Br J Dermatol* **140**:453, 1999
72. Shabtai H et al: L Pruritus in Creutzfeldt-Jakob disease. *Neurology* **46**:940, 1996
73. Krause L , Shuster S: Mechanism of action of antipruritic drugs. *BMJ* **287**:1199, 1983
74. Rukweid R et al: Mast cell mediators other than histamine induce pruritus in atopic dermatitis patients: A dermal microdialysis study. *Br J Dermatol* **142**:1 2000
75. Ruzicka T et al: A short term trial of tacrolimus ointment for atopic dermatitis. *N Engl J Med* **337**: 816, 1997
76. Lindley RP, Payne CMER: Neural hyperplasia is not a diagnostic requirement in nodular prurigo. *J Cutan Pathol* **16**:14, 1989
77. Liang Y et al: Light and electron microscopic immunohistochemical observations of p75 nerve growth factor receptor—Immunoreactive dermal nerves in prurigo nodularis. *Arch Derm Res* **291**:14, 1999
78. Winkelmann RK et al: Thalidomide treatment of prurigo nodularis. *Acta Derm Venereol* **64**:412, 1984
79. Darsow U et al: New aspects of itch pathophysiology: Component analysis of atopic itch using the "Eppendorf itch questionnaire." *Int Arch Allergy Immunol* **124**:326, 2001
80. Bromm B et al: Effects of menthol and cold on histamine-induced itch and skin reactions in man. *Neurosci Lett* **187**:157, 1995

81. Caterina MJ et al: The capsaicin receptor: A heat-activated ion channel in the pain pathway. *Nature* **389**:816, 1997
82. Tang WYM et al: Evaluation on the antipruritic role of transepidermal electrical nerve stimulation in the treatment of pruritic dermatoses. *Dermatology* **199**:237, 1999
83. Wallengren J: Cutaneous field stimulation in the treatment of severe itch. *Arch Dermatol* **137**:1323, 2001
84. Zylicz Z et al: Paroxetine for pruritus in advanced cancer. *J Pain Symptom Manage* **16**:121, 1998.
85. Sanger GJ, Twycross R: Making sense of emesis pruritus 5-HT and 5-HT-3 receptor antagonists. *Progr Pall Care* **4**:7, 1996
86. Metze, D et al: Efficacy and safety of naltrexone, an oral opiate receptor antagonist in the treatment of pruritus in internal and dermatological diseases. *J Am Acad Dermatol* **41**:533, 1999
87. Gilchrest BA et al: Ultraviolet B phototherapy for uremic pruritus. Long-term results and possible mechanism of action. *Ann Intern Med* **91**:17, 1979
88. Balaskas EV et al: Histamine and serotonin in uremic pruritus: Effect of odansetron in CAPD-pruritic patients. *Nephron* **78**:395 1998
89. Bergasa NV et al: Open label trial of oral nalmefene therapy for the pruritus of cholestasis. *Hepatology* **27**:679, 1998
90. Zylicz Z, Krajnik M: Codeine for pruritus in primary biliary cirrhosis. *Lancet* **353**:813, 1999
91. Hishon S et al: The relief of pruritus in primary biliary cirrhosis by hydroxyethyl rutosides. *Br J Dermatol* **105**:457, 1981
92. Maggiore G et al: Phototherapy for pruritus in chronic cholestasis of childhood. *Eur J Pediatr* **139**:90, 1982
93. Matzusaki Y et al: Improvement of biliary enzyme and itching as a result of long-term administration of ursodeoxycholic acid in primary biliary cirrhosis. *Am J Gastroenterol* **85**:15, 1990
94. Duncan JS et al: Treatment of pruritus due to chronic obstructive liver disease. *BMJ* **289**:22, 1984
95. Schworer H, Ramamadori G: Improvement of cholestatic pruritus by odansetron. *Lancet* **341**:1277, 1995
96. Menage H du P et al: The efficacy of psoralen photochemotherapy in aquagenic pruritus. *Br J Dermatol* **127**:163, 1993
97. Kolodny L et al: Danazol relieves refractory pruritus associated with myeloproliferative disorders and other diseases. *Am J Hematol* **51**:112, 1996
98. Muller EW et al: Long-term treatment with interferon-α2b for severe pruritus in patients with polycythemia vera. *Br J Haematol* **89**:313, 1995
99. Lim HW et al: UVB phototherapy is an effective treatment for pruritus in patients infected with HIV. *J Am Acad Dermatol* **37**:414, 1997
100. Berman B et al: Efficacy of pentoxifylline in the treatment of pruritic papular eruption of HIV-infected persons. *J Am Acad Dermatol* **38**:955, 1998

SECTION 8

EPIDERMIS: DISORDERS OF PERSISTENT INFLAMMATION, CELL KINETICS, AND DIFFERENTIATION

CHAPTER 42

Enno Christophers
Ulrich Mrowietz

Psoriasis

Psoriasis is a chronic relapsing disease of the skin characterized by variable clinical features. The cutaneous lesions are usually so distinct that a clinical diagnosis is easy to make. The lesions are classified as erythrosquamous, which indicates that both the vasculature (erythema) and the epidermis (increased scale formation) are involved.

The morphology of the skin lesions varies considerably. Table 42-1 lists the terms commonly used to describe the different morphologic types of the disease (also see Figs. 42-1 through 42-6). Psoriasis vulgaris is the most common type of psoriasis. Circular plaques are predominant on the elbows, knees, lower back, and umbilical area, whereas eruptive (guttate) lesions often are confined to the trunk and proximal extremities.

Psoriatic erythroderma involves the entire body, presenting with generalized erythema and varying degrees of scale.

Psoriasis also may present in a pustular form. There is a generalized form, usually referred to as *pustular psoriasis* (von Zumbusch), and a localized variant, confined to the palms and soles, known as *pustulosis palmaris et plantaris* (PPP; see Chap. 70). In rare instances in psoriasis of the plaque type or guttate psoriasis, pustules may develop after acute relapses (psoriasis with pustules).

The clinical presentation varies depending on a number of factors, which may cause an individual to present with a few localized psoriatic plaques or with generalized skin involvement and the development of pustules. The disease activity is reflected predominantly as scaling in stationary plaques and as inflammation in the eruptive guttate lesions.

Psoriasis can be disabling not only because of skin involvement but also because of concomitant joint disease. Psoriatic arthritis is the only recognized noncutaneous manifestation of the disease and is discussed in detail in Chap. 43.

TABLE 42-1

Terms Describing Morphologic Features of Psoriasis

Annular psoriasis	Gyrate psoriasis
Circinate psoriasis	Inverse psoriasis
Follicular psoriasis	Nummular psoriasis
Generalized psoriasis	Pustular psoriasis
Geographic psoriasis	Serpiginous psoriasis
Guttate psoriasis	

HISTORIC ASPECTS

The earliest descriptions of what appears to represent psoriasis are given at the beginning of medicine in the *Corpus Hippocraticum.* This work was edited in Alexandria 100 years after the death of Hippocrates (460–377 B.C.), who presumably was the author. Hippocrates used the terms *psora* and *lepra* for conditions that can be recognized as psoriasis. Later, Celsus (*ca.* 25 B.C.), who translated the writings of Tiberius Claudius Menekrates (the personal physician of Emperor Tiberius) into Greek, described, among 40 different dermatoses, a form of impetigo that was interpreted by R. Willan (1757–1812) as being psoriasis. Willan separated two diseases as psoriasiform entities, a discoid lepra Graecorum and a polycyclic confluent psora leprosa, which later was called *psoriasis.* In 1841, the Viennese dermatologist Ferdinand von Hebra (1816–1880) unequivocally showed that Willan's lepra Graecorum and psora leprosa were one disease that had caused much confusion because of differences in the size, distribution, growth, and involution of lesions.

EPIDEMIOLOGY

Incidence

Psoriasis is universal in occurrence. In the United States, psoriasis affects about 2 percent of the population, with approximately 150,000 newly diagnosed cases per year. The worldwide incidence varies considerably. Reasons for such variations range from racial to geographic and environmental.[1] For instance, in the Faeroe Islands, 2.8 percent of the population are affected. While inbreeding may contribute to this incidence, the normal positive effect of sunlight on psoriasis also may play a role because the Faeroe Islands are 61° north latitude.[2] Other data

FIGURE 42-1

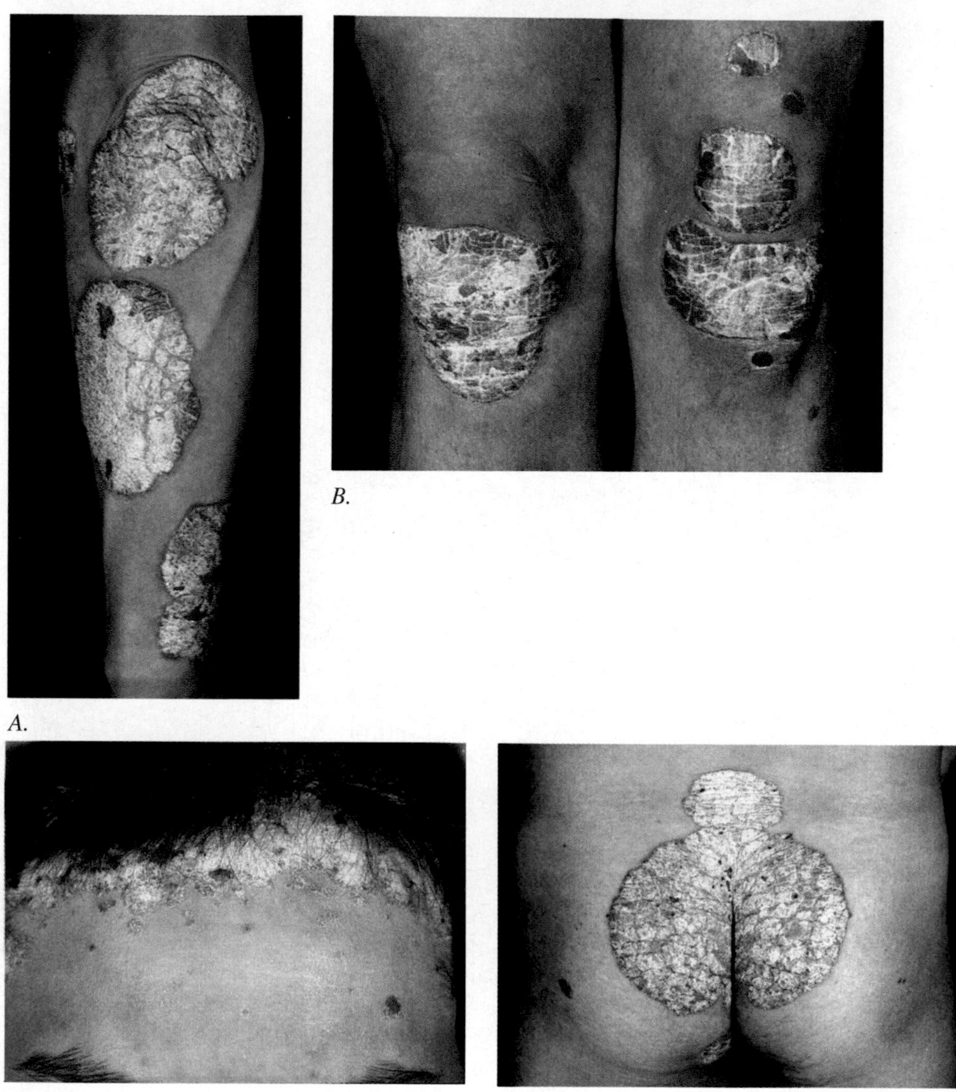

Chronic stationary psoriasis located at typical sites.

demonstrate that the incidence of psoriasis ranges from 0.97 percent in South America to 1.3 percent in Germany, 1.6 percent in Great Britain, 1.7 percent in Denmark, and 2.3 percent in Sweden. Psoriasis is rare in West African and North American blacks. The incidence of the disease is also low in Japanese and Eskimos. Psoriasis is nearly absent in North American Indians, and in an examination of 26,000 South American Indians, not a single case was seen. Psoriasis is equally common in males and females.[1]

Age of Onset

The onset of psoriasis constitutes a lifelong threat. It has been reported to be present at birth and was described recently as having its onset at age 108.[3] As demonstrated by several studies, most patients develop the initial lesions of psoriasis in the third decade of life. First signs appear in males at a mean age of 29 and in females at age 27.[1] A study of the onset of psoriasis in 2400 patients showed a peak incidence at 22.5 years of age; a second peak of onset around age 55 was found in 11.8 percent of the patients[4] (see Fig. 42-5*A*). In a study of psoriasis in 245 children, the mean age of onset was 8.1 years,[5] and in a census study from the Faeroe Islands, the mean age of onset was 12.5 years.[2] An early onset (before age 15) predicts more severe disease relative to the percentage of body surface involved with psoriasis and the response to therapy. Also, the earlier the onset, the greater is the probability of a positive family history of psoriasis.[6]

Mode of Inheritance

The major support for concluding that there is a genetic predisposition to psoriasis comes from studies showing (1) an increased incidence in psoriasis among relatives of affected probands, (2) a proportionally increased incidence of psoriasis in offspring of matings in which one or both parents are afflicted, (3) high rates of concordance for psoriasis among monozygotic twins when one is afflicted, and (4) susceptibility loci located on various chromosomes, including disequilibrium of certain major histocompatibility antigens.[7–9]

Approximately one-third of patients with psoriasis report some relative with the disease.[10] In a recent study it was found that when one parent had psoriasis, psoriasis also developed in 8.1 percent of the offspring. This value increased to 41 percent when both parents had psoriasis. These data are in accordance with a trait of inheritance involving more than one gene.

The incidence of psoriasis has been recorded in 117 monozygotic twins. Of these, 65 percent were concordant for the disease. This percentage contrasts with a 30 percent concordance for psoriasis in 112 dizygotic twins, of whom at least one twin in each pair has psoriasis. Reconsideration of those population-based studies as well as the twin studies confirmed that psoriasis is a heritable disease with a multilocus model of inheritance. Environmental factors are likely to play a role in triggering the disease.

As noted, there is disequilibrium (greater than expected frequency) between certain class I antigens (human leukocyte antigens, or HLAs) of the histocompatibility locus on human cells and psoriasis. The HLA types most frequently reported to be associated with psoriasis are HLA-B13, HLA-Bw57, HLA-Cw6, and HLA-DR7.[8,11]

Mapping of HLA phenotypes in families with psoriasis supports the genetic linkage for psoriasis as well as a link between psoriasis and arthritis.

In a study of 2100 patients with nonpustular psoriasis, evaluation of the age of onset revealed two peaks, one occurring at the age of 16 years in females and 22 years in males and a second near the age of 60 years in both females and males[4] (see Fig. 42-5*A*). Nearly 50 percent of the first-degree family members of patients with early onset were found to be affected, and 85 percent of the patients were HLA-Cw6+. By contrast, only 15 percent of patients with late onset were HLA-Cw6+. Psoriasis in patients with early onset was noted to follow an unstable course, generally with a more severe disease expression.[4]

Generalized pustular psoriasis appears to be in disequilibrium with HLA-B27.[12] This finding contrasts with observations of pustular psoriasis of the palms and soles, in which there is no disequilibrium between the disease and HLA antigens. Patients with psoriasis who also have peripheral arthritis have an association with HLA-B27. This disequilibrium is most marked if spondylitis is present, and this finding may link classic ankylosing spondylitis, Reiter's disease, and psoriasis.

FIGURE 42-2

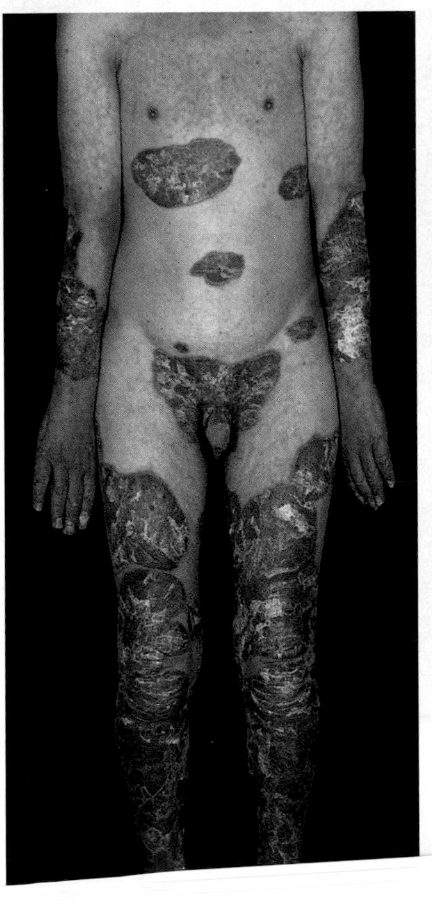

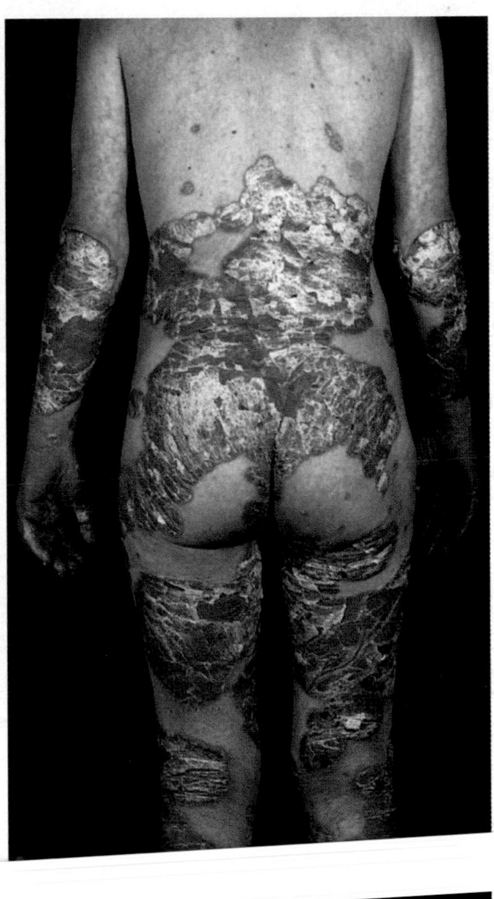

Chronic stationary psoriasis covering large areas of the body.

CLINICAL FEATURES

General Considerations

SKIN Various morphologic forms of psoriasis have been distinguished and given special names (see Table 42-1). Lesions of psoriasis show four prominent features: (1) they are sharply demarcated with clear-cut borders, (2) the surface consists of noncoherent silvery scales, (3) under the scale the skin has a glossy, homogeneous erythema, and (4) there is an Auspitz sign.

The size of a single lesion varies from a pinpoint to plaques that cover large areas of the body. The clinical presentation of psoriasis is better understood when it is realized that disease activity can range from a chronic stationary phase, to a resolving process, to flares of disease that may be associated with numerous sterile pustules.

The Auspitz sign is a specific feature of the erythrosquamous lesion of psoriasis. It is noted when the hyperker[illegible] chanical[illegible] by scra[illegible] within a few seconds after mechanical removal of the scale, small blood droplets appear on the shiny erythematous surface (Fig. 42-7*A–D*). The Auspitz sign has diagnostic value; it is not present in inverse or pustular psoriasis and may help to differentiate psoriasis from other skin conditions with a similar morphology.

In addition to the Auspitz sign, the Koebner phenomenon can be elicited in approximately 20 percent of patients. After nonspecific irritation, psoriatic lesions develop in areas where they were not present previously.

NAILS Nail changes are frequent in psoriasis. Based on a questionnaire to 5600 patients, Farber and Nall[1] reported that fingernails are involved in 50 percent of subjects and toenails in 35 percent. The variety of nail changes ranges from minor defects in the nail plate (pits) to severe alterations of the nail organ (onychodystrophy) and loss of the nail plate when the pustular forms of psoriasis involve the nail.

These morphologic alterations reflect the extent to which the psoriatic process affects the various portions of the nail organ—i.e., the proximal nail fold, nail matrix, nail bed, and hyponychium. The degree of nail involvement depends on the localization of the psoriatic tissue changes at these sites as well as on how long these processes last. Three main morphologic alterations in the structure of the nail are appreciated:

1. Pits are evident within the nail plate. This morphologic pattern apparently is due to defective keratinization of the dorsal side of the proximal nail fold (Fig. 42-8*A*).
2. Yellowish macules beneath the nail plate often extend distally toward the hyponychium. This morphologic pattern appears to be caused by psoriatic processes located in the nail bed (see Fig. 42-8*B*).
3. Severe onychodystrophy results in yellowish keratinous material. This morphologic pattern is believed to be secondary to psoriasis involving the nail matrix (see Fig. 42-8*C*).

In pustular psoriasis, the nail changes consist of subungual pustules of the nail bed or the nail matrix. If major portions of either are affected with this process, loss of the nail plate, or even dystrophy of the matrix (anonychia) can occur (see Fig. 42-8*D*). In pustular psoriasis of the palms and soles, nail changes are rare. Nail changes are more frequent in patients with arthritis.

Clinical Patterns of the Skin Presentation (Table 42-2)

PSORIASIS VULGARIS, CHRONIC STATIONARY PSORIASIS, PLAQUE-TYPE PSORIASIS This clinical pattern is the most frequent. Red scaly lesions, as described earlier, persist for months to years (see Figs. 42-1, 42-3*B*, and 42-9). There is constant production of large amounts of scale with little alteration in shape or distribution of individual plaques. Areas of predilection are the elbows (see Fig. 42-1*A*),

FIGURE 42-3

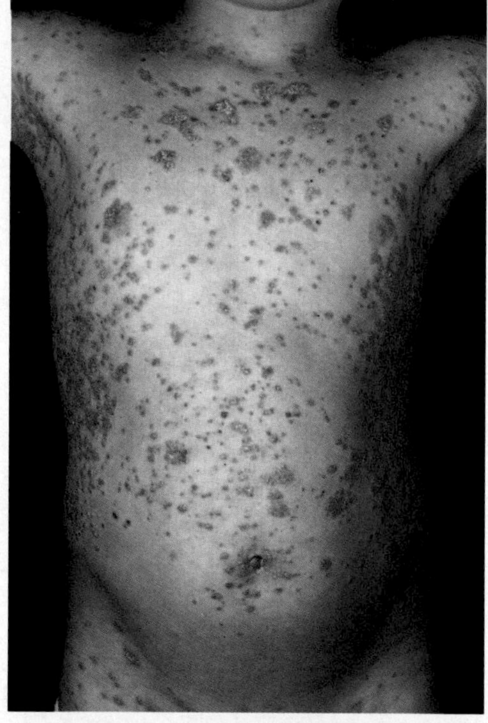

A.

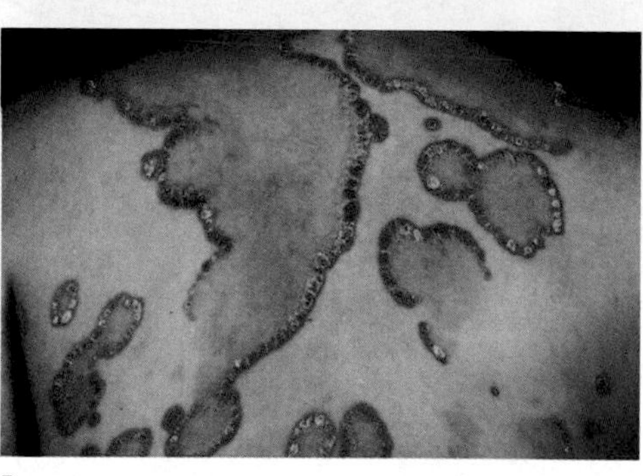

B.

A. Recent onset of eruptive guttate psoriasis showing highly erythematous macules and papules. *B.* Chronic stationary psoriasis presenting as annular lesions.

FIGURE 42-4

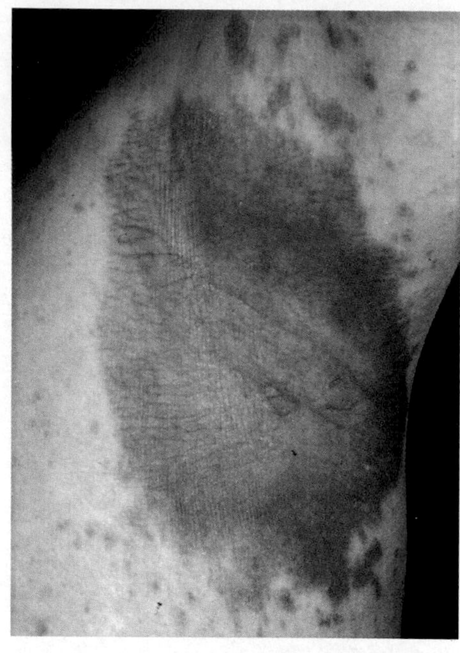

A.

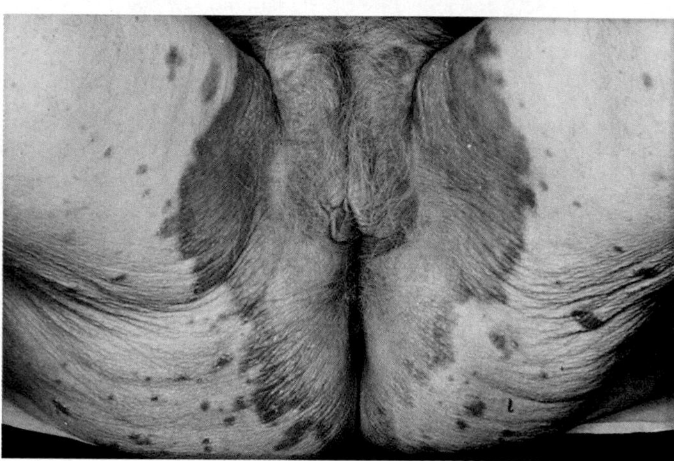

B.

Inverse psoriasis (*A, B*). The skin in the intertriginous areas is highly erythematous, and typical scaling is lacking.

the knees (see Fig. 42-1*B*), the scalp (see Fig. 42-1*C*) and, in particular, the retroauricular region, the lumbar area (Fig. 42-1*D*), and the umbilicus. Single small lesions may become confluent, forming plaques in which the borders resemble a land map (psoriasis geographica) (see Fig. 42-3*B*). Lesions may extend laterally and become circinate because of the confluence of several plaques (psoriasis gyrata). Occasionally there is partial central clearing, resulting in ringlike lesions (annular psoriasis) (see Fig. 42-3*B*).

Psoriasis lesions may be localized in the major skin folds, such as the axillae, the genitocrural region, and the neck (psoriasis inversa) (see Fig. 42-4*A*, *B*). Here, scaling is absent, and the lesions show a glossy, sharply demarcated erythema.

Eruptive (guttate) psoriasis Typically, this pattern (see Fig. 42-3*A*) presents as small (0.5–1.5 cm in diameter) lesions over the upper trunk and proximal extremities. This form is characteristic of psoriasis of an early age of onset and as such is found frequently in young adults. As noted below (see "Trigger Factors" below), streptococcal throat infection frequently precedes the onset or flare of guttate psoriasis. Occasionally, a disseminated macular drug eruption may precede this pattern of psoriasis.

Very active lesions of psoriasis of many types can have pustules that are 1 to 2 mm in diameter and are surrounded by an intensive wall of erythema. This process usually signals an acute exacerbation of disease. Predisposing factors for such an event are bacterial infection, aggressive local therapy, or withdrawal of systemic glucocorticoids (see "Trigger Factors" below).

Psoriatic erythroderma Psoriatic erythroderma (Fig. 42-10) represents the generalized form of the disease that affects all body sites, including the face, hands, feet, nails, trunk, and extremities. Although all the symptoms of psoriasis are present, erythema is the most prominent feature, and scaling usually is less severe compared with chronic stationary psoriasis. Psoriatic erythroderma may have different degrees of disease activity, presenting suddenly as a generalized erythema or evolving gradually from chronic plaque psoriasis into a generalized exfoliative phase. In the latter phase there are usually some areas of uninvolved skin.

Psoriatic erythroderma may be the response to nontolerated topical treatment (e.g., anthralin, ultraviolet B, or UVB), representing a generalized Koebner reaction. Generalized pustular psoriasis may revert to only erythroderma, pustule formation being diminished or absent. This form shows all the features of pustular psoriasis, including fever, malaise, frequent relapses, and relatively high mortality after prolonged courses. There may be complete loss of nail growth due to destruction of the nail matrix. Further descriptions of the effects of exfoliative erythroderma on the body are covered in Chap. 44 and under "Systemic Effects" below.

Generalized pustular psoriasis (von Zumbusch) Pustular psoriasis of the von Zumbusch type (Fig. 42-11) appears as a distinctive acute variant of psoriasis. It is unusual to see other forms of psoriasis on the skin at the same time. Attacks of pustular psoriasis are characterized by fever that lasts several days. A sudden generalized eruption of sterile pustules 2 to 3 mm in diameter parallels the onset of fever. The pustules are disseminated over the trunk and extremities, including the nail beds, palms, and soles. The pustules usually arise on highly erythematous skin, first as patches and then becoming confluent as the disease becomes more severe. In addition to the pustule formation of the nail matrix and loss of the entire nail, the fingertips may become atrophic in patients with prolonged disease. As with other forms of psoriasis, the face usually remains free of lesions. The erythema that surrounds the pustules often spreads and becomes confluent, leading to erythroderma. Characteristically, the disease occurs in waves of fever and pustules. This syndrome is further described below (see "Systemic Effects").

FIGURE 42-5

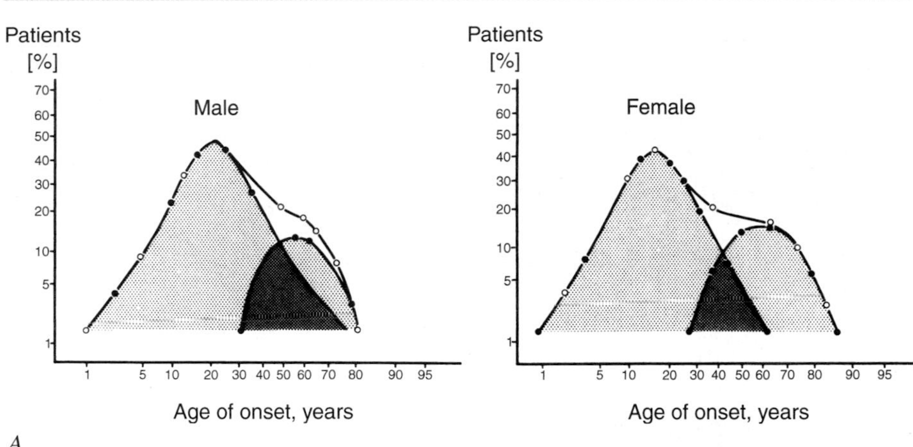

A.

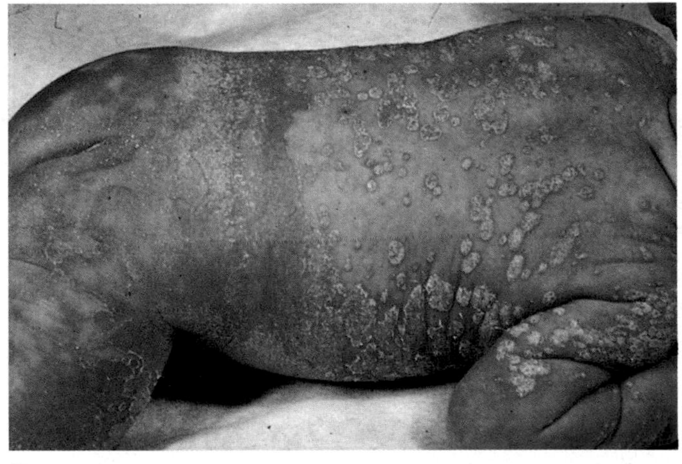

B.

A. Age of patients at the first onset of psoriasis. A total of 2147 patients suffering from various types of psoriasis were examined and the age of onset was recorded. Most patients of both sexes had an early onset [age 16 (F) and 22 (M)], while nearly one-quarter had a late onset (age 56). See original publication for details. (*From Henseler and Christophers,*[1] *with permission.*) *B.* Psoriasis presenting in early infancy.

Annular pustular psoriasis A rare variant of pustular psoriasis is an annular, or circinate, form of the disease (see Fig. 42-11*C*) occurring during episodes of pustular eruptions. Lesions may appear at the onset of pustular psoriasis, with a tendency to spread and form enlarged rings, or they may develop during the course of generalized pustular psoriasis. The main features are pustules on a ringlike erythema that sometimes resembles erythema annulare centrifugum. Histologically, there is mild acanthosis and a neutrophil accumulation with formation of microabscesses.

Identical lesions are found in patients with impetigo herpetiformis, a pustular form of psoriasis associated with pregnancy (see Chap. 142).

Localized pustular psoriasis Localized pustular psoriasis presents as two distinct conditions that must be considered separate from the generalized disease. Systemic symptoms are absent. The two distinct varieties are pustulosis palmaris et plantaris and acrodermatitis continua. They are discussed in Chap. 70.

Quality of Life

Psoriasis represents a lifelong burden for affected patients. A comparative study reported reduction in physical functioning and mental functioning comparable with that seen in cancer, arthritis, hypertension, heart disease, diabetes, and depression.[13] According to a recent survey of the National Psoriasis Foundation, 79 percent of patients with severe psoriasis reported a negative impact on their lives. In terms of treatment, 40 percent felt frustrated with the ineffectiveness of their current therapies.[14] Among the chief complaints of patients with psoriasis are the lowered self-esteem and feelings of being socially outcast. The presence of pruritus and pain can aggravate these symptoms. The increased incidence of arthritis in patients with psoriasis makes arthralgia a frequent complaint (see Chap. 43).

Natural History

Most studies indicate that once psoriasis appears as an early localized disease, it persists throughout life, manifesting at unpredictable intervals.[1] Spontaneous remissions do occur with varying frequencies. In two separate studies involving about 200 patients per study, remission ranged from 17 to 55 percent. In another study of 2800 patients, 29 percent reported a remission. The duration of these remissions ranges from 1 to 54 years. Data relative to permanent remissions, either spontaneous or induced, appear to be unavailable.

FIGURE 42-6

A.

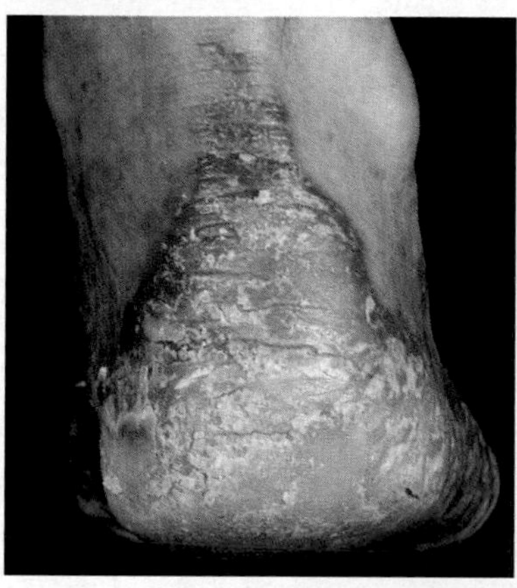

C.

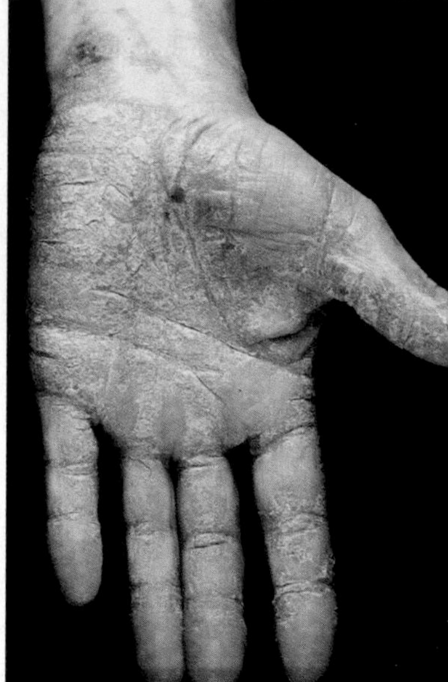

B.

Psoriasis vulgaris of the scalp extending onto the neck (*A*). Psoriatic lesions on palm (*B*) and heel (*C*) skin.

Trigger Factors

External factors may provoke manifestations of psoriatic skin lesions; they may be called *trigger factors.*

Natural incidence studies suggest that environment plays a predisposing role. Hot weather and sunlight are reported to be beneficial, whereas cold weather appears to have an opposite effect. The increased prevalence of psoriasis in the Nordic population of the Faeroe Islands supports this notion.

PHYSICAL TRAUMA: THE KOEBNER PHENOMENON In 1872, Koebner described a patient who, 5 years after developing psoriasis, noted that various traumatic insults to his skin resulted in lesions of psoriasis. Specifically, psoriasis occurred in the precise spots where his horse had bitten him. Shortly thereafter his psoriasis generalized. Koebner hypothesized that there were intervals in the course of psoriasis when skin injury results in disease (Fig. 42-12).

The original description by Koebner suggests that the incidence of the Koebner phenomenon in psoriatic subjects is increased when the disease is active. Patients with the Koebner reaction appear more likely to have developed psoriasis at an early age and to require multiple therapies to control their disease.

INFECTIONS Infections have long been recognized as a trigger for the onset or exacerbation of psoriasis. The frequency with which infections trigger psoriasis varies from a low of 15 percent in a retrospective analysis of clinic charts of 255 patients to a high of 76 percent in mailed questionnaires to over 500 patients. Up to 54 percent of children are reported to exacerbate existing psoriasis during the 2- to 3-week interval after an upper respiratory infection.[5]

Acute guttate psoriasis frequently follows an acute streptococcal infection by 1 to 2 weeks. Among patients with acute guttate psoriasis, 56 to 85 percent have immediately preceding evidence of streptococcal disease. Strep infections may play a role in exacerbating other forms of psoriasis. *Streptococcus pyogenes* (beta-hemolytic streptococci, group A) was isolated in 26 percent of patients with acute guttate psoriasis, 14 percent of patients with guttate flare of plaque psoriasis, and 16 percent of patients with chronic psoriasis.[15] *S. pyogenes* was isolated in 7 percent of the control population. The serotypes did not differ significantly from those of the community. Thus, while streptococcal pharyngitis appears to be a trigger factor, it is not type-specific.[15]

Infection with the human immunodeficiency virus type 1 (HIV-1) may represent another important trigger factor, although the incidence varies considerably.[16] Patients may present with two distinct clinical patterns. One is localized, showing either guttate or large plaques. The other is a more diffuse psoriasiform dermatitis, often associated with palmoplantar keratoderma. The psoriasiform dermatitis may be the first clinical manifestation of HIV infection. Rapid onset of acute eruptive psoriasis, as well as exacerbations in patients with previous chronic stable plaque psoriasis, suggests the possibility of underlying HIV disease.

STRESS Clinical studies support patients' perceptions that psoriasis is made worse by stress in approximately 30 to 40 percent of cases. No personality disorders or traits unique to patients with psoriasis have been found. It is commonly believed that alcohol has an adverse effect on psoriasis, but this impression has not been confirmed. This belief appears to be based on observations of alcoholics who have psoriasis, begin to drink excessive amounts of alcohol, and subsequently have a flare of disease.

ANATOMIC SITES Certain anatomic sites are prone to develop disease and as such can be considered within the realm of trigger factors. In chronic stationary psoriasis, the scalp is involved most frequently, followed by the knees and elbows. Reasons for this pattern are unknown.

DRUGS Beta-adrenergic blockers can exacerbate psoriasis or trigger the development of first lesions. The reported exacerbations of psoriasis associated with antimalarials may have been overemphasized in the past. Lithium is a strong inducer of psoriasis lesions. Certain angiotensin-converting enzyme inhibitors also have been reported as exacerbating drugs in psoriasis.[17]

Systemic Associations

ARTHRITIS AND INFLAMMATORY BOWEL DISEASE The association of arthritis and psoriasis is discussed in Chap. 43. Therapy

FIGURE 42-7

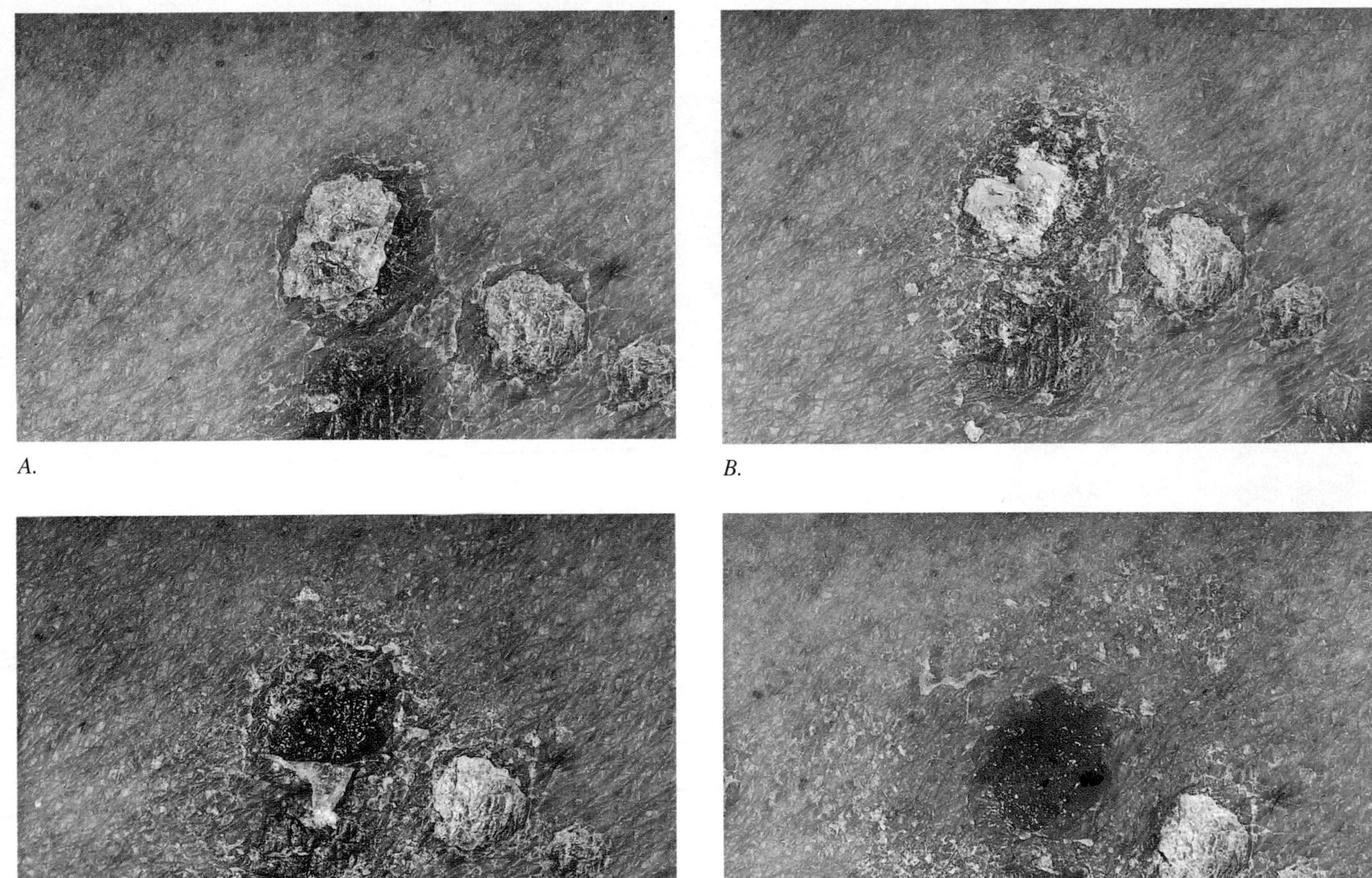

The Auspitz phenomenon in its three phases: *A.* Native psoriatic lesion. *B.* Scratching generates silvery-opaque scale. *C.* Further scratching leads to removal of the scale, and a glossy area is visible. *D.* Further scratching produces blood droplets.

of psoriasis with ultraviolet light leads to improvement in the arthritis. Linkage beyond this (i.e., both diseases being mediated by similar inflammatory processes) remains speculative.

The strong linkage of HLA-B27 to ankylosing spondylitis and ulcerative colitis and the increased frequency of this haplotype in patients with psoriasis and arthritis (about six times normal) suggest that ulcerative colitis should be seen more frequently in patients with psoriasis. Recent studies tend to confirm this impression. The frequency of psoriasis among patients with ulcerative colitis and Crohn's disease is, respectively, 3.8 and 1.6 times normal.[18]

Immunopathology

GENETIC STUDIES Studies conducted in various countries revealed psoriasis as a multifactorial disorder where multiple genes are involved. These are likely to interact with each other as well as with environmental trigger factors. Susceptibility loci located on various chromosomes (see Table 42-3) have been found.[19]

Linkage disequilibrium studies have shown strong association with a gene or genes within the major histocompatibility complex (MHC) within a 12-cM region on chromosome 6p21.3.[20]

In fact, there is a strong association of early-onset psoriasis with class I and II HLA markers—including B13, Bw57, Cw6, and DR7—in contrast to psoriasis of late onset, in which A2 as well as B27 were moderately increased.[4,21] The strongest association was seen in type I psoriasis, with Cw6 being present in over 80 percent of cases.

Extended haplotypes for type I psoriasis were observed by oligonucleotide typing. In addition to Cw6, these consist of DRB1*0701/2, DQA1*0201, and DQB1*0303.[22] Comparison of all HLA loci revealed Cw6 being in linkage disequilibrium with DQB1*0303 as the most powerful disease marker.

The association with HLA-Cw6 is noted worldwide, but only 10 percent of HLA-Cw6+ individuals develop psoriasis. This is likely to be due to the presence of more than one gene necessary to produce disease in addition to the effect of environmental factors.

Whereas HLA-C can be excluded as an psoriasis-causing allele, a gene likely to be responsible for 30 to 50 percent of psoriatic disease expression[20,23] appears to reside within a 300-kb interval centered around the centromeric end of class I MHC beyond HLA-C and toward HLA-A.[19,20] Candidate genes in this region are *corneodesmosin* and *HCR* as well as novel yet unidentified genes in this region.

Patients with early-onset psoriasis (type I) are more likely to carry the *PSORS I* gene. Poststreptococcal guttate psoriasis generally is HLA-Cw6+, indicating that the *PSORS I* gene plays a major role in psoriasis developing at young age.

In addition, HLA-Cw6 is often seen in patients with psoriatic arthritis, and this is more often present as compared with HLA-B27, indicating that HLA-B27 is not the major determinant for psoriatic arthritis.

FIGURE 42-8

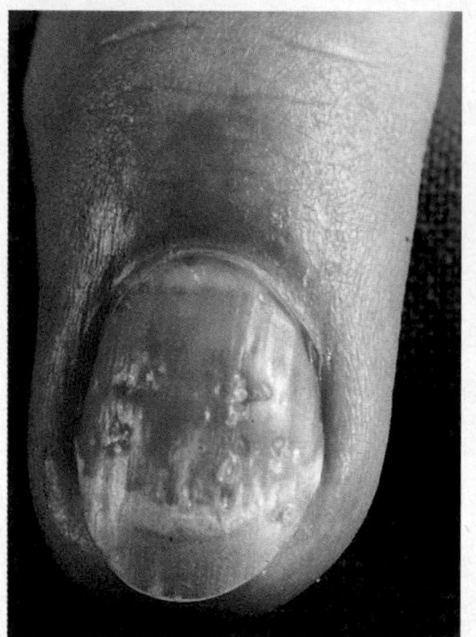

A.

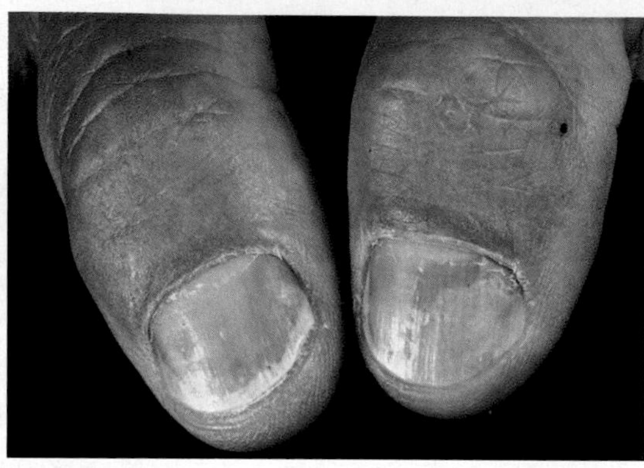

B.

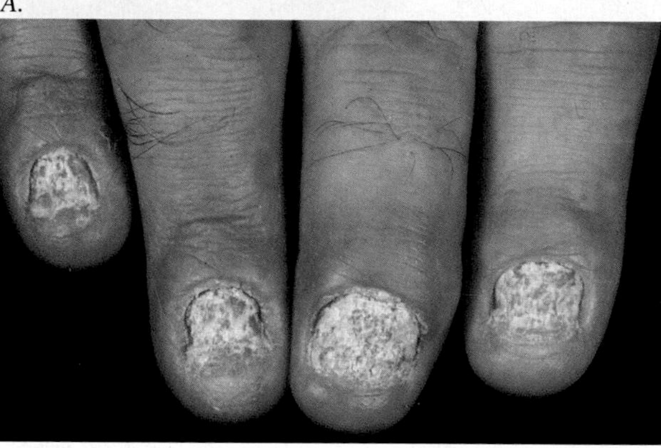

C.

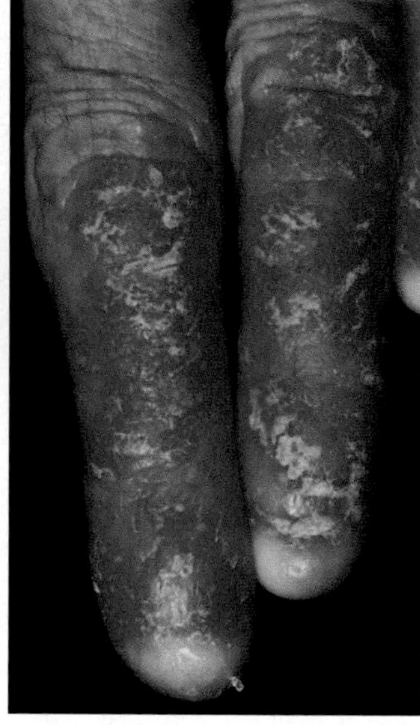

D.

Nail psoriasis shows various features depending on the location of the psoriatic process: *A.* Nail pits. *B.* Characteristic yellowish or brown color known as an *oil spot.* *C.* Involvement of nearly the entire nail bed with onychodystrophy. *D.* Involvement of nearly the entire nail bed followed by loss of nails.

TABLE 42-2

Clinical Classification of Psoriasis

NONPUSTULAR	PUSTULAR
	Pustular psoriasis of von Zumbusch
Psoriasis vulgaris, early and late onset	
Psoriatic erythroderma	Pustulosis palmaris et plantaris
	Pustular psoriasis, annular type
	Acrodermatitis continua
	Impetigo herpetiformis

Evidence for linkage of patients with psoriatic joint disease with a chromosome 17q locus has been presented. This locus is also seen in familial rheumatoid arthritis. Genetic studies on Crohn's disease have found linkage to a candidate locus on chromosome 16. Since the risk for psoriasis is 7 times higher in patients with Crohn's disease, this disease association could indicate a genetic background.

Taking these genetic findings together shows that aside from *PSORS I* in HLA, various non-MHC genes are likely to play a role in modulating disease expression.

Concomitant Diseases

Epidemiologic data reveal a distinct number of diseases associated with psoriasis more often than expected from surveys in nonpsoriatic control individuals. These include (1) arthritis (10–15 times more common), (2) Crohn's disease (4 times more common), and (3) cardiovascular disease, hyperpertension, and diabetes (1.5 times more common). On the other hand, atopy, atopic dermatitis, and urticaria are noted infrequently in psoriasis patients. In addition, the relative paucity of cutaneous infections adds to the distinct pattern of associated disorders in psoriasis.[24]

The frequency of concurrent diseases in patients with psoriasis was reexamined recently in a controlled inpatient study.[24] As a result, a distinct group of systemic disorders—including hypertension, heart failure, obesity, and diabetes, in addition to chronic oropharyngeal infections—was found to be significantly more frequent in psoriasis patients as compared with age-matched control patients suffering from nonpsoriatic skin disorders. In contrast, bacterial and several viral skin infections were reduced significantly.

SYSTEMIC EFFECTS OF PSORIASIS

Beyond the foregoing systemic effects are those associated with pustular psoriasis and exfoliative erythroderma. The physical and laboratory findings associated with exfoliative erythroderma are considerable and are described in greater detail in Chap. 44.

Generalized pustular psoriasis, as described by von Zumbusch, is the form associated with systemic findings. This form of psoriasis appears as waves of sterile pustules on an erythematous skin. Characteristically, short episodes of fever (39–40°C) are followed by another wave of new pustules. In addition to the fever, there are systemic signs of disease, such as weight loss, muscle weakness, leukocytosis, hypocalcemia, and an increased sedimentation rate. These systemic complications may be fatal, usually as a result of the protean manifestations of severe systemic disease, congestive heart failure, and intercurrent infections. The skin symptoms may resolve spontaneously, leading to full recovery.

The cause of this dramatic illness is obscure; however, a number of provoking agents or events are well recognized. They range from local irritating substances, as in von Zumbusch's original case, to pregnancy,

FIGURE 42-9

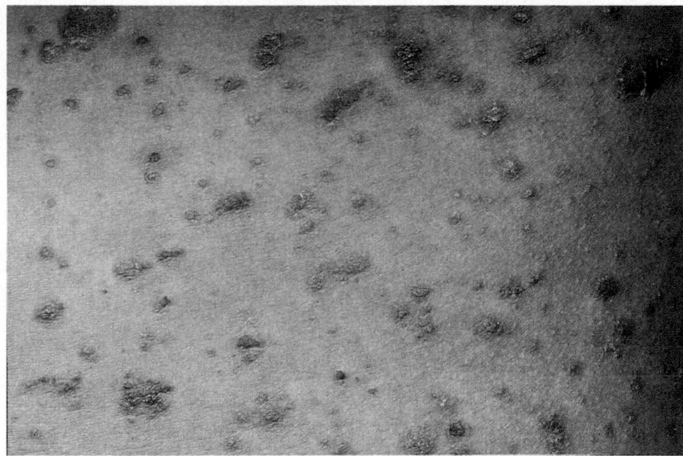

Guttate (eruptive) psoriasis with highly erythematous lesions. These can become confluent within weeks after their first appearance.

oral contraceptives, lithium, infections, hypocalcemia secondary to hypoalbuminemia, and withdrawal from glucocorticoids. In patients with pustular psoriasis, arthropathy is common, as is the HLA-B27 haplotype. The disease is uncommon but well documented in children.

ASSOCIATION WITH MALIGNANCY Studies of approximately 500 patients suggest that patients with psoriasis have a normal risk of systemic cancer and possibly an increased risk of cutaneous cancer.[25] These analyses do not include the risk of developing skin carcinomas in patients undergoing treatments with psoralen plus ultraviolet A (PUVA)[26] (see "Photochemotherapy," below).

PSORIASIS AND OTHER SKIN DISEASES A number of skin diseases are reported to occur concomitantly in patients with psoriasis, and psoriasis may develop in association with preexisting skin diseases. In a study involving more than 2000 patients with atopic dermatitis and 800 with psoriasis, the observed incidence of patients having both diseases was much lower than calculated by their incidence rates.[27] It is suggested that both diseases are mutually exclusive, representing two contrasting types of cutaneous immunopathology.

LABORATORY ABNORMALITIES

Laboratory abnormalities in psoriasis are usually not specific and may not be found in all patients with the exception of those with generalized pustular psoriasis and psoriatic erythroderma (Table 42-4).

Serum uric acid is elevated in up to 50 percent of patients and is mainly correlated with the extent of lesions and the activity of disease. There is an increased risk of developing gouty arthritis. Elevated serum uric acid levels usually cease after therapy.

In severe psoriasis vulgaris, generalized pustular psoriasis, and erythroderma, a negative nitrogen balance can be detected, mainly consisting in a decrease of serum albumin.

C-reactive protein, α_2-macroglobulin, as well as sedimentation rate, can be increased in psoriasis related to disease activity and body involvement. Increased serum IgA levels and IgA immune complexes have been observed in psoriasis, the role of this phenomenon still being unclear.

Bacteriology of Psoriatic Plaques

There are no qualitative differences in the cutaneous bacterial flora when plaques are compared with adjacent normal skin. However, the number of bacteria per unit area is increased by more than two times.[28] This increase can be a problem if the patient with psoriasis is colonized with *Staphylococcus aureus.*

PATHOLOGY

Microscopic changes are present in both the epidermis and the upper dermis of lesions of psoriasis. It is difficult to judge which is more severe and more relevant to the disease. In pustular and guttate psoriasis, the inflammatory features are more prominent than in plaque-type psoriasis.

Chronic (Plaque-Type) Psoriasis

The essential histopathologic features of plaque-type psoriasis (Fig. 42-13) include

1. An epidermis in which epidermal mass is increased three to five times. Whereas the granular layer is constantly absent over the tips of the dermal papillae and parakeratosis is an accompanying feature, a thick granular layer may be seen between the rete ridges, and above these areas keratinization may be normal. Relative to normal, there are many more mitoses in the psoriatic epidermis, with mitotic figures frequently seen above the basal layer (see "Pathogenesis," below).
2. A dermis in which thin, elongated papillae are prominent. These papillae contain dilated, tortuous capillaries embedded in an edematous papillary stroma.
3. A moderate inflammatory infiltrate around the blood vessels consisting of lymphocytes, macrophages, neutrophils, and increased numbers of mast cells. This infiltrate is confined to the papillary dermis.
4. Collections of polymorphonuclear leukocytes, which sometimes extend from the tip of the dermal papillae into the epidermis, where they are associated with focal spongiosis and occasionally cell necrosis. These skin changes result in Munro microabscesses, which are formed from invading leukocytes. In chronic plaque-type psoriasis, the number of neutrophils is sparse compared with that in guttate psoriasis, in which they are more numerous.[28]

Eruptive (Guttate) Psoriasis

Eruptive (guttate) psoriasis, especially when only a few days old, may differ from plaque-type psoriasis in the following features:

1. Epidermal hyperplasia is less marked, and the rete ridges are usually only slightly longer than normal. There may be areas of spongiosis located above the tips of the dermal papillae. There is focal absence of the granular layer.
2. Serum is discharged from the tips of the papillae into the epidermis, and neutrophils accumulate. These cells migrate through the basement membrane individually and sometimes aggregate subcorneally in the suprapapillary areas, forming subcorneal pustules (Fig. 42-14). There may be extravasated erythrocytes in the suprapapillary areas.

FIGURE 42-10

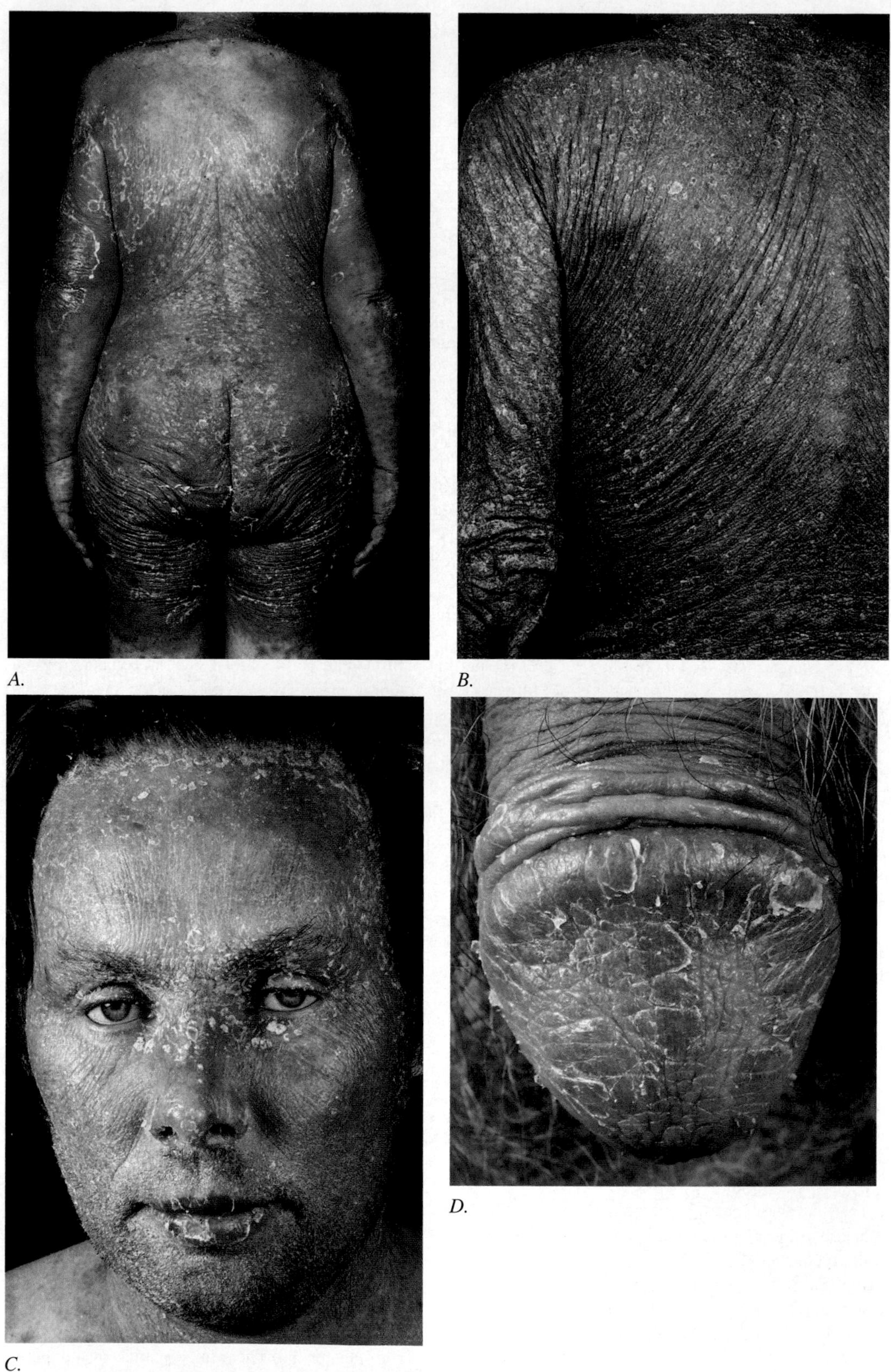

Psoriatic erythroderma. There is generalized erythema and various degrees of scaling in the severe form of psoriasis (*A, B*). The lips (*C*) and the glans penis (*D*) are involved.

FIGURE 42-11

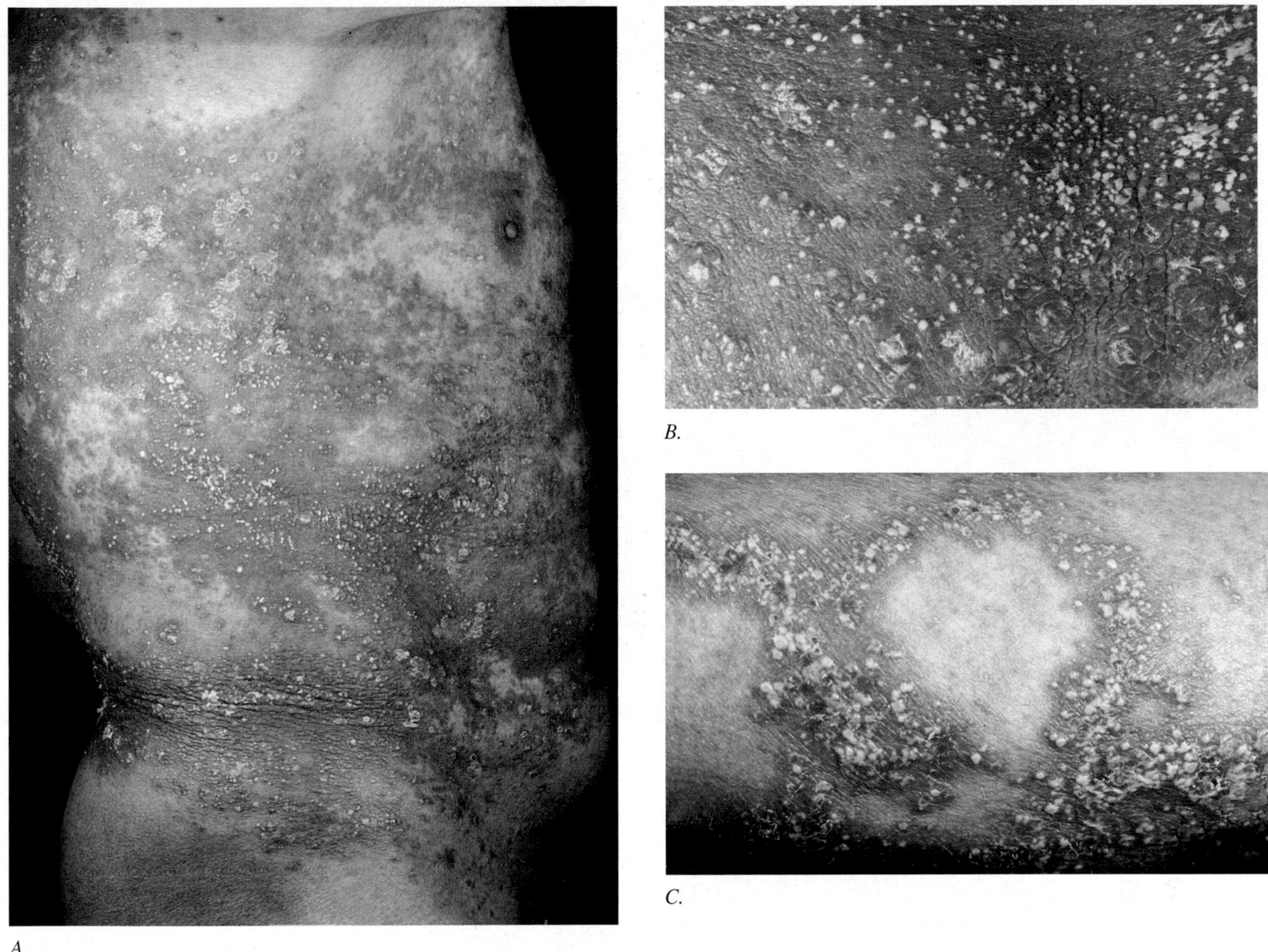

Pustular psoriasis. There are tiny pustules, 1 to 2 mm in diameter, on a highly erythematous slightly indurated skin surface (*A, B*). These pustules may acquire annular shapes (*C*).

The Initial Lesion

Few attempts have been made to examine the earliest skin changes histologically. When pinhead-sized (macular) lesions were examined as the earliest clinical sign of psoriasis, marked edema and round cell infiltrate in the upper dermis were found. These findings are usually confined to the area of one or two papillae. The overlying epidermis soon becomes spongiotic and shows focal loss of the granular layer (see Fig. 42-14). The venules in the upper dermis dilate, and these structures are surrounded by a mononuclear cell infiltrate.

Ultrastructural attempts to analyze the initial tissue changes sequentially revealed mast cell degranulation as well as endothelial activation, followed by macrophage immigration before epidermal changes.

DIAGNOSIS AND DIFFERENTIAL DIAGNOSIS

In patients with typical psoriatic lesions, the features are usually characteristic enough to establish the diagnosis. Difficulties arise when psoriasis is changing its disease activity—i.e., when eruptive, pustular, or erythematous phases are evolving—or when psoriasis is complicated by other diseases. Diagnoses to be considered in the differential diagnosis of psoriasis include eczema, pityriasis rubra pilaris, seborrheic dermatitis, pityriasis lichenoides et varioliformis, candidiasis, tinea, syphilis, cutaneous T cell lymphoma (mycosis fungoides), in situ squamous cell carcinoma (Bowen's disease), and Paget's disease. Thus the morphologic appearance and distribution of a given patient's psoriasis are significant factors in the differential diagnosis, which is further delineated in Table 42-5. In any case, the Auspitz phenomenon provides a diagnostic lead in making the proper diagnosis (see Fig. 42-7).

PATHOGENESIS

Background

Psoriasis is unique because it represents excessive but controlled cellular proliferation and inflammation, both occurring within 0.2 mm of the skin's surface. There is no experimental model, and the pathogenesis is not fully understood.

FIGURE 42-12

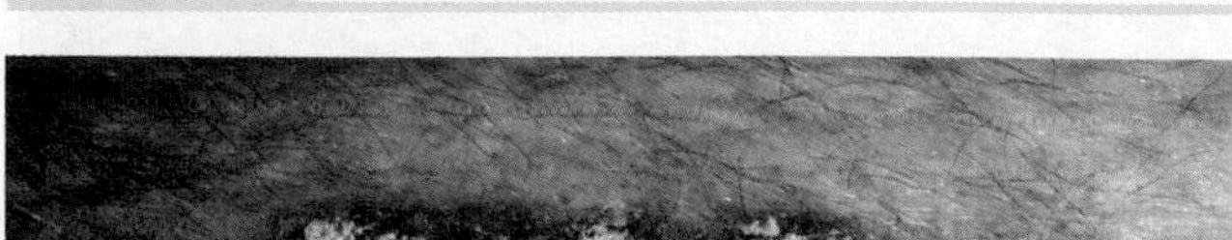

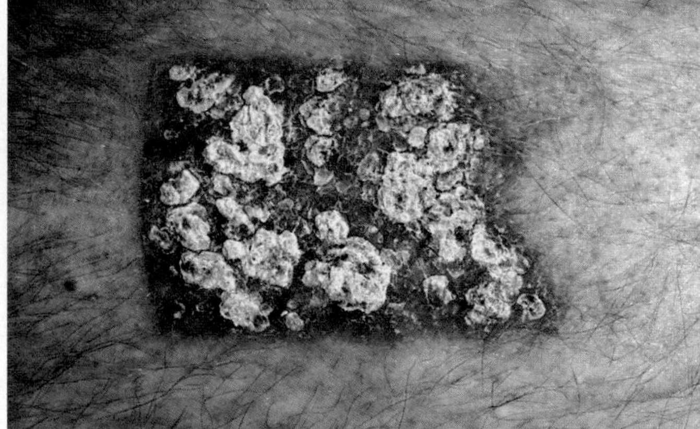

A.

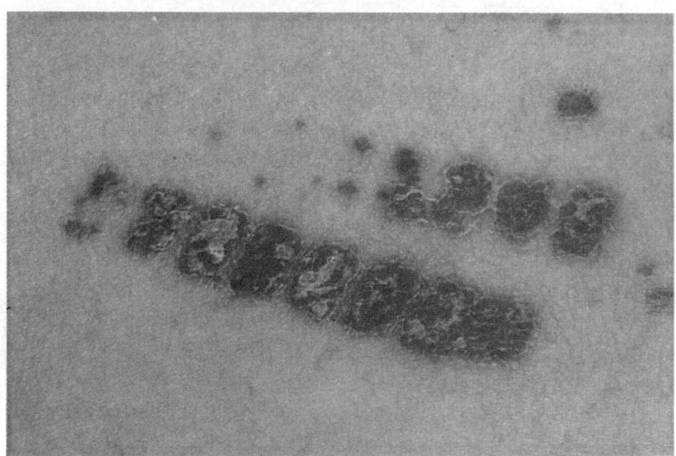

B.

Koebner's phenomenon. As shown (*A*) by the appearance of typical erythematosquamous lesions within a scar or (*B*) after various doses of UVB.

The role of immune mechanisms is documented by a significant number of activated T cells within the altered epidermis and dermis, by macrophages, and by the proven effects of immunosuppressive or immunomodulating therapy. Second, the predominant changes consist of highly increased, persistent keratinocyte proliferation in conjunction with a characteristic inflammatory pattern.

Further, the genetic character represents a hallmark of psoriasis; the inheritance is polygenic with a genetic risk ratio of nearly 10 for first-degree relatives of patients with early-onset psoriasis.[19] It appears that several factors are involved in the pathogenesis of the disease (Fig. 42-15).

KERATINOCYTE PROLIFERATIVE ACTIVITY A characteristic feature of involved skin of psoriatic subjects is hyperproliferation, first defined by Van Scott and Ekel.[29] Currently, there is evidence of more than an eightfold shortening of the epidermal cell cycle (36 h versus 311 h for normal) in involved skin of patients with psoriasis. Further, there is a twofold increase in the proliferative cell population, and 100 percent of the germinative cells of the epidermis appear to enter the growth fraction compared with 60 to 70 percent for normal subjects. These alterations result in a hyperplastic epidermis generating 35,000 cells/mm^2 per day from a proliferative compartment containing approximately 52,000 cells/mm^2 of skin surface. Normal skin produces only 1218 cells/mm^2 per day from a proliferative compartment of 26,000 cells/mm^2.[29] Although there are still no similarly sophisticated studies of uninvolved skin, various investigators have noted significantly altered epidermal proliferation (nearly twice normal) in normal-appearing skin. Additionally, the regeneration response following tape stripping has been noted to be increased in the normal skin of patients with psoriasis.

TABLE 42-3

Genetic Susceptibility Loci in Psoriasis

Locus	Position	Candidate Genes
PSORS1	6p21.3	Corneodesmosin, HCR
PSORS2	17q25	
PSORS3	4q	
PSORS4	1q21	Epidermal differentiation Complex gene cluster
PSORS5	3q	SLC12A8
PSORS6	19p	
PSORS7	1p	

NOTE: HCR, alpha-helix coiled-coil rod homolog gene; SLC12A8, solute carrier family 12 protein A8.

Transplantation studies of human skin to congenitally athymic (nude) mice provide additional insights. These studies demonstrate that epidermal proliferation (as measured by labeling indices) of both uninvolved and involved skin from patients with psoriasis approaches a common mean and that both remain elevated above that of normal skin. In these experiments in which epidermal proliferation of involved and uninvolved skin is elevated, there is no evidence of clinical lesions, i.e., erythema, scale, or induration. Thus excessive epidermal proliferation does not in itself give rise to a lesion of psoriasis.

Immunopathology

IMMUNE SYSTEM As outlined earlier, there are several hints of participation of the immune system in the etiology and pathogenesis of psoriasis. Among the most important are (1) the presence of numerous activated T cells within psoriatic lesions, (2) the antipsoriatic effects of treatment modalities that can reduce cutaneous T cell activation and infiltration, (3) immune-dependent expressions of adhesion molecules on psoriatic keratinocytes, (4) the relative absence of T_H2-related skin disorders, including atopic dermatitis and urticaria,[24] and (5) lymphokine profiles suggesting a T_H1-driven disorder.[30,31]

T Cells Cells prevailing within the psoriatic lesion consist of activated T cells, macrophages, and polymorphonuclear cells. In an early lesion, macrophages are noted within the epidermis, followed by lymphocytes and neutrophils. CD4+ T cells migrate into skin with aggravation of disease as new lesions develop. The majority of CD4+ T cells localize within the affected dermis, whereas those migrating into the epidermis are noted to predominantly consist of the CD8 "killer" phenotype. These T cells appear to be activated, expressing high

TABLE 42-4

Common Laboratory Abnormalities in Psoriasis

Elevated uric acid
Mild anemia
Negative nitrogen balance
Increased α_2-macroglobulin
Immunoglobulin aberrations, increased IgA levels, and increased quantities of immune complexes

FIGURE 42-13

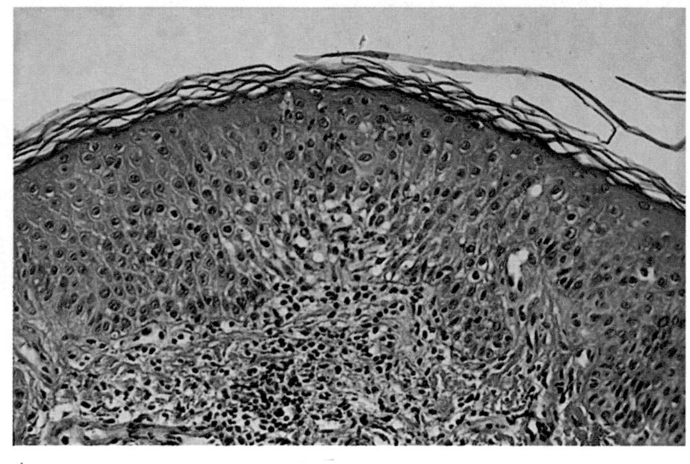

A.

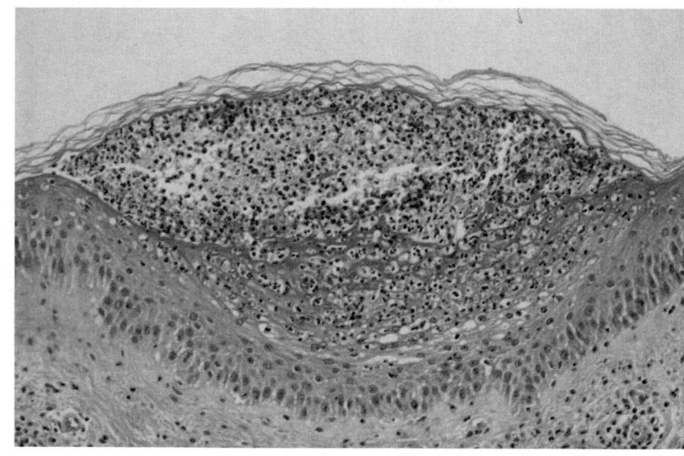

B.

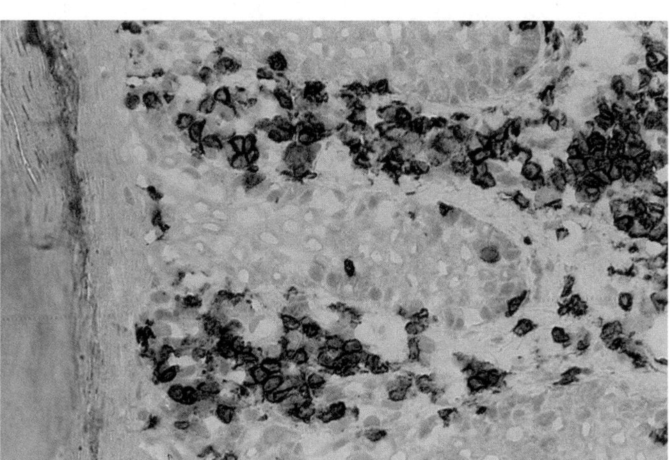

C.

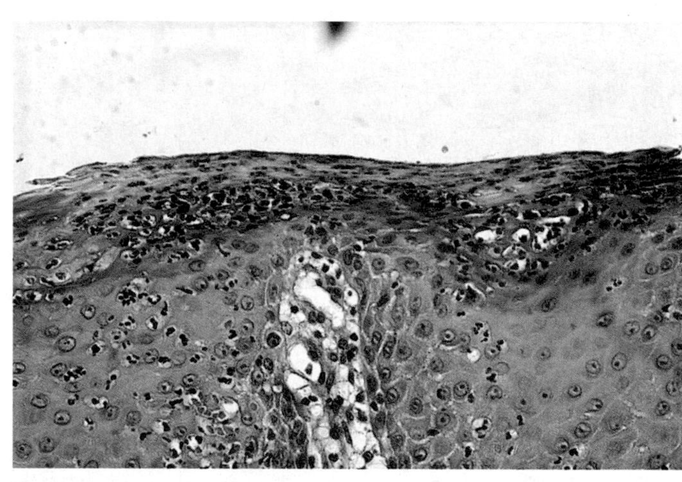

D.

Histopathology of psoriasis. *A.* The earliest changes in psoriasis consist of papillary edema with a marked infiltrate of mononuclear cells, which tend to invade the spongiotic epidermis. Later, neutrophils follow. *B.* Pustular psoriasis with large spongiform abscesses in the subcorneal zone without marked epidermal hyperplasia. *C.* Neutrophils migrating into the stratum corneum form so-called Munro's microabscesses. *D.* In plaque-type psoriasis, large numbers of CD3+ T cells are present and tend to migrate into the affected epidermal portions.

levels of MHC class II molecules as well as CD25 interleukin 2 (IL-2) receptor.[32]

Analysis of the T cell receptor repertoire revealed oligoclonal expansion of T cells derived from lesional psoriatic skin. CD4+ T cells showed significant overrepresentation of Vβ2, Vβ5.1, and Vβ6 T cell receptors as compared with T cells of peripheral blood or normal skin.[33,34] In a longitudinal study it could be demonstrated that the T cell receptor repertoire in lesional skin remains constant during several exacerbations of psoriasis in the same patients.[34] Constant oligoclonal expression of Vβ3 and Vβ13.1 T cell receptors also was found for lesional CD8+ T cells.[35] From these studies, the presence of an antigen responsible for constant oligoclonal T cell expansion may be hypothesized. However, results from other studies reveal that superantigens may not be pathogenetically relevant in chronic plaque-type psoriasis.[36]

T cell migration into psoriatic skin is mediated by receptors on dermal endothelial cells or papillary endothelial cells. In addition, CD4+ CD45 RO+ (memory) T cells selectively bind to papillary endothelial cells, whereas CD8+ T cells localize on high endothelial venules. T cell migration into the skin is stimulated by lipid mediators such as 12[*R*]-hydroxyeicosatetraenoic acid, peptide chemoattractants such as IL-8, MIP-1α and -1β, MCP-1, MCP-2, MCP-3 as well as IP10, and as yet uncharacterized peptides.

Extravasation of T cells, monocytes, and neutrophils follows their adhesion to endothelial cells mediated by adhesion molecules. Within the psoriatic lesion, endothelial cells show increased expression of the intercellular adhesion molecule 1 (ICAM-1) and E-selectin. A subset of T cells expressing cutaneous lymphocyte antigen (CLA) consists of memory T cells preferentially homing to skin. These cells bind to E-selectin, and their number is greatly increased in psoriasis.[37]

Therapies suppressing the immune system are effective in psoriasis Support for the assumption that T cells are fundamentally important in psoriasis comes from therapies known to affect the immune system, experimentally shown by improvement of severe disease following intravenous application of anti-CD3, anti-CD4, and anti-TNF-α monoclonal antibodies. Complete clearing of skin lesions is also obtained by cyclosporine, used as low-dose treatment in severe psoriasis, and by tacrolimus as well as a T cell–selective immunotoxin, DAB_{389}IL-2 or fusion proteins such as alefacept. These drugs are able to selectively suppress T cell–mediated immune responses. In addition, PUVA and UVB are able to deplete affected skin of immune-competent cells, notably T cells, when applied in appropriate doses.[38,39] Furthermore, cure of disease was reported in a patient receiving allogeneic bone marrow transplantation,[40] whereas development of psoriasis was observed in a bone marrow recipient from a psoriatic donor.[41] These

FIGURE 42-14

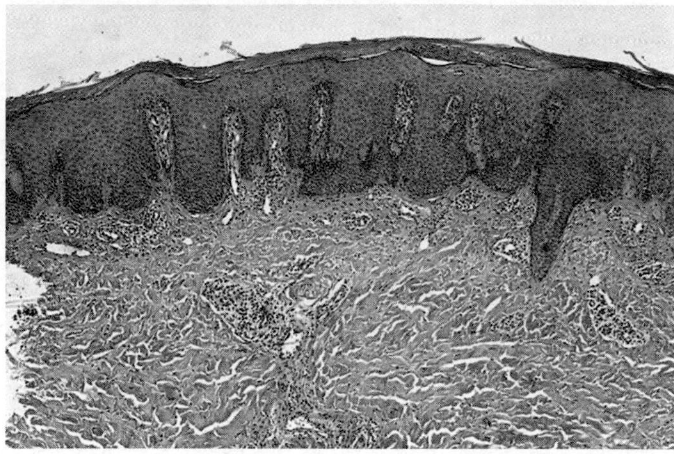

A.

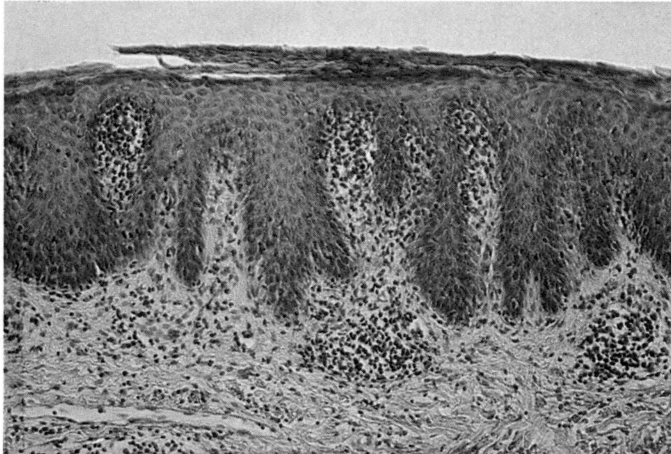

B.

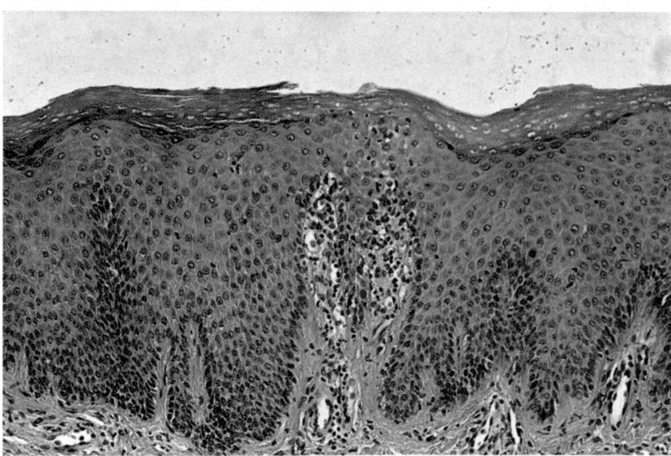

C.

The histology of psoriasis varies depending on the activity of the disease. There is acanthosis and parakeratosis and a lymphohistiocytic infiltrate in the papillary dermis (*A*), which becomes more pronounced (*B*) as the disease activity increases. *C.* Single dermal papillae repeatedly become edematous and infiltrated with neutrophils

TABLE 42-5

Differential Diagnosis of Psoriasis

Type of Psoriasis	Differential Diagnosis
Chronic plaque type	Nummular eczema Mycosis fungoides, plaque stage Tinea corporis
Guttate	Pityriasis rosea Pityriasis lichenoides et varioliformis Syphilis, psoriasiform type Tinea corporis
Erythroderma	Atopic dermatitis Sézary syndrome Drug eruption Generalized contact dermatitis
Intertriginous psoriasis	Candidiasis Contact dermatitis Darier's disease
Nail psoriasis	Tinea unguium Dyskeratosis secondary to injury (trauma, dermatitis, etc.)
Scalp and face	Seborrheic dermatitis
Genitalia	In situ squamous cell carcinoma

observations indicate that depletion of activated T cells from diseased skin correlates with clinical improvement.

GRANULOCYTES Formation of spongiform microabscesses (Munro microabscesses) filled with granulocytes is a hallmark of psoriasis. The presence of these cells in psoriatic lesions is variable and becomes more pronounced with disease activity, e.g., in acute guttate or pustular psoriasis. Ultramicroscopically, degranulation is absent in these cells; instead, they appear to remain intact while migrating in response to chemotactic stimuli. A number of studies recently conducted with isolated peripheral neutrophils revealed signs of activation mostly correlating with disease activity. Expression of ICAM-1 and E-selectin is found on endothelial cells, and both are important for the adhesion of neutrophils, T cell subsets, and monocytes. They are upregulated by IL-1, TNF-α, or lipopolysaccharides. Interestingly, E-selectin is known to be preferentially expressed at sites of chronic inflammation of the skin. It binds skin-homing memory T cells bearing a cutaneous lymphocyte antigen (CLA) as a unique antigen on T cell subsets, which are greatly augmented in psoriasis.[42]

Several cytokines were identified in tissue extracts of patients with psoriasis (Table 42-6). Cytokines isolated and characterized from lesional psoriatic skin include IL-1α and IL-1β, IL-6, and IL-8.[43] An additional set of cytokines is expressed by keratinocytes in culture; their significance is still not well understood.

PROTEASES Another potential mediator system under consideration is the protease-antiprotease system. The demonstration of increased protease activity in lesions of psoriasis has implicated this system as a potential mediator of many of the abnormal findings in psoriasis. Proteases are recognized in other cell systems as important regulators of cell proliferation, and they have the ability to generate inflammatory mediators via the complement cascade.[44] Further, cell surface proteases can be activated or inactivated at a local level, a phenomenon that fits with clinical observations. Without local activation and inactivation, it seems likely that all skin would express disease. The observation that plasminogen activator activity increases in uninvolved skin after transplantation to the nude mouse supports the contention that this is a mediator system.[45]

Another protease, human leukocyte elastase, is greatly increased in psoriatic lesional skin. This enzyme—which shows proteolytic activity

FIGURE 42-15

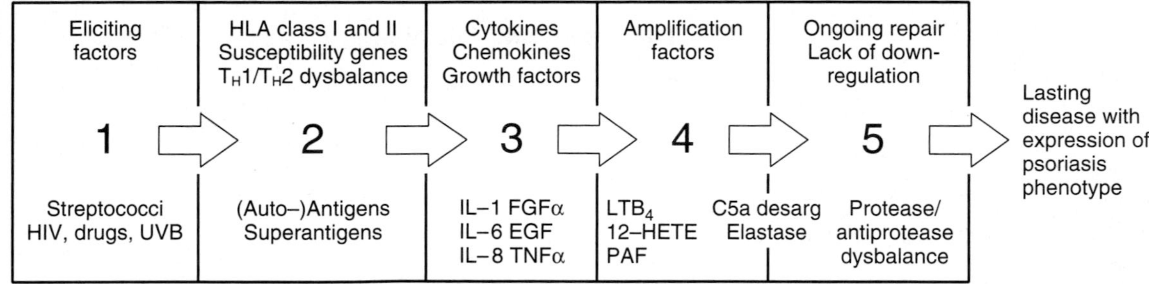

Potential pathogenetic sequence in psoriasis. Noncutaneous eliciting factors may serve as antigens/superantigens or may generate psoriatic "autoantigens." In response to these factors, (1) susceptibility genes are activated, some of which are HLA-associated; (2) the nature of the eliciting factor creates T_H1-T_H2 imbalance within a yet to be defined set of cytokines; (3) possibly by genetic determination, there is a lack of downregulation; with the influx of neutrophils and monocytes/macrophages, lipid mediators are generated with amplifying effects on the inflammatory response; (4) further mediator systems (e.g., proteases) become activated and lead to phenotypical disease expression; and (5) this hypothetical model may become modulated at each phase (1 to 5), whereby the heterogeneity of clinical disease ensues.

toward a variety of substrates, including collagen types III and IV, proteoglycans, and elastin—is normally regulated by antiproteases, one of which was discovered recently in human epidermis.[46] In psoriasis, the presence of excess elastase in an unblocked form suggests increased proteolytic activity within the affected epidermis.

TREATMENT

Various forms of treatment have been developed in the past several decades. They have mostly been developed empirically, and as with all other diseases of unknown cause, new regimens are being tried constantly. Recently, biotechnology has allowed the development of monoclonal antibodies and fusion proteins targeting single epitopes or compounds with relevance in the psoriatic tissue reaction. Furthermore, the experimental administration of recombinant cytokines such as IL-10 showed beneficial effects at least in a subgroup of psoriasis patients. These new-generation therapies will gain importance in the routine treatment of psoriasis in the near future.

There is debate as to whether the aim of any psoriasis therapy should be total clearing of the lesions. Under many circumstances, patients may regard the successful clearing of scaling a sufficient therapeutic response; however, when lesions are present in visible areas such as the hands, complete resolution is necessary.[47] Complete clearing normally needs a much higher therapeutic effort, in particular when patients present with severe, frequently relapsing psoriasis. In these pateints, discussion about the therapeutic goal between dermatologist and patient should define the individual treatment strategy.

TABLE 42-6

Cytokines Detected in Normal Skin and Lesional Psoriatic Skin

Cytokine*	Present in Normal Skin	Changes in Lesional Psoriatic Skin
IL-1α	+	↓↓↓
IL-1β	+	
IL-6	+	↑↑
NAP-1/IL-8	+	↑↑
MGSA/groα	+	↑↑
TNF-α	−	↑
TGF-α	+	↑
IFN-α	−	↑
GM-CSF	+	?
G-CSF	+	?
M-CSF	+	?
MCP-1	+	?

*IL, interleukin; NAP, neutrophil-activating peptide; TNF, tumor necrosis factor; TGF, transforming growth factor; IFN, interferon; GM-CSF, granulocyte-macrophage colony-stimulating factor; G-CSF, granulocyte colony-stimulating factor; M-CSF, monocyte/macrophage colony-stimulating factor; MCAF, monocyte chemotactic and activating factor.

Topical Treatment (See also Chaps. 244 and 251)

ANTHRALIN Anthralin (1,8-dihydroxyanthrone; cignolin, dithranol) was introduced by Galewsky and Unna in 1916. This compound is still a widely used remedy for psoriasis in different vehicles and application modes. A major advantage of anthralin is the lack of any long-term side effects, which allows unlimited reintroduction of the drug as long as therapy is required.

Mode of action Anthralin possesses antiproliferative activity on human keratinocytes. In recent years it has become clear that this compound also exerts strong anti-inflammatory effects mainly on cells of the inflammatory infiltrate. Inhibition of neutrophil and monocyte functions and production and ω-oxidation of leukotriene B_4 from neutrophils have been observed. It was found recently that anthralin induces nuclear transcription factor NF-κB in murine keratinocytes.[48] Since NF-κB is involved in the transcription of proinflammatory cytokines such as IL-6, IL-8, and TNF-α, these findings may be helpful in explaining the irritant properties of anthralin.

Clinical use Chronic plaque-type psoriasis responds best to anthralin treatment. Guttate psoriasis also can be treated effectively.

Classic anthralin therapy starts with low concentrations (0.05–0.1%) incorporated in petrolatum or zinc paste and given once daily. To prevent autooxidation, salicylic acid (1–2%) should be added. The concentration is increased weekly in individually adjusted increments up to about 5% until the lesions resolve.

Short-contact treatment is an alternative mode of application. Higher concentrations of anthralin (1–5%) in water-soluble vehicles are applied to the lesions for a short period of time (usually 10–20 min) and thereafter washed off. Application time is increased weekly until the lesions have cleared. A new galenical formulation (Micanol) reduces local irritation and staining of skin and equipment. A leukoderma-like zone ("pseudoleukoderma") may become visible at the site of treated lesions.

Adverse events Anthralin can cause irritant reactions ("anthralin dermatitis") in susceptible patients or after increasing the concentration too fast. Since anthralin can stain the hair a purple to greenish color, scalp psoriasis should be treated only with great caution.

At higher concentrations, anthralin causes brownish discoloration of the surrounding skin ("anthralin-brown") and of clothing that comes into contact with the compound. Since these oxidation products remain at the upper levels of the stratum corneum, discoloration disappears within days after stopping anthralin application. Removal of stains from clothing, however, is difficult or impossible.

VITAMIN D_3 AND ANALOGUES Since the first report about the beneficial effects of vitamin D_3 in psoriasis by Morimoto et al.,[49] new analogues have been developed to decrease hormonal effects on calcium/phosphate homeostasis and to maintain effects on keratinocyte proliferation and differentiation. Soon after the introduction of the first vitamin D_3 analogue, calcipotriol (also called calcipotriene in some countries), to topical therapy, it became a widely used remedy for plaque-type psoriasis.[50] Another vitamin D_3 analogue, tacalcitol, is available in some countries.[51]

Recently, active hormone 1,25-dihydroxyvitamin D_3 (calcitriol) was registered for topical psoriasis treatment in a number of countries.[52]

Mode of action Vitamin D_3 and its analogues inhibit keratinocyte proliferation and induce terminal differentiation.[53] Anti-inflammatory properties of these compounds include inhibition of nuclear factor NF-κB protein in lymphocytes, leading to a reduced transcription of IL-2.[54] Calcitriol and calcipotriol can inhibit production of IL-6 from cytokine-stimulated human dermal microvascular endothelial cells and reduce the antigen-presenting function of Langerhans cells. Calcitriol is a potent inhibitor of dendritic cell differentiation.[55]

Clinical use Calcitriol, calcipotriol, and tacalcitol are used for plaque-type psoriasis twice or once daily, respectively. Treatment is limited by the area of application and time due to possible effects on calcium/phosphate homeostasis. Calcipotriol is inactivated by salicylic acid; therefore, lesions should not be pretreated with this compound. When calcipotriol is used in combination with ultraviolet (UV) light, application should follow light exposure because of the UV-absorbing properties of calcipotriol.

Adverse effects Local irritation may occur at the beginning of treatment. Some patients develop facial rashes after application of calcipotriol elsewhere on the body.

Changes in calcium and/or phosphate metabolism are rare when application follows the respective guidelines.Calcipotriol has been found to be a safe treatment for children with psoriasis.[56]

TAZAROTENE Tazarotene is a retinoid for topical use that reduces mainly scaling and plaque thickness, with limited effectiveness on erythema. In comparison with other topical drugs for psoriasis, tazarotene has a lower efficacy. However, efficacy can be enhanced by combination with UVB therapy.[57]

TAR The use of tar either as coal tar or wood tar (birch, pine, beech) has a long history in antipsoriatic therapy. These tars contain a great variety of compounds, most of which are not well defined. Very little is known about how tars act in skin. Preparations of 2% to 5% tar in various bases have been shown to be preferentially effective in chronic plaque-type psoriasis. These preparations are nonirritant, and serious side effects are not seen even after long periods of treatment.

TOPICAL GLUCOCORTICOIDS Topical glucocorticoids can be used effectively in psoriasis. They are discussed in detail in Chap. 243.

BLAND EMOLLIENTS Between treatment periods, skin care with bland emollients should be performed in order to avoid dryness, leading to early recurrence, and to prolong therapy-free intervals. The addition of urea (up to 10%) is helpful to improve hydration of the skin and remove scaling of early lesions.

Treatment with Ultraviolet Light

PHOTOCHEMOTHERAPY (PUVA) (See Chap. 266) The use of systemic psoralens plus ultraviolet A (PUVA) to treat psoriasis was introduced in 1974 by Parrish and coworkers.[58] The effectiveness of PUVA in clearing psoriasis has now been widely documented and confirmed by cooperative clinical studies in the United States and in Europe.[59] Treatment consists of oral ingestion of a potent photosensitizer such as 8-methoxypsoralen (8-MOP) or trimethoxypsoralen at a constant dose (0.6–0.8 mg/kg) and variable doses of UVA, depending on the sensitivity of the patient. Approximately 2 h after ingestion of the psoralen, UVA is started, usually at a dose of 1 J/cm^2, adjusting upward for skin type. The UVA dose is increased by suberythematous amounts, generally ranging from 0.5 to 1.5 J/cm^2. The dose of UVA for a given treatment should not lead to brisk erythema. Treatments are performed two or three times a week or, under a more intensive protocol, four times a week.

In most patients, clearing occurs after 19 to 25 treatments, and the amount of UVA needed ranges from 100 to 245 J/cm^2. PUVA results in rapid pigmentation of the skin, making it necessary to increase the dosages of light. Overdosage results in a sunburn type of reaction, which characteristically is more delayed than that seen with UVB; i.e., it occurs 24 to 48 h after treatment. Administration of lower doses of psoralen or UVA, as well as prolonged treatment courses, may demonstrate psoriasis that is nonresponsive and may even result in relapses in patients under treatment.

Psoralens such as 8-MOP intercalate with DNA. With the energy of UVA, psoralens covalently cross-link nucleic acids between opposing strands of duplex regions of DNA. The formation of these cross-linking bifunctional photoadducts leads to irreversible photoinhibition of DNA synthesis and mitosis.[60] This reaction is thought to be important in the hyperproliferative psoriatic epidermis. Because demonstration of interstrand cross-links in treated human epidermis has yet to be shown, mechanisms other than DNA binding need to be considered. Since PUVA was shown to be therapeutically effective in a variety of dermatoses, some of which are not related to hyperproliferation, more than one mode of action appears to be likely.

Side effects and the consequences of overdosage include nausea, dizziness, and headache. Approximately 95 percent of the drug is excreted via the kidneys within 8 h. During this time, cutaneous sensitivity to UV light is increased considerably. Measures for sun protection must be taken during the 8 to 12 h after ingestion of the psoralen. To protect the eyes, UVA-blocking plastic wraparound glasses should be worn outdoors for the 24 h after ingesting psoralen. Indoors, especially in a bright fluorescent light, the same type of protective eyewear is recommended. The psoralen molecule reaches highest concentrations in skin within 2 to 3 h after oral ingestion; the concentration slowly decreases during the following 8 h. During the entire day of treatment, exposure to sunlight should be avoided by wearing protective clothing and taking other appropriate precautions. Since psoralens are found in the lens, ophthalmologic examinations should be performed at yearly intervals.

Long-term side effects are of considerable importance and make it necessary to restrict PUVA to patients with widespread and severe psoriasis. A major early side effect is pruritus, which usually can be managed by the topical use of emollients or low-potency glucocorticoids. Late sequelae include the spectrum of long-term actinic skin damage, e.g., solar elastosis, dry and wrinkled skin, and hyper- and hypopigmentation. PUVA freckles, which may persist for years, represent the potential for the development of skin cancers. Stern et al.[26] analyzed 13,800 patients who had been receiving PUVA therapy and had been followed up for 5.7 years; in this group there was a dose-related increased frequency of squamous cell carcinomas.[26] Patients who have received relatively high dosages of PUVA had a 12.8 times higher incidence of genital squamous cell carcinomas than patients exposed to lower dosages of PUVA. This finding was independent of skin pigmentation, prior tar therapy, or prior x-irradiation.[26] Malignant melanoma risk increases especially in those with more than 250 treatments.[61]

BATH PUVA Another way to deliver the photosensitizer (8-MOP or 5-MOP) to the skin is by addition of these compounds to bath water, first described by Fischer and Alsins in 1976.[62] Major advantages of bath PUVA are the lack of systemic effects, such as gastrointestinal complaints (nausea is present in about 13 percent of patients taking 8-MOP orally), and the overall reduction of UV dose down to one-quarter of that required to obtain therapeutic results similar to those of conventional PUVA, thus reducing the risk of nonmelanoma skin cancer.[63] Furthermore, erythema is less frequent in bath PUVA patients, and eye protection by sunglasses is not required.

Experimental studies have shown that bath PUVA reduces keratinocyte proliferation and suppresses activation of lesional T cells. To reduce the cost of the larger amounts of liquid 8-MOP required when using bath PUVA in a tub (volume of 150–200 L), the employment of a polyethylene sheet bath has been proposed and has been shown to achieve therapeutic results similar to those conventional bathing in a large volume.[64]

BALNEOPHOTOTHERAPY Empirically, it has been known that the combination of salt-water bathing and sunlight exposure is an effective treatment for psoriasis. From studies at the Dead Sea, it became clear that highly concentrated salt water (>20%) together with UVB light is most effective.[65] This therapeutic strategy also was termed *balneophototherapy;* it has become increasingly popular in Europe, where concentrated salt-water baths together with artificial UVB sources are used in psoriasis treatment centers. A possible mechanism of concentrated salt-water bathing is the elution of biologically active peptide mediators and enzymes such as human leukocyte elastase from the inflamed skin.

SELECTIVE UVB THERAPY Treatment with UVB without UVA, also known as *selective UVB phototherapy* (SUP), can be performed as monotherapy or preferably in combination with topical treatments such as glucocorticoids, vitamin D_3 and analogues, tazarotene, or anthralin. SUP is very effective in guttate psoriasis and also improves lesions of the plaque type. Today, narrow-band UVB treatment (311 nm, Philips TL01 bulbs) has become a standard therapy for plaque-type and guttate psoriasis.

Several new aspects of UVB action on the skin have been elucidated. These include depletion of Langerhans cells, decreased leukocyte adhesion to the microvasculature, depletion of intraepidermal T cells, and induction of IL-10 production from macrophages, which acts as an anti-inflammatory mediator.

Systemic Treatment

Systemic treatment of psoriasis is required in cases of severe disease when lesions are widespread or pustular or when psoriasis is in an active phase, with rapid flare-ups after topical courses including UV light. Systemic treatment should be monitored carefully.

METHOTREXATE (See Chap. 256) Methotrexate (MTX) was introduced as an antipsoriatic agent in 1958. It is a widely used systemic regimen for severe forms of psoriasis and most beneficial in pustular forms of the disease. MTX is the drug of choice for severe psoriatic arthritis.

Mechanism of action MTX inhibits DNA synthesis (S phase of the cell cycle) by competing as a substrate for dihydrofolate reductase; originally, it was thought to act primarily on the rapidly dividing basal keratinocytes of the psoriatic lesion. The group of Weinstein[66] demonstrated that proliferating lymphoid cells in psoriatic lesions are over 1000 times more sensitive to the cytotoxic effects of MTX than primary human keratinocytes. It also has been shown that MTX exerts anti-inflammatory effects mediated through intracellular accumulation of 5-aminoimidazole-4-carboxyamide ribonucleotide (AICAR), thereby increasing the release of adenosine. Adenosine exerts anti-inflammatory effects mainly on neutrophils, where an inhibition of adhesion and reactive oxygen intermediate production has been demonstrated. New data suggest that MTX induces apoptosis in activated T cells and keratinocytes.[67,68]

Clinical use Pustular psoriasis and psoriatic arthritis are treated most effectively with MTX. In psoriasis vulgaris of the chronic plaque type, MTX monotherapy is less efficacious and should be combined with topical compounds to achieve clearing of the lesions.

Dosage The usual dosage of MTX is between 10 and 25 mg once a week. The preferred mode of delivery is intravenous or intramuscular in order to obtain best efficacy and to control treatment. MTX can also be given orally using a dosing schedule in which 5 mg is given every 12 h over a 36-h period. This regimen may be as effective as treatment with a once-weekly parenteral dose.

Adverse effects Most commonly nausea, anorexia, fatigue, headaches, and alopecia are encountered as adverse effects. Development of leukopenia and thrombocytopenia indicates serious dysfunction of the bone marrow and may be a sign of MTX overdose. In this case, a folinic acid rescue (25 mg of leucovorin intramuscularly) should be performed, preferably within the first 4 h. In case of renal dysfunction, leucovorin is given repeatedly until renal function improves.

Since MTX is excreted mainly via the kidneys, patients with a history of kidney dysfunction should not be treated with MTX so as to avoid increased kidney toxicity.

A rare but life-threatening side effect of MTX therapy is acute interstitial pneumonitis, which is believed to be a result of a hypersensitivity reaction. Interestingly, in contrast to rheumatoid arthritis therapy, there are only very few reports of pneumonitis in psoriasis patients treated with MTX. Lethality is about 15 percent in rheumatoid arthritis patients treated with the same doses of MTX as are used for psoriasis.

Hepatotoxicity is a major concern with MTX treatment. Patients with a history of liver disease or alcohol abuse must be excluded. The risk of developing liver fibrosis or cirrhosis increases with the overall cumulative MTX dose. Above a cumulative MTX dose of 1.5 g, monitoring of structural liver changes is mandatory.

Control of MTX therapy Routine measurement of hematologic parameters, as well as liver and kidney function, should be performed in MTX-treated patients. A recent study indicates that serial measurement of type III procollagen aminopeptide (PIIINP) is of value in detecting liver damage and may reduce the need for liver biopsy in MTX-treated patients.[69] On the other hand, comparisons of susceptibility to the development of structural liver changes in patients with rheumatoid arthritis and psoriasis reveal a higher risk in psoriasis patients for reasons yet unknown.[70] The dermatologic guidelines for the use of MTX therefore still recommend liver biopsy after a cumulative dose of 1.5 g and thereafter at 1- to 1.5-g intervals.[71]

CYCLOSPORINE (See Chap. 262) Cyclosporine is a cyclic polypeptide that is used widely for the prevention of graft rejection. It is accepted for the treatment of severe psoriasis in many countries.

Mode of action After penetration into the cell by a putative receptor, cyclosporine binds to cyclophilin, a member of the immunophilin group. The cyclosporine-cyclophilin complex binds to the phosphatase calcineurin, thereby blocking its ability to dephosphorylate the cytosolic component of transcription factor NF-AT (nuclear factor of activated T cells). This results in an impaired translocation of the NF-AT component to the nucleus. The nuclear component of NF-AT is required for functional activity to enhance transcription of the IL-2 gene.[72] Other pharmacologic effects of cyclosporine with possible relevance for psoriasis are an inhibition of the antigen-presenting capacity of Langerhans cells and mast cell functions such as degranulation and cytokine production.

Clinical use Multicenter studies have shown that cyclosporine is effective in about 70 percent of patients with severe chronic plaque-type psoriasis when a low-dose regimen (<5 mg/kg per day) is used. Clearing requires several weeks of therapy, which can be maintained continuously.[73] Improvement of nail changes as well as of associated psoriatic arthritis can be seen during long-term therapy. Cyclosporine therapy can be recommended as a short-term intermittent regimen in which the drug is tapered off as soon as major improvement is seen or as long-term continuous treatment in recalcitrant cases. Cyclosporine is also effective in erythrodermic as well as generalized pustular psoriasis.

Despite several attempts to develop ointment formulations, cyclosporine is without effect when used topically.

Dosage The recommended dosage of cyclosporine—arrived at as a result of multicenter studies and consensus meetings—is to start with 2.5 to 3 mg/kg per day divided into two daily doses. This can be increased up to a maximum of 5 mg/kg per day. After clinical response is achieved, the cyclosporine dose can be lowered to the best level for the individual patient.

Adverse effects Among the side effects of cyclosporine, which are dose-related, is impairment of kidney function, which is largely reversible after drug withdrawal; also, hypertension may develop. A rise in serum cholesterol and triglycerides also has been observed. Clinically, hypertrichosis, gingival hyperplasia, tremor, and fatigue may occur. Recent investigations showed that long-term cyclosporine treatment increase the risk for development of skin cancer. This risk is particularly high in patients with a history of PUVA therapy using high doses of UVA.[74]

Control of cyclosporine treatment Control of cyclosporine therapy includes blood pressure measurement and determination of serum creatinine as the most useful parameters for detecting decreased kidney function in clinical practice. If serum creatinine levels rise above 30 percent of individual baseline, the dose of cyclosporine must be reduced. In case of persistently enhanced creatinine values, the drug must be withdrawn. Dermatologic examination is necessary in order to early detect skin malignancies.

RETINOIDS (See Chap. 257) Acitretin, a derivative of vitamin A, is used mainly for the treatment of psoriasis. Best clinical results have been obtained in pustular forms of psoriasis.

Acitretin has replaced formerly used etretinate. The half-life of etretinate is about 100 days and that of acitretin 2 to 3 days. When acitretin was introduced, this short half-life was thought to overcome long-lasting accumulation in the tissues, which meant severe restrictions in the use of etretinate in women due to the risk of teratogenic effects. However, it turned out that a portion of acitretin is reesterified in vivo into *iso*-acitretin and etretinate.[75] Therefore, restrictions on the use of acitretin in women of childbearing age remain the same as for etretinate.

Mechanism of action Retinoids regulate growth and terminal differentiation of keratinocytes, thereby normalizing the hyperproliferative state in psoriasis. After passing the cell membrane, retinoids form complexes with cytosolic binding proteins, which, after translocation into the nucleus, regulate gene transcription through nuclear response elements.

Retinoids also exert some anti-inflammatory effects, such as inhibition of neutrophil functions.

Clinical use Etretinate and acitretin are clinically effective in pustular forms of psoriasis, including generalized pustular psoriasis and PPP. For plaque-type psoriasis, retinoids show lower response rates than other systemic modalities. In combination with PUVA (Re-PUVA), retinoids can improve the clinical effectiveness of acitretin in some cases. After prolonged therapy, retinoids may lead to an improvement in psoriatic arthritis.

Dosage In severe psoriasis vulgaris and psoriatic erythroderma, acitretin is given in a dose of 0.3 to 0.5 mg/kg per day initially, which is increased at 3- to 4-week intervals to 0.75 mg/kg per day. To achieve improvement, treatment over 3 to 4 months is necessary.

Pustular psoriasis requires an initial dose of 1 mg/kg per day of acitretin, which is given until clinical improvement is seen. Thereafter, the dose is lowered gradually to a maintenance dose of about 0.5 mg/kg per day, which is given for 3 to 4 months.

Adverse effects The side effects of etretinate/acitretin therapy are dose-related. The most prominent symptoms are cheilitis, sicca symptoms of the eyes and mouth, generalized pruritus, dryness of the skin, and loss of the stratum corneum of palms and soles, leading to soreness in these areas. There may be considerable hair loss during treatment with acitretin. Muscle and joint pain as well as gastrointestinal complaints also may be present.

An elevation of serum lipids is seen frequently during systemic retinoid treatment, especially in patients with a history of lipid abnormality, obesity, diabetes, smoking, and/or alcohol abuse. Elevations in liver enzymes (SGOT, SGPT, LDH) may occur.

A major concern with the use of systemic retinoids is their high teratogenic potential. Since acitretin is remetabolized into long-lived compounds, use of this drug should be restricted to men and to women with no childbearing potential. If acitretin is given to women of childbearing age, strict contraception is required for the time of therapy and for an additional 2 years after drug withdrawal.

Control of retinoid treatment Liver and kidney function, blood glucose, and serum lipids should be monitored initially at 3-week intervals and later every 2 months. Symptomatic treatment for dry skin, mouth, and eyes should be given.

FUMARIC ACID ESTERS A mixture of fumaric acid monoethyl and dimethyl esters is approved in Germany for systemic treatment of severe psoriasis. Clinical experience exists since 1959 when fuamrates were introduced.

Mode of action Inhibition of TNF-α–induced keratinocyte ICAM-1 expression by dimethylfumarate has been demonstrated. Monomethylfumarate, the main metabolite of dimethylfumarate, was shown to stimulate release of T_H2 cytokines IL-4 and IL-5 from human peripheral blood T cells without changing production of T_H1 cytokines IL-2 and interferon-γ.[76] Dimethylfumarate potently inhibits dendritic cell differentiation.[77] Recently, dimethylfumarate was shown to induce apoptosis is a number of cells, including dendritic cells.[77] Furthermore, this compound inhibits cytokine production by blocking NFκB signaling.[78,79]

Clinical use Fumaric acid esters are used for the treatment of severe psoriasis vulgaris.[80] Multicenter studies have shown that about 70 percent of psoriasis patients respond to therapy.[81] There are reports of long-term use of fumarates, which seems to be possible in patients with recalcitrant psoriasis. Experience with fumarates for the treatment of erythrodermic and pustular psoriasis as well as psoriatic arthritis is very limited.

Adverse effects The most frequently observed adverse effects with fumaric acid ester therapy for psoriasis are gastrointestinal complaints and flush. Symptoms of the first can vary from nausea to severe diarrhea; they are dose-dependent and sometimes limit the use of the drug.

Flush is seen in many different forms from rashes and classical flush to headache-like symptoms that occur irregularly for short periods.

Leukocytopenia and lymphopenia frequently are associated with fumarate therapy. There also may be an increase of eosinophils. In rare cases, impairment of renal function has been observed.

Dosage Fumaric acid ester therapy follows a dosing schedule that begins with a low-strength formulation and is increased weekly for 3 weeks. Then therapy continues with a normal-strength formulation that is increased weekly up to a maximum of 1.29 g/day. Dosage is usually adjusted to an individual level, which can be low in susceptible patients.

Control of fumarate therapy Monitoring of hematologic parameters with particular emphasis on leukocyte and differential counts and of renal function, including urinary protein excretion, is most important. Liver enzymes as well as electrolytes also should be monitored.

SYSTEMIC GLUCOCORTICOIDS Systemic use of glucocorticoids should be restricted to a few selected patients with refractory psoriasis. Although transient improvement can be achieved, this is almost always accompanied by a severe rebound to an even worse situation than before therapy. Transition from psoriasis vulgaris into generalized pustular forms after withdrawal of systemic glucocorticoids can be seen.

EXPERIMENTAL APPROACHES Based on the evidence that psoriasis is a T cell–mediated inflammatory disease, a number of new therapeutic approaches have been developed.[82]

Strategies targeting cellular epitopes on T cells or antigen-presenting cells Targeting activated T cells, which are thought to be of primary importance for the pathogenesis of psoriasis, is a principle adressed in a number of new therapeutic approaches. A fusion protein of IL-2 and diphtheria toxin (DAB_{389}IL-2) was given intravenously to patients with severe psoriasis and led to improvement of only a subgroup of patients.[83] IL-2 signaling pathways also can be abrogated by blockade of IL-2 receptors (CD25, α-chain). Treatment with the specific monoclonal antibody basiliximab was found to be effective in a patient with active psoriasis.[84] However, in an open study in plaque-type psoriasis, the anti-CD25 antibody daclizumab showed only a 30 percent reduction of severity score after 8 weeks of therapy.[85]

Treatment with the fusion protein blocking LFA3-CD2 interaction (alefacept, Amevive) led to improvement of up to 53 percent in the PASI score in a recent study.[86] There is evidence that alefacept treatment preferentially reduces the number of memory T cells (CD45RO+).

Strategies targeting cytokines By using a monoclonal antibody against TNF-α (infliximab, Remicade) or a fusion protein mimicking the TNF-α receptor (etanercept, Enbrel), improvement of lesions can be achieved in plaque-type psoriasis.[87,88]

Strategies using recombinant cytokines Systemic application of human recombinant IL-10 proved to be efficacious at least in a subgroup of patients.[89] This therapy lead to to a variety of changes in T cell function and cytokine secretion in vivo, as demonstrated recently.[90]

OTHER NEW DRUG DEVELOPMENTS

Macrolactams Macrolactams show improvement of lesions by topical use under occlusion, not, however, when applied without oclusion.[91,92] A recent report show a high efficacy in psoriasis within a short time when the macrolactam pimecrolimus (SDZ ASM 981; Elidel) was given orally.

Other New Methods to Treat Psoriasis

Among a variety of newly described methods for treatment of psoriasis, use of the excimer laser may be of future importance. This laser generates light at 308 nm in the UVB range. In a first study it was shown that about four treatments lead to improvement of lesions with a sustained treatment response.[93]

COMBINATION THERAPY A combination of different therapeutic principles may help to speed resolution of the lesions, reduce adverse events, and reduce overall doses when systemic compounds are used.

Several combination regimes have already been established for clinical use, such as topical glucocorticoids with UVB or PUVA, retinoids with PUVA (Re-PUVA), and vitamin D_3 and analogues or tazarotene with UVB.

The combination of coal tar baths, UVB, and anthralin is known as the *Ingram method.* Goeckerman in 1925 introduced the widely used combination of coal tar application followed by suberythemic doses of UV light. Classic anthralin treatment followed by UVB or bath PUVA is also a very effective combination regimen.

More recent studies indicate that combining cyclosporine with calcipotriol or anthralin augments efficacy and reduces cyclosporine dose. Calcipotriol also improves the response to PUVA.

ROTATION TREATMENT To minimize risk to the patient with severe psoriasis requiring systemic treatment, rotation therapy should be performed. Changing between different compounds—with respect to individual risk factors, cumulative dose (for MTX), response, and duration of therapy—should be performed at intervals. Recently published guidelines for rotation therapy may be helpful in scheduling long-term systemic treatment.

REFERENCES

1. Farber EM, Nall ML: The natural history of psoriasis in 5600 patients. *Dermatologica* **148**:118, 1974
2. Lomholt G: *Psoriasis: Prevalence, Spontaneous Course and Genetics: A Census Study on the Prevalence of Skin Diseases on the Faroe Islands.* Copenhagen, GEC Gad, 1963, p 163
3. Buntin DM et al: Onset of psoriasis at age 108. *J Am Acad Dermatol* **9**:276, 1983
4. Henseler T, Christophers E: Psoriasis of early and late onset: Characterization of two types of psoriasis vulgaris. *J Am Acad Dermatol* **13**:450, 1985
5. Nyfors A, Lemholt K: Psoriasis in children: A short review and a survey of 245 cases. *Br J Dermatol* **92**:437, 1975
6. Melski JW, Stern RS: The separation of susceptibility to psoriasis from age of onset. *J Invest Dermatol* **77**:474, 1981
7. Russell TJ et al: Histocompatibility (HL-A) antigens associated with psoriasis. *N Engl J Med* **287**:738, 1972
8. Watson W et al: The genetics of psoriasis. *Arch Dermatol* **105**:197, 1972
9. White SH et al: Disturbance of HL-A antigen frequency in psoriasis. *N Engl J Med* **287**:740, 1972
10. Andresen C, Henseler T: Erblichkeit der Psoriasis. *Hautarzt* **33**:214, 1982
11. Tiilikainen A et al: Psoriasis and HLA-Cw6. *Br J Dermatol* **102**:179, 1980
12. Zachariae H et al: HLA antigens in pustular psoriasis. *Dermatologica* **134**:73, 1977
13. Rapp SR et al: Psoriasis causes as much disability as other major medical diseases. *J Am Acad Dermatol* **41**:401, 1999
14. Krueger G et al: The impact of psoriasis on quality of life: Results of a 1998 National Psoriasis Foundation patient-membership survey. *Arch Dermatol* **137**:280, 2001
15. Chalmers RJG et al: Streptococcal serotypes in patients with guttate psoriasis. *Arch Dermatol* **118**:141, 1982
16. Sadick NS et al: Papulosquamous dermatoses of AIDS. *J AM Acad Dermatol* **22**:1270, 1990
17. Tsankov N et al: Drug-induced psoriasis. Recognition and management. *Am J Clin Dermatol* **1**:159, 2000
18. Yates VM et al: Further evidence for an association between psoriasis, Crohn's disease and ulcerative colitis. *Br J Dermatol* **106**:323, 1982
19. Elder JT et al: The genetics of psoriasis 2001: The odyssey continues. *Arch Dermatol* **137**:1447, 2001
20. Barker JN: Genetic aspects of psoriasis. *Clin Exp Dermatol* **26**:321, 2001
21. Christophers E, Henseler T: Psoriasis type I and type II as subtypes of nonpustular psoriasis, in *Psoriasis,* 2d ed, edited by HH Roenigk, H Maibach. New York, Marcel Dekker, 1990, pp 15–21

22. Schmidt-Egenolf M et al: Oligonucleotide typing reveals association of type I psoriasis with the HLA-DRB1*0701/2, -DQA1*0201, -DQB1*0303 extended haplotype. *J Invest Dermatol* **100**:749, 1993
23. Trembath RC et al: Identification of a major susceptibility locus on chromosome 6p and evidence for further disease loci revealed by a two stage genome-wide search in psoriasis. *Hum Mol Genet* **6**:813,1997
24. Henseler T, Christophers E: Disease concomitance in psoriasis. *J Am Acad Dermatol* **32**:982, 1995
25. Stern R et al: Psoriasis and the risk of cancer. *J Invest Dermatol* **78**:147, 1982
26. Stern RS et al: Cutaneous squamous cell carcinomas in patients treated with PUVA. *N Engl J Med* **310**:1156, 1984
27. Christophers E, Henseler T: Contrasting disease patterns in psoriasis and atopic dermatitis. *Arch Dermatol Res* **279**:S48, 1987
28. Aly R et al: Bacterial flora in psoriasis. *Br J Dermatol* **95**:603, 1976
29. Van Scott EJ, Ekel TM: Kinetics of hyperplasia in psoriasis. *Arch Dermatol* **88**:373, 1963
30. Uyemura K et al: The cytokine network in lesional and lesion-free psoriatic skin is characterized by a T-helper type 1 cell-mediated response. *J Invest Dermatol* **101**:701, 1993
31. Schlaak JF et al: T cells involved in psoriasis vulgaris belong to the Th1 subset. *J Invest Dermatol* **102**:145, 1994
32. Kägi MK et al: Differential cytokine profiles in peripheral blood lymphocyte supernatants and skin biopsies from patients with different forms of atopic dermatitis, psoriasis and normal individuals. *Int Arch Allergy Immunol* **103**:332, 1994
33. Lewis HM et al: Restricted T-cell receptor V_b gene usage in the skin of patients with guttate and chronic plaque psoriasis. *Br J Dermatol* **129**:514, 1993
34. Menssen A et al: Evidence for an antigen-specific cellular immune response in skin lesions of patients with psoriasis vulgaris. *J Immunol* **155**:4078, 1995
35. Chang JCC et al: CD8+ T cells in psoriatic lesions preferentially use T cell receptor V_b3 and/or $V_b13.1$ genes. *Proc Natl Acad Sci USA* **91**: 9282, 1994
36. Boehncke W-H et al: T-cell-receptor repertoire in chronic plaque-stage psoriasis is restricted and lacks enrichment of superantigen-associated V_b regions. *J Invest Dermatol* **104**:725, 1995
37. Babi LFS et al: Migration of skin-homing T cells across cytokine-activated human endothelial cell layers involves interaction of the cutaneous lymphocyte-associated antigen (CLA), the very late antigen-4 (VLA-4), and the lymphocyte function-associated antigen-1 (LFA-1). *J Immunol* **154**:1543, 1995
38. Vallat VP et al: PUVA bath therapy strongly suppresses immunological and epidermal activation in psoriasis: A possible cellular basis for remittive therapy. *J Exp Med* **180**:283, 1994
39. Krueger JG et al: Successful ultraviolet B treatment of psoriasis is accompanied by a reversal of keratinocyte pathology and by selective depletion of intraepidermal *T* cells. *J Exp Med* **182**:2057, 1996
40. Eedy DJ et al: Clearance of severe psoriasis after allogeneic bone marrow transplantation. *BMJ* **300**:908, 1990
41. Gardembas-Pain M et al: Psoriasis after allogeneic bone marrow transplantation. *Arch Dermatol* **126**:1523, 1991
42. Picker LJ et al: Differential expression of homing-associated adhesion molecules by T cell subsets in man. *J Immunol* **145**:3247, 1990
43. Gearing AJH et al: Cytokines in skin lesions of psoriasis. *Cytokine* **2**:68, 1990
44. Fraki JE et al: Correlation of epidermal plasminogen activator activity with disease activity in psoriasis. *Br J Dermatol* **108**:39, 1983
45. Fraki JE et al: Uninvolved skin from psoriatic patients develops signs of involved psoriatic skin after being grafted onto nude mice. *Science* **215**:685, 1982
46. Wiedow O et al: An elastase-specific inhibitor of human skin. *J Biol Chem* **265**:1491, 1990
47. Al Suwaidan SN, Feldman SR: Clearance is not a realistic expectation of psoriasis treatment. *J Am Acad Dermatol* **42**:796, 2000
48. Schmidt KN et al: Anti-psoriatic drug anthralin activates transcription factor NF-κB in murine keratinocytes. *J Immunol* **156**:4514, 1996
49. Morimoto S et al: An open study of vitamin D_3 treatment in psoriasis vulgaris. *Br J Dermatol* **115**:421, 1986
50. Kragballe K et al: Long-term efficacy and tolerability of topical calcipotriol in psoriasis. *Acta Derm Venereol (Stockh)* **71**:475, 1991
51. Gerritsen MJP et al: The effect of tacalcitol [1,24$(OH)_2D_3$] on cutaneous inflammation, epidermal proliferation and keratinization in psoriasis: A placebo-controlled, double-blind study. *Br J Dermatol* **131**:57, 1994
52. Gerritsen MJ et al: Long-term safety of topical calcitriol 3 μg/g ointment *Br J Dermatol* **144**(suppl 58):17, 2001
53. Van de Kerkhof PCM: Biological activity of vitamin D analogues in the skin, with special reference to antipsoriatic mechanisms. *Br J Dermatol* **132**:675, 1995
54. Yu X-P et al: Down-regulation of NF-kappa B protein levels in activated human lymphocytes by 1,25-dihydroxyvitamin D_3. *Proc Natl Acad Sci USA* **92**:10990, 1995
55. Penna G, Adorini L: 1α, 25-dihydroxyvitamin D_3 inhibits differentiation, maturation, activation, and survival of dendritic cells leading to impaired alloreactive T cell activation. *J Immunol* **164**:2405, 2000
56. Oranje AP et al: Topical calcipotriol in childhood psoriasis. *J Am Acad Dermatol* **36**:203, 1997
57. Koo JY: Tazarotene in combination with phototherapy. *J Am Acad Dermatol* **39**:S144, 1998
58. Parrish JA et al: Photochemotherapy of psoriasis with oral methoxsalen and long-wave ultraviolet light. *N Engl J Med* **291**:1207, 1974
59. Henseler T et al: Oral 8-methoxypsoralen photochemotherapy of psoriasis. European PUVA Study: A cooperative study among 18 European centres. *Lancet* **1**:853, 1981
60. Pathak MA et al: Photobiology and photochemistry of furocoumarins (psoralens), in *Sunlight and Man: Normal and Abnormal Photobiologic Responses*, edited by MA Pathak, TB Fitzpatrick. Tokyo, Tokyo University Press, 1974, p 25
61. Stern RS et al: Malignant melanoma in patients treated for psoriasis with methoxsalen (psoralen) and ultraviolet A radiation (PUVA). *N Engl J Med* **336**:1041, 1997
62. Fischer T, Alsins, J: Treatment of psoriasis with trioxsalen baths and dysprosium lamps. *Acta Derm Venereol (Stockh)* **56**:383, 1976
63. Stern RS, Lange R: Non-melanoma skin cancer occurring in patients treated with PUVA five to ten years after first treatment. *J Invest Dermatol* **91**:120, 1988
64. Streit V et al: Treatment of psoriasis with polyethylene sheet bath PUVA. *J Am Acad Dermatol* **35**:208, 1996
65. Abels DJ, Kattan-Byron J: Psoriasis treatment at the Dead Sea: A natural selective ultraviolet phototherapy. *J Am Acad Dermatol* **12**:639, 1985
66. Jeffes EWB III et al: Methotrexate therapy of psoriasis: Differential sensitivity of proliferating lymphoid and epithelial cells to the cytotoxic and growth-inhibitory effects of methotrexate. *J Invest Dermatol* **104**:83, 1995
67. Genestier L et al: Immunosuppressive properties of methotrexate: Apoptosis and clonal deletion of activated peripheral T cells. *J Clin Invest* **102**:322, 1998
68. Heenen M et al: Methotrexate induces apoptotic cell death in human keratinocytes. *Arch Dermatol Res* **290**:240, 1998
69. Zachariae H et al: The value of amino-terminal propeptide of type III procollagen in routine screening for methotrexate-induced liver fibrosis: A 10-year follow-up. *Br J Dermatol* **144**:100, 2001
70. Hassan W: Methotrexate and liver toxicity: Role of surveillance liver biopsy. *Ann Rheum Dis* **55**:273, 1996
71. Roenigk HH et al: Methotrexate in psoriasis: Consensus conference. *J Am Acad Dermatol* **38**:478, 1998
72. Schreiber SL, Crabtree GR: The mechanism of action of cyclosporin A and FK506. *Immunol Today* **13**:136, 1992
73. Mrowietz U et al: Long-term maintenance therapy with cyclosporine and post-treatment survey in severe psoriasis, results of a multicenter study. *J Am Acad Dermatol* **33**:470, 1995
74. Marcil I, Stern RS. Squamous-cell cancer of the skin in patients given PUVA and ciclosporin: Nested cohort crossover study. *Lancet* **358**:1042, 2001
75. Almond-Roesler B, Orfanos CE: *trans*-Acitretin is metabolized back to etretinate: Importance for oral retinoid therapy. *Hautarzt* **47**:173, 1996
76. De Jong P et al: Selective stimulation of T helper 2 cytokine responses by the anti-psoriasis agent monomethylfumarate. *Eur J Immunol* **26**:2067, 1996
77. Zhu K, Mrowietz U: Inhibition of dendritic cell differentiation by fumaric acid esters. *J Invest Dermatol* **116**:203, 2001
78. Vandermeeren M et al: Dimethylfumarate is an inhibitor of cytokine-induced nuclear translocation of NF-kappa B1, but not RelA in normal human dermal fibroblast cells. *J Invest Dermatol* **116**:124, 2001
79. Stoof TJ et al: The antipsoriatic drug dimethylfumarate strongly suppresses chemokine production in human keratinocytes and peripheral blood mononuclear cells. *Br J Dermatol* **144**:1114, 2001
80. Mrowietz U et al: Treatment of severe psoriasis with fumaric acid esters: Scientific background and guidelines for therapeutic use. *Br J Dermatol* **141**:424, 1999
81. Altmeyer P et al: Antipsoriatic effect of fumaric acid derivatives: Results of a multicenter double-blind study in 100 patients. *J Am Acad Dermatol* **30**:977, 1994

82. Krueger IG: The immunologic basis for the treatment of psoriasis with new biologic agents. *J Am Acad Dermatol* **46**:1, 2002
83. Bagel J et al: Administration of DAV_{389} IL-2 to patients with recalcitrant psoriasis: A double-blind, phase II multicenter trial. *J Am Acad Dermatol* **38**:938, 1998
84. Mrowietz U et al: Treatment of severe psoriasis with anti-CD25 monoclonal antibodies. *Arch Dermatol* **136**:675, 2000
85. Krueger JG et al: Successful in vivo blockade of CD25 (high-affinity interleukin 2 receptor) on T cells by administration of humanized anti-Tac antibody to patients with psoriasis. *J Am Acad Dermatol* **43**:448, 2000
86. Ellis CN, Krueger GG: Treatment of chronic plaque psoriasis by selective targeting of memory effector T lymphocytes. *N Engl J Med* **345**:248, 2001
87. Chaudhari U et al: Efficacy and safety of infliximab monotherapy for plaque-type psoriasis: A randomised trial. *Lancet* **357**:1842, 2001
88. Mease PJ et al: Etanercept in the treatment of psoriatic arthritis and psoriasis: A randomised trial. *Lancet* **356**:385, 2000

89. Asadullah K et al: IL-10 is a key cytokine in psoriasis. Proof of principle by IL-10 therapy: A new therapeutic approach. *J Clin Invest* **101**:783, 1998
90. Reich K et al: Response of psoriasis to interleukin-10 is associated with suppression of cutaneous type 1 inflammation, downregulation of the epidermal interleukin-8/CXCR2 pathway and normalization of keratinocyte maturation. *J Invest Dermatol* **116**:319, 2001
91. Mrowietz U et al: The novel ascomycin derivative SDZ ASM 981 is an effective anti-psoriatic compound when used topically under occlusion. *Br J Dermatol* **139**:992, 1998
92. Zonneveld IM et al: Topical tacrolimus is not effective in chronic plaque psoriasis: A pilot study. *Arch Dermatol* **134**:1101, 1998
93. Asawanonda P et al: 308-nm excimer laser for the treatment of psoriasis: A dose-response study. *Arch Dermatol* **136**:619, 2000

CHAPTER 43

Robert Winchester

Psoriatic Arthritis

DEFINITION AND CLASSIFICATION

Psoriatic arthritis is a CD8 T cell–driven autoimmune inflammation that affects the ligaments, tendons, fascia, and spinal or peripheral joints in persons with psoriasis. The pathologic processes in psoriatic arthritis exhibit many parallels to processes found in the skin lesions. Psoriatic arthritis is recognized in about 10 percent of individuals with well-established psoriasis. However in 10 to 15 percent of those with psoriatic arthritis, either the arthritis appears synchronously with the first evidence of skin disease, or no cutaneous involvement is ever detected. In parallel with the skin disease, psoriatic arthritis is exacerbated by physical stress, nonspecific inflammation, or certain infections. Unlike most autoimmune diseases, psoriatic arthritis increases in prevalence and severity in those with advancing AIDS, and special concerns exist about its therapy in this setting.

Psoriatic arthritis is a prototypic major histocompatibility gene complex (MHC) class I-associated autoimmune form of arthritis, in which genetic susceptibility is provided by the MHC class I allele HLA-B27, and additional class I alleles, including those implicated in psoriasis susceptibility. Psoriatic arthritis is classified as one of the seronegative spondyloarthritis group of disorders that includes ankylosing spondylitis, undifferentiated spondylitis, Reiter's syndrome, reactive arthritis, and enteropathic arthritis. These disorders share involvement of the spine (spondylo) and sacroiliac joints and some degree of genetic susceptibility associated with HLA-B27. In particular, many features of the pathogenesis of psoriatic arthritis, including the importance of CD8 T cells, are similar to those of Reiter's syndrome/reactive arthritis and are highly distinct from features of rheumatoid arthritis. The older term "spondyloarthropathy" is falling from use as evidence of the importance of inflammation increases. In addition to synovitis, the spondyloarthritis group of disorders has the singularly distinctive feature of inflammation involving the periarticular structures, particularly tendons and ligaments at their respective points of insertion, which is termed *enthesitis*. This condition results in tendinitis, dactylitis (sometimes graphically termed "sausage digits"), and fasciitis.

Psoriatic arthritis is distinguished from the other spondyloarthritides, such as ankylosing spondylitis, by the limited extent and frequency of spinal involvement, the predominance of peripheral joint involvement, and the relationship to psoriasis. The peripheral joints are involved in a variety of patterns at presentation (Table 43-1), and these patterns are often useful diagnostically as emphasized by Moll and Wright in their classic paper.[1] Indeed, distal interphalangeal joint involvement in an individual with psoriasis is a pattern of joint disease

TABLE 43-1

Patterns of Psoriatic Arthritis

Asymmetric or symmetric peripheral joint involvement
- Distal interphalangeal joint involvement
- Small joints of hands and feet
- Large joints, primarily of legs
- Combination of above (erosive arthritis without osteopenia)

Axial disease
- Spine and sacroiliac joints, with or without peripheral joint involvement

Associated Features
- Tenosynovitis
- Enthesitis
- Onychodystrophy, especially with distal interphalangeal joint involvement
- New bone formation (vertebral squaring, entheses)
- Joint fibrosis and ankylosis
- Osteolysis and mutilating arthritis

that immediately suggests the diagnosis of psoriatic arthritis. However, these patterns are not stable. Over time the disease follows one of two principal patterns of joint involvement: (1) predominant axial disease, the less common form consisting of sacroiliitis with or without peripheral arthritis, and (2) the more common form of peripheral disease without sacroiliitis.[2]

HISTORIC ASPECTS

The identification of psoriatic arthritis in skeletal remains of individuals who sought refuge in ancient Middle Eastern Byzantine monasteries suggests that psoriasis with psoriatic arthritis was one of the forms of biblical "leprosy," attesting to the severe and ancient nature of this condition.[3] The association of arthritis with psoriasis was first formally described in 1818 by Alibert, and was designated psoriasis arthritique by Bazin in 1860. The notion of a distinctive arthritis associated with psoriasis became widely accepted,[4,5] but after World War II psoriatic arthritis was grouped with rheumatoid arthritis as a "rheumatoid variant" or "rheumatoid spondylitis." Subsequently, the distinct nature of psoriatic arthritis was again emphasized, using as criteria the absence of rheumatoid factor and the presence of HLA-B27, enthesitis, and spondylitis.[6–8] Furthermore, whereas rheumatoid arthritis commonly regresses with advancing HIV infection, psoriatic arthritis becomes more prevalent and intense.[9–11]

EPIDEMIOLOGY

Psoriatic arthritis is found in just under 10 percent of individuals with psoriasis,[12,13] but some series report a much higher prevalence that could reflect in part the absence of sensitive and fully developed criteria for diagnosing joint involvement.[14] If the frequency of psoriasis is between 1 and 3 percent, the prevalence of psoriatic arthritis in the general Caucasian population, according to current criteria, would be from 0.05 to 0.24 percent, a value approaching half that of the prevalence of seropositive rheumatoid arthritis and in agreement with recent prevalence studies.[13] A critical review of the syndromic criteria used to diagnose psoriatic arthritis emphasized that all currently used classification/diagnosis criteria have a high specificity but low sensitivity, including those of Moll and Wright, the European Spondyloarthropathy Study Group, and the Amor classification criteria.[15] Importantly, criteria with low sensitivity fail to provide sufficient guidance to the physician for patient diagnosis.

A MODEL OF THE STAGES OF DISEASE PATHOGENESIS

In common with other autoimmune diseases, psoriasis and, subsequently, psoriatic arthritis can be considered to develop in stages, beginning with genetically defined predisposition and ending with overt joint disease (Fig. 43-1). The following sections describe in some detail the stages in the pathogenesis of psoriatic arthritis.

FIGURE 43-1

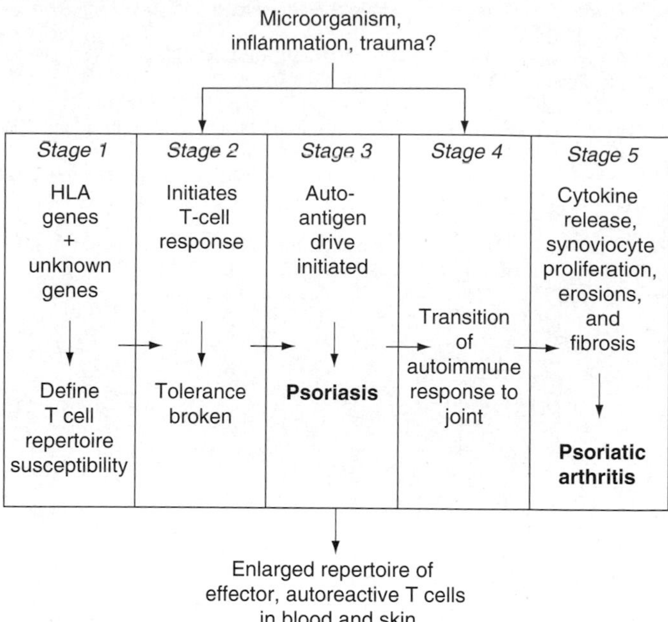

Hypothetical stages in the development of psoriasis or psoriatic arthritis. The first stage is one of genetically defined susceptibility. MHC class I molecules, self-peptides, and other, still unknown genes interact to select a T cell repertoire that has the property of recognizing a self-peptide critical to the pathogenesis of psoriasis or psoriatic arthritis. The second compartment depicts several possible initiation events where the T cell clones selected in stage one are triggered to recognize a self-peptide. This physiologic adaptive immune response is initiated by a specific microorganism or by nonantigen-specific inflammation or trauma. In the third stage, the unlimited amount of self-peptide autoantigen drives the immune response to clonal expansion and an effector phenotype that results in psoriasis. In the fourth stage, these T cell clones acquire the ability to respond to a self-antigen of the joint. In the final stage, these clones acquire the potential to injure the joint by the release of chemokines that recruit and activate monocytes and nonantigen-specific T cells. Multiple inflammatory mechanisms characterize this stage.

Stage One: Genetic Factors Defining Predisposition

Typically, the predisposition phase lasts two or more decades. Germline genes contribute in an important way to the definition of the predisposition to develop psoriasis and psoriatic arthritis, as is shown by the strong familial aggregation of psoriatic arthritis and high twin concordance rates.[16] Psoriatic arthritis or psoriasis was found in 40 percent of first-degree relatives of those with the same disease,[17] a likelihood forty-fold greater than that of their unaffected spouses.[6,18,19] The ratio of familial psoriatic arthritis prevalence to its population prevalence (λ_s) is 20 to 30, being much greater than that for rheumatoid arthritis. Some relatives of a psoriatic arthritis proband may exhibit only typical psoriasis; others may have only an atypical undifferentiated spondyloarthritis; and still others may exhibit classic psoriatic arthritis and psoriasis.[18]

The inheritance of psoriatic arthritis has a mixed pattern found in many autoimmune diseases that either simulates a partially dominant mode of inheritance that is incompletely penetrant[1] or fits a recessive mode.[20] The concordance rate for psoriatic arthritis in both members of an identical twinship is 30 to 40 percent,[16] suggesting that only a third of those with a genetic predisposition actually develop psoriatic arthritis. This finding suggests that the development of psoriatic arthritis depends on nongerm-line–encoded events that could be environmental, involving infection or trauma,[21] or stochastic factors such as T cell repertoire development.

HLA CLASS I GENES INVOLVED IN DETERMINING SUSCEPTIBILITY The first report of a specific allele marking susceptibility to psoriatic arthritis was by Brewerton et al.,[8] who identified a HLA-B27 allele in approximately 20 percent of patients with the peripheral joint involvement of psoriatic arthritis. In addition, the influence of immunogenetic factors on the pattern of joint involvement in psoriatic arthritis was shown by an increase of the frequency of HLA-B27 to approximately 70 percent in patients with spine involvement. These studies have been widely confirmed.[2,19,22] In some populations, additional rare class I alleles, such as HLA-B38 and HLA-B39, are associated with psoriatic arthritis,[23] but not with psoriasis. These alleles appear to be functional alternatives to HLA-B27 in terms of analogous peptide-binding properties, but they do not share ancestral haplotypes with HLA-B27 alleles.

Other class I MHC alleles also have been implicated, including HLA-B13 and HLA-B57. These alleles sharply distinguish psoriatic arthritis from the other spondyloarthritides that do not exhibit any associations of susceptibility with them. The allele group characterized by HLA-Cw6 is found in strong linkage disequilibrium with both HLA-B57 and HLA-B13, but not with HLA-B27, HLA-B38, or HLA-B39; this observation provides the first molecular evidence of potential genetic heterogeneity in psoriatic arthritis (see Chaps. 24 and 42). HLA-Cw6 is present in well over half of all persons with psoriatic arthritis in some studies.[23,24] Alleles encoding HLA-B13 and HLA-B57 are also in strong linkage disequilibrium with the HLA-DR7 and the DQA1*0201 alleles, emphasizing the large genomic distances over which ancestral haplotypes extend. HLA-DR7 and the DQA1*0201 alleles have also been reported at increased frequency in psoriatic arthritis and psoriasis.[25,26] A recent study suggests that the major region determining susceptibility to psoriatic arthritis is centromeric of the HLA-B locus.[27]

At this time, the most probable interpretation of the association of HLA-B27 and the second group of HLA class I alleles, including HLA-B13, HLA-B57, and HLA-Cw6, with the susceptibility to develop psoriasis or psoriatic arthritis, is that these HLA molecules act to select a particular repertoire of CD8 T cells by binding and presenting certain self-peptides during the phase of positive thymic selection of the T cell repertoire. The presence of a T cell repertoire containing clones that can react with a particular self-peptide is a necessary but insufficient condition for psoriatic arthritis.

Stage Two: Triggering of Self-Tolerant T Cells

The second stage of the disease is activation of one or a few clones of CD8 T cells directed to a self-antigen in what is the first part of an adaptive immune response. If tolerization to self in the negative selection phase of repertoire formation were efficient, it would remove all the clones produced in the positive selection phase, because these were all selected on self-peptides. The individuals with psoriatic susceptibility alleles are left with potentially self-reactive CD8 T cells in their repertoire. In some instances, the clone may be in a state termed *clonal ignorance* rather than tolerance, because the provision of appropriate costimulatory signals to the T cells by accessory molecules will result in the response of the T cell clone. The events that trigger the CD8 T cells to become autoreactive are unknown.

Stage Three: Clonal Expansion and the Development of Psoriasis

The third phase of the immunopathogenesis of the immune response leading up to clinical skin disease consists of further substantive CD8 T cell clonal expansion and differentiation to an effector phenotype driven by psoriatic self antigens, as depicted in the third compartment in Fig. 43-1. Typically, the phase of psoriasis without joint involvement lasts nearly another decade until the phase of overt arthritis is precipitated. Detailed aspects of this adaptive immune response are covered in Chap. 42. Ultimately, the number of effector T cell clones with the requisite specificities accumulates to a level capable of initiating a disease-inducing autoimmune response to dermal keratinocytes.

Stage Four: Transition of the Autoimmune Response to the Joint

In a subset of individuals with psoriasis, the autoimmune response advances to involve the joint in what appears to be a similar disease process. There are two alternative possibilities. The autoimmune response affecting the joint is identical to that affecting the skin in terms of peptide recognition, or there is an additional joint-specific immune response that recognizes a peptide distinct from that recognized in keratinocytes. In either case, the development of joint inflammation appears to require a large pool of expanded antigen-reactive CD8 T cell clones with an effector cell phenotype.

Stage Five: Development of Joint Inflammation and Injury

A model for sustained immune stimulation responsible for stage five (Fig. 43-2) envisions a CD8 T cell that cognitively recognizes the specific self-peptide responsible for psoriasis and psoriatic arthritis and responds with activation and proliferation, which drive the inflammatory response responsible for joint inflammation and destruction. A cascade of secondary immune responses occurs in the joint tissue as a result of this drive. Chemokines and cytokines released by this activation (see Chaps. 26 and 27), act on vascular endothelium and monocyte macrophages to affect their pattern of gene expression, and also instigate the nonantigen-specific recruitment of other CD8 T cells and CD4 T cells into the site of inflammation, as well as additional monocytes. These recruited bystander cells, in turn, release additional cytokines that act on synovial lining cells and other cells in the fibroblast lineage to alter their pattern of gene expression, proliferate, and induce new bone formation, in a manner similar to that postulated for their effect on keratinocytes in psoriatic plaques.[28] The combination of cytokines, chemokines, and other proinflammatory factors from these cell types results in joint and tendon inflammation, destruction, and fibrosis.

NATURE OF THE INFLAMMATORY INFILTRATE IN FULLY DEVELOPED PSORIATIC ARTHRITIS

The striking feature in the synovium and joint fluid of patients with psoriatic arthritis is the presence of a small number of very large CD8 T cell clonal expansions with structural features that strongly imply they result from an autoantigen drive.[29,30] These form groups of structurally related clones with the same CDR3 length and the same or homologous CDR3 amino acid sequences. The CD8 T cell clones are derived from an effector precursor pool that is highly expanded in blood ($>$ 20 cell divisions) and could be the population involved in mediating the skin disease. These cells appear to be the CD8 T cells originally selected in the predisposition phase, and they now drive the psoriatic inflammatory process in an autoantigen-driven adaptive immune response (Fig. 43-2). The activation of these cells and their release of chemokines and cytokines are considered to be the basis of the arthritis and enthesitis.

FIGURE 43-2

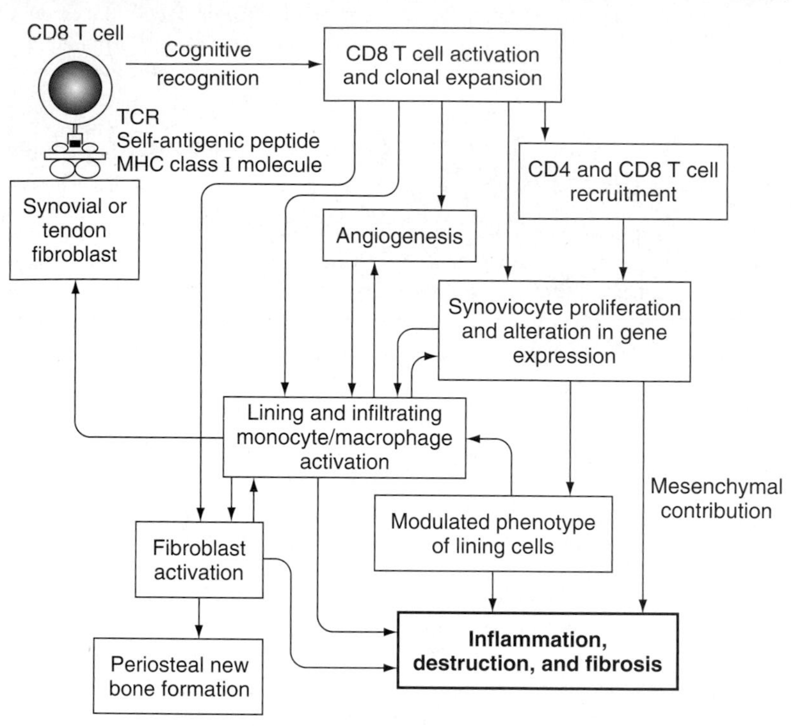

Scheme for pathogenesis of inflammation and tissue destruction in psoriatic arthritis. The process is driven by cognitive recognition of a self-peptide presented to a CD8 T cell by a MHC class I molecule on a joint cell. The ensuing T cell activation and clonal expansion initiates nonantigen-specific recruitment of CD4 and CD8 T cells, angiogenesis, and monocyte recruitment and activation by the release of cytokines and chemokines. The activated cells, in turn, alter patterns of gene expression in cells comprising the joint and related structures. These alterations result in inflammation, fibrosis, new bone formation, erosions, and osteolysis.

The synovium in active arthritis also contains a preponderant infiltrate of polyclonal, nonantigen-specific CD4 T cells (Fig. 43-3), as shown by analysis of the T cell receptor (TCR) β chain (V_β) repertoire at a molecular level.[29,30] These nonantigen-specific T cells arise via recruitment mediated by chemokines, such as monocyte chemotactic protein 1 (MCP-1), which is locally produced in the synovium.[31] Cytokines implicated in the pathogenic process of psoriatic arthritis include interleukin (IL)-6, IL-1β, IL-2, and sIL-2R.[32] T cells in infiltrates elaborate regulated on activation, normal T cell expressed and secreted (RANTES), while macrophages in the lining are gro-α positive, and those in infiltrates are Mig positive.[33] IL-8, a chemokine that could be responsible for the attraction of neutrophils to the joint fluid in psoriatic arthritis is expressed at a high level in the synovial lining cells, and to a lesser extent, in cells located in the perivascular areas. Compared with rheumatoid arthritis synovium, there is markedly less interferon-γ and IL-1 in the psoriatic arthritis synovium. This finding is consistent with the lack of a T_H1 pattern of cytokine production and the dominant role of CD8 T cells.[34] Vascular abnormalities are early histopathologic changes that occur in the psoriatic plaque and are also prominent in the psoriatic synovium; these changes are likely to reflect specific cytokine profiles augmented in the patient with psoriasis. The destruction of cartilage differs from that in rheumatoid arthritis by the presence of minimally elevated levels of aggrecan and greatly increased concentrations of cartilage oligomeric matrix protein.[35]

Other types of bystander-type clonal expansions found in joint fluid are directed to diverse viral and other antigens unrelated to the presumed autoantigens driving the joint disease. These are presumably attracted to the inflammatory milieu and may secondarily contribute to the intensification of arthritis.

The mode of action of methotrexate on the inflammatory T cell infiltrate was recently elucidated by characterization of the T cell repertoire in synovial biopsies of methotrexate-treated patients with full drug-induced remissions.[30] The polyclonal infiltration of predominantly CD4 T cells that dominates the synovium in acute arthritis largely disappears, but the CD8 antigen-driven oligoclonal expansions identified by their sequence remained largely undiminished over 12 to 18 months of therapy. The inability of methotrexate therapy to eliminate the expanded CD8 clones suggests that the methotrexate is suppressive rather than curative. It appears that tumor necrosis factor (TNF) blockade therapy also eliminates major components of the effector pathways of joint inflammation, without significantly altering the lymphocyte populations underlying the autoimmune drive of psoriatic arthritis.[36] Reductions were noted in lining layer thickness, vascularity, and infiltration with neutrophils and macrophages that paralleled the beneficial effect of anti–TNF-α therapy. It is likely that anti-TNF agents exert their beneficial effect largely, if not solely, on the later parts of the inflammatory cascade shown in Fig. 43-2.

CLINICAL MANIFESTATIONS

Onset and Occurrence

Psoriatic arthritis characteristically develops between ages 35 and 45, an average of 10 years after the appearance of psoriasis, but can occur at nearly any age. Onset earlier in adulthood or in childhood is associated with a heightened likelihood of developing destructive arthritis. Typically, early onset psoriatic arthritis occurs in a setting of a strong family history of the disease.[17] The sex ratio parallels that of psoriasis, with a preponderance of females in early childhood, but an essentially equivalent incidence in both sexes in adults.

The onset of arthritis is usually insidious, but occasionally is abrupt, sometimes following a joint injury. In these latter cases, the intensity of the disease may suggest Reiter's syndrome or gout. The subsequent course of posttraumatic psoriatic arthritis is indistinguishable from that of spontaneous onset arthritis.[37] Pitting edema of the hands or feet, sometimes asymmetric, secondary to enthesitis and tenosynovitis has been reported as a first, isolated manifestation of psoriatic arthritis.[38] The development of insidious inflammatory back pain is an important clue to the recognition of axial disease, and this symptom may be the initial manifestation of psoriatic arthritis (Table 43-2). Constitutional features, including fever and malaise, are uncommon and usually are evident only in a fulminant onset with widespread joint disease. However, the erythrocyte sedimentation rate and the serum complement level are commonly elevated, reflecting activation of acute phase reactants by cytokines.[19]

Skin Disease

Susceptibility to the development and severity of arthritis generally increases with the severity of cutaneous involvement. However, remissions and exacerbations of the joint disease correlate poorly with similar changes in the skin disease.[12]

FIGURE 43-3

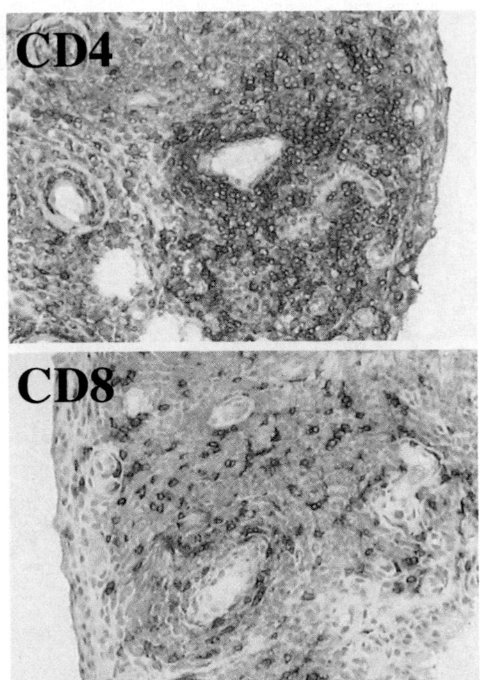

Inflammatory infiltrate of active synovitis in psoriatic arthritis, showing the predominant infiltration of CD4 T cells and somewhat fewer CD8 T cells. (*Courtesy of D. Kane.*)

Joint Disease Patterns and Radiology

The pattern of peripheral joint involvement[2] and the associated findings of nail disease, tenosynovitis, enthesitis, ankylosis, periosteal new bone formation, erosions, osteolysis, and axial involvement provide hallmarks for the recognition of psoriatic arthritis at the bedside and through radiology (Table 43-1; Fig. 43-4). Approximately three-fourths of persons diagnosed with psoriatic arthritis manifest peripheral, usually asymmetric, oligoarthritis that involves the small joints of the hands and feet, the large joints of the legs, or a combination of both small and large joints. When only a few joints are involved, the distribution appears asymmetric. The hand involvement can include stiffness and dactylitis that are attributable to enthesitis as well as synovitis. Dactylitis is strongly suggestive of psoriatic arthritis when it occurs in an individual with psoriasis.[39] Deformity secondary to fibrosis and contractures may occur. The classic pencil-in-cup joint is sometimes seen, consisting of symmetric and conical osteolysis of the proximal head, with enlargement of the base of the distal head by new bone formation. Acral osteolysis and erosions at the tip of the tuft of the digit are characteristic, especially when they involve the hallux. Ankylosis of one or more isolated joints is another distinctive feature due to fibrosis

TABLE 43-2

Inflammatory Back Pain from Spondylitis, Sacroiliitis, or Axial Enthesitis as Initial Manifestation of Psoriatic Arthritis

- Onset before age 40
- Insidious dull, deep buttock or low back pain
- Poorly localized; does not follow nerve root
- Persists > 3 months
- Stiffness/pain on arising in the morning or during sleep
- Improvement with exercise
- Differential diagnosis from mechanical or degenerative spine disease

and new bone formation. Sometimes the initial or only manifestation of psoriatic arthritis is hallux rigidus, implying the subtle nature of joint inflammation and the need for its earlier recognition.

Inflammation of one or many of the distal interphalangeal joints is virtually pathognomonic for psoriatic arthritis or Reiter's syndrome; it need only be distinguished from Heberden's nodes, which occur in a form of osteoarthritis infection, or crystalline arthritides such as gout. In addition to the points of distinction summarized in Table 43-3, the distal interphalangeal joint is rarely, if ever, affected by rheumatoid arthritis. Typically, nail involvement is marked in the digit affected with arthritis, and there may be additional evidence of acral keratodystrophy.

The large joints that are affected in psoriatic arthritis include the hips, knees, and ankles. Often only a single hip or knee joint is involved; the dominant diagnostic considerations in adults include degenerative osteoarthritis or posttraumatic arthritis rather than psoriatic arthritis. Posttraumatic forms of psoriatic arthritis in athletes are particularly challenging to distinguish from purely mechanical injuries. In approximately 5 percent of persons with psoriatic arthritis, the character of the joint injury becomes profoundly destructive with marked osteolysis, resulting in what is sometimes referred to as *arthritis mutilans*. In rare instances this process is generalized, but much more commonly one or a few joints are characterized by destruction out of proportion to the remainder of the illness. Pustular psoriasis or erythroderma is more common among this group.[40]

In occasional patients the sternomanubrial and temporomandibular joints may become involved, in association with extensive typical psoriatic arthritis. Certain syndromes simulate psoriatic arthritis but increasingly appear to be distinct entities; these include the anterior chest wall syndrome of sternomanubrial or costoclavicular involvement, where sternomanubrial disease occurs in isolation; the so-called SAPHO syndrome; and recurrent multifocal osteomyelitis. See reference 41 for a brief review of these entities.

Axial involvement is often most evident in the lower spine and sacroiliac joints. The predisposition to axial involvement is strongly influenced by the presence of HLA-B27. Scattered submarginal syndesmophytes and apophyseal or odontoid erosions without vertebral squaring or ligamentous calcification are found. Sometimes the nonmarginal syndesmophytes become bulky, broad paravertebral excrescences that contrast with the vertically oriented outgrowths of bone in the outer margins of the annulus fibrosus in ankylosing spondylitis.[42,43] Vertebral squaring from new bone formation, apophyseal joint involvement, and ligamentous calcification in the lumbar spine are similar to those found in ankylosing spondylitis. Asymmetric or symmetric sacroiliitis is frequent and is readily identified by computed tomography (CT) or magnetic resonance (MR) imaging. Symphysitis is also present. CT and MR imaging are far more sensitive and specific than conventional x-rays for demonstrating sacroiliitis.[44] By directly imaging changes in the synovium, articular cartilage, and subchondral bone, MR imaging is the most sensitive and specific technique for detecting sacroiliitis and other changes in the axial skeleton.[44]

Whether ascertainment of joint involvement by clinical and classic x-ray procedures in those with psoriasis is adequate has been the subject of several studies with newer imaging modalities such as radionuclide scanning, ultrasonography, and nuclear MR imaging. In a study using MR imaging to examine the frequency of hand involvement in patients with nummular and/or plaque psoriasis who did not have arthritic symptoms, Offidani et al.[45] found that 68 percent of patients with psoriasis had at least one arthritic sign, such as soft-tissue swelling, periarticular effusion, joint effusion–synovial pannus, tendon sheath effusion, bone erosion, subluxation, bone cysts, and subchondral signal intensity abnormalities; by contrast, standard x-rays revealed joint abnormalities in only 32 percent. The ability of magnetic resonance to image

FIGURE 43-4

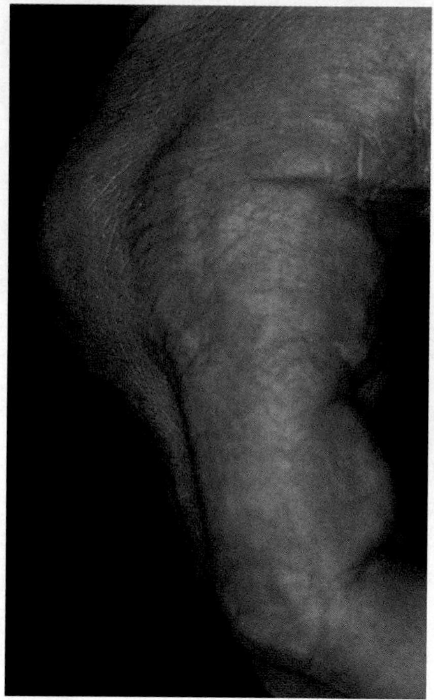

A.

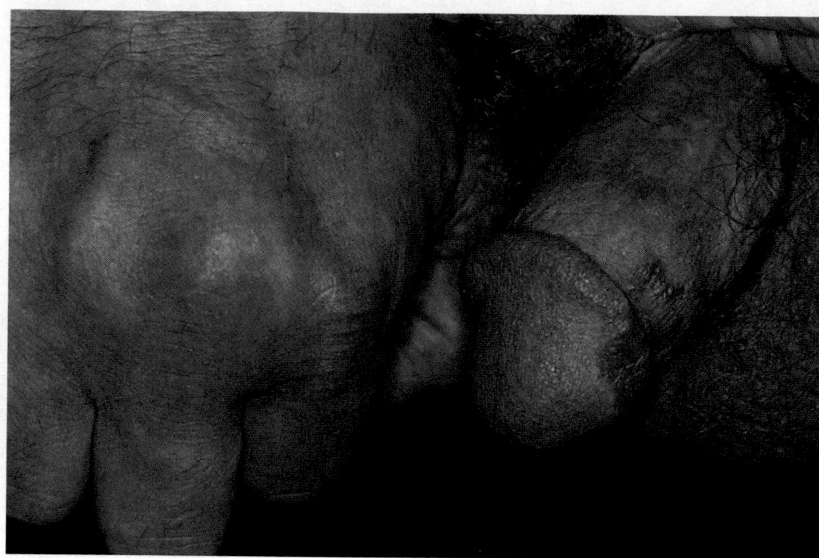

B.

Psoriatic arthritis, acute, monarticular. Arthritis and psoriasis presented coincidentally in a 42-year-old male. *A.* Acute arthritis of the metacarpophalangeal joint. *B.* The patient was unaware of any psoriatic lesions; however, psoriatic lesions were noted on the penis and intergluteal cleft, associated with the development of pits in the fingernails.

ligaments and cartilage is a particular strength, as is its ability to identify tissue edema or small effusions by various types of signal weighting. In a report by Barozzi et al.,[46] ultrasonography was shown to delineate the swelling of the entheses and the peritendinous soft tissues, as well as the distention of adjacent bursae by fluid collections. MR imaging showed the inflammation of the bone adjacent to the insertion as well as the soft tissue changes.

TABLE 43-3

Contrasts between Psoriatic Arthritis and Rheumatoid Arthritis

	Psoriatic Arthritis	Rheumatoid Arthritis
Elevated ESR*	Yes	Yes
Susceptibility alleles	MHC class I	MHC class II
Amelioration with progressive HIV infection	No	Yes
Implied class of lymphocytes driving inflammation	CD8	CD4
Autoantibodies	No	Yes
Immune complexes	No	Yes
Vasculitis	No	Yes
Fibroblastic response	Yes	No
Sacroiliitis	Yes	No
Enthesitis, dactylitis	Yes	No

*ESR, erythrocyte sedimentation rate.

Tenosynovitis and Enthesitis

Tenosynovitis, dactylitis, and enthesitis are hallmarks of psoriatic arthritis and the other spondyloarthritides. They are not found in rheumatoid arthritis. Enthesitis may be quite subtle and is sometimes relatively easy to overlook. It may present only as nonspecific foot pain, "tennis elbow" in the nondominant hand, or isolated posterior tibial tendinitis, which are not considered by the patient to be part of the illness. Enthesitis is commonly widespread and often symmetric, a point that differentiates it from posttraumatic tendon injury. Bone scintigraphy is often useful in identifying the precise location of the sometimes asymptomatic enthesitis.

Nail Disease

Onychodystrophy, nail pitting, subungual keratosis, Beau's lines (ridging), leukonychia, crumbling nail plate, and discoloration are more strongly associated with arthritis than with psoriasis alone, being found in 85 percent of those with arthritis versus 31 percent of those with the isolated cutaneous form of the disease.[47] The most prevalent findings are pitting and onycholysis. Onychodystrophy is closely related to involvement of the distal interphalangeal joint of the same digit, suggesting a broader acral dystrophic state. The appearance of onychodystrophy is closely related in time to the appearance of the arthritis.

Pediatric Psoriatic Arthritis

Psoriatic arthritis in children usually resembles the disease in adults; however, monarticular disease, often presenting in the knee, is much more prevalent, especially during the early stages of disease. Juvenile psoriatic arthritis has a peak incidence with female preponderance between 2 and 4 years of age and a second peak in both sexes beginning at age 11 to 12 years that extends into adulthood. Psoriatic arthritis appears earlier than the other forms of juvenile spondyloarthritides.[48] In contrast to the usual sequence in adults, almost half of juvenile patients presented with arthritis before skin disease, with the interval between the onset of arthritis and psoriasis as long as 8 years.[49] Psoriasis, or a positive family history of psoriasis, usually provides the diagnosis, but if it is absent, diagnosis is often delayed due to the similarities of the disorder with pauciarticular juvenile rheumatoid arthritis. Axial arthritis is common in juvenile spondyloarthritis and is often associated with HLA-B27. Axial involvement is less frequent in juvenile psoriatic arthritis, but when it occurs, it is associated with an increased incidence of HLA-B27. Potentially ominous chronic anterior uveitis, indistinguishable from that seen in young (ages 2 to 4 years) girls with juvenile rheumatoid arthritis, is found in about 15 percent of patients with juvenile psoriatic arthritis and frequently occurs with antinuclear antibodies (ANA).[50] This finding places this subset of juvenile psoriatic arthritis apart from the other juvenile spondyloarthritides, with which it is commonly grouped.[51] The uveitis that occurs in the other spondyloarthritides is typically acute and self-limited, and ANA are not a feature.

The long-term course of juvenile psoriatic arthritis is typically polyarticular with asymmetric involvement of both upper and lower extremities and prominent digital involvement. Criteria have been developed for the classification of childhood psoriatic arthritis where, in addition to the presence of arthritis and psoriasis or a positive family history for these disorders, emphasis is placed on dactylitis, nail pitting, symmetry of arthritis, disease course (oligoarthritis or polyarthritis), ANA, and uveitis.[52] Of five HLA-B27 children reported with what was termed juvenile reactive arthritis after *Salmonella enteritidis* infection, three developed typical psoriasis in the months after the arthritis[53]; this finding emphasizes the interplay between various precipitating events and the development of what is classified as psoriatic arthritis.

Psoriatic Arthritis and HIV Infection

In North America and most of Europe, the considerable earlier problem of psoriasis, psoriatic arthritis, and Reiter's syndrome has abated to some degree in parallel with better antiretroviral therapy and management of other infections; but in some regions of the world these complications of HIV remain a major problem (see ref. 41). The onset of psoriatic arthritis in HIV-infected individuals may appear explosive, with many features indistinguishable from those of Reiter's syndrome, including an antecedent infection with an arthritogenic gram-negative organism, or they may appear in a more insidious manner.[9–11,54] However, the psoriasiform skin disease is usually more severe.[55] The progression of the arthritis takes two general forms: an accumulative pattern evolving to full intensity over several weeks to months, or the more common, milder, intermittent pattern of recrudescences and remissions. The accumulative form is often associated with widespread polyarticular but asymmetric arthritis and is characterized by synovial thickening, erosions, and juxtaarticular osteoporosis. Hand and upper extremity involvement predominates in the accumulative pattern. The intermittent form usually has oligoarticular knee or ankle joint involvement. Severe enthesopathy of the Achilles tendon, plantar fascia, and anterior or posterior tibial tendons may cause some patients to exhibit a characteristic broad-based "AIDS" gait, walking with the feet in inversion and extension in an attempt to diminish pain by distributing weight on the lateral margins. Multidigit dactylitis frequently occurs and, in combination with plantar fasciitis and extensor tenosynovitis, may simulate cellulitis or pedal edema. Whereas synovitis of the knee is prominent, hip disease and shoulder girdle involvement are uncommon. Axial involvement appears to be uncommon, with sacroiliitis only occasionally present.

The cutaneous manifestations overlap those of HIV-associated Reiter's syndrome (see Chap. 182). The rash often resembles widespread pustular psoriasis with a greater tendency for involvement of the groin and intertriginous regions (inverse or sebopsoriasis). A progressive intensification of changes in the distal digits is often very prominent. Acrokeratosis is common, often associated with erythema and periungual pseudoparonychia formation. Severe alterations in the nails of the hands and feet often accompany distal interphalangeal joint (DIP) involvement and are manifested clinically as onychodystrophy with or without subungual hyperkeratoses.

COURSE AND PROGNOSIS

For most patients with psoriatic arthritis, the musculoskeletal manifestations are much milder than those of rheumatoid arthritis. After 8 years of disease, two-thirds of patients with psoriatic arthritis were effectively employed,[56,57] and only 8 percent progressed to an advanced stage of musculoskeletal impairment.[58] However, despite a much greater degree of vitality among those with psoriatic arthritis, evaluation showed quality of life to be diminished as much as in patients with rheumatoid arthritis.[59]

Several patterns of disease progression are evident. For most, the arthritis waxes and wanes in severity, but remains persistently active. About one-fifth of prospectively followed patients experience sustained remissions that last an average of 2.6 years.[60] Among the remainder with persistently active disease, mild but sometimes troublesome localized disease, such as foot pain or recurrent tendinitis or enthesitis, forms a dominant pattern of involvement. For these individuals the overall prognosis is very good. Other patients with psoriatic arthritis progress to fibrous or bony ankylosis of one or a few joints, which may be unnoticed if there are no occupational demands. In yet another pattern, largely asymptomatic axial joint involvement, not ameliorated by any of the specific therapeutic measures, progresses independently of the state of the skin or peripheral joint disease.[61] A few patients with psoriatic arthritis have severe and sustained joint involvement or enthesitis, especially in the HIV-associated form. Persons with hip or knee involvement may eventually require joint replacement.

TREATMENT

Drugs available for treatment of psoriatic arthritis fall into two categories: agents such as nonsteroidal anti-inflammatory drugs (NSAIDs) and sulfasalazine, which have no, or minimal beneficial effect on skin disease; and others, such as etretinate, methotrexate, cyclosporin A, or TNF blockers, which usually benefit both skin and joint disease. The choice among the various agents is dictated by the relative intensity of the cutaneous and articular involvement.

Mild to Moderate Joint Involvement

For most patients with mild to moderate joint involvement or enthesitis, the goals of therapy are the control of inflammation with NSAIDs or analgesics, the maintenance of joint range of motion and function by physical therapy, and the avoidance of potentially injurious extreme joint stress through counseling against repetitive injury. NSAIDs do not appreciably alter the natural history of arthritis, but they do lessen stiffness and pain and thus increase range of motion.

Several biochemical families of NSAIDs or analgesics are available for therapy. Although these agents have some differences in anti-inflammatory efficacy and toxicity, choosing which NSAID to start is mainly dictated by physician experience and the individual response of a patient. Naproxen and indomethacin are traditionally considered representative of NSAIDs with the greatest efficacy in treating spondyloarthritides. Adverse effects shared by all NSAIDs include gastric and renal toxicity; hypersensitivity reactions; central nervous system effects, in particular tinnitus and headache; and coagulation abnormalities. In some patients with psoriasis, NSAIDs induce an idiosyncratic flare of the psoriatic skin lesions, possibly the result of the enhanced production of leukotrienes that occurs with cyclooxygenase inhibition. Most patients have had experience with self-prescribed drugs of this class; and before NSAID therapy is initiated, patients should be asked whether aspirin has caused a flare of psoriasis.

Lack of adequate response to NSAIDs or the presence of progressive or moderate to severe arthritis usually requires additional drug therapy. Intraarticular glucocorticoid injections may relieve an isolated episode of severe synovitis. Injections into the tendon sheaths, usually under ultrasound imaging, may be particularly effective in reducing enthesitis. Systemic glucocorticoid therapy should usually be avoided because of low efficacy coupled with the risks of inciting a transition to pustular psoriasis and a rebound of the skin disease on withdrawal. Sulfasalazine is helpful in reducing clinical parameters of joint disease activity in approximately 30 to 40 percent of patients in extensively documented double blind trials,[62] especially in those with spondylitis.[63] Untoward reactions have been few, mainly a hypersensitivity dermatitis or gastrointestinal intolerance. Parenteral or oral gold salts are rarely used because of their limited efficacy.[62]

Severe Destructive Arthritis

For the treatment of severe destructive arthritis, NSAIDs are supplemented with a more potent anti-inflammatory agent with immunomodulatory properties, such as methotrexate, cyclosporin A, or TNF blockers. The efficacy of both parenteral and, to a lesser degree, oral methotrexate has been extensively documented, and this drug is the current mainstay of therapy for severe arthritis.[64,65] The better-documented efficacy of parenteral methotrexate suggests that this route of administration may be optimal for initial or maintenance therapy in instances of more severe disease.[62] The side effects of methotrexate are discussed in Chaps. 42 and 256. Minimal immune impairment is sometimes encountered, and the uncommon possibility of developing opportunistic infections such as *Pneumocystis carinii* should be kept in mind in the differential diagnosis of pneumonitis developing during methotrexate therapy.

In view of the important role of TNF-α as an effector of inflammation in psoriatic arthritis, the anti–TNF agents etanercept and infliximab are taking a place in the therapy of severe destructive psoriatic arthritis, especially in individuals who do not respond to methotrexate.[66–68] Parallel improvement in skin lesions usually occurs. In one 12-week trial, 73 percent of patients treated with etanercept given subcutaneously twice weekly exhibited an improvement in ACR20 as compared to 13 percent in the placebo group. This is a relatively modest response criteria set, but other less well-controlled studies indicate a greater joint response. Infliximab, administered intravenously at weeks 0, 2, and 6 resulted in marked improvement of arthritis and clearing of some histologic features of inflammation.[36] Considering the central role of TNF-α in the effector arm of the adaptive and innate immune response, blockade of this pathway will subtly impair immunity, as is reflected by instances of activation of latent *Mycobacterium tuberculosis* infection with therapy.[69] The evolving guidelines for use of these blockers should be consulted before therapy is considered. Attention to the development of anti-DNA antibodies and other evidence of autoimmunity with therapy is also warranted.

Cyclosporin A improves both the skin and the joint disease in about 50 percent of patients treated with it. Improvement in skin disease occurs after 2 to 6 weeks of treatment, whereas joint disease took longer to improve.[63,70] Within 4 weeks of discontinuing the drug, exacerbations of both skin and joint disease appeared. Untoward effects of cyclosporin A include usually reversible renal toxicity, with hypertension and azotemia, and the uncommon potential for the development of Epstein-Barr virus-related B cell lymphomas.

The place of DNA antimetabolites in the therapy of psoriatic arthritis has not received extensive analysis. Azathioprine was comparable in efficacy to methotrexate in a randomized trial.[62] Mycophenolate mofetil was used in six patients with psoriatic arthritis with good results.[71] A single report of the notable efficacy of 6-thioguanine in the treatment of psoriasis, associated with the depletion and induction of apoptosis in activated T lymphocytes, suggests that this compound may be beneficial in severe psoriatic arthritis as a complement to the mode of action of methotrexate and TNF blockade.[72]

HIV Infection

In psoriatic arthritis associated with HIV infection, NSAIDs such as naproxen are the first line of therapy. However, in many patients, this drug does not adequately control inflammation, especially the very disabling enthesitis. Etretinate may be particularly useful in the treatment of this form of psoriatic arthritis because it lacks immunosuppressive effects.[73] Methotrexate, although effective in this setting, has been associated with the abrupt development of opportunistic infection and death in individuals with advanced HIV infection.[10] Therefore, methotrexate and similar potentially immunosuppressive agents must be used with caution. Attention should be directed toward monitoring viral levels and overall immunologic competency during such therapy. The use of etanercept to treat psoriatic arthritis associated with HIV infection achieved an excellent clinical response of the skin and joint manifestations, but the drug had to be discontinued because of the development of multiple infections.[74] These observations emphasize the need for considering the presence of HIV infection when instituting immunosuppressive therapy in an individual with recent onset severe psoriatic arthritis.

Surgery and Related Techniques

Arthroscopic synovectomy or intraarticular injection of short-lived radioactive isotopes of elements such as ytterbium are experimental approaches that have been effective in treating instances of severe chronic monarticular synovitis. Because of the enhanced tendency to fibrosis associated with these therapies, anti-inflammatory and physical therapy measures aimed at improving range of motion are important adjuncts to these interventions. Joint replacement and forms of reconstructive therapy are appropriate in situations of advanced joint destruction. Anecdotal reports of the recurrence of psoriatic arthritis in the setting of a fully reconstituted donor marrow suggest that this approach, while promising for rheumatoid arthritis, is not likely to succeed in psoriatic arthritis.[75]

REFERENCES

1. Moll JM, Wright V: Psoriatic arthritis. *Semin Arthritis Rheum* **3**:55, 1973
2. Marsal S et al: Clinical, radiographic and HLA associations as markers for different patterns of psoriatic arthritis. *Rheumatology (Oxford)* **38**:332, 1999
3. Zias, J, Mitchell P: Psoriatic arthritis in a fifth-century Judean Desert monastery. *Am J Phys Anthropol* **101**:491, 1996
4. Hench PS: Arthropathia psoriatica: Presentation of a case. *Proc Staff Meet Mayo Clin* **2**:89, 1927

5. Bauer W et al: The pathology of joint lesions in patients with psoriasis and arthritis. *Trans Assoc Am Physicians* **56**:349, 1941
6. Wright V: Psoriasis and arthritis. *Ann Rheum Dis* **15**:348, 1956
7. Ball J: Enthesopathy of rheumatoid and ankylosing spondylitis. *Ann Rheum Dis* **30**:213, 1971
8. Brewerton DA et al: HL-A 27 and arthropathies associated with ulcerative colitis and psoriasis. *Lancet* **1**:956, 1974
9. Johnson TM et al: AIDS exacerbates psoriasis. *N Engl J Med* **313**:1415, 1985
10. Winchester R et al: The co-occurrence of Reiter's syndrome and acquired immunodeficiency. *Ann Intern Med* **106**:19, 1987
11. Winchester R et al: Implications from the occurrence of Reiter's syndrome and related disorders in association with advanced HIV infection. *Scand J Rheumatol* **74**:89, 1988
12. Hellgren L: Association between rheumatoid arthritis and psoriasis in total populations. *Acta Rheumatol Scand* **15**:316, 1969
13. Shbeeb M et al: The epidemiology of psoriatic arthritis in Olmsted County, Minnesota, USA, 1982. *J Rheumatol* **27**:1247, 2000
14. Gladman DD, Brockbank J: Psoriatic arthritis. *Expert Opin Investig Drugs* **9**:1511, 2000
15. Salvarani C et al: Psoriatic arthritis. *Curr Opin Rheumatol* **10**:299, 1998
16. Gottlieb M et al: Discordance for psoriatic arthropathy in monozygotic twins. *Arthritis Rheum* **22**:805, 1979
17. Rahman P et al: Comparison of clinical and immunogenetic features in familial versus sporadic psoriatic arthritis. *Clin Exp Rheumatol* **18**:7, 2000
18. Moll JMH et al: Associations between ankylosing spondylitis, psoriatic arthritis, Reiter's disease, the intestinal arthropathies and Behçet's syndrome. *Medicine (Baltimore)* **53**:343, 1974
19. Kammer GM et al: Psoriatic arthritis: A clinical, immunologic, and HLA study of 100 patients. *Semin Arthritis Rheum* **9**:75, 1979
20. Swanbeck G et al: A population genetic study of psoriasis. *Br J Dermatol* **131**:32, 1994
21. Moll JMH, Wright V: Familial occurrence of psoriatic arthritis. *Ann Rheum Dis* **22**:181, 1973
22. Gerber LH et al: Human lymphocyte antigens characterizing psoriatic arthritis and its subtypes. *J Rheumatol* **9**:703, 1982
23. Arnett FC, Bias WB: HLA-Bw38 and Bw39 in psoriatic arthritis: Relationships and implications for peripheral and axial involvement. *Arthritis Rheum* **23**:649, 1980
24. Tiilikainen A et al: Psoriasis and HLA-Cw6. *Br J Dermatol* **102**:179, 1980
25. Ikaheimo I et al: Immunogenetic profile of psoriasis vulgaris: Association with haplotypes A2, B13, Cw6, DR7, DQA1*0201 and A1, B17, Cw6, DR7, DQA1*0201. *Arch Dermatol Res* **288**:63, 1996
26. Schmitt-Egenolf M et al: Familial juvenile onset psoriasis is associated with the human leukocyte antigen (HLA) class I side of the extended haplotype Cw6-B57-DRB1*0701-DQA1*0201-DQB1*0303: A population- and family-based study. *J Invest Dermatol* **106**:711, 1996
27. Gonzalez S et al: Polymorphism in MICA rather than HLA-B/C genes is associated with psoriatic arthritis in the Jewish population. *Hum Immunol* **62**:632, 2001
28. Grossman RM et al: Interleukin 6 is expressed in high levels in psoriatic skin and stimulated proliferation of cultured human keratinocytes. *Proc Nat Acad Sci USA* **86**:6367, 1989
29. Costello PJ et al: Psoriatic arthritis joint fluids are characterized by CD8 and CD4 T cell clonal expansions appear antigen driven. *J Immunol* **166**:2878, 2001
30. Curran SA et al: Psoriatic arthritis synovium is characterised by non-antigen-specific T cells that are selectively suppressed by methotrexate therapy. *Arthritis Rheumatol* **44**:S235, 2001
31. Ross EL et al: Localized monocyte chemotactic protein-1 production correlates with T cell infiltration of synovium in patients with psoriatic arthritis. *J Rheumatol* **27**:2432, 2000
32. Wong WM et al: Interleukin-2 is found in the synovium of psoriatic arthritis and spondyloarthritis, not in rheumatoid arthritis. *Scand J Rheumatol* **25**:239, 1996
33. Konig A et al: Mig, GRO alpha and RANTES messenger RNA expression in lining layer, infiltrates and different leucocyte populations of synovial tissue from patients with rheumatoid arthritis, psoriatic arthritis and osteoarthritis. *Virchows Arch* **436**:449, 2000
34. Canete JD et al: Differential Th1/Th2 cytokine patterns in chronic arthritis: Interferon gamma is highly expressed in synovium of rheumatoid arthritis compared with seronegative spondyloarthropathies. *Ann Rheum Dis* **59**:263, 2000
35. Mansson B et al: Release of cartilage and bone macromolecules into synovial fluid: Differences between psoriatic arthritis and rheumatoid arthritis. *Ann Rheum Dis* **60**:27, 2001
36. Baeten D et al: Immunomodulatory effects of anti-tumor necrosis factor alpha therapy on synovium in spondyloarthropathy: Histologic findings in eight patients from an open-label pilot study. *Arthritis Rheum* **44**:186, 2001
37. Punzi L et al: Clinical, laboratory and immunogenetic aspects of post-traumatic psoriatic arthritis: A study of 25 patients. *Clin Exp Rheumatol* **16**:277, 1998
38. Cantini F et al: Distal extremity swelling with pitting edema in psoriatic arthritis: A case-control study. *Clin Exp Rheumatol* **19**:291, 2001
39. Rothschild BM et al: Dactylitis: Implications for clinical practice. *Semin Arthritis Rheum* **28**:41, 1998
40. Koo T et al: Subsets in psoriatic arthritis formed by cluster analysis. *Clin Rheumatol* **20**:36, 2001
41. Winchester R: Psoriatic arthritis and the spectrum of syndromes related to the SAPHO syndrome. *Curr Opin Rheumatol* **11**:251, 1999
42. McEwen C et al: Ankylosing spondylitis and spondylitis accompanying ulcerative colitis, regional enteritis, psoriasis, and Reiter's disease. *Arthritis Rheum* **14**:291, 1971
43. Jones MD et al: Bony overgrowths and abnormal calcifications about the spine. *Radiol Clin North Am* **26**:1213, 1988
44. Luong AA, Salonen DC: Imaging of the seronegative spondyloarthropathies. *Curr Rheumatol Rep* **2**:288, 2000
45. Offidani A et al: Subclinical joint involvement in psoriasis: Magnetic resonance imaging and x-ray findings. *Acta Derm Venereol* **78**:463, 1998
46. Barozzi L et al: Seronegative spondyloarthropathies: Imaging of spondylitis, enthesitis and dactylitis. *Eur J Radiol* **27**(suppl 1):S12, 1998
47. Taggart A, Wright V: Psoriatic arthritis, *in Epidermis: Disorders of Cell Kinetics and Differentiation.* 1990
48. Prieur AM, Chedeville G: Prognostic factors in juvenile idiopathic arthritis. *Curr Rheumatol Rep* **3**:371, 2001
49. Shore A, Ansell BM: Juvenile psoriatic arthritis—An analysis of 60 cases. *J Pediatr* **100**:529, 1982
50. Cabral DA et al: Visual prognosis in children with chronic anterior uveitis and arthritis. *J Rheumatol* **21**:2370, 1994
51. Petty RE: Juvenile psoriatic arthritis, or juvenile arthritis with psoriasis? *Clin Exp Rheumatol* **12**(suppl 10):S55, 1994
52. Roberton DM et al: Juvenile psoriatic arthritis: Followup and evaluation of diagnostic criteria. *J Rheumatol* **23**:166, 1996
53. Kanakoudi-Tsakalidou F et al: Persistent or severe course of reactive arthritis following Salmonella enteritidis infection. A prospective study of 9 cases. *Scand J Rheumatol* **27**:431, 1998
54. Reveille JD et al: Specific amino acid residues in the second hypervariable region of HLA-DQA1 and DQB1 chain genes promote the Ro (SS-A)/La (SS-B) autoantibody responses. *J Immunol* **146**:3871, 1991
55. Duvic M et al: Acquired immunodeficiency syndrome associated psoriasis and Reiter's syndrome. *Arch Dermatol* **123**:1622, 1987
56. Kaarela K et al: Work capacity of patients with inflammatory joint diseases. An eight-year follow-up study. *Scand J Rheumatol* **16**:403, 1987
57. Gladman DD et al: Psoriatic arthritis (PSA)—An analysis of 220 patients. *QJM* **62**:127, 1987
58. Coulton BL et al: Outcome in patients hospitalised for psoriatic arthritis. *Clin Rheum* **8**:261, 1989
59. Husted JA et al: Health-related quality of life of patients with psoriatic arthritis: A comparison with patients with rheumatoid arthritis. *Arthritis Rheum* **45**:151, 2001
60. Gladman DD et al: Remission in psoriatic arthritis. *J Rheumatol* **28**:1045, 2001
61. Hanly JG et al: Psoriatic spondyloarthropathy: A long-term prospective study. *Ann Rheum Dis* **47**:386, 1988
62. Jones G et al: Interventions for psoriatic arthritis. *Cochrane Database Syst Rev* 3, 2000
63. Salvarani C et al: A comparison of cyclosporine, sulfasalazine, and symptomatic therapy in the treatment of psoriatic arthritis. *J Rheumatol* **28**:2274, 2001
64. Zachariae H, Zachariae E: Methotrexate treatment of psoriatic arthritis. *Acta Derm Venereol Suppl (Stockh)* **67**:270, 1987
65. Steinsson K et al: Cyclosporin A in psoriatic arthritis: An open study. *Ann Rheum Dis* **49**:603, 1990
66. Mease PJ et al: Etanercept in the treatment of psoriatic arthritis and psoriasis: A randomised trial. *Lancet* **356**:385, 2000
67. Braun J et al: New treatment options in spondyloarthropathies: Increasing evidence for significant efficacy of anti-tumor necrosis factor therapy. *Curr Opin Rheumatol* **13**:245, 2001
68. Ogilvie AL et al: Treatment of psoriatic arthritis with antitumour necrosis factor-alpha antibody clears skin lesions of psoriasis resistant to treatment with methotrexate. *Br J Dermatol* **144**:587, 2001

69. Keane J et al: Tuberculosis associated with infliximab, a tumor necrosis factor alpha-neutralizing agent. *N Engl J Med* **345**:1098, 2001
70. Mahrle G et al: Anti-inflammatory efficacy of low-dose cyclosporin A in psoriatic arthritis. A prospective multicentre study. *Br J Dermatol* **135**:752, 1996
71. Grundmann-Kollmann M et al: Treatment of chronic plaque-stage psoriasis and psoriatic arthritis with mycophenolate mofetil. *J Am Acad Dermatol* **42**:835, 2000
72. Murphy FP et al: Clinical clearing of psoriasis by 6-thioguanine correlates with cutaneous T-cell depletion via apoptosis: evidence for selective effects on activated T lymphocytes. *Arch Dermatol* **135**:1495, 1999
73. Louthrenoo W: Successful treatment of severe Reiter's syndrome associated with human immunodeficiency virus infection with etretinate. Report of 2 cases. *J Rheumatol* **20**:1243, 1993
74. Aboulafia DM et al: Etanercept for the treatment of human immunodeficiency virus-associated psoriatic arthritis. *Mayo Clin Proc* **75**:1093, 2000
75. Snowden JA et al: Long-term outcome of autoimmune disease following allogeneic bone marrow transplantation. *Arthritis Rheum* **41**:453, 1998

CHAPTER 44

Ming H. Jih
Arash Kimyai-Asadi
Irwin M. Freedberg

Exfoliative Dermatitis

Also referred to as erythroderma, exfoliative dermatitis is an inflammatory skin disease with erythema and scaling that affects nearly the entire cutaneous surface. It may be either primary (idiopathic) or secondary to a variety of drugs or underlying disorders. Primary exfoliative dermatitis has also been referred to as the "red man" or "*l'homme rouge*" syndrome. (See Chap. 138 for a discussion of exfoliative dermatitis associated with drugs; Chap. 157 for a discussion of exfoliative dermatitis associated with cutaneous T cell lymphoma.)

HISTORICAL ASPECTS

The classification of exfoliative dermatitis into Wilson-Brocq (chronic relapsing), Hebra or pityriasis rubra (progressive), and Savill (self-limited) types may have had historical value, but it currently lacks pathophysiologic or clinical utility.

EPIDEMIOLOGY

Exfoliative dermatitis is a rare, yet easily recognized, potentially serious skin condition. Its reported incidence varies widely: from 1 to 71 per 100,000 dermatologic outpatients.[1,2,3] The higher incidences occurred in parts of Asia where the use of traditional medicaments by patients is common. A recent study in the Netherlands found an incidence of 0.9 patients per 100,000 inhabitants.[4] In most case series, men outnumber women in a proportion of two to four men for every one woman, and the mean age is between 40 and 60 years.

ETIOLOGY AND PATHOGENESIS

Although a significant percentage of patients with exfoliative dermatitis have idiopathic disease (approximately 25 percent), the majority of cases result from pre-existing skin diseases, in particular psoriasis (23 percent) and spongiotic disorders (16 percent), cutaneous T cell lymphoma (16 percent), and drug reactions (15 percent).[1–10] A survey of all dermatologists in the Netherlands indicated that, because practitioners refer only a minority of patients to academic centers, the number of idiopathic and malignancy-associated cases may be overestimated in many case series.[4]

The list of drugs that cause exfoliative dermatitis is large and continuously growing (Table 44-1). The association of most of these drugs with exfoliative dermatitis has come from isolated case reports with no clear dose-dependence, although it appears that antiepileptics, cimetidine, lithium, gold, allopurinol, quinidine, and calcium channel blockers may be particularly noteworthy as offending agents. However, it is important to consider all drug exposures, as intradermal and topical ocular preparations have been reported to induce exfoliative dermatitis.

A large number of systemic diseases, malignancies (hematologic or solid tumors), and infections may also play a role (Table 44-2). Exfoliative dermatitis may be the initial manifestation of HIV infection, although drug eruptions are the most common cause of exfoliative dermatitis in HIV-positive patients.[11] In infants with exfoliative dermatitis, seborrheic dermatitis, atopic dermatitis, psoriasis, and staphylococcal scalded skin syndrome are the most common causes. When the condition is congenital, however, the clinician should consider a variety of genetic disorders, in particular Netherton's syndrome and hereditary immunodeficiency syndromes.[12]

In most patients with pre-existing skin diseases, the exfoliative phase follows previous localized disease. For example, psoriatic exfoliative dermatitis can occur in association with the withdrawal of systemic or topical glucocorticoids, the use of systemic medications such as lithium and antimalarials, phototherapy burns, infection, pregnancy, and systemic illnesses in patients with previously limited psoriasis.

Regarding the pathogenesis of exfoliative dermatitis, it is not clear whether dermal inflammation or epidermal dysfunction is primary. Drug- and malignancy-induced exfoliative dermatitis suggests an inflammatory etiology, whereas exfoliative dermatitis in ichthyoses associated with transglutaminase mutations suggests a primary epidermal

TABLE 44-1

Drugs That Cause Exfoliative Dermatitis

Allopurinol*	**Lithium**
Aminoglycosides	Mefloquine
Aminophylline	Mercurials
Amiodarone	Mesna
Amonafide	Methylprednisolone
Ampicillin	Minocycline
Antimalarials	Mitomycin C
Arsenicals	Omeprazole
Aspirin	Penicillin
Aztreonam	Pentostatin
Bactrim	Peritrate and glyceryl trinitrate
Barbiturates	Pheneturide
Bromodeoxyuridine	Phenophthalein
Budesonide	Phenothiazines
Calcium channel blockers	Phenylbutazone
Captopril	**Phenytoin**
Carbamazepine	Phototherapy
Carboplatin	Plaquenil
Cefoxitin	Practolol
Cephalosporins	**Quinidine**
Cimetidine	Ranitidine
Cisplatin	Retinoids
Clodronate	Ribostamycin
Clofazamine	Rifampin
Codeine	St John's wort
Cyanamide	Streptomycin
Dapsone	Sulfasalazine
Dideoxyinosine	Sulfonamide antibiotics
Diflunisal	Sulfonylureas
Diphenylhydantoin	Tar preparations
Ephedrine	Terbinafine
Ethambutol	Terbutaline
Ethylenediamine	Thalidomide
Etretinate	Thiacetazone
Fluorouracil	Thiazide diuretics
GM-CSF	Ticlopidine
Gold	Timolol maleate eyedrops
Herbal medications	Tobramycin
Indeloxazine hydrochloride	Tocainide
Indinavir	Trimetrexate
Interleukin-2	Trovafloxacin
Iodine	Tumor necrosis factor-α
Isoniazid	Vancomycin
Isosorbide dinitrate	Yohimbine
Lansoprazole	Zidovudine
Lidocaine	

*The more commonly implicated agents are listed in bold.

etiology. It is likely that exfoliative dermatitis represents an end-stage inflammatory state that affects the entire integument, in which there is an uncontrolled feedback loop between the epidermis and the dermis.

The epidermis produces significantly elevated amounts of circulating vascular permeability factor/vascular endothelial growth factor in erythrodermic skin, resulting in dermal vascular proliferation and increased vascular permeability.[13] The increases in adhesion molecule expression (VCAM-1, ICAM-1, E-selectin, and P-selectin) seen in exfoliative dermatitis promote chronic dermal inflammation, which may, in turn, promote both epidermal proliferation and epidermal production of inflammatory mediators.[14] The dermal infiltrates may demonstrate either a T_H1 cytokine profile, as in benign reactive exfoliative dermatitis, or a T_H2 cytokine profile, as in Sézary syndrome.[15] This finding is consistent with the fact that a wide range of distinct immunologic processes (e.g., atopic dermatitis and contact dermatitis) may produce exfoliative dermatitis. Alterations in levels of various pro-inflammatory molecules (interleukins 2, 3, and 8; interferon-γ; and ICAM-1) also have occurred with exfoliative dermatitis. However, these changes may be a secondary factor in the exfoliative dermatitis rather than an immunopathogenic cause.

The basic pathophysiology of exfoliative dermatitis involves an increased rate of epidermal turnover. The number of germinative cells and their absolute mitotic rate increase, whereas the transit time of keratinocytes through the epidermis decreases. Consequently, more cellular material is lost from the surface. Because of the rapid cell turnover in exfoliative dermatitis, the stratum corneum retains a number of components that are normally resorbed or metabolized. The desquamated cells show increased amounts of nucleic acids and their degradation products, as well as increased amounts of soluble protein. Although the large amount of protein lost each day has a potentially adverse effect on systemic metabolism (see below), the losses of nucleic acids and other minor constituents are too small to be of metabolic significance.

CLINICAL MANIFESTATIONS

Dermatologic Manifestations

Despite the wide range of underlying dermatologic disorders that may lead to exfoliative dermatitis, the clinical manifestations in all cases are similar. The disease generally starts as erythematous patches resulting from capillary dilation. Over days to weeks, these patches spread until bright red erythema affects the entire skin surface. The epidermis appears thin, giving the skin a shiny appearance.

Desquamation begins a few days after the onset of the erythema and often appears first in flexures. The scales are generally white or yellow and fine, although large platelike sheets of scale may develop, particularly in acute stages and on the palms and soles. As the desquamation progresses, the skin appears dry with a dull scarlet color and a gray hue. It is covered with small laminated scales that exfoliate profusely (Fig. 44-1). In some cases, particularly in the presence of bacterial colonization, there may be profuse moist, adherent crusts, leading to a characteristic musty odor.[11] A purple hue is often evident in dependent areas, and there may be straw-colored exudates.

With time, induration and thickening of the skin from a combination of edema and lichenification may impart a sensation of severe skin tightness to the patient. In mild or early exfoliative dermatitis, the disease may be apparent only by blanching of the skin to demonstrate the mild macular erythema. In darkly pigmented patients, this early sign may be easily overlooked.

Chronic exfoliative dermatitis results in diffuse shedding of hair. The nails become thickened, ridged, dull, and brittle. Subungual hyperkeratosis, distal onycholysis, and splinter hemorrhages are common, and occasionally, the nails may be shed. Paronychia, onycholysis, subungual hyperkeratosis, and Beau lines of the nails may develop.[1] Once these changes develop, they generally overshadow any nail findings of the underlying disease process. "Shoreline" nails, reported to be a specific manifestation of drug-induced exfoliative dermatitis, are characterized by alternating bands of nail plate discontinuity and leukonychia representing periods in which the offending drug was used.[16] Chronic periorbital involvement, resulting in induration and decreased laxity of the eyelids, may lead to ectropion and epiphora. Palmoplantar keratoderma with thick, fissured scales has been reported in up to 80 percent of patients with chronic exfoliative dermatitis, and crusted, seborrheic scaling of the scalp is common.[17] Exfoliative dermatitis does not generally involve mucosal surfaces.

TABLE 44-2

Processes Reported in Association with Exfoliative Dermatitis

Skin Diseases	Systemic Diseases	Genetic Diseases	Malignancies	Infectious Diseases
Actinic reticuloid	C5 deficiency	Chanarin-Dorfman	Adult T cell leukemia	Congenital cutaneous candidiasis
Acute generalized exanthematous pustulosis	Celiac disease	Common variable hypogammaglobulinemia	Anaplastic large cell lymphoma	Congenital syphilis
Atopic dermatitis	Dermatophytosis	Congenital nonbullous ichthyosiform erythroderma	Angioimmunoblastic lymphadenopathy	Dermatomyositis
Bullous pemphigoid	Graft-versus-host disease	Conradi-Hunermann syndrome	B cell lymphoma	Histoplasmosis
Chronic actinic dermatitis	Hepatitis	Epidermolytic hyperkeratosis	Breast carcinoma	Human herpesvirus 6
Contact dermatitis	Postoperative transfusion-related	Essential fatty acid deficiency	Chronic lymphocytic leukemia	Human immunodeficiency virus
Erythema gyratum repens	Reiter syndrome	Holocarboxylase synthetase deficiency	Cutaneous anaplastic large cell lymphoma	Leishmaniasis
Follicular mucinosis	Sarcoidosis	Keratitis-ichthyosis-deafness	Cutaneous lymphoid hyperplasia	Norwegian scabies
Hailey-Hailey disease	Subacute cutaneous lupus	Lamellar ichthyosis	Cutaneous T cell lymphoma	Staphylococcus scalded skin syndrome
Papuloerythroderma of Ofuji	Thyrotoxicosis	Leiner disease	Esophageal carcinoma	Toxic shock syndrome
Paraneoplastic pemphigus	Vogt-Konayagi-Harada syndrome	Lethal congenital erythroderma	Fallopian tube carcinoma	Toxoplasmosis
Pemphigus foliaceus		Maple syrup urine disease	Gastric carcinoma	
Perforating folliculitis		Netherton syndrome	Hodgkin disease	
Pityriasis rubra pilaris		Neutral lipid storage disease	Hypereosinophilic syndrome	
Psoriasis		Omenn syndrome	Liver cancer	
Radiation dermatitis		Secretory IgA deficiency	Lung cancer	
Seborrheic dermatitis		Severe combined immunodeficiency	Malignant histiocytosis	
Senile erythroderma with hyper-IgE		Sjögren-Larsson syndrome	Malignant melanoma	
Stasis dermatitis		Wiskott-Aldrich syndrome	Mastocytosis	
Systemic contact dermatitis			Multiple myeloma	
Toxic epidermal necrolysis			Myelodysplasia	
			Myelomonocytic leukemia	
			Ovarian cancer	
			Prostate cancer	
			Rectal carcinoma	
			Reticulum cell sarcoma	
			Rosai-Dorfman disease	
			Sézary syndrome	
			Thyroid carcinoma	

Occasionally, clinical features may be suggestive of the underlying etiology. Isolated typical psoriatic plaques may remain distinguishable from the surrounding skin changes, and clinical or radiographic evidence of psoriatic arthritis may be present. The violaceous papules and buccal mucosal lesions of lichen planus may be visible. In early cases, nail changes typical of the underlying disease process may be discernible. In exfoliative dermatitis associated with pityriasis rubra pilaris, islands of normal skin, peripheral horny plugs, orange-colored palmoplantar keratoderma, and follicular papules on juxtaarticular extensor surfaces may be evident. The presence of heavily crusted palms and soles with subungual hyperkeratosis should alert the clinician to the possibility of Norwegian scabies. In cases associated with pemphigus foliaceus, crusted patches and erosions may appear on the face and upper trunk. A heliotrope rash, Gottron's papules, periungual telangiectases, and muscle weakness may be seen in erythrodermic dermatomyositis.[18] Papuloerythroderma of Ofuji presents in elderly men as flat-topped red papules that coalesce into generalized erythrodermic plaques, characteristically sparing the abdominal skin folds ("deck chair" sign). Alopecia in infantile exfoliative dermatitis may be a sign of Netherton or Omenn syndromes.[12] In some cases, what initially appears as exfoliative dermatitis rapidly progresses to epidermal necrosis, foretelling toxic epidermal necrolysis, a pathophysiologically different process (see Chap. 58).

Long-term exfoliative dermatitis may resolve with residual dyspigmentation, particularly in darkly pigmented patients. Generalized vitiligo, disseminated pyogenic granulomas, anhidrosis, and xanthomas have been reported to occur after the resolution of exfoliative dermatitis.

Systemic Associations

Axillary and inguinal lymphadenopathy occur in up to 62 percent of patients.[7,9] In general, the lymph nodes are moderately enlarged with a rubbery consistency. The histologic findings are frequently those of dermatopathic lymphadenopathy, with enlarged paracortical areas indicating the proliferation of T lymphocytes, but lacking effacement of the lymph node structure by malignant cells. Hepatomegaly is reported in up to 37 percent of cases; splenomegaly, in up to 23 percent.[7,9] The presence of lymphadenopathy and hepatosplenomegaly, particularly in association with liver dysfunction and fever, may suggest a drug hypersensitivity syndrome or malignancy.

FIGURE 44-1

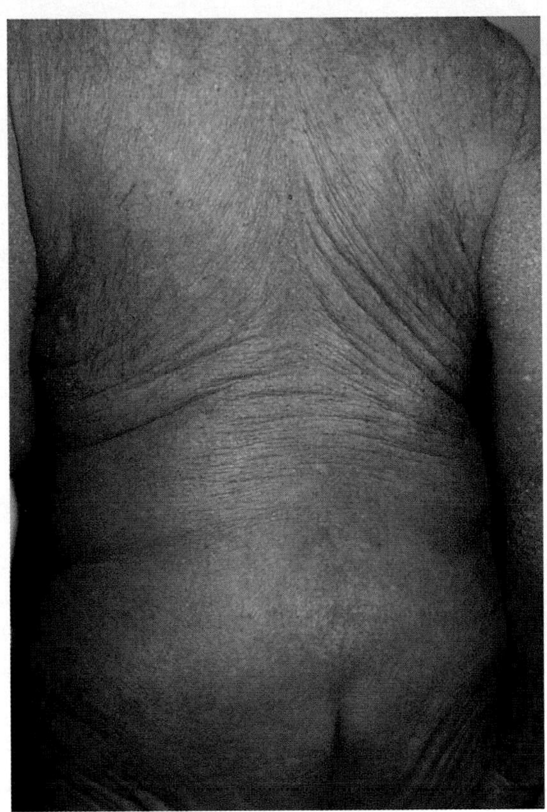

Exfoliative dermatitis.

Patients with exfoliative dermatitis develop poikilothermia, with their core temperatures fluctuating according to the ambient temperature, because the uncontrolled dilation of cutaneous blood vessels results in an increased blood flow to the skin and an inability to compensate for ambient temperature changes. Moreover, the increased transepidermal water loss from the defective cutaneous barrier promotes the evaporation of skin surface fluids, resulting in further heat loss.[10] The dilated dermal vessels provide a low-resistance path for systemic blood flow, occasionally resulting in high-output cardiac failure. This may cause severe cardiac compromise in patients with pre-existing cardiac disease, or it may unmask previous subclinical cardiac insufficiency or coronary artery disease. More common than poikilothermia and high-output cardiac failure, however, are tachycardia and fever, which may develop in up to 80 percent of patients.[9] There is also compensatory hypermetabolism and an elevation of the basal metabolic rate, without an associated abnormality in thyroid function.

Increased fluid losses from both the greater transepidermal water loss and the higher basal metabolic rate may result in dehydration, an elevated blood urea nitrogen level, and renal insufficiency. Normally, approximately 400 mL of water are lost from the skin each day; two-thirds of this amount is diffused directly through the stratum corneum, and the remainder is lost by the evaporation of sweat. Fluid losses are highest when scaling is at its peak, and careful monitoring of intake and output reproducibly demonstrates that extrarenal water losses decrease 5 to 6 days prior to a decrease in scaling. This can provide an objective method of monitoring patients.[19]

The diffuse shedding of scale can result in a protein loss of as much as 20 to 30 g/m^2 per day. This should be contrasted with the 500 to 1000 mg of exfoliated material normally shed from the surface of the glabrous skin each day.[20] On average, psoriatic exfoliative dermatitis results in significantly more protein loss than exfoliative dermatitis from drug reactions and eczema (12.8, 4.2, and 5.6 g/d, respectively).[21] This loss may result in negative nitrogen, potassium, and folate balances. The signs of a negative nitrogen balance include hypoalbuminemia, edema, and loss of muscle mass. Hypoalbuminemia results from decreased synthesis, elevated catabolism to compensate for protein loss, and hypervolemia. Peripheral edema is due to fluid shifts, hypoalbuminemia, and increased capillary permeability. Pulmonary capillary leak syndrome and acute respiratory distress syndrome are rare fatal complications of exfoliative dermatitis. Gynecomastia has been reported in some patients, possibly reflecting a hyperestrogenic state, although the significance of this finding is unclear.[9]

LABORATORY FINDINGS

Laboratory evaluation often reveals anemia (70 percent), lymphocytosis (41 percent), eosinophilia (35 percent), an elevated erythrocyte sedimentation rate (36 percent), and depressed serum protein levels (34 percent).[1,7] Eosinophilia is generally a nonspecific finding, although a highly elevated eosinophil count raises the possibility of underlying Hodgkin's lymphoma. Dehydration may result in abnormal serum electrolyte concentrations and abnormal renal function. Polyclonal gammaglobulinemia appears in approximately 40 percent of patients, and an elevated serum IgE level occurs in up to 80 percent, even in cases not associated with atopic dermatitis.[7,8,17] Decreased counts of lymphocytes, including CD4 cells, may result from lymphocyte sequestration in the skin.[22]

Circulating Sézary cells may be present, but whereas less than 10 percent is considered nonspecific in the setting of exfoliative dermatitis, the presence of 20 percent or more Sézary cells is highly specific for Sézary syndrome.[6,9] In exfoliative dermatitis associated with actinic reticuloid, there is an increased proportion of CD8+ lymphocytes in the skin, whereas in Sézary syndrome there are often clonal, circulating T cell populations and predominantly CD4+ cutaneous infiltrates.[23] Bone marrow biopsies of patients with idiopathic exfoliative dermatitis may demonstrate eosinophilia (32 percent) or benign hyperplasia (20 percent).[17]

PATHOLOGY

Biopsy specimens from patients with exfoliative dermatitis tend to have many nonspecific features, such as hyperkeratosis, parakeratosis, acanthosis, and chronic inflammatory infiltrates. These findings often mask the histologic features of the underlying disease process. Although in some series histologic evaluation was considered to be of no diagnostic benefit,[24] other series have demonstrated that a histologic diagnosis can be made in most cases. The submission of multiple biopsy specimens obtained simultaneously from patients with exfoliative dermatitis enhances the accuracy of histopathologic diagnosis.

In one study, blinded histologic diagnoses were compared with final diagnoses in 56 skin biopsy specimens from 40 patients with exfoliative dermatitis. The histologic and final clinicopathologic diagnoses were consistent in two-thirds of cases, even though the microscopic features were more subtle than those in the underlying diseases.[25] In another study comparing histologic diagnosis with final diagnosis, the mean diagnostic accuracy was 53 percent among a group of dermatopathologists who independently evaluated 56 specimens.[26]

Whereas erythrodermic psoriasis produces diagnostic histologic features in up to 90 percent of patients,[27] the histologic features of erythrodermic cutaneous T cell lymphoma are even more subtle than those of the patch and plaque stages of mycosis fungoides. Even in the presence of a peripheral blood population of clonal T-cells, nonspecific histologic features of chronic dermatitis can occur in one-third of patients with Sézary syndrome.[28] Of note, the presence of a lichenoid infiltrate suggests a lichenoid drug eruption as the etiology.[29]

Direct immunofluorescence studies may be helpful in the diagnosis of exfoliative dermatitis secondary to pemphigus foliaceus, bullous pemphigoid, graft-versus-host disease, and connective tissue disorders. Electron microscopy can be helpful in the evaluation of infantile exfoliative dermatitis, including congenital nonbullous ichthyosiform erythroderma and epidermolytic hyperkeratosis. Premature lamellar body secretion and foci of electron-dense material in the intercellular spaces of the stratum corneum are sensitive and specific markers of Netherton syndrome, permitting early diagnosis before the appearance of hair shaft abnormalities.[30]

TREATMENT AND PROGNOSIS

No matter what the cause of exfoliative dermatitis, the initial treatment is generally similar. It is essential not only to discontinue any suspected offending drug, but also to keep in mind that drugs such as antimalarials and lithium may cause or exacerbate diseases such as psoriasis, and drugs such as phenytoin may cause a clinical picture indistinguishable from that of Sézary syndrome. The patients are more comfortable if they are in a warm, humid environment. Although most patients can be managed as outpatients, some should be admitted to the hospital for monitoring of fluid intake and output, as well as renal function. Careful observation for signs of cardiac failure should be routine. Patients should receive a protein-fortified diet providing approximately 130 percent of the normal balanced diet protein as well as folate supplementation.[21,31]

Supportive skin care with frequent application of bland emollients, soaks, and compresses, as well as mild-to-moderate strength topical glucocorticoid ointments, will usually result in an improvement over 1 to 2 weeks. Patients should avoid irritating topical agents such as tar preparations and anthralin. Because of altered barrier function, there is a possibility of significant systemic absorption with all topical agents. The systemic absorption of up to 20 percent of topically applied hydrocortisone is not uncommon in this condition, and thus, systemic effects may occur even with the topical use of low-potency glucocorticoids.[32] Moreover, erythrodermic patients may develop salicylism from the topical application of preparations that contain salicylic acid. Antihistamines may help control pruritus, and behavioral therapy may help to attenuate scratching.

The systemic administration of appropriate antibiotics may be necessary to control bacterial superinfection. Clinicians should consider antibiotics in all cases, as staphylococcal colonization of the skin may exacerbate exfoliative dermatitis and patients are then at risk for fatal staphylococcal septicemia. As patients with exfoliative dermatitis may contribute to the nosocomial spread of methicillin-resistant *Staphylococcus aureus,* appropriate contact precautions must be employed.[33]

When a patient's medical condition is severe or refractory or when it requires more rapid control of the cutaneous disease, a variety of systemic therapies are available. Cyclosporine, methotrexate, acitretin, and mycophenolate mofetil may be used for psoriatic exfoliative dermatitis; cyclosporine, for spongiotic disease; retinoids, glucocorticoids and extracorporeal photochemotherapy, for pityriasis rubra pilaris; glucocorticoids, for drug hypersensitivity syndrome; and extracorporeal photochemotherapy, for graft-versus-host disease. Cutaneous T cell lymphoma has been treated with glucocorticoids, psoralen plus ultraviolet A, total body electron beam irradiation, interferon-α, systemic chemotherapy, and extracorporeal photochemotherapy. Although acitretin is highly effective in the treatment of ichthyosiform exfoliative dermatitis, the clinician must weigh the benefits against the risks of long-term oral retinoid use, particularly in children. In cases of increased systemic capillary permeability, the administration of parenteral glucocorticoids and intravenous infusions of plasma may be imperative.

When the cause of exfoliative dermatitis is not known, the systemic use of glucocorticoids warrants great caution in order to prevent generalized pustular psoriasis or rebound flares of spongiotic disease. The systemic administration of steroids may also increase fluid retention. Similarly, phototherapy requires great caution, as erythrodermic patients may be exquisitely photosensitive, and a phototoxic reaction may exacerbate their disease.

Some measures may reduce the risk of exfoliative dermatitis. For example, the administration of irradiated blood products can prevent transfusion-related postsurgery exfoliative dermatitis, which is likely a variant of graft-versus-host disease and may be associated with a 90 percent mortality rate. Patients should strictly avoid medications that previously may have caused exfoliative dermatitis, as even topical contact may lead to a recurrence of exfoliative dermatitis. Similarly, erythrodermic systemic contact dermatitis has been reported in patients who have contact allergy to neomycin and who received gentamycin intravenously, and in rhus-allergic patients who took herbal medications, including rhus lacquer.[34,35]

The prognosis of exfoliative dermatitis depends on its cause. Drug-induced cases have the best prognosis, as rapid improvement follows drug discontinuation.[2,7,24] However, toxic epidermal necrolysis and severe drug hypersensitivity reactions associated with hepatotoxicity are associated with a more grave prognosis.[7] Exfoliative dermatitis secondary to underlying skin diseases tends to improve over a few weeks, and as many as two-thirds of patients enter remission.[8] Psoriatic exfoliative dermatitis may recur in up to 20 percent of patients.[36]

Exfoliative dermatitis secondary to cutaneous T cell lymphoma and internal malignancies tends to be more persistent. In these patients, favorable prognostic factors include age less than 65 years, duration of symptoms before diagnosis greater than 10 years, absence of malignant lymph node infiltrates, and the absence of circulating Sézary cells. Depending on the presence or absence of these risk factors, median survival may range from 1.5 to 10.2 years.[37] In a study of 38 patients with exfoliative dermatitis of unknown etiology ("red man" syndrome), 4 patients progressed to mycosis fungoides, and an additional 9 were suspected of having mycosis fungoides. In this group, only one-third of the patients went into complete remission, whereas half of the patients died during the observation period (1 to 23 years).[17]

In the published reports of the past 50 years, the mortality rates associated with exfoliative dermatitis have consistently remained high, ranging from 20 to 60 percent.[5,10,38] Most deaths were in patients with malignancy, severe drug reactions, pemphigus foliaceus, or idiopathic disease; they occurred secondary to pneumonia, underlying malignancy, septicemia, and cardiovascular compromise.[5,10] More recent studies have demonstrated significantly lower mortality rates. In one series of 82 patients, no patient with underlying benign skin disease died, whereas the mortality rate was 25 percent in patients with cutaneous T cell lymphoma, usually from progression of disease, complications of therapy, or bacterial sepsis.[7] In infantile cases, the mortality rate has been reported to be 16 percent.[12]

REFERENCES

1. Sehgal VN, Srivastava G: Exfoliative dermatitis: A prospective study of 80 patients. *Dermatologica* **173**:278, 1986
2. Hasan T, Jansen CT: Erythroderma: A follow-up of fifty cases. *J Am Acad Dermatol* **8**:836, 1983
3. Wong KS et al: Generalised exfoliative dermatitis: A clinical study of 108 patients. *Ann Acad Med Singapore* **17**:520, 1988
4. Sigurdsson V et al: The incidence of erythroderma: A survey among all dermatologists in the Netherlands. *J Am Acad Dermatol* **45**:675, 2001
5. Abrahams I et al: One hundred and one cases of exfoliative dermatitis. *Arch Dermatol* **87**:96, 1963
6. Sigurdsson V et al: Idiopathic erythroderma: A follow-up study of 28 patients. *Dermatology* **194**:98, 1997
7. King LE Jr et al: Erythroderma: Review of 82 cases. *South Med J* **79**:1210, 1986
8. Botella-Estrada R et al: Erythroderma: A clinicopathological study of 56 cases. *Arch Dermatol* **130**:1503, 1994
9. Sigurdsson V et al: Erythroderma: A clinical and follow-up study of 102 patients, with special emphasis on survival. *J Am Acad Dermatol* **35**:53, 1996
10. Nicolis GD, Helwig EB: Exfoliative dermatitis: A clinicopathologic study of 135 cases. *Arch Dermatol* **108**:788, 1973
11. Morar N et al: Erythroderma: A comparison between HIV positive and negative patients. *Int J Dermatol* **38**:895, 1999
12. Pruszkowski A et al: Neonatal and infantile erythrodermas: A retrospective study of 51 patients. *Arch Dermatol* **136**:875, 2000
13. Creamer D et al: Circulating vascular permeability factor/vascular endothelial growth factor in erythroderma. *Lancet* **348**:1101, 1996
14. Sigurdsson V et al: Expression of VCAM-1, ICAM-1, E-selectin, and P-selectin on endothelium in situ in patients with erythroderma, mycosis fungoides, and atopic dermatitis. *J Cutan Pathol* **27**:436, 2000
15. Sigurdsson V et al: Interleukin 4 and interferon-gamma expression of the dermal infiltrate in patients with erythroderma and mycosis fungoides: An immuno-histochemical study. *J Cutan Pathol* **27**:429, 2000
16. Shelley WB, Shelley ED: Shoreline nails: Sign of drug-induced erythroderma. *Cutis* **35**:220, 1985
17. Thestrup-Pedersen K et al: The red man syndrome: Exfoliative dermatitis of unknown etiology. A description and follow-up of 38 patients. *J Am Acad Dermatol* **18**:1307, 1988
18. Nousari HC et al: Paraneoplastic dermatomyositis presenting as erythroderma. *J Am Acad Dermatol* **39**:653, 1998
19. Freedberg IM, Baden HP: The metabolic response to exfoliation. *J Invest Dermatol* **38**:277, 1962
20. Goldschmidt H, Kligman AM: Quantitative estimation of keratin production by the epidermis. *Arch Dermatol* **88**:709, 1963
21. Kanthraj GR et al: Quantitative estimation and recommendations for supplementation of protein lost through scaling in exfoliative dermatitis. *Int J Dermatol* **38**:91, 1999
22. Griffiths TW et al: Acute erythroderma as an exclusion criterion for idiopathic CD4+ T lymphocytopenia. *Arch Dermatol* **130**:1530, 1994
23. Bakels V et al: Differentiation between actinic reticuloid and cutaneous T cell lymphoma by T cell receptor gamma gene rearrangement analysis and immunophenotyping. *J Clin Pathol* **51**:154, 1998
24. Leenutaphong V et al: Erythroderma in Thai patients. *J Med Assoc Thai* **82**:743, 1999
25. Zip C et al: The specificity of histopathology in erythroderma. *J Cutan Pathol* **20**:393, 1993
26. Walsh NM et al: Histopathology in erythroderma: Review of a series of cases by multiple observers. *J Cutan Pathol* **21**:419, 1994
27. Tomasini C et al: Psoriatic erythroderma: A histopathologic study of forty-five patients. *Dermatology* **194**:102, 1997
28. Trotter MJ et al: Cutaneous histopathology of Sézary syndrome: A study of 41 cases with a proven circulating T-cell clone. *J Cutan Pathol* **24**:286, 1997
29. Patterson JW et al: Lichenoid histopathologic changes in patients with clinical diagnoses of exfoliative dermatitis. *Am J Dermatopathol* **13**:358, 1991
30. Fartasch M et al: Altered lamellar body secretion and stratum corneum membrane structure in Netherton syndrome: Differentiation from other infantile erythrodermas and pathogenic implications. *Arch Dermatol* **135**:823, 1999
31. Hild DH: Folate losses from the skin in exfoliative dermatitis. *Arch Intern Med* **123**:51, 1969
32. Aalto-Korte K, Turpeinen M: Quantifying systemic absorption of topical hydrocortisone in erythroderma. *Br J Dermatol* **133**:403, 1995
33. Love JB et al: Exfoliative dermatitis as a risk factor for epidemic spread of methicillin resistant *Staphylococcus aureus*. *Intensive Care Med* **18**:189, 1992
34. Guin JD, Phillips D: Erythroderma from systemic contact dermatitis: A complication of systemic gentamicin in a patient with contact allergy to neomycin. *Cutis* **43**:564, 1989
35. Park SD et al: Clinical features of 31 patients with systemic contact dermatitis due to the ingestion of *Rhus* (lacquer). *Br J Dermatol* **142**:937, 2000
36. Boyd AS, Menter A: Erythrodermic psoriasis: Precipitating factors, course, and prognosis in 50 patients. *J Am Acad Dermatol* **21**:985, 1989
37. Kim YH et al: Prognostic factors in erythrodermic mycosis fungoides and the Sézary syndrome. *Arch Dermatol* **131**:1003, 1995
38. Wilson HTH: Exfoliative dermatitis: Its etiology and prognosis. *Arch Dermatol* **69**:577, 1954

CHAPTER 45

Lowell A. Goldsmith
Howard P. Baden

Pityriasis Rubra Pilaris

Pityriasis rubra pilaris (PRP) refers to a group of chronic disorders characterized by reddish orange, scaling plaques and keratotic follicular papules. Both familial and acquired forms of the disorder have been described. There is a recent extensively referenced review including historical aspects of the disease.[1]

INCIDENCE

The disease is rare, with estimates that it is the presenting problem in from 1 in 5000 to 1 in 50,000 dermatology patients.[2] Both sexes are affected equally. The age incidence curve is at least bimodal with a familial type that starts early in childhood. The acquired type occurs in the fifth and sixth decades.[2]

ETIOLOGY

The familial type has an autosomal dominant mode of inheritance.[3] Vitamin A deficiency and abnormal vitamin A metabolism have been incriminated as an etiologic entity in this disease. This is based primarily on the finding of cutaneous changes suggestive of pityriasis in a group of patients studied by Frazier and Hu in 1931 and thought to be lacking vitamin A. These patients in all likelihood had multiple vitamin deficiencies; attempts to produce keratotic lesions by vitamin A deprivation have been unsuccessful, and there are no data consistent with an abnormality of vitamin A metabolism.

CLINICAL MANIFESTATIONS

Cohen and Prystowsky[4] have reviewed the disease extensively, and a classification of acquired pityriasis rubra pilaris has been proposed by Griffiths.[2,5] Types I and III, the classic types of adult and juvenile onset, are the most common; they seem to be the same disease and have good prognoses. Two cases of a circumscribed childhood form have been described associated with Down's syndrome. The onset is gradual in the familial type and can be more rapid in the acquired type. Redness and scaling of the face and scalp are often seen first, followed by redness and thickening of the stratum corneum of the palms (Fig. 45-1) and soles. The follicular papules so characteristic of the disease soon appear as keratotic follicular plugs surrounded by erythema (Fig. 45-2*B*). The follicular papules are not always present but are very prominent in black South Africans.[6] They are seen most commonly on the dorsal aspects of the proximal phalanges (Fig. 45-2*A*), the elbows, and the wrists. They can occur on other areas of the extremities and even the trunk (Fig. 45-2*B*,*C*) but appear rarely on the face. A more widespread eruption consisting of scaling orange-red plaques is observed on the trunk and extremities (Figs. 45-2C and 45-3) and occasionally on the face. The lesions have sharp borders, and islands of normal skin within them are characteristic (see Fig. 45-3). The lesions may expand and coalesce (Fig. 45-2*C*) and eventually cover the entire body (Figs. 45-2*C* and Fig. 45-3). The scales vary from fine to thick, the latter being particularly common on the palms and soles, which also may fissure and have an intense yellow-orange hue, and may cover the scalp in thick sheets. The disease has been associated with HIV infection; these patients commonly have nodulocystic and pustular acneiform lesions.[7,8]

Dermatomyositis, often associated with internal malignancy, with a PRP eruption, clinically and histologically, has been described and named the *Wong form* of dermatomyositis by some.[9] An association with inflammatory polyarthritis has been reported.[10] A juvenile case with hypogammaglobulinemia and furunculosis also has been reported.[11] The association with neoplasia is probably fortuitous.[12]

Hair and teeth are normal. Nail changes are said to be characteristic, with distal yellow-brown discoloration, subungual hyperkeratosis, nail plate thickening, and splinter hemorrhages,[13] but these findings also can be observed in psoriasis. The changes in mucous membranes include a diffuse whitish appearance of the buccal mucosa[14] as well as lacy white plaques and erosions.[15]

FIGURE 45-1

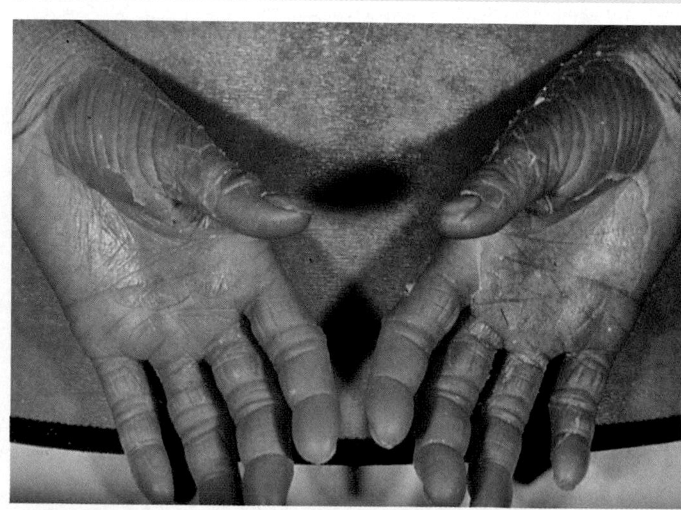

Hyperkeratotic palmar lesions seen in pityriasis rubra pilaris. Characteristically, the palms are smooth and glistening with prominent creases and occasional fissures.

FIGURE 45-2

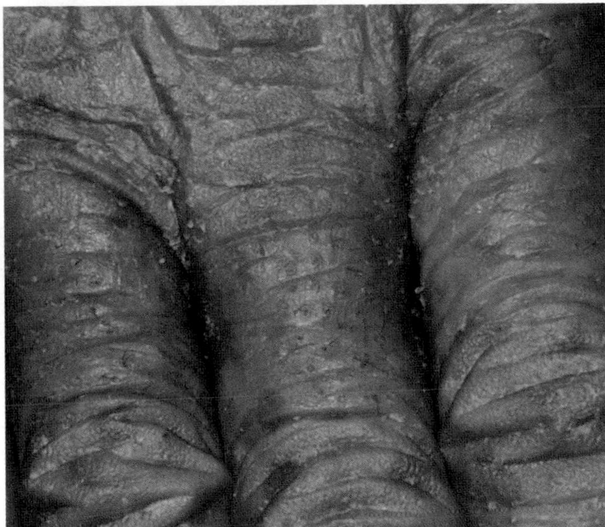

A.

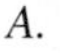

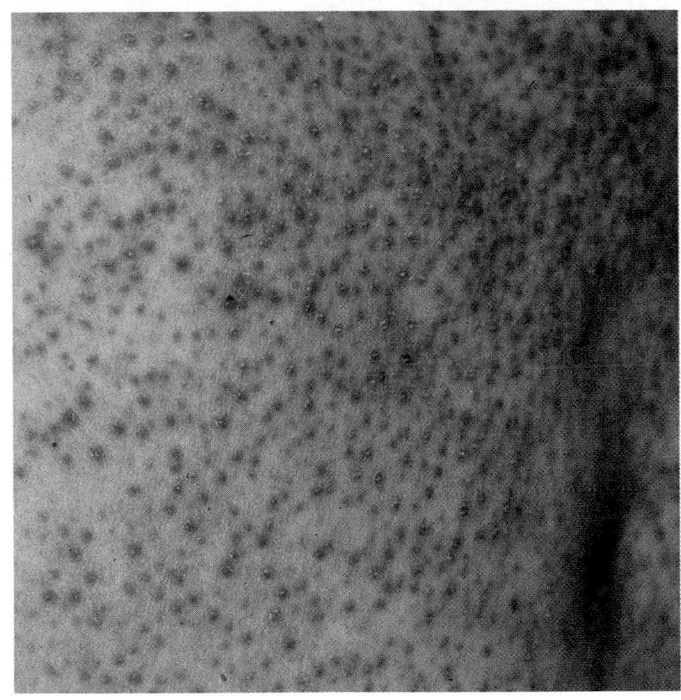

B.

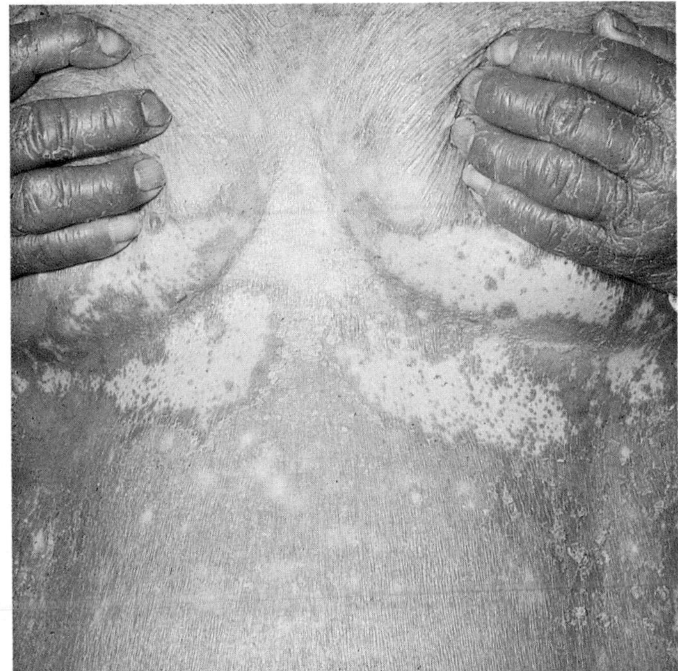

C.

A. Acuminate follicular papules of pityriasis rubra pilaris. (*From Bergeron JR, Stone OJ:* Dermatologica *136:362, 1968, with permission.*) B. Close-up of discrete follicular papules on the trunk. C. Confluent follicular papules of pityriasis rubra pilaris that have formed large orange-red plaques. The lesions have sharp margins and islands of normal skin within them are characteristic.

The familial type often persists throughout life, but the acquired form may have periods of remission. Systemic symptoms are uncommon except when total-body involvement occurs, and then they are similar to those occurring in exfoliative dermatitis, especially with frequent peripheral edema in older patients (see Chap. 44). Pruritus is uncommon.

PATHOLOGY

Hyperkeratosis is the most obvious feature on histologic examination. Parakeratosis is seen around the follicular openings, creating a shoulder effect. Alternating vertical and horizontal parakeratosis in the interfollicular stratum corneum is said to be characteristic. Irregular acanthosis and acantholytic dyskeratosis may accompany a mild chronic inflammatory infiltrate in the upper dermis.

DIFFERENTIAL DIAGNOSIS

When the typical features of follicular hyperkeratosis on the back of the fingers—an orange-colored eruption with spared areas and palmoplantar keratoderma—are observed, the diagnosis can be made with reasonable certainty. This is especially true in patients with a negative family history of psoriasis. Most patients present with fewer diagnostic features, and many of these end up having a clinical course most consistent with psoriasis. Difficulty with diagnosis is especially a problem in the pediatric age group. Even in patients who have a presentation and course consistent with PRP, there may be times when their lesions are more typical of psoriasis. Confusion with psoriasis presents the major diagnostic problem, particularly in early phases of the disease.

FIGURE 45-3

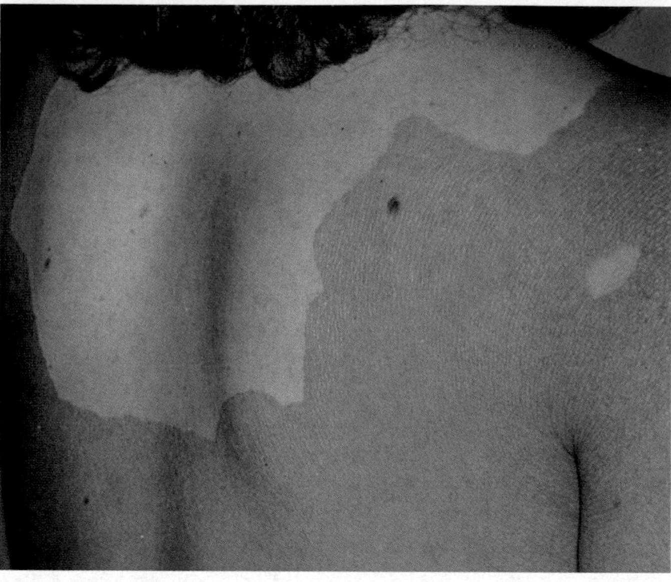

Generalized pityriasis rubra pilaris (large orange plaque). Note areas of sparing, leaving islands of normal skin; this is characteristic but not pathognomonic.

TREATMENT

The use of a keratolytic solution containing propylene glycol and lactic acid under an occlusive plastic dressing for 2 to 4 h followed by a glucocorticoid ointment for 4 to 8 h under an occlusive dressing has proved a valuable mode of therapy in PRP. Isotretinoin also has been reported to be of value,[16] although a recent review suggests that acitretin may be more effective in clearing patients, and today most patients are treated first with acitretin.[17] In the past, megadoses of vitamin A were used.[18] Calcipotriol has been effective.[19] Methotrexate therapy,[20] using the guidelines established for psoriasis, can induce a remission in a significant number of patients; a combination of methotrexate and a retinoid gives even better results.[17] Ultraviolet B (UVB) radiation treatment, as used for psoriasis, has not been helpful, but a retinoid plus psoralen and ultraviolet A (Re-PUVA) can be effective. Narrow-wave-band UVB also worked in connection with acitretin.[21] Unlike psoriasis, PRP does not respond to cyclosporine.

COURSE AND PROGNOSIS

The inherited form of the disorder is persistent throughout life. The acquired disease usually shows remissions and exacerbations, but some patients continue to have trouble for years.[4,22] Some patients with universal involvement are desperate enough to attempt suicide.

REFERENCES

1. Albert MR, Mackool BT: Pityriasis rubra pilaris. *Int J Dermatol* **38**:1, 1999
2. Griffiths WA: Pityriasis rubra pilaris. *Clin Exp Dermatol* **5**:105, 1980
3. Vanderhooft SL et al: Familial pityriasis rubra pilaris. *Arch Dermatol* **131**:448, 1995
4. Cohen PR, Prystowsky JH: Pityriasis rubra pilaris: A review of diagnosis and treatment. *J Am Acad Dermatol* **20**:801, 1989
5. Griffiths WA: Pityriasis rubra pilaris: The problem of its classification. *J Am Acad Dermatol* **26**:140, 1992
6. Jacyk WK: Pityriasis rubra pilaris in black South Africans. *Clin Exp Dermatol* **24**:160, 1999
7. Martin AG et al: Pityriasis rubra pilaris in the setting of HIV infection: Clinical behaviour and association with explosive cystic acne. *Br J Dermatol* **126**:617, 1992
8. Miralles ES et al: Pityriasis rubra pilaris and human immunodeficiency virus infection. *Br J Dermatol* **133**:990, 1995
9. Lupton JR et al: An unusual presentation of dermatomyositis: The type Wong variant revisited. *J Am Acad Dermatol* **43**:908, 2000
10. Conaghan PG et al: The relationship between pityriasis rubra pilaris and inflammatory arthritis: Case report and response of the arthritis to anti-tumor necrosis factor immunotherapy. *Arthritis Rheum* **42**:1998, 1999
11. Castanet J et al: Juvenile pityriasis rubra pilaris associated with hypogammaglobulinaemia and furunculosis. *Br J Dermatol* **131**:717, 1994
12. Sanchez-Regana M et al: Pityriasis rubra pilaris as the initial manifestation of internal neoplasia. *Clin Exp Dermatol* **20**:436, 1995
13. Sonnex TS et al: The nails in adult type 1 pityriasis rubra pilaris: A comparison with Sezary syndrome and psoriasis. *J Am Acad Dermatol* **15**:956, 1986
14. Marshall J: Care of pityriasis rubra pilaris with lesions of buccal mucosa. *Arch Derm Syph* **66**:626, 1952
15. Baden HP, Roth SI: Oral lesions in pityriasis rubra pilaris. *Oral Surg Oral Med Oral Pathol* **25**:691, 1968
16. Goldsmith LA et al: Pityriasis rubra pilaris response to 13-*cis*-retinoic acid (isotretinoin). *J Am Acad Dermatol* **6**:710, 1982
17. Clayton BD et al: Adult pityriasis rubra pilaris: A 10-year case series. *J Am Acad Dermatol* **36**:959, 1997
18. Randel H: Toxic doses of vitamin A for pityriasis rubra pilaris. *Arch Dermatol* **116**:888, 1980
19. Van de Kerkhof PC, Steijlen PM: Topical treatment of pityriasis rubra pilaris with calcipotriol. *Br J Dermatol* **130**:675, 1994
20. Brown J, Perry HO: Pityriasis rubra pilaris: Treatment with folic acid antagonists. *Arch Dermatol* **94**:636, 1966
21. Kirby B, Watson R: Pityriasis rubra pilaris treated with acitretin and narrow-band ultraviolet B (Re-TL-01). *Br J Dermatol* **142**:376, 2000
22. Davidson CL et al: Pityriasis rubra pilaris: A follow-up study of 57 patients. *Arch Dermatol* **100**:175, 1969

CHAPTER 46

Alf Björnberg
Eva Tegner

Pityriasis Rosea

Pityriasis rosea (PR) is an acute, self-limiting skin eruption with a distinctive and constant course. The initial lesion is a primary plaque that is followed after 1 or 2 weeks by a generalized secondary rash with a typical distribution and lasting for about 6 weeks.

HISTORICAL ASPECTS

The literature of the past two centuries records descriptions of disorders apparently identical to the condition now known as pityriasis rosea.[1] The disease has been given many names, such as erythema annulatum (Rayer), herpes tonsurans maculosus et squamosus (Hebra), lichen annulatus serpiginosus (Wilson), pityriasis circiné (Horand), pityriasis disseminé (Hardy), pityriasis marginée et circinée (Vidal), pityriasis rubra aigu disseminé (Bazin), pseudoexanthème erythématodesquamatif (Besnier), roseola annulata (Willan), roseola furfuracea herpetiformis (Behrend), and roseola squamosa (Nicolas and Chapard).

EPIDEMIOLOGY

Prevalence and Incidence

Pityriasis rosea is reported in all races. The prevalence in total populations has been calculated as 0.13 percent in men and 0.14 percent in women, most patients being in the age group of 10 to 43 years. The incidence at different dermatologic centers has varied between 0.3 and 3 percent. In Minnesota, a steady decline has been noted[2]; in Uganda, an increase has been reported[3]; and in Sweden[4] and in eastern Anatolia,[5] no change has been observed.

Sex Distribution

The disease has been reported to be equally common in the two sexes or slightly more common in women.[4]

Age Distribution

Pityriasis rosea is rare in both the very young and the very old. However, it has been described in infants as young as 3 months of age. A feature common to several studies is a steeply rising incidence during childhood to a plateau-like maximum between 10 and 35 years of age, followed by a slow decline.

Seasonal Variations

Pityriasis rosea seems to be prevalent all over the world, irrespective of climate. In temperate zones, it is usually considered to be most common during spring and autumn or during the cool part of the year,[2] but it also has been reported to be common during summer. In a Swedish study, an increase was demonstrated in spring and particularly in autumn, when the "epidemic" accumulation was the result of a successive rise in incidence. The seasonal variation was surprisingly constant from year to year.[4] In Uganda, no peaks of greatly increased incidence have been reported at any time[3]; in Singapore, no monthly variation was observed[6]; whereas in Australia, India, and Malaysia, PR has been found to be most common in the hot, dry season.

ETIOLOGY AND PATHOGENESIS

Infection

The monomorphous clinical picture of PR with its characteristic primary plaque, secondary eruption, and limited course resembles in some respects that of the communicable exanthemas. Like PR, most viral and bacterial infections show increased incidence in autumn and winter, with a decrease in summer. A relationship with recent upper respiratory infection has been recorded.[7]

CLUSTERING Pityriasis rosea has been reported to occur in the same intimate environment,[4] usually in two but also in three or even four people. Physicians' families are included in these reports. When specifically asked, 4 of 108 patients with PR mentioned cases of the disease in their immediate environment.[1] The incidence was higher in people working at or attending educational establishments, and this was considered to support the hypothesis that PR is caused by an infectious agent. A three- to fourfold increase has been demonstrated among dermatologists as compared with ear, nose, and throat surgeons.

TRANSMISSION EXPERIMENTS Most attempts at transmitting PR have failed, but there are interesting accounts of successful transfer of PR with an extract of scales or blister fluid. A typical primary plaque appeared at the site of inoculation after 10 to 15 days and was followed by a classic secondary rash.

The primary plaque sometimes develops at the site of a recent lesion, such as a minor cutaneous infection, flea bite, wasp sting, or smallpox or bacille Calmette-Guérin (BCG) vaccination. A PR-like eruption has been reported after hepatitis B vaccination.[8] This again has raised the question of possible inoculation with an infective agent.

ATTEMPTS TO ISOLATE AN INFECTIVE AGENT Owing to its clinical resemblance to dermatophytosis, PR originally was thought to be a fungal infection. *Staphylococcus albus,* hemolytic streptococci, and spirochetes have all been incriminated. T lymphocytes specific for group A streptococcal antigens occasionally have been demonstrated in PR (as in guttate psoriasis).[9] After inoculation of a suspension of PR scales and biopsy material into the kidney of an African green monkey, a dermatotrophic virus of the picorna series was isolated. The findings in blood, sputum, urine, and feces were normal. Picornavirus-like particles have been seen on electron microscopy.[10] Structures resembling mycoplasma have been detected in ultrastructural studies of the primary plaque.[11]

RECURRENCE Recurrences are regarded as unusual, suggesting lasting immunity after an attack of PR. True recurrence may be seen after several months or years. When specifically looked for, however, recurrence seems to be quite common and may be encountered in 3 percent or more of patients. Multiple recurrences also have been reported.[2] In fact, there seem to be patients with a predisposition to PR who will have 10 or more attacks. During a recurrence, the primary plaque may develop at the same location as before or at another site.

ANTIBODY STUDIES Antistreptolysin titers are normal. *Legionella* antibodies were found in 33 percent of PR patients.[12] No significant rise in titer has been seen in any of the complement-fixation tests for adenovirus; influenza A or B; parainfluenza I, II, or III; or *Mycoplasma.*[13] Antibody studies have yielded no clues with respect to respiratory syncytial virus, ornithosis-psittacosis, herpes-varicella, cytomegalovirus, and Q fever. Antibodies for Epstein-Barr virus early antigen have been demonstrated in a large number of PR patients. Anticytoplasmic IgM antibodies to keratinocytes have been found in the sera of patients with PR, and it was suggested that these induced the development of the secondary eruption.[14] Most other studies on anticutaneous antibodies in PR have yielded negative results. Circulating immune complexes seem unimportant for the development of the secondary rash in PR because no such complexes have been found in the blood or skin. A significant, transient increase in IgD/IgM-bearing cells has been reported during the acute phase of PR in conjunction with a slight increase in the T cell population. A cell-mediated immune mechanism with Langerhans cells involvement may be important.[15–17]

HHV-6 AND HHV-7 Extensive research has been carried out in patients with PR with respect to the newly identified human herpes viruses HHV-6 and HHV-7. The results from different studies, however, are contradictory.[18,19] The virus also has been identified in normal controls. It is thus possible but not yet proved that HHV-6 and HHV-7 play a part in some patients with PR but that other causative agents also may exist. CD-4 serves as the cellular membrane receptor for the lymphotropic HHV-7, as well as for HIV.[20] Interestingly, PR and PR-like eruptions occur in AIDS patients.[21]

Drugs

Many drugs have been reported to cause PR or PR-like rashes. These include arsenic, barbiturates, bismuth, captopril, clonidine, gold, interferon-α, isotretinoin, ketotifen, organic mercurials, methoxypromazine, metronidazole, omeprazole, D-penicillamine, salvarsan, terbinafine, and tripelene amine hydrochloride. Drug-induced PR may be of the classic type, but it often shows atypical features, a protracted course, large lesions, striking resistance to therapy, subsequent marked hyperpigmentation, and transformation to lichenoid dermatitis.

Other Factors

Atopy has been shown to be more common in PR patients than in controls.[2,4] Pityriasis rosea is relatively common in patients with seborrheic dermatitis and acne vulgaris, and dandruff is more common in PR patients than in controls.[4] The quantitative occurrence of *Pityrosporon ovale* is similar in PR patients and controls.[4] Because the distribution of the skin lesions in PR sometimes coincides with the locations of various garments on the body, it has been thought that these precipitate or affect the course of the disease. The proportion of pregnant women with PR has been reported to be high (possibly due to new clothing), but others have been unable to confirm this. Pityriasis rosea–like eruptions have been observed repeatedly after bone marrow transplantation.[22] There is no evidence that PR is a psychosomatic disease.[4]

CLINICAL MANIFESTATIONS

Classic Pityriasis Rosea

The prodromal symptoms of PR have been reported repeatedly as general malaise, nausea, loss of appetite, fever, joint pain, and swelling of lymph nodes (in the acute vesicular form). In a controlled study, headache and gastrointestinal symptoms occurred more frequently in PR patients than in controls.

The primary plaque (plaque primitive, herald patch, primary medallion, mother patch; Fig. 46-1) is seen in 50 to 90 percent of cases. It will, in a few days, reach a diameter of a few centimeters. It is oval or

FIGURE 46-1

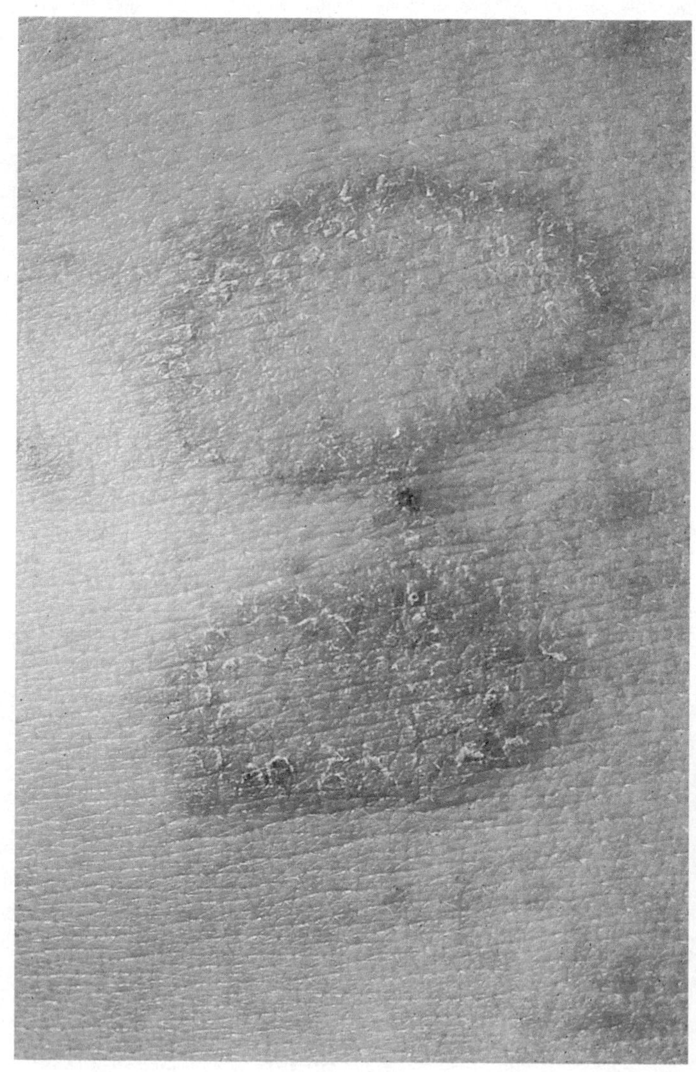

Pityriasis rosea. Double herald patch.

FIGURE 46-2

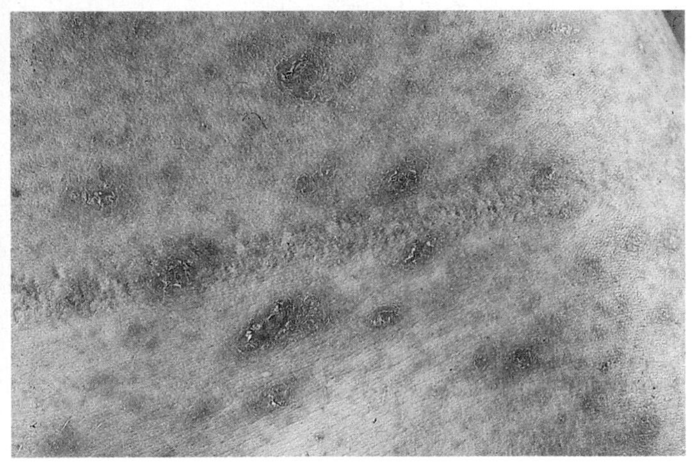

Pityriasis rosea. Generalized eruption. The long axis of the lesions follow the lines of cleavage. Typical marginal collarettes of scale.

FIGURE 46-4

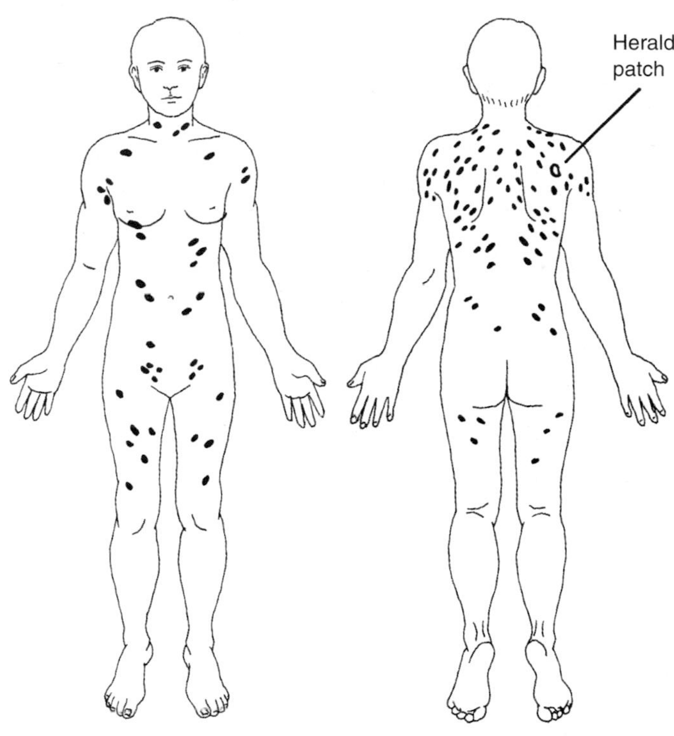

Schematic diagram of the herald patch and typical truncal distribution along the lines of cleavage.

round with a central, wrinkled, salmon-colored area and a darker red peripheral zone, separated by a collarette of fine scaling (Figs. 46-2 and 46-3). When the plaque is irritated, it will have an "eczematous," papulovesicular appearance. The primary plaque is usually situated on the trunk in areas covered by clothes, but sometimes it is on the neck or extremities. Localization to the face or penis is rare. The site of the primary lesion does not differ between men and women.

The interval between the primary and secondary eruption is 2 days to 2 months. Cases have been reported in which the primary and secondary lesions appeared at the same time. The secondary eruption appears in crops at intervals of a few days and reaches its maximum in about 10 days. Occasionally new lesions continue to develop for several weeks. The symmetric eruption is localized mainly to the trunk and adjacent regions of the neck and extremities. The most pronounced lesions extend over the abdomen and anterior surface of the thorax as well as over the back. Lesions distal to the elbows and knees are not uncommon. Two main types of lesion are seen at the classic secondary rash: (1) small plaques resembling primary plaques in miniature, with the two red zones separated by the scaling ring, distributed with their long axes following the lines of cleavage of the skin, forming a "Christmas tree" pattern (Fig. 46-4), and (2) small, red, usually nonscaling papules

FIGURE 46-3

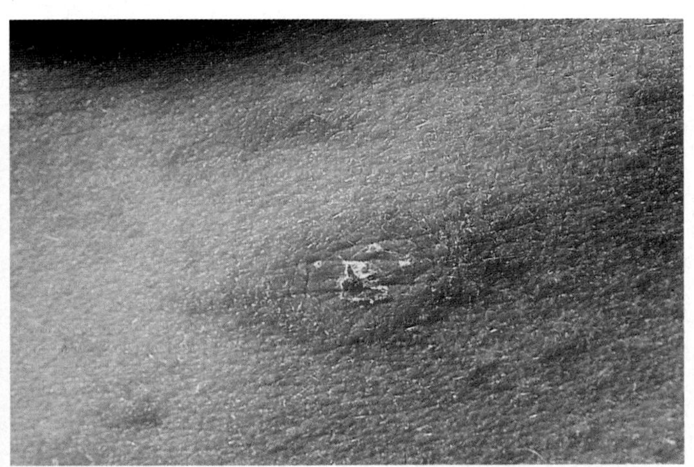

Detail of Fig. 46-2.

that with increasing degrees of inflammation will increase in number and spread peripherally. Both forms may exist concomitantly.

The duration of the secondary eruption varies between 2 and 10 weeks. In severely eczematous or drug-induced rashes, the course may be very protracted (PR perstans).

Itching is severe in 25 percent of patients with uncomplicated PR, slight to moderate in 50 percent, and absent in 25 percent. When PR is irritated, itching is usually prominent.

Atypical Pityriasis Rosea

In about 20 percent of patients, the picture diverges from the classic one. The primary plaque may be missing or present as double or multiple lesions (see Fig. 46-1), often close together. The primary plaque may be the sole manifestation of the disease. The distribution of the secondary rash may be exclusively peripheral (PR inversa). Facial involvement has been reported mainly in children. The vulva may be involved. Localized forms comprise cervicocephalic PR, including the scalp, and the girdle type, affecting the axillae and groins. Unilateral distribution occurs, as well as localization to a small area. The lesions of PR gigantea are fewer than in the small-lesion forms, often develop around the primary plaque, and are not uncommonly confined to a limited region of the trunk; they may be circinate and sometimes confluent, persisting for months (pityriasis circinata et marginata of Vidal).

Enanthema of the mouth may occur exceptionally with or without hemorrhagic patches and even bullae on the tongue and cheeks. The lesions may resemble aphthous ulcers. Nail dystrophy after PR has been reported.

The morphology of the solitary elements of the secondary eruption may be atypical. Macules may lack scaling, papules may be follicular,

FIGURE 46-5

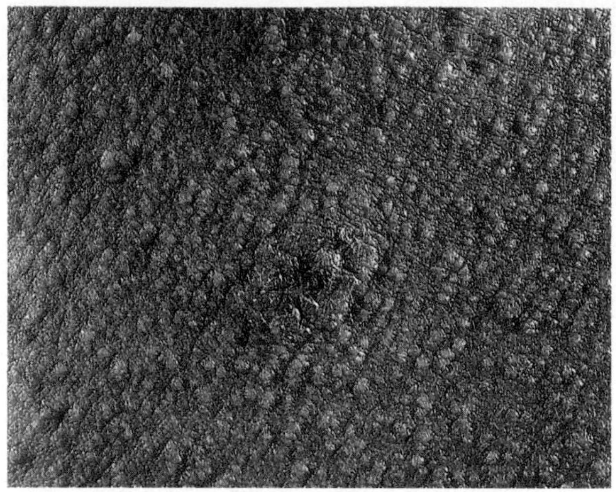

Pityriasis rosea, vesicular type. Even the herald patch is vesicular.

and plaques may be absent or resemble psoriasis. The vesicular type (Fig. 46-5) is uncommon and usually affects children and young adults. It is said to be common in Africa. A purely vesicular form exists, but plaques may occur concomitantly or may develop later within the area of intense vesicular exanthema. The palms and soles sometimes are involved, and the clinical picture may simulate a widespread eczematous eruption. The lesions may be weeping and crusted. A pustular form of PR also exists. PR urticata may, during the first few days, mimic acute urticaria. The whealing is then localized mainly to the borders of the plaques, which tend to become confluent. Purpuric PR is not uncommon, and again, children seem to be predisposed to this form. The hemorrhagic lesions may or may not show scaling, and the skin may be spattered with tiny purpuric spots. A type resembling erythema multiforme also has been described.[23] PR may at the same time show various atypical features, as combined vesicular and purpuric lesions with peripheral localization.

Pigmentary Disturbances

Both hypo- and hyperpigmentation may follow the inflammatory stage. In the black skin of Africans, hyperpigmentation predominates,[3] and intense hyperpigmentation is seen in drug-induced PR. Previous sun tanning may influence the distribution of the secondary rash; the lesions may be confined to the tanned areas, but in some cases, tanning apparently protects the skin from PR lesions.

LABORATORY FINDINGS

The blood picture is usually normal, but leukocytosis, neutrophilia, basophilia, and lymphocytosis have been reported. Slight increases in erythrocyte sedimentation rate, total protein, $alpha_1$ and $alpha_2$ globulins, and albumin also have been observed. Tests for rheumatoid factor, cold agglutinins, and cryoglobulins have been normal.

PATHOLOGY

The histologic findings are similar in the primary plaque and the secondary rash (Figs. 46-6 and 46-7). They are not pathognomonic. Patchy parakeratosis is characteristic, however, and in rare cases may be diffuse. The granular cell layer is reduced or absent. Slight acanthosis occurs. Focal spongiosis rarely may progress to vesiculation. A most impressive sign of PR is the presence of microscopic vesicles, sometimes subcorneal, in a clinically dry lesion. In the papillary dermis there is edema with homogenization of the collagen. A superficial perivascular infiltration consists of lymphocytes, histiocytes, and occasionally eosinophils. The histologic picture may be indistinguishable from that of superficial gyrate erythema.[24] Extravasated erythrocytes may be seen not only in the papillae but also in the epidermis.[25] Other histologic features that have been reported include focal necrosis of epidermal cells; dyskeratotic cells within the upper and middle epidermis with an eosinophilic, homogeneous appearance, suggesting primary damage to the basal cells; multinucleated epidermal giant cells such as are seen in other inflammatory states; focal acantholytic dyskeratosis; and a unique cytolytic degeneration of keratinocytes adjacent to Langerhans cells in the primary plaque.

FIGURE 46-6

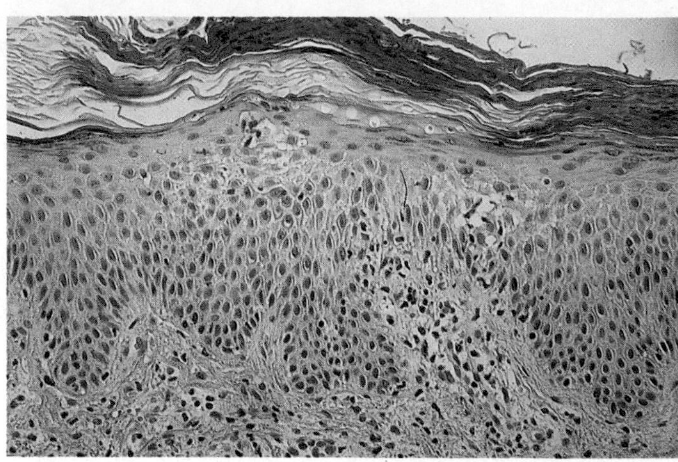

Pityriasis rosea. Patchy parakeratosis, absence of granular layer, slight acanthosis, spongiosis, superficial dermal infiltrate.

In older lesions, the perivascular infiltration is often both superficial and deep, with less spongiosis and more pronounced epidermal hyperplasia.[24] These late lesions may be difficult to distinguish from psoriasis and lichen planus.

FIGURE 46-7

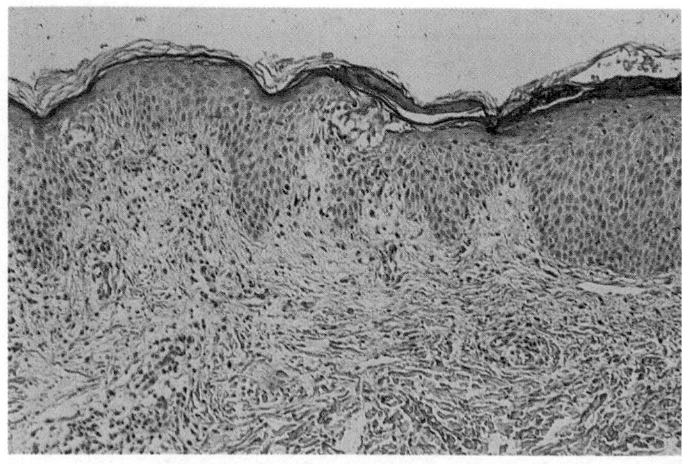

Pityriasis rosea. Absence of granular layer, acanthosis, spongiosis, and discrete inflammatory changes in upper dermis.

DIAGNOSIS AND DIFFERENTIAL DIAGNOSIS

Both the solitary plaque and localized PR gigantea may closely resemble superficial tinea, and widespread eruptions of *Microsporum canis* may simulate generalized PR. Mycologic investigations will be necessary to settle the diagnosis.

"Christmas Tree" Eruptions

Any condition with a "Christmas tree" distribution can be confused with PR. Such conditions include erythema dyschromicum perstans (ashy dermatosis) in its small-lesion form. In ashy dermatosis, slight erythema precedes the characteristic bluish brown patches following the clefts of the skin. The color also differs from the tawny postlesional pigmentation that follows PR and that also fades faster. The histology of erythema dyschromicum perstans, with its hydropic degeneration of the basal cells of the epidermis, is different from that of PR. Classic PR with a primary plaque progressing to typical erythema dyschromicum perstans has been reported. Lichen planus and lichenoid reactions (lichen pigmentosus) with PR distribution often are caused by drugs. Cases have been reported in which lesions characteristic of both PR and lichen planus, both on naked-eye examination and on microscopy, have been present concomitantly. Pityriasis lichenoides may present with a "Christmas tree" pattern on the trunk, but as a rule, typical lesions will be found on the extremities. Histologically, PR can mimic this state. Kaposi's sarcoma may, in the aggressive form associated with HIV infection, show a PR pattern with oval, violaceous papules and nodules chiefly on the arms, neck, and trunk[26] associated with ecchymotic lesions.[27] A variety of papulosquamous dermatoses including PR of the persistent type also may be connected with HIV infection.[21] Histologic examination is necessary.

Annular Eruptions

Pityriasis alba occurs on the face, arms, and thorax in children and young adults. When the skin is irritated, an annular erythema may develop. Pityriasis rosea of the giant annular type may have the same localization, but the course is briefer in PR. Nummular eczema localized to the trunk also can pose difficulties in diagnosis. The lesions are usually round, not oval, and the papulovesicular elements are more prominent than in PR. Again, the course of PR is shorter. Seborrheic dermatitis can present precipitously with annular or figurate lesions on the trunk and arms; it sometimes may simulate localized PR. As a rule, the scalp and face show the typical picture of seborrheic dermatitis, and the course is protracted. Superficial tinea, when acute and with multiple lesions, may resemble PR; mycologic investigation is necessary.

Papular Eruptions

Papular eruptions may be excluded when there is no primary plaque. Various drug eruptions and erythema multiforme of the small-lesion type may have to be considered. The Gianotti-Crosti syndrome can be very difficult to distinguish from inverse papular PR in children. Guttate psoriasis may cause difficulties in differential diagnosis when only a few superficial lesions are present. Histologic examination is not always helpful. Psoriasis runs a chronic course. Secondary syphilis may present with slightly scaling lesions and can mimic papular PR with no primary plaque. Mucosal lesions and enlargement of lymph nodes may occur in both PR and syphilis, but as with involvement of the palms and soles, these are much more common in the latter. Serologic tests for syphilis will differentiate the two.

TREATMENT

Since PR is self-limited, there is no need for active treatment in uncomplicated cases. Water, soap, wool, and sweating may cause irritation and should be avoided in the acute stages. When there is itching, zinc oxide or calamine lotion usually will suffice. In the widespread, severe forms, including vesicular PR, topical glucocorticoids are indicated and, exceptionally, a brief course of an oral glucocorticoid preparation. However, exacerbations with glucocorticoid treatment have been reported.[28] Dapsone has been used in severe vesicular PR. Erythromycin has been shown recently to clear PR in 2 weeks. Complete response was observed in 73 percent of a treatment group and none of a placebo-treated group.[29]

Some therapeutic effect of ultraviolet radiation has been confirmed in controlled studies.[30] A dose large enough to produce erythema and desquamation is necessary. Postinflammatory pigmentation at the site of the PR lesion may follow ultraviolet radiation therapy and has prompted a warning against this form of treatment.

REFERENCES

1. Gibert CM: *Traité Pratique des Maladies de la Peau et de la Syphilis*, 3d ed. Paris, Plon, 1860, p 402
2. Chuang T-Y et al: Pityriasis rosea in Rochester, Minnesota, 1969 to 1978: A 10-year epidemiologic study. *J Am Acad Dermatol* **7**:80, 1982
3. Vollum DI: Pityriasis rosea in the African. *Trans St Johns Hosp Dermatol Soc* **59**:269, 1973
4. Björnberg A, Hellgren L: Pityriasis rosea: A statistical, clinical, and laboratory investigation of 826 patients and matched healthy controls. *Acta Derm Venereol (Stockh)* **42**(suppl 50):1, 1962
5. Harman M et al: An epidemiological study of pityriasis rosea in the eastern Anatolia. *Eur J Epidemiol* **14**:495, 1998
6. Tay YK, Goh CL: One-year review of pityriasis rosea at the National Skin Centre, Singapore. *Ann Acad Med Singapore* **28**:829, 1999
7. Chuang T-Y et al: Recent upper respiratory tract infection and pityriasis rosea: A case-control study of 249 matched pairs. *Br J Dermatol* **108**:587, 1983
8. De Keyser F et al: Immune-mediated pathology following hepatitis B vaccination: Two cases of polyarteritis nodosa and one case of pityriasis rosea-like drug eruption. *Clin Exp Rheumatol* **18**:81, 2000
9. Baker BS et al: Group A streptococcal antigen-specific T lymphocytes in guttate psoriatic lesions. *Br J Dermatol* **128**:493, 1993
10. Metz J: An electronmicroscopic investigation of the pityriasis rosea. *Am J Dermatopathol* **4**:228, 1977
11. Aoshima T et al: Ultrastructural observations of a herald patch in vesicular pityriasis rosea. *Am J Dermatopathol* **5**:273, 1978
12. Gjenero-Margan I et al: Pityriasis rosea (Gibert): Detection of *Legionella micdadei* antibodies in patients. *Eur J Epidemiol* **11**:459, 1995
13. Hudson LD et al: Pityriasis rosea: Viral complement fixation studies. *J Am Acad Dermatol* **4**:544, 1981
14. Takaki Y et al: Immunological studies of pityriasis rosea (Gibert). *J Dermatol (Tokyo)* **4**:37, 1977
15. Parsons JM: Pityriasis rosea update: 1986. *J Am Acad Dermatol* **15**:159, 1986
16. Bos JD et al: Pityriasis rosea (Gibert): Abnormal distribution pattern of antigen presenting cells in situ. *Acta Derm Venereol (Stockh)* **65**:132, 1985
17. Aiba S, Tagami H: Immunohistologic studies in pityriasis rosea: Evidence for cellular immune reaction in lesional epidermis. *Arch Dermatol* **121**:761, 1985
18. Drago F et al: Human herpesvirus 7 in pityriasis rosea. *Lancet* **349**: 1367, 1997
19. Kempf W et al: Pityriasis rosea is not associated with human herpesvirus 7. *Arch Dermatol* **135**:1070, 1999
20. Black JB, Pellett PE: Human herpesvirus 7. *Rev Med Virol* **9**:245, 1999
21. Sadick NS et al: Papulosquamous dermatoses of AIDS. *J Am Acad Dermatol* **22**:1270, 1990
22. Spelman LJ et al: Pityrisis rosea-like eruption after bone marrow transplantation. *J Am Acad Dermatol* **31**:348, 1994
23. Friedman SJ: Pityriasis rosea with erythema multiforme-like lesions. *J Am Acad Dermatol* **17**:135, 1987

24. Ackerman AB: *Histologic Diagnosis of Inflammatory Skin Diseases.* Philadelphia, Lea & Febiger, 1978
25. Panizzon R, Bloch PH: Histopathology of pityriasis rosea (Gibert): Qualitative and quantitative light-microscopic study of 62 biopsies of 40 patients. *Dermatologica* **165**:551, 1982
26. Myskowski PL et al: Kaposi's sarcoma in young homosexual men. *Cutis* **29**:31, 1982
27. Schwartz RA et al: Ecchymotic Kaposi's sarcoma. *Cutis* **56**:104, 1995
28. Leonforte JF: Pityriasis rosea: Exacerbation with corticosteroid treatment. *Dermatologica* **163**:480, 1981
29. Sharma PK et al: Erythromycin in pityriasis rosea: A double-blind, placebo-controlled clinical trial. *J Am Acad Dermatol* **42**:241, 2000
30. Leenutaphong V, Jiamton S: UVB phototherapy for pityriasis rosea: A bilateral comparison study. *J Am Acad Dermatol* **33**:996, 1995

CHAPTER 47

Gary S. Wood
Chung-Hong Hu

Parapsoriasis

Parapsoriasis is a group of disorders characterized by a persistent, scaling, inflammatory eruption. Two clinicopathologic features set the parapsoriasis group apart from other purely inflammatory dermatoses: the relation to malignant lymphoproliferative lesions and the coexistence and/or overlapping of entities in this group. The current, generally accepted classification includes three entities[1]: large-plaque parapsoriasis (LPP), small-plaque parapsoriasis (SPP), and pityriasis lichenoides (Table 47-1). Each of these entities has distinct skin lesions and several morphologic variants. Some authors regard lymphomatoid papulosis as a variant of pityriasis lichenoides, whereas others consider it to be a separate disease. This issue is discussed further in Chaps. 48 and 159.

HISTORICAL ASPECTS

The parapsoriasis group, described and debated for nearly a century, has spawned a confusing nomenclature. In addition to the proliferation of terminologies over the years, many conceptual schemes concern the group's clinical and biologic evolution.

In 1902, Brocq proposed the term *parapsoriasis* to serve as a central link of his grand design encompassing all inflammatory dermatoses.[1] Notably, he subdivided the parapsoriasis group into three forms: guttate, plaque, and lichenoid. In pre-Brocq years, there had been reports describing a number of dermatoses as parapsoriasis, and various morphologic entities were described during the subsequent 50 years. These have been reviewed in detail.[1] Between about 1950 and 1970, the parapsoriasis group was divided into two categories[2]: pityriasis lichenoides and parapsoriasis en plaques. The emphasis was on the potential of parapsoriasis en plaques to evolve into mycosis fungoides. In the 1970s, two observations concerning parapsoriasis en plaques were of importance. First, the distinction between SPP and LPP gained general acceptance,[3] as advanced previously by Degos[4] and Montgomery.[5] The second was the concept that the different types of LPP are all variants of the patch stage of mycosis fungoides.[6]

TABLE 47-1

Classification of Parapsoriasis

1. Large-plaque parapsoriasis—Variants: poikilodermatous, retiform
2. Small-plaque parapsoriasis—Variant: digitate dermatosis
3. Pityriasis lichenoides
   a. Pityriasis lichenoides et varioliformis acuta (Mucha-Habermann)
   b. Pityriasis lichenoides chronica (Juliusberg)
   c. Lymphomatoid papulosis

It has become a generally accepted practice to include the entities listed in Table 47-1 in the parapsoriasis group. There are authors, however, who still prefer to limit the term to LPP and SPP.[7,8] This chapter focuses on these two disorders. Pityriasis lichenoides and lymphomatoid papulosis are discussed in Chaps. 48 and 159, respectively.

EPIDEMIOLOGY

Large-plaque parapsoriasis (LPP) and SPP are, in general, diseases of middle-aged and older people, with a peak incidence in the fifth decade. Occasionally, lesions arise in childhood and may be associated with pityriasis lichenoides. Small plaque parapsoriasis shows a definite male predominance of approximately 3:1. Large plaque parapsoriasis is probably more common in males, but the difference is not as striking as in SPP. Both occur in all racial groups and geographic regions.

Large Plaque Parapsoriasis (LPP)

CLINICAL MANIFESTATIONS Large-plaque parapsoriasis lesions are either oval or irregularly shaped patches or very thin plaques that are asymptomatic or mildly pruritic. They may be well marginated or may blend imperceptibly into the surrounding skin. The size is variable, but typically most lesions are greater than 5 cm in size, often measuring more than 10 cm in diameter. Lesions are stable in size and may increase in number gradually. They are found mainly on the "bathing trunk" and flexural areas (Fig. 47-1). Extremities and the upper trunk, especially the breasts in women, also may be involved. Light red-brown or salmon-pink in color, their surface is covered with small and scanty scales. Lesions may appear finely wrinkled—"cigarette paper" wrinkling. Such lesions exhibit varying degrees of epidermal atrophy.

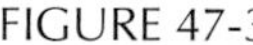

FIGURE 47-1

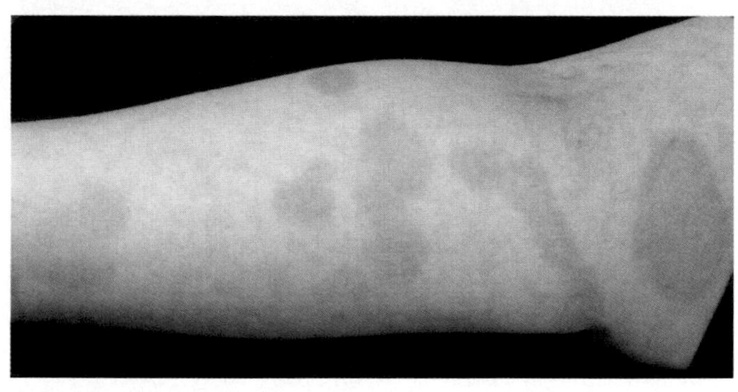

Large-plaque parapsoriasis. Irregularly shaped patches of variable size on the arm of a 16-year-old girl.

Telangiectasia and mottled pigmentation also are observed when the atrophy becomes prominent (Fig. 47-2). This triad of atrophy, mottled pigmentation, and telangiectasia defines the term *poikiloderma* or *poikiloderma atrophicans vasculare,* which also may be seen in certain genodermatoses (Rothmund-Thomson syndrome, Bloom's syndrome, and dyskeratosis congenita) and collagen vascular diseases (dermatomyositis and lupus erythematosus). *Retiform parapsoriasis* refers to a rare variant of LPP that presents as an extensive eruption of scaly macules and papules in a netlike or zebra-stripe pattern that eventually becomes poikilodermatous (Fig. 47-3).

HISTOPATHOLOGIC FEATURES In early LPP lesions, the epidermis is mildly acanthotic and slightly hyperkeratotic with spotty parakeratosis. The dermal lymphocytic infiltrate tends to be perivascular and scattered (Fig. 47-4). In the more advanced lesions one observes an interface infiltrate with definite epidermotropism. These invading lymphocytes may be scattered singly or in groups, sometimes associated with mild spongiosis. In addition, the poikilodermatous lesions show atrophic epidermis, dilated blood vessels, and melanophages (Fig. 47-5). Immunohistologic studies have shown similar features in LPP and early mycosis fungoides, including a predominance of

FIGURE 47-2

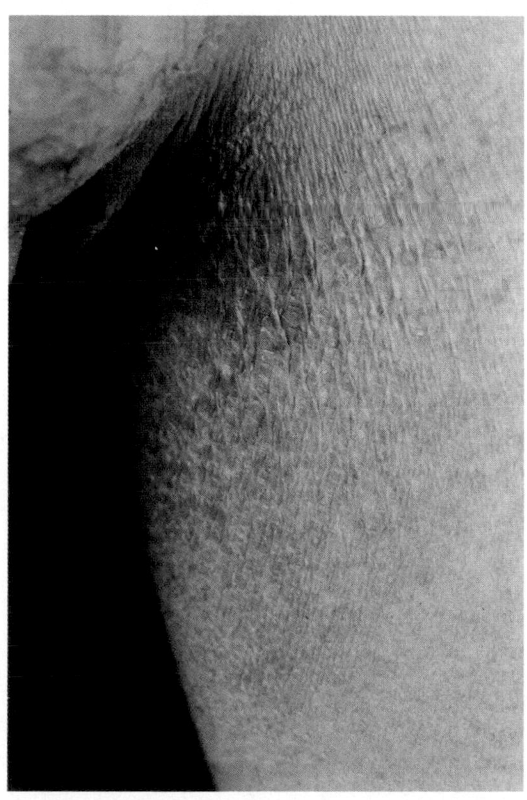

Large-plaque parapsoriasis. Poikilodermatous variant.

FIGURE 47-3

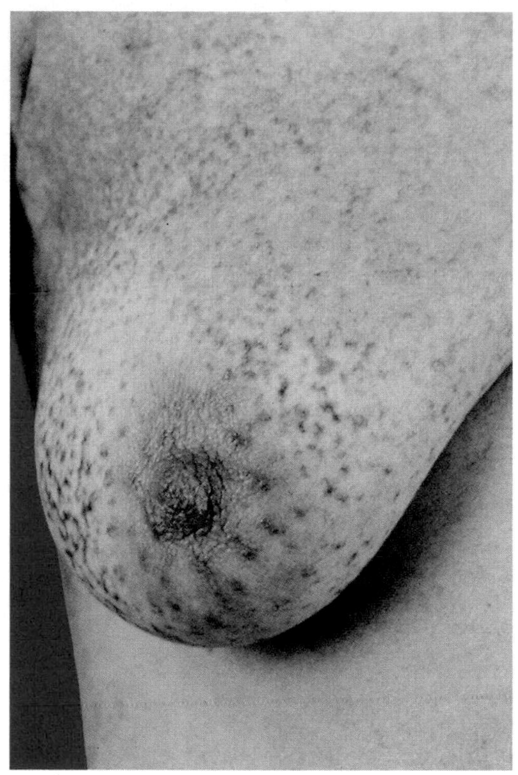

Large-plaque parapsoriasis. Retiform variant.

FIGURE 47-4

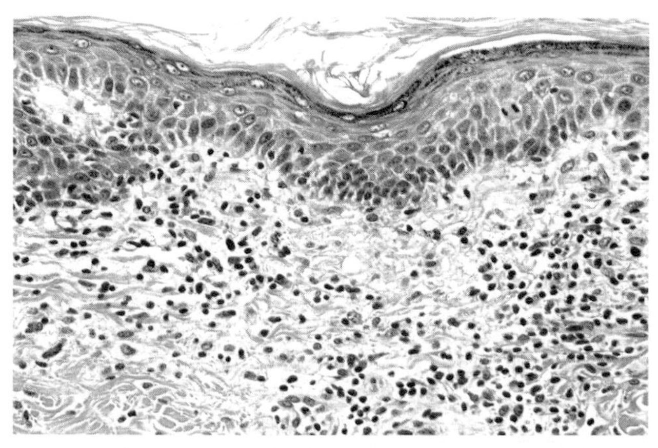

Large-plaque parapsoriasis. Mildly hyperkeratotic and focally parakeratotic epidermis with moderately dense superficial perivascular infiltrate. Lymphoid cells are mostly small, cytologically normal lymphocytes, and there is focal single-cell epidermotropism. (*Courtesy of Helmut Kerl, M.D.*)

FIGURE 47-5

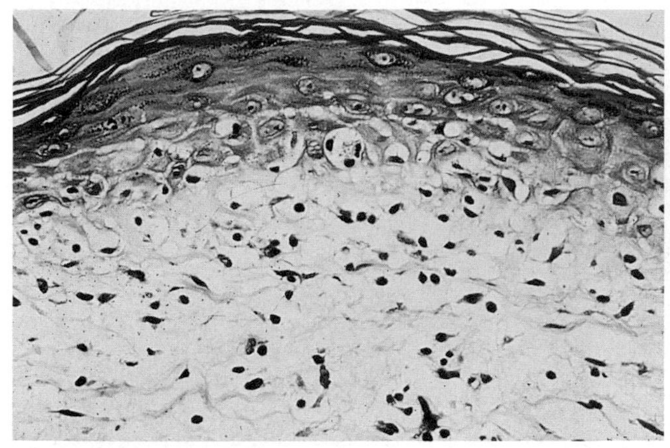

Large-plaque parapsoriasis. Atrophic variant. Sparse superficial lymphoid infiltrate with mild epidermotropism and epidermal atrophy.

CD4+ T cell subsets, frequent CD7 antigen deficiency, and widespread epidermal expression of human leukocyte antigen (HLA-DR).[9–14]

Small Plaque Parapsoriasis (SPP)—Including Digitate Dermatosis

CLINICAL MANIFESTATIONS Small-plaque parapsoriasis characteristically occurs as round, oval, discrete patches or very thin plaques, mainly on the trunk (Fig. 47-6). The lesions measure less than 5 cm in diameter; they are asymptomatic and covered with fine, moderately adherent scales. The general health of the patient is unaffected. A distinctive variant with lesions of the finger shape, known as *digitate dermatosis,*[3] is yellowish or fawn in color (Fig. 47-7). It follows lines of cleavage of the skin and gives the appearance of a hug that left fingerprints on the trunk. The long axis of these lesions often measures greater than 5 cm. *Chronic superficial dermatitis* is a synonym for SPP.[15] Digitate lesions with a yellow hue were referred to in the past as *xanthoerythrodermia perstans.*[1]

HISTOPATHOLOGY Small-plaque parapsoriasis exhibits mild spongiotic dermatitis with focal areas of hyperkeratosis, parakeratosis, scale crust, and exocytosis. In the dermis, there is a mild superficial perivascular lymphohistiocytic infiltrate and dermal edema (Fig. 47-8). There is no progression of the histologic features with time. Immunohistologic studies reveal a predominantly CD4+ T cell infiltrate with nonspecific features resembling those seen in various types of dermatitides.[10]

ETIOLOGY AND PATHOGENESIS

It is likely that a complete understanding of the pathogenesis of parapsoriasis will require a similar comprehension of the pathogenesis of both chronic dermatitis and mycosis fungoides because in many ways parapsoriasis appears to bridge these other disorders (see Chap. 157). The T cells that mediate most inflammatory skin diseases belong to the skin-associated lymphoid tissue (SALT).[17] These T cells express the cutaneous lymphocyte-associated antigen (CLA) and traffic between the skin and the T cell domains of peripheral lymph nodes via the

FIGURE 47-6

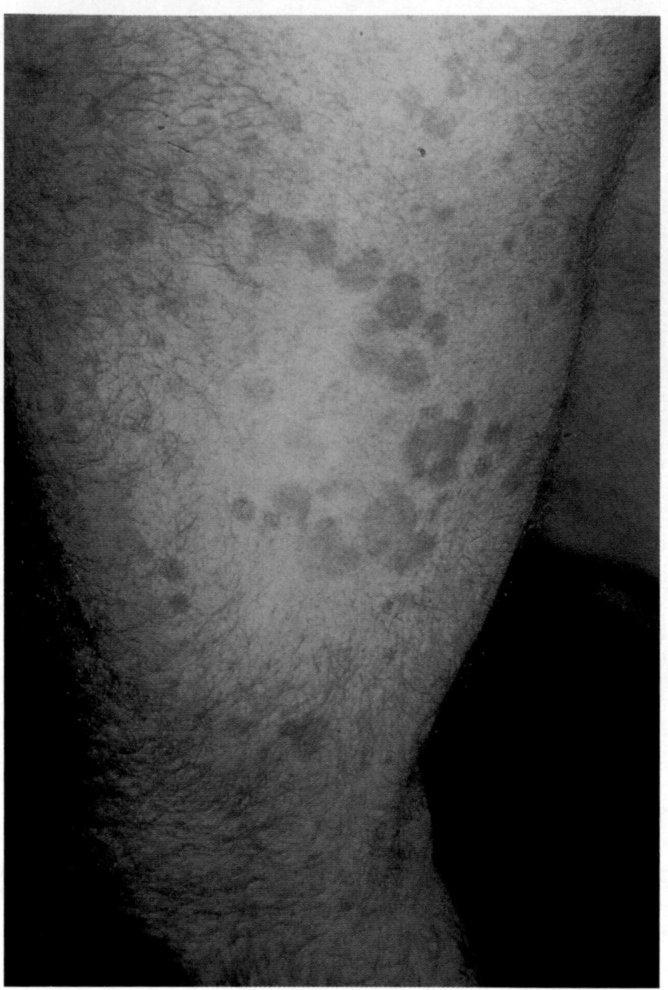

Small-plaque parapsoriasis. Small, discrete patches less than 5 cm in diameter.

lymphatics and bloodstream. Mycosis fungoides has been shown to be a neoplasm of SALT T cells. Sensitive polymerase chain reaction (PCR)–based tumor clonality assays have underscored the SALT nature of mycosis fungoides tumor clones by showing that they can continue to traffic after neoplastic transformation[18] and can even participate in delayed-type hypersensitivity reactions to contact allergens.[19] This implies that rather than being a skin lymphoma per se, mycosis fungoides is actually a SALT lymphoma, i.e., a malignancy of a T cell circuit rather than one particular tissue. Trafficking of mycosis fungoides tumor cells has been detected even in patients with very early stage disease whose lesions were consistent clinicopathologically with LPP.[18] Therefore, it can be said that at least in some cases LPP is a monoclonal proliferation of SALT T cells that have the capacity to traffic between the skin and extracutaneous sites.

This view is also supported by the presence of structural and numerical chromosomal abnormalities in the peripheral blood mononuclear cells of patients with LPP.[20] In this context, LPP can be regarded as the clinically benign end of the mycosis fungoides disease spectrum, which eventuates in transformed large cell lymphoma at its malignant extreme. To say that these diseases belong to the same disease spectrum is not to say that they are biologically equivalent disorders. To lump them all together simply as "mycosis fungoides" would be to ignore their distinctive clinicopathologic features that are likely due to genetic and/or epigenetic differences, such as the *p*53 gene somatic mutations observed in some cases of large cell transformation of mycosis

FIGURE 47-7

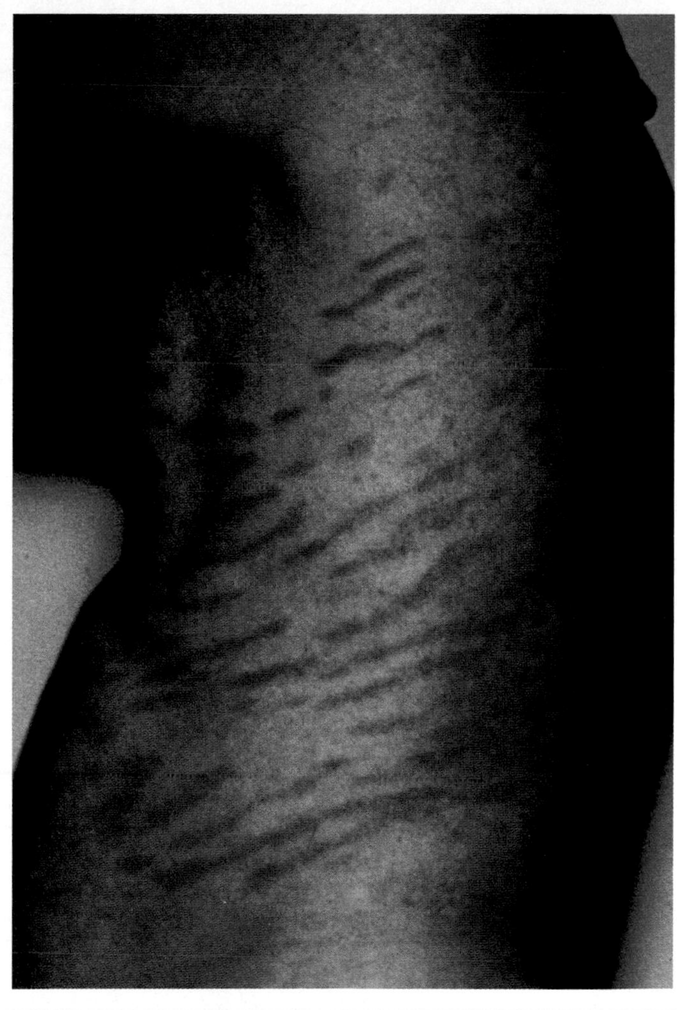

Small-plaque parapsoriasis. Digitate dermatosis variant. Typical "fingerprint" patches on the flank. Note that their length often exceeds 5 cm.

FIGURE 47-8

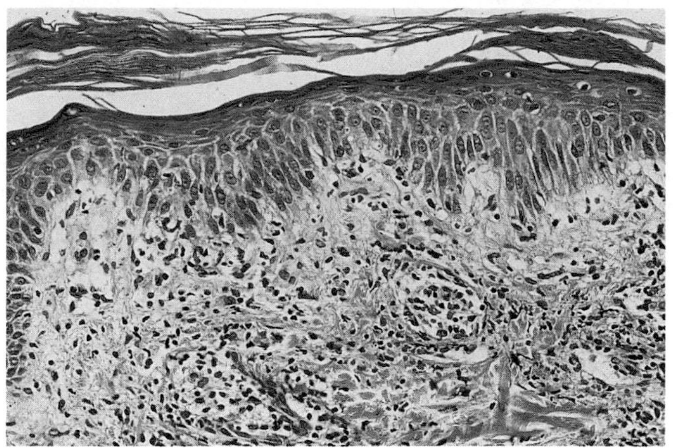

Small-plaque parapsoriasis. Superficial perivascular lymphoid infiltrate, mild spongiosis, parakeratosis, and focal scale crust.

fungoides.[21–23] It is likely that several such differences separate these clinicopathologically defined disorders in a stepwise fashion analogous to the sequential acquisition of somatic mutations that occurs in the colon cancer disease spectrum as colonic epithelial cells progress through normal, hyperplastic, in situ carcinoma, invasive carcinoma, and metastatic carcinoma stages.[24]

A unifying feature of the parapsoriasis group of diseases is that all of them appear to be cutaneous T cell lymphoproliferative disorders; i.e., LPP,[11,12,14,18,25–29] SPP,[12,16] pityriasis lichenoides,[30–32] and lymphomatoid papulosis[12,33–35]; all have been shown to be monoclonal disorders in many cases. In some instances, this has been demonstrated by genomic Southern blot analysis of T cell receptor gene rearrangements, but in others it has required more sensitive PCR-based techniques that are better suited to small skin biopsy specimens containing sparse lymphoid infiltrates. Studies of LPP/early mycosis fungoides, in which PCR-based assays detected monoclonality much more often than genomic Southern blotting,[11,12,14,18,25–29] have suggested a dominant clonal density of roughly 1 to 10 percent. This is less than is seen in more advanced mycosis fungoides, where a dominant clone is consistently demonstrable by genomic Southern blotting and can have a density as high as 50 percent or more. These relationships suggest that progression from LPP through the various stages of the mycosis fungoides disease spectrum is accompanied by an increasing gradient of dominant T cell clonal density resulting from mutations that confer increasing growth autonomy to the neoplastic T cell clone.[36] Interestingly, analysis of peripheral blood has demonstrated that clonal T cells are often detectable in patients with LPP/early mycosis fungoides[28] or SPP,[37] again supporting the systemic SALT nature of these "primary" skin disorders.

It is important to realize that dominant clonality as seen in the parapsoriasis disease group, follicular mucinosis, pagetoid reticulosis (see Chap. 157), and certain other disorders does not equate to clinical malignancy. In fact, most patients with these diseases follow a benign clinical course, in some cases with complete resolution of their disease. In addition, there are other types of chronic cutaneous T cell infiltrates that sometimes exhibit dominant clonality, including primary (idiopathic) erythroderma and nonspecific chronic spongiotic dermatitis. This has given rise to the concept of clonal dermatitis,[25] originally described in the context of clonal nonspecific chronic spongiotic dermatitis but later expanded to include other nonlymphomatous cutaneous T cell infiltrates that harbor occult monoclonal T cell populations. During the past few years, several cases of clonal dermatitis, some of which have progressed to mycosis fungoides, have been identified.[25,29] We suspect that within each disease with a potential for progression to mycosis fungoides, the principal risk may reside within its clonal dermatitis subset because this is the subset within which dysregulation has begun to occur.

The postulated relationships among mycosis fungoides, clonal dermatitis, and selected types of chronic dermatitis are depicted in Fig. 47-9. Each of the entities shown is postulated to be at risk for mycosis fungoides through a clonal dermatitis intermediate. In this model, mycosis fungoides becomes the final common pathway for the clonal evolution of neoplastic T cells emerging from the polyclonal SALT T cell populations present in each of the various precursor diseases.

DIFFERENTIAL DIAGNOSIS

Large-plaque parapsoriasis is distinguished from SPP by the larger size, asymmetric distribution, and irregular shape of its lesions that are less discrete and often poikilodermatous. Large-plaque parapsoriasis may be clinically and histopathologically indistinguishable from the patch stage of mycosis fungoides. Both LPP and SPP are readily distinguished from more advanced infiltrated plaques of mycosis fungoides because

FIGURE 47-9

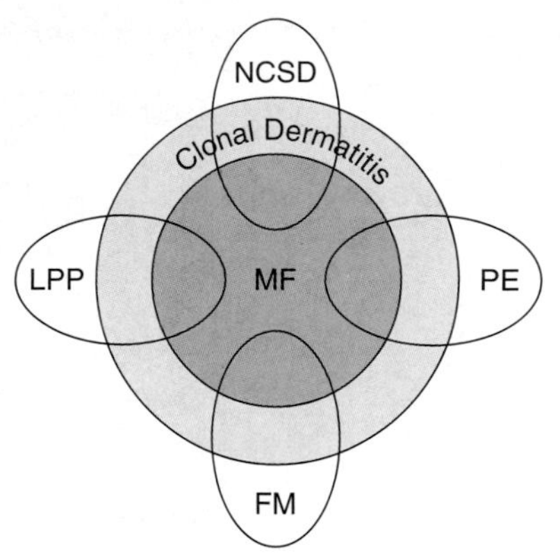

The relationship of clonal dermatitis to mycosis fungoides and various types of chronic dermatitis. The proportions of each entity that represent clonal dermatitis and mycosis fungoides vary with each disease and are not drawn to scale. Abbreviations: MF, mycosis fungoides; NCSD, nonspecific chronic spongiotic dermatitis; PE, primary erythroderma; FM, follicular mucinosis; LPP, large-plaque parapsoriasis.

parapsoriasis lesions are, by definition, not thicker than patches or at most very thin plaques. This is so because the English equivalent of the French term *plaques* is *patches,* i.e., lesions that are essentially flat and devoid of induration or palpable infiltration.[38] Failure to appreciate this important distinction has led to considerable confusion and misuse of the terms *large-plaque* and *small-plaque parapsoriasis* by some individuals. These designations more appropriately might be thought of as large-patch and small-patch parapsoriasis.

The degree to which LPP is differentiated from early mycosis fungoides depends primarily on the histopathologic criteria used to diagnose the latter disorder (see Chap. 157). Unfortunately, there are no universally accepted minimal criteria for the diagnosis of mycosis fungoides; however, one set developed at Stanford University that has proved useful over the years is listed in Table 47-2.[39] Assuming that histopathologic examination does not disclose features diagnostic of some other dermatosis, these criteria allow lesions to be classified into one of four categories: diagnostic of mycosis fungoides, consistent with mycosis fungoides, suggestive of mycosis fungoides, or nonspecific chronic dermatitis. For the practical purposes of clinical management, patients presenting clinically with patch lesions that fall into the first two categories are considered to have unequivocal mycosis fungoides, whereas those in the latter two categories are not. Obviously, the more liberal the histopathologic criteria, the more cases will be considered to be mycosis fungoides. However, there will always be some cases that fail to meet any specific set of criteria, and the designation LPP is a useful term to apply to them because it guides treatment and follow-up and conveys an understanding that the risk of dying from lymphoma is small.

TABLE 47-2

Histopathologic Criteria for Mycosis Fungoides

1. Multiple Pautrier microaggregates
2. Diffuse infiltration of many individual atypical lymphocytes* into the epidermis†
3. A few small intraepidermal clusters of a few atypical lymphocytes
4. A few individual intraepidermal atypical lymphocytes
5. Dense upper dermal bandlike interface infiltrate that includes atypical lymphocytes
6. Mild to moderate polymorphous upper dermal infiltrate that includes atypical lymphocytes and has a focal interface pattern
7. Extension of the infiltrate into the deep dermis

Categories diagnostic of MF: 1; 2; 3 + 4 + 5; 3 + 4 + 6 + 7
Categories consistent with MF: 3 + 5; 3 + 6; 4 + 5; 4 + 6 + 7
Categories suggestive of MF: 3; 4; 5; 6

*Lymphocytes with scant cytoplasm and hyperchromatic, convoluted (cerebriform) nuclei. Cell size may vary.
†Epidermal involvement is characteristically not associated with prominent intercellular edema (spongiosis).
SOURCE: Adapted with minor modifications from the criteria of Alvin J. Cox, M.D., Professor Emeritus of Dermatology and Pathology, Stanford University, with permission.

The clinical and/or histopathologic differential diagnosis of LPP also includes those genodermatoses and collagen vascular diseases exhibiting poikilodermatous features, lichenoid drug eruptions, secondary syphilis, and chronic radiodermatitis. These generally can be distinguished by their associated clinical findings. The histopathologic differentiation among these diseases is included in the discussion of pseudo-mycosis fungoides in Chap. 159.

Small-plaque parapsoriasis, when it presents with its distinctive digitate lesions parallel to skin lines in a truncal distribution, stands out from other types of parapsoriasis. Individual SPP lesions may show some superficial resemblance to pityriasis lichenoides chronica. Small-plaque parapsoriasis is distinguished from psoriasis by the absence of the Auspitz sign, micaceous scale, nail pits, and typical psoriatic lesions involving scalp, elbows, and knees. Histologically, its mild spongiotic dermatitis distinguishes it from both pityriasis lichenoides chronica and psoriasis.

Sometimes patients with mycosis fungoides may exhibit small patches of disease at presentation; however, these lesions typically have histopathologic features at least consistent with mycosis fungoides (as defined in Table 47-2) and generally are associated with larger, more classic lesions of mycosis fungoides elsewhere on the skin. They also may show poikilodermatous features not seen in SPP. Furthermore, the presence of well-developed, moderate to thick small plaques, as seen in some mycosis fungoides patients, is incompatible with the diagnosis of SPP because the latter disorder includes only lesions that are no more than patches or very thin plaques. It is also important to recognize that partially treated or early relapsing lesions of mycosis fungoides may show only nonspecific features that should not be taken as evidence of a pathogenetic link to SPP or any other dermatosis.

TREATMENT

Patients with SPP should be reassured and may be left untreated. The disease may be treated with emollients, topical tar preparations, topical corticosteroids, and/or ultraviolet B (UVB) phototherapy. Response to therapy is variable. Patients should be examined initially every 3 to 6 months and subsequently every year to ensure that the character of the process is stable.

Large-plaque parapsoriasis requires more aggressive therapy: high-potency topical corticosteroids with phototherapy such as UVB, narrowband UVB, or psoralen and ultraviolet A (PUVA). The goal of treatment is to suppress the disorder to prevent possible progression to overt mycosis fungoides. Other methods of treatment, such as topical nitrogen mustard, have been used, particularly for the poikilodermatous type. The patient should be examined carefully every 3 months initially and every 6 months to 1 year subsequently for evidence of progression. Repeated multiple biopsies of suspicious lesions should be performed. Cases that satisfy the clinicopathologic criteria for early mycosis fungoides usually are treated with UVB, narrowband UVB, PUVA, topical nitrogen mustard, or topical carmustine (BCNU). Electron-beam radiation therapy generally is reserved for more advanced, infiltrated lesions of mycosis fungoides.

COURSE AND PROGNOSIS

Both LPP and SPP may persist for years to decades with little change in appearance clinically or histopathologically. Approximately 10 to 30 percent of cases of LPP progress to overt mycosis fungoides.[1,40] In this context, LPP represents the clinically benign end of the mycosis fungoides disease spectrum, with transformation to large cell lymphoma at the opposite extreme. The rare retiform variant is said to progress to overt mycosis fungoides in virtually all cases.[1]

In contrast to the malignant potential of LPP, SPP is a clinically benign disorder. Patients with this disease as defined in this chapter rarely, if ever, develop overt mycosis fungoides as defined in Table 47-2.[15] Despite this fact and what most observers consider to be its nonspecific histopathologic features, some authors favor lumping SPP within the mycosis fungoides disease spectrum as a very early, nonprogressive variant.[41] This issue has been debated at length.[31,42,43]

REFERENCES

1. Lambert WC, Everett MA: The nosology of parapsoriasis. *J Am Acad Dermatol* **5**:373, 1981
2. Ingram JT: Pityriasis lichenoides and parapsoriasis. *Br J Dermatol* **65**:293, 1953
3. Hu C-H, Winkelmann RK: Digitate dermatosis: A new look at symmetrical, small plaque parapsoriasis. *Arch Dermatol* **107**:65, 1973
4. Degos R: *Dermatologie.* Paris, Flammarion, 1953, p 188
5. Montgomery H: *Parapsoriasis in Dermatopathology,* edited by H Montgomery. New York, Harper & Row, 1967, p 337
6. Sánchez JL, Ackerman AB: The patch stage of mycosis fungoides. *Am J Dermatopathol* **1**:5, 1979
7. Lever WF, Schaumburg-Lever G: Parapsoriasis, in *Histopathology of the Skin,* edited by WF Lever, G Schaumburg-Lever. Philadelphia, Lippincott, 1990, p 165
8. Ross S, Sánchez JL: Parapsoriasis: A century later. *Int J Dermatol* **29**:329, 1990
9. Lindae ML et al: Poikilodermatous mycosis fungoides and atrophic large-plaque parapsoriasis exhibit similar abnormalities of T-cell antigen expression. *Arch Dermatol* **124**:366, 1988
10. Ralfkiaer E et al: Phenotypic characterization of lymphocyte subsets in mycosis fungoides: Comparison with large plaque parapsoriasis and benign chronic dermatoses. *Am J Clin Pathol* **84**:610, 1985
11. Kikuchi A et al: Parapsoriasis en plaques: Its potential for progression to malignant lymphoma. *J Am Acad Dermatol* **29**:419, 1993
12. Zelickson BD et al: T-cell receptor gene rearrangement analysis: Cutaneous T cell lymphoma, peripheral T cell lymphoma, and premalignant and benign cutaneous lymphoproliferative disorders. *J Am Acad Dermatol* **25**:787, 1991
13. Buchner SA: Parapsoriasis en plaques: Characterization of the cellular infiltrate using monoclonal antibodies. *Z Hautkr* **63**:423, 1988
14. Menni S et al: Parapsoriasis in two children: A clinical, immunophenotypic, and immunogenotypic study. *Pediatr Dermatol* **11**:151, 1994
15. Samman PD: The natural history of parapsoriasis en plaque (chronic superficial dermatitis) and pre-reticulotic poikiloderma. *Br J Dermatol* **87**:405, 1972
16. Haeffner AC et al: The differentiation and clonality of lesional lymphocytes in small plaque parapsoriasis. *Arch Dermatol* **131**:321, 1995
17. Bos JD (ed): *Skin Immune System.* Boca Raton, FL, CRC Press, 1990
18. Veelken H et al: Molecular staging of cutaneous T cell lymphoma: Evidence for systemic involvement in early disease. *J Invest Dermatol* **104**:889, 1995
19. Veelken H et al: Detection of low-level tumor cell trafficking to allergic contact dermatitis induced by mechlorethamine in patients with mycosis fungoides. *J Invest Dermatol* **106**:685, 1996
20. Karenko L et al: Chromosomal abnormalities in cutaneous T-cell lymphoma and in its premalignant conditions as detected by G-banding and interphase cytogenetic methods. *J Invest Dermatol* **108**:22, 1997
21. Chooback L et al: Overexpression of p53 protein in cutaneous T-cell lymphoma (CTCL): Relationship to large cell transformation (LCT) and disease progression. *J Invest Dermatol* **104**:674, 1995
22. McGregor JM et al: p53 gene mutations in cutaneous T-cell lymphoma. *J Invest Dermatol* **106**:855, 1996
23. Kim BK et al: p53 protein status in cutaneous T-cell lymphoma. *J Cutan Pathol* **24**:107, 1997
24. Fearon ER, Vogelstein B: A genetic model for colorectal tumorigenesis. *Cell* **61**:759, 1990
25. Wood GS et al: Detection of clonal T-cell receptor γ gene rearrangements in early mycosis fungoides/Sézary syndrome by polymerase chain reaction and denaturing gradient gel electrophoresis (PCR/DGGE). *J Invest Dermatol* **103**:34, 1994
26. Bergman R: How useful are T-cell receptor gene rearrangement studies as an adjunct to the histopathologic diagnosis of mycosis fungoides? *Am J Dermatopathol* **21**:498, 1999
27. Simon M et al: Large plaque parapsoriasis: Clinical and genotypic correlations. *J Cutan Pathol* **27**:57, 2000
28. Muche JM et al: Demonstration of frequent occurrence of clonal T cells in the peripheral blood of patients with primary cutaneous T-cell lymphoma. *Blood* **90**:1636, 1997
29. Siddiqui J: Clonal dermatitis: A potential precursor of CTCL with varied clinical manifestations. *J Invest Dermatol* **108**:584, 1997
30. Weiss LM et al: Clonal T-cell populations in pityriasis lichenoides et varioliformis acuta (Mucha-Habermann disease). *Am J Pathol* **126**:417, 1988
31. Shieh S et al: Differentiation and clonality of lesional lymphocytes in pityriasis lichenoides chronica. *Arch Dermatol* **137**:305, 2001
32. Dereure O et al: T-cell clonality in pityriasis lichenoides et varioliformis acuta: A heteroduplex analysis of 20 cases. *Arch Dermatol* **136**:1483, 2000
33. Weiss LM et al: Clonal T-cell populations in lymphomatoid papulosis: Evidence of a lymphoproliferative origin for a clinically benign disease. *N Engl J Med* **315**:475, 1986
34. Kadin ME et al: Clonal composition of T-cells in lymphomatoid papulosis. *Am J Pathol* **126**:13, 1987
35. Chott A et al: The same dominant T cell clone is present in multiple regressing skin lesions and associated T cell lymphomas of patients with lymphomatoid papulosis. *J Invest Dermatol* **106**:696, 1996
36. Wood GS: Lymphocyte activation in cutaneous T-cell lymphoma. *J Invest Dermatol* **105**:105S, 1995
37. Muche JM et al: Demonstration of frequent occurrence of clonal T cells in the peripheral blood but not the skin of patients with small plaque parapsoriasis. *Blood* **94**:1409, 1999
38. Burg G et al: Cutaneous lymphomas consist of a spectrum of nosologically different entities including mycosis fungoides and small plaque parapsoriasis. *Arch Dermatol* **132**:567, 1996
39. Wood GS: The benign and malignant cutaneous lymphoproliferative disorders including mycosis fungoides, in *Neoplastic Hematopathology,* 2d ed, edited by DM Knowles. Baltimore: Williams & Wilkins, 2001, p 1183
40. Lazar AP et al: Parapsoriasis and mycosis fungoides: The Northwestern University experience, 1970 to 1985. *J Am Acad Dermatol* **21**:919, 1989
41. King-Ismael D, Ackerman AB: Guttate parapsoriasis/digitate dermatosis (small plaque parapsoriasis) is mycosis fungoides. *Am J Dermatopathol* **14**:518, 1992
42. Burg G, Dummer R: Small plaque (digitate) parapsoriasis is an abortive cutaneous T-cell lymphoma and is not mycosis fungoides. *Arch Dermatol* **131**:336, 1995
43. Ackerman AB: If small plaque (digitate) parapsoriasis is a cutaneous T-cell lymphoma, even an "abortive" one, it must be mycosis fungoides! *Arch Dermatol* **132**:562, 1996

CHAPTER 48

Mazen S. Daoud
Mark R. Pittelkow

Pityriasis Lichenoides

HISTORIC ASPECTS

Pityriasis lichenoides [Greek, *pityron* ("bran") + *iasis* (condition); Greek *leichen* (lichen-like eruption), *eidos* ("form")] is an uncommon, idiopathic, acquired dermatosis first described by Neisser[1] and Jadassohn[2] in 1894. Based on differences in morphology and temporal evolution and course of the disorder, acute (*acuta*) and chronic (*chronica*) variants have been identified. Pityriasis lichenoides is characterized by evolving groups of erythematous, scaly papules that may either persist for weeks to months (chronica) or erupt and recur in acute exacerbations, often accompanied by vesiculopustular lesions, ulceration, hemorrhage, and crusting (acuta). The original reports by Neisser and Jadassohn included, but did not distinguish between, the acute and chronic forms of the disease. Juliusberg later delineated the chronic form of pityriasis lichenoides and named it pityriasis lichenoides chronica.[3]

The clinical parameters and temporal course of pityriasis lichenoides led Brocq[4] to include it with a group of skin disorders that he had previously described as small-plaque and large-plaque parapsoriasis; he united these under the term *erythrodermies pityriasques en plaques disseminées*. Brocq thought that these heterogeneous dermatoses shared many features, including an unknown etiology, chronic course, lack of symptoms, and poor response to therapy. The prefix *para* (Greek for "alongside of" "near") was used to denote the similarities of these features with those of psoriasis; the terminology was not based on any clinical morphologic resemblance. *Parapsoriasis en gouttes* (Latin guttae, "in drops") was the term Brocq applied to pityriasis lichenoides.

The variable, ill-defined, and confusing terminology and thc lack of clear clinical descriptions to guide early clinicians in the diagnosis of pityriasis lichenoides undoubtedly led Mucha,[5] in 1916, to redescribe acute pityriasis lichenoides as distinct from pityriasis lichenoides chronica, and, in 1925, Habermann designated the condition, *pityriasis lichenoides et varioliformis acuta* (PLEVA).[6] To the present, Mucha-Habermann disease is synonymous with PLEVA. When referring to pityriasis lichenoides chronica, the acronym PLC is often used to distinguish it from PLEVA.

Unfortunately, the classification scheme and terminology that were developed by Brocq at the turn of the century have led to long-standing confusion, and a plethora of alternative terms and abbreviations have subsequently been applied to the acute and chronic forms of pityriasis lichenoides (Table 48-1). Pityriasis lichenoides can be distinguished on clinical and histologic grounds from small- or large-plaque parapsoriasis, and it is widely accepted that pityriasis lichenoides is a distinct and separate entity from plaque-type parapsoriasis. The historic and nosologic perspectives on pityriasis lichenoides and parapsoriasis are intriguing and represent a prime example of the value of accurately defining and carefully assigning dermatologic nomenclature. The reader is referred to several excellent reviews on this subject.[7,8]

The separation of pityriasis lichenoides into two entities, acuta and chronica, remains controversial.[7] There is a rationale for separating these forms when identifying the distinguishing features and, possibly, the different etiologies of the acute and chronic variants of pityriasis lichenoides. However, to recognize that a melding of clinical features can occur and to facilitate establishing a diagnosis, it is prudent to consider pityriasis lichenoides as a single entity with a spectrum of clinical and histologic variations, ranging from PLEVA to pityriasis lichenoides chronica, and including intermediate or overlapping forms of the disease. Expansion of this classification scheme to the more recently defined and dramatic variants includes the acute form of pityriasis lichenoides with ulceronecrosis and hyperthermia (PLUH) first reported by Degos et al.[9] The spectrum extends to the distinctive, and possibly separate, entity lymphomatoid papulosis, which was initially reported by Dupont[10] in 1965, and further characterized and named by McCaulay[11] in 1968 (see Chap. 159).

The relationship between lymphomatoid papulosis and pityriasis lichenoides is still being debated.[7,12–14] Because of the clinical similarities and the histologic presence of atypical lymphocytes in selected cases of pityriasis lichenoides, lymphomatoid papulosis was considered by some investigators as a variant of pityriasis lichenoides with atypical cells.[14] However, other dermatologists believe that the distinctive clinical, histopathologic, and prognostic differences (see below) are sufficient to separate lymphomatoid papulosis from other variants of pityriasis lichenoides. With the tools for molecular genotyping now available, there is evidence that these diseases, or subsets thereof, represent a clonal T cell lymphoproliferative disorder, which may justify reunifying these seemingly disparate conditions.[15–18]

TABLE 48-1

Pityriasis Lichenoides: Alternative Terminology and Abbreviations

Pityriasis Lichenoides et Varioliformis Acuta	Pityriasis Lichenoides Chronica
PLEVA	PLC
PLVA	
Mucha-Habermann disease	Pityriasis lichenoides, Juliusberg
Parapsoriasis lichenoides et varioliformis acuta	Parapsoriasis lichenoides chronica
Parapsoriasis acuta	Parapsoriasis chronica
Acute parapsoriasis	Chronic parapsoriasis
Acute guttate parapsoriasis	Chronic guttate parapsoriasis
Acute pityriasis lichenoides	Chronic pityriasis lichenoides
Parapsoriasis varioliformis	Dermatitis psoriasiformis nodularis

SOURCE: Adapted from Lambert and Everett.[7]

ETIOLOGY AND PATHOGENESIS

Pityriasis lichenoides chronica and PLEVA have no apparent racial or geographic predilection. These dermatoses often affect both children and adults in the early decades of life. Nonetheless, pityriasis lichenoides has been observed at birth through the ninth decade of life for both men and women. A gender difference in incidence has been observed, with variable male predominance in both the pediatric and adult age groups (1.5:1 to 3:1).[19–21] The crude incidence in Brazil of pityriasis lichenoides chronica has been reported as 1:2000; PLEVA is approximately one-third to one-sixth as common.[20]

The etiology of pityriasis lichenoides is unknown. Sporadic outbreaks suggest the possibility of an infectious association. Cases with a history of preceding upper respiratory infection or streptococcal pharyngitis have been reported. The most widely accepted hypothesis invokes an immunologic or "hypersensitivity" reaction to an infectious agent as the underlying mechanism for the development of pityriasis lichenoides. The pathogenic immune reaction includes both immune complex disease and a cell-mediated hypersensitivity response. Elevated circulating immune complexes are found in a high proportion of patients with pityriasis lichenoides.[22] Deposits of IgM and C3 have been identified around blood vessels and at the epidermal basement membrane zone in active cutaneous lesions of PLEVA. Whether the deposition of immunoreactants is the primary event, similar to allergic or leukocytoclastic vasculitis, or represents an epiphenomenon resulting from the inflammatory reaction is unknown. The presence of suppressor rather than helper T lymphocytes in the perivascular spaces in conjunction with Langerhans cells suggests that cell-mediated immune mechanisms may also be important.[23] Furthermore, a reduction of the ratio in circulating T helper (CD4)/T suppressor (CD8) cells also supports this contention.

Southern blot or polymerase chain reaction analysis of T cell receptor gene rearrangements of lesional skin or blood in cases of PLEVA demonstrates the presence of clonal population(s) of T lymphocytes in selected cases, thus identifying PLEVA as a lymphoproliferative rather than an inflammatory process.[16,17] Recently, monoclonal T cell receptor-γ gene rearrangements were detected in skin biopsies from three of six patients with pityriasis lichenoides chronica.[18] Similar findings of clonal T cell population have been observed in a significant percentage of cases of lymphomatoid papulosis.[15] Lymphomatoid papulosis eventuates in lymphoma with some frequency;[15] pityriasis lichenoides, on the other hand, is most often a clinically benign entity and shows no significantly documented association with malignant lymphoma,[17,18,20] except for a few cases.[24] These disparities between PLEVA and lymphomatoid papulosis suggest different causation or an altered biologic ability to control the T cell lymphoproliferative response and accompanying inflammatory reaction that develop in the skin of patients with these dermatoses.

On the other hand, clonality of some cases of pityriasis lichenoides[17,18] gives further support to the theory that PLEVA and pityriasis lichenoides chronica, at least in some cases, should be classified as cutaneous T cell lymphoproliferative disorders. Further evidence exists to support this view. Pityriasis lichenoides chronica is associated with the development of parakeratosis variegata, a type of retiform parapsoriasis, that is a variant of large-plaque parapsoriasis.[7,25]

Moreover, typical cases of pityriasis lichenoides chronica represent a paraneoplastic phenomenon to an underlying non-Hodgkin's lymphoma or to herald malignant lymphoma of the skin.[26] Papular lesions that resemble pityriasis lichenoides clinically were found to represent mycosis fungoides histologically in three children.[27] These findings reinforce the concept that pityriasis lichenoides should be classified with the lymphoproliferative disorders.

There are likely immunogenetic factors that govern the development of the lymphoproliferative process as well as the inflammatory reaction. No specific genetic components have yet been identified; however, the development of pityriasis lichenoides in multiple family members may be informative in eventually uncovering genetic determinants and/or infectious agents involved in the genesis of this dermatosis.

CLINICAL MANIFESTATIONS

The morphologic findings in typical cases of pityriasis lichenoides chronica or acuta are characteristic but can be more protean, depending on whether the acute or chronic forms of the disease manifest independently or simultaneously. Not infrequently, both types of lesions develop concurrently or sequentially, and thus exhibit intermediate features of both variants. Pityriasis lichenoides chronica, the more common form, is characterized by successive crops of asymptomatic, red-brown, oval to round, lichenoid papules that are firm and measure 3 to 10 mm in diameter (Fig. 48-1). The lesions display a centrally adherent, mica-like scale that can be detached by gentle scraping or curettage, revealing a shiny brown, pigmented surface. The scale becomes more evident and less adherent peripherally, sometimes displaying a "collarette" appearance. The papules usually appear on the trunk and proximal extremities and spare the palms, soles, and face; however, lesions may involve these areas, as well as, on occasion, the scalp and mucous membranes. Individual papules may coalesce in a retiform pattern. Rarely, a segmental distribution is observed.[28] As the eruption evolves, the papules flatten and the scale separates spontaneously over the course of 4 to 6 weeks, typically leaving hyperpigmented macules. A transient or more protracted leukoderma may result (Fig. 48-2). New crops of lesions appear while others fade, giving pityriasis lichenoides chronica the characteristic polymorphous appearance with lesions of different age (Fig. 48-3). Scarring is very unusual in pityriasis lichenoides chronica.

In PLEVA, the acute form of pityriasis lichenoides, the cutaneous eruption is usually the first manifestation of the disease; however, low-grade fever, headache, malaise, and arthralgias may occasionally precede or accompany the skin findings. Multiple, disseminated, erythematous, and edematous papules appear and eventually form central vesiculation and, occasionally, pustular or even hemorrhagic necrosis (Fig. 48-4). The vesicles subsequently rupture, leaving crusted erosions or, in the case of severe necrosis, punched-out ulcers that heal with varioliform scars (Fig. 48-5). Hyper- or hypopigmentation may also result. Lesions may be symptomatic and cause pruritus or, occasionally, a burning sensation. They are distributed mainly on the trunk and flexural aspects of the limbs, and usually spare the palms, soles, face, scalp, and mucous membranes, except in rare instances. As in pityriasis lichenoides chronica, a polymorphous appearance of PLEVA results from the presence of many lesions in different stages of development (Fig. 48-6).

Gelmetti et al. found that the duration of the disease in children with lesions confined mainly to distal extremities (peripheral) was longer than those with truncal (central) distribution.[21] The disease in both groups lasted longer than in patients with diffuse lesions. Therefore, these authors recommended classification of pityriasis lichenoides into diffuse, central, or peripheral forms because distribution correlated better with duration of disease than the development of chronic or acute lesions that often coexisted. However, this classification scheme could not be confirmed in a more recent study of pediatric cases.[19]

FIGURE 48-1

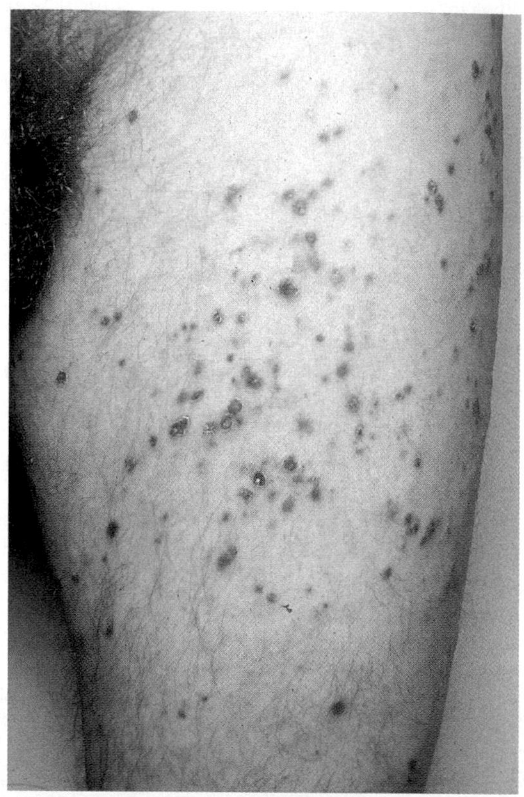

A.

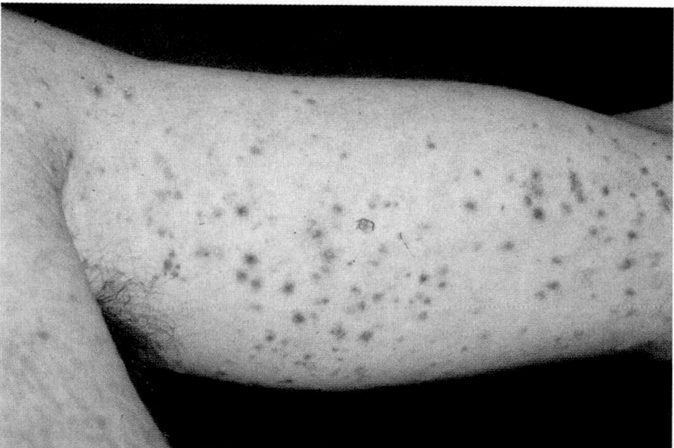

B.

Pityriasis lichenoides chronica. *A.* Clustered red-brown papules, some with fine adherent scale. *B.* Erythematous lesions in various stages of development and involution.

PLUH, the rare hyperacute, ulceronecrotic variant of PLEVA is characterized by the sudden onset of diffuse purpuric papules with necrotic centers measuring from a few millimeters to centimeters. This variant is more destructive, with the development of large necrotic ulcers associated with high fever (40°C/104°F), malaise, myalgias, arthralgias, and gastrointestinal and central nervous system symptoms. PLUH may develop de novo or evolve from either pityriasis lichenoides chronica or PLEVA. Association with Epstein-Barr virus or cytomegalovirus

FIGURE 48-2

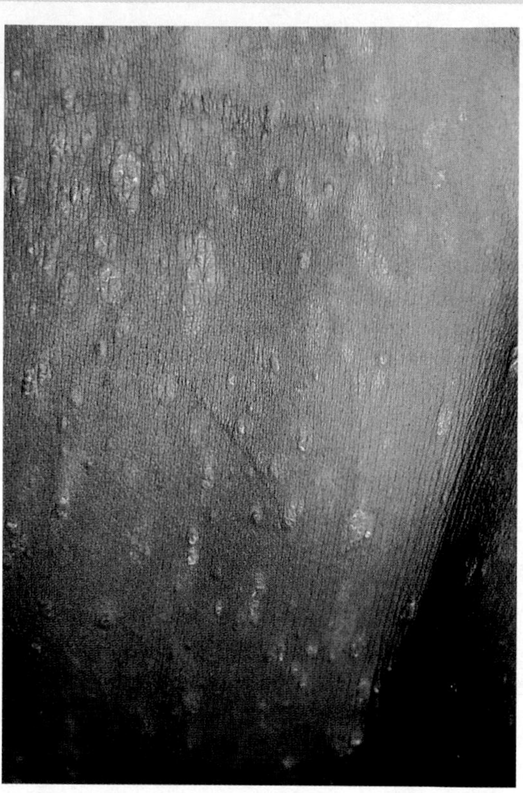

Pityriasis lichenoides chronica. Chronic phase with pink to tan, flat papules (covered by fine, branny scale). Coalescence of papules and secondary hypopigmentation within resolving lesions.

FIGURE 48-3

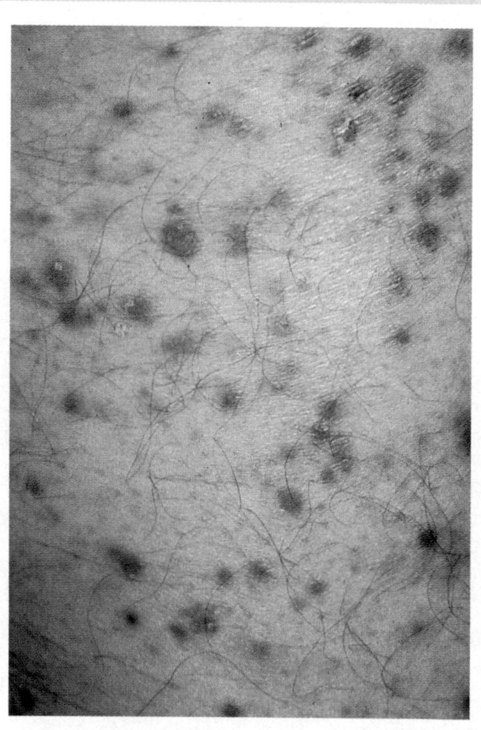

Pityriasis lichenoides chronica. Polymorphous appearance ranging from early erythematous papules to scaling brown-red lesions and tan-brown involuting, flat papules and macules.

FIGURE 48-4

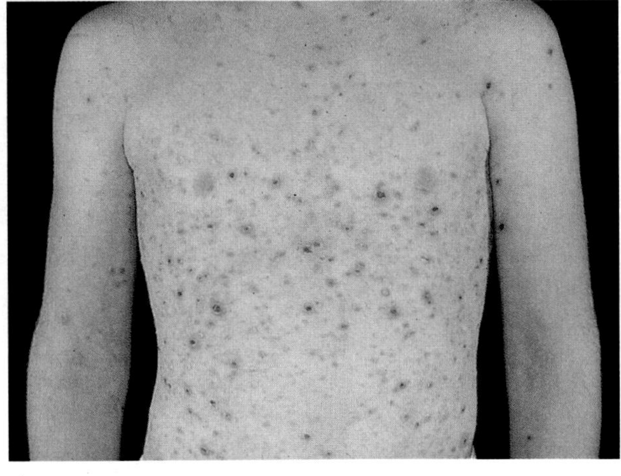

A.

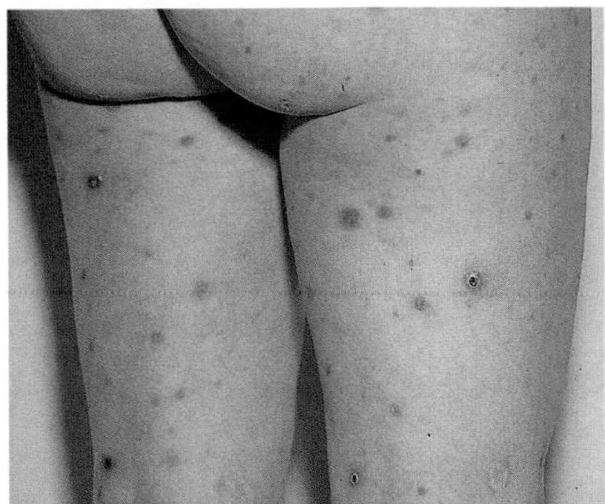

B.

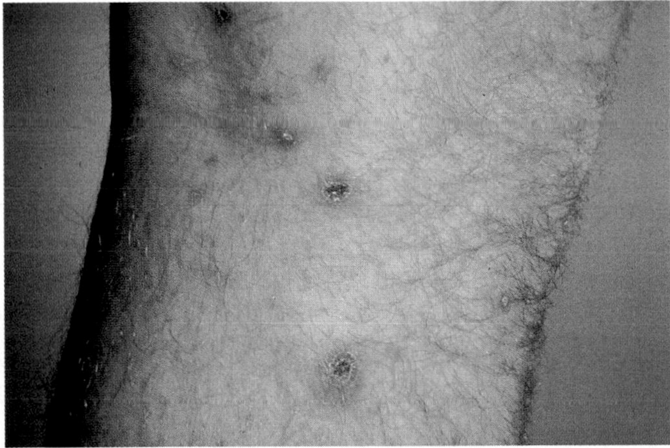

C.

Pityriasis lichenoides et varioliformis acuta. *A.* Adolescent with multiple erythematous papules and crusted lesions in various stages of evolution. *B.* Larger papulovesicular and hemorrhagic, crusted lesions in an adult. Note: Varioliform scars adjacent to active lesions on posterior thigh and leg. *C.* Pustules, crusts, and necrotic-centered papules with erythematous, indurated base.

FIGURE 48-5

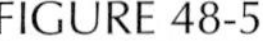

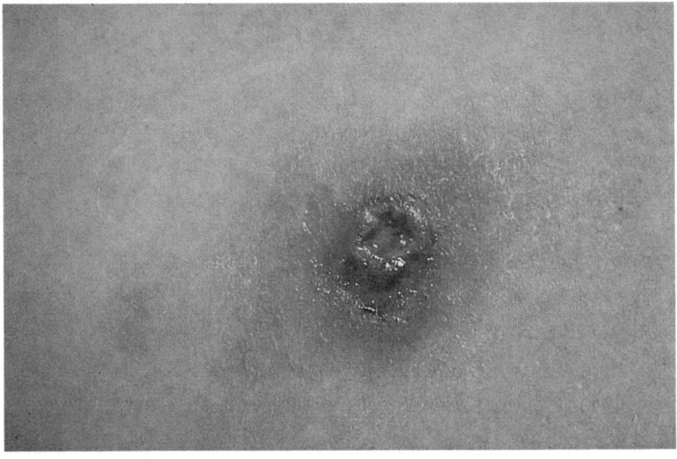

Pityriasis lichenoides et varioliformis acuta. Characteristic varioliform ulcer with raised erythematous collar and central purulent exudate.

infections has been reported. The distribution of lesions is similar to that of PLEVA, with occasional involvement of oral mucosa. Ulcerations are usually larger on the trunk and intertriginous areas, and often become secondarily infected.[29] Ulcers evolve from necrotic lesions that are surmounted by black oyster shell-like crusts (Fig. 48-7). Pruritus and pain are often prominent features. The ulceronecrotic lesions typically resolve with atrophic and dyschromic scars.

In most cases, laboratory findings are not helpful. Occasionally, viral or other infectious agent serologies or direct viral detection by in situ hybridization or polymerase chain reaction methods may be positive. Leukocytosis has been reported in more severe cases of PLEVA and PLUH; erythrocyte sedimentation rate, C-reactive protein, and serum lactic dehydrogenase are elevated. Hyperalbuminemia or increased α_2-globulins may be observed.

FIGURE 48-6

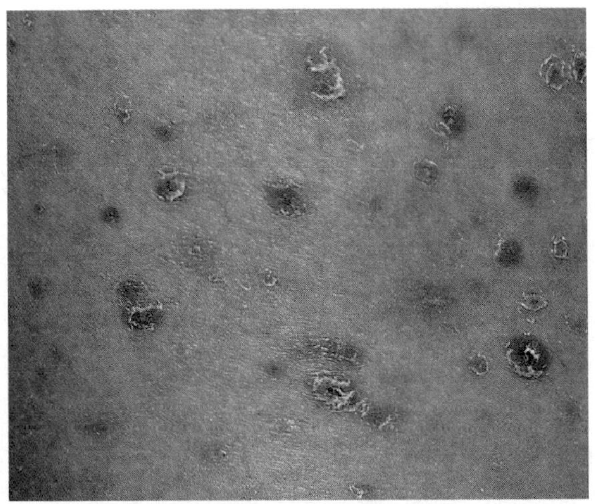

Pityriasis lichenoides et varioliformis acuta. Polymorphous lesions with overlapping features of pityriasis lichenoides chronica. Brown-red scaling lesions, resolving papules with collarette scale, and more prominent erythematous lesions with hemorrhagic crusts.

FIGURE 48-7

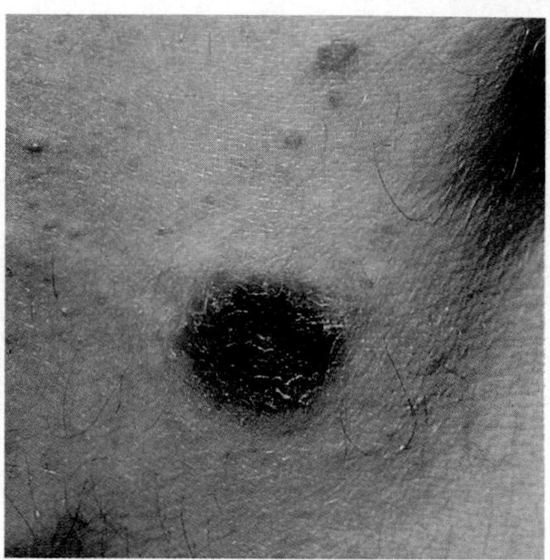

Pityriasis lichenoides, ulceronecrotic, hyperacute variant. Large necrotic eschar with halo erythema developing in febrile patient with antecedent PLEVA.

HISTOPATHOLOGY

The histopathologic findings in PLEVA and pityriasis lichenoides chronica share many features. Microscopic changes correlate with the acute, hyperacute, or chronic variants as well as the stage of the lesions. Dense perivascular lymphocytic inflammation with epidermal exocytosis of lymphocytes, parakeratosis, and focal spongiosis are the most common features in both conditions (Fig. 48-8). Dermal papillary hemorrhage and prominent endothelial swelling are also seen. Features that favor the diagnosis of PLEVA are the dense perivascular lymphocytic infiltrate with fibrinoid necrosis, which has been referred to as "lymphocytic vasculitis," and the presence of basilar epidermal cytoid bodies and epidermal necrosis (Fig. 48-9). Some authors feel that the finding of deeper inflammatory infiltrates favors the diagnosis of PLEVA; however, these differences are a matter of degree. A bandlike lymphocytic infiltrate is more suggestive of pityriasis lichenoides chronica.

The edema and diffuse lymphocytic infiltrate in both the acute and chronic forms of the disease are present in the papillary dermis and mainly around blood vessels. CD8 lymphocytes predominate in the dermis and are also found in the epidermis of patients with PLEVA,[17] whereas CD4 lymphocyte predominance is more common in pityriasis lichenoides chronica.[18] The pathologic findings are typically characteristic for well-developed papules, but older lesions create more difficulty in histologic diagnosis.

In the febrile, ulceronecrotic variant PLUH, pathologic findings are similar to those seen in PLEVA but with prominent fibrinoid necrosis of vessel wall and nuclear dust resembling leukocytoclastic vasculitis.[29] Intravascular thrombus formation and necrosis have been reported. Lymphocytes and other inflammatory cells within walls of blood vessels are also seen.

Immunopathologic findings have been reported in several studies and demonstrate reduced Langerhans cell (CD1) density as well as generalized induction of major histocompatibility complex class II HLA-DR on keratinocytes within the epidermis.[30] Endothelial cells are also HLA-DR+. The T cells in PLEVA show CD3+/CD8+ lymphocyte predominance,[31] whereas CD3+/CD4+ cells are more frequent in pityriasis lichenoides chronica. IgM, C3, and fibrin deposits localize to the perivascular and vascular spaces in the early, acute lesions.[23] Both cellular and humoral immune components show evidence of activation in pityriasis lichenoides.

In summary, differences between PLEVA and pityriasis lichenoides chronica are mainly differences in the depth and density of the inflammatory infiltrates and epidermal changes. The lack of atypical lymphocytes in the infiltrate and the interface (dermal–epidermal) changes distinguish pityriasis lichenoides from lymphomatoid papulosis.

FIGURE 48-8

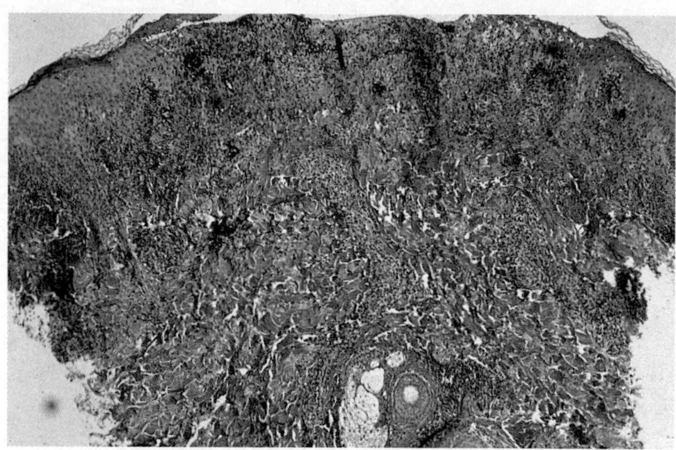

A.

B.

Pityriasis lichenoides et varioliformis acuta. *A.* Ulcerated papule with epidermal necrosis, hemorrhage and superficial and deep perivascular lymphocytic infiltrate. Hematoxylin and eosin (H&E) stain. *B.* Parakeratosis and crust with marked spongiosis and epidermal necrosis. Lymphocyte exocytosis and basal hydropic changes. H& E stain.

DIFFERENTIAL DIAGNOSIS

Pityriasis lichenoides chronica is occasionally difficult to distinguish from small-plaque parapsoriasis. The latter tends to occur in older patients, with male predominance. The characteristic association of papular lesions at different stages of evolution and hypopigmentation differentiates pityriasis lichenoides chronica from small-plaque parapsoriasis, which is characterized by well-defined, slightly scaly, erythematous, yellow or brown macules or thin plaques. Histologically, the

FIGURE 48-9

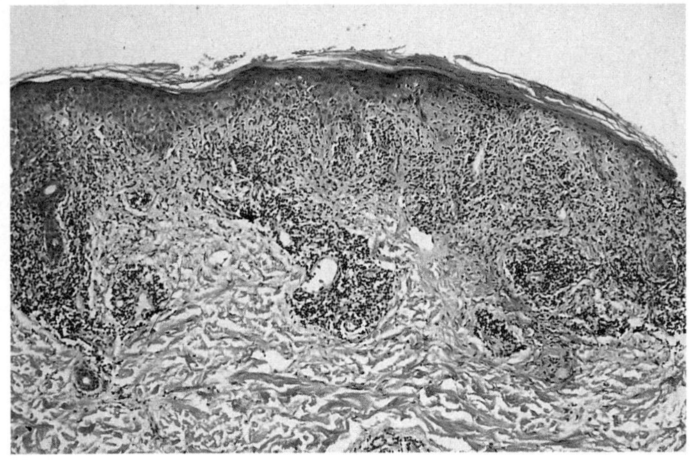

A.

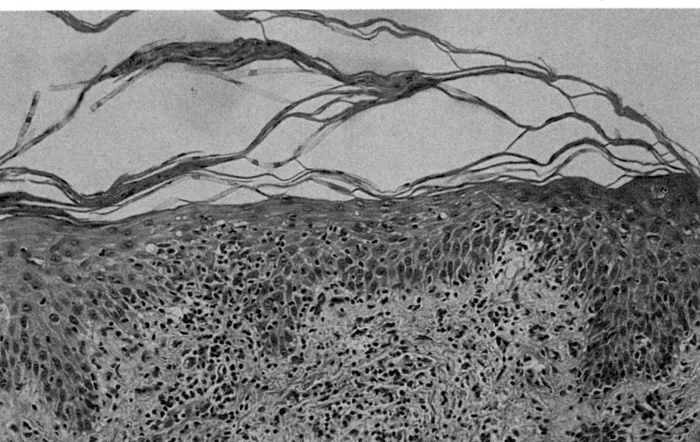

B.

Pityriasis lichenoides chronica. *A.* Compact parakeratosis, lymphocytic exocytosis, occasional eosinophilic necrotic keratinocytes, edema, and diffuse lymphocytic infiltrate localizing to epidermal-dermal interface and perivascular sites within dermis. Hematoxylin and eosin (H&E) stain. *B.* Parakeratosis, spongiosis, and a predominant mononuclear cell infiltrate in the epidermis and dermis with papillary edema. H&E stain.

presence of superficial perivascular lymphohistiocytic infiltrates without interface or epidermal changes is characteristic of parapsoriasis en plaque.

The chronic form of pityriasis lichenoides may resemble guttate psoriasis, pityriasis rosea, or secondary papulosquamous syphilis. Predilection for involvement of different body sites usually distinguishes secondary syphilis from pityriasis lichenoides chronica. The palms and soles, mucous membranes, scalp, and face often show the monomorphous eruption of syphilis, and serologic tests for syphilis are positive. Psoriasis also exhibits a more uniform morphology, with a micaceous scale that is adherent, diffuse, and less cohesive than the scale of pityriasis lichenoides. At the onset, pityriasis lichenoides and pityriasis rosea may mimic one another, but the distinguishing features of the latter include the herald patch, larger lesions, differences in scaling and distribution, and the shorter, self-limited course of the eruption.

PLEVA is usually distinctive and rarely confused with other dermatoses. Cutaneous necrotizing vasculitis or varicelliform secondary syphilis may show papulopustular, vesicular, or hemorrhagic lesions that resemble PLEVA. Syphilides are usually more widespread and monomorphous. Vasculitis shows more prominent leukocytoclastic and necrotizing changes by histologic examination. In children, Gianotti-Crosti syndrome and varicella need to be differentiated from PLEVA.

The presence of grouped papular or self-healing nodular or, occasionally, tumorous lesions that show the characteristic histopathologic changes distinguishes lymphomatoid papulosis from pityriasis lichenoides. Histologically, two types of lymphomatoid papulosis have been described: the nonepidermotropic type A lesion shows a dermal infiltrate composed of CD30+, large, atypical lymphocytes that resemble Reed-Sternberg cells admixed with neutrophils and eosinophils; it is rarely a problem to distinguish it from pityriasis lichenoides. Type B lymphomatoid papulosis differs from pityriasis lichenoides by the predominance of large and hyperchromatic cerebriform mononuclear cells; the presence of a small number of neutrophils, especially in vascular lumina; mitotic figures; and, principally, epidermotropism of lymphocytes. In contrast to pityriasis lichenoides, lymphomatoid papulosis type B usually lacks basal cell vacuolization and epidermal keratinocyte necrosis.

TREATMENT

Various factors prevent comprehensive evaluation of specific therapeutic interventions and the clinical responses and outcomes in pityriasis lichenoides. The unknown etiology of the disease limits current therapies to empiric regimens. The relatively low frequency of the disease and the unpredictability of its course are also limiting factors in evaluating the effectiveness of treatment. However, the unsightly appearance, widespread distribution, symptoms of pruritus, sequelae such as pigment alterations and scarring, and reports of a clonal T cell population in some patients with PLEVA favor treatment of the condition.

Topical steroids and antihistamines are prescribed routinely and may decrease the inflammatory component of the dermatosis but do not significantly influence the course of the disease. Systemic glucocorticoids such as prednisone, 40 to 60 mg/day, are helpful in controlling the cutaneous and systemic symptoms in acute flares of PLEVA and the ulceronecrotic variant PLUH. A variety of antibiotics have been tried, primarily for PLEVA, with variable results. Tetracycline at higher doses (2 g/day for 4 weeks in adults)[32] or erythromycin (2 g/day in adults or 30 to 50 mg/kg per day in children)[33] may yield favorable results. Tapering the antibiotics slowly at the end of the course of treatment may minimize recurrences.

Phototherapy provides the best therapeutic response. Ultraviolet B phototherapy is a useful treatment option.[34,35] Three to five treatment sessions per week over 1.5 to 2 months provides a good response, probably through alteration of local immunity in skin mediated by UVB. PUVA photochemotherapy has also shown therapeutic benefit.[36,37] Relapses following discontinuation of phototherapy are not uncommon. Maintenance PUVA or UVB phototherapy should be considered, ranging from one session per week to one session every 3 weeks. UVAI phototherapy has recently shown efficacy in the treatment of PLEVA and PLC.[38] Sun exposure to induce tanning or simple UVA treatments may be convenient and helpful for the patient in hastening resolution of pityriasis lichenoides.

For more acute and problematic cases of PLEVA, methotrexate in the dose range of 15 to 20 mg per week can be initiated.[39,40] Maintenance therapy with lower doses prevents recurrence. Use of methotrexate is rarely justified in children, however.

For the ulceronecrotic form of pityriasis lichenoides, systemic glucocorticoids, a combination of PUVA and oral methotrexate,[41] intravenous methotrexate, and gamma-globulin[42] reportedly exerts favorable results.

In 1989, a comprehensive review of the existing literature on treatment of pityriasis lichenoides and lymphomatoid papulosis by Lynch revealed that many therapies have shown variable response rates when evaluated independently.[43] This is not surprising given our lack of knowledge on the pathogenesis of pityriasis lichenoides. However, UVB phototherapy, PUVA photochemotherapy, and, for more severe disease, methotrexate offer the most consistent therapeutic responses. This coincides with the known immunomodulating effects of these agents in other inflammatory, papulosquamous skin diseases such as psoriasis. Therefore, in refractory or debilitating cases, oral pharmacologic agents such as cyclosporine[44,45] or retinoids[46] should also be considered as alternative therapeutic interventions.

COURSE AND PROGNOSIS

Pityriasis lichenoides is a chronic immunoreactive or lymphoproliferative dermatosis with the continuous appearance of new lesions that fade over a few weeks. The disease may regress in a few months or, more rarely, persist for years. PLEVA usually has a shorter duration than pityriasis lichenoides chronica. The febrile, ulceronecrotic, and hemorrhagic form, PLUH, usually resolves in a few months; however, a fatal outcome may rarely ensue in elderly, compromised patients.

Pityriasis lichenoides has long been regarded as a benign reactive condition with no malignant potential. The presence of a clonal T cell population and occasional instances of atypical CD30+ cells in a small proportion of cases raises the question of whether these lesions are pityriasis lichenoides or a distinctive form bridging pityriasis lichenoides and lymphomatoid papulosis. Furthermore, there is no strong evidence that clonality in these cases is necessarily a harbinger of lymphoma. The absence of significant systemic involvement and complications portends a generally good prognosis for the various forms of pityriasis lichenoides.

REFERENCES

1. Neisser A: Zur Frage der lichenoiden eruptionen. *Verh Dtsch Dermatol Ges* **4**:4495, 1894
2. Jadassohn J: Über ein eigenartiges psoriasiformes und lichenoides Exanthem. *Verh Dtsch Dermatol Ges* **4**:524, 1894
3. Juliusberg F: Über die pityriasis lichenoides chronica (Psoriasiform lichenoides Exanthem). *Arch Dermatol Syphilol (Wien)* **50**:359, 1899
4. Brocq L: Les parapsoriasis. *Ann Dermatol Syphiligr (Paris)* **3**:433, 1902
5. Mucha V: Über einen der Parakeratosis variegata (Unna) bzw. Pityriasis lichenoides chronica (Neisser-Juliusberg) nahestehenden eigentumlichen Fall. *Arch Dermatol Syphilol* **123**:586, 1916
6. Habermann R: Über die akut verlaufende, nekrotisierende Unterart der Pityriasis lichenoides (Pityriasis lichenoides et varioliformis acuta). *Dermatol Ztschr (Berlin)* **45**:42, 1925
7. Lambert WC, Everett MA: The nosology of parapsoriasis. *J Am Acad Dermatol* **5**:373, 1981
8. Everett MA: Historical aspects of pityriasis lichenoides, in Proceedings of the First International Parapsoriasis Symposium. Rochester, MN, Mayo Foundation, 1989, p 1
9. Degos R et al: Le parapsoriasis ulceronecrotique hyperthermique. *Ann Dermatol Syphiligr* **93**:481, 1966
10. Dupont A: Langsam verlaufende und klinische gutartige Reticulopathie mit höchst maligner histologischer Struktur. *Hautzart* **16**:2824, 1965
11. McCaulay WL: Lymphomatoid papulosis: A continuing self-healing eruption—Clinically benign, histologically malignant. *Arch Dermatol* **97**:23, 1968
12. Rogers M: Pityriasis lichenoides and lymphomatoid papulosis. *Semin Dermatol* **11**:73, 1992
13. Cerroni L: Lymphomatoid papulosis, pityriasis lichenoides et varioliformis acuta, and anaplastic large-cell (Ki−1+) lymphoma. *J Am Acad Dermatol* **37**:287, 1997
14. Black MM: Lymphomatoid papulosis and pityriasis lichenoides: Are they related? *Br J Dermatol* **106**:717, 1982
15. el-Azhary RA et al: Lymphomatoid papulosis: A clinical and histopathologic review of 53 cases with leukocyte immunophenotyping, DNA flow cytometry, and T-cell receptor gene rearrangement studies. *J Am Acad Dermatol* **30**:210, 1994
16. Panhans A et al: Pityriasis lichenoides of childhood with atypical CD30-positive cells and clonal T-cell receptor gene rearrangements. *J Am Acad Dermatol* **35**:489, 1996
17. Dereure O et al: T-cell clonality in pityriasis lichenoides et varioliformis acuta: A heteroduplex analysis of 20 cases. *Arch Dermatol* **136**:1483, 2000
18. Shieh S et al: Differentiation and clonality of lesional lymphocytes in pityriasis lichenoides chronica. *Arch Dermatol* **137**:305, 2001
19. Romani J et al: Pityriasis lichenoides in children: Clinicopathologic review of 22 patients. *Pediatr Dermatol* **15**:1, 1998
20. Rivitti EA: Pityriasis lichenoides: Review of cases seen in two major dermatology centers in Sao Paolo, Brazil, 1977 to 1989, in Proceedings of the First International Parapsoriasis Symposium. Rochester, MN, Mayo Foundation, 1989, p 14
21. Gelmetti C et al: Pityriasis lichenoides in children: A long-term follow-up of 89 cases. *J Am Acad Dermatol* **23**:473, 1990
22. Clayton R et al: Pityriasis lichenoides—An immune complex disease. *Br J Dermatol* **97**:629, 1977
23. Muhlbauer JE et al: Immunopathology of pityriasis lichenoides acuta. *J Am Acad Dermatol* **10**:783, 1984
24. Fortson JS et al: Cutaneous T-cell lymphoma (parapsoriasis en plaque): An association with pityriasis lichenoides et varioliformis acuta in young children. *Arch Dermatol* **126**:1449, 1990
25. Niemczyk UM et al: The transformation of pityriasis lichenoides chronica into parakeratosis variegata in an 11-year-old girl. *Br J Dermatol* **137**:983, 1997
26. Panizzon RG et al: Atypical manifestations of pityriasis lichenoides chronica: Development into paraneoplasia and non-Hodgkin lymphomas of the skin. *Dermatology* **184**:65, 1992
27. Ko JW et al: Pityriasis lichenoides-like mycosis fungoides in children. *Br J Dermatol* **142**:347, 2000
28. Cliff S et al: Segmental pityriasis lichenoides chronica. *Clin Exp Dermatol* **21**:461, 1996
29. Fink-Puches R et al: Febrile ulceronecrotic pityriasis lichenoides et varioliformis acuta. *J Am Acad Dermatol* **30**:261, 1994
30. Wood GS et al: Immunohistology of pityriasis lichenoides et varioliformis acuta and pityriasis lichenoides chronica. *J Am Acad Dermatol* **16**:559, 1987
31. Jang KA et al: Expression of cutaneous lymphocyte-associated antigen and lymphocytes in pityriasis lichenoides et varioliformis acuta an papulosis: Immunohistochemical study. *J Cutan Pathol* **28**:453, 2001
32. Piamphongsant T: Tetracycline for the treatment of pityriasis lichenoides. *Br J Dermatol* **91**:319, 1974
33. Truhan AP et al: Pityriasis lichenoides in children: Therapeutic response to erythromycin. *J Am Acad Dermatol* **15**:66, 1986
34. LeVine MJ: Phototherapy of pityriasis lichenoides. *Arch Dermatol* **119**:378, 1983
35. Tham SN: UV-B phototherapy for pityriasis lichenoides. *Australas J Dermatol* **26**:9, 1985
36. Brenner W et al: Erprobung von PUVA bei verschiedenen Dermatosen. *Hautzart* **29**:541, 1978
37. Powell FC, Muller SA: Psoralens and ultraviolet A therapy of pityriasis lichenoides. *J Am Acad Dermatol* **10**:59, 1984
38. Pinton PC et al: Medium-dose ultraviolet A1 therapy for pityriasis lichenoides et varioliformis acuta and pityriasis lichenoides chronica. *J Am Acad Dermatol* **47**:410, 2002
39. Lynch PJ, Saied NK: Methotrexate treatment of pityriasis lichenoides and lymphomatoid papulosis. *Cutis* **23**:634, 1979
40. Cornelison RL Jr et al: Methotrexate for the treatment of Mucha-Habermann disease. *Arch Dermatol* **16**:507, 1972
41. Lopez-Estebaranz JL et al: Febrile ulceronecrotic Mucha-Habermann disease. *J Am Acad Dermatol* **29**:903, 1993
42. Korppi M et al: Mucha-Habermann disease: A diagnostic possibility for prolonged fever associated with systemic and skin symptoms. *Acta Pediatr* **82**:627, 1993
43. Lynch PJ: Treatment of pityriasis lichenoides and lymphomatoid papulosis, in Proceedings of the First International Parapsoriasis Symposium. Rochester, MN, Mayo Foundation, 1989, p 113
44. Gupta AK et al: Oral cyclosporine in the treatment of inflammatory and noninflammatory dermatoses. *Arch Dermatol* **126**:339, 1990
45. Lim KK et al: Cyclosporine in the treatment of dermatologic disease: An update. *Mayo Clin Proc* **71**:1182, 1996
46. Orfanos CE et al: Current use and future potential role of retinoids in dermatology. *Drugs* **53**:358, 1997

CHAPTER 49

Mazen S. Daoud
Mark R. Pittelkow

Lichen Planus

Lichen planus (Greek *leichen,* "tree moss"; Latin *planus,* "flat") is a unique, common inflammatory disorder that affects the skin, mucous membranes, nails, and hair. The appearance of lichen planus and lichen planus-like or lichenoid dermatoses has been likened to the scurfy, finely furrowed, dry excrescences of the symbiotic vegetation known as lichen. Although this morphologic comparison may be antiquated, lichen planus is a distinctive entity with prototypic "lichenoid" papules that show distinctive color and morphology, develop in typical locations, and manifest characteristic patterns of evolution. Microscopic features, similar to the gross morphology, are distinctive although the microscopic pattern of inflammation and skin response is shared by several dermatoses. The term *lichenoid reaction* is the histologic description used to capsulize the pathologic characteristics of skin diseases resembling lichen planus.

The term *lichen ruber planus* (Latin *ruber,* "red" or "ruddy") has been used to denote the distinctive color of the lesion, but this terminology has largely been abandoned. The *four Ps*—purple, polygonal, pruritic, papule—is the abbreviation often used to recall the constellation of symptoms and skin findings that characterize lichen planus.

HISTORICAL ASPECTS

In 1869, Erasmus Wilson delineated and named the condition leichen (lichen) planus, but the dermatosis was probably described earlier by Hebra as leichen ruber. Kaposi first described a distinctive clinical variant of the disease with blisters, lichen ruber pemphigoides, in 1892. Wickham, in 1895, described the characteristic appearance of whitish striae and punctations that develop atop the flat-surfaced papules. The histologic findings were elaborated by Darier in 1909. Scalp and follicular involvement were reported initially by Graham-Little in 1919.

Lichen planus is classified as a papulosquamous disease, although scaling is not prominent as in psoriasis and other skin diseases included in this category. Lichen planus represents the model for lichenoid reactions. Pinkus[1] formally defined the lichenoid tissue reaction, in 1973, ". . . as one exhibiting epidermal basal cell damage and the chain of histobiologic events resulting from such damage. It is not essential whether damage to the basal cells is primary or is itself due to preceding events in the dermis. This tissue reaction may be called 'lichenoid' because lichen planus is the prototype."

EPIDEMIOLOGY AND GENETICS

The exact incidence and prevalence of lichen planus are unknown, but the overall prevalence is believed to be somewhat less than 1 percent of the general population. Estimates between 0.14 and 0.8 percent have been reported worldwide and approximately 0.44 percent in the United States. No racial predilection has been observed.[2]

At least two-thirds of cases occur between the ages of 30 and 60 years. No sexual predilection is evident. Females are usually affected in their fifties and sixties, whereas males develop lichen planus at a somewhat earlier age. The disease is less common in the very young and the elderly. The development of lichen planus may be affected by seasonal or environmental factors. An increased incidence in the months of December and January or from January to July has been reported.[2]

Fewer than 100 cases of familial lichen planus have been reported. The familial form tends to be more protracted and severe and presents in erosive, linear, or ulcerative patterns or with atypical features affecting young adults and children.[3] Some believe that the familial form represents a separate, unique dermatosis. Different human leukocyte antigen (HLA) haplotypes were reported in familial lichen planus, including HLA-B7, -Aw19, -B18, and -Cw8. In nonfamilial lichen planus HLA-A3, -A5, -A28, -B8, -B16, and -Bw35 are more common.[4] HLA-B8 is more common in patients with oral lichen planus as a sole manifestation, and HLA-Bw35 is more strongly associated with cutaneous lichen planus. In a British population, HLA-B27, -B51, and -Bw57 have been found to be associated with oral lichen planus. Of class II antigens, HLA-DR1, -DR9, and -DQ1 are found more frequently. It must be noted, however, that the ethnicity of the populations composing these studies and the selection of specific anatomic and clinicopathologic types of lichen planus may significantly bias the HLA analyses that have been reported.

ETIOLOGY AND PATHOGENESIS

It is evident that immunologic mechanisms almost certainly mediate the development of lichen planus. No consistent alterations in immunoglobulins have been shown in lichen planus, and humoral immunity most likely is a secondary response in the immunopathogenesis.

Cell-mediated immunity, on the other hand, plays the major role in triggering the clinical expression of the disease. Both CD4+ and CD8+ T cells are found in lesional skin of lichen planus. Progression of disease may lead to preferential accumulation of CD8+ cells. The majority of the lymphocytes in the infiltrate of lichen planus are CD8+ and CD45RO (memory) positive cells and express the $\alpha\beta$ T cell receptor, and in a minority, the $\gamma\delta$ receptor. This later cell subtype is not normally found in healthy skin. These cells are considered responsible for the development of the most characteristic change observed in the lichenoid reaction, namely, apoptosis. The inflammatory process that leads to apoptosis is complex and not fully understood. The epithelial–lymphocyte interaction can be divided into three major stages: antigen recognition, lymphocyte activation, and keratinocyte apoptosis.

Lichen Planus-Specific Antigen Recognition

It is evident that the majority of T cells in the infiltrate of lichen planus, both within the epithelium and adjacent to damaged basal keratinocytes, are activated CD8+ cytotoxic lymphocytes. Evidence from oral lichen planus suggests that CD8+ lesional T cells recognize a lichen planus-specific antigen associated with MHC class I on lesional keratinocytes. The nature of this antigen is unknown. Theoretically, the antigen may be an autoreactive peptide, thus classifying lichen planus as an autoimmune disease. Alternatively, it may represent an exogenous antigen such as an altered protein, drug, contact allergen, viral or infectious agent, or an unidentified immunogenic target.[5]

The role of T helper (CD4) cells in the pathogenesis of lichen planus is not fully defined. T cells may become activated via antigen-presenting cells such as Langerhans cells or accessory cells such as epidermal keratinocytes in association with members of the major histocompatibility complex II and specific cytokines. T helper lymphocytes may also propagate CD8+ cytotoxic lymphocytes through cellular cooperation and release of cytokines.

The nature of antigenic stimulation is not known. Contact sensitizers such as metals could act as haptens and elicit an immunologic response. Enhanced lymphocyte reactivity to inorganic mercury, a component of dental amalgam, has been found in patients with oral lichenoid reactions. Low-grade chronic exposure to mercury, and possibly to other metals such as gold, may stimulate a lymphocytic reaction that manifests as lichen planus. A list of contact chemicals and drugs that can elicit lichenoid reactions is discussed below. The role of infection in the development of lichen planus has been repeatedly raised over the years. Though provocative, no conclusive evidence has molecularly linked lichen planus to any of the following infections or microorganisms: syphilis, herpes simplex virus 2, HIV, amebiasis, chronic bladder infections, hepatitis C virus, *Helicobacter pylori,* and human papillomavirus.

Cytotoxic Lymphocyte Activation

Following antigen recognition, CD8+ T cells are activated. Activated cytotoxic lymphocytes undergo lesional tissue clonal expansion, leading to oligoclonal and occasionally to monoclonal proliferation as detected by analysis of the T cell receptor (TCR)-γ chain gene products.[6]

Activated lymphocytes, both by helper subsets (T_H1 and T_H2) and cytotoxic-suppressor cells, release soluble mediators (cytokines and chemokines), such as interleukin (IL)-2, IL-4, IL-10, interferon (IFN)-γ, tumor necrosis factor (TNF)-α, and transforming growth factor-β1, that attract lymphocytes and regulate their biologic activities within and adjacent to the epithelium. Both pro- and anti-inflammatory cytokines, that is, mixed T_H1 and T_H2 cytokine products, are generated simultaneously. The balance between lymphocytic activation and downregulation determines the clinical behavior of the disease.[7] IFN-γ, produced by T helper cells during the antigen recognition stage, induces keratinocytes to produce lymphotoxin-α and TNF-α, and to upregulate MHC class II, thus increasing interactions with helper T cells. Furthermore, IFN-γ upregulates the expression of intercellular adhesion molecule (ICAM)-1 and vascular cell adhesion molecule (VCAM)-1 by basal keratinocytes, Langerhans cells, and other macrophage–dendritic cells.[8] ICAM-1 is a ligand for the β_2-integrin, leukocyte function-associated antigen (LFA)-1, on the surface of lymphocytes, which further enhances the interaction of these lymphocytes with the antigen-presenting cells.[9] Laminin-5 and collagen types IV and VII, are increased in lesional lichen planus and serve as ligands for β_1-integrin on the surface of lymphocytes, thus allowing for enhanced association of lymphocytes with the basement membrane. Integrin α_3 is present on activated, skin-homing T cells and may localize these effector cells to the epidermal–dermal interface and basement membrane, which contain epiligrin/laminin-5, a ligand for this integrin.[10] This close interaction between lymphocytes and basement membrane targets metalloproteinases produced by lymphocytes to alter extracellular matrix proteins and integrins, and the process eventuates in apoptosis, basement membrane disruption, reduplication, and subepidermal cleft formation (see below). TNF-α upregulates the expression of matrix metalloproteinase (MMP)-9 mRNA in lesional T lymphocytes, thus further enhancing basement membrane disruption (see below).[11]

Keratinocytes also participate in the response by producing IL-1β, IL-4, IL-6, granulocyte-macrophage colony-stimulating factor, and TNF-α. These cytokines further activate tissue macrophages and peripheral blood mononuclear cells[12] and upregulate expression of cell surface adhesion molecules and migration activity. Keratinocyte-produced cytokines also upregulate expression of specific keratin genes. Keratin (K)17, usually restricted to adnexal structures, is variably expressed in the basal and suprabasal layers of the interfollicular epithelium of affected epidermis. K6 and K16 also become detectable in the basal and suprabasal layers. K4 and K13 are reduced in the suprabasal compartment in areas with orthokeratosis, associated with increased production of K1 and K10.[13]

Keratinocyte Apoptosis

The exact mechanisms used by activated cytotoxic T cells to trigger apoptosis of keratinocytes is not completely known. Possible mechanisms include: (1) T cell secreted TNF-α binding to the TNF-α R1 receptor on the keratinocyte surface; (2) T cell surface CD95L (Fas ligand) binding CD95 (Fas) on the keratinocyte; and (3) T cell secreted granzyme B entering the keratinocyte via perforin-induced membrane pores. All these mechanisms may activate the keratinocyte caspase cascade resulting in keratinocyte apoptosis.[5]

Recruited lymphocytes may further contribute to apoptosis via a different mechanism, the loss of a basement membrane-derived cell survival signal that normally prevents the onset of apoptosis. Hence, basement membrane disruption may trigger apoptosis. Principle mediators are the MMPs, a family of zinc-containing endoproteinases that primarily function to degrade connective tissue matrix proteins. The action of these enzymes is also regulated by inhibitors such as tissue inhibitors of metalloproteinases (TIMPs) (see Chap. 17). It has been shown that lesional T cells in lichen planus have higher MMP-9 levels than peripheral blood T cells. Lesional T cell MMP-9 activity increases following stimulation with TNF-α, but not TIMP-1, an inhibitor for MMP-9.[5] These observations suggest that T cell secreted MMP-9 disrupts epithelial basement membranes, blocking cell survival signals to keratinocytes and inducing apoptosis.

Various other environmental, behavioral, or infectious factors have been observed on occasion to be associated with the development or exacerbation of lichen planus. However, no well-established association has been documented between emotional stress, tobacco use, oral or gastrointestinal candidiasis, and development of lichen planus.

CLINICAL MANIFESTATIONS

The classic cutaneous lesion of lichen planus is a faintly erythematous to violaceous, flat-topped, polygonal papule, sometimes showing a small central umbilication (Fig. 49-1). A thin, transparent, and adherent scale may be discerned atop the lesion. Fine, whitish puncta or reticulated networks referred to as *Wickham striae,* named after the dermatologist who described the finding, are present over the surface of many well-developed papules. These are considered to be highly characteristic

FIGURE 49-1

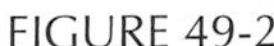

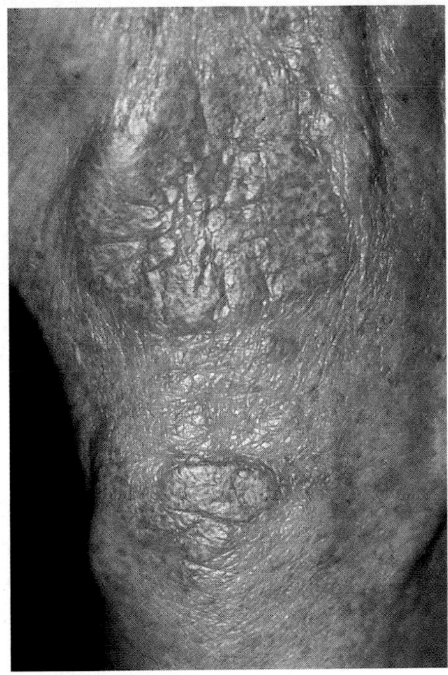

Lichen planus. Variable sized flat-topped, violaceous papules and plaques with Wickham striae involving the extremity.

and are more easily observed after applying oil, xylene, or water and visualizing the lesions with a magnifying lens or a handheld dermatoscope. The surface alteration may result from localized thickening of the keratohyalin-containing cell layers of the stratum granulosum, although a focal increase in the activity of lichen planus may account for the morphologic alteration of Wickham striae.

Lichen planus begins as faintly erythematous macules that form purplish papules over several weeks. Sometimes multiple lesions develop rapidly over a short time, with dissemination following the initial appearance of only a few papules. Further spread of lesions after the initial limited expression occurs in approximately a third of cases. In generalized disease, the eruption often spreads within 1 to 4 months from onset. The initial lesions almost always appear on the extremities, with the lower extremities being somewhat more common.

The lesions are usually distributed symmetrically and bilaterally over the extremities. Lichen planus tends to involve the flexural areas of the wrists, arms, and legs (Fig. 49-2). The thighs, lower back, trunk, and neck may also be affected. Oral mucous membranes and the genitalia are additional sites of involvement (Fig. 49-3). The face is usually spared in typical cases, and palmoplantar involvement is unusual. Inverse lichen planus usually affects the axillae, groin, and inframammary areas.

Lichen planus tends to be quite pruritic, although some patients are completely asymptomatic. The degree of pruritus is generally related to the extent of involvement, with more intense pruritus in generalized cases. An exception is hypertrophic lichen planus, which is more localized but extremely pruritic. Oral involvement is generally asymptomatic unless erosions or ulcers developed. Erosive oral lichen planus is usually extremely painful. In the acute, evolving stages of the disease, scratching, injury, or trauma may induce an isomorphic (Koebner's) response (Fig. 49-4). Lichen planus usually heals with hyperpigmentation, which is more prominent among patients with darker skin color. Hypopigmentation uncommonly develops following resolution of lesions.

Although the clinical and pathologic features of childhood lichen planus are similar to those in adults, scalp, nail, and hair involvement is not common. Mucous membrane involvement, thought to be rare, may occur in up to one-third of patients. The hypertrophic variant occurs in one fourth of children with lichen planus.

FIGURE 49-2

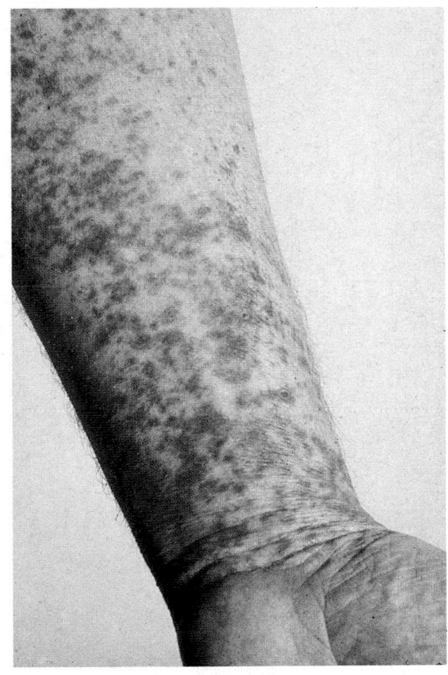

Lichen planus. Dusky violaceous coalescing papules on the flexural aspect of the wrist and forearm.

CLINICAL VARIANTS

Many variations in the clinical presentation have been described and are generally categorized according to (1) the configuration of lesions, (2) the morphologic appearance, or (3) the site of involvement. These variations are patterned by subtle or unknown properties of the disease. The prototypic papule can be altered or modified in configuration, morphology, or anatomic distribution. Table 49-1 reviews and classifies these distinctive variants and other special types of lichen planus that overlap with other dermatoses.

Configuration of Lesions

ANNULAR LICHEN PLANUS Annular lesions occur in approximately 10 percent of cases and commonly develop as arcuate groupings of individual papules that develop rings or peripheral extension of clustered papules with central clearing. They tend to occur in blacks and are more common on the penis and scrotum (Fig. 49-5).[2] Another form of annular lichen planus occurs when larger lesions reach 2 to 3 cm in diameter and become hyperpigmented, with a raised outer rim. This form may occur on the trunk or extremities. Actinic lichen planus, seen in subtropical zones on sun-exposed, dark-skinned young adults and children, is frequently annular in shape.

LINEAR LICHEN PLANUS Papules of lichen planus may develop a linear pattern secondary to trauma (koebnerization) or, uncommonly, as a spontaneous, isolated eruption, usually on the extremities, and rarely

FIGURE 49-3

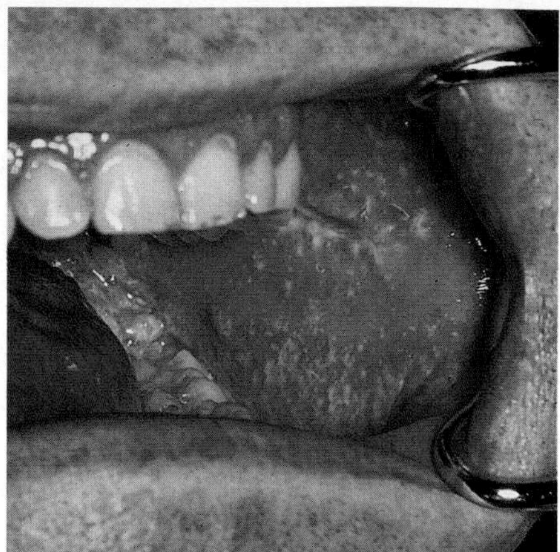

A.

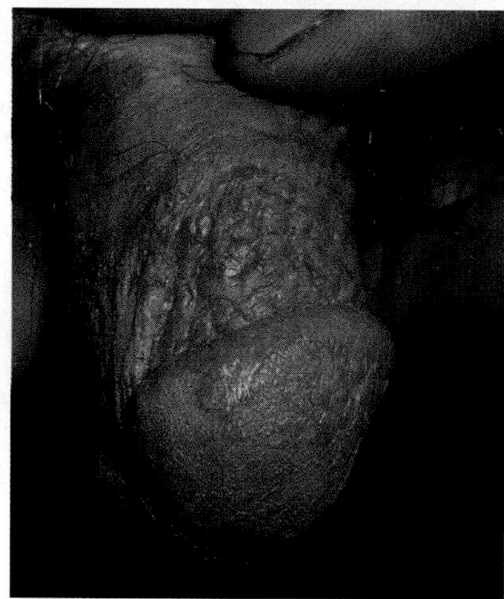

B.

Mucosal lichen planus. *A.* A typical whitish, punctate to reticulated pattern of oral lesions is seen on the buccal mucosa. *B.* Agminate pattern of lesions involving the meatus, glans, and sulcus areas of the penis.

on the face. This linear pattern should be differentiated from nevus unius lateralis and lichen striatus. A zosteriform pattern has also been described,[14] and lichen planus can develop in the site of healed herpes zoster.

Morphology of Lesions

HYPERTROPHIC LICHEN PLANUS Hypertrophic lichen planus (lichen planus verrucosus) usually occurs on the extremities, especially the shins and interphalangeal joints, and tends to be the most pruritic variant. Lesions are thickened and elevated, purplish or reddish-brown in color, and hyperkeratotic. Occasionally, verrucous plaques develop. Lesions may show accentuated and elevated follicular induration and chalklike scale. This variant usually heals with scar formation and hyper- or hypopigmentation. Chronic venous insufficiency is frequently present.

ATROPHIC LICHEN PLANUS The atrophic variant is rare and is characterized by the presence of a few well-demarcated, white-bluish papules or plaques with central superficial atrophy.[2] Sometimes the lesions show more erythema. The lesions are a few millimeters wide but may coalesce to form larger plaques. They are most common on the lower extremities or trunk. The lesions often resemble lichen sclerosus et atrophicus. However, the histologic features are diagnostic.

FIGURE 49-4

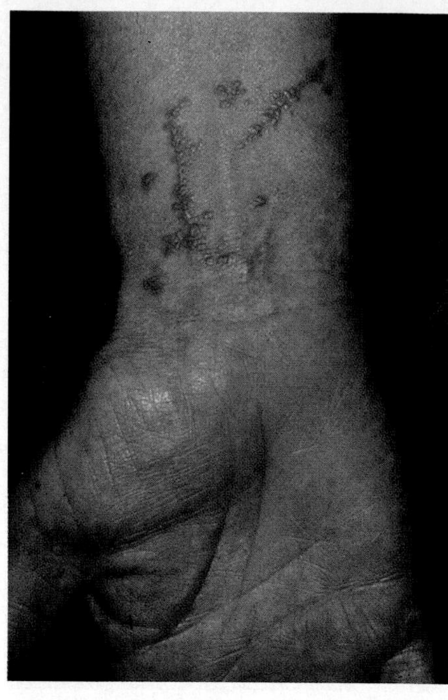

Lichen planus. Linear pattern with Koebner's response adjacent to clustered papules on the flexural wrist.

TABLE 49-1

Classification of Lichen Planus Variants

- Configuration
  - Annular
  - Linear
- Morphology of lesion
  - Hypertrophic
  - Atrophic
  - Vesiculobullous
  - Erosive and ulcerative
  - Follicular
  - Actinic
  - Lichen planus pigmentosus
  - Other rare forms: perforating, guttate, etc.
- Site of involvement
  - Palm and soles
  - Mucous membranes
  - Nails
  - Scalp
- Special forms
  - Drug-induced (lichenoid drug eruption)
  - Lichen planus–lupus erythematosus overlap
  - Lichen planus pemphigoides
  - Keratosis lichenoides chronica
  - Lichen planus and malignant transformation
  - Lichenoid reaction of graft-versus-host disease
  - Lichenoid keratosis
  - Lichenoid dermatitis

FIGURE 49-5

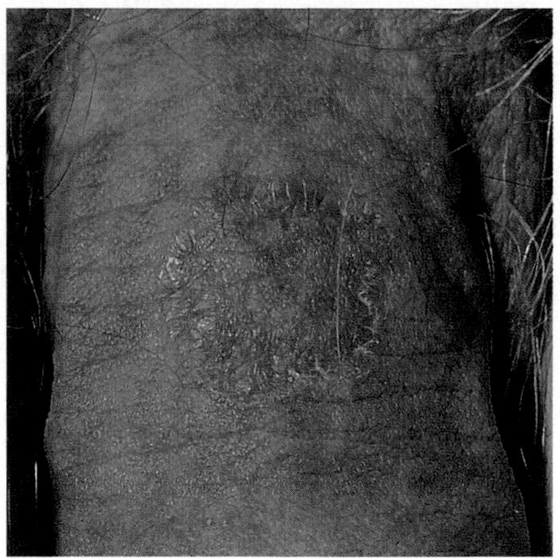

Lichen planus. Annular lesion on the shaft of the penis.

VESICULOBULLOUS LICHEN PLANUS Bullous lichen planus is a rare variant of the disease characterized by the development of vesicles and bullae within the lesions (Fig. 49-6). The bullae, which appear most commonly on the extremities, arise from papules of lichen planus and rarely from normal-appearing skin. They may appear suddenly during an acute flare of disease and are usually associated with mild constitutional symptoms. These lesions usually resolve in a few months. Bulla arising in oral lichen planus can lead to painful erosions. Histologically, the typical changes of lichen planus are seen in conjunction with subepidermal separation. The duration of this variant is no different from that of classic lichen planus. Bullae arising from normal skin are more characteristic of lichen planus pemphigoides and should be differentiated from bullous lichen planus by direct and indirect immunofluorescence (see below).

EROSIVE AND ULCERATIVE LICHEN PLANUS Ulcerative lichen planus is a rare variant presenting with chronic, painful bullae and ulcerations of the feet. Often, cicatricial sequelae are evident (Fig. 49-7). This variant is usually associated with more typical lesions of the nails, mucosal surfaces, and skin, which often aids in establishing the diagnosis. Permanent loss of toenails and cicatricial alopecia of the scalp are common. Because squamous cell carcinoma (SCC) may develop in lesions of ulcerative lichen planus, persistent ulceration should raise suspicions of malignancy, and this potential complication should be

FIGURE 49-6

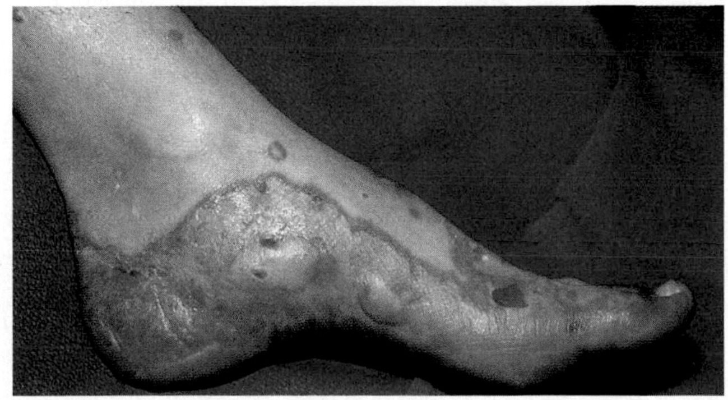

Lichen planus. Vesicles and bullae within violaceous-erythematous papules or plaques of the foot.

FIGURE 49-7

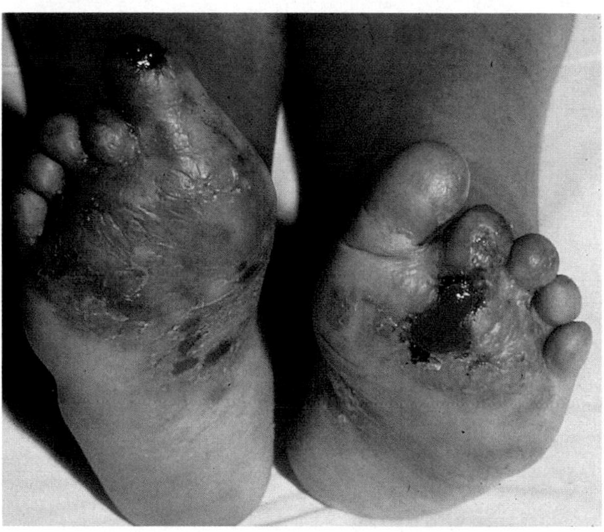

Lichen planus. Ulcerative variant showing erosions, granulation tissue, and scarring of toes and interdigital web space.

ruled out by biopsy. Excision and skin grafting should be considered if conservative therapy is ineffective.[15]

Erosive to ulcerative lesions of lichen planus are also seen with greater frequency in more severe cases of oral lichen planus. Lesions may involve the buccal mucosa, alveolar epithelium, and sulci, and may extend to the posterior pharynx and laryngeal area. Though rare, erosive esophageal disease may result in dysphagia and stenosis.

FOLLICULAR LICHEN PLANUS This form may occur alone or in association with other forms of cutaneous or mucosal lichen planus.[16] The term *lichen planopilaris* has been used to describe this distinctive variant, but other terms include *lichen planus follicularis, peripilaris,* and *acuminatus*. Individual keratotic follicular papules and studded plaques are seen. Sites of predilection include the trunk and medial aspects of the proximal extremities. Follicular lichen planus may affect the scalp with the development of cicatricial alopecia (see "Lichen Planus of the Scalp," below) (Fig. 49-8). The triad of follicular lichen planus of skin (lichen planus spinulosus) and/or scalp, multifocal cicatricial alopecia of the scalp, and nonscarring alopecia of the axillary and pubic areas, has been described as Graham-Little-Piccardi-Lassueur (or Graham-Little-Feldman) syndrome. Sometimes more typical lesions of the skin and nails are seen. Other variants of follicular lichen planus include the pseudopeladic form of Brocq, the lichen planus follicularis tumidus form with oval pseudotumoral plaques of the mastoid area, postmenopausal frontal fibrosing alopecia, and lichen planoporitis, with the lichenoid reaction centered over the acrosyringium and eccrine ducts entering the epidermis.[17]

LICHEN PLANUS PIGMENTOSUS This uncommon variant is characterized by hyperpigmented, dark-brown macules in sun-exposed areas and flexural folds. This entity tends to occur in Latin Americans and other patients with darker-pigmented skin. Histologically, an atrophic epidermis, a vacuolar alteration of the basal cell layer with a scarce lymphohistiocytic lichenoid infiltrate, and pigment incontinence are seen. This variant of lichen planus bears significant similarity to ashy dermatosis or erythema dyschromicum perstans (dermatoses cinecienta) and may represent overlap in the phenotypic spectrum of lichenoid

FIGURE 49-8

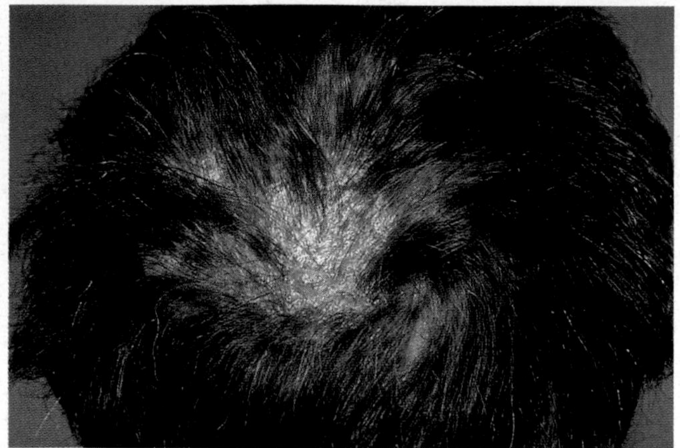

A.

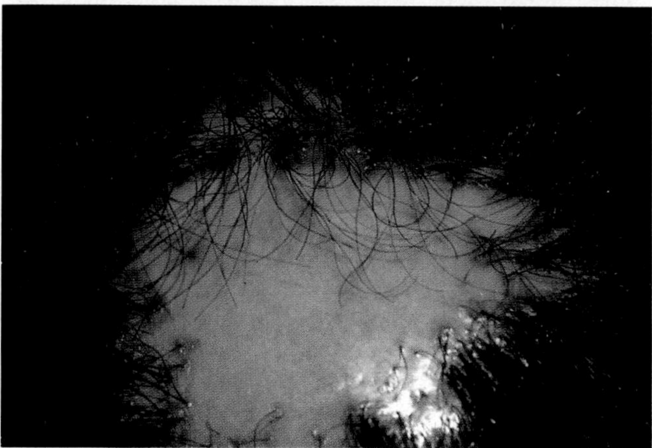

B.

Lichen planus. *A.* Irregular patches of alopecia with violaceous papules and a coalescing plaque of lichen planus within scalp. *B.* Lichen planopilaris resulting in atrophic, scarred, porcelain-colored area centrally, with bordering follicular involvement consisting of dusky erythema, perifollicular hyperkeratosis and scale, and follicular convergence resulting in doll's hair formation.

inflammation in darkly pigmented skin, with ethnic/genetic factors influencing the expression of disease.[18] There are similar histopathologic findings among these diseases. However, distinct clinical, histologic, and immunopathologic differences among these three conditions have been emphasized by some investigators. Erythema dyschromicum perstans may be strongly influenced by environmental agents as well.

The sequela of healing (late waning, resolving) is often slightly atrophic, hyperpigmented skin. In cases where the inflammatory phase was minimal, such as lichen planus "invisible de Gougerot," the pigmentation may be long-lasting and one of the few signs of previously active disease.

ACTINIC LICHEN PLANUS This variant is also known as lichen planus subtropicus, lichen planus tropicus, summertime actinic lichenoid eruption, lichen planus actinicus, lichen planus atrophicus annularis, and lichenoid melanodermatosis. Actinic lichen planus is more common in Middle Eastern countries in spring and summer, where sunlight appears to have a precipitating effect. Exposed areas of the face, dorsal hands and arms, and the nape of the neck are usually affected. Papules are hyperpigmented with violaceous-brown color and a thready, rolled edge showing well-defined borders. Typical lichen planus lesions may be present over the extremities. Pruritus and scaling are minimal.

FIGURE 49-9

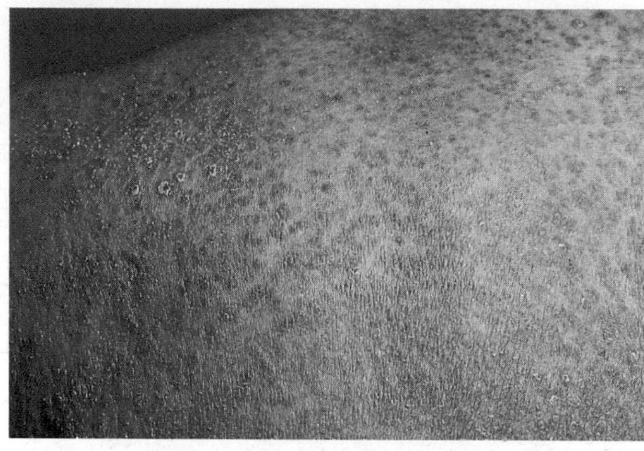

Lichen planus-like eruption. Generalized violaceous papules with superficial scale coalescing to form erythematous variant. History of associated drug exposure leading to lichenoid reaction.

OTHERS A perforating variant has been described. Transepidermal elimination of lichen planus-like inflammatory tissue is observed. Guttate lichen planus is another variant that resembles guttate psoriasis but with the characteristic lichenoid histology. Exfoliative and exanthematous forms are very rare and may represent manifestations of lichenoid drug reactions (Fig. 49-9). The rare entity of invisible lichen planus describes lesions that are not perceptible with visible light illumination but become apparent with Wood's lamp examination. Pruritus is present and biopsy evaluation shows lichenoid histology. This entity may be a minimal variant of lichen planus "invisible de Gougerot."

Site of Involvement

LICHEN PLANUS OF THE SCALP Lichen planopilaris or follicular lichen planus may affect the scalp in a distinctive clinical and histologic pattern. Individual keratotic follicular papules that coalesce and merge over the scalp to form patches are typically seen. Cutaneous, nail, or mucous membrane involvement with lichen planus may also be present. This condition affects women more than men. Patients present with uni- or multifocal hair loss that may be extensive and involve the entire scalp (Fig. 49-10). Perifollicular erythema and acuminate keratotic plugs are characteristic features. Follicular-centered lesions are usually observed under close inspection of the scalp and orifices, particularly at the margins of the alopecic area or within patches still bearing hair.

End-stage disease is characterized by a nondescript scarring alopecia that has led to the use of several clinical terms describing the entity; lichen planopilaris, folliculitis decalvans et atrophicus, lichen spinulosus at folliculitis decalvans, and Graham-Little syndrome are different terms that likely describe the same entity.[16]

Pseudopelade of Brocq is a rare clinical syndrome of scarring alopecia and fibrosis, in which distinct pathologic features are absent. It is generally accepted that pseudopelade of Brocq is the end stage of follicular fibrosis caused by a primary inflammatory dermatosis such as lichen planus, lupus erythematosus, pustular-scarring forms of folliculitis, or fungal infections, including favus, scleroderma, and sarcoidosis.[16]

FIGURE 49-10

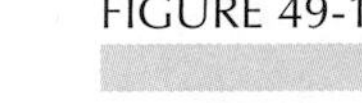

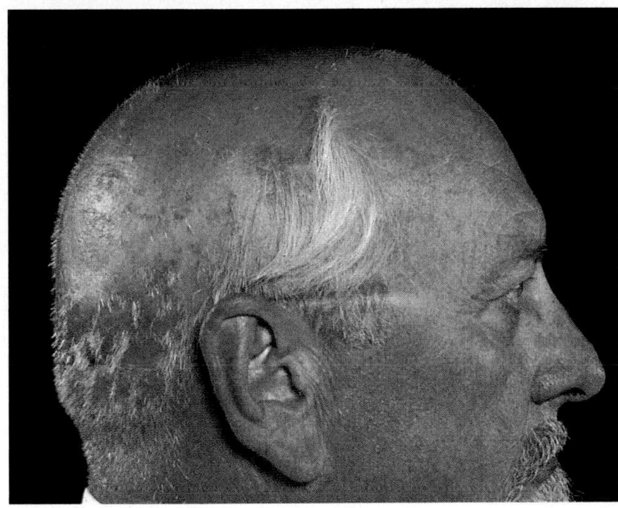

Lichen planus. Extensive hair loss leading to pseudopelade of Brocq appearance. Several remaining tufts of hair showing violaceous erythema and disease activity.

FIGURE 49-11

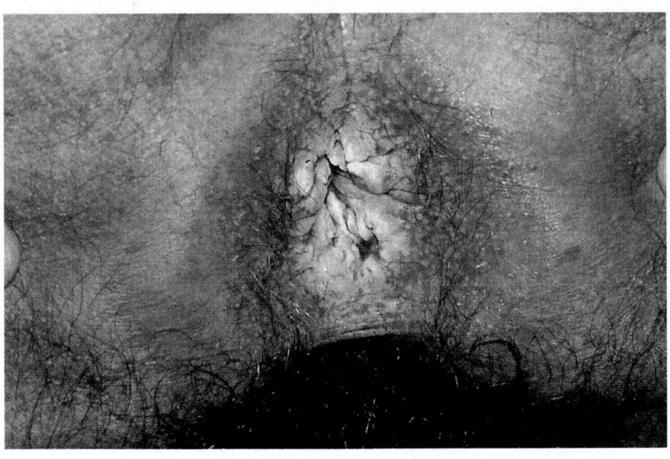

Lichen planus. Perianal leuko- and hyperkeratosis with hypertrophic, folded violaceous epithelium, fissures, and healing biopsy site.

MUCOSAL LICHEN PLANUS Lichen planus can affect the mucosal surfaces of mouth, vagina, esophagus, conjunctiva, urethra, anus, nose, and larynx. Its prevalence is estimated at approximately 1 percent of the adult population. Oral involvement occurs in approximately 60 to 70 percent of patients with lichen planus. It may be the only manifestation in 20 to 30 percent of patients. Oral involvement appears to be the sole manifestation in 15 to 25 percent of patients with lichen planus attending general dermatology clinics, but is far more common in stomatology/mucosal disease specialty referral practices.

Different types of oral lichen planus have been described, including reticular, plaque-like, atrophic, papular, erosive-ulcerative, and bullous forms of the disease.[19] The reticular pattern is considered the most common, but in oral medicine clinics, erosive forms predominate as a consequence of the symptomatology and chronicity. Erosive lichen planus is more common in the elderly and tends to cause a painful, burning sensation. The buccal, gingival, and glossal mucosae are the most commonly affected areas. The palate, floor of the mouth, retromolar pads, and lips may also be affected. Gingival involvement may take the form of gingival stomatitis or desquamative gingivitis, and as a sole presentation, represents 8 to 10 percent of oral lichen planus. Oral lichenoid reaction may be seen on the buccal mucosa adjacent to amalgam dental fillings.[20] Patch tests frequently show positive reactions to mercury, gold, and other metals.[20,21] Because of the prolonged course and associated pain and discomfort, patients with oral lichen planus tend to be depressed, and psychological help should be offered to them.

Bilateral reticular keratotic or atrophic changes of the buccal mucosa and lichenoid atrophic patches over the dorsal tongue have been described in patients with HIV infection. The eruptions usually follow zidovudine or ketoconazole intake. Histologically, liquefaction degradation of basal keratinocytes and epithelial atrophy with lichenoid lymphocytic infiltrate are seen.

Male genitalia are involved in 25 percent of cases, and the glans penis is most commonly affected, with annular lesions frequently present. Female genital involvement consists of patches of leukoplakia or erythroplakia, sometimes with erosions, and, occasionally, as a more generalized desquamative vaginitis. Vaginal adhesions and labial agglutination may result. Anal lesions of mucosal lichen planus present with leukokeratosis, hyperkeratosis, fissuring, and erosions (Fig. 49-11).

A special form of mucosal lichen planus characterized by involvement of vulvar and gingival tissues has been described.[22] The characteristic features include erythema and erosions of the gingivae and tongue and, occasionally, white reticulated plaques, in association with pain and discomfort. Desquamation and erosions of vulva and vagina in association with burning pain, dyspareunia, and vaginal discharge mirror the oral findings.

Conjunctival lichen planus may manifest as cicatricial conjunctivitis. Histologically, irregular thickening with reduplication of the basement membrane is seen. Direct immunofluorescence distinguishes ophthalmic lichen planus from cicatricial pemphigoid.

LICHEN PLANUS OF THE NAILS Nail involvement occurs in 10 to 15 percent of patients.[23] Lichen planus limited to the nails is uncommon, and the initial involvement is followed, in many cases, by the development of typical lesions elsewhere. Lichen planus of nails is infrequent in children. Thinning, longitudinal ridging, and distal splitting of the nail plate (onychoschizia) are the most common findings. Onycholysis, longitudinal striation (onychorrhexis), subungual hyperkeratosis, or even absence (anonychia) of the nail plate can also be seen. Twenty-nail dystrophy (trachyonychia) may represent an isolated nail finding of lichen planus. Psoriasis and alopecia areata can also lead to these distinctive nail changes. Nail loss may result from ulcerative lichen planus involving the nail unit. Pterygium or forward growth of the eponychium with adherence to the proximal nail plate is a classic finding of lichen planus of the nail (Fig. 49-12). An atrophic cicatrizing form of lichen planus with random and progressive nail loss in Asians and blacks has also been reported. The "tenting" or "pup-tent" sign is observed as a result of nail bed involvement that elevates the nail plate and may cause longitudinal splitting.[2]

INVERSE LICHEN PLANUS The inverse pattern occurs only rarely and is characterized by red-brownish, discrete papules and nodules. The eruption occurs mainly in the flexural areas such as axillae, inframammary, groin, and, less likely, the popliteal and antecubital areas. Koebnerized lesions are occasionally present.

PALMOPLANTAR LICHEN PLANUS This acral, localized variant of lichen planus is rare and may create difficulty in diagnosis if it is present as an isolated finding. Very pruriginous, erythematous, scaly plaques with or without hyperkeratosis are characteristic. Lesions are often seen on the internal plantar arch.[24] Yellowish, compact keratotic

FIGURE 49-12

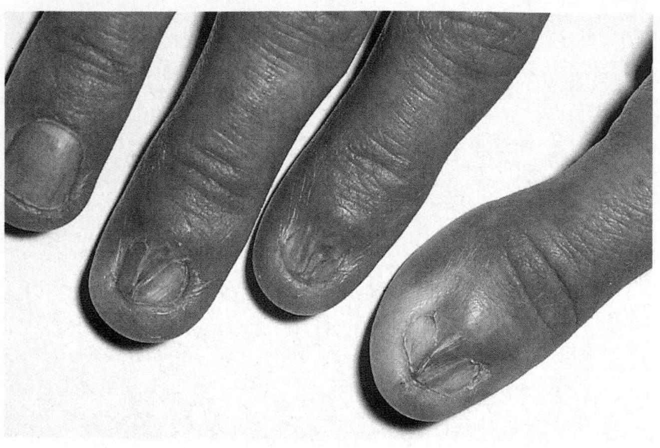

Lichen planus. Classic pterygium formation and tenting of several fingers with loss of nail plates.

papules or papulonodules are seen on the lateral margins of the fingers and hand surfaces; however, they are less likely to affect the fingertips. They appear like callosities with an inflammatory, erythematous halo. The lesions resemble psoriasis vulgaris, warts, calluses, porokeratosis, hyperkeratotic eczema, tinea, or secondary syphilis.[24] Histologically, findings are identical of those of classic lichen planus.

SPECIAL FORMS OF LICHEN PLANUS/LICHENOID ERUPTION

Drug-Induced Lichen Planus

Lichen planus-like or lichenoid eruptions describe a group of cutaneous reactions identical or similar to lichen planus.[25] Lichenoid drug eruptions have been reported after ingestion, contact, or inhalation of certain chemicals (Tables 49-2 and 49-3). A lichenoid drug eruption may be typical or atypical for classic lichen planus, with localized or generalized eczematous papules and plaques and variable desquamation. Lichenoid drug eruptions typically manifest postinflammatory hyperpigmentation and alopecia, and fail to exhibit classic Wickham striae. The eruptions usually appear symmetrically on the trunk and extremities, unlike the flexural distribution of classic lichen planus. A photodistributed pattern is often found, and several drugs frequently induce this reaction (Table 49-4). Mucous membrane involvement is less common and is often associated with specific drugs and chemicals (Table 49-5).

TABLE 49-2

Agents Inducing Lichen Planus and Lichenoid Reactions

	Less-Common Inducers	
Common Inducers	Commonly Prescribed Drugs	Uncommonly Prescribed Drugs
Gold salts	ACE inhibitors	Methyldopa
Beta blockers	Calcium channel blockers	Anti-tuberculosis
Antimalarials	Sulfonylurea hypoglycemic agents	Sulfasalazine
Thiazide diuretics	Nonsteroidal anti-inflammatory drugs	Heavy metals (arsenic, mercury)
Furosemide	Ketoconazole	Lithium
Spironolactone	Tetracycline	Iodides and radiocontrast media
Penicillamine	Phenothiazine derivates	Antimony
		Carbamazepine

TABLE 49-3

Inducers of Lichenoid Drug Eruption—Contact Chemicals

Color film developers
- PPDA (*p*-phenylenediamine)
- IPPD (*p*-isopropylaminodiphenylamine)
- CD_2
- CD_3
- TTS (4-amino-*N*-diethyl-aniline sulfate)
- Antimony trioxide

Dental restorative materials
Musk ambrette
Nickel
Aminoglycoside antibiotics
Gold

SOURCE: With permission from Halevy S, Shai A: Lichenoid drug eruptions. *J Am Acad Dermatol* **29**:249, 1993.

The latency period for development of a lichenoid drug eruption by these agents varies from months to a year or more based on the dosage, host response, previous exposure, and concomitant drug administration. Resolution of the eruptions is quite variable, but most disappear in 3 to 4 months. Resolution of a gold-induced lichenoid eruption may require up to 2 years after discontinuation of the drug. For many inciting drugs, the severity and extent of the eruption influences the rate of clearance. Occasionally, the lichenoid drug eruption disappears or may recur intermittently despite continuation of treatment.

Lichenoid contact dermatitis may result from contact with compounds such as color film developers, dental restoration materials, metals (e.g., mercury, silver, and gold), and aminoglycoside antibiotics.[25] Oral lichenoid drug eruptions related to amalgam seem to be caused by mercury, although gold may be the more common metal sensitizer in oral lichenoid eruptions. Table 49-6 compares the findings in lichen planus and lichenoid during eruptions.

Lichen Planus–Lupus Erythematosus Overlap Syndrome

This rare variant is characterized by lesions that share features of lichen planus and lupus erythematosus. Atrophic plaques and patches with hypopigmentation and a livid red to blue-violet color with telangiectasia

TABLE 49-4

Drugs That Induce Lichenoid Drug Eruption—Photodistributed

5-Fluorouracil
Carbamazepine
Chlorpromazine
Diazoxide
Ethambutol
Pyritinol
Quinine, quinidine
Tetracyclines
Thiazide diuretics and furosemide

SOURCE: With permission from Halevy S, Shai A: Lichenoid drug eruptions. *J Am Acad Dermatol* **29**:249, 1993.

TABLE 49-5

Drugs That Induce Lichen Drug Eruption—Oral Predilection

Allopurinol
Angiotensin-converting enzyme inhibitors
Cyanamide
Dental restorative materials
Gold salts
Ketoconazole
Methyldopa
Nonsteroidal anti-inflammatory drugs
Penicillamine
Sulfonylurea hypoglycemia agents

SOURCE: With permission from Halevy S, Shai A: Lichenoid drug eruptions. *J Am Acad Dermatol* **29**:249, 1993.

and minimal scaling are characteristic. Transient bullae may develop. Classic lesions of lichen planus are not usually seen. Photosensitivity, pruritus, and follicular plugging are also not common. Lesions may develop anywhere, but are most common on the extremities (Fig. 49-13). Some patients with this overlap syndrome may progress to systemic lupus erythematosus. In other instances, laboratory evaluation may reveal only a weak-positive antinuclear antibody. This disease variant is characterized by a prolonged course and lack of response to treatment. Histologically, a lichenoid reaction typical for lichen planus and histologic features of lupus erythematosus are usually present in the same biopsy.[26] By direct immunofluorescence, the most common finding is the presence of cytoids staining with IgG, IgM, and C3 intraepidermally or at the dermal–epidermal junction, as seen in classic lichen planus. Linear to granular deposition of IgM and C3 (as seen in lupus erythematosus, but not in lichen planus) has been observed occasionally. Shaggy deposition of fibrinogen at the basement membrane zone, typical of lichen planus, is sometimes found.[26]

FIGURE 49-13

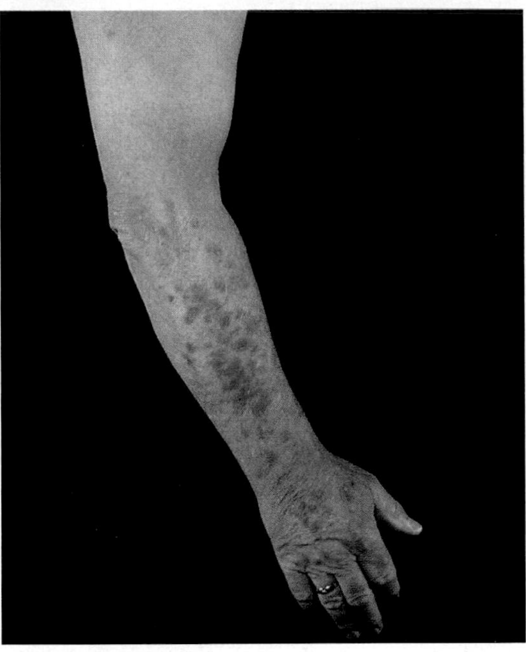

Lichen planus lupus erythematosus overlap syndrome. Lichenoid lesions involving dorsal hand and forearm with direct immunofluorescence evidence of lupus erythematosus.

Lichen Planus Pemphigoides

Lichen planus pemphigoides is characterized by the development of tense blisters atop lesions of lichen planus or the development of vesicles de novo on uninvolved skin (Fig. 49-14). It is important to differentiate this entity from bullous lichen planus, in which blisters develop in lesions of long-standing lichen planus as a result of intense lichenoid inflammation and extensive liquefaction degeneration of basal keratinocytes. The etiology of this variant is not clear. It was proposed that basal cell keratinocyte damage by lymphocytes in lichen planus may unmask hidden antigenic determinants and lead to autoantibody formation and induction of bullous lesions. Histologic findings

FIGURE 49-14

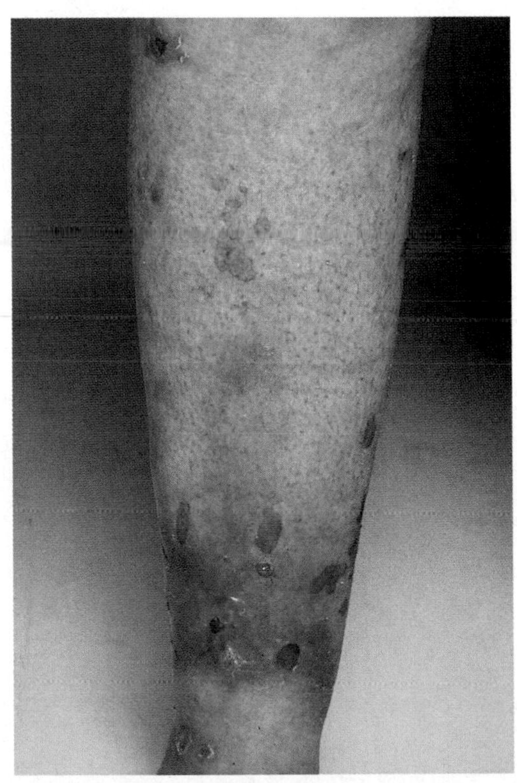

Lichen planus pemphigoides. Lichenoid maculopapular erythema, erosions, and bullae with direct immunofluorescence showing features of bullous pemphigoid. Indirect immunofluorescence also was positive.

TABLE 49-6

Clinical and Histologic Differences between Idiopathic Lichen Planus and Lichenoid Drug Reaction

	Idiopathic Lichen Planus	Lichenoid Drug Eruption
Lesions	Smaller	Larger and scaly
Wickham striae	Usually present	Usually absent
Residual hyperpigmentation	Possible	Common
Alopecia	Uncommon	Common
Predilection	Flexural/extremities	Sun-exposed areas
Mucous membrane involvement	Very common	Less common
Cytoids in granular layer	Very uncommon	Common
Parakeratosis	Not seen	Common

resemble those of lichen planus. Direct immunofluorescence shows linear deposition of IgG and C3 at the dermal–epidermal junction. Sera from these patients react with the epidermal side of NaCl-split human skin. Circulating IgG autoantibodies react to the major noncollagenous extracellular domain (NC16A) of the 180-kDa bullous pemphigoid antigen within the basement membrane zone. Further mapping showed that lichen planus pemphigoides serum reacts with amino acids 46 to 59 of domain NC16A, a protein segment that was previously shown to be unreactive with bullous pemphigoid sera. This newly described epitope is designated MCW-4.[27]

Keratosis Lichenoides Chronica (Nekam's Disease)

Keratosis lichenoides chronica was originally described by Kaposi (as lichen ruber verrucosus et reticularis), but was named after Nekam reported a typical case in 1938. The current descriptive term was introduced in 1972, and the disease is generally felt to represent a special form of lichen planus. Keratosis lichenoides chronica is a rare dermatosis characterized by violaceous papular and nodular lesions, often arranged in a linear and reticulate pattern on the dorsal hands and feet, extremities, and buttocks (Fig. 49-15). The mucous membranes, genitalia, nails, palms, and soles may also be affected. Seborrheic dermatitis-like scaling and telangiectasias of the scalp, face, and neck may develop. Histologically, hyperkeratosis, parakeratosis, and hypergranulosis are seen. The epidermis is usually acanthotic, with mild liquefactive degeneration of basal keratinocytes. A bandlike lymphocytic infiltrate with perivascular and periappendegeal involvement is present. Few plasma cells are seen in the infiltrates. The disease is very refractory to treatment. Photochemotherapy may be helpful, and calcipotriene has shown therapeutic benefit.[28]

FIGURE 49-15

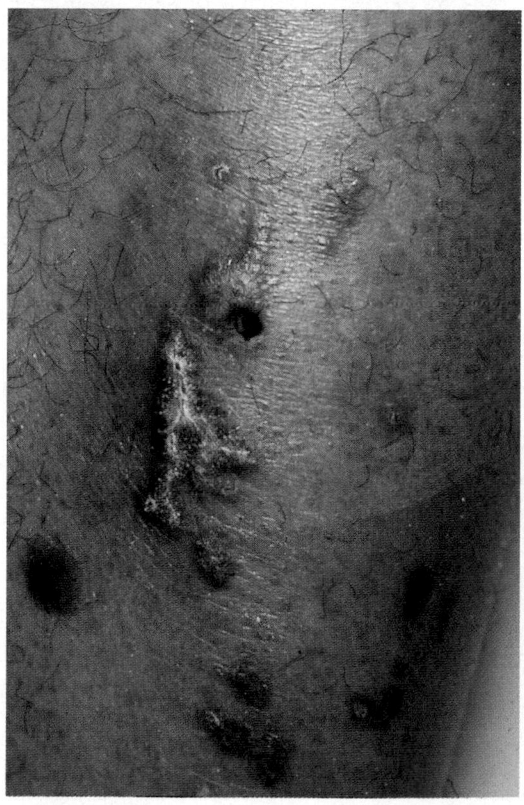

Keratosis lichenoides chronica. Linear to reticulated, hyperpigmented, and hyperkeratotic lesions on the lower leg.

FIGURE 49-16

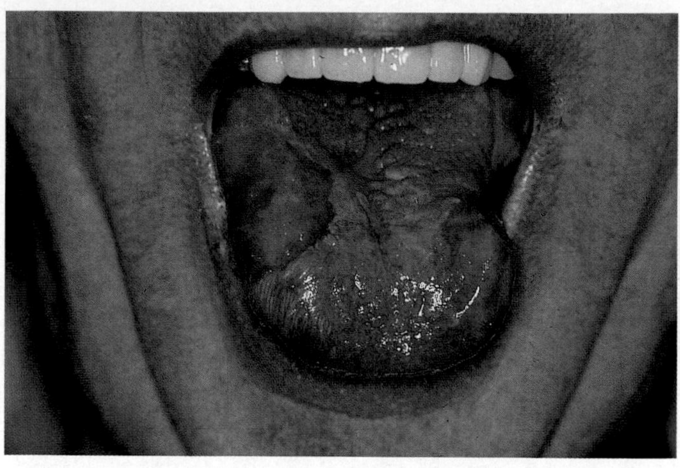

Lichen planus and squamous cell carcinoma. Long-standing oral lichen planus with scarring changes of tongue. Circumscribed erythroplakia and erosion of the right lateral tongue was biopsied and confirmed squamous cell carcinoma.

Lichen Planus and Malignant Transformation

There has been considerable controversy as to whether oral lichen planus inherently harbors malignant potential. It is currently believed that the risk of malignant transformation is fairly low. Risk factors that increase the likelihood of developing oral cancer are long-standing disease, erosive or atrophic types, and tobacco use. It is generally accepted that 0.5 to 5 percent of patients with oral lichen planus develop SCC. The majority of these cases are in situ carcinoma or with microinvasive pattern.[29] The most common site for malignant transformation is the tongue (Fig. 49-16), followed by buccal mucosa, gingiva, and, rarely, the lip. Clinically, the lesions appear as indurated, nonhealing ulcers or exophytic lesions with a keratotic surface in majority of cases. Red atrophic plaques could also be seen and often correlate with SCC in situ. Advanced cases could result in nodal metastases and occasionally death.[29]

The risk of skin malignancy in cutaneous lichen planus is extremely low. Most patients developing SCC in cutaneous lichen planus had a history of either arsenic or x-ray exposure.

Lichenoid Reaction of Graft-Versus-Host Disease

(See also Chap. 118)

Chronic graft-versus-host disease (GVHD) (occurring 100 days after transplant) may present as a lichenoid eruption indistinguishable clinically and histologically from lichen planus. Lichenoid GVHD favors the trunk, buttocks, hips, thighs, palms, and soles. In oral mucosa, xerostomia and oral ulcerations are occasionally seen. Histologically, the findings in lichen planus and oral GVHD are similar, although infiltrating CD3+ T lymphocytes are present in larger numbers in oral lichen planus than in lichenoid lesions of oral GVHD.[30] In a comparative study between those two entities, the number of natural killer cells, Leu-8–positive T cells (homing receptor: CD62L, LECAM), CD25–positive lymphocytes, and the CD4:CD8 ratio were not different. Langerhans cells are often increased in both conditions.

Lichenoid Keratosis

Lichenoid keratoses are brown to red, scaling maculopapules found on sun-exposed skin of extremities. Histologic features of lichen planus are present, with the additional finding of focal parakeratosis. They frequently occur with solar lentigo, seborrheic keratosis, and actinic keratosis, and likely represent an "involuting lichenoid plaque."[31]

Lichenoid Dermatitis

The wide range of disorders and presentations reviewed in this chapter constitute many of the more representative types of lichenoid dermatitis. Additional members of the lichenoid dermatitis group of skin disease include lupus erythematosus, other connective tissue diseases, secondary syphilis, and lymphoproliferative diseases such as lymphomatoid papulosis, mycosis fungoides, and Sézary syndrome.[32] The lymphoproliferative group should be considered carefully in the differential diagnosis of enigmatic lichenoid dermatitis. Special studies, such as direct immunofluorescence, and immunophenotypic and T cell receptor genotypic analyses, are often required to define the underlying pathology manifesting as lichenoid dermatitis more precisely.

ASSOCIATED CONDITIONS

Lichen planus is seen with increased frequency in association with liver diseases such as autoimmune chronic active hepatitis, primary biliary cirrhosis, and postviral chronic active hepatitis.[33] The association with primary biliary cirrhosis is observed regardless of treatment with D-penicillamine, a drug that may cause an exacerbation of lichen planus.

The role of infection in development of lichen planus has been repeatedly raised over the years. Association of lichen planus with syphilis, herpes simplex virus 2, HIV, amebiasis, and chronic bladder infections has been reported.[2] Recently, a more widespread and chronic viral disease, hepatitis C virus (HCV), has been implicated in triggering lichen planus. The prevalence of HCV infection varied between 16 and 29 percent in 517 mainly southern European patients with lichen planus in four different studies.[34,35] On the other hand, many studies from Northern Europe and the United States did not substantiate any link.[36,37] Genetic factors controlling disease susceptibility and prevalence of certain HCV genotypes in certain geographic areas may have significantly influenced these results. A large series of oral lichen planus in the United States found no association with HCV.

Recently, several reports described lichen planus-like eruptions following hepatitis B vaccination.[38]

There is no evidence to link lichen planus to diabetes mellitus, autoimmune diseases, nor internal malignancies. Cases of severe erosive gingivitis and stomatitis with histologic appearance of lichen planus in association with internal malignancies may represent cases of paraneoplastic pemphigus. The pathologic spectrum of findings and target organ involvement in this condition is broad, ranging from lichenoid dermatitis to frank acantholysis, such that a preferred term is *paraneoplastic autoimmune multiorgan syndrome* (PAMS).[39]

LABORATORY FINDINGS

No specific abnormalities of laboratory analyses are seen in lichen planus. The total white blood cell count and lymphocytes may be decreased. This could be related to cytokine activation and local trafficking of cells to skin or other tissue compartments.

Patch tests in patients with oral or cutaneous lichen planus usually reveal positive results in a majority of patients.[20,21] Sensitivity to mercury and gold is often positive in half the cases. Chromate, flavoring agents, acrylate, and thimerosal are common sensitizers.[20,21]

PATHOLOGY

The two major pathologic findings in lichen planus are basal epidermal keratinocyte damage and lichenoid-interface lymphocytic reaction.[1] The epidermal changes include hyperkeratosis, wedge-shaped areas of hypergranulosis, and elongation of rete ridges that resemble a sawtooth pattern (Fig. 49-17). Multiple apoptotic cells or colloid-hyaline (Civatte) bodies are seen at the dermal–epidermal junction. Eosinophilic colloid bodies are present in the papillary dermis. They are PAS-positive and measure about 20 μm in diameter. A bandlike lymphocytic infiltrate is seen in the papillary dermis that abuts the epidermis. Many histiocytes and few plasma cells are seen. Plasma cells are more prominent in mucous membrane specimens. Few eosinophils are seen in drug-induced lichen planus or lichenoid drug eruptions. Melanin pigmentation is invariably present and is more pronounced in older, waning lesions and in dark-skinned individuals. Separation of the epidermis in small clefts (Max Joseph cleft formation) is occasionally seen (Fig. 49-18).

Direct immunofluorescence shows numerous apoptotic cells at the dermal–epidermal junction staining with IgM and, occasionally, with IgG and IgA. Shaggy deposition of fibrinogen at the dermal–epidermal junction is characteristic of lichen planus (Fig. 49-19). Immunocytochemical studies show that the majority of the cells in the infiltrate are T lymphocytes, with scattered B lymphocytes. An increased density of Langerhans cells, dermal dendritic cells, and histiocytes have also been seen, especially in early active lesions.

Different forms of lichen planus share the main pathologic findings and differ by few features. Atrophic lichen planus is characterized by thinning of the epidermis and loss of rete ridges, in contrast to hypertrophic lichen planus, where hyperkeratosis and epidermal hyperplasia are prominent. In the latter, vertical streaking of collagen bundles is found, similar to lichen simplex chronicus. Lichen planus pigmentosus is characterized by the prominent pigment incontinence that extends deeper into the reticular dermis. The inflammatory infiltrate is also less prominent. Psoriasiform acanthosis, vacuolar degeneration, and apoptosis are prominent in keratosis lichenoides chronica. Lichen

FIGURE 49-17

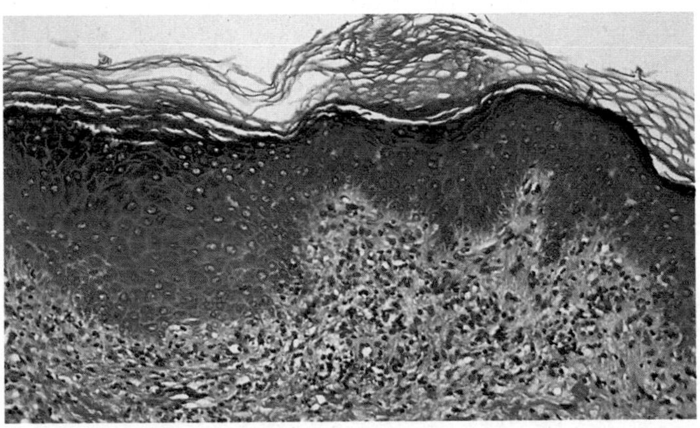

Lichen planus. Typical hyperkeratosis, hypergranulosis, early sawtooth changes and lichenoid interface reaction of classic lichen planus.

FIGURE 49-18

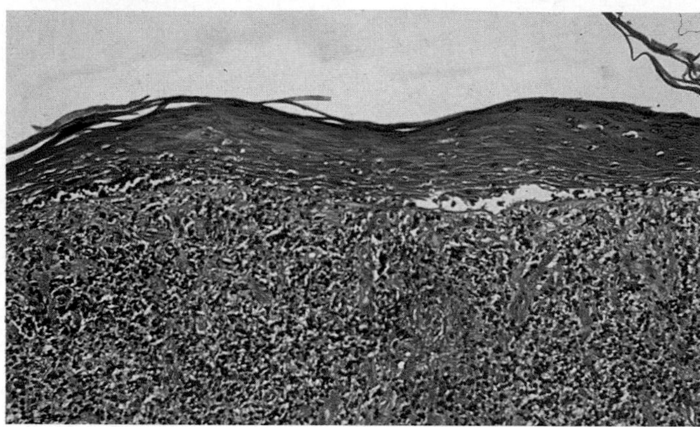

Lichen planus. More extensive epidermal alterations with hydropic changes, thinned epidermis, focal wedge-shaped hypergranulosis, compact orthokeratosis, and pronounced lichenoid inflammation with focal hemorrhage.

planus pemphigoides is characterized by the subepidermal separation and the linear deposition of IgG and C3 along the dermal–epidermal junction. In lichen planopilaris, perifollicular lymphocytic inflammation enveloping the upper third of hair follicle epithelium is usually associated with follicular plugging and hydropic changes of the basal cell layer of the external root sheath. Perifollicular and mid-dermal fibrosis with loss of elastic tissue around follicular epithelium is also found. Classic changes of interface dermatitis as seen in lichen planus are not common in the interfollicular epithelium. Direct immunofluorescence is usually positive in two-thirds of the patients, and should be performed to establish the diagnosis of lichen planopilaris and to rule out other disorders causing cicatricial alopecia, such as lupus erythematosus.[16]

Features that may be seen in lichenoid drug eruptions, but not in lichen planus, include the presence of abundant plasma cells and eosinophils in the infiltrate, focal parakeratosis and hypogranulosis, and the presence of cytoid bodies high in the stratum corneum. Furthermore, lymphocytic infiltration is less dense and not as bandlike as that seen in classic lichen planus.

Lichen planus-like keratosis resembles lichen planus histologically. Lichenoid lymphocytic infiltrates with hyperkeratosis, hypergranulosis, focal acanthosis, and parakeratosis in the absence of keratinocyte atypia are the features of lichen planus-like keratosis.[31] Atypia is present, however, in lichenoid actinic keratosis.

Electron microscopic examination demonstrates basal epidermal alterations with basal lamina interruption and reduplication. Vacuolar changes may be prominent and correlate with tonofilament disruption and loss of desmosome connections. Apoptotic keratinocytes showing typical features of colloid bodies are seen, as well as increased numbers of Langerhans cells, similar to light microscopic changes.

DIAGNOSIS AND DIFFERENTIAL DIAGNOSIS

The appearance of the typical papule of lichen planus is usually sufficient to make the correct diagnosis. Different forms of the disease with various configurations, morphology, or anatomic location are usually associated with more classic lichen planus elsewhere on the body. Careful and thorough skin examination is therefore required. Histopathologic and immunofluorescent evaluation will confirm the diagnosis in cases presenting with atypical lesions.

FIGURE 49-19

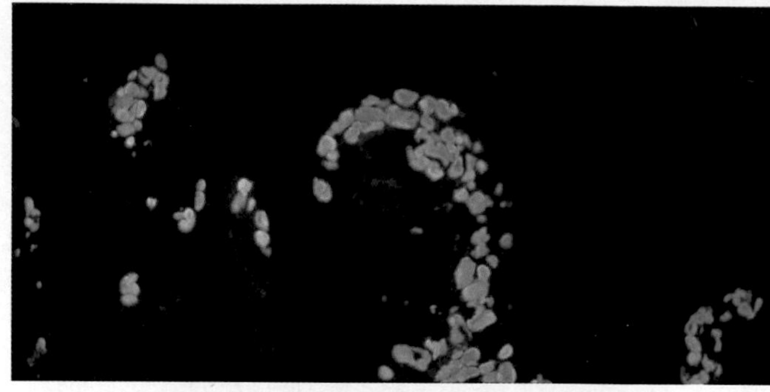

A.

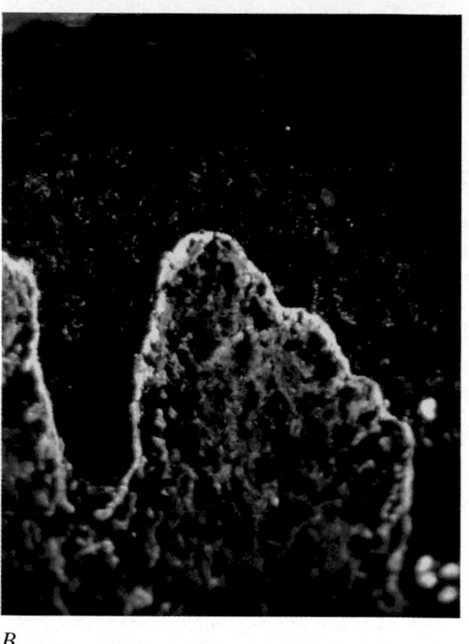

B.

Lichen planus. Direct immunofluorescence examination of involved skin. *A.* Numerous IgM-positive cytoids at the dermal–epidermal junction. *B.* Fibrinogen/fibrin, shaggy pattern at the dermal–epidermal junction.

Other papulosquamous diseases must be differentiated from lichen planus. Psoriasis affecting the penis or the nail may resemble lichen planus; however, classic cutaneous or mucosal lichenoid lesions assist in differentiation. Nail involvement may resemble psoriasis, onychomycosis, or alopecia areata. Genital lesions may resemble psoriasis or seborrheic dermatitis. Lesions of palms and soles should be differentiated from secondary syphilis.

Annular lichen planus may resemble granuloma annulare, but the latter lacks any scale or Wickham striae. Linear lichen planus should be differentiated from nevus unius lateris, lichen striatus, and linear epidermal nevus. Hypertrophic lichen planus may resemble lichen simplex chronicus, prurigo nodularis, lichenoid cutaneous amyloidosis or, on occasion, Kaposi's sarcoma. Atrophic lichen planus may mimic lichen sclerosus et atrophicus. Follicular lichen planus may resemble lichen nitidus and lichen spinulosus. Lichen planopilaris should be differentiated from other causes of cicatricial alopecia such as lupus erythematosus, inflammatory folliculitis, alopecia areata, and cicatricial pemphigoid of Brunsting-Perry. Graham-Little syndrome needs to be distinguished from keratosis follicularis spinulosa decalvans, a genetic disorder with progressive scarring alopecia. Routine histology and direct immunofluorescence findings will separate these disorders.

Severe erosive PAMS-paraneoplastic pemphigus may resemble erosive oral lichen planus and may primarily involve the oral mucosa. Direct and indirect immunofluorescence are usually required to establish the appropriate diagnosis. Oral patches of lichen planus should be differentiated from leukokeratosis, candida infection, lupus erythematosus, mucous patches of secondary syphilis, or traumatic bite line.

Childhood lichen planus should be distinguished from lichen nitidus, lichen striatus, papular acrodermatitis of childhood, and pityriasis lichenoides.

TREATMENT

Management of lichen planus can be challenging and discouraging for both the patient and physician. Lichen planus may be associated with only minor symptoms or may cause considerable discomfort and disability. Hence, treatment options should be assessed for attendant risks and benefits and tailored to the extent and severity of disease. Avoidance of exacerbating drugs, unless necessary, and minimizing trauma to skin and mucosal tissues are routinely recommended.

Various drugs have been proposed for the treatment of cutaneous and oral lichen planus and the majority of these consist of small series of patients or anecdotes. Many of the advocated treatments lack conclusive evidence for efficacy. Many excellent reviews have dealt with this issue.[40,41]

Oral Lichen Planus

GENERAL MEASURES For oral lichen planus, good oral hygiene and regular personal and professional dental care need to be encouraged. Several treatment approaches are useful for oral or mucous membrane lichen planus. Replacement of amalgam or gold dental restorations with composite material is frequently of considerable benefit in patients with oral lichenoid reactions, even in the apparent absence of relevant patch test results. Chronic lesions on the buccal mucosa in contact with metal or other contact sensitizers frequently heal promptly after replacement,[20,21] and, occasionally, lesions at sites distant to oral lesions may also clear following removal of metal restorations. Gingival lesions may respond less favorably. The decision to undergo removal and restoration is often difficult and usually depends on the chronicity, severity, and clinical and patch test evidence for involvement by the metal/prosthesis as well as the level of frustration of the patient.

TOPICAL STEROIDS Topical steroids are the first-line therapy in mucosal lichen planus.[42] A variety of topical glucocorticoids have been shown to be effective. Use of occlusive materials suitable for mucous membranes, such as Orabase, may provide protection and sustained tissue contact with the glucocorticoid, as well as alleviate the discomfort associated with erosive lesions. Fluocinonide in an adhesive gel or base, 0.1% fluocinolone acetonide, and 0.05% clobetasol propionate in Orabase showed good results. Application four to six times a day is recommended. Treatment may be complicated by frequent infections with oral candidiasis. The use of chlorhexidine gluconate mouthwashes and topical anticandidal medications is recommended during therapy.

In some situations where secondary irritation and inflammation of oral tissues appears to be related to colonization of the mouth by candida, an antifungal treatment course (troche or oral) may be indicated.

Topical anesthetics also provide symptomatic benefit for patients who have difficulty with eating and chewing, and is often compounded with topical corticosteroids. Glucocorticoids containing vaginal and rectal suppositories are usually helpful for mucosal involvement in these areas.

Glucocorticoids can be administered by intralesional injections or application under occlusion by a flexible vaginal prosthetic device or cloth strips.

SYSTEMIC GLUCOCORTICOIDS Systemic glucocorticoids provide effectiveness in erosive oral and vulvovaginal lichen planus. Systemic dosing can be used alone, or, more commonly, in conjunction

with topical glucocorticoids. A dose range from 30 to 80 mg/day, tapered over 3 to 6 weeks shows benefit. Relapses are common after dose reduction or discontinuation. Higher doses are often needed for esophageal lichen planus. Oral candidiasis is a common complication.

RETINOIDS Topical retinoic acid (tretinoin gel) has been shown to be effective in erosive as well as plaquelike oral lesions. Irritation often makes this localized approach to therapy less attractive. Isotretinoin gel is also effective, especially in nonerosive oral lesions. Improvement is usually noted after 2 months; however, recurrence is common after discontinuation of therapy. Topical retinoids are often used in conjunction with topical glucocorticoids. Although not proven in clinical trials, this may improve the efficacy and lessen the side effects.

Etretinate orally has been used at 75 mg/day (0.6 to 1.0 mg/kg per day) in erosive oral lichen planus with significant improvement in the majority of patients. Relapses are common following discontinuation of medication.[43] In a double-blind, placebo-controlled study, two-thirds of patients showed marked improvement or complete remission within 8 weeks of instituting acitretin, 30 mg/day.[44] Only the aromatic retinoid acitretin is currently available by prescription following the removal of etretinate from the US market. There is no conclusive data on the efficacy of oral tretinoin or isotretinoin.

CYCLOSPORINE, TACROLIMUS, AND PIMECROLIMUS Topical application of cyclosporine, 100 mg/mL, 5 mL three times daily has shown benefit for oral lichen planus. Application modalities include mouthwashes and manual administration with local massage. Topical cyclosporine washes seem to be effective in oral lichen planus, especially the severe erosive forms,[45] but they do not appear to be better than local glucocorticoid therapy. Lack of effectiveness in a few cases,[46] the high cost of this medication, as well as the lack of a commercial formulation for topical application limits its use. Availability of alternate topical immunosuppressive agents, tacrolimus and pimecrolimus, currently provide useful substitutes to topical cyclosporine. Tacrolimus, a member of the immunosuppressive macrolide family which suppresses T cell activation is effective in erosive mucosal disease, providing rapid relief from pain and burning with minimal side effects.[47] Oral cyclosporine at dose regimens of 3 to 10 mg/kg per day has been used for severe ulcerative disease.

MISCELLANEOUS The polyene antifungal, griseofulvin, has been used empirically for treatment of oral and cutaneous lichen planus; however, it lacks clear effectiveness. Newer antifungal agents (e.g., fluconazole, itraconazole) may be useful in oral lichen planus with evidence of candida overgrowth, especially concomitantly with systemic glucocorticoids.

In one study, hydroxychloroquine at 200 to 400 mg/day for at least 6 months resulted in complete healing of oral erosions of lichen planus.[48] Caution should be used with hydroxychloroquine because antimalarials are implicated as possible inducers of lichen planus.

Thalidomide should be reserved for cases recalcitrant to other remedies. The dose could be started at 50 mg/day and increased gradually to 200 mg/day.[49]

Extracorporeal photochemotherapy (ECP) twice a week for 3 weeks and then tapered has had favorable results. In one study, all seven patients experienced complete remission.[50] Azathioprine, cyclophosphamide, and mycophenolate mofetil have shown benefit in oral lichen planus, but randomized clinical trials are lacking.[41]

Cutaneous Lichen Planus

TOPICAL GLUCOCORTICOIDS A large variety of topical and systemic therapies are available for the treatment of cutaneous lichen planus, and this range of options may be attributed to the chronicity, symptomatology, and variable responsiveness of the dermatosis. Topical glucocorticoids are typically used for limited cutaneous disease.[42] Potent topical glucocorticoids, with or without occlusion, are occasionally beneficial in cutaneous lichen planus.

Intralesional triamcinolone acetonide (5 to 10 mg/mL) is effective in treating oral and cutaneous lichen planus. This may also be used in lichen planus of the nails with injection of the proximal nail fold every 4 weeks. Regression of lesions occurs within 3 to 4 months. For hypertrophic lichen planus, higher concentrations of intralesional glucocorticoid (10 to 20 mg/mL) may be required. Regular and close observation should be performed to monitor for any signs of atrophy or localized hypopigmentation that may develop; treatment should be discontinued promptly with development of these complications.

Systemic glucocorticoids are often useful and effective in doses greater than 20 mg/day (e.g., 30 to 80 mg prednisone) for 4 to 6 weeks with subsequent taper over 4 to 6 weeks. Other regimens include prednisone 5 to 10 mg/day for 3 to 5 weeks. Symptoms are often alleviated, and patients in the early stages of evolution or experiencing a flare have marked benefit and attenuation or aborted progression of disease. However, the rate of relapse following termination of therapy is unknown. In lichen planopilaris, potent topical glucocorticoids in conjunction with oral glucocorticoids, 30 to 40 mg/day, for at least 3 months, seems to be successful; however, relapse typically occurs following discontinuation. Long-term, chronic continuation of oral or injected glucocorticoids is contraindicated in most cases because of the high risk of complications.

RETINOIDS The systemic retinoids demonstrate anti-inflammatory activity and have been used in the treatment of lichen planus. Remission and marked improvement was achieved with 30 mg/day of acitretin for 8 weeks.[44] Oral tretinoin (10 to 30 mg/day) provided complete remission or marked improvement in greater than 90 percent of patients over a period of 1 to 19 months of treatment. Side effects were mild.[51] Low-dose etretinate (10 to 20 mg/day) use has been associated with complete remission of cutaneous, oral, and nail lichen planus after 4 to 6 months of treatment. Prompt beneficial response was noted with the use of 75 mg/day of etretinate,[52] but side effects of retinoids are dose-related and may limit use of higher dose therapeutic regimens. The combination of retinoids and PUVA therapy has not been evaluated.

PHOTOCHEMOTHERAPY PUVA photochemotherapy is usually successful in generalized cutaneous lichen planus. It has been used in conjunction with oral glucocorticoids to hasten the response. In an open study of 75 patients who underwent bath-PUVA therapy with trioxsalen, 65 percent were cured and an additional 15 percent improved; 50 mg of trioxsalen was added to 150 L of water, and the patients were exposed to UVA after 10 min of bathing.[53] During 2- to 5-year follow up, 25 percent of these patients had a relapse. In another study, recurrence rate was higher in patients treated with PUVA than those with placebo. This study indicates that although oral and bath methoxsalen PUVA have a favorable immediate clearing effect, they may prolong the course of the disease.[54] UVA1 phototherapy may also benefit more protracted lichen planus.

IMMUNOSUPPRESSIVE AGENTS Systemic cyclosporine has been used successfully in recalcitrant lichen planus.[55] The administered dose can range from 3 to 10 mg/kg per day. Pruritus usually disappears after 1 to 2 weeks. Clearance of the rash is seen in 4 to 6 weeks. Low doses (1 to 2.5 mg/kg per day) are probably sufficient to achieve remission. Adverse effects on renal function, development of hypertension, and other significant side-effects, as well as relapse after discontinuation of the drug, limit its use to severe cases.[56]

Azathioprine may be useful in recalcitrant, generalized cutaneous lichen planus and in lichen planus pemphigoides.[57] Similar results are seen with mycophenolate mofetil at a dose of 1500 mg twice daily.[58]

MISCELLANEOUS Complete healing was seen in two-thirds of patients with cutaneous and oral lichen planus within 4 months of treatment with dapsone orally at 200 mg/day.[59] Partial improvement was seen in an additional 19 percent of patients. Antimalarials (200 to 400 mg/day) have been reported to be particularly useful in actinic lichen planus.

IFN-α2b has been administered for treatment of generalized lichen planus with improvement, but this biologic response modifier also has been implicated in development or exacerbation of lichen planus.[60]

Thalidomide led to healing in a case of severe acral erosive lichen planus unresponsive to other therapies.[61] Oral metronidazole 500 mg twice daily for 1 to 2 months also reportedly clears the majority of cases of generalized lichen planus.[62]

Based on the benefit in bullous pemphigoid, combination therapy with tetracycline or doxycycline and nicotinamide has been reported as useful in the treatment of lichen planus pemphigoides.[63]

Low molecular weight heparin in low doses has lymphoid antiproliferative and immunomodulatory properties. At a dose of 3 mg weekly, heparin injections have been reported to significantly improve the symptoms of pruritus and activity of the disease. Four to six injections of heparin induced complete regression of lesions within 4 to 10 weeks. Cutaneous involvement and reticulated oral lesions had the best response.[64] Oral lichen planus showed minimal improvement with this regimen.

Skin grafting has been beneficial in the management of ulcerative lichen planus of the feet that is recalcitrant to other treatments. Cyclophosphamide, methotrexate, and phenytoin reportedly are useful but should be reserved for cases refractory to less-toxic drugs.

COURSE AND PROGNOSIS

Lichen planus is an unpredictable disease that typically persists for 1 to 2 years, but which may follow a chronic, relapsing course over many years. The duration varies according to the extent and site of involvement and morphology of lesions. Tompkins reported an average duration of 1 year for patients with cutaneous disease only, 17 months for skin and mucous membrane disease, about 5 years for patients with oral involvement only, and over 8 years for hypertrophic lichen planus.[65] Interestingly, generalized eruptions tend to have a rapid course and heal spontaneously faster than limited cutaneous disease. Lichen planopilaris is one of the most chronic and often progressive disease variants with little potential for hair regrowth following follicular inflammation and destruction.[16] Hypertrophic lichen planus typically follows a protracted, unremitting course.[2] Spontaneous regression is also an uncommon feature of oral lichen planus. The mean duration for oral lichen planus is 5 years. The reticular variant has a better prognosis than erosive disease that does not heal spontaneously. Generally, the duration of disease conforms to the following order: generalized $<$ cutaneous $<$ cutaneous $+$ mucous membrane $<$ mucous membrane $<$ hypertrophic $=$ lichen planopilaris.

Relapse of disease occurs in 15 to 20 percent of cases and tends to occur in the same area as the initial episode. Recurrences are more common in generalized lichen planus and are usually of shorter duration.

Malignant transformation may occur, and SCC usually develops in fewer than 1 percent of persistent oral–mucous lesions on long-term follow-up.[66]

REFERENCES

1. Pinkus H: Lichenoid tissue reactions. *Arch Dermatol* **107**:840, 1973
2. Boyd AS, Nelder KH: Lichen planus. *J Am Acad Dermatol* **25**:593, 1991
3. Mahood JM: Familial lichen planus. *Arch Dermatol* **119**:292, 1983
4. LaNasa G et al: HLA antigen distribution in different clinical subgroups demonstrates genetic heterogeneity in lichen planus. *Br J Dermatol* **132**:897, 1995
5. Sugerman PB et al: Oral lichen planus. *Clin Dermatol* **18**:533, 2000
6. Schiller PI et al: Detection of clonal T cells in lichen planus. *Arch Dermatol Res* **292**:568, 2000
7. Simark-Mattsson C et al: Distribution of interleukin-2, -4, -10, tumor necrosis factor-alpha and transforming growth factor-beta mRNA in oral lichen planus. *Arch Oral Biol* **44**:499, 1999
8. Walton LJ et al: VCAM-1 and ICAM-1 are expressed by Langerhans cells, macrophages and endothelial cells in oral lichen planus. *J Oral Pathol Med* **23**:262, 1994
9. Eversole LR et al: Leukocyte adhesion molecules in oral lichen planus: A T cell-mediated immunopathologic process. *Oral Microbiol Immunol* **9**:376, 1994
10. Wayner EA et al: Epiligrin, a component of epithelial basement membranes, is an adhesive ligand for alpha 3, beta 1 positive T lymphocytes. *J Cell Biol* **121**:1141, 1993
11. Zhou XJ et al: Matrix metalloproteinases and their inhibitors in oral lichen planus. *J Cutan Pathol* **28**:72, 2001
12. Yamamoto T et al: The mechanism of mononuclear cell infiltration in oral lichen planus: The role of cytokines released from keratinocytes. *J Clin Immunol* **20**:294, 2000
13. Bloor BK et al: Gene expression of differentiation-specific keratins (K4, K13, K1, and K10) in oral nondysplastic keratoses and lichen planus. *J Oral Pathol Med* **29**:376, 2000
14. Lutz ME et al: Zosteriform lichen planus without evidence of herpes simplex virus or varicella-zoster virus by polymerase chain reaction. Report of two cases. *Acta Derm Venereol* **77**:491, 1997
15. Stinco G et al: Surgery and cyclosporine in the treatment of erosive lichen planus of the feet. *Eur J Dermatol* **8**:243, 1998
16. Mehregan DA et al: Lichen planopilaris: Clinical and pathologic study of forty-five patients. *J Am Acad Dermatol* **27**:935, 1992
17. Kossard S: Postmenopausal frontal fibrosing alopecia: A frontal variant of lichen planopilaris. *J Am Acad Dermatol* **36**:59, 1997
18. Vega ME et al: Ashy dermatosis versus lichen planus pigmentosus: A controversial matter. *Int J Dermatol* **31**:87, 1992
19. Silverman S, Bahl S: Oral lichen planus update: Clinical characteristics, treatment responses, and malignant transformation. *Am J Dent* **10**:259, 1997
20. Yiannias JA et al: Relative contact sensitivities in oral lichen planus. *J Am Acad Dermatol* **42**:177, 2000
21. Scalf LA et al: Dental metal allergy in patients with oral, cutaneous, and genital lichenoid reactions. *Am J Contact Dermatol* **12**:146, 2001
22. Eisen D: The vulvovaginal-gingival syndrome of lichen planus. The clinical characteristics of 22 patients. *Arch Dermatol* **130**:1379, 1994
23. Tosti A et al: Nail lichen planus: Clinical and pathologic study of twenty-four patients. *J Am Acad Dermatol* **28**:724, 1993
24. Sanchez-Perez J et al: Lichen planus with lesions on the palms and/or soles: Prevalence and clinicopathological study of 36 patients. *Br J Dermatol* **142**:310, 2000
25. Ellgehausen P et al: Drug-induced lichen planus. *Clin Dermatol* **16**:325, 1998
26. Romero RW et al: Unusual variant of lupus erythematosus or lichen planus. Clinical, histopathologic, and immunofluorescence studies. *Arch Dermatol* **113**:741, 1977
27. Zillikens D et al: Autoantibodies in lichen planus pemphigoides reacts with a novel epitope within the C-terminal NC16A domain of BP180. *J Invest Dermatol* **113**:117, 1999
28. Grunwald MH et al: Keratosis lichenoides chronica: Response to topical calcipotriol. *J Am Acad Dermatol* **37**:263, 1997
29. Mignogna MD et al: Clinical guidelines in early detection of oral squamous cell carcinoma arising in oral lichen planus: A 5-year experience. *Oral Oncol* **37**:262, 2001
30. Mattsson T et al: A comparative immunological analysis of the oral mucosa in chronic graft-versus-host disease and oral lichen planus. *Arch Oral Biol* **37**:539, 1992
31. Glaun RS et al: A proposed new classification system for lichenified keratosis. *J Am Acad Dermatol* **35**:772, 1996
32. Oliver GF et al: Lichenoid dermatitis: A clinicopathologic and immunopathologic review of sixty-two cases. *J Am Acad Dermatol* **21**:284, 1989
33. Rebora A: Lichen planus and the liver. *Int J Dermatol* **31**:392, 1992
34. Mignogna MD et al: Oral lichen planus and HCV infection: A clinical evaluation of 263 cases. *Int J Dermatol* **37**:575, 1998
35. Imhof M et al: Prevalence of hepatitis C virus antibodies and evaluation of hepatitis C virus genotypes in patients with lichen planus. *Dermatology* **195**:1, 1997
36. Van Der Meij EH, Van Der Waal I: Hepatitis C virus infection and oral lichen planus: A report from the Netherlands. *J Oral Pathol Med* **29**:255, 2000
37. Ingafou M et al: No evidence of HCV infection or liver disease in British patients with oral lichen planus. *Int J Oral Maxillofac Surg* **27**:65, 1998
38. Usman A et al: Lichenoid eruption following hepatitis B vaccination: First North American case report. *Pediatr Dermatol* **18**:123, 2001
39. Nguyen VT et al: Classification, clinical manifestations and immunopathological mechanisms of the epithelial variant of paraneoplastic autoimmune multiorgan syndrome: A reappraisal of paraneoplastic pemphigus. *Arch Dermatol* **137**:193, 2001
40. McCreary CE, McCartan BE: Clinical management of oral lichen planus. *Br J Oral Maxillofac Surg* **37**:338, 2001
41. Popovsky JL, Camisa C: New and emerging therapies for diseases of the oral cavity. *Dermatol Clin* **18**:113, 2000
42. Lozada-Nur F, Miranda C: Oral lichen planus: Topical and systemic therapy. *Semin Cutan Med Surg* **16**:295, 1997
43. Gorsky M, Ravin M: Efficacy of etretinate (Tegison) in symptomatic oral lichen planus. *Oral Surg Oral Med Oral Pathol* **73**:52, 1992
44. Laurberg G et al: Treatment of lichen planus with acitretin. A double-blind, placebo-controlled study in 65 patients. *J Am Acad Dermatol* **24**:434, 1991
45. Eisen D et al: Effect of topical cyclosporine rinse on oral lichen planus. A double-blind analysis. *N Engl J Med* **323**:290, 1990
46. Jungell P, Malmstrom M: Cyclosporin A mouthwash in the treatment of oral lichen planus. *Int J Oral Maxiofacial Surg* **25**:60, 1996
47. Rozycki TW et al : Topical tacrolimus in the treatment of symptomatic oral lichen planus: A series of 13 patients. *J Am Acad Dermatol* **46**:27, 2002
48. Eisen D: Hydroxychloroquine sulfate (Plaquenil) improves oral lichen planus: An open trial. *J Am Acad Dermatol* **28**:609, 1993
49. Camisa C, Popovsky JL: Effective treatment of oral lichen planus with thalidomide. *Arch Dermatol* **136**:1442, 2000
50. Becherel PA et al: Extracorporeal photochemotherapy for chronic erosive lichen planus. *Lancet* **351**:805, 1998
51. Ott F et al: Efficacy of oral low-dose tretinoin (all-*trans*-retinoic acid) in lichen planus. *Dermatology* **192**:334, 1996
52. Hersle K et al: Severe oral lichen planus: Treatment with an aromatic retinoid (etretinate). *Br J Dermatol* **106**:77, 1982
53. Karvonen J, Hannuksela M: Long term results of topical trioxsalen PUVA in lichen planus and nodular prurigo. *Acta Derm Venereol Suppl (Stockh)* **120**:53, 1985
54. Helander I et al: Long-term efficacy of PUVA treatment in lichen planus: Comparison of oral and external methoxsalen regimens. *Photodermatol* **4**:265, 1987
55. Pigatto PD et al: Cyclosporin A for the treatment of severe lichen planus. *Br J Dermatol* **122**:121, 1990
56. Lim KK et al: Cyclosporine in the treatment of dermatologic disease: An update. *Mayo Clin Proc* **71**:1182, 1996
57. Verma KK et al: Generalized severe lichen planus treated with azathioprine. *Acta Derm Venereol* **79**:493, 1999
58. Nousari HC et al: Successful treatment of resistant hypertrophic and bullous lichen planus with mycophenolate mofetil. *Arch Dermatol* **135**:1420, 1999
59. Kumar B et al: Dapsone in lichen planus [letter]. *Acta Derm Venereol* **74**:334, 1994
60. Hildebrand A et al: Successful treatment of generalized lichen planus with recombinant interferon alfa-2b. *J Am Acad Dermatol* **33**:880, 1995
61. Dereure O et al: Erosive lichen planus: Dramatic response to thalidomide. *Arch Dermatol* **132**:1392, 1996
62. Buyuk AY, Kavala M: Oral metronidazole treatment of lichen planus. *J Am Acad Dermatol* **43**:260, 2000
63. Fivenson DP, Kimbrough TL: Lichen planus pemphigoides: Combination therapy with tetracycline and nicotinamide. *J Am Acad Dermatol* **36**:638, 1997
64. Stefanidou MP et al: Low molecular weight heparin: A novel alternative therapeutic approach for lichen planus. *Br J Dermatol* **141**:1002, 1999
65. Tompkins JK: Lichen planus: Statistical study of 41 cases. *Arch Dermatol* **71**:515, 1955
66. Eisen D: The clinical features, malignant potential, and systemic associations of oral lichen planus: A study of 723 patients. *J Am Acad Dermatol* **46**:207, 2002

CHAPTER 50

Mazen S. Daoud
Mark R. Pittelkow

Lichen Nitidus

Lichen nitidus (Latin nitidus, "shiny" or "glistening") is an uncommon, usually asymptomatic cutaneous eruption first described by Felix Pinkus in 1901 and further characterized by him in 1907.[1,2] The dermatosis consists of small, glistening, flesh-colored to pink or reddish-brown papules that may be limited to the penis, genitalia, abdomen, and extremities or less frequently may occur as a generalized condition. The histopathologic findings are characteristic. Although the condition is often chronic, the prognosis is good, and no clearly associated systemic illnesses have been documented.

EPIDEMIOLOGY

Because the disease is uncommon, accurate epidemiologic characteristics of lichen nitidus have yet to be defined. In general, lichen nitidus is an infrequently occurring dermatosis that has been reported to affect blacks more than Caucasians, although no strong predisposition for any race is clearly evident. Perhaps the relative prominence of pale lesions on dark skin accounts for the reported increased incidence in blacks. A predilection for children, young adults, and males has also been reported in the literature, but, again, these data are not well established. The incidence is estimated to be approximately 3.4 cases per 10,000 population, based on a 25-year survey of skin diseases in blacks.[3] Compared to the more common dermatosis lichen planus, the crude ratio of lichen nitidus to lichen planus is 1.7:100, based on pathologic diagnosis of cases evaluated over several decades at Mayo Clinic.

ETIOLOGY AND PATHOGENESIS

Once considered a tuberculoid reaction, lichen nitidus is currently regarded as a disorder of unknown etiology. The relationship between lichen nitidus and lichen planus has been debated for many years.[4] The coexistence of both diseases in some patients and the observation that the discrete, tiny papules of lichen planus are indistinguishable from those of lichen nitidus were used to support the view that lichen nitidus is a variant of lichen planus. However, most experienced clinicians, as well as research studies, favor the separation of these two diseases as distinct entities based on both clinical and immunodermatopathologic differences and the characteristic and distinctive histologic changes (see below). Table 50-1 summarizes some of these differences and similarities.

TABLE 50-1

Comparison of Features between Lichen Nitidus and Lichen Planus

	LICHEN NITIDUS	LICHEN PLANUS
Incidence	Rare	Common
Lesion		
Size	Usually 1–2 mm	Variable, usually larger
Shape	Round	Polygonal
Color	Flesh, pink, red-brown	Erythematous to violaceous
Wickham striae	Absent	Present
Mucosal changes	Rare	Variably present
Pruritus	Uncommon	Usually present, marked
Histopathology		
Hyperkeratosis	Variable and focal	Usually present
Parakeratosis	Mostly present	Not found
Infiltrate	Focal in 1–3 papillary bodies	Bandlike, extends through many rete ridges
Lymphocytes	Variable	Vast majority of cells
Histiocytes	Variable, almost always present	Almost none
Giant cells	Occasional	None
Dyskeratotic cells	Occasional	Very common
Immunopathology		
Cytoids	Usually negative	IgM and other conjugates
Basement membrane	Usually negative	Fibrinogen, other conjugates
Immunohistochemistry		
CD4+ lymphocytes	Majority of cells	Majority of cells
CD68+ cells	Common	Uncommon

Another etiologic theory of lichen nitidus proposes that an allergen may cause epidermal and dermal antigen-presenting cells (e.g., Langerhans cells) to activate a cell-mediated response, initiate lymphocyte accumulation, and form discrete inflammatory papules. The presence of large numbers of Langerhans cells in the infiltrate supports this theory.[5] Specific cytokines produced by the inflammatory cells influence the immune response and may shift the T lymphocyte response toward the T helper 2 subset (T_H2) that has the potential to produce the superficial dermal granulomas seen in lichen nitidus.[6] Functional impairment in cellular immunity has been reported in generalized lichen nitidus,[7] and lichenoid photoeruptions similar to lichen nitidus were seen in a patient with HIV infection.[8] Rare cases of lichen nitidus associated with atopic dermatitis, Crohn's disease, and juvenile chronic arthritis have been reported. Induction of allergic contact dermatitis by topical application of dinitrochlorobenzene (DNCB) in a patient with lichen nitidus cleared the eruption, presumably by altering the cellular immunity, cellular infiltration, and cytokine expression.[6]

A rare familial presentation of lichen nitidus has been reported, although no genetic factors of the disease have been identified.[9]

CLINICAL MANIFESTATIONS

Lichen nitidus is composed of multiple, discrete, smooth, flat, round papules. Individual papules are 1 to 2 mm in size, flesh-colored to slightly pink or, in blacks, hypopigmented, with a glistening appearance (Fig. 50-1). Sometimes, minimal scale is present or can be elicited by rubbing the surface of the papules. Occasionally, the papules are grouped and the isomorphic or Koebner's phenomenon is observed. Lesions may occur anywhere over the skin surface; however, the most frequent sites of predilection are the flexural surfaces of the arms and the wrists, lower abdomen, breasts, the glans and shaft of the penis, and other areas of the genital region. Rare sites of involvement include mucous membranes, nails, palms, and soles. Rare clinical variants include vesicular, hemorrhagic, spinous follicular, linear, generalized, and actinic types.[10–16]

FIGURE 50-1

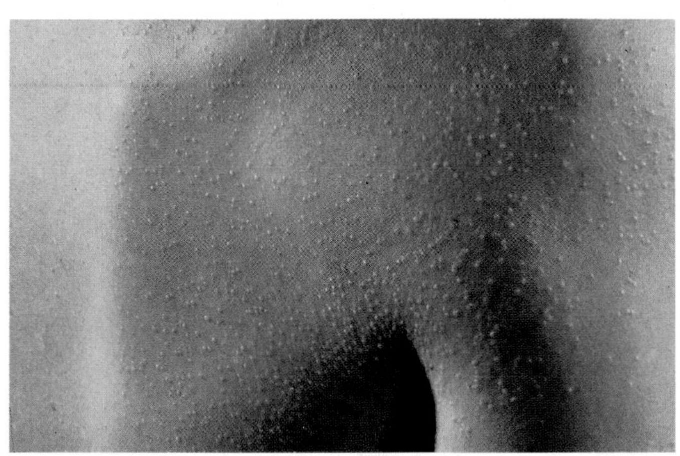

A.

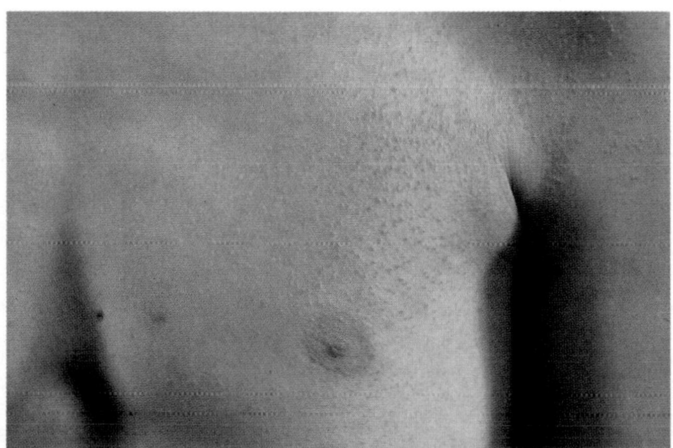

B.

Lichen nitidus. *A.* Pinpoint to pinhead, discrete, dome-shaped papules over upper back, shoulder, and arm. Side-lighting, as performed here, enhances visualization of multiple small lesions. *B.* Individual papules, flesh- to pink-colored over chest and arm, becoming more grouped over anterior axilla.

FIGURE 50-2

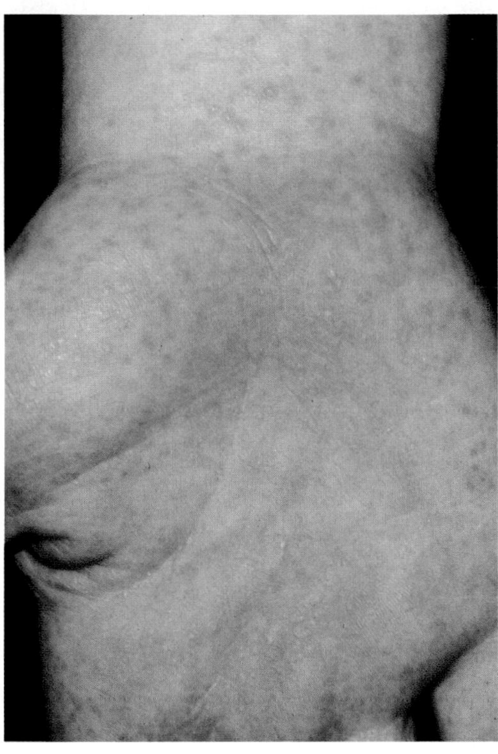

Lichen nitidus. Wrist and palmar involvement with development of hyperkeratotic lesions.

Palmoplantar involvement may manifest several morphologic forms. Bilateral hyperkeratosis of palms and soles with erythema, fissuring, and a texture resembling fine sandpaper has been observed.[13,14] Occasionally, minute keratotic spicules on the palmar surfaces or multiple pinpoint papules that extend to the dorsa of the extremities are observed (Fig. 50-2). Nail abnormalities usually manifest as longitudinal, beaded ridging, and terminal splitting with or without irregular pitting. Lesions of lichen planus may infrequently be present simultaneously.[17] Lichen nitidus is usually asymptomatic; however, pruritus is occasionally present and sometimes intense. There are no constitutional symptoms or systemic abnormalities associated with the disease.

PATHOLOGY

A dense mass of infiltrating lymphohistiocytic cells is situated immediately below the epidermis and results in widening of the papillary dermis with elongation and the appearance of embracement by neighboring rete ridges (Fig. 50-3). Occasionally, two or three papillary spaces merge together as part of the inflammatory infiltrate. The overlying epidermis is thinned and occasionally demonstrates central parakeratosis without hypergranulosis. This is a characteristic diagnostic finding, when observed. Minimal hydropic degeneration with few dyskeratotic cells is usually observed within the basal epidermal layer adjacent to the papillary dermal infiltrate. With the development of hydropic degeneration, basal cell disruption, and epidermal thinning, the epidermis may partially detach from the dermis. Colloid bodies are rarely seen in lichen nitidus, in contrast to their frequent occurrence in lichen planus. The dermal infiltrate is well circumscribed and composed

FIGURE 50-3

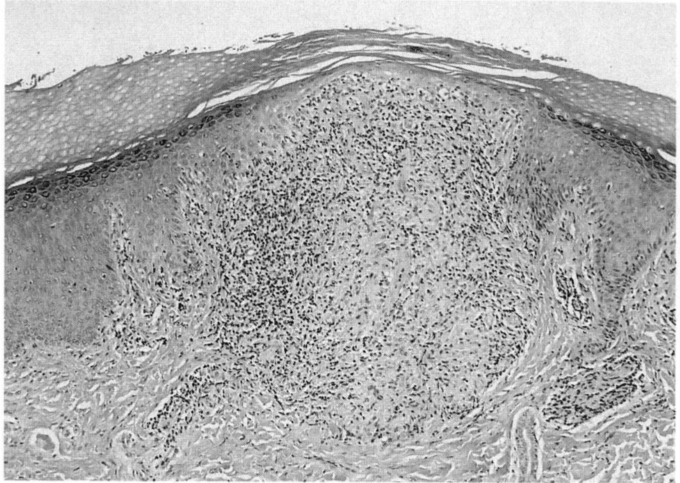

A.

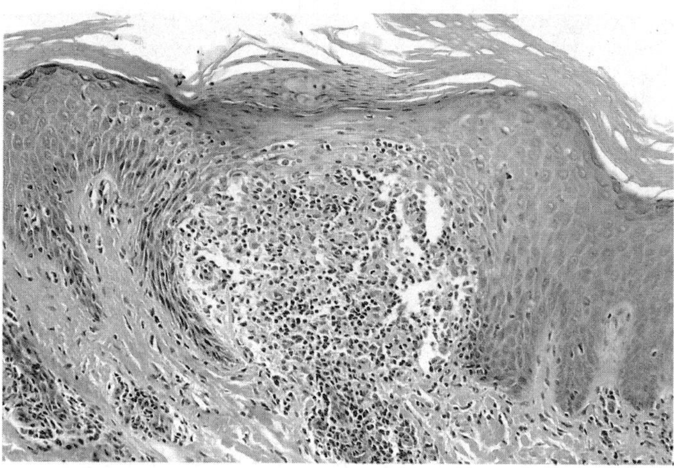

B.

Lichen nitidus. *A.* Distinctive, circumscribed infiltrate of papillary dermis situated directly beneath thinned epidermis. Many histiocytes mingle with lymphocytes that are enveloped by bordering rete ridges. [Hematoxylin and eosin (H & E)] *B.* Central parakeratosis, epidermal thinning, and loss of granular layer with focus of granuloma-appearing, inflammatory cells and reactive, finger-like extensions of epidermis. (H & E).

of closely associated histiocytes, lymphocytes, and occasional foreign body or Touton-type giant cells. Usually, no plasma cells or eosinophils are seen. In some cases, the majority of the cells in the infiltrate are histiocytic. Palmar lesions may show a deep parakeratotic plug. Transepithelial elimination of the inflammatory infiltrate has been described.[5] Purpuric or hemorrhagic lesions are associated with capillary wall degeneration and red blood cell extravasation.[11]

The majority of the cells in the infiltrate are T lymphocytes intermixed with few to many histiocyte–macrophages that stain with CD68, as well as epidermal Langerhans cells and indeterminate cells that express S-100 protein. CD4+ cells predominate over CD8+ T lymphocytes. Many cells in the infiltrate express human leukocyte antigen (HLA)-DR antigen, which implicates them as antigen-presenting cells.[5]

Direct immunofluorescence examination of lichen nitidus is usually negative for deposition of immunoglobulins at the dermal–epidermal junction, in contrast to the vast majority (95 percent) of cases of lichen planus.[18] Cytoids are also not usually observed in lichen nitidus. The results of ultrastructural studies coincide with light microscopic findings and also show activated lymphocyte morphology with convoluted nuclei, resembling Sézary cells.[19]

DIAGNOSIS AND DIFFERENTIAL DIAGNOSIS

The diagnosis of lichen nitidus is easily established based on the characteristic morphology, distribution, and usual lack of symptoms. The pathognomonic microscopic changes seen on skin biopsy will confirm the diagnosis in atypical cases.

The relationship between lichen nitidus and lichen planus has been debated for decades. Immunohistochemical studies show that the majority of cells in the infiltrate of lichen nitidus are T helper (CD4) lymphocytes. However, in contrast to lichen planus, histiocyte–macrophages predominate and form the characteristic granulomatous appearance in lichen nitidus. Fewer cells expressing the skin homing receptor HECA-452 (leukocyte common antigen, LCA) are seen.[4]

Confluent lesions may form plaques that resemble psoriasis, especially if located on the elbows or knees. The plaques, however, are usually brownish and lack the silvery scales seen in psoriasis. Verruca planus can be mistaken for lichen nitidus. However, flat warts are more variable in size, have a more verrucous surface on close examination with a magnifying lens, usually present with fewer lesions than are seen in lichen nitidus, and are less likely to involve multiple anatomic areas. Keratosis pilaris, lichen spinulosus, and papular eczema usually exhibit more keratotic or scaling lesions, unlike the smoother surfaced papules of lichen nitidus. Lichen scrofulosorum usually occurs in young patients with tuberculosis. The lesions are characterized by perifollicular, occasionally keratotic papules and are readily distinguishable from lichen nitidus. Lichenoid syphilitic lesions, bowenoid papulosis, sarcoidosis, and lichen amyloidosis should also be considered in the differential diagnosis.

Palmoplantar involvement of lichen nitidus may be difficult to differentiate from chronic hand eczema; however, the presence of classic lesions of lichen nitidus at other body sites helps to establish the diagnosis.

TREATMENT AND COURSE

Because the disease is asymptomatic and self-limiting, no intervention is required in most cases. Treatment of lichen nitidus is warranted when it is associated with protracted pruritus or when the appearance interferes with the patient's daily activities and outlook. Topical glucocorticoids may yield favorable results. A short course of oral glucocorticoids may also be helpful and hasten resolution of more extensive, generalized, or symptomatic disease. PUVA,[20] UVA/UVB phototherapy and oral glucocorticoids,[21] astemizole,[22] acitretin or etretinate,[14,17] low-dose cyclosporine,[23] and oral itraconazole[24] have also been used successfully when indicated for more problematic disease. One patient with amenorrhea and lichen nitidus responded favorably to estrogen-progesterone combination therapy.[25]

Lichen nitidus is typically a focal, asymptomatic, chronic inflammatory reaction that eventually resolves spontaneously after months to a year in two-thirds of patients or, less frequently, over a few years. Rarely, the eruption may persist indefinitely. New lesions may continue to develop as older lesions resolve. Lesions heal without scar formation or pigmentary abnormalities.

REFERENCES

1. Pinkus F: Verhand. *Berlin Dermat Gessel* **12**:3, 1901
2. Pinkus F: Uber eine neue knotchenformige Hauteruption: Lichen nitidus. *Arch Dermatol Syph* **85**:11, 1907
3. Hazen HH: Syphilis and skin diseases in the American Negro: Personal observations. *Arch Dermatol Syphilol* **31**:316, 1935
4. Smoller BR, Flynn TC: Immunohistochemical examination of lichen nitidus suggests that it is not a localized papular variant of lichen planus. *J Am Acad Dermatol* **27**:232, 1992
5. Wright AL et al: An immunophenotypic study of lichen nitidus. *Clin Exp Dermatol* **15**:273, 1990
6. Kano Y et al: Improvement of lichen nitidus after topical dinitrochlorobenzene application. *J Am Acad Dermatol* **39**:305, 1998
7. Maeda M: A case of generalized lichen nitidus with Koebner's phenomenon. *J Dermatol* **21**:273, 1994
8. Berger TG, Dhar A: Lichenoid photoeruptions in human immunodeficiency virus infection. *Arch Dermatol* **130**:609, 1994
9. Kato N: Familial lichen nitidus. *Clin Exp Dermatol* **20**:336, 1995
10. Jetton RL et al: Vesicular and hemorrhagic lichen nitidus. *Arch Dermatol* **105**:430, 1972
11. Endo M et al: Purpuric lichen nitidus. *Eur J Dermatol* **8**:54, 1998
12. Itami A et al: Perforating lichen nitidus. *Int J Dermatol* **33**:382, 1994
13. Munro CS et al: Lichen nitidus presenting as palmoplanter hyperkeratosis and nail dystrophy. *Clin Exp Dermatol* **18**:381, 1993
14. Lucker GP et al: Treatment of palmoplantar lichen nitidus with acitretin. *Br J Dermatol* **130**:791, 1994
15. Soroush V et al: Generalized lichen nitidus: Case report and literature review. *Cutis* **64**:135, 1999
16. Kanwar AJ, Kaur S: Lichen nitidus actinicus. *Arch Dermatol* **135**:714, 1999
17. Aram H: Association of lichen planus and lichen nitidus. Treatment with etretinate. *Int J Dermatol* **27**:117, 1988
18. Waisman M et al: Immunofluorescent studies in lichen nitidus. *Arch Dermatol* **107**:200, 1973
19. Clauson J et al: Lichen nitidus: Electron microscopic and immunofluorescence studies. *Acta Derm Venereol (Stockh)* **62**:15, 1982
20. Randle HW, Sander HM: Treatment of generalized lichen nitidus with PUVA. *Int J Dermatol* **25**:330, 1986
21. Chen W et al: Generalized lichen nitidus. *J Am Acad Dermatol* **36**:630, 1997
22. Ocampo J, Torne R: Generalized lichen nitidus: Report of two cases treated with astemizole. *Int J Dermatol* **28**:49, 1989
23. Lestringant GG et al: Coexistence of atopic dermatitis and lichen nitidus in three patients. *Dermatology* **192**:171, 1996
24. Libow LF, Coots NV: Treatment of lichen planus and lichen nitidus with itraconazole: Report of six cases. *Cutis* **62**:247, 1998
25. Taniguchi S et al: Recurrent generalized lichen nitidus associated with amenorrhea. *Acta Derm Venereol (Stockh)* **74**:224, 1994

CHAPTER 51

John J. DiGiovanna

Ichthyosiform Dermatoses

The disorders of cornification form a heterogeneous group of diseases characterized by abnormal differentiation (cornification) of the epidermis. The ichthyoses, a member of this group, are distinguished clinically by generalized scaling. The name *ichthyosis* is derived from the Greek *ichthys* meaning "fish," and refers to the similarity in appearance of the skin to fish scale. The ichthyoses themselves are a heterogeneous group of disorders, with both inherited and acquired forms. Early reports of ichthyosis in the Indian and Chinese literature date back to several hundred years B.C., and the condition was discussed by Willan in 1808.[1]

Ichthyosis can present at birth or develop later in life. It can occur as a disease limited to the skin or in association with abnormalities of other organ systems. There are a number of well-defined types of ichthyosis that have characteristic features and can be reliably diagnosed. However, because of the great clinical heterogeneity and the profound effect of the environment on scaling, in certain patients and families, a specific diagnosis can be challenging.

Van Scott, Frost, and Weinstein proposed a classification of the ichthyoses based on differences in rates of epidermal turnover, characterizing them as either disorders of epidermal hyperproliferation or disorders of prolonged retention of the stratum corneum.[2,3] Subsequently, Williams and Elias proposed a classification that lists the disorders of cornification in which clinical, genetic, or biochemical data suggest a distinct disease.[4] Recently, genetic approaches to understanding the inherited disorders of cornification have successfully deciphered the defects underlying several of these genodermatoses.[5-7] A new classification is evolving based on a series of discoveries of the underlying genetic and molecular bases of these disorders. Knowing which gene is mutated directs us to the underlying pathophysiologic process. A listing of the more common and the better understood hereditary ichthyoses according to pattern of inheritance and clinical features is shown in Table 51-1. Grouping these ichthyosiform disorders according to class of disorder (underlying abnormality) facilitates understanding of the clinical phenotypes in terms of underlying mechanism. However, further work is necessary to clearly understand how the gene mutations and resultant protein disruptions result in clinical disease, and, furthermore, how therapeutic interventions can be creatively developed.

CLINICAL PRESENTATION

A specific diagnosis in an individual or family with ichthyosis can help to predict prognosis and is important for genetic counseling. Several features are useful in distinguishing different forms of ichthyosis. These include the age of onset, quality of scale, presence/absence of erythroderma, abnormalities in other parts of the skin (e.g., ectropion,

TABLE 51-1

Features of Selected Ichthyosiform Dermatoses

Mode of Inheritance	Diagnosis	Onset	Characteristic Clinical Features	Associated Features	Etiology: Abnormal			Class of Disorder	Skin Histopathology
					Gene	Protein	Function		
Autosomal dominant	Ichthyosis vulgaris	Infancy/childhood	Fine or centrally tacked-down scale with superficial fissuring. Relative flexural sparing; worse on lower extremities. Hyperlinear palms/soles	Keratosis pilaris; atopy	Unkown	Decrease or absence of filaggrin, or its precursor profilaggrin	Unknown	Unknown	Hyperkeratosis; may have decreased or absent granular layer
Autosomal dominant	Epidermolytic hyperkeratosis (bullous congenital ichthyosiform erythroderma)	Birth	Heterogeneous. May have verrucous, firm, hyperkeratotic (hystrix) spines, often linearly arrayed in flexural creases; blisters; may have erythroderma and/or palmar/plantar keratoderma	Frequent skin infections; characteristic pungent odor	*KRT1, KRT10;* in Vörner type (confined to palms/soles) *KRT 9*	Keratin 1 or 10; in Vörner type, keratin 9	Structural protein abnormality leading to keratin intermediate filament dysfunction–epidermal fragility	Keratin abnormality	Hyperkeratosis; vacuolated degeneration of the epidermal granular (and often deeper) layer; large, irregular keratohyalin granules
Autosomal dominant	Ichthyosis bullosa of Siemens	Birth	Redness and blistering at birth. Later develop hyperkeratosis, accentuated over flexures. Molting: collarette-like lesion where uppermost epidermis has been lost		*KRT2e*	Keratin 2e, which is expressed in superficial epidermis	Structural protein abnormality leading to keratin intermediate filament dysfunction–superficial epidermal fragility	Keratin abnormality	Hyperkeratosis and epidermal vacuolization, similar to epidermolytic hyperkeratosis but confined to the granular layer
Autosomal dominant	Ichthyosis hystrix of Curth and Macklin	Birth	Resembles EHK, varies from palmar/plantar keratoderma to generalized. Thick "porcupine-like" spines. No blistering		*KRT1*—mutation in variable region	Keratin 1	As above for keratin 1	Keratin abnormality	Upper epidermal keratincytes have perinuclear vacuoliza-tion/perinuclear shells of tonofilaments

(*continued*)

TABLE 51-1 (*Continued*)

Mode of Inheritance	Diagnosis	Onset	Characteristic Clinical Features	Associated Features	Etiology: Abnormal Gene	Etiology: Abnormal Protein	Etiology: Abnormal Function	Class of Disorder	Skin Histopathology
Autosomal dominant	Erythrokeratodermia variabilis—generalized type	Birth	Generalized hyperkeratosis and figurate, migratory red patches	Red patches move over min to hours, may be triggered by changes in temperature	*GJB3* or *GJB4*	Connexin 31 or 30.3; connexins form gap junction channels between cells	Abnormal intercellular communication	Connexin abnormality	Hyperkeratosis, acanthosis, papillomatosis, capillary dilitation; epidermis may have "church spire" appearance
	Erythrokeratodermia variabilis—localized type	Variable	Localized hyperkeratotic plaques with figurate, migratory red patches	Hyperkeratotic plaques may be induced by trauma. Considerable intrafamilial variability					
Autosomal dominant/ (recessive has been reported)	Keratitis-Ichthyosis-Deafness (KID) Syndrome	Birth/infancy	Progressive corneal opacification; either mild generalized hyperkeratosis or discrete erythematous plaques, which may be symmetric; neurosensory deafness	Follicular hyperkeratosis, scarring alopecia, dystrophic nails, susceptibility to infection	*GJB2*	Connexin 26; connexins form gap junction channels between cells	Abnormal intercellular communication	Connexin abnormality	Nonspecific
X-linked recessive	X-linked ichthyosis	Birth/infancy	Fine to large scales; comma-shaped corneal opacities on posterior capsule; increased migration of β-lipoproteins on electrophoresis	Cryptorchidism; female carriers may have corneal opacities and delay of onset or progression of labor in affected pregnancies	*STS*	Steroid sulfatase	Abnormal cholesterol metabolism with accumulation of cholesterol sulfate	Lipid metabolism enzyme abnormality	Hyperkeratosis, may have hypergranulosis; nonspecific
X-linked recessive	Chondrodysplasia punctata X-linked (CDPX)	Birth	May begin as erythroderma, linear or whorled atrophic or hyperkeratosis, alopecia, skeletal abnormalities, short stature	Cataracts, deafness	*ARSE*	Arylsufatase E	Ill defined: failure of hydrolylsis of sulfate ester bonds	Lipid metabolism enzyme abnormality	

(*continued*)

TABLE 51-1 (*Continued*)

Features of Selected Ichthyosiform Dermatoses

Mode of Inheritance	Diagnosis	Onset	Characteristic Clinical Features	Associated Features	Etiology: Abnormal Gene	Etiology: Abnormal Protein	Etiology: Abnormal Function	Class of Disorder	Skin Histopathology
X-linked dominant	X-linked dominant chondrodysplasia punctata (Conradi-Hünermann-Happle syndrome) (CDPX2)	Birth	CIE at birth, clears and is replaced by linear hyperkeratosis, follicular atrophoderma and pigmentary abnormalities, stippled calcifications on radiographs	Occurs almost exclusively in females; hair shaft abnormalities, short stature, cataracts	Gene encoding emopamil binding protein (EBP)	EBP—also known as β-hydroxy-steroid-$\Delta^{8,7}$-isomerase	Abnormal cholesterol biosynthesis	Lipid metabolism enzyme abnormality	
Autosomal recessive	Lamellar ichthyosis (LI)	Birth; often collodion presentation	Large, plate-like, brown scale over most of the body; accentuated on lower extremities. Ectropion; alopecia	Heat intolerance	*TGM1;* other genetic loci mapped to 2q33-35 and 19p12-q12	Transglutaminase	Failure to properly cross-link proteins and attach ceramides in formation of stratum corneum	Enzyme abnormality	Hyperkeratosis, acanthosis. Nonspecific
Autosomal recessive	Congenital ichthyosiform erythroderma (CIE)	Birth; often collodion presentation	Fine, white scale; generalized erythroderma	Heat intolerance	*TGM1* in few; mapped to 3p21 and 17p13.2-13.1	Transglutaminase in few	As above	Unknown	Hyperkeratosis, acanthosis, may show parakeratosis. Nonspecific
Autosomal recessive	LI/CIE overlap	Usually birth; often collodion presentation	Heterogenous: scale may be fine to large with various extent of erythroderma	Heat intolerance	Unknown			Unknown	Nonspecific
Autosomal recessive	Netherton's syndrome	Birth; may have collodion presentation	Ichthyosis linearis circumflexa or similar to congenital ichthyosiform erythroderma; trichorrhexis invaginata	Atopy; high serum levels of IgE; may have aminoaciduria	*SPINK5*	LEKTI (a serine protease inhibitor)	Unclear	Protease inhibitor abnormality	Nonspecific
Autosomal recessive	Refsum's disease	Ichthyosis develops in adulthood	Progressive neurologic dysfunction; skeletal, cardiac and renal abnormalities	Retinitis pigmentosa	Most *PAHX; PEX7* also reported	Phytanoyl-CoA hydroxylase (PhyH)	Deficiency of phytanic acid catabolism; results in phytanic acid accumulation	Peroxisomal enzyme abnormality	Lipid-containing vacuoles in basal kertinocytes
Autosomal recessive	Rhizomelic chondrodysplasia punctata (RCDP)		Dwarfism, stippled cartilage calcifications, joint contractures, cataracts, ichthyosis, mental retardation	Low levels red cell plasmalogens; accumulation of phytanic acid	*PEX7*	Peroxin 7	Failure of receptor targeting enzymes to peroxisomes	Peroxisomal biogenesis disorder	

(*continued*)

TABLE 51-1 (*Continued*)

Mode of Inheritance	Diagnosis	Onset	Characteristic Clinical Features	Associated Features	Etiology: Abnormal Gene	Etiology: Abnormal Protein	Etiology: Abnormal Function	Class of Disorder	Skin Histopathology
Autosomal recessive	Sjögren-Larsson syndrome	Ichthyosis apparent at birth	Generalized coarse hyperkeratosis; spastic diplegia; mental retardation; retinal glistening white dots	Short stature, seizures	*FALDH*	Fatty aldehyde dehydrogenase	Fatty aldehyde catabolism	Lipid metabolism enzyme abnormality	Nonspecific
Heterogenous	CHILD syndrome	Birth	Congenital hemidysplasia, ichthyosiform erythroderma, limb defects	Almost exclusively in females	Gene encoding NAD(P)H steroid dehydrogenase-like protein *(NSDHL)*; gene encoding EBP reported	NSDHL (3 β-hydroxysteroid dehydrogenase); EBP reported	Cholesterol biosynthesis	Lipid metabolism enzyme abnormality	
Autosomal recessive	Chanarin-Dorfman syndrome (neutral lipid storage disease)	Birth; may be collodion	Generalized scaling, resembles CIE; variable extracutaneous involvement: cataracts, decreased hearing, psychomotor delay	Neurologic abnormalities	*CGI-58*	Unknown	Unknown	Lipid metabolism enzyme abnormality	Lipid droplets in dermal and epidermal cells and acrosyringia of eccrine ducts
Autosomal recessive	*IBIDS* (trichothiodystrophy, Tay's syndrome)	Ichthyosis apparent at birth, may have collodion presentation	*I*chthyosis, *B*rittle hair, *I*ntellectual impairment, *D*ecreased fertility, Short stature	Hypogonadism; abnormally low sulfur content of hair, hair shaft abnormalities	Unknown	Unknown	Unknown	Unknown	Nonspecific
	PIBI(D)S	Ichthyosis mild and not congential	Similar to IBIDS but with photosensitivity and usually without hypogonadism	Abnormally low sulfur content of hair, hair shaft abnormalities	*ERCC2/XPD* or *ERCC3/XPB*	Helicase components of transcription factor TFIIH	Deficiency in repair of UV induced DNA damage	DNA repair enzyme abnormality	Nonspecific

eclabium) and adnexal structures (e.g., alopecia, hair follicle or shaft abnormality), and involvement of other organ systems. A family pedigree may clarify the pattern of inheritance. However, many autosomal dominant diseases [e.g., *epidermolytic hyperkeratosis (EHK)*] have a high frequency of spontaneous mutation, and the lack of a positive family history does not rule out autosomal dominant inheritance. Alternatively, the presence of parental consanguinity may suggest autosomal recessive inheritance. Light-microscopic features are usually diagnostic in EHK and can be helpful in selected ichthyoses (e.g., Refsum's disease, neutral lipid storage disease, acquired ichthyosis of sarcoidosis), but histopathologic examination may not be useful to distinguish other ichthyoses. The development of ichthyosis in adulthood may be a marker of systemic disease. Acquired ichthyosis is usually mild, resembling ichthyosis vulgaris, and has been associated with malignancy, some medications, AIDS, and sarcoidosis.

ETIOLOGY AND PATHOGENESIS

The fully differentiated end product of the epidermis is the stratum corneum, which is composed of corneocytes ("bricks") surrounded by an intercellular matrix ("mortar"). The corneocyte bricks are protein-enriched, and the intercellular mortar is composed of hydrophobic, lipid-enriched membrane bilayers.[4] The keratin-laden corneocytes are thought to be responsible for the resilience and water retention properties of the stratum corneum, while the matrix is the barrier to water loss. The normal stratum corneum undergoes desquamation in an organized and invisible manner, with individual corneocytes separating from each other and shedding as single cells. Ichthyotic skin has an abnormal quality and quantity of scale, the barrier function of the stratum corneum is compromised, and there may be alterations in the kinetics of epidermal cell proliferation. The stratum corneum can be viewed as a compartment, with thickening of the stratum corneum being the result of cells entering the compartment at an increased rate or leaving (corneocyte disadhesion) too slowly or both.

The process of cornification is complex and not completely understood. Defects in many different aspects and steps of this process can lead to a similar end result: abnormal stratum corneum, scale, and hyperkeratosis. In some of these disorders, the underlying abnormality has been identified. For example, mutations in the genes that encode the epidermal differentiation keratins, keratins 1 and 10, cause EHK.[5] Mutations in the gene encoding transglutaminase-1, an enzyme that catalyzes the cross-linking of proteins and attachment of ceramides during the formation of corneocytes, cause lamellar ichthyosis.[8–11] The observation that key components of this process cause disorders of cornification highlights the importance and complexity of orderly cornification in normal keratinocyte differentiation.

Steroid sulfatase controls the hydrolysis of cholesterol sulfate in corneocytes and is thought to be important in the regulation of corneocyte desquamation. Deficiency of steroid sulfatase causes X-linked ichthyosis.[12,13] The observation that several drugs that lower serum cholesterol (e.g., nicotinic acid, triparanol) can induce ichthyotic skin changes indicates the importance of lipid homeostasis in normal cornification.[14] Further evidence is the identification of mutations in the genes encoding cholesterol biosynthetic enzymes as a cause of X-linked dominant chondrodysplasia punctata and CHILD (congenital hemidysplasia with ichthyosiform erythroderma and limb defects) syndrome. The recent identification of mutations in SPINK5 (*s*erine *p*rotease *in*hibitor, *K*azal type 5), encoding a serine protease inhibitor, confirms a role for protease inhibitors in normal differentiation. The discoveries of connexin abnormalities as causes for erythrokeratodermia variabilis, KID (keratitis, ichthyosis, and deafness) syndrome, and other disorders involving ectodermal tissues highlight the role of intercellular communication for properly functioning skin.[7] These examples demonstrate the complexity of the process of forming a normally functioning stratum corneum and demonstrate that diverse abnormalities can result in similar clinical phenotypes of hyperkeratosis and scaling. Furthermore, our evolving understanding of these mechanisms continues to clarify the multisystem, clinical phenotypes observed in several ichthyosiform disorders.

ICHTHYOSIS VULGARIS

Ichthyosis vulgaris, the most common ichthyosis, is relatively mild. The disease is inherited in an autosomal dominant pattern, and its incidence may be as common as 1 in 250.[15] While infants usually have normal skin, the disease often manifests within the first year.

The scale of ichthyosis vulgaris is usually most prominent on the extensor surfaces of the extremities with flexural sparing (Fig. 51-1). The diaper area tends to be spared. There may be fine, white scale over large areas. Particularly on the lower extremities, which are often the most severely involved area, the scale may be centrally attached, with "cracking" (superficial fissuring through the stratum corneum) at the edges. This turning up at the edges can lead to the skin feeling rough.

A number of other findings are commonly observed in association with ichthyosis vulgaris.[16] Hyperlinear palms are usually present, and some patients may have thickening approaching a keratoderma. Keratosis pilaris is common, even in individuals with mild ichthyosis vulgaris, and usually involves the posterior arms, thighs, and buttocks. Atopy is also frequently observed and can manifest as hay fever, eczema, or asthma. These findings can confound an accurate diagnosis, because hyperlinear palms and keratosis pilaris may be seen in atopic individuals who do not have ichthyosis vulgaris. Rarely, individuals with ichthyosis vulgaris may have hypohidrosis with heat intolerance. There is great variation in the severity of clinical manifestations between affected individuals in the same family (expressivity). The condition usually worsens in climates that are dry and cold and improves in warm, humid environments, where the disease may clear dramatically. By clinical examination, it can sometimes be difficult to distinguish individuals with mild ichthyosis vulgaris from those with simple dry skin (xerosis), because the spectrum of both conditions appears to overlap. In addition, on the basis of skin findings alone, males with severe ichthyosis vulgaris may be difficult to differentiate from those affected with X-linked ichthyosis.[16,17] The histopathologic findings (Fig. 51-2*A*) may be distinctive in specimens taken from areas with the most prominent scaling, showing mild hyperkeratosis and diminished or absent granular layer. Even when the granular layer is present on light microscopy, examination by electron microscopy can show keratohyalin granules that are small, abnormally shaped, and crumbly in appearance.[18] Filaggrin is an epidermal protein, localized to keratohyalin granules, that is thought to be important in the aggregation of keratin intermediate filaments. These filaments form a network, or cell matrix, that gives structural integrity to the epidermal keratinocytes. Biochemical studies of epidermis from patients with ichthyosis vulgaris have shown absence of or decrease in filaggrin and its precursor, profilaggrin. The defective profilaggrin expression may be due to impaired posttranscriptional control.[19]

X-LINKED ICHTHYOSIS

In the 1960s, recessive X-linked ichthyosis was distinguished clinically from other ichthyoses.[15] Shortly thereafter, the syndrome of placental steroid sulfatase deficiency was described in pregnancies with failure to initiate labor as a condition with low maternal urinary estrogens. Because the majority of maternal urinary estrogens are derived from the fetal adrenal and are metabolized by the placenta, low levels can reflect fetal abnormalities or death. However, in this condition, low levels do not indicate severe fetal morbidity. The association between failure to initiate or progress labor and ichthyosis in the male offspring was not appreciated until later.[12,13] Steroid sulfatase hydrolyzes sulfate esters, which include cholesterol sulfate and sulfated steroid hormones.[20] Sulfated fetal adrenal hormones undergo desulfation to estrogens, which are excreted in maternal urine. The absence of steroid sulfatase enzyme in the fetal placenta leads to low maternal urinary estrogens and in some pregnancies, to a failure of labor to initiate or to progress normally. In males with recessive X-linked ichthyosis, steroid sulfatase enzyme activity is decreased or absent in many tissues, including epidermis, stratum corneum, and leukocytes, and in cultured fibroblasts.[21] In addition, cholesterol sulfate, an enzyme substrate, accumulates in the scale. Carrier females have been found to have leukocyte steroid sulfatase levels intermediate between those observed in normal individuals and those in affected males.

FIGURE 51-1

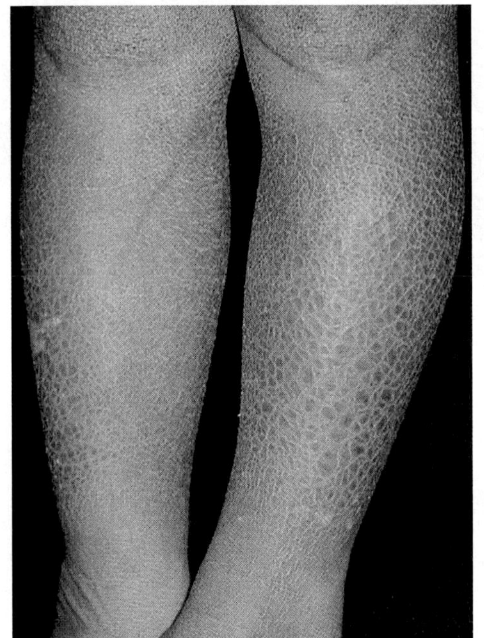

A.

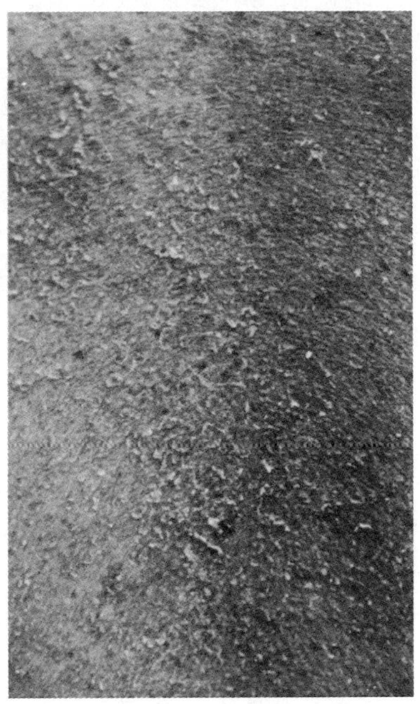

B.

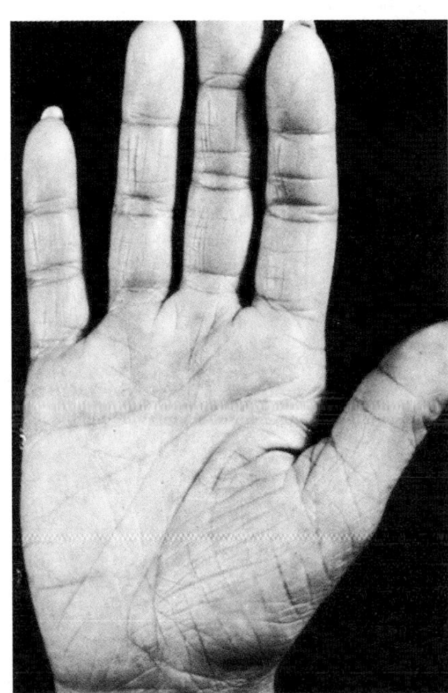

C.

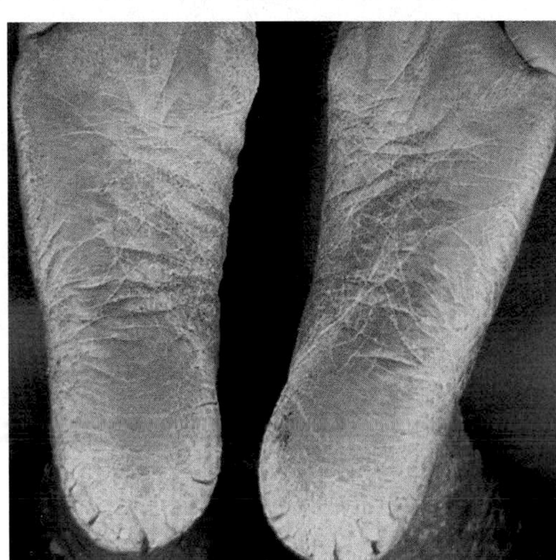

D.

Ichthyosis vulgaris. *A*. Mosaic-like scales are present on the legs. *B*. Back of woman showing fine scales with "pasted-on" appearance. *C*. Palm of 19-year-old girl showing accentuation of palmar markings. *D*. Soles showing marked thickening with splitting of heels.

Recessive X-linked ichthyosis occurs in approximately 1 in 2000 to 6000 males.[15,22] Scaling may begin in the newborn period and is usually most prominent on the extensor surfaces, although there is significant involvement of the flexural areas. While the extent and degree of scaling are variable, X-linked ichthyosis can usually be distinguished from ichthyosis vulgaris on clinical criteria.[15] The latter tends to be associated with hyperlinear palms and soles, keratosis pilaris, and a family history of atopy. X-linked ichthyosis tends to have more severe involvement with larger scale, and comma-shaped, corneal opacities may be present in half of adult patients[23,24] (Fig. 51-3). Corneal opacities do not affect vision and may be present in female carriers.[24] Affected males have an increased risk of cryptorchidism, and independently, they are at increased risk for the development of testicular cancer.[25] Cholesterol sulfate levels are elevated in the serum, epidermis, and scale,[26] and there is increased mobility of β-lipoproteins (low-density lipoproteins) on electrophoresis, a feature that can indicate the diagnosis. Confirmation of the diagnosis is usually made by finding an elevation in serum cholesterol sulfate levels (normal is 80 to 200 μg/dL; X-linked ichthyosis is 2000 to 9000 μg/dL). Steroid sulfatase is one of a group of arylsulfatases located on chromosome Xp22. More than 80 percent of the mutations in X-linked ichthyosis are deletions, explaining the failure to find immunologically detectable enzyme protein in some patients. Deletions that include adjacent sulfatases explain the overlap syndromes involving chondrodysplasia punctata and X-linked ichthyosis.[27]

FIGURE 51-2

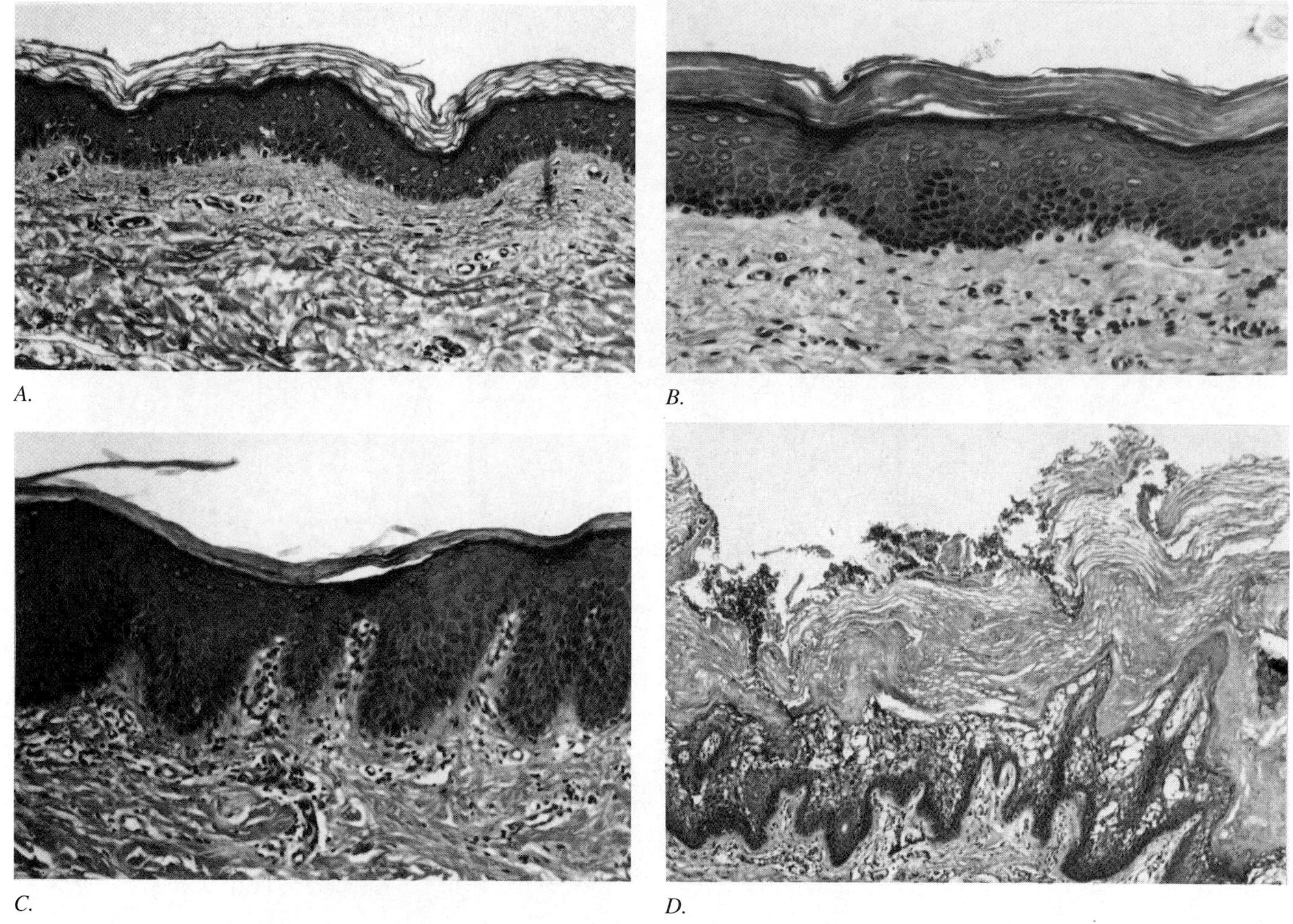

Histopathology. *A.* Ichthyosis vulgaris. Note diminished granular layer. *B.* Lamellar ichthyosis. Thickened stratum corneum composed of compact hyperkeratosis. *C.* Congenital ichthyosiform erythroderma. Hyperkeratosis and acanthosis. *D.* Epidermolytic hyperkeratosis. The stratum corneum is thickened (hyperkeratosis) and there is prominent vacuolar degeneration of suprabasalar epidermis most marked at the granular layer.

In the epidermis, steroid sulfatase catalyzes the hydrolysis of cholesterol sulfate. The identification of steroid sulfatase deficiency in X-linked ichthyosis supports the importance of cholesterol sulfate hydrolysis in normal desquamation. Topical application of cholesterol sulfate in mice can induce a scaling disorder, further supporting the role of cholesterol sulfate hydrolysis in corneocyte disadhesion.

A family was described with an ichthyosis inherited in an X-linked pattern but with normal steroid sulfatase activity and the absence of corneal opacities.[28] This demonstrates heterogeneity within X-linked ichthyosis. Because of its frequent occurrence, steroid sulfatase deficiency accounts for most cases of X-linked ichthyosis, but a normal steroid sulfatase level in a male with ichthyosis does not rule out an X-linked pattern of inheritance.

AUTOSOMAL RECESSIVE ICHTHYOSIS

Congenital ichthyosis can occur alone or as part of a syndrome where it is one component of multiple system abnormalities. When it occurs alone, the term *congenital autosomal recessive ichthyosis* is useful to describe the heterogeneous group of disorders that present at birth with generalized involvement of the skin and lack of manifestations in other organ systems. Autosomal recessive ichthyosis is rare and has been estimated to occur in about 1 in 300,000 persons.[15]

In older literature, nonbullous congenital ichthyosiform erythroderma [*lamellar ichthyosis (LI)*, with autosomal recessive inheritance] was distinguished from bullous congenital ichthyosiform erythroderma (EHK, with autosomal dominant inheritance) based on clinical appearance (bullae) and pattern of inheritance.[2,29] That the term *lamellar ichthyosis* was used interchangeably with *nonbullous congenital ichthyosiform erythroderma* and included a spectrum of phenotypes has led to some confusion. Williams and Elias distinguished LI from nonbullous congenital ichthyosiform erythroderma [usually called *congenital ichthyosiform erythroderma (CIE)*], a milder erythrodermic form.[30] Some patients with LI can be clearly distinguished from those with CIE on the basis of clinical features. LI has large, dark, platelike scale, and while infants may be red at birth, adults have little to no erythroderma (Fig. 51-4). In the more severe, classic presentation of LI, tautness of the facial skin leads to traction on the eyelids and lips, leading to ectropion and eclabium. Scarring alopecia, most prominent at the periphery of the scalp, may be partly due to traction at the hair line. In contrast, CIE has generalized redness and fine, white scale (Fig. 51-5). Patients with classic CIE have little to no ectropion, eclabium, or alopecia. However, many patients do not fit neatly into these two clinical descriptions,[31] in that they have features of both LI and CIE and a clinical phenotype intermediate between both disorders. Therefore,

FIGURE 51-3

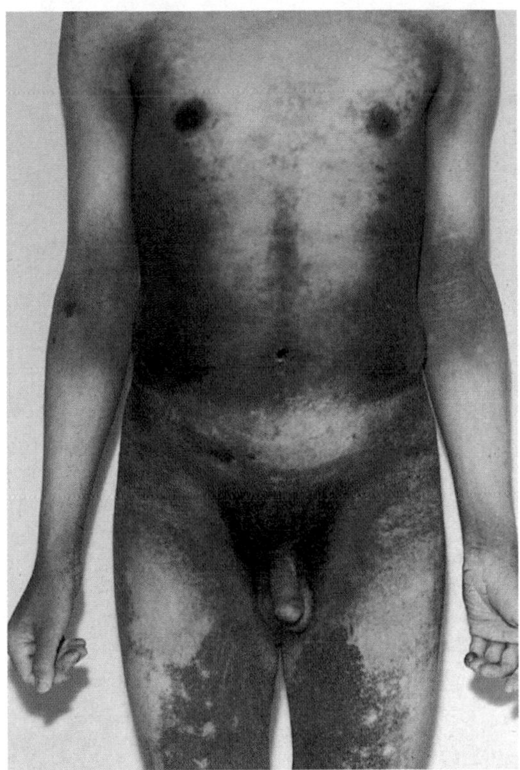

A.

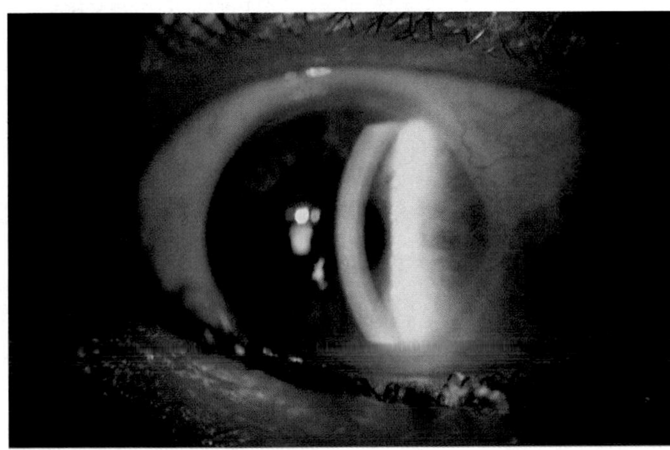

B.

X-linked ichthyosis. *A*. The scales are large and dark and most evident on the flexural areas in this patient. *B*. The blue arc is a cross-section of the cornea as seen by slit-lamp examination. The opacities appear white.

it can be useful to consider these two distinctive presentations as ends of a spectrum, between which lie a gradation of clinical phenotypes with variable degrees of erythema and coarseness of scale. Individual features such as collodion membrane (discussed below), ectropion, and alopecia can occur across the spectrum. The collodion presentation may, over time, evolve into a disease that falls anywhere within the clinical spectrum of severity and can develop into LI, CIE, or have minimal involvement (self-healing collodion baby).[32] So far, attempts to refine the categorization of these disorders by using biochemical and ultrastructural observations have failed to yield a consistent and replicable classification scheme.[33] Identification of the spectrum of specific molecular defects underlying these conditions will undoubtedly help in developing an accurate classification of the disorders.

Most patients with LI or CIE inherit the disease in an autosomal recessive pattern. Rarely, families have been described with similar phenotypes, where the disease is inherited as an autosomal dominant trait.[33] This is an important consideration for genetic counseling.

LAMELLAR ICHTHYOSIS

LI is apparent at birth, and the newborn usually presents encased in a collodion membrane, a translucent covering that desquamates over the subsequent 10 to 14 days (Fig. 51-6). At this time the skin may be red. Over time, the skin develops with large, platelike scales, which appear to be arranged in a mosaic pattern (see Fig. 51-4). In some areas, the scales are centrally attached with raised borders. The scales tend to be largest over the lower extremities where the large, platelike scale separated by superficial cracking can lead to an appearance similar to that of a dry riverbed. During childhood and into adulthood, the degree of erythema may vary, but the severe presentation of classic LI usually has minimal to no erythroderma. Involvement of the palms and soles in LI is variable and ranges from minimal hyperlinearity to severe keratoderma.

The lips and mucous membranes tend to be spared in LI, but the adnexal structures may be compromised by the adherent, firm scale. Thick stratum corneum on the scalp tends to encase hairs and, in conjunction with the tautness of the skin, usually leads to a scarring alopecia, which is most marked at the periphery. The hyperkeratosis can interfere with normal sweat gland function, resulting in hypohidrosis, but the degree of impairment varies between patients. Some patients have severe heat intolerance and must be vigilant to avoid overheating. Treatment with oral retinoids can improve or prevent some sequelae of LI. Patients frequently notice an increase in sweating with improved heat tolerance. While retinoid therapy can cause blepharitis or even conjunctivitis, it is usually well tolerated by patients with LI. Moreover, the ability of systemic retinoid therapy to decrease thick periocular scale can decrease the tendency to develop ectropion. Nevertheless, patients with severe, classic LI usually require careful eye maintenance. Because of the ectropion (see Fig. 51-4), the lids may fail to close fully, particularly during sleep; hydration with liquid tears during the day and ophthalmic lubricants at night can prevent exposure keratitis.

Histopathologic examination typically shows orthokeratotic hyperkeratosis with mild to moderate acanthosis (see Fig. 51-2*C*). Rates of epidermal proliferation are normal or only slightly elevated in patients with LI, in contrast to those with CIE, which has significantly greater labeling indices.

In 1994, genetic linkage studies were performed on a group of families affected with the severe phenotype of classic LI (large, platelike scale; ectropion; and minimal to no erythema). The group included families from the United States and from an inbred Egyptian population. This study found classic LI to be linked to markers on chromosome 14 in the region of the transglutaminase 1 gene locus.[8] The transglutaminases catalyze calcium-dependent cross-linking of proteins through the formation of ε-(γ-glutamyl)lysine isodipeptide bonds. During the formation of the stratum corneum, transglutaminase catalyzes the cross-linking of cellular proteins, mostly involucrin, loricrin, and small proline-rich proteins. The resulting protein complex is deposited on the inner side of the plasma membrane to form the cornified envelope. Transglutaminase also attaches ceramides to cornified envelope proteins, notably involucrin, and thereby is important in the formation of both the protein and lipid components of the stratum corneum.[11]

Subsequently, mutations in *TGM1*, the gene encoding transglutaminase 1, were found in several families with LI, solidifying the role

distinguishable from both classic LI and CIE.[36] An erythrodermic form of autosomal recessive ichthyosis has been linked to chromosome 3.[35]

FIGURE 51-4

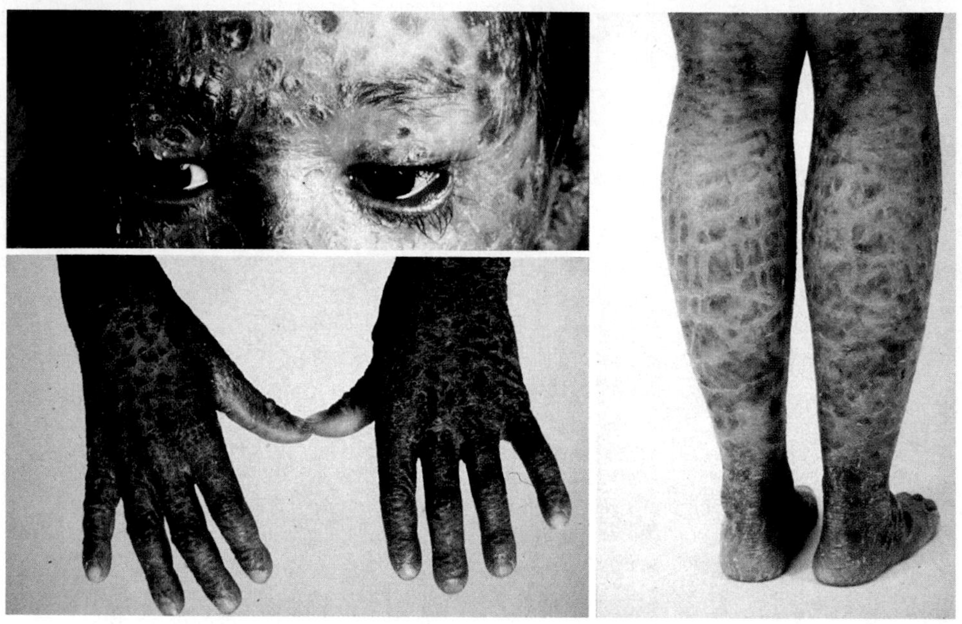

Classic lamellar ichthyosis phenotype. (*Top left*) Ectropion. (*Bottom left, right*) Large, brown, platelike scale. (*From Russell et al.*[8]*, with permission.*)

CONGENITAL ICHTHYOSIFORM ERYTHRODERMA

As with LI, CIE is apparent at birth, and the newborn usually presents with a taut, shiny, collodion membrane (see Fig. 51-6). After shedding of the membrane, the skin of infants with CIE remains red, usually with a fine, white, generalized scale (see Fig. 51-5). On the lower legs, the scale may be larger and darker. The classic presentation of CIE has little to no ectropion, eclabium, or alopecia in contrast to LI. As in LI, there is a wide variation in the ability to sweat, and patients with CIE may have minimal sweating with severe heat intolerance. Mucous membranes are usually spared. Palm/sole involvement is variable. Nails may have ridging, but they are often spared. Dermatophyte infection of the skin and nails is common.

Histopathologic examination shows hyperkeratosis, acanthosis, and often parakeratosis. Studies of epidermal proliferation have shown markedly increased epidermal cell turnover, in contrast to LI. A small subset of patients with CIE have been found to have mutations in *TGM1*, and two siblings with a collodion presentation, CIE, and palmoplantar keratoderma had a mutation in the cornified envelope protein loricrin.[37] In addition, two other genetic loci (3p21 and 17p13.2-13.1) have been found to be associated with CIE.

for transglutaminase 1 in the formation of a normal stratum corneum and its role as a cause of LI.[9,10] In a human skin/immunodeficient mouse xenograph model, transfer of a transglutaminase-1 gene into transglutaminase-1–deficient keratinocytes from LI patients resulted in normalization of transglutaminase expression and epidermal architecture in addition to restoration of cutaneous barrier function.[34] Additional disease-causing loci have been found; however, the responsible genes have not been identified.[35] Further genetic heterogeneity within congenital autosomal recessive ichthyosis was demonstrated with exclusion of *TGM1* as the disease-causing gene in two families with a phenotype of mild redness and fine scale and whose condition was clinically

FIGURE 51-5

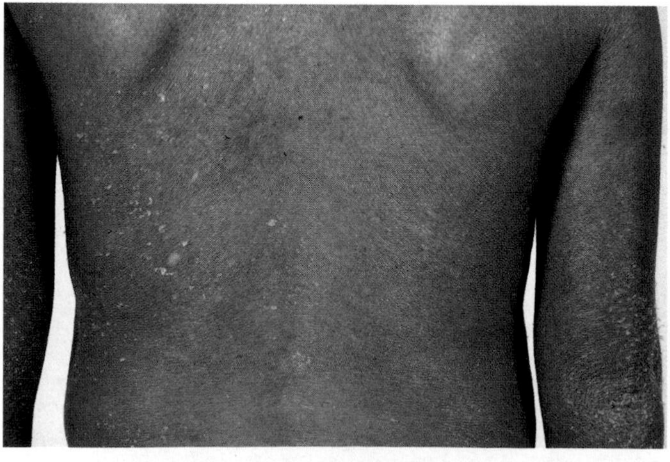

Congenital ichthyosiform erythroderma. Bright, red erythroderma with fine, white scale.

EPIDERMOLYTIC HYPERKERATOSIS

In 1902, Brocq described bullous ichthyotic erythroderma and distinguished the blistering type from the nonblistering type of congenital ichthyotic erythroderma.[38] The original description included three unrelated patients whose clinical manifestations varied. However, this was probably the first description of EHK. Today, the disease is named for the distinctive histopathologic features of vacuolar degeneration of the epidermis (i.e., epidermal lysis) and associated hyperkeratosis. EHK is also known as *bullous congenital ichthyosiform erythroderma,* an earlier descriptive name signifying the blistering, neonatal presentation, scaling, and redness.

EHK is transmitted as an autosomal dominant trait with a prevalence of approximately 1 in 200,000 to 300,000 persons. However, there is a high frequency of spontaneous mutation, and as many as one-half the cases have no family history and represent new mutational events.[29] The disease usually presents at birth with blistering, redness, and peeling (Fig. 51-7). With time, generalized hyperkeratosis may develop, which may or may not be associated with erythroderma. EHK skin usually has a characteristic pungent odor.

In contrast to most other ichthyoses, the histopathologic picture of EHK is distinctive. There are a tremendously thickened stratum corneum and vacuolar degeneration of the upper epidermis, leading to the histologic term *epidermolytic hyperkeratosis* (see Fig. 52-2*D*). The vacuolar degeneration usually involves the upper epidermis and occasionally all of the suprabasilar keratinocytes. Granular cells exhibit dense, enlarged, irregularly shaped masses that appear to be keratohyalin granules.[2] On electron-microscopic examination, clumping of filaments is observed to begin in the first suprabasal layer. These aggregated filaments are clumps of keratin intermediate filaments that contain the terminal differentiation-specific keratins 1 and 10.

There is striking clinical heterogeneity between EHK families. In a study of 52 patients with histologically confirmed EHK from 21 families, the specific clinical features and heterogeneity of this disorder were characterized.[38] Within this group, six clinical phenotypes (Table 51-2) were distinguished (Fig. 51-8). A useful differentiating characteristic was presence versus absence of severe palmar/plantar hyperkeratosis. Three subgroups had *palm/sole (PS types)* hyperkeratosis, while the other three subgroups had *no palm/sole (NPS types)* hyperkeratosis. The subtypes were further distinguished by the presence or absence of erythroderma, quality of scale, extent of involvement, presence of digital contractures, and gait abnormality.

Sporadic EHK due to a postzygotic, spontaneous mutation during embryogenesis can present in a mosaic pattern of skin involvement. Areas of hyperkeratosis alternating with normal skin are often distributed in streaks along Blaschko's lines (Fig. 51-9*A*). These may be limited to a few streaks, or there may be many, with widespread, patchy involvement. Unilateral localization can also occur. This clinical mosaic pattern correlates with underlying genetic mosaicism in that keratin mutations characteristic of EHK, which were found in lesional skin, were absent in normal skin.[39,40] If the germ line is involved, individuals with mosaic EHK can transmit the mutation, which leads to generalized EHK in affected offspring (Fig. 51-9*B*).[40]

FIGURE 51-6

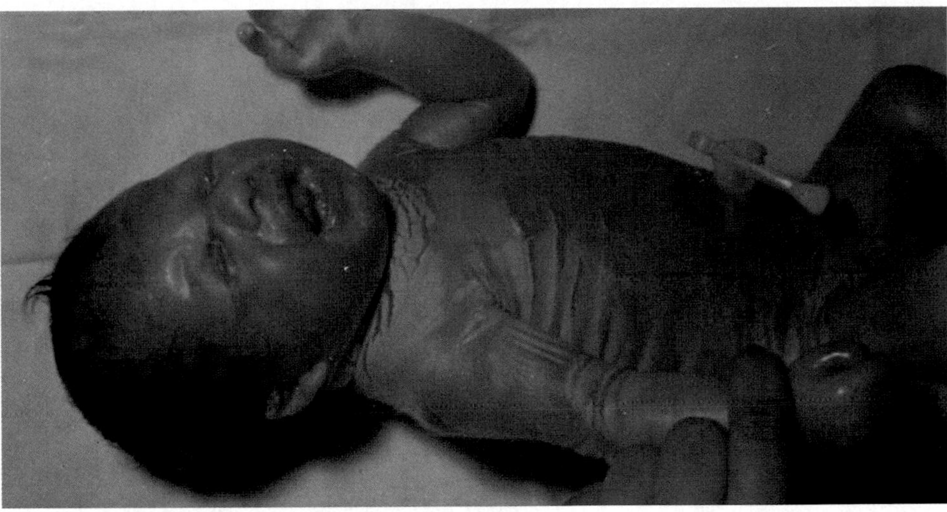

Collodion baby. The infant is 36 h old and is covered with a membrane that shows fissures; note ectropion and eclabium. The condition may develop over time into various clinical phenotypes including lamellar ichthyosis, congenital ichthyosiform erythroderma, and self-healing collodion baby.

FIGURE 51-7

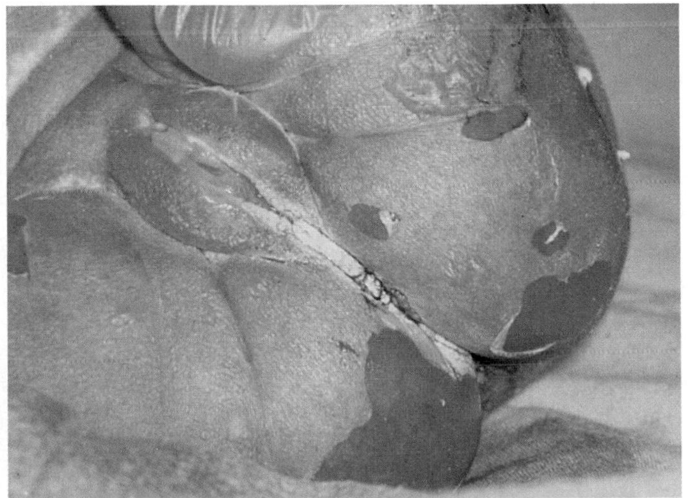

Epidermolytic hyperkeratosis. Newborn showing blistering and erosions.

Genetic linkage studies performed on a large family with a mild type of EHK (PS-1) identified linkage to the cluster of type II (basic) keratin genes located on chromosome 12, implicating keratin 1 in that family as the disease-causing gene.[41] Sequencing the keratin 1 gene in that family identified a mutation that was present in all affected and no unaffected family members.[42] Within keratinocytes, keratin intermediate filaments form an elaborate network that confers structural stability to the cells. In the suprabasilar differentiating keratinocytes, this network is formed by keratins 1 and 10. In EHK, failure of this network leads to keratinocyte fragility (particularly of the upper epidermis), easy blistering, abnormal epidermal kinetics (hyperproliferation), and thickened stratum corneum (hyperkeratosis). Keratin 10 is the coexpressed partner of keratin 1, both of which are required to form keratin intermediate filaments in the cells of the suprabasal layers of the epidermis. It is not surprising, then, that abnormalities in keratin 10 could also cause EHK. To date, a number of EHK families have been studied and found to have mutations in either keratin 1 or 10.[5] Mutations in keratin 9 (a keratin that occurs only in palmar and plantar skin) have been found in families with the type of EHK limited exclusively to the palms and soles (Vörner).[43]

DISORDERS RESEMBLING EPIDERMOLYTIC HYPERKERATOSIS

Ichthyosis bullosa of Siemens is a rare autosomal dominant genodermatosis that is similar in clinical appearance to EHK. Patients are born with redness and blistering. The redness subsides over the subsequent weeks to months, while the skin develops hyperkeratosis, particularly over flexural areas. In some areas there may be a lichenified appearance to the skin. As with EHK, the epidermis is fragile; however, the fragility is more superficial. This can result in loss of the uppermost epidermis (predominantly stratum corneum), yielding a characteristic, collarette-like lesion that has been described as "molting." Histologically, the epidermis shows hyperkeratosis and vacuolization, similar to

EHK but confined to the granular layer. In four families with ichthyosis bullosa of Siemens and two originally diagnosed with EHK but who lacked mutations in keratins K1 and K10, mutations were found in the gene encoding keratin 2e,[44] a differentiation keratin of the suprabasilar epidermis that is expressed in the more superficial epidermal layers.

Ichthyosis hystrix of Curth and Macklin is a rare, autosomal dominant disorder that clinically resembles EHK. Clinical expression varies, even within families, from palmoplantar keratoderma to a severe generalized involvement. There can be widespread patchy, thick, gray-brown hyperkeratosis, most marked at the extensor arms and legs. Patients with extensive involvement resemble those with the NPS-1 type of EHK, with verrucous or porcupine-like (hystrix) hyperkeratosis. However, in contrast to EHK, blistering does not occur. Histologic examination of the epidermis shows acanthosis, papillomatosis, and severe orthokeratotic hyperkeratosis, with frequent binucleate cells. Keratinocytes within the granular and upper spinous layers may have perinuclear vacuolization, and some have prominent perinuclear shells. On electron microscopy, there are concentric, unbroken shells of tonofilaments surrounding the nucleus. Study of a three-generation family with ichthyosis hystrix of Curth and Macklin identified a mutation in the variable tail domain (V2) of the keratin 1 gene. Structural analyses of the resulting keratin 1 abnormality showed a failure of keratin intermediate filament bundling, retraction of the cytoskeleton from the nucleus, and failure of translocation of loricrin to desmosomal plaques.[45]

FIGURE 51-8

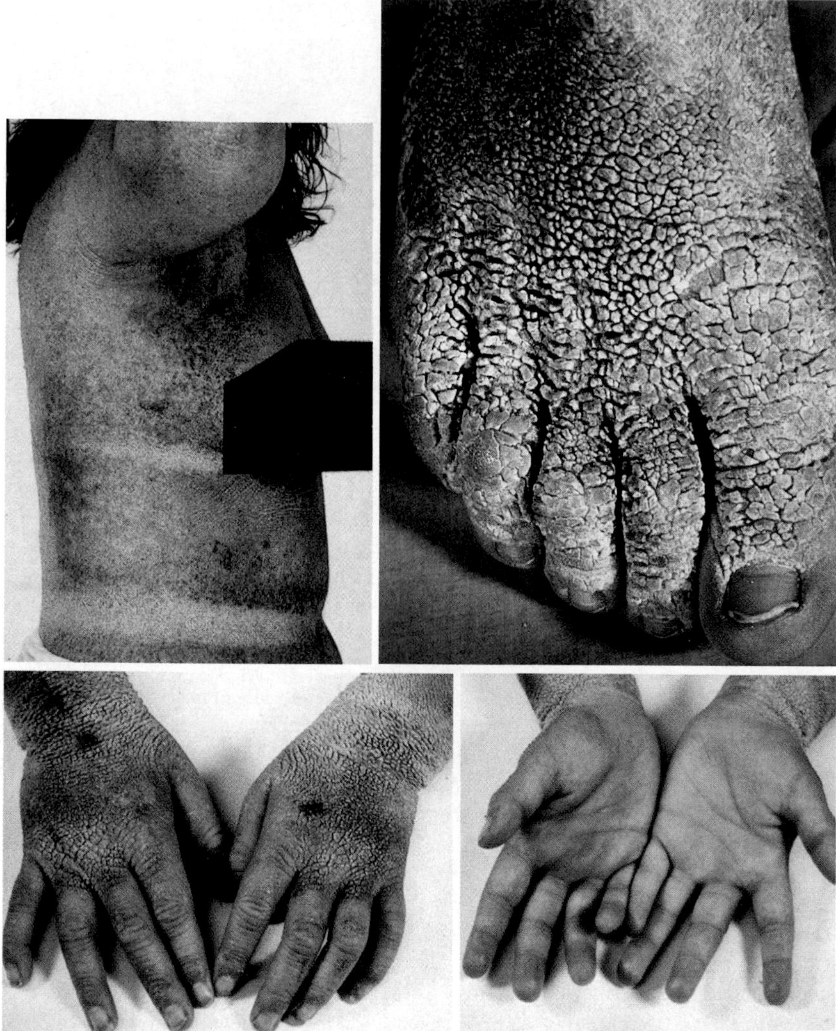

A.

Clinical phenotypes of epidermolytic hyperkeratosis. *A.* NPS-1 (no severe palm/sole hyperkeratosis, type 1). *Top left:* Generalized involvement with thick, brown verrucous hyperkeratosis. *Top right, bottom left:* Hyperkeratosis is arrayed in a characteristic cobblestone or hystrix (porcupine-like) pattern. *Bottom right:* Shows spared palms. *B.* NPS-2 (no severe palm/sole hyperkeratosis, type 2). *Top left, bottom left, bottom right:* Seven-year-old patient with brown hyperkeratosis. Palms are spared. Compared to the verrucous hyperkeratosis in NPS-1, involvement is much milder. *Top right:* Three-year-old patient with blistering and hyperkeratosis, demonstrating hypertrichosis and relative sparing of the skin between the joints. *C.* NPS-3 (no severe palm/sole hyperkeratosis, type 3). *Right:* Generalized erythroderma with white scale and hyperkeratosis. *Left:* Minimal thickening and scale of the palms. *D.* PS-1 (severe palm/sole hyperkeratosis, type 1). *Three left plates:* Palmar and plantar hyperkeratosis with sharp border delineated by a red halo. Blisters are present at the border.Note the relatively smooth surface. *Right plate:* Characteristic involvement at the joints. *E.* PS-2 (severe palm/sole hyperkeratosis, type 2). *Top left, top right:* Hands of a 15-year-old patient with severe palmar hyperkeratosis and contractures. *Right center:* Flank of same patient exhibiting generalized erythroderma and scaling. *Bottom left* (two plates): Hands of a 36-year-old patient with severe palmar hyperkeratosis, contractures, and ainhum-like constricting digital bands. The palmar hyperkeratosis limits spreading of the fingers. *Bottom right:* Eight-year-old boy with generalized redness and peeling. *F.* PS-3 (severe palm/sole hyperkeratosis, type 3). *Top right*: Four-year-old patient with hyperkeratosis in a distinctive cerebriform pattern on the palms and soles (not shown). *Bottom right:* Hyperkeratosis in a cobblestone pattern on the knees. *Left:* Generalized pebbly hyperkeratosis. Note the loss of superficial epidermis on shoulder. (*From DiGiovanna and Bale,*[38] *adapted with permission.*)

ICHTHYOSIS IN THE NEWBORN

A *collodion baby* is the usual presentation of congenital recessive ichthyosis (see Fig. 51-6). The child is born encased in a translucent, parchment-like membrane, which is taut and may impair respiration and sucking. In addition, the birth is often premature, which adds to morbidity. During the first 2 weeks of life, the membrane breaks up and peels off, often leaving fissures, with impairment of the barrier to infection and water loss. This can lead to difficulties in thermal regulation, an increased risk of infection, and hypernatremic dehydration.[46] Newborn care should include careful monitoring of temperature, hydration, and electrolytes and measures to keep the peeling membrane soft and lubricated to facilitate desquamation. The newborn should be in a humidified incubator where the air is saturated with water; wet compresses followed by bland lubricants can be used to further hydrate the membrane and achieve maximum pliability. If, during peeling, residual areas of the membrane are allowed to dry and harden in areas such as the extremities, the taut membrane can constrict and lead to distal swelling. Collodion presentation can develop into a wide spectrum of ichthyotic phenotypes as the child grows. This includes the spectrum of congenital autosomal recessive ichthyosis (severe classic LI, CIE, and intermediate phenotypes) and Netherton's syndrome. In addition, an autosomal recessive, self-healing collodion baby has been described, where the skin clears within the first few weeks and transitions into normal skin thereafter.[32]

A dramatic, severe, and usually fatal presentation of ichthyosis is that of *harlequin ichthyosis* (Fig. 51-10). The child is often premature and born with massive, shiny plates of stratum corneum separated by deep, red fissures that tend to form geometric patterns. There are poorly developed or absent ears and marked ectropion and eclabium. The first report is from the diary of Rev. Oliver Hart, of Charleston, South Carolina, who described these features in 1750.[47] These children are at great risk during the neonatal period and often die shortly after birth. Abnormal water loss through the skin and poor temperature regulation lead to risk of fluid and electrolyte imbalance. The infants are also at risk for infection beginning in the skin, but at the same time, because of poor temperature regulation, do not show the usual signs of infection. Normal respiration may be restricted by the taut skin. Treatment with isotretinoin or etretinate during the newborn period can facilitate desquamation of the membrane.[48,49] Advances in neonatal intensive care together with facilitating desquamation with judicious use of systemic retinoid therapy have led to improvements in survival and to the use of the name "harlequin baby" rather than "harlequin fetus." Some babies have had gastrointestinal disturbances such as poor absorption, leading to failure to thrive and requiring tube feeding. The skin of those who survive the newborn period usually resembles the skin of those with a severe phenotype of CIE.[48,49]

Occurrence of harlequin ichthyosis in consanguineous families suggests autosomal recessive inheritance.[50] However, most cases are sporadic with no evidence of consanguinity, which is also consistent with a new dominant mutation. Therefore, there may be genetic heterogeneity. Studies of epidermal proteins suggest that there may be three types of harlequin ichthyosis. Keratohyalin granules look fairly normal in type 1, are too small to be seen by light microscopy in type 2, and are absent in type 3. In all types, there are no lamellar granules; instead, there are small vesicles that lack internal structure. There is also no evidence of the lipid lamellae that form between granular and cornified cells as a result of discharge of lamellar granule contents into the intercellular space.[51]

FIGURE 51-8 (*Continued*)

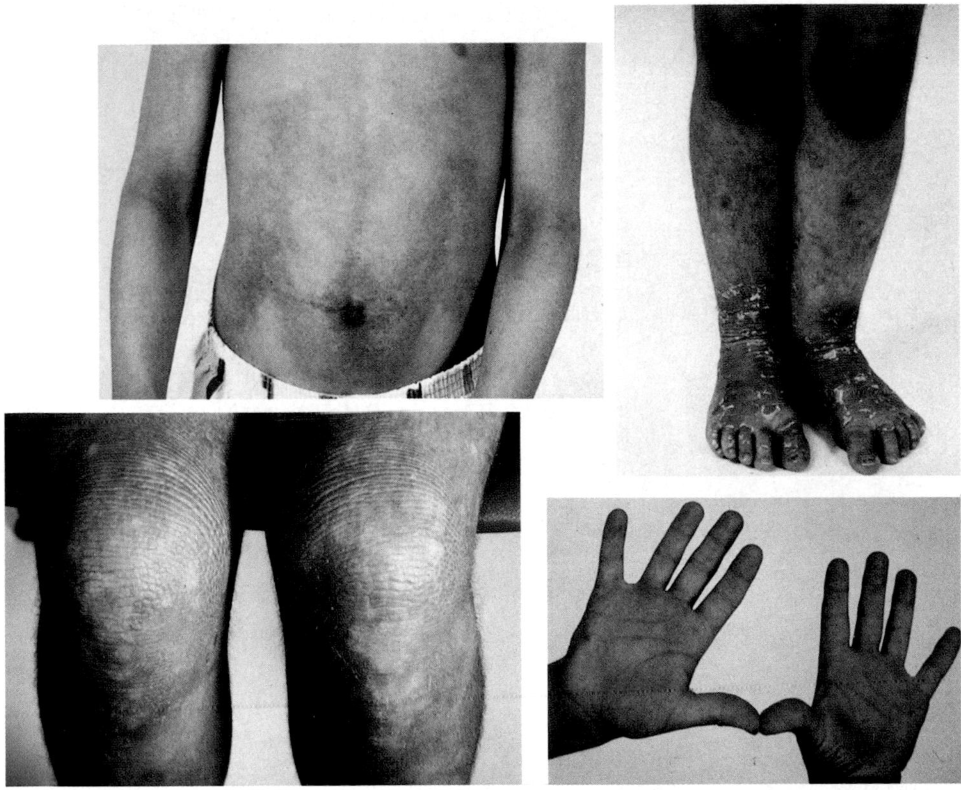

B.

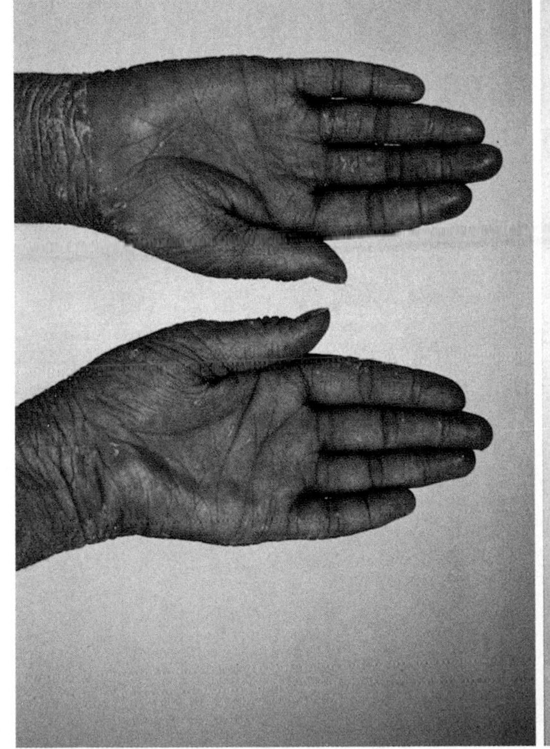

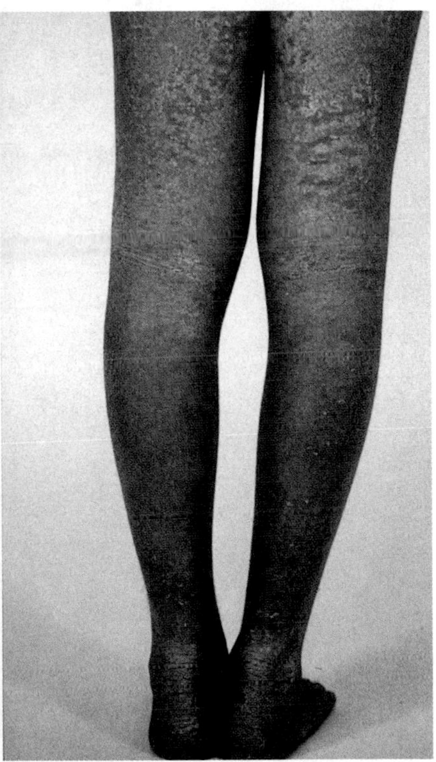

C.

FIGURE 51-8 (*Continued*)

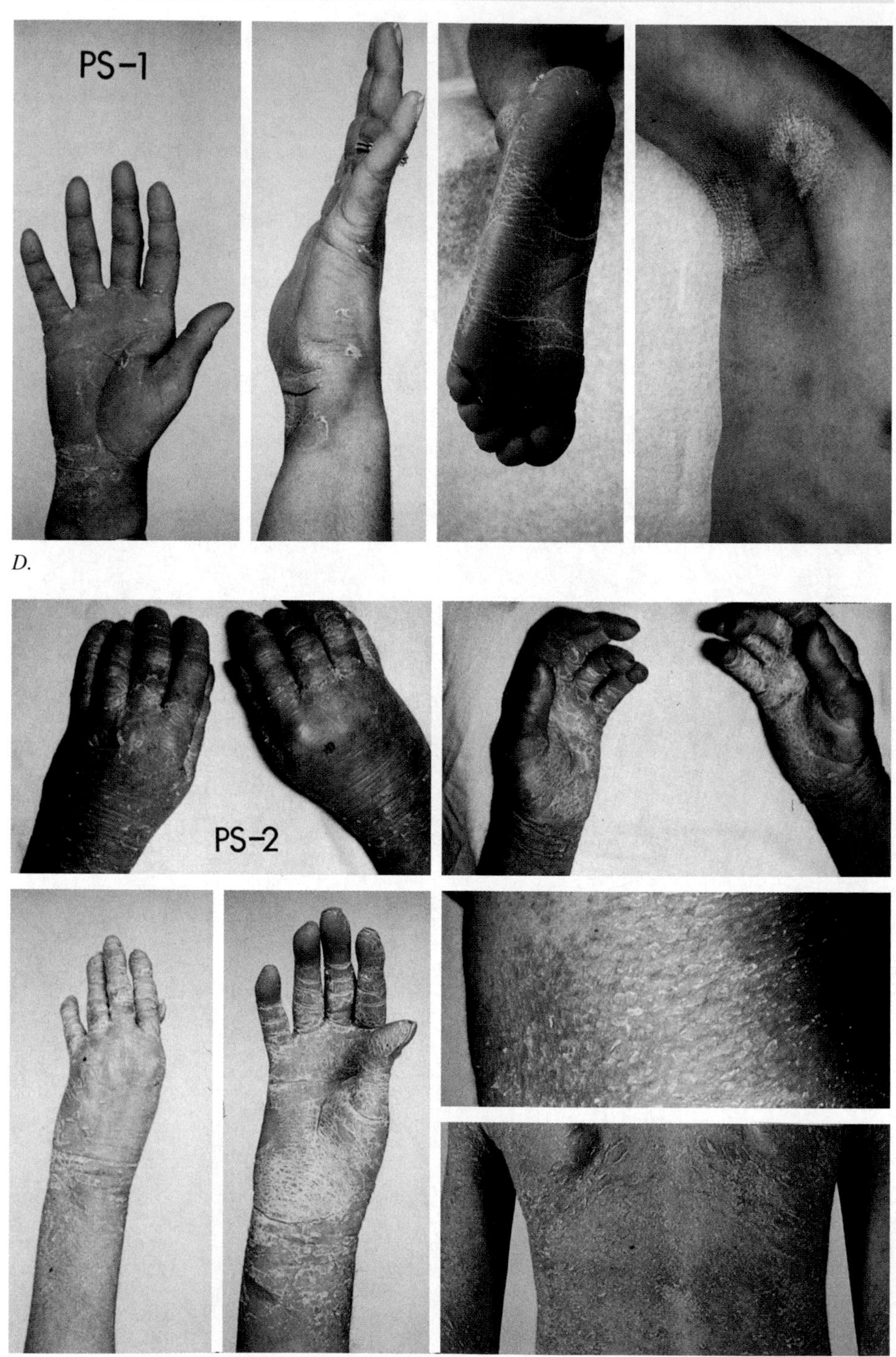

D.

E.

The newborn affected with one of the more severe, generalized types of *EHK* usually has erythema, blistering, widespread erosions, and denuded skin. Because there is a high frequency of new mutations, the disease may be unexpected and the diagnosis may be unknown. Epidermolysis bullosa or staphylococcal scalded-skin syndrome may be suspected, and the infant treated with antibiotics. The newborn may require intensive care with fluid and electrolyte monitoring. Specialized skin care can minimize blistering and enhance healing of erosions and should include lubrication to decrease friction and mechanical trauma, protective padding, and specialized wound dressings. The newborn with extensive erosions is prone to bacterial infection and sepsis, and carefully chosen topical and systemic antibiotics can minimize the extent of infection.

ACQUIRED ICHTHYOSIS

The development of ichthyosis in adulthood can be a manifestation of systemic disease, and it has been described in association with malignancies, drugs, endocrine and metabolic disease, HIV infection, and autoimmune conditions. While Hodgkin's disease is the most common malignancy reported with acquired ichthyosis, non-Hodgkin's lymphomas and a variety of other malignancies have also been observed.[52] The skin involvement may follow the course of malignancy and clear with effective cancer treatment. Acquired ichthyosis is commonly seen in association with AIDS, and ichthyotic or xerotic skin has been observed in up to 30 percent of AIDS patients.[53] A study of HIV-1–positive intravenous drug users found acquired ichthyosis occurred only after profound helper T cell depletion, more frequently with coinfection with *human T cell leukemia/lymphoma virus type II (HTLV-II),* and suggested that it may be a marker for concomitant infection with HIV-1 and HTLV-II.[54]

In acquired ichthyosis occurring in association with sarcoidosis, skin biopsy can be diagnostic, showing noncaseating granulomas in the dermis.[55] Acquired ichthyosis may be a marker of autoimmune disease, occurring with systemic lupus erythematosus, dermatomyositis, mixed connective tissue disease, and eosinophilic fasciitis.[56,57] It has been described in bone marrow transplant recipients, where it may be related to graft-versus-host disease.[58]

While occurrence in association with cholesterol-lowering agents (nicotinic acid, triparanol) highlights the relationship between cholesterol metabolism and normal desquamation, acquired ichthyosis has been observed with a variety of drugs, including butyrophenone (antipsychotic), dixyrazine (major tranquilizer), and nafoxidine (estrogen antagonist).[14]

Confluent and reticulated papillomatosis of Gougerot and Carteaud is an uncommon but distinctive acquired ichthyosiform dermatosis characterized by persistent dark, scaly papules and plaques. Lesions tend to be localized predominantly on the central trunk (intermammary and interscapular regions) where they tend to be confluent and become reticulated towards the periphery (Fig. 51-11).

FIGURE 51-8 (*Continued*)

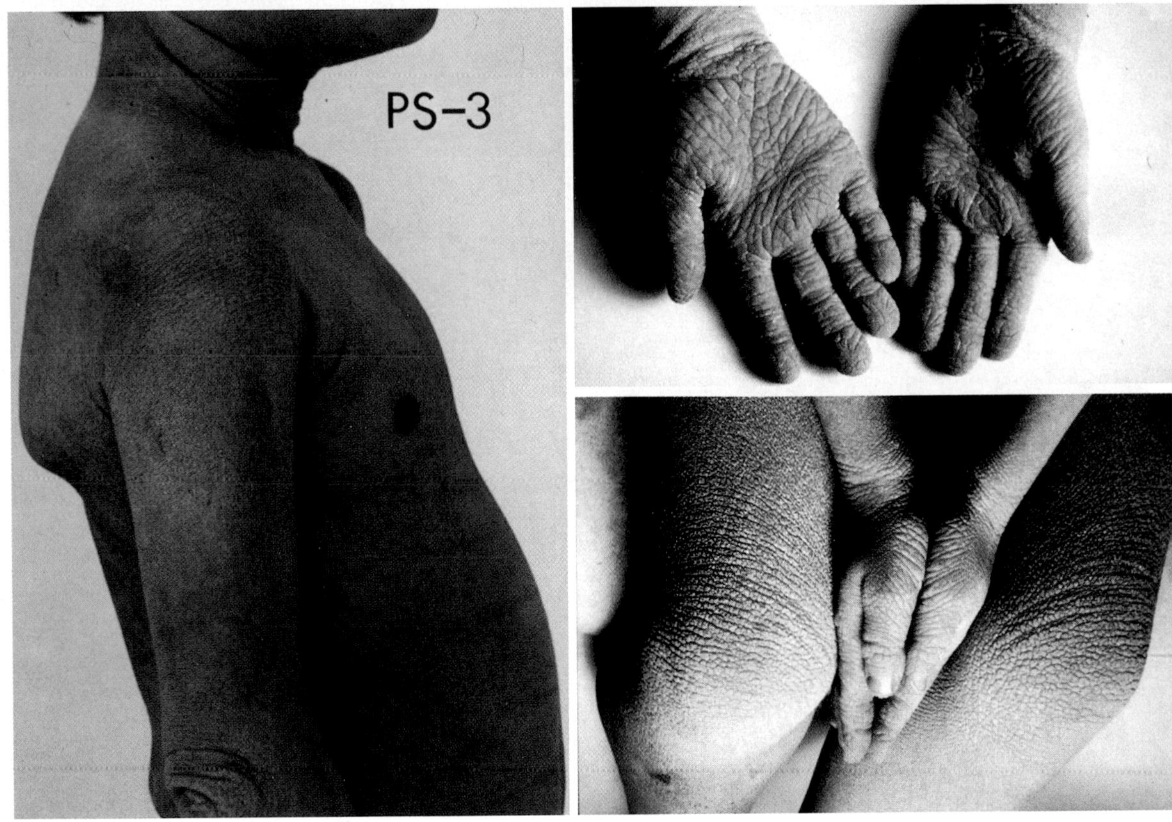

F.

The lesions bear a clinical resemblance to tinea versicolor, a skin infection with Pityrosporum species. A variety of treatment approaches have been reported, including topical (keratolytics, derivatives of vitamin A and D, antimicrobials) and systemic (antibiotics, retinoids) agents. A series of six cases reported responsiveness to various antibiotics including oral minocycline, fusidic acid, clarithromycin, erythromycin, and azithromycin.[59] Minocycline has been suggested as a first-line treatment, and successful retreatment of recurrences supports the concept that this condition is an abnormal response to an infection.[60]

LESS-COMMON ICHTHYOSES

Netherton's syndrome is a rare, autosomal recessive disorder that is characterized by the concurrence of ichthyosis, a structural hair

TABLE 51-2

Clinical Subtypes of Epidermolytic Hyperkeratosis

CHARACTERISTIC	NPS-1	NPS-2	NPS-3	PS-1	PS-2	PS-3
Palm/sole hyperkeratosis	−	−	−	+	+	+
Palm/sole surface	Normal	Normal	Hyperlinear, minimal scale	Smooth	Smooth	Cerebriform
Digital contractures	−	−	−	−	+	−
Scale	Hystrix	Brown	Fine, white	Mild	White scale to peel	Tan
Distribution	Generalized	Generalized	Generalized	Localized	Generalized	Generalized
Erythroderma	−	−	+	−	+	−
Blistering	+	+	+	Localized	+	Neonatal

NOTE: NPS; types without severe palm/sole hyperkeratosis; PS, types with severe palm/sole hyperkeratosis; minus sign, absent; plus sign, present.
SOURCE: From DiGiovanna and Bale,[38] with permission.

FIGURE 51-9

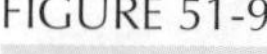

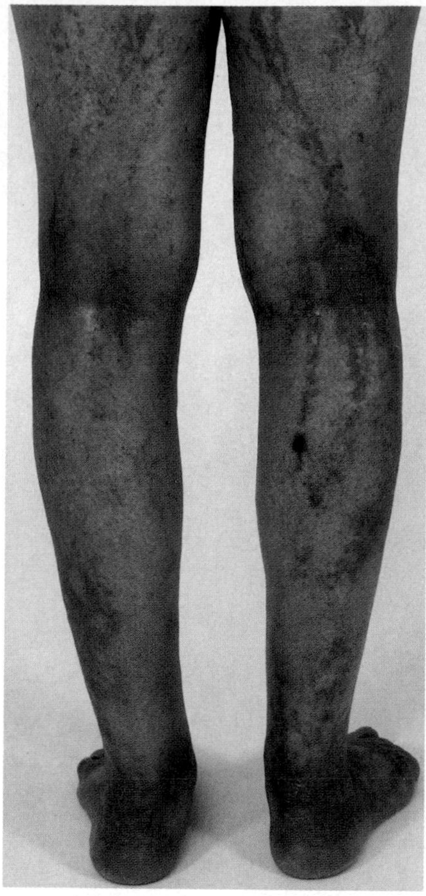

A.

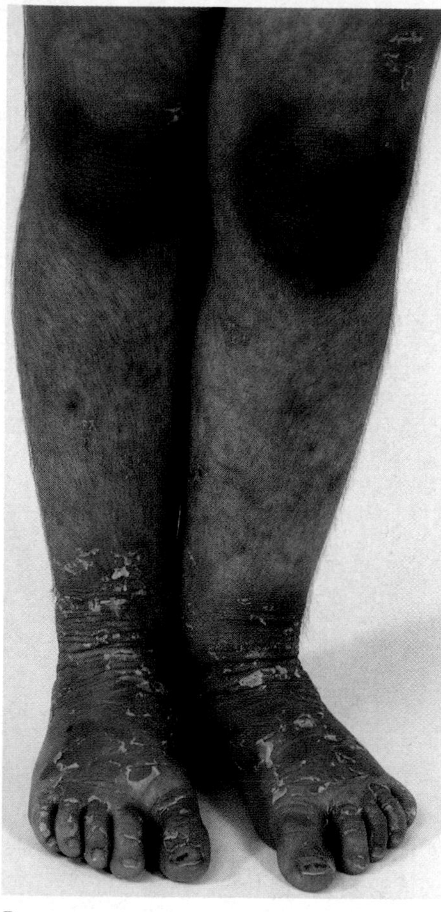

B.

Mosaic epidermolytic hyperkeratosis. *A.* Streaks of hyperkeratosis distributed along Blaschko's lines in a sporadic case due to postzygotic occurrence of new mutation. *B.* Grandchild of patient shown in Panel *A.* Generalized involvement (in this case the NPS-2 clinical phenotype) is transmitted to subsequent generations in an autosomal dominant inheritance pattern.

shaft abnormality, and atopy.[61,62] The usual cutaneous manifestation is *ichthyosis linearis circumflexa,* a distinctive condition of generalized hyperkeratosis and polycyclic and serpiginous erythematous plaques with a characteristic, migratory, double-edged scale at the margins (Fig. 51-12*A*). At birth this may present as generalized erythroderma or a collodion phenotype. Infants and children may have feeding problems, with poor absorption and failure to thrive.[63] With atopic dermatitis, there may be pruritus, and scratching can lead to lichenification at the flexures. In some patients, the ichthyosis resembles LI or CIE.[33,61] Histopathologic examination is not specific and may show features of hyperkeratosis, psoriasis, and atopic dermatitis. Most patients have a specific hair shaft abnormality called *trichorrhexis invaginata,* in which the distal hair segment is telescoped into the proximal one, forming a ball-and-socket–like deformity on microscopic examination (Fig. 51-12*B*). This is also known as "bamboo hair" and is due to abnormal cornification of the internal root sheath. Hair from multiple areas should be examined, because only 20 to 50 percent of hair may be affected, and the characteristic abnormality may be more commonly observed on eyebrow hair.[64] Trichorrhexis nodosa and pili torti may also occur. Atopy in these patients may manifest as atopic dermatitis or asthma, and marked elevations of serum IgE may occur. In some patients, a generalized aminoaciduria, mild developmental delay, and impaired cellular immunity may also be present. Netherton's syndrome has been found to be due to mutations in *SPINK5,* a gene encoding LEKTI (*l*ympho-*e*pithelial *K*azal-*t*ype related *i*nhibitor).[65] LEKTI is a serine protease inhibitor that is predominantly expressed in epithelial and lymphoid tissues, and may be important in the downregulation of inflammatory pathways. This discovery highlights the importance of the regulation of proteolysis in the overlap between epithelial barrier function and the hypersensitivity of atopy. Subsequently, LEKTI was associated with common atopy and atopic dermatitis.[66] Prenatal testing for Netherton's syndrome using molecular data has been successfully accomplished.[67] Tacrolimus ointment, a topical immunosuppressant, is effective in common atopic dermatitis with minimal systemic absorption. However, Netherton's syndrome is complicated by an abnormal skin barrier, allowing increased percutaneous absorption and associated risk for systemic toxic effects. This should be considered when using topical agents such as tacrolimus where monitoring of serum levels may be necessary.[68]

In 1957, Sjögren and Larsson reported on 13 families from north Sweden with a syndrome of congenital ichthyosis, spastic paralysis, and mental retardation. *Sjögren-Larsson syndrome (SLS)* is a rare, autosomal recessive disorder that presents at birth with an ichthyosis that may range from fine scaling to generalized hyperkeratosis. Erythema may be present at birth but tends to gradually clear by 1 year of age. Collodion-like membranes are rarely seen. The ichthyosis manifests as fine scale, large scale, or a thickening of the stratum corneum without scale and may be pruritic. Thickened areas may be yellow to brown in color and have a lichenified appearance with accentuated skin markings. The most involved areas are the sides and back of the neck, lower abdomen, and flexures. Hair, nails, and the ability to sweat are generally normal.[69] During the first 2 to 3 years, neurologic manifestations of spastic diplegia or tetraplegia and mental retardation develop and can be accompanied by speech defects and seizures. A characteristic ophthalmologic finding is the presence of glistening white dots in the macula of the retina; these occur after 1 year of age and may not be present in all patients. Histologic findings of hyperkeratosis, papillomatosis, acanthosis, and a mildly thickened granular layer are nonspecific. Electron-microscopic examination of the skin shows lamellar membranous inclusions in the granular and cornified cells.

Rizzo et al. found deficient *fatty alcohol:NAD oxidoreductase (FAO)* activity in cultured fibroblasts from patients with SLS. FAO is a complex enzyme with two separate proteins that sequentially catalyze the oxidation of fatty alcohol to fatty aldehyde and subsequently to fatty acid. Further work identified the fatty aldehyde dehydrogenase component as the affected component of FAO in SLS. Fatty aldehyde dehydrogenase is a microsomal enzyme that catalyzes the oxidation of medium- and long-chain aliphatic aldehydes derived from metabolism of fatty alcohol, phytanic acid, ether, glycerolipids and leukotriene B4.[70] Mutations found in the fatty aldehyde dehydrogenase gene (FALDH, ALDH10) of three unrelated SLS patients confirmed the role for this enzyme in the etiology of this disorder and the importance of this pathway for normal desquamation.[71]

The identification of decreased fibroblast FAO activity in a family with atypical cutaneous findings (lack of ichthyosis or discrete plaques rather than generalized ichthyosis) has expanded the spectrum of clinical phenotypes associated with abnormal FAO activity.[72]

The *erythrokeratodermias* are a clinically heterogeneous group of disorders characterized by hyperkeratosis and localized erythema. Within a broad spectrum of phenotypes, at least two disorders can be delineated: erythrokeratodermia variabilis and progressive symmetric erythrokeratodermia. There are overlapping clinical features and phenotypic variability within these two designations.

Erythrokeratodermia variabilis, described by Mendes da Costa in 1925, is a rare autosomal dominant disorder that usually presents at birth or during the first year of life. At least two distinct clinical presentations can be distinguished. One type (Fig. 51-13*A*) is characterized by generalized, persistent, brown hyperkeratosis with accentuated skin markings. A second, localized type (Fig. 51-13*B*) has involvement that is limited in extent and characterized by sharply demarcated, hyperkeratotic plaques; these are symmetrically arrayed and remain relatively fixed for months to years. In the localized type, there may be considerable variability between affected family members, and the disorder may not be apparent until later in life. Both types are characterized by striking, sharply demarcated, migratory red patches, which vary in size from a few to many centimeters. These geographic, figurate red patches appear or regress over minutes to hours; some individuals complain of burning at these sites, while in others they are asymptomatic. The red patches develop independently of the hyperkeratosis. Both types of skin lesions may be triggered by trauma to the skin or change in temperature. Palmoplantar hyperkeratosis may be present in either type, but hair, nails, and mucous membranes are unaffected. Histopathologic features are nonspecific and include hyperkeratosis, acanthosis, papillomatosis, and capillary dilatation. Epidermis involved with severe papillomatosis and suprapapillary thinning may result in a "church spire" appearance histologically.

Erythrokeratodermia with ataxia (Giroux-Barbeau type) is an autosomal dominant disorder that presents during infancy with well-defined, symmetric hyperkeratotic plaques and underlying erythema distributed over the extensor surface of the extremities.[73] Skin lesions regress during adulthood while a progressive spinocerebellar ataxia develops. Both the localized type of erythrokeratodermia variabilis and erythrokeratodermia with ataxia have been mapped to a common region (chromosome 1p34-35).[74] Subsequently, Richard et al. found mutations in *GJB3,* the gene encoding connexin 31, in four families with erythrokeratodermia variabilis.[75] Connexins

FIGURE 51-10

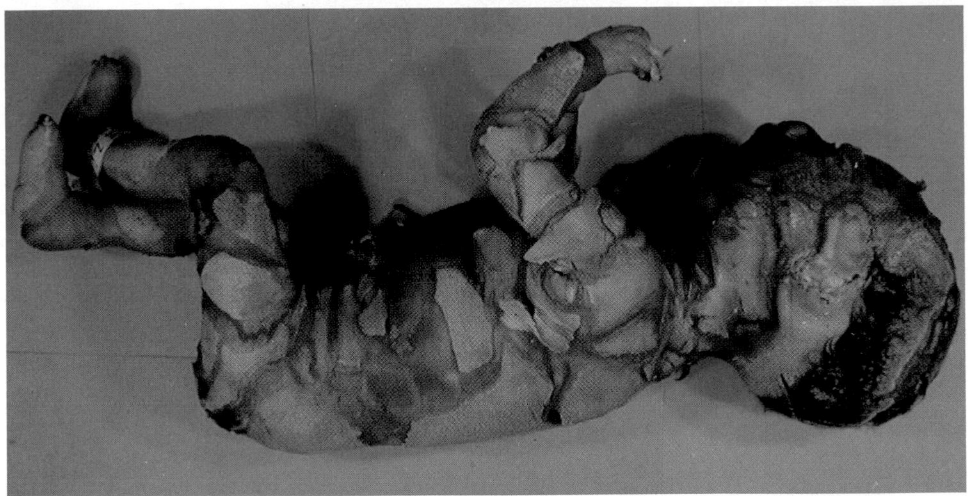

Harlequin ichthyosis. Note rudimentary ears and the distorted appearance as a result of the thick "plates" of stratum corneum. This baby died in a few days.

FIGURE 51-11

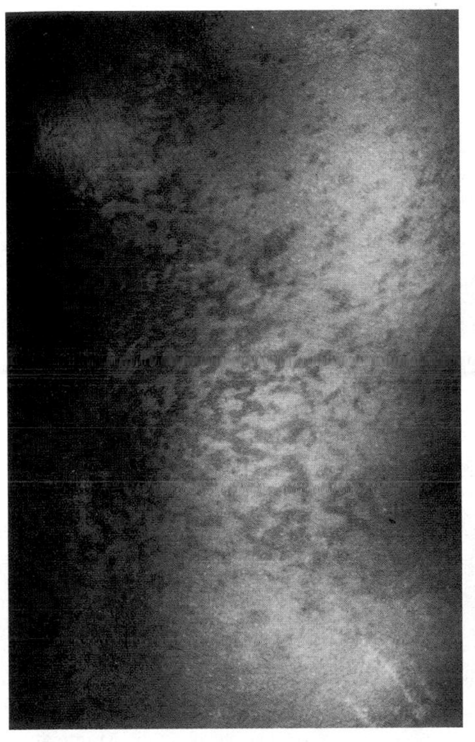

A.

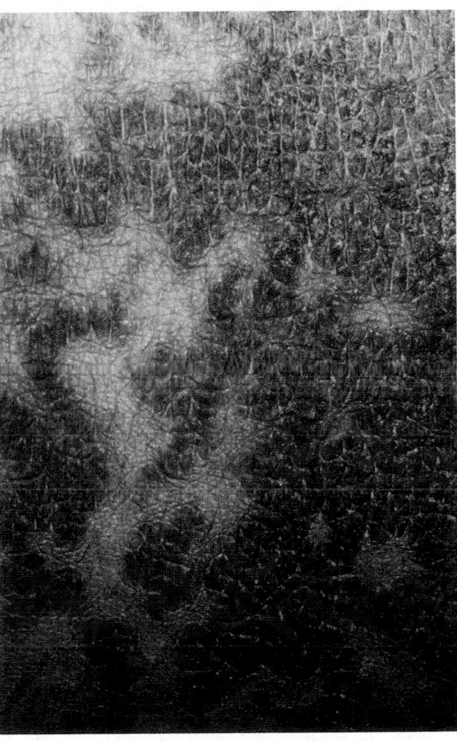

B.

Confuent and reticulated papillomatosis of Gougerot and Carteaud. *A.* Dark, scaly papules and plaques on the trunk which become reticulated towards the periphery. *B.* Close-up view of the distinctive, scaly, reticulated papules and plaques. (*Courtesy of Andrew Montemarano, Do, and Stephen Krivda, MD.*)

FIGURE 51-12

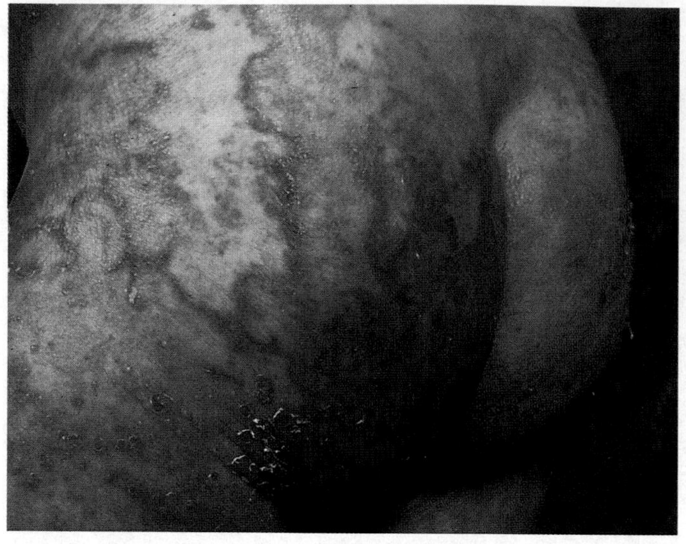

A.

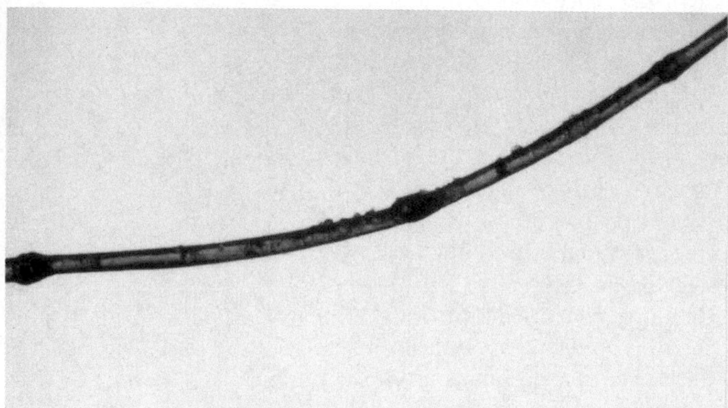

B.

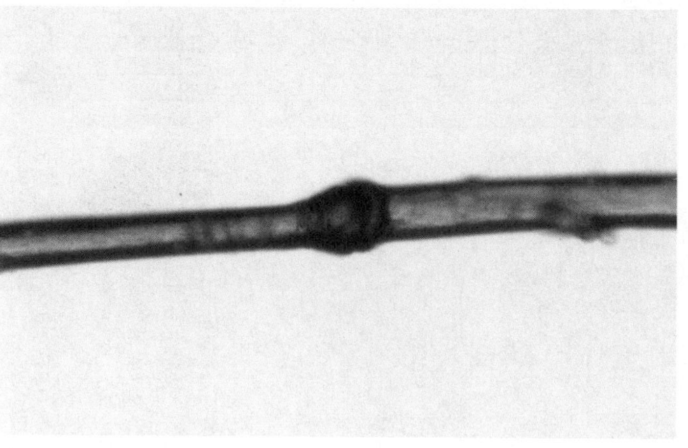

C.

Netherton's syndrome. *A.* Ichthyosis linearis circumflexa showing typical annular lesions. (*Courtesy of James Stroud, MD.*) Bamboo hair shaft (*B*), under higher power (*C*) shows features of trichorrhexis invaginata.

are a family of proteins that form gap junctions, which are important channels for intercellular communication. This intercellular signaling system is crucial for maintaining tissue homeostasis, growth control, development, and synchronized response of cells to stimuli. The identification of connexin mutations as the cause of erythrokeratodermia variabilis implicates this pathway in epidermal differentiation and in the mechanism of skin response to external factors. Different mutations in the same connexin 31 gene (*GJB3*) have been found in other patients with deafness and also in some with peripheral neuropathy. Mutations in the related connexin 30.3 have been found in other families with erythrokeratodermia variabilis.[76]

Progressive symmetric erythrokeratodermia, first described by Darier in 1911, is characterized by well-demarcated, erythematous, hyperkeratotic plaques that are symmetrically distributed over the extremities and buttocks, and often the face.[77] The trunk tends to be spared, but palms and soles may be involved. The plaques appear shortly after birth, progress slowly during the first few years, and then stabilize in early childhood. The plaques usually remain stable in location and appearance but may undergo partial regression at puberty. The variable, migratory erythema that defines erythrokeratodermia variabilis is absent. The disorder is inherited in an autosomal dominant pattern but with incomplete penetrance and variable expressivity. A mutation in the cornified envelope protein loricrin was found in one family.[78]

KID syndrome is a rare disorder characterized by *k*eratitis (with progressive corneal opacification), *i*chthyosis, and *d*eafness (neurosensory). Involvement of multiple ectodermal tissues qualifies KID syndrome as an ectodermal dysplasia. Most cases are compatible with autosomal dominant inheritance. However, occurrence in an inbred sibship suggests the existence of an autosomal recessive form. The disease is characterized by discrete erythematous plaques, and there may be a mild, generalized hyperkeratosis. The distinctive plaques may have a discrete border and a verrucous appearance with crusting and may be conspicuously figurate and symmetric on the face (Fig. 51-14). There may be prominent follicular hyperkeratosis, which can result in a scarring alopecia of the scalp. Several authors have suggested that because the plaques do not scale, this disorder is more accurately designated an erythrokeratodermia rather than an ichthyosis.[79] The nails may be dystrophic and teeth may be small. Auditory evoked potential studies allow detection of the hearing deficit in infancy. Affected individuals can have an increased susceptibility to bacterial, fungal, or viral infections. Squamous cell carcinoma of the skin and tongue have also been reported. In contrast to many other ichthyotic conditions, treatment of these patients with oral retinoids has been reported to be of little benefit and possibly to exacerbate the corneal neovascularization.

FIGURE 51-13

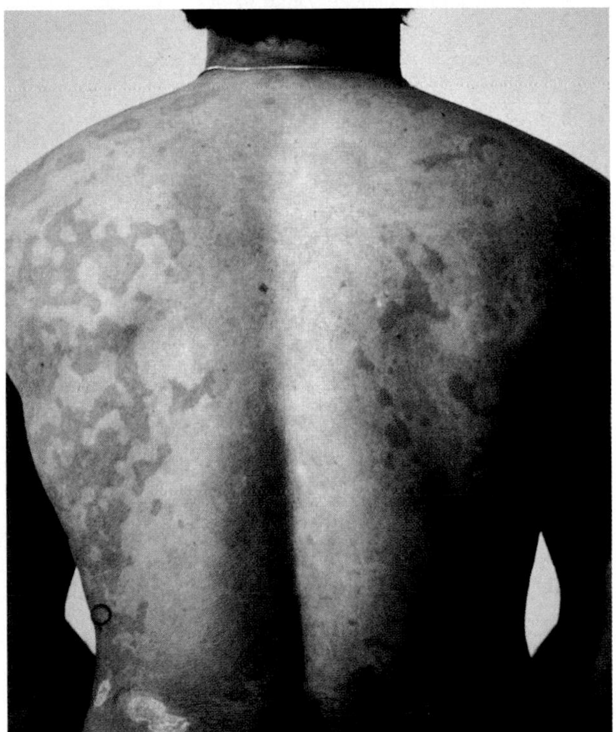

A.

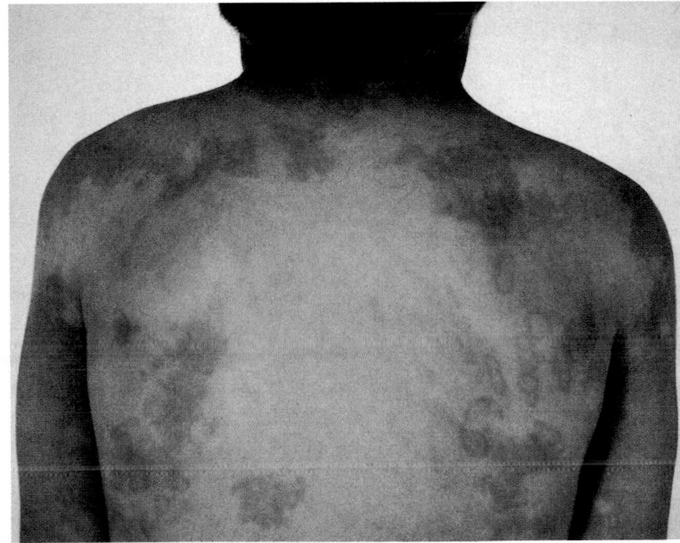

B.

Erythrokeratodermia variabilis. *A.* Generalized type with widespread hyperkeratosis and migratory, figurate, red patches. *B.* Localized type. Sharply demarcated, symmetric, hyperkeratotic plaques and migratory, figurate, red patches.

Richard et al. discovered dominant mutations in *GJB2,* the gene encoding connexin 26 in eight sporadic cases and one family with KID syndrome. Functional studies of cells expressing mutated connexin 26 demonstrated failure of a fluorescent tracer to pass through gap junction channels to neighboring cells, consistent with disruption of intercellular communication.[80] Different mutations in the same gene (*GJB2*) encoding connexin 26 have also been found in a family with a mutilating palmoplantar keratoderma (Vohwinkle's disease) and deafness (without ichthyosis).[81] Connexin proteins aggregate to form gap junction channels, which span the cell membrane between adjacent cells. These channels are flexible structures that are constantly remodeled, and enable a direct cytoplasmic connection that allows the passage of a variety of small particles between cells. The identification of mutations in the genes encoding a variety of connexin proteins has highlighted the role of connexin mediated intercellular communication through gap junctions in the development and maintenance of ectodermal tissues. Connexins 26, 30, and 31 are expressed in the stratified epithelia of the cochlea and epidermis, and abnormalities in these proteins can cause sensorineural hearing impairment and/or skin disorders.[7]

FIGURE 51-14

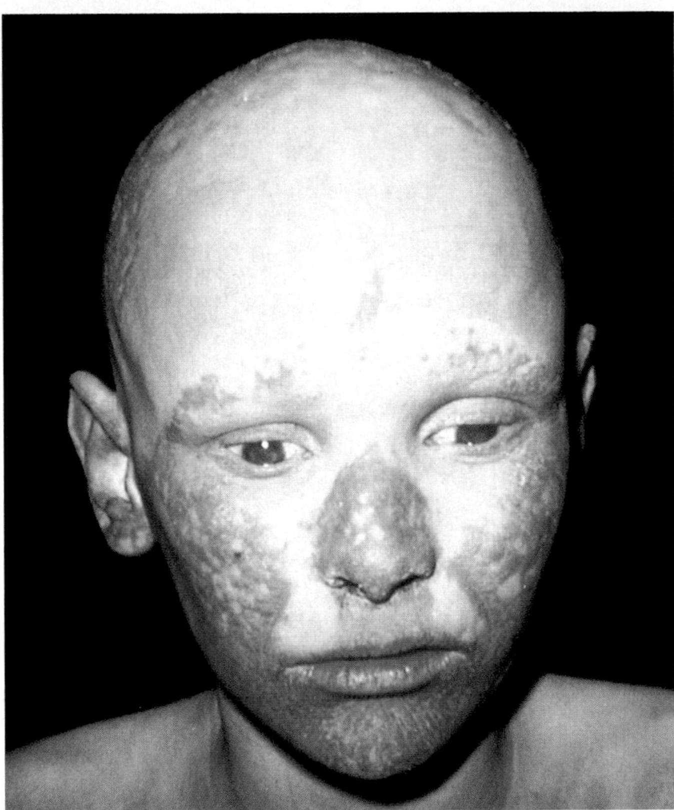

KID syndrome. Discrete, symmetric areas of hyperkeratosis are present on the face. There is a scarring alopecia.

Refsum's disease (heredopathia atactica polyneuritiformis) is a rare, progressive, degenerative disorder of lipid metabolism resulting from the failure to break down dietary phytanic acid and its subsequent accumulation in tissues. This autosomal recessive condition affects mostly the Scandinavians and populations originating from northern Europe. Clinical manifestations include retinitis pigmentosa, peripheral neuropathy, cerebellar ataxia, cranial nerve dysfunction (neural deafness, anosmia), miosis, electrocardiographic abnormalities, cardiomyopathy, renal tubular dysfunction, and skeletal abnormalities (epiphyseal dysplasia). Ichthyosis, which is variable, generally develops in adulthood after the neurologic and ophthalmologic manifestations. Often there are small white scales over the trunk and extremities resembling ichthyosis vulgaris. Routine [hematoxylin and eosin (H&E)] histologic examination shows variably sized vacuoles in the epidermal basal and suprabasal cells, which correspond to lipid accumulation seen with lipid stains of frozen sections.[82]

Phytanic acid (a 20-carbon, branched-chain fatty acid) is derived from a variety of dietary sources including dairy products, ruminant fats, and chlorophyll-containing foods. The disease is caused by a deficiency of phytanoyl-CoA hydroxylase (PhyH), a peroxisomal protein that catalyzes the α-oxidation of phytanic acid. This is the first step in the breakdown of phytanic acid, and PhyH deficiency leads to the accumulation of phytanic acid in the serum and tissues, where it substitutes for the fatty acids normally present. While mutations in *PAHX,* the gene encoding PhyH are responsible for some cases of Refsum's disease,[83] there is genetic heterogeneity.[84] Some affected patients have mutations in the *PEX7* gene, which is the same gene mutated in rhizomelic chondrodysplasia punctata (see below).

Because of the therapeutic effects of systemic retinoid drugs on ichthyosis, it is interesting to note the relationship between phytanoids and retinoids. Phytanic acid and other chlorophyll metabolites bind the *retinoid X receptor (RXR),* as does its natural ligand, 9-*cis*-retinoic acid, and they may be physiologically active in coordinating cellular metabolism through RXR-dependent signaling pathways.[85] Phytanic acid also appears to be a natural ligand for RXRα in that it promotes the formation of an RXRα/RXR response element complex and induces a conformational change similar to that induced by 9-*cis*-retinoic acid. The role of RXR in the pathogenesis of Refsum's disease is unclear.

The diagnosis can be made by detection of elevated levels of plasma phytanic acid. In children who do not have elevated plasma levels of phytanic acid, the diagnosis may be made by measuring PhyH activity in cultured fibroblasts.[86] Treatment includes dietary restriction of foods containing phytanic acid and its precursors and can include plasmapheresis or lipapheresis. In the clinical setting of a delayed onset of ichthyosis in association with neurologic impairment, this disease should be considered since therapy can arrest progression.

Chondrodysplasia punctata is a clinically and genetically diverse group of rare diseases, first described by Conradi, that share the features of stippled epiphyses and skeletal changes. They are characterized by abnormal deposition of calcium in the areas of enchondral bone formation during fetal development and early infancy. Several forms also include ichthyosiform changes. Clinical severity ranges from severe dwarfism and death during infancy to a self-limited radiographic abnormality in others. An autosomal recessive (rhizomelic) type and both X-linked dominant[87] and recessive forms[88] have been described. The validity of the originally described autosomal dominant Conradi-Hünermann type has been questioned, because some reported cases were later shown to belong to the X-linked dominant type, and occurrences previously considered sporadic have subsequently been recognized as resulting from warfarin (Coumadin) anticoagulant embryopathy.[87,89]

Rhizomelic chondrodysplasia punctata (RCDP) (autosomal recessive) is also known as peroxisomal biogenesis disorder complementation group 11 (CG11). It is a rare, multisystem developmental disorder characterized by dwarfism due to symmetric shortening of the proximal long bones (i.e., rhizomelia), specific radiologic abnormalities (i.e., the presence of stippled calcifications of cartilage, vertebral body clefting), joint contractures, congenital cataracts, ichthyosis, and severe mental retardation. Skin changes are present in approximately 25 percent of patients. Patients have low levels of red cell plasmalogens and accumulation of phytanic acid, starting with normal levels at birth and increasing to more than 10 times normal by age 1 year. RCDP is a disorder of peroxisomes, membrane bound multifunctional organelles found in all nucleated cells. Their functions vary with cell type and include a variety of pathways (e.g., hydrogen peroxide based respiration, fatty acid β-oxidation, and lipid and cholesterol synthesis) involving the synthesis and degradation of various compounds. Hereditary human peroxisomal disorders are subdivided into disorders of peroxisome biogenesis, in which the organelle is not formed normally, and those involving a single peroxisomal enzyme. RCDP is one of the group of peroxisome biogenesis disorders, which are characterized by loss of multiple peroxisomal metabolic functions and have been sorted into at least 12 different complementation groups. Many have been found to be due to defects in peroxins, factors required for the import of proteins into the organelle. RCDP is caused by mutations in *PEX7,* a gene that encodes peroxin 7, a receptor required for targeting a subset of enzymes to peroxisomes.[90] Refsum's disease, another peroxisome disorder, exhibits genetic heterogeneity. In Refsum's disease due to mutations in *PAHX,* the gene for PhyH, there is deficiency of the single peroxisomal enzyme PhyH. Refsum's disease can also result from mutations in *PEX7,* and fibroblast cell cultures from those patients show deficiency of several peroxisomal enzymes similar to fibroblasts from patients with RCDP. It is remarkable that different mutations in the same gene can result in such a wide spectrum of clinical disease.

X-linked recessive chondrodysplasia punctata (CDPX) can involve skin (linear or whorled atrophic or ichthyosiform hyperkeratosis, follicular atrophoderma; may begin as erythroderma) (Fig. 51-15), hair (coarse, lusterless, cicatricial alopecia), short stature and skeletal abnormalities, cataracts, and deafness. Curry et al. studied a family who had atypical ichthyosis and elevated cholesterol sulfate in two affected males and identified an X chromosomal deletion (Xp22) that included the gene for steroid sulfatase.[88] There is a cluster of arylsulfatase genes at this location. Mutations in *ARSE,* the gene encoding the enzyme arylsulfatase E, were found in five patients; however, it is possible that the disorder may also be caused by mutations in adjacent arylsulfatase genes.[91] The similarity to warfarin embryopathy suggests that warfarin embryopathy may be due to drug-induced inhibition of the same enzyme.

Happle and coworkers identified X-linked dominant chondrodysplasia punctata (CDPX2) (Conradi-Hünermann-Happle syndrome) as a distinct variant characterized by a mosaic pattern of skin involvement and occurrence almost exclusively in females, with loss of the gene function hypothesized to be lethal to males.[87,92] Affected females have a normal life expectancy and there may be increased disease ex-

FIGURE 51-15

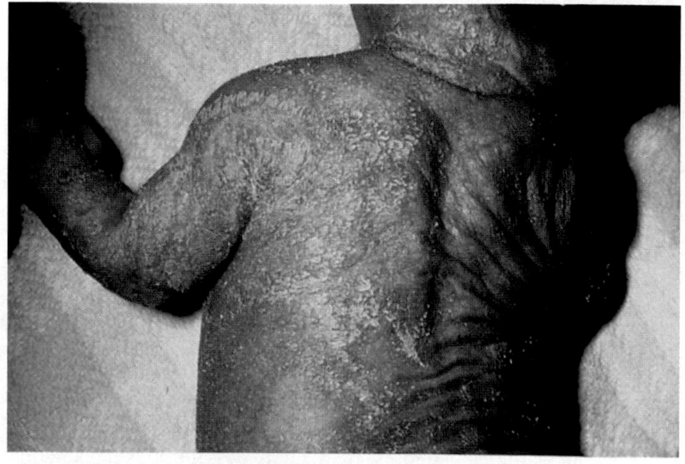

Chondrodysplasia punctata. Newborn child. Generalized erythroderma with scales forming a whorled pattern.

pression in successive generations (anticipation). Occurrence in a male has been observed in association with a 47,XYY karyotype. CDPX2 presents at birth as a congenital ichthyosiform erythroderma that clears over months and is replaced by linear hyperkeratosis, follicular atrophoderma, and pigmentary abnormalities. Happle hypothesized that the linear involvement is due to mosaic X-chromosome inactivation (Lyonization). Hair shaft abnormalities and cicatricial alopecia can also occur. Stippled calcifications are seen in radiographs of areas of endochondral bone formation during childhood but may no longer be visible after puberty. Stature may be short, with asymmetric shortening of the legs. Cataracts occur, usually asymmetrically, in about two-thirds of patients. Histochemical staining for calcium may show calcifications within the epidermis, especially within hair follicles, in young children, which may not be present in older children.[93] Mutations in the gene encoding the emopamil-binding protein (EBP) cause the Conradi-Hünermann-Happle Syndrome. EBP was first identified as a binding target for the drug emopamil, a calcium-channel blocker. It was later found to be 3β-hydroxysteroid-Δ8-Δ7-isomerase that catalyses an intermediate step in the conversion of lanosterol to cholesterol.[94] How this defect causes clinical manifestations is unclear.

The *CHILD syndrome* is a rare disorder consisting of *c*ongenital *h*emidysplasia, *i*chthyosiform erythroderma, and *l*imb *d*efects, which is found almost exclusively in females.[95] The disorder is related to CDPX2, also has skin and skeletal abnormalities, but is distinguished by a sharp midline demarcation of the ichthyosis, with minimal linear or segmental contralateral involvement. Involvement of the right side occurs more frequently than the left. There may be bands of normal skin on the affected side. A case with bilateral involvement has been described. Limb defects occur ipsilateral to the ichthyosis and range from digital hypoplasia to agenesis of the extremity. There may be punctate calcification of cartilage. Unilateral hypoplasia can involve the central nervous system and cardiovascular, pulmonary, renal, endocrine, and genitourinary systems. Studies of kindreds have suggested both an autosomal dominant and recessive inheritance as well as an X-linked dominant form that is lethal in males. Peroxisomal deficiency has been described in a study that showed fibroblasts from involved skin had fewer peroxisomes and accumulated cytoplasmic lipid; ultrastructurally, they accumulated lamellated membrane and vacuolar structures. Subsequently, mutations in either of two peroxisomal genes were found to cause CHILD syndrome. One patient was found to have a mutation in the gene encoding EBP (3β-hydroxysteroid-Δ8-Δ7-isomerase) (the gene underlying CDPX2)[96] and six patients (including one boy) were found to have mutations in NSDHL (*N*AD(P)H *s*teroid *deh*ydrogenase-*l*ike protein) encoding a 3β-hydroxysteroid dehydrogenase.[97] Each enzyme functions in the cholesterol biosynthetic pathway catalyzing intermediate steps in the conversion of lanosterol to cholesterol.

In 1971, Tay described an autosomal recessive disorder characterized by a congenital ichthyosiform erythroderma, growth and mental retardation, progeria-like facies, and brittle hair. This association of *ichthyosis, brittle hair, intellectual impairment, decreased fertility, and short stature* has been given the acronym *IBIDS syndrome* (*Tay's syndrome, trichothiodystrophy*).[98] Newborns may have a collodion presentation, followed by decreasing erythema over weeks and evolution into a generalized ichthyosis, usually without erythema, which varies from fine, translucent scaling to large, dark yellow-brown hyperkeratosis.[98,99] There may be flexural sparing, palmoplantar keratoderma, and dystrophic nails (ridging, splitting). Ectropion usually does not occur. There can be low birth weight, lack of subcutaneous fat (progeria-like facies), short stature, and delayed psychomotor development. Hypogonadism manifests as cryptorchidism in males and impaired sexual maturation in females. An increased susceptibility to infection has been described. Hair is sparse and under microscopic examination shows trichoschisis (transverse fracturing), pili torti, trichorrhexis nodosa (transverse, frayed fractures), and undulating contour of the shaft; under polarization, it has a pattern of alternating bright- and dark-banding (tiger-tail) (Fig. 51-16).[98,100] Banded hairs have abnormally low sulfur content due to a decrease in sulfur-containing amino acids, which led to the term *trichothiodystrophy,* which was coined by Price.

A spectrum of trichothiodystrophy-related syndromes has been recognized.[101] Similar hair and systemic abnormalities but without the ichthyosiform changes have been described as the *BIDS syndrome* (*b*rittle hair, *i*ntellectual impairment, *d*ecreased fertility, and *s*hort stature). A similar constellation of findings, with the addition of photosensitivity, is distinguished as *PIBI(D)S syndrome*.[102] In contrast to IBIDS syndrome, the ichthyosis is mild and not congenital, and hypogonadism is usually absent. There is a relationship with xeroderma pigmentosum in that virtually all PIBI(D)S patients have a deficiency in the nucleotide excision repair (NER) of UV-induced DNA damage that is indistinguishable from that of xeroderma pigmentosum group D, and mutations have been found in the XP group D helicase gene (*ERCC2/XPD*). In a few patients, mutations have been found in the

FIGURE 51-16

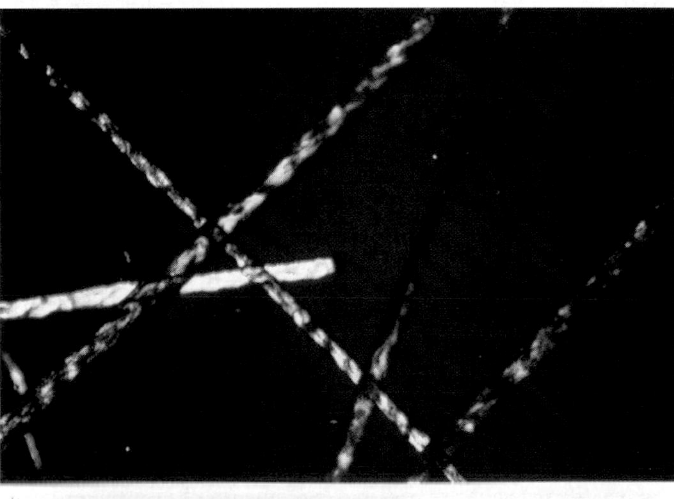

A.

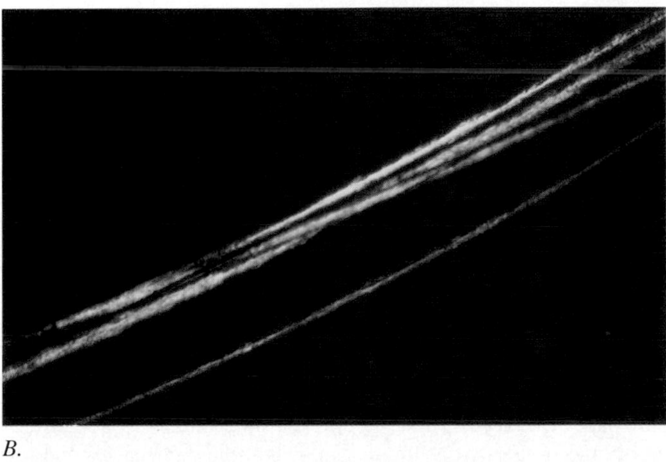

B.

Trichothiodystrophy hair shows tiger-tail banding (*A*) under polarization, which is not observed with normal hair (*B*).

XP complementation group B helicase gene (*ERCC3/XPB*). Although many trichothiodystrophy patients have photosensitivity, in contrast to xeroderma pigmentosum, these photosensitive patients have not been observed to be at high risk for the development of skin cancer. NER is one normal cellular mechanism by which structural DNA damage (e.g., UV induced cyclobutane pyrimidine dimers) is removed and repaired (see Chaps. 35 and 155). TFIIH is involved in the initiation of transcription and in NER, and consists of a complex of proteins including the XPD and XPB proteins. In the vicinity of the damage, these two helicase subunits of TFIIH unwind the DNA in opposite directions.

Chanarin-Dorfman syndrome (neutral lipid storage disease) is an autosomal recessive disorder characterized by accumulation of triglycerides in the cytoplasm of leukocytes, muscle, liver, fibroblasts, and other tissues. Blood lipid levels, however, are normal. To date, approximately 30 patients have been reported, mainly from the Mediterranean basin. The ichthyosis is a generalized fine scaling with variable erythema, resembling congenital ichthyosiform erythroderma. Presentation is often that of a collodion baby with ectropion and eclabion. Extracutaneous involvement, which is variable and may be mild, includes cataracts, decreased hearing, psychomotor delay, myopathy with elevations in serum muscle enzymes, and neurologic abnormalities.

Histopathology of an oil red O or Sudan III stain of frozen sections of the skin shows lipid droplets in dermal cells, in the basal layer (and, to a lesser extent, suprabasally), as well as in the acrosyringia of the eccrine ducts. On electron-microscopic examination there are lipid droplets within the cytoplasm and within lamellar bodies, which disrupt the normal lamellations. These distortions persist after extrusion into the intercellular space.[103] Examination of peripheral blood smears show lipid vacuoles within granulocytes, eosinophils, and monocytes, a feature that may also be present in carriers.[104] Lefèvre et al. identified mutations in the *CGI-58* gene in nine families.[105] CGI-58 belongs to a large family of proteins, most of which are enzymes; however, its exact function has not yet been elucidated.

Multiple sulfatase deficiency is a rare autosomal recessive disorder that is characterized by a deficiency of several sulfatases, which results in the accumulation of sulfatides, glycosaminoglycans, sphingolipids, and steroid sulfates in tissues and body fluids.[106] The activity of both lysosomal (arylsulfatases A and B) and microsomal (arylsulfatase C/steroid sulfatase of X-linked ichthyosis) arylsulfatases is impaired. The disorder is a composite of the clinical features of both metachromatic leukodystrophy and of a mucopolysaccharidosis. Clinical features include neurologic deterioration, skeletal abnormalities, facial dysmorphism, and an ichthyosis resembling that seen in X-linked steroid sulfatase deficiency. This disorder has been proposed to be due to a defect, common to all sulfatases, in posttranslational protein modification that is required for generating a catalytically active enzyme.[107]

The *peeling skin syndrome* is an autosomal recessive disorder characterized by lifelong peeling of the stratum corneum. It may be associated with pruritus, short stature, and easily removed anagen hairs. Low plasma tryptophan levels and aminoaciduria have also been reported.[108] Traupe suggested that there are two types of peeling skin syndrome.[33] Type A, which is noninflammatory and asymptomatic, is characterized by generalized peeling in thin superficial flakes of differing size and shape. On electron microscopy, the intracellular separation occurs in the stratum corneum, that is, within the corneocytes and not between adjacent cells. Intercellular electron-dense globular deposits representing abnormal lipids have been observed localized to the stratum corneum.[109] In contrast, type B presents with congenital ichthyotic erythroderma and evolves into erythematous, scaling, migratory patches. This type is pruritic and may be associated with elevated levels of IgE, aminoaciduria, and short stature. The stratum corneum is easily separated mechanically from the lower epidermis, and histologically the split, which occurs intercellularly, is seen between the stratum corneum and the granular layer. On electron microscopy, electron-dense, irregularly vacuolated bodies have been observed in the granular layer, but observations have been variable.[110] A variant, clinically similar to the inflammatory type B but with associated hair shaft abnormalities has been described.[110]

Rud's syndrome is a poorly characterized disorder, probably of recessive inheritance, that includes epilepsy, mental retardation, infantilism, congenital ichthyosis, and retinitis pigmentosa. Steroid sulfatase deficiency has been reported in some patients. Traupe critically reviewed the literature and suggested that the clinical constellation usually labeled Rud's syndrome is associated steroid sulfatase deficiency (X-linked recessive ichthyosis); because both the neurologic involvement and the ichthyosis are ill defined, the term *Rud's syndrome* should be abandoned.[33]

TREATMENT

Current therapies for the inherited ichthyoses are symptomatic and focus on hydration, lubrication, and keratolysis. Ichthyotic skin, even if thickened, has a decreased barrier function and increased transepidermal water loss. Because pliability of the stratum corneum is a function of its water content, hydration can soften the surface of the skin. In moist, humid climates, most ichthyoses improve, and mild ichthyoses (e.g., ichthyosis vulgaris) may undergo extensive clearing. Moistening the skin with, for example, long baths, can hydrate it. Well-hydrated areas of hyperkeratosis can more easily be thinned with mild abrasives (sponges, buff puffs, pumice stones, etc.). Addition of bath oils or application of lubricants before drying can prolong the hydration and softening. Depending on the ichthyosis and environmental conditions, individual patients may prefer specific lubricating agents, which can take the form of lotions, creams, ointments, oils, or petrolatum. In dry climates and winter months, humidifiers can be used to create a hospitable environment.

Keratolytic agents are used to enhance corneocyte disadhesion and thereby remove scale and thin hyperkeratotic stratum corneum. There are many commercially available keratolytic creams and lotions containing urea, salicylic acid, or α-hydroxy acids (e.g., lactic acid, glycolic acid). Urea may function by its capacity to bind water. Propylene glycol (60% in water), with or without occlusion, can also be effective in scale removal. Occlusion can effectively increase skin hydration and facilitate desquamation; it can also enhance the effect of keratolytic agents. Special care should be taken when using extensive areas of occlusion with keratolytic agents and in individuals who may be heat intolerant. Topical retinoid or vitamin D preparations may also be effective but can be irritating in some patients. The markedly impaired barrier function in ichthyosis should be considered when using topical preparations over large areas of body surface. For example, widespread use of topical salicylic acid preparations can lead to significant absorption, intoxication (e.g., nausea, tinnitus, dyspnea, hallucinations), and even death.[111] Children are at greater risk because they have a greater body surface area per unit weight than adults, a situation that effectively heightens the possibility of developing systemic toxicity from topicals.[33] The abnormal skin barrier should be considered when treating concomitant dermatoses in ichthyosis patients. Topical 0.1% tacrolimus ointment is effective in atopic dermatitis with minimal systemic absorption. However, the atopic dermatitis of Netherton's syndrome is complicated by a defective ichthyotic skin barrier. The defective barrier is associated with increased percutaneous absorption and risk for systemic toxic effects. This should be considered when using topical agents such as tacrolimus, where increased systemic absorption has been observed and monitoring of serum levels may be necessary.[68]

Another risk to children is that in several types of ichthyosis, because of the large turnover of scale, nutritional requirements may be high, and inadequate nutrition can lead to failure to thrive. Some patients with ichthyosis (particularly LI and CIE) have decreased sweating with heat intolerance. It is important for the parents of a newborn with ichthyosis to be aware of the possibility of decreased sweating and to be attentive for signs of heat intolerance, such as flushing and lethargy, particularly during hot weather and, as the child grows, during exercise. Avoiding hot environments and carrying spray bottles with water to moisten the skin and cool it through evaporation can minimize heat stress.

Systemic retinoid therapy with isotretinoin or acitretin can induce dramatic improvement in many ichthyoses and is particularly useful in LI, CIE, and erythrokeratodermia variabilis. The decision to initiate systemic retinoid therapy should be weighed carefully, because once the drug is started, continued benefit usually requires chronic therapy. Treatment of the harlequin newborn with systemic retinoid therapy during the newborn period can be lifesaving due to enhanced desquamation of a constricting membrane.

Fungal infections are common, both of skin and nails, and are often undiagnosed because of the generalized scaling. A high index of suspicion can help diagnose tinea corporis, capitis, or versicolor where the only symptom may be localized pruritus and the only sign a difference in the character of scale or a localized area of alopecia.

The management of epidermolytic hyperkeratosis has acute and chronic aspects and varies with the clinical type. Areas of thick, hard hyperkeratosis, which are not pliable and have a hard rough surface, are prone to mechanical trauma. In patients with the hystrix type of porcupine-like hyperkeratosis, the rough surface causes high traction with objects moving across the skin surface, which tend to catch on the hyperkeratotic horn and peel it off. Topical agents such as lubricants and keratolytics can reduce the thickened, rough areas and help to minimize blistering and erosion. Bacterial infection of the skin is common, often leads to enhanced blistering, and may require frequent therapy with topical and oral antibiotics. In patients with extensive involvement, systemic retinoid therapy can be dramatically effective in decreasing the hyperkeratosis and the frequency of infections. Because these drugs can enhance blistering in epidermolytic hyperkeratosis patients, they should be administered carefully and started at low doses.

PRENATAL DIAGNOSIS

Molecular diagnosis is preferred when possible. Alternative methods, including fetoscopy and fetal skin biopsy, have the disadvantage of not being able to be performed early in pregnancy. Both harbor a risk of fetal mortality. Fetal skin biopsy at approximately 20 to 22 weeks' gestation has been accomplished in LI, CIE, epidermolytic hyperkeratosis, and Sjögren-Larsson syndrome. In harlequin ichthyosis, prenatal diagnosis has been successfully performed by fetal skin biopsy[112] and ultrasonography.[113] When it is possible to do prenatal diagnosis by molecular analysis of a fetal sample, it is optimally performed early in pregnancy. This can be done with chorionic villous sampling or by amniocentesis in disorders where the underlying genetic defect is known and the specific mutation in the family has been identified. If a specific mutation has not been identified, in some circumstances where there is an appropriate family structure, prenatal diagnosis can be done using linkage analysis. Prenatal diagnosis by mutational analysis has been accomplished in epidermolytic hyperkeratosis;[114] lamellar ichthyosis (*TGM1*); Sjögren-Larsson syndrome (*FALDH*); ichthyosis bullosa of Siemens (*K2e*); PIBI(D)S (*ERCC2/XPD, ERCC3/XPB*); autosomal recessive rhizomelic chondrodysplasia punctata (*PEX7*); X-linked chondrodysplasia punctata (arylsulfatase gene cluster at Xp22); and Netherton's syndrome (*SPINK5*).[67] In Sjögren-Larsson syndrome, the diagnosis can be made by assay of enzyme activity in cultured amniocytes, even if the mutation in FALDH is undefined. For autosomal recessive disorders where the mutation is known (e.g., LI and Sjögren-Larsson syndrome), carrier detection may be performed for at-risk relatives.

The National Registry for Ichthyosis and Related Disorders is funded by the National Institutes of Health to identify and enroll individuals affected with the ichthyoses in an effort to improve diagnosis and treatment of these disorders and is located at the University of Washington, Dermatology/Box 356524, Rm.BB1353, 1959 NE Pacific St., Seattle, WA 98195-6524 (Tel: 1-800-595-1265; http://www. skinregistry.org/; e-mail: info@skinregistry.org).

The Foundation for Ichthyosis and Related Skin Types is an organization providing support and information for affected individuals, family members, and friends. It can be reached at F.I.R.S.T., Suite 17, 650 N. Cannon Avenue, Lansdale, PA 19446 (Tel: 215-631-1411; http://www.scalyskin.org/; e-mail: info@scalyskin.org).

REFERENCES

1. Willan R: *On Cutaneous Diseases*. Vol 1., London, Barnard, 1808
2. Frost P, Van Scott EJ: Ichthyosiform dermatoses. Classification based on anatomic and biometric observations. *Arch Dermatol* **94**:113, 1966
3. Frost P: Ichthyosiform dermatoses. *J Invest Dermatol* **60**:541, 1973
4. Williams ML, Elias PM: Genetically transmitted, generalized disorders of cornification. The ichthyoses. *Dermatol Clin* **5**:155, 1987
5. DiGiovanna JJ, Bale SJ: Epidermolytic hyperkeratosis: Applied molecular genetics. *J Invest Dermatol* **102**:390, 1994
6. Bale SJ, DiGiovanna JJ: Genetic approaches to understanding the keratinopathies. *Adv Dermatol* **12**:99, 114, 1997
7. Richard G: Connexins: A connection with the skin. *Exp Dermatol* **9**:77, 2000
8. Russell LJ et al: Linkage of autosomal recessive lamellar ichthyosis to chromosome 14q. *Am J Hum Genet* **55**:1146, 1994
9. Russell LJ et al: Mutations in the gene for transglutaminase 1 in autosomal recessive lamellar ichthyosis. *Nat Genet* **9**:279, 1995
10. Huber M et al: Mutations of keratinocyte transglutaminase in lamellar ichthyosis. *Science* **267**:525, 1995
11. Nemes Z et al: A novel function for transglutaminase 1: attachment of long-chain omega-hydroxyceramides to involucrin by ester bond formation. *Proc Natl Acad Sci USA* **96**:8402, 1999
12. Webster D et al: X linked ichthyosis due to steroid-sulphatase deficiency. *Lancet* **1**:70, 1978
13. Koppe G et al: X-linked ichthyosis. A sulphatase deficiency. *Arch Dis Child* **53**:803, 1978
14. Williams ML et al: Ichthyosis induced by cholesterol-lowering drugs. Implications for epidermal cholesterol homeostasis. *Arch Dermatol* **123**:1535, 1987
15. Wells RS, Kerr CB: Clinical features of autosomal dominant and sex-linked ichthyosis in an English population. *Br Med J* **1**:947, 1966
16. Mevorah B et al: Autosomal dominant ichthyosis and X-linked ichthyosis. Comparison of their clinical and histological phenotypes. *Acta Derm Venereol* **71**:431, 1991
17. Cuevas-Covarrubias SA et al: Accuracy of the clinical diagnosis of recessive X-linked ichthyosis vs ichthyosis vulgaris. *J Dermatol* **23**:594, 1996
18. Anton-Lamprecht I, Hofbauer M: Ultrastructural distinction of autosomal dominant ichthyosis vulgaris and X-linked recessive ichthyosis. *Humangenetik* **15**:261, 1972
19. Nirunsuksiri W et al: Decreased profilaggrin expression in ichthyosis vulgaris is a result of selectively impaired posttranscriptional control. *J Biol Chem* **270**:871, 1995

20. Rose FA: Review: The mammalian sulphatases and placental sulphatase deficiency in man. *J Inherit Metab Dis* **5**:145, 1982
21. Epstein EH Jr, Leventhal ME: Steroid sulfatase of human leukocytes and epidermis and the diagnosis of recessive X-linked ichthyosis. *J Clin Invest* **67**:1257, 1981
22. Lykkesfeldt G et al: Placental steroid sulfatase deficiency: Biochemical diagnosis and clinical review. *Obstet Gynecol* **64**:49, 1984
23. Jay B et al: Ocular manifestations of ichthyosis. *Br J Ophthalmol* **52**:217, 1968
24. Sever RJ et al: Eye changes in ichthyosis. *JAMA* **206**:2283, 1968
25. Lykkesfeldt G et al: Testis cancer. Ichthyosis constitutes a significant risk factor. *Cancer* **67**:730, 1991
26. Epstein EH Jr, Bonifas JM: Recessive X-linked ichthyosis: Lack of immunologically detectable steroid sulfatase enzyme protein. *Hum Genet* **71**:201, 1985
27. Ballabio A et al: Deletion of the distal short arm of the X chromosome (Xp) in a patient with short stature, chondrodysplasia punctata, and X- linked ichthyosis due to steroid sulfatase deficiency. *Am J Med Genet* **41**:184, 1991
28. Robledo R et al: X-linked ichthyosis without STS deficiency: Clinical, genetical, and molecular studies. *Am J Med Genet* **59**:143, 1995
29. Simpson JR: Congenital ichthyosiform erythroderma. *Trans St John's Hosp Derm Soc* **50**:93, 1964
30. Williams ML, Elias PM: Heterogeneity in autosomal recessive ichthyosis. Clinical and biochemical differentiation of lamellar ichthyosis and nonbullous congenital ichthyosiform erythroderma. *Arch Dermatol* **121**:477, 1985
31. Bernhardt M, Baden HP: Report of a family with an unusual expression of recessive ichthyosis. Review of 42 cases. *Arch Dermatol* **122**:428, 1986
32. Frenk E, de Techtermann F: Self-healing collodion baby: Evidence for autosomal recessive inheritance. *Pediatr Dermatol* **9**:95, 1992
33. Traupe H: *The Ichthyoses: A Guide To Clinical Diagnosis, Genetic Counseling, and Therapy*. New York, Springer-Verlag, 1989, page 116
34. Choate KA et al: Corrective gene transfer in the human skin disorder lamellar ichthyosis. *Nat Med* **2**:1263, 1996
35. Fischer J et al: Two new loci for autosomal recessive ichthyosis on chromosomes 3p21 and 19p12-q12 and evidence for further genetic heterogeneity. *Am J Hum Genet* **66**:904, 2000
36. Bale SJ et al: Congenital recessive ichthyosis unlinked to loci for epidermal transglutaminases. *J Invest Dermatol* **107**:808, 1996
37. Matsumoto K et al: Loricrin keratoderma: A cause of congenital ichthyosiform erythroderma and collodion baby. *Br J Dermatol* **145**:657, 2001
38. DiGiovanna JJ, Bale SJ: Clinical heterogeneity in epidermolytic hyperkeratosis. *Arch Dermatol* **130**:1026, 1994
39. Paller AS et al: Genetic and clinical mosaicism in a type of epidermal nevus. *N Engl J Med* **331**:1408, 1994
40. Nazzaro V et al: Epidermolytic hyperkeratosis: Generalized form in children from parents with systematized linear form. *Br J Dermatol* **122**: 417, 1990
41. Compton JG et al: Linkage of epidermolytic hyperkeratosis to the type II keratin gene cluster on chromosome 12q. *Nat Genet* **1**:301, 1992
42. Chipev CC et al: A leucine-proline mutation in the H1 subdomain of keratin 1 causes epidermolytic hyperkeratosis. *Cell* **70**:821, 1992
43. Reis A et al: Keratin 9 gene mutations in epidermolytic palmoplantar keratoderma (EPPK). *Nat Genet* **6**:174, 1994
44. Rothnagel JA et al: Mutations in the rod domain of keratin 2e in patients with ichthyosis bullosa of Siemens. *Nat Genet* **7**:485, 1994
45. Sprecher E et al: Evidence for novel functions of the keratin tail emerging from a mutation causing ichthyosis hystrix. *J Invest Dermatol* **116**:511, 2001
46. Giroux JD et al: Severe hypernatremic dehydration disclosing Netherton syndrome in the neonatal period. *Arch Fr Pediatr* **50**:585, 1993
47. Waring JI: Early mention of a harlequin fetus in America. *Am J Dis Child* **43**:442, 1932
48. Roberts LJ: Long-term survival of a harlequin fetus. *J Am Acad Dermatol* **21**:335, 1989
49. Haftek M et al: A longitudinal study of a harlequin infant presenting clinically as non-bullous congenital ichthyosiform erythroderma. *Br J Dermatol* **135**:448, 1996
50. Unamuno P et al: Harlequin foetus in four siblings. *Br J Dermatol* **116**:569, 1987
51. Milner ME et al: Abnormal lamellar granules in harlequin ichthyosis. *J Invest Dermatol* **99**:824, 1992
52. Schwartz RA, Williams ML: Acquired ichthyosis: A marker for internal disease. *Am Fam Physician* **29**:181, 1984
53. Goodman DS et al: Prevalence of cutaneous disease in patients with acquired immunodeficiency syndrome (AIDS) or AIDS-related complex. *J Am Acad Dermatol* **17**:210, 1987
54. Kaplan MH et al: Acquired ichthyosis in concomitant HIV-1 and HTLV-II infection: A new association with intravenous drug abuse. *J Am Acad Dermatol* **29**:701, 1993
55. Feind-Koopmans AG et al: Acquired ichthyosiform erythroderma and sarcoidosis. *J Am Acad Dermatol* **35**:826, 1996
56. Humbert P, Agache P: Acquired ichthyosis: A new cutaneous marker of autoimmunity. *Arch Dermatol* **127**:263, 1991
57. de la Cruz-Alvarez J et al: Acquired ichthyosis associated with eosinophilic fasciitis. *J Am Acad Dermatol* **34**:1079, 1996
58. Spelman LJ et al: Acquired ichthyosis in bone marrow transplant recipients. *J Am Acad Dermatol* **35**:17, 1996
59. Jang HS et al: Six cases of confluent and reticulated papillomatosis alleviated by various antibiotics. *J Am Acad Dermatol* **44**:652, 2001
60. Montemarano AD et al: Confluent and reticulated papillomatosis: Response to minocycline. *J Am Acad Dermatol* **34**:253, 1996
61. Altman J, Stroud J: Netherton's syndrome and ichthyosis linearis circumflexa. *Arch Dermatol* **100**:550, 1969
62. Hurwitz S et al: Reevaluation of ichthyosis and hair shaft abnormalities. *Arch Dermatol* **103**:266, 1971
63. Stoll C et al: Severe hypernatremic dehydration in an infant with Netherton syndrome. *Genet Couns* **12**:237, 2001
64. Powell J: Increasing the likelihood of early diagnosis of Netherton syndrome by simple examination of eyebrow hairs. *Arch Dermatol* **136**:423, 2000
65. Chavanas S et al: Mutations in SPINK5, encoding a serine protease inhibitor, cause Netherton syndrome. *Nat Genet* **25**:141, 2000
66. Walley AJ et al: Gene polymorphism in Netherton and common atopic disease. *Nat Genet* **29**:175, 2001
67. Sprecher E et al: The spectrum of pathogenic mutations in SPINK5 in 19 families with Netherton syndrome: Implications for mutation detection and first case of prenatal diagnosis. *J Invest Dermatol* **117**:179, 2001
68. Allen A et al: Significant absorption of topical tacrolimus in 3 patients with Netherton syndrome. *Arch Dermatol* **137**:747, 2001
69. Jagell S, Liden S: Ichthyosis in the Sjögren-Larsson syndrome. *Clin Genet* **21**:243, 1982
70. Rizzo WB et al: Fatty aldehyde dehydrogenase: Genomic structure, expression and mutation analysis in Sjögren-Larsson syndrome. *Chem Biol Interact* **130–132**:297, 2001
71. De Laurenzi V et al: Sjögren-Larsson syndrome is caused by mutations in the fatty aldehyde dehydrogenase gene. *Nat Genet* **12**:52, 1996
72. Nigro JF et al: Redefining the Sjögren-Larsson syndrome: Atypical findings in three siblings and implications regarding diagnosis. *J Am Acad Dermatol* **35**:678, 1996
73. Giroux JM, Barbeau A: Erythrokeratodermia with ataxia. *Arch Dermatol* **106**:183, 1972
74. Richard G et al: Linkage studies in erythrokeratodermias: Fine mapping, genetic heterogeneity, and analysis of candidate genes. *J Invest Dermatol* **109**:666, 1997
75. Richard G et al: Mutations in the human connexin gene GJB3 cause erythrokeratodermia variabilis. *Nat Genet* **20**:366, 1998
76. Macari F et al: Mutation in the gene for connexin 30.3 in a family with erythrokeratodermia variabilis. *Am J Hum Genet* **67**:1296, 2000
77. Ruiz-Maldonado R et al: Erythrokeratodermia progressiva symmetrica: Report of 10 cases. *Dermatologica* **164**:133, 1982
78. Ishida-Yamamoto A et al: The molecular pathology of progressive symmetric erythrokeratoderma: A frameshift mutation in the loricrin gene and perturbations in the cornified cell envelope. *Am J Hum Genet* **61**:581, 1997
79. Caceres-Rios H et al: Keratitis, ichthyosis, and deafness (KID syndrome): Review of the literature and proposal of a new terminology. *Pediatr Dermatol* **13**:105, 1996
80. Richard G et al: Missense mutations in *GJB2* encoding connexin-26 cause the ectodermal dysplasia Keratitis-Ichthyosis-Deafness Syndrome. *Am J Hum Genet* **70**:1341, 2002
81. Maestrini E et al: A molecular defect in loricrin, the major component of the cornified cell envelope, underlies Vohwinkel's syndrome. *Nat Genet* **13**:70, 1996
82. Davies MG et al: Epidermal abnormalities in Refsum's disease. *Br J Dermatol* **97**:401, 1977
83. Jansen GA et al: Refsum disease is caused by mutations in the phytanoyl-CoA hydroxylase gene. *Nat Genet* **17**:190, 1997

84. Wanders RJ et al: Refsum disease, peroxisomes and phytanic acid oxidation: A review. *J Neuropathol Exp Neurol* **60**:1021, 2001
85. Kitareewan S et al: Phytol metabolites are circulating dietary factors that activate the nuclear receptor RXR. *Mol Biol Cell* **7**:1153, 1996
86. Poulos A et al: Patterns of Refsum's disease. Phytanic acid oxidase deficiency. *Arch Dis Child* **59**:222, 1984
87. Happle R: X-linked dominant chondrodysplasia punctata. Review of literature and report of a case. *Hum Genet* **53**:65, 1979
88. Curry CJ et al: Inherited chondrodysplasia punctata due to a deletion of the terminal short arm of an X chromosome. *N Engl J Med* **311**:1010, 1984
89. Hosenfeld D, Wiedemann HR: Chondrodysplasia punctata in an adult recognized as vitamin K antagonist embryopathy. *Clin Genet* **35**:376, 1989
90. Motley AM et al: Mutational spectrum in the PEX7 gene and functional analysis of mutant alleles in 78 patients with rhizomelic chondrodysplasia punctata type 1. *Am J Hum Genet* **70**:612, 2002
91. Franco B et al: A cluster of sulfatase genes on Xp22.3: Mutations in chondrodysplasia punctata (CDPX) and implications for warfarin embryopathy. *Cell* **81**:15, 1995
92. Happle R: X-linked dominant ichthyosis. *Clin Genet* **15**:239, 1979
93. Kolde G, Happle R: Histologic and ultrastructural features of the ichthyotic skin in X-linked dominant chondrodysplasia punctata. *Acta Derm Venereol* **64**:389, 1984
94. Becker K et al: Identification of a novel mutation in 3beta-hydroxysteroid-Delta8- Delta7-isomerase in a case of Conradi-Hünermann-Happle syndrome. *Exp Dermatol* **10**:286, 2001
95. Herman GE: X-Linked dominant disorders of cholesterol biosynthesis in man and mouse. *Biochim Biophys Acta* **1529**:357, 2000
96. Grange DK et al: CHILD syndrome caused by deficiency of 3beta-hydroxysteroid-delta8, delta7-isomerase. *Am J Med Genet* **90**:328, 2000
97. Konig A et al: Mutations in the NSDHL gene, encoding a 3beta-hydroxysteroid dehydrogenase, cause CHILD syndrome. *Am J Med Genet* **90**:339, 2000
98. Jorizzo JL et al: Ichthyosis, brittle hair, impaired intelligence, decreased fertility and short stature (IBIDS syndrome). *Br J Dermatol* **106**:705, 1982
99. Happle R et al: The Tay syndrome (congenital ichthyosis with trichothiodystrophy). *Eur J Pediatr* **141**:147, 1984
100. Broughton BC et al: Two individuals with features of both xeroderma pigmentosum and trichothiodystrophy highlight the complexity of the clinical outcomes of mutations in the XPD gene. *Hum Mol Genet* **10**:2539, 2001
101. Itin PH et al: Trichothiodystrophy: update on the sulfur-deficient brittle hair syndromes. *J Am Acad Dermatol* **44**:891, 2001
102. Rebora A, Crovato F: PIBI(D)S syndrome—Trichothiodystrophy with xeroderma pigmentosum (group D) mutation. *J Am Acad Dermatol* **16**:940, 1987
103. Elias PM, Williams ML: Neutral lipid storage disease with ichthyosis. Defective lamellar body contents and intracellular dispersion. *Arch Dermatol* **121**:1000, 1985
104. Srebrnik A et al: Dorfman-Chanarin syndrome. A case report and a review. *J Am Acad Dermatol* **17**:801, 1987
105. Lefevre C et al: Mutations in CGI-58, the gene encoding a new protein of the esterase/lipase/thioesterase subfamily, in Chanarin-Dorfman syndrome. *Am J Hum Genet* **69**:1002, 2001
106. Soong BW et al: Multiple sulfatase deficiency. *Neurology* **38**:1273, 1988
107. Schmidt B et al: A novel amino acid modification in sulfatases that is defective in multiple sulfatase deficiency. *Cell* **82**:271, 1995
108. Aras N et al: Peeling skin syndrome *J Am Acad Dermatol* **30**:135, 1994
109. Silverman AK et al: Continual skin peeling syndrome. An electron microscopic study. *Arch Dermatol* **122**:71, 1986
110. Mevorah B et al: Peeling skin syndrome with hair changes. *Dermatology* **197**:373, 1998
111. Germann R et al: Life-threatening salicylate poisoning caused by percutaneous absorption in severe ichthyosis vulgaris [in German]. *Hautarzt* **47**:624, 1996
112. Suzumori K, Kanzaki T: Prenatal diagnosis of harlequin ichthyosis by fetal skin biopsy; report of two cases. *Prenat Diagn* **11**:451, 1991
113. Watson WJ, Mabee LM Jr: Prenatal diagnosis of severe congenital ichthyosis (harlequin fetus) by ultrasonography. *J Ultrasound Med* **14**:241, 1995
114. Rothnagel JA et al: Prenatal diagnosis of epidermolytic hyperkeratosis by direct gene sequencing. *J Invest Dermatol* **102**:13, 1994

CHAPTER 52

Howard P. Stevens
David P. Kelsell
Irene M. Leigh

The Inherited Keratodermas of Palms and Soles

DEFINITIONS AND CLASSIFICATIONS

The palmoplantar keratodermas (PPKs) are a heterogeneous group of disorders characterized by abnormal thickening of the palms and soles. Autosomal recessive, X-linked, and dominant modes of inheritance as well as acquired forms have all been described. The acquired forms are listed in Table 52-1, and most are discussed in detail elsewhere in this text. Other genodermatoses associated with PPK are listed in Table 52-2. Clinically, three distinct clinical patterns of PPK may be identified[1]:

1. *Diffuse PPK,* which is characterized by an even, thick, symmetric hyperkeratosis over the whole of the palm and sole. This pattern is usually evident at birth or in the first few months of life.
2. *Focal PPK,* in which large, compact masses of keratin develop at sites of recurrent friction, principally on the feet, although also on the palms and other sites. The pattern of calluses in this focal group may be either discoid (nummular) or linear.
3. *Punctate PPK,* in which multiple tiny "raindrop" keratoses involve the palmoplantar surface. They may involve the whole of the palmoplantar surface or may be more restricted in their distribution (i.e., palmar creases). Considerable intra- and interfamily variation is often seen.

Historically, emphasis in clinical diagnosis has been placed on the extent of spread (*transgrediens*) of the keratoderma onto the wrists, dorsa of the hands, knuckles, elbows, and knees. *Transgrediens* is a highly variable feature, even within the same family, and probably represents little more than the normal variation in the extent of ridged skin in that particular patient. Similarly, the progression with age

TABLE 52-1

The Acquired Keratodermas

KERATODERMA	CHAPTER REFERENCE
AIDS-associated	225
Arsenical keratoses	79
Calluses	130
Climacteric keratoderma	144
Corns (clavi)	130
Eczema	125
Human papillomavirus	223
Keratoderma blenorrhagicum	182
Lichen planus	49
Norwegian scabies	238
Paraneoplastic keratoderma	184
Psoriasis	42
Reiter's syndrome	182
Secondary syphilis	228
Tinea pedis	205
Sèzary syndrome	157
Tuberculosis verrucosa cutis	200

(*progrediens*) is unhelpful because many of the keratodermas are induced by physical trauma; thus the severity of the keratoderma may reflect the physical activity of that patient.

The keratodermas additionally are classified into three further subgroups[2] as summarized in Table 52-3:

1. *Simple keratodermas* with only PPK
2. *Complex keratodermas* with PPK associated with lesions of nonvolar skin, hair, teeth, nails, and/or sweat glands, including the ectodermal dysplasias
3. *Syndromic keratodermas* with PPK associated with abnormalities of other organs, including deafness and cancer

The differentiation of the simple PPKs, in which only the skin is involved, from those in which multiple ectodermal structures are involved (derived from the embryonic ectoderm) is important in the classification of the keratodermas. To understand how PPK may be associated with more generalized anomalies, it is useful to consider their embryonic origins in relation to other organ systems that may be involved in these diseases. The ectoderm of the flat trilaminar embryo contributes to the whole of the surface ectoderm, including the epidermis, hair, nails, cutaneous and mammary glands, anterior pituitary gland, enamel of the teeth, inner ear, and lens. In addition, the neuroectoderm-derived structures include the neural crest (cranial and sensory nerves, medulla of adrenal gland, and pigment cells) and the central nervous system (including the retina, pineal body, and posterior pituitary gland).

TABLE 52-2

Other Genodermatoses Associated with Palmoplantar Keratoderma

GENODERMATOSIS	CHAPTER REFERENCE
Basal cell nevus syndrome	82
Congenital bullous ichthyosiform erythroderma	51
Darier-White disease (keratosis follicularis)	54
Epidermodysplasia verruciformis (Lewandowsky-Lutz)	223
Epidermolysis bullosa simplex (Dowling-Meara)	65
Ichthyosis vulgaris (autosomal dominant type)	51
Lamellar ichthyosis (autosomal dominant and recessive type)	51
Pityriasis rubra pilaris (familial type)	45

Although many of the structural proteins found in the specialized palmoplantar epidermis are not palmoplantar-specific, others such as keratin K9 are unique to this site. Keratins K6 and K16 are found in the palmoplantar epidermis, nail plate, hair follicle, oral mucosa, sweat gland, and larynx but not in normal skin. Thus abnormalities of these keratins are likely to be distributed clinically in these sites. Keratin K17 has a limited basal expression in the palmoplantar epidermis but is expressed extensively in the outer hair root sheath and the nails; abnormalities of this keratin are likely in these sites. The codistribution of certain structural proteins with other tissues (e.g., muscle, nerve, and brain) may explain some genetic diseases associated with multiple organ involvement, such as epidermolysis bullosa simplex with muscular dystrophy in which plectin mutations[3] have been identified and connexin mutations associated with PPK and deafness.[4] With our greater understanding of the molecular biologic basis of many of these diseases, a modified clinical classification of the PPKs is evolving.[1,2]

SIMPLE KERATODERMAS

Diffuse PPK

DIFFUSE EPIDERMOLYTIC PPK (PPK cum degeneratione granulosa Vörner, Vörner's epidermolytic PPK)

Clinical features Diffuse epidermolytic PPK is one of the most common patterns of PPK. It is an autosomal dominant condition that presents within the first few months of life. The keratoderma presents as a well-demarcated, symmetric thickening of palms and soles and often has a "dirty" snakeskin appearance due to the underlying epidermolysis (Fig. 52-1). Knuckle pads have been reported rarely, and there may be minimal involvement of the elbows and knees.

Histology There is marked hyperkeratosis, acanthosis, and papillomatosis. Keratinocytes throughout the spinous and granular cell layers show epidermolysis with keratin aggregates and cytolysis. Since epidermolysis is easily missed if the biopsy is performed from the edge of the palm or sole, it is important to biopsy a weight-bearing area or the thenar or hypothenar eminence. A family has been described in whom epidermolysis was associated with a tonotubular cytoskeleton.[5]

Associated malignancy There is no association with malignancy. There was a reported link with breast and ovarian cancer in a French family, but this was a result of two distinct mutations cosegregating in a family, a keratin 9 mutation underlying the PPK and a BRCA1 mutation associated with the cancer susceptibility.

Genetics Keratin 9 mutations have been reported in an increasing number of families.[6] In other families with a milder form of epidermolytic PPK, a keratin 1 mutation has been demonstrated.[7]

Treatment Oral retinoid therapy may be helpful but may lead to desquamation of the whole palmoplantar surfaces, resulting in painful erosions.

DIFFUSE NONEPIDERMOLYTIC PPK (Unna-Thost disease, diffuse orthohyperkeratotic keratoderma, tylosis, keratosis palmoplantaris diffusa circumscripta, keratosis extremitatum progrediens)

Clinical features The keratoderma is inherited as an autosomal dominant condition and is present from infancy. Clinically, there is a well-demarcated, symmetric, often "waxy" keratoderma involving the whole of the palms and soles (Fig. 52-2) with a sharp cutoff at the wrist.

TABLE 52-3

The Complex PPKs

	Inheritance	Malignancy	Nonvolar Skin	Oral	Teeth	Nails	Hair	Neuro	Hearing	Pigment	Cardiac	Ocular
Complex PPK												
The diffuse PPKs												
Erythrokeratoderma veriabilis	AD	–	+	–	–	+/–	–	+/–	+/–	–	–	+/–
PPK of Sybert	AD	–	+	–	–	–	–	–	–	–	–	–
Olmsted syndrome	AD/AR	–	+	+/–	+/–	+	+	–	+/–	–	–	+/–
Congenital poikiloderma with bulla formation	AD	–	+	–	+/–	+/–	–	–	–	–	–	–
The focal PPKs												
Papillon Lefèvre syndrome	AR	–	+/–	+/–	+	+/–	+/–	–	–	–	–	–
Pachyonychia congenital type I	AD	–	+	+	–	+	+/–	–	–	–	–	–
Focal PPK with oral mucosal hyperplasia	AD	–	+	+	–	+	–	–	–	–	–	–
Pachyonychia congenital type II	AD	–	+	+	+ (natal)	+	+/–	–	–	–	–	–
Camissa disease	AD	–	+	–	+/–	+	+	+/–	–	–	–	–
Ectodermal dysplasias												
Clouston's hidrotic ectodermal dysplasia	AD	+/–	+	+	–	+	+	+/–	+/–	–	–	–
Acrokeratotic poikiloderma	AD	–	+	–	–	–	–	–	–	–	+	–
Dermatopathic pigmentosa reticularis	AD	–	+	+	+/–	+/–	+	–	–	+	–	+
Syndromic PPK												
Vohwinkel syndrome	AD	+	–	+/–	+	–	+	+/–	+/–	–	–	–
PPK with esophageal cancer	AD	+	+/–	+/–	–	–	–	–	–	–	–	–
PPK and spastic paraplegia	AD/XL	–	–	–	–	+/–	+	+	–	–	–	–
Diffuse PPK, woolly hair and ARVC (of Naxos)	AR	–	+	–	–	–	+	–	–	–	+	–
Striate PPK, woolly hair and cardiomyopathy	AD/AR	–	+	–	–	–	+	–	–	–	+	–
Keratitis-ichthyosis-deafness (KID) syndrome	AR	–	+	+/–	–	+/–	+	–	+	–	–	+
Corneodermatosseous syndrome	AD	–	–	–	+/–	+/–	–	–	–	–	–	+
Huriez syndrome	AD	+	–	–	–	–	–	–	–	–	–	
Oculocutaneous tyrosinemia	AR	–	+/–	–	–	–	–	–	–	–	–	+
Cardiofaciocutaneous syndrome	AR?	–	+/–	–	+	+/–	+	–	–	+/–	+	+
Eyelid Cysts, PPK, hypodontia, and hypotrichosis	AD	+	+/–	–	+	+/–	+	–	–	–	–	–

AD = autosomal dominant; AR = autosomal recessive; XL = X-linked.

FIGURE 52-1

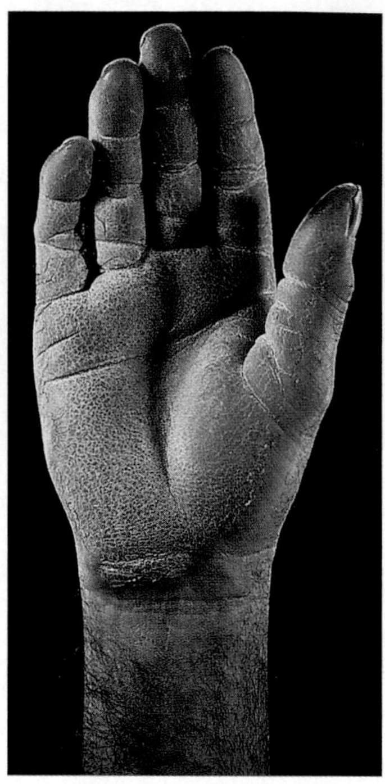

Epidermolytic palmoplantar keratoderma. A "dirty" keratoderma involving the entire palmar surface is demonstrated. (*Courtesy of Royal Hospitals Trust, United Kingdom.*)

FIGURE 52-2

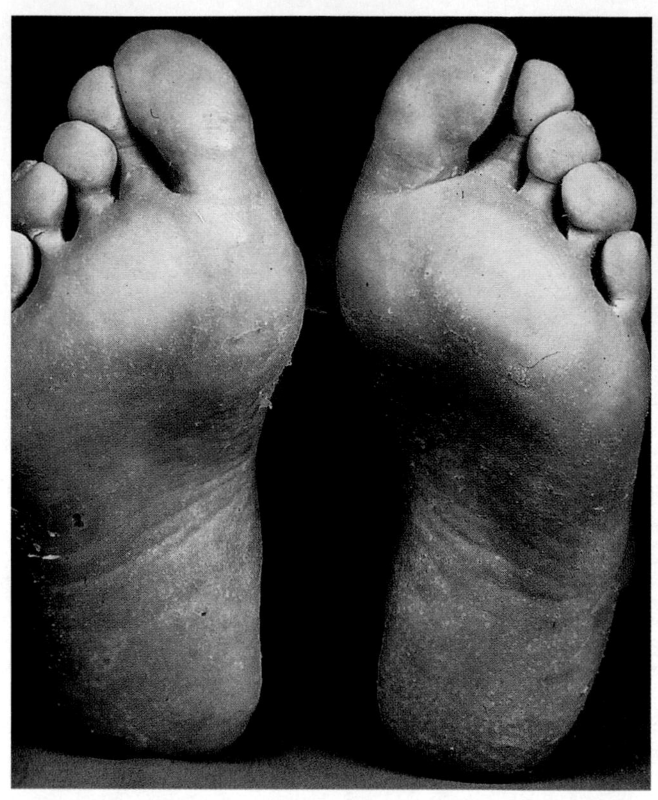

Diffuse nonepidermolytic palmoplantar keratoderma. Note the waxy keratoderma involving the entire plantar surface with involvement of the non-weight-bearing digits. (*Courtesy of Royal Hospitals Trust, United Kingdom.*)

Spread of the hyperkeratosis to the dorsa of the hands and wrists is a variable feature within most pedigrees. The dorsa of the fingers are often involved, with a scleroderma-like thickening of the skin distal to the proximal interphalangeal joint. "Parrot beaking" of the fingernails and widening of the onychocorneal band are characteristic. A "cobblestone" hyperkeratosis of the knuckles may be seen, but the elbows and knees are rarely involved.

Spread of the keratoderma to the dorsum of the hand and to the wrist has led to the attribution of *PPK of Sybert* in some of these families. Secondary dermatophyte infection, leading to maceration and peeling of the palms and soles, is a common complication of this pattern of keratoderma.

Histology The histology of this pattern of keratoderma is nonspecific and is distinguished from epidermolytic PPK by the absence of epidermolysis. The existence of this pattern of PPK has been questioned as a result of reexamination of the histology of the index family of Unna-Thost disease, which has led subsequent authors to suggest that this disease does not exist as a distinct clinical entity.[2]

Genetics Disease in a number of families has now been linked to chromosome region 12q11-q13, which harbors the type II keratin gene cluster. In these families, keratin mutations have been excluded by fine mapping and sequence analysis.[8] However, in one family in which the keratoderma is not restricted to the palmoplantar epidermis, a mutation in the V1 region of keratin 1 has been reported.[9] This region of keratin 1 has been suggested to have a role in keratin-loricrin interactions.

Treatment The disease responds well to oral retinoids. Before starting therapy, it is important to biopsy the thenar or hypothenar eminence to exclude epidermolytic PPK. Long-term treatment with a systemic antifungal agent, itraconazole 100 mg daily, is beneficial in these patients when dermatophyte infection coexists. Topical Whitfield's ointment is a useful keratolytic.

MAL DE MELEDA (Mutilating PPK of the Gamborg-Nielsen type, acral keratoderma, PED [palmoplantar ectodermal dysplasia] type VIII)

Clinical features This autosomal recessive keratoderma presents at birth or in early infancy. The keratoderma is diffuse, symmetrically involving the palms and soles with spread to the dorsa of the hands in a glove-and-stocking distribution. Knuckle pads with elbow and knee hyperkeratosis have been described. Constricting bands (pseudoainhum) around the digits may develop, resulting in loss of function and autoamputation of digits. Koilonychia, subungual hyperkeratosis, longitudinal grooving, onychogryphosis, and leukokeratosis also have been described. Other associations include angular cheilitis, hyperhidrosis, and poor physical development with electroencephalographic anomalies and brachydactyly. A case associated with perioral erythema reported by Brambilla and colleagues may represent a case of Olmsted's syndrome.[10]

Associated malignancy There is no clear association, although there have been four reports of malignant melanomas developing in affected palmoplantar epidermis and a single report of squamous cell carcinoma of affected skin.[1]

Histology The palmoplantar epidermis shows compact orthokeratosis, acanthosis, and hypergranulosis without epidermolysis.

Genetics The disease maps to chromosome 8q24.3, and mutations in the gene encoding SLURP1 have been identified.[11] The protein is thought to be secreted and involved in cell signaling and adhesion.

Treatment Clinical improvement is seen with retinoids, and the pseudoainhum may be treated with either retinoids or Z-plasty to relieve the constriction.

FIGURE 52-3

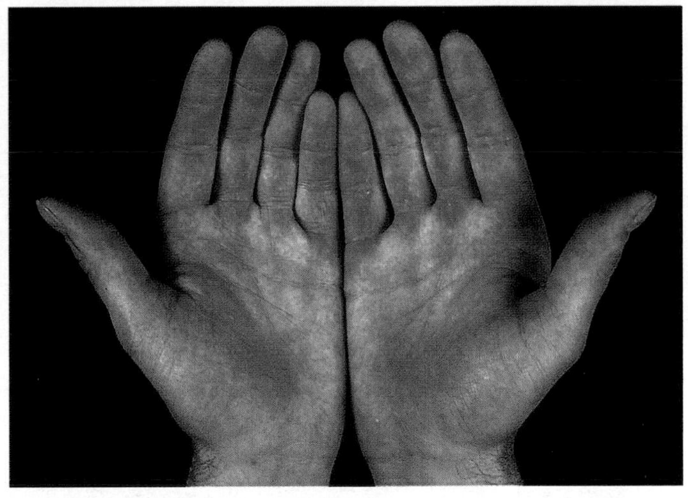

Striate keratoderma. Linear calluses extend up the fingers; this phenotype is highly variable even within the same family. (*Courtesy of Royal Hospitals Trust, United Kingdom.*)

Simple Focal PPK

STRIATE PPK (Brünauer-Fuhs-Siemens type, keratosis palmoplantaris varians, Wachters PPK, acral keratoderma)

Clinical features This is an autosomal dominant keratoderma principally involving the soles with onset in infancy or the first few years of life. The hands may show minimal callous formation; however, with manual labor, a striate pattern of PPK is seen over the palmar aspects of the digits (Fig. 52-3). Elbow and knee involvement is seen variably. Patients also report increased skin fragility, with the skin splitting following trauma, but blistering does not occur. Nails and hair may be variably involved, with ridging of the nails and cuticular hyperkeratosis; woolly hair has been reported in a few individuals.

Histology The histology of the palmar plantar epidermis shows nonspecific changes, with marked hyperkeratosis, acanthosis, and papillomatosis but without any epidermolysis.

Genetics Mutations in two desmosomal proteins have been shown to cause the simple form of striate PPK. These are in the gene for desmoglein 1 on chromosome 18q11-12 or the desmoplakin gene on chromosome 6p21.[12,13] A mutation in the V2 domain of keratin 1 is also associated with striate PPK.[14]

Simple Punctate PPK

KERATOSIS PUNCTATA PALMARIS ET PLANTARIS (Buschke-Fischer-Brauer disease, keratosis papulosa, papulotranslucent acrokeratoderma, keratoderma punctatum, maculosa disseminata, Davis Colley disease)

Clinical features This autosomal dominant PPK with variable penetrance develops at 12 to 30 years of age. Clinically, there are multiple, tiny, punctate keratoses over the entire palmoplantar surfaces, but they begin over the lateral edge of the digits. Lesions are induced by physical trauma and made worse by paring and/or chiropody. The punctate keratoses coalesce into a more diffuse pattern over the pressure points of the sole. Variable nail changes have been described but are an inconsistent part of the phenotype. An association with diverse malignancies in a few families is likely to have occurred by chance.

SPINY KERATODERMA (Punctate keratoderma, punctate porokeratosis of the palms and soles, porokeratosis punctata palmaris et plantaris)

Clinical features This is an autosomal dominant keratoderma of late onset that develops in patients aged 12 to 50 years. Multiple tiny keratotic plugs, mimicking the spines on a music box, involve the entire palmoplantar surfaces.[15] It may be associated with facial sebaceous hyperplasia. Histology shows columnar parakeratosis, which resembles the cornoid lamella of porokeratosis, with a poorly developed granular cell layer.[15]

FOCAL ACRAL HYPERKERATOSIS (Acrokeratoelastoidosis lichenoides, degenerative collagenous plaques of the hands)

Clinical features A late-onset keratoderma, inherited as an autosomal dominant condition, presents with oval or polygonal crateriform papules developing along the border of the hands, feet, and wrists.[16] A more confluent pattern is seen over the palms or soles to give a diffuse pattern. The disease is principally found in black races. Elastorrhexis has been reported.[16]

COMPLEX KERATODERMAS

Complex Diffuse PPK

ERYTHROKERATODERMA VARIABILIS (Progressive symmetric erythrokeratoderma, keratosis palmoplantaris transgrediens et progrediens, keratosis extremitatum progrediens)

Clinical features This keratoderma is inherited in an autosomal dominant fashion. The PPK is evident in infancy and increases in severity throughout childhood. Sharply outlined geographic areas of erythrokeratoderma are distributed symmetrically over the body. Erythematous desquamation of the palms and soles with hyperhidrosis is characteristic, but the disease is not palmoplantar-specific. Spread of the keratoderma to the dorsa of the hands and feet is seen commonly. Associated defects are rare in erythrokeratoderma variabilis (EKV); however, neurologic anomalies (deafness, peripheral neuropathy, decreased tendon reflexes, nystagmus, dysarthria, and cerebellar ataxia) and onychodystrophy have been described.

Histology Histology is not diagnostic and shows only orthohyperkeratosis and acanthosis with a well-preserved granular cell layer. Electron microscopy is normal apart from the stratum granulosum, where a prominent tonofilament-keratohyalin complex envelops a clear cytoplasmic halo around an often-crenellated nucleus.[17]

Genetics EKV has been mapped to the chromosomal region 1p35-p34, and mutations in the genes encoding either connexin 31 (Cx31) or connexin 30.3 (Cx30.3) have been identified in some cases.[18,19] However, a family with a disease with clinical similarities to EKV, progressive symmetric erythrokeratoderma (PSEK), has been described associated with a mutation in loricrin.[20]

Treatment Good results are obtained with oral retinoid therapy.

PPK OF SYBERT (Greither palmoplantar keratoderma, keratosis palmoplantaris transgrediens et progrediens, keratosis extremitatum hereditaria progrediens)

Clinical features PPK of Sybert is an extremely rare autosomal dominant keratoderma with symmetric severe involvement of the whole palmoplantar surface in a glove-and-stocking distribution. Spread of the keratoderma involves elbows and knees.[21] Pseudoainhum formation with amputation of the digits has been described.

Histology The histology of involved skin demonstrates accumulation of lipid-laden cells in the stratum corneum, giving the cells a clear, punctate profile. Amyloid deposition has been noted in the superficial zone of the papillary dermis after treatment with retinoids.

Treatment Good clinical responses have been obtained with systemic retinoids.

OLMSTED SYNDROME (Mutilating palmoplantar keratoderma with periorificial keratotic plaques, polykeratosis of Touraine)

Clinical features With the exception of one family in which a mother and son were affected, suggesting autosomal dominant transmission, all cases are sporadic. Diffuse multilating keratoderma of the palms and soles with flexion deformity of the digits begins in infancy.[22] Constricting bands around the digits lead to autoamputation of the digits. There are progressive perioral, perianal, and perineal hyperkeratotic plaques that may extend to the inner thigh and groin.[22] Alopecia, deafness, nail dystrophy, and dental loss have all been reported. Corneal epithelial dysplasia, leading to corneal scarring and visual impairment, has been reported in one patient, and leukokeratosis has been reported in two patients. Acrodermatitis enteropathica needs to be excluded by measurement of serum zinc levels.

Histology Plantar biopsy demonstrates marked hyperkeratosis without parakeratosis and mild acanthosis with an intact granular layer.

Treatment Skin grafting of the palmar surface has resulted in considerable clinical improvement.[22]

CONGENITAL POIKILODERMA WITH TRAUMATIC BULLA FORMATION, ANHIDROSIS, AND KERATODERMA (Naegeli-Franceschetti-Jadassohn syndrome)

Clinical features This autosomal dominant condition, with onset within the first few years of life, presents with reticulate pigmentation, which may be extensive and not preceded by any inflammation. The pigmentation particularly involves the neck and axilla. A diffuse keratoderma with punctiform and linear accentuations is usually seen, and adermatoglyphia occurs. The hair is normal, but variable nail changes have been described, from almond nails to onychodystrophy. The teeth have enamel defects, are abnormally shaped, and are lost early. Hypohidrosis or anhidrosis is the principal problem, leading to heat intolerance.[23] Since this disorder was considered initially to be a noninflammatory variant of incontinentia pigmenti, transitional cases between the two syndromes have been described.

Histology Skin biopsy typically shows patchy hyperpigmentation of the epidermis and marked secondary pigmentary incontinence, with numerous melanophages, containing melanin granules, in the upper dermis. Eccrine glands appear normal in size and number.[24]

Genetics The disease has been mapped to chromosomal region 17q21-q25.

Complex Focal PPK

PACHYONYCHIA CONGENITA TYPE I (Jadassohn-Lewandowsky syndrome)

Clinical features This autosomal dominant keratoderma principally involves the plantar surfaces. Onset of plantar calluses may be delayed up to 7 years of age. Nail changes may be evident at birth but more commonly develop within the first few months of life (Fig. 52-4). They are characterized by an upward angulation of the distal end of the nail as a result of subungual hyperkeratosis, giving the characteristic "door wedge" distal hyperkeratosis. Calluses develop over the plantar pressure points; palmar calluses are not seen except in manual workers. Blistering may occur on walking. Hair abnormalities and oral, laryngeal, and follicular hyperkeratosis have all been described.

Histology Epidermolysis mirrors the distribution of keratin K6 and K16 within the epidermis. Keratinocyte tonofilament condensation has been described in the palmoplantar epidermis.

Genetics K16 and K6a mutations have been identified in a number of families.[26,27]

FIGURE 52-4

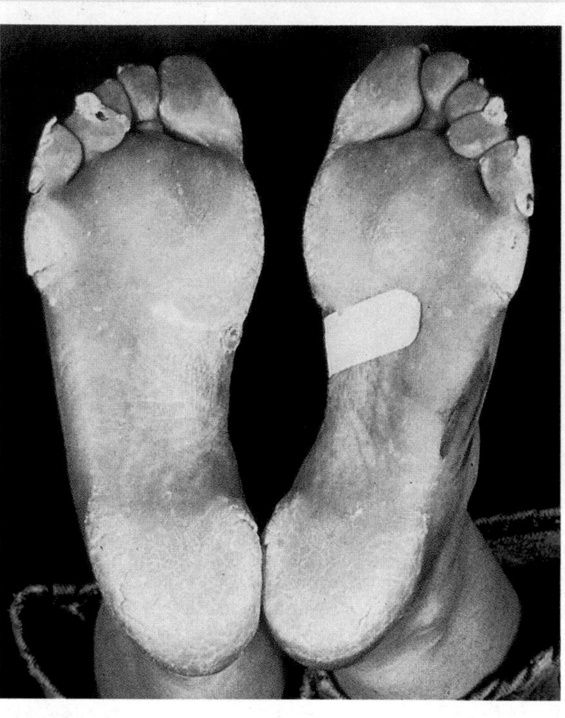

Pachyonychia congenita type I. This figure demonstrates a focal PPK involving most of the plantar surface but with sparing of the non-weight-bearing digits. (*Courtesy of Royal Hospitals Trust, United Kingdom.*)

FOCAL PALMOPLANTAR KERATODERMA WITH ORAL MUCOSAL HYPERKERATOSIS (Keratosis palmoplantaris nummularis, hereditary painful callosity syndrome, keratosis follicularis)

Clinical features This disease represents a clinical overlap syndrome with pachyonychia congenita type I but without the classic nail involvement. It is an autosomal dominant keratoderma in which calluses develop over plantar pressure points. Sparing of palms occurs except in manual workers. Oral hyperkeratosis is seen, particularly involving the labial attached gingiva. The follicular hyperkeratosis evident over the arms and legs becomes less prominent with age. Nail changes range from widening of the onychocorneal band with splinter hemorrhages to the door-wedge subungual hyperkeratosis characteristic of pachyonychia type I. Blistering may occur on walking, thus limiting physical activity. Epidermolysis is a variable feature.[28]

Histology Epidermolysis may or may not be present in the plantar epidermis.

Genetics Mutations in the helix initiation region of keratin K16 have been described.[28]

Treatment Symptomatic chiropody is often beneficial to pare off excess calluses. Oral retinoids may result in rapid improvement but can lead to desquamation of the calluses and markedly increased pain. If used, they should be started at low dosage. Secondary fungal infection of the calluses results in splitting and increased pain. Symptomatic improvement may be obtained from systemic antifungal agents in patients with superimposed fungal infections.

PACHYONYCHIA CONGENITA TYPE II (Jackson-Sertoli syndrome, Jackson-Lawler pachyonychia congenita)

Clinical features This is an autosomal dominant keratoderma presenting with a limited focal plantar keratoderma that may be very minor. Nail changes may be evident at birth but more commonly develop within the first few months of life. The nail changes are characterized by an upward angulation of the distal end of the nail as a result of subungual hyperkeratosis to give the characteristic door-wedge distal hyperkeratosis. Multiple epidermal cysts and steatocystoma are seen. All individuals have woolly scalp hair, and the eyebrows grow straight out, giving a bushy appearance. Natal teeth are seen variably.[26]

Histology Keratin filament aggregation is restricted to sites of keratin K17 and K6b expression, particularly the deep outer hair root sheath and ducts of the sebaceous glands. The exact histology of the cysts seen in both pachyonychia congenita type II and steatocystoma multiplex depends on the part of the pilosebaceous unit involved. Most consist of vellous hair cysts, but epidermal cysts, keratin-filled cysts, and steatocysts also may be seen.

Genetics Mutations in K17 and K6b have been described in a number of families.[26,29]

PAPILLON-LEFÈVRE SYNDROME

Clinical features This autosomal recessive disease develops within the first few months of life. The pattern is focal and involves most of the palmoplantar surface with punctiform accentuation in some areas, particularly along the palmoplantar creases[30] (Fig. 52-5). Spread of the keratoderma to the dorsa of the hands and to the Achilles' tendons, elbows, and knees is found in some cases. Severe periodontitis occurs following eruption of deciduous dentition and recurs with permanent dentition. A subtle, generalized, whitish opalescence of the oral mucosa has been described. Transverse ridging of nails, onychogryphosis, and sheeted follicular hyperkeratosis have all been described. A proneness to infections also has been reported.

Histology The skin lesions show hyperkeratosis with occasional parakeratotic patches, acanthosis, and slight perivascular infiltrates. The periodontal lesions are characterized by pocket formation, with secondary ulceration of the pocket epithelium and a mixed inflammatory cell infiltrate.[30]

FIGURE 52-5

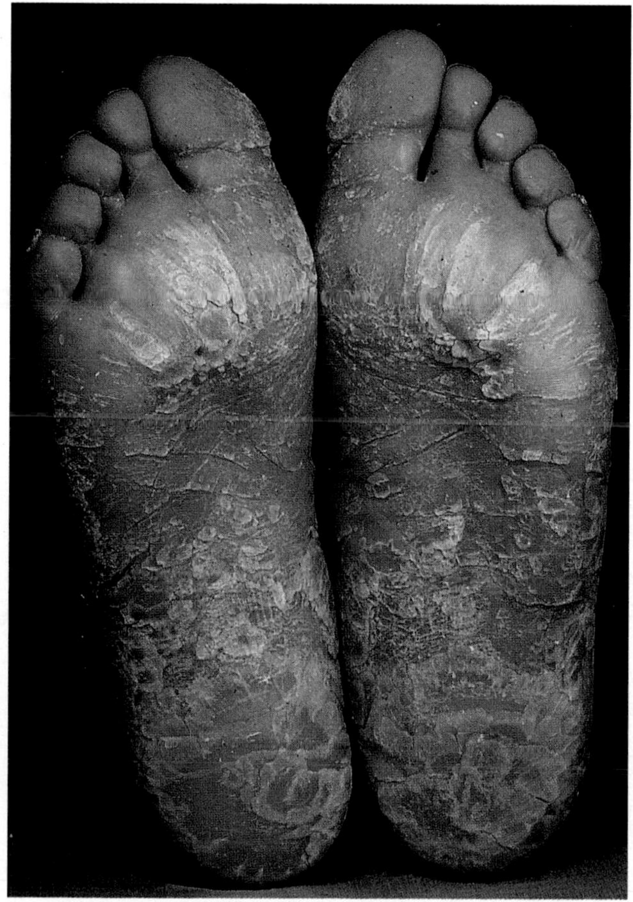

Papillon-Lefèvre syndrome. A complex pattern of keratoderma with focal and punctate lesions involving the sole is demonstrated. (*Courtesy of Royal Hospitals Trust, United Kingdom.*)

Genetics The disease maps to chromosome 11q14-q21, and mutations have been identified in the gene encoding the lysosomal protease cathepsin C.[31]

Treatment Clinical improvement in the severity of the PPK may be observed with the use of systemic retinoids. The loss of the teeth cannot be stopped, but elective extraction of involved teeth may prevent excess bone resorption. Recurrent infections may be serious and require appropriate antibiotic therapy.

Ectodermal Dysplasias

HIDROTIC ECTODERMAL DYSPLASIA (Fischer-Jacobsen-Clouston syndrome, alopecia congenita with keratosis palmoplantaris, keratosis palmaris with drumstick fingers, PPK and clubbing) This entity is discussed in Chap. 53.

ACROKERATOTIC POIKILODERMA (Hyperkeratosis-hyperpigmentation syndrome[32])

Clinical features This is an autosomal dominant keratoderma; patients present with hyperpigmentation at approximately 12 years of age, with the PPK delayed until 15 years of age. The keratoderma has a cobblestoned appearance, with spread to the dorsa of the hands and feet. Poikiloderma is seen, particularly in the sun-exposed areas, and is associated with acral bullae formation and acral lichenoid keratoses. Two families have been described with poikiloderma developing in early childhood associated with a gradual palmoplantar sclerosis and leading to the development of linear or reticulate sclerotic or hyperkeratotic bands with a flexural acral distribution.[33]

DERMATOPATHIC PIGMENTOSA RETICULARIS (Dermatopathia pigmentosa reticularis hypohidotica et atrophica, dermatopathia pigmentosa reticularis hyperkeratotica et mutilans)

Clinical features This is a rare inherited disorder of presumed autosomal dominant inheritance that presents with reticulate hyperpigmentation with truncal accentuation.[34] A number of other associated features have been described, including onychodystrophy, alopecia, adermatoglyphia, pigmentation of the oral mucosa, and ocular abnormalities (lachrymal keratosis, corneal punctae, and pigmentation of Bowman's membrane).[35] Palmoplantar hyperkeratosis with punctiform accentuation is seen, and generalized dry ichthyosis, hypohidrosis, and widespread scattered keratotic lesions have been described.[34] Ainhum formation, traumatic bullae formation, and severe periodontal disease also have been described.

Histology Striking localized pigmentary incontinence with clumps of melanin-filled macrophages and liquefaction degeneration of the basal cell layer are reported. A diffuse hyalinized change of the dermal collagen is a consistent feature.

Syndromic Keratodermas

PALMOPLANTAR KERATODERMA ASSOCIATED WITH ESOPHAGEAL CANCER (Palmoplantar ectodermal dysplasia type III, tylosis)

Clinical features This autosomal dominant keratoderma occurs with late onset. The keratoderma principally is of the focal type involving the plantar pressure points (Fig. 52-6). More diffuse patterns may be seen in some patients, but the non-weight-bearing digits are always spared. The age of onset is usually between 7 and 8 years of age. The palms are usually not involved, but there may be callus formation in manual workers. Oral leukokeratosis often predates the onset of the PPK and involves the buccal mucosa more than the labial attached

FIGURE 52-6

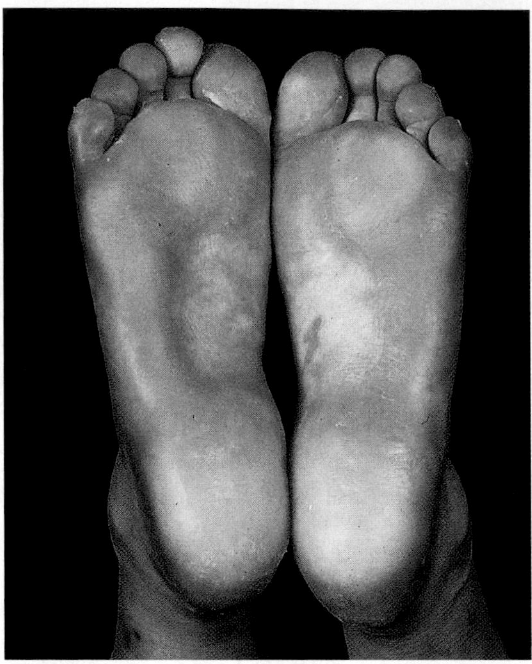

Palmoplantar keratoderma associated with esophageal malignancy. Note the focal PPK involving most of the plantar surface but with sparing of the non-weight-bearing digits. (*Courtesy of Royal Hospitals Trust, United Kingdom.*)

gingival mucosa.[1] Widespread follicular hyperkeratosis is evident, particularly in children. The nails are normal, and this is an important differentiating feature from focal PPK with oral hyperkeratosis.

Associated malignancy The risk of developing esophageal squamous cell carcinoma in these families has been reported as between 40 and 90 percent of those affected by age 65.[1,36] Oral squamous cell carcinomas also have been reported, and there may be an increased incidence of other tumors.

Histology Acanthosis of the sole and palm skin with a prominent granular cell layer and marked hyperkeratosis without parakeratosis are seen. The sweat ducts of the dermis are thickened, and the epithelium is hyperplastic, appearing to occlude the lumen in places.

Genetics In three families, the disease has been mapped to chromosomal region 17q25.[36]

OCULOCUTANEOUS TYROSINEMIA (Tyrosinemia type II, Richer-Hanhart syndrome; see also Chap. 147)

Clinical features This is an autosomal recessive condition with onset between ages 2 and 4 years, when painful circumscribed callosities develop on the pressure points of the palm and sole. Occasionally, calluses also may develop on the elbows and knees. Photophobia and corneal erosions develop within the first few months of life. The corneal erosions may progress to corneal ulceration and glaucoma. Mental retardation develops if patients are not treated.[37]

Histology Histology of the palmoplantar lesions may be helpful diagnostically in demonstrating eosinophilic cytoplasmic inclusions.

Genetics Tyrosine aminotransferase deficiency is the underlying metabolic defect; it results in raised serum tyrosine and phenolic acid metabolites.[38]

Treatment When patients are placed on a low-tyrosine, low-phenylalanine diet, the cutaneous and ocular manifestations disappear.

VOHWINKEL SYNDROME (Keratoma hereditaria multilans[39])

Clinical features This diffuse autosomal dominant keratoderma with onset in early infancy presents with a honeycombed keratoderma involving the palmoplantar surfaces. Flexion contractures and constricting bands of digits, particularly of the fifth digit, result in autoamputation (Fig. 52-7). Spread of the keratoderma occurs with linear and/or starfish keratoses on the extensor surfaces of the elbows, knees, and knuckles. Mild to moderate sensorineural hearing loss is often associated. A diffuse, generalized ichthyosiform dermatosis may be seen in some affected individuals and is specific to the form associated with normal hearing, which is due to loricrin mutations. Nail dystrophy, alopecia, onychogryphosis, and a variety of neurologic abnormalities

FIGURE 52-7

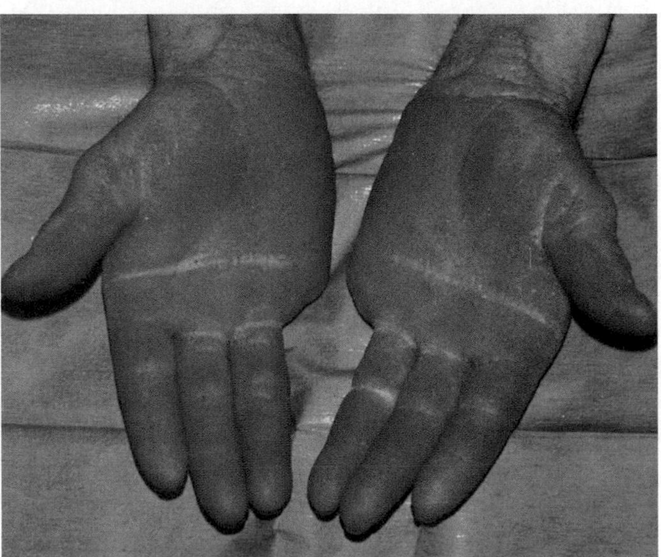

A.

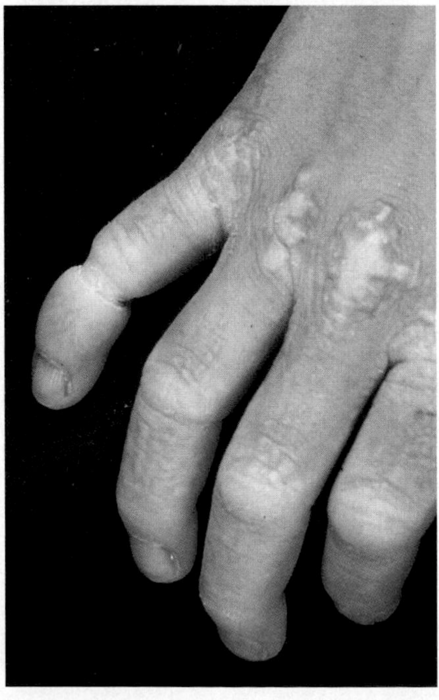

B.

Vohwinkel syndrome. Note the diffuse pattern of keratoderma with pseudoainhum formation. (*Courtesy of Department of Dermatology, University of Heidelberg, Germany.*)

other than sensorineural hearing loss, such as spastic paraplegia, and myopathy have been described.

Histology Histopathology demonstrates the characteristic feature of hyperkeratosis and "round" retained nuclei with hypergranulosis.

Genetics Mutations in the gene encoding the gap junction protein, connexin 26, underlies the classical form of Vohwinkel's syndrome.[40] A mutation in loricrin (a major component of the cornified cell envelope) has been associated with Camisa disease, the variant form of Vohwinkel's with ichthyosis and normal hearing.[41] Other forms of PPK with sensorineural hearing loss have been shown to be due to mitochondrial mutations.[42]

Treatment The keratoderma and pseudoainhum respond well to systemic retinoids.

HURIEZ SYNDROME (PPK with sclerodactyly, scleroatrophic and keratotic dermatosis of limbs, sclerotylosis)

Clinical features This autosomal dominant keratoderma with sclerodactyly presents from birth with a diffuse symmetric keratoderma of the palms and soles. The fingers have a pseudosclerodermatous appearance. Atrophic fibrosis of limb skin also may be seen. Variable nail features have been described, with longitudinal ridging hypoplasia and clubbing.

Associated malignancy Squamous cell carcinoma develops in the atrophic skin in the third to fourth decades,[35] and bowel cancer also has been described in association with this phenotype. An Indian pedigree with "tylosis" and cancer is probably of this type.[43]

Genetics The disease gene has been mapped to chromosomal region 4q23.[44]

DIFFUSE PPK, WOOLLY HAIR AND ARRYTHMOGENIC RIGHT VENTRICULAR CARDIOMYOPATHY (Naxos disease)

Clinical features Both recessive and dominant conditions have been described. The recessive disorder (Naxos disease) has a clear association with cardiomyopathy. The disorder is characterized by the development, during infancy, of a diffuse keratoderma over the plantar pressure points. Other cutaneous anomalies include acanthosis nigricans of the axilla and groin, diffuse xerosis, follicular hyperkeratosis over the zygoma, and palmoplantar hyperhidrosis. Woolly hair over the scalp and short, scanty eyebrows, eyelashes, beard, and axillary and pubic hair are seen. Nails, teeth, and sweat gland function are all normal. Endomyocardial fibrodysplasia with ventricular tachycardia and right ventricular dilatation with right ventricular bands have been reported.[45]

Histology Skin biopsy demonstrates compact hyperkeratosis, hypergranulosis, and acanthosis.

Genetics The recessive disorder maps to chromosomal region 17q21 and is due to mutations in the desmosomal and adherens junction protein plakoglobin.[46]

STRIATE PPK, WOOLLY HAIR AND LEFT VENTRICULAR DILATED CARDIOMYOPATHY

Clinical features Both dominant and recessive forms have been described but only the recessive forms have a clear association with cardiomyopathy. The skin disease presents as a striate PPK with some nonvolar involvement, particularly at sites of pressure or abrasion.[47,48] Cardiologic investigation of a number of affected family members has been reported with the diagnosis of a left ventricular dilated cardiomyopathy often resulting in heart failure during adolescence.

Histology Histology of the skin of patients with the recessive form of the condition reveals large intercellular spaces between suprabasal keratinocytes. Basal cells, however, appeared normal. Electron microscopy of affected palmar skin shows clumping of desmosomes at the sites of cell-cell adhesion.

Genetics The recessive form of the condition maps to chromosomal region 6p24, and mutations in the desmosomal protein desmoplakin have been demonstrated.[48]

KERATITIS-ICHTHYOSIS-DEAFNESS (KID) SYNDROME (Ichthyosiform erythroderma, corneal involvement, and deafness; Desmons' syndrome[49,50])

Clinical features This autosomal recessive disorder with sensorineural deafness presents from birth. Ichthyosiform erythroderma develops with a well-marginated serpiginous outline. Follicular hyperkeratosis, changes perioral furrowed plaques, and oral leukokeratosis have been described. Other changes include a diffuse keratoderma with a reticulate surface, recurrent infections, sensorineural deafness, keratoconjunctivitis and photophobia, hepatitis, mental retardation, and skeletal abnormalities with short stature and pes cavus. Hypotrichosis and nail dystrophy may occur.

Histology Epidermal glycogen deposition has been reported in one patient.

Associated malignancy Multiple cutaneous squamous cell carcinomas are seen.

CORNEODERMATOSSEOUS SYNDROME (CDO syndrome[51])

Clinical features The characteristic features of this autosomal dominant condition with onset in infancy include corneal dystrophy, photophobia, diffuse PPK, distal onycholysis, skeletal abnormalities with brachydactyly, short stature, and medullary narrowing of digits. The teeth are soft and subject to early decay.

PALMOPLANTAR KERATODERMA AND SPASTIC PARAPLEGIA (Charcot-Marie-Tooth disease with PPK and nail dystrophy[52])

Clinical features This autosomal dominant or X-linked dominant keratoderma begins in early childhood with a thick focal keratoderma over the soles and to a lesser extent the palms. Punctate keratoderma has been described in one family.[53] Pes cavus, frontal balding, spastic paraplegia (motor and sensory neuropathy), and mental retardation are reported. Muscular atrophy that develops at approximately 40 years of age starts in the lower legs, with weakness, progressive gait difficulties, and stumbling. Nail dystrophy is an inconsistent feature.[52]

Histology Palmar biopsy shows pronounced orthokeratosis, acanthosis, and regular papillomatosis.

Genetics A mutation in the neurofilament-light gene is associated with Charcot-Marie-Tooth type II and PPK in a single family.[54]

EYELID CYSTS, PALMOPLANTAR KERATOSIS, HYPODONTIA, AND HYPOTRICHOSIS (Schöpf-Schulz-Passarge syndrome[55])

Clinical features This is an autosomal recessive condition with diffuse symmetric PPK. PPK and fragility of the nails begin around age 12. Hair becomes sparse by age 25, and cysts of the eyelid margins occur at age 60. Other changes include facial telangiectasia, early loss of teeth, generalized hypotrichosis, and longitudinal and oblique furrows in nails.

Associated malignancy Multiple squamous cell carcinomas in the area of the palmoplantar keratoderma are reported, as well as eccrine poromas, hypernephroma, and basal cell carcinoma.[55]

Histology Apocrine hidrocystoma of the eyelid margins is one manifestation.

CARDIOFACIOCUTANEOUS SYNDROME[56]

Clinical features This is reported as an autosomal recessive condition, but autosomal dominant transmission cannot be excluded. Typical features include a characteristic "high boxy" craniofacial appearance, psychomotor and growth retardation, and congenital cardiac defects. Various hair defects have been reported with focal PPK. Alopecia, reduced eyebrows and body hair, and curly, woolly, and brittle hair are all described. The skin manifestations include ichthyosis, follicular hyperkeratosis, keratosis pilaris atrophicans faciei, unpleasant body odor, cavernous hemangiomas, café-au-lait spots, and hyperpigmented macules or stripes. The nails are dystrophic, and there is dysplasia of the teeth.

Histology Nonspecific features of ichthyosis with hyperkeratosis of the epidermis and thinning of the granular layer are seen. In one patient, scalp biopsy showed adnexal hyperkeratosis with hyperplasia and dystrophy of sweat ducts. The hair follicles were immature or disrupted by inspissated keratin.

REFERENCES

1. Stevens HP et al: Linkage of an American pedigree with palmoplantar keratoderma and malignancy (palmoplantar ectodermal dysplasia type III) to 17q24: Literature survey and propsed updated classification of the palmoplantar keratodermas. *Arch Dermatol* **132**:640, 1996
2. Hatsell S, Kelsell D: The diffuse palmoplantar keratodermas. *Acta Dermatoven APA* **9**:47, 2000
3. Smith FJD et al: Plectin deficiency results in muscular dystrophy with epidermolysis bullosa. *Nature Genet* **13**:450, 1996
4. Kelsell DP et al: Connexin mutations in skin disease and hearing loss. *Am J Hum Genet* **68**:559, 2001
5. Wevers A et al: Palmoplantar keratoderma with tonotubular keratin. *J Am Acad Dermatol* **24**:638, 1991
6. Reis A et al: Keratin 9 gene mutations in epidermolytic palmoplantar keratoderma (EPPK). *Nature Genet* **6**:174, 1994
7. Hatsell SJ et al: Novel splice site mutation in keratin 1 underlies mild epidermolytic palmoplantar keratoderma in three kindreds. *J Invest Dermatol* **116**:606, 2001
8. Kelsell DP et al: Fine genetic mapping of diffuse non-epidermolytic palmoplantar keratoderma to chromosome 12q11-q13: Exclusion of the mapped type II keratins. *Exp Dermatol* **8**:388, 1999
9. Kimonis V et al: A mutation in the V1 end domain of keratin 1 causes non-epidermolytic palmar-plantar keratoderma. *J Invest Dermatol* **103**:764, 1994
10. Brambilla L et al: Unusual case of Meleda keratoderma treated with aromatic retinoid etretinate. *Dermatologica* **168**:283, 1994
11. Fischer J et al: Mutations in the gene encoding SLURP-1 in mal de meleda. *Hum Mol Genet* **10**:875, 2001
12. Rickman L et al: N-terminal deletion in a desmosomal cadherin causes the autosomal dominant skin disease striate palmoplantar keratoderma. *Hum Mol Genet* **8**:971, 1999
13. Armstrong D et al. Haploinsufficiency of desmoplakin causes a striate subtype of palmoplantar keratoderma. *Hum Mol Genet* **8**:143, 1999
14. Whittock NV et al: Frameshift mutation in the V2 domain of keratin 1 causes the striate form of palmoplantar keratoderma. *J Invest Dermatol* **118**:838, 2002
15. Osman Y et al: Spiny keratoderma of the palms and soles. *J Am Acad Dermatol* **26**:879, 1992
16. Dowd PM et al: Focal acral hyperkeratosis. *Br J Dermatol* **109**:97, 1983
17. MacFarlane AW et al: Is erythrokeratoderma one disorder? A clinical and ultrastructural study of two siblings. *Br J Dermatol* **124**:487, 1991
18. Richard G et al: Mutations in the human connexin gene GJB3 cause erythrokeratodermia variabilis. *Nature Genet* **20**:366, 1998
19. Macari F et al: Mutation in the gene for connexin 30.3 in a family with erythrokeratodermia variabilis. *Am J Hum Genet* **67**:1296, 2000
20. Ishida-Yamamoto A et al: The molecular pathology of progressive symmetric erythrokeratoderma: A frameshift mutation in the loricrin gene and pertubations in the cornified cell envelope. *Am J Hum Genet* **61**:581, 1997
21. Sybert VP et al: Palmar-plantar keratoderma: A clinical, ultrastructural, and biochemical study. *J Am Acad Dermatol* **18**:75, 1988
22. Atherton DJ et al: Mutilating palmoplantar keratoderma with periorificial keratotic plaques (Olmsted syndrome). *Br J Dermatol* **122**:245, 1990
23. Itin PH et al: Natural history of the Naegeli-Franceschetti-Jadassohn syndrome and further delineation of its clinical manifestations. *J Am Acad Dermatol* **28**:942, 1993
24. Sparrow GP et al: Hyperpigmentation and hypohidrosis (the Naegeli-Franceschetti-Jadassohn syndrome): Report of a family and review of the literature. *Clin Exp Dermatol* **1**:127, 1976
25. Whittock NV et al: The gene for Naegeli-Franceschetti-Jadassohn syndrome maps to 17q21. *J Invest Dermatol* **115**:694, 2000
26. McLean WHI et al: Keratin 16 and keratin 17 mutations cause pachyonychia congenita. *Nature Genet* **9**:273, 1995
27. Bowden PE et al: Mutation of a type II keratin gene (K6a) in pachyonychia congenita. *Nature Genet* **10**:363, 1995
28. Shamsher M et al: Novel mutations in keratin 16 gene underlie focal non-epidermolytic palmoplantar keratoderma (NEPPK) in two families. *Hum Mol Genet* **4**:1875, 1995
29. Smith FJD et al: A mutation in human keratin K6b produces a phenocopy of the K17 disorder pachyonychia congenita type 2. *Hum Mol Genet* **7**:1143, 1998
30. Haneke E: The Papillon-Lefèvre syndrome: Keratosis palmoplantaris with periodontopathy. Report of a case and review of the cases in the literature. *Hum Genet* **51**:1, 1975
31. Toomes C et al: Loss-of-function mutations in the cathepsin C gene result in periodontal disease and palmoplantar keratosis. *Nature Genet* **23**:421, 1999
32. Cantú JM et al: A "new" autosomal dominant genodermatosis characterised by hyperpigmented spots and palmoplantar hyperkeratosis. *Clin Genet* **14**:165, 1978
33. Weary PE et al: Hereditary sclerosing poikiloderma: Report of two families with an unusual and distinctive geneodermatosis. *Arch Dermatol* **100**:413, 1969
34. Maso MJ et al: Dermatopathia pigmentosa reticularis. *Arch Dermatol* **126**:935, 1990
35. Gahlen W: Dermatopathia pigmentosa reticularis hypohidotica et atrophica. *Dermatol Wochenschr* **150**:193, 1964
36. Kelsell DP et al: Close mapping of focal non-epidemolytic palmoplantar keratoderma (PPK) locus associated with oesophageal cancer (TOC). *Hum Mol Genet* **5**:857, 1996
37. Goldsmith LA: Tyrosine-induced skin disease. *Br J Dermatol* **98**:119, 1978
38. Natt E et al: Point mutations in the tyrosine aminotransferase gene in tyrosinemia type II. *Proc Natl Acad Sci USA* **89**:9297, 1992
39. Vohwinkel KH: Keratoma hereditarium mutilans. *Arch Derm Syph* **158**:354, 1929
40. Maestrini E et al: A missense mutation in connexin26, D66H, causes mutilating keratoderma with sensorineural deafness (Vohwinkel's syndrome) in three unrelated families. *Hum Mol Genet* **8**:1237, 1999
41. Maestrini E et al: A molecular defect in loricrin, the major component of the cornified cell envelope, underlies Vohwinkel's syndrome. *Nature Genet* **13**:70, 1996
42. Sevior KB et al. Mitochondrial A7445G mutation in two pedigrees with palmoplantar keratoderma and deafness. *Am J Med Genet* **75**:179, 1998
43. Yesudian P et al: Genetic tylosis with malignancy: A study of a South Indian pedigree. *Br J Dermatol* **102**:597, 1980
44. Lee YA et al: A gene for an autosomal dominant scleroatrophic syndrome predisposing to skin cancer (Huriez syndrome) maps to chromosome 4q23. *Am J Hum Genet* **66**:326, 2000
45. Protonotarios N et al: Cardiac abnormalities in familial palmoplantar keratosis. *Br Heart J* **56**:321, 1986
46. McKoy G et al: Identification of a deletion in plakoglobin in arrhythmogenic right ventricular cardiomyopathy with palmoplantar keratoderma and woolly hair (Naxos disease). *Lancet* **355**:2119, 2000
47. Carvajal-Huerta L: Epidermolytic palmoplantar keratoderma with woolly hair and dilated cardiomyopathy. *J Am Acad Dermatol* **39**:418, 1998
48. Norgett EE et al: Recessive mutation in desmoplakin disrupts desmoplakin-intermediate filament interactions and causes dilated cardiomyopathy, woolly hair and keratoderma. *Hum Mol Genet* **9**:2761, 2000
49. Wilson GN et al: Keratitis, hepatitis, ichthyosis, and deafness: Report and review of KID syndrome. *Am J Med Genet* **40**:255, 1991
50. Nazzaro V et al: Familial occurrence of KID (keratitis, ichthyosis, deafness) syndrome: Case reports of a mother and daughter. *J Am Acad Dermatol* **23**:385, 1990
51. Stern JK et al Corneal changes, hyperkeratosis, short stature, brachydactyly, and premature birth: A new autosomal dominant syndrome. *Am J Med Genet* **18**:67, 1984
52. Fitzsimmons JS et al: Four brothers with mental retardation, spastic paraplegia and palmoplantar hyperkeratosis: A new syndrome? *Clin Genet* **23**:329, 1983
53. Powell FC et al: Keratoderma and spastic paralysis. *Br J Dermatol* **109**:589, 1983
54. Mersiyanova IV et al: A new variant of Charcot-Marie-Tooth disease type 2 is probably the result of a mutation in the neurofilament-light gene. *Am J Hum Genet* **67**:37, 2000
55. Monk BE et al: Schöpf-Schulz-Passarge syndrome. *Br J Dermatol* **127**:33, 1992
56. Borradori L, Blanchet-Bardon C: Skin manifestations of cardio-cutaneous syndrome. *J Am Acad Dermatol* **28**:815, 1993

CHAPTER 53

Virginia P. Sybert

Ectodermal Dysplasias

The ectodermal dysplasias (EDs) are a group of inherited disorders that share in common developmental defects involving at least two of the major structures classically held to derive from the embryonic ectoderm—hair, teeth, nails, sweat glands. Freire-Maia and Pinheiro[1] published an exhaustive review and classification system for these disorders using a numeric system of 1 (hair), 2 (teeth), 3 (nail), and 4 (sweat glands) for characterization. This system has little utility in practice, although it did allow for a rational approach to a previously chaotic field. Freire-Maia and Pinheiro laid claim to more than 150 ectodermal disorders in their most recent compilation.[2] This chapter will cover only the most common of these conditions and those whose ectodermal defects are likely to bring them to a dermatologist for diagnosis and medical attention.

The first major step in the algorithm for making a specific diagnosis of an ectodermal dysplasia is the presence of (hidrotic) or absence of (hypohidrotic/anhidrotic) sweating. The involvement of other ectodermal structures and of non-ectodermally derived tissues provide further branching points in a diagnostic hierarchy. Mode of inheritance may differ within a seemingly uniform diagnostic group, and care must be taken in evaluating family members before providing recurrence risks.

Within the last few years, causal genes have been identified in many of the EDs, and this is likely to continue, making any textbook chapter passé before it is printed. The reader is directed to the following resources: *http://www3.ncbi.nlm.nih.gov/Omim* (Victor McKusick's online catalog of Mendelian inheritance in humans) and *http://www.genetests.org* (Roberta Pagon's up-to-date listing of laboratories offering molecular testing). The MIM (Mendelian Inheritance in Man) numbers with each section heading refer to the numbering system in OMIM (Online Mendelian Inheritance in Man). The National Foundation for Ectodermal Dysplasias (*http://www.nfed.org*) is a lay support group that has numerous informative pamphlets for families and physicians, as well as a strong advocacy program for dental care, insurance coverage, and research.

HYPOHIDROTIC ECTODERMAL DYSPLASIA (ANHIDROTIC ECTODERMAL DYSPLASIA; CHRIST-SIEMENS-TOURAINE SYNDROME; MIM 305100)

Historical Aspects

X-linked hypohidrotic ectodermal dysplasia (X-LHED) was described over 200 years ago and enjoys status as a condition referred to by Charles Darwin in his writings on the variation of species. In 1913, Christ characterized it as a congenital ectodermal defect, and Siemens reaffirmed the X-linked nature of inheritance in 1921. In 1936, Touraine published on the wide range of features. In 1944, Felsher suggested the use of the term *hypohidrotic* rather than *anhidrotic* because sweating, while functionally absent, was not absolutely so.

Epidemiology

The disorder occurs in all racial groups and is thought to have an incidence at birth of approximately 1 in 100,000 males.[3]

Etiology/Pathogenesis

The condition results from alterations in the gene *ectodysplasin* (*EDA, EDA1*) located at Xq12-13.[4] The gene codes for a transmembrane protein, ectodysplasin, of 391 amino acids. The gene has alternative splicing forms, the significance of which is not known. More than 50 different mutations in this gene causing X-LHED have been identified. There does not appear to be a correlation between the nature of the mutation and the clinical features[5]; i.e., to date there have been no phenotype:genotype correlations. Inter- and intrafamilial variations occur to a mild degree. Ectodysplasin belongs to the tumor necrosis factor (TNF) family and plays a role in regulation of the formation of ectodermal structures. It forms trimers; is expressed in keratinocytes, the outer root sheath of hair follicles, and sweat glands; and localizes to the lateral and apical surfaces of cells.

Genetics

As is typical of X-linked recessive disorders, expression is full blown in affected males, and carrier females may express no, some, or all the features of the disorder, often in a patchy distribution. The disorder can be inherited from a carrier mother or occur in an affected individual as the result of a de novo mutation. Approximately 70 percent of affected males will have inherited the mutation from a carrier mother. Between 60 and 80 percent of carrier females will express some clinical signs of the disorder; the most frequent are patchy hypotrichosis and hypodontia.

Mutations in an autosomal gene mapped to 2q11q13, *dl* or *downless,* have been implicated in an autosomal dominant form of HED (MIM 129490) and in an autosomal recessive form (MIM 224900)[6] that is clinically similar to X-LHED. Both these entities are much more rare. Mutations in yet another gene, *crinkled,* have been identified recently in autosomal recessive HED.[7] Individuals with autosomal dominant HED appear to have a milder defect in the ability to sweat.

Very recently, certain mutations in the X-linked *NEMO* gene, which causes incontinentia pigmenti in females, have been shown to result in males with HED and immune defects.[8]

Clinical Manifestations

There have been several reviews of a large number of affected individuals over the years, providing the basis for the stated prevalence of clinical features; the most recent appeared in 1987.[9]

FIGURE 53-1

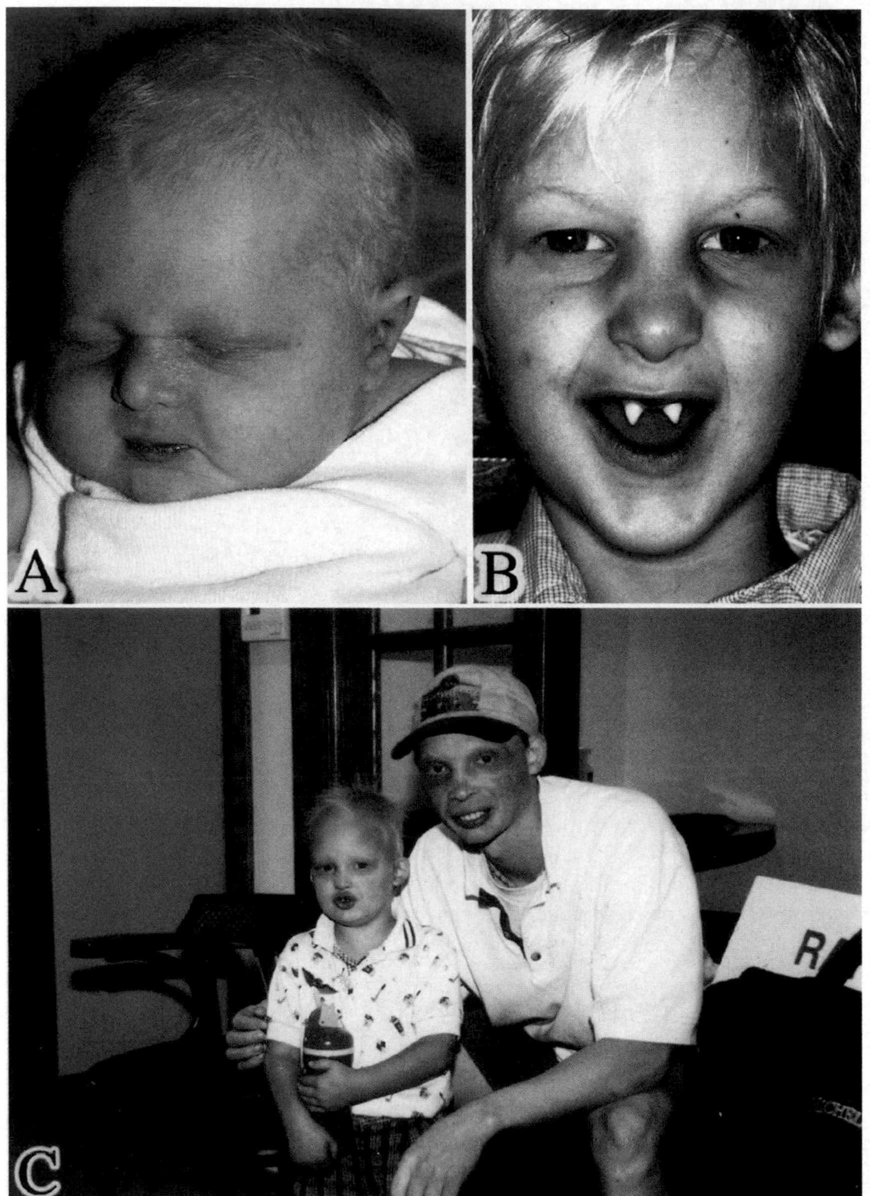

Hypohidrotic ectodermal dysplasia. *A.* Newborn with periorbital wrinkling, beaked nose. Diagnosis would not be suspected unless there was a positive family history. *B.* Peg-shaped teeth; fine periorbital wrinkling can be appreciated. (*From Sybert VP:* Genetic Skin Disorders. *New York, Oxford University Press, 1997.*) *C.* Two unrelated males with X-LHED; adult is wearing dentures; periorbital wrinkling and hyperpigmentation are evident. (*Courtesy of the National Foundation for Ectodermal Dysplasias.*)

DERMATOLOGIC Affected males may present at birth with a collodion membrane or with marked scaling of the skin,[10] similar to congenital ichthyosis. Scalp hair is usually sparse, fine, and blonde. It may thicken and darken at puberty, and secondary sexual hair, especially the beard, may be normal. Other body hair is usually sparse or absent.

The ability to sweat is significantly compromised, and most affected males will have marked heat intolerance. Sweat pores are usually undetectable on physical examination, and fingerprint ridges are effaced. The inability to sweat adequately in response to environmental heat results in an elevation of core temperature and bouts of unexplained high fevers, usually leading to an extensive workup for infectious disease, malignancy, or autoimmune disease before the correct diagnosis is recognized. In older series of patients, mental retardation was reported as a feature of X-LHED. Currently, this is believed to have been due to damage from prolonged high fevers and convulsions and not to be an intrinsic feature of the disorder.

The nails are usually normal; reports of thin, fragile nails are not convincing, and nail dystrophy plays little role in the burden of the disorder.[11] Periorbital wrinkling and hyperpigmentation are typical and often present, albeit unappreciated, at birth (Fig. 53-1*A–C*). Eczema plagues more than two-thirds of affected males and is often difficult to manage. Hyperplasia of sebaceous glands, particularly on the face, can develop over time and appear as small, pearly, flesh-colored to white papules that may resemble milia.

SYSTEMIC ASSOCIATIONS Hypodontia and oligodontia or anodontia are invariable features of X-LHED in affected males. Appreciation of hypoplastic gum ridges can be an early clue to the diagnosis of the disorder. Teeth that do erupt are usually peg-shaped and small (see Fig. 53-1*B*). The facies of the disorder are characterized by frontal bossing and a depressed midface with a saddle nose and full, everted lips. Otolaryngologic manifestations include thick nasal secretions and impaction, ozana, sinusitis, recurrent upper respiratory tract infections and pneumonias, decreased saliva production, hoarse voice, and an increased frequency of asthma. Gastroesophageal reflux and feeding difficulties may be a problem in infancy. Preliminary studies suggest that there may be failure to thrive in infancy and early childhood in as many as 20 to 40 percent of affected boys, with catch-up growth seen later. Although several reviews have suggested that infant mortality may be increased, unbiased confirmatory data are lacking.

Female carriers for X-LHED may be affected as severely as males or show few, if any, signs of the disorder (Fig. 53-2*A*, *B*). Heat intolerance, if present, is usually mild; adult carrier women will comment that they do not sweat much or that they do not like very warm weather, but it is unusual for a female to experience fever due to inability to sweat. Typically, a few teeth may be peg-shaped or missing; scalp hair may be patchy or thin. Careful examination of the skin of carrier females often will reveal a diminution in or patchy distribution of sweat pores. This sometimes can be appreciated readily just by magnification of fingertip pads or may require more sophisticated sweat testing.

VARIANTS As noted earlier, the autosomal dominant and autosomal recessive forms of HED are similar, although the autosomal dominant form may be milder. The X-linked form is by far the most common and always should be the diagnosis of default in a sporadic case.

Pathology

The epidermis is thinned and flattened. There is a reduction in the number of sebaceous glands and hair follicles. Eccrine glands are absent or incompletely developed.

Diagnosis/Differential Diagnosis

The scaling skin at birth may result in a misdiagnosis of congenital ichthyosis. Repeated bouts of fever may be thought to have an infectious source. The diagnosis of HED is recognized readily when expected, such as when an at-risk male is born into a family in which the disorder is known to segregate. Examination for sweat pores and a panorex view of the jaw will lead quickly to the correct diagnosis. In an isolated, fully expressing female, the autosomal dominant and recessive forms of HED need to be considered. Family history, examination of parents, and molecular testing may be helpful. Mothers, especially, always should be examined fully to detect mild manifestations of the X-linked form. Molecular testing is not indicated for clinical diagnosis in most instances.

Treatment

Maintenance of cool ambient temperatures is vital to prevent hyperpyrexia. Most children do well with simple measures such as wet T-shirts, air conditioning in home and school, wet headbands, etc. Occasionally, cooling vests can play a role in allowing a broader range of participation in sports and vigorous physical activity in warm climates.

Dental restoration is of primary importance, and early implementation of dentures and ultimate use of dental implants are mainstays of treatment.

Management of otolaryngologic complications, asthma, and recurrent infections needs to be individualized. The eczema may be quite refractory to care.

The National Foundation for Ectodermal Dysplasias (*www.nfed.org*) has several pamphlets for individuals and professionals dealing with diagnosis and treatment. These are readily available at cost from the organization and are highly recommended.

Although infancy and childhood are complicated by many problems, most individuals with HED lead adult lives that allow them to function successfully in society. Heat intolerance seems to decrease due to the development of some ability to sweat in adolescence or to the development of common sense and adaptation of lifestyle or both.

FIGURE 53-2

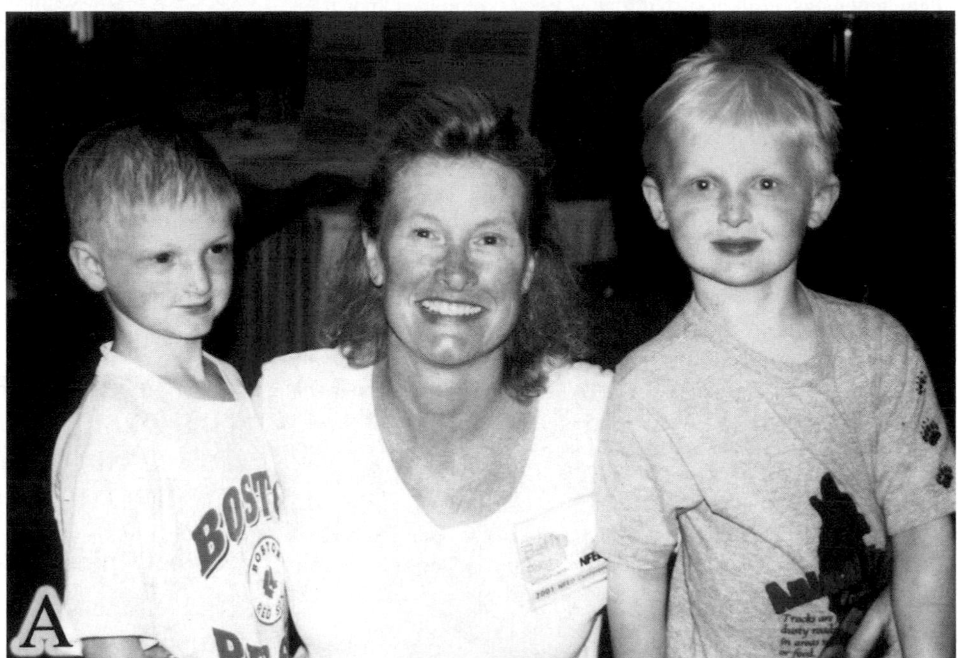

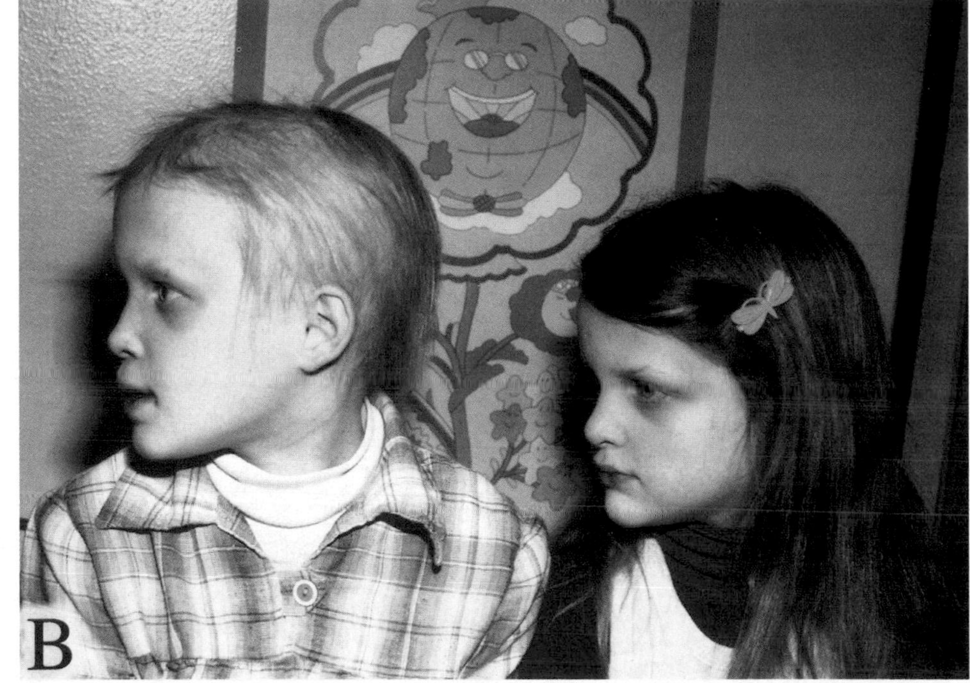

Hypohidrotic ectodermal dysplasia. *A*. Female carrier of X-LHED with two affected sons. (*Courtesy of the National Foundation for Ectodermal Dysplasias.*) *B*. Two sisters with X-LHED manifesting to different degrees. Note periorbital hyperpigmentation, full everted lips, and sculpted noses. (*From Sybert VP: Genetic Skin Disorders. New York, Oxford University Press, 1997.*)

HIDROTIC ECTODERMAL DYSPLASIA (CLOUSTON SYNDROME; MIM 129500)

Historical Aspects/Epidemiology

Clouston[12] first described this disorder in a French-Canadian kindred. It has been reported in other ethnic groups, but the majority of affected individuals can trace their ancestry back to an original French-Canadian settler.

Etiology/Pathogenesis

The disorder is caused by mutations in a connexin gene, *GJB6* or *connexin-30*.[13] Different mutations in the same gene are responsible for a form of nonsyndromic autosomal dominant deafness. Other connexin genes show similar variability in mutation: disease correlations (e.g., mutations in *connexin-31, GJB3*, can cause either erythrokeratodermia variabilis or late-onset autosomal deafness). The pathway by which allelic mutations result in such different diseases is not yet known.

Genetics

HED is autosomal dominant with variable expression (the degree of severity can vary within and between families). Males and females are affected in equal numbers and to equal degree. The gene maps to the centromeric region of the long arm of chromosome 13.

Clinical Manifestations

The scalp hair is wiry, brittle, and pale, and there is often patchy alopecia (Fig. 53-3*A*). This progresses in adult life and may lead to total alopecia. Body and facial hair are affected. The nails may be milky white in infancy and early childhood, gradually thickening and becoming dystrophic. The nail plates in adults are thick, short, slow growing, and separate distally from the nail bed (see Fig. 53-3*C*). Anonychia has been reported. Not all the nails are necessarily affected to the same degree. Progressive palmar/plantar hyperkeratosis is common (see Fig. 53-3*B*). In contrast to hypohidrotic ectodermal dysplasia, sweating is normal, as are the teeth. Oral leukoplakia has been reported. Conjunctivitis and blepharitis, possibly due to poor function of sparse eyelashes, are common.

Pathology

The thickened palms and soles show orthohyperkeratosis with a normal granular layer. On electron microscopy, an increase in the number of desmosomes in the cells of the stratum corneum is found. The hair shows nonspecific changes.

Diagnosis/Differential Diagnosis

The diagnosis is straightforward. The involvement of nails and hair and palmar/plantar thickening, in the absence of other signs of ectodermal dysplasia, are reasonably specific. Other palmar/plantar hyperkeratoses do not have similar hair changes. Orofacial clefting differentiates other forms of autosomal dominant HED, such as ankyloblepharon filiforme adenatum–ectodermal dysplasia–cleft palate (AEC) syndrome or Rapp-Hodgkin syndrome. While the nail changes are similar to those of pachyonychia congenita, the hair changes are distinctive.

Treatment

Occasionally, ablation of the nail matrix is necessary for relief of pain. Wigs may provide cosmetic benefit.

AEC SYNDROME (ANKYLOBLEPHARON FILIFORME ADENATUM-ECTODERMAL DYSPLASIA-CLEFT PALATE; HAY-WELLS' SYNDROME; MIM 106260)

History/Epidemiology

Described first in 1976,[14] Hay-Wells syndrome has been found in ethnically and geographically disparate families.

Etiology/Pathogenesis

The disorder is caused, in at least some families, by mutations in the tumor-suppressor gene *p*63 (also known as *p*51 or *KET*), a gene that has been implicated in the pathogenesis of ectrodactyly–ectodermal

FIGURE 53-3

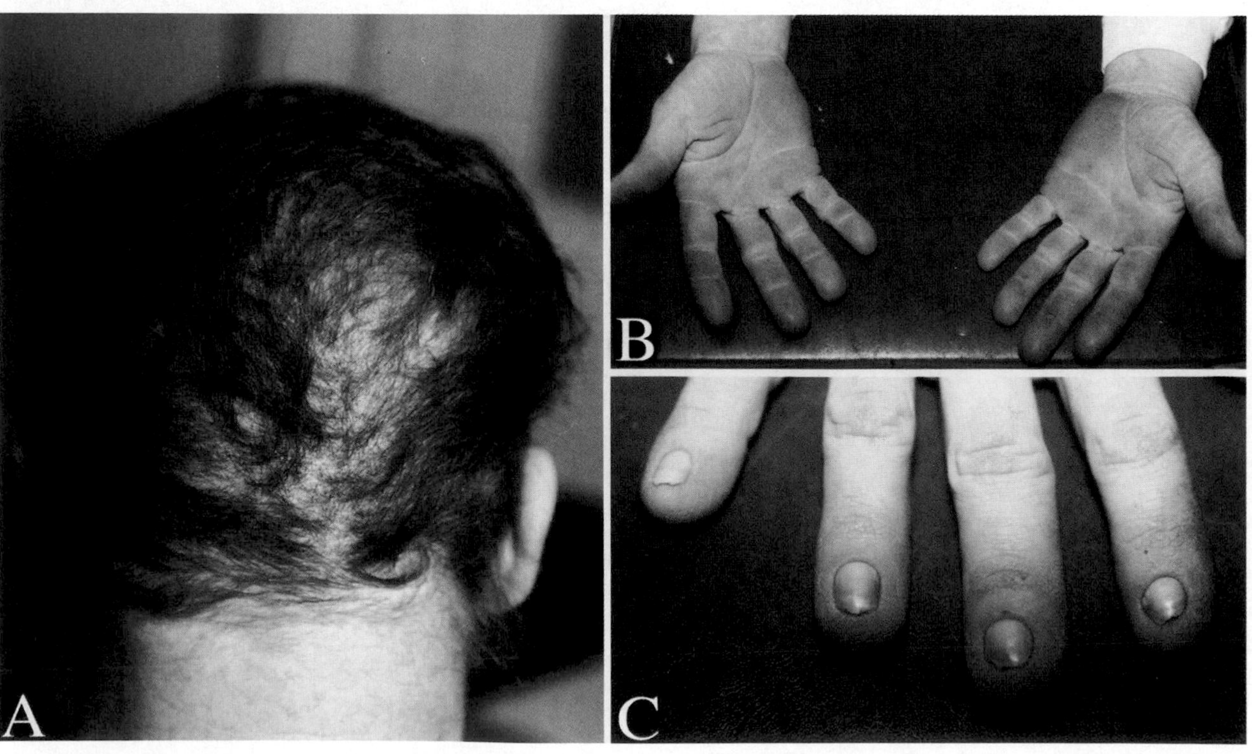

Hidrotic ectodermal dysplasia (Clouston syndrome) *A*. Patchy alopecia in adult. Coarseness of hair can be appreciated. *B*. Palmar hyperkeratosis. *C*. Nail dystrophy.

dysplasia–cleft lip/palate (EEC) syndrome, limb-mammary syndrome, acro-dermato-ungual-lacrimal-tooth (ADULT) syndrome, and other autosomal dominant forms of ectodermal dysplasia. Mutations that cause EEC and AEC cluster in different regions of the gene.[15]

Genetics

AEC syndrome is an autosomal dominant disorder with complete penetrance (if you have the gene, you show clinical evidence of it) and variable expression.

Clinical Features

DERMATOLOGIC Ninety percent of affected infants present at birth with red, cracking, peeling skin and superficial erosions, similar to the appearance of a collodion membrane[11] (Fig. 53-4*A*). This sheds within a few weeks, and the skin underneath is dry and thin. The scalp is almost invariably involved, and many affected individuals are plagued by a chronic erosive dermatitis with abnormal granulation tissue on the scalp (see Fig. 53-4*B*, *C*). Recurrent bacterial infection of the scalp is common. Patchy alopecia is the rule, and the scalp hair that is present is often wiry, coarse, and light in color. Sparseness to absence of body hair is typical. Ankyloblepharon filiforme adnatum—strands of skin between the eyelids—are seen in approximately 70 percent of affected infants (see Fig. 53-4*D*). These may tear spontaneously or require surgical lysis. Lacrimal duct atresia or obstruction is common. The nails may be normal, hyperconvex and thickened, absent, or partially dystrophic, and all changes can be found in a single individual. Sweating is usually normal, although some affected individuals describe subjective heat intolerance. Supernumerary nipples and ectopic breast tissue are seen occasionally, as is mild cutaneous syndactyly of toes two and three.

SYSTEMIC ASSOCIATIONS Cleft palate, with or without cleft lip, occurs in 80 percent of reported cases. There may be hypodontia with missing or misshapen teeth. Malformed auricles have been described in some. Recurrent otitis media and secondary conductive hearing loss are common and may be consequences of the cleft palate rather than primary. Hypospadias has been described in several affected males.

FIGURE 53-4

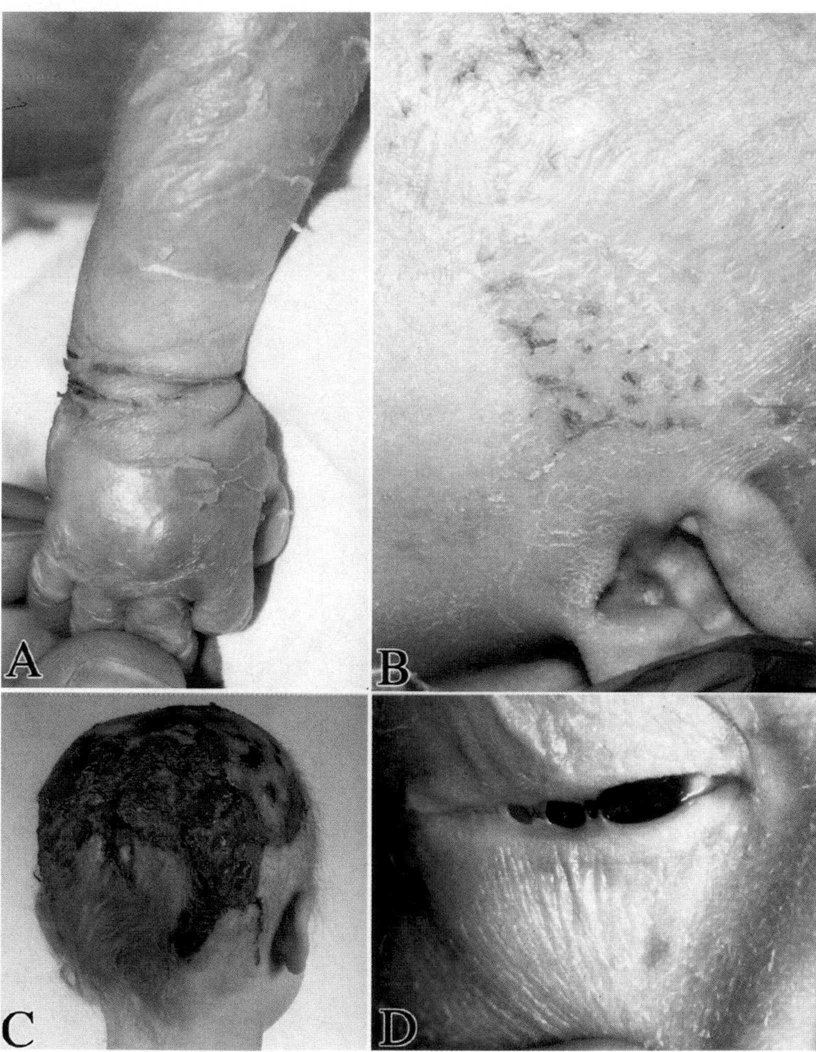

AEC (Hay-Wells) syndrome. *A*. Newborn with peeling collodion membrane. *B*. Superficial erosion and thin skin of scalp in same patient, age 5 days *C*. Abnormal granulation tissue on scalp in older affected female. *D*. Fine strands of tissue (ankyloblepharon filiforme adenatum) between eyelids.

Pathology

Some patients show a decrease in the number of sweat glands. Electron microscopy of hairs shows a defective cuticular structure. There is a decrease in the keratins of the basal and suprabasal layers of the epidermis and disorganized keratin filaments in the stratum corneum.

Diagnosis/Differential Diagnosis

Among the autosomal dominant ectodermal dysplasias associated with clefting, Rapp-Hodgkin syndrome lacks the ankyloblepharon and has a much lower occurrence of scalp involvement. Some argue that it is the same disorder. The EEC syndrome is characterized by bony hand and foot abnormalities not seen in AEC and also lacks the ankyloblepharon. The peeling, eroded skin of the newborn can lead to misdiagnosis of epidermolysis bullosa or congenital ichthyosis. Ankyloblepharon filiforme adnatum can occur in the absence of syndromic associations, and the strands have been seen in several forms of arthrogryposis, in association with chromosomal aneuploidy, and in CHANDS (curly hair, ankyloblepharon, and nail dysplasia syndrome), an autosomal recessive form of ectodermal dysplasia.

Treatment/Prognosis

Light emollients should be used until the collodion membrane sheds. Ankyloblepharon may require surgical lysis. Ongoing ocular hygiene is important. Vigorous and meticulous but gentle scalp care with prompt treatment of infection is extremely important. Grafting of skin to the scalp is not often successful. Clefting will require a team approach for repair and follow-up for secondary issues, such as feeding difficulties, speech defects, orthodontia, and ear infections.

ECTRODACTYLY–ECTODERMAL DYSPLASIA–CLEFT LIP/PALATE (EEC) SYNDROME; SPLIT HAND–SPLIT FOOT–ECTODERMAL DYSPLASIA–CLEFT LIP/PALATE SYNDROME (MIM 129900)

Historical Aspects/Epidemiology

EEC syndrome is an ectodermal dysplasia classified as a multiple congenital anomaly syndrome because it has major involvement of structures other than those derived ectodermally. It was described by Cockayne in 1936 and given its acronym in 1970 by Rudiger and colleagues. EEC syndrome has occurred in all racial groups worldwide.

Etiology/Pathogenesis

Mutations in *p*63, a tumor-suppressor gene mapped to 3q27, have been found in most individuals with EEC syndrome.[16] The gene is expressed widely, including in the basal cells of proliferating epithelial tissues. Mutations in the same gene appear to cause some cases of isolated split hand–split foot disease, limb-mammary syndrome, and Hay-Wells syndrome. There appear to be genotype-phenotype correlations.[17] All alterations identified thus far in Hay-Wells syndrome have been missense mutations in the sterile alpha motif (SAM) domain; in EEC syndrome, the majority of mutations result in single-amino-acid substitutions in the DNA-binding domain.[15] Frameshift mutations in *p*63 cause limb-mammary syndrome, in which ectodermal structures other than the mammary gland often, but not always, appear normal.

Genetics

EEC syndrome is an autosomal dominant disorder with variable expression and reduced penetrance. Intra- and interfamilial differences in severity are common.

Clinical Manifestations

DERMATOLOGIC The ectodermal dysplasia may be quite mild. The hair is usually blond, coarse, and dry (Fig. 53-5*A*). It may be sparse and slow growing. Axillary and pubic hair also may be affected. The nails are dystrophic in about four-fifths of individuals with transverse ridging, pitting, and slow growth (see Fig 53-5*D*). Dry skin and thickening of the palms and soles can occur. Sweating is usually normal.

SYSTEMIC ASSOCIATIONS Hypodontia and premature loss of secondary teeth and the dental abnormalities associated with clefting are

FIGURE 53-5

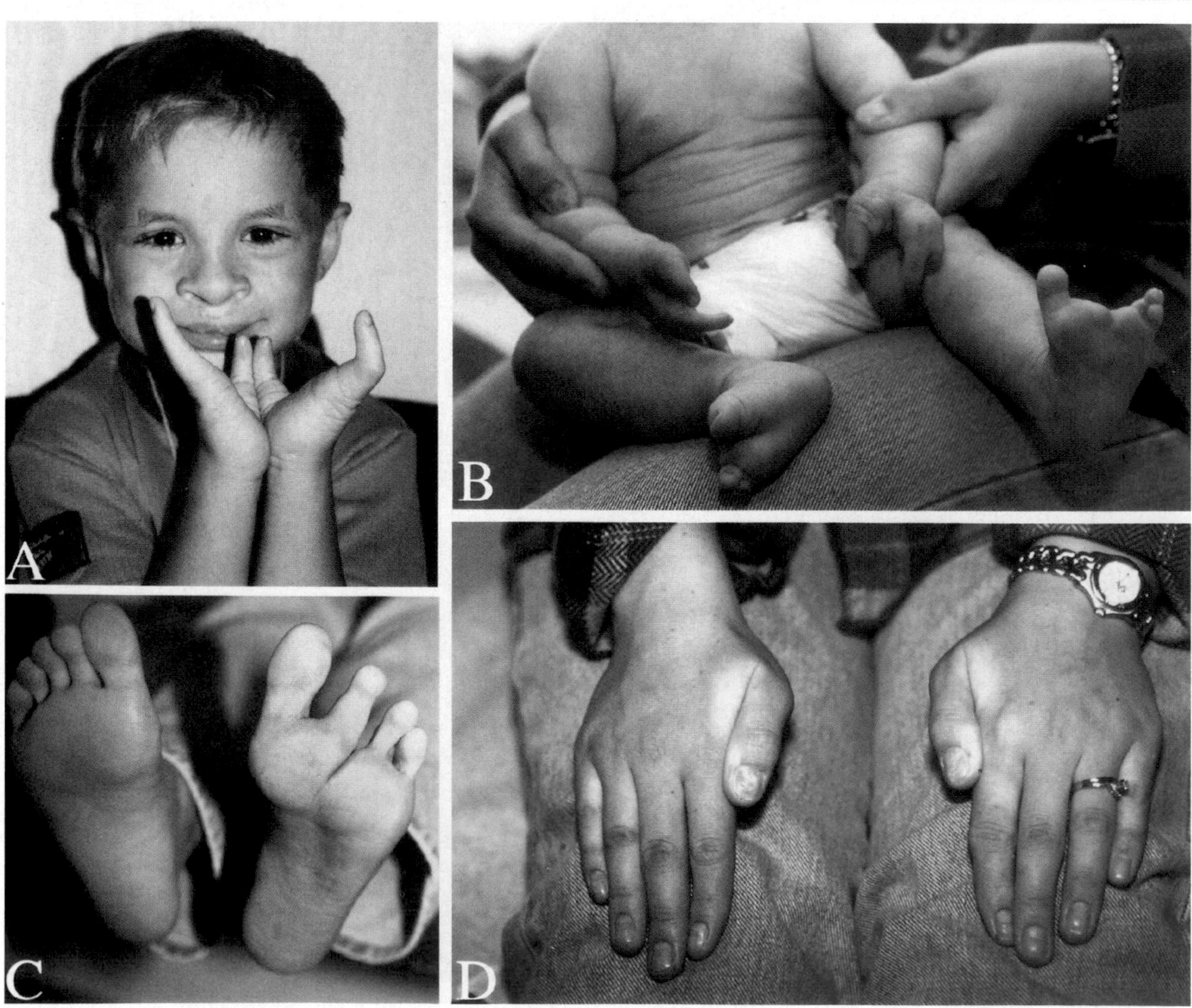

EEC (ectrodactyly–ectodermal dysplasia–clefting) syndrome. *A.* Mild thinness of hair. (*Courtesy of the National Foundation for Ectodermal Dysplasias.*) *B.* Hands and feet of affected infant. *C, D.* Feet and hands of parent of infant in *B* demonstrating variability of expression both among limbs and between family members. Note also the nail dystrophy especially evident on the thumbs.

found in most affected individuals. Lacrimal gland abnormalities are common.

The major distinguishing feature of EEC syndrome is ectrodactyly—abnormal development of the median rays of the hands and feet. The feet are involved more frequently than the hands, and there may be asymmetry of involvement (see Fig. 53-5*B–D*). Cleft palate, with or without cleft lip, occurs in 70 to 100 percent depending on the series.[18,19] Secondary conductive hearing loss is frequent. Genitourinary abnormalities that include hydronephrosis, and structural renal or genital malformations affect a third or more of persons with EEC syndrome. Although mental retardation has been reported, it is not believed to be an inherent feature of the disorder.

Diagnosis/Differential Diagnosis

Among disorders with limb defects that need to be considered in the differential diagnosis of EEC syndrome are the odontotrichomelic syndrome (MIM 273400), in which there are severe absence deformities of the limbs, and aplasia cutis congenita with limb defects (Adams-Oliver syndrome, MIM 100300), which does not have clefting or ectodermal defects other than absence of skin. Other ectodermal dysplasias with clefting include Hay-Wells syndrome, Rapp-Hodgkin syndrome, and limb-mammary syndrome, all of which, in at least some families, appear to be allelic to EEC syndrome. Ectrodactyly with cleft palate without ectodermal dysplasia (ECP syndrome, MIM 129830) also may be a distinct entity. Prenatal diagnosis by ultrasound for detection of limb abnormalities is unreliable; molecular testing may prove useful in some families.

FIGURE 53-6

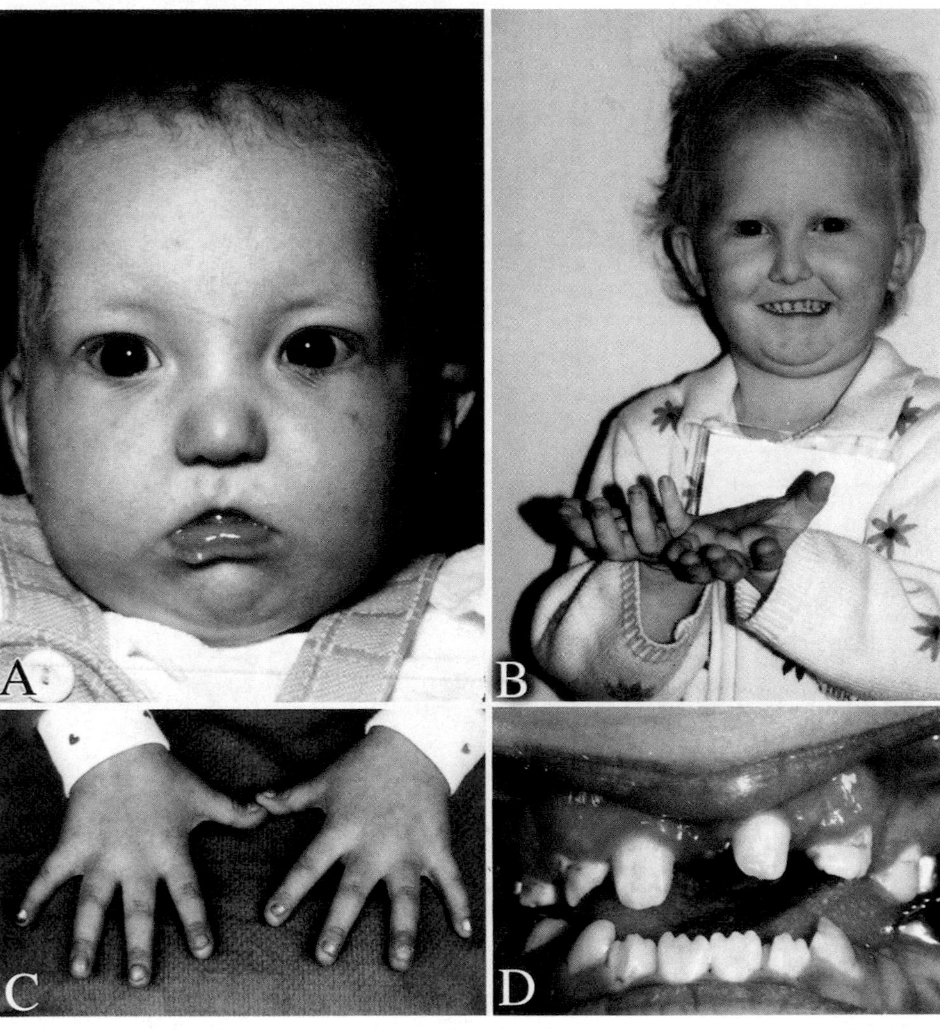

Rapp-Hodgkin syndrome. *A*. Affected infant at 5 months. *B*. Fine, blond, sparse hair; beginnings of nail changes on middle finger of right hand. (*Courtesy of the National Foundation for Ectodermal Dysplasias.*) *C*. Abnormal nails in same patient as *A*, at age 4½ years with thickened and friable nail plates. (*From Sybert VP:* Genetic Skin Disorders. *New York, Oxford University Press, 1997.*) *D*. Abnormal dentition, missing teeth, and peg teeth.

Treatment

As for other ectodermal dysplasias with orofacial clefting and ophthalmologic involvement, management requires a team approach. Similarly, treatment for the limb defects must be individualized. Renal ultrasound and a high index of suspicion for urinary tract problems may be appropriate.

RAPP-HODGKIN SYNDROME (MIM 129400)

Described in 1968,Rapp-Hodgkin syndrome is an autosomal dominant disorder that shares in common with Hay-Wells syndrome cleft palate with or without cleft lip, hypohidrosis usually without episodes of frank hyperpyrexia, abnormal hair with pili torti or pili trianguli et canaliculi and progressive balding, and nail dystrophy.[20,21] The face in Rapp-Hodgkin syndrome is striking, with a short nasal columella and maxillary hypoplasia, thin upper lip, and full lower lip (Fig. 53-6*A*, *B*). The nails are thick and short, worsening with age (see Fig. 53-6*C*). The teeth may be conical and prone to caries (see Fig. 53-6*D*). The lacrimal puncta are aplastic in almost one-third of affected individuals. Hypospadias has been reported in two-fifths of affected males; labial hypoplasia and absence of the opening of the vagina have been reported in a single female. These features are also reminiscent of the EEC syndrome. Rapp-Hodgkin syndrome may prove to be allelic due to mutations in *p63*. Treatment is the same as described for these similar disorders.

TOOTH AND NAIL SYNDROME (WITKOP SYNDROME; HYPODONTIA WITH NAIL DYSGENESIS; MIM 189500)

Historical Aspects/Epidemiology

This is a rare disorder, first described in 1965 and expanded on in 1975.[22]

FIGURE 53-7

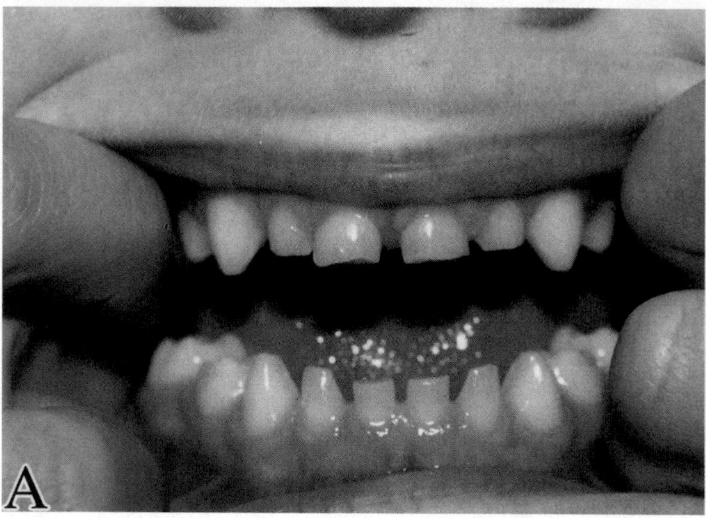

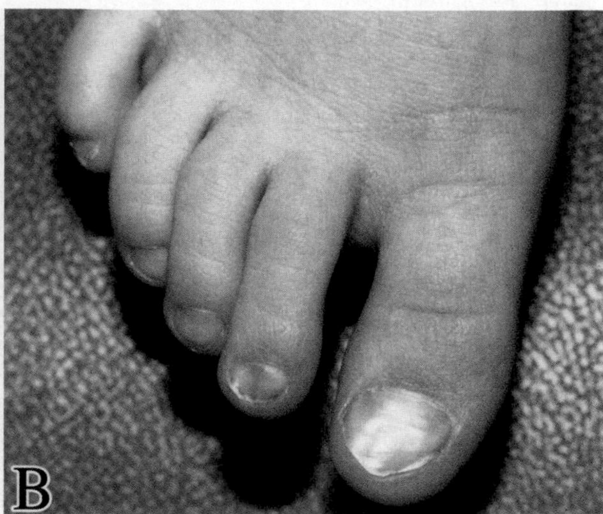

Tooth-nail syndrome. *A*. Primary teeth still in place; failure of adult teeth to erupt. *B*. Dystrophic toenails with flattening of nail plates.

Etiology/Pathogenesis/Genetics

A nonsense mutation in *MSX1*, a gene expressed in the developing teeth and nail beds in mice, has been found in one family with Witkop syndrome.[23] Other mutations in *MSX1* have been associated with isolated tooth agenesis or tooth agenesis with cleft palate. Tooth and nail syndrome is autosomal dominant, with variable expression and intrafamilial variability.

Clinical Manifestations

DERMATOLOGIC The nails are thin, small, and friable and may show koilonychia at birth. Toenails are usually more severely involved than fingernails (Fig. 53-7*B*). Nail changes improve with age and may be unappreciated in affected adults. A few individuals have reported thin, fine hair.

SYSTEMIC ASSOCIATIONS The primary teeth usually are unaffected, although they may be small. The secondary teeth may fail to erupt, and there can be partial or total absence (see Fig. 53-7*A*) The mandibular incisors, second molars, and maxillary canines are missing most often. No other ectodermal structures are affected.

Diagnosis/Differential Diagnosis

This is an easy condition to miss. The nail changes may be subtle. The tooth abnormalities may be mild enough to escape detection by a physician. The lack of associated features, either dermatologic or systemic, readily distinguish Witkop syndrome from other ectodermal dysplasias. There is a presumed autosomal recessive disorder characterized by taurodontia (cone-shaped teeth), absent teeth, sparse hair, and hypoplastic nails that appears similar.

Treatment/Prognosis

The nails usually require no treatment. Restorative dentistry is important.

REFERENCES

1. Freire-Maia N, Pinheiro M: *Ectodermal Dysplasias: A Clinical and Genetic Study*. New York, Liss, 1984
2. Freire-Maia N, Pinheiro M: Ectodermal dysplasias: A clinical classification and a causal review. *Am J Med Genet* **53**:153, 1994
3. Stevenson AC, Kerr CB: On the distribution of frequencies of mutations to genes determining harmful traits in man. *Mutat Res* **4**:339, 1967
4. Kere J et al: X-linked anhidrotic (hypohidrotic) ectodermal dysplasia is caused by a mutation in a novel transmembrane protein. *Nature Genet* **13**:409, 1996
5. Vincent MC et al: Mutational spectrum of the *ED1* gene in X-linked hypohidrotic ectodermal dysplasia. *Eur J Hum Genet* **9**:355, 2001
6. Monreal AW et al: Mutations in the human homologue of mouse *dl* cause autosomal recessive and autosomal dominant hypohidrotic ectodermal dysplasia. *Nature Genet* **22**:366, 1999
7. Headon DJ et al: Gene defect in ectodermal dysplasia implicates a death domain adaptor in development. *Nature* **414**:913, 2001
8. Aradhya S et al: Atypical forms of incontinentia pigmenti result from mutations of a cytosine tract in exon 10 of *NEMO(IKK-γ)*. *Am J Hum Genet* **68**:765, 2001
9. Clarke A et al: Clinical aspects of X-linked hypohidrotic ectodermal dysplasia. *Arch Dis Child* **62**:989, 1987
10. The Executive and Scientific Advisory Boards of the National Foundation for Ectodermal Dysplasias: Scaling skin in the neonate: A clue to the early diagnosis of X-linked hypohidrotic ectodermal dysplasia (Christ-Siemens-Touraine syndrome). *J Pediatr* **114**:600, 1989
11. Sybert V: *Genetic Skin Disorders*. New York, Oxford University Press, 1997
12. Clouston HR: A hereditary ectodermal dysplasia. *Can Med Assoc J* **21**:18, 1929
13. Lamartine J et al: Mutations in *GJB6* cause hidrotic ectodermal dysplasia. *Nature Genet* **26**:142, 2000
14. Hay RJ, Wells RS: The syndrome of ankyloblepharon, ectodermal defects and cleft lip and palate: An autosomal dominant condition. *Br J Dermatol* **94**:277, 1976
15. McGrath JA et al: Hay-Wells syndrome is caused by heterozygous missense mutations in the SAM domain of *p63*. *Hum Mol Gene* **10**:221, 2001
16. Celli J et al: Heterzozygous germline mutations in the *p53* homolog *p63* are the cause of EEC syndrome. *Cell* **99**:143, 1999
17. Van Bokhaven H et al: *p63* gene mutations in EEC syndrome, limb-mammary syndrome and isolated split hand–split foot malformation suggest a genotype-phenotype correlation. *Am J Hum Genet* **69**:481, 2001
18. Buss PW et al: Twenty-four cases of the EEC syndrome: Clinical presentation and management. *J Med Genet* **32**:716, 1995
19. Roelfsema NM, Cobben JM: The EEC syndrome: A literature study. *Clin Dysmorphol* **5**:115, 1996
20. Schroeder HW Jr, Sybert VP: Rapp-Hodgkin ectodermal dysplasia. *J Pediatr* **110**:72, 1987
21. Walpole IR, Goldblatt J: Rapp-Hodgkin hypohidrotic ectodermal dysplasia syndrome. *Clin Genet* **39**:114, 1991
22. Hudson CD, Witkop CJ Jr: Autosomal dominant hypodontia with nail dysgenesis: Report of 29 cases in six families. *Oral Pathol* **39**:409, 1975
23. Jumlongras D et al: A nonsense mutation in *MSX1* causes Witkop syndrome. *Am J Hum Genet* **69**:67, 2001

CHAPTER 54

Lowell A. Goldsmith
Howard P. Baden

Darier-White Disease (Keratosis Follicularis) and Acrokeratosis Verruciformis

DARIER-WHITE DISEASE (KERATOSIS FOLLICULARIS)

Darier-White disease (DWD) is an autosomal dominant disorder with altered keratinization of the epidermis, nails, and mucous membranes. Mutations in a sarcoplasmic endoreticulum Ca^{2+}-ATPase isoform 2 (SERCA2) cause all cases of DWD.[1] Darier and White separately reported the disease in 1889. Although it was suggested initially that the dyskeratotic cell represented an organism, this idea was soon dispelled. White recognized the genetic nature of the disease by discovering that a mother and daughter were affected.

Etiology and Pathogenesis

DWD is not present at birth and usually begins in the first or second decade.[2,3] Males and females are equally affected. Characteristic sites of predilection are the face, forehead, scalp, chest, and the back. Although these sites have many sebaceous glands, lesions also occur commonly in sites without sebaceous glands—the palms and soles—as well as in keratinizing and nonkeratinizing epithelia, such as mucous membranes, cornea, and submandibular glands.[4,5]

DWD is frequently worse in the summer, with heat and humidity as the major factors, and can be exacerbated by ultraviolet B (UVB) light[6] and mechanical trauma, e.g., under the collar of sweaters. The first American patient, described by White in 1889, was well until he entered the Northern army in 1862 at the age of 22, and his eruption appeared under his knapsack after a long march. Lesions have been precipitated by oral lithium and by phenol or ethyl chloride spray.[7] Common complications and causes of exacerbation are bacterial infection and infection with herpes simplex virus, but there are no consistent immunologic abnormalities.[8] The disease does not seem to predispose to cutaneous malignancies, although basal cell carcinomas and one rare sweat gland tumor have been reported.[9] Associated disorders include retinitis pigmentosa[10] and occasional asymptomatic bone cysts.[11] Affective disorders and decreased intelligence have been associated with DWD in recent studies.[12]

Genetics

DWD is inherited as an autosomal dominant trait. New mutations are common, and penetrance is very high, over 95 percent. The largest known pedigree is in upstate New York and southern Pennsylvania.[13] The incidence of DWD is at least 1 in 100,000 in Denmark and has been estimated to be 1 in 36,000 in northeast England.[14] No unique phenotype for genetic homozygotes has been described, and there is no evidence for X-linked or autosomal recessive forms of the disorder. There is no history of anticipation. A diverse set of mutations in Ca^{2+}-ATPase isoform 2 (SERCA2) (see Chap. 5) has been identified, including missense mutations, alternative splicing, deletions, insertions, in-frame exon skipping, frameshift mutations, and premature codon mutations.[15] The locations of these mutations are summarized in Fig. 54-1.

Knockout mice (on a mixed 129/Svj and Black Swiss background) heterozygous for a SERCA2 null mutation developed spontaneous squamous cell carcinoma in the upper digestive tract, oral mucosa, and skin (5 of 14 animals) and hyperkeratosis of a toenail. As discussed below, malignancy is not a common feature of DWD, and this difference between mice and humans deserves further study.[16]

Clinical Manifestations[17]

Multiple discrete, scaling, rough, crusted, pruritic papules that are frequently malodorous and disfiguring characterize DWD. The distribution of lesions in DWD corresponds to the "seborrheic areas" of the body. The chest (Fig. 54-2), back, ears, nasolabial folds, forehead, scalp, and groin are involved commonly. The lesions may first appear as skin-colored papules that are soon covered with a yellowish tan, rough-textured, scaly crust (Fig. 54-3). When this is removed, a pore- or slitlike opening may be seen. The lesions may coalesce into large plaques. At times, these become quite thick, forming hypertrophic warty masses[18] (Figs. 54-4 and 54-5*A*) that are foul smelling, particularly in intertriginous areas, as a result of secondary infection. The hair is normal, although the scalp is frequently covered with thick greasy scales and crusts. Permanent alopecia has been observed as a result of extensive scalp involvement (Fig. 54-6), but this is the exception. Flat wartlike papules may be seen on the dorsa of the feet and hands (Fig. 54-7*B*), and punctate keratoses, either raised or with a central pit, on the palms and soles (see Fig. 54-7*A*). Hypopigmented macules, probably postinflammatory, may be present.[19]

The nails[20] are thin and tend to break distally and show characteristic V-shaped scalloping and subungual thickening (Fig. 54-8). There are longitudinal ridges as well as red and white lines parallel to their long axis. Mucous membrane lesions (Fig. 54-9) appear as white, centrally depressed papules on the mucosae of the cheeks, hard and soft palate, and gums[21] and often present as "cobblestone" lesions. Salivary gland obstruction with histologic changes of DWD in the ductal epithelium has been reported with resulting kerostomia.[22] Rectal mucosal involvement also occurs,[23] and disease localized to the vulva has been reported.[24] Lesions also may be confined to one area of the body in a zosteriform distribution and resemble an epidermal nevus.[25,26] Two cases have been shown to be somatic mosaics with SERCA mutations in affected skin and not in uninvolved skin or peripheral leukocytes.[27] Such mosaic cases have not been reported with familial disease. One

FIGURE 54-1

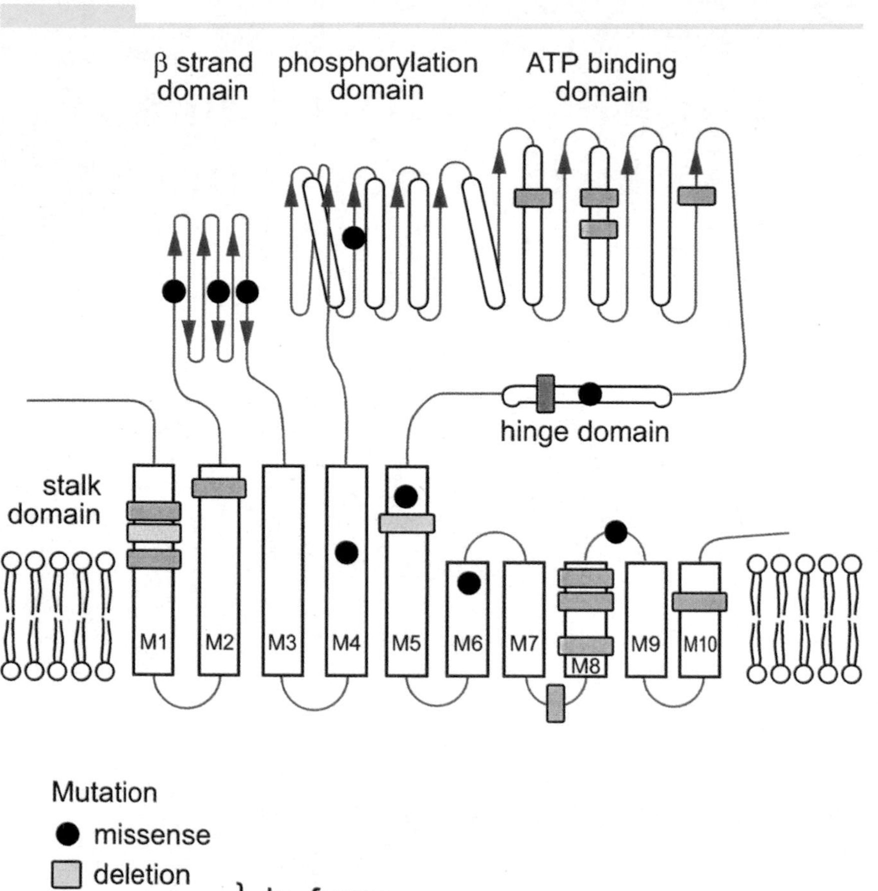

Schematic diagram of the ATP2A2 molecule. Different regions of the molecule have different functional characteristics or functions as indicated. Mutations have been found in most domains. The cell membrane is designated by circles and irregular lines. Ten intramembrane domains are depicted (M1 to M10), and in DWD these domains have missense, deletion, insertion, frameshift, and nonsense mutations as indicated.

case of a Darier like epidermal nevus has been seen in association with Gardner's syndrome that is a mutation of the *APC* (*adenomatous polyposis coli*) gene.[28] Hemorrhagic DWD, often acral, has been reported, characterized by hemorrhagic macules and vesicles[29] (Fig. 54-10); a vesiculobullous form also has been reported.[30] Cutaneous malignancies are reported only rarely with DWD and include two patients with human papilloma virus 16 (HPV-16)–related lesions subungually and on the scrotum.[31,32]

Pathology

Premature and abnormal keratinization and loss of epidermal adhesion with acantholysis characterize the disorder,[33] as do eosinophilic dyskeratotic cells in the spinous layer (corps ronds) and in the stratum corneum (grains). Suprabasal clefts (lacunae) are seen frequently, as are acantholytic cells, and are interpreted as altered adhesion within the epidermis. Papillary overgrowth of the epidermis and hyperkeratosis are common (Figs. 54-11 and 54-12).

Electron microscopic studies show basal cell vacuolization, decreased numbers of desmosomes on the lateral borders of basal cells, separation of tonofilaments from their insertions on the cell membrane, and tonofilaments in large, circular aggregates around the nucleus.[33] The corps ronds contain multiple lamellar bodies, organelles usually associated with the late stages of cornification and epidermal barrier formation (see Chap. 9). The corps ronds have many of the characteristics of apoptotic cells. The lesional morphology led to extensive studies of keratins and cell adhesion proteins, all of which failed to elucidate a primary defect.[34] Cultured DWD keratinocytes show increased locomotion, disorganized growth, and slim intercellular bridges with normal or slightly "immaturely constructed" desmosomes that appear "frail," very widened intercellular spaces, and increased cell dissociation.[35] Burge et al.[36] found increased plasminogen staining in suprabasal cells, in acantholytic cells, and in the keratotic plug.

The identical tissue histopathology seen in the genetic forms of DWD has been described rarely in epidermal nevi,[25] warty dyskeratoma, actinic keratoses, Grover's disease (transient acantholytic disease), after interleukin 4 (IL-4) therapy,[34] and other skin lesions.[38]

Hyperkeratotic papules on the dorsal surface of the hands of DWD patients have a specific histopathology, with a disordered acanthotic epidermis and angular, raised church spire-like epidermal changes.[39] The pathology is consistent with acrokeratosis of Hopf (see below). These lesions are almost always associated with DWD, although there are rare families reported with only acrokeratosis of Hopf.[40]

Hailey-Hailey disease (see Chap. 68) is a disorder of the epidermis in which the lesions are acantholytic but usually lack the extensive dyskeratotic changes seen in DWD. It has been mapped to a different chromosomal location on 3q21-q24[41] and codes for a different sarco/endoplasmic reticulum ATPase, ATP2C1. Transient acantholytic disease (Grover's disease; see Chap. 55) occurs in middle-aged or elderly adults (usually men), has no familial incidence, and often begins after sun exposures. Four patients who were studied did not have

FIGURE 54-2

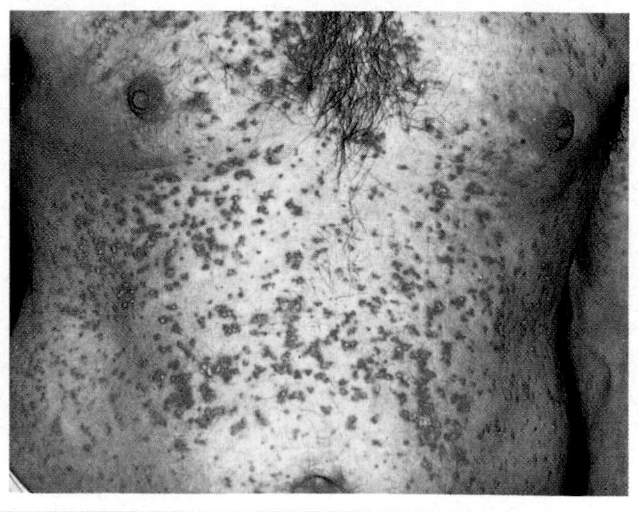

Anterior trunk demonstrating typical distribution of lesions in DWD.

FIGURE 54-3

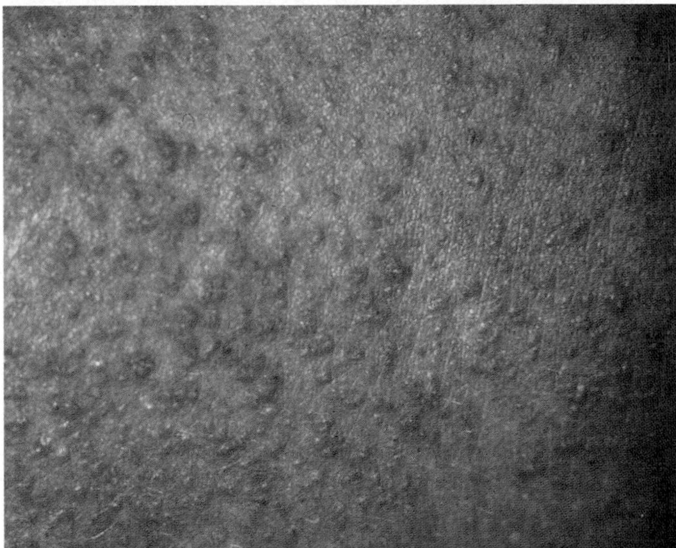

Close-up of keratotic papules in DWD. Some of the papules are associated with hair follicles; others are not.

SERCA2 mutations.[42] SERCA is a complex enzyme with 10 transmembrane domains, an intracellular ATP-binding domain, a phosphorylation domain, and a hinge region (see Fig. 54-1). All regions of the molecule have been mutated in families with DWD. Attempts at genotype-phenotype correlation have been unsuccessful except possibly for the nonspecific association of the acral hemorrhagic form of the disease with transmembrane mutations in a small number of families.

FIGURE 54-4

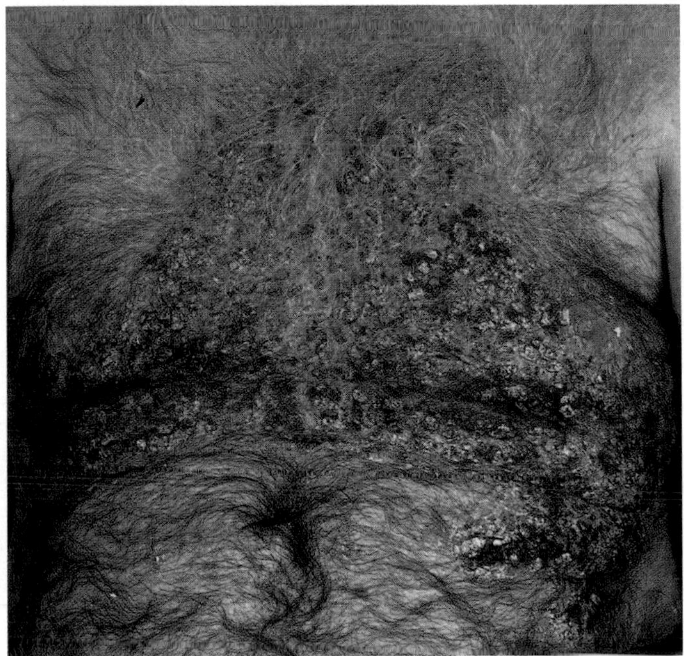

Hypertrophic, eroded, and infected lesion in DWD.

FIGURE 54-5

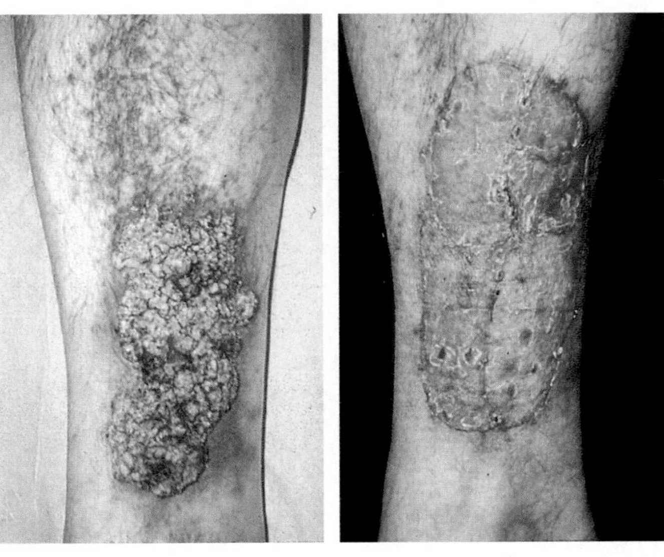

A. *B.*

Hypertrophic lesion of anterior leg (*A*), which has been excised and grafted with permanent remission in grafted site (*B*).

DWD is one of several skin diseases, including Hailey-Hailey disease, desmoplakin-related striate palmoplantar hyperkeratosis, Rubinstein-Tabyi syndrome, and some of the transcription factors associated with DNA repair, in which there is deficiency of one copy of gene and a genetic disease. This is called *haploinsufficiency.*[27] This

FIGURE 54-6

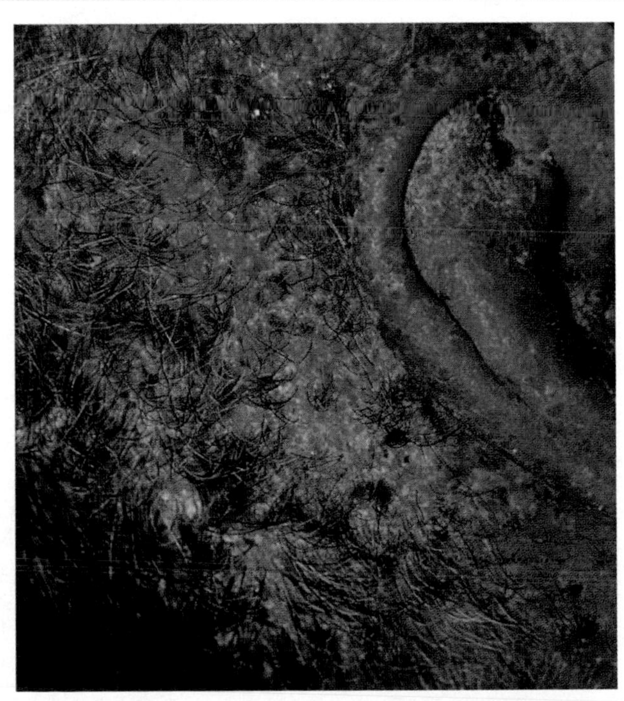

There is extensive involvement of the scalp with heavy crust-scale formation that has led to scarring alopecia.

FIGURE 54-7

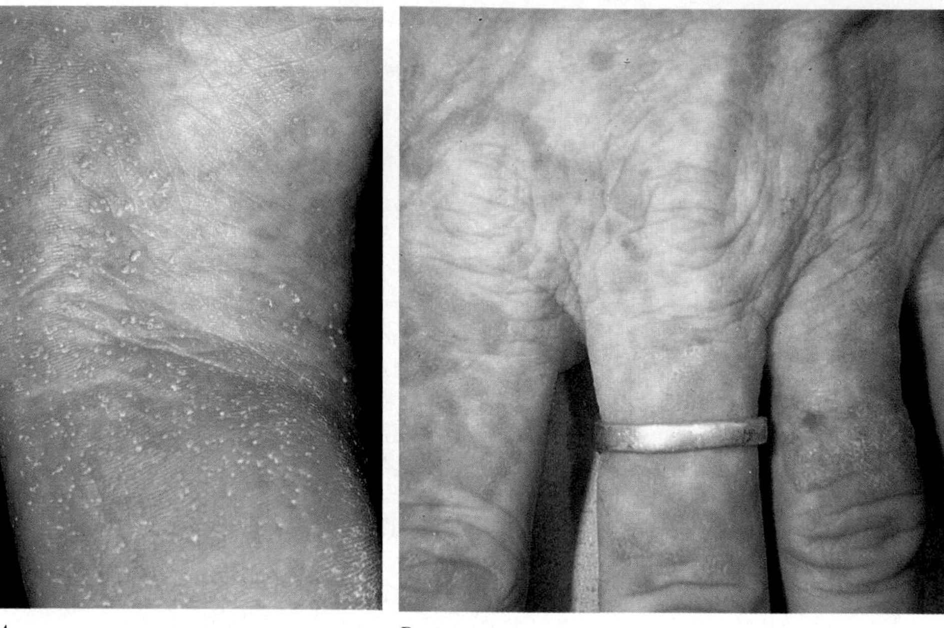

DWD with tiny keratoses of sole (*A*) and dorsum of the hand (*B*). The hand lesions are clinically identical to those of acrokeratosis verruciformis.

is distinct from the usual situation with enzyme defects, in which the heterozygote with one abnomal gene usuallly has a normal phenotype. This suggests that in the complex membrane structures in which these ATPases function, they are not present in great excess so that half the normal gene product, when coupled with another factor such as UVB or mechanical trauma, causes the clinical phenotype.

FIGURE 54-8

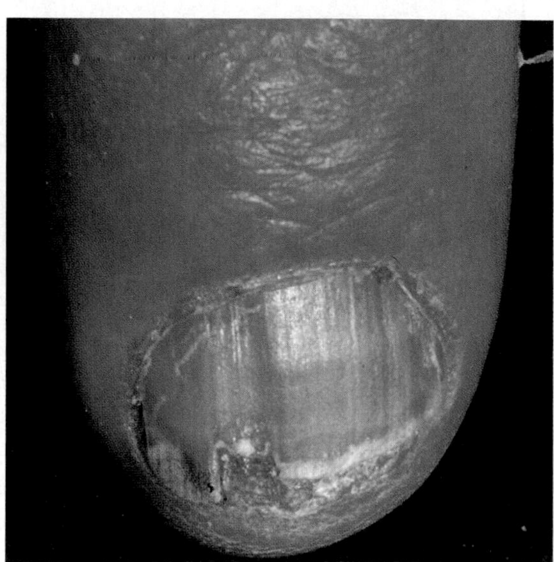

Nails in DWD. Note the subungual keratoses with V-shaped nicks. There are longitudinal ridges as well as red and white lines.

Differential Diagnosis

The history of familial involvement, clinical appearance, and histologic features make the diagnosis certain. Clinical diagnosis of small lesions in adolescence may be difficult and may require biopsy. The condition may be confused with seborrheic dermatitis because of the distribution and waxy appearance of the lesions. Benign familial pemphigus (Chap. 68) and particularly pemphigus foliaceous (Chap. 59) must be considered in the diagnosis but usually can be distinguished on clinical and histologic grounds. The localized and linear form must be differentiated from epidermal nevi with pathologic features. Eruptive forms occurring late in life have been described recently, but these are likely to be examples of transient acantholytic dermatosis.

Treatment

Sunscreens (at least SPF 30) are essential for the management of this disorder, and in those with precipitation by mechanical factors, avoidance of, for example, high sweaters around the neck that may trigger lesions is mandatory.

As with several other genetic disorders affecting the epidermis, the disease is improved by therapy with topical or systemic retinoids, including topical tazarotene and adapalene.[43,44] Systemic isotretinoin remains a reasonable first choice of a systemic therapy. If the disease is not responsive, a trial of acitretin is appropriate. Systemic therapy doses can be modified based on the seasonal variation of the disease. All the safety recommendations concerning systemic retinoids apply to DWD treatment, with the added proviso that therapy will be a long-term, albeit intermittent, process. Tazarotene gel has been effective in children as well as adults.[45] Surgical treatment has been used in the hypertrophic froms of

FIGURE 54-9

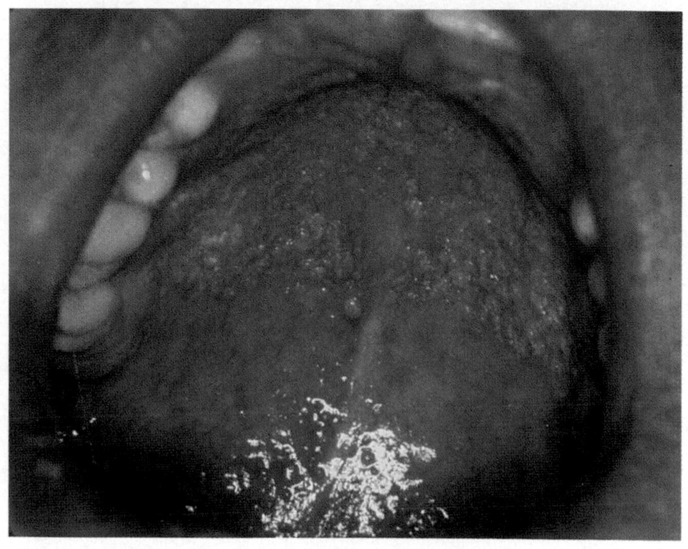

Hard palate demonstrating small "cobblestone-like" papules in DWD.

FIGURE 54-10

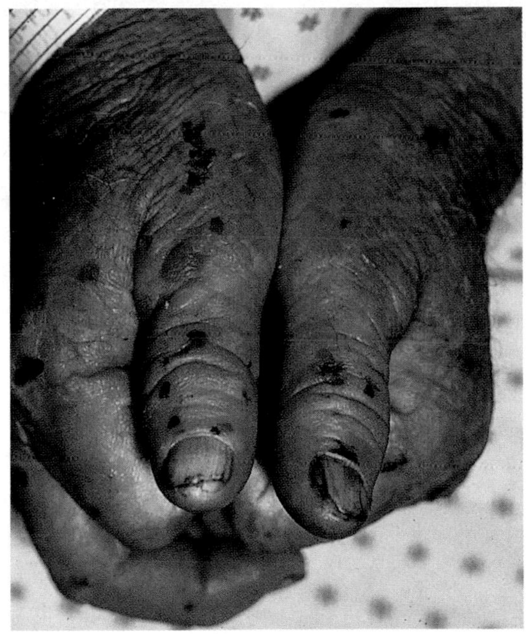

Acral hemorrhagic lesions in a patient with classic DWD.

FIGURE 54-11

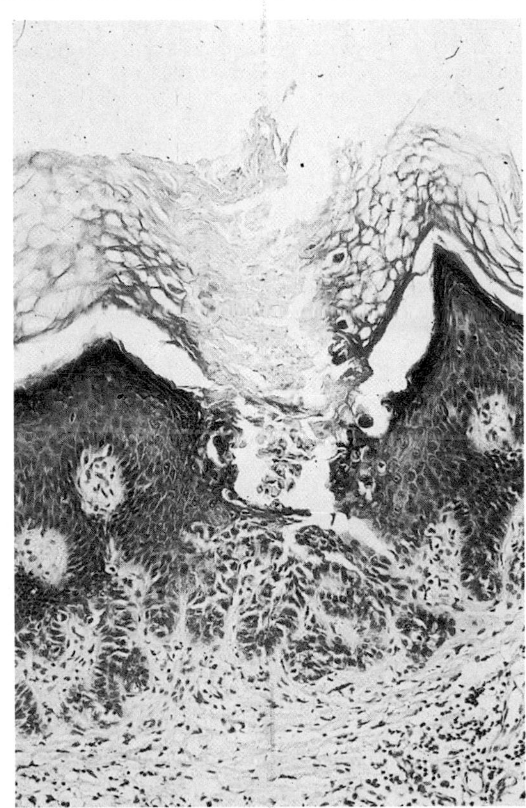

Darier-White disease. The disease is characterized by the downgrowth of narrow cords of epidermal cells from the basal regions and the conjoint exaggeration of the pattern of dermal papillae. There is also faulty cohesion of cells in the epidermal downgrowths, resulting in suprabasal clefts. Above the clefts there is evidence for faulty epidermal differentiation manifested by parakeratotic material and dyskeratotic cells.

FIGURE 54-12

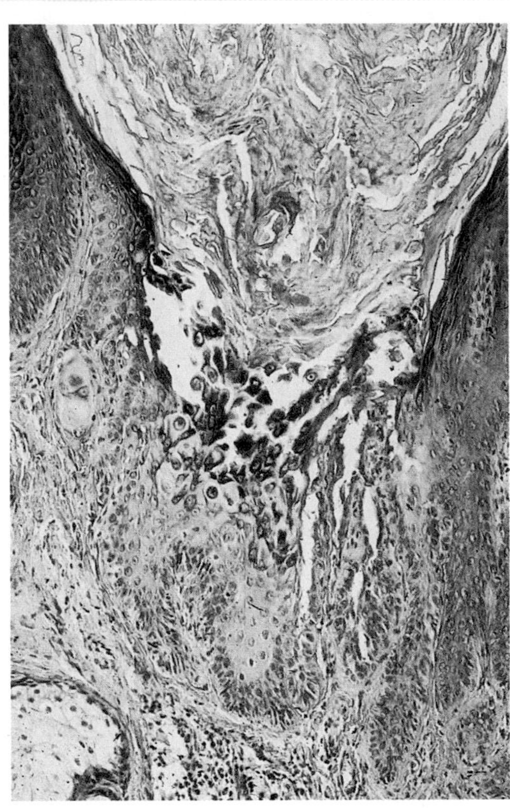

Darier-White disease: intraepidermal clefts and dyskeratotic cells. There are rounded cells with bright eosinophilic cytoplasm and an irregular dark basophilic nucleus; these dyskeratotic cells are commonly observed in DWD.

the disease[46,47] (see Fig. 54-5*B*). Many exacerbations are precipitated by bacterial infection, and appropriate antibiotic therapy can provide dramatic improvement.

ACROKERATOSIS VERRUCIFORMIS[48]

This disease is associated with DWD. Acrokeratosis verruciformis was first described by Hopf in 1931, and the familial nature was reported by Niedelman and McKusick.[40] It is a rare autosomal dominant disorder appearing at birth or in early childhood, although it has been reported to present as late as adulthood. Individual cases are reported with Hailey-Hailey disease, steatocystoma multiplex, and basal cell nevus syndrome, but these may be chance associations.

Clinical Manifestations

The lesions[49] are small, verrucous, flat papules resembling flat warts; they are present predominantly on the dorsa of the hands and feet but may appear on the forearms, knees, and elbows (see Fig. 54-7*B*). They are flesh-colored or reddish brown. Punctate keratoses are present on the palm, and the nail plates may show a variety of changes.

Pathology

Slight papillomatosis is evident, with thickening of the stratum corneum, granular layer, and stratum spinosum.

Differential Diagnosis

Patients with DWD show identical changes (see Fig. 54-7*B*), and on the basis of gross or histologic appearance of the lesions, it may be impossible to separate the conditions,[50] although dyskeratotic cells are not present in acrokeratosis verruciformis.[48] Similar lesions can be seen in epidermodysplasia verruciformis (see Chap. 223), but the histologic appearance distinguishes the two conditions. Verruca plana also has a distinctive histologic picture. The hard nevus of Unna can be differentiated by its late onset, the presence of seborrheic keratoses on the trunk, and the histologic appearance.

Treatment

The only effective therapy is superficial destruction.

Course

The lesions persist but, because of darkening, are more noticeable after prolonged sun exposure.

REFERENCES

1. Sakuntabhai A et al: Mutations in ATP2A2, encoding a Ca^{2+} pump, cause Darier disease. *Nature Genet* **21**:271, 1999
2. Getyler N, Flint A: Keratosis follicularis: A study of one family. *Arch Dermatol* **93**:545, 1966
3. Svendsen I, Albrechtsen B: The prevalence of dyskeratosis follicularis (Darier's disease) in Denmark: An investigation of the heredity in 22 families. *Acta Derm Venereol (Stockh)* **39**:256, 1959
4. Tegner E, Jonsson N: Darier's disease with involvement of both submandibular glands. *Acta Derm Venereol (Stockh)* **70**:451, 1990
5. Blackman HJ et al: Corneal epithelial lesions in keratosis follicularis (Darier's disease). *Ophthalmology* **87**:931, 1980
6. Baba T, Yaoita H: UV radiation and keratosis follicularis. *Arch Dermatol* **120**:1484, 1984
7. Penrod J: Observations on keratosis follicularis. *Arch Dermatol* **82**:367, 1960
8. Halevy S et al: Immunologic studies in Darier's disease. *Int J Dermatol* **27**:101, 1988
9. Latour DL et al: Darier's disease associated with cutaneous malignancies. *J Dermatol Surg Oncol* **7**:408, 1981
10. Itin P et al: Darier's disease and retinitis pigmentosa: Is there a pathogenetic relationship? *Br J Dermatol* **119**:397, 1988
11. Crisp AJ et al: The prevalence of bone cysts in Darier's disease: A survey of 31 cases. *Clin Exp Dermatol* **9**:78, 1984
12. Craddock N et al: Familial cosegregation of major affective disorder and Darier's disease (keratosis follicularis). *Br J Psychiatry* **164**:355, 1994
13. Beck ALJ et al: Darier's disease: A kindred with a large number of cases. *Br J Dermatol* **97**:335, 1977
14. Munro CS: The phenotype of Darier's disease: Penetrance and expressivity in adults and children. *Br J Dermatol* **127**:126, 1992
15. Sakuntabhai A et al: Spectrum of novel ATP2A2 mutations in patients with Darier's disease. *Hum Mol Genet* **8**:1611, 1999
16. Liu LH et al: Squamous cell tumors in mice heterozygous for a null allele of Atp2a2, encoding the sarco(endo)plasmic reticulum Ca^{2+}-ATPase isoform 2 Ca^{2+} pump. *J Biol Chem* **276**:26737, 2001.
17. Burge S: Management of Darier's disease. *Clin Exp Dermatol* **24**:53, 1999
18. Elsbach E, Nater J: The hypertrophic form of Darier's disease. *Dermatologica* **120**:93, 1960
19. Rowley MJ et al: Hypopigmented macules in acantholytic disorders. *Int J Dermatol* **34**:390, 1995
20. Zaias N, Ackerman AB: The nail in Darier-White disease. *Arch Dermatol* **107**:193, 1973
21. Gorlin R, Chaundhry A: The oral manifestation of keratosis follicularis. *Oral Surg* **12**:1468, 1959
22. Graham-Brown RA et al: Darier's disease with salivary gland obstruction. *J R Soc Med* **76**:609, 1983
23. Klein A et al: Rectal mucosa involvement in keratosis follicularis. *Arch Dermatol* **109**:560, 1974
24. Barrett JF et al: Darier's disease localized to the vulva: Case report. *Br J Obstet Gynaecol* **96**:997, 1989
25. Demetree JW et al: Unilateral, linear, zosteriform epidermal nevus with acantholytic dyskeratosis. *Arch Dermatol* **115**:875, 1979
26. O'Malley MP et al: Localized Darier disease: Implications for genetic studies. *Arch Dermatol* **133**:1134, 1997
27. Sakuntabhai A et al: Mosaicism for ATP2A2 mutations causes segmental Darier's disease. *J Invest Dermatol* **115**:1144, 2000
28. Romiti R al: Epidermal naevus with Darier's disease-like changes in a patient with Gardner's syndrome. *J Am Acad Dermatol* **43**:380, 2000
29. Foresman PL et al: Hemorrhagic Darier's disease. *Arch Dermatol* **129**:511, 1993
30. Telfer N: Vesiculo-bullous Darier's disease. *Br J Dermatol* **122**:831, 1990
31. Downs AM et al: Subungual squamous cell carcinoma in Darier's disease. *Clin Exp Dermatol* **22**:277, 1997
32. Orihuela E et al: Developoment of human papillomavirus type 16–associated squamous cell carcinoma of the scrotum in a patient with Darier's disease treated with systemic isotretinoin. *J Urol* **153**:1940, 1995
33. Caulfield J, Wilgram G: An electron microscope study of dyskeratosis and acantholysis in Darier's disease. *J Invest Dermatol* **41**:57, 1963
34. Burge SM, Schomberg KH: Adhesion molecules and related proteins in Darier's disease and Hailey-Hailey disease. *Br J Dermatol* **127**:335, 1992
35. Ishibashi Y et al: Tissue culture of epidermal cells in some acantholytic dermatoses. *Curr Probl Dermatol* **10**:91, 1980
36. Burge SM: Darier's disease: An immunohistochemical study using monoclonal antibodies to proteases. *Br J Dermatol* **121**:613, 1989
37. Mahler SJ et al: Transient acantholytic dermatosis induced by recombinant human interleukin 4. *J Am Acad Dermatol* **29**:206, 1993
38. Ackerman AB: Focal acantholytic dyskeratosis. *Arch Dermatol* **106**:702, 1972
39. Herndon JJ, Wilson J: Acrokeratosis verruciformis (Hopf) and Darier's disease. *Arch Dermatol* **93**:305, 1966
40. Niedelman M, McKusick V: Acrokeratosis verruciformis (Hopf). *Arch Dermatol* **86**:779, 1962
41. Ikeda S et al: Localization of the gene whose mutations underlie Hailey-Hailey disease to chromosome 3q. *Hum Mol Genet* **3**:1147, 1994
42. Powell J et al: Grover's disease, despite histological similarity to Darier's disease, does not share an abnormality in the ATP2A2 gene. *Br J Dermatol* **143**:658, 2000
43. Burge S: Management of Darier's disease. *Clin Exp Dermatol* **24**:53, 1999
44. English JC et al: Effective treatment of localized Darier's disease with adapalene 0.1% gel. *Cutis* **63**:227, 1999
45. Micali G, Nasca MR: Tazarotene gel in childhood Darier disease. *Pediatr Dermatol* **16**:243, 1999
46. Wheeland RG, Gilmore, WA: The surgical treatment of hypertrophic Darier's disease. *J Dermatol Surg Oncol* **11**:420, 1985
47. Toombs EL, Peck GL: Electrosurgical treatment of etretinate-resistant Darier's disease. *J Dermatol Surg Oncol* **15**:1277, 1989
48. Panja RK: Acrokeratosis verruciformis (Hopf): A clinical entity? *Br J Dermatol* **96**:643, 1977
49. Rook A, Stevanovic D: Acrokeratosis verruciformis. *Arch Dermatol* **69**:450, 1957
50. Waisman M: Verruciform manifestations of keratosis follicularis. *Arch Dermatol* **81**:1, 1960

CHAPTER 55

Peter J. Heenan
Christopher J. Quirk

Transient Acantholytic Dermatosis (Grover Disease)

Grover disease (transient acantholytic dermatosis) is a polymorphic, pruritic, papulovesicular dermatosis characterized histologically by acantholysis. Although the disease is predominantly self-limited, the duration ranges from weeks to many months, so the term *transient* is often inappropriate; Grover disease appears to be the best name at present for the condition.

HISTORIC ASPECTS

In 1970,[1] Grover described six patients with an apparently unique pruritic, self-limited, primary acantholytic skin disease that he termed *transient acantholytic dermatosis* (TAD). Chalet et al.[2] reviewed 54 patients and described the clinical and histologic features in more detail, including the four characteristic patterns of acantholysis; a further 24 patients were reported by Heenan and Quirk in 1980.[3] Other sporadic reports of adult-onset papular acantholytic disorders may represent variants of Grover disease.[4–6]

ETIOLOGY AND PATHOGENESIS

Grover's disease is a common disorder that has been reported in many countries. The cause is unknown. The majority of cases have occurred in white males over the age of 40 years.

In several reports, the disease has been linked to excessive sun exposure,[3] heat, sweating,[2–4,7–9] and occlusion of sweat ducts, analogous to miliaria. Other sporadic associations include febrile illness in immunocompromised patients,[8] leukemia,[10,11] lymphoma, solid tumors, and hospitalization,[11] perhaps also related to heat, persistent fever, and sweating. The ultrastructural and light microscopic appearances suggest that disordered keratinization plays an important role in the pathogenesis, with the different patterns of acantholysis perhaps reflecting different stages in development of the lesions.

CLINICAL MANIFESTATIONS

Although some lesions are not pruritic,[12] most patients complain of pruritus of sudden onset, often disproportionate to the extent of the eruption. This eruption may consist of sparse or numerous smooth or warty papules, papulovesicles, eczematous plaques, or shiny, translucent, sometimes excoriated nodules (Figs. 55-1 and 55-2). Bullous lesions have been seen. Commonly affected sites are the trunk, neck, and proximal limbs. The submammary area is a characteristic site. Many

FIGURE 55-1

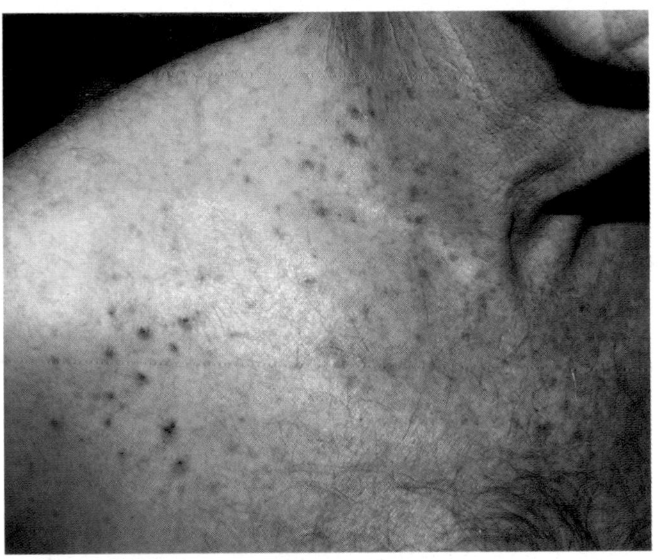

Grover disease. Upper trunk of a 72-year-old man. Multiple discrete polymorphic lesions, including papules and excoriated nodules.

FIGURE 55-2

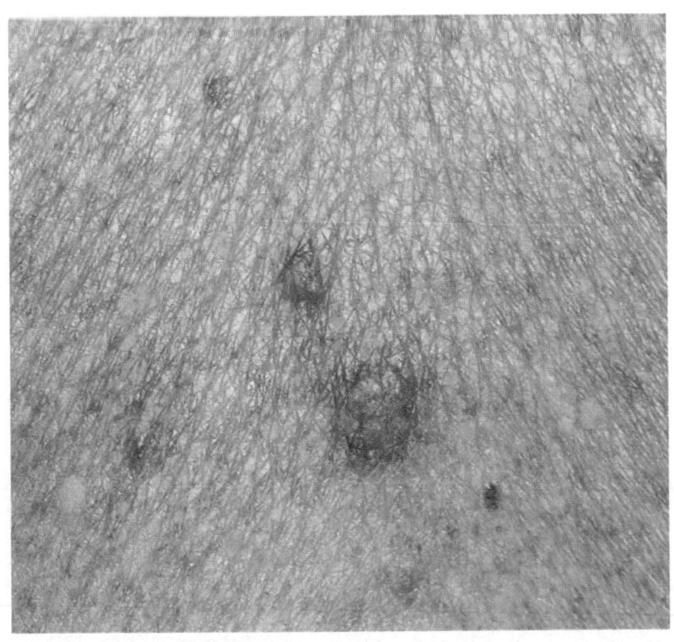

Grover disease: erythematous papules.

cases are transient, but others are persistent.[6] The mean duration in one series was 47 weeks,[3] in another 94 weeks,[11] and in a third series 360 weeks.[13] Reports of a chronic relapsing course are not uncommon.[11] In a retrospective study of 375 cases, Grover showed associations with eczema of various types.[14]

PATHOLOGY

The characteristic acantholysis occurs in four main patterns, described by Chalet et al.[2] as resembling Darier-White disease (keratosis follicularis), pemphigus, Hailey-Hailey disease (familial benign chronic pemphigus), and a spongiotic form with acantholysis (Fig. 55-3). These different patterns may occur singly but are more often seen in combination,

FIGURE 55-3

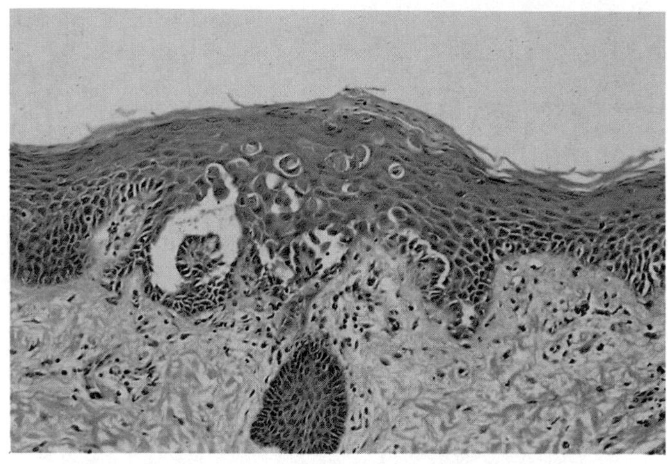

A.

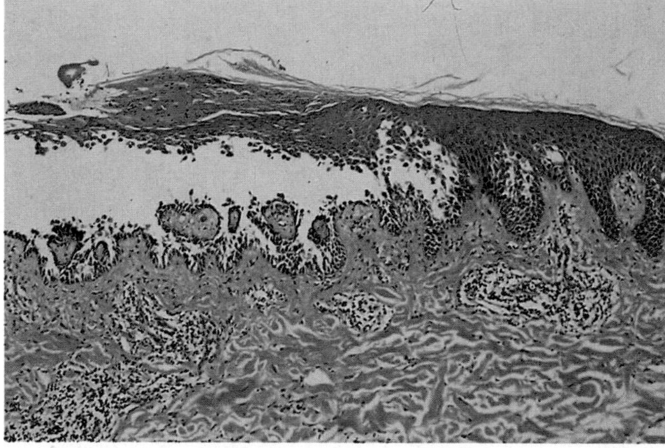

B.

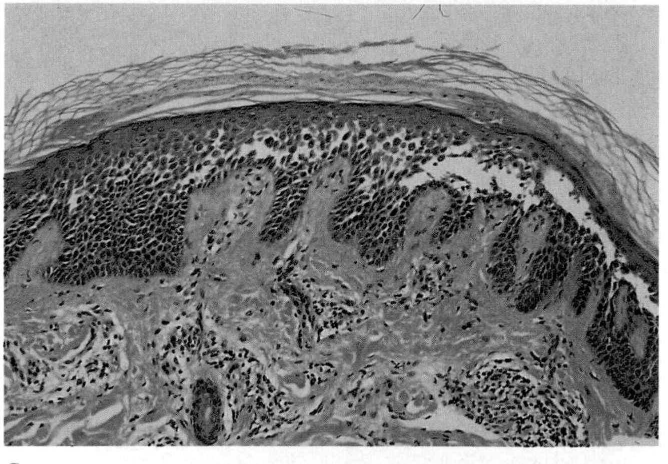

C.

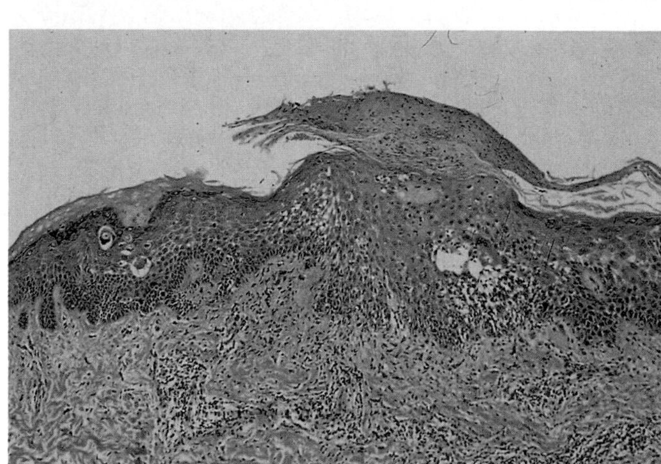

D.

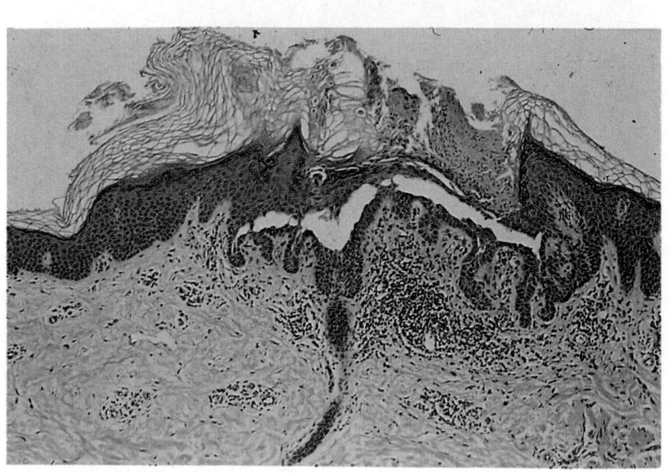

E.

Grover disease: histology. *A.* Darier-White-type lesion with small suprabasal clefts, dyskeratotic cells, and dermal lymphocytic inflammation. *B.* Pemphigus-like lesion with acantholytic cells in a suprabasal cleft. *C.* Hailey-Hailey-like lesion with acantholysis involving most of the stratum malpighii. *D.* Spongiotic lesion with acantholytic cells in the vesicle and a separate focus of dyskeratosis (*left*). *E.* Focus of acantholytic dyskeratosis and suprabasal clefting overlying an eccrine duct.

the Darier-White type being most common overall.[3] The histologic changes typically occupy tiny, circumscribed foci, so several biopsies and multiple sections are often necessary to obtain the representative histologic changes.

The acantholysis usually occurs in a suprabasal location in lesions of the Darier-White and pemphigus types and throughout most layers of the stratum malpighii in those resembling Hailey-Hailey disease, resulting in the formation of small intraepidermal clefts or, infrequently, bullae.[15] Additional epidermal changes include hyperkeratosis, acanthosis, and parakeratosis. These changes tend to be most severe in lesions of the Darier-White type, which sometimes have vertical columns of parakeratosis overlying dyskeratotic, acantholytic foci, whereas other changes are less severe or absent in lesions of the pemphigus type.[3] Lesions are sometimes seen in association with an acrosyringium (see Fig. 55-3*E*), but this association has not been consistently demonstrated.[16] The dermis in most cases contains a superficial perivascular infiltrate of lymphocytes and histiocytes, sometimes with scattered eosinophils.

Immunofluorescence[3,11,17,18] and immunohistochemical[11,19] studies have not demonstrated consistent patterns of positivity. Electron microscopic studies have shown ultrastructural changes resembling those of true Darier-White disease[20] and pemphigus, whereas some differences in detail from Hailey-Hailey disease have been reported.[21]

DIFFERENTIAL DIAGNOSIS

The clinical appearance of many types of papular eruptions may simulate Grover disease. When the papules are scattered, the process may mimic prurigo simplex, miliaria rubra, papular urticaria, folliculitis, scabies, papular eczema, papular infiltrates, or dermatitis herpetiformis. When the papular lesions are so numerous as to be almost confluent, the suspicion of Grover disease is heightened, although some drug eruptions can present a similar appearance. Because of its frequent association with other skin diseases, specifically eczema, dual pathology always should be suspected.[14]

The histologic features of each pattern of acantholysis when seen alone are not specific for Grover disease. Lesions of the Darier-White type are often indistinguishable from those of true Darier-White disease, but tiny foci of dyskeratotic acantholysis with small suprabasal clefts, without an overlying column of parakeratosis, are more typical of Grover disease.[22] The presence of acantholysis within spongiotic vesicles is thought to be a helpful clue to the diagnosis of Grover disease[2] or even unique to this disease.[22] The bland appearance of the pemphigus-like lesions with very few, if any, eosinophils in the dermis helps to distinguish these changes from pemphigus vulgaris, and the distinction is confirmed by negative immunofluorescence. The Hailey-Hailey pattern also occurs only in tiny foci, usually in combination with one or more of the other acantholytic patterns.

The best histologic evidence for the diagnosis of Grover disease is the presence of several different patterns of acantholysis in the same biopsy, occupying very small, circumscribed foci. However, several patterns of acantholysis may occur in association with other acantholytic processes, such as pemphigus vulgaris,[2] so the final diagnosis depends on the correlation of clinical and histologic findings.

TREATMENT

Assessment of efficacy of therapy is difficult because some cases remit spontaneously and others demonstrate a fluctuant course. Avoidance

of heat and sweat-inducing activities is important in achieving clinical improvement; rapid temperature changes often aggravate the condition. Topical glucocorticoids and antipruritics are helpful in controlling the pruritus in mild cases. Systemic glucocorticoids generally are effective in the more severe cases, but relapse is frequent on withdrawal of the drug.

Reports of the successful treatment of other disorders of keratinization, including Darier-White disease, with vitamin A[23] led to its use in Grover disease, with good results in some cases.[24] The synthetic retinoids etretinate, acitretin,[13] and isotretinoin[13,25] have been used in some cases with good effects, but double-blind trials have not been performed with either these drugs or vitamin A. PUVA therapy also has met with some success.[26]

REFERENCES

1. Grover RW: Transient acantholytic dermatosis. *Arch Dermatol* **101**:426, 1970
2. Chalet M et al: Transient acantholytic dermatosis: A reevaluation. *Arch Dermatol* **113**:431, 1977
3. Heenan PJ, Quirk CJ: Transient acantholytic dermatosis. *Br J Dermatol* **102**:515, 1980
4. Heaphy MR et al: Benign papular acantholytic dermatosis. *Arch Dermatol* **112**:814, 1976
5. Gisslen H, Mobacken H: Acute adult-onset Darier-like dermatosis. *Br J Dermatol* **98**:217, 1978
6. Simon RS et al: Persistent acantholytic dermatosis. A variant of transient acantholytic dermatosis (Grover's disease). *Arch Dermatol* **112**:1429, 1976
7. Hu CH et al: Transient acantholytic dermatosis (Grover's disease): A skin disorder related to heat and sweating. *Arch Dermatol* **121**:1439, 1985
8. Horn TD, Groleau GE: Transient acantholytic dermatosis in immunocompromised febrile patients with cancer. *Arch Dermatol* **123**:238, 1987
9. Quarterman MJ, Davis LS: Transient acantholytic dermatosis in a postoperative febrile patient. *Int J Dermatol* **34**:113, 1995
10. Yaffee HS: Possible dysglobulinemia and Grover's disease. *Arch Dermatol* **117**:3, 1981
11. Davis MD et al: Grover's disease: Clinicopathological review of 72 cases. *Mayo Clin Proc* **74**:229, 1999
12. Guana A, Cohen P: Transient acantholytic dermatosis in oncology patients. *J Clin Oncol* **12**:1703, 1994
13. Streit M et al. Transitory acantholytic dermatosis (Grover disease). An analysis of the clinical spectrum based on 21 histologically assessed cases. *Hautarzt* **51**:244, 2000
14. Grover RW, Rosenbaum R: The association of transient acantholytic dermatosis with other skin diseases. *J Am Acad Dermatol* **11**:253, 1984
15. Waisman M et al: Bullous transient acantholytic dermatosis. *Arch Dermatol* **112**:1440, 1976
16. Antley CM et al: Grover's disease: Relationship of acantholysis to acrosyringia. *J Cutan Pathol* **25**:545, 1998
17. Bystryn J-C: Immunofluorescence studies in transient acantholytic dermatosis (Grover's disease). *Am J Dermatopathol* **1**:325, 1979
18. Millns JL et al: Positive cutaneous immunofluorescence in Grover's disease. *Arch Dermatol* **116**:515, 1980
19. Gretzula JC, Penneys NS: Transient acantholytic dermatosis: An immunohistochemical study. *Arch Dermatol* **122**:972, 1986
20. Grover RW, Duffy JL: Transient acantholytic dermatosis: Electron microscopic study of the Darier type. *J Cutan Pathol* **2**:111, 1975
21. Grover RW: Transient acantholytic dermatosis: Electron microscopic study. *Arch Dermatol* **104**:26, 1971
22. Ackerman AB: *Histological Diagnosis of Inflammatory Skin Diseases*. Philadelphia, Lea & Febiger, 1978
23. Porter AD et al: Vitamin A in Darier's disease. *Arch Dermatol* **56**:306, 1947
24. Rohr J, Quirk CJ: Treatment of transient acantholytic dermatosis. *Arch Dermatol* **115**:1033, 1979
25. Helfman RJ: Grover's disease treated with isotretinoin. *J Am Acad Dermatol* **12**:981, 1985
26. Paul BS, Arndt KA: Response of transient acantholytic dermatosis to photochemotherapy. *Arch Dermatol* **120**:121, 1984

CHAPTER 56

Elisabeth Ch. Wolff-Schreiner

Porokeratosis

Porokeratosis is a specific disorder of keratinization that is characterized histologically by the presence of a cornoid lamella—a thin column of closely stacked, parakeratotic cells extending through the stratum corneum. Clinically, the basic lesion is sharply demarcated and hyperkeratotic, and it may be annular with central atrophy, either linear or punctate.

Five clinical variants are recognized (Table 56-1): (1) classic porokeratosis Mibelli; (2) disseminated superficial porokeratosis (DSP) and disseminated superficial actinic porokeratosis (DSAP); (3) porokeratosis palmaris et plantaris disseminata (PPPD); and (4) linear porokeratosis. A fifth form, not listed in the table, is punctate porokeratosis, which is usually associated with the linear or Mibelli variants.

HISTORICAL ASPECTS

Mibelli described the lesions of classic porokeratosis in 1893 as one or more localized, chronically progressive, hyperkeratotic, irregular plaques with central atrophy and a prominent peripheral keratotic ridge. At about the same time, Respighi and, later, Andrews independently described a more superficial, disseminated form.[1] The linear variants were delineated early in the twentieth century. In 1966, Chernosky described DSAP,[2] and in 1971 Guss and associates added disseminated porokeratosis with palmar and plantar involvement (PPPD) to the spectrum.[3] In 1977, punctate porokeratosis was delineated as a minor form, usually associated with the linear or Mibelli variants.[4]

ETIOLOGY AND PATHOGENESIS

The etiology of the different variants of porokeratosis is unknown, but is certainly multifactorial.

Hereditary Factors

The coexistence of various forms of porokeratosis in one patient or in several members of an affected family suggests that the forms are different phenotypic expressions of a common genetic defect. An autosomal dominant mode of inheritance with reduced penetrance has been

TABLE 56-1

Distinguishing Features of Four Types of Porokeratosis

	Classic Porokeratosis (Mibelli)	Disseminated Superficial (Actinic) Porokeratosis (DSP, DSAP)	Porokeratosis Palmaris et Plantaris Disseminata (PPPD)	Linear Porokeratosis
Incidence	Rare	Not rare	Rare	Rare
Inheritance	Autosomal dominant	Autosomal dominant	Autosomal dominant	?
Age of onset	Usually childhood	Third to fourth decades	Childhood to adulthood	Birth to adulthood
Sex predominance, M:F	2:1 to 3:1	1:3	2:1	1:1
Morphology of lesions				
Size (cm)	Variable up to 20	Uniform, usually 0.5–1.0	Uniform, usually 0.5–1.0	Variable, usually 0.5–1.0 coalescent
Height of border (mm)	1–10	<1 (threadlike)	<1	<1 and larger
Furrow in border	Yes	Discrete	Discrete	May be present
Prominence	Quite prominent	Superficial, indistinct	Superficial, but more keratotic	Superficial and prominent
Number of lesions	Only few	Large number	Large number	Few to large number
Distribution of lesions	Localized, anywhere	Generalized (DSP) Sun-exposed skin (DSAP)	Generalized, palms and soles	Localized, linear, unilateral
Palms and soles	Possible	No	Yes	Possible
Mucous membranes	Yes	No	Possible	No
Koebner phenomenon	Reported	Not reported	Not reported	Not reported
Histology (cornoid lamella)	Prominent	Less developed	Less developed	Prominent
Symptomatic	Usually not	37%	37%	Possible
Summer exacerbation	None	48% (DSAP)	25%	Not reported
Malignant degeneration	Reported	Reported	Reported	Reported

SOURCE: Adapted from Guss et al.,[3] with permission.

reasonably well established for porokeratosis Mibelli, PPPD, DSP, and DSAP. A gene locus involved in the phenotypic expression of DSAP has been identified on the long arm of chromosome 12.[5] Linear porokeratosis has been observed in monozygotic twins, is often associated with the disseminated forms of porokeratosis, and has been interpreted as a type 2 segmental manifestation of DSP[6] or DSAP.[7] Sporadic cases may be due to somatic mutations.

All porokeratoses share the cornoid lamella, a thin, parakeratotic column at the periphery of typical lesions. It has been suggested that, at the base of this parakeratotic column, an inherited mutant clone of keratinocytes expands peripherally, leading to the formation of a cornoid lamella between the clonal cells and normal keratinocytes.[8]

Additional Factors

In genetically disposed skin, additional factors are assumed to trigger the clinical manifestations. Irradiation with ultraviolet (UV) light from natural or artificial sources, for example, has induced lesions of DSAP and exacerbations. Additionally, there are increasing numbers of reports of DSP and DSAP in connection with or after organ transplantation,[9,10] bone marrow transplantation,[11] transplant induction therapy,[12] chronic renal[13] and hepatic failure,[14] hepatitis C virus infection with or without hepatocellular carcinoma,[15] HIV infection,[16,17] and various other causes of impaired immunocompetence. It has been suggested that local immunosuppression may explain the promoting effect of UV light.[18] Malignancies rarely arise in porokeratosis lesions in immunosuppressed individuals,[19,20] although profound immunosuppression may facilitate the emergence of abnormal keratinocyte clones and eventually malignant transformation.[16,20,21]

A high rate of abnormal DNA-ploidy[22] and certain phenotypic features indicative of malignant transformation or altered differentiation (i.e., overexpression of p53, decreased mdm2, normal 21Waf1/Cip1 expression;[23,24] abnormal expression of psi-3, cytokeratins, filaggrin, and involucrin) suggest an increased proliferative potential in affected keratinocytes. Cultured fibroblasts from lesional and nonlesional skin may exhibit chromosomal instability[22] and hypersensitivity to x-irradiation.[25] An alternative hypothesis for the hyperproliferative state of keratinocytes in porokeratosis comes from the finding that underneath the epidermis bearing a cornoid lamella there resides an inflammatory mononuclear infiltrate composed of helper T cells, suppressor T cells, and Langerhans cells.[26] Soluble factors released by activated T cells may provide a mitotic stimulus for overlying keratinocytes. The role of the dermis in the pathologic process is further enhanced by the fact that lesions recur after destruction of the epidermis, but not the dermis, and that lesions may develop in predisposed skin after dermal injury.

A hypothetical infectious/transmissible agent has been postulated as an explanation for the high incidence of porokeratoses in transplant recipients, in immunosuppressed patients, and in connection with hepatitis C virus and HIV infection.[27,28]

CLINICAL MANIFESTATIONS

Porokeratosis Mibelli

Lesions of porokeratosis Mibelli start as small, brownish papules that slowly enlarge to form irregular, annular, hyperkeratotic or verrucous plaques. The lesions have a well demarcated, raised hyperkeratotic border that is usually more than 1 mm in height and contains a diagnostic, threadlike groove so that the border resembles a dike split by a longitudinal furrow (Fig. 56-1). The center is usually atrophic, hairless, anhydrotic, and hyper- or hypopigmented. Porokeratosis Mibelli can occur practically anywhere on the body, but preferentially it is

FIGURE 56-1

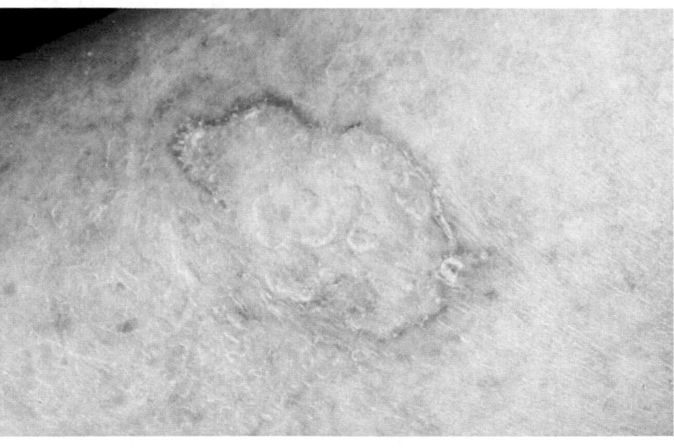

Typical large prominent lesion of porokeratosis Mibelli.

localized to the limbs where lesions may involve palms and soles; lesions can occur on the face, sometimes extending to the lips and the oral mucosa, and in the genital and perigenital region. Porokeratosis Mibelli usually presents as one or a few, generally asymptomatic, lesions from millimeters to several centimeters in diameter, but giant lesions do occur. Malignant degeneration can occur in large lesions of long duration.

Onset is during childhood, and lesions enlarge slowly over the years. Family studies suggest an autosomal dominant mode of inheritance (see Table 56-1).

Disseminated Superficial Porokeratosis and Disseminated Superficial Actinic Porokeratosis

A more generalized process than porokeratosis Mibelli, DSP involves mainly the extremities in a bilateral, symmetric fashion (Fig. 56-2*A*). In about 50 percent of the cases, lesions develop only in sun-exposed areas (DSAP), and patients often offer a history of exacerbations during the summer months with pruritus, burning, or stinging sensations.

Early lesions are small papules, often with a central dell, measuring 1 to 3 mm in diameter. They enlarge over months or years to form superficial, ringlike lesions with a slightly atrophic center, surrounded by a delicate keratotic ridge that is topped by a barely visible furrow (Fig. 56-2*B*). Irregular centrifugal growth and coalescence of lesions may give rise to circinate configurations. Lesions are erythematous, pigmented, or the color of normal skin, and they are typically dry and anhydrotic. Literally hundreds of lesions can be disseminated preferentially over the extensor surfaces of the extremities (see Fig. 56-2*A*); they spare the axillary vaults, inguinal folds, perigenital region, palms, soles and mucous membranes. Involvement of the face is rare in DSP or DSAP.

The course is slowly progressive over years. Disseminated superficial actinic porokeratosis occurs more often in geographic areas with high sun exposure. Irradiation with natural and artificial UV light, photochemotherapy, and phototherapy for psoriasis can lead to exacerbation or persistence of DSAP lesions.

Attempts to induce new lesions by trauma (the Koebner phenomenon) have failed. Autotransplantation of normal skin into a lesion has resulted in re-formation of the lesional ridge within the graft, whereas it disappeared from lesional skin grafted into a normal bed.

FIGURE 56-2

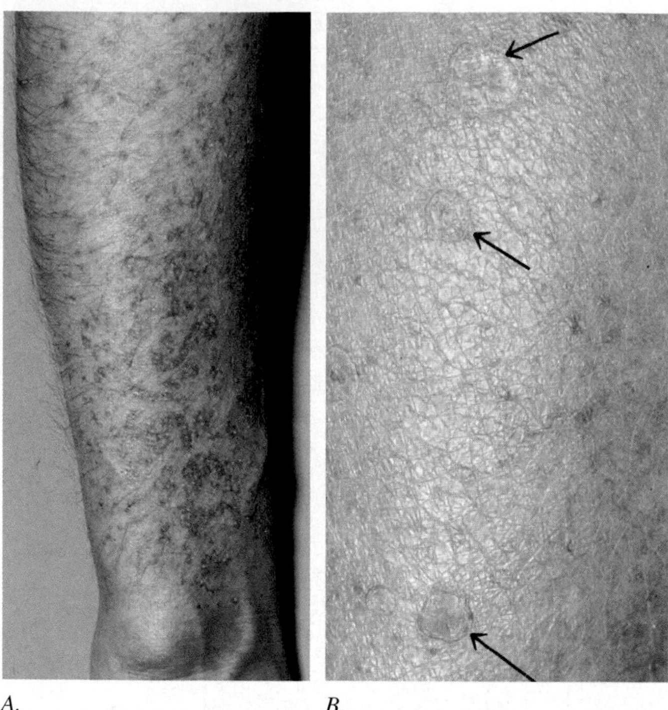

A. Multiple disseminated lesions of superficial actinic porokeratosis on the forearm. *B.* Very discrete, superficial lesions on the forearm in another patient with characteristic furrows in the periphery of lesions (*arrows*).

The disseminated forms of porokeratosis are relatively common. The apparent slight preponderance of female patients is probably not due to genetic factors, but to the fact that women are more likely to seek medical advice than men. Disseminated superficial actinic porokeratosis seems to be extremely rare in blacks. Onset is usually in the third and fourth decades; in no instance has the condition been described in childhood.[5] The mode of inheritance is autosomal dominant with reduced penetrance at a young age (see Table 56-1).

Porokeratosis Palmaris et Plantaris Disseminata

Lesions of PPPD are superficial, small, relatively uniform, and demarcated by a distinct peripheral ridge of no more than 1 mm in height (Fig.56-3). In palmar and plantar lesions, which are generally more hyperkeratotic, the characteristic longitudinal furrow along this ridge may be quite pronounced (Fig. 56-4). Lesions first arise on palms and soles and spread in large numbers over the extremities, the trunk, and other parts of the body, including areas not exposed to sunlight. They can cause pruritus and stinging sensations. Lesions involving the mucous membranes are small, annular or serpiginous, opalescent, asymptomatic, and they can be quite numerous.

Onset is usually during adolescence or early adulthood. Transmitted in an autosomal dominant mode, PPPD affects males twice as often as it affects females (see Table 56-1).

Linear Porokeratosis

In some cases, linear porokeratosis occurs in a unilateral, linear systematized form resembling a linear verrucous epidermal nevus. Clinically, the basic lesions are identical to those of the Mibelli type, including lichenoid papules, annular lesions, hyperkeratotic plaques with central atrophy, and the characteristic peripheral ridge (Fig.56-5). The condition is strictly unilateral. It may involve only one extremity, but may also be present on the other extremity, the trunk, and the face on the same side. On the extremities, lesions are grouped and linearly arranged,

FIGURE 56-3

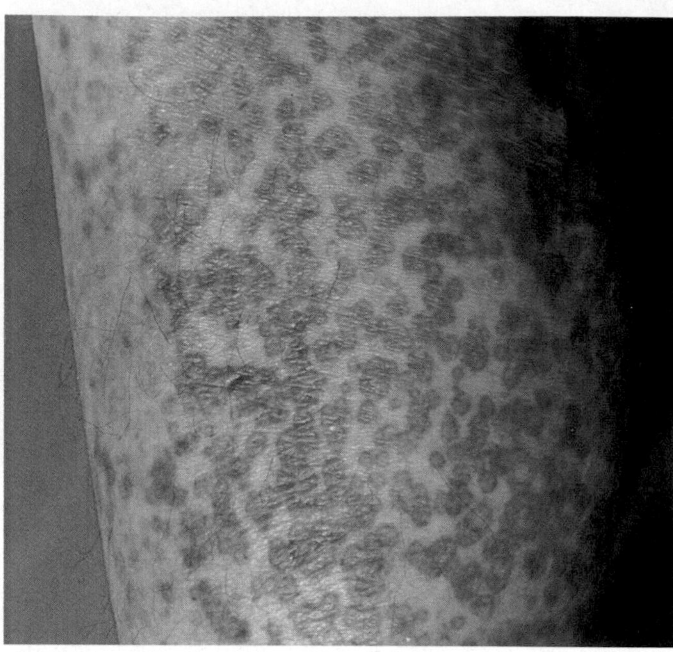

Porokeratosis palmaris et plantaris disseminata. Multiple superficial lesions on the calf. Note similarity to disseminated superficial actinic porokeratosis shown in Fig. 56-2 *A*.

FIGURE 56-4

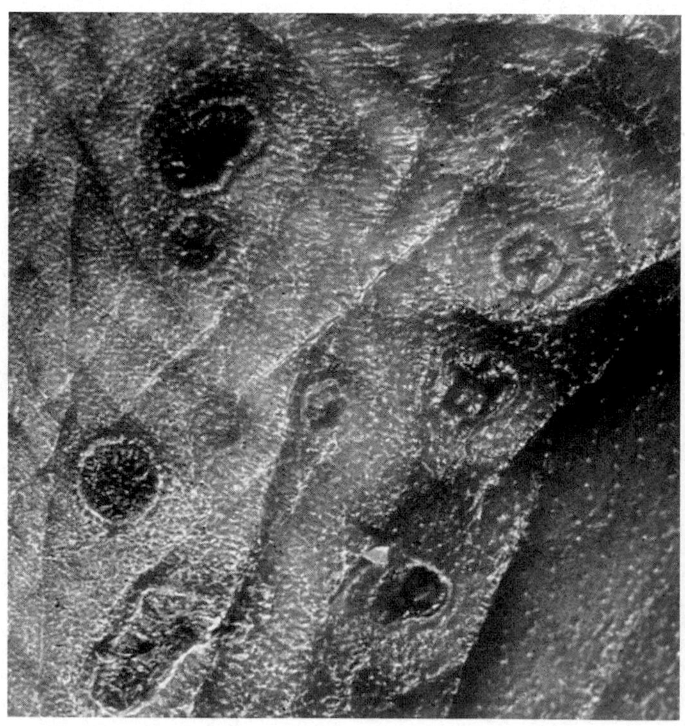

Plantar lesions in porokeratosis palmaris et plantaris disseminata. Note ridge and furrow surrounding the lesions.

FIGURE 56-5

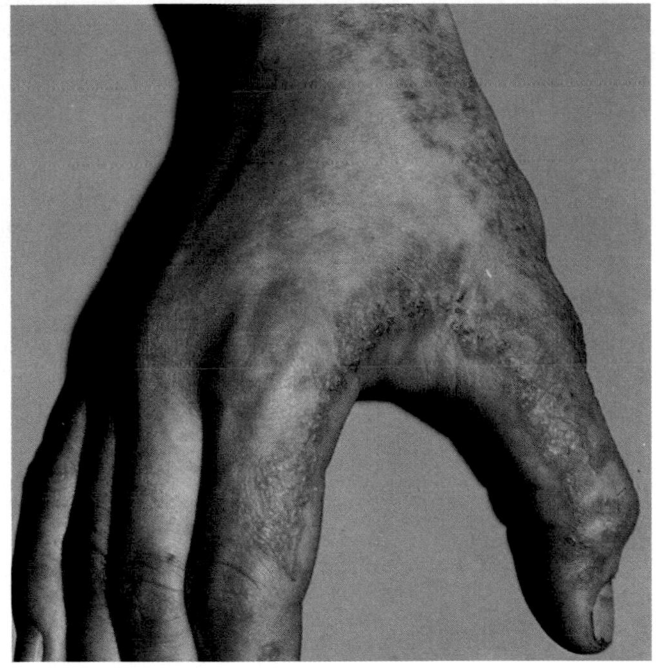

Linear porokeratosis. The similarity to an epidermal nevus is evident.

affecting the distal portion more than the proximal areas; on the trunk, the distribution may be zosteriform. Association with other variants of porokeratosis in one patient or within an affected family is possible. Malignant degeneration has been described.

Onset is usually in infancy and childhood. No definite inheritance pattern has been established (see Table 56-1). In one instance, linear porokeratosis was observed in monozygotic twins.

Punctate Porokeratosis

Usually, punctate porokeratosis is associated with either the Mibelli or linear types. Multiple, minute, and discrete punctate, hyperkeratotic, seedlike lesions surrounded by a thin, raised margin are present on palms and soles. Lesions may occur in a linear arrangement, or they may aggregate to form plaques. Punctate porokeratosis must be differentiated clinically and histopathologically from punctate keratoderma, also referred to as punctate porokeratotic keratoderma or as porokeratosis punctata palmaris et plantaris.

HISTOPATHOLOGY

The histopathologic hallmark common to all clinical variants of porokeratosis is the cornoid lamella,[8] which represents the pathologic substrate for the longitudinal furrow in the keratotic ridgelike border (Fig. 56-6). The cornoid lamella arises in the interfollicular epidermis and may involve the ostia of hair follicles or sweat ducts, which has led to the misnomer porokeratosis.[1] It consists of a tightly packed, thin column of parakeratotic cells extending through the entire thickness of the surrounding orthokeratotic stratum corneum. Below the cornoid lamella the granular layer is missing, and single or clustered dyskeratotic cells and vacuolated keratinocytes lie at its base (Fig.56-7). The adjacent epidermis is hyperkeratotic and acanthotic to a variable degree.

The cornoid lamella occupies an indentation of the epidermis that is generally tilted away from the center of the lesion.[29] The underlying papillary dermis contains a moderately dense inflammatory infiltrate and dilated capillaries. In the center of the lesion, the epidermis is usually atrophic, with areas of liquefaction degeneration in the basal layer, colloid bodies, and flattening of rete ridges. The dermis can be edematous or fibrotic with telangiectasia. Below long-standing lesions of DSP, there may be deposits of amyloid derived from keratinocytes.[30]

FIGURE 56-6

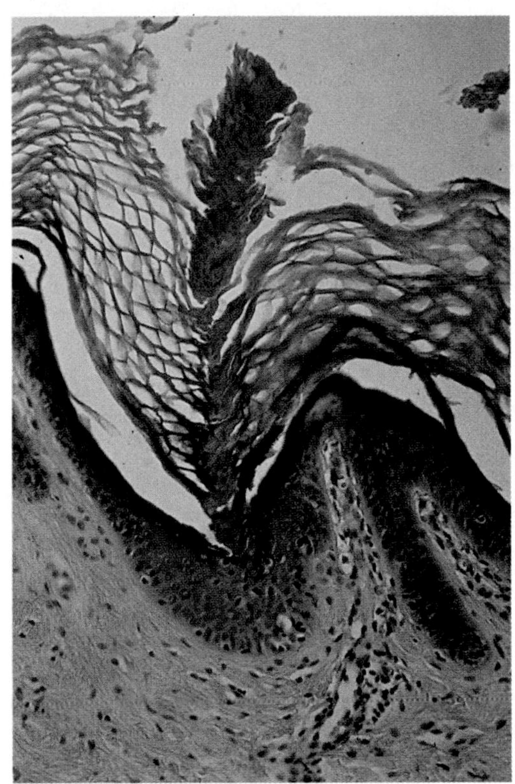

Porokeratosis, margin of lesion. Cornoid lamella arises from a small indentation of the epidermis and extends like a thin column through the entire stratum corneum.

FIGURE 56-7

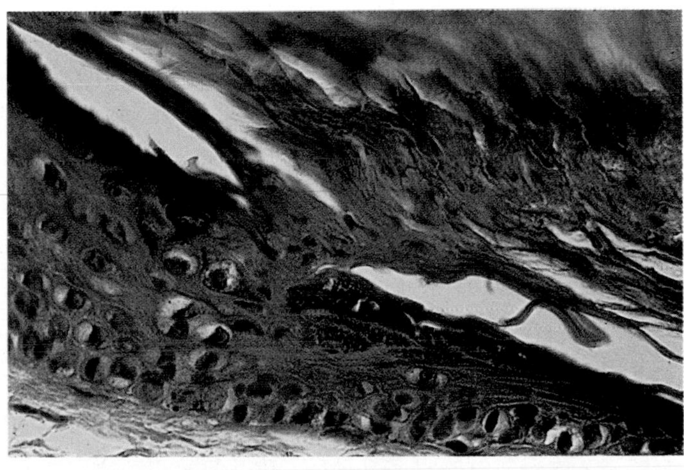

Base of cornoid lamella showing absence of stratum granulosum and vacuolated cells.

In essence, histopathologic changes are similar in all forms of porokeratoses; however, in DSP, DSAP, and PPPD, the cornoid lamella is less pronounced or so minimal as to be difficult to recognize. The ultrastructural findings—vacuolization of keratinocytes, clumping of keratin filaments, and dyskeratosis—are the same in porokeratosis Mibelli, DSP, and DSAP. Large, long-standing, eroded lesions require special attention to malignant transformation.

DIAGNOSIS AND DIFFERENTIAL DIAGNOSIS

Porokeratosis is usually diagnosed with ease, both histopathologically and clinically. The cornoid lamella is the diagnostic criterion for porokeratosis, but the phenomenon of cornoid lamellation can also occur in a number of unrelated diseases, including inflammatory, hyperplastic, and neoplastic conditions. Clinically, the continuous keratotic ridge cleaved by a longitudinal furrow, which surrounds the lesions both in the Mibelli type and in the other variants, is quite diagnostic, as is the localization and distribution of lesions.

Elastosis perforans can appear quite similar to porokeratosis Mibelli, but it consists of erythematous, keratotic papules and lacks the continuous ridge with its furrow. The superficial, disseminated types of porokeratosis may resemble actinic keratoses, stucco keratoses, flat seborrheic keratoses, or flat warts. Small, discrete lesions may be mistaken for lichen sclerosus et atrophicus, lichen planus, acrokeratosis verruciformis, and pityriasis rubra pilaris, but each of these lack the fine, slightly raised, threadlike border. Neoplasic disorders, such as cutaneous T cell lymphoma (CTCL), can mimic lesions of DSAP or porokeratosis Mibelli clinically. Histologically, the lesions lack a cornoid lamella and reveal infiltrates typical of CTCL.

Porokeratosis plantaris discreta is a not uncommon, acquired condition of the soles that is unrelated to the porokeratoses discussed in this chapter.[31] Clinically, it appears as sharply circumscribed, firm nodules up to 0.5 cm in diameter with a yellowish, depressed center surrounded by erythema. There is a central conical plug from which a yellowish, waxy material can be curetted. Lesions occur singly and in groups. They are painful and most often misdiagnosed as calluses or plantar warts. Although a cornoid lamella–like parakeratotic column can be found in these lesions histologically, the condition is unrelated to the porokeratoses. It is thought to be induced by pressure resulting in keratotic plugging of the distal eccrine duct, which produces secondary cystic dilation of the underlying sweat glands.[31]

Punctate keratoderma consists clinically of small, spinelike protruding keratotic excrescences that are limited to the palms, soles, and volar and plantar surfaces of the digits. Histopathologically, these lesions consist of sharply circumscribed spines of densely packed parakeratotic material overlying a shallow pit with a reduced or absent granular layer. In some cases of punctate keratoderma, hereditary transmission as an autosomal dominant trait has been recorded.

TREATMENT

Therapy is disappointing in all forms of porokeratosis, and recurrences can occur with any therapeutic modality. The optimal procedure depends on the size and location of the lesion, the functional and aesthetic requirements, and the age and condition of the patient. Circumscribed lesions of porokeratosis Mibelli or linear porokeratosis may be excised and grafted, destroyed by cryotherapy, electrodesiccation, dermabrasion, CO_2 laser,[32] 585-nm pulsed dye laser,[33] and Nd:YAG laser.[34] Lubrication for superficial lesions and keratolytic treatment of hyperkeratotic variants usually ease symptoms.

Successful treatment has been reported with topical 5-fluorouracil in porokeratosis Mibelli, linear porokeratosis, as well as in DSP and DSAP. In the author's experience, a brisk inflammatory response seems to be a prerequisite for clearing, which can occur as a delayed reaction. Treatment with calcipotriol and topical tacalcitol has been successful in DSAP.[35,36] Oral retinoids have yielded conflicting results: although the results obtained in some patients with DSAP, widespread porokeratosis Mibelli, PPPD, and linear porokeratosis have been excellent, the side effects of oral retinoids and the probability of relapses weeks or months after discontinuation of retinoid therapy require consideration. It has been reported, however, that retinoid therapy causes cytologic atypia to disappear and may have an inhibitory effect on cutaneous carcinogenesis in porokeratotic lesions.[37,38] Therapeutic measures that might increase the malignant potential, such as irradiation, immunosuppression, and excessive UV exposure, should be avoided.

COURSE AND PROGNOSIS

Porokeratotic lesions usually increase in size and number with time. Although this may be an extremely slow process in porokeratosis Mibelli, progression can be quite pronounced in DSP. Eruptions similar to those induced by drugs occur in patients with DSAP after UV exposure.[39] In cases of impaired immunocompetence, fluctuations in severity and remissions may parallel the state of immunocompetence. Thus, sudden aggravation of DSP or DSAP should prompt a search for underlying immunosuppression.[40] Malignant degeneration (squamous cell carcinoma, Bowen's disease, basal cell epithelioma) has occurred; it is more common in large, isolated, long-standing lesions of the Mibelli type of porokeratosis[41] and linear porokeratosis,[42,43] but it also occurs in DSP, DSAP, and PPPD.[38] Statistically, Japanese patients develop earlier, and more often multiple, malignant tumors in lesions of porokeratosis.[41] Widespread metastasis and fatal outcome, as well as soft tissue destruction and mutilation in cases of giant lesions of porokeratosis Mibelli in an acral location, have been reported.[44,45]

REFERENCES

1. Andrews GC: Porokeratosis (Mibelli) disseminated and superficial type. *Arch Dermatol Syphilol* **36**:1111, 1937
2. Chernosky ME: Porokeratosis: Report of twelve patients with multiple superficial lesions. *South Med J* **59**:289, 1966
3. Guss SB et al: Porokeratosis plantaris, palmaris, et disseminata: A third type of porokeratosis. *Arch Dermatol* **104:**366, 1971
4. Rahbari HR et al: Punctate porokeratosis: A clinical variant of porokeratosis of Mibelli. *J Cutan Pathol* **4**:338, 1977
5. Xia JH et al: Identification of a locus for disseminated superficial actinic porokeratosis at chromosome 12q23.2-24.1. *J Invest Dermatol* **114**:1071, 2000
6. Murata Y et al: Type 2 segmental manifestation of disseminated superficial porokeratosis showing a systematized pattern of involvement and pronounced cancer proneness. *Eur J Dermatol* **11**:191, 2001
7. Freyschmidt PP et al: Linear porokeratosis superimposed on disseminated superficial actinic porokeratosis: Report of two cases exemplifying the concept of type 2 segmental manifestation of autosomal dominant skin disorders. *J Am Acad Dermatol* **41**:644, 1999
8. Reed RJ, Leone P: Porokeratosis—A mutant clonal keratosis of the epidermis. *Arch Dermatol* **101**:340, 1970
9. Knoell KA et al: Sudden onset of disseminated porokeratosis of Mibelli in a renal transplant patient. *J Am Acad Dermatol* **41**:830, 1999

10. Kanitakis J et al: Porokeratosis in organ transplant recipients. *J Am Acad Dermatol* **44**:144, 2001
11. Rio B et al: Disseminated superficial porokeratosis after autologous bone marrow transplantation. *Bone Marrow Transplant* **19**:11, 1997
12. Fields LL et al: Rapid development of disseminated superficial porokeratosis after transplant induction therapy. *Bone Marrow Transplant* **15**:993, 1995
13. Hernandez MH et al: Disseminated porokeratosis associated with chronic renal failure: A new type of disseminated porokeratosis? *Arch Dermatol* **136**:1568, 2000
14. Hunt SJ et al: Linear and punctate porokeratosis associated with end-stage liver disease. *J Am Acad Dermatol* **25**:937, 1991
15. Kono T et al: Synchronous development of disseminated superficial porokeratosis and hepatitis C virus–related hepatocellular carcinoma. *J Am Acad Dermatol* **43**:966, 2000
16. Kanitakis J et al: Disseminated superficial porokeratosis in a patient with AIDS. *Br J Dermatol* **131**:284, 1994
17. Rodriguez EA et al: Porokeratosis of Mibelli and HIV infection. *Int J Dermatol* **35**:402, 1996
18. Allen AL, Glaser DA: Disseminated superficial actinic porokeratosis associated with topical PUVA. *J Am Acad Dermatol* **43**:720, 2000
19. Kanitakis J et al: Porokeratosis and immunosuppression. *Eur J Dermatol* **8**:459, 1998
20. Anzai S et al: Squamous cell carcinoma in a renal transplant recipient with linear porokeratosis. *J Dermatol* **26**:244, 1999
21. Bencini PL et al: Porokeratosis and immunosuppression. *Br J Dermatol* **132**:74, 1995
22. Otsuka F M et al: Porokeratosis with large skin lesions: Histologic, cytologic and cytogenetic study of three cases. *Acta Derm Venereol* **71**:437, 1991
23. Nelson C et al: p53, mdm-2, and 21 waf-1 in the porokeratoses. *Am J Dermatopathol* **21**:420, 1999
24. Kawakami T et al: Overexpression of p21Waf1/Cip1 immunohistochemical staining in Bowen's disease, but not in disseminated superficial porokeratosis. *Br J Dermatol* **141**:647, 1999
25. Watanabe R, Otsuka F: Cultured skin fibroblasts derived from three patients with disseminated superficial actinic porokeratosis (DSAP) are hypersensitive to the lethal effects of x-radiation but not to those of ultraviolet (UV) light. *Exp Dermatol* **2**:175, 1993
26. Shumack S et al: Disseminated actinic porokeratosis: A histological review of 61 cases with particular reference to lymphocyte inflammation. *Am J Dermatopathol* **13**:26, 1993
27. Webster GF: Are porokeratoses an infection? *Arch Dermatol* **137**:665, 2001
28. Mizukawa Y, Shiohara T: Onset of porokeratosis of Mibelli in organ transplant recipients: Lack of a search for transmissible agents in these patients. *J Am Acad Dermatol* **44**:143, 2001
29. Crefeld W: Zur Histogenese der Porokeratosis Mibelli. *Z Haut Geschlechtskr* **44**:453, 1969
30. Kim JH et al: Secondary cutaneous amyloidosis in disseminated superficial porokeratosis: A case report. *J Korean Med Sci* **15**:478, 2000
31. Taub J, Steinberg M: Porokeratosis plantaris discreta: A previously unrecognized dermatologic entity. *Int J Dermatol* **9**:83, 1970
32. Rabbin PE, Baldwin HE: Treatment of porokeratosis of Mibelli with CO_2 laser vaporization versus surgical excision with split-thickness skin graft: A comparison. *J Dermatol Surg Oncol* **19**:199, 1993
33. Alster TS, Nanni CA: Successful treatment of porokeratosis with 585 nm pulsed dye laser irradiation. *Cutis* **63**:265,1999
34. Liu HT: Treatment of lichen amyloidosis (LA) and disseminated superficial porokeratosis (DSP) with frequency-doubled Q-switched Nd:YAG laser. *Dermatol Surg* **26**:958, 2000
35. Harrison P, Stollery N: Disseminated superficial actinic porokeratosis responding to calcipotriol. *Clin Exp Dermatol* **19**:95, 1994
36. Bohm M et al: Disseminated superficial actinic porokeratosis: Treatment with topical tacalcitol. *J Am Acad Dermatol* **40**:479, 1999
37. Goldman GD, Milstone LM: Generalized linear porokeratosis treated with etretinate. *Arch Dermatol* **131**:496, 1995
38. Seishima M et al: Squamous cell carcinoma arising from lesions of porokeratosis palmaris et plantaris disseminata. *Eur J Dermatol* **10**:478, 2000
39. Kroiss MM et al: Disseminated superficial porokeratosis induced by furosemide. *Acta Derm Venereol (Stockh)* **80**:52, 2000
40. Levin RM, Heymann WR: Superficial disseminated porokeratosis in a patient with myelodysplastic syndrome. *Int J Dermatol* **38**:138, 1999
41. Otsuka F et al: Porokeratosis large skin lesions are susceptible to skin cancer development: Histological and cytological explanation for the susceptibility. *J Cancer Res Clin Oncol* **119**:395, 1993
42. Sasson M, Krain AD: Porokeratosis and cutaneous malignancy: A review. *Dermatol Surg* **22**:339, 1996
43. Happle R: Cancer proneness of linear porokeratosis may be explained by allelic loss. *Dermatology* **195**:20, 1997
44. Handa S et al: Mutilating lesions in porokeratosis of Mibelli. *Dermatology* **191**:162, 1995
45. Rahbari H et al: Destructive facial porokeratosis. *J Am Acad Dermatol* **33**:1049, 1995

CHAPTER 57

Elisabeth Ch. Wolff-Schreiner

Kyrle Disease and Other Perforating Disorders

KYRLE DISEASE

Definition and Historical Aspects

Kyrle in 1916 described a major dermatosis characterized by numerous up to cherry-sized hyperkeratotic, verrucous, clefted papules and nodules involving almost the entire skin.[1] The histopathologic picture of Kyrle disease was that of a "hyperkeratosis follicularis et parafollicularis in cutem penetrans." Since the original description, the distinctiveness of this rare syndrome has been blurred or questioned altogether.[2] Kyrle disease can be defined as a distinct entity, however; similarly, the syndrome of acquired perforating dermatosis, which is most often misdiagnosed as Kyrle disease, can be delineated.[3]

Etiology and Pathogenesis

The etiology of Kyrle disease is not known. Disease occurrence in siblings suggests a genetic background, possibly an autosomal recessive mode of inheritance.[4] The basic pathogenic event seems to be an uncoupling of epithelial proliferation and differentiation that results in a gradual and progressive lowering of the level of keratinization toward the dermal-epidermal junction.[5] The eventual discontinuity of the basement membrane and direct contact between the partly parakeratotic plug and the dermis lead to granuloma formation and scarring. In Kyrle disease, transepidermal elimination is of no pathogenic significance.

Clinical Findings

Kyrle disease is a chronic, generalized dermatosis that starts most frequently during the third to fifth decades, although the onset may occur in infancy and childhood.[4] It seems to affect females twice as often as males. Kyrle disease preferentially involves the extensor surfaces of the extremities, the scapular region, and the buttocks, but may also involve the axillary vaults,[1] face, hands, and feet.[4] The mucous membranes are invariably spared, although lesions may occur on the vulva and perianal region.[4]

Individual lesions start as pinhead-sized, skin-colored hyperkeratotic papules. As they increase in size, they become more elevated and yellowish brown, with a tightly adherent scale or squamous crust (Fig. 57-1*A*). Older, up to cherry-sized lesions consist of a grayish, verrucous, clefted, cone-shaped horny mass surrounded by a narrow brownish-reddish rim (Figs. 57-1*B* and 57-2). Dense clustering and slow peripheral expansion of grouped lesions result in coalescence and the formation of polycyclic, verrucous growths (Figs. 57-2 and 57-3*A*). The clefted horny mass can be removed easily, leaving an oozing or bleeding crater or a clefted, cup-shaped excavation (see Fig. 57-2). Lesions heal with atrophic scars with spotty hyper- and hypopigmentation. Lesions crop up in an asynchronous fashion so that different stages of development occur side by side (Figs. 57-1*A* and 57-3*B*); recurrences, within or at the periphery of scars, are frequent[1,5] (see Figs. 57-1*A*, 57-3*A*, and 57-3*B*). The eruption is asymptomatic or slightly pruritic. Larger lesions can be mechanically disturbing and tender, particularly after they have been traumatized.

The course of Kyrle disease is extremely chronic over decades. There have been no reports of spontaneous remissions.

Associated Diseases

The small number of authentic cases of Kyrle disease and the notorious problem of distinguishing it from acquired perforating dermatosis (see below) make an evaluation of its association with diabetes difficult. Kyrle original patient was nondiabetic at the time of the first description,[1] but 8 years later had developed diabetes. Several other cases with diabetes are described in the literature; however, the association is statistically not significant.[4] No association exists between Kyrle disease and renal disease.

Histopathology

Serial sectioning of the lesions, essentially parallel to the longitudinal axis of the follicles, makes it possible to appreciate the histopathologic development of Kyrle disease. Lesions occur both in the follicular and interfollicular epidermis and in the acrosyringium.[1] Early lesions reveal a focal thickening of the horny layer with some parakeratotic cells. The epidermis is acanthotic, and the cells of the germinative layer are increased in number, stain more intensely, and are arranged in a somewhat disorderly fashion. In this stage, the papillary dermis is widened, but without inflammatory changes.

In lesions with verrucous hyperkeratosis, the follicular infundibulum or acrosyringium is widely dilated by a funnel-shaped, brightly eosinophilic horny plug (Fig. 57-4*A*). The central portion consists of a parakeratotic column that, at its tip, is in continuity with and seems to emerge from individual or clustered dyskeratotic cells in the underlying epidermis (see Fig. 57-4*A*). These cells have a brightly eosinophilic cytoplasm and darkly staining nuclei, and they retain their normal contacts with the surrounding keratinocytes. Gradually, they merge into the parakeratotic column, and with new dyskeratotic cells developing at its tip, the column approaches the dermal-epidermal junction (Fig. 57-4*B*).

FIGURE 57-1

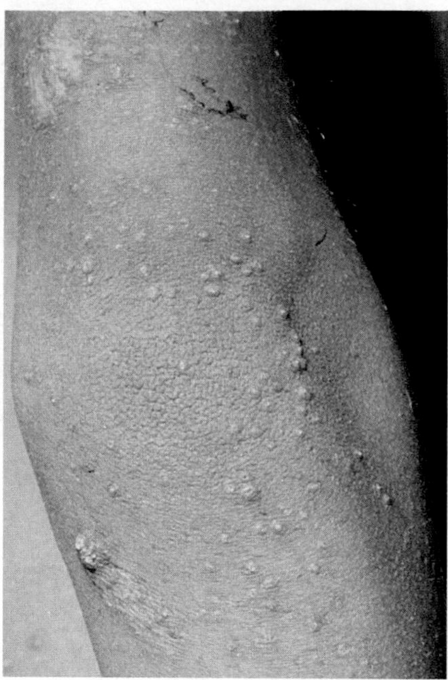

A.

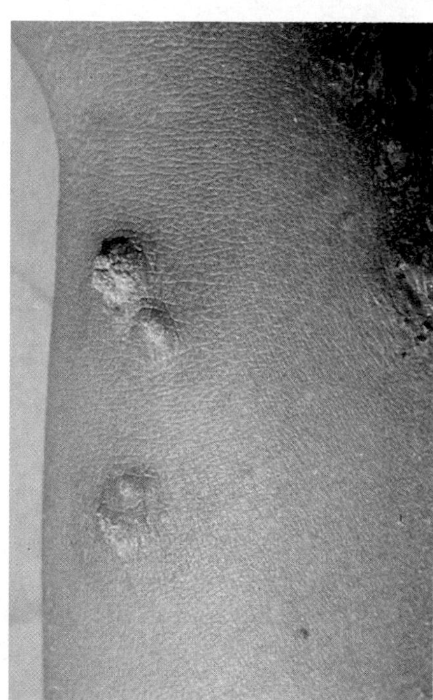

B.

Kyrle disease. *A.* Early lesions: multiple cone-shaped hyperkeratotic papules in a 12-year-old girl. Note atrophic scars with spotty pigmentation. A larger hyperkeratotic nodule is present at the edge of a scar. *B.* Larger lesions with massive, partly clefted hyperkeratoses on the forearm of a 6-year-old boy (brother of the girl in Figs. 57-1*A* and 57-3*A* and *B*).

FIGURE 57-2

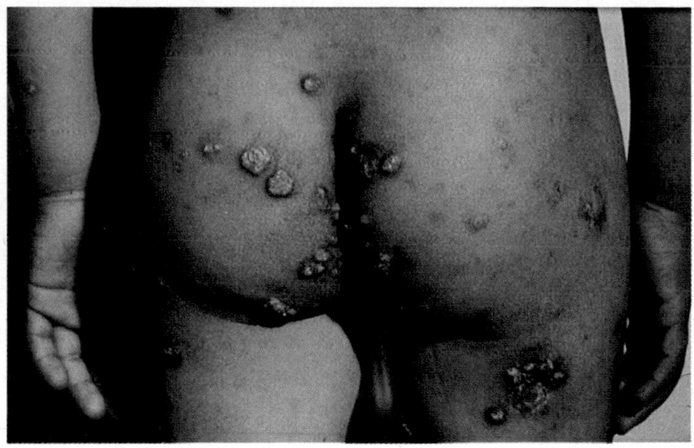

Kyrle disease. Note the protruding, warty, clefted hyperkeratoses, grouping of lesions, and the oozing, hemorrhagic, cup-shaped depression on the right thigh after removal of a hyperkeratotic nodule. Scarring is only minor in this case of short duration.

FIGURE 57-3

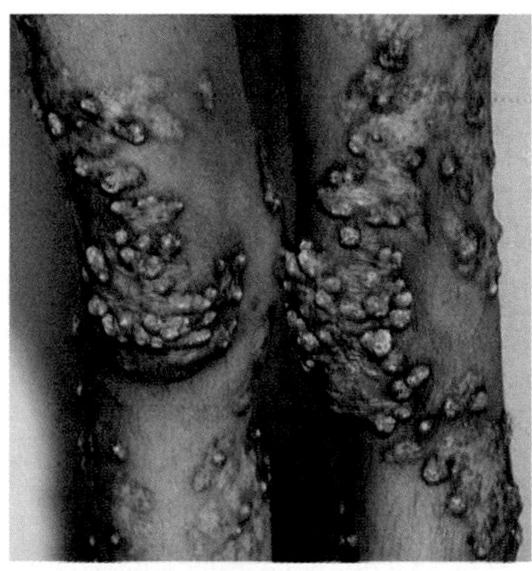

A.

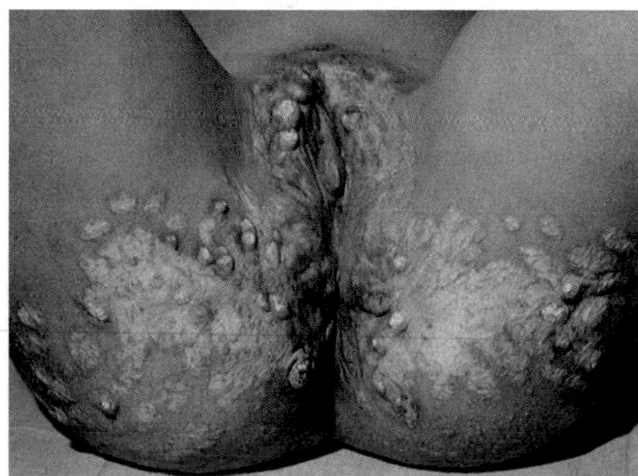

B.

Kyrle disease. *A.* Multiple warty lesions over the knees of the 12-year-old patient shown in Fig. 57-1 *A.* Clefted, verrucous lesions of variable size are grouped or localized in the periphery of atrophic scars with spotty pigmentation. *B.* Anogenital region of the same patient with severe atrophic scarring and a number of large, verrucous lesions, which also involve the labia majora. The vaginal introitus is free of lesions. Note small, early hyperkeratotic papules on the left buttock.

Ultimately establishing contact with the dermis through a focal defect in the basement membrane, the horny plug can reach fairly deep into the dermis.[1,4] The perforation often lies near the opening of the sebaceous gland duct or in eccrine glands in the pit of the acrosyringium.[1] The surrounding epidermis either thins because of the pressure or becomes acanthotic. Before penetration, mononuclear cells invade the dermis below the dyskeratotic cells and the adjacent epidermis (see Fig. 57-4*A*). After penetration, lymphocytes, polymorphonuclear leukocytes, epithelioid cells, and foreign-body giant cells containing eosinophilic fragments of engulfed keratin infiltrate the papillary dermis. In healing lesions, atrophic scar tissue replaces the granuloma.

In the interfollicular epidermis, the histopathologic changes are less dramatic. Lesions are less hyperkeratotic, and perforation, with its severe consequences, occurs less frequently. Clinically, this histopathologic variant corresponds to smaller lesions that grow slowly and regress more readily with no or only mild scarring.[1] Perforation is not obligatory for diagnosis and occurs far less frequently in Kyrle disease than in other perforating disorders (see below). Of importance is the central parakeratotic column that arises from individual cell keratinization and finally establishes direct contact between the keratotic plug and the dermis (Fig. 57-4*B*). Basophilic debris within the follicular compartment is not typical for Kyrle disease.[1]

Differential Diagnosis

Clinically, the early lesions of Kyrle disease can be similar to the early lesions of dyskeratosis follicularis, punctate psoriasis, or keratosis pilaris. The mature exophytic, clefted, verrucous papules or nodules; the distribution pattern, including face, hands, feet, and, eventually, the axillary vaults and perianal-perigenital region; the insignificance of pruritus; and the general lack of an underlying chronic disease allow the clinical differentiation from other perforating disorders. In contrast, acquired perforating dermatosis runs a different clinical course and has an association with certain chronic diseases (see below).

Histopathologically, the differential diagnosis includes all the other perforating diseases. The characteristic keratotic plug, individual cell keratinization in the germinative layer, and the resulting parakeratotic column typical of Kyrle disease do not occur in any of the other perforating dermatoses.

Therapy

No specific therapy for Kyrle disease is known. The small number of authentic cases of the disease makes a comparison of various therapeutic modalities practically impossible.

Kyrle treated his own patient by curetting the hyperkeratoses prior to ultraviolet (UV) irradiation. After a short remission, lesions recurred.[1] The use of high-dose vitamin A, oral retinoids, and a combination of oral retinoids and psoralen plus UVA (Re-PUVA) may have a beneficial effect. Discontinuation of the medication results in prompt recurrence. Topical therapy is unsatisfactory: keratolytics and retinoic acid preparations help to improve the cosmetic appearance; electrocautery, cryotherapy, and CO_2 laser surgery are only temporarily effective.

PERFORATING FOLLICULITIS

Definition and Historical Aspects

In 1968, Mehregan and Coskey described 25 patients with a discrete follicular keratotic eruption involving mainly the hairy parts of the

FIGURE 57-4

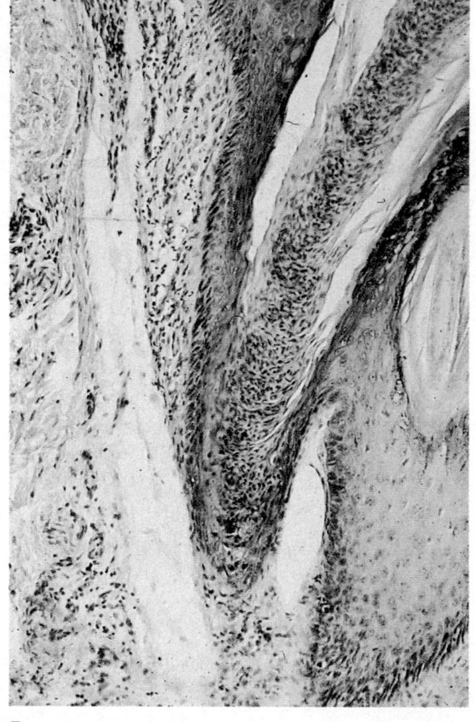

A. B.

Lesions of Kyrle disease before perforation. *A.* Massive hyperkeratosis with central parakeratotic column. At the base of the parakeratotic column, individual cell keratinization can be followed down almost to the basal layer. The surrounding epidermis is acanthotic. (*From Tappeiner et al.,*[4] *with permission of* Hautarzt.) *B.* Higher magnification of the parakeratotic column in the center of a lesion of Kyrle disease.

extremities; they termed the condition perforating folliculitis.[6] Clinically, somewhat similar eruptions have occurred in patients with chronic renal failure with or without hemodialysis and/or diabetes[3] (see "Acquired Perforating Dermatosis," below).

Etiology and Pathogenesis

The etiology of perforating folliculitis is unknown. A perforation of the follicular wall has been considered the initial pathogenic event.[6] Chemical components in textiles (e.g., formaldehyde), as well as curled-up hairs or fragments thereof have been incriminated as the cause of such perforations. Transepidermal elimination, by which dermal components are eliminated through newly formed channels, seems to be coincidental in perforating folliculitis. The fact that the number of new cases has declined since the original description favors an exogenous pathogen.

Clinical Findings

Perforating folliculitis is a chronic, either asymptomatic or mildly pruritic, dermatosis affecting healthy young adults of both sexes. Lesions develop preferentially on the hairy parts of the arms, forearms, thighs, and buttocks as discrete, erythematous, follicular papules 2 to 8 mm in diameter with a central, tightly adherent, whitish keratinous plug that may be pierced by a hair. Removal of the plug leaves a small, bleeding crater. Lesions develop slowly over weeks or months and heal with a hypopigmented spot or a shallow scar. Periods of remission and exacerbation can alternate over months or years.

Histopathology

Early lesions appear as suppurative folliculitis.[7] The infundibular portion of the follicular epithelium is disrupted frequently and early in the course of perforating folliculitis so that the follicular contents spill into the dermis. In fully developed lesions, keratotic material mixed with necrotic debris, inflammatory cells, elastic fibers, and, occasionally, hair-shaft fragments within the follicle or in the adjacent dermis plug a widely dilated hair follicle. A chronic inflammatory infiltrate and foreign-body granuloma with brightly eosinophilic elastic fibers surround perforated follicles. In healing lesions, the follicular epithelium grows in from the periphery of the defect, and the contents of the follicle are sequestrated into the follicular compartment.

Differential Diagnosis

Clinical differential diagnosis of early lesions includes bacterial folliculitis and acne vulgaris. The age of the patient, the distribution pattern, and the presence or absence of other acne lesions are helpful diagnostic hints. Keratosis pilaris is purely keratotic, noninflammatory, and associated with xerosis. The other perforating dermatoses, Kyrle disease, elastosis perforans serpiginosa, reactive perforating collagenosis, and acquired perforating dermatosis vary in their distribution, clinical course, genetic findings, associated chronic diseases, and histopathologic characteristics.

Therapy

No specific treatment for perforating folliculitis is known. Topical keratolytics and tretinoin, systemic isotretinoin, acitretin, and PUVA therapy can prove useful.

ACQUIRED PERFORATING DERMATOSIS

Definition and Historical Aspects

In 1982, White and Hurwitz, together with their colleagues, described several patients whose eruptions were clinically and histopathologically similar to those of perforating folliculitis and who shared a background of chronic renal failure, with or without hemodialysis or peritoneal dialysis, and/or diabetes mellitus.[8,9] Rapini and colleagues delineated this disorder in the setting of chronic renal failure and/or diabetes mellitus under the catch-all term *acquired perforating dermatosis* and postulated a common cause for all these eruptions.[3] Over the last two decades, a number of authorities have supported the concept of acquired perforating dermatosis. However, the condition is not identical to Kyrle disease,[1,5] and the synonymic use of Kyrle disease for acquired perforating dermatosis is incorrect and confusing.[2]

Etiology and Pathogenesis

A causal relationship of acquired perforating dermatosis with pruritus, chronic renal failure, and/or diabetes mellitus is well documented. In the majority of cases, the chronic renal failure is secondary to diabetic nephropathy.[2,10] Acquired perforating dermatosis can precede, accompany, or follow hemodialysis or peritoneal dialysis, and it affects about 10 percent of dialysis patients after a variable duration of chronic renal failure and/or treatment.[9,11] Dialysis does not cause acquired perforating dermatosis,[12] however, as it occurs also after kidney transplantation. In addition, there have been reported associations with chronic active hepatitis,[13] sclerosing cholangitis,[14] liver failure, internal malignancy,[15] hypothyroidism,[13] herpes zoster,[16] and a number of other sporadic diseases.

The term *perforation* is to be understood not as an active process, but as a transepithelial elimination through discontinuities of the basement membrane and the epidermis. Several factors have been incriminated—although none of them proven responsible beyond doubt—in the pathogenesis of acquired perforating dermatosis:

- Mild to severe pruritus in some conditions (e.g., chronic renal failure, chronic liver disease, lymphoma, internal malignancies) leads to superficial traumatization through scratching or rubbing. In combination with poor blood supply because of microangiopathy in long-standing—particularly insulin-dependent—diabetes, this minor trauma may trigger dermal necrosis with elimination of the necrotic material through the epidermis.[17]
- Exocytosis and disintegration of polymorphonuclear cells leading to the release of DNA and proteolytic enzymes may alter collagen or elastic fibers, open up the transepidermal route by alterations and discontinuities of the basement membrane, and precede the sequestration and elimination of cellular debris and degenerated fibers through transepidermal channels.[18,19] There is, however, no consistent evidence for morphologic defects in collagen or elastic fibers below early lesions.[18,20]
- Transepithelial elimination may be a form of foreign-body reaction to altered constituents of the dermis.
- Dermal microdeposits of crystalline substances (i.e., uric acid, hydroxyapatite[12]) may cause an inflammatory reaction, connective tissue degradation, and release of mediators, resulting in epidermal hyperplasia, activation and penetration of mononuclear cells, focal dissolution of the basement membrane, widening of intercellular spaces, and transepidermal elimination of harmful deposits from the dermis.[12]
- In patients with uremia, dysregulation of epithelial differentiation and proliferation caused by defects in the metabolism of vitamins A and D may result in epithelial perforation.[9]
- In patients with diabetes mellitus and uremic nephropathy, the serum level and dermal matrix deposition of fibronectin, an adhesive glycoprotein, are consistently elevated, which may induce physiologically aberrant epithelial turnover or locomotion.[21] Furthermore, macrophages can produce fibronectin and are mobilized as well by it, which may point to a pathogenic role of Langerhans cells.[21]
- The fact that dialysis does not alleviate pruritus and acquired perforating dermatosis may be due to the accumulation of an unidentified, poorly dialysable "uremic" substance.[22]
- Transepidermal elimination of altered dermal components may not be the result of the pathologic process but rather may be secondary to the perforation.[3]

Clinical Findings

The basic lesion of acquired perforating dermatosis is a dome-shaped, umbilicated keratotic papule, 1 to 10 mm in diameter, with a central keratinous plug that can be removed with some force. Lesions are preferentially localized over the extensor surfaces of the extremities, but can also occur on the trunk, neck, face, and, occasionally, the scalp. Lesions can aggregate to form prurigo-like,[3] hyperkeratotic plaques (Fig. 57-5), particularly in patients with severe pruritus who chronically rub

FIGURE 57-5

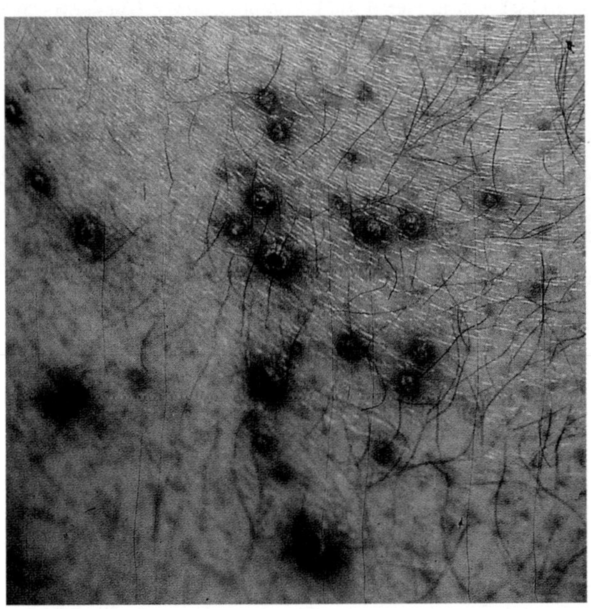

Acquired perforating dermatosis in a 42-year-old patient with diabetes. Note multiple pinhead to pea sized umbilicated papules in various stages of development with central keratotic plugs, as well as grouping of lesions and linear arrangement (Koebner phenomenon).

the itchy lesions. Lesions may develop in scratch marks (Koebner phenomenon; see Fig. 57-5). The course of acquired perforating dermatosis is chronic, with new lesions developing while old ones eventually regress after months without major scarring.

Histopathology

Most commonly, multiple perforations occur within invaginations of the epidermis. It is occasionally possible to identify hair follicles or fragments of hair shafts in association with lesions.[18] Microdeposits of uric acid and hydroxyapatite have appeared in acquired perforating dermatosis–like lesions.[12]

In early lesions, a vigorous suppurative inflammatory reaction takes place at the site of perforation.[7] In older lesions, a more chronic inflammation and foreign-body granuloma are followed by sequestration of necrotic debris and, occasionally simultaneous, elimination of collagen and/or elastic fibers into the necrotic hyperkeratotic plug.[3] In excoriated lesions, collagen bundles in the reticular dermis are continuous with collagen bundles in the necrotic mass through epidermal tunnels. In the healing process, the regeneration of the epidermis, together with the elimination of the necrotic mass, pulls the collagen bundles through the epidermal channels out of the crater.[23] In long-lasting lesions with severe pruritus, a thickened papillary dermis, dome-shaped hyperkeratosis, and irregular epidermal hyperplasia are suggestive of prurigo nodularis.

Differential Diagnosis

Clinically, as well as histopathologically, the other perforating diseases must be excluded before acquired perforating dermatosis can be diagnosed. Diagnostic clues are chronic renal failure, possibly combined with hemodialysis or peritoneal dialysis; diabetes mellitus or another underlying disease; and as a common symptom, pruritus. Histopathologically, multiple perforations, an acutely suppurative early stage, elimination of necrotic material together with elastic and collagen fibers, and a keratotic, intensely basophilic plug are diagnostic.

Therapy

The many therapeutic approaches to acquired perforating dermatosis include lubrication and topical use of keratolytics; topical and/or intralesional use of steroids; topical use of capsaicin or tretinoin;[11] systemic use of isotretinoin;[22] systemic rifampicin;[14] UVB irradiation;[12] PUVA therapy; and, for individual lesions, cryotherapy. It has been suggested that remissions in patients treated with allopurinol result from, besides the uricostatic effect, an immunomodulating and differentiation-promoting effect of allopurinol or the antioxidative effect of allopurinol on glycation and crosslinking of collagen.[24–26] Spontaneous remissions,[27] remissions after cancer surgery,[15] and remissions after cessation of hemodialysis and kidney transplantation have been described.[7–9]

REFERENCES

1. Kyrle J: Über einen ungewöhnlichen Fall von universeller follikulärer und parafollikulärer Hyperkeratose (Hyperkeratosis follicularis et parafollicularis in cutem penetrans). *Arch Dermatol Syphilol (Berlin)* **123**:466, 1916
2. Rapini RP: Perforating disorders, in *Cutaneous Medicine and Surgery: An Integrated Program in Dermatology,* vol 1, edited by KA Arndt, PE Leboit, JK Robinson, BU Winthroub. Philadelphia, WB Saunders, 1996, p 407
3. Rapini RP et al: Acquired perforating dermatosis: Evidence for combined transepidermal elimination of both collagen and elastic fibers. *Arch Dermatol* **125**:1074, 1989
4. Tappeiner J et al: Morbus Kyrle. *Hautarzt* **20**:296, 1969
5. Constantine VS, Carter VH: Kyrle's disease: II. Histopathologic findings in five cases and review of the literature. *Arch Dermatol* **97**:633, 1968
6. Mehregan AH, Coskey RJ: Perforating folliculitis. *Arch Dermatol* **97**:394, 1968
7. White CR Jr: The dermatopathology of perforating disorders. *Semin Dermatol* **5**:359, 1986
8. White CR et al: Perforating folliculitis of hemodialysis. *Am J Dermatopathol* **4**:109, 1982
9. Hurwitz RM et al: Perforating folliculitis in association with hemodialysis. *Am J Dermatopathol* **4**:101, 1982
10. Kawakami T, Saito R: Acquired perforating collagenosis associated with diabetes mellitus: Eight cases that meet Faver's criteria. *Br J Dermatol* **140**:521, 1999
11. Morton CA et al: Acquired perforating dermatosis in a British dialysis population. *Br J Dermatol* **135**:671, 1996
12. Haftek M et al: Acquired perforating dermatosis of diabetes mellitus and renal failure: Further ultrastructural clues to its pathogenesis. *J Cutan Pathol* **20**:350, 1993
13. Faver IR et al: Acquired perforating collagenosis: Report of six cases and review of the literature. *J Am Acad Dermatol* **30**:575, 1994
14. Skiba G et al: Successful treatment of acquired perforating dermatosis with rifampicin in an Asian patient with sclerosing cholangitis. *Liver* **19**:160, 1999
15. Bong JL et al: Reactive perforating collagenosis associated with underlying malignancy. *Br J Dermatol* **142**:390, 2000
16. Lee HN et al: Two cases of reactive perforating collagenosis arising at the site of healed herpes zoster. *Int J Dermatol* **40**:191, 2001
17. Farell AM: Acquired perforating dermatosis in renal and diabetic patients. *Lancet* **349**:895, 1997
18. Patterson JW, Brown PC: Ultrastructural changes in acquired perforating dermatosis. *Int J Dermatol* **31**:201, 1992
19. Zelger B et al: Acquired perforating dermatosis: Transepidermal elimination of DNA material and possible role of leukocytes in pathogenesis. *Arch Dermatol* **127**:695, 1991
20. Beck HI et al: Adult acquired reactive perforating collagenosis: Report of a case including ultrastructural findings. *J Cutan Pathol* **15**:124, 1988
21. Morgan MB et al: Fibronectin and the extracellular matrix in the perforating disorders of the skin. *Am J Dermatopathol* **20**:147, 1998
22. Maurice PD: Acquired perforating dermatosis in renal patients. *Nephrol Dial Transplant* **12**:2774, 1997
23. Yanagihara M et al: The pathogenesis of the transepithelial elimination of the collagen bundles in acquired reactive perforating collagenosis: A light and electron microscopical study. *J Cutan Pathol* **23**:398, 1996
24. Krüger K et al: Erworbene reaktiv perforierende Dermatose. Erfolgreiche Behandlung mit Allopurinol in 2 Fällen. *Hautarzt* **50**:115, 1999
25. Munch M et al: Treatment of perforating collagenosis of diabetes and renal failure with allopurinol. *Clin Exp Dermatol* **25**:615, 2000
26. Querings K et al: Treatment of reactive perforating collagenosis with allopurinol. *Br J Dermatol* **145**:174, 2001
27. Chang P, Fernandez V: Acquired perforating disease: Report of nine cases. *Int J Dermatol* **32**:874, 1993

SECTION 9

EPIDERMIS: DISORDERS OF EPIDERMAL COHESION—VESICULAR AND BULLOUS DISORDERS

CHAPTER 58

Peter O. Fritsch
Ramon Ruiz-Maldonado

Erythema Multiforme, Stevens-Johnson Syndrome, and Toxic Epidermal Necrolysis

The erythema multiforme group of diseases encompasses a number of acute self-limited exanthematic intolerance reactions that share at least two characteristic features: target lesions (stable circular erythemas or urticarial plaques with areas of blistering, necrosis, and/or resolution in a concentric array) and, histologically, satellite-cell (or more widespread) necrosis of the epidermis. These features are the expression of an archetypic polyetiologic reaction pattern of the skin (i.e., a cytotoxic immunologic attack on keratinocytes expressing non-self antigens). Antigens involved are predominantly microbes (viruses) or drugs.

At present, two main subsets are recognized: (1) erythema multiforme—a fairly common, usually mild and relapsing eruption that is most often triggered by recurrent herpes simplex virus (HSV) infection; and (2) the Stevens-Johnson syndrome–toxic epidermal necrolysis complex (SJS–TEN)—an infrequent severe mucocutaneous intolerance reaction that is most often elicited by drugs. Entities that may be grouped very close to the erythema multiforme spectrum are the acute graft-versus-host disease, fixed drug eruption, and erythema multiforme–like disseminated allergic contact dermatitis. The exact relationship among these entities is still a matter of controversy, as are aspects of therapy and management. The pathogenesis is only incompletely understood.

CLASSIFICATION AND HISTORY

No generally accepted classification of the erythema multiforme spectrum exists. Morphology remains the predominant basis for disease definitions, which have been the arena of terminologic disputes for more than a century. Lumping and splitting of entities, introduction of new terms, continued use of discarded ones, and too liberal usage of the term *erythema multiforme* for ill-defined cutaneous eruptions have led to terminologic and conceptual confusion that leaves most of the traditional terms without an unequivocal meaning and jeopardizes the accessibility of the erythema multiforme literature. The confusion can be disentangled only through a review of the historical development.

Descriptions of erythema multiforme date back to antiquity (Celsus). Bateman first described the target lesion in 1814, and Bazin first recognized mucosal involvement and constitutional symptoms in 1862. It was von Hebra who noted the multiform character of erythema multiforme and grouped several then-recognized disorders into a single entity, which he christened erythema exudativum multiforme. Von Hebra's description exactly fits the appearance of what is now known as HSV-associated erythema multiforme, except that he made no reference to oral mucosal involvement. Stevens and Johnson described a severe mucosal disease with "purplish cutaneous macules and necrotic centers" in 1922. In 1950, Thomas proposed that erythema multiforme and the Stevens-Johnson syndrome (SJS) were variants of the same pathologic process, differing only in severity, and that they should be termed erythema multiforme minor and erythema multiforme major, respectively. Although this suggestion was broadly accepted, the term *Stevens-Johnson syndrome* continued to be used as a synonym for erythema multiforme major.

In 1956, Lyell described TEN, again as a separate clinical entity (Lyell's syndrome), as a life-threatening, rapidly evolving mucocutaneous reaction characterized by erythemas, necrosis, and bullous detachment of the epidermis resembling scalding.[1] Lyell's series included not only patients suffering from what would still be called TEN today, but also others with staphylococcal scalded-skin syndrome and generalized fixed drug eruption;[2] thus, the series fueled terminologic disputes for many years. In the following decades, the notion gained ground that, in most or even in all instances, TEN was equivalent to SJS of maximal severity. Lyell himself suggested that the term *toxic epidermal necrolysis* be abandoned,[3] but its use has been retained.

Clearly, the erythema multiforme spectrum has for decades been considered to include the mild "minor" and the less common, but more severe, "major" types of the disorder—the distinctive mark being the presence of mucous membrane involvement—surmounted by the rare devastating TEN. All these categories were interpreted as polyetiologic, with an almost unlimited number of potential causative factors held responsible. It was thought that the milder forms were caused more often by infections; the more severe ones, by drugs. These prototypes were theoretically well defined, but their distinction often proved difficult in practice because of their overlapping features.

Important recent advances have, paradoxically, added to the confusion. It has become clear that mild erythema multiforme is strongly linked to HSV infection.[4] However, HSV-related erythema multiforme cannot simply be equated with "erythema multiforme minor," because it frequently involves mucosal sites (most often oral) that have previously been attributed to "erythema multiforme major." Labeling such cases erythema multiforme major is again confusing,[5,6] because "erythema multiforme major" is firmly engrained as a synonym for SJS.

Clinical and histopathologic observations, mostly by a team of French investigators, have suggested that there are two main morphologic patterns within the erythema multiforme spectrum. The investigators proposed that these patterns be considered different disorders with distinct causes[5–7] (Table 58-1): HSV-related erythema multiforme, characterized by target lesions and a predominantly inflammatory histopathologic pattern, and the primarily drug-related SJS-TEN complex, characterized by atypical or no target lesions at all and a predominantly necrotic histopathologic pattern. Stevens-Johnson syndrome and TEN were taken to differ only in the body surface area (BSA) involved and the severity.

Consensus papers have provided clinical criteria for the entities of the erythema multiforme spectrum that have been widely used in subsequent publications. The basis of the proposed definitions for SJS-TEN is quantitative:[5,7] SJS represents cases of less than 10 percent BSA involvement; TEN indicates more than 30 percent; and those in between are labeled SJS-TEN "overlap." Although somewhat artificial and not particularly simple, this classification is definitely useful for epidemiologic purposes (BSA is a prognostic factor in SJS–TEN) and permits the determination of medication risks. Also, it corresponds to a classification proposed earlier by one of us (R.R.M.).[8]

Several problems remain to be clarified: (1) the issue of overlapping features has not been resolved;[7] (2) the question of whether all instances of erythema multiforme that are not SJS-TEN by clinical criteria are HSV-related has not been properly addressed; (3) it has not been proven that all instances of extensive TEN, in fact, represent variants of SJS (e.g., what has been called "TEN without spots"[5]); and (4) the conditions characterized by mucosal lesions only (formerly "ectodermosis pluriorificialis") find no place in this classification.

We deem it unwise to coin new terms before more is known about the molecular pathophysiology of the conditions concerned. Therefore, we will use the term *erythema multiforme* for all instances of the erythema multiforme spectrum that are not SJS-TEN, and the term *SJS-TEN complex* for both SJS and TEN.

TABLE 58-1

Comparison of Clinical Features of Erythema Multiforme (EM) and Stevens-Johnson Syndrome–Toxic Epidermal Necrolysis (SJS-TEN)

	EM	SJS-TEN
Etiology	HSV (majority)	Drugs (80%–95%)
Course	Acute, self-limited, recurrent	Acute, self-limited, episodic
Prodromes	Absent to moderate	Intensive; skin tenderness
Eruption	Disseminated and symmetric on acral extremities, face	Disseminated with confluence, symmetric on face, neck, trunk
Typical lesions	Fixed plaques, target lesion, blisters; no Nikolsky sign	Macules, flat atypical target lesions, central necrosis; Nikolsky sign
Mucosal involvement	Frequent but mostly mild; usually only oral mucosa	Prominent, severe; 2–3 mucosal sites
Body surface affected	<10%	<10% to >30%
Constitutional symptoms	Absent to moderate	Prominent to severe
Pathology	Satellite-cell necrosis of the keratinocytes, dermoepidermal blister formation, prominent mononuclear-cell infiltrate, edema of papillary dermis	Massive keratinocytic necrosis, sloughing of epidermis, dermal mononuclear infiltrate slight to absent
Internal organ involvement	Absent	Not infrequent
Duration	1–3 weeks	2–6 weeks or more
Complications	None	Septicemia, pneumonia, gastrointestinal hemorrhage, renal failure, heart failure
Mortality rate	0%	1%–50%
Healing	Healing without scarring	Sequelae due to mucosal scarring possible

NOTE: HSV, herpes simplex virus.

ERYTHEMA MULTIFORME

Definition

Erythema multiforme is a self-limited, usually mild and relapsing exanthematic reaction of the skin that is etiologically most often related to recurrent HSV infection. It is clinically characterized by target-shaped, urticarial plaques, and it frequently presents with mucous membrane lesions.

Incidence and Epidemiology

Erythema multiforme is relatively common; it may account for up to 1 percent of dermatologic outpatient visits. The exact incidence is difficult to assess because practically all published series contain cases of SJS and/or erythema multiforme–like cases. Based on our own records, we estimate that erythema multiforme is at least 10 times as frequent as the SJS-TEN complex, for which an incidence of 1.9 cases/million population/year has been reported in Germany.[9] Erythema multiforme may occur in patients of all ages, but it occurs predominantly in adolescents and young adults; it is rare both under the age of 3 years and over the age of 50 years; 75 percent of patients are younger than 40 years. A slight preponderance has been reported both for females and males.[10,11] There is no predominance for ethnic groups or geographic locations. Seasonal clustering in spring is common ("typus annuus"), presumably caused by ultraviolet light provocation of recurrent HSV infection. Erythema multiforme is often recurrent, probably in the majority of the cases.[11] It is impossible at present to determine how often erythema multiforme occurs as a truly single event. Recurrences may occur at short intervals and reappear for many years.

Etiology

Although suspected since the early nineteenth century, it has been recognized only in recent years that HSV infection is the dominant causative factor of erythema multiforme, both in adults and in children.[4,10,12] Both HSV-1 and HSV-2 may trigger erythema multiforme, whereas the closely related varicella-zoster virus shows no such association.

Evidence linking HSV to erythema multiforme is best for recurrent erythema multiforme, as clinical lesions of recurrent HSV infection precede an outbreak of erythema multiforme in about 80 percent of patients.[12] In situ hybridization and the polymerase chain reaction have demonstrated HSV-DNA in the epidermal cells (not in the dermis) of erythema multiforme lesions in up to 90 percent of patients,[13,14] even in individuals without obvious preceding HSV infection.[15] In addition, immunofluorescence and immune histochemistry have demonstrated HSV-specific antigens in lesional skin. Most patients with recurrent erythema multiforme are seropositive for HSV, and it is occasionally possible to recover HSV from circulating immune complexes.[16] Peripheral blood mononuclear cells from patients with HSV infection and those with HSV-related erythema multiforme exhibit a similarly skewed T cell receptor response on stimulation with HSV antigen, indicating a specific immune response against HSV in both conditions.[17] Proof for the pathogenetic relevance of HSV infection derives from the fact that the prophylactic administration of acyclovir can effectively prevent recurrent HSV-associated erythema multiforme;[18] this is also true for many patients with no clinical evidence of HSV infection. There are no data at present, however, to prove that nonrecurring erythema multiforme is as strongly related to HSV as recurring erythema multiforme.

It is a matter of terminology (and therefore controversy) whether cases should be classified as erythema multiforme if they fulfill the clinical criteria, but do not show evidence of preceding HSV infection. There is little doubt that such eruptions exist, but it is unclear how frequent they are; they may occur more often in nonrecurrent erythema multiforme. The evidence for causative factors other than HSV infection is only circumstantial. Published reports implicate hepatitis B and C virus, as well as other viral infections.[19,20] Progesterone may elicit chronic recurrent erythema multiforme that responds to tamoxifen treatment[21] and oophorectomy. Drugs are a rare cause of erythema multiforme with mucous membrane lesions.[7] It may, of course, be argued whether these eruptions were truly erythema multiforme or mere imitators; moreover, subclinical HSV infection generally cannot be ruled out. Other problems are idiopathic cases, in which neither HSV infection nor any other cause can be uncovered. Such cases are fairly common under routine circumstances, but are even found in studies that specifically looked for HSV infection.[21] Many such cases respond to prophylactic acyclovir treatment and are thus likely to have been triggered by subclinical HSV infection; some, however, are resistent.[21]

Erythema multiforme–like dermatitic eruptions result from contact sensitization to sulfonamides, antihistamines, dinitrochlorobenzene (DNCB), diphencyprone (DPCP), rosewood, *Rhus,* primula, tea tree oil, cutting oils, cinnamon, and other substances; these rashes should be viewed as only imitators of erythema multiforme, despite clinical and histopathologic similarities.[22]

Pathogenesis

The current belief is that erythema multiforme is a cell-mediated immune reaction leading to the destruction of keratinocytes expressing HSV antigens. However, many aspects of the underlying pathomechanisms are not known.

Although erythema multiforme lesions can exhibit viral antigens and DNA, attempts at viral cultures almost invariably fail, and electron microscopy cannot detect intact virions. Therefore, erythema multiforme lesions are not sites of regular HSV replication, as can be suspected from their histopathologic appearance. This paradox has been partially resolved:[14] no viable HSV particles are present in epidermal keratinocytes; there are only DNA fragments, most often encoding viral DNA polymerase. Fragments of DNA persisted for 1 to 3 months in the epidermis after healing (as in acute HSV lesions); viral polymerase RNA, however, was identified only in fresh, not in healed erythema multiforme lesions. These data suggest that transcription and translation are limited, and that the development of erythema multiforme lesions may be associated with the expression of viral polymerase (and/or additional antigens), stimulating a specific immune response.

Obviously, HSV-DNA reaches distant cutaneous locations from a site of active replication via the bloodstream. Immune complexes may mediate hematogenous transport;[16] more importantly, however, peripheral blood mononuclear cells, which contained HSV-DNA in more than 60 percent of patients during acute erythema multiforme episodes, may be the transport vehicle.[13] The use of this vehicle may explain viral DNA fragmentation: monocytes are nonpermissive for HSV replication, which may lead to DNA damage.[14] Upregulation of adhesion molecules greatly increases binding of HSV-containing mononuclear cells to endothelial cells; HLA-class I and adhesion molecule upregulation in endothelial cells may account for the dermal inflammatory response.[23] The reason that viral DNA fragments home to the specific predilection sites of erythema multiforme—or elicit the formation of lesions there (HSV-DNA has been recovered from apparently healthy control skin[13])—is a matter of speculation. Precipitating factors such as ultraviolet light may play a role: sun exposure is known to trigger erythema multiforme ("light-sensitive" erythema multiforme), and the lesions are often confined to sun-exposed areas. At times, erythema multiforme may even assume the clinical appearance of polymorphous light eruption and juvenile spring eruption.[24]

Cytotoxic effector cells (CD8+ T lymphocytes), which predominate in the rather scarce inflammatory infiltrate within the epidermis, carry out the immunologic attack on HSV-expressing epidermal keratinocytes. These induce apoptosis of individual scattered keratinocytes, leading to satellite-cell necrosis in early lesions or to more widespread necrosis in older ones.[25] Exocytosis of these cells into the epidermis is facilitated by strong expression of intercellular adhesion molecule 1 (ICAM 1) in the basal layer and pockets of the spinous layer, which may be caused by interferon-γ released from dermal CD4+ T lymphocytes.[26] Neighboring epidermal cells are HLA-DR-positive.[4]

In comparison to SJS-TEN, erythema multiforme displays much less striking epidermal necrosis, but more intense dermal inflammation, which is mediated chiefly by CD4+ T lymphocytes and monocytes,[27] and is responsible for the wheal-like clinical appearance of the typical target lesions. Inflammation is associated with microvascular damage that is likely to be caused by HSV-containing mononuclear cells binding to the endothelium.[23] The explanation for these obvious differences in pathology may lie in the observation that skin lesions of HSV-related erythema multiforme express interferon-γ, but not tumor necrosis factor–α (TNF-α), whereas the reverse is true for drug-induced SJS-TEN.[28] The two subsets thus appear to be "mechanistically" different, and erythema multiforme may have a delayed type hypersensitivity component that is absent from SJS-TEN.

As recurrent HSV infection is common and erythema multiforme episodes are much less so, it is obvious that HSV-related erythema multiforme must be linked to a specific predisposition. Clinically, HSV lesions associated with erythema multiforme are not different from those without such an association.[11] One report indicated not differences between the specific immune responses of patients suffering from recurrent HSV infection with associated erythema multiforme and those of patients without such an association.[29] Increased frequencies of certain HLA antigens were described in association with HSV-related erythema multiforme, particularly HLA-Bw62 (B15), -B35, and -DR53.[30] Kämpgen and colleagues demonstrated significant associations with the DR4 and DQw3 alleles; the relative risk for DQw3 was 44.2.[31]

There was no such correlation in patients with recurrent HSV infection without associated erythema multiforme.

Clinical Manifestations

As noted in Table 58-1, prodromal symptoms are absent in most cases of erythema multiforme. If present, they are mild, variable, and nonspecific, merely suggesting an upper respiratory infection (e.g., cough, rhinitis, low-grade fever).

The skin rash arises abruptly. In most patients, all lesions appear within 3 days; but in some, several crops follow each other during one episode of erythema multiforme. Up to hundreds of lesions may form, most in a symmetric, acral distribution on the extensor surfaces of the extremities (dorsa of hands and feet, elbows, and knees) and the face; they appear less often on palms and soles, thighs, buttocks, and trunk (Fig. 58-1). Lesions often first appear acrally and then spread in a centripetal manner. Mechanical (Koebner phenomenon) and actinic (predilection of sun-exposed sites) factors appear to influence the distribution of lesions. Zosteriform hemicorporeal and linear distribution along Blaschko's lines of erythema multiforme lesions may occur.[32] Although patients occasionally report burning and itching, the eruption is usually symptomless.

As the name implies, the clinical picture of erythema multiforme is variable, but the rash is usually monomorphous in a given patient. Variability results from the variable morphologic expression along a scale of severity of a single prototypic lesion. Typically, this lesion is a highly regular, circular, wheal-like erythematous papule or plaque that is stable (i.e., of fixed position and persistent for 1 week or more); it measures from a few millimeters to about 2 cm and may expand slightly over 24 to 48 hours. While the periphery remains erythematous and edematous, the center becomes violaceous and dark; inflammatory activity may regress or relapse in the center, thus giving rise to concentric rings of color change (Fig. 58-1*A*). Often, the center turns purpuric and/or necrotic or transforms into a tense vesicle or bulla. The result is the classic target or iris lesion (Fig. 58-1*A*).

According to the proposed classification, typical target lesions consist of at least three concentric components: (1) a dusky central disk, or blister; (2) more peripherally, a ring of pale edema; and (3) an erythematous halo.[5,7] Not all lesions of erythema multiforme are typical: some display two rings only ("raised atypical targets"), but none are flat, which is the typical lesion of SJS-TEN. In some patients with erythema multiforme, most lesions are livid vesicles overlying a just slightly darker central portion, encircled by an erythematous margin (Fig. 58-1*C*). Larger lesions may have a central bulla and a marginal ring of vesicles (herpes iris of Bateman; Fig. 58-1*B*).

Mucosal lesions are present in up to 70 percent of patients,[11] almost exclusively limited to the oral cavity and most often only a few. Predilection sites are the lips, palate, and gingivae. On the lips, identifiable target lesions may form; otherwise, vesicles, erosions, and crusting are evident. Extensive, painful oral involvement with only few skin lesions occasionally occurs. Cervical lymphadenopathy is usually present in these patients. "Ectodermosis pluriorificialis" is a rare occurrence characterized by severe involvement of two or three mucosal sites in the absence of skin lesions. Its place within the erythema multiforme spectrum is not quite clear, but its often relapsing nature suggests that it is HSV-related.

In most cases, erythema multiforme affects well under 10 percent of the BSA. Rare instances of extensive skin lesions and prominent involvement of the oral mucosa (at times called "bullous erythema multiforme" or "erythema multiforme major"—see "Classification and History," above) may be difficult to distinguish from SJS-TEN.

Patients with erythema multiforme are afebrile, physical examination is normal, and there are no reports of joint or muscular complaints or lymphadenopathy, except in patients with mucosal erosions.

Course and Prognosis

Erythema multiforme runs a mild course in most cases, and each individual attack subsides within 1 to 4 weeks. Recovery is complete, and there are no sequelae (not even in mucosal lesions), except for transient hypo- or hyperpigmentation in some cases. The condition does not progress to SJS-TEN. Recurrences are common and may occur in the majority of cases. In one report on a large series of patients with recurrent erythema multiforme, the mean number of attacks was 6 per year (range, 2 to 36), and the mean total duration of disease was 9.5 years; in 33 percent, the condition persisted for more than 10 years.[10] Up to 50 recurrences have been described in a single patient.[21] The severity of episodes in patients with recurrent erythema multiforme is highly variable and unpredictable. The frequency of episodes and cumulative duration of disease are not correlated with the severity of attacks. The frequency and severity of recurrent erythema multiforme tend to improve spontaneously over time (after 2 years or more), parallel to the improvement of recurring HSV infection.

RELATIONSHIP TO RECURRENT HSV INFECTION In more than 70 percent of patients with recurrent erythema multiforme, an episode of recurrent HSV infection precedes the rash; the association with herpes labialis predominates (9:1) over that with genital herpes, or that with herpes in other locations. The average interval is 8 days (range, 2 to 17);[10] the duration of the lag period appears to be specific for individual patients. In a small number of patients, HSV recrudescence and erythema multiforme may occur simultaneously. Not all episodes of erythema multiforme are preceded by clinically evident HSV infection, and not all HSV episodes are followed by erythema multiforme. Episodes of recurrent HSV infection may precede the development of HSV-related erythema multiforme for many years.

CONTINUOUS AND PERSISTENT ERYTHEMA MULTIFORME A small fraction of patients experience a prolonged series of overlapping attacks of erythema multiforme; this constellation has been labeled "continuous erythema multiforme"[21] and has been connected to the systemic administration of glucocorticoids. Similar rare cases with widespread and therapy-resistant lesions have been described as "persistent erythema multiforme."[33] It is doubtful that all these cases truly represent erythema multiforme.

Pathology

Early lesions of erythema multiforme exhibit lymphocyte accumulations at the dermal-epidermal interface, with exocytosis into the epidermis, scattered keratinocyte necrosis with lymphocytes attached to the necrotic keratinocyte (satellite-cell necrosis), spongiosis, vacuolar degeneration of the basal layer, and focal junctional and subepidermal cleft formation (Fig. 58-2). Epidermal necrosis is more extensive in central portions and older lesions. The papillary dermis is often highly edematous with a dense mononuclear cell infiltrate, which is more abundant in older lesions than in fresh lesions. The vessels are ectatic with swollen endothelial cells; there may be extravasated erythrocytes and eosinophils. Advanced lesions show subepidermal blisters and frank epidermal necrosis (Fig. 58-3). Immunofluorescence findings are nonspecific. In late lesions, melanophages may be prominent.

The histopathologic appearance of erythema multiforme is different from that of SJS-TEN, in which dermal inflammation is moderate to absent and epidermal necrosis is much more pronounced.[27,34,35] Formerly interpreted as expressions of the variability of the erythema multiforme spectrum[36] or as consecutive stages in the dynamic evolution of

FIGURE 58-1

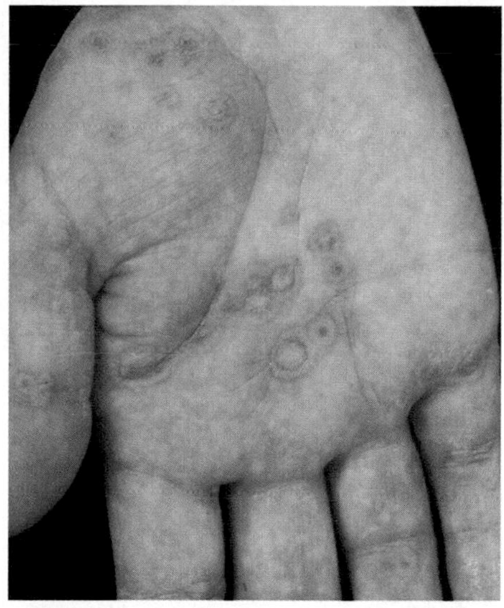

A.

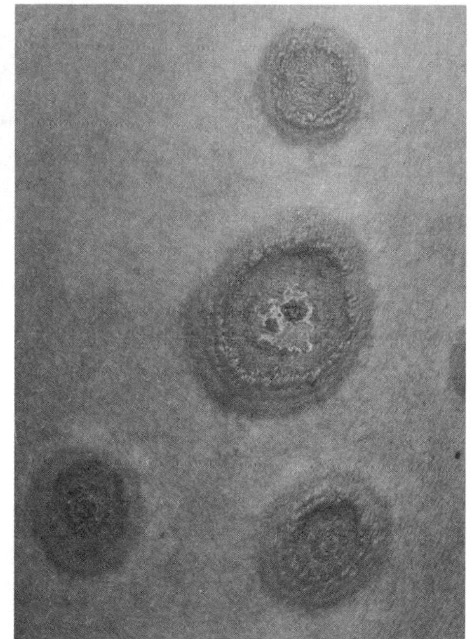

B.

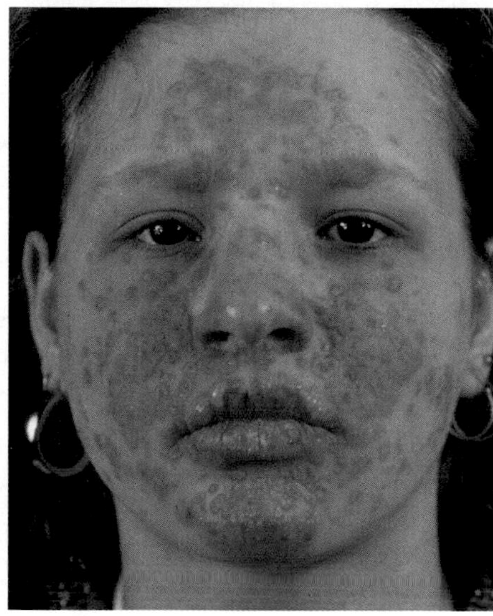

C.

Erythema multiforme. *A*. Papular, urticarial, and vesicular target lesions in acral distribution. *B*. Herpes iris of Bateman. *C*. Vesicular and target lesions of erythema multiforme.

target lesions,[37] these differences have been demonstrated in very early lesions of the respective entities and thus appear to be inherent features. Still, the histopathologic appearances are somewhat overlapping and do not allow the distinction of erythema multiforme from SJS-TEN in all instances.[38]

Laboratory Investigations

Laboratory findings are usually normal in patients with erythema multiforme. In more severe cases, an elevated erythrocyte sedimentation rate, moderate leukocytosis, acute phase proteins, and mildly elevated liver transaminase levels may occur.

Differential Diagnosis

In typical cases, erythema multiforme is easily identifiable because of its characteristic appearance, stability, and symmetric acral distribution of the target lesions. At times, however, atypical cases display features of a variety of other skin conditions (Table 58-2). A disorder frequently mistaken for erythema multiforme is acute annular urticaria, which is often drug-induced; this disorder is characterized by annular polycyclic, concentric, or arcuate urticarial lesions that extend peripherally, leaving central ecchymotic violaceous areas, thus mimicking target lesions. Histologically, only slight edema and minimal perivascular infiltrates are found. "Target purpura" (acute hemorrhagic edema of infancy) is a manifestation of leukocytoclastic vasculitis in infants and small children; it is characterized by symmetric erythematous and purpuric concentric rings in acral locations, similar to target lesions, that spontaneously resolve in about a week. Erythema multiforme–like lesions are sometimes found in lupus erythematosus ("Rowell's syndrome").[39] It may sometimes be difficult to distinguish mucosal lesions from pemphigus vulgaris and herpetic gingivostomatitis. Disseminated contact dermatitis may exhibit lesions that mimic target lesions closely, both clinically and histologically.[22]

Treatment

In most cases, erythema multiforme causes little discomfort and regresses spontaneously within about 2 weeks. Symptomatic treatment with shake lotions, topical steroids, analgesics, and antihistamines has little impact on the course, but may reduce subjective symptoms. Liquid antacids, topical glucocorticoids, and local anesthetics relieve

FIGURE 58-2

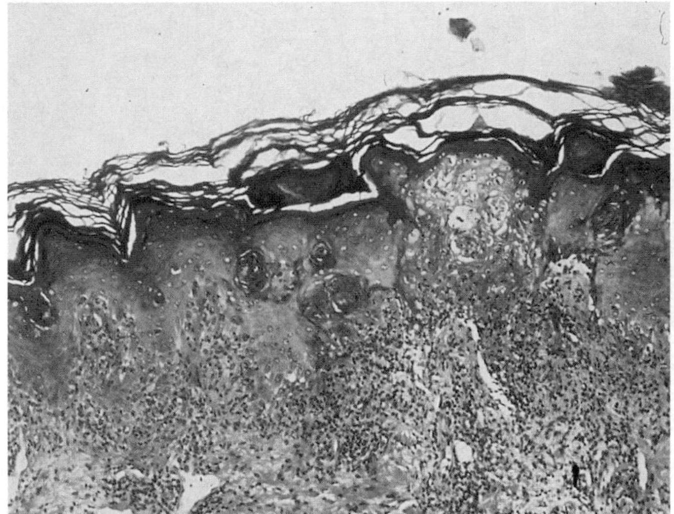

A.

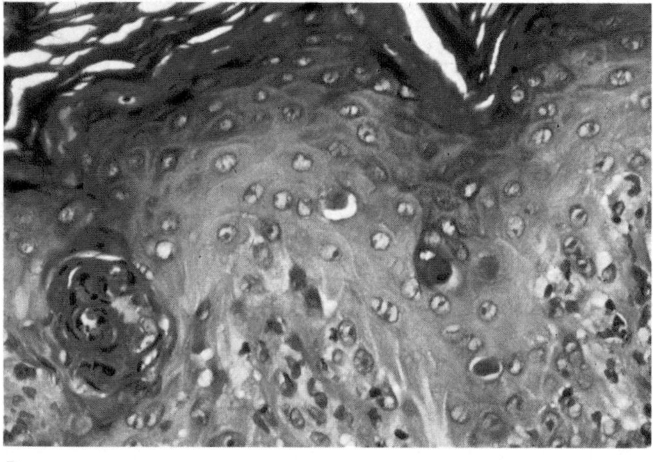

B.

Histopathology of erythema multiforme (early lesion). *A*. An intense lymphohistiocytic infiltrate fills the mid-dermis and obliterates many blood vessels. The dermal papillae are edematous and contain material with the staining properties of fibrin. There is subepidermal cleft formation and circumscribed necrosis of the epidermis. *B*. High-power magnification of scattered keratinocyte necrosis.

symptoms of painful mouth erosions. The systemic administration of glucocorticoids is unnecessary and may even have worsened some cases.

In recurrent erythema multiforme, early treatment of HSV infection with oral acyclovir (200 mg five times per day for 5 days) or its derivatives with better bioavailability (e.g., valacyclovir or pencyclovir) may prevent erythema multiforme, but often it comes too late. In such cases, continuous administration of low-dose acyclovir (400 to 800 mg per day) or valacyclovir (500 mg per day) for a 6-month period is indicated. This regimen is highly effective in preventing episodes of both HSV infection and erythema multiforme as long as it is continued, even in patients in whom HSV is not the obvious precipitating factor.[10] Attacks recur after withdrawal, but generally tend to be less frequent and less severe. As alternatives for patients who do not respond to this treatment, dapsone, antimalarials, and even azathioprine and thalidomide have been advocated.

FIGURE 58-3

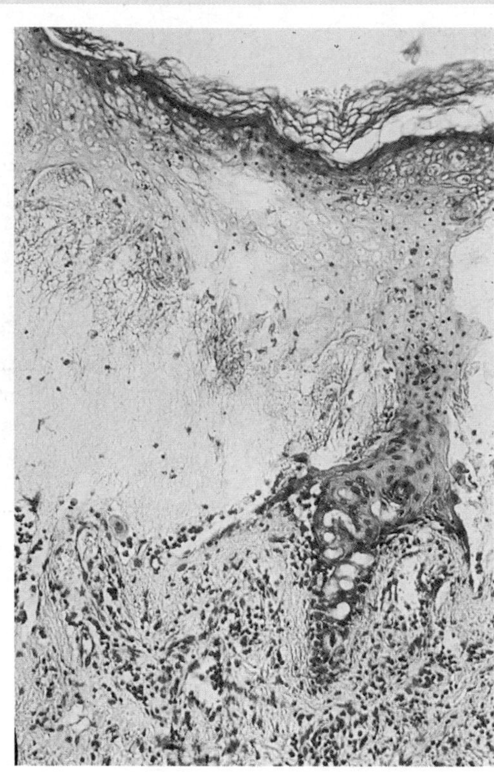

Erythema multiforme: advanced lesions with subepidermal blister and epidermal necrosis.

STEVENS-JOHNSON SYNDROME AND TOXIC EPIDERMAL NECROLYSIS

Definition

Stevens-Johnson syndrome and toxic epidermal necrolysis are severe, episodic, acute mucocutaneous reactions that are most often elicited by drugs and occasionally elicited by infections. They are closely related or identical, differing only in the extent of BSA involved (see above).[5,7] Both are characterized by rapidly expanding, often irregular macules ("atypical target lesions") and involvement of more than one mucosal site (oral, conjunctival, and anogenital). In TEN, the rash coalesces to widespread dusky erythema, necrosis, and detachment of the epidermis resembling scalding. Constitutional symptoms and internal organ involvement occur often and may be severe. In principle, SJS and TEN are self-limited; the mortality rate in TEN is significant,

TABLE 58-2

Differential Diagnosis of Erythema Multiforme

Urticaria
Urticarial vasculitis
Figurate erythemas
Acute febrile neutrophilic dermatosis (Sweet's syndrome)
Disseminated lesions of contact dermatitis
Bullous pemphigoid, linear IgA dermatosis, herpes gestationis
Lupus erythematosus

however, and sequelae may develop because of mucosal scarring. It is currently impossible to draw an absolutely sharp line of distinction between SJS-TEN and the more severe forms of erythema multiforme.

Incidence and Epidemiology

The incidence of SJS-TEN is estimated at 2 to 3 cases per million population per year in Europe and the United States.[9,40,41] In Germany, it was found to be 1.9 cases per million population per year; the relative proportions of SJS, "SJS-TEN overlap," and TEN were 3:2:1.[9] Stevens-Johnson syndrome–toxic epidermal necrolysis occurs worldwide and affects females about twice as frequently as males.[41] The disorder appears most often in adults, but also occurs in children.[8] It typically occurs sporadically, but epidemics have followed the mass use of drugs.[42] In most cases, SJS-TEN is a single event; after reexposure to the culprit drug, it takes a more severe course.[43] The incidence is increased up to three orders of magnitude in the HIV-infected population.[44] An association of SJS-TEN with the HLA-A29 and -B12 (relative risk, 13.4), and with the HLA-B12 and DR7 haplotypes, has been found.[45] Population-based and case-control studies on SJS-TEN have been initiated in the United States and Europe to clarify pending issues of epidemiology and drug etiology.[46,47]

Etiology

Although SJS-TEN has a polyetiologic reaction pattern, drugs are clearly the leading causative factor (80 to 95 percent of patients with TEN, more than 50 percent of those with SJS; see Table 58-3), and only a minority of cases appear to be linked to infection, vaccination, or graft-versus-host disease. In a small percentage of patients with SJS-TEN (less than 5 percent for TEN), neither drugs nor other potential causes become apparent (idiopathic SJS-TEN). The lack of appropriate diagnostic in vitro and skin tests hampers the identification of the responsible trigger factors. Circumstantial evidence, therefore, usually serves as the only criterion.

Uncertainty still exists about the relative risk of SJS-TEN associated with individual drugs and the role of accompanying factors. Obviously, the many case reports or retrospective studies in which more than 100 drugs have been found to elicit SJS-TEN do not provide this information.[40,41] Similarly, population-based studies that correlate the

TABLE 58-3

Drugs Associated with Stevens-Johnson Syndrome and Toxic Epidermal Necrolysis

Drugs Most Frequently Associated*	Drugs Also Associated
Sulfadoxine	Cephalosporins
Sulfadiazine	Fluoroquinolones
Sulfasalazine	Vancomycin
Co-trimoxazole	Rifampin
Hydantoins	Ethambutol
Carbamazepine	Fenbufen
Barbiturates	Tenoxicam
Benoxaprofen†	Tiaprofenic acid
Phenylbutazone	Diclofenac
Isoxicam†	Sulindac
Piroxicam	Ibuprofen
Chlormezanone	Ketoprofen
Allopurinol	Naproxen
Amithiozone	Thiabendazole
Aminopenicillins	

*Together these drugs account for approximately two-thirds of the cases attributed to drugs in large series in France, Germany, and the United States.
†This drug is no longer marketed.
SOURCE: Roujeau et al.[49]

incidence of SJS-TEN with the number of drug users or the daily drug dose consumed in a certain population, do not supply reliable data because of the rarity of SJS-TEN.[46] To solve this problem, investigators have begun prospective case-control studies to compare the drugs taken by index patients to those taken by controls. The relative risks and the influence of cofactors such as age, gender, region, multiple drug intake, or underlying diseases can thus be calculated by multivariate analysis. Initial results have been published,[47,48] but more are to follow.

Although the list of causative drugs may vary from country to country and over time because of differences in drug use, three groups are cited as the most common triggers in all surveys and reviews: antibacterial sulfonamides, anticonvulsants, and nonsteroidal anti-inflammatory drugs (NSAIDs). Antimalarials, allopurinol, and a few others follow a close second.

Sulfa drugs, particularly long-acting sulfonamides and co-trimoxazole, appear to elicit SJS-TEN most often, with an estimated incidence of 1 to 10 per 100,000 users;[48] the relative risk is 172. Particularly aggressive cases have occurred in HIV-infected patients in the context of *Pneumocystis carinii* infection and malaria prophylaxis. Anticonvulsive drugs such as phenytoin, carbamazepine, and phenobarbital may carry relative risks from 11 to 15.[48] Carbamazepine may elicit SJS-TEN most frequently (14 per 100,000 users).[49] Hydantoins are considered the main cause of TEN in children.[5] Valproic acid, often used as an alternative for hydantoins, has an equally high relative risk.[49] Severe SJS-TEN has developed in patients who received phenytoin simultaneously with cranial irradiation.[50] There have been several cases of SJS-TEN due to the new anticonvulsant lamotrigine.[51] Nonsteroidal anti-inflammatory drugs such as butazone and oxicam derivatives have often been reported as inciting drugs; isoxicam, for instance, was withdrawn in France following 13 cases of TEN.[40] The case-control study confirmed the association for oxicam derivatives (relative risk, 18) and, to a lesser degree, for propionic acid derivatives (relative risk, 4.5). Pyrazolones and salicylates, formerly often thought to cause SJS-TEN, had only low relative risks.[48]

Allopurinol and chlormezanone (a tranquilizer unrelated to benzodiazepines) are important causes of SJS-TEN in developed countries,[48,52] whereas antituberculosis drugs play an important role in Third World countries.[53] Antibiotics have been more often suspected than actually shown to be causative, however, relevant risks may exist for cephalosporins, tetracyclines, aminopenicillins, quinolones, and imidazole antifungals.[49] In recent years, antiretroviral drugs, such as nevirapine and protease inhibitors, emerged as important causes of SJS-TEN.[54] A variety of other agents, such as hormones, chinine-containing beverages, airborne and contact allergens, and toxins, have been reported to cause SJS-TEN. In 3 of 20 cases of TEN observed in Singapore, Chinese herbs were found to be responsible.[55]

It is a problem in determining the etiology of SJS-TEN that drugs taken during the prodromal phase to alleviate symptoms cannot be distinguished from those that actually caused the disease. The often listed antibiotics, pyrazolones, and salicylates may be such drugs. The same possibly holds true for systemic glucocorticoids, which were found to be associated with a surprisingly high relative risk of 12.[48]

The significance of individual predisposing factors that may promote SJS-TEN has not been fully elucidated. Familial occurrence is rarely a feature of SJS-TEN, but there may be a genetic susceptibility, as documented by the association with certain HLA haplotypes. Synergistic effects (e.g., viral infection and drug intake[56]) and drug interactions are likely to play roles in many cases; in one study, patients had taken a mean of 4.4 drugs prior to the onset of TEN.[57] Physical factors such as ultraviolet light and x-rays may precipitate drug-induced SJS-TEN, with the skin lesions being of maximal intensity at the sites of exposure.[50,57] Also, SJS-TEN appears to occur preferentially in patients with multiple accompanying diseases, particularly those that activate the immune system, such as collagen vascular diseases, neoplasia and lymphoma, and acute graft-versus-host disease; it may even follow vaccination.[58]

Infectious agents play a much less prominent role in the etiology of SJS-TEN. The most thoroughly documented cases were caused by *Mycoplasma pneumoniae,*[59] which has been isolated from the lesions of SJS-TEN. Less well documented cases have been linked to histoplasmosis, adenovirus infections, hepatitis A, infectious mononucleosis, coxsackievirus B5, varicella-zoster virus, gram-negative septicemia, milker's nodules, and yersiniosis. The link to other infectious agents is more tenuous.

Acute graft-versus-host disease is an obviously rare cause of SJS-TEN, but its incidence in allogeneic bone marrow recipients is high (9 of 152, according to one survey[60]). The relationship between acute graft-versus-host disease and TEN is difficult to assess because the skin lesions that appear in patients with these conditions are nearly indistinguishable, both clinically and histologically; differences pertain more to type and severity of internal organ involvement (e.g., gastrointestinal tract, liver) than to skin symptoms. Also, bone marrow allograft recipients are subject to factors that in their own right (or synergistically) may precipitate TEN (e.g., x-rays, cytotoxic drugs, cytomegalovirus infection). It is clear, however, that TEN may result from acute graft-versus-host disease independently from drug intake: it was observed in a patient with thymus hypoplasia who took no drugs,[61] and it can be reproduced in an animal model for acute graft-versus-host disease.[62] Among patients with acute graft-versus-host disease, TEN has been shown to have a 100 percent mortality rate.

Identification of the provocative agent rests mainly on history; skin testing and in vitro tests are usually not helpful,[63] and exposure tests are ethically unacceptable. Exceptional reports describe positive intracutaneous and patch tests with positive lymphocyte transformation tests,[52] or increased lymphocyte susceptibility to cytotoxic killing by liver microsome–induced drug intermediates[64] in patients with drug-induced TEN.

Pathogenesis

The pathomechanisms of SJS-TEN are only partially understood. There are similarities to the pathomechanisms of HSV-related erythema multiforme, but important differences have become apparent. Like erythema multiforme, SJS-TEN is viewed as a cytotoxic immune reaction aimed at the destruction of keratinocytes expressing foreign (drug-related) antigens. The characteristic lag between exposure and disease onset (1 to 45 days; mean, 14), which tends to be much briefer at repeated exposure, also suggests an immune pathogenesis. Drug-specific activation of T cells (including both CD4+ and CD8+) has been shown in vitro on peripheral blood mononuclear cells of patients with bullous drug eruptions;[65] a high production rate of interleukin (IL)-5, in addition to that of other cytokines, was noted. As in HSV-related erythema multiforme, epidermal injury is based on the induction of apoptosis.[25] Furthermore, in both conditions, memory CD4+ lymphocytes appear to dominate dermal mononuclear cells, whereas CD8+ cytotoxic cells (and large granular lymphocytes) were prevalent in the epidermis.[66] In both conditions, epidermal keratinocytes express ICAM-1 and class II major histocompatibility complex (MHC) antigens; Langerhans cells are notably reduced or absent.[67]

It has always puzzled investigators how the relatively few cytotoxic cells present in the epidermis of patients with SJS-TEN may induce an epidermal injury far in excess of that of erythema multiforme, which features many more such effector cells. Paquet and colleagues demonstrated that in contrast to erythema multiforme, inflammatory cells in SJS-TEN contain large numbers of activated macrophages and factor XIII+ dendrocytes.[27,68] Furthermore, there is a drastic overexpression of TNF-α (less so of IL-6) in the epidermis with SJS-TEN,[69] while only minute amounts of this cytokine occur in erythema multiforme. As TEN blister fluid contains viable CD8+ lymphocytes and high amounts of TNF-α,[70,71] it appears likely that TNF-α plays an important role in epidermal destruction by inducing apoptosis directly, by attracting cytotoxic effector cells, or both.[28] The source of TNF-α may be both macrophages and keratinocytes; mutual stimulation is likely. Interestingly, physical factors that precipitate or accentuate drug-induced SJS-TEN are known to stimulate TNF-α expression in keratinocytes (ultraviolet light and x-rays).

The nature of the antigens that drive the cytotoxic cellular immune reaction is not well understood. It has been proposed that drugs or their metabolites act as haptens and render keratinocytes antigenic by binding to their surfaces.[72,73] Obviously, the drug-modified peptide may be presented on both MHC I and MHC II molecules.[64] Shear and colleagues linked cutaneous drug eruptions to a defect of the detoxification systems (in both liver and skin):[73] aromatic drug metabolism by cytochrome P_{450} leads to the formation of reactive hydroxylamines from sulfonamides or arene oxides from aromatic anticonvulsants that bind to cell constituents if not rapidly detoxified by epoxide hydrolases. Genetically determined defective detoxification may thus result in direct toxicity or alteration of the antigenic properties of keratinocytes. This attractive hypothesis gains support from the association of SJS-TEN with the carbamazepine or hydantoin hypersensitivity syndromes,[74] the association of sulfonamide-triggered SJS-TEN with the slow acetylator phenotype,[75] preliminary results of in vitro cytotoxicity assays,[76] and the overproportional occurrence in HIV-infected patients who are deficient in glutathione, an important scavenger of toxic compounds.[77] It has been hypothesized that the cytotoxic assault may be directed at viral antigens that persist in the skin.[78] High amounts of mRNA for inducible nitric oxide synthase have been detected in the inflammatory infiltrate of SJS-TEN;[78] nitric oxide, which is known to induce apoptosis and necrosis, may thus have a role in the pathogenesis of SJS-TEN. Although drug-induced SJS-TEN occasionally occurs in animals, no animal model is available at present.

Autoantibodies against desmoplakin I and II have been detected in a subset of SJS.[79] In these cases, suprabasal acantholysis was present, while the clinical disease was no different from that manifested in other patients with SJS who lacked these antibodies.

Clinical Manifestations

In at least half of the patients, SJS-TEN begins with a nonspecific prodrome of 1 to 14 days (see Table 58-1): fever, malaise, headache, rhinitis, cough, sore throat, chest pain, vomiting, diarrhea, myalgias, and arthralgias. Patients often feel ill and receive antimicrobial and anti-inflammatory treatment that later may cause difficulties in determining the offending factor. The onset of disease is sudden; cases vary within wide limits in terms of length of the lag period between exposure and onset of the eruption, rapidity of evolvement, BSA involved and degree of confluence, prominence of mucous membrane involvement, accompanying constitutional symptoms, and internal organ involvement.

A macular, often morbilliform rash appears first on the face, neck, chin, and central trunk areas; it may then spread to the extremities and the rest of the body. The individual lesions may have dusky centers reminiscent of target lesions, or they may be mere roundish, irregularly shaped and moderately well defined pale livid macules (Fig. 58-4). They are often larger than target lesions, flat, and tender, and exhibit a positive Nikolsky sign (Figs. 58-4*B*, 58-5*A*, and 58-5*C*); some form flaccid and occasionally hemorrhagic blisters. Despite these obvious differences from erythema multiforme, occasional raised atypical, or even typical, target lesions may appear. The lesions rapidly increase in number and size, usually reaching maximal disease expression within

FIGURE 58-4

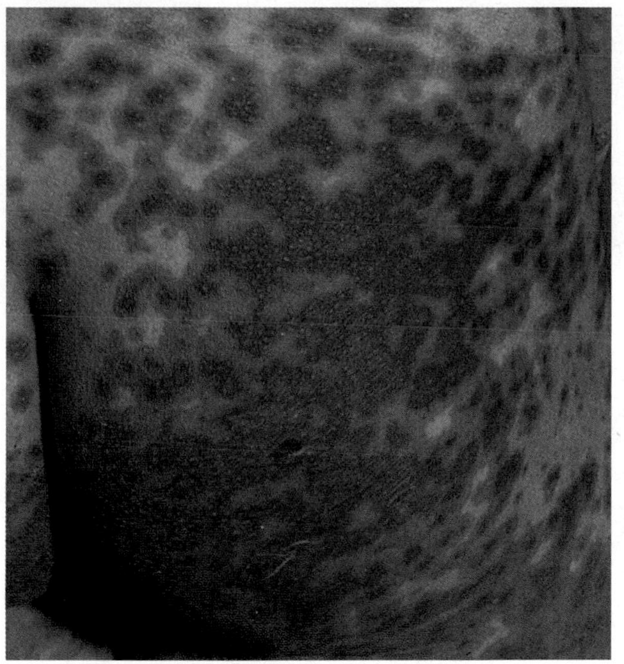

A.

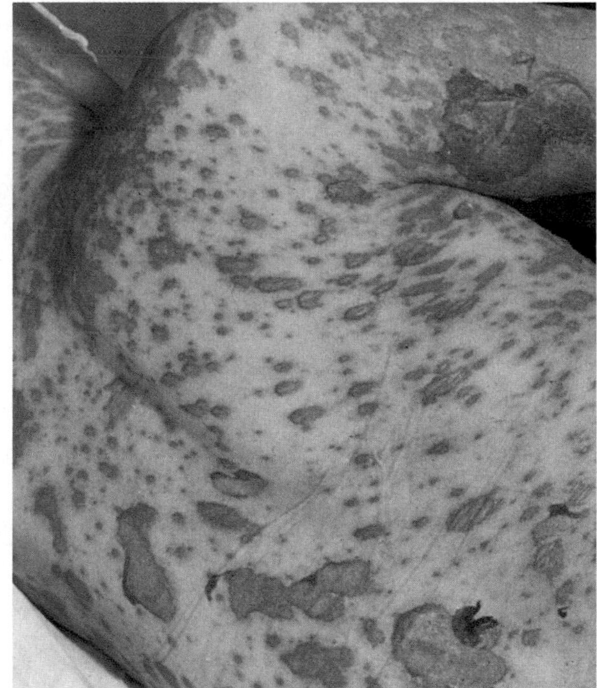

B.

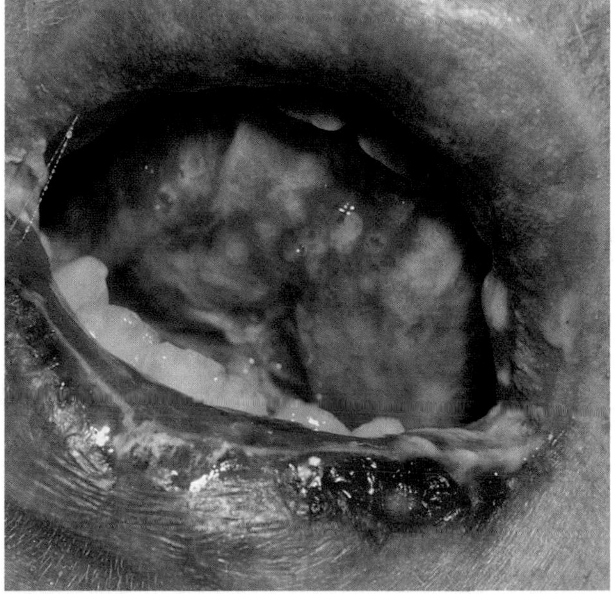

C.

Stevens-Johnson syndrome. *A.* Initial stage: partially confluent erythematous lesions with dusky centers, presenting as flat atypical target lesions. Note the positive Nikolsky sign. *B.* Advanced stage: generalized macular eruption with detachment of necrotic epidermis. *C.* Extensive necrosis and erosions of the lips and oral mucosa.

4 to 5 days; however, new crops may emerge considerably later if a long-acting drug is the inciting agent.

There is a striking tendency for coalescence; confluence is only partial, limited to the predilection sites (face, neck, chest) in SJS, but widespread to total in TEN (see Fig. 58-5). Areas of confluence represent extensive, diffuse erythemas; individual macular lesions remain discernible in the periphery. Within such lesions, the epidermis becomes loose and easily detached following minimal frictional trauma. Large flaccid blisters form; the blister roofs turn necrotic and rupture easily. Sheets of necrotic epidermis slide off the face and at pressure points such as the back and shoulders, leaving intensely red, oozing erosions (see Fig. 58-5*C*). Denudation may involve 10 to 90 percent of the BSA. In severe cases of TEN, prominent involvement of the skin appendages may lead to shedding of the finger- and toenails, as well as loss of the eyebrows and cilia (see Fig. 58-5*B*).

Mucous membrane lesions parallel or even precede the rash. The oral cavity (buccal mucosa, palate) and the vermilion border of the lips (see Figs. 58-4*C* and 58-5*B*) are almost invariably affected; less often, the bulbar conjunctiva and anogenital mucosae. All three sites are involved in approximately 40 percent of cases.[11] Signs that herald lesions are sore and burning sensations of the conjunctivae, lips, and buccal mucosa; edema; and erythema; following these signs are blisters that rupture and become extensive, hemorrhagic dull red erosions coated by grayish-white pseudomembranes (necrotic epithelium and fibrin; see Fig. 58-4*C*) or shallow aphthous-like ulcers. Massive hemorrhagic crusts cover the lips. Oral lesions are severely painful and cause eating and breathing difficulties and hypersalivation. The process may extend to the gingiva, tongue, pharynx, nasal cavity, and even to the larynx, esophagus, and respiratory tree. Otitis media may develop. Conjunctival involvement features inflammation and chemosis, vesiculation

FIGURE 58-5

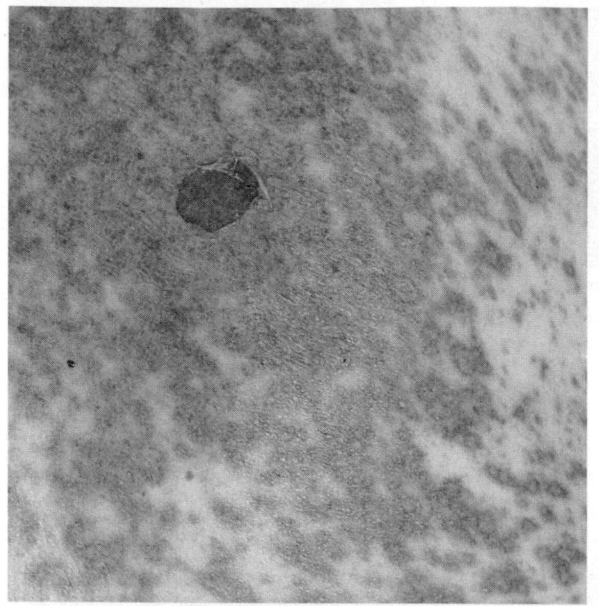

A.

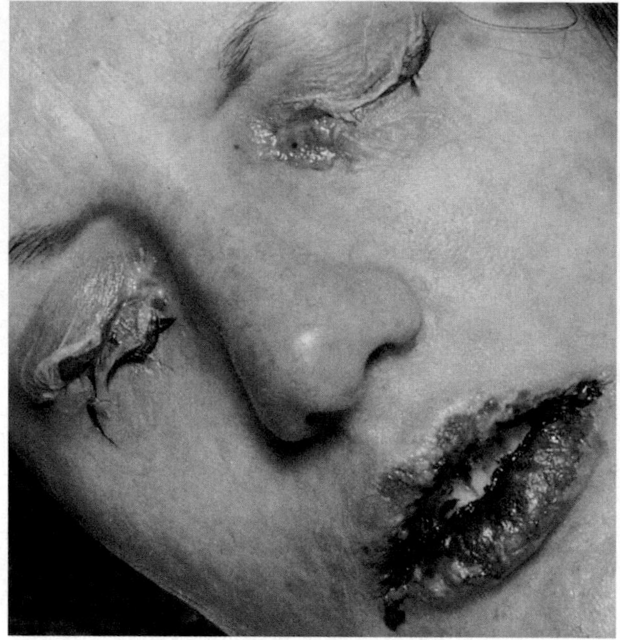

B.

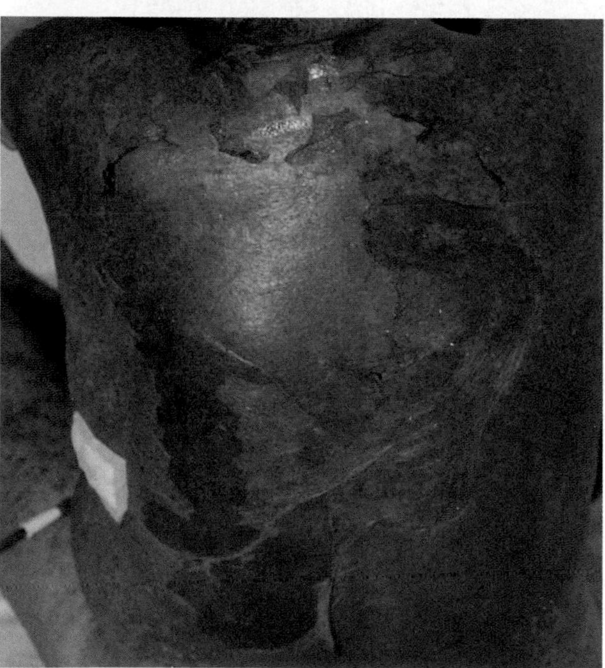

C.

Toxic epidermal necrolysis. *A.* Confluent morbilliform eruption; note the positive Nikolsky sign. *B.* Diffuse erythema of the face with shedding of the cilia and epidermis of the eyelids, severe erosions, and hemorrhagic crusting of the lips. *C.* Diffuse generalized shedding of the epidermis of the entire back reminiscent of scalding.

and painful erosions, and bilateral lacrimation. Less common are purulent conjunctivitis with photophobia and/or pseudomembranes, corneal ulceration, anterior uveitis, and panophthalmitis. Genital involvement most often includes painful hemorrhagic bullous-erosive or purulent lesions of the fossa navicularis and glans penis, or of the vulva and vagina, and may lead to urinary retention and phimosis. Anal erosions are less frequent.

TEN WITHOUT SPOTS In a small minority of cases, TEN does not arise from confluent lesions of SJS, but presents with primary, ill-demarcated, diffuse erythemas that are rapidly progressive and may become erythrodermic. Mucous membranes may sometimes remain unaffected. A trickle of such cases have been recorded through the decades, but TEN without spots is still an ill-defined entity. It affects predominantly elderly females. The same drugs that trigger SJS-TEN may trigger TEN without spots, but "idiopathic" cases occur more often. The majority of cases of TEN caused by the graft-versus-host reaction represent this type of TEN, and the prognosis may be worse than that of SJS-TEN. Differentiation from generalized fixed drug eruption is difficult; it rests mainly on the presence of prominent systemic signs in TEN.

EXTRACUTANEOUS SYMPTOMS Constitutional signs of SJS-TEN include fever, arthralgias, weakness, and prostration. Internal organ involvement is rare in SJS, but may be severe in TEN, most often affecting the respiratory and gastrointestinal tracts. Tracheal and bronchial symptoms include breathing difficulties, sloughing of the respiratory tract mucosa leading to persistent cough, bronchial obstruction and expectoration of bronchial casts, adult respiratory distress syndrome, tracheitis, patchy pulmonary disease, bronchopneumonia, and pneumothorax.[80] Less commonly, ileal involvement, diarrhea, abdominal pain, esophageal and gastrointestinal bleeding, excretion of necrotic intestinal epithelium, colonic perforation, melena, and hepatitis have been reported.[81] Toxicity, dehydration, and water and electrolyte imbalance may proceed to hemodynamic shock, pulmonary edema, mental obtusion, confusion, coma, and seizures. Myocarditis and myocardial infarction are common in fatal cases, although they are generally uncommon. Except for microalbuminuria, renal complications are rare; if present, they are more often linked to septicemia or septic shock than to TEN. Acute tubular necrosis, membranous glomerulonephritis, and renal failure have been described.[82]

LATE COMPLICATIONS Skin lesions heal with transitory hyper- and/or hypopigmentation. Scarring does not usually appear except in extensive cases with secondary infection, where contractures, alopecia, and anonychia may develop. Scarring is a characteristic and frequent (up to 30 percent in TEN) late complication of mucosal lesions; it is most serious in the eyes, as symblepharon, synechiae, entropion and ectropion, trichiasis, corneal opacities or scarring, and pannus formation potentially result in blindness. Lesions of the lips and oral mucosa usually resolve without sequelae, but esophageal, bronchial, vaginal, urethral, and anal strictures develop at times. A Sjögren-like syndrome may develop as the result of damage to the salivary and lacrimal glands.

Course

Following the outbreak, SJS-TEN enters a phase of progression that usually lasts 4 to 5 days, but can be more protracted. Progression may halt at any point of BSA involvement (from 10 to close to 100 percent), and the patient enters a plateau phase that again may take from a few days up to 2 weeks, depending on the severity of SJS-TEN and the physical constitution of the patient. It is during this phase that the hazard of systemic complications is highest. A lightening of the erythema, lessening of oozing and skin tenderness, and transformation of the detached epidermis into dry blackish parchment-like squames heralds the phase of regression. Reepithelialization may take several weeks.

Pathology

In contrast to the only scanty signs of inflammation in both epidermis and dermis, epidermal necrosis is prominent in SJS-TEN. Epidermal injury may appear as satellite-cell necrosis in early stages and progresses to more extensive eosinophilic necrosis of the basal and suprabasal layers; subepidermal separation may be evident (Fig. 58-6). In TEN, there is total thickness necrosis and sloughing of the epidermis. There is a moderately dense to sparse mononuclear cell infiltrate in the papillary dermis, with exocytosis into the epidermis. Spongiosis and dermal edema are most often absent. Neutrophils and nuclear dust are occasionally evident.

In severe SJS-TEN, extensive fibrinoid necrosis may occur in several internal organs, including the stomach, spleen, trachea, and bronchi. Despite the frequency of pulmonary radiologic abnormalities, the pathology in uncomplicated cases is limited to sparse mononuclear cell infiltrates.

Laboratory Investigations

An elevated erythrocyte sedimentation rate accompanies SJS-TEN; in addition, patients may develop moderate leukocytosis, fluid-electrolyte imbalance, microalbuminuria, hypoproteinemia, elevation of liver transaminase levels, and anemia. In the acute phase, patients with TEN may have a transient decrease of peripheral CD4+ T lymphocyte counts, accompanied by reduced allogeneic and natural-killer–cell cytotoxicity, which return to normal after 7 to 10 days. These laboratory abnormalities resemble, to some degree, those found in second-degree burn injuries; however, they are usually less severe. Neutropenia, which

FIGURE 58-6

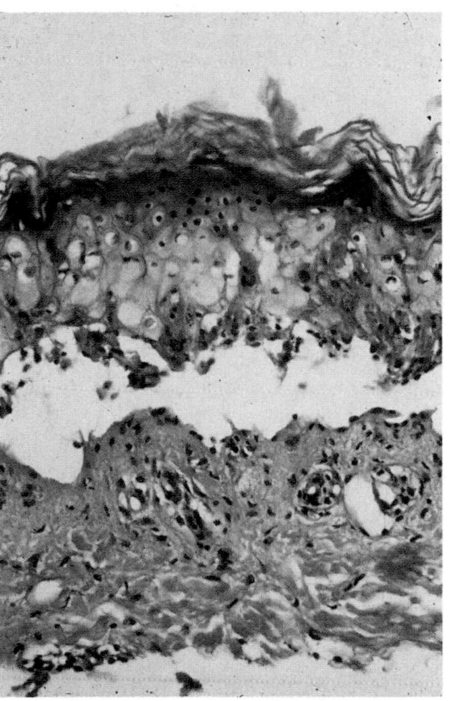

A.

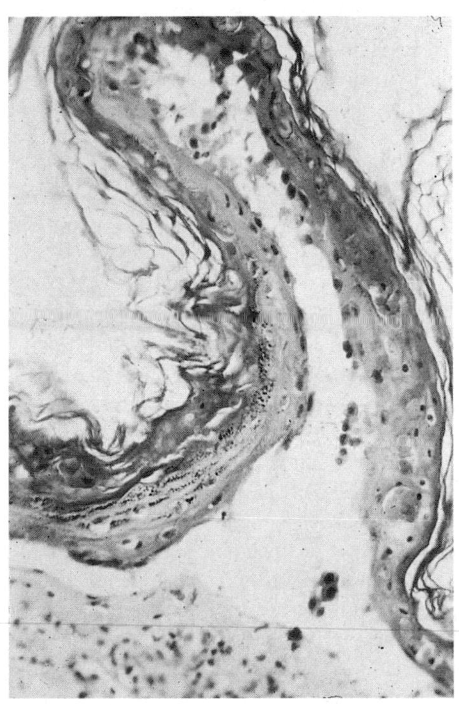

B.

Histologic appearance of TEN. *A.* Eosinophilic necrosis of the epidermis in the peak stage, with little inflammatory response in the dermis. Note cleavage in the junction zone. *B.* The completely necrotic epidermis has detached from the dermis and folded like a sheet.

TABLE 58-4

Differential Diagnosis of Stevens–Johnson Syndrome (SJS) and Toxic Epidermal Necrolysis (TEN)

SJS	TEN
Erythema multiforme	Staphylococcal scalded-skin syndrome
Viral exanthems	Generalized fixed drug eruption
Ampicillin rash	Burns, cauterization, etc.
Morbilliform drug eruptions	Toxic erythroderma
Fixed drug eruption	
Acute graft-versus-host disease	

occurs in a minority of cases, is regarded as an unfavorable prognostic sign.[11] Eosinophilia may be found in some cases. Circulating immune complexes have been demonstrated in several reports, but are not, in general, accompanied by complement consumption. Renal abnormalities such as proteinuria and elevated blood urea nitrogen levels occur in about 5 percent of cases.[11] A host of other laboratory findings may become abnormal as involvement of internal organs or secondary infection occurs.

Differential Diagnosis

Most often, SJS-TEN is a straightforward diagnosis. Difficulties may arise in two situations: (1) in viral or drug-induced macular exanthems, in which it is difficult to predict whether they will proceed to SJS-TEN, or (2) in other eruptions characterized by widespread erythema and detachment of the skin.

Table 58-4 lists other entities to be considered in the differential diagnosis. Macular morbilliform eruptions, for example, may be morphologically indistinguishable from the initial SJS-TEN lesions that are not yet confluent or necrotic. The lesions are not tender, do not exhibit a positive Nikolsky's sign, and lack prominent involvement of mucous membranes, however. (For a comparison of the clinical features of SJS-TEN with those of erythema multiforme, see Table 58-1.)

MULTILOCULAR OR GENERALIZED BULLOUS FIXED DRUG ERUPTION A classic differential diagnosis of SJS-TEN, multilocular or generalized bullous fixed drug eruption appears in many series of patients with SJS-TEN, particularly those with recurrences. The main points of distinction are its primary lesions, which are large erythemas (faintly discernible even after confluence), most often irregularly distributed and of a characteristic purplish-livid color, at times with flaccid blisters; the rarity of mucous membrane involvement; and the paucity of constitutional symptoms. Histopathology is similar to that of SJS-TEN, except for the more pronounced inflammation and a marked edema of the papillary dermis. Often, history reveals milder prior episodes following intake of the culprit drugs. Generalized bullous fixed drug eruption takes a much milder course than SJS-TEN. Recovery is rapid and complete, without sequelae.

Drug-induced linear IgA dermatosis mimicking SJS-TEN has been observed.[83]

STAPHYLOCOCCAL SCALDED-SKIN SYNDROME A disorder unrelated to SJS-TEN, staphylococcal scalded-skin syndrome is caused by staphylococcal epidermolysin toxinemia and characterized by subcorneal acantholysis. It occurs almost exclusively in children and may be confused with SJS-TEN because of a resemblance to scalding that is common to both. A wide range of clinical criteria (e.g., absence of mucosal lesions and of internal organ involvement) facilitate the differential diagnosis. In ambiguous cases, the diagnosis can be rapidly made by exfoliative cytology or frozen sections of biopsy material (see Chap. 195).

PHYSICAL AND CHEMICAL INJURY The diagnosis of physical and chemical injury, such as scalding and burns, solar erythema, and chemical burns (e.g., kerosene or paraffin burns) is clear if a history is available, but may be difficult in unconscious patients. Injury by exogenous agents displays an artificial distribution pattern, mucous membranes are only rarely involved, and there is no antecedent macular rash. If necrosis arises, it tends to involve deeper layers, including the skin appendages, whereas it is purely epidermal in SJS-TEN.

Treatment

The fate of patients depends on rapid referral to a specialized center experienced in the management of SJS-TEN and in general skin care (i.e., to a dermatology center with inpatient facilities), if available. Under no circumstances may a patient with SJS-TEN be treated on an ambulatory basis because supportive care and constant supervision are no less important than are active therapeutic measures. This is true, even though in the initial stages of SJS-TEN, patients may feel fairly well or even euphoric and may be unwilling to be admitted to the hospital. Although widely claimed, referral to an intensive care unit or to a burn center is not mandatory except when disease is extensive or complications are severe. If properly treated, SJS-TEN is linked to many fewer systemic symptoms than second-degree burns of the same BSA. Furthermore, the literature does not support the conclusion that mortality rates are higher in dermatologic wards than in intensive care units.

The management of SJS-TEN rests on three cornerstones: (1) identification and elimination of the provocative agent (i.e., withdrawal of the offending drug or treatment of the underlying infection, if available), (2) active therapy, and (3) supportive measures. There are no generally accepted regimens or treatment guidelines for SJS-TEN, and no controlled therapeutic trials have ever been published. This is because SJS-TEN is an infrequent and life-threatening disease of high clinical variability that requires complex treatment and individually adapted care.

WITHDRAWAL OF THE SUSPECTED OFFENDING DRUGS Obviously, the causative drug should rapidly be identified and withdrawn. Prompt withdrawal of all non–life-sustaining drugs in patients with incipient SJS-TEN may reduce the death risk by about 30 percent per day.[83] This measure, however, does not immediately halt disease progression. At present, the detection of the most likely culprit is a matter of empirical calculation based on a careful history of drug intake with special focus on recent drug use, its relation to the development of symptoms, and prior episodes of SJS-TEN. The most likely offending drug is one that has been newly administered in the past 4 weeks and is known as a risk drug for SJS-TEN. The intake of multiple drugs, drugs newly administered for the treatment of prodromal symptoms (i.e., antimicrobials, analgesics, or NSAIDs), drug interactions, and infections may obscure matters.

ACTIVE SUPPRESSION OF DISEASE PROGRESSION A number of anti-inflammatory and/or immunosuppressive treatment modalities have been proposed to have beneficial effects on SJS-TEN. The lack of controlled trials and the lack of a clear-cut distinction between progression and peak phases in many of the single case reports and small (usually heterogeneous) patient series described in the literature mars the evidence, however. Thus, there is currently no consensus regarding which, if any, therapeutic measure will shorten the natural course of the disease. Furthermore, many of the treatment modalities bear potential harmful side effects that clinicians must weigh against the benefits. As a consequence, many clinicians rely only on supportive measures. This view, which is unique in the context of an acute immune system–mediated life-threatening disease, must be attributed to a much too far-reaching and unjustified equation of SJS-TEN with burn injuries. Burns result from a single thermal trauma, whereas TEN is an immunological-cytotoxic attack that may progress for more than a week (not just 3 to 4 days, as often claimed), depending on detoxification and excretion of the offending agent. It should be the treatment strategy of this early phase to halt disease progression and thus limit the extent of skin and mucosal necrosis and reduce the severity of sequelae.

Glucocorticoids The systemic administration of glucocorticoids has been the mainstay of the treatment of SJS-TEN for a long time, but has come into disrepute in the past years. The scientific community is divided over their use; fervent supporters fiercely oppose those who condemn glucocorticoids and even consider them "detrimental."[56,73,84] The discussion arose because glucocorticoids, if given for longer than the phase of progression, clearly increase the risk of infection and thus may contribute to mortality. Surgical intensive care specialists who were striving to shape the treatment of SJS-TEN according to the principles of the management of burns, where the systemic administration of glucocorticoids is obviously not indicated, adopted this position. The argument was expanded by the assumption that glucocorticoids, in principle, have no effect on disease progression. Additional observations supported this idea: mortality rates do not differ significantly between countries where physicians commonly use glucocorticoids (e.g., Germany: 80 percent use glucocorticoids) and those where physicians are reluctant to use them (e.g., France: 20 percent use glucocorticoids), and SJS-TEN may arise in patients who are on long-term, albeit low-dose, glucocorticoid treatment for other reasons.[86] Mortality rates are highly different in published series, however, ranging from zero to more than 50 percent, both with and without the use of steroids. Long-term sequelae were apparent in 7 of 11 children with TEN who were not treated by the systemic administration of glucocorticoids.[87]

If steroids do curb disease progression in the initial phase, which may be expected in an immune system–mediated disease, they do not shorten the peak and regression phases. Obviously, they must be used with utmost caution. If given, relatively high initial doses are required (1 to 2 mg/kg methyl prednisolone per day given orally), and rapid tapering is indicated as soon as disease progression halts. They should be given only as part of a total program (see below) if the physical condition of the patient permits. It is absolutely unacceptable to consider steroids as the only measure.

Immunoglobulins Recently, the intravenous administration of pooled human immunoglobulins (IVIG) has emerged as a promising strategy for blocking the progression of SJS-TEN, based on the immunoglobulins' content of antibodies against Fas ligand that are capable of preventing apoptotic cell death in vitro.[88] In the original study, 10 patients were treated, with IVIG dosages ranging from 0.2 to 0.75 g/kg body weight per day for 4 consecutive days. In all patients, rapid decrease of disease progression and evidence of recovery were observed. Similar favorable results have been reported since in a number of cases.[89,90] Pending adequately sized controlled studies, however, this very expensive treatment should be reserved for clinical trials. Although IVIG has a good safety profile, nephropathy is a rare but dangerous side effect that may result in renal failure.

Plasmapheresis and Hemodialysis Scattered and partially contradictory reports suggest that the removal of the causative drug, its metabolites, or other toxic molecules from the circulation may stop progression of SJS-TEN.[91,92] In the absence of formal proof and in view of the stress on the patient associated with the treatments, these strategies are not recommended at the present time.

Cyclophosphamide Cyclophosphamide is an inhibitor of cell-mediated cytotoxicity. Although it has been used successfully in a small number of patients with TEN, it is a potent immunosuppressive agent and has itself been the cause of several cases of SJS-TEN.

Cyclosporine Again, several case reports suggest the efficacy of cyclosporine in SJS-TEN.[93] It has been suggested that cyclosporine interacts with TNF-α metabolism.[64]

N-***Acetylcysteine*** Along with *S*-adenosyl-L-methionine, *N*-acetylcysteine may act through replenishing cells with antioxidant capacity and by inhibiting cytokine (TNF-α)–mediated immune reactions.[94] The evidence as to its use in SJS-TEN is sporadic.

Thalidomide The rationale for the experimental use of thalidomide, a known inhibitor of TNF-α, was the hypothesized pivotal role of this cytokine in the genesis of SJS-TEN.[69] Yet, in a randomized placebo controlled study, the thalidomide group exhibited a significantly higher mortality rate than the control group, and the study had to be discontinued.[95] (See also Chap. 264.) It remains unclear whether this outcome was due to paradoxical enhancement of TNF-α production or effects, or to IL-2–mediated T cell stimulation.

MAINTENANCE OF HEMODYNAMIC EQUILIBRIUM, PROTEIN AND ELECTROLYTE HOMEOSTASIS The rationale for treating patients with TEN in burn units would be to apply the therapeutic principles of burn injuries (i.e., rigorous adjustment of fluid, protein, and electrolyte balance; control of infection; and early surgical debridement of skin lesions). This rationale is questionable because, despite the clinical similarities, the pathomechanisms of SJS-TEN are totally different from those of burn injuries. The main difference is the virtual absence of vascular damage in SJS-TEN; consequently, edema and loss of fluid into the interstitial tissues are not a prominent feature. There is also much less loss of fluid to the outside, as tense and large blisters form only rarely. Water loss in SJS-TEN mainly occurs through evaporation from erosions and is thus highest in the peak phase. Metabolic acidosis is not a regular feature. All of these factors cooperate to render the fluid and electrolyte imbalances associated with SJS-TEN much less drastic and of later onset than those associated with burns. Hemodynamic shock is a possibility, but it is rare and occurs primarily in unsatisfactory clinical settings and in patients with cardiovascular or metabolic compromise. Also, second-degree burn injuries are more painful than SJS-TEN.

Blood pressure, hematocrit, and levels of blood gases, electrolytes and serum proteins must be monitored and adjusted appropriately. Fluid replacement regimens are recommended only when required. Central venous lines (as well as urinary catheters) should not routinely be inserted.

ANTIBIOTIC/ANTIMICROBIAL TREATMENT It is universally agreed that infections pose the most important threat for patients with SJS-TEN. Bacterial and fungal cultures should therefore be taken two to three times per week from skin and mucosal erosions, blood, and sputum; oral and genital mucosae should be repeatedly inspected for infection with HSV or *Candida*. In many series, patients received antibiotics only when clinical symptoms of infection were already present and the causative organism identified. This is probably due to the reluctance of many clinicians to use antibiotics prophylactically or to their fear of introducing a further drug into a patient with drug intolerance. Clinicians should take into account, however, the fact that antibiotics are only rarely the offending drug in SJS-TEN and that those with a known risk of severe cutaneous reactions are easily avoidable. It has been the strategy of our group (P.O.F.) to start prophylactic antibiotic treatment (sodium penicillin, 2×10 million units per day) from the beginning, and to adjust the antibiotic according to the cultured organism; pursuing this strategy, the mortality rate of patients with TEN has been kept to less than 10 percent in our institution throughout the past two decades.

SUPPORTIVE TREATMENT

Skin Loose sheets of detached epidermis may be cautiously removed, but early aggressive debridement as performed in burn patients is not indicated because the necrosis is only superficial and represents no obstacle for reepithelialization. As a rule, spontaneous reepithelialization is rapid. Erosions should be covered with gauze or hydrocolloid dressings. Sulfonamide-containing topicals should be avoided. When topical antibiotics or antiseptics are used, the possibility of systemic absorption has to be considered. Fresh-frozen or cryopreserved cadaver allograft and porcine xenograft skin, as well as biosynthetic dressings, have been advocated, but their value is questionable because—unlike burn injuries—SJS-TEN leaves the dermis largely uninvolved and reepithelialization is not a problem.

Eyes In the acute phase of conjunctival involvement, lubricants, steroid and antibiotic drops should be applied several times a day. Lid-globe adhesions should be cautiously removed twice daily with a glass rod to avoid occlusion of the fornices; care must be taken not to strip pseudomembranes, which may lead to bleeding and increased conjunctival scarring.[96]

Respiratory Tract Supportive pulmonary care includes postural drainage and, if necessary, cautious suctioning.

Alimentation Patients with SJS-TEN are often unable to eat and drink because of their oral and/or esophageal mucosal involvement, or their poor general condition. Local anesthetics, as a mouthwash before the meals, may be helpful. A high-calorie and high-protein diet or intravenous administration is recommended, although the risk of septicemia associated with intravenous lines must be taken into account.

Prognosis

The prognosis for patients with SJS-TEN depends on the severity of disease and the quality of medical care. The mortality rate is low (less than 1 percent) for SJS,[7] and it ranges from 5 to 50 percent for TEN. Old age, extensive skin lesions, neutropenia, impaired renal function, and intake of multiple drugs appear to be unfavorable prognostic signs. A recently proposed severity-of-illness score for TEN identified seven independent risk factors:[97]

1. Age over 40 years
2. Malignancy
3. Tachycardia more than 120 beats per minute
4. Initial epidermal detachment of more than 10 percent
5. Serum urea level greater than 10 mmol/L
6. Serum glucose level greater than 14 mmol/L
7. Bicarbonate level less than 20 mmol/L

Excellent agreement was found between expected and actual mortality.

Fatal outcome is most often the result of septicemia (e.g., *Staphylococcus aureus, Pseudomonas, Candida*), pneumonia, gastrointestinal hemorrhage, myocardial infarction, and cardiac insufficiency. Much more rarely, it results from renal insufficiency and hemodynamic shock.[98] Recovery is slow; it may require 3 to 6 weeks or more, depending on the presence of complications. Healing occurs with a tendency for scar and stricture formation at mucosal sites.

REFERENCES

1. Lyell A: Toxic epidermal necrolysis: An eruption resembling scalding of the skin. *Br J Dermatol* **68**:355, 1956
2. Lyell A: Toxic epidermal necrolysis (the scalded skin syndrome): A reappraisal. *Br J Dermatol* **100**:69, 1979
3. Lyell A: Requiem for toxic epidermal necrolysis. *Br J Dermatol* **122**:837, 1990
4. Huff JC: Erythema multiforme and latent herpes simplex infection. *Semin Dermatol* **11**:207, 1992
5. Bastuji-Garin S et al: Clinical classification of cases of toxic epidermal necrolysis, Stevens-Johnson syndrome and erythema multiforme. *Arch Dermatol* **129**:92, 1993
6. Roujeau JC: The spectrum of Stevens-Johnson syndrome and toxic epidermal necrolysis. *J Invest Dermatol* **102**:28S, 1994
7. Assier H et al: Erythema multiforme with mucous membrane involvement and Stevens-Johnson syndrome are different disorders with distinct causes. *Arch Dermatol* **131**:539, 1995
8. Ruiz-Maldonado R: Acute disseminated epidermal necrolysis types 1, 2, and 3: Study of sixty cases. *J Am Acad Dermatol* **13**:623, 1985
9. Rzany B et al: Epidemiology of erythema exsudativum multiforme majus, Stevens-Johnson syndrome, and toxic epidermal necrolysis in Germany (1990–1992): Structure and results of a population-based registry. *J Clin Epidemiol* **49**:769, 1996
10. Schofield JK et al: Recurrent erythema multiforme: Clinical features and treatment in a large series of patients. *Br J Dermatol* **128**:542, 1993
11. Brice SL et al: Erythema multiforme, in *Current Problems in Dermatology*, edited by WL Weston. Chicago, Year Book, 1990
12. Howland WW et al: Erythema multiforme: Clinical histopathologic and immunologic study. *J Am Acad Dermatol* **10**:438, 1984
13. Brice SL et al: Examination of non-involved skin, previously involved skin and peripheral blood for herpes simplex virus DNA in patients with recurrent herpes-associated erythema multiforme. *J Cutan Pathol* **21**:408, 1994
14. Imafuku S et al: Expression of herpes simplex virus DNA fragments located in epidermal keratinocytes and germinative cells is associated with the development of erythema multiforme. *J Invest Dermatol* **109**:550, 1997
15. Weston WL et al: Herpes simplex virus in childhood erythema multiforme. *Pediatrics* **89**:32, 1992
16. Kazmierowski JA et al: Herpes simplex antigen in immune complexes of patients with erythema multiforme. *JAMA* **247**:2547, 1982
17. Imafuku S et al: T cell repertoire usage in herpes simplex infections and erythema multiforme. *J Invest Dermatol* **104**:565, 1995
18. Tatnall FM et al: A double blind placebo controlled trial of continuous acyclovir therapy in recurrent erythema multiforme. *Br J Dermatol* **132**:267, 1995
19. Dumas V et al: Recurrent erythema multiforme and chronic hepatitis C: Efficacy of interferon alpha. *Br J Dermatol* **142**:1248, 2000
20. Loche F et al: Erythema multiforme associated with hepatitis B immunization. *Clin Exp Dermatol* **25**:167, 2000
21. Leigh IM et al: Recurrent and continuous erythema multiforme—Clinical and immunological study. *Clin Exp Dermatol* **10**:58, 1985
22. Puig L et al: Erythema multiforme–like eruption due to topical contactants: Expression of adhesion molecules and their ligands and characterization of the infiltrate. *Contact Dermatitis* **33**:329, 1995
23. Larcher C et al: Interaction of HSV-1 infected peripheral blood mononuclear cells with cultured dermal microvascular endothelial cells: A potential model for the pathogenesis of HSV-1 induced erythema multiforme. *J Invest Dermatol* **116**:150, 2001
24. Wolf P et al: Recurrent post-herpetic erythema multiforme mimicking polymorphic light and juvenile spring eruption: Report of two cases in young boys. *Br J Dermatol* **131**:364, 1994
25. Inachi S et al: Epidermal apoptotic cell death in erythema multiforme and Stevens-Johnson syndrome: Contribution of perforin-positive cell infiltration. *Arch Dermatol* **133**:845, 1997
26. Bennion SD et al: In three types of interface dermatitis, different patterns of expression of intercellular adhesion molecule-1 (ICAM-1) indicate different triggers of disease. *J Invest Dermatol* **105**:71S, 1995
27. Paquet P et al: Erythema multiforme and toxic epidermal necrolysis: A comparative study. *Am J Dermatopathol* **19**:127, 1997
28. Kokuba H: Herpes simplex virus–associated erythema multiforme: Interferon-gamma is expressed in HAEM lesions and tumor necrosis factor-alpha in drug-induced erythema multiforme lesions. *J Invest Dermatol* **113**:808, 1999
29. Brice SL et al: The herpes-specific immune response of individuals with herpes-associated erythema multiforme compared with that of individuals with recurrent herpes labialis. *Arch Dermatol Res* **285**:193, 1993
30. Schofield JK et al: Recurrent erythema multiforme: Tissue typing in a large series of patients. *Br J Dermatol* **131**:532, 1994
31. Kämpgen E et al: Association of herpes simplex virus induced erythema multiforme with the human leukocyte antigen Dqw3. *Arch Dermatol* **124**:1372, 1988
32. Micalizzi C, Farris A: Erythema multiforme along Blaschko's lines. *J Eur Acad Dermatol Venereol* **14**:203, 2000
33. Drago F et al: Persistent erythema multiforme: Report of two new cases and review of the literature. *J Am Acad Dermatol* **33**:366, 1995

34. Cote B et al: Clinicopathological correlation in erythema multiforme and Stevens-Johnson syndrome. *Arch Dermatol* **131**:1268, 1995
35. Rzany B et al: Histopathological and epidemiological characteristics of patients with erythema exsudativum multiforme majus, Stevens-Johnson syndrome and toxic epidermal necrolysis. *Br J Dermatol* **135**:6, 1996
36. Orfanos CE et al: Dermal and epidermal types of erythema multiforme. *Arch Dermatol* **109**:682, 1974
37. Ackerman AB et al: Erythema multiforme exudativum: Distinctive pathological process. *Br J Dermatol* **84**:554, 1971
38. Hering O et al: The dermal type of erythema multiforme: A rare variant of Stevens-Johnson syndrome or cases of clinical misclassification? *Acta Derm Venereol* **77**:217, 1997
39. Rowell NR et al: Lupus erythematosus and erythema multiforme–like lesions. *Arch Dermatol* **88**:176, 1963
40. Roujeau JC et al: Toxic epidermal necrolysis (Lyell syndrome): Incidence and drug etiology in France, 1981–1985. *Arch Dermatol* **126**:37, 1990
41. Schopf E et al: Toxic epidermal necrolysis and Stevens-Johnson syndrome: An epidemiologic study from West Germany. *Arch Dermatol* **127**:839, 1991
42. Hernborg A: Stevens-Johnson syndrome after mass prophylaxis with sulfadoxine for cholera in Mozambique. *Lancet* **1**:1072, 1985
43. Correia O et al: Evolving pattern of drug-induced toxic epidermal necrolysis. *Dermatology* **186**:32, 1993
44. Rzany B et al: Incidence of Stevens-Johnson syndrome and toxic epidermal necrolysis in patients with the acquired immunodeficiency syndrome in Germany. *Arch Dermatol* **129**:1059, 1993
45. Roujeau JC et al: Genetic susceptibility to toxic epidermal necrolysis. *Arch Dermatol* **123**:1171, 1987
46. Kaufman DW: Epidemiologic approaches to the study of toxic epidermal necrolysis. *J Invest Dermatol* **102**:31S, 1994
47. Kelly JP et al: An international collaborative case-control study of severe cutaneous adverse reactions (SCAR): Design and methods. *J Clin Epidemiol* **48**:1099, 1995
48. Roujeau JC et al: Medication use and the risk of Stevens-Johnson syndrome or toxic epidermal necrolysis. *N Engl J Med* **333**:1600, 1995
49. Roujeau JC et al: Severe adverse reactions to drugs. *N Engl J Med* **331**:1272, 1994
50. Duncan KO et al: Stevens-Johnson syndrome limited to multiple sites of radiation therapy in a patient receiving phenobarbitural. *J Am Acad Dermatol* **40**:493, 1999
51. Bushan M et al: Prolonged toxic epidermal necrolysis due to lamotrigine. *Clin Exp Dermatol* **39**:621, 2000
52. Auböck J et al: Asymptomatic hyperuricaemia and allopurinol induced toxic epidermal necrolysis. *BMJ* **290**:1969, 1985
53. Nanda A et al: Drug-induced toxic epidermal necrolysis in developing countries. *Arch Dermatol* **126**:125, 1990
54. Fagot JP et al: Nevirapine and the risk of Stevens-Johnson syndrome or toxic epidermal necrolysis. *AIDS* **15**:1843, 2001
55. Chan HL: Toxic epidermal necrolysis in Singapore, 1989 through 1993: Incidence and antecedent drug exposure. *Arch Dermatol* **131**:1212, 1995
56. Chosidow O et al: Drug rashes: What are the targets of cell mediated cytotoxicity? *Arch Dermatol* **130**:627, 1994
57. Fritsch PO, Sidoroff A: Drug-induced Stevens Johnson syndrome/toxic epidermal necrolysis. *Am J Clin Dermatol* **1**:349, 2000
58. Ball R et al: Stevens-Johnson syndrome and toxic epidermal necrolysis after vaccination: Reports to the vaccine adverse event reporting system. *Pediatr Infect Dis J* **20**:219, 2001
59. Tay YK et al: *Mycoplasma pneumoniae* infection is associated with Stevens-Johnson syndrome, not erythema multiforme (von Hebra). *J Am Acad Dermatol* **35**:757, 1996
60. Villada G et al: Toxic epidermal necrolysis after bone marrow transplantation: Study of nine cases. *J Am Acad Dermatol* **23**:870, 1990
61. McCarty JR et al: Toxic epidermal necrolysis from graft-vs-host disease: Occurrence in a patient with thymic hypoplasia. *Am J Dis Child* **132**:282, 1978
62. Streilein JW et al: An analysis of graft-vs-host disease in Syrian hamsters. I. The epidermolytic syndrome: Description and studies on its procurement. *J Exp Med* **132**:163, 1970
63. Wolkenstein P et al: Patch testing in severe cutaneous adverse drug reactions, including Stevens-Johnson syndrome and toxic epidermal necrolysis. *Contact Dermatitis* **35**:234, 1996
64. Friedmann PS et al: Investigation of mechanism in toxic epidermal necrolysis induced by carbamazepine. *Arch Dermatol* **130**:598, 1994
65. Mauri-Hellweg D et al: Activation of drug-specific CD4+ and CD8+ T cells in individuals allergic to sulfonamides, phenytoin and carbamazepine. *J Immunol* **155**:462, 1995
66. Redondo P et al: Drug-induced hypersensitivity syndrome and toxic epidermal necrolysis: Treatment with *N*-acetylcysteine. *Br J Dermatol* **136**:645, 1997
67. Correia O et al: Cutaneous T-cell recruitment in toxic epidermal necrolysis: Further evidence of CD8+ lymphocyte involvement. *Arch Dermatol* **129**:466, 1993
68. Villada G et al: Immunopathology of toxic epidermal necrolysis: Keratinocytes, HLA-DR expression, Langerhans cells, and mononuclear cells. An immunopathologic study of five cases. *Arch Dermatol* **128**:50, 1992
69. Paquet P et al: Macrophages and tumor necrosis factor alpha in toxic epidermal necrolysis. *Arch Dermatol* **130**:505, 1994
70. Paquet P, Pierard GE: Soluble fractions of tumor necrosis factor-alpha, interleukin-6 and of their receptors in toxic epidermal necrolysis: A comparison with second-degree burns. *Int J Mol Med* **1**:459,1998
71. Le Cleach L et al: Blister fluid T lymphocytes during toxic epidermal necrolysis are functional cytotoxic cells which express human natural killer (NK) inhibitory receptors. *Clin Exp Immunol* **119**:225, 2000
72. Paquet P et al: Immunoregulatory effector cells in drug-induced toxic epidermal necrolysis. *Am J Dermatopathol* **22**:413, 2000
73. Shear NH et al: Differences in metabolism of sulfonamides predisposing to idiosyncratic toxicity. *Ann Intern Med* **105**:179, 1986
74. Roujeau JC: Drug-induced toxic epidermal necrolysis: II. Current aspects. *Clin Dermatol* **11**:493, 1993
75. Conger LA et al: Dilantin hypersensitivity reaction. *Cutis* **57**:223, 1996
76. Wolkenstein P et al: A slow acetylator genotype is a risk factor for sulphonamide-induced toxic epidermal necrolysis and Stevens-Johnson syndrome. *Pharmacogenetics* **5**:255, 1995
77. Wolkenstein P et al: Metabolic predisposition to cutaneous adverse drug reactions: Role in toxic epidermal necrolysis caused by sulfonamides and anticonvulsants. *Arch Dermatol* **131**:544, 1995
78. Lerner LH et al: Nitric oxide synthase in toxic epidermal necrolysis and Stevens-Johnson syndrome. *J Invest Dermatol* **114**:196, 2000
79. Födinger D et al: Autoantibodies to desmoplakin I and II in patients with erythema multiforme. *J Exp Med* **181**:169, 1995
80. McIvor RA et al: Acute and chronic respiratory complications of toxic epidermal necrolysis. *J Burn Care Rehabil* **17**:237, 1996
81. Michel P et al: Ileal involvement in toxic epidermal necrolysis (Lyell syndrome). *Dig Dis Sci* **38**:1938, 1993
82. Blum L et al: Renal involvement in toxic epidermal necrolysis. *J Am Acad Dermatol* **34**:1088, 1996
83. Hughes AP, Callen JP: Drug-induced linear IgA bullous dermatosis mimicking toxic epidermal necrolysis. *Dermatology* **202**:138, 2001
84. Garcia-Doval I et al: Toxic epidermal necrolysis and Stevens-Johnson syndrome: Does early withdrawal of causative drugs decrease the risk of death? *Arch Dermatol* **136**:323, 2000
85. Tripathi A et al: Corticosteroid therapy in an additional 13 cases of Stevens-Johnson syndrome: A total of 67 cases. *Allergy Asthma Proc* **21**:101, 2000
86. Guibal F et al: Characteristics of toxic epidermal necrolysis in patients undergoing long-term glucocorticoid therapy. *Arch Dermatol* **131**:669, 1995
87. Sheridan RL et al: Long-term consequences of toxic epidermal necrolysis in children. *Pediatrics* **109**:74,2002
88. Viard I et al: Inhibition of toxic epidermal necrolysis by blockade of CD95 with human intravenous immunoglobulin. *Science* **282**:490, 1998
89. Morici MV et al: Intravenous immunoglobulin therapy for children with Stevens-Johnson syndrome. *J Rheumatol* **27**:2494, 2000
90. Stella M et al: Toxic epidermal necrolysis treated with intravenous high-dose immunoglobulins: Our experience. *Dermatology* **203**:45,2001
91. Egan CA et al: Plasmapheresis as an adjunct treatment in toxic epidermal necrolysis. *J Am Acad Dermatol* **40**:458, 1999
92. Furubake A et al: Lack of significant treatment effect of plasma exchange in the treatment of drug-induced toxic epidermal necrolysis. *Intensive Care Med* **25**:1307,1999
93. Arevalo JM et al: Treatment of toxic epidermal necrolysis with cyclosporin A. *J Trauma* **48**:473,2000
94. Redondo P et al: *N*-acetylcysteine inhibits production of tumor necrosis factor-alpha and interleukin-1 beta;. *Arch Intern Med* **156**:1238, 1996
95. Wolkenstein P et al: Randomized comparison of thalidomide versus placabo in toxic epidermal necrolysis. *Lancet* **352**:1586, 1998
96. Lehmann SS: Long-term ocular complication of Stevens-Johnson syndrome. *Clin Pediatr* **38**:425, 1999
97. Bastuj-Garin S et al: Scorten: A severity-of-illness score for toxic epidermal necrolysis. *J Invest Dermatol* **115**:149, 2000
98. Avakian R et al: Toxic epidermal necrolysis: A review. *J Am Acad Dermatol* **25**:69, 1991

CHAPTER 59

John R. Stanley

Pemphigus

DEFINITION AND CLASSIFICATION

The term *pemphigus* refers to a group of autoimmune blistering diseases of skin and mucous membranes that are characterized histologically by intraepidermal blisters due to acantholysis (i.e., separation of epidermal cells from each other) and immunopathologically by in vivo bound and circulating IgG directed against the cell surface of keratinocytes. The nosology of this group of diseases is outlined in Table 59-1. Essentially, pemphigus can be divided into four major types: vulgaris, foliaceus, paraneoplastic (see Chap. 60), and IgA pemphigus (see Chap. 69). In pemphigus vulgaris, the blister occurs in the deeper part of the epidermis, just above the basal layer, and in pemphigus foliaceus, also called superficial pemphigus, the blister is in the granular layer.[1]

HISTORICAL ASPECTS

The history of the discovery of pemphigus, and its various forms, is covered in Lever's classic monograph *Pemphigus and Pemphigoid.*[1] Both pemphigus vulgaris and pemphigus foliaceus display a spectrum of disease. Various points along these spectra have been given unique names, but because the presentation of these diseases is fluid, patients' disease usually crosses these artificial designations over time. Thus, patients with pemphigus vulgaris may present with more localized disease, one form of which is called pemphigus vegetans of Hallopeau. This may become slightly more extensive and may merge into pemphigus vegetans of Neumann. Finally, with more severe disease, full-blown pemphigus vulgaris may appear. Similarly, patients with pemphigus foliaceus may present with more localized disease, represented by pemphigus erythematosus. However, these patients will often go on to more widespread pemphigus foliaceus.

TABLE 59-1

Classification of Pemphigus

TYPE	FORM
Pemphigus vulgaris	Pemphigus vegetans: localized Drug-induced
Pemphigus foliaceus	Pemphigus erythematosus: localized Fogo selvagem: endemic Drug-induced
Paraneoplastic pemphigus	
IgA Pemphigus	Subcorneal pustular dermatosis Intraepidermal neutrophilic IgA dermatosis

The discovery by Beutner and Jordon in 1964 of circulating antibodies against the cell surface of keratinocytes in the sera of patients with pemphigus vulgaris pioneered our understanding that pemphigus vulgaris is a tissue-specific autoimmune disease of skin and mucosa. Ultimately, their work led the way to the discoveries of autoantibodies in other autoimmune bullous diseases of the skin.[2]

EPIDEMIOLOGY

Several retrospective surveys of patients with pemphigus vulgaris and/or pemphigus foliaceus allow certain general conclusions regarding the epidemiology of pemphigus[1,3–7]. The prevalence of pemphigus of both types in men and women is about equal. The mean age of onset of disease is about 50 to 60 years; however, the range is broad, and disease may start in the elderly and in children.

Incidence and Prevalence

The exact incidence of disease and the prevalence of pemphigus vulgaris compared with that of pemphigus foliaceus depend very much on the population studied. Pemphigus vulgaris is more common in Jews and probably in people of Mediterranean descent. This same ethnic predominance does not exist for pemphigus foliaceus. Therefore, in areas where the Jewish population predominates, the incidence of pemphigus, as well as the ratio of pemphigus vulgaris to pemphigus foliaceus cases, tends to be higher. For example, in Jerusalem, the incidence of pemphigus vulgaris has been estimated to be 1.6 per 100,000 population, whereas in Finland, where there are very few Jews and people of Mediterranean origin, the incidence is much lower, 0.76 per million population. In addition, in New York and Los Angeles, the ratio of pemphigus vulgaris to pemphigus foliaceus cases is about 5 to 1, whereas in Finland, it is about 0.5 to 1. In France, the incidence of pemphigus vulgaris is 1.3 cases per million population per year and that of pemphigus foliaceus is 0.5 cases per million per year.

Fogo Selvagem

Also called endemic pemphigus foliaceus, fogo selvagem is a disease that is clinically, histologically, and immunopathologically the same as sporadic pemphigus foliaceus in any individual patient, but its epidemiology is unique.[8] Fogo selvagem is endemic in the rural areas of Brazil, especially along inland riverbeds. The geographic distribution of disease clustering is similar to that of a black fly, *Simulium nigrimanum,* thought by natives to be a vector of this disease. A study of potential environmental risk factors has also implicated the bite of this black fly, showing it to be significantly more frequent among those with the disease compared to an age-, sex-, and occupation-matched control population with unrelated dermatoses.[9] The prevalence in some rural areas of Brazil is as high as 3.4 percent.[10]

Fogo selvagem occurs often in children and young adults, unlike sporadic pemphigus foliaceus, which is a disease of mostly middle-aged and older patients. Also unlike pemphigus foliaceus, fogo selvagem occurs not infrequently in genetically related family members, although it is not contagious. This fact probably implies a common exposure, as well as susceptibility. There is no known racial or ethnic predominance, and anyone moving into an endemic area may be susceptible to disease. Finally, the development of the rural endemic areas of Brazil decreased the incidence of disease. Certainly, this fascinating disease holds clues to the triggering mechanism for the autoimmune response.

ETIOLOGY AND PATHOGENESIS

Electron Microscopy

Ultrastructural studies of the blisters in pemphigus have focused on the appearance of desmosomes, because these are the most prominent cell-to-cell adhesion junctions in stratified squamous epithelia. Early studies of pemphigus vulgaris lesions seemed to demonstrate early dissolution of cell-to-cell membrane contacts between intact desmosome junctions, with later separation and disappearance of the desmosomes.[11] However, other studies have suggested that dissolution of desmosomes or failure to form them might result in the blisters.[12] For example, biopsies of uninvolved skin from patients with pemphigus vulgaris show disruption of desmosomes and decreased numbers of desmosomes. Further, the addition of pemphigus vulgaris serum to cultured keratinocytes affects desmosome structure by causing the retraction of the tonofilaments that normally attach to desmosomal plaques.[13]

Similarly, in lesions of pemphigus foliaceus, electron microscopy was reported to show abnormalities in desmosome structure in early acantholysis.[14] The earliest of these changes seemed to be retraction of tonofilaments from the desmosome-dense plaque. Later, there was a decrease or absence of desmosomes. These electron microscopic studies are difficult to interpret regarding the time course of events, but they all indicate that, at least in some stage of acantholysis, desmosomes are destroyed.

Immunopathology

IMMUNOFLUORESCENCE The hallmark of pemphigus is the finding of IgG autoantibodies against the cell surface of keratinocytes. These autoantibodies were first discovered in patients' sera by indirect immunofluorescence and soon thereafter were discovered by direct immunofluorescence of patients' skin.[15] Essentially all patients with active pemphigus vulgaris or pemphigus foliaceus have a positive finding on a direct immunofluorescence test for IgG on the cell surface of keratinocytes in perilesional skin (Fig. 59-1*A*).[16] The diagnosis of pemphigus should be seriously questioned if the test result of direct immunofluorescence is negative. Depending on the substrate used for indirect immunofluorescence, more than 80 percent of patients with pemphigus have circulating antiepithelial cell surface IgG (Fig. 59-1*B*).[17] Patients with early localized disease and those in remission are most likely to have negative findings on an indirect immunofluorescence test.

Patients with pemphigus vulgaris and those with pemphigus foliaceus display similar direct and indirect immunofluorescence findings with IgG on the cell surface of epidermal cells throughout the epidermis. Therefore, it is not possible to differentiate the two diseases by the pattern of immunofluorescence. The substrate used to detect pemphigus antibody binding in indirect immunofluorescence greatly influences the sensitivity of the test, however. In general, monkey esophagus is more

FIGURE 59-1

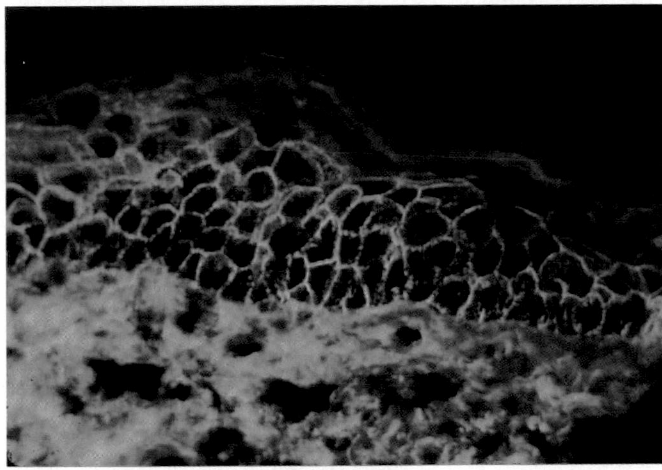

A.

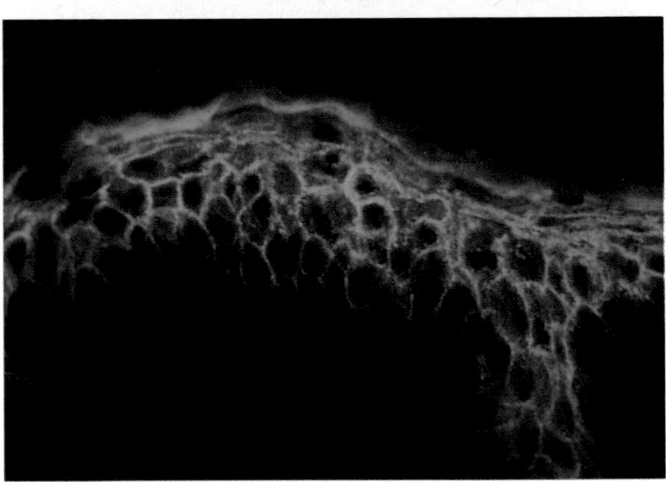

B.

Immunofluorescence in pemphigus. *A.* Direct immunofluorescence for IgG of perilesional skin from a patient with pemphigus vulgaris. Note cell surface staining throughout the epidermis. *B.* Indirect immunofluorescence with the serum from a patient with pemphigus foliaceus on normal human skin. Note IgG on the cell surface throughout the epidermis.

sensitive for detecting pemphigus vulgaris antibodies, and guinea pig esophagus is a superior substrate for detecting pemphigus foliaceus antibodies.[17]

There is a positive, but imperfect, correlation between the titer of circulating anti–cell surface antibody and the disease activity in pemphigus vulgaris and in pemphigus foliaceus.[18] Although this correlation may hold in general, and although patients in remission often show serologic remission with negative direct and indirect immunofluorescence findings,[19,20] disease activity in individual patients does not necessarily correlate with antibody titer. Therefore, in the day-to-day management of these patients, following disease activity is much more important than following antibody titer.

Recently, antigen-specific enzyme-linked immunosorbent assays have been shown to be more sensitive and specific (e.g., they can differentiate pemphigus vulgaris from pemphigus foliaceus) than immunofluorescence, and their titer correlates much better than that of indirect immunofluorescence with disease activity.[21,22]

Pemphigus erythematosus is a localized form of pemphigus foliaceus with a characteristic direct immunofluorescence finding of immunoreactants, usually IgG and C3, at the basement membrane zone of erythematous facial skin. These immunoreactants are in addition to the epidermal cell surface IgG.[23]

PEMPHIGUS ANTIGENS Immunologic evidence and molecular cloning have demonstrated that pemphigus antigens are desmogleins, transmembrane glycoproteins of desmosomes (organelles important in cell-to-cell adhesion). Immunoelectron microscopy has localized both pemphigus vulgaris and pemphigus foliaceus antigens to the cell surface of keratinocytes in desmosomal junctions.[24–26]

Characterization of pemphigus antigens at a molecular level has confirmed that they are molecules in desmosomes. Immunoprecipitation and immunoblotting studies with extracts from cultured keratinocytes or epidermis have demonstrated that pemphigus foliaceus antigen (as well as the fogo selvagem antigen) is desmoglein 1, a 160-kDa transmembrane glycoprotein of desmosomes.[27–29]

Molecular cloning of the cDNA encoding pemphigus vulgaris antigen identified it as desmoglein 3, another desmoglein isoform encoded by a separate gene.[30] All patients with pemphigus vulgaris have anti–desmoglein 3 antibodies, and some of these patients also have anti–desmoglein 1 antibodies.[21,31] Patients with pemphigus vulgaris that affects predominantly mucous membranes tend to have only anti–desmoglein 3 antibodies, while those with mucocutaneous disease usually have both anti–desmoglein 3 and anti–desmoglein 1 antibodies.[32–34] The dual antibody status of some patients with pemphigus vulgaris is in contrast to the single antibody status of pemphigus foliaceus patients, who have antibodies against only desmoglein 1.

Desmogleins 1 and 3 are closely related members of the cadherin supergene family. The original members of this family (e.g., E-cadherin) have been shown to be transmembrane, calcium-dependent, homophilic cell adhesion molecules. Presumably, the desmogleins fulfill similar functions in desmosomes. Pemphigus foliaceus and pemphigus vulgaris sera bind calcium-sensitive, conformational epitopes on desmogleins 1 and 3, respectively, suggesting that they might interfere with a calcium-sensitive adhesion function.[35,36] Although other cell surface molecules, such as acetylcholine receptors, may modulate adhesion, their direct involvement in the pathophysiology of pemphigus is controversial.[37–39]

Pathophysiology of Acantholysis

Pemphigus autoantibodies both from patients with pemphigus vulgaris and from those with pemphigus foliaceus are pathogenic. The occurrence of neonatal pemphigus vulgaris demonstrates that maternal IgG can cross the placenta and cause disease.[40] However, neonatal pemphigus foliaceus is very rare.[41]

Essentially, neonatal pemphigus vulgaris results from the passive transfer of IgG to the fetus. Similar experimental passive transfer studies show that pemphigus vulgaris and pemphigus foliaceus IgG cause acantholysis at the suprabasilar and granular layers of the epidermis, respectively, when added to skin in organ culture.[42,43] Antibody-induced acantholysis in this system occurs without the participation of complement or inflammatory cells.

Further compelling evidence of autoantibody-mediated pathology in pemphigus comes from studies of the passive transfer of pemphigus vulgaris and pemphigus foliaceus IgG to neonatal mice. These mice develop blisters and erosions that clinically and histologically mimic the corresponding type of pemphigus.[44,45] Complement fixation is not necessary to produce disease, and, consistent with this observation, even monovalent Fab′ immunoglobulin fragments are pathogenic in these mice.[45,46]

Additional studies have shown that the pathology-causing autoantibodies in pemphigus are those directed against desmogleins 1 and 3. IgG that is affinity-purified from pemphigus vulgaris sera on the extracellular domain of desmoglein 3 can cause suprabasilar acantholysis, the typical histologic finding of pemphigus vulgaris lesions, when injected into neonatal mice.[47,48] Furthermore, the extracellular domain of desmoglein 3 can adsorb out of pemphigus vulgaris sera antibodies pathogenic in neonatal mice.[49] Similarly, the extracellular domain of desmoglein 1 can adsorb out all pathogenic antibodies from pemphigus foliaceus sera, and antibodies affinity-purified on desmoglein 1 are pathogenic.[50] Finally, an active animal model of pemphigus vulgaris has been established by immunizing mice that are not tolerant of desmoglein 3 (i.e., mice whose desmoglein 3 gene has been deleted) in order to generate an immune response against desmoglein 3.[51] After the passive transfer of lymphocytes from these immunized mice to normal mice, the latter develop clinically and histologically typical lesions of pemphigus vulgaris and have anti–desmoglein 3 antibodies in their skin and sera.

These data strongly suggest that pemphigus vulgaris and pemphigus foliaceus autoantibodies against desmogleins 3 and 1, respectively, cause the blister formation in these diseases. Recent data indicate that they do so by interfering with a cell-to-cell adhesion function of these desmogleins or with their role in desmosome assembly. If indeed the pathophysiology of pemphigus arises from such antibodies directly inhibiting the function of desmoglein, interfering with the function of the desmoglein in some other way should result in a process that mimics pemphigus. This hypothesis was recently tested by genetically engineering a mouse with a targeted deletion of the desmoglein 3 gene.[52] The phenotype of this mouse closely resembled that of patients with pemphigus vulgaris, with suprabasilar blisters developing in the oral mucosa and skin. These data, then, are consistent with the idea that autoantibodies directly cause a loss of adhesion of keratinocytes.

Another line of evidence that inactivation of desmogleins causes the blistering of pemphigus comes from studies of bullous impetigo and staphylococcal scalded-skin syndrome, which are caused by exfoliative toxin released by *Staphylococcus aureus*. Desmoglein 1 is the specific receptor for exfoliative toxin. The enzyme proteolytically cleaves desmoglein 1, resulting in blisters identical to those seen in pemphigus foliaceus.[53] Thus, inactivation of desmoglein 1 can cause blisters identical to those seen in pemphigus foliaceus, which suggests that the anti–desmoglein 1 antibodies in pemphigus foliaceus patients also inactivate desmoglein 1.

Although the anti-desmoglein antibodies in pemphigus may directly inactivate desmogleins in desmosomes, it is also possible that they interfere with the incorporation of the desmoglein into desmosomes. In this way, they may ultimately deplete the desmosome of their particular desmoglein target.[54]

If depletion or inactivation of desmoglein isoforms results in blistering, then why do blisters in pemphigus vulgaris and pemphigus foliaceus have specific tissue localizations that do not necessarily correlate with the sites at which the antibodies bind by immunofluorescence? In pemphigus foliaceus, for example, the anti–desmoglein 1 antibodies bind throughout the epidermis and mucous membranes,[55] yet blisters occur only in the superficial epidermis. This apparent paradox has been explained by desmoglein compensation, as outlined in Figure 59-2. The concept of desmoglein compensation originates in the assumptions that autoantibodies against one desmoglein isoform inactivate only that isoform and that another isoform co-expressed in the same area can compensate in adhesion.[56,57] Desmoglein compensation also explains why neonatal pemphigus foliaceus is so unusual, even though the anti–desmoglein 1 antibodies cross the placenta; in neonatal skin, as opposed to adult skin, desmoglein 3 is co-expressed with desmoglein 1 in the superficial epidermis.[58] The validity of desmoglein compensation has been proven by the demonstration that transgenic mice with forced expression of desmoglein 3 in the superficial epidermis are protected against blistering by passive transfer of pemphigus foliaceus IgG.[58]

Abnormal Immune Response and Immune Response Genes

Compared to a matched population, patients with pemphigus vulgaris have a markedly increased frequency of certain class II major histocompatibility complex (MHC) antigens. Among Ashkenazi Jews with pemphigus vulgaris, the serologically defined HLA-DR4 haplotype is predominant, whereas in other ethnic groups with pemphigus vulgaris, the DQ1 allele is more common.[59] However, the association with disease susceptibility becomes even more striking in an analysis of these MHC alleles at a genetic level to determine the amino acid sequence of the cell surface molecules that they encode. Patients with the DR4 serotype almost all have an unusual allele called DRB1*0402, and patients with the DQ1 serotype almost all have a rare allele called DQB1*0503. The protein chains encoded by these alleles vary from those encoded by the alleles found in HLA-DR4 and DQ1 controls without disease in only a few amino acids.

These MHC alleles encode cell surface molecules that are necessary for antigen presentation to the immune system; therefore, it is hypothesized that the disease-associated MHC class II molecules allow presentation of desmoglein 3 peptides to T cells. Consistent with this hypothesis is the finding that certain peptides from desmoglein 3, predicted to fit into the DRB1*0402 peptide-binding pocket, were able to stimulate T cells from patients.[60] Furthermore, in this binding pocket, if one of the negatively charged amino acids specific for the DRB1*0402 subtype of DR4 was changed to a positively charged amino acid (characteristically present in other subtypes of DR4) by site-directed mutagenesis, then the desmoglein 3 peptide could no longer be effectively presented to the T cells. Other studies have confirmed that the immune response in pemphigus is restricted to certain desmoglein peptides and immune response genes coding for antigen presentation molecules.[61–63] These studies suggest that certain populations are susceptible to pemphigus vulgaris because of the genetics of their immune response genes.

FIGURE 59-2

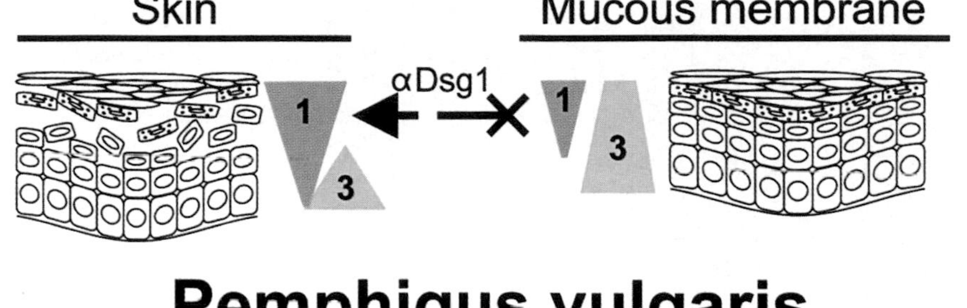

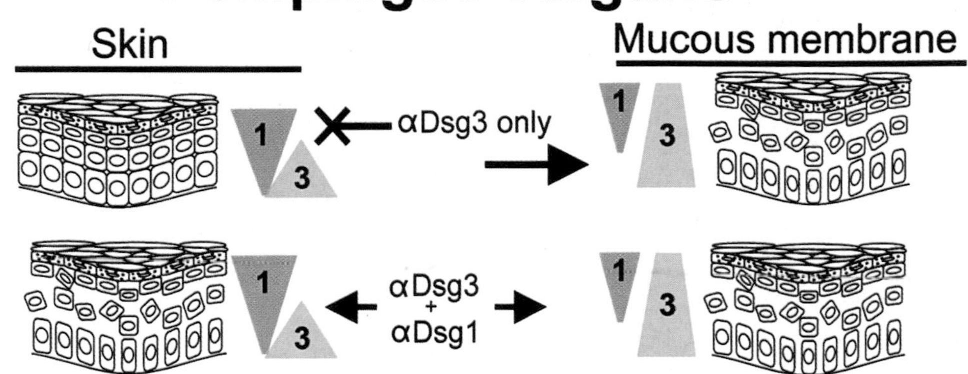

Desmoglein compensation. Triangles represent the distribution of desmoglein (Dsg) 1 and 3 in skin and mucous membranes. Anti-Dsg1 antibodies in pemphigus foliaceus cause acantholysis only in the superficial epidermis of skin. In the deep epidermis and in mucous membranes, Dsg3 compensates for antibody-induced loss of function of Dsg1. In early pemphigus vulgaris, antibodies are present only against Dsg3, which cause blisters only in the deep mucous membrane where Dsg3 is present without compensatory Dsg1. However, in mucocutaneous pemphigus, antibodies against both Dsg1 and Dsg3 are present, and blisters form in both mucous membrane and skin. The blister is deep probably because antibodies diffuse from the dermis and interfere first with the function of desmosomes at the base of the epidermis.

CLINICAL MANIFESTATIONS

Pemphigus Vulgaris

SKIN The skin lesions in pemphigus vulgaris are rarely pruritic, but are often painful.[1] The primary lesion of pemphigus vulgaris is a flaccid blister, which may occur anywhere on the skin surface (Fig. 59-3*A*). Usually, the blister arises on normal-appearing skin, but it may develop on erythematous skin. Even new blisters are usually flaccid or become so within a short time. Because these blisters are fragile, intact blisters may be sparse. The most common skin lesions that occur in these patients are erosions, often painful, subsequent to broken blisters. These erosions are often quite large, as they have a tendency to spread at their periphery (Fig. 59-4*A*). The clinician can elicit this characteristic finding in pemphigus patients with active blistering by applying lateral pressure to normal-appearing skin at the periphery of active lesions. The result is a shearing away of the epidermis, a phenomenon known as the Nikolsky sign (Fig. 59-4*B*). This sign is not specific for pemphigus vulgaris or pemphigus foliaceus, but is evident in other active blistering diseases, such as bullous pemphigoid and erythema multiforme.

In certain patients, erosions have a tendency to develop excessive granulation tissue and crusting (Fig. 59-5); that is, these patients display more vegetating lesions. This type of lesion tends to occur more frequently in intertriginous areas, in the scalp, or on the face (Fig. 59-5*A*). In pemphigus vegetans of Hallopeau, vegetating lesions are present from the outset of disease (Fig. 59-5*B*). Before the advent of effective therapy for pemphigus, the prognosis for these patients was not as grave as that for patients with the more usual type of pemphigus vulgaris. In other patients (e.g., those with pemphigus vegetans of Neumann), ordinary pemphigus vulgaris erosions may tend to develop vegetations.

FIGURE 59-3

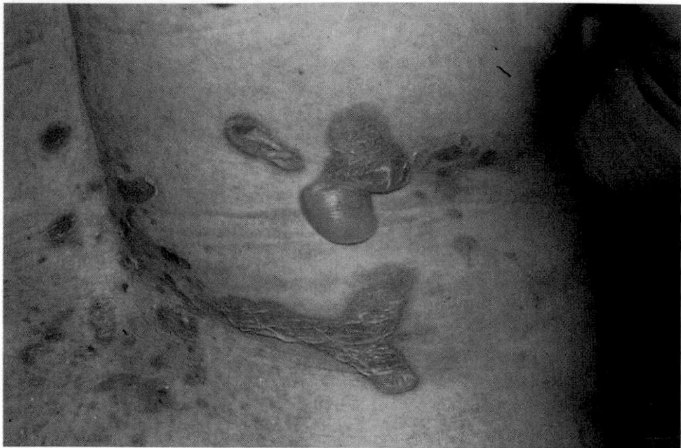

A.

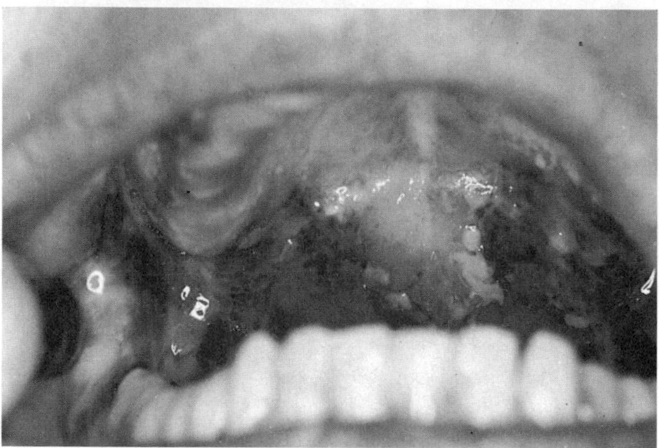

B.

Pemphigus vulgaris. *A.* Flaccid blisters. (*Courtesy of Lawrence Lieblich, MD.*) *B.* Oral erosions.

The vegetating type of response may also appear in certain lesions that tend to be resistant to therapy and remain for long periods of time in one place. Thus, vegetating lesions seem to be one reactive pattern of the skin to the autoimmune insult of pemphigus vulgaris, with certain areas of the skin showing more of a tendency to form vegetations.

MUCOUS MEMBRANES In the majority of patients, painful mucous membrane erosions are the presenting sign of pemphigus vulgaris and may be the only sign for an average of 5 months before skin lesions develop.[3] The mucous membranes most often affected are those of the oral cavity, which is involved in almost all patients with pemphigus vulgaris and is often the only area involved (Fig. 59-3*B*). Intact blisters are rare, probably because they are fragile and break easily. Scattered and often extensive erosions may appear on any part of the oral cavity, although they perhaps occur most frequently on the buccal mucosa. These erosions may spread to involve the pharynx and larynx with subsequent hoarseness. Often, these erosions are so uncomfortable that the patient is unable to eat or drink adequately.

Mucous membranes in other areas may also be involved with painful erosions; these include conjunctiva, anus, penis, vagina, and labia.[64] Even the esophagus has been reported to be involved in unusual cases.[65]

Pemphigus Foliaceus

SKIN The characteristic clinical lesions of pemphigus foliaceus are scaly, crusted erosions, often on an erythematous base.[1,66] In more localized and early disease, these lesions are usually well demarcated and scattered in a seborrheic distribution, including the face, scalp, and upper trunk (Fig. 59-6*A*). The primary lesions of small flaccid blisters are often inconspicuous and difficult to find. Disease may stay localized for years, or it may rapidly progress to sometimes generalized involvement, resulting in an exfoliative erythroderma (Fig. 59-6*B*). Exposure to sun and/or heat may exacerbate disease activity. Patients with pemphigus foliaceus often complain of pain and burning in the skin lesions. In contrast to patients with pemphigus vulgaris, those with pemphigus foliaceus only very rarely, if ever, have mucous membrane involvement, even with widespread disease.

The colloquial term for Brazilian endemic pemphigus, *fogo selvagem* (Portuguese for "wild fire"), takes into account many of the clinical aspects of this disease: the burning feeling of the skin, the exacerbation of disease by the sun, and the crusted lesions that make the patients appear as if they had been burned.

PEMPHIGUS ERYTHEMATOSUS Also known as Senear-Usher syndrome, pemphigus erythematosus is simply the localized form of pemphigus foliaceus. Typical scaly and crusted lesions of pemphigus foliaceus occur across the malar area of the face and in other seborrheic areas. Pemphigus erythematosus may remain localized for years, or it may evolve into more generalized pemphigus foliaceus. If there is a unique aspect of pemphigus erythematosus, it is the immunopathology noted earlier. In addition, many patients with pemphigus erythematosus show serologic findings suggestive of systemic lupus erythematosus, especially the presence of antinuclear antibodies, although few patients have been reported to actually have the two diseases concurrently.[67]

Neonatal Pemphigus

Infants born to mothers with pemphigus vulgaris may display clinical, histologic, and immunopathologic signs of pemphigus.[40] The degree of involvement varies from none to severe enough to result in a stillbirth. If the infant survives, disease tends to remit as maternal antibody is catabolized. Mothers with pemphigus foliaceus may also transmit their autoantibodies to the fetus, but, as discussed earlier, neonatal pemphigus foliaceus occurs only rarely.[68,69] Neonatal pemphigus should be distinguished from pemphigus vulgaris and pemphigus foliaceus that occur in childhood, which are similar to the autoimmune diseases seen in adults.[70]

Drug-Induced Pemphigus

Although there are sporadic case reports of pemphigus associated with the use of several different drugs, the association with penicillamine, and perhaps captopril, is the most significant.[71] The prevalence of pemphigus in penicillamine users is estimated to be about 7 percent. Pemphigus foliaceus (including pemphigus erythematosus) is more common than pemphigus vulgaris in these penicillamine-treated patients, although either may occur. The findings of direct and indirect immunofluorescence are positive in most of these patients. Three patients with drug-induced pemphigus foliaceus and one with drug-induced pemphigus vulgaris have been shown to have autoantibodies to the same molecules involved in sporadic pemphigus, namely, desmoglein 1 and desmoglein 3, respectively.[72] Therefore, by immunofluorescence and immunochemical determinations, these patients with drug-induced pemphigus resemble those with sporadic disease.

Both penicillamine and captopril contain sulfhydryl groups that may interact with the sulfhydryl groups in desmoglein 1 and/or 3, thereby causing pemphigus either by directly interfering with these adhesion molecules or, more likely, by modifying them so that they become more antigenic. The use of these drugs may also lead to a more generalized dysregulation of the immune response, allowing production of other autoantibodies such as those resulting in myasthenia gravis. Most, but not all, patients with drug-induced pemphigus go into remission after they stop taking the offending drug.

FIGURE 59-4

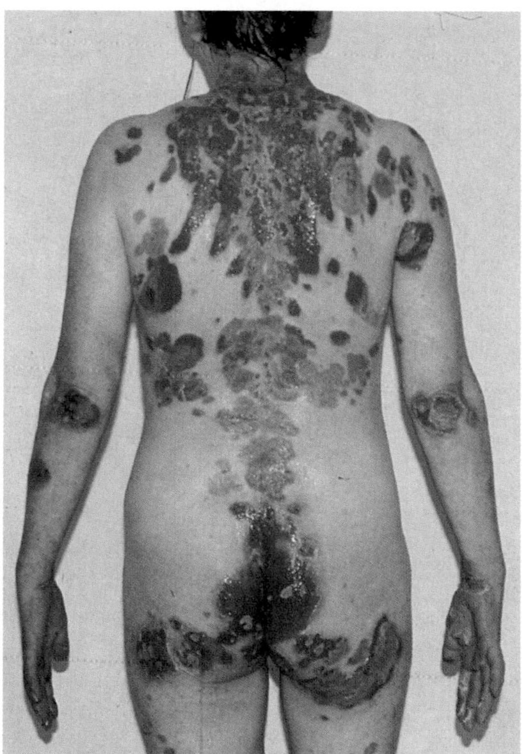

A.

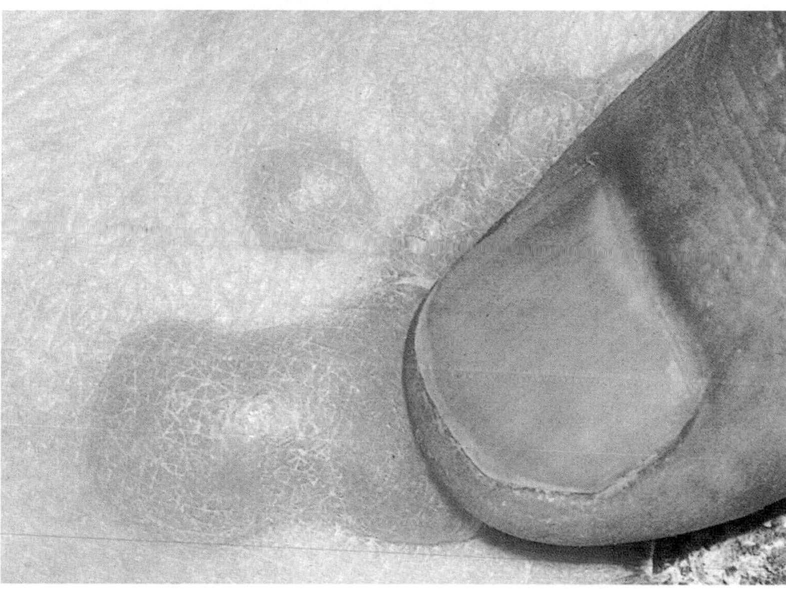

B.

Pemphigus vulgaris. *A*. Extensive erosions due to blistering. Almost the entire back is denuded. Note intact, flaccid blisters at the lower border of eroded lesions. *B*. The bulla has been extended following pressure with the finger (Nikolsky's sign).

Associated Diseases

Myasthenia gravis and/or thymoma have been associated with pemphigus vulgaris and pemphigus foliaceus.[73] Approximately one-half of associated pemphigus cases are vulgaris; one-half, foliaceus or erythematosus. Most of these data, however, were reported before the recognition of paraneoplastic pemphigus as a distinct entity. Therefore, although thymoma may clearly be associated with pemphigus vulgaris and pemphigus foliaceus, it may also be associated with paraneoplastic pemphigus (see Chapter 60). The course of myasthenia gravis and the course of pemphigus seem independent of each other. Likewise, the thymic abnormality may either precede or follow the onset of pemphigus. Thymic abnormalities include benign or malignant thymoma and thymic hyperplasia. Irradiation of the thymus or thymectomy, while clearly beneficial for myasthenia gravis, may not improve the pemphigus disease activity. Although this association is reported in at least 30 cases, the finding of thymoma or myasthenia gravis in a patient with pemphigus vulgaris or pemphigus foliaceus is still unusual.

Although very uncommon, pemphigus vulgaris or pemphigus foliaceus has been associated with bullous pemphigoid in the same patient.[74] Finally, pemphigus vulgaris has rarely evolved into pemphigus foliaceus, and vice versa, as determined by clinical, histologic and immunochemical criteria.[75]

PATHOLOGY

Pemphigus Vulgaris

The characteristic histopathologic finding in pemphigus vulgaris is a suprabasilar blister with acantholysis (Fig. 59-7). Just above the basal cell layer, epidermal cells lose their normal cell-to-cell contacts and form a blister. Often, a few rounded up (acantholytic) keratinocytes are in the blister cavity. The basal cells stay attached to the basement membrane, but may lose the contact with their neighbors; as a result, they may appear to be a "row of tombstones." Usually, the upper epidermis (from one or two cell layers above the basal cells) remains intact, as these cells maintain their cell adhesion. Pemphigus vegetans shows not only suprabasilar acantholysis, but also papillomatosis of the dermal papillae and downward growth of epidermal stands into the dermis, with hyperkeratosis and scale-crust formation. In addition, pemphigus vegetans lesions may show intraepidermal abscesses composed of eosinophils.[1] Early pemphigus vulgaris lesions may show eosinophilic spongiosis.[76]

Pemphigus Foliaceus

The histopathology of early blisters in pemphigus foliaceus patients demonstrates acantholysis (loss of cell-to-cell contact) just below the stratum corneum and in the granular layer (Fig. 59-8*A*). The stratum corneum is often lost from the surface of these lesions. The deeper epidermis, below the granular layer, remains intact. Another frequent finding is subcorneal pustules, with neutrophils and acantholytic epidermal cells in the blister cavity (Fig. 59-8*B*). These histologic findings are indistinguishable from those seen in bullous impetigo. Pemphigus

FIGURE 59-5

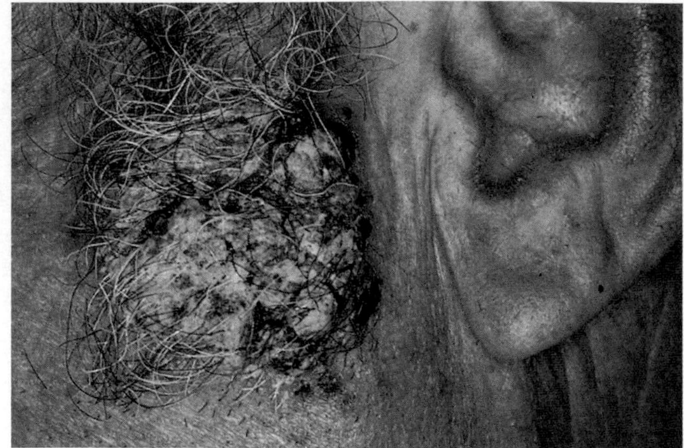

A.

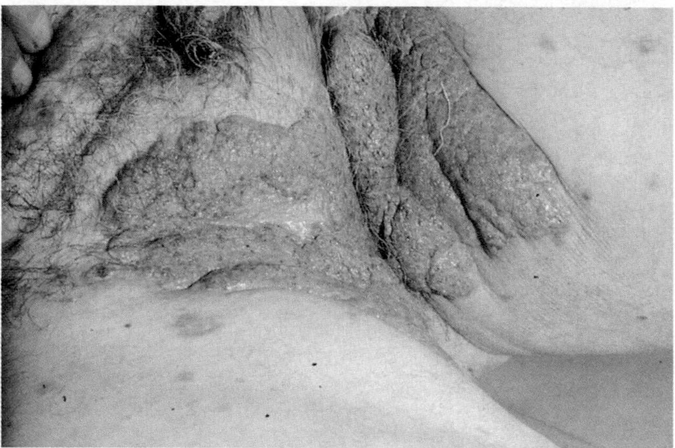

B.

A. Crusted, vegetating lesions in pemphigus vulgaris. *B.* Extensive, vegetating granulomatous lesions in pemphigus vegetans.

FIGURE 59-6

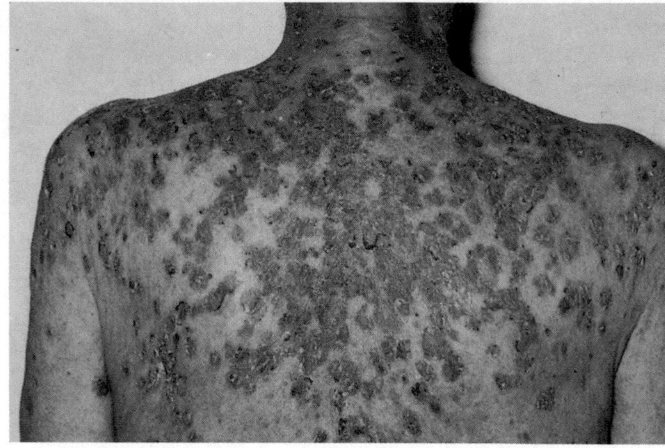

A.

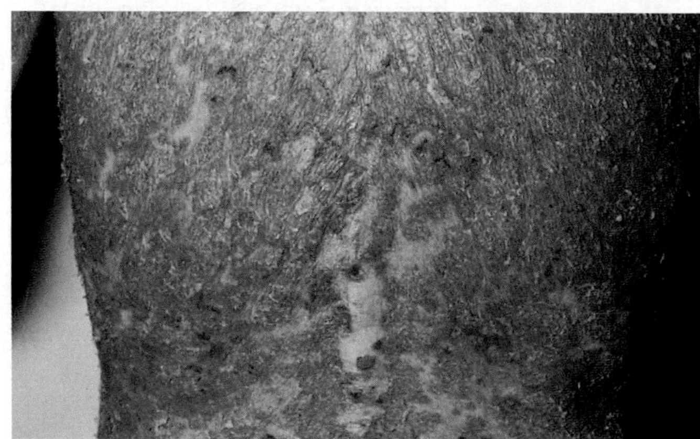

B.

Pemphigus foliaceus. *A.* Scaly, crusted lesions on upper back. *B.* Exfoliative erythroderma due to confluent lesions.

erythematosus has histologic findings identical to those of pemphigus foliaceus. As in pemphigus vulgaris lesions, very early pemphigus foliaceus lesions may show eosinophilic spongiosis.[76]

TREATMENT AND PROGNOSIS

Before the advent of glucocorticoid therapy, pemphigus vulgaris was almost invariably fatal, and pemphigus foliaceus was fatal in about 60 percent of patients. Pemphigus foliaceus was almost always fatal in elderly patients with concurrent medical problems.[77]

The systemic administration of glucocorticoids and the use of immunosuppressive therapy have dramatically improved the prognosis for patients with pemphigus; however, pemphigus is still a disease associated with a significant morbidity and mortality.[78,79] Infection is often the cause of death, and by causing the immunosuppression necessary in the treatment of active disease, therapy is frequently a contributing factor.[80] With glucocorticoid and immunosuppressive therapy, the mortality (from disease or therapy) of pemphigus vulgaris patients followed

FIGURE 59-7

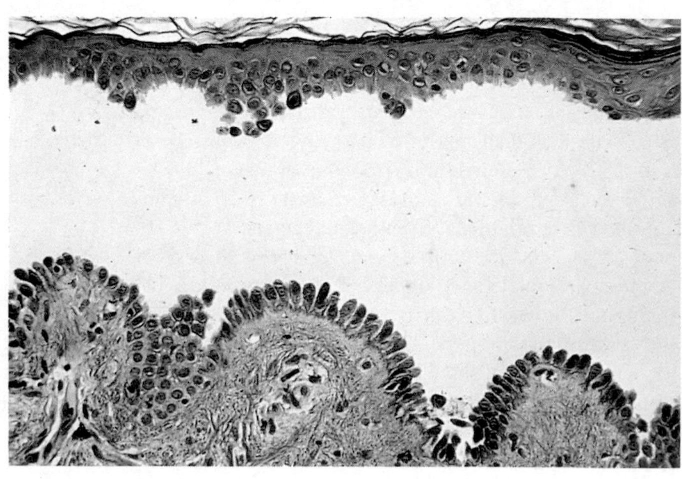

Histopathology of pemphigus vulgaris. Suprabasilar acantholysis. The row of tombstones. ×250.

FIGURE 59-8

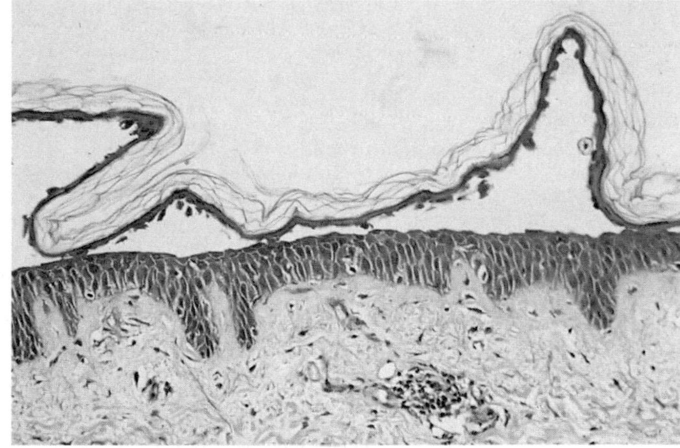

A.

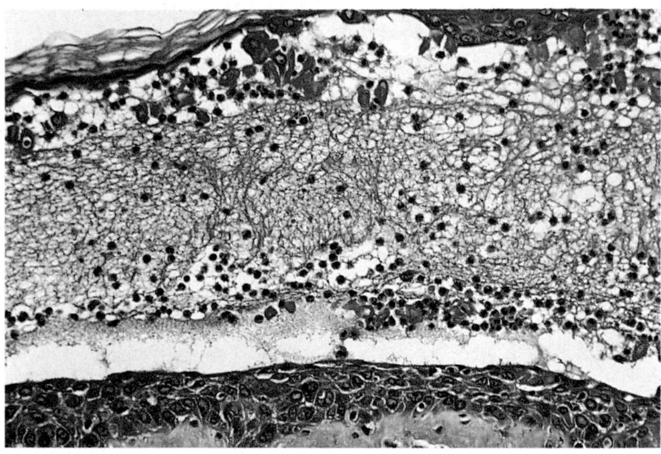

B.

Histopathology of pemphigus foliaceus. *A*. Acantholysis in the granular layer. ×250. *B*. Subcorneal pustule with acantholysis. ×250.

from 4 to 10 years is about 10 percent or less whereas that of pemphigus foliaceus is probably even less.

It is generally agreed that pemphigus vulgaris, even if initially limited in extent, should be treated at its onset, because it will ultimately generalize, and the prognosis without therapy is very poor. In addition, it is probably easier to control early disease than widespread disease, and mortality may be higher if therapy is delayed.[81]

Because pemphigus foliaceus may be localized for many years, and the prognosis without systemic therapy may be good, patients with this type of pemphigus do not necessarily require treatment with systemic therapy; the use of topical glucocorticoids may suffice. When the disease is active and widespread, however, the therapy for pemphigus foliaceus is, in general, similar to that for pemphigus vulgaris.

The systemic administration of glucocorticoids, usually prednisone, is the mainstay of therapy for pemphigus. At one time, primarily before adjuvant immunosuppressive therapy was available, very high initial doses of prednisone were recommended for therapy. Now, however, few authorities recommend such high doses, and many feel that intermediate or low doses, especially if used in combination with immunosuppressive therapy and, if necessary, with tolerance of some residual disease activity, result in fewer complications and decreased mortality.[6,80,82,83] Once disease activity is controlled, tapering prednisone to an alternate-day dosage will decrease the incidence of glucocorticoid side effects.

Although there are no controlled studies, most authors feel that immunosuppressive agents, such as mycophenolate mofetil, azathioprine, and cyclophosphamide, have a steroid-sparing effect, decrease the incidence of side effects of therapy, and may increase the numbers of remissions.[20,77,78,83,84] Treatment regimens often begin with both an immunosuppressive agent and prednisone in moderate to intermediate doses, depending on disease activity, although some authors suggest first determining if the disease responds to a course of glucocorticoids alone.[20,79,83] In any case, if there are contraindications to glucocorticoid use, if the glucocorticoids do not control the disease, or if the dosage low enough to minimize the risk of steroid complications is not effective, the patient should receive adjuvant therapy, usually consisting of immunosuppressive agents.

Results obtained by using prednisone and immunosuppressive agents to treat patients with pemphigus vulgaris, although not controlled, have been impressive. For example, in a series of 29 patients treated with prednisone and azathioprine, about 50 percent went into clinical and serologic remission and continued off therapy for a mean follow-up of 4 years.[20] Many of these patients were considered cured. Only 1 patient in this study died because of complications of therapy. The disease activity of most of the other patients was well controlled.

Mycophenolate mofetil, in particular, has been shown to have a rapid effect in lowering pemphigus antibody titers and to decrease disease activity, even in patients whose disease is unresponsive to azathioprine.[84] As it probably has fewer adverse reactions than azathioprine, it may ultimately replace azathioprine as a first-line agent in treating these patients.

Early localized pemphigus vulgaris may be treated with relatively low-dose prednisone (e.g., 40 mg) either given initially on alternate days or rapidly tapered to alternate-day dosage, often with an immunosuppressive agent.[85]The decision to use immunosuppressive agents in young patients must take into account the potential increased incidence of malignancies that might be associated with the use of these drugs, as well as the risks of infertility (especially associated with cyclophosphamide) and teratogenicity. In some patients, especially those who are elderly with limited disease or those in whom glucocorticoids are contraindicated, immunosuppressive agents alone may be used.[86] Because patients may die from complications of therapy, it is important to monitor all patients closely for potential side effects, such as infection; diabetes; leukopenia; thrombocytopenia; anemia; gastrointestinal ulcer disease; and bleeding, liver and renal function abnormalities, high blood pressure, electrolyte disturbances, and osteoporosis.

There are additional, innovative therapies that are usually used when more standard treatment is not effective. For example, the intravenous, pulse administration of methylprednisolone, 250 to 1000 mg given over about 3 h every 24 h for 4 to 5 consecutive days, can result in long-term remissions and decrease the total dose of glucocorticoids necessary to control disease.[87] Although the purpose of this therapy is to decrease the incidence of complications of long-term steroid use, it can result in all the usual glucocorticoid complications, as well as cardiac arrhythmias and anaphylaxis, and its use is controversial.[88] Intravenous pulse therapy with cyclophosphamide, with or without pulse therapy with glucocorticoids, has also been reported to result in remissions of pemphigus vulgaris.[89] Pulses of cyclophosphamide, given intravenously, are thought to allow a decrease in the daily oral dosage and thereby cut down on the side effects.

Plasmapheresis is another therapy for severe pemphigus, especially if the disease is unresponsive to a combination of prednisone and immunosuppressive agents. Although one controlled study found it to be ineffective,[90] other studies have found that it both reduces serum levels of pemphigus autoantibodies and controls disease activity.[91] For maximum effectiveness, it is probably necessary to perform plasmapheresis on patients taking immunosuppressive agents to prevent the antibody-rebound phenomenon that can follow the removal of IgG. Another creative approach to therapy has been to synchronize plasmapheresis and pulse therapy with cyclophosphamide to cause maximum cytotoxicity when pathogenic B cell clones might be proliferating as a result of the loss of the negative feedback of IgG on antibody production.[92] However, whether this approach is any better than simply using plasmapheresis in patients on continual immunosuppressive therapy is not known.

Another method of suppressing autoantibody production is the intravenous use of gamma globulin. It is probably ineffective in pemphigus when used alone, but may be useful as adjuvant therapy in those whose condition is failing to respond to more conventional therapy.[93]

Other potential therapies for pemphigus, used less frequently than those that have been discussed, include immunoablative therapy without stem cell rescue; the administration of cyclosporine, gold, antimalarials, or dapsone; and extracorporeal photochemotherapy.[78,94]

All in all, there has been a tremendous advance in the armamentarium of therapies for pemphigus since the time before the development of glucocorticoids when pemphigus vulgaris was a fatal disease. Thanks to these advances, the "row of tombstones" seen in the pathology of pemphigus vulgaris no longer alludes to its prognosis.

REFERENCES

1. Lever WF: *Pemphigus and Pemphigoid.* Springfield, IL, Charles C Thomas, 1965
2. Beutner EH, Jordon RE: Demonstration of skin antibodies in sera of pemphigus vulgaris patients by indirect immunofluorescent staining. *Proc Soc Exp Biol Med* **117**, 505, 1964
3. Krain LS: Pemphigus: Epidemiologic and survival characteristics of 59 patients, 1955–1973. *Arch Dermatol* **110**:862, 1974
4. Pisanti S et al: Pemphigus vulgaris: Incidence in Jews of different ethnic groups, according to age, sex, and initial lesion. *Oral Surg Oral Med Oral Pathol* **38**:382, 1974
5. Rosenberg FR et al: Pemphigus: A 20-year review of 107 patients treated with corticosteroids. *Arch Dermatol* **112**:962, 1976
6. Hietanen J, Salo OP: Pemphigus: An epidemiological study of patients treated in Finnish hospitals between 1969 and 1978. *Acta Derm Venereol (Stockh)* **62**:491, 1982
7. Bastuji-Garin S et al: Comparative epidemiology of pemphigus in Tunisia and France: Unusual incidence of pemphigus foliaceus in young Tunisian women. *J Invest Dermatol* **104**:302, 1995
8. Diaz LA et al: Endemic pemphigus foliaceus (fogo selvagem): II. Current and historical epidemiological aspects. *J Invest Dermatol* **92**:4, 1989
9. Lombardi C et al: Environmental risk factors in endemic pemphigus foliaceus (fogo selvagem). The Cooperative Group on Fogo Selvagem Research. *J Invest Dermatol* **98**:847, 1992
10. Warren SJ et al: The prevalence of antibodies against desmoglein 1 in endemic pemphigus foliaceus in Brazil. The Cooperative Group on Fogo Selvagem Research. [Comments]. *N Engl J Med* **343**:23, 2000
11. Hashimoto K, Lever WF: An electron microscopic study on pemphigus vulgaris of the mouth and the skin with special reference to the intercellular cement. *J Invest Dermatol* **48**:540, 1967
12. Grando SA et al: Ultrastructural study of clinically uninvolved skin of patients with pemphigus vulgaris. *Clin Exp Dermatol* **16**:359, 1991
13. Caldelari R et al: A central role for the armadillo protein plakoglobin in the autoimmune disease pemphigus vulgaris. *J Cell Biol* **153**:823, 2001
14. Wilgram GF et al: An electron microscopic study of acantholysis and dyskeratosis in pemphigus foliaceus. *J Invest Dermatol* **43**:287, 1964
15. Beutner EH et al: Autoantibodies in pemphigus vulgaris. *JAMA* **192**:682, 1965
16. Judd KP, Lever WF: Correlation of antibodies in skin and serum with disease severity in pemphigus. *Arch Dermatol* **115**:428, 1979
17. Harman KE et al: The use of two substrates to improve the sensitivity of indirect immunofluorescence in the diagnosis of pemphigus. *Br J Dermatol* **142**:1135, 2000
18. Krasny SA et al: Specificity and sensitivity of indirect and direct immunofluorescent findings in the diagnosis of pemphigus, in *Immunopathology of the Skin,* 3rd ed, edited by EH Beutner et al. New York, Wiley, 1987, p 207
19. O'Loughlin S et al: Fate of pemphigus antibody following successful therapy: Preliminary evaluation of pemphigus antibody determinations to regulate therapy. *Arch Dermatol* **114**:1769, 1978
20. Aberer W et al: Azathioprine in the treatment of pemphigus vulgaris: A long-term follow-up. *J Am Acad Dermatol* **16**:527, 1987
21. Ishii K et al: Characterization of autoantibodies in pemphigus using antigen-specific enzyme-linked immunosorbent assays with baculovirus-expressed recombinant desmogleins. *J Immunol* **159**:2010, 1997
22. Amagai M et al: Usefulness of enzyme-linked immunosorbent assay using recombinant desmogleins 1 and 3 for serodiagnosis of pemphigus. *Br J Dermatol* **140**:351, 1999
23. Chorzelski T et al: Immunopathological investigations in the Senear-Usher syndrome (coexistence of pemphigus and lupus erythematosus). *Br J Dermatol* **80**:211, 1968
24. Rappersberger K et al: Immunomorphological and biochemical identification of the pemphigus foliaceus autoantigen within desmosomes. *J Invest Dermatol* **99**:323, 1992
25. Karpati S et al: Pemphigus vulgaris antigen, a desmoglein type of cadherin, is localized within keratinocyte desmosomes. *J Cell Biol* **122**:409, 1993
26. Shimizu H et al: Pemphigus vulgaris and pemphigus foliaceus sera show an inversely graded binding pattern to extracellular regions of desmosomes in different layers of human epidermis. *J Invest Dermatol* **105**:153, 1995
27. Koulu L et al: Human autoantibodies against a desmosomal core protein in pemphigus foliaceus. *J Exp Med* **160**:1509, 1984
28. Stanley JR et al: A monoclonal antibody to the desmosomal glycoprotein desmoglein 1 binds the same polypeptide as human autoantibodies in pemphigus foliaceus. *J Immunol* **136**:1227, 1986
29. Stanley JR et al: Antigenic specificity of fogo selvagem autoantibodies is similar to North American pemphigus foliaceus and distinct from pemphigus vulgaris autoantibodies. *J Invest Dermatol* **87**:197, 1986
30. Amagai M et al: Autoantibodies against a novel epithelial cadherin in pemphigus vulgaris, a disease of cell adhesion. *Cell* **67**:869, 1991
31. Eyre RW, Stanley JR: Identification of pemphigus vulgaris antigen extracted from normal human epidermis and comparison with pemphigus foliaceus antigen. *J Clin Invest* **81**:807, 1988
32. Ding X et al: Mucosal and mucocutaneous (generalized) pemphigus vulgaris show distinct autoantibody profiles. *J Invest Dermatol* **109**:592, 1997
33. Amagai M et al: The clinical phenotype of pemphigus is defined by the anti-desmoglein autoantibody profile. *J Am Acad Dermatol* **40**:170, 1999
34. Miyagawa S et al: Late development of antidesmoglein 1 antibodies in pemphigus vulgaris: correlation with disease progression. *Br J Dermatol* **141**:1084, 1999
35. Eyre RW, Stanley JR: Human autoantibodies against a desmosomal protein complex with a calcium-sensitive epitope are characteristic of pemphigus foliaceus patients. *J Exp Med* **165**:1719, 1987
36. Amagai M et al: Conformational epitopes of pemphigus antigens (Dsg1 and Dsg3) are calcium dependent and glycosylation independent. *J Invest Dermatol* **105**:243, 1995
37. Stanley JR et al: Pemphigus: Is there another half of the story? *J Invest Dermatol* **116**:489, 2001
38. Grando SA et al: Pemphigus: An unfolding story. *J Invest Dermatol* **117**:990, 2001
39. Stanley JR et al: Pemphigus: An unfolding story. [Reply]. *J Invest Dermatol* **117**:994
40. Chowdhury MMU, Natarajan S: Neonatal pemphigus vulgaris associated with mild oral pemphigus vulgaris in the mother during pregnancy. *Br J Dermatol* **139**:500, 1998
41. Rocha-Alvarez R et al: Pregnant women with endemic pemphigus foliaceus (fogo selvagem) give birth to disease-free babies. *J Invest Dermatol* **99**:78, 1992
42. Schiltz JR, Michel B: Production of epidermal acantholysis in normal human skin in vitro by the IgG fraction from pemphigus serum. *J Invest Dermatol* **67**:254, 1976
43. Hashimoto K et al: Anti-cell surface pemphigus autoantibody stimulates plasminogen activator activity of human epidermal cells. *J Exp Med* **157**:259, 1983
44. Anhalt GJ et al: Induction of pemphigus in neonatal mice by passive transfer of IgG from patients with the disease. *N Engl J Med* **306**:1189, 1982
45. Rock B et al: Monovalent Fab′ immunoglobulin fragments from endemic pemphigus foliaceus autoantibodies reproduce the human disease in neonatal Balb/c mice. *J Clin Invest* **85**:296, 1990
46. Anhalt GJ et al: Defining the role of complement in experimental pemphigus vulgaris in mice. *J Immunol* **137**:2835, 1986
47. Amagai M et al: Autoantibodies against the amino-terminal cadherin-like binding domain of pemphigus vulgaris antigen are pathogenic. *J Clin Invest* **90**:919, 1992

48. Ding X et al: The anti-desmoglein 1 autoantibodies in pemphigus vulgaris sera are pathogenic. *J Invest Dermatol* **112**:739, 1999
49. Amagai M et al: Absorption of pathogenic autoantibodies by the extracellular domain of pemphigus vulgaris antigen (Dsg3) produced by baculovirus. *J Clin Invest* **94**:59, 1994
50. Amagai M et al: Antigen-specific immunoabsorption of pathogenic autoantibodies in pemphigus foliaceus. *J Invest Dermatol* **104**:895, 1995
51. Amagai M et al: Use of autoantigen-knockout mice in developing an active autoimmune disease model for pemphigus. *J Clin Invest* **105**:625, 2000
52. Koch PJ et al: Targeted disruption of the pemphigus vulgaris antigen (desmoglein 3) gene in mice causes loss of keratinocyte cell adhesion with a phenotype similar to pemphigus vulgaris. *J Cell Biol* **137**:1091, 1997
53. Amagai M et al: Toxin in bullous impetigo and staphylococcal scalded-skin syndrome targets desmoglein 1. *Nature Med* **6**:1275, 2000
54. Aoyama Y, Kitajima Y: Pemphigus vulgaris-IgG causes a rapid depletion of desmoglein 3 (Dsg3) from the triton X-100 soluble pools, leading to the formation of Dsg3-depleted desmosomes in a human squamous carcinoma cell line, DJM-1 cells. *J Invest Dermatol* **112**:67, 1999
55. Rivitti EA et al: Pemphigus foliaceus autoantibodies bind both epidermis and squamous mucosal epithelium, but tissue injury is detected only in the epidermis. The Cooperative Group on Fogo Selvagem Research. *J Am Acad Dermatol* **31**:954, 1994
56. Shirakata Y Lack of mucosal involvement in pemphigus foliaceus may be due to low expression of desmoglein 1. *J Invest Dermatol* **110**:76, 1998
57. Mahoney MG et al: Explanation for the clinical and microscopic localization of lesions in pemphigus foliaceus and vulgaris. *J Clin Invest* **103**:461, 1999
58. Wu H et al: Protection of neonates against pemphigus foliaceus by desmoglein 3. *N Engl J Med* **343**:31, 2000
59. Wucherpfennig KW, Strominger JL: Selective binding of self peptides to disease-associated major histocompatibility complex (MHC) molecules: A mechanism for MHC-linked susceptibility to human autoimmune diseases. [Comment]. *J Exp Med* **181**:1597, 1995
60. Wucherpfennig KW et al: Structural basis for major histocompatibility complex (MHC)-linked susceptibility to autoimmunity: Charged residues of a single MHC binding pocket confer selective presentation of self-peptides in pemphigus vulgaris. *Proc Natl Acad Sci USA* **92**:11935, 1995
61. Lin MS et al: Development and characterization of desmoglein-3 specific T cells from patients with pemphigus vulgaris. *J Clin Invest* **99**:31, 1997
62. Hertl M et al: Heterogeneous MHC II restriction pattern of autoreactive desmoglein 3 specific T cell responses in pemphigus vulgaris patients and normals. *J Invest Dermatol* **110**:388, 1998
63. Hertl M et al: Recognition of desmoglein 3 by autoreactive T cells in pemphigus vulgaris patients and normals. *J Invest Dermatol* **110**:62, 1998
64. Hodak E et al: Conjunctival involvement in pemphigus vulgaris: A clinical, histopathological and immunofluorescence study. *Br J Dermatol* **123**:615, 1990
65. Trattner A et al: Esophageal involvement in pemphigus vulgaris: A clinical, histologic, and immunopathologic study. *J Am Acad Dermatol* **24**:223, 1991
66. Perry HO, Brunsting LA: Pemphigus foliaceus. *Arch Dermatol* **91**:10, 1965
67. Amerian ML, Ahmed AR: Pemphigus erythematosus: Senear-Usher syndrome. *Int J Dermatol* **24**:16, 1985
68. Eyre RW, Stanley JR: Maternal pemphigus foliaceus with cell surface antibody bound in neonatal epidermis. *Arch Dermatol* **124**:25, 1988
69. Avalos-Diaz E et al: Transplacental passage of maternal pemphigus foliaceus autoantibodies induces neonatal pemphigus. *J Am Acad Dermatol* **43**:1130, 2000
70. Kanwar AJ et al: Further experience with pemphigus in children. *Pediatr Dermatol* **11**:107, 1996
71. Mutasim DF et al: Drug-induced pemphigus. [Review]. *Dermatol Clin* **11**:463, 1993
72. Korman NJ et al: Drug-induced pemphigus: Autoantibodies directed against the pemphigus antigen complexes are present in penicillamine and captopril-induced pemphigus. *J Invest Dermatol* **96**:273, 1991
73. Patten SF, Dijkstra JW: Associations of pemphigus and autoimmune disease with malignancy or thymoma. [Review]. *Int J Dermatol* **33**:836, 1994
74. Korman NJ et al: Coexistence of pemphigus foliaceus and bullous pemphigoid: Demonstration of autoantibodies that bind to both the pemphigus foliaceus antigen complex and the bullous pemphigoid antigen. *Arch Dermatol* **127**:387, 1991
75. Ishii K et al: Development of pemphigus vulgaris in a patient with pemphigus foliaceus: antidesmoglein antibody profile shift confirmed by enzyme-linked immunosorbent assay. *J Am Acad Dermatol* **42**:859, 2000
76. Emmerson RW, Wilson-Jones E: Eosinophilic spongiosis in pemphigus. *Arch Dermatol* **97**:252, 1968
77. Carson PJ et al: Influence of treatment on the clinical course of pemphigus vulgaris. *J Am Acad Dermatol* **34**:645, 1996
78. Stanley JR: Therapy of pemphigus vulgaris. *Arch Dermatol* **135**:76, 1999
79. Bystryn JC, Steinman NM: The adjuvant therapy of pemphigus: An update. [Review]. *Arch Dermatol* **132**:203, 1996
80. Ahmed AR, Moy R: Death in pemphigus. *J Am Acad Dermatol* **7**:221, 1982
81. Seidenbaum M et al: The course and prognosis of pemphigus: A review of 115 patients. *Int J Dermatol* **27**:580, 1988
82. Ratnam KV et al: Pemphigus therapy with oral prednisolone regimens: A 5-year study. *Int J Dermatol* **29**:363, 1990
83. Fine JD: Management of acquired bullous skin diseases. [Comments]. [Review]. *N Engl J Med* **333**:1475, 1995
84. Enk AH, Knop J: Mycophenolate mofetil is effective in the treatment of pemphigus vulgaris. *Arch Dermatol* **135**:54, 1998
85. Lever WF: Pemphigus and pemphigoid. *J Am Acad Dermatol* **1**:2, 1979
86. Lever WF, Schaumburg Lever G: Immunosuppressants and prednisone in pemphigus vulgaris: therapeutic results obtained in 63 patients between 1961 and 1975. *Arch Dermatol* **113**:1236, 1977
87. Werth VP: Treatment of pemphigus vulgaris with brief, high-dose intravenous glucocorticoids. *Arch Dermatol* **132**:1435, 1996
88. Roujeau JC: Pulse glucocorticoid therapy: The 'big shot' revisited. *Arch Dermatol* **132**:1499, 1996
89. Pasricha JS et al: Dexamethasone-cyclophosphamide pulse therapy for pemphigus. *Int J Dermatol* **34**:875, 1995
90. Guillaume JC et al: Controlled study of plasma exchange in pemphigus. *Arch Dermatol* **124**:1659, 1988
91. Turner MS et al: The use of plasmapheresis and immunosuppression in the treatment of pemphigus vulgaris. *J Am Acad Dermatol* **43**:1058, 2000
92. Euler HH et al: Synchronization of plasmapheresis and pulse cyclophosphamide therapy in pemphigus vulgaris. *Arch Dermatol* **123**:1205, 1987
93. Engineer L et al: Analysis of current data on the use of intravenous immunoglobulins in management of pemphigus vulgaris. *J Am Acad Dermatol* **43**:1049, 2000
94. Hayag MV et al: Immunoablative high-dose cyclophosphamide without stem cell rescue in a patient with pemphigus vulgaris. *J Am Acad Dermatol* **43**:1065, 2000

CHAPTER 60

Grant J. Anhalt
H. Carlos Nousari

Paraneoplastic Pemphigus

Paraneoplastic pemphigus is an autoimmune disorder that is almost invariably linked to an underlying lymphoproliferative disorder. These features define it: (1) Painful stomatitis and a polymorphous cutaneous eruption with lesions that may be blistering, lichenoid or resemble erythema multiforme. (2) Histologic findings that reflect the variability of the cutaneous lesions, showing acantholysis, lichenoid or interface change. (3) Direct immunofluorescence demonstrating deposition of IgG and complement in the epidermal intercellular spaces, and often granular/linear complement deposition along the epidermal basement membrane zone. (4) Serum autoantibodies that bind the cell surface of skin and mucosae in a pattern typical for pemphigus, but in addition, bind to simple, columnar, and transitional epithelia. (5) These serum autoantibodies identify desmogleins 1 and 3, but additionally identify members of the plakin family of epithelial proteins, such as desmoplakins, envoplakin, and periplakin. The disease is associated in the majority of cases with non-Hodgkin's lymphoma, chronic lymphocytic leukemia and Castleman's disease. Treatment of the autoimmune disease is difficult and most patients die from complications of the disease, including pulmonary involvement with respiratory failure.

HISTORICAL ASPECTS

In December 1990, Anhalt et al. published observations based on five cases that defined a previously unrecognized autoimmune mucocutaneous disease linked to underlying lymphoproliferative neoplasms, and proposed the term *paraneoplastic pemphigus* to describe this syndrome.[1] Since then, numerous cases have been reported that verified the essential features of the disease as first described, with some important additions and clarifications. It is clear that this syndrome of paraneoplastic pemphigus (PNP) was not a "new" disease. Based on a retrospective literature review, it is apparent that cases of paraneoplastic pemphigus were identified over the years. These cases, however, were often characterized as atypical cases of pemphigus vulgaris,[2] as unusual cases of erythema multiforme with pemphigus-like antibodies,[3] or as an unusual paraneoplastic bullous disease without further clarification.[4]

EPIDEMIOLOGY

The incidence of the disease is unknown, but it is less common than pemphigus vulgaris or foliaceus. In a recent analysis of adverse event reporting in 100,000 patients with known non-Hodgkin's lymphoma and chronic lymphocytic leukemia, there were 12 cases of paraneoplastic pemphigus (Nagy S and Anhalt GJ, manuscript in preparation). Of note, only three of these cases were identified by the reporting physician as such, and the remainder were identified by retrospective data analysis. That implies that the majority of cases are still not properly diagnosed. The commonest misdiagnoses applied in this series were erythema multiforme, Stevens-Johnson syndrome, toxic epidermal necrolysis, and drug reaction.

ETIOLOGY AND PATHOGENESIS

In almost all cases, this syndrome is associated with a limited number of lymphoproliferative neoplasms. The approximate frequency of specific neoplasms has been estimated, based upon 140 cases of PNP diagnosed by our laboratory and confirmed by immunoprecipitation demonstration of the characteristic autoantibody profile, to be 44 percent non-Hodgkin's lymphoma (NHL), 19 percent chronic lymphocytic leukemia (CLL), 16 percent Castleman's disease (giant follicular hyperplasia), 8 percent thymoma (malignant and benign), 7 percent sarcomas that are retroperitoneal and often poorly differentiated, 4 percent Waldenström's macroglobulinemia, and in 2 percent no identified neoplasm. The majority of cases are associated with NHL and CLL, but the disproportionate representation of Castleman's disease is notable because of the rarity of this disorder. The association with Castleman's is even more striking in pediatric cases, where it is the underlying neoplasm in almost all cases.[5] Prior to the description of paraneoplastic pemphigus there were many cases of Castleman's disease associated with atypical forms of pemphigus, and we suspect most were cases of PNP.[6] Archived clinical material was available from one such case, which subsequently confirmed that the patient had autoantibodies specific for PNP.[7]

Almost without exception, more common cancers, such as adenocarcinomas of breast, bowel, and lung, or basal cell and squamous cell carcinoma of skin have not been associated with PNP. There are a few reports of PNP occurring with tumors such as squamous cell carcinoma, but most of these diagnoses have not been confirmed by immunochemical testing, so the association remains unproven.

The mechanisms by which these tumors induce autoimmunity against epithelial proteins remains speculative. One hypothesis states that the tumors constitutively or anomalously express epithelial proteins. These proteins are targeted by the antitumor immune response that cross-reacts with normal constitutive epithelial proteins of the host. This mechanism occurs in several neurologic paraneoplastic syndromes.[8] This antitumor immune response may be initiated by reactivity against plakin proteins, and the antitumor immune response may cross react with normal constitutive proteins of epithelia.

Alternate mechanisms are also possible, for it has been observed that treatment with cytokines may induce PNP,[9] raising the possibility of more complex interactions between the tumor cells and the immune system. There is some evidence that dysregulated cytokine production by tumor cells drives the development of autoimmunity. Patients with PNP have evidence of markedly elevated levels of interleukin 6 (IL-6).[10] It has been observed that in a subset of cases of non-Hodgkin's lymphomas,[11] CLL, and Castleman's tumors, the tumor cells will secrete massive amounts of IL-6 in vitro. IL-6 is known to promote B cell differentiation and to drive immunoglobulin production, and dysregulated IL-6 production has been implicated in certain autoimmune diseases. Castleman tumors are known to be associated with other autoimmune phenomena such as myasthenia gravis and autoimmune cytopenias, and these patients also have high serum levels of IL-6. Symptoms attributable to Castleman tumors are routinely reversed by complete excision of the affected node(s), and, coincidentally, serum IL-6 levels revert to normal. Administration of anti-IL-6 monoclonal antibodies will also effectively reverse systemic manifestations of Castleman's disease.[12]

Almost all patients have autoantibodies against desmogleins, demonstrable by enzyme-linked immunosorbent assay (ELISA), and when the desmoglein autoantibodies from these patients are injected into neonatal mice, acantholytic skin lesions are induced.[13] However, none of features of the disease that suggest cell-mediated autoimmunity[14] are recreated by immunoglobulin injections. No other internal organs are involved, and there is no lymphocyte-mediated cell damage. This is also an indication that humoral immunity alone will reproduce features of acantholysis, but passive transfer of autoimmune cells from these patients may be necessary to reproduce the complete spectrum of the disease in animals.

CLINICAL FEATURES

Dermatologic

The most constant clinical feature of the disease is the presence of intractable stomatitis (Fig. 60-1). This is the earliest presenting sign, and after treatment it is the one feature that persists throughout the course of the disease and is extremely resistant to therapy. This stomatitis consists of erosions and ulcerations that can affect all surfaces of the oropharynx. The lesions differ from those seen in pemphigus vulgaris in that they show more necrosis and lichenoid change. They also preferentially localize to the lateral borders of the tongue, and characteristically extend onto and involve the vermilion of the lips. Occasionally, oral lesions are the only manifestation of the disease.[15]

The cutaneous lesions of paraneoplastic pemphigus are quite variable, and different morphologies may occur in an individual patient according to the stage of the disease. The initial patients reported with the syndrome had episodes of waves of blistering affecting the upper trunk, head and neck, and proximal extremities. These lesions consisted of blisters that ruptured easily leaving erosions. The blisters on the extremities were sometimes quite tense, resembling those seen in bullous pemphigoid, or they had surrounding erythema, clinically resembling erythema multiforme. On the upper chest and back, confluent erosive lesions can develop, producing a picture resembling toxic epidermal necrolysis (TEN). The similarity of the mucocutaneous features to erythema multiforme/TEN explains why this is the most common differential diagnosis for PNP. However, it is important to note that erythema multiforme/TEN are self-limited events that evolve and resolve over several weeks, whereas PNP is a relentlessly progressive disease that continuously evolves over months.

Cutaneous lichenoid eruptions are very common and they may be the only cutaneous signs of the disease,[16] or may develop in lesions that had previously been blistered. When cutaneous lichenoid lesions are present, severe stomatitis is also invariably present. In the chronic form of the disease and after treatment, this lichenoid eruption may predominate over blistering on the cutaneous surface. Both blisters and

lichenoid lesions affecting the palms and the soles as well as the paronychial tissues are common, and help to distinguish this from pemphigus vulgaris in which acral and paronychial lesions are uncommon.

VARIANTS There are a small number of patients that appear to have PNP, but who do not have demonstrable circulating autoantibodies. These patients tend to have predominantly lichenoid skin and mucosal lesions, but behave in every other way like antibody-positive patients, and have the same underlying neoplasms. Because the definition of the disease relies so heavily on demonstration of the specific autoantibody markers, further study is required to know how to classify these patients.

The disease has also been identified in a horse[17] and a dog.[18] In animal species, the disease has the same associated neoplasms and clinical outcomes.

SYSTEMIC ASSOCIATIONS

PNP is the only form of pemphigus that has involvement of nonstratified squamous epithelium. Approximately 30 to 40 percent of cases will develop pulmonary injury, often with a fatal outcome.[19] The earliest symptoms are progressive dyspnea associated initially with an absence of findings on chest radiography. Pulmonary functions studies show airflow obstruction, involving large and small airways. Inflammation of the large airways evolves, and is evidenced by endoscopic biopsy showing acantholysis of bronchial respiratory epithelium. Pulmonary function deteriorates in most cases despite immunosuppressive therapy, and radiologic, histologic and functional changes characteristic of bronchiolitis obliterans develop.[20]

LABORATORY FINDINGS

The key finding is the serologic identification of polyclonal IgG autoantibodies against plakin proteins and, in most cases, desmogleins 1 and 3.[21] The plakins are a group of sequence-related proteins that form the intracellular plaque of desmosomes and hemidesmosomes, and mediate attachment of cytoskeletal intermediate filaments to transmembrane adhesion molecules such as the desmogleins. Autoantibodies against these proteins are the most characteristic surrogate markers for the disease. The pattern of antigens recognized by individual patients shows considerable variability, but the most characteristic and consistently recognized plakin antigens are envoplakin[22] and periplakin[23] (210 and 190 kDa, respectively). Next most frequently detected are antibodies against desmoplakin I and desmoplakin II (250 and 210 kDa, respectively). Less commonly, patients recognize bullous pemphigoid Ag 1 (230 kDa), plectin and plakoglobin. The identity and frequency of an antigen band at 170 kDa is not well defined. PNP patients may also have clinical and serologic evidence of other autoimmune phenomena such as myasthenia gravis and autoimmune cytopenias (Figs. 60-2 and 60-3).

To screen for PNP autoantibodies, one can test for IgG autoantibodies by indirect IF reactive with rodent urinary bladder epithelium. A positive result implies the presence of plakin autoantibodies; however, the sensitivity and specificity of this serologic test are only about 75 percent and 83 percent, respectively.[24] More specific and sensitive tests include immunoblotting against epidermal cell extracts that can effectively detect antibodies against envoplakin, periplakin, and desmoplakin, and

FIGURE 60-1

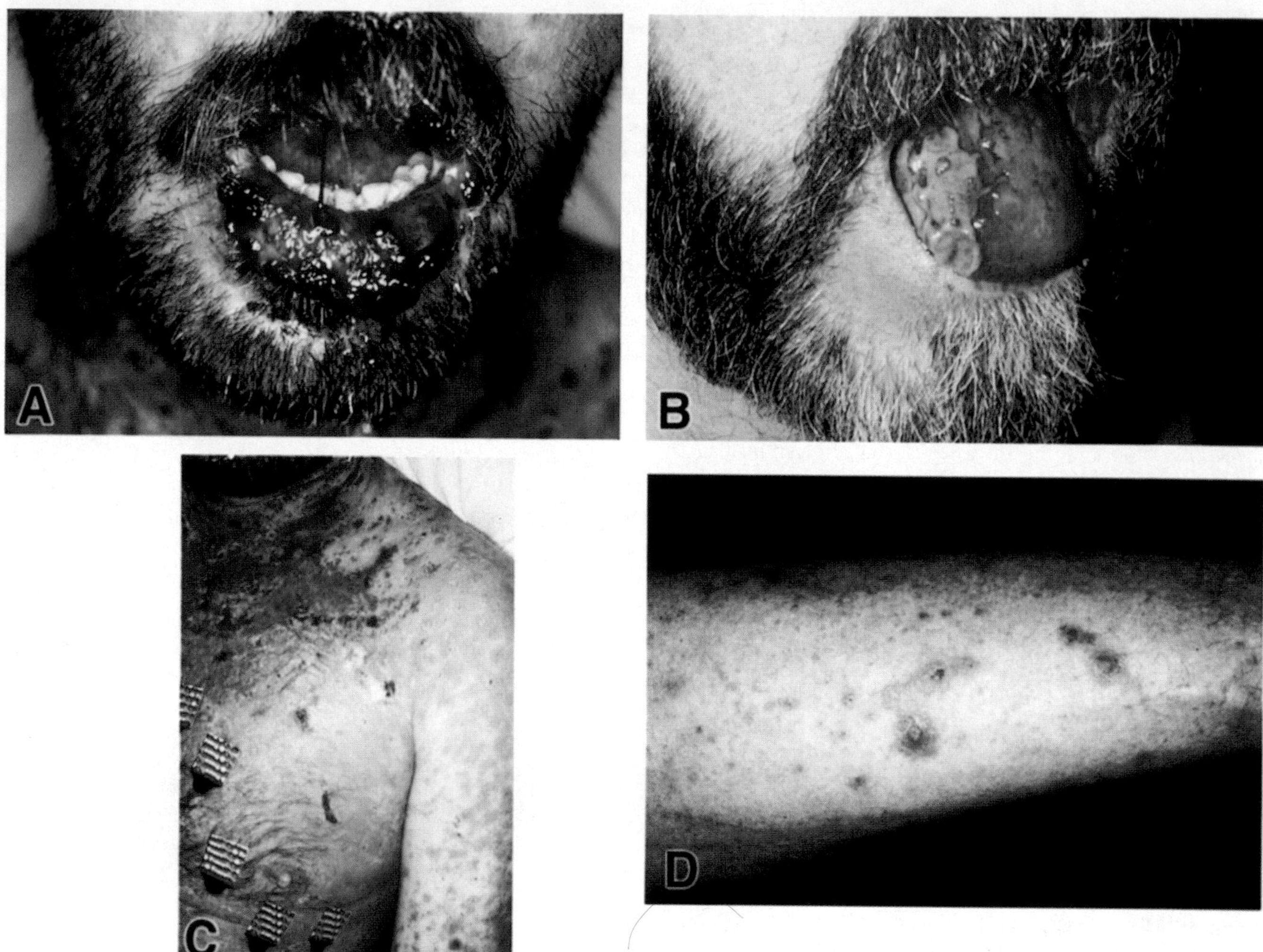

A. Extensive erosions involving the vermillion of the lips in a patient presenting with paraneoplastic pemphigus and an occult lymphoma. The characteristic severe stomatitis, accompanied by polymorphous cutaneous lesions are the most consistent features of the disease. *B.* Painful ulcerations tend to localize to the lateral border of the tongue. *C.* Lesions of the trunk from the same patient pictured in *A.* Erythematous macules and papules coalesce, and become erosive on the upper chest as the cutaneous lesions evolve. *D.* Lesions from the forearm of the same patient. These lesions clinically resemble erythema multiforme, but biopsy will show a mix of individual cell necrosis, interface change and acantholysis.

immunoprecipitation, using radiolabeled keratinocyte extracts, which can detect antibodies against any of the plakin proteins.

The PNP autoantibody profile is more complex than that observed in pemphigus vulgaris or foliaceus, where there are autoantibodies produced only against the desmogleins. The humoral immunity in PNP may represent an example of epitope spreading in which patients develop autoantibodies against structurally related plakin proteins and structurally unrelated transmembrane cell surface protein (the desmogleins) that are physically linked to the plakin proteins in the desmosome and hemidesmosome.[25]

PATHOLOGY

The histopathology of PNP is distinctive from pemphigus vulgaris and foliaceus for two reasons. First, because the lesions can be clinically very polymorphous, there is substantial variability in the histologic findings.[26,27] Second, findings due to cell-mediated cytotoxicity are frequently observed.

Biopsy of oral lesions is difficult to interpret because the mucositis is extremely severe and many biopsies will yield nonspecific changes of inflammation and ulceration. If one can biopsy perilesional epithelium, a lichenoid mucositis with variable degrees of individual cell necrosis and suprabasilar acantholysis can be observed.

When evaluating biopsies from skin lesions, one must recognize that lesions with different clinical morphologies will yield differing histologic findings. In noninflammatory cutaneous blisters, suprabasilar acantholysis is expected to be more prominent than the interface/lichenoid change (see Fig. 60-2*A*). When erythematous macules and papules are sampled, interface and lichenoid dermatitis will be predominant (see Fig. 60-2*B* and *C*). Lesions with a mixed clinical pattern will also show mixed histologic features of concomitant suprabasilar acantholysis and interface/lichenoid dermatitis.

There is also variability of the interface and lichenoid dermatitis observed. The spectrum of changes can include: (1) individual keratinocyte necrosis with lymphocytic infiltration into the epidermis, reminiscent of that seen in erythema multiforme or graft versus host disease; (2) vacuolar interface change with sparse lymphocytic infiltrate of the basilar epithelium, resembling cutaneous lupus erythematosus

FIGURE 60-2

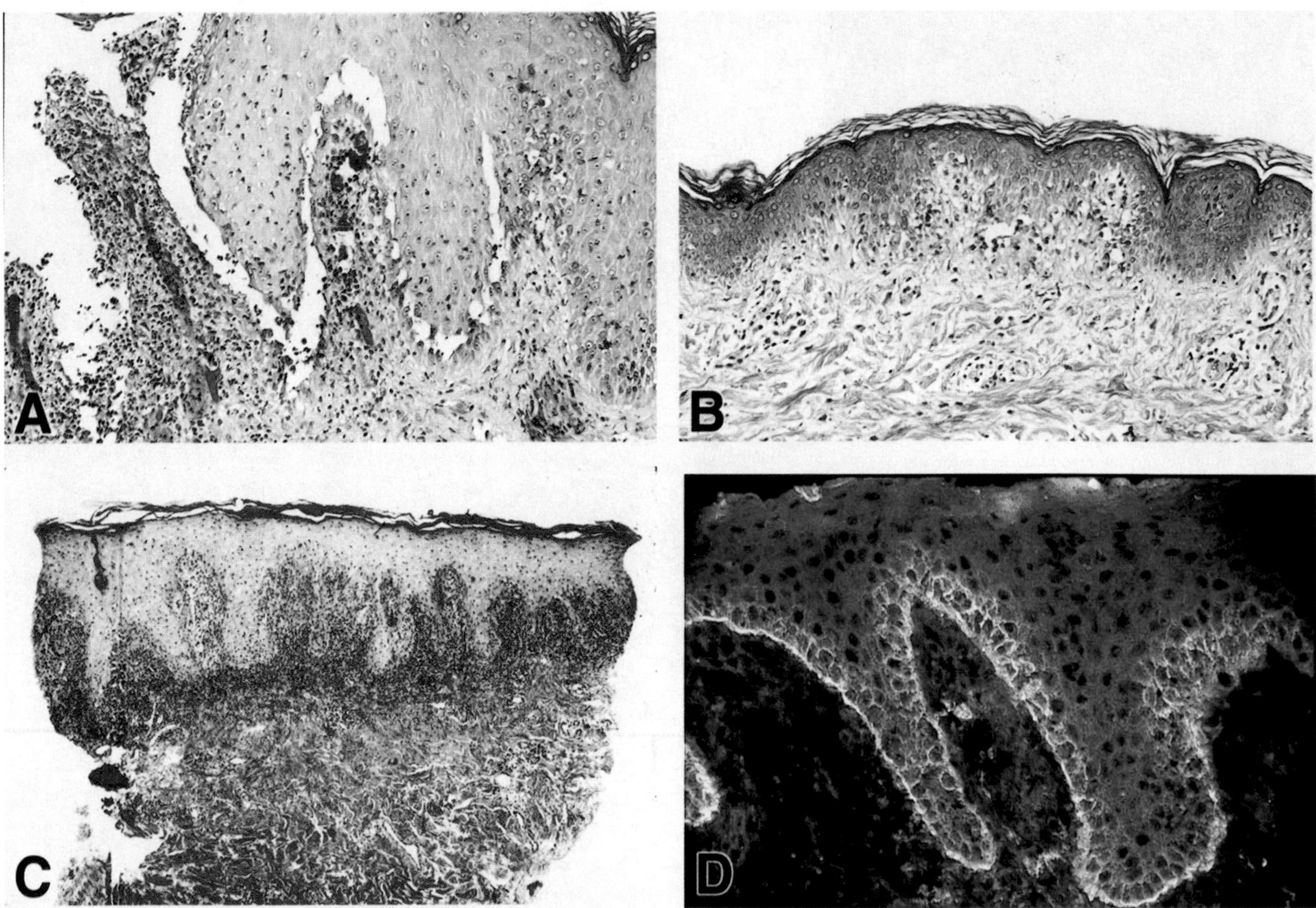

A. Histopathology of a blistering cutaneous lesion in PNP. This demonstrates the characteristic presence of vacuolar interface change and suprabasilar acantholysis. [hematoxylin and eosin (H&E), 200×] *B.* Macular and papular lesions may show just vacuolar interface change. (H&E, 100×) *C.* Lichenoid lesions demonstrate lichenoid infiltrates on histologic exam. (H&E, 40×) The presence of these varied histologic findings help differentiate PNP from pemphigus vulgaris. *D.* Direct immunofluorescence can be negative in a significant number of cases, but when positive, the most characteristic changes are those of deposition of IgG and complement components on both the surface of basilar and suprabasilar keratinocytes and along the epidermal basement membrane zone. (Immunofluorescence with fluoresceinated anti-IgG, 200×)

or dermatomyositis; and (3) a thick lichenoid band along the dermal–epidermal junction similar to that seen in lichen planus. Although most of the specimens show a complex overlap of histologic patterns, there is a relatively good correlation between the clinical and the predominant histologic pattern.

The histopathologic variability of this disease may be related to the fact that it is a presumed antitumor immune response. If this speculation is correct, one would expect to observe a combination of both humoral and cell-mediated immunity that is aberrantly directed against normal epithelium. In such a setting, one would expect to see changes of the sort described above. This degree of cell-mediated immunity is not seen in pemphigus vulgaris or foliaceous; hence the unique histopathologic features, and, presumably, the unique clinical features, as well.

IMMUNOPATHOLOGY

Patients should have evidence of IgG autoantibodies bound to the cell surface of affected epithelium by direct immunofluorescence. However, false negatives are more common in PNP than in pemphigus vulgaris and repeated biopsies may be necessary to demonstrate this finding. In a minority of cases, one might also see a combination of both cell surface and basement membrane zone deposition of IgG and complement components, but the absence of this combined cell surface/basement membrane zone staining does not negate the diagnosis.

DIAGNOSIS AND DIFFERENTIAL DIAGNOSIS

Not all patients demonstrate all of the five criteria that were originally proposed to define the disease. The following represent the minimal criteria for diagnosis of PNP with a high degree of confidence:

1. Painful, progressive stomatitis, with preferential involvement of the tongue. This finding is so consistent that the diagnosis should not be considered if stomatitis is absent.
2. Histologic features of acantholysis, lichenoid, or interface dermatitis. Although acantholysis is most readily detected in oral lesions, the necrosis and secondary inflammation makes this difficult to detect without repeated biopsies. Some patients never develop skin lesions. Some show only lesions that clinically and

FIGURE 60-3

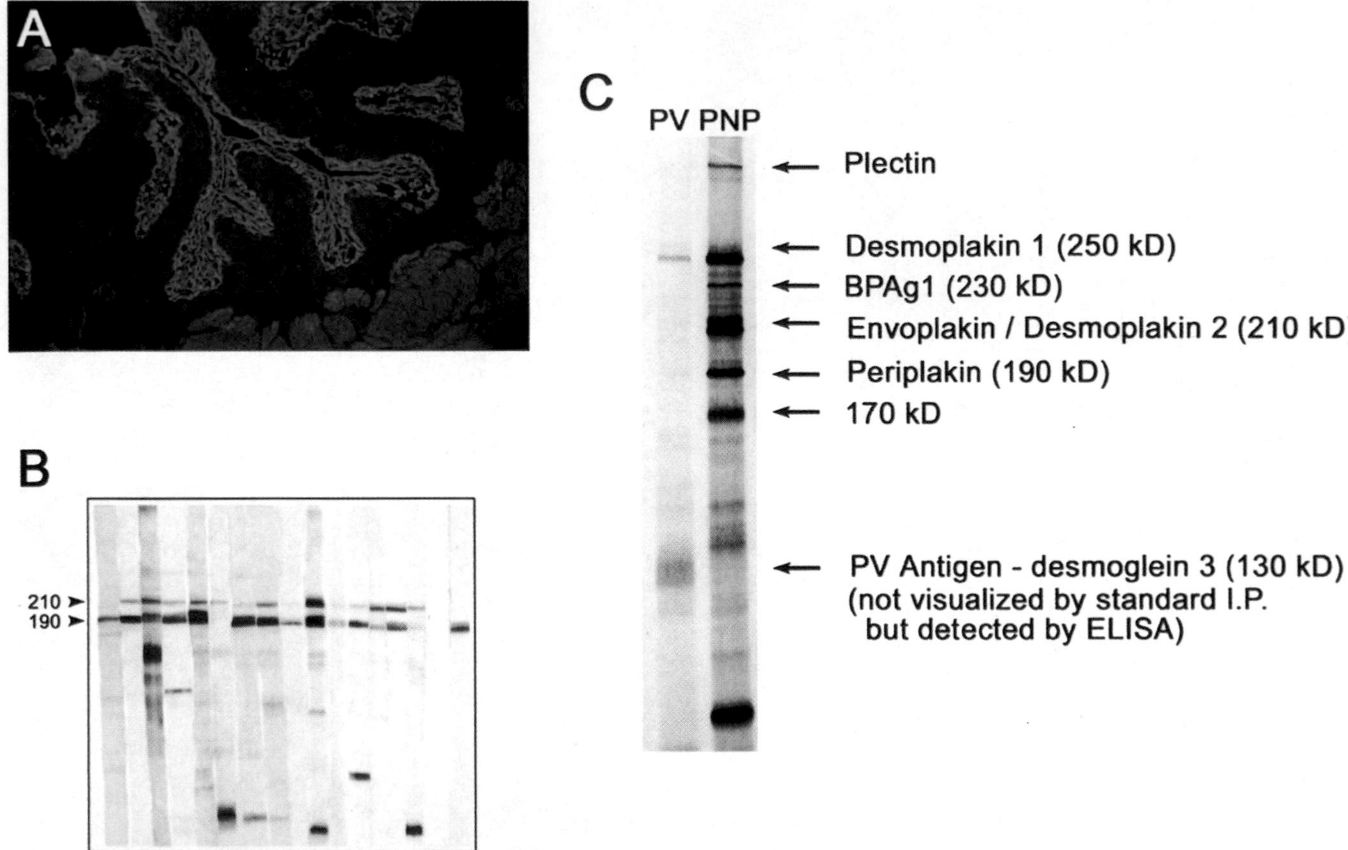

Diagnosis of PNP depends upon the demonstration of anti-plakin antibodies. **(A)** This can be accomplished by indirect immunofluorescence of patient serum on rodent urinary bladder demonstrating binding of IgG to the cell surface of transitional epithelial cells. A positive result implies the presence of anti-plakin antibodies. This technique, although easily performed, has the lowest sensitivity and specificty. **(B)** Immunoblotting against epidermal cell extracts is much more sensitive and specific. This shows detection of envoplakin (210 kD) and/or periplakin (190 kD) in 15 patients with PNP. Lane 16 is a normal control and lane 17 shows a monoclonal antibody against periplakin. This technique employs denatured antigen extracts, so it does not reliably detect some of the PNP antigens, but antibodies against the most characteristic plakin antigens, envoplakin and periplakin are easily detected. **(C)** Immunoprecipitation using radiolabeled, non-denatured epidermal extracts and serum from a patient with PNP and pemphigus vulgaris. In this case, the PNP patient's serum identifies all of the plakin antigens. Envoplakin and desmoplakin II migrate as a doublet at 210 kD. This technique is the most sensitive and specific test for demonstration of anti-plakin antibodies in PNP, but has limited availability. Although this technique readily detects the anti-plakin antibodies, desmoglein 3 is not always efficiently identified, and this is best shown by using ELISA.

histologically are lichenoid or resemble erythema multiforme. Direct immunofluorescence (IF) is very frequently negative, and the serologic markers for the disease are so specific that demonstration of tissue bound autoantibodies is not an essential criteria.

3. Demonstration of anti-plakin autoantibodies. These are the key serologic markers for the entity. Positive indirect IF on rodent bladder is readily available, but not highly reliable. Immunochemical techniques are much more precise and should demonstrate, at a minimum, autoantibodies against periplakin and/or envoplakin.[28] Patients with PNP should have a positive indirect IF test on monkey esophagus, and have antibodies against desmoglein 3 by ELISA, but this will not discriminate PNP from pemphigus vulgaris.
4. Demonstration of an underlying lymphoproliferative neoplasm. Approximately two-thirds of cases arise in the context of known malignant disease, most often NHL or CLL. In approximately one-third of cases, there is no known neoplastic lesion at the time the mucocutaneous disease develops. These cases tend to be associated with Castleman's disease, abdominal lymphoma, thymoma, or retroperitoneal sarcomas. In most cases, the occult neoplastic lesion can be detected by the investigations shown in Table 60-1. The most effective radiologic investigation is computed tomography of chest, abdomen, and pelvis, which will detect most of these neoplasms.

TABLE 60-1

Recommended Investigations for Suspect Paraneoplastic Pemphigus

- Biopsy skin or mucosa for H&E, direct immunofluorescence, serum for indirect immunofluorescence on monkey esophagus and rodent bladder epithelium
- Serum for immunoblotting or immunoprecipitation against epidermal extracts
- Complete blood count, chemistry panel, serum protein electrophoresis
- Examine liver, spleen, lymph nodes, and abdomen for organomegaly or masses
- Computed tomography of chest, abdomen and pelvis

Differential Diagnosis

The major differential diagnosis for patients with only oral involvement should include pemphigus vulgaris, oral lichen planus, and major aphthous stomatitis. Those with more lichenoid skin lesions and mucositis can closely resemble extensive lichen planus. Patients with skin and oral involvement most closely resemble erythema multiforme, TEN, or pemphigus vulgaris. There are a small number of patients with recurrent erythema multiforme major that have antibodies against desmoplakins, and will therefore have a positive indirect IF on bladder epithelium. These cases are distinguished from PNP because they do not have an underlying malignancy, and they do not have antibodies against the plakin proteins envoplakin and periplakin, which are more specific for PNP.[29]

TREATMENT AND PROGNOSIS

Systemic Treatment

Individuals with benign or encapsulated tumors such as Castleman's tumors or thymoma should have them surgically excised, for if the entire lesion can be excised, the disease generally improves substantially or goes into complete remission.[30] The remission of the autoimmune disease may take 1 to 2 years after surgery, so continued immunosuppression during this period is required. The usual treatment involves combined use of prednisone, 0.5 mg/kg, cyclosporine 5 mg/kg, and oral cyclophosphamide 2 mg/kg, tapering as symptoms improve. In pediatric cases with respiratory disease, the persistent autoimmunity immediately postsurgery can cause ongoing pulmonary injury, and lung transplantation might be required for long-term survival.[31]

In patients with malignant neoplasms, there is no consensus regarding a therapeutic regimen that is consistently effective. Although there are a couple of individual reports of long-term survivors,[32] almost all patients with NHL or CLL will succumb in a period of 1 month to 2 years after diagnosis. Oral corticosteroids in a dose of 0.5 to 1 mg/kg will produce partial improvement, but not complete resolution of lesions. Although cutaneous lesions respond more quickly to therapy, the stomatitis is generally quite refractory to any form of therapy. In addition to corticosteroids, many other agents have been tried in individual cases, but none have proven to be particularly effective. Methods that have been tried and that have generally failed include immunosuppression with cyclophosphamide or azathioprine, gold, dapsone, plasmapheresis, and photopheresis. A subset of patients, usually with CLL as an underlying neoplasm, have responded to a combination of prednisone, 0.5 to 1 mg/kg per day and cyclosporine, 5 mg/kg per day.[33] Additional treatment with intermittent pulse cyclophosphamide to control the underlying CLL was also used in many of these cases, and this also may have contributed to the good outcome. Some patients have shown improvement after treatment with rituximab in combination with prednisone and cyclophosphamide.[34] It is not known why PNP is so refractory to the type of immunosuppressive treatments that usually work well in pemphigus vulgaris and other autoimmune diseases.

In those patients who do succumb, death has been attributed in individual cases to multiple factors including sepsis, gastrointestinal bleeding, "multiorgan failure," and respiratory failure. Patients with autoimmune disease associated with B cell neoplasms are known to have a high frequency of autoimmune cytopenias, and some fatal episodes of sepsis are suspect to have occurred because of sudden and unexplained neutropenia, possibly due to this mechanism. Respiratory failure is a common terminal event. The development of shortness of breath with obstructive disease progressing to bronchiolitis obliterans is a terminal pathway in most cases. Because these patients have autoantibodies that react with desmoplakins, and because desmoplakins are present in respiratory epithelium, respiratory failure may be due to autoantibody-mediated injury to bronchial epithelium, with plugging of terminal bronchioles, resulting in airflow obstruction and ventilation/perfusion abnormalities. Additionally, direct damage to alveolar epithelium could cause a diffusion barrier and subsequent intractable hypoxia. These mechanisms are speculative at present. The pulmonary injury does not respond to medical treatment, and the development of shortness of breath and hypoxia in a patient with this syndrome is an ominous prognostic sign.

In patients with malignant neoplasms there is no definite correlation between tumor burden and the activity of the autoimmune syndrome. Treatment of the primary malignancy does not affect the activity of the autoimmune disease. It seems that once the process in initiated by the malignancy, the autoimmunity progresses independently. An example of the disconnect between tumor burden and autoimmunity is found in the case reported by Fullerton et al.[19] in which paraneoplastic pemphigus occurred after successful autologous bone marrow transplantation for non-Hodgkin's lymphoma. This patient was free of detectable tumor burden at the time of his death, but died from pulmonary injury secondary to paraneoplastic pemphigus. It is notable that the patient underwent autologous bone marrow transplantation, and therefore received his own memory T cells, or possibly individual malignant lymphoid cells that were not detectable by routine autopsy methods.

REFERENCES

1. Anhalt GJ et al: Paraneoplastic pemphigus: An autoimmune mucocutaneous disease associated with neoplasia. *N Engl J Med* **323**:1729, 1990
2. Redon J et al: Pemphigus associated with giant lymph node hyperplasia. *Br Med J* **287**:176, 1983
3. Matsuoka LY et al: Epidermal autoantibodies in erythema multiforme. *J Am Acad Dermatol* **21**:677, 1989
4. Panielieyva GA: Paraneoplastic bullous dermatoses. *Vestn Dermatol Venerol* **2**:50, 1990
5. Mimouni D et al: Paraneoplastic pemphigus in children and adolescents. *Br J Dermatol* **147**:725, 2002
6. Tagami H et al: Severe erosive stomatitis and giant lymph node hyperplasia of retroperitoneum (Castleman's tumor). *Dermatologica* **157**:138, 1978
7. Plewig G et al: Castleman tumor, lichen ruber und pemphigus vulgaris: Paraneoplastiche assoziation immunologischer erkrankungen? *Hautarzt* **41**:662, 1990
8. Kornguth SE: Neuronal proteins and paraneoplastic syndromes. *N Engl J Med* **321**:1607, 1989
9. Kirsner RS et al: Treatment with alpha interferon associated with the development of paraneoplastic pemphigus. *Br J Dermatol* **132**:474, 1995
10. Nousari HC et al: Elevated levels of interleukin-6 in paraneoplastic pemphigus. *J Invest Dermatol* **112**:396, 1999
11. Yee C et al: A possible autocrine role for interleukin-6 in two lymphoma cell lines. *Blood* **74**:798, 1989
12. Beck JT et al: Alleviation of systemic manifestations of Castleman's disease by monoclonal anti–interleukin-6 antibody. *N Engl J Med* **330**:602, 1994
13. Amagai M et al: Antibodies against desmoglein 3 (pemphigus vulgaris antigen) are present in sera from patients with paraneoplastic pemphigus and cause acantholysis in vivo in neonatal mice. *J Clin Invest* **102**:775, 1998
14. Reich K et al: Graft-versus-host disease-like immunophenotype and apoptotic keratinocyte death in paraneoplastic pemphigus. *Br J Dermatol* **141**:739, 1999
15. Bialy-Golan A et al: Paraneoplastic pemphigus: Oral involvement as the sole manifestation. *Acta Derm Venerol* **76**:253, 1996
16. Stevens SR et al: Paraneoplastic pemphigus presenting as a lichen planus pemphigoides-like eruption. *Arch Dermatol* **129**:866, 1993
17. Williams MA et al: Paraneoplastic bullous stomatitis in a horse. *J Am Vet Med Assoc* **207**:331, 1995
18. de Bruin A et al: Periplakin and envoplakin are target antigens in canine and human paraneoplastic pemphigus. *J Am Acad Dermatol* **40**:682, 1999
19. Fullerton SH et al: Paraneoplastic pemphigus with immune deposits in bronchial epithelium. *JAMA* **267**:1550, 1992

20. Nousari HC et al: The mechanism of respiratory failure in paraneoplastic pemphigus. *N Engl J Med* **340**:1406, 1999
21. Ohyama M et al: Clinical phenotype and anti-desmoglein autoantibody profile in paraneoplastic pemphigus. *J Am Acad Dermatol* **44**:593, 2001
22. Kim SC et al: cDNA cloning of the 210-kDa paraneoplastic pemphigus antigen reveals that envoplakin is a component of the antigen complex. *J Invest Dermatol* **109**:365, 1997
23. Mahoney MG et al: The members of the plakin family of proteins recognized by paraneoplastic pemphigus antibodies include periplakin. *J Invest Dermatol* **111**:308, 1998
24. Helou J et al: Accuracy of indirect immunofluorescent testing in the diagnosis of paraneoplastic pemphigus. *J Am Acad Dermatol* **32**:44, 1995
25. Craft J, Fatenetad S. Self antigens and epitope spreading in systemic autoimmunity *Arthritis Rheum* **40**:1374, 1997
26. Horn TD, Anhalt GJ: Histologic features of paraneoplastic pemphigus. *Arch Dermatol* **128**:1091, 1991
27. Mehregan DR et al: Paraneoplastic pemphigus: A subset of patients with pemphigus and neoplasia. *J Cutan Pathol* **20**:203, 1993
28. Kiyokawa C et al: Envoplakin and periplakin are components of the paraneoplastic pemphigus antigen complex. *J Invest Dermatol* **111**:1236, 1998
29. Foedinger D et al: Autoantibodies to desmoplakin I and II in patients with erythema multiforme. *J Exp Med* **181**:169, 1995
30. Jansen T, Plewig G: Castleman tumor, lichen ruber and pemphigus vulgaris: Paraneoplastic association of immunologic disease (letter)? *Hautarzt* **42**:727, 1991
31. Chin AC et al: Paraneoplastic pemphigus and bronchiolitis obliterans associated with a mediastinal mass: A rare case of Castleman's disease with respiratory failure requiring lung transplantation. *J Pediatr Surg* **36**:E22, 2001
32. Camisa C et al: Paraneoplastic pemphigus: A report of three cases including one long-term survivor. *J Am Acad Dermatol* **27**:547, 1992
33. Ståhle-Backdähl M et al: Paraneoplastic pemphigus: A report of two patients responding to cyclosporine. *Eur J Dermatol* **5**:671, 1995
34. Borradori L et al: Anti-CD20 monoclonal antibody (rituximab) for refractory erosive stomatitis secondary to CD20(+) follicular lymphoma-associated paraneoplastic pemphigus. *Arch Dermatol* **137**:269, 2001

CHAPTER 61

John R. Stanley

Bullous Pemphigoid

Bullous pemphigoid is a subepidermal blistering skin disease, usually occurring in the elderly, that is characterized by large, tense blisters and the immunopathologic findings of C3 (the third component of complement) and IgG at the epidermal basement membrane zone. Mucous membranes are spared in most cases, with the exception of nonscarring bullae or erosions of the oral mucous membranes in a minority of patients.

Walter Lever was a pioneer in classifying bullous pemphigoid as a disease different from pemphigus with its own distinctive clinical and histologic features.[1] This was important because at the time pemphigus vulgaris usually was fatal, whereas bullous pemphigoid had a comparatively good prognosis. This classification of bullous pemphigoid and pemphigus was confirmed and fully justified by the distinctive immunopathologic features of these diseases discovered about 12 years later.[2,3]

EPIDEMIOLOGY

The majority of patients with bullous pemphigoid are over 60 years old at the age of onset.[4] Although bullous pemphigoid does occur rarely in children,[5] reports earlier than about 1970 (when the use of immunofluorescence for diagnosis became more widespread) were inaccurate because these most likely included children with chronic bullous disease of childhood, which is now differentiated from bullous pemphigoid by the presence of IgA, rather than IgG, at the basement membrane zone. There is no known ethnic, racial, or sexual predilection for developing bullous pemphigoid. The incidence of bullous pemphigoid is estimated to be 7 per million per year in both France and Germany.[6,7]

ETIOLOGY AND PATHOGENESIS

Electron Microscopy

Ultrastructural studies demonstrate that early blister formation in bullous pemphigoid occurs in the lamina lucida, between the basal cell membrane and the lamina densa.[8] With blister formation, there is loss of anchoring filaments and hemidesmosomes. With degranulation of infiltrating leukocytes, there is fragmentation and ultimate loss of the lamina densa.[9] In addition, degranulation of mast cells near the epidermal basement membrane has been observed both by light and electron microscopy.[10]

Immunopathology

Direct immunofluorescence of perilesional skin from pemphigoid patients reveals immunoreactants deposited in a linear pattern at the epidermal basement membrane.[2,3] C3 is detected in almost all patients, sometimes as the sole immunoreactant; however, IgG is also detected in most patients.[11–13] (Fig. 61-1*A*).

Indirect immunofluorescence indicates that about 70 to 80 percent of patients with bullous pemphigoid have circulating IgG that binds to the basement membrane of normal stratified squamous epithelia, such as human epidermis or monkey esophagus[11–14] (Fig. 61-1*B*). Most patients with circulating anti–basement membrane IgG also have anti–basement membrane IgE in their sera.[15,16] If the immunofluorescence substrate is incubated first in 1 *M* NaCl to separate the epidermis from the dermis at the lamina lucida, then an even higher percentage of

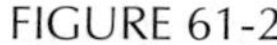

FIGURE 61-1

A.

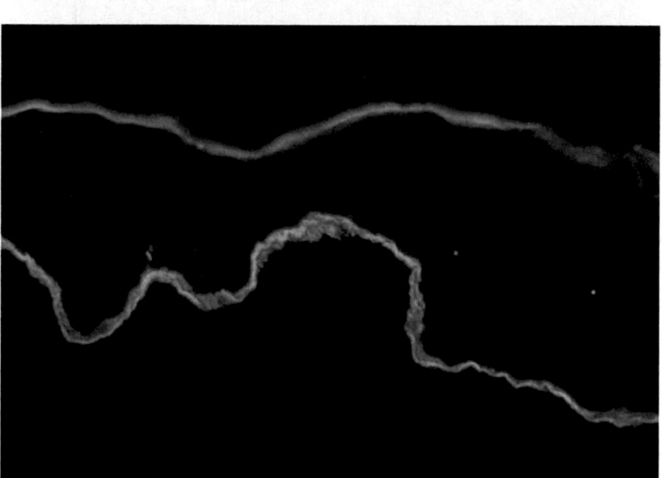

B.

Immunofluorescence in bullous pemphigoid. *A.* Direct immunofluorescence of perilesional skin shows a linear band of C3 (×340). *B.* Indirect immunofluorescence shows a linear pattern of IgG binding to the epidermal basement membrane of normal skin (×340).

FIGURE 61-2

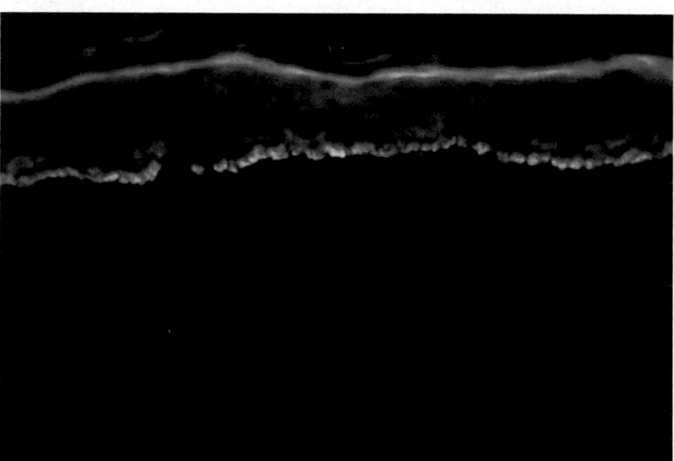

A.

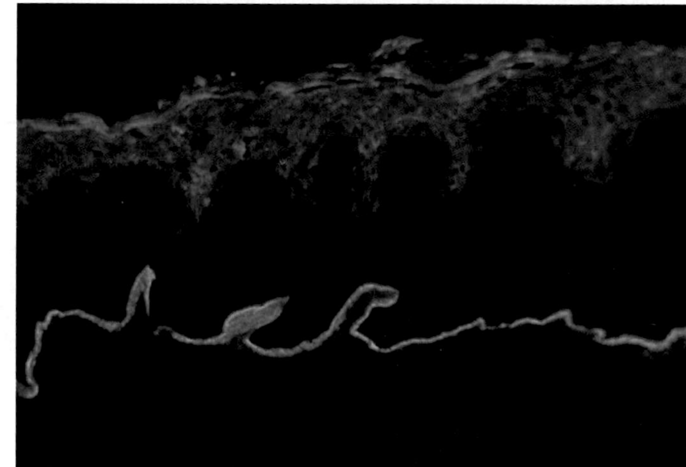

B.

Indirect immunofluorescence on normal skin previously incubated in 1 *M* NaCl. *A.* IgG from bullous pemphigoid serum binds to the roof of the artificial blister (×330). *B.* IgG in epidermolysis bullosa acquisita serum binds to the base (×215).

patients will have detectable circulating antibody.[17,18] Besides being more sensitive, the other advantage of this 1 *M* NaCl-split substrate is that bullous pemphigoid antibodies bind to the roof of the artificially induced blister (i.e., the bottom of the basal cells) and thus can be differentiated from the antibodies of patients with epidermolysis bullosa acquisita; their antibodies bind the base (i.e., dermal side) (Fig. 61-2). In contrast to pemphigus, in bullous pemphigoid the indirect immunofluorescence antibody titer does not usually correlate with disease extent or activity[19].

In addition to C3, other components of both the classical and alternative complement pathways and the complement regulatory protein β1H are deposited at the epidermal basement membrane zone in bullous pemphigoid patients.[20–22] Furthermore, activated complement components are found in the blister fluid of these patients, and in vitro complement fixation immunofluorescence assays indicate the ability of bullous pemphigoid sera to fix complement components of the classical and alternative pathways to the epidermal basement membrane. These studies suggest that bullous pemphigoid IgG causes complement activation by the classical pathway, with activation of the alternative pathway by the C3 amplification mechanism.

Pemphigoid Antigens

Immunoelectron microscopic studies have localized bullous pemphigoid antigen in the hemidesmosome, an organelle important in anchoring the basal cell to the basement membrane.[23,24] Autoantibodies bind both inside the cell to the plaque of the hemidesmosome and outside the cell to the extracellular face of the hemidesmosome.

Molecular characterization of bullous pemphigoid antigen by immunochemical methods revealed the unexpected finding that autoantibodies from these patients bind two distinct molecules.[25] Essentially all bullous pemphigoid patients have antibodies against a 230-kDa molecule.[26] Cloning of the cDNA encoding this molecule (now called *BPAG1* or *BPAG1e)* indicated that it belongs to a gene family that includes desmoplakin I, a desmosome plaque protein that is important in anchoring keratin intermediate filaments to the desmosome.[27,28] BPAG1e has been localized ultrastructurally to the plaque of the hemidesmosome, exactly where keratin intermediate filaments insert.[29] Further proof that the function of BPAGle is to anchor keratin intermediate filaments to the hemidesmosome was obtained by analysis of a mouse that was genetically engineered with a targeted deletion of this molecule.[30] This mouse showed fragility of basal cells due to collapse of the keratin filament network but no epidermal-dermal adhesion defect, suggesting that bullous pemphigoid antibodies do not act by inhibiting the function of BPAG1e. In fact, since BPAG1e is inside the cell, it is unclear if patient autoantibodies normally have access to it. Interestingly, an alternatively spliced form of BPAG1e is expressed in neural tissue. Now termed BPAG1n, this form stabilizes the cytoskeleton of sensory nerves,[31,32] just as BPAG1e stabilizes the cytoskeleton of epidermal cells.

Immunochemical studies have revealed that almost all patients with bullous pemphigoid, as well as patients with herpes gestationis, also have autoantibodies against a 180-kDa molecule now called BPAG2 or *type XVII collagen*.[33–35] The cDNA encoding the BPAG2 molecule has been cloned, and the expressed protein is a transmembrane molecule with a collagenous extracellular domain.[36] Antibodies against BPAG2 localize it as a transmembrane molecule at the hemidesmosome, and cell biologic studies indicate that its cytoplasmic domain targets it to that location.[37,38] The extracellular domain of BPAG2 has been localized to anchoring filaments.[39] The autoantibodies from most patients with bullous pemphigoid (as well as those from patients with herpes gestationis) recognize a particular epitope in a small noncollagenous region of BPAG2 that is just outside the membrane.[40,41] As discussed below, antibodies against this epitope are capable of mediating subepidermal blister formation in neonatal mice. In addition, antibody titers against this epitope, as determined by enzyme-linked immunoassay, correlate with disease activity.[16] Further evidence that BPAG2 mediates epidermal-dermal adhesion comes from analysis of the gene defect in patients with the genetic subepidermal blistering disease *generalized atrophic benign epidermolysis bullosa*. These patients have recessively inherited mutations in the *BPAG2* gene that result in a missing or dysfunctional protein.[42]

Not only patients with bullous pemphigoid and herpes gestationis but also patients with linear IgA disease, cicatricial pemphigoid, and lichen planus pemphigoides have antibodies against BPAG2 or its metabolic products.[43]

Pathophysiology of Lesion Production

Autoantibodies, particularly those against BPAG2, detected in patients with bullous pemphigoid are probably pathogenic. Bullous pemphigoid IgG injected into rabbit cornea fixes to the basement membrane and causes subepithelial blister formation.[44] Furthermore, it has been demonstrated that antibodies against BPAG2 can induce disease by passive transfer to neonatal mice.[45] In these studies, antibodies were raised in rabbits against the epitope on mouse BPAG2 that corresponds to the epitope that most human bullous pemphigoid and herpes gestationis sera recognize. Passive transfer of these rabbit antibodies to neonatal mice induces blisters with histology very similar to that of bullous pemphigoid lesions. In this model, complement, neutrophils, and neutrophil elastase are necessary for anti-BPAG2 induction of blister formation.[46] In vitro studies with normal human skin sections indicate that the bullous pemphigoid IgG is capable of activating complement by the classical pathway, thereby causing leukocyte adherence to the basement membrane, with degranulation and resulting dermal-epidermal separation.[47]

The preceding immunopathologic observations are consistent with proposed pathophysiologic explanations for blister formation in bullous pemphigoid.[48] The initial step in blister formation is postulated to be antibody binding to the bullous pemphigoid antigen. Fixation of IgG to the basement membrane activates the classical complement cascade and probably also the C3 amplification mechanism. Activated complement components cause chemotaxis of leukocytes as well as degranulation of mast cells. Mast cell products cause chemotaxis of eosinophils through mediators such as eosinophil chemotactic factor of anaphylaxis. Finally, leukocyte and mast cell proteases result in dermal-epidermal separation. For example, eosinophils, the predominant inflammatory cell at the basement membrane in bullous pemphigoid lesions, produce a gelatinase that cleaves the collagenous extracellular domain of BPAG2, probably contributing to blister formation.[49]

In light of identification of the bullous pemphigoid antigens as components of the hemidesmosome, it also must be considered that antibodies may interfere directly with the function of this organelle, thought to be important in anchoring the basal cells to the basement membrane. In this regard, a mechanism of blister formation in which antibodies against BPAG2 interfere with hemidesmosome formation has been proposed.[50]

As in most autoimmune diseases, the cause of the induction of autoantibody production in bullous pemphigoid remains obscure, although the overexpression of the class II major histocompatability complex (MHC) allele *DQβ1*0301* in bullous pemphigoid patients suggests that presentation of BPAG2 peptides to the immune system in a way that causes disease is restricted to individuals with certain immune response genes.[51]

CLINICAL MANIFESTATIONS

Skin and Mucous Membrane Involvement

The skin lesion characteristic of bullous pemphigoid is a large, tense blister arising on normal skin or on an erythematous base[4] (Fig. 61-3*A*). These lesions are most common on the lower abdomen, inner or anterior thighs, and flexor forearms, although they may occur anywhere. The bullae usually are filled with clear fluid but may be hemorrhagic. Eroded skin from ruptured blisters usually shows a good tendency to reepithelialize, and unlike pemphigus vulgaris, these erosions do not tend to expand at the periphery. However, new, discrete vesicles may form at the edge of old, resolving lesions. The lesions of bullous pemphigoid do not scar. There is usually, but not always, marked pruritus.

Sometimes the erythematous component predominates, and patients may present with urticarial lesions, especially early in the course of disease (see Fig. 61-3*B*). The erythematous component also can appear serpiginous, with peripheral blisters, and may be quite extensive (Fig. 61-4). Resolution usually occurs from the center and may be accompanied by hyperpigmentation.

Mucous membrane lesions occur in about 10 to 35 percent of patients and are almost always limited to the oral mucous membranes, especially the buccal mucosa.[4,11] Intact blisters or, more usually, erosions are seen. These do not scar and usually are not extensive. Unlike erythema multiforme, the vermillion border of the lips is involved rarely.

In addition to the characteristic clinical findings described earlier, there have been descriptions of bullous pemphigoid with unusual presentations.[52] In all these cases, the diagnosis has been confirmed by immunofluorescence findings. For example, lesions in bullous pemphigoid sometimes are localized, most commonly to the lower legs.[53] These patients with localized disease have antibodies against the same pemphigoid antigens described earlier[54,55] and they may go on to generalized bullous pemphigoid or remain localized for years. There is a specific type of localized pemphigoid described in childhood in which blisters and erosions are limited to the vulvar and perivulvar area.[56] As in other forms of localized pemphigoid and childhood pemphigoid, antibodies from this disease bind the pemphigoid antigens.[5,56] Not infrequently, especially early in disease, patients may have only urticarial

FIGURE 61-3

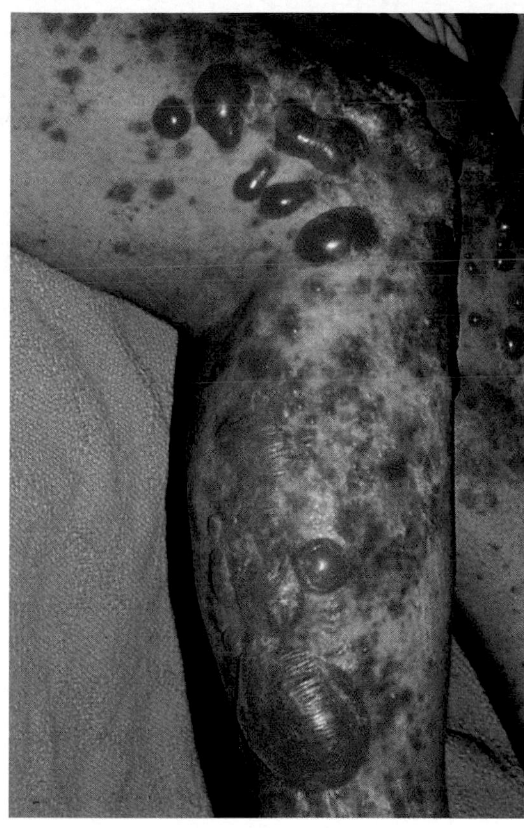

A.

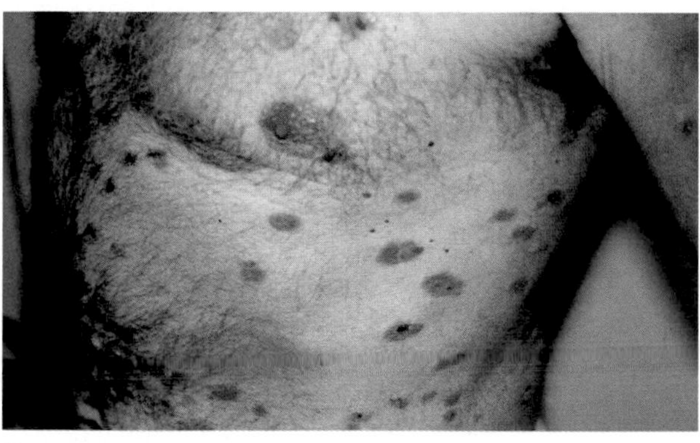

B.

Bullous pemphigoid. *A.* Large, tense bullae and erythematous macules on the thighs and lower legs. (*Courtesy of James Fitzpatrick, MD.*) *B.* Urticarial lesions of bullous pemphigoid.

FIGURE 61-4

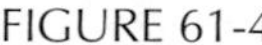

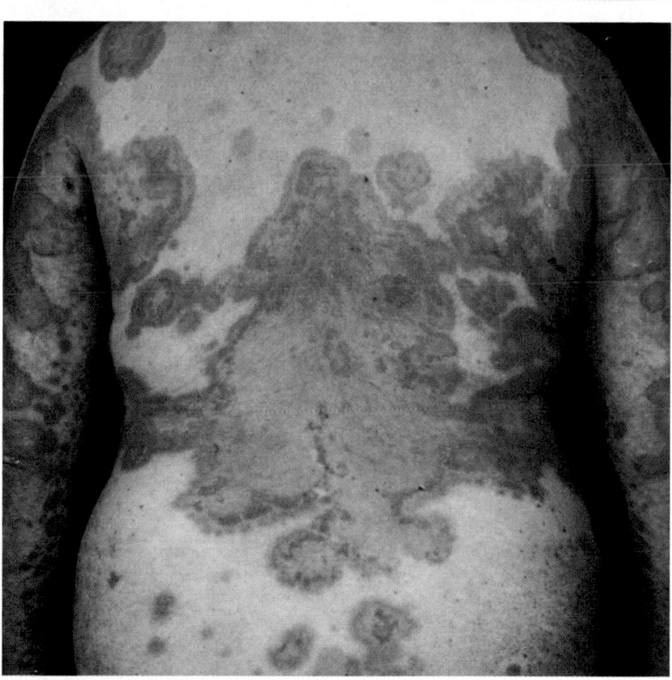

A.

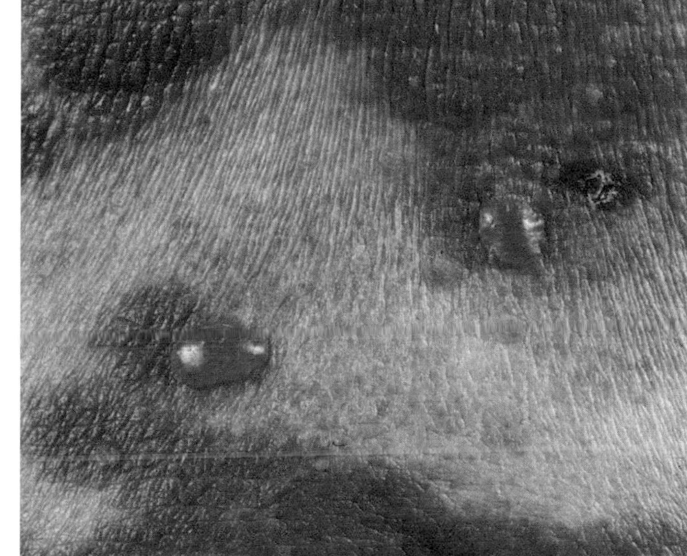

B.

Bullous pemphigoid. *A.* Extensive urticarial, inflammatory plaques with central regression and hyperpigmentation. *B.* Large, tense bullae and erythematous urticarial-type lesions.

and eczematous lesions without bullae. Other less usual presentations include erythroderma, prurigo nodularis-like or vegetating lesions, and dyshidrotic dermatitis-like lesions. Again, the antibodies from these patients show typical immunofluorescence localization and bind the pemphigoid antigens.[57–60]

Precipitating Factors

Most cases of bullous pemphigoid occur sporadically without any obvious precipitating factors. However, there are several reports of precipitation of bullous pemphigoid by ultraviolet (UV) light, either UVB or psoralens with UVA, and radiation therapy.[61–64]

Laboratory Abnormalities

In addition to the immunopathologic features described earlier, almost one-half of patients will have elevated total serum IgE, levels of which are positively correlated with IgG anti–basement membrane zone immunofluorescence titers.[13,65,66] Furthermore, elevated levels of IgE correlate with the presence of pruritus.[13] Finally, about one-half of patients have peripheral blood eosinophilia, sometimes marked, but not correlated with serum IgE levels.[13,67]

Associated Diseases

There have been many case reports of bullous pemphigoid associated with malignancy. However, bullous pemphigoid occurs in elderly patients, as does malignancy, and case-control studies suggest that there is no increase, or a very small increase, in the incidence of malignancy in patients compared with age-matched controls.[68–70] However, there may be an increased incidence of malignancy in bullous pemphigoid patients with negative indirect immunofluorescence as compared with those with positive indirect immunofluorescence.[11,71] Whether this increase means that in indirect immunofluorescence–negative patients with bullous pemphigoid there is an overall increased incidence of malignancy compared with age-matched controls is not known. Most authors agree that, other than a general physical examination and good review of systems, an extensive screening workup for an asymptomatic malignancy is not indicated for a bullous pemphigoid patient.

The coexistence of bullous pemphigoid and lichen planus, referred to as *lichen planus pemphigoides,* has been well documented.[72] These cases show typical clinical, histologic, and immunopathologic features of both diseases. It is postulated that anti–basement membrane zone antibodies develop as a consequence of the damage induced by the T cell lymphocytic infiltrate at the basement membrane in lichen planus. Some authors have reported an association of bullous pemphigoid with various other autoimmune diseases, including pemphigus.[73–76] These associations occur only rarely. Finally, there may be a slight increased incidence of psoriasis in bullous pemphigoid patients as compared with age-matched controls.[77,78]

FIGURE 61-5

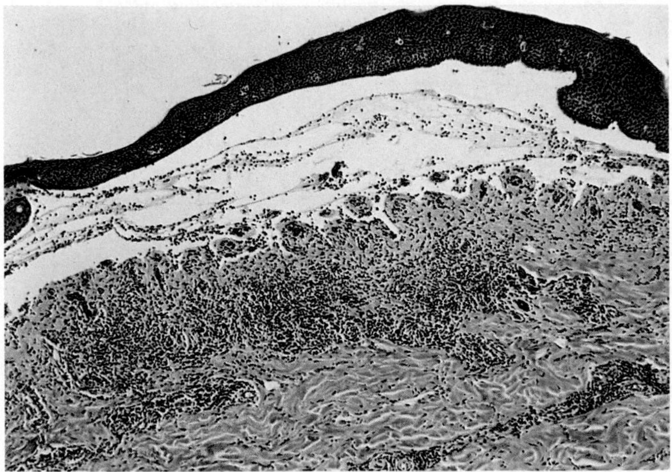

A.

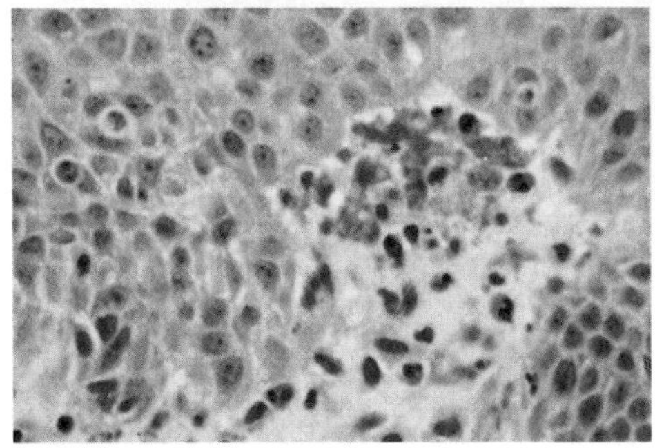

B.

Histopathology of bullous pemphigoid. *A.* Subepidermal blister with an inflammatory cell infiltrate, containing eosinophils, in the superficial dermis. *B.* Degranulating eosinophils at the epidermal basement membrane and eosinophilic spongiosis.

PATHOLOGY

Biopsy of an early small blister is most diagnostic. Histology of such a biopsy will show a subepidermal blister without epidermal necrosis and a superficial dermal infiltrate consisting characteristically of lymphocytes, histiocytes, and eosinophils[4] (Fig. 61-5*A*). The degree of the infiltrate ranges from intense to sparse, but it characteristically contains some eosinophils. Biopsies from blisters arising on erythematous bases tend to have more extensive infiltrates. Eosinophils are also seen often in the blister cavity. Neutrophils may be seen in the infiltrate, but in contrast to histologic findings in dermatitis herpetiformis, they seldom form microabscesses in the papillary tips. Urticarial lesions may show only a superficial dermal infiltrate of lymphocytes, histiocytes, and eosinophils with papillary dermal edema. Histology of these urticarial lesions also may display degranulating eosinophils at the dermal-epidermal junction, with early separation of individual basal cells from the basement membrane and/or eosinophilic spongiosis[79] (See Fig. 61-5*B*).

DIFFERENTIAL DIAGNOSIS

Bullous pemphigoid can be differentiated easily from most other blistering diseases, such as linear IgA disease, chronic bullous disease of childhood, dermatitis herpetiformis, erythema multiforme, and pemphigus, by histology and immunofluorescence. The most difficult diseases to differentiate from bullous pemphigoid are epidermolysis bullosa acquisita (EBA) and cicatricial pemphigoid.[80,81] EBA usually can be distinguished by clinical criteria if it presents as a noninflammatory mechanobullous disease (see Chap. 67). However, occasionally it may present as an inflammatory disease that may be similar clinically and histologically to bullous pemphigoid.[80] By routine direct and indirect immunofluorescence, these diseases also may show indistinguishable findings. However, EBA may be distinguished from bullous pemphigoid by indirect or direct immunofluorescence on skin incubated in 1 *M* sodium chloride to cause a split in the lamina lucida, as discussed earlier[82] (see Fig. 61-2). Immunoelectron microscopy also distinguishes these diseases because the IgG in EBA is below the lamina densa on the anchoring fibrils,[83] whereas the IgG in bullous pemphigoid is closely associated with the basal cell hemidesmosomes. Finally, autoantibodies from EBA patients bind type VII collagen.[84]

As opposed to bullous pemphigoid, cicatricial pemphigoid usually manifests clinical activity predominantly, if not exclusively, on mucous membranes (see Chap. 62). Cicatricial pemphigoid is characterized by desquamative gingivitis as well as inflammation and scarring of conjunctiva. If there is blistering of the skin, it may be transient or may result in scarring. Large, tense blisters, which are characteristic of bullous pemphigoid, are usually not seen in cicatricial pemphigoid.

TREATMENT AND PROGNOSIS

Bullous pemphigoid, even without therapy, is often a self-limited disease, but it may last from several months to many years. Lever[4] reported that 8 of 30 adults with bullous pemphigoid, before the advent of glucocorticoid therapy, went into remission after about 15 months (range 3–38 months) of active disease. Eight of these patients, all above 65 years of age, died with bullous pemphigoid as a contributing cause of death, whereas none of 16 adult patients less than 65 years of age died. A more recent study of bullous pemphigoid patients, mean age 79, showed a 17 and 31 percent mortality at 3 and 6 months, respectively, mainly from sepsis and cardiovascular disease.[85] Old age (>86 years old), poor general health, and generalized disease were associated with poor prognosis, as might be expected. Other authors feel that these mortality rates are higher than their experience and that of previous reports of approximately 20 percent at 1 year and 30 percent at 3 years.[86] Thus bullous pemphigoid is a potentially fatal disease mostly in the elderly, whose health already may be fragile.

About one-half of treated patients will go into remission within about 2.5 to 6 years; however, in individual patients, disease may continue for 10 years or more.[11,13] Clinical remission with reversion of direct and indirect immunofluorescence to negative has been noted in patients, even those with severe generalized disease, treated with oral glucocorticoids alone or with azathioprine.[12,13]

Localized bullous pemphigoid often can be treated successfully with topical glucocorticoids alone.[12,13,87] More extensive disease, which is often more difficult to control than less extensive disease,[12] is usually treated with oral prednisone.[87] However, a study from France has shown that potent topical steroids are effective in both moderate and severe bullous pemphigoid.[88] In elderly patients, the complications of systemic glucocorticoid therapy (such as osteoporosis, diabetes, and immunosuppression) may be especially severe.[89] Therefore, it is important (1) to try to minimize the total dose and duration of therapy with prednisone and (2) to attempt to either treat initially with or taper rapidly to alternate-day therapy. In addition, immunosuppressive agents such as azathioprine (and less often methotrexate or cyclophosphamide) often are used for their potential steroid-sparing effects.[87,90–92] However, one study found that if systemic glucocorticoids are given at rather high dosage for 4 weeks without taper, the addition of azathioprine does not add appreciable benefit.[93] Therefore, the beneficial effects of azathioprine probably reside in its steroid-sparing effects.[90] In elderly patients, these immunosuppressives may be used during initial therapy and even may be used without accompanying prednisone in limited disease. However, to bring widespread disease under rapid control, systemic glucocorticoids often are necessary because their effect is usually rapid (within days), whereas immunosuppressives take at least 4 to 6 weeks to show any effect. High-dose "pulse" therapy with intravenous methylprednisolone also has been reported to be effective in rapidly controlling active blister formation in bullous pemphigoid.[94]

Sulfones may be effective in a minority of patients. Dapsone and sulfapyridine have been reported to control disease activity in 15 to 44 percent of bullous pemphigoid patients.[95–97]

An increasing number of reports have described successful treatment of some bullous pemphigoid patients with tetracycline and nicotinamide or variations on this theme, such as erythromycin and nicotinamide or tetracycline alone.[98–100] In small numbers of patients, other therapies reported to be effective include mycophenolate mofetil[101,102] (which may provide a less toxic alternative for azathioprine), leflunomide,[103] chlorambucil,[104] plasmapheresis,[105] and intravenous gammaglobulin.[106]

REFERENCES

1. Lever WF: Pemphigus. *Medicine* **32**:1, 1953
2. Jordon RE et al: Basement zone antibodies in bullous pemphigoid. *JAMA* **200**:751, 1967
3. Beutner EH et al: Autoantibodies in pemphigus vulgaris. *JAMA* **192**:682, 1965
4. Lever WF: *Pemphigus and Pemphigoid.* Springfield, Ill.: Charles C. Thomas, 1965

5. Trüeb RM et al: Childhood bullous pemphigoid: Report of a case with characterization of the targeted antigens. *J Am Acad Dermatol* **40**:338, 1999
6. Bernard P et al: Incidence and distribution of subepidermal autoimmune bullous skin diseases in three French regions. Bullous Diseases French Study Group. *Arch Dermatol* **131**:48, 1995
7. Zillikens D et al: Incidence of autoimmune subepidermal blistering dermatoses in a region of central Germany. *Arch Dermatol* **131**:957, 1995
8. Lever WF: Pemphigus and pemphigoid. *J Am Acad Dermatol* **1**:2, 1979
9. Schaumburg-Lever G et al: Electron microscopic study of bullous pemphigoid. *Arch Dermatol* **106**:662, 1972
10. Wintroub BU et al: Morphologic and functional evidence for release of mast-cell products in bullous pemphigoid. *New Engl J Med* **298**:417, 1978
11. Person JR, Rogers RS 3d: Bullous and cicatricial pemphigoid: Clinical, histopathologic, and immunopathologic correlations. *Mayo Clin Proc* **52**:54, 1977
12. Ahmed AR et al: Bullous pemphigoid. *Arch Dermatol* **113**:1043, 1977
13. Hadi SM et al: Clinical, histological and immunological studies in 50 patients with bullous pemphigoid. *Dermatologica* **176**:6, 1988
14. Beutner EH et al: The immunopathology of pemphigus and bullous pemphigoid. *J Invest Dermatol* **51**:63, 1968
15. Parodi A, Rebora A: Serum IgE antibodies bind to the epidermal side of the basement membrane zone splits in bullous pemphigoid (letter). *Br J Dermatol* **126**:526, 1992
16. Dopp R et al: IgG4 and IgE are the major immunoglobulins targeting the NC16A domain of BP180 in bullous pemphigoid: Serum levels of these immunoglobulins reflect disease activity. *J Am Acad Dermatol* **42**:577, 2000
17. Gammon WR et al: Differentiating anti-lamina lucida and anti-sublamina densa anti-BMZ antibodies by indirect immunofluorescence on 1.0 *M* sodium chloride separated skin. *J Invest Dermatol* **82**:139, 1984
18. Kelly SE, Wojnarowska F: The use of chemically split tissue in the detection of circulating anti-basement membrane zone antibodies in bullous pemphigoid and cicatricial pemphigoid. *Br J Dermatol* **118**:31, 1988
19. Sams WM Jr, Jordon RE: Correlation of pemphigoid and pemphigus antibody titres with activity of disease. *Br J Dermatol* **84**:7, 1971
20. Jordon RE, Bushkell LL: The complement system in pemphigus, bullous pemphigoid and herpes gestationis. *Int J Dermatol* **18**:271, 1979
21. Carlo JR et al: Demonstration of the complement regulating protein, B1H, in skin biopsies from patients with bullous pemphigoid. *J Invest Dermatol* **73**:551, 1979
22. Dahl MV et al: Deposition of the membrane attack complex of complement in bullous pemphigoid. *J Invest Dermatol* **82**:132, 1984
23. Mutasim DF et al: Definition of bullous pemphigoid antibody binding to intracellular and extracellular antigen associated with hemidesmosomes. *J Invest Dermatol* **92**:225, 1989
24. Shimizu H et al: Demonstration of intra- and extracellular localization of bullous pemphigoid antigen using cryofixation and freeze substitution for postembedding immunoelectron microscopy. *Arch Dermatol Res* **281**:443, 1989
25. Stanley JR: Cell adhesion molecules as targets of autoantibodies in pemphigus and pemphigoid, bullous diseases due to defective epidermal cell adhesion. *Adv Immunol* **53**:291, 1993
26. Stanley JR et al: Characterization of bullous pemphigoid antigen: A unique basement membrane protein of stratified squamous epithelia. *Cell* **24**:897, 1981
27. Stanley JR et al: Isolation of cDNA for bullous pemphigoid antigen by use of patients' autoantibodies. *J Clin Invest* **82**:1864, 1988
28. Green KJ et al: Comparative structural analysis of desmoplakin, bullous pemphigoid antigen and plectin: Members of a new gene family involved in organization of intermediate filments. *Int J Biol Macrobiol* **14**:145, 1992
29. Tanaka T et al: Production of rabbit antibodies against carboxy-terminal epitopes encoded by bullous pemphigoid cDNA. *J Invest Dermatol* **94**:617, 1990
30. Guo L et al: Gene targeting of BPAG1: Abnormalities in mechanical strength and cell migration in stratified epithelia and neurologic degeneration. *Cell* **81**:233, 1995
31. Brown A et al: The mouse dystonia musculorum gene is a neural isoform of bullous pemphigoid antigen 1. *Nature Genet* **10**:301, 1995
32. Yang Y et al: An essential cytoskeletal linker protein connecting actin microfilaments to intermediate filaments. *Cell* **86**:655, 1996
33. Labib RS et al: Molecular heterogeneity of the bullous pemphigoid antigens as detected by immunoblotting. *J Immunol* **136**:1231, 1986
34. Haase C et al: Detection of IgG autoantibodies in the sera of patients with bullous and gestational pemphigoid: ELISA studies utilizing a

baculovirus-encoded form of bullous pemphigoid antigen 2. *J Invest Dermatol* **110**:282, 1998
35. Zillikens D et al: A highly sensitive enzyme-linked immunosorbent assay for the detection of circulating anti-BP180 autoantibodies in patients with bullous pemphigoid. *J Invest Dermatol* **109**:679, 1997
36. Giudice GJ et al: Cloning and primary structural analysis of the bullous pemphigoid autoantigen BP180. *J Invest Dermatol* **99**:243, 1992
37. Ishiko A et al: Human autoantibodies against the 230-kD bullous pemphigoid antigen (BPAG1) bind only to the intracellular domain of the hemidesmosome, whereas those against the 180-kD bullous pemphigoid antigen (BPAG2) bind along the plasma membrane of the hemidesmosome in normal human and swine skin. *J Clin Invest* **91**:1608, 1993
38. Borradori L et al: The localization of bullous pemphigoid antigen 180 (BP180) in hemidesmosomes is mediated by its cytoplasmic domain and seems to be regulated by the beta4 integrin subunit. *J Cell Biol* **136**:1333, 1997
39. Masunaga T et al: The extracellular domain of BPAG2 localizes to anchoring filaments and its carboxyl terminus extends to the lamina densa of normal human epidermal basement membrane (see comments). *J Invest Dermatol* **109**:200, 1997
40. Giudice GJ et al: Bullous pemphigoid and herpes gestationis autoantibodies recognize a common non-collagenous site on the BP180 ectodomain. *J Immunol* **151**:5742, 1993
41. Zillikens D et al: Tight clustering of extracellular BP180 epitopes recognized by bullous pemphigoid autoantibodies. *J Invest Dermatol* **109**:573, 1997
42. McGrath JA et al: A homozygous deletion mutation in the gene encoding the 180-kDa bullous pemphigoid antigen (BPAG2) in a family with generalized atrophic benign epidermolysis bullosa. *J Invest Dermatol* **106**:771, 1996
43. Zillikens D et al: Autoantibodies in lichen planus pemphigoides react with a novel epitope within the C-terminal NC16A domain of BP180. *J Invest Dermatol* **113**:117, 1999
44. Anhalt GJ et al: Pathogenic effects of bullous pemphigoid autoantibodies on rabbit corneal epithelium. *J Clin Invest* **68**:1097, 1981
45. Liu Z et al: A passive transfer model of the organ-specific autoimmune disease, bullous pemphigoid, using antibodies generated against the hemidesmosomal antigen, BP180. *J Clin Invest* **92**:2480, 1993
46. Liu Z et al: A critical role for neutrophil elastase in experimental bullous pemphigoid. *J Clin Invest* **105**:113, 2000
47. Gammon WR et al: An in vitro model of immune complex-mediated basement membrane zone separation caused by pemphigoid antibodies, leukocytes, and complement. *J Invest Dermatol* **78**:285, 1982
48. Sams WM Jr, Gammon WR: Mechanism of lesion production in pemphigus and pemphigoid. *J Am Acad Dermatol* **6**:431, 1982
49. Stahle-Backdahl M et al: 92-kD gelatinase is produced by eosinophils at the site of blister formation in bullous pemphigoid and cleaves the extracellular domain of recombinant 180-kD bullous pemphigoid autoantigen. *J Clin Invest* **93**:2022, 1994
50. Kitajima Y et al: Internalization of the 180 kDa bullous pemphigoid antigen as immune complexes in basal keratinocytes: An important early event in blister formation in bullous pemphigoid. *Br J Dermatol* **138**:71, 1998
51. Yancey KB, Egan CA: Pemphigoid: Clinical, histologic, immunopathologic, and therapeutic considerations. *JAMA* **284**:350, 2000
52. Provost TT et al: Unusual subepidermal bullous diseases with immunologic features of bullous pemphigoid. *Arch Dermatol* **115**:156, 1979
53. Person JR et al: Localized pemphigoid. *Br J Dermatol* **95**:531, 1976
54. Domloge-Hultsch N et al: Autoantibodies from patients with localized and generalized bullous pemphigoid immunoprecipitate the same 230-kD keratinocyte antigen. *Arch Dermatol* **126**:1337, 1990
55. Schumann H et al: A child with localized vulval pemphigoid and IgG autoantibodies targeting the C-terminus of collagen XVII/BP180. *Br J Dermatol* **140**:1133, 1999
56. Farrell AM et al: Childhood vulval pemphigoid: a clinical and immunopathological study of five patients. *Br J Dermatol* **140**:308, 1999
57. Strohal R et al: Nonbullous pemphigoid: Prodrome of bullous pemphigoid or a distinct pemphigoid variant? *J Am Acad Dermatol* **29**:293, 1993
58. Borradori L et al: Localized pretibial pemphigoid and pemphigoid nodularis. *J Am Acad Dermatol* **27**:863, 1992
59. Chan LS et al: Pemphigoid vegetans represents a bullous pemphigoid variant: Patient's IgG autoantibodies identify the major bullous pemphigoid antigen. *J Am Acad Dermatol* **28**:331, 1993
60. Korman NJ, Woods SG: Erythrodermic bullous pemphigoid is a clinical variant of bullous pemphigoid. *Br J Dermatol* **133**:967, 1995
61. Cram DL, Fukuyama K: Immunohistochemistry of ultraviolet-induced pemphigus and pemphigoid lesions. *Arch Dermatol* **106**:819, 1972
62. Thomsen K, Schmidt H: PUVA-induced bullous pemphigoid. *Br J Dermatol* **95**:568, 1976
63. Koerber WA Jr et al: coexistent psoriasis and bullous pemphigoid. *Arch Dermatol* **114**:1643, 1978
64. Knoell KA et al: Localized bullous pemphigoid following radiotherapy for breast carcinoma. *Arch Dermatol* **134**:514, 1998
65. Baba T et al: An eosinophil chemotactic factor present in blister fluids of bullous pemphigoid patients. *J Immunol* **116**:112, 1976
66. Arbesman CE et al: IgE levels in sera of patients with pemphigus or bullous pemphigoid. *Arch Dermatol* **110**:378, 1974
67. Bushkell LL, Jordon RE: Bullous pemphigoid: A cause of peripheral blood eosinophilia. *J Am Acad Dermatol* **8**:648, 1983
68. Stone SP, Schroeter AL: Bullous pemphigoid and associated malignant neoplasms. *Arch Dermatol* **111**:991, 1975
69. Lindelof B et al: Pemphigoid and cancer. *Arch Dermatol* **126**:66, 1990
70. Venning VA, Wojnarowska F: The association of bullous pemphigoid and malignant disease: A case control study. *Br J Dermatol* **123**:439, 1990
71. Hodge L et al: Bullous pemphigoid: The frequency of mucosal involvement and concurrent malignancy related to indirect immunofluorescence findings. *Br J Dermatol* **105**:65, 1981
72. Stingl G, Holubar K: Coexistence of lichen planus and bullous pemphigoid. *Br J Dermatol* **93**:313, 1975
73. Callen JP: Internal disorders associated with bullous disease of the skin. *J Am Acad Dermatol* **3**:107, 1980
74. Chorzelski TP et al: Coexistence of pemphigus and bullous pemphigoid. *Arch Dermatol* **109**:849, 1974
75. Leibovici V et al: Coexistence of pemphigus and bullous pemphigoid. *Int J Dermatol* **28**:259, 1989
76. Ishiko A et al: Combined features of pemphigus foliaceus and bullous pemphigoid: Immunoblot and immunoelectron microscopic studies (letter). *Arch Dermatol* **131**:732, 1995
77. Grattan CEH: Evidence of an association between bullous pemphigoid and psoriasis. *Br J Dermatol* **113**:281, 1985
78. Kirtschig G et al: Acquired subepidermal bullous diseases associated with psoriasis: A clinical immunopathological and immunogenetic study. *Br J Dermatol* **135**:738, 1996
79. Crotty C et al: Eosinophilic spongiosis: A clinicopathologic review of seventy-one cases. *J Am Acad Dermatol* **8**:337, 1983
80. Gammon WR et al: Epidermolysis bullosa acquisita: A pemphigoid-like disease. *J Am Acad Dermatol* **11**:820, 1984
81. Venning VA et al: Mucosal involvement in bullous and cicatricial pemphigoid: A clinical and immunopathological study. *Br J Dermatol* **118**:7, 1988
82. Gammon WR et al: Direct immunofluorescence studies of sodium chloride–separated skin in the differential diagnosis of bullous pemphigoid and epidermolysis bullosa acquisita. *J Am Acad Dermatol* **22**:664, 1990
83. Karpati S et al: In Situ localization of IgG in epidermolysis bullosa acquisita by immunogold technique. *J Am Acad Dermatol* **26**:726, 1992
84. Woodley DT et al: Epidermolysis bullosa acquisita antigen is the globular carboxyl terminus of type VII procollagen. *J Clin Invest* **81**:683, 1988
85. Roujeau JC et al: High risk of death in elderly patients with extensive bullous pemphigoid. *Arch Dermatol* **134**:465, 1998
86. Korman NJ: Bullous pemphigoid: The latest in diagnosis, prognosis, and therapy (letter, comment). *Arch Dermatol* **134**:1137, 1998
87. Fine JD: Management of acquired bullous skin diseases (see comments). *New Engl J Med* **333**:1475, 1995
88. Joly P et al: A comparison of oral and topical cortieosteroids in patients with bullous pemphigoid. *N Engl J Med* **346**:321, 2002
89. Savin JA: The events leading to the death of patients with pemphigus and pemphigoid. *Br J Dermatol* **101**:521, 1979
90. Burton JL et al: Azathioprine plus prednisone in treatment of pemphigoid. *BMJ* **2**:1190, 1978
91. Paul MA et al: Low-dose methotrexate treatment in elderly patients with bullous pemphigoid. *J Am Acad Dermatol* **31**:620, 1994
92. Heilborn JD et al: Low-dose oral pulse methotrexate as monotherapy in elderly patients with bullous pemphigoid. *J Am Acad Dermatol* **40**:741, 1999
93. Guillaume JC et al: Controlled trial of azathioprine and plasma exchange in addition to prednisolone in the treatment of bullous pemphigoid. *Arch Dermatol* **129**:49, 1993
94. Siegel J, Eaglstein WH: High-dose methylprednisolone in the treatment of bullous pemphigoid. *Arch Dermatol* **120**:1157, 1984
95. Person JR, Rogers RS III: Bullous pemphigoid responding to sulfapyridine and the sulfones. *Arch Dermatol* **113**:610, 1977
96. Venning VA et al: Dapsone as first line therapy for bullous pemphigoid. *Br J Dermatol* **120**:83, 1989

97. Bouscarat F et al: Treatment of bullous pemphigoid with dapsone: Retrospective study of thirty-six cases. *J Am Acad Dermatol* **34**:683, 1996
98. Berk MA, Lorincz AL: The treatment of bullous pemphigoid with tetracycline and niacinamide: A preliminary report. *Arch Dermatol* **122**:670, 1986
99. Fivenson DP et al: Nicotinamide and tetracycline therapy of bullous pemphigoid. *Arch Dermatol* **130**:753, 1994
100. Kolbach DN et al: Bullous pemphigoid successfully controlled by tetracycline and nicotinamide. *Br J Dermatol* **133**:88, 1995
101. Bohm M et al: Bullous pemphigoid treated with mycophenolate mofetil. *Lancet* **349**:541, 1997
102. Nousari HC et al: Successful therapy for bullous pemphigoid with mycophenolate mofetil. *J Am Acad Dermatol* **39**:497, 1998

103. Nousari HC, Anhalt GJ: Bullous pemphigoid treated with leflunomide: A novel immunomodulatory agent. *Arch Dermatol* **136**:1204, 2000
104. Milligan A, Hutchinson PE: The use of chlorambucil in the treatment of bullous pemphigoid. *J Am Acad Dermatol* **22**:796, 1990
105. Roujeau JC et al: Plasma exchange in bullous pemphigoid. *Lancet* **2**:486, 1984
106. Engineer L, Ahmed AR: Role of intravenous immunoglobulin in the treatment of bullous pemphigoid: Analysis of current data. *J Am Acad Dermatol* **44**:83, 2001

CHAPTER 62

Kim B. Yancey

Cicatricial Pemphigoid

Cicatricial pemphigoid is a rare chronic autoimmune subepithelial blistering disease characterized by erosive lesions of mucous membranes and skin that result in scarring of at least some sites of involvement.[1–3] Lesions commonly involve the oral mucosa and the conjunctivae. Other sites that may be affected include the nasopharyngeal, laryngeal, esophageal, genital, and rectal mucosae. Skin lesions are present in about one-third of patients; tend to predominate on the scalp, face, and upper trunk; and usually consist of a few scattered erosions or tense blisters on an erythematous or urticarial base. Cicatricial pemphigoid is typically chronic and progressive; it may result in serious complications. Immunopathologic studies of perilesional mucosa and skin demonstrate in situ deposits of immunoreactants in epithelial basement membranes. Circulating anti–basement membrane autoantibodies can be detected in the sera of some but not all patients. Studies have shown that a variety of different autoantigens are recognized by autoantibodies in patients with cicatricial pemphigoid. These and other findings have led to the idea that cicatricial pemphigoid is not a single nosologic entity but rather a disease phenotype that develops as a consequence of mucosal injury arising from different mechanisms.

HISTORICAL ASPECTS

Cicatricial pemphigoid has been referred to by a variety of designations based largely on its site of involvement. Examples of such terminology include *desquamative gingivitis, ocular pemphigus,* and *benign mucous membrane pemphigoid.* Currently, such designations are thought to be confusing or somewhat misleading (e.g., pemphigus in this context is a misnomer, and this disorder is hardly benign given the extent of morbidity it can cause). Moreover, some designations (e.g., *desquamative gingivitis*) are limited when the potential spectrum of this chronic disease is considered.

EPIDEMIOLOGY

Cicatricial pemphigoid is rare, occurring in perhaps 1 person per million annually. Females are affected 1.5 to 2 times as often as males. Cicatricial pemphigoid is a disease with a mean age of onset in the early to middle 60s. Although there is no known racial or geographic predilection, some forms have been associated with certain immunogenetic haplotypes.[5–8] Specifically, the *HLA-DQB1*0301* allele has been shown to be significantly increased in frequency in patients with oral, ocular, and generalized bullous pemphigoid[5,8]; amino acid residues at positions 57 and 71–77 of the DQB1 protein may represent a specific disease susceptibility marker for these patients.[6,7]

ETIOLOGY AND PATHOGENESIS

Electron Microscopy

Ultrastructural studies found that blisters of skin and mucous membranes in patients with cicatricial pemphigoid develop within the lamina lucida.[9] The basal lamina may appear partially or completely destroyed in older lesions. A generally held impression is that blisters form below those of bullous pemphigoid, since scarring is more common in patients with this disease. Reports of patients with blisters in the sublamina densa region may represent mucosal-predominant forms of epidermolysis bullosa acquisita (see below).

Immunofluorescence Microscopy

Direct immunofluorescence microscopy of normal-appearing perilesional tissue from patients with cicatricial pemphigoid shows continuous deposits of immunoreactants in epithelial basement membranes.[2,10] The most commonly detected immunoreactants are IgG and C3

FIGURE 62-1

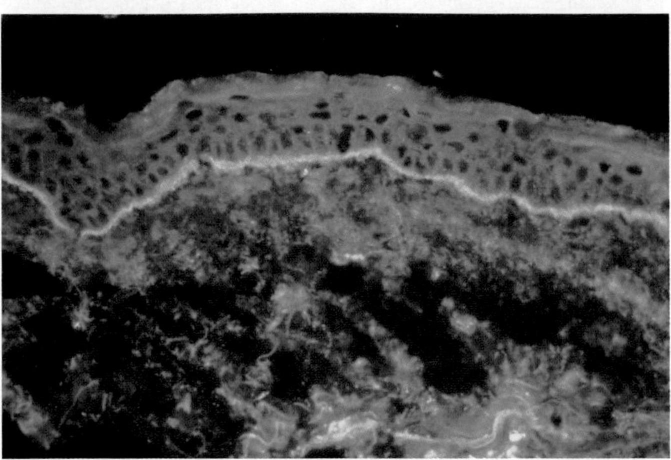

Direct immunofluorescence microscopy of normal-appearing perilesional skin from a patient with cicatricial pemphigoid shows continuous linear deposits of C3 in the epidermal basement membrane.

(Fig. 62-1); the predominant subclass of these autoantibodies is IgG_4.[11] IgA, IgM, and/or fibrin are found in some patients.[12] One study of skin and mucosal samples from 10 patients found immunoreactants more commonly in perilesional mucosal biopsies, suggesting that mucous membranes are the preferred biopsy site for direct immunofluorescence microscopy studies.[10] Splitting tissue samples with 1 *M* NaCl increases the sensitivity of direct immunofluorescence microscopy and facilitates identification of immunoreactants as well as their relative distribution within epithelial basement membranes.[13]

Indirect immunofluorescence microscopy studies using intact skin or mucosa often find low-titer IgG (and/or IgA) anti–basement membrane autoantibodies in patients with cicatricial pemphigoid.[2,14] Studies employing 1 *M* NaCl split skin as a test substrate substantially increase the detection of such autoantibodies.[15–17] In such studies, IgG (and/or IgA) binding is usually directed against the epidermal side of 1 *M* NaCl split skin, although combined epidermal and dermal or exclusively dermal binding can occur. In fact, this heterogeneity in autoantibody binding patterns was one of the first clues that cicatricial pemphigoid is associated with different autoantibody systems. While some studies have suggested that the use of human mucosal tissue substrates increases the likelihood of detecting autoantibodies in patients with cicatricial pemphigoid, other studies have not obtained similar results.[1,10] Recent studies found that patients with both IgG and IgA anti–basement membrane autoantibodies had a worse prognosis as defined by requirements for medications to control disease as well as overall clinical severity score.[18,19]

Autoantigens

Recent studies have shown that autoantibodies from patients with cicatricial pemphigoid may recognize a variety of different antigens present in epithelial basement membranes (Table 62-1). Some of these autoantigens are relatively well characterized, whereas others are identified only on the basis of their molecular weight and reactivity with autoantibodies present in the sera of patients with this phenotype. Several well-characterized patient subsets are reviewed briefly below.

Many cicatricial pemphigoid patients who have circulating IgG that binds the epidermal side of 1 *M* NaCl split skin have autoantibodies reactive with bullous pemphigoid antigen 2 (BPAG2), a 180-kDa type II transmembrane protein associated with hemidesmosomes in basal keratinocytes.[20–22] Autoantibodies in such patients typically bind the distal extracellular domain of BPAG2 alone or in association with reactivity to an epitope situated near the plasma membrane of basal keratinocytes.[21] The latter, the NC16A domain of BPAG2, is also targeted by IgG autoantibodies from patients with bullous pemphigoid and pemphigoid gestationis.[23] Interestingly, immunoelectron microscopy studies have shown that anti-BPAG2 IgG from patients with cicatricial pemphigoid localizes within the lower lamina lucida near its junction with the lamina densa,[22] a site that corresponds to the localization of the distal extracellular domain of BPAG2 in epidermal basement membrane.[24,25] This observation may explain the greater likelihood of scar formation in patients with this disease rather than those with bullous or gestational pemphigoid.

In contrast to the patients just described, some cicatricial pemphigoid patients have IgG autoantibodies directed exclusively against the dermal side of 1 *M* NaCl split skin. Some of these patients have IgG autoantibodies that bind the superior surface of the lamina densa at its interface with the lamina lucida and immunoprecipitate a set of disulfide-linked polypeptides produced by human keratinocytes.[26,27] Because the protein that was identified initially as this autoantigen was at the time termed *epiligrin,* this form of disease was called *antiepiligrin cicatricial pemphigoid.*[16] Subsequent studies showed that epiligrin is identical to laminin-5 ($\alpha_3\beta_3\gamma_2$) and that these patients' autoantibodies usually bind the alpha subunit of this protein.[28] Because this subunit is immunologically cross-reactive with the alpha subunit of laminin-6 ($\alpha_3\beta_1\gamma_1$), these patients' autoantibodies recognize this protein as well.[29,30]

Examples of other cicatricial pemphigoid autoantigens that appear to be restricted to certain sites of disease or represent rare variants are briefly summarized below. Sera from some patients with ocular cicatricial pemphigoid have been shown to bind a 205-kDa protein in extracts of epithelial cell lines and also isolate a cDNA clone corresponding to the cytoplasmic domain of integrin subunit β_4 (a component of hemidesmosomes in basal keratinocytes).[31,32] Recent in vitro studies have shown that such autoantibodies may be pathogenic (see below).[33] Although less well characterized, a 168-kDa polypeptide in extracts of mucosal tissue was found to be specifically reactive with autoantibodies from cicatricial pemphigoid patients with oral involvement.[34] This antigen is not apparently related to bullous pemphigoid antigen 1, BPAG2, or laminin-5. Patients with a mucosal-predominant form of epidermolysis bullosa acquisita are often

TABLE 62-1

Autoantigens in Patients with Cicatricial Pemphigoid

Antigen	Size (kDa)	Localization	References
BPAG2*	180	Hemidesmosome-anchoring filament complexes	20, 21, 22
Laminin-5	440–400†	Interface of lamina lucida and lamina densa	16, 26, 28
Integrin subunit β_4	205	Hemidesmosome-anchoring filament complexes	31, 32
M168	168	Lamina lucida	34
Type VII collagen	290	Anchoring fibrils	35, 36

*BPAG2, bullous pemphigoid antigen 2.
†Like other laminin isoforms, laminin 5 ($\alpha_3\beta_3\gamma_2$) is a large heterotrimer. Most patients who have IgG against this protein target its alpha subunit.

indistinguishable from patients with cicatricial pemphigoid.[35] Like other patients with epidermolysis bullosa acquisita, these individuals have circulating and/or in situ deposits of IgG against type VII collagen in anchoring fibrils.[3,36] Other patients with the cicatricial pemphigoid phenotype have IgA anti–basement membrane autoantibodies. While IgA from some of these patients has been shown to bind BPAG2, autoantigens identified in other patients have not been characterized (or shown to be relevant to disease pathophysiology).[14,37,38]

Disease Pathophysiology

The immunopathologic findings in patients with cicatricial pemphigoid have suggested that autoantibodies in these patients (like those in patients with pemphigus or bullous pemphigoid) are pathogenic. However, for most autoantibody systems associated with cicatricial pemphigoid, additional study is required to confirm this hypothesis. As noted earlier, BPAG2 is the major autoantigen in cicatricial pemphigoid patients with IgG autoantibodies that bind the epidermal side of 1 *M* NaCl split skin. Such sera typically bind the distal extracellular domain of this protein alone or in association with its more proximal NC16A epitope.[21] Passive-transfer studies have shown that experimental antibodies directed against the murine homologue of the NC16A portion of human BPAG2 elicit subepidermal blisters in neonatal mice with clinical, histologic, and immunopathologic features like those seen in patients with bullous pemphigoid.[39] However, it remains to be determined if antibodies against the distal extracellular portion of BPAG2 elicit mucosal-predominant scarring lesions in experimental animals that mimic those seen in patients with cicatricial pemphigoid.

Recent studies showed that passive transfer of anti–laminin-5 IgG to neonatal mice induced subepidermal blisters of skin and mucous membranes with the same clinical, histologic, and immunopathologic features as those seen in patients with antiepiligrin cicatricial pemphigoid.[40] Anti–laminin-5 IgG induced the same lesions in complement- or mast cell–deficient mice, suggesting that such antibodies may elicit epidermal detachment in vivo in a noninflammatory and perhaps direct manner.[40] Moreover, recent studies showed that injection of IgG from patients with this form of cicatricial pemphigoid into human skin grafts on immunodeficient mice elicited noninflammatory subepidermal blisters, confirming that these patients' autoantibodies are pathogenic in vivo.[41]

Using a human conjunctival organ culture system, investigators showed that antibodies against integrin subunit β_4 elicited subepithelial blister formation in vitro—a finding suggesting that such antibodies are pathogenic in humans in vivo.[33] As is true for disease that predominates on skin, epidermolysis bullosa acquisita affecting mucous membranes is thought to be mediated by anti-type VII collagen autoantibodies. This hypothesis awaits experimental confirmation.

CLINICAL MANIFESTATIONS

Mucous Membranes

The mouth is the most frequent site of involvement in patients with cicatricial pemphigoid; it is often the first site affected. Lesions in the mouth often involve the gingiva, buccal mucosa, and palate (Figs. 62-2 and 62-3); other sites such as the alveolar ridge, tongue, and lips are also susceptible.[4,42] The most frequent oral manifestation is desquamative gingivitis. Other lesions may present as tense blisters that rupture easily or as mucosal erosions that form as a consequence of epithelial fragility. Lesions in the mouth may result in a delicate white pattern of reticulated scarring. In severe disease, adhesions may develop between the buccal mucosa and the alveolar process, around the uvula and tonsillar fossae, and between the tongue and the floor of the mouth. Gingival involvement can result in tissue loss and dental complications (e.g., caries, periodontal ligament damage, and loss of bone mass and teeth). Disease may be limited to the mouth.

Ocular involvement in patients with cicatricial pemphigoid is common and may become sight-threatening.[43] Ocular lesions typically manifest as conjunctivitis that progresses insidiously to scarring. Early ocular disease can be quite subtle and nonspecific. Although disease is usually bilateral, it often begins unilaterally and progresses to both

FIGURE 62-2

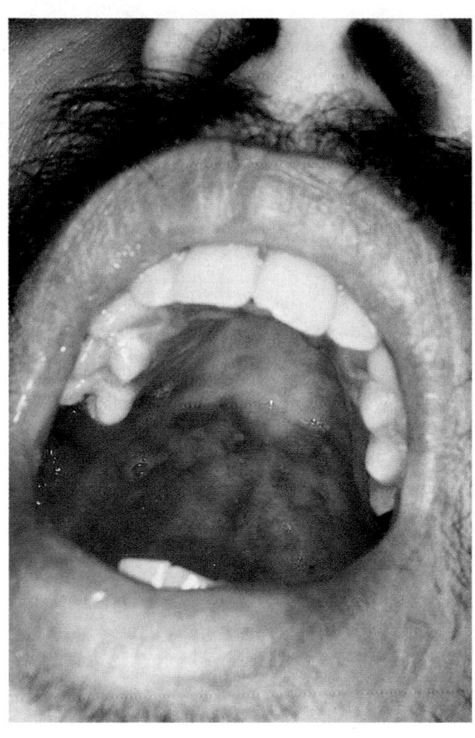

Cicatricial pemphigoid. Erosive lesions on the hard palate.

FIGURE 62-3

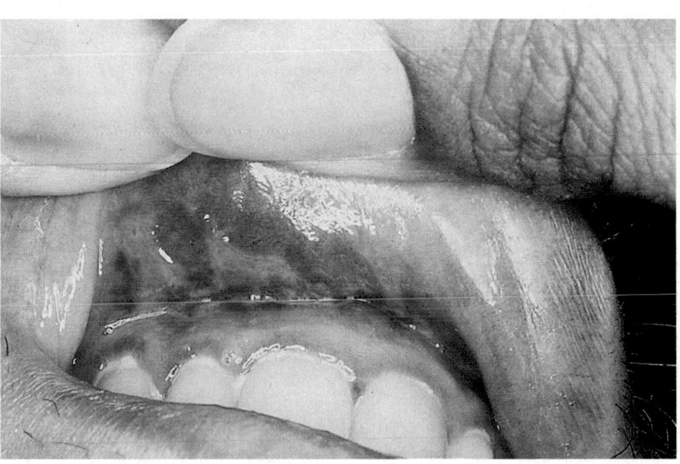

Cicatricial pemphigoid. Denuded sites on the oral mucosa.

eyes within several years. Patients may complain of burning, dryness, or a foreign-body sensation in one or both eyes; frank blisters on conjunctival surfaces are rarely seen. Early disease is best appreciated by slit-lamp examination. Because disease may be localized to the upper tarsal conjunctiva, it may escape detection without eversion of the eyelids. Chronic ocular involvement can result in scarring characterized by shortened fornices, symblephara (i.e., fibrous tracts between bulbar and palpebral conjunctival surfaces), and in severe disease, ankyloblephara (i.e., fibrous tracts fusing the superior and inferior palpebral conjunctivae with obliteration of the conjunctival sac). Conjunctival scarring also can cause entropion and trichiasis (i.e., in-turning of the eyelashes) that results in corneal irritation, superficial punctate keratinopathy, corneal neovascularization, corneal ulceration, and blindness. Additional ocular complications include scarring of lacrimal ducts, decreased tear secretion, and loss of mucosal goblet cells leading to decreased tear mucus content and unstable tear films. It is very important for patients with suspected ocular involvement to be examined by an ophthalmologist because early disease may be subtle, is only identified by slit-lamp examination, and can result in severe complications. Cicatricial pemphigoid may be limited to the eyes.

Other mucous membranes that may be involved by cicatricial pemphigoid include the nasopharyngeal, laryngeal, esophageal, genital, and rectal mucosae. Nasopharyngeal lesions can result in discharge, epistaxis, excessive crust formation, impaired airflow, chronic sinusitis, scarring, and tissue loss. Laryngeal involvement may present as hoarseness, sore throat, or loss of phonation. Chronic laryngeal erosions, edema, and scarring may result in supraglottic stenosis and airway compromise that eventually necessitates tracheostomy.[44] Esophageal involvement may result in stricture formation, dysphagia, odynophagia, weight loss, and/or aspiration. Moreover, it has been suggested that esophageal dysfunction and gastroesophageal reflux may elicit or exacerbate laryngeal disease and/or bronchospasm in such patients. Although involvement of the genital and/or rectal mucosae in patients with cicatricial pemphigoid is rare, it can be a source of substantial pain and morbidity. Rare cases of urethral stricture, vaginal stenosis, and anal narrowing have developed as a consequence of this disease.

Skin

The skin is involved in 25 to 35 percent of patients with cicatricial pemphigoid. The most frequently affected areas are the scalp, head, neck, and upper trunk. Lesions typically consist of small vesicles or bullae situated on erythematous and/or urticarial bases. Lesions rupture easily and are often seen as small, crusted papules or plaques. In general, the extent and number of cutaneous lesions are small. Skin lesions sometimes recur in the same areas.

Systemic Associations

A cohort of 35 patients with antiepiligrin cicatricial pemphigoid was reported to have an increased relative risk for solid cancer.[45] Ten patients in this cohort had solitary solid cancers (three lung, three gastric, two colon, two endometrial); eight patients developed cancer after the onset of cicatricial pemphigoid (six within a year, seven within 14 months). The time between blister onset and cancer diagnosis was approximately 14 months in 9 of the 10 patients. Eight patients in this cohort died as a consequence of their cancer; all deaths occurred within 21 months. This form of cicatricial pemphigoid appears to have a relative risk for malignancy that approximates that for adults with dermatomyositis; as is true for the latter, the risk for cancer appears to be particularly high in the first year of disease.

VARIANTS

Brunsting-Perry Pemphigoid

In 1957, Brunsting and Perry described seven patients with locally recurrent and scarring subepidermal blistering lesions of the head or neck that for many years was thought to be a form of cicatricial pemphigoid.[46] Although these patients were elderly, had subepithelial bullous lesions that scarred, and demonstrated deposits of immunoreactants in their epidermal basement membranes like other patients with cicatricial pemphigoid, Brunsting-Perry pemphigoid predominated in men and lacked mucous membrane involvement. Recently, patients with the same clinical, histologic, and immunopathologic features have been reported to have autoantibodies directed against bullous pemphigoid antigens or type VII collagen.[3,47] Identification of similar patients with blister planes beneath the lamina densa further suggests that some individuals with this phenotype represent localized forms of epidermolysis bullosa acquisita. Additional study will clarify this variant further.

Ocular Cicatricial Pemphigoid

Some patients have disease that is limited to conjunctival mucous membranes, and several series have segregated patients on the basis of this finding.[5,6,8,48] Additional studies hopefully will determine if there is further heterogeneity among these patients in respect to their autoantibody systems, pathophysiology, and/or response to treatment.

PATHOLOGY

Although light microscopy studies of lesional skin or mucosa from patients with cicatricial pemphigoid often are nonspecific, they characteristically show a subepidermal blister and a dermal leukocytic infiltrate composed of lymphocytes and histiocytes as well as variable numbers of neutrophils and eosinophils. Plasma cells often are seen in mucosal lesions, whereas eosinophils and neutrophils are seen most commonly in skin lesions. Biopsies of older lesions may be relatively "cell poor" and correlate with the noninflammatory character of such sites clinically. Light microscopy studies of older lesions often show fibroblast proliferation and lamellar fibrosis (i.e., fibrosis characterized by collagen bundles ordered parallel to the surface epithelium).

DIFFERENTIAL DIAGNOSIS

The diagnosis of cicatricial pemphigoid is suggested when patients present with bullous or erosive lesions of mucous membranes and demonstrate continuous deposits of immunoreactants in epithelial basement membranes of perilesional tissue. The distinction of cicatricial pemphigoid from other autoimmune bullous diseases such as pemphigus vulgaris, bullous pemphigoid, epidermolysis bullosa acquisita, and linear IgA dermatosis can be difficult and may require specialized immunopathologic studies and/or immunoelectron microscopy. In contrast to cicatricial pemphigoid, lesions in patients with pemphigus vulgaris form as a consequence of acantholysis and show deposits of immunoreactants on the surfaces of keratinocytes. Lesions in patients with bullous pemphigoid dominate on the skin, consist of large, tense blisters or vesicles situated on urticarial and/or erythematous bases, and (except in rare cases, e.g., excoriation) do not scar. Circulating IgG autoantibodies in patients with bullous pemphigoid bind BPAG1 and BPAG2 and by immunoelectron microscopy localize to hemidesmosomal plaques and the portion of the lamina lucida adjacent to plasma membranes of basal keratinocytes. In epidermolysis bullosa acquisita, lesions can resemble those seen in patients with bullous pemphigoid or present as dermolytic erosions on areas exposed to pressure or trauma. IgG autoantibodies in patients with epidermolysis bullosa acquisita are directed against type VII collagen in anchoring fibrils.[36] As noted previously, mucosal-predominant forms of this disease do exist, are important to recognize, and often represent management challenges. Some forms of linear IgA dermatosis clinically resemble bullous pemphigoid or dermatitis herpetiformis, whereas others dominate on mucous membranes. These patients are distinguished by continuous deposits of IgA in their epidermal basement membranes and (in many cases) circulating IgA anti–basement membrane autoantibodies. Because immunofluorescence microscopy, immunoblotting, and immunoelectron microscopy studies have demonstrated that a number of different proteins in the lamina lucida or sublamina densa region are targeted by autoantibodies in these patients, mucosal forms of linear IgA dermatosis are considered heterogeneous and incompletely characterized at present.

Other disorders that must be differentiated from cicatricial pemphigoid include lichen planus, erythema multiforme, lupus erythematosus, paraneoplastic pemphigus, lichen sclerosus, and—in the case of ocular disease—cicatrizing conjunctivitis that results from chronic use of certain ophthalmologic preparations (e.g., pilocarpine, guanethidine, or ephedrine used in the treatment of glaucoma or idoxuridine used as an antiviral). It also has been reported that some cases of ocular cicatricial pemphigoid develop after an acute episode of severe ocular inflammatory injury secondary to Stevens-Johnson syndrome.[49] Interestingly, the time between Stevens-Johnson syndrome and the onset of ocular cicatricial pemphigoid in these patients can range from a few months to more than 30 years.

TREATMENT AND PROGNOSIS

Cicatricial pemphigoid is typically a chronic and progressive disorder, although involvement may be limited to a given anatomic site (e.g., the mouth, the conjunctivae) for many years. Cicatricial pemphigoid rarely goes into spontaneous remission; its treatment is largely tempered by its severity and sites of involvement. Scarring can only be prevented in these patients; it never is completely reversed. The following overview is representative of most treatment regimens. Mild lesions of the oral mucosa and skin sometimes can be treated effectively with topical glucocorticoids. Mouthwash (dexamethasone 100 μg/mL, 5 mL per rinse) used in a "swish and spit" regimen for 5 min two to three times each day is one approach. Topical glucocorticoids in a gel or occlusive base (e.g., Orobase) applied two to four times each day is another. These agents are particularly effective before bed because oral secretions diminish during sleep. Because it is difficult to maintain contact of topical agents with mucous membranes (and because lesions often are localized to the gingiva), customized delivery trays to occlude topical glucocorticoids over lesional sites in the mouth are also useful.[50] This approach also facilitates interactions with professionals who can manage other complications in these patients (e.g., dental complications). For oral disease resistant to topical glucocorticoids, these agents can (in some instances) be administered intralesionally.

A number of reports have suggested that dapsone (50–150 mg by mouth daily) may be effective.[43,51] Others have found that cicatricial pemphigoid does not respond to this agent. In severe cases, systemic glucocorticoids can be administered alone (e.g., 20–60 mg of prednisone by mouth each morning) or in combination with dapsone. Because of potentially severe complications, ocular, laryngeal, and/or esophageal involvement requires aggressive management by teams of physicians familiar with specialized care of these organ systems. For mild or moderate ocular involvement, systemic glucocorticoids (e.g., 20–40 mg of prednisone by mouth each morning) alone or in conjunction with daily dapsone may be effective. Patients whose ocular disease is complicated by trichiasis may benefit from permanent epilation, although this decision is best made by an ophthalmologist. For severe disease affecting the ocular, pharyngeal, or urogenital epithelia, a combination of systemic glucocorticoids and an immunosuppressive drug is indicated. In such cases, cyclophosphamide (1–2 mg/kg per day) is often used in conjunction with daily prednisone (1 mg/kg per day). In this regimen, daily prednisone is tapered gradually over approximately 6 months, and the patient is maintained on cyclophosphamide alone for an additional 6 to 12 months. Such combined regimens have had success in halting the progression of severe ocular disease, limiting scarring, and producing long-term remissions. In an effort to avoid adverse effects and complications produced by prolonged treatment with immunosuppressive agents, attempts have been made to treat patients with intravenous immunoglobulin (i.e., IVIG, 2–3 g/kg of body weight administered over 2–3 days every 2–6 weeks for 4–6 months).[52] Additional experience with this agent is required to confirm preliminary results suggesting potential utility.

Involvement of the nasopharynx or esophagus potentially has severe complications and requires aggressive and specialized care. Nasal lesions often benefit from twice-daily irrigation of nasal passages with saline or tap water as well as the use of topical emollients. Esophageal involvement requires medical management to avert dysphagia, pain, tissue loss, and secondary complications such as gastroesophageal dysfunction, stricture formation, aspiration, laryngeal irritation, or bronchospastic pulmonary disease. All patients with cicatricial pemphigoid require long-term follow-up because of the possibility for this chronic disease to relapse.

REFERENCES

1. Lever WF: *Pemphigus and Pemphigoid.* Springfield, IL, Charles C Thomas, 1965
2. Bean SF et al: Cicatricial pemphigoid: Immunofluorescence studies. *Arch Dermatol* **106**:195, 1972
3. Fleming TE, Korman NJ: Cicatricial pemphigoid. *J Am Acad Dermatol* **43**:571, 2000
4. Laskaris G et al: Bullous pemphigoid, cicatricial pemphigoid, and pemphigus vulgaris: A comparative clinical survey of 278 cases. *Oral Surg Oral Med Oral Pathol* **54**:656, 1982
5. Ahmed RA et al: Association of DQw7 (*DQB1*0301*) with ocular cicatricial pemphigoid. *Proc Natl Acad Sci USA* **88**:11579, 1991
6. Yunis JJ et al: Common major histocompatibility complex class II markers in clinical variants of cicatricial pemphigoid. *Proc Natl Acad Sci USA* **91**:7747, 1994
7. Delgado JC et al: A common major histocompatibility complex class II allele *HLA-DQB1*0301* is present in clinical variants of pemphigoid. *Proc Natl Acad Sci USA* **93**:8569, 1996
8. Chan LS et al: Significantly increased occurrence of *HLA-DQB1*0301* allele in patients with ocular cicatricial pemphigoid. *J Invest Dermatol* **108**:129, 1997
9. Bernard P et al: Studies of cicatricial pemphigoid autoantibodies using direct immunoelectron microscopy and immunoblot analysis. J Invest Dermatol 94:630, 1990
10. Fine JD et al: Immunofluorescence and immunoelectron microscopic studies in cicatricial pemphigoid. *J Invest Dermatol* **82**:39, 1984
11. Hsu R et al: Noncomplement fixing, IgG_4 autoantibodies predominate in patients with antiepiligrin cicatricial pemphigoid. *J Invest Dermatol* **109**:557, 1997
12. Leonard JN et al: The relationship between linear IgA disease and benign mucous membrane pemphigoid. *Br J Dermatol* **110**:307, 1984
13. Gammon WR et al: Immunofluorescence studies of sodium chloride-separated skin in the differential diagnosis of bullous pemphigoid and epidermolysis bullosa acquisita. *J Am Acad Dermatol* **22**:664, 1990

14. Sarret Y et al: Salt-split human skin substrate for the immunofluorescent screening of serum from patients with cicatricial pemphigoid and a new method of immunoprecipitation with IgA antibodies. *J Am Acad Dermatol* **24**:952, 1991
15. Kelly S, Wojnarowska F: The use of chemically split tissue in the detection of circulating anti–basement membrane zone antibodies in bullous pemphigoid and cicatricial pemphigoid. *Br J Dermatol* **118**:31, 1988
16. Domloge-Hultsch N et al: Anti-epiligrin cicatricial pemphigoid: A subepithelial bullous disorder. *Arch Dermatol* **130**:1521, 1994
17. Lazarova Z, Yancey KB: Reactivity of autoantibodies from patients with defined subepidermal bullous diseases against 1 mol/L NaCl-split skin. *J Am Acad Dermatol* **35**:398, 1996
18. Setterfield J et al: Mucous membrane pemphigoid: A dual circulating antibody response with IgG and IgA signifies a more severe and persistent disease. *Br J Dermatol* **138**:602, 1998
19. Setterfield J et al: Cicatricial pemphigoid: Serial titres of circulating IgG and IgA anti–basement membrane antibodies correlate with disease activity. *Br J Dermatol* **140**:645, 1999
20. Bernard P et al: The major cicatricial pemphigoid antigen is a 180-kDa protein that shows immunologic cross-reactivities with the bullous pemphigoid antigen. *J Invest Dermatol* **99**:174, 1992
21. Balding SD et al: Cicatricial pemphigoid autoantibodies react with multiple sites on the BP180 extracellular domain. *J Invest Dermatol* **106**:141, 1996
22. Bedane C et al: Bullous pemphigoid and cicatricial pemphigoid autoantibodies react with ultrastructurally separable epitopes on the BP180 ectodomain: Evidence that BP180 spans the lamina lucida. *J Invest Dermatol* **108**:901, 1997
23. Giudice GJ et al: Bullous pemphigoid and herpes gestationis autoantibodies recognize a common non-collagenous site on the BP180 ectodomain. *J Immunol* **151**:5742, 1993
24. Hirako Y et al: Demonstration of the molecular shape of BP180, a 180-kDa bullous pemphigoid antigen and its potential for trimer formation. *J Biol Chem* **271**:13739, 1996
25. Masunaga T et al: The extracellular domain of BPAG2 localizes to anchoring filaments and its carboxyl terminus extends to the lamina densa of normal human epidermal basement membrane. *J Invest Dermatol* **109**:200, 1997
26. Domloge-Hultsch N et al: Epiligrin, the major human keratinocyte integrin ligand, is a target in both an acquired autoimmune and an inherited subepidermal blistering skin disease. *J Clin Invest* **90**:1628, 1992
27. Shimizu H et al: Autoantibodies from patients with cicatricial pemphigoid target different sites in epidermal basement membrane. *J Invest Dermatol* **104**:370, 1995
28. Kirtschig G et al: Anti–basement membrane autoantibodies in patients with antiepiligrin cicatricial pemphigoid bind the α subunit of laminin 5. *J Invest Dermatol* **105**:543, 1995
29. Chan LS et al: Laminin 6 and laminin 5 are recognized by autoantibodies in a subset of cicatricial pemphigoid. *J Invest Dermatol* **108**:848, 1997
30. Lazarova Z et al: Anticpiligrin cicatricial pemphigoid represents an autoimmune response to subunits present in laminin 5 ($\alpha_3\beta_3\gamma_2$). *Br J Dermatol* **139**:791, 1998
31. Mohimen A et al: Detection and partial characterization of ocular cicatricial pemphigoid antigens on COLO and SCaBER tumor cell lines. *Curr Eye Res* **12**:741, 1993
32. Tyagi S et al: Ocular cicatricial pemphigoid antigen: Partial sequence and biochemical characterization. *Proc Natl Acad Sci USA* **93**:14714, 1996
33. Chan RY et al: The role of antibody to human beta$_4$ integrin in conjunctival basement membrane separation: Possible in vitro model for ocular cicatricial pemphigoid. *Invest Ophthalmol Vis Sci* **40**:2283, 1999
34. Ghohestani RF et al: Identification of a 168-kDa mucosal antigen in a subset of patients with cicatricial pemphigoid. *J Invest Dermatol* **107**:136, 1996
35. Luke ML et al: Mucosal morbidity in patients with epidermolysis bullosa acquisita. *Arch Dermatol* **135**:954, 1999
36. Woodley DT et al: The epidermolysis bullosa acquisita antigen is the globular carboxyl terminus of type VII collagen. *J Clin Invest* **81**:683, 1988
37. Egan CA et al: Characterization of the antibody response in oesophageal cicatricial pemphigoid. *Br J Dermatol* **140**:859, 1999
38. Egan CA et al: The immunoglobulin A antibody response in clinical subsets of mucous membrane pemphigoid. *Dermatology* **198**:330, 1999
39. Liu Z et al: A passive transfer model of the organ-specific autoimmune disease, bullous pemphigoid, using antibodies generated against the hemidesmosomal antigen, BP180. *J Clin Invest* **92**:2480, 1993
40. Lazarova Z et al: Passive transfer of anti-laminin 5 antibodies induces subepidermal blisters in neonatal mice. *J Clin Invest* **98**:1509, 1996
41. Lazarova Z et al: Human anti-laminin 5 autoantibodies induce subepidermal blisters in an experimental human skin graft model. *J Invest Dermatol* **114**:178, 2000
42. Rogers RS et al: Desquamative gingivitis: Clinical, histopathologic, immunopathologic, and therapeutic observations. *J Am Acad Dermatol* **7**:729, 1982
43. Foster CS: Cicatricial pemphigoid. *Trans Am Ophthalmol Soc* **84**:527, 1986
44. Lazor JB et al: Management of airway obstruction in cicatricial pemphigoid. *Laryngoscope* **106**:1014, 1996
45. Egan CA et al: Antiepiligrin cicatricial pemphigoid and relative risk for cancer. *Lancet* **357**:1850, 2001
46. Brunsting LA, Perry HO: Benign pemphigoid? A report of seven cases with chronic, scarring, herpetiform plaques about the head and neck. *Arch Dermatol* **75**:489, 1957
47. Joly P et al: Brunsting-Perry cicatricial pemphigoid: A clinical variant of localized acquired epidermolysis bullosa? *J Am Acad Dermatol* **28**:89, 1993
48. Chan LS et al: Immune-mediated subepithelial blistering diseases of mucous membranes. *Arch Dermatol* **129**:448, 1993
49. Chan LS et al: Ocular cicatricial pemphigoid occurring as a sequelae of Stevens-Johnson syndrome. *JAMA* **266**:1543, 1991
50. Aufdemorte TB et al: Modified topical steroid therapy for the treatment of oral mucous membrane pemphigoid. *Oral Surg Oral Med Oral Pathol* **59**:256, 1985
51. Tauber J et al: Systemic chemotherapy for ocular cicatricial pemphigoid. *Cornea* **10**:185, 1991
52. Foster CS, Ahmed AR: Intravenous immunoglobulin therapy for ocular cicatricial pemphigoid: A preliminary study. *Ophthalmology* **106**:2136, 1999

CHAPTER 63

Caroline L. Rao
Russell P. Hall, III

Linear IgA Dermatosis and Chronic Bullous Disease of Childhood

Linear IgA dermatosis is a rare immune-mediated blistering skin disease that is defined by the presence of homogeneous linear deposits of IgA at the cutaneous basement membrane (Fig. 63-1). Although in the original description of patients with linear IgA dermatosis it was considered to be a manifestation of dermatitis herpetiformis (DH), it has now been clearly separated from DH on the basis of its immunopathology, immunogenetics, and lack of consistent association with a gluten-sensitive enteropathy.[1–3] Patients with linear IgA dermatosis can present with phenotypic characteristics suggestive of epidermolysis bullosa acquisita (EBA), DH, bullous pemphigoid, lichen planus, or cicatricial pemphigoid.[1–4]

These different clinical presentations appear to result from the IgA binding to different epidermal antigens. Chronic bullous disease of childhood (CBDC) is a rare blistering disease that occurs predominantly in children younger than 5 years of age and has an identical pattern of homogeneous linear IgA deposits at the epidermal basement membrane.[5,6] Recent studies have demonstrated that in some patients CBDC and linear IgA dermatosis represent different presentations of the same disease process.[7,8]

FIGURE 63-1

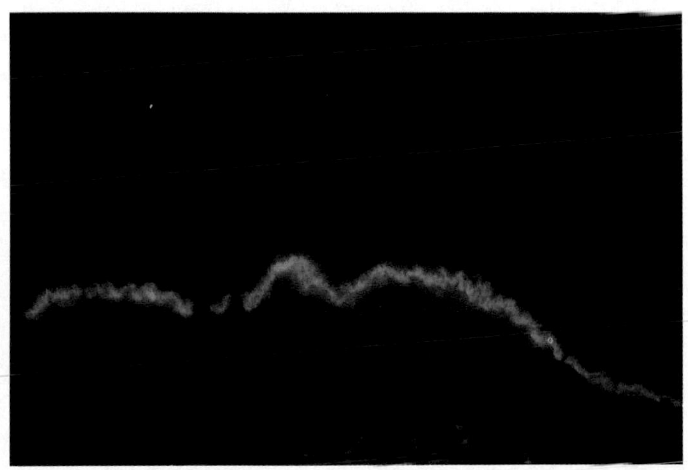

Direct immunofluorescence of normal-appearing perilesional skin from a patient with linear IgA dermatosis. A homogeneous band of IgA is present at the dermal-epidermal junction.

EPIDEMIOLOGY

Linear IgA dermatosis occurs most often after puberty, with most patients presenting after the fourth decade of life.[2,9,10] A slight predominance of females has been noted in several studies.[2,9] In contrast, CBDC presents most often before the age of 5 years.[9] As in patients with linear IgA dermatosis, there is a slight female predominance in patients with CBDC.[6,9]

Evaluation of the HLA association in patients with linear IgA dermatosis and CBDC has yielded conflicting results. Some investigators have found an increased frequency of the human histocompatibility antigen HLA-B8 in patients with linear IgA dermatosis, whereas others have found no increased frequency.[11–14] In CBDC, an increased frequency of HLA-B8 has been noted, with up to 76 percent of patients expressing HLA-B8.[9] Recently, Collier et al.[13] demonstrated an increased frequency of B8, DR3, and DQ2 in CBDC that was not seen in adults with linear IgA dermatosis. These authors suggested that these haplotypes may have a role in earlier disease presentation. In addition, the *TNF2* allele was found with increased frequency in both adults and children with linear IgA disease when compared with normal subjects. There was, however, no increase seen in either adults or children when compared with HLA−DR3+ controls.

ETIOLOGY AND PATHOGENESIS

Immunopathology

Linear IgA dermatosis and CBDC are defined by the presence of a homogeneous linear band of IgA at the dermal-epidermal basement membrane. A minority of patients in both groups have additional deposits of other immunoreactants, most often IgG and occasionally the third component of complement (C3).[9] Since IgA is the predominant immunoglobulin of the secretory immune system, numerous investigators have attempted to determine if the IgA present in the skin of these patients is of mucosal origin. Characterization of the IgA subclass in the skin has revealed almost exclusively IgA1 and not the subclass most often associated with mucosa, IgA2.[14–16] In addition, neither secretory piece nor J chain, both of which are present in secretory IgA, have been found in the IgA present in the skin of patients with linear IgA deposits.[17] Although these data have led to suggestions that the IgA is not of mucosal origin, the true origin of the IgA deposits in the skin of these patients is not known.

Initially it was thought that patients with linear IgA dermatosis and CBDC rarely had circulating IgA antibodies against the epidermal basement membrane. Indirect immunofluorescence, using 1 *M* NaCl-split normal human skin as a substrate, demonstrates that the majority of patients with CBDC have low-titer circulating antibodies against the epidermal side of the split skin.[9,18] Circulating low-titer IgA antibodies directed against the epidermal basement membrane also have been found in adults with linear IgA dermatosis.[9,18] Others have reported binding of these antibodies to the dermal side of normal human split skin, suggesting that more than one antigen may be the target for the IgA anti–basement membrane antibodies.[18]

Immunoelectron microscopic studies have been performed to determine the exact location of the IgA in the skin of patients with both linear IgA dermatosis and CBDC. Immunoelectron microscopy of the skin of patients with linear IgA deposits has revealed three distinct patterns of immunoreactants. In some patients with linear IgA dermatosis, the IgA deposits are found in the lamina lucida region of the basement membrane zone, similar to the location of immunoreactants present in the skin of patients with bullous pemphigoid.[19,20] A second pattern of IgA deposition has been detected in which the IgA deposits are present at and below the lamina densa in a pattern similar to that seen in EBA.[19–21] Prost et al.[20] have described a third pattern of immunoreactants in some patients with linear IgA dermatosis in which the IgA deposits are found both above and below the lamina densa. In a similar manner, immunoelectron microscopic studies of patients with CBDC have shown the IgA immunoreactants to be in either the lamina lucida or a sublamina densa location.[21,22] These findings further support the possibility that multiple antigens may be involved as the targets in both adults and children with linear IgA deposits in the skin.

Although the relatively low titer of IgA antibodies against the basement membrane present in the sera of patients with both linear IgA dermatosis and CBDC has complicated the search for specific antigenic targets for the IgA, several investigators have made significant observations regarding the antigenic targets in these diseases. Zone et al.[23] studied sera from patients who had circulating IgA antibodies that bound to the epidermal side of 1 *M* NaCl-split normal human skin, as shown by indirect immunofluorescence. Using immunoblotting, they found that serum IgA from these patients bound to a 97-kDa protein present in both dermal and epidermal extracts of normal human skin. Specificity was demonstrated by eluting IgA from the 97-kDa protein and demonstrating that it bound in the same location in skin as the serum IgA. In a similar manner, these authors eluted IgA that had bound to normal human skin and demonstrated that it also bound to the 97-kDa protein. Zone et al.[7] also have demonstrated similar findings in patients with CBDC who have IgA antibodies that bind to the epidermal side of split skin, as shown by indirect immunofluorescence. Immunoelectron microscopy revealed that the 97-kDa antigen is present in the lamina lucida, below the hemidesmosome of normal human skin, in a location similar to where the IgA is localized in patients with CBDC and linear IgA dermatosis.[24]

Subsequently, Zone et al.[25] determined that the 97-kDa linear IgA bullous disease antigen is identical to a portion of the extracellular domain of the 180-kDa bullous pemphigoid antigen (BPAG2 or collagen XVII), which is essential in anchoring basal keratinocytes to the epidermal basement membrane. The antigen consists of a 180-kDa transmembrane protein and 120-kDa portion that corresponds to the collagenous ectodomain. Roh et al.[26] and Schumann et al.[27] have reported that autoantibodies in patients with linear IgA dermatosis recognize the soluble 120-kDa ectodomain of type XVII collagen. The 120-kDa antigen target is not unique to linear IgA dermatosis because it is also the antigen targeted by autoantibodies in some patients with cicatricial pemphigoid and bullous pemphigoid. This may explain in part the overlap in clinical and histologic features of these conditions.[26,27]

Wojnarowska et al.[28] also have identified a possible target antigen in patients with linear IgA dermatosis and CBDC. They studied the sera of patients in whom the IgA bound to the epidermal side of 1 *M* NaCl-split skin on routine indirect immunofluorescence. Using immunoblot techniques, they found that IgA in the sera of some patients with these diseases bound to a 285-kDa protein and that the protein was not the 230-kDa bullous pemphigoid antigen or type VII collagen, the EBA antigen.[28] These investigators have not shown, however, that the IgA that binds the 285-kDa protein in vitro is able to bind to skin in a pattern similar to that seen in tissue from patients. The reasons for the differences between these two suggested antigenic targets of the IgA from these patients is not known, and further studies are needed to resolve these findings.

In addition to the two target antigens noted earlier, additional proteins have been detected that bind IgA from some patients with linear IgA dermatosis or CBDC. Smith et al.[29] have identified a 45-kDa protein that binds IgA from patients with a clinical phenotype most suggestive of cicatricial pemphigoid but who have linear IgA deposits at the epidermal basement membrane. In patients with linear IgA dermatosis and IgA antibodies that bind to the dermal side of 1 *M* NaCl-split normal human skin, the IgA has been shown to bind to the EBA antigen, type VII collagen.[30] The antibody from at least one of these patients bound to a different region of the EBA antigen than the region recognized by the sera of most patients with EBA. This suggests that the difference in the binding site in patients with linear IgA diseases, compared with those with EBA, may account for the clinical differences seen in these two groups of patients.[28]

In summary, a number of different antigenic targets have been identified in patients with linear IgA diseases. The specific antigen detected appears to be related to the clinical phenotype, the cutaneous localization of the immunoreactants, and at the current time the laboratory performing the study. Further analysis that takes into account the clinical phenotype, molecular characterization of the antigens, and the continued exchange of sera and other reagents should allow for the more precise characterization of the antigens involved in patients with linear IgA dermatosis and CBDC.

CLINICAL MANIFESTATIONS

Cutaneous Manifestations

The clinical manifestations of linear IgA dermatosis are heterogeneous and often indistinguishable from those seen in patients with DH.[2,9,10,31] Patients may present with combinations of annular or grouped papules, vesicles, and bullae (Figs. 63-2 and 63-3). Typically, these lesions are distributed symmetrically on extensor surfaces, including elbows, knees, and buttocks. Lesions most often are very pruritic, resulting in numerous crusted papules (Fig. 63-4). The clinical presentation can be difficult to distinguish from that seen in patients with DH. However, the degree of pruritus seen in patients with linear IgA dermatosis is variable and, in general, less severe than that seen in patients with DH. Some patients with linear IgA dermatosis present with larger bullae, in a pattern more consistent with that seen in patients with bullous pemphigoid, or occasionally with cutaneous findings similar to those seen in patients with EBA.

The clinical presentation of CBDC is characterized most often by the development of tense bullae, often on an inflammatory base.[4] These lesions occur most frequently in the perineum and perioral region and often may occur in clusters, giving a "cluster of jewels" appearance (Figs. 63-5, 63-6, and 63-7). New lesions sometimes appear around the

FIGURE 63-2

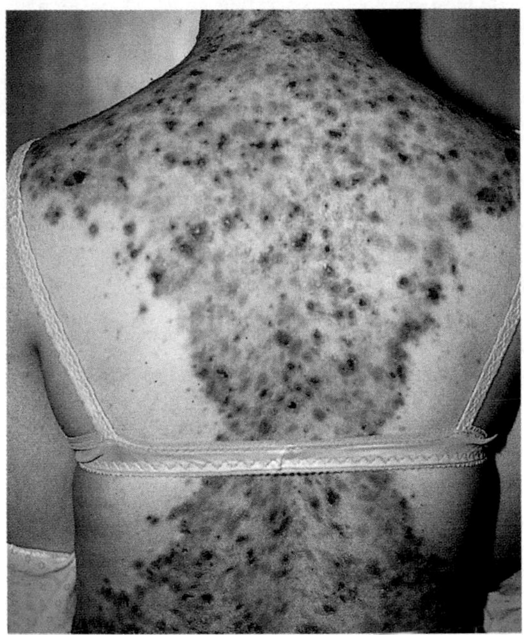

Patient with linear IgA dermatosis with crusted erosions, papules, and vesicles on the back and neck.

periphery of previous lesions, with a resulting "collarette" of blisters. Patients often report significant pruritus and/or a burning of the skin with the development of skin lesions. Patients with CBDC often present with the acute development of large numbers of tense blisters, which may rupture and become secondarily infected.

Rarely, patients with linear IgA dermatosis may present with an acute febrile illness with arthritis, arthralgias, and generalized malaise.[33] The presence of multiple papules and vesicles in a patient with systemic signs and symptoms has led to the evaluation of these patients for systemic infections, including viral infections. Routine direct immunofluorescence, however, has revealed linear deposits of IgA, and these patients have responded to conventional therapy.

FIGURE 63-3

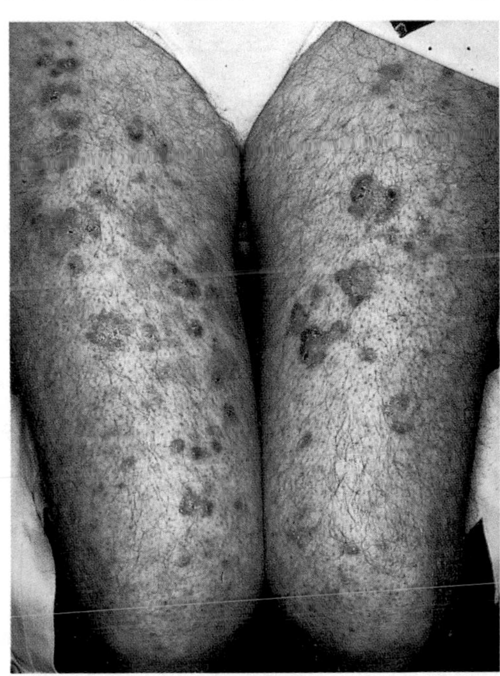

Patient with linear IgA dermatosis with annular erythematous plaques on the thighs.

FIGURE 63-4

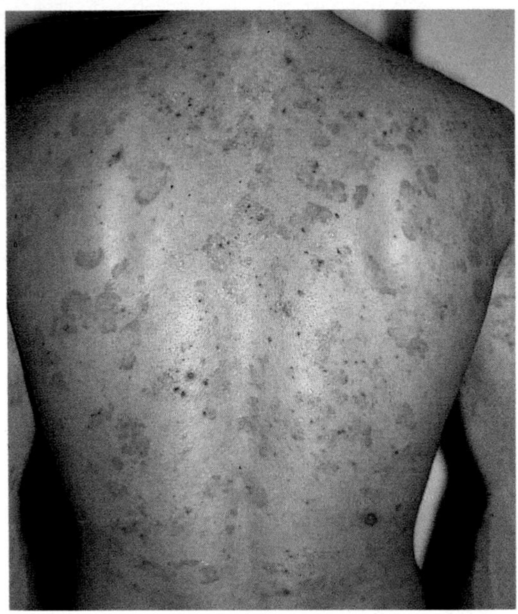

Patient with linear IgA dermatosis with grouped urticarial papules on the back with scattered crusted erosions.

Mucosal Involvement

Mucosal involvement is an important clinical manifestation seen in patients with linear IgA dermatosis and CBDC. This involvement can range from largely asymptomatic oral ulcerations and erosions to severe

FIGURE 63-5

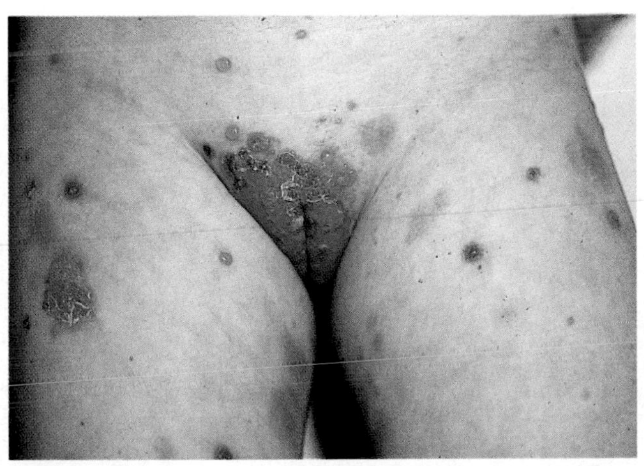

Patient with chronic bullous disease of childhood. Tense bullae and crusted papules are present on the abdomen, with a clustering of bullae noted in the perineal region.

FIGURE 63-6

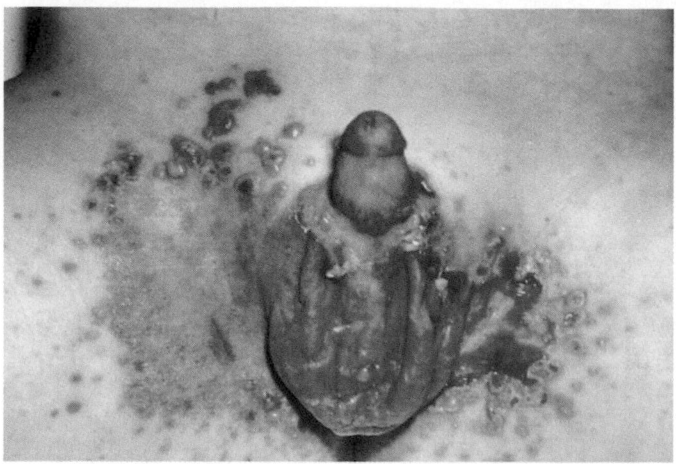

Chronic bullous disease of childhood. Tense blisters on erythematous bases in the pubic and inguinal areas.

oral disease alone as well as to severe conjunctival and oral disease typical of that seen in cicatricial pemphigoid.[9,35,36] Oral lesions may occur in up to 70 percent of patients with linear IgA disease.[9] Although most patients with linear IgA dermatosis and mucosal involvement have significant cutaneous disease, cases have been reported in the literature in which the presenting and predominant clinical manifestations are lesions of the mucous membranes.[35,37] These patients may present with desquamative gingivitis and oral lesions consistent with those seen in patients with cicatricial pemphigoid. Patients also may present with conjunctival disease and scar formation typical of that seen in patients with cicatricial pemphigoid. It appears likely that the different clinical manifestations seen in patients with linear IgA deposits will relate to the difference in antigenic targets.

FIGURE 63-7

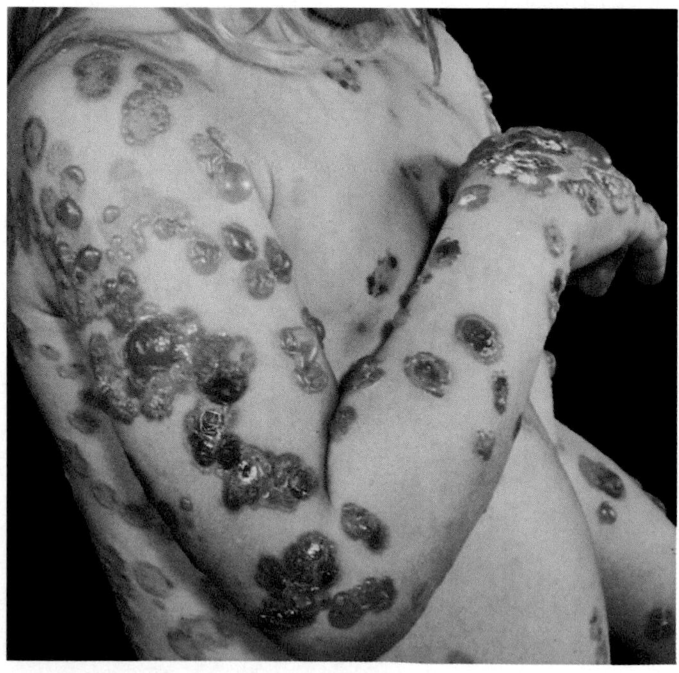

Extensive chronic bullous disease of childhood. Note tense and flaccid blisters without notable inflammation.

Disease Associations

The similar clinical presentation of many patients with linear IgA disease to that seen in patients with DH led to the investigation of patients with linear IgA disease for an associated gluten-sensitive enteropathy. Although some investigators have found evidence of minimal inflammatory changes in the small bowel of patients with linear IgA disease, numerous investigators have failed to show that the majority of patients with linear IgA disease have significant evidence of the villous atrophy characteristically seen in patients with DH.[1,38] In addition, the clinical manifestations of linear IgA disease have not been controlled by the use of a gluten-free diet.[39] Circulating autoantibodies against tissue transglutaminase, which occur in high frequency in patients with untreated gluten-sensitive enteropathy and DH, have not been found in most patients with linear IgA diseases.[40] Recently, Egan et al.[41] reported a patient with linear IgA dermatosis and well-documented gluten-sensitive enteropathy. This patient responded to a gluten-free diet with normalization of small bowel mucosal and control of the skin disease. In addition, this patient's skin disease flared with reinstitution of gluten in the diet. This case and documentation in the literature that a minority of patients with linear IgA disease have minimal changes of small bowel mucosal consistent with that seen in gluten-sensitive enteropathy suggest that there may be a subset of linear IgA patients who have an associated gluten-sensitive enteropathy and that their skin disease may respond to a gluten-free diet.[39,41]

Other conditions have been reported in association with CBDC. Baldari et al.[42] reported a case of CBCD occurring after acute mononucleosis. These authors suggest that this virus may have a role in initiation of the disease through immune stimulation. CBDC also has been reported in association with chronic granulomatous disease in the setting of *Paecilomyces* lung infection.[43] The relationship between these conditions and CBDC has yet to be established.

Linear IgA disease has been associated with the administration of a variety of drugs. Case reports have described patients with the relatively acute onset of clinical, histologic, and immunopathologic findings consistent with linear IgA disease who have been taking a variety of drugs, including vancomycin, lithium, furosemide, atorvastatin, captopril, and diclofenac. The mechanism of this interaction is not known. However, it is clear that some drugs can induce linear IgA deposits in the skin and the associated skin disease.

Linear IgA disease also has been associated rarely with a variety of malignancies. Patients with linear IgA disease have been reported with both lymphoid and nonlymphoid malignancies.[44,45] Godfrey et al.[44] reported three cases of lymphoid malignancies in 70 patients with linear IgA disease followed for a mean of 8.5 years. This represented an increase over the predicted number of 0.2 cases in an age- and sex-matched population. No increase in the rate of nonlymphoid malignancies was seen. These findings suggest a small risk of lymphoid malignancy in these patients. However, larger population-based studies need to be done to confirm these findings.

PATHOLOGY

Routine histopathology of an early lesion in patients with linear IgA dermatosis and CBDC reveals a subepidermal bulla with collections of neutrophils along the basement membrane, often accumulating at the papillary tips (Fig. 63-8). A mild lymphocytic infiltrate may be present around the superficial dermal blood vessels without any

FIGURE 63-8

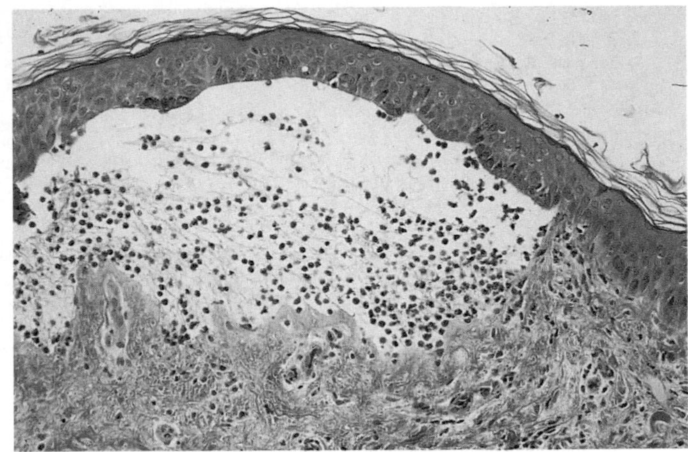

Histopathology of lesional skin from a patient with linear IgA dermatosis showing a subepidermal blister filled with neutrophils. (*Courtesy of Kim B.Yancey, MD.*)

evidence of neutrophilic vasculitis. Occasionally, the inflammatory infiltrate is composed of eosinophils, but most frequently neutrophils are the major component of the subepidermal inflammation.[9,46,47] Electron microscopic examination of the blisters found in patients with both linear IgA dermatosis and CBDC has revealed that the blister forms either within the lamina lucida or in a sublamina densa location.[19,22]

Most often the histopathology seen in linear IgA disease is difficult to distinguish from that seen in patients with DH. Smith et al.[46] reported that patients with linear IgA disease tended to have fewer papillary microabscesses and a more diffuse infiltrate of neutrophils at the basement membrane zone. However, Blenkinsopp et al.[47] found no significant difference between the histopathology found in patients with linear IgA disease and those with DH. In general, the histopathology of blisters in linear IgA disease, CBDC, and DH is virtually indistinguishable.

DIFFERENTIAL DIAGNOSIS

Linear IgA dermatosis often closely mimics the clinical pattern seen in patients with DH. Some patients may have findings that resemble those seen in patients with bullous pemphigoid, cicatricial pemphigoid, or EBA. In a similar manner, patients with CBDC must be differentiated from those with DH of childhood and childhood bullous pemphigoid. The findings of linear IgA deposits at the basement membrane by direct immunofluorescence, most often in the absence of IgG and the third component of complement (C3), can distinguish this disease from bullous pemphigoid, cicatricial pemphigoid, and EBA, whereas granular IgA deposits are found at the basement membrane in patients with DH.

TREATMENT AND PROGNOSIS

Adults with linear IgA dermatosis have an unpredictable course.[2,9] Many patients have disease that continues for years, with few, if any, episodes of remission. Occasionally, patients may have a spontaneous remission with loss of clinical features of the disease and disappearance of the linear IgA deposits in the skin. Patients with severe mucosal disease, especially of the eyes, may have persistent problems with symblepharon formation and resulting structural problems with the eyelids and cornea, even after active blistering has remitted.

Patients with linear IgA disease most often respond dramatically to dapsone or sulfapyridine. This response usually occurs within 24 to 48 h, in a manner similar to that seen with DH; as such, it is not a helpful diagnostic sign for linear IgA disease.[2,9,10] While most patients are well controlled with dapsone or sulfapyridine alone, some patients require low-dose prednisone therapy to suppress blister formation.[9,10] The majority of patients with linear IgA disease cannot control their skin disease with a gluten-free diet.[39]

CBDC is most often a self-limited disease, with most children going into remission within 2 years of the onset of the disease.[5,6,9] Occasionally, the disease persists well into puberty but often is less severe than the initial eruption. Patients with CBDC respond in a similar dramatic fashion to dapsone or sulfapyridine.[4] Many children, however, require the addition of relatively small doses of prednisone to bring the disease under control.[5,6] Isolated case reports suggests that some patients with CBDC may respond to antibiotics, including sulphonamides, dicloxacillin, and erythromycin.[48,49] However, spontaneous remission in these patients cannot be ruled out.

REFERENCES

1. Lawley TJ et al: Small intestinal biopsies and HLA types in dermatitis herpetiformis patients with granular and linear IgA skin deposits. *J Invest Dermatol* **74**:9, 1980
2. Leonard JN et al: Linear IgA disease in adults. *Br J Dermatol* **107**:301, 1982
3. Chorzelski TP et al: Immunofluorescence studies in the diagnosis of dermatitis herpetiformis and its differentiation from bullous pemphigoid. *J Invest Dermatol* **56**:373, 1971
4. Cohen DM et al: Linear IgA disease histopathologically and clinically masquerading as lichen planus. *Oral Surg Oral Med Oral Pathol Oral Radiol Endod* **88**:196, 1999
5. Chorzelski TP, Jablonska S: IgA linear dermatosis of childhood (chronic bullous disease of childhood). *Br J Dermatol* **101**:535, 1979
6. Jablonska S et al: Linear IgA bullous dermatosis of childhood (chronic bullous dermatosis of childhood). *Clin Dermatol* **9**:393, 1992
7. Zone JJ et al: Antigenic specificity of antibodies from patients with linear basement membrane deposition of IgA. *Dermatology* **189**(suppl):64, 1994
8. Dmochowski M et al: Immunoblotting studies of linear IgA disease. *J Dermatol Sci* **6**:194, 1993
9. Wojnarowska F et al: Chronic bullous disease of childhood, childhood cicatricial pemphigoid and linear IgA disease of adults: A comparative study demonstrating clinical and immunopathologic overlap. *J Am Acad Dermatol* **19**:792, 1988
10. Chorzelski TP et al: Linear IgA bullous dermatosis of adults. *Clin Dermatol* **9**:383, 1992
11. Venning VA et al: HLA type in bullous pemphigoid, cicatricial pemphigoid and linear IgA disease. *Clin Exp Dermatol* **14**:283, 1989
12. Sachs JA et al: A comparative serological and molecular study of linear IgA disease and dermatitis herpetiformis. *Br J Dermatol* **118**:759, 1988
13. Collier PM et al: Adult linear IgA disease and chronic bullous disease of childhood: The association with human lymphocyte antigens Cw7, B8, DR3 and tumour necrosis factor influences disease expression. *Br J Dermatol* **141**:867, 1999
14. Wojnarowska F et al: Chronic bullous disease of childhood and linear IgA disease of adults are IgA1-mediated diseases. *Br J Dermatol* **131**:201, 1994
15. Flotte TJ et al: Immunopathologic studies of adult linear IgA bullous dermatosis. *Arch Pathol Lab Med* **109**:457, 1985
16. Hall RP, Lawley TJ: Characterization of circulating and cutaneous IgA immune complexes in patients with dermatitis herpetiformis. *J Immunol* **135**:1760, 1985
17. Leonard JN et al: Evidence that the IgA in patients with linear IgA disease is qualitatively different from that of patients with dermatitis herpetiformis. *Br J Dermatol* **110**:315, 1983
18. Wojnarowska F et al: The localization of the target antigens and antibodies in linear IgA disease is heterogeneous and dependent on the methods used. *Br J Dermatol* **132**:750, 1995

19. Karpati S et al: Ultrastructural immunogold studies in two cases of linear IgA dermatosis: Are there two distinct types of this disease? *Br J Dermatol* **127**:112, 1992
20. Prost C et al: Diagnosis of adult linear IgA dermatosis by immunoelectron microscopy in 16 patients with linear IgA deposits. *J Invest Dermatol* **92**:39, 1989
21. Bhogal B et al: Linear IgA bullous dermatosis of adults and children: An immunoelectron microscopic study. *Br J Dermatol* **117**:289, 1987
22. Dabrowski J et al: The ultrastructural localization of IgA deposits in chronic bullous disease of childhood (CBDC). *J Invest Dermatol* **72**:291, 1979
23. Zone JJ et al: Identification of the cutaneous basement membrane zone antigen and isolation of antibody in linear immunoglobulin A bullous dermatosis. *J Clin Invest* **85**:812, 1990
24. Ishiko A et al: 97-kDa linear IgA bullous dermatosis (LAD) antigen localizes to the lamina lucida of the epidermal basement membrane. *J Invest Dermatol* **106**:739, 1996
25. Zone JJ et al: IgA Antibodies in chronic bullous diseases of childhood react with a 97-kDa basement membrane zone protein. *J Invest Dermatol* **106**:1277, 1996
26. Roh JY et al: The 120-kDa soluble ectodomain of type XVII collagen is recognized by autoantibodies in patients with pemphigoid and linear IgA dermatosis. *Br J Dermatol* **143**:104, 2000
27. Schumann H et al: The shed ectodomain of collagen XVII/BP180 is targeted by autoantibodies in different blistering skin diseases. *Am J Pathol* **156**:685, 2000
28. Wojnarowska F et al: Identification of the target antigen in chronic bullous disease of childhood and linear IgA disease of adults. *Br J Dermatol* **124**:157, 1991
29. Smith EP et al: Identification of a basement membrane zone antigen reactive with circulating IgA antibody in ocular cicatricial pemphigoid. *J Invest Dermatol* **101**:619, 1993
30. Hashimoto T et al: A case of linear IgA bullous dermatosis with IgA anti-type VII collagen autoantibodies. *Br J Dermatol* **134**:336, 1996
31. Peters MS, Rogers RS: Clinical correlations of linear IgA deposition at the cutaneous basement membrane zone. *J Am Acad Dermatol* **20**:761, 1989
32. Marsden RA et al: A study of benign chronic bullous dermatosis of childhood and comparison with dermatitis herpetiformis and bullous pemphigoid occurring in childhood. *Clin Exp Dermatol* **5**:159, 1980
33. Leigh G et al: Linear IgA dermatosis with severe arthralgia. *Br J Dermatol* **119**:789, 1988
34. Blockmans D et al: Linear IgA dermatosis: A new cause of fever of unknown origin. *Neth J Med* **47**:214, 1995
35. Leonard JN et al: The relationship between linear IgA disease and benign mucous membrane pemphigoid. *Br J Dermatol* **110**:307, 1984
36. Kelly SE et al: A clinicopathological study of mucosal involvement in linear IgA disease. *Br J Dermatol* **119**:161, 1988
37. Porter SR et al: Linear IgA disease manifesting as recalcitrant desquamative gingivitis. *Oral Surg Oral Med Oral Pathol* **74**:179, 1992
38. deFranchis R et al: Small-bowel involvement in dermatitis herpetiformis and in linear IgA bullous dermatosis. *J Clin Gastroenterol* **5**:429, 1983
39. Leonard JN et al: Experience with a gluten-free diet in the treatment of linear IgA disease. *Acta Derm Venereol (Stockh)* **67**:145, 1987
40. Rose C et al: Circulating autoantibodies to tissue transglutaminase differentiate patiens with dermatitis herpetiformis from those with linear IgA disease. *J Am Acad Dermatol* **41**:957, 1999
41. Egan CA et al: Linear IgA bullous dermatosis responsive to gluten-free diet. *Am J Gastroenterol* **96**:1927, 2001
42. Baldari U et al: Chronic bullous disease of childhood following Epstein-Barr virus seroconversion: A case report. *Clin Exp Dermatol* **21**:123, 1996
43. Smitt JH et al: Chronic bullous disease of childhood and a *Paecilomyces* lung infection in chronic granulomatous disease. *Arch Dis Child* **77**:150, 1997
44. Godfrey K et al: Linear IgA disease of adults: Association with lymphoproliferative malignancy and possible role of other triggering factors. *Br J Dermatol* **123**:447, 1990
45. McEvoy MT, Connolly SM: Linear IgA dermatosis: Association with malignancy. *J Am Acad Dermatol* **22**:59, 1990
46. Smith SB et al: Linear IgA bullous dermatosis v dermatitis herpetiformis: Quantitative measurements of dermoepidermal alterations. *Arch Dermatol* **120**:324, 1984
47. Blenkinsopp WK et al: Histology of linear IgA disease, dermatitis herpetiformis and bullous pemphigoid. *Am J Dermatopathol* **5**:547, 1983
48. Powell J et al: Mixed immunobullous disease of childhood: a good response to antimicrobials. *Br J Dermatol* **144**:769, 2001.
49. Siegfried EC et al: Chronic bullous disease of childhood: Successful treatment with dicloxacillin. *J Am Acad Dermatol* **39**:797, 1998

CHAPTER 64

Stephen I. Katz

Pemphigoid Gestationis (Herpes Gestationis)

Pemphigoid gestationis (PG) is a rare, pruritic, polymorphic, inflammatory, subepidermal, bullous dermatosis of pregnancy and the postpartum period. Since it is unrelated to any known viral infection and has characteristics of bullous pemphigoid, the former name, *herpes gestationis* (HG), has been abandoned in favor of PG. Its incidence has been roughly estimated to be 1 in 1700[1] to 1 in 10,000 deliveries.[2] Definitive diagnosis can be made with specific immunopathologic studies.

ETIOLOGY AND PATHOGENESIS

The etiology of PG is unknown. It is not related to herpes group viruses. The consistent finding of C3 deposition at the basement membrane zone of lesional and normal-appearing skin, in addition to the usual findings of an avidly complement-fixing IgG antibody (HG factor) in the serum, points to a role for immunologic mechanisms. One can postulate that the IgG antibodies are initiated in response to an antigenic stimulus peculiar to pregnancy, perhaps in the amnion.[3] These antibodies, as well as T cells, have specificity for a 14-amino-acid stretch of the ectodomain of the 180-kDa antigen (BPAG2, BP180, or type XVII collagen) that is a hemidesmosomal protein.[4–6] The antibodies bind to an extracellular site located near the membrane-spanning domain of this protein.[5–7] Once deposited at the basement membrane zone, these antibodies activate the complement cascade, which in turn generates an inflammatory response and the cutaneous features of inflammation that are morphologically recognized as PG. IgG_1 and IgG_3 are the major subclasses of immunoglobulin that target the antigen.[8] These IgG antibodies can, in most cases, cross the placenta—hence the occasional genesis of the transient blistering or papular disease in the infant. The infant's catabolism of the maternal IgG rapidly terminates the immunologic assault on the infant's skin. An animal model using passive transfer of antibodies to the extracellular domain of BP180 has demonstrated that mice injected with these antibodies develop subepidermal blisters that mimic those in bullous pemphigoid and PG.[9]

Ultrastructurally, the C3 and the IgG are deposited along the lamina lucida and on the dermal side of the basal cell plasma membranes.[10] Necrosis of basal cells occurs in both early lesional skin and in many areas of normal-appearing skin.[10]

Hormonal factors undoubtedly play an important role in the pathogenesis of PG. The onset in pregnancy or very shortly thereafter, the postpartum flares, the associated exacerbations with hormone-producing tumors,[11] and the oral contraceptive exacerbation of the disease in patients whose diagnoses have been verified immunologically are all well documented. To date, however, an immunologically verified PG-like dermatosis has not been reported from the use of oral contraceptive agents in patients without a prior history of PG.

CLINICAL MANIFESTATIONS

Pemphigoid gestationis usually presents as an extremely pruritic papulovesicular eruption on the abdomen but may involve other areas, including the palms, soles, chest, back, and face.[10,12] Mucosal surfaces usually are spared. Lesions vary from erythematous, edematous papules to large, tense bullae (Fig. 64-1), with many intermediate forms including small vesicles, confluent papules and vesicles, and urticaria-like plaques (Fig. 64-2) with and without grouped vesicles, bullae, erosions, and crusts. Although the more severe cases show a combination of many of these lesions (Fig. 64-3), milder cases may present only with moderate pruritus and a few erythematous papules or isolated edematous plaques 1 to 2 cm in diameter[12,13] (see Fig. 64-2).

Pemphigoid gestationis usually begins from the fourth to the seventh month of pregnancy, but the onset has been reported during the first trimester and in the immediate postpartum period.[12,14,15] Postpartum exacerbations as well as flares with the first few menstrual periods are common. Although the disease is self-limited for a particular episode, it may or may not recur in subsequent pregnancies; if it does, it is likely to begin earlier. PG may be exacerbated by the use of estrogen- or progesterone-containing medications.[12]

Fetal prognosis has been sought in several studies. One review of fetal and maternal risk factors in 41 immunologically verified cases revealed significant fetal death and premature deliveries,[14] and another series of 11 evaluable cases showed one intrauterine death.[16] Some studies have suggested that there is no increase in fetal mortality,[15,17,18] whereas others have indicated an increase in prematurity and small-for-gestational-age infants.[19] Less than 5 percent of babies are born with urticarial, vesicular, or bullous lesions.[12,14] These lesions almost always resolve spontaneously during the first several weeks.

FIGURE 64-1

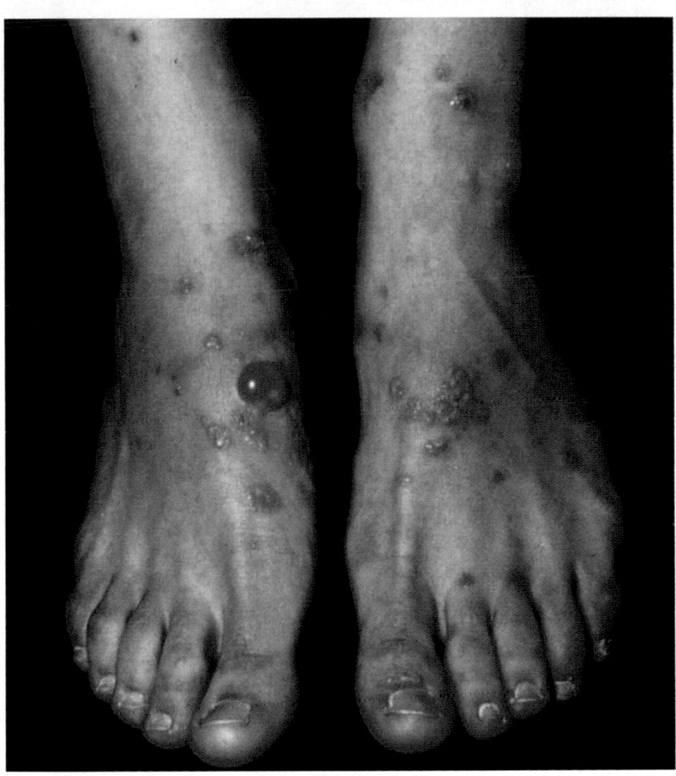

Herpes gestationis. Polymorphic lesions on dorsa of feet.

HISTOPATHOLOGY

The histopathologic features are variable. Both superficial and deep dermal vascular plexuses usually are surrounded by an infiltrate (of varying intensity) composed of lymphocytes, histiocytes, eosinophils, and occasionally a few neutrophils. Eosinophil infiltration is thought by some to be the most constant histopathologic feature.[20,21] There is edema of the dermal papillae and epidermis together with characteristic foci of basal cell necrosis over the tips of the dermal papillae.[22] Some authors have suggested that liquefaction degeneration or a variable degree of spongiosis represents the most constant epidermal finding and that dermal infiltration by eosinophils is the single most consistent finding in PG.[15] Vesicular lesions show subepidermal blister formation in a bulbous teardrop shape, although sections cut through the lateral extensions of the blisters at times may appear to show intraepidermal vesicles (Fig. 64-4). Although the findings may be characteristic, they are not diagnostic of PG.

IMMUNOLOGIC FEATURES

Direct Immunofluorescence Studies

The examination of peribullous and urticarial lesions or of normal-appearing skin in PG consistently has demonstrated heavy, homogeneous linear deposition of C3 along the basement membrane zone (Fig. 64-5) with concomitant IgG deposition in approximately 30 to

FIGURE 64-2

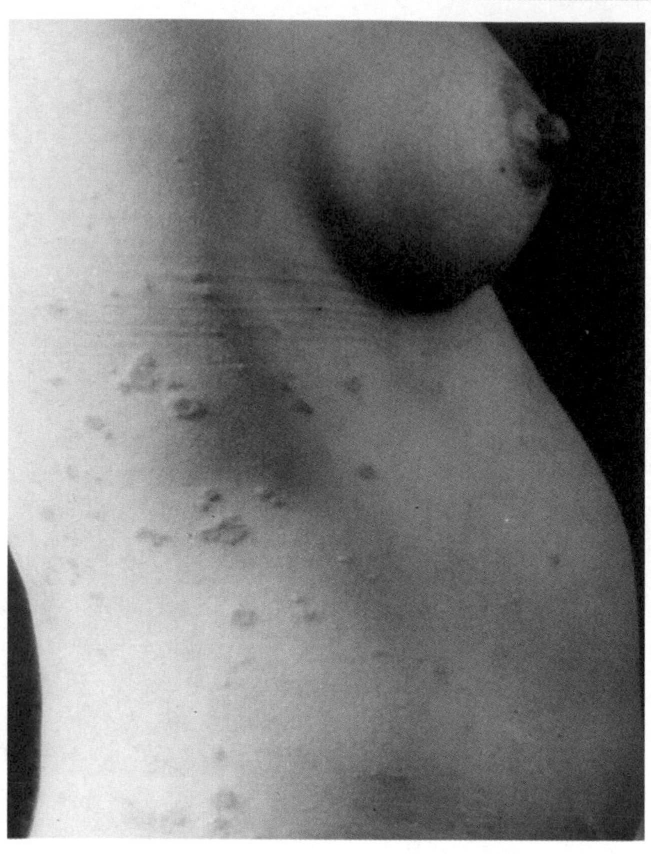

Herpes gestationis. Urticarial papules and plaques on the trunk.

40 percent of patients. When monoclonal antibodies are used, IgG_1 may be detected in the skin basement membrane zone of all patients.[23] IgA and IgM deposition have been noted infrequently. Properdin and, less frequently, properdin factor B, components of the alternative complement pathway, also may be detected along the basement membrane zone. C1q and C4, components of the classical complement pathway, have been detected less frequently, and C5 deposition also has been reported. The heavy deposition of C3 at the basement membrane zone of skin, however, is the diagnostic hallmark in patients with PG.[24–26] The immunofluorescence findings may persist in these patients' skin for several months and for as long as a year after lesions have resolved.

Similar direct immunofluorescence findings have been noted in infants born of affected mothers. The C3 deposition has been noted in clinically normal as well as affected infants' skin.

FIGURE 64-3

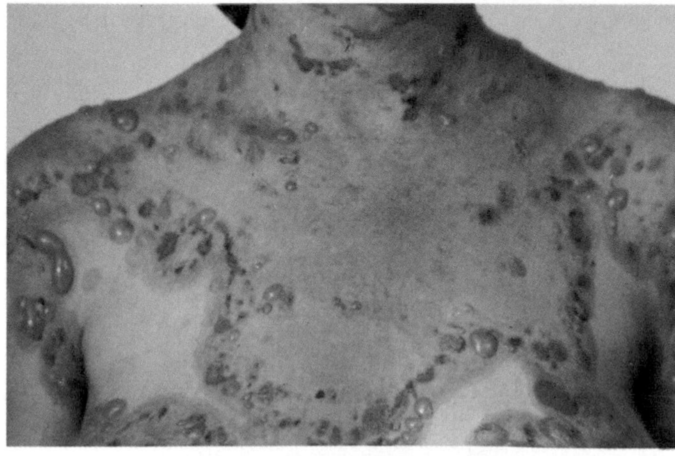

Herpes gestationis. Erythematous urticarial and bullous lesions on the chest and shoulders.

FIGURE 64-4

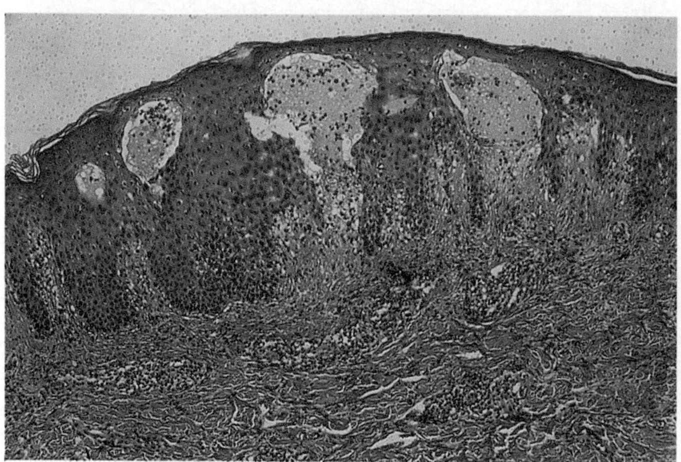

Herpes gestationis. Subepidermal vesicle formation; dermal edema; infiltrate consisting of lymphocytes, histiocytes, eosinophils, and a few neutrophils; and focal basal cell necrosis. Note bulbous, teardrop-like vesicles.

Indirect Immunofluorescence Studies

Using routine indirect immunofluorescence techniques, IgG serum anti–basement membrane antibodies are detected in only about 20 percent of patients with PG,[14] whereas ELISA and immunoblotting assays will detect autoantibodies in greater than 71 percent of sera.[27,28] However, when monoclonal antibodies are used, almost all sera have been shown to contain an IgG_1 anti–basement membrane zone antibody.[23] Several reports have indicated the presence of a serum complement-fixing factor in many, but not all, patients with PG.[14,24–26] This factor,

FIGURE 64-5

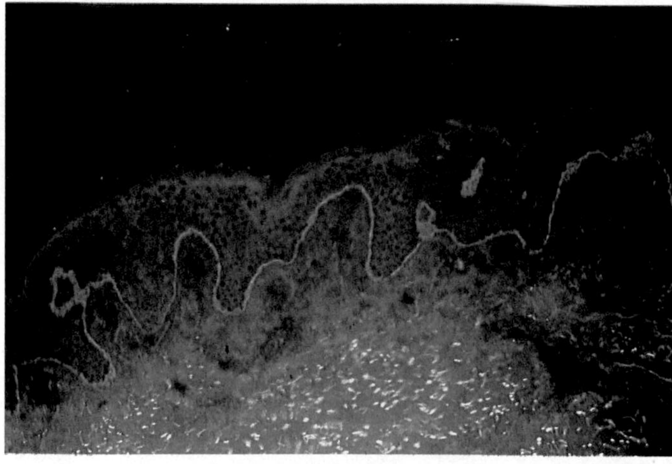

Herpes gestationis. Linear deposition of C3 along the basement membrane zone.

termed the *HG factor,* is an avid complement-fixing IgG antibody (presumably IgG_1) frequently present in the sera of patients in such low concentrations as to escape detection by routine indirect immunofluorescence techniques. The HG factor binds to amniotic epithelial basement membrane[3] and also has been detected in cord sera of some infants born of affected mothers.

IMMUNOGENETIC STUDIES

A genetic predisposition has been proposed for PG in that there is a marked increase in the HLA-B8, -DR3, and -DR4 genotypes in affected patients,[29] particularly with DRB1*0301 and DRB1*0401/ 040X.[30] Complement polymorphism studies also have demonstrated a 90 percent frequency of the C4 null allele in patients with a history of HG.[31]

DIFFERENTIAL DIAGNOSIS

The disease most often confused with PG is pruritic urticarial papules and plaques of pregnancy (PUPPP), an eruption that begins on the abdomen (usually in striae), manifests as papules and plaques (often with blanched halos), usually occurs late in pregnancy, and is severely pruritic[32] (see Chap. 142). In PUPPP, there are no immunoreactants seen at the dermal-epidermal junction. Differentiation of PG from other dermatoses of pregnancy is discussed elsewhere (see Chap. 142).

The tendency for the vesicles and bullae to group and the intense pruritus in PG have erroneously promoted the idea that PG is related to, or identical with, dermatitis herpetiformis (see Chap. 67). Another source of confusion is erythema multiforme (see Chap. 58). However, these two diseases, erythema multiforme and dermatitis herpetiformis, should be easily distinguished from PG by routine direct immunofluorescence techniques. In dermatitis herpetiformis, IgA deposition occurs along the basement membrane zone of perilesional and normal-appearing skin; in erythema multiforme, immunoglobulin and complement may be seen only in the superficial blood vessels.

The possible relation between PG and bullous pemphigoid is unresolved. The features suggesting a close relationship between PG and bullous pemphigoid are (1) the morphologic similarity of the cutaneous lesions in the two diseases, (2) the similar direct immunofluorescence findings, (3) the persistence of PG in rare patients, and most important, (4) the very close relationship, if not the identity, of the PG antigen with the 180-kDa bullous pemphigoid antigen.[4–6] There are several dissimilar features, however, that necessitate caution in proposing a common etiology between HG and bullous pemphigoid. These are (1) the patient population at risk, (2) the provocative factors (i.e., estrogens or progesterones), (3) the almost universal tendency toward remission following and between pregnancies, (4) the complement-fixing ability of the anti–basement membrane antibody in PG, which frequently exceeds the anti–basement membrane antibody titer (by comparison, the anti–basement membrane antibody titer of bullous pemphigoid sera frequently exceeds the complement-fixing titer), and (5) ultrastructural studies suggesting that blister formation in bullous pemphigoid occurs between the lamina densa and the basal cell membrane, whereas in PG the separation may occur at the level of the degenerated basal cells.[10]

TREATMENT

The treatment of PG is designed to suppress blister formation and to relieve the intense pruritus. These goals usually can be achieved by giving

20 to 40 mg of prednisone per day in the morning; however, the itching may be so severe that divided doses may be required. Exacerbations of the pruritus and blistering commonly occur at parturition and may then require an increase in prednisone. The prednisone is tapered gradually during the postpartum period, but exacerbations at the time of menses may demand a temporary increase in dosage. This is true for most patients; however, a few patients do not require systemic prednisone and can be managed with antihistamines and topical steroids or emollients.[12] At the other extreme, some individuals, after parturition, require azathioprine in addition to the prednisone for control of their disease.

Infants born of affected mothers who have received high doses of prednisone should be examined carefully by a neonatologist for evidence of adrenal insufficiency. This complication is rare but is theoretically possible if continuous large doses of glucocorticoids are employed for several months prior to birth to control the mother's disease. The cutaneous lesions noted in such infants are of a transient nature requiring no therapy.

REFERENCES

1. Roger D et al: Specific pruritic diseases of pregnancy: A prospective study of 3192 pregnant women. *Arch Dermatol* **130**:734, 1994
2. Kolodny RG: Herpes gestationis: A new assessment of incidence, diagnosis and fetal prognosis. *Am J Obstet Gynecol* **104**:39, 1969
3. Ortonne JP et al: Herpes gestationis factor reacts with the amniotic epithelial basement membrane. *Br J Dermatol* **117**:147, 1987
4. Morrison LH et al: Herpes gestationis autoantibodies recognize a 180-kDa human epidermal antigen. *J Clin Invest* **81**:2023, 1988
5. Giudice GJ et al: Bullous pemphigoid and herpes gestationis autoantibodies recognize a common non-collagenous site on the BP180 ectodomain. *J Immunol* **151**:5742, 1993
6. Lin MS et al: Identification and characterization of epitopes recognized by T lymphocytes and autoantibodies from patients with herpes gestationis. *J Immunol* **162**:4991, 1999
7. Bedane C et al: Bullous pemphigoid and cicatricial pemphigoid autoantibodies react with ultrastructurally separable epitopes on the BP180 ectodomain: Evidence that BP180 spans the lamina lucida. *J Invest Dermatol* **108**:901, 1977
8. Chimanovitch I et al: IgG_1 and IgG_3 are the major immunoglobulin subclasses targeting epitopes within the NC16A domain of BP180 in pemphigoid gestationis. *J Invest Dermatol* **109**:140, 1999
9. Liu Z et al: A passive transfer model of the organ-specific autoimmune disease, bullous pemphigoid, using antibodies generated against the hemidesmosomal antigen, BP180. *J Clin Invest* **92**:2480, 1993
10. Yaoita H et al: Herpes gestationis: Ultrastructure and ultrastructural localization of in vivo–bound complement. Modified tissue preparation and processing for horseradish peroxidase staining of skin. *J Invest Dermatol* **66**:383, 1976
11. Halkier-Sorensen L et al: Herpes gestationis in association with neoplasma malignum generatisatum: A case report. *Acta Derm Venereol (Stockh)* **120**:96, 1985
12. Jenkins RE et al: Clinical features and management of 87 patients with pemphigoid gestationis. *Clin Exp Dermatol* **24**:255, 1994
13. Ogilvie P et al. Pemphigoid gestationis without blisters. *Hautartz* **51**:25, 2000
14. Lawley T et al: Fetal and maternal risk factors in herpes gestationis. *Arch Dermatol* **114**:552, 1978
15. Shornick JK et al: Herpes gestationis: Clinical and histologic features of twenty-eight cases. *J Am Acad Dermatol* **8**:214, 1983
16. Mcrchaoui J et al: Obstetrical prognosis of gestational pemphigoid: Study of a series of 13 cases and review of the literature. *J Gynecol Obstet Biol Reprod (Paris)* **21**:963, 1992
17. Holmes RC et al: A comparative study of toxic erythema of pregnancy and herpes gestationis. *Br J Dermatol* **106**:499, 1982
18. Harrington CI, Bleehan SS: Herpes gestationis: Immunopathological and ultrastructural studies. *Br J Dermatol* **100**:389, 1979
19. Shornick JK, Black MM: Fetal risks in herpes gestationis. *J Am Acad Dermatol* **26**:63, 1992
20. Shornick JK: Herpes gestationis. *J Am Acad Dermatol* **17**:539, 1987

21. Borrego L et al: Polymorphic eruption of pregnancy and herpes gestationis: Comparison of granulated cell proteins in tissue and serum. *Clin Exp Dermatol* **24**:213, 1999
22. Hertz KC et al: Herpes gestationis: A clinicopathologic study. *Arch Dermatol* **112**:1543, 1976
23. Kelly SE et al: The distribution of IgG subclasses in pemphigoid gestationis: PG factor is an IgG1 autoantibody. *J Invest Dermatol* **92**:695, 1989
24. Provost TT, Tomasi TB Jr: Evidence for complement activation via the alternate pathway in skin diseases: I. Herpes gestationis, systemic lupus erythematosus and bullous pemphigoid. *J Clin Invest* **52**:1779, 1973
25. Katz SI et al: Herpes gestationis: Immunopathology and characterization of the HG factor. *J Clin Invest* **57**:1434, 1976
26. Jordon RE et al: The immunopathology of herpes gestationis: Immunofluorescent studies and characterization of HG factor. *J Clin Invest* **57**:1426, 1976
27. Giudice GJ et al: Development of an ELISA to detect anti-BP180 autoantibodies in bullous pemphigoid and herpes gestationis. *J Invest Dermatol* **102**:878, 1994
28. Murakami H et al: Analysis of antigens recognized by autoantibodies in herpes gestationis: Usefulness of immunoblotting using a fusion protein representing and extracellular domain of the 180-kDa bullous pemphigoid antigen. *J Dermatol Sci* **13**:112, 1996
29. Shornick JK et al: High frequency of histocompatibility antigens HLA-DR3 and -DR4 in herpes gestationis. *J Clin Invest* **68**:553, 1981
30. Shornick JK et al: Class II MHC typing in pemphigoid gestationis. *Clin Exp Dermatol* **20**:123, 1995
31. Shornick JK et al: Complement polymorphism in herpes gestationis: Association with C4 null allele. *J Am Acad Dermatol* **29**:545, 1993
32. Lawley T et al: Pruritic urticarial papules and plaques of pregnancy. *JAMA* **241**:1696, 1979

CHAPTER 65

M. Peter Marinkovich
Paul A. Khavari
G. Scott Herron
Eugene A. Bauer

Inherited Epidermolysis Bullosa

EPIDERMOLYSIS BULLOSA AS A DISEASE ENTITY

Epidermolysis bullosa (EB) refers to a group of inherited disorders that involve the formation of blisters following trivial trauma. The most obvious signs are vesicles and bullae within the skin and mucous membranes; however, internal organs may also be involved and clinical heterogeneity is a manifestation of a variety of heritable molecular defects. Marked skin and mucosal fragility causing painful vesicles and bullae define this disease. Abnormal wound repair responses that eventuate into chronic erosions, scarring, and invasive carcinoma are common. Although the milder phenotypes share several of these features, the most severe recessively inherited forms are mutilating, multiorgan disorders that threaten both the quality and length of life.

A number of early studies identified the major subtypes of EB. Epidermolysis bullosa was known to be distinct from pemphigus since the time of von Hebra and the term *epidermolysis bullosa hereditaria* was first coined by Koebner. Hallopeau was the first to distinguish between simplex (nonscarring) and dystrophic (scarring) forms of the disease, while Weber and Cockayne, Dowling and Meara, and Koebner each described unique forms of epidermolysis bullosa simplex. Hoffman, Cockayne, Touraine, Pasini, and Bart provided much of the information about subtypes of dystrophic epidermolysis bullosa. Herlitz described epidermolysis bullosa letalis which was later found to be a part of the third major category of epidermolysis bullosa, the junctional form. The application of electron microscopy toward diagnosis of epidermolysis bullosa led to the studies of Pearson[1] and collaborators who classified the patients not only on the basis of clinical findings but also on the existence of ultrastructural changes. Recent major advances have led to the identification of specific protein and genetic abnormalities in most types of epidermolysis bullosa patients. These studies permitted an improved understanding of the biologic basis of epidermolysis bullosa and, finally, a classification of epidermolysis bullosa based on molecular etiology that will provide a rational approach to future specific therapy.

THE DERMAL EPIDERMAL BASEMENT MEMBRANE

Overview (See also Chap. 16)

Epidermolysis bullosa arises from defects associated with basal keratinocytes and the dermal–epidermal basement membrane zone (BMZ). Many tissues, such as the skin and cornea, which are subjected to external disruptive forces, contain a complex BMZ composed of a group of specialized components that combine together to form anchoring complexes (Fig. 65-1). At the most superior aspect of the BMZ, keratin-containing intermediate filaments of the basal cell cytoskeleton insert upon electron-dense condensations of the basal cell plasma membrane termed *hemidesmosomes*. Anchoring filaments span the lamina lucida connecting hemidesmosomes with the lamina densa and anchoring filaments. At the most inferior aspect of the BMZ, type VII, collagen-containing anchoring fibrils extend from the lamina densa into the papillary dermis and combine with the lamina densa and anchoring plaques, trapping interstitial collagen fibrils. Thus the cutaneous BMZ connects the extensive basal cell cytoskeletal network with the abundant network of interstitial collagen fibrils in the dermis.[2,3]

Keratin Filaments (See also Chap. 7)

Keratins are obligate heteropolymers composed of pairs of acidic and basic monomers. The keratin pair 5 and 14 assemble together to form the extensive intermediate filament network of the basal cell cytoskeleton.[4] Keratins contain a central α-helical rod with several nonhelical interruptions, as well as nonhelical carboxyl- and amino-terminal regions. The regions of highest conservation among the keratins are located on the ends of the keratin rod in the helix boundary motifs. Extensive mutagenesis studies suggest that helical regions near the ends of the central rod are important in keratin filament elongation, whereas the nonhelical domains may be important in forming lateral associations. As noted, keratin intermediate filaments insert into the hemidesmosomes.

FIGURE 65-1

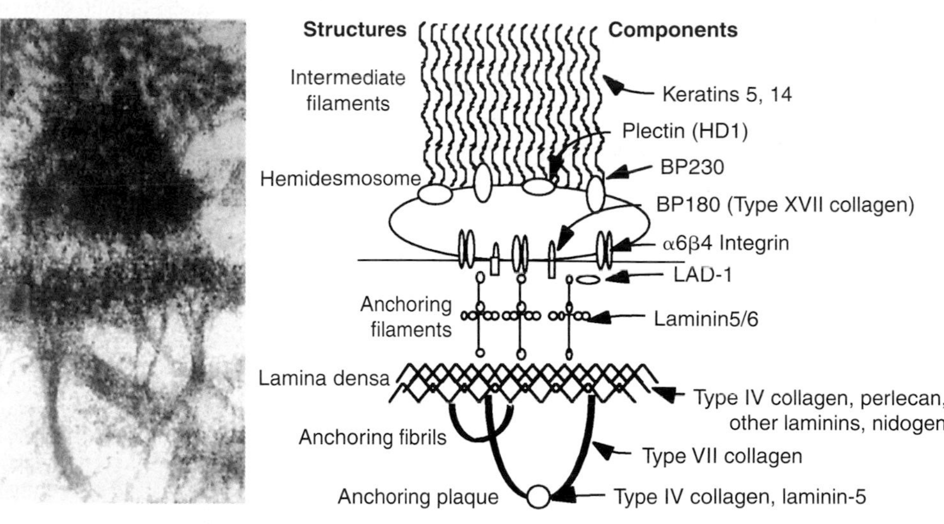

The ultrastructural elements of the dermal–epidermal basement membrane, as shown in the electron micrograph on the *left*, are correlated with the known molecular composition of this structure, as shown in the schematic on the *right*.

Hemidesmosomes (See also Chap. 16)

Hemidesmosomes contain intracellular proteins including plectin and BP230. *Plectin* (also termed *HD1* and *IFAP 300*) is a 500-kDa protein that is believed to act as an intermediate filament binding protein. It is possible that plectin also interacts with microfilaments, as plectin contains a domain with similarity to the actin-binding domain of spectrin.[5] BP230, also known as BPAG1, is a 230-kDa protein that has homology both to desmoplakin[6] and to plectin. Several splicing variants of BPAG1 are of vital importance in the nervous system.[7] BP230 localizes to a region referred to as the inner plate on the cytoplasmic surface of the hemidesmosome and, like HD1, is suspected to function in the connection between hemidesmosomes and intermediate filaments. BP230 negative transgenic mice lack a hemidesmosomal inner plate and the connection between hemidesmosomes and intermediate filaments is severed, creating a cytoplasmic zone of mechanical fragility just above the hemidesmosomes.[8] In these mice, neither hemidesmosome stability nor cell substratum adhesion appear to be weakened. Consequently, neither BP230 nor HD1/plectin appears to be essential for hemidesmosome assembly.

Anchoring Filaments (See also Chap. 16)

Hemidesmosomes also contain the transmembrane proteins *type XVII collagen* (also termed *BPAG2*)[9] and $\alpha 6\beta 4$ integrin.[10] The cytoplasmic portions of these molecules make up part of the hemidesmosome dense plaque, whereas the extracellular portions of these molecules make up portions of the anchoring filament and probably contribute to the structure known as the subbasal dense plate that underlies hemidesmosomes in the lamina lucida region. β_4 integrin is known to combine with only the α_6 subunit, whereas the α_6 subunit can combine either with the β_4 integrin or with the β_1 integrin. Both the $\alpha_6\beta_1$ or $\alpha_6\beta_4$ integrin combinations act as receptors for laminins and $\alpha_6\beta_4$ integrin appears specifically to act as a receptor for laminin 5.[11] $\alpha_6\beta_4$ integrin plays a central role in hemidesmosome formation in that transgenic mice lacking the β_4 integrin show skin devoid of hemidesmosomes with severe deficits in cell adhesion.[12] The β_4 integrin contains an especially large cytoplasmic domain that is suspected to function in the interaction with other proteins of the hemidesmosomal plaque.

Type XVII collagen (BPAG2, type XVII collagen) is a collagenous protein with a type II transmembrane orientation. Based on electron microscopy and cross-linking studies, type XVII collagen assembles into a triple-helical homotrimer and contains three main regions: an intracellular amino-terminal globular head, a central rod, and an extracellular flexible tail.[13] Type XVII collagen associates with laminin 5 and $\alpha_6\beta_4$ integrin in adhesion structures termed *stable-anchoring contacts* formed by keratinocytes in vivo. These structures are thought to represent pre-hemidesmosomes.[14] Type XVII collagen undergoes processing in keratinocyte cultures.[15] LAD-1, the autoantigen in linear IgA bullous dermatosis[15,16] (see Chap. 63) is a 120-kDa protein that was recently shown, by peptide sequencing, to contain the exodomain of type XVII collagen.[17] Thus LAD-1 appears to be the processed product of the type XVII collagen exodomain.[19]

In addition to $\alpha_6\beta_4$ integrin and type XVII collagen, anchoring filaments contain the molecules laminin 5 and laminin 6. Like all members of the family of laminin proteins,[20] laminin 5 is a large heterotrimeric molecule, containing α_3, β_3, and γ_2 chains.[21,22] The first laminins to be described contained three short arms and one long arm, forming a cross shape as shown by rotary shadowing analysis. In contrast, laminin 5 contains truncations of each short arm.[23–25] Because of these short arm truncations, laminin 5 cannot self-polymerize with other laminins or bind to nidogen. Instead, laminin 5 forms a disulfide bonded attachment to laminin 6,[26] the other known anchoring filament laminin[27] that contains α_3, β_1 and γ_1 chains, laminin 5. Laminin 5 also undergoes processing of its γ_2 and α_3 chains,[22] which may be mediated by bone morphogenic protein 1,[28] plasmin,[29] matrix metalloproteinase 2,[30] or membrane-type matrix metalloproteinase 1.[31] The γ_2 chain short arm appears important in the assembly of laminin 5 into basement membrane.[32] The antigen recognized by monoclonal antibody (MAb) 19-DEJ-1[33] also localizes to anchoring filaments; however, this protein remains incompletely characterized.

Anchoring Fibrils (See also Chap. 16)

Type VII collagen is the major constituent of anchoring fibrils. Analysis of the deduced amino acid sequence of type VII collagen[34] reveals the presence of a long central collagenous region characterized by repeating Gly-X-Y sequences that contains a number of noncollagenous interruptions, including a 39–amino-acid noncollagenous segment in the center of the helix that corresponds to the "hinge region" predicted by biochemical studies.[35,36] These interruptions account for the flexibility of the type VII collagen molecule, and explain its ability to loop around and entrap dermal matrix molecules, in order to provide its function of stabilizing the basement membrane to the underlying papillary dermis.[37] A 50-kDa component of anchoring fibrils has also been identified that appears to localize to the insertion sites of anchoring fibrils to the lamina densa.[38]

Primary sequence analysis has determined that the 145-kDa N-terminal end of type VII collagen contains the largest noncollagenous domain. This domain inserts onto the lamina densa and anchoring plaques. Type IV collagen, the most abundant component of these structures, binds to type VII collagen NC-1 domain. A direct interaction between anchoring filaments and anchoring fibrils has been demonstrated by studies that demonstrate a specific interaction between the anchoring filament component laminin 5 and type VII collagen NC-1 domain.[39,40] Type VII collagen appears to interact with the β_3 chain on laminin 5.[41] Like all collagens, type VII collagen assembles into a triple helix. Because only one chain of type VII collagen, the α_1 chain, has been identified, one gene codes for an entire molecule. Type VII collagen triple helices are joined together at their processed NC-2 globular domains to form antiparallel dimers.[37,42] Anchoring fibrils may derive from lateral associations of the antiparallel dimers.

DISEASE DESCRIPTIONS

Table 65-1 presents a simplified classification of EB based on the ultrastructural level within which the cleavage plane of the blister occurs. Thus, for the practitioner, the current diagnostic "gold standard" for grouping EB remains electron microscopy, although immunomapping of basement membrane antigens adjacent to the tissue split provides complementary data. The three disease groups are (1) epidermolytic or EB simplex (EBS), (2) junctional EB (JEB), and (3) dermolytic or dystrophic EB (DEB). Within each of these groups there are several distinct types of EB based on clinical, genetic, histologic, and biochemical evaluation.[43] Table 65-2 shows these different subclassifications of EB.

EB Simplex

Epidermolytic EB is defined by the occurrence of intraepidermal blistering; the vast majority of cases are due to keratin gene mutations. However, there is considerable phenotypic variation among different subgroups (Table 65-3).[44] At least 11 distinct forms of EBS exist, 7 of which are dominantly inherited. The four most common EBS types are dominantly inherited and include generalized EBS (Koebner), localized EBS (Weber-Cockayne), EBS of the Ogna variety found in Norwegian kindreds, and the herpetiform EBS of Dowling-Meara. All these varieties share the common features of heat-sensitive formation of serous or serosanguineous, nonscarring vesicles and bullae.

TABLE 65-1

Classification of Epidermolysis Bullosa (EB)

Blister Location	Disease Group	Inheritance
Intraepidermal	EB simplex	Autosomal dominant* Autosomal recessive
Basement membrane zone	Junctional EB	Autosomal recessive
Sublamina densa	Dystrophic EB	Autosomal recessive Autosomal dominant

*The vast majority of EB simplex patients are from autosomal dominant kindreds.

GENERALIZED EBS In the Koebner variant of generalized EBS onset is at birth to early infancy with a predilection for hands, feet, and extremities. Palmar-plantar hyperkeratosis and erosions may be present (Fig. 65-2). Nails, teeth and oral mucosa are usually spared but if they are affected, the changes are minimal compared to recessive junctional or dystrophic EB.

LOCALIZED EBS The Weber-Cockayne subtype of EBS is characterized by onset in childhood or later in life, and this variant is the most common form of EBS. The disease may not present itself until adulthood, when thick-walled blisters on the feet or hands occur after excessively strenuous exercise, such as during athletic competition or in the military. Hyperhidrosis of the palms and soles is common. Secondary infection of blistered lesions on the feet is the most common complication of this disorder.

EB HERPETIFORMIS The onset of Dowling-Meara EBS is at birth with a generalized distribution. Oral mucosa is often involved with variable lesions in infancy. A pronounced inflammatory phase with transient milium formation may occur in infancy; however, blisters are nonscarring by early childhood (Fig. 65-3*A*). Spontaneous grouped or "herpetiform"' blisters occur on the trunk and proximal extremities and heal without scarring (Fig. 65-3*B*). Nails may shed and regrow with dystrophy. A distinctive feature is that heat does not appear to exacerbate the blistering in EB herpetiformis as it does in the Koebner and Weber-Cockayne forms. After the age of 6 or 7 years, hyperkeratosis of the palms and soles may develop. Laryngeal involvement[45] and pyloric atresia[46] have also been reported in patients with severe forms of EB herpetiformis.

EBS OF OGNA Onset in infancy is common with seasonal blistering (summer) on the acral areas. Small hemorrhagic and serous blisters occur primarily on the extremities. Healing occurs without scarring. All patients described thus far have come from Norway and a genetic linkage to erythrocyte glutamic-pyruvic transaminase (GPT) may help to explain the tendency toward easy bruising and hemorrhagic blisters which characterize Ogna EBS.

EBS WITH MUSCULAR DYSTROPHY This rare clinical entity is the first and only epidermolytic EB described that is not caused by a keratin gene mutation.[47] It presents as generalized intraepidermal blistering similar to EBS of Koebner; however, an adult onset muscular dystrophy is associated with the disease.

Molecular Pathology of EBS

Most of the patients with EB simplex analyzed at the genetic level have been found to be associated with mutations of the genes coding for keratins 5 and 14.[48] The level of separation of the skin in these patients is at the mid-basal cell, shown in Fig. 65-4, associated with variable intermediate filament clumping. Hemidesmosomes and other BMZ structures are normal by electron microscopy. The majority of keratin gene mutations associated with epidermolysis bullosa simplex are dominantly inherited due to abnormalities in the multimeric assembly of keratin filaments. There is a smaller subset of patients with recessively inherited disease of varying severity.[49,50]

Mutations coding for the most conserved regions of keratins 5 and 14, the helix boundary domains,[51] correlate with the most severe forms of epidermolysis bullosa simplex, such as the Dowling-Meara subtype, which exhibits intermediate filament clumping. On the other hand, milder types of disease, such as the Weber-Cockayne subtype, are associated with mutations coding for regions of keratins 5 and 14 that are less conserved. Mutations that code for a specific region of the amino terminus of keratin 5 are associated with mottled pigmentation in certain epidermolysis bullosa simplex patients,[52] although significance of this mutation and its association with pigmentary abnormalities remains unclear.[53,54] This condition is distinct from the large melanocytic nevi that can be seen in all three EB types.[55]

A small group of patients with recessive EB simplex have been shown to have associated muscular dystrophy and they have been shown to harbor mutations in the gene coding for HD1/plectin.[47,56,57] In these patients, the level of blistering is just above the hemidesmosome and complete disruption of the connection between the cytoskeleton and hemidesmosome is observed ultrastructurally. The mutations associated with this disease thus far are homozygous and produce premature termination codons which result in lack of expression of plectin. Plectin is normally expressed in a wide range of tissues, including muscle. While the mechanism of muscular dystrophy in plectin-deficient patients is unknown, it has been observed that disorganization of muscle sarcomeres occurs in the absence of plectin. It is possible that absence of plectin's spectrin-like domain, which may normally interact with actin filaments in muscle, may be a key factor in the muscle pathology.[58]

TABLE 65-2

Clinical Heterogeneity of Epidermolysis Bullosa (EB)

EPIDERMOLYTIC	JUNCTIONAL	DERMOLYTIC
Generalized EBS (Koebner)	JEB gravis (Herlitz)	Generalized RDEB (Hallopeau-Siemens)
Localized EBS (Weber-Cockayne)	JEB mitis	Localized RDEB
EB herpetiformis (Dowling-Meara)	JEB-pyloric atresia	Dominant DEB (Cockayne-Touraine)
EBS (Ogna)	GABEB	Dominant DEB albopapuloid (Pasini)
Muscular dystrophy-EBS	Localized JEB	

EBS, EB simplex; GABEB, generalized atrophic benign EB; JEB, junctional EB; RDEB, recessive dystrophic EB.

TABLE 65-3

Clinical Phenotype–Molecular Defect Correlations in Epidermolysis Bullosa

DISEASE*	GENES†	PROTEINS	REFERENCE
EBS-DM	KRT5, 14	Keratins 5, 14	4, 43
EBS-WC	KRT5, 14	Keratins 5, 14	4, 43
EBS-K	KRT5, 14	Keratins 5, 14	4, 43
Recessive EBS-MD	PLEC1	Plectin	47, 56
Recessive EBS-K	KRT14	Keratins 14	49, 50
JEB-lethal	LAMA3, B3, C2	Laminin 5 $\alpha_3, \beta_3, \gamma_2$	63, 64, 65
JEB-PA	ITGA6, B4	Integrin $\alpha_6\beta_4$	71
GABEB	COL17A1, LAMB3	BP180, Laminin	62, 68, 69, 70
DDEB	COL7A1	Type VII collagen	37, 77
RDEB	COL7A1	Type VII collagen	37, 77

*Disease categories reflect clinical phenotyes of individual EB patients studied in selected references.
†Genes indicated represent candidate genes identified by DNA mutation analysis as correlating with disease phenotype. Examples of genetic defects include: KRT5 or 14 heterozygous missense or in-frame deletions in dominant forms of EBS; KRT5 or 14 homozygous missense or premature termination codons (PTC) in recessive EBS; PLEC1 homozygous in-frame deletion or PTC in EBS-MD; LAMA3, B3, C2 homozygous PTC in Herlitz JEB; ITGA6 or B4 heterozygous PTC/in-frame deletion or homozygous PTC in JEB-PA; COL17A1 heterozygous PTC/missense or homozygous PTC in GABEB; COL7A1 heterozygous gly substitution in DDEB; COL7A1 homozygous PTC or gly substitution in RDEB-HS; COL7A1 homozygous missense or gly substitution or heterozygous PTC/gly substitution in RDEB mitis.
DDEB, dominant dystrophic EB; EBS-DM, EB simplex, Dowling-Meara type; EBS-K, EB simplex, Koebner type; recessive EBS-MD, EB simplex associated with muscular dystrophy; EBS-WC, EB simplex, Weber-Cockayne type; GABEB, generalized atrophic benign EB; JEB-lethal, junctional EB, Herlitz type; JEB-PA, JEB associated with pyloric atresia; RDEB, recessive dystrophic EB.

Junctional EB

Of all EB types, JEB shows the most genetic variation with at least seven different basement membrane components serving as candidate genes in this disorder (Table 65-3). All patients with JEB share the common histopathologic feature of blister formation within the lamina lucida of the BMZ either as part of stable anchoring complexes (i.e., hemidesmosomes) or anchoring filaments. This trait is inherited in an autosomal recessive manner and represents a spectrum of clinical phenotypes, depending on the type of genetic lesion present and a variety of environmental factors.

There are at least six clinical subtypes of JEB; however, three principal forms are most common. Herlitz disease, JEB gravis or lethal JEB are synonymous terms used to describe patients presenting with the most severe phenotypic disease. A more indolent form of JEB is termed *mitis JEB* and a third, relatively mild form is called *generalized atrophic benign EB* (GABEB) (Table 65-2).

JEB GRAVIS Patients with Herlitz EB often do not survive infancy and death rates are estimated at 40 percent the first year of life. The majority of patients succumb by 5 years of age. This makes Herlitz disease the most lethal of all EB subtypes. Generalized blistering is observed at birth (Fig. 65-5) with severe and clinically distinctive periorificial granulation tissue, which can also occur in nonlethal subtypes (Fig. 65-6). Nails are usually lost early and are dystrophic when present. Teeth are dysplastic due to enamel defects and most mucosal surfaces are involved with chronic erosions. Scalp lesions consisting of chronic nonhealing erosions with hyperplastic granulation tissue are common.

Associated systemic findings in severe cases include the entire spectrum of epithelial blistering with respiratory, gastrointestinal, and genitourinary organ systems involved. Tracheolaryngeal blistering, stenosis, or obstruction are commonly associated with Herlitz disease, and hoarseness in early infancy is an ominous sign. Marked growth retardation and a refractory, mixed anemia complicate management. Patients usually die of sepsis, multiorgan system dysfunction, and inanition.

A rare and distinct clinical variant of lethal JEB is that type presenting at birth with severe junctional blistering associated with pyloric and/or duodenal atresia. These patients exhibit extreme mucosal and cutaneous fragility due to integrin mutations in either the *ITGA6* or *ITGB4* genes.[59] Patients diagnosed as junctional EB with pyloric atresia (JEB-PA) may also have various urologic abnormalities, including hydronephrosis and nephritis. JEB with pyloric stenosis has also been reported in association with hydronephrosis.

JEB MITIS Some patients present at birth with moderate junctional disease or present with severe JEB but survive infancy and clinically improve with age. Hoarseness is usually mild or absent. Scalp and nail lesions are prominent and periorificial nonhealing erosions commonly

FIGURE 65-2

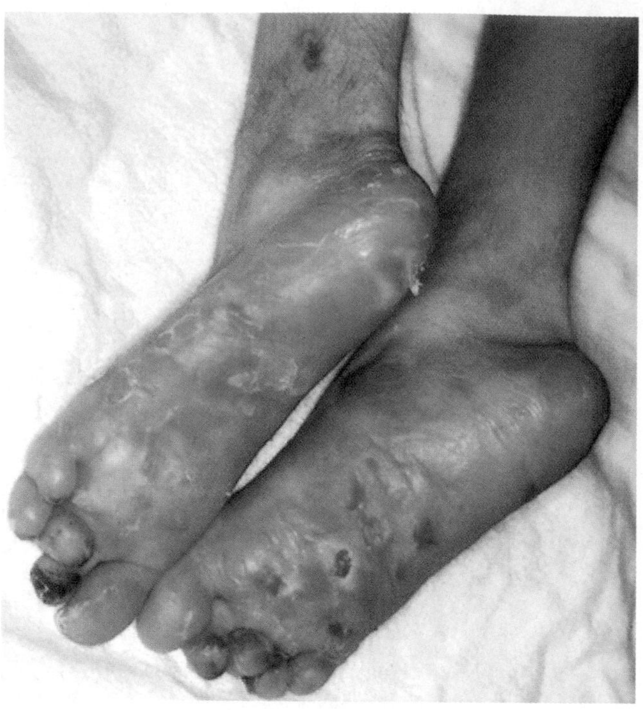

Generalized EBS: clinical appearance. Note the typical blisters of the feet with hyperkeratosis and callus formation.

FIGURE 65-3

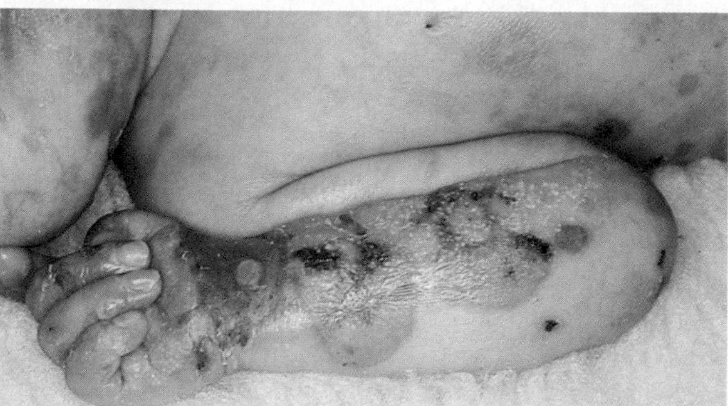

A.

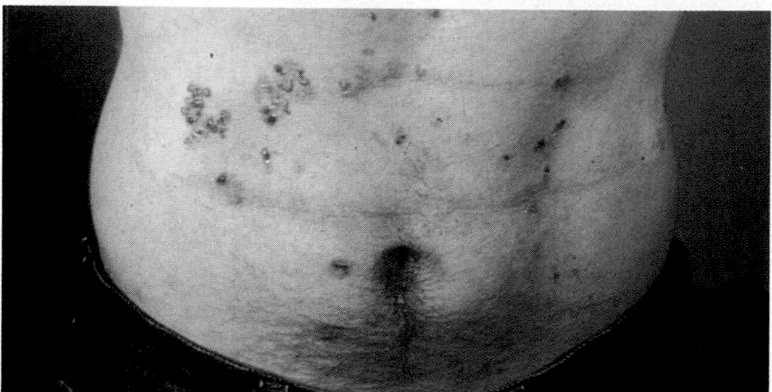

B.

Epidermolysis bullosa herpetiformis. *A.* Clinical appearance in newborn. Note the extensive erosions and milia. *B.* Clinical appearance in an adult male. Note the grouped vesicles.

characterize this disease in children between the ages of 4 and 10 years. Although the disease process is debilitating, patients who present in this way may be designated as having *nonlethal JEB* or *JEB mitis*. Several of these patients have heterozygous laminin 5 mutations with one allele of a single laminin 5 subunit representing a premature termination codon and the other a missense mutation or an in-frame splicing mutation. There are other rare variants of nonlethal JEB that present with localized junctional blistering of the extremities or intertriginous areas.

GENERALIZED ATROPHIC BENIGN EB A separate form of nonlethal JEB also presents at birth with generalized cutaneous involvement.[60,61] Variable-sized bullae occur, predominantly on the extremities; however, the trunk, scalp, and face are also involved. Survival to adulthood is the rule with persistent serous or serosanguineous bullae and chronic erosions of the extremities, trunk, and scalp. Blistering activity is particularly pronounced with increased ambient temperature. Nail dystrophy can be severe and a nonscarring alopecia (Fig. 65-7) with atrophic scarring of healed blisters are distinctive features of this EB subtype. Mucous membrane involvement of the oral cavity is mild and enamel defects contribute to dystrophic dentition. Blistering improves with age but the dental abnormalities and atrophic scalp lesions persist into adulthood. Overall growth is normal and anemia is rarely seen. In contrast to Herlitz disease, GABEB patients have a normal life span.

Molecular Pathology of JEB

Molecular diagnostic analysis has shown that different patients with JEB can carry mutations in any of the three laminin 5 subunits (i.e., α_3, β_3, γ_2).[62–64] However, about 80 percent of laminin 5 mutations can be traced to one of two recurrent nonsense mutations in the *LAMB3* gene making prenatal testing for laminin 5 lesions easier than other EB candidate genes.[65] In the letalis patients, all of the mutations so far detected have been those producing a premature termination codon, resulting in absence of expression of laminin-5. The combination of severe skin involvement and mucosal fragility since birth, hoarseness, absence of laminin 5 expression, and premature termination codons in both alleles of a laminin 5 subunit are the best indicators of Herlitz EB.

In the JEB variant GABEB, blistering occurs in the lamina lucida region and abnormalities of hemidesmosomes/anchoring filaments are usually present (see Fig. 65-4). Some patients with GABEB display a reduced but still positive expression of laminin 5.[62,66,67] Mutation-induced disruption of the connection of laminin 5 to other BMZ ligands such as type VII collagen or laminin 6 may provide an explanation for the patient's phenotype. Thus, partial loss of laminin 5 function leads to a more benign phenotype, whereas total loss of laminin 5 function leads to a lethal phenotype.

While laminin 5 mutations underlie a subset of GABEB patients, the majority of these patients have abnormalities of the hemidesmosomal protein type XVII collagen. A number of mutations of the gene coding for type XVII collagen[68,69] have been described in GABEB patients, including premature termination codon mutations, missense mutations, and a glycine substitution mutation. Of interest, one mosaic GABEB patient was identified who demonstrated well-defined areas of blistering associated with absence of type XVII collagen expression as well as areas of nonblistering skin associated with normal type XVII collagen expression. Careful analysis of the patient's keratinocytes revealed reversion of one of the two alleles of the mutation, most likely due to a mitotic gene conversion involving nonreciprocal exchange of parental allele DNA.[70]

Mutations of the genes coding for the β_4 and α_6 integrin are also associated with JEB;[71] in this group of diseases, pyloric atresia is present, and separation of the skin occurs at the level of the hemidesmosome region. Often fragments of the basal cell cytoplasm are found associated with the base of the split. In these patients, hemidesmosomes are almost absent or rudimentary at best, and the level of separation is such that fragments of the basal cell plasma membrane remain adherent to the base of the blister. The skin ultrastructure in patients with $\alpha_6\beta_4$ defects is remarkably similar to the β_4 integrin knockout mice described above. Nonlethal cases have been characterized which appear to result from a partial loss of function of β_4 integrin.[72] Interestingly, nonlethal JEB can sometimes ameliorate itself through alterations in mRNA splicing.[73,74]

FIGURE 65-4

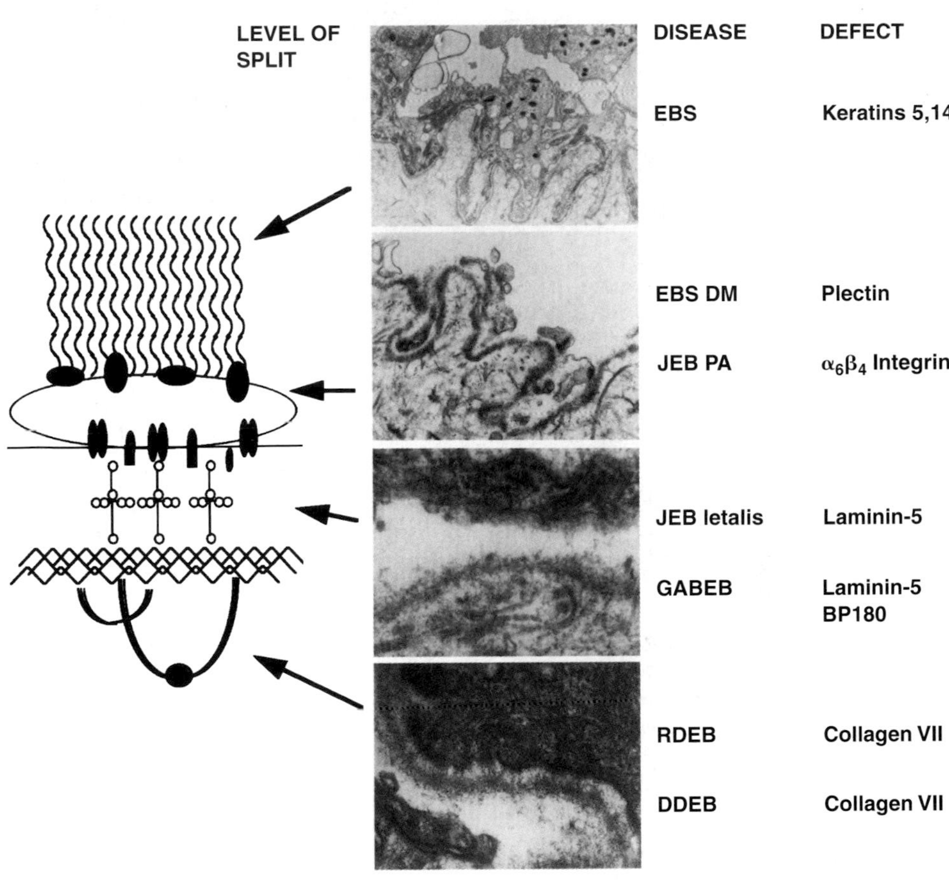

Representation of cutaneous basement membrane zone with examples of ultrastructural abnormalities observed in EB skin. The figure depicts four subtypes of EB based upon their respective levels of cleavage within the BMZ and examples of the candidate gene defect correlated with each blistering disorder (see text for details).

DYSTROPHIC EB

Dystrophic EB (DEB) is a "dermolytic" disease and healing after blister formation is usually accompanied by scarring and milium formation. There are four principal subtypes of heritable DEB and all share the common pathogenetic features of subepidermal blistering due to anchoring fibril type VII collagen mutations (Tables 65-2 and 65-3); however, several rarer forms also exist. The main types, which are separated on clinical grounds, include dominant DEB of Cockayne-Touraine; dominant DEB of the albopapuloid or Pasini variant; localized recessive DEB; and generalized recessive DEB (Table 65-2).

DOMINANT DEB In Cockayne-Touraine disease blistering is usually acral with nail dystrophy and onset in infancy or early childhood. Healing occurs with milia and scar formation, which may be hypertrophic or hyperplastic. Oral lesions are uncommon and teeth are usually normal.

The Pasini variant of DEB is usually seen at birth and blistering is more extensive with atrophic scarring and milium formation. Flesh-colored, scarlike papular lesions appear spontaneously on the trunk in the absence of obvious trauma and are called *albopapuloid lesions*. As these same lesions have been observed in other subtypes of EB, the specificity of this sign is debatable. Later in life, blisters are located primarily on the extremities but occasionally may be generalized. Dystrophic or absent nails are common; however, mucosal surfaces and teeth are often minimally affected.

RECESSIVE DEB The clinical phenotypes of recessive DEB (RDEB) include a wide spectrum of disease severity. A localized, less severe form, often called *RDEB-mitis,* occurs at birth and usually involves the acral areas with atrophic scarring of the joint surfaces and nail dystrophy but little mucosal involvement. The mild subtype of localized recessive DEB makes it clinically indistinguishable from some forms of localized dominant DEB.

Severe recessive DEB is a mutilating disease, known also as the Hallopeau-Siemens (HS) variant. Generalized blistering is present at birth and progression during infancy and childhood (Fig. 65-8) results in remarkable scarring, shown in Fig. 65-9*A*. Acquired syndactyly leading to "mitten-like" deformities of the hands and feet are the rule and the scarring process may extend proximally to involve the entire extremity in flexion contracture (Fig. 65-9*B*). Milia formation may be considerable (Fig. 65-10). Nails, teeth, and scalp are affected. Most mucosal surfaces are invariably involved with recurrent blisters and erosions leading to esophageal strictures and webbing, urethral and anal stenosis, phimosis and ocular surface scarring. Malnutrition, growth retardation, and chronic mixed anemia are common.

Perhaps the most devastating complication of HS-RDEB is the high risk of developing aggressive squamous cell carcinomas in areas of chronic erosions. In more than 50 percent of HS-RDEB, patients develop these "scar" carcinomas by 30 years of age and many of these die of metastatic disease.

Molecular Pathology of DEB

Abnormalities of anchoring fibrils are present in DEB patients ranging from subtle changes in some patients with dominant disease, to absence

FIGURE 65-5

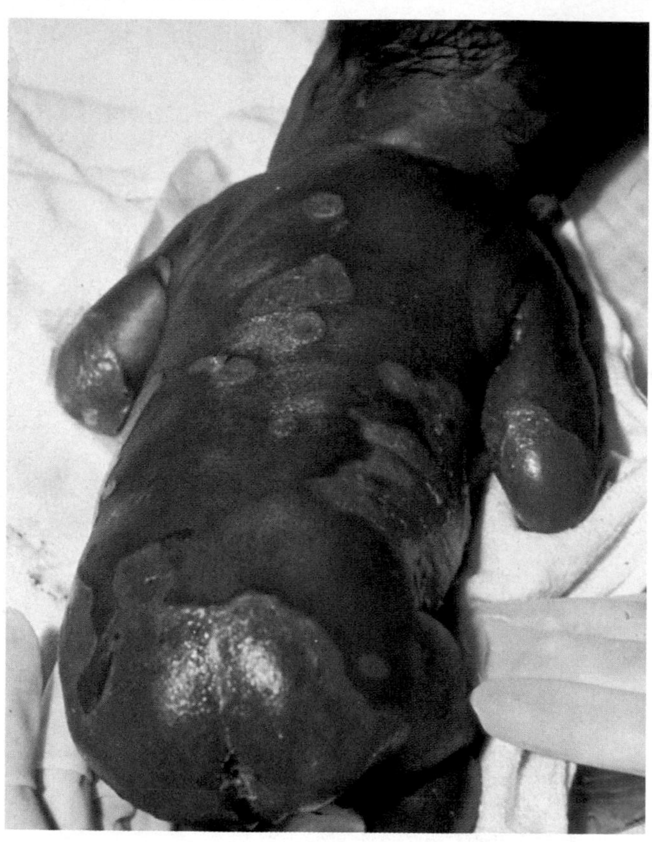

Junctional epidermolysis bullosa (Herlitz variant): clinical appearance in a newborn. Note the extensive erosion.

FIGURE 65-6

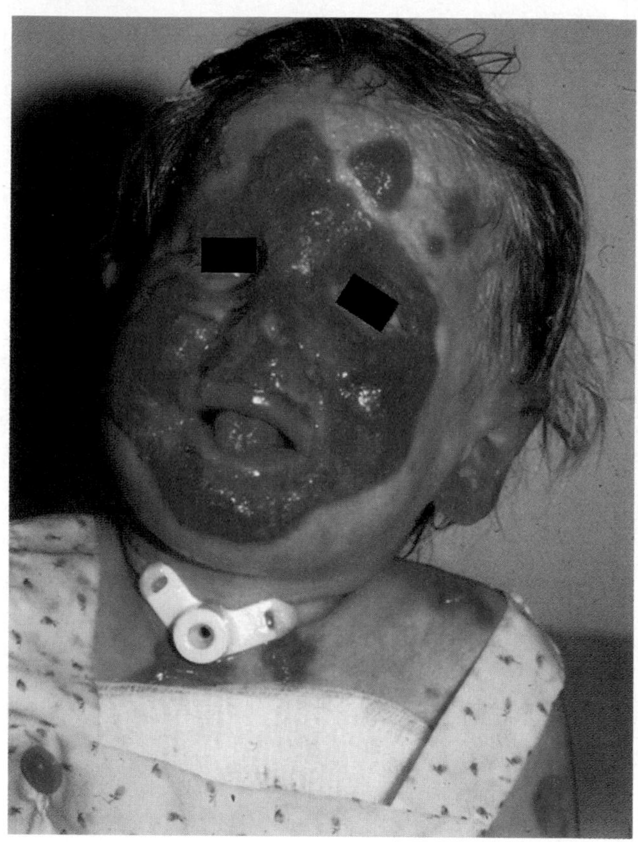

Junctional epidermolysis bullosa (Herlitz variant): clinical appearance in a child with typical periorificial involvement and exuberant granulation tissue. Severe laryngeal involvement necessitated tracheostomy.

of anchoring fibrils in patients with the severe recessive form of this disease. A sublamina densa plane of blister cleavage is present (Fig. 65-4). These observations correlate with indirect immunofluorescent microscopic analysis of DEB patients that demonstrates varying degrees of linear basement membrane staining in patients with dominant disease and totally absent staining in severe patients with recessive disease. In some patients, there is a cytoplasmic retention of type VII collagen that can be demonstrated in patient biopsy sections and analysis of patient keratinocytes.[75]

In all cases thus far, dystrophic EB is associated with mutations of the gene coding for type VII collagen (COL7A1) (Table 65-3). In the recessive forms, mutations usually cause premature termination codons that result in lack of type VII collagen in tissue. It is known that mRNAs bearing premature stop codons show accelerated turnover.[76] In addition, truncated proteins that are secreted would not assemble into anchoring filaments and may also show accelerated turnover. Either or both of these mechanisms can explain the lack of detectable type VII collagen in the tissue of individuals with severe RDEB associated with mutations that produce premature termination codons.[37,77,78]

Generally, *COL7A1* mutations that do not cause premature termination codons produce less-severe disease. For example, mutations that produce glycine substitutions of the triple-helical region interfere with triple-helical assembly of the type VII collagen molecule. These types of mutations are present in many patients with milder dominant forms of this disease.[79–86] In these patients, type VII collagen molecules may not be able to assume the proper conformation needed to polymerize into anchoring fibrils. Other *COL7A1* mutations are associated with

FIGURE 65-7

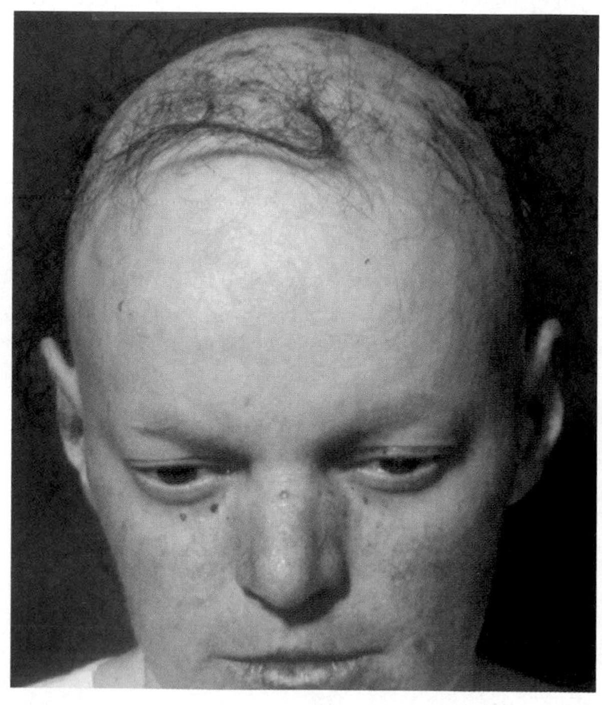

Junctional epidermolysis bullosa (generalized atrophic benign variant): clinical appearance. Note the typical alopecia.

FIGURE 65-8

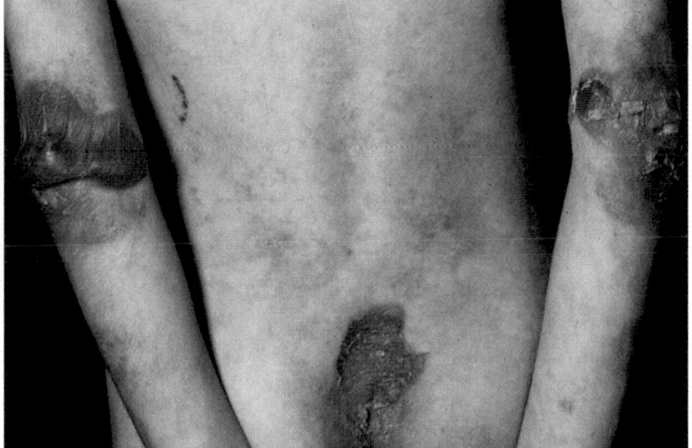

Recessive dystrophic epidermolysis bullosa. Note the flaccid blisters and erosions over elbows and sacral region.

impaired secretion of type VII collagen, resulting in intracellular accumulation of this molecule.[87–90] In one study, DEB patient mutations that involve the area of the gene coding for the type VII collagen NC2 domain were shown to interfere with NC2 processing and the assembly of anchoring fibrils.[91]

APPROACH TO THE PATIENT

Diagnosis

Technological advances in our approach to EB patient diagnosis have provided new insights into clinical phenotype-genotype correlations.[3] This approach integrates multiple analytic steps and unifies EB disease classification, course, genetic counseling and management options (Fig. 65-11). Each step in this approach utilizes our previous clinical experience with EB patients, detailed understanding of the molecular components of the cutaneous basement membrane and rapid advances in DNA mutation detection and gene transfer technology.

Ideally, the clinician will provide EB patient tissue samples that can be divided into several pieces: one for hematoxylin-and-eosin (H&E) light microscopy, one for immunofluorescence microscopy, one for electron microscopy and another for cell culture. Blood samples or buccal swabs are usually obtained from the nuclear family members for genetic analysis. In the majority of cases, not all diagnostic steps are necessary to arrive at a final diagnosis; however, the information provided by these studies is helpful for eventual development of targeted gene transfer and ultimately gene therapy of the EB patient.

Provisional diagnosis is made by a combination of patient history/physical exam and histopathology at the light microscope level on perilesional skin biopsy (Fig. 65-12). For example, EB simplex can often be classified at this stage and in the vast majority of cases a dominant family history is obtained. However, when no family history is given (or available), a recessive pattern should be considered, especially if the epidermolytic disease is severe or associated with extracutaneous disorders (e.g., muscular dystrophy). When a junctional cleavage pattern is recognized, recessive disease is the rule.

FIGURE 65-9

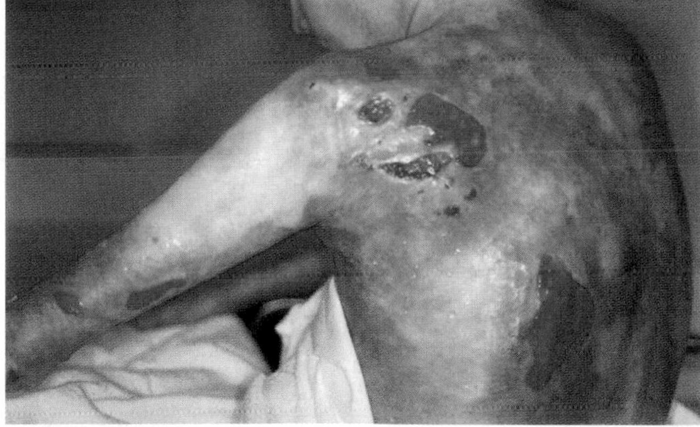

A.

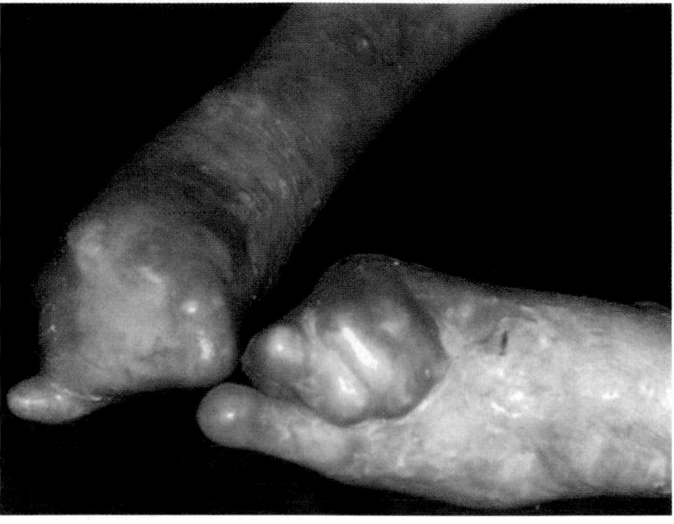

B.

A. Recessive dystrophic epidermolysis bullosa (Hallopeau-Siemens variant): clinical appearance. Note the extensive full thickness erosions, ulcers, and thick scarring. *B.* Note "mitten" deformity of fingers and nail loss.

Because light microscopy cannot distinguish junctional from dermolytic EB, ultrastructural analysis is required to provide definitive information about both blister location and alterations of basal keratinocyte anchoring complexes. However, the use of new immunodiagnostic reagents is often comparable to ultrastructural studies and in many cases these reagents provide more precise information about specific EB candidate gene product dysfunction. For example, immunofluorescence microscopy may show absence or diminished expression of a specific basement membrane component and this information helps to guide the search for genetic defects in EB candidate genes.

After a provisional diagnosis is made, several additional steps may be required, especially in cases where the mode of inheritance and/or previous diagnostic clues are unclear. For instance, often the clinical severity in patients with localized forms of RDEB makes them indistinguishable from those having mild dominant dystrophic forms or even localized, mild junctional EB. Furthermore, ultrastructural analysis may show only subtle alterations in anchoring complexes and immunofluorescence of skin may show normal expression of all EB candidate gene products at the BMZ, making the diagnosis even more difficult.

FIGURE 65-10

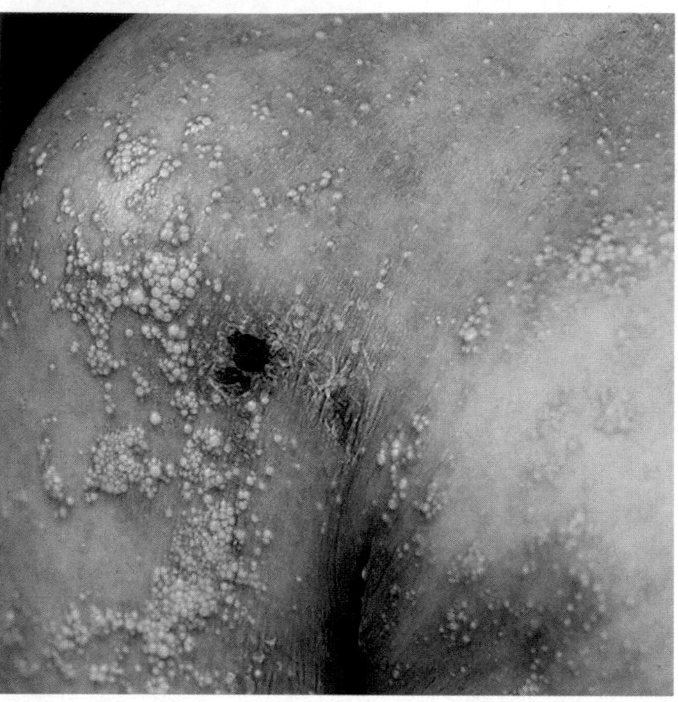

Extensive milia formation in previously blistered areas in recessive dystrophic epidermolysis bullosa.

In these cases, the combination of clinical signs, modern immunodiagnostic analysis and mutational studies are required to classify the EB type. A distinction between mild dominant dystrophic EB and recessive dystrophic EB can be made by mutation analysis. The presence of a single mutant *COL7A1* allele in both the proband and one parent or affected sibling confirms the former diagnosis, whereas, the latter diagnosis would be applicable if two mutant alleles were found (i.e., compound heterozygous or homozygous). In the absence of any *COL7A1* mutations, one of the many JEB candidate genes may harbor missense mutations or a combination of missense and nonsense mutations (Fig. 65-12).

Establishing cell cultures from biopsy specimens serves multiple purposes (Fig. 65-12). Easily cultured proband fibroblasts can be grown to provide DNA for mutation analysis. If keratinocytes can be grown, they can be immortalized to provide large amounts of biochemical and genetic material for subsequent analyses. Both immunofluorescence microscopy and immunoblotting (Western) can be performed on keratinocyte culture media to confirm the results of tissue analysis. Northern blot hybridization confirms diminished or absent mRNA levels. This information is essential to implement gene therapy efforts utilizing ex vivo protocols (see below).

Genetic Counseling

Genetic information provided by mutation analyses on EB candidate genes provides an immediate benefit to families of EB patients. Siblings of a proband with recessive EB at reproductive age who contemplate having a child often want to know whether or not they carry a mutant allele. Most importantly, prenatal diagnosis of EB in affected families is now a genetic-based protocol provided the original proband has had mutational analysis or identification of the defective gene. Fetal skin biopsies and fetoscopy with their increased risk of pregnancy loss can now be avoided by analysis of either chorionic villus sampling as early as 8 to 10 weeks or amniocentesis in the second trimester.[92] The development of highly informative intragenic and flanking polymorphic DNA markers in EB candidate genes together with rapid screening of genetic "hotspots" makes genetic screening of at risk pregnancies a viable option.[93,94] Coupling of the technique of in vitro fertilization with EB prenatal diagnosis, preimplantation diagnosis has now been successfully performed for EB cases.[95]

THERAPY

Therapy for EB is tailored to the severity and extent of skin involvement and consists of supportive skin care, supportive care for other organ systems in indicated subtypes, and use of systemic therapies in an attempt to alter disease progression. Because of the involvement of multiple organ systems in severe EB subtypes, a multidisciplinary approach to patient care is often required. In most cases, the triad of wound management, nutritional support, and infection control are key to management of all EB patients.

Supportive Skin Care

Comprehensive topical therapy is a mainstay of treatment in EB, with avoidance of trauma a central goal. In EBS, maintenance of a cool environment and the use of soft, well-ventilated leather shoes is advisable. Blistered skin can be treated with modified Dakin's or simple saline compresses followed by topical antibiotics; in inflamed lesions the limited use of topical steroids may produce some degree of relief as well. Topical treatment for patients severely affected with junctional or dystrophic EB with the use of nonadhering dressings, such as Exu-Dry or Omniderm, over Vaseline or Aquaphor is extremely helpful in providing symptomatic relief. Gentle bathing and cleansing in modified Dakin's solution is best followed by application of a protective emollient and nonadherent dressing. In addressing the chronic hypertrophic granulation tissue seen in the periorificial regions of the face in JEB (Fig. 65-6), the use of keratinocyte autografts may be worthy of consideration. Such autografts, however, have demonstrated no significant benefit in the treatment of nonhypertrophic granulation tissue wounds in RDEB. In dystrophic epidermolysis bullosa, use of finger splinting and appropriate hand protection against trauma is indicated. Management of cutaneous infections is an important part of EB patient care. Systemic antibiotic therapy is frequently indicated for cutaneous wound infection and chronic wound colonization is managed best by regular cleansing with modified Dakin's solution and topical antibiotics as needed.

Surgical treatment is often required in the management of patients with dystrophic EB[96] and surgical intervention benefits from specialized anesthesia care.[97] Surgical release of fused digits followed by splinting is a therapeutic option for severely affected patients; however, therapy may require repetition at periodic intervals.[96,98,99] Surgery to correct limb, perioral, and perineal contractures may also be required; however, recurrence is common in dystrophic EB.[100,101] Patients with RDEB frequently develop squamous cell carcinoma[102,103] and prompt treatment of these tumors is indicated because they may develop metastases. Surgical excision is an important first-line modality, with radiation therapy limited by poor tumor response and impaired site healing.[104]

Care for Extracutaneous Involvement

Severe cases of JEB and DEB can involve multiple organ systems and require a multidisciplinary patient care approach. An additional source of support for patients and families include several important organizations that assist with patient education and support including Dystrophic Epidermolysis Bullosa Research Association (DEBRA) and Epidermolysis Bullosa Medical Research Foundation. A pediatric dentist is often of great help in managing the dental conditions with the use of a very soft brush and water pulsation devices preferable to hard brushing. Nutritional supplementation somewhat similar to that required for burn victims is important and a blenderized diet should be used for all patients with esophageal symptoms. Treatment of hematologic problems, primarily iron deficiency anemia, is important as is the overall nutritional support of these patients. Gastrointestinal involvement in DEB and JEB can include dysphagia with stricture formation requiring surgical release most common in RDEB and DDEB. Additional gastrointestinal procedures such as dilatation and gastrostomy may be indicated in those who suffer from severe involvement of the upper gastrointestinal system.[105] For the treatment of constipation seen in EB patients, increased fluid and fiber intake and stool softeners may be of value. In patients with airway involvement, there is danger of pulmonary aspiration. Ocular involvement in epidermolysis bullosa may include corneal abrasions and stromal scarring in junctional and dystrophic EB. Significant eye involvement should be managed with the assistance of an ophthalmologist to prevent clouding of the corneal stroma and serious visual compromise.

Systemic Therapies

Systemic therapies have not been effective in ameliorating the fundamental bullous tendency in EB patients. Historically, tetracycline and phenytoin have been used in the past for this disorder but are not current mainstays of treatment. Antimalarials and retinoids have also been used; however, the utility of these agents has not been definitively established. Systemic corticosteroids have not proven useful in these disorders.

Future Potential Therapies

Future potential therapies include protein and gene therapy as well as the use of tissue engineered skin equivalents. In the former case, the missing or defective protein is produced by recombinant methods and applied directly to blistered skin. This may be of most utility in proteins such as laminin 5 chains that do not require complex processing or transmembrane cellular anchorage. In the case of gene therapy, delivery of genes targeted to restore normal protein expression is the goal. Recent genomic expression profiling model studies have suggested that gene transfer may effect normalization of gene expression more broadly than protein transfer.[106] Successful corrective gene delivery was recently achieved in human EB tissue in the immune-deficient model system

FIGURE 65-11

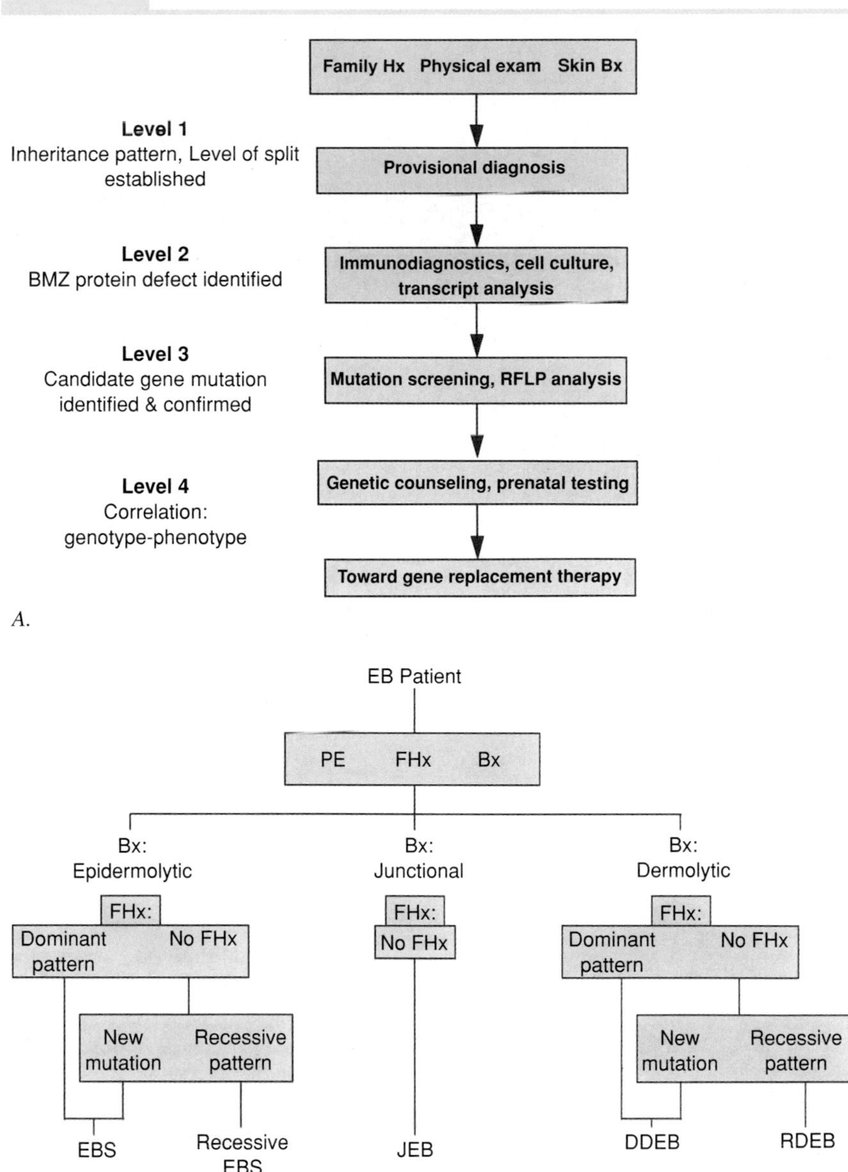

Key points in establishing a provisional diagnosis for an EB patient involve clinical clues in combination with the level of blister formation within the cutaneous basement membrane. Inheritance patterns guide the clinician to an accurate provisional diagnosis. While spontaneous mutations in EB candidate genes are rarely found, they should not be overlooked when the family history shows no evidence of EB.

Diagrammatic overview of the approach toward molecular diagnosis EB patients. Clinical encounter with unknown patient manifesting mechanobullous disease characteristics requires detailed family history, physical exam and skin biopsy to assess first level, provisional diagnosis. Second level of diagnostic work-up requires analysis of EB candidate gene defect by immunofluorescence microscopy of skin biopsy, and/or immunoblotting and candidate gene transcript analysis from EB patient's cultured keratinocytes. When a provisional diagnosis is correlated with an EB candidate gene product defect, the next level of analysis is performed by screening proband DNA for mutations in the specific candidate gene identified. In most circumstances, confirmation of a homozygous or heterozygous mutation is performed on nuclear family DNA via restriction fragment length polymorphism (RFLP; if the genetic defect involves a restriction enzyme site) or allele-specific oligonucleotide hybridization. Complete knowledge of the genetic defect will allow correlation of clinical phenotype and highest level EB patient care via genetic counseling, prenatal testing services and ultimately gene replacement.

FIGURE 65-12

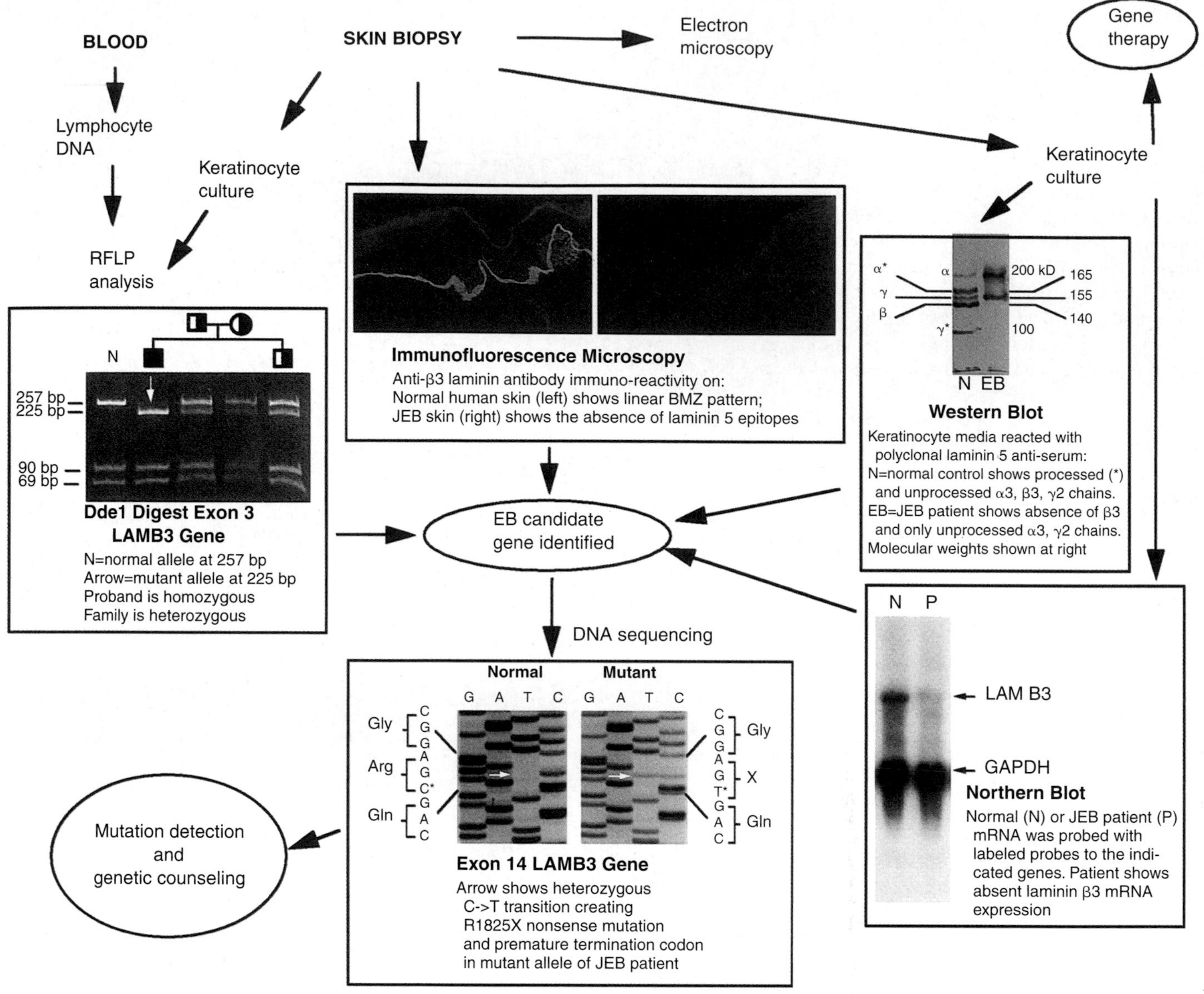

Examples of methodology used in the molecular diagnosis of EB: analysis of a Herlitz variant junctional EB patient at the protein, mRNA, and DNA levels. Lack of expression of EB candidate gene product (i.e., laminin 5 β_3 chain) is demonstrated by both immunofluorescence microscopy on skin biopsy and by Western blotting of patient-derived keratinocyte culture media. Transcript analysis by Northern blot hybridization shows decreased LAMB3 mRNA levels from the same keratinocytes. All three analyses point to identification of LAMB3 as the candidate gene responsible for skin fragility in this Herlitz patient and suggest that the mutation(s) in the LAMB3 gene results in functionally null alleles inherited from both parents. Sequence analysis of patient DNA demonstrates that one allele harbors a C→T transition in exon 14 of the LAMB3 gene, converting an arginine at position 1825 to a premature termination codon (AGT), confirming a compound heterozygous state. Further mutation detection analysis can identify the other LAMB3 mutant allele and provide data for genetic counseling in the family.

Detection of common DNA mutations found in the LAMB3 gene can be performed directly on DNA derived from either lymphocytes or cultured skin cells using restriction fragment length polymorphism (RFLP) techniques. In a different junctional EB case the restriction enzyme, Dde1, is used to digest LAMB3 exon 3 from the proband and family DNA. The normal state shows three digestion products (bands at 257, 90, and 69 base pairs), whereas the proband (*solid square*) shows a new band at 225 bp with no 257 bp band. The unaffected sister and both parents show heterozygosity of this Dde1 RFLP. Such information can be used to identify the EB candidate gene for subsequent DNA mutation analysis.

Information derived from molecular diagnostic analyses can be used directly to design therapeutic gene delivery strategies for individual EB patients.

described below for both laminin 5 and Type XVII collagen.[107,108] Thus, genetic therapies may be of significant utility in the future. In the case of tissue-engineered skin, application of skin equivalents recently demonstrated some promise in wound healing and in improvement of quality of life,[109] and thus represents an area of future investigation.

DISEASE MODELS

A number of new models have recently been developed to facilitate the study and development of therapy for epidermolysis bullosa. Some of these models use mouse genetic approaches to produce entirely murine tissue models.[110] These include transgenic mouse models with skin targeted expression of *trans*-dominant molecules[111]—including inducible-disease phenotype models.[112] These include dominant-negative basal keratins in models of epidermolysis bullosa simplex. Murine knockout models have also been used, including knockout of basal keratin genes in a model of the same disorder and of the α_6 and β_4 integrins, laminin 5, and type VII collagen.[12,113–116] These targeted gene disruptions in mice have accurately recapitulated the blistering phenotype of the corresponding human disorders. These murine genetic models have been of great utility in clarifying our understanding of the pathogenesis of this group of disorders and in providing disease models for development of potential future therapies.

In addition to such purely murine tissue models, human skin/mouse chimeras have been generated in an attempt to produce true human tissue models of epidermolysis bullosa. These chimeras have either used full thickness grafting of EB patient skin or epidermis regenerated on skin composites and sheets from EB keratinocytes grown in culture.[117] Immune-deficient SCID (severe combined immunodeficiency disease) and nude mice readily accept such xenografts and the grafted EB skin retains the clinical and molecular characteristics of the patient donor. This approach has been reported for recessive dystrophic EB due to mutations in type VII collagen, and for benign junctional EB due to mutations in type XVII collagen. Because human epidermis differs dramatically from mouse epidermis in tissue architecture, these in vivo models of human tissue in EB may be of special utility in development of models for gene therapy of these disorders. In addition to gene therapy applications, these models are attractive for attempts at protein therapy, as in the case of topical laminin 5, in some subtypes of JEB.

REFERENCES

1. Pearson RW: Studies on the pathogenesis of epidermolysis bullosa. *J Invest Dermatol* **39**:551, 1962
2. Burgeson RE, Christiano AM: The dermal–epidermal junction. *Curr Opin Cell Biol* **9**:651, 1997
3. Marinkovich MP: Update on inherited bullous dermatoses. *Dermatol Clin* **17**:473, 1999
4. Fuchs E, Cleveland DW: A structural scaffolding of intermediate filaments in health and disease. *Science* **279**:514, 1998
5. Wiche G: Domain structure and transcript diversity of plectin. *Biol Bull* **194**:381, 1998
6. Stanley JR: Pemphigus and pemphigoid as paradigms of organ-specific, autoantibody-mediated diseases. *J Clin Invest* **83**:1443, 1991
7. Leung CL et al: The BPAG1 locus: Alternative splicing produces multiple isoforms with distinct cytoskeletal linker domains, including predominant isoforms in neurons and muscles. *J Cell Biol* **154**:691, 2001
8. Guo LL, Degenstein L et al: Gene targeting of BPAG1: Abnormalities in mechanical strength and cell migration in stratified squamous epithelia and severe neurological degeneration. *Cell* **81**:233, 1995
9. Giudice GJ et al: Cloning and primary structural analysis of the bullous pemphigoid autoantigen BP180. *J Invest Dermatol* **99**:243, 1992
10. Sonnenberg A et al: Integrin $\alpha_6\beta_4$ complex is located in hemidesmosomes, suggesting a major role in epidermal cell-basement membrane adhesion. *J Cell Biol* **113**:907, 1991
11. Niessen CM et al: The $\alpha_6\beta_4$ integrin is a receptor for both laminin and kalinin. *Exp Cell Res* **211**:360, 1995
12. Dowling J et al: Beta4 integrin is required for hemidesmosome formation, cell adhesion and cell survival. *J Cell Biol* **134**:559, 1996
13. Hirako Y et al: Demonstration of the molecular shape of BP180, a 180-kDa bullous pemphigoid antigen and its potential for trimer formation. *J Biol Chem* **271**:13739, 1996
14. Carter WG et al: Distinct functions for integrins $\alpha_3\beta_1$ in focal adhesions and $\alpha_6\beta_4$/bullous pemphigoid antigen in a new stable-anchoring contact (SAC) of keratinocytes: Relation to hemidesmosomes. *J Cell Biol* **111**:3141, 1990
15. Schäcke H et al: Two forms of collagen XVII in keratinocytes. A full-length transmembrane protein and a soluble ectodomain. *J Biol Chem* **273**:25937, 1998
16. Zone JJ et al: Identification of the cutaneous basement membrane antigen in linear IgA bullous dermatosis. *J Clin Invest* **85**:812, 1990
17. Marinkovich MP et al: LAD-1, the linear IgA bullous dermatosis autoantigen, is a novel 120-kDa anchoring filament protein synthesized by epidermal cells [published erratum appears in *J Invest Dermatol* 106:1343, 1996]. *J Invest Dermatol* **106**:734, 1996
18. Zone JJ et al: The 97-kDa linear IgA bullous disease antigen is identical to a portion of the extracellular domain of the 180-kDa bullous pemphigoid antigen, BPAg2. *J Invest Dermatol* **110**:207, 1998
19. Schumann H et al: The shed ectodomain of collagen XVII/BP180 is targeted by autoantibodies in different blistering skin diseases. *Am J Pathol* **156**:685, 2000
20. McGowan KA, Marinkovich MP: Laminins and human disease. *Microsc Res Tech* **51**:262, 2000
21. Rousselle P et al: Kalinin: An epithelium-specific basement membrane adhesion molecule that is a component of anchoring filaments. *J Cell Biol* **114**:567, 1991
22. Marinkovich MP et al: The anchoring filament protein kalinin is synthesized and secreted as a high molecular weight precursor. *J Biol Chem* **267**:17900, 1992
23. Gerecke DR et al: Hemidesmosomes, anchoring fibrils, in *Extracellular Matrix Assembly and Structure*, edited by RP Mecham, DE Birk, PD Yurchenko. San Diego, Academic Press, 1994, p 417
24. Ryan MC et al: Cloning of the gene encoding the α_3 chain of the adhesive ligand epiligrin. Expression in wound repair. *J Biol Chem* **269**:22779, 1994
25. Kallunki P et al: A truncated laminin chain homologous to the β_2 chain: Structure, spatial expression, and chromosomal assignment. *J Cell Biol* **119**:679, 1992
26. Champliaud MF et al: Human amnion contains a novel laminin variant, laminin 7, which, like laminin 6, covalently associates with laminin 5 to promote stable epithelial-stromal attachment. *J Cell Biol* **132:1**189, 1996
27. Marinkovich MP et al: The dermal–epidermal junction of human skin contains a novel laminin variant. *J Cell Biol* **119**:695, 1992
28. Amano S et al: Bone morphogenetic protein 1 is an extracellular processing enzyme of the laminin 5 gamma 2 chain. *J Biol Chem* **275**:22728, 2000
29. Goldfinger LE et al: The α_3 laminin subunit, $\alpha_6\beta_4$ and $\alpha_3\beta_1$ integrin coordinately regulate wound healing in cultured epithelial cells and in the skin. *J Cell Sci* **112:2**615, 1999
30. Giannelli G et al: Induction of cell migration by matrix metalloprotease-2 cleavage of laminin-5. *Science* **277**:225, 1997
31. Koshikawa N et al: Role of cell surface metalloprotease MT1-MMP in epithelial cell migration over laminin-5. *J Cell Biol* **148**:615, 2000
32. Gagnoux-Palacios L et al: The short arm of the laminin gamma 2 chain plays a pivotal role in the incorporation of laminin 5 into the extracellular matrix and in cell adhesion. *J Cell Biol* **153**:835, 2001
33. Fine JD et al: 19-DEJ-1, a hemidesmosome-anchoring filament complex associated monoclonal antibody. Definition of a new skin basement membrane antigenic defect in junctional and dystrophic epidermolysis bullosa. *Arch Dermatol* **125**:520, 1989
34. Parente MG et al: Human type VII collagen: cDNA cloning and chromosomal mapping of the gene (COL7A1) on chromosome 3 to dominant dystrophic epidermolysis bullosa. *Am J Hum Genet* **24**:119, 1991
35. Burgeson RE et al: The structure and function of type VII collagen. *Ann N Y Acad Sci* **580**:32, 1990
36. Bachinger HP et al: The relationship of the biophysical and biochemical characteristics of type VII collagen to the function of anchoring fibrils. *J Biol Chem* **265**:10095, 1990
37. Bruckner-Tuderman L et al: Biology of anchoring fibrils: Lessons from dystrophic epidermolysis bullosa. *Matrix Biol* **18**:43, 1999
38. Gayraud B et al: Characterization of a 50-kDa component of epithelial basement membranes using GDA-J/F3 monoclonal antibody. *J Biol Chem* **272**:9531, 1997
39. Chen M et al: Interactions of the amino-terminal noncollagenous (NC1) domain of type VII collagen with extracellular matrix components. *J Biol Chem* **272**:14516, 1997
40. Rousselle P et al: Laminin 5 binds the NC-1 domain of type VII collagen. *J Cell Biol* **138**:719, 1997
41. Chen M et al: NC1 domain of type VII collagen binds to the beta3 chain of laminin 5 via a unique subdomain within the fibronectin-like repeats. *J Invest Dermatol* **112**:177, 1999
42. Chen M et al: The carboxyl terminus of type VII collagen mediates antiparallel-dimer formation and constitutes a new antigenic epitope for EBA autoantibodies. *J Biol Chem* **27**:27, 2001

43. Fine JD et al: Revised classification system for inherited epidermolysis bullosa: Report of the Second International Consensus Meeting on diagnosis and classification of epidermolysis bullosa. *J Am Acad Dermatol* **42**:1051, 2000
44. Horn HM, Tidman MJ: The clinical spectrum of epidermolysis bullosa simplex. *Br J Dermatol* **142**:468, 2000
45. Shemanko CS et al: Laryngeal involvement in the Dowling-Meara variant of epidermolysis bullosa simplex with keratin mutations of severely disruptive potential. *Br J Dermatol* **142**:315, 2000
46. Morrell DS et al: Congenital pyloric atresia in a newborn with extensive aplasia cutis congenita and epidermolysis bullosa simplex. *Br J Dermatol* **143**:1342, 2000
47. McLean WH et al: Loss of plectin causes epidermolysis bullosa with muscular dystrophy: cDNA cloning and genomic organization. *Genes Dev* **10**:1724, 1996
48. Epstein E: Finding the mutations causing hereditary diseases of the skin. *Prog Dermatol* **26**:1, 1992
49. Rugg EL et al: A functional "knockout" of human keratin 14. *Genes and Development* **8**:2563, 1994
50. Jonkman MF et al: Effects of keratin 14 ablation on the clinical and cellular phenotype in a kindred with recessive epidermolysis bullosa simplex. *J Invest Dermatol* **107**:764, 1996
51. Coulombe PA: The cellular and molecular biology of keratins: Beginning a new era. *Curr Opin Cell Biol* **5**:17, 1993
52. Uttam J et al: The genetic basis of epidermolysis bullosa simplex with mottled pigmentation. *Proc Natl Acad Sci USA* **93**:9079, 1996
53. Irvine AD et al: Molecular confirmation of the unique phenotype of epidermolysis bullosa simplex with mottled pigmentation. *Br J Dermatol* **144**:40, 2001
54. Moog U et al: Epidermolysis bullosa simplex with mottled pigmentation: Clinical aspects and confirmation of the P24L mutation in the KRT5 gene in further patients. *Am J Med Genet* **86**:376, 1999
55. Bauer JW et al: Large melanocytic nevi in hereditary epidermolysis bullosa. *J Am Acad Dermatol* **44**:577, 2001
56. Gache Y et al: Defective expression of plectin/HD1 in epidermolysis bullosa simplex with muscular dystrophy. *J Clin Invest* **97**:2289, 1996
57. Dang M et al: Novel compound heterozygous mutations in the plectin gene in epidermolysis bullosa with muscular dystrophy and the use of protein truncation test for detection of premature termination codon mutations. *Lab Invest* **78**:195, 1998
58. Uitto J et al: Plectin and human genetic disorders of skin and muscle. The paradigm of epidermolysis bullosa with muscular dystrophy. *Exp Dermatol* **5**:237, 1996
59. Gil SG et al: Junctional epidermolysis bullosis: Defects in expression of epiligrin/nicein/kalinin and integrin beta 4 that inhibit hemidesmosome formation. *J Invest Dermatol* **103**:31S, 1994
60. Hashimoto I et al: Epidermolysis bullosa hereditaria with junctional blistering in an adult. *Dermatologica* **152**:72, 1976
61. Hintner H, Wolff K: Generalized atrophic benign epidermolysis bullosa. *Arch Dermatol* **118**:375, 1982
62. McGrath JA et al: Altered laminin 5 expression due to mutations in the gene encoding the β_3 chain in generalized atrophic benign epidermolysis bullosa. *J Invest Dermatol* **104**:467, 1995
63. McGrath JA et al: A recurrent homozygous nonsense mutation within the LAMA3 gene as a cause of Herlitz junctional epidermolysis bullosa in patients of Pakistani ancestry: Evidence for a founder effect. *J Invest Dermatol* **106**:781, 1996
64. Aberdam D et al: Herlitz's junctional epidermolysis bullosa is linked to mutations in the gene (LAMC2) for the $\gamma 2$ subunit of nicein/kalinin (LAMININ-5). *Nat Genet* **6**:299, 1994
65. Kivirikko S et al: Mutational hotspots in the LAMB3 gene in the lethal (Herlitz) type of junctional epidermolysis bullosa. *Hum Mol Genet* **5**:231, 1996
66. Cserhalmi-Friedman PB et al: Molecular basis of non-lethal junctional epidermolysis bullosa: Identification of a 38-base pair insertion and a splice site mutation in exon 14 of the LAMB3 gene. *Exp Dermatol* **7**:105, 1998
67. Pulkkinen L et al: LAMB3 mutations in generalized atrophic benign epidermolysis bullosa: Consequences at the mRNA and protein levels. *Lab Invest* **78**:859, 1998
68. McGrath JA et al: Mutations in the 180-kD bullous pemphigoid antigen (BPAG2), a hemidesmosomal transmembrane collagen (COL17A1), in generalized atrophic benign epidermolysis bullosa. *Nat Genetics* **11**:83, 1995
69. Jonkman MF: Hereditary skin diseases of hemidesmosomes. *J Dermatol Sci* **20**:103, 1999
70. Jonkman MF et al: Revertant mosaicism in epidermolysis bullosa caused by mitotic gene conversion. *Cell* **88:5**43, 1997
71. Vidal F et al: Integrin beta 4 mutations associated with junctional epidermolysis bullosa with pyloric atresia. *Nat Genet* **10**:229, 1995
72. Inoue M et al: A homozygous missense mutation in the cytoplasmic tail of beta4 integrin, G931D, that disrupts hemidesmosome assembly and underlies non-Herlitz junctional epidermolysis bullosa without pyloric atresia? *J Invest Dermatol* **114**:1061, 2000
73. Chavanas S et al: Splicing modulation of integrin beta4 pre-mRNA carrying a branch point mutation underlies epidermolysis bullosa with pyloric atresia undergoing spontaneous amelioration with aging. *Hum Mol Genet* **8**:2097, 1999
74. Gache Y et al: Genetic bases of severe junctional epidermolysis bullosa presenting spontaneous amelioration with aging. *Hum Mol Genet* **10**:2453, 2001
75. Smith LT, Sybert VP: Intra-epidermal retention of type VII collagen in a patient with recessive dystrophic epidermolysis bullosa. *J Invest Dermatol* **94**:261, 1990
76. Cui Y et al: Identification and characterization of genes that are required for the accelerated degradation of mRNAs containing a premature translational termination codon. *Genes Dev* **9**:423, 1995
77. Uitto J et al: Molecular basis of the dystrophic and junctional form of epidermolysis bullosa: Mutations in the type VII collagen and kalinin (laminin-5) genes. *J Invest Dermatol* **103**:39S, 1994
78. Christiano AM et al: Premature termination codons in the type VII collagen gene (COL7A1) underlie severe, mutilating recessive dystrophic epidermolysis bullosa. *Genomics* **21**:160, 1994
79. Christiano AM et al: Dominant dystrophic epidermolysis bullosa: Identification of a Gly→Ser substitution in the triple-helical domain of type VII collagen. *Proc Natl Acad Sci USA* **91**:3549, 1994
80. Nordal EJ et al: Generalized dystrophic epidermolysis bullosa: Identification of a novel, homozygous glycine substitution, G2031S, in exon 73 of COL7A1 in monozygous triplets. *Br J Dermatol* **144**:151, 2001
81. Jonkman MF et al: Dominant dystrophic epidermolysis bullosa (Pasini) caused by a novel glycine substitution mutation in the type VII collagen gene (COL7A1). *J Invest Dermatol* **112**:815, 1999
82. Lee JY, Li C, Chao SC, et al., A de novo glycine substitution mutation in the collagenous domain of COL7A1 in dominant dystrophic epidermolysis bullosa. *Arch Dermatol Res* **292**:159, 2000.
83. Masunaga T et al: Combination of novel premature termination codon and glycine substitution mutations in COL7A1 leads to moderately severe recessive dystrophic epidermolysis bullosa. *J Invest Dermatol* **114**:204, 2000
84. Rouan F et al: Novel and de novo glycine substitution mutations in the type VII collagen gene (COL7A1) in dystrophic epidermolysis bullosa: Implications for genetic counseling. *J Invest Dermatol* **111**:1210, 1998
85. Tasanen K et al: Collagen XVII is destabilized by a glycine substitution mutation in the cell adhesion domain Col15. *J Biol Chem* **275**:3093, 2000
86. Terracina M et al: Compound heterozygosity for a recessive glycine substitution and a splice site mutation in the COL7A1 gene causes an unusually mild form of localized recessive dystrophic epidermolysis bullosa. *J Invest Dermatol* **111**:744, 1998
87. Sakuntabhai A et al: Deletions within COL7A1 exons distant from consensus splice sites alter splicing and produce shortened polypeptides in dominant dystrophic epidermolysis bullosa. *Am J Hum Genet* **63**:737, 1998
88. Hammami-Hauasli N et al: Some, but not all, glycine substitution mutations in COL7A1 result in intracellular accumulation of collagen VII, loss of anchoring fibrils, and skin blistering. *J Biol Chem* **273**:19228, 1998
89. Chen M et al: The recombinant expression of full-length type VII collagen and characterization of molecular mechanisms underlying dystrophic epidermolysis bullosa. *J Biol Chem* **277**:2118, 2002
90. Hatta N et al: Spontaneous disappearance of intraepidermal type VII collagen in a patient with dystrophic epidermolysis bullosa. *Br J Dermatol* **133**:619, 1995
91. Bruckner-Tuderman L et al: Immunohistochemical and mutation analyses demonstrate that procollagen VII is processed to collagen VII through removal of the NC-2 domain. *J Cell Biol* **131**:551, 1995
92. Marinkovich MP et al: Prenatal diagnosis of Herlitz junctional epidermolysis bullosa by amniocentesis. *Prenat Diagn* **15**:1027, 1995
93. Uitto J, Pulkkinen L: Molecular complexity of the cutaneous basement membrane zone. *Mol Biol Rep* **23**:35, 1996
94. McGrath JA et al: First trimester DNA-based exclusion of recessive dystrophic epidermolysis bullosa from chorionic villus sampling. *Br J Dermatol* **134**:734, 1996

95. Cserhalmi-Friedman PB et al: Preimplantation genetic diagnosis in two families at risk for recurrence of Herlitz junctional epidermolysis bullosa. *Exp Dermatol* **9**:290, 2000
96. Terrill PJ et al: Experience in the surgical management of the hand in dystrophic epidermolysis bullosa. *Br J Plast Surg* **45**:435, 1992
97. Iohom G, Lyons B: Anaesthesia for children with epidermolysis bullosa: A review of 20 years' experience. *Eur J Anaesthesiol* **18**:745, 2001
98. Ladd AL et al: Surgical treatment and postoperative splinting of recessive dystrophic epidermolysis bullosa. *J Hand Surg [Br]* **21**:888, 1996
99. Glicenstein J et al: The hand in recessive dystrophic epidermolysis bullosa. *Hand Clin* **16**:637, 2000
100. Terrill PJ et al: The surgical management of dystrophic epidermolysis bullosa (excluding the hand). *Br J Plast Surg* **45**:426, 1992
101. Vozdvizhensky SI, Albanova VI: Surgical treatment of contracture and syndactyly of children with epidermolysis bullosa. *Br J Plas Surg* **46**:314, 1993
102. McGrath JA et al: Epidermolysis bullosa complicated by squamous cell carcinoma: report of 10 cases. *J Cutan Pathol* **19**:116, 1992
103. Newman C et al: Squamous cell carcinoma secondary to recessive dystrophic epidermolysis bullosa. A report of 4 patients with 17 primary cutaneous malignancies. *J Dermatol Surg Oncol* **18**:4, 1992
104. Bastin KT et al: Radiation therapy for squamous cell carcinoma in dystrophic epidermolysis: Case reports and literature review. *Am J Clin Oncol* **20**:55, 1997
105. Ergun GA et al: Gastrointestinal manifestations of epidermolysis bullosa. A study of 101 patients. *Medicine (Baltimore)* **71**:121, 1992
106. Robbins PB et al: Impact of laminin 5 beta3 gene versus protein replacement on gene expression patterns in junctional epidermolysis bullosa. *Hum Gene Ther* **12**:1443, 2001
107. Seitz CS et al: BP180 gene delivery in junctional epidermolysis bullosa. *Gene Ther* **6**:42, 1999
108. Robbins PB et al: In vivo restoration of laminin 5 beta 3 expression and function in junctional epidermolysis bullosa. *Proc Natl Acad Sci USA* **98**:5193, 2001
109. Falabella AF et al: Tissue-engineered skin (Apligraf) in the healing of patients with epidermolysis bullosa wounds. *Arch Dermatol* **136**:1225, 2000
110. Rothnagel JA et al: Transgenic models of skin diseases. *Arch Dermatol* **129**:1430, 1993
111. Vassar R et al: Mutant keratin expression in transgenic mice causes marked abnormalities resembling a human genetic skin disease. *Cell* **64**:365, 1991
112. Cao T et al: An inducible mouse model for epidermolysis bullosa simplex: Implications for gene therapy. *J Cell Biol* **152**:651, 2001
113. Peters B et al: Complete cytolysis and neonatal lethality in keratin 5 knockout mice reveal its fundamental role in skin integrity and in epidermolysis bullosa simplex. *Mol Biol Cell* **12**:1775, 2001
114. Heinonen S et al: Targeted inactivation of the type VII collagen gene (Col7a1) in mice results in severe blistering phenotype: A model for recessive dystrophic epidermolysis bullosa. *J Cell Sci* **112**:3641, 1999
115. Georges-Labouesse E et al: Absence of integrin alpha 6 leads to epidermolysis bullosa and neonatal death in mice. *Nat Genetics* **13(3):**370, 1996
116. Ryan MC et al: Targeted disruption of the LAMA3 gene in mice reveals abnormalities in survival and late stage differentiation of epithelial cells. *J Cell Biol* **145**:1309, 1999
117. Kim YH et al: Recessive dystrophic epidermolysis bullosa phenotype is preserved in xenografts using SCID mice: Development of an experimental in vivo model. *J Invest Dermatol* **98**:191, 1992

CHAPTER 66

David T. Woodley
Mei Chen
W. Ray Gammon
Robert A. Briggaman

Epidermolysis Bullosa Acquisita

Epidermolysis bullosa acquisita (EBA) is a chronic subepidermal blistering disease associated with autoimmunity to the collagen (type VII collagen) within anchoring fibril structures that are located at the dermal-epidermal junction. Although it is an acquired disease that usually begins in adulthood, it was placed in the category epidermolysis bullosa (EB) approximately 100 years ago because physicians were struck by how similar the lesions were to those seen in children with hereditary dystrophic forms of EB.

HISTORICAL ASPECTS

Two cases of a blistering disease with adult onset and features highly reminiscent of hereditary dystrophic EB were reported by Elliott in 1895. These clinical features included skin fragility, erosions, blisters, and a healing response characterized by scarring and the formation of milia cysts. In the early decades of the twentieth century, other similar case reports appeared. It is not certain if all these early reports were of EBA patients as defined today, but the existence of an acquired form of EB was recognized.

In the early 1970s, Roenigk et al.[1] summarized the EBA world literature, reported three new cases, and suggested the first diagnostic criteria: (1) a negative family and personal history for a previous blistering disorder, (2) an adult onset of the eruption, (3) spontaneous or trauma-induced blisters that resemble those of hereditary dystrophic EB, and (4) the exclusion of all other bullous diseases.

It was thought that immunofluorescence studies would separate EBA from other primary subepidermal bullous diseases such as bullous pemphigoid (BP), cicatricial pemphigoid (CP), and herpes gestationis. In 1973, however, Kushniruk[2] showed that patients with EBA had IgG deposits at the dermal-epidermal junction just like patients with BP. This observation was confirmed by Gibbs and Minus[3] and by Nieboer et al.[4] Some EBA patients also had an anti–basement membrane autoantibody circulating in their plasma. Therefore, it became obvious that both indirect and direct immunofluorescence studies could be identical in EBA and BP patients.

In the early 1980s, Nieboer et al.[4] and Yaoita et al.[5] showed that while EBA and BP have identical immunofluorescence findings, they could be separated by immunoelectron microscopy. The IgG deposits in EBA are located within and below the lamina densa area of the basement membrane zone, whereas BP immune deposits are within hemidesmosomes and high in the lamina lucida (see Chap. 61). The ability to separate EBA from the BP group has become more relevant with the observations of Gammon et al.,[6] Dahl,[7] and others[8–11] that EBA does not always have the "classical" presentation of a mechanobullous EB-like disease and may present with a clinical syndrome highly reminiscent of BP, Brunsting-Perry pemphigoid, or CP.

ETIOLOGY AND PATHOGENESIS

The etiology of EBA is unknown, but most of the evidence suggests an autoimmune etiology. Direct immunofluorescence of perilesional skin biopsies from EBA patients reveals IgG deposits at the dermal-epidermal junction.[2–5] EBA antibodies bind to type VII collagen within anchoring fibrils.[12,13] Anchoring fibrils are wheat stack–like structures that emanate from the lamina densa in a perpendicular fashion and stretch about 200 to 300 nm into the papillary dermis, where they associate with globular structures called *anchoring plaques* that contain type IV collagen, a component shared with the lamina densa zone of the basement membrane zone between the epidermis and dermis (see Chap. 16).

Anchoring fibrils anchor the epidermis and its underlying basement membrane zone to the papillary dermis. Patients with hereditary forms of dystrophic EB (see Chap. 65) and EBA have decreased numbers of anchoring fibrils in their dermal-epidermal junction.[14] This paucity of anchoring fibrils is associated with two similar clinical phenotypes, EBA and dystrophic forms of heretitary EB, because both diseases are characterized by skin fragility, subepidermal blisters, milia formation, and scarring. While both EBA and hereditary forms of dystrophic EB are etiologically unrelated in terms of their underlying pathogenesis, they share the common feature of decreased anchoring fibrils. In the case of dystrophic forms of hereditary EB, the cause of decreased or absent anchoring fibrils is a genetic defect in the gene that encodes for type VII collagen alpha chains that ultimately results in small, nonfunctional or decreased anchoring fibrils.[15] The gene coding for type VII collagen is located on the short arm of chromosome 3, approximately 21 cM from zero.[16] The gene defects involved in hereditary forms of dystrophic EB have been identified at variable locations, but the severity of the disease appears to correlate with the degree of type VII collagen and anchoring fibril perturbations.[17] In EBA, the IgG autoantibodies binding to the type VII collagen alpha chains result in decreased anchoring fibrils, but the pathway leading to this reduction is unknown. It may be that type VII collagen alpha chains that are newly synthesized but decorated with EBA autoantibodies cannot form triple-helical structures and stable anchoring fibrils. Healed burn wounds that have been covered with cultured keratinocyte sheets also have decreased numbers of anchoring fibrils within the first year after transplantation, and this is associated with spontaneous blister formation, shortened suction blistering times, and skin fragility.[18] These observations provide indirect evidence that anchoring fibrils play a role in maintaining adherence between the epidermis and dermis.

The type VII collagen alpha chain has a molecular mass between 250 and 320 kDa, and the collagen consists of a homotrimer of three identical alpha chains (see Chap. 16). Each alpha chain consists of a large globular noncollagenous amino terminus called the *noncollagenous 1* (NC-1) *domain* that is approximately half the entire mass of the alpha chain. Next, there is a helical domain with typical glycine-X-Y repeats. At the carboxyl terminus is a second globular noncollagenous domain, NC-2, that is much smaller than NC-1. Most EBA autoantibodies recognize four predominant antigenic epitopes within the NC-1 domain and do not recognize the helical or NC-2 domains.[19,20] There may be something intrinsically "antigenic" about the NC-1 domain because the available monoclonal antibodies that have been generated against type VII collagen (anti–C-VII antibodies) specifically recognize only NC-1 subdomains.

Type VII collagen has affinity for fibronectin, a large glycoprotein in the papillary dermis.[21] The interaction between fibronectin and type VII collagen may play a role in adhering the basement membrane beneath the epidermis onto the dermis. Lapiere et al.[22] and Chen et al.[23] have identified two fibronectin-binding sites within the type VII collagen alpha chain. One of these is within the NC-1 domain where EBA autoantibodies are targeted.[23] Therefore, it is conceivable that when EBA autoantibodies bind to type VII collagen, the interaction between type VII collagen and fibronectin is abrogated and results in poor epidermal-dermal adherence.

Further evidence for the pathogenic role of EBA antibodies also comes from the observation that when patients with systemic lupus erythematosus (SLE) develop autoantibodies to the EBA antigen, they develop widespread skin blisters and fall into a subset of SLE called *bullous SLE*.[24] This "experiment of nature" also suggests that EBA autoantibodies are pathogenic and capable of inducing disadherence between the epidermis and dermis. Nevertheless, consistent induction of blisters in an animal by the passive transfer of EBA IgG autoantibodies into the animal has not been achieved despite numerous attempts.[25]

Although EBA is not a genetic disease with a Mendelian inheritance pattern, some EBA patients may have a genetic predisposition to autoimmunity.[26] African American patients in the southeastern part of the United States who have either EBA or bullous SLE have a high incidence of the HLA-DR2 phenotype. The calculated relative risk for EBA in HLA-DR2+ individuals is 13.1 in these patients. These results also suggest that EBA and bullous SLE are immunogenetically related and that either the HLA-DR2 gene is involved with autoimmunity to anchoring fibril collagen or is some sort of a marker for some other gene that exists in linkage disequilibrium with it.[26]

CLINICAL MANIFESTATIONS

The common denominator for patients with EBA is autoimmunity to type VII (anchoring fibril) collagen.[10,13] Although the clinical spectrum of EBA is still being defined, there are at least five clinical presentations: (1) a classical presentation, (2) a BP-like presentation, (3) a CP-like presentation, (4) a presentation reminiscent of Brunsting-Perry pemphigoid with scarring lesions and a predominant head and neck distribution, and (5) a presentation reminiscent of linear IgA bullous dermatosis or chronic bullous disease of childhood (see Chap. 63).

Classical Presentation

The classical presentation (Figs. 66-1 and 66-2*A*) is of a noninflammatory bullous disease with an acral distribution that heals with scarring and milia formation. This presentation is reminiscent of porphyria cutanea tarda (PCT) (see Chap. 149) when it is mild and of the hereditary form of recessive dystrophic EB when it is severe (see Chap. 65). The classical form of EBA is thus a mechanobullous disease marked by skin fragility. These patients have erosions, tense blisters within non-inflamed skin, and scars over trauma-prone surfaces such as the backs of the hands, knuckles, elbows, knees, sacral area, and toes (Figs. 66-3 and 66-2*A*). Some blisters may be hemorrhagic or develop scales, crusts, or erosions. The lesions heal with scarring and frequently with

FIGURE 66-1

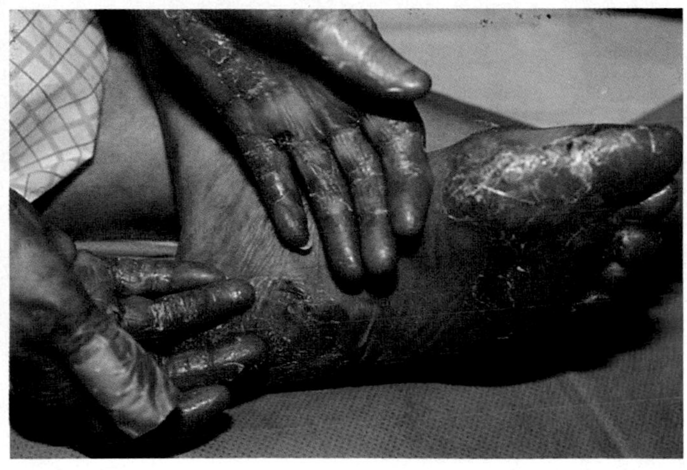

A patient with EBA who has severe blistering, erosions, scarring, and milia formation on trauma-prone areas of her skin.

the formation of pearl-like milia cysts within the scarred areas. Although this presentation may be reminiscent of PCT, these patients do not have other hallmarks of PCT, such as hirsutism, a photodistribution of the eruption, or scleroderma-like changes, and their urinary porphyrins are within normal limits. A scarring alopecia and some degree of nail dystrophy may be seen.

Although the disease is usually not as severe as that of patients with hereditary forms of recessive dystrophic EB, EBA patients with the classical form of the disease may have many of the same sequelae, such as scarring, loss of scalp hair, loss of nails, fibrosis of the hands and fingers, and esophageal stenosis.[27]

Bullous Pemphigoid–like Presentation

A second clinical presentation of EBA is of a widespread, inflammatory vesiculobullous eruption involving the trunk, central body, and skin folds in addition to the extremities.[6] The bullous lesions are tense and surrounded by inflamed or even urticarial skin. Large areas of inflamed skin may be seen without any blisters and only erythema or urticarial plaques. These patients often complain of pruritus and do not demonstrate prominent skin fragility, scarring, or milia formation. This clinical constellation is more reminiscent of BP (Figs. 66-2*B* and 66-4) than a mechanobullous disorder. Like BP, the distribution of the lesions may show an accentuation within flexural areas and skin folds.

Cicatricial Pemphigoid–like Presentation

Both the classical and BP-like forms of EBA may have involvement of mucosal surfaces. However, EBA also may present with such predominant mucosal involvement that the clinical appearance is reminiscent of CP[7] (Fig. 66-2*C*). These patients usually have erosions and scars on the mucosal surfaces of the mouth, upper esophagus, conjunctiva, anus, or vagina with or without similar lesions on the glabrous skin.

Brusting-Perry Pemphigoid–like Presentation

Brunsting-Perry cicatricial bullous pemphigoid is a chronic recurrent vesiculobullous eruption localized to the head and neck and characterized by residual scars, subepidermal bullae, IgG deposits at the dermal-epidermal junction, and minimal or no mucosal involvement (see Chap. 62). The antigenic target for the IgG autoantibodies, however, has not been defined. Nevertheless, a patient reported with this constellation of findings had IgG autoantibodies directed to anchoring fibrils below the lamina densa.[11] We have seen three additional patients with the features of Brunsting-Perry pemphigoid and autoantibodies directed to type VII collagen (unpublished observations). Therefore, it appears that EBA patients may present with a clinical phenotype of Brusting-Perry pemphigoid (Fig. 66-2*D*).

IgA Bullous Dermatosis–like Presentation

This form of EBA is manifested by a subepidermal bullous eruption, a neutrophilic infiltrate, and linear IgA deposits at the basement membrane zone when viewed by direct immunofluorescence (DIF). It may resemble linear IgA bullous dermatosis (LABD), dermatitis herpetiformis, or chronic bullous disease of childhood (CBDC) and may feature tense vesicles arranged in an annular fashion and involvement of mucous membranes[28–33] (see Chap. 63). The autoantibodies are usually IgA, IgG, or both.

The diagnosis of these subepidermal blistering cases with IgA anti-C-VII antibodies showing linear IgA deposition at the basement membrane zone is disputable. Some clinicians regard the patients as having purely LABD,[30] whereas others regard them as having a subset of EBA.[31] In a recent study,[32] 20 EBA patients' sera were evaluated for serum IgA anti-C-VII antibodies by immunoblotting. This study showed that low titers of IgA anti-C-VII antibodies were detected in 80 percent of patients in addition to IgG antibodies.

Childhood EBA is a rare disease. It has a variable presentation with 5 of 14 patients reviewed presenting with an LABD-like disease, 5 with BP-like disease, and 4 with the classical type.[33] Eleven of 14 had mucosal involvement, and all had deposits of IgG, as well as other immunoreactants, at the basement membrane zone by DIF. Indirect immunofluorescence (IIF) was positive in 10 of 14 patients' sera, and the predominant serum antibody was of the IgG class. Although mucosal involvement is frequent and severe in childhood EBA, the overall prognosis and treatment are more favorable than in EBA.[29,33]

According to the authors' experience, about 25 percent of patients with EBA may present with a BP-like clinical appearance. The disease of some of these patients eventually will smolder into a more noninflammatory mechanobullous form. However, both the classical and BP-like forms of the disease may coexist in the same patient[27] (Fig. 66-4). The clinical phenotype of EBA that is reminiscent of pure CP occurs in fewer than 10 percent of all EBA cases.

A number of published reports suggest that EBA may be associated with various systemic diseases[1,34] such as inflammatory bowel disease, SLE, amyloidosis, thyroiditis, multiple endocrinopathy syndrome, rheumatoid arthritis, pulmonary fibrosis, chronic lymphocytic leukemia, thymoma, diabetes, and other diseases in which an autoimmune pathogenesis has been implicated. At the University of North Carolina, Stanford, and Northwestern, with a combined experience of following over 60 EBA patients, it appears that inflammatory bowel disease is the systemic disease most frequently associated with EBA.[35]

PATHOLOGY

Routine histologic examination of lesional skin obtained from EBA patients shows a subepidermal blister and a clean separation between the epidermis and dermis. The degree of inflammatory infiltrate within the dermis usually reflects the degree of inflammation of the lesion observed by the clinician. Lesions that are reminiscent of recessive dystrophic EB or PCT usually have a notable scarcity of inflammatory cells

FIGURE 66-2

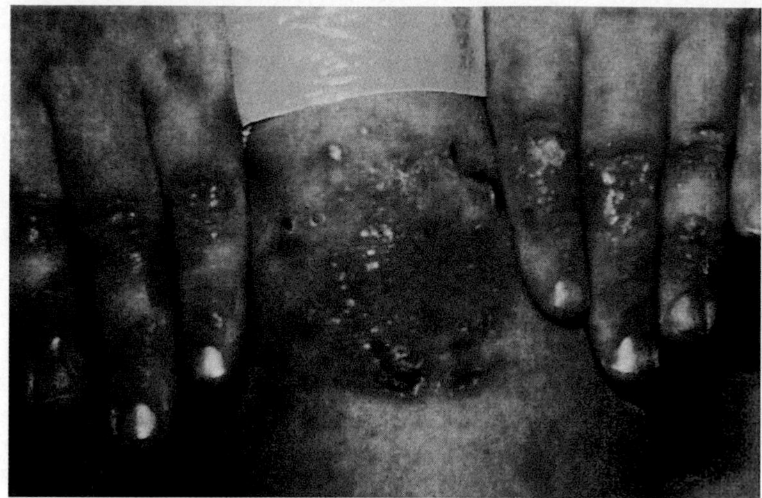

A.

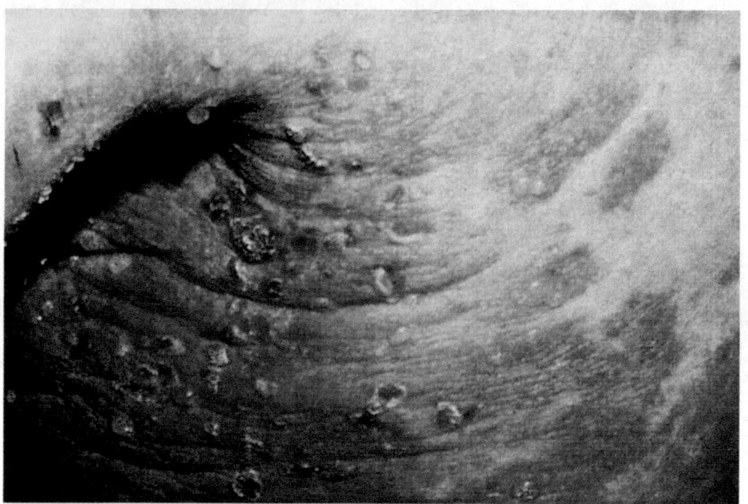

B.

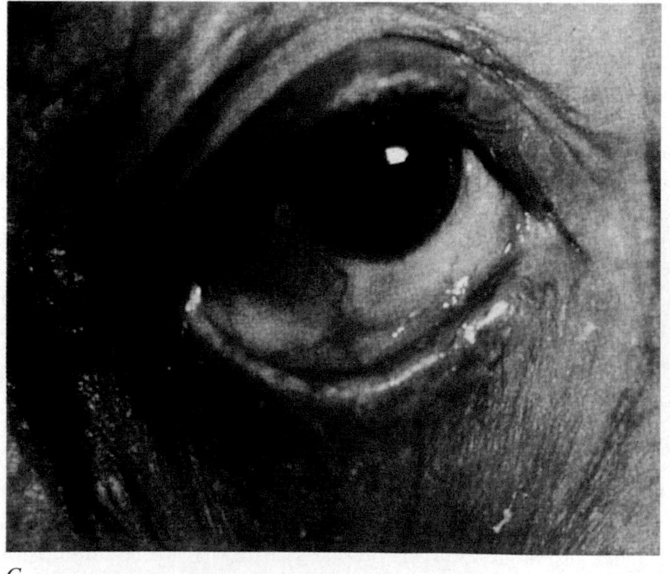

C.

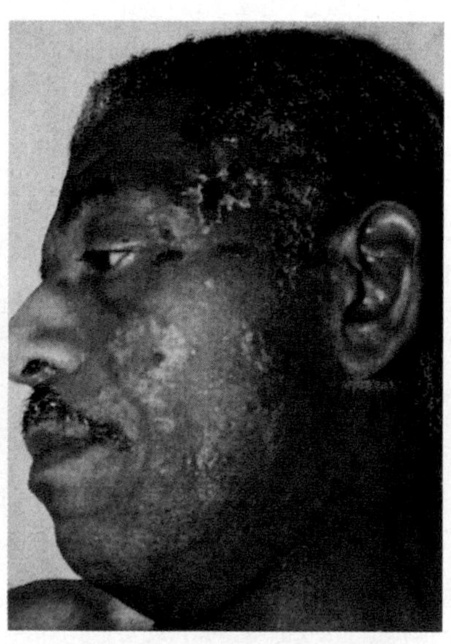

D.

A. Classical presentation of EBA with scarring and milia over trauma-prone areas of skin. *B.* Bullous pemphigoid–like presentation of EBA with a widespread inflammatory vesiculobullous dermatosis. *C.* Cicatricial pemphigoid–like presentation of EBA with a mucosal-centered bullous scarring eruption. *D.* Brunsting-Perry pemphigoid–like presentation of EBA with bullous and scarring lesions predominantly on the head and neck.

FIGURE 66-3

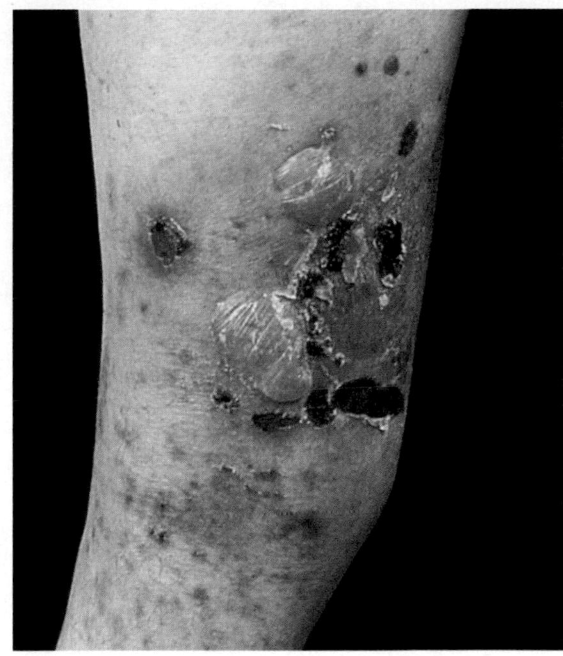

An EBA patient with involvement of the leg. Note bullae, crusts, and scarring at site of trauma.

within the dermis. Lesions that are clinically reminiscent of BP usually have significantly more inflammatory cells within the dermis, and these cells may be a mixture of lymphocytes, monocytes, neutrophils, and eosinophils. The histology of EBA skin specimens obtained from BP-like lesions may be difficult to distinguish from BP itself.

Ultrastructural studies of EBA skin have demonstrated a paucity of anchoring fibrils and an amorphous, electron-dense band just beneath the lamina densa.[8] Despite the sub–lamina densa deposits, EBA blisters frequently separate above the immune deposits within the lamina lucida.[36] The lamina lucida is the Achilles' Heel of the cutaneous basement membrane zone and is more susceptible to disadherence than the sub–lamina densa zone. Briggaman et al.[37] have shown that the entire cutaneous basement membrane zone is susceptible to degradation by a number of proteolytic enzymes that exist within inflammatory cells. Therefore, the cleavage plane of the blister is not a good way to discriminate EBA from other subepidermal bullous diseases.

FIGURE 66-4

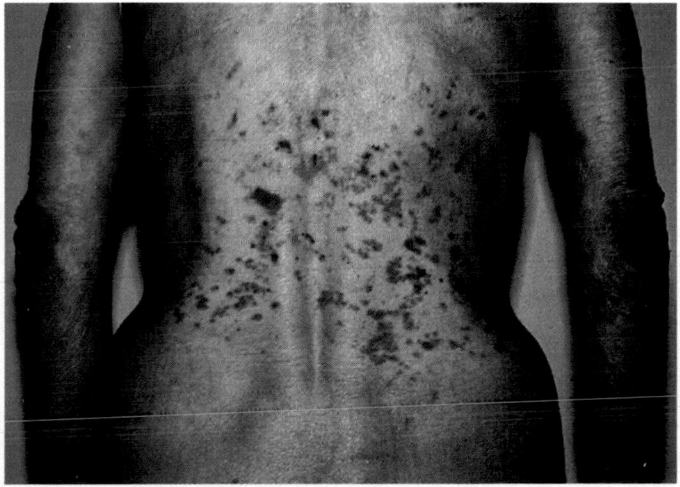

An EBA patient demonstrating two presentations of the disease: the classical mechanobullous presentation with erosions, scarring, and milia over the elbows and the more inflammatory BP-like lesions on her trunk.

IMMUNOLOGIC PARAMETERS

Routine Immunofluorescence

Patients with EBA have IgG deposits within the dermal-epidermal junction of their skin.[2,5] This is best detected by DIF of a biopsy specimen obtained from a perilesional site (Fig. 66-5). IgG is the predominant immunoglobulin class, but deposits of complement, IgA, IgM, factor B, and properdin also may be detected. The DIF staining demonstrates an intense linear fluorescent band at the dermal-epidermal junction. Yaoita et al.[5] have suggested that a positive DIF and IgG deposits within the sub–lamina densa zone are necessary criteria for the diagnosis of EBA.

Patients with PCT, which may mimic EBA clinically, frequently have IgG and complement deposits at the dermal-epidermal junction similar to those of EBA patients (see Chap. 149). However, the DIF feature that distinguishes PCT from EBA is that PCT skin also demonstrates immune deposits around the dermal blood vessels.

Patients with EBA may have autoantibodies in their blood directed against the dermal-epidermal junction.[12] These antibodies can be detected by IIF of the patient's serum on a substrate of monkey or rabbit esophagus or human skin and will stain the dermal-epidermal junction in a linear fashion that may be indistinguishable from bullous pemphigoid sera.

Immunoelectron Microscopy

The localization of the immune deposits within the dermal-epidermal junction of the skin of EBA patients by immunoelectron microscopy is the "gold standard" for the diagnosis. As demonstrated by Nieboer

FIGURE 66-5

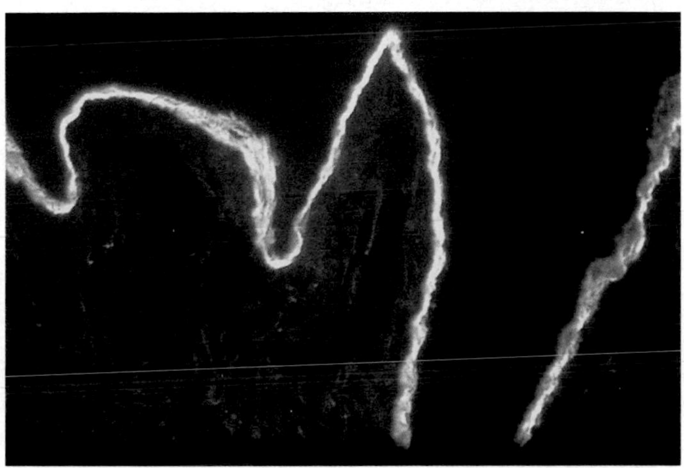

Direct immunofluorescence staining for IgG deposits in perilesional skin of an EBA patient. Note the dense deposits within the dermal-epidermal junction (the epidermis is on top in this section).

et al.[4] and Yaoita et al.,[5] patients with EBA have immune deposits within the sub–lamina densa zone of the cutaneous basement membrane zone. This localization is clearly distinct from the deposits in BP, which are higher up in the hemidesmosome area or lamina lucida area of the basement membrane. It is also distinct from CP, which has antigenic targets confined to the lamina lucida (see Chaps. 61 and 62).

Indirect Salt-Split Skin Immunofluorescence

When human skin is incubated in 1 *M* NaCl, the dermal-epidermal junction fractures cleanly through the lamina lucida zone.[38] This fracture places the BP antigen on the epidermal side of the split and all other basement membrane structures on the dermal side of the separation. Salt-split skin substrate can be used to distinguish EBA and BP sera.[39] If the serum antibody is IgG and labels the epidermal roof, the patient does not have EBA, and BP should be considered. If, on the other hand, the antibody labels the dermal side of the separation, the patient usually has either EBA or bullous SLE. The latter can be ruled out by other serology and by clinical criteria.

It was thought that only EBA and bullous SLE gave dermal labeling when salt-split skin immunofluorescence technology was used. It was also thought that the dermal fluorescent pattern on salt-split skin was indicative of immune deposits localized within the lamina densa or sub–lamina densa space, whereas epidermal-roof labeling was seen when deposits were localized within hemidesmosomes or the lamina lucida space. These conclusions are not correct and need modification with the advent of new knowledge about several new blistering disorders. The first new disease is found in a subset of CP patients who have autoantibodies against laminin-5, a noncollagenous component of anchoring filaments within the lamina lucida compartment.[40] The second is a BP-like disease in which the patients have autoantibodies to a 105-kDa lamina lucida glycoprotein that is unrelated to laminin-5.[41] In both diseases, the immune deposits are within the lower lamina lucida, and salt-split skin immunofluorescence gives a dermal-floor pattern of staining identical to EBA. As shown by Ceilley et al.,[42] this is so because laminin-5 and the 105-kDa protein go down with the dermis when the skin basement membrane zone is fractured by salt. The third newly discovered disease that gives dermal staining by salt-split skin immunofluorescence is a subepidermal blistering disease associated with renal insufficiency reported by Ghohestani and colleagues.[43] In this disease, the IgG autoantibodies are directed against the $\alpha5$ chain of type IV collagen, a component of the lamina densa zone of the basement membrane zone. In Table 66-1, these subepidermal bullous diseases that can give dermal fluorescence by salt-split skin immunofluorescence are summarized.

Direct Salt-Split Skin Immunofluorescence

Perilesional skin incubated in cold 1 *M* NaCl is fractured through the dermal-epidermal junction, which effectively places the BP antigen (and any associated immune deposits) on the epidermal roof and the EBA antigen (and any associated immune deposits) on the dermal floor of the separation.[44] If the patient has EBA, immune deposits are detected on the dermal side of the separation by a routine DIF method employing fluorescein-conjugated anti–human IgG.

TABLE 66-1

Subepidermal Autoimmune Bullous Diseases That Show Dermal Fluorescence on Immunofluorescent Analysis of Salt-Split Skin

1. Epidermolysis bullosa acquisita
2. Bullous SLE
3. Anti–laminin-5 cicatricial pemphigoid
4. p105 pemphigoid (Chan's disease)
5. Anti–type IV collagen bullous disease (Ghohestani's disease)

Western Immunoblotting

Antibodies in EBA sera will bind to a 290-kDa band in Western blots of human skin basement membrane proteins containing type VII collagen, whereas sera from all other primary blistering diseases will not.[12] This band is the alpha chain of type VII collagen. Often a second band of 145 kDa will be labeled with EBA antibodies. This band is the amino-terminal globular NC1 domain of the type VII collagen alpha chain, which is rich in carbohydrate and contains the antigenic epitopes of EBA autoantibodies, bullous SLE autoantibodies, and monoclonal antibodies against type VII collagen.[12,45]

Enzyme-Linked Immunosorbent Assay

Chen et al.[23] have produced milligram quantities of recombinant, purified, posttranslationally modified NC1 in stably transfected human cells and have used this NC1 to develop an enzyme-linked immunosorbent assay (ELISA) for autoantibody detection in EBA patients and in patients with bullous SLE.[46] This new ELISA is more sensitive than immunofluorescence and Western blotting, and yet it is very specific for antibodies to type VII collagen.

DIAGNOSIS

The diagnostic criteria developed by Yaoita et al.[5] for the diagnosis of EBA still stand. These criteria, with slightly updated modifications, are as follows:

- A bullous disorder within the clinical spectrum outlined earlier
- No family history of a bullous disorder
- Histology showing a subepidermal blister
- Deposition of IgG deposits within the dermal-epidermal junction, i.e., a positive DIF of perilesional skin
- IgG deposits localized to the lower lamina densa and/or sub–lamina densa zone of the dermal-epidermal junction when perilesional skin is examined by direct immunoelectron microscopy

Alternatives for the last item are indirect or direct salt-split skin immunofluorescence, Western blotting, and ELISA (see above).

TREATMENT

EBA is a very difficult disease to treat. EBA patients are refractory to high doses of systemic glucocorticoids, azathioprine, methotrexate, and cyclophosphamide, especially when they have the classical mechanobullous form of the disease. These agents are somewhat helpful in controlling EBA when it appears as an inflammatory BP-like disease. Some EBA patients improve on dapsone, especially when neutrophils are present in their dermal infiltrate.

Cyclosporine, an immunosuppressive agent that is used chiefly in organ transplantation, has been shown to be beneficial in EBA.[47,48] However, the long-term toxicity of this drug limits its use.

There are now three independent reports of EBA patients responding to high doses of colchicine.[49] This is often used as a first-line drug because its side effects are relatively benign compared with other therapeutic choices. Diarrhea is a common side effect of colchicine, however, which makes it difficult for many patients to achieve a high enough dose to control the disease. Moreover, because of this side effect, we are hesitant to try colchicine in EBA patients who also have inflammatory bowel disease. In addition, there are patients who do not respond to colchicine.[49] Colchicine is a well-known microtubule inhibitor, but it also appears to have properties that have the potential to inhibit antigen presentation to T cells, which could downregulate autoimmunity.[50]

Photophoresis has been used in Sézary syndrome, mycosis fungoides, and a variety of autoimmune bullous diseases (see Chap. 266). Photophoresis had a dramatic effect on one EBA patient in a life-threatening situation,[51] and in three other EBA patients it improved some clinical parameters and remarkably lengthened the suction blistering times of the patients, suggesting an improvement in their dermal-epidermal adherence.[52]

Intravenous immunoglobulin has been used in dermatomyositis, an entity in which autoimmunity may play a role. Intravenous immunoglobulin has been reported to be effective in some patients with EBA.[53] The mechanism by which gamma globulin may invoke a positive response in EBA is unknown.

Supportive therapy is warranted in all patients with EBA. This includes instruction in open wound care and strategies for avoiding trauma. Patients should be warned not to overwash or overuse hot water or harsh soaps and to avoid prolonged or vigorous rubbing of their skin with a washcloth or towel. In some patients it appears that prolonged sun exposure may aggravate or promote new lesions on the dorsal hands and knuckles. Avoidance of prolonged sun exposure and the use of sunscreens may be helpful. The patient should be educated to recognize localized skin infections and to seek medical care and antibiotic therapy promptly when they occur.

REFERENCES

1. Roenigk HH et al: Epidermolysis bullosa acquisita: Report of three cases and review of all published cases. *Arch Dermatol* **103**:10, 1971
2. Kushniruk W: The immunopathology of epidermolysis bullosa acquisita. *Can Med Assoc J* **108**:1143, 1973
3. Gibbs RB, Minus HR: Epidermolysis bullosa acquisita with electron microscopical studies. *Arch Dermatol* **111**:215, 1975
4. Nieboer C et al: Epidermolysis bullosa acquisita: Immunofluorescence, electron microscopic and immunoelectron microscopic studies in four patients. *Br J Dermatol* **102**:383, 1980
5. Yaoita H et al: Epidermolysis bullosa acquisita: Ultrastructural and immunological studies. *J Invest Dermatol* **76**:288, 1981
6. Gammon WR et al: Epidermolysis bullosa acquisita: A pemphigoid-like disease. *J Am Acad Dermatol* **11**:820, 1984
7. Dahl MGC: Epidermolysis bullosa acquisita: A sign of cicatricial pemphigoid? *Br J Dermatol* **101**:475, 1979
8. Richter BJ, McNutt NS: The spectrum of epidermolysis bullosa acquisita. *Arch Dermatol* **115**:1325, 1979
9. Provost TT et al: Unusual sub-epidermal bullous diseases presenting as an inflammatory bullous disease. *Arch Dermatol* **115**:156, 1979
10. Woodley DT: Epidermolysis bullosa acquisita. *Prog Dermatol* **22**:1, 1988
11. Kurzhals G et al: Acquired epidermolysis bullosa with the clinical features of Brunsting-Perry cicatricial bullous pemphigoid. *Arch Dermatol* **127**:391, 1991
12. Woodley DT et al: Identification of the skin basement membrane autoantigen in epidermolysis bullosa acquisita. *N Engl J Med* **310**:1007, 1984
13. Woodley DT et al: The epidermolysis bullosa acquisita antigen is the globular carboxyl terminus of type VII procollagen. *J Clin Invest* **81**:683, 1988
14. Ray TL et al: Epidermolysis bullosa acquisita and inflammatory bowel disease. *J Am Acad Dermatol* **6**:242, 1982
15. Christiano AM et al: A common insertion mutation in COLA1 in two Italian families with recessive dystrophic epidermolysis bullosa. *J Invest Dermatol* **106**:679, 1996
16. Parente MG et al: Human type VII collagen: cDNA cloning and chromosomal mapping of the gene. *Proc Natl Acad Sci USA* **88**:6931, 1991
17. Shimizu H: Molecular basis of recessive dystrophic epidermolysis bullosa: Genotype/phenotype correlation in a case of moderate clinical severity. *J Invest Dermatol* **106**:119, 1996
18. Woodley DT et al: Burn wounds resurfaced by cultured epidermal autografts show abnormal reconstitution of anchoring fibrils. *JAMA* **259**:2566, 1988
19. Lapiere J-C et al: Epitope mapping of type VII collagen: Identification of discrete peptide sequences recognized by sera from patients with acquired epidermolysis bullosa. *J Clin Invest* **92**:1831, 1993
20. Jones DA et al: Immunodominant autoepitopes of type VII collagen are short, paired peptide sequences within the fibronectin type III homology region of the non-collagenous (NC1) domain. *J Invest Dermatol* **104**:231, 1995
21. Woodley DT et al: Specific affinity between fibronectin and the epidermolysis bullosa acquisita antigen. *J Clin Invest* **179**:1826, 1987
22. Lapiere J-C et al: Type VII collagen specifically binds fibronectin via a unique subdomain within the collagenous triple helix. *J Invest Dermatol* **103**:637, 1994
23. Chen M et al: Interactions of the amino-terminal noncollagenous (NC1) domain of type VII collagen with extracellular matrix components. *J Biol Chem* **272**:14516, 1997
24. Gammon WR et al: Evidence that antibasement membrane zone antibodies in bullous eruption of systemic lupus erythematosus recognize epidermolysis bullosa acquisita autoantigens. *J Invest Dermatol* **84**:472, 1985
25. Barradori L et al: Passive transfer of autoantibodies from a patient with mutilating epidermolysis bullosa acquisita induces specific alterations in the skin of neonatal mice. *Arch Dermatol* **131**:590, 1995
26. Gammon WR et al: Increased frequency of HLA DR2 in patients with autoantibodies to EBA antigen: Evidence that the expression of autoimmunity to type VII collagen is HLA class II allele associated. *J Invest Dermatol* **91**:228, 1988
27. Stewart MI, Woodley DT: Acquired epidermolysis bullosa and associated symptomatic esophageal webs. *Arch Dermatol* **127**:373, 1991
28. Park SB et al: Epidermolysis bullosa aquisita in childhood: A case mimicking chronic bullous dermatosis of childhood. *Clin Exp Dermatol* **22**:220, 1997
29. Callot-Mellot C et al: Epidermolysis bullosa aquisita in childhood. *Arch Dermatol* **133**:1122, 1997
30. Hashimoto T et al: A case of linear IgA bullous dermatosis with IgA anti-type VII collagen autoantibodies. *Br J Dermatol* **134**:336, 1996
31. Bauer JW et al: Ocular involvement in IgA-epidermolysis bullosa acquisita. *Br J Dermatol* **141**:887, 1999
32. Lee CW: Serum IgA autoantibodies in patients with epidermolysis bullosa acquisita: A high frequency of detection. *Dermatology* **200**:83, 2000
33. Edwards S et al: Bullous pemphigoid and epidermolysis bullosa acquisita: Presentation, prognosis and immunopathology in 11 children. *Pediatr Dermatol* **15**:184, 1998
34. Burke WA et al: Epidermolysis bullosa acquisita in a patient with multiple endocrinopathies syndrome. *Arch Dermatol* **122**:187, 1986
35. Chan L, Woodley DT: Pemphigoid: Bullous and cicatricial, in *Current Therapy in Allergy, Immunology and Rheumatology*, 5th ed, edited by LM Lichtenstein, AS Fauci. St. Louis, Mosby, 1996, p 93
36. Fine JD et al: The presence of intra-lamina lucida blister formation in epidermolysis bullosa acquisita: Possible role of leukocytes. *J Invest Dermatol* **92**:27, 1989
37. Briggaman RA et al: Degradation of the epidermal-dermal junction by proteolytic enzymes from human skin and human polymorphonuclear leukocytes. *J Exp Med* **160**:1027, 1984
38. Woodley DT et al: Localization of basement membrane components after dermal-epidermal junction separation. *J Invest Dermatol* **81**:149, 1983
39. Gammon WR et al: Differentiating anti-lamina lucida and antisublamina dense anti-BMZ antibodies by direct immunofluorescence on 1.0 *M* sodium chloride separated skin. *J Invest Dermatol* **84**:215, 1984
40. Domloge-Hultsch N et al: Antiepiligrin cicatricial pemphigoid: A subepithelial bullous disorder. *Arch Dermatol* **130**:1521, 1994
41. Chan LS et al: A newly identified 105-kDa lower lamina lucida autoantigen is an acidic protein distinct from the 105-kDa gamma 2 chain of laminin 5. *J Invest Dermatol* **105**:75, 1995
42. Ceilley E et al: Labeling of fractured human skin with antibodies to BM 600/nicein, epiligrin, kalinin and other matrix components. *J Dermatol Sci* **5**:97, 1993
43. Ghohestani RF et al: The $\alpha 5$ chain of type IV collagen is the target of IgG autoantibodies in a novel autoimmune disease with subepidermal blisters and renal insufficiency. *J Biol Chem* **275**:16002, 2000
44. Gammon WR et al: Direct immunofluorescence studies of sodium chloride–separated skin in the differential diagnosis of bullous pemphigoid and epidermolysis bullosa acquisita. *J Am Acad Dermatol* **22**:664, 1990

45. Woodley DT et al: Epidermolysis bullosa acquisita antigen, a new major component of cutaneous basement membrane, is a glycoprotein with collagenous domains. *J Invest Dermatol* **86**:668, 1986
46. Chen M et al: Development of an ELISA for rapid detection of anti–type VII collagen autoantibodies in epidermolysis bullosa acquisita. *J Invest Dermatol* **108**:68, 1997
47. Connolly SM, Sander HM: Treatment of epidermolysis bullosa acquisita with cyclosporin. *J Am Acad Dermatol* **16**:890, 1987
48. Crow LL et al: Clearing of epidermolysis bullosa acquisita on cyclosporin A. *J Am Acad Dermatol* **19**:937, 1988
49. Cunningham BB et al: Colchicine for epidermolysis bullosa (EBA). *J Am Acad Dermatol* **34**:781, 1996
50. Mekori YA et al: Inhibition of delayed hypersensitivity reaction by colchicine: Colchicine inhibits interferon-gamma-induced expression of HLA-DR on an epithelial cell line. *Clin Exp Immunol* **78**:230, 1989
51. Miller JL et al: Remission of severe epidermolysis bullosa acquisita induced by extracorporeal photochemotherapy. *Br J Dermatol* **133**:467, 1995
52. Gordon K et al: Treatment of refractory epidermolysis bullosa acquisita with extracorporeal photochemotherapy. *Br J Dermatol* **136**:415, 1997
53. Meier F et al: Epidermolysis bullosa acquisita: Efficacy of high dose intravenous immunoglobulins. *J Am Acad Dermatol* **29**:334, 1993

CHAPTER 67

Stephen I. Katz

Dermatitis Herpetiformis

Dermatitis herpetiformis (DH) is characterized by an intensely itchy, chronic papulovesicular eruption that usually is distributed symmetrically on extensor surfaces. The disease can be clearly distinguished from the other subepidermal blistering eruptions by histologic, immunologic, and gastrointestinal criteria. The prevalence of DH in various Caucasian populations varies between 10 and 39 per 100,000 persons.[1–3] It may start at any age, including childhood; however, the second, third, and fourth decades are the most common. After presentation, DH persists indefinitely, although with varying severity. Most patients have an associated gluten-sensitive enteropathy (GSE) that is usually asymptomatic.

HISTORICAL ASPECTS

In 1884, Louis Duhring first described the clinical features and natural history of a polymorphous pruritic disorder that he called *dermatitis herpetiformis.*[4] Not all of his patients would now be considered to have DH, since Duhring probably included patients with bullous pemphigoid. In 1888, Brocq described patients with a very similar disorder and called it *dermatite polymorphe prurigineuse.*[5] In addition, he analyzed Duhring's report and excluded several types of patients from the diagnosis. Since that time, several important discoveries have been made. In 1940, Costello[6] demonstrated the efficacy of sulfapyridine in the treatment of DH. In the early 1960s, Pierard and Whimster[7] and MacVicar et al.[8] found that early lesions of DH are characterized by neutrophilic microabscesses in the dermal papillae. In 1967, Cormane[9] found that the skin of DH patients contained granular immunoglobulin deposits in dermal papillary tips, and in 1969, van der Meer[10] extended these studies and found that the most regularly detected immunoglobulin deposited in DH is IgA. The association between DH and intestinal abnormalities was first observed by Marks et al.[11] in 1966. Fry et al.[12] and Shuster et al.[13] identified the intestinal findings as a GSE. In 1973, Fry et al.[14] demonstrated that strict adherence to a gluten-free diet would improve the skin disease as well as reverse the intestinal abnormality, as occurs in celiac disease. Katz et al.[15] identified a strong association between DH and certain histocompatibility antigens in 1972. In 1979, Chorzelski et al.[16] distinguished those patients with linear IgA deposits from those with granular IgA deposits and defined a distinct entity. In 1999, Dieterich et al.[17] identified antibodies to tissue transglutaminases in the sera from DH patients. Distinguishing between various types of transglutaminases enabled Sardy et al.[18] in 2002 to demonstrate that epidermal transglutaminase is the dominant autoantigen in DH.

ETIOLOGY AND PATHOGENESIS

Gluten, a protein found in wheat, barley, and rye, plays a critical role in the pathogenesis of DH. Oats, long thought to contain gluten and play a role in inducing DH lesions, has been shown to be devoid of toxicity in patients with DH.[19,20] In 1966, Marks et al.[11] first noted a gastrointestinal abnormality in patients with DH. Shortly thereafter it was shown that the lesion was reversible by avoidance of the dietary protein gluten.[12,13] Initially, the intestinal abnormality was thought to be present in 60 to 75 percent of DH patients. However, this view has been modified in two ways. First, the diagnostic criteria for DH have now been delineated more precisely, and second, it can be shown that certain patients without apparent gastrointestinal pathology can be "induced" to develop gastrointestinal lesions by subjecting them to a large gluten intake; such patients have been said to have *latent celiac sprue.*[21] Thus most patients with DH have a gastrointestinal abnormality similar (if not identical) to celiac disease, however minimal that may be when the patient is ingesting a normal gluten load. As in celiac disease, there is an increased density of intraepithelial (gut) T cells with a gamma/delta T cell receptor in the jejunum of patients with DH.[22] The finding that T cell lines from patients with DH produce significantly more interleukin 4 (IL-4) than those from patients with GSE suggests that different cytokine patterns may play a role in the varied clinical manifestations of these two diseases.[23] Increased serum IL-2 receptor levels may reflect an ongoing immune response in the gastrointestinal tract.[24]

The GSE seen in DH patients probably relates to the IgA deposits that are found in the skin of these patients, although a direct relationship has not been demonstrated. It has long been thought that IgA deposits may represent complexes of immunoglobulin and gastrointestinally derived antigens, and recent studies have strongly suggested that this may be the case. It is known that patients with both GSE and DH have antibodies to transglutaminases (TGs) that are thought to be the major autoantigens in these diseases.[17] There appears to be a predilection for the autoantibodies to bind to epidermal TG in DH, whereas the predilection is for autoantibodies to bind tissue TG in GSE.[18] The epidermal TG autoantibody probably binds to the TG in the gut and circulates as an immune complex and deposits in skin.[18]

Whether the IgA skin deposits play a role in the pathophysiology of blister formation is not known. The finding of IgA and complement in almost all skin sites, not only in lesional skin, makes one postulate that if IgA (either alone or as a part of an immune complex) does play a role, additional factors are still needed to explain the initiation of lesions. With these additional factors, IgA activates complement, probably via the alternative pathway, with the subsequent chemotaxis of neutrophils that release their enzymes and produce the tissue injury known as DH. Alternatively, it may be that after neutrophils arrive at the site of immune complex formation, they release factors such as cytokines or proteases that induce basal keratinocytes to produce collagenases or stromelysin-1 that contributes to the formation of blisters.[25,26] Other studies have suggested that T cells may play a role in the pathogenesis of the skin lesions[27]; however, no specific T cell responses to gluten have been detected.[28]

It has been known for some time that iodides, administered orally, can exacerbate or elicit eruptions of DH, and this has, in former times, been used for diagnostic purposes. The availability of immunopathologic techniques for the detection of IgA deposits in skin has made such provocation tests obsolete.

CLINICAL MANIFESTATIONS

The primary lesion of DH is either an erythematous papule, an urticaria-like plaque, or most commonly, a vesicle (Figs. 67-1, 67-2, and 67-3). Large bullae occur infrequently. Vesicles, especially if they occur on the palms, may be hemorrhagic. The continual appearance and disappearance of lesions may result in hyperpigmentation and hypopigmentation. Patients may present with only crusted lesions, and a thorough search may not reveal a primary lesion. The herpetiform (herpes-like) grouping of lesions is often present in some areas (see Figs. 67-1 and 67-3), but patients also may have many individual nongrouped lesions.

Symptoms vary considerably from the usually severe burning and itching in most patients to the almost complete lack of symptoms in a rare patient. Most patients usually can predict the eruption of a lesion as much as 8 to 12 h before its appearance because of localized stinging, burning, or itching.

The usual symmetric distribution of lesions on elbows, knees, buttocks, shoulders, and sacral areas is seen in most patients at one time or another (see Figs. 67-1 through 67-4). Although these regions are affected most commonly, most patients will have scalp lesions and/or lesions in the posterior nuchal area. Another commonly affected area is the face and facial hairline. Mucous membrane lesions are uncommon, as are lesions on the palms and soles.

FIGURE 67-1

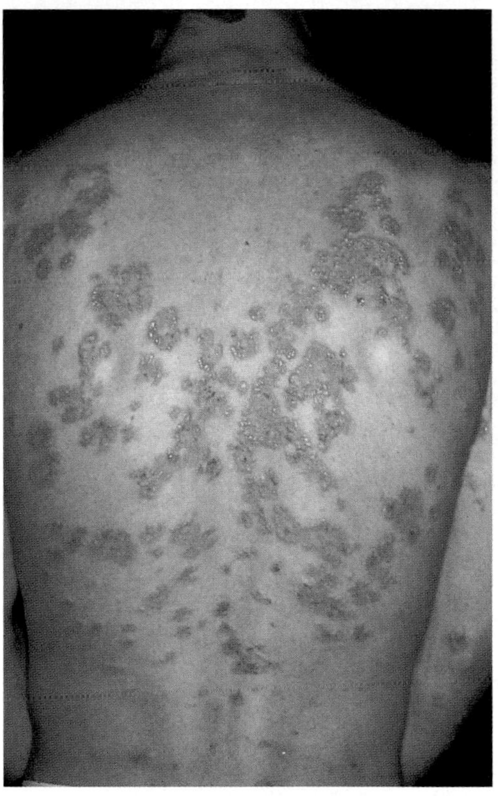

Dermatitis herpetiformis. Extensive eruption with grouped papules, vesicles, and crusts on the back.

LABORATORY FINDINGS

In Vivo Bound IgA and Complement

After Cormane[9] demonstrated that both perilesional and uninvolved skin of patients with DH contained granular (or fibrillar) immunoglobulin deposits located in dermal papillary tips, van der Meer[10] found that the most regularly detected immunoglobulin class in DH skin was

FIGURE 67-2

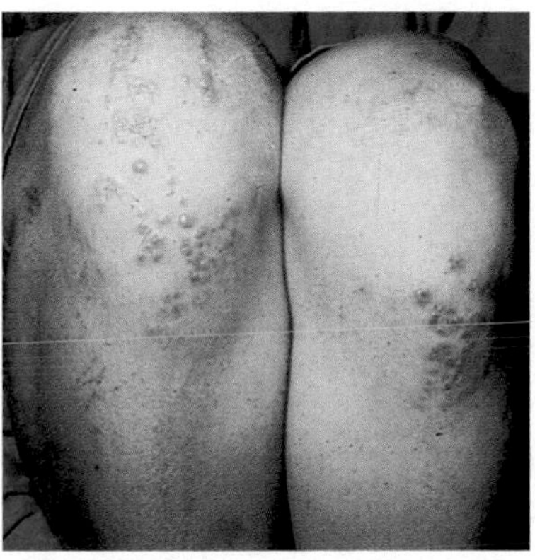

Dermatitis herpetiformis. Papules, vesicles, and crusts on knees.

FIGURE 67-3

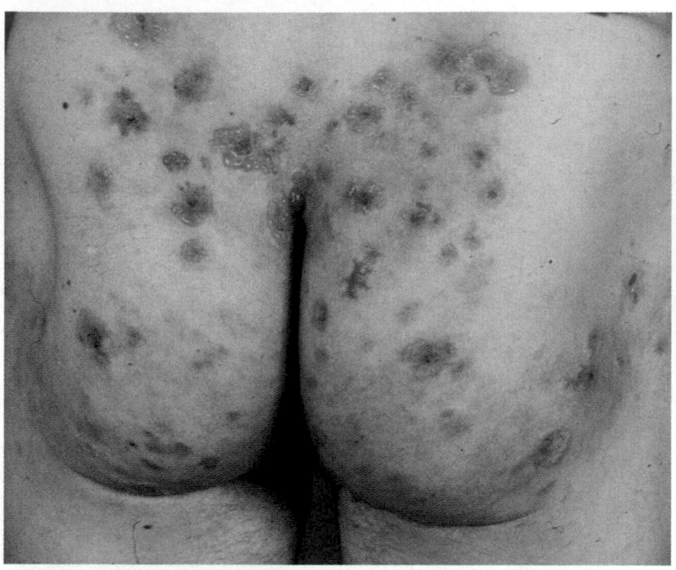

Dermatitis herpetiformis. This patient has many firm-topped vesicles and bullae, some erosions, and residual hyperpigmentation. Some of the vesicles are arranged in an annular pattern.

IgA (Fig. 67-5). Seah and Fry[29] were able to detect IgA deposits in the skin of each of 50 patients studied, with only 2 patients requiring a second biopsy for IgA detection. Others have failed to find IgA in a very small minority of patients who, on other grounds, are considered to have DH.[30]

FIGURE 67-4

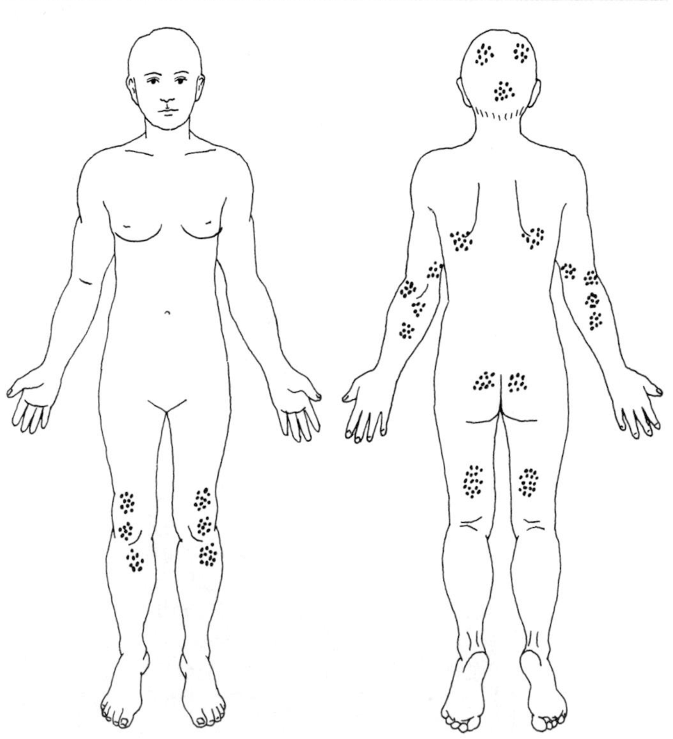

Dermatitis herpetiformis. Pattern of distribution.

FIGURE 67-5

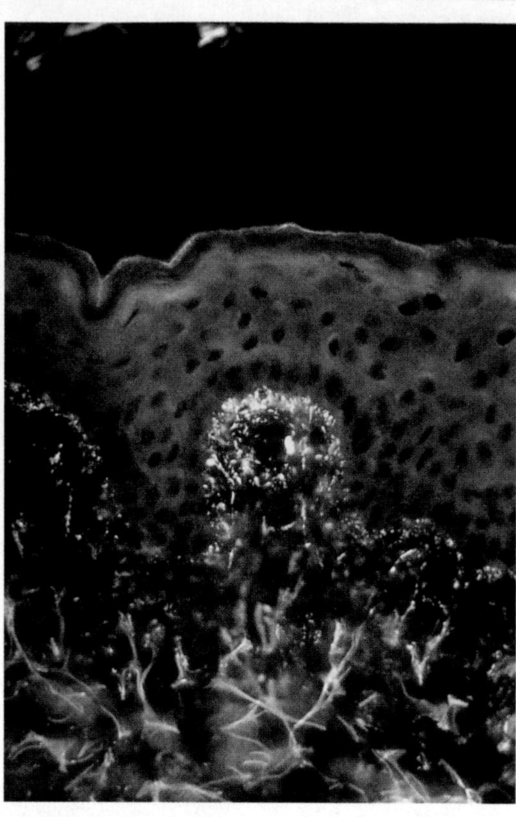

Dermatitis herpetiformis. Direct immunofluorescence showing granular dermal papillary deposits of IgA.

Granular IgA deposits in normal-appearing skin are the most reliable criteria for the diagnosis of DH.[29–31] These IgA deposits are unaffected by treatment with drugs but may decrease in intensity or disappear after long-term adherence to a gluten-free diet.[32,33] The IgA deposits are not uniformly intense throughout the skin and may be detected more easily in normal-appearing skin near active lesions.[34] In DH, other immunoglobulins sometimes are bound to the skin in the same areas as the IgA.[29] IgA deposits also may be seen in the skin of patients with bullous pemphigoid, scarring pemphigoid, Henoch-Schönlein purpura, and alcoholic liver disease, although in different patterns of distribution than those seen in DH.

Because of the IgA skin deposits and the association between DH and GSE (celiac disease), several groups have studied the IgA subclasses in DH. IgA_1 is the predominant (or exclusive) subclass that has been identified in the skin of DH patients.[35,36] Most IgA_1 is produced in the bone marrow, whereas most IgA_2 is produced at mucosal sites. This does not negate the possibility that the IgA_1 in skin may still be of mucosal origin.

The third component of complement (C3) is frequently found in the same location as IgA. The presence of C3 in both perilesional and normal-appearing skin is not affected by treatment with dapsone (diaminodiphenyl sulfone),[37] but C3 may not be detectable after treatment with a gluten-free diet.[33,38] C5 and components of the alternative complement pathway also may be seen in areas corresponding to the IgA deposits. The C5-C9 membrane attack complex, which is formed as the terminal event in complement activation, is also seen in normal-appearing and perilesional skin of patients.[39]

The exact site of the IgA deposits in DH skin has been studied by immunoelectron microscopy. Early studies indicated that IgA is preferentially associated with bundles of microfibrils and with anchoring fibrils of the papillary dermis immediately below the basal lamina.[40,41]

More recent studies, however, have indicated that some or almost all of the IgA deposits are related to nonfibrillar components of skin and other connective tissues.[42,43] There is also no agreement as to whether the IgA deposits in DH colocalize to fibrillin, a major component of the elastic microfibrillar bundles.

Serum Studies

Antireticulin antibodies of the IgA and IgG classes have been detected in the sera of 17 to 93 percent of patients with DH and in higher percentages of patients with other diseases, especially celiac disease.[45] Thyroid microsomal antibodies[46] and antinuclear antibodies also have been detected in increased incidence in the sera of patients with DH. Putative immune complexes have been detected in the sera of 25 to 40 percent of patients.[47,48]

Chorzelski et al.[49] have described an IgA antibody that binds to an intermyofibril substance (endomysium) of smooth muscle. The nature of this antigen has been identified recently by the studies of Sardy et al.,[18] who showed that these IgA autoantibodies have specificity for transglutaminases, particularly epidermal-specific transglutaminases.

IMMUNOGENETIC FINDINGS

There is a marked increase in the incidence of certain major histocompatibility complex antigens in patients with DH. Worldwide studies have found that 77 to 87 percent of DH patients have HLA-B8[31,50] (compared with 20–30 percent of normal individuals). In addition, the class II major histocompatibility complex antigens HLA-DR and -DQ are associated with DH even more frequently than is HLA-B8.[51,52] Park et al.[53] reported that more than 90 percent of patients expressed Te24, which was later shown to be similar to HLA-DQw2, and this finding has been confirmed by others. Molecular studies indicate that susceptibility to DH is not associated with a unique HLA-DQw2 molecule.[54] Virtually all patients with DH have genes that encode the HLA-DQ ($\alpha 1$*0501, $\beta 1$*02) or the HLA-DQ ($\alpha 1$*03, $\beta 1$*0302) heterodimers, a pattern identical to that seen in celiac disease.[54–56] This strong association between susceptibility genes and DH and GSE is important clinically and pathophysiologically in that there is a strong concordance of these two diseases in monozygotic twins.[57] Furthermore, first-degree relatives of both DH and GSE patients are often (4–5 percent) affected with one or the other of these diseases.[58]

PATHOLOGY

The histology of an early skin lesion (clinically nonvesicular) is characterized by dermal papillary collections of neutrophils (microabscesses), neutrophilic fragments, varying numbers of eosinophils, fibrin, and at times, separation of the papillary tips from the overlying epidermis (Fig. 67-6). In addition, in such early lesions, the upper and middle dermal blood vessels are surrounded by a lymphohistiocytic infiltrate as well as some neutrophils and an occasional eosinophil.[7,8] At times, early lesions may be difficult or impossible to differentiate from those of linear IgA disease (see Chap. 63), the bullous eruption of lupus erythematosus (see Chap. 171), bullous pemphigoid (see Chap. 61), or the neutrophil-rich form of epidermolysis bullosa acquisita (see Chap. 66). The histology of older lesions shows subepidermal vesicles that may be impossible to differentiate from other subepidermal bullous eruptions, such as bullous pemphigoid, erythema multiforme (see Chap. 58), bullous drug eruption, and pemphigoid gestationis (see Chap. 64). Immunofluorescent localization and ultrastructural studies of the site

FIGURE 67-6

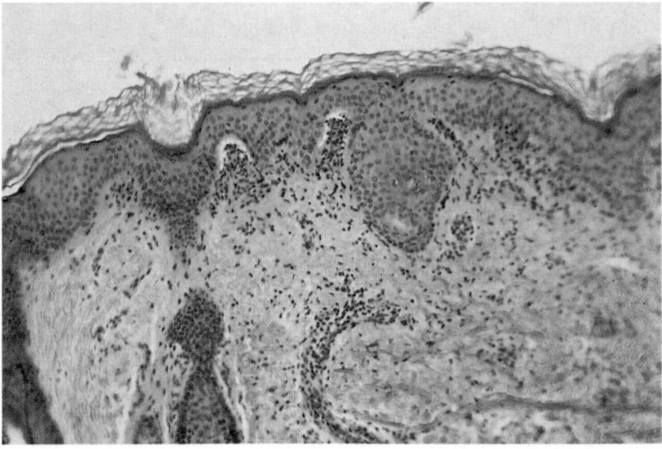

A.

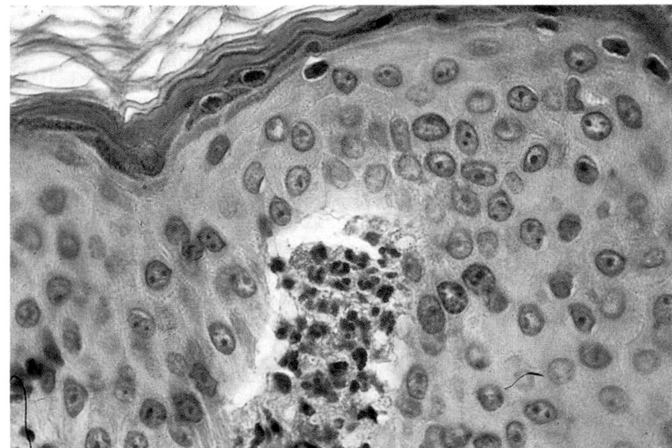

B.

Dermatitis herpetiformis. Biopsy of an early lesion showing dermal papillary collections of neutrophils and eosinophils and subepidermal vesiculation at low (*A*) and high (*B*) magnification.

of blister formation in DH have demonstrated that the blister forms above the lamina densa—within the lamina lucida.[59,60] This is thought to occur because the lamina lucida is the most vulnerable component of the dermal-epidermal junction.

ASSOCIATED PROBLEMS

Gastrointestinal Manifestations

It is now well accepted that most, if not all, DH patients have an associated gastrointestinal abnormality that is caused by gluten sensitivity.[30,31,61] The pathology of the GSE associated with DH and that in celiac disease (GSE unassociated with DH) is essentially the same, although the lesion in the latter is usually much more severe; this applies to the epithelial cell derangement as well as to the character of the lymphoplasmacytic infiltrate. In addition, the distribution of the gastrointestinal lesion in the small intestine is, as a general rule, more widespread in celiac disease. The functional changes in the bowel and clinical sequelae encountered in the GSE associated with DH and those encountered in celiac disease are similar but again differ in degree, those in the latter being more severe. Thus in DH one observes steatorrhea (20–30 percent of patients), abnormal D-xylose absorption (10–33 percent of patients), and occasional anemia secondary to iron or folate deficiency. In patients not taking dapsone or related drugs, the latter is usually due to malabsorption. Studies using elemental diets (see below) in the treatment of DH have questioned the critical role attributed to gluten in the pathogenesis of this disease. In addition to the small intestinal lesion, patients with DH have an increased incidence of achlorhydria and atrophic gastritis.[62,63] Reports of pernicious anemia and antibodies to gastric parietal cells are thus likely to be due to more than chance.

Malignancy

Leonard et al.[64] have reported an increased frequency of malignancies, especially gastrointestinal lymphomas, and Collin et al.[65] have reported a significant increase in non-Hodgkin's lymphomas in patients with DH. A combined retrospective study from both these groups suggests a protective role for a gluten-free diet against gastrointestinal lymphomas.[66]

Other Diseases

In addition to celiac disease, atrophic gastritis, and pernicious anemia (see above), DH patients have a higher incidence of other autoimmune diseases such as thyroid disease, insulin-dependent diabetes, lupus erythematosus, Sjögren's syndrome, and vitiligo.[46,67,68] This predilection for associated autoimmune diseases may be due to the high frequency of the 8.1 ancestral haplotype in these DH patients.[69]

DIAGNOSIS

DH may be confused with numerous other conditions because of its pleomorphic manifestations and the occasional lack of diagnostic lesions. Erythema multiforme, neurotic excoriations, scabies, eczema, papular urticaria, transient acantholytic dermatosis, pemphigoid, herpes gestationis, and various other dermatoses can be differentiated easily on the basis of histologic and immunologic criteria. Linear IgA disease may be more difficult to differentiate clinically and histologically, but it is distinctive immunologically. A high index of suspicion is very helpful in that even in the absence of primary lesions, DH can be diagnosed based on the typical in vivo–bound granular IgA deposits in normal-appearing skin.

TREATMENT

Sulfones

Diaminodiphenyl sulfone (dapsone), sulfoxone (diasone—not available in the United States), and sulfapyridine provide prompt improvement in symptoms and signs of the disease. Symptoms may abate in as few as 3 h or as long as a few days after the first pill is taken, and new lesions no longer erupt after 1 to 2 days of treatment. Exacerbations occur from hours to days after cessation of treatment. This response to therapy was, for a long time, the most important element in making a diagnosis. The preferred treatment for an adult is dapsone at an initial dosage of 100 to 150 mg per day (this usually can be taken at one time of day). An occasional patient may require 300 to 400 mg of dapsone for initial improvement. Patients should be instructed to take the minimal dose required to suppress signs and symptoms. Not all patients require daily treatment; in rare cases, 25 mg weekly is sufficient. Sulfapyridine, in a dosage of 1 to 1.5 g daily, is particularly useful in patients intolerant of dapsone, in elderly patients, and in those with cardiopulmonary problems. The pharmacology, mechanism(s) of action, adverse effects, and monitoring of dapsone are discussed in Chap. 254. It is important to know that nonsteroidal anti-inflammatory drugs often exacerbate DH, even in patients taking dapsone.[70]

Gluten-Free Diet

EFFECT ON THE SMALL INTESTINE There is no doubt that the intestinal lesion in DH responds to dietary gluten withdrawal. The time course of the response in adults with DH is the same as that in adults with celiac disease.

EFFECT ON THE SKIN DISEASE Strict adherence to a gluten-free diet will, after variable periods of time (from 5 months to 1 year), reduce or completely eliminate the requirement for medication in most, but not all, patients. The most extensive early study by Fry et al.[14] has been confirmed by several groups. However, it is only the very highly motivated patient who can adhere to the diet, which requires counseling by an individual who is very familiar with its use.

Elemental Diet

Studies in small numbers of DH patients have indicated that elemental diets (composed of free amino acids, short-chain polysaccharides, and small amounts of triglycerides) can be very beneficial in alleviating the skin disease within a few weeks.[71,72] The beneficial effect on the skin disease may be achieved even if the patient ingests large amounts of gluten.[72] Unfortunately, elemental diets are difficult to tolerate for long periods.

REFERENCES

1. Reunala T, Lokki J: Dermatitis herpetiformis in Finland. *Acta Derm Venereol (Stockh)* **58**:505, 1978
2. Moi H: Incidence and prevalence of dermatitis herpetiformis in a county in central Sweden, with comments on the course of the disease and IgA deposits as diagnostic criterion. *Acta Derm Venereol (Stockh)* **64**:144, 1984
3. Smith JB et al: The incidence and prevalence of dermatitis herpetiformis in Utah. *Arch Dermatol* **128**:1608, 1992
4. Duhring L: Dermatitis herpetiformis. *JAMA* **3**:225, 1884
5. Brocq L: De la dermatite herpétiforme de Duhring. *Ann Dermatol Syphiligr* (second series):9, 1888
6. Costello M: Dermatitis herpetiformis treated with sulfapyridine. *Arch Dermatol Syphilol* **41**:134, 1940
7. Pierard J, Whimster I: The histological diagnosis of dermatitis herpetiformis, bullous pemphigoid and erythema multiforme. *Br J Dermatol* **73**:253, 1961
8. MacVicar DN et al: Dermatitis herpetiformis, erythema multiforme and bullous pemphigoid: A comparative histopathological and histochemical study. *J Invest Dermatol* **41**:289, 1963
9. Cormane RH: Immunofluorescent studies of the skin in lupus erythematosus and other diseases. *Pathol Eur* **2**:170, 1967
10. van der Meer JB: Granular deposits of immunoglobulins in the skin of patients with dermatitis herpetiformis: An immunofluorescent study. *Br J Dermatol* **81**:493, 1969
11. Marks J et al: Small bowel changes in dermatitis herpetiformis. *Lancet* **2**:1280, 1966
12. Fry L et al: Small-intestinal structure and function and haematological changes in dermatitis herpetiformis. *Lancet* **2**:729, 1967
13. Shuster S et al: Coeliac syndrome in dermatitis herpetiformis. *Lancet* **1**:1101, 1968
14. Fry L et al: Clearance of skin lesions in dermatitis herpetiformis after gluten withdrawal. *Lancet* **1**:288, 1973

15. Katz SI et al: HL-A8: A genetic link between dermatitis herpetiformis and gluten-sensitive enteropathy. *J Clin Invest* **51**:2977, 1972
16. Chorzelski TP et al: Linear IgA bullous dermatosis, in *Immunopathology of the Skin,* 2d ed, edited by EH Beutner, TP Chorzelski, and S Jablonska. New York, Wiley, 1979, p 315
17. Dieterich W et al: Antibodies to tissue transglutaminase as serologic markers in patients with dermatitis herpetiformis. *J Invest Dermatol* **113**:133, 1999
18. Sardy M et al: Epidermal transglutaminase (Tgase 3) is the autoantigen of dermatitis herpetiformis. *J Exp Med* **195**:1, 2002
19. Hardman CM et al: Absence of toxicity of oats in patients with dermatitis herpetiformis. *New Engl J Med* **337**:1884, 1997
20. Reunala T et al: Tolerance to oats in dermatitis herpetiformis. *Gut* **43**:490, 1998
21. Weinstein WM: Latent celiac sprue. *Gastroenterology* **66**:489, 1974
22. Savilahti E et al: Density of gamma/delta T cells in the jejunal epithelium of patients with coeliac disease and dermatitis herpetiformis is increased with age. *Clin Exp Immunol* **109**:464, 1997
23. Hall RP et al TCR Vb expression in the small bowel of patients with dermatitis herpetiformis and gluten-sensitive enteropathy. *Exp Dermatol* **9**:275, 2000
24. Ward MM et al: Soluble interleukin-2 receptor levels in patients with dermatitis herpetiformis. *J Invest Dermatol* **97**:568, 1991
25. Airola K et al: Urokinase plasminogen activator is expressed in basal keratinocytes before interstitial collagenase, stromelysin-1, and laminin-5 in experimentally induced dermatitis herpetiformis lesions. *J Invest Dermatol* **108**:7, 1997
26. Salmela MT et al: Parallel expression of macrophage metalloelastase (MMP-12) in duodenal and skin lesions of patients with dermatitis herpetiformis. *Gut* **48**:496, 2001
27. Garioch JJ et al: T cell receptor V beta expression is restricted in dermatitis herpetiformis skin. *Acta Derm Venereol (Stockh)* **77**:184, 1997
28. Baker BS et al: Absence of gluten-specific T lymphocytes in the skin of patients with dermatitis herpetiformis. *J Autoimmun* **8**:75, 1995
29. Seah PP, Fry L: Immunoglobulins in the skin in dermatitis herpetiformis and their relevance in diagnosis. *Br J Dermatol* **92**:157, 1975
30. Marks JM: Dogma and dermatitis herpetiformis. *Clin Exp Dermatol* **2**:189, 1978
31. Katz SI et al: Dermatitis herpetiformis: The skin and the gut. *Ann Intern Med* **93**:857, 1980
32. Leonard J et al: Gluten challenge in dermatitis herpetiformis. *New Engl J Med* **308**:816, 1983
33. Reunala T: Gluten-free diet in dermatitis herpetiformis: II. Morphological and immunological findings in the skin and small intestine of 12 patients and matched controls. *Br J Dermatol* **98**:69, 1978
34. Zone JJ et al: Deposition of granular IgA relative to clinical lesions in dermatitis herpetiformis. *Arch Dermatol* **132**:912, 1996
35. Hall RP, Lawley TJ: Characterization of circulating and cutaneous IgA immune complexes in patients with dermatitis herpetiformis. *J Immunol* **135**:1760, 1985
36. Barguthy FS et al: Identification of IgA subclasses in skin of patients with dermatitis herpetiformis. *Int Arch Allergy Appl Immunol* **85**:268, 1988
37. Katz SI et al: Effect of sulfones on complement deposition in dermatitis herpetiformis and on complement-mediated guinea pig reactions. *J Invest Dermatol* **67**:688, 1976
38. Ljunghall K, Tjernlund U: Dermatitis herpetiformis: Effects of gluten-restricted and gluten-free diet on dapsone requirement and on IgA and C3 deposits in uninvolved skin. *Acta Derm Venereol (Stockh)* **63**:129, 1983
39. Dahlbäck K et al: Vitronectin colocalizes with Ig deposits and C9 neoantigen in discoid lupus erythematosus and dermatitis herpetiformis, but not in bullous pemphigoid. *Br J Dermatol* **120**:725, 1989
40. Yaoita H: Identification of IgA binding structures in skin of patients with dermatitis herpetiformis. *J Invest Dermatol* **71**:213, 1978
41. Stingl G et al: Ultrastructural localization of immunoglobulins in dermatitis herpetiformis. *J Invest Dermatol* **67**:507, 1976
42. Karpati S et al: Dermatitis herpetiformis bodies. *Arch Dermatol* **126**:1469, 1990
43. Karpati S et al: Ultrastructural binding sites of endomysial antibodies from sera of patients with dermatitis herpetiformis and coeliac disease. *Gut* **33**:191, 1992
44. Dahlbäck K, Sakai L: IgA immunoreactive deposits colocal with fibrillin immunoreactive fibers in dermatitis herpetiformis. *Acta Derm Venereol (Stockh)* **70**:194, 1990
45. Hällström O: Comparison of IgA-class reticulin and endomysium antibodies in caeliac disease and dermatitis herpetiformis. *Gut* **30**:1225, 1989
46. Zettinig G et al: Dermatitis herpetiformis is associated with atrophic but not with goitrous variant of Hashimoto's thyroiditis. *Eur J Clin Invest* **30**:53, 2000
47. Zone JJ et al: Circulating immune complexes of IgA type in dermatitis herpetiformis. *J Invest Dermatol* **75**:152, 1980
48. Hall RP et al: IgA containing circulating immune complexes in dermatitis herpetiformis, Henoch-Schönlein purpura, systemic lupus erythematosus and other diseases. *Clin Exp Immunol* **40**:431, 1980
49. Chorzelski TP et al: IgA class endomysium antibodies in dermatitis herpetiformis and coeliac disease. *Ann NY Acad Sci* **420**:325, 1983
50. Reunala T et al: Histocompatibility antigens and dermatitis herpetiformis with special reference to jejunal abnormalities and acetylator phenotype. *Br J Dermatol* **94**:139, 1976
51. Keuning JJ et al: HLA-DW3 associated with coeliac disease. *Lancet* **1**:506, 1976
52. Thomsen M et al: Association of Ld-8a and Ld-12a with dermatitis herpetiformis. *Tissue Antigens* **7**:60, 1976
53. Park MS et al: The 90% incidence of HLA antigen (Te24) in dermatitis herpetiformis. *Tissue Antigens* **22**:263, 1983
54. Otley CC et al: DNA sequence analysis and restriction fragment length polymorphism (RFLP) typing of the HLA-DQw2 alleles associated with dermatitis herpetiformis. *J Invest Dermatol* **97**:318, 1991
55. Spurkland A et al: Dermatitis herpetiformis and celiac disease are both primarily associated with the HLA-DQ (α1*0501, β1*02) or the HLA-DQ (α1*03, β1*0302) heterodimers. *Tissue Antigens* **49**:29, 1997
56. Balas A et al: Absolute linkage of celiac disease and dermatitis herpetiformis to HLA DQ. *Tissue Antigens* **50**:52, 1997
57. Hervonen K et al: Concordance of dermatitis herpetiformis and celiac disease in monozygotous twins. *J Invest Dermatol* **115**:990, 2000
58. Hervonen K et al: First-degree relatives are frequently affected in coeliac disease and dermatitis herpetiformis. *Scand J Gastroenterol* **37**:51, 2002
59. Klein GF et al: Junctional blisters in acquired bullous disorders of the dermal-epidermal junction zone: Role of the lamina lucida as the mechanical locus minoris resistentiae. *Br J Dermatol* **109**:499, 1983
60. Smith JB et al: The site of blister formation in dermatitis herpetiformis is within the lamina lucida. *J Am Acad Dermatol* **27**:209, 1992
61. Fry L et al: The small intestine in dermatitis herpetiformis. *J Clin Pathol* **27**:817, 1974
62. O'Donoghue DP et al: Gastric lesion in dermatitis herpetiformis. *Gut* **17**:185, 1976
63. Stockbrugger H et al: Autoimmune atrophic gastritis in patients with dermatitis herpetiformis. *Acta Derm Venereol (Stockh)* **56**:111, 1976
64. Leonard JN et al: Increased incidence of malignancies in dermatitis herpetiformis. *BMJ* **286**:16, 1983
65. Collin P et al: Malignancy and survival in dermatitis herpetiformis: A comparison with coeliac disease. *Gut* **38**:528, 1996
66. Lewis HM et al: Protective effect of gluten-free diet against development of lymphoma in dermatitis herpetiformis. *Br J Dermatol* **135**:363, 1996
67. Fry L: Dermatitis herpetiformis. *Baillieres Clin Gastroenterol* **9**:371, 1995
68. Reunala T, Collin P: Diseases associated with dermatitis herpetiformis. *Br J Dermatol* **136**:315, 1997
69. Price P et al: The genetic basis for the association of the 8.1 ancestral haplotype (A1, B8, DR3) with multiple immunopathological diseases. *Immunol Rev* **167**:257, 1999
70. Griffiths CEM et al: Dermatitis herpetiformis exacerbated by indomethacin. *Br J Dermatol* **112**:443, 1985
71. Zeedijk N et al: Dermatitis herpetiformis: Consequences of elemental diet. *Acta Derm Venereol (Stockh)* **66**:316, 1986
72. Kadunce DP et al: The effect of an elemental diet with and without gluten on disease activity in dermatitis herpetiformis. *J Invest Dermatol* **97**:175, 1991

CHAPTER 68

Robin A.C.
Graham-Brown

Familial Benign Pemphigus (Hailey-Hailey Disease)

Familial benign pemphigus (FBP), or "Hailey-Hailey disease," is a rare blistering disorder, first described by the Hailey brothers in 1939[1] and characterized by recurrent vesicles and erosions, particularly involving flexural areas.

ETIOLOGY

The sexes are equally affected by FBP, which is inherited in an autosomal dominant manner, but because only 70 percent of patients have a clear family history, there must be some variability in gene penetrance.

Lesions are frequently precipitated by friction and infection with various bacteria. Yeasts and viruses also appear to play a role in some patients.

The major underlying pathologic process in FBP is acantholysis and the changes appear in isolated keratinocyte cultures,[2] indicating a fundamental defect in the keratinocytes themselves. Cell adhesion is abnormal,[3–7] the fragility occurring in the adhesion complex.[8–11] The gene responsible for upregulation of P-cadherin has been reported[12] to be located on chromosome 3, the location being 3q21-q24.[13–15] It has been established that the genetic abnormality for FBP lies in *ATP2C1,* which encodes an adenosine triphosphate (ATP)-powered calcium pump.[16,17]

CLINICAL MANIFESTATIONS

Signs first appear from the age of 11 or older, with most patients first experiencing lesions in the third or fourth decade. Most individuals have disease of relatively limited extent,[18] although widespread and severe involvement can occur.[19] The most commonly affected sites are the axillae (Fig. 68-1), groins (Fig. 68-2), intertriginous areas such as the inframammary folds, and the neck; nearly half the patients in the largest series reported to date recalled that their first lesions appeared on the sides of the neck.[18] Lesions may also occur on the trunk and in the antecubital and popliteal fossae. Seborrheic dermatitis-like involvement of the scalp has also been described.[20]

Mucosal surfaces are only rarely involved, but lesions have been reported in the mouth,[21] esophagus,[22] larynx,[23] and the perianal and vulvovaginal areas.[24–26] Genital lesions may resemble warts.[27]

Longitudinal white streaks may appear in the nails.[18,28]

Individual lesions consist primarily of flaccid vesicles and blisters on an erythematous background, but because of friction and secondary infection, it is more common to find eroded plaques in the sites of predilection, with a highly characteristic fissured appearance (Fig. 68-3). Crusting, scaling, and hypertrophic, vegetative changes may also occur. The involved areas tend to extend peripherally before stabilizing, often producing annular or serpiginous shapes. Recurrence is very common.

Most patients remain healthy, but they complain of significant discomfort and some find that the condition severely restricts their work and leisure activities.[18] Many patients are also aware of an unpleasant odor arising from the diseased areas, and notice that external friction by clothing, adhesive bandages, and even electrocardiographic electrodes may induce lesions. Sunlight has been reported either to improve or exacerbate FBP, while deterioration has been noted either with stress or premenstrually.[18] Occasionally a severe exacerbation with a generalized systemic disturbance and varicelliform vesicular pustules may be associated with widespread infection with herpes simplex virus.[29]

PATHOLOGY

Light microscopy reveals suprabasal cleavage, acantholysis, and intercellular edema (Fig. 68-4). The appearance has been likened to

FIGURE 68-1

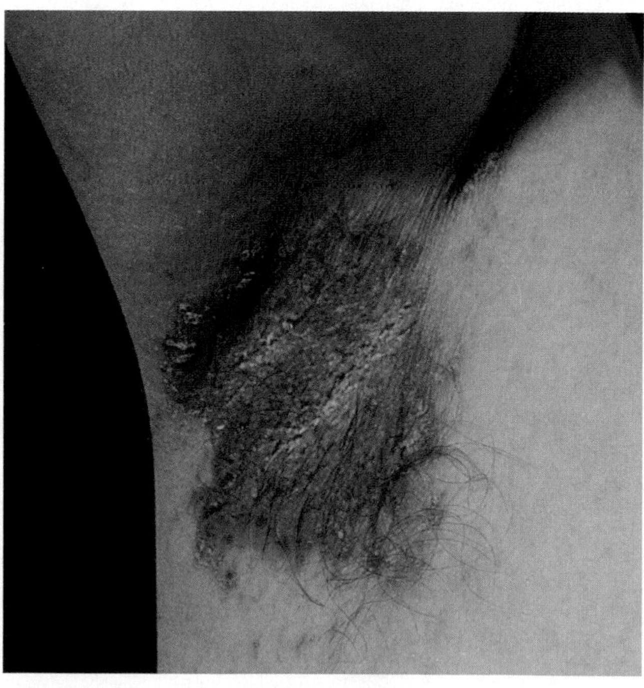

Familial benign pemphigus. Sites of predilection are the intertriginous areas, especially the axillae.

FIGURE 68-2

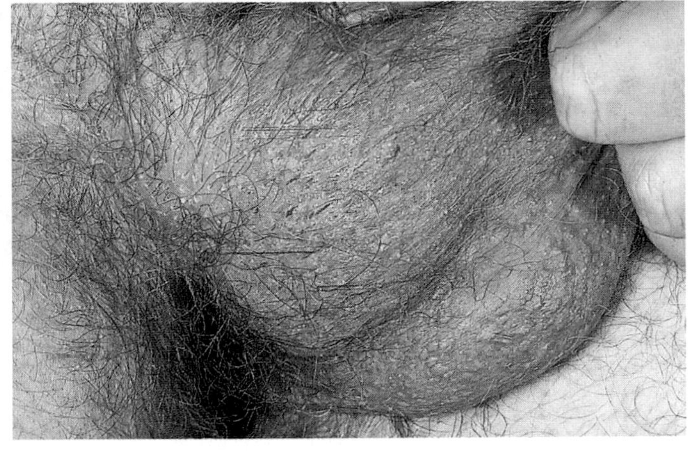

A site commonly involved is the groin as illustrated here. Erosions on an erythematous base give rise to the highly characteristic, tiny, fissured lesions on scrotum.

that of a "dilapidated brick wall";[30] it is often indistinguishable from pemphigus vulgaris. Occasionally, however, a few dyskeratotic cells, similar to the corps ronds of Darier's disease, are seen in the granular layer. Both direct and indirect immunofluorescence for intercellular antibodies is negative. The electron microscopic changes are consistent with a defect of desmosomal adhesion: there is separation of tonofilaments from desmosomes and a reduction of visible desmosomes on the cell surfaces; electron-dense material is seen around the nucleus.[3,4]

FIGURE 68-3

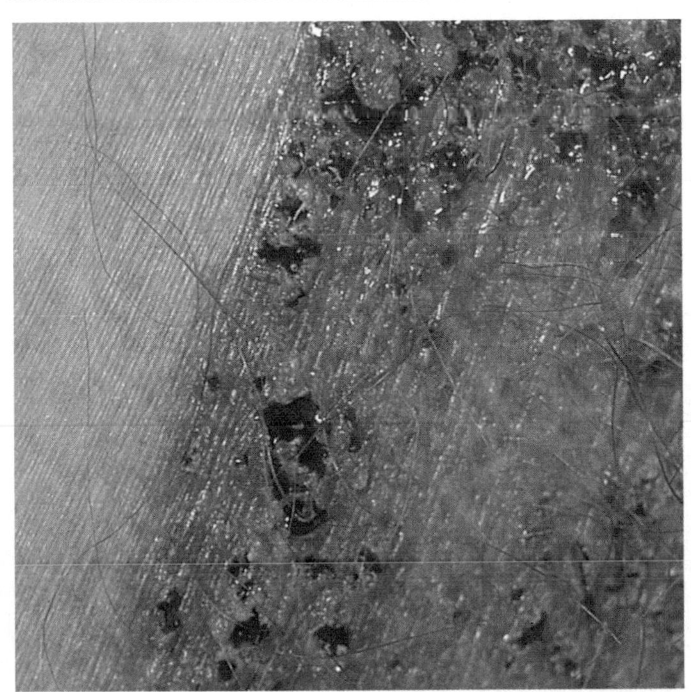

Familial benign pemphigus. Erosions are present on an erythematous base in the axilla of this patient.

FIGURE 68-4

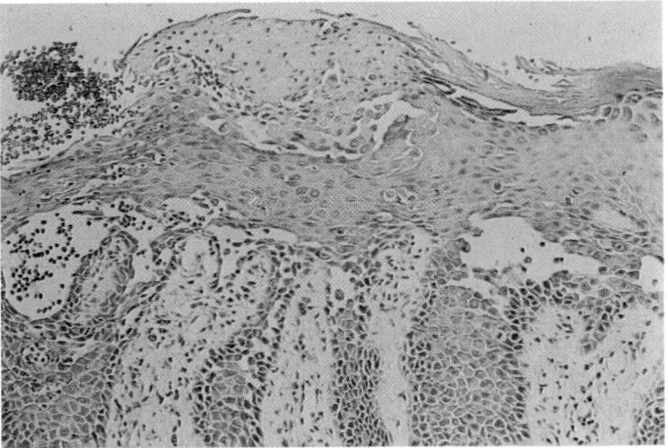

A.

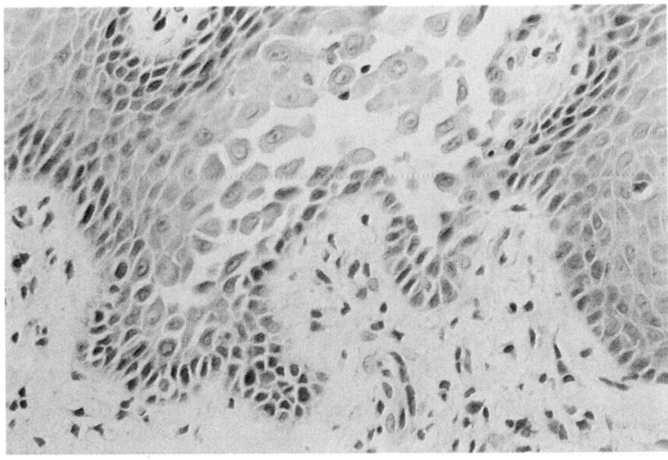

B.

Familial benign pemphigus. Suprabasal bulla formation with acantholysis is seen. *A.* The resulting partial adherence of the epidermal keratinocytes has been likened to a "dilapidated brick wall." *B.* Few dyskeratotic cells are seen in the lower power view.

DIFFERENTIAL DIAGNOSIS

The diagnosis of FBP is often delayed with genital and perianal lesions particularly leading to diagnostic confusion with other disorders. FBP must be distinguished clinically from chronic bacterial or fungal infections and intertrigo. Because anti-infective agents may improve FBP, the diagnosis can be made only on biopsy. Pemphigus vulgaris or vegetans can be confused with FBP both clinically and histologically, but these disorders generally affect wider areas, including the mouth. Immunofluorescence will provide further differentiation. Histologically, Darier's disease and the transient acantholytic dermatosis of Grover can produce similar appearances. Lesions of Darier's disease, however, generally show less-marked acantholysis, while evidence of dyskeratosis, in the form of grains and corps ronds, is much more striking. Clinical distinction is generally straightforward, with Darier's disease typically producing warty papules in the "seborrheic" areas. Darier's disease and FBP have, however, been described in the same individual.[31] As a consequence, it was suggested that there may be genetic overlap between the two disorders, but this is not the case,[32] although both diseases are associated with mutations in calcium pump protein. Grover's disease also shows more limited cleavage and acantholysis but greater dyskeratosis than FBP.

TREATMENT

Simple anti-infective agents, administered either topically or systemically, reduce the severity of exacerbations and remain the mainstay of treatment. Topically, tetracyclines, fusidic acid, and imidazoles are all useful, while systemically, tetracyclines seem to work better than most. It may be best to combine anti-infective therapy with topical glucocorticoids, as 86 percent of patients in Burge's series found them helpful, especially if started immediately at the onset of discomfort.[18] Generally, moderate to potent agents are required, although some patients find weaker glucocorticoids useful. A few patients seem to benefit from short courses of systemic glucocorticoids to control major exacerbations, but this may result in a rebound of the disease when the drugs are withdrawn.[19]

Responses have also been described with a number of other therapeutic modalities. Superficial (Grenz) rays have been reported to induce remission in several patients,[20] but very few centers now have the equipment needed. Dapsone and topical and systemic cyclosporine have been reported to be successful in a few patients.[33–36] Methotrexate[37] and retinoids[18] have also been used to treat resistant disease. Gonadotrophin-releasing hormone analogue therapy followed by oophorectomy virtually abolished FBP in a patient with marked premenstrual flares.[38] If secondary infection with herpes simplex is suspected, appropriate antiviral therapy should be instituted.

Finally, there may be a place for surgical approaches to disease of limited extent. Surgical excision and grafting have been advocated,[39] although there may be recurrences, especially around the edges of the treated areas or upon further friction or trauma. Patients have also been treated with dermabrasion[40] and carbon dioxide laser vaporization.[41]

COURSE

The usual pattern of disease activity is of frequent exacerbations with temporary periods of quiescence. In some patients, lesions appear almost continuously. Some, however, report prolonged remissions; in general, the condition becomes less troublesome with age.

REFERENCES

1. Hailey H, Hailey H: Familial benign chronic pemphigus. *Arch Dermatol Syphilol* **39**:679, 1939
2. Regnier LM et al: Histological defects of chronic benign familial pemphigus expressed in tissue culture. *Arch Dermatol Res* **281**:538, 1990
3. Wilgram GF et al: An electron microscopic study of acantholysis and dyskeratosis in Hailey and Hailey's disease. *J Invest Dermatol* **39**:373, 1962
4. Gottlieb SK, Lutzner MA: Hailey-Hailey disease: An electron microscopic study. *J Invest Dermatol* **54**:368, 1970
5. Ishibashi Y et al: The nature and pathogenesis of dyskeratosis in Hailey-Hailey's disease and Darier's disease. *J Dermatol* **11**:335, 1984
6. Setoyama M et al: Desmoplakin I and II in acantholytic dermatoses: Preservation in pemphigus vulgaris and pemphigus erythematosus and dissolution in Hailey-Hailey's disease and Darier's disease. *J Dermatol Sci* **2**:9, 1991
7. Burge SM, Garrod DR: An immunohistochemical study of desmosomes in Darier's disease and Hailey-Hailey disease. *Br J Dermatol* **124**:242, 1991
8. Hashimoto K et al: Junctional proteins of keratinocytes in Grover's disease, Hailey-Hailey's disease and Darier's disease. *J Dermatol* **22**:159, 1995
9. Metze D et al: Involvement of the adherens junction-actin filament system in acantholytic dyskeratosis of Hailey-Hailey disease. A histological, ultrastructural, and histochemical study of lesional and non-lesional skin. *J Cutan Pathol* **23**:211, 1996
10. Cooley JF et al: Hailey-Hailey disease keratinocytes: Normal assembly of cell-cell junctions in vitro. *J Invest Dermatol* **107**:877, 1996
11. Burge SM, Schomberg KH: Adhesion molecules and related proteins in Darier's disease and Hailey-Hailey disease. *Br J Dermatol* **127**:335, 1992
12. Hakuno M et al: Upregulation of P-cadherin expression in the lesional skin of pemphigus, Hailey-Hailey disease and Darier's disease. *J Cutan Pathol* **28**:277, 2001
13. Ikeda S et al: Localization of the gene whose mutations underlie Hailey-Hailey disease to chromosome 3q. *Hum Mol Genet* **3**:1147, 1994
14. Peluso AM et al: Narrowing of the Hailey-Hailey disease gene region on chromosome 3q and identification of one kindred with a deletion in this region. *Genomics* **30**:77, 1995
15. Richard G et al: Hailey-Hailey disease maps to a 5 cM interval on chromosome 3q21-q24. *J Invest Dermatol* **105**:357, 1995
16. Hu Z et al: Mutations in ATP2C1, encoding a calcium pump, cause Hailey-Hailey disease. *Nat Genet* **24**:61, 2000
17. Subra KR et al: Hailey-Hailey disease is caused by mutations in ATP2C1 encoding a novel Ca(2+) pump. *Hum Mol Genet* **9**:1131, 2001
18. Burge SM: Hailey-Hailey disease: The clinical features, response to treatment and prognosis. *Br J Dermatol* **126**:275, 1992
19. Marsch WC, Stütgen G: Generalized Hailey-Hailey disease. *Br J Dermatol* **99**:553, 1978
20. Marren P, Burge SM: Seborrhoeic dermatitis of the scalp: A manifestation of Hailey-Hailey disease in a predisposed individual? *Br J Dermatol* **126**:294, 1992
21. Botvinick I: Familial benign chronic pemphigus with oral mucous membrane lesions. *Cutis* **12**:371, 1973
22. Kahn D, Hutchnison E: Esophageal involvement in familial benign chronic pemphigus. *Arch Dermatol* **109**:718, 1974
23. Schneider W et al: Zur Frage der schleimhautbeteiligung beim pemphigus benignus familiaris chronicus. *Arch Klin Exp Dermatol* **225**:74, 1966
24. Wilkin JK: Chronic benign familial pemphigus: Minimal involvement mimicking chronic perianal candidiasis. *Arch Dermatol* **114**:136, 1978
25. Vaclavinkova Y, Neumann E: Vaginal involvement in familial chronic benign pemphigus (morbus Hailey-Hailey). *Acta Derm Venereol Suppl (Stockh)* **62**:80, 1982
26. Evron S et al: Familial benign chronic pemphigus appearing as leukoplakia of the vulva. *Int J Dermatol* **23**:556, 1984
27. Langenberg A et al: Genital benign chronic pemphigus (Hailey-Hailey disease) presenting as condylomas. *J Am Acad Dermatol* **26**:951, 1992
28. Kirtshig G et al: Leukonychia longitudinalis als ein Leitsymptom des Morbus Hailey-Hailey. *Hautarzt* **43**:451, 1992
29. Flint ID et al: Eczema herpeticum in association with familial benign chronic pemphigus. *J Am Acad Dermatol* **28**:257, 1993
30. Haber H, Russell B: Sisters with familial benign chronic pemphigus (Gougerot, Hailey and Hailey). *Br J Dermatol Syph* **62**:458, 1950
31. Ganor S, Sagher F: Keratosis follicularis (Darier) and familial benign chronic pemphigus (Hailey-Hailey) in the same patient. *Br J Dermatol* **77**:24, 1965
32. Welsh EA et al: Hailey-Hailey disease is not allelic to Darier's disease. *J Invest Dermatol* **102**:992, 1994
33. Sire DJ, Johnson BL: Benign familial chronic pemphigus treated with dapsone. *Arch Dermatol* **103**:262, 1971
34. Jitsukawa K et al: Topical cyclosporine in chronic benign familial pemphigus (Hailey-Hailey disease). *J Am Acad Dermatol* **27**:625, 1992
35. Ormerod AD et al: Benign familial pemphigus responsive to cyclosporin: A possible role for cellular immunity in pathogenesis. *Br J Dermatol* **124**:299, 1991
36. Berth-Jones J et al: Benign familial chronic pemphigus (Hailey-Hailey disease) responds to cyclosporin. *Clin Exp Dermatol* **20**:70, 1995
37. Fairris GM et al: Methotrexate for intractable benign familial chronic pemphigus. *Br J Dermatol* **115**:640, 1986
38. James MP, Williams RM: Benign familial pemphigus-premenstrual exacerbation suppressed by goserelin and oophorectomy. *Clin Exp Dermatol* **20**:54, 1995
39. Shelley WB, Randall P: Surgical eradication of familial benign chronic pemphigus from the axillae. *Arch Dermatol* **100**:275, 1969
40. Zachariae H: Dermabrasion of Hailey-Hailey disease. *J Am Acad Dermatol* **27**:136, 1992
41. Don PC et al: Carbon dioxide laser abrasion: A new approach to management of familial benign chronic pemphigus (Hailey-Hailey disease). *J Dermatol Surg Oncol* **13**:1187, 1987

CHAPTER 69

Herbert Hönigsmann
Franz Trautinger
Klaus Wolff

Subcorneal Pustular Dermatosis (Sneddon-Wilkinson Disease)

Subcorneal pustular dermatosis (SPD) is a rare, chronic, recurrent, pustular eruption characterized histopathologically by subcorneal pustules that contain abundant neutrophils. The condition was originally described in 1956 by Sneddon and Wilkinson,[1] who separated SPD from other previously unclassified pustular eruptions. Up to 1966, when the first comprehensive review appeared, more than 130 cases had been reported, but not all fulfilled the clinical and histopathologic criteria required for this diagnosis.[2] A considerable number of additional cases have since appeared in the literature, and a subtype clinically resembling SPD with intraepidermal IgA deposits has been recognized[3] (SPD-type IgA pemphigus).

INCIDENCE

There is no racial predilection. Most of the reported cases have been in whites, but the disease has also been observed in Africans, Japanese, and Chinese. The condition is more common in women and in persons older than 40 years of age, but SPD may occur at any age.[2] A pustular eruption that is clinically and histologically similar to the human disease, which also responds to dapsone treatment, has been observed in dogs.[4]

ETIOLOGY

The cause of SPD is unknown. Cultures of the pustules consistently fail to reveal bacterial growth. The role of trigger mechanisms such as preceding or concomitant infections, though repeatedly discussed, has remained speculative. Immunologic mechanisms have been implicated in the pathogenesis, and in a subset of patients, whose disease clinically resembled SPD, intraepidermal IgA deposits have been detected. Some of these patients also had circulating IgA antibodies against the same sites within the epidermis. Desmocollin I has been described to be the target of these antibodies.[3,5] Although the pathogenetic role of IgA in intraepidermal pustule formation remains elusive, these findings led to the concept of a separate disease clinically and histopathologically similar to SPD with intraepidermal IgA deposits. This condition has been designated subcorneal pustular dermatosis type IgA pemphigus and is clinically indistinguishable from classical SPD.[6]

The occasional association of SPD with certain other diseases may represent more than a mere coincidence. Increased serum IgA has been detected in a number of patients, and the disease has been reported to occur in cases of IgA-paraproteinemia and IgA multiple myeloma.[7–10] In addition, SPD is associated with pyoderma gangrenosum,[11,12] ulcerative colitis,[13] and Crohn's disease.[14] On the other hand, pyoderma gangrenosum is not uncommon in patients with inflammatory bowel disease, paraproteinemia, and myeloma. Whether or not the coexistence of these conditions reflects common pathogenetic mechanisms remains to be clarified, but an additional common denominator linking these disorders is their response to sulfone and sulfonamide therapy.

Further associations reported to date include IgG paraproteinemia,[15,16] CD30+ anaplastic large-cell lymphoma,[17] non–small-cell lung cancer,[18] apudoma,[19] rheumatoid arthritis,[20,21] hyperthyroidism,[22] and mycoplasma pneumoniae infection.[23]

CLINICAL FEATURES

The primary lesions are small, discrete, flaccid pustules or vesicles that rapidly turn pustular and usually arise in crops within a few hours on clinically normal or slightly erythematous skin. In dependent regions, pus characteristically accumulates in the lower half of the pustule; as the pustules usually have the tendency to coalesce, they often, but not always, form annular, circinate, or bizarre serpiginous patterns. After a few days the pustules rupture and dry up to form thin, superficial scales and crusts, closely resembling impetigo. Peripheral spreading and central healing leave polycyclic, erythematous areas in which new pustules arise as others disappear (Fig. 69-1). There is no atrophy or scarring, but an occasional brownish hyperpigmentation may mark previously affected sites. Variable intervals of quiescence, lasting from a few days to several weeks, may be followed by the sudden development of new lesions. The eruptions tend to occur symmetrically, affecting mainly the axillae, groins, abdomen, submammary areas, and the flexor aspects of the limbs. In rare cases, the face,[24] palms, and soles[2,25] may be involved. Scalp and mucous membranes invariably remain free of lesions. Episodic itching and burning represent subjective symptoms in a small number of patients, but there are no systemic symptoms or abnormalities in routine laboratory parameters.

HISTOPATHOLOGY

The hallmark of the disease is a strictly subcorneal pustule filled with polymorphonuclear leukocytes,[1] with only an occasional eosinophil.[2] Acantholysis is not involved in pustule formation, but a few acantholytic cells may be found in older lesions (secondary acantholysis). Surprisingly, the epidermal layers underlying the pustule exhibit little pathology, and, apart from a variable number of migrating leukocytes, there is little evidence of spongiosis or cytolytic damage to the epidermal cells. The dermis contains a perivascular infiltrate composed of neutrophils and rarely mononuclear cells and eosinophils (Fig. 69-2).

In a subset of patients, direct immunofluorescence reveals intraepidermal IgA deposits.[15] In these cases, IgA is usually present in a pemphigus-like intercellular pattern, either in the entire epidermis or

FIGURE 69-1

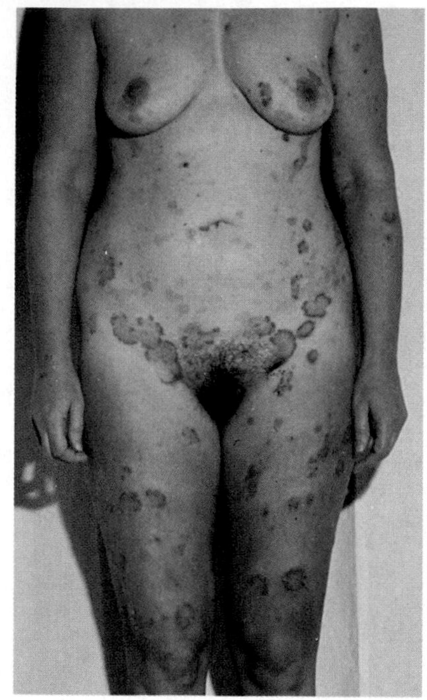

A.

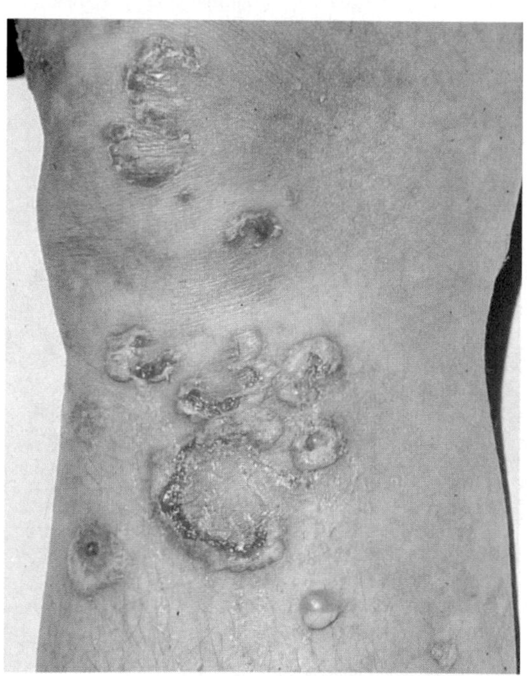

B.

Subcorneal pustular dermatosis. *A.* Typical distribution. Note accentuated involvement of groins and abdomen. Hyperpigmented macules mark previously affected areas. *B.* Close-up showing coalescence of pustules, which form annular and circinate patterns. Lesions of different developmental stages are seen side by side. At the lower right, newly formed pustule with characteristic hypopyon formation.

confined to its upper layers. By indirect immunofluorescence, circulating IgA antibodies directed against the intercellular substance of the epidermis were detected in single cases.

FIGURE 69-2

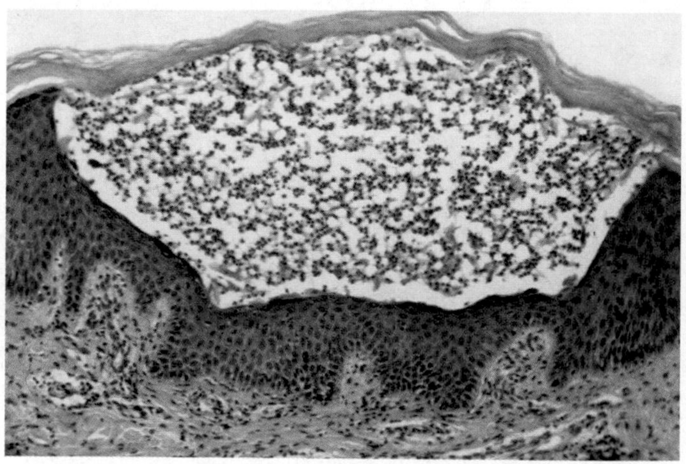

Subcorneal pustular dermatosis. Strictly subcorneal pustule filled with polymorphonuclear leukocytes, the underlying epidermal layers exhibiting only slight edema and some migrating leukocytes. There is a mild inflammatory infiltrate around dermal blood vessels (33×).

Ultrastructural examination of paralesional skin has shown cytolysis of keratinocytes confined to the granular layer;[26] the formation of pustules has been regarded as a secondary event caused by invasion and subcorneal accumulation of leukocytes.

DIAGNOSIS AND DIFFERENTIAL DIAGNOSIS

SPD must be differentiated from impetigo contagiosa, dermatitis herpetiformis, pemphigus foliaceus, glucagonoma syndrome, and acute generalized pustulosis. An early localized eruption of SPD may be clinically and histologically indistinguishable from impetigo, but the distribution pattern of the lesions, the absence of bacteria in the pustules, the ineffectiveness of topical and systemic antibiotic therapy, and the course of the disease lead to the correct diagnosis. Dermatitis herpetiformis is a papulovesicular eruption with subepidermal vesicle formation; it is highly pruritic, affecting primarily the extensor surfaces. In a high percentage of the patients, there are changes in the jejunal mucosa, a phenomenon not as yet observed in SPD. The typical pattern of IgA deposits in the dermal papillae as revealed by direct immunofluorescence, which is diagnostic for dermatitis herpetiformis, is not found in SPD.

Occasionally, lesions of pemphigus foliaceus may be misdiagnosed on clinical examination and, if acantholysis is not very prominent, can be mistaken for SPD histologically. However, SPD either fails to exhibit the immunofluorescence pattern typical for pemphigus or presents with intraepidermal IgA deposits (SPD type IgA pemphigus, see above). Generalized pustular psoriasis (von Zumbusch type) may sometimes present differential diagnostic difficulties. Systemic symptoms (fever, malaise, leukocytosis), the presence of spongiform pustules within the epidermis, and the failure of pustular psoriasis to respond to sulfones represent reliable criteria to distinguish it from SPD. The necrolytic migratory eruption of glucagonoma syndrome can be differentiated by its distribution, lack of actual pustule formation, erosions of the lips and oral mucosa, and, histologically, necrobiosis of the upper epidermis. Biochemically, excess levels of glucagon are diagnostic. Acute generalized pustulosis is a widespread pustular eruption, with predilection of the distal parts of the extremities, that histologically exhibits leukocytoclastic vasculitis. Juvenile bullous pemphigoid and erythema multiforme should not give rise to confusion.

TREATMENT

The drugs of choice are the sulfones, such as dapsone in a dose of 50 to 150 mg daily. The response is slower and less dramatic than in dermatitis herpetiformis, but complete remission is most often obtained. In some patients, the treatment may be withdrawn after several months, although in others it may have to be continued for years; the minimal effective dose to suppress disease should be determined in these patients. Sulfapyridine (1.0 to 3.0 g daily) is also beneficial; systemic corticosteroids are less effective, although they can suppress generalized flares when given in large doses. Obviously, the long-term use of potentially dangerous drugs in the treatment of a benign disease should be carefully considered. Retinoids, PUVA, and UVB have been reported to induce remissions, but this awaits confirmation.[27–30] Responses to colchicine, cyclosporine, and topical tacalcitol (1α-$24R$–dihydroxyvitamin D_3) have been anecdotally reported, and a combination of antitumor necrosis factor α antibody followed by retinoids reportedly results in remission.[31]

COURSE AND PROGNOSIS

SPD is a benign condition. Without treatment, attacks recur over many years and remissions are variable, lasting from a few days to several weeks. Despite the protracted course and the occasional involvement of large areas of the skin, the general health of the patient is not impaired. However, one of our own cases who had SPD, pyoderma gangrenosum, and IgA paraproteinemia of more than 20 years' duration died of septicemia with staphylococcal abscesses in the lungs, liver, and spleen.

REFERENCES

1. Sneddon IB, Wilkinson DS: Subcorneal pustular dermatosis. *Br J Dermatol* **68**:385, 1956
2. Wolff K: A contribution to the nosology of subcorneal pustular dermatosis (Sneddon-Wilkinson) [in German]. *Arch Klin Exp Dermatol* **224**:248, 1966
3. Robinson ND et al: The new pemphigus variants. *J Am Acad Dermatol* **40**:649, 1999
4. Kalaher KM, Scott DW: Subcorneal pustular dermatosis in dogs and in human beings: Comparative aspects. *J Am Acad Dermatol* **22**:1023, 1990
5. Hashimoto T et al: Human desmocollin 1 (Dsc1) is an autoantigen for the subcorneal pustular dermatosis type of IgA pemphigus. *J Invest Dermatol* **109**:127, 1997
6. Reed J, Wilkinson J: Subcorneal pustular dermatosis. *Clin Dermatol* **18**:301, 2000
7. Lautenschlager S et al: Subcorneal pustular dermatosis at the injection site of recombinant human granulocyte-macrophage colony-stimulating factor in a patient with IgA myeloma. *J Am Acad Dermatol* **30**:787, 1994
8. Takata M et al: Subcorneal pustular dermatosis associated with IgA myeloma and intraepidermal IgA deposits. *Dermatology* **189**:111, 1994
9. Vaccaro M et al: Subcorneal pustular dermatosis and IgA lambda myeloma: An uncommon association but probably not coincidental. *Eur J Dermatol* **9**:644, 1999
10. Stone MS, Lyckholm LJ: Pyoderma gangrenosum and subcorneal pustular dermatosis: Clues to underlying immunoglobulin A myeloma. *Am J Med* **100**:663, 1996
11. Scerri L et al: Pyoderma gangrenosum and subcorneal pustular dermatosis, without monoclonal gammopathy. *Br J Dermatol* **130**:398, 1994
12. Kohl PK et al: Pyoderma gangrenosum followed by subcorneal pustular dermatosis in a patient with IgA paraproteinemia. *J Am Acad Dermatol* **24**:325, 1991
13. Miyakawa K et al: Vesiculopustular dermatosis with ulcerative colitis. Concomitant occurence of circulating IgA anti-intercellular and anti-basement membrane zone antibodies. *Eur J Dermatol* **5**:122, 1995
14. Delaporte E et al: Subcorneal pustular dermatosis in a patient with Crohn's disease. *Acta Derm Venereol* **72**:301, 1992
15. Lutz ME et al: Subcorneal pustular dermatosis: A clinical study of ten patients. *Cutis* **61**:203, 1998
16. Yamamoto T et al: A variant of subcorneal pustular dermatosis with monoclonal IgG gammopathy of undetermined significance. *Eur J Dermatol* **5**:640, 1995
17. Guggisberg D, Hohl D: Intraepidermal IgA pustulosis preceding a CD30+ anaplastic large T-cell lymphoma. *Dermatology* **191**:352, 1995
18. Buchet S et al: Pustulose sous-cornee associee a un carcinome epidermoide du poumon. *Ann Dermatol Venereol* **118**:125, 1991
19. Villey MC et al: Apudoma and subcorneal pustular dermatosis (Sneddon-Wilkinson disease). *Dermatology* **185**:269, 1992
20. Roger H et al: Subcorneal pustular dermatosis associated with rheumatoid arthritis and raised IgA: Simultaneous remission of skin and joint involvements with dapsone treatment. *Ann Rheum Dis* **49**:190, 1990
21. Butt A, Burge SM: Sneddon-Wilkinson disease in association with rheumatoid arthritis. *Br J Dermatol* **132**:313, 1995
22. Taniguchi S et al: Subcorneal pustular dermatosis in a patient with hyperthyroidism. *Dermatology* **190**:64, 1995
23. Winnock T et al: Vesiculopustular eruption associated with Mycoplasma pneumoniae pneumopathy. *Dermatology* **192**:73, 1996
24. Lotery HE et al: Subcorneal pustular dermatosis involving the face. *J Eur Acad Dermatol Venereol* **12**:230, 1999
25. Haber H, Wells GC: Subcorneal pustular dermatosis of the soles. *Br J Dermatol* **71**:253, 1959
26. Metz J, Schröpl F: Ultrastructural investigations of subcorneal pustular dermatosis [in German]. *Arch Klin Exp Dermatol* **236**:190, 1970
27. Bauwens M et al: Subcorneal pustular dermatosis treated with PUVA therapy. A case report and review of the literature. *Dermatology* **198**:203, 1999
28. Marliere V et al: Successful treatment of subcorneal pustular dermatosis (Sneddon-Wilkinson disease) by acitretin: Report of a case. *Dermatology* **199**:153, 1999
29. Cameron H, Dawe RS: Subcorneal pustular dermatosis (Sneddon-Wilkinson disease) treated with narrowband (TL-01) UVB phototherapy. *Br J Dermatol* **137**:150, 1997
30. Orton DI, George SA: Subcorneal pustular dermatosis responsive to narrowband (TL-01) UVB phototherapy. *Br J Dermatol* **137**:149, 1997
31. Voigtländer C et al: Infliximab (antitumor herpes factor α antibody). A novel, highly effective treatment of recalcitrant subcorneal pustular dermatosis (Sneddon-Wilkinson disease). *Arch Dermatol* **137**:1521, 2001

CHAPTER 70

Enno Christophers
Ulrich Mrowietz

Pustular Eruptions of Palms and Soles

Pustular eruptions of the palms and soles include pustulosis palmaris et plantaris (PPP; synonym: pustular psoriasis of the Barber type), acrodermatitis continua (Hallopeau's disease), and infantile acropustulosis (Table 70-1). The entities present with chronic and persistent eruptions of sterile, purulent vesicles. The sites of predilection are the thickened skin of the palms and soles, and the unifying histologic feature in all of these conditions is the presence of sterile pustules within the epidermis.

PUSTULOSIS PALMARIS ET PLANTARIS

PPP is a chronic recurrent pustular dermatosis localized on the palms and soles only. Histologically, it is characterized by intraepidermal vesicles filled with neutrophils.

For historical reasons this condition has been given different designations. The terms pustulosis palmaris et plantaris, persistent palmoplantar pustulosis, and pustular psoriasis of the extremities have been used synonymously. Controversy has arisen as to whether the so-called pustular bacterid of Andrews should be considered as a distinct entity.[1] In 1935, Andrews and Machacek described 15 patients with recurrent purulent vesicles on the hands and feet that clinically and histologically resembled the condition previously described as pustular psoriasis of hands and feet by Barber.[2] The presence of foci of bacterial infection, mainly of the teeth and tonsils, together with the absence of signs of overt psoriasis, prompted the authors to question the psoriatic nature of these changes. The term pustular bacterid was chosen for the condition because a close association with bacterial infections was assumed. Because clinically and histologically these conditions cannot be distinguished with certainty and evidence for the pathogenic role of bacteria is scarce, we use the term pustulosis palmaris et plantaris for this condition.

Epidemiology

The disease has a worldwide distribution. It is a rare condition, but the exact incidence is not known. At the Department of Dermatology in Stockholm, 272 patients were seen during a 10-year period.[3]

Females show a higher incidence than males, with a ratio of approximately 3:1. Onset of the disease occurs mostly between the ages of 20 and 60; rarely, the condition occurs after the sixth decade of life, and in 10 percent of the patients the onset is before the age of 20 years.[2] In a group of 272 patients with PPP, a positive family history of psoriasis was recorded in 25 percent of the patients.[3] Other studies have shown psoriasis to be associated with palmoplantar pustules in less than 10 percent of patients.[4] HLA typing of patients with PPP reveals no increased frequency of any of the known psoriasis-linked alloantigens.[4] In a Japanese survey, PPP was found in 4.7 percent of patients with spondyloarthropathies.[5]

Etiology

The cause of PPP is not known. In some patients, the association with psoriasis elsewhere on the body is striking, but others may show palmoplantar pustules in the absence of other cutaneous changes. The association of PPP with Sweet's syndrome[6] suggests that PPP is a response pattern in genetically predisposed patients to neutrophil activation.[7]

An imbalance of the protease/antiprotease system in the skin consisting of decreased antileukoprotease (elafin/SKALP) activity in pustular psoriasis has been discussed as a possible mechanism of pustule formation.[8] Exacerbation of PPP has been observed after patch testing with metals and was accompanied by elevated leukotriene by levels in plasma and pustules.[9]

In a long-term survey from Japan, the incidence of PPP was found to be positively correlated to heavy smoking (>20 cigarettes per day), tonsillitis, and seasonal factors such as high humidity and high temperature.[10] A normal proliferative response of peripheral blood mononuclear cells to a streptococcal preparation in PPP patients has

TABLE 70-1

Pustular Eruptions of Palms and Soles

	Sterile Pustules on Palms and Soles	Age	Cutaneous Atrophy	Associated Disease	Histology
Pustulosis palmaris et plantaris (PPP)	Yes	Adults	Absent	Psoriasis, SAPHO* syndrome	Spongiform pustule, neutrophils
Acrodermatitis continua (Hallopeau)	Yes	Adults	Present	Pustular psoriasis, von Zumbusch type	Spongiform pustule, neutrophils
Infantile acropustulosis	Yes	Infants	Absent	Absent	Subcorneal pustule, neutrophils, some eosinophils

*Synovitis, acne, pustulosis, hyperostosis, and osteitis.

been described as a distinct feature from the reduced responses observed in patients with psoriasis vulgaris.[11]

Clinical Features

The primary lesions are pustules of nearly equal size measuring 2 to 4 mm in diameter. Crops of pustules usually arise within a few hours on the normal-appearing palmar and plantar skin (Fig. 70-1). Single lesions then become surrounded by an erythematous ring. Rarely, the

pustules extend to the dorsa of the fingers, the feet, or over the volar wrists (Fig. 70-1*C*). Episodes of new pustular eruptions occur at varying intervals and remain strictly confined to the sites of predilection.

As pustules become older, their yellow color changes to dark brown, so that in untreated PPP, the lesions show various shades of color (Fig. 70-1*C* and *D*). Dried pustules are shed within approximately 8 to 10 days.

FIGURE 70-1

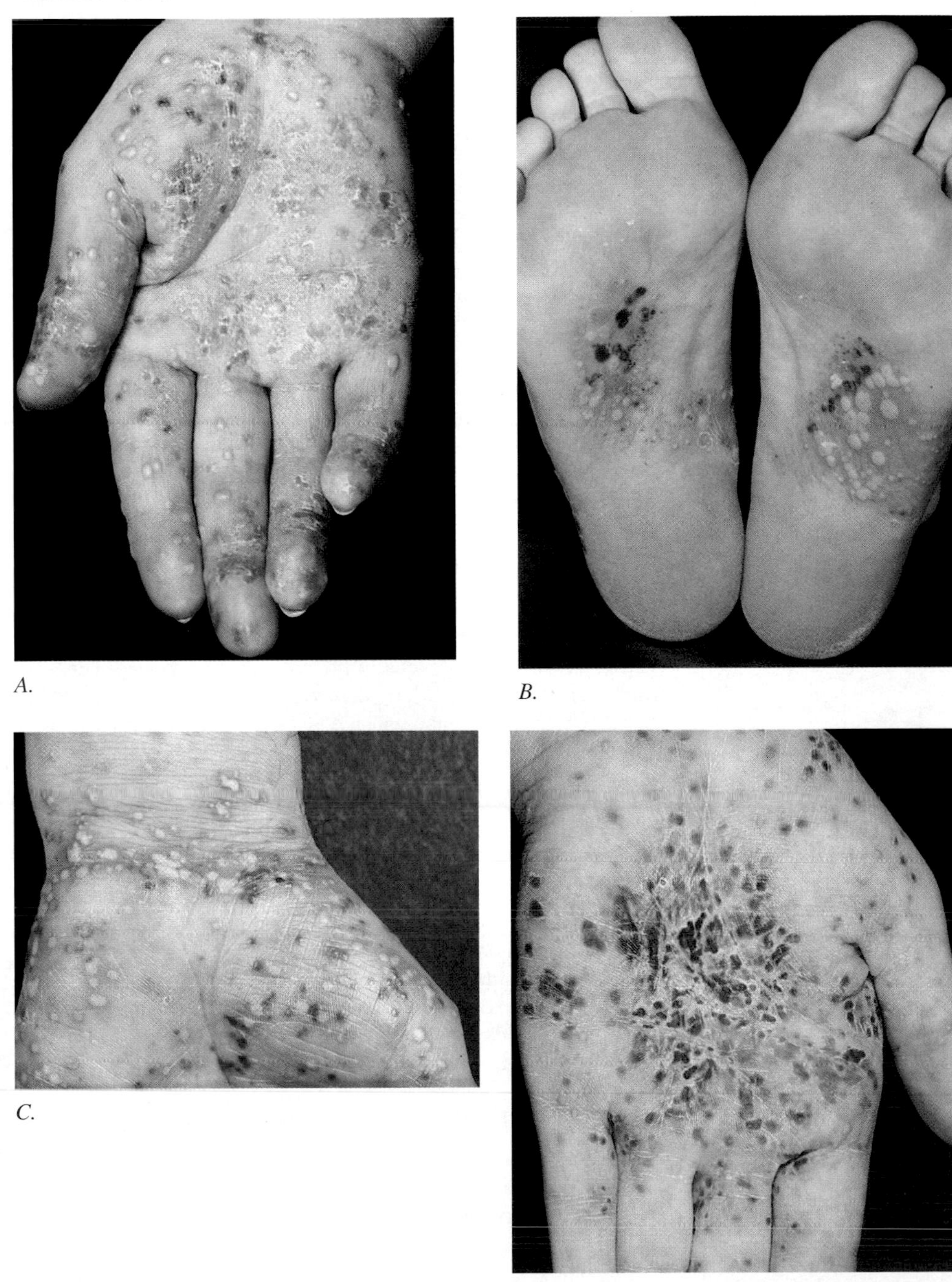

A. *B.* *C.* *D.*

Pustulosis palmaris et plantaris. *A* and *B*. Groups of pustules measuring 1 to 3 mm in diameter occur on erythematous skin on palms and soles. Both feet and both hands are normally affected symmetrically. *C* and *D*. Lesions may occasionally spread beyond the predilection sites and pustules may appear on the wrists. Within several days after pustule formation, lesions dry, flatten, and acquire a brownish color. This may be followed by eczematous changes with scaling and fissuring.

There are no symptoms other than some itching or a burning sensation, which may precede new crops of lesions. While the eruptions occasionally occur unilaterally, most patients show symmetric involvement, and hands and soles are usually equally affected.[2]

As remission begins, fewer pustules are produced, but the skin may remain erythematous and hyperkeratotic, resembling eczema. Remissions last for weeks or months until pustulation again occurs.

PPP is frequently noted in patients with chronic recurrent multifocal osteomyelitis as well as with noninfectious inflammatory bone lesions. An association of PPP and osteoarthritis of the anterior chest wall was first described in Japan.[12] As reported by Swedish authors, involvement of the manubriosternal joint is present in 6 percent and of the sternoclavicular joints in 10 percent of patients.[13] Scintigraphic investigations showed sternocostoclavicular joint involvement to be present in 16 of 73 patients.[14] For this condition, the term *SAPHO syndrome* (synovitis, acne, pustulosis, hyperostosis, osteitis) has been established.[15] Clinical manifestations of SAPHO syndrome are similar whether they occur in relation to severe acne (mostly acne conglobata) or PPP (see also Chap. 98). The primary lesion consists of a sterile abscess containing neutrophils. The site of predilection is the anterior chest wall. SAPHO syndrome can be associated with pseudoinfectious arthritis. Involvement of the sacroiliac joints may be present.[16]

Histopathology

Histologically there is an intraepidermal cavity filled with polymorphonuclear leukocytes associated with spongiform changes within the surrounding epidermis (Fig. 70-2). Compacted collections of neutrophils may be seen within the stratum corneum, and a variably dense mononuclear infiltrate with some neutrophils is found around the dilated vessels of the upper dermis.

Sequential histologic studies of the various stages of pustule formation reveal that spongiosis of the epidermis due to the invasion of mononuclear cells is the first step in pustule formation.

Laboratory Findings

The lesions of PPP are sterile; a moderately increased white blood cell count may occasionally be observed, but all other laboratory tests are normal.

FIGURE 70-2

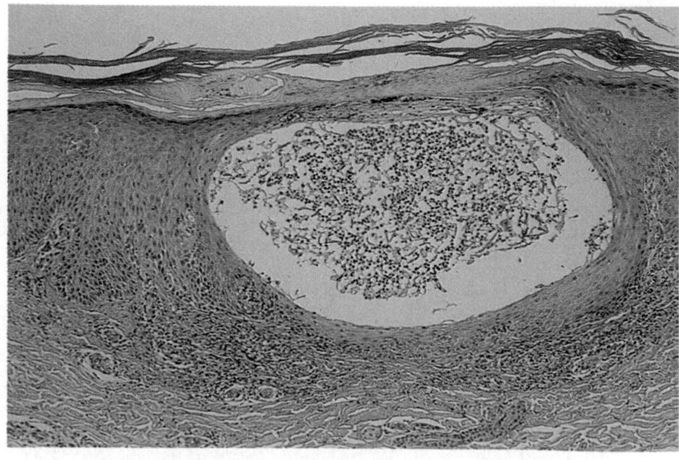

Histologically, there are spongiform pustules and a moderate lymphohistiocytic infiltrate.

Diagnosis and Differential Diagnosis

PPP is a distinct entity. The course of the disease, together with the characteristic morphology and the occasional association with psoriasis elsewhere on the body, permit the proper diagnosis. The disease must be differentiated from "dyshidrotic" eczematous dermatitis (pompholyx), especially when pustules due to secondary infection are present (see Chap. 125). In this condition, the onset is also acute, but clear vesicles of various sizes are scattered on the palms, soles, and volar and interdigital aspects of the fingers. These may coalesce and secondarily become pustular because of secondary bacterial infection; in such cases, the signs of inflammation will become more prominent. Tinea of the palms and soles only rarely shows the presence of pustules of equal size and symmetry. Similarly, pustules developing in infected scabies lack the features mentioned previously. Bacterial cultures or demonstration of hyphae or mites will clearly separate these entities from PPP. Biopsies will further demonstrate spongiform pustule formation as a distinctive sign.

Treatment

Pustular palmoplantar psoriasis is difficult to treat and attempts to clear the affected sites rapidly by conventional measures are usually not very rewarding.

When erythema and hyperkeratosis are prominent, potent or superpotent topical steroids under occlusion will provide relief. Treatment with either topical or systemic psoralen plus ultraviolet irradiation (PUVA) usually leads to clearing and may produce long-lasting remissions. Antipsoriatic remedies such as dithranol or ultraviolet radiation have been used with variable success.

Methotrexate (15 to 25 mg per week) may be given for severe forms; this procedure will reduce pustulation as long as methotrexate is given and for a short time thereafter.

Therapeutic success has been obtained with etretinate.[17] At a daily dose of 25 to 50 mg orally, this drug effectively prevents the formation of new pustules and rapidly clears the skin. Relapses will occur when patients are taken off the drug. Acitretin, which has now replaced etretinate in most countries, is equally effective. The recommended dose is 1 mg/kg per day initially. After improvement is seen, the dose is tapered down to 0.5 mg/kg per day, which is given for several weeks to months. Because of their teratogenic potential, systemic retinoids should be given to women of childbearing age only with great caution, if at all.

Systemic steroids are of questionable value. Withdrawal is usually followed by a rebound. Therefore, the use of systemic steroids in PPP is not recommended.

Low-dose cyclosporine is an effective regimen to treat recalcitrant PPP. Treatment may be short-term (<3 months), followed by topical therapy after major improvement is achieved, or long-term, with continuous treatment in severe cases.[18,19]

Colchicine, known as a potent inhibitor of leukocyte motility, has also been reported to be effective clinically in suppressing pustulation.[20]

Combination and Sequential Treatment

In difficult-to-treat dermatoses, such as PPP, the combination of different regimens is superior to monotherapy. Established combinations for PPP include potent or superpotent steroids together with bath or cream PUVA.

In some patients, topical vitamin D_3 or analogues such as calcipotriol/calcipotriene are effective in maintaining improvement achieved with topical steroids before. Tazarotene may also be tried after steroid pretreatment.

Systemic therapy should always be combined with topicals to speed-up time of improvement and to reduce dosage of the systemic treatment.

Prognosis

The disease tends to pursue a chronic course with remissions lasting up to a few months. In one series, most cases showed remissions lasting for 5 to 10 years.

ACRODERMATITIS CONTINUA

Acrodermatitis continua is a rare, sterile, pustular eruption of the fingers or toes that slowly extends proximally. Continuous pustulation may cause nail destruction and atrophy of the distal phalanx. Synonyms are pustular acrodermatitis, acrodermatitis continua suppurativa Hallopeau, dermatitis perstans, and dermatitis repens Crocker.

In 1888, Crocker[21] described a relapsing bullous and pustular eruption on hands and feet; this was further delineated by Hallopeau.[22] Dermatitis continua is now classified as a form of acropustular psoriasis.

Clinical Features

The disease most often begins at the tips of one or two fingers (Fig. 70-3), less often on the toes. The nail folds are affected very early, and trauma is thought to play an initiating role. The first signs consist of small pustules, which, on bursting, leave an erythematous, shiny area in which new pustules develop. These then tend to coalesce, forming polycyclic lakes of pus. As the disease extends proximally the affected area shows either glossy erythema or a crusted, keratotic, and fissured surface with newly formed pustules underneath (see Fig. 70-3). Pustulation of the nail bed and the nail matrix almost always occurs and quite often leads to loss of the nail plate or severe onychodystrophy (see Fig. 70-3). Acrodermatitis continua of long duration may show complete destruction of the nail organ and thus lead to anonychia. The skin becomes shiny and severely atrophic, and there is atrophic thinning of the distal part of the phalanx.

The disease may remain confined to the original site, sometimes up to several years, but more often it spreads proximally to cover the hand, dorsum of forearm, or foot. In such instances more than one extremity is involved.

As in pustular psoriasis, lesions may occur elsewhere on the body. Especially during long courses of acrodermatitis continua, pustulation may extend to involve the entire body skin, being indistinguishable from the von Zumbusch type of pustular psoriasis. In such cases, systemic reactions with fever, leukocytosis, a high sedimentation rate, and malaise occur (see also Chap. 42).

Histopathology

The main histopathologic feature of acrodermatitis continua is a subcorneal cavity filled with polymorphonuclear neutrophils. Epidermal cell necrosis and spongiosis do not occur, but the roof and shoulder zones adjacent to the pustule show aggregated leukocytes between the epidermal cells, forming spongiform pustules of Kogoj. There is a moderate lymphohistiocytic infiltrate in the upper dermis, together with focal edema.

Lesions of long duration show severe atrophy of the papillary dermis and thinning of the epidermis.

Laboratory Findings

Systemic abnormalities are absent, and laboratory tests are usually noncontributory. The pustules are sterile. In advanced cases, x-ray films may reveal atrophy of the distal phalanx and arthropathy of the interphalangeal joints.

FIGURE 70-3

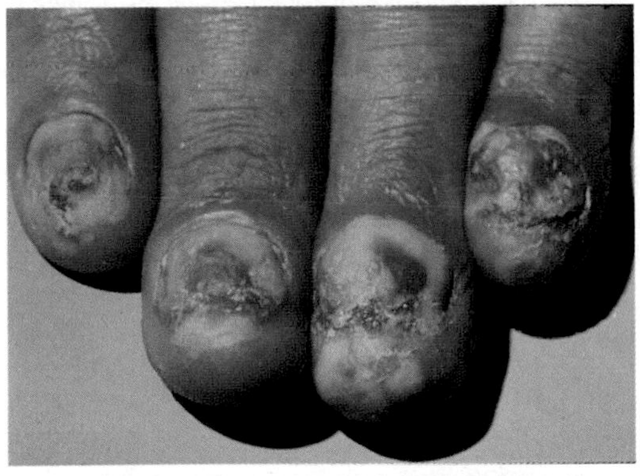

A.

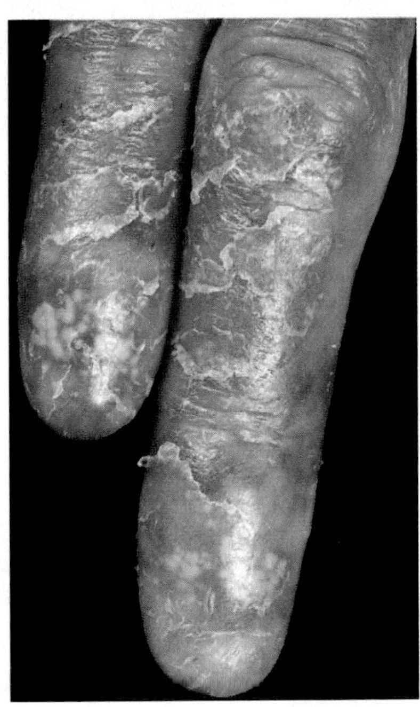

B.

A. Acrodermatitis continua demonstrating acral pustule formation and subungual lakes of pus with destruction of the nail plate. *B.* Repeated eruptions lead to nail loss and severe atrophy. Note pustulation within the atrophic epidermis of the distal phalanges.

Diagnosis and Differential Diagnosis

Acrodermatitis continua at an early stage must be differentiated from acute paronychia caused by bacteria or fungi. Cultures and smears will help rule out infectious causes. The distal localization and the tendency of the pustules to become confluent, forming denuded, erythematous, or crusted lesions, distinguishes acrodermatitis continua from PPP or pustular dyshidrotic eczema. Atrophy and loss of nails do not occur in these conditions. Contact dermatitis with secondary infection and pustulation has less clearly defined margins, runs a different clinical course, and lacks the persistence typical for acrodermatitis continua.

Treatment

As in pustular psoriasis, no specific drug brings about lasting remissions. Potent or superpotent topical steroids, preferentially under occlusion, are useful in blocking pustulation. Caution is advised in cases already showing atrophy. PUVA suppresses the eruption of new pustules and can be employed for long periods as maintenance treatment (see Chap. 266).

Treatment with a combination of systemic acitretin and local calcipotriol/calcipotriene was successful in one patient in a left/right comparison.[23] In recalcitrant patients, dapsone may be tried.[24]

In principle, regimens used for treatment of PPP may also be used for therapy of acrodermatitis continua. The therapeutic result lasts as long as the drugs are given, and relapses occur after withdrawal.

Course and Prognosis

Acrodermatitis continua shows a chronic course with a tendency of the lesions to spread proximally. Spontaneous improvement is rare, and episodes of acute pustulation occur without apparent cause. The development of pustules at other sites, or even the eruption of generalized pustular psoriasis, supports the idea that acrodermatitis continua is a variant of psoriasis.

INFANTILE ACROPUSTULOSIS

This entity is discussed in Chap. 143.

REFERENCES

1. Andrews GC, Machacek GF: Pustular bacterids of the hands and feet. *Arch Dermatol Syphilol* **32**:837, 1935
2. Barber HW: Acrodermatitis continua vel perstans (dermatitis repens) and psoriasis pustulosa. *Br J Dermatol* **42**:500, 1930
3. Hellgren L, Mobaken H: Pustulosis palmaris et plantaris. *Acta Derm Venereol Suppl (Stockh)* **51**:284, 1971
4. Ward JM, Barnes RMR: HLA antigens in persistent palmoplantar pustulosis and its relationship to psoriasis. *Br J Dermatol* **99**:477, 1978
5. Hukuda S et al: Spondyloarthropathies in Japan: Nationwide questionnaire survey performed by the Japan Ankylosing Spondylitis Society. *J Rheumatol* **28**:554, 2001
6. Gambichler T et al: Sweet's syndrome with eruptions of pustulosis palmaris. *J Eur Acad Dermatol Venereol* **14**:327, 2000
7. Van de Kerkhof PCM: Pustulosis palmaris et plantaris. *J Eur Acad Dermatol Venereol* **14**:248, 2000
8. Kuijpers ALA et al: Skin-derived antileukoprotease (SKALP) is decreased in pustular forms of psoriasis: A clue to the pathogenesis of pustule formation? *Arch Dermatol Res* **288**:641, 1996
9. Nakamura K et al: Exacerbation of pustulosis palmaris et plantaris after topical application of metals accompanied by elevated levels of leukotriene B_4 in pustules. *J Am Acad Dermatol* **42**:1021, 2000
10. Akiyama T et al: The relationships of onset and exacerbation of pustulosis palmaris et plantaris to smoking and focal infections. *J Dermatol* **22**:930, 1995
11. Takahashhi K et al: Normal proliferative responses of peripheral blood mononuclear cells to streptococcal preparation OK-432 in patients with pustulosis palmaris et plantaris constitute a distinct feature from the reduced responses observed in those with psoriasis vulgaris, pustular psoriasis and acrodermatitis continua of Hallopeau. *J Dermatol* Sci **25**:87, 2001
12. Sasaki T: A case with osteomyelitis of the bilateral clavicles associated with pustulosis palmaris et plantaris. *Rinsho Sei Keigara* **2**:333, 1967
13. Bergdahl K et al: Pustulosis palmoplantaris and its relation to chronic recurrent multifocal osteomyelitis. *Dermatologica* **159**:37, 1979
14. Hradil E et al: Skeletal involvement in pustulosis palmo-plantaris with special reference to the sternocostoclavicular joints. *Acta Derm Venereol Suppl (Stockh)* **68**:65, 1988
15. Benhamou CL et al: Synovitis-acne-pustulosis-hyperostosis-osteomyelitis syndrome (SAPHO): A new syndrome among the spondyloarthropathies? *Clin Exp Rheumatol* **6**:109, 1988
16. Kahn MF, Chamot AM: SAPHO syndrome. *Rheum Dis Clin North Am* **18**:225, 1992
17. Reymann F: Two years' experience with Tegison treatment of pustulosis palmo-plantaris and eczema keratoticum manuum. *Dermatologica* **164**:209, 1982
18. Meinardi MMHM et al: Oral cyclosporin A is effective in clearing persistent pustulosis palmaris et plantaris. *Acta Derm Venereol Suppl (Stockh)* **70**:77, 1990
19. Erkko P et al: Double-blind placebo-controlled study of long-term low-dose cyclosporin in the treatment of palmoplantar pustulosis. *Br J Dermatol* **139**:997, 1998
20. Takigawa M et al: Treatment of pustulosis palmaris et plantaris with oral doses of colchicine. *Arch Dermatol* **118**:458, 1982
21. Crocker HR: *Diseases of the Skin*. London: HK Lewis; 1888
22. Hallopeau H: Sur une asphyxie locale des extrémités avec polydactylite suppurative chronique et pussées éphéméres des dermatite pustuleuse disséminées et symmétriques. *Ann Dermatol Syphiligr (Paris)* **1**:420, 1890
23. Kuijpers AL et al: Acrodermatitis continua of Hallopeau: Response to combined treatment with acitretin and calcipotriol ointment. *Dermatology* **192**:357, 1996
24. Nikkels AF et al: Breaking the relentless course of Hallopeau's acrodermatitis by dapsone. *Eur J Dermatol* **9**:126, 1999

SECTION 10

DISORDERS OF EPIDERMAL APPENDAGES AND RELATED DISORDERS

CHAPTER 71

Elise A. Olsen

Hair

As with abnormalities of other organ systems, hair disorders can represent either a primary or secondary dysfunction and can be related to exogenous or endogenous causes. Hair is unique when compared to other organ systems, however, in that it undergoes repetitive planned obsolescence and rebirth, laying open the possibility of clinical disorders based on cycling abnormalities. Further difficulties arise when the type and/or amount of hair in a given body area deviates from the expected norm. The end result of any of these abnormalities, either hair loss or overgrowth, often leads to major psychological problems for patients.

This section on hair abnormalities reviews the primary causes of hair loss and hair overgrowth and defines the significant pathophysiologic and clinical features and therapeutic options of each.

HAIR CYCLE (See also Chap. 12)

Knowledge of the hair cycle is vital to understanding hair problems. The duration and rate of growth of the anagen (growth) phase normally vary at different body sites, in different individuals, and at various ages, and determine the ultimate length of hair in that area.[1] Catagen is the transitional portion of the cycle between anagen and telogen and is short-lived (2 to 4 weeks) in duration. Telogen duration also varies greatly in different body sites, but interindividual variability appears more limited. In a normal scalp, telogen is assumed to last 3 to 4 months and anagen to last 3-plus years. With age, there is both a diminution in anagen duration and an increase in the time interval between two anagen cycles.[2] At any given time, ~90 percent of the scalp hair is in anagen and 10 percent in telogen; this is subject to some seasonal variability.[3]

At the end of anagen, each hair bulb moves from its location in the subcutaneous tissue or dermis (depth of location is determined by whether the follicle is terminal or vellus) to a more superficial location by means of shrinkage and remolding of that portion of the follicle below the "bulge" where the arrector pili muscle inserts. The concentric layers of the inner root sheath, which anchor the hair shaft in the follicle, are only present to the bottom of the isthmus of the follicle, the region to which the hair bulb ascends in telogen (Fig. 71-1). Consequently, the hair shaft in telogen is no longer anchored securely in the tissue, as it was in anagen, and it may be dislodged with the gentle traction of shampooing, combing, brushing, etc. The recapitulation of the anagen follicle and initiation of growth of a new anagen hair leads to the shedding of any remaining telogen hair in the follicular canal (see Fig. 12-5).

FIGURE 71-1

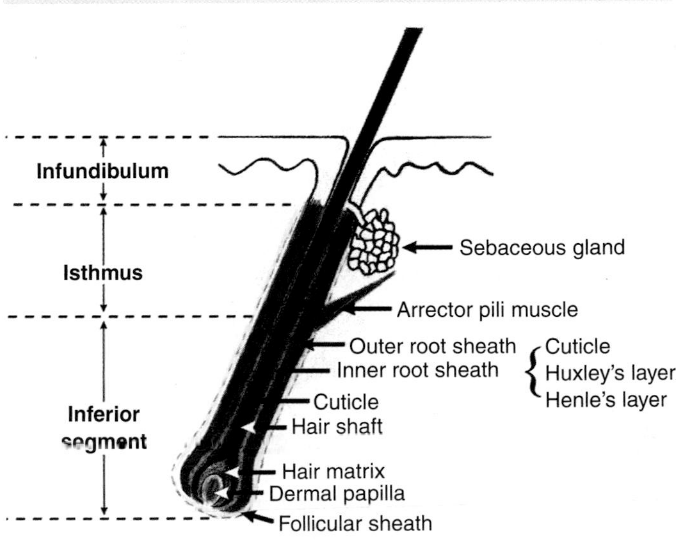

Diagram of a normal anagen hair follicle.

DIAGNOSTIC TECHNIQUES

Techniques to Assess Cycling Abnormalities

There are several tools for determining aberrations of scalp hair cycling. The first is the *hair pull,* which should be done on every patient with a complaint of hair loss. This simple technique involves manually grasping a group of 50 to 100 scalp hairs and applying gentle traction from the base to the terminal ends and repeating this in various areas of the scalp.[4] Normally, in the author's experience, only three to five hairs *total* are dislodged on six to eight such hair pulls *if* the hair has been shampooed regularly: shedding of more than three to five hairs *per* hair pull is pathologic. This is a subjective test and results normally will vary slightly in any given patient depending upon the physician performing the test, each of whom may exert different degrees of traction on different sizes of hair clumps. In the case of increased shedding, the proximal ends of the hairs so obtained should be evaluated microscopically to determine whether there is an intact hair shaft and bulb, indicating either an effluvium (Latin, "a flowing out") or hair breakage. The hair bulbs should be further evaluated to determine whether they are normal telogen (indicating a physiologic aberration) versus dystrophic telogen or anagen hairs (indicating a pathologic process).

There is little reason to do a *hair pluck* today. This momentarily painful technique involves applying a clamp or needle holder to the base of 50 to 100 hairs and quickly pulling the hairs out en masse. Although this technique, which is used in a *trichogram,* allows one to determine an anagen/telogen ratio by inspection of the proximal hair bulbs, it fails to give critical information about the type of hair being shed.

A third means of determining specifics regarding the hair cycle is the *phototrichogram.*[5] In this technique, hairs are clipped very short or shaved in a given target area and comparative photographs are taken of the target area at baseline and again 2 to 3 days later. As only the anagen hairs will have increased their length on subsequent follow-up (normal hair growth is ~ 1 cm/month), this technique can be used to determine (1) the percentage of hairs in anagen based on the number of longer hairs compared to total hairs and (2) with sophisticated cameras and computer software, the hair growth rate. To be reliable, a phototrichogram requires locating the same precise target site at each time point, standardized photography, and standardized hair counting by image analysis. A related procedure, called a *hair window,* involves clipping or shaving the hairs in a given area and having the patient return anywhere from 3 to 30 days later to evaluate regrowth. Without photography, this is a gross technique for assessing the potential for regrowth in a given area, and does not yield reliable information regarding the specifics of cycling in the target area.

Biopsy

A biopsy of the scalp may or may not help with the diagnosis of a particular hair disorder. The information it delivers about cycling aberrations is merely confirmatory to that obtained by other simpler, less expensive means, and the diagnosis of hair shaft abnormalities cannot be made by a scalp biopsy. The real value of a scalp biopsy is the insight it can offer into mechanisms of alopecia. A 4-mm punch biopsy is preferred to a 3-mm one because of the ease of laboratory preparation and accumulated quantifying data on normal scalp in the larger specimen. The biopsy should be taken in the direction of the follicle growth and to a sufficient depth to contain the follicular bulbs in anagen (generally into the subcutaneous tissue). Vertical sectioning of the biopsy specimen gives an immediate overview of the anatomy of the tissue from the epidermis down to the fat, but unless multiple step sections are taken, the view is limited to a snapshot of a few follicles. Horizontal (or transverse) sectioning of the specimen gives a simultaneous overview of many follicles.[6] This latter technique requires sectioning at several different levels of the skin because the terminal portion of the hair follicles will be at different depths depending on the type (terminal versus vellus) of hair and part of the cycle (anagen versus telogen) they are in, and because the pathology may lie anywhere along the length of the follicle. Once appropriate sectioning is done, however, all the follicles in a given horizontally sectioned biopsy can be viewed simultaneously, giving a much greater amount of information than is available from a similar number of vertical sections.

Hair Shaft Evaluation

The preferred hairs to examine in patients with a complaint of shedding are those gently pulled from the scalp. This avoids the two major problems of a hair pluck: physical distortion of the hair shaft by a clamp and the distortion of all anagen hair bulbs so obtained. The proximal portions of the collected hairs should be lined up on a slide in a drop of cyanoacrylic glue, a coverslip applied, and the hairs viewed under light microscopy. Telogen hairs have a cornified rounded-up bulb without an attached root sheath (Fig. 71-2*A*). Anagen hairs are recognized clinically by their pigmented, somewhat distorted, malleable bulb.

FIGURE 71-2

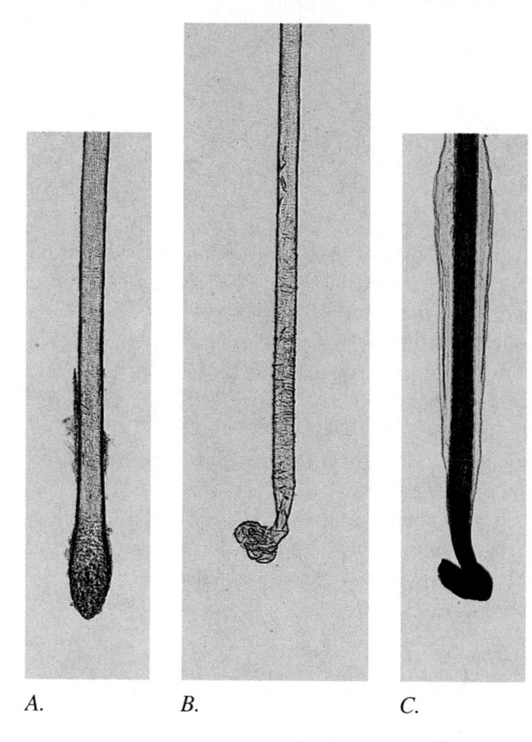

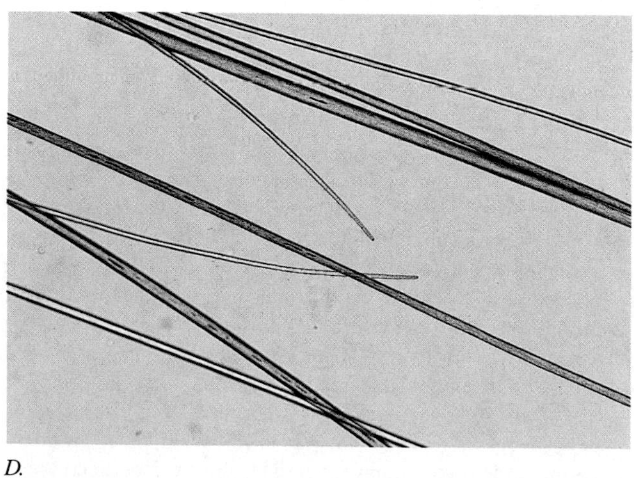

A. Normal telogen hair obtained by hair pull. *B.* Loose anagen hair obtained by hair pull; note the ruffled cuticle. *C.* Proximal end of normal anagen hair obtained by hair pluck. *D.* Distal ends of newly regrowing anagen hairs; note the tapered tips and comparative diameter with established anagen hairs.

Anagen hairs should not normally be found in a hair *pull* except in very young children—in this case, anagen hairs with an attached ruffled cuticle, so-called *loose anagen hairs* (Fig. 71-2*B*), may be found in small numbers, probably secondary to poor hair shaft anchoring to the root sheath.[7] Comparison with a normal anagen hair obtained by hair *pluck* is shown in Fig. 71-2*C*.

In those in whom the hair appears to be breaking off, "not growing," or unruly, the distal portion of the hair shaft should be evaluated. If a fungal infection is suspected, potassium hydroxide (KOH) instead of glue should be placed on the slide and the proximal hair examined for spores and hyphae. The proximal hairs may need to be plucked from the scalp in this case. In other situations, where a hair shaft disorder is suspected, a gentle hair pull should be used to obtain hairs, but if no hairs are forthcoming, then hairs should be cut, not plucked, for evaluation. A newly growing anagen hair will have a tapered distal tip (Fig. 71-2*D*) rather than the blunt distal end of hairs that have been cut or trimmed or in which the ends are intrinsically broken. Most hair shaft abnormalities can be diagnosed by light microscopic examination, although some types will require further examination by scanning electron microscopy to confirm findings only suggested by light microscopy (e.g., longitudinal grooving). Polariscopic examination should be performed if trichoschisis (a particular pattern of hair breakage) is seen under light microscopy in order to evaluate potential trichothiodystrophy (sulfur-deficient hair).

The etiology of brittle hair can be further pursued by direct amino acid analysis of whole-hair hydrolysates and electrophoretic characterization of the main classes of proteins in hair (generally defined by their cysteine content and designated ultrahigh-, high-, and low-cysteine or ultrahigh, high-, and low-sulfur proteins).

ALOPECIA

To begin a discussion of hair loss or aberrant hair growth, it is useful to have a means of organizing, rather than merely cataloguing the myriad causes of alopecia. Deciding whether the hair loss is diffuse (global) or focal (patchy or localized) can facilitate differentiation of the types of alopecia. The following pathophysiologic categories can aid in further defining the diffuse hair loss: (1) failure to produce or continue to produce a normal hair *follicle;* (2) aberrations in the production of a normal hair *shaft;* (3) aberration of the normal hair cycle; and (4) destruction of the hair follicle. Determining whether the hair loss is a destructive or a nondestructive process (clinically suggested by observing whether follicular openings are preserved in areas of hair loss) can further narrow the differential diagnosis. An approach that uses the aforementioned diagnostic tools to aid in assignment of the hair loss process to one of these categories is given in Table 71-1.

Diffuse (Global) Hair Loss

FAILURE OF FOLLICLE PRODUCTION There has been a recent explosion of knowledge, largely fueled by null mutant rodent models, regarding the genetic causes of diffuse alopecia presenting in infancy and childhood. The most notable finding is the abnormality of the human homologue of the mouse hairless (*hr*) gene, which causes *congenital universal atrichia* and *atrichia with papular lesions*.[8–10] The atrichia may be present from birth or develop over the first year of life: this is concordant with an abnormality in recapitulation of the anagen follicle after the first pelage as seen in hairless knockout mice. The patients with atrichia with papular lesions develop follicular cysts, generally 3 to 18 years after the alopecia (Fig. 71-3). The hairless gene product is a putative multifunctional transcription factor and the gene locus is on chromosome 8p12. A similar clinical phenotype with universal hair loss during the first year of life and cutaneous cysts years later but

TABLE 71-1

Differential Diagnosis of Hair Loss

- Diffuse (global) hair loss
  - Nonscarring
    - Failure of follicle production
      - Congenital universal atrichia
      - Atrichia with papular lesions
      - Hereditary vitamin D-resistant rickets
    - Hair shaft abnormality
      - Hair breakage
      - Unruly hair
    - Abnormality of cycling (shedding)
      - Telogen effluvium
      - Anagen effluvium
      - Loose anagen syndrome
      - Alopecia areata
- Focal hair loss
  - Nonscarring
    - Production decline
      - Triangular alopecia
      - Pattern hair loss
    - Hair breakage
      - Trichotillomania
      - Traction alopecia
      - Tinea capitis
      - Primary or acquired hair shaft abnormality
    - Unruly hair
      - Hair shaft abnormality
    - Abnormality of cycling
      - Alopecia areata
      - Syphilis
    - Scarring hair loss

FIGURE 71-3

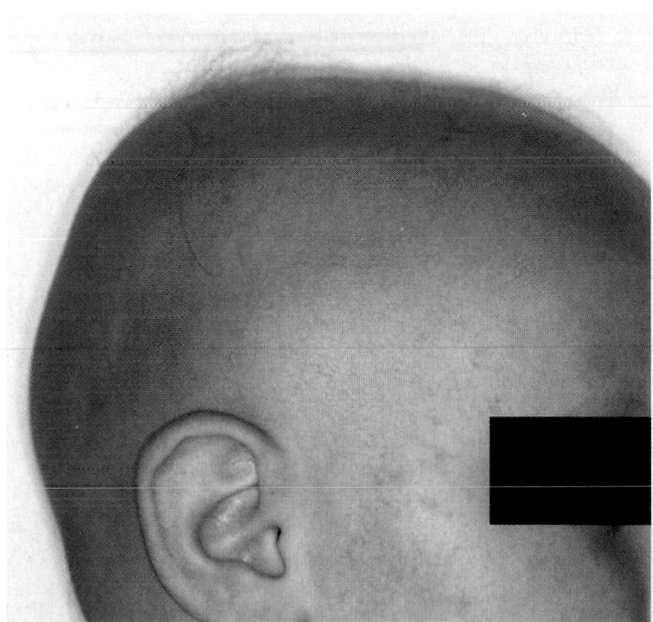

Atrichia with papular lesions. (Photograph courtesy of Abraham Zlotogorski, MD.)

accompanied by rachitic bones is seen in *hereditary vitamin D-resistant rickets*.[11] This condition is secondary to mutations in the vitamin D receptor, probably in the zinc finger domain, which, like the *hr* gene, acts as a transcription factor. Patients previously diagnosed with alopecia universalis (alopecia areata) at birth or few months of age may, in fact, have one of the conditions noted above, particularly if the universal hair loss is persistent and/or familial.

HAIR SHAFT ABNORMALITIES Diffuse hair loss in infancy is more commonly one of hypotrichosis than total atrichia and may be secondary to abnormal production of a subset of hair follicles and/or hair shafts. Most of the hereditary alopecias do not occur alone but in the company of a constellation of other anomalies, most frequently bone, central nervous system, or eye. Freire-Maia has suggested a classification system for those hereditary disorders of ectodermally derived tissue that demonstrate a primary abnormality of two of the following: hair, teeth, nails, or eccrine glands: these are termed *type A ectodermal dysplasias*.[12] An abnormality of one of these four major anomalies plus one other "ectodermal" sign is termed *type B ectodermal dysplasia*. Those ectodermal dysplasias that involve hair have been further catalogued in the available detail by Olsen using the classification system of type A ectodermal dysplasias.[13] Most reported syndromes that involve hair are also discussed and regularly updated, including genetic information, in McKusick's *Mendelian Inheritance in Man*.[14] These three sources facilitate the diagnosis of hereditary childhood alopecias.

Hair shaft abnormalities can be primary and hereditary or secondary to external factors. Some hair shaft abnormalities represent common endpoints to various forms of trauma or inherent shaft weaknesses, and some are specific to a particular constellation of findings or inherent make-up of the hair shaft. Hair shaft abnormalities can be divided into those associated with hair breakage and those associated with unruly hair.

Hair shaft abnormalities associated with hair breakage

TRICHORRHEXIS NODOSA The most common defect of the hair shaft leading to hair breakage is *trichorrhexis nodosa*.[15] Mechanical or chemical damage triggers this response, which can occur in normal hair, but occurs much more readily in inherently weak hair. Microscopically, the affected hair develops a breach in the cuticle, with eventual separation and fraying of the exposed cortical fibers leading to a nodal swelling.[16] The fibers then fracture and the shaft breaks with the resultant appearance of a splayed paintbrush or fanlike array (Fig. 71-4). Trichorrhexis nodosa may be congenital or acquired.

Congenital trichorrhexis nodosa may be present at birth or may appear within the first few months of life. Although it might occur as an isolated defect or, rarely, with follicular hyperkeratosis or teeth/nail defects,[15] the occurrence of congenital trichorrhexis nodosa should lead to a search for an underlying metabolic disorder. Patients with *argininosuccinic aciduria*, primarily those with the late-onset form (occurring at >2 years of age),[15] have associated hair defects. In this condition, in which absence of the enzyme argininosuccinase leads to an accumulation of the nitrogenous waste precursor argininosuccinic acid, brittle lusterless hair develops along with psychomotor retardation and ataxia. The diagnosis is established by finding acidosis, hyperammonemia, and low serum arginine.[17] Citrulline (the normal precursor of argininosuccinic acid in the urea cycle) accumulates in the condition *citrullinemia*, which is caused by a defect in the enzyme argininosuccinic acid synthetase. In this condition, the hair is brittle and both trichorrhexis nodosa and pili torti (another common hair shaft defect) may be present.[15,18] Affected infants have an associated dermatitis that may be widespread but more pronounced in the perioral and diaper area. Patients with *Menkes syndrome*, caused by a defect in copper efflux,[19] and *trichothiodystrophy*, caused by a defect in the synthesis of the ultrahigh- and high-sulfur proteins integral to hair,[20] both have trichorrhexis nodosa apparent on microscopic examination of the associated brittle hair.

FIGURE 71-4

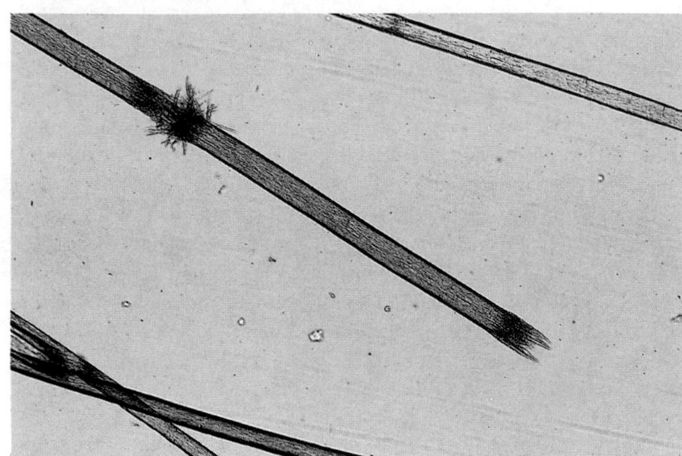

Trichorrhexis nodosa.

Acquired trichorrhexis nodosa may be either distal or proximal. Proximal breakage appears most commonly in African-American women, usually after repetitive chemical or hot-comb straightening.[15] Distal trichorrhexis nodosa is more commonly secondary to excessive brushing, back-combing, or sporadic use of permanent waves.

Treatment of trichorrhexis nodosa, congenital or acquired, is by avoidance of chemical or physical trauma to the hair.

TRICHOSCHISIS The break in *trichoschisis* is a clean transverse fracture through the entire hair shaft at a location where there is a focal absence of cuticle (Fig. 71-5*A*). Trichoschisis is usually, but not specifically, a marker for the sulfur-deficient hair of *trichothiodystrophy*, in which the hairs of the scalp, eyelashes, and brows are short and brittle.[15] The hair abnormality of trichothiodystrophy identifies a group of autosomal recessive disorders in which acronyms or eponyms identify particular constellations of extratrichologic neuroectodermal abnormalities (Table 71-2). In affected individuals, the hair cystine

FIGURE 71-5

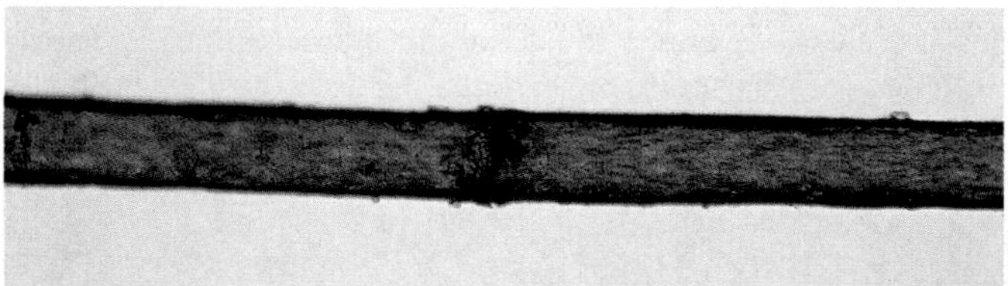

A.

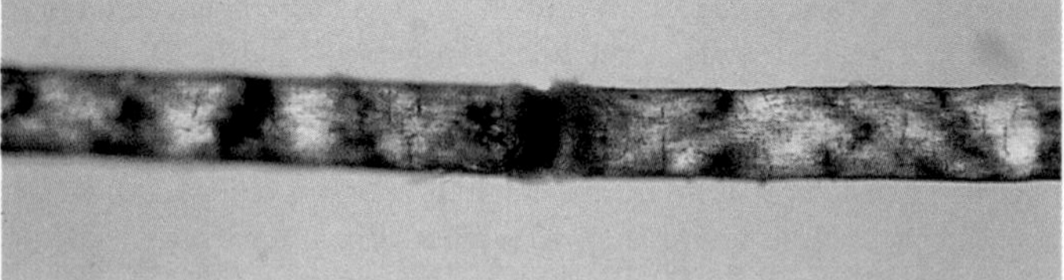

B.

Trichothiodystrophy. *A.* Hair shaft with trichoschisis without polarization (light micrograph ×100). *B.* Hair shaft with polarization (light micrograph ×100). (*From Whiting,*[15] *with permission.*)

TABLE 71-2

Trichothiodystrophy

	Brittle Hair	Brittle Nails	Intellectual Impairment	Decreased Fertility	Short Stature	Ichthyosis	Photo-sensitivity	Neutropenia	Other Findings
Trichoschisis	+								
Trichoschisis/ onychodystrophy	+	+							
Sabinas syndrome	+	+	+	+					Astigmatism, pale optic discs, retinopathy
BIDS (Amish brittle hair syndrome)	+	+	+	+	+				Quadriplegia, seizures, microcephaly, ataxia
IBIDS [Tay syndrome, Pollitt syndrome (SIBIDS)]	+	+	+	+	+	+			Abnormal teeth, tongue plaques, cataract, VSD, osteosclerosis
PIBIDS	+	+	+	+	+	+	+		Xeroderma pigmentosum
Onychotrichodysplasia, neutropenia, mental retardation (ONMR)	+	+	+		+	+		+	Recurrent infections, folliculitis, conjunctivitis
Marinesco-Sjögren syndrome	+	+	+		+				Ataxia, dysarthria, cataracts, abnormal teeth (primarily neuroectodermal)

SOURCE: Modified from Table 6–3 in Whiting DA: Hair shaft defects, in *Disorders of Hair Growth: Diagnosis and Treatment,* Edited by EA OLSEN 1994.

content is less than half normal, primarily from a major reduction and altered composition of the ultrahigh-sulfur matrix proteins.[20] Polariscopic examination of affected hairs characteristically shows alternating light and dark bands, presumably secondary to variations in sulfur content[15] (Fig. 71-5*B*). Sulfur and/or amino acid analysis of the hair is diagnostic.

Patients with trichothiodystrophy, particularly the 50 percent with associated photosensitivity, may have a defect in excision repair of ultraviolet damage but without an increased risk of skin cancer.[21] Recent data support correlation of mutations in the DNA repair and transcription gene *ERCC2* locus with the nucleotide excision repair characteristics of both trichothiodystrophy and xeroderma pigmentosa.[22] No treatment is currently available, but photosensitive patients should be tested for their cellular response to ultraviolet radiation and encouraged to practice sun protection.

PILI TORTI The short and brittle hairs in patients with *pili torti,* when viewed through a microscope, appear flattened and twisted through 90° to 360°.[15] The twisting must be differentiated from the normal twisting seen in Negroid hair and in the pubic/axillary hairs of other races; the hairs are distinguished by the multiple irregular intervals of twisting along an otherwise straight hair shaft (Fig. 71-6*A*).

As with trichorrhexis nodosa, pili torti does not signify a particular abnormality but can be seen in many different syndromes and in the presence of other hair shaft abnormalities. Hereditary pili torti as an isolated finding, usually autosomal dominant, but potentially autosomal recessive or sporadic, is present at birth or develops over the first 2 years of life (Fig. 71-6*B*). Clinically, the patient may have patchy alopecia with coarse stubble or longer broken hairs. The hair abnormality may improve after puberty.

FIGURE 71-6

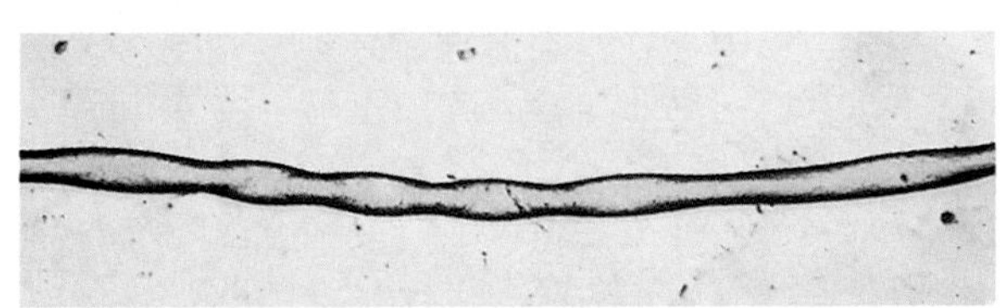

A.

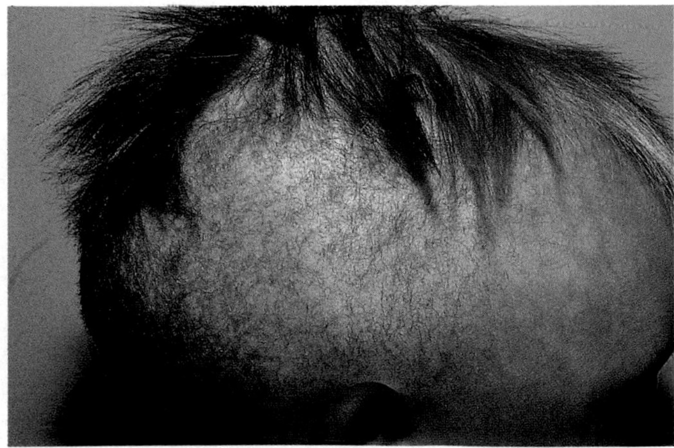

B.

Pili torti. *A.* Irregularly spaced 180° twists in hair shaft. (*From Whiting,*[15] *with permission.*) *B.* Brittle broken hair typical of congenital pili torti.

TABLE 71-3

Causes of Telogen Effluvium

- Endocrine
  - Hypo- or hyperthyroidism
  - Postpartum
  - Peri- or postmenopausal state
- Nutritional
  - Biotin deficiency
  - Caloric deprivation
  - Essential fatty acid deficiency
  - Iron deficiency
  - Protein deprivation
  - Zinc deficiency
- Drugs (only those with incidence >1% noted here)
  - Angiotension-converting enzyme inhibitors
  - Anticoagulants
  - Antimitotic agents (dose dependent)
  - Benzimidazoles
  - Beta blockers
  - Interferon
  - Lithium
  - Oral contraceptives
  - Retinoids
  - Valproic acid
  - Vitamin A excess
- Physical stress
  - Anemia
  - Surgery
  - Systemic illness
- Psychological stress

Pili torti, or a facsimile best characterized as "twisting hair dystrophy,"[23] may occur with other abnormalities (Table 71-3). Particularly notable is the association of pili torti with *Menkes' syndrome* or *trichopoliodystrophy*. Infants with Menkes' syndrome develop sparse, depigmented brittle hairs that show pili torti or trichorrhexis nodosa on microscopic examination.[15] The affected child characteristically has pale, lax skin, and mental and neurologic impairment secondary to degeneration of cerebral, cerebellar, and connective tissue.[24] In this X-linked recessive disorder, the defective gene, *MKN* or *ATP7A,* which maps to Xq13.3, encodes a copper-translocating membrane protein ATPase that prevents effective copper transport and leads to the accumulation of intracellular copper in some tissues.[19] The excessive intracellular copper inappropriately triggers the synthesis of metallothionein, whose normal function is to chelate copper to prevent cellular toxicity. This further deprives the copper-requiring enzymes of the copper needed for normal function.[25] A low serum level of ceruloplasmin is diagnostic. Copper replacement is ineffective in preventing the inevitable progressive and lethal neurologic decline, but copper-histidine given immediately postpartum may prevent or ameliorate the severe neurodegeneration.[26]

TRICHORRHEXIS INVAGINATA *Trichorrhexis invaginata* ("bamboo hair") is a distinctive hair shaft abnormality that may occur sporadically, either in normal hair or with other hair shaft abnormalities, or regularly as a marker for Netherton's syndrome. The primary defect appears to be abnormal keratinization of the hair shaft in the keratogenous zone, allowing intussusception of the fully keratinized and hard distal shaft into the incompletely keratinized and soft proximal portion of the shaft.[27] This leads to the typical "ball-and-socket" deformity (Fig. 71-7) or, if fracture of the shaft occurs, a golf tee-shaped distal end of the shaft.

Netherton's syndrome (see Chap. 51) is an autosomal recessive inherited disorder consisting of a triad of ichthyosis, atopic diathesis, and trichorrhexis invaginata.[15] Affected hairs are generally short and

FIGURE 71-7

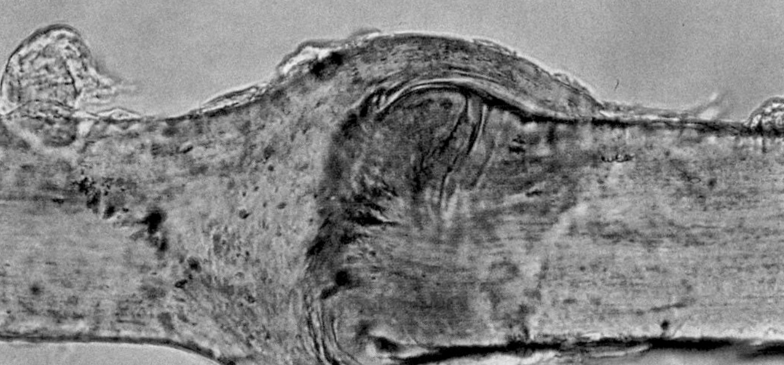

Trichorrhexis invaginata (light micrograph ×400). *(From Whiting,[15] with permission.)*

brittle and may be irregularly distributed over the scalp; this may lead to potential sampling errors on hair shaft evaluation. The ichthyosis is usually polycyclic ichthyosis linearis circumflexa but may be lamellar ichthyosis or even ichthyosis vulgaris or X-linked ichthyosis. The atopic diathesis may include erythroderma. Recurrent infections, short stature, and mental retardation are rarely reported with Netherton's syndrome. The Netherton's syndrome gene product is LEKTI, a serine protease inhibitor; the gene (*SPINK5*) locus is chromosome 5q32.[28] Retinoids and phototherapy may be of value, although the condition may improve spontaneously over time.

MONILETHRIX The hair abnormality of *monilethrix* is distinctive, with extremely short, brittle hairs emerging from keratotic follicular papules[29] (Fig. 71-8*A*). The onset may be delayed until patients are in their teens, and the loss may be localized or diffuse. Microscopically, hairs show elliptical nodes with a regular periodicity of 0.7 to 1 mm.[15] Between the nodes, the hair shaft is constricted, and it is in these areas that the hair usually fractures (Fig 71-8*B*). The disorder is caused by mutations in the genes for type II hair keratins hHb1 or hHb6 in the type II keratin gene cluster on chromosome 12q13.[30,31] Both hHb1 and hHb6 are expressed in the hair cortex cells with the abnormality in the helix termination or initiation motifs.[30]

Most cases of monilethrix are of autosomal dominant inheritance, with variable expressivity—the hair defect can be mild and localized to the occiput.[15,31] The hair defect may occur alone or in association with keratosis pilaris, physical retardation, syndactyly, cataracts, and nail/teeth abnormalities. Retinoids and topical minoxidil may be useful treatments, although this condition may also improve spontaneously with age.

Hair shaft abnormalities associated with unruly hair

UNCOMBABLE HAIR SYNDROME The distinctive hair of patients with *uncombable hair syndrome* may present any time from infancy to puberty. The slow-growing, silvery blonde, "spun-glass" hair is generally unmanageable and disorderly but not unduly fragile[15,32] (Fig. 71-9*A*). The condition may be autosomal dominant or sporadic. Under light microscopy, the hair appears normal or may have some suggestion of a longitudinal groove or ribbon-like flattening (Fig. 71-9*B*). Scanning electron microscopy confirms a longitudinal groove, and the hair may, if viewed on cross-section, show a kidney bean or triangular shape, which accounts for the alternate term of *pili trianguli et canaliculi*. The longitudinal groove in the hair shaft is not specific to this syndrome but can be seen in normal hair, in other etiologies of unruly hair, and in several types of ectodermal dysplasia.[15] The defect may be secondary to an abnormal configuration of the inner root sheath, which keratinizes before the hair shaft and thus determines its shape.[32] Biotin supplementation has been advocated in one case report,[33] but generally there is no effective treatment for the syndrome.

FIGURE 71-8

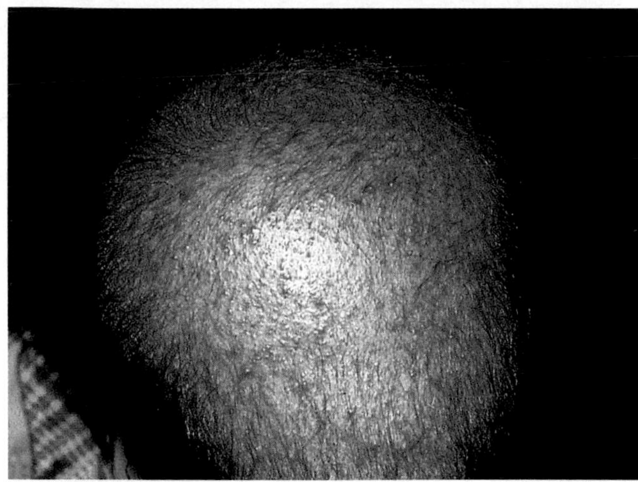

A.

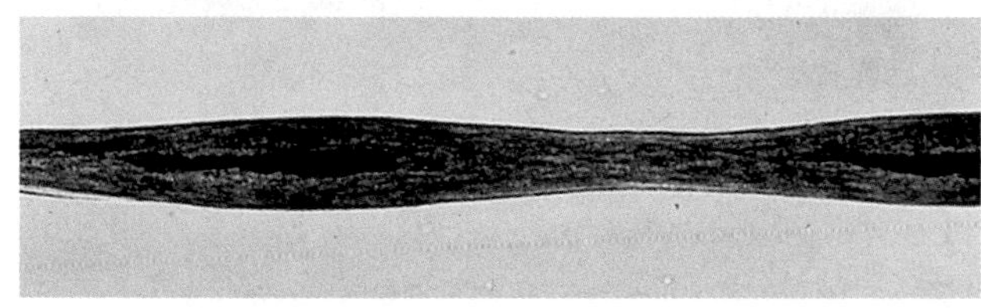

B.

Monilethrix. *A*. Keratotic papules in areas of alopecia. *B*. Typical beaded appearance of hair as seen under light microscopy (×40). *(From Whiting,[15] with permission.)*

WOOLY HAIR *Wooly hair* is the presence of Negroid hair on the scalp of persons of non-Negroid background. Microscopically, the hairs are tightly coiled. The unruly hair presents at birth or in infancy, usually as a solitary problem inherited in an autosomal dominant fashion.[34] However, two families with either autosomal dominant or autosomal recessive inheritance and associated palmoplantar keratoderma and cardiac abnormalities have been reported.[35] A sporadic variant has been reported with fine white-blond hair (Fig. 71-10). *Diffuse partial wooly hair,* a recently described autosomal dominant condition, presents in young adulthood with two distinct populations of scalp hair, one straight and the other very curly.[36] The curly hairs are thinner than normal hairs, which may contribute to the clinical appearance of a reduction in hair density.

MARIA-UNNA TYPE OF HEREDITARY HYPOTRICHOSIS This autosomal dominant condition is unusual in that the hair abnormality varies with age. The scalp hair in *Maria-Unna type of hereditary hypotrichosis* is sparse or absent at birth, with variable coarse, wiry hair regrowth in childhood, and potential loss again at puberty.[37] Body hair is sparse to absent. Light microscopic examination of the hairs shows irregular twisting, and scanning electron microscopic examination shows longitudinal ridging and cuticle peeling. Diffuse follicular hyperkeratosis and facial milia-like lesions may be present. A distinct gene in chromosomal region 8p21 close to the hairless (*hr*) locus has been noted.[38]

FIGURE 71-9

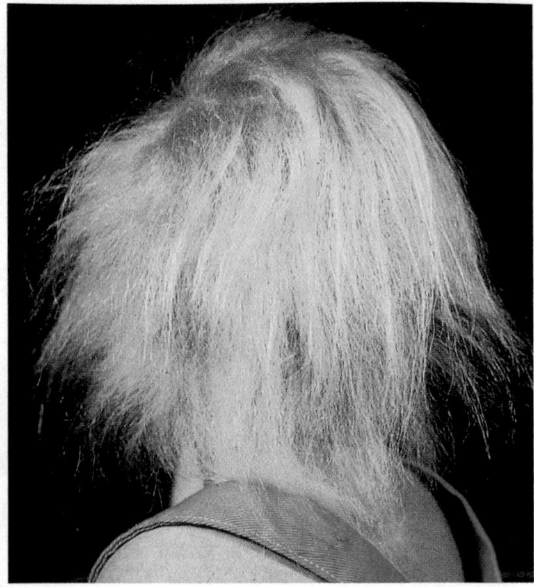

A.

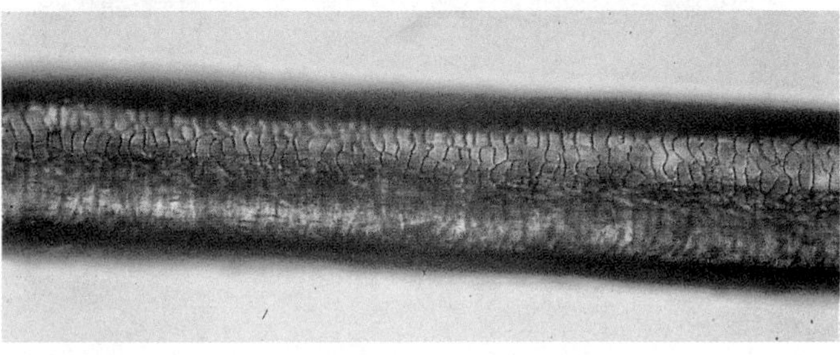

B.

Uncombable hair syndrome. *A.* Typical clinical picture. *(Photograph courtesy of Vera H. Price, MD.)* *B.* Longitudinal groove seen in uncombable hair syndrome (light micrograph ×400). *(From Whiting,[15] with permission.)*

FIGURE 71-10

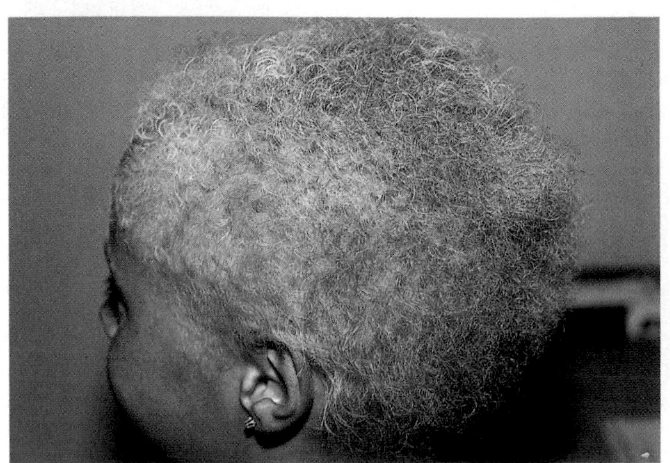

Sporadic recessive wooly hair.

Hair shaft abnormalities unassociated with breakage or unruly hair There are a few specific abnormalities of the shaft that should be noted here because of their frequency. The hair in *pili annulati,* an autosomal dominant (occasionally sporadic) condition, shows alternating light and dark bands both clinically and under light microscopy secondary to air-filled spaces in the cortex.[39] Cuticle folding and holes in the cortex are seen with electron microscopy.[15] Clinically, the hair in *pseudo pili annulati* shows a similar light microscopic picture, but the condition is nonhereditary and is not associated with any hair shaft cortex abnormality.[40] The cause of the latter appears to be periodic flattening of the hair shaft that causes light to be reflected as bright bands.

Both conditions appear primarily in blond hair and are not associated with hair breakage. With transverse illumination, the banding in pili annulati is seen in whatever way light strikes the hair, whereas pseudo pili annulati is seen only when the hair is rotated into certain positions.[39]

ABNORMALITIES OF HAIR CYCLING

Telogen effluvium This common type of hair loss may occur at any age and represents a precipitous shift of a percentage of anagen hairs to telogen. Telogen effluvium is a reaction pattern to a variety of physical or mental stressors; the most common causative factors are given in Table 71-3. Any drug can potentially cause telogen effluvium, although some classes of drugs routinely cause this.

The clinical increase in scalp hair shedding (over a normal of 50 to 100 hairs per day) usually begins as the first group of anagen hairs to be thrown prematurely into telogen finally completes telogen and moves once again into anagen, 3 to 4 months after the inciting event. If the inciting cause is removed the shedding will resolve over the next several months as the percentage of hairs in telogen return to normal; however, the hair density may take 6 to 12 months to return to baseline. In a significant number of patients, no obvious cause is found for telogen effluvium, and the increased shedding, and concomitantly the decreased density, of the scalp hair may become chronic.[41] Telogen effluvium is always potentially reversible and does not lead to total scalp hair loss, as the percentage of hairs in telogen rarely goes beyond 50 percent (Fig. 71-11).

Anagen effluvium The daily loss of some telogen hairs is entirely normal, but it is always abnormal to shed anagen hairs. The term *anagen effluvium,* as currently used to describe the pathologic loss of anagen hairs, is somewhat misleading because the abnormal anagen hairs in this condition are usually broken off rather than shed. The anagen hairs in *loose anagen syndrome,* however, are shed in toto.

The classic and easily recognizable causes of anagen effluvium of the scalp are radiation therapy to the head and systemic chemotherapy,

FIGURE 71-11

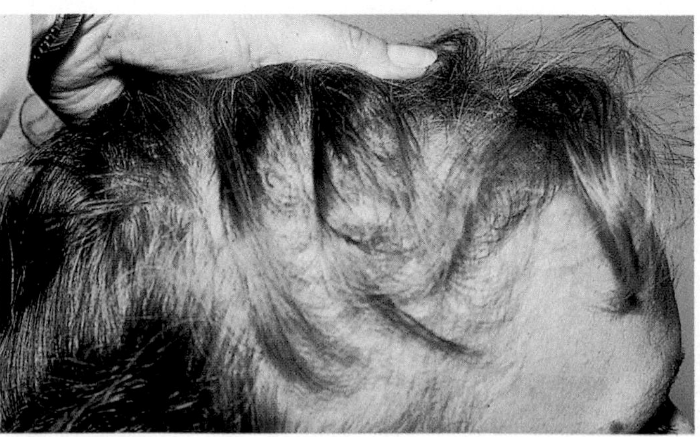

Telogen effluvium.

especially with alkylating agents. These agents can impair or totally disrupt the anagen cycle. The net result is either anagen hairs that break off within the follicle or at the level of the scalp secondary to a weak point in the hair shaft and are then shed without roots, or dystrophic anagen hairs that are easily dislodged from the usual follicular moorings. Replacement with a normal pelage usually occurs rapidly after discontinuation of chemotherapy although high-dose busulfan as part of the preparatory treatment for bone marrow transplantation may lead to permanent alopecia.[42] Regrowth after radiation therapy depends on type, depth, and dose-fractionation.[43]

In the absence of these obvious causes of anagen disruption, one must consider exposure to toxic agents. *Mercury intoxication,* through either chronic industrial exposure, consumption of polluted water or seafood, or inadvertent exposure to mercury-containing antiseptics or fungicides, can lead to hair loss with or without other symptoms, especially neurologic ones.[44] Diagnosis is by documenting elevated mercury levels in hair, blood, or urine. *Boric acid intoxication* may be through exposure to household pesticides or ingestion of some common household products in which boric acid is a preservative. Patients may develop hair loss along with gastrointestinal, central nervous system, and renal symptoms, a hemorrhagic diathesis, and exfoliation or bullae.[43,45] Blood boric acid levels are elevated in affected patients.

Thallium poisoning has the most dramatic associated hair loss, with complete epilation occurring 2 to 3 weeks after intoxication.[46] Acutely, patients experience primarily neurologic symptoms including irritability, dysesthesia, ataxia, convulsions and coma. Blood and urine levels are positive at the time of acute poisoning.

Toxic exposure to colchicine and ingestion of certain plants can lead to anagen loss.[43] Severe *protein malnutrition* may also lead to anagen effluvium. Arsenic exposure does not cause hair loss; instead, arsenic is concentrated in the hair, which facilitates a diagnosis long after intoxication may have occurred.

Loose anagen syndrome This recently described syndrome has been primarily described in fair-haired children who have easily dislodgable hair (Fig. 71-12*A*).[47,48] However, *loose anagen syndrome* can occur in adults and may be familial. This condition can be, and probably previously was, misdiagnosed as telogen effluvium if the shed hair roots are not examined microscopically. The hair loss may be inapparent except when traumatic pulling or extraction easily dislodges clumps of hair; this is particularly so in the parents of affected children, who themselves may have a mild, but previously unrecognized, variant of the condition that clinically may appear indistinguishable from a mild persistent telogen effluvium. The hair may also present with unruliness, occasionally causing confusion with uncombable hair syndrome or wooly hair (Fig. 71-12*B*). Microscopically, the proximal shed hair shows a normal anagen bulb, with a ruffled cuticle but without the usual attached root sheath[7] (see Fig. 71-2*B*). A scalp biopsy, which is unnecessary for diagnosis, may show premature and abnormal keratinization of the inner root sheath, with clefts between the inner and outer sheath and the hair shaft. The hair loss may improve with age, and gentle handling decreases shedding.

FIGURE 71-12

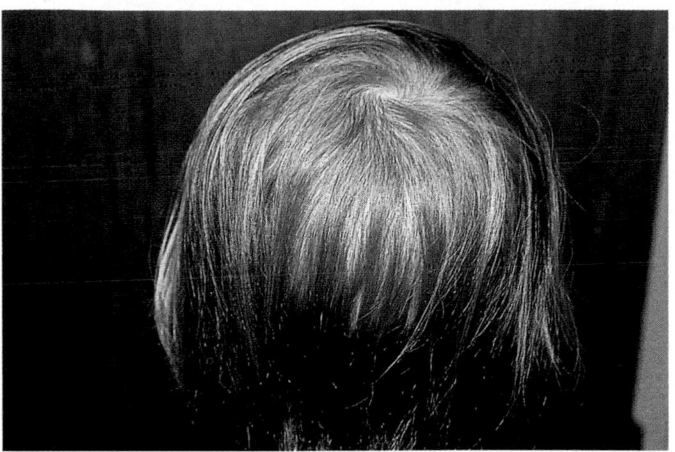

A.

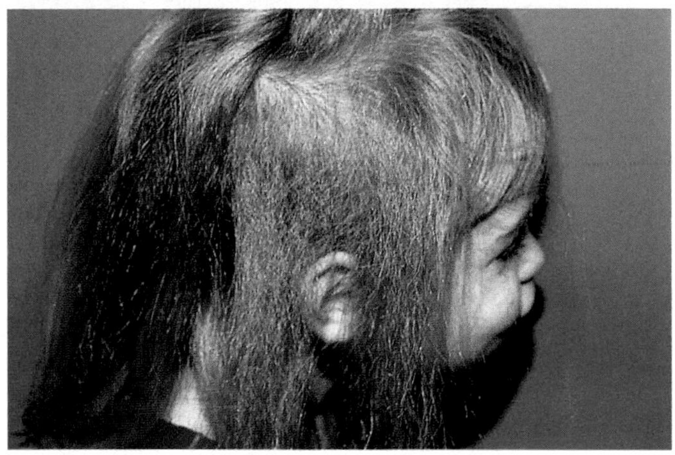

B.

Loose anagen syndrome. *A*. Diffuse hair loss. *B*. Unruly hair. (From Olsen,[7] with permission.)

Alopecia areata At any given time, approximately 0.2 percent of the population has alopecia areata and approximately 1.7 percent of the population will experience an episode of alopecia areata during their lifetime.[49,50] Clinically, patients with alopecia areata may have patchy or confluent hair loss on the scalp and/or body (Fig. 71-13*A*). *Alopecia totalis* refers to the total absence of terminal scalp hair, and *alopecia universalis* refers to the total loss of terminal body and scalp hair.[51] *Ophiasis* refers to a bandlike pattern of hair loss over the periphery of the scalp (Fig 71-13*B*). Hair loss may also be diffuse, mimicking anagen effluvium (Fig. 71-13*C*).

The scalp appears normal in alopecia areata. In affected areas, anagen is abruptly terminated prematurely and affected hairs move prematurely into telogen, with resultant often precipitous hair shedding. The near pathognomonic "exclamation point" hairs may be present, particularly at the periphery of areas of hair loss (Fig. 71-14). These short broken hairs, whose distal ends are broader than the proximal ends, illustrate their inherent sequence of events: follicular damage in anagen and then a rapid transformation to telogen. White or graying hairs are frequently spared and probably account, in cases of fulminant alopecia areata, for the mysterious phenomenon of "going gray overnight." There is an increased incidence of autoimmune diseases in patients with alopecia areata, particularly thyroid-related disease,[52] and there is a higher prevalence of pigmentary defects in patients with alopecia areata.[53] Nails in patients with alopecia areata may show fine pitting or, less commonly, mottled lunula, trachyonychia, or onychomadesis.[54]

A scalp biopsy is generally unnecessary to establish the diagnosis of alopecia areata, except in the uncommon presentation of diffuse shedding in which telogen or anagen effluvium is also a consideration. Typically, a biopsy of involved scalp shows a peribulbar, perivascular, and outer root sheath mononuclear cell infiltrate of T cells and macrophages.[55] Follicular dystrophy, including abnormal pigmentation and matrix degeneration, may also be present.[56]

The pathogenesis of alopecia areata is still obscure, although most authors tend to classify alopecia areata as an autoimmune disease. As opposed to normal hairs, strong major histocompatibility complex

FIGURE 71-13

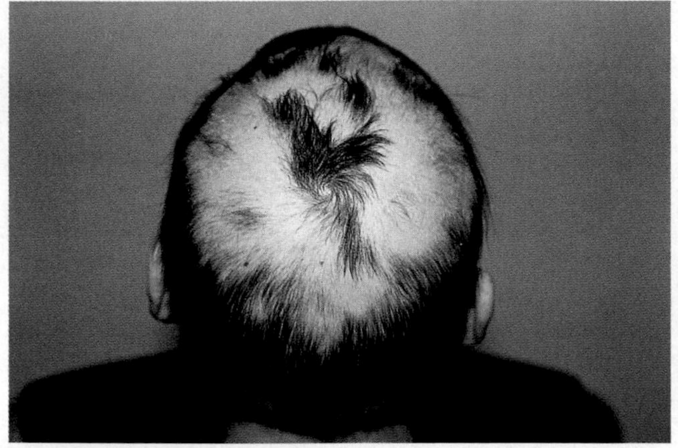

A.

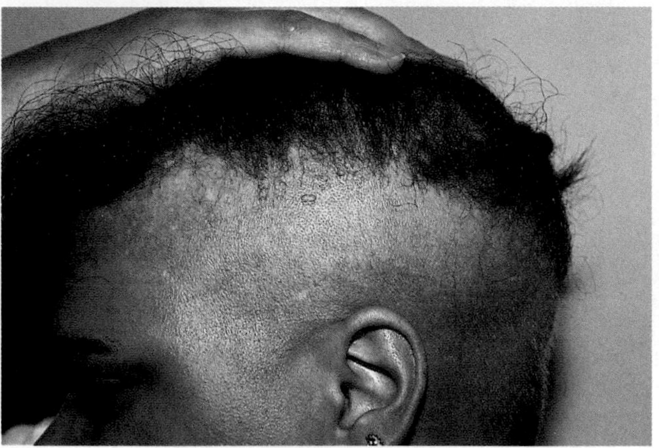

B.

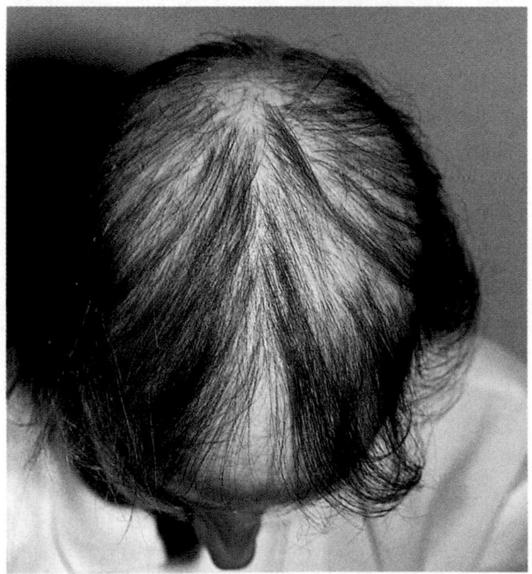

C.

A. Extensive patchy alopecia areata. *B*. Ophiasis pattern of alopecia areata. *C*. Diffuse pattern of loss in alopecia areata. (*Reprinted with permission from Hardinsky MK: Alopecia areata, in* Disorders of Hair Growth: Diagnosis and Treatment, *edited by EA Olsen. New York, McGraw-Hill, 1994.*)

FIGURE 71-14

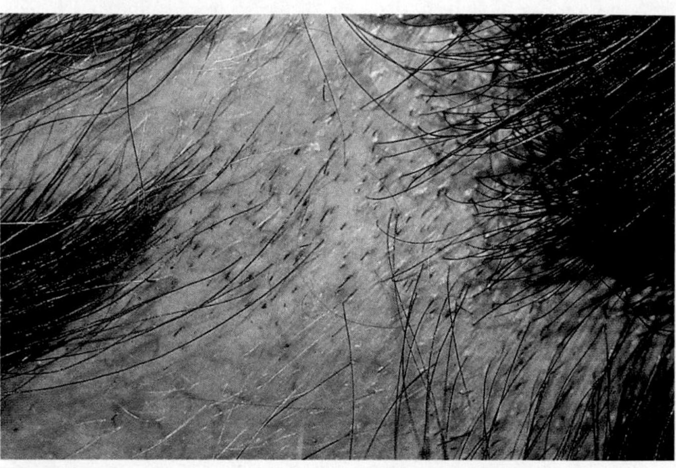

Exclamation mark hairs of alopecia areata. (*From Olsen EA: Clinical tools for assessing hair loss, in Disorders of Hair Growth: Diagnosis and Treatment, edited by EA Olsen, New York, McGraw-Hill, 1994, with permission.*)

(MHC) class I and class II immunoreactivity are found in lesional alopecia areata follicles, which also display aberrant expression of adhesion molecules known to direct hematopoietic cell migration.[54] One potential explanation for the failure of repression of MHC expression necessary for autoimmunity to develop in alopecia areata is the release of cytokines by certain stimuli, including trauma, neurogenic inflammation, or infectious agents. The elusive follicular autoantigens so exposed may be of keratinocyte or melanocyte origin, but the almost exclusive attack on melanogenically active anagen follicles makes this a particularly attractive hypothesis. That there is a genetic association with both susceptibility to and severity of alopecia areata is clearly shown by recent human leukocyte antigen (HLA) studies.[57]

Spontaneous remission is common in patchy alopecia areata, but is less so with alopecia totalis or universalis.[52] Spontaneous or treatment-related regrowth is also adversely affected by the location of hair loss (ophiasis pattern is particularly recalcitrant), the age of onset (children younger than 5 years old with alopecia totalis or universalis have the worse prognosis), association of atopy, and duration of hair loss in a given area.[52,58] Current treatment is not, at this point, directed at the etiology of alopecia areata but rather at the resulting inflammatory infiltrate and (presumably) the growth inhibitory factors produced by this response. Relapse is common, both acutely and over a lifetime.

Treatment of alopecia areata is with either immunosuppressives (local or systemic) or with irritants/immunogens, and is generally tailored to the severity of the disease.[54] For localized patchy alopecia areata, intralesional steroids given at 4- to 6-week intervals are usually effective, with the main side effect being local dermal/subcutaneous atrophy related to the depth and concentration of injected steroid. Topical glucocorticoids classes I to V are also effective but take several months for initiation of hair growth, rather than the weeks for intralesional steroids. Side effects of topical steroids are generally limited to acne/hypertrichosis on the face from inadvertent transfer from the scalp and local epidermal atrophy with the more potent steroids. Systemic steroids, particularly short courses (less than 8 weeks) of tapering doses, are often used either alone or in conjunction with topical agents. In this setting, acne and weight gain are commonly seen side effects.[59] PUVA is another immunosuppressant treatment that may be effective in alopecia areata, particularly in patients with extensive scalp and body hair loss. Between 30 and 80 treatments may be necessary before hair induction occurs, and there is an increased risk of photodamage/photoaging and skin cancer with PUVA use.[60]

The immunostimulation of topical irritants, especially anthralin, or topical immunogens (diphencyprone, squaric acid dibutylester) can be very effective in alopecia areata, but their use runs the risk of intolerable irritation if the dose titration is inappropriate. The particular mechanism of action of contact dermatitis that makes it a treatment for alopecia areata is purely speculative at this time, but it may include enhanced clearance of the putative follicular antigens through recruitment of new T cells and antigenic competition and interference with the initial or continued production of proinflammatory cytokines by the follicular keratinocytes.[61]

Five percent topical minoxidil, as a nonspecific hair growth promoter, may be a useful drug as a single agent or as an adjuvant with topical anthralin.[62] There is a low incidence of local dryness/irritation and facial hypertrichosis with topical minoxidil. Although rare, the potential for systemic effects of topical minoxidil, particularly in young children, must be considered and the total amount applied kept to the recommended $\leq$ 2 mL/day.

Patients with alopecia areata need psychological support and physical means of camouflaging their hair loss. The latter often requires the use of a wig, which should be considered an integral part of treatment in patients with extensive scalp hair loss. The National Alopecia Areata Foundation is an excellent source of information for patients (www.naaf.org).

Focal Hair Loss

NONSCARRING HAIR LOSS

Production decline

TRIANGULAR (TEMPORAL) ALOPECIA *Triangular alopecia* may be congenital but usually appears in childhood as a focal patch of hair loss. The hair loss either may be complete or fine vellus hairs may remain.[13,63] The underlying scalp is normal. The temporal region is a common location, and the hair loss is frequently bilateral (Fig. 71-15). Histologically, the affected area shows a transition from terminal to vellus hair. The alopecia is usually persistent.

PATTERN HAIR LOSS The term androgenetic alopecia was previously applied to both men and women with a very common, potentially reversible scalp hair loss that generally spares the "Hippocratic wreath" portion of the scalp. The hair loss condition in men and women has in common miniaturization and shortening of anagen duration of affected hairs and, consequently, an increased percentage of affected hairs in telogen.[64,65] Men with this type of alopecia tend to have somewhat synchronous behavior of hairs in the four different regions of the top of the scalp (vertex, mid, frontal, and bitemporal) along with potentially profound degrees of miniaturization leading to recognizable patterns of hair loss (Fig. 71-16).[65] In men, this male pattern baldness is hereditary (probably autosomal dominant) and androgen dependent, specifically dihydrotestosterone-related.[64,66]

FIGURE 71-15

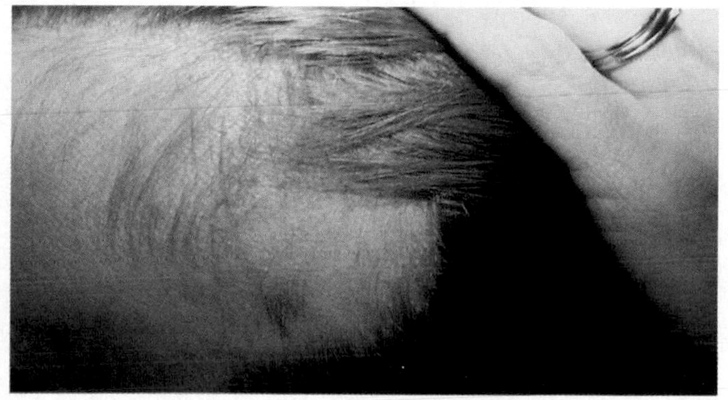

Triangular alopecia.

FIGURE 71-16

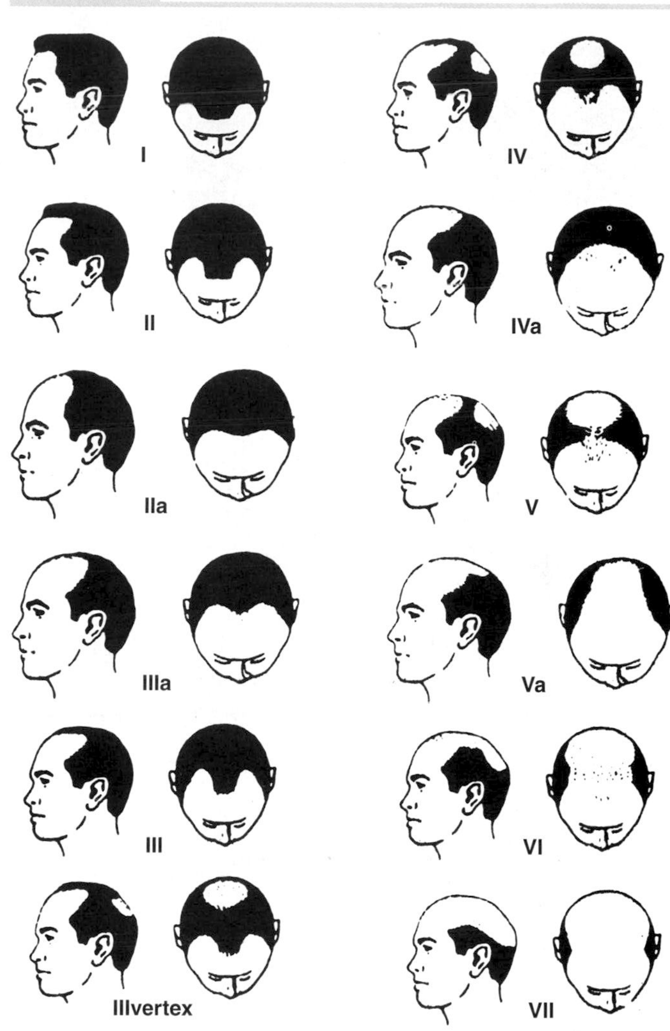

Hamilton-Norwood classification of pattern hair loss in men. *(From Olsen,[illegible] with permission.)*

Women, on the other hand, have lesser degrees of miniaturization of terminal hairs in affected areas and, hence, rarely any "balding" when compared to men. Patterning is less obvious then in men, although three patterns of hair loss do exist in women (Fig. 71-17*A*, *B*).[65] Not all women with pattern hair loss have proven androgen-dependence. Women with profound hyperandrogenemia, which is usually tumor related, may develop a Hamilton pattern of hair loss or severe diffuse central scalp hair loss, and women with other stigmata of hyperandrogenemia/hypersensitivity, such as those with polycystic ovarian syndrome, may present with pattern hair loss in the second to third decades.[65] The majority of women with pattern hair loss, however, have no increase in serum androgens, no other signs/symptoms of androgen hypersensitivity, and do not respond to androgen inhibition with reversal of hair loss.[64,65] Therefore, the preferred more encompassing "umbrella" term for this hair loss in women is *female pattern hair loss*. Subcategories of "early onset female pattern hair loss with or without androgen excess" and "late postmenopausal onset female pattern hair loss with or without androgen excess"[65] will allow sorting out of the genetic (e.g., polycystic

FIGURE 71-17

Male Pattern (Hamilton)

Diffuse (Ludwig)

Frontal Accentuation (Olsen)

A.

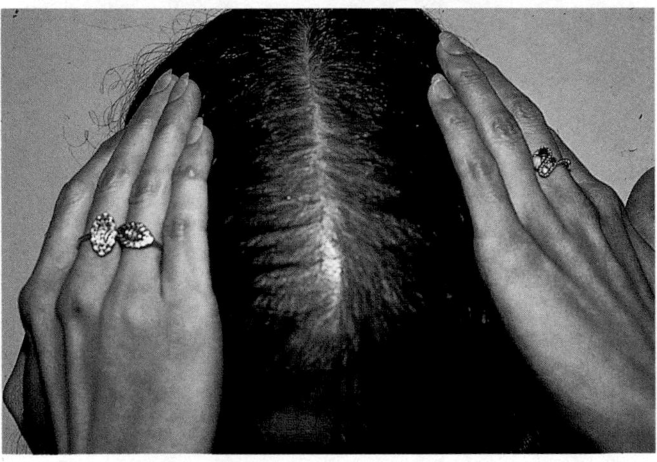

B.

Pattern hair loss in women. *A.* Different phenotypic expressions. *B.* Characteristic frontal accentuation.

ovarian syndrome and early male pattern baldness appear genetically linked)[67] and cellular mechanisms of these various subtypes.

Androgen-mediated hair growth (or loss) requires formation of an androgen-androgen receptor complex, which then binds to the androgen-response element DNA-binding site leading, in turn, to transcription of certain protein(s).[64] Androgens are 19-carbon steroid structures (Fig. 71-18), that are normally produced by both adrenal glands and gonads. The most potent androgens (testosterone, dihydrotestosterone, and androstenediol) are those with a 17-hydroxy group, as this moiety is necessary for high-affinity androgen receptor binding. The weaker 17-ketosteroids, such as dehydroepiandrosterone and androstenedione, assume importance by their interconversion by 17-OH steroid dehydrogenase to more potent androgens at the end-organ site, including the hair follicle. The enzyme 5α-reductase converts testosterone to dihydrotestosterone, which has greater affinity and avidity for the androgen receptor.[68] Two isozymes of 5α-reductase, called 5αR1 and 5αR2, have been cloned and their corresponding genes are located on chromosomes 5 and 2 respectively.[66] Although type I 5α-reductase appears to be more ubiquitously distributed in skin, particularly in the sebaceous gland, 5α-reductase type 2 is found in the outer root sheath[69] and dermal papillae of hair follicles, but is differentially expressed in various tissues.[64] That 5α-reductase type 2 is involved in male pattern baldness is suggested by the absence of balding in men with 5α-reductase type 2 deficiency;[66] the increased expression of 5α-reductase in balding versus nonbalding scalp;[70] the results in animal models of androgenetic alopecia showing reversal of hair loss with type 2 but not type 1 5α-reductase inhibitors;[64] and the response of men with male pattern baldness to finasteride, an inhibitor of 5α-reductase type 2.[71]

Effective treatment of pattern hair loss in both men and women can include both medical and surgical approaches. Topical minoxidil (2% and 5%) is a nonspecific hair-growth promoter affecting anagen induction, duration, and size of hair shaft. Although the mechanism of action in hair growth promotion is unclear, its calcium channel opener activity appears to be important.[64] The medication should be applied to the scalp twice a day, with the earliest clinical response seen at 4 to 6 months and generally a maximum response at 1 year.[64] About 20 to 25 percent of persons so treated will have notable clinical regrowth, although most patients will experience at least a stabilization of loss.[72] There is slight risk of facial hypertrichosis and of irritation/allergic contact dermatitis, secondary to either the minoxidil or propylene glycol. Both side effects are more frequent with the 5% versus the 2% preparation.[64] Whether the facial hypertrichosis is from inadvertent transfer from the scalp or secondary to a local reaction to low levels of serum minoxidil is not clear.

Surgical treatment of pattern hair loss has undergone dramatic improvement in recent years[73] (see Chap. 277). It is based on the premise of "donor dominance" whereby hairs from a nonandrogen-dependent site (occiput) can be successfully transplanted to a bald androgen-dependent site. Cosmetic coverage is currently limited by the amount and density of available occipital donor hair and the expertise of the surgeon. Ideally, male candidates for this procedure should be those in whom final resculpturing of the frontal hair line has naturally occurred. A combination of minigrafts (1.5- to 2.5-mm grafts) and micrografts (one to two hairs each graft) of donor hair are used more frequently now than the once standard 4-mm plugs to fill in areas of baldness. The micrografts are particularly useful because they do not require removal of a plug of tissue into which to insert the graft; rather, a small hole or incision can be made to accommodate a single or a few donor hairs. Micrografting is the surgical treatment of choice in women with pattern hair loss, who, unlike men, never develop baldness and for whom the use of standard hair transplants means sacrificing terminal hair when a recipient plug of tissue is removed.

For women with pattern hair loss, at least those who have documented androgen excess or androgen hypersensitivity, the use of medications that block either the production of or the cellular utilization of androgens may be helpful. Although the systemic antiandrogens spironolactone (in doses $\geq$ 100 mg daily),[74] flutamide (in doses of 250 to 500 mg bid to tid),[75] and cyproterone acetate[76] have shown some effectiveness in women with pattern hair loss, none of these have been studied in large placebo-controlled trials or with stratification of women by presence or absence of hyperandrogenism. This is especially important today because there is a lower threshold, given our knowledge of coincident insulin resistance, to identify polycystic ovarian syndrome, a potential cause of hyperandrogenism and concomitant pattern hair loss.

Spironolactone is a potassium-sparing diuretic whose main side effects are hyperkalemia, irregular menses, and breast tenderness/bloating. Flutamide users must be monitored for potential hepatotoxicity. Because both drugs can cause feminization of a male fetus, they should be used only in women of non-childbearing potential or in those women of childbearing potential who are using effective contraception, preferably combination oral contraceptive pills. Cyproterone acetate (CPA) is marketed outside the United States in conjunction with ethinyl estradiol, either in a reversed sequential regimen of 100 mg CPA on days 5 to 15 and 50 μg ethinyl estradiol on days 5 to 25, or in a low-dose combined formulation of 2 mg CPA and 50 μg ethinyl estradiol on days 5 to 25. Side effects are similar to those of oral contraceptive pills.[64] Topical antiandrogens, which theoretically could also be used in men, are not commercially available at this time.

Men with androgenetic alopecia may use a systemic 5α-reductase inhibitor without the biologic concerns of emasculinization seen with systemic antiandrogens since there is neither a decrease in testosterone levels nor any effect on androgen-receptor binding. In men with androgenetic alopecia, placebo- controlled studies of the type 2 5α-reductase inhibitor finasteride have shown increased hair growth in ~50 percent of men at 1 year and 66 percent by 2 years.[71] The placebo-treated group, by comparison, had hair growth in 7 percent at 1 year and a progressive decline at 2 years that continued over a 5-year follow-up.[77] Sexual adverse events (1.8 percent of those on 1 mg finasteride versus 1.3 percent of those on placebo) were the only significant side effects and generally cleared, either on or off treatment.[71]

FIGURE 71-18

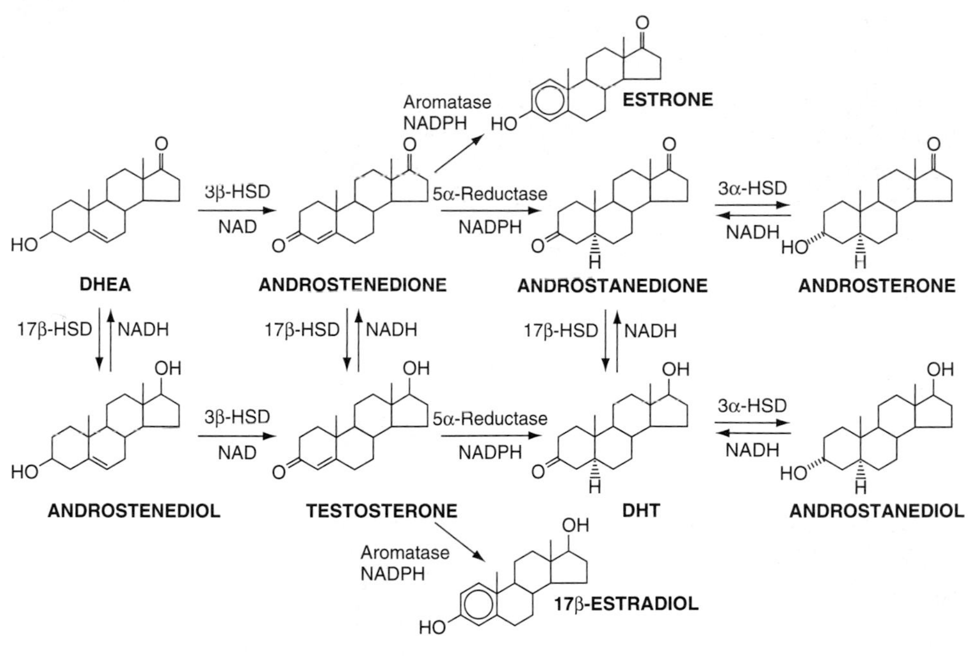

Androgen pathway. (*From Kaufman,*[66] *with permission.*)

Hair breakage

TRICHOTILLOMANIA *Trichotillomania* (Greek, "hair pulling madness") is a common, but difficult to manage, cause of focal scalp hair loss. It is classified as an impulse control disorder in which patients pull, pluck, or cut their hair.[78,79] The clinical presentation is usually quite distinctive, with a confluence of very short sparse hairs within an otherwise normal area of the scalp (Fig. 71-19*A*, *B*). Microscopic examination of the ends of cut or plucked hairs generally reveals either the tapered tips of newly regrowing anagen hairs or bluntly cut hairs. (A hair pull here is usually negative because the telogen hairs have generally all been dislodged) The differential diagnosis includes alopecia areata and tinea capitis, and because patients generally deny any role in the hair loss, these usually need to be definitively ruled out. A scalp biopsy can be diagnostic, showing the characteristic increase in the number of catagen hairs (rarely seen in biopsies of normal scalp), trichomalacia, and melanin within the follicular canal secondary to traumatic hair removal and the absence or sparsity of a perifollicular inflammatory infiltrate.[80,81]

Treatment of these patients is challenging. Children with trichotillomania may have a form of habit tic, which can be broken by mere acknowledgment of the problem or behavior modification. Adolescents and adults with this condition, who tend to be primarily females, are usually particularly reluctant to accept the diagnosis and often require psychological intervention and/or medication to help modify their behavior.[78,79] Clomipramine may be particularly effective.

TRACTION ALOPECIA *Traction alopecia* is caused by inadvertent prolonged traction on the scalp by the physical pressure of tight braids, certain hair styles (e.g., pony tail), foam rollers, etc (Fig. 71-20). While potentially reversible, the hair loss may be persistent if the traction is unrelenting over months to years.

TINEA CAPITIS (See also Chap. 205) *Tinea capitis* is a very common cause of hair breakage or loss, particularly in children. Typically, there is either a seborrheic dermatitis presentation, with or without erythema of the scalp (Fig. 71-21*A*), or a noninflammatory "black dot ring-worm" presentation, with broken hairs filling, but not projecting from, follicular orifices (Fig. 71-21*B*). Less commonly, tinea capitis can present as a pyoderma-like kerion.

The etiologic agent(s) of tinea capitis varies in different parts of the world. Currently in the United States, in which the condition is far more prevalent in African Americans and Hispanics than in Caucasians, the usual fungal isolate is *Trichophyton tonsurans.*[82] This is an endothrix infection and KOH examination of affected hairs shows arthrospores and hyphae interspersed among the keratin fibers of the hair shaft. To establish a diagnosis, hairs should be cultured as well as examined after KOH preparation, since a positive yield by KOH alone is dependent on the amount of inflammation and may vary from 29 to 66 percent.[83] Only ectothrix fungal infections fluoresce under Wood's light.

Treatment of tinea capitis must be by the systemic route, and contacts must be sought and treated to prevent reinfection. Asymptomatic carriers are common. Treatment is with griseofulvin, terbinafine, or one of the newer azoles.[82,84,85] Griseofulvin, 20 to 25 mg/kg per day of the microsized product (or 10 to 15 mg/kg of the ultramicrosized product), is given with a fat-containing meal until the culture is negative (generally 6 to 10 weeks).[82] Griseofulvin is fungistatic. Terbinafine, an allylamine, is not significantly affected by food and is fungicidal: doses of 62.5 to 250 mg qd for 4 weeks (62.5 mg/day for those weighing $<$20 kg, 125 mg/day for those weighing 20 to 40 kg, 250 mg/day for those weighing $>$ 40 kg) are effective. The azoles, itraconazole at 100 mg qd, or fluconazole 6 to 8 mg/kg for 4 to 6 weeks are effective alternative treatments. Both latter drugs inhibit the cytochrome P_{450} system so drug–drug interactions should be considered. Fluconazole

FIGURE 71-19

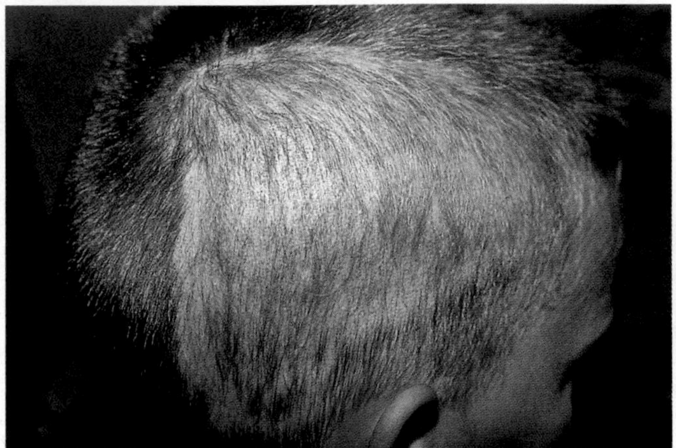

A.

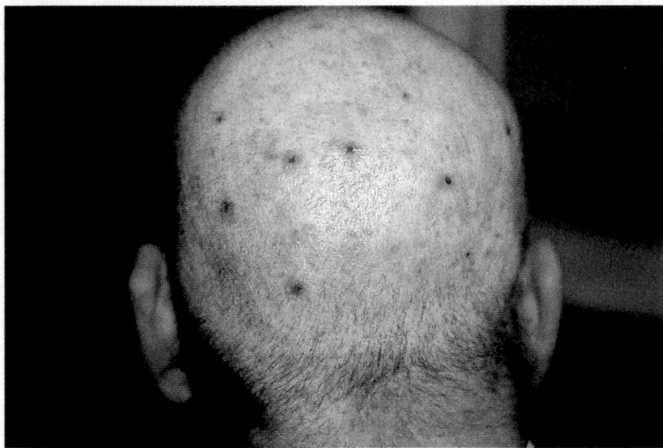

B.

Trichotillomania. *A*. Bizarre pattern of localized hair loss in a boy. *B*. Extensive hair loss in a woman.

FIGURE 71-20

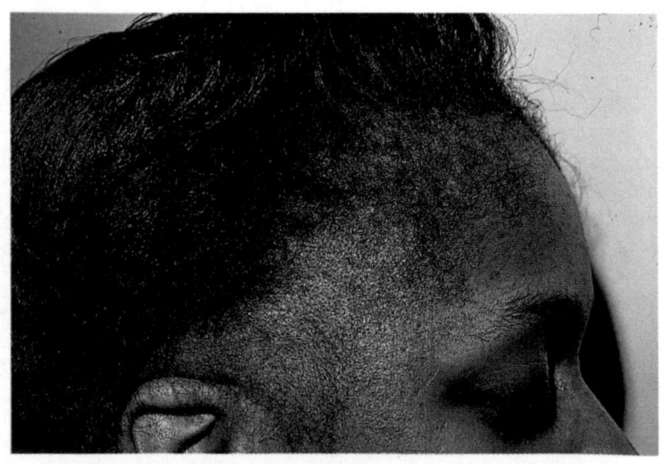

Traction alopecia.

FIGURE 71-21

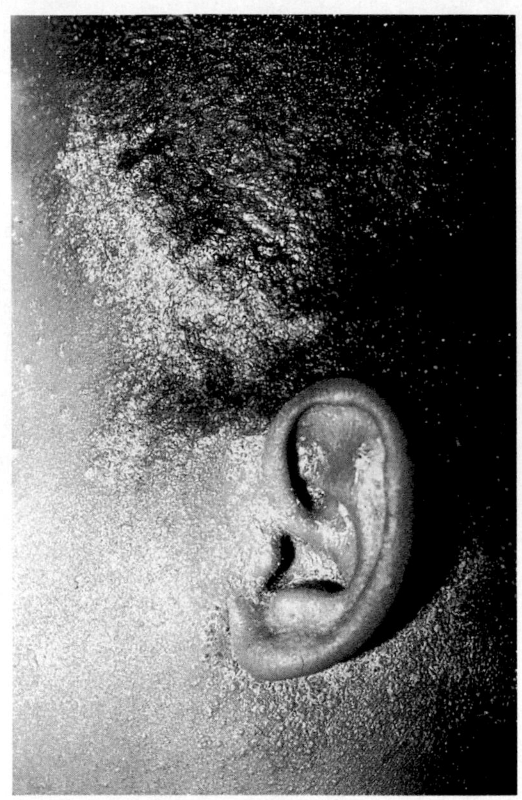

A.

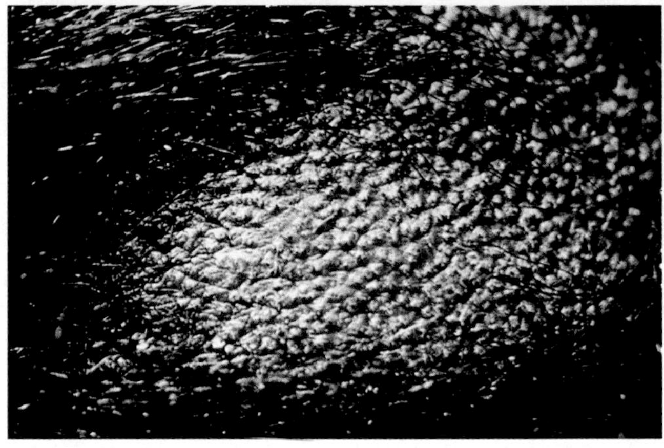

B.

Tinea capitis. *A*. Endothrix infection caused by *Trichophyton tonsurans* presenting as seborrheic dermatitis. *B*. Endothrix infection caused by *T. tonsurans*. Note "black dots" of broken, infected hairs within the follicular canals. (*Reprinted with permission from DeVillez RL: Infections, physical, and inflammatory causes of hair and scaly abnormalities, in* Disorders of Hair Growth: Diagnosis and Treatment, *edited by EA Olsen. New York, McGraw-Hill, 1994, pp 71–90.*)

bioavailability is not affected by food. Topical sporicidal agents, such as selenium sulfide or ketoconazole, help to limit the spread of infectious spores.

Primary or acquired localized hair shaft abnormalities

ACQUIRED LOCALIZED TRICHORRHEXIS NODOSA *Acquired localized trichorrhexis nodosa* may be seen in hair that is subject to repetitive rubbing, such as with lichen simplex chronicus or trichotillomania. It may also present in focal areas secondary to trauma from chemical or heat processing of hair. *Acquired pili torti* may present as a focal patch of fragile hair. This is usually secondary to trauma or some underlying, potentially scarring, scalp abnormality.[15] Hypervitaminosis in patients with anorexia nervosa or retinoids have also been associated with acquired pili torti. *Bubble hair* is a recently recognized and very distinctive abnormality of the hair shaft and is characterized by rows of bubbles seen microscopically within localized areas of brittle hair.[86] Exposure to prolonged high temperatures from curling irons or hair dryers are the usual causative factors, and the defect is completely reversible.

Unruly hair

WOOLY HAIR NEVUS *Wooly hair nevus* is a nonhereditary focal condition which usually appears within the first 2 years of life but can occur as late as adolescence.[87] Fifty percent of cases have an associated epidermal, verrucous, or pigmented nevus, although not necessarily immediately under the affected hair.[15] There may be associated ocular abnormalities, such as persistent papillary membrane or retinal abnormality. Spontaneous improvement in the hair may occur with age.

ACQUIRED PROGRESSIVE KINKING This condition has been primarily reported in postpubescent males with androgenetic alopecia.[88] It presents with gradual curling and darkening of the frontal, temporal, auricular, and vertex hairs. Microscopically, affected hairs show kinks and twists, with or without longitudinal grooving.

Abnormality of cycling

ALOPECIA AREATA As noted previously, alopecia areata can (and usually does) present as focal hair loss.

SYPHILIS Hair loss may be one or the sole cutaneous manifestation of *secondary syphilis.* This may present as a patchy "moth-eaten" alopecia or as generalized thinning (Fig. 71-22). A scalp biopsy may show either a superficial and deep perivascular mixed lymphocytic/macrophage/plasma cell infiltrate, a peribulbar perifollicular lymphocytic infiltrate mimicking alopecia areata, or a noninflammatory telogen effluvium picture.[89,90] Serologic testing should be positive, and treatment with appropriate antibiotics will reverse the hair loss.

Scalp conditions associated with focal hair loss Most eczematous conditions of the scalp do not cause hair loss, the exception being pityriasis amiantacea, severe scalp psoriasis and malignancies such as cutaneous T cell lymphoma or histiocytosis X. In *pityriasis amiantacea,* thick tenaciously adherent scale infiltrates and surrounds the base of a group of scalp hairs[91] (Fig. 71-23). The condition may mimic psoriasis clinically, but, in contradistinction to psoriasis, the hair in involved areas is dislodged on attempts to physically remove the scale. Removal of the scale in this manner can lead to scarring alopecia. The condition usually presents in children, is best treated with keratolytics, and usually improves with age.

FIGURE 71-22

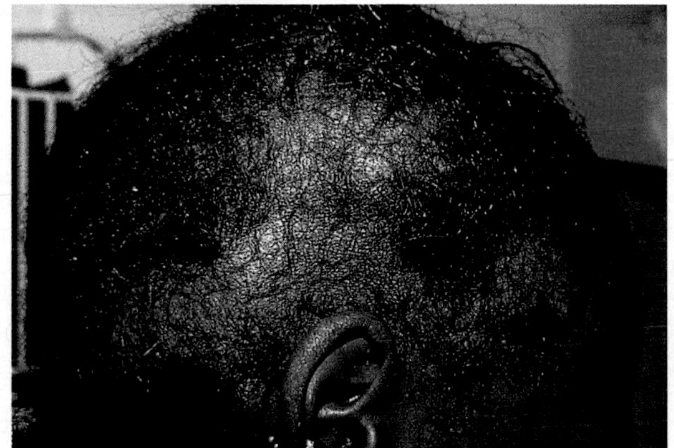

Alopecia of secondary syphilis.

FIGURE 71-23

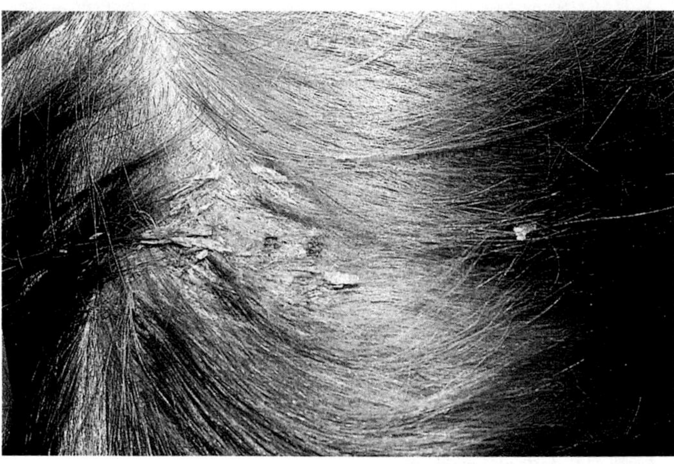

Pityriasis amiantacea. Note area of patchy alopecia after manual removal of adherent scale.

CICATRICIAL ALOPECIA (DESTRUCTION OF THE FOLLICLE)

The term *cicatricial or scarring alopecia* implies the potential of permanent destruction of the hair follicle. Clinically, there is effacement of follicular orifices, always in a patchy or focal distribution. A biopsy is confirmative, showing replacement of follicles with fibrotic stellae and either fibrosis or hyalization of surrounding collagen.[92–94] Although some cases of cicatricial alopecia are due to physical or developmental causes (e.g., pressure or aplasia cutis congenita), or to the hair follicle being secondarily involved in a destructive process (e.g., "kerion" fungal infection or metastatic/primary neoplasm), most patients seeking medical attention have a primary cicatricial alopecia. Although these conditions have a common endpoint, they have varied clinical and histologic features and virtually no therapies able to turn the process completely off.

There is direct evidence in the mouse, and indirect evidence in the human, that compromising the integrity of the sebaceous gland and/or bulge is important in the development of the scarring process in the primary cicatricial alopecias.[95] Selective destruction of the stem cell region in mice and graft versus host disease,[96] in which an inflammatory infiltrate involves the stem cells, can lead to follicular destruction. Moreover, alopecia areata, in which the inflammation spares the stem cell area, does not lead to permanent hair loss. In the asebia mouse, which lacks one gene responsible for normal sebum production, the hair follicle is destroyed when the shaft is unable to exit the follicle properly.[95] Other animals with sebaceous gland pathology also develop cicatricial alopecia.

A new classification system based on the type of inflammatory infiltrate on biopsy (Table 71-4) along with recommended standardization of biopsy site, processing and pathology parameters, and cataloguing of clinical findings,[97] will help us to identify and evaluate significant differences between these entities. The primary cicatricial alopecias are presented in keeping with this classification system.

Primary cicatricial alopecia

LUPUS ERYTHEMATOSUS (See also Chap. 171) *Chronic cutaneous lupus erythematosus* may present in the scalp, usually with erythema,

TABLE 71-4

Proposed Working Classification of Primary Cicatricial Alopecia

Lymphocytic
- Chronic cutaneous lupus erythematosus
- Lichen planopilaris (LPP)
  - Classic LPP
  - Frontal fibrosing alopecia
  - Graham Little Syndrome
- Classic pseudopelade (Brocq)*
- Central centrifugal cicatricial alopecia**
- Alopecia mucinosa
- Keratosis follicularis spinulosa decalvans

Neutrophilic
- Folliculitis decalvans
- Dissecting cellulitis/folliculitis (*perifolliculitis abscedens et suffodiens*)

Mixed
- Folliculitis (acne) keloidalis
- Folliculitis (acne) necrotica
- Erosive pustular dermatosis

Nonspecific†

*Clinically discrete, smooth, flesh-tone or white areas of alopecia without follicular hyperkeratosis or perifollicular inflammation

**Cicatricial alopecia starting in the central scalp and progressing centrifugally. This entity has previously been referred to by other terms (i.e., follicular degeneration syndrome, pseudopelade in African-Americans, central elliptical pseudopelade in caucasians) but we are suggesting this more descriptive term which embraces all previous entities.

†Nonspecific cicatricial alopecia is defined as an idiopathic scarring alopecia with inconclusive clinical and histopathological findings. This category may include the end stage of a variety of inflammatory cicatricial alopecias such as lichen planopilaris and folliculitis decalvans.

atrophy and variable hypopigmentation and/or follicular plugging (Fig. 71-24). Patients may have no other clinical lesions nor serologic evidence of lupus erythematosus. Scalp biopsy is generally confirmative, showing vacuolar degeneration of the basal cell layer, a perivascular and periadnexal lymphoid infiltrate, increased dermal mucin and sebaceous gland loss.[92] Direct immunofluorescence studies most commonly demonstrate granular deposits of IgG and C3 at the dermal–epidermal junction and at the junction of the dermis and follicular epithelium. Potentially effective treatments include topical, intralesional, and systemic steroids, antimalarials, systemic retinoids, and thalidomide.[93,98]

FIGURE 71-24

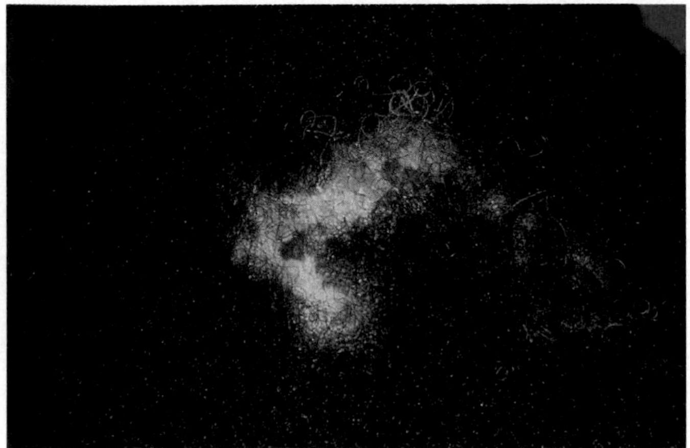

Lupus erythematosus.

FIGURE 71-25

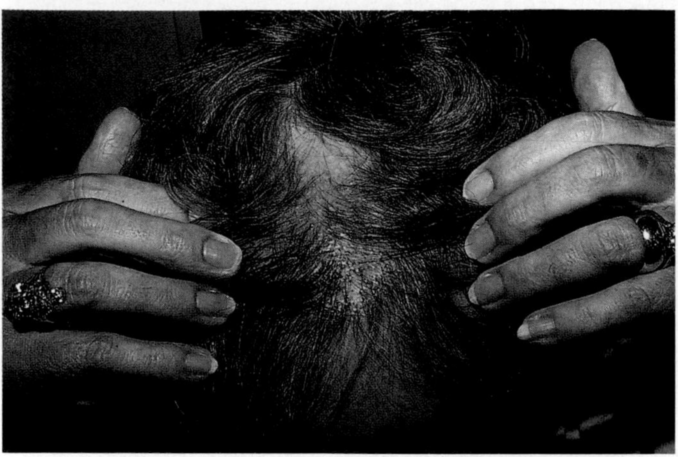

Lichen planopilaris.

LICHEN PLANOPILARIS Areas of active alopecia in *lichen planopilaris* are clinically distinguished by perifollicular erythema and/or a violaceous discoloration of the scalp (Fig. 71-25). Keratotic follicular papules may be evident. Evidence of lichen planus may be present elsewhere, and this should be sought to help confirm the diagnosis. Histologically, there is a perifollicular lymphoid, often bandlike, infiltrate primarily in the infundibular and isthmus portions of the follicle, with or without the presence of adjacent colloid bodies. The typical overlying histologic changes of lichen planus may or may not be present; these include sawtooth rete ridges, interface dermatitis, hypergranulosis, and Civatte bodies.[99] Immunofluorescence findings consist of globular deposits of IgM adjacent to follicular epithelium and patchy or linear fibrogen deposits along the basement membrane zone. Glucocorticoids are the mainstay of treatment.

Lichen planopilaris histologically can be seen in two other disparate conditions. *Graham-Little syndrome* is characterized by lichen planus-like lesions and a follicular "spines"/keratosis pilaris-like picture that develop in areas of alopecia on the scalp, eyebrows, axillary, and pubic areas.[92] *Frontal fibrosing alopecia* is a term given to the frontotemporal hairline recession and eyebrow loss in postmenopausal women that is associated with perifollicular erythema, especially along the hairline.[100] Scalp biopsy is indistinguishable from lichen planopilaris. Topical and intralesional steroids, topical and systemic retinoids, and hormone replacement therapy do not prevent the hair loss progression; oral steroids and chloroquine have been demonstrated to slow the progression in a few patients.

A lichenoid inflammatory infiltrate has also been seen in a progressive inflammatory (perifollicular erythema and follicular keratosis) scarring alopecia limited to the area of pattern hair loss.[101] There appears to have some overlap with frontal fibrosing alopecia.

PSEUDOPELADE OF BROCQ In clinical terms, *pseudopelade of Brocq* implies flesh- to pink-colored, irregularly shaped alopecia that may begin in a moth-eaten pattern with eventual coalescence into larger patches of alopecia[102] (Fig. 71-26). There has been considerable debate as to the specificity of this diagnosis versus an assignation of the term to describe all noninflammatory scarring alopecias, including the end-stage of a variety of initially inflammatory conditions. Histologically, the lesions are characterized by a perifollicular and perivascular lymphocytic infiltrate primarily at the level of the follicular infundibulum, loss of sebaceous epithelium, and fibrotic streams into the subcutis without interface or follicular plugging changes.[103] Elastin stains may distinguish pseudopelade (persistent elastic fibers around the midshaft of the follicle) from lichen planopilaris and lupus erythematosus (loss of

FIGURE 71-26

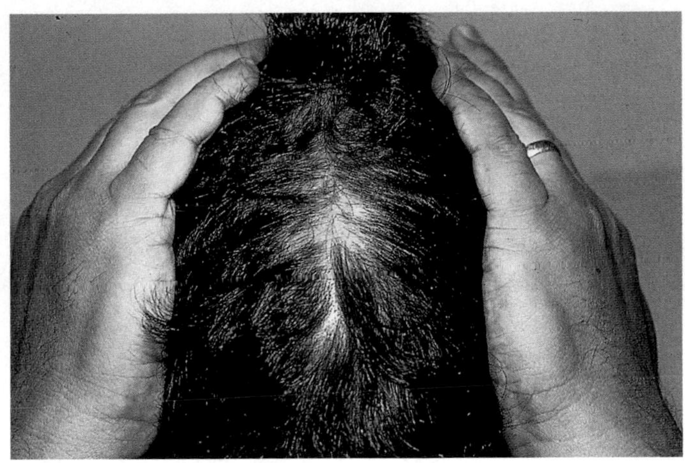

Pseudopelade of Brocq.

elastic fibers in this location).[104] Direct immunofluorescence is negative in the majority of cases. It is unclear what treatment specifically helps.

CENTRAL CENTRIFUGAL CICATRICIAL ALOPECIA Recently, a subset of cicatricial alopecia has been identified in African Americans and given the name of *central centrifugal cicatricial alopecia* (CCCA).[97] This condition has also been called hot comb alopecia, follicular degeneration syndrome, and central centrifugal scarring alopecia, the latter meant to be an umbrella term for follicular degeneration syndrome as well as other causes of central scalp hair loss.[105] Affected patients with CCCA show follicular loss primarily over the crown, with little in the way of either bogginess or tautness to the scalp (Fig. 71-27). Inflammation has been reported more commonly in affected men than in affected women.[106] Histologically, the earliest and most distinctive change is premature desquamation of the inner root sheath with later changes including migration of the hair shaft through the outer root sheath, a mononuclear infiltrate primarily at the isthmus, and, finally, loss of the follicular epithelium and replacement with fibrous tissue.[106] Although tight braiding, hot combs, and hair straightening agents are often invoked as causative or at least contributory factors and their use discouraged in CCCA, this has not been definitely proven. The distribution of CCCA overlaps that of pattern hair loss but the sex distribution is tremendously skewed toward women.

FIGURE 71-27

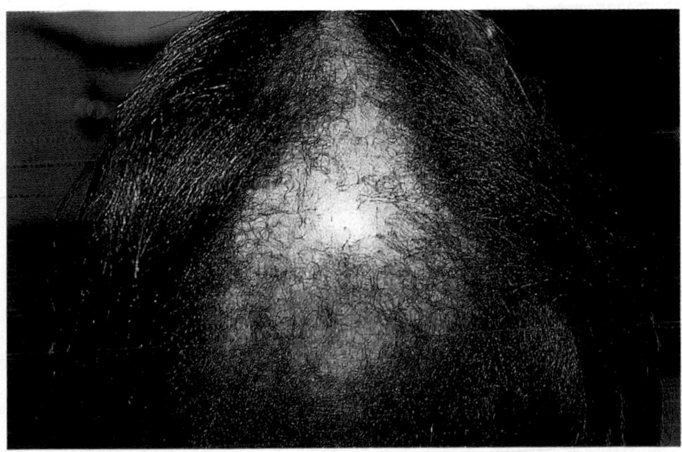

Central centrifugal cicatricial alopecia.

FIGURE 71-28

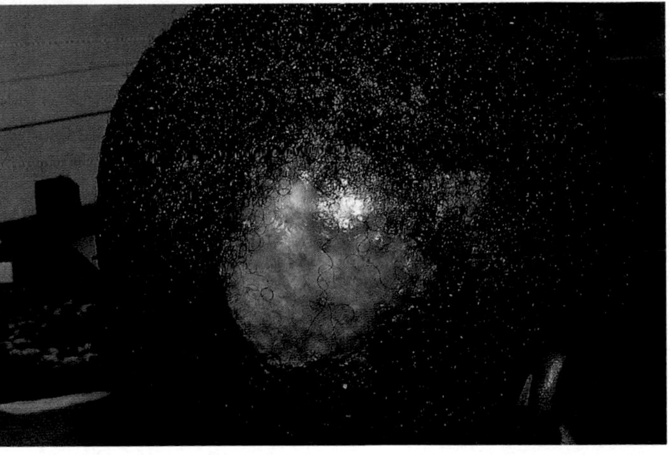

Folliculitis decalvans.

ALOPECIA MUCINOSA *Alopecia mucinosa* generally presents, but not exclusively, as erythematous plaques or flat patches without hair primarily on the scalp and face.[94] Biopsy reveals prominent follicular, epithelial and sebaceous gland mucin, and perifollicular lymphohistiocytic infiltrate without concentric lamellar fibrosis.[92,94]

KERATOSIS FOLLICULARIS SPINULOSA DECALVANS Keratosis follicularis spinulosa decalvans (KFSD) is an X-linked disorder with the gene located at Xp22.13–p22.2.[107] Female carriers are frequently affected. The disorder is characterized by follicular hyperkeratosis, scarring alopecia of the scalp, absence of eyebrows and sometimes eyelashes, severe photophobia, and resulting corneal dystrophy. Onset is in early childhood and the symptoms decrease with age. Histopathologically, there is plugging of the pilosebaceous orifices with keratinaceous debris, and superficial and deep perivascular and periappendageal infiltrate of lymphocytes and plasma cells. Retinoids may be useful in treatment.

FOLLICULITIS DECALVANS *Folliculitis decalvans* is an inflammatory alopecia that leads to bogginess or induration of involved parts of the scalp along with pustules, erosions, crusts, and scale[108] (Fig. 71-28). Predictably, *Staphylococcus aureus* is usually cultured from these pustules, but whether this is a primary or secondary process is unclear. Histologically, early lesions show an acute suppurative folliculitis with neutrophils and eosinophils, later mixed with lymphocytes and histocytes.[92,93] Loss of sebaceous epithelium and perifollicular fibrosis is common.[92] Systemic antibiotics with or without rifampin, systemic and/or topical steroids, and systemic retinoids may also be helpful.[108]

DISSECTING FOLLICULITIS *Dissecting folliculitis* or *perifolliculitis capitis abscedens et suffodiens of Hoffman* is another inflammatory condition of the scalp that can lead to scarring alopecia. African Americans are primarily affected. This condition begins with deep inflammatory nodules, primarily over the occiput, that progress to coalescing regions of boggy scalp (Fig. 71-29). Sinus tracts may form and dislodge purulent material. As in folliculitis decalvans, *S. aureus* is the most common bacterial isolate. Biopsy of early lesions shows follicular plugging and suppurative follicular or perifollicular abscesses with a mixed inflammatory infiltrate of neutrophils, lymphocytes, plasma cells, or eosinophils.[92–94] Later, foreign-body giant cells, granulation tissue, and, finally, scarring with sinus tracts occur. Control is difficult to attain, but systemic steroids, systemic antibiotics, dapsone, or

FIGURE 71-29

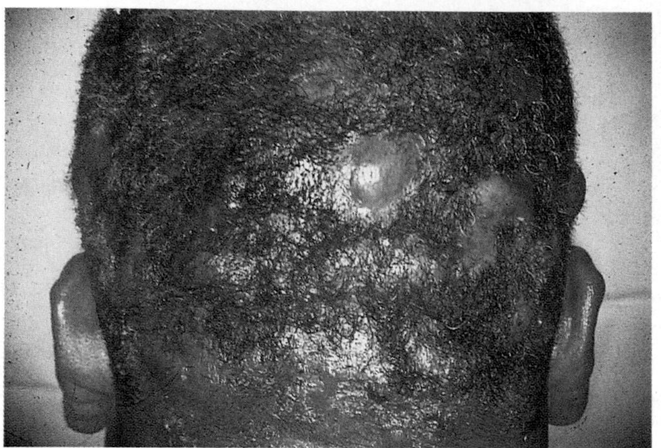

Dissecting folliculitis.

retinoids[109] are useful therapies. Surgical incision and drainage, excision with grafting, and/or x-ray epilation are occasionally used for refractory cases.

ACNE KELOIDALIS *Acne keloidalis (nuchae)* is a destructive scarring folliculitis that occurs almost exclusively on the occipital scalp of African Americans, primarily men (Fig. 71-30). The clinically distinctive lesions begin as follicular pustules and papules and progress to persistent firm papules or coalesce into hairless keloid-like plaques.[110] On histopathologic examination of an early lesion, there is follicular dilatation and a mixed peri-infundibular infiltrate that goes into follicular rupture and foreign body granulomas, loss of sebaceous glands, and lamellar fibroplasia. Treatment with systemic antibiotics, topical and/or intralesional steroids, and cryosurgery is usually helpful.

ACNE NECROTICA The primary lesion in acne necrotica is a pruritic or painful erythematous follicular-based papule that develops central necrosis and crusting and heals with a varioliform scar.[111] The lesions are concentrated on the nose, forehead and anterior scalp but may spread, primarily to the trunk. The course is chronic. Pathology is characterized by follicular dilatation, an early mixed lymphocytic/neutrophilic infiltrate in the peri-infundibulum, and later a lymphocytic/plasmacytic perivascular and perifollicular infiltrate. Lymphocytic exocytosis and individual cell necrosis of keratinocytes within the outer root sheath and surrounding epidermis go on to confluent necrosis of the central follicle. Treatment with tetracycline is generally helpful and *cis*-retinoic acid may be of value.[111]

FIGURE 71-30

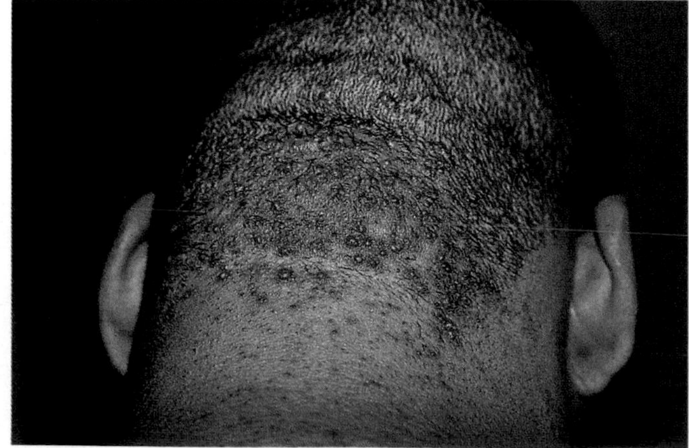

Acne keloidalis.

FIGURE 71-31

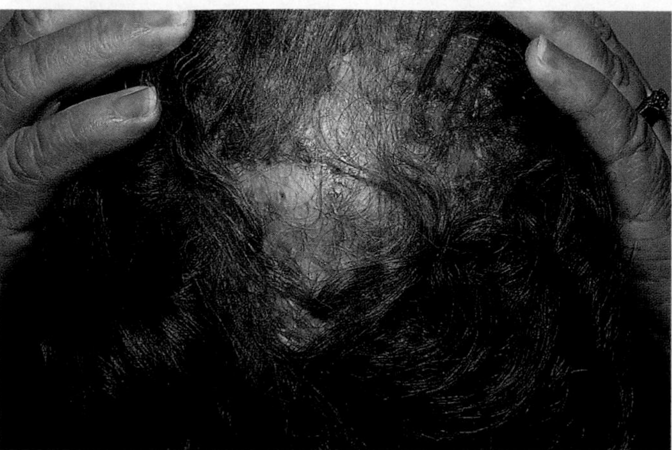

Pustular dermatosis of the scalp.

EROSIVE PUSTULAR DERMATOSIS Erosive pustular dermatosis of the scalp presents with pustules, erosions, and crusts on the scalp of primarily older Caucasean females (Fig. 71-31).[112] On biopsy, there is a lymphoplasmacytic infiltrate ± foreign body giant cells and pilosebaceous atrophy. These lesions have a slow but progressive course. Multiple organisms, both bacterial and fungal, have been cultured but these probably represent secondary colonization; patients do not generally respond to antibacterial or antifungal drugs. Potent topical steroids, zinc sulfate, or isotretinoin may be helpful.

Secondary Cicatricial Alopecia Cicatricial alopecia may present as a hereditary or development problem, alone or as part of a syndrome. Examples of the latter are Conradi-Hünermann chondrodysplasia punctata; incontinentia pigmenti; ankyloblepharon, ectodermal defect, cleft lip or palate (AEC) syndrome; Hallermann-Streiff syndrome; and generalized atrophic benign epidermolysis bullosa.[13]

The most common congenital cicatricial alopecia is *aplasia cutis congenita,* which is the congenital focal absence of epidermis with or without absence of other layers of the skin.[13] Hair follicles in the involved areas are variably affected. The condition may present at birth as an ulceration, crust, scar, or parchment-like membrane (Fig. 71-32). Eighty-five percent of aplasia cutis congenita presents on the scalp, and 70 percent of affected patients have only a single lesion. The lesions are usually small and round but can be large and extend to the dura or meninges. Aplasia cutis congenita may occur alone or in conjunction with various other abnormalities. Unless the lesions of aplasia cutis congenita are very large, no specific treatment is needed.

EXCESS HAIR

Hirsutism refers to hair growth in women in areas of the body where hair growth is under androgen control and in which normally only postpubescent males have terminal hair growth. These areas include the moustache, beard, chest, escutcheon, and inner thigh.

FIGURE 71-32

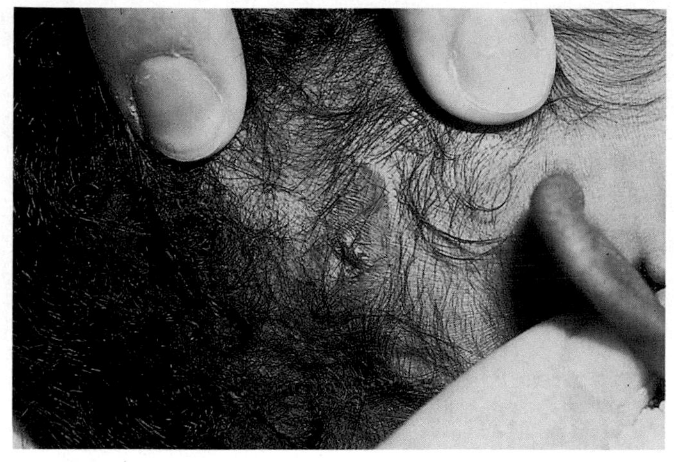

Aplasia cutis congenita. (*Photograph courtesy of Neil Prose, MD.*)

Hypertrichosis specifically refers to hair density or length beyond the accepted limits of normal for a particular age, race, or sex. The excess hair may be generalized or localized and may consist of lanugo, vellus, or terminal hair.

Hirsutism

Table 71-5 lists the causes of hirsutism. Most cases of hirsutism secondary to hyperandrogenism are associated with irregular menses or amenorrhea. There may be evidence of other cutaneous androgen-sensitive disorders such as acne and female pattern hair loss, or cutaneous clues to a related systemic problem such as acanthosis nigricans seen with insulin-resistant diabetes. Virilization is uncommon and should lead one to consider an underlying androgen-producing tumor.

For endogenous causes of hirsutism, a simple screening test of serum free or total testosterone will often determine whether further testing is necessary. Elevation of testosterone levels well above the upper limits of normal indicates the necessity of screening for an

TABLE 71-5

Hirsutism

- Androgen secreting tumors
  - Adrenal
    - Adenoma
    - Adenocarcinoma (rare)
    - Ectopic ACTH-secreting tumor (rare)
  - Ovarian
    - Gonadal stromal tumor
    - Thecoma
    - Lipoid tumor
- Functional androgen excess
  - Adrenal enzyme deficiencies (congenital adrenal hyperplasia)
    - Early onset 21-hydroxylase deficiency
    - Late-onset 21-hydroxylase deficiency
    - 11β-hydroxylase deficiency
    - 3β-ol dehydrogenase deficiency
  - Cushing's syndrome
  - Polycystic ovarian disease
    - With or without adrenal contribution
    - Hyperthecosis
- "Idiopathic" hirsutism
- Medication/drug use

SOURCE: Hughes CL: Hirsutism, in *Disorders of Hair Growth: Diagnosis and Treatment*, Edited by EA Olsen. New York, McGraw-Hill, 1994, p β44.

ovarian or adrenal tumor. Far more common is the mild elevation of androgens in an otherwise healthy woman, which is most commonly secondary to either polycystic ovarian syndrome (PCOS) or late-onset congenital adrenal hyperplasia (CAH). PCOS is multifactorial, with a pituitary and gonadal component, as well as hyperinsulinemia that may lead to increased production of androgen, decreased production of estrogen, and anovulation.[113,114] The most common cause of late-onset CAH is 21-hydroxylase deficiency with overproduction of 17-hydroxyprogesterone.[64] 3β-Hydroxylase and 11β-hydroxylase deficiency may also present with late-onset hirsutism; overproduction of 17-hydroxypregnenolone and 11-deoxycortisol, respectively, occur with these enzyme deficiencies. The diagnosis of late-onset CAH, while suggested by an elevated level of dehydroepiandrosterone and testosterone, can only be established by a cosyntropin-stimulation test showing the expected rise in the specific steroid hormone that builds up immediately behind the enzyme blockade or deficiency.[64] Women with hyperprolactinemia may have an increase in functional androgens through adrenal overproduction and through a decrease in sex hormone-binding globulin (SHBG) caused by a diminution of ovarian estrogen production; a prolactin level is diagnostic.[115]

The effective treatment of hirsutism depends on the cause, but the mainstays of treatment are oral contraceptive pills, both for their direct effect on lowering androgen production and indirect effect on lowering androgen bioavailability by increasing SHBG, and for their contraceptive effect when used with antiandrogens or 5α-reductase inhibitors. Antiandrogens, such as spironolactone, flutamide, or cyproterone acetate (see discussion of antiandrogens in "Pattern Hair Loss," above), are particularly useful in hirsutism as is finasteride.[116] There are marginal differences in efficacy between these agents but all generally take 6 to 12 months for sufficient miniaturization of terminal hairs to occur to be clinically significant. Treatment of congenital adrenal hyperplasia may also be accomplished through the use of low-dose dexamethasone. Hyperprolactinemia may be treated directly with either medical (bromocriptine) or surgical treatment of the hyperprolactinoma, and/or an antiandrogen may be utilized.

Hypertrichosis

GENERALIZED HYPERTRICHOSIS: INHERITED *Congenital hypertrichosis lanuginosa* presents as a confluent, generalized overgrowth of silvery blonde to gray lanugo hair at birth or in early infancy. It is rare (1 in 1 billion) and thought to occur as an autosomal dominant trait with variable expressivity. In most cases, other than possibly anomalous dental eruptions, children are otherwise healthy. The hair may persist, increase, or decrease with age.[117]

There are several other congenital disorders associated with generalized hypertrichosis, but none that are so evenly distributed as congenital hypertrichosis lanuginosa. These are noted in Table 71-6.[118] Patients with the autosomal dominant *Ambras syndrome* or *hypertrichosis universalis congenita* present with much longer, thicker hair, with accentuation over the entire face, ears, and shoulders.[119] Associated facial dysmorphism and dental anomalies are common. Members of the five-generation family described with *congenital generalized hypertrichosis* also have excess terminal hair on the face and upper body, more severe in men than women in keeping with the X-linked dominant inheritance.[120] Patients with the autosomal dominant (rarely autosomal recessive) *gingival fibromatosis* frequently have hypertrichosis, mostly on the face, eyebrows, limbs, and upper back, along with seizures and oligophrenia.[118] Hypertrichosis may be delayed until puberty although gingival fibromatosus in this situation usually appears with the emergence of the primary, versus secondary, teeth.

TABLE 71-6

Causes of Generalized Hypertrichosis

Congenital/hereditary
- Congenital hypertrichosis lanuginosa
  - Ambras syndrome
  - Congenital generalized hypertrichosis
- With gingival fibromatosis
  - Hereditary gingival fibromatosis with generalized hypertrichosis
  - Zimmermann-Laband syndrome
  - Ramon syndrome
- Brachmann-de Lange syndrome
- Wiedemann's syndrome
- Cantu's generalized hypertrichosis with osteochondrodysplasia
- Hurler's syndrome
- Reticular ichthyosiform erythroderma
- Donahue syndrome (Leprachaunism)
- Buntinex syndrome
- Barbar-Say syndrome
- Pivnick syndrome
- Jalili syndrome
- Coffin-Siris syndrome
- Gorlin's syndrome
- Hyperkinetic circulatory disorder
- Schinzel-Giedion syndrome
- Lawrence-Seip syndrome
- Generalized smooth muscle hamartoma
  - Michelin-Tire syndrome

Acquired
- Acquired hypertrichosis lanuginosa (malignancy)
- Drugs
  - Minoxidil
  - Diazoxide
  - Phenytoin sodium
  - Cyclosporine
  - PUVA
  - Topical steroids
  - Streptomycin
  - Acetazolamide
  - Oxadiazolopyrimidine
  - Fenoterol
- Porphyria
  - Porphyria cutanea tarda
  - Hepatoerythropoietic porphyria
  - Variegate porphyria
  - Erythropoietic porphyria
- POEMS syndrome
- Juvenile dermatomyositis
- Hypothyroidism
- Acrodynia
- Malabsorption syndromes
- CNS-related problems or trauma
  - After encephalitis
  - Multiple sclerosis
  - Schizophrenia
  - Head injury
  - Hyperostosis interna
  - Anorexia nervosa

SOURCE: Reprinted with permission from Olsen EA: Hypertrichosis, in *Disorders of Hair Growth: Diagnosis and Treatment,* Edited by EA Olsen. New York, McGraw-Hill, 2003[118].

ACQUIRED GENERALIZED HYPERTRICHOSIS There are few more ominous signs in dermatology than the onset of generalized hypertrichosis without an obvious drug-related explanation. *Acquired hypertrichosis lanuginosa* almost always signals an underlying malignancy or is a harbinger of one to develop in the near future (Fig. 71-33).[121]

FIGURE 71-33

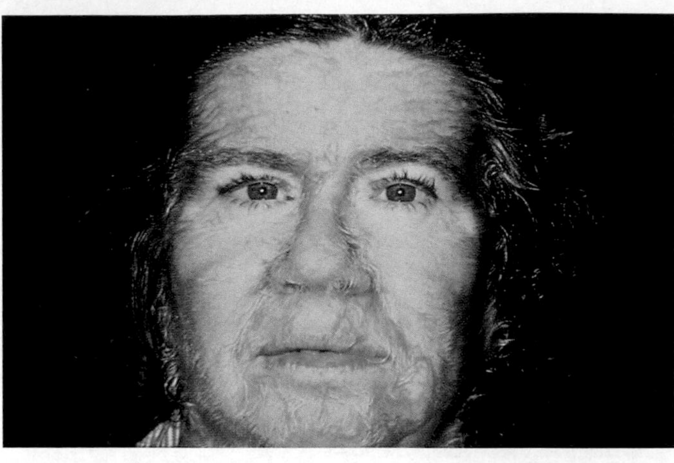

Acquired hypertrichosis lanuginosa. (*From Olsen,*[118] *with permission.*)

There are several drugs that routinely cause generalized hypertrichosis (see Table 71-6).[118] Oral minoxidil, a piperidinopyramidine derivative that is a potassium channel opener and antihypertensive agent when used systemically, causes hypertrichosis in 80 percent of patients, most prominently over the face, shoulders, and extremities. Diazoxide, a benzothiadiazine used primarily in malignant hypertension or idiopathic hypoglycemia of infancy, leads to lanugo-like hypertrichosis of the face, trunk, and extremities in 1 to 20 percent of adults but in almost 100 percent of children. Dilantin use leads to terminal hair hypertrichosis in 5 to 12 percent of patients, again first over the extremities, trunk, and face. Cyclosporine, a cyclic undecapeptide of fungal origin and an immunosuppressive agent, causes terminal hair hypertrichosis in 40 to 95 percent of patients, with a more diffuse distribution of excess hair, but primarily over the upper body (Fig. 71-34).[122,123]

FIGURE 71-34

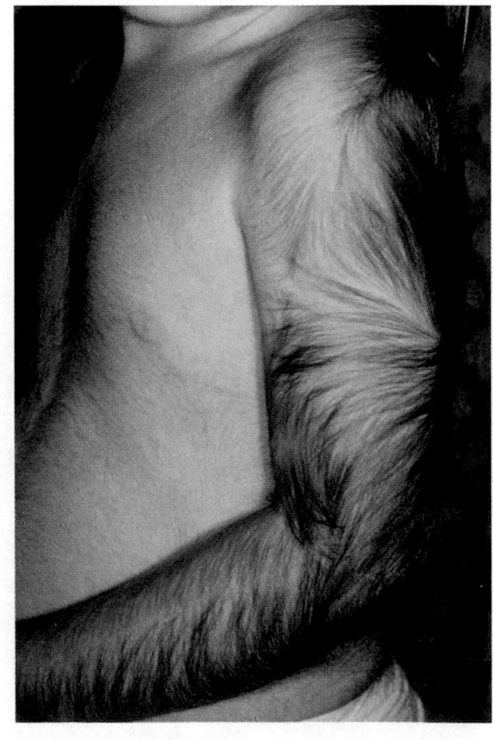

Cyclosporine-related hypertrichosis.

TABLE 71-7

Causes of Localized Hypertrichosis

Congenital/hereditary
- Middorsum hypertrichosis with underlying neuroectodermal abnormality
  - Spina bifida oculta
  - Traction (e.g., meningocoele manqué)
  - Diastematomyelia
- Familial cervical hypertrichosis
- Hairy elbows
- Anterior cervical hypertrichosis
- Hairy pinna
- Trichomegaly alone
- Congenital smooth muscle hamartoma
- Winchester syndrome
- Nevoid hypertrichosis
- Stiff skin syndrome
- Congenital pigmented nevus
- Hemimaxillofacial dysplasia

Acquired
- Becker's nevus
- Melorheostatic scleroderma
- Postmorphea
- Reflex sympathetic dystrophy
- Osteosclerotic myeloma
- Scrotal hair in male infants
- Drugs
  - Interferon
  - Sodium tetradecyl sulfate
  - Topical latanoprost
  - Topical minoxidil
- Undercasts
- Irritants (topical)
- Repeated trauma
  - Pressure (e.g., sack bearers, costaleros)
  - Lichen simplex chronicus
  - Biting
  - Insect bites
- Stasis/lymphedema
- Congenital A-V fistula
- Denervated areas
- Chronic osteomyelitis
- Site of immunizations
  - Smallpox
  - Diphtheria-tetanus
- Chickenpox
- HIV
- Periphery burned area
- Kala-azar (eyelashes)

SOURCE: Reprinted with permission from Olsen EA, Hypertrichosis, in *Disorders of Hair Growth: Diagnosis and Treatment,* Edited by EA Olsen. New York, McGraw-Hill, 2003.[118]

Both diazoxide and cyclosporine are also associated with gingival hyperplasia.

Certain medical illnesses are associated with widespread, although not confluent, hypertrichosis. They are listed in Table 71-6.

Localized Hypertrichosis Table 71-7 lists the conditions associated with localized hypertrichosis. These are generally either inherited, developmental, or secondary to irritation or trauma.

Treatment of Hypertrichosis

Removal of the inciting cause should be the prime approach to treatment and usually leads to regression of the hypertrichosis. However, in situations where that is not possible, one must either help the patient deal psychologically with the physical anomaly and/or use means of either temporarily or permanently removing the hair. Depilatories, plucking, waxing, and shaving are all means of temporarily removing hair but, with the exception of shaving, may be associated with irritation and/or pseudofolliculitis barbae. Potentially, electrolysis can permanently remove unwanted hair, but this technique varies widely in effectiveness depending on the training of the electrologist, the type of machine, the pulse frequency, the intensity and duration applied, and the probe used.[1] Two main types of electrolysis are in general use, thermolysis (AC current) with destruction of the hair by local heat production and "the blend," a combination of thermolysis and galvanic (DC current) which produces destruction of the hair by local production of caustic lye and H_2 gas. Potential, but ultimately controllable, side effects of electrolysis are pain, scarring, infection, and folliculitis.

Recently, several different kinds of laser have been approved for removal of hair.[1] The lasers selectively target the hair follicle, either by targeting a chromophore that is a natural component of the follicle, such as melanin, or one that is introduced into the follicle. The ruby (694 nm), alexandrite (755 nm), and semiconductor diode (800 nm) lasers, as well as a flash-lamp device with filters able to deliver light of >590 nm, each target melanin in the hair shaft and cause selective thermal injury.[1] The limiting factor in selecting melanin as the target is the concomitant absorption by epidermal melanin with both potential epidermal injury and a diminution in energy dispersal down the hair follicle. The Q-switched neodymium:yttrium-aluminum-garnet (Nd:Yag) laser with a wavelength of 1064 nm does not target melanin; instead, it targets a topically applied carbon-based material that leads to both thermal and mechanical damage to the follicle. All of the aforementioned lasers induce temporary hair removal. None of these techniques has been proven to lead to complete and permanent hair removal, although those that target melanin clearly can lead to a long-term reduction in terminal hair density, much apparently due to miniaturization, versus destruction, of the follicles.[124] A more experimental treatment is photodynamic therapy based on a topical photosensitizer (aminolevulinic acid), and subsequent exposure to red light, which causes selective follicular damage by the synthesis of the potent photosensitizer, protoporphyrin.[1]

CONCLUSION

The range of abnormalities in hair disorders mirrors the complexities of hair production. The astute clinician is able to diagnose hair disorders by a combination of clinical clues, microscopic evaluation of hairs, a biopsy of the affected area, and confirmatory laboratory tests. Treatment efficacy mirrors diagnostic accuracy although we are currenly woefully short of treatment to help those patients with herediary disorders of hair follicle or shaft production. As we come to better understand the genetic and molecular controls on hair growth, earlier diagnosis and implementation of effective directed treatments for the primary disorders of hair loss or overgrowth will become possible.

REFERENCES

1. Olsen EA: Methods of hair removal. *J Am Acad Dermatol* **40**:143, 1999
2. Courtois M et al: Ageing and hair cycles. *Br J Dermatol* **132**:86, 1995
3. Randall VA, Ebling FJG: Seasonal changes in human hair growth. *Br J Dermatol* **124**:146, 1991
4. Olsen EA: Clinical tools for assessing hair loss, in *Disorders of Hair Growth: Diagnosis and Treatment,* edited by EA Olsen. New York, McGraw-Hill, 2003
5. Olsen EA: Current and novel methods for assessing efficacy of hair growth promoters in pattern hair loss. Accepted for publication. *J Am Acad Dermatol* **48**:253, 2003
6. Solomon AR: The transversely sectioned scalp biopsy specimen: The technique and the algorithm for its use in the diagnosis of alopecia. *Adv Dermatol* **9**:127, 1994

7. Olsen EA et al: The presence of loose anagen hairs obtained by hair pull in the normal population. *J Invest Dermatol* **4**:258, 1999
8. Pantelleyev AA et al: The role of the hairless (*hr*) gene in the regulation of hair follicle catagen transformation. *Am J Pathol* **155**:159, 1999
9. Ahmad W et al: Genomic organization of the human hairless gene (*hr*) and identification of a mutation underlying congenital atrichia in an Arab Palestinian family. *Genomics* **56**:144, 1999
10. Zlotogorski A et al: Clinical and molecular diagnostic criteria of congenital atrichia with papular lesions. *J Invest Dermatol* **117**:1662, 2001
11. Miller J et al: Atrichia caused by mutations in the vitamin D receptor gene is a phenocopy of generalized atrichia caused by mutations in the hairless gene. *J Invest Dermatol* **117**:612, 2001
12. Freire-Maia N: Ectodermal dysplasias. *Hum Hered* **21**:309, 1971
13. Olsen EA: Hair loss in childhood, in *Disorders of Hair Growth: Diagnosis and Treatment,* edited by EA Olsen. New York, McGraw-Hill, 2003
14. McKusick VA ed: *Mendelian Inheritance in Man.* Maryland, Johns Hopkins University, 1998
15. Whiting DA: Hair shaft defects, in *Disorders of Hair Growth: Diagnosis and Treatment,* edited by EA Olsen. New York, McGraw-Hill, 2003
16. Dawber RPR, Comaish S: Scanning electron microscopy of normal and abnormal hair shafts. *Arch Dermatol* **101**:316, 1970
17. Batshaw ML et al: New approaches to the diagnosis and treatment of inborn errors of urea synthesis. *Pediatrics* **68**:290, 1981
18. Goldblum OM et al: Neonatal citrullinemia associated with cutaneous manifestations and arginine deficiency. *J Am Acad Dermatol* **14**:321, 1986
19. Davies K: Cloning the Menkes disease gene. *Nature* **361**:98, 1993
20. Gillespie JM, Marshall RC: Effect of mutations on the proteins of wool and hair, in *The Biology of Wool and Hair,* edited by GE Rogers, PJ Reis, KA Ward, RC Marshall. London, Chapman & Hall, 1989, p 257
21. Price VH et al: Trichothiodystrophy: Sulfur-deficient brittle hair as a marker for a neuroectodermal symptom complex. *Arch Dermatol* **116**:1375, 1990
22. Takayama K et al: Defects of the DNA repair and transcription gene ERCC2(XPD) in trichothiodystrophy. *Am J Hum Genet* **58**:263, 1996
23. Sinclair RD et al: *Handbook of Diseases of the Hair and Scalp.* Oxford, Blackwell Science, 1999, p 161
24. Kaler SG: Menkes disease. *Adv Pediatr* **41**:263, 1994
25. Leone A et al: Menke's disease: Abnormal metallothionein gene regulation in response to copper. *Cell* **40**:301, 1985
26. Tümer Z et al: Early copper-histidine treatment for Menkes disease. *Nat Genet* **12**:11, 1996
27. Ito M et al: Pathogenesis in trichorrhexis invaginata (bamboo hair). *J Invest Dermatol* **83**:1, 1984
28. Chavanas S et al: Mutations in SPINK5, encoding a serine protease inhibitor, cause Netherton syndrome. *Nat Genet* **25**:141, 2000
29. Gilchrist TC: A case of monilethrix with an unusual distribution. *J Cutan Genito-Urinary Dis* **16**:157, 1898
30. Korge BP et al: Identification of novel mutations in basic hair keratins hHb1 and hHb6 in monilethrix: Implications for protein structure and clinical phenotype. *J Invest Dermatol* **113**:607, 1999
31. Birch-Machin MA et al: Mapping of monilethrix to the type II keratin gene cluster at chromosome 12q13 in three new families, including one with variable expressivity. *Br J Dermatol* **137**:339, 1997
32. Mallon ME et al: Cheveux incoiffables—Diagnostic, clinical and hair microscopic findings, and pathogenic studies. *Br J Dermatol* **131**:608, 1994
33. Shelley WB, Shelley ED: Uncombable hair syndrome: Observation on response to biotin and occurrence in siblings with ectodermal dysplasia. *J Am Acad Dermatol* **13**:97, 1985
34. Hutchinson PE et al: Woolly hair: Clinical and genetic aspects. *Trans St John's Hosp Dermatol Soc* **60**:160, 1974
35. Tosti A et at: Wooly hair, palmoplantar keratoderma and cardiac abnormalities: Report of a family. *Arch Dermatol* **130**:522, 1994
36. Guidetti MS et al: Diffuse partial woolly hair. *Acta Derm Venereol (Stockh)* **75**:141, 1995
37. Solomon LM et al: Hereditary trichodysplasia: Marie Unna's hypotrichosis. *J Invest Dermatol* **57**:389, 1971
38. Cichon S et al: A distinct gene close to the hairless locus on chromosome 8p underlies Marie Unna type hypotrichosis in a German family. *Br J Dermatol* **143**:811, 2000
39. Price VH: Structural anomalies of the hair shaft, in *Hair and Hair Diseases,* edited by CE Orfanos, R Happle. Berlin, Springer-Verlag, 1990, p 363
40. Price VH et al: Pseudopili annulati: An unusual variant of normal hair. *Arch Dermatol* **102**:354, 1970
41. Whiting DA: Chronic telogen effluvium. *Dermatol Clin* **14**:723, 1996
42. Ljungman P et al: Busulfan concentration in relation to permanent alopecia in recipients of bone marrow transplants. *Bone Marrow Transplant* **15**:869, 1995
43. Sinclair R et al: Anagen hair loss, in *Disorders of Hair Growth: Diagnosis and Treatment,* edited by EA Olsen. New York, McGraw-Hill, 2003
44. Elhassani SB: The many faces of methylmercury poisoning. *J Toxicol* **19**:875, 1982
45. Stein KM et al: Toxic alopecia from ingestion of boric acid. *Arch Dermatol* **108**:95, 1973
46. Bank WJ et al: Thallium poisoning. *Arch Neurol* **26**:456, 1972
47. Price VH, Gummer CL: Loose anagen syndrome. *J Am Acad Dermatol* **20**:249, 1989
48. Baden HP et al: Loose anagen hair as a cause of hereditary hair loss in children. *Arch Dermatol* **128**:1349, 1992
49. Safavi K: Prevalence of alopecia areata in the First National Health and Nutrition Examination Survey. *Arch Dermatol* **128**:702, 1992
50. Price VH: Alopecia areata: Clinical aspects. *J Invest Dermatol* **96**:68S, 1991
51. Olsen EA et al: Alopecia areata investigational assessment guidelines. *J Am Acad Dermatol* **40**:242, 1999
52. Muller SA, Winkelman RK: Alopecia areata. An evaluation of 736 patients. *Arch Dermatol* **88**:290, 1963
53. Paus R et al: Is alopecia areata an autoimmune response against melanogenesis-related proteins exposed by abnormal MHC Class I expression in the anagen hair bulb? *Yale J Biol Med* **66**:541, 1994
54. Hordinsky MK: Alopecia areata, in *Disorders of Hair Growth: Diagnosis and Treatment,* edited by EA Olsen. New York, McGraw-Hill, 2003
55. Headington JT: The histopathology of alopecia areata. *J Invest Dermatol* **96**:69S, 1991
56. Tobin DJ et al: Ultrastructural observations on the hair bulb melanocytes and melanosomes in acute alopecia areata. *J Invest Dermatol* **94**:803, 1990
57. Colombe BW et al: HLA class II alleles in long standing alopecia totalis/universalis and long standing patchy alopecia areata differentiate these two clinical groups. *J Invest Dermatol* **104**:4S, 1995
58. Ikeda T: A new classification of alopecia areata. *Dermatologica* **131**:421, 1965
59. Olsen EA et al: Systemic steroids with or without 2% topical minoxidil in the treatment of alopecia areata. *Arch Dermatol* **128**:1457, 1992
60. Claudy AL, Gagnaire D: PUVA treatment of alopecia areata. *Arch Dermatol* **119**:975, 1983
61. Shapiro J: Topical immunotherapy in the treatment of chronic severe alopecia areata. *Dermatol Clin* **11**:611, 1993
62. Fiedler VC et al: Treatment-resistant alopecia areata: Response to combination therapy with minoxidil plus anthralin. *Arch Dermatol* **126**:756, 1990
63. Trakimas C et al: Clinical and histologic findings in temporal triangular alopecia. *J Am Acad Dermatol* **31**:205, 1994
64. Olsen EA: Pattern hair loss, in *Disorders of Hair Growth: Diagnosis and Treatment,* edited by EA Olsen. New York, McGraw-Hill, 2003
65. Olsen EA: Female pattern hair loss. *J Am Acad Dermatol* **45**:S70, 2001
66. Kaufman KD: Androgen metabolism as it affects hair growth in androgenetic alopecia. *Dermatol Clin* **14**:697, 1996
67. Carey AH et al: Polycystic ovaries and premature male pattern baldness are associated with one allele of the steroid metabolism gene CYP17. *Hum Mol Genet* **3**:1873, 1994
68. Zhou Z-X et al: Specificity of ligand-dependent androgen receptor stabilization: Receptor domain interactions influence ligand dissociation and receptor stability. *Mol Endocrinol* **9**:208, 1995
69. Bayne EK et al: Immunohistochemical localization of types 1 and 2 5α-reductase in human scalp. *Br J Dermatol* **141**:481, 1999
70. Sawaya ME, Price VH: Different levels of 5α-reductase type I and II, aromatase and androgen receptor in hair follicles of women and men with androgenetic alopecia. *J Invest Dermatol* **109**:296, 1997
71. Kaufman KD et al: Finasteride in the treatment of men with androgenetic alopecia. *J Am Acad Dermatol* **39**:578, 1998
72. Price VH, Menefee E: Quantitative estimation of hair growth: Comparative changes in weight and hair count with 5% and 2% minoxidil, placebo and no treatment, in *Hair Research for the Next Millenium,* edited by D van Neste, VA Randall. Amsterdam, Elsevier Science BV, 1996, p 67
73. Unger WS: Surgical approach to hair loss, in *Disorders of Hair Growth: Diagnosis and Treatment,* edited by EA Olsen. New York, McGraw-Hill, 2003

74. Rushton DH et al: Quantitative assessment of spironolactone treatment in women with diffuse androgen-dependent alopecia. *J Soc Cosmet Chem* **42**:317, 1991
75. Cusan L et al: Treatment of hirsutism with the pure antiandrogen flutamide. *J Am Acad Dermatol* **23**:462, 1990
76. Dawber RPR et al: Oral antiandrogen treatment of common baldness in women. *Br J Dermatol* **107**(suppl 22):20, 1982
77. The Finasteride Male Pattern Hair Loss Study Group: Long-term (5-year) multinational experience with finasteride 1 mg in the treatment of men with androgenetic alopecia. *Eur J Dermatol* **12**:38, 2002
78. Rothbaum BO, Ninan PT: The assessment of trichotillomania. *Behav Res Ther* **32**:651, 1994
79. Stein DJ et al: Trichotillomania and obsessive-compulsive disorder. *J Clin Psychiatry* **56**:28, 1995
80. Muller SA: Trichotillomania: A histopathologic study in sixty-six patients. *J Am Acad Dermatol* **23**:56, 1990
81. Mehregan AH: Trichotillomania: A clinicopathologic study. *Arch Dermatol* **102**:129, 1970
82. Elewski BE: Tinea capitis: A current perspective. *J Am Acad Dermatol* **42**:21, 2000
83. Gan VN et al: Epidemiology and treatment of tinea capitis: Ketoconazole vs. griseofulvin. *Pediatr Infect Dis J* **6**:46, 1987
84. Roberts J, Devillez R: Infectious, physical, and inflammatory causes of hair and scalp abnormalities, in *Disorders of Hair Growth: Diagnosis and Treatment,* edited by EA Olsen. New York, McGraw-Hill, 2003
85. Jones TC: Overview of the use of terbinafine (Lamisil) in children. *Br J Dermatol* **132**:683, 1995
86. Detwiler SP et al: Bubble hair: A case caused by an overheating hair dryer and reproducibility in normal hair with heat. *J Am Acad Dermatol* **30**:54, 1994
87. Reda AM et al: Wooly hair nevus. *J Am Acad Dermatol* **22**:377, 1990
88. Esterly NB et al: Acquired progressive kinking of the hair. *Arch Dermatol* **125**:813, 1989
89. Cuozzo DW et al: Essential syphilitic alopecia revisited. *J Am Acad Dermatol* **32**:840, 1995
90. Jordaan HF, Louw M: The moth-eaten alopecia of secondary syphilis. *Am J Dermatopathol* **17**:158, 1995
91. Bettencourt MLS, Olsen EA: Pityriasis amiantacea: A report of two cases in adults. *Cutis* **64**:187, 1999
92. Whiting DA: Cicatricial alopecia: A review of clinico-pathological findings and treatment and a clinico-pathological examination of 358 cases using horizontal and vertical sections of scalp biopsies. *Clin Dermatol* **19**:211, 2001
93. Bergfeld WF, Elston DM. Primary cicatricial alopecia (and other causes of permanent alopecia), in *Disorders of Hair Growth: Diagnosis and Treatment,* edited by EA Olsen. New York, McGraw-Hill, 2003
94. Templeton SF, Solomon AR: Scarring alopecia: A classification based on microscopic criteria. *J Cutan Pathol* **21**:97, 1994
95. Stenn K et al: Hair follicle biology, the sebaceous gland and scarring alopecias. *Arch Dermatol* **135**:973, 1999
96. Sale GE: Does graft versus host disease attack epithelial stem cells? *Mol Med Today* **2**:114, 1996
97. Olsen EA et al: Summary of NAHRS sponsored workshop on cicatricial alopecia, Duke University Medical Center, Feb 10–11, 2001. *J Am Acad Dermatol* Accepted for publication
98. George SJ: Lichen planopilaris treated with thalidomide. *J Am Acad Dermatol* **45**:965, 2001
99. Mehregan DA et al: Lichen planopilaris: Clinical and pathologic study of forty-five patients. *J Am Acad Dermatol* **22**:935, 1992
100. Kossard S et al: Postmenopausal frontal fibrosing alopecia: A frontal variant of lichen planopilaris. *J Am Acad Dermatol* **36**:59, 1997
101. Zinkernagel MS, Trüeb RM: Fibrosing alopecia in a pattern distribution. *Arch Dermatol* **136**:205, 2000
102. Brocq L et al: Recherches sur l'alopecie atrophiante, variete pseudopelade. *Ann Dermatol Syphil* **6**:97, 1905
103. Braun-Falco O et al: Pseudopelade of Brocq. *Dermatologica* **172**:18, 1986
104. Pinkus H: Differential patterns of elastic fibres in scarring and non-scarring alopecia. *J Cutan Pathol* **5**:93, 1978
105. Sperling LC et al: A new look at scarring alopecia. *Arch Dermatol* **136**:235, 2000
106. Sperling LC et al: Follicular degeneration syndrome in men. *Arch Dermatol* **130**:763, 1994
107. Oosterwijk JC et al: Refinement of the localization of the X linked keratosis follicularis spinulosa decalvans (KFSD) gene in Xp22.13-p22.2. *J Med Genet* **32**:736, 1995
108. Bronzena SJ et al: Folliculitis decalvans—Response to rifampin. *Cutis* **42**:512, 1988
109. Bjellerup M, Wallengran J: Familial perifolliculitis capitis abscedens et suffodiens in two brothers successfully treated with isotretinoin. *J Am Acad Dermatol* **23**:752, 1990
110. Sperling LC et al: Acne keloidalis is a form of primary scarring alopecia. *Arch Dermatol* **136**:479, 2000
111. Kossard S et al: Necrotizing lymphocytic folliculitis: The early lesion of acne necrotica (varioliformis). *J Am Acad Dermatol* **16**:1007, 1987
112. Caputo R, Veraldi S: Erosive pustular dermatosis of the scalp. *J Am Acad Dermatol* **28**:96, 1993
113. Hatch R et al: Hirsutism: Implications, etiology, and management. *Am J Obstet Gynecol* **140**:815, 1981
114. Barbieri RL et al: The role of hyperinsulinemia in the pathogenesis of ovarian hyperandrogenism. *Fertil Steril* **50**:197, 1988
115. Glickman SP et al: Multiple androgenic abnormalities, including elevated free testosterone, in hyperprolactinemic women. *J Clin Endocrinol Metab* **55**:251, 1982
116. Wong IL et al: A prospective randomized trial comparing finasteride to spironolactone in the treatment of hirsute women. *J Clin Endocrinol Metab* **80**:233, 1995
117. Partridge JW: Congenital hypertrichosis lanuginosa: Neonatal shaving. *Arch Dis Child* **62**:623, 1987
118. Olsen EA: Hypertrichosis, in *Disorders of Hair Growth: Diagnosis and Treatment,* edited by EA Olsen. New York, McGraw-Hill, 2003
119. Baumeister FAM et al: Ambras syndrome: Delineation of a unique hypertrichosis universalis congenita and association with a balanced pericentric inversion (8) (p11.2;q22). *Clin Genet* **44**:121, 1993
120. Figuera LE et al: Mapping of the congenital generalized hypertrichosis locus to chromosome x q24-q27.1. *Nat Genet* **10**:202, 1995
121. Hovenden A: Acquired hypertrichosis lanuginosa associated with malignancy. *Arch Intern Med* **147**:2013, 1987
122. European Multicentre Trial Group: Cyclosporin in cadaveric renal transplantation: One year follow-up of a multicentre trial. *Lancet* **2**(2):986, 1983
123. Bencci PL et al: Cutaneous lesions in 67 cyclosporine treated renal transplant recipients. *Dermatologica* **172**:24, 1986
124. Dierickx CC et al: Permanent hair removal by normal mode ruby laser. *Arch Dermatol* **134**:837, 1998

CHAPTER 72

Robert Baran
Antonella Tosti

Nails

PATTERNS OF DISRUPTION OF THE COMPONENTS OF THE NAIL UNIT[1]

The diagnosis of disorders of the nail unit is based mainly on the sites of primary and secondary pathology. This chapter is based upon such an approach. The biology of the nail unit is presented in Chap. 13 and surgery of the nail is described in Chap. 280.

Variations in General Contour

Clubbing is defined as increased transverse and longitudinal nail curvature. It is made up of hypertrophy of the soft tissue components of the digit's pulp; hyperplasia of the fibrovascular tissue at the base of the nail, allowing the plate to be "rocked"; and local cyanosis. In normal individuals, the opposition of the dorsum of two fingers from opposite hands delineates a diamond-shaped "window" formed at the base of the nail beds (Fig. 72-1). Early clubbing obliterates this window and creates a prominent distal angle between the ends of the nails (Fig. 72-2). Almost 80 percent of cases are caused by intrathoracic disorders (Table 72-1).

In addition to clubbing, *hypertrophic pulmonary osteoarthropathy* is associated with acromegalic limb changes, pseudoinflammatory symmetric large joint arthropathy, bilateral proliferative periostitis, peripheral cyanosis and paresthesia, local pain, and swelling. The distal digit disorders may be relieved by treating the underlying disease. When only the lower limbs are affected, the condition results from aortofemoral bypass grafts, reversed patent ductus, or aortointestinal fistula, all of which may be complicated by infection. Pachydermoperiostosis is a rare type of idiopathic hypertrophic osteoarthropathy.

In *koilonychia* (spoon nails) (Fig. 72-3), the nail is concave with raised edges. Involvement of the first three fingernails suggests an occupational origin of the deformity. Koilonychia is physiologic in early infancy. Iron-deficiency anemia associated with Plummer-Vinson's syndrome is rarely observed in association with spoon nails.

In *transverse overcurvature,* the nail may be tile-shaped or, more often, it displays an increase in curvature along the nail bed (pincer or

FIGURE 72-1

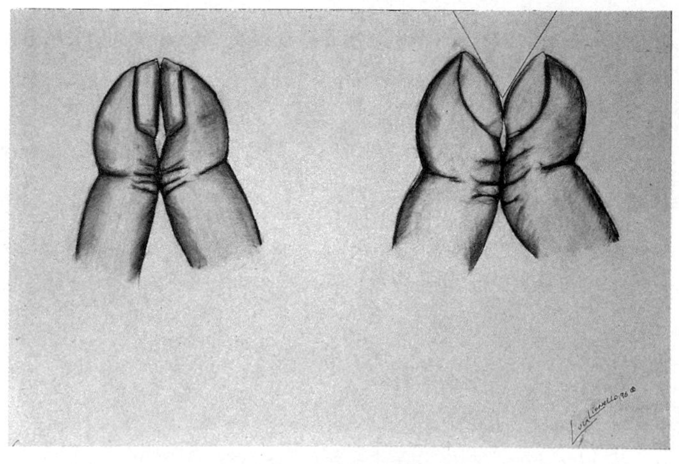

Opposition of the dorsum of two fingers from opposite hands in normal individuals.

FIGURE 72-2

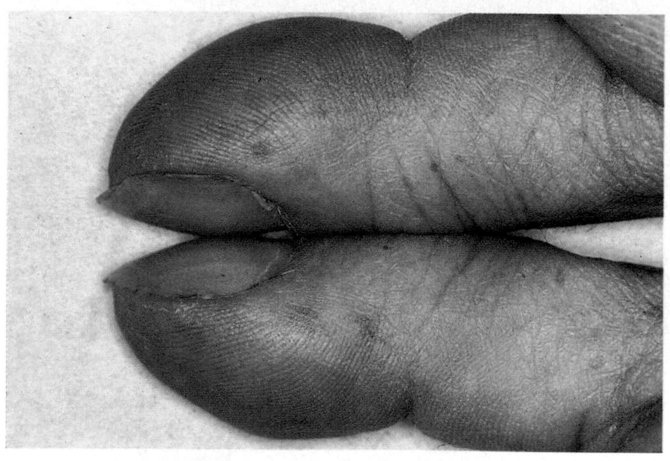

Early clubbing.

TABLE 72-1

Causes of Clubbing

Cardiovascular disorders	Aortic aneurysm* Congenital cardiopathy†
Bronchopulmonary conditions‡	Intrathoracic neoplams Chronic intrathoracic suppurative disease
Gastrointestinal disorders	Inflammatory bowel disease Gastrointestinal neoplasms Liver disorders Multiple polyposis Bacillary and amoebic dysentery
Chronic methemoglobinemia	

*Unilateral
†With cyanosis
‡Associated with hypertrophic osteopathy

FIGURE 72-3

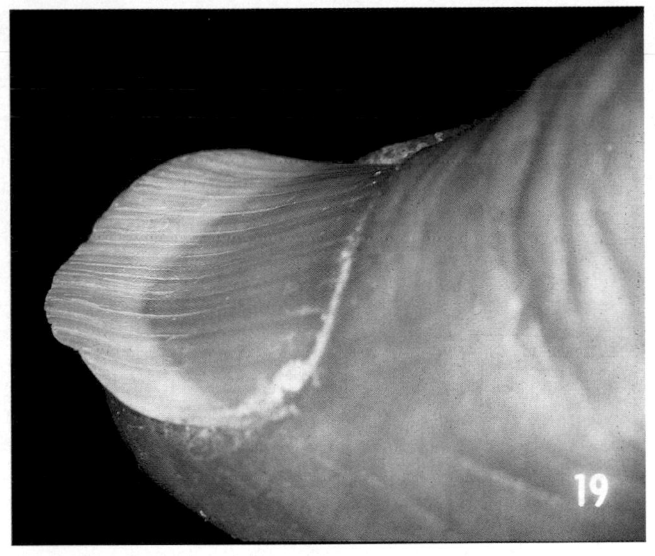

Koilonychia.

trumpet nail). Overcurvature may extend to the point of encompassing a cone of nail bed soft tissue, which can be extremely painful.

In *racquet nail* (Fig. 72-4), the width of the nail bed and nail plate is greater than their length. The racquet thumb is usually inherited as an autosomal dominant trait due to premature obliteration of the epiphyseal line.

Anonychia implies the absence of all or part of one or several nails, which may be congenital (with underlying bone abnormalities) or acquired (e.g., through lichen planus).

Variations in Nail Surface

There are various causes of grooves, ridges, and pits, including local trauma to the nail matrix and acute febrile systemic disease. Poor nutrition to the matrix leads to a defective band of nail formation resulting in a *transverse groove* of thin nail plate (Beau's line) (Fig. 72-5). Recurrent disease will produce recurrent transverse grooves separated by normal nail. The depression may extend all the way to the nail plate, leading to temporary loss of nail. By measuring the position of the transverse grooves, it is possible to date previous illness. Transverse

FIGURE 72-4

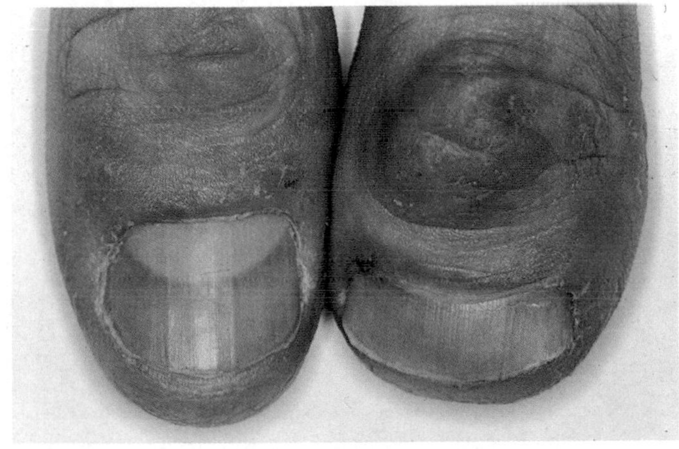

Racquet nail.

FIGURE 72-5

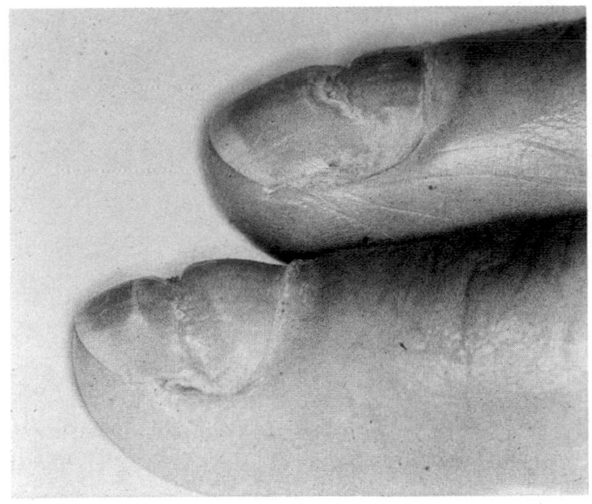

Beau's lines.

grooves are sometimes found in psoriasis. These should be differentiated from "wash-board" nails in which there is also a longitudinal depression usually affecting one or both thumb nails; this commonly results from habitually pushing back the cuticle.

Longitudinal ridges are small rectilinear projections extending from the proximal nail fold to the free edge of the nail. They may be interrupted at regular intervals, giving rise to a beaded appearance. A *longitudinal groove* may run all or part of the length of the nail. *Median canaliform dystrophy of Heller* (Fig. 72-6) is the most distinctive nail surface anomaly. It may be split in the midline with a fir-tree-like appearance of backwards-angled ridges. Thumbs, which are most commonly involved, show usually an enlarged lunula resulting probably from pressure on the base of the nail repeatedly exerted.

A single, wide groove, or *canal,* develops from pressure, permanent or intermittent, on the matrix; it is caused by a tumor-like myxoid cyst (Fig. 72-7). *Ridging* is pronounced in old age, lichen planus, rheumatoid arthritis, peripheral vascular disease, and Darier's disease.

Pits are punctate depressions in the nail, arranged in haphazard or regular patterns. They are characteristic of psoriasis (Fig. 72-8) but may also be found in alopecia areata or in eczema.

FIGURE 72-6

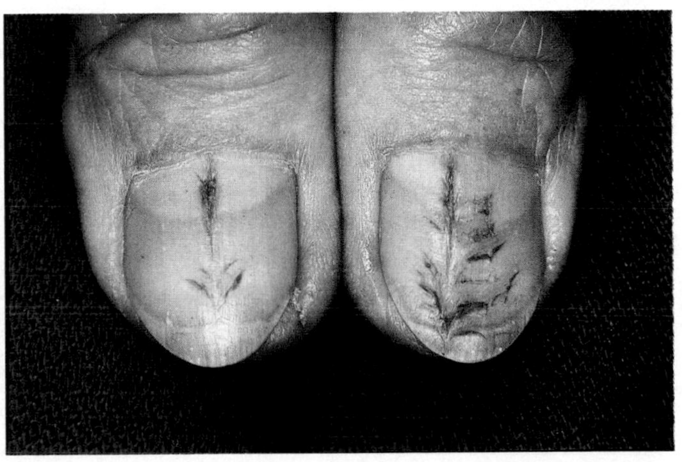

Median canaliform dystrophy of Heller.

FIGURE 72-7

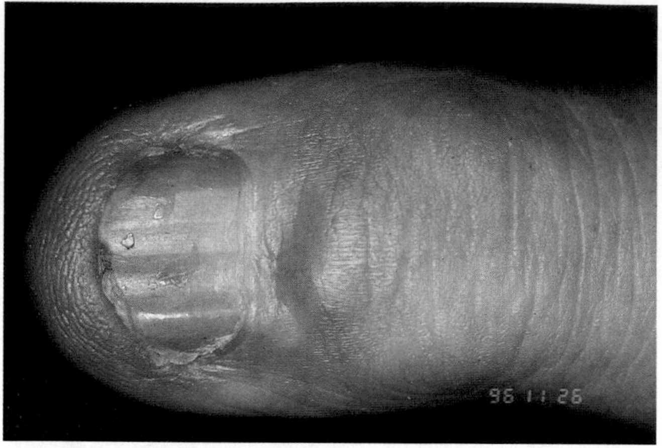

Canal developed from permanent pressure on the matrix due to myxoid cyst.

Trachyonychia (rough nail) is observed in dermatologic diseases as a 20-nail dystrophy or in single finger nails, resulting from external chemical treatment.

Variations in Nail Color

The term *chromonychia* indicates an abnormality in color of the substance and/or the surface of the nail plate and/or subungual tissues. Examination of abnormal nails should be done with the fingers completely relaxed and not pressed against a surface. To differentiate between discoloration of the nail plate itself and the vascular nail bed, the finger tip should be blanched to determine whether the color changes. If the pigment originates from the blood vessels (e.g., in methemoglobinemia), it will usually disappear. If the pigmentation is not altered in the blanching test, it may be obliterated by a penlight pressed against the pulp, meaning that the pigment is deposited in the nail bed; the exact position of the discoloration can then more easily be identified. All digits are usually involved when pigmentation is a result of systemic absorption of a chemical through the skin. When the cause is endogenous, the discoloration often corresponds to the shape of the lunula (Fig. 72-9). By contrast, when the discoloration follows the shape of the *proximal nail fold (PNF),* it is caused by an external contactant (Fig. 72-10). In that case, finger pressure producing blanching does not alter the pigmentation, nor does a penlight placed against the finger pulp. The discoloration can sometimes be removed by scraping or cleaning the nail plate with a solvent such as acetone. To determine if the color is within the nail, a piece of nail should be excised and examined while it is immersed in water. In deeper or subungual impregnation of the nail keratin, microscopic studies (KOH; PAS stain) may be indicated.

FIGURE 72-8

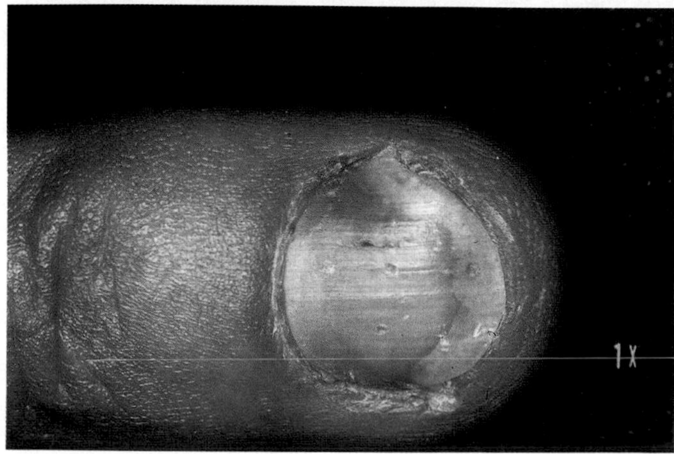

Pits associated with onycholysis.

FIGURE 72-9

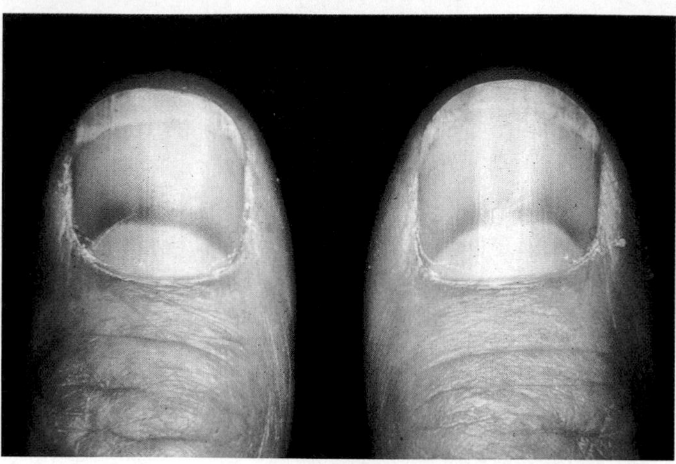

Argyria. The discoloration distal to the lunula corresponds to its shape.

LEUKONYCHIA

True leukonychia This white discoloration of the nail is attributable to matrix dysfunction and presents five patterns: (1) total leukonychia (usually inherited); (2) subtotal leukonychia, when the distal portion of the nail appears normally pink; (3) transverse leukonychia, in which there is a 1- to 2-mm wide transverse arcuate band (Fig. 72-11) reflecting a systemic disorder when several nails are involved; (4) punctate leukonychia, in which white spots result, usually

FIGURE 72-10

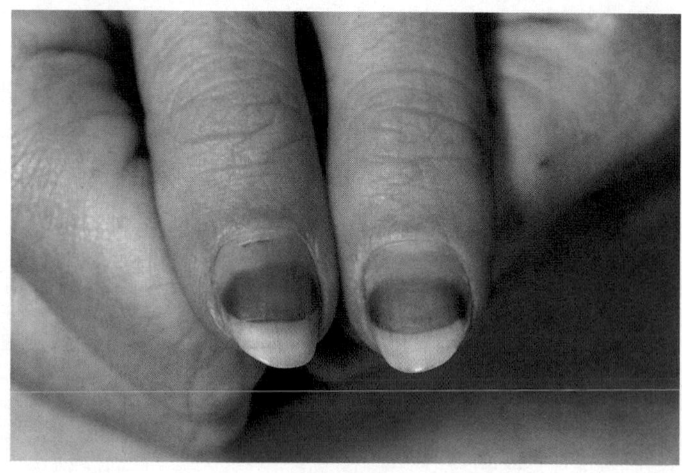

External contactant. The discoloration follows the shape of the proximal nail fold.

FIGURE 72-11

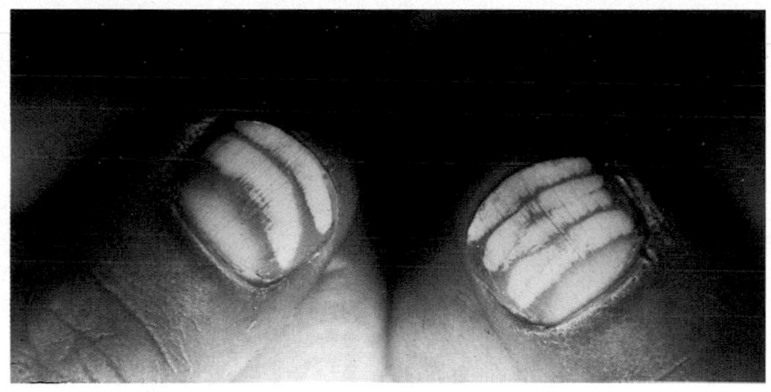

Transverse true leukonychia.

from minor trauma (manicure); and (5) longitudinal leukonychia, which may be associated with Darier's disease.

Pseudoleukonychia This term is used when the nail plate alteration has an external origin, such as in onychomycosis or in keratin granulations observed after nail enamel applications.

Apparent leukonychia The white appearance of the nail is due to changes in the underlying tissue and may present as the following:

1. *Terry's nail* (Fig. 72-12), in which the white discoloration stops suddenly 1 to 2 mm from the distal edge, leaving a pink-brown area 0.5 to 3.0 mm wide. This condition, which involves all nails uniformly, is associated with cirrhosis of the liver, chronic congestive heart failure, or adult-onset diabetes mellitus.
2. *Half-and-half nail* with the two parts showing a sharp demarcation. The proximal area is dull white, and the distal area (20 to 60 percent of the total length) is brownish. It has been reported in uremic patients.
3. *Muehrcke's paired, narrow white bands* (Fig. 72-13) parallel the lunula in the nail bed and are commonly associated with hypoalbuminemia or following chemotherapy.

SPLINTER HEMORRHAGES These longitudinal hemorrhages in the distal nail bed conform to the pattern of subungual vessels. Emphasis has recently been given to their association with the antiphospholipid syndrome. Proximal splinter hemorrhages have been reported in bacterial endocarditis, trichinosis, and onychomatricoma. They may be seen following external trauma.

FIGURE 72-12

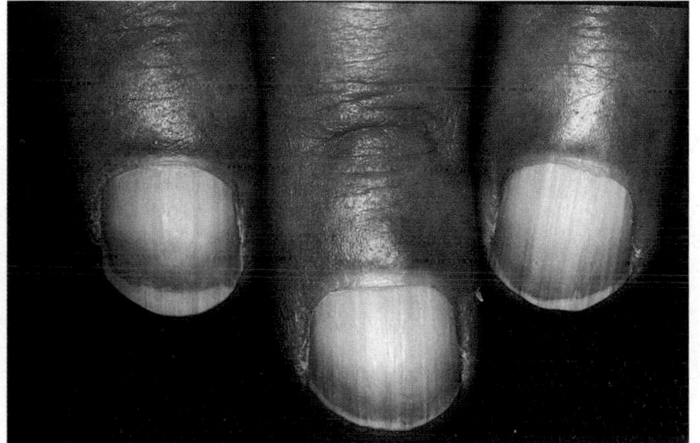

Apparent leukonychia: Terry's nail.

FIGURE 72-13

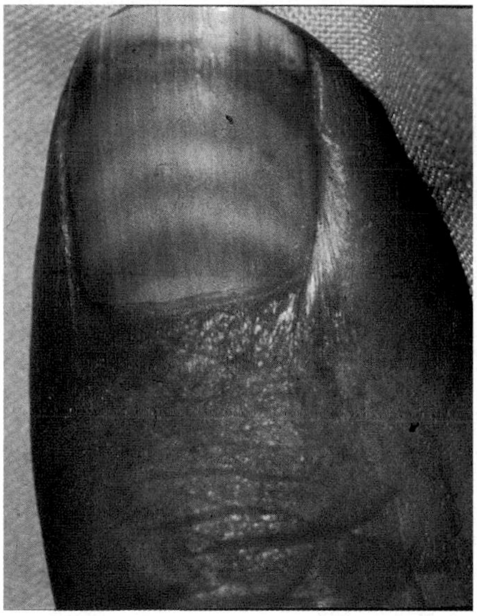

Apparent leukonychia: Muehrcke's paired, narrow white bands.

Variations in Direction of Nail Growth

ONYCHOGRYPHOSIS (Fig. 72-14) In this disorder, the nail is severely distorted, thickened, opaque, brownish, spiraled, and without attachment to the nail bed. The nail of the great toe is particularly vulnerable; it is often shaped like a ram's horn or an oyster. Nail keratin is produced by the nail matrix at uneven rates, with the faster-growing side determining the direction of the deformity. Onychogryphosis is usually caused by pressure from footwear in the elderly. In rare cases, it may be produced by acute trauma, and rarely it is inherited as an autosomal dominant trait. Hemionychogryphosis with lateral deviation of the nail plate often results from congenital malalignment of the big toenail.

MALALIGNMENT OF THE NAIL PLATE Congenital malalignment of the nail of the great toe (Fig. 72-15)[2] is often misdiagnosed even

FIGURE 72-14

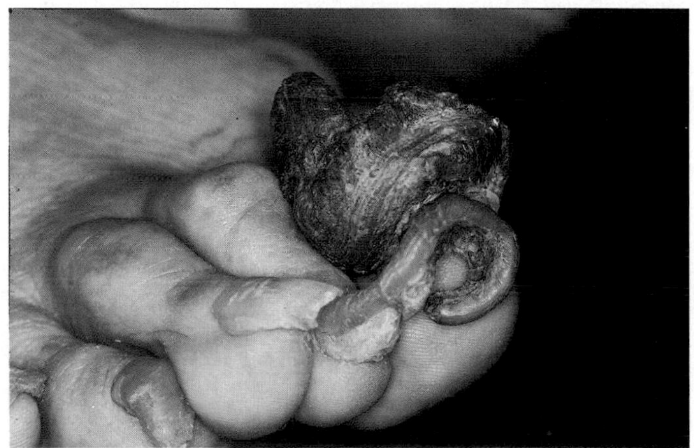

Onychogryphosis.

FIGURE 72-15

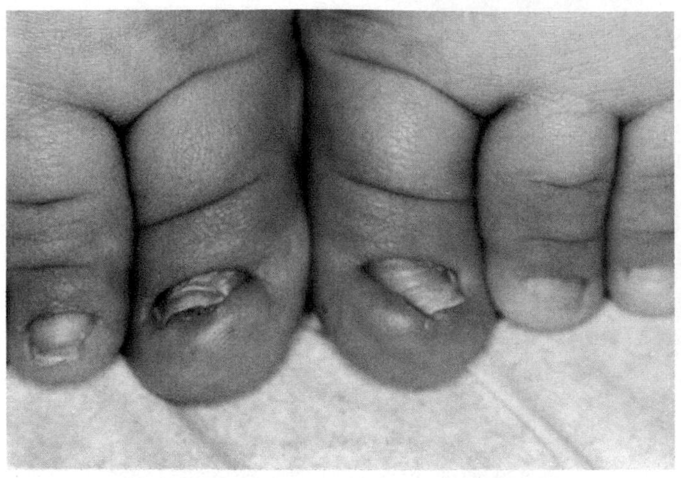

Malalignment of the great toe nails.

though it is a common condition. It consists of a lateral deviation of the long axis of nail growth relative to the distal phalanx. This would be of minor importance if it were not for local complications that may arise both in infancy and adulthood. Some cases of this inherited condition have, however, a tendency to improve spontaneously. Photographic surveys should be made at regular intervals to monitor the need for possible surgery which rotates the nail plate. Acquired traumatic malposition may follow acute trauma. Broad lateral longitudinal surgical excision of the nail apparatus may also cause malalignment of the remaining nail. Acquired traumatic malposition may follow acute trauma.

HOOK NAIL This reflects bowing of the nail bed due to a lack of support from the short bony phalanx.

Pathologic Reactions in Periungual Tissue

ABNORMALITIES IN PARONYCHIAL TISSUE The proximal nail fold (PNF) adheres tightly to the dorsum of the nail plate, and its free border, producing the cuticle, seals the proximal nail groove. The PNF can become acutely or chronically inflamed.

Acute paronychia may follow any break in the skin. The infection starts in the paronychium at the side of the nail, with local redness, swelling, and pain. If it does not show clear signs of response to penicillinase-resistant antibiotics within 2 days, partial avulsion of the base of the nail plate should be performed.

Chronic paronychia is a separate disorder prevalent in individuals whose hands are subjected to moist local environments and is often due to contact dermatitis. It manifests as a red, semicircular indurated cushion around the base of the nail, which is detached from the distal portion of the PNF that has lost its cuticle. This is followed by secondary retraction of the paronychial tissue. From time to time, the persistent low-grade inflammation may flare into subacute painful exacerbations. This causes disturbances of the nail plate that may produce discolored, cross-ridged lateral edges, reflecting *Candida* invasion.

Dorsal pterygium (Fig. 72-16) consists of a gradual shortening of the proximal nail groove, leading to progressive thinning of the nail plate and secondary fissuring caused by the fusion of the PNF to the matrix and subsequently to the nail bed. The portions of the divided nail plate progressively decrease in size as the pterygium widens. After several years, the pathologic process results in total loss of the nail, with permanent atrophy and sometimes scarring in the nail area. Pterygium is characteristic of lichen planus. It may also follow severe bullous dermatoses, radiotherapy, trauma, or digital ischemia. Rarely, it is congenital.

FIGURE 72-16

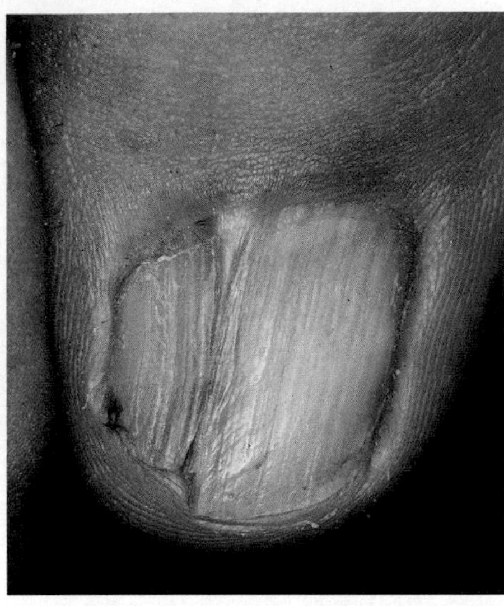

Dorsal pterygium.

Ventral pterygium (Fig. 72-17) is a distal extension of the hyponychial tissue that is anchored to the undersurface of the nail, thereby obliterating the distal groove. Several conditions can cause ventral pterygium including: scleroderma associated with Raynaud's phenomenon, causalgia of the median nerve, trauma, and a reaction to a formaldehyde-containing nail cosmetic. Congenital forms exist.

FAULTY ATTACHMENT OF NAIL PLATE AND SOFT TISSUE *Nail shedding,* which is the spontaneous separation of the nail from the matrix, is called *onychomadesis* and is usually latent (Fig. 72-18). The nail plate shows a transverse split but continues growing for some time because there is no disruption in its attachment to the nail bed. Growth ceases when the nail is cast off after losing this connection. The process termed *onychoptosis defluvium,* or alopecia unguium, is sometimes a component of alopecia areata, even though it is confined to the nails. *Onycholysis* (Fig. 72-19) refers to the detachment of the nail from its bed starting at its distal and/or lateral attachment. The nail plate–nail bed separation extends proximally along a convex line, creating a subungual space that gathers dirt and keratin debris. The grayish-white color is due to the presence of air beneath the nail, but the color may vary according the etiology.

FIGURE 72-17

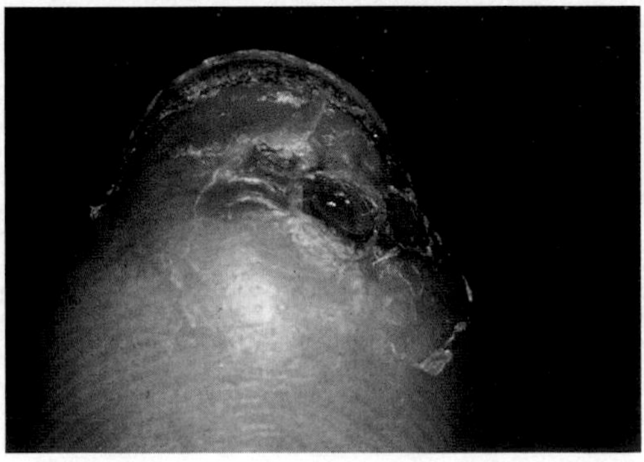

Ventral pterygium.

FIGURE 72-18

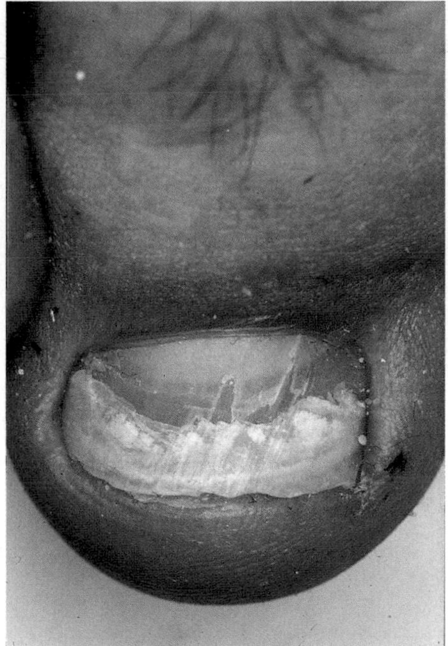

Latent onychomadesis.

Variation in Consistency

Hard nails are a major characteristic of the pachyonychia congenita syndrome. *Soft nail* disease may be congenital (unusual) or acquired, occupational contact with water and chemicals being the most common cause. *Brittle nails* may be divided into three types, in isolation or combination:

1. Splitting, more often single than multiple, sometimes associated with shallow parallel furrows, called *onychorrhexis,* and running along the dorsum of the nail.
2. Lamellar, splitting involving either the free edge, following frequent water immersion, or the proximal surface of the nail associated with lichen planus, or oral retinoids therapy.
3. Transverse splitting and breaking of the lateral edge close to the free margin.

FIGURE 72-19

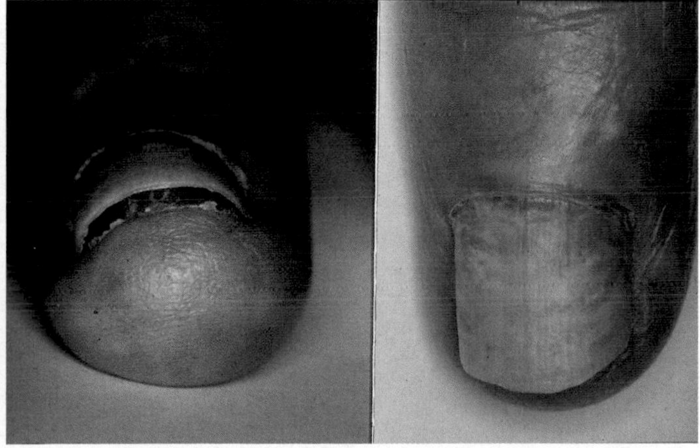

Onycholysis.

The dorsum of the nail may be friable in superficial onychomycosis as well as following nail enamel use. Friability may extend throughout the entire nail in advanced psoriasis and onychomycosis.

NAIL ABNORMALITIES IN DERMATOLOGIC DISORDERS

PSORIASIS Nail abnormalities are seen in 10 to 55 percent of adults with psoriasis. They are less common in children (7 to 13 percent). Psoriasis limited to the nails is quite frequent.

The following nail abnormalities are highly suggestive for a diagnosis of psoriasis: irregular pitting, salmon patches of the nail bed, and onycholysis. All these nail abnormalities are almost exclusively found in the fingernails. Nail pitting results from the presence of easily detachable parakeratotic cells in the superficial layers of the nail plate. This nail abnormality indicates a disturbance in the maturation and keratinization of the proximal nail matrix. In psoriasis, pits are typically deep, large, irregular in size, and randomly distributed. Salmon patches appear as yellow or salmon-pink areas, irregular in size and shape, visible through the transparent nail plate. They result from a psoriatic involvement of the nail bed.

The term *onycholysis* describes the distal or lateral detachment of the nail plate from the nail bed. Onycholysis may be a consequence of inflammatory, traumatic, or neoplastic conditions that involve the nail bed. In psoriasis, the onycholytic area is characteristically surrounded by an erythematous margin that marks its proximal border (Figs. 72-8 and 72-20). In addition to these three clinical signs, which are very useful for diagnosis, psoriasis of the nail produces other nail abnormalities that are not diagnostic, including splinter hemorrhages, nail bed hyperkeratosis, thickening and crumbling of the nail plate, and chronic paronychia. In the absence of skin lesions or typical nail signs, the differential diagnosis of nail psoriasis includes the disorders listed in Table 72-2.

When psoriasis is limited to the toenails, the differential diagnosis from onychomycosis may be very difficult, because toenail psoriasis most commonly produces massive subungual hyperkeratosis and onycholysis clinically indistinguishable from those of onychomycosis

FIGURE 72-20

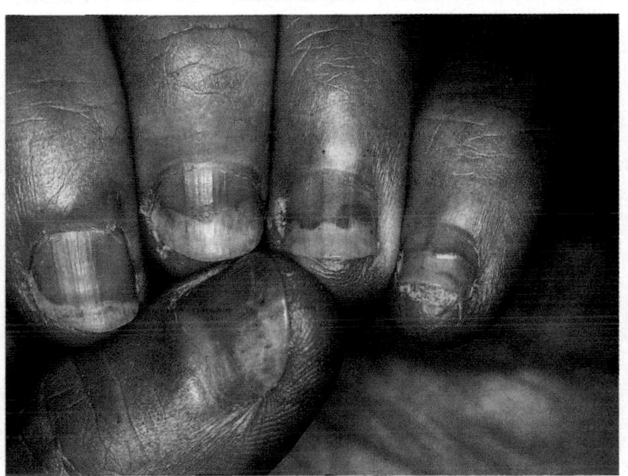

Nail psoriasis. Onycholysis and salmon patches of the nail bed.

TABLE 72-2

Differential Diagnosis of Nail Psoriasis

Contact dermatitis
Inflammatory linear verrucous epidermal nevus
Keratoderma
Keratoderma blennorrhagica
Keratotic scabies
Lichen planus
Onychomycosis
Parakeratosis pustulosa
Pityriasis rubra pilaris
Reiter's disease

(Fig. 72-21). Psoriasis and onychomycosis actually are also frequently associated because psoriatic nails are more susceptible to fungal invasion than healthy nails.

Nail psoriasis is difficult to treat.[3] Patients must be instructed to avoid traumas that may trigger or worsen their condition (Koebner's phenomenon). When onycholysis is present, the detached nail plate should be removed. Systemic administration of methotrexate or cyclosporin A may improve the nail changes, but these drugs are not recommended in the absence of extensive skin psoriasis. Intralesional steroid injections (10 mg/mL) are effective but very painful. Retinoids and PUVA are scarcely effective and may even worsen the nail changes. Topical application of creams containing steroids and salicylic acid, and/or topical application of calcipotriol ointment may be useful. Because nail psoriasis is frequently associated with psoriatic arthropathy (Fig. 72-22), a rheumatological evaluation is advisable.

PUSTULAR PSORIASIS/HALLOPEAU'S ACRODERMATITIS CONTINUA This condition frequently involves the nails and the periungual tissues. The disease, which is most frequently localized to one digit (usually a finger), typically shows a chronic course with periodic episodes of painful acute inflammation. In the acute phase, the affected digit shows severe inflammatory changes with pustular lesions of the nail bed and periungual skin (Fig. 72-23). In the chronic phase, the nail bed and the periungual tissues show erythema and scaling. The nail plate is onycholytic or absent. The condition often

FIGURE 72-21

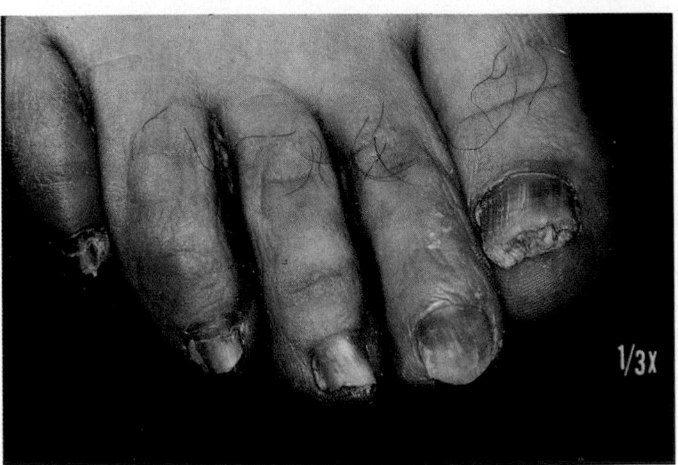

Toenail psoriasis showing massive nail bed hyperkeratosis.

FIGURE 72-22

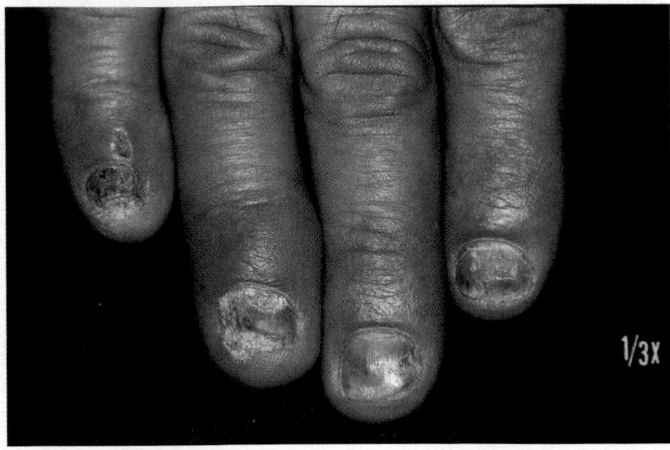

Nail psoriasis associated with psoriatic arthropathy.

improves with topical calcipotriol. Systemic retinoids may be useful in severe cases.[4]

PARAKERATOSIS PUSTULOSA This condition, which is exclusively seen in children, usually involves one finger, most commonly the thumb or the index finger. The affected nail shows subungual hyperkeratosis and onycholysis, which are usually more marked on one side of the nail (Fig. 72-24). Erythema and scaling of the fingertip is typical, but not always present. Parakeratosis pustulosa is possibly a variety of psoriasis and some children develop typical nail psoriasis later in life. The disease usually regresses spontaneously at puberty.

LICHEN PLANUS Nail involvement occurs in about 10 percent of patients with lichen planus. Lichen planus limited to the nails is uncommon but not exceptional. It may be observed in children.[5]

FIGURE 72-23

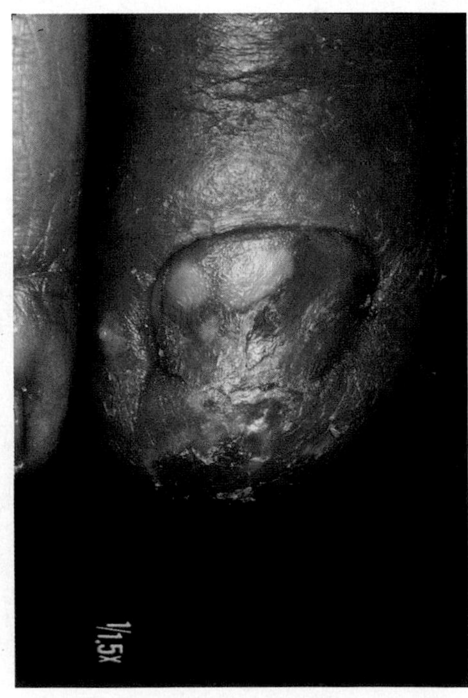

Hallopeau's acrodermatitis. Pustular lesions of the nail bed.

FIGURE 72-24

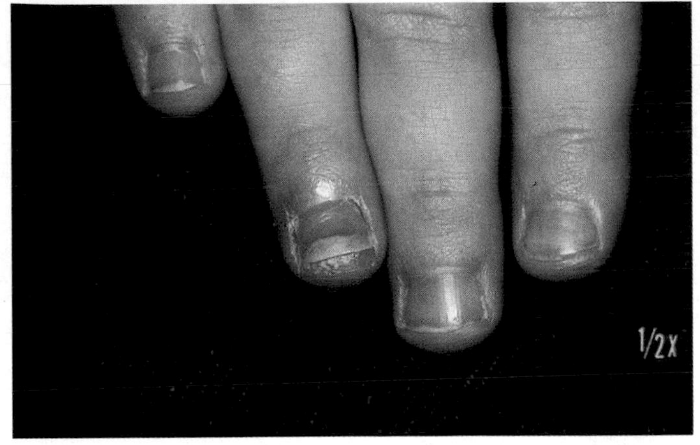

Parakeratosis pustulosa. This child has psoriasiform nail lesions associated with fingertip scaling of one digit.

Lichen planus of the nail matrix is a harmful condition because it frequently produces diffuse nail scarring (Fig. 72-25). Nail abnormalities that are highly suggestive of lichen planus include dorsal pterygium and diffuse nail thinning and splitting. Pterygium appears as an extension of the skin of the proximal nail fold that expands distally to adhere to the nail bed (Fig. 72-25). Although lichen planus is the most common cause of nail pterygium, this lesion may be a consequence of nail matrix destruction by other conditions, including trauma, digital ischemia, and bullous disorders. Nail thinning and splitting are consequences of diffuse and mild involvement of the nail matrix by lichen planus. The nail plate is diffusely or partially thinned and presents longitudinal ridging and splitting (Fig. 72-26). Nail bed lichen planus produces subungual hyperkeratosis and onycholysis. Yellow-nail–like changes are not uncommon in toenails and may also affect fingernails. In children, nail lichen planus may present with atypical features such as trachyonychia or idiopathic atrophy of the nails.[6] Differential diagnosis of these clinical features include traumatic nail lesions, tumors that compress the nail matrix, age-related nail changes, systemic amyloidosis, and lichen striatus.

The definitive diagnosis of nail matrix lichen planus requires a nail biopsy. Except for trachyonychia, treatment of nail lichen planus is mandatory, because if left untreated, it may produce diffuse nail scarring (Fig. 72-26). Systemic (triamcinolone 0.5 to 1 mg/kg IM every 30 days) or intralesional steroids are effective. Acitretin is also effective.

FIGURE 72-25

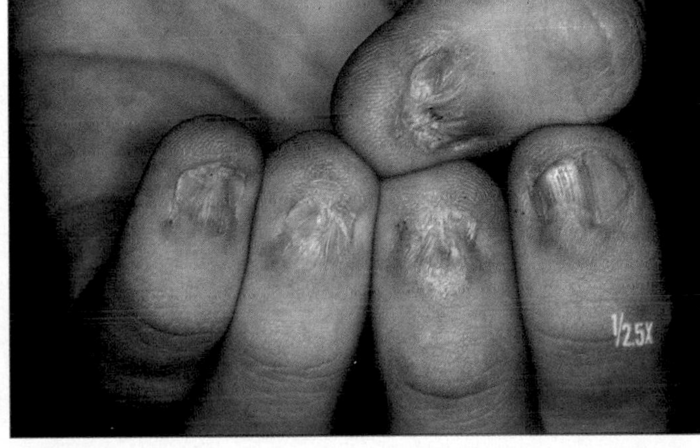

Severe nail scarring due to lichen planus.

FIGURE 72-26

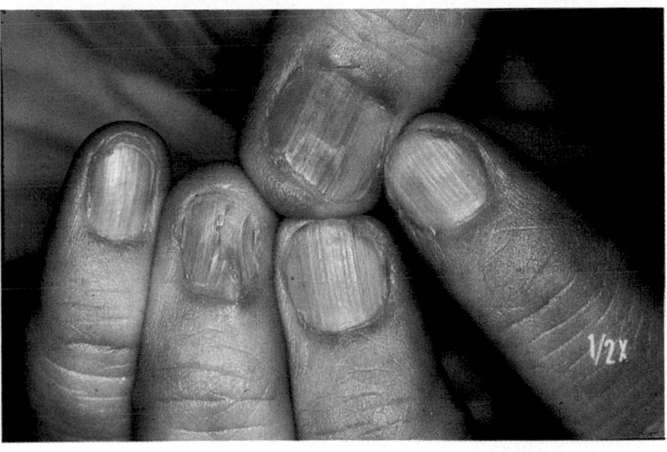

Diffuse nail thinning and onychorrhexis due to lichen planus.

ALOPECIA AREATA Nail abnormalities are frequent in patients with alopecia areata, particularly in children. They may precede or follow the onset of the disease and usually regress spontaneously. The changes include geometric pitting, mottled erythema of the lunulae, and trachyonychia. Pits are usually small, superficial, and regularly distributed in a geometric pattern.

Trachyonychia observed in 20-nail dystrophy describes nail roughness caused by excessive longitudinal striations. This nail sign is not exclusive to alopecia areata because it can also be a sign of other inflammatory disorders such as lichen planus, psoriasis, eczema, and pemphigus vulgaris.[7] The affected nails may be opaque (sandpapered nails) (Fig. 72-27) or, less frequently, have a shiny appearance (Fig. 72-28). Trachyonychia is more frequent in children, where it may be an isolated sign (idiopathic trachyonychia).

DARIER'S DISEASE The nail abnormalities are diagnostic and consist of longitudinal subungual white and red streaks. White streaks are

FIGURE 72-27

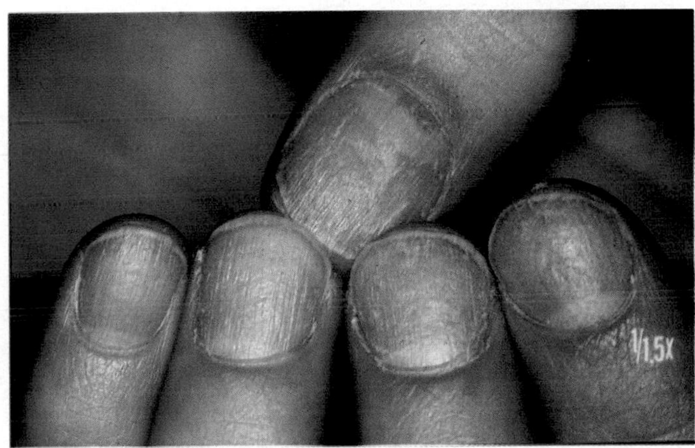

Trachyonychia. Sandpapered nails.

FIGURE 72-28

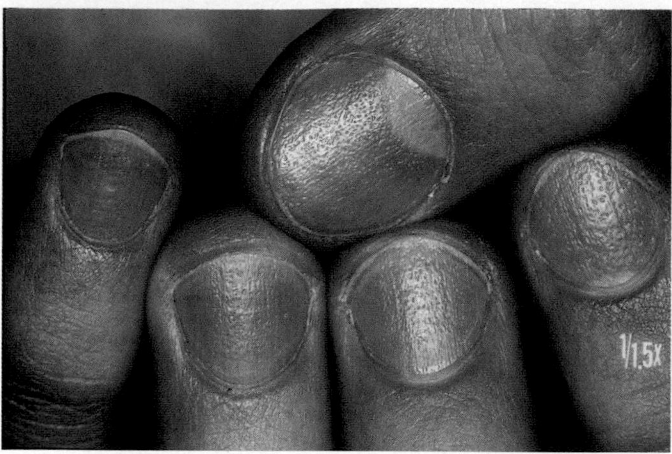

Shiny appearance in 20-nail dystrophy. Multiple superficial pits distributed in a regular pattern.

associated with V-shaped distal notching due to wedge-shaped hyperkeratotic papules of the distal nail bed (Fig. 72-29).

CONTACT DERMATITIS Irritant and allergic contact dermatitis may occasionally be localized to the nail, where they most commonly affect the proximal nail fold and the hyponychium.

Contact dermatitis of the proximal nail fold is responsible for chronic paronychia and nail plate surface abnormalities, such as irregular pitting and Beau's lines. These are caused by mild involvement of the adjacent proximal nail matrix. Contact dermatitis of the hyponychium produces severe subungual hyperkeratosis and nail bed splinter hemorrhages (Fig. 72-30). The differential diagnosis includes onychomycosis, psoriasis, parakeratosis pustulosa, pityriasis rubra pilaris, and keratoderma.

FIGURE 72-29

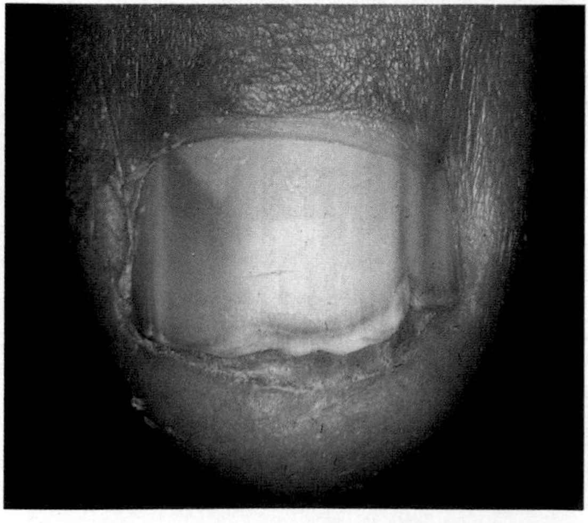

Darier's disease. Red and white streaks with distal V-shaped notches.

FIGURE 72-30

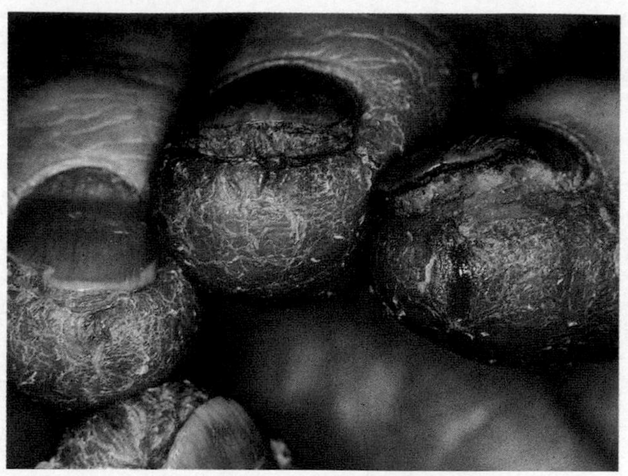

Contact dermatitis of the hyponychium and distal tip with severe subungual hyperkeratosis.

NAIL ABNORMALITIES ASSOCIATED WITH GENERAL MEDICAL CONDITIONS[7]

Examination of the nails may sometimes offer a clue for the diagnosis of systemic conditions. Nail signs that may indicate a systemic illness are listed in Table 72-3.

Collagen disorders

PROXIMAL NAIL FOLD CAPILLARY ABNORMALITIES Proximal nail fold capillaries can easily be examined using a portable ophthalmoscope.

In systemic sclerosis and dermatomyositis, proximal nail fold capillaries are limited due to the presence of avascular areas. Enlarged capillary loops are present (Fig. 72-31).

In systemic lupus erythematosus, capillary density is normal, but capillary loops are tortuous and meandering.

CLUBBING Clubbing may be associated with joint effusion and periosteal bone formation. Clubbing or hypertrophic osteoarthropathy may be a consequence of a large number of diseases that involve tissues with a vagus nerve supply (see Table 72-1).

TABLE 72-3

Nail Signs in Systemic Illness

Beau's lines—onychomadesis	High fever Peripheral nerve injury Surgery Drugs
Koilonychia	Sideropenic anemia
Proximal splinter hemorrhages	Bacterial endocarditis Trichinosis Vasculitis
Periungual erythema	"Collagen" disease HIV infection HCV infection
Lichenoid nail changes with hemorrhages	Systemic amyloidosis

FIGURE 72-31

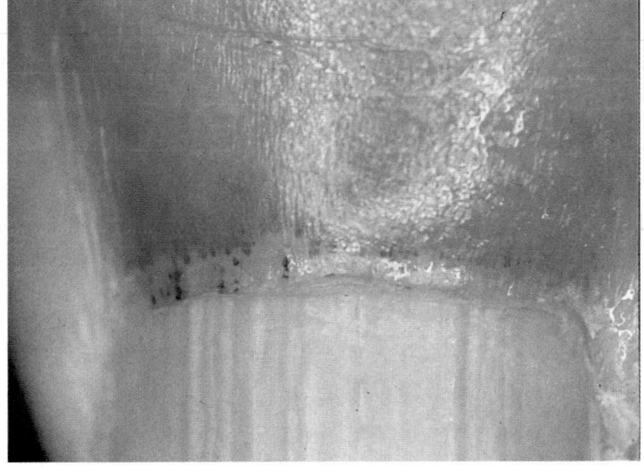

Systemic sclerosis. Avascular areas and enlarged capillaries.

TABLE 72-4

Systemic Causes of Acroosteolysis

Neurologic disorders	Peripheral neuropathies
	Diabetes
	Leprosy
	Carpal tunnel syndrome
	Cervical rib
	Myelopathies
	Tabes dorsalis
	Syringomyelia
Vascular disease	Atherosclerosis
	Perniosis
	Buerger's disease
	Raynaud's disease
	Systemic sclerosis

ACROOSTEOLYSIS Destructive changes in the distal phalangeal bone may be associated with minimal skin changes or with ischemic skin lesions that may result in digital necrosis (Fig. 72-32). The affected digits usually show bulbous fingertips with soft tissue thickening and pseudo-clubbing. Shortening of the distal phalanges causes the nails to appear abnormally broad (acquired racquet nails). Acroosteolysis results from a wide variety of systemic and localized disorders that produce impaired phalangeal perfusion (Table 72-4).

ACROKERATOSIS PARANEOPLASTICA OF BAZEX This condition is characterized by psoriasiform changes of hands, feet, ears, and nose. Involvement of the nails and periungual tissues is characteristic, nail lesions being indistinguishable from nail psoriasis (Fig. 72-33). Acrokeratosis paraneoplastica of Bazex occurs in association with malignant epitheliomata of the upper respiratory or digestive tract and may precede the diagnosis of the tumor.

YELLOW NAIL SYNDROME This condition is typically characterized by an arrest in the nail growth. Fingernails and toenails are hard and excessively curved from side to side and show a diffuse pale yellow to dark yellow-green discoloration. Cuticles are absent. Secondary onycholysis is frequent (Fig. 72-34). In typical cases, the nail changes are associated with lymphedema and respiratory tract involvement. Yellow nail syndrome may occasionally be a paraneoplastic sign. The nail changes may benefit from treatment with high dosages of vitamin E combined with systemic itraconazole or fluconazole.

PSEUDO-INFLAMMATORY CHANGES Digital ischemia frequently produces massive swelling, erythema, and pain of the nails and periungual tissues, which resemble acute paronychia. The affected digit, however, is cold. Digital metastases may also produce an acute paronychia-like picture.

MELANONYCHIA Multiple bands of longitudinal melanonychia may be a consequence of pharmacologic treatment and numerous systemic diseases including AIDS, Addison's disease, Cushing's syndrome, hyperthyroidism, folic acid or vitamin B_{12} deficiency (Fig. 72-35). Transverse melanonychia is frequently observed in patients undergoing anticancer chemotherapy.

DRUG-INDUCED NAIL CHANGES Drugs may produce a large number of nail abnormalities.[7,8] Usually, several nails are

FIGURE 72-32

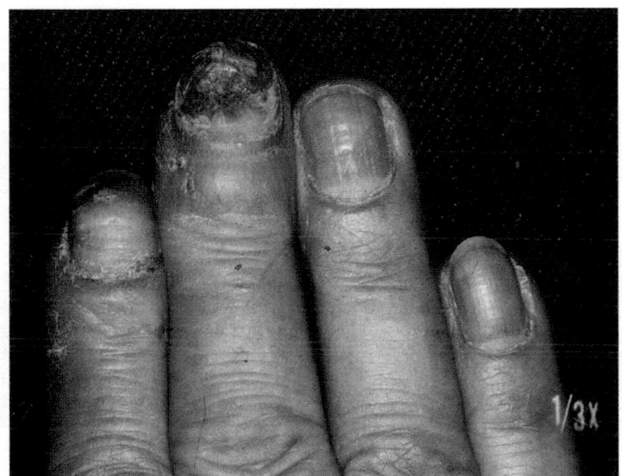

Necrotic nail lesions and acroosteolysis in a patient with carpal tunnel syndrome.

FIGURE 72-33

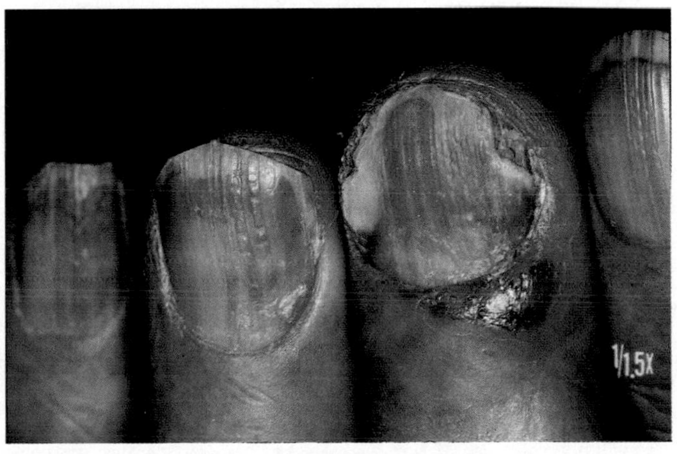

Psoriasiform nail lesions due to Bazex' syndrome.

FIGURE 72-34

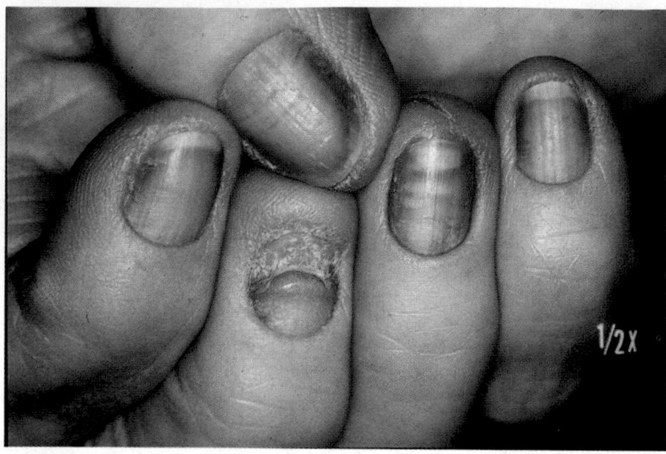

Yellow nail syndrome. Transverse overcurvature with loss of cuticle.

simultaneously affected and the nail changes regress after withdrawal of the drug. Table 72-5 lists the most common nail changes induced by drugs.

HEREDITARY AND CONGENITAL NAIL DISORDERS[9]

Nail defects occurring between the ninth and twentieth week of fetal life are called *embryopathies*. They include abnormalities of the nail matrix (absence, reduction, position, or function) and/or nail bed (hereditary partial onycholysis, pachyonychia congenita). *Fetopathies* occur after 20 weeks of gestation (malformations due to drugs).

The term *hereditary ectodermal dysplasia* is used to cover a heterogeneous group of primary epidermal disorders in which one of the following signs occur: hypotrichosis, hypodontia, onychodysplasia, and anhidrosis, plus at least one sign affecting other structures of epidermal origin (see Chap. 53).

FIGURE 72-35

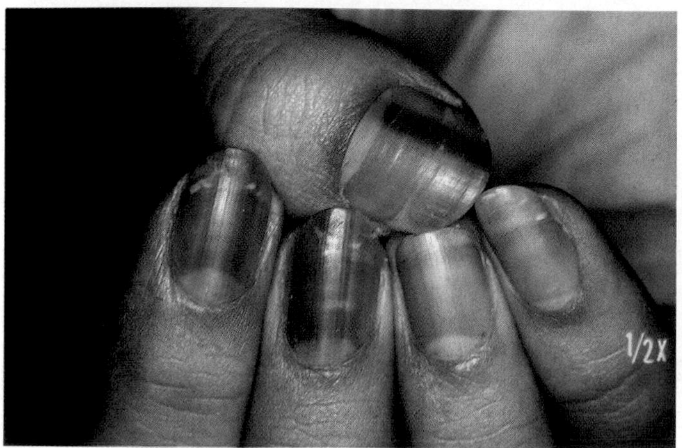

Multiple bands on longitudinal melanonychia in a patient with AIDS.

TABLE 72-5

Drug-Induced Nail Changes

Drugs	Symptom
Retinoids	Nail brittleness Pseudopyogenic granuloma
Azidothymidine (AZT)	Melanonychia
Indinavir	Paronychia/pyogenic granuloma
β-Blockers	Digital ischemia
Antineoplastic	Melanonychia Onycholysis/photoonycholysis Apparent leukonychia Beau's lines Onychomadesis
PUVA therapy	Melanonychia Photoonycholysis

In the *nail-patella syndrome,* there is an association of nail changes, triangular lunula, and usually partial nail loss (Fig. 72-36), with the severity of the defects decreasing from the thumb to the fifth finger. Skeletal abnormalities, such as an absent or hypoplastic patella, iliac horns, and kidney involvement with collagen-like fibrils in the glomerular basement membrane, are also found.

In *pachyonychia congenita,* an autosomal dominant keratin disorder, thickening of the nail and subungual hyperkeratosis appear in infants up to 6 months of age, but late onset has also been reported. Jadassohn-Lewandowsky syndrome is characterized by hyperkeratosis of palms and soles, follicular keratosis, and oral leukoplakia, as well as a striking increase in thickness of the distal portion of the nail and yellow to brown discoloration with pinched margins and upward tilt of distal tips (Fig. 72-37). This may interfere with the coordination of finger movement, sometimes leading to ablation of the nail matrix and bed.

Nail changes in dystrophic and junctional forms of *epidermolysis bullosa (EB)* are common, but although they strongly suggest the disease, they are not pathognomonic. They result from abnormalities of the nail matrix and nail bed, associated with the pathogenetic alterations of the dermal-epidermal junction that occur in EB. In addition, secondary trauma in the areas of dermal-epidermal separation and chronic inflammation of the nail matrix are probably contributory factors, even in nonscarring forms of EB.

FIGURE 72-36

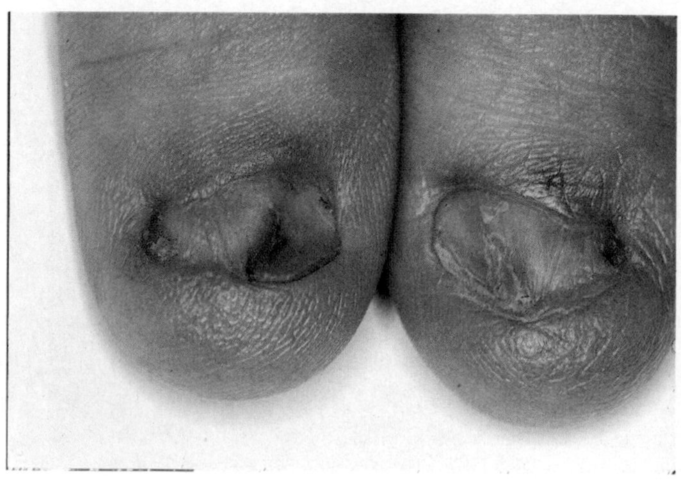

Partial nail loss in nail-patella syndrome.

FIGURE 72-37

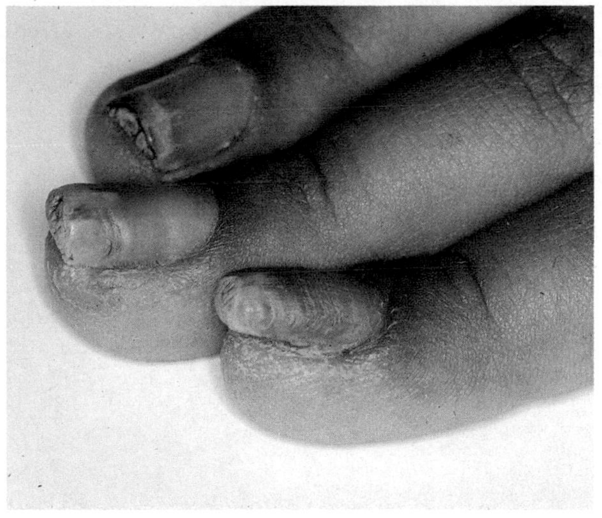

Pachyonychia congenita.

FIGURE 72-38

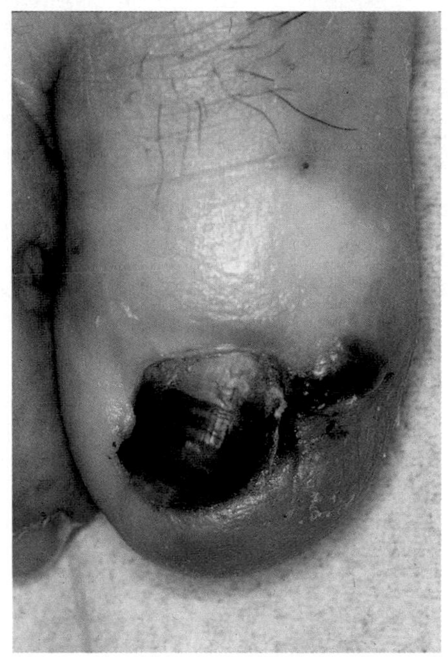

Keratin implantation cyst following surgery for ingrown toenail.

TUMORS INVOLVING THE NAIL AREA[10]

Epithelial Tumors

Warts are benign, fibroepithelial tumors that are caused by human papilloma viruses (HPV) of different types, most frequently HPV-1, HPV-2, and HPV-4, but other HPV types have also been isolated from the nail region. Periungual and subungual warts are mildly contagious and probably caused by inoculation of HPV DNA into the skin after biting or picking. Periungual warts are circumscribed keratotic papules with a rough verrucous surface; they sometimes exhibit fissures and clefts that may cause pain and give rise to secondary bacterial infections. The warts may merge to form larger, plaquelike tumors. When extending under the nail plate, they may raise the plate, causing discoloration, loss of transparency, or splitting and breaking of the plate. Any pressure may then be painful. Even bone erosion from subungual warts has been observed. Injection of bleomycin is one of the best treatments.

Keratin implantation cysts (Fig. 72-38), which are lined with epidermis and filled with keratin, are occasionally observed under the nail. They are most commonly due to trauma that causes a laceration of the nail bed and start to grow after the patient has already forgotten the injury. Depending on the location in the nail apparatus, the keratin cyst may appear as a large subungual tumor raising the nail plate or causing a bulbous enlargement of the terminal phalanx. Intraosseous epidermal cysts may lead to spontaneous fracture and may mimic a bone tumor or intraosseous metastasis. An x-ray is mandatory and will show a sharply demarcated, round defect. Cysts lined with matrix epithelium and filled with keratin-like nail substance have been observed after incomplete removal of the lateral matrix horn.

Onychomatricoma (Fig. 72-39) is a recently described distinctive tumor of the nail matrix.[11] The clinical criteria for diagnosis include a longitudinal band of yellow thickening of the nail plate, increased transverse curvature of the nail, and splinter hemorrhages in the proximal portion of the nail. Histologically the tumor is characterized by filiform epithelial projections in the center of which traumatic clefts or parakeratotic columns are visible.

Keratoacanthomas (Fig. 72-40) are benign, but rapidly growing, locally aggressive tumors, which sometimes occur on the nail apparatus.[12] Keratoacanthomas in this site differ from those of the skin. The most frequent location is the hyponychium or the lateral nail groove from which the lesion may grow under the nail plate. Keratoacanthomas usually start as small, painful nodules visible under the nail plate margin. They may achieve a diameter of 1 to 2 cm within 4 to 8 weeks. Whereas the typical dome shape is not usually seen, there is almost always a central keratotic plug that tends to be extruded upon pressure on

FIGURE 72-39

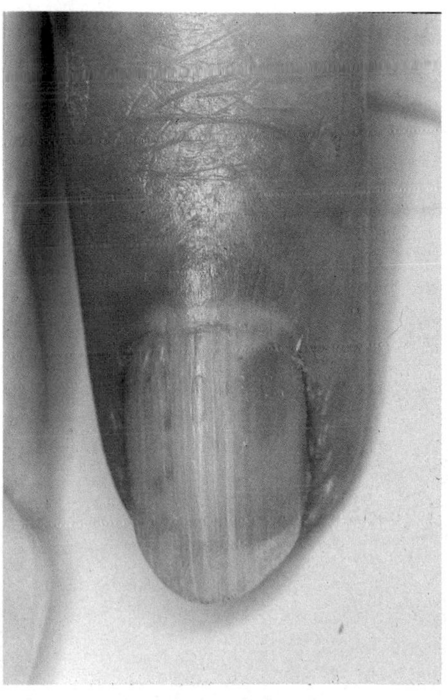

Onychomatricoma. Longitudinal xanthonychia.

FIGURE 72-40

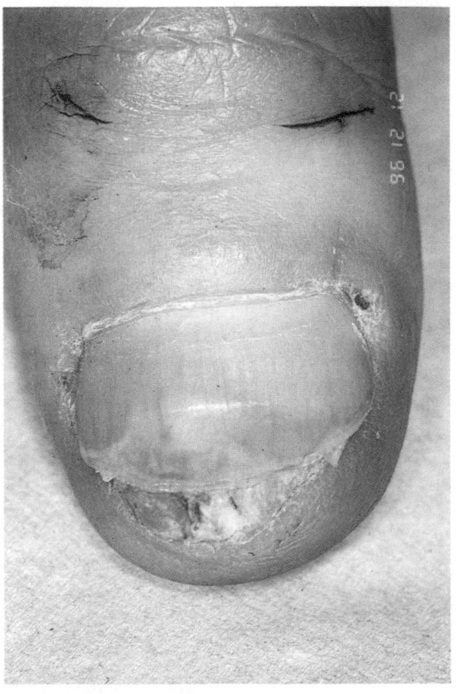

Distal subungual keratoacanthoma.

the surrounding tissue. Pain is a very typical symptom of subungual keratoacanthoma. The subungual tumors reported in adolescents or young adults in incontinentia pigmenti are probably true keratoacanthomas.

Fibrous Tumors

Fibrous tumors encompass a wide spectrum of clinical manifestations although the histology is quite uniform.

ACQUIRED PERIUNGUAL FIBROKERATOMA (See Fig. 72-41) This presents as an asymptomatic nodule with a hyperkeratotic tip and a narrow base, occurring mostly in the periungual area. The fibrokeratoma often emerges from beneath the PNF, grows on the nail,

FIGURE 72-41

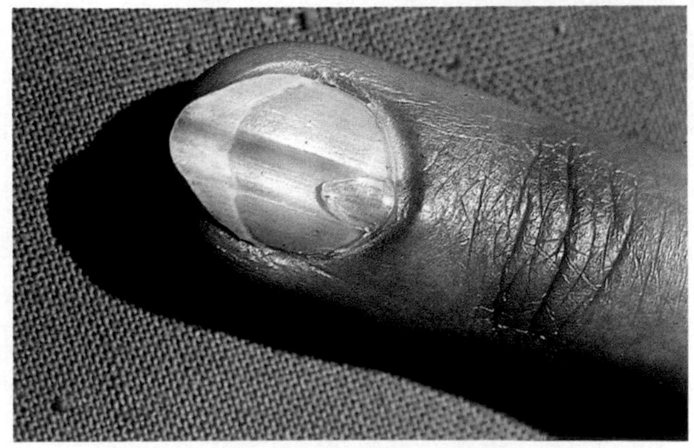

Acquired fibrokeratoma causing a sharp longitudinal depression.

FIGURE 72-42

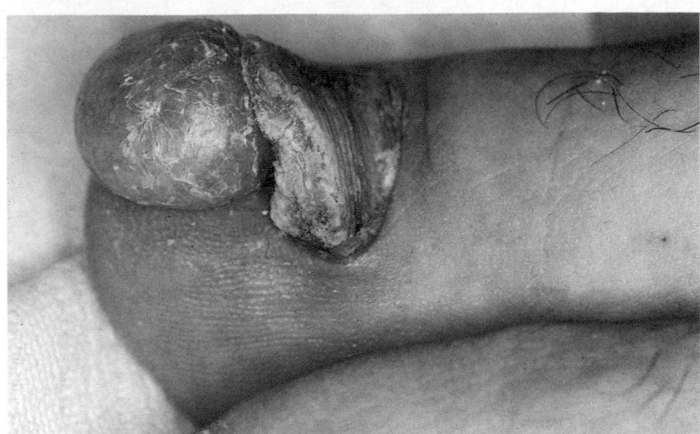

Distal subungual fibroma lifting up the nail plate.

and causes a sharp longitudinal depression. Such fibrokeratomas may present as double and even triple lesions. The hyperkeratotic tip is not present in the "garlic-glove" fibroma.

KOENEN'S TUMOR Koenen's periungual fibromas develop in 50 percent of tuberous sclerosis cases. They appear in patients between 12 and 14 years of age and increase progressively in size and number with age. The tumors may be either small, round, smooth, flesh-colored, and asymptomatic, or they may be slightly hyperkeratotic at the tip, resembling fibrokeratoma. Excessively large tumors involving the nail bed are often painful.

FIBROUS DERMATOFIBROMAS (See Fig. 72-42) Fibromas develop as painless slow-growing nodular tumors, spherical or oval in shape and firm or rubbery, in consistency, in any epidermal tissue. They may move freely or remain fixed. In the distal nail bed, they lift the nail plate. Nail dystrophy usually results in a longitudinal depression as pressure is exerted on the nail matrix.

INFANTILE DIGITAL FIBROMATOSIS (See Fig. 72-43) These round, smooth, dome-shaped, shiny, firm, tense, reddish or livid red

FIGURE 72-43

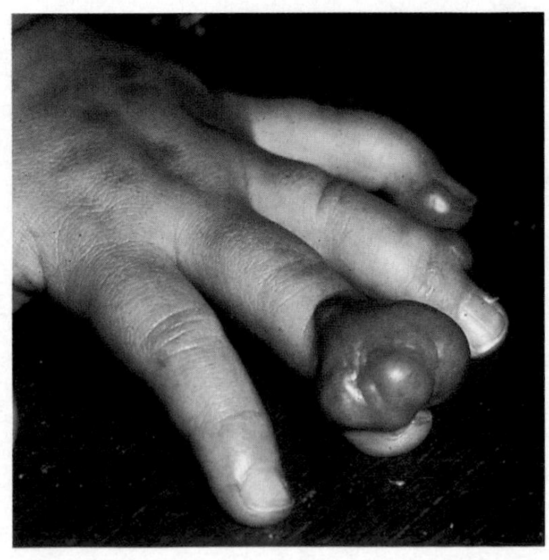

Infantile digital fibromatosis.

FIGURE 72-44

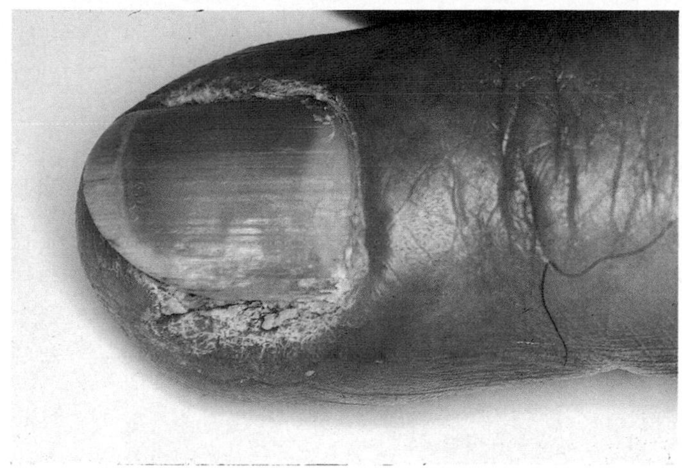

Bowen's disease involving the lateral nail groove.

dermal nodules are usually located on the dorsal and axial surfaces of the fingers and toes, but spare the thumbs and the great toes.

They may be present at birth or develop during infancy. Multiple lesions occur in 50 percent of patients. The tumors may cause considerable distortion of the distal digit, but spontaneous resolution is the rule, which may be hastened by cryosurgery.

EPIDERMOID CARCINOMAS (Bowen's disease and squamous cell carcinomas) (see Fig. 72-44). Bowen's disease is a carcinoma developing into frankly invasive squamous cell carcinoma. Because the clinical picture does not permit a distinction to be made between carcinoma in situ and invasive carcinoma, the term *epidermoid carcinoma* was coined for these lesions in the nail region. The etiology of epidermoid carcinomas has recently been linked to HPV-16, HPV-34, and HPV-35, but arsenic may also play a role.

Bowen's disease occurs most frequently in males between 50 and 70 years of age. The fingers, mainly the first three, are most frequently affected. When a toe is involved, it is usually the great toe. The lesion grows slowly and is resistant to conservative therapy. In most cases, it presents as a circumscribed plaque, with a warty surface extending from the nail groove both under and around the nail. Nail dystrophy develops when the matrix is affected. Because involvement of the nail bed causes onycholysis, the overlying nail plate should be cut away to permit evaluation of the extent of nail bed involvement. Erosions, oozing, bleeding, and development of a tumor mass indicate malignant degeneration. Bowen's disease of the nail may be pigmented, causing longitudinal melanonychia. It may mimic ungual fibrokeratoma and occur on several digits.

Carcinoma cuniculatum is a rare variant of squamous cell carcinoma, with low biologic malignancy. Diagnosis requires histologic examination of the entire surgical specimen.

METASTASES (See Fig. 72-45) More than 120 cases of metastases to the nail apparatus and finger tip have been reported. Most lesions are bone metastases. Frequent symptoms are swelling, pseudo-clubbing, redness, nail dystrophy, pulsating pain, or acute paronychia-like symptoms, with pain being much less intense than expected from the clinical findings. Osteolysis is usually seen radiographically. Bronchial carcinoma is by far the most frequent to metastasize to the fingertip, with breast carcinoma being second.

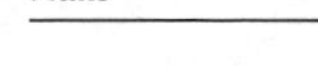

FIGURE 72-45

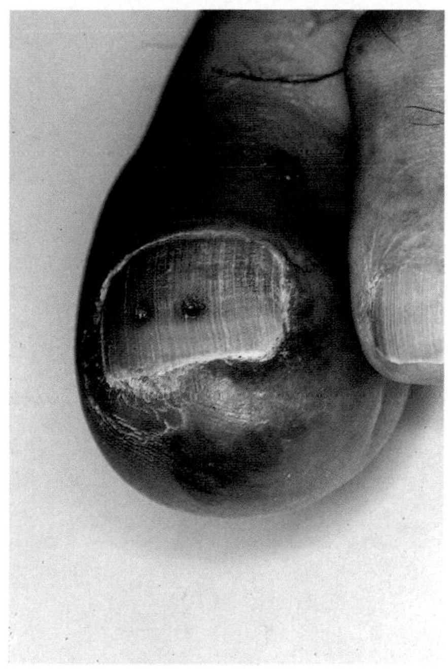

Bronchial carcinoma metastasis to the distal phalanx.

Vascular Tumors

Pyogenic granuloma (Fig. 72-46) is an eruptive hemangioma that is usually seen following trauma. A small bluish-red nodule develops rapidly on the periungual skin. The lesion becomes necrotic, developing an oozing appearance with a collarette of macerated white epithelium.

FIGURE 72-46

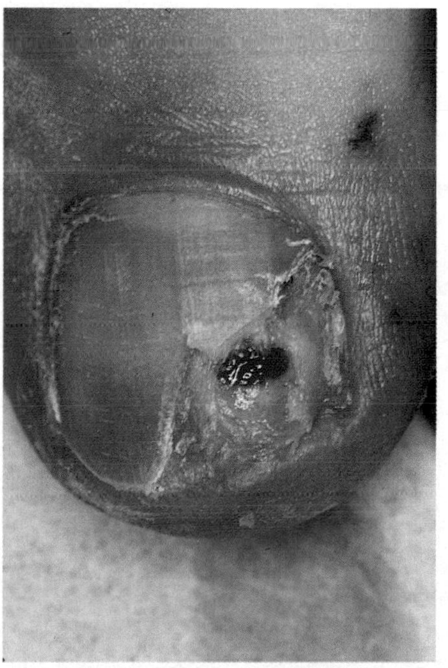

Pyogenic granuloma involving the nail bed.

FIGURE 72-47

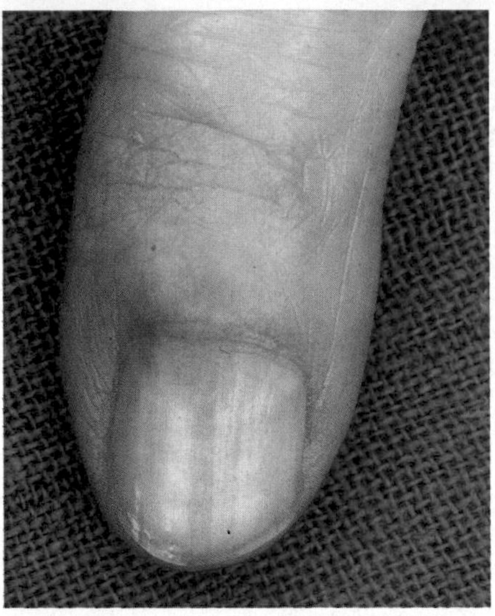

Glomus tumor. Longitudinal red streak.

Onycholysis occurs when the hyponychium is involved. Injury penetrating the nail plate may cause pyogenic granuloma in the nail bed or even the matrix. Complete removal of the tumor should always be accompanied by histologic examination of the specimen to rule out amelanotic melanoma.

Glomus tumor (Fig. 72-47) presents as a classic triad of symptoms: pain, tenderness, and temperature sensitivity. In typical cases, there is a reddish spot in the nail bed, sometimes with a distal fissured nail plate. Although the use of magnetic resonance imaging (MRI)[13] to detect small tumors is not necessary, MRI is most useful in recurrent tumors, not only because the original may have been missed by surgery, but also because multiple glomus tumors may occur in the same digit.

FIGURE 72-48

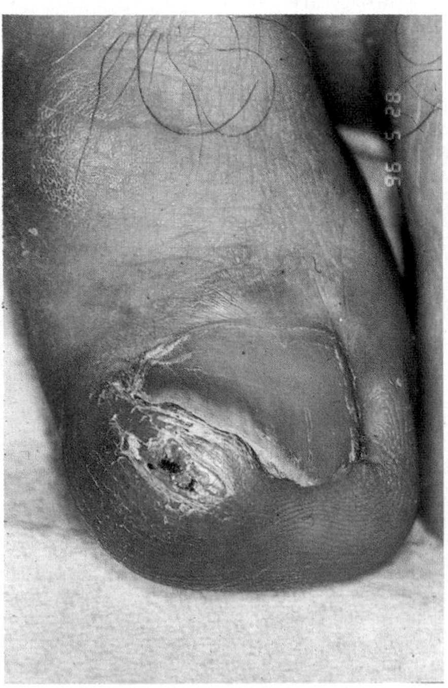

Exostosis.

FIGURE 72-49

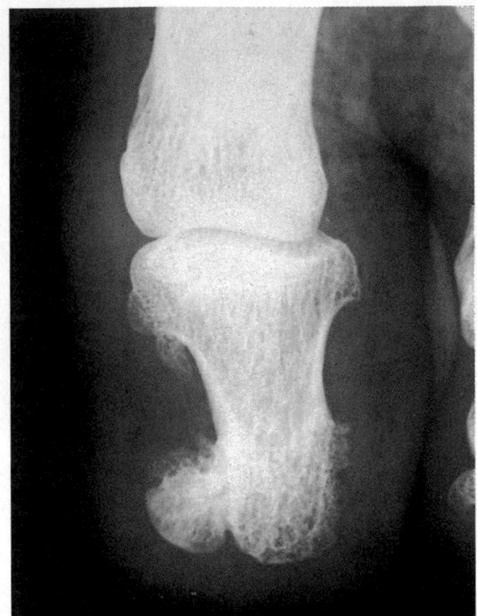

X-ray of patient with exostosis.

Osteocartilaginous Tumors

Exostosis (Fig. 72-48) and *osteochondroma* commonly occur on toes and rarely on fingers. Trauma appears to be the main cause of these reactive lesions. They are often painful and may elevate the nail plate

FIGURE 72-50

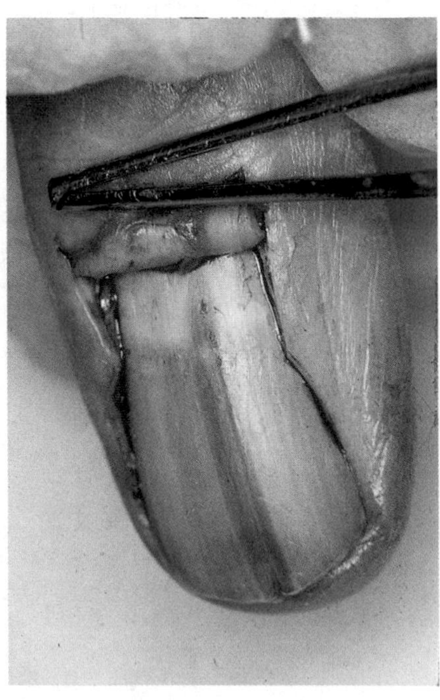

Isolated longitudinal melanonychia.

FIGURE 72-51

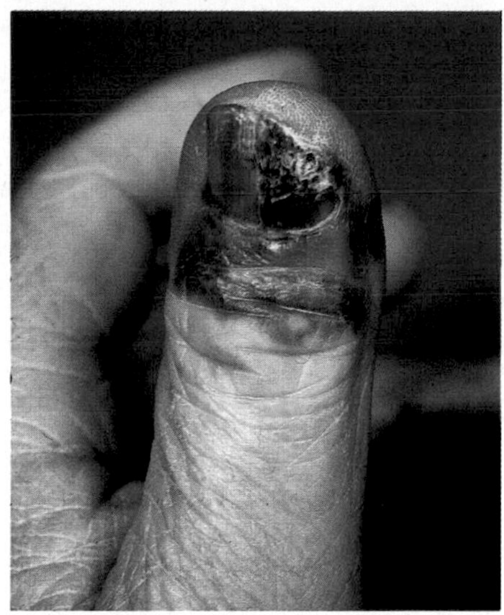

Melanonychia with distal fissure and pigmentation of the proximal nail fold (Hutchinson's sign).

or cause an ingrown nail, especially on the great toe. Palpation reveals a bone-hard tumor, which should be confirmed by x-ray (Fig. 72-49). Exostoses in the nail region are infrequently seen in the multiple exostosis syndrome. *Enchondroma* of the terminal phalanx is rare. It may result in a painful, bulbous enlargement of the finger tip, clubbing, nail deformation, and discoloration, or even an apparent paronychia. X-ray reveals a sharply delimited radiolucent defect.

Degenerative Lesions

Myxoid cysts (see Fig. 72-7) are much more frequent on fingers than toes. The tumor begins as an asymptomatic smooth swelling that slowly enlarges to about the size of a bean. Its consistency varies from soft to firm, cystic to fluctuant. It is usually located on one side of the midline, but tumors may appear beneath the nail matrix and nail bed. A space-occupying lesion in the PNF may compress the matrix, thereby interfering with nail plate formation. This may result in a longitudinal depression running the length of the nail or in a series of irregular transverse grooves that suggest alternating intermittent episodes of decompression and refilling of the cystic tumor. Heberden's nodes and osteoarthritis of distal joints are present in most cases. Transillumination reveals the cystic nature of the tumor and rules out a giant cell tumor on the dorsum of the distal digit. Surgical treatment involves exposure of the DIP joint, removal of all osteophytes with a rongeur, and preservation of the cyst wall.[14]

Melanocytic Lesions[15]

Isolated *longitudinal melanonychia* (Fig. 72-50) is a diagnostic problem because it may be of trivial etiology or represent a malignant melanoma, especially in white patients. The clinician should be suspicious and always take a proper biopsy when an area of longitudinal melanonychia suddenly becomes darker or wider; occurs in either the first, second, or third digits; demonstrates blurred borders; or is accompanied by nail dystrophy and/or periungual pigmentation (Hutchinson's sign) (Fig. 72-51). Multiple bands of longitudinal melanonychia may be a consequence of drug treatment or numerous systemic diseases including AIDS (Fig. 72-35). Addison's disease, Cushing's syndrome, or hyperthyroidism may result from folic acid or vitamin B_{12} deficiency. *Transverse melanonychia* is frequently observed in patients treated with cytotoxic drugs.

Between 2 and 3 percent of *melanomas* in caucasians occur in the nail, whereas in blacks the figure is about 20 percent. About a quarter of melanomas of the nail are amelanotic, presenting initially as nail dystrophy, indolent tumor nodules, or chronic granulation tissue.

REFERENCES

1. Baran R et al: Physical signs, in *Baran & Dawber's Diseases of the Nails and Their Management,* 3rd ed, edited by R Baran, RPR Dawber, D De Berker, E Haneke, A Tosti. Oxford, Blackwell Scientific, 2001, p 48
2. Baran R: Significance and management of congenital malalignment of the big toenail. *Cutis* **58**:181, 1996
3. De Berker D: Management of nail psoriasis. *Clin Exp Dermatol* **25**:357, 2000
4. Piraccini BM et al: Pustular psoriasis of the nails: Treatment and long-term follow-up of 46 patients. *Br J Dermatol* **144**:1000, 2001
5. Tosti A et al: Nail lichen planus in children: Clinical features, response to treatment and long-term follow-up. *Arch Dermatol* **137**:1027, 2001
6. Tosti A et al: Idiopathic trachyonychia (twenty-nail dystrophy): A pathological study of 23 patients. *Br J Dermatol* **131**:866, 1994
7. Tosti A et al: The nail in systemic diseases and drug-induced changes, in *Baran & Dawber's Diseases of the Nails and Their Management,* 3rd ed, edited by R Baran, RPR Dawber, D De Berker, E Haneke, A Tosti. Oxford, Blackwell Scientific, 2001, p 223
8. Piraccini BM et al: Drug induced nail disorders, incidence, management and prognosis. *Drug Safety* **21**:187, 1999
9. Juhlin L et al: Hereditary and congenital nail disorders, in *Baran & Dawber's Diseases of the Nails and Their Management,* 3rd ed, edited by R Baran, RPR Dawber, D DE Berker, E Haneke, A Tosti. Oxford, Blackwell Scientific, 2001, p 370
10. Baran R et al: Tumours of the nail apparatus and adjacent tissues, in *Baran & Dawber's Diseases of the Nails and Their Management,* 3rd ed, edited by R Baran, RPR Dawber, D De Berker, E Haneke, A Tosti. Oxford, Blackwell Scientific, 2001, p 515
11. Perrin C et al: Onychomatricoma: Clinical and histopathologic findings in 12 cases. *J Am Acad Dermatol* **39**:560, 1998
12. Baran R et al: Distal digital keratoacanthoma. Two cases with a review of the literature. *J Dermatol Surg* **27**:5, 2001
13. Drapé JL et al: Imaging of tumors of the nail unit, in *Nail Surgery,* edited by E Krull, EG Zook, R Baran, E Haneke. Philadelphia, Lippincott, Williams & Wilkins, 2001, p 319
14. De Berker D et al: Ganglion of the distal interphalangeal joint (myxoid cyst) therapy by identification and repair of the leak of joint fluid. *Arch Dermatol* **137**:607, 2001
15. Goettmann-Bonvallot S et al: Longitudinal melanonychia in children. A clinical and histopathologic study of 40 cases. *J Am Acad Dermatol* **41**:17, 1999

CHAPTER 73

Diane M. Thiboutot
John S. Strauss

Diseases of the Sebaceous Glands

ACNE VULGARIS

Acne vulgaris is a self-limited disease, seen primarily in adolescents, involving the sebaceous follicles. Most cases of acne are pleomorphic, presenting with a variety of lesions consisting of comedones, papules, pustules, nodules, and, as sequelae to active lesions, pitted or hypertrophic scars. Although classically classified as a sebaceous gland disease, it is actually a process that involves the pilosebaceous unit.

Anatomy of the Sebaceous Gland

In the human fetus, sebaceous glands develop in the thirteenth to fifteenth week of gestation from bulges on the developing hair follicles. When fully formed, the glands remain attached to the hair follicles by a duct through which sebum flows into the follicular canal and eventually to the skin surface. Sebaceous glands are associated with hair follicles all over the body. Only the palms and soles, which have no hair follicles, are totally devoid of sebaceous glands. Sebaceous glands known as *Fordyce spots* are sometimes present in the oral epithelium. In this location, the sebaceous ducts open directly to the surface.

Sebaceous glands are unilobular or multilobular and vary considerably in size, even in the same individual and in the same anatomic area. Fordyce spots are visible to the unaided eye because of their large size (up to 2 to 3 mm) and the transparency of the oral epithelium. On the external body surface, most glands are only a fraction of a millimeter in size. The largest glands and the greatest density of glands are found on the face and scalp. The hairs associated with the large glands in these areas are often tiny, and it has been suggested that the total structures be more properly termed *sebaceous follicles* rather than hair follicles.

Physiology of the Sebaceous Gland

The sebaceous glands exude lipids by disintegration of entire cells, a process known as *holocrine secretion*. The stages of this process are evident in the histology of the gland (Fig. 73-1).[1] The outermost cells, just inside the basement membrane, are small, nucleated, and devoid of lipid droplets. This layer contains the dividing cells that replenish the gland as cells are lost in the process of lipid excretion. As cells are displaced into the center of the gland, they begin to produce lipid, which accumulates in droplets. Eventually the cells become greatly distended with lipid droplets and the nuclei and other subcellular structures disappear. As the cells approach the sebaceous duct, they disintegrate and release their contents. Only neutral lipids reach the skin surface. Proteins, nucleic acids, and the membrane phospholipids are digested and apparently recycled during the disintegration of the cells. Sebaceous gland activity is high at birth but then declines to become almost nonexistent in children between ages 2 and 6 years. At about age 7, sebum secretion begins to increase and continues to do so well into the teens.[2] From the twenties on, there is a decline of approximately 23 percent per decade in men and approximately 32 percent per decade in women.[3] There is great individual variation and overlap between the sexes, although males have higher values, on average, than females.

FIGURE 73-1

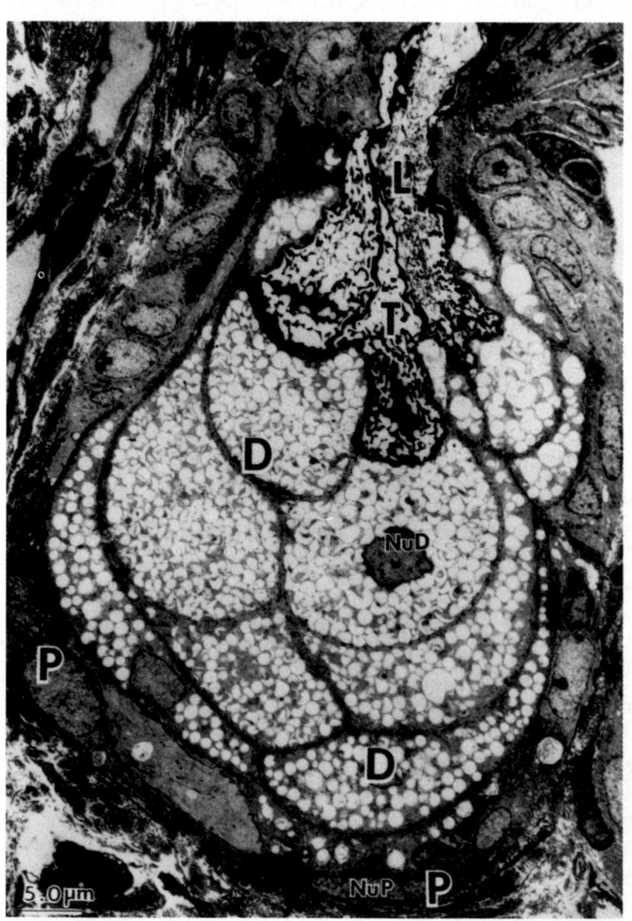

Electron micrograph of a rabbit sebaceous gland stained with uranyl acetate-lead citrate. The peripheral cells (P) contain ellipsoidal nuclei (NuP) and no lipid droplets. As the cells differentiate (D), lipid droplets accumulate and the nuclei (NuD) become irregularly shaped. In the terminally differentiated cells (T), near the lumen (L) of the sebaceous duct, all subcellular structures appear to break down. (*From Ito et al.,*[1] *with permission. Copyright by Williams & Wilkins, 1984.*)

FIGURE 73-2

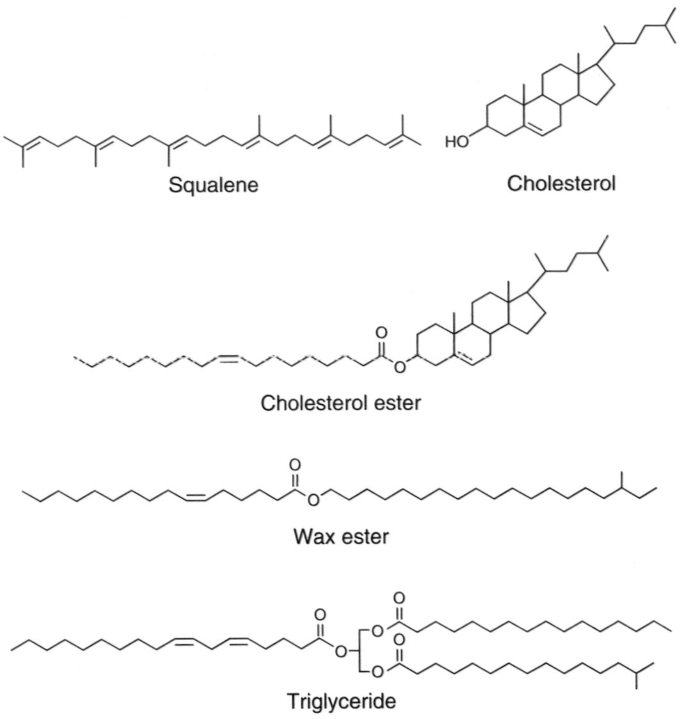

Human sebaceous gland lipids. The structures of the cholesterol ester, wax ester, and triglyceride are representative of the many species that are present. Two sebaceous-type unsaturated fatty acid moieties are shown: sapienic acid (16:1Δ6) (in the wax ester structure); and sebaleic acid (18:2Δ5,8) (in the triglyceride structure). Anteiso branching is shown in the alcohol moiety of the wax ester, and iso branching is shown in the triglyceride.

Lipid Composition of Sebum

Human sebum, as it leaves the sebaceous gland, contains squalene, cholesterol, cholesterol esters, wax esters, and triglycerides (Fig. 73-2). During passage of sebum through the hair canal, bacterial enzymes hydrolyze some of the triglycerides, so that the lipid mixture reaching the skin surface contains free fatty acids and small proportions of mono- and diglycerides in addition to the original components. The wax esters and squalene distinguish sebum from the lipids of human internal organs, which contain no wax esters and little squalene. Squalene that is synthesized in internal tissues is quickly converted to lanosterol and eventually to cholesterol. Human sebaceous glands, however, appear to be unable to cyclize squalene to sterols.

The patterns of unsaturation of the fatty acids in the triglycerides, wax esters, and cholesterol esters also distinguish human sebum from the lipids of other organs. The "normal" mammalian pathway of desaturation involves inserting a double bond between the ninth and tenth carbon of stearic acid (18:0) to form oleic acid (18:1Δ9). A Δ6 double bond can be added only after the Δ9 double bond is in place. However, in human sebaceous glands, the predominant pattern is the insertion of a Δ6 double bond into palmitic acid (16:0). The resulting sapienic acid (16:1Δ6) (Fig. 73-2) is the major fatty acid of adult human sebum. Elongation of the chain by two carbons and insertion of another double bond between the fifth and sixth carbon gives sebaleic acid (18:2Δ5,8) (Fig. 73-2), a fatty acid thought to be unique to human sebum.

Sebaceous fatty acids and alcohols are also distinguished by chain branching. Methyl branches can occur on the next to last (penultimate) carbon of a fatty acid chain (iso branching), on the third from the last (antepenultimate) carbon (anteiso branching), or on any even-numbered carbon (internal branching). Examples of these unusual unsaturated and branched-chain moieties are included in the lipid structures in Fig. 73-2.

Factors Regulating Sebaceous Gland Size and Sebum Production

The exact mechanisms underlying the regulation of human sebum production have not been defined. Clearly, sebaceous glands are regulated by androgens and retinoids, but recently, other factors, such as melanocortins, peroxisome proliferator-activated receptors (PPARs), and acyl-CoA:diacylglycerol acyl transferase (DGAT), have been postulated to play a role as well.

Androgens

It has long been recognized that sebaceous glands require androgenic stimulation to produce significant quantities of sebum. Individuals with a genetic deficiency of androgen receptors (complete androgen insensitivity) have no detectable sebum secretion.[4] However, there is still a question as to which androgen is physiologically significant. Although the most powerful androgens are testosterone and its end-organ reduction product dihydrotestosterone (DHT), levels of testosterone do not parallel the patterns of sebaceous gland activity. For example, testosterone levels are many-fold higher in males than in females, with no overlap between the sexes, while average rates of sebum secretion are only slightly higher in males than in females, with considerable overlap between the sexes. Also, sebum secretion starts to increase in children during adrenarche, a developmental event that precedes puberty by about 2 years.

The weak adrenal androgen, dehydroepiandrosterone sulfate (DHEAS), might be a significant regulator of sebaceous gland activity through its conversion to testosterone and dihydrotestosterone in the sebaceous gland. Levels of DHEAS are high in newborns, very low in 2- to 4-year-old children, and start to rise when sebum secretion starts to increase. In adulthood, DHEAS levels show considerable individual variation, but are only slightly higher in men than in women on the average. There is a decline in DHEAS levels in both sexes starting in early adulthood and continuing throughout life, this decline parallels the decline of sebum secretion. DHEAS is present in the blood in high concentration. The enzymes required to convert DHEAS to more potent androgens are present in sebaceous glands.[5] These include 3β-hydroxysteroid dehydrogenase, 17β-hydroxysteroid dehydrogenase and 5α-reductase. Each of these enzymes exists in two or more isoforms that exhibit tissue-specific differences in their expression. The predominant isozymes in the sebaceous gland include the type 1 3β-hydroxysteroid dehydrogenase, the type 2 17β-hydroxysteroid dehydrogenase and the type 1 5α-reductase.

Retinoids

Isotretinoin (13-*cis*-retinoic acid) is the most potent known pharmacologic inhibitor of sebum secretion. Significant reductions in sebum production can be observed as early as 2 weeks after use.[6] Histologically, sebaceous glands are markedly reduced in size and individual sebocytes appear undifferentiated lacking the characteristic cytoplasmic accumulation of sebaceous lipids. The mechanism by which 13-*cis*-retinoic acid lowers sebum secretion is unknown. It does not interact with any of the known retinoid receptors. Isotretinoin may serve as a prodrug for the synthesis of all-*trans*-retinoic acid or 9-*cis*-retinoic acid, which do interact with retinoid receptors, however, it has greater sebosuppressive action than do all-*trans*- or 9-*cis*-retinoic acid.[7] Unfortunately 13-*cis*-retinoic acid is teratogenic, so there is a continuing need for a nonteratogenic retinoid or retinoid-like compound that would inhibit human sebaceous glands.

Melanocortins

Melanocortins include melanocyte-stimulating hormone (MSH) and adrenocorticotropic hormone (ACTH). In rodents, melanocortins increase sebum production. Transgenic mice deficient in the melanocortin-5 receptor have hypoplastic sebaceous glands and reduced sebum production.[8] The melanocortin-5 receptor has been identified in human sebaceous glands where it may play a role in the modulation of sebum production.[9] Further experimentation however is required to test this hypothesis.

Peroxisome Proliferator Activated Receptors

Peroxisome proliferator activated receptors (PPARs) are orphan nuclear receptors that are similar to retinoid receptors in many ways. Each of these receptors form heterodimers with retinoid X receptors in order to regulate the transcription of genes involved in a variety of processes, including lipid metabolism and cellular proliferation and differentiation. Rat preputial cells serve as a model for human sebocytes.[10] In rat preputial cells, agonists of the PPAR-γ receptor, such as drugs of the thiazolidinedione class, increase lipid accumulation.[11] The PPAR-γ receptor is strongly expressed in human sebaceous glands, where it may play a role in mediating sebum production.[12]

Acyl-CoA:Diacylglycerol Acyltransferase (DGAT)

Acyl-CoA:diacylglycerol acyltransferase an enzyme involved in the final step of triglyceride synthesis, was recently shown to be important in sebaceous gland homeostasis in mice.[13] The absence of DGAT leads to sebaceous gland atrophy and changes in the composition of surface lipid. This effect does not appear to be mediated through androgens, and did not occur in the absence of leptin, a peptide hormone secreted by adipocytes. The importance of these findings in human sebaceous gland activity remains to be determined.

Epidemiology of Acne

Acne is sufficiently common that it often has been termed physiologic. Mild degrees of acne are often seen at birth, probably resulting from follicular stimulation by adrenal androgens, and mild cases may continue in the neonatal period. However, it is not until puberty that acne becomes a common problem. Acne is often an early manifestation of puberty; in the very young patient the predominant lesions are comedones. In girls, the occurrence of acne may precede menarche by more than a year. The greatest number of cases is seen during the middle-to-late teenage period; subsequently, the incidence decreases. However, particularly in women, acne may persist through the third decade or even later. Acne seems to be familial, but owing to the high prevalence of the disease this has been extremely difficult to assess. Nodulocystic acne has been reported to be more common in white males than in black males,[14] and one group of investigators has found that acne is more severe in patients with the XYY genotype.[15]

Etiology and Pathogenesis of Acne

Although the basic cause of acne is unknown, there is considerable information on the various factors concerned in its pathogenesis. Acne is a multifactorial disease, developing in the sebaceous follicles. Its pathophysiology centers on the interplay of follicular hyperkeratinization, colonization with *P. acnes* bacteria, increased sebum production, and inflammation.

FIGURE 73-3

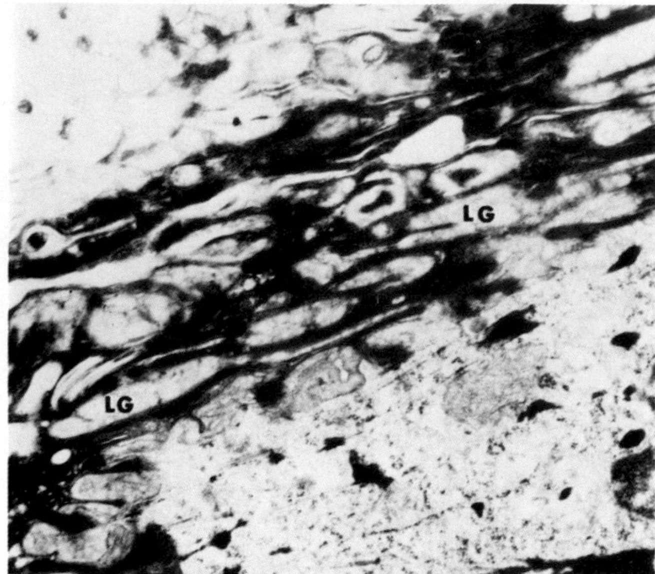

A.

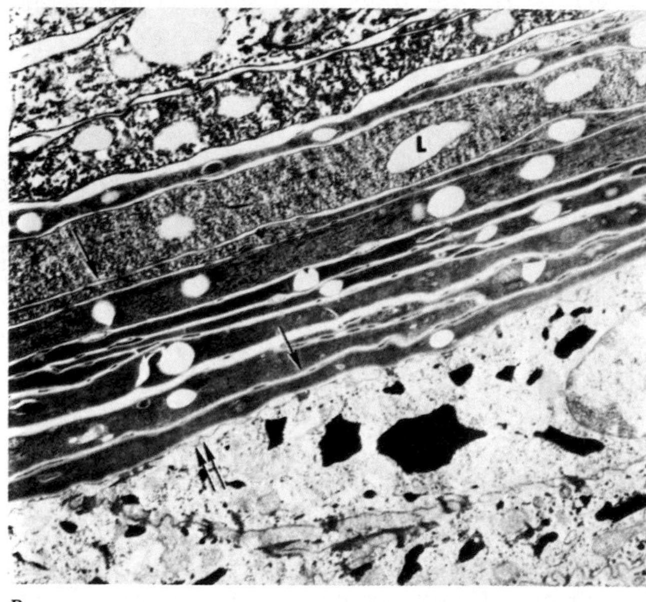

B.

A. High magnification of the keratinized layer in the proximal infundibulum of a normal sebaceous follicle. The cornified cells are thin and filamentous, and the cell membranes are indistinct. Large clusters of lamellar granules (LG) fill the intracellular spaces. (×15,258) *B.* High magnification of the infundibular region of an early comedo from the face. The keratinized cells have thickened cell margins (*single arrows*), and many layers accumulate. In comparison with the normal follicle (see Fig. 73-3*A*), there are fewer small clusters of lamellar granules (*double arrows*) at the junction of the granular and cornified layers. Note intracellular lipid inclusions (L). (×8493). (*From Knutson,[16] with permission.*)

FOLLICULAR HYPERKERATINIZATION The primary change in the sebaceous follicle in acne is an alteration in the pattern of keratinization within the follicle.[16] Normally, the keratinous material in the follicle is loosely organized (Fig. 73-3*A*). On the ultrastructural level, there are many lamellar granules and relatively few keratohyaline granules. The initial changes in comedo formation are observed in the lower portion of the follicular infundibulum. The keratinous material becomes more dense, the lamellar granules are less numerous, keratohyaline granules are increased, and some of the cells contain amorphous material, which is probably lipid, generated during the process of keratinization (Fig. 73-3*B*). Kinetic studies demonstrate that there is an increase in cellular turnover in comedones.

The initiating factor in comedo formation still has not been definitely identified. Follicular hyperkeratinization may relate to a local deficiency of linoleic acid, production of interleukin-1 within the follicle, or, possibly, the effects of androgens on follicular keratinization. Downing et al.[17] advanced the theory that the decreased concentrations of linoleic acid that accompany the high sebum secretion rate found in patients with acne result in a localized essential fatty acid deficiency of the follicular epithelium. This, in turn, theoretically induces follicular hyperkeratosis and decreased epithelial barrier function, both of which are characteristic of the essential fatty acid deficiency syndrome.

Investigators have developed models using human infrainfundibular segments to study the process of follicular hyperkeratinization. Guy et al. found that the addition of 1 ng/mL of interleukin (IL)-1α to infrainfundibular segments caused hypercornification similar to that seen in comedones.[18] This could be blocked by addition of an IL-1 receptor antagonist. These authors suggest that changes in sebum secretion or composition could lead to the release of IL-1 by follicular keratinocytes, which, in turn, may stimulate comedogenesis.

Androgens are known to regulate the development of the sebaceous gland and sebum production. In addition, androgens may play a role in the follicular hyperkeratinization seen in acne. Indirect evidence in support of this latter hypothesis includes these observations: (1) androgen receptors have been localized to the outer root sheath of the infrainfundibular region of follicles;[19] (2) the formation of follicular casts is reduced in patients treated with antiandrogens;[20] and (3) each of the key enzymes involved in androgen metabolism has been identified in follicles.[21] No direct effect of androgens on follicular hyperkeratinization has been demonstrated, however. Additional studies are needed to determine whether androgens modulate follicular hyperkeratinization.

PROPIONIBACTERIUM ACNES The predominant organism in the follicular flora is the anaerobic pleomorphic diphtheroid *Propionibacterium acnes*. In 11- to 15-year-olds, practically no *P. acnes* are found in individuals without acne, whereas in patients with acne, the geometric mean of *P. acnes* organisms is 114,800 per square centimeter.[22] Similar differences are found in 16- to 20-year-old groups, but in older individuals the number of organisms is the same in those with and without acne. It is generally accepted that *P. acnes* are important in the pathogenesis of acne. While the initial impression was that inflammation resulted from the production of free fatty acids, and it was shown that *P. acnes* was the main source of follicular lipases, *P. acnes* also produces other extracellular enzymes such as proteases and hyaluronidases, which may be important in the inflammatory process. Furthermore, there are other ways in which *P. acnes* may produce inflammation.[23] The organism has been shown to secrete chemotactic factors[24] and chemotactic activity has been found in comedones.[25] The dialyzable, low molecular weight chemotactic factor does not require serum complement for activation, and, because of its small size, it can probably escape from the follicle and attract polymorphonuclear leukocytes. If the polymorphonuclear leukocytes enter the follicle, they can ingest *P. acnes* organisms, resulting in the release of hydrolytic enzymes, which, in turn, may be of importance in producing follicular epithelial damage.[26] In addition, the classical and alternative complement activation pathways are stimulated by *P. acnes,* possibly also contributing to the inflammatory response.[27]

The host response may also be important. Circulating antibodies to *P. acnes* are elevated in patients with severe acne.[28] Whether this has a direct effect is not proved, but it has been shown that the *P. acnes* induction of lysosomal hydrolases by polymorphonuclear leukocytes is anti-*P. acnes* antibody dependent.[26] There is other evidence of changes in the immune response as demonstrated by increased response to *P. acnes* injections in patients with acne.[29]

SEBUM PRODUCTION A connection between acne and high rates of sebum secretion is supported by at least three types of evidence: (1) children do not get acne during the age range from approximately 2 to 6 years, when sebum secretion is extremely low; (2) average rates of sebum secretion are higher in individuals with acne than in those without acne;[30] and (3) treatments that reduce sebum secretion (such as estrogen or 13-*cis*-retinoic acid) improve acne.[31,32] It is unclear, however, why elevated rates of sebum secretion lead to acne. The triglyceride fraction of sebum, which is unique to humans, is probably responsible for acne. The bacterial population of the follicle hydrolyzes triglycerides to fatty acids, which eventually appear on the skin surface. In the past, the free fatty acid fraction of sebum was considered to be important in the causation of inflammation, but in recent years, it has become evident that there are probably other more important causes of inflammation, as discussed below.

Most studies have failed to detect any changes in the composition of sebum in patients with acne as compared to age-matched controls. However, there is a significant decrease in the levels of linoleic acid in patients with acne, and there is an inverse relationship between sebum secretion and the linoleic acid concentration of sebum. Linoleic acid cannot be synthesized in mammalian tissues, and so the linoleate concentration in human sebum depends on the quantity of this essential fatty acid with which each cell is endowed and the extent to which this initial endowment is diluted by subsequent endogenous lipid synthesis in sebaceous cells. In individuals with high rates of sebum secretion, the fatty acids of the skin surface may contain only about 0.5 percent linoleate.[2] During passage through the follicle, some of the linoleate-deficient fatty acids may percolate through the follicular wall and dilute the linoleate necessary for a healthy epithelium. Although this mechanism is speculative, the involvement of follicular bacteria and free fatty acids in acne is supported by the fact that when the bacterial population is reduced with oral antibiotics, free fatty acids are reduced and acne may thus be alleviated.

Clinical Manifestations of Acne

The primary site of acne is the face and to a lesser degree the back, chest, and shoulders. On the trunk, lesions tend to be numerous near the midline. The disease is characterized by a great variety of clinical lesions. Although one type of lesion may be predominant, close observation usually reveals the presence of several types of lesions (Fig. 73-4). The lesions may be either noninflammatory or inflammatory. The noninflammatory lesions are comedones, which may be either open (blackheads) or closed (whiteheads). The open comedo appears as a flat or slightly raised lesion with a central dark-colored follicular impaction of keratin and lipid. The closed comedones, in contrast to the open comedones, may be difficult to visualize. They appear as pale, slightly elevated, small papules and do not have a clinically visible orifice. Stretching of the skin is an aid in detecting the lesions. Because the closed comedones are potential precursors for the large inflammatory lesions, they are of considerable clinical importance. Although comedones are the primary lesions of acne, they are not unique in this disease as they may be seen under other conditions (e.g., so-called senile comedones, which are common, particularly in the periorbital area of older persons, and comedones that are seen in atrophic skin resulting from x-ray therapy).

The inflammatory lesions vary from small papules with an inflammatory areola to pustules to large, tender, fluctuant nodules (Figs. 73-4, 73-5, and 73-6). Some of the large nodules were previously called "cysts" and the term *nodulocystic* has been used to describe severe cases of inflammatory acne. True cysts are rarely found in acne, and this term should be abandoned and the term *severe nodular acne* used instead (Fig. 73-6). Whether the lesion appears as a papule, pustule, or

FIGURE 73-4

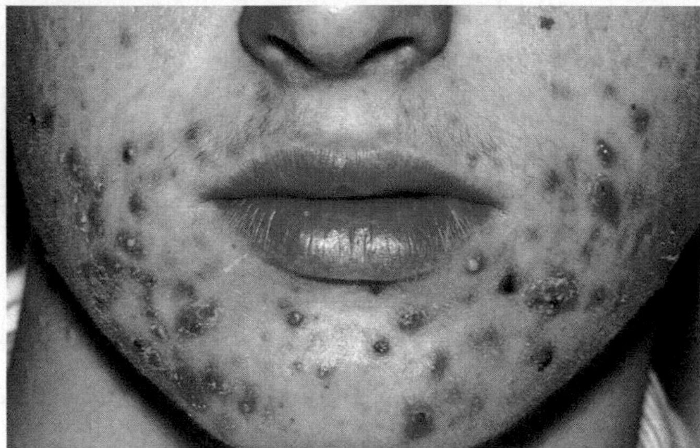

A.

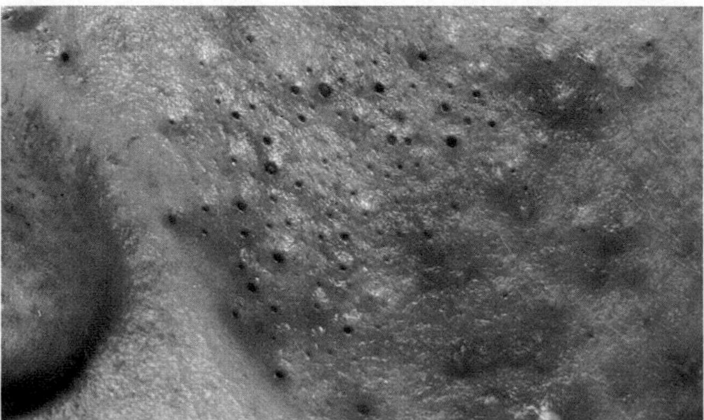

B.

Acne vulgaris, mild to moderate. *A.* Close-up of the lower face with comedones, papules, pustules, and scars. *B.* Close-up of the cheek, showing large open comedones, and inflammatory papules and pustules that become confluent, forming an erythematous plaque.

nodule depends on the extent and location of the inflammatory infiltrate in the dermis.

In addition to the above-described lesions, patients may have scars of varying size (Fig. 73-7). The characteristic scar of acne is a sharply punched-out pit. These are ordinarily single, but where inflammation has been marked, the pits may have multiple openings. Less commonly, broader pits may occur, and in rare instances, especially on the trunk, the scars may be hypertrophic.

It has been mentioned that seborrheic dermatitis is commonly seen in association with acne, but there does not appear to be any relation between these two diseases.

Diagnosis and Differential Diagnosis

Although one type of lesion may predominate, the diagnosis of acne vulgaris is usually made from the finding of a mixture of lesions of acne (comedones, pustules, papules, and nodules) on the face, back, or chest. Diagnosis is usually easy, but acne may be confused with folliculitis, rosacea, and the various miscellaneous acneiform disorders that are discussed subsequently. Lupus miliaris disseminatus faciei may also have a similar appearance.

Laboratory Findings

In general, laboratory workup is not indicated for patients with acne unless hyperandrogenism is suspected. There are numerous clinical studies relating acne to elevated serum levels of androgens in both adolescents and adults. Varying results have been obtained based on the patient population studied and the methodology used. Among 623 prepubertal girls followed over time, girls with acne had increased levels of DHEAS as compared to aged-matched controls without acne.[33] DHEAS can serve as a precursor for testosterone and dihydrotestosterone. Elevated serum levels of androgens have been found in cases of severe cystic acne[34] and in acne associated with a variety of endocrine conditions, including congenital adrenal hyperplasia (11β- and 21β-hydroxylase deficiencies), ovarian or adrenal tumors, and polycystic ovarian disease. In the majority of acne patients, however, serum androgens are within the normal range. Several studies indicate that the mean serum levels of DHEAS, testosterone, or dihydrotestosterone may be higher (but still within the normal range) in patients affected with acne as compared to normal controls.[35] It should be stressed that most of these studies involved older patients with treatment-resistant acne, and that other investigators, using a younger age group, either have not demonstrated increased androgens[36,37] or have shown that if increased blood androgens are found, the levels, at most, are variable. At this time, a potential androgen excess should be considered, particularly in older female patients who have treatment-resistant acne. However, there is no evidence that there are endocrinologic changes in all patients with acne. For this reason, it is thought that the local production of androgens within the skin may correlate more directly with the development of acne,[38] and it has been shown that the skin possesses each of the enzymes required to convert precursor DHEAS into more potent androgens.[21,39] Focus is also centering on the role of 5α-reductase in acne. Testosterone is converted to dihydrotestosterone by the action of 5α-reductase. Skin biopsies from men and women with acne have demonstrated increased 5α-reductase activity when compared to normal controls.[40] Two isozymes of 5α-reductase have been identified that differ in their tissue localization.[41] The type 1 isozyme is active in human sebaceous glands and is more active in glands from areas that are prone to acne such as the face, when compared to areas of the skin not predisposed to acne.[42]

Hyperandrogenism should be considered to be a contributing factor to the development of acne in female patients whose acne is severe, sudden in its onset, or associated with hirsutism or irregular menstrual periods. A medical history and physical examination directed toward eliciting any symptoms or signs of hyperandrogenism should be performed. The patient should be asked about the frequency and character of her menstrual periods and whether her acne flares with changes in her menstrual cycle. Hyperandrogenism can also result in deepening of the voice or an increase in libido. In addition to acne, other skin signs of endocrine diseases associated with hyperandrogenism include hirsutism, male pattern alopecia, acanthosis nigricans, and truncal obesity.

Acne can also result from the administration of exogenous androgens such as testosterone, other anabolic steroids, gonadotrophins, glucocorticoids, and ACTH. The latter two agents are the cause of steroid acne, an entity to be described later.

Many patients report that their acne flares during periods of stress. Although objective data are limited, stress is known to increase the output of adrenal steroids, which may affect the sebaceous gland. It has been shown that patients with acne have a greater increase in urinary glucocorticoid levels after corticotropin administration.

Excess androgens may be produced by either the adrenal gland or ovary. The laboratory workup should include measurement of serum DHEAS, total testosterone, free testosterone, and the luteinizing hormone (LH) to follicle-stimulating hormone (FSH) ratio. Testing should be obtained in the luteal phase of the menstrual cycle (within 2 weeks prior to the onset of menses), and patients on oral contraceptives will need to discontinue their medication for at least 1 month prior to testing. The above tests can be used to screen for the source of the

FIGURE 73-5

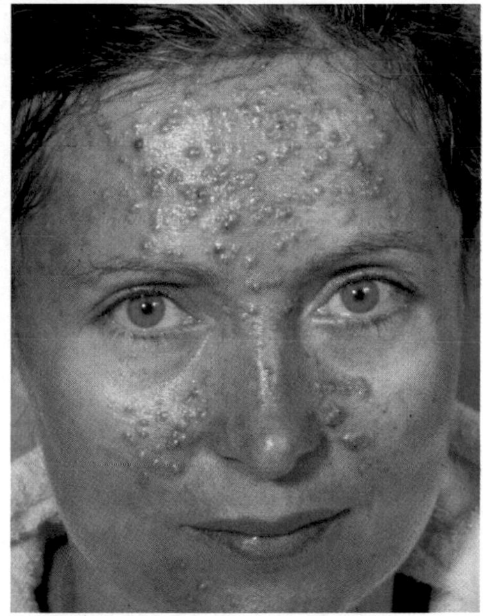

A.

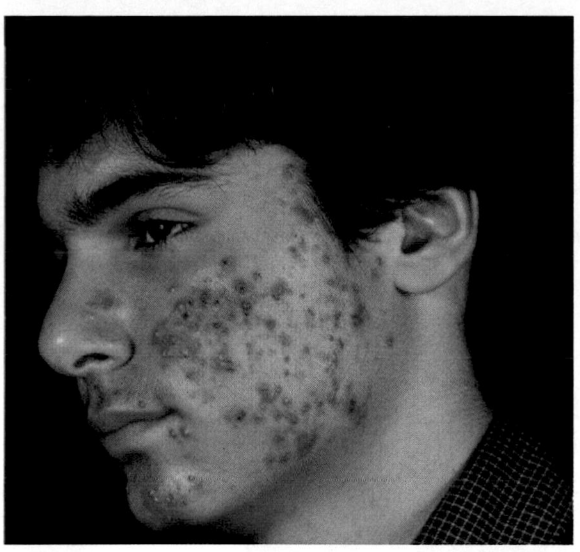

B.

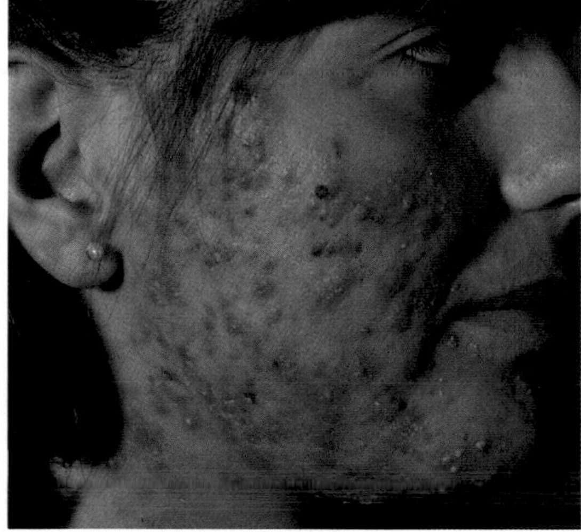

C.

Acne vulgaris, nodular, moderate to severe. *A.* Many papules and nodules are seen on the forehead and cheeks with little scarring apparent at this time. *B.* Nodular acne with scars on the cheek. *C.* Larger nodules on the cheek and chin with significant scarring.

hyperandrogenism. Values of DHEAS in the range of 4000 to 8000 ng/mL may be associated with congenital adrenal hyperplasia. Patients with a serum level of DHEAS > 8000 ng/mL could have an adrenal tumor and should be referred to an endocrinologist for further evaluation. An ovarian source of excess androgens can be suspected in cases where the serum total testosterone is > 150 ng/dL. Serum total testosterone in the range of 150 to 200 ng/dL or an increased LH/FSH ratio (greater than 2.0) can be found in cases of polycystic ovary disease. Greater elevations in serum testosterone may indicate an ovarian tumor, and appropriate referral should be made. There is a significant amount of variability in an individual's serum androgen levels. In cases in which abnormal results are obtained, it may be wise to repeat the test before proceeding with therapy or additional testing.

Pathology

As already stated, acne develops in the sebaceous follicles, and the primary lesion is the comedo. Comedo development starts in the midportion of the follicle as an expanding mass of lipid-impregnated keratinous material, resulting in thinning and ballooning-out of the follicular wall. Gradually, more keratinous material accumulates, and, as it does, further thinning and dilatation of the follicular wall occur. At the same time, the sebaceous glands begin to atrophy and are replaced by undifferentiated epithelial cells. The fully formed comedo has a thin wall and a minimal number of sebaceous cells, if they can be found at all. The open comedo has a patulous orifice, and the keratinous material is arranged in a lamellar concentric fashion (Fig. 73-8). With lipid stains, it can be shown that the keratin is permeated by lipid. Diphtheroid bacteria are also present. In cross section, the keratinous material consists of whorls of lamellar material centered on appendageal structures such as the hairs. In fact, most comedones contain multiple hairs. The closed comedo differs from the open comedo in that the keratinous material is not as compact and the follicular orifice is narrow and not distended (Fig. 73-9).

The fully developed open comedo is not usually the site of inflammatory changes, unless it is traumatized by the patient. The developing microcomedo and, to a lesser degree, the closed comedo are the major sites for the development of inflammatory lesions. The initial event appears to be escape of lipid through an edematous comedo wall, with the development of a cellular reaction in the adjacent dermis. Once

FIGURE 73-6

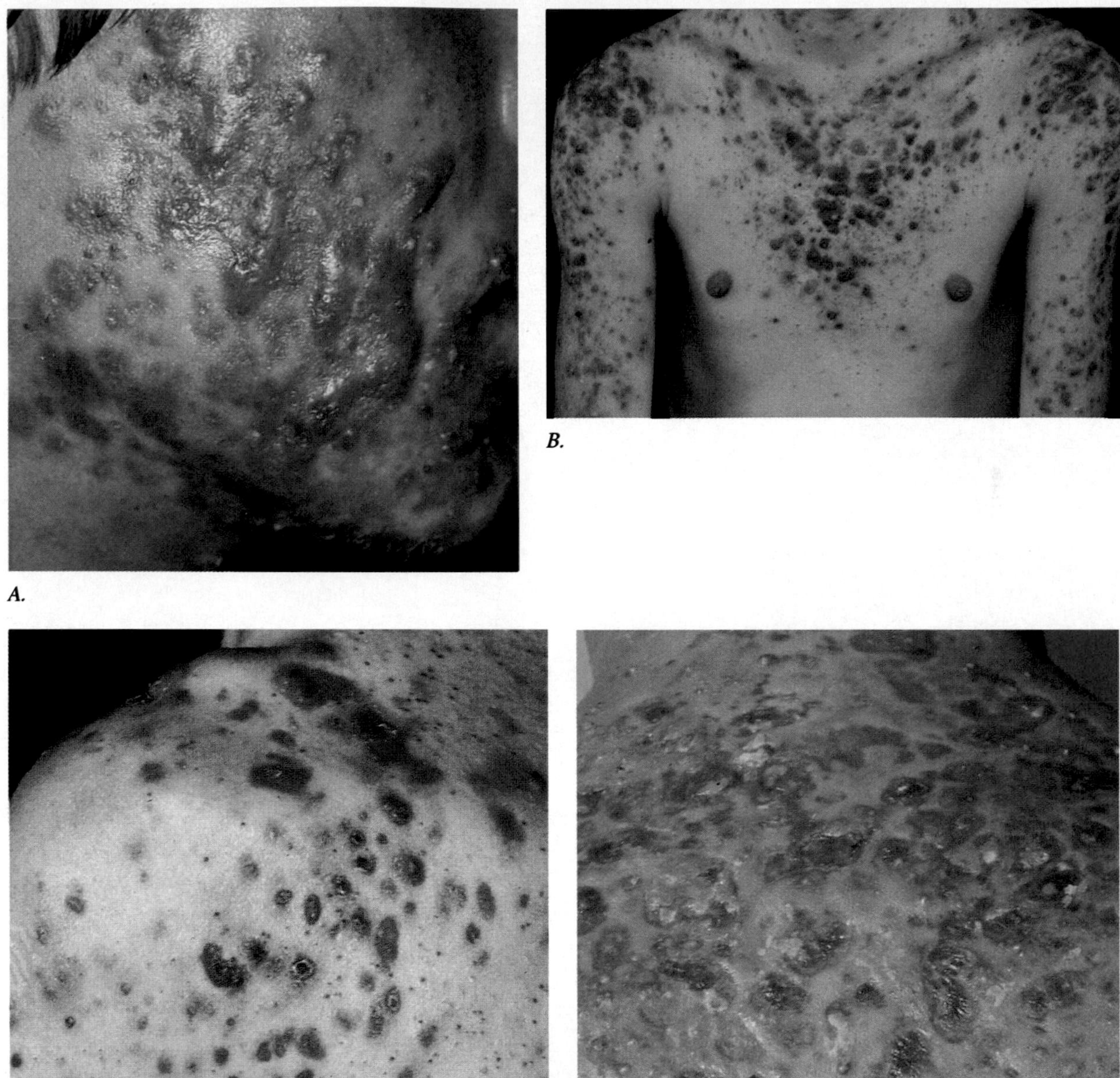

Acne vulgaris, nodular, severe. *A.* Large confluent nodules formed by confluence of smaller lesions with interconnecting channels, associated with atrophic and hyperplastic scars. *B.* Extensive nodules on the chest and arms with severe scarring. *C.* Close-up of nodules, crusted ulcers, and scars on the shoulder. *D.* Severe nodular acne of the back with little residual normal uninvolved skin.

complete rupture has occurred, the entire contents of the comedo are extruded into the dermis (Fig. 73-10). This reaction is much greater, and giant cells are common, reflecting the escape of the keratinous material. Within the inflammatory infiltrate, gram-positive diphtheroid bacteria with the morphologic characteristics of *P. acnes* may be observed free and within polymorphonuclear leukocytes. Depending upon the site and extent of inflammation, these ruptured lesions may appear as a pustule, a nodule, or as a nodule surmounted by a pustule.

It should be realized that the skin is always attempting to repair itself, and sheaths of cells will grow out from the epidermis or appendageal structures in an attempt to encapsulate the inflammatory reaction. This encapsulation may be complete so that the inflammatory infiltrate appears to be within the follicle, but often it is far from complete, and further rupture may occur leading to multichanneled tracts, as can be seen in many acne scars. Fibrous contraction also contributes to scar formation.

FIGURE 73-7

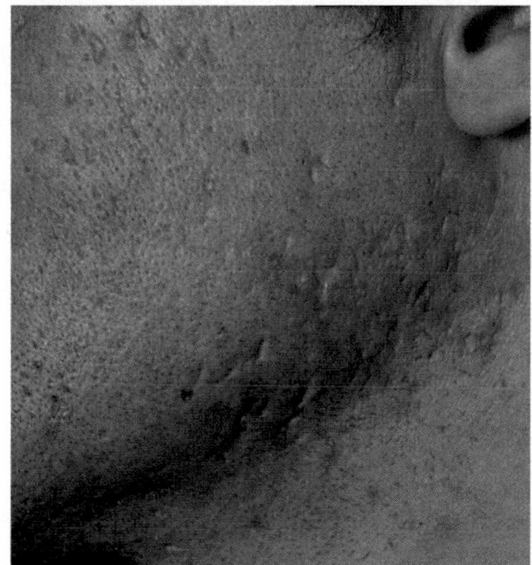

A.

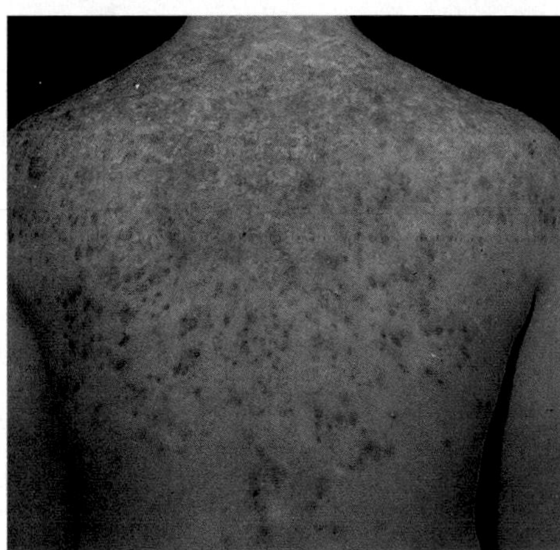

B.

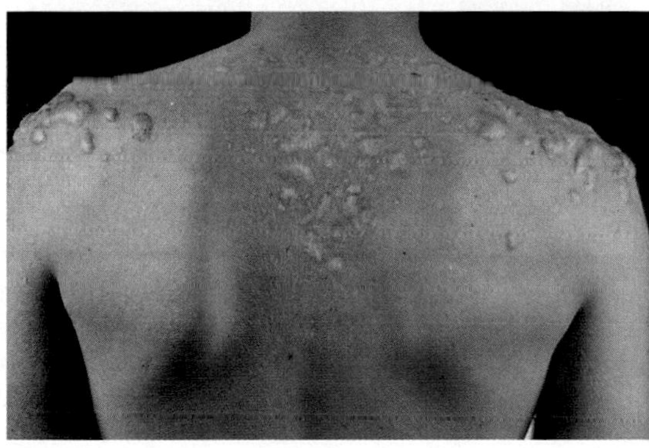

C.

Acne vulgaris, scarring. *A.* "Punched out" and "ice-pick" scars are seen on the cheek as a residual of burned-out nodular acne. *B.* Extensive atrophic scarring of the back associated with recent nodular acne. *C.* Severe hypertrophic scarring of the back in a patient with history of nodular acne.

Treatment

There may be great fluctuations in the natural course of acne; furthermore, the response to placebo therapy is considerable. Therefore, the determination of the therapeutic efficacy of medications used in acne is not a simple task, and it is possible to find many favorable therapeutic

FIGURE 73-8

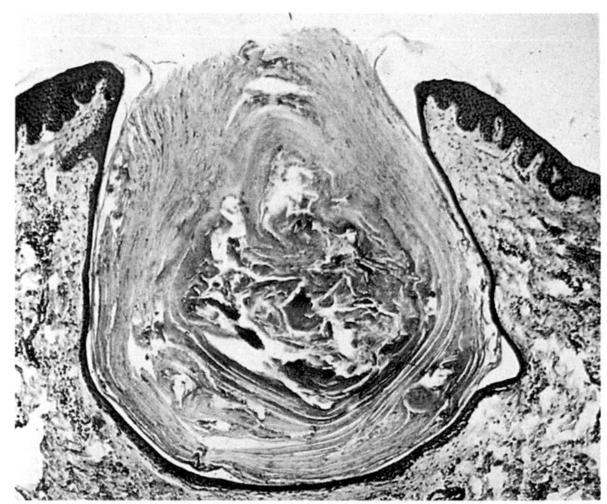

Open comedo. The mouth of the follicle is widely dilated. The comedo is composed of a lamellar keratinous mass impregnated with lipid. Bacteria are also present. The sebaceous glands have undergone atrophy. *(From Strauss and Kligman,[80] with permission.)*

reports for agents that are obviously of little value in the treatment of acne. In this section, no attempt is made to be all-inclusive; only the more commonly used or useful modalities are discussed.

In general, there are four major principles governing the therapy of acne, and the individual therapeutic modalities listed below are related to these principles, where possible. These principles are: (1) correct the altered pattern of follicular keratinization; (2) decrease sebaceous gland activity; (3) decrease the follicular bacterial population, particularly the *P. acnes* population, and inhibit the production of extracellular inflammatory products (either directly or indirectly) by inhibiting the bacterial organisms; and (4) produce an anti-inflammatory effect. The

FIGURE 73-9

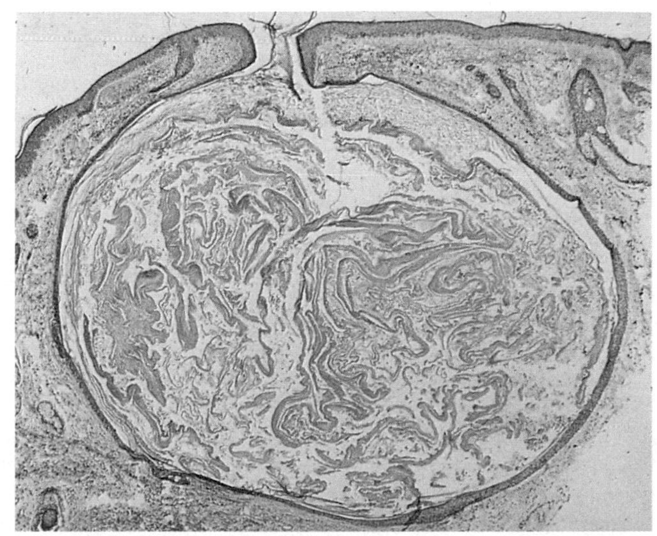

Closed comedo. The structure of the lesion is similar to that of the open comedo. However, the orifice is small, and the contents of the comedo are not as compact. *(From Strauss and Kligman,[80] with permission.)*

FIGURE 73-10

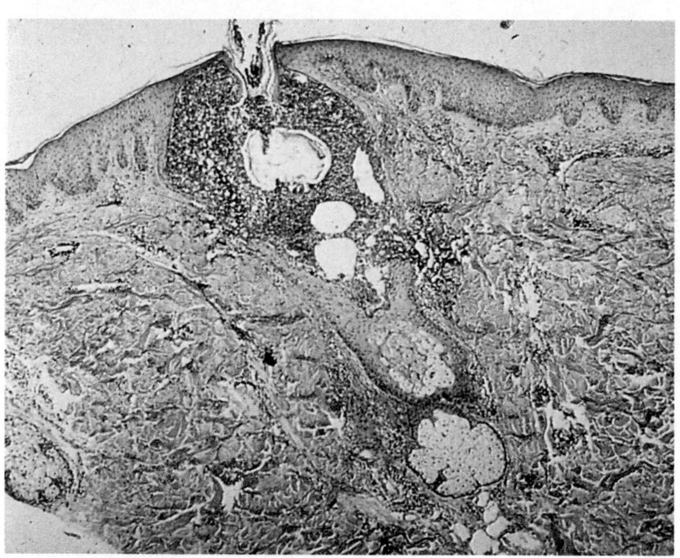

Pustule following rupture of a sebaceous follicle. The original walls of the follicle can be seen at the follicular orifice. New strands of epithelial cells are migrating from the epidermis to encapsulate the inflammatory mass, making the inflammatory material appear to be within the follicle.

first of these treatment principles, namely, changing the altered pattern of follicular keratinization, should be the primary form of therapy in noninflammatory acne; the rest of the modalities are primarily designed for use in inflammatory acne. Nonetheless, because altered follicular keratinization is the starting point for the development of inflammatory acne, therapy directed at this abnormality also should be of value in inflammatory acne.

LOCAL THERAPY

Cleansing There is no evidence that either surface sebum or surface bacteria aggravates acne. Therefore, in order for a soap or topical antibacterial agent to be of aid in the therapy of acne, the topical agent would have to remove the lipids or the bacteria (or both) from within the follicle. Certainly, the action of a soap will not remove open or closed comedones. Any dermatologist can readily describe cases of acne that he or she has seen in compulsive washers. It would appear that washing as a therapeutic measure is often overemphasized, but many acne patients do not have a pronounced seborrhea, and washing or cleansing to remove this excessive oil, if not overdone, provides subjective benefit.

Topical agents Topical therapy of acne has undergone periodic change. Many years ago, empirical reliance was placed on the use of sulfur- and resorcinol-containing products, and to a degree, they are still used in the over-the-counter market. Their mechanism of action has not been defined. Products containing salicylic acid, a keratolytic agent, have also enjoyed some popularity. However, the major topical agents now in use are retinoids and antimicrobials such as benzoyl peroxide and topical antibiotics.

Topical retinoids, such as tretinoin and tazarotene, and agents with retinoid activity, such as adapalene, are used extensively for their comedolytic activity. These agents can be irritants; in general, the order of irritancy increases as one progresses from the use of cream preparations to gels to the solution. Most patients can use low-potency tretinoin or adapalene cream daily without developing an irritant reaction. Patients must also be cautioned about sun exposure, because an exaggerated burn may follow what previously was an easily tolerated sun exposure. Unlike tretinoin, adapalene and tazarotene are specific for a subset of retinoic acid receptors (RARs). These two drugs selectively activate RAR-β and RAR-γ, but not RAR-α receptors. The binding of these agents to nuclear retinoic acid receptors affects the expression of genes involved in cell proliferation, cell differentiation, and inflammation. At the cellular level, the result may be a modification of several acne pathogenic factors, including corneocyte accumulation and cohesion, and inflammation. Topical retinoids are comedolytic, and reversal of the altered pattern of follicular keratinization has been seen at an ultrastructural level. Epidermal cell turnover is increased in comedones. Salicylic acid is also comedolytic but is not as effective as topical retinoids.

Benzoyl peroxide preparations are among the most common topical medications prescribed by dermatologists, and benzoyl peroxide is a major therapeutic agent in the over-the-counter acne market. Benzoyl peroxide is a powerful antibacterial agent, and its effect is probably related to a decrease in the bacterial population and an accompanying decrease in the hydrolysis of triglycerides. Benzoyl peroxide preparations are available in both lotion and gel forms, the latter generally being considered more active. The compound can produce significant dryness and irritation, and allergic contact dermatitis has occurred, but this is an uncommon event. Topical antibiotics are also used for the treatment of acne, the most popular preparations containing erythromycin or clindamycin. These two agents have also been used in combination preparations with benzoyl peroxide. Increased levels of *P. acnes* resistance have been reported in patients who are being treated with antibiotics. However, the development of resistance is less likely in patients who are treated with a combination of benzoyl peroxide/erythromycin or clindamycin.[43] Therefore, these combination products are preferable over topical antibiotics alone.

Another topical agent is a cream containing 20% azelaic acid. Azelaic acid is a naturally occurring dicarboxylic acid found in cereal grains. It is available as a topical cream, which is effective in inflammatory and comedonal acne. The activity of azelaic acid against inflammatory lesions may be greater than its activity against comedones. Azelaic acid is applied twice daily and its use is reported to have fewer local side effects than topical retinoids. In addition, it may help to lighten postinflammatory hyperpigmentation.

Because comedolytic agents, such as topical retinoids or salicylic acid, and antimicrobial agents, such as benzoyl peroxide or antibiotics, have different modes of action, they are often used together in an individual patient. However, they should be applied at separate times.

SYSTEMIC THERAPY Over the years, many different agents have been used systemically. The major systemic modalities that are currently being used include antibiotics and antibacterial agents, hormones, and an oral synthetic retinoid.

Antibiotics and antibacterial agents Currently, the broad-spectrum antibiotics are widely used in the treatment of acne. Although the oral administration of tetracycline does not alter sebum production, it does decrease the concentration of free fatty acids while the esterified fatty acid content increases. This decrease in free fatty acids is seen with dosages ranging from 250 mg/day to 1 g/day. The free fatty acids are probably not the major irritants in sebum, but their level is an indication of the metabolic activity of the organism and its secretion of other proinflammatory products. The decrease in free fatty acids may take several weeks to become evident. This, in turn, is reflected in the clinical course of the disease during antibiotic therapy, as several weeks are often required for maximal clinical benefit. The effect, then, is one of prevention; the individual lesions require their usual time to undergo resolution. However, the fact that a decrease in free fatty acids does occur strengthens the rationale for the use of tetracycline. Tetracycline may act through direct suppression of the number of *P. acnes,* but part of its action may also be due to its anti-inflammatory activity. Decreases in free fatty acid formation also have been reported with erythromycin, demethylchlortetracycline, clindamycin, and minocycline.

Most studies support the efficacy of tetracycline and its derivatives in the treatment of acne. In clinical practice, tetracycline is usually given initially in dosages of 500 mg/day to 1000 mg/day. While the dose is often decreased as improvement occurs and may be continued at a level of 250 mg/day or less, there is increasing concern that this may generate resistant strains. Tetracycline should be taken on an empty stomach to promote absorption. Erythromycin has been used in the past in patients who have difficulty in taking tetracycline on an empty stomach, but there is increasing evidence of the development of erythromycin-resistant strains of *P. acnes* from both the topical and systemic use of erythromycin. Therefore, it is wise to limit the use of oral erythromycin to those cases where tetracyclines are contraindicated, that is, in pregnant women and young children.

Increasingly, doxycycline and minocycline are being used as alternatives for tetracycline or in tetracycline-unresponsive cases. These two drugs appear to be more effective than tetracycline, and drug resistance is less likely to occur, especially with minocycline. Doxycycline should be administered in dosages of 50 to 100 mg twice daily. The major disadvantage of the use of doxycycline is that it can produce photosensitivity reactions, and patients should be switched to another antibiotic, if possible, during the summer months. Minocycline is given in divided dosages at a level of 100 mg/day to 200 mg/day. Patients on minocycline should be monitored carefully as the drug can cause blue-black pigmentation, especially in the acne scars, as well as the hard palate, alveolar ridge, and anterior shins. Minocycline-induced autoimmune hepatitis and a systemic lupus erythematosus-like syndrome have been reported during minocycline therapy, but to date, these side effects are very rare.[44,45] Oral clindamycin has been used in the past, but because of the potential of pseudomembranous colitis, it is now rarely used for acne.

Although long-term, low-dosage antibiotic therapy is often continued for many months, very few side effects have been observed. Tetracyclines have an affinity for rapidly mineralizing tissues and are deposited in developing teeth, where they may cause irreversible yellow-brown staining; also, tetracyclines have been reported to inhibit skeletal growth in the fetus. Therefore, they should not be administered to pregnant women, especially after the fourth month of gestation, or to babies. The tetracyclines also should not be given to children younger than 8 years of age. The only safe antibiotic to administer to pregnant women or children is erythromycin.

A rare complication, but one that can easily be missed, is the development of a gram-negative folliculitis.[46] With prolonged antibiotic therapy, gram-negative organisms may proliferate in the anterior nares and spread out onto the surrounding skin. The physician should be alerted to this diagnosis if there is a sudden flare with pustules or nodules in a patient who is otherwise improving. Two types of lesions are seen. Most commonly there are multiple pustules with an intense inflammatory areola. This type of lesion is often caused by *Enterobacter* or *Klebsiella*. The patient may also have deep indolent nodules from which *Proteus* organisms are most often isolated. Culture confirmation is necessary, and antibiotic therapy should be governed by the results of sensitivity studies. Ampicillin is often the antibiotic of choice. Patients who do not show a response to antibiotics should be treated with a full course of isotretinoin (see below).

Tetracycline in dosages ranging from 1500 mg/day to 3500 mg/day has been used in patients with very severe acne. The results of this form of therapy are encouraging, particularly because the treated patients have otherwise been resistant to therapy. Patients under treatment with high-dose tetracycline should be carefully monitored with frequent laboratory evaluation.

Trimethoprim-sulfamethoxazole combinations are also effective in acne. In general, because the potential for side effects is greater with their use, they should be used only in patients with severe acne who do not respond to other antibiotics. If trimethoprim-sulfamethoxazole is used, the patient must be monitored for potential hematologic suppression approximately monthly.

Hormonal therapy of acne Sebum secretion is increased by agents with androgenic activity, including synthetic anabolic steroids, and decreased by agents that counteract or interfere with androgen action, namely estrogens and antiandrogens. The goal of hormonal therapy is to counteract the effects of androgens on the sebaceous gland. This can be accomplished with the use of estrogens, antiandrogens, or agents designed to decrease the endogenous production of androgens by the ovary or adrenal gland, including oral contraceptives, glucocorticoids, or gonadotropin-releasing hormone (GnRH) agonists.

ESTROGENS Any estrogen given in sufficient amounts will decrease sebum production. The dose of estrogen required to suppress sebum production, however, is greater than the dose required to suppress ovulation. Although some patients will respond to lower-dose agents containing 0.035 to 0.050 μg of ethinyl estradiol or its esters, higher doses of estrogen are often required.[47] If estrogen therapy is indicated and if the physician is unfamiliar with its usage or side effects, it is best to work with a gynecologist. Breast examinations and Pap smears are recommended for women receiving estrogen therapy. The incidence of more serious side effects such as clotting and hypertension that follow the use of estrogens is, fortunately, rare in young healthy females. Nevertheless, the physician and patient should be aware of the possibilities, and the risk/benefit ratio should be carefully considered before undertaking estrogen therapy.

Although the use of estrogen therapy for acne has decreased dramatically since oral isotretinoin has been available, there are specific patients in whom its use is still appropriate. As mentioned below, estrogens can be used in combination with glucocorticoids.

ORAL CONTRACEPTIVES With the use of estrogen-progestin-containing oral contraceptives rather than estrogen alone, side effects such as delayed menses, menorrhagia, and premenstrual cramps are uncommon. However, other side effects such as nausea, weight gain, spotting, breast tenderness, amenorrhea, and melasma can occur. The third-generation progestins, desogestrel, norgestimate, and gestodene (not available in the United States), have the lowest intrinsic androgenic activity.[48] Two oral contraceptives are currently FDA approved for the treatment of acne (Ortho Tri-Cyclen and Estrostep). Ortho Tri-Cyclen is a triphasic oral contraceptive comprised of a norgestimate-ethinyl estradiol (35 μg) combination.[49] In an effort to reduce the estrogenic side effects of oral contraceptives, preparations with lower doses of estrogen (20 μg) have been developed and are being studied for the treatment of acne. Estrostep contains a graduated dose of ethinyl estradiol (20 to 35 μg) in combination with norethindrone acetate.[50] An oral contraceptive containing a low dose of estrogen (20 μg) in combination with levonorgestrel (Alesse) has also demonstrated efficacy in acne.[51] Side effects from oral contraceptive use include nausea, vomiting, abnormal menses, weight gain, and breast tenderness. Rare but more serious complications include thrombophlebitis, pulmonary embolism, and hypertension.

GLUCOCORTICOIDS Because of their anti-inflammatory activity, high-dose systemic glucocorticoids may be of benefit in the treatment of acne. In practice, their use is usually restricted to the severely involved patient. Furthermore, because of the potential side effects, these drugs are ordinarily used for limited periods of time, and recurrences are common after therapy is discontinued. Prolonged use may result in the appearance of steroid acne. Glucocorticoids in low dosages are also indicated in those female patients who have an elevation in serum DHEAS associated with an 11- or 21-hydroxylase deficiency or in other individuals with demonstrated androgen excess. Low-dose prednisone (2.5 mg or 5 mg) or dexamethasone can be given orally at bedtime to suppress adrenal androgen production.[34] The combined use of glucocorticoids and estrogens has been used in recalcitrant acne in women, based upon the inhibition of sebum production by this combination.[52] The mechanism of action is probably related to a greater reduction of plasma androgen levels by combined therapy than is produced by either drug alone.

GONADOTROPIN-RELEASING HORMONE AGONISTS GnRH agonists act on the pituitary gland to disrupt its cyclic release of gonadotropins. The net effect is suppression of ovarian steroidogenesis in women. These agents are used in the treatment of ovarian hyperandrenogenism. GnRH agonists have demonstrated efficacy in the treatment of acne and hirsutism in females both with and without endocrine disturbance.[53] Their use, however, is limited by their side-effect profile, which includes menopausal symptoms and bone loss.

ANTIANDROGENS Cyproterone acetate is a progestational antiandrogen that blocks the androgen receptor. It is combined with ethinyl estradiol in an oral contraceptive formulation that is widely used in Europe for the treatment of acne. Cyproterone acetate is not available in the United States. Spironolactone functions both as an androgen receptor blocker and inhibitor of 5α-reductase. In doses of 50 to 100 mg twice a day, it has been shown to reduce sebum production and to improve acne.[54] Side effects include potential hyperkalemia, irregular menstrual periods, breast tenderness, headache, and fatigue. As an antiandrogen, there is a risk of feminization of a male fetus if this medication is taken by a pregnant female. Risk to a fetus and the symptoms of irregular menstrual bleeding can be alleviated by combining spironolactone treatment with an oral contraceptive. Flutamide, an androgen receptor blocker, has been used at doses of 250 mg twice a day in combination with oral contraceptives for treatment of acne or hirsutism in females.[55] Liver function tests should be monitored as cases of fetal hepatitis have been reported.[56] Pregnancy should be avoided. Use of flutamide in the treatment of acne may be limited by its side effect profile.

ENZYME INHIBITORS The development of 5α-reductase inhibitors, such as finasteride, that block the conversion of testosterone to DHT in the prostate suggested the possibility of an approach to interfering with androgen action on the sebaceous glands that would be appropriate for use in males. However, finasteride does not inhibit sebum secretion.[4] Its lack of action is attributed to the existence of two different 5α-reductases, with the enzyme in the prostate being blocked by the drug while that in the skin is unaffected.[42,57] Specific inhibitors of the type 1 5a-reductase are being developed.[58] If these agents reduce sebum production, they may be efficacious in the treatment of acne.

ISOTRETINOIN (See also Chap. 257) The use of the oral retinoid, isotretinoin, has revolutionized the management of severe treatment-resistant acne.[59] Isotretinoin, like vitamin A, produces side effects, but, as discussed below, these are not usually severe enough to necessitate interruption of therapy in most cases. The remarkable aspects of isotretinoin therapy are the completeness of the remission in almost all cases and the longevity of the remission, which lasts for months to years in the great majority of patients.

Isotretinoin therapy, for all practical purposes, is always accompanied by side effects that may mimic those seen in the chronic hypervitaminosis A syndrome.[60] Thus, side effects related to the skin and mucous membranes are most common. Cheilitis of varying degrees is found in almost all cases. Other side effects that are likely to be seen in over 50 percent of patients are dryness of the mucous membranes, xerosis, conjunctivitis, and pruritus. Side effects seen with lesser degrees of frequency include bone and joint pain; thinning of hair; headache and accompanying symptoms associated with increased intracranial pressure; palmoplantar desquamation; and nausea and vomiting. The laboratory abnormalities that have occurred include elevations in triglycerides, erythrocyte sedimentation rate, platelet count, liver function tests, and white blood cells in the urine and decreases in red blood cell parameters, white cell counts, and high-density lipoprotein levels. The elevation of triglycerides, which is dose-related, is of particular concern because it is often accompanied by a decrease in the high-density lipoprotein levels, which may increase the risk of coronary artery disease. There are also reports of the development of bony hyperostoses after isotretinoin therapy, but these are more likely to be seen in patients who receive the drug for longer periods of time in higher dosages for diseases of keratinization.[61]

The issue of isotretinoin and psychiatric effects has come to the forefront. From 1982 to May 2000, 37 cases of suicide, 110 cases of hospitalized depression, suicidal ideation or suicide attempt, and 284 cases of nonhospitalized depression in patients on isotretinoin were reported to the FDA's Adverse Event Reporting System.[62] In one population-based cohort study comparing isotretinoin users with oral antibiotic users, the relative risk for development of depression or psychosis was approximately 1.0, indicating no increased risk.[63] Further studies are needed to resolve this issue of causality. Until then, a careful review for signs and symptoms of depression and suicidal ideation should be performed in all patients for whom isotretinoin therapy is considered, and the patients must be carefully monitored during therapy.

Studies show that some of the side effects are dosage related. These same studies demonstrate that clinical results can be obtained with dosages as low as 0.1 mg/kg per day. However, with such dosages, the incidence of relapses after therapy is greater. The recommended daily dosage of isotretinoin is in the range of 0.5 to 1 mg/kg per day. Because back and chest lesions show less of a response than facial lesions, dosages as high as 2 mg/kg per day may be necessary in those patients who have very severe trunk involvement. Patients with severe acne, particularly those with granulomatous lesions, will often develop marked flares of their disease when isotretinoin is started. Therefore, the initial dosing should be low, even below 0.5 mg/kg per day. These patients often need pretreatment for 1 to 2 weeks with prednisone (40 to 60 mg per day), which may have to be continued for the first 2 weeks of therapy. Isotretinoin is usually given for 20 weeks, but the length of the course of treatment is not absolute; in patients who have not shown an adequate response, therapy can be extended, if necessary. Some improvement is usually seen for 1 to 2 months after isotretinoin is discontinued, so that total clearing is not a necessary endpoint for determining when to discontinue therapy. Approximately 10 percent of patients treated with isotretinoin require a second course of the drug. The likelihood for repeat therapy is increased in patients younger than 16 to 17 years of age. It is best to allow at least 2 to 3 months between courses of isotretinoin. Studies suggest that the chances of inducing a long-term remission are greatest if the patient has received a total dose of 120 to 150 mg/kg of isotretinoin during a course of therapy.[64]

Isotretinoin should be used only in those patients with severe acne. Furthermore, laboratory monitoring is indicated. It is appropriate to obtain a baseline complete blood count and liver function tests, but the greatest attention should be paid to following serum triglyceride levels. Baseline values for serum triglycerides should be obtained and repeated at 3 to 4 weeks and 6 to 8 weeks of therapy. If the values are normal at 6 to 8 weeks, there is no need to repeat the test during the remaining course of therapy unless there are risk factors. If serum triglycerides increase above 500 mg/dL, the levels should be monitored frequently. Levels above 700 to 800 mg/dL are a reason for interrupting therapy or treating the patient with a lipid-lowering drug such as gemfibrozil. Eruptive exanthemas or pancreatitis can occur at higher serum triglyceride levels.

In rare instances, exuberant granulation tissue has appeared in some lesions. If this occurs, the dosage of drug may have to be decreased or the drug may have to be discontinued. Glucocorticoids may have to be administered either systemically or intralesionally to control the granulation tissue.

The greatest concern during isotretinoin therapy is the risk of the drug being administered during pregnancy and thereby inducing teratogenic effects in the fetus.[65,66] The drug is not mutagenic; its effect is on organogenesis. Therefore, the production of retinoic embryopathy occurs very early in pregnancy, with a peak near the third week of gestation.[65,66] Theoretically, based on animal studies and the pharmacokinetics of the drug, there should be more safety in the use of isotretinoin than either vitamin A or etretinate.[67,68] However, that is not the case, and a significant number of fetal abnormalities have been reported after the use of isotretinoin. For this reason, it should be emphasized that isotretinoin should be given only to patients who have not responded to other therapy. Furthermore, women who are of childbearing age must be fully informed of the risk of pregnancy. The patient must either avoid sexual exposure totally or should employ two highly effective contraception techniques such as the use of an oral contraceptive and condoms with a spermicidal jelly. Contraception must be started at least 1 month before isotretinoin therapy. The patient must have a negative serum pregnancy test at the time when therapy is decided upon and on the second or third day of the next menstrual period or 11 days after the last unprotected intercourse in a woman who is amenorrheic. The woman must thoroughly understand the contraception techniques she is using and continue them throughout the course of isotretinoin and for 1 month after stopping treatment. No more than 1 month's supply of drug should be given to a female patient so that she can be counseled on a monthly basis on the hazards of pregnancy during isotretinoin therapy. The pregnancy test should be repeated monthly to maintain patient awareness. The manufacturer and the FDA have recently instituted a verification process requiring that authorization stickers be affixed to prescriptions to insure that pregnancy-prevention procedures are followed.

As stated above, retinoic acid embryopathy results from the effect of isotretinoin on early organogenesis. Therefore, because the drug is not mutagenic, there is no risk to a fetus conceived by a male who is taking isotretinoin. Although it may seem obvious, it is important to remind men who are taking isotretinoin not to give any of their medication to female companions under any circumstances.

The mechanism of action of isotretinoin is not completely known. The drug produces profound inhibition of sebaceous gland activity, and this undoubtedly is of great importance in the initial clearing.[69,70] In some patients, sebaceous gland inhibition continues for at least a year, but in the majority of patients, sebum production returns to normal after 2 to 4 months.[69] Thus, this action of the drug cannot be used to explain the long-term remissions. The *P. acnes* population is also decreased during isotretinoin therapy, but this decrease is not often long lasting.[70,71] Isotretinoin has no inhibitory effect on *P. acnes* in vitro. Therefore, the effect on the bacterial population is probably indirect, resulting from the decrease in intrafollicular lipids necessary for organism growth. Isotretinoin also has anti-inflammatory activity and probably has an effect on the pattern of follicular keratinization. Once again, it has not been demonstrated that these effects are long lasting. Thus, while the drug may influence the course of severe acne through several different mechanisms, the explanation for the long-term remissions remains obscure.

DIET Currently, there is little enthusiasm for the elimination of various foods such as shellfish, chocolate, sweets, milk, and fatty foods from the diet of patients with acne. There is no evidence to support the value of elimination of these foods, although some patients will attest to flares of their disease after ingestion of certain foods. This is especially true with chocolate. Because patients will cling to their beliefs, it is best to restrict those dietary agents that they feel produce flares.

PHYSICAL THERAPY Superficial x-ray therapy, ultraviolet light therapy, and cryotherapy have been used extensively in the past for the treatment of acne. Superficial x-ray therapy was helpful in that it produced temporary suppression of the sebaceous glands, but the hazards associated with this procedure, including thyroid carcinoma, far outweigh the gains, and it is rarely, if ever, used now. There is no proof that ultraviolet light therapy is effective, other than the masking produced by the tan, and cryotherapy is rarely used.

ACNE SURGERY This modality, used for the removal of comedones and superficial pustules, aids in bringing about involution of individual acne lesions. Acne surgery was a mainstay of therapy in the past. However, with the advent of comedolytic agents such as topical vitamin A acid, it is not needed as often. Its use is primarily restricted to those patients who do not respond to comedolytic agents. Even in those patients, the comedones are removed with greater ease and less trauma if the patient is treated first with topical vitamin A acid or a similar topical agent for 3 to 4 weeks. This pretreatment should be done in all patients who are going to undergo mechanical comedo removal.

Acne surgery is helpful only when properly done, and inaccurate placement of the comedo extractor may serve only to push the inflammatory material further into the skin. Therefore, it is inadvisable to have the patient do acne surgery at home. The Unna type of comedo extractor, which has a broad flat plate and no narrow sharp edges, is preferable. The removal of open comedones does not materially influence the course of the disease because these lesions do not become inflammatory. However, it is desirable to remove them for cosmetic purposes. In contrast, closed comedones should be removed to prevent their rupture. Unfortunately, the orifice of closed comedones is often very small, and usually the material contained within the comedo can be removed only after the orifice is gently enlarged with a no. 25 needle or other suitable sharply pointed instrument.

INTRALESIONAL GLUCOCORTICOIDS Intralesional injection of glucocorticoids, either by the use of a syringe or by the use of an automatic needleless injector, usually dramatically decreases the size of deep nodular lesions. The injection of 0.05 to 0.25 mL per lesion of a triamcinolone acetate suspension (2.5 to 10 mg/mL) is recommended as the anti-inflammatory agent. This is a very useful form of therapy in the patient with nodular acne, but it often has to be repeated every 2 to 3 weeks. A major advantage is that it can be done without incising or draining the lesions, thus avoiding the possibility of scar formation.

Course and Prognosis

The age of onset of acne varies considerably. It may start as early as 6 to 8 years of age or it may not appear until the age of 20 or later. The course is one of several years' duration followed by spontaneous remission, the cause of which is unknown. While most patients will clear by their early twenties, some have acne extending well into the third or fourth decades. The extent of involvement varies, and spontaneous fluctuations in the degree of involvement are the rule rather than the exception. In the northern sections of the United States, where seasonal differences are great, relative clearing occurs in the summer for reasons that are not understood. Also, in women there is often a fluctuation in association with menses, with a flare just before the onset of menstruation. This flare is not due to a change in sebaceous gland activity as there is no increase in sebum production in the luteal phase of the menstrual cycle.

The prognosis of acne vulgaris is favorable, and almost all cases undergo spontaneous resolution as mentioned above. The only physical sequela is scarring which, with proper care, can often be minimized. Several different procedures are available to correct the scarring. Dermabrasion, laser resurfacing and deeper chemical peels seek to reduce the variability of the skin surface area and smooth out pitted complexions. The scar may be treated by superficial peeling with agents such as phenol or trichloroacetic acid, but it is unlikely that the technique will eliminate more than the most superficial scars. For discreet, depressed scars, soft tissue augmentation can be temporarily beneficial. Filler substances used include bovine collagen, autologous fat, silicone, and dermal grafts. Hypersensitivity to xenographic fillers should be ruled out prior to their use. For larger hypertrophic or aggregated pitted scars, full thickness surgical excision may result in improved scar placement and a better cosmetic outcome.

Many scars are erythematous, and the redness may be decreased by treatment with a pulsed dye laser. However, the most definitive treatment for scars is the use of deep abrasive therapy with motor-driven brushes or wheels to remove the epidermis and upper dermis down to the level of the scars. Potential patients for dermabrasive therapy must be carefully screened. Because the sebaceous glands are suppressed by the administration of isotretinoin, procedures such as dermabrasion or laser resurfacing, which are dependent upon intact appendageal structures for resurfacing, should be delayed at least 6 months. It should be noted that emotionally unstable individuals are poor risks because they likely will blame their appearance for their underlying difficulties. The improvement from dermabrasion is unlikely to solve these difficulties, and such patients are often not satisfied with the results. Persistent erythema, hyperpigmentation or hypopigmentation may follow dermabrasion or resurfacing, and, very rarely, hypertrophic scarring may occur. When deep scars exist, more than one dermabrasion may be necessary. For all these reasons, the patient must give considerable thought to the pros and cons before undertaking this surgical procedure. If there is no medical contraindication to dermabrasion, the decision to undergo the procedure should rest with the patient and not with the physician.

It is important, however, to look beyond the physical scarring, for, as has been stated, there is no disease that has caused more insecurity and feelings of inferiority than acne.[72] Indeed, acne is perceived by adolescents as having negative personal and social consequences.[73] The psychiatric morbidity associated with acne can assume many varied forms, including impaired self-image and self-esteem, social impairment, depression, or even anger.

MISCELLANEOUS TYPES OF ACNE

In the past, acne was divided into various minor subgroups on the basis of the predominant lesions. Thus, there are references to, for example, comedonal, papular, and pustular acne. As stated earlier, this classification has limited value because close scrutiny usually discloses an admixture of lesions. Nevertheless, there are a few varieties of acne that warrant presentation as separate entities.

Neonatal Acne

An acneiform eruption may occur in newborns or infants. This is often seen on the nose and adjacent portions of the cheeks. The appearance of acne at this time is probably related to the glandular development that occurs during fetal life. Clearing usually occurs, even without treatment. Recent studies suggest that neonatal cephalic pustulosis, a condition confused with neonatal acne, may be due to an inflammatory reaction against Malassezia species.[74] Acne can also start after birth and persist for a few months. This is called *infantile acne*.

Acne Excoriée des Jeunes Filles

Mild acne may be accompanied by extensive excoriations. As a result of the depth of the lesions, linear scarring may occur in these patients. Because this is most frequently seen in young adult women, the above name has been used to describe these cases. Excoriated acne is usually very difficult to treat and may even require supportive psychotherapy.

Steroid Folliculitis

Following administration of glucocorticoids or corticotropin, a folliculitis may appear. This is very uncommon in children but may occur in any adult as early as 2 weeks after steroids are started. Similar lesions may follow the prolonged application of topical glucocorticoids to the face. For this reason, topical glucocorticoids have no place in the treatment of acne, and their use on the face, in general, should be limited. The pathology of steroid acne is that of a focal folliculitis with a neutrophilic infiltrate in and around the follicle. On histologic examination, hyperkeratinization is not a prominent feature, which is consistent with the clinical findings. This type of acne clearly differs from acne vulgaris in its distribution and in the type of lesions observed. The lesions, which are usually all in the same stage of development, consist of small pustules and red papules. In contrast to acne vulgaris, they appear mainly on the trunk, shoulders, and upper arms, with lesser involvement of the face. Postinflammatory hyperpigmentation may occur, but comedones, cysts, and scarring are unusual.

Halogen Acne

Iodides and bromides may induce an acneiform eruption similar to that observed with steroids. With iodides, in particular, inflammation may be marked. The iodine content of iodized salt is low and, therefore, it is extremely unlikely that enough iodized salt could be ingested to cause this type of acne. Rather, when it occurs, it is due to ingestion of halogen-containing sedatives, expectorants, drugs, vitamins, and the like.

Miscellaneous Drugs

Acne resembling steroid acne has been reported after the use of isonicotinic acid hydrazide, and there is a report that patients in whom inactivation of this drug is slow are prone to develop this type of acne.[75] Acne also occurs in patients taking diphenylhydantoin, and it has been reported in individuals taking lithium carbonate.

Occupational Acne

Several different groups of industrial compounds may cause acne. These include coal tar derivatives, insoluble cutting oils, and chlorinated hydrocarbons (chlornaphthalenes, chlordiphenyls, and chlordiphenyloxides). Acne from these agents tends to be quite inflammatory and, in addition to large comedones, is characterized by papules, pustules, large nodules, and true cysts. Tar acne is often accompanied by hyperpigmentation. The lesions of industrial acne are not restricted to the face and, in fact, are more common on covered areas where intimate contact with clothing saturated with the offending compound is maintained. Because the cutting oils are so widely used, they are the most common cause of industrial acne. However, the chlorinated hydrocarbons have posed a more difficult problem because of the severity of the disease induced with these compounds. Many cases have occurred as the result of massive exposure in industrial accidents.[76]

Tropical Acne

Acne vulgaris may flare, and a severe folliculitis may develop, in tropical climates. These skin conditions are a major cause of dermatologic disability in the Armed Forces. Tropical acne, which occurs mainly on the trunk and buttocks, has many deep, large, inflammatory nodules with multiple draining areas. It resembles acne conglobata (see below). The pathogenesis of this type of acne is unknown, although secondary infection with coagulase-positive staphylococci almost always ensues. Systemic antibiotics must be given, but often more important is the necessity to remove the patient to a cooler environment.

Acne Aestivalis

This monomorphous eruption consists of multiple, uniform, red, papular lesions and is reported to occur after sun exposure. It is referred to as *Mallorca acne* because it occurred in many Scandinavians after they had been in southern Europe. Almost all cases have occurred in women, mainly 20 to 30 years old. The lesions are common on the shoulders, arms, neck, and chest. Histologically, the lesions resemble steroid acne in that they show a focal follicular destruction with neutrophilic infiltrate. Comedones are not part of the clinical or histologic picture. The pathogenesis is unknown.

Acne Cosmetica

In the past, various cosmetic compounds were found to induce comedo formation when applied to the external ear canal of rabbits, and cosmetics were considered to be a major cause of adult acne in women. However, new guidelines for interpretation of assays using the rabbit ear model for comedogenesis are now available[77] and cosmetic companies are testing their compounds adequately for comedogenicity before marketing. Consequently, with the exception of very greasy, occlusive products, cosmetics are infrequent etiologic agents for acne.

Pomade Acne

This form of acne is seen most often in black men and women. Some of the pomade that is applied to the scalp is also applied to the forehead and is responsible for the development of multiple, closely packed comedones close to the hairline. If the pomade is spread over greater areas of the face, the lesions themselves may be more extensive and may appear on areas such as the cheek. Pomades are comedogenic in the rabbit ear canal model.

Acne Mechanica

Acneiform eruptions have been observed after repetitive physical trauma to the skin such as rubbing. This can occur from clothing (belts and straps) or sports equipment (football helmets and shoulder pads). It has been induced by occluding the skin with adhesive tape. These extrinsic factors probably produce flares of preexisting acne, and it is uncertain whether they can produce acne in otherwise uninvolved skin. Probably the most common location to see this form of acne is on the forehead and the chin area in those wearing football helmets.

Acne with Facial Edema

Acne may uncommonly be associated with a peculiar inflammatory edema of the mid-third of the face. The edema is unresponsive to high-dose oral antibiotics, but sometimes responds to oral glucocorticoids, often in combination with isotretinoin. However, recurrences are common when glucocorticoids are stopped.

Acne Conglobata

This is a highly inflammatory disease with comedones, nodules, abscesses, and draining sinus tracts. Healing occurs with severe scarring, which is often keloidal in nature. This type of acne is rare and usually starts in adult life.

EPIDEMIOLOGY Males predominate, but a few cases have been reported in females. There may be an antecedent history of acne vulgaris, but this is not invariable.

ETIOLOGY AND PATHOGENESIS Acne conglobata is generally considered to be a separate entity from acne vulgaris because of its occurrence at a later age and its chronic unremitting course. Its true pathogenesis is unknown, but because of the frequent recovery of coagulase-positive staphylococci, and sometimes β-hemolytic streptococci, it is often considered to be a true pyoderma.

CLINICAL MANIFESTATIONS The patients with acne conglobata have a mixture of comedones, papules, pustules, nodules, abscesses, and scars on the back, buttocks, chest, and, to a lesser extent, on the abdomen, shoulders, neck, face, upper arms, and thighs. The comedones often have multiple openings. The inflammatory lesions are large, tender, and dusky-colored. The draining lesions discharge a foul-smelling serous, purulent, or mucoid material. Subcutaneous dissection with the formation of multichanneled sinus tracts is common. Healing results in an admixture of depressed and keloidal scars.

LABORATORY FINDINGS Although some lesions may be sterile or show only the presence of resident coagulase-negative staphylococci and anaerobic diphtheroids, is common to isolate coagulase-positive staphylococci. Occasionally, β-hemolytic streptococci are found. The presence of a chronic infection may be reflected by the presence of a normochromic, normocytic anemia, an elevated white blood count with an increased percentage of polymorphonuclear leukocytes, and an increased sedimentation rate. There is no evidence that these patients have decreased γ-globulins; in fact, γ-globulins may be elevated. The fasting blood sugar and glucose tolerance tests are normal.

PATHOLOGY This disease is highly inflammatory, resulting in the destruction of the normal architecture of the appendageal structures. Where follicles can be identified, there is a dense perifollicular inflammatory infiltrate of lymphocytes, polymorphonuclear leukocytes, and plasma cells. Abscess formation is common. Many proliferating tongues of epithelial cells permeate the inflammatory masses, leading eventually to the formation of interconnecting sinus tracts.

DIAGNOSIS AND DIFFERENTIAL DIAGNOSIS The highly inflammatory nature of the lesions, their distribution on the trunk, and the usual age of onset are aids in establishing the diagnosis and differentiating this disease from cystic acne vulgaris. Acne conglobata may also be confused with tropical acne, acne fulminans, and chloracne. Because lesions may occur in the axillary and inguinal regions, the disease may resemble hidradenitis suppurativa. In fact, acne conglobata, hidradenitis suppurativa, and perifolliculitis capitis abscedens et suffodiens of the scalp are often seen in the same patient.

TREATMENT The management of these patients is very difficult and the effect of treatment is often temporary. Several medications have been used including intensive high-dose therapy with antibiotics governed by in vitro antibiotic sensitivity studies, intralesional glucocorticoids, systemic glucocorticoids, x-ray therapy, surgical debridement, surgical incision, and surgical excision. The use of isotretinoin has produced dramatic results in some of these patients. In severe cases, dosages as high as 2 mg/kg per day for a 20-week course may be necessary. However, because severe flares may occur when isotretinoin is started, the initial dose should be 0.5 mg/kg per day or less, and systemic glucocorticoids are often required either before initiating isotretinoin therapy or as concomitant therapy.

COURSE AND PROGNOSIS This disease tends to run a recalcitrant, chronic course, and patients often have emotional disturbances. However, the prognosis is much better now as isotretinoin can be used to control the active disease, although in many instances significant scarring may remain. Slow-growing, well-differentiated squamous cell carcinoma has been reported in the lesions of acne conglobata.[78] To date, no metastases have been reported. Spondyloarthropathy has also been reported.[79]

Acne Fulminans

This catastrophic disease has also been called *acute febrile ulcerative acne*. It is characterized by the sudden appearance of massive, inflammatory, tender lesions of the back and chest that rapidly become ulcerative and heal with scarring. The disease is reported to occur exclusively in teenage boys. The face is often not involved. The patients are febrile, have a leukocytosis of 10,000 to 30,000/mm^3 white blood cells, and usually have polyarthralgia, myalgia, and other systemic symptoms. X-ray examination may disclose the presence of osteolytic areas in parts of bone tenderness. Although this disease is often classified with acne conglobata, there are basic differences. The onset of acne fulminans is more explosive; nodules and polyporous comedones are less common; the face is not involved as frequently and the neck is usually spared; ulcerative and crusted lesions are unique; and systemic symptoms are more common. Systemic glucocorticoid therapy, along with intensive use of oral antibiotics and intralesional glucocorticoids, is the treatment regimen required for these patients. Isotretinoin is also of benefit in these patients, but in order to prevent explosive flares, systemic glucocorticoids must be started before isotretinoin and continued during the first few weeks of isotretinoin therapy. The initial dosing of isotretinoin must also be small. The daily dose of glucocorticoids should be slowly decreased as tolerated.

Steatocystoma Multiplex

This is a disorder characterized by multiple, varying sized, cystic lesions of the trunk.

EPIDEMIOLOGY Both men and women may be affected. The disease starts in early adult life. It is familial and has been said to be inherited as a dominant characteristic.

ETIOLOGY AND PATHOGENESIS The exact pathogenesis of these lesions is unknown. It has been proposed that this is a cystic sebaceous nevus, and it has also been proposed that the lesions are a result of blockage of the follicular orifice. Relationship to the development of the sebaceous glands is indicated by their location in the midline and the appearance of the lesions at puberty.

CLINICAL MANIFESTATIONS The cutaneous lesions appear chiefly on the upper anterior trunk. They may also be found on the back, arms, forearms, thighs, and scrotum. The individual lesions vary from 1 to 2 mm up to 1 to 2 cm in diameter. They may be flesh-colored or distinctly yellow. The lesions are soft and freely movable. The contents may be either a clear oily liquid or a cheesy white material. There are no systemic manifestations. No laboratory abnormalities have been reported.

PATHOLOGY Serial sections will disclose the presence of a follicular duct that is filled with keratinous material. The cysts are filled with keratin and lipid. Usually, however, there is much less keratin than is found in keratinous cysts. The follicular wall is atrophic, but appendageal remnants may be visible. Some of the cells of the cyst walls may show lipid differentiation. Lanugo hairs may be seen. The surrounding dermis is compressed by the expanding lesions.

DIAGNOSIS AND DIFFERENTIAL DIAGNOSIS The appearance of the multiple cystic lesions, varying in size, particularly on the anterior chest, is essential for diagnosis. Any confusion with solid epithelial tumors or infiltrates into the skin can be eliminated by incising one of the lesions.

TREATMENT None is indicated, but the lesions can be drained by incision or aspiration. They may be excised, although the number of lesions usually precludes any significant overall improvement.

COURSE AND PROGNOSIS The number of lesions, as well as their size, may increase slowly. Except for the cosmetic appearance, this disease poses no threat to the person's health. Malignant degeneration has not been reported.

REFERENCES

1. Ito M: New findings on the proteins of sebaceous glands. *J Invest Dermatol* **82**:381, 1984
2. Stewart ME, Steele WA et al: Changes in the relative amounts of endogenous and exogenous fatty acids in sebaceous lipids during early adolescence. *J Invest Dermatol* **92**:371, 1989
3. Jacobsen E: Age-related changes in sebaceous wax ester secretion rates in men and women. *J Invest Dermatol* **85**:483, 1985
4. Imperato-McGinley J et al: The androgen control of sebum production. Studies of subjects with dihydrotestosterone deficiency and complete androgen insensitivity. *J Clin Endocrinol Metabol* **76**:524, 1993
5. Chen W et al: Cutaneous androgen metabolism: Basic research and clinical progress *J Invest Dermatol,* **119**:992, 2002
6. Stewart M et al: Effect of oral 13-*cis*-retinoic acid at three dose levels on sustainable rates of sebum secretion and on acne. *J Am Acad Dermatol* **8**:532, 1983
7. Hommel L et al: Sebum excretion rate in subjects treated with oral all-*trans*-retinoic acid. *Dermatology* **193**:127, 1996
8. Chen W et al: Exocrine gland dysfunction in MC5-R deficient mice: Evidence for coordinated regulation of exocrine gland function by melanocortin peptides. *Cell* **91**:789, 1997
9. Thiboutot D et al: The melanocortin-5 receptor is expressed in human sebaceous glands and rat preputial cells. *J Invest Dermatol* **115**:614, 2000
10. Laurent S et al: Growth of sebaceous cells in monolayer culture. *In Vitro Cell Dev Biol* **28A**:83, 1992
11. Rosenfield RL et al: Rat preputial sebocyte differentiation involves peroxisome proliferator-activated receptors. *J Invest Dermatol* **112**:226, 1999
12. Rosenfeld RK, Deplewski D, Greene ME: Peroxisome proliferator-activated receptors and skin development. *Horm Res* **54**:269, 2000
13. Chen H et al: Leptin modulates the effects of acyl CoA: diacylglycerol acyltransferase deficiency on murine fur and sebaceous glands. *J Clin Invest* **109**:175, 2002
14. Wilkins JWJ, Voorhees JJ: Prevalence of nodulocystic acne in white and Negro males. *Arch Dermatol* **102**:631, 1970
15. Voorhees JJ: Nodulocystic acne as a phenotypic feature of the XYY genotype. *Arch Dermatol* **105**:913, 1972
16. Knutson D: Ultrastructural observations in acne vulgaris: The normal sebaceous follicle and acne lesions. *J Invest Dermatol* **62**:288, 1974
17. Downing D, Stewart M et al: Essential fatty acids and acne. *J Am Acad Dermatol* **14**:221, 1986
18. Guy R, Green M et al: Modeling of acne in vitro. *J Invest Dermatol* **106**:176, 1996
19. Choudhry R, Hodgins M et al: Localization of androgen receptors in human skin by immunohistochemistry: Implications for the hormonal regulation

of hair growth, sebaceous glands and sweat glands. *J Endocrinol* **133**:467, 1991
20. Cunliffe W, Forster R: Androgen control of the pilosebaceous duct? *Br J Dermatol* **116**:449, 1987
21. Hay JB, Hodgins MB: Distribution of androgen metabolizing enzymes in isolated tissues of human forehead and axillary skin. *J Endocrinol* **79**:29, 1978
22. Leyden JJ: Propionibacterium levels in patients with and without acne vulgaris. *J Invest Dermatol* **65**:382, 1975
23. Webster G: Mechanisms of *Propionibacterium acnes*-mediated inflammation in acne vulgaris. *Semin Dermatol* **1**:299, 1982
24. Puhvel SM, Sakamoto M: The chemoattractant properties of comedonal components. *J Invest Dermatol* **71**:324, 1978
25. Tucker SB: Inflammation in acne. Leukocyte attraction and cytotoxicity by comedonal material. *J Invest Dermatol* **74**:21, 1980
26. Webster GF: Polymorphonuclear leukocyte lysosomal release in response to *Propionibacterium acnes* in vitro and its enhancement by sera from inflammatory acne patients. *J Invest Dermatol* **74**:398, 1980
27. Webster GF: Complement activation in acne vulgaris. Consumption of complement by comedones. *Infect Immun* **26**:183, 1979
28. Puhvel SM: Study of antibody levels to Corynebacterium acnes. *Arch Dermatol* **99**:421, 1964
29. Kersey P: Delayed skin test reactivity to *Propionibacterium acnes* correlates with severity of inflammation in acne vulgaris. *Br J Dermatol* **103**:651, 1980
30. Harris HH: Sustainable rates of sebum secretion in acne patients and matched normal control subjects. *J Am Acad Dermatol* **8**:200, 1983
31. Strauss JS et al: The effect of androgens and estrogens on human sebaceous glands. *J Invest Dermatol* **39**:139, 1962
32. Farrell L et al: The treatment of severe cystic acne with 13-*cis*-retinoic acid. *Am Acad Dermatol* **3**:602, 1980
33. Lucky AW et al: Acne vulgaris in premenarchal girls. *Arch Dermatol* **130**:308, 1994
34. Marynick SP et al: Androgen excess in cystic acne. *N Engl J Med* **308**:981, 1983
35. Lucky A et al: Plasma androgens in women with acne vulgaris. *J Invest Dermatol* **81**:70, 1983
36. Levell MJ: Acne is not associated with abnormal plasma androgens. *Br J Dermatol* **120**:649, 1989
37. Sultan C: Free and total plasma testosterone in men and women with acne. *Acta Derm Venereol* **66**:301, 1986
38. Lookingbill DP et al: Tissue production of androgens in women with acne. *J Am Acad Dermatol* **12**:481, 1985
39. Simpson NB et al: The relationship between the in vitro activity of 3β-hydroxysteroid dehydrogenase delta$^{4-5}$-isomerase in human sebaceous glands and their secretory activity in vivo. *J Invest Dermatol* **81**:139, 1983
40. Sansone G, Reisner RM: Differential rates of conversion of testosterone to dihydrotestosterone in acne and in normal human skin—A possible pathogenic factor in acne. *J Invest Dermatol* **56**:366, 1971
41. Jenkins EP, Andersson S et al: Genetic and pharmacological evidence for more than one human steroid 5α reductase. *J Clin Invest* **89**:293, 1992
42. Thiboutot D, Harris G et al: Activity of the type 1 5α-reductase exhibits regional differences in isolated sebaceous glands and whole skin. *J Invest Dermatol* **105**:209, 1995
43. Eady E, Bojar R et al: The effects of acne treatment with a combination of benzoyl peroxide and erythromycin on skin carriage of erythromycin-resistant propionibacteria. *Br J Dermatol* **134**:107, 1996
44. Gough A: Minocycline-induced autoimmune hepatitis and systemic lupus erythematosus-like syndrome. *BMJ* **312**:169, 1996
45. Goulden V: Safety of long-term high-dose minocycline in the treatment of acne. *Br J Dermatol* **134**:693, 1966
46. Leyden JJ: Gram-negative folliculitis: A complication of antibiotic therapy in acne vulgaris. *Br J Dermatol* **88**:533, 1973
47. Strauss JS, Kligman AM: Effect of cyclic progestin-estrogen therapy on sebum and acne in women. *JAMA* **190**:815, 1964
48. Speroff L, DeCherney A: Evaluation of a new generation of oral contraceptives. *Obstet Gynecol* **81**:1034, 1993
49. Lucky AW et al: Effectiveness of norgestimate and ethinyl estradiol in treating moderate acne vulgaris. *J Am Acad Dermatol* **37**:746, 1997
50. Maloney M et al: Use of a low-dose oral contraceptive containing norethindrone acetate and ethinyl estradiol in the treatment of moderate acne vulgaris. *Clin J Women's Health* **1**:124, 2001
51. Thiboutot D et al: A randomized, controlled trial of a low-dose contraceptive containing 20 μg of ethinylestradiol and 100 μg of levonorgestrel for acne treatment. *Fertil Steril* **76**:461, 2001
52. Pochi P, Strauss J: Sebaceous gland inhibition from combined glucocorticoid-estrogen treatment. *Arch Dermatol* **112**:1108, 1976
53. Faloia E, Filipponi S et al: Treatment with a gonadotropin-releasing hormone agonist in acne or idiopathic hirsutism. *J Endocrinol Invest* **16**:675, 1993
54. Goodfellow A, Alaghband-Zadeh J et al: Oral spironolactone improves acne vulgaris and reduces sebum excretion. *Br J Dermatol* **111**:209, 1984
55. Cusan L: Treatment of hirsutism with the pure antiandrogen flutamide. *J Am Acad Dermatol* **23**:462, 1990
56. Wysowski D, Freiman J et al: Fatal and nonfatal hepatotoxicity associated with flutamide. *Ann Int Med* **118**:860, 1993
57. Russell DW, Wilson JD: Steroid 5α-reductase: Two genes/two enzymes. *Annu Rev Biochem* **63**:25, 1994
58. Chen W et al: The 5 alpha-reductase system and its inhibitors. Recent development and its perspective in treating androgen-dependent skin disorders. *Dermatology* **193**:177, 1996
59. Peck GL: Prolonged remissions of cystic acne with 13-*cis*-retinoic acid. *N Engl J Med* **300**:329, 1979
60. Windhorst DB, Nigra T: General clinical toxicity of oral retinoids. *J Am Acad Dermatol* **6**:675, 1982
61. Pittsley RA, Yoder FW: Retinoid hyperostosis: Skeletal toxicity associated with long-term administration of 13-*cis*-retinoic acid for refractory ichthyosis. *N Engl J Med* **308**:1012, 1983
62. Wysowski D et al: An analysis of reports of depression and suicide in patients treated with isotretinoin. *J Am Acad Dermatol* **45**:515, 2001
63. Jick S et al: Isotretinoin use and risk of depression, psychotic symptoms, suicide and attempted suicide. *Arch Dermatol* **136**:1231, 2000
64. Lehucher C, Weber-Buisset M: Isotretinoin and acne in practice: A prospective analysis of 188 cases over 9 years. *Dermatology* **186**:123, 1993
65. Stern RS: Isotretinoin and pregnancy. *J Am Acad Dermatol* **10**:851, 1984
66. Lammer EJ: Retinoic acid embryopathy. *N Engl J Med* **310**:1023, 1984
67. Kamm JJ: Toxicology, carcinogenicity, and teratogenicity of some orally administered retinoids. *J Am Acad Dermatol* **6**:652, 1982
68. Brazzell RK, Colburn WA: Pharmacokinetics of the retinoids isotretinoin and etretinate. A comparative review. *J Am Acad Dermatol* **6**:643, 1982
69. Strauss JS, Stranieri AM: Changes in long-term sebum production from isotretinoin therapy. *J Am Acad Dermatol* **6**:751, 1982
70. Leyden JJ, McGinley KJ: Effect of 13-*cis*-retinoic acid on sebum production and *Propionibacterium acnes* in severe nodulocystic acne. *Arch Dermatol* **272**:331, 1982
71. Weismann A: Reduction of bacterial skin flora during treatment with 13-*cis*-retinoic acid. *Arch Dermatol* **270**:179, 1981
72. Koo J: The psychological impact of acne: Patient's perceptions. *J Am Acad Dermatol* **32**:S26, 1995
73. Krowchuk D et al: The psychosocial effects of acne on adolescents. *Pediatr Dermatol* **8**:332, 1991
74. Niamba P et al: Is common neonatal cephalic pustulosis (neonatal acne) triggered by Malassezia sympodialis? *Arch Dermatol* **134**:995, 1998
75. Cohen LK: Isoniazid-induced acne and pellagra: Occurrence in slow inactivators of isoniazid. *Arch Dermatol* **109**:377, 1974
76. Dunagin WG: Cutaneous signs of systemic toxicity due to dioxins and related chemicals. *J Am Acad Dermatol* **10**:689, 1984
77. Strauss JS: American Academy of Dermatology Invitational Symposium on Comedogenicity. *J Am Acad Dermatol* **20**:272, 1989
78. Dillon JS, Spjut HJ: Epidermoid carcinoma occurring in acne conglobata. *Ann Surg* **159**:451, 1964
79. Ellis BI: Acne-associated spondyloarthropathy: Radiographic features. *Radiology* **162**:541, 1987
80. Strauss JS, Kligman AM: The pathologic dynamics of acne vulgaris. *Arch Dermatol* **82**:779, 1968

CHAPTER 74

Gerd Plewig
Thomas Jansen

Rosacea

The disease was originally called *acne rosacea,* an inappropriate term that invites confusion with acne vulgaris and is best abandoned. Papules and pustules occur in the central region of the face against a livid erythematous background with telangiectases. Later, there may occur diffuse hyperplasia of connective tissue with enlarged sebaceous glands. The disease evolves in stages. The early signs are recurrent episodes of blushing that finally become persistent dark red erythema, particularly on the nose and cheeks, often before the age of 20 years. These persons are the so-called flushers and blushers. Rosacea is common in the third and fourth decades and peaks between the ages of 40 and 50 years. In the worst cases, nonpitting edema (fibrosis), particularly of the nose (rhinophyma), may develop after many years. Early diagnosis and appropriate management are required to minimize patient discomfort and psychological distress.

OCCURRENCE

Rosacea is a relatively common disease, especially in fair-skinned people of Celtic or northern European heritage, hence the term *curse of the Celts.*[1] It is rarer in dark-skinned people, particularly so with American and African blacks.[2] The disease is estimated to affect at least 5 percent of Americans, or some 13 million people. Although it is said that women are more often affected than men in earlier stages (3:1 ratio), men develop the tissue and sebaceous gland hyperplasia leading to rhinophyma much more frequently. Although rosacea tends to be milder in women, it can lead to severe emotional distress owing to its chronic course.

The importance of sun-damaged skin in rosacea cannot be stressed enough.[3] Rosacea is always associated with solar elastosis and often with heliodermatosis. This is a consistent background on which rosacea is superimposed. However, an increase in ultraviolet sensitivity has not been demonstrated in rosacea patients, nor is the disease more common in outdoor workers.

There is also a wide spectrum of rosacea manifestations. Especially in young patients there may be a history of acne giving rise to variants of two independent facial diseases that are difficult to recognize and treat. It is important to realize that rosacea and acne can coexist, though normally rosacea begins and reaches its peak incidence decades after acne declines.

PATHOGENESIS

Although the precise etiology of rosacea remains a mystery, various factors have been suspected to contribute to this condition.[4,5] None of them, however, has been definitely confirmed. Rosacea patients are constitutionally predisposed to flushing and blushing. Migraine headaches have been shown to be two or three times more common in rosacea patients than among age- and sex-matched control subjects, suggesting the possibility of a more generalized vascular pathogenesis. The fact that vasomotor lability is especially pronounced during menopause and that a significant number of rosacea patients are perimenopausal women supports this hypothesis.[5] Experimental studies show that the involved skin responds normally to various vasoactive chemicals, with facial blood vessels maintaining their capacity for dilatation and constriction. The basic abnormality seems to be a microcirculatory disturbance of the function of the facial angular veins directly involved in the brain-cooling vascular mechanism.[6]

An hypothesis holds that rosacea is preceded by degenerative changes of the perivascular, and possibly vascular, collagen and elastic tissues in inherently susceptible individuals exposed to climatic factors.[4] These dermal changes are believed to lead to small vessel dilatation resulting in flushing, telangiectases, and erythema. Eventually, the dilated vessels become incompetent with perivascular leakage of potentially inflammatory substances.

Different mediators, including the neurotransmitter peptide substance P, histamine, serotonin, and prostaglandins, have been proposed to be involved in the erythematous response. It is also possible that none of these is responsible but that the reaction is triggered by another, still unknown mechanism.

The presence of microorganisms has also been examined as a potential contributing factor to rosacea, but results have been inconclusive. *Demodex folliculorum* mites are merely commensals and do not, in contrast to former belief, play a significant part in the pathogenesis of rosacea, although an inflammatory reaction to the mites may be important in this condition.[7] This is different from *Demodex folliculorum* folliculitis (demodicosis, demodicidosis). Some reports suggest that patients with rosacea have an increased prevalence of *Helicobacter pylori* infection, although other reports fail to confirm this association.[8] Eradication of *H. pylori* has been occasionally associated with an improvement of rosacea symptoms. Study results are inconsistent, but it has been suggested that *H. pylori* synthesizes gastrin, which may stimulate flushing.

Rosacea is considered by some authors as a seborrheic disease. Many patients with rosacea, however, do not show signs of excessive sebaceous activity although others do. One report says that there is no significant association between rosacea and seborrhea. It is not a primary disease of sebaceous follicles in contrast to acne vulgaris. Comedones are absent and the initial findings are not related to follicles, though papulopustules are follicular bound.

No acceptable evidence of genetic predisposition has been reported so far, although more than one case in a family is often encountered.

CLINICAL FINDINGS

Rosacea is a centrofacial disease. It is principally localized on the nose, cheeks, chin, forehead, and glabella. Rarer localizations, which are usually overlooked, are the retroauricular areas, the V-shaped area of the chest, the neck, the back, the balded scalp, and even the limbs (extrafacial rosacea).[9]

The hallmarks of rosacea are livid red erythema and telangiectases, preceded by episodes of flushing, papules, and pustules. Comedones are notably absent. If present, they are of different origin, such as concomitant solar comedones (Favre-Racouchot's disease), acne vulgaris, or contact acne (acne cosmetica). In severe cases, papules are numerous enough to be confluent. Granulomatous changes can emerge in later stages, sometimes receiving special designations such as *lupoid rosacea*. Rhinophyma and other phymas are the ultimate tissue reaction, particularly in men.

For didactic as well as for therapeutic reasons, rosacea is classified into stages, which may develop successively (Table 74-1).[1] In some affected individuals, there is progression through all stages, but this succession does not necessarily occur.

Episodic Erythema (The Rosacea Diathesis)

Rosacea patients characteristically react with erythema on the central areas of the face, less often the neck and the V-shaped area of the chest. These individuals are constitutionally predisposed to flushing and blushing, evoked by numerous nonspecific stimuli such as ultraviolet radiation, heat, cold, chemical irritation, strong emotions, alcoholic beverages, hot drinks, and spices. Flushing is more intense and lasts longer than in those who tend to blush when embarrassed. Eventually flushing and blushing lead to permanent erythema.

Stage I

The erythema persists for hours and days, hence the old description *erythema congestivum*. Telangiectases become progressively more prominent, forming sprays on the nose, nasolabial folds, cheeks, and glabella. Most of these patients complain of sensitive skin that stings and burns after application of a variety of cosmetics, fragrances, and certain sunscreens. Trauma from abrasives and peeling agents readily induces long-lasting erythema.

TABLE 74-1

Rosacea: Classification and Key Features

Stages in rosacea
- Episodic erythema: the rosacea diathesis
- Stage I. Persistent moderate erythema with scattered telangiectases
- Stage II. Persistent erythema, numerous telangiectases, papules, and pustules
- Stage III. Persistent deep erythema, dense telangiectases forming sprays of vessel especially on the nose; papules, pustules, nodules with variable plaquelike edema

Variants of rosacea
- Persistent edema of rosacea
- Ophthalmic rosacea
- Lupoid or granulomatous rosacea
- Steroid rosacea
- Gram-negative rosacea
- Rosacea conglobata
- Rosacea fulminans
- Phymas in rosacea
  - Rhinophyma
  - Gnathophyma
  - Metophyma
  - Otophyma
  - Blepharophyma

Stage II

Dome-shaped inflammatory papules less than 0.5 to 1.0 mm in size, with or without pustules, crop up and persist for weeks. Some papules show a small pustule at the apex, justifying the term *papulopustular*. The lesions are always follicular in origin; vellus and sebaceous follicles are involved. Although patients with concomitant acne may exhibit comedones, comedones should be considered part of an acne process unrelated to rosacea. Spacious sebaceous follicles contain cheesy follicular filaments, which can easily be expressed as a pasty wormlike material. The deeper inflammatory lesions may heal with scarring, but scars are small and tend to be shallow. Facial pores become more prominent. If there has been much solar exposure for decades, the stigmata of photodamaged skin become superimposed, such as elastosis, solar comedones, and heliodermatosis. The papulopustular attacks become increasingly frequent. Finally, rosacea may extend over the entire face and also the scalp (Fig. 74-1). Itchy follicular pustules of the scalp are typical. These either contain the normal bacterial flora or are sterile.

Stage III

A small proportion of the patients go on to develop the worst expressions of the disease, namely large inflammatory nodules, furunculoid infiltrations, and tissue hyperplasia. These derangements occur particularly on the cheeks and nose, less often on the chin, forehead, or ears (Fig. 74-2). The facial contours become coarse, thickened, and irregular. Although patients may not appreciate the coarsened appearance, the change becomes evident when photographs from previous years are reviewed. Finally, the patient shows inflamed and thickened edematous skin with large pores, resembling the surface of an orange (*peau d'orange*). These features are caused by inflammatory infiltration, connective tissue hypertrophy with masses of collagen deposition, diffuse sebaceous gland hyperplasia, and overgrowth of individual sebaceous glands forming dozens of yellowish umbilicated papules on cheeks, forehead, temples, and nose. Along with folds and ridges the appearance may mimic leonine facies in leprosy or leukemia. The ultimate deformities are the phymas, such as rhinophyma (Figs. 74-3 and 74-4).

VARIANTS OF ROSACEA

Classic rosacea is easily recognized; the variants of rosacea are easily overlooked or misdiagnosed.

Persistent Edema of Rosacea

This feature is uncommon and the diagnosis is often missed. The literature hardly mentions this distressing condition referred as rosaceous lymphedema, chronic upper facial erythematous edema, or Morbihan's disease.[10] A hard nonpitting edema is found on the areas involved, mainly on the forehead, glabella, upper eyelids, nose, or cheeks (Fig. 74-5). Subjective complaints are slight, except for the deformed facial contours. This unusual manifestation may lead to other irrelevant diagnoses that delay proper treatment, such as streptococcal cellulitis. A similar edema, although rare, may occur in acne vulgaris and in Melkersson-Rosenthal's syndrome, or without any of these disorders.

FIGURE 74-1

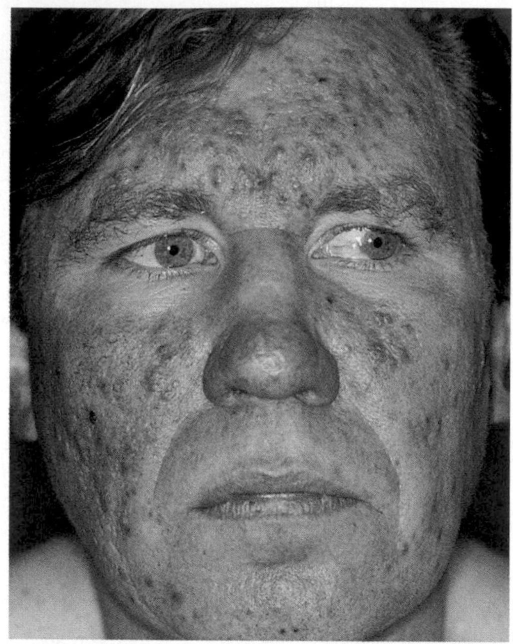

A.

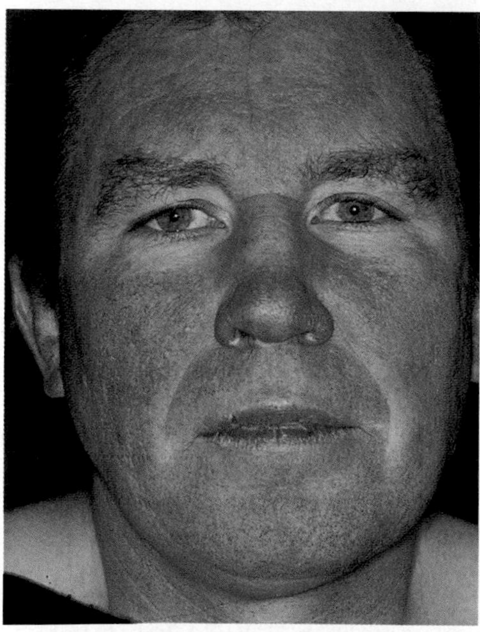

B.

A. Rosacea, stage II. Persistent erythema, telangiectases, numerous papules, pustules, and bulbous nose. Before therapy. *B.* After 12 weeks of isotretinoin treatment (0.5 mg/kg body weight per day, monotherapy). There was no recurrence in 2 years.

This edema develops on the background of chronic inflammation from any cause, including bacterial infection.

Ophthalmic Rosacea (Ocular Rosacea)

The exact prevalence of ocular involvement in patients with rosacea is unknown, although it has been reported to be as low as 3 percent and as

FIGURE 74-2

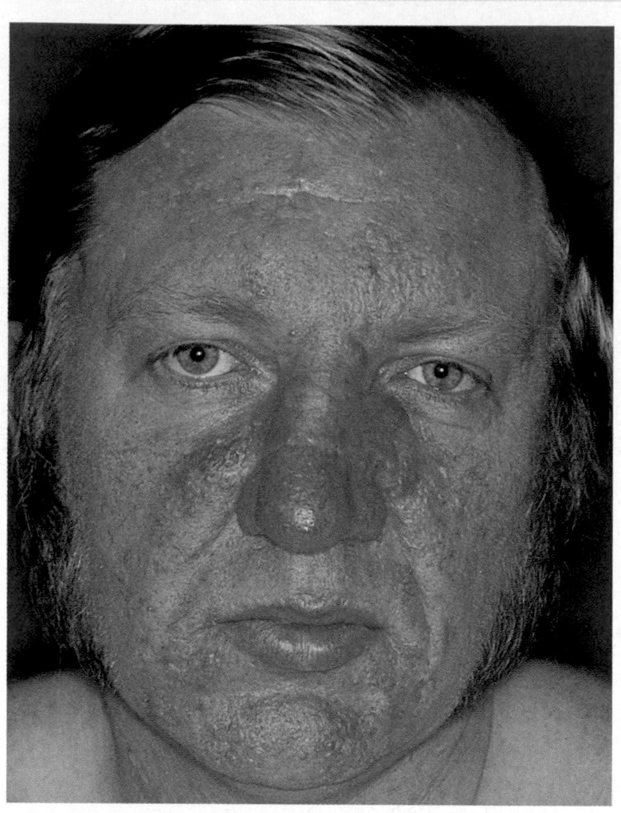

Rosacea, stage III. Persistent erythema, papules, pustules, rhinophyma, plaquelike edema and phymas of the perinasal zone.

FIGURE 74-3

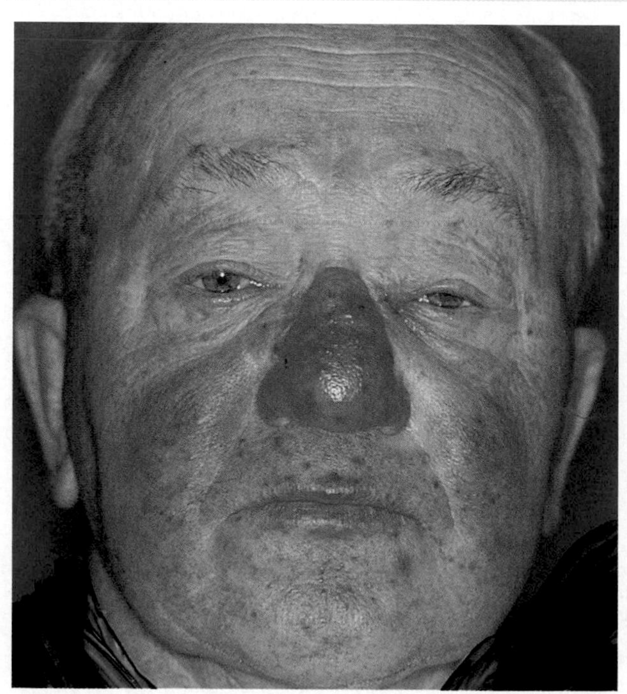

Rosacea, stage III. Persistent deep erythema, papules, rhinophyma, and persistent edema of cheeks. Ophthalmic rosacea with blepharitis and conjunctivitis.

FIGURE 74-4

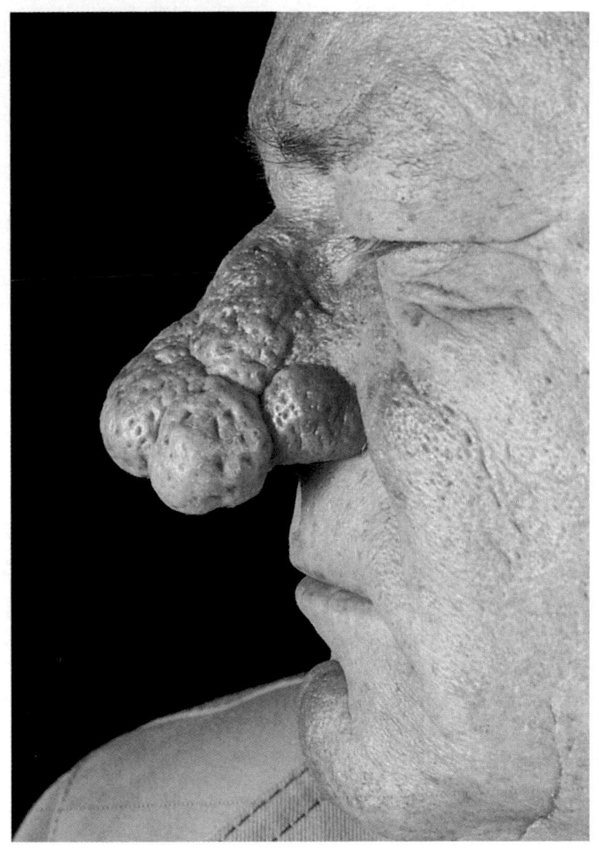

Rosacea, stage III. Severe rhinophyma. Persistent, deep erythema and edema of the forehead (metophyma), cheeks, and chin (gnatophyma).

high as 58 percent. The disease may begin in the eye and escape diagnosis for a long time, even years, and be accompanied by inappropriate treatments. Ophthalmic manifestations may develop prior to cutaneous manifestations in up to 20 percent of patients with ophthalmic rosacea.

FIGURE 74-5

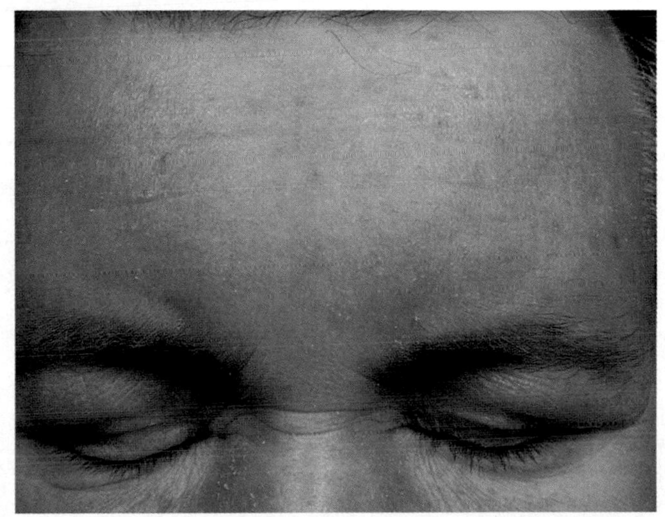

Persistent edema of rosacea. This patient had stage II rosacea, which quickly responded to oral tetracyclines, but the nonpitting edema on forehead, eyelids, and cheeks (not shown) did not respond.

TABLE 74-2

Ophthalmic Rosacea: Clinical Spectrum

Lid	Blepharitis
	Chalazion, meibomian gland plugging
Conjunctiva	Conjunctival hyperemia
	Conjunctivitis
	Keratoconjunctivitis sicca
Sclera	Scleritis, episcleritis
Iris	Iritis, iridocyclitis, hypopyoniritis
Cornea	Superficial punctate keratopathy
	Corneal thinning, ulceration, perforation
	Corneal neovascularization, scarring
	Blindness

Approximately half of these patients develop skin lesions first, and a minority develop both manifestations simultaneously. The ophthalmic complications are independent of the severity of facial rosacea. However, there is a strong correlation between the degree of eye involvement and tendency to flushing.

The ophthalmic signs are variable including blepharitis, conjunctivitis, iritis, iridocyclitis, hypopyoniritis, and even keratitis (Table 74-2; Fig. 74-3).[11–13] The term *ophthalmic rosacea* (ophthalmorosacea) covers all these signs, also discourteously referred to as rabbit eyes.

Rosacea keratitis has an unfavorable prognosis, and in extreme cases can lead to blindness because of corneal opacity. The most frequent eye sign, which may never progress, is chronically inflamed margins of the eyelids, with scales and crusts, quite similar to seborrheic dermatitis, with which it is often confused. Pain and photophobia may be present. It is instructive to ask rosacea patients how their eyes react to bright sunlight. All patients with progressive rosacea should be seen by an ophthalmologist for a thorough examination to detect other subclinical complications. Indeed, such rosacea patients are ideally managed by the cooperative efforts of the dermatologist and the ophthalmologist.

Lupoid or Granulomatous Rosacea

Some patients develop epithelioid (lupoid) granulomas in a diffuse pattern.[14] Clinically, dozens of brown-red papules or little nodules are seen on a diffusely reddened, thickened skin, frequently involving the lower eyelids. Diascopy with a glass spatula or slide reveals the infiltrations. Histopathologic examination reveals perifollicular and perivascular noncaseating epithelioid granulomas. These histopathologic features lead to earlier designations such as *rosacea-like tuberculid of Lewandowsky* and *micropapular tuberculid.*

The course is chronic and unremitting. The diagnosis is often missed. Differential diagnosis includes lupoid perioral dermatitis, lupoid steroid rosacea, small nodular sarcoidosis, and lupus miliaris disseminatus faciei.

Steroid Rosacea

When a rosacea patient is erroneously treated for a prolonged time with topical corticosteroids, the disorder may at first respond, but inevitably the signs of steroid atrophy emerge with thinning of the skin and marked increase in telangiectases.[15,16] The complexion becomes dark red with a copper-like tone. Soon the surface becomes studded with follicular, round, deep-seated papulopustules, firm nodules, and even secondary comedones. The appearance is shocking with a flaming red, scaling, papule-covered face (Fig. 74-6). Steroid rosacea is a pitiable, avoidable

FIGURE 74-6

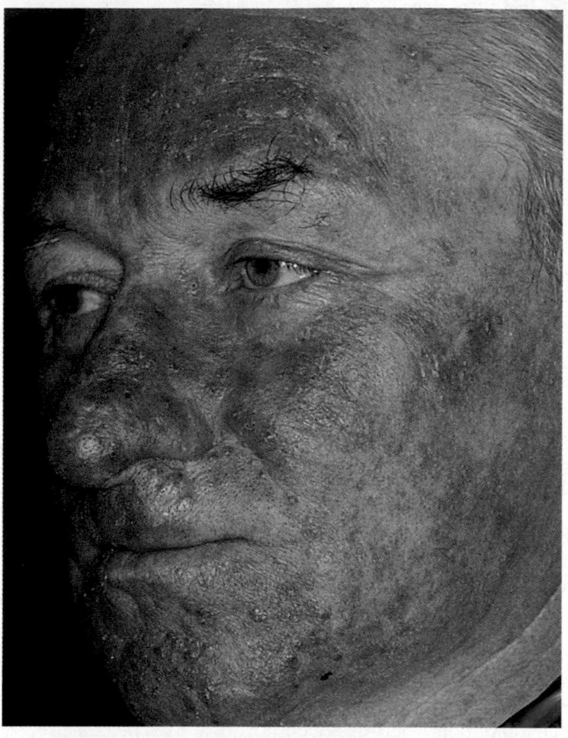

Steroid rosacea. The patient was treated for a long time with topical glucocorticoid preparations. Flaming red, atrophic facial skin, papulopustules, and edema. Withdrawal of the steroid caused an uncomfortable exacerbation of rosacea.

condition that, in addition to disfigurement, is accompanied by severe discomfort and pain. Withdrawal of the steroid is inevitably accompanied by exacerbation of the disease, a trying experience for patient and physician.

Gram-Negative Rosacea

The process has only recently been described among gram-negative infections,[17] and is not likely to be diagnosed unless one has been informed of its existence. Clinically it looks like stage II or III rosacea. Multiple tiny yellow pustules (type I) or deep-seated nodules (type II) on the perioral or perinasal region increase suspicion. Neither oral antibiotics nor topical metronidazole will control the disease. The diagnosis rests on demonstration of gram-negative organisms by culturing the contents of several pustules and the nares. The disease is analogous to gram-negative folliculitis, which sometimes develops on top of acne vulgaris as a result of long-term oral antibiotic administration. The organisms are the same: *Klebsiella, Escherichia coli, Pseudomonas, Acinetobacter* (type I), and *Proteus* (type II), as well as others.

Rosacea Conglobata

Rarely a patient with severe rosacea shows a reaction which mimics acne conglobata with hemorrhagic nodular abscesses and indurated plaques (Fig. 74-7).[1] It may be provoked by the oral intake of halogen-containing preparations. The course is progressive and chronic. This variant seems to occur mainly in women. Diagnosis is based on recognizing preexisting rosacea, confinement to the face, and no other signs of acne conglobata on back, shoulders, chest, or extremities.

FIGURE 74-7

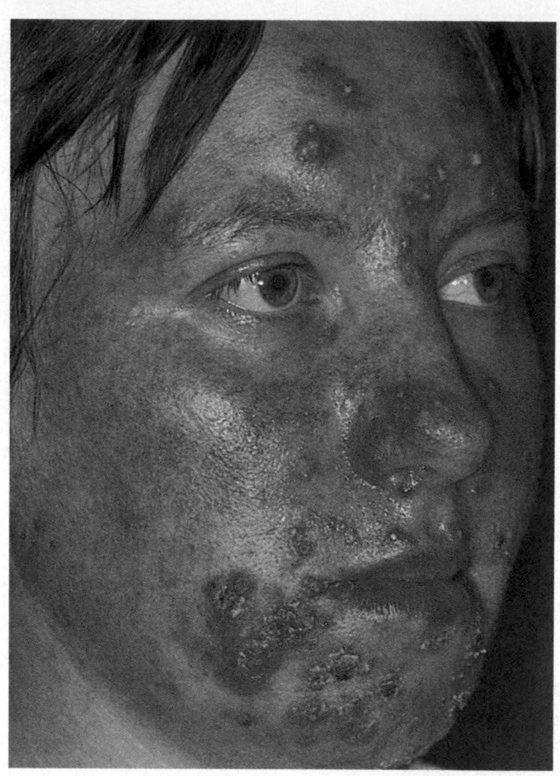

Rosacea conglobata. Purple red skin with intractable episodes of flushing and blushing. Hemorrhagic fluctuating nodules, papules, and pustules. The disease is limited to the face.

Rosacea Fulminans

This variant was first described by O'Leary and Kierland under the designation *pyoderma faciale*. It has been a matter of controversy ever since.[18] One can say with certainty that it is not a variant of acne conglobata; neither is it pyoderma. We interpret it as an extreme form of rosacea conglobata with sudden onset occurring almost exclusively in postadolescent women. In analogy to its acne-counterpart, acne fulminans, we opt to call it *rosacea fulminans*.[19]

This is a conglobate, nodular disease springing up abruptly on the face (Fig. 74-8).[20] Once seen, it is never forgotten. Large coalescent nodules and confluent draining sinuses occupy most of the face. The main locations are the chin, cheeks, and forehead. Ripe abscesses form with multiple pustules riding on top of the carbunculoid nodules. The face is diffusely reddened. Seborrhea is a constant feature but may be overlooked. When questioned closely, patients will often describe the development of extreme oiliness before or concomitant with the explosion. The disease is both embarrassing and debilitating.

The history is uniform. The skin is ferociously attacked within a few weeks. Prior acne or rosacea is usually denied. However, we perceived a connection to rosacea because after the stormy blowup, signs of rosacea often make their appearance. Some patients, too, have been flushers and blushers.

Its etiology remains obscure. Often blamed, but unproven, is a severe emotional trauma, such as the death of a family member, divorce, loss of a lover, accidents, and the like. Other patients lack such stress situations. There is a definite association with pregnancy[19] and inflammatory bowel diseases (Crohn's disease, ulcerative colitis)[21,22] in a significant number of patients.

The prognosis is excellent. Once the disease has been brought under control it does not recur, though the rosacea diathesis or mild stages of rosacea become progressively more noticeable.

FIGURE 74-8

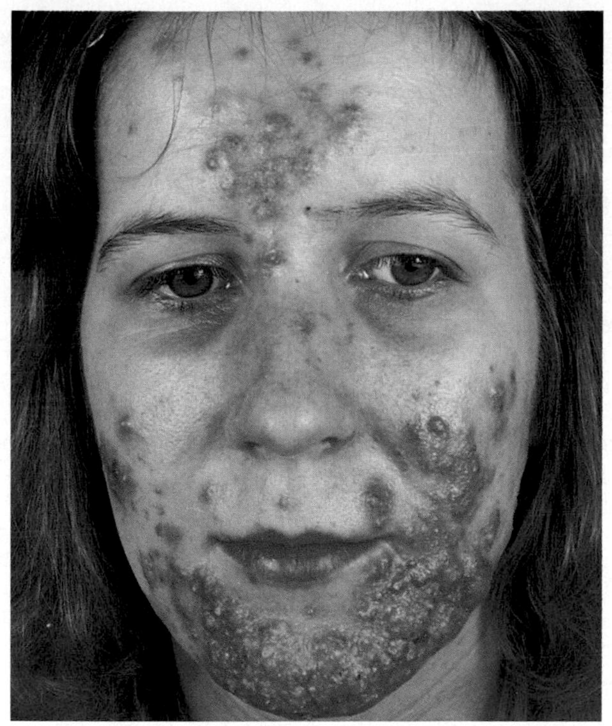

Rosacea fulminans. Large coalescent nodules and abscesses limited to the face attacked this woman within a few weeks.

PHYMAS IN ROSACEA

Phyma is the Greek word for swelling, mass, or bulb. Phymas occur in various areas of the face and ears. Rhinophyma is the most common form; other phymas can cause difficulties in diagnosis.

Rhinophyma

It occurs almost exclusively in men. Fortunately, only a few rosacea patients develop this complication. The bulbous nose develops over many years as a result of progressive increase in connective tissue, sebaceous gland hyperplasia, ectatic veins, and chronic deep inflammation. Rhinophyma may accompany stage III rosacea; in other patients surprisingly the signs of rosacea in the rest of the face may be rather mild. Four variants of rhinophyma are recognizable.[23,24]

GLANDULAR FORM The nose is enlarged mainly because of enormous lobular sebaceous gland hyperplasia. The surface is pitted, with deeply indented and mildly distorted follicular orifices. The tumorous expansions of the nose are often asymmetric and of varying size. Humps and sulci occur. Sebum excretion is increased. Compression by the fingers yields a white pasty substance consisting of an amalgam of corneocytes, sebum, bacteria, and *Demodex folliculorum* mites.

FIBROUS FORM Diffuse hyperplasia of the connective tissue dominates this picture. A variable amount of sebaceous gland hyperplasia may be seen.

FIBROANGIOMATOUS FORM The nose is copper-red to dark red, greatly enlarged, edematous, and covered by a network of large, ectatic veins. Pustules are frequently present.

ACTINIC FORM Nodular masses of elastic tissue distort the nose. These are rather similar to the elastomas that occur in older individuals who have markedly photodamaged skin as a result of overexposure to sunlight. This variety is mainly observed in subjects of Celtic origin who burn easily and tan poorly.

Phymas in other locations

- Gnathophyma (Greek *gnathos,* jaw) involves swelling of the chin.
- Metophyma (Greek *metopon,* forehead) refers to cushion-like swellings on the forehead above the saddle of the nose.
- Otophyma (Greek *ota,* ear) is a cauliflower-like swelling of one or both ears.
- Blepharophyma (Greek *blepharon,* lid) refers to chronic swelling of eyelids, mainly due to sebaceous gland hyperplasia.

HISTOPATHOLOGY

The histopathologic changes of rosacea vary according to the stage and quality of the disease.[25] They are often not diagnostic, resembling other chronic disorders. Skin damage by sunlight is a rather constant background feature, hence often severe elastosis is prominent and may be quite marked.

In stage I rosacea, there are mainly ectatic venules and lymphatics, slight edema, and sparse lymphatic perivascular infiltration. Moderate hyperplasia of the elastic tissue is present with increased curled, thickened elastic fibers.

In stage II rosacea, there is increasing lymphohistiocytic perivascular and perifollicular infiltration. Intrafollicular collections of neutrophils are often found, invariably when pustules are observed. The infiltrate likewise surrounds sebaceous ducts and glands. The veins are thickened and grossly dilatated. Elastosis is more advanced.

In stage III rosacea, there is diffuse expansion of the connective tissue, accompanied by hyperplasia of sebaceous follicles with long, distorted follicular canals, and large, irregular sebaceous lobules. Epithelialized tunnels undermine the hyperplastic tissue and are filled with inflammatory debris. The elastotic changes are prominent, often evident as amorphous masses of degenerated elastic tissue.

Demodex folliculorum mites are often found in all types of rosacea within the follicular infundibula and sebaceous ducts.

Epithelioid granulomas of the noncaseating type with multiple foreign body multinucleated cells are the histopathologic equivalent of lupoid rosacea. *Demodex folliculorum* mites may be involved in the pathogenesis of this condition.

Persistent edema of rosacea is characterized by mild edema in the middle and deep dermis, ectatic lymph vessels, and occasionally a sparse to dense lymphohistiocytic perivascular infiltrate. There are remarkably many mast cells throughout the fibrotic-thickened dermis.

Multiple abscesses with pseudoepitheliomatous hyperplasia, widespread necrosis, and lakes of granulocytes are characteristic of rosacea fulminans.

Immunofluorescence and immunohistochemical techniques have not contributed to the histopathologic identification of rosacea. In some studies, deposition of immunoglobulins and complement at the dermoepidermal junction has been observed by immunofluorescent staining.

DIFFERENTIAL DIAGNOSIS

Rosacea is a clinical diagnosis, because there is no specific laboratory test to confirm the diagnosis. Many disorders share similar characteristics with rosacea, such as acne vulgaris, seborrheic dermatitis, lupus erythematosus, dermatomyositis, perioral dermatitis, sarcoidosis, polymorphous light eruption, and Haber's syndrome. The episodic facial flushing of the carcinoid syndrome may resemble that of rosacea, but the 24-h urinary excretion of 5-hydroxyindoleacetic acid is normal in rosacea.

TREATMENT

Rosacea is a treatable disease. Sometimes treatment is difficult. Caring for rosacea patients requires a dedicated clinician and a compliant patient. Treatment schedules are determined by the stage and severity of the disease.[1]

Topical

Rosacea patients have a skin that is unusually vulnerable to chemical and physical insults. All sources of local irritation, such as soaps, alcoholic cleansers, tinctures, astringents, abrasives, and peeling agents must be avoided. Only mild soaps or cleansers are advised. Protection against sunlight must be emphasized.[1,5]

Antibiotics, as used in acne, are sometimes effective. Topical tetracyclines, clindamycin, and erythromycin, usually in concentrations from 0.5% to 2.0%, are commercially available. Erythromycin and clindamycin[26] seem to be superior. Tetracycline is effective orally, but a disappointment topically. An inhibition of chemotaxis or inflammatory cells or a direct effect on vascular endothelium may be responsible for its action.

Metronidazole has become an important addition to the antirosacea repertoire. The observation that topical metronidazole was comparable in its effects to oral tetracycline (250 mg bid) led to placebo-controlled double-blind clinical studies demonstrating its effectiveness.[27] In many countries throughout the world there is a 0.75% gel, cream, or lotion, as well as a 1% cream available. It is applied once or twice daily and has its greatest effect on papules and pustules, and reduces erythema to a lesser degree. It does not alter telangiectases or flushing. Topical metronidazole may be used as monotherapy or, in more severe forms, in combination with oral antibiotics. One study found that 0.75% metronidazole gel rapidly reduced inflammatory lesions during the first 3 weeks of treatment, potentially allowing quick tapering and discontinuation of oral medication. Long-term use of 0.75% metronidazole gel has been shown to keep rosacea in remission. A study involving 88 patients whose rosacea was initially controlled with a combination of oral tetracycline and metronidazole found that more than 80 percent of those patients given metronidazole remained in remission after 6 months, while 40 percent of those patients given placebo relapsed.[28] The mechanism by which metronidazole ameliorates the inflammatory lesions and erythema of rosacea may be related to anti-inflammatory or immunosuppressive actions of the drug.

Imidazoles are also gaining popularity with the treatment of rosacea. The authors' personal experience, although not substantiated by appropriate clinical trials, is best with ketoconazole cream applied once or twice daily. The imidazoles are anti-inflammatory agents, affect gram-positive bacteria, and, above all, are well tolerated by most rosacea patients with sensitive skin.

Old-time remedies should not be forgotten, even though their use is not supported by evidence-based trials. Drying lotions fall into this category, with a very thin application at night recommended. Lotions with 2% to 5% sulfur have been used successfully.[29] Because they are messy, we no longer use them. Other topical medications proven effective for treating rosacea include sulfacetamide sodium 10% lotion, as well as sulfacetamide sodium 10% and sulfur 5% lotion, which may be tinted or tint free.[30] They are used in a similar fashion and for the same purpose as metronidazole.

Retinoids are worth a trial. In an uncontrolled clinical study, women with rosacea used 0.025% tretinoin cream over a period of several months.[31] After a predictable early exacerbation of symptoms, the patients then appeared to develop hardening and side effects diminished. Gratifying long-term results were reported, including a reduction in erythema. Alternative topical retinoids may prove easier to use. There is preliminary evidence that 0.2% isotretinoin in a bland cream is helpful. It is less irritating than tretinoin, and suppresses inflammatory lesions in stage II and III rosacea. No data exist for adapalene, which seems to be the least irritating of all topical retinoids.

In a clinical study, 20% *azelaic acid* cream was more effective than its vehicle cream in reducing the number of inflammatory lesions and degree of erythema associated with rosacea. In a recent study, 20% azelaic acid cream gave results comparable to 0.75% metronidazole cream with the added benefit of increased patient satisfaction.[32] The efficacy of azelaic acid in rosacea may be due to the anti-inflammatory properties of this compound.

As stated earlier, *Demodex folliculorum* mites are not considered to play an etiologic role in rosacea, although massive infestation of *Demodex folliculorum* mites may sometimes aggravate the condition. Nevertheless, it is good to check for mites. This is best done with the skin-surface biopsy technique of placing a drop of cyanoacrylate on a glass slide that is covered with immersion oil and analyzed with the 10 or 20 × objective in the light microscope.[7] The mites are hard to control with any of the antiparasitic drugs such as lindane (γ-hexachlorocyclohexane), crotamiton, permethrin, or benzyl benzoate. The effect of treatment on the mite population can be monitored by cyanoacrylate skin-surface biopsies.

Sunscreens, preferably of the broad spectrum UVA plus UVB and infrared type, with a skin protection factor (SPF) of 15 or higher are always recommended to rosacea patients and should be used every day of the year. The sunscreens with a base of micronized zinc oxide or titanium oxide are nonirritating and work well for anyone with the sensitive skin of rosacea, but they leave sometimes an opaque hue on the skin, especially in the spacious facial pores. For this reason patients often turn away from these products.

Glucocorticoids should never be used. The only exception is with rosacea conglobata and rosacea fulminans. In these patients, short courses of oral and topical glucocorticoids are a reasonable option because of their anti-inflammatory properties.

Systemic

ANTIBIOTICS The most agreeable feature of rosacea is that it generally responds well to oral antibiotics. Tetracycline-HCl, oxytetracycline, doxycycline, and minocycline are usually quite effective in controlling papulopustular rosacea and even reducing erythema.[33] It is important to start with full doses, for example, 1.0 to 1.5 g tetracycline-HCl or oxytetracycline per day. Likewise 50 mg of minocycline (our own choice) or doxycycline twice daily can be given. If tetracyclines are ineffective or not tolerated, erythromycin or other macrolides such as clarithromycin[34] or azithromycin[35] may be used. As soon as full control of papulopustules is achieved, usually after 2 to 3 weeks, maintenance doses of 250 to 500 mg tetracycline-HCl or oxytetracycline, or 50 mg minocycline or doxycycline per day or every other day are generally sufficient. Rosacea patients often know how to titrate disease activity and vary dosage accordingly. Some get by with 250 mg tetracycline-HCl every other day. The patient's input should be encouraged and antibiotic usage should be carefully monitored. The disease has exacerbations and remissions and topical drugs may be sufficient during inactive periods. Some patients seem to become "addicted" to oral antibiotics and find ways to get them without prescription. Tetracycline therapy is mandatory for ophthalmic rosacea.

ISOTRETINOIN (13-*CIS*-RETINOIC ACID) This drug is exceptionally effective, although accompanied by far greater risks than tetracyclines (Fig. 75-1).[36] Before using it, one has to consider indications, contraindications, and all risks. Isotretinoin may be appropriate for all forms of severe or therapy-resistant rosacea, especially the variants which are unresponsive to antibiotics, such as lupoid rosacea, stage III rosacea, rosacea conglobata, gram-negative rosacea,[36] and rosacea fulminans.[19,20] It is particularly helpful in patients who have oily, wide-pored skin and multiple, often many dozens of sebaceous gland hyperplasias. Furthermore, all forms of phymas are worthwhile indications. The dose required for the control of severe rosacea varies. Tailored doses are recommended.

The standard dose of isotretinoin is lower than in acne, namely 0.2 to 0.5 mg/kg body weight per day. Side effects on the eyes make this low dose unbearable for some patients. Ophthalmic rosacea may get worse, complaints of dry eyes can increase, and so can blepharitis. This may lead to the inability to use contact lenses. The standard dose is only used in rosacea fulminans, or preoperatively for a couple of months to shrink rhinophyma before surgical reduction of the bulbous nose.

More recent studies demonstrate the efficacy of low-dose isotretinoin in the treatment of rosacea.[37] In this schedule, initially 10 mg or 20 mg daily (not adjusted to body weight) are used. This dose is helpful in many forms of the disease, especially stage III rosacea, lupoid rosacea, and persistent edema in rosacea. After 1 to 2 months, this is further reduced to 10 mg every other day or even to two or three of seven days per week. Side effects on the eyes are minimal. Duration of therapy is longer as with the standard dose, for about 6 months. The cumulative dose, however, is very low.

The usual precautions apply as in the therapy of acne. Isotretinoin is a teratogen and is contraindicated for women of childbearing age unless the patient meets all the requirements printed in detail in the package insert.

Laboratory monitoring includes liver transaminases, bilirubin, cholesterol, and triglycerides before therapy and at monthly or bimonthly intervals thereafter.

METRONIDAZOLE This is a synthetic nitroimidazole-derivative antibacterial and antiprotozoal agent for the treatment of infections caused by *Trichomonas vaginalis, Entamoeba histolytica,* and several anaerobic organisms. The usual dose is 500 mg twice daily for 6 days.

Oral metronidazole is generally effective in all types of rosacea, including stage II and III.[38] However, it may require 20 to 60 days to achieve control with a daily dose of 500 mg. The use of oral metronidazole is limited by concerns over adverse systemic effects and toxicity with long-term therapy, and it is not approved for rosacea treatment. Consequently, oral metronidazole is a second-line drug that may be tried when other methods are not working. It is very helpful for the treatment of *Demodex* folliculitis, even its worst form, such as *Demodex*-associated abscesses and furunculoid nodules. The dose is 750 to 1500 mg daily in divided doses for 10 to 14 days.

CLONIDINE In a limited clinical trial, the vasoconstrictor clonidine has been able to reduce flushing in rosacea, but subdepressor doses, which do not cause a decrease in blood pressure, have little or no effect. It is not our choice.

NADOLOL The betablocker nadolol has been used with variable success to reduce flushing in rosacea. It has significant side effects and is therefore best reserved for intractable cases. It is not our choice.

SPIRONOLACTONE An uncontrolled study of 13 male rosacea patients showed promising results.[39] There was improvement in itching and erythema from the low dose of 50 mg spironolactone daily given over a 4-week period. It is postulated that the observed improvement may be due to an inhibitory effect on epidermal cytochrome P_{450}. Further studies are required to confirm these observations. It is not our choice.

Miscellaneous

FACIAL MASSAGE This has long been recommended and is the so-called Sobye's massage with twice daily gentle circular massage given for several minutes to nose, cheeks, and forehead. Its value is uncertain, and controlled studies are lacking. The mechanism of action may be accelerated lymphatic drainage with reduction of edema. It is not our choice.

DIET IN ROSACEA There is no specific rosacea diet. Dietary limitations relate only to factors that provoke erythema, flushing, and blushing, such as alcoholic beverages, hot drinks, and spicy food. Patients should be encouraged to discover which dietary items are troublesome and to avoid them.

CAMOUFLAGE Women may benefit from the use of a coverup makeup that has a green tint to help mask the underlying telangiectatic erythema of the skin.

SURGICAL TREATMENT This is a very successful approach in rhinophyma. Excellent cosmetic results can be obtained, and the patients brought back into society. A variety of techniques are available, including scalpel or razor modeling; electrocoagulation;[40] cryosurgery;[41] elevation of the intact epidermis with débridement of excess tissue below it with the original epidermis used to cover the wound to maintain a most natural skin surface; argon laser; CO_2 laser;[40] Neodynium:YAG laser,[42] Erbium:YAG laser;[43] and others. Much depends on the training and preferences of the physician. Low-dose oral isotretinoin may be used successfully before the surgical procedure to shrink down the bulbous portions, and it can be continued postoperatively for many months.[44,45] Unfortunately, information was published that isotretinoin causes unsightly hypertrophic scarring when used close to surgical techniques. We use oral isotretinoin directly before and after the surgical procedure.

Obliteration of ectatic vessels, particularly on the nose, can be achieved by intravascular insertion of a fine diathermy needle or by argon or pulsed dye lasers. In expert hands, these physical modalities work satisfactorily.

Special Situations

OPHTHALMIC ROSACEA Management of the ophthalmic disease requires both systemic and topical treatment, including lid hygiene, lubrication, and, occasionally, short-term topical corticosteroids.

ROSACEA FULMINANS This variant requires special care.[19,20] Treatment starts with oral glucocorticoids such as prednisolone 1.0 mg/kg body weight per day for 7 to 10 days to suppress the inflammatory process. Then isotretinoin is added at 0.2 to 0.5 mg, rarely

1.0 mg per kg body weight per day, with a slow tapering of the glucocorticoid over the next 2 to 3 weeks. Isotretinoin is continued until all inflammatory lesions have disappeared. This may require 3 to 4 months. Draining abscesses should not be incised. Concomitant treatment in the first 2 weeks may consist of warm compresses and topical application of a potent glucocorticoid cream. Besides rosacea conglobata, this is the only indication for topical and systemic glucocorticoids in the treatment of rosacea, and the steroids should never be used for more than 2 or 3 weeks.

PERSISTENT EDEMA OF ROSACEA Treatment has been highly unsatisfactory so far. Our tentative recommendation is low-dose isotretinoin, 0.1 to 0.2 mg/kg body weight per day over a period of 2 to 6 months. This drug is combined with ketotifen, 1 to 2 mg per day, which is a potent H_1-antagonist and possesses antiallergic activities by inhibition of mediator release from mast cells. Preliminary results are encouraging.[46] Clofazimine may be worth a trial, at a dosage of about 100 mg four times weekly.

REFERENCES

1. Jansen T: Rosacea, in *Acne and Rosacea,* edited by G Plewig, AM Kligman. 3rd ed. Berlin, Springer, 2000, p 455
2. Rosen T, Stone MS: Acne rosacea in blacks. *J Am Acad Dermatol* **17**:70, 1987
3. Logan RA, Griffiths WAD: Climatic factors and rosacea, in *Acne and Related Disorders,* edited by R Marks, G Plewig. London, Dunitz, 1989, p 311
4. Marks R: Rosacea: Hopeless hypotheses, marvelous myths and dermal disorganization, in *Acne and Related Disorders,* edited by R Marks, G Plewig. London, Dunitz, 1989, p 293
5. Wilkin JK: Rosacea: Pathophysiology and treatment. *Arch Dermatol* **130**:359, 1994
6. Brinnel H et al: Rosacea: Disturbed defense against brain overheating. *Arch Dermatol Res* **281**:66, 1989
7. Forton F, Seys B: Density of *Demodex folliculorum* in rosacea: A case-control study using standardized skin-surface biopsy. *Br J Dermatol* **128**:650, 1993
8. Jones M: *Helicobacter pylori* in rosacea: lack of an association. *Arch Dermatol* **134**:511, 1998
9. Dupont C: How common is extrafacial rosacea? *J Am Acad Dermatol* **14**:839, 1986
10. Jansen T, Plewig G: Morbus Morbihan. *Akt Dermatol* **22**:161, 1996
11. Akpek EK et al: Ocular rosacea: patient characteristics and follow-up. *Ophthalmology* **104**:1863, 1997
12. Meschig R et al: Ophthalmological complications of rosacea, in *Acne and Related Disorders,* edited by R Marks, G Plewig. London, Dunitz, 1989, p 321
13. Quarterman MJ et al: Ocular rosacea: Signs, symptoms, and tear studies before and after treatment with doxycycline. *Arch Dermatol* **133**:49, 1997
14. Helm KF et al: A clinical and histopathologic study of granulomatous rosacea. *J Am Acad Dermatol* **25**:1038, 1991
15. Jansen T et al: Steroidrosazea. *Akt Dermatol* **21**:129, 1995
16. Leyden JJ et al: Steroid rosacea. *Arch Dermatol* **110**:619, 1974
17. Neubert U et al: Bacteriologic and immunologic aspects of gram-negative folliculitis: A study of 46 patients. *Int J Dermatol* **38**:270, 1999
18. Jansen T, Plewig G: An historical note on pyoderma faciale. *Br J Dermatol* **129**:594, 1993
19. Plewig G et al: Pyoderma faciale: A review and report of 20 additional cases: Is it rosacea? *Arch Dermatol* **128**:1611, 1992
20. Jansen T et al: Diagnosis and treatment of rosacea fulminans. *Dermatology* **188**:251, 1994
21. Jansen T, Plewig G: Fulminating rosacea conglobata (rosacea fulminans) and ulcerative colitis. *Br J Dermatol* **137**:830, 1997
22. Romiti R et al: Rosacea fulminans in a patient with Crohn's disease: A case report and review of the literature. *Acta Derm Venereol (Stockh)* **80**:127, 2000
23. Aloi F et al: The clinicopathologic spectrum of rhinophyma. *J Am Acad Dermatol* **42**:468, 2000
24. Jansen T, Plewig G: Clinical and histological variants of rhinophyma, including nonsurgical treatment modalities. *Facial Plast Surg* **14**:241, 1998
25. Marks R et al: Histopathology of rosacea. *Arch Dermatol* **100**:683, 1969
26. Wilkin JK, DeWitt S: Treatment of rosacea: Topical clindamycin versus oral tetracycline. *Int J Dermatol* **32**:65, 1993
27. Dahl MV et al: Once-daily topical metronidazole cream formulations in the treatment of the papules and pustules of rosacea. *J Am Acad Dermatol* **45**:723, 2001
28. Dahl MV et al: Topical metronidazole maintains remissions of rosacea. *Arch Dermatol* **34**:679, 1998
29. Blom I, Hornmark AM: Topical treatment with sulfur 10 percent for rosacea. *Acta Derm Venereol (Stockh)* **64**:358, 1984
30. Lebwohl MG, Medansky RS: The comparative efficacy of sodium sulfacetamide 10% sulfur 5% (Sulfacet-R) lotion and metronidazole 0.75% (MetroGel) in the treatment of rosacea. *J Geriatr Dermatol* **3**:183, 1995
31. Kligman AM: Topical tretinoin for rosacea: A preliminary report. *J Dermatol Treat* **4**:71, 1993
32. Maddin S: A comparison of topical azelaic acid 20% cream and topical metronidazole 0.75% cream in the treatment of patients with papulopustular rosacea. *J Am Acad Dermatol* **40**:961, 1999
33. Wereide K: Long-term treatment of rosacea with oral tetracycline. *Acta Derm Venereol (Stockh)* **49**:176, 1968
34. Torresani C et al: Clarithromycin versus doxycycline in the treatment of rosacea. *Int J Dermatol* **36**:942, 1997
35. Elewski BE: A novel treatment for acne vulgaris and rosacea. *J Eur Acad Dermatol Venereol* **14**:424, 2000
36. Plewig G et al: Action of isotretinoin in acne, rosacea, and gram-negative folliculitis. *J Am Acad Dermatol* **6**:766, 1982
37. Erdogan FG et al: Efficacy of low-dose isotretinoin in patients with treatment-resistant rosacea. *Arch Dermatol* **134**:884, 1998
38. Saihan EM, Burton JL: A double-blind trial of metronidazole versus oxytetracycline therapy for rosacea. *Br J Dermatol* **102**:443, 1980
39. Aizawa H, Niimura M: Oral spironolactone therapy in male patients with rosacea. *J Dermatol* **19**:293, 1992
40. Greenbaum SS et al: Comparison of CO_2 laser and electrosurgery in the treatment of rhinophyma. *J Am Acad Dermatol* **18**:363, 1988
41. Sonnex TS, Dawber RP: Rhinophyma-treatment by liquid nitrogen spray cryosurgery. *Clin Exp Dermatol* **11**:284, 1986
42. Wenig BL, Weingarten RT: Excision of rhinophyma with Nd:YAG laser: A new technique. *Laryngoscope* **103**:101, 1993
43. Orenstein A et al: Treatment of rhinophyma with Er:YAG laser. *Lasers Surg Med* **29**:230, 2001
44. Irvine C et al: Isotretinoin in the treatment of rosacea and rhinophyma, in *Acne and Related Disorders,* edited by R Marks, G Plewig. London, Dunitz, 1989, p 301
45. Rödder O, Plewig G: Rhinophyma and rosacea: Combined treatment with isotretinoin and dermabrasion, in *Acne and Related Disorders,* edited by R Marks, G Plewig. London, Dunitz, 1989, p 335
46. Jansen T, Plewig G: The treatment of rosaceous lymphoedema. *Clin Exp Dermatol* **22**:57, 1997

CHAPTER 75

Ronald Marks

Perioral Dermatitis

DEFINITION

Perioral dermatitis (POD) is a relatively common inflammatory disorder of facial skin of unknown cause in young women in which small papules and pustules occur around the mouth.

HISTORICAL ASPECTS

This disorder seems to have appeared in the second half of the twentieth century, as the first reports of a disease with its characteristic clinical picture appeared in the 1950s. Unfortunately, the various names used and the lack of clinical criteria for inclusion of patients make some aspects of the history somewhat uncertain.

It is generally accepted that the report of Frumess and Lewis, in 1957,[1] of what they termed light-sensitive seborrhcid was the first description of the condition. Mihan and Ayres[2] subsequently gave the condition the name "perioral dermatitis", which has stuck, although other names were used, such as "rosacea-like dermatosis."[3] Definitive descriptions were presented by Cochran and Thomson[4] and Wilkinson et al.[5]

CLINICAL FEATURES

This disorder is consistent in its clinical presentation. Characteristically, it first appears around the external nares and the superior end of the nasolabial folds or around the lip commissures (Fig 75-1). The eruption then spreads around the mouth leaving a clear and uninvolved zone immediately adjacent to the lips. When severe and/or long-standing, the condition travels up at the sides of the nose and may even involve the glabella. A variant has been described in which the disorder occurs predominantly around the eyes. This is known as *periocular perioral dermatitis* (Fig 75-2).[6]

The lesions of POD are typically small papules (or micropapules) but some lesions seem to be surmounted by tiny pustules, and pustules may occur independently. Unlike rosacea, there is little in the way of persistent erythema or telangiectasia, although there may be a background faint pink flush on the affected skin. The papules themselves are a shade of red. Generally, POD causes little in the way of symptoms apart from some mild soreness. The condition, nonetheless, causes considerable distress because of the perceived cosmetic disability.

POD is easily differentiated from rosacea because the latter disorder occurs on facial convexities and is characterized by persistent erythema and telangiectasia. It is often confused with seborrheic dermatitis, but the scaling in this disease and the occurrence of dandruff, as well as affected areas occurring elsewhere over the skin in seborrheic dermatitis, should enable the distinction to be made from POD. The age group affected may also lead the dermatologist to consider the possibility of acne. However, the different distributions of rash over the face, and

FIGURE 75-1

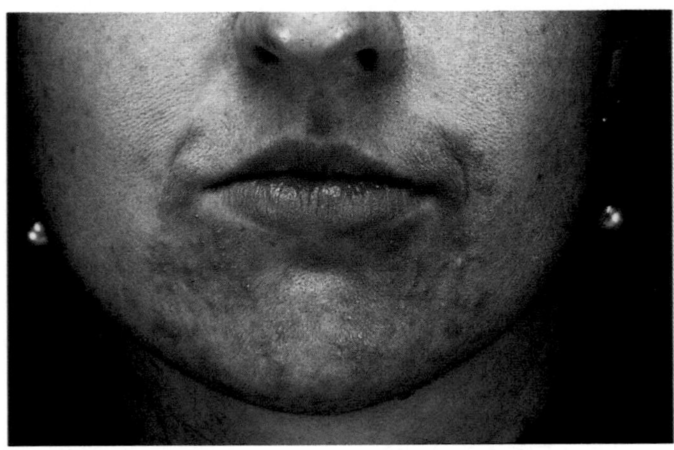

Typical perioral dermatitis: The eruption is confined to the nasolabial folds and the skin of the chin.

FIGURE 75-2

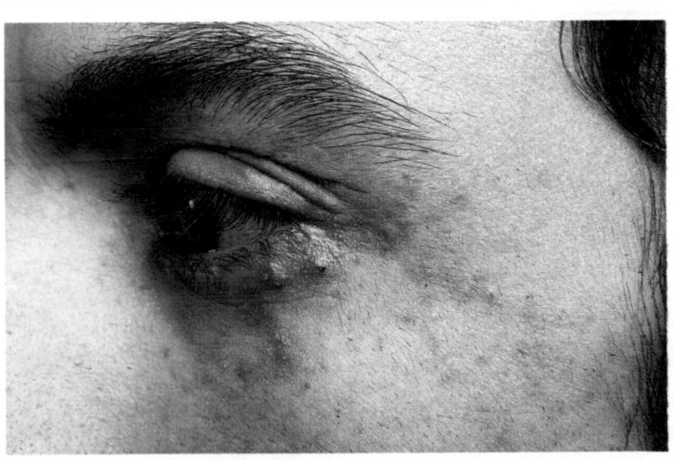

Periocular perioral dermatitis: There are a number of small papules and papular pustules around the eye.

the presence in acne of lesions on the upper trunk, of comedones and seborrhea serve to distinguish these two conditions.

The term dermatitis is really a misnomer and it is important to differentiate forms of "true" dermatitis from POD. One form of dermatitis that is quite distinctive and sometimes mistaken for POD is "lip-licking cheilitis," which is seen predominantly in the 7- to 15-year-old age group. In this disorder, the rash is caused by the repeated licking of the skin around the mouth and is marked by a scaling, pink band around the mouth. Curiously, there is often a spared 1 to 2 mm zone immediately adjacent to the vermilion of the lips just as in perioral dermatitis. Allergic contact dermatitis to lip cosmetic can also result in a "circumoral" dermatitis,[7] but this is quite uncommon.

COURSE AND PROGNOSIS

The condition usually arises spontaneously over the course of a week or two. In nearly every patient, there is a striking dependency on topical corticosteroids. A frequently heard story is that the patient presents with the earliest signs of the rash and is given a potent or moderately potent topical corticosteroid. The condition then shows some improvement but when an attempt is made to stop treatment the condition dramatically worsens after a few days. This happens every time the steroid preparation is stopped. In fact, the condition tends to be doggedly persistent and there does not seem to be any tendency to spontaneous remission. Fortunately, the correct treatment with antibiotics cures the condition (see below).

EPIDEMIOLOGY

The condition is mainly a disease of women aged 15 to 25 years, but occasionally it is seen in children.[8–11] There is no validated data on the frequency of the disease, and it may well be that the incidence varies in different countries. In the United Kingdom, it seemed at one time to be a very common disorder in routine dermatologic practice but then in the 1980s, it seemed to vanish and became quite uncommon. However, it showed a resurgence in the 1990s. The same sequence does not seem to have been the case in the United States and some other countries from which reports of studies and case reports continue to appear.[12]

PATHOLOGY

There have been few studies of the pathologic appearances of POD, presumably because of the reluctance of clinicians to biopsy facial skin of young women. However, a 3- or 4-mm diameter punch biopsy rarely produces a significant scar in inflamed facial skin if no sutures are inserted. Our study[13] of 26 patients demonstrated eczematous changes predominantly, with most of the spongiotic change being focused in the external root sheaths of the follicles. In this investigation, there did not appear to be any similarity to the pathologic changes noted in rosacea. Ramelet,[14] however, stated that in his series of 30 cases, the changes were most like those of rosacea. In one series of POD in children,[9] a granulomatous reaction was a consistent finding and this often appeared to emanate from follicular rupture.

THE CAUSE OF PERIORAL DERMATITIS

As yet no convincing explanation to account for the disease has emerged. The striking predominance in women, the relationship with topical corticosteroids, and the curious sudden appearance of the disorder in the 1960s and 1970s have been difficult to fit together into any rational hypothesis. The early view that it was light induced has not been sustained and most writers on the topic have focused on either an infective cause or the result of some form of topical application.

Both *Candida* and fusiform bacteria have been considered as etiological agents, but supporting evidence has not been forthcoming.[15,16] The *Demodex* mite has also been accused of causing the eruption.[17] Cosmetics have been often considered as evocative agents of the condition. If this is the case, then physical occlusion[12] or some form of irritation may be responsible, as allergic contact dermatitis does not seem likely because patch tests to various cosmetic agents have been consistently negative.[18] Contact with bristly male chin stubble[15]has been discussed as a cause, but has been hotly denied as a possibility by some patients. Fluoride-containing toothpaste[19–23] and/or fluoridation of water supplies has been blamed, but neither has received further support.

Most attention has been given to potent topical corticosteroids, particularly fluorinated topical corticosteroids as causative agents.[24,25] It is certainly the case that many subjects develop a strange dependency on the use of these steroids and flare when they stop using them, but this is a long way from saying that they actually cause the disorders. It has to be borne in mind that a small number of patients vigorously deny ever having used topical corticosteroids.

MANAGEMENT OF PATIENTS WITH PERIORAL DERMATITIS

Most patients are anxious and depressed by the time they reach the dermatologist because of the succession of ineffective treatments they have had. Strong reassurance concerning the eventual successful outcome is needed. At the start of treatment, all topical corticosteroids should be stopped and the patient should be warned that a flare of the rash will almost certainly develop within a few days, but will only last for a few days. Some have suggested that a weak corticosteroid such as hydrocortisone should be given during this period, but this doesn't stop the flare or alleviate the symptoms in most patients. It is probably better to experience the flare "cold turkey" using just an emollient and continuing to take oral tetracycline (see below).

Most patients respond to oral tetracycline, either tetracycline[18] itself or to one of the more recent analogues, such as minocycline, doxycycline or lymecycline. These drugs should be given in full dosage until the patient starts to respond—usually a 3- or 4-week period—and then reduced to half dosage until the rash has completely resolved. Usually treatment can be stopped after 8 to 10 weeks. Recurrences are very uncommon and, luckily, there are no sequelae. The mode of action of the tetracyclines does not appear to be purely antimicrobial and is yet another of the mysteries associated with POD.

Other oral antibiotics such as erythromycin have been used and have been claimed as successful. Topical metronidazole,[26,27] topical erythromycin, and topical tetracycline[28] have all been used, but it is rare that such therapies are required.

REFERENCES

1. Frumess GM, Lewis HM: Light-sensitive seborrheid. *Arch Dermatol* **75**:245, 1957
2. Mihan R, Ayres S Jr: Perioral dermatitis. *Arch Dermatol* **89**:803, 1964

3. Weber G: Rosacea-like dermatitis: Contraindication or intolerance to strong steroid. *Br J Dermatol* **86**:253, 1972
4. Rosacea-like dermatitis [editorial]. *BMJ* **3**:545, 1969
5. Wilkinson DS et al: Perioral dermatitis. *Br J Dermatol* **101**:245, 1979
6. Fisher AA: Periocular dermatitis akin to the perioral variety. *J Am Acad Dermatol* **15**:642, 1986
7. Hayakawa R et al: Lipstick dermatitis due to C18 aliphatic compounds. *Contact Dermatitis* **4**:215, 1987
8. Bruyngeel DP: A child with perioral dermatitis. *Contact Dermatitis* **1**:43, 1987
9. Frieden IJ et al: Granulomatous perioral dermatitis in children. *Arch Dermatol* **125**:369, 1989
10. Gianotti F et al: Particuliere dermatitie peri-orale infantile. Observation su 5 cas. *Bull Soc Fr Dermatol Syphiligr* **77**:341, 1970
11. Manders M, Lucky AW: Perioral dermatitis in childhood. *J Am Acad Dermatol* **27**:688, 1992
12. Malik R, Quirk CJ: Topical applications and perioral dermatitis. *Australas J Dermatol* **41**:54, 2000
13. Marks R, Black MM: Perioral dermatitis: A histopathological study of 26 cases. *Br J Dermatol* **84**:242, 1971
14. Ramelet AA, Delacretaz J: Histopathological study of perioral dermatitis. *Dermatologica* **47**:163, 361, 1981
15. Buck A, Kalkoff KW: Zur Nachweis von Fusobakterien aus Effloreszenzen der perioralen dermatitis. *Hautarzt* **22**:433, 1971
16. Beetz HM et al: Uber die bedeutung von bakterien bei den sogenannter periorale dermatitis. *Hautarzt* **24**:220, 1973

17. Ayres S Jr, Ayres S III: Demodectic eruptions (demodicidosis) in the human. *Arch Dermatol* **83**:816, 1961
18. Marks R: Perioral dermatitis, in *Common Facial Dermatoses*. Bristol, England, John Wright, 1976, p 25
19. Epstein E: Fluoride toothpastes as a cause of acne-like eruptions. *Arch Dermatol* **112**:1033, 1976
20. Saunders MA: Fluoride toothpastes: A cause of acne-like eruptions. *Arch Dermatol* **111**:793, 1975
21. Kocsard E, King RH: Perioral dermatitis. *Australas J Dermatol* **13**:49, 1972
22. Sainio EL, Kanerva L: Contact allergens in toothpaste. *Contact Dermatitis* **33**:100, 1995
23. Ferlito TA: Tartar control toothpastes and perioral dermatitis. *J Clin Orthod* **26**:43, 1992
24. Sneddon IB: Iatrogenic dermatitis. *BMJ* **4**:49, 1969
25. Verbov J, Abell E: Iatrogenic dermatitis. *BMJ* **4**:621, 1969
26. Veien NK et al: Topical metronidazole in treatment of perioral dermatitis. *J Am Acad Dermatol* **24**:258, 1991
27. Miller SR, Shalita AR: Topical metronidazole gel for the treatment of perioral dermatitis in children. *J Am Acad Dermatol* **31**:847, 1994
28. Wilson RG: Topical tetracycline in the treatment of perioral dermatitis. *Arch Dermatol* **115**:637, 1979

CHAPTER 76

Lowell A. Goldsmith

Disorders of the Eccrine Sweat Glands

Disorders of sweating can occur for many different reasons, including dysfunction of the sweat centers; changes in preganglionic efferent sympathetic pathways; alterations in sympathetic ganglia or postganglionic sympathetic fibers; responses to pharmacologic receptors; and abnormalities in the secretory function of the sweat gland or the sweat duct. Generalized hypohidrosis results in heat intolerance in adults and fever "of unknown etiology" in infants. Acquired generalized hypohidrosis can result in compensatory hyperhidrosis in the areas of the skin with normal sweat gland function. Very frequently it is the compensatory hyperhidrosis, not the underlying hypohidrosis, that brings the patient to the physician's office.

Tables 76-1 and 76-2 summarize the differential diagnoses of patients with hyperhidrosis and anhidrosis, both generalized and localized.

IN VIVO METHODS OF STUDYING SWEAT GLAND FUNCTION

Visualization of Sweat

Sweat (actually the water in sweat) is readily visualized by an iodine-starch reaction.[1] The one-step method involves applying iodinated starch powder (prepared by adding 0.5 to 1 g of iodine crystals to 500 g of soluble starch in a tightly capped bottle) to the skin with large cotton balls, a body powder applicator, or an atomizer. In addition, iodine-impregnated imprint papers can be made by exposing about 100 sheets of ordinary copy machine paper to 1 g of iodine crystals in an airtight jar for 1 week or longer. The imprints can be photocopied for storage.

The most informative measure of sweat gland function that can be determined in vivo is the maximal sweat rate. Higher sweat rates are associated with larger sweat glands and greater pharmacologic sensitivity.[2] Methods for determining the maximal sweat rate include using a water vapor analyzer, collecting the sweat under mineral oil, and using an anaerobic bag method.

VISUAL EXAMINATION OF THE SKIN

When sweat from patients with cystic fibrosis is dried, it forms fernlike crystals, whereas sweat from healthy individuals does not have this characteristic. Similarly, the skin of an infant with cystic fibrosis is much saltier than normal skin, as detected when the infant is kissed.

The urea content of sweat increases with increasing serum levels of urea. In uremia, the evaporation of sweat with high concentrations of urea results in the deposition of urea in the solid state on the skin. This is commonly referred to as "uremic frost."

TABLE 76-1

Generalized and Localized Hyperhidrosis

Hyperhidrosis of a relatively large area (>100 cm^2 or generalized)
- In patients with a past history of spinal cord injuries
  - Autonomic dysreflexia
  - Orthostatic hypotension
  - Posttraumatic syringomyelia
- Associated with peripheral neuropathies
  - Familial dysautonomia (Riley-Day syndrome)
  - Congenital autonomic dysfunction with universal pain loss
  - Exposure to cold
- Associated with probable brain lesions
  - Episodic with hypothermia (Hines and Bannick syndrome)
  - Episodic without hypothermia
  - Olfactory
- Associated with intrathoracic neoplasms or lesions
- Associated with systemic medical problems
  - Pheochromocytoma, Parkinson's disease, thyrotoxicosis, diabetes mellitus, congestive heart failure, anxiety, menopausal state, etc.
- Due to drugs or poisoning
- Night sweats
- Compensatory

Hyperhidrosis of relatively small area (<100 cm^2)
- Idiopathic unilateral circumscribed hyperhidrosis
- Reported association with blue rubber bleb nevus, glomus tumor,
  - POEMS syndrome, burning feet syndrome
  - (Goplan's), causalgia, pachydermoperiostosis, pretibial myxedema
- Gustatory sweating associated with
  - Encephalitis, syringomyelia
  - Diabetic neuropathies, herpes zoster
  - Parotitis, parotid abscesses, thoracic sympathectomy
  - Auriculotemporal or Frey's syndrome

Miscellaneous
- Lacrimal sweating
- Harlequin syndrome
- Palm, sole, and axillary hyperhidrosis (emotional)

Chromhidrosis is the secretion of colored sweat. Several dyes, when injected intravenously, are secreted in eccrine sweat.[3] Colored eccrine sweat has been described in various situations, but in all probability, the sweat is colorless when secreted but immediately becomes colored after reaching the surface, for example, blue sweat noted in copper workers and in those exposed to dye powders (e.g., bromophenol blue or quinazarin).

HYPERHIDROSIS OF RELATIVELY LARGE AREAS (See Table 76-1)

Hyperhidrosis Associated with Past Spinal Cord Injuries

Some patients with a past history of spinal cord injuries experience episodes of profuse sweating months or years after the injuries. The areas of hyperhidrosis are not explained by the sensory or sympathetic dermatomes. The episodes include hyperhidrosis associated with autonomic dysreflexia,[4,5] hyperhidrosis triggered by orthostatic hypotension,[5] and posttraumatic syringomyelia.[6,7]

TABLE 76-2

Generalized and Localized Anhidrosis

Hypohidrosis or anhidrosis (AH) of relatively large area
- Due to poral occlusion
  - Papulosquamous, dermatitic, or ichthyosiform lesions
  - Xerosis (incl. xerosis of atopics)
  - Acquired generalized AH (= tropical anhidrotic asthenia?)
  - Sweat retention syndrome
- Due to absence of the sweat gland
  - Anhidrotic ectodermal dysplasia (Christ-Siemens-Touraine syndrome)
- Due to paucity, atrophy, or dysfunction of the sweat gland
  - Systemic sclerosis
  - Fabry disease
- Due to impaired autonomic function
  - Congenital sensory neuropathy type IV (= congenital insensitivity to pain with AH)
  - Progressive segmental AH with Adie's tonic pupils (Ross's syndrome)
  - Progressive isolated segmental AH without tonic pupils
  - Autonomic insufficiency syndrome (postural hypotension and AH)
  - Chronic idiopathic anhidrosis—diabetic neuropathy
  - Others: Guillain-Barré, Fabry

Anhidrosis or hypohidrosis of relatively small area
- Damage to the glands by infection, trauma, tumors, morphea, scars, or inflammatory infiltrate
- Denervation
  - Incontinentia pigmenti
  - Dermatomal vitiligo
- Miscellaneous
  - Follicular atrophoderma (Bazex syndrome)
  - Hypomelanosis of Ito

HYPERHIDROSIS ASSOCIATED WITH AUTONOMIC DYSREFLEXIA This syndrome occurs in paraplegic patients with spinal cord lesions at or above T6. Following stimuli such as distention of the bowel or bladder, visceral inflammation, or skin irritation, there is episodic profuse sweating (on the face, neck, and upper trunk), vasodilatation (flushing of the face and congestion of the nasal passages), and throbbing headaches and other signs of sympathetic hyperactivity, such as piloerection and hypertension, and of hyperparasympathetic hyperactivity, such as bradycardia with vasodilatation.[4] The mechanism of hyperhidrosis in autonomic dysreflexia (usually but not always above the spinal cord lesions) is not well understood. The beneficial effect of oral propoxyphene-HCl and propantheline bromide on hyperhidrosis in autonomic dysreflexia has been reported in a few patients.[4]

A similar condition occurs in quadriplegic patients. Upon switching from a supine to a tilted or upright position, a sudden spell of dizziness due to orthostatic hypotension is followed within 5 to 10 min by rising blood pressure; profuse sweating on the face, neck, upper chest, and arms; chattering of teeth; piloerection; blurred vision; and agitation. Fludrocortisone acetate, 0.3 mg daily, may control sweating in such patients.[5]

HYPERHIDROSIS DUE TO POSTTRAUMATIC SYRINGOMYELIA The patients may or may not be paraplegic due to injuries to the spinal cord. In most cases, hyperhidrosis may be the only initial symptom.[7] The onset of hyperhidrosis lags months to many years behind trauma. Because the syrinx (a fluid-filled cavity in the spinal cord) develops above and/or below the level of transaction, hyperhidrosis can occur above and/or below the lesion.

Hyperhidrosis Associated with Peripheral Neuropathies

FAMILIAL DYSAUTONOMIA (RILEY-DAY SYNDROME OR HEREDITARY SENSORY NEUROPATHY TYPE III) Hyperhidrosis has been reported in some patients with familial dysautonomia and is caused by mutations in the *IKAP* gene (the IKK complex associated protein forms a scaffold for the complex which includes the NFκB-inducing complex).[7,8] Riley-Day syndrome, a recessively inherited disorder is usually seen in Ashkenazi Jews. Hyperhidrosis is probably due to the increased excitability of the sweat center[9] and is usually episodic. The diagnostic criteria include the lack of an axon reflex flare following intradermal histamine injection (indicating peripheral panneuropathy); the absence of fungiform papillae on the tongue; miosis of the pupil following instillation of 2.5% methacholine (normal subjects do not respond; miosis means hypersensitivity of the parasympathetic nerves); diminished deep-tendon reflexes; a lack of overflow tears; failure to thrive; a generalized reduction in pain sensation; mild mental retardation; and an erythematous mottling of the skin upon heat exposure.[10] Congenital autonomic dysfunction with universal pain loss is a similar syndrome in those not of Ashkenazi Jewish descent.

PERIPHERAL MOTOR NEUROPATHY WITH AUTONOMIC DYSFUNCTION The onset of profuse sweating in the neck and the thorax was reported in two sisters with this condition.[11] Sweating is aggravated by cold weather or nervousness. These patients also noted slowly progressive muscular weakness and muscular hypertrophy (due to demyelination of motor nerves), distal cyanosis, orthostatic hypotension, and esophageal achalasia, but they lacked sensory neuropathy.

Hyperhidrosis Associated with Brain Lesions

A variety of lesions in the brain can cause episodes of profuse sweating; they may be separated into two major groups: those associated with hypothermia and those not associated with hypothermia.

EPISODIC HYPOTHERMIA WITH HYPERHIDROSIS (HINES AND BANNICK SYNDROME) Hyperhidrosis in the Hines and Bannick syndrome[12] begins at anytime from 9 months to 38 years of age. Episodes of profuse sweating are triggered on awakening or standing up and are preceded by a feeling of warmth, tingling, and flushing of the face, during which time the body temperature decreases to between 24° to 31°C (75° to 88°F). Sweating lasts only 5 min in some patients, but it may persist for as long as several hours in others. Hyperhidrosis in these patients is most likely due to the episodic decrease of the hypothalamic temperature set point (diencephalic epilepsy or hypothalamic storm) by diencephalic lesions or malformations such as agenesis of the corpus callosum, heterotopias, microgyria, parencephalia, malformation of cranial nerves and brainstem nuclei, cholesteatoma, lipoma, or surgical manipulation of the anterior hypothalamus.[13] Anticonvulsants and oxybutynin have been used for control of hypothermia and hyperhidrosis with variable success.

GENERALIZED HYPERHIDROSIS NOT ASSOCIATED WITH HYPOTHERMIA Hyperhidrosis has been reported in rare patients with episodic hypertension and hypothalamic-pituitary dysfunction after a brain injury and after a cerebrovascular accident in the region of the hypothalamus.

OLFACTORY HYPERHIDROSIS Profuse facial sweating precipitated by perfume smells, but not by gustatory or mental stimuli, was reported in a 42-year-old woman[14] and was successfully treated with amitriptyline.

Hyperhidrosis Associated with Intrathoracic Neoplasms or Lesions

PAROXYSMAL UNILATERAL HYPERHIDROSIS ASSOCIATED WITH INTRATHORACIC NEOPLASMS Abnormal thoracic sympathetic activity due to encroachment of tumors (pulmonary adenocarcinoma, bronchial carcinoma, mesothelioma, etc.), osteomas, or cervical ribs on the sympathetic trunk, or postganglionic fibers can cause ipsilateral hyperhidrosis.[15] Sweating is usually spontaneous and profuse on the face, neck, and chest.

Generalized Hyperhidrosis Associated with Systemic Medical Problems

Increased sweating has been reported in diabetes mellitus, hypoglycemia, congestive heart failure, thyrotoxicosis, hyperpituitarism, anxiety, dumping syndrome, carcinoid, alcohol and drug withdrawal, and the menopausal state. At 34°C (93°F) a significantly higher rate of sweating than normal is seen in patients with thyrotoxicosis. Sweating is a feature of growth hormone excess and is decreased in growth hormone deficiency in males.[16] Growth hormone administered to adults with growth hormone deficiency did not increase sweating.[16] In Parkinson's disease, an increase in pharmacologic sweating was reported, and other studies[17] have noted a combination of patchy areas of anhidrosis and areas of hyperhidrosis. The symptomatic triad of excessive and inappropriate paroxysmal sweating, tachycardia, and pounding headaches (associated with increased blood pressure), almost assures the diagnosis of pheochromocytoma.[18]

Hyperhidrosis Associated with Drugs or Poisoning

Excessive diaphoresis has also been reported as a side effect of antidepressants such as cyclobenzapine and fluoxetine. Acrodynia, a form of mercury poisoning, occurred in a child exposed to paint fumes in a home recently painted with a brand of house latex paint containing mercury.[19]

NIGHT SWEATS (NOCTURNAL DIAPHORESIS) Night sweats are occasionally associated with tuberculosis; endocarditis; lymphoma; hyperthyroidism; diabetes mellitus; hypoglycemia due to insulinoma; systemic vasculitis; pheochromocytoma; carcinoid syndrome; drug withdrawal; dysautonomic states; other chronic infectious diseases; acromegaly; and Prinzmetal's angina pectoris.

NIGHT SWEATS ASSOCIATED WITH HODGKIN'S DISEASE Hodgkin's disease is characterized by the triad of fever, sweating, and weight loss; in many patients, night sweats may be the only symptom.[20] The increased sweating in this disease may be due to a fluctuating fever and instability of the thermoregulatory hypothalamic center. In fact, the sudden drop of body temperature was found to coincide with the onset of profuse night sweats. The excessive production of interleukin-1 (IL-1) by activated macrophages is implicated as the cause of the temperature instability.[20] IL-1 is known to induce an abrupt increase in the synthesis of prostaglandin E_2 in the preoptic anterior hypothalamic region, causing an elevation of the temperature "set point."

Compensatory Hyperhidrosis

Compensatory hyperhidrosis describes the occurrence of hyperhidrosis on the trunk and legs after thoracic sympathectomy for the treatment of palmar hyperhidrosis, facial hyperhidrosis in patients with generalized sweat retention syndrome, or distal anhidrosis due to diabetic

FIGURE 76-1

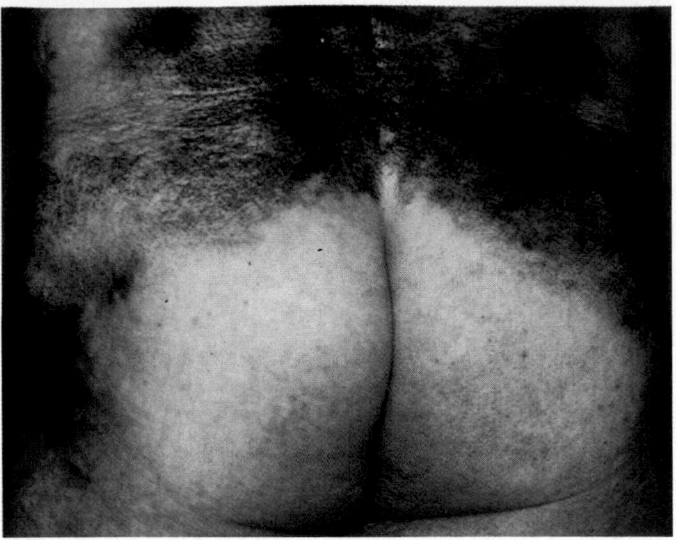

Compensatory hyperhidrosis in a patient with herniation of intervertebral disk at L1–L2 with subsequent partial sensory and motor neuropathy of the buttock and legs. The patient complained of excessive spontaneous sweating on the trunk and face, and although his skin was dry in our clinic, brief exposure to a sauna induced sweating on the trunk but not on the buttock and legs. The dark areas are hyperhidrotic areas visualized by the one-step iodinated starch method. Note that the buttock and legs are completely anhidrotic with a sharp cut-off line.

neuropathy (Fig. 76-1). Sweating in such a patient is usually triggered by thermal stimuli or by physical exercise and is presumably due to the increased thermoregulatory need for the remaining functional sweat glands. The most frequent causes of anhidrosis in such patients include diabetes mellitus, lesions in the spinal cord or sympathetic trunk, and widespread poral occlusion in atopic dermatitis or in extensive miliaria.

LOCALIZED HYPERHIDROSIS

Idiopathic Unilateral Circumscribed Hyperhidrosis

The involved area in unilateral circumscribed hyperhidrosis is usually sharply demarcated and no larger than $10 \times 10\,cm^2$. It occurs mainly on the face and upper extremities of otherwise healthy individuals[21] (see Fig. 76-2). Profuse sweating, which is usually precipitated by heat, lasts 15 to 60 min. In some patients, mental or gustatory (in the case of facial hyperhidrosis) stimulation also triggers sweating. There is no accompanying sensory or motor neuropathy, flushing of the face, headaches, excessive salivation, lacrimation, vasodilation, or piloerection. The pathogenesis of circumscribed hyperhidrosis is unknown. Sweating may be partially controlled by local application of 25% aluminum salts or topical anticholinergic agents or by systemic clonidine (which inhibits central sympathetic outflow). Local injections of botulism toxin to the affected area may also control the sweating (see Chap. 276). As a last resort, total excision of the affected area should be considered.

FIGURE 76-2

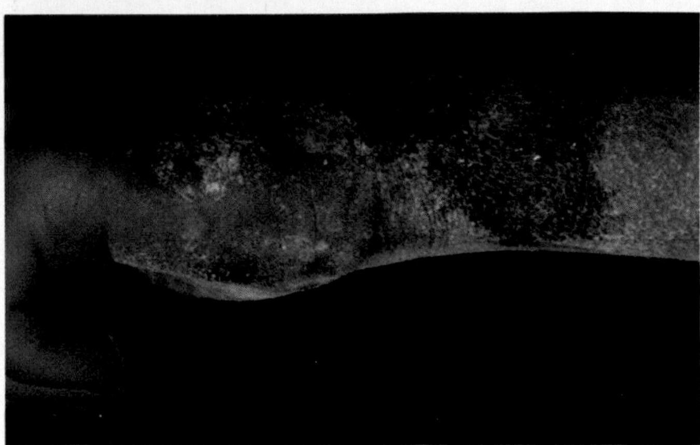

Idiopathic unilateral circumscribed hyperhidrosis in a 7-year-old boy visualized by the conventional Minor's iodine starch method (the skin was painted with tincture of iodine, air-dried, and sprayed with starch). Hyperhidrosis was precipitated by heat. Over the following 2 years, the hyperhidrosis gradually improved without treatment.

Localized Hyperhidrosis Associated with Cutaneous Diseases

Localized hyperhidrosis has been reported to occur in the skin over a blue rubber bleb nevus (presumably due to axon-reflex sweating after manipulation of the painful lesion), in the perilesional skin of a glomus tumor (presumably due to increased local temperature and/or pain), and in POEMS (polyneuropathy, organomegaly, endocrinopathy, M protein, and skin changes) syndrome, Goplan's disease (burning-feet syndrome), causalgia, pachydermoperiostosis, and painful pretibial myxedema.

Gustatory Sweating

GUSTATORY SWEATING DUE TO HYPERACTIVITY OF SYMPATHETIC FUNCTION Gustatory sweating on the face and neck can occur in association with encephalitis or syringomyelia or the invasion of the cervical sympathetic trunk by a tumor.[22] Gustatory sweating occurs in 73 percent of patients after an upper dorsal sympathectomy and is explained by pre- and postganglionic sympathetic regeneration with collateral sprouting into, or aberrant synapsing with, the superior cervical ganglion.[23] Thus ipsilateral gustatory sweating can occur in the presence of other signs of Horner's syndrome (full Horner's syndrome includes ipsilateral anhidrosis, ptosis, miosis, and enophthalmos), but sweating is more intense in their absence.[24] Gustatory sweating rarely occurs in diabetic neuropathy.

AURICULOTEMPORAL (OR FREY'S) SYNDROME Frey's syndrome occurs in 37 to 100 percent of patients 1 month to 5 years after parotid gland surgery or injury to the preauricular region. This syndrome most frequently results from injury to the auriculotemporal nerve, which carries sensory fibers from the skin, parasympathetic fibers to the salivary glands, and sympathetic fibers to the sweat glands in the preauricular region (Fig. 76-3). According to the misdirection hypothesis, the severed parasympathetic fibers in the auriculotemporal nerve regenerate and migrate into the postganglionic sympathetic fibers to reach the sweat glands as well as the blood vessels in the preauricular region. When the greater auricular nerve is damaged together with the parotid gland, the parasympathetic fibers regenerating from the damaged parotid gland migrate into the distal segment of the greater auricular nerve to innervate the sweat glands in the infraauricular area. Gustatory sweating in Frey's syndrome is usually mild, i.e., only

FIGURE 76-3

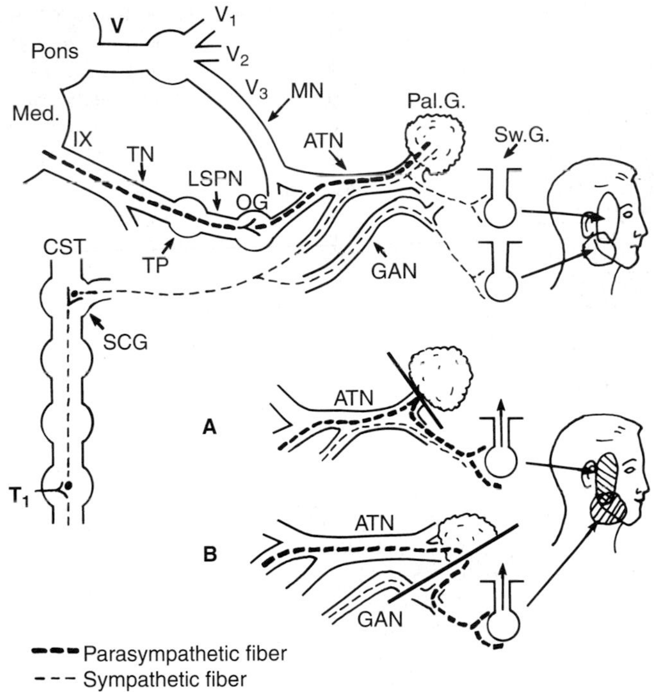

Illustration of parotid secretomotor and sudomotor neural pathway. ATN, auriculotemporal nerve; CST, cervical sympathetic trunk; GAN, greater auricular nerve; IX, glossopharyngeal nerve; LSPN, lesser superficial petrosal nerve; Med., medulla oblongata; MN, mandibular nerve; OG, otic ganglion; Pal. G, parotid gland; SCG, superior cervical ganglion; Sw.G, sweat gland; T1, first thoracic nerve; TN, tympanic nerve (or Jacobson's nerve); TP, tympanic plexus; V, trigeminal nerve. *A* and *B*. The most widely held "misdirection" hypothesis on the pathogenesis of Frey's syndrome, i.e., injury to the parotid gland and/or auriculotemporal nerve (as indicated by a diagonal line), causes misdirection of its parasympathetic fibers toward the sweat glands in the preauricular area (*A*). When both the greater auricular nerve (GAN) and the parotid gland are severed, the regenerating parasympathetic fibers from the ATN migrate into the GAN to reach the sweat glands, causing gustatory sweating in the infraauricular area. (*From Sato et al.,*[1] *with permission.*)

10 percent of the patients may require treatment. Topical scopolamine cream (3 to 5%) and 20% aluminum chloride in ethanol have been used with variable success. Injecting alcohol around the auriculotemporal nerve may eliminate symptoms for several months. Tympanic neurectomy and an interpositional fascial graft may offer permanent relief. Gustatory sweating secondary to parotitis or parotid abscess is a variant of Frey's syndrome.

Lacrimal Sweating

Lacrimal sweating refers to continuous profuse sweating in the right supraorbital region associated with Raeder's syndrome (Horner's syndrome plus temporal and frontal headache).[25] The etiology of this rare condition is unknown, but the nature of Horner's syndrome suggests that it is due to the localized neuropathy of sympathetic fibers supplying the orbital area.

Harlequin Syndrome

Five patients, aged 27 to 64 years, suddenly developed onset of unilateral facial flushing and sweating.[26] Brainstem infarct was suspected in one patient; occlusion of the anterior radicular artery due to strenuous exertion (with consequent damage to the third thoracic segment) was suspected in the other four patients. The flushing side showed increased sympathetic activity (which was abolished by ipsilateral stellate ganglionectomy), whereas contralateral sympathetic activity was found to be deficient. Sweating was aggravated by heat or exercise in all the patients, but in four of the five patients, gustatory stimuli also triggered sweating. Thus, the contralateral anhidrotic side with absent sympathetic activity may be the primary abnormality, and the ipsilateral hyperhidrosis (with sympathetic hyperactivity) may be compensatory in nature.

EMOTIONAL SWEATING

Hyperhidrosis of the Palms and Soles

Excessive sweating of the palms and soles occurs during mental stress and may be associated with tachycardia and vasomotor instability. Palmar hyperhidrosis interferes with occupations in which instruments and tools are handled. Increased moisture may be an accessory factor in contact dermatitis by leaching out sensitizing chemicals from solid objects in contact with the skin.

The hypothalamic sweat center controlling the palms and soles (and the axillae in some patients) is distinct from the rest of the hypothalamic sweat centers and receives nervous inputs from the cerebral cortex but not from the thermosensitive elements and is activated predominantly by emotional stimuli. Thus, sweating on the palms and soles does not occur during sleep or sedation, nor is it augmented in a warm environment. Patients with hyperhidrosis of the palms and soles show electroencephalographic (EEG) abnormalities such as sharp wave bursts when challenged by hyperventilation, and their frontal cortexes are hyperperfused.[27] These patients have less reflex bradycardia than control subjects in response to the Valsalva maneuver or facial immersion, but a higher degree of cutaneous vasoconstriction in response to finger immersion in cold, suggesting that they have increased sympathetic outflow passing through the T2–T3 ganglia.[28] Excessive palmoplantar sweating lowers the skin temperature of the hands and fingers by excessive evaporative cooling, which further increases the sympathetic outflow and aggravates the hyperhidrosis. Successful treatment of the palmoplantar hyperhidrosis elevates the palmar skin temperature by 2.5°C (4.5°F) which may also help to alleviate the vicious cycle of sympathetic reflex.

Tap water iontophoresis is an effective, safe, and inexpensive therapeutic modality for palmoplantar hyperhidrosis (Fig. 76-4).[29] Local injection of botulinum toxin is an effective treatment for palmar hyperhidrosis[30] and for axillary hyperhidrosis as measured in a double-blind placebo trial.[31] This therapy shows measurable improvement in the quality of life of the infected individual.[32] The biology of botulinum toxin is discussed in Chap. 8 and its clinical use is reviewed in Chap. 276.

Hyperhidrosis of the Axillae

Patients with excessive axillary sweating rarely emit a pungent axillary odor, supporting the notion that the apocrine glands but not the apoeccrine glands are responsible for the axillary odor. The important role of the axillary apoeccrine sweat glands to the overall axillary wetness is discussed in Chap. 8. The emotional nature of the axillary sudomotor function (supplied mainly by the fourth thoracic ganglion) is similar to that on the palms and soles except that axillary sweat glands also respond to thermal stimuli to varying extents. Only 25 percent of patients with axillary hyperhidrosis also have palmoplantar hyperhidrosis.

FIGURE 76-4

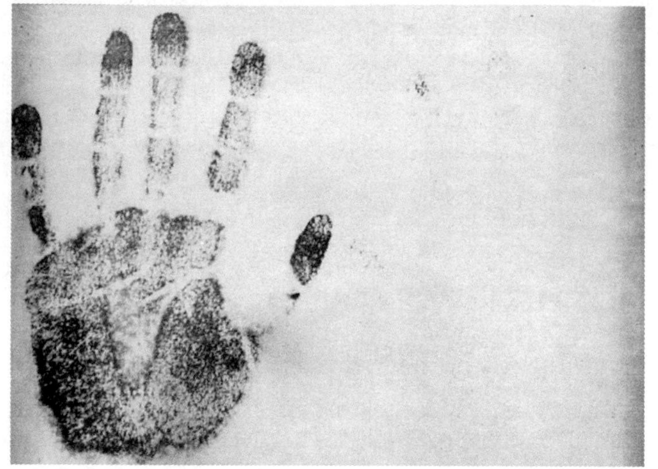

Successful treatment of hyperhidrosis with tap water iontophoresis. The right palm was treated for 30 min daily for 7 days at 20 mA by anodal current, whereas the left palm was only immersed in water. The right foot was connected to a cathodal electrode. The sweat prints were taken using an iodine-impregnated paper.

Unlike palmar sweating, axillary sweating is relatively well controlled by topical application of 25% aluminum chloride in alcohol solution applied at bedtime, with or without subsequent occlusion with a plastic film.[33] Botulinum toxin is also an effective treatment. Thoracic sympathectomy (usually second through fourth thoracic ganglia) should be considered only as the last resort. Treatment with systemic anticholinergic (atropine-like) drugs should be discouraged because of the excessive side effects (e.g., excessive dryness of the mouth, failure of accommodation). Local application of anticholinergics has been disappointing.

HYPOHIDROSIS (ANHIDROSIS) OF RELATIVELY LARGE AREAS

Anhidrosis can result from poral occlusion, congenital or acquired absence of sweat glands, damage to sweat gland function by inflammation of the skin, or dysfunction of sympathetic nerves in neuropathies. Anhidrosis can involve relatively large areas or very small areas of the skin (Table 76-2). The anhidrotic ectodermal dysplasias are discussed in Chap. 53.

Hypo- or Anhidrosis due to Poral Occlusion

Delivery of sweat to the skin surface is hindered to varying extents in papulosquamous lesions, dermatophytosis, ichthyosiform erythroderma, and the xerotic skin of atopic patients.[34] Following sunstroke, patients may suddenly develop generalized anhidrosis and heat intolerance that may last as long as 6 years. Biopsy revealed atrophic and vacuolar changes of the sweat secretory cells. This disorder may be a variant of tropical anhidrotic asthenia.

Hypohidrosis due to Atrophy, Paucity, or Dysfunction of the Sweat Gland

Atrophy of the sweat gland is seen in systemic sclerosis, systemic lupus erythematosus, or Sjögren's syndrome.

Hypohidrosis due to Impaired Autonomic Function

CONGENITAL INSENSITIVITY TO PAIN WITH ANHIDROSIS (HEREDITARY SENSORY NEUROPATHY TYPE 4 WITH ANHIDROSIS) This autosomal recessive disorder is characterized by generalized anhidrosis, mental retardation, self-mutilation, painless ulcers, fractures, and episodes of high fever. Skin bruises may suggest a diagnosis of child abuse. In the skin, there is a lack of unmyelinated fibers and a marked reduction in the number of myelinated nerves in sweat glands. The glands are unresponsive to local injection of pilocarpine. Mutations in the high affinity tyrosine kinase receptor for nerve growth factors is the molecular etiology of the syndrome.[35]

PROGRESSIVE SEGMENTAL ANHIDROSIS WITH TONIC PUPILS (ROSS SYNDROME OR HOLMES-ADIE SYNDROME WITH ANHIDROSIS) Ross syndrome affects both males and females, with the age of onset ranging from 3 to 50 years.[36] Patients usually present with heat intolerance and irregular segmental areas of anhidrosis on the trunk and/or the extremities and hyporeflexia. Examination shows tonic pupils, anisocoria, sluggish reaction to light, and abnormal constriction by 2.5% methacholine. The symptoms are generally ascribed to postganglionic denervation of the parasympathetic fibers that travel with the third cranial nerve. The absence of deep-tendon reflexes in the extremities is also seen consistently. The mechanism of anhidrosis in these patients is unknown.

PROGRESSIVE ISOLATED SEGMENTAL ANHIDROSIS One patient had anhidrosis without tonic pupils, sensory neuropathy, or areflexia.[37] The anhidrotic areas remained responsive to intradermal cholinergic agents for several months but became unresponsive 2 years later. The authors concluded that the anhidrosis in their patient was due to denervation of preganglionic sympathetic fibers.

CHRONIC IDIOPATHIC ANHIDROSIS Eight patients reported by Low et al.[38] showed generalized anhidrosis of from 1 to 10 years duration without orthostatic hypotension. Some of these patients showed mild anisocoria, sluggish pupillary response to light and accommodation, and an abnormal pupillary response to cocaine (indicative of mild postganglionic sympathetic failure). Five of them showed electrophysiologic evidence of mild peripheral somatic sensory nerve involvement. Recovery from anhidrosis occurred in one patient. The age of onset of their symptoms ranged from 18 to 60 years. The histology of the sweat glands was apparently normal. Thus, chronic idiopathic anhidrosis could be a forme fruste or stage of acute panautonomic neuropathy. Fisher and Maibach[39] reported five patients with postural hypotension, of whom two had generalized anhidrosis and one had localized anhidrosis.

DIABETIC NEUROPATHY WITH ANHIDROSIS Autonomic neuropathy is a frequent complication of diabetes mellitus that often accompanies, or even precedes, the first signs of more commonly recognized sensorimotor polyneuropathy.[40] Diabetic neuropathy commonly involves distal sensorimotor neuropathy, painful thoracolumbar monoradiculopathy, and polyradiculopathy. Of 51 patients with diabetic neuropathy, 48 presented with unequivocal abnormalities of thermoregulatory sweating.[41] Compensatory hyperhidrosis may accompany diabetic anhidrosis.

OTHER ANHIDROSIS DUE TO NEUROPATHIES Anhidrosis of the lower limbs is seen in 12 percent of patients with Guillain-Barré syndrome.[42] In Fabry's disease, extensive deposition of ceramide trihexoside in the peripheral and central autonomic nerves, the dorsal root ganglia, and the peripheral sensory nerves results in pandysautonomia and sensory neuropathy[43] and deposition of lamellar lipid granules in the ductal and secretory cells. Thus, whether the sweat gland itself is rendered inactive by the lipid deposition or whether the anhidrosis is secondary to peripheral and central autonomic dysfunction remains to be determined.

LOCALIZED HYPOHIDROSIS

Localized hypohidrosis can occur whenever sweat glands are damaged by surgery or trauma, scar formation, cutaneous neoplasms, irradiation, infection, inflammation of the skin, granulomatous lesions, scleroderma, or vasculitis. Delivery of sweat to the skin surface may be impaired in a variety of dermatoses and papulosquamous diseases, presumably because of poral occlusion. Blister formation with sweat gland necrosis has been reported during intoxication with barbiturates, methadone, diazepam, carbon monoxide, amitriptyline, and clorazepate.[44] Moss and Ince[45] observed the absence of sweating in the hypopigmented streaks and patches on the legs, arms, and scalp of 10 women with incontinentia pigmenti. Skin biopsy revealed a lack of eccrine sweat glands and hair follicles in the anhidrotic, hypopigmented lesions. Koga[46] reported that hypohidrosis occurs only in dermatomally distributed vitiligo and not in the nondermatomal type. Anhidrosis of the face and neck has been reported in members of a family with "follicular atrophoderma, basal cell carcinoma, and hypotrichosis," a rare X-linked, dominantly inherited syndrome.[47] The hypomelanotic regions in hypomelanosis of Ito are anhidrotic.[47] Disorders with congenital absence of sweat glands may not have active cutaneous vasodilatation that can contribute to poor heat transfer to the skin and increased core temperature.

SWEAT RETENTION SYNDROMES (See Table 76-3)

Miliaria

When the free flow of eccrine sweat to the skin surface is obstructed and sweat is retained within the skin, a variety of signs and symptoms result.[48,49] Based on clinical and histopathologic findings, miliaria is subdivided into four groups: (1) miliaria crystallina; (2) miliaria rubra; (3) miliaria pustulosa; and (4) miliaria profunda. Every clinical type of miliaria has been produced experimentally in the laboratory.[48,49]

Miliaria crystalline (sudamina) consists of superficial, subcorneal, noninflammatory vesicles (Fig. 76-5) that easily rupture when rubbed with a finger.

Miliaria rubra (prickly heat) results when obstructed sweat migrates into the living layers of the epidermis as well as the upper dermis, causing pruritic inflammatory papules around the sweat pores. This disorder is especially common in infants, but also occurs in adults after repeated episodes of sweating in a hot, humid environment. The eruption usually subsides within a day after the patient moves to a cool environment. Anhidrosis associated with miliaria, however, takes 2 weeks (the time needed to repair the affected epidermal sweat duct unit by epidermal turnover) to recover completely. Some of the eruptions of miliaria rubra become pustular, resulting in miliaria pustulosa. A recent epidemic called miliaria rubra occurred in miners working underground in a metalliferous mine in Australia. The miners were exposed to groundwater and had lesions on the lower legs; in addition one-quarter of the miners had folliculitis.[50]

TABLE 76-3

Sweat Retention Syndromes

Miliarias
- Miliaria crystallina (sudamina)
- Miliaria rubra (prickly heat)
- Miliaria pustulosa
- Miliaria profunda

Tropical anhidrotic asthenia

? Transient acantholytic dermatosis (Grover's)

? Dyshidrosis (pompholyx)

FIGURE 76-5

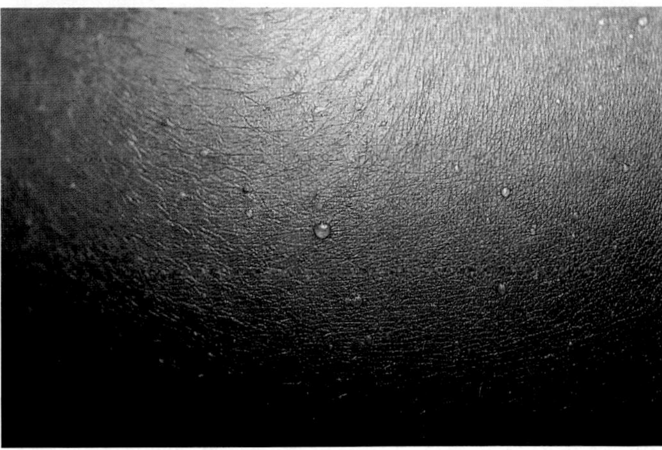

Miliaria crystallina. Note the delicate, droplike vesicles without erythema.

Miliaria profunda results when the sweat leaks into the dermis. During exposure to intense heat or after local injection of cholinergic agents, the affected skin can be uniformly covered with multiple discrete, flesh-colored papules that resemble gooseflesh. Ductal blockade at various levels is the immediate cause of miliaria. However, investigators do not agree on why the sweat escapes the duct at different levels (causing different subgroups of miliaria) nor on what causes the ductal blockade and/or ductal leakage at different levels. It is puzzling that the morphologic evidence of ductal blockade—such as keratin rings, PAS-positive proteins, or clusters of microorganisms—is rarely seen by light microscopic observation of miliarial lesions. Thus, Holzle and Kligman[49] speculated that the keratin rings and PAS-positive proteins are the consequence but not the cause of ductal damage. The role of resident organisms has long been suspected as the leading predisposing factor in miliaria.[51] Indeed, there was a linear correlation between the severity of miliaria rubra and the number of cocci in experimental miliaria under a plastic film. The development of experimental miliaria could be markedly suppressed by pretreatment of the skin with hexachlorophene or pyrithione.[49]

Tropical Anhidrotic Asthenia

Tropical anhidrotic asthenia,[51] which is frequently seen in military troops engaged in hot, humid environments, is a postmiliarial hypohidrosis.[52] Upon deployment in tropical theaters, most troops first develop extensive miliaria. However, a few weeks later, some troops develop persistent widespread hypohidrosis and heat intolerance without clinically visible miliaria. Keratin plugs are noted in the sweat pores. Their sweating recovers partially after a week in a cool environment or after desquamation by exposure to ultraviolet light. This condition may lead to the chronic extensive form of miliaria profunda.

Transient Acantholytic Dermatosis (Grover's Disease) (See Chap. 55)

The edematous and excoriated papules and vesicles that appear predominantly on the trunk often occur after excessive heat, heavy sweating, or sweating accompanying malignancy.[53]

Eccrine Hidradenitis

Neutrophilic infiltration of sweat glands occurs after treatment with several chemotherapeutic agents[54] and occurs on the palms and soles associated with local pseudomonas infection.[55]

Heat Hyperpyrexia and Heat Stroke

Heat hyperpyrexia and heat stroke are states of thermoregulatory failure of sudden onset that are characterized by general anhidrosis, hyperpyrexia [rectal temperature greater than 40.5°C (105°F)], and disturbances of the central nervous system. The exact cause of this disorder is unknown. The picture is generally one of environmental stress too severe for the thermoregulatory system, which suddenly collapses. Whether the anhidrosis is primary and the central nervous system pathology is secondary to the hyperpyrexia or vice versa is unclear. In some cases, dehydration, with its depression of the sweat rate, appears to be an initiating factor. The presence of local defects of the sweat glands (e.g., miliaria, profunda, ectodermal dysplasia) that interfere with thermoregulation may be a contributory factor. It appears, however, that the syndrome can occur as a result of hyperpyrexia per se—from heat stress too severe to be compensated for—without any primary defect of the sweat glands or any significant alteration of body fluids. Destructive lesions of the hypothalamus have been described in some cases coming to autopsy. In the late stages, there may also be petechial hemorrhages in many organs in association with thrombocytopenia; in some cases, other coagulation defects such as fibrinogenopenia are present. Destructive lesions in the brain outside the hypothalamus, hepatic and renal changes, as well as adrenal hemorrhages have been noted. In the early stages, sweating may still be present and the patient rational, but the rectal temperature may be greater than 40.5°C (105°F). Within minutes, anhidrosis, mental confusion, coma, and/or seizures may appear. The diagnosis should be suspected from the clinical setting of activity in extreme heat and rectal temperature greater than 40.5°C (105°F); it should be accepted with the additional presence of anhidrosis, hot, dry skin, and any degree of central nervous system manifestations. If untreated, the disorder is uniformly fatal. In treated cases, the mortality is approximately 35 percent.

Heat stroke is an acute medical emergency. Primary attention should be given to lowering the body temperature by any means available, ideally by immersion in ice or very cold water. Because some cutaneous vasoconstriction will occur with vigorous cooling, even in the presence of hyperpyrexia, chlorpromazine, which inhibits this response, has been advised by many. In view of possible adrenal hemorrhages, the administration of adrenal steroids is probably desirable. Rectal temperature should be lowered to less than 39°C (102°F) before efforts are reduced. The patient should then be placed in a relatively cool environment. General medical management of possible renal or hepatic disorders should be maintained. Some instability of thermoregulation may persist for several days to weeks. Mental and neurologic aberrations may persist and improve slowly only after several months. Permanent sequelae such as ataxia are not infrequent.

REFERENCES

1. Sato K et al: Biology of the eccrine sweat gland: II. Hyperhidrosis and hypohidrosis. *J Am Acad Dermatol* **20**:713, 1989
2. Sato K, Sato F: Individual variations in structure and function of human eccrine sweat gland. *Am J Physiol* **245**:R203, 1983
3. Hurley H, Witkowski J: Dye clearance and eccrine sweat secretion in human skin. *J Invest Dermatol* **36**:259, 1961
4. Canaday BR, Stanford RH: Propantheline bromide in the management of hyperhidrosis associated with spinal cord injury. *Ann Pharmacother* **29**:489, 1995
5. Khurana RK: Orthostatic hypotension-induced autonomic dysreflexia. *Neurology* **37**:1221, 1987
6. Ottomo M, Heimburger RF: Alternating Horner's syndrome and hyperhidrosis due to dural adhesions following cervical spinal cord injury: Case report. *J Neurosurg* **53**:97, 1980
7. Slaugenhaupt SA et al: Tissue-specific expression of a splicing mutation in the IKBKAP gene causes familial dysautonomia. *Am J Hum Genet* **68**:598, 2001
8. Anderson SL et al: Familial dysautonomia is caused by mutations of the IKAP gene. *Am J Hum Genet* **68**:753, 2001
9. Green M, Behrendt H: Sweat gland reactivity to local thermal stimulation in dysautonomia. *Am J Dis Child* **130**:816, 1976
10. Axelrod FB, Pearson J: Congenital sensory neuropathies. Diagnostic distinction from familial dysautonomia. *Am J Dis Child* **138**:947, 1984
11. Lisker R et al: Peripheral motor neuropathy associated with autonomic dysfunction in two sisters: new hereditary syndrome? *Am J Med Genet* **9**:255, 1981
12. Hines EA, Bannick EG: Intermittent hypothermia with disabling hyperhidrosis: Report of a case with successful treatment. *Mayo Clin Proc* **9**:705, 1935
13. LeWitt PA et al: Episodic hyperhidrosis, hypothermia, and agenesis of corpus callosum. *Neurology* **33**:1122, 1983
14. Eedy DJ, Corbett JR: Olfactory facial hyperhydrosis responding to amitriptyline. *Clin Exp Dermatol* **12**:298, 1987
15. Pleet DL et al: Paroxysmal unilateral hyperhidrosis and malignant mesothelioma. *Arch Neurol* **40**:256, 1983
16. Sneppen SB et al: Sweat secretion rates in growth hormone disorders. *Clin Endocrinol (Oxf)* **53**:601, 2000
17. Aminoff MJ, Wilcox CS: Assessment of autonomic function in patients with a Parkinsonian syndrome. *Br Med J* **4**:80, 1971
18. Bravo EL, Gifford RW: Current concepts. Pheochromocytoma: Diagnosis, localization and management. *N Engl J Med* **311**:1298, 1984
19. Agocs MM et al: Mercury exposure from interior latex paint. *N Engl J Med* **323**:1096, 1990
20. Gobbi PG et al: Night sweats in Hodgkin's disease. A manifestation of preceding minor febrile pulses. *Cancer* **65**:2074, 1990
21. Cunliffe WJ et al: Localized unilateral hyperhidrosis—A clinical and laboratory study. *Br J Dermatol* **86**:374, 1972
22. McGibbon BM, Paletta FX: Further concepts in gustatory sweating. *Plast Reconstr Surg* **49**:639, 1972
23. Kurchin A et al: Gustatory phenomena after upper dorsal sympathectomy. *Arch Neurol* **34**:619, 1977
24. Bronshvag MM: Spectrum of gustatory sweating, with especial reference to its presence in diabetics with autonomic neuropathy. *Am J Clin Nutr* **31**:307, 1978
25. van Weerden TW et al: Lacrimal sweating in a patient with Reader's syndrome. *Clin Neurol Neurosurg* **81**:119, 1979
26. Lance JW et al: Harlequin syndrome: The sudden onset of unilateral flushing and sweating. *J Neurol Neurosurg Psychiatr* **51**:635, 1988
27. Momose T et al: *N*-isopropyl I-123 p-iodoamphetamine brain scans with single photon emission computed tomography: Mental sweating and EEG abnormality. *Radiat Med* **4**:46, 1986
28. Shih CJ et al: Autonomic dysfunction in palmar hyperhidrosis. *J Auton Nerv Syst* **8**:33, 1983
29. Levit F: Simple device for treatment of hyperhidrosis by iontophoresis. *Arch Dermatol* **98**:505, 1968
30. Shelley WB et al: Botulinum toxin therapy for palmar hyperhidrosis. *J Am Acad Dermatol* **38**:227, 1998
31. Naumann M, Lowe NJ: Botulinum toxin type A in treatment of bilateral primary axillary hyperhidrosis: Randomised, parallel group, double-blind, placebo-controlled trial. *BMJ* **323**:596, 2001
32. Swartling C et al: Botulinum A toxin improves life quality in severe primary focal hyperhidrosis. *Eur J Neurol* **8**:247, 2001
33. Brandrup F, Larsen PO: Axillary hyperhidrosis: Local treatment with aluminum chloride hexahydrate 25% in absolute ethanol. *Acta Derm Venereol* **58**:461, 1978
34. Sulzberger MB, Hermann F: *The Clinical Significance of Disturbances in the Delivery of Sweat.* Springfield, IL, CC Thomas, 1954
35. Mardy S et al: Congenital insensitivity to pain with anhidrosis (CIPA): Effect of TRKA (NTRK1) missense mutations on autophosphorylation of the receptor tyrosine kinase for nerve growth factor. *Hum Mol Genet* **10**:179, 2001
36. Heath PD et al: Ross syndrome and skin changes. *Neurology* **32**:1041, 1982
37. Faden AI et al: Progressive isolated segmental anhidrosis. *Arch Neurol* **39**:172, 1982

38. Low PA et al: Chronic idiopathic anhidrosis. *Ann Neurol* **18**:344, 1985
39. Fisher DA, Maibach HI: Postural hypotension and anhidrosis. The autonomic insufficiency syndrome. *Arch Dermatol* **102**:527, 1970
40. Kennedy WR, Navarro X: Sympathetic sudomotor function in diabetic neuropathy. *Arch Neurol* **46**:1182, 1989
41. Fealey RD et al: Thermoregulatory sweating abnormalities in diabetes mellitus. *Mayo Clin Proc* **64**:617, 1989
42. Singh NK et al: Assessment of autonomic dysfunction in Guillain-Barré syndrome and its prognostic implications. *Acta Neurol Scand* **75**:101, 1987
43. Cable WJ et al: Fabry disease: Impaired autonomic function. *Neurology* **32**:498, 1982
44. Herschthal D, Robinson MJ: Blisters of the skin in coma induced by amitriptyline and clorazepate dipotassium. Report of a case with underlying sweat gland necrosis. *Arch Dermatol* **115**:499, 1979
45. Moss C, Ince P: Anhidrotic and achromians lesions in incontinentia pigmenti. *Br J Dermatol* **116**:839, 1987
46. Koga M: Vitiligo: A new classification and therapy. *Br J Dermatol* **97**:255, 1977
47. Steijlen PM et al: Sweat testing in hypomelanosis of Ito: Divergent results reflecting genetic heterogeneity. *Eur J Dermatol* **10**:217, 2000

48. Lobitz WC, Dobson RL: Miliaria. Sweat retention syndrome. *Pediatr Clin North Am* **3**:791, 1965
49. Holzle E, Kligman AM: The pathogenesis of miliaria rubra. Role of the resident microflora. *Br J Dermatol* **99**:117, 1978
50. Donoghue AM, Sinclair MJ: Miliaria rubra of the lower limbs in underground miners. *Occup Med (Lond)* **50**:430, 2000
51. O'Brien JP: The etiology of poral closure: An experimental study of miliaria rubra, bullous impetigo and related diseases of the skin. I: An histological review of the causation of miliaria. *J Invest Dermatol* **15**:95, 1950
52. Sulzberger MB, Griffin TB: Induced miliaria, postmiliarial hypohidrosis, and some potential sequelae. *Arch Dermatol* **99**:145, 1969
53. Hu CH et al: Transient acantholytic dermatosis (Grover's disease). A skin disorder related to heat and sweating. *Arch Dermatol* **121**:1439, 1985
54. Fitzpatrick JE: The cutaneous histopathology of chemotherapeutic reactions. *J Cutan Pathol* **20**:1, 1993
55. Fiorillo L et al: The pseudomonas hot-foot syndrome. *N Engl J Med* **345**:335, 2002

CHAPTER 77

Mazen S. Daoud
Charles H. Dicken

Disorders of the Apocrine Sweat Glands

The apocrine sweat glands are members of the apocrine system, which also includes the mammary glands, ceruminous (wax) glands of the ear canal, and glands of Moll in the eyelid. The apocrine sweat glands are usually found in the axillae, anogenital area, and mammary areola, and are scattered over the skin of trunk, face, and scalp. Four disorders of the apocrine sweat glands are considered in this chapter: apocrine bromhidrosis, apocrine chromhidrosis, Fox-Fordyce disease, and hidradenitis suppurativa.

APOCRINE BROMHIDROSIS

Apocrine bromhidrosis, also known as bromidrosis or osmidrosis, is a disorder characterized by excessive or abnormal body odor arising from the apocrine glands.[1] It should be differentiated from the less common eccrine bromhidrosis, which may be keratinogenic, metabolic, or exogenous.

Epidemiology

The disease usually affects young adults after puberty; blacks more than whites or Asians. There is no occupational or geographic predisposition. The problem is more intense in the summer because of increased eccrine sweating that augments apocrine sweating. Poor personal hygiene may aggravate the problem. Axillary hyperhidrosis may actually cause a decrease in the odor because the eccrine sweat flushes away the apocrine sweat. A positive family history is present in the majority of cases reported from the Far East.

Plantar bromhidrosis is seen in young males and middle-aged adults. There is no racial or sexual predisposition. The process is not seasonal, because volar sweating is induced by emotional not thermal stimulation. Intertriginous eccrine bromhidrosis is more prominent in the summer.

Etiology and Clinical Features

In males, the most abundant odor component is known to be ϵ-3-methyl-2-hexenoic acid, which is liberated from nonodorous apocrine secretions by axillary bacteria. Other materials include short-chain fatty acids and ammonia. ϵ-3-Methyl-2-hexenoic acid is carried to the skin surface bound to two proteins, apocrine secretion odor-binding proteins-1 (ASOB1) and -2 (ASOB2). Both male and female subjects appear to have the same proteins. Partial sequence data obtained from the N-terminus of ASOB1 suggested that it shares homology with the α chain of apolipoprotein J.[2] Local bacterial flora in the axillary area, whose growth is supported by warmth and moisture, increase apocrine odor production. Leyden et al. demonstrated that aerobic diphtheroids are capable of producing axillary odor.[1] However, bacterial contamination of apocrine sweat may not be the sole cause of apocrine bromhidrosis. Not all family members of a person afflicted with bromhidrosis have the disease, even when they harbor axillary bacteria and live in the same environment. Increased apocrine sweat production as documented by increased number and size of apocrine glands in affected versus normal individuals has been suggested as a possible cause.[3]

The role of androgens is also important. High levels of 5α-reductase has been detected in apocrine glands, and the concentration of dihydrotestosterone has been found to be higher than that of testosterone in the nuclear fraction of the skin of patients with osmidrosis.[4] Apocrine glands express type I 5α-reductase mRNA almost exclusively.

Patient complaints vary based on cultural and geographic location. In the Far East, patients complain of the apocrine odor (bromhidrosis) rather than the excessive sweating, because odorous sweat is considered the greater social embarrassment. In much of the Western world, both hyperhidrosis and bromhidrosis are usually equal complaints. The appearance of axillary skin in patients with bromhidrosis is normal. No laboratory abnormalities are reported.

Eccrine bromhidrosis results from bacterial action on keratin softened by sweating. The soles of the feet are the most common location affected. A similar mechanism is responsible for odor production in other intertriginous areas. Physical examination is essentially normal in these areas except when intertrigo, erythrasma, or candidiasis develop.

Pathology

In these patients, increased numbers of apocrine glands have been found as compared to controls, and the apocrine to eccrine ratio is significantly higher.[3] The apocrine glands are several times larger than the eccrine glands, a feature not seen in patients without excessive sweating. No significant inflammation in the apocrine glands is seen.

Diagnosis

The diagnosis of bromhidrosis is a clinical one. The definition of "normal" odor is a subjective and poorly defined term that varies among races. Hurley reported that the presence of axillary odor is a normal finding in all postpubertal individuals, and bromhidrosis is an accentuation of the axillary odor.[5] In the Asian population, the presence of even a faint odor is considered diagnostic of bromhidrosis.[3] Furthermore, although recognizing an odor-producing chemical is possible using chromatographic or spectroscopic methods, these methods cannot differentiate normal odor from one caused by bromhidrosis. Some individuals may have olfactory limitations to the perception of a single or a broad range of odors, and hence the definition of cutaneous odor is highly variable.

Trimethylaminuria gives rise to a "fishy" odor. It affects patients who have deficient trimethylamine oxidase in the liver or a defective demethylation mechanism; they are unable to metabolize the absorbed trimethylamine produced by intestinal bacteria after ingestion of choline- and lecithin-containing food such as fish, eggs, liver, and kidney. Accumulation of trimethylaminuria in the urine, sweat, and mucosa of the mouth and respiratory tract gives rise to the characteristic odor.

Treatment

The control of axillary bromhidrosis may be accomplished by reducing bacterial flora and apocrine sweat of the axilla. Cleansing with antibacterial soap and the use of topical antibacterial agents, deodorants, perfumes, and antiperspirants should always be recommended. Careful, regular axillary hygiene should be followed. Systemic antibiotics are not helpful. Attention should be paid to odor arising from dried sweat on clothing.

Reduction of eccrine sweating using aluminum chloride may help reduce the local bacterial flora but will not reduce apocrine sweat production. One useful treatment is 20% aluminum chloride in anhydrous ethanol applied at bedtime, with or without occlusion; it may be used on two consecutive nights, then every three to seven nights thereafter. Local radiation treatment and adrenergic nerve sympathectomy are not justifiable.

A variety of surgical techniques have been described in the treatment of bromhidrosis. Excision of subcutaneous tissue, with preservation of the overlying skin, provides good clinical response and minimal complications and avoids contraction of the skin.[6]

Surgical removal of axillary skin and subcutaneous tissue by simple excision can also be done; however, tightness of the axillary fossa may develop.

Ultrasonic surgical aspiration of axillary apocrine glands with endoscopic confirmation is highly effective.[7] Ultrasound energy liquefies fat and sweat glands via cavitation, but minimally affects blood vessels and nerves, which minimizes side effects. Superficial ultrasound-assisted lipoplasty removes the apocrine glands located in the dermis and dermosubcutaneous junction.[8] The frequency-doubled, Q-switched Nd:YAG laser has been reported to be an effective, noninvasive treatment for axillary bromidrosis.[9]

Similar therapeutic measures are used for treatment of eccrine bromhidrosis. Iontophoresis of tap water produces an antiperspirant effect on volar skin when used two to three times a week until there is reduction in sweating, after which maintenance treatment is employed every 3 to 4 weeks. Treatment of secondary intertrigo, candidiasis, and erythrasma is essential.

Course and Prognosis

The course of bromhidrosis is chronic, and spontaneous resolution is not likely. It should be emphasized that patients with bromhidrosis may find it a most distressing and embarrassing problem; if untreated, these patients may develop significant psychological symptoms.

APOCRINE CHROMHIDROSIS

Apocrine chromhidrosis refers to the secretion of colored sweat by the apocrine glands. It is a localized disease affecting apocrine-bearing skin and may be of two clinical varieties, axillary and facial. Areolar involvement has also been described.[10] The responsible pigment is produced inside the apocrine glands, in contrast to false or extrinsic chromhidrosis, in which local bacteria, fungi, or dyes may color apocrine sweat.

Historical Aspects

Yonge first described facial chromhidrosis in 1709. The apocrine origin of the secretion was established in 1954 by Shelley and Hurley,[11] who also described axillary apocrine chromhidrosis in detail, surveyed the world literature, and designated the lipofuscins as the responsible pigment.

Epidemiology

Apocrine chromhidrosis is not seen until after puberty, when apocrine secretory function is activated. Slow regression of the disease is noted with advanced age, in parallel with the regression of apocrine glands. The disease is more common in blacks than whites. There is no sexual, occupational, or geographic predisposition, and seasonal or climatic variations exert little or no influence on these conditions.

Etiology and Pathogenesis

The pigment responsible is apparently one or more of the lipofuscins, which are found in chromhidrotic apocrine sweat in higher concentrations or in a higher state of oxidation than in the normal secretion. No systemic or acquired metabolic or dietary alteration has been detected

FIGURE 77-1

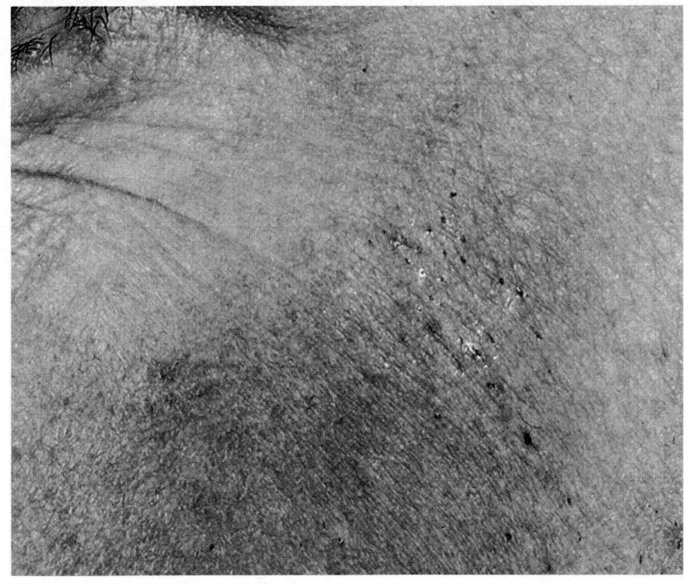

Black sweat produced in a patient with facial apocrine chromhidrosis after gentle squeezing of the cheeks.

that could account for the production of these colored apocrine lipofuscins. Dietary restriction or overloading of carotenoids does not seem to alter the pigment production. No other systemic or pathologic findings accompany the disease.

Clinical Manifestations

Apocrine chromhidrosis is usually seen in one of two major skin areas, the axillae or the face (Fig. 77-1). Axillary apocrine chromhidrosis is rarely a clinical problem, and it is often observed only by the affected person. Staining of the undershirt is the usual complaint, the most common color being yellow; much less frequently, it is green, blue, blue-black, or brown-black. The quantities of apocrine sweat seen are comparatively small, with each droplet at a follicular orifice representing 0.001 mL or less. The droplets are odorless, dry quickly, and fluoresce under UV radiation (360 nm). In general, very light- or very dark-colored apocrine sweat does not fluoresce. Emotional and local physical stimuli appear to excite apocrine sweat.

Facial apocrine chromhidrosis is a rare variant; it is seen on the cheeks and malar eminences most commonly but the forehead and eyelids may also be involved. Concomitant chromhidrosis in other apocrine-bearing skin areas is not present. Onset of colored sweating may be preceded by an aura of warmth or a prickling sensation and is usually prompted by emotional excitation such as anger, fear, or pain. Local physical stimulation will induce the appearance of these colored droplets. Most patients will be able to express the secretion mechanically. The color is usually dark blue or black and is situated at follicular orifices. When dried, the secretion results in adherent, deeply colored flecks. The skin of the affected region is otherwise normal. No pertinent laboratory abnormalities are present.

Pathology

The apocrine glands are normal in size and morphology. Increased numbers of lipofuscin granules are seen in the cytoplasm of the secretory cells. Many granules are seen on unstained slides. Schmorl stain may be positive. Autofluorescence of an unstained paraffin-embedded histologic section has been demonstrated microscopically using a UV excitation wavelength of 360 nm (as used in routine immunofluorescence microscopy).[12] A yellow-green color is seen by examining clothing fibers from an area of staining. The staining is much less intense than the blue-green staining from normal clothing fibers.[12]

Diagnosis and Differential Diagnosis

The history and physical examination suggest the diagnosis of apocrine chromhidrosis. Induction of apocrine sweat by emotional, pharmacologic, or mechanical stimulation confirms the diagnosis. The presence of lipofuscin granules in apocrine cells and the characteristic fluorescence usually also confirm the diagnosis. Patients with ochronosis may have brown-colored sweat. Confirmation by qualitative urinalysis for homogentisic acid is recommended in all patients with chromhidrosis. Contamination of sweat from *Corynebacteria, Piedraia* organisms, or from paint or clothing dye should be ruled out.

Treatment and Course

There is no satisfactory therapy for apocrine chromhidrosis. Capsaicin depletes the neuron of substance P, an important transmitter in apocrine sweat production, and has been used successfully in the treatment of chromhidrosis.[10] The disease is chronic and tends to fade gradually but slowly with age.

FOX-FORDYCE DISEASE

Fox-Fordyce disease is a chronic, pruritic, papular eruption, mainly in women, with a strict localization to areas bearing apocrine glands. Synonyms that have been used for this condition include apocrine miliaria and chronic itching papular eruption of the axillae and pubes. The disease was first described by Fox and Fordyce in 1902.[13]

Epidemiology

The exact incidence of the disease is not known. The majority of patients are women (90 percent), usually between the ages of 15 and 35 years. The disease does not occur before puberty, and cases after menopause are rare. No racial predilection is known. Seasonal, geographic, climatic, and occupational influences are of no significant importance in the development of the disease.

Etiology and Pathogenesis

The fundamental etiologic factors in Fox-Fordyce disease are unknown. The distribution, clinical course, and histopathologic findings clearly indicate a disease of apocrine glands. Since its description, many theories have attributed the disease to emotional, hormonal, and structural factors. Keratinous obstruction of the distal portion of the apocrine duct seems an early finding. Retention of sweat results in rupture of the intraepidermal portion of the apocrine duct, producing a microvesicle. A localized inflammatory reaction around the vesicle then becomes prominent. Dilatation of the apocrine duct results from accumulation of sweat in the distal parts. The reason for the rupture of the intraepidermal duct is unknown. A genetic predisposition for the development of the disease is possible; and the disease has been reported in family members of affected patients and in identical twins. Although clinical improvement is seen in pregnant women during the third trimester of pregnancy, a documented endocrine dysfunction has never been established.

FIGURE 77-2

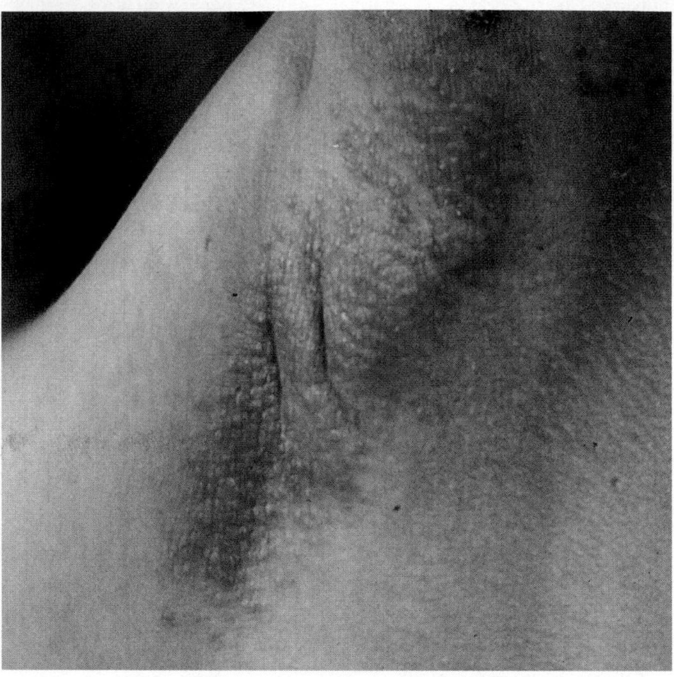

Classic follicular papules in axilla of a patient with Fox-Fordyce disease.

Clinical Manifestations

Fox-Fordyce disease is characterized by discrete, flesh-colored, perifollicular papules with a dome-shaped contour and an occasional central punctum. The process often affects the axillae (Fig. 77-2), pubic area, labia, perineum, areola, presternal skin, umbilicus, and medial thighs. The eruption is usually pruritic and worse in the summer, and it improves with the use of oral contraceptives. Paroxysmal exacerbations are seen after emotional or physical stimulation of the apocrine glands. In a few cases where the majority of the apocrine glands are affected, the apocrine sweat odor may disappear.

Pathology

Obstruction of the outer portion of the apocrine duct and follicular orifice is seen. Dilatation of the proximal portion of the duct causes spongiosis and vesiculation of the intraepidermal portion of the duct and spongiosis of the adjacent epidermis. An inflammatory reaction is seen, composed of lymphocytes and occasional histiocytes and rare eosinophils. Epidermal acanthosis and mucinous deposition in the follicular epithelium are not uncommon. A lymphocytic inflammatory infiltrate is often seen in the upper dermis.

Because serial sectioning is often necessary to see the characteristic pathologic changes of Fox-Fordyce disease, transverse serial sectioning of biopsy specimens seems to be more effective and efficient in establishing the diagnosis.[14]

Diagnosis and Differential Diagnosis

The diagnosis of Fox-Fordyce disease is often made based on the clinical features, morphology, and distribution of the lesions. The lesions are perifollicular papules, confined to the "apocrine areas" of the body, and commonly associated with reduction in sweat odor. Pruritus, often exacerbated with emotional, physical, or pharmacologic stimuli, is often characteristic and this aids in establishing the diagnosis. A 2- or 3-mm punch biopsy will confirm the diagnosis. Serial sectioning may be needed to show the characteristic findings. The differential diagnosis includes lichen planus, lichen nitidus, infective folliculitis, chronic dermatitis, and syringomas. These disorders can be excluded based on the clinical and certainly the pathologic features.

Treatment

The treatment of Fox-Fordyce disease is often difficult. Temporary relief is seen during treatment; however, flares are noted after discontinuation. Clindamycin solution twice a day has been associated with reduction of burning and itching and should be considered as the initial step. Tretinoin cream 0.1% is safe and occasionally effective in reducing the associated pruritus. However, it has minimal effect on the papules themselves. Destructive methods have been used, such as the use of an epilation needle inserted into the superficial part of the follicular orifice and short pulses of electrodesiccation current to destroy the obstructing epithelium. Estrogens and oral contraceptives are occasionally efficacious; however, the response may be slow. Topical glucocorticoid gels may be tried. Systemic glucocorticoids may bring immediate, but temporary, relief to the pruritus. X-ray therapy and surgical excision are not justified.

Course and Prognosis

Fox-Fordyce disease is a chronic, rarely remitting disease that may improve spontaneously during pregnancy. Complications such as folliculitis may develop secondary to intense pruritus. Hidradenitis suppurativa may be associated with the disease.

HIDRADENITIS SUPPURATIVA

Hidradenitis suppurativa is a chronic, inflammatory, scarring disease of the apocrine sweat gland–bearing skin. The disease is characterized by the presence of multiple abscesses, fibrosis, and sinus tracts. A number of synonyms are used to indicate hidradenitis suppurativa such as apocrinitis, hidradenitis axillaris, and abscess of the apocrine sweat gland.

Hidradenitis suppurativa was first described by Velpeau in 1839. Verneuil suggested that the etiology was abscess formation of sweat glands.[15] Histologic features of hidradenitis suppurativa were first described in 1939.[16]

Epidemiology

The disease occurs in both sexes, usually in the second or third decade, and affects women more than men. The disease is rare before puberty. No racial predilection is described. The prevalence of hidradenitis suppurativa is estimated at 4 percent of women in the general population. The prevalence was 1 percent in the general Danish population and 4 percent in a selected group of young adults attending a sexually transmitted diseases clinic.[17] The different age groups examined and differences in diagnostic specificities may account for the variable prevalence estimates.

Etiology and Pathogenesis

The pathogenesis of hidradenitis suppurativa is unknown. The anatomic location of the disease in the axilla, groin, perianal, and inframammary areas suggests a disorder of apocrine glands. It has been suggested that occlusion of the apocrine duct may lead to severe dilatation and apocrine gland inflammation, with ensuing bacterial growth and neutrophilic inflammation of the duct and surrounding tissue, and later fibrosis and sinus tract formation.

Follicular occlusion is another possibility.[18] The clinical similarity of hidradenitis suppurativa to, and its frequent association with, the follicular occlusion–related diseases, such as acne conglobata and dissecting cellulitis of the scalp, suggests that hidradenitis suppurativa may share the same pathogenesis. Follicular occlusion is a prominent feature in all biopsy specimens from patients with hidradenitis suppurativa.[19] At a later stage, apocrine glands may become inflamed due to direct continuity of the apocrine glands to the follicular infundibulum. Apoeccrine glands, whose secretory coils show decapitation secretion with a straight intradermal duct opening directly onto the surface of the skin, remain intact until dermal fibrosis distorts the opening duct, causing irritation by the apocrine sweat.[19]

The role of androgens or other hormones in hidradenitis seems unclear. Obesity, a common finding in hidradenitis suppurativa, is known to alter sex hormone metabolism, leading to an androgen-excess state. Excess androgens can lead to coarsening of the hair shaft and hence to follicular occlusion.[19] Women with hidradenitis suppurativa tend to have a shorter menstrual cycle and a longer duration of menstrual flow, suggesting a possible hormonal influence. However, the incidence of acne, hirsutism, and irregular menstrual periods—signs of a hyperandrogenic state—is not different from that in the general population. There is no difference in the levels of plasma androgens between hidradenitis suppurativa patients and controls.[20] However, cyclic variations during the menstrual cycle, with amelioration of the disease during the estrogen-elevation phase and flares during the estrogen fall phase, have been reported.[20] Furthermore, improvement is noted during pregnancy, and flares may be seen postpartum. A familial form of hidradenitis suppurativa with autosomal dominant inheritance may exist. An insufficiently sensitive disease definition, a variable degree of gene penetrance and possibly a hormonal influence on gene expression may explain the reduced risk to first-degree relatives, which falls short of the expected 50 percent mark.[21]

The significance of bacterial findings in hidradenitis suppurativa is controversial. In one study, bacterial culture was positive in all cases for at least one bacterial species.[22] This motivates a reevaluation of the significance of bacteria in the progress of hidradenitis suppurativa. It is of interest to note that cigarette smoking was found to be a major triggering factor.[23]

Clinical Manifestations

Patients with hidradenitis suppurativa are usually otherwise healthy. Obesity is common, as are follicular occlusive diseases, such as acne conglobata, and dissecting cellulitis of the scalp. The early lesion is a tender, red dermal abscess measuring about 0.5 to 2 cm. The lesion may resemble an inflamed epidermoid cyst. The abscess gradually increases in size and may open to the surface, discharging purulent or seropurulent material, if untreated. The inflammation subsides gradually; however, recurrent episodes of inflammation in the same abscess or others is the rule. Inflammatory abscesses may appear at other anatomic areas at the same time. Fibrosis eventually becomes prominent, and healing appears incomplete (Fig. 77-3). In advanced stages, bands of scar tissue and bridging fibrosis develop that may restrict the mobility of the tissue (Fig. 77-4). Three clinical stages of hidradenitis suppurativa were described by Hurley[24] and are summarized in Table 77-1.

The axillae, buttocks, inguinal, perianal, mammary, and inframammary areas are the most commonly affected. The abdominal wall, chest, scalp, and lower extremities may also be involved. Although apocrine sweating is absent in chronic cases, the lesions have a foul smell secondary to bacterial overgrowth and colonization. Sinus tracts are often seen, draining minimal purulent discharge. Perianal hidradenitis

FIGURE 77-3

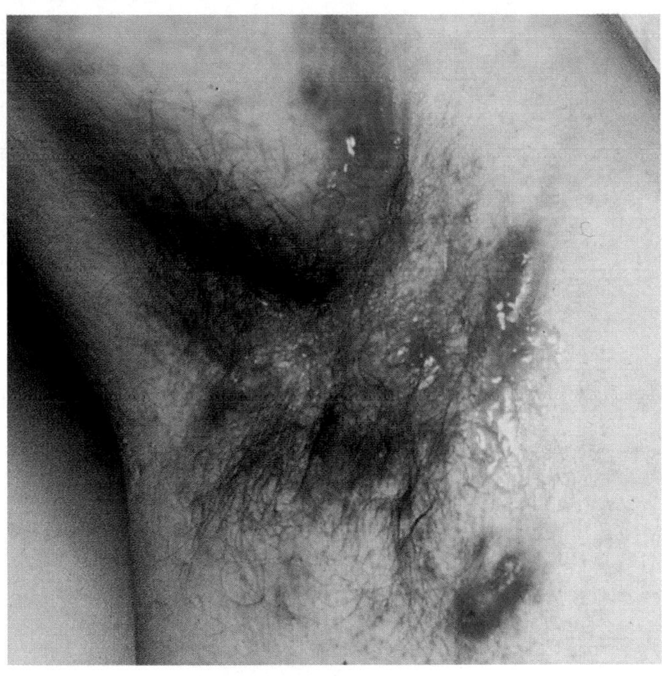

Multiple abscesses in the axilla of a patient with stage I hidradenitis suppurativa. No fibrosis is yet present in the involved area.

can extend to involve the anus and rectum. Sinus tract formation and anal canal fibrosis can lead to stricture formation. Urethral and vaginal fistulas may develop with deep vaginal involvement. Mild arthritis of axial and peripheral type may be seen in acute flares. Laboratory evaluation reveals occasional elevation of white blood cells. Staphylococcus aureus and coagulase-negative staphylococci are the most common species cultured from skin lesions.[22] Other aerobic bacteria include *Streptococcus pyogenes, Pseudomonas aeruginosa,* and *Escherichia coli*. The most frequently isolated anaerobes are *Peptostreptococcus* and *Provotella* species.[25]

Pathology

The histologic findings in hidradenitis suppurativa cover a wide spectrum of changes. Follicular plugging and poral occlusion are prominent features. Occasionally, large cystic spaces are seen, filled with keratin material and hair shafts and lined by stratified squamous epithelium, resembling epithelial cysts. Fibrosis is often seen in the dermis and may occasionally extend to the subcutaneous tissue. Various degrees of inflammation and fibrosis are seen, according to the stage of the disease. Folliculitis and perifollicular inflammation are common and seen in approximately two-thirds of cases, with or without follicular occlusion. The inflammatory cells are composed of neutrophils, lymphocytes, plasma cells, and occasional eosinophils. Areas of frank dermal abscess are seen. Active inflammation around sweat glands is less common than that around hair follicles. Apocrine gland destruction by neutrophilic infiltrates is seen occasionally in the axilla.[19] Apocrinitis, originally suggested as the typical histologic appearance of hidradenitis suppurativa, is seen in a minority of cases.[26] Foreign body-type granulomas around hair follicles and sinus tracts are occasionally seen. The presence of epithelioid granulomas in the dermis away from areas of inflammation is a rare finding (5 percent) and should alert the clinician to the possibility of coexisting Crohn's disease or sarcoidosis.

FIGURE 77-4

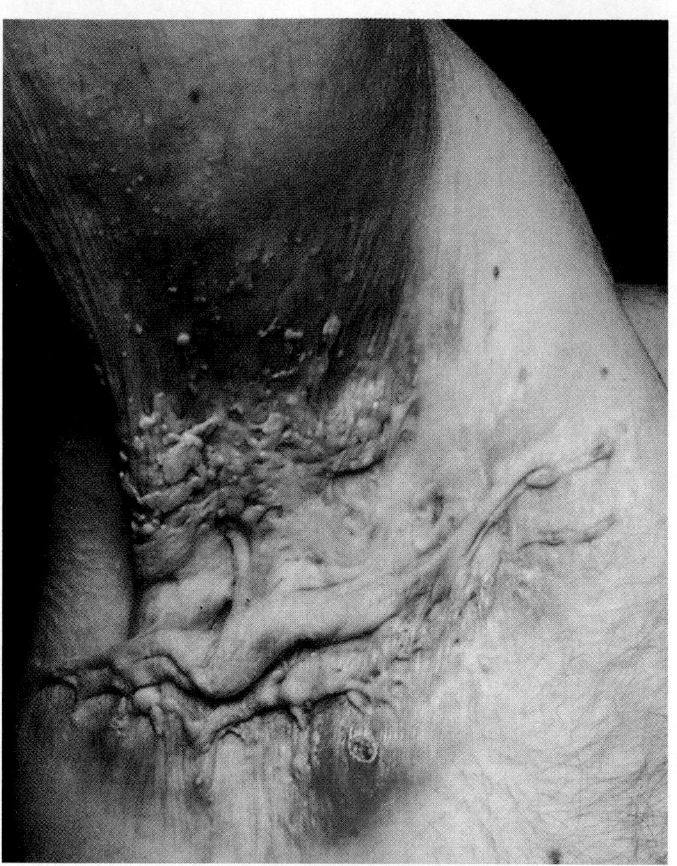

Multiple interconnected sinus tracts with severe fibrosis representing end-stage hidradenitis suppurativa. A new abscess is present at the edge of the axilla.

Diagnosis and Differential Diagnosis

Any inflammatory, abscess-like swelling of the apocrine gland–bearing skin should be regarded as possible hidradenitis suppurativa. A solitary abscess in the early stages resembles a carbuncle, lymphadenitis, or an infected epidermoid cyst. In the vaginal area, it resembles an infected Bartholin cyst. Multiple abscesses in different apocrine gland–bearing skin areas should present no difficulty in establishing the diagnosis. The distribution and characteristic scarring, sinus tracts, and partial healing of infected abscesses are usually diagnostic. Other dermatoses that produce fistulas and sinuses should be included in the differential diagnosis, such as tuberculosis, actinomycosis, tularemia, and cat-scratch disease. In the inguinal area, lymphogranuloma venereum, granuloma inguinale, Crohn's disease, and ulcerative colitis should be excluded.

TABLE 77-1

Clinical Staging of Hidradenitis Suppurativa

Stage I	Solitary or multiple isolated abscess formation without scarring or sinus tracts
Stage II	Recurrent abscesses, single or multiple widely separated lesions, with sinus tract formation and cicatrization
Stage III	Diffuse or broad involvement across a regional area with multiple interconnected sinus tracts and abscesses

Adapted and reprinted with permission from Hurley.[27]

Treatment

Treatment of hidradenitis suppurativa is very difficult. Medical management is recommended in early stages; however, a surgical approach is preferred if scarring and sinus tract formation have developed.

For early disease, intralesional triamcinolone acetonide (5 to 10 mg/mL) may help. Incision and drainage are helpful if spontaneous rupture is imminent. In these situations, drainage and intralesional glucocorticoid injections can be done simultaneously. Bacterial culture of the drained material should be done, and antibiotics should be selected based on sensitivity. Concomitant use of antibiotics is recommended. Minocycline, ciprofloxacin, cephalosporins, clindamycin, or semisynthetic penicillins can be used in the usual doses for soft tissue infections. Isotretinoin may be helpful in some patients. The dose is 1 mg/kg/day as in acne patients; however, higher dosages or longer duration may be needed. The response rate is less than 50 percent. Once significant fibrosis ensues, retinoids are less effective. If inflammation is severe, a short course of systemic glucocorticoids (daily prednisone 40 to 60 mg to be tapered over 2 to 3 weeks) is often needed.

A regimen of 100 mg of cyproterone acetate from days 5 to 14 and 50μg of ethinylestradiol from days 5 to 25 of each menstrual cycle can be helpful.[27]

Local care includes gentle cleansing with antiseptic soaps or cleansers and application of warm compresses with saline or Burow's solution. Some have advocated the use of 6.25% aluminum chloride hexahydrate in absolute ethanol as an antiperspirant and antibacterial agent. Also suggested are avoidance of tight fitting clothing and roll-on antiperspirant deodorants, which can produce frictional trauma and exacerbation of the disease. Topical clindamycin is often used between flare ups.

If scarring develops in conjunction with inflammation, exteriorization is preferred. The aim of the procedure is to destroy the tracts and drain the abscessed area. Fibrotic tracts are explored by soft probes, and complete destruction of granulation tissue and epithelial cells is attempted, even from the smallest pockets. Curettage and electrofulguration of the base are used to destroy residual infected tissue. The wound is then covered with sterile gauze and cleaned twice daily with warm compresses and topical antibiotic ointments. The use of oral antibiotics is recommended on an individual basis. The wound usually heals in 4 to 8 weeks, and the scar is usually smooth and acceptable. This procedure can be performed in all locations except the perianal area, where the risk of traumatizing the anal sphincter is high. Simple excision and primary closure can be done for smaller lesions, but recurrences are more likely.

In severe, stage III disease, complete removal of the affected area is often required. Wide local excision and healing by second intention is considered the surgical treatment of choice.[28] Large wounds in the genital area are best covered with synthetic dressings, with healing by second intention. Negative pressure dressing can secure skin grafts firmly to the wound bed after radical excision. These dressings are simple to apply and are highly effective.[29] Large defects of the axilla can be repaired by advancement or transposition of an island flap from the lateral thoracic wall, pedicled on two or three nourishing vessels arising from the lateral thoracic or thoracodorsal vessels.[30] The use of CO_2 laser ablation of lesions, by vaporizing the tissue in layers until all of the macroscopically abnormal tissue has been removed, could spare normal tissue.[31]

Course and Prognosis

Hidradenitis suppurativa is a chronic disease that progresses relentlessly despite treatment, but the early stages may be curable with proper diagnosis and treatment. The psychological impact of the disease exceeds the systemic complications. Patients with advanced disease are often depressed and socially isolated.[32] Secondary infection of the lesions, which causes a foul smelling odor, adds to the misery of some patients.

Septicemia is a rare event. Restricted mobility, secondary to extensive scarring, and fistula formation are common complications. Urethral and rectal fistulas and strictures are uncommon, and squamous cell carcinoma is a rare complication of long-standing disease. The majority of cases develop on the buttocks and perianal areas. Squamous cell carcinoma arising from hidradenitis suppurativa usually behaves aggressively, with local invasion, distant metastasis, and high mortality. Other rare complications include amyloidosis, interstitial keratitis, and anemia.

REFERENCES

1. Leyden JJ et al: The microbiology of human axilla and its relationship to axillary odor. *J Invest Dermatol* **77**:413, 1981
2. Spielman AL et al: Identification and immunohistochemical location of protein precursors to human axillary odors in apocrine glands and secretion. *Arch Dermatol* **134**:813, 1998
3. Bang YH et al: Histopathology of apocrine bromhidrosis. *Plast Reconst Surg* **98**:288, 1996
4. Sato T et al: Predominance of type I 5-alpha-reductase in apocrine sweat glands of patients with excessive or abnormal odour derived from apocrine sweat (osmidrosis). *Br J Dermatol* **139**:806, 1998
5. Hurley HJ: Diseases of the apocrine sweat glands, in *Dermatology,* 3d ed, vol 2, edited by SL Moschella, HJ Hurley. Philadelphia, Saunders, 1992, p 1495
6. Wang HJ et al: Surgical management of axillary bromidrosis—a modified Skoog procedure by an axillary bipedicle flap approach. *Plast Reconstr Surg* **98**:524, 1996
7. Chung S et al: Ultrasonic surgical aspiration with endoscopic confirmation for osmidrosis. *Br J Plast Surg* **53**:212, 2000
8. Park S: Very superficial ultrasound-assisted lipoplasty for the treatment of axillary osmidrosis. *Aesth Plast Surg* **24**:275, 2000
9. Kunachak S et al: Noninvasive treatment of bromidrosis by frequency-doubled Q-switched Nd:YAG laser. *Aesth Plast Surg* **24**:198, 2000
10. Saff DM et al: Apocrine chromhidrosis involving the areola in a 15-year-old amateur figure skater. *Pediatr Dermatol* **12**:48, 1995
11. Shelley WB, Hurley HJ Jr: Localized chromhidrosis: Survey. *Arch Dermatol* **69**:449, 1954
12. Cox NH et al: Autofluorescence of clothing as an adjunct in the diagnosis of apocrine chromhidrosis. *Arch Dermatol* **128**:275, 1992
13. Fox GH, Fordyce JA: Two cases of a rare papular disease affecting the axillary region. *J Cutan Genitourinary Dis* **120**:1, 1902
14. Stashower ME et al: Fox-Fordyce disease: Diagnosis with transverse histologic sections. *J Am Acad Dermatol* **42**:89, 2000

15. Verneuil AS: Etudes sur les tumours de la peau: De quelque maladies des glands sudoripares. *Arch Gen Med* **94**:693, 1854
16. Brunsting HA: Hidradenitis suppurativa: Abscess of the apocrine sweat glands. *Arch Dermatol Syphil* **39**:108, 1939
17. Jemec GBE et al: The prevalence of hidradenitis suppurativa and its potential precursor lesions. *J Am Acad Dermatol* **35**:191, 1996
18. Yu CCW, Cook MG: Hidradenitis suppurativa: A disease of follicular epithelium, rather than apocrine glands. *Br J Dermatol* **122**:763, 1990
19. Attanoos RL: The pathogenesis of hidradenitis suppurativa: A closer look at apocrine and apoeccrine glands. *Br J Dermatol* **133**:254, 1995
20. Barth JH et al: Endocrine factors in pre- and postmenopausal women with hidradenitis suppurativa. *Br J Dermatol* **134**:1057, 1996
21. Von Der Werth JM et al: The clinical genetics of hidradenitis suppurativa revisited. *Br J Dermatol* **142**:947, 2000
22. Lapins J et al: Coagulase-negative staphylococci are the most common bacteria found in cultures from the deep portions of hidradenitis suppurativa lesions, as obtained by carbon dioxide laser surgery. *Br J Dermatol* **140**:90, 1999
23. Konig A et al: Cigarette smoking as a triggering factor of hidradenitis suppurativa. *Dermatol* **198**:261, 1999
24. Hurley HJ: Axillary hyperhidrosis, apocrine bromhidrosis, hidradenitis suppurativa and familial benign pemphigus: Surgical approach, in *Dermatologic Surgery, Principles and Practice,* edited by RA Roenigk, HH Roenigk Jr. New York, Marcel Dekker, 1989, p 735
25. Brook I, Frazier EH: Aerobic and anaerobic microbiology of axillary hidradenitis suppurativa. *J Med Microbiol* **48**:103, 1999
26. Jemec GBE: Histology of hidradenitis suppurativa. *J Am Acad Dermatol* **34**:994, 1996
27. Sawers RS et al: Control of hidradenitis suppurativa in women using combined antiandrogen (cyproterone acetate) and oesterogen therapy. *Br J Dermatol* **115**:269, 1986
28. Banerjee AK: Surgical treatment of hidradenitis suppurativa. *Br J Dermatol* **79**:863, 1992
29. Elwood ET, Bolitho DG: Negative pressure dressings in the treatment of hidradenitis. *Ann Plastic Surg* **46**:49, 2001
30. Schwabegger AH et al: The lateral thoracic fasciocutaneous island flap for treatment of recurrent hidradenitis axillaris suppurativa and other axillary skin defects. *Br J Plast Surg* **53**:676, 2000
31. Lapins J et al: Surgical treatment of chronic hidradenitis suppurativa: CO_2 laser stripping–secondary intention technique. *Br J Dermatol* **131**:551, 1994
32. Von der Werth JM, Jemec GB: Morbidity in patients with hidradenitis suppurativa. *Br J Dermatol* **144**:809, 2001

CHAPTER 78

Peter Fritsch

Follicular Syndromes with Inflammation and Atrophy

Follicular keratosis is a characteristic reaction pattern of the ostioinfundibular portion of the hair follicles. It is defined by orthohyperkeratotic follicular plugs that distend the ostia and may protrude from the orifices, rendering the skin surface rough to touch, at times even "nutmeg-grater–like." This phenomenon is exceedingly common, and it may be found either as an isolated symptom or associated with a broad spectrum of pathologic conditions. Clinical expression is highly variable, ranging from very subtle to conspicuous; this may explain the very discrepant data on the prevalence which range from 1 percent[1] to 44 percent.[2] Several overlapping clinical entities have been described. Ordinarily, the horny plugs do not impair hair growth or lead to follicular atrophy; those few entities in which they do are classified under the term *keratosis follicularis atrophicans* (see below).

Keratosis pilaris (synonym: keratosis follicularis, lichen pilaris) (KP) is the most common type of follicular keratosis.[3] KP is a harmless but fairly stable eruption of grouped keratotic follicular papules which may be localized to the predilection sites (extensor and lateral aspects of the proximal extremities, buttocks, less often face, neck and trunk) or, infrequently, generalized. A subtle erythema may rim the affected follicle, particularly in skin damaged by chronic exposure to cold (chilblain, cutis marmorata). KP arises in the first decade of life, reaches a peak at adolescence and tends to ameliorate or to subside in the subsequent decades.[4] In a mild form, KP may be found in up to half of the population, thus it is often viewed as a "physiological" condition. KP is of unknown cause; there is no racial predilection, and it appears to be transmitted in an autosomal dominant mode.

Association of KP is most often found with autosomal dominant ichthyosis vulgaris (up to 75 percent[2]) and the ichthyosis-like phenotype that often accompanies dry skin and atopy.[2,5] Interestingly, KP is not a feature of patients with atopic dermatitis who lack the ichthyosis-like phenotype.[2] Association with other disorders of keratinization is less common. KP can also be caused or aggravated by a number of metabolic disturbances such as malnutrition,[6] scurvy,[7] hypovitaminosis B_2 and A (phrynoderma), hypothyroidism, hyperandrogenism, hypercorticism, diabetes and obesity,[8] renal insufficiency, and others. It may also be found in Noonan's and Down's syndrome.[3]

Lichen spinulosus is an uncommon variant of KP that is characterized by sudden appearance of patches of spiny follicular keratoses in children that tend to resolve spontaneously. Another rare variant is erythromelanosis follicularis faciei et colli.

Keratosis pilaris atrophicans (KPA), in contrast, includes a group of phenotypically related, rare disorders that show keratotic follicular papules like KP but, in addition, have nonpurulent inflammation of variable degree, and atrophic end stages characterized by irreversible hair loss and/or atrophic depressions similar to pitted scars.[9,10] All of these disorders appear to be hereditary, to have their onset early in life, and to have disease activity that tends to relent after puberty while atrophy remains. KPA most conspicuously affects the face and scalp, but KP of the ordinary type is a common associated finding on the rest of the body (which then often proves more persistent than the usual type KP). In most cases, KPA is a disorder of the skin only and is mainly of cosmetic relevance, but rare associations with a variety of developmental defects have been reported.

CLASSIFICATION

Attempts at classification are still predominantly based on clinical criteria. Three categories of KPA are generally accepted: the more localized entities of keratosis pilaris atrophicans faciei (KPAF) and atrophoderma vermiculatum (AV) and the generalized keratosis follicularis spinulosa decalvans (KFSD) of Siemens. It has been a matter of debate whether these categories are manifestations or stages of a single process,[9,11] or, instead, independent clinical entities.[12] Heterogeneity of KPA is most likely in view of the different modes of inheritance, significant clinical differences, and the results of gene mapping hitherto available.

Both KPAF and AV are fairly well defined entities with little overlap. Early stage KFSD, however, is similar to KPAF and differs only by its tendency for more widespread expansion and involvement of the scalp later on. Confusion has arisen because KFSD has variously been lumped with similar but different genodermatoses such as the keratosis-ichthyosis-deafness (KID) syndrome[13,14] and the ichthyosis follicularis-alopecia-photophobia (IFAP) syndrome.[15,16] Moreover, KFSD may be heterogeneous in itself; most patients in published cases were members of several large kinships in which the disease phenotype appears fairly homogenous.[17–21] Many of the unrelated cases, however, do not conform to this "classic" type of KFSD (e.g., see Refs. 9 and 11). According to Oranje et al,[12] a more intensely inflammatory phenocopic variant should be distinguished, which they term *folliculitis spinulosa decalvans*.

HISTORICAL ASPECTS

Keratosis Pilaris Atrophicans Faciei

In 1878, Erasmus Wilson described a syndrome characterized by erythematous follicular papules of the eyebrows, cheeks, back, and arms, which began in childhood and eventually led to complete alopecia of the eyebrows; he called it *folliculitis rubra*.[22] Later, several other synonyms were introduced to describe the same condition, including ulerythema ophryogenes (from the Greek *ule,* "scar," and *ophrys,* "eyebrow"),[23] *lichen pilaire ou xerodermie pilaire symmetrique de la face,*[24] and others.

Keratosis Follicularis Spinulosa Decalvans

This name was given by Siemens, in 1926, to an inflammatory follicular syndrome in a Bavarian family, that included scarring alopecia of the scalp, specific eye symptoms, and hyperkeratosis of the palms and soles.[17] X-linked dominant inheritance was proposed. This pedigree was later traced by Thelen.[25] In 1950, Jonkers[18] traced the pedigree of a family in the Netherlands with this disease, which had been briefly described by Lameris in 1905.[26] This latter kinship is now the largest one published so far.[19] Other large kinships with KFSD have been reported from Finland[20] and from Great Britain.[21]

Atrophoderma Vermiculatum

In 1896, Unna introduced the term *ulerythema acneiforme* to describe follicular red papules of the cheeks that eventually progress to reticulate atrophy.[27] Synonyms introduced later include *acne vermoulante,*[28] *atrophodermie vermiculée des joues avec kératoses folliculaires,*[29] *honeycomb atrophy,*[30] and others.

EPIDEMIOLOGY

All categories of KPA are rare, AV and KFSD exceedingly so. KPAF is the most common, but no estimates on its prevalence are available. Familial incidence in all types of KPA has been documented (besides many sporadic cases, particularly in AV). For KPAF and AV, no sex predilection is apparent, and autosomal dominant transmission is likely. KFSD is an X-linked trait; thus most patients are males, but female carriers may also be severely affected.[11,12,31]

ETIOLOGY AND PATHOGENESIS

The disorders that make up KPA are genodermatoses of unknown etiology. In the Dutch pedigree, the gene for KFSD has been mapped to Xp22.13-p22.2, in the region of the genes for X-linked juvenile retinoschisis, the Coffin-Lowry syndrome, and hypophosphatemic rickets.[32] Linkage to the same locus was confirmed for the English family,[33] but in a smaller kinship reported by Harth,[31] the gene could not be tracked to the candidate region, suggesting genetic heterogeneity of KFSD.[34] The gene loci of KPAF and AV are still unknown. KPAF has been observed associated with deletions of 18p in a number of cases,[35–37] and an involvement of the *LAMA1* (laminin α_1 chain) gene has been hypothesized.[38]

The pathogenesis is not well understood. The primary pathogenetic event appears to be abnormal keratinization of the ostioinfundibulum of the hair follicle, resulting in horny plugs that dilate the follicular ostium and may protrude in a spinelike manner. From early stages on, inflammatory infiltrates appear around the follicle. These later mediate perifollicular fibrosis, atrophy, and destruction of the hair bulb. Inflammation, fibrosis, and shrinkage are deeper and more intense in AV, leading to a scarlike reticulate remodeling of the skin surface that is absent in KPAF and KFSD.

Atrophy and inflammation may not be caused simply by pressure from the horny plugs and, later on, by a foreign-body reaction to keratin. The size of follicular horny plugs in common type KP is not necessarily smaller but still does not lead to intense inflammation and scarring. More specific pathomechanisms may thus be anticipated.[11] It is likely that this undefined atrophogenic property of KPA (or at least of KFSD) is common to all hair follicles, even though alopecia becomes apparent first and most conspicuously in the face and scalp, and KP of the rest of the body is indistinguishable from that of the nonscarring type. Follicular atrophy is slow to develop; it does not usually affect all follicles of the face and scalp even in full-blown cases of KFSD; on the other hand, body hair is typically sparse in these cases, and inflammation can on occasion also be found in the seemingly common type of KP.[3,11]

Inflammation is of varying degree in all categories of KPA. In some instances, it is a purely histopathologic sign; in others, it manifests as a visible erythema.

FIGURE 78-1

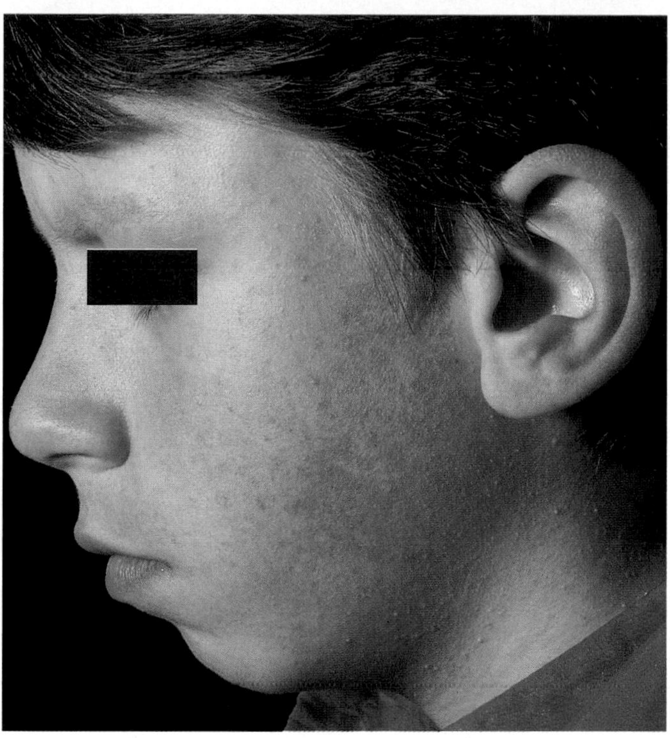

Keratosis pilaris atrophicans faciei (KPAF) (ulerythema ophryogenes) in an 11-year-old boy. Note follicular papules of eyebrows, cheek, and neck; sparsity of lateral eyebrow; and perifollicular erythema.

CLINICAL FEATURES

Keratosis Pilaris Atrophicans Faciei (MIM 604093)

In KPAF, the process begins in the lateral third of the eyebrows a few months after birth, with follicular papules surrounded by an erythematous halo (Fig. 78-1). The skin of the eyebrows may appear diffusely inflamed. There is a gradual loss of hair from the follicles during childhood that may eventually involve the entire eyebrow. The follicular pores appear dilated; their number diminishes over the years. Pitlike scarring and remodeling of the skin surface is absent. The process may progress to involve the cheeks and forehead, where it is less conspicuous because hair loss is not readily detected. KPAF is often accompanied by KP of the extensor sites of the extremities. Progression appears to cease after puberty. The likely mode of inheritance is autosomal dominant.

KPAF has been seen with other ectodermal defects or with multiple congenital abnormalities.[39,40] Mertens studied 15 patients from 5 families with KPAF and found most patients to have an atopic diathesis.[41] Five cases of Noonan's syndrome associated with KPAF were described by Pierini,[10] and woolly hair may be found in patients with KPA with and without Noonan's syndrome.[42,43]

Keratosis Follicularis Spinulosa Decalvans (MIM 308800)

KFSD is more widespread but morphologically similar to KPAF. It begins in infancy with numerous horny follicular plugs and milia on the nose and cheeks and later on the eyebrows, scalp, neck, and body (Fig. 78-2*A*). Erythema is variable and often very faint.[12] Scarring alopecia of the scalp, eyebrows, and eyelashes becomes apparent in childhood and progresses until puberty. It is often restricted to patches and rarely proceeds to full baldness. Remnant hairs of the eyelashes typically protrude in different directions. Facial lanugo hair is absent. There is KP of the body that resembles that of the nonatrophic type, but many hair follicles appear empty (Fig. 78-2*B*). Axillary and pubic hair thinning is frequently observed. Patches of eczema, particularly of the scalp, may be seen. Ichthyosiform scaling of the interfollicular epidermis is typically absent. After puberty, progression slowly subsides.

Associated features include palmoplantar keratoderma, with predilection for the calcaneal region, and the unusual sign of high cuticles.[19] Photophobia is a regular feature caused by subepithelial opacities in the Bowman's membrane.[44] Conjunctivitis and corneal vascularization (circular pannus) are infrequently combined. Another cause of corneal dystrophy may be hardened secretions of the meibomian glands forming hard prickles. Photophobia is found predominantly in children; it improves after puberty, similar to the skin symptoms. Visual prognosis is good. KFSD is not associated with other physical or mental disturbances. As rare exceptions, combinations have been described with aminoaciduria[45] and with Noonan's syndrome.[46] There are no abnormalities of the cutaneous microbial flora.[11]

X-linked dominant mode of inheritance has been shown. Therefore, the most severe manifestations are found in males. Female carriers mostly show only dry skin and KP. Not infrequently, however, they may present the full clinical picture,[9,21,31] which is interpreted as nonrandom X-chromosome inactivation.[12]

Variant cases published as KFSD,[9–11] and put together by Oranje et al.[12] under the tentative term *folliculitis spinulosa decalvans,* are also characterized by KPA but differ in several aspects: more pronounced

FIGURE 78-2

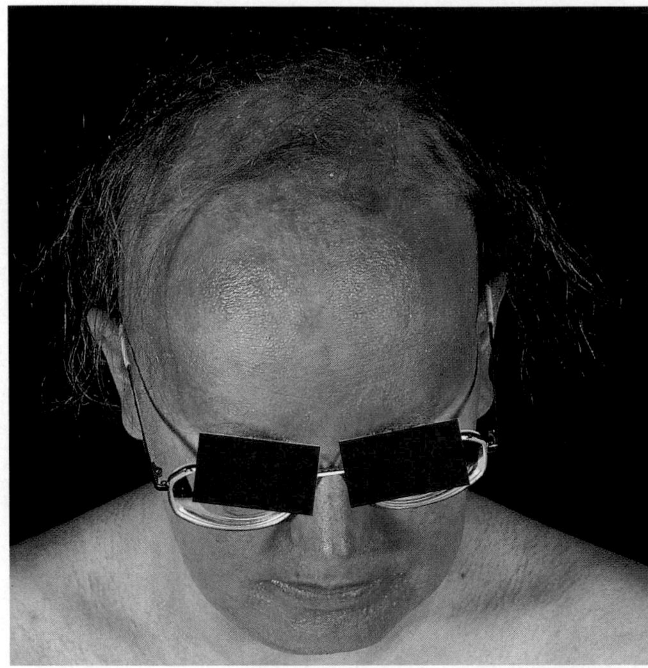

A.

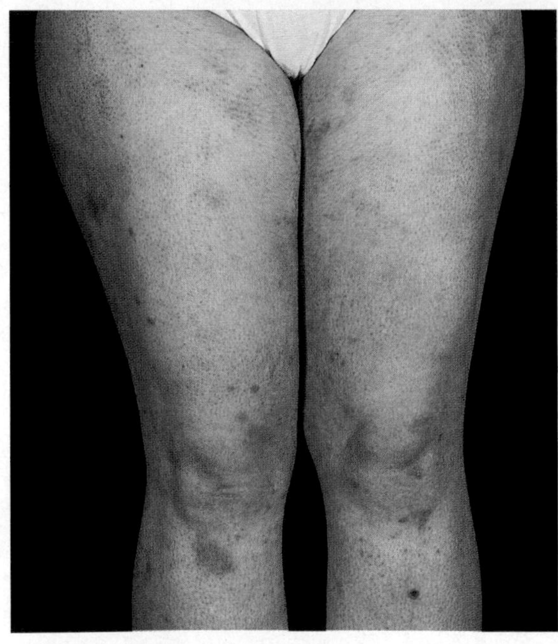

B.

Keratosis follicularis spinulosa decalvans (KFSD) in a 25-year-old female. *A.* Scarring alopecia, generalized follicular papules, and diffuse erythema of the face. *B.* Keratosis pilaris of the thighs.

inflammation and extensive erythema, pustule formation particularly of the scalp, crusting, and desquamation. An increased incidence of atopic dermatitis has been reported.[11] After puberty, the process fails to ameliorate; but rather, it gets worse. The mode of inheritance is likely to be autosomal dominant. This disorder must be distinguished from folliculitis decalvans.

FIGURE 78-3

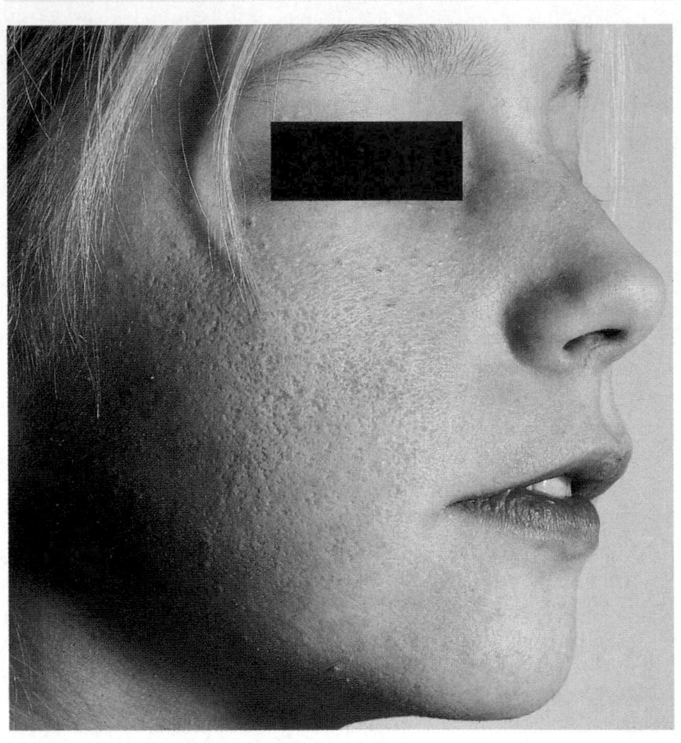

Atrophoderma vermiculatum (AV) in a 10-year-old girl. Note multiple confluent, atrophic, pitlike depressions of the cheek.

Atrophoderma Vermiculatum (MIM 209700)

AV is set apart clinically from KPAF and KFSD by its later age of onset (between 5 and 12 years; some cases have been noted to begin at puberty or in adulthood) and by its morphologic hallmark, which is scarlike atrophic pits of the cheeks. It begins with erythematous follicular keratotic plugs, papules, and milia, which transform into conspicuous pitlike depressions separated by narrow epidermal ridges, lending the area a reticulate "honeycomb-like" or "worm-eaten" aspect. The pits are irregular in shape—approximately 1 mm in depth and up to 2 mm^2 in size. At times, they may extend to the upper lip, ears, and forehead (Fig. 78-3). Through the thinned epidermis of the pits, an erythematous blush may be seen. Eyebrows, eyelashes, and scalp are notably spared. The cheeks appear to be waxy and shiny and firmer on palpation than the surrounding skin. AV is typically symmetric, but unilateral occurrence has been reported.[47] Again, the progression of AV subsides after puberty. Most authors favor an autosomal dominant trait,[48] but autosomal recessive inheritance has also been considered.[12]

Associations of AV have occasionally been reported with various minor or major developmental anomalies such as epidermal cysts and folliculitis decalvans, birefringent hairs, mongolism, Eisenmenger complex and intraauricular septal defect,[49] and the Rombo syndrome (an autosomal dominant condition similar to the Bazex syndrome, with milia, hypotrichosis, basal cell carcinomas).[50]

PATHOLOGY

The histologic picture[11,51] depends on the stage of the process, which may be different in neighboring hair follicles. Early inflammatory papules reveal acanthotic, hypergranulotic infundibula dilated by compact keratin plugs that contain dystrophic or twisted hairs. There is a lymphocytic infiltrate with neutrophils around the upper (in AV also the lower) portions of the appendages. More advanced stages show mixed lymphohistiocytic infiltrates with multinucleated giant cells, often around keratinous debris or naked hair particles; atrophy or absence of the hair bulbs; and deposition of collagen. End-stage biopsies exhibit the nonspecific findings of cicatricial alopecia: sclerosis of dermal collagen and atrophy of rete ridges and sebaceous glands. In the only electron-microscopic study of KFSD hitherto published, an increase of abnormally rounded keratohyalin granules, precocious appearance of the cornified envelope, and delayed desmosome dissolution were found in the infundibular epithelium.[52] Immunofluorescence was reported negative by Maroon et al.[53]

DIFFERENTIAL DIAGNOSIS

All types of KPA must principally be distinguished from the nonatrophic KP. Early KPAF may be misinterpreted as patches of seborrheic or atopic dermatitis. KFSD must be distinguished from atopic dermatitis associated with lichen pilaris and thinning of the lateral eyebrow (Hertoghe's sign).

The KID syndrome is similar to KFSD because of its extensive horny plugs in hair follicles and sweat gland pores, sparse hair, and variable degree of erythema. It is distinguished by the absence of follicular scarring and by its associated features: neurosensory deafness, vascularizing keratitis, and reticulated palmoplantar hyperkeratosis obliterating the dermatoglyphics.

The IFAP syndrome (described in 1909 by MacLeod as "ichthyosis follicularis"[54]) shares several features with KFSD: generalized keratosis pilaris, eye symptoms, hair loss, and an X-linked inheritance.[16,55] In contrast, the alopecia is nonscarring and universal, and keratosis pilaris is noninflammatory and exhibits extensive spiny horn plugs; there is also ichthyosis of the interfollicular epidermis in some body regions, and associated features such as severe photophobia and failure to thrive.

Atrichia with papular lesions is a developmental defect of the pilosebaceous system characterized by complete loss of hair in the first months of life and formation of extensive papules and horny plugs that histologically resemble trichoepitheliomas.

AV may resemble acne infantum (but does not have pustules) and acneiform eruptions such as those found in children exposed to the chloracnegen 2,3,7,8-tetrachlorodibenzo-*p*-dioxin in the industrial accident in Seveso, Italy.[56] After puberty, AV may be indistinguishable from acne scars (although these are rarely as localized as AV). Nevus comedonicus may be morphologically similar but is usually unilateral and follows the Blaschko lines.

TREATMENT, COURSE, AND PROGNOSIS

No effective therapy is available for reversing the course of these syndromes. Temporary symptomatic treatment, including emollients, topical steroids, tretinoin, and keratolytic agents, may be of limited value. Topical and systemic antibiotics are ineffective. Hair transplantation may be helpful in scalp alopecia. Dermabrasion and/or collagen implants may prove useful in treatment of the facial pits. Pulsed tunable dye laser treatment was found to improve the erythematous component of KPAF but not the follicular keratoses.[57] Systemic retinoids were found to be ineffective in KFSD by some authors[11,52] but helpful by others.[58–60] At any rate, possible therapeutic benefits must be weighed against the toxicity of chronic therapy.

REFERENCES

1. Fung WK, Lo KK: Prevalence of skin disease among school children and adolescents in a student health service center in Hong Kong. *Pediatr Dermatol* **17**:440, 2000
2. Mevorah B et al: The prevalence of accentuated palmoplantar markings and keratosis pilaris in atopic dermatitis, autosomal dominant ichthyosis and control dermatological patients. *Br J Dermatol* **112**:679, 1985
3. Lateef A, Schwartz RA: Keratosis pilaris. *Cutis* **63**:205, 1999
4. Poskitt L, Wilkinson JD: Natural history of keratosis pilaris. *Br J Dermatol* **130**:711, 1994
5. Yosipovitch G et al: High body mass index, dry scaly leg skin and atopic conditions are highly associated with keratosis pilaris. *Dermatology* **201**:34, 2000
6. Forman L: Keratosis pilaris. *Br J Dermatol* **66**:279, 1954
7. Hilty N et al: Skorbut bei Trisomie 21. *Hautarzt* **42**:464, 1991
8. Yosipovitch G et al: The prevalence of cutaneous manifestations in IDDM patients and their association with diabetes risk factors and microvascular complications. *Diabetes Care* **21**:506, 1998
9. Rand R, Baden H: Keratosis follicularis spinulosa decalvans. Report of two cases and literature review. *Arch Dermatol* **119**:22, 1983
10. Pierini DO, Pierini AM: Keratosis pilaris atrophicans faciei (ulerythema ophryogenes): A cutaneous marker in Noonan's syndrome. *Br J Dermatol* **100**:409, 1979
11. Baden HP, Byers HR: Clinical findings, cutaneous pathology and response to therapy in 21 patients with keratosis pilaris atrophicans. *Arch Dermatol* **130**:469, 1994
12. Oranje AP et al: Keratosis pilaris atrophicans. One heterogeneous disease or a symptom in different clinical entities? *Arch Dermatol* **130**:500, 1994
13. Britton H et al: Keratosis follicularis spinulosa decalvans: An infant with failure to thrive, deafness and recurrent infections. *Arch Dermatol* **114**:761, 1978
14. Morris J et al: Generalized spiny hyperkeratosis, universal alopecia, and deafness: A previously undescribed syndrome. *Arch Dermatol* **100**:692, 1969
15. Martino F et al: Child with manifestations of dermotrichic syndrome and ichthyosis follicularis-alopecia-photophobia (IFAP) syndrome. *Am J Med Genet* **44**:233, 1992
16. Hamm H et al: Further delineation of the ichthyosis follicularis, atrichia, and photophobia syndrome. *Eur J Pediatr* **150**:627, 1991
17. Siemens HW: Keratosis follicularis spinulosa decalvans. *Arch Dermatol Syphilol* **151**:384, 1926
18. Jonkers GH: Hyperkeratosis follicularis en cornea degenerative. *Ned Tijdschr Geneeskd* **94**:1464, 1950
19. van Osch LDM et al: Keratosis follicularis spinulosa decalvans: A family study of seven male cases and six female carriers. *J Med Genet* **29**:36, 1992
20. Kuokkanen K: Keratosis follicularis spinulosa decalvans in a family from northern Finland. *Acta Derm Venereol Suppl (Stockh)* **51**:146, 1971
21. Herd RM, Benton EC: Keratosis follicularis decalvans: Report of a new pedigree. *Br J Dermatol* **134**:138, 1996
22. Wilson E: *Lectures on Dermatology*. London, J & A Churchill, 1878, p 217
23. Taenzer P: Ueber das Ulerythema ophryogenes, eine noch nicht beschriebene hautkrankheit. *Monatsschr Prakt Dermatol* **8**:197, 1889
24. Brocq L: Lichen pilaire ou xérodermie pilaire symetrique de la face. *Ann Dermatol Syphiligr (Paris)* **10**:339, 1889
25. Thelen L: Keratosis folliculitis spinulosa decalvans (Siemens). *Z Haut Geschlechtskr* **66**:56, 1940
26. Lameris HJ: Ichthyosis follicularis. *Ned Tijdschr Geneeskd* **41**:1524, 1905
27. Unna PG: Ulerythema acneiforme, in *Histopathology of Diseases of the Skin,* translated from German by N Walker. Edinburgh, Clay, 1896, p 1084
28. Thieberge G: Acne vermoullante, in *La Pratique Dermatologique,* vol 1, edited by E Besnier, Brocq L, Jacquet L. Paris, Masson et Cie, 1900, p 207
29. Darier J: Atrophodermie vermiculée des joues avec kératoses folliculaires. *Bull Soc Fr Dermatol Syphiligr* **27**:345, 1920
30. Savatard L: Honeycomb atrophy. *Br J Dermatol* **55**:259, 1943
31. Harth W et al: Keratosis follicularis spinulosa decalvans: The complete syndrome in a female. *Z Hautkr* **67**:1080, 1992
32. Oosterwijk JC et al: Refinement of the localization of the X-linked keratosis follicularis spinulosa decalvans (KFSD) gene in Xp22.13-p22.2. *J Med Genet* **32**:736, 1995
33. Porteous M et al: Keratosis follicularis spinulosa decalvans: Confirmation of linkage to Xp22.13-p22.2. *J Med Genet* **35**:336, 1998

34. Oosterwijk JC et al: Molecular genetic analysis of two families with keratosis follicularis spinulosa decalvans: Refinement of gene localization and evidence for genetic heterogeneity. *Hum Genet* **100**:520, 1997
35. Zouboulis CC et al: Ulerythema ophryogenes and keratosis pilaris in a child with monosomy 18p. *Pediatr Dermatol* **11**:172, 1994
36. Nazarenko SA et al: Keratosis pilaris and ulerythema ophryogenes associated with an 18p deletion caused by a Y/18 translocation. *Am J Med Genet* **95**:179, 1999
37. Horsley SW et al: Del(18p) shown to be a cryptic translocation using a multiprobe FISH assay for subtelomeric chromosome rearrangements. *J Med Genet* **35**:722, 1998
38. Zouboulis C et al: Keratosis pilaris/ulerythema ophryogenes and 18p deletion: Is it possible that the LAMA1 gene is involved? *J Med Genet* **38**:127, 2001
39. Davenport DD: Ulerythema ophryogenes: Review and report of a case: Discussion of relationship to certain other skin disorders and association with internal abnormalities. *Arch Dermatol* **89**:74, 1964
40. Burnett JW et al: Ulerythema ophryogenes with multiple congenital abnormalities. *J Am Acad Dermatol* **18**:437, 1988
41. Mertens RLJ: Ulerythema ophryogenes and atopy. *Arch Dermatol* **97**:662, 1968
42. McHenry PM et al: The association of keratosis pilaris atrophicans with hereditary woolly hair. *Pediatr Dermatol* **7**:202, 1990
43. Snell JA, Mallory SB: Ulerythema ophryogenes in Noonan syndrome. *Pediatr Dermatol* **7**:77, 1990
44. Franceschetti A et al: Manifestations cornéennes dans la keratosis follicularis spinulosa decalvans (Siemens). *Ophthalmologica* **133**:259, 1957
45. Grosshans E et al: Keratosis follicularis spinulosa decalvans et aminoacidurie. *Ann Dermatol Venereol* **105**:433, 1978
46. Grob JJ et al: Les signes cutanées du syndrome de Noonan. A propos d'une observation avec ulérythème ophryogène, kératose pilaire et sudorale disséminée et alopécie progressive. *Ann Dermatol Venereol* **115**:303, 1988
47. Arieta E, Milgram-Sternberg Y: Honeycomb atrophy on the right cheek. *Arch Dermatol* **124**:1001, 1988
48. Frosch PJ, Brumage MR: Atrophoderma vermiculatum. Case reports and review. *J Am Acad Dermatol* **18**:538, 1988
49. Kooij R, Venter J: Atrophodermia vermiculata with unusual localization and associated congenital anomalies. *Dermatologica* **118**:161, 1959
50. Michaelsson G et al: The Rombo syndrome: A familial disorder with vermiculate atrophy, milia, hypotrichosis, trichoepitheliomas, basal cell carcinomas, and peripheral vasodilation with cyanosis. *Acta Derm Venereol Suppl (Stockh)* **61**:497, 1981
51. Brazelli V, Borroni G: Aspetti istologici e tardivi dell'atrophodermia vermiculata. *G Ital Derm Venereol* **125**:185, 1990
52. Puppin D et al: Keratosis follicularis spinulosa decalvans: Report of a case with ultrastructural study and unsuccessful trial of retinoids. *Dermatologica* **184**:133, 1992
53. Maroon M et al: Keratosis pilaris and scarring alopecia. *Arch Dermatol* **128**:397, 1992
54. MacLeod JMH: Three cases of "ichthyosis follicularis" associated with baldness. *Br J Dermatol* **21**:165, 1909
55. Konig A, Happle R: Linear lesions reflecting lyonization in women heterozygous for IFAP syndrome (ichthyosis follicularis with atrichia and photophobia). *Am J Med Genet* **85**:365, 1999
56. Gianotti F: Chloracné au tétrachloro-2,3,7,8-dibenzo-*p*-dioxide chez les enfants. *Ann Dermatol Venereol* **104**:825, 1977
57. Clark SM et al: Treatment of keratosis pilaris atrophicans with the pulsed tunable dye laser. *J Cutan Laser Ther* **2**:151, 2000
58. Richard G, Harth W: Keratosis follicularis spinulosa decalvans. Therapie mit Isotretinoin und Etretinat im entzündlichen Stadium. *Hautarzt* **44**:529, 1993
59. Fritsch P, Sidoroff A: Safety of retinoids and indications for use. *Curr Opin Dermatol* **1**:207, 1993
60. Layton AM, Cunliffe WJ: A case of ulerythema ophryogenes responding to isotretinoin. *Br J Dermatol* **129**:945, 1993

CHAPTER 79

Karynne O. Duncan
David J. Leffell

Epithelial Precancerous Lesions

A precancerous or premalignant lesion is one that has a strong likelihood of transforming into a malignancy. There is much debate about the validity of the concept of "precancerous" lesions.[1–4] The lesions discussed in this chapter are those that clinically have a demonstrated potential to become invasive carcinomas and that histopathologically demonstrate atypia confined to the epidermis. The focus is only on the precancerous keratinocyte lesions and not on those of other epithelial cells such as the melanocyte, Merkel, and appendageal cells. Discussion of malignancies and premalignancies associated with these cells can be found in Chaps. 92, 93, 86, and 85, respectively.

A common feature of all premalignant epithelial tumors listed in Table 79-1 is that they all have the potential to become invasive squamous cell carcinoma (SCC). These precancerous lesions and SCC are considered by many to represent a continuum of disease with dysplasia at one end of the spectrum and invasive carcinoma at the other.[5]

ACTINIC KERATOSES

Actinic keratoses (AKs) are cutaneous neoplasms consisting of proliferations of cytologically aberrant, epidermal keratinocytes that develop in response to prolonged exposure to ultraviolet radiation. The concept of a precancerous keratosis was first presented by Dubreuilh in the late 1800s.[5] AKs were first identified and named "keratoma senilis" by Freudenthal in 1926.[6] In 1958, Pinkus further characterized these lesions and coined the term *actinic keratosis*.[7] These lesions have also been called solar keratoses and senile keratoses. *Actinic keratosis* literally means a condition (*-osis*) of excessive horny (*kerat-*) tissue induced by a ray of light (*aktis*), presumably ultraviolet light. AKs have historically been considered precancerous or premalignant lesions, with a potential for developing into squamous cell carcinomas. In recent years, however, there has been an effort to redefine AKs as malignant neoplasms, as these lesions are essentially intraepithelial squamous cell carcinomas in evolution. Although not all AKs become SCCs, AKs are essentially the initial lesion in a disease continuum that progresses to squamous cell carcinoma. This concept of a progression along a spectrum is analogous to that of cervical carcinoma, where cervical intraepithelial neoplasia is the initial, "precancerous" lesion.

TABLE 79-1

Precancerous Keratinocytic Lesions

- Actinic keratoses
- Arsenical keratoses
- Thermal keratoses
- Hydrocarbon keratoses
- Chronic radiation keratoses
- Chronic scar keratoses
- Reactional keratoses
- PUVA keratoses
- Viral keratoses
  - Bowenoid papulosis
  - Epidermodysplasia verruciformis
- Bowen's disease
- Erythroplasia of Queyrat
- Erythroplakia
- Leukoplakia

Actinic keratoses are clinically important lesions, not only because of their potential to develop into SCC, but because they are one of the strongest predictors that an individual may subsequently develop SCC or basal cell carcinoma (BCC) of the skin.[8,9] With the increasing incidence and prevalence of these nonmelanoma skin cancers (NMSCs), as discussed in Chaps. 80 and 81, persons with AKs are the perfect candidates for close longitudinal observation for prevention and early treatment.

Epidemiology

Actinic keratoses are lesions commonly encountered in dermatology practice. After acne vulgaris and dermatitis, AKs are the third most common reason for patients to see a dermatologist.[10] In a recent survey of outpatient visits between 1990 and 1994, it was estimated that of 127 million office visits, 14.6 million (11.5 percent) were for the evaluation and management of AKs.[11] Data on the prevalence of AKs (proportion of people in a population who have at least one AK) come primarily from studies in Australia, where AKs and NMSCs are more common than anywhere else in the world.[12] Studies outside of Australia are more limited and have reported AK prevalence rates ranging from 11 percent in persons older than age 21 in County Galway, Ireland, to 25 percent in a high-risk group of outdoor workers in Maryland, USA.[13,14] Studies of the incidence (proportion of people in a population who develop a new AK in a specific time period) of AKs are even more limited, with one such study from Australia reported to date.[15] In that study, 59 percent of the people had at least one AK and 41 percent were lesion free. At the 12-month visit, 60 percent of people from the former group had developed new AKs, whereas only 19 percent of people from the latter group had developed new AKs.

Various risk factors have been identified for the expression of AKs, with the two major groups being individual susceptibility and cumulative ultraviolet radiation exposure. One of the most important susceptibility risk factors is age, as all the epidemiologic studies indicate that AKs increase in prevalence with increasing age, ranging from <10 percent in white adults aged 20 to 29 years to 80 percent in similar adults aged 60 to 69 years. Males appear to have more AKs than females in most epidemiologic studies, reflecting assumed greater cumulative sun exposure in males compared to females.[12] This sex differential is more pronounced at younger ages. Other individual susceptibility risk factors include a phenotype of fair skin that easily burns and freckles, while rarely tans; blue or light-colored eyes; and red or blond hair.[10,12] Another individual risk factor is immunosuppression, as it is well known that organ transplant recipients are at increased risk of developing AKs and SCCs. Lastly, individuals with certain genetic syndromes are at greater risk of developing AKs, namely albinism and xeroderma pigmentosum, and possibly Rothmund-Thomson and Bloom's syndromes.

Cumulative exposure to ultraviolet radiation, including tanning beds, is the other major risk factor for developing AKs. Evidence that sun exposure plays a role in the development of AKs is seen in the fact that over 80 percent of all AKs are distributed on chronically sun-exposed areas of the body, such as the scalp, head, neck, forearms, and dorsal hands.[12] Variables that affect a person's cumulative ultraviolet radiation exposure include one's age, gender, occupation, recreational activities, and place of residence. As stated above, AKs increase in prevalence the older the individual. Intuitively, the older the individual, the greater is the cumulative exposure to ultraviolet radiation. In addition to this factor, the age at which a person received the greatest amount and intensity of exposure to ultraviolet radiation appears to be a risk factor, with such exposure in childhood apparently posing the greatest risk. In migration studies from Australia, British immigrants who moved to Australia before the age of 20 had fewer AKs than the native white Australians early in life, but they equaled the native Australians in later years. British immigrants who moved to Australia after the age of 20 years never developed the same number of AKs as the native Australians or the early British immigrants.[16]

Etiology and Pathogenesis

In the past decade tremendous strides have been made in understanding the scientific basis of AKs and nonmelanoma skin cancer. Although genetic and environmental factors may play a role in the development of AKs and SCC, it has long been recognized that the most important contributing factor is chronic exposure to ultraviolet radiation, namely sunlight exposure. Ultraviolet radiation is responsible for the development of AK, and eventually SCC, in two ways: first, it causes mutations in cellular DNA that, when unrepaired, lead to unrestrained growth and tumor formation, and, second, it acts as an immunosuppressant to prevent tumor rejection.[17] Carcinogenesis is discussed in great depth in Chaps. 36 to 38.

It has become evident with recent studies involving the molecular biology of skin cancer that ultraviolet radiation–induced mutations in the tumor-suppressor gene *p53* play a pivotal role in the initiation of AKs and their development into SCC. *p53*, in general, is the most commonly mutated tumor-suppressor gene and is present in greater than 50 percent of all human cancers.[17] Ziegler et al. identified mutation hot spots in the *p53* gene in human NMSCs and demonstrated that the *p53* mutations, which are present in more than 90 percent of SCCs, are also present in AKs.[18] Normal *p53* gene activity produces a protein that is a transcription factor whose targets include genes that regulate the cell cycle. This protein acts to ensure that cells do not proliferate uncontrollably and to ensure that abnormal, mutated cells are destroyed so that they cannot divide and continue to pass along the mutation to daughter cells. This latter process of controlled cell suicide is also known as apoptosis, and it is one of the most important mechanisms by which cancer cells are kept in check in the human body. Several animal and human-based experiments have proven the role of ultraviolet radiation in causing unique mutations in *p53*, and in causing apoptosis in the skin.[19] While keratinocytes with normal functioning *p53* are undergoing apoptosis in the presence of repeated exposure to sunlight, the *p53*-mutated clone of keratinocytes is dividing and expanding into the space left behind by these dying cells. At some point, repeated exposure to sunlight may result in a second UVB-induced mutation in the *p53* gene (second hit or progression) with resultant malignant transformation and the development of the AK clone into SCC (Fig. 79-1).

Prevention

It is widely believed that, because most AKs are related to exposure to ultraviolet radiation, preventive measures aimed at limiting the amount and intensity of sun exposure, especially in childhood and adolescence, should prove effective in decreasing their prevalence. The best prevention is avoidance of the sun, especially mid-day when the intensity is greatest. As this is often impractical, the next best preventive measures are wearing protective clothing, such as tightly woven, long-sleeved pants and shirts, and wide-brimmed hats, and the use of a high sun protection factor (SPF) sunscreen. Sunscreens reduce the frequency of tumors induced experimentally in animals exposed to ultraviolet radiation and reduce the development of AKs in humans.[20]

There is some evidence that adhering to a diet low in fat may decrease the incidence of AKs.[21] Oral retinoids are effective in preventing NMSC and AKs, especially in high-risk patients such as organ transplant recipients and patients with xeroderma pigmentosum, but they are only effective as long as the patient is taking the medication. The combination of low dose 13-*cis*-retinoic acid (10 mg every other day) with topical tretinoin has been advocated as prophylaxis of both AKs and NMSC in renal transplant recipients.[22]

Clinical Manifestations

The typical person who presents with AKs is an elderly, fair-skinned, light-eyed individual who has a history of significant sun exposure, who burned and freckled rather than tanned, and who has significant solar elastosis on examination (Fig. 79-2). AKs, however, can be seen in younger individuals if they have sustained sufficient sun exposure over their lives. As mentioned earlier, AKs (80 percent) are typically found on chronically sun-exposed sites of the body, such as the head, neck, forearms, and dorsal hands.[10] The majority are found on the upper limbs (approximately 65 percent).[12] The typical AK lesion, sometimes called the erythematous AK, presents most commonly as a 2- to 6-mm erythematous, flat, rough or scaly papule. It is usually easier felt than seen. AKs can vary in size, and sometimes reach up to several centimeters in diameter. They are most often found amongst a background of solar elastosis, with dyspigmentation, yellow discoloration, ephelides, telangiectases, and sagging skin being prominent. At times the number and confluence of AKs is so great that the patient appears to have a rash.

In addition to the typical erythematous AK, there are several other clinical subtypes. The hypertrophic AK (HAK) presents as a thicker, scaly, skin-colored, gray or erythematous, rough papule or plaque

(Fig. 79-3). It can be found on any chronically sun-exposed site on the body, but has a propensity for the dorsal hands and arms. A typical erythematous AK can progress into a HAK. At times, it is difficult to clinically distinguish a HAK from a SCC and a biopsy is necessary.

Cutaneous horn, also known as cornu cutaneum, refers to a reaction pattern and not a particular lesion (Fig. 79-4). In reference to AKs, a cutaneous horn is a type of HAK that presents with a conical hypertrophic protuberance emanating from a skin-colored to erythematous papular base. In classic definitions of a cutaneous horn, the height is at least one-half of its largest diameter. Thirty-eight to 40 percent of all cutaneous horns represent AKs.[23] In fact, on examination of biopsy specimens, the base of a cutaneous horn can be a number of different lesions, such as AK, SCC, seborrheic keratosis, filiform verruca vulgaris, trichilemmoma, keratoacanthoma, or BCC. The most common underlying lesion in elderly, fair-skinned persons is a HAK.

Actinic cheilitis represents confluent AKs on the lips, most often the lower lip (Fig. 79-5). Persons with this condition present with red, scaly, chapped lips, and at times erosions or fissures may be present. The vermilion border of the lip is often indistinct, and focal hyperkeratosis and leukoplakia may also be seen. Individuals with this condition often complain of persistent dryness and cracking of the lips, and the diagnosis of actinic cheilitis should always be suspected in elderly patients with such complaints. Persistent ulcerations or indurated areas on the lip require biopsy to ensure that SCC is not present.

Unusual variants of AK include the pigmented AK, spreading pigmented AK, proliferative AK, and conjunctival AK. The pigmented AK presents as a flat, tan to brown-colored, scaly papule. Clinically, it is difficult to distinguish from a solar lentigo. Spreading pigmented AK is a particular lesion that is often found on the face or scalp. It is typically a large lesion, often reaching greater than 1 cm in diameter, and presents as scaly, verrucous or smooth plaque with variable colors. Proliferative AK is seen as an expanding, red, oval, scaly plaque that often reaches a up to 4 cm in diameter. It has poorly defined borders. Conjunctival AK is classified as a type of pinguecula or pterygium. It appears as a wedge-shaped, opaque thickening near the limbus, and it may extend onto the cornea from the scleral conjunctiva.

FIGURE 79-1

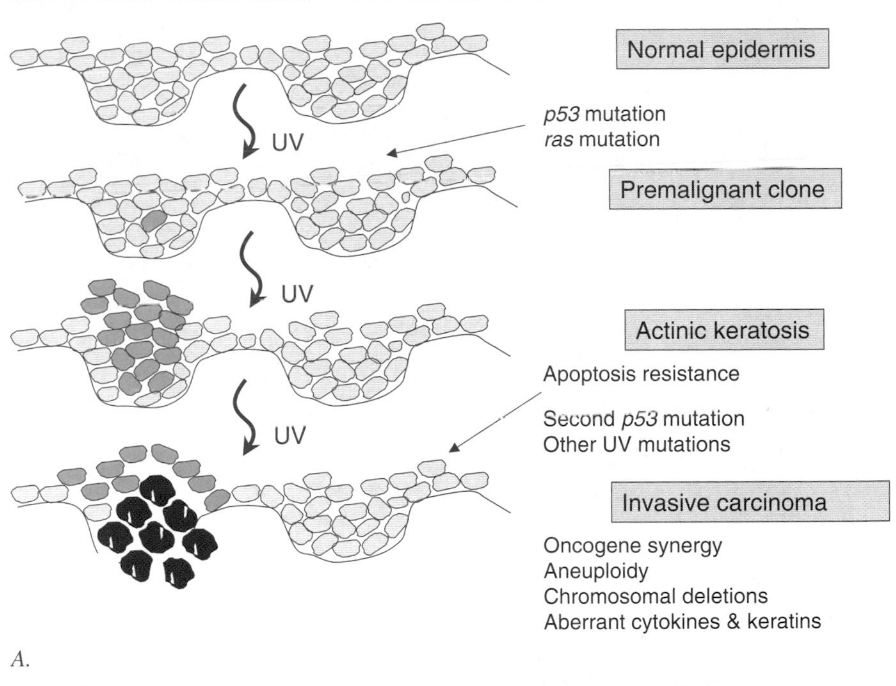

A.

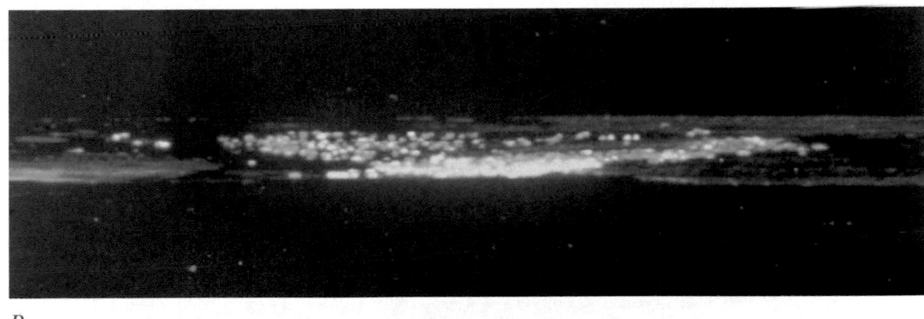

B.

A. Diagram demonstrating the development of clonal expansion of ultraviolet-mutated p53 gene in epithelium. In the multistage model of carcinogenesis, UV-induced mutations provide selective growth advantage of neighboring cells leading to clonal expansion. *(Adapted from Grossman D, Leffell DJ: The molecular basis of nonmelanoma skin cancer. Arch Dermatol 133:1263, 1997). B.* Confocal microscopy revealing expansion of UV-induced clone of abnormal keratinocytes in sun-damaged skin. (*Courtesy Jonason et al: Frequent clones of p53-mutated keratinocytes in normal human skin. Proc Natl Acad Sci USA 93:1402, 1996*)

Pathology

The typical erythematous AK has characteristic architectural and cytologic histopathologic features. All of the abnormalities are confined to the epidermis, although dermal solar elastosis is usually present and an inflammatory dermal infiltrate may also be seen. The classic histopathologic findings include foci of atypical, pleomorphic keratinocytes in the basal cell layer, protruding as buds into the papillary dermis. The basal cell layer appears more basophilic because of the crowding of the atypical keratinocytes. Overlying these foci of abnormal cells one sees irregular acanthosis, hyperkeratosis, and parakeratosis. There is notable sparing of the adnexal epithelium, with orthokeratosis overlying these structures, thus giving rise to the characteristic pattern of alternating orthokeratosis and parakeratosis. Cytologically, there is an increased nuclear to cytoplasmic ratio in the atypical keratinocytes.

Just as there are clinical variants of AKs, there are histopathologic variants as well. These histopathologic variants all share the classic features of the AK as described above, but with some additional findings. In HAK, the hypertrophic areas consist of solid hyperkeratosis and parakeratosis. Cutaneous horns that represent AKs demonstrate similar but more exaggerated changes than the HAK with massive tiers of hyperkeratosis and parakeratosis. The base of such a cutaneous horn shows the typical histopathologic changes of an AK. An atrophic AK has very mild hyperkeratosis and a thinned epidermis that is devoid of rete ridges. Bowenoid AK is a histopathologic variant that demonstrates full epidermal dysplasia, but unlike true Bowen's disease or SCC in situ, there is no involvement of the adnexal

FIGURE 79-2

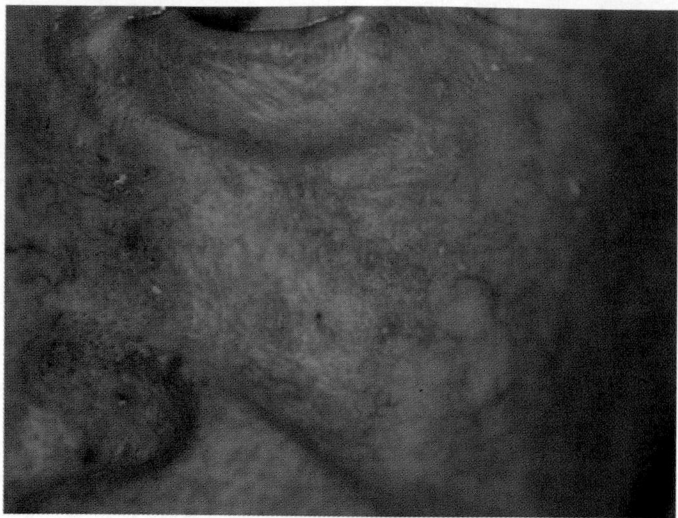

Severe solar damage of the face revealing telangiectasias as well as actinic keratoses at different stages in development, including the flat, pink macules and hyperkeratotic papules.

epithelium. In proliferative AK there is exaggerated proliferation of the budlike downgrowths of atypical keratinocytes into the papillary dermis. Although difficult to distinguish from SCC at times, these proliferative budlike downgrowths are contiguous with the epidermis in the proliferative AK, unlike in true SCC.

FIGURE 79-3

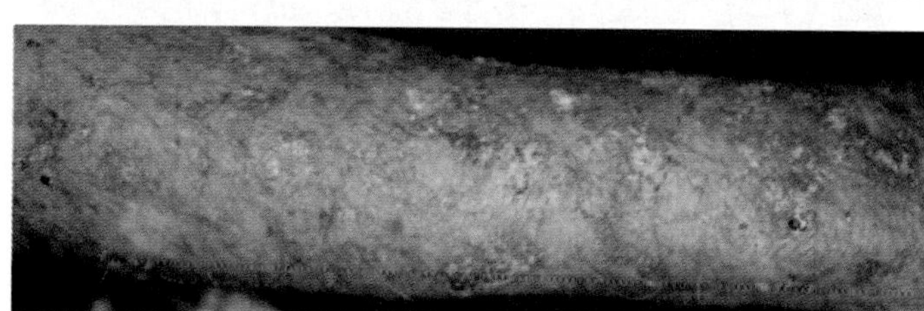

A.

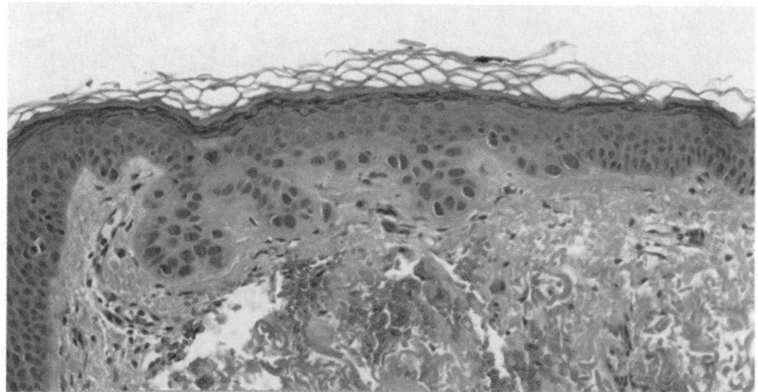

B.

A. Severe solar damage of the dorsal arm demonstrating hypertrophic actinic keratoses and AKs. *B.* Histopathology of actinic keratoses demonstrates atypical cells along basal layer with sparing of adnexal epithelium.

FIGURE 79-4

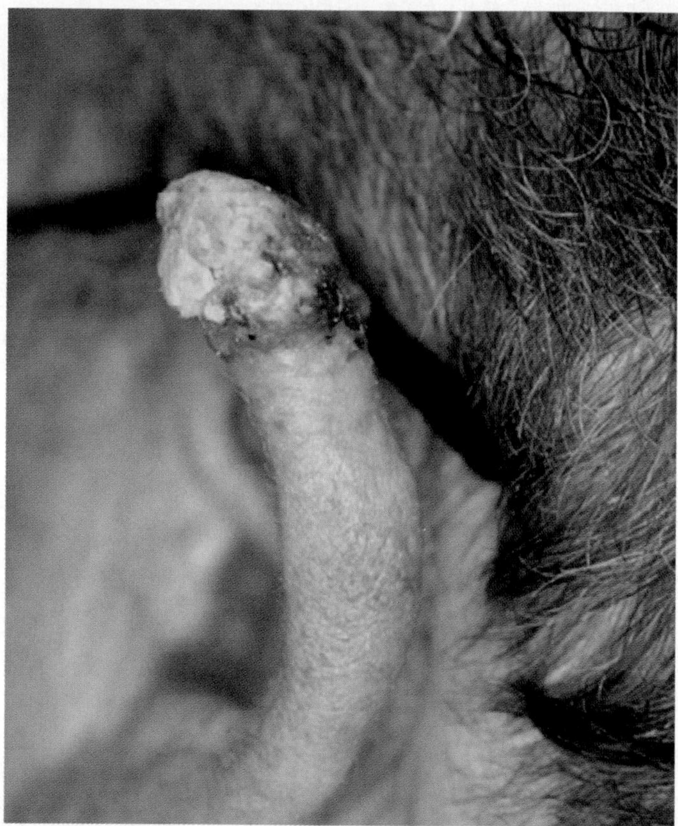

A.

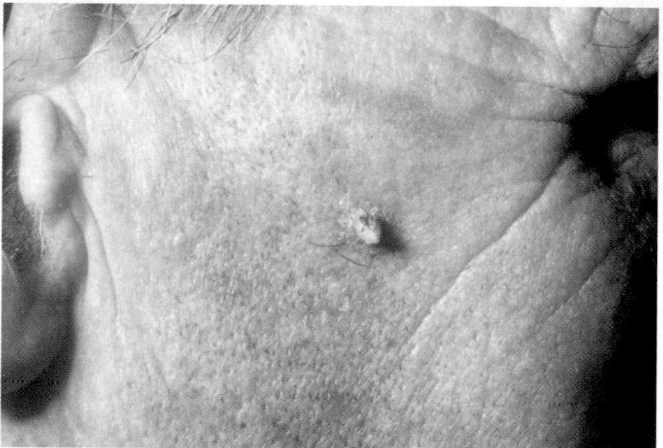

B.

A. Cutaneous horn of the ear. Only biopsy will confirm whether this is an actinic keratosis or a squamous cell carcinoma. *B.* Cutaneous horn of the cheek.

In the pigmented AK one sees excessive amounts of melanin, especially in the basal cell layer. In the spreading pigmented AK variant, in addition to the typical AK histopathologic findings, one may see increased melanin in melanocytes and in the atypical keratinocytes. Lichenoid AKs are characterized by a dense, bandlike lymphohistiocytic infiltrate at the dermal–epidermal junction with basal cell liquefactive degeneration and occasional Civatte bodies. In the acantholytic AK variant there are clefts of lacunae directly above the atypical keratinocytes, reminiscent of the changes seen in Darier's disease. The acantholysis in an acantholytic AK is a result of the anaplastic changes occurring in the lower epidermis. Separation of cells and acantholytic

FIGURE 79-5

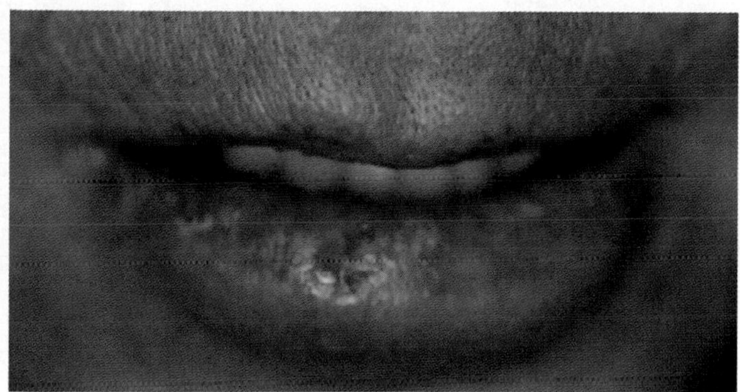

Actinic cheilitis of the lower lip in a young man with a marine occupation. The patient is at risk for developing SCC of the lip. Preventative treatment of the actinic cheilitis can include laser, cryosurgery, and topical treatment.

cells within the clefts are also seen. The clear cell variant of AK results from an excess of cytoplasmic glycogen, resulting histopathologically in marked vacuolation of the epidermis.

Two different histopathologic reaction patterns may be seen in AKs, namely epidermolytic hyperkeratosis (EHK) and the pattern known as intraepidermal epithelioma of Borst-Jadassohn. In an otherwise classic histopathologic AK, one may find incidental changes consistent with EHK. The findings of EHK in these AKs most commonly are focal and isolated and have no clinical importance. Some authors consider the intraepidermal epithelioma of Borst-Jadassohn to be a specific lesion,[24] but other authors[25] believe this entity actually represents a type of reaction pattern found in a variety of lesions, such as AK, Bowen's disease, clonal seborrheic keratosis, intraepidermal malignant eccrine poroma, mammary and extramammary Paget's disease, intraepidermal junctional nevus, and malignant melanoma in situ. The pattern so-named is that of an intraepidermal neoplasm characterized by nests of different types of typical or atypical cells.

An important point to remember about making the diagnosis of AK histopathologically is that if the physician has a strong clinical suspicion of SCC or BCC and the initial cuts reveal AK, it is prudent to section more deeply into the block of tissue to ensure that an SCC or BCC is not missed. A recent study found that additional diagnostic findings were present on step sections in 23 of 69 specimens (33 percent) initially diagnosed histopathologically as AK. Of these additional findings, 13 percent were that of Bowen's disease, 4 percent basal cell carcinoma, and 3 percent invasive SCC. Three variables that correlated with the discovery of malignancy on step sections were ulceration on the first level, a clinical diagnosis of skin cancer, and a history of skin cancer confirmed previously by biopsy examination.[26]

Diagnosis and Differential Diagnosis

The diagnosis of AK is accurately made by clinical examination in most instances when the examiner is familiar and skilled in making such diagnoses. In practice, very few AKs are histopathologically confirmed, hence little data exist on the accuracy of clinical diagnosis. In a clinical referral setting, accurate clinical diagnosis is greater than that found in the general community setting. One study from a referral setting revealed a diagnostic accuracy of 94 percent, based on the correct histopathologic diagnosis of 34 of 36 clinically suspect, typical AKs.[27] Two studies out of community-based settings reported a diagnostic accuracy of only 80 percent when random clinically diagnosed AKs were confirmed histopathologically.[12,20]

The clinical features of typical erythematous AKs are not unique to these lesions. The differential diagnosis includes other common lesions, such as benign lichenoid keratosis, seborrheic and irritated seborrheic keratoses, verruca vulgaris, Bowen's disease, SCC, keratoacanthoma, basal cell carcinoma, porokeratosis, discoid lupus erythematosus, large cell acanthoma, psoriasis, and other variants of cheilitis. Of the clinical AK variants, pigmented AKs are difficult to distinguish from solar lentigos, spreading pigmented AKs from lentigo maligna or a large seborrheic keratosis, HAK from SCC, and cutaneous horns from the many entities they may represent.

Clinically, the greatest dilemma is in trying to distinguish an AK from a SCC, as the latter portends a more serious prognosis and requires different treatment from an AK. There are no reliable criteria for distinguishing between the two entities, but findings of induration, larger size, ulceration, bleeding, rapid growth, and recurrence or persistence after treatment should make the diagnosis of SCC more suspect.

Histopathologically, actinic keratoses can be confused with benign lichenoid keratoses, as both can show vacuolar alteration of the basal cell layer. Closer inspection, however, reveals that in benign lichenoid keratoses there is no cellular atypia of the keratinocytes as seen in AKs. An atrophic AK can be mistaken for cutaneous lupus erythematosus, as both can demonstrate epidermal thinning and basal cell liquefaction. In cutaneous lupus, however, other classic features of the disease should also be present, such as follicular plugging and a patchy periappendageal infiltrate. Lastly, a pigmented AK may be confused histopathologically with lentigo maligna, but the latter usually has more flattening of the epidermis, an increased number of melanocytes, atypical melanocytes, and normal keratinocytes.

Prognosis and Treatment

In discussing the prognosis of AKs, there are basically three outcomes to consider. An AK can persist, regress, or undergo malignant transformation to invasive SCC. Which path any given AK may take is impossible to predict. The relative risk of progression to SCC depends upon factors related to the AK itself, in addition to individual patient characteristics, such as immune status. Several studies have attempted to determine the risk for the progression of AKs to SCC, but most of them are inadequate in one respect or another. The range of risk for progression of AK to SCC in the literature varies from <1 percent[28] up to 20 percent.[29] The problems with these studies are that they did not predict the malignant transformation risk for an individual AK, the follow-up periods were relatively short, patients were younger than the average person with SCC, and the initial diagnoses of AK were made clinically rather than being confirmed histopathologically.

Another way to approach this question of malignant transformation risk is to look at the percentage of SCCs that arise from preexisting AKs. One such study estimated that 60 percent of SCCs arose from a previous AK,[28] while others have found that in 100 percent of histopathologically confirmed SCCs, an AK was found at the periphery or within the confines of the existing SCC.[30] In terms of which AKs will spontaneously regress, clinical prediction is again impossible for an individual lesion. One study found that up to 25 percent of AKs remitted over a 1-year period, especially if sun exposure was limited during that time.[15] Another study found that more AKs regressed in individuals who routinely wore sunscreen.[20]

In addition to these three basic outcomes for an individual lesion, AKs are also sensitive clinical markers for predicting the future development of NMSC in a given person. The presence of AKs on an individual serves as a marker for chronic sun damage and identifies a high-risk group of people who are at risk for developing SCC, BCC, and, to a lesser extent, melanoma.

The estimate of metastases arising from actinically derived SCC has ranged from 1 to 2 percent up to 6 percent. The risk of metastases is much higher in actinically derived SCC of the lip, perhaps up to 20 percent.[31]

The inability to predict which AK will persist, regress, or become malignant makes treatment of these lesions equally confusing. Although some clinicians have argued that because of the low malignant transformation risk, treatment of AKs is unnecessary, most dermatologists now advocate the treatment of these lesions to avoid any chance of progression to invasive SCC.[32]

There are many available treatments that are extremely effective in eliminating AKs; in fact, cure rates of greater than 90 percent are not uncommon with many of these treatments. Which treatment a physician chooses depends on individual patient characteristics as well as size, location, and number of AKs present.

The most common treatment method for AKs in the United States is cryosurgery, with liquid nitrogen (–195.8°C [–320.4°F]) being the most common cryogen (see Chap. 278). When liquid nitrogen is applied to the affected skin, the temperature of the treated area is lowered to approximately –50°C (–58°F) and the atypical keratinocytes of the AK are destroyed. Liquid nitrogen can be applied in several ways, most commonly via cotton tip application or by using a spray device. Cure rates of up to 98.8 percent have been reported when employing liquid nitrogen cryosurgery for the treatment of AKs.

Curettage, with or without electrosurgery, is another commonly used treatment for AKs. This approach and cryosurgery, account for roughly 80 percent of all treatments for AKs in the United States.[33] A curette is used to mechanically scrape away the atypical keratinocytes of the AK. Electrosurgery may or may not be employed to further destroy atypical cells and to provide hemostasis. Minimal use of cautery enhances the final cosmetic result and optimizes healing. A local anesthetic is needed for this procedure, and other hemostatic agents, such as aluminum chloride and ferric subsulfate, can be used to stop the bleeding if electrosurgery is not used. Patients can expect some discomfort with injection of the local anesthetic, and the treated area will take a few weeks to completely heal. Typically, the patient will have to care for the treated lesion at home by keeping it clean and covered with a small bandage and antibiotic ointment. This technique is ideal for patients with relatively few AK lesions. It is also beneficial for treatment of lesions after biopsy and for the treatment of hypertrophic AKs. Potential side effects include infection, scarring, and dyspigmentation.

Another frequently employed treatment for AKs is the use of the topical chemotherapy agent 5-fluorouracil (5-FU) (see Chap. 249). Its use has been estimated at 3.6 percent of office visits for AKs.[33] This agent blocks the methylation reaction of deoxyuridylic acid to thymidylic acid, and thus interferes with the synthesis of DNA and RNA.[34] Although many different treatment regimens have been used with topical 5-FU, the standard, FDA-approved method consists of twice-daily application of 5-FU to the entire affected region, typically for 2 to 4 weeks. Spot treatment of specific lesions is not recommended. There is also some evidence that concurrent or pretreatment with topical tretinoin for AKs on the forearms and dorsal hands is more effective than topical 5-FU alone in these areas. Treatment should be continued until the treated area demonstrates erythema, erosion, crusting, and necrosis, according to the treatment guidelines. Different strengths (1%, 2%, 5%) and vehicles (gel or cream base) for topical 5-FU are available, and the choice of which one to use depends on physician preference, individual patient characteristics, and the number and location of AKs being treated.

Physicians who prescribe topical 5-FU should spend time with the patient educating him or her about the proper application and the expected outcomes. Written handouts with similar information are also quite helpful for the patient to take home. Patients should expect discomfort, pruritus, and burning at the sites of application, as well as erythema, erosion, crusting, and ulceration (Fig. 79-6). These and other adverse reactions to 5-FU are discussed in Chap. 249. Regions of the skin that seemingly had no visible evidence of AKs may also become quite inflamed during treatment, as the 5-FU is uncovering incipient AKs in these treated areas. If such outcomes are achieved with good patient compliance, cure rates of greater than 90 percent can be expected. Much lower cure rates are seen when patient compliance is poor and the expected end points are not reached. Thus, topical 5-FU therapy is best reserved for those patients who can tolerate the normal, expected effects of the medication. It is ideal for compliant patients who have numerous AKs in a given region of the body, such as the face or arms. It is not very effective for treating hypertrophic AKs. Recurrence of AKs following treatment with 5-FU is commonly reported in the literature, with recurrence rates of 25 to 75 percent being seen with follow-up periods extending beyond 12 months.

FIGURE 79-6

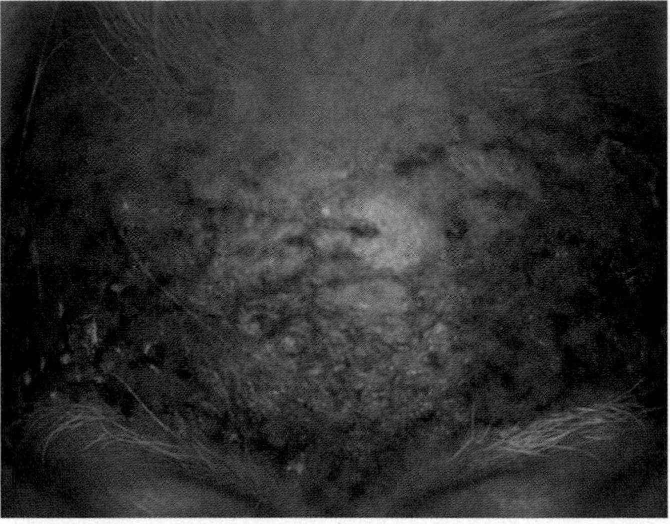

A.

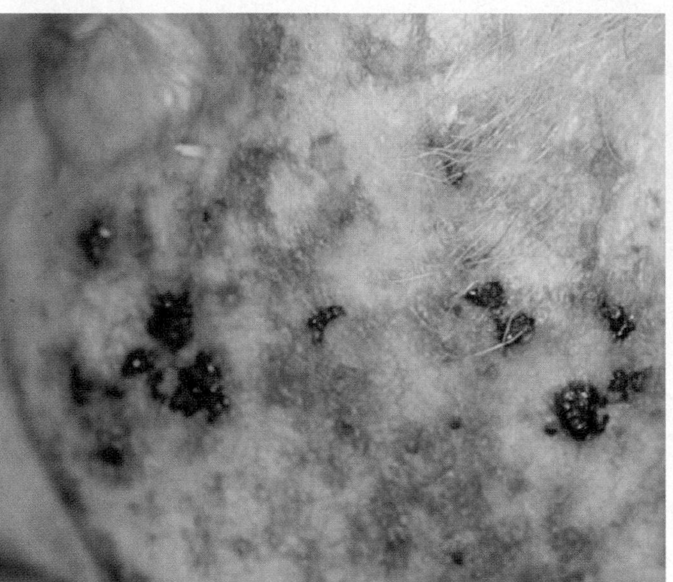

B.

A. Erythema and crusting secondary to treatment with 5-fluorouracil *B.* Superficial hemorrhage in patient on Coumadin who was treated with 5-FU.

Less-common treatments for AKs include dermabrasion, chemical peels, cryopeels, laser therapy, and photodynamic therapy (PDT). These techniques are also highly effective in curing AKs when performed by skilled clinicians. Dermabrasion is an older technique that is quite effective in the treatment and prophylaxis of AKs. It is not a widely used modality because it is more difficult to learn than other, previously discussed alternative treatments. There also is the risk of exposure to blood splatter for the practitioner. Local anesthetics are necessary and the healing time can be prolonged (several weeks) if large areas are treated. Persistent erythema, activation of herpes simplex infection, scarring, dyspigmentation, and bacterial infection are potential side effects. It is ideal for patients with severe photodamage and multiple AKs, who frequently require repeated treatments of their AKs.

Medium-depth chemical peels with Jessner's solution and 35% trichloroacetic acid have reported efficacy rates of 75 percent at 1-month follow-up in one study, with equal efficacy to topical 5-FU therapy at 12-month and 32-month follow-ups.[35,36] Such medium-depth chemical peels typically require a one-time application with minimal discomfort for the patient. Local anesthetics are not routinely administered prior to the peel. Patients can expect erythema and mild desquamation lasting up 1 to 2 weeks following the procedure. Prolonged erythema and activation of herpes simplex infection are potential side effects, and scarring and infection are rare in the hands of skilled clinicians. This treatment modality is ideal for patients with diffuse solar damage and numerous AKs, but it is not effective for treating hypertrophic AKs. As with treatment with 5-FU, recurrence of AKs 1 or more years following treatment is common, with efficacy rates of 25 percent (1-year follow-up)[35] and 75 percent (3-year follow-up).[36]

Cryopeeling consists of extensive liquid nitrogen cryosurgery to the areas of discrete AKs as well as to the surrounding normal-appearing skin. Like dermabrasion, chemical peels, laser, and PDT, it requires further training to master the technique, but once mastered is quite easy to perform. Cryopeeling is a one-time application procedure, in which patients experience mild discomfort and burning. Topical and local anesthetics are often used. Postprocedure erythema, swelling, blistering, and peeling can be expected, and at-home care of the skin with daily cleanings and the application of topical petrolatum is necessary for 1 to 2 weeks. Efficacy has been reported to be equal to or slightly better than 5-FU for extensive AKs.

This procedure is ideal for patients with widespread actinic damage and for diffuse actinic cheilitis.

Laser therapy for the treatment and prophylaxis of AKs is a recently explored option. The carbon dioxide (CO_2) laser in preliminary, small series studies has been reported to be effective in clearing multiple facial AKs, with no recurrence reported at 6 to 24 months in one study.[37] Operation of the CO_2 laser requires training and experience for adequate results with minimal complications. It requires local or general anesthesia and sedation and the recovery time is longer than the other treatment modalities previously discussed. Persistent erythema is a common problem, often lasting up to 3 months following the procedure. Dyspigmentation, scarring, and infection are also potential complications. A pilot study[38] evaluated the erbium:YAG laser for the treatment of diffuse AKs in five patients, noting that clearance rates of 86 to 96 percent were found at 3 months' follow-up. In general, laser therapy is best reserved for patients with diffuse AKs and for the treatment of actinic cheilitis. Thicker lesions can also be treated with CO_2 laser because of its ability to make several, deeper passes in the skin.

PDT of AKs is another treatment modality that is gaining popularity in the treatment of AKs. Topical PDT was approved by the FDA in 1999. With PDT, topical 5-aminolevulinic acid (5-ALA) is applied directly to targeted AKs on the skin. It accumulates preferentially in the more rapidly proliferating, dysplastic cells and is converted to the photosensitizer, protoporphyrin IX (PP IX) via enzymes involved in the heme biosynthetic pathway. When the 5-ALA treated skin is then exposed to a light source that includes the absorption spectrum of PP IX (400 to 730 nm), PP IX is photoactivated with the resultant generation of reactive oxygen intermediates, which leads to the destruction of the cells. Both laser and nonlaser light sources have been used in studies of PDT for the treatment of AKs. Cure rates of 88 percent have been reported after a single cycle of PDT using a nonlaser blue light source,[39] and cure rates equivalent to 3 weeks of topical 5-FU have also been reported.[40] This technique requires a one- or two-time application of the topical 5-ALA followed by exposure to the light source several hours later. Patients experience some discomfort, including burning and stinging of the treated areas, primarily during exposure to the light source. This discomfort is tolerable and dissipates completely within 72 h, in most cases. Precise indications for PDT in the treatment of AKs have not been established, and longer-term follow-up studies with this therapy are lacking. Nonetheless, it may prove to be a viable treatment option in patients with multiple, non-HAKs who cannot tolerate or be compliant with topical 5-FU.

Uncommon treatments for AKs include excision, interferon, topical immune response modifiers, oral and topical retinoids, α-hydroxy acids, and salicylic acid. Excision can be completely curative, but such a procedure involving full-thickness excision is rarely needed and may be considered therapeutically excessive. Interferon is also highly effective, but costly. Topical immune response modifiers, such as imiquimod, were recently investigated as potential treatment options for AKs.[41] Topical retinoids, α-hydroxy acids, and salicylic acid are questionably effective as sole modalities for the treatment of AKs, but agents such as topical tretinoin have been advocated as adjuncts to other treatment approaches and as prophylaxis against the recurrence of AKs following treatment. Topical masoprocol is rarely used because of concerns about sensitization.

ARSENICAL KERATOSES

Arsenical keratoses (ArKs) are precancerous lesions found in association with chronic arsenicism. These lesions have the potential to develop into invasive SCC. Arsenic is a ubiquitous element that has no color, taste, or odor. It has the potential to cause characteristic acute and chronic syndromes in persons exposed to it, and such exposures are typically obscure because of medicinal, occupational, and environmental sources. Detecting acute and chronic arsenicism is important, because the acute form can be fatal and the chronic form is associated with a variety of cutaneous and internal malignancies. ArKs are associated with chronic arsenicism.

History and Epidemiology

The medicinal benefits and poisoning potential of arsenic date back to ancient times. Arsenic was introduced into the United States Pharmacopoeia in 1850 and, prior to its discontinuation around 1965, it was used medicinally in the United States and Europe in the form of Fowler's solution, Donovan's solution, and Asiatic pills for various illnesses such as psoriasis, asthma, and syphilis. Medicinal exposure is now basically limited to the treatment of tropical diseases, such as African trypanosomiasis. Arsenic in opium has been and is still used for medicinal and pleasure purposes in India, and inorganic arsenic is still found in some traditional Chinese herbal preparations.[42]

Arsenic exposure can occur in a variety of occupations, either by direct exposure to arsenic or through indirect exposure via contaminated water and landfills. In 1973, it was estimated that more than 1.5 million workers in the United States were potentially exposed to arsenic in the workplace.[43] Occupations that are at risk for exposure include the mining, smelting, agricultural, computer microchip, forestry, electroplating, semiconductor, and glassmaking industries. Environmental exposure is often obscure and insidious, as latent periods of up to 50 years may occur before manifestations of chronic arsenicism appear. Arsenic is routinely found in soil, and it is found in much higher levels in the well water of certain regions where smelting and mining activities predominate, such as Taiwan, Sweden, and Argentina.[42] Other routes of environmental exposure include some illegally produced alcoholic beverages and the burning of pressure-treated lumber that has been pretreated with chromium-copper-arsenate. In all forms of medicinal, occupational, and environmental exposures, longer duration of exposure and higher cumulative doses are associated with a higher risk for the development of ArKs.

The association between arsenic exposure and skin cancer was first noted by Paris in 1822.[44] Arsenical keratoses were first described on the palms and soles of individuals in the late 1800s. In 1898, Dubreuilh categorized ArKs as precancerous lesions.[5] The relationship of arsenic ingestion to palmar and plantar ArKs and to skin cancer has been documented in several studies that involved wide-scale exposure to known sources of arsenic.[15] In particular, chronic arsenicism and an increased risk of skin cancer has been attributed to drinking water that contains greater than 0.6 mg of arsenic per liter.[43] The United States Environmental Protection Agency has set a maximum arsenic contaminant level at 50 μg/L.[45] Ingestion of as little as 400 mL of Fowler's solution is associated with signs of chronic arsenicism.[42] A compilation of the results of 12 reports that linked malignancy with the ingestion of inorganic arsenic found that skin cancer occurred in 70 percent and an internal malignancy in 6.3 percent of ingesters.[46]

Etiology and Pathogenesis

Arsenic is present as either organic or inorganic compounds as well as in three potential oxidative states: metalloid, trivalent, or tetravalent. Trivalent arsenicals are the most common and hazardous to humans. The toxicity of these compounds depends on the accumulation of arsenic in target tissues and its metabolism and elimination. Organic arsenicals are excreted rapidly and trivalent inorganic arsenicals are the most acutely and chemically toxic compounds. Because arsenic is metabolized and detoxified in the liver via methylation, those patients with preexisting liver disease may be at greater risk for arsenic-related toxicity.

The mechanisms of arsenic-induced ArKs and malignancy are not fully understood. Arsenic reacts with the sulfhydryl groups in certain tissue proteins and subsequently affects many different enzymes that are essential to cellular metabolism. Arsenic has been found to cause chromosomal mutations, chromosomal breaks, sister chromatid exchanges, and mutations in *p53*.[47,48]

Clinical Manifestations

Arsenical keratoses typically begin as pinpoint papules that are easier felt than seen. They develop into small, 2 to 10 mm, punctate, yellow, keratotic papules most commonly seen on the palms and soles in areas of constant pressure or repeated trauma (Fig. 79-7). They preferentially arise on the thenar and lateral borders of the hands, the sides of fingers, and sometimes on the dorsal aspects of the fingers, overlying the joints. Although unusual, ArKs can be found on more widespread body areas such as the trunk, extremities, eyelids, and genitalia. ArKs may also present as slightly elevated, erythematous, scaly or pigmented plaques. ArKs on the palms and soles are more likely to be seen in individuals with chronic arsenicism caused by medicinal exposure, in comparison to occupational exposure. Also, individuals with arsenical-related

FIGURE 79-7

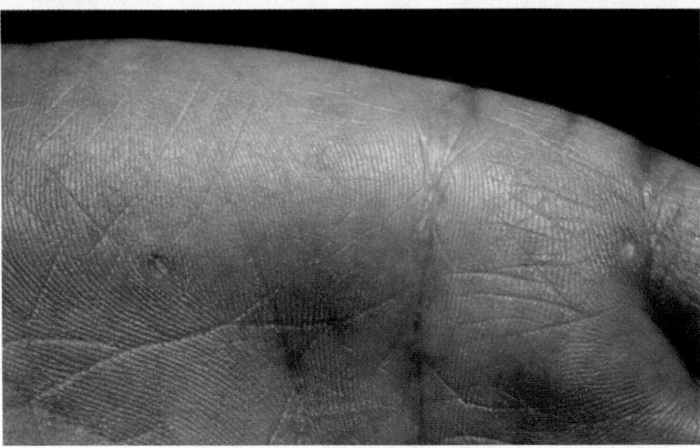

A.

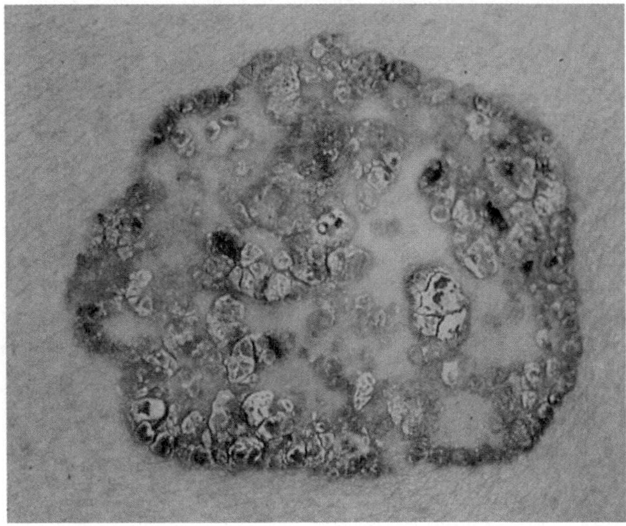

B.

A. Arsenical keratoses of the palm. (*Courtesy of James E. Fitzpatrick, MD, University of Colorado, Deptartment of Dermatology.*) *B.* Arsenical in situ squamous cell carcinoma.

cancer are more likely to have palmar and plantar ArKs. The mean latency periods for ArKs varies considerably from 9 to 30 years.[49]

Other cutaneous neoplasms associated with chronic arsenicism include Bowen's disease, BCC, and SCC. Mean latency periods for the development of Bowen's disease and SCC can also be as long as 40 years.[49] With arsenic as the carcinogen rather than ultraviolet radiation, these neoplasms, like the ArKs, are distributed in a more widespread, random, and nonphotodamaged distribution. Arsenical Bowen's disease often begins as a small flesh- to pink-colored papule with a thick horny layer or crust. When this crust is removed, the underlying skin appears erythematous and oozing. Over time, unlike the relatively stable ArKs, these lesions increase in size, forming nodular and plaquelike lesions that often group together. Approximately one-third of patients have multiple lesions of Bowen's disease.[42]

Arsenic-induced BCCs are also usually multiple and the majority are of the superficial type, although small nodular BCC are sometimes seen. These BCCs are found in a random, scattered distribution, primarily on the trunk and in hair-bearing regions. Clinically, the superficial BCCs are often indistinguishable from Bowen's disease. Arsenic-related SCC can arise de novo or from malignant transformation of ArKs and Bowen's disease. In one study, 55 percent of SCCs arose from preexisting ArKs or Bowen's disease.[49] Patients with SCC are more likely to have been exposed to arsenic later in life as compared to those without SCC.[49] They also are more likely to have multiple lesions of Bowen's disease and more numerous palmar and plantar ArKs. The majority of SCCs have been found on the distal extremities of the hands and feet, and it has been hypothesized that irritation and trauma in these areas may increase the risk of malignant transformation. Clinically, ArKs that show progression to SCC often present with pain, bleeding, fissuring, and later ulceration. They tend to gradually expand in diameter, forming a large erosion or ulceration, and they sometimes reach sizes up to 20 cm.

Other signs of chronic arsenicism include hyperpigmentation primarily affecting the nipples, axillae, groin, and other pressure points. Within these hyperpigmented patches, one often sees small areas of hypopigmentation, resembling raindrops. Diffuse alopecia of the scalp may be present. Longer term, patients may develop "blackfoot disease," which is a peripheral vascular disease affecting the lower extremities that eventually results in gangrene. Hepatic cirrhosis can also be seen. A variety of internal malignancies have also been associated with chronic arsenicism, with long lag periods of 20 to 50 years reported. The internal malignancies linked with chronic arsenicism include lung, urinary tract, hepatic, hepatic angiosarcoma, leukemia, and lymphoma.

Histopathology

The histopathology of ArKs is essentially the same as for actinic keratoses. No reliable histopathologic criteria can distinguish between the two. Some cases of ArKs are characterized by marked vacuolation of the epithelial cells and keratin horn formation. Also, solar elastosis is usually absent and a chronic dermal lymphocytic infiltrate is commonly seen. Likewise, arsenic-related Bowen's disease, BCC, and SCC are histopathologically similar to their non–arsenic-induced counterparts.

Diagnosis and Differential Diagnosis

Arsenical keratoses may be mistaken for other types of punctate keratoses, such as disseminated punctate keratoderma, Darier's disease, corns, and verruca vulgaris. Disseminated punctate keratoderma usually appears earlier in life. It has also been reported that on removal of the keratinous plugs in punctate keratoderma, small crater-like pits are left behind, whereas no pits are seen on removal of the keratin plugs in ArKs. Darier's disease presents with characteristic lesions elsewhere. Corns are usually not so numerous and not so common on the hands. Warts often demonstrate evidence of thrombosed capillaries on removal of the surface keratin.

A diagnosis of ArKs and chronic arsenicism should be considered when numerous characteristic keratoses are seen on the palms and soles or when multiple lesions of Bowen's disease, SCC, or BCC are found on an individual, especially when these lesions are in non–sun-exposed regions of the body. In most patients with such neoplasms, palmar and plantar keratoses will also be present. Such patients should be questioned about previous occupations, living conditions, environmental, and medicinal exposures to elicit a history of potential arsenic exposure anywhere from 10 to 40 years previously. One should biopsy any changing ArK or erythematous nodule or plaque on the body to ensure that Bowen's disease, BCC, or progression to SCC are not present.

Prognosis and Treatment

Arsenical keratoses and arsenical-induced Bowen's disease tend to persist for many years, and the chance of progression into invasive SCC is believed to be relatively rare. Invasive SCC that arises in ArK, however, is more locally aggressive and has a greater chance of metastases when compared to SCC arising in AK.[42] In lesions of arsenical-induced Bowen's disease, locally invasive SCC has been seen histopathologically in up to 20 percent of cases. Once invasive SCC has occurred in Bowen's disease, it is said that at least one-third will demonstrate evidence of metastases unless adequate treatment is provided.[50]

Management of patients with chronic arsenicism and ArKs should include regularly scheduled total-body skin examinations and general physical examinations, possibly on an every 6-month basis.[49] Because the exact incidence of internal malignancies associated with chronic arsenicism is unknown, there is no standard protocol for the evaluation of potential internal malignancies. Exhaustive evaluations for such malignancies have not been recommended. Biannual detailed history taking and physical examinations, yearly chest radiographs, and selective tests when clinically indicated are probably reasonable recommendations.

Treatment of ArKs likewise is not standard and not mandatory, and treatment of these lesions is sometimes initiated to relieve the associated discomfort hat some patients experience. Available localized treatment options include surgical excision, cryosurgery, electrodesiccation and curettage, CO_2 laser, and topical chemotherapy with 5-FU, although success with 5-FU in treating ArKs is less than the success with AKs.[42] PDT with 5-ALA has also been used to treat these lesions. Oral retinoids may be useful in reducing the hyperkeratosis associated with ArKs.

THERMAL KERATOSES

Thermal keratoses (TKs) are keratotic lesions produced in the skin by exposure to infrared radiation. They have the potential to develop into SCC. Various sources of heat are implicated in causing these lesions and several classic syndromes have been reported. Most notable are the kangri basket cancers in Kashmir, the kang cancers in China, the railway cancers in Britain, and the peat fire cancers in Ireland. The kangri is a pot that contains a type of fuel, such as charcoal, that is held against the thigh or lower abdomen as a source of warmth. In Kashmir, the malignancies arose in the skin over the lower abdomen and thighs, where the baskets were in contact with the body. The skin overlying the greater trochanters is where the cancers developed in the Chinese and Tibetans. Heat was reported to be responsible for cancer of the skin overlying the shins of railway-engine drivers in England. In Ireland, more than 150 women were reported to have lesions of erythema ab igne and SCC on the lower legs. These women all reported many years of sitting close to an open fire of burning peat to stay warm. Because peat is a less-efficient fuel than coal, these women had to sit closer to the source to attain adequate warmth. The men did not experience the same cutaneous effects because they primarily wore thick, longer trousers. In the United States, TKs, Bowen's disease, and the development of SCC have been noted in persons exposed long-term to coal and wood-burning stoves used as sources for heat and cooking.[51] The incidence and prevalence of thermal keratoses is not known. Likewise, the pathogenesis of these lesions is not fully understood and the percentage of TKs that will progress to invasive SCC is also unknown.

Clinical Manifestations

Prolonged exposure to infrared radiation and to sources of heat can clinically produce the characteristic lesion of erythema ab igne that manifests as an erythematous to brownish, fixed, thick, reticulated patch on the skin overlying the area that has been chronically exposed to heat. It differs from livedo reticularis in that it is more brownish in color, usually nonblanchable, and fixed. The sites of predilection are the back and abdomen from exposure to hot water bottles and heating pads or blankets, and the lower legs from exposure to fires or heating units as sources of warmth. After many years of such exposures, thermal keratoses may appear within these patches of erythema ab igne. SCC in situ within such patches has also been reported, and like solar-induced AKs, progression to invasive SCC from TKs can also occur. Clinically, TKs present as hyperkeratotic papules and plaques.

Histopathology

The histopathology of thermal keratoses is similar to that of AKs, including alternating hyperkeratosis and parakeratosis, keratinocyte atypia, sparing of the appendageal units, and interestingly, even dermal elastosis and vascular ectasia. In one study, biopsy specimens from erythema ab igne without apparent TKs showed evidence of keratinocyte atypia.[52] Merkel cell carcinoma has also been reported to arise alongside SCC within a patch of erythema ab igne.

Diagnosis and Differential Diagnosis

Hyperkeratotic papules or plaques that develop within a long-standing patch of erythema ab igne should be biopsied to confirm the diagnosis and to rule-out progression to SCC. Erythema ab igne should be distinguished from acute burn scars, the latter of which may also harbor scar keratoses and SCC. Potentially, erythema ab igne and ulcerated TKs or SCC on the lower extremities could be confused with periarteritis nodosa, which presents most often on the lower extremities with livedo reticularis, nodules, and ulceration.

Prognosis and Treatment

There is a paucity of information in the literature regarding the risk of progression of TK to invasive SCC and the general prognosis of thermal SCC. Similarly, little is written about the treatment of these lesions. Surgical excision, electrodesiccation and curettage, cryosurgery, and possibly laser therapy appear to be reasonable therapeutic options. Patients with erythema ab igne should be counseled about the need to discontinue exposure to whatever heat source they have been in contact with and they should be followed long-term with physical examinations to identify early changes suggestive of TK or SCC.

HYDROCARBON KERATOSES

Hydrocarbon keratoses (HKs), also known as tar keratoses, pitch keratoses, and tar warts, are precancerous keratotic skin lesions that occur primarily in persons who are exposed occupationally to polycyclic aromatic hydrocarbons (PAHs). SCC and keratoacanthomas have also been linked to such exposures. PAHs are produced by the incomplete combustion and distillation of coal, natural gas, and oil shale. They are found in tar, fuel oils, lubricating oils, oil shale, and bitumen.[44] Workers at risk for exposure to such compounds include workers in tar distillation, shale extraction, and workers exposed to creosotes, which are one of the main distillate fractions of coal tars and coal tar pitches.[53] Creosotes are used extensively as wood preservatives. Roofers, asphalt workers, road pavers, and highway maintenance workers are exposed to PAHs from fumes formed during the heating of bitumen.[53] Other groups of workers at risk for exposure to coal tar products include railway workers, brick masons, and diesel engineers.[44] Lastly, persons exposed to mineral oils, cutting oils, and coolants also are at risk for the development of HKs and SCC.[53]

The most infamous occupational exposure to PAHs was that of the chimney sweeps who developed scrotal SCC.[54] Mule spinners have also been reported to develop SCC of the scrotal skin.[44] Mule spinners frequently have their thighs and scrotum in contact with an oil-covered bar on the mule, which is a machine used to spin cotton.

Etiology and Pathogenesis

Hydrocarbon keratoses, SCCs, and keratoacanthomas develop in persons whose skin is exposed to PAHs over long periods of time. The risk of these precancerous and cancerous lesions is associated with dermal exposure to PAHs; inhalation of PAHs is not associated with skin cancers, although lung cancer is noted with such exposures.[53] PAHs are known carcinogens that damage DNA and potentially cause mutations in the *p53* gene, at least in lung cancers.[54] Ultraviolet radiation exposure has been considered a cofactor in the development of HKs and related skin cancers, but a recent study found that the majority of HKs and SCC in a large group of tar refinery workers developed in non–sun-exposed regions of the body, thus questioning this belief.[55] The duration of exposure before the development of HKs ranges from 2.5 to 45 years.[56]

Clinical Manifestations

Hydrocarbon keratoses present as small, oval to round, gray, flat papules that are easily removed without residual bleeding. These papules can then become larger in size, more verrucous in appearance, and eventually may develop into invasive SCC. Sites of predilection include the face, nostril rims, upper lip, forearms, volar wrists, dorsal feet, lower legs, vulva, and scrotum.[55] Of note, the lesions on the nostril rims, upper lip, genitalia, and forearms are not the typical sun-exposed sites of the body. Thus, keratoses or malignancies in these regions should prompt the physician to inquire about potential occupational hazardous exposures. Other cutaneous findings related to PAH skin exposure include patchy hyperpigmentation, acne, and telangiectases in sites of exposure. The presence of acneiform lesions on the forearms and thighs should alert one to the possibility of PAH exposure. Facial features associated with long-term tar exposure include periocular fibromas, brownish or slate-gray discoloration, comedones, and hair follicle plugs.[55]

PAHs have also been reported to cause internal malignancies, such as lung and bladder cancers.[53]

Histopathology

Hydrocarbon keratoses histopathologically appear similar to AKs and ArKs, as previously described. Often, in HKs, there is more of a progression to full-thickness atypia, or a bowenoid form. In early HKs, it has been said that distinction between benign and malignant epidermal changes can be difficult.

Diagnosis and Differential Diagnosis

Hydrocarbon keratoses, with their grayish keratotic appearance, may be mistaken for verruca vulgaris lesions, stucco keratoses, or even ArKs. A high index of suspicion is needed to make the diagnosis of HKs, as histopathologically they are difficult to distinguish from AKs and ArKs. The distribution of the lesions and other cutaneous findings of tar skin can aid in the diagnosis and lead one to further, pointed questioning of the patient. Once a diagnosis of HK has been made, closer examination for SCC or KAs should ensue and a good history and physical examination to detect signs of internal malignancy may be warranted, based on the type of occupational exposure. Examination of the scrotal and vulvar regions is essential.

Prognosis and Treatment

The exact risk of a HK progressing to SCC is unknown. Most recommendations in the literature are for biopsy and surgical removal of HKs, especially on the vulvar and scrotal regions and mucosal surfaces, where the risk of early metastasis from SCC is greater. Cryosurgery and electrodesiccation with curettage are probably reasonable treatment options for HKs on other cutaneous sites. Prevention is the key for workers exposed to PAHs in their occupations. Long-term follow-up of individuals with previous known PAH exposures is essential for early diagnosis and treatment of lesions and for the potential early detection of internal malignancy if at risk.

CHRONIC RADIATION KERATOSES

Chronic radiation keratoses (CRKs) are precancerous keratotic lesions that may arise on the skin many years after exposure to ionizing radiation. They have been described in persons exposed to x-ray therapy, including grenz-ray therapy for benign skin disorders, such as acne vulgaris and tinea capitis; medical personnel, dentists, and physicians who have administered x-rays over many years;[44] other professionals who handle radioactive materials in their workplace; on the fingers of persons who unknowingly wore gold rings contaminated by radioactivity (Fig. 79-8);[57] survivors of the atomic bomb in Japan;[58] and in the unfortunate victims of nuclear accidents such as the one in Chernobyl, Ukraine.[59] For the purpose of the following discussion, radiation refers to ionizing radiation, thus excluding the ultraviolet and infrared spectrums of radiation.

Clinical Manifestations

The primary neoplasms resulting in the skin from ionizing radiation include CRK, BCC, and SCC. Cutaneous sarcomas rarely occur. Chronic radiation keratoses and BCC are more commonly seen than SCC, but any given CRK can potentially evolve into invasive SCC. The site and penetration of the ionizing radiation determine which type of tumor develops, as palms, soles, and mucosal surfaces are said to favor CRK. The neoplasms that develop are often multiple, healing poorly and frequently recurring.[44] CRKs usually develop within areas of chronic radiation dermatitis or in persistent ulcerations arising in such chronically damaged areas of the skin. They appear as hyperkeratotic papules or plaques. The latency period from time of exposure to the development of CRKs and radiation-induced skin cancers is typically long, having been reported to range up to 56 years. The development of these tumors is inversely proportional to the radiation dose. Patients exposed to ionizing radiation are also at risk for the development of other internal malignancies, such as breast, bone, soft tissue, uterus, larynx, pharynx, thyroid, and maxillary sinus.[44]

FIGURE 79-8

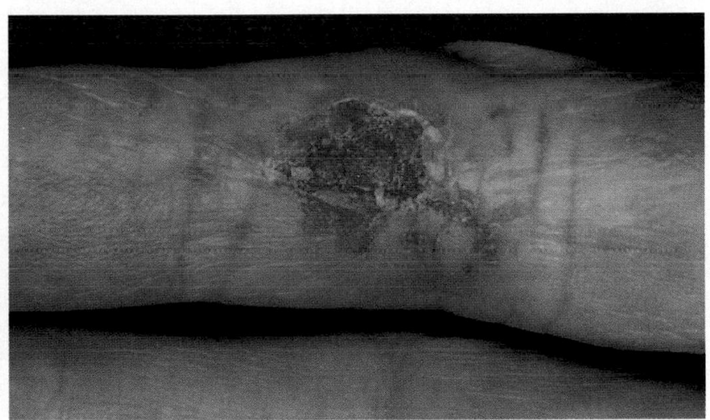

Chronic radiation keratoses on finger of an older dentist.

Pathology

Chronic radiation keratoses histopathologically display keratinocyte dyskeratosis with hyperchromatic nuclei and abnormal mitoses. The dermis often demonstrates findings consistent with chronic radiation changes, such as hyalinization of the collagen bundles, thickening and occlusion of deep dermal blood vessels, and destruction of the pilosebaceous units.

Prognosis and Treatment

The development of CRKs should be taken seriously, as they have the potential to develop into invasive SCC. Once radiation-induced invasive SCC develops, it has the ability to be quite aggressive with a higher potential for metastasis than does actinically induced SCC. The percentage of CRKs that will develop into SCC is unknown. It is recommended that CRKs be removed promptly and that surgical excision is often the recommended treatment of choice. Persons with ionizing radiation exposure should be followed with skin examinations at regular intervals for the rest of their life, as the latency period for the development of cutaneous neoplasms is quite long, and the number of skin cancers in such patients tends to increase with time after irradiation. Evaluation for the development of other high-risk internal malignancies should also be considered in the long-term follow-up of these patients. Lastly, these patients should be counseled regarding the avoidance of other potential carcinogens, such as ultraviolet radiation.

CHRONIC SCAR KERATOSES

Chronic scar keratoses (CSKs), also known as chronic cicatrix keratoses, are precancerous keratotic lesions that arise in long-standing scars. Chronic scar keratoses can arise in a number of different chronic scarring processes, such as chronic ulcers, burn scars, pilonidal sinuses, draining sinuses, chronic osteomyelitis, vaccination scars, chronic hidradenitis suppurativa, old frostbite scars, and scarring acne vulgaris.

History and Epidemiology

In 1828, Jean-Nicholas Marjolin described chronic ulcers that arose from scar tissue, without referring to them as malignant.[60] Today, the term Marjolin's ulcer is synonymous with malignant transformation of chronic ulcers, sinus tracts, and burn scars, although the term is used most frequently to describe malignant changes within burn scars. It is estimated that 2 percent of burn scars will undergo malignant degeneration. Most burn scar carcinomas are SCCs, but cases of BCC, melanoma, sarcoma, and malignant fibrous histiocytoma have also been reported.[61] Two types of Marjolin's ulcer have been described: an acute form and a chronic form. The acute type develops within 1 year from the time of injury, while the chronic form develops more than 1 year after the injury.[62] The average latency period from injury to onset of malignancy for the chronic form is 36 years, with a range of 1 to 75 years.[63] The latency period is inversely proportional to the patient's age at the time of the burn injury.

Etiology and Pathogenesis

The pathogenesis of a premalignant keratosis or a carcinoma arising in a chronic scar is not known. Proposed mechanisms for malignant degeneration within a burn scar include production of a carcinogenic toxin with the burn injury; immunologic privilege within scarred tissue allowing unchecked tumor growth; chronic irritation leading to malignancy; multistep carcinogenesis involving initiation, promotion, and progression; and burn-induced DNA damage leading to malignant transformation. Characteristics of the burn scar that predispose to malignant transformation include a prolonged healing phase, repetitive trauma, and rejected graft site.

Clinical Manifestations

Chronic scar keratoses present as hyperkeratotic papules, plaques, or erosions within the scarred skin. In terms of burn scars, two clinical types of carcinoma have been described. The more common presentation is of a flat, ulcerative, indurated lesion with elevated borders and surrounding induration. The less-common type is the exophytic, papillomatous lesion resembling granulation tissue.[62] Bleeding, pain, and a foul odor may also be present. Typically, chronic and recurrent ulcerations have been present in the burn scar prior to malignant degeneration and the malignancy often develops at an ulcer margin. One important fact about burn scar carcinomas is that usually only a portion of the ulcer undergoes malignant transformation. The remaining ulcer persists as a nonhealing wound, and thus false-negative results from biopsies of the ulcer are quite high.[61] Sites of predilection for burn scar carcinomas are the extremities and in areas overlying joints, presumably because of repeated trauma in these areas.

Pathology and Diagnosis

Histopathologically, most scar keratoses range in pattern from several atypical keratinocytes to full epidermal thickness atypia or in situ SCC. The majority of burn scar carcinomas are of the well-differentiated squamous cell type. Histopathologic diagnosis may be confused with pseudoepitheliomatous hyperplasia, a benign reactionary process. Any persistent lesion, erosion, or ulceration within a scar should be biopsied. In addition, in terms of burn scar carcinomas, because only a portion of the ulcer may be malignant, multiple biopsies or excisional biopsies are recommended if the suspicion of carcinoma is high, so as not to miss the diagnosis.

Prognosis and Treatment

Chronic scar keratoses may show a gradual progression to in situ carcinoma and frank SCC. Prompt diagnosis of these lesions is important because once overt, invasive SCC develops in a scar, it can quickly become aggressive and the risk for metastasis is high. In terms of burn scar carcinoma, the metastatic rate is estimated at approximately 35 percent, much higher than actinically induced SCC.[62] Lesions occurring on the lower extremities have the highest rates of metastases, averaging 50 percent,[64] while those on the head, neck, and upper extremities fare better. Lymph node metastasis on presentation is the single most important prognostic indicator.

Burn scar carcinoma may be prevented by meticulous burn wound care, early skin grafting, prompt treatment of infections, avoiding contractures, and by early excision of any degenerative changes within the scarred area. Large full-thickness burns are also probably best managed surgically, and not allowed to heal by secondary intention. Treatment of chronic scar keratoses should include prompt destruction of the lesion or excision of the entire area, with step sections through the specimen to ensure a malignancy has not been missed. Excision with wide margins (at least 2 cm) is the treatment of choice for burn scar carcinoma.[62,64] Initial skin grafting is preferred over the use of a skin flap to cover the wound defect. If the latter is to be used, a waiting period of 12 months is recommended so as not to obscure the possibility of a recurrence.[64] Radiation therapy and topical chemotherapy have not been beneficial in the treatment of these lesions.[52,64]

REACTIONAL KERATOSES

Reactional keratoses (RKs) are premalignant keratotic lesions that may arise in a variety of long-standing, nonscarring, inflammatory processes such as cutaneous lupus erythematosus, necrobiosis lipoidica, porokeratosis, erythema elevatum diutinum, granuloma inguinale, epidermolysis bullosa variants, pemphigus vulgaris, lichen sclerosis, lichen planus, and chronic deep fungal infections. Clinically, RKs present as hyperkeratotic papules or plaques. As with other precancerous keratotic lesions, a continuum from RK to SCC in situ to invasive SCC may be seen. Once invasive SCC has developed, there is a significant risk of metastatic disease developing, similar to that of scar keratoses. The main diagnosis to consider in the clinical and histologic differential is pseudoepitheliomatous hyperplasia.

PUVA KERATOSES

PUVA keratoses are precancerous keratotic lesions that arise in individuals exposed to psoralen plus ultraviolet A (UVA) light therapy for the treatment of a variety of cutaneous conditions. Although UVA on its own does not appear to be significantly mutagenic to humans, the combination of UVA with psoralen is associated with a dose-dependent increased risk of premalignant keratoses and other cutaneous malignancies, such as SCC, melanoma, and possibly Merkel cell carcinoma (see Chap. 265).

VIRAL KERATOSES

Viral keratoses, otherwise known as warts, are one of the most common keratotic lesions in humans. These lesions are caused by infection with the human papillomavirus (HPV).

Bowenoid Papulosis

Bowenoid papulosis is characterized clinically by the presence of pigmented verrucous papules and plaques primarily on the genitalia of predisposed individuals, and histopathologically by the presence of SCC in situ–like changes (Fig. 79-9). Genital lesions that histopathologically resembled SCC in situ were first described by Lloyd, in 1970, as multicentric pigmented Bowen's disease of the groin.[65] In 1977, Kopf et al.[66] described multiple bowenoid papules of the penis. In 1979, Wade et al. coined the term *bowenoid papulosis of the genitalia*.[67] Other terms used for this condition include pigmented penile papules with carcinoma in situ changes, genital keratinocytic dysplasia, and penile carcinoma in situ associated with HPV infection.

Bowenoid papulosis (BP) is caused by infection with HPV and numerous HPV types have been linked to BP, including types 16, 18, 31 to 35, 39, 42, 48, and 51 to 54 (see Chap. 223). HPV 16 is the most

FIGURE 79-9

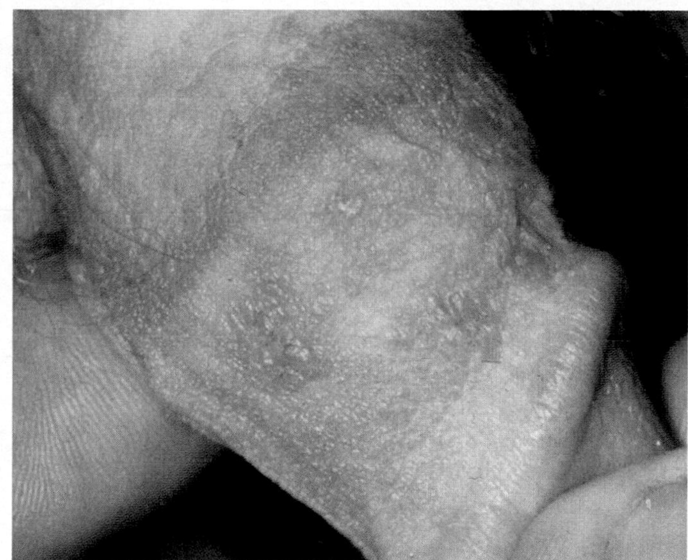

Bowenoid papulosis of the penis. (*Courtesy of James E. Fitzpatrick, MD, University of Colorado, Deptartment of Dermatology.*)

common, and types 16, 18, and 33 are considered the most oncogenic. Typically, BP presents in sexually active young males and females with multiple reddish-brown to violaceous-colored papules. Many are verrucous and, at times, the small papules coalesce into larger plaques. Sites of predilection include the penis in males and the external genitalia in females. Several reports of extragenital locations have also been described, typically on the neck and chin. The clinical differential diagnosis includes condyloma acuminata and, in fact, most lesions of BP are clinically diagnosed as condyloma acuminata. Unlike BP, typical anogenital Bowen's disease presents as a slowly enlarging pink plaque in most cases. Seborrheic keratoses and melanocytic nevi may sometimes be confused clinically with BP.

Histopathologically, the epidermis is usually hyperplastic with atypia, disordered maturation, scattered mitotic figures, and dyskeratotic keratinocytes. BP and Bowen's disease can usually be distinguished histopathologically by the fact that BP usually lacks the full-thickness epidermal atypia that is present in Bowen's disease. In BP, the atypical keratinocytes are randomly scattered throughout the epidermis and the acrotrichia are typically spared. In Bowen's disease the acrotrichia are usually involved.

The course of BP is variable, ranging from spontaneous regression to persistence of lesions to transformation into Bowen's disease and invasive SCC. Patients with BP and their sexual partners should be followed and examined periodically because of the risk of developing SCC and cervical and vulvar neoplasia.[68] Patients with persistent disease should probably undergo testing for an altered immune status. Treatment of BP is recommended and it typically responds well to local therapy, although recurrences are common. Therapeutic options include local destructive measures such as electrodesiccation and curettage, CO_2 laser, neodymium:YAG laser, cryosurgery, and excision. Topical tretinoin, topical 5-FU and low-dose interferon-α have also been beneficial.

Epidermodysplasia Verruciformis

Epidermodysplasia verruciformis (EV) is an autosomal recessive genetic disease that manifests in childhood with disseminated flat, wartlike papules. These patients also appear to have a defect in their cellular immunity (see Chap. 223). Histopathologically, the wartlike lesions of EV display hyperkeratosis, hypergranulosis, and acanthosis. The keratinocytes are vacuolated and appear pale blue-gray on staining with hematoxylin and eosin. This blue-gray pallor is most pronounced in the granular layer of the epidermis, and the vacuolated keratinocytes are typically arranged in clusters or columns. As the lesions progress to atypia, the nuclei of the keratinocytes become larger, more hyperchromatic, and cellular maturation is disordered. Changes of in situ SCC and SCC may eventually be seen.

HPV and Cutaneous Malignancy in Immunosuppressed and Immunocompetent Hosts

The role of HPV as an etiologic agent in the development of premalignant and malignant neoplasms in immunosuppressed and immunocompetent individuals is less clear (see Chap. 223).

BOWEN'S DISEASE

Bowen's disease (BD) is a form of squamous cell carcinoma in situ that was originally described in 1912 by John T. Bowen, a Boston dermatologist.[69] It affects both skin and mucous membranes and has the potential to progress into invasive SCC.

Epidemiology

Bowen's disease may occur at any age in adults, but it is rarely seen in individuals before the age of 30 years. The typical patient with BD is older than 60 years of age. The disease is said to occur with an equal incidence in men and women, although most studies report a slight preponderance in women.[70] Bowen's disease can be found on any body site, including both sun-exposed and non–sun-exposed regions of the body, and it appears to have a predilection for sun-exposed surfaces such as the head and neck, and for the lower legs of women, in particular. The exact incidence of BD in the United States is unknown, but in one population study from Hawaii, the incidence was estimated at 142 per 100,000 persons.[71] Lesions of BD are usually solitary but may be multiple in up to 10 to 20 percent of individuals.

Etiology and Pathogenesis

A number of different factors have been implicated in the etiology of BD, including a history of significant sun exposure, arsenic exposure, ionizing radiation, immunosuppression, and certain types of HPV. The age group and sites of predilection of BD suggest the association with sun exposure. Bowen's disease is also rare in more heavily pigmented individuals and it has been described with increased frequency in patients undergoing PUVA therapy. The association with arsenic exposure has already been discussed and it is seen commonly in organ transplant recipients after years of immunosuppression from medication. Infection with HPV has been implicated in causing certain subtypes of BD. In particular, HPV 16 has been detected in many cases of anogenital BD and in some cases of finger and periungual BD.[72]

Clinical Manifestations

Bowen's disease typically presents as a discrete, slowly enlarging, pink to erythematous, thin plaque with well-demarcated, irregular borders and overlying scale or crust (Fig. 79-10). Hyperkeratotic and verrucous surface changes may be seen, and a pigmented variant of BD has

FIGURE 79-10

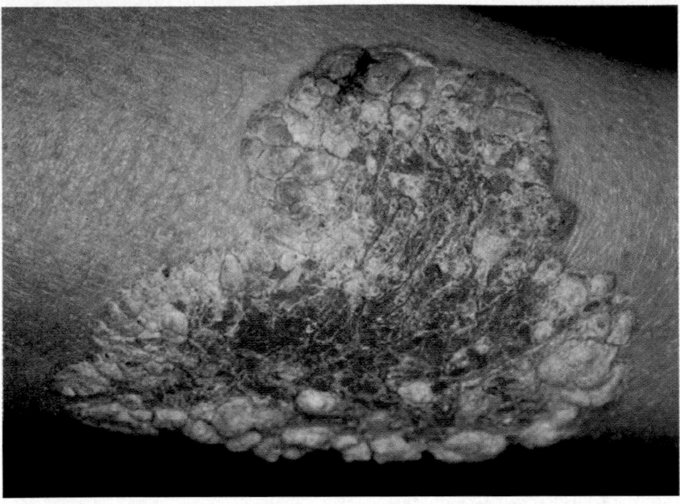

Large plaque of Bowen's disease of the leg.

been reported in less than 2 percent of cases.[73] Individual lesions may measure up to several centimeters in diameter, and multiple lesions are not uncommon. As previously mentioned, sites of predilection include sun-exposed areas such as the head and neck and lower legs in women, although any body site may be affected.

A few clinical variants of BD deserve special mention. Intertriginous BD can present as an oozing, erythematous, dermatitic plaque or as a pigmented patch or plaque. Bowen's disease involving the periungual region may appear as an erythematous, scaly, thin plaque around the cuticular margin, a crusted erosion, nail discoloration or onycholysis, a verrucous plaque, or as destruction of the nail plate. Bowen's disease of mucosal surfaces can present as verrucous or polypoid papules and plaques, erythroplakia, or as a velvety erythematous plaque. These last two entities are discussed separately below.

Pathology

The epidermis displays full-thickness atypia, including the intraepidermal portions of the adnexal structures. Involvement spans from the stratum corneum down through the basal cell layer, although the basement membrane remains intact (Fig. 79-11). Characteristically, parakeratosis and hyperkeratosis are present as is acanthosis with complete disorganization of the epidermal architecture. At times the hyperkeratosis and parakeratosis are so pronounced that a cutaneous horn is present. Throughout the epidermis are numerous, atypical, pleomorphic, hyperchromatic keratinocytes producing the characteristic "windblown" appearance. These cells are sometimes vacuolated and have a prominent pale-staining cytoplasm, reminiscent of the cells in Paget's disease. There is loss of maturation and polarity of these cells, in addition to numerous mitotic figures. Individually keratinized cells with large, rounded, eosinophilic cytoplasm and hyperchromatic nuclei can be found in the epidermis, as can multinucleated cells. These atypical cells also are seen throughout the pilosebaceous units, within the acrotrichia, follicular infundibula, and sebaceous glands. The upper dermis is typically infiltrated by numerous chronic inflammatory cells, including lymphocytes, plasma cells, and histiocytes.

Several histopathologic subtypes of BD can be seen. Psoriasiform BD displays parakeratosis and marked acanthosis with broad, sometimes fused, epidermal rete ridges. Atrophic BD, like the atrophic AK, demonstrates a thinned epidermis, but in addition there is full-thickness atypia and lack of maturation, as well as adnexal involvement. The acantholytic BD shows marked acantholysis in the epidermis. Epidermolytic BD has changes of incidental EHK present. The phenomenon of intraepidermal epithelioma of Borst-Jadassohn, namely nesting of the atypical cells within the epidermis, can also be seen.

FIGURE 79-11

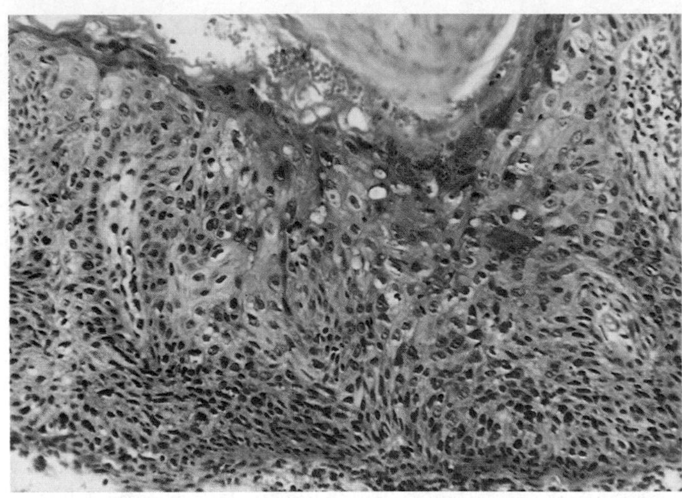

Bowen's disease showing full-thickness atypia of epithelium.

Diagnosis and Differential Diagnosis

Clinically, BD is most often mistaken for superficial BCC, patches of dermatitis, psoriasis or lichen planus, AK, benign lichenoid keratosis, irritated seborrheic keratosis, or amelanotic melanoma. More hyperkeratotic or verrucous lesions of BD may be difficult to clinically distinguish from viral warts, seborrheic keratoses and SCC, and pigmented BD lesions can be mistaken for melanoma. Superficial BCC can usually be distinguished by its raised, subtle, translucent border.

Histopathologically, BD must be differentiated from Paget's disease, pagetoid melanoma in situ, bowenoid papulosis, and podophyllin-induced changes of a wart. Both Paget's disease and BD may share the findings of vacuolated cells, but in contrast with BD, Paget's disease shows no dyskeratosis. Also, the material present in the Paget's cells is PAS-positive and diastase resistant, while the PAS-positive material sometimes present in the BD cells is glycogen and therefore PAS-labile. Lastly, staining for carcinoembryonic antigen is positive in Paget's disease but negative in BD. Pagetoid melanoma in situ can be difficult at times to histopathologically distinguish from BD. In BD, the intercellular desmosomal bridges should be identifiable between the atypical keratinocytes, and S-100 staining is positive in melanoma cells but negative in BD and Paget's disease. Bowenoid papulosis lacks the full-thickness epidermal atypia present in BD. Podophyllin applied topically to skin lesions causes metaphase arrest with resultant bizarre keratinocyte formation and sometimes a pattern of pseudoepitheliomatous hyperplasia. These changes typically resolve after a few days to a week.[74]

Prognosis and Treatment

The risk of BD progressing to invasive SCC has been estimated at approximately 5 percent.[75,76] Once invasive SCC occurs in BD, it has also been estimated that approximately 33 percent may metastasize unless adequate therapy is initiated.[76] These risk estimates were drawn from retrospective case series, and are far in excess of the experience of the senior author of this chapter.

The presence of BD on any given individual is a marker for the high risk of developing a subsequent NMSC.[77] In studies addressing the association between BD and the risk of other NMSCs, approximately 30 to 50 percent of patients had either previous or subsequent NMSC. Another recent study estimated the incidence ratio for subsequent NMSC to be 4.3.[77] Previous studies have also purported that the presence of BD is a marker for internal malignancy, although a significant number of other studies have been unable to uphold this association. Critical analysis and meta-analysis of these past studies do not support the routine investigation for internal malignancy in persons with BD. The one exception to this position is in cases of BD related to previous arsenic exposure, in which the possibility of internal malignancy is real, as previously discussed. Also, BD involving the vulvar region in females has been associated with an increased risk of uterine, cervical, and vaginal cancer.[50,78]

A number of different modalities are available for the treatment of BD including excision, Mohs micrographic surgery, electrodesiccation and curettage, cryosurgery, topical chemotherapy with 5-FU, topical immune response modifiers, laser therapy, radiotherapy, and PDT. Although some of these modalities have better reported cure rates than others, no one treatment is right for all forms of BD. Therapy has to be guided by the size and location of the BD, in addition to individual patient characteristics, such as age and healing capability.

Surgical excision is generally regarded as the treatment of choice for most BD lesions if the lesion's size and location permit such a procedure. The rationale for recommending excision is twofold: first, to remove the entire lesion for histopathologic confirmation in order to rule-out invasive SCC; and second, to ensure complete removal of the lesion, including appendageal involvement. One retrospective study compared excision with a cure rate of 95 percent, to standard cryosurgery (34 percent cure rate) and topical 5-FU (14 percent cure rate).[50] Mohs micrographic surgery is regarded by many as the treatment of choice for BD of the nail bed and periungual region.[79]

Cure rates of 60 to 95 percent have been reported for curettage alone, with cure rates of 80 to 90 percent achieved with combination curettage and cautery regimens.[80] The length of follow-up in many of these studies was not reported. Curettage for superficial or extensive lesions of BD is ideal because of the avoidance of wound closure issues and the relative simplicity and speed of the procedure. Lower cure rates are expected with this procedure, however, because of the possibility of missing BD involving the appendages.

Properly administered cryosurgery can be quite effective in treating BD, especially in difficult to excise lesions, and in elderly individuals who may not tolerate more time-consuming surgery. It is a convenient, cost-effective, and widely available procedure. Two sets of investigators reported cure rates of 96 to 97 percent with cryosurgery, although their techniques used were not clearly defined (see Chap. 278).

Topical 5-FU chemotherapy has been used to treat BD in several studies, although most of these studies were small case series of 10 to 20 patients. Cure rates of 66 to 92 percent have been reported, with the highest cure rates being achieved when treatment included a margin of normal skin around the lesion and the treatment continued for 6 to 16 weeks.[80,81] Recurrences are not uncommon, with one study finding a 14 percent recurrence rate.[50] This treatment modality may play a role in cases of multiple, small, thin lesions of BD, when surgery is not an option.

Another topical agent that was recently explored as a treatment for BD is the immune response modifier drug imiquimod. A recent study investigating the daily application of 5% imiquimod cream on clinically noninfiltrated patches of BD for 16 weeks reported a cure rate of 93 percent, with no clinical recurrence at a 6-month follow-up.[82] Local irritation and bacterial superinfection were the most significant

side effects. Further studies on imiquimod as a treatment for BD need to be undertaken before it is accepted as mainstream therapy for this disease.

Lasers used to treat BD include the CO_2 argon, and Nd:YAG lasers. Laser ablation of BD appears to be most beneficial for lesions in difficult to treat sites, such as the finger or genitalia. These modalities are of little use if deep follicular involvement with BD is present. Published results with these modalities are limited. Radiotherapy using various techniques and regimens report cure rates of 89 to 100 percent with average follow-up between 6 months and 6 years.[80] It is advantageous for managing large or multiple lesions, especially in elderly patients who may not tolerate surgical procedures or in patients who tend to form hypertrophic scars or keloids. The main drawback of ionizing radiation therapy of BD is the problem with healing. In fact, healing after radiotherapy of BD lesions on the lower legs is so poor, that it is not recommended at these sites.

PDT, which was previously discussed under treatment modalities for AKs, is another newer, currently investigational treatment option for BD. Initial clinical clearance rates of approximately 90 percent have been reported in multiple studies, with recurrence rates of 0 to 11 percent being reported at 12-month follow-ups.[83] Longer term follow-up is needed with this modality, but it may ultimately play a role in treating larger or multiple lesions of BD, especially in difficult areas, such as the lower legs, where healing with other modalities is generally poor.

ERYTHROPLASIA OF QUEYRAT

Erythroplasia of Queyrat (EQ) is an in situ SCC (Bowen's disease) affecting the mucosal surfaces of the penis in uncircumcised males. This condition was described by Queyrat, in 1911, as "erythroplasie du gland."[84] The term *erythroplasia of Queyrat*, rather than simply SCC in situ or BD, is preferred for this condition because it is clinically distinct, presenting as a well-demarcated, shiny, velvety, bright-red plaque. EQ occurs in uncircumcised males between the ages of 20 and 80, although the majority of cases are seen between the third and sixth decades. Risk factors for developing this condition in uncircumcised males include poor hygiene, smegma, heat, friction, trauma, and genital herpes simplex virus infection.[85] HPV subtypes 16 and 8 have also been identified in a number of EQ lesions.[85]

Clinically, EQ presents as a glistening, red, velvety plaque on the glans penis, the prepuce, or the urethra (Fig. 79-12). It begins as a solitary plaque in approximately 50 percent of cases, and as multiple plaques in the remainder of cases.[50] Affected males complain of localized pain, pruritus, difficulty retracting the foreskin over the glans, bleeding, and crusting. Histopathologically, EQ is similar to BD as previously described. In addition, there may also be epidermal hypoplasia and many more plasma cells in the dermal infiltrate, as often seen in other processes affecting mucosal surfaces. The clinical differential diagnosis includes other benign inflammatory conditions such as psoriasis, lichen planus, lichen sclerosus, candidiasis, plasma cell balanitis (Zoon's balanitis), lymphogranuloma venereum, granuloma inguinale, syphilis, and drug eruptions. If the diagnosis of EQ is under consideration, a biopsy should be performed.

Lesions of EQ persist and enlarge slowly, and they typically have been present for several years (an average of 3.4 years in one study[86]) before a biopsy is taken. Progression of EQ to invasive SCC is more common than in other lesions of BD, and is said to occur in up to 33 percent of cases.[85] Once invasive SCC has occurred, approximately 20 percent of patients will display evidence of regional lymph node or

FIGURE 79-12

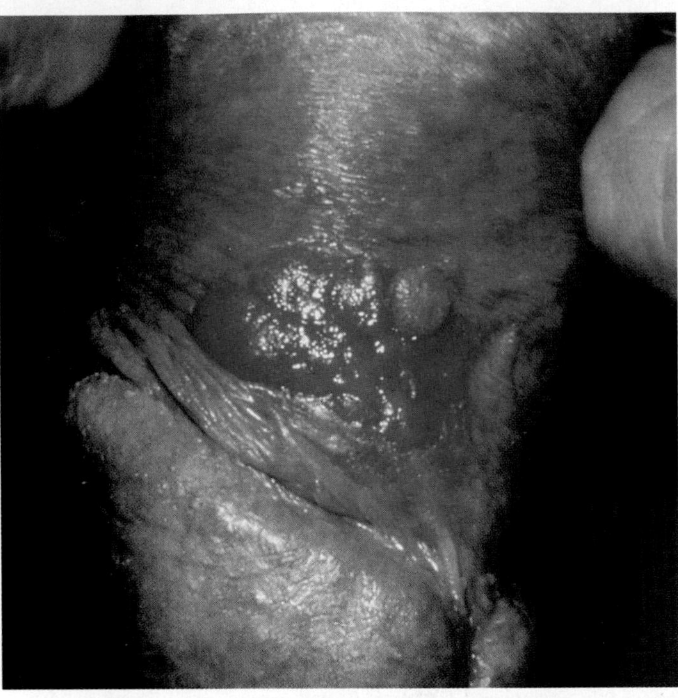

Erythroplasia of Queyrat. (*Courtesy of James E. Fitzpatrick, MD, University of Colorado, Department of Dermatology.*)

more distant metastases.[50] Prevention of EQ in uncircumcised males may be maximized by adhering to good personal hygiene regimens, and early circumcision may also reduce the incidence of this disease. Several treatment options are available, including excision, Mohs micrographic surgery, CO_2 laser, and topical 5-FU.

ERYTHROPLAKIA (ERYTHROPLASIA)

Erythroplakia, also known as erythroplasia, is a clinical term used to describe a red macule or patch on a mucosal surface that cannot be clinically or histopathologically categorized as any other known disease entity caused by inflammatory, vascular, or traumatic factors. Histopathologically, it typically displays either findings of SCC in situ or focal areas of invasive SCC, and thus is considered a precancerous lesion in most instances. Erythroplakia can involve any mucosal surface, but most commonly, in more than half of all cases, it refers to lesions in the oral mucosa. Of all oral precancerous lesions, it is considered to be the most dangerous, carrying the greatest risk of progressing to or harboring invasive carcinoma.

Erythroplakia is an uncommon lesion in the oral cavity, and it is said to be one of the least commonly diagnosed lesions among the group of oral lesions that may or may not become malignant.[87] Typically, erythroplakia is found in males who have a history of tobacco use and/or alcohol use. In fact, more than 80 percent of patients with intraoral carcinoma in situ are males, the majority of whom are older than 50 years of age.[88] It is not known precisely how alcohol and tobacco together induce carcinoma, but the synergistic effect of the two substances in causing intraoral carcinoma is well regarded.

Clinical Manifestations

Erythroplakia of the oral mucosa is found either intraorally or on the vermilion surface of the lower lip. Intraorally, the most common sites involved include the lateral and ventral tongue, floor of the mouth, and soft palate. Erythroplakia presents as a subtle, asymptomatic, erythematous macule or patch. Most often it is less than 1.5 cm in its widest diameter, but lesions up to 4 cm in diameter have been described.[87] It characteristically is sharply demarcated from the surrounding pink mucosa, and its surface is most often smooth and homogeneous in color. On occasion lesions of erythroplakia demonstrate a pebbled or stippled surface change. On palpation it is said to have a velvety feel. Erythroplakia is commonly seen in association with leukoplakia, termed erythroleukoplakia. Overwhelmingly, it is the red patches of erythroleukoplakia that most likely contain or will develop into a malignancy.

Pathology and Diagnosis

Histopathologic examination of a lesion of erythroplakia usually reveals findings of SCC in situ (Bowen's disease), occasionally with areas of focal dermal invasion. Partial or sampling biopsies of erythroplakia may unfortunately miss these focal areas of invasive SCC. The use of toluidine blue to aid in the diagnosis and to help in choosing the best site for biopsy can be quite helpful. Mashberg and Samit's technique is the most widely used one.[89] This metachromatic dye selectively stains areas of dysplastic epithelium, and its topical administration to subtle lesions can help outline the lesion. Because inflammatory lesions can give false-positive results with this technique, potential irritants should be eliminated at least 2 weeks prior to the staining. Sites that stain positively on two successive visits should be biopsied, as should all clinically suspicious lesions regardless of the results of staining. In general terms, any erythroplakia lesion should be biopsied if the etiology is not obvious or if it does resolve over a period of several weeks.

Differential Diagnosis

Erythroplakia is a diagnosis of exclusion, so the onus is on the clinician to rule out all other erythematous oral lesions before the term erythroplakia can be applied. Other entities that should be considered in the differential diagnosis include acute and chronic mechanical trauma, thermal or chemical injury, candidiasis, lichen planus, chronic contact or allergic dermatitis, submucosal hemorrhage, and various forms of glossitis.

Prognosis and Treatment

The rate at which in situ carcinoma of the oral cavity progresses to invasive SCC is not known. The transformation rate for treated cases has ranged from 14 to 50 percent, with an average of 26 percent.[87] In high-risk individuals, such as heavy smokers or drinkers, up to 80 percent of erythroplakia lesions on biopsy may contain focal areas of invasive carcinoma.[89] The definitive treatment is controversial. For early dysplastic or in situ carcinoma lesions of erythroplakia, simple excision or Mohs micrographic surgery is ideal because the entire lesion can be removed with histopathologic confirmation of the diagnosis. Other modalities, such as laser ablation, cryosurgery, and electrocoagulation, have also been used. Regardless of the treatment method used to remove the lesion, all patients should be followed at regular intervals to evaluate for the development of a second primary lesion in the oral cavity or aerodigestive tract. Carcinogenic stimuli, such as tobacco and alcohol, should be discontinued.

LEUKOPLAKIA

Leukoplakia is a fixed, predominantly white lesion of the mucosa, which cannot be clinically or histopathologically characterized as any other disease. Leukoplakia is most often seen on the oral and anogenital mucosal surfaces. Some lesions are benign and others will transform into cancer. Like erythroplakia, leukoplakia should be considered a clinical diagnosis until a definitive histopathologic diagnosis has been determined following biopsy. It, too, is associated with alcohol and tobacco use, in addition to chronic trauma and infection. Leukoplakia with premalignant and malignant potential is also seen in the genetic disease dyskeratosis congenita. Because of the various factors contributing to the formation of the process, it can affect any age range.

Clinical Manifestations

Leukoplakia associated with carcinogenesis typically occurs in an older male, in the fifth to seventh decades of life. A history of long-standing tobacco use and/or alcohol abuse is not uncommon. Premalignant or malignant leukoplakia lesions are most likely to be found on the floor of the mouth, lateral and ventral tongue, and soft palate. Lesions in these sites are much less likely to be caused by trauma or infection, and they carry a higher risk of premalignancy and malignancy. In fact, it has been estimated that leukoplakic lesions in these anatomic sites have an approximate 40 percent risk of being malignant or premalignant.[90] As a general group, oral leukoplakias carry a 5 to 25 percent risk of harboring some form of dysplasia or malignancy.[90]

Clinically, leukoplakia presents as an asymptomatic, asymmetric white plaque. It cannot be easily rubbed off. It may have overlying roughness or a granular surface or it may be soft and smooth. Some lesions that also have concomitant areas of redness are termed *erythroleukoplakia*. This latter lesion carries a more ominous prognosis, because the risk of premalignancy or malignancy being present in the erythematous portion of the lesion is much greater.

Pathology

As previously mentioned, the majority of leukoplakic lesions, unlike the erythroplakias, do not show malignant or premalignant histopathologic changes. These more common, reactive leukoplakias exhibit hyperkeratosis, acanthosis or epithelial atrophy, and chronic inflammation.[90] Focal areas of candidiasis may also be seen. Some of the leukoplakias, however, do reveal histopathologic dysplasia, SCC in situ, or frank invasive SCC.

Diagnosis and Differential Diagnosis

In general, leukoplakia should be biopsied to determine the true histopathologic diagnosis. As mentioned earlier, leukoplakia on the floor of the mouth, lateral and ventral tongue, and soft palate carry a much greater risk of being malignant or premalignant and thus should be carefully evaluated, biopsied, and probably removed completely regardless of the histopathologic diagnosis.[90] Other conditions that may present with oral or mucosal white plaques include oral white sponge nevus, lichen planus, candidiasis, syphilis, lichen sclerosus, leukoedema, smoker's keratosis, Darier's disease, and cheek biting.

Prognosis and Treatment

In general, the prognosis for reactive leukoplakias is quite good. For all leukoplakias the risk of progression to malignant SCC is approximately 4 percent, and even higher in the high-risk anatomic sites.[91] In a series of 782 patients with oral or lip leukoplakia followed on a regular basis, 2.4 percent developed SCC in 10 years and 4 percent developed SCC in 20 years.[90] Patients should be followed closely, at regular intervals, and reevaluated should the leukoplakia persist or recur following adequate intervention. Treatment depends on the site. Lesions at low-risk sites, such as the buccal mucosa, hard palate, and gingival mucosa can be followed closely if the histopathologic features are benign or reactive. Lesions on high risk sites, such as the floor of the mouth, lateral and ventral tongue, and soft palate should be removed completely. Surgical excision or Mohs micrographic surgery are treatment options. Other therapeutic approaches for known premalignant lesions include topical 5-FU, laser ablation, and cryosurgery. Patients should also be advised to discontinue tobacco use and alcohol consumption.

REFERENCES

1. Cockerell CJ: Histopathology of incipient intraepidermal squamous cell carcinoma ("actinic keratosis"). *J Am Acad Dermatol* **42**:S11, 2000
2. Freeman RG et al: What is the boundary that separates a thick actinic keratosis from a thin squamous cell carcinoma? *Am J Dermatopathol* **6**:301, 1984
3. Yantsos VA et al: Incipient intraepidermal cutaneous squamous cell carcinoma: A proposal for reclassifying and grading solar (actinic) keratoses. *Semin Cutan Med Surg* **18**:3, 1999
4. Heaphy MR, Ackerman AB: The nature of solar keratosis: A critical review in historical perspective. *J Am Acad Dermatol* **43**:138, 2000
5. Dubreuilh W: Des hyperkeratoses circonscrites, in *Third International Congress of Dermatology. Official Transactions*, edited by JJ Pringle. London, Waterlow and Sons, 1898, p 125
6. Freudenthal W: Verruca senilis und keratoma senile. *Arch f Dermat u Syph (Berlin)* **158**:529, 1926
7. Pinkus H: Keratosis senilis: A biologic concept of its pathogenesis and diagnosis based on the study of normal epidermis and 1730 seborrheic and senile keratoses. *Am J Clin Pathol* **29**:193, 1958
8. Marks R et al: The relationship of basal cell carcinomas and squamous cell carcinomas to solar keratoses. *Arch Dermatol* **1224**:1039, 1988
9. Green A, Battistutta D: Incidence and determinants of skin cancer in a high-risk Australian population. *Int J Cancer* **46**:356, 1990
10. Salasche SJ: Epidemiology of actinic keratoses and squamous cell carcinoma. *J Am Acad Dermatol* **42**:S4, 2000
11. Feldman SR et al: Most common dermatologic problems identified by internists, 1990–1994. *Arch Intern Med* **158**:726, 1998
12. Frost CA, Green AC: Epidemiology of solar keratoses. *Br J Dermatol* **131**:455, 1994
13. O'Beirn SF et al: Skin cancer in county Galway, Ireland, in *Proceedings of the Sixth National Cancer Conference*. Philadelphia, JB Lippincott, 1970, p 2811
14. Vitasa BC et al: Association of nonmelanoma skin cancer and actinic keratosis with cumulative solar ultraviolet exposure in Maryland waterman. *Cancer* **65**:2811, 1990
15. Marks R et al: Spontaneous remission of solar keratoses: The case for conservative management. *Br J Dermatol* **115**:649, 1986
16. Marks R et al: The role of childhood sunlight exposure in the development of solar keratoses and nonmelanoma skin cancer. *Med J Aust* **152**:62, 1990
17. Grossman D, Leffell DJ: The molecular basis of nonmelanoma skin cancer. *Arch Dermatol* **133**:1263, 1997
18. Ziegler A et al: Sunburn and p53 in the onset of skin cancer. *Nature* **372**:773, 1994
19. Leffell DJ: The scientific basis of skin cancer. *J Am Acad Dermatol* **42**:S18, 2000
20. Thompson SC et al: Reduction of solar keratoses by regular sunscreen use. *N Engl J Med* **329**:1147, 1993
21. Black HS et al: Effect of a low-fat diet on the incidence of actinic keratosis. *N Engl J Med* **330**:1272, 1995
22. Rook AH et al: Beneficial effect of low-dose systemic retinoid in combination with topical tretinoin for the treatment and prophylaxis of premalignant and malignant skin lesions in renal transplant recipients. *Transplantation* **59**:714, 1995

23. Yu RCH et al: A histopathological study of 643 cutaneous horns. *Br J Dermatol* **24**:449, 1991
24. Cruces Prado MJ, de la Torre C: Jadassohn's intraepidermal epithelioma. *Dermatologica* **168**:10, 1984
25. Steffan C, Ackerman AB: Intraepidermal epithelioma of Borst-Jadassohn. *Am J Dermatopathol* **7**:5, 1985
26. Carag HR et al: Utility of step sections: Demonstration of additional pathological findings in biopsy samples initially diagnosed as actinic keratosis. *Arch Dermatol* **136**:471, 2000
27. Ponsford MW et al: The prevalence and accuracy of diagnosis of nonmelanotic skin cancer in Victoria. *Australas J Dermatol* **24**:79, 1983
28. Marks R et al: Malignant transformation of solar keratosis to squamous cell carcinoma. *Lancet* **1**:795, 1988
29. Montgomery H, Dörffel J: Verruca senilis und keratoma senile. *Arch f Dermatol u Syphilol (Berlin)* **166**:286, 1932
30. Lober BA et al: Actinic keratosis is squamous cell carcinoma. *J Am Acad Dermatol* **43**:881, 2000
31. Boddie AW Jr et al: Squamous carcinoma of the lower lip in patients under 40 years of age. *South Med J* **70**:711, 715, 1977
32. Drake LA et al: Guidelines for the care of actinic keratoses. *J Am Acad Dermatol* **32**:95, 1995
33. Feldman SR et al: Destructive procedures are the standard of care for treatment of actinic keratoses. *J Am Acad Dermatol* **40**:43, 1999
34. Eaglstein WH et al: Fluorouracil: Mechanism of action in human skin and actinic keratoses, I: Effect on DNA synthesis in vivo. *Arch Dermatol* **101**:132, 1970
35. Lawrence N et al: A comparison of the efficacy and safety of Jessner's solution and 35% trichloroacetic acid vs 5% fluorouracil in the treatment of widespread facial actinic keratoses. *Arch Dermatol* **131**:176, 1995
36. Witheiler DD et al: Long-term efficacy and safety of Jessner's solution and 35% trichloroacetic acid vs 5% fluorouracil in the treatment of widespread actinic keratoses. *Dermatol Surg* **23**:191, 1997
37. Trimas SJ et al: The carbon dioxide laser: An alternative for the treatment of actinically damaged skin. *Dermatol Surg* **23**:885, 1997
38. Jiang B et al: YAG laser for the treatment of actinic keratoses. *Dermatol Surg* **26**:437, 2000
39. Jeffes EW et al: Photodynamic therapy of actinic keratoses with topical aminolevulinic acid hydrochloride and fluorescent blue light. *J Am Acad Dermatol* **45**:96, 2001
40. Kurwa HA et al: A randomized paired comparison of photodynamic therapy and topical 5-fluorouracil in the treatment of actinic keratosis. *J Am Acad Dermatol* **41**:414, 1999
41. Stockfleth E et al: Successful treatment of actinic keratosis with imiquimod cream 5%: A report of 6 cases. *Br J Dermatol* **144**:1050, 2001
42. Schwartz RA: Arsenic and the skin. *Int J Dermatol* **36**:241, 1997
43. Blejer HP, Wagner W: Case study 4: Inorganic arsenic-ambient level approach to the control of occupational cancerigenic exposures. *Ann N Y Acad Sci* **271**:179, 1976
44. Travis LB, Arndt KA: Occupational skin cancer. *Postgrad Med* **79**:211, 1986
45. Col M et al: Arsenic-related Bowen's disease, palmar keratosis, and skin cancer. *Environ Health Perspect* **107**:687, 1999
46. Jackson R Grainge JW: Arsenic and cancer. *Can Med Assoc J* **113**:396, 1975
47. Pershagen G: The carcinogenicity of arsenic. *Environ Health Perspect* **40**:93, 1981
48. Hsu C-H et al: Mutational spectrum of p53 gene in arsenic-related skin cancers from the blackfoot disease endemic area of Taiwan. *Br J Can* **80**:1080, 1999
49. Wong SS et al: Cutaneous manifestations of chronic arsenicism: Review of 17 cases. *J Am Acad Dermatol* **38**:179, 1998
50. Graham JH: Selected precancerous skin and mucocutaneous lesions, in *Neoplasms of Skin and Malignant Melanoma*. Chicago, Year Book Medical Publishers, 1976, p 69
51. Arrington JH III, Lockman DS: Thermal keratoses and squamous cell carcinoma in situ associated with erythema ab igne. *Arch Dermatol* **115**:1226, 1979
52. Shahrad P, Marks R: The wages of warmth: Changes in erythema ab igne. *Br J Dermatol* **97**:179, 1977
53. Boffetta P et al: Cancer risk from occupational and environmental exposure to polycyclic aromatic hydrocarbons. *Cancer Causes Control* **8**:444, 1997
54. Pott P: Chirurgical works of Percivall Pott, in *Cancer Scroti*. Dublin, James Williams, 1775, p 403
55. Letzel S, Drexler H: Occupationally related tumors in tar refinery workers. *J Am Acad Dermatol* **39**:712, 1998
56. Götz H: Tar keratosis, in *Cancer of the Skin: Biology-Diagnosis-Management*, edited by Andrade R, Gumport SL, Popkin GL, Rees TD. Philadelphia, WB Saunders, 1976, p 492
57. Helm KF et al: Radiation keratosis associated with exposure to a gold ring. *Cutis* **57**:435, 1996
58. Yamada M et al: Prevalence of skin neoplasms among the atomic bomb survivors. *Radiat Res* **146**:223, 1996
59. Peter RU et al: Chronic cutaneous damage after accidental exposure to ionizing radiation: The Chernobyl experience. *J Am Acad Dermatol* **30**:719, 1994
60. Marjolin JN: Ulcere, in *Dictionnaire de Medecine,* vol 21. Paris, Bechet, 1828, p 31
61. Phillips TJ et al: Burn scar carcinoma. *Dermatol Surg* **22**:561, 1998
62. Dupree MT et al: Marjolin's ulcer arising in a burn scar. *Cutis* **62**:49, 1998
63. Arons MS et al: Scar tissue carcinoma: A clinical study with special references to burn scar carcinoma. *Ann Surg* **161**:170, 1965
64. Novick M et al: Burn scar carcinoma: A review and analysis of 46 cases. *J Trauma* **17**:809, 1977
65. Lloyd KM: Multicentric pigmented Bowen's disease of the groin. *Arch Dermatol* **101**:48, 1970
66. Kopf AW, Bart RS: Tumor conference. No 11. Multiple bowenoid papules of the penis: A new entity? *J Dermatol Surg Oncol* **3**:265, 1977
67. Wade TR et al: Bowenoid papulosis of the genitalia. *Arch Dermatol* **115**:306, 1979
68. Obalek S et al: Bowenoid papulosis of the male and female genitalia: Risk of cervical neoplasia. *J Am Acad Dermatol* **14**:433, 1986
69. Bowen JT: Precancerous dermatoses. A study of two cases of chronic atypical epithelial proliferation. *J Cutan Dis* **30**:241, 1912
70. Kossard S, Rosen R: Cutaneous Bowen's disease: An analysis of 1001 cases according to age, sex, and site. *J Am Acad Dermatol* **27**:406, 1992
71. Reizner GT et al: Bowen's disease (squamous cell carcinoma in situ) in Kauai, Hawaii: A population-based incidence report. *J Am Acad Dermatol* **31**:596, 1994
72. McGrae JD et al: Multiple Bowen's disease of the fingers associated with HPV type 16. *Int J Dermatol* **32**:104, 1993
73. Ragi G et al: Pigmented Bowen's disease and review of 420 Bowen's disease lesions. *J Dermatol Surg Oncol* **14**:765, 1988
74. Civatte J: Pseudo-carcinomatous hyperplasia. *J Cutan Pathol* **12**:214, 1985
75. Peterka ES et al: An association between Bowen's disease and cancer. *Arch Dermatol* **84**:623, 1961
76. Kao GF: Carcinoma arising in Bowen's disease. *Arch Dermatol* **122**:1124, 1986
77. Jaeger AB et al: Bowen disease and risk of subsequent malignant neoplasms. A population-based cohort study of 1147 patients. *Arch Dermatol* **135**:740, 1999
78. Ragnarsson B et al: Carcinoma in situ of the vulva: Long-term prognosis. *Acta Oncol* **26**:277, 1987
79. Sau P et al: Bowen's disease of the nail bed and periungual area. A clinicopathologic analysis of seven cases. *Arch Dermatol* **130**:204, 1994
80. Ball SB, Dawber RPR: Treatment of cutaneous Bowen's disease with particular emphasis on the problem of lower leg lesions. *Australas J Dermatol* **39**:63, 1998
81. Sturm HM: Bowen's disease and 5-fluorouracil. *J Am Acad Dermatol* **1**:1513, 1979
82. Mackenzie-Wood A et al: Imiquimod 5% cream in the treatment of Bowen's disease. *J Am Acad Dermatol* **44**:462, 2001
83. Morton CA et al: Photodynamic therapy for large or multiple patches of Bowen disease and basal cell carcinoma. *Arch Dermatol* **137**:319, 2001
84. Queyrat L: Erythroplasie du gland. *Bull Soc Fr Dermatol Syphiligr* **22**:378, 1911
85. Wieland U et al: Erythroplasia of Queyrat: Coinfection with cutaneous carcinogenic human papillomavirus type 8 and genital papillomaviruses in a carcinoma in situ. *J Invest Dermatol* **115**:396, 2000
86. Graham JH, Helwig EB: Erythroplasia of Queyrat: A clinicopathologic and histochemical study. *Cancer* **32**:1396, 1973
87. Bouquot JE, Ephros H: Erythroplakia: The dangerous red mucosa. *Pract Periodontics Aesthet Dent* **7**:59, 1995
88. Bouquot JE: Epidemiology, in *Pathology of the Head and Neck*, edited by DR Gnopp. New York, Churchill Livingstone, 1987, p 263
89. Mashberg A, Samit A: Early detection, diagnosis, and management of oral and oropharyngeal cancer. *Cancer* **39**:67, 1989
90. Summerlin DJ: Precancerous and cancerous lesions of the oral cavity. *Dermatol Clin* **14**:205, 1996
91. Silverman S Jr et al: Oral leukoplakia and malignant transformation. A follow-up study of 257 patients. *Cancer* **53**:563, 1984

CHAPTER 80

Douglas Grossman
David J. Leffell

Squamous Cell Carcinoma

Cutaneous squamous cell carcinoma (SCC) is a malignant neoplasm derived from suprabasal epidermal keratinocytes. These and basal cell cancers are the nonmelanoma skin cancers that represent the most common malignancies in humans. While basal cell carcinoma (BCC) (discussed in Chap. 81) is thought to arise de novo, SCC probably evolves in most cases from precursor lesions of actinic keratosis (AK) and Bowen's disease (SCC in situ) (see Chap. 79). This chapter focuses on clinical aspects of invasive SCC. Cutaneous SCC represents a broad spectrum of disease ranging from easily managed, superficially invasive cancer to highly infiltrative, metastasizing tumors that can result in death. The clinical presentation can be variable despite the existence of easily identified typical lesions. The cellular and molecular aspects of SCC carcinogenesis are discussed elsewhere (see Chaps. 36 to 38).

HISTORICAL ASPECTS

Recognition of nonmelanoma skin cancer dates back to biblical times. Although precise clinical descriptions were documented centuries ago, distinctions between SCC and BCC were not fully appreciated until the late nineteenth century with advances in tissue preparation, staining, and microscopy. Percivall Pott was likely the first to describe the malignant nature of SCC in 1775.[1] His descriptions of "soot warts" in adolescent British chimney sweeps led to the early appreciation of an occupational carcinogen and the promulgation of the original occupational safety laws. Additional occupational associations with SCC were later revealed, most of which involved chronic exposure of factory workers to hydrocarbons in the form of coal tar or lubricating oils.[2] So-called mule spinner's disease was named for the oiled turning axle of the cotton spinning machine (mule) straddled by workers who later developed genital SCC.[3] The French surgeon Jean-Nicholas Marjolin, in 1828, first described SCC arising in traumatic scars, and subsequently SCC associated with burn scars was termed *Marjolin's ulcer*.[4] Arsenic, once commonly found in drinking water and fumes released in copper smelting, was recognized as a significant skin carcinogen in the early 1800s.[5] Sir Jonathan Hutchinson, in 1887, famously reported that medicinal arsenic in the form of potassium arsenite (Fowler's solution), then a treatment for psoriasis and asthma, caused skin tumors.[6] X-ray exposure was associated with SCC in the early 1900s in technicians operating roentgen machines,[7] and later in patients treated with grenz rays for a variety of benign conditions including psoriasis, acne, and hirsutism.[8] Today, it is ultraviolet (UV) radiation, rather than these occupational hazards, that is the predominant factor in the development of SCC (see Chap. 38).[9]

In light of these associations, the precursor lesions of SCC were initially called hydrocarbon keratoses, scar keratoses, burn keratoses, arsenical keratoses, radiation keratoses, and solar keratoses, among other names. These terms are generally of historical interest and seldom used today, with the exception of solar (actinic) keratosis (AK) because it is the most common.

EPIDEMIOLOGY

Incidence

The precise incidence of BCC and SCC is unknown because these cutaneous malignancies are generally not documented by the National Cancer Institute or most state registries. Conservative estimates for the year 2001 are well over 1 million cases in the United States, including approximately 200,000 cases of SCC.[10] Although less common than BCC, SCC carries a risk of metastasis and thus accounts for the majority of the several thousand deaths attributable to nonmelanoma skin cancer each year. By comparison, cutaneous melanoma accounts for only 50,000 cases, but approximately 10,000 deaths, annually.[11] Similar trends for SCC have been noted in Australia[12] and the Caribbean.[13]

SCC is strongly associated with *advanced age,* with a sharp increase in incidence after age 40.[14] Today, the lifetime risk of SCC among whites is approximately 15 percent, almost double that of two decades ago. Increased exposures to UV radiation (through increased use of tanning salons, more time spent outdoors, changes in clothing style, and ozone depletion) and increased longevity have been suggested as possible causes for the increase in disease. It is likely that this trend will continue as a result of further depletion of the ozone layer and the increasing age of the US population. The increased incidence of SCC over the past several decades has been paralleled by a 20 percent decrease in mortality, attributed largely to increased public awareness and aggressive treatment of high-risk lesions.[15] Following a diagnosis of SCC, patients have a 44 to 50 percent cumulative risk of developing another nonmelanoma skin cancer (18 to 30 percent risk of SCC) in the subsequent 3 to 5 years.[16] In addition, these patients are at increased risk for extracutaneous cancers.[17]

Demographics

Squamous cell cancer is twice as common in men than in women, probably a result of greater lifetime UV exposure in men. Similarly, longer hairstyle and use of lipstick may account for less-frequent SCC on the ears and lips of women. There is an inverse relationship between *skin pigmentation* and SCC incidence, largely because of the protective effect of eumelanin. Thus, persons with white skin, blue eyes, fair complexion, red hair, and Celtic ancestry who tan poorly are at greatest risk. Increased pigmentation is not only associated with a lower incidence of SCC, but also an inversion in the BCC to SCC ratio. When American blacks are compared with whites, the incidence of SCC decreases 30-fold and the BCC to SCC ratio falls to 0.8 to 1.[14] Tanzanian albinos all

TABLE 80-1

Predisposing Factors for SSC

Precursor lesions (AK, Bowen's disease)
UV exposure
Ionizing radiation
Environmental carcinogens
Immunosuppression
Scars
Burns or chronic heat exposure
Chronic scarring or inflammatory dermatoses
Human papilloma virus
Genodermatoses (albinism, xeroderma pigmentosum, porokeratosis, epidermolysis bullosa)

develop SCC by young adulthood, and the ratio of BCC to SCC is only 0.2 to 1. Asians and Polynesians, with intermediate skin pigmentation, have correspondingly intermediate levels of SCC. A gene involved in melanogenesis, encoding melanocortin-1 receptor (MC1R), is a major determinant of skin pigmentation and hair color. The MC1R gene is highly polymorphic, with more than 20 variants described.[18] Several variant MC1R alleles are associated with increased risk of SCC that was independent of skin type and hair color.

ETIOLOGY AND PATHOGENESIS

Predisposing Factors

There are a number of factors, including both acquired and genetic skin conditions, that may predispose to SCC (Table 80-1). Patients often demonstrate a multiplicity of factors that together are sufficient to induce SCC development. Thus, a given skin site may be exposed to both UV radiation and another environmental carcinogen.

PRECURSOR LESIONS Most SCCs develop from precursor lesions such as AKs or Bowen's disease (see Chap. 79).

UV EXPOSURE UV radiation is considered the predominant risk factor for SCC. Importantly there is a linear correlation between the incidence of SCC and UV exposure. The incidence of SCC has been reported to double with each 8- to 10-degree decline in geographic latitude, and is highest at the equator.[19] World War II veterans stationed in the Pacific developed much higher rates of SCC than did their colleagues who served in Europe.[20] Similarly, SCC is more prevalent in Japanese people who emigrated to Hawaii than in those who remained in Japan.[21] Excessive UV radiation appears to be more related to the development of SCC than BCC. Rates of SCC rise more rapidly than those of BCC with increasing UV exposure,[22] and UV-induced skin cancers in mice are almost exclusively SCCs rather than BCCs.[23] Moreover, in patients receiving long-term PUVA for psoriasis there is an associated 30-fold increase in nonmelanoma skin cancer, most of which are SCCs.[24]

IONIZING RADIATION There is a strong association of SCC with ionizing radiation (Fig. 80-1), as described above. In a recent survey of SCC patients, the association with radiotherapy was observed only among those whose skin was likely to sunburn (see Chap. 79).

FIGURE 80-1

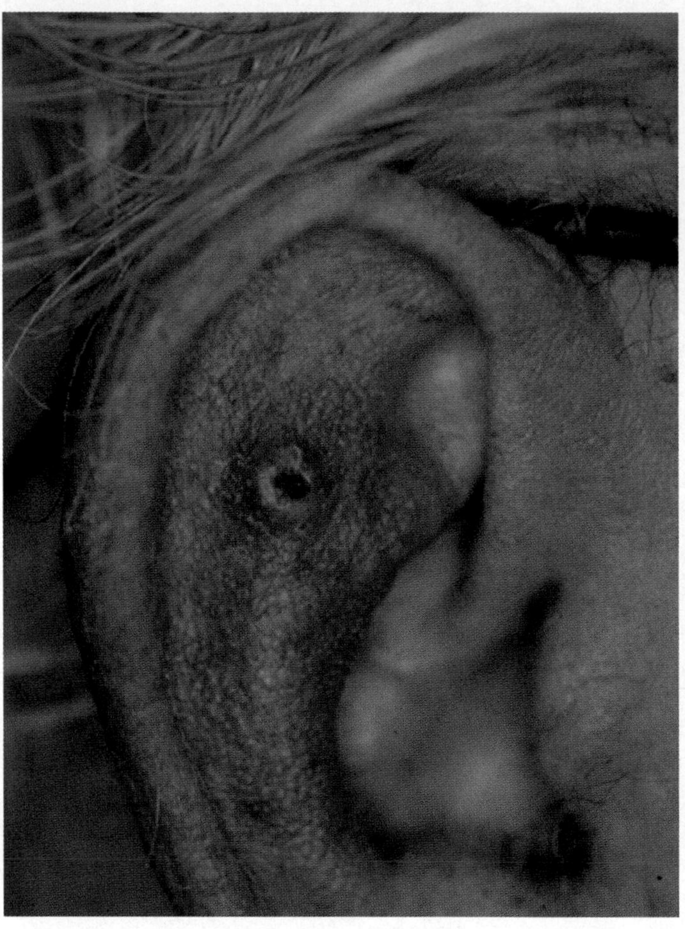

Papular SCC of the ear. The differential diagnosis includes chondrodermatitis nodularis helicis, which, unlike SCC, is associated with pain.

ENVIRONMENTAL CARCINOGENS There are numerous occupational and environmental carcinogens, such as arsenic and aromatic hydrocarbons, that predispose to SCCs. With the exception of 3-methylcholanthrene and anthramine, chemical carcinogens generally produce SCCs rather than BCCs.[25] Exposures to insecticides and herbicides have also been associated with SCCs. In addition, smoking and alcohol use are strongly associated with SCCs of the oral cavity.

IMMUNOSUPPRESSION Chronic immunosuppression may lead to an increase in SCCs, primarily on sun-exposed sites.[26] An 18-fold increase in SCC has been reported in renal transplant patients;[27] these tend to appear 3 to 7 years after the onset of chronic immunosuppressive therapy, with corticosteroids, azathioprine, and cyclosporine most frequently implicated. With the increase in the total number of organ transplant patients, management of SCCs in this population is becoming more important. In patients with leukemia and lymphoma, SCCs are both increased and more aggressive.[28] Although multiple SCCs have been described in HIV patients, advanced HIV infection has generally not been associated with an increased incidence of SCC, possibly because many patients do not live long enough to develop them.

SCARS AND UNDERLYING DISEASES Historically, SCC has been associated with both burn scars and chronic ulcers as noted above, although this is seldom seen today. Also rare but reported is the development of SCCs in the context of *chronic infections*, particularly those associated with draining sinuses and scarring, such as perianal pyoderma, osteomyelitis, chromomycosis, hyalohyphomycosis, granuloma inguinale, lupus vulgaris, and leprosy. Chronic *inflammatory processes*, particularly those associated with scarring, such as venous ulcer, snake-bite ulcer, discoid lupus erythematosus, oral lichen planus, morphea, lichen sclerosis et atrophicus, pilonidal cyst, acne conglobata, hidradenitis suppurativa, Hailey-Hailey disease, dissecting folliculitis of the scalp, and necrobiosis lipoidica, can all give rise to SCCs. An exception is vaccination scars, which are associated with BCCs rather than SCCs. SCCs have also been observed in transplanted skin, epidermal cyst, dental cyst, and dermoid cyst.

THERMAL FACTORS Chronic heat exposure can lead to SCCs. The role of thermal radiation in the development of skin cancer has long been recognized in many cultures, where common practices include placing hot ashes under the clothes to keep warm in winter or smoking opium while lying on heated beds. SCCs are increased in persons who habitually sit in front of heating stoves, and at sites of erythema ab igne (see Chap. 79).

HUMAN PAPILLOMA VIRUS There is a role for human papilloma virus (HPV) infection in some types of SCC. Verrucous carcinoma appears to be associated with several HPV types, as noted below. Head and neck and periungual SCCs are frequently associated with HPV type 16. Patients with epidermodysplasia verruciformis are chronically infected with HPV, most commonly type 5, and one-third of these patients ultimately develop SCCs (see Chaps. 79 and 223).

GENODERMATOSES A variety of heritable diseases predispose to SCC development. Patients with oculocutaneous albinism develop predominantly SCCs (rather than BCCs) at an early age. Xeroderma pigmentosum, a disorder of DNA repair, is also characterized by early onset development of SCCs. SCCs have been reported to develop in the Mibelli, disseminated superficial actinic, and palmaris et plantaris disseminata forms of porokeratosis (see Chap. 56), and in oral lesions of dyskeratosis congenita. As noted above, lesions of epidermodysplasia verruciformis can degenerate into SCCs. Finally, patients with the dystrophic form of epidermolysis bullosa are at increased risk for SCC.

Molecular Aspects

Like most cancers, the development of SCC from normal keratinocytes begins with mutations in the cellular DNA and genomic instability. Alterations in gene expression lead to loss of growth controls, penetration of the basement membrane and ultimately invasion into surrounding tissue. Along the pathway to SCC, keratinocytes become resistant to apoptosis (programmed cell death) and immune attack.

GENETIC ALTERATIONS Most analyses of genetic alterations in SCCs have been performed in cases of oral or head and neck SCCs. Chromosomal deletions (loss of heterozygosity) commonly involve chromosomes 3, 9, 11, and 17; the regions most commonly identified include 9p21 and 17p13 where the p16 I^{NK4A} and p53 tumor suppressors are respectively located.[29] Similar genetic lesions were found in a study of young patients (younger than 40 years old).[30] It is unclear whether these genetic markers will serve as useful prognostic indicators.

p53 IN THE DEFENSE AGAINST SKIN CANCER Apoptosis of keratinocytes that have sustained UV-induced DNA damage, termed *sunburn cells,* requires the *p53 tumor suppressor* and represents a key protective mechanism against skin cancer by removing premalignant cells that have acquired mutations.[31] In keratinocytes, UV radiation upregulates p53,[32] which delays cell-cycle progression until DNA damage can be repaired, or facilitates cell elimination by apoptosis.[33] Compromise of p53 function could undermine this apoptosis-based defense mechanism, giving UV-damaged cells a selective advantage to survive additional cycles of UV exposure.[34] Further impairment of p53 and other genes through additional UV-induced mutations may then lead to even greater resistance to apoptosis, increased proliferation, and ultimately development of SCC. The increased susceptibility of p53-deficient mice to UV-induced SCC[35] highlights this protective role of p53.

***p53* MUTATIONS IN SCC** Consistent with this scenario, mutations in the *p53* gene are a common finding in SCC. In most cases, these are C→T single base and CC→TT tandem transition mutations at dipyrimidine sequences, that is, "UVB signature" mutations.[36] Most SCCs exhibit loss of heterozygosity with respect to *p53* and isolated mutations on the remaining allele. In one study, the *p53*-apoptosis pathway was disrupted in 50 percent of oral SCC.[37] With respect to SCC precursors, *p53* mutations have been found in up to 75 percent of AKs and SCCs in situ[38] lesions. Interestingly, while different *p53* mutations were found in separate AKs, all cells within a single precursor lesion have the same mutation.[31] *p53* mutations can also be detected in keratinocytes from clinically normal sun-exposed skin.[39] *p53*-mutated keratinocytes occur in clonal patches that are larger and more frequent in sun-exposed skin.[40] These findings substantiate a clonal basis for UV-induced SCC and suggest that *p53* mutation is an early event in the development of SCC.

In addition to mutation, p53 can be compromised in keratinocytes infected with HPV. The E6 protein encoded by oncogenic HPV types binds p53 and targets it for rapid degradation, disabling the p53-apoptosis pathway. This is a primary mechanism by which HPV infection predisposes to SCC (see Chap. 223).

OTHER APOPTOTIC REGULATORS IN SCC In addition to p53, dysregulation of other apoptotic regulatory proteins has been described in SCC. In a study of vulvar SCC, expression of the apoptotic inhibitor *Bcl-2* correlated with metastasis.[41] Similarly, in esophageal SCC, expression of the apoptotic inhibitor *Bcl-XL* correlated with tumor invasion and metastasis.[42] In SCC of the tongue, low apoptotic index and decreased expression of the proapoptotic *Bax* correlated significantly with poor prognosis, whereas low *Bcl-2* expression was associated with a favorable clinical outcome.[43] Expression of the antiapoptotic *BAG-1* was associated with nodal metastasis in oral SCC.[44] Consistent with these observations, transgenic mice expressing Bcl-2 and Bcl-XL in the skin exhibit increased susceptibility to chemical-induced tumorigenesis. In addition to these Bcl-2 family members, the inhibitor of apoptosis protein *survivin* is expressed both in SCC and precursor lesions,[45] and in one study its expression correlated with aggressive tumor phenotype.[46]

IMMUNE EVASION Working with UV-induced SCCs in mice, Kripke and colleagues first demonstrated the importance of immunosuppression in UV-induced SCC in the 1970s (see Chap. 38). They found that while UV-induced SCC was promptly rejected when transplanted into genetically identical recipient mice, the transplanted tumors grew rapidly and rejection did not occur if recipient mice were first treated with a subcarcinogenic dose of UV. These experiments suggested that UV radiation not only induced SCC, but also impaired the ability of host animals to mount protective immune responses against foreign tumor antigens. While immunosuppressed patients are at great risk for SCC, as discussed above, the development and progression of SCC in all individuals requires some level of continuous local and perhaps systemic immunosuppression to prevent tumor rejection.

PREVENTION

Those at risk for SCC, namely persons with a prior history of nonmelanoma skin cancer or any of the predisposing conditions discussed above, should be monitored closely. They should receive complete skin examinations on a regular basis.

Sun Protection

The most effective preventive measure is protection from sun exposure. It is likely that adequate sun protection beginning in early childhood could prevent most SCCs.[47] This requires establishing patterns of behavior, at an early age, such as repeated application of sunscreen, wearing hats and protective clothing, and avoiding the sun during the hours of peak intensity. However, the role of sun prevention in childhood should not be construed to mean that sun protection later in life will be of no benefit. There is evidence that aggressive sun protection throughout life can prevent the development of SCC precursor lesions and cancers themselves.

Treatment of Precursor Lesions

Treatment of precursor lesions is expected to reduce the incidence of SCC. Several options are available for treatment of AK (see Chap. 79). Isolated lesions can often be effectively removed by liquid nitrogen cryotherapy. For patients with many AKs, or areas of skin with a multitude or confluence of lesions, topical chemotherapy using 5-fluorouracil is an option. More information on this topic can be found in Chap. 79.

Other Preventive Measures

A number of additional preventive measures can be taken that may reduce the incidence of SCC in individual patients. For example, the use of condoms can prevent transmission of HPV and may thereby reduce the risk of genital SCC. Decreased alcohol consumption and smoking cessation is likely to reduce the risk of oral SCC. Several years ago there was great interest in both retinoids and interferons as systemic chemopreventive agents. Low-dose etretinate (10 mg per day) has been used successfully in renal transplant patients.[48] A more recent recommendation is Accutane (10 mg every day or every other day) in addition to topically applied tretinoin.[49] Topical application of a DNA repair enzyme in liposomes was recently shown in an experimental trial to reduce the incidence of new AK in xeroderma pigmentosum patients.[50] Finally, topical immunologic modifiers are showing promise as a new class of agents that may stimulate the endogenous cutaneous immune system to destroy malignant cells.

CLINICAL MANIFESTATIONS

In white men and women, the majority of SCCs arise on sun-exposed areas such as the head, neck, and dorsal hands. SCC of the legs is more common in women.[51] In blacks, on the other hand, SCC tends to be distributed equally on sun-protected and exposed areas.[52] SCC typically presents in solitary fashion, arising from precursor lesions as noted above. An exception is in immunosuppressed patients, who may manifest eruptive SCCs.

FIGURE 80-2

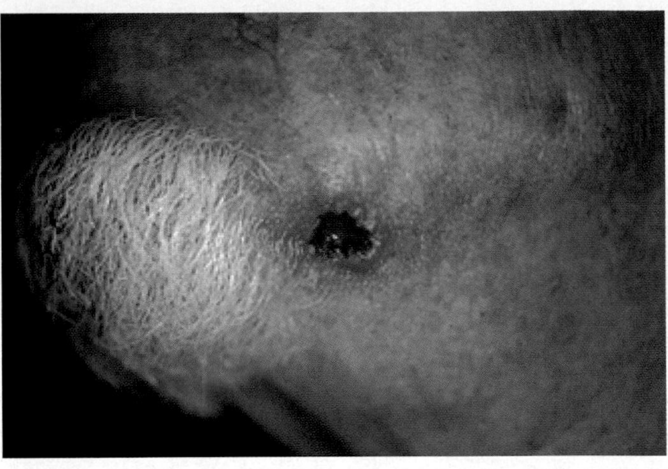

Ulcerative SCC of the jaw. In this region, extension of the cancer can invade the marginal mandibular nerve.

Development from Precursor Lesions

AKs often occur as a multiplicity of lesions, ranging in size from pinpoint to over 2 cm, and the borders are usually ill defined. A dry adherent scale gives them a rough gritty texture. By contrast, lesions of *Bowen's disease* are usually solitary, sharply demarcated scaling papules or plaques, often initially mistaken for eczema, psoriasis, or lichen simplex. These disorders are often pruritic, whereas Bowen's disease is usually not. In sun-protected sites, Bowen's disease may have a noneczematous appearance. For example, it may appear verrucous in the anogenital area, nail bed, and eyelid, and as a dark patch or oozing erythematous plaque in intertriginous areas. These precursor lesions are usually asymptomatic, and the development of tenderness, induration, erosion, increased scale, or enlarging diameter may herald evolution into SCC. Typically a patient with multiple AKs may present with a single lesion that gradually becomes more prominent than the rest (Fig. 80-1), or with a solitary, persistent, nonpruritic, scaling patch that is unresponsive to topical steroids.

SCC Morphologies

A firm, flesh-colored or erythematous, keratotic papule or plaque is most common (Fig. 80-1), but SCCs may also be pigmented. Other presentations include an ulcer (Fig. 80-2), a smooth nodule (Fig. 80-3), and a thick cutaneous horn. SCC may also be verrucous or present as

FIGURE 80-3

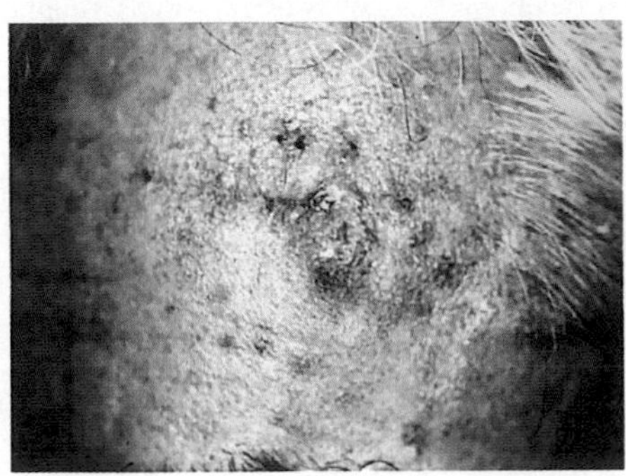

Nodular SCC of the forehead. This lesion is recurrent and can be seen arising in the previous surgical scar. It should be considered high risk.

FIGURE 80-4

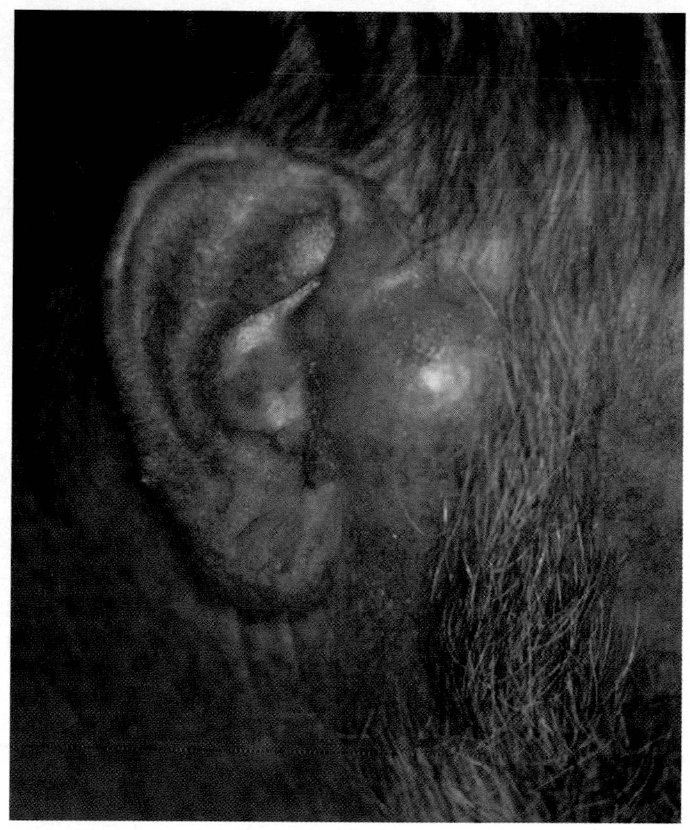

Preauricular mass resulting from metastasis of cutaneous SCC. Involvement of the parotid gland can result from metastasis of SCC in the temple and ear region.

an abscess, particularly if in a periungual location. The margins may be indistinct. With enlargement, there is usually increased firmness and elevation. Progressive tumor invasion ultimately results in fixation to underlying tissues. Especially in the head and neck region, an enlarged lymph node nearby that is firm and nontender may indicate tumor metastasis (Fig. 80-4).

Oral SCC

SCC of the oral cavity usually occurs in patients with a long history of cigarette smoking, chewing tobacco, or alcohol use, but recently it has been documented in younger adults without these traditional risk factors. There is a male predominance, and the palate and tongue are the most common sites. Oral SCC most commonly evolves from lesions of erythroplakia and is usually asymptomatic (see Chap. 79). Distinct patterns include a persistent rough red patch or granular velvety red plaque that ultimately becomes firm and nodular. Surprisingly, the risk of transformation to SCC does not appear to correlate with the degree of epithelial dysplasia.[53] The floor of the mouth, ventrolateral tongue, and soft palate are considered high-risk sites. It may also present as a peritonsillar abscess.

Lower Lip

SCC of the lower lip begins as a roughened papule of actinic cheilitis or scaly leukoplakia, with slow progression to a tumor nodule (Fig. 80-5). Clinical clues associated with evolving SCC include persistent lip chapping with localized scale or crust, red and white blotchy atrophic vermillion lip, indistinct or "wandering" vermillion border,

FIGURE 80-5

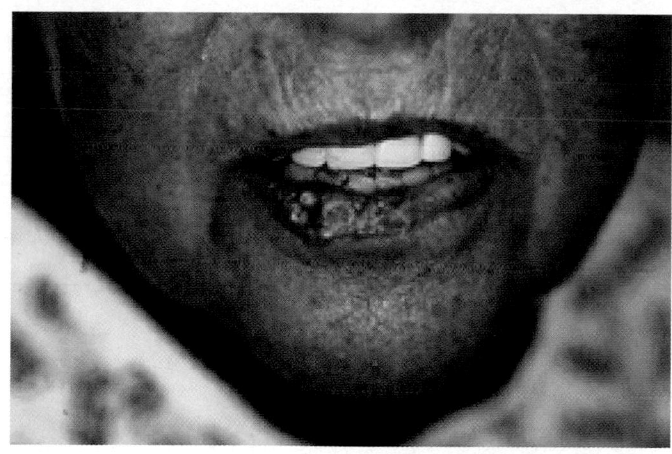

SCC of the lower lip develops in the setting of chronic solar exposure and actinic cheilitis. Metastasis to draining lymph nodes can occur.

and small fissuring or ulceration within an area of indurated actinic cheilitis. Symptoms of underlying pain or altered sensation should be investigated as a potential sign of perineural invasion.

Genital SCC

SCC of the *vulva* most commonly occurs on the anterior labia majora, beginning as a small warty nodule or an erosive erythematosus plaque. These lesions may be asymptomatic, but more often are associated with pruritus or bleeding. Lesions of lichen sclerosus are another common precursor of SCC of the vulva. SCC of the *cervix* is associated with HPV, most commonly type 16. SCC of the *scrotum* begins as a small pruritic verrucous lesion that becomes friable with increasing size. SCC of the *penis* usually occurs in uncircumcised males, and, although very uncommon in Western countries, may account for 10 percent of cancers in places where genital hygiene is poor. A distinct precursor of penile SCC is erythroplasia of Queyrat, characterized by a velvety red plaque. In addition to lack of circumcision, penile SCC has also been associated with history of condyloma and phimosis and lichen sclerosus et atrophicus. Once thought to be a common location for SCC following long-term PUVA therapy, this complication can be avoided by shielding the genitalia during treatment, and this association is rarely seen today. Perianal SCC may also occur (Fig. 80-6).

Scar SCC

SCCs arising in scars typically begin decades after injury with skin breakdown and persistent erosion. Most commonly this occurs on the lower extremities at sites of chronic pyogenic or venous stasis ulcers. Gradually there is acquisition of nodularity, although detection is often delayed because of concealment by surrounding indurated scar tissue. In the case of SCC developing in chronic sinuses, however, nodularity may not be present. The development of increased pain, drainage, or bleeding alone should raise concern and warrant further investigation.

Keratoacanthoma

The hallmark of this tumor is rapid growth, up to several centimeters in weeks, and then gradual involution over a period of months in most cases (see Chap. 83). The typical presentation is in an elderly patient on

FIGURE 80-6

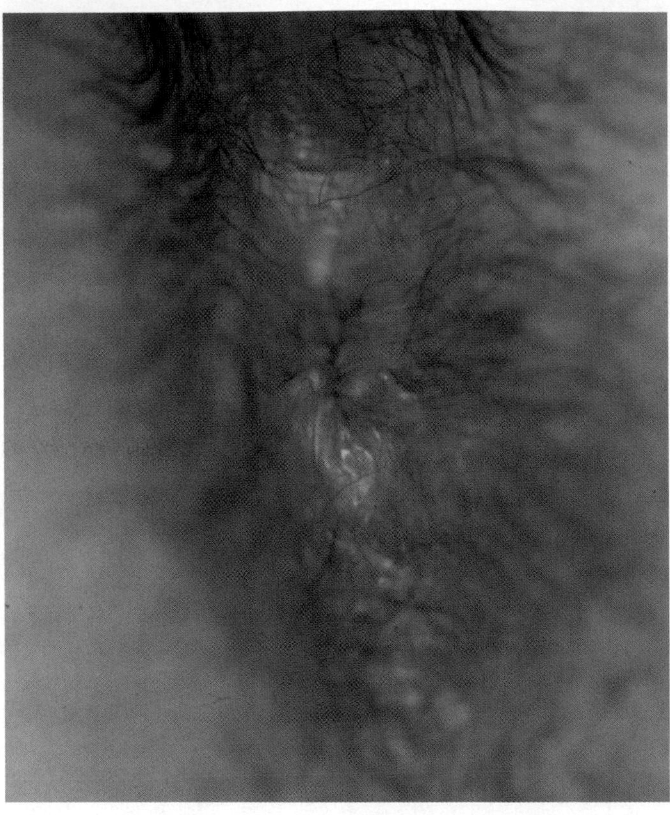

Perianal SCC in situ. Identification of these lesions requires thorough proctoscopic exam and monitoring for invasive SCC.

a sun-exposed site, particularly an extremity. Morphologically, keratoacanthoma is usually a large, smooth, dome-shaped, verrucous nodule with a central keratotic crater. Although historically viewed as a benign neoplasm because of its tendency toward spontaneous resolution, the keratoacanthoma can be locally destructive and aggressive and must be viewed as a clinical subtype of SCC. This tumor may occur in association with sebaceous neoplasms and gastrointestinal malignancies in the Muir-Torre syndrome.

Verrucous Carcinoma

This form of SCC encompasses several clinical entities all characterized by slow-growing exophytic tumors with cauliflower-like appearance that develop at sites of chronic irritation.[54] They may be clinically mistaken for giant warts. Four subtypes are recognized based on site of occurrence. Type I consists of oral tumors on the buccal mucosa of elderly male tobacco chewers, and have been referred to as *oral florid papillomatosis*. Representing 2 to 12 percent of all oral cancers, they are most commonly found on the buccal mucosa, tongue, gingiva, and floor of the mouth. Type II is the *anogenital type,* as described by Buschke and Loewenstein. It occurs on the glans penis of young uncircumcised males, the scrotum, perianally in both sexes, and, less commonly, on the female genitalia. Type III, also known as *epithelioma cuniculatum,* is a malodorous tumor often found on the plantar feet of elderly men (Fig. 80-7). It usually involves the skin underlying the first metatarsal head and tends to form draining sinuses that are caniculated (like rabbit burrows) in appearance. Finally, type IV occurs at other

FIGURE 80-7

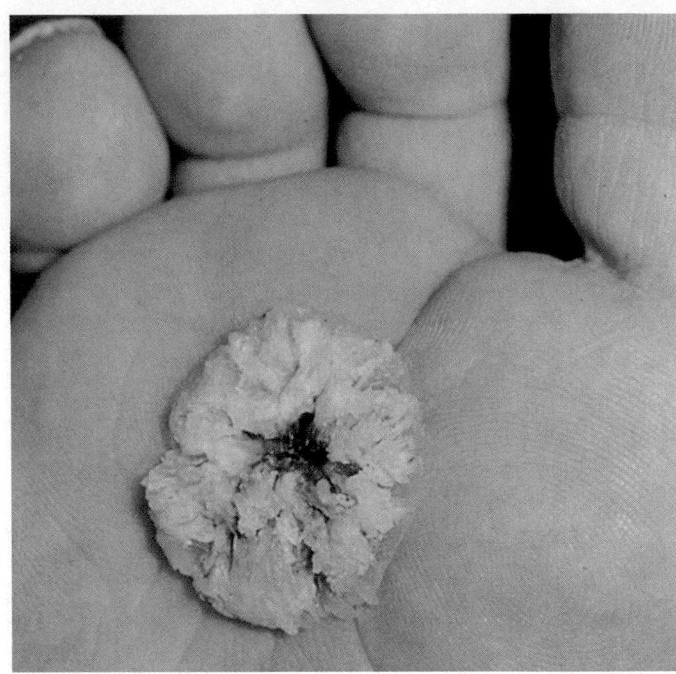

Epithelioma cuniculatum, verrucous carcinoma of foot.

sites including the scalp, trunk and extremities. Detection of HPV type 6, 11, 16, and 18 sequences in epithelioma cuniculatum and type 11 sequences in oral verrucous carcinoma raises the possibility that these tumors evolve from verruca vulgaris.

Metastatic SCC

Metastatic SCC in the skin can have a variety of presentations. It may be signaled by a palpable lymph node near the treatment site of a prior SCC. On the other hand, it may present as large keratotic papules or nodules resembling the primary lesion (Fig. 80-8). Metastatic SCC on the skin may be the first sign of internal malignancy, initially presenting in the skin as clusters of firm pink or red papules that may be keratotic centrally.

FIGURE 80-8

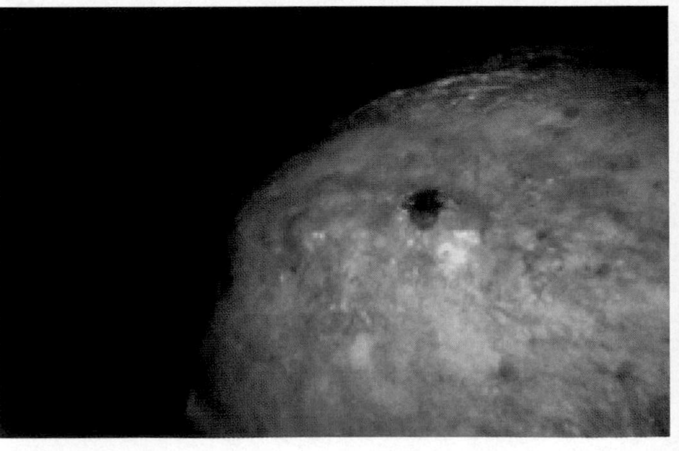

SCC metastatic to skin.

FIGURE 80-9

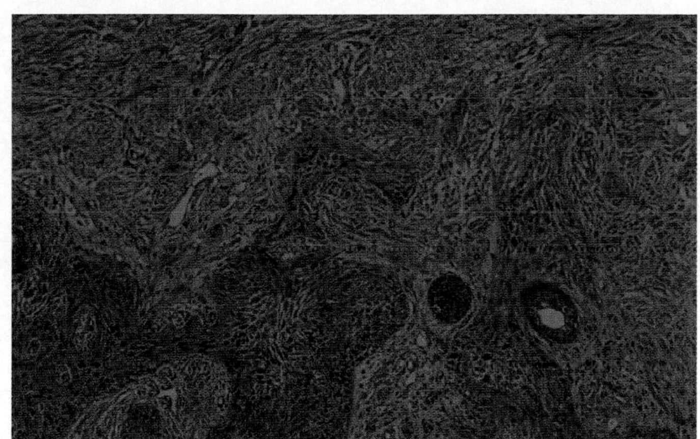

A.

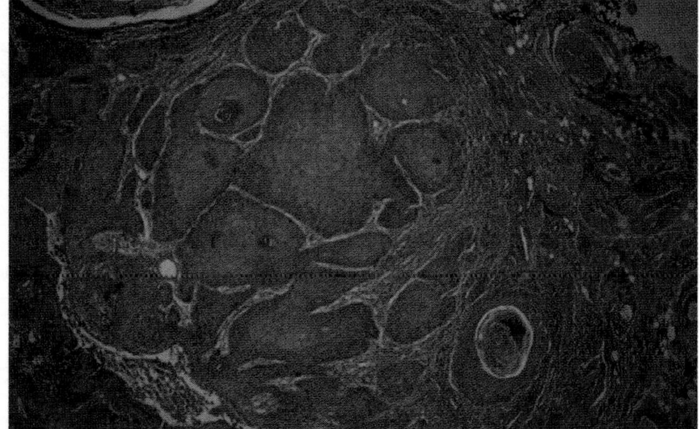

B.

A. Low-power magnification of SCC demonstrating invasive cancer. *B.* SCC demonstrating atypical keratinocytes and foci of keratinization.

HISTOPATHOLOGY

GENERAL CONSIDERATIONS

The hallmark of invasive SCC is the extension of atypical keratinocytes beyond the basement membrane and into the dermis (Fig. 80-9). The absence of a connection between tumor cells and the epidermis should raise concern for metastatic SCC, although this may simply reflect undermining from adjacent tumor. In every case, it is important to note clues that may indicate a precursor lesion or particular etiology. For example, the presence of solar elastosis and keratinocyte atypia at the margins would suggest that the SCC is actinically derived. On the other hand, the presence of scar tissue may indicate recurrent disease or a sinister scar-associated SCC. These considerations have important implications for treatment and prognosis, as discussed below.

Basic Features

The tumor may appear as single cells, small groups or nests of cells, or a single mass. The inferior border may broadly impose on the dermis, or be represented by individual foci of microinvasion. Invasive tumor is usually confined to the dermis, and subcutaneous involvement is unusual. There are typically varying proportions of normal-appearing and atypical squamous cells, the latter characterized by increased mitoses, aberrant mitotic figures, nuclear hyperchromasia, and loss of intercellular bridges. Squamous differentiation is seen as foci of keratinization in concentric rings of squamous cells called *horn pearls*. Loss of differentiation is associated with decreased keratin production.

TABLE 80-2

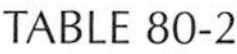

Broders' Grading System for SSC

Grade	% Undifferentiated Cells	Other Features
1	<25	Keratinization
2	<50	
3	<75	
4	>75	Atypia, loss of intracellular bridges

Grading

Histologic grading of SCC is based on degree of cellular differentiation. Low-grade tumors are comprised of uniform cells, resembling mature keratinocytes, with intracellular bridges and keratin production. High-grade SCC, by contrast, is characterized by atypical cells, loss of intracellular bridges, and minimal or absent keratin production. Another feature of higher-grade tumors is a less-distinct demarcation between malignant cells and adjacent normal stroma. In 1932, Broders[55] introduced a formal grading system based on keratinocyte differentiation that is still used today. Tumors are graded on a scale of 1 to 4 based on increasing percentages of undifferentiated cells (Table 80-2). In addition to grade, the depth of penetration, tumor thickness, and hair follicle involvement should also be reported.

Histologic Subtypes

There are many histologic subtypes of SCC.[56] In the *adenoid* (or pseudoglandular) SCC, there is a tubular microscopic pattern and keratinocyte acantholysis. In *clear cell* SCC, the keratinocytes appear clear as a result of hydropic cytoplasmic swelling and accumulation of lipid vacuoles. *Spindle cell* SCC reveals spindle-shaped atypical cells. *Signet-ring cell* SCC is a rare variant characterized by concentric rings composed of keratin and large vacuoles corresponding to markedly dilated endoplasmic reticulum. In addition, a *basaloid* variant has been described. In *verrucous carcinoma,* the superficial component resembles verruca vulgaris with prominent acanthosis and papillomatosis, while the deeper component extends downward, displacing collagen bundles. Finally, *keratoacanthoma* reveals a symmetric keratin-filled crater, with the epidermis on each side extending over to form a distinct lip.

DIAGNOSIS AND DIFFERENTIAL DIAGNOSIS

Making the Diagnosis

The diagnosis of SCC is always made by skin biopsy. Any persistent, enlarging or nonhealing lesion, particularly if on a sun-exposed site, warrants biopsy evaluation. It is important that the biopsy be of sufficient depth so that invasive SCC can be distinguished from in situ disease. If a lesion is flat or minimally elevated (less than 1 mm),

FIGURE 80-10

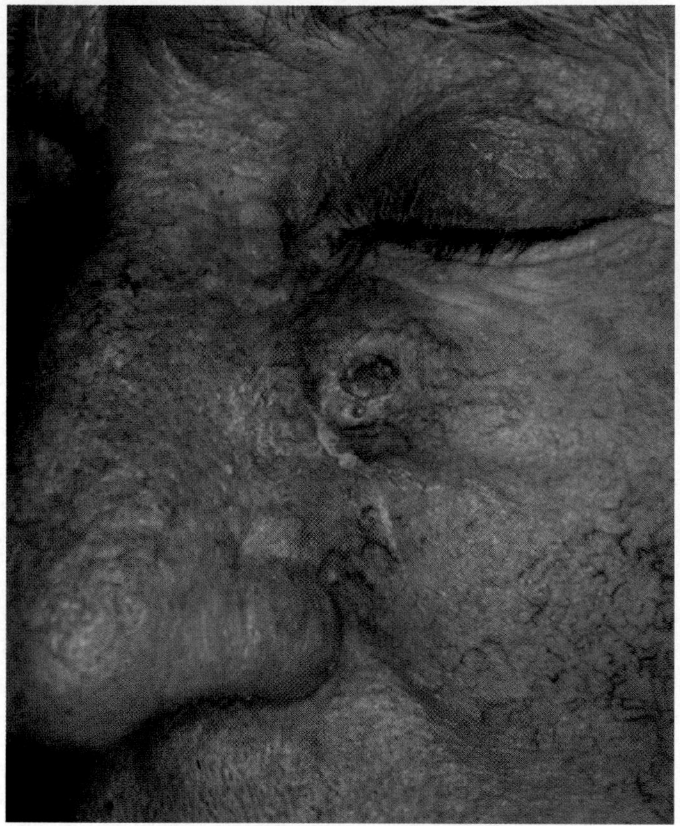

A.

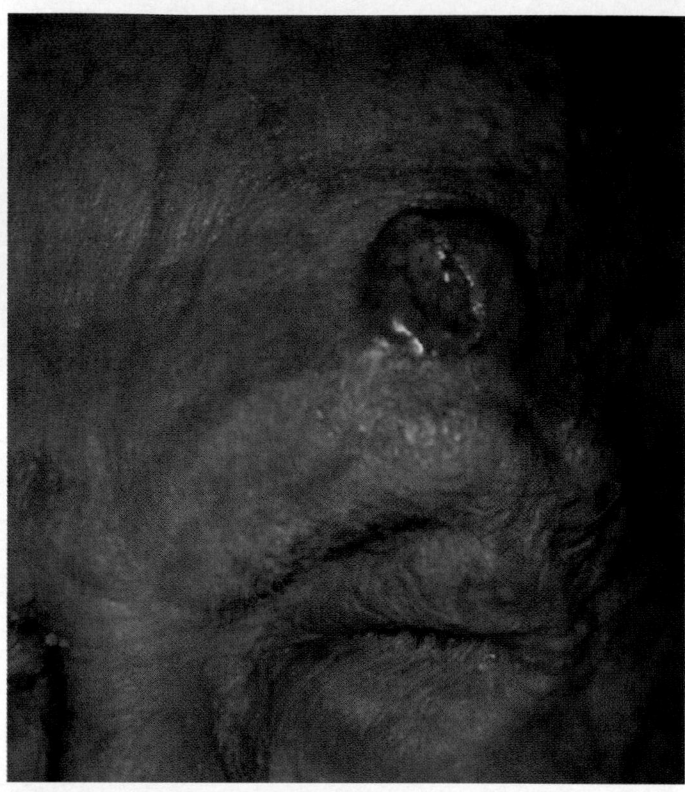

B.

A. Infiltrative SCC demonstrating retraction of underlying tissue of the left cheek, where extension might involve infraorbital nerve. *B.* SCC of left side of forehead, where extension to bone with invasion might lead to death.

the superficial shaving technique minimizes wound size and scarring, and is usually adequate. For elevated lesions, the punch technique or a deep shave excision should be used to ensure that a specimen of adequate depth is taken. Because the diagnosis of keratoacanthoma depends largely on overall architecture, excisional biopsy or an incisional ellipse through the entire lesion is recommended. A tangential excision through the deep dermis also usually suffices.

Differential Diagnosis

Clinically, the differential diagnosis of SCC is long, but can be narrowed based on lesion morphology. For verrucous or scaly lesions, benign considerations include wart, seborrheic keratosis, AK, melanocytic nevus, pyogenic granuloma, eccrine poroma, and deep fungal infections such as chromomycosis. The entity "erosive pustular dermatosis of the scalp" is a benign condition often initially mistaken for SCC. Other malignant verrucous lesions include atypical fibroxanthoma, BCC, Bowen's disease, verrucous melanoma, Merkel cell carcinoma, and, of course, metastatic SCC. Pigmented SCC in particular may mimic melanoma. For ulcerative lesions, additional diagnoses include trauma, BCC, and herpes virus infection (either herpes simplex virus or varicella-zoster virus).

Histologically, the differential diagnosis of well-differentiated SCC includes verruca vulgaris and inverted follicular keratosis. In addition, reactive epidermal hyperplasia (pseudoepitheliomatous hyperplasia) secondary to mycosis, halogenated drug eruptions (bromoderma and iododerma), and even mechanical trauma can mimic SCC. In these hyperplasias, however, the keratinocytes usually remain well differentiated; the margins of the proliferating epidermis are often pointed or irregular, rather than bulbous; there is leukocyte invasion with occasional keratinocyte disintegration; and granulomas or intraepidermal abscesses may be present.[57] Some adenoid SCC may demonstrate a pseudovascular pattern, with erythrocytes in pseudovascular spaces, and may be confused with angiosarcoma; these tumors do not express factor VIII antigens or bind ulex agglutinin. Clear cell SCC may simulate adnexal tumors with sebaceous differentiation or sebaceous carcinoma. Distinguishing spindle cell SCC from atypical fibroxanthoma is difficult. The differential diagnosis of poorly differentiated SCC also includes fibrosarcoma, Merkel cell carcinoma, and melanoma. In most cases, SCC can be distinguished from these others by special stains for various cytokeratins, but, in difficult cases, electron microscopy may be needed to establish the diagnosis.[56] In general, SCC does not stain for melanocyte (S-100, HMB-45) or smooth muscle (vimentin, actin) markers.

RECURRENCE AND METASTASIS

SCC, like BCC, may cause local tissue destruction, but it also has significant potential for metastasis. Metastases, when they occur, are generally to regional lymph nodes, and are detected 1 to 3 years after initial diagnosis and treatment.[19] In many cases, metastasis is preceded by local recurrence at the site of the primary lesion. Historically, the reported rate of metastasis for SCC ranges from 0.5 to 6 percent,[58,59] and tends to occur with tumors that are large, recurrent, and involve deep structures or cutaneous nerves (Fig. 80-10).

TABLE 80-3

High-Risk SSC

Diameter greater than 2 cm
Depth greater than 4 mm and Clark level IV or V
Tumor involvement of bone, muscle, nerve
Location on ear, lip
Tumor arising in scar
Broders grade 3 or 4
Patient immunosuppression
Absence of inflammatory infiltrate

High-Risk Lesions

In a classic study, Rowe et al.[60] reviewed all major series of SCC dating back to 1940 to determine risk factors associated with recurrence and metastasis. Table 80-3 summarizes the characteristics of "high-risk" lesions. With respect to *size*, tumors less than 2 cm in diameter are low-risk, with an overall metastatic rate of roughly 1 percent. In one study,[61] the metastatic rate increased to 9.2 percent and 14.3 percent for tumors of 2 to 5 cm and greater than 5 cm, respectively. With respect to *depth and invasion*, tumors less than 4 mm deep and Clark levels I to III have limited metastatic potential, while close to half of those greater than 4 mm and Clark levels IV or V were metastatic in some series.[61,62] Tumor involvement of bone, nerve, or muscle tissue is highly associated with metastasis. With respect to *anatomic site*, SCC of the ear has the highest rate of recurrence (18.7 percent), while lip SCC has the highest rate of metastasis (13.7 percent), with half of lip metastases present at time of initial diagnosis.[60] All SCCs *arising in scars* are high-risk, with metastatic rates approaching 40 percent in some series.[63] By contrast, SCCs arising in actinically damaged skin are of considerably lower risk, with an average metastatic rate of 5.2 percent.[60] *Poorly differentiated* SCCs (Broders' grade 3 or 4) demonstrate a recurrence rate of 28.6 percent and metastatic rate of 32.8 percent, as compared to 13.6 percent and 9.2 percent, respectively, for well-differentiated tumors.[60] The prognosis is particularly poor for spindle cell SCCs.[64] *Immune status* is another important consideration, as one study[65] found that 23 percent of patients with metastatic SCC were immunosuppressed. A heavy *inflammatory response* appears to be a favorable prognostic sign, as absence of infiltrate has been correlated with higher rates of recurrence and metastasis.

TREATMENT

Table 80-4 summarizes the variety of treatment modalities available for SCCs. Treatment selection is largely directed by assessment of tumor risk for recurrence and metastasis, as discussed above. Ablative techniques such as electrodesiccation and curettage, liquid nitrogen cryotherapy, carbon dioxide laser, intralesional chemotherapy, and photodynamic therapy are superficial, do not allow histologic margin control, and thus are generally inappropriate for invasive SCCs. An exception may be the use of topical 5-fluorouracil for conjunctival SCCs.[66]

TABLE 80-4

Treatment of SCC

Nonexcisional ablative techniques (in situ disease only, or special circumstances)
Mohs surgery
Conventional surgical excision
Radiation

TABLE 80-5

Indications of Mohs Surgery

Infiltrative SCC
Poorly defined clinical margins
Lip, ear, nail bed, nasal tip, eyelid, genitalia
History of radiation at site
Involvement of nerve, bone, muscle
Immunosuppressed patient
Recurrent or large SCC
Verrucous carcinoma
SCC arising from chronic scarring conditions

Surgical Excision

Conventional surgical excision is viewed by most as the treatment of choice for primary SCCs. Recommended margins are 4 mm for low-risk lesions or SCCs with a depth less than 2 mm; for lesions with depth greater than 6 mm or diameter greater than 1 cm, margins of 6 mm or Mohs microscopically controlled surgery (MMCS) are recommended.[67] MMCS is recommended in specific circumstances when the highest cure rate and minimal tissue destruction are desired (Table 80-5). Specifically, cases involving deeply infiltrative tumor; history of radiation at the site; involvement of underlying structures (nerve, bone, muscle); immunosuppression; recurrent or large tumor; poorly defined clinical margins; sites with high recurrence rates (lip, ear, nail bed); and sites important for tissue preservation (nasal tip, lip, eyelid, ear, genitalia) should strongly be considered for Mohs surgery.[68] Additional indications include verrucous carcinomas and high-risk SCCs such as those arising from chronic scarring conditions.

Radiation

Radiation can be used for superficially invasive to moderate-risk lesions, and serves as an important adjuvant to excisional surgery in treating residual microscopic disease and prophylaxis against metastatic disease. It has been shown to be particularly useful for SCCs of the external auditory canal.[69] Radiotherapy is not advised for verrucous carcinoma, in which there is an associated low rate of anaplastic transformation. Radiation may also be used as adjuvant therapy in cases where perineural SCC was identified on surgical pathology specimens but treatment failures occur.

Recurrence Rates

In their extensive review noted above, Rowe et al.[60] also assessed responses to treatment. They reported increasing combined rates of recurrence with each of the following treatment modalities (for primary cancers): MMCS (3.1 percent), electrodesiccation and curettage (3.7 percent), excisional surgery (8.1 percent), and radiation (10 percent). A recent review of MMCS for SCC with 4-year follow-up reported a cure rate of 92 percent.[70] The surprisingly low rate of recurrence for electrodesiccation and curettage likely reflects its judicious use for low-risk lesions. Similarly, the recurrence rates for both MMCS and excisional surgery may be somewhat skewed by their use for high-risk lesions. For lip SCC, the overall recurrence rate was 2.3 percent for Mohs surgery as compared to 10.5 percent for other modalities; for ear SCC, the recurrence rates were 5.3 percent and 18.7 percent, respectively.[60] For all recurrent tumors, cure rates were 76.7 percent with excision, as compared to 90 percent with Mohs surgery.[60] For low-risk SCCs, overall recurrence rates were 1.9 percent with Mohs surgery versus 16.5 percent with all other modalities.[60] Overall 5-year survival rates for metastatic SCCs were 26.8 percent,[60] with poorer outcomes among patients with lip lesions[71] and those treated with surgery alone (and no radiation).

Treatment of High-Risk Lesions

Management of high-risk lesions is reviewed elsewhere.[72] Oral 5-fluorouracil has been used for aggressive lesions refractory to conventional treatments.[73] Additional treatments, including beta-carotene, interferon, and retinoids, have been employed with variable results. High-risk lesions may require formal staging. Computed tomography or magnetic resonance imaging may be useful in the detection of advanced perineural involvement of head and neck SCC.[74] Sentinel lymphadenectomy has been combined with MMCS.[75] Involvement of lymph nodes may warrant radical lymph node dissection and radiation therapy. Elective cervical lymphadenectomy may be indicated for high-risk lesions of the lip.[76] In cases of negative clinical lymph node examination, further intervention may still be indicated if the tumor is considered sufficiently high-risk.

Patient Follow-up

Following a diagnosis of SCC, all patients should be considered at high risk for developing additional lesions of SCC as well as BCC. They should be seen at regular intervals, ranging between 3 and 12 months, depending on the degree of prior lesion risk, status of precursor lesions, and individual patient compliance. A complete skin examination should be performed at each visit, including examination of the oral mucosa. In addition, sites of previous lesions and treatments should be assessed for signs of recurrence. Finally, a lymph node exam is indicated to monitor for metastatic disease.

REFERENCES

1. Pott P: *Chirurgical Observations Relative to the Cataract, the Polypus of the Nose, the Cancer of the Scrotum, and Different Kinds of Ruptures, and Mortification of the Toes and Feet.* London: Hawes, Clark & Collins, 1775
2. Waterhouse JA: Cutting oils and cancer. *Ann Occup Hyg* **14**:161, 1971
3. Waldron HA et al: Scrotal cancer in the West Midlands 1936–76. *Br J Indus Med* **41**:437, 1984
4. Horton CE et al: The malignant potential of burn scars. *Plast Reconstr Surg* **22**:348, 1958
5. Neubauer O: Arsenical cancer: A review. *Br J Cancer* **1**:192, 1947
6. Hutchinson J: Arsenic cancer. *Br Med J* **2**:1280, 1887
7. Traenkle HL: X-ray-induced skin cancer in man. *Natl Cancer Inst Monogr* **10**:423, 1963
8. Dabski K, Stoll HL Jr: Skin cancer caused by grenz rays. *J Surg Oncol* **31**:87, 1986
9. Alam M, Ratner D: Cutaneous squamous-cell carcinoma. *N Engl J Med* **344**:975, 2001
10. Boring CC et al: Cancer statistics, 1994. *CA Cancer J Clin* **44**:7, 1994
11. Jemal A et al: Recent trends in cutaneous melanoma incidence among whites in the United States. *J Natl Cancer Inst* **93**:678, 2001
12. Marks R: Epidemiology of non-melanoma skin cancer and solar keratoses in Australia: A tale of self-immolation in Elysian fields. *Australas J Dermatol* **38**(Suppl 1):S26, 1997
13. Kennedy C, Bajdik CD: Descriptive epidemiology of skin cancer on Aruba: 1980–1995. *Int J Dermatol* **40**:169, 2001
14. Miller DL, Weinstock MA: Nonmelanoma skin cancer in the United States: Incidence. *J Am Acad Dermatol* **30**:774, 1994
15. Weinstock MA: Nonmelanoma skin cancer mortality in the United States, 1969 through 1988. *Arch Dermatol* **129**:1286, 1993
16. Marcil I, Stern RS: Risk of developing a subsequent nonmelanoma skin cancer in patients with a history of nonmelanoma skin cancer: A critical review of the literature and meta-analysis. *Arch Dermatol* **136**:1524, 2000
17. Hemminki K, Dong C: Subsequent cancers after in situ and invasive squamous cell carcinoma of the skin. *Arch Dermatol* **136**:647, 2000
18. Rees JL, Healy E: Melanocortin receptors, red hair, and skin cancer. *J Investig Dermatol Symp Proc* **2**:94, 1997
19. Johnson TM et al: Squamous cell carcinoma of the skin (excluding lip and oral mucosa). *J Am Acad Dermatol* **26**:467, 1992
20. Ramani ML, Bennett RG: High prevalence of skin cancer in World War II servicemen stationed in the Pacific theater. *J Am Acad Dermatol* **28**:733, 1993
21. Chuang TY et al: Nonmelanoma skin cancer in Japanese ethnic Hawaiians in Kauai, Hawaii: An incidence report. *J Am Acad Dermatol* **33**:422, 1995
22. Vitaliano PP, Urbach F: The relative importance of risk factors in nonmelanoma carcinoma. *Arch Dermatol* **116**:454, 1980
23. Winkleman RK et al: Squamous cell carcinoma produced by ultraviolet light in hairless mice. *J Invest Dermatol* **40**:217, 1963
24. Stern RS, Lange R: Non-melanoma skin cancer occurring in patients treated with PUVA five to ten years after first treatment. *J Invest Dermatol* **91**:120, 1988
25. Miller SJ: Etiology and pathogenesis of basal cell carcinoma. *Clin Dermatol* **13**:527, 1995
26. Markey AC: Etiology and pathogenesis of squamous cell carcinoma. *Clin Dermatol* **13**:537, 1995
27. Gupta AK et al: Cutaneous malignant neoplasms in patients with renal transplants. *Arch Dermatol* **122**:1288, 1986
28. Weimar VM et al: Aggressive biologic behavior of basal- and squamous-cell cancers in patients with chronic lymphocytic leukemia or chronic lymphocytic lymphoma. *J Dermatol Surg Oncol* **5**:609, 1979
29. Scully C et al: Genetic aberrations in oral or head and neck squamous cell carcinoma 3: Clinicopathological applications. *Oral Oncol* **36**:404, 2000
30. Jin YT et al: Genetic alterations in oral squamous cell carcinoma of young adults. *Oral Oncol* **35**:251, 1999
31. Ziegler A et al: Sunburn and p53 in the onset of skin cancer. *Nature* **372**:773, 1994
32. Wang Y et al: Differential regulation of p53 and Bcl-2 expression by ultraviolet A and B. *J Invest Dermatol* **111**:380, 1998
33. Vogelstein B, Kinzler KW: p53 function and dysfunction. *Cell* **70**:523, 1992
34. Leffell DJ, Brash DE: Sunlight and skin cancer. *Sci Am* **275**:52, 1996
35. Li G et al: Induction of squamous cell carcinoma in p53-deficient mice after ultraviolet irradiation. *J Invest Dermatol* **110**:72, 1998
36. Wikonkal NM, Brash DE: Ultraviolet radiation induced signature mutations in photocarcinogenesis. *J Investig Dermatol Symp Proc* **4**:6, 1999
37. Stoll C et al: Prognostic significance of apoptosis and associated factors in oral squamous cell carcinoma. *Virchows Arch* **436**:102, 2000
38. Campbell C et al: p53 mutations are common and early events that precede tumor invasion in squamous cell neoplasia of the skin. *J Invest Dermatol* **100**:746, 1993
39. Nakazawa H et al: UV and skin cancer: Specific p53 gene mutation in normal skin as a biologically relevant exposure measurement. *Proc Natl Acad Sci U S A* **91**:360, 1994
40. Jonason AS et al: Frequent clones of p53-mutated keratinocytes in normal human skin. *Proc Natl Acad Sci U S A* **93**:14025, 1996
41. Hantschmann P, Kurzl R: Regulation of apoptosis in squamous cell carcinoma of the vulva. *J Reprod Med* **45**:633, 2000
42. Matsumoto M et al: Clinical significance and prognostic value of apoptosis related proteins in superficial esophageal squamous cell carcinoma. *Ann Surg Oncol* **8**:598, 2001
43. Xie X et al: The prognostic value of spontaneous apoptosis, Bax, Bcl-2, and p53 in oral squamous cell carcinoma of the tongue. *Cancer* **86**:913, 1999
44. Shindoh M et al: BAG-1 expression correlates highly with the malignant potential in early lesions (T1 and T2) of oral squamous cell carcinoma. *Oral Oncol* **36**:444, 2000
45. Grossman D et al: Expression of the apoptosis inhibitor, survivin, in nonmelanoma skin cancer and gene targeting in a keratinocyte cell line. *Lab Invest* **79**:1121, 1999
46. Lo Muzio L et al: Expression of the apoptosis inhibitor survivin in aggressive squamous cell carcinoma. *Exp Mol Pathol* **70**:249, 2001
47. Marks R et al: The role of childhood exposure to sunlight in the development of solar keratoses and non-melanocytic skin cancer. *Med J Aust* **152**:62, 1990
48. Rook AH et al: Beneficial effect of low-dose systemic retinoid in combination with topical tretinoin for the treatment and prophylaxis of premalignant and malignant skin lesions in renal transplant recipients. *Transplantation* **59**:714, 1995
49. Rook AH, Shapiro M: Cutaneous squamous-cell carcinoma. *N Engl J Med* **345**:296, 2001
50. Yarosh D et al: Effect of topically applied T4 endonuclease V in liposomes on skin cancer in xeroderma pigmentosum: A ran-

domised study. Xeroderma Pigmentosum Study Group. *Lancet* **357**:926, 2001

51. Bernstein SC et al: The many faces of squamous cell carcinoma. *Dermatol Surg* **22**:243, 1996
52. Mora RG, Perniciaro C: Cancer of the skin in blacks. I. A review of 163 black patients with cutaneous squamous cell carcinoma. *J Am Acad Dermatol* **5**:535, 1981
53. Saito T et al: Development of squamous cell carcinoma from pre-existent oral leukoplakia with respect to treatment modality. *Int J Oral Maxillofac Surg* **30**:49, 2001
54. Schwartz RA: Verrucous carcinoma of the skin and mucosa. *J Am Acad Dermatol* **32**:1, 1995
55. Broders AC: Practical points on the microscopic grading of carcinoma. *N Y State J Med* **32**:667, 1932
56. Lohmann CM, Solomon AR: Clinicopathologic variants of cutaneous squamous cell carcinoma. *Adv Anat Pathol* **8**:27, 2001
57. Freeman RG: On the pathogenesis of pseudoepitheliomatous hyperplasia. *J Cutan Pathol* **1**:231, 1974
58. Katz AD et al: The frequency and risk of metastases in squamous cell carcinoma of the skin. *Cancer* **10**:1162, 1957
59. Lund HZ: How often does squamous cell carcinoma of the skin metastasize? *Arch Dermatol* **92**:635, 1965
60. Rowe DE et al: Prognostic factors for local recurrence, metastasis, and survival rates in squamous cell carcinoma of the skin, ear, and lip. Implications for treatment modality selection. *J Am Acad Dermatol* **26**:976, 1992
61. Breuninger H et al: Microstaging of squamous cell carcinomas. *Am J Clin Pathol* **94**:624, 1990
62. Friedman HI et al: Prognostic and therapeutic use of microstaging of cutaneous squamous cell carcinoma of the trunk and extremities. *Cancer* **56**:1099, 1985
63. Novick M et al: Burn scar carcinoma: A review and analysis of 46 cases. *J Trauma* **17**:809, 1977
64. Petter G, Haustein UF: Histologic subtyping and malignancy assessment of cutaneous squamous cell carcinoma. *Dermatol Surg* **26**:521, 2000
65. Dinehart SM et al: Immunosuppression in patients with metastatic squamous cell carcinoma from the skin. *J Dermatol Surg Oncol* **16**:271, 1990
66. Midena E et al: Treatment of conjunctival squamous cell carcinoma with topical 5-fluorouracil. *Br J Ophthalmol* **84**:268, 2000
67. Brodland DG, Zitelli JA: Surgical margins for excision of primary cutaneous squamous cell carcinoma. *J Am Acad Dermatol* **27**:241, 1992
68. Drake LA et al: Guidelines of care for Mohs micrographic surgery. American Academy of Dermatology. *J Am Acad Dermatol* **33**:271, 1995
69. Hashi N, et al: The role of radiotherapy in treating squamous cell carcinoma of the external auditory canal, especially in early stages of disease. *Radiother Oncol* **56**:221, 2000
70. Turner RJ et al: A retrospective study of outcome of Mohs' micrographic surgery for cutaneous squamous cell carcinoma using formalin fixed sections. *Br J Dermatol* **142**:752, 2000
71. Veness MJ et al: Squamous cell carcinoma of the lip. Patterns of relapse and outcome: Reporting the Westmead Hospital experience, 1980–1997. *Australas Radiol* **45**:195, 2001
72. Salasche SJ, Cheney ML: Recognition and management of the high-risk cutaneous squamous cell carcinoma. *Curr Probl Dermatol* **5**:141, 1993
73. Cartei G et al: Oral 5-fluorouracil in squamous cell carcinoma of the skin in the aged. *Am J Clin Oncol* **23**:181, 2000
74. Williams LS et al: Perineural spread of cutaneous squamous and basal cell carcinoma: CT and MR detection and its impact on patient management and prognosis. *Int J Radiat Oncol Biol Phys* **49**:1061, 2001
75. Weisberg NK et al: Combined sentinel lymphadenectomy and Mohs micrographic surgery for high-risk cutaneous squamous cell carcinoma. *J Am Acad Dermatol* **43**:483, 2000
76. Zitsch RP 3rd et al: Cervical lymph node metastases and squamous cell carcinoma of the lip. *Head Neck* **21**:447, 1999

CHAPTER 81

John A. Carucci
David J. Leffell

Basal Cell Carcinoma

Basal cell carcinoma (BCC) is a malignant neoplasm derived from nonkeratinizing cells that originate in the basal layer of the epidermis. If left untreated, BCC can become invasive and may result in substantial tissue damage. Metastasis is a rare event.

EPIDEMIOLOGY

BCC is the most common cancer in humans. It is estimated that 900,000 new cases occur per year in the United States.[1] BCC is more common in elderly individuals, but is becoming increasingly common in people younger than 50 years of age.[2,3] The malignancy accounts for approximately 75 percent of all nonmelanoma skin cancers and almost 25 percent of all cancers diagnosed in the United States.[4] The tumor characteristically develops on sun-exposed skin of lighter skinned individuals with 30 percent occurring on the nose.[3] Men are affected slightly more often than are women. Levi et al. report that the incidence of BCC rose steadily in the Swiss Canton of Vaud between 1976 and 1998 to levels in males of 75.1/100,000 and in females 66.1/100,000.[5] A recent study of nonmelanoma skin cancers in Aruba supports these findings.[6] In that study, BCC was the most common type of skin cancer diagnosed between 1980 and 1995. Tumors were more frequent in patients older than 60 years of age and 57% were in men. The greatest percentage of cases occurred on the nose (20.9 percent) followed by other sites on the face (17.7 percent).

Risk factors for BCC have been well characterized and include ultraviolet light (UVL) exposure, light hair and eye color, northern European ancestry, and inability to tan.[7] Although some investigators suggested a potential link between BCC and internal malignancies, this relationship remains to be defined.[8,9] Bower et al.[10] recently reported that individuals with BCC had a threefold increased risk for melanoma, but no increased risk for any other type of cancer. Conversely, an increased risk for BCC has been reported in patients with a history of melanoma.[11]

ETIOLOGY AND PATHOGENESIS

The pathogenesis of BCC involves exposure to UVL, particularly the ultraviolet B (UVB) spectrum (290 to 320 nm) that induces mutations in tumor-suppressor genes.[3,7,12–14] Other studies indicate that intermittent brief holiday exposures may place patients at higher risk than occupational exposure.[15] Ramani and Bennett reported a significant increased incidence of BCCs in World War II servicemen stationed in the Pacific theater as compared to those stationed in Europe.[16] This suggests that several months or years of intense exposure to UVL may have deleterious long-term effects. Other factors that appear to be involved in the pathogenesis include mutations in regulatory genes,[17] exposure to ionizing radiation,[18] and alterations in immunosurveillance.[14]

The observation that BCC incidence is increased following radiation therapy (XRT) for conditions including neuroblastoma, tinea capitis, and acne vulgaris, suggests a role for this type of radiation in the etiology of some forms of this cancer.[18,19] Although XRT is no longer used in the treatment of benign conditions, it is notable that the latency period between treatment and recurrence may be as long as 40 years. Ron et al.[19] studied more than 10,000 patients radiated for tinea capitis and found a fourfold increase in skin cancers over nonirradiated controls. BCC accounted for 98 percent of tumors observed in this study.

The propensity to develop multiple BCCs may be inherited. Included among heritable conditions predisposing to the development of this epithelial cancer are the nevoid basal call carcinoma syndrome (NBCCS),[20] Bazex syndrome,[21] Rombo syndrome,[22] and unilateral basal cell nevus syndrome.[23] Patients with NBCCS may develop hundreds of BCCs and may exhibit a broad nasal root, borderline intelligence, jaw cysts, palmar pits, and multiple skeletal abnormalities (see Chap. 82). Recent studies indicate an association with mutations in the *PTCH* regulatory gene, which functions as a tumor-suppressor gene.[24] Mutations in the same gene, have been identified in sporadic nonfamilial BCC.

Bazex syndrome is transmitted in an x-linked dominant fashion.[21] Patients present with multiple BCCs, follicular atrophoderma, dilated follicular ostia with ice-pick scars, hypotrichosis, and hypohidrosis. In contrast, Rombo syndrome is transmitted in an autosomal dominant fashion.[22] Patients present with vermiculate atrophoderma, milia, hypertrichosis, trichoepitheliomas, BCCs, and peripheral vasodilation. Hypohidrosis is not a feature of Rombo syndrome. Linear basal cell nevus has been described including congenital, unilateral comedones and epidermoid cysts with basal cell proliferations that are thought to be basaloid follicular hamartomas.[23]

The role of the immune system in the pathogenesis of skin cancer is not completely understood. Immunosuppressed patients with lymphoma or leukemia,[25] and patients who have received an organ transplant,[26] have a marked increase in the incidence of squamous cell carcinoma (SCC), but only a slight increase in the incidence of BCC. Interestingly, Bastiaens et al.[27] found that transplant recipients developed more BCCs on the trunk and arms than did nonimmunosuppressed patients. Patients with HIV develop BCCs at the same rate as immunocompetent individuals, based on similar risk factors.[28] Immunosuppressed chronic alcoholics tend to develop infiltrative BCCs with increased frequency.[29]

A potential link between UVL and immunosurveillance has been suggested by Nickoloff and colleagues who demonstrated that UVL-induced BCC tumor cells express Fas ligand (CD95L).[14] They further showed that these cells were associated with CD95-bearing T cells undergoing apoptosis. This represents a potential mechanism by which UVL might facilitate the avoidance by the tumor cells of cytotoxic T lymphocytes.

CLINICAL MANIFESTATIONS

Presentation

The presence of any friable, nonhealing lesion should raise the suspicion of skin cancer. Frequently, BCC is diagnosed in patients who state that the lesion bled briefly, then healed completely only to recur. BCC usually develops on sun exposed areas of the head and neck but can occur anywhere on the body. Features include translucency, ulceration, telangiectasias, and the presence of a rolled border. Characteristics may vary according to clinical subtypes, which include nodular, superficial, morpheaform, and pigmented BCC and fibroepithelioma of Pinkus.

Basal Cell Carcinoma Subtypes

NODULAR BCC Nodular BCC is the most common clinical subtype of BCC (Fig. 81-1*A* and *B*). It occurs most commonly on the sun-exposed areas of the head and neck[30] and appears as a translucent papule or nodule depending on duration. There are usually telangiectasias and often a rolled border. Larger lesions with central necrosis are referred to by the historical term of "rodent ulcer" (Fig. 81-2). The differential diagnosis of nodular BCC includes dermal nevus and amelanotic melanoma.

PIGMENTED BCC Pigmented BCC is a subtype of nodular BCC that exhibits increased melanization. Pigmented BCC appears as a hyperpigmented, translucent papule which may also be eroded (Fig. 81-3). The differential diagnosis includes nodular melanoma.

SUPERFICIAL BCC Superficial BCC occurs most commonly on the trunk[30] and appears as an erythematous patch (often well-demarcated) that resembles eczema (Fig. 81-4). An isolated patch of eczema that does not respond to treatment should raise suspicion for superficial BCC.

MORPHEAFORM BCC Morpheaform BCC is an aggressive growth variant of BCC with a distinct clinical and histologic appearance. Lesions of morpheaform BCC may have an ivory white appearance and may resemble a scar (Fig. 81-5). Thus, the appearance of scar tissue in the absence of trauma or previous surgical procedure or the appearance of atypical appearing scar tissue at the site of a previously treated skin lesion should alert the clinician to the possibility of morpheaform BCC and the need for biopsy.

FIBROEPITHELIOMA OF PINKUS Fibroepithelioma of Pinkus (FEP) classically presents as a pink papule, usually on the lower back.[31] It may be difficult to distinguish from amelanotic melanoma.

BIOLOGICAL BEHAVIOR

Local Invasion

The greatest danger of BCC results from local invasion. In general, BCC is a slow-growing tumor that invades locally rather than metastasizes.[32] The rate of doubling is estimated to be between 6 months and 1 year.[32]

FIGURE 81-1

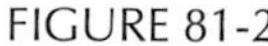

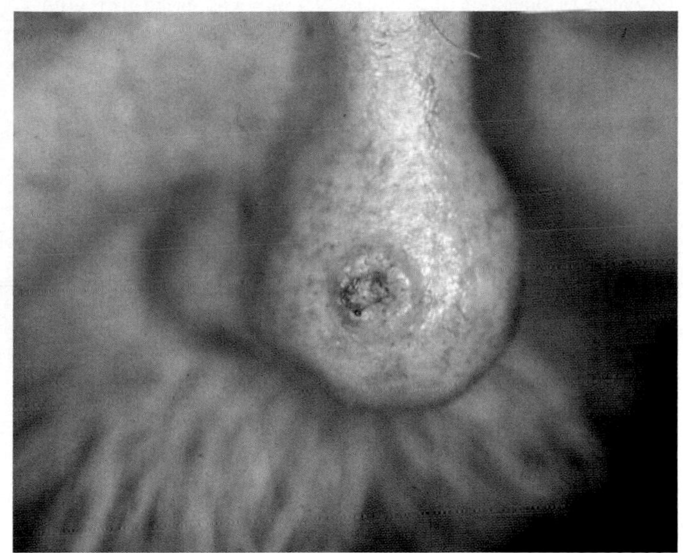

A.

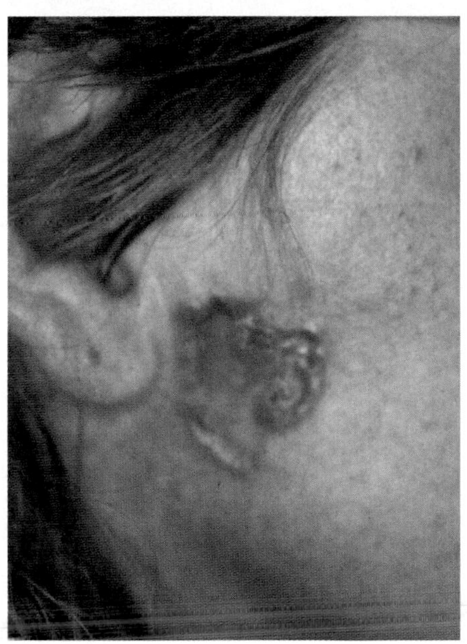

B.

A. Basal cell carcinoma, nodular type. *B.* An ulcerated nodular basal cell carcinoma.

If left untreated, the tumor will progress to invade subcutaneous tissue, muscle, and even bone. Anatomic fusion planes appear to provide a low resistance path for tumor progression. Tumors along the nasofacial or retroauricular sulcus may be extensive. In one informative case, a patient documented the progression of his own tumor with photographs over a 27-year period.[33] The lesion, which encompassed an entire side of the face, including the maxillary sinus, apparently doubled over a 10-year period and grew rapidly in the 2 years prior to admission. This scenario occurs in the context of physical or psychiatric disability that interferes with judgment or access to health care. In another case,[34] a 35-cm BCC on the back of a 65-year-old man recurred after wide local excision and XRT, and compressed the spinal cord. There have been two other reported cases of BCC causing spinal cord compression. Extension to the central nervous system (CNS) has been described by Schroeder et al.[35] who report cerebral invasion from BCC on the scalp in a 51-year-old woman 4 years after resection of a recurrent parietal BCC that had extended to bone and dura mater.

FIGURE 81-2

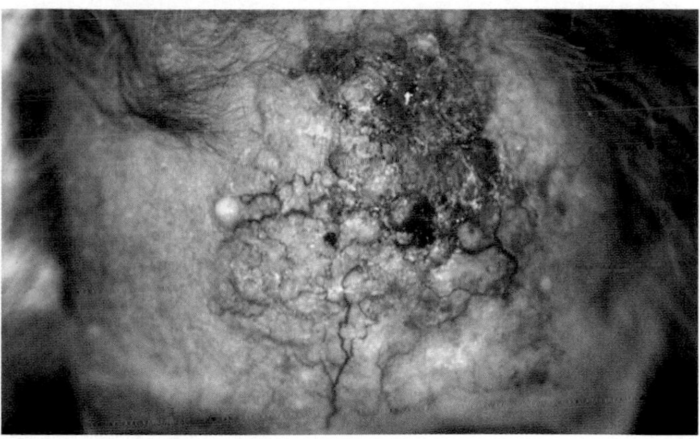

Basal cell carcinoma, rodent ulcer type. Extensive local tissue destruction is seen in this lesion.

Perineural Invasion

Perineural invasion is uncommon in BCC and occurs most often in histologically aggressive or recurrent lesions. In one series, Niazi and Lamberty identified perineural invasion in less than 0.2% of cases.[36] In that series, perineural BCC was seen most often with recurrent tumors located in the preauricular and malar areas. Ratner et al.[37] showed a higher incidence in their study (3.8 percent). Perineural spread may

FIGURE 81-3

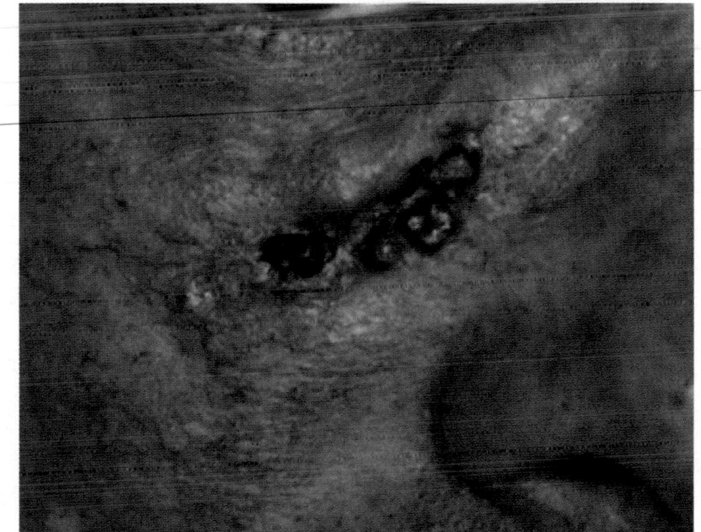

Pigmented basal cell carcinoma. This lesion may resemble a malignant melanoma.

FIGURE 81-4

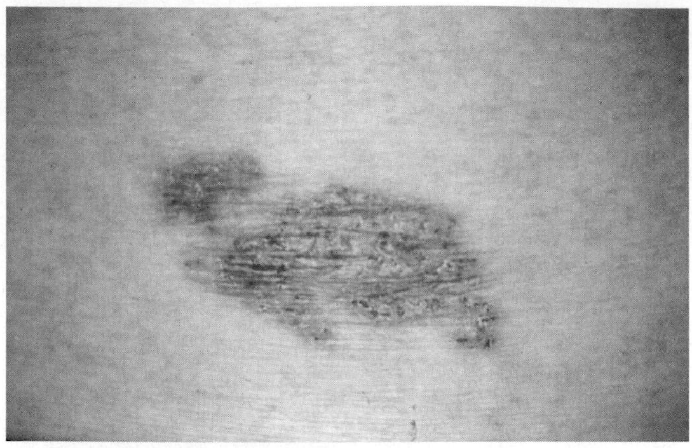

Superficial basal cell carcinoma. The well-demarcated plaque with a rolled edge characteristically occurs on the trunk.

present with pain, paresthesias, weakness, or paralysis. Cranial nerve involvement has been reported.[38] The presence of focal neurologic symptoms at the site of a previously treated skin cancer should raise concern about nerve involvement.

Metastasis

Metastasis of BCC occurs only rarely with rates varying from 0.0028 to 0.55 percent.[39–41] Involvement of lymph nodes and lungs were most common. Domarus et al.[42] reported five cases of metastatic BCC in which perineural or intravascular invasion had been noted in three of the five cases. Squamous differentiation was not observed in the primary tumors in the cases they presented, but was noted in two of five cases of metastatic cancer. Overall, squamous differentiation was present in 15 percent of the primary or metastatic tumors from the 170 cases reviewed. Perineural invasion was present in 5 of 12 cases of metastatic BCC reported by Lo et al.[43]

FIGURE 81-5

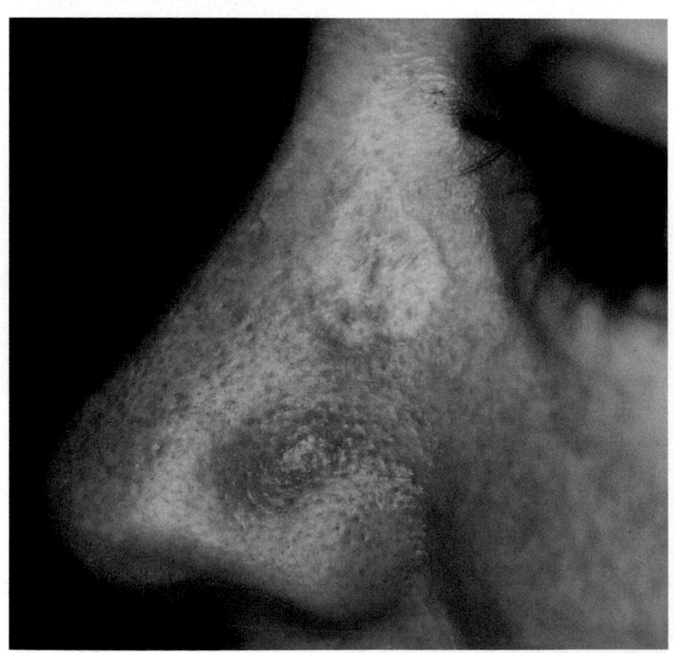

Morpheaform basal cell carcinoma. This lesion may resemble a scar and may be difficult to detect. It may, therefore, attain a considerable size before diagnosis.

DIAGNOSIS

Diagnosis of BCC is accomplished by accurate interpretation of the skin biopsy. The preferred biopsy methods include shave biopsy, which is often sufficient, and punch biopsy. The use of a sterilized razor blade, which can be precisely manipulated by the operator to adjust the depth of the biopsy is often superior to the use of a no. 15 scalpel for shave biopsies. A punch biopsy may be useful for flat lesions of morpheaform BCC or for diagnosis of recurrent BCC occurring in a scar.

HISTOPATHOLOGY

Histopathology varies somewhat with subtype, but most BCCs share some common histologic features.[44] The malignant basal cells have large nuclei and relatively little cytoplasm. Although the nuclei are large they may not appear atypical. Usually, mitotic figures are absent. Frequently, retraction of stroma from tumor islands is present, creating peritumoral lacunae that are helpful in histopathologic diagnosis.

Nodular BCC

Nodular BCC accounts for half of all BCCs and is characterized by nodules of large, basophilic cells and stromal retraction (Fig. 81-6).[44] The term micronodular BCC is used to describe tumors with multiple microscopic nodules less than 15 μm in size.

Pigmented BCC

Pigmented BCC shows histologic features similar to nodular BCC but with the addition of melanin.[44] Approximately 75 percent of BCCs contain melanocytes but only 25 percent contain large amounts of melanin. The melanocytes are interspersed between tumor cells and contain numerous melanin granules in their cytoplasm and dendrites. Although the tumor cells contain little melanin, numerous melanophages populate the stroma surrounding the tumor.

Superficial BCC

Superficial BCC is characterized microscopically by buds of malignant cells extending into the dermis from the basal layer of the epidermis.[44] The peripheral cell layer shows palisading. There may be epidermal atrophy and dermal invasion is usually minimal. This histologic subtype is encountered most often on the trunk and extremities, but may also appear on the head and neck. There may be a chronic inflammatory infiltrate in the upper dermis.

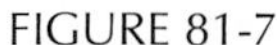

FIGURE 81-6

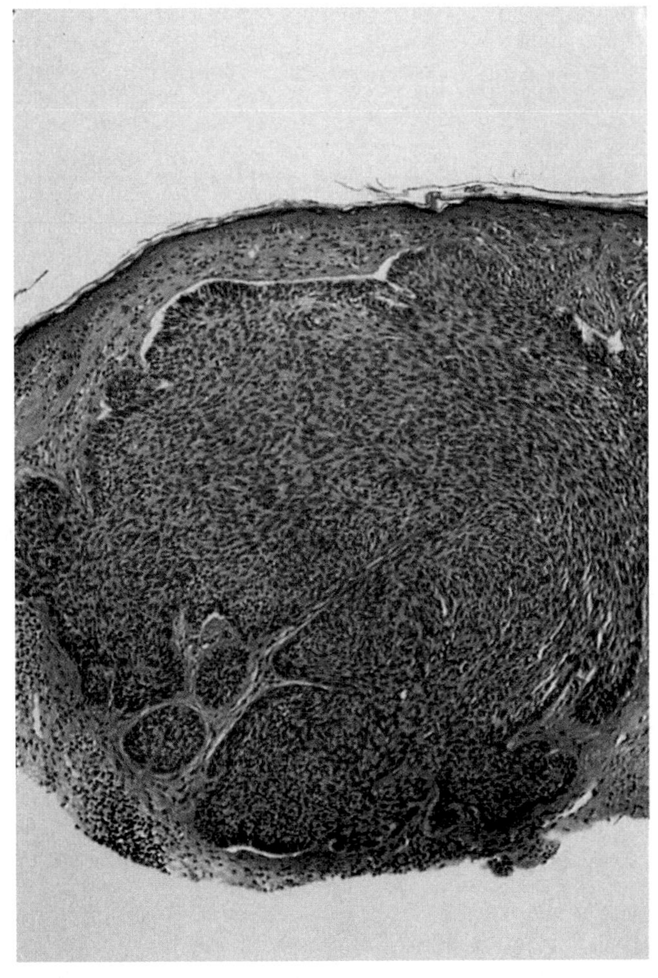

Nodular basal cell carcinoma. Palisading is evident at the periphery of tumor nodules.

FIGURE 81-7

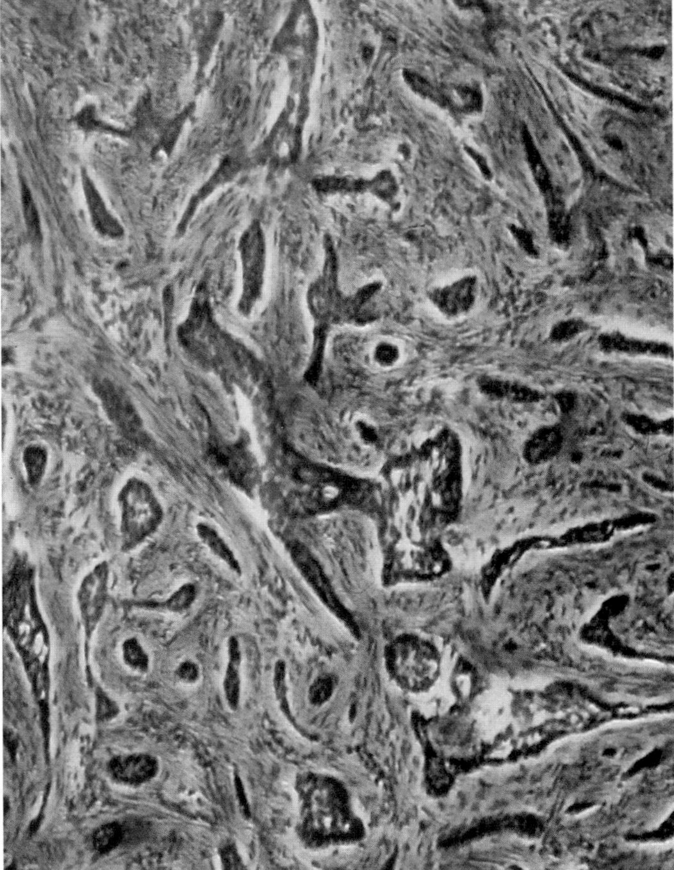

Infiltrative basal cell carcinoma. Small, spiky groups of cells are suggestive of aggressive behavior.

Morpheaform BCC

Morpheaform or infiltrative BCC consists of strands of tumor cells embedded within a dense fibrous stroma.[44] Tumor cells are closely packed and in some cases, only one cell thick. Strands of tumor extend deeply into the dermis. The cancer is often larger than the clinical appearance indicates (Fig. 81-7). Recurrent BCC may also demonstrate infiltrating bands and nests of cancer cells embedded within the fibrous stroma of scar (Fig. 81-8).

Fibroepithelioma of Pinkus

In FEP, long strands of interwoven basiloma cells are embedded in fibrous stroma.[31] Histologically, FEP shows features of reticulated seborrheic keratoses and superficial BCC.

TREATMENT

Management is guided by anatomic location and histology. Approaches include Mohs micrographic surgery (MMS), standard surgical excision, destruction by various modalities, and topical chemotherapy. The best chance to achieve cure is through adequate treatment of primary BCC because recurrent tumors are more likely to recur and to cause further local destruction.

Mohs Micrographic Surgery (see Chap. 279)

MMS offers superior histologic analysis of tumor margins while permitting maximal conservation of tissue, when compared to standard excisional surgery.[45] In a series reviewed by Rowe et al., the recurrence rate for primary BCCs treated by MMS was approximately 1 percent.[46] This was superior to other modalities including standard excision (10 percent), curettage and desiccation (C&D) (7.7 percent), XRT (8.7 percent), and cryotherapy (7.5 percent). Recurrent BCC treated by MMS recurred with a rate of 5.6 percent, which was again superior to other modalities including excision (17.6 percent), XRT (9.8 percent), and C&D (40 percent). MMS is the treatment of choice for morpheaform, poorly delineated, incompletely removed, and otherwise high-risk primary BCC. It is the preferred treatment for recurrent BCC[47] and for any BCC that occurs at a site where tissue conservation is desired. MMS is particularly useful in high-risk anatomic sites including the embryonic fusion planes represented by the nasofacial junction and retroauricular sulcus (Table 81-1).

FIGURE 81-8

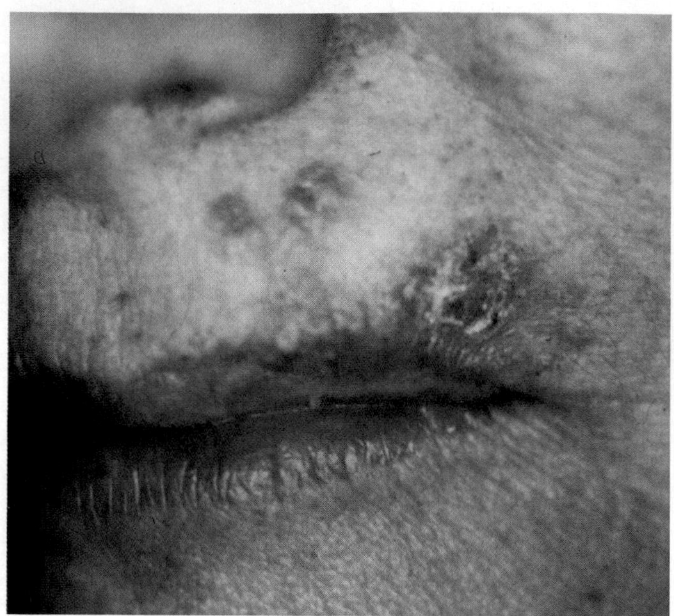

A.

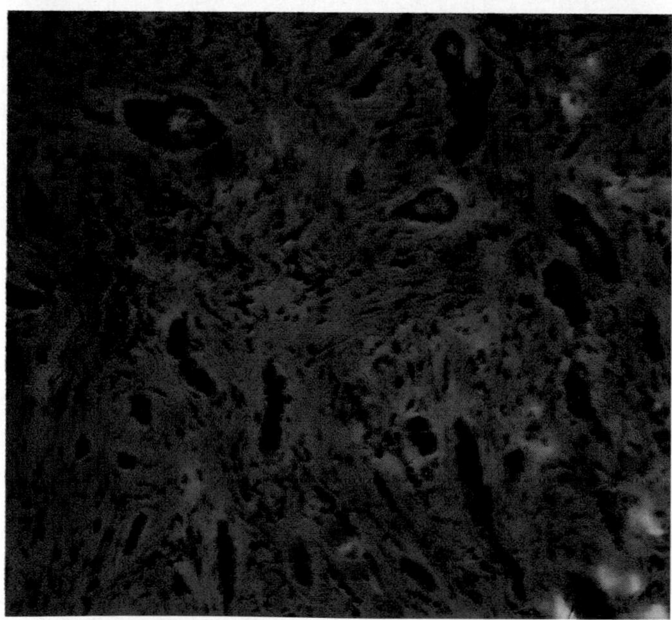

B.

Recurrent basal cell carcinoma. *A.* Recurrence within a scar may be difficult to detect clinically and may be widely infiltrative. *B.* Recurrent basal cell carcinoma demonstrates deeply infiltrative nests of tumor cells.

Standard Excision

Compared with nonexcisional techniques, standard surgical excision offers the advantage of histologic evaluation of the removed specimen. Although standard excision is appropriate for many BCCs, cure rates for standard excisional surgery are inferior to MMS in cases of primary morpheaform BCC, recurrent BCC, and tumors located in high-risk anatomic sites.[46,47] Wolf and Zitelli[48] demonstrated that margins of 4 mm were adequate in 95 percent of nonmorpheaform BCC less than 2 cm in diameter when treated by standard excision. Johnson et al.[49] reported a 96.7 percent cure rate when the excision included a 2-mm margin beyond the area defined by curettage. Tumor was present in 64 of 403 curette margins and in 12 of 403 excision margins. The histologic subtype was aggressive in 11 of 12 cases with positive excision margins. Margins of 5 mm are necessary for primary morpheaform BCC or recurrent BCC. Excision of primary BCC should extend to fat to ensure adequate tumor removal.

TABLE 81-1

Indications for Mohs Micrographic Surgery in Basal Cell Carcinoma

Recurrent tumor
Primary tumor
- With aggressive histologic pattern
- In site with high risk of recurrence (perioral, periorbital, nasolabial, nasal ala)
- >2 cm diameter
- With ill-defined clinical margin
- Where tissue conservation is important (nasal tip and alae, lips, eyelid, fingers and toes, genitalia)

Curettage and Desiccation

C&D is one of the most frequently used treatment modalities for BCC. That C&D is operator dependent was shown by Kopf et al., who identified a significant difference in cure rate between patients treated by private practitioners (94.3 percent) and those treated by residents (81.2 percent).[50] Spiller and Spiller showed a cure rate of 97 percent in 233 patients.[51] Cure rate decreased as a function of primary lesion size: for lesions less than 1.0 cm the cure rate was 98.8 percent; 95.5; for lesions between 1.0 and 2.0 cm; and 84 percent for lesions greater than 2.0 cm. Recurrences were noted most often on the forehead, temple, ears, nose, and shoulders. C&D is not recommended for large primary BCC, morpheaform BCC, or recurrent BCC.

Cryosurgery

Cryosurgery is another destructive modality that has been used in the treatment of BCC.[52] Two freeze-thaw cycles with a tissue temperature of –50°C (–58°F) are required to destroy BCC. In addition, a margin of clinically normal tissue must be destroyed to eradicate subclinical extension. Cryosurgery lacks the benefit of histologic confirmation of tumor removal. Kuflik and Gage[53] reported 99 percent cure rates in 628 patients followed for 5 years. Complications of cryosurgery may include hypertrophic scarring and postinflammatory pigmentary changes. Another serious potential adverse outcome is tumor recurrence obscured by fibrous scar tissue. Any recent change in a cryosurgery scar after normal healing is completed should raise the suspicion of recurrent BCC.

Topical Treatment

IMIQUIMOD Imiquimod is a recent addition to the nonsurgical options for treating BCC. It is a biologic response modifier that elicits local cytokine production including interferon (IFN)-α and interleukin (IL)-12. It is currently indicated for the treatment of condyloma. Beutner et al.[54] showed clearing of BCC with 10 to 16 weeks of treatment. In a phase II study by Marks et al., clearance rates of 69.7 percent, 73.3 percent, 87.9 percent, and 100 percent were achieved with once daily application three times per week, twice daily application three times per week, and once daily and twice daily application of imiquimod over 6 weeks.[55] Severe local reactions, including erythema, edema, pain, vesicles, ulceration, and scabbing, were observed frequently (up to 100 percent with twice daily treatment). Importantly, no patients discontinued therapy. Follow-up studies are necessary to determine the correct role of this modality.

5-FLUOROURACIL 5-Fluorouracil (5-FU), a topically applied chemotherapeutic agent used in the treatment of actinic keratoses, has also been used to treat BCCs. In one series, Epstein showed a 5-year recurrence rate of 21 percent, which was reduced to 6 percent when curettage was performed initially.[56] 5-FU is metabolized by dihydropyrimidine dehydrogenase (DHD) and is contraindicated in patients deficient in that enzyme.[57] The use of 5-FU to treat BCC should be carefully considered and should include an evaluation of the risk of recurrence and treatment failure.

PHOTODYNAMIC THERAPY Photodynamic therapy (PDT) involves the activation of a photosensitizing drug by visible light to produce activated oxygen species that destroy the constituent cancer cells.[58] Exogenous δ-aminolevulinic acid increases intracellular production of the endogenous photosensitizer protoporphyrin type IX, which preferentially accumulates in tumor cells. Morton et al.[59] reported an 88 percent initial clearance of 40 large (>2 cm) BCCs after 1 to 3 treatments. The range of follow up was between 12 and 60 months. Clearance rates of 95 percent were reported by Varma et al. when tumors larger than 1.5 cm were excluded.[60]

RADIATION THERAPY In cases in which surgery is contraindicated, XRT can be considered. XRT may be useful in the treatment of primary BCC or in cases where postsurgical margins are positive for cancer.[61] Advantages include minimal patient discomfort and avoidance of an invasive procedure in a patient unwilling or unable to undergo surgery. Potential disadvantages include lack of histologic verification of tumor removal, prolonged treatment course, cosmesis that may worsen over time, and predisposition to aggressive and extensive recurrences. Local control rates of 93 to 97 percent have been reported;[62] however, cosmesis has been rated inferior to results achieved surgically.[63]

SPECIAL MANAGEMENT ISSUES

Incompletely Excised Basal Cell Carcinoma

Based on data from the 1960s suggesting that 50 to 70 percent of incompletely excised BCCs do not recur, some physicians adopted a "wait and see" approach.[64] In some cases, flap and graft repair may have been performed prior to confirmation of negative margins, thus distorting the anatomy. This confounds identification of positive margins for definitive treatment. Incomplete resection was addressed by Robinson and Fisher,[65] who reported on 994 consecutive patients referred for treatment of recurrent BCC that had been incompletely excised. Of these, only 32 were referred for MMS for complete tumor removal at the time the original operating surgeon received the pathologic confirmation of positive excision margins. Of the remaining 962 recurrent BCCs, the nose was the most common anatomic site (43 percent) and flap repair was the most common form of reconstruction (52 percent). Based on the potentially lengthy interval to definitive therapy for recurrence, it seems prudent to recommend MMS for the treatment of incompletely excised BCC. Patients unable to undergo reexcision should be evaluated for XRT.

Neurotropic Basal Cell Carcinoma

Perineural invasion by BCC is a rare event (<0.2 percent).[36] When perineural invasion is detected, every effort should be made to clear the tumor, preferably by MMS. We suggest that patients with microscopic evidence of perineural invasion be evaluated for adjunctive XRT after surgery. Control rates of 50 percent were reported by McCord et al. in patients with gross perineural disease treated with XRT alone or in combination with surgery.[66] Five-year control rates of 78 percent were achieved in patients with microscopic perineural disease treated by XRT alone or in combination with surgery.[67]

Metastatic Basal Cell Carcinoma

Although exceedingly rare, the possibility of metastatic disease exists and may need to be addressed.[32,42,43] If nodal disease is suspected on surgical exam, lymph node biopsy and imaging studies, as well as evaluation by medical and surgical oncologists, are indicated. Suspicion for distant metastatic disease must be followed up with appropriate imaging studies and consultation. Platinum-based chemotherapy has been used with modest results in metastatic BCC.[68]

COURSE AND PROGNOSIS

When treated appropriately the prognosis for most patients with BCC is excellent. Control rates as high as 99 percent have been achieved by MMS.[46] Although tumor control rates for primary tumors are high, patients must be monitored for recurrence and development of new primary BCCs. The risk for development of a second primary BCC ranges from 36 to 50 percent.[69] We recommend periodic full-body skin examinations and counseling about sun protection for any patient with a history of BCC. This is especially important because patients with a history of BCC are at increased risk for melanoma.

The prognosis for patients with recurrent BCC is still favorable, although recurrent tumors are more likely to recur again and to behave aggressively. Patients with a history of recurrent disease must be monitored more frequently for the development of further recurrences and new primary tumors. For the rare patient with metastatic disease prognosis is poor with mean survival of 8 to 10 months from diagnosis.

REFERENCES

1. Miller DLW, Weinstock MA: Nonmelanoma skin cancer in the United States: Incidence. *J Am Acad Dermatol* **30**:744, 1994
2. Roudier-Pujol C et al: Basal cell carcinoma in young adults: Not more aggressive than in older patients. *Dermatology* **199**:119, 1999
3. Gloster HM Jr, Brodland DG: The epidemiology of skin cancer. *Dermatol Surg* **22**:217, 1996
4. Strom SS, Yamamura Y: Epidemiology of nonmelanoma skin cancer. *Clin Plast Surg* **24**:627, 1997
5. Levi F et al: Trends in skin cancer incidence in Vaud: An update, 1976–1998. *Eur J Cancer Prev* **10**:371, 2001
6. Kennedy C, Bajdik CD: Descriptive epidemiology of skin cancer in Aruba: 1980–1995. *Int J Dermatol* **40**:169, 2001
7. Van Dam R et al: Risk factors basal cell carcinoma of the skin in men: Results from the health professionals follow up study. *Am J Epidemiol* **150**:459, 1999
8. Levi F et al: Incidence of invasive cancers following basal cell skin cancer. *Am J Epidemiol* **135**:722, 1998
9. Karagas MR et al: Occurrence of other cancers among patients with prior basal cell and squamous cell skin cancer. *Cancer Epidemiol Biomarkers Prev* **7**:157, 1998
10. Bower CPR et al: Basal cell carcinoma and risk of subsequent malignancies: A cancer registry based study in southwest England. *J Am Acad Dermatol* **42**:988, 2000
11. Kroumpouzos G et al: Risk of basal and squamous cell carcinoma in persons with prior cutaneous melanoma. *Dermatol Surg* **26**:547, 2000

12. Lindgren G et al: Basal cell carcinoma of the eyelids and solar ultraviolet radiation exposure. *Br J Ophthalmol* **82**:1412, 1998
13. Gailani MR et al: Relationship between sunlight exposure and a key genetic alteration in basal cell carcinoma [see comments]. *J Natl Cancer Inst* **88**:349, 1996
14. Gutierrez-Steil C et al: Sunlight-induced basal cell carcinoma tumor cells and ultraviolet-B–irradiated psoriatic plaques express Fas ligand (CD95L). *J Clin Invest* **101**:33, 1998
15. Naldi L et al: Host-related and environmental risk factors for cutaneous basal cell carcinoma: Evidence from an Italian case control study. *J Am Acad Dermatol* **42**:446, 2000
16. Ramani ML, Bennett RG: High prevalence of skin cancer in World War II servicemen stationed in the Pacific theater. *J Am Acad Dermatol* **28**:733, 1993
17. Gailani MR et al: The role of the human homologue of *Drosophila* patched in sporadic basal cell carcinomas [see comments]. *Nat Genet* **14**:78, 1996
18. Karagas MR et al: Risk of basal cell and squamous cell skin cancers after ionizing radiation therapy. For The Skin Cancer Prevention Study Group. *J Natl Cancer Inst* **88**:1848, 1996
19. Ron E et al: Radiation induced carcinomas of the head and neck. *Radiat Res* **125**:318, 1991
20. Gorlin RJ: Nevoid basal cell carcinoma syndrome. *Dermatol Clin* **13**:113, 1995
21. Goeteyn M et al: The Bazex-Dupre-Christol syndrome. *Arch Dermatol* **130**:337, 1994
22. Ashinoff R et al: Rombo syndrome: A second case report and review. *J Am Acad Dermatol* **28**:1011, 1993
23. Bleiberg J, Brodkin RH: Linear basal cell nevus with comedones. *Arch Dermatol* **100**:187, 1969
24. Wicking C et al: Mutations of the human homolog of *Drosophila* patched in the nevoid basal cell carcinoma syndrome. *Cell* **85**(6):841, 1996
25. Ramsay HM et al: Multiple basal cell carcinomas in a patient with acute myeloid leukaemia and chronic lymphocytic leukaemia. *Clin Exp Dermatol* **24**:281, 1999
26. Espana A et al: Skin cancer in heart transplant recipients. *J Am Acad Dermatol* **32**:458, 1995
27. Bastiaens MT et al: Differences in age, site distribution, and sex between nodular and superficial basal cell carcinoma indicate different types of tumors. *J Invest Dermatol* **110**:880, 1998
28. Lobo DV et al: Nonmelanoma skin cancers and infection with the human immunodeficiency virus. *Arch Dermatol* **128**:623, 1992
29. Oram Y et al: Histologic patterns of basal cell carcinoma based upon patient immunostatus. *Dermatol Surg* **21**:611, 1995
30. McCormack C et al: Differences in age and body site distribution of the histological subtypes of basal cell carcinoma. A possible indicator of differing causes. *Arch Dermatol* **133**:593, 1997
31. Pinkus H: Epithelial and fibroepithelial tumors. *Arch Dermatol* **91**:24, 1963
32. Miller SJ: Biology of basal cell carcinoma (Part I). *J Am Acad Dermatol* **24**:1, 1991
33. Sherman JE, Talmor M: Slow progression and sequential documentation of a giant basal cell carcinoma of the face. *Surgery* **130**:90, 2001
34. Fogarty GB, Ainslie J: Recurrent basal cell carcinoma causing spinal cord compression. *Aust N Z J Surg* **71**:129, 2001
35. Schroeder M et al: Extensive cerebral invasion of a basal cell carcinoma of the scalp. *Eur J Surg Oncol* **27**:510, 2001
36. Niazi ZB, Lamberty BG: Perineural infiltration in basal cell carcinomas. *Br J Plast Surg* **46**:156, 1993
37. Ratner D et al: Perineural spread of basal cell carcinomas treated with Mohs micrographic surgery. *Cancer* **88**:1605, 2000
38. Carlson KC, Roenigk RK: Know your anatomy: Perineural involvement of basal and squamous cell carcinoma on the face. *J Dermatol Surg Oncol* **16**:827, 1990
39. Raszewski RL, Guyuron B: Long-term survival following nodal metastases from basal cell carcinoma. *Ann Plast Surg* **24**:170, 1990
40. Christian MM et al: Metastatic basal cell carcinoma presenting as unilateral lymphedema. *Dermatol Surg* **24**:1151, 1998
41. Berti JJ, Sharata HH: Metastatic basal cell carcinoma to the lung. *Cutis* **63**:165, 1999
42. Domarus H, Stevens PJ: Metastatic basal cell carcinoma. *J Am Acad Dermatol* **10**:1043, 1984
43. Lo JS et al: Metastatic basal cell carcinoma: Report of twelve cases with a review of the literature [see comments]. *J Am Acad Dermatol* **24**:715, 1991
44. Rippey JJ: Why classify basal cell carcinomas? *Histopathology* **32**:393, 1998
45. Vuyk H, Lohuis PJ: Mohs micrographic surgery for facial skin cancer. *Clin Otoloaryngol* **26**:265, 2001
46. Rowe DE et al: Long-term recurrence rates in previously untreated (primary) basal cell carcinoma: Implications for patient follow-up. *J Dermatol Surg Oncol* **15**:315, 1989
47. Rowe DE et al: Mohs surgery is the treatment of choice for recurrent (previously treated) basal cell carcinoma. *J Dermatol Surg Oncol* **15**:424, 1989
48. Wolf DJ, Zitelli JA: Surgical margins for basal cell carcinoma. *Arch Dermatol* **123**:340, 1987
49. Johnson TM, Swanson NA: Combined curettage and excision: A treatment method for primary basal cell carcinoma. *J Am Acad Dermatol* **24**:613, 1991
50. Kopf AW et al: Curettage-electrodesiccation treatment of basal cell carcinomas. *Arch Dermatol* **113**:439, 1977
51. Spiller W, Spiller RF: Treatment of basal cell epithelioma by curettage and electrodesiccation. *J Am Acad Dermatol* **11**:808, 1984
52. Kuflik EG: Cryosurgery updated. *J Am Acad Dermatol*; **31**:925, 1994
53. Kuflik E, Gage AA: The five-year cure rate achieved by cryosurgery for skin cancer. *J Am Acad Dermatol* **26**:283, 1992
54. Beutner KR et al: Therapeutic response of basal cell carcinoma to the immune response modifier imiquimod 5% cream. *J Am Acad Dermatol* **41**:1002, 1999
55. Marks R et al: Imiquimod 5% cream in the treatment of superficial basal cell carcinoma: Results of a multicenter 6-week dose-response trial. *J Am Acad Dermatol* **44**:807, 2001
56. Epstein E: Fluorouracil paste treatment of thin basal cell carcinomas. *Arch Dermatol* **121**:207, 1985
57. Johnson MR et al: Life-threatening toxicity in a dihydropyrimidine dehydrogenase deficient patient after treatment with topical 5-fluorouracil. *Clin Cancer Res* **8**:2006, 1999
58. Fritsch C et al: Photodynamic therapy in dermatology. *Arch Dermatol* **134**:207, 1998
59. Morton CAWC et al: Photodynamic therapy for large or multiple patches of Bowen disease and basal cell carcinoma. *Arch Dermatol* **137**:319, 2001
60. Varma SWH et al: Bowen's disease, solar keratoses, and superficial basal cell carcinomas treated by photodynamic therapy using a large-field incoherent light source. *Br J Dermatol* **144**:567, 2001
61. Halpern JN: Radiation therapy in skin cancer. A historical perspective and current applications. *Dermatol Surg* **23**:1089, 1997
62. Morrison WHGA, Kian Ang K: Radiation therapy for nonmelanoma skin carcinomas. *Clin Plast Surg* **24**:719, 1997
63. Petit JYAM et al: Evaluation of cosmetic results of a randomized trial comparing surgery and radiotherapy in the treatment of basal cell carcinoma of the face. *Plast Reconstr Surg* **105**:2544, 2000
64. Gooding CAWG, Yatsuhashi M: Significance of marginal extension in excised basal cell carcinoma. *N Engl J Med* **273**:923, 1965
65. Robinson JKFS: Recurrent basal cell carcinoma after incomplete resection. *Arch Dermatol* **136**:1318, 2000
66. McCord MW et al. Skin cancer of the head and neck with clinical perineural invasion. *Int J Radiat Oncol Biol Phys* **47**:89, 2000
67. McCord MW et al: Skin cancer of the head and neck with incidental microscopic perineural invasion. *Int J Radiat Oncol Biol Phys* **43**:591, 1999
68. Moeholt K et al: Platinum-based cytotoxic therapy in basal cell carcinoma—A review of the literature. *Acta Oncol* **35**:677, 1996
69. Czarnecki D: The prognosis of patients with basal and squamous cell carcinoma of the skin. *Int J Dermatol* **37**:656, 1998

CHAPTER 82

Ervin Epstein, Jr.

Basal Cell Nevus Syndrome

The basal cell nevus syndrome (BCNS; nevoid basal cell carcinoma syndrome, Gorlin syndrome, [*MIM* 109400]) is a rare autosomal dominant abnormality with a panoply of phenotypic abnormalities that can be divided into developmental anomalies and postnatal tumors, especially basal cell carcinomas (BCCs).[1] Although individual aspects had been reported previously, their syndromic association was appreciated widely first in the late 1950s.[2,3] As in many dominant conditions, new mutations are common, and so patients frequently have no affected ancestors or siblings.

ETIOLOGY AND PATHOGENESIS

Genetic Abnormality[4]

The BCNS is caused by mutations in the *PATCHED1* (*PTCH1*) gene.[5,6] This gene is the human homologue of the *Drosophila patched* (*ptc*) gene, which is essential for the establishment of normal body and limb patterning in the developing fly embryo. Efforts to identify this gene began in the mid-1980s when it became apparent that (1) the appearance of BCCs in small numbers at an older age in sporadic cases and in larger numbers at a younger age in patients with BCNS is reminiscent of differences in sporadic and hereditary cases of retinoblastoma;[7] (2) BCCs follow the Knudson "two-hit" model for familial cancers; and (3) a tumor-suppressor gene important in the common sporadic BCCs might be identified by study of the rare BCNS. Numerous laboratories participated in efforts to identify the BCNS gene, and its cloning enabled verification of the prediction that the same gene is mutated in BCCs by two somatic "hits" in sporadic cases or by one somatic hit plus the inheritance of one defective allele in BCNS patients. Mutations in *PTCH1* have been identified in other sporadic tumors as well, including those known to be present in greater-than-expected numbers in BCNS patients (e.g., medulloblastomas and meningiomas). Screening has identified *PTCH1* somatic mutations in a minority of BCCs and constitutional mutations in less than 100 percent of BCNS patients, but it is likely that much or all of at least the latter "failure" is due simply to insensitivity/incompleteness of the screening methods used thus far. The *PTCH1* gene resides on chromosome 9q, and no family with BCNS has been reported in which the causative gene does not map to this site.

PTCH1 Function

The best-investigated function of the PTCH1 protein is its role as a participant in the hedgehog signaling pathway. Genetic and biochemical evidence indicates that PTCH1 protein inhibits this signaling pathway by inhibiting the function at the cell periphery of smoothened (SMO) protein and that the extracellular ligand hedgehog alleviates this inhibition. Signaling by SMO results in the activation of the GLI family (particularly GLI1 and GLI2) of transcription factors. SMO signaling proceeds through interacting proteins including the serine kinase FUSED, suppressor of FUSED, protein kinase A, and Costal 2 (no vertebrate homologue identified). Both the predicted 7-transmembrane protein structure and more direct biochemical evidence indicate that SMO can function as a G protein-coupled receptor.[8] Classically (i.e., circa mid-1990s), PTCH1 inhibition of SMO function was considered to be mediated by direct binding of PTCH1 protein to SMO protein, and, indeed, PTCH1, SMO, and hedgehog proteins all can be found bound to each other.[9,10] More recently, however (i.e., since circa 2000), the alternative view that PTCH1 protein controls SMO functioning by indirect means has gained more credence. Indeed, both PTCH1 and SMO protein appear, in large measure, not to be present at the cell surface, and abrogation of PTCH1 inhibition may be accompanied by activating changes (e.g., in phosphorylation) and translocation of SMO to the cell surface, where it is active in signaling.[11–13] Binding of hedgehog (HH) to PTCH1 protein, on the other hand, removes PTCH1 from the cell surface, with internalization of HH–PTCH1 complexes.

Activation of GLI, likely controlled in part by proteolytic processing and its inhibition and by localization to the nucleus, enhances the expression of hedgehog target genes. Clearly these include PTCH1 protein itself, so that there is a negative feedback loop in which decreased PTCH1 protein function leads to increased PTCH1 mRNA expression and, if the mRNA is of normal sequence, increased PTCH1 protein and dampening of the pathway signaling. Also upregulated are mRNA species encoding HIP (hedgehog-interacting protein, a cell surface protein that binds hedgehog protein with an avidity equal to that of PTCH1 but of currently unknown function) and GLI1. BCCs essentially all have increased mRNA for these three genes, providing evidence that hedgehog signaling dysregulation is pivotal to BCC carcinogenesis. However, it is far from certain how hedgehog signaling dysregulation causes the failure of differentiation and continued proliferation that characterize this tumor. One candidate for part of that mechanism is the upregulation of platelet-derived growth factor receptor (PDGFR)-α expression with consequent activation of ras and of the mitogen-activated protein kinase (MAPK) pathway.[14]

One paper also reports a separate and novel function of PTCH1 protein—its binding of cyclin B1.[15] This sequestration would be expected to keep the cyclin out of the nucleus, and binding of hedgehog to PTCH1 appears to prevent this interaction and hence to allow progression of the cell cycle from S to G1. Similarly, loss of PTCH1 protein function might in part abrogate the S/G2 checkpoint and help to account for cell-cycle abnormalities in BCCs.[16]

Mutations of SMO protein have been identified in approximately 10 percent of BCCs, and these mutations appear to render SMO protein resistant to PTCH1 inhibition. Indeed, experimental transfection of cells with mutant SMO sequences can transform them to a malignant phenotype.[17] This finding that BCCs may have upregulation of HH target gene expression due to mutations in either PTCH1 or in SMO argues that it is the upregulation of hedgehog signaling rather than the specific mutation that is crucial to BCC formation. Consistent with this is the finding that mutations in the gene encoding SUFU, an intracellular inhibitor of hedgehog signaling that helps keep GLI out of the nucleus, have been reported to underlie formation of medulloblastomas.[18]

The identification of these molecular abnormalities in BCCs for the first time has permitted the development of mouse models of this tumor. Previous insults to mouse skin—ultraviolet or ionizing radiation or carcinogenic chemicals—have produced papillomas and carcinomas of the squamous, but not basal cell, lineage. Models in which mice spontaneously develop BCC-like tumors include those with epidermal overexpression of hedgehog,[19] of mutant SMO,[17] or of GLI1[20] or GLI2.[21] In addition, *ptc1*+/− mice, which, like BCNS patients, have one instead of two functioning alleles of *PTCH1*, develop not only BCCs and related tumors but also develop plantar pits, medulloblastomas, and rhabdomyosarcomas, as do BCNS patients. The mouse BCCs (mimicking BCCs in BCNS patients) occur spontaneously in low numbers and in small sizes but in much higher numbers and of greater size in mice exposed to ultraviolet or ionizing radiation.[22,23]

PTCH1 normally is expressed not only postnatally but also, in vertebrates as well as in insects, during development. Experimental models with abnormalities of the hedgehog signaling pathway cause significant developmental anomalies in mice and flies. The resemblance of some of these anomalies to those characteristic of BCNS implies that aberrant prenatal activation of the hedgehog signaling pathway is a sufficient explanation for the developmental anomalies of the BCNS, even if the precise pathogenic mechanisms have yet to be elucidated.

FIGURE 82-1

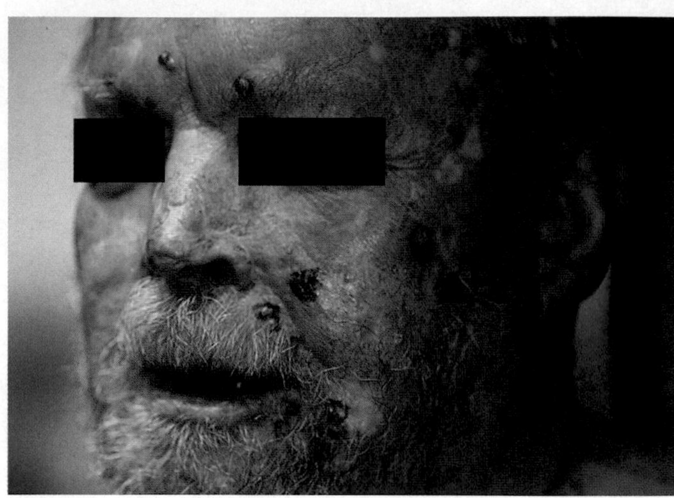

Face of man with severe scarring from growth and treatment of multiple BCCs. Note multiple outlined new BCCs despite extensive and frequent surgery.

CLINICAL FEATURES

Patients with BCNS sustain multiple abnormalities, none of which are unique to this syndrome.[1,24–26] The three abnormalities traditionally considered to be most characteristic of the syndrome are BCCs, pits of the palms and soles, and cysts of the jaw.

BCCs in patients with the BCNS cannot be distinguished individually from those in sporadic cases, which is not surprising in view of the similar pathogenesis in familial and sporadic cases. What is distinguishing is their appearance in large numbers starting at an early age. They may be banal-appearing and confused grossly with nevocytic nevi—hence the name *basal cell nevus*. They may also have a translucent, papulonodular appearance more characteristic of sporadic basal cell carcinomas and may invade locally, and even, rarely, metastasize, causing the patient's death. Although the ratio of sun-protected to sun-exposed BCCs may be higher in BCNS than in sporadic cases, sunlight clearly accelerates BCC formation in BCNS patients, and darkly pigmented BCNS patients may have few to no BCCs (Figs. 82-1 to 4).

Palmoplantar pits are small defects in the stratum corneum and may be pink or, if dirt has accumulated, dark in color (Fig. 82-5). Jaw cysts often are the first detectable abnormality, and they may be asymptomatic and therefore diagnosed only radiologically. However, they also may erode enough bone to cause pain, swelling, and loss of teeth (see Chap. 112).

Tissue overgrowth, which also is a feature of hedgehog signaling pathway activation in *Drosophila*, often is manifested by an overall body size larger than that of other family members; limbs may be particularly long, giving a marfanoid appearance, and a large head circumference (at least in probands) and frontal bossing are often described.

Table 82-1 lists the phenotypic abnormalities that have been reported often enough that they probably are true components of the syndrome. Variation in clinical severity is typical even within a single kindred, and this heterogeneity is likely due to both environmental differences (e.g., exposure to ultraviolet and ionizing radiation) and genetic background differences.

PATHOLOGY

Histologic examination cannot differentiate abnormalities that arise sporadically from those that arise in the context of BCNS.

FIGURE 82-2

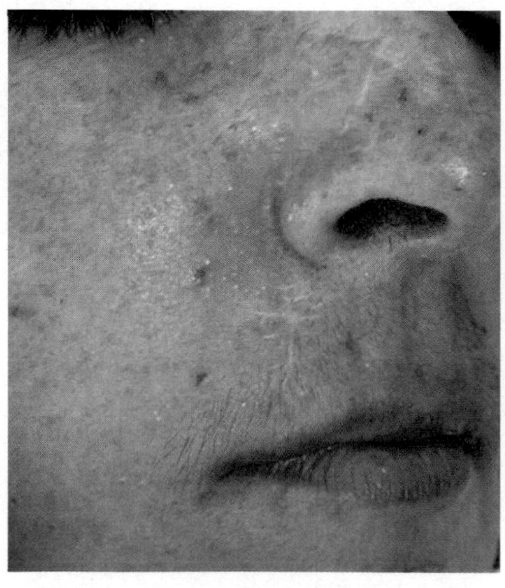

Face of woman with BCNS with less severe scarring with multiple milia.

FIGURE 82-3

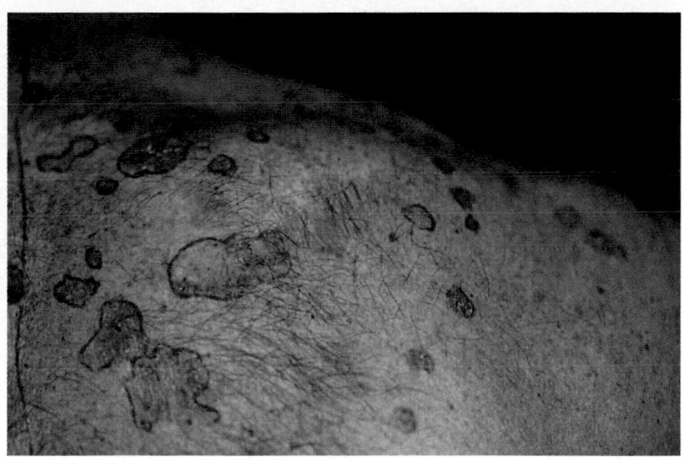

Upper back of man with BCNS with innumerable BCCs, some of which are nodular and most of which are flat, erythematous patches.

FIGURE 82-5

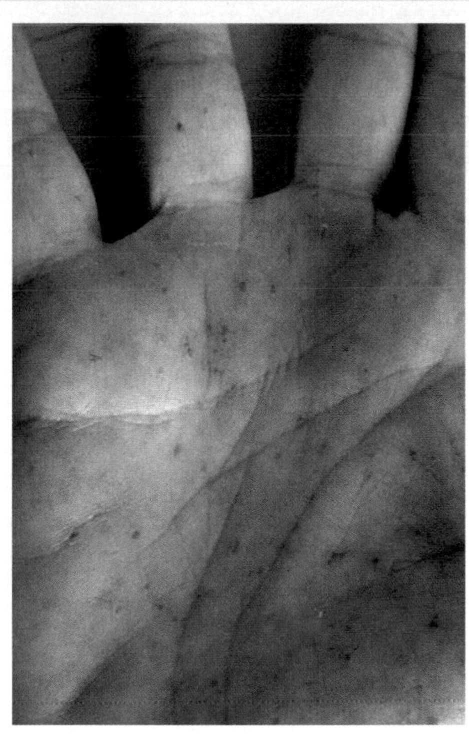

Unusually florid palmar pits in a patient with BCNS.

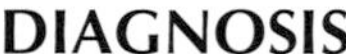

DIAGNOSIS

Because the individual abnormalities are not unique to BCNS patients, it is possible to diagnose the BCNS clinically only when multiple, typical defects are present. The severity of abnormalities may differ markedly among members of a single kindred, and diagnostic certainty may be difficult for individuals even if they belong to a kindred with known BCNS. Generally, the diagnosis is suggested to the dermatologist in a patient with multiple BCCs arising at an unexpectedly early age and in unexpectedly large numbers. Further evaluation should include (1) questions about whether other family members have had abnormalities consistent with the BCNS (although perhaps 25 to 30 percent of patients with BCNS have no affected ancestors) and whether the patient is taller and heavier than his or her relatives; (2) examination for palmoplantar pits and skin cysts and assessment of body and head size; and (3) radiologic evaluation for jaw cysts (which often appear around the start of the second decade and which frequently recur following surgery[27]), calcification of the falx (which occurs in nearly all adults with BCNS[28] and which may be present in early childhood in BCNS patients, thus suggesting the diagnosis of BCNS in patients with early onset medulloblastomas[29]), and abnormalities of the ribs, spine, and phalanges (flame-shaped lucencies), each of which are present in one-third to one-half of BCNS patients (Fig. 82-6). Kimonis and colleagues have proposed a set of major and minor criteria for presumptive diagnosis of BCNS (Table 82-2).[25] Identification of *PTCH1* gene mutations eventually should become the "gold standard" for diagnosis.

FIGURE 82-4

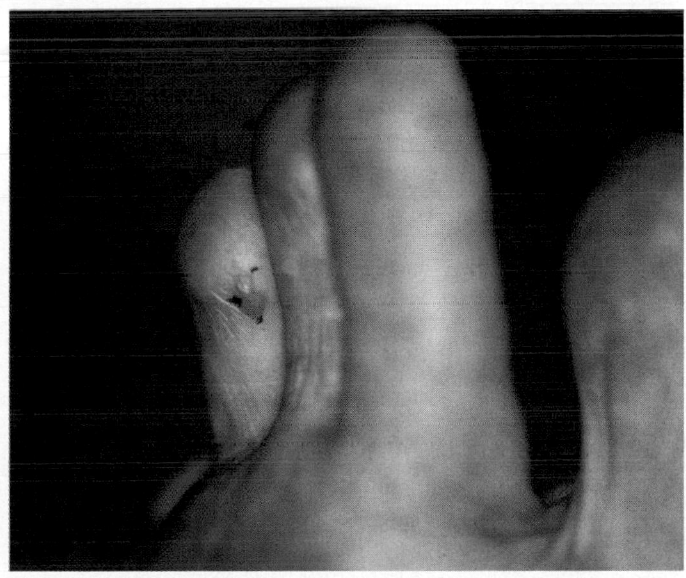

BCC on toe of a patient with BCNS, illustrating that the whole skin surface of BCNS patients is susceptible to BCC formation.

Differential Diagnosis

Several very rare syndromes that include the development of multiple BCCs have been described. These include Bazex-Dupre-Christol syndrome,[30] the Rombo syndrome,[31] and a family with BCCs, milia, and coarse, sparse hair.[32] Hair abnormalities are present in all three syndromes; a finding of interest in view of the often-repeated suggestion that BCCs arise from hair follicles rather than from interfollicular epidermis. The exact nosologic relationships among these three syndromes are uncertain, but patients with the BCNS have normal hair, and all three syndromes seem quite different from the BCNS.

Patients with chronic arsenic ingestion may have multiple BCCs; their dyschromia and lack of other phenotypic abnormalities

TABLE 82-1

Diagnostic Findings in Adults with Basal Cell Nevus Syndrome

DEVELOPMENTAL	HYPER/NEOPLASTIC
Frequency ≥ 50 percent	
Enlarged occipitofrontal circumference (macrocephaly, frontoparietal bossing, in index cases only?)	Multiple basal cell carcinomas
High-arched palate	Odontogenic keratocysts of jaws
Palmar or plantar pits	Epidermal cysts of skin
Rib anomalies (e.g., splayed, fused, partially missing, bifid)	
Spina bifida occulta of cervical or thoracic vertebrae	
Calcified diaphragma sellae (bridged sella, fused clinoids)	
Hyperpneumatization of paranasal sinuses	
Frequency 15 to 49 percent	
Calcification of tentorium cerebelli and petroclinoid ligament	Calcified ovarian fibromas
Short fourth metacarpals	Pseudocystic lytic lesion of bones (hamartomas)
Kyphoscoliosis or other vertebral anomalies	
Lumbarization of sacrum	
Narrow sloping shoulders	
Prognathism	
Pectus excavatum or carinatum	
Strabismus (exotropia)	
Frequency < 14 percent but not random	
Inguinal hernia (?)	Medulloblastoma
True ocular hypertelorism	Meningioma
Ovarian fibrosarcoma	Lymphomesenteric cyst
Marfanoid build	Cardiac fibroma
Anosmia	Fetal rhabdomyoma
Agenesis of corpus callosum	
Cyst of septum pellucidum	
Cleft lip and/or palate	
Low-pitched female voice	
Polydactyly, postaxial in hands or feet	
Sprengel deformity of scapula	
Syndactyly	
Congenital cataract, glaucoma, coloboma of iris, retina, optic nerve, medullated retinal nerve fibers	
Subcutaneous calcifications of skin (possibly underestimated frequency)	
Minor kidney malformations	
Hypogonadism in male subjects	
Mental retardation	

SOURCE: Adapted from Gorlin,[1] with permission.

TABLE 82-2

BCNS Diagnostic Criteria

MAJOR CRITERIA	MINOR CRITERIA
1. More than 2 BCCs or 1 BCC prior to the age of 20 years	1. Macrocephaly determined after adjustment for height
2. Odontogenic keratocysts of the jaw proven by histology	2. Congenital malformations: cleft lip or palate, frontal bossing, "coarse face," moderate or severe hypertelorism
3. Three or more palmar and/or plantar pits	3. Skeletal abnormalities: Sprengel deformity, marked pectus deformity, or marked syndactyly of the digits
4. Bilamellar calcification of the falx cerebri (if younger than 20 years old)	4. Radiologic abnormalities: bridging of the sella turcica; rib anomalies such as bifid or splayed ribs; vertebral anomalies such as hemivertebrae, fusion, or elongation of the vertebral bodies; modeling defects of the hands and feet; or flame-shaped lucencies of the hands or feet
5. Fused, bifid, or markedly splayed ribs	5. Ovarian fibroma
6. First-degree relative with BCNS	6. Medulloblastoma
7. *PTC* gene mutation in normal tissue	

SOURCE: Modified from Kimonis et al.[25]

FIGURE 82-6

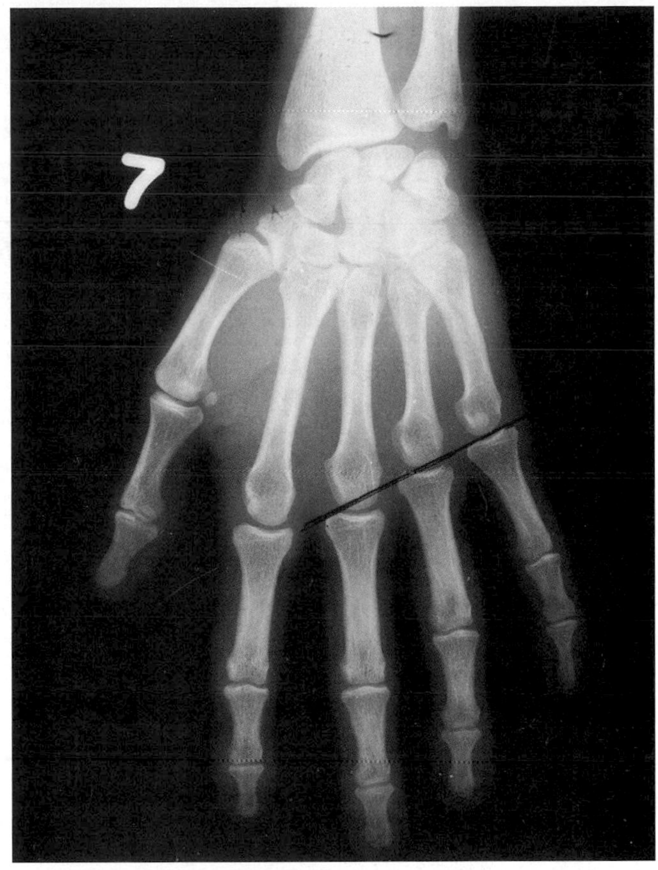

A.

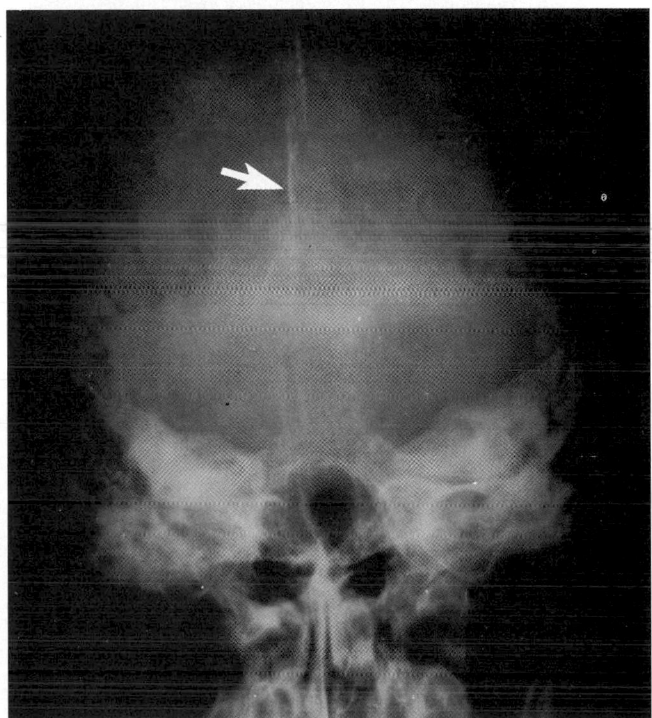

B.

Basal cell nevus syndrome. *A.* Short fourth, metacarpal (Albright's sign). A line drawn through the distal ends of the fifth and fourth metacarpals intersects the third metacarpal proximal to its end. *B.* Lamellar calcification of the flax (*arrow*).

differentiate them from BCNS patients (Chap. 81). Patients with xeroderma pigmentosa develop multiple BCCs but are readily differentiated from BCNS patients by their severe photosensitivity and other phenotypic abnormalities (Chap. 155). Finally, patients with a marked propensity to develop multiple BCCs, sometimes sporadically and rarely following therapeutic irradiation (e.g., for Hodgkin's disease), occasionally produce diagnostic confusion, and it is not known whether their defect is related to the hedgehog pathway, to DNA repair, to an unknown toxin, and/or to undescribed mechanisms.

TREATMENT

Therapy must be directed at the individual lesions as they arise, and the most important aspect of management is frequent examination, enthusiastic counseling about avoidance of sun exposure, and early treatment of small tumors. Clinicians caring for BCNS patients generally become confident enough of their clinical acumen that they treat tiny BCCs, for example, with cryotherapy, without histopathologic confirmation, because obtaining tissue for the latter produces more scarring. Other nonsurgical approaches often of real benefit are topical treatment with 5-fluorouracil (with or without occlusion, depending upon the degree of inflammation produced) or with imiquimod.[33] Oral therapy with retinoids also may be of real therapeutic value, but often only at a dose that causes severe side effects. Because the key is to convince the patient to accept frequent treatments, minimization of discomfort and of scarring is a major concern.

X-irradiation of BCCs should be avoided if possible, because enhanced radiation-induced carcinogenesis (e.g., in the skin of the portals of irradiation of childhood medulloblastomas) is characteristic of BCNS (Fig. 82-7).

FIGURE 82-7

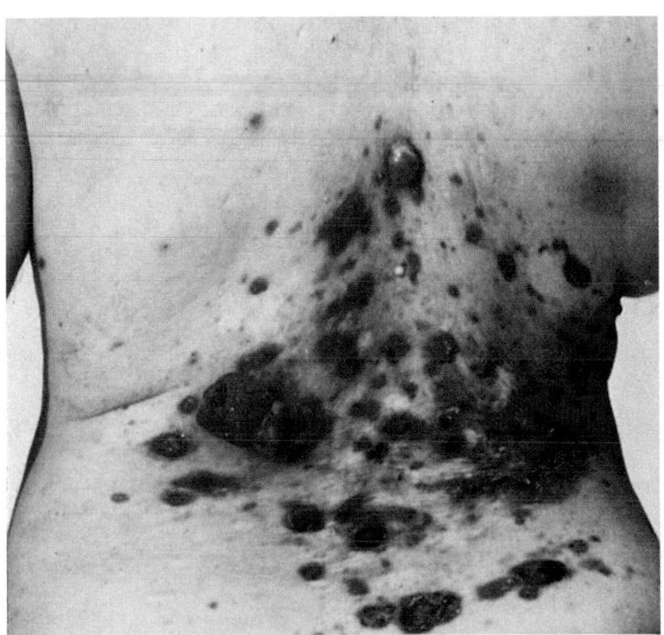

Basal cell nevus syndrome. Multiple, large, fungating basal cell carcinomas arising in a portion of the lower back treated years earlier with superficial x-ray for therapy of basal cell carcinomas.

Genetic counseling is appropriate. Half of the children of affected individuals are expected to develop the BCNS, and prenatal diagnosis is potentially achievable for many families if they desire this option.

REFERENCES

1. Gorlin RJ: Nevoid basal cell carcinoma syndrome. *Medicine* **66**:98, 1987
2. Howell JB, Caro MR: Basal cell nevus: Its relationship to multiple cutaneous cancers and associated anomalies of development. *Arch Dermatol* **79**:67, 1959
3. Gorlin RJ, Goltz RW: Multiple nevoid basal-cell epithelioma, jaw cysts and bifid ribs: A syndrome. *N Engl J Med* **262**:908, 1960
4. Bale AE, Yu K-P: The hedgehog pathway and basal cell carcinomas. *Hum Mol Genet* **10**:757, 2001
5. Hahn H et al: Mutations of the human homologue of *Drosophila* patched in the nevoid basal cell carcinoma syndrome. *Cell* **85**:841, 1996
6. Johnson RL et al: Human homologue of *patched*, a candidate gene for the basal cell nevus syndrome. *Science* **272**:1668, 1996
7. Howell JB: Nevoid basal cell carcinoma syndrome: Profile of genetic and environmental factors in oncogenesis. *J Am Acad Dermatol* **11**:98, 1984
8. DeCamp DL et al: Smoothened activates Galphai-mediated signaling in frog melanophores. *J Biol Chem* **275**:26322, 2000
9. Stone D et al: The tumour-suppressor gene *patched* encodes a candidate receptor for Sonic hedgehog. *Nature* **384**:129, 1996
10. Marigo V et al: Biochemical evidence that Patched is the hedgehog receptor. *Nature* **384**:176, 1996
11. Ingham PW et al: Patched represses the hedgehog signaling pathway by promoting modification of the smoothened protein. *Curr Biol* **10**:1315, 2000
12. Denef N et al: Hedgehog induces opposite changes in turnover and subcellular localization of patched and smoothened. *Cell* **102**:521, 2000
13. Alcedo J et al: Posttranscriptional regulation of smoothened is part of a self-correcting mechanism in the hedgehog signaling system. *Mol Cell* **6**:457, 2000
14. Xie J et al: A role of PDGFR alpha in basal cell carcinoma proliferation. *Proc Natl Acad Sci U S A* **98**:9255, 2001
15. Barnes EA et al: Patched1 interacts with cyclin B1 to regulate cell cycle progression. *EMBO J* **20**:2214, 2001
16. Fan H, Khavari PA: Sonic hedgehog opposes epithelial cell cycle arrest. *J Cell Biol* **147**:71, 1999
17. Xie J et al: Activating SMOOTHENED mutations in sporadic basal-cell carcinoma. *Nature* **391**:90, 1998
18. Taylor MD et al: Mutations in *SUFU* predispose to medulloblastoma. *Nat Genet* **31**:302, 2002
19. Oro AE et al: Basal cell carcinomas in mice overexpressing Sonic hedgehog. *Science* **276**:817, 1997
20. Nilsson M et al: Induction of basal cell carcinomas and trichoepitheliomas in mice overexpressing GLI-1. *Proc Natl Acad Sci U S A* **97**:3438, 2000
21. Grachtchouk M et al: Basal cell carcinomas in mice overexpressing GLI2 in skin. *Nat Genet* **24**:216, 2000
22. Aszterbaum M et al: Ultraviolet and ionizing radiation enhance the growth of BCCs and trichoblastomas in patched heterozygous knockout mice. *Nat Med* **5**:1285, 1999
23. Hahn H et al: Rhabdomyosarcomas and radiation hypersensitivity in a mouse model of Gorlin syndrome. *Nat Med* **4**:619, 1998
24. Shanley S et al: Nevoid basal cell carcinoma syndrome: Review of 118 affected individuals. *Am J Med Genet* **50**:282, 1994
25. Kimonis VE et al: Clinical manifestations in 105 persons with nevoid basal cell carcinoma syndrome. *Am J Med Genet* **69**:299, 1997
26. Lo Muzio L et al: Nevoid basal cell carcinoma syndrome. Clinical findings in 37 Italian affected individuals. *Clin Genet* **55**:34, 1999
27. Meara JG et al: The odontogenic keratocyst: A 20-year clinicopathologic review. *Laryngoscope* **108**:280, 1998
28. Ratcliffe JF et al: The diagnostic implication of falcine calcification on plain skull radiographs of patients with basal cell naevus syndrome and the incidence of falcine calcification in their relatives and two control groups. *Br J Radiol* **68**:361, 1995
29. Stavrou T et al: Intracranial calcifications in childhood medulloblastoma: Relation to nevoid basal cell carcinomas syndrome. *Am J Neuroradiol* **21**:790, 2000
30. Goeteyn M et al: The Bazex-Dupre-Christol syndrome. *Arch Dermatol* **130**:337, 1994
31. Ashinoff R et al: Rombo syndrome: A second case report and review. *J Am Acad Dermatol* **28**:1011, 1993
32. Oley CA et al: Basal cell carcinomas, coarse sparse hair, and milia. *Am J Med Genet* **43**:799, 1992
33. Kagy MK, Amonette R: The use of imiquimod 5% cream for the treatment of superficial basal cell carcinomas in a basal cell nevus syndrome patient. *Dermatol Surg* **26**:577, 2000

CHAPTER 83

Lorenzo Cerroni
Helmut Kerl

Keratoacanthoma

Keratoacanthoma is a common epithelial tumor of the skin characterized by rapid growth, histopathologic features similar to those of cutaneous squamous cell carcinoma, and a tendency toward spontaneous regression in absence of treatment. The exact nosology and classification of keratoacanthoma are a matter of debate. Some authors regard keratoacanthoma as a benign cutaneous tumor that is the prototype of the "pseudomalignant" tumors of the skin, whereas others maintain that it truly represents a malignant neoplasm and should be regarded as a peculiar variant of cutaneous squamous cell carcinoma.

HISTORICAL ASPECTS

The first description of solitary keratoacanthoma was provided by Sir Jonathan Hutchinson in 1889, who called this tumor "crateriform ulcer of the face."[1] Based on histopathologic features, he classified the lesion as a form of epithelial cancer. MacCormac and Scarff, in 1936, underlined the peculiar clinical features of this rapidly growing, self-healing tumor.[2] The term *keratoacanthoma* was officially first adopted in 1950 by Rook and Whimster.[3] They acknowledged that the designation keratoacanthoma was used by G.B. Dowling in London since the 1940s, and that Walter Freudenthal had coined the term keratoacanthoma in 1936, in order to underline its remarkable histopathologic aspects.[4]

Several other terms have been used to define lesions showing identical clinicopathologic features—molluscum sebaceum; molluscum pseudocarcinomatosum; kyste sébacé atypique; tumor-like keratosis; keratocarcinoma; self-healing primary squamous cell carcinoma; verrucome aveque adenite; button epithelioma; and idiopathic cutaneous pseudoepitheliomatous hyperplasia are some of the many names proposed in the past for keratoacanthoma.[4,5]

In addition to the solitary type of keratoacanthoma, a number of other variants have been described in the literature. Ferguson-Smith, in 1934, reported on a young patient presenting with multiple self-healing squamous cell carcinomas of the skin, a condition that later would be renamed as "multiple keratoacanthomas of the Ferguson-Smith type."[6] The occurrence of thousands of lesions in a single patient, today known as "multiple keratoacanthomas of the Grzybowski type," was reported by Grzybowski in 1950.[7] In 1961, Fisher published the first report on digital keratoacanthoma, pointing at the destructive features of the disease.[8] Another rare variant, today described as "keratoacanthoma centrifugum marginatum," a term that was coined in 1962 by Miedzinski and Kozakiewicz,[9,10] was first described by Puente Duany in 1958.[10]

EPIDEMIOLOGY

Keratoacanthoma is a relatively common neoplasm, but its exact incidence is unknown. The tumor is more frequent in light-skinned persons, and rarer in dark-skinned persons and in Japanese. The relative frequency in comparison with squamous cell carcinoma of the skin is controversial, but most studies show a lower incidence of keratoacanthoma than of squamous cell carcinoma. Discordant results may be explained, at least in part, by differences in classification of these lesions.

Studies on gender distribution reveal that both sexes are affected equally, possibly with a slight predilection for men. Keratoacanthoma occurs mostly in adult life, with a peak between ages 55 and 65 years; it has been observed rarely in younger patients. The familial type of keratoacanthoma occurs often during adolescence, and a neonatal case has been reported.[11] Although the incidence was thought to remain stable after a peak in the sixth decade, a study conducted in a defined population in Hawaii revealed that keratoacanthoma increases with age, in a fashion similar to that observed for cutaneous basal and squamous cell carcinomas.[12]

RELATIONSHIP TO SQUAMOUS CELL CARCINOMA

The authors of earlier reports considered keratoacanthoma to be a form of epithelial cancer of the skin, and named it accordingly. However, since the introduction of the concept of keratoacanthoma as a benign, self-healing neoplasm distinct from squamous cell carcinoma, the relationship between these two epithelial tumors has been the subject of debate. In their paper published in 1950, Rook and Whimster wrote, "This disease is evidently not cancerous or precancerous."[3] On the other hand, Kwittken, in 1975, stated, "I have come to the firm conclusion that all of these lesions are malignancies and that the formerly accepted concept of a self-healing squamous cell carcinoma of the skin is a correct one,"[13] and in 1979, even Rook amended his initial concept by writing, "... transformation from keratoacanthoma to squamous cell carcinoma occurs frequently."[4] Cases of typical keratoacanthoma with metastases have been observed,[14] and four possible explanations for this phenomenon have been suggested: an initial misdiagnosis of keratoacanthoma; the presence of both keratoacanthoma and squamous cell carcinoma in the same lesion; the malignant transformation of keratoacanthoma into squamous cell carcinoma; and, finally, the possibility that keratoacanthoma may be a peculiar variant of squamous cell carcinoma.[15] The debate is not settled yet, and some authors still maintain that keratoacanthoma represents a benign epithelial tumor, distinct from squamous cell carcinoma,[16] whereas others hold that it is a variant of squamous cell carcinoma with tendency to spontaneous regression, but with the potential for giving distant metastases and killing the patients.[17] Two recent studies based on large numbers of cases underlined the impossibility of reliably differentiating keratoacanthoma from squamous cell carcinoma using histopathologic criteria alone.[18,19] Other investigations pointed at similarities among squamous cell carcinoma and keratoacanthoma in the expression of oncogenetic and cell-cycle–regulating proteins as well as regarding the presence of trisomy 7 in a subset of tumors in both groups, thus suggesting a close relationship between these two entities.[20–23] On the other hand, recent publications on loss of heterozygosity, and on expression of angiotensin type 1 receptor and of desmogleins 1 and 2 showed clear-cut differences among keratoacanthomas and squamous cell carcinomas, revealing different phenotypes of the two tumors.[24–26] In short, at present, and in spite of the great amount of clinical and experimental data collected over the decades, the exact nosology of keratoacanthoma is not clear.

The authors of this chapter believe that keratoacanthoma represents a peculiar variant of squamous cell carcinoma, based on the rare but well known potential for distant metastases, and the capability for local destruction of important structures.

ETIOLOGY AND PATHOGENESIS

Different etiologic factors are probably involved in the development of keratoacanthomas in different patients, and it seems likely that these different factors act synergistically to induce the onset of a lesion in a given patient. The role of chronic UV light exposure in the etiology of keratoacanthoma is well documented by the frequent occurrence on sun-exposed areas, as well as by the presence of keratoacanthomas in patients with xeroderma pigmentosum and after prolonged PUVA treatment. In patients with multiple keratoacanthomas, PUVA treatment accelerates the development of the tumors,[27] but the risk for keratoacanthoma after therapy with PUVA seems lower than that for squamous or basal cell carcinoma.[28] An etiologic link to UV light has been confirmed also by experimental studies in mice.

The relationship of keratoacanthoma to chemical carcinogens has been well documented in humans and in several animals.[29] In fact, the incidence of keratoacanthoma is higher in industrial towns, and among industrial workers coming in contact with pitch, mineral oils, and tar. Chemical carcinogens may act in conjunction with UV rays to induce the onset of keratoacanthomas. Smokers seem also to be more affected than nonsmokers.[29]

Keratoacanthomas have been reported at the site of injury, thus suggesting an infectious etiology, at least in some cases. The association with trauma is also documented by the report of cases occurring after skin grafting, at both the donor and the recipient sites, and at the site of arterial puncture and vaccination.[5,30] The role of human papilloma virus

(HPV) remains controversial. Recently, evidence of HPV infection was documented by the highly sensitive polymerase chain reaction (PCR) technique,[31] but other studies failed to detect viral material within lesions of keratoacanthoma.[32] Some studies found an association with HPV type 25, and HPV-19 and HPV-48 have been isolated in a lesion arising in a HIV-patient.[33,34] Several other types of HPV have been linked to keratoacanthoma, including types 6, 9, 14, 16, 19, 35, 37, 58, and 61.

Genetic factors probably play a major role in the familial type of keratoacanthoma. In the other variants of keratoacanthoma, it seems likely that genetic aspects interplay with other etiologic factors (i.e., UV rays, trauma, infections) by providing the genetic predisposition for the development of keratoacanthoma, in a fashion similar to that documented for basal and squamous cell carcinomas of the skin. Keratoacanthomas are commonly observed in patients with Muir-Torre syndrome, suggesting that the genetic defect(s) of this syndrome also plays a role in the development of keratoacanthoma.[35,36] In addition, keratoacanthomas have been observed in patients affected by a variety of skin diseases including psoriasis, lupus erythematosus, lichen planus, atopic dermatitis, herpes zoster, acne conglobata, and pemphigus foliaceus, among others.[5]

Keratoacanthomas also have been observed in patients under immunosuppression as a result of bone marrow transplantation, cyclosporine treatment, or infection with HIV, thus suggesting that immunosuppression may play an etiologic role in some cases. In these patients, most lesions of keratoacanthoma tested for presence of HPV proved positive, suggesting that immunosuppression may contribute by decreasing the immune response against possible causative agents.[37] Similarly, UV light may act not only by direct carcinogenesis, but also by virtue of the local immunosuppression caused by sun exposure (see Chap. 38).

Clinical and experimental evidence indicates that most keratoacanthomas derive from the epithelium of the hair follicles. In 1961, Ghadially suggested that type 1 tumors derive from the upper part of the hair follicle and give rise to lesions with a bud-shaped pattern, whereas types 2 and 3 tumors derive from the more proximal portion of the hair follicle or from the hair bulb (see below), thus giving rise to lesions that are characterized by a dome-shaped or a berry-shaped morphology.[30] Although it seems likely that most, if not all, keratoacanthomas on hair-bearing skin derive from hair follicles, keratoacanthomas may occur at times on mucous membranes and in the subungual region, suggesting that the presence of hair follicles is not essential for their development. The onset of keratoacanthomas on the oral mucosa has been explained by the association with ectopic sebaceous glands, but it seems much more reasonable to postulate that in non–hair-bearing skin, keratoacanthomas derive from surface epithelium, as was suggested by Eversole et al.[38] It must be added, however, that some authors, based on differences in keratoacanthoma behavior (tendency to persist, local destructiveness), suggested that keratoacanthomas arising on the oral mucosa and ungual bed may represent a different tumor altogether, rather than a variant of keratoacanthoma.

Little is known about the pathogenesis of keratoacanthoma, and about the exact mechanisms inducing regression in the absence of any treatment. Studies on p53 oncoprotein expression and p53 gene mutations revealed expression of p53 oncoprotein in the great majority of tested cases, and association with a point mutation in the p53 gene in slightly more than 10 percent of these cases, suggesting a possible role of p53 gene in the development of some keratoacanthomas.[21] Cyclins regulating the cell cycle and mitotic activity may also play a role in the evolution of keratoacanthoma.[23] Microsatellite instability has been detected in about 30 percent of keratoacanthomas in Muir-Torre syndrome, but in less than 10 percent of cases of sporadic keratoacanthoma, suggesting that microsatellite instability does not play a role in this variant of the disease.[35,39] The rapid growth and regression of keratoacanthoma suggested to some an analogy to the normal cycle of the hair follicle, in which rapid growth is followed by slow involution.[30] However, it seems likely that regression in keratoacanthoma is not only due to its follicular derivation, but is also related to tumor and host factors.[40] Activated T-helper lymphocytes and increased numbers of Langerhans cells are present within the reactive inflammatory infiltrate of keratoacanthomas. Recently, the antiapoptotic *bcl-2* protein, the growth regulatory cytokine oncostatin M, and the cyclin-dependent kinase inhibitor p27 have been suggested to play a role in the regression of keratoacanthoma.[22,41,42]

No genetic markers have been identified for solitary keratoacanthoma, the most common form of the disease. Multiple keratoacanthomas of the Ferguson-Smith type show a familial distribution, and are transmitted in an autosomal dominant fashion. The gene responsible for this syndrome is localized to chromosome 9q. The majority of the cases have been described in some Scottish families, and in these patients, the syndrome is thought to be caused by a single genetic mutation that occurred before 1790.[43]

CLINICAL MANIFESTATIONS

Keratoacanthomas occur mostly on sun-exposed skin of the face, forearms, and dorsal aspects of the hands (Fig. 83-1). Actinic damage is commonly found in the surrounding skin. In most instances, they are located on hairy skin, but lesions with similar clinicopathologic aspects have been described in the oral cavity, the subungual region, the genital mucosa, and the conjunctiva.

The stereotypic example of keratoacanthoma is represented by a solitary lesion growing rapidly within a few weeks, and subsequently showing a slow involution over a period of a few months. Three clinical stages have been described: proliferative, mature, and resolving.[5] Lesions in the proliferative stage are rapidly enlarging erythematous papules that grow up to a dimension of 1 to 2 cm or more. In this stage the lesions are symmetric, firm, and show a smooth surface. In the mature stage there are symmetric, firm, erythematous or skin-colored nodules with a central keratotic core (Fig. 83-2). The central part can appear crateriform if the keratotic core is removed. Ghadially divided mature keratoacanthomas into three main morphologic types: type 1, or bud-shaped; type 2, or dome-shaped; and type 3, or berry-shaped.[30] Regressing lesions are characterized by a keratotic, partly necrotic nodule that becomes progressively flat upon elimination of the keratotic plug, eventually leaving an hypopigmented scar (Fig. 83-3).

FIGURE 83-1

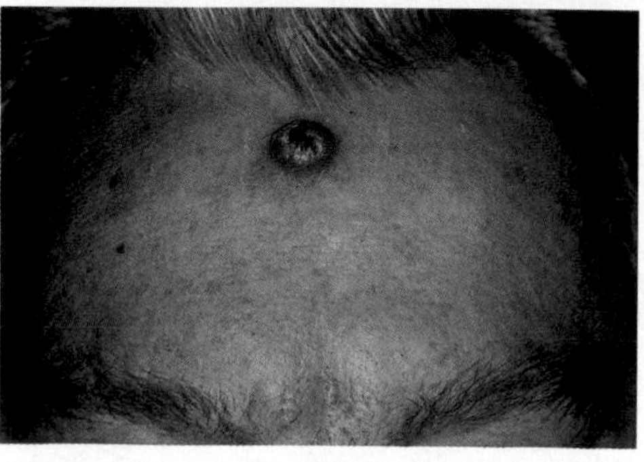

Keratoacanthoma on the forehead of a 64-year-old woman.

FIGURE 83-2

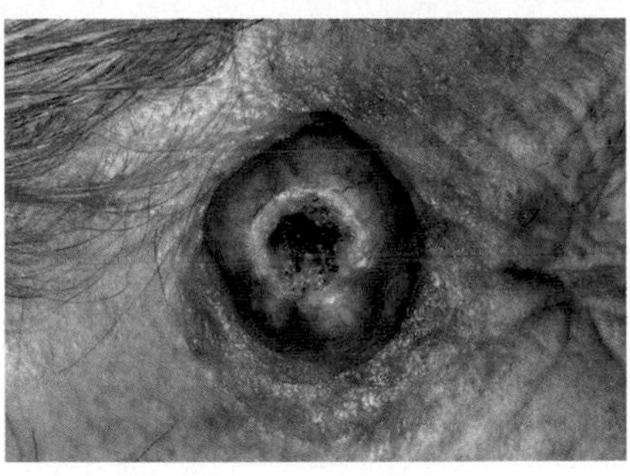

Mature keratoacanthoma on the temple of a 93-year-old woman. Note central keratotic core giving a white-yellowish appearance to the superficial part of the lesion.

Systemic Associations

Keratoacanthomas may be associated with multiple internal cancers in patients with Muir-Torre syndrome and the related hereditary nonpolyposis colorectal cancer syndrome. Patients with multiple keratoacanthomas should always be evaluated for the presence of typical traits of Muir-Torre syndrome where cutaneous sebaceous tumors and low-grade visceral malignancies can be observed (most commonly carcinomas of the gastrointestinal tract, but also carcinomas of the lung and genitourinary system, and, occasionally, colonic polyps). It has been suggested that at least some of the patients with multiple keratoacanthomas of the Ferguson-Smith type may have an incomplete form of the Muir-Torre syndrome.

Keratoacanthomas may also occur in patients with xeroderma pigmentosum (see Chap. 155), and rarely in patients with lymphomatoid papulosis (see Chap. 159).

Variants

Several variants of keratoacanthoma have been described, and different morphologic types of keratoacanthoma have been observed in a single patient.[44]

GIANT KERATOACANTHOMA In some instances, keratoacanthomas may reach dimensions of several centimeters (Fig. 83-4), and even a tumor reaching 15 cm in its diameter has been observed. Giant keratoacanthomas show a predilection for the nose and the dorsum of the hands. In some cases, the growth of the tumor may be associated with destruction of underlying tissues (Fig. 83-5).

FIGURE 83-3

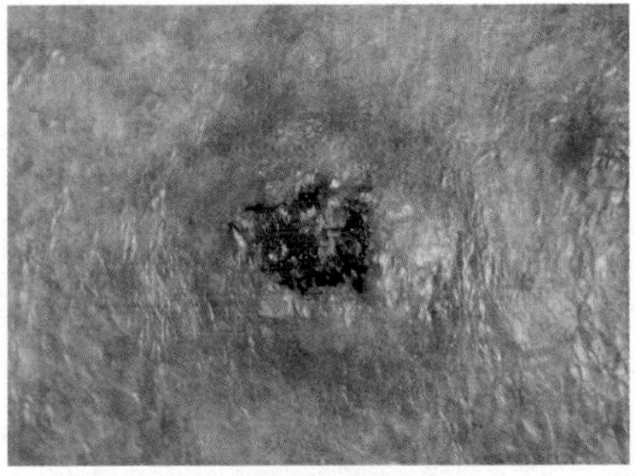

Regressing keratoacanthoma on the lower leg of a 59-year-old man. There is a whitish flattened plaque with superficial ulceration in the center.

FIGURE 83-4

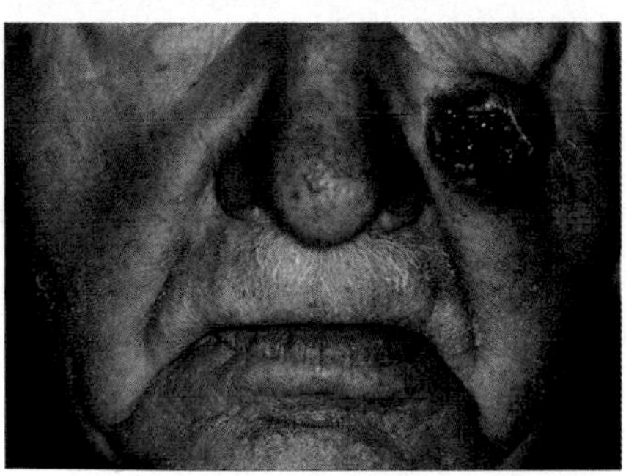

Giant keratoacanthoma on the cheek of a 91-year-old man. The tumor is asymmetric and reveals ulceration with necrosis.

KERATOACANTHOMA CENTRIFUGUM MARGINATUM Keratoacanthoma centrifugum marginatum is characterized by multiple tumors growing on a localized area, usually on the face, trunk, or extremities (Fig. 83-6). Tumors are annular, polycyclic, or circular in morphology. The area affected may reach 20 cm in diameter, and resolution may be slower than in solitary keratoacanthoma.

MULTIPLE KERATOACANTHOMAS OF THE FERGUSON-SMITH TYPE This is a familial form of keratoacanthoma that affects both sexes with approximately equal severity, which is characterized by the appearance of multiple, sometimes hundreds of keratoacanthomas, each with the clinicopathologic aspects of a solitary keratoacanthoma. The disorder is inherited in an autosomal dominant manner, and the majority of the cases have been described in a few Scottish families. Patients develop keratoacanthomas during adolescence and early adulthood, but onset during childhood is not infrequent. It has been suggested that at least some of these patients may have an incomplete form of the Muir-Torre syndrome.

GENERALIZED ERUPTIVE KERATOACANTHOMAS OF GRZYBOWSKI This variant is characterized by the presence of hundreds to thousands of tiny follicular keratotic papules disseminated all over the body, with predominance on sun-exposed areas. Facial involvement is usually severe, and coalescence of lesions around the eyes may cause ectropion. The mucosal regions (oral, genital) may be affected, whereas palms and soles are usually not involved. The age

FIGURE 83-5

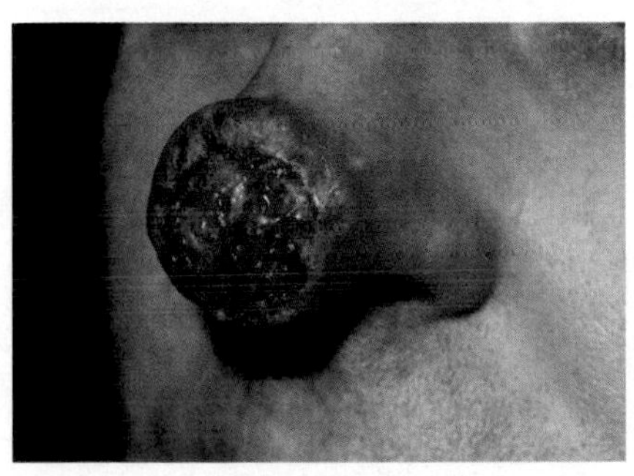

Giant keratoacanthoma on the tip of the nose of a 52-year-old man. Note the destructive appearance of the tumor.

FIGURE 83-6

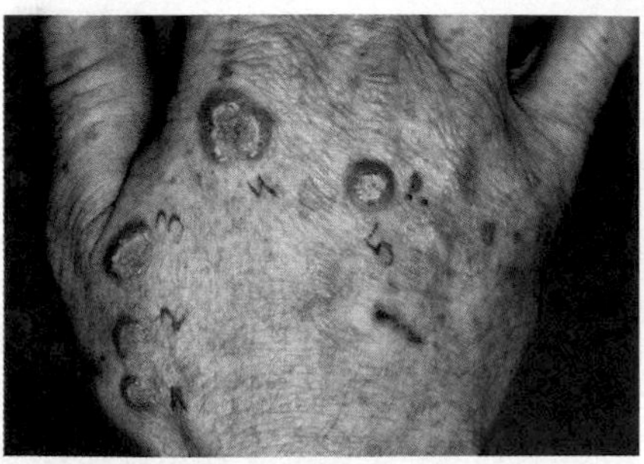

Multiple keratoacanthomas with an annular arrangement and central, keratin-filled craters on the back of the hand (keratoacanthoma centrifugum marginatum). This 42-year-old male patient also had lupus erythematosus.

of onset is similar to that of solitary keratoacanthoma, and clustering in families has not been observed.

SUBUNGUAL KERATOACANTHOMA Subungual keratoacanthoma (Fig. 83-7) differs from the other types of keratoacanthoma by being persistent and often causing destruction of the underlying bone. The tumor originates in the distal nail bed separating the nail plate from the nail bed, and can grow rapidly causing destruction of the entire phalanx. The predilection sites are the thumb, index, and middle fingers. Pain is a common symptom. Many authors consider subungual keratoacanthoma to be distinct from solitary keratoacanthoma because of the absence of hair, the common lack of tendency to spontaneous regression, and the destructive growth pattern. However, in patients with multiple keratoacanthomas at other sites, tumors involving the nails have been observed, suggesting a relationship between the two types.

KERATOACANTHOMA OF THE MUCOSAL REGIONS Keratoacanthomas have been described in the oral mucosa, the conjunctiva, the nasal mucosa, and the genital mucosa. In fact, involvement of the oral and genital mucosa is common in the generalized eruptive keratoacanthomas of the Grzybowski type. Keratoacanthomas arising on mucosal regions, especially on the oral mucosa, present clinically as slowly growing crateriform lesions that tend to persist for many months or years.

FIGURE 83-7

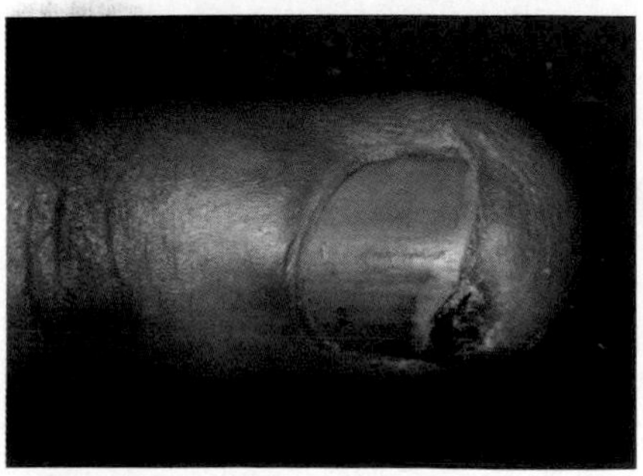

Subungual keratoacanthoma in a 38-year-old woman. A small keratotic tumor can be observed on the distal portion of the nail bed.

PATHOLOGY

The histopathologic diagnosis of keratoacanthoma rests mainly on the silhouette of the tumor as assessed at scanning magnification; inadequate specimens (i.e., punch biopsies, shaving biopsies, curettage) do not allow a diagnosis and differentiation from squamous cell carcinoma. Two large studies on the histopathologic criteria for diagnosis of keratoacanthoma recently emphasized the overlapping features between this tumor and squamous cell carcinoma, which render differentiation very difficult or even impossible in given cases.[18,19]

The histopathologic features of keratoacanthoma depend on the stage of evolution of the tumor. In early, proliferative lesions, the epithelium is markedly hyperplastic, and the central keratotic plug is not as pronounced as in fully developed lesions. The lesion has an overall symmetrical aspect (Fig. 83-8). Although atypical cells do not represent the majority of the cells in typical keratoacanthoma, there may be atypical keratinocytes and mitoses, especially at the lower margin of the tumor. Nests of epithelial cells may detach from the main tumor mass and be found in the superficial reticular dermis. Fully developed, mature lesions are characterized by a large central core of keratin surrounded by a well-differentiated proliferation of squamous epithelium that in some cases may resemble squamous cell carcinoma (Fig. 83-9*A*). The epidermis at both sides of the central core extends over the keratotic area in a fashion that has been described as "lipping" or "buttressing," giving a distinct crateriform appearance to the lesion. Nests and strands of keratinocytes may be found apart from the main bulk of the tumor, but usually do not extend lower than the level of sweat glands. Especially in keratoacanthomas originating from the epithelium of the hair follicles, intraepithelial microabscesses are often present. Cytomorphologically, large keratinocytes with eosinophilic cytoplasm are commonly observed, together with atypical cells and mitoses (Figure 83-9*B*). An inflammatory infiltrate containing lymphocytes, plasma cells, histiocytes, eosinophils, and neutrophils is a common feature, and in some instances may be conspicuous. Neurotropism and even vascular invasion can be observed in otherwise typical keratoacanthomas, but the prognosis does not seem to be affected by these histopathologically worrisome features (Fig. 83-9*C*).[16] In resolving lesions, the thickness of the epithelial proliferation decreases, and the tumor becomes more flattened and less crateriform (Fig. 83-10*A*). Atypical cells and mitoses are usually not observed at this stage. Granulomatous inflammation and fibrosis of the superficial dermis, eventually resulting in a scar, are a common feature of resolving lesions (Fig. 83-10*B*).

HISTOPATHOLOGIC VARIANTS Subungual keratoacanthomas often are more vertically oriented and do not show the typical epithelial "lipping" over the central keratotic plug, and reveal a greater number of dyskeratotic cells. Neutrophils within the epithelium are not observed,

FIGURE 83-8

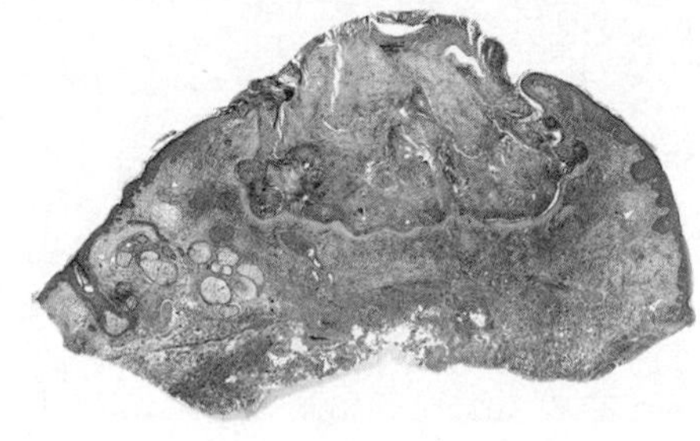

Keratoacanthoma (earlier stage) showing a symmetric epithelial tumor with a central keratotic crater surrounded by epithelial lipping.

FIGURE 83-9

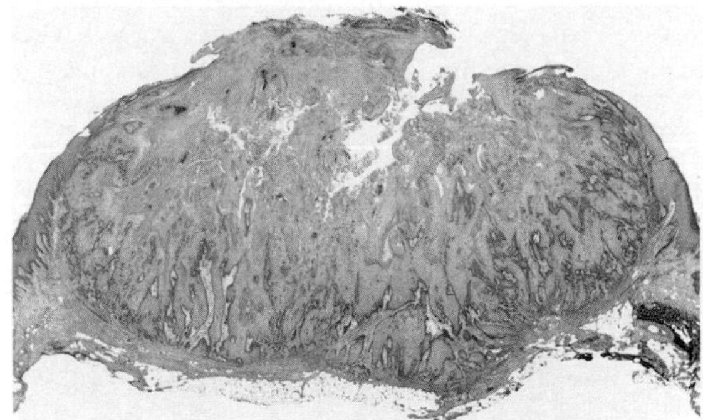

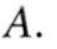

A.

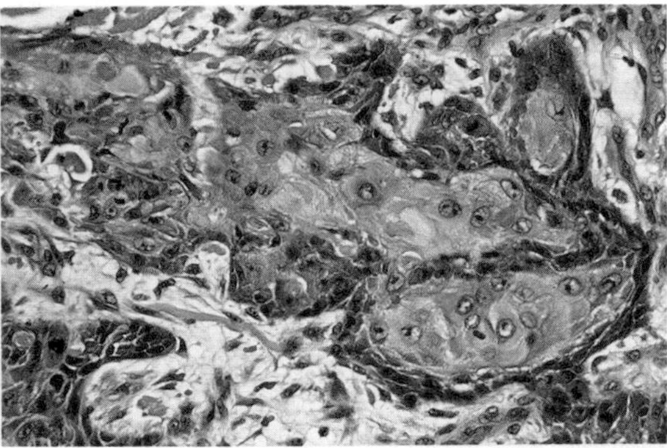

B.

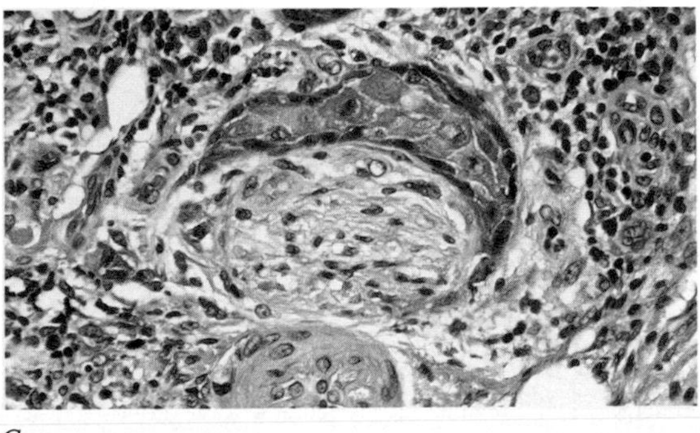

C.

Mature keratoacanthoma. *A.* Low-power magnification revealing a symmetric lesion with a central keratotic core. *B.* Tumor complexes with large eosinophilic cells admixed with atypical cells and a few mitoses. *C.* Perineural growth of tumor cells (neurotropism).

and there is no fibrosis. The absence of fibrosis also characterizes keratoacanthomas arising on mucous membranes. Keratoacanthomas in patients with Muir-Torre syndrome may show the concomitant presence of sebaceous proliferation. Multiple keratoacanthomas of the Ferguson-Smith type differ in that the lateral demarcation is less definite, the cells may be more pleomorphic and atypical, and the amount of central keratin may be less pronounced than in solitary keratoacanthoma.

DIAGNOSIS AND DIFFERENTIAL DIAGNOSIS

Diagnosis and differential diagnosis of keratoacanthoma rest on clinicopathologic features of the lesions. The clinical differential diagnosis of fully developed keratoacanthomas includes mainly squamous cell carcinoma, and it may be impossible to tell these two entities apart on clinical grounds only. Rarely, differential diagnosis includes other cutaneous lesions such as common warts, molluscum contagiosum, and prurigo nodularis. Lesions located at the tip of the nose may clinically resemble metastatic carcinoma. Subungual lesions should be differentiated from subungual warts and from other tumors arising on the nail bed. Regressing tumors may simulate clinically a regressing lesion of lymphomatoid papulosis and/or anaplastic large cell lymphoma.

FIGURE 83-10

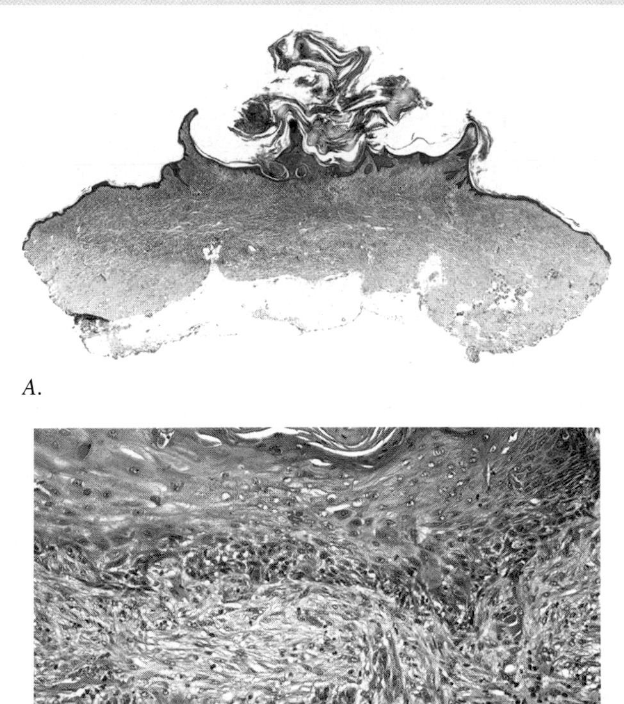

A.

B.

Regressing keratoacanthoma. *A.* Low-power magnification showing a symmetric, flattened lesion with inflammatory infiltrate and fibrosis. *B.* Proliferation of fibroblasts in the papillary dermis.

Histopathologic differential diagnosis mainly includes squamous cell carcinoma and differentiation among the two neoplasms may be impossible in a given case. Features in favor of a diagnosis of keratoacanthoma are the presence of a relatively symmetric, flasklike epithelial neoplasm with a central core of keratin and epithelial "lipping," as well as the lack of prominent atypia and mitotic figures. Although several immunohistochemical stains may be helpful in the differential diagnosis of keratoacanthoma versus squamous cell carcinoma, the utility of immunohistologic markers for differentiation of keratoacanthoma from squamous cell carcinoma is controversial. Staining for proliferative cells with the antibody MIB-1 (Ki-67 antigen) shows a peripheral pattern in keratoacanthoma, as opposed to a more diffuse pattern in squamous cell carcinoma.

TREATMENT AND PROGNOSIS

Keratoacanthomas show a tendency to spontaneous regression, and in typical cases, an acceptable therapeutic option may be to adopt the so-called watchful waiting strategy. However, because of the uncertainty regarding the exact nosology of this tumor, as well as the difficulty to differentiate it clinically from squamous cell carcinoma, complete conservative excision is advisable in most cases, especially in those of solitary keratoacanthoma. Biopsies by shaving or curettage are being increasingly performed for keratoacanthoma. If done so that architecture is preserved, these techniques are acceptable. These surgical methods, however, in most instances do not allow a definitive histopathologic diagnosis because the complete architectural features of the lesion are missed. Punch biopsies never allow differentiation of keratoacanthoma from well-differentiated squamous cell carcinoma, and should be avoided. For diagnostic purposes, a longitudinal biopsy that includes normal skin at both margins of the lesion as well as the underlying fat tissues is acceptable. However, whenever possible, a simple complete surgical excision should be performed. Special surgical techniques, such as Mohs micrographic surgery, have been adopted for difficult cases, for instance for recurrent lesions, giant lesions, or lesions of keratoacanthoma centrifugum marginatum, that may cover a large area of the body.[45] Therapy by laser vaporization, electrodesiccation, and cryosurgery with liquid nitrogen do not allow the histopathologic verification of the clinical diagnosis. Curettage followed by electrodesiccation or cryosurgery has been used in many instances, with a relative low rate of recurrences.[46]

Keratoacanthomas have been treated by radiotherapy with excellent results.[47] This type of treatment is particularly indicated for lesions that can be difficult to manage surgically, and for lesions of large dimensions. Several different types of radiotherapy have been employed, including electron beam, orthovoltage radiation, and superficial x-ray. Intralesional application of chemotherapeutic agents has also proven therapeutically successful.[5,48] Methotrexate, bleomycin, and 5-fluorouracil have been used with success by intralesional injection, and 5-fluorouracil has been applied also topically. Some keratoacanthomas have been treated by intralesional injection of interferon alfa-2a,[49] and others have been successfully treated with intralesional application of triamcinolone. Successful topical treatment has been performed with podophyllin, either alone or in combination with other treatment modalities. However, podophyllin is also capable of inducing keratoacanthomas. Multiple keratoacanthomas have been treated successfully with oral retinoids in several cases, but larger studies have not been performed.[50] Systemic treatments include chemotherapy with methotrexate, cyclophosphamide, or 5-fluorouracil.

A new, promising treatment option for keratoacanthoma of both solitary and multiple types is represented by photodynamic therapy with δ-aminolevulinic acid (see Chap. 266). The treatment is simple, and has been shown to achieve good therapeutic and cosmetic results.[51,52] Topical imiquimod is presently being evaluated.

Preventive measures against the development of keratoacanthomas are similar to those applied for basal and squamous cell carcinoma of the skin. In predisposed subjects (i.e., fair skin, history of multiple actinic keratoses, basal and/or squamous cell carcinomas, Muir-Torre syndrome), avoidance of direct sun exposure should be achieved, and skin protection creams applied.

Prognosis

Solitary keratoacanthoma behaves as a benign tumor in the majority of the cases, but lymph node and visceral metastases have been observed in a small number of patients. There are no clear-cut features to predict the biologic behavior of a given tumor, but persistent and recurrent lesions should be managed by complete surgical excision. Histopathologic features that are associated with a poor prognosis in common squamous cell carcinoma, such as neurotropism and vascular invasion, do not seem to have prognostic implications in keratoacanthomas.[16] Ungual keratoacanthomas do not show a tendency to spontaneous regression, and often are the cause of massive bone destruction.[53] In spite of aggressive local behavior, however, distant metastases have not been observed in ungual and mucosal types of keratoacanthoma.

REFERENCES

1. Hutchinson J: The crateriform ulcer of the face: a form of acute epithelial cancer. *Trans Pathol Soc London* **40**:275, 1889
2. MacCormac H, Scarff RW: Molluscum sebaceum. *Br J Dermatol* **48**:624, 1936
3. Rook A, Whimster I: Le Kerato-Acanthome. *Arch Belg Dermatol Syphiligr* **6**:137, 1950
4. Rook A, Whimster I: Keratoacanthoma: A thirty-year retrospect. *Br J Dermatol* **100**:41, 1979
5. Schwartz RA: Keratoacanthoma. *J Am Acad Dermatol* **30**:1, 1994
6. Ferguson-Smith J: A case of multiple primary squamous celled carcinomata of the skin in a young man, with spontaneous healing. *Br J Dermatol Syph* **46**:267, 1934
7. Grzybowski MA: A case of peculiar generalized epithelial tumours of the skin. *Br J Dermatol Syph* **62**:310, 1950
8. Fisher AA: A distinctive destructive digital disease. *Arch Dermatol* **83**:1030, 1961
9. Miedzinski F, Kozakiewicz J: Das Keratoakanthoma centrifugum—eine besondere Varietät des Keratoakanthoms. *Hautarzt* **13**:348, 1962
10. Puente Duany N: Squamous cell pseudoepithelioma (keratoacanthoma): A new clinical variety, gigantic, multiple, and localized. *Arch Dermatol* **91**:505, 1958
11. Kumar V et al: Multiple keratoacanthoma with neonatal onset in a girl. *Pediatr Dermatol* **16**:411, 1999
12. Chuang TY et al: Keratoacanthoma in Kauai, Hawaii. The first documented incidence in a defined population. *Arch Dermatol* **129**:317, 1993
13. Kwittken JA: A histologic chronology of the clinical course of the keratocarcinoma (so-called keratoacanthoma). *Mt Sinai J Med* **42**:127, 1975
14. Hodak E et al: Solitary keratoacanthoma is a squamous-cell carcinoma: Three examples with metastases. *Am J Dermatopathol* **15**:332, 1993
15. Goldenhersh MA, Olsen TG: Invasive squamous cell carcinoma initially diagnosed as a giant keratoacanthoma. *J Am Acad Dermatol* **10**:372, 1984
16. Godbolt AM et al: Keratoacanthoma with perineural invasion: a report of 40 cases. *Australas J Dermatol* **42**:168, 2001
17. Choonhakarn C, Ackerman AB: Keratoacanthomas: a new classification based on morphologic findings and on anatomic site. *Dermatopathol Pract Concept* **7**:7, 2001
18. Sanchez-Yus E et al: Solitary keratoacanthoma: A self-healing proliferation that frequently becomes malignant. *Am J Dermatopathol* **22**:305, 2000
19. Cribier B et al: Differentiating squamous cell carcinoma from keratoacanthoma using histopathological criteria. Is it possible? A study of 296 cases. *Dermatology* **199**:208, 1999
20. Cheville JC et al: Trisomy 7 in keratoacanthoma and squamous cell carcinoma detected by fluorescence in situ hybridization. *J Cutan Pathol* **22**:546, 1995
21. Perez MI et al: p53 oncoprotein expression and gene mutations in some keratoacanthomas. *Arch Dermatol* **133**:189, 1997
22. Tran TA et al: Comparison of oncostatin M expression in keratoacanthoma and squamous cell carcinoma. *Mod Pathol* **13**:427, 2000
23. Tran TA et al: Comparison of mitotic cyclins and cyclin-dependent kinase expression in keratoacanthoma and squamous cell carcinoma. *J Cutan Pathol* **26**:391, 1999
24. Waring AJ et al: Loss of heterozygosity analysis of keratoacanthoma reveals multiple differences from cutaneous squamous cell carcinoma. *Br J Cancer* **73**:649, 1996
25. Takeda H, Kondo S: Differences between squamous cell carcinoma and keratoacanthoma in angiotensin type-1 receptor expression. *Am J Pathol* **158**:1633, 2001
26. Krunic AL et al: Immunohistochemical staining for desmogleins 1 and 2 in keratinocytic neoplasms with squamous phenotype: actinic keratosis, keratoacanthoma and squamous cell carcinoma of the skin. *Br J Cancer* **77**:1275, 1998
27. Penmetcha M et al: Failure of PUVA in lichen myxedematosus: Acceleration of associated multiple keratoacanthomas with development of squamous carcinoma. *Clin Exp Dermatol* **12**:220, 1987
28. Henseler T et al: Skin tumors in the European PUVA study. Eight-year follow-up of 1643 patients treated with PUVA for psoriasis. *J Am Acad Dermatol* **16**:108, 1987

29. Ghadially FN et al: The etiology of keratoacanthoma. *Cancer* **16**:603, 1963
30. Ghadially FN: The role of the hair follicle in the origin and evolution of some cutaneous neoplasms of man and experimental animals. *Cancer* **14**:801, 1961
31. Hsi ED et al: Detection of human papillomavirus DNA in keratoacanthomas by polymerase chain reaction. *Am J Dermatopathol* **19**:10, 1997
32. Lu S et al: Known HPV types have no association with keratoacanthomas. *Arch Dermatol Res* **288**:129, 1996
33. Payne D et al: Human papillomavirus DNA in nonanogenital keratoacanthoma and squamous cell carcinoma of patients with HIV infection. *J Am Acad Dermatol* **33**:1047, 1995
34. Gassenmaier A et al: Human papillomavirus 25-related DNA in solitary keratoacanthoma. *Arch Dermatol Res* **279**:73, 1986
35. Honchel R et al: Microsatellite instability in Muir-Torre syndrome. *Cancer Res* **54**:1159, 1994
36. Burgdorf WH et al: Muir-Torre syndrome. Histologic spectrum of sebaceous proliferations. *Am J Dermatopathol* **8**:202, 1986
37. Stockfleth E et al: Identification of DNA sequences of both genital and cutaneous HPV types in a small number of keratoacanthomas of nonimmunosuppressed patients. *Dermatology* **198**:122, 1999
38. Eversole LR et al: Intraoral and labial keratoacanthoma. *Oral Surg Oral Med Oral Pathol* **54**:663, 1982
39. Langenbach N et al: Assessment of microsatellite instability and loss of heterozygosity in sporadic keratoacanthomas. *Arch Dermatol Res* **291**:1, 1999
40. Ramselaar CG, van der Meer JB: The spontaneous regression of keratoacanthoma in man. *Acta Derm Venereol* **56**:245, 1976
41. Hu W et al: Expression of the cyclin-dependent kinase inhibitor p27 in keratoacanthoma. *J Am Acad Dermatol* **42**:473, 2000
42. Sleater JP et al: Keratoacanthoma: a deficient squamous cell carcinoma? Study of bcl-2 expression. *J Cutan Pathol* **21**:514, 1994
43. Ferguson-Smith MA et al: Multiple self-healing squamous epithelioma. *Birth Defects* **7**:157, 1971
44. Schaller M et al: Multiple keratoacanthomas, giant keratoacanthoma and keratoacanthoma centrifugum marginatum: Development in a single patient and treatment with oral isotretinoin. *Acta Derm Venereol* **76**:40, 1996
45. Larson PO: Keratoacanthomas treated with Mohs' micrographic surgery (chemosurgery). A review of forty-three cases. *J Am Acad Dermatol* **16**:1040, 1987
46. Kingman J, Callen JP: Keratoacanthoma: a clinical study. *Arch Dermatol* **120**:736, 1984
47. Donahue B et al: Treatment of aggressive keratoacanthomas by radiotherapy. *J Am Acad Dermatol* **23**:489, 1990
48. Melton JL et al: Treatment of keratoacanthomas with intralesional methotrexate. *J Am Acad Dermatol* **25**:1017, 1991
49. Somlai B, Hollo P: Die Anwendung von Interferon alpha (IFN alpha) in der Keratoakanthombehandlung. *Hautarzt* **51**:173, 2000
50. Street ML et al: Multiple keratoacanthomas treated with oral retinoids. *J Am Acad Dermatol* **23**:862, 1990
51. Calzavara-Pinton PG: Repetitive photodynamic therapy with topical delta-aminolevulinic acid as an appropriate approach to the routine treatment of superficial non-melanoma skin tumours. *J Photochem Photobiol B* **29**:53, 1995
52. Radakovic-Fijan S et al: Efficacy of topical photodynamic therapy of a giant keratoacanthoma demonstrated by partial irradiation. *Br J Dermatol* **141**:936, 1999
53. Baran R, Goettmann S: Distal digital keratoacanthoma: A report of 12 cases and a review of the literature. *Br J Dermatol* **139**:512, 1998

CHAPTER 84

Shane G. Silver
Vincent C.Y. Ho

Benign Epithelial Tumors

Benign epithelial tumors are exceedingly common. Unfortunately, a good classification for these tumors is lacking. For discussion purposes, we have divided the benign epithelial tumors into various groups based upon their histology (Table 84-1). Although lesions grouped in this manner represent seemingly divergent clinical entities, such a classification helps us with our understanding of these diseases by linking possible common etiologic factors and aberrant cellular mechanisms.

SEBORRHEIC KERATOSIS

Synonyms: Senile wart, senile keratosis, seborrheic verruca, basal cell papilloma. Seborrheic keratoses are benign skin tumors. They are exceedingly common and most people will develop at least one such lesion in their lifetime. Seborrheic keratoses are most commonly found in the over-30 age group. These lesions can appear on any part of the body except the mucous membranes. When multiple and occurring on the trunk, seborrheic keratoses can be seen in a "Christmas tree" pattern, lying with their long axis along skin folds, or Blaschko's lines.

Seborrheic keratoses typically begin as flat, sharply demarcated, brown macules. As they progress, they become polypoidal, with an uneven surface. The usually dull or lackluster surface commonly shows a "warty" topography with multiple plugged follicles and fronds (Fig. 84-1). Follicular prominence is one of the hallmarks of seborrheic keratoses. This can either be caused by pale follicular plugs within a darker lesion, or by black or brown plugs within a pale lesion. Seborrheic keratoses typically have a "stuck-on" appearance secondary to their somewhat polypoidal morphology (Fig. 84-2). Colors of these lesions can vary from a pale brown with pink tones to dark brown or black. Some seborrheic keratoses can be almost white (see "Stucco Keratosis" later in this chapter).

A clinical variant of the typical seborrheic keratosis described above is the small polypoidal lesion commonly called *skin tags*. Distinct from smooth skin tags, these small, furrowed, rough-surfaced polyps appear most commonly around the neck, under the breast, or in the axillae. They seem to have a predilection for points of chronic trauma. They show a surface morphology, similar to that of the classic seborrheic keratosis, but their diameter is frequently only 1 to 2 mm, with a height above the skin of sometimes more than 3 mm. These lesions may spontaneously disappear by dropping off.

TABLE 84-1

Overview

- Seborrheic keratosis
  - Common seborrheic keratosis
  - Reticulated seborrheic keratosis
  - Stucco keratosis
  - Clonal seborrheic keratosis
  - Irritated seborrheic keratosis
  - Seborrheic keratosis with squamous atypia
  - Melanoacanthoma (pigmented seborrheic keratosis)
  - Dermatosis papulosa nigra
  - Sign of Leser-Trélat
- Epidermal nevi
  - Linear verrucous epidermal nevus-localized, systematized
  - Nevus unius lateris
  - Ichthyosis hystrix
  - Inflammatory linear verrucous epidermal nevus (ILVEN)
  - Nevus sebaceous of Jadassohn
  - Nevus comedonicus
  - Eccrine nevus
  - Apocrine nevus
  - Becker's nevus
  - White sponge nevus
  - Epidermal nevus syndrome
- Lichen Striatus
- Clear cell acanthoma
- Warty dyskeratoma
- Acanthoma fissuratum
- Cysts of epithelial origin
  - Epidermoid cyst
  - Trichilemmal cyst
  - Milium
  - Steatocystoma multiplex
  - Dermoid cyst
  - Branchial cyst
  - Preauricular cyst and sinus

Seborrheic keratoses are an annoyance. Lesions around the neck can catch on clothing, as can lesions around the waist. Others can grow to become cosmetically undesirable, whether on the face or on the trunk. Many can cause concern because of confusion with nevi, and the thought that the lesion is becoming a malignant melanoma. Conversely, dysplastic nevi or malignant melanomas can lurk in a forest of seborrheic keratoses and be undetected until a late stage, posing a significant danger.

Etiology

The etiology of seborrheic keratoses is unknown. In patients with a great number of seborrheic keratoses, there may be a positive family history. This may well reflect a genetic propensity. Seborrheic keratoses have sometimes been blamed on sun exposure. Yeatman et al. reported a higher prevalence of seborrheic keratoses on sun-exposed areas when taking into account skin surface area.[1] There is a propensity for the large type of seborrheic keratoses to develop in areas of intermittent sun exposure, such as the back and anterior chest.

Because of the verrucous appearance of seborrheic keratoses, human papilloma virus (HPV) has also been suggested as a possible etiology. In a study, 173 seborrheic keratoses were compared with 173 normal skin samples from nongenital sites for the presence of HPV. All specimens derived from normal skin were negative, whereas 34 of 173 seborrheic keratoses specimens were positive for HPV.[2]

FIGURE 84-1

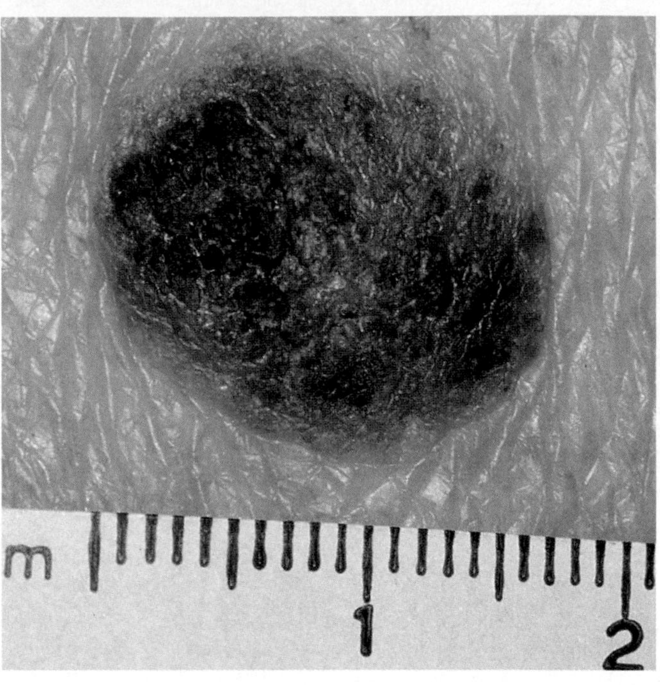

Seborrheic keratosis (basal cell papilloma) showing lackluster surface and "stuck-on" appearance.

Epidermal growth factors (EGF) are implicated in the development of seborrheic keratoses. The eruptive appearance of multiple seborrheic keratoses (the sign of Leser-Trélat) in association with various internal malignancies and with concomitant acanthosis nigricans, another epidermal hyperplastic phenomenon, suggests the possibility that

FIGURE 84-2

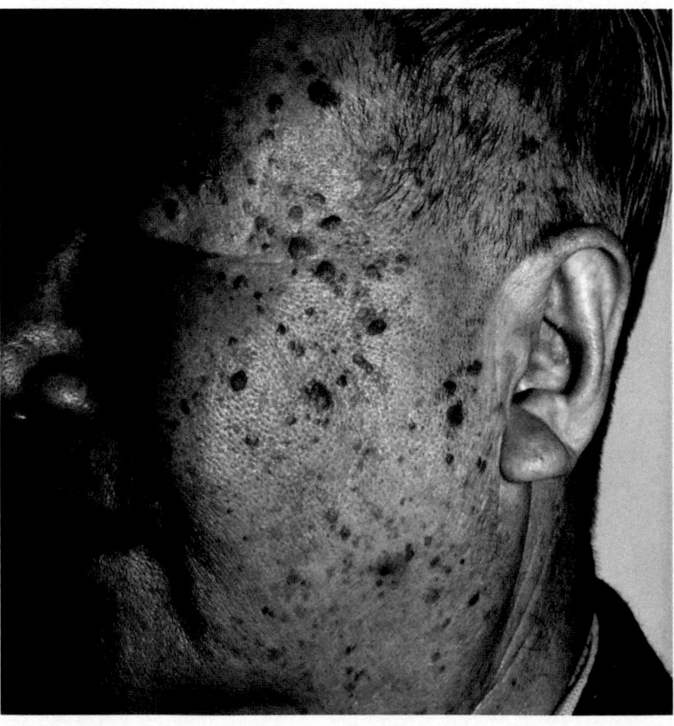

Multiple small seborrheic keratoses.

FIGURE 84-3

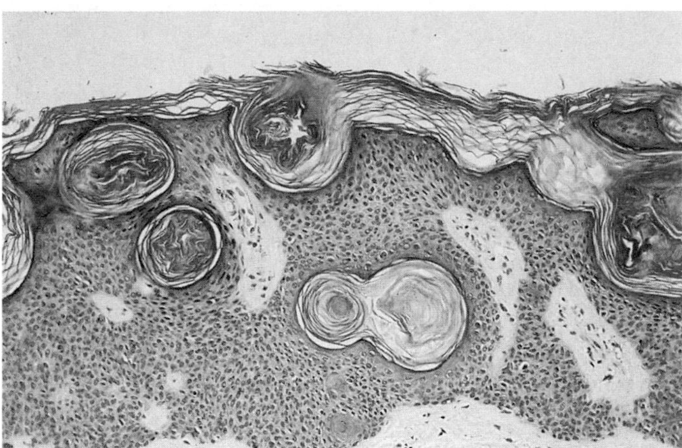

Seborrheic keratosis (basal cell papilloma) showing a papillomatous acanthotic epidermis consisting of basaloid cells.

a tumor-derived circulating growth factor or humoral factor may be involved in the pathogenesis of these lesions. Ellis et al.[3] described a patient with cutaneous melanoma, acanthosis nigricans, and the sign of Leser-Trélat. This patient had increased EGF receptors and urinary transforming growth factor (TGF)-α. After excision of the melanoma, TGF-α and EGF receptors decreased to normal.[3,4] Melanocytic hyperplasia is commonly seen in seborrheic keratoses. It has been suggested that melanocytes or melanocyte-derived growth factors may have a role in the development of seborrheic keratoses. However, a causal relationship has not been determined.

Clinicopathologic Variants

There are several histologic and sometimes clinically distinct forms of seborrheic keratoses.[5]

COMMON SEBORRHEIC KERATOSIS *Synonyms:* Basal cell papilloma, solid seborrheic keratosis. This is considered the classic lesion. The configuration is mushroom-like, with sharply demarcated hyperplastic epidermis overhanging the surrounding skin. The tumor consists of uniform basaloid cells. Keratin cysts are often prominent, and may be follicular or extrafollicular (Fig. 84-3). Melanocytes are often present in considerable numbers, and their pigment production results in the color of the darker lesions. Pigment transfer to the keratinocytes appears to be fairly normal.

RETICULATED SEBORRHEIC KERATOSIS *Synonym:* Adenoid seborrheic keratosis. Thin cords of basaloid cells descend from the base of the epidermis. Keratin cysts are embraced by these thin strands of cells (Fig. 84-4). A fine eosinophilic collagen stroma wraps these cords and can form much of the lesion.

STUCCO KERATOSIS *Synonyms:* Hyperkeratotic seborrheic keratosis, digitate seborrheic keratosis, serrated seborrheic keratosis, verrucous seborrheic keratosis. Stucco keratoses present as multiple 3- to 4-mm skin-colored or gray-white papules presenting symmetrically on the lower legs. Church-spire–like projections of the epidermal cells around a collagen core thrust upward into a basket-weave type of hyperkeratosis. The vacuolated keratinocytes seen in verruca vulgaris are not seen in this lesion, although clinically it can resemble a small viral wart.

FIGURE 84-4

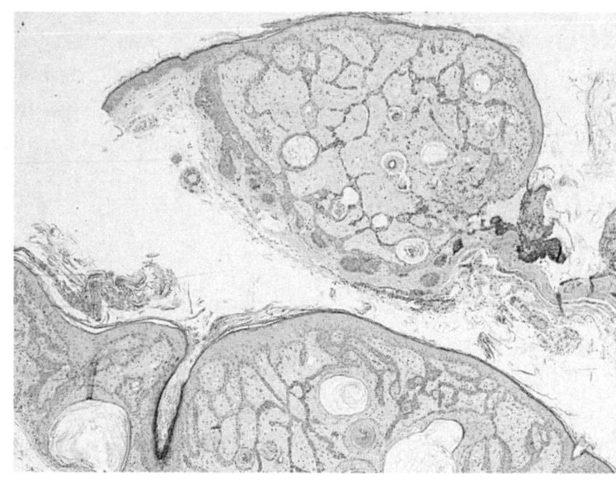

Reticulated seborrheic keratosis showing reticulated cords of basaloid cells descending from the base of the epidermis.

CLONAL SEBORRHEIC KERATOSIS Nests, usually but not always well defined, of round, loosely packed cells, are present within the epidermis (Fig. 84-5). Although the predominant cell is the keratinocyte, the nests may contain large numbers of melanocytes. The keratinocytes vary in size.

IRRITATED SEBORRHEIC KERATOSIS *Synonym:* Inflamed seborrheic keratosis, basosquamous cell acanthoma. Eczematous changes can occur in and around an otherwise typical seborrheic keratosis. The cause of this eczematous reaction is unknown. Trauma may play a role, but in most instances there is no apparent antecedent event. Histologically, an irritated seborrheic keratosis shows, apart from inflammatory changes, many whorls or eddies of eosinophilic flattened squamous cells arranged in an onionskin fashion. These resemble poorly differentiated keratin pearls in squamous cell carcinoma, but can be distinguished by their large number, small size, and circumscribed configuration. Keratinocytes within an irritated seborrheic keratosis show a higher degree of keratinization or more complete maturation

FIGURE 84-5

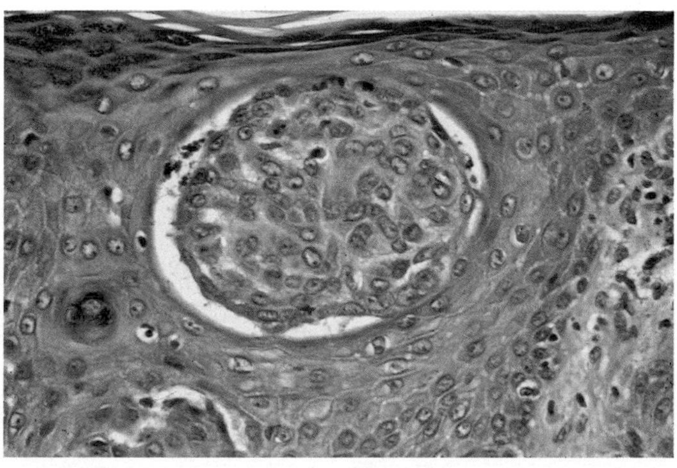

Clonal seborrheic keratosis showing round nests of keratinocytes and some melanocytes.

as compared with the common seborrheic keratosis; the mechanism for this phenomenon is unknown.

SEBORRHEIC KERATOSIS WITH SQUAMOUS ATYPIA Cellular atypia and dyskeratosis can be seen in some seborrheic keratoses. These lesions can closely mimic Bowen's disease or invasive squamous cell carcinoma. It is not known what causes these changes, whether they are a result of irritation/activation, or whether they are precursors of squamous cell carcinoma. It seems prudent to completely remove these lesions.

MELANOACANTHOMA *Synonym:* Pigmented seborrheic keratosis. Melanoacanthoma is more than a darkly pigmented seborrheic keratosis. Within the lesion there is a striking proliferation of dendritic melanocytes. These melanocytes are engorged with melanin, whereas the surrounding keratinocytes contain hardly any melanin. The melanocytes may proliferate as nests, extending from the basal layer into the superficial layers of the epidermis. This lesion has no malignant potential.

DERMATOSIS PAPULOSA NIGRA These small facial papules, originally described in African Americans, but seen in darker-skinned people of many other races, appears to be a variant of seborrheic keratosis. They resemble tiny melanoacanthomas. They have the histologic appearance of a common seborrheic keratosis but are smaller.

Skin Cancer Association

Basal cell carcinomas and other common skin cancers have been reported, rarely, in association with seborrheic keratoses.[6,7] In a study of 4310 tumors clinically diagnosed as seborrheic keratoses, 60 (1.4 percent) proved to be squamous cell carcinoma in situ.[7] In another study of 108 seborrheic keratoses, a 4.6 percent incidence of associated squamous cell carcinoma was reported.[6] Malignant melanoma in association with seborrheic keratoses has rarely been reported.[8] It has been suggested that basal cell carcinoma, squamous cell carcinoma, and melanomas associated with seborrheic keratoses may arise from the basaloid cells, spinous cells, and melanocytes that comprise seborrheic keratoses.[9] Most likely, however, malignant associations with seborrheic keratoses represent a collision phenomenon. Prudence, however, dictates that seborrheic keratoses that have undergone rapid growth or are clinically atypical be biopsied and that lesions demonstrating cellular atypia be completely removed.

The Sign of Leser-Trélat

Multiple eruptive seborrheic keratoses, also known as the *sign of Leser-Trélat,* have been mentioned in association with multiple internal malignancies.[10] The most frequent associations are adenocarcinoma of the stomach, colon, and breast. This sign has also been reported with a variety of other tumors, including lymphoma, leukemia, and melanoma.[10] It has also been mentioned in associations with hyperkeratosis of the palms and soles associated with malignant disease[11] and with acanthosis nigricans.[3,10] Evidence to support the presumed relationship of seborrheic keratoses to malignant disease is meager. Most of the cancers described in association with seborrheic keratoses are common cancers. Seborrheic keratoses are also common. Proving an uncommon causal relationship between a common cancer and a common skin sign is difficult.

The phenomenon of eruptive seborrheic keratoses, may represent an inflammatory dermatosis centered around skin papillomas and seborrheic keratoses making them suddenly more prominent. Indeed, it is common clinical experience to see an increase in the prominence of seborrheic keratoses in patients with generalized dermatitis from any cause. Chemotherapy, in particular cytarabine, can cause inflammation of seborrheic keratoses, especially when associated with the sign of Leser-Trélat (Fig. 84-6).[12] Malignant acanthosis nigricans is present in 35 percent of patients with the sign of Leser-Trélat, suggesting a similar mechanism of action.[3,4] However, the true relationship of multiple eruptive seborrheic keratoses to internal malignant disease remains to be defined.

FIGURE 84-6

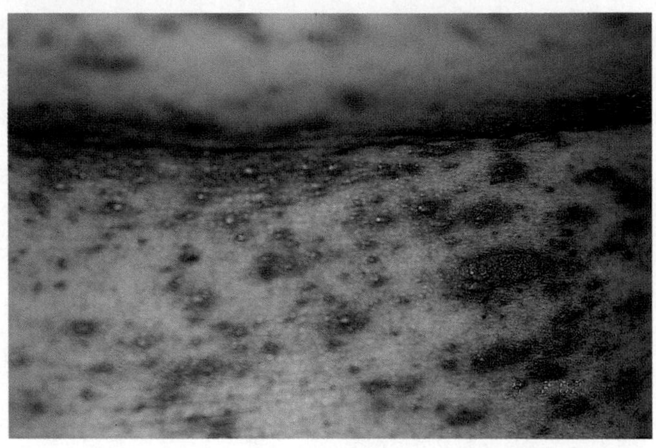

Inflamed seborrheic keratoses occurring during cytarabine therapy.

Treatment

Lesions that are symptomatic or cosmetically bothersome to the patient can be treated. Cryotherapy is probably the treatment of choice for the majority of lesions. A freeze to a 1-mm diameter around the lesion using either a cotton applicator or spray usually produces an excellent response. Should there be a residual lesion, or should the lesion recur, repeat treatment may be given. Following cryotherapy, postinflammatory hypopigmentation or hyperpigmentation may develop. Although usually temporary, these pigmentary changes may persist in darker-skinned patients and can be most disturbing.

Other treatment modalities include electrodesiccation followed by the easy removal of the lesion with a curette, or curettage followed by light electrodesiccation. Laser therapy using a pigmented lesion laser is also effective, and when used to treat flat seborrheic keratoses, may carry a lower risk of postinflammatory pigmentation or scarring as compared to cryotherapy or electrodesiccation. Surgical excision is also effective, but is usually not the treatment of choice in view of the adverse effect of scarring. Less-common treatment modalities used for giant seborrheic keratoses include topical fluorouracil and dermabrasion.[13,14]

One of the greatest dangers posed by treating a "seborrheic keratosis" other than by surgical excision is that the treated lesion could be a dysplastic melanocytic lesion or a malignant melanoma. It is strongly recommended that if the lesion is not absolutely typical of a seborrheic keratosis, it should be submitted for histologic examination.

EPIDERMAL NEVUS

Epidermal nevi, are hamartomatous proliferations developing from embryonic ectoderm, which gives rise to many structures in the skin, including keratinocytes, apocrine glands, eccrine glands, hair follicles, and sebaceous glands. Therefore, epidermal nevi may be classified into a number of variants depending on the clinical appearance (morphology), extent of involvement, and the predominant epidermal structure in the lesion (Table 84-2).[15] There is considerable overlap between these variants and rigid categorization is not advisable. The term nevus is used here to denote a developmental defect; there is no proliferation of nevocellular nevus cells (melanocytes) in the lesion.

TABLE 84-2

Classification of Epidermal Nevi

Epidermal Nevus Variant	Predominant Structure	Morphology	Extent
Verrucous epidermal nevus	Surface epidermis	Verrucous	
Localized			Localized
Systematized			Widespread
Nevus unius lateris			Widespread unilateral
Ichthyosis hystrix			Widespread bilateral
Inflammatory linear verrucous epidermal nevus		Inflamed	Localized
Nevus sebaceous	Sebaceous glands	Yellow verrucous	Localized, rarely diffuse
Nevus comedonicus	Hair follicles	Grouped comedones	Localized, rarely diffuse
Eccrine nevus	Eccrine sweat glands	Nondescript papule	Localized
Apocrine nevus	Apocrine sweat glands	Nondescript papule	Localized
Becker's nevus	Surface epidermis Hair follicles, +smooth muscles, melanization	Pigmented, hairy	Localized
White sponge nevus	Mucosal epithelium	Gray-white plaque	Localized or diffuse

Epidemiology

The incidence of epidermal nevi is estimated to be 1 per 1000 live births.[16] The majority occur sporadically and affect both sexes equally; familial cases have been described.[16] Most epidermal nevi are present at birth or infancy, but rarely do they appear as late as puberty.[16] In one study of 131 cases,[15] 60 percent were present at birth, and more than 80 percent had onset of their epidermal nevi in the first year of life; the remainder developed the lesion between the ages of 1 and 7 years with the exception of one patient whose onset was at 14 years; all the epidermal nevi on the head were present at birth. There are rare reports of adult onset of epidermal nevi, with the oldest patient being a 60-year-old woman.[17] Such late-developing epidermal nevi probably represent lesions that have always been present subclinically, but recent growth resulted in clinical recognition.

VERRUCOUS EPIDERMAL NEVUS *Synonyms:* Linear verrucous epidermal nevus, linear epidermal nevus.

Clinical features Verrucous epidermal nevi are characterized by closely set, skin-colored, brown, or gray-brown verrucous papules, which may coalesce to form well-demarcated papillomatous plaques (Fig. 84-7). A linear configuration is common, especially for lesions on a limb (Fig. 84-8). Such lesions may appear to follow skin tension lines, or Blaschko's lines.

Verrucous epidermal nevi may be localized or diffuse. An epidermal nevus with diffuse or extensive distribution is called a *systematized epidermal nevus*. When the lesions are distributed on one-half of the body, it is termed *nevus unius lateris* (Fig. 84-9). *Ichthyosis hystrix* refers to an

FIGURE 84-7

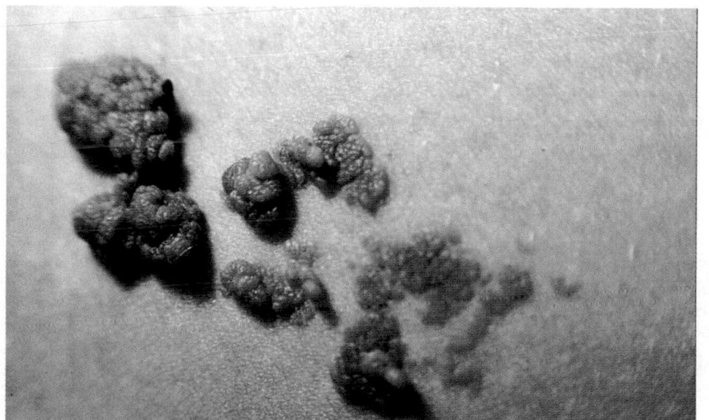

Verrucous epidermal nevus.

FIGURE 84-8

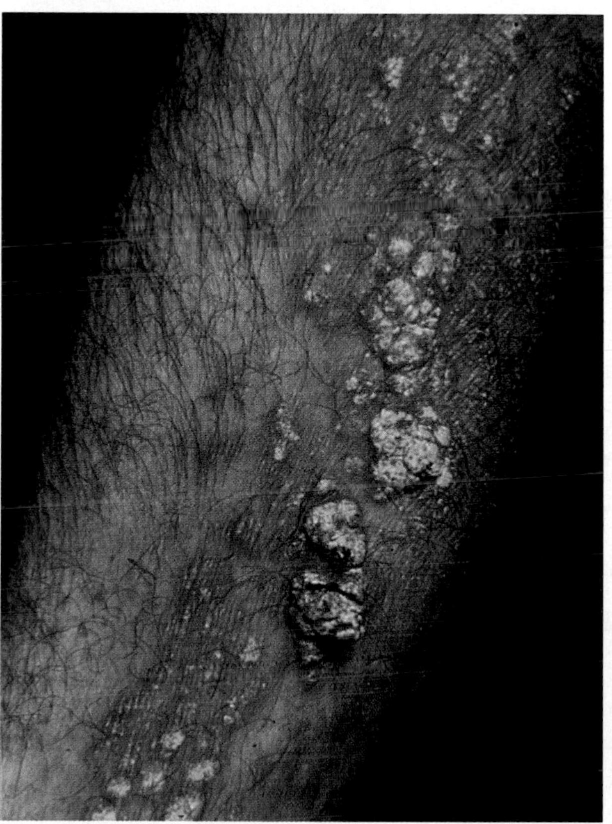

Verrucous epidermal nevus showing linear configuration.

FIGURE 84-9

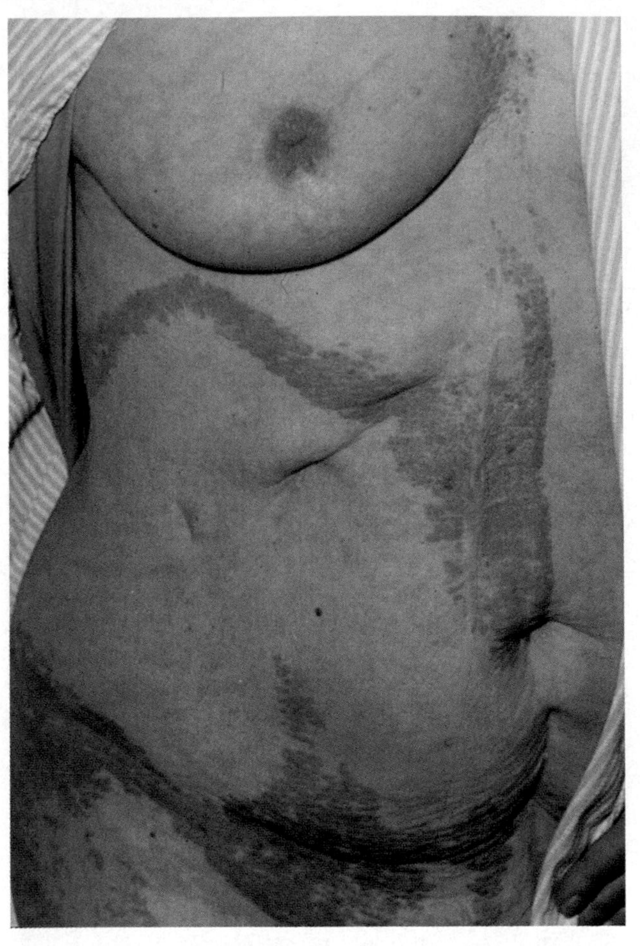

Nevus unius lateris. Epidermal nevus affecting one-half of body.

epidermal nevus with extensive bilateral distribution. In these systematized nevi, the lesions on the limbs are usually linear in configuration, while those on the trunk tend to form wavy, transverse bands.

FIGURE 84-10

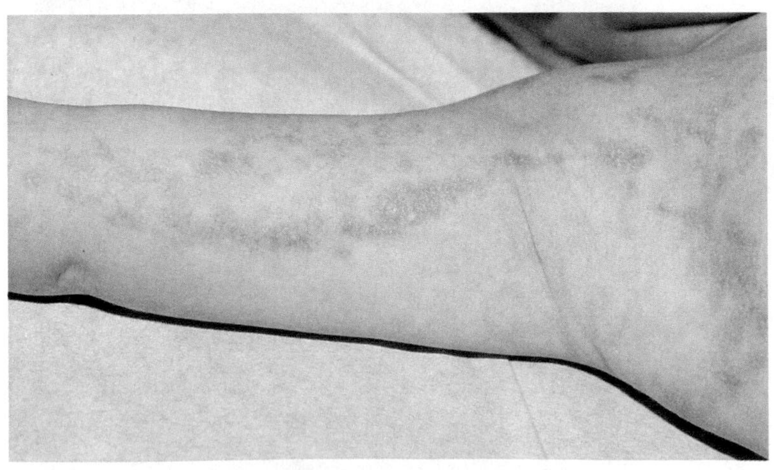

Inflammatory linear verrucous epidermal nevus (ILVEN) showing erythema and scaling.

Inflammatory linear verrucous epidermal nevus (ILVEN), as the name implies, is an inflammatory variant of epidermal nevus. The lesion is pruritic and shows clinical signs of inflammation, namely, erythema, scaling, and crusting (Fig. 84-10).

Course and complications A verrucous epidermal nevus may enlarge slowly during childhood. By adolescence, the lesion usually reaches a stable size and further extension is unlikely.[16] In Rogers' series of 131 cases, only 16 percent of the epidermal nevi present at birth showed extension, as compared to 65 percent of lesions of later onset; extension rarely lasts for more than 2 years.[15] Epidermal nevi may be associated with other cutaneous lesions, most commonly, café au lait macules, congenital hypopigmented macules, and congenital nevocellular nevi.[15] Epidermal nevi, especially if extensive, may be associated with developmental abnormalities in other systems (see later discussion on epidermal nevus syndrome). Rarely, basal cell and squamous cell carcinomas have been reported to develop in an epidermal nevus; this malignant transformation should be suspected when sudden localized growth, nodules or ulcers appear.[18] Malignant transformation of verrucous epidermal nevi usually occurs in long-standing, extensive lesions in middle-aged to elderly patients. The youngest reported case of malignant transformation was in a 17-year-old woman. Epidermal nevi in intertriginous areas may become macerated and secondarily infected.

There have been isolated reports of generalized epidermolytic hyperkeratosis developing in offspring of parents with epidermal nevi.[19] Paller et al. investigated three patients with the rare subgroup of segmental epidermal nevi displaying histopathologic features of epidermolytic hyperkeratosis (see below), each of whom had offspring with generalized epidermolytic hyperkeratosis.[20] Affected parents demonstrated mutations in one of the two K10 (keratin) alleles from lesional, but not normal, skin. The identical K10 mutation was found in each of their offspring. Each parent demonstrated genetic mosaicism, defined as the presence of two genetically distinct cell lines arising from a postzygotic mutation during embryogenesis.[21] Therefore, mosaicism is exemplified by epidermal nevi displaying epidermolytic hyperkeratosis and offspring of such patients may develop generalized epidermolytic hyperkeratosis.

Pathology There is hyperkeratosis, acanthosis and papillomatosis with (Fig. 84-11) elongated rete ridges. The histologic picture is essentially that of a benign papilloma. Epidermolytic hyperkeratosis, characterized by compact hyperkeratosis, vacuolization of the upper and middle prickle cell layer, and large keratohyaline granules within or outside the cells may be seen, most frequently in ichthyosis hystrix but also in localized epidermal nevi. The ILVEN lesion shows a dermal chronic inflammatory infiltrate in the dermis in addition to the above findings. Furthermore, the characteristic feature of alternating areas of hyperkeratosis with a thickened granular layer and parakeratosis without a granular area may be present.[22]

Differential diagnosis Verrucous epidermal nevi should be differentiated from other linear hyperkeratotic or verrucous lesions, namely, incontinentia pigmenti (verrucous stage), lichen striatus, linear porokeratosis, linear Darier's disease, linear lichen planus, and linear psoriasis. The latter two conditions are considered by some authors to be lichenoid and psoriasiform variants of linear epidermal nevus.[23] Linear porokeratosis is distinguished by its pathognomonic cornoid lamellae. The history of an antecedent vesicular stage and the transient nature of the linear verrucous lesions of incontinentia pigmenti allow differentiation of this condition from an epidermal nevus; histologically, incontinentia pigmenti shows eosinophilic exocytosis, dyskeratosis, basal layer vacuolization, and pigment incontinence, which are absent in an epidermal nevus. Lichen striatus may be difficult to exclude clinically and histologically from ILVEN. Their differentiation is important from a prognostic point of view as lichen striatus

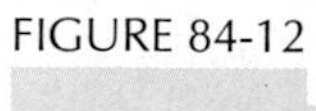

FIGURE 84-11

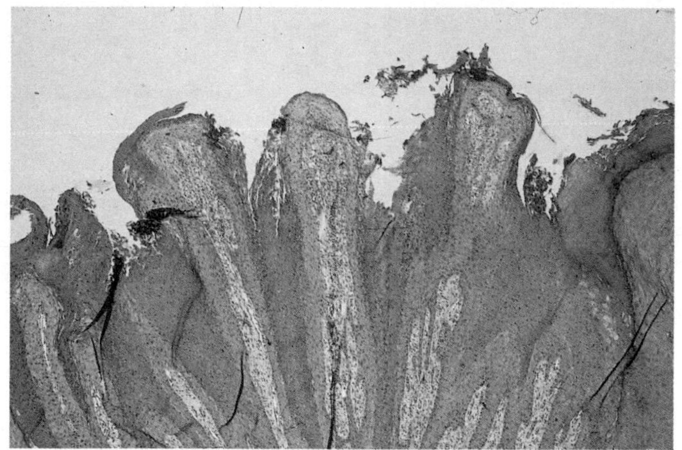

Epidermal nevus showing hyperkeratosis, acanthosis, papillomatosis, and elongation of rete ridges.

is self-limited, whereas ILVEN persists indefinitely. Lichen striatus is asymptomatic, whereas ILVEN is usually pruritic; histologically, lichen striatus shows little or no acanthosis and may have a lichenoid inflammatory infiltrate.

Treatment Excision is the most reliable treatment. However, this may not be practical or advisable if the epidermal nevus is very extensive or at sites not amenable to simple surgery. The excision should extend to the deep dermis, otherwise, the lesion will recur. Therefore, the patient should be advised that scarring is to be expected. Alternative treatments include laser,[24] electrofulguration, cryotherapy, dermabrasion, and chemical peels with trichloroacetic acid or phenol. These treatments usually remove the superficial portion of the nevus and recurrence is common. Topical treatments include podophyllin, retinoic acid, anthralin, calcipotriol, or alpha-hydroxy acids, and are relatively ineffective.[25,26] Occasionally, using combination topical therapy will lead to higher efficacy.[25] Systemic retinoids can produce a partial but usually temporary response in some patients with extensive disease. Success with antipsoriatic treatments is not surprising as some argue that ILVEN represents true linear psoriasis or superimposed psoriasis.[27] Because epidermal nevi are associated with a small risk of malignant transformation, suspect areas of any lesion should be biopsied. If malignancy is confirmed, the entire lesion must be excised.

NEVUS SEBACEOUS *Synonym:* Nevus sebaceous of Jadassohn, organoid nevus.

Clinical features This usually presents as a solitary lesion at birth or early childhood. It has a predilection for the scalp where it presents as a solitary patch or a slightly elevated yellowish plaque with alopecia. Less commonly, nevus sebaceous may be found on the face, neck, or trunk, or, rarely, in the oral cavity.[28] The well-developed lesion, with its characteristic yellow or yellow-brown color, linear configuration and verrucous surface is quite distinctive (Fig. 84-12). However, in early childhood, the lesion may be quite flat and inconspicuous; the characteristic appearance may not develop until puberty. Nevus sebaceous occurs sporadically; familial nevus sebaceous has been described but is exceedingly rare.[29]

Course and complications Nevus sebaceous appears to be under some hormonal control and frequently enlarges during puberty. The lesion can be raised at birth, flatten in childhood, and become raised again during puberty. Further extension after puberty is uncommon. Systemic abnormalities may develop in association with a nevus sebaceous (see "Epidermal Nevus Syndrome" below). This is more common in patients with multiple or extensive lesions. Another significant complication is the development of secondary benign and malignant tumors. It is believed that nevus sebaceous arises from pluripotential primary epithelial germ cells and these cells have the capacity to differentiate into various epithelial tumors. Early reports indicate an increased risk of basal cell carcinomas (6.5 to 50.0 percent) developing within lesions of nevus sebaceous (Fig. 84-13).[30] However, two recent studies of 596 and 154 patients found the incidence of basal cell carcinoma to be quite low (0.0 to 0.8 percent) and it appears that most lesions diagnosed as basal cell carcinoma were most likely trichoblastomas.[31,32] Mutations

FIGURE 84-12

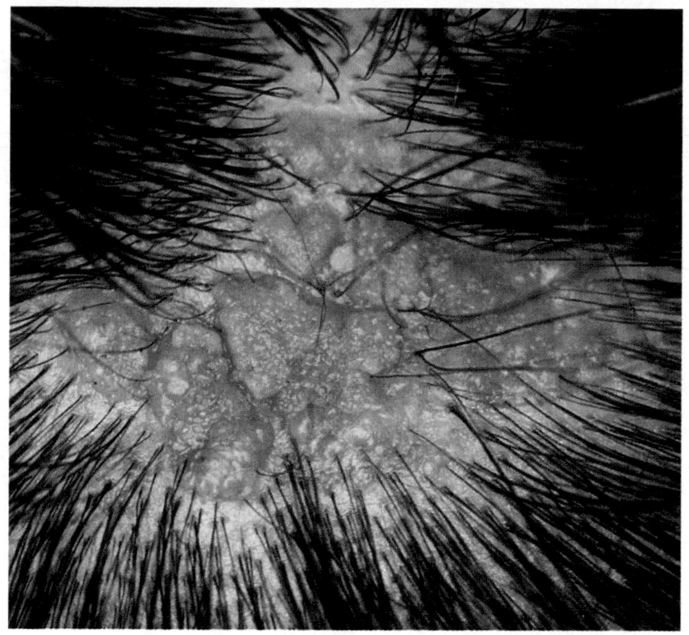

Nevus sebaceous.

FIGURE 84-13

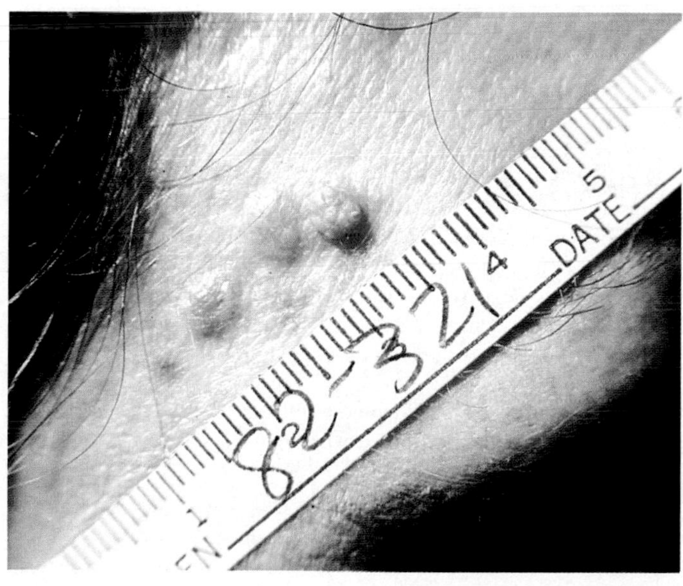

The development of basal cell carcinoma in a nevus sebaceous.

FIGURE 84-14

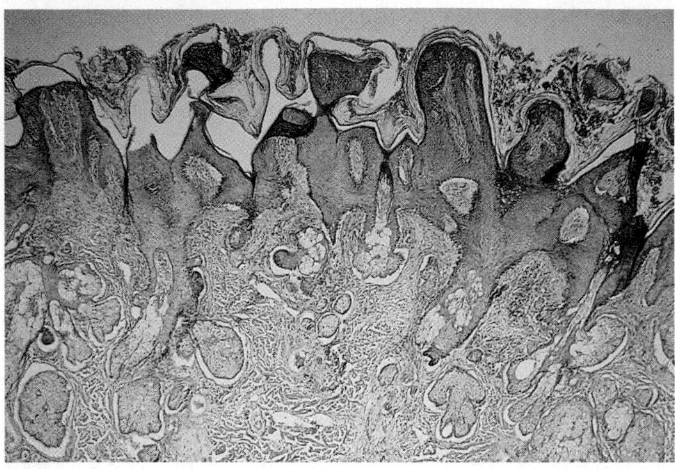

Nevus sebaceous showing epidermal hyperplasia and increased numbers of sebaceous glands and apocrine glands in the dermis.

in the patched gene within nevus sebaceous has been postulated to be the cause of the increased incidence of basal cell carcinoma.[33] The patched gene mutation is also associated with both sporadic basal cell carcinomas and the basal cell nevus syndrome. In studies in which trichoblastoma was not discussed, syringocystadenoma papilliferum proved to be the most common benign neoplasm developing in lesions of nevus sebaceous (8 to 19 percent).[31,32] Less-common associations include sebaceous epithelioma, hidradenoma, syringoma, chondroid syringoma, trichilemmoma, and desmoplastic trichilemmoma, proliferating trichilemmal tumor.[34,35] The development of squamous cell carcinoma, apocrine carcinoma, and malignant eccrine poroma has been reported but is rare.[30]

Pathology The epidermis shows papillomatous hyperplasia. In the dermis, there are increased numbers of mature sebaceous glands and apocrine glands are often found in the deep dermis (Fig. 84-14). Frequently, small hair follicles and buds of basaloid cells that may represent malformed hair germs are present. In early childhood, the sebaceous glands in nevus sebaceous are underdeveloped and the histologic finding may only consist of immature hair structures.

Differential diagnosis In a well-developed lesion, nevus sebaceous is easy to diagnose and should not be confused with other conditions. Although some authors make a distinction between an epidermal nevus with a predominant sebaceous component and a nevus sebaceous, this may well be a matter of semantics. In early childhood, when the lesion is not well developed, the differential diagnosis should include other congenital causes of localized alopecia such as aplasia cutis and congenital triangular alopecia.

Treatment Prophylactic surgical excision of a nevus sebaceous is controversial as a consequence of recent articles demonstrating a low incidence of basal cell carcinoma and other tumors.[31,32] Some investigators feel that nevus sebaceous should be excised because of malignant potential and cosmetic considerations. Others suggest that surgical excision should only be performed when clinical signs suggestive of a secondary tumor develop.[31,32]

NEVUS COMEDONICUS Synonym: Comedo nevus.

Clinical features Many authors believe that nevus comedonicus is a hamartoma of the pilosebaceous follicle, with normal development of keratin but incomplete development of terminal hair and sebaceous glands.[36] As with other epidermal nevi, nevus comedonicus may be present at birth or develop in early childhood. It is characterized by closely set papules that have in their centers dilated follicular orifices, which are filled with keratotic plugs, thus resembling comedones (Fig. 84-15). The lesion most commonly occurs on the face, neck, upper arm, and chest, often in a linear configuration. Nevus comedonicus is usually a solitary, circumscribed plaque; rarely, the nevus may be systematized.[36]

FIGURE 84-15

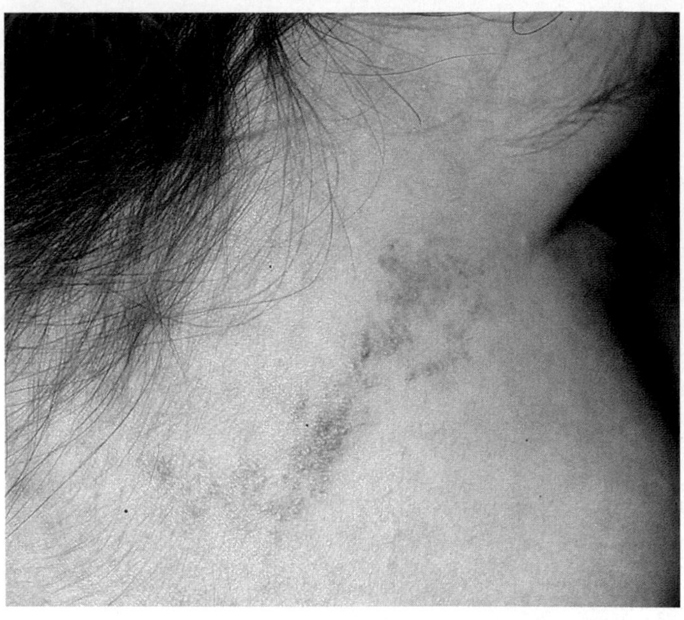

Nevus comedonicus consisting of closely set comedone-like papules.

Course and complications Spontaneous resolution has not been reported. Nevus comedonicus is usually asymptomatic but may become inflamed. Pustules, cysts, and scarring may develop, resembling acne vulgaris. Rarely, developmental defects of the central nervous system, eyes, bone, and skin have been associated with nevus comedonicus syndrome. This is considered a variant of the epidermal nevus syndrome.

Pathology There are multiple dilated pilosebaceous follicles filled with keratinous plugs. Occasionally, the follicular epithelial wall may show epidermolytic hyperkeratosis.

Differential diagnosis Acne vulgaris, acne neonatorum, nevus sebaceous, and linear Darier's disease are included. Nevus comedonicus is differentiated from acne vulgaris by its circumscribed (unilateral) distribution and its early onset and persistence.

Treatment Nevus comedonicus is usually treated for aesthetic purposes or because of recurrent inflammation. Topical retinoic acid treatment may be helpful in some cases. A patient with extensive nevus comedonicus responded dramatically within 1 month to a once-daily application of 12% ammonium lactate lotion. Individual comedones may be manually extracted. Lesions with recurrent inflammation and cyst formation may be treated with intralesional corticosteroids, incision and drainage, or systemically with antibiotics and isotretinoin. Destructive treatment methods include laser resurfacing and dermabrasion. Definitive treatment by surgical excision may offer good cosmetic results.

ECCRINE NEVUS Eccrine nevus is very rare. There are three types of presentation: the first is a circumscribed area of hyperhidrosis;[37] the second is a solitary pore that discharges a mucoid substance;[38] the third is a small skin colored plaque that often has a linear configuration.[39]

Histologically, eccrine nevi may show an increase in size or number of eccrine secretory coils. In some cases, there is eccrine duct hyperplasia consisting of thickening of the walls and dilatation of the lumina. The epidermis overlying the lesion may show basaloid proliferation.[5]

A variant of eccrine nevus, known as eccrine angiomatous hamartoma, presents as skin-colored or violaceous nodules or plaques; hyperhidrosis may not be apparent. Histologically, there are increased numbers of eccrine structures and increased capillaries.[5]

Treatment is by excision if desirable.

APOCRINE NEVUS Apocrine nevus is an extremely rare lesion that is composed of hyperplastic mature apocrine glands. Apocrine nevi do not show uniform clinical appearance. Clinical presentations have included solitary nodules on the scalp,[40] bilateral soft axillary masses, and multiple small firm papules on the chest. Histologically, numerous mature apocrine glands extend from the reticular layer of the dermis to the subcutis. Basaloid proliferation of the epidermis resembling basal cell carcinoma may be seen.[40]

Treatment is by excision if desirable.

EPIDERMAL NEVUS SYNDROME *Synonyms:* Schimmelpenning's syndrome, Feuerstein and Mims syndrome, Solomon's syndrome. Epidermal nevus syndrome refers to a disease complex consisting of the association of an epidermal nevus with various developmental abnormalities of the skin, eyes, nervous, skeletal, cardiovascular, and urogenital systems. As mentioned earlier, epidermal nevi are classified according to their predominant component, which includes *nevus sebaceous* (sebaceous glands), *nevus comedonicus* (hair follicles), and *nevus verrucous* (keratinocytes). Therefore, the generic term *epidermal nevus syndrome* traditionally refers to any one of these entities, when associated with abnormalities in other organ systems.[41] However, some authors present strong arguments that *epidermal nevus syndrome* encompasses several distinct syndromes (see below).[42]

Epidemiology Epidermal nevus syndrome is believed to occur sporadically, but there have been some reports of autosomal dominant transmission, which has not been substantiated.[16] Both sexes are affected equally. Ages of diagnosis ranges from birth to 40 years.[16] Although the exact incidence of epidermal nevus syndrome is unknown, a study of 119 cases of epidermal nevi showed that 33 percent of patients showed one or more extracutaneous abnormalities, 16 percent showed two or more abnormalities, 10 percent showed three or more abnormalities, and 5 percent showed five or more abnormalities.[15]

Clinical features Solomon and Esterly[16] provided a detailed account of the spectrum of epidermal nevi seen in the epidermal nevus syndrome. They described seven types of lesions. The majority of patients had nevus unius lateris; 20 percent of patients had ichthyosis hystrix; and another 20 percent had what the authors termed the *acanthotic form* of epidermal nevus. These lesions presented as large, unilateral, brown, slightly scaly patches. About 10 percent of patients had linear nevus sebaceous involving the scalp and face. Localized linear verrucous nevus and a velvety epidermal nevus in the axilla similar to acanthosis nigricans were seen in a minority of cases. Some patients had a mixture of several types of lesions.

Table 84-3 lists the mucocutaneous changes other than epidermal nevus that may be seen in patients with epidermal nevus syndrome.[15,16,43] Hemangiomas and pigmentary changes are found in 10 to 20 percent of patients. Less-common findings are hair abnormalities, dental abnormalities in association with mucosal epidermal nevi, and dermatomegaly. This last condition involves an increase in skin thickness, warmth, and hairiness. As discussed earlier, various cutaneous tumors may develop within the epidermal nevus.

A wide range of skeletal abnormalities has been reported (Table 84-4).[15,16,43,44] The incidence of skeletal changes have ranged from 15 to 70 percent. Solomon and Esterly classified the osseous changes into primary and secondary effects. Primary changes include

TABLE 84-3

Cutaneous Findings in Epidermal Nevus Syndrome

Epidermal nevus	Cutaneous malignancies
Hemangioma	Keratoacanthoma
Pigmentary changes	Basal cell carcinoma
Café-au-lait spots	Squamous cell carcinoma
Hypopigmentation	Syringocystadenoma papilliferum
Melanocytic nevi	Other adnexal tumors
Dermatomegaly	

bone deformities and cysts, and secondary bone changes include atrophies and hypertrophies. In several patients, bone deformities have resulted from hypophosphatemic vitamin D resistant rickets, thought to be induced by epidermal nevi producing a potent phosphaturic factor. In one such case report, after excision of the epidermal nevus the hypophosphatemia resolved.[45]

Neurologic abnormalities occur in 15 to 50 percent of cases (Table 84-5).[15,16,43] Mental retardation, seizures, and cognitive development delay are the most common findings. These may be associated with cerebrovascular malformations, cortical atrophy, hydrocephalus, and intracranial calcifications. Central nervous system abnormalities are reported to be associated with epidermal nevi on the head,[46] but this has been disputed.[15]

From 9 to 30 percent of patients with epidermal nevus syndrome have ocular abnormalities (Table 84-6);[15,16,43,47] the most common abnormalities are colobomas and choristomas. A coloboma is defined as an absence or functional defect of ocular tissue; most commonly, the iris, ciliary body, or choroid. A choristoma is a congenital overgrowth of normal tissue in an abnormal location. Choristomas include dermoid, lipodermoid, single-tissue choristoma and complex choristoma. Table 84-7 lists the other uncommon abnormalities associated with this syndrome.[15]

As in isolated epidermal nevi, malignant transformation may occur within the epidermal nevi in patients with epidermal nevus syndrome. This occurrence is most common in those with nevus sebaceous. Perhaps less well known is the association of visceral malignancies with the epidermal nevus syndrome. The following tumors are reported to occur at a higher frequency and at an earlier age in patients with epidermal nevus syndrome: tumors of the genitourinary system (Wilm's tumor, nephroblastoma, metastatic transitional cell carcinoma of the bladder, and rhabdomyosarcoma of the bladder); tumors of the gastrointestinal tract (hepatic adenoma, salivary gland adenocarcinoma, and carcinoma

TABLE 84-4

Skeletal Findings in Epidermal Nevus Syndrome

Bone cysts
Bone hyperplasia or hypertrophy
Chondroblastoma
Asymmetry of skull
Short stature
Brachydactylia
Kyphosis
Scoliosis
Spina bifida
Syndactyly, polydactyly, chinodactyly
Vitamin D–resistant rickets

TABLE 84-5

Neurologic Findings in Epidermal Nevus Syndrome

Cerebrovascular accidents	Encephalocele
Cerebrovascular malformations and neoplasias	Hemiparesis
Cortical atrophy	Hydrocephalus
Cortical blindness	Mental retardation
Cranial nerve palsies	Seizures (generalized focal infantile spasms)
Delayed milestones	Spinal cord stenosis
Macrocephaly	

of the esophagus and stomach); and tumors of the central nervous system (astrocytoma, mixed glioma, and meningioma). Breast carcinoma, mandibular ameloblastoma, chondroma, odontoma, and endometrioma are other tumors associated with epidermal nevus syndrome.[41] However, these associations have not been confirmed by case-controlled studies.

Recently, Happle[42,48] proposed that the epidermal nevus syndrome is not a single entity; rather, it consists of at least six distinct diseases that differ in genetic origin but which share the common feature of mosaicism, including Schimmelpenning's syndrome; nevus comedonicus syndrome; pigmented hairy epidermal nevus syndrome; Proteus syndrome; congenital hemidysplasia, ichthyosiform dermatitis, and limb defects (CHILD) syndrome; and phacomatosis pigmentokeratotica (see Chap. 188 for more information).

Management Patients with extensive epidermal nevi or those with epidermal nevi and systemic abnormalities should be suspected of having the epidermal nevus syndrome. Evaluation and management of patients with epidermal nevus syndrome requires a multidisciplinary team approach involving the dermatologist, pediatrician, ophthalmologist, neurologist, plastic surgeon, and orthopedic services. These patients require a careful history with particular attention given to developmental history, attainment of milestones, history of seizures, and abnormalities of the bones, eyes, and urinary tract. Thorough mucocutaneous, neurologic, ophthalmologic, and orthopedic examinations are necessary. Depending on the findings on history and physical examination, further investigations may be indicated. These may include biopsy of the epidermal nevus, electroencephalography, computed tomography, magnetic resonance imaging, intravenous pyelography, and radiographic evaluation of bones. A regular follow-up program should be set up for the patient.

TABLE 84-6

Ocular Findings in Epidermal Nevus Syndrome

Astigmatism
Lipodermoid
Bilateral cataracts
Blocked tear duct
Choristomas
Colobomas of lid, iris, choroid retina
Corneal opacity and pannus formation
Cortical blindness
Ectopic lacrimal glands
Extension of epidermal nevus to eyelid, conjunctiva, or sclera
Micro- or macrophthalmia
Nystagmus
Oculomotor dysfunction
Optic nerve hypoplasia
Ptosis
Strabismus

TABLE 84-7

Miscellaneous Abnormalities Associated with the Epidermal Nevus Syndrome

Urogenital	Others
Horseshoe kidneys	Teratoma
Undescended testes	Choanal atresia
Testicular adenomas	Pyloric stenosis
Double ureters	Hernia
Vascular	
Aneurysms	
Arteriovenous malformations	
Coarctations	
Patent ductus arteriosus	
Renal artery stenosis	

LICHEN STRIATUS

Synonym: BLAISE (Blaschko linear acquired inflammatory skin eruption). Lichen striatus is a self-limited linear dermatosis most commonly seen in children.

Etiology and epidemiology Lichen striatus commonly presents in children between 5 to 15 years of age. However, a study of 61 children by Kennedy et al. found the mean age to be 3 years.[49] Lichen striatus is rarely present in adults. Females are more commonly affected than males, with a ratio of 2:1. The etiology of lichen striatus is unknown but reports of its occurrence in siblings, atopic individuals, and in the spring and summer support genetic, infectious, and environmental factors.[49–51]

Clinical features Lichen striatus presents as a sudden eruption of discrete pink, red, or skin-colored 1- to 3-mm flat-topped papules distributed in a linear configuration commonly following the lines of Blaschko. Individual papules are either smooth or have a very fine scale. The papules coalesce into a 1- to 3-cm wide band, which gradually, over a few weeks, progresses unilaterally on an upper or lower extremity with occasional extension onto the trunk. It is usually asymptomatic but some patients may experience mild pruritus. Nail involvement of lichen striatus is uncommon and presents as nail plate thinning with longitudinal ridging and splitting. It is usually associated with typical skin lesions; however, rarely, lichen striatus may be limited to the nails.[52]

Course and complications Lichen striatus may progress over a few weeks, and then remain stable for months, eventually regressing within 1 year. Postinflammatory hypopigmentation or hyperpigmentation may persist for years. Nail involvement also improves spontaneously.

Pathology Epidermal changes consists of hyperkeratosis, focal parakeratosis, mild spongiosis with lymphocyte exocytosis, and a few necrotic keratinocytes. Within the dermis there is a superficial and deep perivascular infiltrate, with either focal or lichenoid patterns at the dermal–epidermal junction and appendageal involvement. Colloid bodies are present in 50 percent of cases.[53]

Differential diagnosis Lichen striatus is diagnosed based on history and physical exam. Other dermatoses presenting in a linear configuration are lichen planus, psoriasis, porokeratosis, lichen nitidus, Darier's disease and ILVEN. ILVEN may be distinguished from lichen striatus by its appearance at birth or early infancy, associated pruritus, lack of spontaneous regression, and histologically having alternating parakeratosis and orthokeratosis with acanthosis and mild superficial lymphocytic infiltrate.

Treatment Treatment is not necessary as lichen striatus undergoes spontaneous regression and is usually asymptomatic. For patients with mild pruritus, topical steroids may be useful.

CLEAR CELL ACANTHOMA

Synonyms: Degos' acanthoma, pale cell acanthoma. Clear cell acanthoma is a benign epidermal tumor characterized histologically by clear, glycogen-containing epidermal cells.

Etiology and pathogenesis It was postulated that clear cell acanthoma was of sweat duct origin, but Penneys et al., found no carcinoembryonic antigen (CEA) positivity and felt that a sweat duct origin was unlikely.[54] The expression of involucrin and epithelial membrane antigen suggests that clear cell acanthoma is derived from surface epithelium.[55] The etiology of clear cell acanthoma, however, remains unknown. Ohnishi and Watanabe[56] suggest that the pattern of cytokeratin expression is similar to that found in inflammatory dermatosis, suggesting that there is a relationship with psoriasis, lichen planus, or discoid lupus. Finch et al. reported a case of clear cell acanthoma developing within a psoriatic plaque, which supports this theory.[57]

Epidemiology Clear cell acanthoma is an uncommon tumor occurring in adults, most commonly presenting between 50 and 70 years of age. There is no sexual predilection.

Clinical features The typical lesion is a slowly growing, sharply marginated, dome-shaped nodule or small plaque, with a "stuck on" appearance. There is frequently a wafer-like peripheral collarette scale. The color varies from pink to brown; a rare, pigmented variant has been reported.[58] The surface is often moist and may show red vascular puncta giving an erythematous appearance. Blanching is almost complete with pressure. It is usually approximately 1 to 2 cm in diameter, but a variant named *giant clear cell acanthoma* may be as large as 5 cm. Clear cell acanthoma is usually solitary; multiple lesions ranging in number from several to more than 100 have been reported but are rare. The most common location is the legs, although it has been reported to occur on the trunk, face, and back.[59]

Pathology This exo-endophytic epidermal tumor is sharply circumscribed. The acanthotic epidermis consists of slightly enlarged malpighian cells with strikingly clear cytoplasm (Fig. 84-16). The "clear cell" appearance is due to glycogen deposition in the cells as verified by PAS staining. The epidermis is commonly infiltrated by abundant numbers of neutrophils, which may form microabscesses in the parakeratotic stratum corneum. A well-formed granular layer is absent. There are dilated superficial capillaries accounting for the characteristic red color and red puncta of this lesion.

FIGURE 84-16

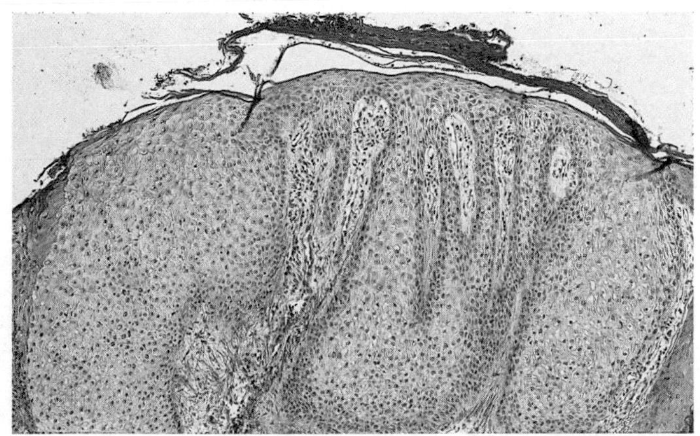

Clear cell acanthoma showing a well-circumscribed epidermal tumor composed of clear (glycogen-rich) cells.

Differential diagnosis The clinical differential diagnosis may include an irritated seborrheic keratosis, hemangioma, dermatofibroma, basal cell carcinoma, squamous cell carcinoma, amelanotic melanoma, and pyogenic granuloma.

Treatment, course, and prognosis Clear cell acanthoma does not show spontaneous regression. This benign tumor can be removed by simple excision or curettage and electrofulguration. Complete resolution with good cosmetic results following liquid nitrogen cryotherapy has been reported.[60] This mode of therapy may be suitable for patients with large lesions, multiple lesions, or lesions over bony prominences or for patients on anticoagulant therapy for whom surgery may be difficult.

WARTY DYSKERATOMA

Synonym: Isolated dyskeratosis follicularis. Warty dyskeratoma is a benign, usually solitary tumor characterized clinically as a crateriform keratotic nodule and histologically by acantholytic dyskeratosis.

Etiology and pathogenesis The etiology and pathogenesis of warty dyskeratoma are unknown. Its derivation from the pilosebaceous unit has been proposed, but the observation that warty dyskeratoma can occur on the oral mucosa argues against this proposal. Smoking may be a predisposing factor to warty dyskeratoma.

Epidemiology The exact incidence of this lesion is unknown. It is not common. There is no sexual predisposition.

Clinical features Warty dyskeratoma usually occurs as a solitary papule or nodule with a central keratotic plug. Rarely, multiple warty dyskeratomas have been reported.[61] The lesion may be skin-colored to red-brown. It most commonly occurs on the face, scalp, or neck; lesions on other locations, including the oral mucosa, have been reported. The lesion grows slowly and, after reaching the usual size of 1 to 2 cm, persists indefinitely.

Pathology The tumor is well circumscribed and appears as a cup-shaped invagination of the acanthotic epidermis (Fig. 84-17). The center of this invagination is filled with a keratotic plug. Within this cavity are many acantholytic dyskeratotic cells. Numerous pseudovilli (dermal papillae lined with basal cells) project up from the base of the invagination. Corps ronds (acantholytic dyskeratotic cells with central basophilia, pyknotic nuclei surrounded by a clear halo) and grains (parakeratotic cells surrounded by homogeneous eosinophilic material) are commonly found.

Treatment, course, and prognosis This benign tumor may be treated by saucerization or elliptical excision, which allows for histologic examination of the entire lesion. Untreated, the lesion persists indefinitely.

ACANTHOMA FISSURATUM

Synonyms: Granuloma fissuratum, spectacle frame acanthoma. Acanthoma fissuratum is a localized thickening of the skin in response to pressure caused by an eyeglass frame.

FIGURE 84-17

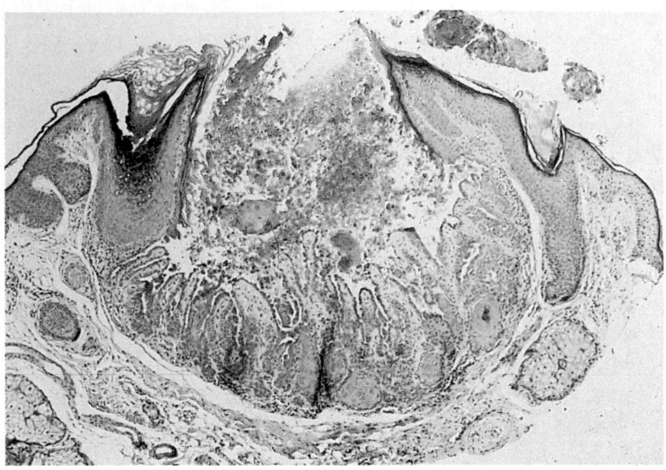

Warty dyskeratoma showing cup-shaped invagination of the acanthotic epidermis and acantholysis.

Clinical features Acanthoma fissuratum is usually unilateral and may occur on any of the pressure points of the eyeglass frame: retroauricular fold, superior auricular crease, or bridge of the nose. The lesion is a red-brown nodule with a central depressed groove where the eyeglass frame rests on the skin[62] (Fig. 84-18): This groove may be fissured, ulcerated, and crusted; it may or may not be tender.

Pathology The epidermis is acanthotic and may even show pseudoepitheliomatous hyperplasia. In the center, the epidermis may be atrophic or degenerated, beneath which the collagen appears hyalinized. There is a variable degree of perivascular infiltration of plasma cells, histiocytes, and lymphocytes.

FIGURE 84-18

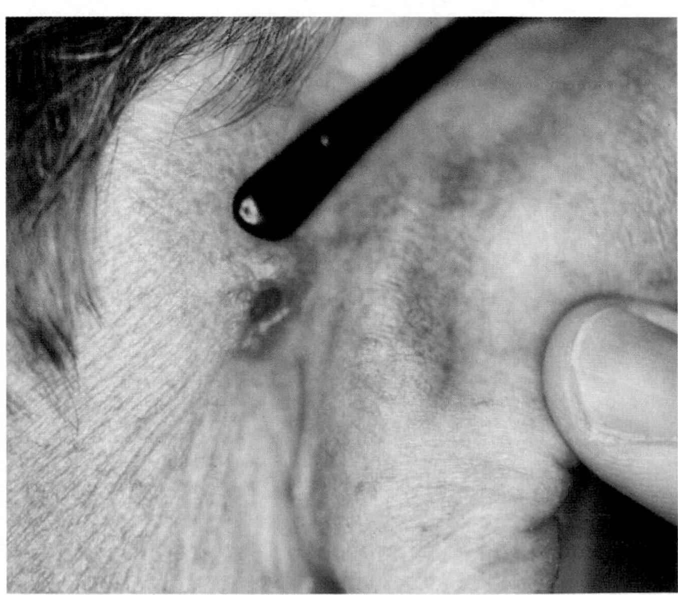

Acanthoma fissuratum due to excessive pressure from eyeglasses.

Differential diagnosis The common clinical differential diagnosis includes basal cell carcinoma, squamous cell carcinoma, and chondrodermatitis nodularis helicis. Recognition that the lesion is related to external pressure should lead to the correct diagnosis. If in doubt, histologic examination provides easy distinction.

Treatment, course, and prognosis The lesion can be expected to slowly resolve if the excessive pressure on the affected area caused by ill-fitting spectacle frames can be relieved. Otherwise, the lesion may become thicker or pressure necrosis and ulceration may ensue.

CYSTS OF EPIDERMAL ORIGIN

EPIDERMOID CYST *Synonyms:* Epidermal cyst, epithelial cyst, keratin cyst, sebaceous cyst (a misnomer). An epidermoid cyst is a keratin-containing cyst lined by surface epidermis.

Etiology and pathogenesis An epidermoid cyst is the result of the proliferation of surface epidermal cells within the dermis. Production of keratin within a circumscribed space results in a cyst. Epidermoid cysts may arise from occlusion of pilosebaceous follicles, from implantation of epidermal cells into the dermis following penetration injury, and from trapping of epidermal cells along embryonal fusion planes. The first mechanism is the most common, and it is widely believed that the epidermal lining of the cyst is derived from the follicular infundibulum. Ohnishi et al.[63] have recently confirmed that the cytokeratin profile of epidermal cysts is the same as the follicular infundibulum. The theory of epidermal cells trapped along fusion planes explains reports of intracranial, intraabdominal, and testicular epidermoid cysts.[64,65] Several reports show the presence of human papillomavirus types 57 and 60 in palmoplantar epidermoid cysts.[66]

Epidemiology Epidermoid cysts are rare in children but common in adults. Both sexes are affected equally. Patients with Gardner's syndrome and nevoid basal cell carcinoma syndrome may have many lesions.

Clinical features An epidermoid cyst presents as a 1- to 5-cm intradermal or subcutaneous, dome-shaped protuberance, which is freely

FIGURE 84-19

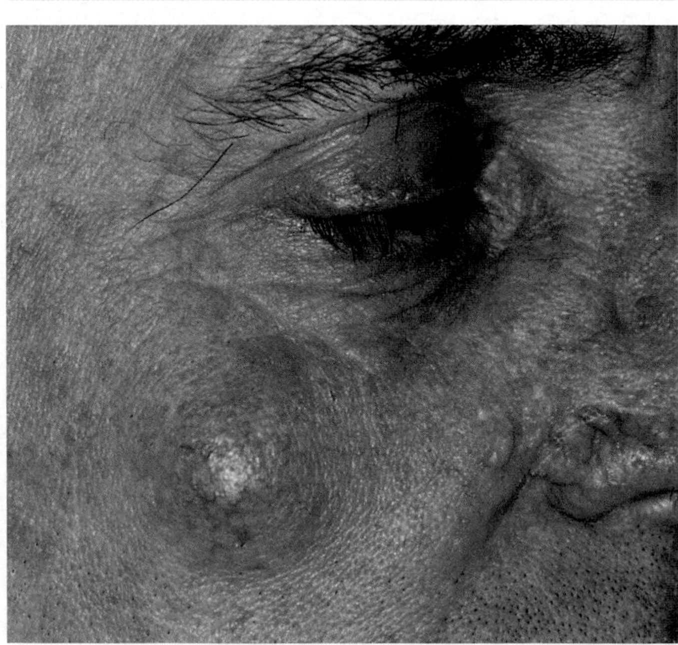

Epidermoid cyst presenting as a dome-shaped protuberance of the skin.

mobile over underlying structures (Fig. 84-19). Some cysts may be tethered to the epidermis, and there may be a central punctum from which cheesy keratinous material may be expressed, representing the plugged orifice of the pilosebaceous follicle. Cysts that are superficially located may appear yellowish or white. Epidermoid cysts are most commonly found on the face, neck, chest, and upper back, where the sebaceous glands are most numerous and active. Cysts secondary to traumatic implantation usually occur on the palms or soles or on the buttocks.

Complications Epidermoid cysts are slow-growing and are usually not symptomatic. Some cysts may become inflamed and secondarily infected. This occurs most frequently on the face and neck in association with acne vulgaris. Rupture of an inflamed epidermoid cyst induces a foreign-body inflammatory response in the dermis. Dystrophic calcification of the cyst contents may also occur, but this is rarely detected clinically. In a study of the microbiology of infected epidermal cysts Brook[67] found 192 of 231 clinically infected epidermoid cysts yielded bacterial growth, of which 44 percent had aerobic organisms, 30 percent had anaerobic organisms, and 26 percent had mixed growth. The predominant aerobic bacteria were *Staphylococcus aureus* (81 isolates), group A *Streptococcus* (9 isolates), and *Escherichia coli* (7 isolates). The predominant anaerobic organisms were *Peptostreptococcus* species (85 isolates) and *Bacteroides* species (55 isolates). Anaerobic organisms were isolated more frequently in perirectal, vulvovaginal, and head infections and less frequently in trunk and extremity lesions. This study highlights the polymicrobial nature and the predominance of anaerobes in cyst abscesses. There have been rare reports of basal cell carcinoma,[68] Bowen's disease,[69] and squamous cell carcinoma[70] developing in epidermoid cysts. Some of these reported cases may represent pseudoepitheliomatous hyperplasia or a proliferating trichilemmal tumor rather than malignant transformation.

Pathology The cyst is lined by a true epidermis composed of several layers of stratified squamous epithelium and a granular layer. Within the cyst is keratinous material arranged in laminated layers (Fig. 84-20). An epidermal cyst may contain melanocytes; as a result pigmentation is more commonly seen in dark-skinned individuals. A foreign body-type reaction with multinucleated giant cells may be found in the dermis surrounding the cyst in response to spillage of cyst contents.

Differential diagnosis The typical epidermoid cyst can usually be diagnosed clinically with confidence, especially if there is a central punctum through which the characteristic cheesy keratinous material can be expressed. Epidermoid cysts are clinically indistinguishable from pilar cysts; cysts on the trunk are usually epidermoid while those on the scalp are pilar in origin. Steatocystoma, especially the simplex variant, may cause diagnostic confusion, but typically it contains a yellow oily fluid rather than the cheesy-white keratinous debris seen in an epidermoid cyst. A lipoma may resemble an epidermoid cyst but may be differentiated by its soft consistency.

FIGURE 84-20

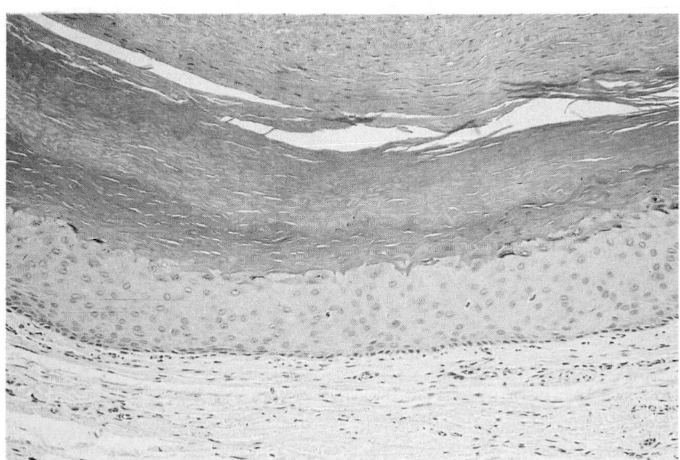

Epidermoid cyst lined by stratified epithelium with a granular layer. Within the cyst, the keratinous material is arranged in laminated layers.

Treatment An inflamed noninfected cyst can be treated by intralesional triamcinolone 5 mg/mL. A fluctuant, probably infected cyst should be incised, drained, and cultured; if there is no improvement, antibiotic treatment should be started. The initial antibiotic therapy should be directed against *S. aureus,* as this is the most common pathogen; the antibiotic treatment can be modified according to culture and sensitivity results. Removal of the cyst is usually best deferred until the inflammation and infection have subsided. A cyst that has never been inflamed can usually be easily enucleated through a simple incision. A cyst with a history of previous inflammation and scarring as a result may need to be carefully dissected out. To prevent recurrence, the entire epidermal lining should be removed or destroyed.

TRICHILEMMAL CYST *Synonym:* Pilar cyst. A trichilemmal cyst is a keratin-containing cyst, most commonly located on the scalp, which is derived from the lower portion of the hair follicle.

Etiology and pathogenesis The trichilemmal cyst wall is derived from the outer root sheath from the lower portion of the isthmus of the hair follicle located between the arrector pili muscle and the orifice of the sebaceous duct. As a result of this origin, the squamous epithelium undergoes abrupt homogeneous keratinization without the interposition of a granular layer. Leppard et al. illustrated features of an autosomal dominant mode of inheritance from pedigrees of patients with trichilemmal cysts.[71]

FIGURE 84-21

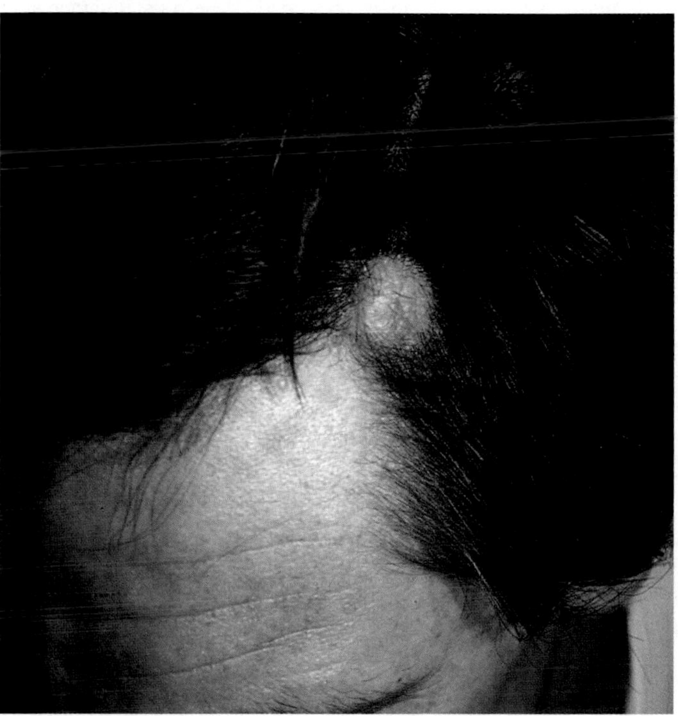

A trichilemmal (pilar) cyst on the scalp.

FIGURE 84-22

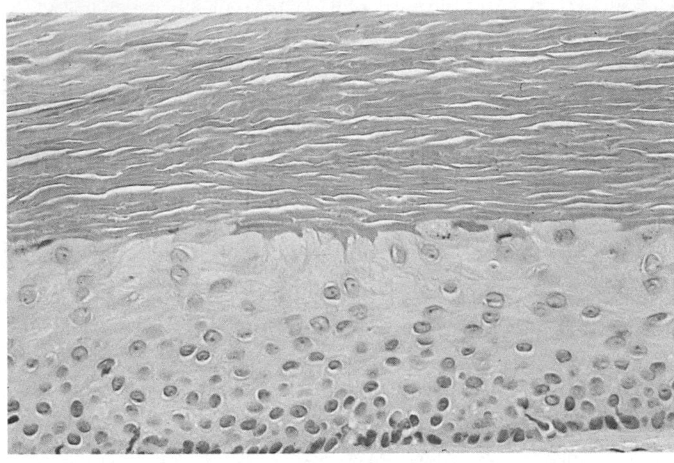

Trichilemmal cysts showing an epithelial lining that lacks a granular layer.

FIGURE 84-23

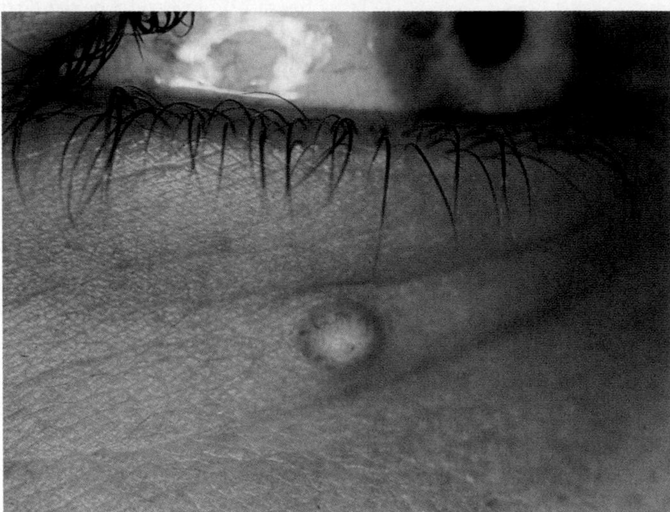

Primary milium. A 3.0-mm, hard, seedlike white papule.

Epidemiology Trichilemmal cysts account for 10 to 20 percent of keratinous cysts seen in surgical pathology. They are reportedly more common in women and usually present in middle age. They occur in 5 to 10 percent of the population.

Clinical features Trichilemmal cysts are smooth, mobile, firm dermal nodules. They are located in areas of dense hair follicle concentrations; therefore, 90 percent occur on the scalp (Fig. 84-21).[71] Occasionally, lesions may form on the face, neck, and trunk. Patients usually have multiple lesions; more than 70 percent of patients have several lesions and 10 percent of patients have more than 10 lesions.[71]

Complications Trichilemmal cysts may become inflamed and may suppurate, but this is uncommon. Rarely, the cyst may fuse with the epidermis to form a marsupialized cyst. Proliferating trichilemmal cyst (also known as proliferating trichilemmal tumor) may develop from an ordinary trichilemmal cyst.[71] This condition is usually seen in elderly women and is clinically recognized as a progressively enlarging lobulated mass that may ulcerate and resemble a squamous cell carcinoma. Although considered biologically benign, it may be locally aggressive. Very rarely, malignant transformation (malignant proliferating trichilemmal cyst) may occur, and this is heralded by rapid enlargement of a nodule.[72,73]

Pathology A trichilemmal cyst is lined by epidermal cells that tend to be cuboidal, with indistinct intercellular bridges. The peripheral cell layer often shows palisading. There is no granular layer (Fig. 84-22). The cyst contains homogeneous eosinophilic keratinous material; foci of calcification may develop. A proliferating trichilemmal cyst shows a well-demarcated lobular squamous epithelial tumor. Characteristically, the epithelium in the center of the lobule changes abruptly into eosinophilic amorphous keratin, indicating trichilemmal keratinization. Infiltrative margins with a loss of a periodic acid-Schiff–reactive basement membrane and stromal desmoplasia suggest malignant transformation.[73]

Differential diagnosis See "Epidermoid Cyst," above.

Treatment Treatment is the same as that for an epidermoid cyst. An uncomplicated trichilemmal cyst can usually be removed easily. A proliferating trichilemmal cyst must be excised with a narrow margin to ensure complete removal.

MILIUM A milium is a small, superficial keratin cyst.

Etiology and pathogenesis Milia are common skin tumors classified as either primary or secondary. Primary milia are believed to be derived from the lowest portion of the infundibulum of vellus hairs. Secondary milia may represent retention cysts following injury to the skin and are believed to be derived from a hair follicle, sweat duct, sebaceous duct, or epidermis. Secondary milia may be seen in blistering dermatoses, after dermabrasion or 5-fluorouracil treatment, and in areas of chronic glucocorticoid-induced atrophy.[74]

Epidemiology Milia are very common and most of the time are not brought to medical attention. They are commonly found on the skin and mucosa of term infants. They also commonly occur in adults and show no sexual predisposition.

Clinical features Milia are clinically distinct. They are superficial, pearly white, globoid papules, generally only 1 to 2 mm in diameter (Fig. 84-23). Primary milia arise most commonly on the face, especially on the eyelids and cheeks. Milia in the newborn also have a predilection for the face, especially the nose. They may also appear elsewhere on the body and on mucosae (palate and gingiva). Milia on the palate are known as Epstein's pearls. A rare subtype of primary milia, called milia en plaque, occurs in middle-aged individuals and consists of grouped milia on an erythematous, indurated plaque, commonly located around the ears. Secondary milia are morphologically identical to primary milia; they are scattered within the affected areas. Rare cases of eruptive milia in which large numbers of lesions develop acutely on the face and trunk have been reported.[75]

Pathology The pathology of milia is identical to that of an epidermoid cyst, differing only in size. On serial section, a primary milium may be connected to a vellus hair follicle by an epithelial pedicle. Similarly, a secondary milium may show connection to its "parent" epithelial structure.

Treatment Spontaneous resolution of congenital milia is common and they do not require treatment. Milia arising later in life persist and can easily be expressed with a comedone extractor after incision with a no. 11 scalpel blade or a needle. When there are many lesions, they may be treated by light electrodesiccation of the surface of the lesions; the keratin core may extrude after the charred epidermal surface sloughs off.

FIGURE 84-24

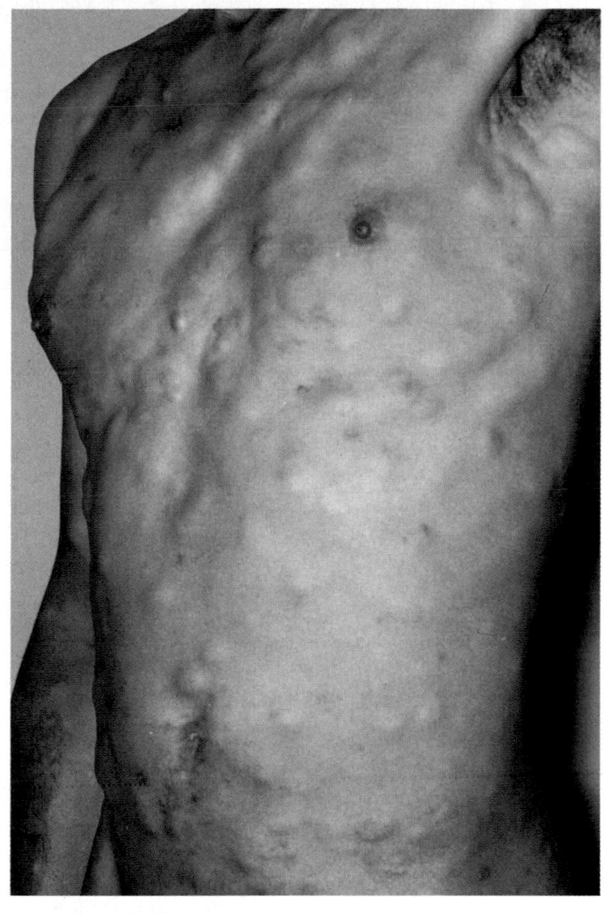

Steatocystoma multiplex. Multiple yellow cystic lesions on the trunk.

STEATOCYSTOMA MULTIPLEX *Synonyms:* Sebocystomatosis, epidermal polycystic disease. Steatocystoma multiplex is characterized by the presence of multiple dermal cysts that contain sebum and are lined by an epithelium containing sebaceous follicles.

Etiology and pathogenesis This is an autosomal dominant disorder; however, in some cases, no familial pattern can be established. Steatocystoma also occurs as a solitary lesion known as steatocystoma simplex, which has no hereditary tendency.

Epidemiology Both steatocystoma multiplex and simplex are uncommon. The condition usually begins in adolescence or early adulthood and persists indefinitely. Both sexes are affected equally.

Clinical features Patients present with many smooth, firm, dermal cystic papules and nodules adherent to the overlying skin (Fig. 84-24). The trunk and proximal extremities are most commonly involved, but lesions may appear anywhere, including the scrotum. Lesions vary from a few millimeters to several centimeters in diameter. The deeper lesions are skin-colored; superficial ones often appear yellow. When punctured, the cysts discharge a characteristic oily or creamy fluid. The lesions are usually asymptomatic; some may become inflamed, suppurate, and heal with scarring. Multiple lesions can be associated with pachyonychia congenita.

Pathology The cyst is situated in the mid-dermis. The cyst wall is convoluted with a peripheral layer of palisaded basal cells. The luminal surface of the wall is lined by a thick, homogeneous, eosinophilic layer (Fig. 84-25). There is no granular layer. Sebaceous glands are characteristically present in the cyst wall. The cystic cavity may contain small hairs.

FIGURE 84-25

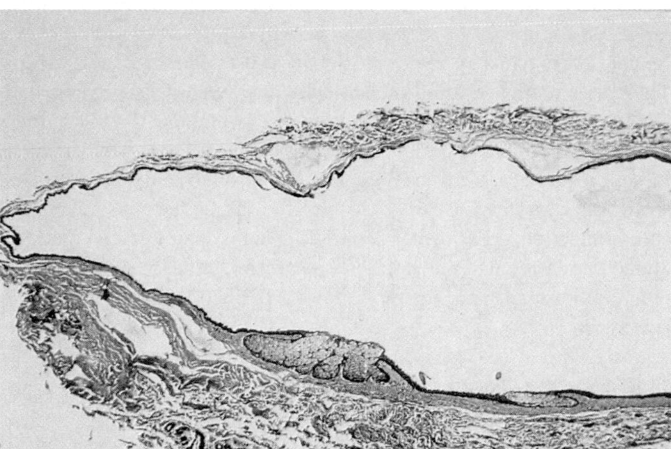

Steatocystoma multiplex. Sebaceous glands are present in the cyst wall.

Differential diagnosis The main differential diagnoses include "epidermoid cyst" (discussed earlier) and eruptive vellus hair cysts. Eruptive vellus hair cyst, which can be clinically indistinguishable from steatocystoma multiplex, are of both sporadic and autosomal dominant inheritance, most commonly presenting in adolescents as asymptomatic smooth papules and nodules on the anterior chest and extremities. It is histologically distinctive from steatocystoma multiplex. In a vellus hair cyst the cyst wall has several layers of mature squamous cells with a well-defined granular layer. The lumen is filled with laminated and amorphous keratinous material and numerous fragments of vellus hair. Sebaceous glands are situated close to the cyst, but rarely within the cyst wall. There are reports demonstrating that steatocystoma multiplex and eruptive vellus hair cysts may be variants of one entity.[76]

Treatment The multiplicity of lesions of steatocystoma multiplex usually precludes surgical excision. Recent reports of 1- to 3-mm incisions at the domes of lesions and removal of cyst walls with artery forceps have offered both excellent cosmetic results and long lasting remissions.[77] Inflamed lesions may be excised or treated with incision and drainage and/or intralesional glucocorticoids. Other attempts of treatment with aspiration, isotretinoin, cryotherapy, and CO_2 laser have had variable success.

DERMOID CYST A dermoid cyst is a cyst that is lined by an epidermis containing various epidermal appendages.

Etiology and pathogenesis Dermoid cysts develop from sequestration of epithelium along lines of embryonic fusion.

Epidemiology Dermoid cysts are rare, the estimated incidence is about 0.002 to 0.005 percent of births.[78] They may first be noted at birth or in early childhood. The sexes are affected equally.

Clinical features As expected, these lesions are found along embryonal fusion planes. The most common locations are the lateral third of the eyebrows, the nose, and the scalp. Nasal dermoid cysts may have a sinus tract that opens on the skin of the nose anywhere between the base of the columella and the glabella, with the distal one-third of the nasal dorsum being the most common site. A cheesy material may be expressed from the sinus, and tufts of hair may project from it.[79] Cystic swellings may appear anywhere along the sinus tract. Uncommon locations include the neck, sternum, scrotum, perineal raphe, and sacrum.[79] The cysts are usually subcutaneous and freely mobile, although they may occasionally be fixed to the periosteum. They are smooth and firm in consistency. They enlarge slowly and may reach sizes ranging from 1 to 4 cm or more in diameter.

Complications Dermoid cysts can become inflamed and infected. Infection may be introduced iatrogenically through aspirations or biopsies. This may lead to serious complications if there is intracranial communication.[80] Periocular dermoids usually do not extend intracranially, but dermoids in the midline frontal (including nasal dermoids), temporal-parietal, and occipital regions frequently have intracranial extensions.[81]

Pathology The cyst is lined by epidermis and the cyst wall contains various mature skin appendages; namely, hair follicles, sweat glands, and sebaceous glands. Hairs are often present within and projecting into the cyst cavity.

Differential diagnosis The differential diagnosis includes other cysts of epithelial origin, glioma, encephalocele, hemangioma, rhabdomyosarcoma, and fibrosarcoma. The early onset of the lesion and the location should help distinguish a dermoid cyst from other cysts of epithelial origin.[81] A hemangioma has a purple to bluish hue. Rhabdomyosarcomas and fibrosarcomas are hard and rapidly growing. When the lesion is located on the neck, thyroglossal duct cyst, bronchial cyst, and ectopic thyroid should be considered. It is important to differentiate a nasal dermoid cyst from an extranasal glioma or an encephalocele because the latter two lesions may connect with the subarachnoid space. Extranasal glioma is a rare benign tumor of heterotopic brain tissue thought to arise from abnormal sequestration of normal elements during development. It may present at birth as a firm, red-to-purple protrusion at the root of the nose. A useful differentiating feature is that glioma is almost always eccentric and not midline. An encephalocele is a herniation of cranial contents through a skull defect; it may show size fluctuation or spontaneous pulsation; hypertelorism is frequently seen.

Treatment Treatment of a dermoid cyst is by excision.[82] Any possible underlying sinus tract should be explored and excised to prevent recurrence. Careful preoperative evaluation is essential to delineate any intracranial extension. When appropriate, consultations with otolaryngology or facial plastic surgery and neurosurgery services should be obtained. Imaging studies include magnetic resonance imaging or computed tomography as well as polytomography of the base of the skull.[81,82]

BRANCHIAL CYST *Synonym:* Branchial cleft cyst. A branchial cyst is an epithelial cyst that arises from incomplete obliteration of the branchial clefts in embryologic development.

Etiology and pathogenesis Branchial cysts usually arise from incomplete closure of the second branchial cleft and rarely from the third branchial clefts. The cysts are derived from the sequestrated remains of the cleft membrane. Most appear to be sporadic cases, but pedigrees showing autosomal dominant inheritance have been reported.

Epidemiology This is a rare disorder.

Clinical features Asymptomatic sinuses or fistulas present in infancy, drain internally to the pharynx and/or externally through the skin of the neck along the middle to lower third of the anterior edge of the sternocleidomastoid muscle. Branchial cleft cysts occur in childhood or early adulthood as a result of occlusion of the sinus tract. They most frequently present after an upper respiratory tract infection as a painful, warm, erythematous inflammatory mass, deep to the anterior border of the sternocleidomastoid muscle. Most are unilateral, but 10 percent are bilateral. They may have a mucoid discharge and may become infected.

Pathology The cysts and sinuses are lined by stratified squamous epithelium. The wall commonly contains lymphoid tissue with germinal centers.

Treatment Complete excision is recommended at diagnosis, as recurrent infections are common. Infected cysts and sinus tracts should be treated with warm compresses and systemic antibiotics.

PREAURICULAR CYST AND SINUS *Synonyms:* Ear pits, congenital auricular fistula. A preauricular cyst or sinus is an epithelial cyst or sinus in the preauricular region; it arises from incomplete fusion of the first two branchial arches.

Etiology and pathogenesis During Embryonic development, six tubercles from the first two branchial arches produce the tragus and pinna. Their incomplete fusion results in epithelium-lined pouches. These become epithelial cysts known as preauricular cysts. The cysts tunnel to the surface of the skin, forming preauricular sinuses.

Epidemiology Preauricular cysts and sinuses are common, occurring in 1 percent of the population. Familial cases with autosomal dominant inheritance have been described.

Clinical features Most cases are asymptomatic and bilateral, and the lesions are noted incidentally as bilateral cystic swellings or pits just anterior to the superior auricular crease; the pits represent the openings of the preauricular sinuses. Sometimes, the lesions may present as infected cysts draining pus through the preauricular sinuses to the surface of the skin.

Complications The majority of preauricular cysts and sinuses are uncomplicated. Sometimes, secondary infection may occur. Rarely, other developmental anomalies of the ear and branchial arches may coexist. Deafness has been associated with this disorder.[83]

Pathology The cysts and sinus tracts are lined by stratified squamous epithelium.

Treatment Asymptomatic lesions require no treatment. Secondarily infected lesions should be treated with antibiotics. Excision should be delayed until the infection has subsided.

CHONDRODERMATITIS NODULARIS HELICIS*

Chondrodermatitis nodularis helicis (CNH) usually occurs as a single, less than 1 cm diameter, exquisitely tender eroded nodule on the free border of the helix of the ear.

Etiology and Pathogenesis[84,85]

The pinnae are exposed to constant mechanical and environmental trauma (e.g., pressure, sun, wind, and extremes of temperature), leading to thinning of the skin and cartilage, to loss of elastic tissue, and to degenerative vascular and connective tissue changes. Anatomically, there is no subcutaneous tissue in the lateral ear for thermal or mechanical protection; the blood supply to the pinna is through relatively small blood vessels. Minor trauma may precipitate damage and inadequate blood supply may prevent tissue repair.

---

*Portions of this chapter are modified from the chapter by K. Arndt in the fourth edition of this text.

FIGURE 84-26

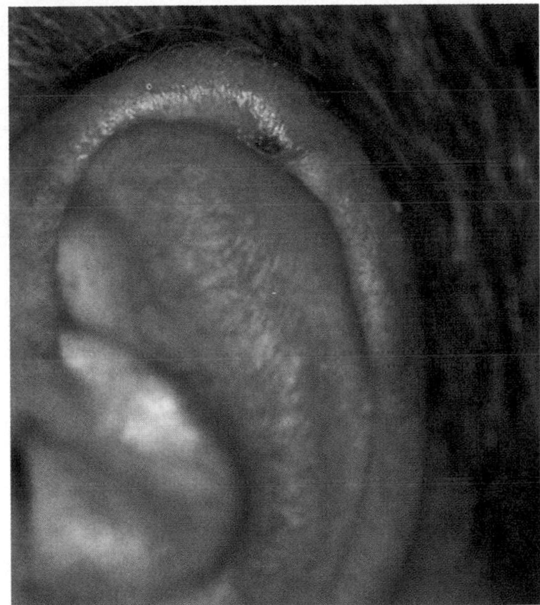

Painful nodule of the ear: a typical lesion of chondrodermatitis nodularis helicis.

Goette suggested that CNH represents an actinically induced, necrobiotic granuloma with secondary epithelial changes leading to transepidermal elimination of degenerated connective tissue.[85] Factors supporting this concept include: CNH is most common in the middle-aged and the elderly, darkly pigmented patients are affected less frequently, and often there is solar elastosis at the periphery of the lesion. Biopsies frequently show transepidermal elimination of necrobiotic material through overlying epidermal channels, slits, or erosions.

Whether inflammation proceeds outward from primarily damaged perichondrium or inward from injured epidermis or dermis is unknown.

Epidemiology[86]

CND is most common in adult males over 50 years old. Women account for approximately 10 percent of the total cases.

Clinical Features

CNH nodules usually appear spontaneously, enlarge quickly to less than 1 cm, and then remain stationary unless altered by infection or trauma. Lesions are firm, well-defined, round to oval with sloping margins, either embedded in the skin or elevated several millimeters. They range from 3 to 20 mm in diameter (average 4 to 7 mm) and have a flat or dome-shaped surface covered with an adherent scale (Fig. 84-26). The surrounding skin is gray-white, or waxy and translucent. A narrow inflammatory areola may surround the nodule. The right ear is more commonly involved than the left and helical lesions are more common in women.

Spontaneous pain or tenderness is almost always the initial presenting complaint, but is often intensified by pressure or cold. The discomfort is described as intense and stabbing, paroxysmal or continuous, and is momentary or lasts several hours. The pain may be temporarily relieved by removal of the crust. A history of ulceration or drainage is frequent. There is no relation to systemic disease.

Elderly women often have multiple lesions that are only slightly, if at all, painful. These resolve spontaneously and may be a variant of CNH. The nodules are larger, more rounded, and always directly attributable to trauma such as from the constant friction of a nun's headpiece.

Spontaneous remission is rare. With treatment, remissions of months to years may occur, but the disease generally continues to be active indefinitely unless adequately treated.

Basal cell and squamous cell carcinomas are commonly confused with CNH. Actinic keratosis, keratoacanthoma, and warts may present a similar appearance, as, to a lesser degree, do clavus, tophus, rheumatoid or rheumatic nodules, and discoid lupus erythematosus. Relapsing polychondritis presents painful areas on the ears but is otherwise dissimilar.

Pathology[84,85]

The epidermis shows well-localized acanthosis with either a central depression or an erosion covered by a hyperkeratotic parakeratotic scale. The acanthotic region is often penetrated by a channel filled with necrotic dermal debris. In the dermis there is intense edema, fibrinoid degeneration, necrolysis of the collagen, and ingrowth of richly vascularized granulation tissue. Lymphocytes, plasma cells, and histiocytes are present, as are epithelioid cells. Elastic tissue is diminished or absent in areas of inflammation. The thickened and layered perichondrium shows an infiltrate continuous with granulation tissue in the dermis. Cartilage may be altered but is frequently normal. Calcification and ossification of the distal chondral laminae have been described.

Treatment

Relief of pressure with custom or commercially available foam rubber pillows, with a depression for the ear, is often effective for symptomatic relief. High-potency topical corticosteroids are occasionally effective and should be tried first. Single or multiple intralesional injections of corticosteriods will often cause lesions to regress or disappear (triamcinolone acetonide, 10 to 40 mg/mL, 0.2 to 0.5 mL).[87] Carbon dioxide laser surgery is useful in clearing lesions.[88] Ablation of lesions with a defocused carbon dioxide laser beam may lead to smooth asymptomatic scars that remain painless for long periods of time. The definitive treatment, excisional surgery or cartilage excision, eliminates the mechanical squeezing of the dermis by removing the pathologic tissue, relieves pain by cutting the nerves, and reduces the amount of projecting rim of helical cartilage, although recurrence occurs.[89,90]

REFERENCES

1. Yeatman JM et al: The prevalence of seborrhoeic keratoses in an Australian population: Does exposure to sunlight play a part in their frequency? *Br J Dermatol* **137**:411, 1997
2. Tsambaos D et al: Detection of human papillomavirus DNA in nongenital seborrhoeic keratoses. *Arch Dermatol Res* **287**:612, 1995
3. Ellis DL et al: Melanoma, growth factors, acanthosis nigricans, the sign of Leser-Trélat, and multiple acrochordons. A possible role for alpha-transforming growth factor in cutaneous paraneoplastic syndromes. *N Engl J Med* **317**:1582, 1987
4. Heaphy MR Jr et al: The sign of Leser-Trélat in a case of adenocarcinoma of the lung. *J Am Acad Dermatol* **43**:386, 2000
5. Lever W, Schaumberg-Lever G: *Histopathology of the Skin*. Philadelphia, Lippincott, 1997
6. Sloan JB, Jaworsky C: Clinical misdiagnosis of squamous cell carcinoma in situ as seborrheic keratosis. A prospective study. *J Dermatol Surg Oncol* **19**:413, 1993

7. Rao BK et al: The relationship between basal cell epithelioma and seborrheic keratosis. A study of 60 cases. *J Dermatol Surg Oncol* **20**:761, 1994
8. Zabel RJ et al: Malignant melanoma arising in a seborrheic keratosis. *J Am Acad Dermatol* **42**:831, 2000
9. Cascajo CD et al: Malignant neoplasms associated with seborrheic keratoses. An analysis of 54 cases. *Am J Dermatopathol* **18**:278, 1996
10. Schwartz RA: Sign of Leser-Trélat. *J Am Acad Dermatol* **35**:88, 1996
11. Millard LG, Gould DJ: Hyperkeratosis of the palms and soles associated with internal malignancy and elevated levels of immunoreactive human growth hormone. *Clin Exp Dermatol* **1**:363, 1976
12. Williams JV et al: Chemotherapy-induced inflammation in seborrheic keratoses mimicking disseminated herpes zoster. *J Am Acad Dermatol* **40**:643, 1999
13. Tsuji T, Morita A: Giant seborrheic keratosis on the frontal scalp treated with topical fluorouracil. *J Dermatol* **22**:74, 1995
14. Pepper E: Dermabrasion for the treatment of a giant seborrheic keratosis. *J Dermatol Surg Oncol* **11**:646, 1985
15. Rogers M et al: Epidermal nevi and the epidermal nevus syndrome. A review of 131 cases. *J Am Acad Dermatol* **20**:476, 1989
16. Solomon LM, Esterly NB: Epidermal and other congenital organoid nevi. *Curr Probl Pediatr* **6**:1, 1975
17. Adams BB, Mutasim DF: Adult onset verrucous epidermal nevus. *J Am Acad Dermatol* **41**:824, 1999
18. Ichikawa T et al: Squamous cell carcinoma arising in a verrucous epidermal nevus. *Dermatology* **193**:135, 1996
19. Reddy BS et al: Generalized epidermolytic hyperkeratosis in a child born to a parent with systematized epidermolytic linear epidermal nevus. *Int J Dermatol* **36**:198, 1997
20. Paller AS et al: Genetic and clinical mosaicism in a type of epidermal nevus. *N Engl J Med* **331**:1408, 1994
21. Happle R: Mosaicism in human skin. Understanding the patterns and mechanisms. *Arch Dermatol* **129**:1460, 1993
22. Dupre A, Christol B: Inflammatory linear verrucose epidermal nevus. A pathologic study. *Arch Dermatol* **113**:767, 1977
23. Brownstein MH et al: Lichenoid epidermal nevus: "Linear lichen planus." *J Am Acad Dermatol* **20**:913, 1989
24. Baba T et al: Successful treatment of dark-colored epidermal nevus with ruby laser. *J Dermatol* **22**:567, 1995
25. Kim JJ et al: Topical tretinoin and 5-fluorouracil in the treatment of linear verrucous epidermal nevus. *J Am Acad Dermatol* **43**:129, 2000
26. Bohm I et al: Successful therapy of an ILVEN in a 7-year-old girl with calcipotriol [in German]. *Hautarzt* **50**:812, 1999
27. Ozkaya-Bayazit E et al: Pustular psoriasis with a striking linear pattern. *J Am Acad Dermatol* **42**:329, 2000
28. Morency R, Labelle H: Nevus sebaceus of Jadassohn: A rare oral presentation. *Oral Surg Oral Med Oral Pathol* **64**:460, 1987
29. Sahl WJ Jr: Familial nevus sebaceus of Jadassohn: Occurrence in three generations. *J Am Acad Dermatol* **22**:853, 1990
30. Chun K et al: Nevus sebaceus: Clinical outcome and considerations for prophylactic excision. *Int J Dermatol* **34**:538, 1995
31. Cribier B et al: Tumors arising in nevus sebaceus: A study of 596 cases. *J Am Acad Dermatol* **42**:263, 2000
32. Jaqueti G et al: Trichoblastoma is the most common neoplasm developed in nevus sebaceus of Jadassohn: A clinicopathologic study of a series of 155 cases. *Am J Dermatopathol* **22**:108, 2000
33. Xin H et al: The sebaceous nevus: a nevus with deletions of the PTCH gene. *Cancer Res* **59**:1834, 1999
34. Hunt SJ et al: Desmoplastic trichilemmoma: Histologic variant resembling invasive carcinoma. *J Cutan Pathol* **17**:45, 1990
35. Rahbari H, Mehregan AH: Development of proliferating trichilemmal cyst in organoid nevus. Presentation of two cases. *J Am Acad Dermatol* **14**:123, 1986
36. Cestari TF et al: Nevus comedonicus: Case report and brief review of the literature. *Pediatr Dermatol* **8**:300, 1991
37. Parslew R, Lewis-Jones MS: Localized unilateral hyperhidrosis secondary to an eccrine naevus. *Clin Exp Dermatol* **22**:246, 1997
38. Herzberg J: Ekkrines syringocystadenoma. *Arch Klin Exp Dermatol* **214**:600, 1962
39. Imai S, Nitto H: Eccrine nevus with epidermal changes. *Dermatologica* **166**:84, 1983
40. Civatte J et al: Apocrine nevus. Study of 2 cases. *Ann Dermatol Syphiligr* **101**:251, 1974
41. Hodge JA et al: The epidermal nevus syndrome. *Int J Dermatol* **30**:91, 1991
42. Happle R: Epidermal nevus syndromes. *Semin Dermatol* **14**:111, 1995
43. Eichler C et al: Epidermal nevus syndrome: Case report and review of clinical manifestations. *Pediatr Dermatol* **6**:316, 1989
44. Chow MJ, Fretzin DF: Epidermal nevus syndrome: Report of association with chondroblastoma of bone. *Pediatr Dermatol* **6**:358, 1989
45. Ivker R et al: Hypophosphatemic vitamin D-resistant rickets, precocious puberty, and the epidermal nevus syndrome. *Arch Dermatol* **133**:1557, 1997
46. Baker RS et al: Neurologic complications of the epidermal nevus syndrome. *Arch Neurol* **44**:227, 1987
47. Mansour AM et al: Ocular choristomas. *Surv Ophthalmol* **33**:339, 1989
48. Happle R et al: Phacomatosis pigmentokeratotica: A melanocytic-epidermal twin nevus syndrome. *Am J Med Genet* **65**:363, 1996
49. Kennedy D, Rogers M: Lichen striatus. *Pediatr Dermatol* **13**:95, 1996
50. Di Lernia V et al: Lichen striatus and atopy. *Int J Dermatol* **30**:453, 1991
51. Patrizi A et al: Simultaneous occurrence of lichen striatus in siblings. *Pediatr Dermatol* **14**:293, 1997
52. Tosti A et al: Nail lichen striatus: Clinical features and long-term follow-up of five patients. *J Am Acad Dermatol* **36**:908, 1997
53. Zhang Y, McNutt NS: Lichen striatus. Histological, immunohistochemical, and ultrastructural study of 37 cases. *J Cutan Pathol* **28**:65, 2001
54. Penneys NS et al: Clear cell acanthoma: Not of sweat gland origin. *Acta Derm Venereol* **61**:569, 1981
55. Hashimoto T et al: Two cases of clear cell acanthoma: An immunohistochemical study. *J Cutan Pathol* **15**:27, 1988
56. Ohnishi T, Watanabe S: Immunohistochemical characterization of keratin expression in clear cell acanthoma. *Br J Dermatol* **133**:186, 1995
57. Finch TM, Tan CY: Clear cell acanthoma developing on a psoriatic plaque: Further evidence of an inflammatory aetiology? *Br J Dermatol* **142**:842, 2000
58. Langer K et al: Pigmented clear cell acanthoma. *Am J Dermatopathol* **16**:134, 1994
59. Langtry JA et al: Giant clear cell acanthoma in an atypical location. *J Am Acad Dermatol* **21**:313, 1989
60. Betti R et al: Successful cryotherapic [sic] treatment and overview of multiple clear cell acanthomas. *Dermatol Surg* **21**:342, 1995
61. Griffiths TW et al: Multiple warty dyskeratomas of the scalp. *Clin Exp Dermatol* **22**:189, 1997
62. Cerroni L et al: Acanthoma fissuratum. *J Dermatol Surg Oncol* **14**:1003, 1988
63. Ohnishi T, Watanabe S: Immunohistochemical observation of cytokeratins in keratinous cysts including plantar epidermoid cyst. *J Cutan Pathol* **26**:424, 1999
64. Walsh C, Rushton HG: Diagnosis and management of teratomas and epidermoid cysts. *Urol Clin North Am* **27**:509, 2000
65. Talacchi A et al: Assessment and surgical management of posterior fossa epidermoid tumors: Report of 28 cases. *Neurosurgery* **42**:242, 1998
66. Egawa K et al: Human papillomavirus 57 identified in a plantar epidermoid cyst. *Br J Dermatol* **138**:510, 1998
67. Brook I: Microbiology of infected epidermal cysts. *Arch Dermatol* **125**:1658, 1989
68. Delacretaz J: Keratotic basal-cell carcinoma arising from an epidermoid cyst. *J Dermatol Surg Oncol* **3**:310, 1977
69. Shelley WB, Wood MG: Occult Bowen's disease in keratinous cysts. *Br J Dermatol* **105**:105, 1981
70. Lopez-Rios F et al: Squamous cell carcinoma arising in a cutaneous epidermal cyst: Case report and literature review. *Am J Dermatopathol* **21**:174, 1999
71. Leppard BJ, Sanderson KV: The natural history of trichilemmal cysts. *Br J Dermatol* **94**:379, 1976
72. Sau P et al: Proliferating epithelial cysts. Clinicopathological analysis of 96 cases. *J Cutan Pathol* **22**:394, 1995
73. Lopez-Rios F et al: Proliferating trichilemmal cyst with focal invasion: Report of a case and a review of the literature. *Am J Dermatopathol* **22**:183, 2000
74. Tsuji T et al: Milia induced by corticosteroids. *Arch Dermatol* **122**:139, 1986
75. Cairns ML, Knable AL: Multiple eruptive milia in a 15-year-old boy. *Pediatr Dermatol* **16**:108, 1999
76. Kiene P et al: Eruptive vellus hair cysts and steatocystoma multiplex. variants of one entity? *Br J Dermatol* **134**:365, 1996
77. Adams BB et al: Steatocystoma multiplex: a quick removal technique. *Cutis* **64**:127, 1999

78. Nocini PF et al: Dermoid cyst of the nose: A case report and review of the literature. *J Oral Maxillofac Surg* **54**:357, 1996
79. Brownstein MH, Helwig EB: Subcutaneous dermoid cysts. *Arch Dermatol* **107**:237, 1973
80. Crawford R: Dermoid cyst of the scalp: intracranial extension. *J Pediatr Surg* **25**:294, 1990
81. Thomson HG: Common benign pediatric cutaneous tumors: Timing and treatment. *Clin Plast Surg* **17**:49, 1990
82. Fornari M et al: Surgical treatment of intracranial dermoid and epidermoid cysts in children. *Childs Nerv Syst* **6**:66, 1990
83. Fourman P, Fourman J: Hereditary deafness in a family with ear-pits. *Br Med J* **2**:1354, 1955
84. Shuman R, Helwig EB: Chondrodermatitis nodularis chronica helicis. *Am J Clin Pathol* **24**:126, 1954
85. Goette DK: Chrondrodermatitis nodularis chronica helicis: A perforating necrobiotic granuloma. *J Am Acad Dermatol* **2**:148, 1980
86. Newcomer VD et al: Chondrodermatitis nodularis chronica helicis: Report of 94 cases and survey of literature, with emphasis on pathogenesis and treatment. *Arch Dermatol Syphilol* **68**:241, 1953
87. Cox NH, Denham PF: Intralesional triamcinolone for chondrodermatitis nodularis: A follow-up study of 60 patients. *Br J Dermatol* **146**:712, 2002
88. Taylor MB: Chondrodermatitis nodularis chronca helicis. Successful treatment with the carbon dioxide laser. *J Dermatol Surg Oncol* **18**:862, 1992
89. Zimmerman MC: Chondrodermatitis nodularis chronica helicis: A nondeforming surgical cure for painful nodules of the ear. *Arch Dermatol* **78**:41, 1958
90. Hudson-Peacock MJ et al: The long-term results of cartilage removal alone for the treatment of chondrodermatitis nodularis. *Br J Dermatol* **141**:703, 1999

CHAPTER 85

Steven Kaddu
Helmut Kerl

Appendage Tumors of the Skin

GENERAL CONSIDERATIONS

Appendage tumors of the skin show differentiation toward epithelial components of normal (embryonal or mature) adnexal structures (i.e., apocrine, eccrine, hair follicle, and sebaceous units) (Table 85-1).[1–6] They may occur as solitary or multiple lesions. Solitary lesions generally reveal no distinctive clinical features. Their anatomic distribution, however, often reflects areas with high densities of corresponding normal cutaneous adnexa. Appendage tumors arising as multiple lesions frequently display a characteristic distribution. They are often inherited as autosomal dominants and may be associated with other cutaneous and extracutaneous pathology.

Histopathology is the most important tool for diagnosis and classification of appendage skin tumors. Diagnosis is based mainly on assessment of architectural and cytomorphologic characteristics as well as estimation of the predominant direction and level of differentiation towards normal adnexa.[1–6] Diagnostic criteria are apparent in the vast majority of cases on routine hematoxylin and eosin (H&E)-stained sections, although they may be absent or less prominent in different areas of the same tumor. A careful and adequate sampling of the specimen is, therefore, essential.

Immunohistologic analyses are occasionally necessary for interpretation of the tumors (Table 85-2). Interestingly, there is a significant overlap of immunohistologic features among tumors with ductal differentiation (apocrine and eccrine tumors), and certain visceral malignancies. In our experience, ultrastructural studies are of limited value in routine diagnosis of these tumors.

Recently, cytogenetic and molecular studies have shed some light on the pathogenesis of several cutaneous appendage tumors. For instance, *p53* mutations have been detected in a number of neoplasms, suggesting a possible etiologic role for UV light exposure.[7] Mutation of the human homologue of *Drosophila patched (PTC)* gene is considered to be the molecular defect in follicular appendage tumors arising in patients with the basal cell nevus (Gorlin) syndrome (i.e., trichoblastoma and basal cell carcinoma; see Chap. 82).[8] Germ-line mutations have consistently been reported in other familial syndromes, suggesting a role of these aberrations in pathogenesis. For example, mutations of *PTEN*, a tumor-suppressor gene, have been identified in tumors from patients with Cowden's (multiple hamartoma) syndrome[9] (see Chap. 184). Microsatellite instability as well as mutations of the *hMSH2* and *hMLH1* mismatch repair genes have also been detected in neoplasms from patients with Muir-Torre syndrome[10] (see Chap. 184).

PRINCIPLES OF DIAGNOSIS

Apocrine and eccrine tumors are characterized histopathologically by the presence, at least focally, of features of ductal differentiation. The ductal structures in apocrine neoplasms display "apocrine" secretion ("decapitation" or "pinching"), while those of eccrine tumors are lined by a flattened epithelium.[1] Follicular tumors show a range of morphologic features that recapitulate specific portions of normal hair and hair follicle[3] such as the infundibulum, isthmus, stem, and bulb (see Chap. 71). The finding of matrical cells reflects differentiation towards follicular bulbs. Trichohyalin granules and blue-gray corneocytes indicate differentiation towards the inner root sheath. Differentiation toward the outer root sheath is manifested by the presence of either clear columnar cells aligned in a palisade (outer root sheath differentiation at the bulb), subtly cornified cells with pink cytoplasm (outer root sheath differentiation at the stem), or fully cornified cells with red cytoplasm ("tricholemmal keratinization") which corresponds to outer root sheath

TABLE 85-1

Classification of Appendage Tumors of the Skin

Tumors with Apocrine Differentiation	Tumors with Eccrine Differentiation	Tumors with Follicular Differentiation	Tumors with Sebaceous Differentiation
Cysts	*Cysts*	*Cysts*	*Cysts*
Hidrocystoma	Hidrocystoma	Epidermal cyst	Steatocystoma
Moll's gland cyst		Hybrid follicular cyst	
		Keratocyst	
		Pigmented follicular cyst	
		Tricholemmal cyst	
		Vellus hair cyst	
Hamartomas	*Hamartomas*	*Hamartomas*	*Hamartomas*
Apocrine nevus	Eccrine hamartoma	Basaloid follicular hamartoma	Folliculo-sebaceous cystic hamartoma
Supernumerary nipple		Hair follicle nevus	Fordyce's spots and Montgomery's tubercles
		Linear unilateral basal cell nevus	Nevus sebaceus
		Neurofollicular hamartoma	
		Nevus comedonicus	
		Nevus sebaceus	
Hyperplasias	*Hyperplasias*	*Hyperplasias*	*Hyperplasias*
Fibroadenoma of the breast	Mucinous syringometaplasia	—	Sebaceous hyperplasia and rhinophyma
	Syringolymphoid hyperplasia		
Benign Neoplasms	*Benign Neoplasms*	*Benign Neoplasms*	*Benign Neoplasms*
Adenoma of the nipple	Cylindroma	Desmoplastic trichoepithelioma	Mantleoma
Hidradenoma papilliferum	Eccrine syringofibroadenoma	Dilated pore (Winer)	Reticulated acanthoma
Mixed tumor	Hidradenoma	Fibrofolliculoma	Sebaceoma
Reticulated acanthoma	Poroma	Fibrous papule	
Syringocystadenoma papilliferum	Spiradenoma	Inverted follicular keratosis	
	Syringoma	Lymphadenoma (cutaneous)	
	Tubular adenoma	Panfolliculoma	
		Pilar sheath acanthoma	
		Pilomatricoma	
		Proliferating pilar tumor	
		Trichoadenoma	
		Trichoblastoma	
		Trichodiscoma	
		Trichoepithelioma	
		Trichofolliculoma	
		Tricholemmoma	
		Tumor of follicular infundibulum	
Malignant Neoplasms	*Malignant Neoplasms*	*Malignant Neoplasms*	*Malignant Neoplasms*
Adenoid cystic carcinoma	Aggressive digital papillary adenoma and adenocarcinoma	Basal cell carcinoma with follicular (and sebaceous) differentiation	Sebaceous carcinoma (and neoplasms in Muir-Torre syndrome)
Apocrine adenocarcinoma	Cylindrocarcinoma	Pilomatrical carcinoma	
Ductal carcinoma	Eccrine carcinoma	Tricholemmal carcinoma	
Extramammary Paget's disease	Hidradenocarcinoma		
Hidradenocarcinoma papilliferum	Microcystic adnexal carcinoma		
Malignant mixed tumor	Polymorphous sweat gland carcinoma		
Mucinous carcinoma	Porocarcinoma		
Signet-ring cell carcinoma	Spiradenocarcinoma		
Syringocystadenocarcinoma papilliferum			

differentiation at the isthmus. Sebaceous tumors reveal areas with sebocytes and tubular structures.[2] Notably, some tumors may display one or more lines of differentiation.

Determination of whether an appendage neoplasm is benign or malignant requires assessment of architectural and cytomorphologic characteristics. Great care is, however, necessary when applying traditional morphologic criteria of malignancy such as asymmetry, poor circumscription, and presence of epithelial aggregations with prominent atypia and mitotic activity. Some malignant and aggressive neoplasms (e.g., microcystic adnexal carcinoma) show deceptively bland appearances. Furthermore, there are certain neoplasms whose malignant potential is not always predictable on morphologic grounds.

PRINCIPLES OF CLASSIFICATION

The number of current classifications of appendage tumors of the skin indicate how little consensus exists about their grouping and their etiology and pathogenesis.[1–6] There is also no unanimity among authors as to whether particular tumors are truly neoplasms, hyperplasias or hamartomas. In this chapter, we have categorized appendage tumors of the skin as cysts, hamartomas, hyperplasias, and benign or malignant neoplasms, and have arranged them alphabetically (Table 85-1). A *cutaneous cyst* is defined as an epithelium-lined, round or oval sac-like lesion. The term *cutaneous hamartoma* refers to a possibly

TABLE 85-2

Immunohistochemical Findings in Appendage Tumors of the Skin

Tumors	Carcinoembryonic Antigen (CEA)	Cytokeratin 5/6	Epithelial Membrane Antigen (EMA)	Gross Cystic Disease Fluid Protein (GCDFP)	Pancytokeratin	S-100	Vimentin
Tumors with apocrine differentiation	±	+	+	+	+	–	–
Tumors with eccrine differentiation	±	+	+	±	+	±	±
Tumors with follicular differentiation	–	+	±	–	+	–	–
Tumors with sebaceous differentiation	–	+	+	–	+	–	–

–, No reaction; ±, weak reaction; +, strong reaction

embryologic malformation characterized by an abnormal arrangement of "normal" cutaneous tissues. *Cutaneous hyperplasia* represents an increase in number of normal cells but with relatively normal arrangement in the skin. A *benign* neoplasm has no potential to metastasize. A *malignant* neoplasm possesses the potential for local destruction and metastasis.

PRINCIPLES OF THERAPY

A diagnostic biopsy of a suspicious lesion and a correct diagnosis is usually the first step in appropriate management of patients with appendage skin tumors. A number of tumor-related and patient-related factors influence the choice of treatment. Tumor-related factors include the type, size, and anatomic location. Patient-related factors include life expectancy, comorbid conditions, and cosmetic concerns.

Specific treatment of benign appendage tumors is sometimes unnecessary. In some cases, removal of the tumor is indicated for cosmetic reasons only. Treatment of choice for the majority of benign appendage tumors and relatively nonaggressive, malignant appendage neoplasms is excisional surgery. A variety of superficial ablative techniques (electrodesiccation and curettage and cryotherapy) have proved to be effective in selected patients. A number of other alternative treatment options, including the use of systemic retinoids, laser, and photodynamic therapy, have also been advocated for use in some cases. However, these alternative therapies are still considered investigational because of lack of sufficient data regarding their efficacy and side effects.

Treatment of malignant appendage tumors aims mainly at eradication of the cancer, and preservation or restoration of normal function, as well as cosmesis. High-risk patients with tumors known to have a high rate of recurrence or metastasis most frequently require wide excisional surgery, Mohs micrographic surgery, and/or radiotherapy. Notably, sentinel node biopsy is sometimes valuable in staging of patients with eccrine and apocrine carcinomas.

APPENDAGE TUMORS WITH APOCRINE DIFFERENTIATION

Appendage tumors with ductal differentiation (sweat gland tumors) have traditionally been divided into apocrine and eccrine. However, over the years, it has become increasingly recognized that distinction between apocrine and eccrine is not always possible, as classic features of apocrine differentiation are sometimes observed in tumors traditionally categorized as eccrine.

Generally, the anatomic distribution of apocrine tumors reflects that of normal glands manufacturing apocrine secretion which are confined to the head and neck, axillae, and genital or perianal skin. The vast majority of apocrine tumors are benign.[1] Malignant neoplasms show varied and diverse morphologic features and biologic potential.

Cysts

HIDROCYSTOMA Hidrocystoma (cystadenoma) is a relatively common cystic lesion that shows features of either apocrine (apocrine type) or eccrine (eccrine type) differentiation. It presents mostly in middle-aged or elderly individuals as a solitary, small- to medium-sized, skin-colored, reddish or bluish cystic nodule situated on the head or neck, especially around the eyes[1,4–6,11] (Fig. 85-1*A*). Men and women are equally affected. Unusual presentations include multiple lesions, giant tumors (up to 7 cm), and lesions occurring in childhood. Hidrocystoma occasionally develops within a nevus sebaceus (see Chap. 84). Multiple hidrocystomas localized to borders of the upper and lower eyelids bilaterally may represent a feature of ectodermal dysplasia.

Histopathology There is an unilocular or occasionally a multilocular cyst located in the dermis. The epithelial lining displays either features of apocrine (decapitation secretion) or eccrine (single or double layered, cuboid often flattened epithelium) differentiation.[1] Prominent papillations protruding into the lumen are noted in a subset of cases (Fig. 85-1*B*). Secretory products contain lipofuscin, melanin, and/or hemosiderin.

Treatment of choice in solitary lesions is simple surgical excision. Multiple lesions may be removed using a carbon dioxide laser, electrodesiccation, or surgery with blepharoplasty.

MOLL'S GLAND CYST Moll's gland cyst is a cystic dilatation of Moll's glands, which are modified apocrine glands located on the eyelids. The lesion presents mainly as a solitary, dome-shaped cystic tumor located on the inner or outer canthus of the eyelid.[1]

Histopathology The histology is essentially similar to that of apocrine hidrocystoma.

Hamartomas

APOCRINE NEVUS Apocrine nevus is a rare hamartoma that consists of proliferation in the dermis of normal appearing apocrine glands. Two variants are recognized: a type occurring as a part of nevus sebaceus and an extremely rare type arising independently (pure apocrine nevus). Pure apocrine nevus presents as a unilateral or bilateral, soft, lobulated dermal mass in the axilla or as a circumscribed area on the scalp.[1,4–6,11] Cases of apocrine nevus occurring as multiple, firm papules on the chest have been reported.[12]

FIGURE 85-1

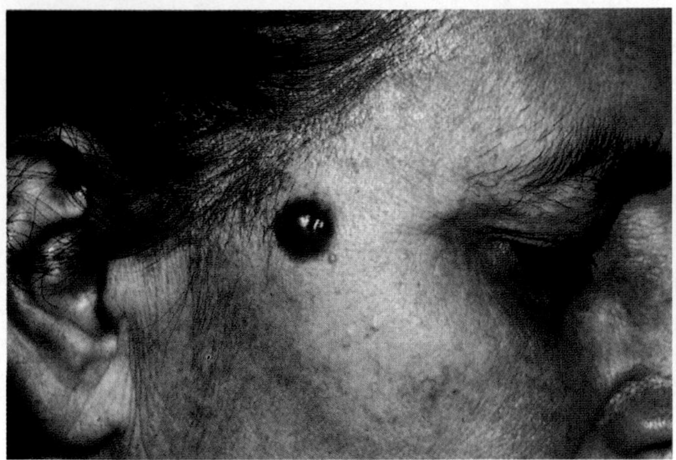

A.

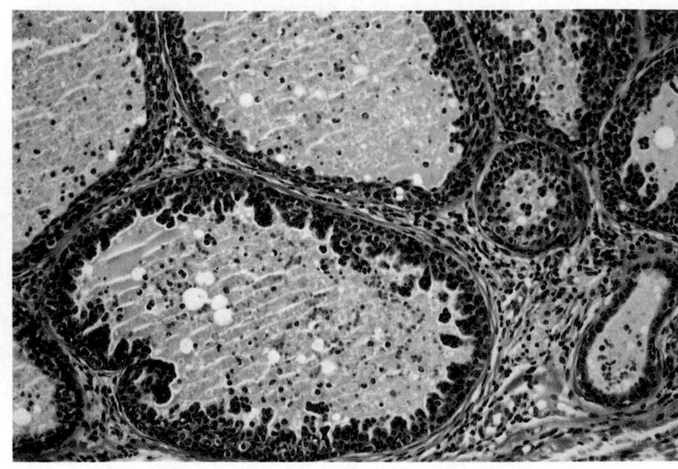

B.

Apocrine hidrocystoma. *A.* Reddish-brown to bluish cystic nodule. *B.* Multilocular tumor with papillary projections ("apocrine secretion").

Histopathology There are numerous, discrete, closely spaced tubular structures in the dermis and/or the subcutaneous fat. The tubules are lined by typical apocrine glandular epithelium and contain a homogeneous or vacuolated pink material (apocrine secretion). An apocrine nevus developing within a preexisting nevus sebaceus usually arises in the deeper portion, sometimes in association with a syringocystadenoma papilliferum or trichoblastoma.[13]

SUPERNUMERARY NIPPLE This condition is characterized by the presence of solitary or multiple rudimentary nipples developing along the embryonal milk line. Lesions present mainly in young individuals.[1] Males and females are equally affected. Most cases are sporadic but some lesions show a genetic transmission. Supernumerary nipples occur commonly as solitary, asymptomatic, soft, brown papules with a dimple, resembling dermatofibromas, fibromas, or melanocytic nevi. Less frequently, patients show supernumerary nipples with an appearance of an areola (polythelia areolaris), a patch of hair (polythelia pilosa), or a subcutaneous mass with or without areola. Rare cases present as a pedunculated or dermal mass in the axilla or vulva. Supernumerary nipples have also been reported in association with adenoma of the nipple (erosive adenomatosis)[1,14] and with renal abnormalities, including renal cell carcinoma.

Histopathology There is usually an exophytic or dome-shaped lesion consisting of variable components of a normal nipple, including sebaceous lobules and ducts (Montgomery's tubercles). A rudimentary vellus follicle, various lactiferous ducts, dilated venules, and fascicles of smooth muscle can be observed.

Treatment is by simple surgical excision.

Hyperplasia

FIBROADENOMA Fibroadenoma represents the most common cause of a breast mass in women younger than 25 years of age. Rarely, the tumor arises along the embryonic milk line or in other locations.[1,15] Although previously generally considered to be a benign neoplasm, fibroadenoma is now widely regarded as a form of hyperplasia of normal breast lobules. The etiology is unknown, but the condition probably results from a proliferation of breast tissue in response to excessive circulating estradiol over progesterone. Lesions commonly present as single or multiple firm, rubbery, smooth, mobile, painless infiltrates ranging up to 2 cm in diameter. Patients occasionally show bilateral tumors. Smaller lesions are being increasingly discovered on routine mammography. A subset of cases presents as large or giant tumors measuring 15 to 20 cm in diameter. These lesions represent mainly a distinctive juvenile type that arises in teenage females and grows rapidly, often leading to extensive stretching of the skin and distortion of the nipple.

Histopathology Histopathologic examination reveals a variably hyalinized or mucinous, fibrous stroma surrounding a proliferation of ductal structures with apocrine secretion.

Treatment is by complete local surgical excision. Conservative management without surgery has also been proposed.[15]

Benign Neoplasms

ADENOMA OF THE NIPPLE Adenoma of the nipple (florid papillomatosis, erosive adenomatosis, papillary adenoma) is a rare, benign neoplasm currently thought to originate from terminal lactiferous ducts and subareolar breast tissue. Peak incidence is in the fifth decade in women; however, the lesion may present at any age. Men are occasionally affected. Patients sometimes complain of pain or an itchy, burning sensation within the lesion. Clinically, there is usually a unilateral enlargement and/or induration of the nipple which contains a palpable, firm, subareolar nodule.[1,5,6,11] The surface is occasionally erythematous, ulcerated or crusted, and may ooze a serous, serosanguineous or bloody discharge. The overall clinical appearance is often indistinguishable from that of mammary Paget's disease. Bilateral tumors have been reported. The lesion has also been observed to develop in association with a supernumerary nipple.[14]

Histopathology An endophytic proliferation of tubular structures in the dermis with a verrucous or ulcerated surface is usually found. Some of the tubular structures exhibit cystic dilations with discrete papillations. They are lined by an inner apocrine secretory epithelium and an outer myoepithelial layer, and are separated by a fibrous stroma.

Treatment of choice is complete surgical excision. Persistence or recurrences are common. Mohs micrographic surgery and cryosurgery may be useful in the treatment of some patients.

HIDRADENOMA PAPILLIFERUM Hidradenoma papilliferum (papillary hidradenoma) is a relatively uncommon benign neoplasm, which usually occurs as a unilateral, small (up to 1 cm in diameter), asymptomatic, skin-colored nodule on the vulva or perineum of adult

FIGURE 85-2

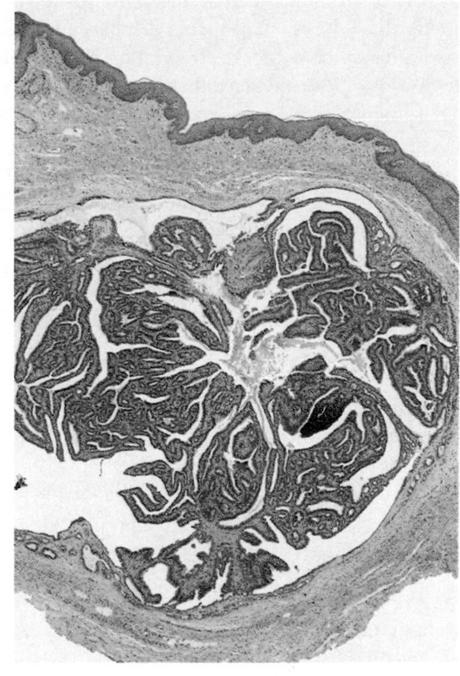

Hidradenoma papilliferum. Cystic tumor with papillary and glandular areas.

women.[1,4–6,11] There are, however, a few reports of similar neoplasms arising on the eyelid[16] and external auditory canal.

Histopathology Histopathologic examination reveals a partly solid or solid-cystic lesion, usually without an epidermal connection. The tumor shows a complex pattern with anastomosing papillary structures and tubules as well as some glandular areas (Fig. 85-2). The papillary structures are interconnected with each other resulting in a trabecular pattern. The epithelial lining consists of an inner layer of tall and columnar cells with an eosinophilic cytoplasm and features of decapitation secretion. A thin, outer myoepithelial layer is frequently present.

Treatment is by simple surgical excision. In perianal tumors, consultation with a colorectal surgeon is advised to assure preservation of a normal sphincter function. One patient with a fatal, metastasizing squamous carcinoma arising in a hidradenoma papilliferum has been reported.[17]

MIXED TUMOR OF THE SKIN Mixed tumor of the skin (chondroid syringoma) represents a group of adnexal neoplasms with ductal differentiation and a fibromyxochondroid stroma.[1,4–6,11] Features of either apocrine (apocrine type) or eccrine (eccrine type) differentiation predominate in individual cases. Skin lesions present usually as solitary, firm, nonulcerated nodules measuring from 2 mm to several centimeters in diameter, situated on the head and neck[18] (Fig. 85-3*A*). They commonly show a shiny or a waxy surface. Middle-aged and elderly individuals, and preferentially men, are commonly affected. Mixed tumors may occasionally develop on a variety of other anatomic sites, including genitalia.

Histopathology There is a well-circumscribed dermal and/or subcutaneous lesion composed of elongated, partly ramifying tubular structures and/or complex solid nests as well as cords (Fig. 85-3*B*). The epithelial component is typically embedded in a stroma consisting of a variable admixture of spindled and stellate cells, mucin, as well as chondroid material. The apocrine type reveals, at least focally, small tubular lumina and cystic structures with apocrine secretion. A homogenous material is sometimes noted within the cystic cavities. Foci of polygonal, plasmacytoid, pale and clear cells may be observed. Occasional cases display follicular and sebaceous differentiation, fat metaplasia, and/or collagenous spherulosis.[1,19] The eccrine type is characterized by tubulocystic spaces attached to solid elements, resembling the tadpole configuration seen in syringomas. Notably, some mixed tumors reveal atypical histologic features, including an infiltrative margin, satellite tumor nodules, and tumor necrosis. These atypical histologic appearances do not generally correspond with aggressive potential.

Treatment is by complete surgical excision. To date, there are no convincing reports of malignant transformation of benign mixed tumor in the literature.[1,5]

RETICULATED ACANTHOMA The term *reticulated acanthoma* was recently suggested for a group of benign tumors that

FIGURE 85-3

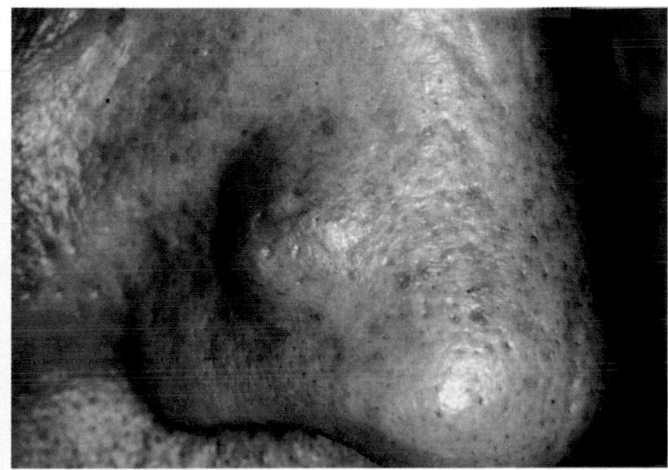

A.

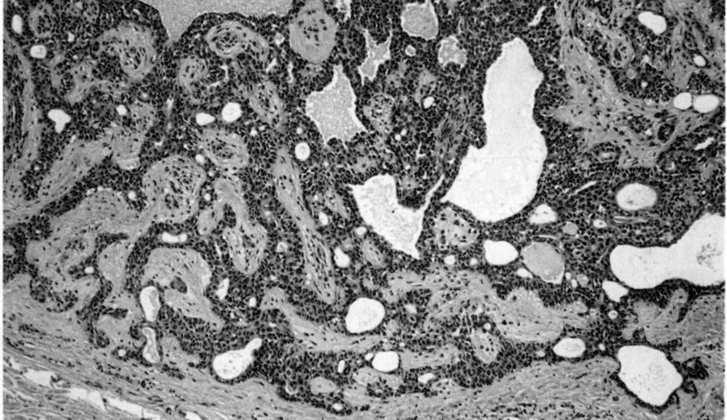

B.

Mixed tumor. *A.* Mixed tumor on the nose. *B.* Solid cords and tubular structures in a background of a fibromyxoid stroma.

histopathologically show a reticulated pattern and an epithelial component with multidirectional differentiation toward folliculosebaceous, apocrine, and sometimes eccrine units.[1] In the past, similar tumors have been described under a number of different names, including "poroma with follicular, sebaceous, and apocrine differentiation," "complex poroma-like adenoma," "combined polymorphic epidermal and adnexal tumor," "benign cutaneous adnexal tumor with combined folliculosebaceous, apocrine, and eccrine differentiation," and "sebocrine adenoma."[1] Reticulated acanthomas with prominent sebaceous differentiation are probably identical to tumors previously termed "superficial epithelioma with sebaceous differentiation" or "benign sebaceous neoplasm with prominent epidermal component."[2] The clinical appearance of reticulated acanthoma is not distinctive. Lesions occur as solitary, asymptomatic hyperkeratotic plaques and nodules on the face, trunk, and extremities. They are often suspected to be seborrheic keratosis or basal cell carcinoma.

Histopathology Usually, a broad superficial lesion confined to the papillary dermis and composed of cords and anastomosing columns of epithelial cells with a distinctive reticulated pattern is observed. Epithelial columns in individual lesions reveal variable features of apocrine, sebaceous, and/or follicular differentiation, and occasionally eccrine differentiation.

Treatment is by simple surgical excision.

SYRINGOCYSTADENOMA PAPILLIFERUM The exact nosologic status of syringocystadenoma papilliferum among tumors with ductal differentiation is still debatable. Most authors consider it to be a benign tumor,[5,6] while others categorize it as a hamartoma.[1] The lesion develops either independently or arises in association with a nevus sebaceus.[13] Solitary syringocystadenoma papilliferum occurs as a single, papillomatous, verrucous, sometimes erosive plaque or nodule measuring 1 to 3 cm in diameter, situated on the head and neck of adults[1,4–6,11] (Fig. 85-4*A*). A small fistula discharging a clear, bloody or malodorous fluid may be noted. Less common presentations include childhood tumors, lesions located on unusual anatomic sites (e.g., chest, upper arms, and thighs) and lesions arising as multiple or linearly arranged cutaneous nodules.

Histopathology There is a crateriform epidermal invagination with the upper portion lined by squamous epithelium and the lower portion lined by apocrine epithelium (Fig. 85-4*B*). The surrounding epidermis usually reveals papillomatosis, hypergranulosis and hyperkeratosis. Foci with variously sized papillations covered by a squamous epithelium are frequently observed within the epidermal invagination. In the dermis, cystic structures with villous projections exhibiting apocrine secretion may be present. The lesion is often surrounded by a variable lymphoplasmacytic infiltrate. Syringocystadenoma papilliferum arising in nevus sebaceus sometimes coexists with trichoblastomas.[13]

Treatment of choice is surgical excision. Carbon dioxide laser may be effective in removing tumors on anatomic sites unfavorable to surgical excision. Syringocystadenocarcinoma papilliferum may develop from long-standing syringocystadenoma (see below).

FIGURE 85-4

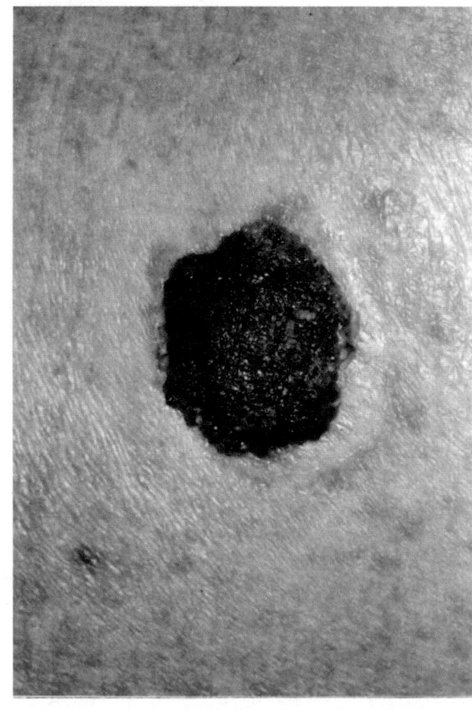

A.

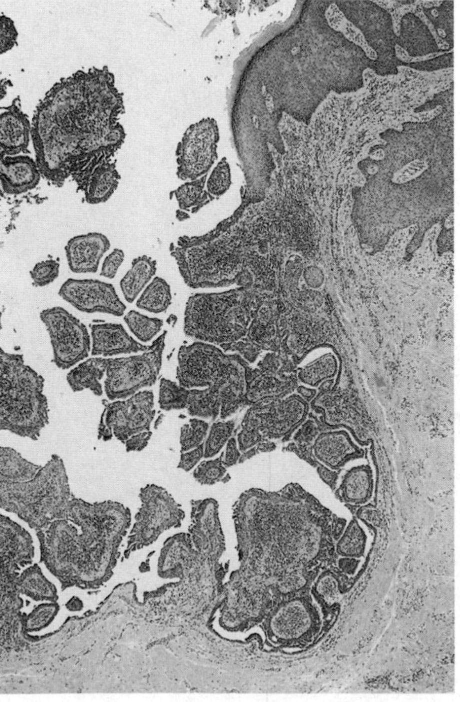

B.

Syringocystadenoma papilliferum. *A*. Erosive nodule on the forehead. *B*. Epidermal invagination with papilliferous projections.

Malignant Neoplasms

ADENOID CYSTIC CARCINOMA Adenoid cystic carcinoma occurs as either a primary cutaneous neoplasm or as an extracutaneous tumor, especially in the salivary glands. Primary cutaneous adenoid cystic carcinoma presents in adults as a solitary, slowly growing, asymptomatic or slightly painful, firm, papule or nodule, with predilection for the scalp.[1,4–6,11,20] Rare patients show multiple nodules. The tumor has occasionally been reported on other anatomic sites, including the trunk and upper extremities.

Histopathology Lesions consist of irregularly shaped, variously sized, asymmetric aggregations of basaloid neoplastic cells arranged in solid, tubular, and/or sieve-like patterns within the dermis. Extension to the subcutis is sometimes noted. Some areas of the tumor reveal cystic spaces with mucin. Foci with authentic tubules exhibiting apocrine secretion are noted in sections. Neoplastic cells are mainly monomorphous, and display round, hyperchromatic nuclei with inconspicuous nucleoli. Mitotic figures are rare. Perineural involvement is a common finding.

Treatment is by surgical excision with adequate margins. The tumor sometimes recurs after excision and rarely metastasizes.

APOCRINE ADENOCARCINOMA Apocrine adenocarcinoma (apocrine carcinoma) is a rare, poorly documented, aggressive adnexal neoplasm. Lesions present predominantly in adults as either solitary or multiple nodules and plaques measuring 2 to 8 cm in diameter, situated in the axilla or anogenital area.[1,4,11] Occasional cases may involve the fingers, nipples, or chest. Lesions occasionally develop in association with nevus sebaceus, apocrine hamartoma or extramammary Paget's disease.[1,21]

Histopathology Histopathologic examination reveals a dermal/subcutaneous nonencapsulated tumor with infiltrative margins. The epithelial component shows variable papillary, solid or mixed, patterns. Foci of partly anastomosing tubular structures exhibiting apocrine (decapitation) secretion and infiltrating cords of neoplastic cells can be observed. Neoplastic cells display variable pleomorphism and mitotic activity, as well as abundant, sometimes granular or vacuolated, eosinophilic cytoplasm. It is particularly important to differentiate apocrine adenocarcinoma from cutaneous metastases from other organs, especially from the breast.

Treatment is by surgical excision with adequate margins. Regional lymph node metastases and fatal visceral metastases have been recorded.[22]

DUCTAL CARCINOMA The term *ductal carcinoma* has been suggested to denote a rare type of malignant sweat gland carcinoma characterized by prominent, closely packed tubular structures with either apocrine or eccrine features.[1,23] Tumors present usually as solitary, asymptomatic nodules in the axilla of elderly individuals, preferentially of men.[23] Occasional cases arise as multiple lesions or are situated on unusual sites, including face, scalp, sternal region, and nipple. Tumors developing within a preexisting nevus sebaceus have been reported.[21]

Histopathology There is a deep dermal and/or subcutaneous proliferation composed of numerous, closely packed, tubular structures, sometimes with cystic and solid aggregations of neoplastic cells. The tubular and solid elements are composed of atypical neoplastic cells with abundant eosinophilic cytoplasm, hyperchromatic nuclei and frequent mitotic figures. Features of apocrine or eccrine differentiation can be observed in individual cases.[1,23]

Treatment is by surgical excision with adequate margins. Recurrences are common. Metastases especially to regional lymph nodes, lungs, and to other organs can be found.

EXTRAMAMMARY PAGET'S DISEASE
See Chap. 87.

HIDRADENOCARCINOMA PAPILLIFERUM This is a rare malignant appendage tumor that most often arises from a preexisting, usually long-standing, benign hidradenoma papilliferum.[1,24] It presents mainly in middle-aged women as a solitary, small, often ulcerated nodule in the anogenital region, and rarely in the axilla. Most lesions are asymptomatic, but a few patients complain of slight pain or a brownish, watery discharge. Lesions have occasionally been observed in association with extramammary Paget's disease.[25]

Histopathology Histopathologically, unlike hidradenoma papilliferum, this malignant tumor often shows asymmetry and high cellularity. It consists of tubules and cystic cavities with features of apocrine differentiation, surrounded by compressed fibrous stroma. Papillations with a central fibrovascular tissue core are noted projecting in the cyst cavities.

Treatment is by local surgical excision. Fatal metastases, often initially involving lymph nodes, have been recorded. Sentinel node biopsy may be valuable in staging of these patients.

MALIGNANT MIXED TUMOR This malignant counterpart of benign mixed tumor appears mainly to develop de novo.[1,5,26] Moreover, it also shows predilection for the trunk and extremities,[1,5,27] anatomic sites not usually involved by benign mixed tumors. Malignant mixed tumor presents in middle-aged adults, preferentially women, as a solitary, occasionally painful, firm or cystic, nonulcerated cutaneous or subcutaneous nodule measuring 2 to 10 cm in diameter.[1,4–6,11,27]

Histopathology The tumor shows lobulated epithelial aggregations with tubular structures, cords and solid elements. The epithelial component is surrounded by a fibrous stroma with myxomatous and cartilaginous areas. Neoplastic cells display polygonal, plasmacytoid, or cuboidal appearances with variable pleomorphism and scattered mitotic figures. Tubular structures show either apocrine (apocrine type) or eccrine differentiation (eccrine type). The apocrine type is characterized by foci of elongated tubules lined by two or more layers of epithelial cells displaying apocrine (decapitation) secretion. The eccrine type reveals small, round tubules lined by a single layer of flattened, atypical epithelial cells. Foci of ossification may be noted. A recognizable component of a benign mixed tumor is usually not present.

Treatment of choice is total surgical excision. Local and distant metastases, especially to lymph nodes are common. Some authors advocate prophylactic removal of regional lymph node chains.[5] Adjuvant radiotherapy may facilitate long-term survival.

MUCINOUS CARCINOMA Primary mucinous carcinoma of the skin (colloid, gelatinous, or adenocystic carcinoma) is a rare, low-grade carcinoma with close morphologic resemblance to mucinous carcinoma of the breast. It presents as a solitary, slowly growing, soft to firm, grayish, reddish, or bluish, smooth-surfaced nodule measuring up to 3 cm in diameter.[1,4–6,11,28] Lesions tend to occur in older adults on the head, and particularly around the eyelids.[28] Men are more commonly affected than women. Occasional tumors arise on the scalp, axilla, and trunk. Scalp tumors may occur as a patch of alopecia.

Histopathology There are solid and cystic aggregations of neoplastic cells within the dermis, often with extension to the subcutis, embedded in large pools of mucin. Mucinous areas are typically separated by fibrous septae. Focal areas with a cribriform pattern, and tubular as well as glandular structures may be noted. Neoplastic cells are usually round, oval, or polygonal. They show abundant, often eosinophilic and/or vacuolated, cytoplasm and small, moderately pleomorphic nuclei. Malignant satellites may be found in adjacent tissues. Occasional cases reveal signs of neuroendocrine differentiation or show features mimicking mammary carcinoma and Paget's disease. Mucinous areas stain positive with PAS, mucicarmine, and colloidal iron. Tumor cells express low molecular weight cytokeratin, S-100 protein, and carcinoembryonic antigen (CEA).

Treatment is by wide surgical excision. Recurrences have been reported in about 28 percent of cases.[28] Metastases are rare, and involve mostly regional lymph nodes.

SIGNET-RING CELL CARCINOMA Primary carcinoma of the skin with signet-ring cell morphology occurs either as an eyelid lesion or as an expression of mammary or extramammary Paget's disease.[1,4,5,11,29] Signet-ring cell carcinoma of the eyelid presents mainly in older adults, preferentially in males as a solitary nodule or a as diffuse eyelid swelling.[29] The lower eyelids are most commonly involved.

Histopathology Histopathologic examination shows closely packed, variably shaped dermal/subcutaneous aggregations of atypical neoplastic cells arranged in solid nests, and sometimes in cords and strands. They reveal, at least focally, neoplastic cells with eccentric nuclei and vacuolated cytoplasm (signet-ring cells). The cytoplasm of these cells stains positive for sialic acid-containing mucins (PAS, Alcian blue, and mucicarmine stains). Apart from signet-ring cells, a subset of neoplastic cells display abundant foamy cytoplasm, reminiscent of lipidized histiocytes. Sections of the lesions occasionally show small tubular structures. An inflammatory infiltrate composed of lymphocytes is usually noted within the tumor. A fibrotic or partially sclerotic stroma commonly surrounds the lesion.

Treatment of choice is total surgical excision. Tumors frequently recur locally. Fatal metastases have been reported.[29]

SYRINGOCYSTADENOCARCINOMA PAPILLIFERUM This rare neoplasm usually arises in a long standing syringocystadenoma papilliferum, and occasionally in a nevus sebaceus.[1,11,30,31] The tumor preferentially involves the scalp of adult women. A few cases have been reported on the chest. Patients may give a history of sudden enlargement of long-standing clusters of skin-colored or yellowish, sometimes ulcerated, papules or nodules.[31]

Histopathology Syringocystadenocarcinoma papilliferum superficially resembles syringocystadenoma papilliferum on scanning magnification. However, the malignant tumor is characteristically asymmetric and poorly circumscribed, and frequently shows extension deeply into the subcutis. It consists mainly of papillations which project above the skin surface into cystic cavities. The cystic cavities are lined by two layers of epithelium with crowded atypical cells and numerous mitotic figures. Tubular structures with apocrine secretion are noted in some sections.

Treatment of choice is surgical excision. The neoplasm occasionally gives rise to regional lymph node metastases.[31]

APPENDAGE TUMORS WITH ECCRINE DIFFERENTIATION

Eccrine tumors show a wider anatomic distribution than do apocrine tumors.[32] This is due to the broader distribution of normal eccrine glands in virtually all topographic sites, in contrast to normal apocrine glands, which are confined to the head and neck, axillae, genital, and perineal skin.

Histopathologically, eccrine tumors comprise a large spectrum of lesions with differentiation to various portions of normal eccrine apparatus, including intraepidermal (acrosyringium), dermal, and secretory ducts.[32] There are no uniform criteria for diagnosis. The most important feature is the tendency to form lumina with a flattened epithelium. Distinction from apocrine tumors is not always straightforward as the ducts of each gland type are similar and "decapitation" can be observed in certain tumors traditionally classified as "eccrine."

Cyst

HIDROCYSTOMA See appendage tumors with apocrine differentiation.

Hamartoma

ECCRINE HAMARTOMA The term *eccrine hamartoma* is employed for a number of conditions characterized by an increase in size and/or number of normal intradermal eccrine ducts and coils, including eccrine nevus, eccrine angiomatous hamartoma, and porokeratotic eccrine ostial and dermal duct nevus.[11,32]

Eccrine nevus usually presents as a solitary, well-circumscribed area of hyperhidrosis. A few cases occurring as linear papules and multiple plaques have been reported. Eccrine angiomatous hamartoma commonly shows a solitary, flesh-colored, hyperhidrotic, painful papule or plaque appearing at birth or during childhood.[33,34] A few cases arising as multiple, symmetrically located lesions have been reported. Porokeratotic eccrine ostial and dermal duct nevus typically presents as congenital, keratotic papules and plaques located on the distal extremities. Lesions may show a linear arrangement.

Histopathology There is an increase in size and/or number of normal eccrine ducts and coils in the dermis. Eccrine angiomatous hamartoma, in addition, reveals a proliferation of small blood vessels, sometimes with an admixture of nerve fibers and/or fatty tissue. Porokeratotic eccrine ostial and dermal duct nevus displays a comedo-like dilatation and hyperplasia of the acrosyringium, as well as parakeratotic cornoid lamella-like plugs within the sweat gland pores and ducts.

Most patients require no specific treatment. Surgical excision is indicated for painful eccrine angiomatous hamartomas. Carbon dioxide laser therapy has been employed in some cases of porokeratotic eccrine ostial and dermal duct nevus.[33]

Hyperplasias

MUCINOUS SYRINGOMETAPLASIA Mucinous syringometaplasia is a rare benign, presumably reactive condition. Lesions present as slowly growing verrucous plaques on acral sites, particularly on palms and soles.[32] They commonly resemble viral warts.[35]

Histopathology There is an epidermal invagination with one or several ductlike structures that are lined by a stratified squamous epithelium alternating with mucin-containing goblet cells. A prominent papillary dermis commonly surrounds the lesion.

Treatment is by surgical excision.

SYRINGOLYMPHOID HYPERPLASIA Syringolymphoid hyperplasia is a chronic skin condition that may present either as an isolated lesion or in association with cutaneous T-cell lymphoma.[36] Patients usually show patches of hairless, anhidrotic, reddish-brown papules with pseudofollicular hyperkeratosis. Males are preferentially affected.

Histopathology Hyperplastic eccrine structures are surrounded by a dense lymphocytic infiltrate with "syringotropism." Lesions associated with mycosis fungoides occasionally reveal a perifollicular lymphocytic infiltrate and follicular mucinosis.

Careful follow-up with biopsy of persistent lesions is recommended in apparently idiopathic cases in order to exclude lymphoma.

Benign Neoplasms

CYLINDROMA Two main clinical forms of cylindroma are recognized, namely a common, solitary type and a less-frequent form showing multiple lesions. Solitary cylindromas occur as slowly growing, asymptomatic or painful, skin-colored, reddish or bluish papules, nodules, or tumors on the head and neck region of adults.[4–6,11,32] Women are more commonly affected than men.

Multiple cylindromas are often familial and inherited as an autosomal dominant trait, mainly in the setting of Brooke-Spiegler syndrome (familial cylindromatosis). Multiple cylindromas occur as numerous papules, nodules, or variously sized tumors distributed mostly on the scalp, and sometimes on the face or trunk. They show a tendency to confluence, and may cover the entire scalp (so-called turban tumors; Fig. 85-5*A*) or display a linear arrangement. Rarely, patients reveal widespread nodules, a clinical picture that mimics neurofibromatosis. Patients with Brooke-Spiegler syndrome show multiple cylindromas and trichoepitheliomas, occasionally in association with multiple basal cell adenomas of the parotid glands, milia, organoid nevi, basal cell carcinomas, and spiradenomas. The susceptibility gene has been mapped to chromosome 16q12-q13 and has features of a recessive oncogene/tumor-suppressor gene.[37]

Histopathology There is usually a well-circumscribed dermal and/or subcutaneous lesion composed of irregularly shaped tumor islands and cords of basaloid cells arranged in a jigsaw puzzle-like pattern (Fig. 85-5*B*). Islands of basaloid cells are surrounded by a prominent rim of uniformly thickened PAS-positive basement membranes. They consist of two types of basaloid cells, namely, a central population with

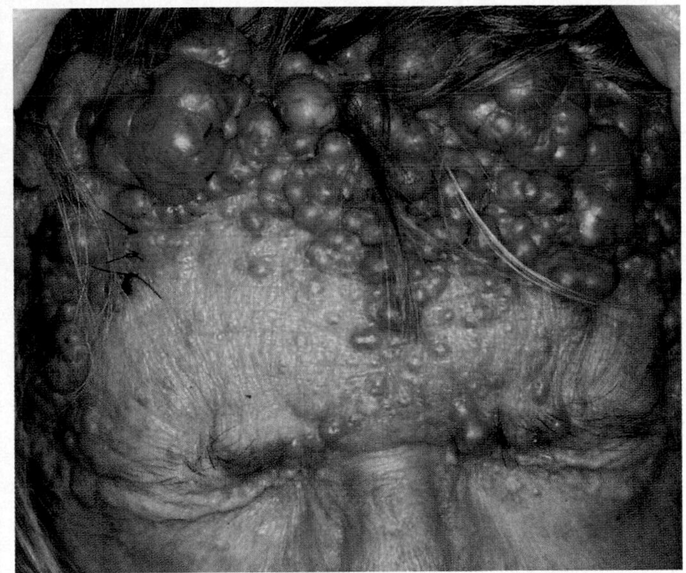

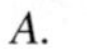

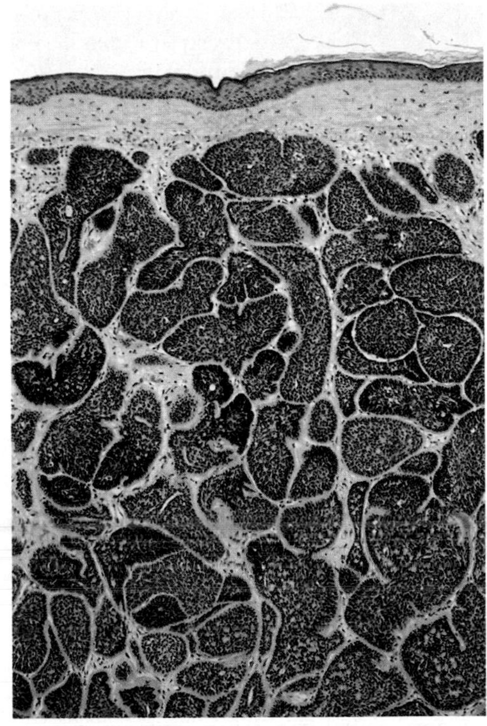

B.

A. Cylindroma or turban tumor. *B*. Cylindroma with irregularly shaped aggregations of basaloid cells arranged in a "jigsaw puzzle" pattern.

large nuclei and abundant cytoplasm and a peripheral population with smaller nuclei, arranged in a palisade at the periphery.

Cylindromas may recur if incompletely excised. Local aggressive behavior and malignant transformation has occasionally been observed, especially in long standing turban tumors of the scalp.[38]

ECCRINE SYRINGOFIBROADENOMA Eccrine syringofibroadenoma (acrosyringeal nevus) is a rare, benign tumor that usually presents as a solitary, slowly growing, skin-colored to reddish nodule or plaque on the face, trunk, and distal extremities of adults.[11,32,39] Rarely, familial cases have been recorded. A few patients show confluent lesions

("syringofibradenomatosis"), especially in association with venous insufficiency. Some lesions arise in association with diabetes mellitus, hidrotic ectodermal dysplasia, or periocular, and ocular, abnormalities.

Histopathology Histopathologic examination reveals interconnected cords and columns of predominantly basaloid cells, extending from beneath the epidermis into the upper dermis. Foci with tubular structures resembling eccrine ducts are frequently observed. A highly vascular, edematous stroma commonly surrounds the epithelial component.

Surgical removal is often not necessary except for cosmetic reasons.

HIDRADENOMA Hidradenoma (eccrine acrospiroma) presents mainly in adults, preferentially in women as a slowly growing, firm, solitary, smooth-surfaced, usually bluish-red, movable dermal and/or subcutaneous papule or nodule.[4–6,11,32] Lesions are located mostly on the scalp, face, trunk, and abdomen, and occasionally on the extremities (Fig. 85-6*A*). Unusual presentations include childhood neoplasms, large or rapidly growing lesions,[40] painful and/or ulcerated lesions, as well as pedunculated tumors.

Histopathology A nodular, solid or solid-cystic lesion in the dermis, sometimes with extension to the subcutis can be observed (Fig. 85-6*B*). The epithelial component consists of closely packed aggregations of round, fusiform or polygonal cells with either eosinophilic or clear cytoplasm. Individual lesions show a variable cellular composition. Clear cells predominate in about one-third of cases. Mitotic figures are sometimes noted within the epithelial component, a feature that does not generally indicate malignancy. The cystic spaces are often filled with mucin. Lesions frequently show some ductal structures with features of either eccrine or apocrine differentiation. The tumors are commonly surrounded by a variably fibrous, vascularized, or hyalinized stroma, occasionally with myxoid or chondroid changes. Unusual findings include the presence of mucinous syringometaplasia, oncocytic cells, squamoid cells, melanin pigmentation, and an increased number of melanocytes.

Treatment is by complete surgical excision. Hidradenoma shows a high rate of local recurrence and may rarely undergo malignant transformation.[41]

POROMA The term *poroma* refers to a group of cutaneous appendage tumors composed of cells (cuticular and poroid cells) similar to those of the acrosyringium. Poromas are traditionally subcategorized histopathologically based on their location in relation to the epidermis into three main variants, namely, hidroacanthoma simplex, eccrine poroma, and dermal duct tumor.[4–6,32] Some authors add poroid hidradenoma to this group.[32] There are also reports of "poromas" with differentiation towards the folliculosebaceous–apocrine unit.

Clinically, hidroacanthoma simplex presents mostly in middle-aged and elderly individuals, preferentially in women as a solitary, hyperkeratotic plaque, with predilection for the extremities. Eccrine poroma occurs commonly as a solitary, slowly growing, skin-colored or pigmented, sometimes bright red, itchy or painful, pedunculated, sessile papule or nodule, situated mostly on the soles and palms of adults. Unusual presentations of eccrine poroma include trunk, head, and neck lesions, and rapidly growing giant tumors. Eccrine poromas may occasionally arise in association with a variety of cutaneous conditions, including hypohidrotic ectodermal dysplasia, chronic radiation dermatitis, and Bowen's disease. Dermal duct tumor is usually observed in adults, revealing a solitary, skin-colored or pigmented papule or plaque on the head and neck region.

Histopathology Hidroacanthoma simplex shows sharply demarcated aggregations of cuboid to ovoid cells confined to the epidermis. Eccrine poroma reveals aggregations of uniform basaloid cells that

FIGURE 85-6

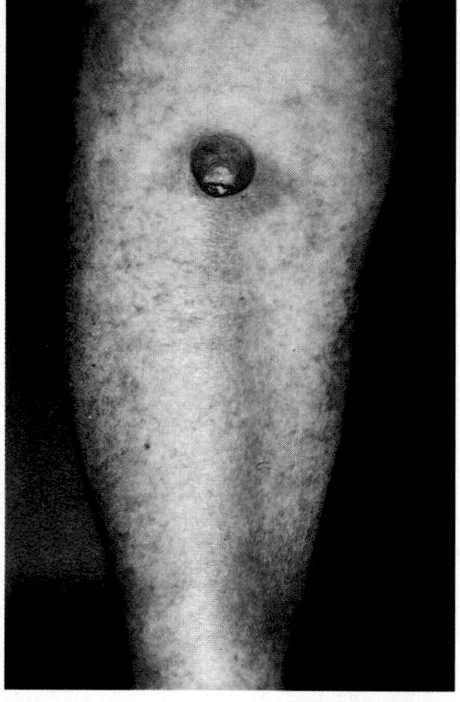

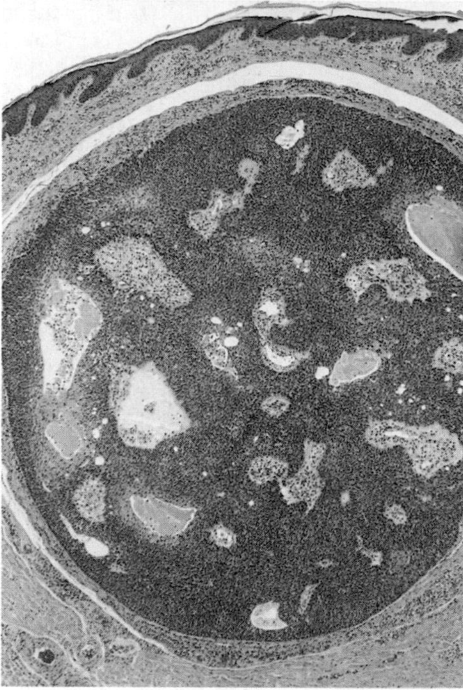

A. B.

Hidradenoma. *A.* Dome-shaped nodule on the leg. *B.* Well-circumscribed, dermal nodule composed of two cell types.

radiate from the basal layer of the epidermis into the dermis (Fig. 85-7). Dermal duct tumor consists of several, sharply circumscribed, mainly dermal nodules composed of poroid and cuticular cells. Ductal structures are frequently observed. Poroid hidradenoma is characterized by intradermal, solid, and cystic aggregations of poroid cells.

Treatment of choice is total surgical excision. Eccrine poroma is rarely observed to precede the development of porocarcinoma.

FIGURE 85-7

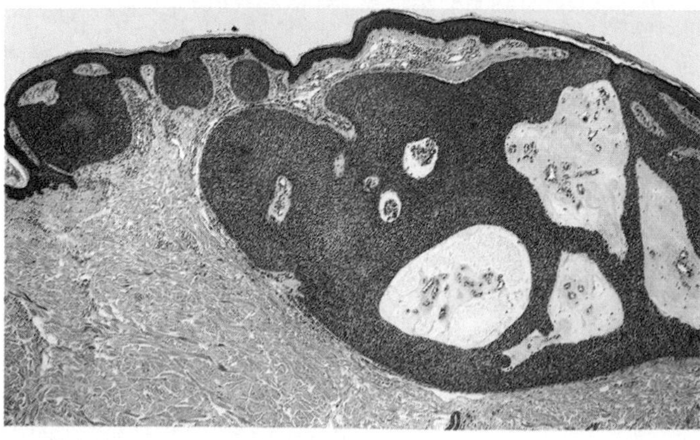

Eccrine poroma. Nodular aggregations of basaloid cells extend from the epidermis into the superficial dermis.

SPIRADENOMA Spiradenoma presents usually as a solitary, slowly growing, sometimes painful, reddish-brown, intradermal or deeply subcutaneous nodule on the head and trunk of young and middle-aged adults[4–6,11,32,42] (Fig. 85-8*A*). A subset of lesions arises in the setting of Brooke-Spiegler syndrome, in association with multiple cylindromas and trichoepitheliomas. Unusual presentations include childhood neoplasms, relatively large or giant tumors, pedunculated tumors, ulcerated lesions, and cutaneous nodules arranged in a linear or zosteriform pattern.

Histopathology There are one or several, well-circumscribed, basophilic nodules in the dermis, sometimes with extension to the subcutis. Nodules show epithelial cell aggregates arranged in sheets and cords or in a trabecular pattern (Fig. 85-8*B*). They consist of two types of cells, namely small, dark-staining basaloid cells located at the periphery, and larger cells with a pale nucleus situated mostly in the center. Tubular or cystic structures are occasionally noted within the epithelial aggregations. Some areas of the tumor contain a PAS-positive hyaline material. The surrounding fibrous stroma occasionally reveals prominent vessels with telangiectasia and edematous or hemorrhagic changes. Additional findings in individual cases include squamous eddies, small cysts, and a variable lymphocytic infiltrate within tumor nests. Cylindromatous areas are observed in a subset of lesions.

Treatment of choice is complete surgical excision. Malignant transformation has been reported in a few patients.[38]

SYRINGOMA Syringoma is a benign neoplasm with differentiation toward eccrine acrosyringium. It presents as numerous, small, firm, smooth, skin-colored, or slightly yellowish papules situated on the face, particularly around the lower eyelids of adults[4–6,11,32] (Fig. 85-9*A*). Women are more commonly affected. Lesions sometimes develop in other anatomic sites, including the vulva and penis, the dorsum of the fingers, axillae, lower abdomen, umbilicus, and buttocks, as well as scalp. Scalp lesions often present as nonscarring alopecia. Syringomas occasionally show a unilateral, linear, or bathing-trunk type distribution. Familial cases have been recorded. There appears to be an increased frequency of syringomas in patients with Down's syndrome. Eruptive syringomas represent a distinctive, occasionally familial form presenting mainly in pubescent or adolescent girls as successive crops of numerous, disseminated, sometimes confluent papules. These lesions tend to involve the upper half of the body, particularly the anterior aspect of the neck, chest, trunk, axillae, inner aspects of the upper arms, and umbilical area.

Histopathology Numerous epithelial aggregations of small, solid nests, cords, and tubular structures focally with a tadpole shape in the upper half of the dermis can be observed (Fig. 85-9*B*). The epithelial areas are commonly surrounded by thickened, closely packed collagen bundles. Tubular structures show an inner layer of luminal cells with one or two rows of peripheral cells. They sometimes contain a homogenous or eosinophilic, PAS-positive and diastase-resistant material. Sections of the lesions sometimes reveal cystic structures filled with cornified cells. A distinctive clear cell variant with an epithelial

FIGURE 85-8

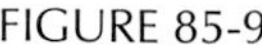

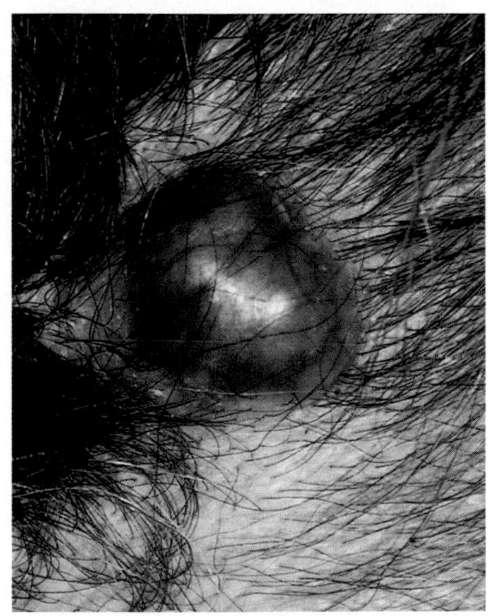

A.

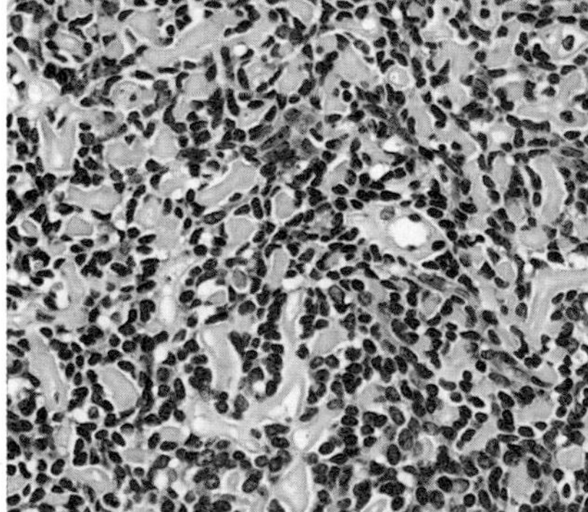

B.

Spiradenoma. *A.* Reddish-brown tumor on the scalp. *B.* Tumor cells arranged in a trabecular pattern. Note hyaline material in the background.

lining consisting of cells having large amounts of cytoplasmic glycogen has been described. This variant is most commonly found in patients with diabetes mellitus.

Treatment is usually unnecessary. Some patients seek removal of the lesions because of cosmetic concerns. Surgery generally produces less-satisfactory cosmetic results. Alternative therapeutic approaches may include dermabrasion, electrodesiccation with curettage, and laser resurfacing.[43]

FIGURE 85-9

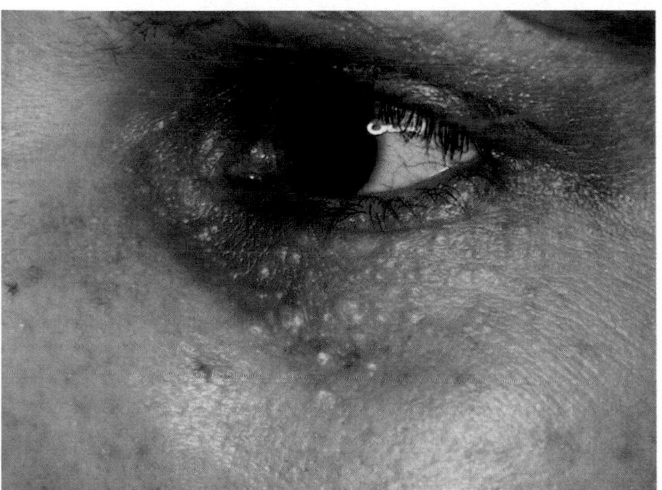

A.

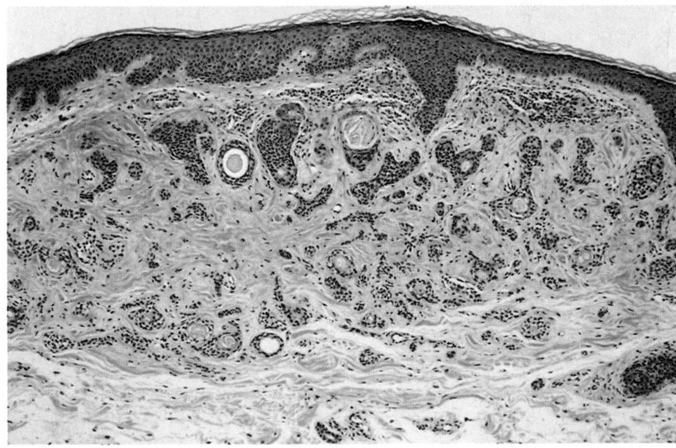

B.

Syringoma. *A.* Multiple, small papules on the periorbital skin of a young woman. *B.* Solid, tubular, and cystic structures in the upper dermis. Note "tadpole"-like morphology of tumor lobules.

TUBULAR ADENOMA The term *tubular adenoma* defines a group of benign appendage tumors histopathologically characterized mainly by numerous cystic, dilated, and branching tubular structures in the dermis surrounded by a compressed fibrous stroma.[11,32,44] Lesions show either eccrine (tubular eccrine adenoma) or apocrine (tubular apocrine adenoma) differentiation. They are found in middle-aged adults as solitary, slowly growing, well-circumscribed nodules, situated mostly on the extremities. Black women appear to be preferentially affected. Unusual presentations include their occurrence during childhood, large tumors, and lesions with verrucous or eroded surfaces. Some cases arise in association with a preexisting nevus sebaceus or a syringocystadenoma papilliferum.

Histopathology There is a relatively well-circumscribed dermal nodule consisting of numerous cystic, dilated and branching tubules, surrounded by compressed or focally hyalinized fibrous tissue. The tubules usually display an inner layer with intraluminal papillations. Tubular lumina are often filled with homogeneous, eosinophilic material or necrotic debris. Features of apocrine or eccrine differentiation are observed in individual cases. Occasional lesions reveal areas with clear or squamous cell changes.

Treatment is by simple surgical excision. Tubular adenomas sometimes recur after surgical excision but malignant transformation has not been observed.

Malignant Neoplasms

AGGRESSIVE DIGITAL PAPILLARY ADENOMA AND ADENOCARCINOMA Aggressive digital papillary adenoma and adenocarcinoma are rare neoplasms characterized mainly by an acral localization and a tendency to recur after excision.[1,4,11,45] Aggressive digital papillary adenoma represents the less-aggressive end of the spectrum. *Aggressive digital papillary adenocarcinoma* is the term reserved for more aggressive tumors with a potential for metastasis. The neoplasms present mainly in middle-aged adults, preferentially white males, as single, painless, flat or slightly elevated, often ulcerated, crusted or bleeding nodules measuring up to 2 cm in diameter. The volar surface of the fingers and toes and the adjacent parts of the palms and soles are predominantly involved. Adherence to underlying deeper tissues is often apparent.

Histopathology There is usually a dermal/subcutaneous lobular proliferation of ductal and glandular structures with focal solid and cribriform zones.[45] Epithelial components are separated by a fibrocollagenous stroma. Ductal structures show variable dilatations forming cystic spaces in which several intraluminal papillary projections are present. Solid and ductal structures are composed mainly of polygonal cells. Additional findings in individual cases include areas of squamous metaplasia and spindle cells, as well as features of apocrine as well as sebaceous differentiation. An inflammatory infiltrate consisting predominantly of lymphocytes and plasma cells is sometimes noted. Aggressive digital papillary adenocarcinoma commonly reveals cellular atypia, pleomorphism, and focal necrosis, as well as an infiltrative growth with involvement of deeper soft tissues, blood vessels, and sometimes bone. Immunohistochemical studies have shown positivity of neoplastic cells for CEA, S-100, and cytokeratins,[45] and in the malignant variant for ferritin.

Treatment is by surgical excision. Approximately 50 percent of aggressive digital papillary adenomas recur locally. In one study, metastases were recorded in 7 of 17 cases of aggressive digital papillary adenocarcinoma.[45] Metastases involve mainly the lungs (71 percent of cases), but have occasionally been observed in other tissues such as lymph nodes, brain, skin, bone, and kidney.

CYLINDROCARCINOMA Cylindrocarcinoma is a very rare malignant appendage tumor with a tendency for local destructive growth and the potential to metastasize. It presents in middle-aged and elderly individuals (mean age 66 years) as a rapidly growing ulcerated or bleeding nodule on the scalp.[27,32,46] Women are more commonly affected than men. There is often a family history of cylindromas or a history of previous excision of a benign cylindroma.

Histopathology The vast majority of cylindrocarcinomas show a remnant of a benign cylindroma (see above). The cylindrocarcinomatous areas consist of irregularly shaped, poorly circumscribed, focally confluent nests and cords of atypical basaloid cells. Neoplastic cells reveal two distinctive populations, namely, small cells located mostly at the periphery and solid nests of larger cells in the center. Unlike benign cylindromas, cylindrocarcinomas reveal only small foci of the jigsaw puzzle-like arrangement, and sometimes show no thickened basement membrane. Tumors often display areas of geographic necrosis.

Treatment is by surgical excision. Local recurrences are sometimes observed. Metastases, particularly to lymph nodes and occasionally to other internal organs, including liver, lung, and bone, have occasionally been reported.

FIGURE 85-10

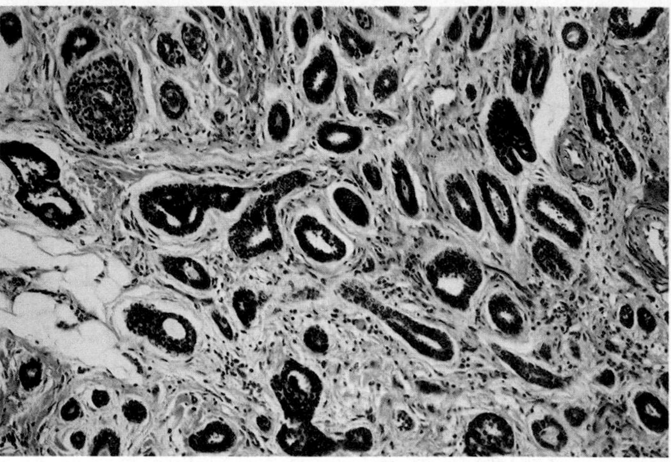

Eccrine carcinoma with nests and tubular structures. Note focal syringomatous features.

ECCRINE CARCINOMA Eccrine carcinoma is a term used for a group of rare, malignant eccrine neoplasms with a great diversity in histomorphologic features and wide differences in biologic behavior.[5,11,23,32] The common histopathologic denominator is the presence of variable areas of basaloid cells with tubular structures. These tumors have previously been described under different names, including basal cell tumor with eccrine differentiation (eccrine epithelioma), syringoid carcinoma, and eccrine syringomatous carcinoma. Lesions show no distinctive clinical features. They present as slowly growing, solitary, nodules, plaques, and tumors on the scalp, extremities, or trunk of older adults.

Histopathology There is a wide spectrum of histopathologic features. Some tumors show confinement to the dermis, whereas oth ers reveal involvement of the subcutis and deeper soft tissues. Lesions may display relatively well-differentiated features with areas of clear-cut ductal differentiation. A subset of lesions exhibit anapl astic fea tures with only subtle signs of ductal differentiation. Relatively well-differentiated tumors are characterized by basaloid aggregations arranged in strands, solid nests, and dilated or branching tubular structures (Fig. 85-10). Foci with syringomatous features may be present. Perineural invasion is a common finding.

Treatment is by wide surgical excision. Local recurrences are common. Lymph node and distant metastases are observed in some patients. Sentinel node biopsy may be valuable in diagnosis of lymph node metastases.

HIDRADENOCARCINOMA Hidradenocarcinoma (clear cell hidradenocarcinoma, malignant clear cell hidradenoma, solid-cystic hidradenocarcinoma, malignant acrospiroma, malignant clear cell myoepithelioma, clear cell eccrine carcinoma) is an exceedingly rare tumor. It presents as an ulcerated nodule on the head/neck, trunk, and extremities of middle-aged or elderly individuals[1,11,32,41] (Fig. 85-11). Many cases are probably malignant from inception, but exceptional hidradenocarcinomas have been associated with a component of a benign hidradenoma.

Histopathology There is usually a nonencapsulated dermal/subcutaneous nodule consisting of irregularly shaped lobules of predominantly large, atypical, polygonal cells with eosinophilic cytoplasm. Foci of clear cells are frequently observed. Sections of the lesions often reveal cords and nests of tumor cells infiltrating the surrounding tissues. Mitotic figures are frequent. Individual lesions show ductal structures with either eccrine or apocrine differentiation. Areas

FIGURE 85-11

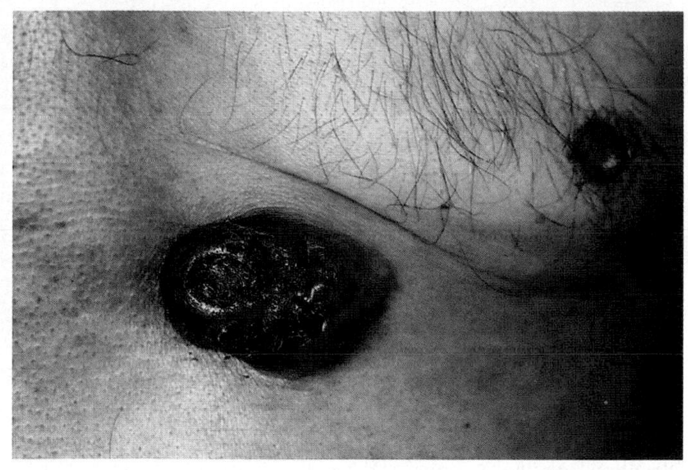

Hidradenocarcinoma. Large ulcerated tumor.

with basaloid or squamoid features are noted in some cases. Tumors arising within long-standing nodular hidradenomas reveal a separate, distinctive component of a "benign" nodular hidradenoma.

Treatment of choice is wide surgical excision. Local recurrences are frequent. Lymphatic spread and distant metastases have been recorded.

MICROCYSTIC ADNEXAL CARCINOMA Microcystic adnexal carcinoma (syringomatous carcinoma, sclerosing sweat duct carcinoma) is a rare, locally aggressive tumor with a high potential for local recurrences. It presents usually in elderly individuals as a solitary, slowly growing, firm, indurated plaque on the face, particularly around the upper lip and orbit.[1,4,5,11] For reasons that are unclear, the tumor tends to occur on the left side of the face. Lesions may occasionally be found on extrafacial locations, including the nipple, axilla, and lower extremities. Patients sometimes complain of a burning sensation and numbness within the lesion, probably as a result of perineural involvement. The skin surface is often normal, atrophic or scaly. Unusual presentations include tumors arising in relatively young individuals, and ulcerated lesions. A few cases have developed in previously therapeutically irradiated facial areas.

Histopathology There is a large, ill-defined dermal-subcutaneous component composed of islands of basaloid keratinocytes, some of which contain horn cysts. The epithelial aggregates are focally embedded in a desmoplastic stroma. In the superficial portion, ducts and glandlike structures lined by a two-cell layer, sometimes filled with homogeneous, eosinophilic material, predominate. The deeper portion reveals individual, thin strands of cells with a tendency to dissect collagen bundles and skeletal muscle, and to involve perineural spaces. Despite these findings, cytologic atypia and mitotic figures are only rarely noted. Lesions sometimes show involvement of underlying fascia or skeletal muscle. Sections in some cases may display foci with clear cells, sebaceous differentiation, and/or amyloid deposition.

Treatment of choice is wide surgical excision. Local recurrences are common (about 50 percent of cases), and may develop several years after initial diagnosis and therapy. Prolonged follow-up is therefore usually necessary. A more favorable cure rate (up to 89 percent) has been achieved with Mohs micrographic surgery. Regional and distant metastases are rare.[47]

POLYMORPHOUS SWEAT GLAND CARCINOMA This is a rare tumor characterized by a distinct, but varied, morphologic appearance, and a low-grade malignant behavior.[11,48] Patients are usually middle-aged women (mean age, 60 years) presenting a single, slowly growing, or long-standing nodule situated on the extremities.

Histopathology There is a highly cellular proliferation of epithelial cells with a variety of growth patterns, including solid, trabecular, tubular, pseudopapillary, and cylindromatous. The lesion is often surrounded by a stroma with hemorrhagic, hyalinized, and/or cystic changes.

Treatment is by surgical excision. Recurrences and metastases, especially to regional lymph nodes, have been observed.

POROCARCINOMA Porocarcinoma, the malignant counterpart of eccrine poroma, is a rare, potentially aggressive neoplasm. It presents in elderly individuals as a partially ulcerated, verrucous plaque or polypoid tumor on the lower extremities.[4–6,11,32,49,50] Patients may show lesions on other anatomic sites, including the head and neck,[49] trunk, upper extremities, and vulva. There is frequently a history of a long-standing nodule, suggesting malignant transformation of an eccrine poroma or hidroacanthoma simplex. Occasional cases present as multiple cutaneous nodules or rapidly growing tumors. Rarely, porocarcinoma arises in a nevus sebaceus. Some cases have been observed in association with a range of unrelated cutaneous and systemic conditions including, extramammary Paget's disease, chronic radiation, sarcoidosis, pernicious anemia, chronic lymphocytic leukemia, Hodgkin's disease, and visceral carcinomas. Of note is a peculiar presentation of epidermotropic and nonepidermotropic cutaneous metastases of porocarcinoma as numerous, skin-colored to reddish/purple, papules or nodules. These may be accompanied by lymphedema caused by lymphatic involvement.

Histopathology Histopathologically, primary porocarcinoma reveals either a carcinomatous area with an adjacent benign eccrine poroma or a hidroacanthoma simplex component, or a carcinomatous area only. The lesion is characterized by sharply circumscribed nests and islands of atypical basaloid cells within the epidermis. The underlying dermis is variably involved by irregularly shaped nests with neoplastic cells displaying striking atypia and mitotic activity. Epithelial aggregations reveal, at least focally, features of ductal differentiation ranging from variably mature eccrine ducts to focal intracytoplasmic lumina.[50] Areas of necrosis, perineural, and lymphatic/vascular invasion are occasionally present. Some cases reveal clear cell, squamous cell, and/or spindle cell differentiation. A small subset of cases (up to 15 percent) occurs as "in situ" porocarcinoma. Additional findings may include foci of cornification, melanin pigmentation, and colonization by melanocytes. Immunohistologic studies show positivity of tumor cells for CEA, cytokeratin, and epithelial membrane antigen (EMA), and negativity for S-100.

Treatment is by wide local surgical excision. Previous studies suggest a generally poor prognosis with frequent local recurrences (up to 20 percent of cases), lymph node metastases, and occasionally distant metastases. Distant metastases have been observed in a number of internal organs, including the lung, breast, mediastinum, peritoneum, and liver. Metastatic porocarcinoma is very resistant to adjunctive chemotherapy or radiation, and such patients have a high mortality rate (up to 67 percent).[49] However, there is now mounting evidence that porocarcinoma may not be as aggressive as previously thought.[50]

SPIRADENOCARCINOMA Spiradenocarcinoma is a rare, malignant, appendage tumor that usually arises on long-standing benign spiradenoma and sometimes behaves aggressively.[11,32,51] It presents mainly in middle-aged and elderly individuals as a single, large, nodule on the extremities, trunk, or abdomen. Occasional lesions arise on the head and neck. Patients sometimes give a history of a long-standing cutaneous nodule that had grown slowly for several years, but that recently rapidly enlarged in size with a change in color, ulceration, or bleeding. One case of spiradenocarcinoma developing in a scar after a previous excision of a benign spiradenoma has been recorded.[52]

Histopathology The tumor usually shows a carcinomatous area, representing spiradenocarcinoma, in association with a typical, benign spiradenoma. The carcinomatous area is characterized by aggregations of atypical basaloid or squamous cells focally arranged in sheets and showing an infiltrative pattern.[52] Unlike the benign spiradenoma component, spiradenocarcinoma exhibits a less-conspicuous two-cell population. Neoplastic cells display nuclear hyperchromasia and pleomorphism, and an increased mitotic activity. Areas of *necrosis en masse* are often present. Additional findings in individual cases include foci with features of ductal, clear cell, rhabdomyoblastic, and osteosarcomatous differentiation. Immunohistologically, tumor cells show positivity for epithelial markers, and occasionally for S-100.

Treatment is by wide surgical excision. Patients sometimes develop local recurrences and/or lymph node involvement. Fatal metastases have been reported in about 20 percent of cases.[27] Radiation, systemic chemotherapy, and hormonal treatment with tamoxifen have been used for metastatic disease.

APPENDAGE TUMORS WITH FOLLICULAR DIFFERENTIATION

The follicular cysts, hamartomas, and neoplasms reviewed in this section show predominantly histopathologic features that resemble different portions of a normal hair follicle, hair shaft and/or perifollicular fibrous sheath. They exhibit a wide range of morphologic features and may display variable degrees of differentiation. Consequently, uniform diagnostic criteria do not exist for a number of entities.[3–6,11]

Cysts

EPIDERMAL CYST Epidermal (epidermoid, infundibular, epithelial) cyst is the most common type of follicular cyst. It presents usually as a solitary, mobile, skin-colored, white or yellowish nodule on the head and neck or trunk of young and middle-aged adults.[53] It is discussed in Chap. 84.

Multiple epidermal cysts may be a feature of Gardner's syndrome.[4,5,53] Gardner's syndrome, caused by mutations in the *adenomatous polyposis coli (APC)* gene, is a rare, inherited autosomal dominant trait characterized by multiple epidermal cysts and pilomatricomas, soft-tissue proliferations (fibromatosis, lipomas, leiomyomas), multiple craniofacial osteomas, bilateral pigmented ocular fundus lesions (congenital hypertrophy of the retinal epithelium), and intestinal (colorectal) polyposis. If intestinal (colorectal) polyposis is undetected or untreated, virtually all patients develop colonic carcinoma at a young age. The cutaneous cysts frequently predate the intestinal polyps.

HYBRID CYST Hybrid cysts present usually as solitary, cystic nodules situated on the head and neck.[4,54] Tumors occur in all age groups.

Histopathology There is a cystic lesion displaying a mixed type of epithelial lining with a stratified squamous epithelium in its upper portion and outer sheath differentiation with tricholemmal cornification in its lower portion.

KERATOCYST Cutaneous keratocysts present typically in patients with basal cell nevus syndrome[53,55](see Chap. 82). The cutaneous keratocysts show similar histopathologic features to the jaw keratocysts of patients with this syndrome. They have been observed on the trunk and extremities.

Histopathology Histopathologic examination shows a cystic structure with a corrugated or festooned configuration. The epithelial lining reveals several layers of squamous epithelium without a granular zone. A lanugo hair is observed within the cyst cavity of some lesions.

PIGMENTED FOLLICULAR CYST Pigmented follicular cyst shows differentiation toward the infundibular portion of the hair follicle. It presents usually as a solitary, relatively small (0.4 to 1.5 cm), pigmented papule/nodule situated on the head and neck region of adult males.[4,53,56]

Histopathology There is a cystic structure filled with numerous, heavily pigmented hair shafts. The cyst is lined by a stratified squamous epithelium.

TRICHOLEMMAL CYST Tricholemmal (sebaceous, trichilemmal, isthmus-catagen, pilar) cyst is a relatively common lesion characterized by outer root sheath differentiation at the level of the follicular isthmus and tricholemmal cornification.[4–6,53] Lesions present as solitary, cutaneous/subcutaneous nodules on the scalp of adults, preferentially of women. Some patients show multiple, occasionally familial tumors. Familial tricholemmal cysts are inherited in an autosomal dominant fashion.[57] The lesion is discussed in detail in Chap. 84.

VELLUS HAIR CYST Vellus hair cysts show differentiation toward the infundibular portion of the hair follicle and typically contain numerous vellus hairs. Lesions are either sporadic or inherited in an autosomal dominant fashion. Multiple, small (1- to 3-mm), asymptomatic, pigmented, reddish or grayish papules distributed on the chest, abdomen, and axilla (eruptive vellus hair cysts) may be observed.[5,6,53] The face, neck, and extremities are occasionally involved. Familial cases present most commonly at birth or in early infancy. Sporadic lesions tend to develop in the first or second decades of life. Eruptive vellus hair cysts may be associated with steatocystoma multiplex, trichostasis spinulosa, anhidrotic ectodermal dysplasia,[58] and pachyonychia congenita, as well as some neurologic disorders.

Histopathology Histopathologic examination reveals a cystic structure located in the middle or upper dermis. It is lined by a stratified squamous epithelium with focal features of outer root sheath differentiation at the level of the follicular isthmus and tricholemmal cornification. Several transversely and obliquely sectioned vellus hair shafts and keratin material are present within the cystic lumen.

Eruptive vellus hair cysts are difficult to treat surgically. Patients may benefit from therapy with isotretinoin, pulsed carbon dioxide and erbium: YAG-laser ablation.[59] Spontaneous regression has occasionally been observed.

Hamartomas

BASALOID FOLLICULAR HAMARTOMA Basaloid follicular hamartoma occurs either as a solitary, nonhereditary tumor or as multiple, hereditary lesions.[60,61] Familial, multiple, basaloid follicular hamartomas manifest as numerous, small (1 to 2 mm in diameter), flesh-colored papules located predominantly over the central face, and occasionally on the scalp, neck, and shoulders. Lesions have been reported in association with myasthenia gravis, alopecia, hypohidrosis, facial sclerosis, or cystic fibrosis.[60,61] Solitary forms of basaloid follicular hamartoma are commonly found on the face and scalp. Localized linear and unilateral variants have also been documented. The exact nature of solitary and multiple basaloid follicular hamartomas and their relationship to basal cell carcinoma is still controversial. Some authors believe these lesions represent a distinctive type of basal cell carcinoma.[3]

Histopathology Histopathologic examination shows anastomosing strands of basaloid cells with numerous epidermal connections. Central areas of epithelial aggregations occasionally reveal cells with a squamoid appearance. Features of follicular differentiation including horn cysts, rudimentary germs, and follicular papillae are variably present.

HAIR FOLLICLE NEVUS Hair follicle nevi have been reported in all age groups.[3,11,62] They occur as slightly dome-shaped, skin-colored papules and nodules on hair-bearing skin, particularly on the face.[62] Cases with a linear arrangement have been documented. A number of specific conditions have been included as variants of hair follicle nevus by different authors, namely the so-called faun-tail, a cutaneous lesion characterized by the presence of a patch of hairs arising over the lower sacral area, hair follicles arising on the palms and soles, and Becker's pigmented hairy nevus.[11,63] There is currently disagreement as to whether "hair follicle nevus" ("congenital vellus hamartoma") represents a distinct entity or a variant of trichofolliculoma.[3]

Histopathology The upper dermis reveals a well-circumscribed area with numerous closely packed mature vellus follicles. Hair follicles are surrounded by prominent sheaths of perifollicular connective tissue. Clefts are usually observed bordering the perifollicular connective tissue. Some lesions display sebaceous lobules.

Treatment of choice is surgical excision.

LINEAR UNILATERAL BASAL CELL NEVUS Linear unilateral basal cell nevus presents at birth or in infancy as numerous, cutaneous papules or nodules distributed unilaterally, sometimes in a zosteriform fashion. Lesions often show comedone plugs and closely resemble nevus comedonicus. One patient with diffuse osteoma cutis, unilateral anodontia, and abnormal bone mineralization has been reported.[64]

Histopathology Histopathologic features simulate those of basal cell carcinoma. Lesions are characterized by a lattice-like pattern of basaloid cells attached to the undersurface of the epidermis. Hints of follicular differentiation are usually present.

NEUROFOLLICULAR HAMARTOMA Neurofollicular hamartoma is a rare hamartoma characterized by a proliferation of spindle cells and hyperplastic pilosebaceous units. Lesions present as solitary, small (up to 7 mm in diameter), pale papules on the face, particularly around the nose, of children and adults.[65]

Histopathology There are hyperplastic pilosebaceous units in the dermis surrounded by a stroma composed of spindle cells. The spindle cells are arranged mainly in broad, haphazard fascicles. Immunohistologically, the spindle cells show variable positivity for S-100.

NEVUS COMEDONICUS Nevus comedonicus is a follicular hamartoma characterized by contiguous structures that resemble aberrant infundibula.[3] Patients show grouped, unilateral, linear, or segmentary arranged dark papules with keratin-plugs situated on the face and neck.[3,6,11] The condition is fully discussed in Chap. 84.

NEVUS SEBACEUS Nevus sebaceus (organoid nevus, pilosyringosebaceous nevus) is a hamartoma that presents mostly at birth or in early childhood as a yellowish plaque on the scalp, face, neck, and trunk.[3–6,11,13,66] Nevus sebaceus is discussed in Chap. 84.

Benign Neoplasms

DESMOPLASTIC TRICHOEPITHELIOMA Desmoplastic trichoepithelioma (sclerosing epithelial hamartoma) is a relatively uncommon tumor that presents as a small (up to 1 cm in diameter), asymptomatic firm, oval, oblong, or annular papule or plaque on the face (Fig. 85-12), particularly around the angle of the lip.[3–6,11] Plaques often reveal a raised border and depressed center. The tumor shows a predilection for young and middle-aged adults. Women are about three times more commonly affected than men. Familial cases of solitary or multiple lesions have been reported.

FIGURE 85-12

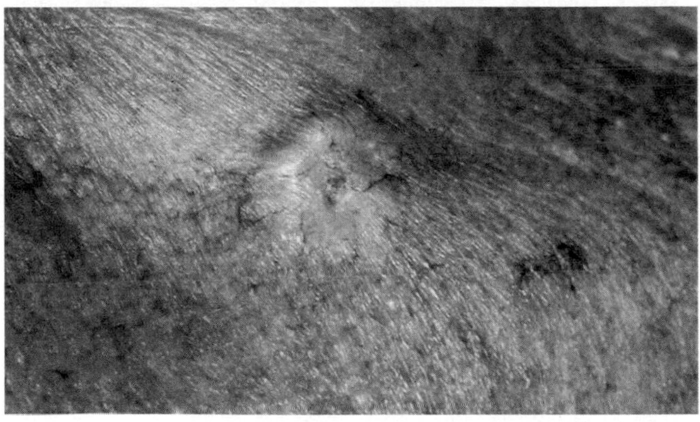

Desmoplastic trichoepithelioma located on the infraorbital region.

Histopathology Histopathologic examination reveals a relatively well circumscribed lesion in the upper two-thirds of the dermis, rarely with extension to the lower dermis and subcutis. It is composed of basaloid aggregations arranged predominantly in columns and cords and admixed with infundibulocystic structures, surrounded by a dense, hypocellular desmoplastic stroma. A focal connection to the epidermis is usually observed. Additional features in some lesions include foci of sebaceous cells, shadow ("ghost") cells, foreign-body granulomas, calcification, and ossification. A subset of cases are associated with a dermal melanocytic nevus.

Treatment is by local surgical excision.

DILATED PORE OF WINER Although classified as a neoplasm in this section, there is currently some debate as to whether dilated pore represents a type of follicular (infundibular) cyst or a neoplastic process.[3,5,6,67] The lesion presents usually as a solitary, comedo-like, keratin-filled structure on the head and neck of elderly individuals.[67] In some cases lesions arise in the setting of cystic acne or actinic damage.

Histopathology A single or several contiguous, markedly dilated infundibula are observed in the upper dermis, sometimes with extension to the lower dermis. The epithelial lining reveals focal acanthosis and finger-like projections radiating into the surrounding dermis. Dilated infundibula contain cornified cells arranged in basket-weave and laminated patterns. Heavy pigmentation of the epithelium can be observed in some cases.

Treatment is by local surgical excision.

FIBROFOLLICULOMA Fibrofolliculoma is a rare tumor that presents usually as multiple, small papules measuring 2 to 4 mm in diameter, situated on the head and neck, upper trunk, and arms.[3,5,6] Fibrofolliculomas commonly develop in middle-aged individuals. Multiple, familial fibrofolliculomas occurring in association with trichodiscomas, perifollicular fibromas, and skin tags are a feature of Birt-Hogg-Dubé syndrome.[68] Patients with this syndrome show a tendency to develop colonic polyposis and a range of internal neoplasms (e.g., renal carcinoma). Rare examples of fibrofolliculoma occur as solitary lesions.

Regarding pathogenesis, fibrofolliculoma has traditionally been considered to represent a distinct follicular adnexal neoplasm. However, some authors recently suggested that this lesion may indeed be a type of hamartoma with sebaceous differentiation, closely related to trichodiscoma.[3] This hypothesis is based on chronological considerations and frequent occurrence of both fibrofolliculomas and trichodiscomas in patients with Birt-Hogg-Dubé syndrome. According to these authors, both fibrofolliculoma and trichodiscoma represent temporal stages in the development of a single pathologic tumor, called "mantleoma." The term *mantleoma* reflects the likely derivation of this tumor from the sebaceous mantle, a well-described but little known part of the sebaceous gland cycle (see below).

Histopathology Fibrofolliculoma is characterized by a dome-shaped lesion with a central, relatively well-formed hair follicle displaying a single or several, contiguous, dilated, keratin-filled infundibula. The infundibula are connected to several thin, focally anastomosing epithelial strands that extend in a radial fashion into the connective tissue. The lesion is often surrounded by a well-circumscribed fibrillary collagenous or mucinous stroma with scant or no elastic tissue.

Treatment of choice in solitary lesions is by surgical excision. Carbon dioxide laser can be useful in removal of multiple lesions. Patients should be screened for other features of Birt-Hogg-Dubé syndrome.

FIBROUS PAPULE Fibrous papule (perifollicular fibroma) presents mainly as a solitary papule or as several dome-shaped, skin-colored, pigmented, or reddish lesions situated on the face, particularly around the nose of adults.[3,5,6,11] Multiple fibrous papules occurring in association with fibrofolliculomas and trichodiscomas are a feature of Birt-Hogg-Dubé syndrome.[68] Currently, there is some disagreement as to whether fibrous papule represents a neoplastic process or a hamartoma.[3]

Histopathology A dome-shaped or polypoid lesion consisting of one or more poorly formed hair follicles, surrounded by cellular fibrous stroma is observed in the upper dermis. The epidermis sometimes reveals an increased number of large, single melanocytes located along the dermal–epidermal junction. There is usually a proliferation of small vessels within the dermis. Spindle- and stellate-shaped, sometimes multinucleated fibrocytes can be found within the stroma.

Treatment of choice is surgical excision. Carbon dioxide laser is useful in removing multiple lesions.

INVERTED FOLLICULAR KERATOSIS Inverted follicular keratosis presents as an asymptomatic, small (3 to 10 mm in diameter), solitary papule or nodule on the face of middle-aged and older individuals.[3–6,11] Most lesions are located around the cheek and upper lip. Males are two to three times more commonly affected than females. Because of the wartlike morphology, it was recently suggested that inverted follicular keratosis may represent a manifestation of human papillomavirus infection rather than a true neoplasm.[3]

Histopathology Histopathologic examination reveals an endophytic or exophytic–endophytic lesion consisting of several large epithelial lobules extending into the dermis. Four distinctive histopathologic patterns are recognized, namely, papillomatous, keratoacanthoma-like, solid, and cystic. The center of the epithelial lobules is composed of squamous cells focally arranged in a whorled pattern (squamous eddies). The periphery is sometimes occupied by basaloid cells. Additional features in some lesions include foci of tricholemmal differentiation, mucinous areas with spongiosis, and melanin pigmentation. A mild lymphohistiocytic inflammatory infiltrate often surrounds the lesion.

Treatment is by surgical excision.

LYMPHADENOMA Cutaneous lymphadenoma (adamantinoid trichoblastoma) is a rare appendage tumor that is currently classified as a peculiar variant of trichoblastoma.[3] The neoplasm presents mainly in adults in the fourth to fifth decades as a solitary, skin-colored nodule situated on the head and neck.[3,4,11,69] The usual clinical diagnosis is basal cell carcinoma.

FIGURE 85-13

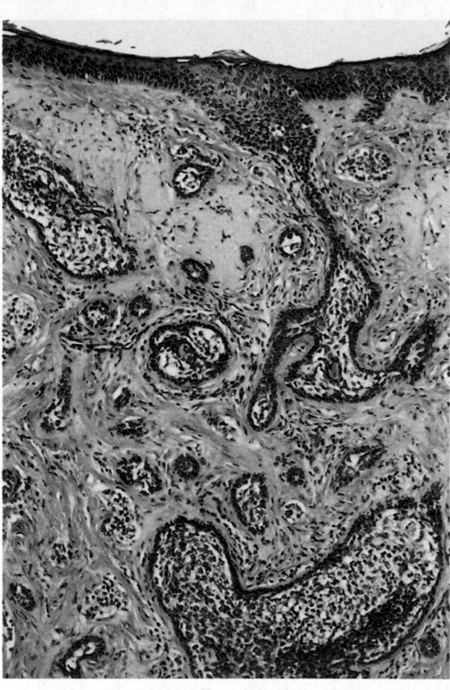

Lymphadenoma. Multiple, variably sized basaloid lobules in the dermis. Note the prominent palisading of nuclei at the periphery and the lymphoid cells within the lobules.

Histopathology There are multiple, variably sized lobules in the dermis composed of basaloid cells, surrounded by a fibrous stroma. The basaloid lobules display focal palisading of nuclei at the periphery. An infiltrate of T and B lymphocytes is typically observed within the basaloid lobules, with focal sprinkling of the lymphocytes in the stroma (Fig. 85-13). Some cases reveal adamantinoid features. Epithelial aggregations in individual lesions display variable signs of follicular and sebaceous differentiation.

Treatment is by surgical excision. Local recurrences or metastases have not been observed.

PANFOLLICULOMA This is a recently described benign neoplasm that shows differentiation toward portions of both the upper and lower segments of a normal hair follicle.[3] The tumor reveals several morphologic similarities to trichoblastoma. Clinically, cystic, skin-colored or reddish, dome-shaped papules, situated on the head, trunk, and lower limbs of adults can be found.

Histopathology The tumor is characterized by several closely packed, solid, solid-cystic, or cystic aggregations of epithelial cells in the dermis, sometimes extending into the subcutis. They are surrounded by a fibrous stroma with focal clefts between the stroma and adjacent "normal" dermis or subcutaneous fat. Neoplastic cells reveal a spectrum of morphologic features reflecting bulbar, stem, isthmic, and infundibular differentiation. These include the presence of germinative and matrical cells (bulb), cells with trichohyline granules and blue-gray corneocytes (inner root sheath), and cells with abundant pale and clear cytoplasm (outer root sheath). Cystic structures are lined by infundibular epithelium with a granular zone and filled with blue-gray corneocytes arranged in basket-weave, laminated, and compact patterns.

Treatment is by surgical excision.

PILAR SHEATH ACANTHOMA Pilar sheath acanthoma is characterized by a small (5 to 10 mm in diameter), solitary, skin-colored papule situated on the head and neck, particularly around the upper lip.[3–6,70] A central, occasionally keratin plugged pore is often present. Middle-aged and elderly individuals are commonly affected.

Histopathology There is a crateriform depression in the epidermis representing a widely dilated, keratin-filled infundibulum or closely set infundibula, contiguous at the base with numerous epithelial lobules of pink keratinocytes. The epithelial lobules radiate into the dermis, sometimes with involvement of the subcutis. They are surrounded by a narrow rim of fibrous tissue. The epithelium shows similar features to those of the isthmus of a normal hair follicle. Small infundibulocystic structures, tubular structures and foci of sebaceous differentiation (ducts or sebaceous lobules) are variably observed in individual cases.

Treatment is by surgical excision.

PILOMATRICOMA Pilomatricoma (calcifying epithelioma of Malherbe) is a relatively common appendage tumor that predominantly shows differentiation towards the matrical portion of a normal hair follicle at the level of the bulb. Lesions present usually as solitary, skin-colored or pigmented cystic or firm nodules on the head and neck (Fig. 85-14*A*) and upper extremities of children and young persons.[3–6,11] Some tumors arise in older adults. Unusual clinical features include rapidly growing tumors, lesions associated with overlying striae or anetodermic changes, and neoplasms arising in a nevus sebaceus. A few patients present with multiple lesions (usually fewer than five in number). Multiple pilomatricomas have also been reported in patients with Gardner's syndrome.[4,53] Gardner's syndrome is described in the earlier section on epidermal cysts.

Histopathology Pilomatricoma shows a spectrum of morphologic features which mainly reflect different evolutionary stages.[71] Early and well-developed pilomatricomas reveal variably sized, round to oval cystic lesions lined by a basaloid epithelium at the periphery and filled in the center with masses of eosinophilic, faulty hair matrix material containing "shadow" ("ghost") cells (Fig. 85-14*B*). Basaloid (matrical) cells show monomorphous round nuclei with one or more distinctive nucleoli, and variable numbers of mitotic figures. Foci of squamoid epithelium are sometimes noted within the epithelial lining. Regressing pilomatricomas display haphazardly arranged foci of basaloid cells and shadow cells, as well as an inflammatory infiltrate with multinucleated histiocytic giant cells. Granulation tissue is sometimes noted. Old pilomatricomas reveal no basaloid component but show irregularly shaped, partially confluent masses of shadow cells with foci of calcification or ossification. Melanin deposition, transepidermal elimination, and extramedullary hematopoiesis have been described in some pilomatricomas. A peculiar variant with relatively large areas of basaloid cells and small foci of shadow cells ("proliferating pilomatricoma") is occasionally observed in older adults.

Treatment of choice is surgical excision. Some lesions show spontaneous regression. Local recurrences may occasionally develop after surgical excision. A case of malignant transformation has been described.[72]

PROLIFERATING PILAR TUMOR Proliferating pilar tumor was previously reported under different names including proliferating trichilemmal cyst, pilar tumor, proliferating trichilemmal tumor, invasive pilomatrixoma, trichochlamydocarcinoma, giant hair matrix tumor, trichilemmal pilar tumor, and proliferating follicular cystic neoplasm. Clinically, lesions present as solitary, slowly growing, cystic or lobulated nodules and tumors on the scalp and trunk, as well as on the extremities of older adults.[3,5,11] Women are approximately two times more commonly affected than men. A few patients show multiple, sometimes familial, lesions. Occasional tumors may be ulcerated or occur as relatively large extracranial masses (up to 25 cm in diameter) (Fig. 85-15). Rarely, the neoplasm has been reported in association with nevus sebaceus or basaloid follicular hamartoma.

The exact nature of proliferating pilar tumor is still debatable. Traditionally, the tumor has been regarded as a benign follicular neoplasm. There are, however, several well-documented reports demonstrating that proliferating pilar tumor is capable of undergoing frank carcinomatous transformation, even with development of distant metastases. This has prompted some authors to advance the view that proliferating pilar tumor represents a low-grade type of squamous cell carcinoma ("proliferating tricholemmal cystic squamous carcinoma").[3]

Histopathology Histopathologic examination usually reveals a sharply circumscribed, round or oval, cystic neoplasm occupying the

FIGURE 85-14

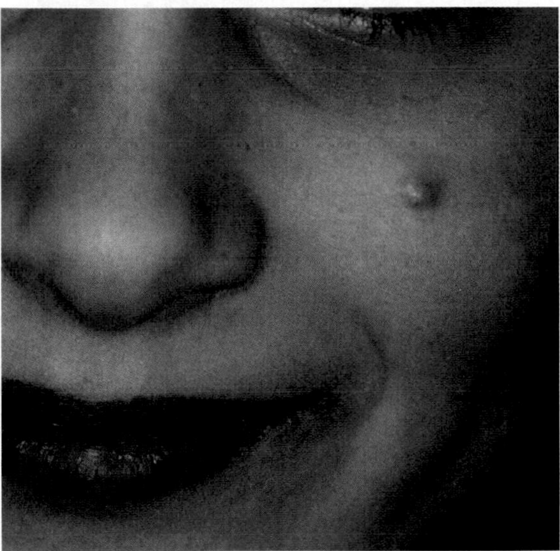

A.

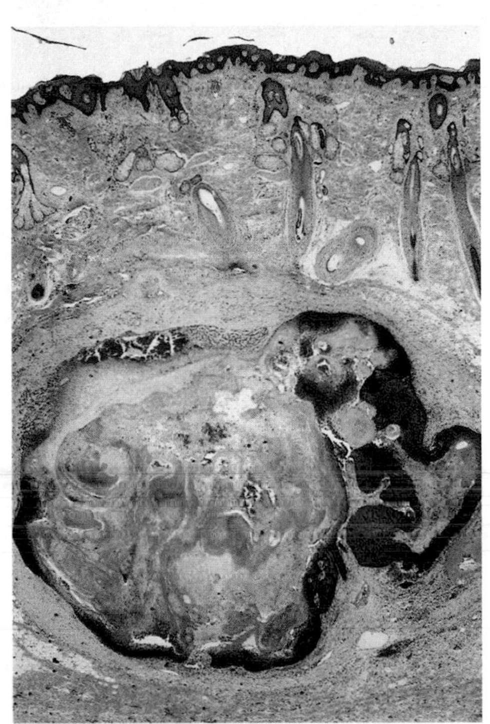

B.

Pilomatricoma. *A.* A tumor in a young girl. *B.* Cystic lesion lined focally at the periphery by basaloid epithelium and filled with masses of eosinophilic, cornified material with shadow cells.

FIGURE 85-15

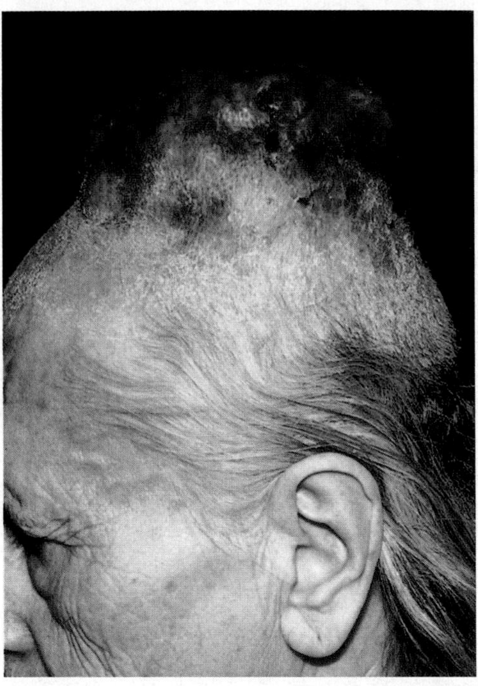

Proliferating pilar tumor. Ulcerated giant nodule on the scalp.

lower dermis and subcutis. There is an epithelial component lining nearly the whole lesion, and extending within it in a radial fashion. The epithelium forms several partially interconnecting solid and cystic lobules. A zone of fibrous stroma with clefts between the stroma and surrounding normal tissue encompasses the tumor. Tumor nests are composed mainly of squamous cells with some areas of clear cells containing glycogen. A characteristic feature is the presence, in the center of lobules, of tricholemmal cornification; that is, abrupt formation of compact eosinophilic keratin without granular layer interposition. Foci with keratohyaline granules, small horn pearls and squamous eddies, calcification, stromal calcium deposition, ossification, and shadow cells, as well as a palisading arrangement of the nuclei at the periphery of the lobules are observed in individual tumors. Some lesions reveal a lymphohistiocytic inflammatory infiltrate with foreign-body granulomas. A small subset of cases exhibits rather "atypical" features with numerous mitoses and dyskeratotic cells, edema and cystic degeneration, tumoral necrosis, and local infiltration of tumor cells into the stroma and galea, as well as underlying cranium. These changes are mainly suggestive of aggressive behavior.

Treatment is by complete excision. Local recurrences and metastatic spread have been observed even in histopathologically typical cases. Accurate follow-up is recommended in all patients.

TRICHOADENOMA Trichoadenoma (of Nikolowski) is a rare follicular tumor that some authors consider a neoplastic process, while other authors consider it a malformation.[3–6,11] Lesions are commonly found in adults and present as solitary, slowly growing, grayish nodules measuring up to 1.5 cm in diameter. They are mainly situated on the face and trunk.

Histopathology A dome-shaped, sharply defined, nodule composed of numerous, round to oval, infundibulocystic structures is observed in the dermis. Involvement of the subcutis may be noted in some cases. Infundibulocystic structures are lined by a squamous epithelium with a clear-cut basal layer, spinous zone and granular layer. They contain corneocytes arranged in a laminated pattern. A conspicuous collagenous stroma often surrounds the tumor cell nests. A subset of cases shows prominent verrucous hyperplasia of the epidermis.

Treatment is by surgical excision.

TRICHOBLASTOMA Headington first introduced the name "trichoblastoma" in 1970, in a classification of neoplasms of the hair germ.[73] In his classification, tumors of the hair germ were divided into trichoblastomas, trichoblastic fibromas, and trichogenic trichoblastomas, based on their stromal characteristics. Ackerman et al. now suggest using the term *trichoblastoma* to embrace all benign appendage tumors whose common histopathologic denominator is the presence of an epithelial component consisting predominantly of follicular germinative (basaloid) cells.[3] Trichoblastomas are best subdivided according to the predominant morphologic pattern into large nodular (including pigmented), small nodular (including adamantinoid or lymphadenoma), retiform (giant solitary trichoepithelioma), cribriform (classic trichoepithelioma), racemiform (nonclassic trichoepithelioma), and columnar (desmoplastic trichoepithelioma) variants.[3] Exact subclassification is difficult in some lesions because of the presence of more than one predominant morphologic pattern. Here we focus mainly on "conventional" trichoblastomas. Other specific variants, including lymphadenoma and trichoepitheliomas, are discussed elsewhere in this chapter.

Clinically, trichoblastomas present as solitary, nonulcerated, skin-colored to brown or bluish-black papules/nodules situated mostly on the head and neck, particularly on the scalp and face of adults. Lesions sometimes develop on extremities or trunk. They are frequently initially suspected to be basal cell carcinomas or dermal nevi. Trichoblastomas are also commonly observed in association within a preexisting nevus sebaceus[13,74] (Fig. 85-16*A*), or may occasionally coexist with a basal cell carcinoma.[3]

Histopathology Lesions are characterized by several, dermal/subcutaneous, smooth-bordered aggregations of basaloid (germinative) cells arranged in different morphologic patterns including, cribriform, nodular, racemiform, and retiform. Epithelial aggregations are surrounded by a variable sclerotic or partly hyalinized stroma. They typically reveal peripheral palisading and several foci with rudimentary follicular papillae and germs (Fig. 85-16*B*). The basaloid cells are relatively monomorphous and exhibit dark-staining nuclei with large prominent nucleoli and scanty, pale, or eosinophilic cytoplasm. A few mitotic figures and single necrotic cells are sometimes noted. Additional findings in some cases include heavy melanin pigmentation, horn cysts, and amyloid deposits.

Treatment is by complete excision.[3]

TRICHODISCOMA Trichodiscoma is a rare tumor that presents as multiple, asymptomatic, small, skin-colored papules situated on the face, arms, trunk, and sometimes the legs.[3,5,6,11] Multiple, trichodiscomas may be inherited in an autosomal dominant fashion in the setting of Birt-Hogg-Dubé syndrome[68] (see above). Recently, the cutaneous lesions in this syndrome (fibrofolliculomas and trichodiscomas) have been interpreted as different developmental stages of one single tumor with sebaceous differentiation, called "mantleoma."

Histopathology Histopathologic examination reveals a well-circumscribed, nonencapsulated, dome-shaped nodule in the dermis consisting of a zone of loose, finely fibrillar connective tissue with bundles of collagen, fibrocytes, and venules. The lesion is encircled by collarettes of infundibular epithelium that are focally continuous with epithelial cords radiating into the stroma. The epithelial cords sometimes contain sebaceous cells. A hair follicle or nerve fibers may be noted at the edge.

Treatment of choice in solitary lesions is by surgical excision. Carbon dioxide laser is useful in removal of multiple lesions. Patients should be screened for other features of Birt-Hogg-Dubé syndrome.

FIGURE 85-16

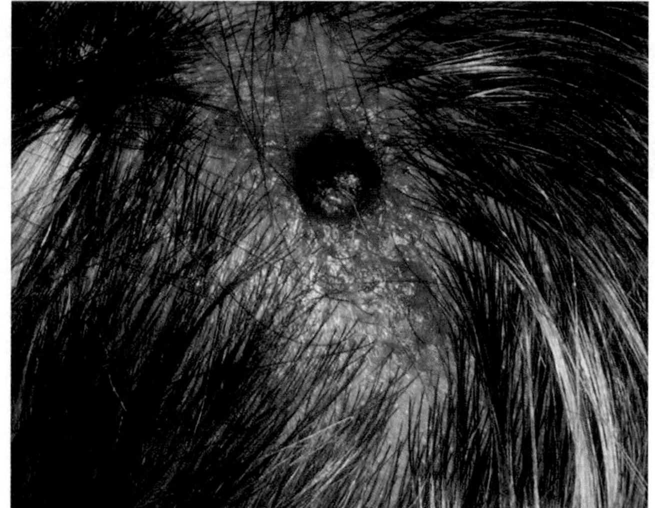

A.

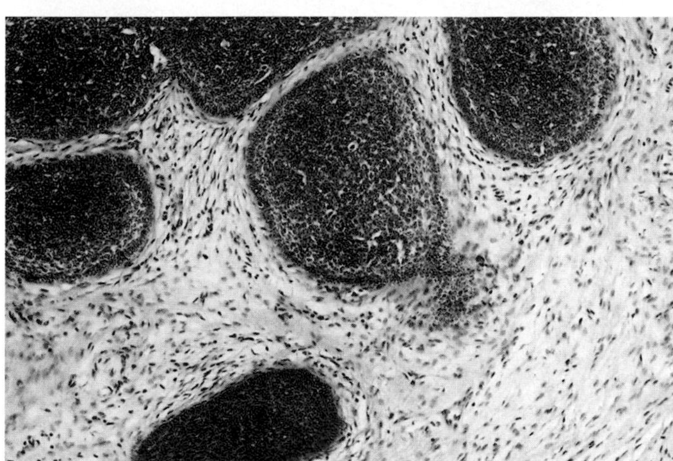

B.

Trichoblastoma. *A.* Pigmented type arising in a nevus sebaceous. *B.* Nodular aggregations of basaloid cells surrounded by abundant fibrous stroma. Note prominent peripheral palisading of nuclei and a focus with a follicular germ and papilla.

TRICHOEPITHELIOMA Trichoepithelioma shows a spectrum of histopathologic features reflecting mainly differentiation toward hair and hair follicle, particularly follicular germs.[3–6,11] These include aggregations of basaloid (follicular germinative) cells arranged in a cribriform or lacelike reticular pattern, conspicuous germs and follicular papillae, small horn cysts, and fibrotic stroma. This neoplasm is therefore best regarded as a distinct variant of trichoblastoma described above.

Three distinctive forms of trichoepitheliomas are recognized, namely solitary, multiple, and desmoplastic.[3] Desmoplastic trichoepithelioma was discussed earlier.

Solitary trichoepithelioma occurs mainly as a small (5 to 8 mm in diameter), skin-colored papule situated on the face, especially around the nose, upper lip, and cheeks of adults.[3–6,11] Occasional lesions develop on the trunk, neck, scalp, and lower extremities.

Multiple trichoepitheliomas present usually in adolescents as numerous, small papules distributed on the face, with predilection for the area around the nasolabial folds, forehead, chin, and preauricular area (Fig. 85-17*A*). A few patients reveal plaques, nodules, or tumors due to coalescing of several lesions. Multiple trichoepitheliomas are mostly transmitted as an autosomal dominant trait in patients with Brooke-Spiegler (epithelioma adenoides cysticum) syndrome. In this syndrome, patients show predisposition for developing multifocal cylindromas, spiradenomas, and milia.[75] Multiple trichoepitheliomas have also rarely been associated with a number of other systemic conditions, including Rombo's syndrome (atrophoderma, milia, hypotrichosis, basal cell carcinomas, and peripheral vasodilatation),[76] systemic lupus erythematosus, and myasthenia gravis.

FIGURE 85-17

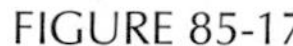

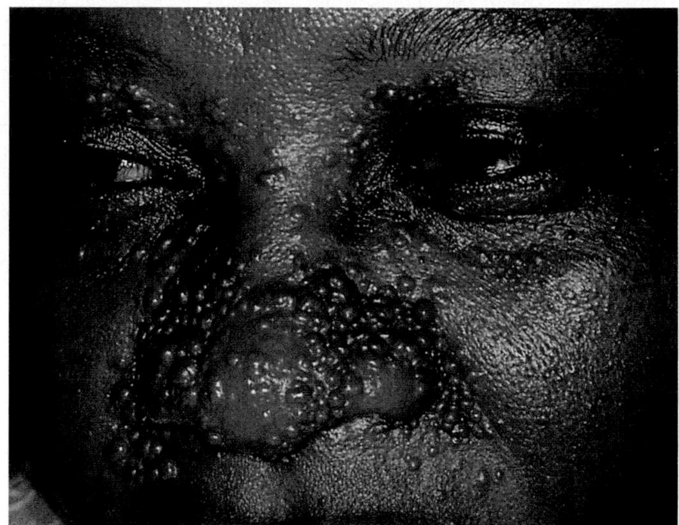

A.

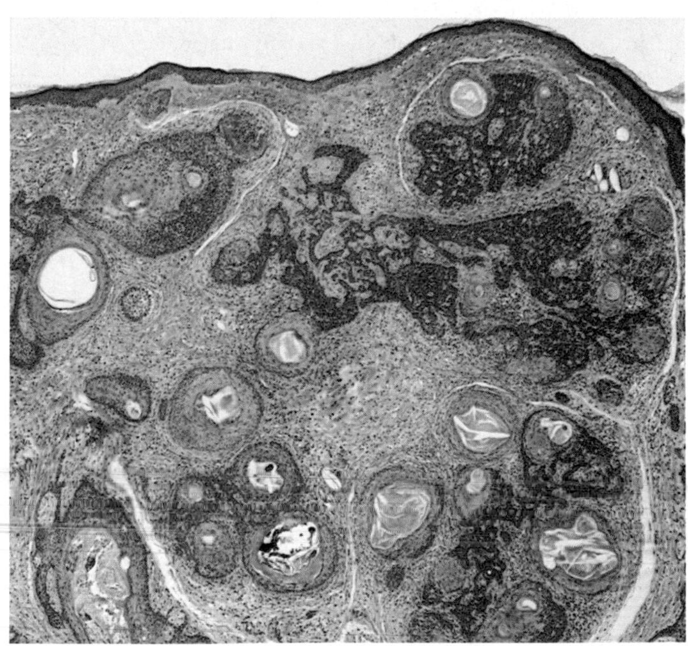

B.

Trichoepithelioma. *A.* Multiple familial type. *B.* Well-circumscribed, multilobular dermal tumor consisting of solid and branching basaloid aggregations admixed with horn cysts, surrounded by abundant fibrous stroma. Note a focal cribriform pattern.

Histopathology There is a dome-shaped, sharply circumscribed lesion composed of aggregations of relatively monomorphic basaloid (germinative) cells in the upper dermis, surrounded by abundant fibrous stroma with intrastromal clefts (Fig. 85-17*B*). The basaloid aggregations are mainly arranged in a cribriform pattern, but may show other architectural patterns, including nodular, racemiform, and retiform. They typically reveal peripheral palisading and several foci with rudimentary follicular papillae and germs. In some lesions, other findings include infundibulocystic structures, shadow cells, sebaceous glands, amyloid, calcification, melanin pigmentation, and mucin deposition. A lymphohistiocytic infiltrate with small foreign-body granulomas is sometimes present.

Surgery is usually effective in removing solitary lesions. However, surgical treatment of multiple trichoepitheliomas is generally disappointing. Alternative therapies have included cryotherapy, electrodesiccation, and carbon dioxide laser.

TRICHOFOLLICULOMA Trichofolliculoma is a rare tumor which presents mainly in adults as a small, solitary, dome-shaped papule or nodule situated on the face, particularly around the nose.[3–6,11] A central, dilated keratin plugged ostium with vellus hair(s) is often present (Fig. 85-18). Trichofolliculoma has been regarded by different authors either as a neoplastic process or as a hamartoma (hair follicle nevus).

Histopathology The lesion is basically centered on one, or less frequently on several contiguous, variably dilated, primary follicles lined by infundibular and isthmus type epithelium and opening to the skin surface. Numerous, smaller, secondary (vellus) follicles bud from the wall of the central follicle in a radial fashion. The central follicle is commonly filled with cornified cells and sometimes contains vellus hairs. The secondary follicles often reveal differentiation toward germinative epithelium or formation of hair. They are surrounded by a prominent fibrous stroma. Individual tumors display variable features of outer root sheath differentiation at the isthmus with tricholemmal cornification and basaloid matrical, as well as sebaceous, differentiation. Sebaceous trichofolliculoma represents a distinctive variant with large sebaceous follicles connecting to the central cavity.

Treatment is by surgical excision.

TRICHOLEMMOMA Tricholemmoma (trichilemmoma) shows mainly differentiation toward the outer root (tricholemmal) sheath of a normal hair follicle at the level of the bulb. Lesions present usually in adults as solitary, small (3 to 8 mm in diameter), asymptomatic, keratotic, or smooth-surfaced papules on the face, particularly around the nose and upper lip.[3–6,11] Some cases arise in association with nevus sebaceus.[74] Multiple facial tricholemmomas represent an important cutaneous marker for Cowden's syndrome, which is discussed in Chap. 184. Patients with Cowden's syndrome show a tendency to develop particular internal malignancies, especially involving the breast, colon and thyroid. A tumor-suppressor gene (designated *PTEN/MMAC1*) has been demonstrated to play a causative role.[9] Recently, based mainly on the wartlike morphology, some authors have proposed tricholemmoma to represent an old viral wart.[3]

FIGURE 85-18

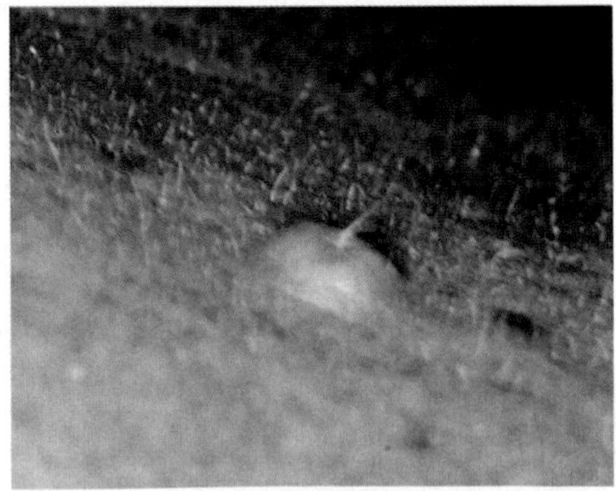

Trichofolliculoma. Papule on the forehead with a hair emanating from its central pore.

Histopathology Lesions show a lobular, folliculocentric, exoendophytic proliferation of polygonal, pale-staining, glycogen-containing squamoid cells. The epidermal surface often reveals parakeratosis with scale crusts, and sometimes a cutaneous horn (tricholemmal horn). The periphery of the lobules is bordered by columnar cells arranged in a palisade. Foci with small squamous eddies are occasionally observed within the center of tumor lobules. A conspicuous basement membrane usually surrounds the lesions. Desmoplastic tricholemmoma represents a special variant with prominently hyalinized or desmoplastic stroma.[77]

Treatment is by surgical excision.

TUMOR OF THE FOLLICULAR INFUNDIBULUM Despite its name, tumor of the follicular infundibulum shows mainly differentiation toward the isthmus of a normal hair follicle, rather than the infundibulum. Lesions present as solitary, small (5 to 10 mm in diameter), asymptomatic, smooth or keratotic papules on the head and neck of middle-aged and elderly individuals.[3,5,11] A small subset of cases occur as multiple lesions (infundibulomatosis, eruptive infundibulomas). Tumors developing in association with Cowden's syndrome or with a preexisting nevus sebaceus have been reported.

Histopathology There is a horizontally oriented, platelike tumor in the upper dermis with an epithelial component showing multifocal connections to the epidermis or hair follicles. The epithelium typically reveals a fenestrated pattern with interconnecting cords and columns. Infundibulocystic structures are focally present. Cells display small, monomorphic nuclei and abundant, pale to pink-staining cytoplasm. The tumors are sometimes surrounded by a collagenous stroma with a network of elastic fibers. Variable areas with single necrotic cells, clear cells, rudimentary papillae and germs, ductal structures, and features of sebaceous differentiation are observed in some cases.

Treatment is by surgical excision.

Malignant Neoplasms

BASAL CELL CARCINOMA WITH FOLLICULAR DIFFERENTIATION

See Chap. 81.

PILOMATRICAL CARCINOMA Pilomatrical carcinoma (matrical carcinoma) is rare tumor that is found in older adults on the head and neck, and occasionally on the trunk.[3–6,11] Clinical appearances are generally not distinctive. Most cases probably develop de novo, but malignant transformation from a benign pilomatricoma has been reported.[72]

Histopathology Histopathologic examination shows irregularly sized and variously shaped cutaneous/subcutaneous epithelial islands of basaloid (matrical and supramatrical) cells with conspicuous foci of shadow cells (Fig. 85-19). The basaloid cells reveal nuclear atypia and mitoses, as well as areas of geographic necrosis. Involvement of vascular lumina, subjacent deep soft tissues, and bone may be observed.

Treatment of choice is surgical excision with adequate margins.[72] Pilomatrical carcinoma is mainly locally aggressive, but distant metastases, especially to lungs, bones, and lymphatics have rarely been reported.

FIGURE 85-19

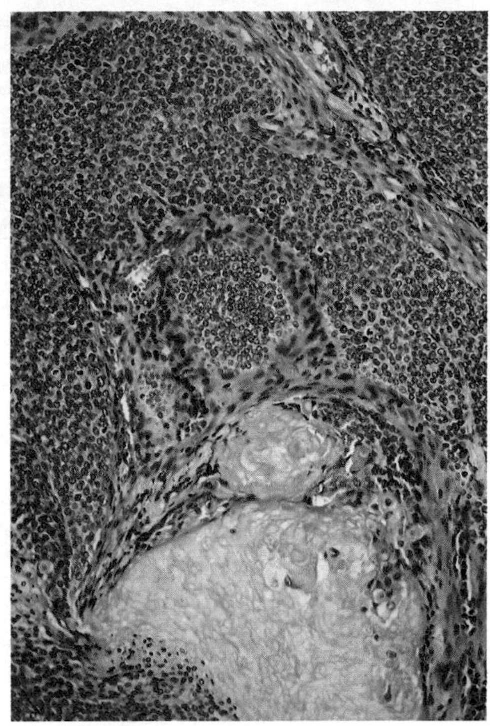

Pilomatrical carcinoma. Irregular aggregations of atypical basaloid cells continuous with an area of cornified material containing shadow cells.

TRICHOLEMMAL CARCINOMA This is an extremely rare tumor that presents mainly in elderly individuals as a solitary, slowly growing, sometimes indurated, papule, plaque, or nodule situated on sun-exposed, hair-bearing areas.[5,11] Lesions are mostly located on the face, scalp, auricular skin, and extremities. They are most frequently initially suspected to be basal cell carcinomas or squamous cell carcinomas.

Histopathology There is a predominantly dermal tumor composed of several epithelial aggregations arranged in various growth patterns including solid, lobular, and trabecular. Focal connections to the epidermis and pilosebaceous structures are noted in some sections. Most lesions show prominent atypia and a high mitotic activity. Epithelial aggregations exhibit, at least focally, features of outer root sheath differentiation, including neoplastic cells with abundant, clear cytoplasm, and focal tricholemmal cornification. Peripheral nuclear palisading may be observed in some tumor nests.

Treatment of choice is surgical excision with adequate margins. The tumor usually behaves in an indolent fashion, but a few patients have shown local recurrences. So far, no cases of distant metastases have been reported.

APPENDAGE TUMORS WITH SEBACEOUS DIFFERENTIATION

Apart from sebaceus hyperplasia, sebaceous tumors appear to be less common and to show less morphologic diversity than other types of appendage tumors. Terminology is still controversial. Benign sebaceous neoplasms were conventionally divided into sebaceous hyperplasia, sebaceous adenoma, and sebaceous epithelioma, and malignant sebaceous neoplasms into basal cell carcinoma with sebaceous differentiation and sebaceous carcinoma.[5,6] Recently, the existence of sebaceous epithelioma as a distinctive neoplasm was challenged.[2] The term *sebaceoma* has been recommended for the most common benign neoplasm with sebaceous differentiation, whose malignant counterpart is sebaceous carcinoma. Furthermore, it has been proposed that sebaceous adenoma represents a superficial sebaceous carcinoma rather than a benign neoplasm. This section adopts this classification.

Cyst

STEATOCYSTOMA
See Chap. 84.

Hamartomas

FOLLICULOSEBACEOUS CYSTIC HAMARTOMA Folliculosebaceous cystic hamartoma is a cutaneous hamartoma that is comprised of follicular, sebaceous, and mesenchymal elements. Lesions present as solitary, long-standing, asymptomatic papules or nodules measuring 0.5 to 2 cm or more in diameter, situated on the head and neck.[11,78] The face, especially the region around the nose, is mainly involved. Some lesions show a slightly depressed area with a centrally located crateriform pore.

Histopathology A dome-shaped nodule with a mature infundibular structure to which numerous rudimentary hair follicles and/or sebaceous units are attached is observed. The follicular structure is typically surrounded by abundant fibrous and elastic tissue. Adipocytes, nerves, and blood vessels are frequently found within the stroma.

Treatment is by simple surgical excision.

FORDYCE'S SPOTS (FORDYCE'S DISEASE) AND MONTGOMERY'S TUBERCLES Fordyce's spots and Montgomery's tubercles represent the occurrence of sebaceous glands on the lips and buccal mucosa, and on breast areola, respectively.[2] Despite the ectopic locations, both conditions reveal sebaceous glands with a "normal" histopathologic appearance and are therefore best regarded as hamartomas.

Clinically, Fordyce's spots present as tiny white or yellowish, focally grouped papules on the lip near the vermilion or on a buccal mucosa of adults. Rare lesions develop on the genital mucosa. Montgomery's tubercles arise as tiny papules distributed in a circle near the periphery of the breast areola of adult women. They have not been described in men.

Histopathology Fordyce's spots show similar features to those in Montgomery's tubercles. They consist of a single sebaceous gland or lobule located in the upper submucosa or dermis, respectively. Some lesions reveal no accompanying sebaceous duct.

NEVUS SEBACEUS
See Chap. 84.

Hyperplasia

SEBACEOUS HYPERPLASIA AND RHINOPHYMA Sebaceous hyperplasia presents commonly as solitary or multiple, small (less than 3 mm in diameter), yellowish, papules on the face, particularly on the forehead of middle-aged individuals.[2,4–6,11] Lesions often reveal a central dell. Males are more commonly affected than females. Clinically, lesions are often suspected to be basal cell carcinomas. Unusual presentations of sebaceous hyperplasia include linear and zosteriform lesions, giant and diffuse tumors, and lesions confined to the areola or genital (vulva) region. Rare cases show a familial pattern.

Rhinophyma is currently widely considered to represent a special form of sebaceous hyperplasia[2] and is discussed in Chap. 74.

Histopathology Both sebaceous hyperplasia and rhinophyma reveal large mature sebaceous lobules clustered around discrete, often dilated, infundibula and located mainly in the upper dermis. The infundibulum is sometimes filled with debris and bacteria, and may contain a vellus hair. In addition, rhinophyma often reveals striking telangiectases in the upper dermis and features of folliculitis as well as granulomatous perifolliculitis. Old rhinophyma lesions are characterized by severe dermal fibrosis and scarring.

Treatment of choice is surgical excision. However, a variety of treatment options have previously been tried, including oral isotretinoin, electrodesiccation, CO_2 laser surgery, cryosurgery, and shave excision with curettage.

Benign Neoplasms

MANTLEOMA Mantleoma (see also fibrofolliculoma discussed earlier) is a recently described benign tumor that shows differentiation toward the sebaceous mantle.[3] The sebaceous mantle is a well-recognized, but poorly documented, part of the sebaceous gland cycle. In the resting phase, the sebaceous mantle represents cords of undifferentiated cells that project from the infundibulum of a hair follicle and droop down aside the follicle. Cyclically, vacuolated sebocytes appear at the terminus of these cords, singly, then in groups, and finally as fully developed sebaceous lobules and glands. Sebaceous glands probably involute to become undifferentiated mantles.

Mantleomas occur either as solitary or as multiple tumors.[3,11] Solitary mantleomas appear to be sporadic. They present as small papules on the face, frequently mimicking basal cell carcinomas or dermal nevi. As far as multiple mantleomas are concerned, it was recently proposed that both fibrofolliculomas and trichodiscomas arising in patients with Birt-Hogg-Dubé syndrome actually represent different developmental stages of mantleoma. Multiple mantleomas in these patients occur as numerous, small papules located mainly on the head and neck, as well as the trunk.

Histopathology Mantleomas show various histopathologic features. Some lesions consist only of cords and columns of undifferentiated epithelial cells that radiate from an infundibulum. Other lesions reveal interconnected cords with sebocytes and sebaceous ductal structures.

Treatment of solitary lesions is by surgical excision. Management of multiple mantleomas is that of multiple fibrofolliculomas and trichodiscomas.

RETICULATED ACANTHOMA See the earlier section on tumors with apocrine differentiation.

SEBACEOMA Sebaceoma represents the most common benign neoplasm with sebaceous differentiation. It presents usually as a solitary, slowly growing, asymptomatic, yellowish papule or small nodule on the face and scalp of older individuals[2,75] (Fig. 85-20*A*). Women appear to be more commonly affected than men. Occasional tumors arise in association with nevus sebaceus or seborrheic keratosis.

Histopathology Lesions are centered in the dermis and consist of relatively symmetric, well-circumscribed, and smoothly bordered lobular aggregations of epithelial cells with focal connections to preexisting infundibula.[2,79] Involvement of the subcutis is observed in some cases. Epithelial aggregations are composed of basaloid cells with relatively monomorphous nuclei, admixed with variable foci of discernible sebocytes and sebaceous ductal structures (Fig. 85-20*B*). Some cases reveal entirely immature sebocytes, that is, cells with small monomorphous nuclei and scant cytoplasm, but without vacuoles. Other cases display a variable mixture of immature and mature sebocytes with highly vacuolated abundant cytoplasm and nuclei exhibiting scalloped borders. Scattered mitoses are observed in some cases. Additional features may include a "ripple-like" pattern, and cystic as well as ductlike structures containing sebaceous secretion.

Treatment of choice is simple surgical excision. Electrodesiccation, curettage, and cryotherapy are effective in some cases.

FIGURE 85-20

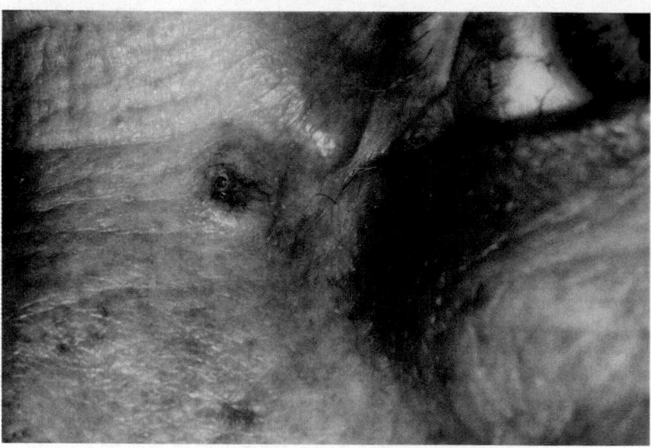

A.

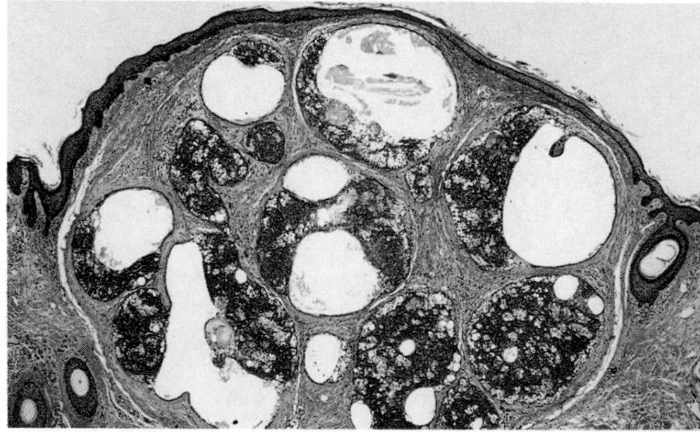

B.

Sebaceoma. *A.* Yellowish nodule near the inner canthus of the eye. *B.* Well-circumscribed tumor composed of basaloid aggregations, admixed with sebocytes and ductal, as well as cystic structures.

Malignant Neoplasms

SEBACEOUS CARCINOMA AND NEOPLASMS IN MUIR-TORRE SYNDROME Sebaceous carcinoma represents a spectrum of rare malignant appendage tumors with sebaceous differentiation and with a potential for aggressive behavior.[2,4–6,11,79] They have traditionally been divided into ocular and extraocular types. Of these, the ocular type is the commonest.

Ocular type of sebaceous carcinoma usually presents in older adults as a small, solitary, papule or nodule on the eyelid, particularly around the Meibomian glands and glands of Zeiss of the upper eyelid.[2] Women are more commonly affected than men. Patients may give a history of radiation. Lesions are often suspected to be chalazions. Rare cases have been observed in young individuals infected with human immunodeficiency virus.

Extraocular sebaceous carcinoma occurs mostly as a yellowish, firm, often ulcerated nodule on the head and neck of elderly individuals. Other anatomic sites, such as the foot and genital regions (labia and penis), may occasionally be involved. Lesions often mimic pyogenic granuloma, hemangioma, or squamous cell carcinoma.

Sebaceous carcinoma represents an important cutaneous marker of Muir-Torre syndrome[80] (see Chap. 184). In this syndrome, the tumors occur as single or multiple, skin-colored, yellowish or reddish-brown, sometimes ulcerated papules with the appearance of sebaceus hyperplasia and nodules, situated commonly on the face. They may coexist with keratoacanthomas and/or epidermal cysts. There is still controversy regarding the nature of sebaceous tumors arising in patients with Muir-Torre syndrome. Previous examples have mostly been considered as benign neoplasms ("sebaceous adenomas" or sebaceomas) and less commonly as sebaceous carcinomas. Based mainly on morphology, some authors recently proposed that the vast majority of sebaceous tumors arising in these patients are, in fact, sebaceous carcinomas.[79]

Histopathology Sebaceous carcinoma is characterized by an asymmetric lesion centered in the dermis, and consisting of variously sized and irregularly shaped aggregations of neoplastic cells.[2,79] Involvement of the subcutaneous tissue and/or underlying muscle is observed in some cases. Neoplasms may be relatively well-differentiated with prominent sebaceous lobules and/or sebaceous ductal structures or show undifferentiated features with neither readily discernible cytoplasmic vacuoles nor ductal differentiation. The nuclei of the neoplastic cells, especially along the periphery of the tumor nests tend to be crowded and pleomorphic, and may exhibit marked atypia, as well as increased mitotic figures. Sections often reveal areas with geographic necrosis. A peculiar variant with cystic features may be difficult to differentiate from sebaceoma.

Treatment of choice is surgical excision with adequate margins. Radiation therapy may be effective in some patients with eyelid neoplasms. Up to one-third of patients with ocular type of sebaceous carcinoma show lymph node metastases, particularly to the preauricular and cervical nodes, and the 5-year mortality rate is about 20 percent. Histopathologic features suggestive of a poor prognosis include the presence of vascular and lymphatic invasion, orbital extension, poor differentiation, an infiltrative growth pattern, and large tumor size. In contrast to ocular tumors, extraocular sebaceous carcinoma very rarely reveals nodal or visceral metastases. Sebaceous carcinomas arising in Muir-Torre syndrome, like visceral malignancies in these patients, also seem to be less aggressive than their ocular counterpart, which is unassociated with the syndrome.[80]

REFERENCES

1. Requena L et al: *Neoplasms with Apocrine Differentiation.* Philadelphia, Lippincott-Raven, Ardor Scribendi, 1997
2. Steffen C, Ackerman AB: *Neoplasms with Sebaceous Differentiation.* Philadelphia, Lea & Febiger, 1994
3. Ackerman AB et al: *Neoplasms with Follicular Differentiation.* New York Ardor Scribendi, 2001
4. Hurt MA, Santa Cruz DJ: Adnexal tumors, in *Diagnostic Histopathology of Tumors*, 2d ed, edited by CDM Fletcher. Edinburgh, Churchill Livingstone, 2000, p 1378
5. Wick MR, Swanson PE: *Cutaneous Adnexal Tumors: A Guide to Pathologic Diagnosis.* Chicago, ASCP Press, 1991
6. Maize JC et al: Adnexal tumors, in *Cutaneous Pathology*, edited by JC Maize. Philadelphia, Churchill-Livingstone, 1998, p 483
7. Biernat W et al: p53 Mutations in sweat gland carcinomas. *Int J Cancer* **76**:317, 1998
8. Aszterbaum M et al: Ultraviolet and ionizing radiation enhance the growth of BCCs and trichoblastomas in patched heterozygous knockout mice. *Nat Med* **5**:1285, 1999
9. Stambolic V et al: Negative regulation of PKB/Akt-dependent cell survival by the tumor suppressor PTEN. *Cell* **95**:29, 1998
10. Kruse R et al: Is the mismatch repair deficient type of Muir-Torre syndrome confined to mutations in the hMSH2 gene? *Hum Genet* **98**:747, 1996
11. Weedon D: Tumors of cutaneous appendages, in *Skin Pathology.* New York, Churchill-Livingstone, 1997, p 713
12. Vakilzadeh F et al: Fokale dermale Hypoplasie mit apokrinen Naevi und streifenfoermiger Anomalie der Knochen. *Arch Dermatol Res* **256**:189, 1976
13. Cribier B et al: Tumors arising in nevus sebaceus: A study of 596 cases. *J Am Acad Dermatol* **42**:263, 2000
14. Civatte J et al: Adenomatose érosive sur mamelon surnuméraire. *Ann Dermatol Venereol* **104**:777, 1977
15. Wilkinson S et al: Fibroadenoma of the breast: A follow-up of conservative management. *Br J Surg* **76**:390, 1989
16. Santa Cruz DJ et al: Hidradenoma papilliferum of the eyelid. *Arch Dermatol* **117**:55, 1981
17. Shenoy YMV: Malignant perianal papillary hidradenoma. *Arch Dermatol* **83**:965, 1961
18. Hirsch P, Helwig EB: Chondroid syringoma. Mixed tumor of the skin, salivary gland type. *Arch Dermatol* **84**:835, 1961
19. Requena L et al: Apocrine type of cutaneous mixed tumor with follicular and sebaceous differentiation. *Am J Dermatopathol* **14**:186, 1992
20. Cooper PH et al: Primary cutaneous adenoid cystic carcinoma. *Arch Dermatol* **120**:774, 1984
21. Domingo J, Helwig EB: Malignant neoplasms associated with nevus sebaceus of Jadassohn. *J Am Acad Dermatol* **1**:545, 1979
22. Warkel RL: Selected apocrine neoplasms. *J Cutan Pathol* **11**:437, 1984
23. Urso C et al: Histologic spectrum of carcinomas with eccrine ductal differentiation (sweat-gland ductal carcinomas). *Am J Dermatopathol* **15**:435, 1993
24. Bannatyne P et al: Vulvar adenosquamous carcinoma arising in a hidradenoma papilliferum with rapidly fatal outcome: Case report. *Gynecol Oncol* **35**:395, 1989
25. Weilburg RD et al: Paget's disease of the vulva associated with adenocarcinoma developing in a hidradenoma papilliferum. *Am J Obstet Gynecol* **98**:294, 1967
26. Metzler G et al: Malignant chondroid syringoma: Immunohistopathology. *Am J Dermatopathol* **18**:83, 1996
27. Santa Cruz DJ: Sweat gland carcinomas: A comprehensive review. *Semin Diagn Pathol* **4**:38, 1987
28. Wright JD, Font RL: Mucinous sweat gland adenocarcinoma of eyelid: A clinicopathologic study of 21cases with histochemical and electron microscopic observations. *Cancer* **44**:1757, 1979
29. Jakobiec FA et al: Primary infiltrating signet ring carcinoma of the eyelids. *Ophthalmology* **90**:291, 1983
30. Ishida-Yamamoto A et al: Syringocystadenocarcinoma papilliferum: Case report and immunohistochemical comparison with its benign counterpart. *J Am Acad Dermatol* **45**:755, 2001
31. Numata M et al: Syringadenocarcinoma papilliferum. *J Cutan Pathol* **12**:3, 1985
32. Abenoza P, Ackerman AB: *Neoplasms with Eccrine Differentiation.* Philadelphia, Lea & Febiger, 1990
33. Leung CS et al: Porokeratotic eccrine ostial and dermal duct naevus with dermatomal trunk involvement: Literature review and report on the efficacy of laser treatment. *Br J Dermatol* **138**:684, 1998
34. Morrell DS et al: Eccrine angiomatous hamartoma: A report of symmetric and painful lesions of the wrists. *Pediatr Dermatol* **18**:117, 2001
35. Trotter MJ et al: Mucinous syringometaplasia: A case report and review of the literature. *Clin Exp Dermatol* **20**:42, 1995
36. Tannous Z et al: Syringolymphoid hyperplasia and follicular mucinosis in a patient with cutaneous T-cell lymphoma. *J Am Acad Dermatol* **41**:303, 1999
37. Biggs PJ et al: The cylindromatosis gene (cyld1) on chromosome 16q may be the only tumour-suppressor gene involved in the development of cylindromas. *Oncogene* **12**:1375, 1996
38. Galadari E et al: Malignant transformation of eccrine tumors. *J Cutan Pathol* **14**:15, 1987
39. Mehregan AH et al: Eccrine syringofibroadenoma (Mascaro). Report of two cases. *J Am Acad Dermatol* **13**:433, 1985
40. Hunt SJ et al: Giant eccrine acrospiroma. *J Am Acad Dermatol* **23**:663, 1990
41. Hernandez-Perez E, Cestoni-Parducci R: Nodular hidradenoma and hidradenocarcinoma. A 10-year review. *J Am Acad Dermatol* **12**:15, 1985
42. Mambo NC: Eccrine spiradenoma: Clinical and pathologic study of 49 tumors. *J Cutan Pathol* **10**:312, 1983
43. Frazier CC et al: The treatment of eruptive syringomas in an African American patient with a combination of trichloroacetic acid and CO_2 laser destruction. *Dermatol Surg* **27**:489, 2001

44. Rulon DB, Helwig EB: Papillary eccrine adenoma. *Arch Dermatol* **113**:596, 1977
45. Kao GF et al: Aggressive digital papillary adenoma and adenocarcinoma. A clinicopathological study of 57 patients, with histochemical, immunopathological, and ultrastructural observations. *J Cutan Pathol* **14**:129, 1987
46. Gerretsen AL et al: Cutaneous cylindroma with malignant transformation. *Cancer* **72**:1618, 1993
47. Carroll P et al: Metastatic microcystic adnexal carcinoma in an immunocompromised patient. *Dermatol Surg* **26**:531, 2000
48. Suster S, Wong TY: Polymorphous sweat gland carcinoma. *Histopathology* **25**:31, 1994
49. Snow SN, Reizner GT: Eccrine porocarcinoma of the face. *J Am Acad Dermatol* **27**:306, 1992
50. Robson A et al: Eccrine porocarcinoma (malignant eccrine poroma): A clinicopathologic study of 69 cases. *Am J Surg Pathol* **25**:710, 2001
51. Fernandez-Acenero MJ et al: Malignant spiradenoma: Report of two cases and literature review. *J Am Acad Dermatol* **44**:395, 2001
52. Granter SR et al: Malignant eccrine spiradenoma (spiradenocarcinoma): A clinicopathologic study of 12 cases. *Am J Dermatopathol* **22**:97, 2000
53. Weedon D: Cysts and sinuses, in *Skin Pathology*. New York, Churchill-Livingstone, 1997, p 425
54. Brownstein MH: Hybrid cyst: A combined epidermoid and trichilemmal cyst. *J Am Acad Dermatol* **9**:872, 1983
55. Barr RJ et al: Cutaneous keratocysts of nevoid basal cell carcinoma syndrome. *J Am Acad Dermatol* **14**:572, 1986
56. Requena CL, Sanchez Yus E: Pigmented follicular cyst. *J Am Acad Dermatol* **21**:1073, 1989
57. Leppard BJ et al: Hereditary trichilemmal cysts. Hereditary pilar cysts. *Clin Exp Dermatol* **2**:23, 1977
58. Kose O et al: Anhidrotic ectodermal dysplasia with eruptive vellus hair cysts. *Int J Dermatol* **40**:401, 2001
59. Kageyama N, Tope WD: Treatment of multiple eruptive hair cysts with erbium: YAG laser. *Dermatol Surg* **25**:819, 1999
60. Shimizu H et al: A case of generalized hair follicle hamartoma associated with diffuse sclerosis of the face. *Br J Dermatol* **143**:1103, 2001
61. Brownstein MH: Basaloid follicular hamartoma: Solitary and multiple types. *J Am Acad Dermatol* **27**:237, 1992
62. Davis DA, Cohen PR: Hair follicle nevus: case report and review of the literature. *Pediatr Dermatol* **13**:135, 1996
63. Headington JT: Tumors of the hair follicle. A review. *Am J Pathol* **85**:479, 1976
64. Aloi FG et al: Unilateral linear basal cell nevus associated with diffuse osteoma cutis, unilateral anodontia, and abnormal bone mineralization. *J Am Acad Dermatol* **20**:973, 1989
65. Sangueza OP, Requena L: Neurofollicular hamartoma. A new histogenetic interpretation. *Am J Dermatopathol* **16**:150, 1994
66. Mehregan A, Pinkus H: Life history of organoid nevi: Special references to nevus sebaceus of Jadassohn. *Arch Dermatol* **91**:574, 1965
67. Steffen C: Winer's dilated pore: the infundibuloma. *Am J Dermatopathol* **23**:246, 2001
68. Toro JR et al: Birt-Hogg-Dubé syndrome: A novel marker of kidney neoplasia. *Arch Dermatol* **135**:1195, 1999
69. Santa Cruz DJ et al: Cutaneous lymphadenoma. *Am J Surg Pathol* **15**:101, 1991
70. Smolle J, Kerl H: Das "pilar sheath acanthoma": Ein gutartiges follikulaeres Hamartom. Dermatologica **167**:335, 1983
71. Kaddu S et al: Morphological stages of pilomatricoma. *Am J Dermatopathol* **18**:333, 1996
72. Sassmannshausen J, Chaffins M: Pilomatrix carcinoma: A report of a case arising from a previously excised pilomatrixoma and a review of the literature. *J Am Acad Dermatol* **44**:358, 2001
73. Headington JT: Differentiating neoplasms of hair germ. *J Clin Pathol* **23**:464, 1970
74. Kaddu S et al: Basaloid neoplasms in nevus sebaceus. *J Cutan Pathol* **27**:327, 2000
75. Weyers W et al: Spiradenomas in Brooke-Spiegler syndrome. *Am J Dermatopathol* **15**:156, 1993
76. Ashinoff R et al: Rombo syndrome: A second case report and review. *J Am Acad Dermatol* **28**:1011, 1993
77. Hunt SJ et al: Desmoplastic trichilemmoma: Histologic variant resembling invasive carcinoma. *J Cutan Pathol* **17**:45, 1990
78. Templeton SF: Folliculosebaceous cystic hamartoma: A clinical pathologic study. *J Am Acad Dermatol* **34**:77, 1996
79. Ackerman AB et al: Sebaceoma versus sebaceous carcinoma, in *Differential Diagnosis in Dermatopathology,* edited by AB Ackerman. Philadelphia, Ardor Scribendi, 2001, p 134
80. Schwartz RA, Torre DP: The Muir-Torre syndrome: A 25-year retrospect. *J Am Acad Dermatol* **33**:90, 1995

CHAPTER 86

Helmut Kerl
Rainer Hofmann-Wellenhof

Cutaneous Neuroendocrine Carcinoma: Merkel Cell Carcinoma

In 1875, Friedrich S. Merkel (1845–1919) discovered unusual clear-staining cells at the dermal–epidermal junction and in the basal epidermis that were intimately associated with myelinated nerve fibers. He named these previously undescribed cells, which later became known as Merkel cells, "Tastzellen" (touch cells).

In 1972, Toker[1] reported five cases of skin neoplasms with a prominent "trabecular" architectural pattern. Subsequent reports[2] pointed out that the cells of trabecular carcinomas displayed striking ultrastructural similarities to the Merkel cell. Further immunocytochemical and biochemical investigations indicated that this group of skin carcinomas expressed features of neuroendocrine and epithelial differentiation[3–5] and the term *cutaneous neuroendocrine carcinoma* (neuroendocrine skin carcinoma) was proposed.[6]

In recent years, numerous publications dealing with cutaneous neuroendocrine carcinomas have appeared under various designations.

FIGURE 86-1

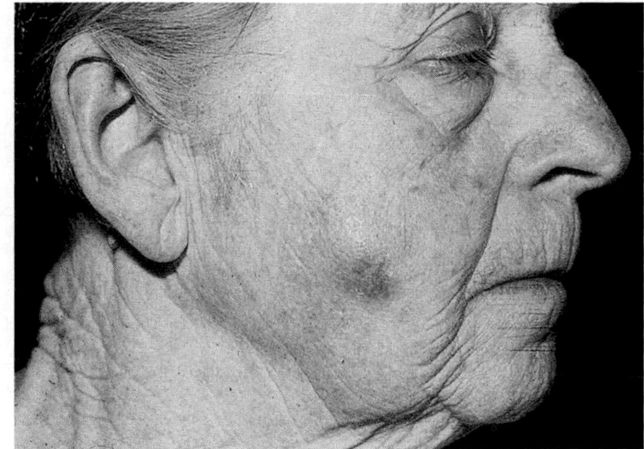

A.

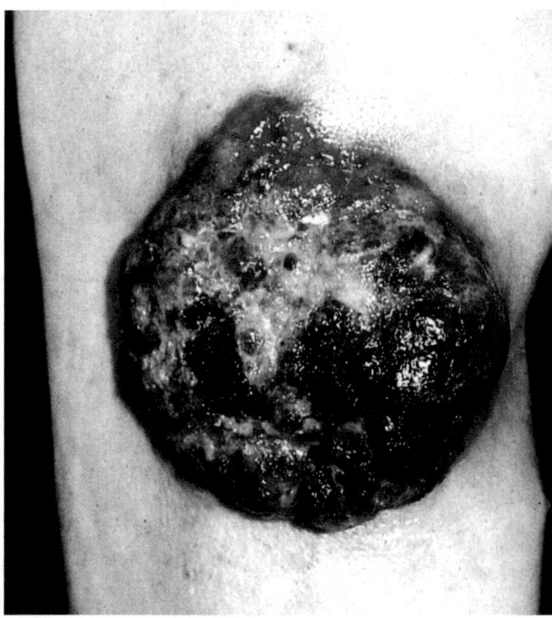

B.

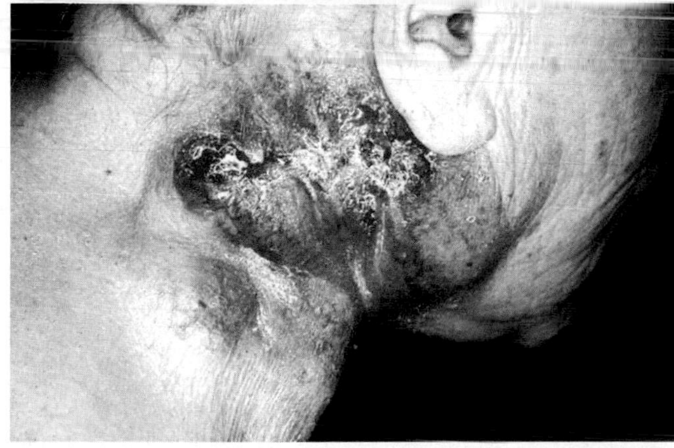

C.

Clinical features of cutaneous neuroendocrine carcinoma. *A.* Erythematous nodule on the cheek. *B.* Ulcerated tumor on the right upper arm. *C.* Large ulcerated masses with involvement of lymph nodes on the neck.

Cases termed *primary neuroepithelial tumor of the skin, primary small cell carcinoma of the skin, primary cutaneous carcinoid, cutaneous APUD-oma,* and *adult neuroblastoma* seem to represent cutaneous neuroendocrine carcinomas.

CLINICAL FEATURES

More than 50 percent of cutaneous neuroendocrine carcinomas arise in the head (face) and neck region, followed by the extremities, buttocks, and trunk. The patients range in age from 15 to 97 years. Most patients, however, are in their seventh or eighth decade, with an average of 65 years at diagnosis. The sex distribution is approximately equal.[5,7–9]

Clinically, pink, bluish-red, or reddish-brown cutaneous-subcutaneous nodules are observed. The overlying skin is usually intact (Fig. 86-1*A*). The tumors range in size from 0.5 to 5 cm, but sometimes large ulcerated masses are found (Fig. 86-1*B* and *C*). The majority of cutaneous neuroendocrine carcinomas are solitary. In a few reports multifocal or even disseminated lesions have been described. The neoplasms grow rapidly within 1 year, but there may be a longer duration of the lesions before diagnosis.

The association of cutaneous neuroendocrine carcinoma with squamous cell carcinoma, adnexal neoplasms, basal cell carcinoma, actinic keratosis, and Bowen's disease in the same anatomic area has been documented.[5]

A relationship between cutaneous neuroendocrine carcinoma and concomitant clinical endocrinopathies [increased levels of adrenocorticotropic hormone (ACTH) and calcitonin in the serum] has been found, but this is extremely rare. The tumors have also been described in young patients with congenital ectodermal dysplasia, Cowden's disease, and in patients with B cell lymphoma.[7,9] The cause of cutaneous neuroendocrine tumors is still unknown. Some authors postulate that UV radiation may lead to the development of these tumors. Two cases developed in an area of erythema ab igne, and one case occurred in an irradiation site.[8,9] Merkel cell carcinomas have been found to have an increased incidence among immunosuppressed patients.[10,11]

HISTOLOGIC FEATURES

The histologic features of cutaneous neuroendocrine carcinomas are variable.[2,12] Two main architectural patterns are found: (1) a nodular and/or diffuse pattern mimicking malignant lymphoma (Fig. 86-2); (2) sheets of cells forming nests, cords, and trabeculae (Fig. 86-3). Frequently, a mixed pattern with features of both the nodular/diffuse and trabecular forms is observed. The epidermis is usually spared. Rarely, epidermotropism with pagetoid growth of tumor cells can be present. The tumors involve the dermis and extend into the subcutaneous fat.

The neoplastic cells are uniform in size with round or oval nuclei and have evenly dispersed chromatin, small nucleoli, and sharply defined nuclear membranes. Cytoplasm is scanty and amphophilic (Fig. 86-4). The cells show various degrees of intercellular adhesion. Necrotic areas, scattered pyknotic nuclei, and numerous mitotic figures are frequently evident. Occasionally, pseudorosettes or Homer-Wright rosettes (Fig. 86-5*A*), myxoid stroma, spindle cell proliferation, eccrine differentiation, or the collision of cutaneous neuroendocrine and squamous-

FIGURE 86-2

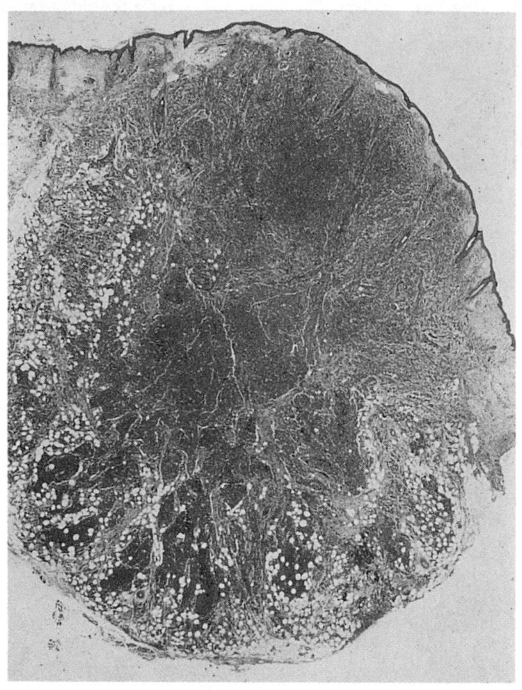

Histologic features of cutaneous neuroendocrine carcinoma. The scanning magnification illustrates a nodule with deep extension into the subcutaneous fat (H&E).

cell carcinoma (Fig. 86-5*B*) are found.[5] A dense lymphocytic infiltrate can also often be observed. Some authors described the Azzopardi phenomenon (DNA-deposition in intratumoral blood vessels) in cutaneous neuroendocrine carcinoma.[13] Gould et al.[6] have recognized three

FIGURE 86-3

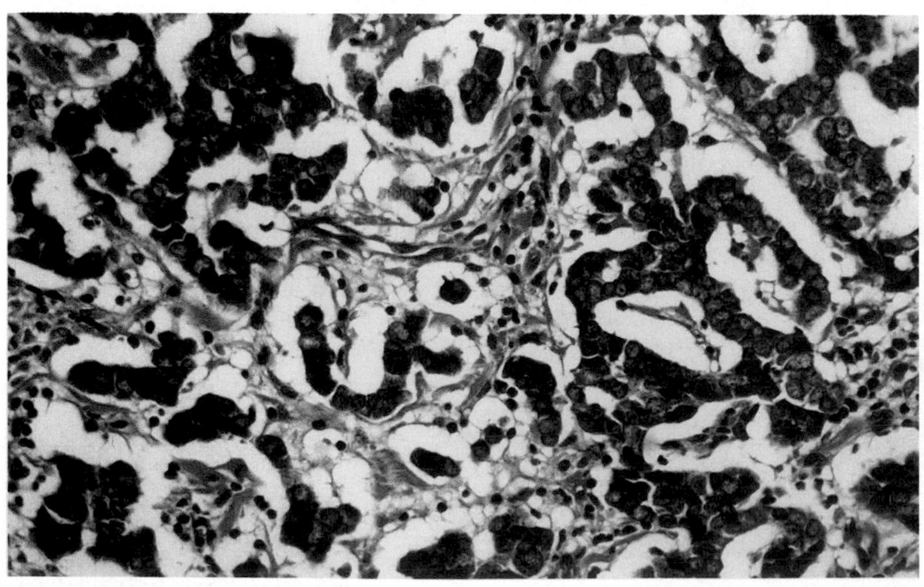

Cutaneous neuroendocrine carcinoma. Trabecular pattern (H&E).

FIGURE 86-4

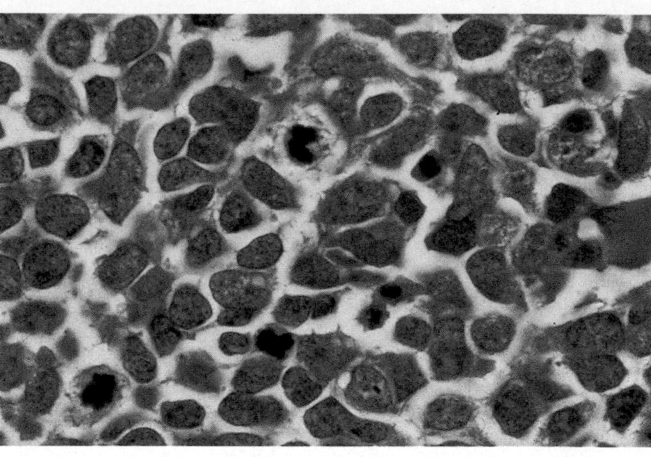

Cutaneous neuroendocrine carcinoma. Cytomorphologic details. Loosely cohesive monomorphic cells with frequently round nuclei and a narrow cytoplasm. Note the scattered pyknotic nuclei and mitotic figures (H&E).

variants of cutaneous neuroendocrine carcinoma: a trabecular, an intermediate, and a small cell type that mimics oat-cell carcinoma of the lung at other sites.

ULTRASTRUCTURAL FEATURES

Electron microscopy plays a key role in the recognition of cutaneous neuroendocrine carcinoma.[2,6,14] The tumor cells exhibit variable numbers of peripherally arranged, membrane-bound, dense-core neurosecretory granules (Fig. 86-6) measuring 80 to 150 nm in diameter. The neurosecretory granules are frequently concentrated in cytoplasmic processes. Further typical ultrastructural features are bundles in concentric configuration or bundles of 10-nm intermediate-sized filaments in juxtanuclear location (fibrous bodies). Intercellular junctions resembling primitive desmosomes or adherent-type junctions are occasionally present.

IMMUNOHISTOLOGIC, BIOCHEMICAL, AND MOLECULAR FEATURES

Neuron-specific enolase is the most constant marker found in cutaneous neuroendocrine carcinoma. The tumor cells have epithelial and neural properties because coexpression of cytokeratin filaments (simple epithelial cytokeratins 8, 18, 19, and 20) and neurofilaments (neurofilament L- and M-polypeptides) can be observed[3–6] (Fig. 86-7). The characteristic staining pattern displays a ringlike appearance or paranuclear discoid, plaque- and ball-like profiles that correlate well with the electron microscopically detectable perinuclear accumulations of intermediate-sized filaments. Further

FIGURE 86-5

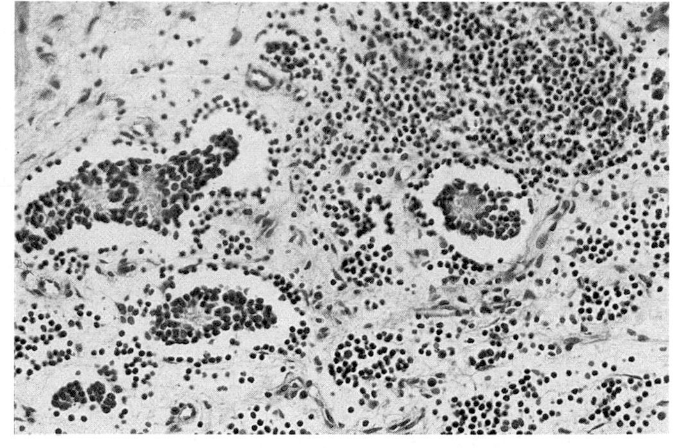

A.

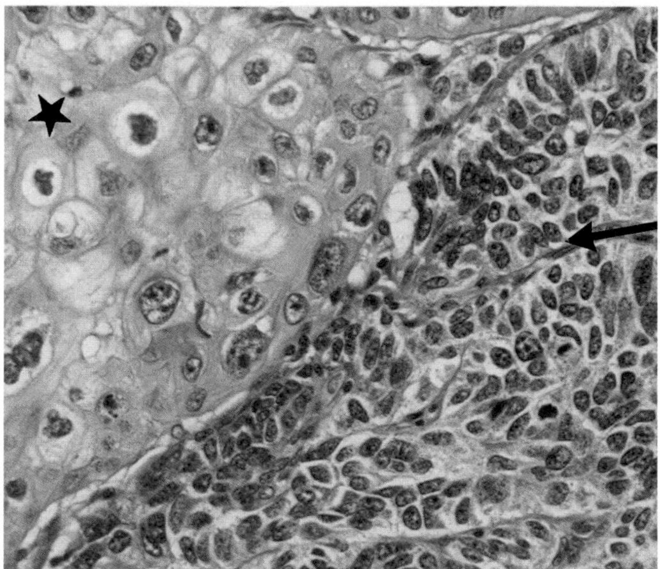

B.

A. Cutaneous neuroendocrine carcinoma. Area of a tumor containing Homer-Wright neural rosettes with central fibrillary cores (H&E). *B.* Coexistence of cutaneous neuroendocrine carcinoma (*arrow*) and squamous-cell carcinoma (*star*) (H&E).

evidence for epithelial differentiation of cutaneous neuroendocrine carcinomas is represented by positive reactions for epithelial membrane antigen and desmoplakin. Chromogranin A/B, synaptophysin, and peripherin, which are very important markers for the diagnosis of neuroendocrine tumors, are also present in cutaneous neuroendocrine carcinomas.[5] The tumors can contain several neuropeptides including calcitonin, bombesin, gastrin, met-enkephalin, substance P, ACTH, vasoactive intestinal polypeptide, neural cell adhesion molecule, and protein gene product 9.5. The expression of these substances is, however, inconstant. S-100 protein, glial fibrillary acidic protein, actin, and vimentin are usually not detectable in cutaneous neuroendocrine carcinomas.[12]

The bcl-2 protein, which may assume oncogenic function by blocking apoptosis, is expressed in cutaneous neuroendocrine tumors, whereas the p53 protein and the cell adhesion protein CD44 are only found in some cases.[15–18]

Cytogenetic analysis of neuroendocrine tumors revealed changes in chromosome 1 most frequently. Genes located on chromosomes 3, 6, 18, and 20 may also play an important role in the development of these tumors.[19]

The diagnosis of cutaneous neuroendocrine carcinoma can be made reliably by the immunohistologic demonstration of neuron-specific enolase, chromogranin A, and the characteristic paranuclear globular coexpression of the simple epithelial cytokeratins and neurofilament proteins.

DIFFERENTIAL DIAGNOSIS

Several primary and metastatic neoplasms should be considered in the differential diagnosis of cutaneous neuroendocrine carcinomas, namely, amelanotic malignant melanoma, malignant lymphoma (especially lymphoblastic type), neuroblastoma, Ewing's sarcoma, peripheral neuroepithelioma, adnexal neoplasms, lymphoepithelioma-like carcinoma of the skin, and skin metastases. Malignant melanoma is S-100– and HMB-45–positive, whereas malignant lymphomas react positively with common leukocyte antigen. Neuroblastomas are neurofilament- and neuron-specific enolase-positive, but, in contrast to cutaneous neuroendocrine carcinoma, they are keratin-negative. Adnexal neoplasms reveal keratin positivity and are neurofilament- and neuron-specific enolase-negative. Problems arise in the differential diagnosis of skin metastases from neuroendocrine tumors of internal origin, especially pulmonary neuroendocrine neoplasms. Cytokeratin 20 (Fig. 86-8) and thyroid transcription factor-1 are useful markers to distinguish between primary cutaneous neuroendocrine carcinoma and a metastatic pulmonary neuroendocrine tumor.[20] The characteristic paranuclear ring- or plaquelike neurofilament- and cytokeratin-staining pattern in cutaneous neuroendocrine carcinoma may provide an additional clue in the differential diagnosis.

Integrin expression may help to distinguish cutaneous neuroendocrine carcinomas of the skin from primitive peripheral neuroectodermal tumors.[21]

HISTOGENESIS

The histogenesis of cutaneous neuroendocrine carcinomas remains unresolved.[4–6,12,13] Merkel cells and cutaneous neuroendocrine carcinomas have similar ultrastructural features. Furthermore, Merkel cells and the cells of cutaneous neuroendocrine carcinomas both express neuron-specific enolase, low molecular weight cytokeratins, neurofilaments, and other markers.

On the other hand, cutaneous neuroendocrine carcinomas possibly may have no histogenetic relationship to Merkel cells, and the arguments for this assumption are that (1) most cases of cutaneous neuroendocrine carcinoma arise in the dermis and subcutaneous tissue without obvious epidermal involvement or contact with the outer root sheath of hair follicles where Merkel cells are normally located; (2) Merkel cells seem to predominate in the skin of palms, digits, and dorsa of the feet, a distribution that is completely different from that of cutaneous neuroendocrine carcinoma; and (3) proliferating Merkel cells are absent in normal skin.

FIGURE 86-6

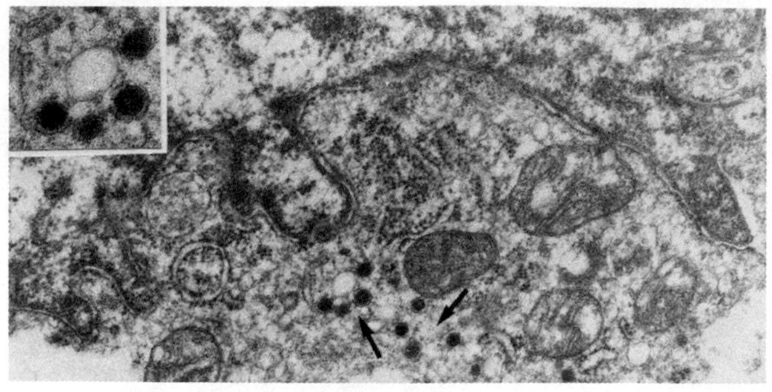

Electron micrograph of cutaneous neuroendocrine carcinoma. Cytoplasm of neoplastic cell displaying abundant organelles. The arrows denote neurosecretory granules. 38,000×. Inset: Higher magnification to better illustrate the dense-core neurosecretory granules.

FIGURE 86-7

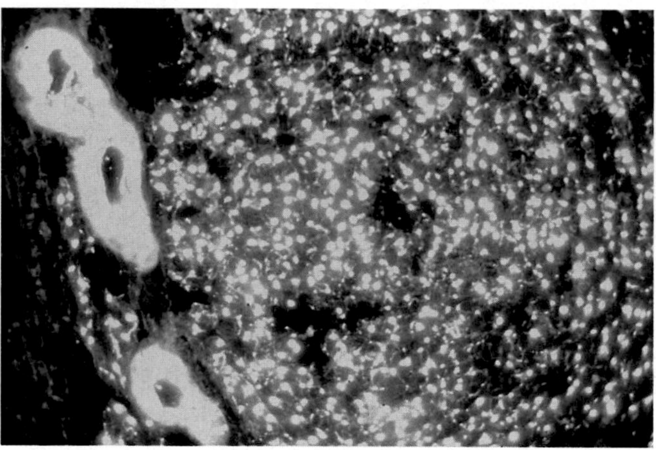

A.

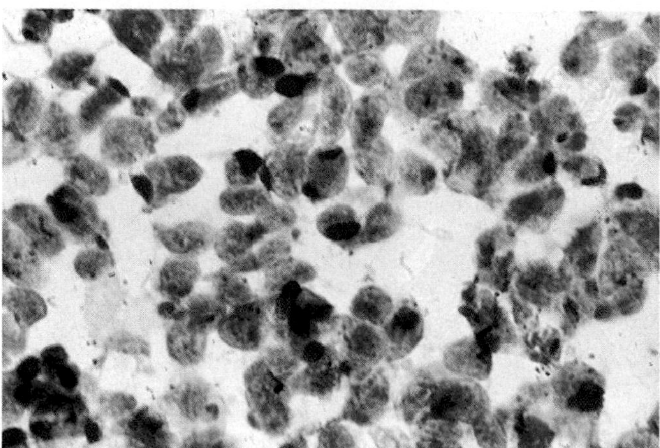

B.

Immunohistologic features of cutaneous neuroendocrine carcinoma. *A.* Strong fluorescence of paranuclear cytokeratin accumulations in tumor cells. Note the positive reaction in epithelial structures (eccrine glands). Indirect immunofluorescence. *B.* Tumor cells staining with monoclonal antibodies against neurofilaments. Note the discoid pattern. PAP-technique.

FIGURE 86-8

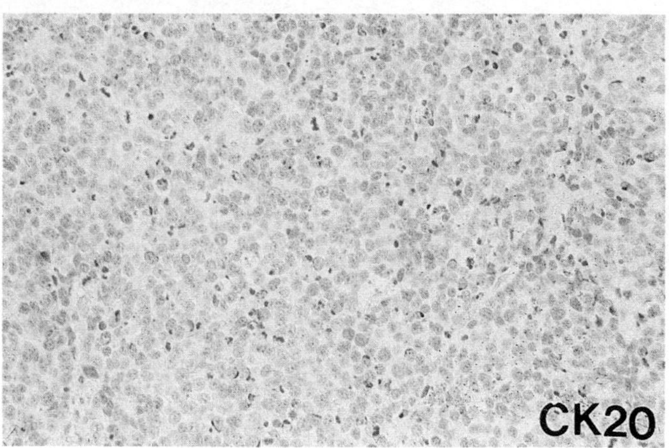

Cutaneous neuroendocrine carcinoma. Anticytokeratin 20 is a useful antibody to distinguish between cutaneous neuroendocrine carcinoma and metastatic small cell carcinoma of the lung in which CK 20 is usually absent. PAP-technique.

Cutaneous neuroendocrine carcinomas may be of epithelial origin, having undergone neuroendocrine differentiation, or the neoplasms may be derived from pluripotent epidermal stem cells.[5,12] Alternatively, cutaneous neuroendocrine carcinomas could also arise from or differentiate toward dermal neuroendocrine cells. There is some similarity between cutaneous neuroendocrine carcinomas and gastrointestinal carcinoids, which probably originate from subepithelial stromal cells that have migrated downward into the stroma from the epithelial layer.[4]

PROGNOSIS AND TREATMENT

Cutaneous neuroendocrine carcinomas are aggressive high-grade malignant tumors with local recurrences and metastases as common features. The overall survival rates are: 1 year, 88 percent; 2 years, 72 percent; and approximately 55 percent at 3 years. The 5-year survival rate varies between 64 and 30 percent.[8,9] Depending on the length of follow-up, 40 percent of patients develop local recurrences following surgical excision. Recurrent tumor can be observed in the previous excisional scar and surrounding it in a satellite-like fashion. Regional nodal metastases are found in 50 to 60 percent of patients, and distant metastases develop in 30 to 40 percent of patients. Sites for distant metastases are lungs, liver, bones, brain, deep lymph node groups (retroperitoneum), and other locations. Spontaneous regression of cutaneous neuroendocrine carcinoma has been rarely documented.

Management of cutaneous neuroendocrine carcinoma is based on a thorough clinical evaluation for evidence of distant metastases, careful palpation of regional lymph nodes, and a close, regular follow-up for evidence of recurrent tumor or regional lymphadenopathy. No standard treatment protocol for cutaneous neuroendocrine carcinoma exists.[22]

Different therapeutic regimens are appropriate according to the clinical presentation, and patients can be categorized into various stages of tumor spread (Table 86-1).

For primary treatment, wide local excision (1- to 2-cm margin) of the tumor and sentinel lymph node biopsy should be performed.[23] In addition, radiation therapy should be administered to the surgical bed and the draining lymph nodes.[24] Radiation therapy can be used

TABLE 86-1

Treatment of Cutaneous Neuroendocrine Carcinoma

Stage I: Localized disease	Surgery Sentinel lymph node biopsy Radiotherapy
Stage II: Regional lymph node metastases	Surgery Radiotherapy Chemotherapy
Stage III: Disseminated disease	Chemotherapy Innovative: α-interferon, cytokines, Bcl-2 antisense oligonucleotides

prophylactically as well as for recurrent disease and nodal metastases. Chemotherapy has been used especially for patients with metastatic cutaneous neuroendocrine carcinoma.[22,25] The combination of drugs that are active against small cell carcinoma of the lung is recommended.[25] Other treatment possibilities include local hyperthermia, hyperthermic limb perfusion chemotherapy, the somatostatin analogue octreotide, blood stem cell transplantation, cytokines, direct intralesional administration of recombinant human tumor necrosis factor, or perhaps, in the future, Bcl-2 antisense oligonucleodides.[8,26–28]

REFERENCES

1. Toker C: Trabecular carcinoma of the skin. *Arch Dermatol* **105**:107, 1972
2. Frigerio B et al: Merkel cell carcinoma of the skin: The structure and origin of normal Merkel cells. *Histopathology* **7**:229, 1983
3. Kerl H et al: New immunocytochemical observations in cutaneous neuroendocrine carcinoma (Merkel cell tumor). *J Invest Dermatol* **84**:541, 1984
4. Höfler H et al: The intermediate filament cytoskeleton of cutaneous neuroendocrine carcinoma (Merkel cell tumour). Immunohistochemical and biochemical analyses. *Virchows Arch* **406**:339, 1985
5. Walsh NMG: Primary neuroendocrine (Merkel cell) carcinoma of the skin: Morphologic diversity and implications thereof. *Hum Pathol* **32**:680, 2001
6. Gould VE et al: Neuroendocrine (Merkel) cells of the skin: Hyperplasias, dysplasias, and neoplasms. *Lab Invest* **52**:334, 1985
7. Ratner D et al: Merkel cell carcinoma. *J Am Acad Dermatol* **29**:143, 1993
8. Haag ML et al: Merkel cell carcinoma. Diagnosis and treatment. *Dermatol Surg* **21**:669, 1995
9. Tai PT et al: Merkel cell carcinoma of the skin. *J Cutan Med Surg* **4**:186, 2000

10. Penn I et al: Merkel's cell carcinoma in organ recipients: Report of 41 cases. *Transplantation* **68**:1717, 1999
11. An KP et al: Merkel cell carcinoma in the setting of HIV infection. *J Am Acad Dermatol* **45**:309, 2001
12. Moll I: Merkelzellkarzinom, in *Histopathologie der Haut*, edited by H Kerl, C Garbe, L Cerroni, HH Wolff. Berlin, Springer, 2002
13. Sibley RK et al: Primary neuroendocrine (Merkel cell?) carcinoma of the skin. *Am J Surg Pathol* **9**:95, 1985
14. Mount SL et al: Neuroendocrine carcinoma of the skin (Merkel cell carcinoma). An immunoelectron-microscopic case study. *Am J Dermatopathol* **16**:60, 1994
15. Moll I et al: Differences of bcl-2 protein expression between Merkel cells and Merkel cell carcinoma. *J Cutan Pathol* **23**:109, 1996
16. Penneys NS et al: CD44 expression in Merkel cell carcinoma may correlate with the risk of metastasis. *J Cutan Pathol* **21**:22, 1994
17. Van Gele M et al: Mutation analysis of P73 and TP53 in Merkel cell carcinoma. *Br J Cancer* **82**:823, 2000
18. Feinmesser M et al: Expression of the apoptosis-related oncogenes bcl-2, bax, and p53 in Merkel cell carcinoma: Can they predict treatment response and clinical outcome? *Hum Pathol* **30**:1367, 1999
19. Leonard JH et al: Deletion mapping on the short arm of chromosome 1 in Merkel cell carcinoma. *Cancer Detect Prev* **24**:620, 2000.
20. Leech SN et al: Merkel cell carcinoma can be distinguished from metastatic small cell carcinoma using antibodies to cytokeratin 20 and thyroid transcription factor 1. *J Clin Pathol* **54**:727, 2001
21. Perrin C et al: VLA and $alpha_6beta_4$ integrin expression in neuroendocrine carcinomas of the skin (their xenografts on nude mice and a corresponding primary culture). *J Cutan Pathol* **23**:223, 1996
22. Medina-Franco H et al: Multimodality treatment of Merkel cell carcinoma: Case series and literature review of 1024 cases. *Ann Surg Oncol* **8**:204, 2001
23. Rodrigues LK et al: Early experience with sentinel lymph node mapping for Merkel cell carcinoma. *J Am Acad Dermatol* **45**:303, 2001
24. Meeuwissen JA et al: The importance of postoperative radiation therapy in the treatment of Merkel cell carcinoma. *Int J Radiat Oncol Biol Phys* **31**:325, 1995
25. Voog E et al: Chemotherapy for patients with locally advanced or metastatic Merkel cell carcinoma. *Cancer* **85**:2589, 1999
26. Olieman AF et al: Hyperthermic isolated limb perfusion with tumor necrosis factor alpha, interferon gamma, and melphalan for locally advanced nonmelanoma skin tumors of the extremities: a multicenter study. *Arch Surg* **134**:303, 1999
27. Waldmann V et al: Transient complete remission of metastasized Merkel cell carcinoma by high-dose polychemotherapy and autologous peripheral blood stem cell transplantation. *Br J Dermatol* **143**:837, 2000
28. Schlagbauer-Wadl H et al: Bcl-2 antisense oligonucleotides (G3139) inhibit Merkel cell carcinoma growth in SCID mice. *J Invest Dermatol* **114**:725, 2000

CHAPTER 87

S. M. Connolly

Mammary and Extramammary Paget's Disease

Mammary and extramammary Paget's disease are rare intraepidermal adenocarcinomas with similar clinical features that mimic inflammatory or infectious conditions. Whereas mammary Paget's disease is most often associated with an underlying carcinoma of the breast, extramammary Paget's disease is a heterogenous condition representing either an intraepidermal adenocarcinoma in situ with potential to become invasive, or pagetoid spread of an underlying adnexal tumor or of a regional internal malignancy.

HISTORICAL ASPECTS

In 1874, Sir James Paget described 15 women with a chronic eczematous eruption of the nipple and areola in whom carcinoma developed in the underlying mammary gland. Almost all cases of mammary Paget's disease (MPD) are associated with an underlying intraductal breast carcinoma. In 1889, Crocker described extramammary Paget's disease (EMPD), involving the penis and scrotum with histologic features similar to the cases defined by Paget. The origin of the tumor cells was thought to be from underlying adnexal structures. Although the clinical and histologic features of MPD are generally accepted and the frequent association with underlying breast carcinoma recognized, the source of the neoplastic cells in EMPD has been controversial.

EPIDEMIOLOGY

MPD accounts for 2 to 3 percent of neoplastic conditions affecting the breast and presents at the median age of 56 years, which is 5 to 10 years higher than the overall peak age of incidence of invasive breast carcinoma.[1,2] The average duration of symptoms prior to diagnosis is 6.5 months but may be many years, which reflects an inappropriate delay in diagnosis. Males rarely develop MPD.

EMPD is rare and usually develops in the seventh decade.[3] There is a predilection for areas with a high density of apocrine glands, including the vulva, perianal region, male genitalia, and axillae. Vulvar involvement is most common, yet accounts for only 2 percent of all primary vulvar neoplasms. Occurrence in sites with modified apocrine glands, such as the eyelid and external auditory canal, and rare ectopic or mucosal cases have been noted.[3] Simultaneous anogenital and axillary involvement can occur, as can MPD and EMPD.[2–5]

ETIOLOGY AND PATHOGENESIS

The proportion of cases of MPD in which an associated in situ or invasive ductal breast carcinoma can be identified is high (82 to 92 percent) and supports the epidermotropic theory of origin. The in situ transformation theory was proposed to explain those cases in which there is no underlying mammary carcinoma or when there is cancer remote from the nipple–areola complex. The Paget's cells are purported to arise as malignant cells in the nipple epithelium independent from any other pathologic process.[3,6]

Heregulin-α is a motility factor produced and released by normal nipple epidermal keratinocytes. Heregulin receptors are expressed by Paget's cells. Binding of heregulin-α to the receptor complex on Paget's cells was recently shown to result in chemotaxis of the breast cancer cells, which migrate into the overlying epithelium.[7] There may be other mechanisms. A "field" effect in the duct system harboring intraductal carcinoma and the adjacent epidermis may play a role in the tumor cell spread in the epidermis as well as in the ductal system.[8]

Whereas MPD is highly associated with an underlying breast carcinoma, approximately 25 percent of EMPD cases are associated with neoplastic disease in adnexal structures or in organs with a contiguous lining. The current theory is that EMPD arises as an intraepithelial neoplasm in most cases.[2,9] The origin of the cell is either from intraepidermal cells of the apocrine gland ducts or from pluripotent keratinocyte stem cells. These cases are often referred to as "primary" EMPD. "Secondary" EMPD refers to cases in which there is epithelial spread from an underlying neoplasm either arising in the adnexal structures or from an organ with a contiguous epithelium.[2] Most vulvar EMPD is of the primary type, but endometrial, endocervical, and vaginal, as well as vulvar, urethral, and bladder carcinoma can be associated.[2,9] EMPD of the male genitalia is thought to be more frequently associated with internal malignancy of the genitourinary tract.[10] Perianal EMPD is less common than the vulvar form of the disease. It is associated with colorectal or anal adenocarcinoma in 70 to 80 percent of cases and is more often thought to be secondary. Although there are rare reports of distant tumors arising without direct epithelial connection to the affected epidermis such as ovarian, renal cell, breast, or hepatocellular carcinoma, there is no clear evidence that the Paget's cells arise from these.

CLINICAL MANIFESTATIONS

MPD presents as a unilateral, sharply demarcated, erythematous or scaly patch on the nipple or areola with variable extension to surrounding skin (Fig. 87-1). It can be exudative with vesicles occurring as an early manifestation; bleeding, ulceration, or nipple invagination reflecting adherence to underlying tumor tend to be late findings. Pruritus, pain, and tenderness are early and prominent symptoms in approximately 25 percent of cases. In 82 to 92 percent of cases, tumor cells have spread to the skin of the nipple and areola from an underlying invasive or ductal carcinoma in situ.[2] A palpable breast mass is noted in approximately 50 percent of cases of MPD.[6] Although the carcinoma is more often centrally located, it may be peripheral. It is said to be more commonly multifocal.[11,12] If palpable, the carcinoma is more often invasive (90 to 94 percent) and axillary metastases are present in one-half to two-thirds of these. If it is not palpable, ductal carcinoma in situ is more likely.

FIGURE 87-1

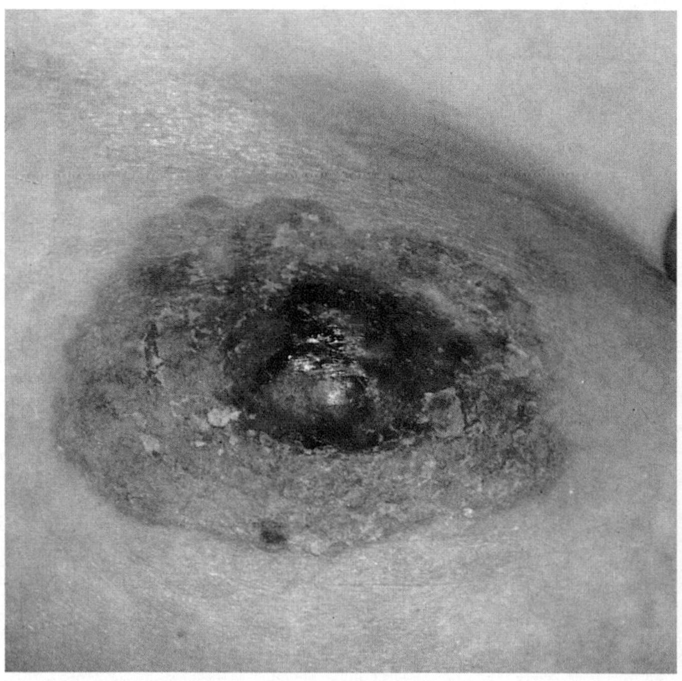

Paget's disease of the nipple. On the nipple and the areola mammae is a sharply demarcated erythematous area with scaling and an erosive moist surface. There is slight superficial induration.

FIGURE 87-2

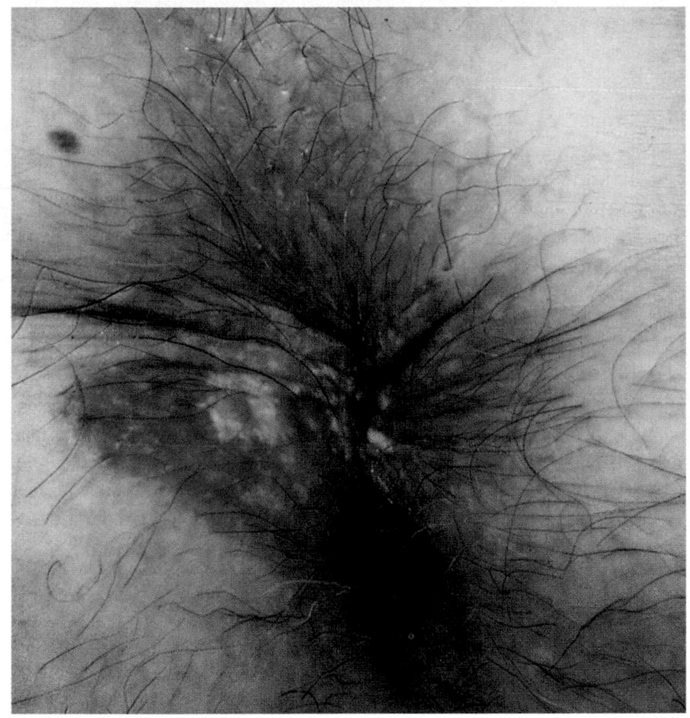

Perianal Paget's disease presenting as a moist superficially eroded patch. (*Courtesy of Robert Spencer, M.D.*)

Bilateral MPD with underlying intraductal carcinoma identified in one breast, development of MPD in a supernumerary nipple associated with an underlying intraductal carcinoma in the ectopic breast, MPD in a supernumerary nipple without associated carcinoma, and MPD developing after conservative management of breast cancer are among the unusual presentations of MPD.

EMPD also presents as moist superficially eroded or erythematous scaly patches. Gray-white eczematous patches are also a common presentation; hypopigmented macules, ulceration, crusting, or a palpable tumor may be present (Fig. 87-2). Pruritus is frequently present in EMPD; bleeding, oozing, tenderness, or a burning sensation can occur. Symptoms may be present for months to many years.

LABORATORY FINDINGS

Evaluation of MPD or EMPD begins with cutaneous biopsy to establish the diagnosis. Mammography is indicated in all cases of MPD but may be normal. The incidence of abnormal radiographic findings varies from 24 to 97 percent.[1] Mammography does not discriminate between ductal carcinoma in situ and invasive disease; it is more likely to detect changes suggestive of malignancy if there is a palpable mass (97 percent) as compared to cases without a palpable mass (50 percent). The tumor may be a significant distance from the nipple and multifocal disease may not be appreciated radiographically.[6,9,11,12] Occasionally, a lesion invisible on mammography may be identified by ultrasonography or by magnetic resonance imaging; ^{99m}Tc MIBI prone scintimammography may be useful.[6]

Because EMPD of the female and male genitalia or perianal skin may be associated with underlying neoplasms of the genitourinary or gastrointestinal tracts, a thorough general physical examination, along with laboratory and radiographic testing, with emphasis on the region adjacent to the site of EMPD, is indicated. Evaluation of the breasts is indicated because of the rare association of EMPD and MPD. Examination of the axillae should not be overlooked because of the rare simultaneous occurrence of axillary and anogenital EMPD.

PATHOLOGY

MPD and EMPD are characterized by distinctive intraepithelial neoplastic proliferative cells with abundant pale-staining cytoplasm and large atypical nuclei apparent on routine hematoxylin and eosin histologic sections (Fig. 87-3). Mitoses are often present and Paget cells may be distributed singly or in clusters in the epithelium with variable extension into hair follicles and sweat gland ducts. Intercellular bridges are not appreciated on light microscopy. The epithelium is variably hyperkeratotic or hypokeratotic, acanthotic, or eroded and ulcerated. A dermal mixed inflammatory infiltrate is usually present.

In MPD, Paget's cells do not invade the dermis from the epidermis but can extend into the outer root sheath; underlying lactiferous ducts often show adenocarcinoma, which can invade the surrounding stroma. In primary EMPD, Paget's cells may be present in the outer root sheath but are also found in sebaceous, apocrine, or eccrine gland structures; they can form glandular and ductal structures in the epidermis and adnexal epithelium. Unless there is disruption of the basement membrane

FIGURE 87-3

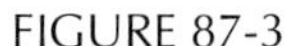

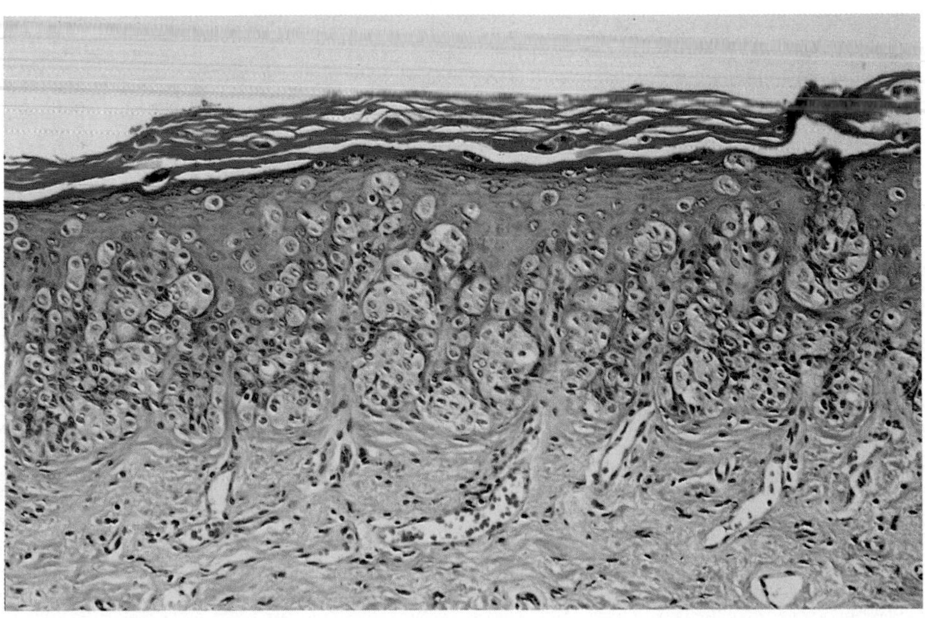

Neoplastic Paget's cells are randomly dispersed throughout the epidermis and readily appreciated on this hematoxylin and eosin section. Paget's cells have distinctive pale-staining cytoplasm when compared to surrounding keratinocytes.

with extension of Paget's cells into the dermis, EMPD is in situ. In secondary EMPD, Paget's cells extend from an underlying adenocarcinoma arising in the adnexal structures or from a local organ with contiguous epithelium. Careful histologic examination is key and immunohistochemistry may assist in identification of secondary EMPD.

Sialomucin, a nonsulfated acid mucopolysaccharide, is found in the cytoplasm of Paget's cells. It stains with colloidal iron, Alcian blue at a pH of 2.5, and mucicarmine, PAS, and aldehyde fuchsin at a pH of 1.7. It is resistant to diastase and bovine testicular hyaluronidase. Mucin stains more frequently and more extensively in EMPD than in MPD, but mucin stains can be negative because of patchy distribution of mucin and skip areas.

IMMUNOHISTOCHEMISTRY

Immunohistochemistry is helpful in the diagnosis of Paget's disease and may clarify the cellular origin.[2] Certain markers may be helpful in determining whether an internal malignancy might be associated with EMPD. Immunohistochemistry has not permitted differentiation of intraepidermal in situ disease from that arising from an adnexal structure.

Cytokeratins are fibrous proteins present in almost all epithelia. Cytokeratin 7 is a sensitive marker for MPD and EMPD.[13] It is not specific; some mammary gland-related clear cells (Toker cells) and Merkel cells are stained.[14] It is an excellent marker for intraepithelial and invasive Paget's cells and distinguishes hyperplastic and malignant squamous cells. Cytokeratin 20, which is present in gastrointestinal and urothelial carcinoma, is found more frequently in EMPD from pagetoid spread of extracutaneous carcinoma than in primary EMPD; immunophenotypes other than cytokeratin 7+/cytokeratin 20– in Paget's cells suggest underlying regional internal malignancy.[15]

Gross cystic disease fluid protein-15 (GCDFP-15), a marker of apocrine epithelial cells is strongly expressed in vulvar and perianal Paget's disease without an underlying internal malignancy, and less frequently in those with a malignancy.[16–18] Normal, metaplastic, and carcinomatous apocrine epithelium is stained and, hence, GCDFP-15 does not exclude a dermal apocrine tumor.

Most cases of EMPD stain strongly for carcinoembryonic antigen, whereas MPD is positive in approximately 35 percent of cases. S-100 may be expressed in 25 percent of MPD, and, rarely, in EMPD. It is best used along with HMB-45 to differentiate Paget's disease from malignant melanoma. MPD and EMPD are HMB-45 negative.[2]

The histologic differential diagnosis of Paget's cells includes those conditions characterized by spread of cells singly or in clusters throughout the epithelial layers. Thus, superficial spreading malignant melanoma, Bowen's disease, mycosis fungoides, Langerhans cell histiocytosis, pagetoid Spitz nevus, clear cell papulosis, Merkel cell carcinoma with pagetoid intraepidermal invasion, eccrine porocarcinoma, sebaceous carcinoma, clear cells of Toker, and pagetoid dyskeratoses are other considerations.[19]

DIAGNOSIS AND DIFFERENTIAL DIAGNOSIS

The key to diagnosis of MPD or EMPD is a high index of suspicion and confirmation with skin biopsy. Any eczematous or thickened area in regions with a high density of apocrine glands that does not resolve promptly with what is deemed appropriate therapy must be considered as possible Paget's disease. The clinical differential diagnosis of MPD includes dermatitis, benign intraductal papilloma, frictional hyperkeratosis of the nipple, erosive adenomatosis, Hailey-Hailey disease, and pemphigus. Fungal, viral, or bacterial infections are frequent misdiagnoses. Identification of MPD in individuals who have other active dermatoses, such as psoriasis, is difficult. Bowen's disease, basal cell carcinoma, metastatic carcinoma, malignant melanoma, mammary duct ectasia with chronic nipple discharge associated with eczematoid nipple-areola changes, hyperplasia of Toker cells, and leiomyomas of the nipple are other considerations that might arise.[4–6]

The differential diagnosis in the anogenital area is similarly broad and includes candidiasis, dermatitis, psoriasis, seborrheic dermatitis, lichen sclerosus et atrophicus, lichen simplex chronicus, lichen planus, necrolytic migratory erythema, histiocytosis, erythroplasia of Queyrat, malignant melanoma, and periorificial tuberculosis.[3] Axillary EMPD may be mistaken for dermatitis, psoriasis, or candidiasis. Histochemical and immunohistochemical techniques have improved our ability to differentiate Paget's disease.

TREATMENT AND PROGNOSIS

Mastectomy has been the standard therapy for MPD.[6] In patients with a palpable mass there is a higher risk of axillary node metastasis as the mass is often invasive and mastectomy remains the standard. Pathologic findings of the mass and axillary staging direct therapy.[12] Patients with MPD with a palpable mass have a greater incidence of invasive carcinoma, multifocal lesions, and nodal metastases and worse survival.[11]

Controversy exists in cases in which disease is apparently confined to the nipple. Breast-conserving therapies currently considered include nipple excision alone, central segmentectomy alone, or radiation with or without resection.[2,6,20–22] However, selecting patients with disease amenable to these approaches without mastectomy is difficult and can be associated with understaging and high rates of recurrence.[11]

Patients with MPD and no palpable mass have 5- and 10-year survival rates of 90 to 100 percent following mastectomy as compared to survival rates of 20 to 60 percent at 5 years and 9 to 40 percent at 10 years for those with palpable disease.[1] MPD in the male breast has a poor prognosis with a 20 to 30 percent 5-year survival rate.[23]

Primary EMPD is managed at any site by surgical excision. Other modalities that have been employed include radiation, electrodesiccation and curettage, cryosurgery, Mohs micrographic technique, topical 5-fluorouracil, photodynamic therapy (PDT), and CO_2 laser. Because this condition can often be multifocal and extend beyond the visible clinical margin, recurrence or residual disease are frequently seen. Long-term follow-up is required because of this and the associated risk of late progression to invasive disease. Recurrence rates for vulvar EMPD range from 15 percent with vulvectomy, 27 percent with the Mohs technique, and 43 percent with wide local excision; perianal disease recurs in 28 percent of patients after Mohs and in 50 percent of patients after wide local excision.[24]

Efforts to better define the extent of disease in EMPD have included preoperative topical 5-fluorouracil application to delineate extent of disease prior to Mohs micrographic surgery. Multiple punch biopsies prior to therapy to define margins have also been used. PDT has been used to guide margins of the involvement prior to destruction by CO_2 laser or as an adjunctive therapy for residual disease after radiation or wide local excision.[24–27] PDT has also been combined with the Mohs technique to minimize tissue loss and decrease risk of recurrence in EMPD.[24] The multimodal approach of PDT, Mohs technique, and cytokeratin 7 staining of Mohs sections holds the promise of lower recurrence rates. (O'Connor WJ, personal communication).

Prognosis for primary intraepithelial EMPD is excellent; patients require long-term follow-up because of the multifocal nature of the condition and high recurrence rate. In a large series of cases of vulvar EMPD, there was a 12 percent prevalence rate of invasive disease and a 4 percent prevalence rate of associated vulvar adenocarcinoma.[9] EMPD at any site has a worse prognosis in the presence of dermal invasion. Depth of invasion may be a prognostic factor but requires further confirmation.[17,18,27] If there is lymphatic invasion with lymph node metastases present, the prognosis is poor.[22] If EMPD is associated with an underlying regional internal malignancy, the prognosis and therapy are directed by the underlying carcinoma.

REFERENCES

1. Jamali FR et al: Paget's disease of the nipple-areola complex. *Surg Clin North Am* **76**:365, 1996
2. Lloyd J, Flanagan AM: Mammary and extramammary Paget's disease. *J Clin Pathol* **53**:742, 2000
3. Lupton GP, Graham JH: Mammary and extramammary Paget's disease, in *Cancer of the Skin*, edited by RJ Friedman DS Rigel, AW Kopf, MN Harris, D Baber. Philadelphia, WB Saunders, 1991, p 217
4. Heyman WR: Extramammary Paget's disease. *Clin Dermatol* **11**:83, 1993
5. Popiolek DA et al: Synchronous Paget's disease of the vulva and breast *Gynecol Oncol* **71**:17, 1998
6. Sakorafas GH et al: Paget's disease of the breast. *Cancer Treat Rev* **27**:9, 2001
7. Schelfout VRJ et al: Pathogenesis of Paget's disease: Epidermal heregulin-α, motility factor, and the HER receptor family. *J Natl Cancer Inst* **92**:622, 2000
8. Mai KT: Morphological evidence for field-effect as a mechanism for tumor spread in mammary Paget's disease. *Histopathol* **35**:567, 1999
9. Fanning J et al: Paget's disease of the vulva: Prevalence of associated vulvar adenocarcinoma, invasive Paget's disease, and recurrence after surgical excision. *Am J Obstet Gynecol* **180**:24, 1999
10. Allen SJR et al: Paget's disease of the scrotum: A case exhibiting positive prostate specific antigen staining and associated prostatic adenocarcinoma. *Br J Dermatol* **4**:689, 1998
11. Yim JH et at: Underlying pathology in mammary Paget's disease. *Ann Surg Oncol* **4**:287, 1997
12. Kollmorgen DR et al: Paget's disease of the breast: A 33-year experience. *J Am Coll Surg* **187**:171, 1998
13. Smith KJ et al: Cytokeratin 7 staining in mammary and extramammary Paget's disease. *Mod Pathol* **10**:1069, 1997
14. Lundquist K et al: Intra-epidermal cytokeratin 7 expression is not restricted to Paget's cells but is also seen in Toker cells and Merkel cells. *Am J Surg Pathol* **23**:212, 1999
15. Ohnishi T, Watanabe S: The use of cytokeratins 7 and 20 in the diagnosis of primary and secondary extramammary Paget's disease. *Br J Dermatol* **142**:243, 2000
16. Kohler S, Smoller BR: Gross cystic disease fluid protein-15 reactivity in extramammary Paget's disease without associated internal malignancy. *Am J Dermatopathol* **18**:118, 1996
17. Goldblum JR, Hart WR: Vulvar Paget's disease: A clinicopathologic and immunohistochemical study of 19 cases. *Am J Surg Pathol* **21**:1178, 1997
18. Goldblum JR, Hart WR: Perianal Paget's disease—A histologic and immunohistochemical study of 11 cases with and without associated rectal carcinoma. *Am J Surg Pathol* **22**:170, 1998
19. Kohler S et al: The differential diagnosis of Pagetoid cells in the epidermis. *Mod Pathol* **11**:79, 1998
20. Bijker N et al: Breast-conserving therapy for Paget disease of the nipple: A prospective European Organization for Research and Treatment of cancer study of 61 patients. *Cancer* **91**:472, 2001
21. Pierce LJ et al: The conservative management of Paget's disease of the breast with radiotherapy. *Cancer* **80**:1065, 1997
22. DeVita VT Jr: Cancers of the skin, in *Cancer, Principles and Practice of Oncology* edited by VT DeVita, Jr, S Hellman, SA Rosenberg. New York, Lippincott Raven, 1997, p 1565
23. Desai DC et al: Paget's disease of the male breast. *Am Surgeon* **62**:1068, 1996
24. Zollo JD, Zeitouni NC: The Roswell Park Cancer Institute experience with extramammary Paget's disease. *Br J Dermatol* **142**:59, 2000
25. Becker-Wegerich PM et al: Carbon dioxide laser treatment of extramammary Paget's disease guided by photodynamic therapy. *Br J Dermatol* **138**:169, 1998
26. Henta T et al: Photodynamic therapy for inoperable vulval Paget's disease using delta-aminolevulinic acid: Successful management of a large skin lesion. *Br J Dermatol* **141**:347, 1999
27. Crawford D et al: Prognostic factors in Paget's disease of the vulva; a study of 21 cases. *Intl J Gynecol Pathol* **18**:351, 1999

SECTION 12

DISORDERS OF MELANOCYTES

CHAPTER 88

Thomas B. Fitzpatrick
Jean-Paul Ortonne

Normal Skin Color and General Considerations of Pigmentary Disorders

SKIN COLOR

The varieties of normal skin color in humans range from people of "no color" (pale white) to "people of color" (light brown, dark brown, and black). Skin color is a blend resulting from the skin chromophores *red* (oxyhemoglobin), *blue* (deoxygenated hemoglobin), *yellow-orange* (carotene, an exogenous pigment), and *brown* (melanin). Melanin, however, is the major component of skin color (Fig. 88-1); it is the presence or absence of melanin in melanosomes in melanocytes and melanin in keratinocytes that is responsible for *epidermal* pigmentation, and the presence of melanin in macrophages or melanocytes in the dermis (Fig. 88-2) that is responsible for *dermal* pigmentation. A scholarly treatise on skin has been published that[1] integrates the various aspects of skin color from an historical standpoint.

FIGURE 88-1

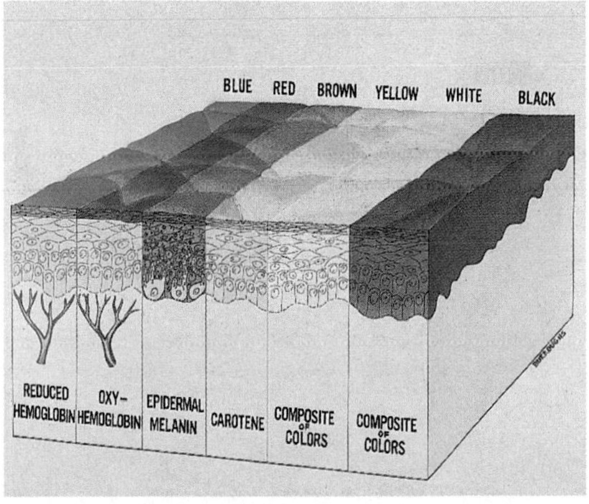

Components of normal skin color include red (oxyhemoglobin), blue (deoxyhemoglobin), brown (melanin), and yellow (carotene).

Melanocytes are the sole site of melanin formation; they are specialized dendritic cells present in normal skin only in the hair matrix and at the epidermal-dermal junction (see Chap. 11). All melanocytes are derived from the neural crest (melanoblasts), with the single exception of melanocytes in the retinal pigment epithelium (RPE); these do not migrate from the neural crest but arise from the outer layer of the optic cup. Melanocytes are normally found in humans in the skin (hair matrix and at the dermal-epidermal junction), in all the mucous membranes, the uveal tract, the RPE, and in the stria vascularis of the inner ear. In certain peoples, such as Asians, American Indians, African Americans, and some Caucasians, melanocytes are normally present at birth in the dermis, usually located in the lumbosacral areas in the so-called Mongolian spot (see Chap. 90). Melanocytes in the epidermis are not

FIGURE 88-2

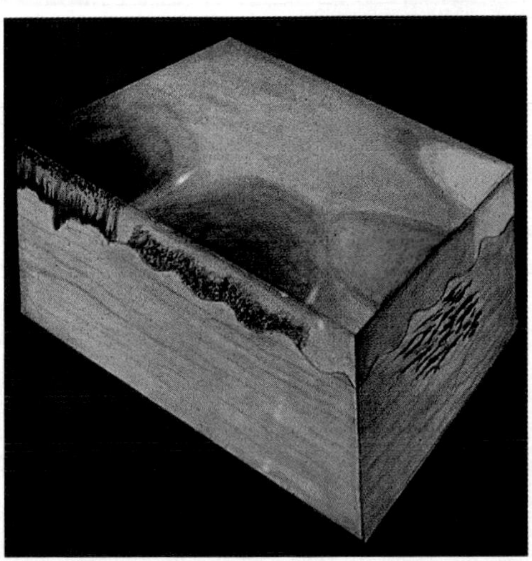

Expressions of abnormalities of melanin pigmentation: white (hypopigmentation); brown (epidermal hyperpigmentation); and blue (dermal pigmentation).

FIGURE 88-3

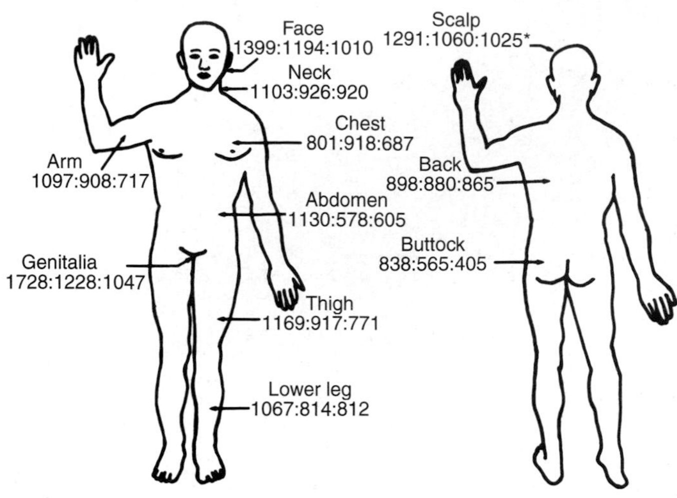

Comparison of average number of melanocytes in the epidermal skin of various body surfaces in three age groups (per mm²).

FIGURE 88-4

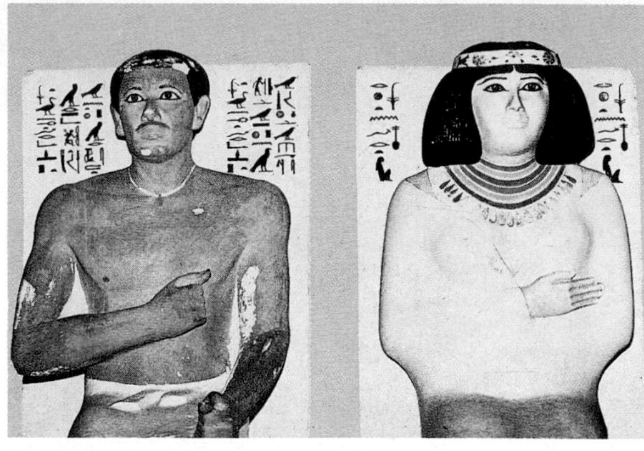

Impact of sun exposure on skin color; tanned Egyptian male reflects considerable sun exposure (facultative color), while Egyptian woman who remains indoors remains pale (constitutive color).

equally distributed throughout the skin, but there are essentially equal numbers of melanocytes in skin of various colors (Fig. 88-3).

Constitutive and Facultative Skin Color and Skin Phototype

Two types of normal melanin pigmentation form the basis for normal skin color. *Constitutive* skin color (also called basic skin color) is the genetically determined color (light brown, medium brown, and dark brown) or absence of color (white) in skin unexposed to solar irradiation; this is found in habitually sun-shielded areas such as the buttocks and inner upper arms. *Facultative* skin color is the skin color that results from an increase in the intensity of skin color as a result of ultraviolet radiation (UVR) exposure and reflects the genetically predetermined capacity of the skin to darken in response to UVR (Fig. 88-4). "White" people are dissimilar in their capacity to tan. This is the basic premise of the system of *skin phototypes* (Table 88-1). The phenotype (hair and eye color) is not a reliable guide to *sunburn sensitivity* because the "white" population is a mix of various skin phototypes: although persons with white skin with freckling and red hair have a limited or no capacity to tan, this failure to tan can also be present in persons who have brown eyes and dark hair. Because of the unreliability of the phenotype, a system of *skin phototypes* (SPT) was developed, in 1975,[2,3] to provide a basis for estimating the dose of UVA in the use of psoralen photochemotherapy.

The term "fair" skin is frequently used by epidemiologists to describe white skin. This can be very misleading because, in fact, persons with SPTs I, II, and II are regarded together as "fair" and have virtually the same degree of "whiteness," yet this term would include three very different SPTs, each with a different capacity to tan; a "fair" skin person with SPT III can become very tanned, while "fair" persons with SPT I cannot tan at all, even after multiple exposures, and persons with SPT II can tan only minimally. This is truly a spectrum of skin pigment. At one end of the spectrum are persons with oculocutaneous albinism and SPTs I and II who have limited tanning potential who are, in fact, melanocompromised. At the other end of the spectrum are persons who are melanocompetent (SPT IV) who have a full tanning potential without sunburn (Table 88-1).

Skin phototyping can used to counsel these persons about risk of sun exposure; skin phototypes I, II, and III are at risk for developing photodamage of all types: dermatoheliosis (wrinkling, solar lentigo, actinic keratosis), nonmelanoma skin cancer, and cutaneous malignant melanoma. For example, the *p-16 Leiden* (Holland) carriers in the familial atypical mole malignant melanoma (FAMMM) with skin phototype I run the highest risk of developing melanoma.

The degree of tanning response is genetically determined and is the logical basis for the division of normal skin into SPTs. Once UVR exposure is discontinued, the facultative color spontaneously recedes to constitutive levels until further melanogenic influences are introduced. Although the degree of facultative skin color is genetically determined, endocrine changes that occur in pregnancy and in Addison's disease may also result in facultative pigmentation. Thus, the fluctuation in skin color is a combined result of genetics, UV irradiation, and hormonal influences; disorders of melanin pigmentation must always be considered against this background.

TABLE 88-1

Classification of Skin Phototypes (SPT)

SPT	Reaction To Moderate* Sun Exposure	Skin Color
	MELANOCOMPROMISED	
I	Burn and no tan	Pale white
II	Burn and minimal tan	Pale white
III	Burn then tan well	White
	MELANOCOMPETENT	
IV	Tan, no burn	Light brown
V	Tan, no burn	Brown
VI	Tan, no burn	Dark brown

*Thirty minutes unprotected sun exposure, i.e., without sunscreen, in peak season (spring or summer) depending on the latitude.

The extent of genetic control of facultative skin color change is unknown. However, the degree of facultative color change is not directly related to constitutive skin color because the constitutive skin colors for SPTs I to III are quite similar and there is considerable variability in the intensity of the tanning response that can be induced in white persons. This variation in response can be graded by personal history.

The additive interaction of three or four genic pairs is probably adequate to account for the variation in skin color between the very fair-skinned individual and the very dark. These few interacting loci may be responsible for the variation in constitutive skin color over the globe.

Besides the polygenic series responsible for constitutive skin color, there are other genes that, as in albinism, act individually partly or completely to dilute melanin pigmentation. There appear to be two basic genetic influences: (1) those responsible for the phenotype of melanoblasts programmed to undergo differentiation, and (2) those responsible for the capability of melanoblasts to survive and to differentiate in embryonic life. The genetic influences in humans may well be as complex as those in mice, in which more than 100 genes at about 62 loci influence skin and hair color (see also Chap. 11). If one envisions a scheme in which an increasing number of genes are operative in the process of melanoblast migration and differentiation with the final controlling genes expressed in specific cutaneous zones (dermatomes), one may view the numerous melanin disorders as expressions of different genic defects operative at various levels; many such chromosomal defects have been identified (e.g., albinism, piebaldism, and Waardenburg's syndrome; see Chaps. 89 and 90).

Melanin Pigmentation and Ultraviolet Radiation

Ultraviolet radiation (UVR) is, at the same time, a powerful stimulus to melanin pigmentation and a destructive agent on the melanocytes. UVR can stimulate skin melanocytes to increase epidermal melanin content, which then functions as a very effective density photoprotective filter of UVR. In contrast, mutations caused by UVR (principally UVB) result in disfiguring changes related to pigmentation (actinic leukoderma, solar lentigo) and induce fatal malignancies (malignant melanoma in white persons). Visible melanin pigmentation in human skin is directly related to the number of, melanization of, transfer of, and degradation of the metabolic unit and specific organelle of melanocytes, the melanosome (see Chap. 11). The production, size, degree of melanization, and transfer to keratinocytes of melanosomes are all under genetic control. UVR (both UVB and UVA) elicits a response in direct relation to the tanning potential of the epidermal melanin unit (the melanocyte and its cluster of keratinocytes.)

In cultured melanocytes from different skin phototypes, melanin content is five times higher in SPTs IV to VI than in SPTs I to III, and the melanocytes maintain their phenotype according to their original skin phototype.[4] After UVB irradiation a stronger induction of endonuclease sensitive sites was found for melanocytes with a lower level of total melanin and a high content of pheomelanin. By measuring the clone-forming ability in different melanocyte cultures after UVB irradiation, significant better survival was found in case of the cells with the higher melanin content.[4]

Visibly equivalent UVB and UVA tans are not equally protective; the UVA tan is much less protective. This is because while UVA increases melanin pigmentation, it is virtually limited to the basal cell layer; UVB results in melanin that is distributed throughout the epidermis. A UVA tan is photoprotective, however, against vascular damage and inflammation. UVA tanning but not UVB tanning is prevented by vascular occlusion, presumably because it is oxygen dependent. Most interesting is the observation that the action spectra for delayed tanning and erythema differ on the basis the SPT. In SPTs I and II, the action spectra for erythema and tanning are the same, while in SPTs III and IV, the action spectra separate in the longer UV-wave range (UVA) and it is therefore possible using UVA to develop tanning without burning.[5]

Eumelanin, Pheomelanin, and Neuromelanin

(See also Chap. 11)

Melanocytes produce two chemically distinct types of melanin pigments: *eumelanin* and *pheomelanin*. These pigments can be quantitatively analyzed by acidic permanganate oxidation or by reductive hydrolysis with hydriodic acid to form pyrrole-2,3,5-tricarboxylic acid or aminohydroxyphenylalanine, respectively. About 30 coat color genes in mice have been cloned, and functions of many of those genes have been elucidated. However, little is known about the interacting functions of these loci.

Three types of melanin in humans have been demonstrated. *Eumelanin* (brown-black melanin) is found in ellipsoidal melanosomes, which impart brown-black color to skin, eye, and hair. *Pheomelanin* (yellow-red melanin), found in spherical melanosomes, is the basis for yellow-red hair and has also recently been found in basal layer melanocytes. *Neuromelanin* is the black pigment formed within nerve cells (e.g., the substantia nigra) that is formed by an enzymatic pathway different from that responsible for eumelanin or pheomelanin synthesis; therefore, in albinism, the pigment in the substantia nigra is unchanged. The concept of mixed melanins (eumelanin and pheomelanin) arises from evidence that melanins cannot be easily characterized as purely eumelanin or purely pheomelanin. For example, small amounts of pheomelanin are probably present in most melanocytes; red hair, however, may only contain pheomelanin.

The melanocortin-1 receptor (MC1R), a seven-pass transmembrane G protein coupled receptor, is a control site in melanogenesis and skin pigmentation. It has been ascertained that variants of the *MC1R* gene are common in individuals with red hair and fair skin. Loss-of-function mutations in *MC1R* result in a switch from eumelanin to pheomelanin production. The shade of red hair frequently differs in heterozygotes from that in homozygotes/compound heterozygotes, and there is also evidence for a heterozygote effect on beard hair color, SPT, and freckling. There appears to be evidence for a dosage effect of *MC1R* variants on hair as well as skin color.[6] This area of research is expanding rapidly and recently it was shown that *MC1R* has a clear heterozygote effect on SPT, with up to 30 percent containing loss-of-function mutations.[7]

Hormonal Control of Melanin Pigmentation

Tsatmali et al.[8] have summarized the role of hormones in melanin pigmentation. They state that melanin pigmentation of the skin is regulated by locally produced MSH-α rather than that of pituitary origin. MSH-α acts as a paracrine and/or autocrine mediator of UV-induced pigmentation. However, the predominant MSH-α in human skin is desacetyl MSH-α and, compared to the acetylated form, is a relatively weak agonist at the human MC1R. By acting as a partial agonist desacetyl MSH-α may even oppose the actions of acetylated MSH-α and other MC1R agonists. The most abundant MC1R agonist in human epidermis is adrenocorticotropic hormone (ACTH)1-17. This proopiomelanocortin (POMC) peptide, which is produced by keratinocytes, is more potent than acetylated MSH-α in stimulating melanogenesis in human melanocytes and, in contrast to the latter, produces a biphasic dose-response curve. This is probably a consequence of its activation of both the CAMP and inositol 1,4,5-triphosphate (IP_3)/diacylglycerol (DAG) signaling pathways. MSH-α peptides, on the other hand, selectively activate the CAMP pathway. Compared with MSH-α, ACTH1-17 could have a more important role as a paracrine mediator of melanogenesis and other melanocytic processes. However, ACTH1-17 is not the only POMC peptide in the skin and may interact with related peptides at the MC1R. These interactions are likely to represent important determinants of melanocyte function and skin pigmentation. For example, Bastiaens et al.[9] have reported that nearly all individuals with ephelides (freckles) are carriers of at least one *MC1R* gene variant and suggest that *MC1R* gene variants are necessary to develop ephelides.

Melanocytes and the Epidermal Melanin Unit

Melanin pigment is synthesized in specialized cytoplasmic organelles called *melanosomes,* which contain the principal pigment-synthesizing enzyme *tyrosinase* (see Chap. 11). It is the presence of melanized melanosomes within the keratinocytes that imparts skin color. The number, melanin content, and location of these melanosomes determine the various hues of human skin and hair color. Melanosomes are synthesized in melanocytes, transferred to keratinocytes, and transported to the epidermal surface. Melanin formation cannot occur in melanosomes that have been transferred to keratinocytes.

The *epidermal melanin unit* (Fig. 88-5) is the functional unit responsible for the orderly process of melanin synthesis. This multicellular unit is composed of a melanocyte and an associated cluster of about 36 keratinocytes and is the focal point for the control of melanin metabolism within the mammalian epidermis. When melanosomes are confined to the melanocytes at the epidermal-dermal junction and the melanosomes are not transferred to keratinocytes, a dilution of the normal skin color results (hypomelanosis secondary to "transfer block" as in postinflammatory hypomelanosis).

Melanin in Perspective

Melanin is not biodegradable, similar to plastic polymers, and it is surprising that the world is not covered with melanin! Nature in its economy must have regarded melanin as an important polymer, most probably because of its role in protection of the skin and the eye, from damaging radiant energy, especially ultraviolet. Certainly the earliest hominids did not have a use for melanin in photoprotection as their skin was white and the protection against radiant energy was provided by dark pigmented hair. As the hair was lost early in the evolution of *Homo sapiens,* the naked white skin developed a melanized epidermis as a shield against damaging UVR. Quevedo et al. summarized the evolution of melanin pigmentation and the role of climate and sunlight.[10] It was suggested that melanin pigmentation was related to human fitness, acting in natural selection during evolution. Before man used clothing, pigment protected the skin against solar radiation in a particular environment. The variations in skin color can be regarded as adaptive and related to the level of ultraviolet. As hominids moved outside of the tropics, melanin depigmentation decreased to permit synthesis of previtamin D_3.[11] There is a strong correlation between absolute latitude and UV radiation levels.

FIGURE 88-5

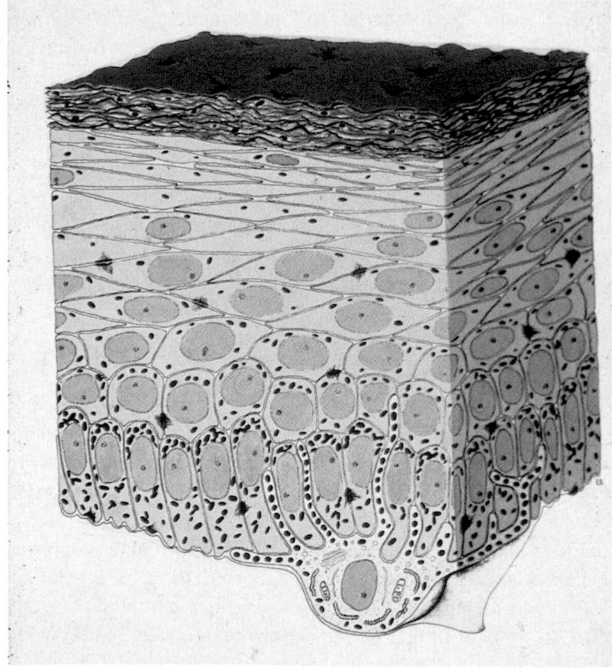

A.

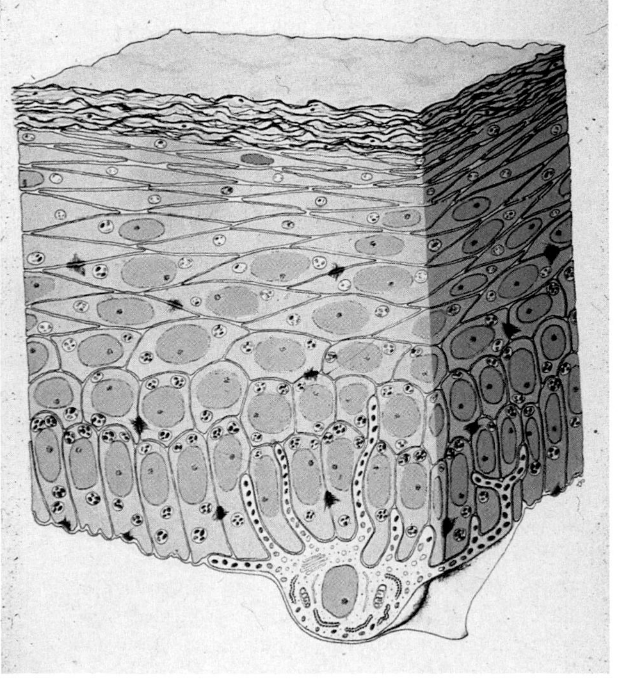

B.

Epidermal melanin unit. This multicellular unit is composed of a melanocyte and a cluster of approximately 36 keratinocytes to which melanosomes are transferred. In melanocompetent individuals, there is a higher density of melanosomes, which are distributed as single large organelles (*A*), whereas in melanocompromised skin, melanosomes are smaller, occur as multiples in membrane-limited vesicles (melanosome complexes), and undergo gradual degradation (*B*).

Melanized epidermis acts as a shield for vulnerable cells of the epidermis and dermis, reducing the penetration of UVB and UVA radiation into the skin. There is an inverse relationship between melanin density of the skin and sun-induced skin damage: skin cancer and dermatoheliosis (photoaging). Melanin absorbs UVR, acts as a biologic electron exchange polymer, quenching free radicals that are generated by UVR, and preventing the inactivation of superoxide dismutase.[12] The protective role of melanin against skin cancer is the basis of the marked reduction in photoaging and skin cancer (basal cell carcinoma, squamous cell carcinoma, and malignant melanoma) in populations with high levels of constitutive melanin pigmentation such as SPTs IV, V, and VI. We call these *melanocompetent* in contrast to light SPTs I, II, and III that we call *melanocompromised.* Not only is there a higher melanin density in the melanocompetent but the melanosomes remain as single large organelles while in melanocompromised skin the melanosomes are smaller, occurring in membrane-limited vesicles and undergo gradual degradation into small, electron-dense particles (see Fig. 88-5); this aggregation in keratinocytes is related to the size of the melanosomes; small melanosomes are aggregated and large melanosomes that occur in heavily melanized skin are nonaggregated, and thus provide a better shield against penetration of ultraviolet.[13] Norlund et al.[14] recently produced a summary of the pigmentary system.

DIAGNOSIS OF MELANIN PIGMENTARY DISORDERS

Classification of Disorders of Melanin Pigmentation

There are three categories of melanin pigmentary disturbances: (1) hypomelanosis (*leukoderma,* white or lighter than the individual's normal color);[14] (2) brown hypermelanosis (*melanoderma*); and (3) gray, slate, or blue hypermelanosis (*ceruloderma*). Figure 88-6 provides a visual example of these and gives selected examples in certain general categories, based on the number of melanocytes and/or the amount of melanin.

Clinicopathologic Classification based on the Number of Melanocytes and/or the Amount of Melanin

(see also Chap. 90)

Hypomelanoses or leukodermas may be subdivided based on the increase, reduction, or absence of melanocytes and/or melanin. Vitiligo is an example of a *melanocytopenic* disorder in which melanocytes are absent. This stands in contrast to albinism, which is one of the *melanopenic* disorders, in which a normal number of melanocytes is present but the melanin content of melanosomes is reduced. Nonmelanotic disorders are those pigmentary aberrations in which melanin pigmentation is unaffected but rather the pigmentary abnormality is caused by a chromophore other than melanin (minocycline, chlorpromazine). Disorders of hyperpigmentation may be called *melanotic* when the number of melanocytes is normal but the amount of melanin is increased (e.g., Addison's disease, melasma), or *melanocytotic* when the number of melanocytes is increased (oculodermal melanocytosis nevus of Ota). The intent of this classification is to categorize the pigmentary disorders according to an increase or decrease of melanin or of melanocytes.

Diseases with alterations in melanin pigmentation are not as common as the most frequent skin disorders (e.g., acne, psoriasis, eczema, verrucae), so that physicians are generally less familiar with pigmentary disorders. Furthermore, many pigmentary disorders are difficult to identify, as the diagnosis requires specialized knowledge and the use of special techniques. In parts of the world where the majority of the indigenous population has brown or black skin, pigmentation disorders (especially vitiligo, melasma, and postinflammatory hyperpigmentation) are a major reason for seeking a dermatologic consultation.

Establishing the correct diagnosis requires a good history, a detailed physical examination, the use of special lighting techniques, and sometimes a biopsy of the abnormally pigmented skin as well as of the normally pigmented skin.

Clinical History in Diagnosis of Melanin Pigmentary Disorders

Variations in normal skin color often confound the recognition of melanin disorders; diffuse brown hypermelanosis in SPTs II or III may be fairer than diffuse hypopigmentation of SPTs V or VI (see Chap. 90). The intensity of coloration in the normal skin of a white person originating ethnically from one of the Mediterranean countries may be no different from that in abnormally pigmented skin of an Anglo-Saxon with Addison's disease. There are two clues, however, that suggest abnormal diffuse brown hypermelanosis: (1) change in the intensity of skin color and (2) the appearance, for the first time, of pigmentation in sites that are normally pigmented in some persons with dark brown or black skin, such as the axillae, the palmar creases, and, especially, the mucous membranes (buccal mucosa and gums). In addition, the patient may observe that his or her summer tan has not faded over the winter

FIGURE 88-6

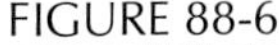

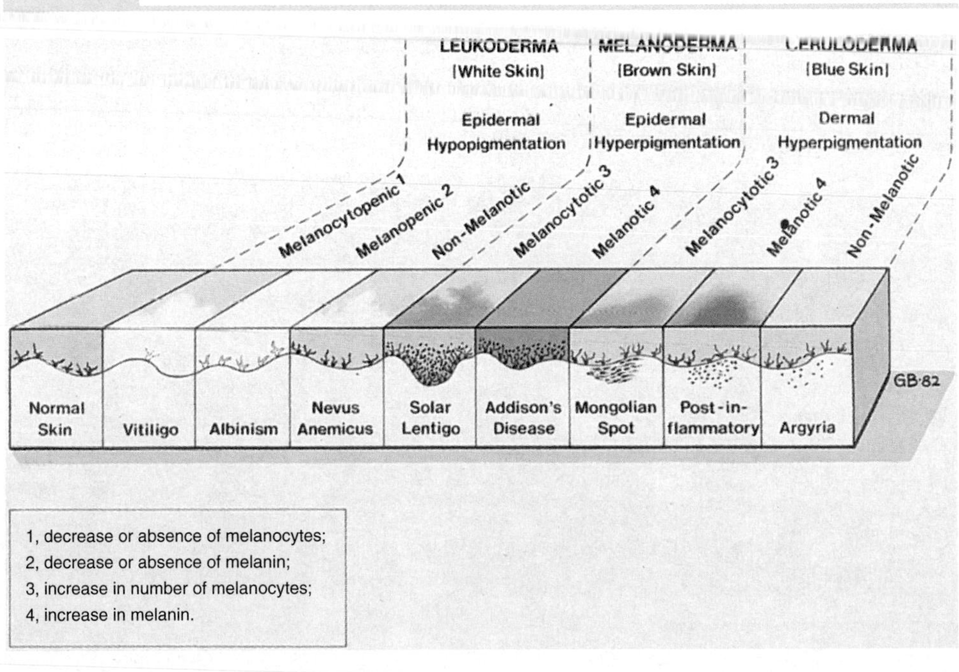

Clinicopathologic classification of pigmentary disorders.

FIGURE 88-7

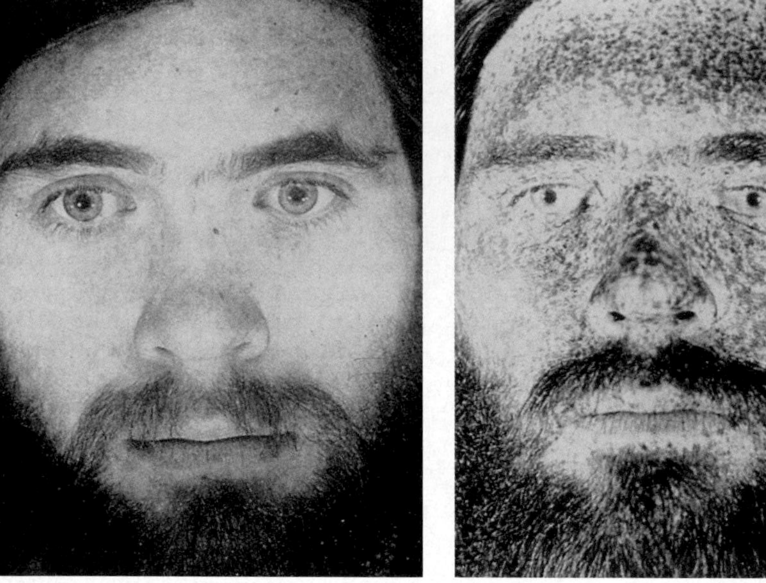

A. Photograph taken with conventional lighting. *B.* Accentuation of epidermal changes (freckling in this case) under examination with a Wood's lamp.

so that persons who see the patient only from time to time may observe that the skin has darkened abnormally. The determination of normal pigmentation involves consideration of many factors. This requires knowledge of the patient's basic or constitutive skin color. A certain degree of pigmentary dilution obvious in the darker-skinned white persons may not identifiable in the light-skinned white persons such as the Celtic people (Scotland, Ireland, Wales, Cornwall, French Briton). Proper assessment depends upon history and physical examination, often aided by established and newer auxiliary investigational techniques.

FIGURE 88-8

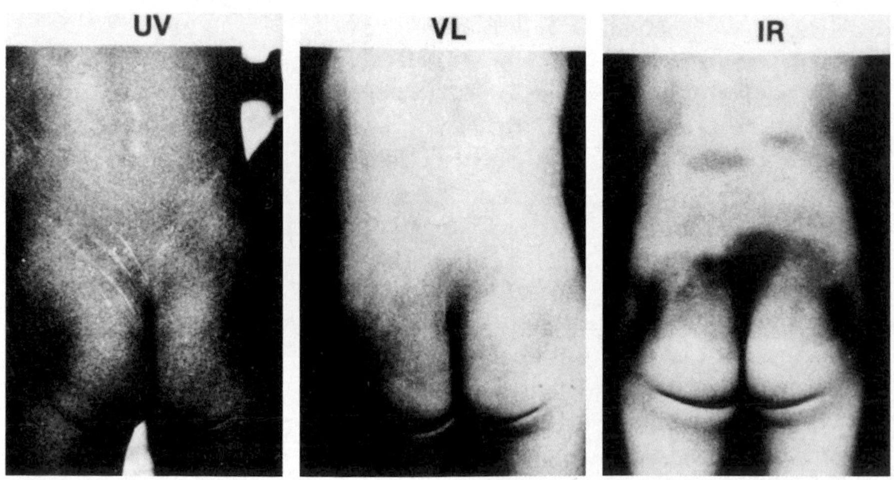

Infrared (IR) photography for dermal pigmentation. With dermal melanoses, there is no accentuation with UV light as compared to room or visible (VL) light; however, accentuation is apparent with special IR photography.

History of onset and evolution of the pigmentary change are also important. Are the lesions congenital, as in piebaldism or nevus depigmentosus, or are they acquired, as in vitiligo or hypomelanosis of Ito? Not all congenital pigmentary disorders, particularly hypomelanoses, are obvious at birth. In a fair-skinned child not exposed to sunlight in the first year or years of life, hypopigmented lesions, which are, in fact, congenital, may be thought to be acquired, inasmuch as a white infant born in the late fall may not become tanned for at least a year. For example, the white macules in tuberous sclerosis may not be apparent until the skin is tanned after sun exposure, providing contrast between normal tanned skin and the hypomelanotic macule.

Physical Examination in Diagnosis of Melanin Pigmentary Disorders

(See Chap. 90)

In examination of the skin for hypo- or hyperpigmented macules, it is helpful to view the patient in a slightly darkened room in order to accentuate the contrast. Furthermore, it is important that the examiner take the few moments required to become dark adapted.

Distribution of lesions may be useful; vitiligo and piebaldism have typical distribution patterns. Furthermore, segmental or dermatomal distribution of hypomelanosis suggests segmental vitiligo, nevus depigmentosus, or, rarely, tuberous sclerosis. The *size* of lesions may be useful, as very small or confetti macules, for example, may occur with chemical leukoderma, tuberous sclerosis, tinea versicolor, vitiligo, or idiopathic guttate hypomelanosis. The presence of sharp, discrete margins in vitiligo macules distinguishes vitiligo from pityriasis alba and postinflammatory hypermelanosis. *Scales* on white lesions, although minimal in pityriasis alba and in tinea versicolor, may be a clue to the disease. History of an antecedent or concomitant eruption may suggest a postinflammatory hyper- or hypomelanosis. The presence of other cutaneous abnormalities, such as a shagreen patch and adenoma sebaceum in a patient with the typical lance-ovate hypomelanotic macules of tuberous sclerosis, may provide additional clues. In patients from areas with endemic leprosy, including the southern United States, all hypomelanotic macules should be tested for hypesthesia.

Diagnosis of more diffuse and widespread, ill-defined melanin disorders may be particularly difficult. The patient with Addison's disease may be unaware of the pigment darkening, especially of axillae, palmar creases, may only complain that their summer tan did not fade.

The Wood's Light in Diagnosis of Melanin Pigmentary Disorders

The use of the Wood's lamp facilitates diagnosis of epidermal pigmentary disorders because it helps to define the extent and level (dermal or epidermal) of the pigmentary change (Fig. 88-7). Hypomelanoses appear whiter;

TABLE 88-2

Investigation of Melanin Pigmentary Disorders

I. Clinical aspects
  A. History
    1. Onset of lesion, or first appearance (at birth, infancy, or later in life)
    2. Relation to season, exposure to sunlight or ultraviolet radiation, drug ingestion, occupation
    3. Constitutional symptoms: "chronic illness" syndrome (malaise, weight loss, weakness)
    4. Systems review
    5. Family history (especially for genetic disorders, piebaldism, neurofibromatosis, tuberous sclerosis, etc.)
  B. Physical examination
    1. Type of lesion
       Usually macule with brown or blue color, or loss of color (leukoderma). Check for anesthesia in white macules. If generalized, can be brown or blue color, or loss of color (leukoderma).
    2. Shape of individual lesions
       Ash leaf and confetti macules in tuberous sclerosis; isomorphic phenomenon in vitiligo
    3. Arrangement of multiple lesions
       Linear or segmented lesions in nevus depigmentosus
    4. Distribution pattern
       Dermatomal pattern in tuberous sclerosis and nevus depigmentosus; symmetric in vitiligo; characteristic sites of involvement in vitiligo, melasma, Addison's disease.
  C. Special clinical aids
    1. Magnification with hand lens (7 to 10×)
    2. Illumination
       a. Oblique lighting (to detect depression or elevation of lesions, e.g., morphea)
       b. Subdued lighting (important for better visualization of both hyperpigmented and hypopigmented macules; accentuates the contrast)
       c. Wood's lamp (in a totally dark room, wait for dark adaptation)
    3. Epiluminescence skin microscopy
       The epiluminescence microscope, called a dermatoscope, uses wide-field objective lenses with a focal distance of 10 to 15 cm. For routine observations 10 × magnification is sufficient. The lower epidermis and dermis can be examined by applying oil to the skin surface and then applying a glass slide for compression to make the stratum corneum transparent. The dermatoscope can be equipped with a camera for documentation purposes or incorporated into a computer system, which allows for digitalization of images obtained and for storage and retrieval of data for purposes of comparison. Patterns of epidermal–dermal pigmentation can be readily visualized, and irregular patterns are seen in dysplastic nevi, primary malignant melanoma, pigmented basal cell carcinoma, etc. (see Chaps. 92 and 93).

II. Histologic aspects
  A. Hematoxylin and eosin (H&E). In H&E-stained sections there may be no evidence of melanin or melanocytes. For the study of cutaneous pigmentation, there are two techniques of value: the "dopa reaction" and the silver stain. Upon staining with H&E, melanocytes are seen as "clear" cells resulting from shrinkage of the cytoplasm (a fixation artifact), whereas upon staining with silver or dopa, they appear as dendritic cells wedged between the basal cells of the epidermis.
  B. Dopa reaction requires fresh tissue with partial fixation in 5% formaldehyde for 45 min and is done by soaking thin sections of skin in a solution of 3,4-dihydroxyphenylalanine (dopa). Melanocytes stain dark because the tyrosinase enzyme they contain converts the colorless dopa into dopa melanin
  C. Silver stains demonstrate the presence of melanin, via their (1) argyrophilic and (2) argentaffin properties.
    1. Silver nitrate binds to melanin and, upon reduction, stains black.
    2. The Masson-Fontana stain, using ammoniate silver nitrate, leads to the release of black silver when the phenolic groups present in the melanin reduce the silver salt. Stains melanin in keratinocytes and melanocytes.
    3. Immunochemical stains for melanocytes
       a. S100-sensitive but not specific; also stains Langerhans cells, dermal dendrocytes, and nerves.
       b. HMB 45 is less sensitive but more specific than S100.
       c. Mart-1 is more specific than HMB 45 and very specific for melanocytes. Some adrenal tumors have been found to stain positively; thus, it is not absolutely specific if evaluating a metastatic tumor.

III. Specialized laboratory methods
  A. Split dopa histochemical technique. To count the melanocytes per millimeter or to study the perikaryon and dendrites of the melanocytes, whole mounts of the epidermis are prepared by obtaining a small split-skin graft and separating the epidermis from the dermis by sodium bromide. The epidermal sheet is incubated in a dopa solution and mounted afterwards on a microscopic slide. Unlike Masson-Fontana stains, this is specific for melanocyte.
  B. Electron microscopy
    1. Standard section to enumerate melanosomal characteristics or number per dendrite as in tuberous sclerosis.
    2. Transmission electron microscopy using ultrathin sections and freeze-fracture replicas; x-ray microanalysis which demonstrates elements (e.g., copper) by the measurement of energy dispersion in the electron microscope.
    3. Scanning electron microscopy.
  C. Cell culture methods to study the behavior, proliferation, and cell surface receptors of melanocytes in culture are now available. Also, functional studies concerning the susceptibility of melanocytes to external stimuli (e.g., UV radiation, hormones and drugs) can be performed with these culture techniques.
  D. Physical methods
    1. Spectrophotometry
    2. Electron spin resonance (ESR) signal analysis

epidermal hypermelanoses become accentuated, but dermal melanoses (which in visible light can be brown, gray, or blue) are not enhanced and, in fact, may become less apparent. Furthermore, Wood's lamp examination facilitates distinction of melanocytopenic disorders that are amelanotic (such as vitiligo or piebaldism) from melanopenic macules that are off-white to tan, as found in tuberous sclerosis, pityriasis alba, or postinflammatory hypomelanosis. To use the Wood's light in assessing hypermelanoses, it is useful to *first* grade the hyperpigmentation in visible light, and then to estimate the grade of pigmentary change under the Wood's lamp. A café au lait macule or ephelide will be graded 2 in visible light but will increase to grade 3 under the Wood's lamp (Fig. 88-7); by contrast, a Mongolian spot will be grade 2 in visible light and will remain grade 2 or less with the Wood's lamp (Fig. 88-8). The use of infrared film makes it possible to detect whether the pigmentation is dermal. An important caveat is that this technique is not useful in persons with brown skin because of optical factors that vitiate dermal melanin. Because this technique requires the use of a camera and special equipment, it is not as practical as the Wood's lamp.

Histology and Transmission Electron Microscopy as Diagnostic Tools (See Table 88-2)

Histologic study provides several levels of information. Standard hematoxylin and eosin (H&E) preparations may confirm the presence or absence of melanocytes; it is also possible to assess the amount of pigment that has been transferred to the keratinocytes and thereby to identify the "transfer-block" hypomelanoses. Split-dopa preparations are used to count the number of melanocytes. The dopa histochemical test also provides information about the number, size, and dendritic quality of identifiable melanocytes. Study of abnormalities of the melanin pathway is facilitated with the electron microscope. Some melanin disturbances have typical if not characteristic electron microscopic features. For example, melanin pigmentary disorders may result from or be associated with (1) decreased or absent melanocytes (vitiligo), (2) abnormal formation or melanization of melanosomes (as in albinism), or (3) failure of transfer of melanosomes from melanocytes to keratinocytes (eczematous dermatitis).

REFERENCES

1. Holubar K, Schmidt C: *Sun and Skin.* Vienna, Verlag der Osterreichischen Ärztekammer, 1994, p 47
2. Fitzpatrick TB: Soleil et peau. *J Med Esthet* **2**:33, 1975
3. Pathak MA, Fitzpatrick TB: Preventative treatment of sunburn, dermatoheliosis and skin cancer with sun-protective agents, in *Dermatology in General Medicine,* 4th ed, edited by TB Fitzpatrick, AZ Eisen, K Wolff, IM Freedberg, KF Austen. New York, McGraw Hill, 1993, p 1689
4. De Leeuw SM, et al: Melanin content of cultured human melanocytes and UV-induced cytotoxicity. *J Photochem Photobiol B* **61**:106, 2001
5. Parrish JA et al: Erythema and melanogenesis action spectrum of normal human skin. *Photochem Photobiol* **36**:187, 1982
6. Flanagan N et al: Pleiotropic effects of the melanocortin 1 receptor (MC1R) gene on human pigmentation. *Hum Mol Genet* **9**:2531, 2000
7. Rees JL: The melanocortin 1 receptor (MC1R): More than just red hair. *Pig Cell Res* **13**:135, 2000
8. Tsatmali M et al: Skin POMC peptides: Their actions at the human MC-1 receptor and roles in the tanning response. *Pig Cell Res* **13:**125, 2000
9. Bastiaens M et al: The melanocortin-1-receptor gene is the major freckle gene *J Hum Mol Genet,* **10:**1701, 2001
10. Quevedo et al: Role of light in human skin color variation. *Am J Phys Anthropol* **43:**393, 1975
11. Jablonski NG, Chaplin G: The evolution of human coloration. *J Hum Evol* **39:**57, 2000
12. Pathak MA: Functions of melanin and photoprotection by melanin in melanin: Its role in human photoprotection, in *Melanin Its Role in Human Photoprotection,* edited by L Zeise, MR Chedekel, TB Fitzpatrick. Overland Park, KS, Valdenmar Publishing, 1995, p 125
13. Wolff K et al: Experimental pigment donation in vivo. *J Ultrastruct Res* **47**:400, 1974
14. Nordlund JJ et al: *The Pigmentary System.* New York, Oxford University Press, 1998, p 1025

CHAPTER 89

Philippe Bahadoran
Jean-Paul Ortonne
Richard A. King
William S. Oetting

Albinism

Albinism refers to genetic abnormalities of melanin synthesis associated with a normal number and structure of melanocytes.[1,2] Reduced melanin synthesis in the melanocytes of the skin, hair, and eyes is termed *oculocutaneous albinism* (OCA), and hypopigmentation primarily involving the retinal pigment epithelium of the eyes is termed *ocular albinism* (OA).[1] The precise definition of albinism includes specific changes in the development and function of the eyes and the optic nerves, and the ocular changes are necessary to make the diagnosis.[3] Changes in the auditory system are also found in the brain in albinism, but they produce no hearing loss.[4] A generalized reduction in skin pigment without ocular changes should be referred to as *cutaneous hypopigmentation* rather than albinism or cutaneous albinism.

The characteristic changes in the development and function of the eyes and optic nerves, common to all types of OCA and OA, include nystagmus,[3] reduced melanin in the retinal pigment epithelium associated with foveal hypoplasia, reduced visual acuity, and misrouting of the optic nerves at the chiasm[3,5] (Table 89-1). These ocular changes are present only in individuals with albinism with one exception. In X-linked OA, 80 to 90 percent of obligate female heterozygotes without skin changes do have observable changes in ocular pigment that are related to X-chromosome inactivation.[6]

OCULOCUTANEOUS ALBINISM

Classification of Albinism

Classification of OCA should be based on the genetic locus involved. Indeed, there is a range of phenotypes of OCA associated with mutations at each of the responsible loci. On the other hand, mutations at different loci can result in closely related, if not similar, phenotypes. This classification will be used in this chapter and is summarized in Tables 89-2 and 89-3.

Inheritance of OCA

All types of OCA characterized to date are autosomal recessive in inheritance. There are no phenotypic changes with obligate heterozygotes except as noted earlier. Rare families with OCA having dominant inheritance have been described. X-linked OA is produced by mutations of a gene on the short arm of the X chromosome.

Prevalence of OCA

Oculocutaneous albinism is the most common inherited disorder of generalized hypopigmentation, with an estimated frequency of 1:20,000 in most populations.[1] Four different types of OCA have been described up to now. OCA1 and OCA2 are the most frequent types and account for approximately 40 and 50 percent, respectively, of OCA worldwide. OCA3 and OCA4 are far less frequent.

Oculocutaneous Albinism Type 1

Oculocutaneous albinism type 1 (OCA1; MIM 203100), one of the two most common types of albinism, is produced by loss of function of the melanocytic enzyme tyrosinase resulting from mutations of the *TYR* gene. Classic OCA, with a total absence of melanin in the skin, hair, and eyes, is the most obvious type of OCA1, but the spectrum of OCA1 is broad and includes the development of moderate to nearly normal amounts of cutaneous melanin over time (Fig. 89-1). Null mutations are associated with a total loss of function and no pigment formation (OCA1A), whereas "leaky" mutations result in an enzyme that retains some function and is associated with some pigment formation (OCA1B). Most individuals affected with a type of OCA1 have white hair, milky white skin, and blue eyes at birth, and this helps distinguish this type from other OCA types.

OCA1 PHENOTYPES (See Table 89-2)

OCA1A In OCA1A, or the classic tyrosinase-negative OCA, there is a complete inability to synthesize melanin in skin, hair, and eyes, resulting in the characteristic "albino" phenotype. Affected individuals are born with white hair and skin and blue eyes, and there are no changes as they mature.[2] The phenotype is the same in all ethnic groups and at all ages (Fig. 89-2). The hair may develop a slight yellow tint due to denaturing of the hair protein related to sun exposure and/or shampoo

TABLE 89-1

Ocular System Changes in Albinism

Reduction in iris pigment
Reduction in retinal pigment
Foveal hypoplasia
Misrouting of the optic fibers at the chiasm
Nystagmus
Alternating strabismus

TABLE 89-2

Classification of Albinism: Clinical Phenotypes

Type	Subtypes	Clinical Phenotypes
OCA1	OCA1A	Tyrosinase-negative OCA
	OCA1B	Minimal pigment OCA
		Platinum OCA
		Yellow OCA
		Temperature-sensitive OCA
		Autosomal recessive OA (some)
OCA2		Tyrosinase-positive OCA
		Brown OCA (most cases)
		Autosomal recessive OA (some)
		Prader-Willi's and Angelman's syndromes
OCA3		Rufous/red OCA
		Brown OCA (one case)
OCA4		
HPS	HPS1	Hermansky-Pudlak syndrome
	HPS2	
	HPS3	
	HPS4	
CHS		Chediak-Higashi syndrome
OA1		X-linked OA, Nettleship-Falls type

ABBREVIATIONS: OCA: oculocutaneous albinism; OA: ocular albinism.

use. The irides are translucent, appear pink early in life, and often turn a gray-blue color with time. No pigmented lesions develop in the skin, although amelanotic nevi can be present. The architecture of skin and hair bulb melanocytes is normal. The melanosomes show a normal surrounding membrane and normal internal matrix formation (stage I and II premelanosomes) (see Chap. 11).

OCA1B The OCA1B phenotype is produced by mutations that result in an enzyme that retains some function. The variation in the phenotype of OCA1B can be from minimal hair pigment to near-normal skin and hair pigment.[5] Mutations coding for enzyme with differing amounts of residual activity are the primary cause of this variation, and a moderate amount of residual activity can lead to near-normal cutaneous pigmentation and the mistaken diagnosis of OA.

The original OCA1B phenotype was called "yellow albinism" because the affected individuals had this hair color. The hair color is the result of pheomelanin synthesis. OCA1B includes several previously described OCA types, including minimal-pigment OCA,[7] platinum OCA,[2] temperature-sensitive OCA,[8] and autosomal recessive ocular albinism (AROA).

Most individuals with OCA1B have very little or no pigment at birth and develop varying amounts of melanin in the hair and skin in the first or second decade of life (see Fig. 89-1 and 89-3). In some cases the melanin develops within the first year. The hair color changes to light yellow, light blond, or golden blond first and eventually can turn dark blond or brown in adolescents and adults. The irides can develop light-tan or brown pigment, sometimes limited to the inner third of the iris, and iris pigment can be present on globe transillumination. Some degree of iris translucency, as demonstrated by slit-lamp examination, is usually present. Many individuals with OCA1B will tan with sun exposure, although it is more common to burn without tanning. Pigmented lesions (nevi, freckles, lentigines) develop in the skin of individuals who have developed pigmented hair and skin.

One of the more interesting variations of OCA1B is the temperature-sensitive phenotype.[8] Scalp hair color is white at birth and remains white or slightly yellow. Axillary hair remains white, whereas arm and leg hair pigments. The skin remains white and does not tan. Analysis of

FIGURE 89-1

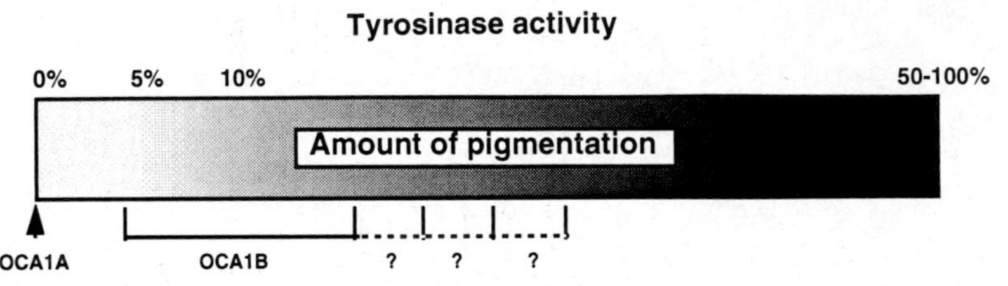

Pigment spectrum in OCA1 related to tyrosinase gene mutations that are associated with different amounts of residual enzyme function.

tyrosinase from scalp and leg hair bulbs of the originally described proband showed that the enzyme was temperature-sensitive, losing activity above 35°C.[8] As a result, melanin synthesis occurred in the cooler but not the warmer areas of the body, such as the arms and legs, in a pattern similar to the Siamese cat and the Himalayan mouse.

MOLECULAR PATHOGENESIS OF OCA1 (See Table 89-3) Analyses of DNA from individuals with OCA1A have shown a large number of different mutations in the *TYR* gene. These mutations include missense, nonsense, frameshift, splice site, and deletion mutations.[5,9,10] Most individuals with OCA1 are compound heterozygotes with different mutant maternal and paternal alleles. Missense mutations in the *TYR* gene are distributed into four clusters of the coding region, suggesting functional domains of the encoded protein. Two of the clusters are in the copper-binding regions, a third cluster is 3′ of the copper B–binding region, and a fourth cluster is near the amino-terminus of the protein. Missense mutations in the copper-binding regions would be expected to cause hypopigmentation through impairment or loss of enzymatic activity of tyrosinase.[9,10] Frameshift mutations have been identified in OCA1, and analysis of the flanking sequences shows that these mutations tend to occur in repetitive sequences, as in other mammalian genes. The identified frameshift mutations lead to a premature stop codon, and the abnormal protein would be expected to have reduced stability, altered processing, or loss of enzyme function.[9,10]

Recently it was shown that different types of mutant tyrosinase, including deletion mutants that destroy catalytic function, and missense mutants that have a temperature-sensitive phenotype, were retained and degradated in the endoplasmic reticulum compartment. This suggests that regardless of the type of mutation, most *TYR* gene mutants may not be transported properly to melanosomes.[11–13] Considering the large variety of *TYR* gene mutations observed in OCA1, more work is required to assess the relative, contribution of the aforementioned mechanisms, e.g., loss of enzymatic activity or lack of transport to melanosomes, in the genesis of hypopigmentation in OCA1.

Oculocutaneous Albinism Type 2

Individuals with albinism who have pigmented hair and eyes have long been identified, particularly in the African and African American populations, and have been described with a variety of terms such as *partial albinism, incomplete albinism,* or *imperfect albinism.*[14] The identification of mutations of the *P* gene in humans has now provided a molecular basis of this type of albinism, which is called *oculocutaneous albinism type 2* (OCA2; MIM 203200).[15,16] From the standpoint of melanin synthesis, the defect in OCA2 appears to involve a reduction in eumelanin synthesis primarily, with less effect on pheomelanin synthesis.[17] OCA2 is the most common type of OCA in the world primarily because of its high frequency in equatorial Africa.[18,19] OCA2 has been described in most populations.

OCA2 PHENOTYPES (See also Table 89-2) In Caucasian individuals, the amount of hair pigment present at birth or developing with time varies from minimal in northern Europeans (particularly Scandinavians) to moderate in southern European or Mediterranean individuals. The hair can be very lightly pigmented at birth, having a light yellow or blond color, or more pigmented with a definite blond, golden blond, or even red color. Furthermore, the normal delayed maturation of the pigment system and sparse hair early in life in many normally pigmented northern European individuals (i.e., very blond children who develop dark blond or brown hair with maturation) can make the distinction between OCA1 and OCA2 difficult in the first few months of life. Many such persons would not be recognized as having albinism if the visual changes were absent.

The skin is creamy white and does not tan. The iris color is blue-gray or lighted pigmented, and the amount of translucency correlates

FIGURE 89-2

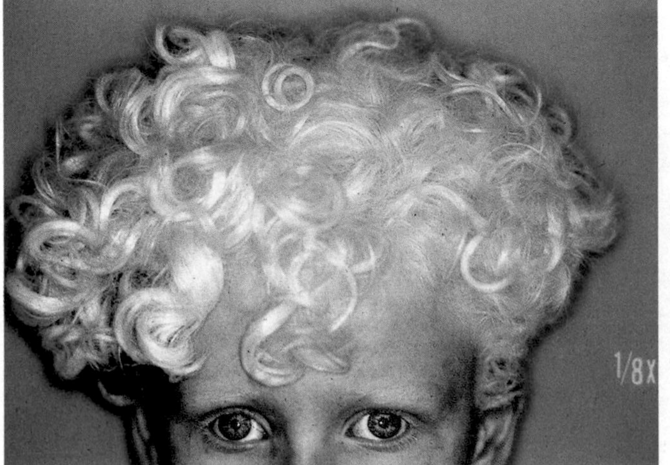

OCA1A with no hair or skin pigment, demonstrating iris translucency.

FIGURE 89-3

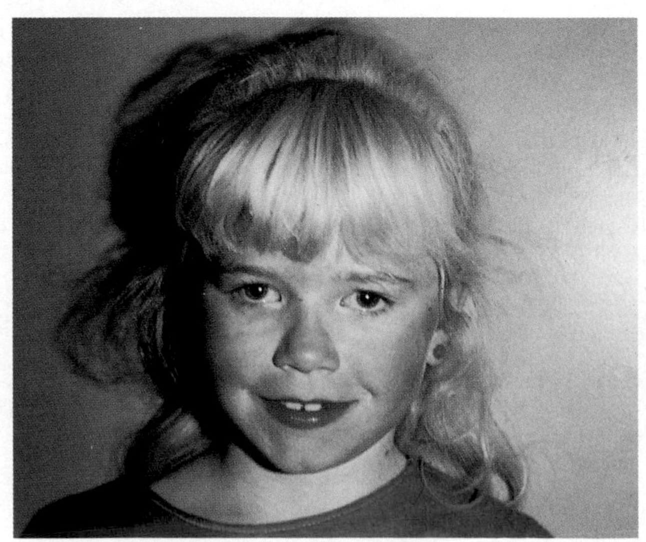

OCA1B with golden blond scalp hair and tan.

FIGURE 89-4

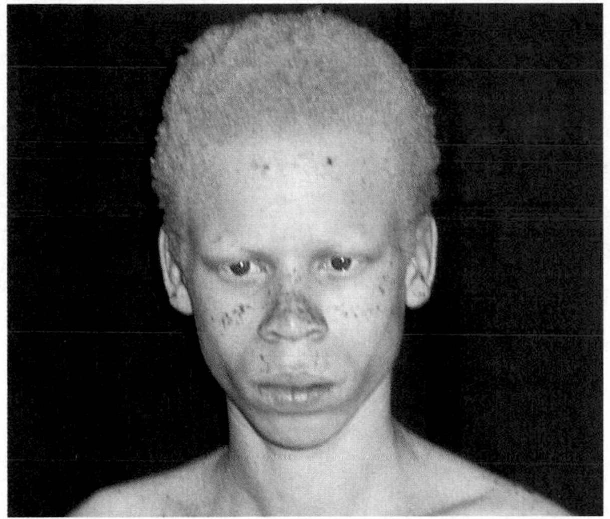

OCA2 with yellow hair, white skin, and freckles in an African individual (classic tyrosinase-positive OCA phenotype).

with the development of iris pigment. With time, pigmented nevi and lentigines may develop, and pigmented freckles are seen in areas with repeated sun exposure. The hair in Caucasian individuals may slowly turn darker through the first two or more decades of life.

In African and African American individuals, there is a distinct OCA2 phenotype[14,18] (Fig. 89-4). Hair is yellow at birth and remains so throughout life, although the color may turn darker. Hair color can turn lighter in older individuals, and this probably represents the normal graying with age. The skin is creamy white at birth and changes little with time. No generalized skin pigment is present, and no tan develops with sun exposure, but pigmented nevi, lentigines, and freckles often develop. The irides are blue-gray or lightly pigmented. This phenotype may be related to the existence of a single common deletion mutation of the *P* gene in Africans and African Americans with OCA2.[14,18,19] The development of lentigines or ephelides, well-demarcated pigmented patches usually on sun-exposed areas of the skin, may be evidence of a separate genetic susceptibility because these lesions only develop in some OCA2 families and not in others. The presence of ephelides is associated with a lower risk of skin cancer in South African individuals.

BROWN OCA Brown OCA has been described in the African and African American populations in which the amount of eumelanin in the skin and hair is reduced but not absent.[20] Recent studies have shown that brown OCA is associated with heterozygosity for *P* gene alleles, one of which is null and the other having partial function.[19,21]

In African and African American individuals with the brown OCA phenotype, the hair and skin color are light brown and the irides are gray to tan at birth[19,21] (Fig. 89-5). With time, there is little change is skin color, but the hair may turn darker, and the irides may accumulate more tan pigment. The skin generally does not burn but may darken with sun exposure. Affected individuals are recognized as having albinism rather than a variation in normal pigmentation because of the ocular changes present. The iris has punctate and radial translucency, and moderate retinal pigment is present. Visual acuity ranges from 20/60 to 20/150. The brown OCA phenotype has not been described in Caucasian individuals and is most likely part of the OCA2 phenotypic range that is being recognized.

PRADER-WILLI'S AND ANGELMAN'S SYNDROMES While it is clear that the *P* gene is not involved directly in these syndromes, Prader-Willi's and Angelman's syndromes often are associated with hypopigmentation, and this appears to be related to OCA2 and the *P* gene, at least to a certain extent.

FIGURE 89-5

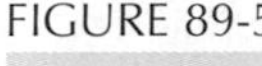

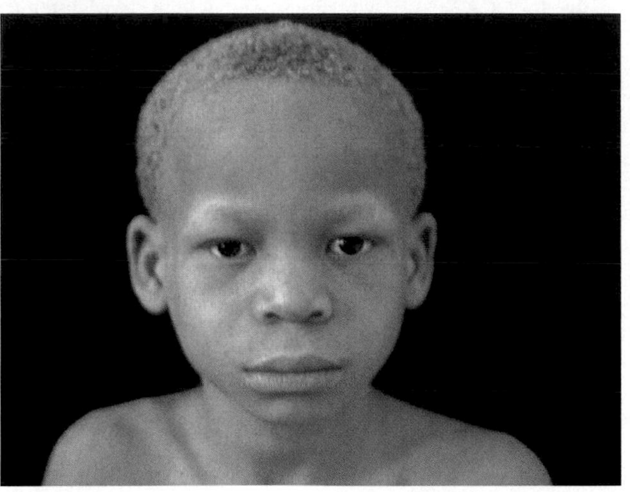

OCA2 with brown hair and skin in an African individual (brown OCA phenotype).

Prader-Willi's syndrome Prader-Willi's syndrome is a developmental syndrome that includes neonatal hypotonia, hyperphagia and obesity, hypogonadism, small hands and feet, and mental retardation associated with characteristic behavior. Approximately 70 percent of individuals with Prader-Willi's syndrome have an interstitial deletion on the long arm of the paternal chromosome 15, and most of those without a deletion of the paternal chromosome 15 have uniparental disomy for the maternal chromosome.

Many individuals with Prader-Willi's syndrome are hypopigmented but do not have the typical ocular features of albinism[23]; however, individuals with Prader-Willi's syndrome can have typical features of OCA.[24,25] For those without OCA, the hypopigmentation is characterized by having hair and skin that are lighter than unaffected family members. Childhood nystagmus and strabismus are common but often do not persist into adult life. The irides are pigmented with some translucency on globe transillumination, and retinal pigment is reduced in amount. Foveal hypoplasia usually is not present, but the fovea may not appear entirely normal.[26] Visual evoked potential studies have revealed optic tract misrouting similar to that found in albinism in some individuals with Prader-Willi's syndrome and hypopigmentation,[26] but this is not a universal finding. Some individuals with Prader-Willi's syndrome have typical OCA2 with cutaneous hypopigmentation and all ocular features of albinism.[15,24]

Angelman's syndrome Angelman's syndrome is a complex developmental disorder with developmental delay and severe mental retardation, microcephaly, neonatal hypotonia, ataxic movements, and inappropriate laughter. Approximately 70 percent of individuals with Angelman's syndrome have an interstitial deletion of the long arm of the maternal chromosome 15. Many without a deletion have uniparental disomy for the paternal chromosome 15.

In Angelman's syndrome, the hypopigmentation is characterized by light skin and hair.[22] Nystagmus or strabismus may be present early in life, and iris translucency and reduced retinal pigment may be present. No analysis of optic nerve formation is available. As in Prader-Willi's syndrome, individuals with Angelman's syndrome who have typical OCA2 features have been described.[19]

MOLECULAR PATHOGENESIS OF OCA2 (See also Table 89-3) Mutations of the *P* gene, which maps to chromosome 15q, are responsible for OCA2.[16,19,25] Mutations of mouse pink-eyed dilution (*p*) gene, the murine homologue of the human *P* gene, result in hypopigmentation of the coat and the eyes, and many alleles have been identified at this locus. As expected, a number of mutations of the human *P* gene are associated with human OCA2.[15,19,24,27]

In sub-Saharan Africa, a single 2.7-kb deletion allele accounts for 60 to 90 percent of mutant *P* alleles and is associated with a common haplotype, suggesting a common founder. It has been estimated that this single mutation is associated with 25 to 50 percent of all mutant *P* alleles in African Americans. However, other diverse mutant alleles have been described in this population and in Africans. In an American group with African heritage, the Brandywine, Maryland isolate, 1 in 85 individuals has OCA2 and is homozygous for the 2.7-kb deletion allele of the *P* gene. Thus it is likely that this 2.7-kb deletion allele accounts for the distinct OCA2 phenotype in Africans and African Americans.[19]

OCA2 also has been reported at high frequencies in specific Native American groups. Individuals within this population presumably have mutations in the *P* gene. However, it cannot be excluded that mutations in another gene lead to a similar phenotype in individuals and groups for which no molecular data are yet available. Many diverse mutations in the *P* gene have been reported in individuals with OCA2 from diverse ethnic backgrounds. The missense mutations described to date in the *P* gene do not seem to cluster in any specific region, as observed for tyrosinase.[19]

A model system in which to test for *P* allele function has been described. The assay for this system is complementation of the hypopigmentation of *P* mutant melanocytes by the expression of a transfected copy of the human *P* gene. A normal *P* gene restores pigmentation, whereas the expression of a transfected copy of an OCA2 allele does not.[28]

There has been considerable progress in the last few years in understanding of the *P* gene product function. It was suggested, based on the observation that melanocytes from mice lacking expression of the p protein pigmented in the presence of high concentrations of tyrosine, that the p protein may play a role in tyrosine transport. However, it has been demonstrated clearly that tyrosine transport is normal in *P* mutant melanocytes. These data, though apparently conflicting, are consistent with the possibility that the p protein mediates conditions favorable for tyrosinase activity. Recently it has been shown that melanosomes from p protein–deficient melanocytes have an abnormal pH. Melanosomes in cultured melanocytes derived from wild-type mice are typically acidic, whereas melanosomes from p protein–deficient mice are nonacidic. In light of these observations, it is likely that the p protein regulates the acidic pH of melanosomes. Whether or not acidic conditions directly enhance tyrosinase activity in mammalian melanosomes in vivo is still an open question. An alternate possibility is that the acidic conditions mediated by the p protein favor the normal biogenesis of melanosomes, including the correct targeting of other melanosomal proteins such as tyrosinase.[19]

The mechanism for the hypopigmentation in Prader-Willi's and Angelman's syndromes has not been fully explained. Most patients who are hemizygous for the *P* gene in the context of a large deletion of 15q are hypopigmented regardless of their remaining *P* gene allele.[19,20] These observations are difficult to resolve with the recessive nature of both human *P* and mouse *p* mutations. Thus hypopigmentation in hemizygous Prader-Willi's or Angelman's syndrome may reflect the presence of other genetic determinants of pigmentation in the chromosome 15 region of the *P* gene rather than an altered maternal *P* allele. Further analysis of this phenomenon will be easier now that the function of the gene product of the *P* locus is being determined.

Patients with Prader-Willi's syndrome or Angelman's syndrome truly associated with OCA2 have been found to have a typical deletion of one homologue of the *P* gene in the context of Prader-Willi's syndrome or Angelman's syndrome and inheritance of a mutation on the another homologue, making them compound heterozygotes for *P* gene mutations, which result in their albinism.[19]

AUTOSOMAL RECESSIVE OCULAR ALBINISM Families in which male and female children of normally pigmented parents had the ocular features of albinism but did not appear to have significant cutaneous hypopigmentation were identified as having AROA. It now appears that the designation AROA is not correct. The affected individuals may have nearly normal cutaneous pigmentation, but their albinism is associated with mutations of the *tyrosinase* or *P* genes and actually represents part of the spectrum of OCA1B and OCA2 (see Table 89-2).

Oculocutaneous Albinism Type 3

The human phenotypic variations associated with genetic alterations of the *TYRP1* gene, which encodes tyrosinase-related protein 1, have been identified. Individuals with oculocutaneous albinism type 3 (OCA3; MIM 203290) present with minimal pigment reduction in the skin, hair, and eyes. This form of albinism was referred to previously as rufous and possibly some forms of brown albinism. The function of Tyrp1 in the human melanocyte is not well characterized yet.

OCA3 PHENOTYPES (See also Table 89-2) An African-American newborn twin boy with a mutation of the *TYRP1* gene had light brown skin, light brown hair, and blue/gray irides, whereas his fraternal twin brother had normal pigmentation.[30] The affected twin also had nystagmus, and the clinical presentation of this patient was felt to be consistent with brown OCA. Melanocyte cultures from the patient had only 7 percent of the amount of insoluble melanin as a result of compromised tyrosinase activity.[30] This family was lost to follow-up, so the ultimate phenotype of the affected child was unknown. Meanwhile, it has been shown that brown-African OCA is a subtype of OCA2. Thus the aforementioned patient represents the brown OCA phenotype classified under OCA3.

Mutations of the *TYRP1* gene also were found in a substantial number of individuals with rufous OCA in the South African population.[31,32] The rufous OCA phenotype in South African individuals includes red or reddish brown skin, ginger or reddish hair, and hazel or brown irides.[33] The ocular changes are not always present, and many do not have iris translucency, nystagmus, strabismus, or foveal hypoplasia. Furthermore, no misrouting of the optic nerves has been demonstrated by a visual evoked potential, suggesting either that this is not a true type of albinism, as strictly defined in this chapter, or that the hypopigmentation is not sufficient to consistently alter optic nerve development.[33] Hair bulb and skin melanocytes show eumelanosomes and pheomelanosomes in various stages of melanization. This is consistent with the red color coming from pheomelanin synthesis, since pheomelanosomes are absent in normally pigmented black skin and hair bulbs.[33] The described phenotype in New Guinea includes reddish brown skin, deep mahogany hair, reddish brown to brown irides with some translucency, and normal retinal pigment and foveal development.[34] Congenital nystagmus is present in this population but does not segregate specifically with the red phenotype. The phenotype for *TYRP1*-related OCA in the Caucasian and the Asian populations is unknown.

MOLECULAR PATHOGENESIS OF OCA3 (See also Table 89–3) The *TYRP1* gene was mapped to chromosome 9p. The first *TYRP1* gene mutation, identified both in the twin boy described as having brown OCA and in South African individuals with rufous OCA, was a single-base deletion at codon 368 (1104delA) producing a frameshift and a premature stop codon in exon 6 and a slightly truncated TYRP1 molecule. The second *TYRP1* mutation, identified in the rufous OCA

TABLE 89-3

Classification of Albinism: Genetic Loci

Disease	Chromosome	Gene Focus	Protein	Murine Locus
Oculocutaneous albinism type 1	11q21	*TYR*	Tyrosinase (TYR)	*albino (c)*
Oculocutaneous albinism type 2	15q11.2–q12	*P*	Pink protein (P)	*pink eyed dilution (p)*
Oculocutaneous albinism type 3	9p23	*TYRP1*	Tyrosinase-related protein1 (TYRP1)	*brown (b)*
Oculocutaneous albinism type 4	5p	*MATP*	Membrane-associated transporter protein (MATP)	*underwhite (uw)*
Hermansky-Pudlak syndromes				
Type 1	10q24	*HPS1*	?	*pale-ear (ep)*
Type 2	15q15	*AP3B1*	Beta-3 subunit of adaptor protein 3 complex (AP3B1)	*pearl (pe)*
Type 3	3q24	*HPS3*	?	*cocoa (coa)*
Type 4	?	*HPS4*	?	*light-ear (le)*
Chediak-Higashi syndrome	1q43	*LYST*	Lysosome trafficking (LYST)	*beige (bg)*

population, was a single-base substitution at codon 166 (S166X) resulting in the alteration of a serine to a premature stop codon in exon 3 and a truncated Tyrp1 molecule. Two additional nonpathologic mutations also were identified.[30–32]

In the African population, the *TYRP1* and *P* gene mutations appear to be responsible, respectively, for the rufous and brown OCA phenotypes.[19,21,30–32] This suggests that the African American individual first described with the 1104delA *TYRP1* gene mutation[30] actually has rufous rather than brown OCA. Alternatively, the phenotypic similarity between *P* mutant and *TYRP1* mutant brown OCA may result from modification by genetic background and/or mixed ancestry between the two types.

A more comprehensive analysis to identify polymorphisms of the human *TYRP1* gene was performed to determine the role of variation in *TYRP1* sequences and resulting variation in amino acids to changes in pigmentary phenotype. However, evaluation of 100 Caucasian individuals of varying hair color did not result in identification of amino acid variations in the *TYRP1* gene.[32]

The pathogenesis of OCA3 is poorly understood because the normal role of Tyrp1 in human melanocytes is still unclear. It is now generally accepted that in the murine system, the Tyrp1 protein functions as DHICA oxidase. However, this enzymatic activity should be interpreted cautiously because in a recent study it has not been observed for human Tyrp1 protein. Besides, it has been demonstrated that human tyrosinase itself, in contrast to mouse tyrosinase, has DHICA oxidase activity. Therefore, though logical, the role of human Tyrp1 as a DHICA oxidase cannot be stated unequivocally. Tyrosinase, Tyrp1, and Dct are type 1 membrane-bound melanosomal glycoproteins with similar structural features. All three are believed to interact with one another in melanosomes to form a melanogenic protein complex; it was shown that Tyrp1 has an important function of stabilizing tyrosinase in melanosomes. Very recently it was demonstrated that Tyrp1 and tyrosinase also form a complex in the endoplasmic reticulum and that a mutation in each of them results in the retention and degradation of both in the endoplasmic reticulum and markedly slows down their transport to melanosomes. This suggests that abnormal trafficking of wild-type tyrosinase elicited by mutant Tyrp1 could be an important etiologic factor of OCA3.[31,35]

Oculocutaneous Albinism Type 4

Oculocutaneous albinism type 4 (OCA4; MIM 606574) is a new clinical form of oculocutaneous albinism that has been described very recently in a patient of Turkish descent presenting with generalized hypopigmentation and ocular abnormalities within the phenotypic range commonly associated with OCA2. No mutations were detected in the *P* gene alleles, but a splice-acceptor-site mutation was found in exon 2 of a gene called *MATP* (membrane-associated transporter protein) located on chromosome 5p. 100 The murine orthologue of the *MATP* gene is the *uw* (underwhite) gene.[36,37] *uw/uw* mice have a light-beige outer fur, very white underfur, and pink eyes at birth, which darken with age.[38] The severity of hypopigmentation among *uw* alleles is correlated with melanosomal size, shape, melanin content, and maturity.[36] Mutations in the fish orthologue of mouse and human *MATP* genes have been detected in the medaka fish,[39] which has a generalized hypopigmentation.

The human, murine, and fish *MATP* genes share several common features. The encoded proteins are predicted to span the membrane 12 times. They contain a conserved sucrose transporter signature sequence, suggesting an important functional role for this motif. In addition, melanosome anomalies have been observed in the medaka fish and in the *uw* mouse. These data indicate that Matp plays a critical role in vertebrate pigmentation and suggest that Matp may be a component of the melanosomal membrane, presumably mediating the transport of a molecule required for melanogenesis or for another melanosome function.[36–39]

Autosomal Dominant OCA

Several families have been described with autosomal dominant expression of OCA or cutaneous hypopigmentation, but characterization is incomplete, and most do not meet the strict criteria for albinism.[40] The characterization of dominant OCA must await the careful evaluation of families with a clear autosomal dominant expression of OCA.

TYPES OF OCA IN WHICH THE PRIMARY DEFECT IS NOT LIMITED TO THE MELANOCYTE

The two disorders included in this section, the Hermansky-Pudlak syndrome (HPS; MIM 203300) or, more correctly, syndromes and the Chediak-Higashi syndrome (CHS; MIM 214500), are now considered hallmark disorders of the biogenesis of lysosome-related organelles/secretory lysosomes (LROs/SOs). LROs/SOs, a newly recognized type of intracellular vesicle, play an important role in different cell types, Melanosomes in melanocytes and dense bodies in platelets are typical examples of LROs/SOs.[41,42] This concept is fully consistent with the multiple clinical manifestations of HPS and CHS. It also explains the locus heterogeneity of HPS because many different gene products are required for LRO/SO biogenesis. Consequently, these diseases and their causative genes have become of immense interest to researchers in cellular biology.

Hermansky-Pudlak Syndrome (See also Table 89-2)

HPS is a complex disorder that presents with OCA, a bleeding diathesis, and a ceroid lipofuscin–like lysosomal storage in a variety of tissues.[43,44] HPS is autosomal recessive in inheritance. Although HPS reflects a process that affects not only melanocytes but also platelets and other tissues, the pigmentry disorder is similar to the primary OCA types described earlier, and ocular features of HPS are the same as those found with other types of OCA. HPS is rare in most populations, except in the Caribbean island of Puerto Rico, particularly in the northwestern region, where the majority of patients are found with an incidence of 1:1800. HPS is not found on other Caribbean islands but is frequent in one long-isolated mountain village in the Swiss Valais.[43,44]

HPS PHENOTYPES The clinical manifestations of HPS are colored by the ethnic background of affected patients, as well as by the causative locus. HPS is a pigmenting type of OCA in that cutaneous and ocular pigments develop in many affected individuals, and the amount of pigment that forms is quite variable.[43–46] (Fig 89-6).

In Puerto Rico, affected individuals have hair color that varies from white to yellow to brown.[43–47] Skin color is creamy white and definitely lighter than in normally pigmented individuals in this population. Albinism in HPS is associated with quantitatively reduced and qualitatively abnormal melanosomes in skin and hair melanocytes.[43–47] Freckles can be present in the sun-exposed regions, often coalescing into large areas that look like normal dark skin pigment, but tanning does not occur. Pigmented nevi are common. Iris color varies from blue to brown, and all the ocular features of albinism are present.[47] Typically, HPS patients are legally blind, with a visual acuity of 20/200 or worse, but occasionally, a patient has an acuity as high as 20/50.[47] The presence of OCA may not be obvious in a Puerto Rican individual with brown hair, skin pigment in exposed areas, and brown eyes unless the cutaneous pigmentation is compared with that of unaffected family members, who generally are darker in pigment, and unless the ocular features of albinism are recognized.

FIGURE 89-6

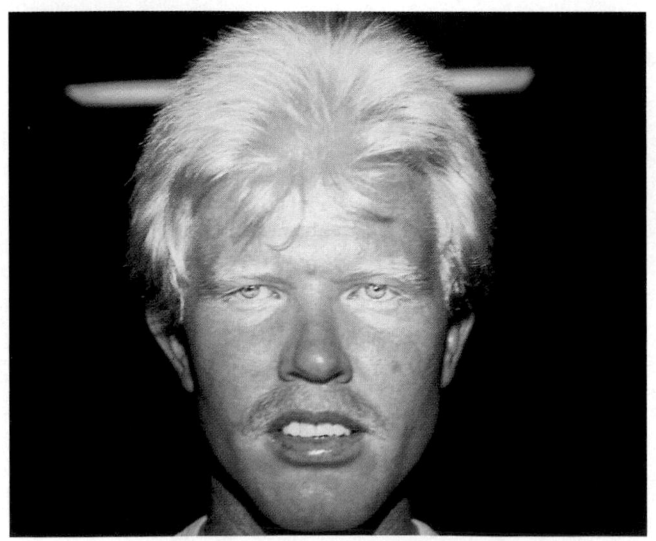

Hermansky-Pudlak syndrome in Puerto Rican individual.

Affected individuals have been identified in other populations, and the phenotype shows the same degree of variation in pigmentation as is found in Puerto Ricans. Hair color varies from white to brown, and this correlates somewhat with the ethnic group. The skin is white and does not tan. Eye color varies from blue to pigmented.

The bleeding diathesis in HPS usually produces mild hemorrhagic episodes. The first sign in HPS patients usually consists of excess bruising beginning at the time of ambulation Episodes of epistaxis are frequent but offen remit during adolescence. Other events that result in excess bleeding include dental extractions, surgeries, acute colitis, menstrual periods, and child birth. Fatalities due to bleeding are rare.[47] The cause of bleeding is absence of platelet dense granules, making the disease a platelet storage pool deficiency. Dense granules are intracellular LROs/SOs that contain ADP, ATP, serotonin, calcium and polyphosphates and disgorge their contents on stimulation. Released components, ADP in particular, cause aggregation of surrounding platelets, contributing to clot formation. HPS patients have a normal or increased platelet count but an attenuated secondary aggregation response. The bleeding time is often but not always prolonged. Absence of dense bodies, which confirms the diagnosis of HPS, is demonstrable by wet-mount electron microscopy.

The most severe clinical manifestations of HPS are related to the pulmonary and intestinal changes. Interstitial pulmonary fibrosis has been described in many individuals with HPS; in particular, patients with HPS1 disease (see below) are at increased risk for developing pulmonary fibrosis. The etiology of the fibrosis is unknown.[47] Approximately 15 percent of HPS patients, whether Puerto Rican or non–Puerto Rican, suffer from granulomatous colitis.[47] The distal colon is involved most often by this complication, and the colitis of HPS resembles Crohn's disease. The etiology of the colitis is unknown.[43,44,47]

HPS is associated with accumulation of ceroid lipofuscin–like materials in the lysosomes of many cell types, suggesting lysosomal dysfunction.[43,44] Average survival of HPS patients is 30 to 50 years, with death usually resulting from restrictive lung disease or, less frequently, hemorrhage or colitis.

MOLECULAR PATHOGENESIS OF HPS (See also Table 89-3) HPS can be caused by mutations in any one of four genes *HPS1, HPS2, AP3B1, or HPS4.* This reflects, in part, the situation in mice, where at least 15 different genes cause hypopigmentation and platelet storage pool deficiency. Consequently, the identification of additional genes in HPS patients is possible.[43–46]

Hermansky-Pudlak syndrome type 1 (HPS1; MIM 604982) The *HPS1* gene (chromosome 10q23) is the first identified HPS gene[43,44] and a major cause of HPS in Puerto Rican patients. The *HPS1* gene codes for a 79.3-kDa protein with no significant homology to any other known proteins. It has been proposed that the Hps1 complex is involved in the biogenesis of early melanosomes, but its specific role remains to be determined.

In melanotic cells, the Hps1 protein is contained in two distinct high-molecular-weight complexes distributed between uncoated vesicles, early stage melanosomes, and the cytosol. The Hps1 protein does not seem to be associated with lysosomes, consistent with the mild and indirect lysosomal defects observed in HPS1 patients cells. The mouse pale-ear (*ep*) locus is the homologue to the human *HPS1* locus.[43,44,48]

Hermansky-Pudlak syndrome type 2 (HPS2; MIM 603401) Mutations in the *AP3B1* gene (chromosome 15q15), causing HPS2 disease, have been found in three individuals in two families.[49,50] Patients with

HPS2 display characteristic clinical findings. They have mild OCA, a mild bleeding diathesis, persistent neutropenia, and possibly recurrent childhood infections. Pulmonary function tests are borderline low.

AP3B1 codes for the β_{3A} subunit of adaptor complex 3 (AP-3), one of four known adaptor complexes. AP-3 interacts with tyrosinase, and tyrosinase is not targeted properly to melanosomes in *AP3B1*-deficient melanocytes.[44] These data suggest that in melanocytes, AP-3 mediates the trafficking of tyrosinase, and presumably other melanosomal proteins, from an intracellular site to melanosomes. The same may stand true for the transport of transmembrane proteins to LROs/SOs in the other cell types involved in HPS2. The mouse pearl (*pe*) locus is the homologue to the human *HPS2* locus.[43,44]

Hermansky-Pudlak syndrome type 3 (HPS3; MIM 606118) Recently, a third HPS-causing gene, *HPS3* (chromosome 3q24), was isolated in a population of HPS patients from central Puerto Rico who were devoid of mutations in *HPS1*.[45] Among these patients, one Puerto Rican–Italian patient inherited the common Puerto Rican 3904-bp deletion from his father, whereas no mutation was detected in the coding region of his maternal allele. In the other non–Puerto Rican patients, however, other *HPS3* mutations gave rise to HPS3 disease. Five patients were Ashkenazi Jews, three of whom were homozygous for a 1303+1G→A splice-site mutation that causes skipping of exon 5 and decreases the amount of mRNA. The other two were heterozygous for the 1303+1G→ A mutation and for either a 1831+2T→ G or a 2621 − 2A→G splicing mutation. The finding of a common mutation in *HPS3* among patients of Ashkenazi Jewish descent is important because it suggests a founder effect in this population and shows a need for a heightened awareness of the possibility of HPS among Ashkenazi Jews, particularly those with some degree of albinism or platelet storage pool deficiency. Another patient, of German-Swiss descent, was a compound heterozygous for a 2729+1G→C splicing mutation removing exon 14 and decreasing HPS3 mRNA and an R397W missense mutation involving an arginine residue conserved from mice to humans. The last patient, of Irish-English descent, was heterozygous for an 89-bp insertion between exons 16 and 17 resulting from abnormal splicing and a yet unidentified mutation. The HPS3 disease associated with severe *HPS3* mutations, such as splicing mutations, is relatively mild. Hence it cannot be excluded that the diagnosis of HPS3 is overlooked in some patients, and additional studies are needed to assess the exact importance of the *HPS3* locus in non–Puerto Rican patients. Patients with less severe mutations, such as missense mutations, may be indistinguishable from normal individuals.[51]

Hermansky-Pudlak syndrome type 4 (HPS4; MIM 606118) Very recently, a fourth HPS-causing gene, *HPS4*, was isolated in a number of non–Puerto Rican individuals and thus appears potentially as an important HPS locus in this subset of patients. The Hps4 protein is a 72.7-kDa polypeptide unrelated to any known proteins. Preliminary data suggest that Hps4 functions in the same pathway of organelle biogenesis as Hps1, but its specific function is currently unknown. The mouse light ear (*le*) locus is the homologue to the human *HPS4* locus.[46]

Chediak-Higashi Syndrome

CHS PHENOTYPE Chediak-Higashi syndrome (CHS; MIM 214500) is a rare autosomal recessive disorder characterized by severe immunologic defects, hypopigmentation, bleeding tendency, progressive neurologic dysfunction, and the presence of giant peroxidase-positive lysosomal granules in peripheral blood granulocytes.[52] As with HPS, the hypopigmentation is the result of a primary defect that affects many other cell types than the melanocyte. The skin, hair, and eye pigments are reduced or diluted in CHS. The affected individuals often do not have obvious albinism, and the hypopigmentation may be noted only when compared with that of other family members. Hair color is light brown to blond, and the hair has a metallic silver-gray sheen. The skin is creamy white to slate gray. Iris pigment is present, and nystagmus and photophobia may be present or absent. Histologic studies of the eye in CHS have shown reduced iris pigment, a marked reduction in retinal pigment granules, and infiltration of the choroid with reticuloendothelial cells. Visual evoked potential studies show misrouting of the optic fibers in a pattern that is similar to that seen in individuals with OCA1 and OCA2. It should be noted that children with CHS have many serious medical problems and that the hypopigmentation is usually not a medical concern. Most patients with CHS die young unless they undergo allogenic bone marrow transplantation because of the so-called accelerated phase, consisting of a lymphoproliferative syndrome with hemophagocytosis and infiltration of most tissues by activated T lymphocytes. About 10 to 15 percent of patients exhibit a much milder clinical phenotype and survive to adulthood but develop progressive and often fatal neurologic dysfunction. Very rare patients exhibit an intermediate adolescent CHS phenotype, presenting with severe infections in early childhood but a milder course by adolescence and no accelerated phase.

Cells from patients with CHS and from beige mice contain giant intracellular vesicles that cluster around the nucleus. Affected vesicles are lysosomes and LROs/Sos, such as melanosomes, platelet dense granules, and cytolytic granules. The susceptibility to bacterial infections appears to be the result of the abnormal granules in the neutrophils and other cells.[52] The hypopigmentation also arises from the formation of abnormal granules. Giant melanosomes form in the melanocyte. As a result, the melanosomes (and their contained melanin) stay centralized in the cell and do not transfer to surrounding keratinocytes, the result being hypopigmentation of the skin and hair. The pigment granules in the hair shaft are large and have an irregular shape when compared with those in normally pigmented hair from an unaffected individual, and this observation has been used to make a prenatal diagnosis of CHS.

MOLECULAR PATHOGENESIS OF CHS (See also Table 89-3) The beige (*bg*) mouse was proposed as a model of CHS. The mouse *beige* gene[53] and its human orthologue, the *LYST* (lysosomal regulator trafficking) gene (chromosome 1q)[52,53] have now been identified and cloned.[52,54] It has been hypothesized that the Beige/CHS protein is involved in vesicular transport, and this would explain the defective vesicular transport to and from lysosomes and the aberrant compartmentalization of lysosomal and granular enzymes. Most *LYST* gene alterations published so far result in a truncated protein because of frameshift or nonsense mutations, suggesting that missense substitutions in the *LYST* gene may result in a milder phenotype.[55,56] Indeed, very recently, mutation analysis of 21 unrelated patients with the childhood, adolescent, and adult forms of CHS showed that patients with severe childhood CHS had only functionally null mutant *CHS1* alleles, whereas patients with the adolescent and adult forms of CHS also had missense mutatnt alleles that likely encode Chs1 polypeptides with partial function. These results suggest an allelic genotype-phenotype relationship among the various clinical forms of CHS.[57]

The *beige* gene encodes a 400-kDa cytosolic protein that is expressed in most mouse tissues. Most data available to date on the function of the Lyst protein arise from immunologic studies. Cultured mouse fibroblasts in which the Beige protein is overexpressed have smaller than normal lysosomes, suggesting that the Beige protein could control lysosomal fission.[58] CHS T cells have defective peptide loading and MHC class II molecules, endosomal sorting, and altered surface expression of cytotoxic T lymphocyte–associated antigen 4 (CTLA-4). These data suggest alternatively that the Lyst protein could control membrane targeting of the proteins present in LROs/SOs.[59,60] However, in cytotoxic T lymphocyte (CTL) clones derived from CHS patients, it was shown that the initial steps of secretory lysosome formation are normal but that these organelles subsequently fuse together during cell maturation to form the giant secretory lysosomes.[61] Additional studies are needed to shed more light on these apparently conflicting data.

OCULAR ALBINISM

OA, albinism in which the hypopigmentation is primarily localized to the eye, is less common than OCA. It is important to note that the hypopigmentation in OA is clinically limited to the eye, but changes in the cutaneous pigment system also may be present when the ultrastructure of these tissues is analyzed.

OA1: X-Linked Recessive OA

OA1 PHENOTYPES (See also Table 89-2) Ocular albinism type 1 (OA1, X-linked ocular albinism of the Nettleship-Falls type; MIM 300500) is the most common form of OA, with an estimated prevalence of about 1:50,000. Affected males have normal generalized skin and hair pigment. The irides are blue to brown, and all the optic system changes of albinism are present.[62] In African American males, iris color is brown, and iris translucency can be minimal. The skin of Caucasian individuals with OA1 appears normally pigmented, whereas that of African American individuals with darker skin may have scattered hypopigmented macules; these are rarely seen in the skin of Caucasian individuals.

Approximately 80 percent of obligate heterozygous females can be detected clinically because of ocular pigment changes that result from X inactivation. These include a variegated pattern of retinal pigment and punctate areas of iris translucency. A small number of heterozygous females have ocular changes of albinism, including nystagmus and reduced acuity, that are thought to be the result of nonrandom patterns of X inactivation.

In OA1 melanocytes in the skin and hair follicles, as well as those of the iris and retina, contain large melanosomes called *giant melanosomes, macromelanosomes,* or *melanin macroglobules* along with normal melanosomes.[63] The giant melanosomes are also found in the tissues of obligate heterozygous females.

Molecular Pathogenesis of OA1

The gene for OA1 was mapped to the Xp22.3-Xp22.2 region. The analysis of mutations in patients with OA1 indicates that approximately 50 percent of independent mutations responsible for the disorder are represented by partial or complete deletions of the *OA1* gene, frameshift, splice site, and nonsense mutations. All these mutations presumably lead to gene inactivation. Numerous missense mutations also have been identified along the coding region of the gene.[60–65] Recent data indicate that many missense mutations of the *OA1* gene observed in OA1 determine endoplasmic reticulum retention and altered glycosylation of the OA1 protein, thus impairing its proper targeting to melanosomes.[66] Conformational changes in the tertiary structure, rather than lack of *N*-glycosylation per se, are likely to be the cause of this misrouting.[67]

The *OA1* gene sequence predicts a protein of 404 amino acids with several transmembrane domains and several potential *N*-glycosylation sites. It has been confirmed that the *OA1* gene product is an integral membrane glycoprotein.[68,69] In human pigment cells, the OA1 protein was localized to melanosomes.[68] However, in a murine system oa1 was localized to late endosome/lysosomes rather than to melanosomes.[69] It was found that OA1 displays structural homology with G protein–coupled seven transmembrane domain receptors (GPCR) and interacts with heterotrimeric G proteins.[70] Since the other known members of the GPCR family are localized to the plasma membrane, OA1 would be the first example of intracellular GPCR identified in a mammalian system. It was proposed that this putative OA1 receptor may represent a "sensor" of a yet unidentified intramelanosomal ligand regulating organelle biogenesis and maturation through activation of heterotrimeric G proteins on the cytoplasmic side of the melanosomal membrane.[70]

DIAGNOSIS OF ALBINISM

The determination of the specific type of albinism can be made with the family history and clinical examination. For OCA, the family history is usually negative, or there is an affected sibling of either sex, indicative of autosomal recessive inheritance.

Children with OCA1 are almost always born with white hair. Many develop pigmented hair, skin, and irides with time (OCA1B), whereas many have white hair and skin with blue eyes all their lives (OCA1A). If hair pigment is present at birth, then the most likely diagnosis is OCA2. For both OCA1 and OCA2, the child is often identified because of the lack of visual attention and the concern for vision. In northern European families, the cutaneous hypopigmentation at birth or early in life is often similar to that of the parents and relatives, and the first concern is raised when it appears that the child is not tracking well or has developed nystagmus.

The presence of strabismus and nystagmus is sufficient to indicate misrouting of the optic fibers at the chiasm. Specialized hematologic tests such as a platelet count, bleeding time, and platelet aggregation or ultrastructure analysis are reserved for individuals with albinism who have a bleeding problem such as easy bruising, recurrent expistaxis, or heavy menstrual bleeding (HPS).

Molecular testing is available in several laboratories and does allow a precise diagnosis to be made at the gene level. In general, this is not necessary for the proper care of a child or adult with albinism. However, it has been proposed recently to screen for HPS among patients who have some degree of hypopigmentation. The rationale for this is that (1) the phenotype of HPS can be extremely mild with respect to both pigmentation and bleeding, (2) as the genotype-phenotype relationship in HPS is becoming clearer, strategies for the molecular diagnosis of patients with HPS are becoming better defined, and (3) identification of patients with a bleeding diathesis among those with hypopigmentation could improve the proper care of these patients. Finally, all patients should be encouraged to participate in research protocols when available because a great deal of the new information on albinism has come from these studies. A mutation database for genes involved in OCA and OA is available at *http://www.cbc.umn.edu/ifpcs/micemut.htm*.

MANAGEMENT OF ALBINISM

All individuals with albinism should be under the care of an ophthalmologist and should have annual examinations until adult life. Most are hyperopic or myopic, and many have significant astigmatism; refractive correction aids in their visual attentiveness and performance.

Protection from ultraviolet radiation of the sun and care by a dermatologist are necessary for individuals with OCA who have little or no skin and hair pigment. This care is the same as that necessary for individuals without albinism who have type I or II skin and includes the use of sunscreens, hats, and long sleeves, as well as sun avoidance.

REFERENCES

1. King RA et al: Albinism, in *The Metabolic and Molecular Bases of Inherited Disease,* 7th ed, edited by CR Scriver, AL Beaudet, WS Sly, D Valle. New York, McGraw-Hill, 1995, p 4353
2. Witkop CJ Jr: Inherited disorders of pigmentation. *Clin Dermatol* **3**:70, 1985
3. Creel DJ et al: Visual anomalies associated with albinism. *Ophthal Pediatr Genet* **11**:193, 1990
4. Garber SR et al: Auditory system abnormalities in human albinos. *Ear Hear* **3**:207, 1982
5. Summers CG et al: Diagnosis of oculocutaneous albinism with molecular analysis. *Am J Ophthalmol* **121**:724, 1996
6. Schnur RE et al: Phenotypic variability in X-linked ocular albinism: Relationship to linkage genotypes. *Am J Hum Genet* **55**:484, 1994
7. King RA et al: Minimal pigment: A new type of oculocutaneous albinism. *Clin Genet* **29**:42, 1986
8. King RA et al: Temperature-sensitive tyrosinase associated with peripheral pigmentation in oculocutaneous albinism. *J Clin Invest* **87**:1046, 1991
9. Oetting WS, King RA: Molecular basis of albinism: Mutations and polymorphisms of pigment genes associated with albinism. *Hum Mutat* **13**:99, 1999
10. Oetting WS: The tyrosinase gene and oculocutaneous albinism type 1 (OCA1): A model for understanding the molecular biology of melanin formation. *Pigment Cell Res* **13**:320, 2000
11. Berson JF et al: A common temperature-sensitive allelic form of human tyrosinase is retained in the endoplasmic reticulum at the nonpermissive temperature. *J Biol Chem* **275**:12281, 2000
12. Halaban R et al: Endoplasmic retioulum retention is a common defect associated with tyrosinase-negative albinism. *Proc Natl Acad Sci USA* **97**:5889, 2000
13. Toyofuku K et al: The molecular basis of oculocutaneous-albinism type 1 (OCA1): Sorting failure and degradation of mutant tyrosinases results in a lack of pigmentation, *Biochem J* **355**:259, 2001
14. Okoro AN: Albinism in Nigeria: A clinical and social study. *Br J Dermatol* **92**:485, 1975
15. Rinchik EM et al: A gene for the mouse pink-eyed dilution locus and for human type II oculocutaneous albinism. *Nature* **361**:72, 1993
16. Gardner JM et al: The mouse pink-eyed dilution gene: Association with human Prader-Willi and Angelman syndromes. *Science* **257**:1121, 1992
17. Barsh GS: The genetics of pigmentation: From fancy genes to complex traits. *Trends Genet* **12**:299, 1996
18. King RA et al: Albinism in Nigeria with delineation of new recessive oculocutaneous type. *Clin Genet* **17**:259, 1980
19. Brilliant MH: The mouse *p* (*pink-eyed dilution*) and human *P* genes, oculocutaneous albinism type 2 (OCA2), and melanosomal pH. *Pigment Cell Res* **14**:86, 2001
20. King RA et al: Brown oculocutaneous albinism: Clinical, ophthalmological, and biochemical characterization. Ophthalmology **92**:1496, 1985
21. Kerr R et al: Identification of *P* gene mutations in individuals with oculocutaneous albinism is sub-Saharan Africa. *Hum Mutat* **15**:166, 2000
22. King RA et al: Hypopigmentation in Angelman syndrome. *Am J Med Genet* **46**:40, 1993
23. Wiesner GL et al: Hypopigmentation in the Prader-Willi syndrome. *Am J Hum Genet* **40**:431, 1987
24. Lee S-T et al: Mutations of the *P* gene in oculocutaneous albinism, ocular albinism, and Prader-Willi Syndrome. *N Engl J Med* **330**:529, 1994
25. Rinchik EM et al: A gene for the mouse pink-eyed dilution locus and for human type II oculocutaneous albinism. *Nature* **361**:72, 1993
26. Creel DJ et al: Abnormalities of the central visual pathways in Prader-Willi syndrome associate with hypopigmentation. *N Engl J Med* **314**:1606, 1986
27. Stevens G et al: An intragenic deletion of the *P* gene is the common mutation causing tyrosinase-positive oculocutaneous albinism in southern African Negroids. *Am J Hum Genet* **56**:586, 1995
28. Sviderskaya EV et al: Complementation of hypigmentation in *p* mutant (*pink-eyed dilution*) mouse melanocytes by normal human *P* cDNA, and defective complementation by *OCA2* mutant sequences. *J Invest Dermatol* **108**:30, 1997
29. Spritz RA et al: Hypopigmentation in the Prader-Willi syndrome correlates with *P* gene deletion but not with haplotype of the hemizygous *P* allele. *Am J Med Genet* **71**:57, 1997
30. Boissy RE et al: Mutation in and lack of expression of tyrosinase-related protein 1 (TRP-1) in melanocytes from an individual with brown oculocutaneous albinism: A new subtype of albinism classified as OCA3. *Am J Hum Genet* **48**:1145, 1996
31. Manga P et al: Rufous oculocutaneous albinism in southern African blacks is caused by mutations in *TYRP1* gene. *Am J Hum Genet* **61**:1095, 1997
32. Sarangarajan R, Boissy RE: Tyrp1 and oculocutaneous albinism type 3, *Pigment Cell Res* **14**:437, 2001
33. Kromberg JGR et al: Red or rufous albinism in southern Africa. *Ophthal Pediatr Genet* **11**:229, 1990
34. Hornabrook RW et al: Congenital nystagmus among the red-skins of the highlands of Papua New Guinea. *Br J Ophthalmol* **64**:375, 1980
35. Toyofuku K et al: Oculocutaneous albinism types 1 and 3 are ER retention diseases: Mutation of tyrosinase of *TYRP1* can affect the processing of both mutant and wild-type proteins. *FASEB J* **15**:2149, 2001
36. Newton JM et al: Mutations in the human orthologue of the mouse *underwhite* gene (*uw*) underlie a new form of oculocutaneous albinism, OCA4. *Am J Hum Genet* **69**:981, 2001
37. Du J, Fisher DE: Identification of *Aim-1* as the *underwhite* mouse mutant and its transcriptional regulation by MITF. *J Biol Chem* **277**:402, 2002
38. Lehman A et al: The *underwhite* (*uw*) locus acts autonomously and reduces the production of melanin. *J Invest Dermatol* **115**:601, 2000
39. Fukamachi S et al: Mutations in the gene encoding B, a novel transporter protein, reduces melanin content in medaka. *Nature* Genet **28**:381, 2001
40. Fitzpatrick TB et al: Dominant oculocutaneous albinism. *Br J Dermatol* **91**(suppl 10):23, 1974
41. Marks MS, Seabra MC: The melanosome: Membrane dynamics in black and white. *Nature Rev Mol Cell Biol* **2**:738, 2001
42. Blott EJ, Griffiths GM: Secretory lysosomes. *Nature Rev Mol Cell Biol* **3**:122, 2002
43. Spritz RA: Hermansky-Pudlak syndrome and pale-ear: Melanosome making for the millennium. *Pigment Cell Res* **13**:15, 2000
44. Huizing M et al: Hermansky-Pudlak syndrome and related disorders of organelle formation. *Traffic* **1**:823, 2000
45. Anikster Y et al: Mutations of a new gene causes a unique form of Hermansky-Pudlak syndrome in a genetic isolate of central Puerto Rico. *Nature Genet* **28**:376, 2001
46. Suzuki T et al: Hermansky-Pudlak syndrome is caused by mutations in *HPS4,* the human homolog of the mouse light-ear gene. *Nature Genet* **30**:321, 2002
47. Gahl WA et al: Genetic defects and clinical characteristics of patients with a form of oculocutaneous albinism (Hermansky-Pudlak syndrome). *N Engl J Med* **338**:1258, 1998
48. Gardner JM et al: The mouse pale ear (*ep*) mutation is the homologue of Hermansky-Pudlak syndrome (HPS). *Proc Natl Acad Sci USA* **94**:9238, 1997
49. Dell'Angelica E et al: Altered trafficking of lysosomal proteins in Hermansky-Pudlak syndrome due to mutations in the beta3A subunit of the AP-3 adaptor. *Mol Cell* **3**:11, 1999.
50. Shotelersuk V et al: A new variant of Hermansky-Pudlak syndrome due to mutations in a gene responsible for vesicle formation. *Am J Med* **108**:423, 2000
51. Huizing M et al: Hermansky-Pudlak syndrome type 3 in Ashkenazi Jews and other non–Puerto Rican patients with hypopigmentation and platelet storage-pool deficiency. *Am J Hum Genet* **69**:1022, 2001
52. Spritz RA: Molecular genetics of Hermansky-Pudlak and Chediak-Higashi syndromes. *Platelets* **9**:21, 1998
53. Barbosa MDFS et al: Identification of the homologous beige and Chediak-Higashi syndrome genes. *Nature* **382**:262, 1996
54. Nagle DL et al: Identification and mutation analysis of the complete gene for Chediak-Higashi syndrome. *Nature Genet* **14**:307, 1996
55. Barbosa MD et al: Identification of mutations in two major isoforms of mRNA of the Chediak-Higashi syndrome gene in humans and mouse. *Hum Mol Genet* **6**:1091, 1997
56. Certain S et al: Protein truncation test of *LYST* reveals heterogeneous mutations in patients with Chediak-Higashi syndrome. *Blood* **95**:979, 2000
57. Karim MA et al: Apparent genotype-phenotype correlation in childhood, adolescent, and adult Chediak-Higashi syndrome. *Am J Med Genet* **108**:16, 2002
58. Perou CM: The Beige/Chediak-Higashi protein encodes a widely expressed cytosolic protein. *J. Biol Chem* **272**:29790, 1997
59. Faigle W et al: Deficient peptide loading and MHC class II endosomal sorting in a human genetic immunodeficiency syndrome: The Chediak-Higashi syndrome. *J Cell Biol* **141**:1121, 1998
60. Barrat FJ et al: Defective CTLA-4 cycling pathway in Chediak-Higashi syndrome: A possible mechanism for deregulation of T lymphocyte activation. *Proc Natl Acad Sci USA* **96**:8645, 1999
61. Stinchcombe JC et al: Secretory lysosome biogenesis in cytotoxic T lymphocytes from normal and Chediak-Higashi syndrome patients. *Traffic* **1**:435, 2000

62. O'Donnell FE, Green WR: The eye in albinism, in *Clinical Ophthalmology*, vol 4, edited by TD Duane. Philadelphia, Lippincott, 1989, p 1
63. Garner A, Jay BS: Macromelanosomes in X-linked ocular albinism. *Histopathology* **4**:243, 1980
64. Rosenberg T, Schwarz M: X-linked ocular albinism: Prevalence and mutations—a national study. *Eur J Hum Genet* **6**:570, 1998
65. Schnur R et al: OA1 deletions and mutations in X-linked ocular albinism. *Am J Hum Genet* **62**:800, 1998
66. d'Addio M et al: Defective intracellular transport and processing of OA1 is a major cause of ocular albinism type 1. *Hum Mol Genet* **9**:3011, 2000
67. Shen B, Orlow SJ: The ocular albinism type 1 gene product is a *N*-glycoprotein but glycosylation is not required for its subcellular distribution. *Pigment Cell Res* **14**:485, 2001
68. Schiaffino MV et al: The ocular albinism type 1 gene is a membrane glycoprotein localized to melanosomes. *Proc Natl Acad Sci USA* **93**:9055, 1996
69. Samaweera P et al: The mouse ocular albinism 1 gene product is an endolysosomal protein. *Exp Eye Res* **72**:312, 2001
70. Schiaffino MV et al: Ocular albinism: Evidence for a defect in an intracellular signal transduction system. *Nature Genet* **23**:108, 1999

CHAPTER 90

Jean-Paul Ortonne
Philippe Bahadoran
Thomas B. Fitzpatrick
David B. Mosher[†]
Yoshiaki Hori[†]

Hypomelanoses and Hypermelanoses

HYPOMELANOSES

Pigmentary disturbances (Table 90-1) may be congenital or acquired, circumscribed or generalized, and partially or completely hypomelanotic (having reduced melanin pigmentation). The term *hypomelanosis* refers to reduction in melanin compared with that individual's normal skin, whereas *amelanosis* signifies total absence of melanin. The term *depigmentation* implies loss of preexisting melanin pigmentation. History and physical examination usually can quickly establish the diagnosis or at least limit the differential. A congenital generalized hypomelanosis may only be appreciated by comparison with unaffected first-generation family members; an acquired generalized amelanosis results from the progressive destruction of melanocytes characteristic of vitiligo and chemical leukoderma. Morphologic and metabolic pathways leading to hypomelanosis and amelanosis are shown in Fig. 90-1. Circumscribed or localized hypomelanoses represent islands of disease amidst clinically normal skin. These also may be amelanotic and progressive (vitiligo, chemical leukoderma); amelanotic, congenital, and stable [piebaldism, Waardenburg's syndrome (WS)]; hypomelanotic and progressive (tinea versicolor, postinflammatory); or hypomelanotic and stable (tuberous sclerosis, nevus depigmentosus).

Circumscribed hypomelanotic macules may have certain features that facilitate diagnosis; these include size, shape, hue, array, and additional features. Confetti or 1- to 2-mm macules may be seen in vitiligo, chemical leukoderma, and tuberous sclerosis. The lesions of pityriasis alba and postinflammatory leukoderma are larger but have fuzzy, indistinct margins, unlike the sharp margins observed with idiopathic guttate melanosis and often tinea versicolor. Scalloped or convex borders are seen in vitiligo or chemical leukoderma. The lance-ovate shape is characteristic of the white macule of tuberous sclerosis. Vitiligo and piebald macules are milk- or chalk-white as opposed to the off-white color seen with nevus depigmentosus, tuberous sclerosis, or postinflammatory leukoderma. A dermatomal, quasi-dermatomal to segmental array of macules can be caused by vitiligo (milk-white), nevus depigmentosus (off-white), tuberous sclerosis (usually with fairly discrete macules), hypermelanosis of Ito. Vitiligo, tinea versicolor, and chemical depigmentation typically involve numerous macules, whereas nevus depigmentosus and tuberous sclerosis are usually characterized by only a few scattered lesions. Vitiligo typically involves extensor surfaces, periorificial skin, anterior shins, flexor wrists, and lower back, whereas piebaldism involves the central forehead and the midarms and legs, sparing the dorsal spine in a cephalocaudal direction. Symmetry is often found with vitiligo, piebaldism, WS, and chemical leukoderma. Isolated hypomelanotic macules with raised erythematous borders suggest tinea versicolor or inflammatory vitiligo, anesthesia suggests leprosy, telangiectasia suggests lupus erythematosus, and hyperpigmented macules suggest piebaldism, pinta, or repigmenting vitiligo. Other features may be observed. Scaling is typical of pityriasis alba and tinea versicolor.

Thus, with attention to the variability of extent of hypomelanosis, history of evolution, attention to hue, and awareness of ancillary features, the differential diagnosis usually can be quickly narrowed down. In fair-skinned individuals, the Wood's lamp is always useful.

Clinicopathologic Correlation in Hypomelanoses

The color or hue of the hypomelanotic macules has a limited clinicopathologic correlation with the defect in melanization (see Fig. 90-1). Melanocytopenic (brilliant or milk-white due to the reflection of incident light) macules may arise because of absence or loss of melanocytes. Melanopenic disorders arise because of failure of normal melanocyte or epidermal melanin unit function.

[†]Deceased.

TABLE 90-1

Hypopigmentation: Clinicopathologic Classification of Disorders

Etiologic Factors	Melanocytopenic (Melanocytes Decreased or Absent)	Melanopenic (Melanin Decreased or Absent)	Nonmelanotic (No Melanin Defect)
Chemical	Catechols (certain)	Arsenicals	
	Monobenzylether of hydroquinone	Chloroquine	
	Para-substituted phenols (certain)	Glucocorticoids	
	Sulfhydryls	Hydroxychloroquine	
		Hydroquinone	
		Mercaptoethylamines	
		Retinoids	
Endocrine		Addison's disease	
		Hypopituitarism	
		Hypothyroidism	
Genetic	Ataxia telangiectasia	Albinism (see Chap. 87)	Nevus anemicus
	Piebaldism	Type I oculocutaneous albinism (OCA)	
	Vitiligo	A Tyrosinase negative	
	Alezzandrini's syndrome	B Yellow	
	Idiopathic	MP Minimal pigment	
	Vogt-Koyanagi-Harada syndrome	TS Temperature sensitive	
	Waardenburg's syndrome	Type II OCA	
	Woolf's syndrome	Tyrosinase positive	
	Xeroderma pigmentosum	Unclassified	
	Ziprkowski-Margolis syndrome	Type III OCA	
		Type IV OCA	
		Chediak-Higashi syndrome	
		Cross-McKusick-Breen syndrome	
		Griscelli's syndrome	
		Hermansky-Pudlak syndrome	
		Rufous	
		BADS syndrome*	
		Canities, premature	
		Fanconi's syndrome	
		Histidinemia	
		Homocystinuria	
		Horner's syndrome	
		Hypomelanosis of Ito and mosaicism	
		Menkes' steely hair	
		Nevus depigmentosus	
		Tuberous sclerosis	
Inflammatory	Actinic reticuloid	Leprosy	Woronoff's ring
	Mycosis fungoides	Pityriasis alba	
	Onchocerciasis	Postinflammatory	
	Pityriasis lichenoides chronicus	Discoid lupus	
	Pinta	Eczema	
	Yaws	Psoriasis	
		Post-Kala-azar	
		Sarcoidosis	
		Syphilis	
		Endemic	
		Secondary	
		Tinea versicolor	
Metabolic		Alpert's syndrome	
		Chromosomal 5p defect	
		Osteopathic striae	
		Prolidase deficiency	
Neoplastic	Halo nevus	Melanoma	
	Leukoderma acquisitum centrifugum	Halo around primary or metastatic lesions	
Nutritional	Vitamin B_{12} deficiency	Chronic protein loss	
		Kwashiorkor	
		Malabsorption	
		Nephrosis	
		Ulcerative colitis	

(*continued*)

TABLE 90-1 (*Continued*)

Hypopigmentation: Clinicopathologic Classification of Disorders

Etiologic Factors	Melanocytopenic (Melanocytes Decreased or Absent)	Melanopenic (Melanin Decreased or Absent)	Nonmelanotic (No Melanin Defect)
Physical	Burns Ionizing Thermal UV Trauma	Postdermabrasion Postlaser	
Miscellaneous	Alopecia areata Scleroderma	Canities Horner's syndrome Idiopathic guttate hypomelanosis Vagabond's leukoderma	Anemia Edema

*BADS, black lock, oculocutaneous albinism, deafness of the sensorineural type.

MELANOCYTOPENIC DISORDERS

1. Failure of migration of melanoblasts to the skin (piebaldism, WS)
2. Failure of differentiation and/or survival of melanoblasts into melanocytes (piebaldism, WS)
3. Failure of mitotic division of melanocytes (? vitiligo)

MELANOPENIC DISORDERS

1. Defect of synthesis of functional tyrosinase (albinism)
2. Failure of biogenesis of melanosomal matrix
3. Defect in tyrosinase transport
4. Failure of normal melanosome formation [tuberous sclerosis, Chédiak-Higashi syndrome (CHS)]
5. Failure of melanization of melanosomes (albinism, hypomelanosis of Ito, idiopathic guttate hypomelanosis, tinea versicolor)
6. Defective transport or transfer of melanosomes [CHS, pityriasis alba, postinflammatory hypomelanosis, Griscelli's syndrome (GS)]
7. Alteration in degradation of melanosomes (CHS, nevus depigmentosus, pityriasis alba, postinflammatory hypomelanosis, tinea versicolor)
8. Alteration in melanin removal related to loss of stratum corneum

In time it is expected that there will be more specificity between a particular pathophysiologic defect and a certain hypomelanotic disorder.

Generalized Hypomelanoses Attributed to Heritable/Congenital Factors

ALBINISM (See Chap. 89)

HISTIDINEMIA Histidinemia is characterized by fair skin, blue eyes, and fair to reddish hair.[1]

HOMOCYSTINURIA (See Chap. 147) Reversible hypopigmentation in homocystinuria is the result of tyrosinase inhibition by homocyst(e)ine; this likely results from the interaction of homocyst(e)ine with copper at the active site of tyrosinase. Affected individuals with classic homocystinuria have fine blond hair, blue eyes, and fair skin; however, fewer than half the reported patients have blond hair,[1] and there are even rare reports of patients with black or dark brown hair. Reversal of hypopigmentation of hair has been reported with pyridoxine supplementation in some patients with cystathionine synthetase deficiency.[2]

MENKES' SYNDROME (See Chap. 71) Decreased cutaneous pigmentation has been noted in some patients and is due to tyrosinase deficiency. The hair is sparse, wiry, and depigmented. Normally colored hair at birth fades to an ivory-white by 6 weeks of age.

PHENYLKETONURIA (See Chap. 147) *Phenylketonuria* (PKU) is an autosomal recessive disorder characterized by pigmentary dilution involving skin, hair, and eyes and attributed to a large number of mutations at the phenylalanine hydroxylase locus. Mental retardation is the most significant consequence of untreated or undertreated PKU.

Clinical features PKU is characterized by blond hair, blue eyes, and fair skin; these changes may be so subtle that they become apparent only by comparison with other unaffected family members. While hair color may vary from light blond to dark brown, in most series blond hair predominates. In the Japanese, however, PKU is associated with dark brown hair, clearly lighter in color than the black hair normally found in this race. Between 64 and 93 percent of patients have blue eyes, and most PKU patients have such fair skin that they sunburn easily, though some patients tan mildly. Melanocytes are present in normal to increased numbers; however, there is a reduction in the number of mature melanosomes.

Pathogenesis of hypomelanosis PKU results from a deficiency in *phenylalanine hydroxylase* (PAH), which is the enzyme that catalyzes the conversion of phenylalanine to tyrosine. Hypomelanosis in PKU patients has been attributed to impaired tyrosine metabolism due to hyperphenylalaninemia. Tyrosinase, the key enzyme in the melanogenesis pathway is competitively inhibited by increased amounts of L-phenylalanine, thus reducing melanin production. In addition, phenylalanine competitively inhibits tyrosine uptake by melanocytes in a melanoma cell line. Hypomelanosis of skin and hair can be prevented by a strict low-phenylalanine diet from early infancy. Phenylketonuria is caused by deficiency of phenylalanine hydroxylase, resulting in a decreased conversion of phenylalanine into tyrosine. A mouse model of PKU has been developed. These mice show behavioral abnormalities and pronounced hypomelanosis. Reversal of hypopigmentation by adenovirus-mediated transfer of human PAH cDNA, suggests the feasibility of gene therapy for PKU and demonstrates that the correction of hyperphenylalaninemia and the increased conversion of phenylalanine into tyrosine reverse hypomelanosis.

Treatment Dietary therapy with a low-phenylalanine diet is the treatment of choice. Hair color normally darkens with dietary restriction and again lightens if the dietary restrictions are relaxed.

GRISCELLI'S SYNDROME Griscelli's syndrome is an uncommon disorder transmitted as an autosomal recessive trait and characterized by hypomelanosis of the skin and hair and immunodeficiency.[3] Although pigmentary dilution of the skin may be seen, hypomelanosis in GS may be limited to an abnormal appearance of the hair, described as silvery gray or grayish golden. Histologic and ultrastructural studies show large pigment clumps within hair shafts and an accumulation of melanosomes in melanocytes with poorly pigmented adjacent keratinocytes. Numerous mature melanosomes are arranged in a perinuclear distribution in melanocytes, whereas few or no melanosomes are observed at the tips of dendrites. Frequent pyogenic infections and acute episodes of fever, hepatosplenomegalia, neutropenia, and thrombopenia are common features of GS. Immune deficiency in GS is associated with a profound impairment of B cell and T cell immunity and with impaired natural killer (NK) cell function. Early death is the usual outcome. Many GS patients have neurologic involvement, including intracranial hypertension, cerebellar signs, bulbar poliomyelitis, encephalopathy, hemiparesis, hypotonia, seizures, and psychomotor retardation, with or without immune abnormalities. A hemophagocytic syndrome and uncontrolled T lymphocyte and macrophage activation syndrome leading to death has been observed. Mutations in the *myosin Va* gene have been identified in GS patients exhibiting primarily neurologic impairment without immune defects (GS1). In contrast, mutations in another gene, *RAB27A,* have been found in patients with immune defects (GS2). These findings demonstrate that GS consists of at least two different disorders. Rab27a protein is not expressed in brain tissue. Direct interaction between Rab27a and myosin Va have been demonstrated. Several other syndromes may be closely related to GS.[4] *Elejalde's syndrome,* also called *melanosomal disease,* is characterised by silvery hair and severe dysfunction of the central nervous system (seizures, severe hypotonia, mental retardation). The pigmentary abnormality in Elejalde's syndrome seems different from that of GS. In Elejalde's syndrome, melanosomes are apparently transferred to basal keratinocytes. Mutations analysis of the *MYO Va* gene in Elejalde's patients would be extremely interesting.

FIGURE 90-1

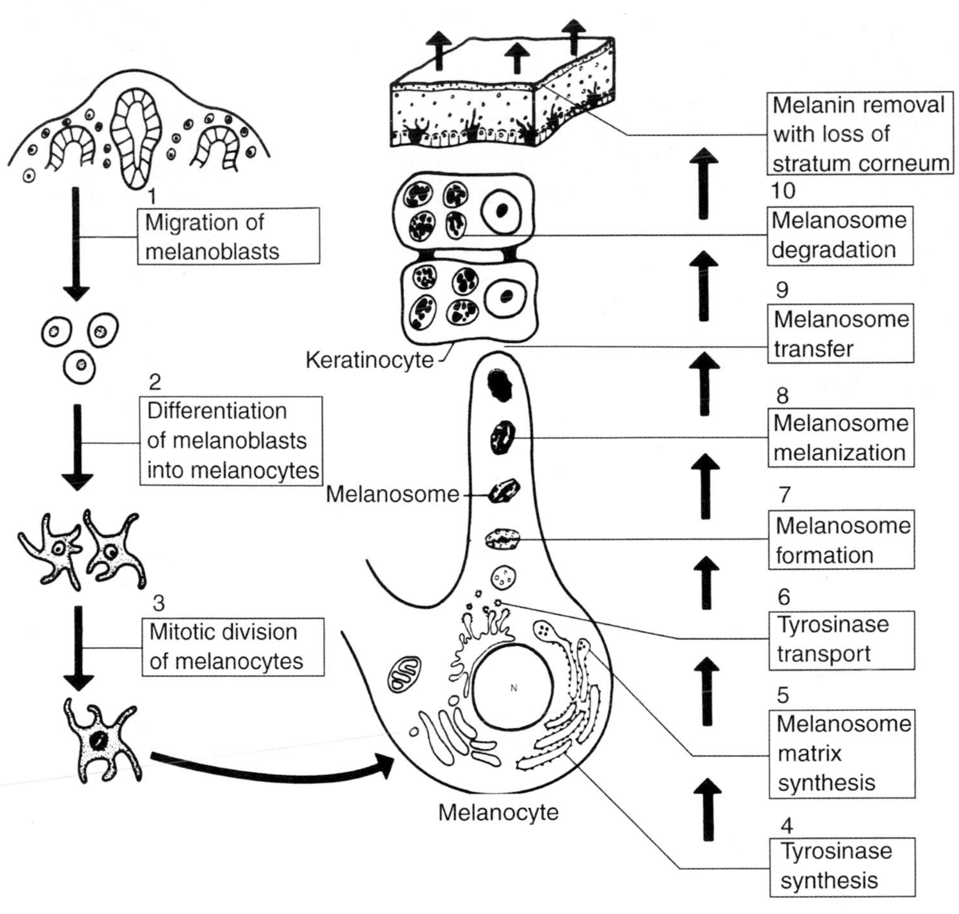

Morphologic and metabolic pathway of melanin hypopigmentation.

Circumscribed Melanocytopenic Hypomelanoses Attributed to Heritable/Congenital Factors

VITILIGO Vitiligo is a specific, common, often heritable, acquired disorder characterized by well-circumscribed milky-white cutaneous macules devoid of identifiable melanocytes. It carries a risk for ocular abnormalities, particularly iritis.[1,5,6]

Psychosocial implications of vitiligo Vitiligo, particularly in brown and black peoples and in Caucasian persons who can tan deeply [*skin phototype* (SPT) IV; see Chap. 88] may be a psychosocial disaster.

Incidence Across the globe, vitiligo is a relatively common cause of leukoderma; although studies have demonstrated an incidence of 0.14 to 8.8 percent, the likely incidence is between 1 and 2 percent. All races are affected. Both sexes are affected equally; the female prevalence in some studies probably can be attributed to greater concern (and greater willingness to express concern) about a cosmetic defect. Vitiligo appears to be observed more commonly in sun-exposed areas and in darker skin types. About 85 percent of patients tan well, and only 15 percent sunburn in constitutively normal skin. SPT IV is the prevalent skin type among Caucasian vitiligo patients. Normal hair color may be black, brown, blond, or red, and the eyes may be blue, hazel, or brown. Black to dark-brown hair and brown iris color seem more common than expected. Vitiligo may develop at any age; onset has been reported from birth to 81 years of age. Congenital vitiligo is very rare, however. The peak age of onset in all series was between 10 and 30 years; in 50 percent of cases, the age of onset fell within the first two decades of life.

Etiology Although vitiligo is generally recognized as a single entity, the etiology is complex. There appears to be a certain genetic predisposition and a number of potential precipitating causes.

Heritability (Fig. 90-2) Familial cases of vitiligo are common, strongly suggesting a genetic basis for this disorder. It is likely, however, that vitiligo is not transmitted in a simple Mendelian autosomal dominant or recessive pattern. The transmission is more complex, most likely polygenic with variable expression. Many studies on the relationship between the human leukocyte antigen (HLA) system and vitiligo showed variable findings. An association between the catalase gene (*CAT*) and vitiligo has been suggested.[7] A novel gene named *VIT1*, possibly associated with vitiligo, has been identified recently by differential display. The involvement of the GTP cyclohydrolase I gene (*GTPCH*), which encodes a key enzyme of the biopterin pathway, has been ruled out. The exact genetic defects in vitiligo remain to be elucidated, and the vitiligo susceptibility genes have not yet been identified.

FIGURE 90-2

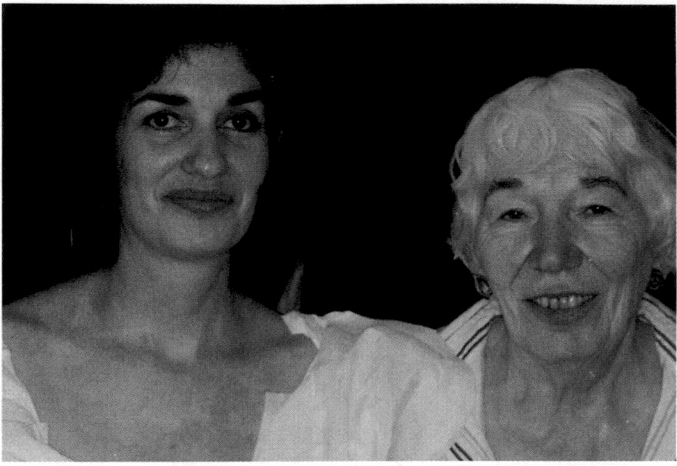

Vitiligo (familial vitiligo). Vitiligo in mother and daughter. The daughter has typical generalized vitiligo, but the mother's condition has evolved to vitiligo universalis.

Precipitating factors Vitiligo patients often can attribute the onset of their disease to a specific life event, crisis, or illness. Many can relate it to loss of a job, death of a close family member, an accident, or a severe systemic disease. In some, the onset follows a physical injury such as a cut or abrasion; this development of vitiligo congruent with a site of injury is referred to as the *Koebner phenomenon* and is characteristic of at least a third of vitiligo patients. Many patients related onset to sun exposure; this may cause koebnerization in predisposed individuals. In darker-skinned individuals who have lost their previous summer tans, a single sun exposure may darken normally pigmented skin to reveal amelanotic macules not previously apparent. Gradual tanning of normal skin also reveals previously inapparent preexisting vitiligo macules that no longer tan.

Clinical features

TYPICAL MACULE OF VITILIGO The typical vitiligo macule has a chalk- or milk-white color, is round to oval in shape, has slightly brushed to fairly distinct, often scalloped margins, measures from several millimeters or many centimeters in diameter, and usually lacks other epidermal changes (Fig. 90-3). There are several variations on the typical vitiligo macule, however. *Trichrome vitiligo* (Fig. 90-4) refers to the presence of an intermediate color; this is a uniform tan coloration that is a narrow to broad interface between the normally pigmented skin and the typical vitiligo macule. An occasional vitiligo macule may be entirely off white to tan (tan being the third color). A trichrome lesion naturally evolves to a typical white vitiligo macule, albeit not at a predictable rate.

Quadrichrome refers to the fourth color; this is a macular perifollicular or marginal hyperpigmentation seen in some cases of repigmenting vitiligo (especially in darker skin phototypes). The macules of hyperpigmentation vary from one to several millimeters in diameter. *Pentachrome vitiligo* (white, tan, brown hyperpigmented, blue-gray hyperpigmented, and normal) also may be observed. Blue vitiligo corresponds to vitiligo macules occurring in sites of postinflammatory hypermelanosis.

Inflammatory vitiligo has an erythematous, raised border similar to that seen in tinea versicolor. Erythema of the entire macule of vitiligo occurs following sun exposure, but a vitiligo macule itself does not clinically resemble an inflammatory dermatosis. *Confetti macules,* which are typical in color but only 1 to 2 mm in diameter, may occur randomly or may be perifollicular. There may be one, several, or up to hundreds of macules that may be small to large in size, even in a single patient. As vitiligo naturally evolves over time, the macules enlarge, coalesce, and impart a scalloped appearance to the interface of the normal and vitiligo skin. When vitiligo becomes very extensive so that little normal pigment remains, the remaining islands of normal pigmentation have concave borders (as if the whole process were evolving) (see Fig 90-4), which is a diagnostic clue that distinguishes this process

FIGURE 90-3

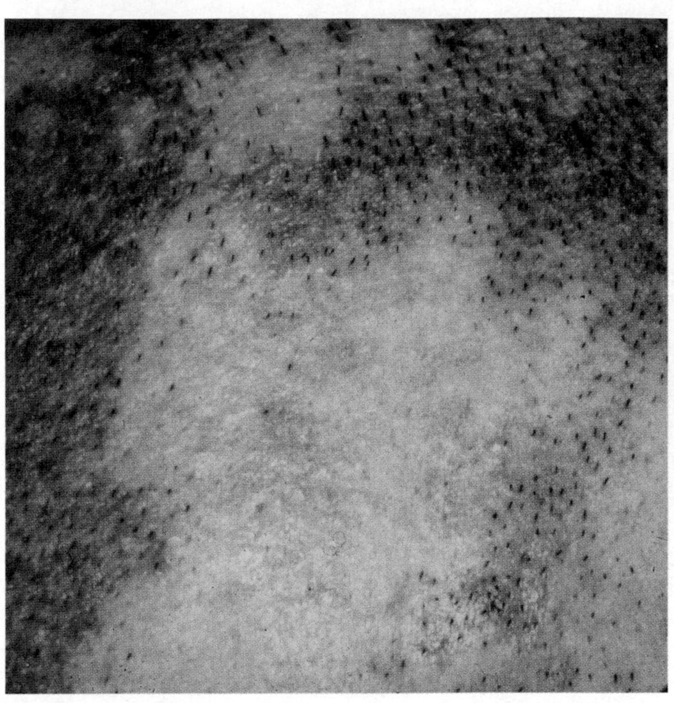

Vitiligo. Scalloping of the border of the remaining normal pigmentation suggests that the evolving hypopigmentation is invading the normally pigmented skin. Note that in this case (beard area) vitiligo is associated with alopecia areata.

FIGURE 90-4

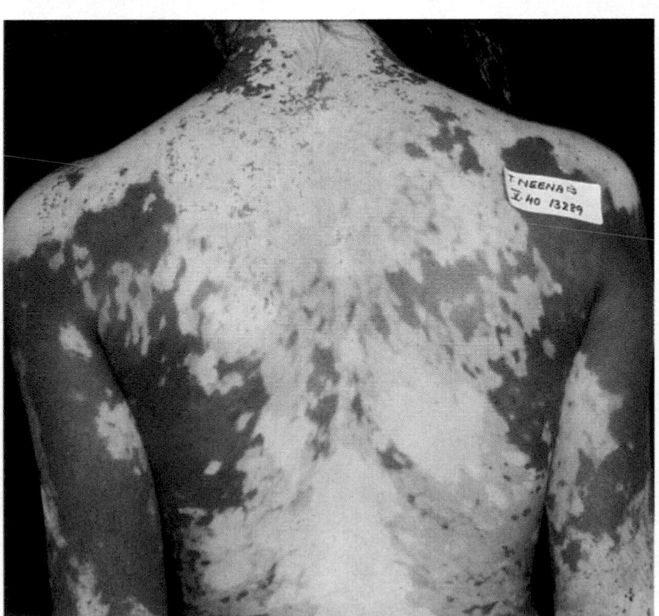

Vitiligo. Trichrome vitiligo displays three colors—white, light tan, and normal brown. The light tan area is metastable and will evolve to the amelanosis typical of vitiligo.

FIGURE 90-5

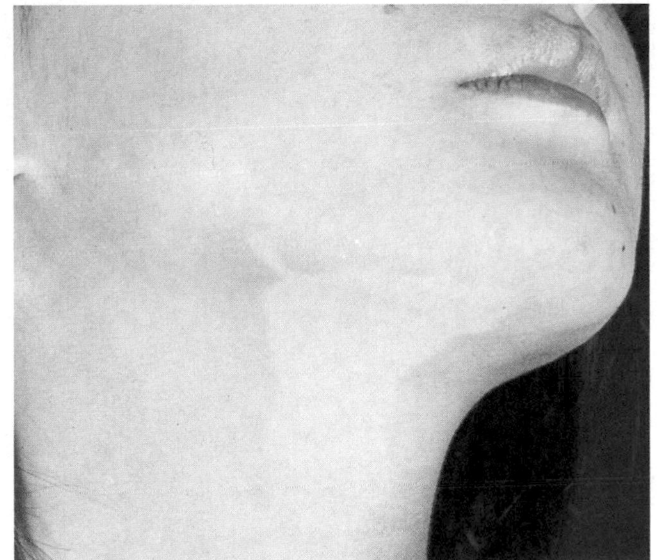

Segmental vitiligo. Distribution is unilateral and quasidermatomal. Evolution is very unusual outside the generally involved dematome(s): rarely generalized vitiligo develops at a later date.

from hyperpigmented macules on normal, extremely fair skin. In actively repigmenting vitiligo, the margins lose their impressionistic character and become surrealistically sharp and again convex (representing foci of melanocytes migrating into vitiligo skin).

Types of Vitiligo The following types represent the most characteristic patterns of vitiligo: focal, segmental, generalized, and universal.

Focal vitiligo (see Fig. 90-3) is an isolated macule or a few scattered macules; by vague convention, the macules are limited in both size and number. Twenty percent of children with vitiligo have the focal pattern.

Segmental vitiligo (Fig. 90-5) is characterized by unilateral macules in a dermatomal or quasi-dermatomal distribution. This should be considered a special type of vitiligo that has a stable course and is unlikely to be associated with thyroid disease or with other vitiligo-associated diseases. Segmental vitiligo tends to be earlier in onset and more stable than generalized vitiligo and is not familial. Involved patients are unlikely to develop remote or contralateral lesions. Koebnerization is not characteristic. Five percent of adults but more than 20 percent of children with vitiligo are found to have this pattern. The trigeminal area is the most common single site of involvement (>50 percent); the neck and trunk are involved in 23 and 17 percent, respectively. Up to 13 percent may have multiple sites of involvement. Nearly half are associated with poliosis (white hairs; see below). In various studies, from 5 to 28 percent of patients have been noted to have the segmental pattern.

Generalized vitiligo (Fig. 90-6) is the most common type of vitiligo and is characterized by few to many widespread macules. These macules are often symmetrically placed (Fig. 90-7*A*) and involve extensor surfaces; the most common extensor surfaces include interphalangeal joints, metacarpal/metatarsal interphalangeal joints, elbows, and knees. Other surfaces involved include volar wrists, malleoli, umbilicus, lumbosacral area, anterior tibia, and axillae. Vitiligo macules may be periorificial and involve the skin around the eyes, nose, ears, mouth, and anus. Periungual involvement may occur alone or with certain mucosal surfaces (lips, distal penis, nipples); the latter is lip-tip vitiligo (Fig. 90-7*B*). Acrofacial vitiligo involves distal digits and periorificial facial areas. Universal vitiligo (vitiligo universalis) (Fig. 90-8) describes such widespread vitiligo that there are few remaining normal macules of pigmentation; this type has been associated with the multiple endocrinopathy syndrome.

The general array of macules in generalized vitiligo is often remarkably symmetric, sometimes seemingly mirror image, but asymmetry is

FIGURE 90-6

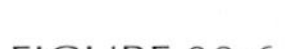

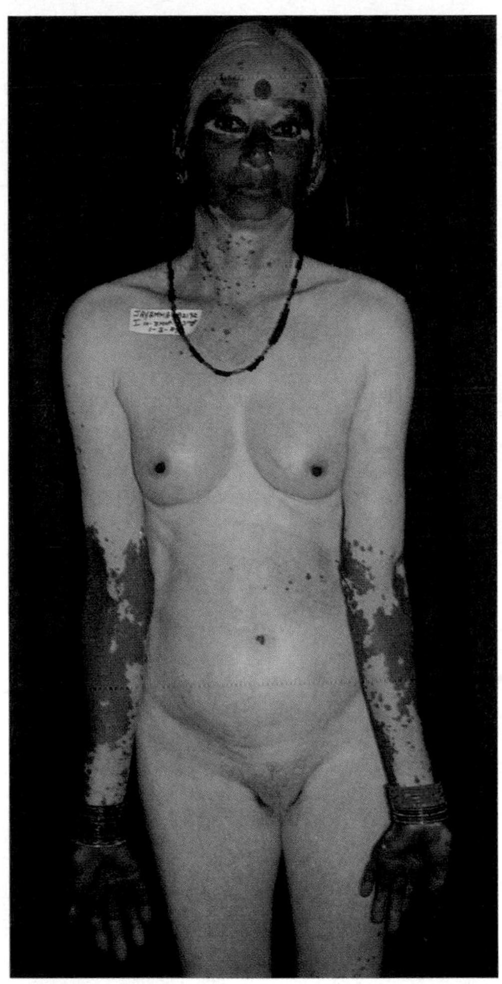

Vitiligo. Generalized vitiligo in a patient with very extensive involvement. Note symmetry.

not unusual. An artifactual or atypically shaped macule may represent koebnerization and is a macule of vitiligo that corresponds exactly to the area of injury; a laceration will leave a macule of linear depigmentation, and a burn will leave an amelanotic lesion conforming to the exact area burnt. Shoulder-strap, waistband, and collar areas—areas frequently rubbed by clothing—seem particularly common sites. Involvement of bony prominences also may represent koebnerization. Mucosal involvement is not infrequent; the genitalia, nipples, lips, and gingiva may be involved. Involvement of the palms and soles, once considered rare, can now be said to be rather common, although often unapparent without Wood's lamp examination, particularly in a fair-skinned individual.

Other Cutaneous Abnormalities Vitiligo may be associated with leukotrichia, prematurely gray hair, halo nevi, and alopecia areata. Depigmented hairs are found commonly in isolated vitiligo macules; leukotrichia (poliosis) has been reported in 9 to 45 percent of vitiligo patients. From one to all of the hairs in a macule may be white. Depigmented scalp hair occurs with or without an underlying vitiligo macule. Extensive white hair may be a marker for poor prognosis in repigmentation, but this may not apply for very small macules. Aside from macular leukotrichia, premature graying of hair (canities) occurs in up to 37 percent (see Chap. 91). Halo nevi appear relatively commonly. There may be one to many halo nevi. Confluence of these lesions in the stage of

FIGURE 90-7

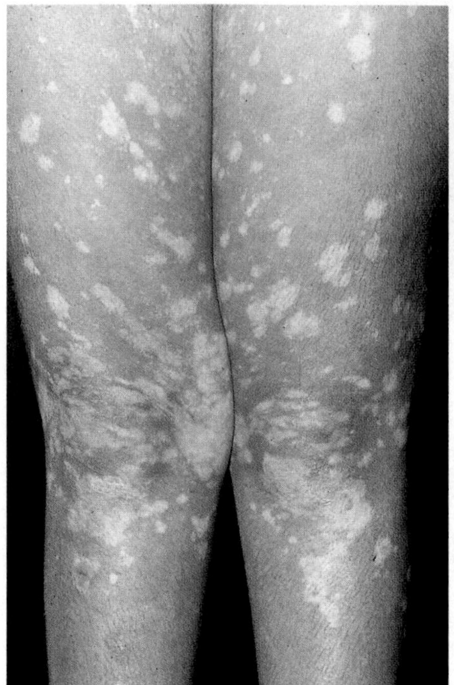

A.

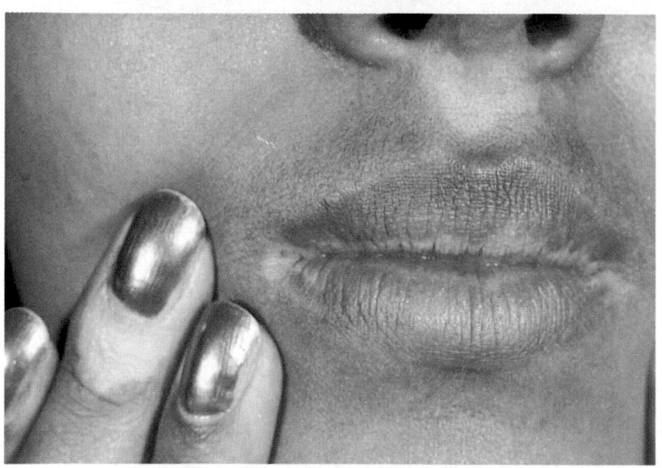

B.

Vitiligo. Characteristic types and features. *A.* Symmetry. There is often nearly mirror-image symmetry as in this 14-year-old Indian girl. *B.* Lip-tip vitiligo. The coexistent involvement of the distal digits and the lips is a common subtype of vitiligo that also includes involvement of the areolae and the penis.

disappearance of the nevus leaves a typical vitiligo-like macule with scalloped borders. Alopecia areata has been reported in up to 16 percent of vitiligo patients (see Fig. 90-3).

OCULAR ABNORMALITIES Vitiligo patients normally have no ophthalmologic complaints (except for the Vogt-Koyanagi-Harada syndrome, see below), but may have iris and retinal pigmentary abnormalities. Careful examination has revealed choroidal abnormalities in up to 30 percent and evidence of iritis in 5 percent. Visual acuity is normally unaffected.

FIGURE 90-8

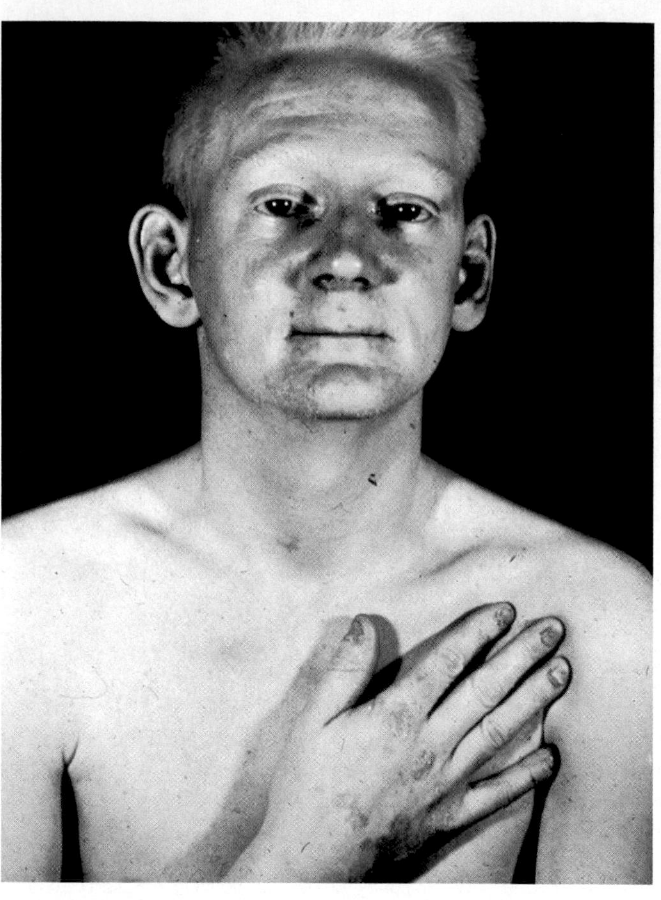

Vitiligo (vitiligo universalis). This patient, who developed total body vitiligo at the age of 9, also has Addison's disease, hypothyroidism, and cutaneous moniliasis. (Note onychomycosis of fingernails.)

OTIC ABNORMALITIES Clinically significant hearing difficulties are not observed. However, deafness has been described in a cluster of patients on a small island where inbreeding and vitiligo are very common. In an audiometric study, no abnormalities implicating ear melanocytes could be found in a group of 93 vitiligo patients.

SYSTEMIC DISEASE ASSOCIATIONS Many authors have reported an association of vitiligo and thyroid dysfunction, either hyper- or hypothyroidism. Taking into account the high incidence of thyroid disease in the population, it is difficult to draw definitive conclusions about the association of vitiligo with thyroid dysfunction or the presence of thyroid antibodies in vitiligo patients, and this association is now questioned. Also, the validity of an association of vitiligo and diabetes mellitus is not obvious from the available data. Incidental association of vitiligo and Addison's disease, pernicious anemia, lymphomas, leukemias, and HIV infections has been reported. An increased incidence (13 percent) of vitiligo in patients with autoimmune polyendocrinopathy, candidiasis–ectodermal dystrophy (APECED), has been established. The gene mutated in this syndrome is called *AIRE* (autoimmune regulator). This association suggests that vitiligo, at least in a subset of patients, is an autoimmune disease. Diabetes mellitus, both juvenile- and adult-onset types, occurs in 1 to 7.1 percent of vitiligo patients, and conversely, vitiligo occurs in 4.8 percent of diabetic patients. The incidence of Addison's disease in vitiligo is said to be 2 percent but is likely much less common. Adrenal cortical and steroid cell antibodies do not appear increased in vitiligo patients.

Pernicious anemia, although uncommon, occurs with increased frequency in vitiligo patients. The multiple endocrinopathy syndrome is found particularly among those with extensive vitiligo.

Histology The current consensus is that no identifiable melanocytes are present in vitiligo macules. A recent report that melanocytes are not absent in lesional skin of long-duration vitiligo illustrates the dynamic nature of the melanocyte loss in vitiligo. The number of melanocytes in trichrome vitiligo, decreased in light-brown skin compared with perilesional normal skin and in vitiligo skin compared with light-brown skin, confirms the centrifugal progression of vitiligo lesions. In the dermis, few lymphocytes may be present in the upper dermis in involved macules and in inflammatory vitiligo with raised and erythematous borders. Melanin may be present in dermal macrophages in darker skin types.[8]

Vitiligo affects the entire epidermal melanin unit. Indeed, cytoplasmic vacuolization and/or the presence of extracellular granular material that may be derived from the cytoplasm of altered keratinocytes has been reported in the adjacent normal-appearing skin but also in the perilesional skin and rarely in the lesional hypomelanotic skin. The Langerhans' cell (LC) density in vitiligo macules has been variably reported as increased, normal, or decreased. The differences in the density of epidermal LCs in the various zones of trichrome vitiligo strongly suggest the involvement of LCs in the pathogenesis of this disorder. In addition, functional impairment of LCs has been documented in vitiligo skin. Repigmentation with PUVA is characterized by activation of inactive melanocytes from the middle and lower outer root sheath; this is followed by proliferation, division, migration, and maturation of melanocytes along with movement from the surface of the outer root sheath to the dermal-epidermal junction, where these appear as active melanocytes.

Pathogenesis An undisputable fact in the pathogenesis of vitiligo is that there are no melanocytes present in the fully evolved white macules. Theories on the pathogenesis therefore center on mechanisms for the destruction of melanocytes. Traditionally, there have been three hypotheses to explain vitiligo[9]: the neural hypothesis, the self-destruct hypothesis, and the immune hypothesis.

NEURAL HYPOTHESIS The neural hypothesis[10] was based initially on anecdotal observations suggesting that stress and severe emotional trauma may initiate or precipitate vitiligo. The common embryologic origin of melanocytes, the nervous system, and the dermatomal distribution of segmental vitiligo are additional arguments put forward to support this view. Local physiologic abnormalities reflecting possible neuromediated aberrations have been reported in vitiligo patients. Direct contact between cutaneous free nerve endings and epidermal melanocytes has been demonstrated in vitiligo. The discovery of a wide range of neuropeptides in the skin and the demonstration that some of them are able to regulate melanocyte differentiation (melanogenesis, dendricity) have given more strength to the neural hypothesis. An increased immunoreactivity of neuropeptide Y (NPY) or an altered balance of nerve growth factor receptors and calcitonin gene–related peptide have been observed in vitiligo skin. Alterations of the catecholamine pathway, increased catechol-*o*-ethyltransferase and monoamino oxidase activities, and increased expression of β_2-adrenoreceptors have been described in vitiligo skin. These alterations are said to induce melanocyte dysfunction and melanocyte injury by promoting the production of melanocytotoxic compounds and by decreasing the natural detoxification-decreasing systems of melanocytes. At present, however, the role of the nervous system in vitiligo, if any, is poorly defined. Clinical evidence is misleading, since the so-called dermatomal or polydermatomal distribution of segmental vitiligo is, in fact, pseudodermatomal.

THE SELF-DESTRUCT HYPOTHESIS According to the self-destruct hypothesis initially put forward by A. B. Lerner, melanocytes in vitiligo have lost an intrinsic protective mechanism that eliminates toxic intermediates or metabolites in the melanogenesis pathway. This pathway is still not identified. The toxic potential of a large number of melanin precursors is well established. Chemicals such as monomethyl- and monobenzyl-ether of hydroquinone induce vitiligo-like hypomelanosis that is clinically and histologically indistinguishable from vitiligo. It has been suggested that the melatonin receptor and melatonin could play a key role in vitiligo. Indeed, melatonin is known to stimulate the melanogenic pathway without production of melanins, leading to an accumulation of toxic intermediate metabolites of the melanogenesis pathway. According to this hypothesis, these toxic products lead to melanocyte and keratinocyte injury with release of specific cellular proteins that initiate a secondary autoimmune reaction. However, this interesting theory is without any substantial experimental basis. The presence of melatonin receptors on melanocytes has not been demonstrated, and the role of melatonin in melanogenesis, if any, is unknown. Several reports provide evidence for increased oxidative stress in the entire epidermis of vitiligo patients.[11] The presence of high epidermal H_2O_2 levels in vitiligo has been demonstrated, and low epidermal catalase levels in involved and uninvolved skin of vitiligo patients have been found. These findings suggest a major stress arising from increased epidermal H_2O_2 generation in vitiligo. Indeed, normal human melanocytes show an increased sensitivity to hydroperoxide in vitro. Protection of these cells against H_2O_2 cytotoxicity can be achieved in vitro by adding catalase to the culture medium. Several pathways could be involved in the overproduction of H_2O_2 in vitiligo. The first is an abnormality in tetrabiopterin metabolism leading to an overproduction of metabolites of this pathway, $6BH_4$ (6*R*)-L-erythro-5,6,7,8-tetrahydro- and $7BH_4$ (7*R*)-L-erythro-5,6,7,8-tetrahydrobiopterin. This accumulation of 6- and 7-BH_4 is detectable clinically by a characteristic yellow-green or bluish fluorescence on Wood's light examination. The defective recycling of 6-BH_4 in vitiligo skin may lead to the formation of H_2O_2. Overproduction of H_2O_2 in vitiligo is claimed to result also from increased catecholamine biosynthesis in association with increased levels of monoamine oxidase A from inhibition of thioredoxin/thioredoxin reductase by calcium and increased nitric oxide synthase activities.

THE AUTOIMMUNE HYPOTHESIS The putative association of vitiligo with autoimmune diseases has suggested an immunologic basis for vitiligo.[12] This concept is now strongly supported by many recent studies. Involvement of humoral immunity was first demonstrated by the findings of circulating antibodies to melanocytes. The vitiligo antibodies are predominantly directed to various melanocyte antigens, including tyrosinase, tyrosinase-related protein 1, and tyrosinase-related protein 2. More recently, autoantibodies to a transcription factor called *SOX10* have been found in vitiligo associated with polyglandular dysfunction (APECED) and in a small number of patients with isolated vitiligo. The level of these antibodies has been claimed to correlate with the disease activity and the extent of the cutaneous involvement. These vitiligo antibodies have the ability to kill human melanocytes in vitro. The best evidence that vitiligo antibodies play a role in melanocyte destruction is the observation of the disappearance of melanocytes from normal human skin engrafted onto nude mice injected with vitiligo patient sera. Evidence for a role of cellular immunity in vitiligo is even stronger. In marginal skin from progressing lesions of inflammatory and generalized vitiligo, an infiltrate of skin-homing (CLA+) cytotoxic T cells expressing granzyme/perforin is often found close to the remaining melanocytes. This infiltrate is composed of CD8+ T cells, CD4+ T cells, and subsets of macrophages, and this correlates with the increased numbers of CLA+ MART-1–reactive CD8+ T cells in the peripheral blood of patients with progressive vitiligo. In vitro, direct analysis of cutaneous T cells from margins of vitiligo macules demonstrates that they have a T_H1 phenotype with a secretory repertoire including interferon-γ and tumor necrosis factor α (TNF-α). These specific cytotoxic T cells react against the melanocyte differentiation antigens Melan-A/MART-1, tyrosinase, and gp100 in vitiligo patients. These CD4+ and particularly CD8+ T cells are associated with the destruction of melanocytes during active disease.[13] It is still unknown whether these specific immune abnormalities are a cause or an effect of the disease, whether they damage melanocytes or aggravate melanocyte injury initiated by other causes, or are an irrelevant epiphenomenon. However, the presence of HLA-A2–restricted melanocyte-specific CLA+ CD8+ T lymphocytes is related to disease activity. Furthermore, melanocyte-associated vitiligo-like depigmentation is observed following successful immunotherapy of melanoma patients, with peptide-pulsed dendritic cells triggering tumor peptide–specific cytotoxic T cell responses.

OTHER THEORIES Besides these three prevailing hypothesis, other possible pathomechanisms have been proposed: an intrinsic defect of the structure and function of the rough endoplasmic reticulum in vitiligo melanocytes,[14] a deficiency in a melanocyte growth factor, a viral origin, a dysregulation of melanocyte apoptosis, and a primary disturbance of T lymphocytes resulting in the development of "forbidden" clones of autoreactive lymphocytes in the epidermis.[9]

ANIMAL MODELS Several animal models of vitiligo have been identified in horses, swine, and mice.[15] The most interesting model is the Smyth chicken. These birds develop a delayed partial or total feather hypomelanosis. They also express many of the associated disorders presented by patients with vitiligo, including ocular depigmentation and uveitis, alopecia areata–like trait, autoimmune thyroiditis, and sometimes spontaneous repigmentation. The etiology of hypomelanosis in the Smyth chicken appears to include an inherent defect in the melanocytes followed by an autoimmune reaction involving antibody-producing B cells. Indeed, elimination of the humoral immune system in the Smyth chicken by neonatal bursectomy results in a significant decrease in the expression and severity of the feather amelanosis.

From the available data, it is likely that the loss of epidermal and follicular melanocytes in vitiligo may be the result of several different pathogenic mechanisms. A convergence theory suggests that genetic factors, stress, accumulation of toxic compounds, infection, autoimmunity, mutations, altered cellular environment, and impaired melanocyte migration and proliferation can all contribute to the phenomenon.[16] Present knowledge strongly suggests an immune pathogenesis, at least in a subgroup of vitiligo patients. However, the concept that the disorder we call vitiligo does not represent a single entity but constitutes a syndrome composed of a variety of different diseases is still valid.[6]

Diagnosis The diagnosis of generalized vitiligo in a patient with progressive, acquired chalk-white macules in typical sites is normally straightforward. Few such acquired conditions are so patterned and symmetric as vitiligo can be. Wood's lamp examination may be required to visualize macules in patients with lighter SPTs and to identify macules in sun-protected areas.

The differential diagnosis of generalized vitiligo includes the following:

Chemical leukoderma: History of exposure to certain phenolic germicides, confetti macules
Leprosy: Endemic area, anesthetic macules, off-white color
Lupus erythematosus: Atypical distribution, inflammation, atrophy, positive immunofluorescence
Melanoma-associated leukoderma: Different distribution, may disappear completely, may have melanocytes
Piebaldism: Congenital, white forelock, stable, large hyperpigmented macules, different distribution
Pityriasis alba: Slight scaling, fuzzy margins, off-white color, ill-defined border
Postinflammatory hypomelanosis: Off-white macules, ill-defined border, history of psoriasis, eczema in same areas
Tinea versicolor: Fine scales with fluorescence under Wood's lamp, positive KOH
Tuberous sclerosis: Congenital, white macules, occasional segmental and confetti macules, stable
Waardenburg's syndrome: Widely spaced inner canthi, heterochromia, broadened nasal root, deafness

Segmental vitiligo is confined to one unilateral quasi-dermatomal distribution, and the following should be excluded:

Nevus depigmentosus: Unusually congenital, stable to progressive, hypomelanotic as opposed to amelanotic
Tuberous sclerosis: Usually associated with typical white ash-leaf macules or confetti macules elsewhere; hypomelanotic, not amelanotic
Idiopathic guttate hypomelanosis: Porcelain-white macule, discrete margins, may be slightly depressed

A solitary white macule or several white to off-white macules often present a challenge because they may be the presenting stage in the evolution of any of the processes listed above.

In some instances, a biopsy may be helpful, but standard histologic studies cannot distinguish a vitiligo macule from one of chemical leukoderma, piebaldism, or WS. Biopsy is useful to establish diagnoses such as lupus erythematosus, leprosy, and tinea versicolor. The presence of melanin or melanocytes in a biopsy cannot be assumed to exclude a diagnosis of vitiligo because trichrome vitiligo, marginal (vitiligo) skin, and repigmenting macules of vitiligo also demonstrate melanocytes.

Once the diagnosis has been established, testing for vitiligo-associated diseases is indicated.

Natural course The natural course of vitiligo is unpredictable. Focal vitiligo, although stable for a time, may be a precursor of generalized vitiligo. The natural course of common vitiligo is often one of abrupt onset, followed by progression for a time; then a period of stability follows and may last for some time, even decades. This may be followed later by a period of more rapid evolution. Total spontaneous regression is rare, and evolution to vitiligo universalis is unusual, although not rare. The most common course is one of gradual evolution of existing macules and periodic development of new ones. Segmental vitiligo, on the other hand, is usually very stable. The period of evolution is often less than a year, after which there is little extension or regression; significant spontaneous repigmentation is unusual.

Treatment While there are several options in the management of vitiligo, most patients require reassurance and an understanding of their affliction. In an increasingly sophisticated world, many patients present with a certain level of knowledge of their options. All patients should be encouraged to use sunscreens to protect the vitiliginous areas, reassured that the use of cosmetic coverup is perfectly acceptable, and educated about the benefits and risks of attempts at repigmentation and depigmentation.[17,18] Additional information is available through support groups, printed brochures, and the Internet.

Professional counseling should be offered to those particularly distressed over their appearance. Patients suffering untoward life disruption in personal or professional relationships particularly should be encouraged to seek help.

Sunscreens offer both protection from sunburn reaction with possible resulting koebnerization and attenuation of facultative tanning of normally pigmented skin; were the latter successful, the contrast between vitiligo macules and normal skin remains minimal, as is the case in the winter months or on habitually unexposed areas of skin. Opaque sunblocks with a *sun protection factor* (SPF) of over 30, containing ZnO and/or TiO_2, are most suited for this purpose (see Chap. 247). Daily use of opaque sunscreens alone may be adequate management for those who are melanodeficient (tan weakly).

Cosmetics, including conventional makeups, dyes, and "self-tanning" preparations, provide quick and practical solutions that are perfectly adequate for many patients. Certain specialized, thicker cosmetics are readily available and can be custom mixed to match most skin colors. Because cosmetics do rub off, they may be of limited value for the lower neck and wrists (rub off on clothing) and hands (because of handshaking). These areas may be better covered with dyes or self-tanning agents or one of the many cosmetic stains, respectively. A formulation containing 5% dihydroxyacetone in an oil-in-water emulsion base is practical and well accepted in vitiligo patients. However, the stains are usually modestly satisfactory at best and do tend to wash off. Patients need to be reassured that none of these preparations will cause their vitiligo to progress, nor will they preclude success of other options.

Repigmentation involves any attempt to reverse the depigmentation and to reestablish normal pigmentation in established macules of vitiligo. Systematic review of the literature reveals that only a few randomized clinical trials have been performed on vitiligo therapies. All current attempts should be viewed as treatments or quasi-remissive techniques and not as a cure. Current available options include topical glucocorticoids for limited vitiligo, topical PUVA for focal and segmental types, PUVA-grafting (see below) for refractory segmental vitiligo or stable vitiligo, narrow-band ultraviolet B (UVB) therapy and oral PUVA for segmental or generalized vitiligo. All forms of treatment require a certain commitment from patients and should be undertaken with the full understanding of the advantages and limitations of each approach (discussed below). A meta-analysis of the literature concludes that class 3 glucocorticoids and UVB therapy are the most effective and safest therapies for localized and generalized vitiligo, respectively.[18]

Topical glucocorticoids have proven effective for isolated macules in some cases, but overall results tend to be disappointing. Hydrocortisone may be used for isolated macules in sensitive areas such as the face and axillae and for children. More potent topical steroids generally are more successful. However, with the most potent topical steroids, the approach should be daily application for 3 weeks, skip a week, and repeat to avoid local glucocorticoid side effects. If there has been no response after 2 months, treatment should be abandoned. If treatment is to be continued, monitoring every 2 months for signs of atrophy is prudent; irreversible striae may develop on the legs after as little as 4 months of continuous treatment. Topical steroids may be used in conjunction with other modalities.

PUVA is indicated in patients for whom no other option is satisfactory and in patients who understand its limitations (see Chap. 266 and Fig. 90-9). Concurrent topical calcipotriol potentiates the efficacy of PUVA in the treatment of vitiligo whereas calcipotriol monotherapy is uneffective.

Narrow-band UVB is presently considered a treatment of choice for vitiligo.[19] Narrow-band fluorescent tubes (e.g., Philips TL-01/100 W) with an emission spectrum of 311 nm are used for this therapy. For a detailed discussion of PUVA and narrow-band UVB for vitiligo, see Chaps. 266 and 265, respectively. *Focused microphototherapy* delivers UVB light with a spectrum of 280 to 315 nm only on the hypomelanotic skin. About 25percent of patients have excellent results. Unfortunately, this therapy requires expensive equipment and trained personal and therefore will not be available for many patients.

Numerous *surgical techniques* have been reported to be successful in repigmentation,[20] but it should be noted that no controlled studies are available. Regardless of the surgical technique, segmental vitiligo is the best candidate for surgical intervention. Vitiligo, which always carries the risk of koebnerization, may be considered suitable for surgical interaction in those cases in which the vitiligo is limited in area and has been stable for some time (2 years). In most cases, pretreatment with PUVA will establish those islands of inapparent melanocytes capable of repigmenting and define sites that have no ability to repigment. The

FIGURE 90-9

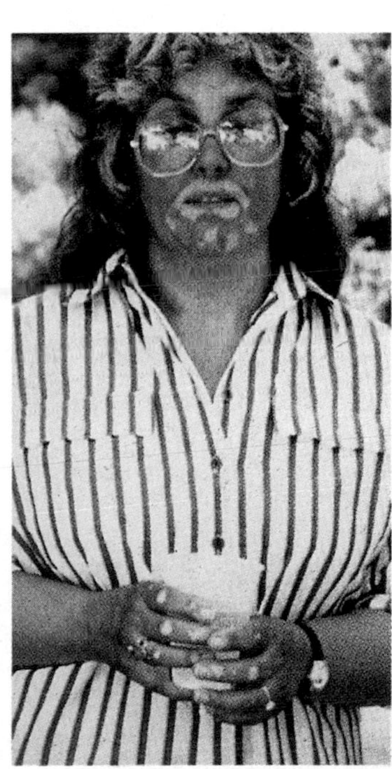

A.

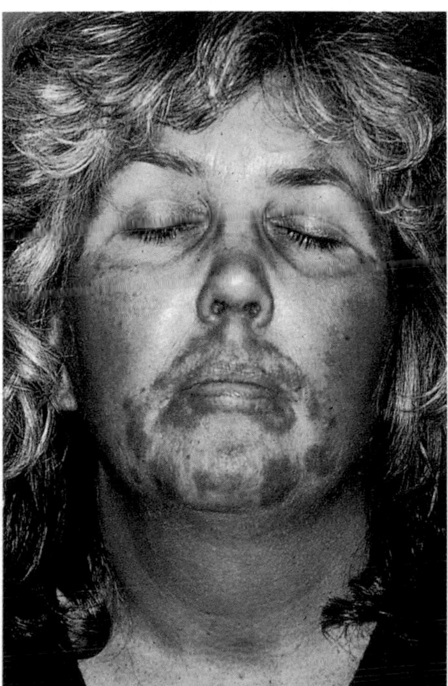

B.

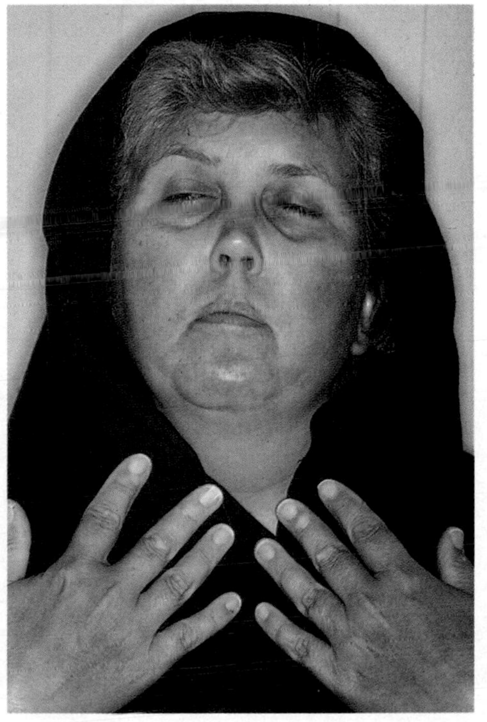

C.

PUVA treatment of vitiligo. *A.* Typical symmetric periorificial vitiligo with characteristic involvement of the skin overlying the interphalangeal joints. *B.* After treatment there is marked hyperpigmentation, often seen in darker skin types. *C.* After discontinuation of treatment, the hyperpigmentation has faded, but the facial macules have remained filled in. A remarkable amount of repigmentation was also noted on the hands.

minigrafting test described by Falabella and colleagues is particularly useful in predicting success (or failure) in minigrafting of stable vitiligo; in all patients, the results demonstrate to the patient the expected cosmetic appearance of the graft and donor sites. The patient and the physician together then may decide if proceeding with extensive grafting will likely be satisfactory.

Various surgical techniques have been described. Transplantation of cultured autologous melanocytes to depigmented macules has led to excellent results, but the method is tedious. Up to 6 to 8 months are required for an excellent color blend. The grafts are generally stable over the 1 to 2 years of follow-up. Falabella reported that even the dorsal hands can be grafted successfully.[20] Cryostorage of excess cultured melanocytes is a source of melanocytes for future procedures.

FIGURE 90-10

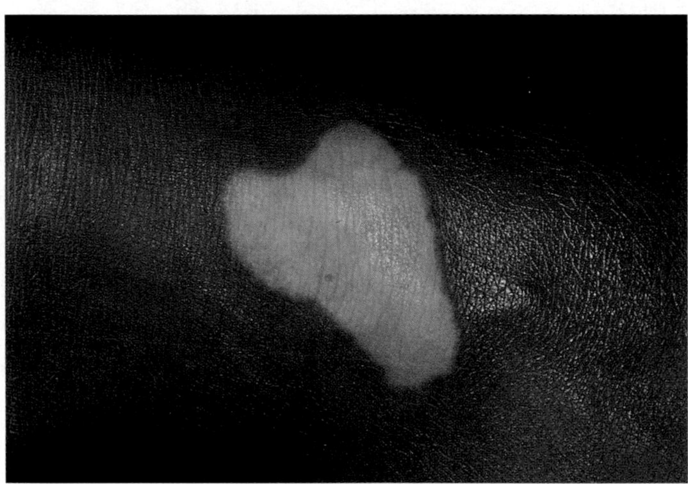

A.

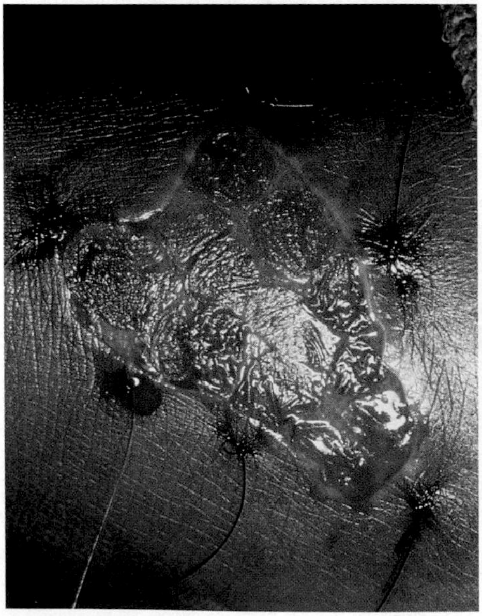

B.

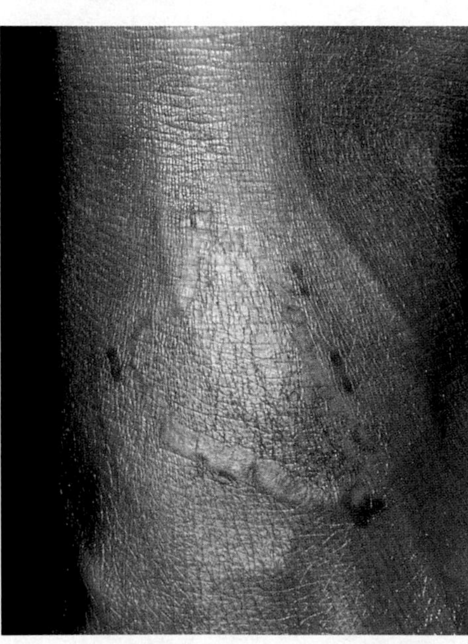

C.

Vitiligo. Treatment with grafting. *A.* Vitiligo macule unresponsive to PUVA. *B.* Same macule after grafts have been placed; pigmentation begins to spread outward from the graft site. *C.* Repigmentation of the macule. PUVA may sometimes be required after grafting to complete the repigmentation. (*Courtesy of WL Morison, MD, and J. Skouge, MD.*)

Minigrafting with 1- to 2-mm punch grafts or split-skin grafts may be most practical for isolated small macules. Placement of four 1.5-mm grafts per square centimeter is a practical technique; pigment spread beyond the graft site should be visible within a month. PUVA may be required to complete the repigmentation (Fig. 90-10). Hyperpigmentation and pebbling may be observed but generally will reverse over time. Patients with stable vitiligo without koebnerization seem to be the best surgical candidates; reversal of leukotrichia also has been observed. Permanent dermal micropigmentation using a nonallergic iron oxide pigment can be used to cover recalcitrant areas of vitiligo.[21]

OTHER THERAPIES *Multivitamin therapy* (folic acid/vitamin B_{12}/Vitamin C) has been reported to show repigmentation, particularly in children. *Melagenina* (placental therapy) generally has proven disappointing outside of Cuba, where it was first described. Likewise, *phenylalanine/UVA* (PAUVA) generally has been inconsistent. The combination of *calcium, pseudocatalase,* and *UVB* has been reported to result in repigmentation even of such refractory areas as the dorsal hand; this improved response plus the relevance of this therapy to new understanding of the disease makes this approach particularly exciting. However, this open study has not yet been confirmed. Oral administration of compounds such as ubiquinone, tocopherol, selenium, and methionine in vitiligo patients is common practice among dermatologists. No controlled study demonstrating the efficacy of antioxidant therapy is yet available.

Depigmentation is another option (Table 90-2) for those with extensive vitiligo and/or in those who have failed PUVA, for whom PUVA is not an option, or who have rejected it (Fig. 90-11). Bleaching, which implies destruction of residual melanocytes with *monobenzylether of hydroquinone* (MBEH) 20% cream is a permanent, irreversible process. Application of MBEH may be associated with satellite depigmentation; therefore, MBEH cannot be used selectively to bleach just limited areas of normal pigmentation; the risk of distant and remote macules of depigmentation is very real. The patient may elect to treat all residual pigmentation or just selected cosmetically bothersome areas. Successful bleaching with MBEH requires twice-daily application for 2 to 3 months before improvement is observed and 9 to 12 months before complete depigmentation is achieved. Up to 50 percent of patients may complain of erythema, dryness, burning, and pruritus, particularly on the face; these symptoms may be diminished by reducing the frequency of use or by mixing the MBEH with an emollient. Contact dermatitis restricted to normally melanized skin occurs in nearly 15 percent of users.[22] Between 90 and 95 percent of patients will be fully bleached in a year. Maintenance applications are not required. However, although this depigmentation is

TABLE 90-2

Monobenzylether of Hydroquinone Therapy of Vitiligo

- Criteria for selection
  - Absolute
    - PUVA failure (or unable/unwilling to treat with PUVA)
    - Patients who can accept the expected irreversible, universal nature of treatment
    - Dark-skinned patients who are prepared to become totally white
    - Patients who will use effective sunblock and avoid midday sunlight
  - Relative
    - Older than 40 years
    - Extensive vitiligo (often > 40%)
    - Fair-skinned (melanodeficient) skin types
- Side effects of therapy
  - Acute
    - Cutaneous irritation
    - Satellite depigmentation
    - Remote depigmentation
    - Contact dermatitis
    - Focal resistant macules (unusual)
    - Rare rapid repigmentation following cessation of use
  - Chronic
    - None expected
    - Occasional focal repigmentation in sun-interactive skin

normally considered to be irreversible, an occasional patient will observe focal repigmentation following sun exposure, which requires reapplication of MBEH for a month or more. Assiduous avoidance of midday sun and routine use of high-SPF opaque sunblocks usually minimize this risk. There have been no long-term untoward effects from the use of MBEH.

Some patients who have bleached may wish to attenuate the chalk-white appearance of their skin; this may be achieved by daily ingestion of 30 to 60 mg of beta-carotene; the intensity of the color may be adjusted by increasing or decreasing the dose.

TREATMENT OF VITILIGO IN CHILDREN There is a particular challenge in the treatment of vitiligo in children, for the complex parent-child relationship may bear heavily on what is asked of the dermatologist. The compelling principle is to segregate the needs of the child from those of the parent. Often it is the parent, not the child, who is concerned; in this case it is the parental worries that must be addressed. In some regions, support groups are available and can be quite helpful.

FIGURE 90-11

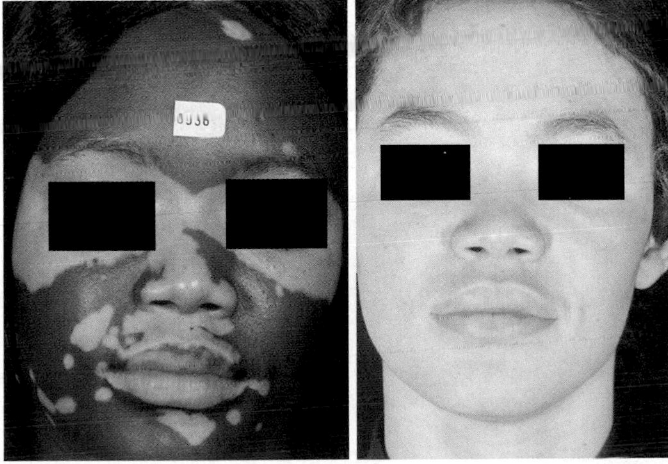

A. *B.*

Vitiligo. Treatment of "normal" skin by depigmentation with 20% monobenzylether of hydroquinone. *A.* Dark-skinned patient with extensive vitiligo before therapy. *B.* Permanent depigmentation after a year of application of 20% monobenzylether of hydroquinone cream. The patient has remained uniformly depigmented for over 15 years.

Sunscreens and cover-up are the initial steps. The next is topical steroids, which may take weeks to be effective. In certain cases of limited vitiligo, topical psoralens may be considered. Narrow-band UVB therapy is the treatment of choice for children (over 6 years). Oral psoralens may be considered after maturity of the ocular lens can be reasonably assured (about age 10). The specifics of each approach are the same as for adults.

VOGT-KOYANAGI-HARADA SYNDROME (VKHS) VKHS is a rare multisystem disease characterized by vitiligo, poliosis, uveitis, dysacousia, and alopecia. While Vogt-Koyanagi syndrome was associated with anterior uveitis and Harada with posterior uveitis and retina detachment, there is enough crossover of features that all these cases may be grouped as one syndrome, VKHS.

Clinical Features Classic VKHS appears in three phases. The first is the meningoencephalitic phase, which begins with the prodrome of fever, malaise, headache, nausea, and vomiting. The degree of involvement is variable, but confusion, psychosis, hemiparesis, paraplegia, aphasia, syncope, generalized muscle weakness, dysphagia, and nuchal rigidity follow. Personality changes and paresis have been known to persist, although neurologic sequelae are unusual. The second phase—the ophthalmic-auditory phase—may appear rapidly and last for 10 or more years. Common features include decreased visual acuity, photophobia, and eye irritation, as well as headache, eye pain, and low-grade fever. Anterior uveitis is usually accompanied by complaints of ocular pain, whereas posterior uveitis is usually less symptomatic but may be associated with retinal detachment, which can be permanent. Dysacousia, which is usually bilateral, occurs in 50 percent of patients. The convalescent phase starts as uveitis begins to abate and is characterized by alopecia, poliosis, and vitiligo. Up to 90 percent may have poliosis, 73 percent alopecia, and 63 percent or less have leukoderma. The macules of hypomelanosis appear with or after the eye symptoms and resemble vitiligo; these are symmetric, may enlarge centrifugally, and seem principally to involve the head, eyelids, neck, and shoulders. Poliosis is usually observed after the onset of alopecia, which is patchy or diffuse. The poliosis may affect the scalp, eyebrows, and eyelashes.

Histology In established macules the most consistent abnormality is absence of melanocytes, as in vitiligo. There are reports of edema and vasodilatation in the dermis, pigment-laden macrophages, and a lymphocytic infiltrate. Histopathologic studies of the skin taken a month after the onset of ocular symptoms reveal a mononuclear infiltrate of a slightly edematous dermis; these are mostly T lymphocytes, but a small number of B cells have been noted. The infiltrate is particularly concentrated around hair follicles and sweat glands. The CD4/CD8 ratio is 3:1.

Diagnosis Diagnosis is based on the presence of ocular and CNS abnormalities, the otic abnormalities being less common and more subtle. Vitiligo with poliosis or canities is the major diagnosis to be excluded. Diagnosis is critical because treatment of the eye abnormalities with steroids may prevent progression to blindness.

Treatment Systemic glucocorticoids are used for eye involvement. Treatment options for skin depigmentation are the same as for vitiligo; abundant poliosis remains an indicator of a poor prognosis for repigmentation.

ALEZZANDRINI'S SYNDROME Alezzandrini's syndrome has been reported in five patients; the syndrome includes facial vitiligo, poliosis, deafness, and unilateral tapetoretinal degeneration.

PIEBALDISM Piebaldism is an uncommon, autosomal dominant, congenital, stable leukoderma characterized by a white forelock and vitiligo-like amelanotic macules, usually containing a few normally pigmented or hyperpigmented macules. The incidence of piebaldism is estimated to be less than 1 in 20,000 persons. Both males and females are equally affected, and no race is spared.[23]

Clinical features The typical piebald macule is chalk or milk white like that of vitiligo and may have feathered margins. The classic pattern for piebaldism (Fig. 90-12) includes a central macule with a white forelock; the lateral trunk, sparing the dorsal spine; and the midarms and legs, sparing the hands, feet, and periorificial areas so characteristic of vitiligo. In up to 90 percent of cases of classic piebaldism, there is a congenital white forelock arising from a triangular, elongated, or diamond-shaped, midline, usually symmetric white macule of the forehead (see Fig. 90-12*A*). This white macule extends to the medial eyebrows, which are often white; the eyelashes also may be depigmented. Amelanotic macules are apparent elsewhere in characteristic symmetric patterns; in 10 to 20 percent of patients with piebaldism, these macules may be the only expression of the disorder. The most characteristic depigmented sites are the anterior abdomen extending to the chest and dorsally to the back with sparing of the midline (see Fig. 90-12*B*), mid-upper arms to wrists, midthighs to midcalves, occasionally the face, in addition to the typical macule associated with the white forelock. Mucosal involvement also has been observed. The hands, upper arms, shoulders, upper thighs, and feet to midcalves usually remain normally pigmented. Hyperpigmented macules within the amelanotic macules and on normally pigmented skin are characteristic of piebaldism. Most hyperpigmented macules are less than 1 cm in diameter, although larger macules have been described. These macules are darker than the normal skin color, are not uniformly pigmented, and have a characteristic electron microscopic appearance. They may appear over time or follow sun or artificial UVA exposure. Partial repigmentation of piebald macules has been reported, as has complete depigmentation.

Piebaldism variants Although patients with piebaldism are generally otherwise normal, occasional patients also have heterochromic irides or deafness. *Woolf's syndrome* is considered a distinct autosomal recessive syndrome characterized by piebaldism with deafness. Interstitial chromosome 4 deletions have been found in several piebald patients with mental retardation. Other variants of piebaldism include X-linked occipital white forelock, white forelock and osteopathic striae, and X-linked autosomal recessive white forelock with blue striae, ocular hypertelorism, epicanthal folds, high arched palate, atrial septal defect, syndactyly, and other problems.

Histology In established macules, the most consistent abnormality is absence of melanin, and melanocytes as in vitiligo.

Pathogenesis Animal model systems provide additional insight suggesting defective melanoblast differentiation or survival. Dominant white spotting, a mouse equivalent of human piebaldism, has been shown to result from deletions or point mutations of the *kit* protooncogene, which encodes the tyrosine kinase transmembrane cellular receptor for mast/cell stem growth factor. In piebaldism, the human homologue of this gene, located on chromosome 4q12.8, is mutated. This affects most patients, but those without *KIT* mutations have no abnormality of the gene encoding SLF itself. Phenotypic variations are a function of the site of the *KIT* gene mutation.[23]

Diagnosis Vitiligo is the major diagnosis to be excluded (Table 90-3). Congenital onset, stable typical pattern, hyperpigmented macules in normal and depigmented skin, and an autosomal dominant inheritance pattern establish the diagnosis of piebaldism. Uncommonly, heterochromia without deafness or lateral displacement of the inner canthus will suggest a variant of piebaldism instead of Waardenburg's syndromes (WS) (see below). Deafness and piebaldism without the other features of WS is Woolf's syndrome. Audiometry should be considered for patients with piebaldism.

Treatment Autologous minigrafts or use of autologous cultured melanocytes has potential because there is no risk of koebnerization in the donor sites as in vitiligo; however, the scope of potential grafting

FIGURE 90-12

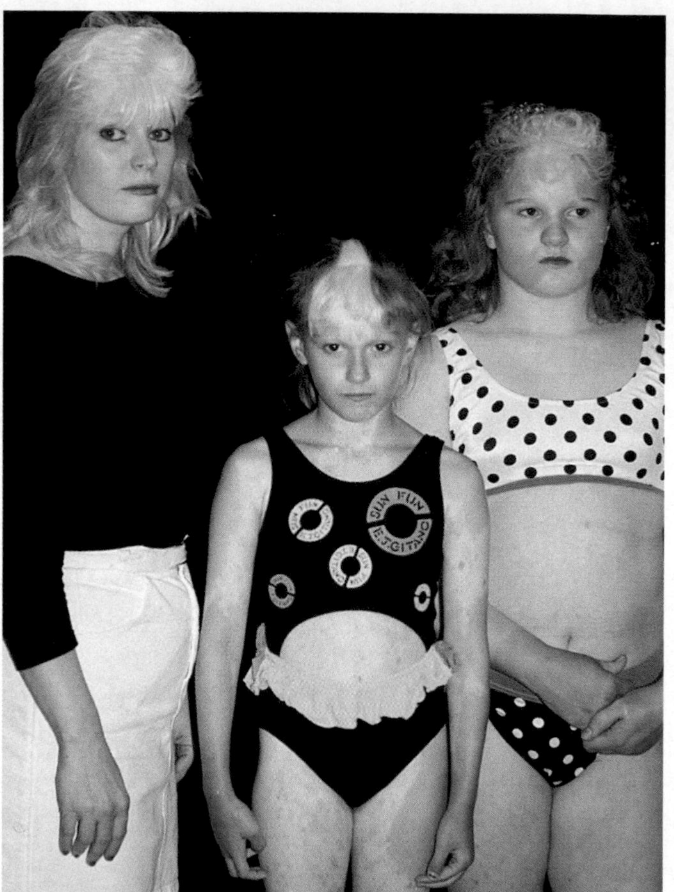

A.

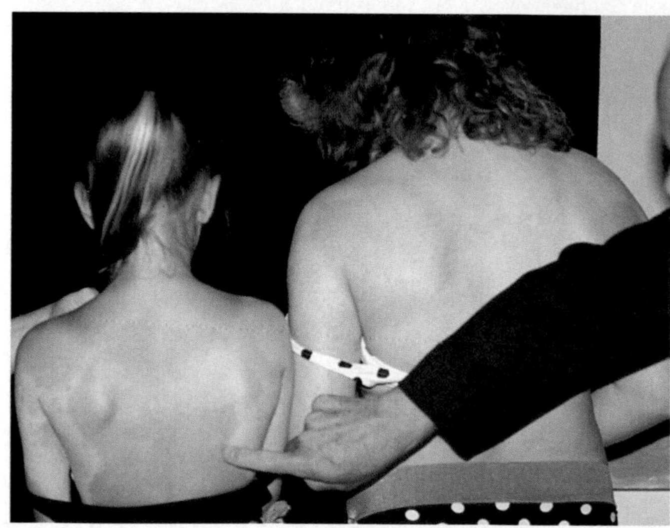

B.

Piebaldism. *A.* Autosomal dominant inheritance pattern is shown by involvement of a mother and two daughters, all of whom have the typical white forelock. *B.* Dorsal sparing of involvement with piebald macules is particularly apparent; the central back is normally unaffected.

TABLE 90-3

Comparative Features of Vitiligo, Piebaldism, and Waardenburg's Syndrome

	Vitiligo	Piebaldism	Waardenburg's Syndrome
Age of onset	Birth to old age; half by age 20; rarely congenital	Birth	Birth
Course	Chronic, progressive; occasional limited improvement	Chronic, stable	Chronic, stable
Color	Milk-white	Milk-white	Milk-white
Size/shape	Millimeters to centimeters; round, scalloped margins	Few to several centimeters irregular	Few to several millimeters
Distribution	Symmetric, periorificial, extensor limbs/digits, periungual	Central forehead with white forelock, mid trunk sparing dorsal spine, mid arms/legs sparing hands/feet	Face, neck, trunk, dorsal hands
Wood's lamp	Enhances contrast	Enhances contrast	Enhances contrast
Special features	Trichrome, occasional segmental pattern	Hyperpigmented macules in white macules/normal skin	None
Other skin changes	Scattered poliosis, halo nevi, alopecia areata	Poliosis	White forelock, eyebrow hyperplasia
Extracutaneous	Hypo/hyperthyroidism, diabetes mellitus, rarely others	None; variants—Woolf's; X-linked	Heterochromic irides, broad nasal root, deafness
Histology of white macule	Melanocytes absent; lymphocytes in active lesions	Melanocytes absent, spherical melanosomes in hyperpigmented macules	Melanocytes absent
Treatment options	Topical steroids, topical PUVA, oral PUVA, 20% MBEH cream to remove normal skin color	20% MBEH cream to remove normal skin color	20% MBEH cream to remove normal skin color
Medical significance	Associated with thyroid disease, diabetes, Addison's disease, pernicious anemia, multiple endocrinopathy syndrome	None	Deafness
Special studies	TSH, FBS (some cases), ANA (for PUVA)	Audiometry (Woolf's)	Audiometry
Major diagnostic clues	Acquired nature, typical patterns	White forelock, autosomal dominance, typical pattern	Cluster or partial cluster of typical features in patient with poliosis, deafness, and a positive family history

NOTE: TSH, thyroid-stimulating hormone; FBS, fasting blood sugar; ANA, antinuclear antibodies.

required is often daunting. Bleaching with MBEH has proved successful in several patients (personal observations), but the process appears to take much longer than the year usually required for vitiligo.

WAARDENBURG'S SYNDROME This is a rare autosomal dominant disorder that is characterized by lateral displacement of the inner canthi and of lacrimal puncta, prominence of the nasal root and of the medial eyebrows, congenital deafness, heterochromic irides, white forelock, and hypomelanotic macules (Fig. 90-13). Variable expression and penetrance create confusion about adequate criteria for the diagnosis of WS. Spontaneous occurrences of WS are seen and may not be unusual. WS has been reported widely; the incidence ranges from 1 in 20,000 in Kenya to 1 in 40,000 in the Netherlands. It may be the cause of deafness in up to 3 percent of the deaf.[23]

Four types of WS have been isolated. Type I (WS1) is associated with dystopia canthorum, and most commonly with cutaneous pigmentary changes and with white forelock. Type II (WS2) is associated with a high incidence of congenital sensorineural hearing loss (familial; 77 percent) and heterochromia (47 percent) but not with dystopia canthorum.

WS1 and WS3 are caused by mutation of *PAX3* that encodes a transcription factor expressed during embryonic development of the melanocyte system. Type II WS or Klein-Waardenburg syndrome is heterogeneous, being caused by mutations in the microphthalmia (*MITF*) gene in some but not all affected families. Patients with WS4, also called *Waardenburg-Shah syndrome,* have mutations in *SOX10,* a gene encoding a transcription factor that plays an essential role in the development of neural crest–derived human cell lineages. A mutation in the endothelin-3 gene has been described in a patient with Waardenburg-Shah syndrome. Types I, II, and III WS are inherited in an autosomal dominant manner, whereas WS4 is an autosomal recessive condition. Molecular genetic analyses have shown that WS1 and WS3 are allelic variants, whereas WS2 and WS4 are distinct entities.

Clinical features A dappled appearance of the skin, white forelock, and premature graying of hair, eyebrows, and cilia are the pigmentary changes found in WS. White forelock, found in from 17 to 58 percent, is present at birth or appears soon thereafter but may disappear over time; it is usually associated with amelanosis. The hypopigmented macules resemble those of piebaldism but may be localized or generalized and symmetrically or asymmetrically arrayed. Forehead, neck, anterior chest, abdomen, anterior knees and arms, and dorsal hands are the most commonly involved sites. The hair within the white macules is usually white. The fundi may be hypopigmented.

FIGURE 90-13

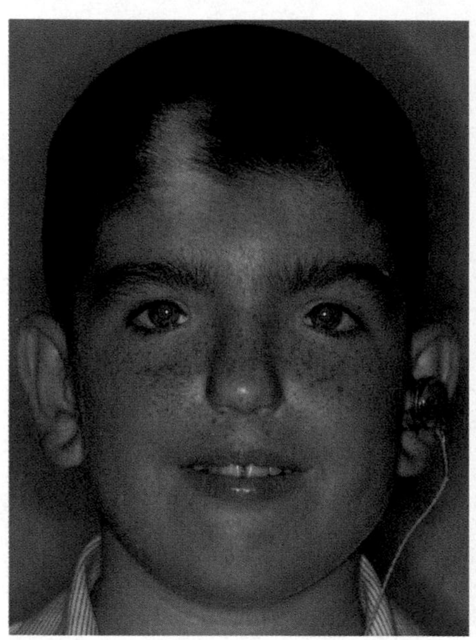

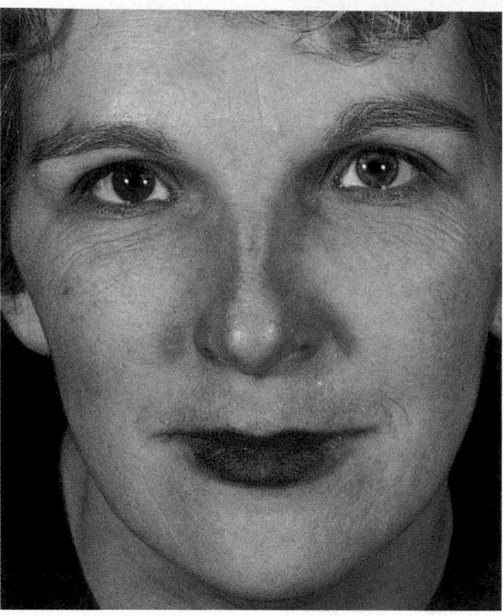

A. B.

Waardenburg's syndrome. *A.* This 15-year-old boy displays the white forelock (which often disappears entirely), broadened nasal root, wide-spaced inner canthi, and hearing deficit. *B.* Heterochromia is particularly apparent in this woman (note one blue and one brown eye).

Other features of WS (See also Chap. 188) Nearly all patients (99 percent) have laterally displaced medial canthi, but the interpupillary distance remains normal. Hypopigmented irides are seen in 87 percent of blacks and 81 percent of Caucasians. Waardenburg found a broad nasal root in 78 percent. Eyebrow hyperplasia with confluence of normally colored medial eyebrows is reported in 17 to 69 percent. Fundal pigmentary abnormalities may occur in about half of patients, but visual acuity is unaffected. Deafness is reported in 9 to 38 percent. Various other CNS and ocular abnormalities have been observed but may be incidental.

Variants of WS A few cases of pseudo-WS have been described, with congenital unilateral eyelid ptosis, heterochromia or isohypochromia, congenital deafness, fair hair with scattered white scalp hairs, dystopia canthorum, and broad nasal root. In another family, several features of WS (except dystopia canthorum) were associated with foveal hypoplasia, iris translucency, and hyperopia-extropia amblyopia. The association of cutaneous white hair, blue irides, macules of retinal depigmentation, a black temporooccipital lock, and aganglionosis of the gut has been reported as a new neural crest syndrome with autosomal recessive inheritance and likely represents an additional example of WS with some unusual clinical features.

Histology and electron microscopy of white macules Melanocytes are absent from the depigmented skin. Reduced numbers of melanocytes are found at the margins of the depigmented macules.

Pathogenesis WS is considered to be one of the neural crest disorders. Melanoblasts fail to migrate, fail to differentiate, and fail to survive. Since nerve cells also may fail to migrate properly, deafness may occur.

Diagnosis The presence of three or more of the classic features usually establishes the diagnosis. Woolf's syndrome (piebaldism with deafness) must be excluded (see above). Rozychi's syndrome is characterized by typical leukoderma, congenital deafness, muscle wasting, and achalasia. Fisch's syndrome includes deafness, early graying of hair, and sometimes partial heterochromia but not laterally displaced inner canthi. Tietz's syndrome is characterized by deaf-mutism, eyebrow hyperplasia, blue eyes, and a generalized cutaneous hypomelanosis characterized histologically by an absence of melanin. The hair is light blond and the eyes are blue, but other features of WS or of albinism are absent. An autosomal dominant inheritance pattern has been suggested.

Treatment No treatment of the pigmentary dilution is available. Spontaneous disappearance of the white forelock does occur, and spontaneous repigmentation and contraction of the white macules have been reported. Early diagnosis and management of the hearing defect is important for normal social and mental development and for genetic counseling.

ZIPRKOWSKI-MARGOLIS SYNDROME (ZMS) ZMS is a curious, rare, X-linked recessive syndrome that occurs in males. The ZMS gene has been localized at Xg26.3-q27.1. ZMS is characterized by deaf-mutism, heterochromic irides, and piebald-like hypomelanosis of the skin and hair. Although the skin appears totally amelanotic at birth, hyperpigmented macules, which are round, oval, or geographic, develop mainly on the extremities and trunk (Fig. 90-14) but rarely on the scalp, where the hair is usually white. Even in the pigmented macules, the hair remains white. The number of melanocytes is equal in the pigmented and amelanotic skin; the dopa reaction is strongly positive in the former and weakly positive in the latter.

TUBEROUS SCLEROSIS (TS) (See also Chap. 189) White macules are found in 79 to 98 percent of tuberous sclerosis patients. Most lesions have been assumed to be present at birth but are relatively unapparent in fair-skinned individuals not examined with the Wood's lamp. However, delayed onset has been demonstrated in longitudinal studies; in one study of 479 Japanese patients, white spots were noted in 82 percent at 1 year and 100 percent at 2 years. Four types of hypopigmented macules are recognized: lance-ovate macules, polygonal macules, confetti spots, and hypomelanosis in dermatomal distribution. Poliosis may occur. The average lesion is 1 to 3 cm in diameter, but macules may vary from 4 mm to 12 cm; 89 percent are larger than 1 cm. The long axis of the lance-ovate macules (Fig. 90-15) is usually axial on the extremities and transverse on the trunk. Confetti macules (2 to 3 mm) (Fig. 90-16) occurr symmetrically from the wrists to the elbows and from the ankles to the knees. Dermatomal patterns (Fig. 90-17) also may occur zarely but usually only in conjunction with other typical macules. The margins of the lesions are usually fairly discrete, and the color of the lesions is dull to off-white or milk-white, unlike the pure white of vitiligo macules. Wood's lamp examination may be particularly useful to find hypomelanotic macules not readily apparent. The white macules may fade in adulthood. Poliosis also occurs with or independently of hypomelanotic macules. Macular hypopigmentation of the retina and of the iris also have been described.[24]

Histology of hypopigmented macules The hypopigmented macules of tuberous sclerosis are characterized by a normal to reduced

FIGURE 90-14

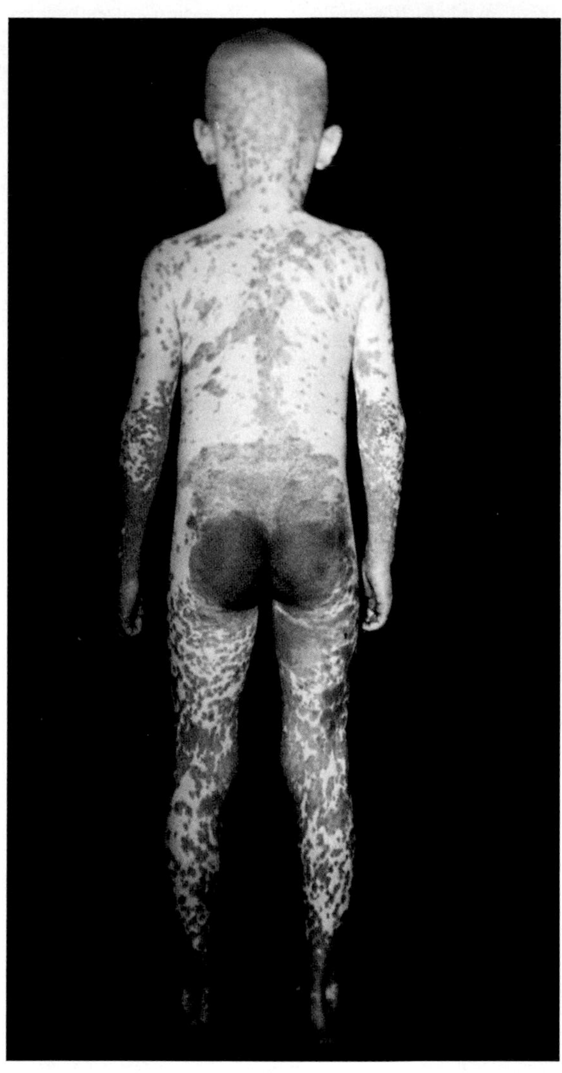

Ziprkowski-Margolis syndrome. Round, oval, or geographic hyperpigmented macules develop in congenitally amelanotic skin. The scalp involvement seen here is unusual.

FIGURE 90-15

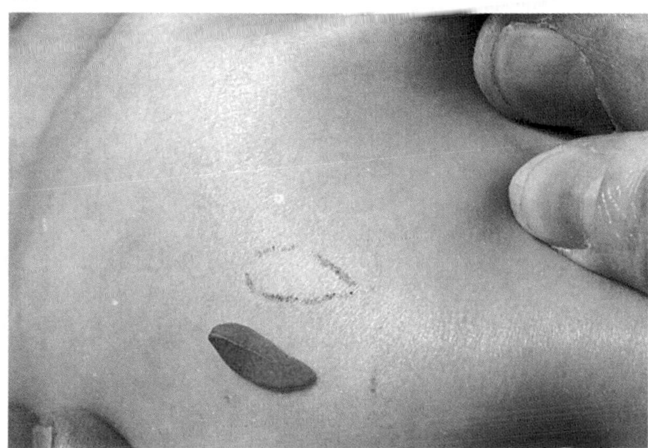

Tuberous sclerosis (TS). Ash-leaf spot. The lance-ovate macule in TS is exactly the shape of a mountain ash leaf. This type of white macule is the most typical of TS but not the most common.

FIGURE 90-16

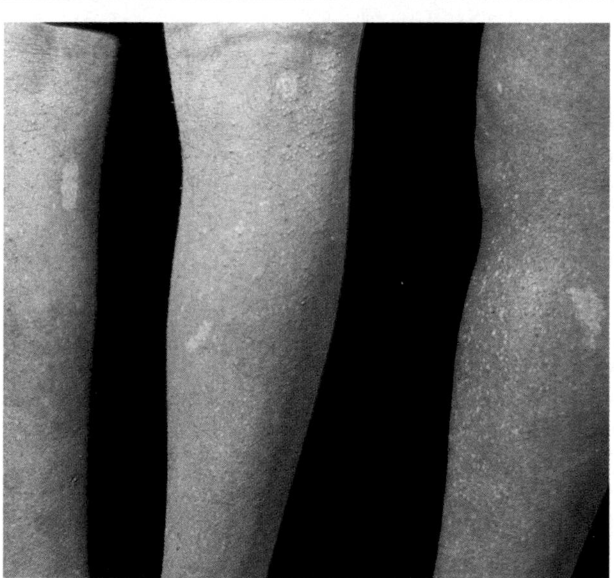

Tuberous sclerosis (TS). Numerous ash-leaf spots in a mother and her son with TS. Note the myriad of scattered tiny white macules, 1 to 2 mm in diameter, on the legs. These are highly characteristic of TS; the "confetti-like" hypomelanotic macules are now regarded as a "presumptive" feature of TS and are an indication for performing imaging studies.

FIGURE 90-17

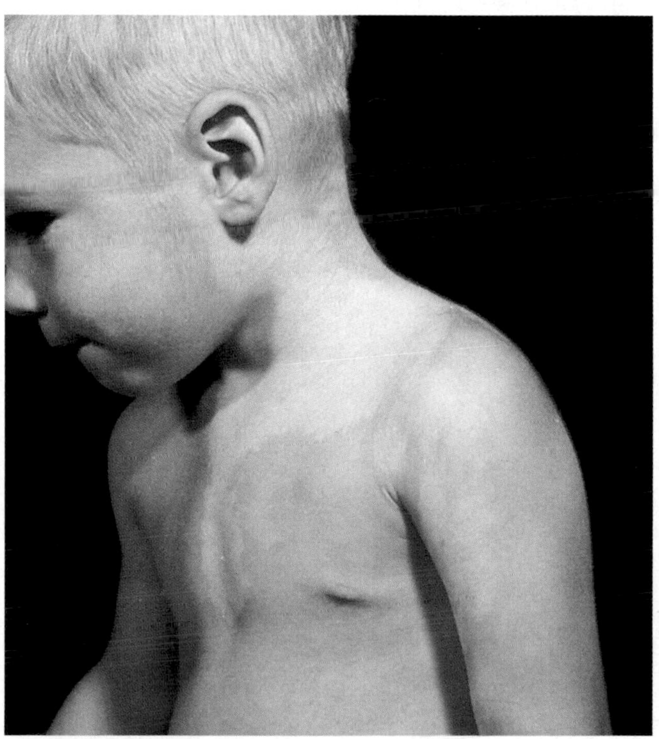

Tuberous sclerosis. Segmental hypomelanosis. This shoulder macule could be mistaken for nevus depigmentosus, which is similarly off-white.

TABLE 90-4

Precis of the Diagnosis of Tuberous Sclerosis

In infancy, tuberous sclerosis (TS) may be suspected by pathognomonic white spots and seizures. In young children with TS there may or may not be angiofibromata, shagreen patches, and mental retardation; however, white spots are present in 95% patients. The positive identification of TS in persons with typical white spots at any age depends on imaging.

History	
Skin signs	White macules, present at birth in 79 to 98%, persist throughout life. Angiofibromata and shagreen patches, present in 21 to 80%, usually appear in childhood during the first 4 years. They are not present at birth.
Constitutional symptoms	Seizures
Appearance of patient	Mental retardation or *normal* intelligence
Physical examination	
Skin	
Type of lesion	Macules—not pure white but off-white Papules/nodules—red and skin-color Plaques—shagreen patch—skin-color
Shape, size, arrangement of lesions	White macules; polygonal (thumb-print) 0.5–2.0 cm, and lance-ovate (ash-leaf); with the long axis 1.0–12.0 cm, average 3–4 cm; scattered, discrete, never grouped Angiofibromatous papules (many) 1–2 mm or nodules (few) 1.0 cm on the face Plaques (shagreen patches), usually isolated, soft, single or rarely multiple
Distribution of lesions	White macules occur on the trunk (56%), lower extremities (32%), upper extremities (7%), and head and neck (5%) Angiofibromatous papules on the face Shagreen patches most often on the posterior trunk or buttocks
Associated systems involved	Central nervous system (tubers producing seizures), eye (gray or yellow retinal plaques, 50% incidence), heart (benign rhabdomyomas), kidney, liver, thyroid, testes, and gastrointestinal (hamartomas of mixed-cell type)
Laboratory and special examinations	
Dermatopathology	
Light and electron microscopy	Decreased number of melanocytes, decreased dopa reaction, decreased melanosome size, and melanization
Wood's lamp examination	Hypomelanosis, a dull white or off-white, but not as white as vitiligo
Imaging	CT scan for detection of location, size, and shape of calcifications and for presence of gliomas; especially necessary in children with white spots and seizures and in parents (of childbearing age) of TS patients with or without skin signs, seizures, or mental retardation Magnetic resonance is especially useful for hydrated lesions and may permit classification of tubers
Differential diagnosis	White spots; vitiligo, piebaldism, nevus depigmentosus, postinflammatory leukoderma

number of melanocytes, which have poorly developed dendrites and which contain small and poorly melanized melanosomes.

Other cutaneous manifestations Adenoma sebaceum is a misnomer because the lesions are angiofibromas that appear as small (up to 0.3 cm) reddish brown or flesh-colored, shiny papules located centrofacially, particularly on the sides of the nose and the medial portions of the cheeks and are dealt with in Chaps. 189 and 102 (Fig. 102-8). In these lesions there is a proliferation of dense collagen surrounding appendages and ectatic blood vessels (see Fig. 102-9). Other lesions are shagreen patches, flat, slightly elevated, skin-colored, or brownish plaques present in up to 80 percent and usually appearing in childhood during the first 4 years. These lesions occur on the trunk and buttocks and are not present at birth. Angiofibromas also occur in the nail folds and at subungual sides, and these lesions are called *Koenen tumors*. These periungual fibromas develop in 50 percent of tumorous sclerosis cases, appear between the ages 12 and 14, and increase progressively in size and number with age. The tumors are small, round, and flesh-colored and may be hyperkeratotic, resembling fibrokeratoma (see Chap. 189).

Diagnosis A précis of the diagnosis of TS is given in Table 90-4. The diagnosis of TS is a clinical one based on primary, secondary, and tertiary criteria. Hypomelanotic macules are the earliest clinical sign of TS. They can be detected in patient of all ages including neonates and are identified most clearly with the use of a Wood's light. The ash-leaf shaped hypomelanotic macules is most characteristic of TS. Congenital confetti macules are also particularly significant but have been found in other disorders (multiple endocrine neoplasia type 1).

In a patient with three or more typical white lance-ovate or "thumb-print" macules or confetti macules, seizures, and mental retardation, the diagnosis is readily apparent and a pediatric neurologist should be consulted.

Diagnostic difficulties arise when there are fewer than three macules, where there are no other features of TS, or when the issue of subclinical TS must be resolved. If occurring alone, hypomelanotic macule are not sufficient for diagnosis. The true incidence of solitary white macules in the general population is uncertain. One study of 4412 neonates found no white macules. In another study, 98 percent of congenital white spots resolved. These lesions obviously did not represent TS, but the study did not incorporate use of Wood's lamp and there was no long-term follow-up. In a large series of babies, all of those with three or more hypomelanotic macules were mentally retarded, of the eight with two macules, one had seizures and two had frank TS. None of the 60 with a solitary white macules had other clinical features of TS.

Whether or not a solitary white macule is an expression of heterogeneity remains unresolved; isolated hypomelanotic macules have been found in apparently unaffected parents of affected children. While hypopigmented macules may represent secondary or tertiary criteria for diagnosis, the presence of white macules with or without CNS findings may require exclusion of the diagnosis of TS. Cranial CT scan may diagnose calcified subependymal glial nodules, and MRI may show cerebral cortical and subcortical lesions, which are not always pathognomonic. Compared with CT scans, MRI findings more closely correlate with the severity of neurologic impairment. Echocardiograms are sensitive, especially in those under 2 years of age. Abdominal ultrasound identifies renal disease in infancy and adolescence. Distinguishing between spontaneous and heritable TS can be difficult. Examination of first-degree family members with the Wood's lamp is helpful if white macules are found, but since these macules may fade with time, the absence of adult white macules does not exclude familial TS. No consensus has emerged with regard to radiologic screening of first-degree relatives of affected patients.

Differential diagnosis The differential diagnosis is that of stable congenital hypomelanotic macules (Table 90-5). The difficulties are underscored by a recent study that found hypopigmented macules (resembling those of TS) such as streaks or round to oval off-white macules to be common in apparently normal individuals.

The diagnosis of TS should be considered in every newborn with seizures and/or mental retardation. Wood's lamp examination is essential, particularly in fair-skinned individuals.

Treatment There is no treatment for the white macules of TS.

HYPOMELANOSIS AND CUTANEOUS MOSAICISM These include two different entities, hypomelanosis of Ito (HI) and phylloid hypomelanosis.

Hypomelanosis of Ito[25,26] This disorder is also termed *incontinentia pigmenti achromians* or *pigmentary mosaicism of the Ito type.* It is characterized by randomly distributed hypomelanotic macules with a bizarre whorled and streaked marble-cake configuration (Fig. 90-18). These lesions consist of bilateral or unilateral streaks corresponding to the lines of Blaschko.[27] On the back, the lesions resemble an inverted Christmas tree. Any part of the body, including the face, may be involved. The lesions present at birth become recognizable during the natal period or early childhood. Other types of pigmentary patterns such as a checkerboard arrangement likewise have been described. HI is often associated with extracutaneous anomalies (75 percent). They include CNS abnormalities (seizures, mental or motor retardation, microcephaly, hypotony, hyperkinesias, ataxia, and deafness), ophthalmologic abnormalities (ptosis, nonclosure of the upper lid, symblepharon, dacryostenosis, strabismus, nystagmus,

TABLE 90-5

Comparative Features of Nevus Depigmentosus, Tuberous Sclerosis, and Hypomelanosis of Ito

	Nevus Depigmentosus	Tuberous Sclerosis	Hypomelanosis of Ito
Age of onset	Birth, rarely early childhood	Birth	Early childhood
Heredity	Nonhereditary	Some hereditary, many sporadic	Some hereditary, many sporadic
Course	Chronic, stable in most, progressive in others	Chronic, may fade or disappear	Evolves, stabilizes, and often reverses
Color	Off-white	Off-white	Off-white
Size/Shape	Quasidermatomal	Lance-ovate, thumb-print, segmental, confetti	Swirls and parallel streaks of hypomelanosis
Distribution	Unilateral on trunk or extremities	Trunk, arms, legs; three or more lesions usually	Trunk and limbs
Wood's lamp	Increased contrast	Increased contrast	Increased contrast
Special features	Nevoid pattern	Ash-leaf spots, confetti macules	"Marble cake" pattern in many
Other skin changes	None	Adenoma sebaceum, shagreen patches, fibromata	Occasional atrophy
Extracutaneous features	None	Seizures, mental retardation, cerebral calcification, rhabdomyomas (heart), bone lesions, renal hamartomas	>75% with abnormalities of CNS, eyes, hair, musculoskeletal system, or internal organs, mental retardation in over 60%, seizures in over 50%
Histology	Normal number of melanocytes; may be melanosomal aggregates in melanocytes; fewer melanosomes in keratinocytes	Normal to decreased numbers of melanocytes; decreased melanization of melanosomes; fewer stage III and IV melanosomes	Decreased numbers of poorly dendritic melanocytes; decreased numbers and size in melanocytes and keratinocytes
Treatment (white macules)	None	None	None
Medical significance	None	Up to 25% autosomal dominant; risk of seizures, mental retardation	Many autosomal dominant; high risk of multiple abnormalities, many significant
Special studies	None	CT scan, MRI, echocardiography, neurologic evaluation	Neurologic and ophthalmologic evaluation
Major diagnostic clues	Unilateral distribution of congenital off-white macules in healthy individuals	Presence of white macules in newborn with seizures and mental retardation; presence of ash-leaf spots not characteristic of other disorders	Acquired, swirled, streaked hypomelanosis in patient with seizures, retardation, and multiple musculo-skeletal abnormalities

FIGURE 90-18

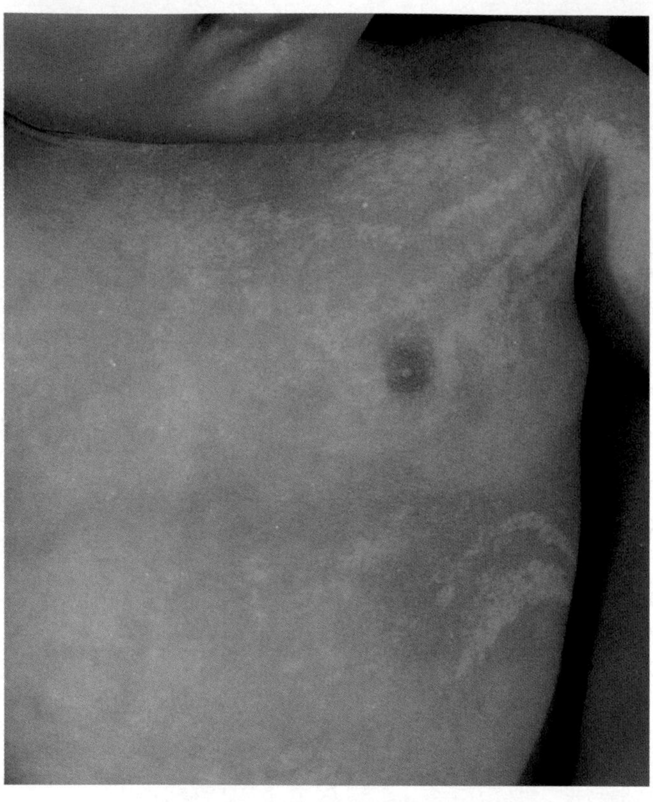

Hypomelanosis of Ito. Over 75 percent of patients will have abnormalities of the eyes, musculoskeletal system, and/or nervous system. Swirls of hypomelanosis on the chest of an infant who had similar lesions on the back.

FIGURE 90-19

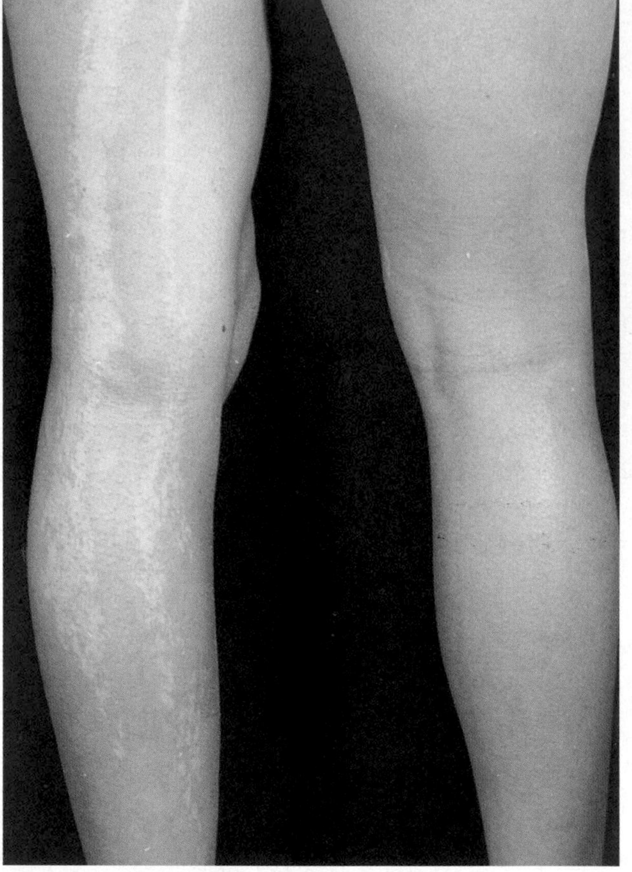

Nevus depigmentosus. This congenital nevoid off-white stable hypomelanosis, unlike segmental vitiligo, does not usually change in size or color over time. This linear nevus depigmentosus involves one leg posteriorly.

corneal opacification, cataracts, myopia, amblyopia, microphthalmia, iridal heterochromia, scleral melanosis, patchy hypopigmented fundi, and retinal degeneration), enamel changes and other dental defects, and skeletal defects (short stature, pectus carinatum or excavatum, scoliosis, syndactyly, polydactyly, brachydactyly, clinodactyly, asymmetry of limbs, and facial asymmetry). HI is a cutaneous sign of many different forms of genomic mosaicism. Indeed, karyotypic abnormalities of different chromosomes are found in lymphocytes and fibroblasts and rarely kératinocytes. Mosaicism affecting melanocytes has not yet been demonstrated. Histologic and ultrastructural studies show rounded melanocytes with reduced or absent dendrites and slightly decreased epidermal melanin pigmentation.

DIAGNOSIS The clinical picture is characteristic enough to suggest the diagnosis when the whorled pattern is present (see Table 90-5).

Phylloid hypomelanosis[28] This newly recognized disorder is characterized by round or oval hypomelanotic macules resembling the asymmetric leaves of a begonia or oblong lesions. A mosaic trisomy 13 or translocation trisomy 13 has been found in the peripheral blood lymphocytes of a majority of patients with this phylloid hypomelanotic pattern. All patients had CNS defects: mental retardation, absence of corpus callosum, conductive hearing loss, choroidal and retinal coloboma, craniofacial defects, as well as brachydactyly, camptodactyly, and other skeletal abnormalities. In contrast to HI which is a cutaneous sign of many different forms of genomic mosaicism, phylloid hypomelanosis appears to be a cytogenetically rather uniform neurocutaneous phenotype.

Nevus depigmentosus Whether nevus depigmentosus (ND) is a distinct entity or a manifestation of cutaneous mosaicism is still a matter of debate. ND occurs equally among males and females and can affect any ethnic group. Three clinical forms of ND are described: an isolated, circular or rectangular macule or, less commonly, a dermatomal or quasi-dermatomal pattern (Fig 90-19) or a systematized (unilateral whorls or streaks) form. The hypomelanotic lesions remains stable throughout life. ND occurs most commonly on the trunk and proximal extremities. ND typically does not cross the midline. Rare reports of associated findings (seizures, mental retardation, limb hypertrophy) have been reported. Several authors believe that HI and ND belong to cutaneous mosaicism. Cytogenetic abnormalities in ND patients have not yet demonstrated.

INCONTINENTIA PIGMENTI (IP) (See Chaps. 143 and 188) IP is a syndrome characterized by skin lesions that are arranged in a linear pattern.[29] This uncommon X-linked dominant disorder, generally lethal in males, has three stages: vesiculobullous, verrucous, and hyperpigmented. However, in about 13 percent there is a fourth stage, that of swirls of hypopigmentation, consisting of atrophic hypo- or amelanotic bands of streaks that fail to tan with sun exposure. In addition, these lesions are hypohydrotic and hairless. Hypomelanosis is a late manifestation of the disease, observed most commonly in adults. Hypomelanosis involves mainly the back but also the abdomen and the limbs. The pathogenesis of these lesions is not understood. Hypomelanotic lesions of IP share with HI the streaky distribution and the frequent occurrence of extracutaneous abnormalities. However in HI, hypomelanotic lesions are either recognized at birth or become visible during the neonatal period or early childhood.[29]

ATAXIA TELANGIECTASIA (See Chap. 191) Ataxia telangiectasia may be associated with premature graying of hair and with hypomelanotic macules. Vitiligo-like leukoderma has been reported in a few patients.

XERODERMA PIGMENTOSUM (See Chap. 155) Hypopigmented lesions 1 to 5 mm in diameter have been reported in patients with xeroderma pigmentosum. No melanocytes are present in the centers of the lesions, and decreased numbers of melanocytes are found at the margins. These melanocytes in both normally sun-exposed and unexposed areas of skin are bizarre in that they are characterized by melanin macroglobules, melanosomes aggregated in autophagic vacuoles, abnormal melanin deposition, and few melanosomes in upper-level keratinocytes alone.

PREUS SYNDROME The association of growth retardation, dolichocephaly, cataracts, high arched palate, small, widely spaced teeth, generalized hypopigmentation (tyrosinase positive), psychomotor retardation, and hypochromic anemia has been reported in two siblings of consanguineous parents. An additional patient has been reported with additional features (coxa valga, generalized osteoporosis). This disorder appears to be distinct from the oculocerebral hypopigmentation described by Cross.[4]

MISCELLANEOUS DISORDERS Circumscribed hypomelanosis also has been described in the focal dermal hypoplasia syndrome (linear or reticular pattern), in punctate keratosis of palms and soles, and in ectodermal dysplasia.

Hypomelanosis Associated with Nutritional Disorders

KWASHIORKOR (See Chap. 145) In kwashiorkor, the depigmentation, which may precede other features by weeks, begins on the face. A shiny erythema is followed by raised plaques that gradually darken until they assume a shiny black appearance. Exfoliation may be followed by depigmentation; the latter patches may repigment with hypermelanosis. The lesions are most common on sites of pressure. A generalized pallor also may occur. Red-brown to gray or golden hair is common. The hypopigmentation has been attributed to disruption of normal melanogenesis. The hypomelanosis and dyschromic hair are reversible with dietary correction.

SELENIUM DEFICIENCY Two children with selenium deficiency following long-term parenteral nutrition developed pigmentary dilution of the hair and skin. After 6 months of selenium replacement, the two children with decreased pigmentation became dark-skinned, and their hair color changed from blond to dark brown. A third child's hair, which had been blond, also became darker. The mechanism by which selenium contributes to hair and skin color changes is as yet unknown.

Hypomelanosis Associated with Endocrinopathies

Numerous endocrinopathies have been associated with pigmentary dilution (see Chap. 169).

Hypopituitarism is associated with reversible hypomelanosis secondary to decreased MSH and ACTH production. Depigmentation of the extensor hands and feet has been reported in a patient with adrenal insufficiency secondary to defective corticotropin-releasing factor; since ACTH levels were not increased, the pigmentary abnormality was attributed to presumed decreased MSH levels. Most cases of selective ACTH deficiency are not associated with hypopigmentation, however.

Hypogonadism may be associated with pallid skin. One male eunuch tanned poorly until after testosterone therapy; he then tanned deeply in sun-exposed areas. Orchiectomy has been reported to decrease melanin pigmentation of the skin in men.

Hypomelanosis Secondary to Physical Trauma[30]

Hypomelanosis may result from a multitude of types of trauma, including thermal injury, physical injury, hypothermia and freezing, and x-ray, ionizing, and UV irradiation. X-rays have long been known to cause depigmentation. Epilating doses of x-rays have been shown to result in regrowth of white hair. This appears to result from the loss of functioning melanocytes.

Hypomelanoses Resulting from Chemical Exposure

CHEMICAL LEUKODERMA[31,32] Chemical leukoderma is an acquired hypomelanosis arising from repeated exposure to specific chemical compounds, particularly certain phenol derivatives and sulfhydryl compounds. Awareness of chemical leukoderma dates from a report of a vitiligo-like leukoderma appearing among tannery workers exposed to monobenzylether of hydroquinone (MBEH), which was being used as an antioxidant. Chemical compounds reported to cause chemical leukoderma are listed in Table 90-6. Exposure may be reasonably widespread. MBEH, for example, is found not only in disinfectants and germicides but also in rubber-covered wire dish trays, adhesive tape, hatbands, contraceptive diaphragms, rubber finger cots, rubber clothing, rubber aprons, powdered rubber condoms, rubber dolls, neoprene, and fabric-lined rubber gloves; all of the latter have been implicated in production of chemical leukoderma. Previously unsuspected by-products of rubber processing have been shown to be parasubstituted phenols,

TABLE 90-6

Chemicals Implicated in Causing Chemical Leukoderma

Phenols/catechols	Miscellaneous/unclassified
Alkyl phenol	Ammoniated mercury
Butylated hydroxytoluene	Arsenic
Catechol	Benzoyl peroxide
Dihydroxyphenylmethane	Brilliant lake red R
Hydroquinone	Carmustine (BCNU)
4-Isopropylcatechol	Chloroquine
Methylcatechol	Cinnamic aldehyde
Monobenzylether of hydroquinone	Dinitrochlorobenzene (DNCB)
Monoethylether of hydroquinone	Eserine
Monomethylether of hydroquinone	Fluorouracil
p-Tertiary amylphenol	Glucocorticoids
p-Tertiary butylcatechol	Guanonitrofuracin
p-Tertiary butylphenol	Thiotepa
Tretinoin	
Sulfhydryls	
β-Mercaptoethylamine HCl	
β-Mercaptoethylamine HCl	
β-Metcaptopropylamine HCl	
N-(2-Mercaptoethyl)-dimethylamine	
Sulfanolic acid	

which may be implicated in chemical leukoderma. Certain medications may cause pigmentary dilution. Topical tretinoin can cause subtle hypomelanosis and reversal of hyperpigmentation. Intralesional cortiosteroids also can cause ill-defined hypomelanosis. Benzoyl peroxides (acne preparations) bleach hair. Cinnamic aldehyde, once in toothpaste, has been shown to cause a vitiligo-like leukoderma. Soymilk and two soymilk-derived proteins (soybean trypsin inhibitor and Bownran-birk protease inhibitor) inhibit the protease-activated receptor 2 (PAR-2) that regulates pigmentation via keratinocyte-melanocyte interactions. This inhibition of PAR-2 blocks melanosome transfer and thus induces skin depigmentation. The use of PAR-2 inhibitors could lead to new class of depigmenting agents.[33]

Clinical features The leukoderma attributed to MBEH and other substances resembles that of vitiligo (Fig. 90-20). Hypomelanotic macules are milk-white and appear not only at the site of contact with the offending compound but also remotely. Remote or satellite lesions are guttate or confetti macules. A prior irritant or contact eruption is not required for the leukoderma to develop. In early stages, the leukoderma may be reversible if the chemical exposure is stopped.

In contrast to leukoderma due to MBEH, which is vitiligo-like and sharply defined, hypomelanosis due to hydroquinone usually does not have sharp margins (Fig. 90-20*B*) and is usually a more subtle, ill-defined hypomelanosis. Complete depigmentation and satellite depig-

FIGURE 90-20

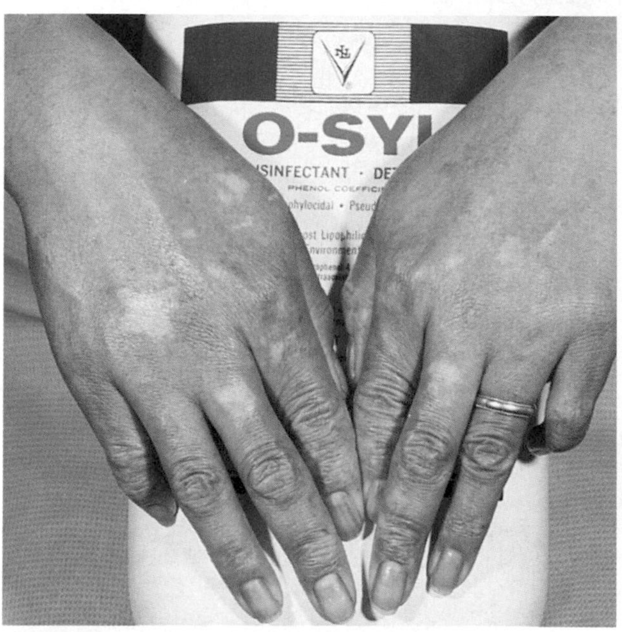

A.

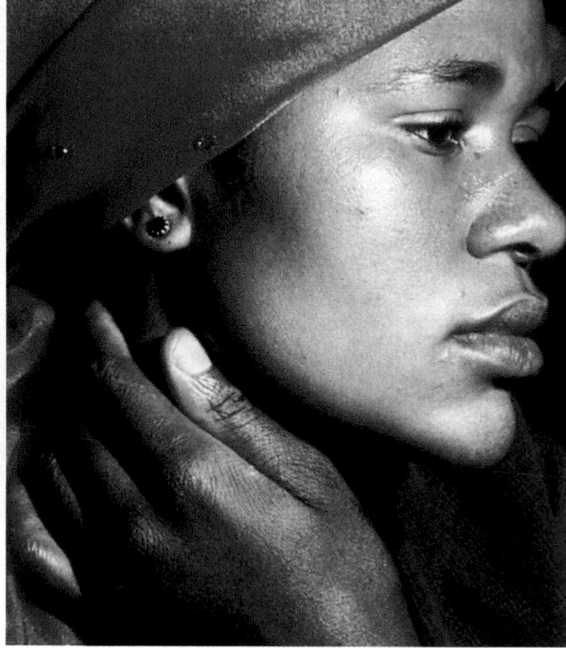

B.

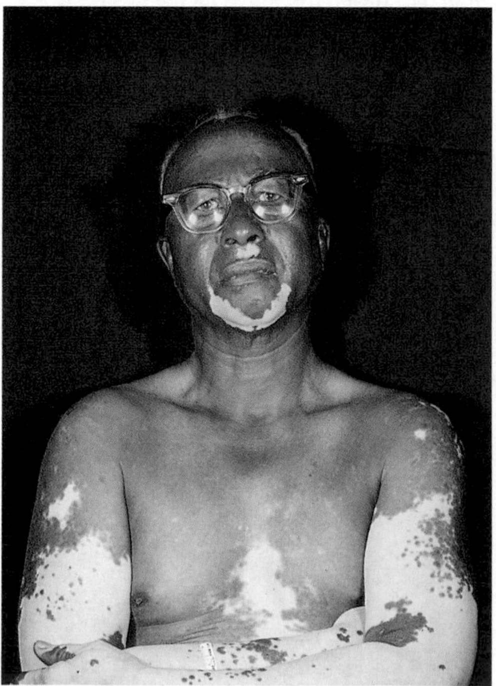

C.

Chemical leukoderma. *A.* O-Syl (a phenolic disinfectant)–induced chemical leukoderma that mimics vitiligo clinically. Repeated exposure is required to depigment, but antecedent clinical inflammation is not observed. *B.* Reversible hypomelanosis of the face in a South African woman after several weeks application of topical hydroquinone. Note color contrast of face to that of (untreated) hand. *C.* African American factory worker depigmented from repeated exposure to monobenzylether of hydroquinone.

mentation do not occur. Hydroquinone has been used for many years to lighten the skin to an acceptable cosmetic color.

Histology Chemical leukoderma has no typical diagnostic features to distinguish it from vitiligo; typically, melanocytes are absent, and there are no dermal or other epidermal changes in established macules. Histologic evidence of melanocyte disruption and destruction may be noted in evolving lesions.

Pathophysiology There are many possible mechanisms involved in cutaneous depigmentation induced by chemicals. These include selective action on the melanocyte through free-radical formation, competitive inhibition of tyrosinase, inhibition of oxidation of tyrosine to dopa synthesis, interference with premelanosome or melanosome synthesis, interference with tyrosinase synthesis by combining with melanocytic ribosomes, interference with transfer of melanosomes from melanocytes to keratinocytes by inhibition of arborization of melanocytic dendrites, and reduction of melanin present in melanosomes. Sulfhydryls may be cytotoxic agents that alter or block melanin formation through inhibition of tyrosinase or promote the production of phaeomelanins and their colorless metabolites rather than eumelanogenesis.

Diagnosis Chemical leukoderma always should be in the differential diagnosis of vitiligo (Table 90-7) or any other acquired, circumscribed, progressive amelanosis. The site of the initial leukoderma should correspond to the area of primary and repeated chemical exposure. A presumptive diagnosis may be made on the basis of history of repeated exposures to known or suspected leukoderma-producing agents (see Table 90-6); leukoderma that follows an untoward single exposure to a chemical may result in postinflammatory leukoderma or koebnerization in a patient with a vitiligo diathesis. Unfortunately, there is no definitive test or histology to distinguish vitiligo from chemical leukoderma. Despite isolated reports of abnormal thyroid studies or hepatosplenomegaly, most patients with chemical leukoderma are healthy.

Treatment Established chemical leukoderma is irreversible if the offending chemical is not eliminated soon enough. Early localized cases may be reversed by discontinuing the offending chemical and, if necessary, by topical or oral PUVA; as with vitiligo, established acral and mucosal macules are usually refractory to repigmentation. Discontinuation of the exposure is mandatory; surveillance of the environment to exclude others at risk is equally prudent. Hydroquinone-induced leukoderma is usually spontaneously reversible, particularly with small amounts of solar irradiation. The subtle hypomelanosis secondary to topical tretinoin is also slowly reversible on discontinuation of the preparation. Hypopigmentation secondary to topical steroids is also usually spontaneously reversible, but that secondary to intralesional glucocorticoids may be amelanotic and persistent, particularly in patients of SPT V and VI.

POSTINFLAMMATORY HYPOMELANOSIS A number of inflammatory dermatoses may be associated with or may resolve to leave hypomelanotic macules corresponding to the cutaneous sites of involvement. This is seen commonly with atopic dermatitis, eczematous dermatitis, and psoriasis but also less commonly with chronic guttate parapsoriasis, pityriasis lichenoides chronica, alopecia mucinosa, mycosis fungoides, discoid lupus erythematosus, lichen planus, lichen striatus, and seborrheic dermatitis.[34]

Clinical features Most cases of postinflammatory hypomelanosis are clinically similar regardless of the preexisting inflammatory dermatosis. The macules are tan to off-white with indiscrete margins and always correspond to sites of prior eruption (Fig. 90-21). The hypomelanosis immediately follows resolution of the primary process and starts to fade over weeks to months, particularly in sun-exposed areas.

Pathogenesis This process is considered to result from a melanosome transfer block. In eczema, the defect may result from edema, whereas markedly increased epidermal turnover may be responsible in psoriasis. In T cell lymphoma, there are degenerative changes in melanocytes and spherical melanosomes.

Diagnosis The diagnosis rests on the observation or the history of the associated dermatosis. When the diagnosis is unclear, biopsy of a hypomelanotic lesion may reveal histologic evidence of the underlying dermatosis.

Treatment Treatment is normally that of the underlying disorder. Once the inflammatory process has resolved, normally constitutive skin color is slowly reestablished. This may be facilitated by solar exposure; the color of macules will not normalize, however, so long as the inflammatory process is present.

TABLE 90-7

Comparative Features of Chemical Leukoderma and Vitiligo

	Chemical Leukoderma	Vitiligo
Age of onset	Usually adulthood	Acquired from birth to old age, half by age 20
Course	Chronic	Chronic progressive, occasional improvement
Color	White to off-white	Milk-white
Size/shape	Confetti macules; vitiligo-like	Millimeters to centimeters; round, scalloped margins
Distribution	Hands, arms, face most common; remote macules	Symmetric, periorificial, extensor limbs/digits
Wood's lamp	Enhanced contrast	Enhanced contrast
Special features	None	Trichrome; occasional segmental pattern
Other skin changes	None	Scattered leukotrichia, halo nevi, alopecia areata
Systemic disease	None	Hypo-/hyperthyroidism, diabetes mellitus, rarely others
Histology	Melanocytes absent; like vitiligo	Melanocytes absent; lymphocytes in active lesions
Treatment options	Identify and remove chemical exposure; PUVA	Topical steroids, topical PUVA, oral PUVA, MBEH
Medical importance	None	Associated with thyroid disease, diabetes, Addison's disease, pernicious anemia, multiple endocrinopathy syndrome
Special studies	None	T_4, TSH, FBS, ANA/Ro/La (prior to PUVA)
Major diagnostic clues	Vitiligo-like melanosis in worker exposed to para-substituted phenolic compounds	Acquired nature, pattern of depigmentation

NOTE: T_4, tetraiodothyronine; TSH, thyroid-stimulating hormone; FBS, fasting blood sugar.

FIGURE 90-21

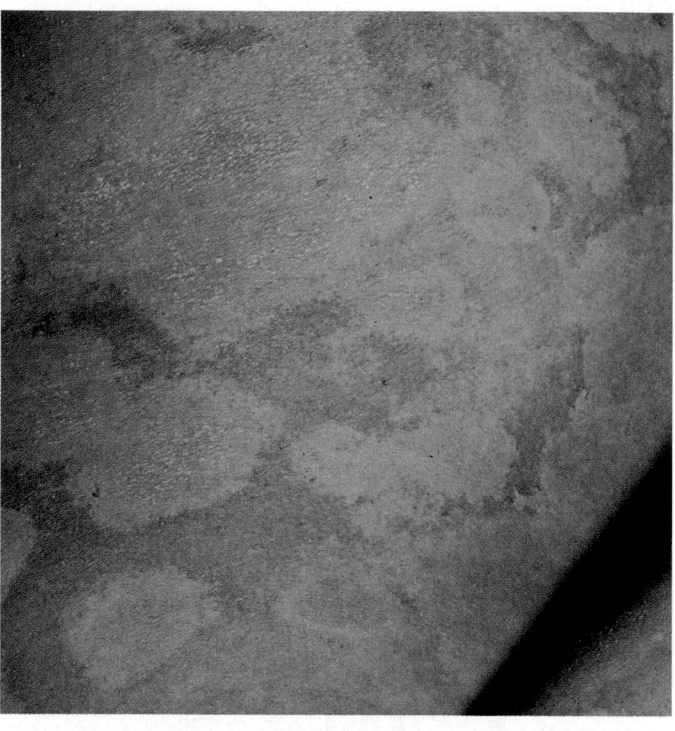

Postinflammatory hypomelanosis (psoriasis). The hypomelanotic lesions correspond exactly to the antecedent eruption. There is some residual psoriasis within the lesions.

MYCOSIS FUNGOIDES (See Chap. 157) Hypopigmentation in mycosis fungoides has been reported in patients of darker skin types. The eruption clinically resembles tinea versicolor, generalized pityriasis alba, postinflammatory hypopigmentation, or vitiligo (including trichrome vitiligo). Involvement tends to be more central than acral. Onset may, however, occur in the teens. Histologically, hypopigmented mycosis fungoides lacks epidermal atrophy and demonstrates moderate to marked exocytosis resembling pagetoid reticulosis. The number of melanocytes is generally reduced, and reduced numbers of melanosomes in keratinocytes suggested a transfer block. PUVA therapy is very effective. Topical nitrogen mustard and topical carmustine are also effective.

PITYRIASIS ALBA Pityriasis alba is a common hypomelanosis that occurs in all races, although it is considered more common, perhaps just more obvious, in blacks.

Clinical features Pityriasis alba is generally a disorder of young children and affects males and females equally. The typical macule is pale pink or light brown with very indistinct margins. The subtle erythema fades over weeks to leave an off-white to tan-white macule with a powdery scale (Fig. 90-22). The face, particularly the midforehead, malar ridges, and around the eyes and mouth, is the most commonly involved area, but macules on the neck, trunk, back, limbs, and scrotum do occur. Macules vary from 5 to 30 mm or larger. While only 2 or 3 lesions are usually present, from 1 to over 20 are possible. Usually pityriasis alba is asymptomatic, but some patients complain of burning or itching. The macules, once present, are usually stable and then gradually disappear with age; however, persistence into adulthood has been reported. *Pigmenting pityriasis alba* is a variant in which there is a central bluish coloration of involved macules. The histology is nonspecific.

FIGURE 90-22

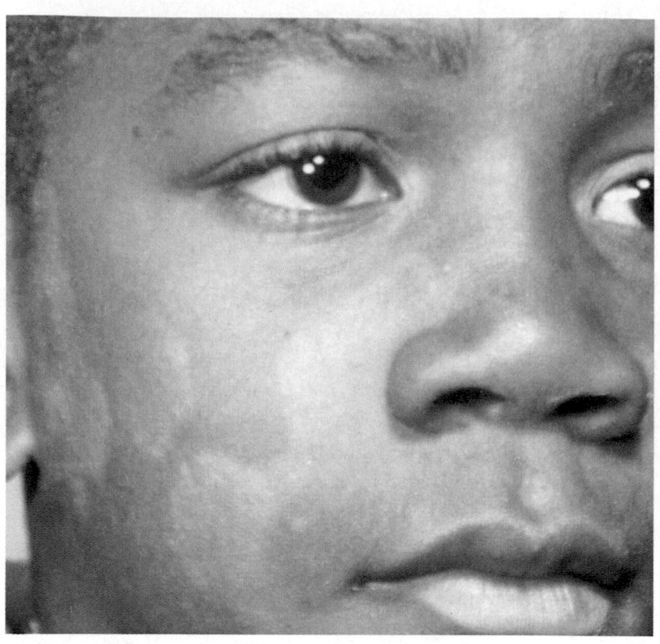

Pityriasis alba. The lesions are typically hypomelanotic, finely scaling, and have indistinct borders. Spontaneous resolution is typical but slow.

Pathogenesis Pityriasis alba is probably an eczematous dermatosis with hypomelanosis resulting from postinflammatory changes and ultraviolet screening effects of the hyperkeratotic and parakeratotic epidermis.

Diagnosis The absence of a positive scraping readily excludes tinea versicolor. The tan color, indistinct margins, and appearance under Wood's lamp examination exclude vitiligo.

Treatment Treatment of pityriasis alba is often not satisfactory, but the condition is self-limited. Topical glucocorticoids are useful. PUVA has been found to be effective for extensive pityriasis alba.

Hypomelanosis Associated with Infection[35]

TINEA VERSICOLOR (See Chap. 206) Tinea versicolor is caused by the lipophilic yeast *Malassezia furfur*. The typical lesion is a round, scaling hypomelanotic macule that is occasionally raised and may have erythematous raised margins (Fig. 90-23). Individual macules are several millimeters to a centimeter in diameter. Macules may increase in number and in size so that they may become confluent; this imparts a scalloped appearance to the border. The macules occur typically on the upper back and chest but also may occur on the upper arms, neck, and face, especially in patients living in the tropics. Tan, hyperpigmented and erythematous macules may precede and/or coexist with hypopigmented macules; these have features otherwise similar to the white macules. The disease is chronic, although as the summer tan fades, the lesions may become less obvious. In contrast to vitiligo, tinea versicolor has fine, often barely perceptible, dustlike scales.

Pathogenesis It has been suggested that the depigmentation in tinea versicolor results from inhibition of tyrosinase by C_9 and C_{11} dicarboxylic acids, such as azelaic acid, which are formed by cultures of this lipophilic yeast and which, in cultures, inhibit tyrosinase activity. For diagnosis and treatment, see Chap. 206.

TREPONEMATOSES (See Chap. 229)

Clinical features Hypochromia is commonly a late feature of pinta. Secondary lesions, or *pintides,* are usually erythematous or copper-colored, then slate-blue, and finally mottled with both hypo- and

FIGURE 90-23

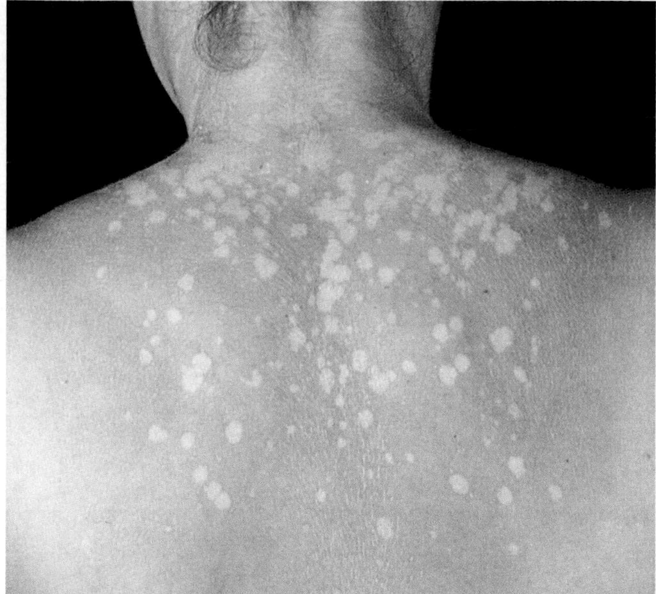

A.

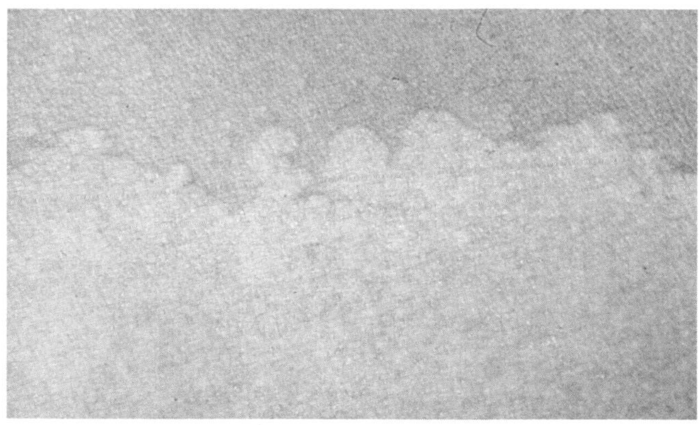

B.

Tinea versicolor. *A.* Typical macules are round, very well circumscribed, have fine scale, and are off-white to tan in color. Typical distribution involves the upper back and upper chest. Involvement of the lower arms and legs and of the face is unusual. *B.* Confluent macules create scalloped borders. This is a characteristic pattern of macules of tinea versicolor.

hyperpigmentation. Macules occur symmetrically over bony prominences, namely, elbows, knuckles, knees, ankles, and flexor wrists. The margins are distinct and may be outlined with peripheral hypermelanosis. Lesions are usually milk-white (Fig. 90-24). For histology, pathogenesis, diagnosis, and treatment, see Chap. 229.

Depigmentation in Bejel (nonvenereal syphilis) is an uncommon feature of the late stage and may resemble pinta. Early use of penicillin may result in repigmentation. The primary lesion of yaws, at the site of inoculation, may heal to leave atrophic hypochromic or achromic scars that occasionally have dark halos. Rarely, lenticular or hypochromic macules occur in secondary yaws. Most commonly, the hypomelanosis follows the tertiary stage of the disease; lesions are symmetrically placed and particularly involve the anterior wrists (with a triangular macule pointing dorsally), dorsal hands, small joints over the extensor hands, and less commonly, the feet. Lesions are depigmented and tend to enlarge centrifugally. Treatment in the infectious stages prevents the characteristic late leukoderma (see Chap. 229).

FIGURE 90-24

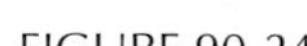

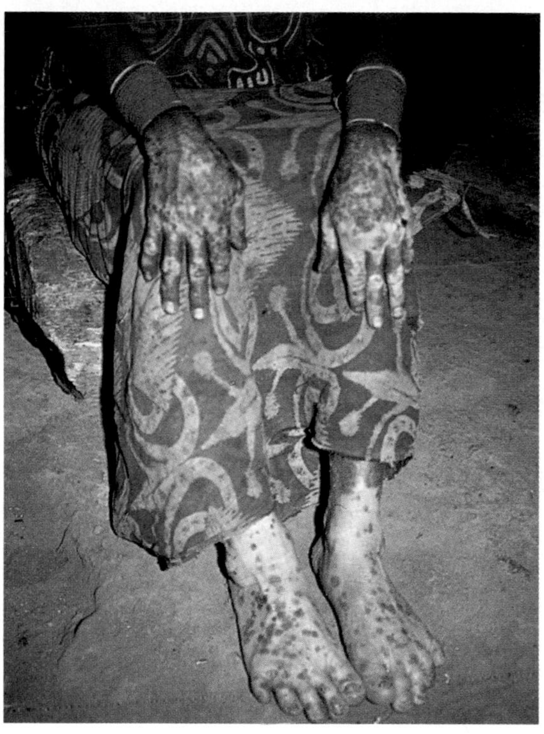

Pinta. The hypomelanosis in pinta is a vitiligo-like hypomelanosis that occurs later in the disease and is associated with deep blue to slate-gray areas of hyperpigmentation.

ONCHOCERCIASIS (See Chap. 236) The depigmentation is a late feature and usually involves the pretibial skin—usually bilaterally; the groin and the pelvic and axillary areas less commonly may become depigmented. This hypomelanosis gives the patient a leopard-like appearance. Repigmentation from the margins occurs in some cases. Melanocytes are absent in the later stages.

POST KALA-AZAR (See Chap. 235) The lesions begin as pinpoint hypopigmented macules and gradually enlarge to a centimeter or so in diameter. The most common sites are the chest, back, arms, anterior thighs, and neck; the skin from the waist to the feet is conspicuously spared. In later stages, the lesions become raised. The lesions are asymptomatic. The hypomelanosis is generally irreversible, even with treatment.

LEPROSY (See Chap. 202) The presence of anesthetic hypomelanotic macules is virtually diagnostic. The numbers of such lesions vary from a solitary lesion (Fig. 90-25) to a few in indeterminate and tuberculoid leprosy to many in borderline and lepromatous leprosy. Lesions are most common in the brachial and lumbar plexus areas of skin; they are usually small, except in the lepromatous type, which is characterized by large lesions. Tuberculoid lesions are well delineated, as may be the lesions in indeterminate leprosy, but borderline and lepromatous lesions have ill-defined margins.

Hypomelanosis Associated with Tumors

Tumors have been associated with leukoderma in two different instances, the halo nevus, and a much more insidious process, melanoma-associated leukoderma.

FIGURE 90-25

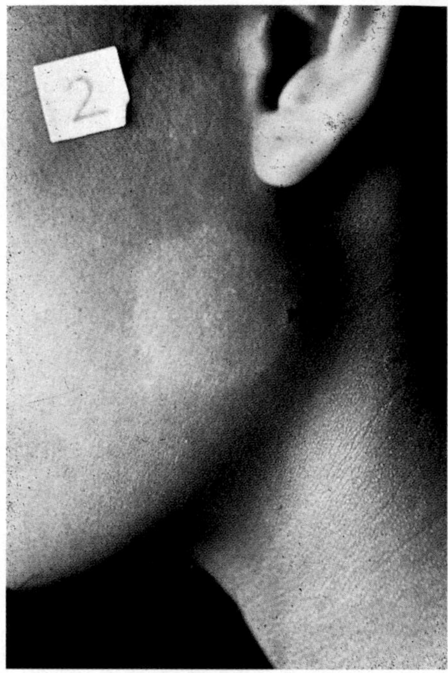

A characteristic off-white hypomelanotic and anesthetic macule of leprosy.

HALO NEVI (See Chap. 91) Halo nevus, also referred to as *Sutton's nevus* or *leukoderma acquisitum centrifigum,* is a nevus surrounded by a macule of leukoderma.

MELANOMA-ASSOCIATED LEUKODERMA (See Chap. 93) Several types of hypomelanosis may be associated with melanoma, and any type of melanoma may be associated with hypomelanosis. The first type, analogous to halo nevus, is associated with a primary melanoma; it has an eccentrically placed irregular halo. The second type is a remote leukoderma, well distant from the primary lesion. The third type is vitiligo-like (Fig. 90-26*A*). Halos also may develop around metastatic lesions (Fig. 90-26*B*). In addition, leukoderma may develop at sites distant from the tumor or its metastases. The prevalence has been suggested to be from 1.3 to 20 percent of melanoma patients. Among 42 reported cases, the time of onset of the melanoma and of the leukoderma were fairly close. In many, the depigmentation appeared between several months and 5 years after the appearance of the tumor, but usually in patients older than 40 years of age. In two cases, the leukoderma came first, and none of the patients had a family history of vitiligo. Most cases are associated with visceral or lymph node involvement.

Clinical features Melanoma-associated leukoderma is a diffuse vitiligo-like macular hypomelanosis or depigmentation. It develops distant from the melanoma, is frequently first observed on the trunk, and may spread to the extremities. It may be symmetric or asymmetric. The hypomelanosis may be mottled (hypomelanotic) or milk-white, as in vitiligo (amelanotic) (see Fig. 90-26*A*). Spontaneous repigmentation may occur. Uveitis also may be observed. Histologically, there is an absence of melanocytes in established lesions or reduced numbers of melanocytes with very stubby dendrites in earlier lesions.

Pathogenesis Strong evidence suggests that melanoma-associated hypomelanosis is the visible consequence of a cellular antitumoral response. The hypomelanosis infiltrates lymphocytes and most exclusively T lymphocytes, and most are CD8+. These CD8+ T cells have a clonal or oligoclonal T cell receptor profile, and they specifically recognize differentiation antigens shared by normal melanocytes and melanoma cells.[36]

FIGURE 90-26

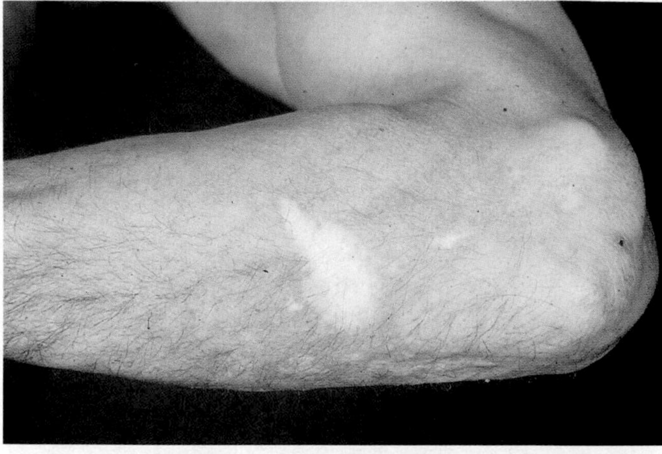

A.

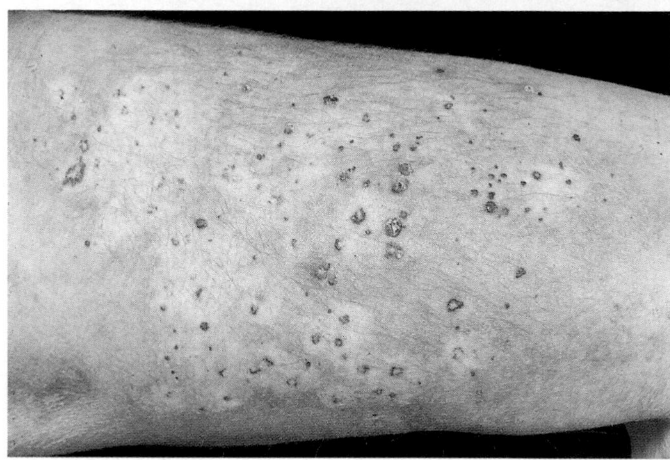

B.

Melanoma-associated leukoderma. *A.* This hypomelanosis may resemble vitiligo clinically and be characterized by an absence of melanocytes. It may be associated with a favorable prognosis. *B.* These macules in a different patient developed after the patient developed metastases to the skin. They surround the individual metastases.

Hypomelanoses—Idiopathic, Circumscribed

IDIOPATHIC GUTTATE HYPOMELANOSIS (IGH) IGH is a common acquired, discrete hypomelanosis particularly affecting the extremities in darker-skinned individuals.[37]

Clinical features IGH is probably found in all races but is simply most apparent in darker-skinned ones. Males and females are equally affected. Typical lesions are very discrete, well-circumscribed, porcelain-white macules (Fig. 90-27), occasionally containing black dots. The lesions are usually round but may be stellate; they average about 5 mm in diameter but may be from 1 mm to about 2 cm in diameter. The lesions number from few to many, may increase in number and in size with age, and are most common in sun-exposed areas of the extremities, particularly the anterior lower legs, but are not observed on the face. The lesions are asymptomatic and irreversible.

Histology and electron microscopy The most consistent histologic abnormalities include flattening of the dermal-epidermal junction, a moderate to marked reduction of the melanin granules in the basal

FIGURE 90-27

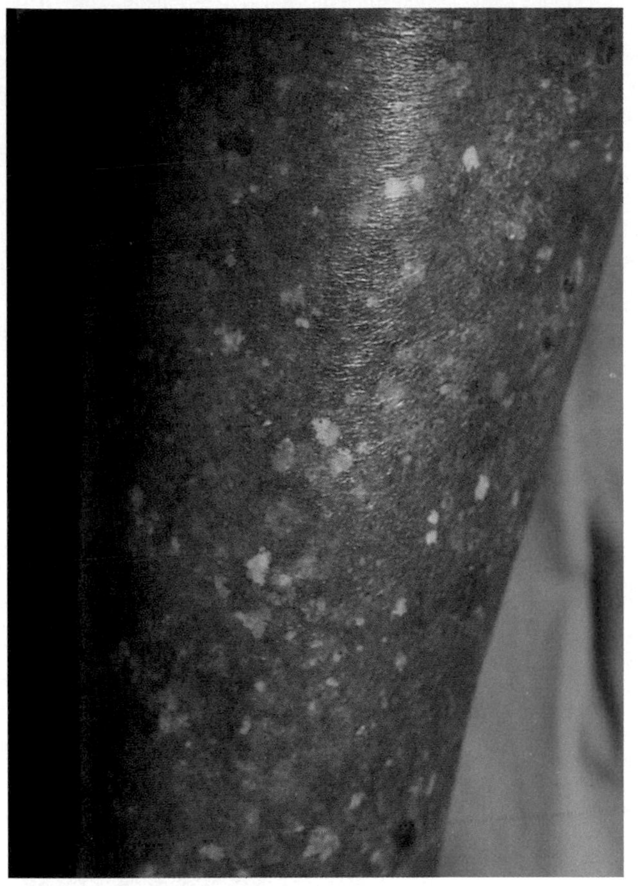

Idiopathic guttate hypomelanosis. Lesions on the leg of an African American individual.

and prickle cell layers, epidermal atrophy, and basket-weave hyperkeratosis. Changes in collagen and elastic fibers are less common. There is a moderate reduction in the number of melanocytes, and they have stubby dendrites.

Pathogenesis There appear to be two general types of IGH. The first is the actinic type. The second is a nonactinic familial type, which does not necessarily occur on sun-exposed areas and is found particularly on the trunk, especially in individuals of SPT VI. A genetic predisposition is possible.

Diagnosis Clinically, the lesions must be distinguished from vitiligo, tinea versicolor, tuberous sclerosis, chemical depigmentation, and postinflammatory hypomelanosis. Careful examination with a hand lens reveals the very sharp, discrete margins and porcelain-colored smooth surface not found in entities other than IGH.

Treatment The cosmetic significance of lesions of IGH, particularly in darker-skinned individuals, should not be minimized. However, reports of successful treatment of IGH are few. Improvement may be achieved with intralesional triamcinolone, with or without small grafts in the center of the hypopigmented lesions; permanency remains to be established, however. Cryotherapy has given mixed results. PUVA has not proved successful.

Confetti Leukoderma

Confetti leukoderma refers to small, 1- to 3-mm hypopigmented cutaneous macules. These may be found as macular lesions in vitiligo, *leukoderma punctatum* in patients undergoing PUVA therapy (see below), tuberous sclerosis, chemical leukoderma, tinea versicolor, IGH,

and photoaging. Perifollicular hypopigmentation may be observed in vitiligo, tinea versicolor, Grover's disease, and Darier's disease. A few patients with multiple endocrine neoplasia type 1 have been observed to have confetti-like hypomelanotic macules; these macules are more likely on the neck and trunk, whereas those of tuberous sclerosis are found on the extremities. Confetti hypomelanosis also may present as small raised papules in disseminated hypopigmented keratoses. *White lentiginosis* is a very unusual disorder characterized by flat to raised keratotic and depigmented macules of the trunk. Histologically, features include a lentiginous hyperplasia of the epidermis with elongated club-shaped rete ridges and a loss of epidermal pigmentation with abnormal keratinization.

Miscellaneous Types of Hypomelanosis

HEMODIALYSIS Widespread acquired hypopigmentation of the hair and skin has been described in uremia patients undergoing maintenance hemodialysis.

PIGMENTARY DEMARCATION LINES Futcher's or Voigt's lines, known as *pigmentary demarcation lines,* are abrupt transitions from deeply pigmented skin to lighter-pigmented skin (Fig. 90-28) commonly found in African Americans and darker-skinned Caucasians. Pigmentary demarcation lines have been noted in up to 10 percent of Caucasians and 4 percent of Japanese; they are often present at birth or develop in early childhood and tend to darken with time.

PROGRESSIVE MACULAR HYPOMELANOSIS OF THE TRUNK A condition frequently observed in the West Indies is characterized by a progressively spreading macular hypomelanosis of the trunk and

FIGURE 90-28

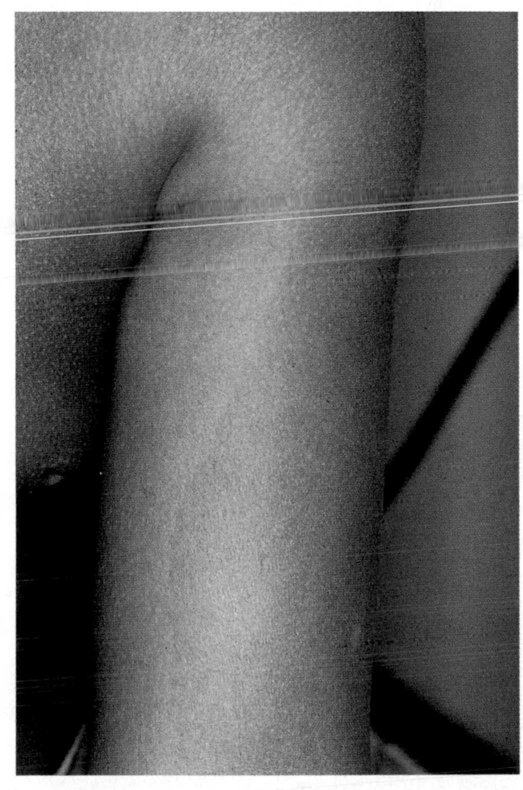

Pigmentary demarcation line. These lines are often barely perceptible and not unusual in darker-skinned phototypes.

is found mainly in females from 18 to 25 years of age. Microscopic examination of the hypochromic macules reveals a slight reduction in epidermal melanin. Ultrastructural examination of the macules shows a switch from type IV single melanosomes to small, aggregated type I to III melanosomes. These findings suggest that this disorder may result from a variation in melanosome size and distribution. This disorder does not respond to treatment but does regress spontaneously within 3 to 4 years.

SARCOIDOSIS (See Chap. 183) Only a few cases have been described in the literature. Hypopigmented sarcoidosis appears to be more common in dark-skinned individuals. Spontaneous or PUVA-induced repigmentation of the hypopigmented macules of sarcoidosis may occur.[38]

SCLERODERMA[39] (See Chap. 173) A vitiligo-like hypomelanosis has been described with scleroderma. The lesions are located primarily on the upper trunk and distal extremities and are amelanotic with perifollicular sparing; this resembles repigmenting vitiligo except for the additional presence of atrophy.

VAGABOND'S LEUKODERMA Vagabond's leukoderma is actually a leukomelanoderma found in older, ill-kempt men and women with a history of poor hygiene, inadequate diet, and chronic alcohol abuse. Depigmented macules are found in diffuse, light-brown, hyperpigmented patches around the waist and groin, on the buttocks, in the axillae, over the back, and on the back of the neck. The arms, legs, and face are usually less dramatically involved. Vagabond's leukoderma has been attributed to multiple ectoparasitic infections. Dietary management and good hygiene usually reverse the pigmentary abnormalities.

Hypomelanosis of Hair Alone (Canities)

There are numerous entities, besides physiologic aging, associated with graying or whitening of the hair as a predominant pigmentary abnormality. This may be expressed as diffuse graying, or canities, or as focal hypomelanosis, or poliosis. The entities to be considered in this section are associated with canities and/or poliosis but not with hypomelanosis of the skin. They include many genetic syndromes such as Fanconi's syndrome, myotonia dystrophica, Rothmund-Thomson syndrome, Seckel's syndrome, Böök's syndrome (bicuspid aplasia, premature whitening of hair, and hyperhidrosis transmitted as an autosomal dominant trait), Fisch syndrome (early graying of hair and deafness without the typical features of WS), and premature aging syndromes (Werner's syndrome, progeria). Diffuse pigmentary dilution of hair may accompany acquired disorders such as nutritional deficiency, iron deficiency, zinc deficiency, kwashiorkor, pernicious anemia, celiac disease, ulcerative colitis, and necrotizing enterocolitis. Numerous medications and chemicals have been associated with hypomelanosis of hair. Both chloroquine and hydroxychloroquine may cause hypopigmentation of scalp hair, especially in blondes; eyelids and eyelashes also may be affected. Mephenesin also has been reported to cause reversible lightening of hair color. Triparanol and valproic acid have been associated with lightening of hair in isolated cases.[40]

PHYSIOLOGIC GRAYING OF HAIR Graying of hair is a normal concomitant of aging. While graying is more readily apparent in those with black hair, fair-haired individuals appear totally gray earlier. Clinically, graying begins at the temples, spreads to the vertex, and slowly involves the entire scalp. Beard and body hair become gray later, but axillary, pubic, and chest hair may remain pigmented even in old age. While graying is ultimately irreversible, temporary reversal even to darker than the preexisting hair color may follow inflammation, particularly folliculitis. Histochemically, there is a gradual loss of melanocytes. Animal models do provide some insight. Bcl-2–deficient mice demonstrate hypopigmented hair that turns gray during the second hair cycle. In these animals, an accelerated disappearance of follicular melanocytes by apoptosis mimics the loss of melanocytes in human senile gray and white hair. In the light mouse, a mutation in the tyrosinase-related protein gene (*Trp1*) results in hairs pigmented only at their tips. This phenotype is due to premature death of melanocytes, mediated through the inherent cytotoxicity of pigment production. Premature aging with early graying is observed in DNA repair and transcription abnormalities resulting from a mutation in *XPD,* a gene encoding a DNA helicase.

SUDDEN WHITENING OF HAIR There is no known physiologic mechanism to explain abrupt depigmentation of established hairs. Rather, this is an expression of alopecia areata in which the pigmented hairs are lost selectively. Regrowth also may be white and be characterized by a total absence of melanocytes or by reduced numbers of melanocytes with poorly developed dendritic processes. Degenerative melanocytes have been observed only in the presence of adjacent keratinocytes showing necrosis.

Hypopigmentation Unrelated to Melanin Pigmentation

NEVUS ANEMICUS (Fig. 90-29) Nevus anemicus is an uncommon congenital, localized vascular malformation observed more frequently

FIGURE 90-29

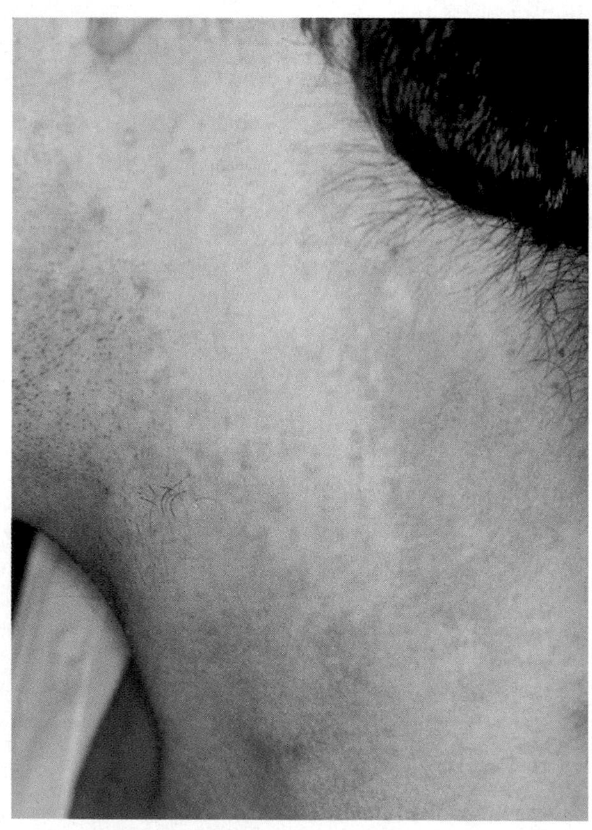

Nevus anemicus. This entity is a pharmacologic nevus; unlike melanocytic disorders, pressure over the lesion with a glass slide causes the lesion to become inapparent; nevus anemicus becomes invisible under the Wood's lamp but becomes more prominent after rubbing, which induces vasodilatation only in the adjacent uninvolved skin. (*Courtesy of RA Johnson, MD.*)

in women than in men. Most lesions occur on the chest, but involvement of the face and extremities also occurs. The typical macule appears to be off-white, not totally colorless, but is capable of exhibiting a delayed tanning reaction. Wood's lamp examination does not accentuate nevus anemicus, unlike true hypomelanoses. Pressure on the lesion from a glass slide makes the lesion inapparent. Finally, friction or cold or heat application fails to induce erythema in the leukoderma areas. The histology is normal, and the vascular structures are normal by electron microscopy. The defect of nevus anemicus may be at the motor endplate or at the smooth muscle effector cells of the blood vessels or arises from a focal increased blood vessel sensitivity to catecholamines.

BIER SPOTS Bier spots are small, light macules usually found on the arms and legs of young adults. The intervening skin may seem erythematous but blanches with pressure so that the light macules disappear. This is a benign physiologic vascular anomaly of no significance.

WORONOFF'S RING Woronoff's ring is a hypomelanotic ring surrounding psoriatic lesions under treatment secondary to vascular rather than melanin-related changes.

HYPERMELANOSES

Epidermal Hypermelanoses

Epidermal hypermelanosis refers to brown hyperpigmentation that results from increased melanin in the epidermis. This is generally caused by increased melanin production by existing melanocytes (melanotic hyperpigmentation) and less often by increased proliferation of active melanocytes (melanocytotic hyperpigmentation).

Epidermal hypermelanosis also may be categorized by pattern. There may be diffuse hypermelanosis or localized circumscribed lesions like café-au-lait macules, or the lesions may be multiple. Multiple lesions may be, scattered, isolated, discrete macules like ephelides, reticulated macules like Dowling-Degos disease, or ill-defined ones like postinflammatory lesions. Lesions may have particularly characteristic anatomic locations such as the face in melasma and hands in acral melanoses.

Some hypermelanoses can present with a banding pattern. These lesions are described with various terms such as *agminated, linear, segmental, zosteriform,* or *following Blaschko lines.* Typical examples include partial unilateral lentiginosis, linear whorled hypermelanosis, segmentary neurofibromatosis, McCune-Albright syndrome, speckled lentiginous nevus, or stage IV IP. Beyond these clinical aspects, there is growing evidence that most, if not all, entities that fall into this category are caused by a common mechanism of somatic mosaicism. The same concept probably stands true for hypomelanoses presenting with a banding pattern, such as hypomelanosis of Ito, nevus depigmentosus, or stage III incontinentia pigmenti (see above). A clinicopathologic classification of epidermal hypermelanoses is given in Table 90-8.

MELANOCYTOTIC EPIDERMAL HYPERMELANOSES Lentigines are small, usually less than 5 mm in diameter, circumscribed, brown to dark-brown to black, variegated to uniformly colored macules. They may be found as isolated macules in sun-exposed areas or as multiple lesions on any cutaneous surface, including the palms and soles. Lentigines are characterized histologically by basilar hyperpigmentation with melanocyte proliferation in elongated epidermal rete ridges. Syndromes with multiple lentigines in a characteristic nonrandom pattern are known as *lentiginoses*. Some lentiginoses have a defined set of associated extracutaneous anomalies.

Lentigo simplex (See also Chap. 91) *Lentigo simplex* is the term applied to isolated lentigines found on any cutaneous site irrespective of UV exposure (Fig. 90-30). Apart from some lentiginoses, there is no known genetic predisposition for lentigo simplex. Lentigo simplex also can occur on the oral and genital mucosa. In the nail, lentigo simplex is a possible cause of melanonychia striata longitudinalis.

Lentigo senilis (actinica) (See also Chaps. 91 and 134) *Lentigo senilis et actinica,* more commonly known as *senile* or *actinic lentigo* or *solar lentigo,* is the term applied to lentigines induced by UV radiation (Fig. 90-31). The prevalence of actinic lentigines is correlated with low-grade phototype and increasing age. They are present in 90 percent of Caucasians older than 60 years. Sun-exposed areas, especially the face and hands, are involved. Their diameters range from less than 1 mm to a few centimeters. They are usually light brown, occasionally black. They may persist with minimal or no fading in the absence of sun exposure. They differ from ephelides, which generally occur in Caucasian children and fade or disappear when sun exposure is discontinued. Specific variants include ink-spot lentigo, PUVA lentigo, sunbed lentigo. Ink-spot lentigo is a variant characterized by its jet-black color and reticulated border. PUVA lentigines are found in patients receiving extensive PUVA. Sunbed lentigines have been described after the use of UVA sunbeds.

Eruptive lentiginosis Eruptive lentiginosis is the widespread occurrence of several hundred lentigines over a few months to years, usually in adolescents and young adults, in the absence of systemic abnormalities. This is different from *eruptive nevi.*

Partial unilateral lentiginosis Partial unilateral lentiginosis (PUL) is a rare pigmentary disorder characterized by numerous lentigines arranged in a group and involving one-half of the body. PUL is diagnosed mostly in young people, and it can even be present at birth. There is no known inheritance pattern. Histologically, most of the cases have a lentigo pattern, but some patients have a "jentigo" pattern (some small nests of melanocytes at the dermal-epidermal junction) in addition. It is generally admitted that PUL has no commonly associated abnormalities.

Multiple hypotheses exist concerning the pathogenesis of PUL, with as yet no clear-cut answer. Some cases of PUL may be a form of segmental neurofibromatosis. In other cases, PUL may represent the incomplete expression of a lentiginosis syndrome. These possibilities are all consistent with the more general view that PUL reflects somatic mosaicism.[41]

Inherited-pattern lentiginosis in blacks Generalized lentiginosis has been described in 10 adult black patients with onset during infancy or early childhood and familial clustering in an autosomal pattern in patients, without somatic abnormalities. Face, lips, extremities, buttocks, and palmoplantar but not mucosal surfaces were involved.

Laugier-hunziker syndrome Laugier-Hunziker syndrome is characterized by early to midlife appearance of macular hyperpigmentation of the lips and buccal mucosa and often of the palms and soles. Other cutaneous surfaces may be involved, and hyperpigmented nail streaks may be present. Patients are otherwise healthy.

Leopard syndrome (See Chap. 166) LEOPARD syndrome (OMIM 151100, Moynahan's syndrome) is an uncommon autosomal dominant syndrome. The features of the full syndrome include lentigines, ECG conduction defects, ocular hypertelorism, pulmonary stenosis, abnormal genitalia, growth retardation, and deafness. Lentigines are first noted in infancy, evolve until adulthood, and are distributed with no particular pattern all over the body except mucous membranes. Variable expression is common, as illustrated by a family in which five of six members exhibited only lentigines, whereas the sixth member had lentigines with most other features. Linkage analysis suggests that the LEOPARD syndrome is not linked to the neurofibromatosis-1 (NF-1) gene.[42]

TABLE 90-8

Epidermal Hypermelanoses: Clinicopathologic Classification of Disorders

Epidermal Factors	Melanocytotic (Increase in Number of Melanocytes)	Melanotic (Increase in Melanin)	
Heritable or developmental	Lentigines Moynahan's syndrome Centrofacial neurodysraphic lentiginosis Peutz-Jegher syndrome PUVA Sotos' syndrome	Café-au-lait macule Neurofibromatosis Albright's syndrome Silver-Russell syndrome Westerhof's syndrome Watson's syndrome Bloom's syndrome Gastrocutaneous syndrome Becker's melanosis Nevus spilus Ephelides (freckles) NAME/LAMB syndrome Ichthyosis nigricans	Neurocutaneous melanosis Familial periorbital hyperpigmentation Familial progressive hyperpigmentation Dowling-Degos disease Dyskeratosis congenita Fanconi's syndrome Human chimera Acropigmentation of Dohi Reticulate acropigmentation of Kitamura Dermatopathia pigmentosa reticularis POEMS syndrome Carbon baby syndrome
Metabolic		Porphyria cutanea tarda Hemochromatosis Hepatolenticular degeneration Gaucher's disease Niemann-Pick disease	
Endocrine		Melasma ACTH- and MSH-producing tumors Exogenous ACTH therapy Pregnancy Addison's disease Estrogen therapy Carney's complex syndrome	
Chemical and drug		Arsenicals Busulfan Photochemical agents (psoralens, tar) Berloque dermatitis	5-Fluorouracil, systemic Cyclophosphamide Nitrogen mustard, topical Bleomycin
Nutritional		Kwashiorkor Pellagra Sprue Vitamin B_{12} deficiency	
Physical	Lentigo, solar Ultraviolet (radiation tanning)	Ultraviolet radiation (suntanning) Thermal radiation Alpha, beta, gamma ionizing radiation Trauma (e.g., chronic pruritus)	
Inflammation and infection		Postinflammatory melanosis (exanthems, drug eruptions) Lichen planus Lupus erythematosus, discoid	Lichen simplex chronicus Atopic dermatitis Psoriasis
Neoplastic		Melanoma Mastocytosis Acanthosis nigricans with adenocarcinoma and lymphoma	Tinea versicolor
Miscellaneous	Lentigines, eruptive Lentigo, senilis	Scleroderma, systemic Chronic hepatic insufficiency Whipple's syndrome Cronkhite-Canada syndrome	

CARNEY COMPLEX (See Chap. 166) Carney complex (CNC; OMIM 160980) is an autosomal dominant disorder characterized by spotty pigmentation, cardiac and cutaneous myxomas, and endocrine hyperactivity Subjects with LAMB syndrome (*l*entigines, *a*trial myxoma, *m*ucocutaneous myxomas, *b*lue nevi) or NAME syndrome (*n*evi, *a*trial myxomas, *m*yxoid neurofibromata, *e*phelides) have the same characteristics that are now called CNC. The most common presentation of CNC is that of lentigines (see Fig. 166-3) with cardiac myxoma. Early appreciation of cutaneous lesions and their significance allows patients and primary relatives to be screened. Spotty skin pigmentation can be cutaneous and/or mucocutaneous. Lentigines and blue nevi usually predominate. Ephelides, if present, may be profuse in number. Junctional nevi and compound nevi also may be present. Myxomas affect the heart, skin, and breast; tend to be multiple in each affected

FIGURE 90-30

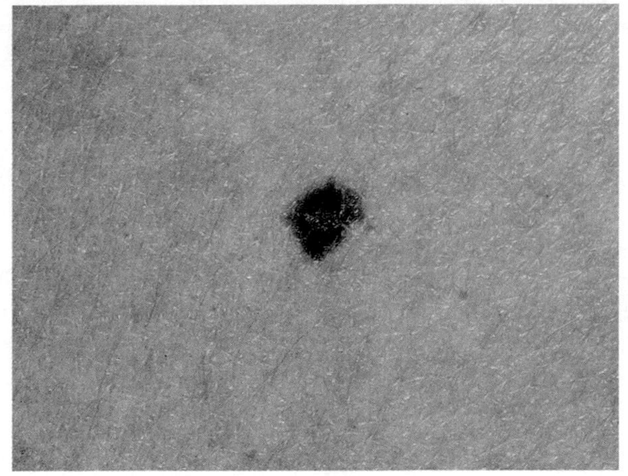

Lentigo simplex, a slightly irregular dark brown to black spot, level with the skin.

organ; and recur commonly after excision. More than 65 percent of patients with the complex have cardiac myxomas. Skin myxomas are present in 33 percent of patients. An occult cardiac myxoma always should be suspected in the presence of multiple cutaneous myxomas. Breast myxoid mammary fibroadenomas occur in 25 percent of female patients. There are several manifestations of endocrine hyperactivity in CNC. Cushing's syndrome, due to the rare primary pigmented adrenocortical disease, is present in 20 percent of patients. Acromegaly, due to growth hormone–secreting pituitary adenomas, is present in 10 percent of patients. Testicular tumors, predominantly of the rare, large cell, calcifying Sertoli cell type, occur in 30 to 50 percent of affected males. Schwannomas, of the rare psamommatous melanotic type, are present in 14 percent of patients, of which approximately 10 percent are malignant, extensively metastatic, and fatal. The pigmented lesions in Peutz-Jeghers syndrome (PJS) (see below) are the same as in CNC, and both syndromes include the rare, large cell, calcifying Sertoli cell of the testis. However, PJS patients often have ovarian tumors and exhibit numerous blue nevi but lack cardiac and cutaneous myxomas. Conversely, ovarian tumors have been described in CNC, and blue nevi are commonly singular.[43]

FIGURE 90-31

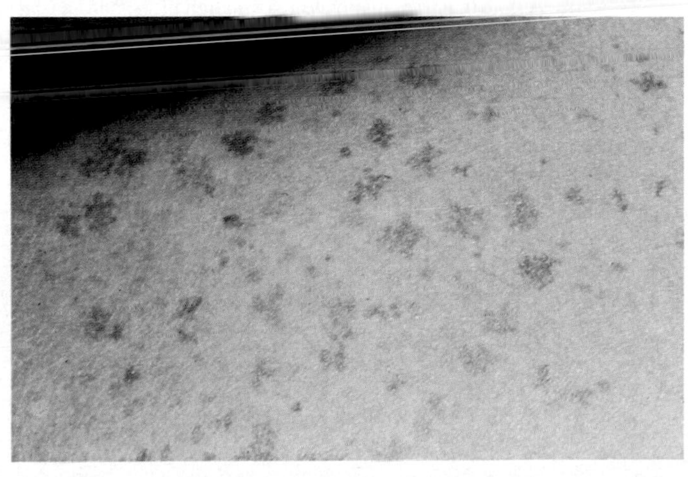

Actinic or solar lentigines are induced by UV radiation. They are usually light brown, sharply defined, and irregular in outline, and occur on sun-exposed sites in light skin phototypes. Here they are shown on the shoulder of a 50-year old male who had sustained repeated sunburns during adolescence.

CNC is a disorder of neural crest, mesenchymal, and endocrine tissues. It was demonstrated that the *PRKAR1A* gene, located on 17q22-24, is mutated in about half of CNC kindreds. *PRKAR1A* is a tumor-suppressor gene, as demonstrated by loss of heterozygosity at the 17q22-24 locus in tumors associated with the complex. The *PRKAR1A* gene codes for the type 1 alpha regulatory subunit of PKA. A second locus, at chromosome 2p16, to which most but not all of the remaining kindreds map, is also involved in the molecular pathogenesis of CNC tumors. Despite the known genetic heterogeneity in the disease, phenotypic difference between patients with *PRKAR1A* mutations and those without has not been detected.[44]

Peutz-Jeghers syndrome Peutz-Jeghers syndrome (PJS; OMIM 175200) is an autosomal dominant disorder characterized by macular mucocutaneous pigmentation and hamartomatous polyps of the gastrointestinal tract.[45] Hyperpigmentation is usually the first sign of the disorder and develops in infancy or childhood. Macules are most common on the buccal mucosa and are dark brown, blue, or blue-brown in color. They are usually 10 to 15 mm in diameter and may resemble freckles but may be larger and resemble café-au-lait macules. They are usually found on the face, dorsal hands and feet (Fig. 90-32*A*), and, around the mouth, eyes, umbilicus, and anus. Mucosal lesions typically occur on the lips, palate, and tongue (Fig. 90-32*B*). The diagnosis of PJS is important because of the presence of hamartomatous gastrointestinal polyps. Although most polyps are benign, there is a 2 to 3 percent risk for malignant transformation. In addition to gastrointestinal malignancies, which may arise from normal mucosa as well as from polyps, patients with PJS are predisposed to develop other types of cancer.

Two acquired conditions that share features with PJS are Cronkhite-Canada syndrome and Laugier-Hunziker syndrome. In the former, there are hyperpigmented macules and gastrointestinal polyposis, but the macules affect the skin and not the mucosa. In addition, there is nail dystrophy and alopecia, and the onset is generally over age 50. In latter, there are hyperpigmented macules of the lips and oral mucosa but no gastrointestinal polyps.

The *LKB1/STK11* gene, located on 19p13, is mutated in approximately half of PJS kindreds and codes for a novel serine threonine kinase. *LKB1/STK11* is a tumor-suppressor gene, more precisely a mediator of p53-dependent cell death.[46]

Centrofacial neurodysraphic lentiginosis Centrofacial neurodysraphic lentiginosis (OMIM 151000) is a rare neurocutaneous syndrome characterized by lentigines limited to the medial face, neuropsychiatric problems, and dysraphic malformations. There seems to have been no report of this syndrome for nearly 30 years.[47]

Arterial dissection with lentiginosis This familial syndrome of multiple lentigines and arterial dissection (OMIM 600459) was reported in two families. Cystic necrosis of the arterial media was found in some cases, an interesting finding considering that melanocytes and arterial media both originate from neural crest cells.

Bannayan-Riley-Ruvalcaba syndrome The term *Bannayan-Riley-Ruvalcaba* (BRR; OMIM 153480) *syndrome* has been proposed to encompass the clinical overlap of three conditions previously described as separate entities and each inherited in an autosomal dominant fashion. They are the Riley-Smith, Bannayan-Zonana, and Ruvalcaba-Myhre-Smith syndromes. BRR syndrome is a hamartoma syndrome, with macrocephaly, multiple lipomas, and vascular malformations as hallmark features. Pigmented lesions of the glans penis were noted in some patients and were presented as café-au-lait macules or lentigines. The latter diagnosis is supported by histology. As predicted by some clinical overlap between the two entities, it was demonstrated that BRR syndrome can result from mutations in the tumor-suppressor

FIGURE 90-32

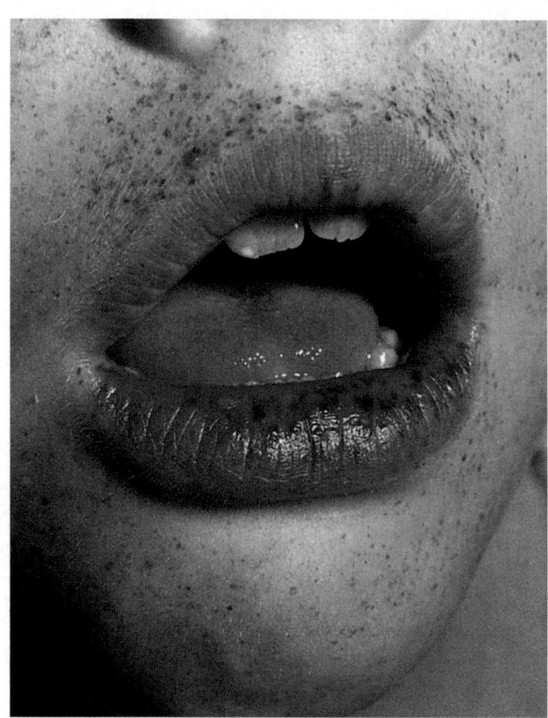
A.

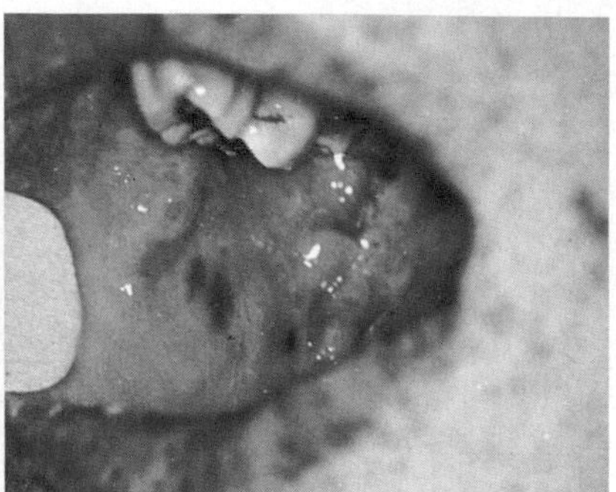
B.

Peutz-Jeghers syndrome. *A.* Lentigines, which are dark brown to gray-blue, appear on the lips, around the mouth, and on the fingers. Lip macules may, over time, disappear. *B.* Macules of the buccal mucosa are blue to blue-black and are pathognomonic; unlike lip lesions, these do not tend to disappear with time.

gene *PTEN,* implicated in Cowden's syndrome[47] (see Chap. 184). The genetic etiology of BRR syndrome is heterogeneous because many patients have no mutations in the *PTEN* gene.

Tay's syndrome This autosomal recessive disorder of multiple lentigines, vitiligo, café-au-lait macules, premature canities, growth and mental retardation, cirrhosis, hypersplenism, and multiple skeletal defects was reported in two Malaysian sisters.

Faces syndrome Faces syndrome, with unique facial features, anorexia, cachexia, and eye and skin anomalies affecting three family members, has been reported as a new hereditary condition. The cutaneous pigmentary changes include multiple lentigines and café-au-lait macules.

MELANOTIC EPIDERMAL HYPERMELANOSES Melanotic epidermal hyperpigmentation may be local, with isolated individual lesions such as café-au-lait macules or Becker's nevus, or occur in a widespread small (ephelides), patterned (periorbital melanosis, reticular melanosis, acromelanosis), or widespread and diffuse (postinflammatory, drug) distribution. Melanotic hypermelanoses are characterized histologically by increased epidermal melanin and a normal number of melanocytes.

Isolated melanotic epidermal hypermelanoses

CAFÉ-AU-LAIT MACULES Café-au-lait macules (CALMs) are discrete, uniformly pale brown, well-circumscribed, less than one to several centimeter large macules. They are characterized by serrated or irregular margins (Fig. 90-33). They appear at or soon after birth and tend to disappear with age. CALMs are common cutaneous findings. Isolated CALMs occur in up to 10 to 20 percent of the normal population. Their size usually ranges from 5 to 15 mm in adults. Ninety-eight percent of normal young adults who have CALMs have fewer than three. CALMS also can be markers for multisystem disease, in particular, neurofibromatosis (see Chap. 190), where they may be associated with intertrigmous "freckling" and neurofibromas.[48]

Unless no adult relatives with CALMS and no other stigmata of NF-1 can be found in two generations, a young child with multiple CALMS should be evaluated thoroughly and followed closely because CALMS can be the only manifestation of NF-1 at this age.

MCCUNE-ALBRIGHT SYNDROME McCune-Albright syndrome (MAS; OMIM 174.800), also known as *Albright's syndrome,* is characterized in its complete form by the triad of bone lesions termed *polyostotic fibrous dysplasia,* a hyperfunctioning endocrine system, and cutaneous lesions of light-brown pigmentation.[50] Most cases of MAS are sporadic. The pigmented lesions may be present at birth, but most develop in infancy. Sites of predilection include the head, trunk, sacral area, and buttocks. The lesions are unilateral and do not cross the midline. They are usually large with irregular jagged borders, differing from the regular smooth-bordered macules usually observed in NF (Fig. 90-34). The bony lesions of polyostotic fibrous dysplasia and the pigmented macules often occur in the same distribution. Precocious puberty and hyperthyroidism are the most common endocrinopathies observed in MAS. Molecular genetics studies indicate that MAS is a disorder of mosaicism, resulting from postzygotic somatic mutations in the *GNAS1* gene that encodes for the alpha subunit of the stimulatory G proteins.

BLOOM'S SYNDROME (See Chap. 155) Cardinal features of this syndrome include congenital facial telangiectatic erythema, photosensitivity, short stature, and predispositon to malignancy. Café-au-lait macules are present in roughly 50 percent of patients. The gene for Bloom's syndrome, *BLM,* encodes for a DNA helicase.

SILVER-RUSSELL SYNDROME Cardinal features of this syndrome include prenatal-onset growth restriction, small triangular face, body asymmetry, and a characteristic small triangular face. Café-au-lait macules are present in roughly 30 percent of patients; they are usually one or two in number. However, there can be considerable variability in the clinical expression of this syndrome.[51] The disorder is also genetically heterogeneous, but only chromosomes 7 and 17 have been consistently implicated in patients with a verified diagnosis.[52]

WATSON'S SYNDROME Watson's syndrome (OMIM 193520) is a rare autosomal dominant syndrome consisting of multiple CALMs, intertriginous freckling, short stature, mental deficiency, and pulmonary stenosis. Linkage analysis suggests that this disorder is an allelic variant of NF-1.[53]

WESTERHOF'S SYNDROME Congenital hypermelanotic and hypomelanotic macules were described in three generations of a family. The pattern suggested autosomal dominant inheritance. Some affected family members also showed growth and mental retardation.

BECKER'S NEVUS Becker's nevus is a common/acquired focal epidermal melanotic hypermelanosis. The reported incidence in males

FIGURE 90-33

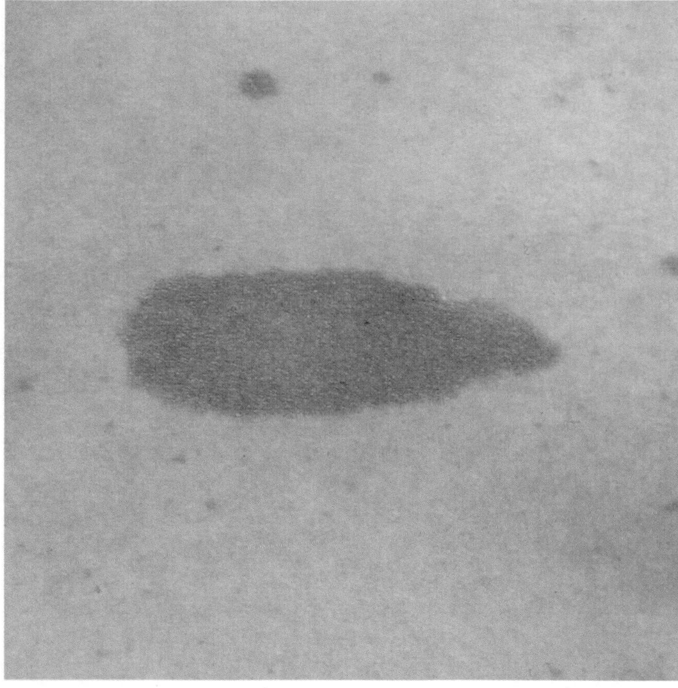

A.

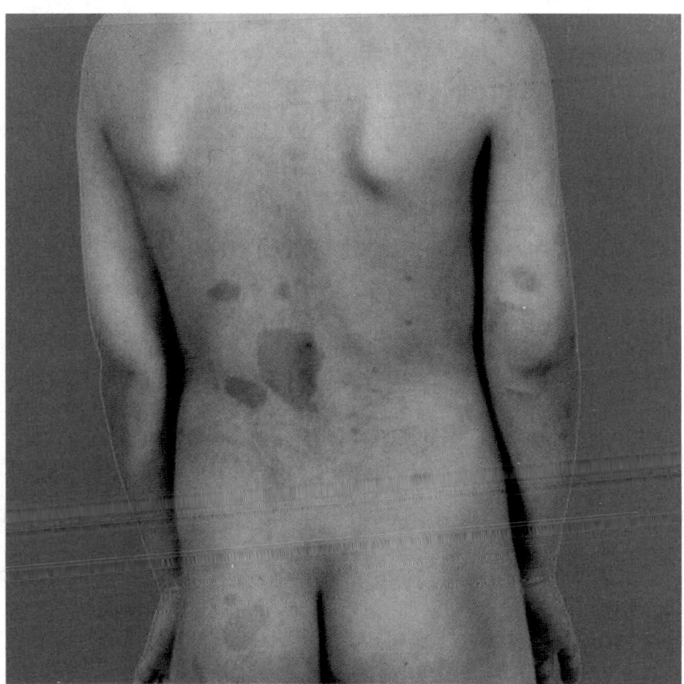

B.

Café-au-lait macules (CALMs) are uniformely pale-brown, sharply defined macules. *A.* Isolated CALMs occur in up to 10 to 20 percent of the population. *B.* CALMs are also a marker for multisystem disease, in particular neurofibromatosis where they are associated with intertriginous freckling and neurofibromas.

is 1 in 200, much less in females. The nevus typically appears at about the time of puberty as a unilateral, several centimeter large, hyperpigmented, irregular patch. It involves the upper part of the trunk, especially the shoulder, submammary area, and back (Fig. 90-35).

FIGURE 90-34

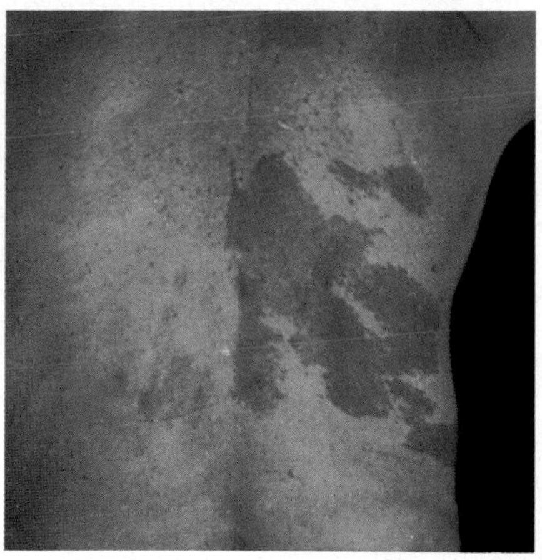

Albright's syndrome. The melanotic macules are indistinguishable from café-au-lait macules in neurofibromatosis.

The color, most often light brown, is uniform and rarely fades over time. The jagged margins are sharply demarcated. Although the lesion is macular, there is a palpable quality, particularly in the center. A variable amount of hypertrichosis occurs (see Fig. 90-35). The hairs are darker and coarser than normal. Tissue hypoplasia, such as shortening of an arm or reduced breast development, rarely may underlie Becker's nevus. Spina bifida also has been associated. In addition to epidermal melanotic hyperpigmentation, histology shows acanthosis, papillomatosis, thickening of the dermis, and smooth muscle hyperplasia. Becker's nevus is considered as an organoid nevus with epidermal melanocytic and dermal components.[54]

NEVUS SPILUS/SPECKLED LENTIGINOUS NEVUS Nevus spilus/speckled lentiginous nevus (NS/SLN) presents as a circumscribed, usually lightly pigmented macule containing scattered, usually more darkly pigmented spots. The Greek root *spilos* means "spot," hence the term of *nevus spilus*. NS/SLN can appear on any area of the body. Background pigmentation in NS/SLN is often 3 to 6 cm in diameter, but

FIGURE 90-35

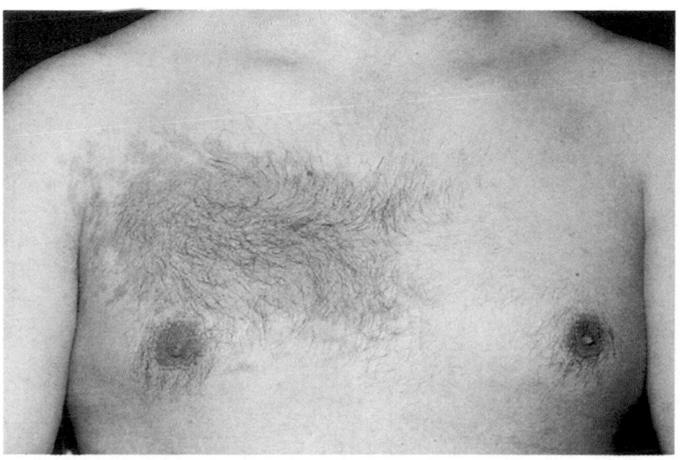

Becker's nevus (pigmented hairy hamartoma). This acquired reticulate lesion is usually flat or raised. Neck and trunk locations are common sites. Up to 50 percent demonstrate hypertrichosis.

FIGURE 90-36

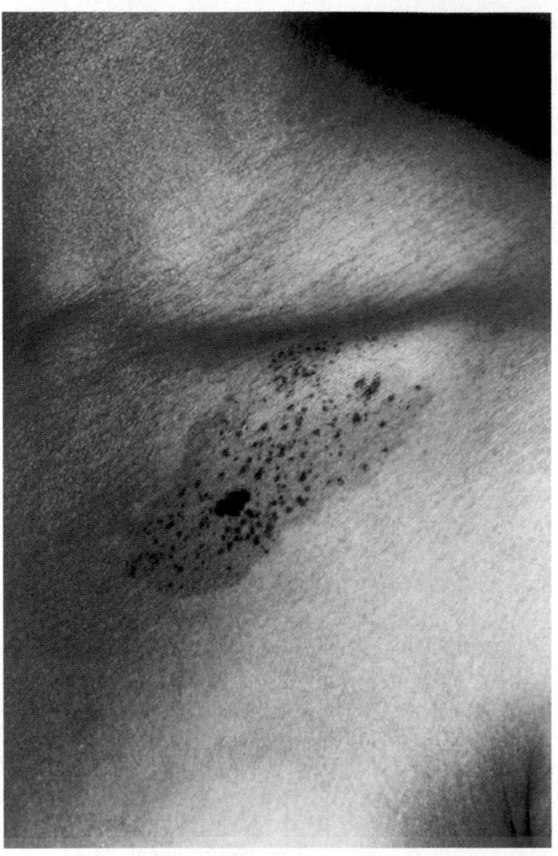

Nevus spilus. A café-au-lait macule sprinkled with melanotic macules that are either lentigines or common nevi.

FIGURE 90-37

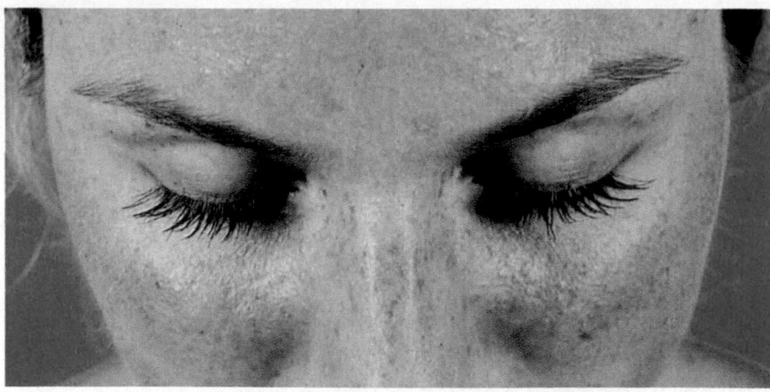

Ephelides. Typical small, flat, medium brown macules in sun-exposed areas of skin.

it can vary from 1 to over 60 cm. Histopathology is consistent with lentigo. There is a wide spectrum of clinical findings when it comes to the spots, including red to brown to blue to black macules and papules (Fig. 90-36). Their size is often 2 to 3 mm in diameter but can range from 1 to 9 mm. Accordingly, histopathology ranges from lentigines to junctional, compound, and dermal nevi to Spitz and blue nevi. Most commonly, the shape of an NS/SLN is oval, but there are clinical variants: blocklike with a sharp demarcation at the midline, linear (and the linear lesions may follow the lines of Blaschko), extensive over large areas of the body, and lastly, a divided form involving both eyelids.[55]

LINEAR AND WHORLED HYPERMELANOSIS Linear and whorled hypermelanosis (LWH), also classified as a variety of other names such as *zebra-like hyperpigmentation,* is characterized by linear streaks of hyperpigmentation along Blaschko's lines.[56] The pigmentary anomalies become apparent in infancy or early childhood and usually remain stable, but they may either increase in extent or fade over time. Histopathology suggests melanotic hypermelanosis in most cases, but melanocytotic hypermelanosis and less often pigmentary incontinence also have been reported.

Although the general opinion was that LWH is not typically associated with extracutaneous anomalies, there have been many case reports to suggest the contrary. The concept that LWH is a disorder of mosaicism has been supported recently by molecular genetics studies.[57,58] Striking homologies exist between HI and LWH. In addition, several patients have been reported who display bands of both hypo- and hyperpigmentation, making the distinction between HI and LWH somewhat blurred. In some cases, it is difficult to know with certainty whether the cells producing the "background" skin tone or those producing the distinctly hued bands are the genetically abnormal ones, making the putative distinction between HI and LWH even less clear. Emerging opinion is that a revised nomenclature should group HI and LWH as a single entity including hypopigmentation or hyperpigmentation along the lines of Blaschko, possible association with extracutaneous anomalies in approximately 30 percent of patients, and somatic mosaicism in a yet-indetermined but probably several different genes involved in human pigmentation.

Widespread epidermal melanotic hyperpigmentation

EPHELIDES Ephelides, or freckles, are small, usually less than 0.5 cm in diameter, discrete brown macules that appear on sun-exposed skin (Fig. 90-37). They occur commonly in the Caucasian population, more frequently in fair-skinned individuals with red or light-blond hair. Ephelides appear early in childhood and partly vanish with age. Fair skin, red hair, and ephelides are indicators for an increased risk of melanoma and nonmelanoma skin cancer. The melanocortin-1 receptor gene is the major ephelide gene.[59] Ephelide-like pigmented macules may be found in neurofibromatosis, progeria, Moynahan's syndrome, and xeroderma pigmentosum.

MELASMA Melasma is a common acquired symmetric hypermelanosis characterized by irregular light-brown to gray-brown macules and patches on sun-exposed areas of the skin (Fig. 90-38). It is far more common in women and in persons with high-grade phototype. The major etiologic factors in the pathogenesis of melasma include genetic influences, exposure to UV radiation, and female sex hormones. A melasma-like facial hyperpigmentation also has been described in relation with HIV infection.[60] Melasma is generally considered as an epidermal melanotic hyperpigmentation. However, it was suggested recently that an increased number of melanocytes may account for the epidermal hyperpigmentation of melasma.[61] The pathogeny of melasma is not yet fully understood. A recent study suggests that a high expression of α-MSH in the lesional keratinocytes of melasma plays a key role in the hyperpigmentation of melasma skin.[62]

Successful treatment of melasma involves the triad of sunblocks, bleach, and time (Fig. 90-38). The sunscreen must be an opaque formulation; however, use of a broad-spectrum formulation with an SPF of more than 30 plus coverup is adequate. Without daily use of opaque sunscreen, treatment will fail. Topical hydroquinone 2% to 4%, alone or in combination with tretinoin 0.05% to 0.1%, is an established bleaching treatment (see Fig. 90-38*B*). Possible side effects of hydroquinone are allergic sensitization and exogenous ochronosis. Topical azelaic acid 15% to 20% has also been used. Kojic acid, alone or in combination with glycolic acid or hydroquinone, has shown good results.[63]

FIGURE 90-38

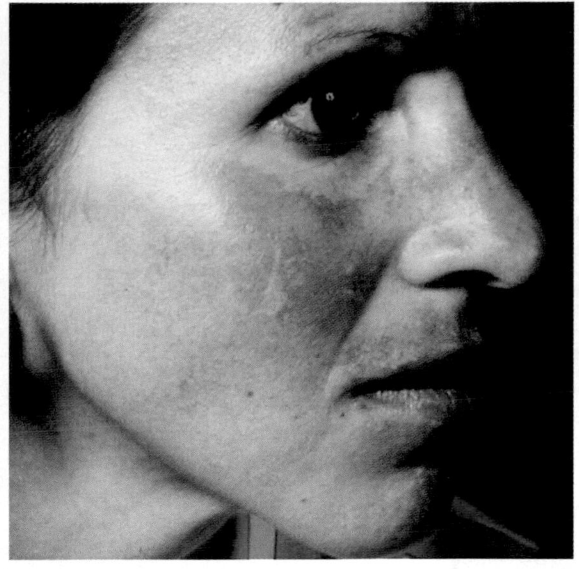

A.

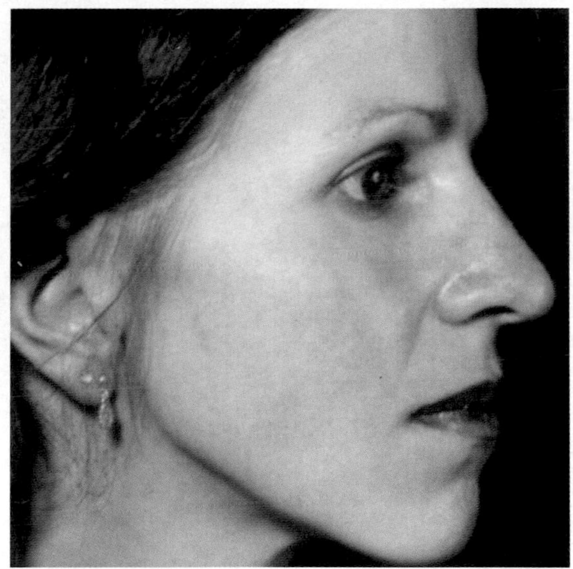

B.

Melasma. *A*. Typical blotchy, macular pigmentation bilaterally on the cheeks, upper lip, and bridge of the nose. *B*. Excellent cosmetic result after 10 weeks of treatment with 4% hydroquinone and tretinoin.

For epidermal melasma, normally up to 2 months are required to begin to initiate response and up to 6 months to complete the process. Dermal melasma does not respond to the preceding formulation and at the present time cannot be treated; coverup with opaque cosmetics is the only management option. Mixed-type melasma will improve only to the extent that there is a treatable epidermal component. Laser treatments do not offer promise.

Patients taking oral contraceptives should understand that successful treatment of their melasma may not be possible as long as the oral contraceptive is continued. Treatment of melasma during pregnancy or breast feeding is not advised.

ACQUIRED BRACHIAL CUTANEOUS DYSCHROMATOSIS Acquired brachial cutaneous dyschromatosis (ABCD) is a common acquired bilateral hypermelanosis characterized by gray-brown patches with geographic borders, occasionally interspersed with hypopigmented macules, on the dorsum of the forearms. It is observed most often in postmenopausal Caucasian women. Histologic findings are melanotic epidermal hyperpigmentation and dermal elastosis. Civatte's poikiloderma is observed in nearly 50 percent of patients.[64]

TAR MELANOSIS Tar melanosis also has been called *melanodermatitis toxica*. This is an entity found mainly in workers exposed to tar and other hydrocarbons, which also may be present in cosmetics. It likely follows a photosensitivity reaction. Erythema, edema, vesiculation, and pruritus are found most often on the face or dorsal hands. The late stage features a reticulate hyperpigmentation with hyperkeratosis. Histology shows edema, follicular hyperkeratosis, reduction of basal layer pigmentation, pigment-laden macrophages, and lymphocytic perivascular infiltrate.

PELLAGRA (See Chap. 145) Chronic pellagra may be characterized by eczema-like lesions, thickening, fissuring, and striking hyperpigmentation of the dorsal hands, neck area, nasal bridge, and scalp. These changes are most prominent over bony prominences. A leukomelanoderma also may be present. Niacin deficiency is associated with photosensitivity and susceptibility to mechanical trauma.

POSTINFLAMMATORY HYPERPIGMENTATION In many instances, hyperpigmentation follows resolution of specific eruptions. Certain rashes, such as contact dermatitis to poison ivy or primula, atopic dermatitis, etc., are particularly likely to result in postinflammatory hyperpigmentation. These pigmentary changes, which are characteristically discrete macules with hazy, feathered margins, correspond exactly with the primary eruption (Fig. 90-39) and may persist for months.

FIGURE 90-39

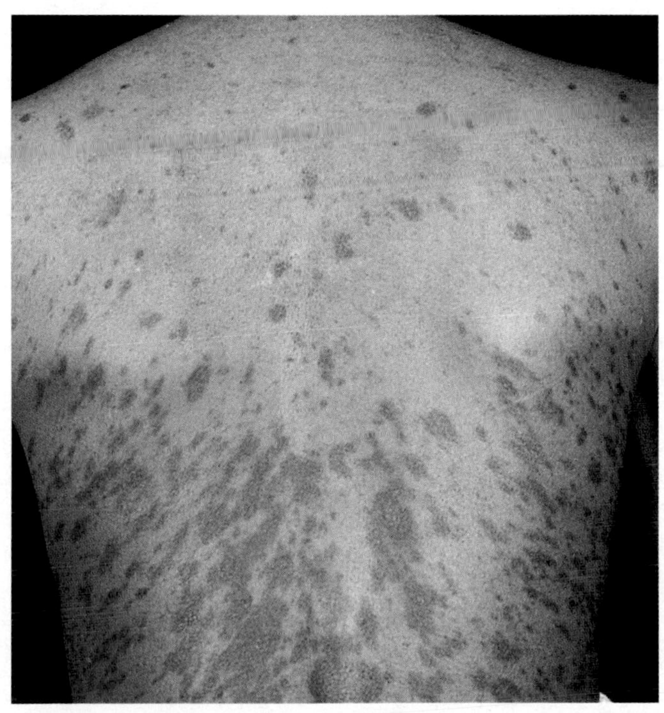

Postinflammatory hyperpigmentation. Epidermal hyperpigmentation corresponds to areas of resolved primary eruption.

FIGURE 90-40

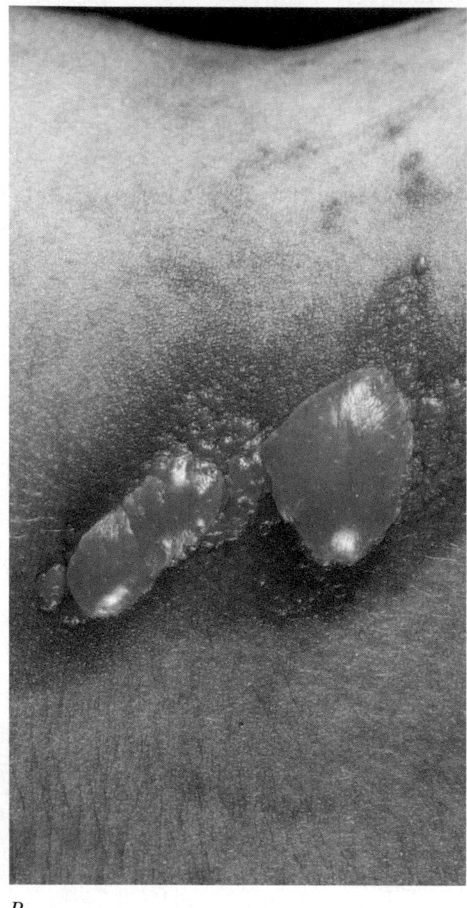

A. B.

Berloque dermatitis. *A.* Cutaneous photosensitization developed following application of a 5-methoxypsoralen–containing perfume; after sun exposure, the hyperpigmentation developed. *B.* A similar reaction due to furocoumarin present in a plant (phytophotodermatitis). After inflammation and bullous eruption have subsided, pigmentation as in (*A*) will develop.

Tinea Versicolor (See Chap. 206) In tinea versicolor, hyperpigmented macules are not as common as the hypopigmented macules, but they are by no means unusual. The brown lesions are otherwise analogous to the white lesions in size, distribution, scaling, and in response to topical therapy.

Photocontact Dermatitis (See Chap. 136) Photocontact dermatitis is caused by application of photosensitising compounds such as psoralens. Psoralens can be found in plants or in perfumes. The first stage of photocontact dermatitis is an inflammatory bullous eruption 24 to 48 h after contact (Fig. 90-40*B*). It is mostly observed after contact with certain plants and subsequent sun exposure, hence the term *phytophotodermatitis* (see Chap. 136). The second stage is a macule of brown hyperpigmentation 7 to 10 days after the first stage, often with discrete margins and streaking. This is also called *berloque dermatitis* (see Fig. 90-40*A*).

Cronkhite-Canada Syndrome Cronkhite-Canada syndrome (CCS; OMIM 175.500), also known as *intestinal polyposis with hyperpigmentation,* is a rare sporadic syndrome mostly reported in Japanese patients. There are many cutaneous manifestations. A common feature is development of a diffuse hyperpigmentation affecting all parts of the integument. Patchy hair loss that progresses to almost complete alopecia is common. The fingernails become thin and brittle and later are shed from the ends of the fingers. The main extracutaneous features are polyps that form throughout the intestinal tract. Loss of fluid from the polyp results in diarrhea and malabsorption.[65]

Dyschromatosis Universalis Hereditaria Dyschromatosis universalis hereditaria (DUH; OMIM) has been reported almost exclusively in Asian families. It shows an autosomal dominant pattern of inheritance. The pigmentary features of DUH generally appear during infancy or early childhood. Pinpoint to pea-sized hyperpigmented and hypopigmented macules form the striking reticulated pattern characteristic of this syndrome (Fig. 90-41). They are distributed over the entire integument, especially on the trunk, abdomen, and limbs. The face is involved rarely. Palms and soles are spared usually. Nails, hair, teeth, and mucous membranes are unaffected.[66]

Familial Periorbital Hyperpigmentation Periorbital hyperpigmentation, or dark circles around the eyes, is a common finding in otherwise healthy people. This form of hyperpigmentation also was described as an autosomal dominant disorder. Clinical expression is variable. The hyperpigmentation usually starts during childhood in the lower eyelids and progresses with age to involve the entire periorbital area.[67]

Familial Progressive Hyperpigmentation This rare dermatosis, inherited mostly in an autosomal dominant manner, also was reported under different terms. The salient clinical finding is intense pigmentation that is variably described as jet black, dark brown, or bronze. Patchy hyperpigmentation occurs at birth or develops in early infancy. The initial site of involvement is usually the face or groin. Generally, the pigment becomes diffusely distributed due to coalescence of the pigmented macules. The pigmentation involves the palms, soles, lip, oral mucosa, and conjunctivae. The cornea may be affected as well.[68]

Reticular melanotic hypermelanoses

Dowling-Degos Disease Dowling-Degos disease (OMIM 179.850), or reticular pigmented anomaly of the flexures, is a rare genodermatosis characterized by an acquired reticular macular hyperpigmentation that initially affects the axillae and groin and later involves intergluteal and inframammary folds, neck, trunk, and arms. Onset is in early adult life and is slowly progressive. Both sexes are involved. Histologically, there are pigmented filiform epidermal projections involving the follicular infundibulum as well as the epidermis. There is no increase in the number of melanocytes. The main concentration of melanin is in the keratinocytes of the elongated rete ridges, particularly near the lower tips.

This entity is separate from acanthosis nigricans because Dowling-Degos disease has no papillomatosis, has elongation of the rete ridges that does not resemble that of acanthosis nigricans, and has a follicular anomaly not found in acanthosis nigricans.

Dyskeratosis Congenita Dyskeratosis congenita (DKC) is a rare genodermatosis characterized by reticulate hyperpigmentation,

FIGURE 90-41

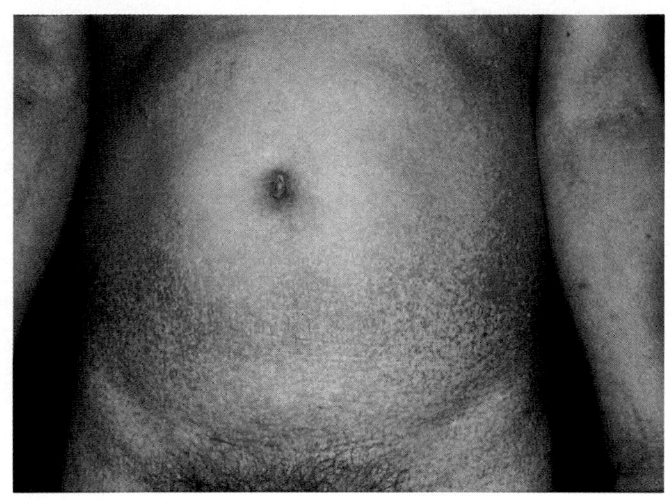

Dyschromatosis universalis. (*Courtesy of Y Tomita, MD.*)

nail atrophy, hyperkeratosis and atrophy of palms and soles, and leukokeratosis of the mucosal surfaces. X-linked chromosomal pattern and autosomal dominant inheritance have been described. The complete syndrome, which also includes mucosal lesions and pancytopenia, is not apparent until the second or third decade of life. Mucosal lesions on the oral, vaginal, urethral, and conjunctival epithelia present as whitish plaques. Mucosal malignancy is a frequent complication. Pancytopenia occurs in over a third of patients and may be responsible for death.

DKC is the gene responsible for X-linked dyskeratosis congenita. Dyskerin is a *DKC1* gene product. The pathology of DKC is a defect in telomerase maintenance that may limit the proliferative capacity of epithelial and blood cells.[69]

TERC is the gene responsible for autosomal DKC. The *TERC* gene product is known to interact with *DYSKERIN,* the gene mutated in X-linked DKC.[70]

DKC may be confused with Fanconi's syndrome, which is associated with short stature, aplasia or hypoplasia of the thumbs, and a reduced number of carpal bones. In Fanconi's syndrome, the skin is hyperpigmented in multiple patches, particularly the trunk, neck, axillae, and groin. This pigmentation is present in the first few years of life—earlier than in dyskeratosis congenita.

Acromelanoses

DIFFUSE ACROMELANOSIS Diffuse acromelanosis consists of diffuse hyperpigmentation of the fingers that is not in a reticular pattern. It is found in many races, may be autosomal dominant, and is first expressed in early childhood. It evolves and may extend to the flexor creases of larger joints. This pigmentary pattern is particularly common in darker races.

RETICULATED ACROPIGMENTATION OF DOHI Reticulate acropigmentation of Dohi is the localized form of dyschromatosis universalis hereditaria, hence the term *dyschromatosis symmetrica hereditaria.* This rare disorder is often familial and has been reported mostly in Asian and Brazilian populations. It presents generally during infancy or early childhood as symmetrical pinpoint to pea-sized hyperpigmented and hypopigmented macules on the back of the hands and feet.[71]

RETICULATE ACROPIGMENTATION OF KITAMURA Reticulate acropigmentation of Kitamura is an autosomal dominant pigmentary disorder that is characterized by reticulate freckle-like hyperpigmentation (which darkens over time) beginning on the dorsal hands and subsequently spreading over the body. These slightly depressed brown macules may be associated with palmar pits and breaks in the epidermal rete ridge pattern. Two-thirds of the cases reported have been from Japan, but other cases have been reported from Iran, Great Britain, western India, Ghana, and elsewhere. Unlike reticulate acropigmentation of Dohi, white macules are not observed. Histologic features include epidermal atrophy and an increased number of epidermal melanocytes. Increased melanocyte activity is also apparent.

Diffuse melanotic hypermelanoses *Diffuse* or *widespread epidermal melanotic hypermelanosis* refers to the marked accentuation of normal areas of melanin pigmentation all over but often with particular accentuation in certain areas, particularly over the pressure points (vertebrae, knuckles, elbows, knees, and the like), in the body folds, in the palmar creases, in recent scars, and in some cases in the mucous membranes. This also may be referred to as *addisonian hyperpigmentation* and may result from a number of factors. Because these pigmentary changes may reflect a variety of disease entities and may occur in normal persons of all races, comparative observations are required to identify any abnormality. A congenital, diffuse, mottling syndrome may occur rarely; it features many light- and dark-brown macules that are irregular in size and shape and up to 2 cm in diameter. Proximal nail beds are also partly pigmented.

ADDISON'S DISEASE (See Chap. 169) Addison's disease is rare (1 in 100,000), resulting from primary adrenocortical insufficiency and affecting all ages and both sexes equally. The disease becomes apparent after physical or metabolic stress. Weakness is the prominent symptom, first reported after stress; later on, patients report chronic weakness, fatigue, and weight loss. Nausea and vomiting are frequent complaints; there may be orthostatic hypotension with dizziness and syncope. Hyperpigmentation occurs as a change in the intensity of pigmentation in normally pigmented areas especially or as the development of new areas of pigmentation, e.g., gingival or buccal mucous membrane. Pigmentation also develops in new scars; around the eyes, nipples, and creases of the palms; over bony prominences; and in the linea nigra (abdomen), axillae, and the anogenital areas. Linear streaks of pigmentation are found in the nail plate (a normal finding in brown- and black-skinned persons). Gray scalp hair may darken as the disease progresses. Axillary hair may be decreased or absent. The hyperpigmentation results from the melanogenic action of α-MSH.

OTHER CAUSES OF ADDISONIAN-LIKE HYPERPIGMENTATION Other causes of addisonian-like hyperpigmentation are listed in Table 90-9. In Nelson's syndrome, involving adrenalectomized individuals with functioning pituitary adenomas, there are often darkening of hair, multiple lentigines, and pigmented nail bands. The hyperpigmentation in hyperthyroidism may spare mucosal surfaces and be associated with eyelid hyperpigmentation (see Chap. 169).

In Siemerling-Creuzfeldt disease (leukodystrophy, hyperpigmentation, and adrenal atrophy), which is inherited, unaffected carriers may

TABLE 90-9

Diseases Associated with Addisonian-like Hyperpigmentation

Addison's disease	Hyperthyroidism
ACTH administration	Lymphoma, particularly Hodgkin's disease
ACTH-producing tumors (Nelson's syndrome)	Pheochromocytoma
Acromegaly	POEMS syndrome
AIDS	Porphyria cutanea tarda
Carcinoid	Schilder's disease
Cirrhosis	Scleroderma
Cushing's syndrome	Siemerling-Creuzfeldt disease
Hepatolenticular degeneration	Still's disease

show increased pigmentation at an early age. Death occurs in early life to the midfifties.

The generalized hypermelanosis observed in 90 to 98 percent of cases of hemochromatosis (see also Chap. 164) may be bronze, blue gray, or brown black and may be accentuated in sun-exposed areas of skin. The changes are attributed to deposition of melanin (brown) and hemosiderin (blue black). Cutaneous and mucous membrane involvement, seen in 15 to 25 percent, may resemble Addison's disease and may precede cirrhosis and associated (diabetes mellitus by years. Hyperpigmentation also may involve genitalia, flexor folds, scars, and nipples. Other cutaneous signs include atrophy, ichthyosis-like changes, alopecia, koilonychia, onychonychia, palmar erythema, spider angiomas, and leukonychia.[72] Biopsy sections stained with potassium ferrocyanide demonstrate hemosiderin around sweat glands and cutaneous blood vessels. Color abnormalities increase with exacerbations and decrease with remissions. The siderosis is more likely to be affected by treatment than is the hypermelanosis.

Universal Acquired Melanosis—The Carbon Baby Several such cases have been reported. In general, the hyperpigmentation begins between birth and 2 to $2^1/_2$ years, is observed initially on the face or groin, and over the years spreads gradually over the entire body. The palms, soles, and mucous membranes display a mottled or homogeneous dark hyperpigmentation that gradually may become less uniform and mottled, even with white patches.

POEMS Syndrome The POEMS syndrome is a rare plasma cell dyscrasia characterized by the combination of polyneuropathy, organomegaly (involving liver, spleen, lymph nodes), endocrinopathies (diabetes mellitus, gynecomastia, impotence, oligomenorrhea/ amenorrhea, and hyperthyroidism), M protein, and skin changes. Abnormal pigmentation of the skin, either generalized or localized, is observed in 98 percent of patients. The hyperpigmentation is diffuse, but there may be accentuation over extensor surfaces, the back, neck, and axillae. The hyperpigmentation may ameliorate with effective treatment of the plasmacytoma.[73]

Miscellaneous Conditions *Whipple's intestinal lipodystrophy* may be associated with hyperpigmentation in up to a third of cases. Cutaneous but not mucosal hyperpigmentation may be found in *primary biliary cirrhosis;* this occurs in sun-exposed areas, resembles a deep tan, and disappears as the cirrhosis improves (see also Chap. 164).

Porphyria cutanea tarda is associated with a diffuse generalized brown hypermelanosis accentuated in sun-exposed areas; this is associated with facial hirsutism and other characteristic features (see Chap. 149). *Renal failure* is often associated with hyperpigmentation (see Chap. 165).

Hyperpigmentation in vitamin B_{12} deficiency, in which hyperpigmentation is accentuated over the knuckles, is associated with loss of hair, and it reverses with vitamin B_{12} therapy. Folate deficiency also may be associated with hyperpigmentation (see Chap. 145).

Progressive systemic sclerosis may give an intensely brown hyperpigmentation without significant induration of the skin. Hypermelanosis also may be associated with local scleroderma or morphea (see Chap. 173).

Hyperpigmentation due to drugs/chemical agents A number of drugs have been reported to cause epidermal hyperpigmentation in various patterns. These are listed in Table 90-10.

Dermal Hypermelanoses

Dermal hyperpigmentation, or ceruloderma, results from the presence of pigment in the dermis (Table 90-11). Because of the Tyndall effect, dermal pigment is perceived as blue, gray, blue gray, or gray brown and is distinctive from normal skin color in all skin phototypes. Unlike epidermal hypermelanosis, comparison with normal skin color is rarely required to establish that an abnormality exists. Although dermal pigment disorders are rather rare among Caucasians, they are observed commonly in East Indians and Asians. The Wood's lamp is not useful as a diagnostic tool; infrared photography accentuates dermal pigmentation but not epidermal pigmentation. Skin biopsy may be required to identify the presence of melanin, iron, or exogenous pigment in the dermis. Clinicopathologic classification of dermal hypermelanoses is given in Table 90-11.

TABLE 90-10

Drug-Induced Hyperpigmentation

Generalized types of hyperpigmentation
- Addisonian
  - ACTH
  - Busulfan (sun-exposed areas)
  - 5-Fluorouracil
- Diffuse
  - Carmustine
  - Clofazimine
  - Cyclophosphamide
  - Dibromomannitol
  - Mechlorethamine
  - Procarbazine
  - Tetracosactide (cosyntropin)

Patterned types of hyperpigmentation
- Linear
  - Bleomycin
  - Zidovudine
- Palms, soles (diffuse)
  - Cyclophosphamide
  - Dibromomannitol
  - Doxorubicin (also palmar creases)
  - Procarbazine
- Around small joints
  - Bleomycin (knuckles)
  - Doxorubicin (interphalangeal joints)
- Melasma-like
  - Estrogen
  - Estrogen-progesterone
  - Mephenytoin
  - Phenytoin

PATHOGENESIS OF DERMAL HYPERPIGMENTATION The pathogenesis of dermal hyperpigmentation is based on several possible mechanisms. Dermal hyperpigmentation may result from melanin in the dermis attributed to (1) *dermal melanotic hyperpigmentation,* that is, melanin formed in the epidermis by epidermal melanocytes and transferred to the dermis, (2) *dermal melanocytotic hyperpigmentation,* that is, melanin formed in dermal melanocytes, or (3) *nonmelanin dermal pigmentation,* attributed to pigment other than melanin deposited in the dermis.

The phenomenon of epidermal melanin incontinence is a reaction pattern common to a number of diseases of diverse etiologies and associated with dermal melanosis. Although there may be slight variations, the common sequence in these diverse entities appears to be (1) a targeted attack on the melanosome-containing keratinocytes, (2) loss of nuclei from basal keratinocytes to form anucleate, aggregated, filamentous, eosinophilic masses (Civatte bodies), (3) movement of the Civatte bodies, often containing melanosomes, into the dermis either inside macrophages or in some unknown manner as free bodies to remain as extracellular masses in the dermal connective tissue or to be phagocytosed by macrophages.

CIRCUMSCRIBED DERMAL MELANOCYTOTIC HYPERPIGMENTATION Circumscribed dermal melanoses are generally developmental or heritable, localized to one area or general area of the body, and particularly common among Asians.

TABLE 90-11

Dermal Hypermelanoses: Clinicopathologic Classification of Disorders

Etiologic Factors	Melanocytotic (Increase in Number of Melanocytes)	Melanotic (Increase in Melanin)	Nonmelanotic (No Melanin Defect)	
Heritable or developmental	Mongolian spot (dermal melanocytosis) Nevus of Ota and nevus of Ito Blue melanocytotic nevus Carleton-Biggs syndrome Levene's syndrome	Incontinentia pigmenti Franceschetti-jadassohn syndrome		
Metabolic		Hemochromatosis Macular amyloidosis	Alkaptonuria Ochronosis	
Endocrine		Melasma, dermal (female facial melanosis)		
Chemical and drug		Fixed drug eruption	Heavy metals Mercury Silver Bismuth Arsenic Gold Lead Iron	Antimalarials Oral contraceptives Phenothiazine Minocycline PCB poisoning Amiodarone Tattoos
Nutritional		Chronic nutritional deficiency		
Physical		Erythema ab igne		
Inflammation and infection		Pinta (exposed areas) Erythema dyschromicum perstans Riehl's melanosis Postinflammatory (occupational contact)		
Neoplasms	Melanoma metastases	Slate-gray dermal pigmentation with melanoma and melanogenuria		

Mongolian spots or congenital dermal melanocytosis The term *Mongolian spot,* or *congenital dermal melanocytosis* (CDM), applies to specific blue-gray macules commonly observed among Asians and Polynesians, although occasionally they are seen in Caucasians and blacks.

CLINICAL FEATURES CDM is almost always located on the lumbosacral skin or on the buttocks. The lesions are macular with distinct margins and blue black in color, although with variations in intensity (Fig. 90-42). The lesions are characteristically a few centimeters in diameter but may be large enough to cover the entire lower back and buttocks. In typical CDM, the dermal melanocytes appear microscopically at the fetal age of 3 months, and the pigmentation appears at the fetal age of 7 months. The natural course of CDM is to disappear in childhood.

CLINICAL VARIANTS Several variants of typical CDM appear to exist. The so-called persistent Mongolian spot is said to occur in 3 to 4 percent of Japanese adults. Aberrant Mongolian spots occur not on the common sites of the buttocks and lumbosacral areas but in less common regions such as the face or extremities; when they occur on the face, they may be confused with nevus of Ota (oculodermal melanocytosis). The latter almost always has a mottled appearance composed of blue-black, slate-gray, or brown macules and is acquired in early childhood or young adulthood, whereas CDM is congenital. Persistent aberrant Mongolian spots may be called *macular-type blue nevi*. The value of laser treatment is uncertain.

Nevus of Ota (oculodermal melanocytosis) (See Chap. 91) Nevus of Ota is usually congenital but may appear in early childhood or in puberty. It is usually characterized by unilateral, flat, blue-black or slate-gray macules intermingled with small, flat brown, spots occurring most characteristically in the skin innervated by the first and second branches of the trigeminal nerve (Fig. 90-43). Mucosa, conjunctivae, and tympanic membranes may be involved. This disorder, which is not hereditary, is said to occur in up to 0.8 percent of dermatologic outpatients in Japan but also occurs in Chinese, blacks, East Indians, and Caucasians. Women are affected five times as frequently as men.

Hyperpigmentation in the involved areas of cornea, iris, optic nerve, fundus, extraocular muscles, retrobulbar fat, and periosteum may occur. Similar involvement may be located on the hard palate, pharynx, nasal mucosa, buccal mucosa, and tympanic membrane of the involved side.

COURSE AND TREATMENT Nevus of Ota does not improve with time. There have been a large number of reported cases of melanoma development in nevus of Ota. Selective photothermolysis with the Q-switched ruby laser is a safe and effective treatment. Multiple treatments increase the response rate.

Acquired circumscribed dermal facial melanocytosis Hori's nevus, or acquired circumscribed dermal melanocytosis of the face, is characterized by blue-brown macules that occur bilaterally on the forehead, temples, eyelids, malar areas, nasal alae, and nasal root of middle-aged Japanese women. These macules are clinically very similar to classic nevus of Ota. The lesions usually are noted in the fourth or fifth decade of life in Japanese women and do not extend to ocular or mucosal surfaces.

Nevus of Ito Initially described by Ito in 1954, nevus of Ito is analogous to nevus of Ota and may in fact coexist in the same patient. With nevus of Ito, the cutaneous involvement occurs in the distribution of the lateral supraclavicular and lateral brachial nerves. Except for the fact that the involvement is more diffuse and less mottled, the pigmentary change is the same as that of the nevus of Ota.

FIGURE 90-42

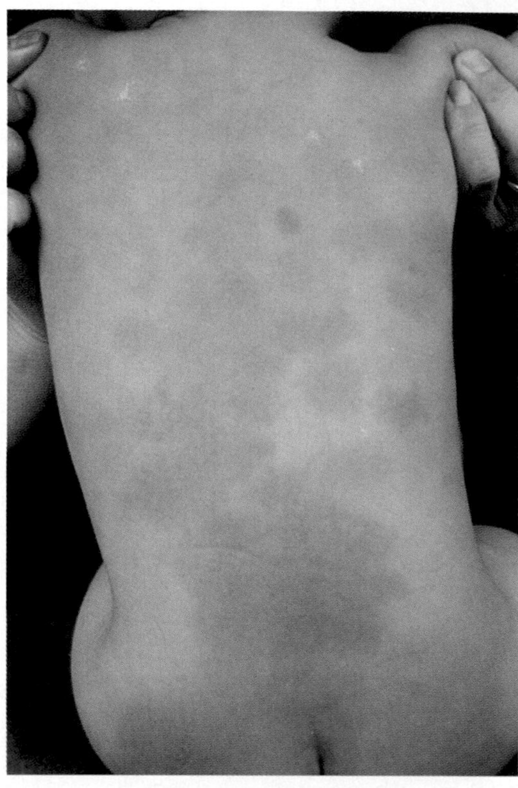

Classic Mongolian spot in the lumbosacral region, and aberrant or extrasacral Mongolian spots on the back.

Diffuse dermal melanocytotic hyperpigmentation Extensive blue pigmentation of the skin involving the forehead, nose, lips iris, sclera, vestibule of the mouth, and trunk has been reported twice.[74]

CIRCUMSCRIBED DERMAL MELANOTIC HYPERPIGMENTATION Each of these disorders has characteristic features, some of which are presented in greater detail in other sections of this chapter or elsewhere in this book.

Incontinentia pigmenti (See above and Chaps. 143 and 188) Of the three stages of evolution of IP, hyperpigmentation is observed only in the third stage and is characterized by whorls and streaks of hyperpigmentation over the trunk and extremities (Fig. 90-44). The pigmentary macules are bizarre, macular, brown, dirty brown to slate gray, and intensity in color up to age 2 and then begin to fade gradually through adolescence and early adulthood. Up to 14 percent of patients will develop hypopigmentation.

Franceschetti-Jadassohn syndrome This condition, affecting a father and two daughters, is a distinct entity that has been described only in one Swiss family. The pigmentary anomaly, which occurs without antecedent inflammation, begins at 2 years of age and is characterized by reticular brown, dirty-brown, slate-gray, or gray-brown pigmentation on the trunk and upper extremities. Yellowing of teeth, hyperkeratosis of palms and soles, hyperhidrosis, and heat intolerance also have been observed.

Dermatophathia pigmentosa reticularis This is characterized by macular pigmentation that develops in infancy and forms a reticulate network, particularly on the trunk, neck, shoulders, and thighs. This may be a variant of the Franceschetti-Jadassohn syndrome. Nail dystrophy and alopecia, as well as palmoplantar keratoderma and ainhum-like constriction, have been described.

Macular amyloidosis (See Chap. 148) The macular variety of amyloidosis is characterized by brownish gray, reticulated pigmentation that may or may not be associated with pruritus. Macular amyloidosis is more common in females than in males and is frequently noted in individuals from Central or South America and from Mediterranean countries and in Asiatic peoples. There are occasional reports of non-Mediterranean Europeans and rare ones of blacks. The average age of onset is under 30 years.

Clinically, the common sites of occurrence are the upper back (interscapular areas), buttocks, chest (over the clavicles, on the ribs), breast, and extremities (shins, forearms). The eruption is usually symmetric and is often observed to arise at sites where the skin comes in contact with clothing; the latter observation has given support to the theory that cutaneous amyloidosis is a postinflammatory process, possibly related to friction, or localized lichenification (see Chap. 148).

Dermal Melanoses from Chemical or Pharmacologic Agents

Numerous chemical or pharmacologic agents may result in dermal pigmentation of a local or widespread nature. Perhaps most fascinating is the very localized repetitive type, the fixed drug eruption.

FIXED DRUG ERUPTION (See Chap. 138) This is a reddish brown to slate-gray cutaneous macule that may be localized or generalized. The most typical cases flare repeatedly in the same area following ingestion or injection of a particular medication. The initial phase of erythema, edema, and/or desquamation may be followed by a spontaneously resolving vesiculobullous eruption and finally by hyperpigmentation.

WIDESPREAD/DIFFUSE DERMAL MELANOSES RELATED TO DRUGS Numerous medications have been implicated in diffuse blue-gray coloration of the skin; in some cases these represent drug bound to melanin and in others drug alone. Particularly implicated has been long-term use of chlorpromazine, other phenothiazines, hydrochlorothiazide, and minocycline. This blue-gray coloration may involve any normally sun-exposed area but occurs especially on the forehead, malar eminences, and nose. Although the initial color is brown, repeated sun exposure leads to a slate-gray or violaceous hue. With chlorpromazine (Fig. 90-45), blue-gray pigmentation has been reported in 1 to 15 percent of those taking 800 to 2000 mg daily for over a year. Pigment deposition also has been described in the kidney, heart, skeletal muscle, brain, eye, and reticuloendothelial system. The eye changes are restricted to the lens.

There is evidence to implicate melanin in chlorpromazine-related hyperpigmentation. An additional chromophore, a polymer of chlorpromazine, also has been implicated. This stems from the discovery of electron-dense bodies without recognizable internal structure in endothelial cells in the dermis and alongside the melanosomes within the phagocytic lysosomes.

Thiazides, tetracyclines, and amiodarone cause a photosensitivity-related hyperpigmentation. As with chlorpromazine, melanin is not the only pigment implicated.

Amiodarone, a drug given for cardiac diseases, induces a low-grade photosensitivity. Clinical findings include dusky-red erythema and later slate blue-gray pigmentation in sun-exposed areas of the face and hands (Fig. 90-46). The course of evolution is subtle in that some patients gradually develop pigmentary changes without clinically apparent phototoxicity, whereas others express a dusky-red erythema of the face and dorsal hands within 30 to 120 min of sun exposure. This reaction lasts 1 to 2 days.

FIGURE 90-43

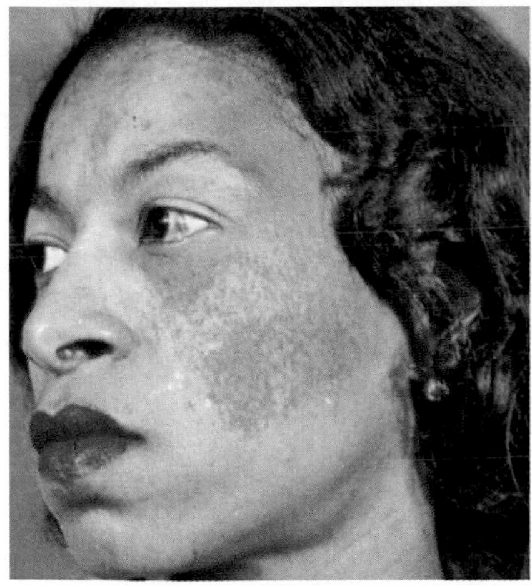

A.

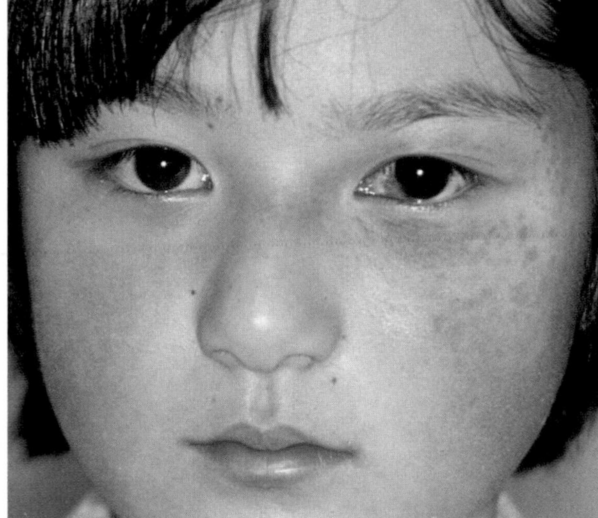

C.

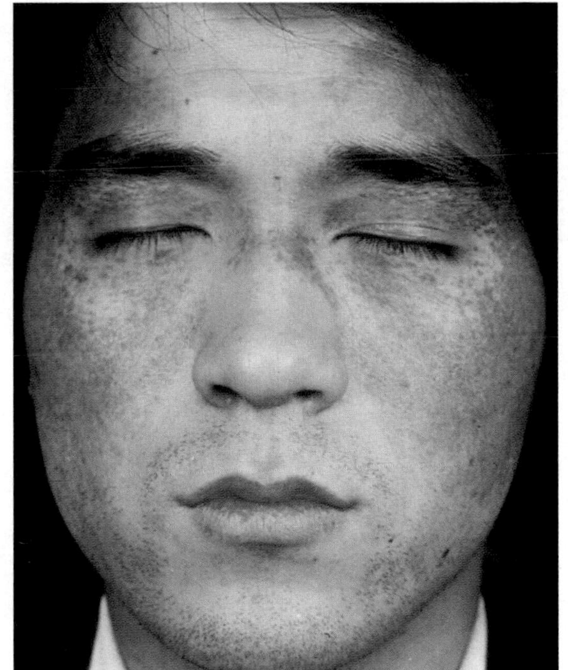

B.

Nevus of Ota. *A.* Nevus of Ota in an African American; this pigmentation is not usually congenital but rather develops at puberty and does not disappear. Both epidermal and dermal components may coexist. *B.* Bilateral type. *C.* Unilateral type with ocular involvement.

FIGURE 90-44

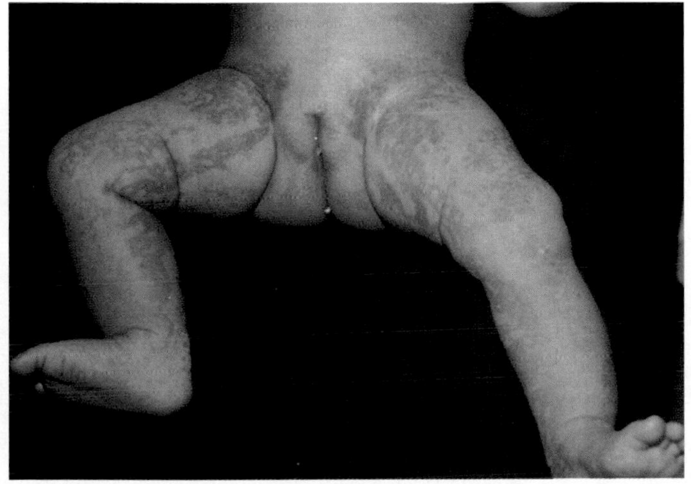

Incontinentia pigmenti. The pigmentary stage shows bizarre swirls of gray-brown hypermelanosis over the trunk and extremities.

FIGURE 90-45

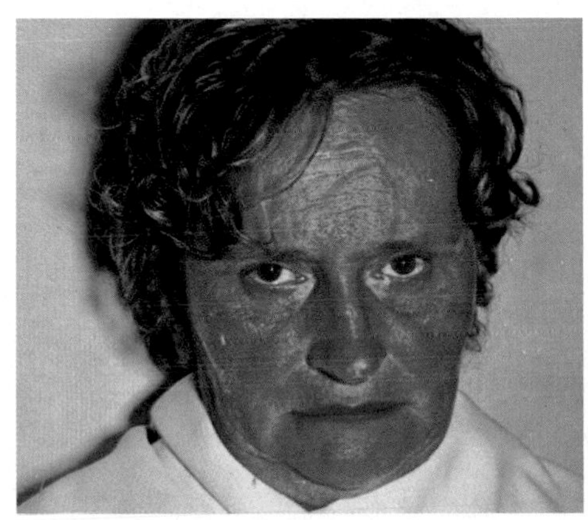

Chlorpromazine pigmentation. Purple pigmentation in a schizophrenic patient after prolonged high dosage of chlorpromazine.

FIGURE 90-46

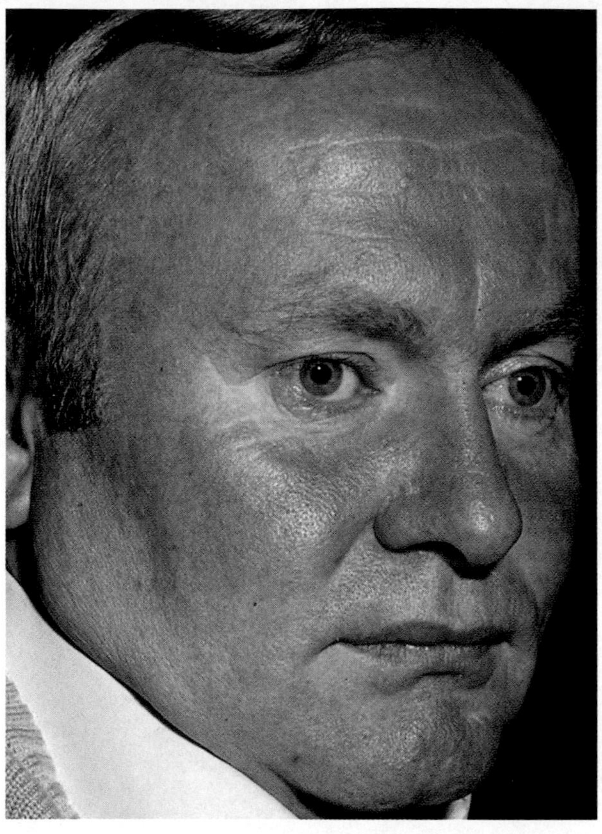

Amiodarone hyperpigmentation. This patient exhibits a striking amiodarone-induced, slate-gray pigmentation of the face. The blue color (ceruloderma) is due to the deposition of a brown pigment in the dermis, contained in macrophages and endothelial cells.

Histopathologic studies reveal a perivascular dermal lymphohistiocytic infiltrate. Brown granular pigment is noted in histiocytes, endothelial cells, and circulating neutrophils. Large amounts are found in dermal macrophages. The pigment occurs as electron-dense, compact, and lamellated granules in lysosomes.[75]

The pathogenesis of the photosensitivity involves incorporation of amiodarone into cell membranes that then absorb UVA so as to induce a phototoxic injury to erythrocytes, macrophages, and lymphocytes.

Systemic complications include pulmonary fibrosis, pneumonitis, hepatotoxicity, thyroid disturbances, neuropathy, and myopathy.

The subtle phototoxicity may persist for 12 to 24 months after discontinuation of the drug as the drug is slowly eliminated from lysosomal membranes. Resolution of the pigmentation required 33 months in one patient who was followed very carefully.[75]

Imipramine hyperpigmentation also has been described. In a reported case, the hyperpigmentation followed ingestion of 150 mg/day for 5 years, occurred in sun-exposed areas, and returned slowly to normal after discontinuation of the drug for a year. The color of the iris also was reported to be darkened. Histologic studies showed doubly refractile golden-yellow granules in the papillary dermis, and electron microscopy revealed many phagocytosed melanosomes and other separate electron-dense inclusions in histiocytes, phagocytes, fibroblasts, and dermal dendrocytes. The electron-dense granules were considered to be imipramine or its metabolites.[76]

FIGURE 90-47

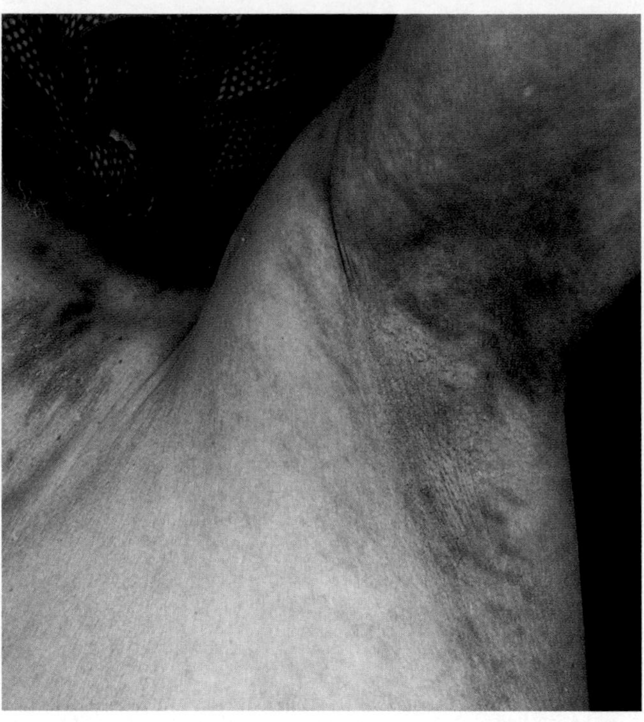

Erythema dyschromicum perstans (ashy dermatosis). Eruption often begins with erythematous macules that rapidly evolve to blue-gray macules.

Dermal Hypermelanosis Secondary to Infectious Diseases

Pinta is a treponematosis caused by *Treponema carateum;* it was first described in 1757 by Alzate y Raminez, who was a missionary priest who lived in the area of the volcano Jorulla and ministered to many people with blue spots on the skin. The blue-gray pigmentation arises in the third phase of pinta and generally in previously involved areas, particularly the face, waistline, and trochanteric areas (see Chap. 229 and Fig. 90-24).

Idiopathic Circumscribed Dermal Melanoses

Erythema dyschromicum perstans (EDP) is an idiopathic, acquired, generalized, macular, ashen–gray-blue hypermelanosis (Fig. 90-47) that occurs in otherwise healthy individuals. The lesions begin in the first or second decade as erythematous macules that gradually assume a slate-gray hue. Usually the lesions are flat, although there may be a thin, raised, erythematous border like "a thin piece of string." The macules of EDP may vary in size from a few millimeters to many centimeters, may enlarge slowly, and may coalesce to be as large as half the trunk. No effective treatment is available.

RIEHL'S MELANOSIS This is a reticular black to brown-violet pigmentation of the face (Fig. 90-48). Because most of the patients with Riehl's melanosis are middle-aged women, the term *female facial melanosis* also has been used. The pigmentary change occurs not only on the face but sometimes on the neck, dorsal hands, and forearms. Although the etiology remains unsettled, Riehl's melanosis may be a result of contact sensitivity or photocontact dermatitis related to a chemical, particularly fragrance, found in cosmetics.[77]

FIGURE 90-48

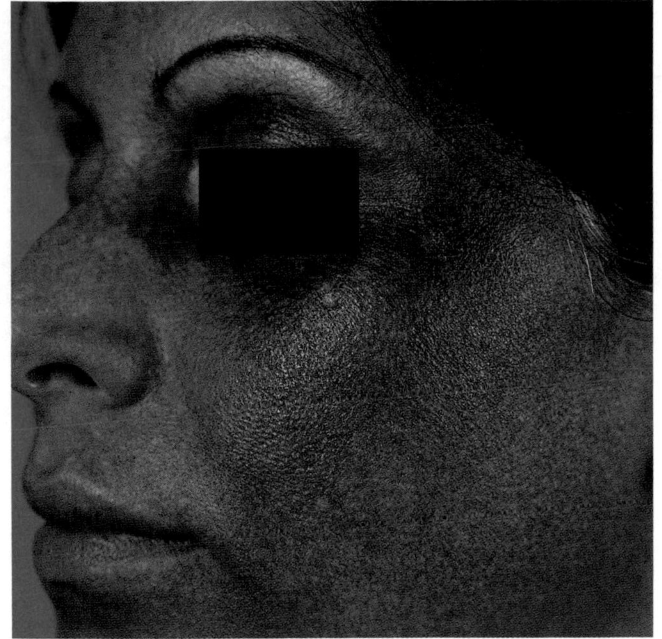

Riehl's melanosis. In this patient the mottled and disfiguring hyperpigmentation resulted from the chronic application of undefined cosmetics to the face.

ERYTHEMA AB IGNE (HEAT-INDUCED CIRCUMSCRIBED DERMAL MELANOSIS) Erythema ab igne is a reticular hypermelanosis that has a livedo reticularis pattern (Fig. 90-49). The process is thought to arise from repeated heat exposure, such as from a heating pad. There may be certain predisposing factors, particularly a combination of venous stasis, aging, and heat injury.[78]

Diffuse Dermal Melanotic Hypermelanoses

Widespread or diffuse slate-gray coloration may be secondary to chronic nutritional deficiency and to widespread metastatic melanoma. *Chronic nutritional deficiency* may give an ashen coloration accompanied by generalized scaling or eczematous or psoriasiform dermatitis. *Metastatic melanoma* and *melanogenuria* present with a generalized blue-gray cutaneous discoloration, sometimes accentuated in sun-exposed areas of skin (Fig. 90-50). The color varies from gray to brown with a metallic tint. This rare change is secondary to dermal melanin, and individually metastatic melanoma cells[79] and can develop in as little as 2 months.

FIGURE 90-49

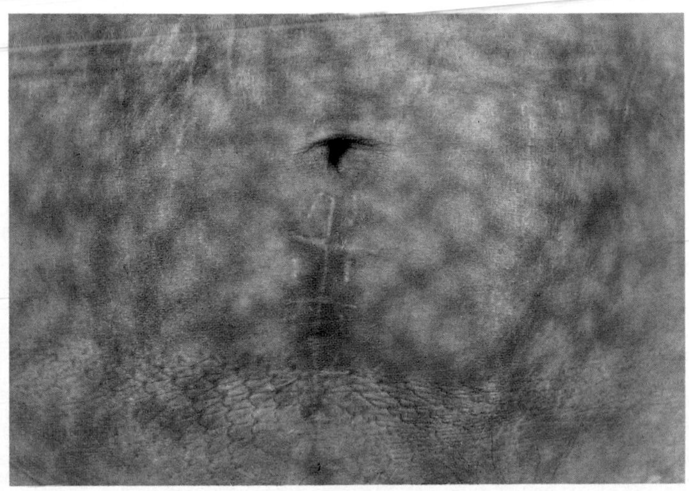

Reticular hyperpigmentation (erythema ab igne) resulting from repeated applications of a heating pad over several years.

FIGURE 90-50

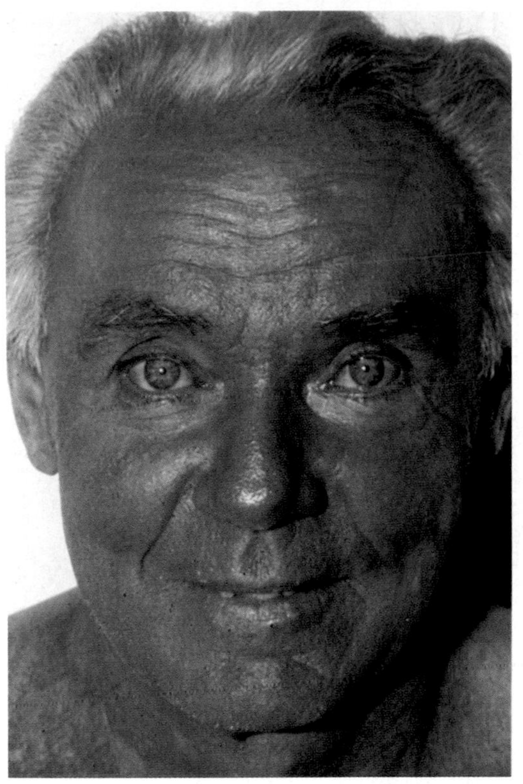

Metastatic melanoma-associated, slate-gray, dermal pigmentation involving the entire body. There was melanogenuria and at autopsy all internal organs were found to be black.

Nonmelanin Dermal Hyperpigmentation

Drugs, heavy metals, and other exogenous agents may deposit in the dermis to give rise to a blue-gray pigmentation that clinically mimics dermal melanosis. Drugs that may lead to dermal pigmentation include minocycline, hydroquinone, and antimalarials. Heavy metals include mercury, silver, bismuth, arsenic, gold, and lead. Ochronosis, or alkaptonuria, is one disease entity that gives rise to nonmelanin ceruloderma.

CERULODERMA DUE TO OCHRONOSIS (See Chap. 147) Clinically alkaptonuria, or ochronosis, presents as faint, uniform blue or blue-gray color of the pinnae, tip of the nose, sclera, costochondral junctions, axillae, and overlying extensor tendons of the hands. A butterfly pattern on the face, involvement of the axillae and genitalia, and uncommonly, diffuse involvement may occur. The facial pigmentation actually may result from myriads of circumscribed blue macules. Fingernails may be affected, nevi may darken, the sclerae may have pigment granules, and the tympanic membranes may be involved.

PIGMENTATION DUE TO HEAVY METALS *Argyria* results from deposition of silver in the skin to give rise to blue to slate-gray

FIGURE 90-51

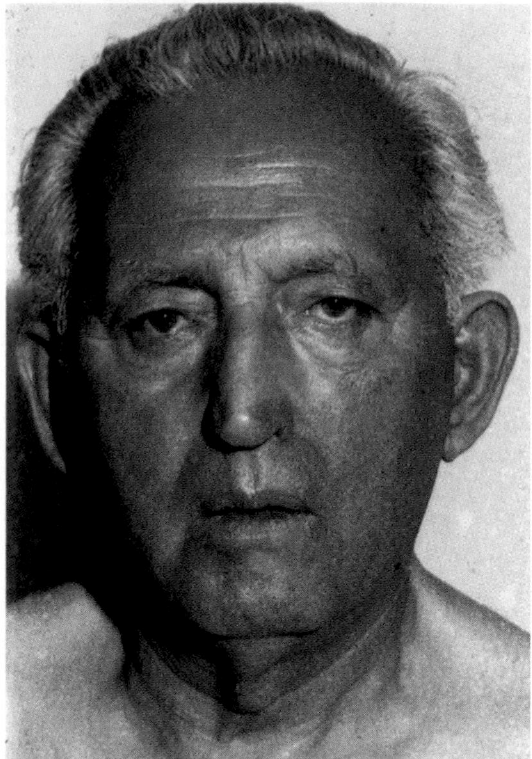

A.

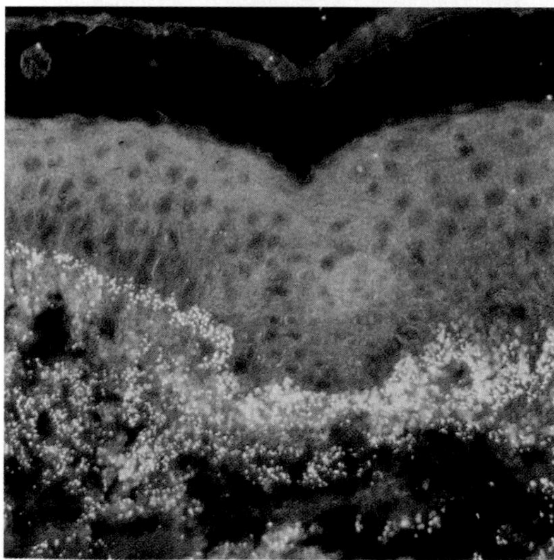

B.

Argyria. *A.* Blue to slate-gray coloration, particularly in sun-exposed areas. Note that this is a mix of gray and tan. This patient had taken medication containing silver salts for chronic gastritis. *B.* Dark-field microscopy reveals refractile silver granules scattered throughout the dermis.

coloration, particularly in sun-exposed areas (Fig. 90-51*A*). The degree of pigmentation is proportional more to the silver exposure than to sun exposure. Histologically, there are small, uniform, refractile granules scattered throughout the dermis, particularly about the sweat glands and in the papillary dermis; melanin also may be increased in the epidermis and in dermal chromatophores (see Fig. 90-51*B*).

Arsenic gives a bronze color, prominent on the trunk; melanin is also implicated. Bismuth and lead may both give generalized pigmentation and a gingival pigment line. Bismuth also may pigment the conjunctivae and oral mucosa; small granules are found in the papillary and reticular dermis. *Chrysoderma* is a rare consequence of parenteral gold administration and is prominent around the eyes and in sun-exposed areas. Biopsy shows round to oval, black, irregularly sized granules in dermal histiocytes and around vessels. Isolated macules occasionally may be present over sites of intramuscular gold injection.

Mercury exposure causes pigmentation of skin from topical administration and gingival hyperpigmentation from systemic administration. The pigment is present in the upper dermis around capillaries and associated with elastic fibers or collagen fibers; melanin also may be increased in the basal layer and be found in dermal macrophages.

Tattoos result from the deliberate introduction of exogenous pigments into skin in a decorative fashion. Traumatic entry of foreign substances (e.g., graphite from a lead pencil) may result in permanent tattooing. Biopsy shows pigment-laden macrophages. Common sources of adventitial tattooing include abrasions induced by falls from bicycles and motorcycles (blacktop and asphalt) and chemicals such as gunpowder.

NONMELANIN PIGMENTATION DUE TO DRUGS Chloroquine, if taken for protracted periods of time, may be associated with ceruloderma, particularly on the shins. Clofazimine may cause both increased basilar melanin and brown pigment in dermal macrophages. Clinically, however, clofazimine-induced discoloration appears orange-red. Hydroxyurea may cause ceruloderma of the back and pressure points. Minocycline is a tetracycline derivative frequently used for acne vulgaris. Dermal pigmentation (Fig. 90-52) may follow ingestion of from 100 to 200 mg/day for 1 to 3 years, although cases have been described from lower doses and shorter courses. The blue-gray, dirty coloration develops in acne scars, on the anterior lower legs and feet, on the gingiva and hard palate, and around the eyes. Circumscribed lesions are the most common, but generalized and diffuse ceruloderma may occur, as can pigmentation of the conjunctivae and the teeth. The brown pigment in the dermal macrophages is composed of iron and sulfur. Gradual resolution over months to years follows discontinuation of the drug.

Exogenous ochronosis secondary to phenol applied to a leg ulcer was first reported in 1912. Hydroquinone-induced ochronosis by topical application was reported in up to 35 percent of African blacks using a 6% to 8% preparation. The complication has been seen in American blacks allegedly using only 2% hydroquinone. Histopathologic studies reveal yellow-brown banana-shaped fibers in the papillary dermis. Colloid degeneration and elastosis are also seen. Also, the condition requires the presence of melanocytes because it does not occur in vitiligo skin. The course is chronic, and the treatment is disappointing.

Mixed Hypermelanoses and Leukomelanodermas

A number of different disorders are characterized clinically by features of both epidermal and dermal hyperpigmentation (mixed hypermelanoses) or by features of both hypo- and hyperpigmentation (leukomelanodermas).

MIXED HYPERMELANOSES In the following entities there may be a mixture of dermal (blue) and epidermal (brown) hyperpigmentation. In general, the changes are randomly mixed. These disorders have been discussed above.

- Dermatopathia pigmentosa reticularis
- Hemochromatosis
- Melasma. There is a dermal component, particularly in Latinos, Africans, and African-Americans.

FIGURE 90-52

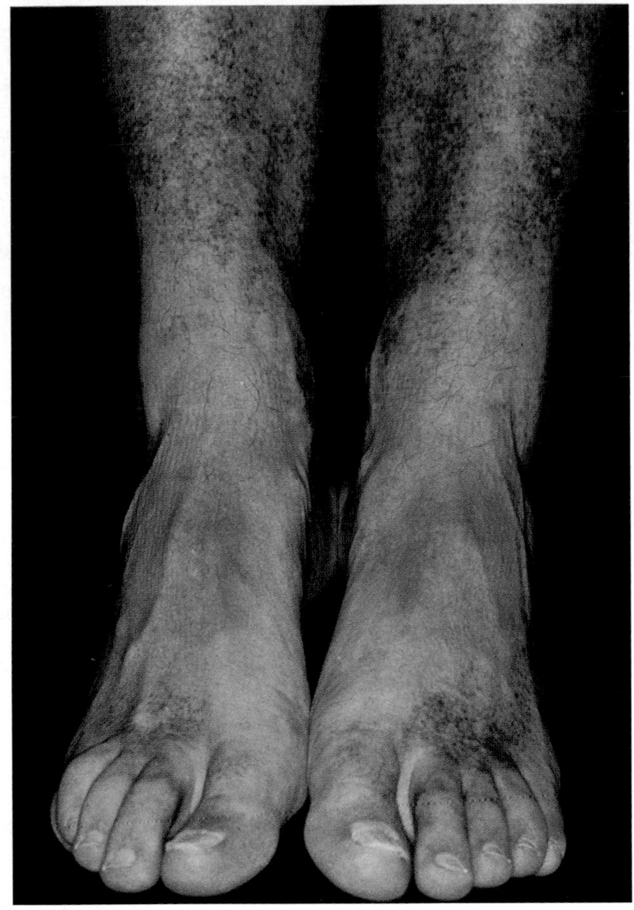

Minocycline pigmentation. Blue-gray coloration follows long-term moderate to high-dose ingestion and may first be observed in old scars, on the lateral face, anterior lower legs, or the gingiva.

- Nevus of Ota. The dermal component is usually clinically dominant.
- Postinflammatory hypermelanosis. The relative risk of a dermal component increases with increasing skin phototype.
- Tar melanosis. The dermal component is dominant.

HYPERMELANOSES WITH HYPOMELANOSIS The following are disorders associated primarily with hyperpigmentation but sometimes may have hypopigmentation as a feature. They have been discussed above.

- Acropigmentation of Dohi. Acral hypo- and hyperpigmented macules are found.
- Dyschromatosis. Hyper- and hypopigmented macules are intermixed.
- Linear inherited hypermelanosis. Mixed swirls of hyper- and hypopigmentation are found.
- Tay's syndrome. Vitiligo, café-au-lait macules, and lentigines are found.
- Tinea versicolor. Usually there are more hypopigmented than hyperpigmented macules, which are otherwise morphologically similar.
- Westerhof's syndrome. This is an autosomal dominant syndrome with congenital hyper- and hypopigmented macules.

HYPOMELANOSES (LEUKODERMAS) WITH HYPERPIGMENTATION The following entities are disorders associated primarily with hypopigmentation but sometimes may have also a hyperpigmentation feature. They have been discussed above or are dealt with in other chapters.

- Chemical leukoderma. Confetti macules are often found within a hyperpigmented background.
- Piebaldism. Thumbprint hyperpigmented macules appear in amelanotic macules and at times on normal skin.
- Pinta. Epidermal and dermal melanosis is characteristic of the late stage.
- Postinflammatory leukoderma. Particularly lupus erythematosus and lichen planus may be characterized by leukomelanoderma with the hyperpigmentation at the margins. In lichen planus, the hyperpigmentation may be dermal.
- Repigmenting vitiligo. Brown hyperpigmented macules may be found at the margins and around hair follicles.
- Scleroderma. Macules may resemble repigmenting vitiligo or postinflammatory leukoderma.
- Secondary syphilis. Leukomelanoderma may be postinflammatory.
- Tinea versicolor. Macules may be red, white, or brown, always in characteristic shapes and locations.
- Vagabond's leukoderma. Hyperpigmented macules are found particularly in the groin, buttocks, axillae, on the back of the neck, and over the back.
- Xeroderma pigmentosum. Hyperpigmented and hypopigmented macules are generally apparent in sun-exposed areas.
- Yaws. Dark halos may occur around achromic macules.
- Ziprkowski-Margolis syndrome. Hyperpigmented macules appear after birth within white macules.

XANTHODERMAS (YELLOW SKIN COLOR)

Xanthoderma, or yellow skin color, can arise from exogenous (quinacrine, beta-carotene, picric acid) or endogenous (secondary carotenemia, bilirubin) pigments. *Bronze baby syndrome* is a rare complication of phototherapy of icteric infants. During the treatment, the skin shows a grayish brown discoloration; direct hyperbilirubinemia develops, and urine and serum turn dirty gray. This syndrome is probably induced by the photooxidation products of bilirubin.

Carotenemia develops following ingestion of large amounts of fruits and vegetables that contain carotene (oranges, mangoes, apricots, carrots, and all green vegetables) and in patients taking synthetic beta-carotene. The yellow skin color is most prominent on the palms and soles and behind the ears. Carotenemia occurs in about 10 percent of patients with diabetes mellitus and in hypothyroidism. An idiopathic or benign essential carotenemia also has been described.

Jaundice arises from increased levels of bilirubin that deposits in the dermis and in the sclerae because of the affinity of bilirubin for elastic tissue. In patients with high levels of conjugated bilirubin, the skin color may assume a greenish hue because of the oxidation of bilirubin to green biliverdin. The sclerae are also yellow (see Chap. 164).

Quinacrine pigmentation produces a greenish yellow color that does not involve the sclerae. Because quinacrine does not produce retinopathy, as do chloroquine and hydroxychloroquine, it is used in the treatment of extensive discoid lupus erythematosus and polymorphous light eruption. Administration of beta-carotene simultaneously appears to produce a more cosmetically acceptable yellowing than quinacrine alone.

Xanthoma planum is a circumscribed, macular, yellow pigmentation found especially on the upper arms; widespread normolipemic generalized planar xanthoma may be associated with multiple myeloma (see Chap. 150).

REFERENCES

1. Ortonne JP et al: *Vitiligo and Other Hypomelanosis of Hair and Skin.* New York, Plenum, 1983
2. Nagasaki Y et al: Reversal of hypopigmentation in phenylketonuria mice by adenovirus-mediated gene transfer. *Pediatr Dermatol* **45**:465, 1999
3. Huizing M et al: Hermansky-Pudlak syndrome and related disorders of organelle formation. *Traffic* **1**:823, 2000
4. Bahadoran P et al: Hypomelanosis, immunity, central nervous system: No more "and," not the end. *Am J Med Genet* **116A**:334, 2003
5. Hann SK, Nordlund JJ: Definition of vitiligo, in *Vitiligo,* edited by SK Hann, JJ Nordlund. London, Blackwell Science, 2000, p 3
6. Nordlund JJ, Ortonne JP: Vitiligo and depigmentation, in *Current Problems in Dermatology,* St Louis, edited by WL Weston et al. Mosby–Year Book, 1992
7. Bradley CA et al: Genetic association of the catalase gene (CAT) with vitiligo susceptibility. *Pigment Cell Res* **15**:62, 2002
8. Boissy RE: Histology of vitiliginous skin, in *Vitiligo,* edited by SK Hann, JJ Nordlund. London, Blackwell Science, 2000, p 23
9. Ortonne JP, Bose SK: Vitiligo: Where do we stand? *Pigment Cell Res* **6**:61, 1993
10. Orecchia GE: Neural pathogenesis, in *Vitiligo,* edited by SK Hann, JJ Nordlund. London, Blackwell Science, 2000, p 142
11. Schallreuter KU et al: Biochemical theory of vitiligo: A role of pteridines in pigmentation, in *Vitiligo,* edited by SK Hann, JJ Nordlund. London, Blackwell Science, 2000, p 151
12. Bystryn JC: Theories on the pathogenesis of depigmentation: Immune hypothesis, in *Vitiligo,* edited by SK Hann, JJ Nordlund. London, Blackwell Science, 2000, p 129
13. Das PK et al: A symbiotic concept of autoimmunity and tumour immunity: Lessons from vitiligo. *Trends Immunol* 22:130, 2001
14. Boissy RE: The intripsic (genetic) theory for the cause of vitiligo, in *Vitiligo,* edited by SK Hann, JJ Nordlund. London, Blackwell Science, 2000, p 123
15. Lamoureux L, Boissy RE: Animal models, in *Vitiligo,* edited by SK Hann, JJ Nordlund. London, Blackwell Science 2000, p 281
16. Le Poole IC et al: Review of the etiopathomechanism of vitiligo: A convergence theory. *Exp Dermatol* **2**:145, 1993
17. Njoo MD, Westerhof W: Vitiligo: Pathogenesis and treatment. *Am J Clin Dermatol* **2**:167, 2001
18. Njoo MD et al: Management of vitiligo: Results of a questionnaire among dermatologists in the Netherlands. *Int J Dermatol* **38**:866, 1999
19. Westerhof W, Nieuweboer-Krobotova L: Treatment of vitiligo with UV-B radiation vs topical psoralen plus UV-A. *Arch Dermatol* **133**:1525, 1997
20. Falabella R: Surgical therapies for vitiligo, in *Vitiligo,* edited by SK Hann, JJ Nordlund. London, Blackwell Science, 2000, p 193
21. Halder RM: Micropigmentation, in *Vitiligo,* edited by SK Hann, JJ Nordlund. London, Blackwell Science, 2000, p 202
22. Mosher DB et al: Monobenzylether of hydroquinone: A retrospective study of treatment of 18 vitiligo patients and a review of the literature. *Br J Dermatol* **97**:669, 1977
23. Spritz RA: Piebaldism, Waardenburg syndrome, and related disorders of melanocyte development. *Semin Cutan Med Surg* **16**:15, 1997
24. Jimbow K: Tuberous sclerosis and guttate leukodermas. *J Cutan Med Surg* **16**:30, 1997
25. Ruiz Maldonado R et al: Hypomelanosis of Ito: Diagnostic criteria and report of 41 cases. *Pediatr Dermatol* **9**:1, 1992
26. Küster W et al: Hypomelanosis of Ito and mosaicism, in *The Pigmentary System: Physiology and Pathophysiology,* edited by JJ Nordlund, RE Boissy, VJ Hearing, RA King, J-P Ortonne. New York, Oxford University Press, 1998, p 594
27. Loomis CA: Linear hypopigmentation and hyperpigmentation including mosaicism. *J Cutan Med Surg* **16**:44, 1997
28. Happle R: Phylloid hypomelanosis and mosaic trisomy 13: A new etiologically defined neurocutaneous syndrome. *Hautarzt* **52**:3, 2001
29. Francis JS, Sybert VP: Incontinentia pigmenti. *J Cutan Med Surg* **16**:54, 1997
30. Lacour JP: Physical agents, in *The Pigmentary System: Physiology and Pathophysiology,* edited by JJ Nordlund, RE Boissy, VJ Hearing, RA King, J-P Ortonne. New York, Oxford University Press, 1998, p 627
31. Jimbow K, Jimbow M: Chemical and pharmacologic agents, in *The Pigmentary System: Physiology and Pathophysiology,* edited by JJ Nordlund, RE Boissy, VJ Hearing, RA King, J-P Ortonne. New York, Oxford University Press, 1998, p 621
32. Miyamoto L, Taylor JS: Chemical leukoderma, in *Vitiligo,* edited by SK Hann, JJ Nordlund. London, Blackwell Science, 2000, p 269
33. Paine C et al: An alternative approach to depigmentation by soybean extracts via inhibition of the PAR-2 pathway. *J Invest Dermatol* **116**:587, 2001
34. Ruiz Maldonado R, Orozco-Covarrubias M: Postinflammatory hypopigmentation and hyperpigmentation. *Semin Cutan Med Surg* **16**:36, 1997
35. Lacour JP: Infectious hypomelanoses, in *The Pigmentary System: Physiology and Pathophysiology,* edited by JJ Nordlund, RE Boissy, VJ Hearing, RA King, J-P Ortonne. New York, Oxford University Press, 1988, p 629
36. Le Gal FA et al: Direct evidence to support the role of antigen-specific CD8+ T cells in melanoma-associated vitiligo. *J Invest Dermatol* **117**:1464, 2001
37. Ortonne JP, Perrot H: Idiopathic guttate hypomelanosis. *Arch Dermatol* **116**:664, 1980
38. Mitchell IC et al: Ulcerative and hypopigmented sarcoidosis. *J Am Acad Dermatol* **15**:1062, 1986
39. Ortonne JP, Perrot H: Scleroderma: Ultrastructural study of the melanin pigmentary disturbances of the skin. *Clin Exp Dermatol* **5**:13, 1980
40. Castanet J, Ortonne JP: Hair pigmentation, in *Hair and Its Disorders: Biology, Pathology and Management,* edited by FM Camacho, VA Randall, VH Price. Amsterdam, Martin Dunitz, 2000, p 49
41. Trattner A, Metzker A: Partial unilateral lentiginosis. *J Am Acad Dermatol* **29**:963, 1993
42. Cullen MK: Leopard syndrome, in *The Pigmentary System: Physiology and Pathophysiology,* edited by JJ Nordlund, RE Boissy, VJ Hearing, RA King, JP Ortonne. New York, Oxford University Press, 1998, p 770
43. Cullen MK: Carney complex, in *The Pigmentary System: Physiology and Pathophysiology,* edited by JJ Nordlund, RE Boissy, VJ Hearing, RA King, JP Ortonne. New York, Oxford University Press, 1998, p 781
44. Stratakis CA et al: Clinical and molecular features of Carney complex: Diagnostic criteria and recommendations for patient evaluation. *J Clin Endocrinol Metab* **86**:4041, 2001
45. Esterly NB et al. Peutz-Jeghers syndrome, in *The Pigmentary System: Physiology and Pathophysiology,* edited by JJ Nordlund, RE Boissy, VJ Hearing, RA King, JP Ortonne. New York, Oxford University Press, 1998a, p 790
46. Karuman P et al: The Peutz-Jegher gene product is a mediator of p53-dependent cell death. *Mol Cell* **7**:1307, 2001
47. Marsh DJ et al: *PTEN* mutation spectrum and genotype-phenotype correlations in Bannayan-Riley-Ruvalcaba syndrome suggest a single entity with Cowden syndrome. *Hum Mol Genet* **8**:1461, 1999
48. Esterly NB et al: Neurofibromatosis, in *The Pigmentary System: Physiology and Pathophysiology,* edited by JJ Nordlund, RE Boissy, VJ Hearing, RA King, JP Ortonne. New York, Oxford University Press, 1998, p 741
49. Ruggieri M, Huson SM: The clinical and diagnostic implications of mosaicism in the neurofibromatoses. *Neurology* **56**:1433, 2001
50. Esterly NF et al: Polyostotic fibrous dysplasia (McCune-Albright syndrome), in *The Pigmentary System: Physiology and Pathophysiology,* edited by JJ Nordlund, RE Boissy, VJ Hearing, RA King, JP Ortonne. New York, Oxford University Press, 1998, p 748
51. Price SM et al: The spectrum of Silver-Russell syndrome: A clinical and molecular genetic study and new diagnostic criteria. *J Med Genet* **36**:837, 1999
52. Hitchins MP et al: Silver-Russell syndrome: A dissection of the genetic aetiology and candidate chromosomal regions. *J Med Genet* **38**:810, 2001
53. Esterly NF et al: Watson's syndrome, in *The Pigmentary System: Physiology and Pathophysiology,* edited by JJ Nordlund, RE Boissy, VJ Hearing, RA King, JP Ortonne. New York, Oxford University Press, 1998, p 753
54. Happle R, Koopman RJ: Becker nevus syndrome. *Am J Med Genet* **68**:357, 1997
55. Bolognia JL: Speckled lentiginous nevus, in *The Pigmentary System: Physiology and Pathophysiology,* edited by JJ Nordlund, RE Boissy, VJ Hearing, RA King, JP Ortonne. New York, Oxford University Press, 1998, p 958
56. Loomis CA: Linear hypopigmentation including mosaicism. *Semin Cutan Med Surg* **16**:44, 1997
57. Verghese S et al: Mosaic trisomy 7 in a patient with pigmentary anomalies. *Am J Med Genet* **87**:371, 1999
58. Komine M et al: Linear and whorled nevoid hypermelanosis: A case with systemic involvement and trisomy 18 mosaicism. *Br J Dermatol* **146**:500, 2000
59. Bastiaens M et al: The melanocortin-1-receptor gene is the major freckle gene. *Hum Mol Genet* **10**:1701, 1975
60. Bahadoran P: Hyperpigmentation associated with human immunodeficiency virus infection, in *The Pigmentary System: Physiology and Pathophysiology,* edited by JJ Nordlund, RE Boissy, VJ Hearing, RA King, JP Ortonne. New York, Oxford University Press, 1998, p 859
61. Kang WH et al: Melasma: Histopathological characteristics in 56 Korean patients. *Br J Dermatol* **146**:228, 2002

62. Im S et al: Increased expression of a melanocyte-stimulating hormone in the lesional skin of melasma. *Br J Dermatol* **146**:165, 2002
63. Perez Bernal A et al: Management of facial hyperpigmentation. *Am J Clin Dermatol* **1**:261, 2000
64. Rogioletti F, Rebora A: Acquired brachial cutaneous dyschromatosis: A common pigmentary disorder of the arm in middle-aged women. *J Am Acad Dermatol* **42**:680, 2000
65. Nordlund JJ: Cronkhite-Canada syndrome, in *the Pigmentary System: Physiology and Pathophysiology,* edited by JJ Nordlund, RE Boissy, VJ Hearing, RA King, JP Ortonne. New York, Oxford University Press, 1998, p 865
66. Im S: Dyschromatosis universalis hereditaria, in *The Pigmentary System: Physiology and Pathophysiology,* edited by JJ Nordlund, RE Boissy, VJ Hearing, RA King, JP Ortonne. New York, Oxford University Press, 1998, p 724
67. Esterly NB et al: Periorbital hyperpigmentation, in *The Pigmentary System: Physiology* and Pathophysiology, edited by JJ Nordlund, RE Boissy, VJ Hearing, RA King, JP Ortonne. New York, Oxford University Press, 1998, p 804
68. Esterly NB et al: Familial progressive hyperpigmentation, in *The Pigmentary System: Physiology and Pathophysiology,* edited by JJ Nordlund, RE Boissy, VJ Hearing, RA King, JP Ortonne. New York, Oxford University Press, 1998, p 713
69. Mitchell JR et al: A telomerase component is defective in the human disease dyskeratosis congenital. *Nature* **402**:551, 1999
70. Vulliany T et al: The RNA component of telomerase is mutated in autosomal dominant dyskeratosis congenita. *Nature* **413**:432, 2001
71. Im S et al: Reticulated acropigmentation of Dohi, in *The Pigmentary System: Physiology and Pathophysiology,* edited by JJ Nordlund, RE Boissy, VJ Hearing, RA King, JP Ortonne. New York, Oxford University Press, 1998, p 733
72. Chevrant-Breton J et al: Cutaneous manifestations of idiopathic hemochromatosis. *Arch Dermatol* **113**:161, 1977
73. Fedderson RM et al: Plasma cell dyscrasia: A case of POEMS syndrome with a unique dermatologic presentation. *J Am Acad Dermatol* **21**:1061, 1989
74. Bashito HM et al: General dermal melanocytosis. *Arch Dermatol* 117:791, 1981
75. Rappersberger K et al: Morphological changes in peripheral blood cells and skin in amiodarone-treated patients. *Br J Dermatol* **114**:189, 1986
76. Hashimoto K et al: Imipramine hyperpigmentation: A slate-gray discoloration caused by long-term imipramine administration. *J Am Acad Dermatol* **25**:357, 1991
77. Nakayama H et al: Pigmented cosmetic dermatitis. *Int J Dermatol* **15**:673, 1976
78. Sharood P, Marks R: The wages of warmth: Changes in erythema ab igne. *Br J Dermatol* **97**:179, 1977
79. Kourad K, Wolff K: Pathogenesis of diffuse melanosis secondary to malignant melanoma. *Br J Dermatol* **91**:635, 1974

CHAPTER 91

James M. Grichnik
Arthur R. Rhodes
Arthur J. Sober

Benign Hyperplasias and Neoplasias of Melanocytes

Benign melanocytic proliferative lesions form a spectrum of disorders ranging from a simple increase in epidermal melanocyte number to extensive cutaneous infiltration of melanocytic cells exhibiting various states of differentiation. In this chapter these lesions will be separated into the *melanocytic hyperplasias,* a term used to indicate increased normal melanocytes in the basal layer of the epidermis, and *melanocytic neoplasias,* a term used to describe the presence of melanocytic cells in epidermal nests within the dermis or in other tissues.

The specific molecular events causing melanocytic hyperplasias and neoplasias remain poorly defined. Simple hyperplasias are likely to be the result of an alteration of normal melanocytic homeostatic mechanisms leading to the accumulation of increased numbers of differentiated melanocytes in the epidermis. These alterations could be due to a primary melanocytic defect (such as an ultraviolet-induced mutation) or to homeostatic signaling changes in the local environment. Melanocytic neoplasias may be the result of aberrant melanocytic differentiation due to the presence of melanocytic cells lacking normal melanocytic differentiation (referred to as *nevomelanocytes*). Normal melanocytic differentiation occurs in a stepwise manner from a subpopulation of neural crest–derived cells. It is possible that aberrant differentiation from this population of neural crest cells is responsible for the diverse variety of melanocytic neoplasias.

The extent of melanocytic hyperplasia can be quite variable, ranging from lesions in which the increased melanin content is notable but the increase in melanocyte number is marginal to lesions in which accumulation of melanocytes is marked. The point at which a melanocytic hyperplasia becomes a neoplasia is artificially defined as the point at which three or more melanocytic cells form a nest (or theque) in the epidermis or defined as clonally derived based on genetic composition. The presence of melanocytic cells in the dermis also is sufficient to define a melanocytic neoplasia. The extent of melanocytic proliferation, spectrum and type of differentiation, location of cells, and age of the lesion may all affect the clinical and histopathologic features.

Until discrete molecular markers are defined, definitive subclassification of these melanocytic lesions is not possible. This heterogeneous group of disorders is currently loosely subgrouped based on clinical features, time of appearance, and microscopic characteristics. The benign melanocytic hyperplasias described in this chapter include lentigo simplex, combination lesions with lentigo simplex (agminated lentigines and nevus spilus), and solar lentigines. The neoplasias described include common acquired nevomelanocytic nevi (including halo nevi and excluding dysplastic/atypical nevi), epithelioid/spindle cell nevomelanocytic nevi, blue nevi, and congenital nevomelanocytic nevi.

HYPERPLASIAS

A well-defined hyperpigmented lesion with an increased number of individual melanocytes confined to the epidermal compartment is a lentigo (plural, lentigines, derived from Latin *lens,* meaning "lentil"). Although separated into simplex and solar lentigines, a number of subtypes exist with varying degrees of melanocytic and/or keratinocytic abnormalities. While the primary defect may be melanocytic in some lentigines, it is possible that the melanocytic hyperplasia is merely a secondary response to abnormal keratinocytic function (or some other local abnormality) in others. Other lesions in which epidermal melanocytic hyperplasia may be noted and some overlap may exist with lentigines include café-au-lait macules, seborrheic keratoses, melasma, and inflammatory/cytokine-induced proliferation.

Lentigo Simplex

Lentigo simplex (Fig. 91-1) is an acquired or congenital hyperpigmented macule consisting of intraepidermal melanocytic hyperplasia and increased melanin formation. Lentigo simplex lesions may be isolated or multiple and present on skin, nails, and mucous membranes. Multiple lentigines may be associated with systemic disorders.

HISTORICAL ASPECTS There has been a continual debate regarding the nosologic differentiation between lentigo and nevomelanocytic nevus. Early treatises by Darier, Scholtz, and Kissmeyer included lentigo among the nonelevated nevi. Zeisler and Becker in 1936 and Lund and Kraus in 1962 defined lentigo as an entity separate and distinct from nevomelanocytic nevus.

EPIDEMIOLOGY The frequency of lentigo simplex in children and adults has not been determined. Lentigo simplex is the most common histopathologic pattern of darkly pigmented lesions excised from acral sites of darkly pigmented races.[1] Pigmented nail bands in up to 20 percent of Japanese may have histopathologic features of lentigo simplex.[2]

ETIOLOGY AND PATHOGENESIS The increased density of melanocytes in lentigines is presumably due to an underlying developmental or intrinsic defect in melanocyte homeostasis. In some lentigines, the presence of melanin macroglobules in melanocytes and keratinocytes suggests that defects affecting melanization pathways are also involved. The presence of lentigo simplex in association with somatic abnormalities in such diverse conditions as Peutz-Jeghers syndrome, LEPOARD syndrome, and LAMB/myxoma syndrome suggests that lentigo development may be influenced by a number of different genetic factors.

CLINICAL MANIFESTATIONS Lentigo simplex usually is a sharply circumscribed, light-brown or dark-brown macule (see Fig. 91-1). There appears to be no relation between sun exposure and appearance of lentigo simplex. Lentigo simplex may appear as early as the first decade and may occur anywhere on skin or mucous membranes.

Generalized lentigines may occur as an isolated phenomenon without known familial aggregation and present at birth, during infancy, or during adulthood. Familial clustering in an autosomal pattern also has been noted. A number of syndromes are recognized (reviewed in Chap. 90). In Moynahan's (LEOPARD) syndrome, lentigines are present at birth or shortly thereafter and may increase in number during childhood; they occur on both sun-exposed and sun-protected sites, including genitalia, conjunctiva, oral mucosa, palms, and soles. In Peutz-Jeghers syndrome, numerous lentigines may be present at birth or appear during early childhood. Oral mucosa is almost always involved. Other common sites of involvement in Peutz-Jeghers syndrome include lips, nose, eyelids, anus, nail bed, and dorsal and ventral surfaces of hands and feet. Oral pigmentation usually persists in Peutz-Jeghers syndrome, whereas cutaneous lentigines usually fade after puberty. The myxoma syndromes (also referred to as LAMB and NAME syndromes) are also associated with mucocutaneous lentigines (see also Chaps. 90 and 166). Lentigines in this syndrome occur mainly on the face and genitalia as tan to black macules (see Fig. 91-1). In centrofacial lentiginosis, the presence of pigmented macules is restricted to a horizontal band across the central face. The lesions appear in the first year of life, increase in number during the first decade, and then fade in later life.

PATHOLOGY Lentigo simplex consists of intraepidermal melanocytic hyperplasia in the basal layer of elongated epidermal rete ridges without nest formation (Fig. 91-2). At one end of the lentigo spectrum are lesions more similar to café-au-lait lesions, in which the melanocyte number may not be significantly increased but pigmentary differences are marked, and at the other end of the spectrum the increased number of melanocytes is sufficient to begin forming nests bordering on a junctional nevus.

FIGURE 91-1

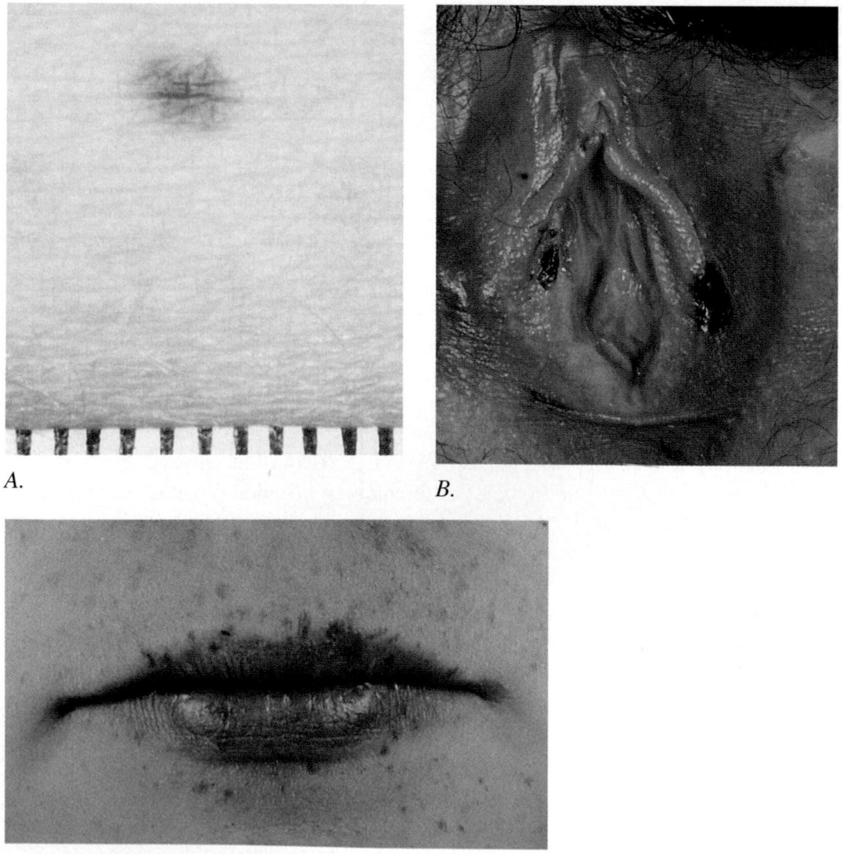

A.

B.

C.

Lentigo simplex. *A.* Isolated acquired lentigo simplex on the abdomen of a 42-year-old white man who has dysplastic nevi and a family history of melanoma. *B.* Acquired darkly pigmented lentigines on the vulva of a 13-year-old white girl who has LAMB (myxoma syndrome). *C.* Multiple lentigines on the lips of the same patient.

FIGURE 91-2

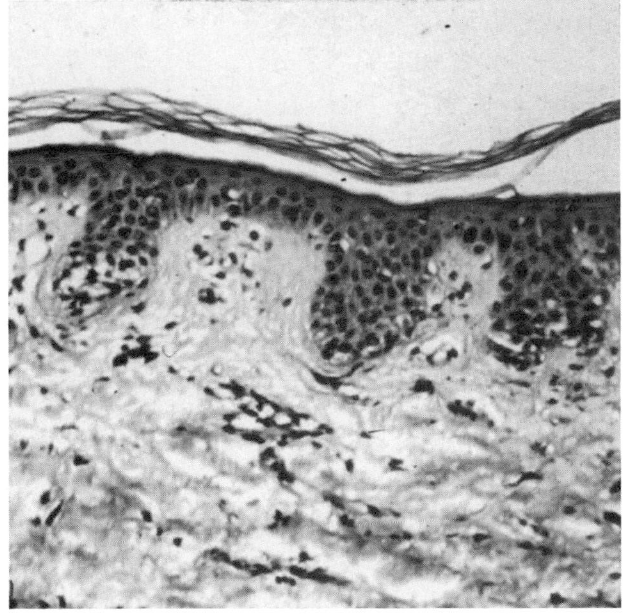

A.

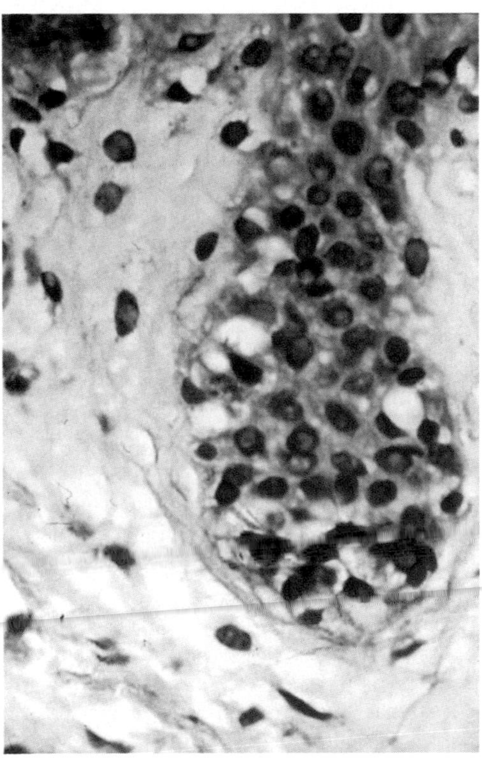

B.

Histopathologic features of lentigo. Lentigo simplex (*A*) and higher magnification (*B*). There is hyperpigmentation and increased numbers of melanocytes without nest formation. The solar lentigo also demonstrates keratinocytic hyperplasia and bulbous rete pegs.

Further, depending on the degree of keratinocytic hyperplasia, distinct separation from solar lentigo may not be possible in some lesions based on histopathologic interpretation. Giant pigment granules (melanin macroglobules) may occur in lentigo simplex in isolation and in association with multiple-lentigines (LEOPARD) syndrome.

DIAGNOSIS AND DIFFERENTIAL DIAGNOSIS Lentigo simplex should be differentiated from solar lentigines, junctional nevomelanocytic nevi, dysplastic melanocytic nevi, café-au-lait macules, and melanoma (Table 91-1).

TREATMENT There is no need to treat benign-appearing lentigo simplex. However, lesions that are significantly unusual, irregular, asymmetric, or changing in shape should be examined histopathologically for melanocytic dysplasia or melanoma. Wood's lamp examination is useful in defining margins of lentigo simplex.

COURSE AND PROGNOSIS The natural history of isolated lentigo simplex is not known. Once developed, the lesions are presumed to be relatively stable. There is no convincing evidence that lentigo simplex evolves to a nevomelanocytic nevus. As with any process in which melanocytes are present (including normal skin), it is possible for melanoma to evolve in a lentigo, but an elevated risk has not been demonstrated conclusively.

Combined Lesions of Lentigo Simplex

Multiple lentigines may appear in localized patches of skin, suggesting an underlying developmental abnormality. Two patterns will be reviewed that may represent different ends of a similar spectrum: numerous lentigines appearing together as an isolated group on otherwise normal-appearing skin (agminated lentigines) and a patch with features consistent with lentigo or café-au-lait macule with internal nevomelanocytic and/or melanocytic hyperplastic foci (nevus spilus).

Agminated Lentigines

Agminated lentigines may be defined as a circumscribed grouping of small pigmented macules arranged in a small or large group, often in a segmental pattern, each macule consisting of a lentiginous epidermal proliferation of melanocytes. Other names for this entity include *unilateral lentigines, partial unilateral lentiginosis, lentiginous mosaicism, segmental lentiginosis,* and *zosteriform lentiginous nevus.* Cases reported under the name of *zosteriform lentiginous nevus* also include examples of nevus spilus.

HISTORICAL ASPECTS A segmental distribution of lentigines was reported by McKelway in 1904. Since then, at least 11 cases of this pigmentary anomaly have been reported under the various names listed earlier.

EPIDEMIOLOGY The population prevalence of this disorder is unknown, but it is believed to be rare. There does not appear to be a racial or gender predilection.

ETIOLOGY AND PATHOGENESIS Chromosomal mosaicism confined to neural crest melanoblasts may have some role in this disorder.

CLINICAL MANIFESTATIONS Agminated lentigines first become manifest at birth or early childhood as small, circumscribed, light-brown macules, 2 to 10 mm in diameter, confined to a localized area of the body, often in a segmental distribution (Fig. 91-3) and frequently in a curvilinear or swirled pattern. While there are usually no associated disorders, agminated lentigines may occur with somatic abnormalities, including cerebrovascular hypertrophy, neuropsychiatric disturbance, rigid cavus foot, epidermal nevus, and ocular involvement.

This clinical and microscopic definition of nevus spilus has been illustrated in multiple case reports under the same or different names.

TABLE 91-1

Differential Diagnosis of Brown Macule/Patch

BROWN MACULES	BROWN PATCHES
Lentigo simplex	Lentigo simplex
Café-au-lait macule	Café-au-lait macule
Solar lentigo	Solar lentigo
PUVA lentigo	Becker's melanosis
Solar lentigines in xeroderma pigmentosum	Atypical lentigo simplex
Sunbed lentigines	Lentigo maligna
Genital lentiginosis	Nevus spilus*
LEOPARD syndrome	Benign pigmented keratosis*
Cardiac myxoma syndrome (LAMB, NAME)	Large cell acanthoma*
Peutz-Jeghers syndrome	Melanoma on acral and mucosal sites*
Agminated lentigines	Nevomelanocytic nevus, junctional type*
Centrofacial lentiginosis	Dysplastic melanocytic nevus*
Generalized lentigines	
Scar lentigo	
Atypical lentigo simplex	
Lentigo maligna	
Nevus spilus*	
Pigmented actinic keratosis*	
Melanoma on acral and mucosal sites*	
Nevomelanocytic nevus, junctional type*	
Dysplastic melanocytic nevus*	

*May have elevated component (papule/plaque).

PATHOLOGY Histopathologic studies reveal increased numbers of melanocytes in elongated epidermal rete ridges, similar to lentigo simplex, without nests of nevomelanocytes or cellular inflammation.

DIAGNOSIS AND DIFFERENTIAL DIAGNOSIS Agminated lentigines may be confused with nevus spilus and other varieties of pigmented macules (see Table 91-1). Wood's lamp examination may be required to differentiate agminated lentigines from nevus spilus because it can help differentiate the background pigmentation in the latter and its absence in the former.

TREATMENT Until the long-term course of agminated lentigines is known, it may be prudent to recommend periodic examinations to detect the earliest signs of possible atypical evolution.

COURSE AND PROGNOSIS The long-term course and malignant potential of agminated lentigines are unknown.

Nevus Spilus

Nevus spilus (derived from Greek *spilos,* meaning "spot") is defined as a circumscribed macule/patch of tan pigmentation including scattered, more darkly pigmented melanocytic or nevomelanocytic macular and/or papular elements. Cases fitting the gross and microscopic description of nevus spilus have been called *speckled lentiginous nevus* and *zosteriform lentiginous nevus.*

HISTORICAL ASPECTS In older terminology, *nevus spilus* referred to a solitary, hairless, melanotic macule that was not associated with von Recklinghausen's neurofibromatosis or McCune-Albright syndrome. This term is still being used by some authors to describe uncharacterized macular hyperpigmentation. Nevus spilus was redefined by Ito and Hamada in 1952[3] and reemphasized by Cohen et al. in 1970[4] to be a circumscribed tan macule in which more darkly pigmented, raised and/or flat, melanocytic or nevomelanocytic elements are distributed.

EPIDEMIOLOGY Nevus spilus occurs in less than 0.2 percent of newborns, 1 to 2 percent of white school children, and 2 percent of white adults. There are no prevalence data in darkly pigmented persons. There does not appear to be a gender predilection.[5]

ETIOLOGY AND PATHOGENESIS Nevus spilus may be postulated to represent a localized defect in neural crest melanoblasts. Genetic and environmental factors also may play a role. Hypothetically, the development of a nevus spilus may be a multistep process involving a primary genetic defect creating the hyperpigmented macule/patch coupled with a secondary intrinsically (growth factor) or extrinsically (UV light) mediated event leading to the development of focal individual melanocytic neoplasms.

CLINICAL MANIFESTATIONS Rarely, nevus spilus may be present at birth. More commonly, the lesion becomes evident during infancy or early childhood. More darkly pigmented, flat or raised speckles are usually present when the lesion is first recognized, but new speckles may appear over time. The tan macular background pigmentation ranges from less than 1 cm to greater than 10 cm in diameter (Fig. 91-4). Although nevus spilus may occur anywhere, lesions have been noted primarily on the torso and extremities. A divided nevus spilus of the eyelid has been reported.[6] Lesions may be localized or have a segmental distribution. Giant varieties of nevus spilus may occur. Nevus spilus has been associated with other anomalies of vascular, central nervous system, or connective tissue origin. Multiple granular tumors and nevus flammeus have been associated with a giant nevus spilus.

PATHOLOGY The tan background pigmentation usually consists of increased numbers of melanocytes in a lentiginous epidermal pattern. Routine and electron microscopic studies of nevus spilus may demonstrate melanin macroglobules in some cases. The flat, dark speckles of nevus spilus usually demonstrate lentiginous melanocytic hyperplasia, whereas the raised elements usually contain collections of nevomelanocytes in the epidermis and/or dermis. The speckled elements of nevus spilus also may consist of epithelioid and/or spindle cell nevi, nevi with dysplastic features, or blue nevi.

DIAGNOSIS AND DIFFERENTIAL DIAGNOSIS Nevus spilus can be differentiated from simple café-au-lait macules, relatively flat and hairless varieties of large congenital nevi, Becker's melanosis, and other varieties of lentigines (see Table 91-1) largely based on clinical features. The internal hyperpigmented or occasionally hypopigmented foci of nevus spilus may require biopsy to determine the nature of the associated melanocytic proliferation, which could be lentigo, junctional or compound nevus, epithelioid/spindle cell nevus, blue nevus, dysplastic nevus, or melanoma.

TREATMENT No standard guidelines for management of patients with nevus spilus exist. Clinical appearance (typical or atypical), history of stability or instability of pigmented elements, congenital or noncongenital onset, perceived risk of developing melanoma, and cosmetic concerns are considerations when determining whether to excise or recommend periodic clinical evaluation. Atypical-appearing new and/or unstable elements in nevus spilus should be evaluated by histopathologic examination to exclude melanoma. A nevus spilus with dysplastic or congenital features may have a greater risk of developing melanoma.[7,8]

COURSE AND PROGNOSIS There are insufficient data to be certain of the natural history of nevus spilus or to comment specifically about its malignant potential; however, caution must be exercised for affected individuals. There are at least 12 well-documented cases of melanoma developing in contiguity with nevus spilus, some cases ending in metastatic disease and death. When viewed as a risk marker for melanoma, nevus spilus shows a trend for being more common in melanoma cases than in controls. Kopf et al.[5] detected nevus spilus in 5 (4.8 percent) of 105 white adults with melanoma compared with 14 (2.3 percent) of 601 dermatology outpatients, but overmatching bias in the control group could not be excluded.

FIGURE 91-3

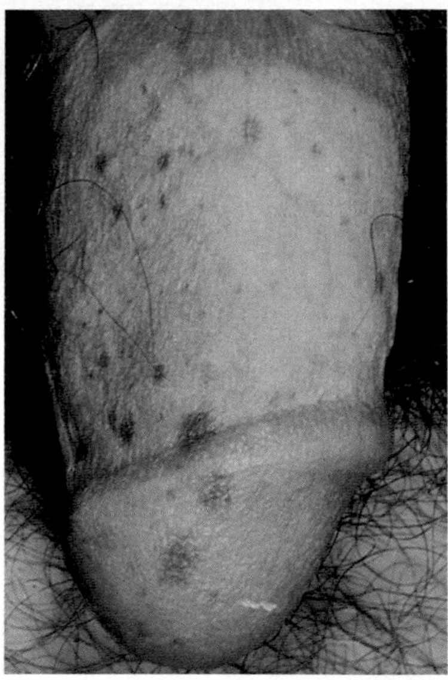

A.

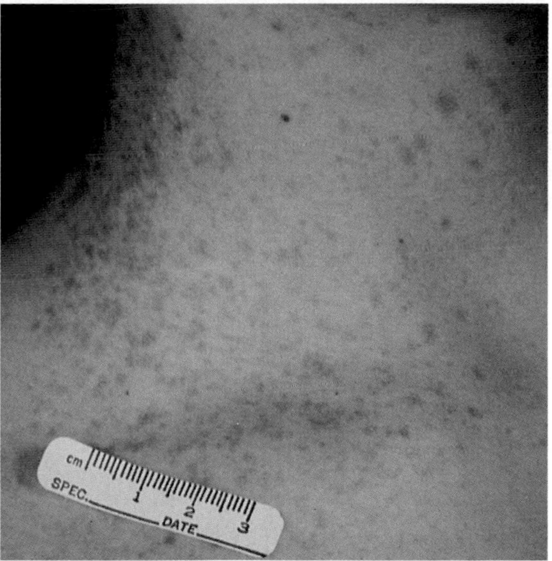

C.

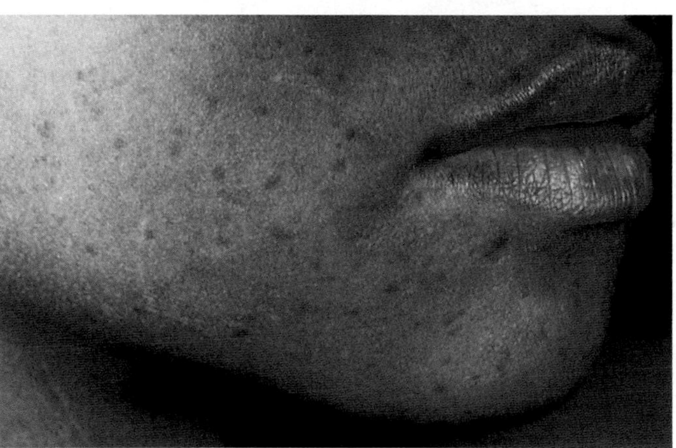

B.

Agminated lentigines. *A.* Grouping of small light brown macules, present since age 14 years, on the right side of the shaft and glans penis of a 17-year-old healthy white male. *B.* Grouping of small, light brown macules, present for at least 6 years, on the right cheek of a healthy 10-year-old African-American male. *C.* Grouping of small light brown macules, present since age 2 years, on the right neck and supraclavicular area of a 13-year-old healthy white female.

Solar Lentigo

Solar lentigo is a circumscribed pigmented macule occurring singly or as multiple lesions induced by natural or artificial sources of ultraviolet (UV) radiation (Figs. 91-5 and 91-6). Outdated synonyms for solar lentigo include *sun-induced freckle, lentigo senilis,* and *senile lentigo.* Solar lentigines are separated from simplex lentigines based on the clinical characteristics suggesting UV light as the precipitating factor and histopathologic characteristics suggesting a pronounced keratinocytic proliferative response. Specific defects involved are not yet known, but the primary defects could be either melanocytic or keratinocytic.

A distinction is made between a freckle (ephelis) and a solar lentigo. Freckle (derived from Middle English, *freken*) and ephelis (plural, ephelides; derived from the Greek) also refer to circumscribed, pigmented macules on sun-exposed skin. Freckles are common on the central face and often first noted in early childhood, presumably developing after significant sun-exposure. Ephelides are said to fade or even disappear when sun exposure is discontinued. Unfortunately, there are no longitudinal studies of ephelides or solar lentigines that document gross morphologic or time-course differences that would reliably allow a clinical distinction between ephelides and solar lentigines. According to dopa studies on epidermal sheets, ephelides were reported to show increased melanogenesis but decreased melanocyte number, which infers a different pathologic basis.[9,10] Studies in dopa-incubated tissue sections suggest that melanocytes are increased in ephelides in children and young adults, similar to solar lentigines.[11,12]

HISTORICAL ASPECTS In 1950, Cawley and Curtis[13] called attention to solar lentigo as a unique lesion that appears mostly in older individuals and consists of a localized proliferation of intraepidermal melanocytes in elongated epidermal rete ridges. In 1963, Hodgson[14] confirmed the proliferation of melanocytes in solar lentigo using routine and dopa histochemical studies. Montagna et al.[15] emphasized the concurrent proliferation of melanocytes and keratinocytes in solar lentigo in the elderly. Solar lentigines also may occur in healthy white children and young adults even in the first several decades of life.

EPIDEMIOLOGY The prevalence of solar lentigines is correlated directly with increasing age, and they are present in 90 percent of white people over 60 years of age.[14] Solar lentigines are common in individuals who sunburn easily and fail to tan, whereas they are uncommon among people who have darkly pigmented skin.[16]

FIGURE 91-4

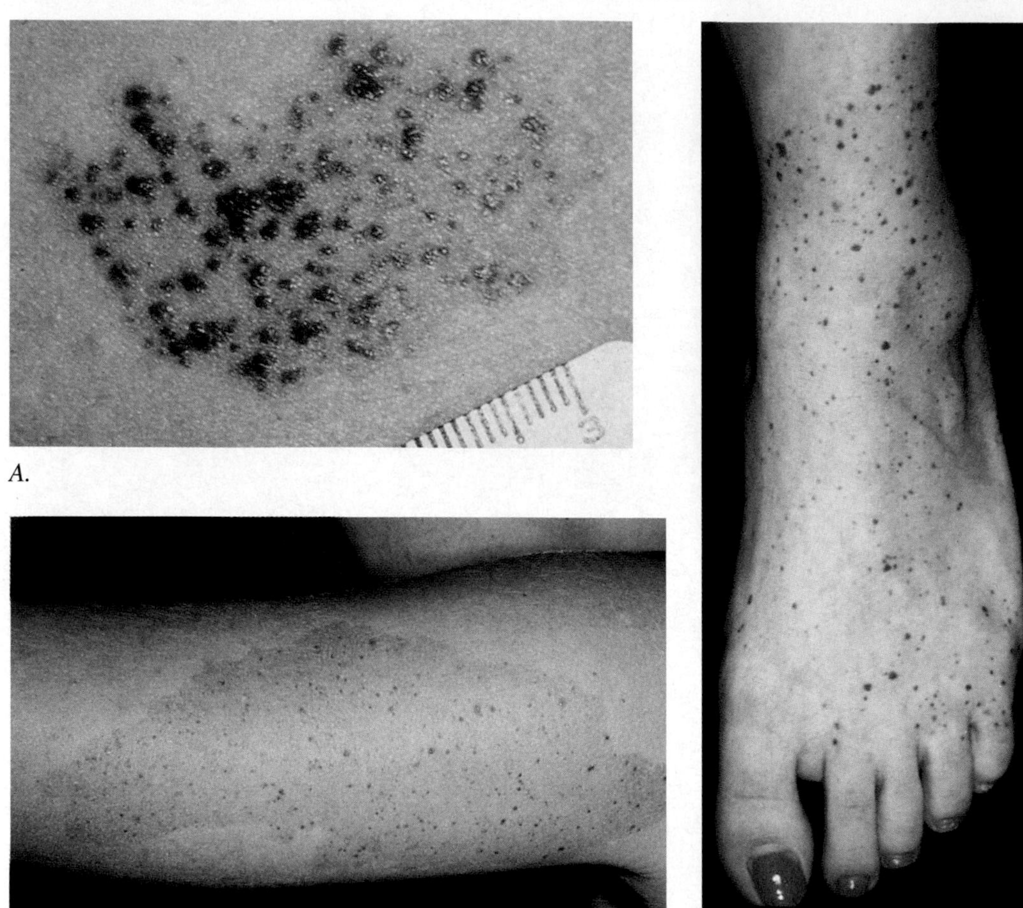

Nevus spilus. *A.* Acquired nevus spilus of indeterminate duration on the abdomen of a 29-year-old white woman. *B.* Nevus spilus appearing first at age 3 years on the ankle and foot of a 25-year-old white woman *C.* Congenital nevus spilus on the arm of a 10-year-old white male.

Lentigines may be induced by photochemotherapy (PUVA lentigo), occurring in 40 to 50 percent of patients an average of 5.7 years after starting therapy, their frequency and severity directly attributable to the total number of treatments[16] (Fig. 91-6) (see also Chap. 266). Darkly pigmented skin is associated with the lowest risk for PUVA-induced or solar-induced lentigines.[16] Lentigines have been associated with UVA tanning bed use.[17]

Lesions similar in gross and microscopic appearance to solar lentigo occur in children and young adults. They may appear within the first 5 years of life, tend to aggregate in families, and are significantly associated with red hair; their location and density correlate with sun sensitivity and sun exposure. The presence of freckles has been associated with a 2.5-fold increase in the rate of sunburn susceptibility and poor tanning response and a 3-fold greater likelihood of a lower minimal erythema dose in people who mostly burn and tan minimally or not at all.[18] The presence of dense sun-induced freckling increases the estimated risk for melanoma by three- to fourfold[19] (Table 91-2).

ETIOLOGY AND PATHOGENESIS Solar lentigines are thought to represent a marker of intermittent high-intensity UV radiation, cumulative UV radiation, and/or a unique susceptibility to the proliferative, stimulatory, and/or mutagenic effects of UV radiation. Sun-exposed skin consistently reveals a twofold greater melanocytic density compared with nonexposed skin. In addition, experimental repeated UV radiation exposure is known to increase epidermal melanocyte number.[20] However, the acute hyperplastic response normally decreases by 2 months after UV radiation is discontinued.[20] It is possible that a mutation in a UV radiation–induced lentigo results in proliferation and enhanced pigment production in response to UV radiation, but this lesion remains persistent, unlike normal skin. It is possible that there is a genetic susceptibility to the development of solar lentigo in response to acute or chronic UV radiation and that melanocytes in these circumscribed proliferations are permanently altered.

The minimal *freckling dose* to single exposures of experimental UVB radiation (320 mm) is 6 to 10 times the minimal erythema dose, and susceptibility to experimental induction of freckles appears to be restricted to people who already have the freckling tendency.[10] Phototoxic doses of photochemotherapy may lead to the development of lentigines 6 to 8 months later.[21] Lentigines that develop in patients receiving chronic photochemotherapy for psoriasis may persist 1 to 2 years or longer after therapy is discontinued,[16] and cellular atypia of epidermal melanocytes in these lentigines also may persist. In addition to the total dose of UV radiation received during photochemotherapy, individual susceptibility factors to lentigo development include race, age, and burning/tanning response to sunlight.[16]

Disorders with increased sensitivity to UV light such as xeroderma pigmentosum (XP), in which the melanoma incidence rate in the first two decades of life is several orders of magnitude greater than

FIGURE 91-5

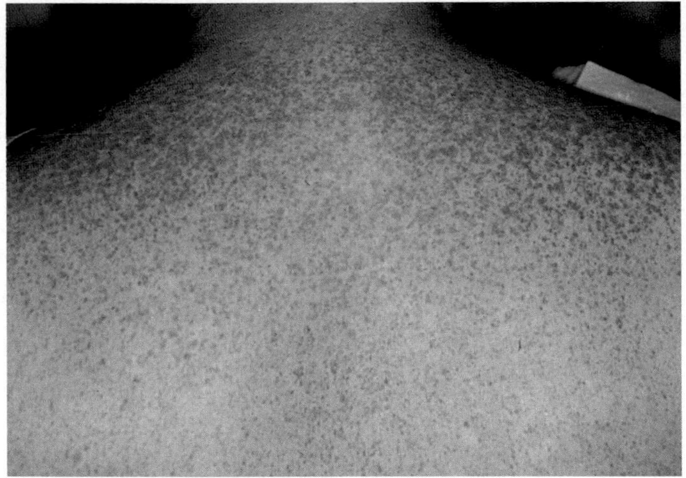

A.

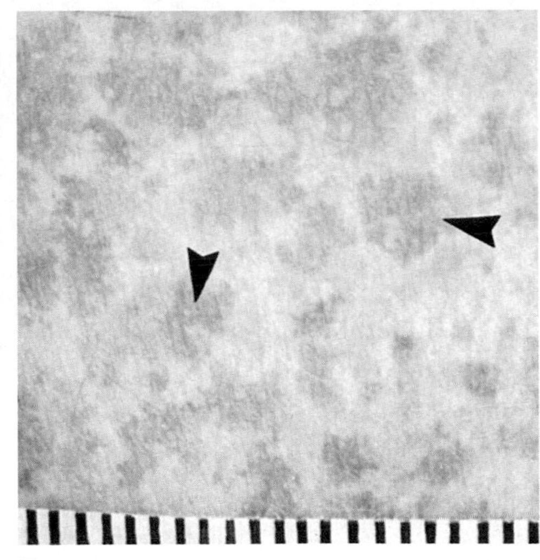

B.

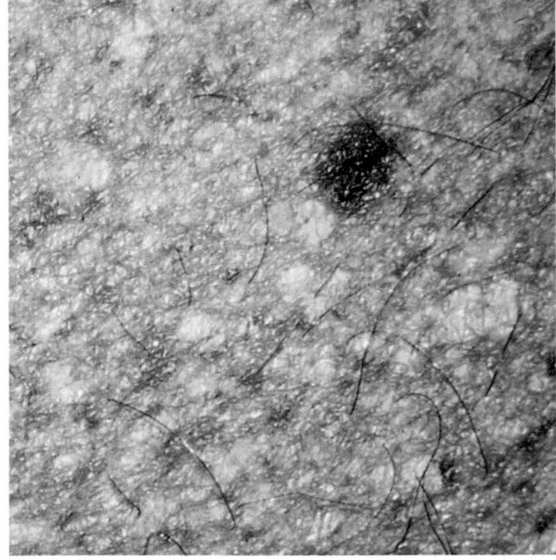

C.

Solar lentigo. *A.* Uncountable solar lentigines on the back of a 30-year-old white man, appearing initially during early childhood following multiple sunburns. *B.* High magnification of lentigines in (*A*) showing light-brown macules with markedly irregular outlines. *C.* Solar lentigines on sun-damaged dorsal hand skin (hypopigmentation, wrinkling, and telangiectasia) of an elderly white man.

expected, is associated with hyperpigmented macules on light-exposed skin within the first 5 years of life (see Chap. 155). These lesions demonstrate hyperplasia of variably atypical epidermal melanocytes (i.e., atypical lentigines) and persist despite sun avoidance. The lesions in XP are presumed to reflect hypermutability of melanocytes related to an impaired capacity to repair UV radiation–induced damage.[22] Lentigo maligna melanoma was the predominant melanoma type in one series of XP patients from Japan,[23] suggesting an association between this tumor subtype, sensitivity to UV radiation, and the presence of UV radiation–induced atypical solar lentigines.

CLINICAL MANIFESTATIONS Solar lentigo occurs as a circumscribed pigmented macule on skin exposed to natural sunlight or artificial sources of UV radiation, usually in the presence of similar lesions in the same location (see Fig. 91-5). Lesions may be tiny (<1 mm) or large (up to a few centimeters in diameter), with a tendency to confluence in severely sun-damaged skin and with smooth or markedly irregular outlines. Lesions are usually light brown, but varieties of solar lentigo are jet black, similar to an ink stain. When examined by dermoscopy (epiluminescence microscopy), the pigmented pattern in solar lentigo is reticulated.[12] Lentigines in patients receiving photochemotherapy and in individuals who have XP are often darkly and/or irregularly pigmented. Although solar lentigo usually occurs on sun-exposed skin, identical-appearing lesions may occur on sun-protected sites (including the penis and buttocks) that have been exposed to photochemotherapy (see Fig. 91-6).

The oral-labial melanotic macule has gross morphologic characteristics similar to solar lentigo (Fig. 91-7), but its relation to a sun-sensitive phenotype or excessive sun exposure has not been well documented.

PATHOLOGY Solar lentigo shows elongated epidermal rete ridges with club-shaped or budlike extensions, frequent branching and fusing of rete ridges, a thinned or atrophic epidermis between rete ridges, and increased numbers of epidermal melanocytes without nesting (see Fig. 91-2). The microscopic appearance suggests a concurrent proliferation of keratinocytes and melanocytes.[15] There is a scant to moderate perivascular mononuclear cell infiltrate in the dermis, usually associated with scattered melanin-laden macrophages.

Electron microscopic studies of solar lentigo reveal abundant melanosome complexes in keratinocytes, the complexes being generally larger than complexes in keratinocytes in adjacent skin.[15] Compared with melanocytes in sun-protected skin, melanocytes in solar lentigo reveal increased activity manifested by marked dopa reactivity (suggesting increased tyrosinase activity), elongated dendrites, large numbers of normal-appearing melanosomes, enlarged perikarya with well-developed rough endoplasmic reticula, numerous mitochondria, and hypertrophic Golgi complexes.[24] Melanin macroglobules also have been noted.[25]

FIGURE 91-6

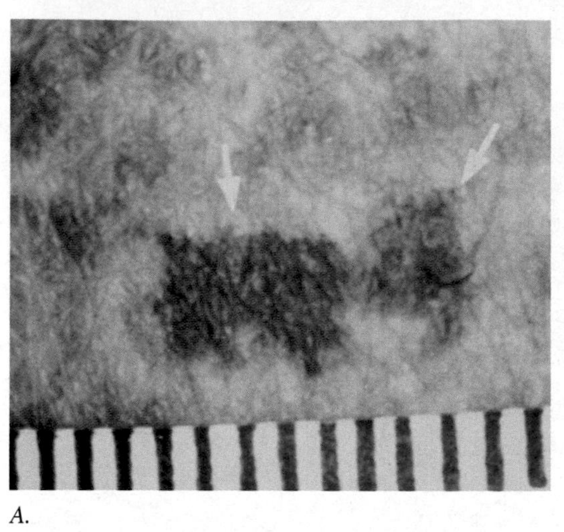

A.

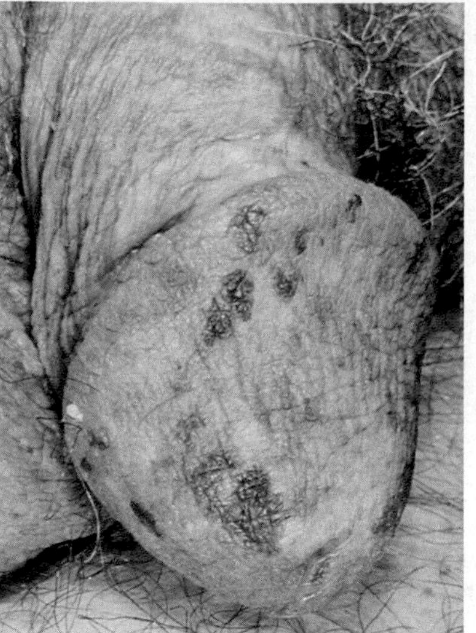

B.

Photochemotherapy (PUVA)–induced lentigines on the buttock (*A*) and penis (*B*) of a 57-year-old white man who had received PUVA for psoriasis several times per week for 5 years. The PUVA lentigines appeared between 1 to 2 years after PUVA therapy was begun. The current recommendation is to shield the male genitalia during PUVA therapy to prevent epithelial tumors of the penis and scrotum.

Pathologic features of photochemotherapy-induced lentigo (PUVA lentigo) include increased numbers of melanocytes in elongated epidermal rete ridges, with large cell bodies and sometimes atypical cellular morphologic features, dendrites often extending high into the epidermis, and melanocytes frequently residing above the epidermal basal unit.[12] Melanocytes in PUVA lentigo occasionally manifest autophagocytosis, sharply invaginated nuclear contours, nuclear pseudoinclusions, double nuclei, striking melanosomal alterations, and melanin macroglobules; melanosomes in keratinocytes of PUVA lentigines are often large and single instead of small and compound as in solar lentigines.[24] Cosmetic UVA tanning also induces lentigines, and cellular atypia has been reported.

Histopathologic characteristics of the labial melanotic macule (labial lentigo) are similar to those of solar lentigo, showing melanocytic hyperplasia but without cellular atypia. The presence of melanocytic hyperplasia in labial melanotic macule is not a uniform finding in all studies.

TABLE 91-2

Risk Factors for the Development of Cutaneous Melanoma

Risk Factor	Relative Risk*
1. New mole or mole that has changed or is changing	Very high†
2. Adulthood (≥15 years vs. <15 years)	88
3. Unique mole and/or prominent mole pattern	
a. Dysplastic mole(s), prior melanoma, and familial melanoma	500
b. Dysplastic mole(s) and familial melanoma, no prior melanoma	148
c. Dysplastic mole(s), no familial melanoma or prior melanoma	7–27
d. Congenital mole	2–21
e. Lentigo maligna	10
f. 50 moles ≥2 mm diameter	4–54
g. 12 moles ≥5 mm diameter	41
h. 5 moles ≥5 mm diameter	7–10
4. Caucasian race vs. black	20
5. Prior cutaneous melanoma	9
6. Cutaneous melanoma in first-degree blood relative	8
7. Immunosuppression	4
8. Sun-induced freckles (marked)	4
9. Sun sensitivity	3

*Degree of estimated increased risk for people who have the risk factor compared to people who do not have the risk factor. A relative risk of 1.0 implies no increased risk.
†Risk estimated roughly to be increased tenfold to four hundredfold based on theoretical prevalence of a "new mole or a mole that has changed or is changing" in the general population compared with the same risk factor in the population of patients who have melanoma.
SOURCE: Adapted from Rhodes,[100] modified with additional data from text.

DIAGNOSIS AND DIFFERENTIAL DIAGNOSIS Other lesions that may be confused with solar lentigo include relatively "flat" varieties of seborrheic keratosis, lentigo simplex, junctional nevomelanocytic nevus, pigmented actinic keratosis, and large-cell acanthoma (see Table 91-1). Solar lentigines not apparent in visible light may be visualized using Wood's lamp illumination in a completely darkened examination room.

TREATMENT Solar lentigo usually requires no therapy, but more important, its presence indicates sensitivity and/or excessive exposure to UV radiation. Cosmetically displeasing lesions may resolve for as long as a year after light application of liquid nitrogen or other superficial destructive techniques. Bleaching creams containing hydroquinone are usually not effective. It may be possible to prevent further solar lentigines by reducing sun exposure. This may be accomplished through avoidance, protective clothing, and sunscreens. Optimally, these

FIGURE 91-7

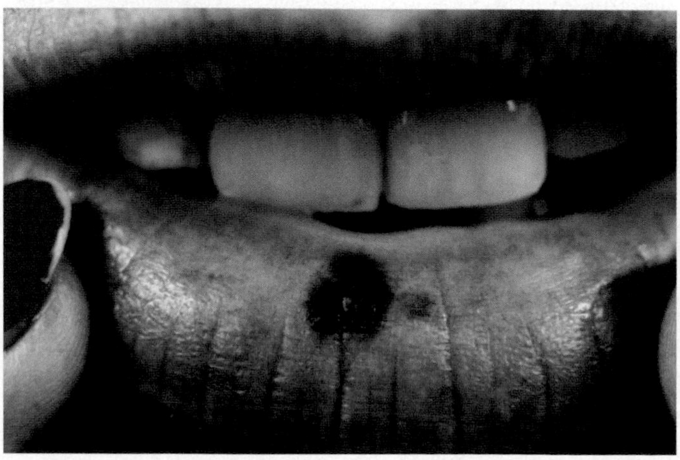

Labial melanotic macule, appearing 5 years earlier, on the lower lip of a 26-year-old white woman.

measures should be initiated during early childhood and continued throughout life.

COURSE AND PROGNOSIS Solar lentigines may appear at any time of life. A solar lentigo may enlarge, darken, and become stable over time, but longitudinal studies of solar lentigines are lacking. It is possible that once formed, solar lentigines may persist indefinitely or fade slightly with time. Solar lentigines may be a heterogeneous population that includes lesions that fade and lesions that do not fade after UV radiation avoidance.

It has been proposed that some varieties of lichenoid keratosis (see Chap. 79) evolve from solar lentigo and that spontaneous resolution of lichenoid keratosis may cause regression of the associated lentigo.[26] This hypothesis has not been confirmed in longitudinal studies.

The long-term course of atypical varieties of PUVA lentigo is unknown, but it is clear that PUVA lentigines (see Fig. 91-6) may persist 1 to 2 years or longer after therapy is discontinued[16] and that cellular atypia of epidermal melanocytes in these lesions may persist as well. It is also clear that these patients may be at increased risk for melanoma[27] and should be followed periodically for life.

The presence of dense solar lentigines in adults is associated with an estimated two- to fourfold increased risk for epithelial skin cancer and two- to sixfold increased risk for melanoma.[24] Lentigo maligna (see Chap. 93) may masquerade as a lentigo early in its development or, alternatively, may evolve from a preexisting solar lentigo. A solar lentigo not matching the patient's other lentigines and/or enlarging/darkening out of step should be examined histopathologically or followed closely.

NEOPLASIAS

The benign melanocytic neoplasias include lesions in which nevomelanocytes are noted to be present in nests in the epidermis and/or present in locations other than the epidermis. The nevomelanocytes forming these lesions often do not demonstrate normal melanocytic differentiation and hence their name *nevomelanocytes*. The extent of melanocytic proliferation, spectrum and type of differentiation, location of cells, and age of the lesion all may influence clinical and histopathologic features. This section will focus on the spectrum of benign melanocytic neoplasias, excluding atypical (dysplastic) melanocytic nevi, nevus of Ota/Ito, and dermal melanocytosis (Mongolian spot) (see Chaps. 90 and 92). Cutaneous melanoma is covered separately in Chap. 93.

Common Acquired Nevomelanocytic Nevus

Nevomelanocytic nevus is a collection of nevomelanocytes in the epidermis (junctional), dermis (intradermal), or both areas (compound). Other names include *nevus cell nevus, nevocellular nevus, nevocytic nevus, soft nevus, neuronevus, pigmented nevus, pigmented mole, common mole, melanocytic nevus, hairy nevus, cellular nevus,* and *benign melanocytoma. Dysplastic* melanocytic nevi usually are acquired nevi (see Chap. 92).

EPIDEMIOLOGY Common (also called *typical*) acquired nevomelanocytic nevi (Fig. 91-8) develop after birth, slowly enlarge symmetrically, stabilize, and persist or regress later in life. The majority of common acquired nevi appear to develop during the second and third decades of life, although some lesions may appear in the first 6 to 12 months of life.

A number of studies have quantitated the number of typical acquired nevi in different age groups. In 432 European whites between the ages of 4 days and 96 years, nevi that were 3 mm in diameter or larger were detected in females and males, respectively, at median numbers of 0 and 2 in the first decade, 16 and 10 in the second decade, 24 and 16 in the third decade, 19 and 10 in the fourth decade, 12 and 15 in the fifth decade, 12 and 4 in the sixth decade, and 3.5 and 2 in the seventh through the ninth decades.[28] In a series of Australian whites, the average number of nevi per person peaked at 43 for males and 27 for females during the second and third decades, respectively, and decreased to very few in the sixth and seventh decades.[29] A similar age-related prevalance rate for nevi has been documented in other countries. A difference in

FIGURE 91-8

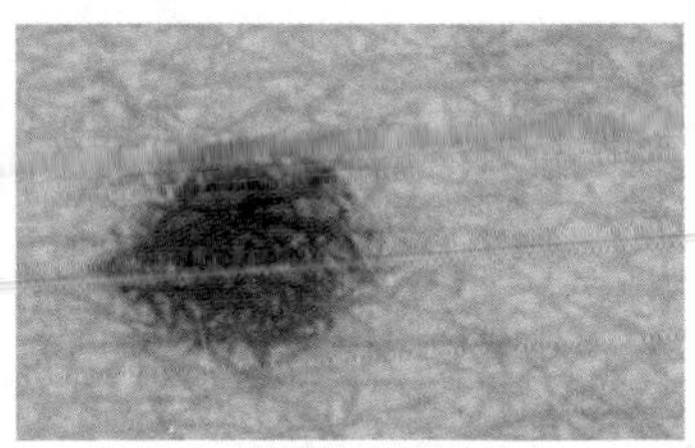
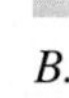
A.

B.

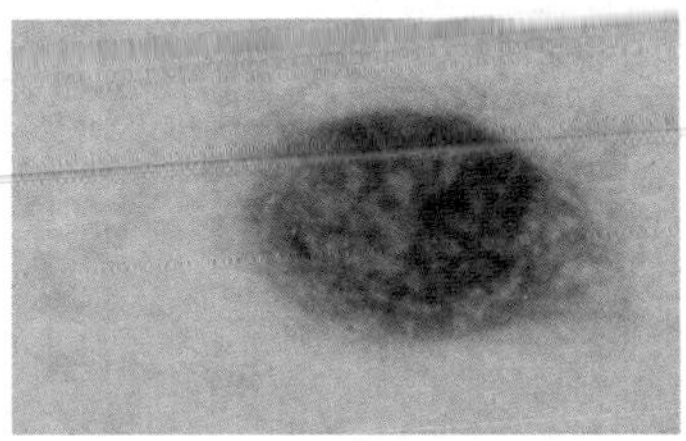
C.

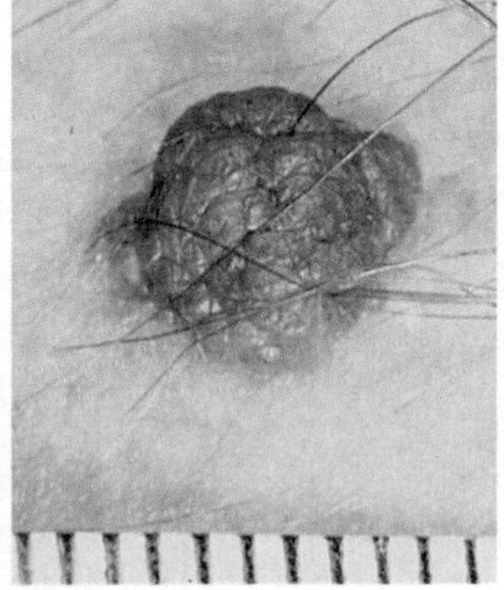
D.

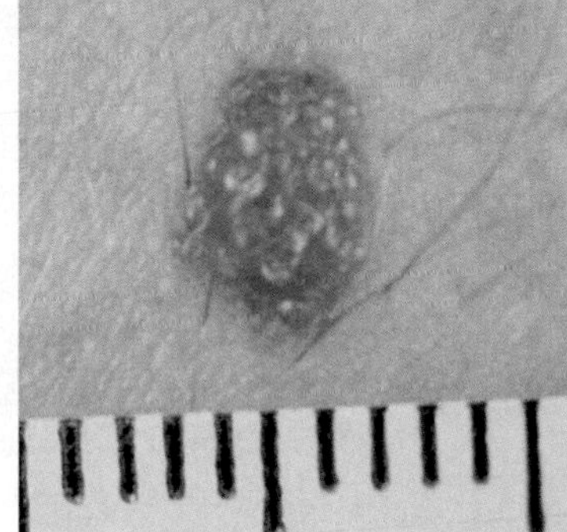
E.

Typical acquired nevomelanocytic nevi. *A.* Junctional nevus on the chest of a 25-year-old white woman. *B.* Junctional nevus, present and stable for 6 years but darkening and enlarging in the past 6 months, on the left thigh of a 27-year-old Chinese woman. *C.* Dermal nevus on the abdomen of a 27-year-old white woman. *D.* Compound nevus (primarily dermal) on the shoulder of a 32-year-old white man. *E.* Compound nevus on the back of a 22-year-old white man. Scale in millimeters.

frequency distribution of nevi according to gender is not clear, although most series show a close to equal prevalence in males and females.

The prevalence of nevi varies according to race. In blacks, the overall prevalence of nevi (regardless of size) tends to be higher in those with lighter skin versus those with darker skin.[1] When prepubertal whites were examined for nevi, a significant association for excess nevi was documented for pale skin, blue or green eyes, blond or light-brown hair, and a tendency to sunburn, but not a tendency to freckle.[30] Other studies show variable relationships to these same parameters.

Environmental exposure to UV light appears to be a critical exacerbating factor for the development of melanocytic nevi. In an Australian study, mole density has been shown to increase with increasing sun intensity in the northern parts of the continent.[31] Further, the use of UV blocking sunscreens has been shown to decrease the number of new moles in children.[32]

Genetics plays a role in nevus development. There is evidence that the size, frequency, and distribution patterns of acquired nevi tend to aggregate in families. This observation is well documented for atypical nevi in the setting of familial cutaneous melanoma (see Chap. 92) and congenital nevi. Correlation coefficients for total nevus counts were significantly higher in 153 monozygotic versus 199 dizygotic twin pairs in Australia (0.94 versus 0.64).[33] In studies of children younger than 12 years of age in Queensland, a history of melanoma in a child's first- or second-degree relative was associated with an increase in total nevi and an increase in large nevi (>5 mm).[30]

ETIOLOGY AND PATHOGENESIS There has been a continual debate as to the origin of nevi. Although many theories have been proposed and some supporting data are available, the critical events leading to nevus development remain a mystery. A number of hypotheses have been proposed. These include (1) transformation from epidermal melanocytes and subsequent deposition/migration into the dermis, (2) dual origin, i.e., nevomelanocytes in the epidermis and upper dermis being derived from epidermal melanocytes, and nevomelanocytes in the lower dermis being derived from Schwann cells of nerves, (3) hamartomatous change affecting many cell types, and (4) benign neoplastic proliferation originating from a defect in melanoblast/neural crest cells.

Evidence for the first hypothesis includes the demonstration of basement membrane around nevomelanocytes in the dermis based on routine, ultrastructural, and immunohistologic features, suggesting structural contiguity of dermal nevomelanocytes with epidermis.[34] These studies would suggest that nevomelanocytes extend down from the epidermis along with the basement membrane.

Evidence for the second hypothesis is based on differences in differentiation of nevomelanocytes. This includes positive staining by a monoclonal antibody to the Schwann cell–associated antigen for nevomelanocytes in the lower dermis and negative staining for nevomelanocytes in the epidermis and upper and middle dermis. Moreover, nevomelanocytes in the epidermis and papillary dermis commonly resemble epithelioid cells, aggregate in nests, demonstrate tyrosinase activity but not cholinesterase activity, stain weakly for neuron-specific enolase, and contain melanin. Nevomelanocytes in the deep dermis tend to resemble fibroblasts or Schwann cells or form concentrically arranged and loosely layered structures becoming nevic corpuscles that resemble Meissner corpuscles, are usually disposed as single cells, demonstrate minimal tyrosinase activity, have abundant cholinesterase activity, and commonly stain positively for neuron-specific enolase. This hypothesis would suggest that the phenotypic differences in the nevomelanocytes are due to different origins (melanocytes and Schwann cells).

Evidence for the third hypothesis includes changes in the associated epidermis, including lentiginous, seborrheic, or epidermal nevus type patterns, and aberrations of appendageal and neurovascular structures, particularly in congenital nevi. These findings reinforce the notion that nevomelanocytic nevi are benign hamartomas involving multiple tissue elements.

The fourth hypothesis is based on the existence of defective melanoblasts that may lead to defective differentiation. Neural crest–derived melanoblasts migrate to the dermis and basal layer of the epidermis before 40 days of estimated gestational age. These cells are thought to take up residence in the epidermis and/or superficial dermis (or the deep dermis, panniculus, and adnexal structures in the case of congenital nevi). Melanocytic "precursor" cells have been shown to be present in adult human skin.[35] Theoretically, these cells could aberrantly proliferate and differentiate, giving rise to melanocytic neoplasms. Depending on the defect, timing, and local tissue influences, a variety of different melanocytic neoplasias could be created. This fourth hypothesis is supported by data showing that human acquired nevi are clonal.[36–38]

CLINICAL MANIFESTATIONS Common acquired nevi vary considerably in their gross appearance. In general, appearance to the naked eye is orderly; i.e., lesions have a homogeneous surface and coloration pattern, round or oval shape, regular outlines, and relatively sharp border (Fig. 91-8). Common acquired nevi may be papillomatous, dome-shaped, pedunculated, or flat-topped and usually are flesh-colored, pink, or brown. More elevated acquired nevi tend to be more lightly pigmented, and flatter acquired nevi tend to be more darkly pigmented. More elevated and less pigmented lesions tend to have a prominent intradermal nevus component, whereas flatter and darker lesions have a more prominent junctional melanocytic or nevomelanocytic component and a less prominent dermal component. Very dark brown and black are unusual colors for common acquired nevi in lightly pigmented people. In contrast, dark pigmentation is usual for common acquired nevi in people who have darkly pigmented skin. Very dark brown and black in nevi on acral and mucosal surfaces and nail apparatus should be viewed with suspicion regardless of constitutive skin color. Blue, gray, red, and white areas in a nevus are not typical features and ought also to be viewed with suspicion. The surfaces of nevi may reveal hair that is less than, equal to, or greater than that of surrounding skin. Hair in nevi may be coarser, longer, and darker than that in surrounding skin. Lesions on palms and soles are usually hairless. Size, shape, skin markings, and hair quality of nevi in darkly pigmented races are similar to those in whites.

Pigmented nevi of the nail apparatus may be a dark or light brown, extending from the nail matrix to the distal edge of the nail plate (Fig. 91-9); extension of the pigmentation onto the skin of the nail fold

FIGURE 91-9

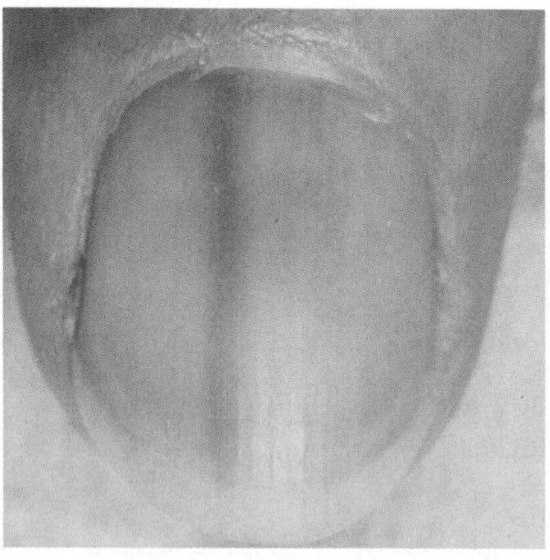

Acquired melanocytic nevus of the nailbed in a 32-year-old white man. Note the lack of involvement of proximal nail fold.

or beyond the distal nail groove should be considered suspicious for melanocytic dysplasia or melanoma. Nevi on palms and soles, even compound nevi, may not distort the skin surface, perhaps because of a thickened stratum corneum in these sites.

Relatively large and numerous nevi are common in Turner's syndrome and Noonan's syndrome and in persons who have atypical nevi. Multiple studies demonstrate that prominent numbers of nevi indicate an increased melanoma risk. Tucker et al.[39] noted a 3.4 (95% CL: 2.0–5.7) adjusted relative risk for melanoma in patients with 100 nevi or more (>2 mm and <5 mm) compared with those with fewer than 25 nevi. The relative risk was increased to 12 (95% CI: 4.4–31) for patients with 10 or more atypical nevi compared with patients without atypical nevi. Absence of direct site specificity of nevi and melanoma suggests that nevus proneness per se indicates a general melanoma risk,[40] largely independent of hair and eye color and overall sun exposure.[41] Other traits, including skin color and freckles, may be multiplicative to the number of nevi in increasing melanoma risk.[42]

PATHOLOGY Nevomelanocytes in the epidermis have a nuclear size similar to or larger than nuclei of epidermal melanocytes. Nevomelanocytes are arranged in nests surrounded by a smooth perimeter of epidermis and separated from nevomelanocytes by a retraction artifact (Fig. 91-10). Nevomelanocytes have abundant pale-staining eosinophilic cytoplasm and may have pseudopodic or dendritic extensions that are more evident when dopa histochemistry is used for visualization. Nuclei of nevomelanocytes are pale-staining, characterized as vacuolated or reticulated; a nucleolus is usually visible.[43] Epidermal melanocytes between junctional theques of nevomelanocytes in typical nevomelanocytic nevi are disposed as single cells, with overall numbers and cell size equal to or slightly greater than that in adjacent sun-exposed skin[11] (see Fig. 91-10). The overlying epidermis is often normal in appearance but may be thickened in a lentiginous pattern (elongated and club-shaped rete ridges), with an appearance similar to seborrheic keratosis complete with horn cysts or epidermal verrucous hyperplasia similar to epidermal nevus.

The dermal component of nevi has an orderly progression from top to bottom, with larger epithelioid cells above (epidermis and superficial papillary dermis) blending into a pattern of smaller cells in the deeper dermis. Nevomelanocytes in epidermis and upper papillary dermis frequently resemble epithelial cells, with an oval or cuboidal shape, a well-outlined cytoplasm that is homogeneous in character, a nucleus not much larger than nuclei of basal keratinocytes, and a visible nucleolus. Nevomelanocytes in the epidermis and superficial dermis frequently contain melanin, but the dopa histochemical reaction in nevomelanocytes in the epidermis and dermis is usually minimal.[11] Nevomelanocytes in the middle or deep dermis are usually smaller than nevomelanocytes in the superficial dermis or epidermis and frequently resemble lymphoid cells. Nevomelanocytes in the deep dermis may be round or oval and often resemble Schwann cells or fibroblasts when they are singly disposed and may be difficult to differentiate from fibroblasts unless they are disposed in sheets, cords, or patchy aggregates[44] (see Fig. 91-10). Usually, dermal nevomelanocytes are interposed among collagen bundles, and there is no distinct rim of collagen or retraction artifact between surrounding collagen and cellular aggregates.

Features that suggest atypicality of nevomelanocytes in the dermis are nests or fascicles "pushing" and compressing collagen in the reticular dermis, lack of maturation with descent into the deep dermis, persistence of pigment production in the deep dermis, irregularity of size and shape of cells, frequent mitotic figures, and desmoplasia or fibrosis in the dermis. Nevomelanocytes in the dermis of typical acquired nevi have a monotonous similarity one to another within the same anatomic level and an overall symmetry of architecture from top to bottom and side to side.

Inflammatory cellular infiltrates in typical, stable acquired nevi are usually scanty[43] or absent. Melanin-laden macrophages are usually apparent in the superficial papillary dermis of nevi, their number usually proportional to degree of melanin production.[43] Blood vessel proliferation, eosinophilic fibrosis, and lamellar fibroplasia (features frequently

FIGURE 91-10

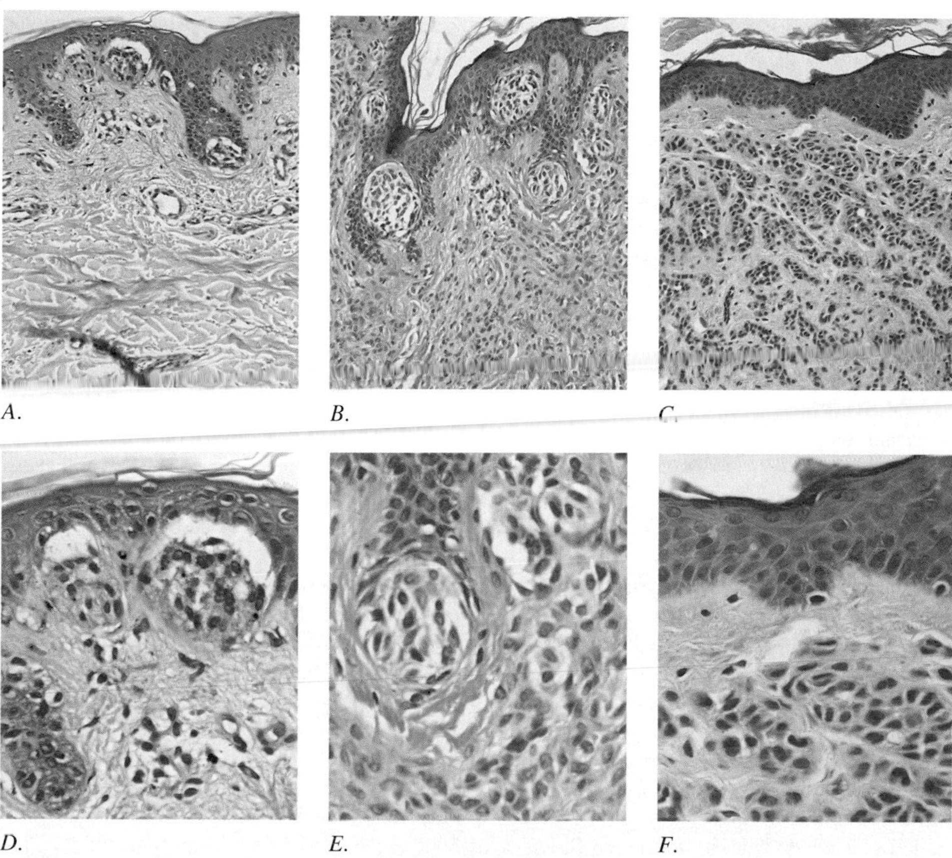

Histopathologic features of acquired nevi. Junctional nevus (*A*) and higher magnification (*D*). Compound nevus (*B*) and higher magnification (*E*). Intradermal nevus (*C*) and higher magnification (*F*). Well-formed nests of nevomelanocytes are present in the junctional and compound nevi. Sheets and cords of nevocytes are present in the dermis of the compound and intradermal nevi. A Grenz zone free of nevomelanocytes is present just below the epidermis in the intradermal nevus (*C* and *F*).

seen in atypical melanocytic nevi) are usually not prominent in typical acquired nevi. Langerhans cell density overlying typical acquired nevi and atypical nevi is increased compared with adjacent skin.

Intradermal nevi that have few or no junctional nests frequently have a Grenz zone relatively free of nevomelanocytes just below the epidermis (see Fig. 91-10). Multinucleated nevomelanocytes occur occasionally and may be interpreted as a sign of benignity. Nevomelanocytes in the deep dermis may be disposed within a collagenous framework that is loose, pale, and wavy in formations called *neuroid tubes,* similar to a neurofibroma; they may be disposed in concentrically arranged whorls resembling Meissner's tactile corpuscles; and they may be spindle-shaped and embedded in loosely arranged connective tissue (neural nevi). Both neural nevi and neurofibromas show nonspecific cholinesterase activity. Myelin basic protein is detected in various neural tumors but not in melanocytic or nevomelanocytic tumors, and melanosomes are present in nevomelanocytes but not in neurofibromas or nerve tissue. Cutaneous neural lesions may be distinguished from melanocytic tumors by the presence of myelin basic protein and neurofilaments and the absence of vimentin.

The balloon cell nevus is composed of peculiar foam cells comprising a portion or all of a given lesion. In addition to clear cells with single basophilic nuclei, multinucleated balloon cells and multinucleated giant cells are seen frequently. Electron microscopic studies suggest that the vacuolization of the nevomelanocytes is due to enlargement and destruction of melanosomes. There appears to be no distinguishing gross features of balloon cell nevi.

The *combined nevus* refers to the in-contiguity association of different types of melanocytic nevi. These lesions include the combined compound nevus (acquired or congenital)–blue nevus and compound nevus–spindle cell and/or epithelioid cell nevus.

Recurrent melanocytic nevus (pseudomelanoma) is the name given to recurrent lesions following incomplete removal of a benign nevomelanocytic nevus.[45] Pseudomelanoma is said to be relatively common after superficial destructive procedures (i.e., shave biopsy or dermabrasion). A markedly atypical clinical and histopathologic appearance may accompany this recurrence, making these lesions worrisome for possible melanoma. Clinically, the recurrent nevus is confined to the scar but may be markedly irregular. Histopathologically, the recurrent lesions often demonstrate the presence of melanocytic hyperplasia in a lentiginous or junctional pattern (often to a greater extent than the original nevus). Moderate nuclear atypia may be present in 12 percent of recurrent nevi, mitotic figures in 8 percent, and pagetoid scattering in 3 percent, raising concern about the potential biologic behavior of some recurrent lesions. Other studies suggest that deliberate trauma to benign nevi in the form of incisional biopsy was not associated with atypical melanocytic changes.[46]

Various findings have been identified in nevi that may suggest modes of regression or elimination of melanocytic elements. Some of the findings include neuroid, fibrous, mucinous, and fatty degeneration.[47] The presence of nevomelanocytes in the stratum corneum[48] suggests transepidermal elimination. Psamomma bodies and amyloid bodies, present occasionally in nevi, also may be related to degeneration or regression. Fibrosis may occur as an age-related phenomenon, whereas true desmoplasia appears to be a reactive process or functional transformation by the nevomelanocytes. Follicular mucinosis has been reported in nevi in at least two cases. Spicules of bone are observed occasionally in nevi, possibly related to reactive metaplasia, trauma, or infection.

There may be histopathologic artifacts in nevomelanocytic nevi. Shrinkage clefts may resemble lymphatics or vascular spaces, prominent in the midportion of nevi and particularly in areas with hemorrhage. Separation of sheets of nevomelanocytes into parallel rows may be caused by improper cutting. Local anesthesia injection directly into the nevus also may be associated with artifactural changes.

DIAGNOSIS AND DIFFERENTIAL DIAGNOSIS It may be difficult to differentiate relatively flat nevomelanocytic nevi that are pale brown from solar lentigo, lentigo simplex, or café-au-lait macules without resorting to oblique lighting, which usually will reveal at least some skin surface distortion in nevomelanocytic nevi. Dermoscopy also may be useful and may reveal a number of diagnostic patterns in nevi, including reticular, globular, cobblestone, and parallel patterns.[49,50] Clinically, a nevomelanocytic nevus must be differentiated from melanoma, blue nevus, pigmented fibrous histiocytoma (dermatofibroma), Kaposi's sarcoma, pigmented basal cell carcinoma, pigmented actinic keratosis, benign pigmented keratosis, mastocytoma, seborrheic keratosis, epidermal nevus, Becker's melanosis, common wart, molluscum contagiosum, subungual hematoma, supernumerary nipple, pigmented spindle cell and/or epithelioid cell nevus, sclerosing hemangioma, appendage tumor, pyogenic granuloma, and large cell acanthoma. Nevus spilus has melanocytic or nevomelanocytic pigmented elements within a lighter background of lentigo simplex. The differentiation between typical acquired nevomelanocytic nevus and acquired atypical melanocytic nevus (or cutaneous melanoma) is discussed in Chaps. 92 and 93. Nevomelanocytic nevi that are nonpigmented or pink must be distinguished from other nonpigmented tumors, such as basal cell carcinoma, fibrous papule, wart, dermal mucinosis, clear cell acanthoma, and a variety of appendageal tumors.

TREATMENT The vast majority of acquired nevomelanocytic nevi require no treatment. Indications for removal of benign-appearing lesions may include cosmetic concerns or continual irritation that could be mistaken for a changing mole. Lesions with features worrisome for melanoma need to be excised. These features are addressed in detail in Chaps. 92 and 93. Dermoscopy may be used to differentiate benign and potentially malignant features. A photographic medical record can play a critical role in identifying changes that might not have been detected otherwise.[51]

Complete removal of nevi is best accomplished by elliptical excision. Leaving a partially excised nevus, regardless of the initial pathology, is fraught with potentially alarming consequences of repigmentation and/or regrowth (pseudomelanoma).[45] Incisional biopsy, even for melanoma, is necessary at times, particularly for lesions that cannot be excised easily and that require histopathologic diagnosis. Destructive modes of therapy (electrodesiccation, cryotherapy, dermabrasion, and laser) should be considered very carefully if used in the management of melanocytic and nevomelanocytic nevi. They have the definite disadvantage of not providing tissue for histopathology. Although dermabrasion has been used to eliminate pigmentation of nevomelanocytic nevi, residual nevus cells in the dermis are to be expected, cosmetic outcome is often unpredictable, and recurrence with worrisome clinical features may complicate future management. Laser treatment of melanocytic and nevomelanocytic lesions has the theoretical risk of malignant transformation, but there is no proof for this.

COURSE AND PROGNOSIS Typical acquired nevi have not been followed systematically from their inception to resolution or regression. Therefore, dynamic evolution of acquired nevi must be surmised from static information or short-term follow-up studies.

It has been stated that during the early years of life, virtually all nevomelanocytic nevi are composed primarily of junctional theques,[52] that nevomelanocytes in these junctional theques eventually push their way to the dermis and finally lose their epidermal contact as they continue to grow into the dermis and become intradermal nevi, and that in the intermediate stage of this process there are junctional theques in the epidermis and sheets and nests of nevomelanocytes in the dermis (i.e., compound nevi).[53] This argument suggests that because nevi in adults are primarily of the dermal type and because nevi in children are primarily of the junctional type, nevi evolve by a process of nevus cells from the epidermis "dropping down" into the dermis (*Abtropfung*).[52] The precise nature of the "dropping down" process has not been defined.

FIGURE 91-11

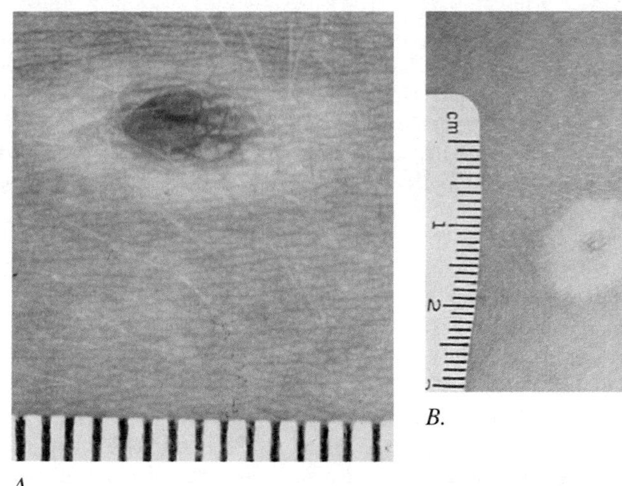

A. B.

Acquired halo nevomelanocytic nevus. *A.* Acquired halo nevus on the chest of a 16-year-old white boy whose maternal grandmother had melanoma. *B.* Acquired halo nevi on the back of a 6-year-old white boy who has dysplastic nevi in the hairy scalp and a history of melanoma in his maternal grandmother. Scale in millimeters.

It is likely that acquired nevi evolve through a life cycle, first becoming apparent after infancy in the vast majority of cases, peaking in number during the second and third decades of life, and then disappearing by the seventh to ninth decades.[28,29,47] Regression of nevi is believed to occur by neuroid, fibrous, mucinous, or fatty degeneration.[47] The formation of cylindrical neuroid structures in aging nevi suggests an end stage in differentiation and not a source of origin of intraepidermal nevi. Transepidermal elimination of nevomelanocytes occurs rarely,[48] in 0.13 percent of cases in one study.[54] Rarely, nevomelanocytes have been documented to show spontaneous disappearance. Nevi also may involute during the course of inflammatory halo depigmentation (halo nevi).

There may be relatively sudden changes in nevi that are unrelated to malignant transformation. Any single nevus that is noted to suddenly change independently should be cause for concern. Causes of sudden changes in a nevus (color, surface, or size, with or without pain, itching, ulceration, or bleeding) over days or weeks include cystic dilatation of a hair follicle, epidermal cyst formation, folliculitis, abscess formation, trauma, hemorrhage, and, in the case of a pedunculated nevus, strangulation and thrombosis. These benign causes of sudden change may require close observation until resolution occurs over the course of 7 to 10 days (in the case of trauma or inflammation) or histopathologic examination. Cases have been described of the eruptive appearance of nevi after blistering skin disease, immunosuppression, or chemotherapy.

The vast majority of acquired nevi are harmless, growing in proportion to body growth, with physiologic spurts of enlargement during early childhood and puberty. Melanoma risk appears to be related to the number and size of nevi; patients with numerous nevi, atypical nevi, and a personal or family history of melanoma should be considered for periodic surveillance examinations (see Table 91-2).

Halo Nevomelanocytic Nevus

The halo nevus is defined as a nevomelanocytic nevus surrounded by a halo of depigmentation (Figs. 91-11 and 91-12). This lesion should not be considered a unique melanocytic neoplasia but rather a reaction pattern that may occur around any melanocytic neoplasm. This phenomenon often, but not always, indicates the onset of involution and subsequent regression of the melanocytic nevus. Other names for this phenomenon include *leukoderma acquisitum centrifugum, Sutton's nevus, leukopigmentary nevus, perinevoid vitiligo, and perinevoid leukoderma.* The halo phenomenon may be associated with acquired and congenital nevomelanocytic nevi as well as with melanoma and nonmelanocytic tumors.

EPIDEMIOLOGY Of 8298 whites aged 12 to 16 years, there were 51 males (1.2 percent) and 22 females (0.5 percent) who had one or more halo nevi, for an overall prevalence rate of 0.9 percent.[56] In one large series of halo nevus,[57] individuals ranged in age from 3 to 42 years (mean age 15 years), the vast majority of cases occurring before age 20 years. No race is spared. The most common condition associated with halo nevus is vitiligo, occurring in 18 to 26 percent of patients. Halo nevus may be associated with poliosis, Vogt-Koyanagi-Harada syndrome (see Chap. 90), pernicious anemia, and a personal or family history of melanoma (including ocular melanoma). Halo nevus has been reported after exposure to external depigmenting agents.

ETIOLOGY AND PATHOGENESIS Pathogenesis of the halo phenomenon is poorly understood. Available evidence suggests that both humoral and cellular factors may be responsible for nevus destruction.

Lymphocytes isolated from patients with halo nevus or melanoma, but not patients with vitiligo or normal controls, show enhanced

FIGURE 91-12

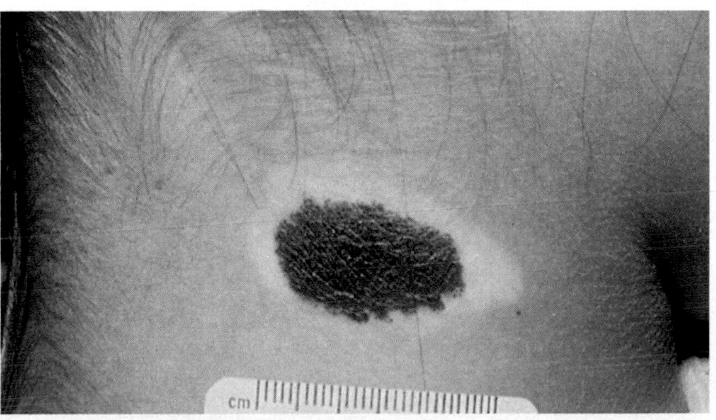

Halo congenital nevomelanocytic nevus on the neck of a 4-year-old female of a black African-American mother and white father. This child also had scattered areas of vitiligo-like depigmentation in other sites. A 3-year follow-up after excision of the nevus revealed almost total repigmentation of the widely scattered previously depigmented areas.

cell killing of human melanoma cells in culture.[58] A cytoplasmic antibody has been demonstrated against melanoma in patients with resolving halo nevus but not in patients who have vitiligo without halo nevus or in patients with Spitz or ordinary nevi.[59] These lymphocyte and serologic abnormalities do not indicate the exact sequence of events in the halo phenomenon, nor whether these abnormalities are primary or secondary. Reed et al.[60] postulate atypicality of nevomelanocytes as the initiating factor for the immune response, which may cross-react with normal epidermal melanocytes and typical nevomelanocytes.

Sinclair swine may provide an animal model for halo nevus because melanocytic tumors associated with metastatic disease in these animals are similar to human melanoma, and regression of tumors is associated with surrounding depigmentation as a concomitant event that follows an inflammatory cellular infiltrate in the tumors. A second process that may provide some insight into factors involved in melanocytic interactions with the immune system is a process that results in the development of an eczematous dermatitis presenting as a red halo around nevi (halo dermatitis). Unlike halo nevi, regression of the nevus does not usually occur, and the eczematous changes clear over the course of several months.

CLINICAL MANIFESTATIONS The typical halo nevus has a pink or brown central nevomelanocytic nevus surrounded by a symmetric round or oval halo of depigmented skin. The central nevus may be small, in the case of typical acquired nevus, or large, in the case of acquired dysplastic or congenital nevus (see Figs. 91-11 and 91-12). The halo of depigmentation is variable in size, usually a radial zone 0.5 to 5 cm around the central lesion. Under Wood's lamp, which may be required to visualize depigmentation in lightly pigmented individuals, the perinevic halo is seen as depigmented with sharply defined borders. White hairs may be seen in hair-bearing depigmented areas. Alopecia areata surrounding halo nevus has been reported.

The number of halo nevi per person may be one or many, multiple lesions occurring in 25 to 50 percent of patients. For patients who have multiple lesions, only a few nevi are usually affected, but as many as 90 halo nevi have been reported in a single person. Any nevus in any anatomic site may be involved, but the posterior torso is involved most commonly. Lesions are usually asymptomatic. UV radiation may cause redness and even blistering in the perinevic halo.

The typical history for halo nevus is that depigmentation appears around a preexisting nevus. Time for full evolution to depigmentation of the halo is not known, but patients report the phenomenon occurring over days to weeks, with little change occurring in the halo thereafter. A trichrome appearance of the halo has been reported. Occasionally, the depigmented halo may show transient redness as the initial manifestation. The central nevus may remain unchanged, or it may change from one or more shades of brown to variegations of brown and red or totally red or pink. The central nevus may persist or eventually flatten and disappear. Disappearance may take months to years. Areas of depigmentation that remain after the central nevus disappears may remain stationary for many years or repigment after months to years. There are nevi in which the nevus fails to involute, and repigmentation of the depigmented halo may occur. Occasionally, congenital nevi associated with halo phenomenon may show clinical regression of surface pigmentation overlying the nevus.

PATHOLOGY The usual histopathologic findings in a halo nevus are the central nevomelanocytic nevus, a dermal lymphocytic infiltrate associated with the nevus, and a depigmented zone totally or almost totally devoid of epidermal basal unit dopa-reactive melanocytes. In early-regressing lesions, the nevus is associated with a marked cellular infiltrate, but there is little or no destruction of nevomelanocytes. In later lesions, there is cytolysis of nevomelanocytes, portions of which are evident in macrophages. In the most regressed lesions, there is vitiligo-like loss of pigmentation, total absence of nevomelanocytes, and few or no inflammatory cells. The histopathologic appearance of a given halo nevus depends on the stage of evolution.

Epidermal melanocytes in the depigmented halo initially show detachment from the basal layer, autophagocytosis of preformed melanosomes, vacuolization of melanosomes, pyknotic nuclei, and abnormal cytoplasmic features. Remaining melanocytes in the depigmented halo show only a few melanosomes in very early stages of formation. In the completely depigmented halo, epidermal melanocytes are absent, and numerous Langerhans cells occupy the epidermal basal layer. Epidermal keratinocytes in the depigmented halo are devoid of melanosomes, degenerative changes are sometimes seen, and the epidermis also may be infiltrated by a few lymphocytes and nerve fibers. The dermis below the depigmented halo is usually devoid of inflammation.

The central nevus may be purely junctional or purely dermal, but the most common pathology is compound. The inflammatory infiltrate is usually located in a bandlike pattern beneath the nevus and/or intermixed with dermal nevomelanocytes. Immunohistochemical staining for S100 protein (or other melanocytic markers) may help to identify the nevomelanocytes in the inflammatory infiltrate. The inflammatory infiltrate is composed mainly of lymphocytes, plasma cells, and histiocytes. Mast cells are scarce, and eosinophils and neutrophils are not usually evident. The lymphocytes appear to be antigenically stimulated, and 80 percent are T lymphocytes, whereas B lymphocytes are scarce or absent. The T cells appear to belong to the CD8+ population.[61]

DIAGNOSIS AND DIFFERENTIAL DIAGNOSIS Diagnosis of halo nevus is usually clinical, based on the presence of an acquired or congenital nevus surrounded by macular depigmentation. The halo phenomenon may be associated with nevi exhibiting a wide spectrum of histopathologic cellular atypia. Tumors associated with the halo phenomenon include congenital nevomelanocytic nevus, atypical melanocytic nevus, melanoma, Spitz nevus, histiocytoma, molluscum contagiosum, flat wart, seborrheic keratosis, basal cell epithelioma, neurofibroma, congenital dermal melanocytosis (Mongolian spot), and miscellaneous conditions such as blue nevus, lichen planus, sarcoidosis, psoriasis, and angioma. An atypical gross appearance of the central nevus or an asymmetric halo of depigmentation around a suspicious nevus, particularly in adults, should raise suspicion for melanocytic dysplasia or melanoma. The depigmented halo associated with melanoma tends to be irregular and surrounds the tumor asymmetrically, but this is not always the case.

TREATMENT Patients who have benign-appearing, centrally placed nevi within a symmetric halo of depigmentation should have a mucocutaneous examination in visible and Wood's light to exclude melanoma, dysplastic melanocytic nevi, and vitiligo. Although a benign-appearing nevus associated with halo depigmentation need not be removed, it is reasonable to recommend periodic examination of affected individuals for dysplastic melanocytic nevi, vitiligo, and melanoma. Atypical-appearing central nevi, presence of an asymmetric halo, eccentric placement of a melanocytic lesion in the halo, or the setting of atypical melanocytic nevi and/or melanoma (personal or family) should suggest the need for histopathologic examination for melanoma. Coverup or sunscreens should be recommended for sun-exposed areas of depigmentation to prevent acute burn, chronic actinic damage, and carcinogenesis.

COURSE AND PROGNOSIS For a given halo nevus, the central tumor may persist unchanged, become less pigmented over time, or flatten and disappear totally. Areas of depigmentation may persist unchanged for months or years or repigment totally. New halo nevi may appear over time. Dysplastic nevi, melanoma, and vitiligo may occur more frequently in individuals with halo nevus.

Epithelioid Cell and/or Spindle Cell Melanocytic Nevus

Epithelioid cell and/or spindle cell (EC-SC) melanocytic nevi are unique, usually acquired, usually benign melanocytic tumors differing grossly and histopathologically from typical acquired nevomelanocytic nevi; they are often alarming in their clinical presentation and sufficiently bizarre histopathologically as to cause diagnostic confusion for melanoma. Other terms for EC-SC nevus include *Spitz tumor, nevus prominens et pigmentosus, pseudomelanoma, spindle and epithelioid cell nevus, nevus of large spindle and/or epithelioid cells, and compound melanocytoma.* The previously used terms *Spitz's juvenile melanoma, benign juvenile melanoma,* and *prepubertal melanoma* should not be employed. Use of the adjective *juvenile* (i.e., juvenile melanoma) is misleading because EC-SC nevi are not restricted to children. Use of the term *melanoma* to describe the EC-SC nevus is unfortunate because EC-SC nevi usually (although not always) have a benign course. The term *benign,* when applied to melanoma, is likely to confuse both patients and physicians. The term *epithelioid cell* and/or *spindle cell melanocytic nevus* characterizes these tumors as melanocytic in origin, usually composed of epithelioid cells and/or spindle cells, not confined to children, and not guaranteeing a benign course.

HISTORICAL ASPECTS Examples of melanocytic tumors having gross and microscopic features resembling melanoma but behaving in a benign manner were described by Darier and Civatte in 1910 and Miescher in 1933. The tumor was named *juvenile melanoma* by Spitz in 1948,[62] *benign juvenile melanoma* by Kopf and Andrade in 1966,[63] and *EC-SC nevus* by Helwig in 1975.[64] The pigmented spindle cell tumor was reported as a variant of EC-SC nevus by Reed et al.[60] in 1975 and Sagebiel et al.[65] in 1984.

EPIDEMIOLOGY An annual incidence rate of 1.4 cases per 100,000 individuals in Australia for EC-SC nevus has been estimated compared with 25.4 per 100,000 individuals for cutaneous melanoma during the same time interval.[66] Among melanocytic nevi excised in children, 1 to 8 percent of cases are interpreted as EC-SC nevus.[65] In a case series of 308 patients with EC-SC nevi reported by Allen,[67] 15 percent of lesions occurred in adolescents and adults, the oldest patient being 56 years of age. There appears to be no gender predilection for EC-SC nevus. Published cases have been described primarily in whites. EC-SC nevus may be pigmented more frequently in adults than in children.

ETIOLOGY AND PATHOGENESIS It may be presumed that EC-SC nevi are derived from the same progenitor cells giving rise to epidermal melanocytes and nevomelanocytes. Except for a single report of multiple tumors in identical twin boys,[63] genetic factors have not been investigated systematically. The role of trauma in the histogenesis of EC-SC nevi is speculative. One case is reported to have arisen at the site of bacille Calmette-Guérin (BCG) vaccination. There are unique aberrations of genes occurring on chromosome 11 in some cases of EC-SC nevi.[68]

CLINICAL MANIFESTATIONS EC-SC nevus may present in one of the following ways: (1) a pink or tan, smooth-surfaced elastic papule that flattens easily with external pressure (Fig. 91-13), (2) a lightly pigmented blue papule, often with telangiectasias on the surface, resembling a fibrous histiocytoma or keloid, (3) a darkly pigmented, usually smooth-surfaced, firm papule (Fig. 91-14), (4) multiple agminated lesions consisting of red, red-brown, brown, or dark-brown papules or nodules, with a fine stippled surface (Fig. 91-15), often occurring in the early years of life within a background of congenital (sometimes acquired) macular pigmentation or occasionally a hypopigmented plaque, (5) single or multiple lesions developing in a large congenital nevomelanocytic nevus, or (6) eruptive widespread lesions in the absence of background macular pigmentation or large congenital nevomelanocytic nevus.

FIGURE 91-13

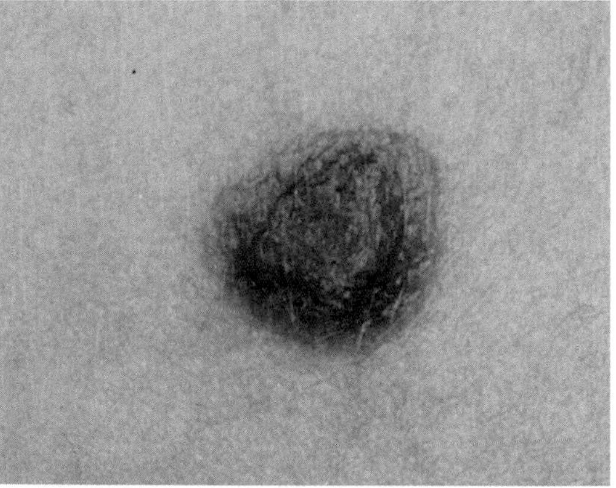

A.

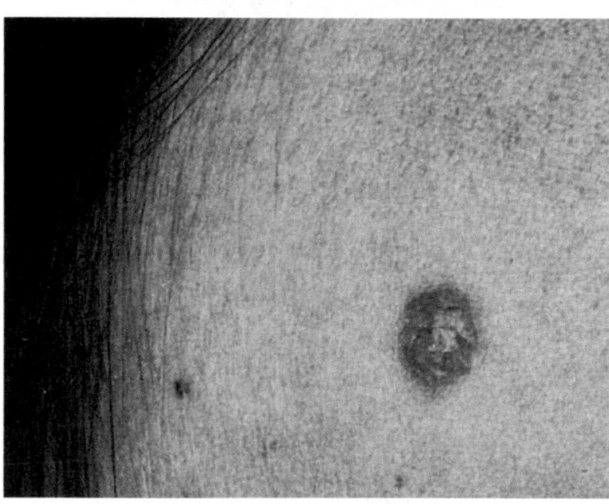

B.

Acquired epithelioid cell and/or spindle cell nevus, predominantly epithelioid cell type. *A.* Pink plaque, which appeared de novo over an 8-week period, becoming more elevated with time, in the preauricular area of a 4-year-old white boy. *B.* Dome-shaped pink papule, which appeared de novo over a 2-week interval 4 months before, on the forehead of a 5-year-old white boy.

The most common variety of EC-SC nevus is the solitary, asymptomatic, pink or red, hairless, firm, dome-shaped, verrucous, or smooth-surfaced telangiectatic papule or nodule (see Fig. 91-13). Infrequently, lesions may have a polypoid or pedunculated shape. Borders may be indefinite and/or irregular or smooth and sharply demarcated. Although the surface is commonly smooth or verrucous, lesions may have a scaly, stippled, crusted, or (rarely) eroded surface. Translucent varieties of EC-SC nevus have been described. Very darkly pigmented lesions constitute a minority of EC-SC nevi, up to 7 percent of cases.[62,63,69] EC-SC nevi are usually asymptomatic, but pruritus, tenderness, and/or bleeding may occur.[63] A halo of depigmentation has been associated with several cases of EC-SC nevus.[57,70]

FIGURE 91-14

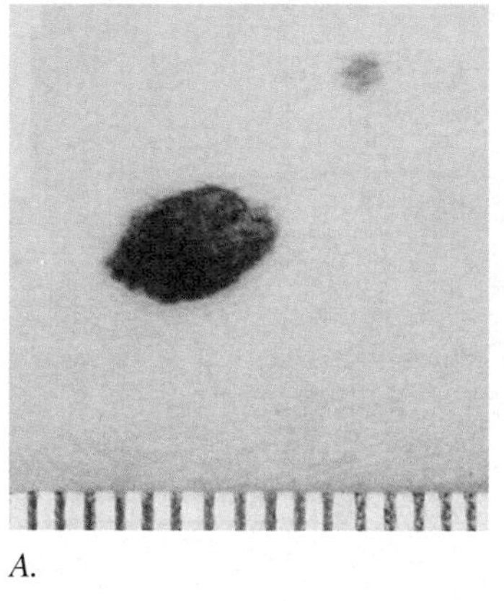

A.

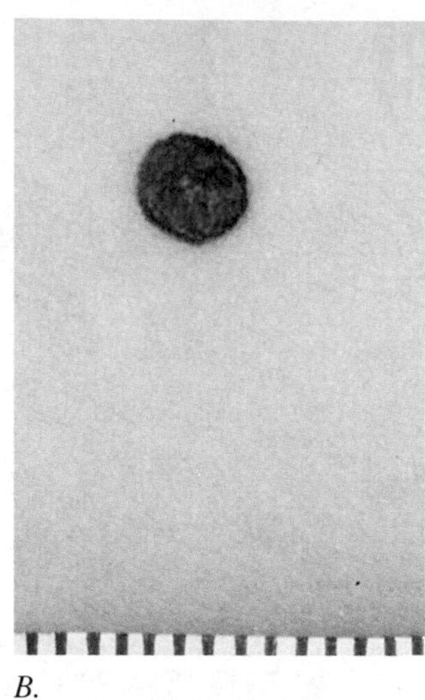

B.

Acquired epithelioid cell and/or spindle cell nevus, predominantly pigmented spindle cell type. *A.* Very dark brown plaque appearing over several weeks on the posterior thigh of a 22-year-old white woman. *B.* Very dark bluish plaque appearing de novo 3 months previously on the back of an 8-month-old white (Hispanic) boy. Scale in millimeters.

The diameter of EC-SC nevi ranges from several millimeters to several centimeters, the average being 8 mm in one series.[63] In 73 percent of patients in one series,[66] the tumor was 6 mm or less in greatest diameter, and in 94 percent of patients, the tumor was less than 10 mm in diameter. Most cases are described as superficial papules or nodules, although subcutaneous involvement may occur.[62] The duration of solitary EC-SC nevus before presentation is usually less than 9 months. Lesions usually show an increase in radial size over time, some gradual and others rapid.[62] In one series of 43 patients,[63] the anatomic location included the head or neck in 18, upper extremities in 9, torso in 9, and lower extremities in 7. The EC-SC nevus tends to spare palms, soles, and mucous membranes.

The *deep penetrating nevus* may be considered a variety of EC-SC nevus, combined nevus, or a unique dermal nevomelanocytic dysplasia. These lesions are said to be darkly pigmented, blue-black papules or nodules. Lesions are mostly on the head and neck or upper extremities, 2 to 9 mm in diameter, and occurring predominantly in the first four decades of life, including childhood.

PATHOLOGY Although the bizarre histopathologic features and frequent occurrence of dermal inflammation may cause diagnostic confusion, EC-SC nevus usually can be differentiated from melanoma. EC-SC nevus in children and adults is histopathologically similar.

Although EC-SC nevus usually has nested melanocytic elements in the epidermis and dermis (Fig. 91-16), the tumor may be restricted to either anatomic zone. Melanocytic elements are usually arranged in well-circumscribed nests, although there may be permeation of the epidermis by single cells or small groups of cells. In those cases with epidermal nests, artifactual clefts are usually seen above the nests in half the cases, a finding rarely observed in melanoma.[66] The epidermis is usually hyperplastic, with elongated and bulbous pegs and knobs extending into the dermis, although thinning and even ulceration may occur rarely. The dermal inflammatory cell infiltrate may be slight or marked, bandlike, and mainly at the base or patchy around blood vessels

FIGURE 91-15

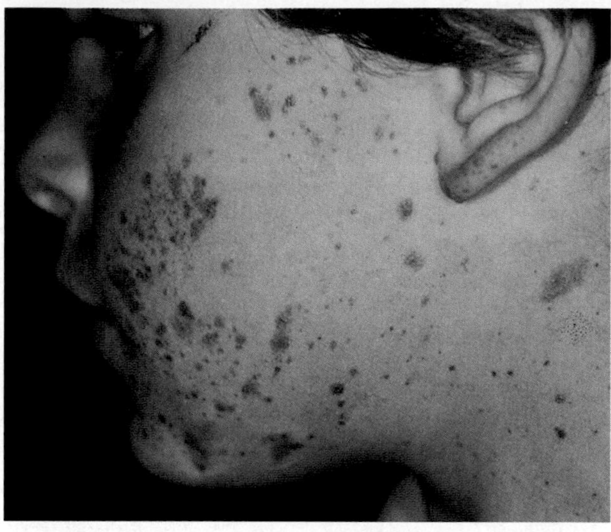

A.

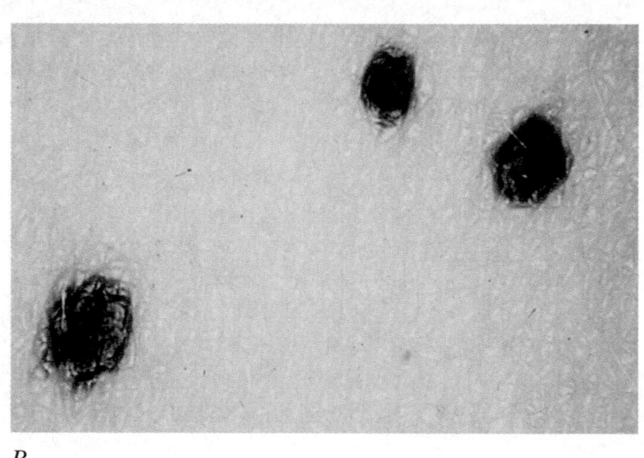

B.

Agminated (grouped) epithelioid cell and/or spindle cell nevi. *A.* Numerous grouped pink papules and plaques, appearing at age 6 months, on the face of a 4-year-old white boy. *B.* Multiple black papules, appearing suddenly several years before, on the anterior torso of a 13-year-old white girl.

and/or intermixing with tumor cells. Although melanin was observed in all 13 patients described by Spitz,[62] in other studies melanin was moderate in 10 percent of patients and heavy in 5 percent.[70] Subtypes of EC-SC nevus may be heavily pigmented.

Spindle cells predominate in 45 to 54 percent of EC-SC nevi, epithelioid cells in 21 percent, and a relatively equal combination of cell types in 24 to 34 percent.[70,71] The pigmented spindle cell nevus described by Reed et al.[60] and later by others[65,72] as a variant of EC-SC nevus is usually a sharply circumscribed, uniformly darkly pigmented papule or plaque (see Fig. 91-14) consisting of compact and aggregated spindle-shaped, pigment-producing melanocytes (see Fig. 91-16), distinguished from melanoma by its uniform nuclei, uniform cellular detail, and distinctive pattern of growth. In a review of 91 pigmented spindle cell nevi by Sagebiel et al.,[65] cells were predominantly spindle in 74 percent and mixed spindle cell and epithelioid cell in 26 percent of patients. Almost all cases of pigmented spindle cell nevus have a lymphohistiocytic host response. Spindle cells extend down eccrine ducts in 40 percent and involve hair follicles in 22 percent of patients.[65] There are atypical variants of pigmented spindle cell nevi in which there are architectural alterations and striking cellular atypia.[72]

Unlike ordinary nevi and melanomas, melanocytic cells in EC-SC nevi are large, often twice the size of epidermal basal keratinocytes,[62] with prominent mononuclear or multinucleated giant cells in the epidermis and/or dermis (see Fig. 91-16). Mitoses, usually few in number, are detected in half the cases,[70] whereas atypical mitoses are uncommon in EC-SC nevus. In contrast to melanoma, the melanocytic cells in EC-SC nevi show progressive maturation with increasing depth, becoming smaller and more similar to ordinary nevomelanocytes,[62,70] with the overall distribution of cells in the dermis being wedge-shaped, with narrowing of the wedge toward the subcutaneous fat.

Coalescent eosinophilic globules (Kamino bodies), PAS-positive and diastase-resistant (resembling colloid bodies), have been reported in 60 percent of EC-SC nevi[73] (see Fig. 91-16). Similar globules may be detected in 2 percent of melanomas and 0.9 percent of typical acquired nevi, but the globules are smaller in size, more difficult to find, single rather than coalescent, and commonly PAS-negative.[73]

A histopathologic diagnosis of EC-SC nevus depends on the presence of multiple histopathologic features, none of which have been subjected to systematic testing for predictive value. Features believed to distinguish EC-SC nevi from melanomas include presence in the former of bizarre mononuclear and multinucleated giant cells, maturation of tumor cells with increasing depth (as reflected in mean nuclear size and DNA content), prominent coalescent eosinophilic globules, and artifactual clefts of junctional nests and absence of atypical mitoses, nuclear pleomorphism, prominent upward spread of nevomelanocytes as single cells or small nests in the epidermis, or hyperchromasia of tumor cells. Favoring the diagnosis of melanoma (and a potential for metastasis) are deep dermal invasion, intense melanin production in the dermis, arrangement of epithelioid cells in contiguous aggregates, atypical mitoses, and lack of cellular maturation with increasing tumor depth.

FIGURE 91-16

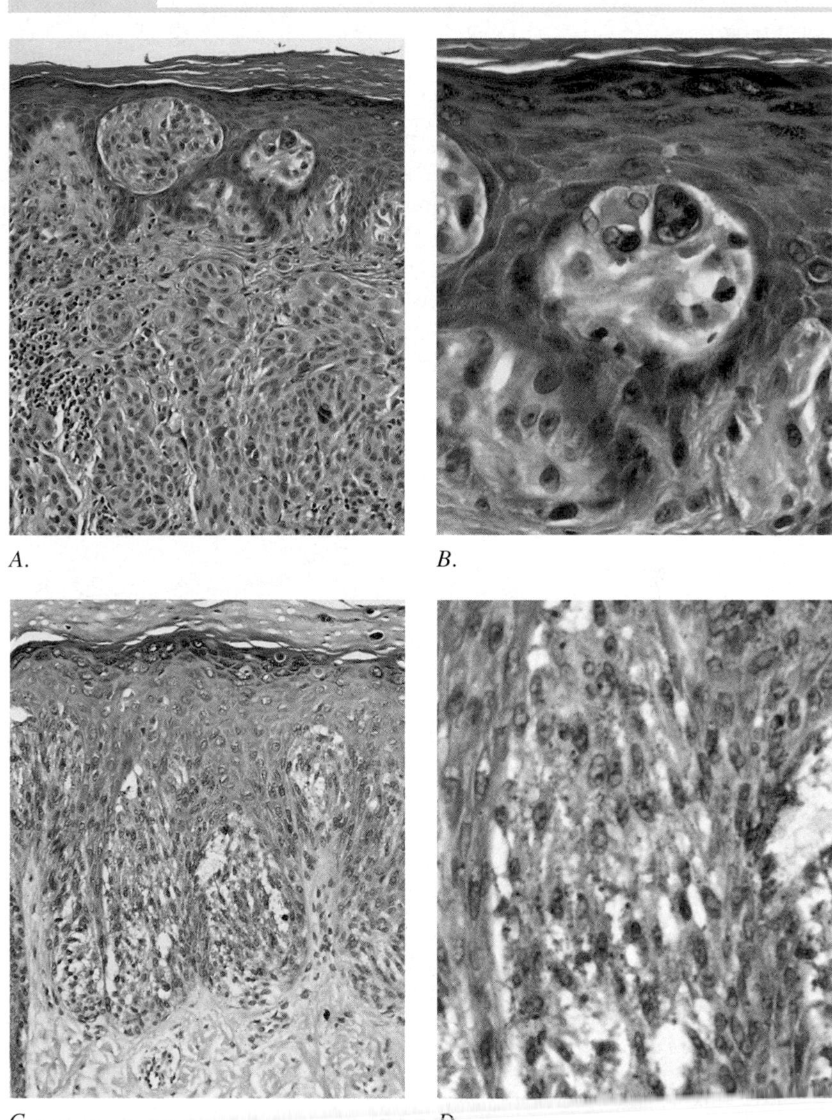

Histopathologic features of acquired epithelioid and/or spindle cell nevi. Epithelioid Spitz nevus (*A*) and higher magnification of the intraepidermal component revealing eosinophilic cytoplasmic changes in several cells (*B*). Pigmented spindle cell nevus (*C*) and higher magnification of the intraepidermal component (*D*) revealing pigmented spindle shaped cells.

DIAGNOSIS Nonpigmented varieties of EC-SC nevi (see Fig. 91-13) may resemble amelanotic melanoma, juvenile xanthogranuloma, hemangioma, pyogenic granuloma, molluscum contagiosum, dermal nevomelanocytic nevus, solitary mastocytoma, granuloma, clear cell acanthoma, insect bite reaction, and dermatofibroma. Pigmented varieties of EC-SC nevus (see Figs. 91-14 and 91-15) may appear similar to melanoma, dysplastic melanocytic nevus, fibrous histiocytoma, sclerosing hemangioma, appendage tumor, keloid, and unusual varieties of acquired junctional and compound nevus called *hypermelanotic nevus*.[74] Warty variants of EC-SC nevi may be confused for verrucca vulgaris, seborrheic keratosis, and epidermal nevus.

TREATMENT Complete excision with a clear margin of normal skin is generally sufficient treatment for EC-SC nevi. Given the difficulty of confidently excluding the possibility of melanoma, a wider margin of normal skin may be prudent for histopathologically worrisome lesions.[75] Incompletely excised lesions may recur in as many as 7 to 16 percent of patients. Management of patients who have numerous EC-SC nevi requires individual judgment and periodic examination for new or unstable lesions.

COURSE AND PROGNOSIS The natural history of the EC-SC nevus is unknown because lesions are usually singular, and histopathologic confirmation is required to establish the diagnosis. It is possible that some lesions regress spontaneously. A concern is that some varieties of EC-SC nevus may progress to melanoma or represent melanoma at the outset.[75] Tumors believed to have histopathologic features similar to EC-SC nevus occasionally may metastasize.[75] The pigmented spindle cell nevus variant of EC-SC nevus is said to have a benign course in most cases but prospective studies of intact lesions are not available.

Blue Nevus

The blue nevus consists of an acquired or congenital blue, blue-gray, or blue-black papule, nodule, or plaquelike aggregate of aberrant dermal melanocytes actively producing melanin. Three types of blue nevus are recognized: (1) common blue nevus, (2) cellular blue nevus, and

(3) combined blue nevus–nevomelanocytic nevus. The cellular blue nevus differs from the common blue nevus in that it is usually larger, more elevated, more aggressive locally, and occasionally associated with lymph node "benign metastasis." Melanoma may develop in a cellular blue nevus. Other names for blue nevus include *benign mesenchymal melanoma, blue neuronevus, chromatophoroma, melanofibroma, blue nevus of Jadassohn-Tieche, pilar neurocristic hamartoma,* and *dermal melanocytoma.*

HISTORICAL ASPECTS The blue nevus was described by Tieche in 1906, but similar lesions had been described earlier as chromatophoromas by Riecke and as melanofibromas by Kreibich. The cellular blue nevus was classified originally as a variant of melanoma by Darier in 1925 and reclassified as a variant of blue nevus by Allen in 1949.[54] A malignant variant of cellular blue nevus has been described as an entity separate from both melanoma and cellular blue nevus. Tuthill et al.[76] defined a unique presentation of grouped blue nevi with peripilar arrangement of pigment-laden cells called *pilar neurocristic hamartoma.* An atypical variant of peripilar blue nevus has been called *bizarre blue nevus.*

FIGURE 91-17

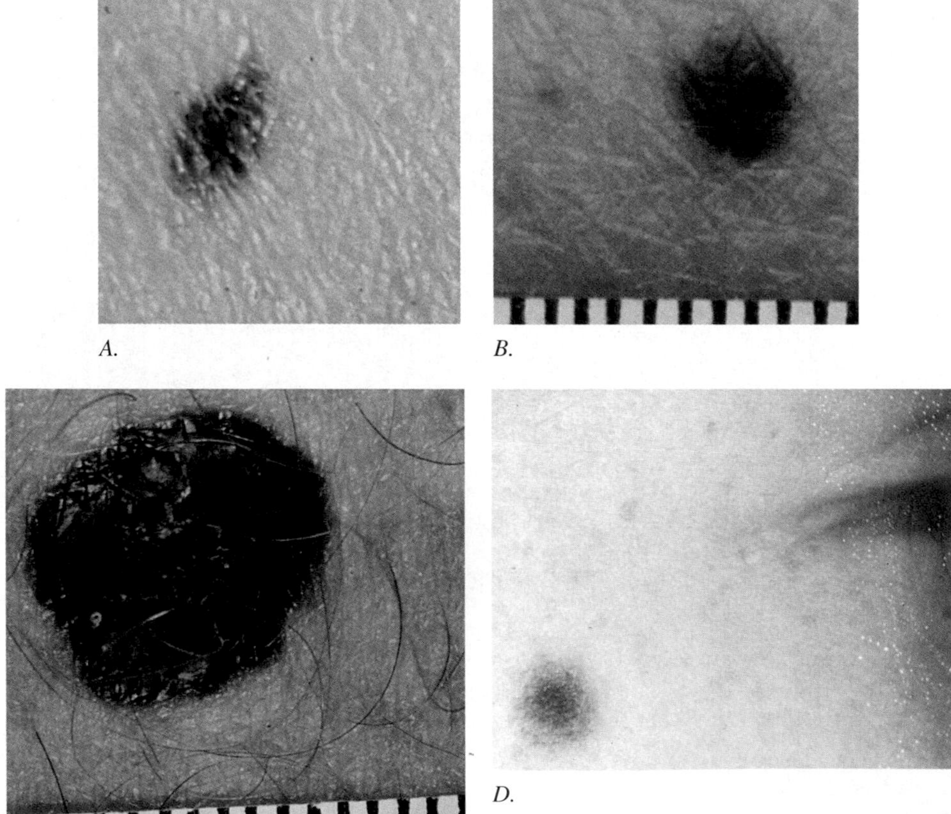

Blue nevus. *A.* Common blue nevus appearing as an acquired blue-gray papule on the shoulder of an 18-year-old white woman. *B.* Common blue nevus appearing as an acquired blue-gray papule on the buttock of an 62-year-old white man. *C.* Cellular blue nevus appearing as a congenital blue papule on the low back of a 30-year-old white man. *D.* Combined common blue nevus–nevomelanocytic nevus appearing as a brown papule with a blue-gray center on the cheek of a 12-year-old white boy, beginning as a pinpoint dot at age 1 year and enlarging slowly over time. Scale in millimeters.

EPIDEMIOLOGY Blue nevi are present in fewer than 1 in 3000 newborns, in about 1 in 1000 during the first 5 years of life, and in 1 to 2 percent of white school children, 3 percent of Japanese adults, and 0.5 to 4 percent of healthy white adults. They are said to be uncommon in darkly pigmented persons. The vast majority of blue nevi are single, small, deep-blue macules or papules about 1 to 2 mm in diameter.

Multiple blue nevi may be associated with lentigines, cardiac myxoma, and mucocutaneous myxomas (LAMB syndrome). Blue nevi have been associated with nodular mastocytosis, and a histogenic relationship has been claimed for melanocytes and mast cells. Blue nevi have been reported to occur in oral mucosa, uterine cervix, vagina, spermatic cord, prostate, and lymph nodes.

ETIOLOGY AND PATHOGENESIS Although a Schwann cell or endoneural origin is postulated for blue nevi based on ultrastructural features and cholinesterase activity, a melanocytic origin is suggested by the presence of obvious melanin synthesis in common blue nevi and ultrastructural evidence of melanin synthesis in cellular blue nevi. The common blue nevus is believed to represent an ectopic accumulation of melanin-producing melanocytes in the dermis during their migration from the neural crest to sites in the skin, i.e., a normal melanocyte with an abnormal location and abnormal function. An origin from melanocytes in hair follicles is also believed possible. An additional hypothesis is that common blue nevi and cellular blue nevi represent benign neoplasms, each resulting from an abnormal melanoblast derived from the neural crest. The causative factor in eruptive blue nevi has been attributed to sun exposure,[77] although other etiologies are possible.

CLINICAL MANIFESTATIONS Common blue nevi are usually acquired, solitary, asymptomatic blue, blue-gray, or blue-black papules, usually less than 10 mm in diameter (Fig. 91-17). The blue-gray color of blue nevi is an optical effect of dermal melanin viewed through the overlying skin. The longer wavelengths of visible light penetrate the deep dermis and are absorbed by black dermal melanin, but the shorter (blue) wavelengths do not penetrate deeply enough to be absorbed by melanin and are thus reflected back to the observer's eye, giving a blue-gray cast to the deeply situated melanin. Common blue nevi occur anywhere, but about half the reported cases present on the dorsa of hands and feet. Usually, the common blue nevus is singular, but rarely, lesions may be multiple and agminated or arranged in large plaques consisting of multiple solitary papules or nodules with intervening areas of blue discoloration. The large plaque blue nevus (pilar neurocristic hamartoma) may be apparent at birth or later in childhood and occasionally is associated with a background of lentigo simplex (nevus spilus). The common blue nevus occasionally may have a target-like appearance, with a blue-gray central nodule, a flesh-colored or hypopigmented surrounding area, and a blue-black rim. The target blue nevus occurs mostly on the hands and feet but also on the back and perianal area. Hypopigmented blue nevi with only minimal identifiable melanin pigment have been reported. Common blue nevi occasionally may have satellite lesions that may be mistaken for melanoma metastasis.[78]

Cellular blue nevi are blue-gray or blue-brown nodules or plaques 1 to 3 cm in diameter, occasionally larger (see Fig. 91-17). Their surface is usually smooth but may be irregular. About half the cases are located on the buttocks or sacrum. Rare giant varieties of congenital blue nevus occur, often with multiple satellite lesions. Cellular blue nevi may develop in association with congenital nevomelanocytic nevi, occasionally with target appearance.

Combined blue nevus–nevomelanocytic nevus (see Fig. 91-17) and a compound variant of blue nevus are usually diagnosed clinically as atypical nevi or suspected melanomas. These lesions are blue brown and/or blue black, variable in size, and have a smooth or slightly irregular elevated surface.

Malignant blue nevus may develop in contiguity with a cellular blue nevus, nevus of Ota (see Chap. 90), combined congenital blue nevus–nevus of Ota, or de novo. Malignant blue nevus presents as an expanding dermal nodule with or without ulceration. There is some dispute as to whether malignant blue nevus should be considered a separate entity from melanoma or simply referred to as a melanoma developing in a blue nevus.

PATHOLOGY In common blue nevi, dermal melanocytes appear as melanin-containing fibroblast-like cells grouped in irregular bundles admixed with melanin-containing macrophages, ultimately associated with excessive fibrous tissue in the middle or upper reticular dermis, occasionally extending downward to subcutaneous fat or upward to papillary dermis (Fig. 91-18). Elongated melanin-producing dermal melanocytes in common blue nevi usually lie with their long axis parallel to the epidermis. Except in the case of combined blue nevus–nevomelanocytic nevus, the epidermis in common blue nevi appears normal. In the combined blue nevus–nevomelanocytic nevus, there is a blue nevus associated with a typical nevomelanocytic nevus or EC-SC nevus. A close histopathologic association between blue nevi and nevomelanocytic nevi has been noted in 1 percent of melanocytic nevi excised for histopathologic examination. The compound variant of blue nevus is remarkable for hyperplasia of dendritic melanocytes in the epidermis and common blue nevus in the dermis.

Pathology of the plaquelike blue nevus (pilar neurocristic hamartoma) reveals a peripilar grouped arrangement of mostly spindle cells containing varying amounts of melanin, patterns of a common blue nevus and a Mongolian spot, and presence of abnormal (granular) melanosomes. There are other varieties of plaquelike blue nevi with subcutaneous cellular nodules with a range of histologic appearances from dermal melanosis to common blue and cellular blue nevi.[79]

In cellular blue nevi, there is usually a component of a common blue nevus plus fascicles of spindle-shaped cells with ovoid nuclei and abundant pale cytoplasm with little or no melanin, and often epithelioid cells, present in the dermis and often in subcutaneous fat in nests, bundles, and neuroid forms with little or no intervening stroma (see Fig. 91-18). Epithelioid cell and amelanotic varieties of the cellular blue nevus have been described. Epithelioid blue nevi have been reported with[80] or without[81] an association with cardiac myxoma. Histopathologic diagnosis may be difficult when the common blue nevus component and melanin production are sparse or inapparent. Ultrastructural studies combined with dopa histochemistry demonstrate that cells of cellular blue nevi are capable of melanin production, and therefore, the cells are melanocytes and not Schwann cells. Atypical melanosomes may be seen in cellular blue nevi. Some varieties of cellular blue nevi stain for CD-34, suggesting an origin from cells derived from the neural crest.[82] Differentiation between a cellular blue nevus and a melanoma that has developed in a cellular blue nevus may be difficult. Occasionally, small groups of well-differentiated melanocytes are present in the marginal sinus or parenchyma of lymph nodes draining the anatomic site of the cellular blue nevus, making it difficult to differentiate true metastasis from pseudometastasis. It is believed that "inert" deposits of melanocytes in the capsules and peripheral sinuses of lymph nodes draining some varieties of cellular blue nevus are transported passively. An alternative hypothesis is that these cellular deposits represent ectopic embryologic rests. The malignant blue nevus may be regarded as a variant of melanoma, distinguished from cellular blue nevus by invasiveness, cellular atypia, pleomorphism, atypical mitoses, and areas of necrosis. There are atypical variants of cellular blue nevi that are intermediate in histopathologic appearance between typical cellular blue nevi and melanoma.[83]

DIAGNOSIS AND DIFFERENTIAL DIAGNOSIS Blue nevus may be confused clinically with sclerosing hemangioma, dermatofibroma, histiocytoma, glomus tumor, primary or metastatic melanoma, pyogenic granuloma, pigmented spindle cell nevus, and traumatic tattoo. There are acquired variants of macular dermal melanocytosis that may cause confusion for blue nevus. Mongolian spots, nevus of Ota, and nevus of Ito are also accumulations of melanin-producing melanocytes, but unlike typical blue nevus, these forms of dermal melanocytosis are usually broad in extent and macular.

TREATMENT A common blue nevus that is stable for many years in an adult usually requires no therapy. Sudden appearance of a blue nodule, expansion of a preexisting blue nodule, a congenital blue nodule, or a relatively large blue nodule or plaque greater than 10 mm in diameter demands histopathologic examination. Excision should include subcutaneous fat to ensure complete removal of deep dermal melanocytes, which are frequently present in the subcutaneous tissue of cellular blue nevus. The large plaque blue nevus (pilar neurocristic hamartoma) requires consideration for excision or periodic evaluation for suspicious change. Cellular blue nevus should be evaluated for excision because of its malignant potential.

COURSE AND PROGNOSIS The natural evolution has not been studied for common blue nevi or cellular blue nevi. It is likely that once established, blue nevi remain unchanged or possibly regress over time. More than a dozen cases of melanoma have been noted to evolve in cellular blue nevus.

Congenital Neyomelanocytic Nevus

Congenital nevomelanocytic nevi (CNNs; synonyms: *garment nevus, nevus pigmentosus et pilosus, giant nevus, verrucous nevus,* and *giant pigmented nevus*) are nevomelanocytic nevi apparent at birth. However, there are also rare varieties of relatively large nevomelanocytic nevi (>1.5 cm) that appear for the first time between 1 month and 2 years of life, according to parental observations and corroborated by photographs (tardive congenital nevi).

HISTORICAL ASPECTS In 1832, a giant "waist coat and drawers" nevus was described by Alibert. In 1861, Rokitansky described a patient with a giant CNN and leptomeningeal hyperpigmentation. The malignant potential of giant CNN was documented as early as 1879 by Jablokoff and Klein, and there were at least 53 cases by 1959.[84] The malignant potential of smaller varieties of CNN was illustrated in 1982 based on historic and histopathologic association compared with expected association based on chance and body-surface-area considerations.[85] Staged excisions of very large CNNs were reported

FIGURE 91-18

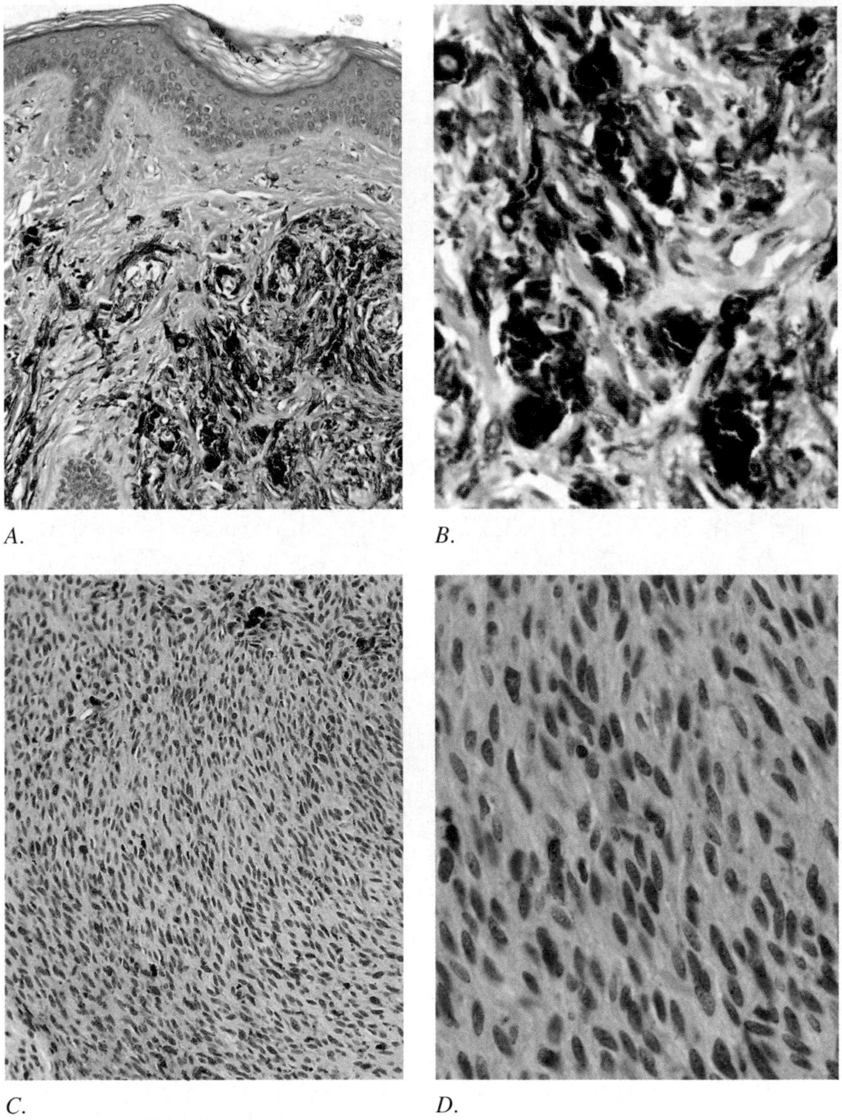

A. B.

C. D.

Histopathologic features of common and cellular blue nevi. Common blue nevus (*A*) and higher magnification of the dermal component (*B*) revealing heavily pigmented, elongated melanocytes. Cellular blue nevus (*C*) and higher magnification (*D*) revealing sheets of melanocytes with ovoid nuclei.

by Baker in 1878 and later by Morestin in 1915 and Roy in 1925. The histopathologic appearance of very large CNNs was reviewed in detail by Reed et al.[86] in 1965. Microscopic similarities between large and small varieties of CNN and differences from acquired nevi have been noted.[44]

EPIDEMIOLOGY Some 2.5 percent of newborns have pigmented lesions,[87] but only 1 percent have a biopsy-confirmed nevomelanocytic nevus. The most reliable prevalence rate for CNN in a homogeneous racial group was obtained by biopsying all pigmented lesions in 841 white infants examined within 72 h of birth; of 21 infants with pigmented lesions, 7 babies (0.83 percent of 841) had a biopsy-confirmed nevomelanocytic nevus.[87] Many other series have yielded equivalent results. The vast majority of CNNs noted at birth are small and singular, and no gender predilection has been demonstrated.

ETIOLOGY AND PATHOGENESIS The congenital divided nevus of the eyelid (Fig. 91-19) is an important natural experiment, for it reflects the probable time of development of CNN in utero.[88] Because of the contiguous nature of this lesion on the upper and lower eyelids,[5] it may be presumed that the nevus was already in place during or after eyelid fusion but before the eyelids split. The eyelids form at between 5 and 6 weeks in utero, begin to fuse at about 8 to 9 weeks, and reopen during the sixth uterine month. Because melanocytes begin to appear in fetal skin before 40 days' estimated gestational age, it is likely that CNNs form after that time but before the sixth uterine month. Familial aggregation has been demonstrated for both large and small varieties of CNN (Fig. 91-20). This observation is remarkable considering that CNNs of 99 mm or more in diameter occur in only 1 of every 20,000 newborns, and CNNs with a garment distribution occur in only 1 of every 500,000 newborns. Discordance for giant CNNs has been demonstrated for identical twins in at least three cases and for nonidentical twins in two cases. It is likely that developmental and genetic mechanisms play some role in CNN development.

CLINICAL MANIFESTATIONS Although CNNs are on average larger than acquired nevi, there is no specific size limitation that can be used to predict reliably wheather a given nevus is congenital or acquired for lesions less than 1.5 cm in diameter. Nevi attaining a diameter of 1.5 cm or more are likely to be congenital, atypical, or melanomas.

There is no completely satisfactory way to separate CNNs as small or large. Definitions based on ease of removal and absolute size are most popular. CNNs may be defined as small if they can be excised easily and the wound defect closed primarily without significant deformity and without using skin flaps or grafts (see Fig. 91-20). Based on these practical definitions, otherwise "small" CNNs in noncritical sites (such as the torso or buttocks) might be regarded as "large" in critical anatomic sites (such as the face, digits, or genitalia). Arbitrary size criteria to categorize CNNs as small, large, or giant also have been based on the diameter or surface area of a given lesion. *Giant* has been variously defined as a lesion as large as the patient's palm for the face or neck (and twice that area for other anatomic sites), 30 percent of the body surface (Fig. 91-21), or 900 cm^2 in adults (or smaller if it involves a major anatomic area). Others have arbitrarily divided CNNs according to the largest diameter as small (<1.5 cm), medium (1.5–19.9 cm), and large (≥ 20 cm). Lesions that are regarded as small or medium in the newborn period may be designated medium or large, respectively, by late childhood or adulthood, given that CNNs appear to grow in proportion to the affected anatomic site.[89]

The overall appearance of CNNs and acquired nevi is similar (see Figs. 91-12, 91-19, 91-20 and 91-21). In general, CNNs are usually round or oval, and skin markings distort the skin surface at least slightly when assessed by oblique lighting. The outlines of CNNs are usually smooth, regular, and sharply demarcated (see Figs. 91-12 and 91-21). At birth, some CNNs have coarse and long hairs, whereas others are relatively hairless; coarse, long, darkly pigmented hair may appear within the first year or two of life or be delayed for several years. Lesions may have a smooth, pebbly, rugose, verrucous, cerebriform, or grossly lobular surface (see Fig. 91-21).

FIGURE 91-19

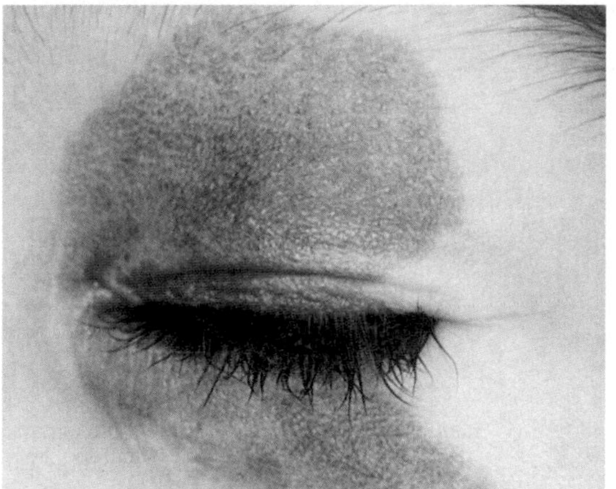

Congenital divided nevomelanocytic nevus of the eyelid. The nevus is contiguous when the eyelids are closed, suggesting that the lesion was formed in the developing fetus before the eyelids split, i.e., before 24 weeks.

CNNs with a cerebriform appearance may present as cutis verticis gyrata.

CNNs usually have a uniform pigmentation pattern consisting of medium- or dark-brown speckles symmetrically disposed in a tan or light-brown field or a reticular pattern when assessed by dermoscopy. Other patterns are similar to those described for acquired nevi. Unique varieties of CNNs may have an atypical appearance, striking for their haphazard, very dark-brown, black, or blue-black pigmentation or discontinuous pigmentation and poorly demarcated and/or irregular outlines, often associated with atypical histopathologic features. Very darkly pigmented CNNs are distinctly uncommon in whites and should suggest the possibility of atypical histopathologic features. In darkly pigmented infants, CNNs are usually even more darkly pigmented.

FIGURE 91-20

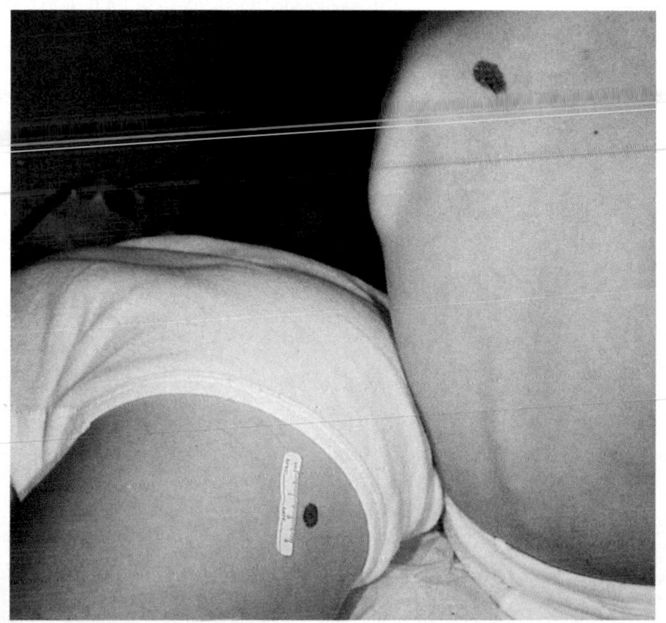

Familial aggregation of small congenital nevomelanocytic nevi. Note small congenital nevus on the thigh of a 3-year-old white boy and on the back of his 5-year-old male sibling.

FIGURE 91-21

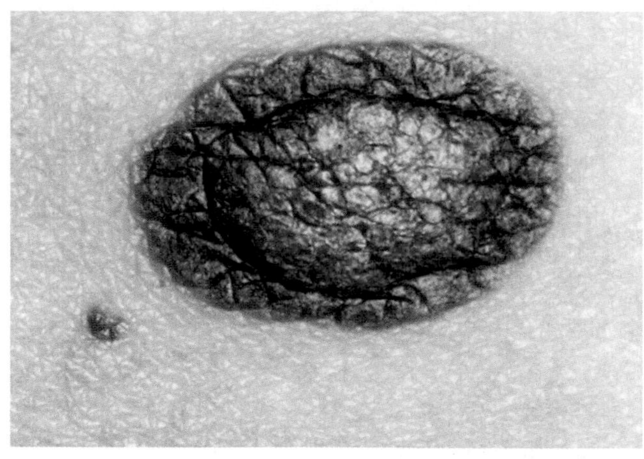

Small congenital nevomelanocytic nevus, 12 mm in diameter. Note regular configuration, heavy regular pigmentation, and slightly corrugated surface.

While small CNNs usually occur as single lesions, giant CNNs often present as single, very large lesions or multiple smaller CNNs (Fig. 91-22). CNNs may have a delayed onset, often appearing during infancy and as late as early childhood. Histopathologically, these late lesions nonetheless show all the features of CNNs (see below). In giant CNNs nevomelanocytes have been found in regional lymph nodes without further evidence of progressive metastatic disease.

There is a significant association between neurofibromatosis and giant CNNs. In a study by Crowe et al.,[90] 3 of 223 patients with neurofibromatosis had extensive CNNs. In his monograph on neurofibromatosis, von Recklinghausen described 1 of 28 patients as having a giant CNN. Tumors indistinguishable from neurofibroma in the absence of von Recklinghausen's neurofibromatosis may develop in association with giant varieties of CNN.

CNNs of the head or neck area or posterior midline may be associated with underlying cranial and/or spinal leptomeningeal melanocytosis. This phenomenon may be asymptomatic or may give rise to communicating or noncommunicating hydrocephalus, seizures, focal neurologic deficits, mental retardation, or even melanoma. CNNs need not be giant to be associated with this underlying disorder. Symptomatic leptomeningeal melanocytosis carries a poor prognosis, even in the absence of malignant degeneration. Both small and large varieties of CNNs have been associated with loss of pigmentation, halo depigmentation (see Fig. 91-12), and even regression.

The relationship between melanoma and large CNNs is well documented. The risk of melanoma development is proportional to the size of the congenital nevus,[91] with clear evidence of increased risk in patients with congenital nevi that involve over 5 percent of the body surface.[41] The cumulative 5-year risk has been calculated to be 2.3 percent[93] and 5.7 percent.[94] The lifetime risk of melanoma for patients with very large CNNs has been estimated to be at least 6.3 percent, based on a questionnaire follow-up study of 151 persons with CNNs examined between 1915 and 1973 in Denmark.[95] Melanoma may develop in large CNNs at any time, but the diagnosis of melanoma was established in the first 3–5 years of life in about half of published cases in which patients ultimately developed melanoma in association with giant CNN.

FIGURE 91-22

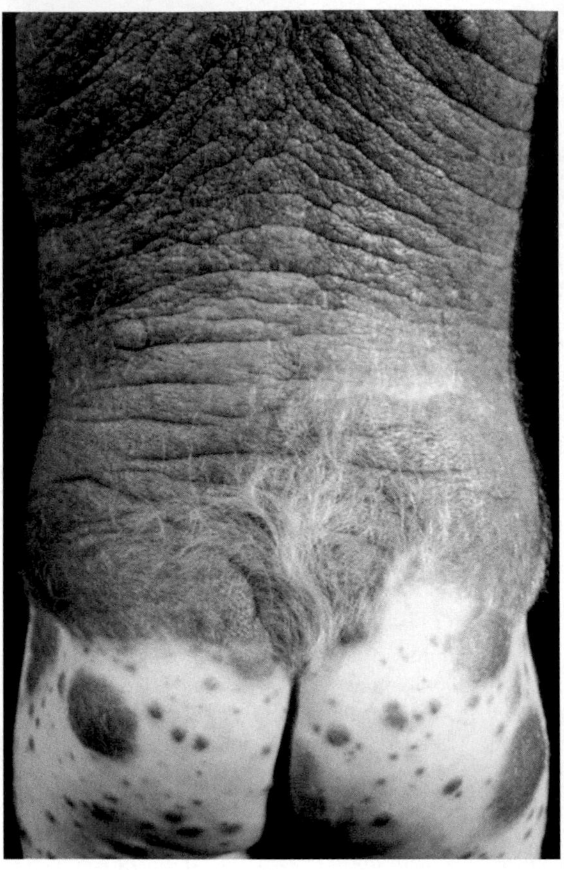

Giant congenital nevomelanocytic nevus. The lesion involves the entire back; the surface is pebbly; rugose, in areas even cerebriform, and there is hypertrichosis in the sacral region. There are also multiple smaller CNNs on the buttocks, thighs, and elsewhere on the body. Most of these were not present at birth but developed during infancy.

Malignant degeneration of large CNNs may be associated with the relatively sudden appearance of a dermal or subcutaneous nodule, very dark pigmentation, itching, pain, bleeding, or ulceration. Often, CNN-associated melanomas appear to have evolved in nonepidermal locations.[86] Therefore, early detection of melanoma in association with a giant CNN may be difficult and not recognized until a dermal nodule or metastatic disease appears. The prognosis for patients who develop melanoma in association with giant CNNs is usually grave.[86] Unlike melanoma in general, there is no racial predilection for melanoma developing in a giant CNN. There have been multiple cases of lethal melanoma developing in association with giant CNNs in black children.

A causal association between small CNNs and melanoma is more difficult to establish than for large CNNs. When histopathologic features were studied, 6 to 8 percent of primary melanomas were found to be in contiguity with nevi that had microscopic features characteristic of CNN.[96,97] These findings support the concept of melanoma evolution even in small congenital nevi, given the expected chance association based on body-surface-area considerations.[85]

PATHOLOGY CNNs are characterized by the presence of nevomelanocytes in the epidermis as well-ordered theques and/or nevomelanocytes in the dermis as sheets, nests, cords, and/or single cells. Although histopathologic features are cited as being useful in distinguishing nevi as congenital or acquired, there are no known features with absolute specificity and sensitivity. The histopathologic features of very large CNNs may be divided into nevomelanocytic, neuroid, epithelioid cell and/or spindle cell, dermal melanocytic, and mixed types.

In the nevomelanocytic type of large CNN, the histopathologic appearance may be identical to typical acquired nevi, with nevomelanocytes in the epidermis as well-defined theques and/or nevomelanocytes in the papillary dermis as sheets, cords, or nests. CNNs are more likely than acquired nevi to have nevomelanocytes in the lower two-thirds of the reticular dermis or deeper and to be associated with nevomelanocytes in appendageal and neurovascular structures in the reticular dermis (Fig. 91-23). There may be preferential involvement of one or more epithelial structures in CNN, such as eccrine ducts, and these structures may be abundant and malformed. Veins may be preferentially involved, with an "inflammatory" appearance showing nevomelanocytes within and around blood vessel walls. Subendothelial protrusion by nevomelanocytes in lymphatic vessels may be prominent. Arrector pili may be malformed, large, and infiltrated by nevomelanocytes.

FIGURE 91-23

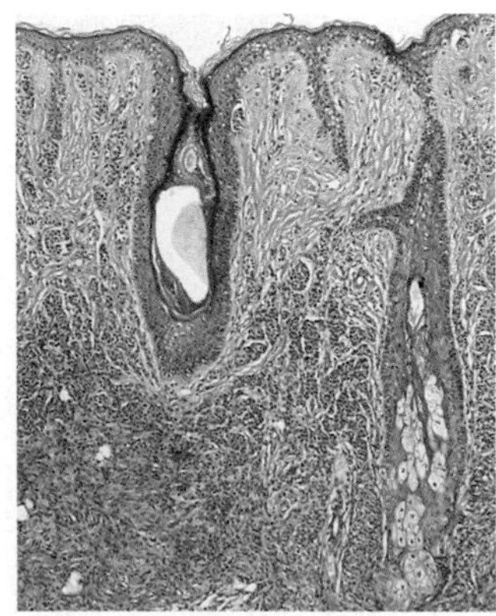

A.

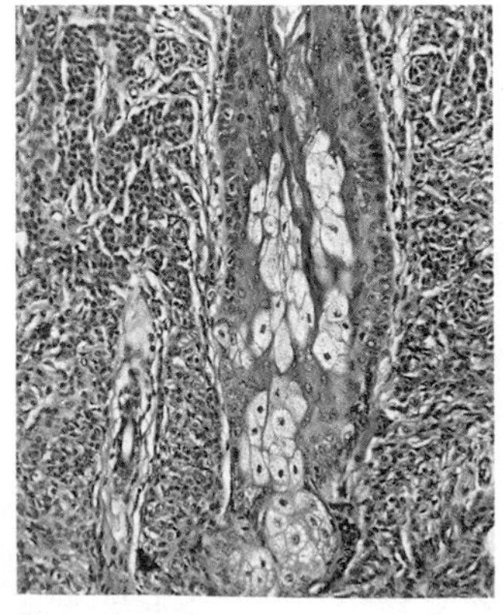

B.

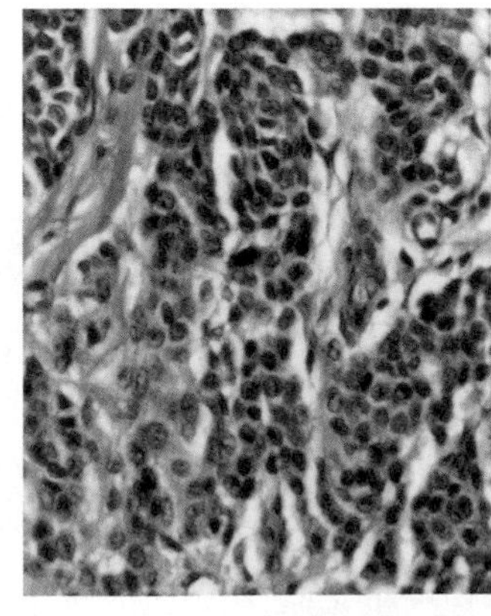

C.

Histopathologic features of congenital nevomelanocytic nevus. Nevomelanocytes in the low-magnification image (*A*) reveal dense accumulation in the lower two-thirds of the dermis; at medium magnification (*B*), these cells encroach on dermal adnexal structures (follicular and eccrine); and (*C*) higher magnification reveals dense collections of small nevomelanocytic cells.

Hair follicles are often quite large and frequently associated with abundant melanin in the hair bulb. Nevomelanocytes in the deep reticular dermis may be distributed as single cells or as a single-file array insinuating among collagen bundles, sheets of cells, or combinations of patterns.

In the neuroid type of giant CNN, melanocytic elements take on the appearance of Wagner-Meissner corpuscles (lames foliacée), a palisaded arrangement of cells around a cellular mass of homogeneous material (Verocay body), and sheathing of nerves by neuroid tissue (neuroid tubes). The neuroid type of nevus may be responsible for lobulation and redundancy of tissue (pachydermatous or cerebriform appearance) due mainly to the production of connective tissue elements, reticulin, collagen, and sometimes mucinous stroma. The neuroid type of giant CNN may take on the appearance of a pigmented neurofibroma and may be associated with congenital anomalies of bone (club foot, spina bifida, and atrophy) as well as with a "neurosarcomatous" morphologic variant of melanoma.

In the spindle cell and/or epithelioid cell type of giant CNN, the dermis may be infiltrated in whole or in part by nests or sheets of epithelioid cells and/or spindle cells. Unlike the usual variety of acquired epithelioid cell and/or spindle cell nevus, the epithelioid and spindle cell elements in CNN may involve deep reticular dermis, often intermixing with neuroid elements and ordinary nevomelanocytes. The epithelioid cell and/or spindle cell elements in giant CNN may have atypical cellular and architectural features, making differentiation from melanoma extremely difficult. In some cases, large epithelioid cells may comprise superficial papillary zones of the nevus, and smaller nevomelanocytes may appear in the same lesion in deeper zones of the reticular dermis, with a Grenz zone separating the two elements.

In the dermal melanocytic type of giant CNN, the appearance may be that of a giant blue nevus, or the lesion may have elements of blue nevus (either common or cellular type). Heavily pigmented spindle-shaped melanocytes may occur alone or may be intermixed with nevomelanocytes in the reticular dermis or deeper.

Unique to the very large CNN is the occasional presence of nevomelanocytes within the substance of muscle, bone, placenta, umbilical cord, cranium, and dura mater. Very extensive CNN may be intermixed with elements of vascular malformation, hemangiomas, increased numbers of mast cells, cartilage, calcification, and even bone. There may be sparse mononuclear cell infiltrates associated with some giant CNNs. In addition to melanoma, associated tumors developing in CNN include schwannoma, neuroid tumor, lipoma, rhabdomyosarcoma, neurofibroma, sebaceous nevus, blue nevus, epithelioid cell and/or spindle cell nevus, hemangioma, lymphangioma, and mastocytoma. A possible explanation of mixed neoplasms containing melanocytic and neuronal elements in CNN is that the neural crest is the origin not only of melanoblasts, Schwann cells, and sensory ganglia but also of bone, muscle, blood vessels, and fat.

Small CNNs may have a histopathologic appearance similar to large CNNs. When CNNs are compared with acquired nevi, CNNs are significantly more likely to show nevomelanocytes in the lower reticular dermis and to involve dermal appendages and neurovascular structures. The positive predictive value of nevomelanocytes in the midreticular dermis or deeper for diagnosing nevi as congenital may be estimated to be 76 to 97 percent based on available sensitivity and specificity data and a prevalence rate for CNNs of 50 percent of melanocytic tumors selected for excision at a pediatric hospital.[44] However, some CNNs cannot be distinguished microscopically from acquired nevi.

DIAGNOSIS AND DIFFERENTIAL DIAGNOSIS The differential diagnosis of CNN includes other pigmented lesions apparent at birth, including Mongolian spot, café-au-lait macule, lentigo simplex, nevus spilus, epidermal nevus, nevus sebaceous, arrector pili (smooth muscle) hamartoma, and "congenital" Becker's nevus. To experienced examiners, congenital pigmented lesions that are not melanocytic usually can be distinguished from CNN based on clinical examination alone. In some cases, a small biopsy may be required to confirm the presence of nevomelanocytes, particularly in relatively lightly pigmented and flat varieties of CNN. In lightly pigmented individuals, very dark pigmentation or haphazard pigmentation in a nevus (with or without irregular and/or poorly demarcated outlines) should suggest the possibility of intraepidermal melanocytic dysplasia, pigmented spindle cell nevus, or melanoma. An ulcerated surface, a nodule, or discontinuous pigmentation in a CNN should suggest the possibility of intraepidermal melanocytic dysplasia or melanoma. Any nevomelanocytic lesion that is 1.5 cm or greater in diameter (and is not a dysplastic melanocytic nevus or melanoma) is likely to be a CNN.

TREATMENT The treatment of CNNs, large and small, depends on the perceived risk of melanoma plus cosmetic and functional considerations. Strongly stated positions on both sides of the issue are reflected in clinical practice. The results from a questionnaire survey of academic and nonacademic dermatologists in 1984[98] revealed that (1) a clear majority referred their patients with very large CNNs for plastic surgical evaluation, (2) infants with very large CNNs usually were treated by 12 months of age, (3) an incidence of conversion to melanoma of 0.1 percent or greater warranted prophylactic removal of small CNNs, (4) about half the respondents excised small varieties of CNN in children and adults, and (5) fewer than 40 percent of dermatologists stated that they observe small CNNs rather than excise.

The most important consideration of CNN management relates to the perceived malignant potential. While there is disagreement about the exact frequency of association between CNN and melanoma, most students of the controversy would agree that at least some melanomas develop in CNNs, large and small. Melanoma may arise in very large CNNs even in the first several years of life. Therefore, excision of very large CNNs should be considered as early as possible, but it is probably prudent to wait until after the first 6 months of life to reduce surgical and anesthetic risks. Management of patients with very large CNNs must be individualized. Extensive involvement of the body surface, with little or no normal skin available for graft sites, may necessitate abandoning efforts at prophylactic excision and accepting lifelong surveilance to detect the earliest signs of malignant change. It may be impossible to remove every nevomelanocyte in very large CNNs, particularly when there is involvement of vital structures or deep anatomic zones. The treatment goal is to remove as much of the nevus as possible while preserving function and improving cosmetic appearance. Tissue expansion and artificial skin replacement are invaluable in repairing large wound defects. Other indications for surgical excision of very large CNNs include chronic pruritus, ulceration, and infection. In at least one case, infection of a puritic giant CNN resulted in sepsis and death. Unlike surgical excision, dermabrasion and other modes of destructive therapy do not address the malignant potential of CNN; nevomelanocytes may still be left behind in the dermis (if present initially), and the cosmetic results associated with destructive therapy are unpredictable. Melanoma has been reported following dermabrasion of large CNNs. Partial excision of a giant CNN resulting in "pseudomelanoma" has been described after laser treatment of a CNN.

The approach to small CNNs needs to be considered carefully. It appears that the risk of melanoma development depends on CNN size, and therefore, smaller lesions appear to have less risk. However, due to the smaller size, complete excision of small congenital nevi may be relatively straightforward, resulting in excellent cosmetic results. The risks and benefits need to be weighed carefully. The following considerations should be made when managing patients who have small CNNs. First, all CNNs should be documented at birth, preferably in the form of high-quality photographs that can be used to aid follow-up by parents and physicians. Follow-up will be complicated by the natural evolutionary changes that take place in a nevus during body growth (i.e., surface, size, color, and hair). Therefore, periodic updates of photographs may be warranted. A physician experienced in gross morphologic examination and histopathologic correlation should help to determine management decisions. Second, small CNNs should be considered for prophylactic excision. However, given the risk of general anesthesia for lesions perceived to be at low risk during the first decade of life, it is appropriate to consider waiting until the child is old enough to tolerate local anesthesia. Careful surveillance without excision may be an option depending on gross appearance, size, location, cosmetic and functional deficits (or improvement) resulting from excision, and general health issues. Third, atypical-appearing CNNs should be considered for immediate prophylactic excision because even small CNNs may give rise to melanomas during infancy and early childhood. Fourth, during follow-up, suspicious changes in color, surface, or size would require urgent evaluation.

COURSE AND PROGNOSIS CNNs do not remain static after their appearance at birth. Lesions in fully grown individuals should remain stable, but CNNs have a dynamic evolution during body growth.[99] With few exceptions, CNNs generally expand in direct proportion to growth of a given anatomic zone, although disproportionately rapid area expansion of some congenital nevi may occur during early infancy.[89] In a 12-year follow-up of seven CNNs observed (and biopsied) in the newborn period, Nickoloff et al.[99] confirmed a two- to eightfold increase in size in five patients and no increase in size in two.

CNNs at birth usually distort the skin surface at least slightly when assessed by oblique lighting and may become more elevated over time. Surface pigmentation also may change. Lightly pigmented CNNs may become more darkly pigmented, and darkly pigmented CNNs eventually may become less pigmented. Relatively hairless CNNs at birth may develop long, dark, coarse hair or may maintain a relatively normal hair density. Very large CNNs may demonstrate fading of surface pigmentation over time. CNNs also may develop a halo of depigmentation (see Fig.91-12), potentially heralding spontaneous regression. Loss of pigmentation has been associated with regression of underlying nevomelanocytes and the replacement with sclerosis in some cases. Although acquired nevi are believed to regress with old age, there are no natural history studies to document this phenomenon for CNNs or acquired nevi.

REFERENCES

1. Coleman WP et al: Nevi, lentigines, and melanomas in blacks. *Arch Dermatol* **116**:548, 1980
2. Tasaki K: On band or linear pigmentation of the nails. *Jpn J Dermatol* **33**:568, 1983
3. Ito M, Hamada Y: Nevus spilus en nappe. *Tohoku J Exp Med* **55**:44, 1952
4. Cohen HJ et al: Nevus spilus. *Arch Dermatol* **102**:433, 1970
5. Kopf AW et al: Congenital nevus-like nevi, nevi spili, and cafe-au-lait spots in patients with malignant melanoma. *J Dermatol Surg Oncol* **11**:275, 1985
6. Sato S et al: Divided nevus spilus and divided form of spotted grouped pigmented nevus. *J Cutan Pathol* **6**:507, 1977
7. Rhodes AR, Mihm MC Jr: Origin of cutaneous melanoma in a congenital dysplastic nevus spilus. *Arch Dermatol* **126**:500, 1990
8. Grinspan D et al: Melanoma on dysplastic nevus spilus. *Int J Dermatol* **36**:499, 1997
9. Breathnach AS: Melanocyte distribution in forearm epidermis of freckled human subjects. *J Invest Dermatol* **29**:253, 1957
10. Wilson PD, Kligman AM: Experimental induction of freckles by ultraviolet-B. *Br J Dermatol* **106**:401, 1982
11. Rhodes AR et al: Increased intraepidermal melanocyte frequency and size in dysplastic melanocytic nevi and cutaneous melanoma: A comparative quantitative study of dysplastic melanocytic nevi, superficial spreading melanoma, nevocellular nevi, and solar lentigines. *J Invest Dermatol* **80**:452, 1983
12. Rhodes AR et al: The PUVA-induced pigmented macule: A lentiginous proliferation of large, sometimes cytologically atypical, melanocytes. *J Am Acad Dermatol* **9**:47, 1983
13. Crawley EP, Curtis AC: Lentigo senilis. *Arch Dermatol Syphilol* **62**:635, 1950
14. Hodgson C: Senile lentigo. *Arch Dermatol* **87**:197, 1963
15. Montagna W et al: A reinvestigation of solar lentigines. *Arch Dermatol* **116**:1151, 1980
16. Rhodes AR et al: The PUVA lentigo: An analysis of predisposing factors. *J Invest Dermatol* **81**:459, 1983
17. Kadunce DP et al: Persistent melanocytic lesions associated with cosmetic tanning bed use: "Sunbed lentigines." *J Am Acad Dermatol* **23**:1029, 1990
18. Azizi E et al: Skin type, hair color, and freckles are predictors of decreased minimal erythema ultraviolet radiation dose. *J Am Acad Dermatol* **19**:32, 1988
19. Mackie-RM: Personal risk-factor chart for cutaneous melanoma. *Lancet* **2**:487, 1989
20. Szabo G: Photobiology of melanogenesis: Cytological aspects with special reference to differences in racial coloration, in *Advances in Biology of the Skin,* vol 8, edited by W Montagna, F Hu. Oxford, England, Pergamon, 1967, p 379
21. Konrad K et al: Ultrastructure of poikiloderma-like pigmentary changes after repeated experimental PUVA overdosage. *J Cutan Pathol* **4**:219, 1977
22. Kraemer KH et al: Reduced DNA repair in cultured melanocytes and nevus cells from a patient with xeroderma pigmentosum. *Arch Dermatol* **125**:263, 1989
23. Takebe H et al: Melanoma and other skin cancers in xeroderma pigmentosum patients and mutation in their cells. *J Invest Dermatol* **92**:236S, 1989
24. Nakagawa H et al: Morphologic alterations of epidermal melanocytes and melanosomes in PUVA lentigines: A comparative ultrastructural investigation of lentigines induced by PUVA and sunlight. *J Invest Dermatol* **82**:101, 1985
25. Rhodes AR et al: Sun-induced freckles in children and young adults: A correlation of clinical and histopathologic features. *Cancer* **67**:1990, 1991
26. Barranco VP: Multiple benign lichenoid keratosis simulating photodermatoses: Evolution from senile lentigines and their spontaneous resolution. *J Am Acad Dermatol* **13**:201, 1985
27. Stern RS: The risk of melanoma in association with long-term exposure to PUVA. *J Am Acad Dermatol* **44**:755, 2001
28. MacKie RM et al: The number and distribution of benign pigmented moles (melanocytic naevi) in a healthy British population. *Br J Dermatol* **113**:167, 1985
29. Nicholls EM: Development and elimination of pigmented moles, and the anatomical distribution of primary malignant melanoma. *Cancer* **32**:191, 1973
30. Green A et al: Melanocytic nevi in schoolchildren in Queensland. *J Am Acad Dermatol* **20**:1054, 1989
31. Kelly JW et al: Sunlight: A major factor associated with the development of melanocytic nevi in Australian schoolchildren. *J Am Acad Dermatol* **30**:40,1994
32. Gallagher RP et al: Broad-spectrum sunscreen use and the development of new nevi in white children: A randomized controlled trial. *JAMA* **283**:2955, 2000
33. Zhu G et al. A major quantitative trait locus for mole density is linked to the familial melanoma gene CDKN2A: A maximum likelihood combined linkage and association analysis in twins and their sibs. *Am J Hum Genet* **65**:483, 1999
34. Lea PJ, Pawlowski A: Human melanocytic naevi. *Acta Derm Venereol (Stockh)* 127(suppl):5, 1986
35. Grichnik JM et al: KIT expression reveals a population of precursor melanocytes in human skin. *J Invest Dermatol* **106**:967, 1996
36. Robinson WA et al: Human acquired naevi are clonal. *Melanoma Res* **8**:499, 1998
37. Harada M et al: Clonality in nevocellular nevus and melanoma: An expression-based clonality analysis at the X-linked genes by polymerase chain reaction. *J Invest Dermatol* **109**:656, 1997
38. Hui P et al: Assessment of clonality in melanocytic nevi. *J Cutan Pathol* **28**:140, 2001
39. Tucker MA et al: Clinically recognized dysplastic nevi: A central risk factor for cutaneous melanoma. *JAMA* **277**:1439, 1997
40. Weinstock MA et al: Moles and site-specific risk of nonfamilial cutaneous malignant melanoma in women. *J Natl Cancer Inst* **81**:948, 1989

41. Swerdlow AJ et al: Benign melanocytic nevi as a risk factor for malignant melanoma. *Br Med J* **292**:1555, 1986
42. Seykora J, Elder D: Dysplastic nevi and other risk markers for melanoma. *Semin Oncol* **23**:682, 1996
43. Rhodes AR et al: Dysplastic melanocytic nevi: A reproducible histologic definition emphasizing cellular morphology. *Mod Pathol* **2**:306, 1989
44. Rhodes AR et al: A histologic comparison of congenital and acquired nevomelanocytic nevi. *Arch Dermatol* **121**:1266, 1985
45. Kornberg R, Ackerman AB: Pseudomelanoma: Recurrent melanocytic nevus following partial surgical removal. *Arch Dermatol* **111**:1588, 1975
46. Curley RK et al. Effect of incisional biopsy on subsequent histology of melanocytic nevi. *Br J Dermatol* **123**:503, 1990
47. Stegmaier OC: Natural regression of the melanocytic nevus. *J Invest Dermatol* **23**:413, 1959
48. Kantor GR, Wheeland RG: Transepidermal elimination of nevus cells: A possible mechanism of nevus involution. *Arch Dermatol* **123**:1371, 1987
49. Pehamberger H et al: In vivo epiluminescence microscopy of pigmented skin lesions: I. Pattern analysis of pigmented skin lesions. *J Am Acad Dermatol* **17**:571, 1987
50. Steiner A et al: In vivo epiluminescence microscopy of pigmented skin lesions: II. Diagnosis of small pigmented skin lesions and early detection of maligant melanoma. *J Am Acad Dermatol* **17**:584, 1987
51. Kelly JW et al: A high incidence of melanoma found in patients with multiple dysplastic naevi by photographic surveillance. *Med J Aust* **167**:191, 1997
52. Unna PG: *Histopathology of the Diseases of the Skin,* 1st ed, translated by N Walker. New York, MacMillan, 1896, p 1129
53. Allen AC: A reorientation on the histogenesis and clinical significance of cutaneous nevi and melanomas. *Cancer* **2**:28, 1949
54. Gartmann H: Transepidermale Ausscheidung von Nävus- und Melanomzellen. *Hautarzt* **33**:495, 1982
55. Richert S et al: Widespread eruptive dermal and atypical melanocytic nevi in association with chronic myelocytic leukemia: case report and review of the literature. *J Am Acad Dermatol* **35**:326, 1996
56. Larsson P-A, Liden S: Prevalence of skin disease among adolescents 12–16 years of age. *Acta Derm Venereol (Stockh)* **60**:415, 1980
57. Kopf AW et al: Broad spectrum of leukoderma acquisitum centrifugum. *Arch Dermatol* **92**:14, 1965
58. Mitchell MS et al: Comparison of cell-mediated immunity to melanoma cells in patients with vitiligo, halo nevi, or melanoma. *J Invest Dermatol* **75**:144, 1980
59. Copeman PS et al: Immunologic associations of the halo nevus with cutaneous melanoma. *Br J Dermatol* **88**:127, 1973
60. Reed RJ et al: Common and uncommon melanocytic nevi and borderline melanomas. *Semin Oncol* **2**:119, 1975
61. Zeff RA et al: The immune response in halo nevi. *J Am Acad Dermatol* **37**:620, 1997
62. Spitz S: Melanomas of childhood. *Am J Pathol* **3**:591, 1948
63. Kopf AW, Andrade R: Benign juvenile melanoma, in Yearbook of Dermatology 1965–1966, edited by AW Kopf, R Andrade. Chicago, Year Book, 1966, p 7
64. Helwig EB: Malignant melanoma in children, in *Neoplasms of the Skin and Malignant Melanoma*. Chicago, Year Book, 1976, p 11
65. Sagebiel RW et al: Pigmented spindle cell nevus: Clinical and histologic review of 90 cases. *Am J Surg Pathol* **8**:645, 1984
66. Weedon D, Little JH: Spindle and epithelioid cell nevi in children and adults: A review of 211 cases of Spitz nevus. *Cancer* **40**:217, 1977
67. Allen AC: Juvenile melanomas. *Ann NY Acad Sci* **100**:29, 1963
68. Bastian BC et al. Chromosomal gains and losses in primary cutaneous melanomas detected by comparative genomic hybridization. *Cancer Res* **58**:2170, 1998
69. Kernan JA, Ackerman LV: Spindle cell nevi and epithelioid cell nevi (so-called juvenile melanomas) in children and adults. *Cancer* **13**:612, 1960
70. Harvell JD et al: Spitz's nevi with halo reaction: A histopathologic study of 17 cases. *J Cutan Pathol* **24**:611, 1997
71. Gartmann H, Ganser M: Der Spitz-Naevus: Spindelzellen- und/oder Epitheloidzellnaevus-eine klinishe Analyse von 652 Tumoren. *Z Hautkr* **60**:22, 1984
72. Barnhill RS et al: The histologic spectrum of pigmented spindle cell nevus: A review of 120 cases with emphasis on atypical variants. *Hum Pathol* **22**:52, 1991
73. Kamino H et al: Eosinophilic globules in Spitz's nevus: New findings and a diagnostic sign. *Am J Dermatopathol* **1**:319, 1979
74. Cohen LM et al: Hypermelanotic nevus: Clinical histopathologic, and ultrastructural features in 316 cases. *Am J Dermatopathol* **19**:23, 1997
75. Barnhill RL et al: Atypical Spitz nevi/tumors: Lack of consensus for diagnosis, discrimination from melanoma, and prediction of outcome. *Hum Pathol* **30**:513, 1999
76. Tuthill RJ et al: Pilar neurocristic hamartoma: Its relationship to blue nevus and equine melanotic disease. *Arch Dermatol* **118**:592, 1982
77. Betti R et al: Agminate and plaque-type blue nevus combined with lentigo, associated with follicular cyst and eccrine changes: A variant of speckled lentiginous nevus. *Dermatology* **195**:387, 1997
78. Kang DS, Chung KY: Common blue perivascular dissemination resulting in clinical resemblance to malignant melanoma. *Br J Dermatol* **141**:992, 1999
79. Busam KJ et al: Large plaque-type blue nevus with subcutaneous cellular nodules. *J Cuttan Pathol* **24**:92, 2000
80. Carney JA, Ferreiro JA: The epithelioid blue nevus. A multicentric familial tumor with important associations, including cardiac myxoma and psammomatous melanotic schwannoma. *Am J Surg Pathol* **20**:259, 1996
81. Moreno C et al: Epithelioid blue nevus: A rare variant of blue nevus not always associated with the Carney complex. *J Cutan Pathol* **27**:218, 2000
82. Smith K et al: CD-34 positive cellular blue nevi. *J Cutan Pathol* **28**:145, 2001
83. Tran TA et al: Cellular blue nevus with atypia (atypical cellular blue nevus): A clinicopathologial study of nine cases. *J Cutan Pathol* **25**:252, 1998
84. Russel JL, Reyes RC: Giant pigmented nevi. *JAMA* **171**:2083, 1959
85. Rhodes AR et al: The malignant potential of small congenital nevocellular nevi: An estimate of association based on a histologic study of 234 primary cutaneous melanomas. *J Am Acad Dermatol* **6**:230, 1982
86. Reed WB et al: Giant pigmented nevi, melanoma, and leptomeningeal melanocytosis: A clinical and histopathological study. *Arch Dermatol* **91**:100, 1965
87. Walton RG et al: Pigmented lesions in newborn infants. *Br J Dermatol* **95**:389, 1976
88. Ribuffo D et al: Divided nevus of the eyelid: A case report. *Ophthalmic Plast Reconstr Surg* **12**:186, 1996
89. Rhodes AR et al: Congenital nevomelanocytic nevi: Proportionate area expansion during infancy and early childhood. *J Am Acad Dermatol* **34**:51, 1996
90. Crowe FW et al: *A Clinical, Pathological, and Genetic Study of Multiple Neurofibromatosis.* Springfield, IL, Charles C Thomas, 1956, p 181
91. Marghoob AA et al: Large congenital melanocytic nevi and the risk for the development of malignant melanoma: A prospective study. *Arch Dermatol* **132**:170, 1996
92. Swerdlow AJ et al: The risk of melanoma in patients with congenital nevi: A cohort study. *J Am Acad Dermatol* **32**:595, 1995
93. Bittencourt FV et al: Large congenital melanocytic nevi and the risk for development of malignant melanoma and neurocutuaneous melanosis. *Pediatrics* **106**:736, 2000
94. Egan CL et al: Cutaneous melanoma risk and phenotypic changes in large congenital nevi: A follow-up study of 46 patients. *J Am Acad Dermatol* **39**:923, 1998
95. Lorentzen M et al: The incidence of malignant transformation in giant pigmented nevi. *Scand J Plast Reconstr Surg* **11**:163, 1977
96. Harly S, Walsh N: A new look at melanomas. Am J Dermatopathol **18**:137, 1996
97. Betti R: Small congenital nevi associated with melanoma: Case reports and considerations. *J Dermatol* **27**:583, 2000
98. Sweren RJ: Management of congenital nevocytic nevi: A survey of current practices. *J Am Acad Dermatol* **11**:629, 1984
99. Nickoloff BJ et al: Immunohistologic patterns of congenital nevocellular nevi. *Arch Dermatol* **122**:1263, 1986
100. Rhodes AR: Public education and cancer of the skin: What people need to know about melanoma and nonmelanoma skin cancer. *Cancer* **75**:613, 1995

CHAPTER 92

Hensin Tsao
Arthur J. Sober

Atypical Melanocytic Nevi

Recognition of nonmalignant melanocytic and nevomelanocytic tumors is important because of their pathogenic relationship to cutaneous melanoma. A history of a preexisting pigmented lesion at the site of primary melanoma may be elicited in 18 to 85 percent of patients, while histologic remnants of nevus cells can be observed in 18 to 72 percent of melanoma cases.[1] Because the majority of adults have one or more pigmented lesions, it is important to identify melanocytic and nevomelanocytic hyperplasias that have an increased risk of developing melanoma from those pigmented lesions that carry little or no enhanced melanoma risk.

Atypical melanocytic nevi (AMN) are acquired, usually irregular-appearing, melanocytic tumors (Figs. 92-1 and 92-2), characterized histologically by architectural and/or cytologic atypia. AMN are important because they are potential histiogenic precursors of melanoma and markers of increased melanoma risk. Other names that have been used for AMN include atypical nevus, atypical mole, B-K mole (B and K represent family names of two kindreds in which atypical nevi aggregated with familial melanoma), Clark's nevus (after the late Dr. Wallace H. Clark, Jr.), and dysplastic nevus.

The older designation for AMN—"dysplastic nevus"—is derived from the Greek roots *dys* and *plasis* and refers to abnormal tissue development. Although the term *dysplasia* is frequently used in the cancer context, it can also refer to abnormally formed states with no tendency for neoplasia (e.g., ectodermal dysplasia, enamel dysplasia). Given ambiguities in its definition, a 1992 National Institutes of Health Consensus Development Panel recommended against the use of dysplastic nevus as a diagnosis.[2] The clinical lesions should be described as *atypical moles* while the microscopic patterns should be designated *nevi with architectural disorder* with varying amounts of cellular atypia. Although the diagnosis of AMN is suspected for atypical-appearing melanocytic lesions, histologic confirmation is encouraged to establish the diagnosis because not all atypical-appearing melanocytic lesions have an atypical histology. Table 92-1 delineates some clinical characteristics that can help to distinguish acquired typical between atypical nevi.

FIGURE 92-1

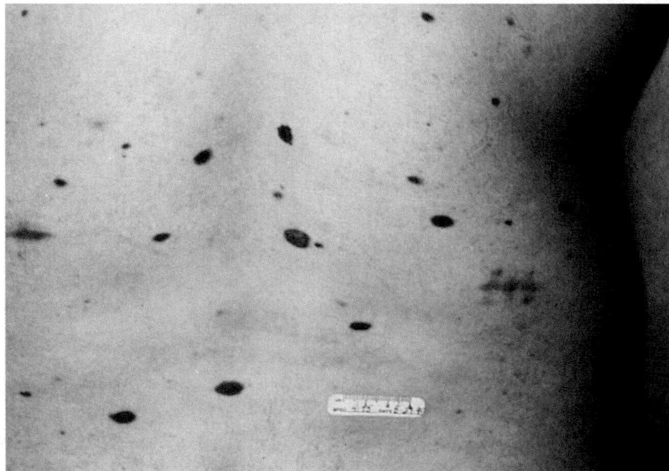

A.

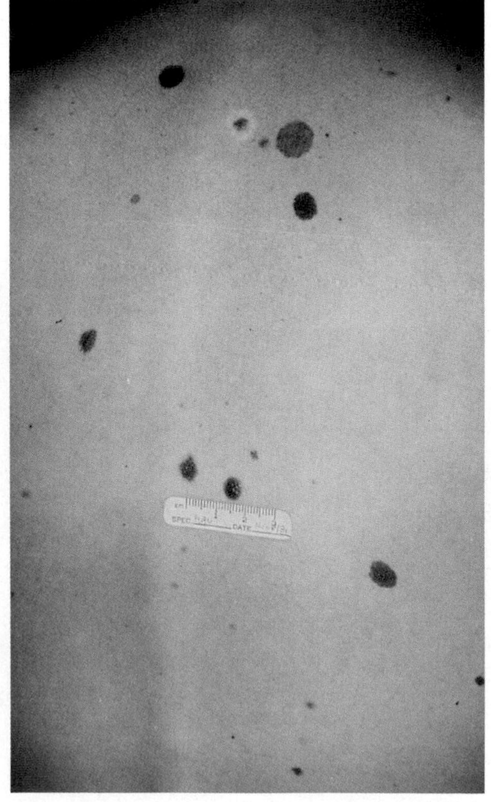

B.

Multiple acquired atypical melanocytic nevi on the back of a healthy 30-year-old white man who has no personal or family history of melanoma (*A*), and on the back of a 13-year-old white female who has no personal or family history of melanoma but whose father has multiple atypical nevi (*B*). Note associated halo nevus in (*B*). (*Courtesy of Arthur R. Rhodes, MD.*)

FIGURE 92-2

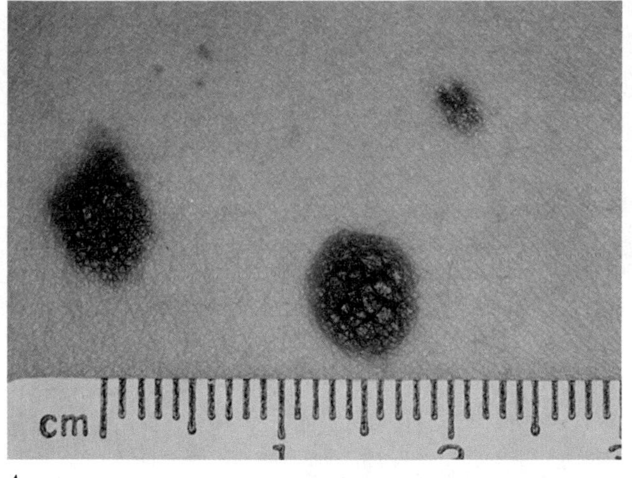

A.

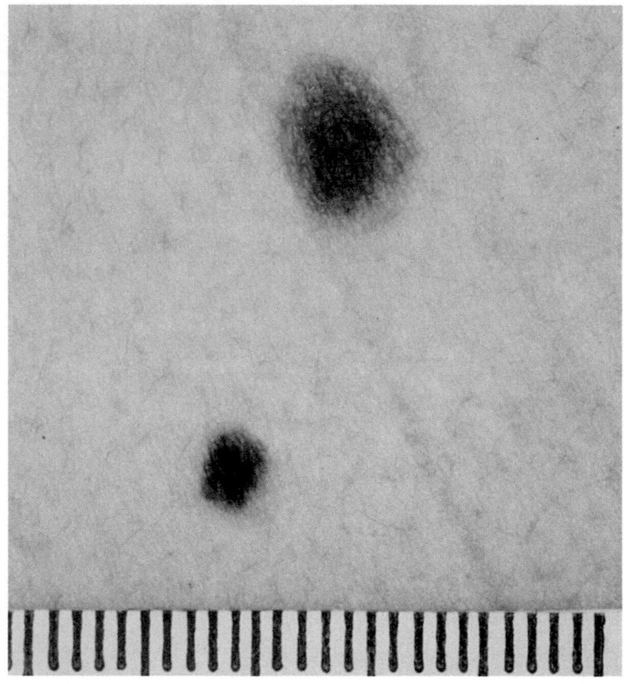

B.

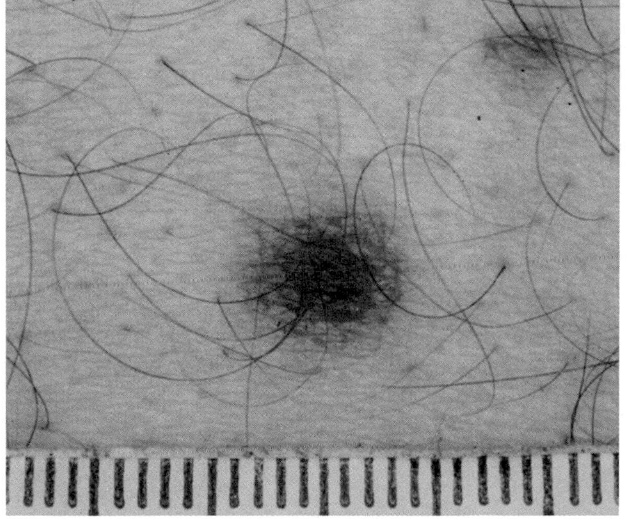

C.

Acquired atypical melanocytic nevi. Atypical compound nevi (*A* to *E* and *G* to *I*) and atypical junctional nevus (*F*). These nevi are striking for irregular and/or dark pigmentation or "fried egg" appearance, irregular and/or sharp or poorly demarcated outlines, relatively large size, and relatively "flat" surface relative to breadth. Scale in millimeters. (*Courtesy of Arthur R. Rhodes, MD.*)

HISTORICAL ASPECTS Although the concept of AMN as a precursor to melanoma has been popularized as an entity sui generis only in the last several decades,[3–6] reports of such lesions date back to the 1800s when Norris[7] described a family in which two members developed cutaneous melanoma and other family members had "many moles on various parts of their bodies." The numerous moles in the family described by Norris may very well have been AMN. Munro[8] showed the gross and microscopic appearance of what we now know to be AMN as early as 1974, in association with a family history of melanoma. Formerly, AMN were described grossly and histologically by other names, including "intraepidermal melanoma" and "atypical" or "active" junctional nevi.[9] The first published reports formally delineating the presence of AMN as a marker for and precursor of cutaneous melanoma were described in the setting of familial cutaneous melanoma–B-K mole syndrome and familial atypical multiple mole melanoma (FAMMM) syndrome.[3,10,11]

EPIDEMIOLOGY Earlier reports suggested that approximately 30,000 people in the United States belong to AMN/familial melanoma kindreds.[12] Although AMN were originally described in these melanoma-prone kindreds, subsequent studies have documented its presence in the general population. In Australia and New Zealand, the prevalence rate is approximately 5 to 9 percent.[13,14] In Germany, 2.2 percent of 500 white males aged 16 to 25 years had histologically documented AMN.[15] In Sweden, clinically identified AMN were detected in 69 of 379 white adults (18 percent) aged 30 to 50 years, while only 30 of these or 8 percent of the total had histopathologically determined AMN.[16] In the United States, up to 17 percent of the healthy population is reported to harbor at least one AMN.[17,18] In France, 63 out of 295 healthy individuals (24 percent) had at least one "clinically atypical nevus" but only 5 had "clinically very atypical nevus."[19] The marked variation in prevalence among various populations and the extraordinarily high rates in some groups may relate to true population heterogeneity, the marked variation of gross and/or microscopic definitions used for ascertainment, or differences in the amount of sun exposure in various regions of the world.

ETIOLOGY AND PATHOGENESIS Intraepidermal melanocytic dysplasia in AMN has been interpreted by some as a block in nevocellular differentiation.[20] Evidence for this abnormal differentiation in

FIGURE 92-2 (*Continued*)

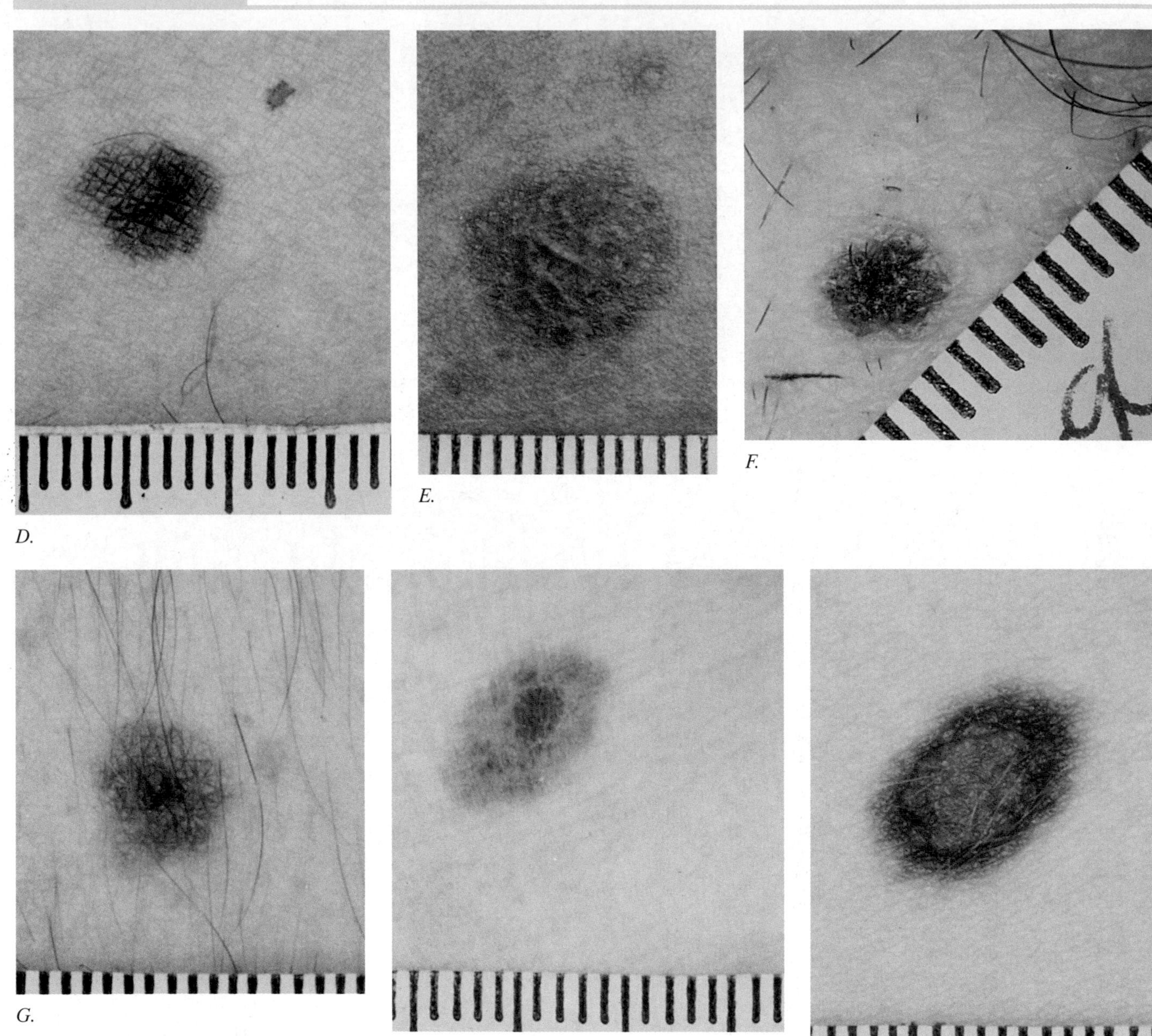

D. E. F. G. H. I.

AMN includes the relatively large clinical lesions, deranged melanogenesis associated with increased pheomelanin content and abnormal melanosomes, enlarged cell bodies, increased dopa-positivity, and the associated disordered proliferation of melanocytes, inflammatory host response, and unique mesenchymal features.[20–23] As with most neoplastic processes, AMN most likely result from an interaction between genetics and the environment.

Many advances have been made in the molecular characterization of FAMMM kindreds. Initial genetic analysis of these families suggested an autosomal dominant mode of inheritance with a possible locus on chromosome 1.[24] Subsequent mapping of the FAMMM locus by using the National Cancer Institute kindreds suggested a locus for familial cutaneous melanoma and AMN on chromosome 1p36.[25] This localization, however, could not be confirmed in other melanoma-prone kindreds around the world.[26–28] Cannon-Albright et al. eventually identified a melanoma susceptibility locus on chromosome 9p21,[29] thereby setting the groundwork for the isolation of *CDKN2A* (also designated p16) as a melanoma predisposition gene from this chromosomal region.[30,31] Subsequent genetic analysis of *CDKN2A* in chromosome 9p–linked families showed a high rate of germ-line mutations.[32] In this study,[32] the mutations appeared to cosegregate with the melanoma phenotype, but not with the atypical mole phenotype. Thus, other unidentified loci may be responsible for AMN susceptibility. Somatic analyses of sporadic AMN have shown evidence of allelic deletion on chromosomes 1 and 9,[33–35] although confirmation of deleterious mutations of any specific gene in AMN is still lacking. Inconsistencies between the localization data and phenotype point to significant genetic heterogeneity among the FAMMM kindreds. Evidence suggests that the chromosome 1p36 locus may contribute to both cutaneous melanoma and AMN, while the chromosome 9p locus only determines melanoma susceptibility.[36,37]

TABLE 92-1

Comparison of Acquired Typical Nevomelanocytic Nevus and Acquired Atypical Melanocytic Nevus (AMN) in White Adults*†

Feature	Acquired Typical Nevomelanocytic Nevus	Acquired Atypical Melanocytic Nevus	Comments
Age at onset	Usually after the first 6–12 months of life; usually evident by age 20 years	Probably the same as typical nevus; usually evident by age 20 years	Affected people with AMN may develop new lesions throughout life; there are dysplastic varieties of congenital nevus
Initial appearance	Begin as tiny pigmented specks; skin surface distorted under oblique lighting	Probably the same as typical nevus; one or more relatively large acquired nevi should suggest the diagnosis in children	A large number of relatively large nevi should raise concern for the presence of AMN regardless of age
Anatomic distribution	Any site affected; relative sparing of sun-protected sites	Any site affected, even sun-protected sites; "horse collar" area most heavily involved	The scalp may be the first site of presentation for AMN in children
Number	Few or many; up to 15% of white adults have none	One or many	Only one is required to develop melanoma
Size	Vast majority <5 mm in greatest diameter	No lower limit on size, but usually ≥ 5 mm in diameter	Size is the best dependable criterion for excluding the diagnosis of AMN (or melanoma)
Coloration pattern, naked eye	Orderly and symmetric distribution of usually no more than two shades of brown	Disorderly and haphazard display of usually more than two shades of brown and/or very darkly pigmented	Very darkly pigmented AMN may be difficult to differentiate from pigmented spindle cell nevus and melanoma
Coloration pattern, dermoscopy‡	Medium or dark brown speckles symmetrically distributed in tan or light brown and/or pink field and/or brown reticular pattern; dermal nevi are usually pale brown or flesh-colored with typical vascular pattern	Light, medium, dark brown, and commonly very dark brown hues distributed haphazardly, often mixed with pink; very dark brown may predominate; pigment pattern obscured to some degree.	Discontinuous pigmentation (one portion light and the other dark, or a dark area asymmetrically placed in a lighter field) should suggest a focus of cellular atypia; pink color may indicate epithelioid cell dysplasia in AMN
Shape	Round or oval	Round, oval, or misshapen	Nodular melanoma may be round or oval
Outline	Smooth, regular, well demarcated	Irregular and/or poorly demarcated ("fuzzy")	A smooth and well-demarcated outline does not exclude AMN or melanoma
Surface (assessed by oblique lighting)	Slight distortion in junctional nevus; obviously elevated (dome-shaped, pedunculated, or flat-topped) in dermal and compound nevus	Plaque or papule with minimal ("pebbly") or obvious surface distortion; "flare" of macular pigmentation may surround a papule or plaque	Melanocytic dysplasia may be macular on acral or mucosal surfaces or on sun-damaged skin

*There are insufficient data to characterize dysplastic nevi in darkly pigmented races.
†Atypical nevi may not be sufficiently evolved to establish the diagnosis before puberty.
‡Pigment pattern assessed using 10× magnification of the brightly illuminated mineral oil–covered lesion surface, called epiluminescence microscopy or dermoscopy.

Although strong epidemiologic data support an association between cutaneous melanoma and excessive ultraviolet radiation (UVR) exposure (reviewed in Ref. 38), the role of sunlight in the induction of AMN is not well established. Many studies report a higher mole density on intermittently sun-exposed sites (upper arms, upper back) as compared to sun-protected (lower back, buttocks) and chronically irradiated (head and neck) sites.[39–42] For total mole development, these anatomic patterns argue against a direct dose effect by the sun. Furthermore, the prevalence of AMN and anatomic distribution of AMN appear to be even less sun-related than common acquired nevi.[40,43,44] The direct effects of ultraviolet exposure on AMN nevomelanocytes are also unclear. Stierner et al. irradiated 11 AMN patients and 22 healthy subjects with UVB irradiation over 17 days and found no abnormal melanocytic UV response in the AMN patients.[45] However, Noz et al. observed a higher rate of DNA damage after UVB irradiation in nevus cells from AMN when compared with nevus cells from common acquired nevi and melanocytes from neonatal foreskin.[46] On the other hand, cyclobutane thymine dimers, a marker of genomic UV injury, do not occur with increased frequency in UV-irradiated AMN melanocytes when compared with UV-irradiated neonatal foreskin melanocytes.[47] Thus, the role of UVR in the pathogenesis of AMN remains speculative.

Analyses of nonmelanocytes from patients with AMN have revealed genetic instability in response to genotoxic stress. In fibroblast cultures, excision repair of UVR-induced thymine dimers was altered adversely within the first hour after UVR (but was normal by 90 min) in seven of eight patients who had AMN (with or without a personal or family history of melanoma).[48] In response to γ-irradiation, skin fibroblasts from members of FAMMM kindreds with AMN show significantly more chromatid breaks and gaps.[49] Based on an analysis of Giemsa-banded karyotypes of peripheral blood lymphocytes, there appears to be a significant excess of apparently random chromosome abnormalities (major and minor structural and numerical abnormalities, i.e., general chromosomal instability) in subjects with AMN in the presence or absence of a personal history of melanoma, as compared to spouse controls and unaffected blood relatives.[50]

Other carcinogens besides UVR have been used to create models of AMN progression in animals. Topical application of 7,12-dimethylbenzanthracene (DMBA) elicits intraepidermal melanocytic hyperplasia and cutaneous melanomas in both Weiser-Maple guinea pigs[51] and albino guinea pigs.[52] The biological relationship, however, of these hyperplastic lesions to AMN is unknown.

In summary, the etiology of AMN remains elusive. Although no recurrent mutational targets have been detected in these melanocytic lesions, there is some indication that cells from AMN patients may be genetically unstable. Moreover, the interaction between AMN and melanomas within FAMMM kindreds is complex; that is, melanoma patients within these families may lack AMN and vice versa. At the current time, the extant information does not support the involvement of a single gene in both AMN and cutaneous melanoma or a direct effect by UVR.

CLINICAL MANIFESTATIONS Reliable clinical criteria are not available to predict with absolute certainty the presence of intraepidermal melanocytic dysplasia in a given melanocytic nevus, although general characteristics may be helpful in distinguishing dysplastic nevi from typical nevi (see Table 92-1 and Figs. 92-1, 92-2, and 92-3). Because the term "dysplastic nevus" is still frequently used by dermatopathologists, it is not uncommon for clinicians to designate moles with atypical features as AMN and for pathologists to define lesions with melanocytic dysplasia as "dysplastic nevi."

The 1992 NIH Consensus Panel defined atypical moles as "acquired pigmented lesions of the skin whose clinical and histologic appearances are different from those of typical common moles."[2] In general, AMN are larger than common moles, have macular and/or papular components, have ill-defined or irregular borders, and exhibit variegation in color that ranges from tan to dark brown or black. These lesions tend to occur on the trunk, although they can also appear on sun-protected areas such as the buttocks. Maiweg et al. found that 96 percent of AMN have at least one of the following four criteria: irregular border, irregular pigmentation, greatest diameter >5mm, and black-colored areas.[53] Although these features can also be found in melanomas, pigmented lesions that lack at least one of these features are unlikely to be AMN.

AMN are often different from one another in the same individual, and AMN in different people may have a variable appearance. Lesions may barely distort the skin surface or have obvious "cobblestoning" of the surface when viewed with oblique lighting. Some lesions have a "fried-egg" appearance, with a central raised component and a more macular pigmented flare that blends imperceptibly into adjacent skin. Other varieties of AMN are very darkly pigmented throughout, distorting the skin surface minimally, and sharply demarcated or

FIGURE 92-3

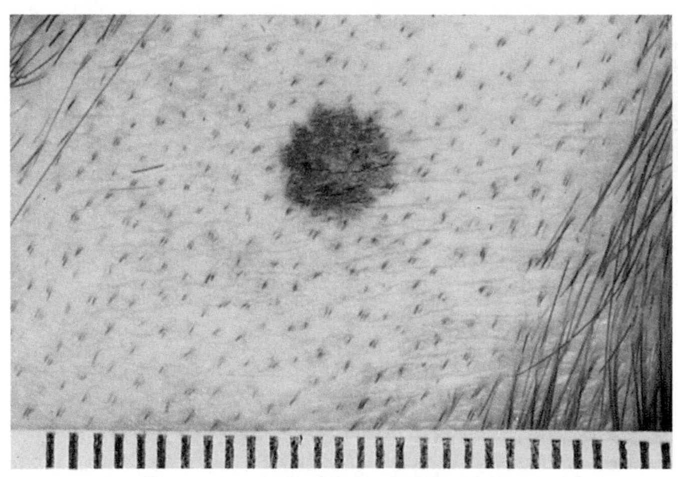

A.

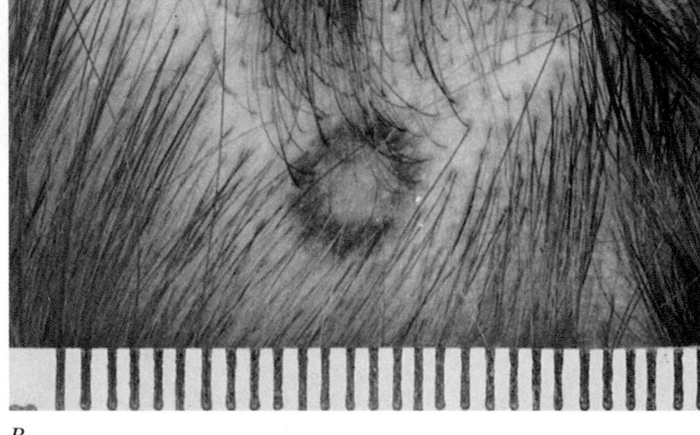

B.

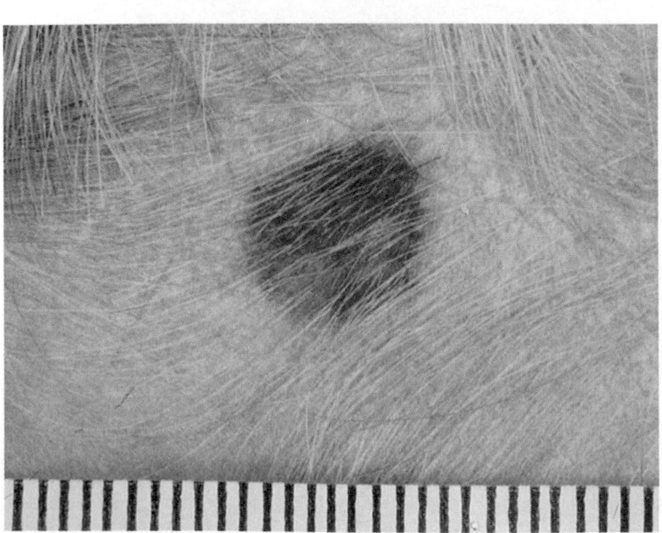

C.

Acquired atypical compound nevi on the scalp (*A* to *C*). (*Courtesy of Arthur R. Rhodes, MD.*)

blending into surrounding skin. Some lesions are sharply demarcated with an irregular border, distorting the skin surface as an obviously raised plaque (Figs. 92-2 and 92-3). Atypical histologic features should be suspected in melanocytic tumors that have very dark pigmentation and/or haphazard disposition of multiple hues (shades of brown, pink, and flesh tone) or a target appearance, irregular and/or poorly demarcated outlines, and relatively large size (5 mm or larger) (Figs. 92-2 and 92-3). The presence of pink hue with or without pigmentation in a relatively large nevus correlates with the presence of epithelioid cell dysplasia.[54]

Surface topography and size are useful parameters in assessing AMN. Although AMN usually distort the skin surface to some degree when assessed by oblique lighting and a macular component is usually present, melanocytic dysplasia in a given lesion cannot be excluded based on topographic features. For instance, lentigo maligna and melanocytic dysplasias on acral and mucosal surfaces need not distort the skin surface. Although nevi less than 4 mm in greatest diameter rarely exhibit melanocytic dysplasia,[54] size alone cannot be used to exclude melanocytic dysplasia. Likewise, location also cannot be used to exclude melanocytic dysplasia. In melanoma-prone families (or in any patient with AMN or melanoma), hidden areas such as the scalp (Fig. 92-3) must be examined carefully for AMN, for such sites may be the source of lethal melanoma, even in children.[55] There are also several case reports of AMN disposed in quadrant distribution.[56,57]

People with AMN may have a few to hundreds of lesions (Fig. 92-1). Population-based AMN counts in different countries have yielded varying results. For instance, Augustsson et al. found that more than 15 percent of residents from the city of Gothenburg, Sweden, had more than 100 AMN,[16] whereas Grob et al. found that only 5 percent of a French health-center population had more than 1 AMN.[19] There are several possibilities for these discrepancies. The stringency of criteria used to diagnose AMN is often different between studies. The Swedish study defined AMN as a nevus ≥5 mm plus at least two of the following: an ill-defined or irregular border, speckled pigmentation, erythema, or a pebbled surface,[16] whereas the French investigators defined AMN as a nevus with any three of the following: ill-defined border, irregular border, irregularly distributed pigmentation, diameter 5 mm or greater, background erythema, and accentuated skin markings.[19] Moreover, there is limited interobserver agreement as to the presence of these atypical clinical features. In one study, four physicians (two oncologists, one internist, one dermatologist) were asked to evaluate a fixed panel of 156 AMN lesions and to identify AMN features within these lesions. Among the clinical features assessed, the examiners noted macular components in 86 to 96 percent of lesions, asymmetry in 47 to 80 percent of lesions, irregular borders in 55 to 80 percent of lesions, ill-defined borders in 40 to 84 percent of lesions, and haphazard color in 41 to 74 percent of lesions.[58] This wide range of values suggests that different observers have different interpretations of "irregular borders" and "irregular pigment." Because of the low concordances, some clinicians have advocated using more quantitative measures, such as total numbers or maximal sizes of nevi, rather than the subjective determinations of atypia,[59] when assessing melanoma risk. Finally, the AMN individuals participating in these various studies originated from clinics in a single institution[17,19,60–62] or from multiple institutions[18] to randomly selected individuals in a given location.[16] A healthy control population in a case-controlled series is different from a residential population because the latter would also include melanoma patients and persons at high risk for developing cutaneous melanoma.

Although the characteristic appearance of AMN may not be evident until puberty, AMN may occur in young children.[55] Significantly more lesions with a histologically confirmed diagnosis of AMN occur in individuals 20 years of age or older. Children who have a prominent mole pattern but without obvious AMN should be reexamined periodically until at least age 20 years. If AMN are not apparent by age 20 years and prominent moles are not evident, it is unlikely that an individual has the AMN trait, at least in the setting of familial melanoma.[63] Unlike common acquired nevi, AMN remain dynamic throughout adult life. New AMN develop in about 20 percent of individuals over 50 years of age, while nearly 50 percent of all AMN undergo some kind of change. The change may represent an increase or decrease in extent of clinical atypia or a disappearance of the mole altogether.[64]

Given the relatively ill-defined criteria for AMN and the dynamic nature of these lesions, adjunctive measures have been added to clinical practice for surveillance of AMN. One such tool is dermoscopy (i.e., epiluminescence microscopy). Although many dermoscopic features of melanoma have been described (see Chap. 93), dermoscopic features of AMN are not quite as straightforward and are not equally well delineated.[65] However, they are distinct enough to make a diagnosis in most cases.[65] There is usually some distortion of the dermoscopic pigment network in AMN, but other dermoscopic features of melanoma are lacking. In melanoma, the pigment pattern is widely spaced and associated with black globular pigment accumulations, pigment streaming and pseudopods, gray haze, gray-blue areas, and areas of pigment loss.[65] Recently, a dermoscopic classification of AMN was devised based on 829 AMN from 23 patients (Fig. 92-4*A* to *L*). The utility of this classification scheme will ultimately depend upon the reproducibility of these results and the correlation between dermoscopic findings and histology.[66]

There are also no agreed upon clinical criteria for classifying individuals with AMN. At least three different, but related, systems exist. The NIH Consensus Panel defined the FAMMM syndrome as (1) occurrence of melanoma in one or more first- or second-degree relatives, (2) large numbers of moles (often >50), some of which are atypical and often variable in size, and (3) moles that demonstrate certain distinct histologic features.[2] The *classic atypical moles syndrome* is defined by the presence of (1) more than 100 nevi, (2) one or more nevi ≥8 mm in greatest diameter, and (3) one or more nevi with clinically atypical features.[67] The *atypical mole syndrome* has also been scored on a point system. One point is assigned for each of these features: (1) two or more pigmented lesions of the iris; (2) more than 100 nevi larger than 2 mm in diameter (or >50 nevi in patients older than 50 years or younger than 20 years); (3) two or more clinically atypical moles; (4) moles on the anterior aspect of the scalp; and (5) moles abnormally distributed (e.g., one on the buttocks or two or more on the dorsum of the foot). Affected individuals are said to have the "atypical mole syndrome" phenotype if they score 3 or more points.[68] All of these systems are arbitrary and have not been fully tested for melanoma risk.

PATHOLOGY Histologic features required to diagnose AMN have not been tested sufficiently for sensitivity, specificity, and predictive value. Therefore, diagnostic criteria are not universally accepted. Nevertheless, sufficient data are available to make a histologic diagnosis until universally accepted criteria are available.

Elder et al.[69] outlined diagnostic features for AMN as *absolute* (necessary for the diagnosis) and *relative* (frequently associated). These criteria have been modified slightly as follows: *Absolute* histologic criteria include (1) a proliferation of intraepidermal melanocytes disposed singly and/or in irregular nests in the epidermal basal unit or slightly above, in a lentiginous epidermal pattern (elongated, club-shaped, and/or fused rete ridges), and (2) variable and discontinuous cellular atypia of melanocytes (Fig. 92-5*A* to *C*). *Relative* histologic criteria include (1) lymphohistiocytic infiltrates in the dermis, with or without melanin-laden macrophages; (2) a dermal mesenchymal response consisting of concentric eosinophilic fibrosis (condensed papillary dermal collagen abutting epidermal rete ridges), lamellar fibroplasia (delicate collagen fibrils and elongated fibroblasts parallel to the epidermal surface, situated at the tips of epidermal rete ridges), and/or

FIGURE 92-4

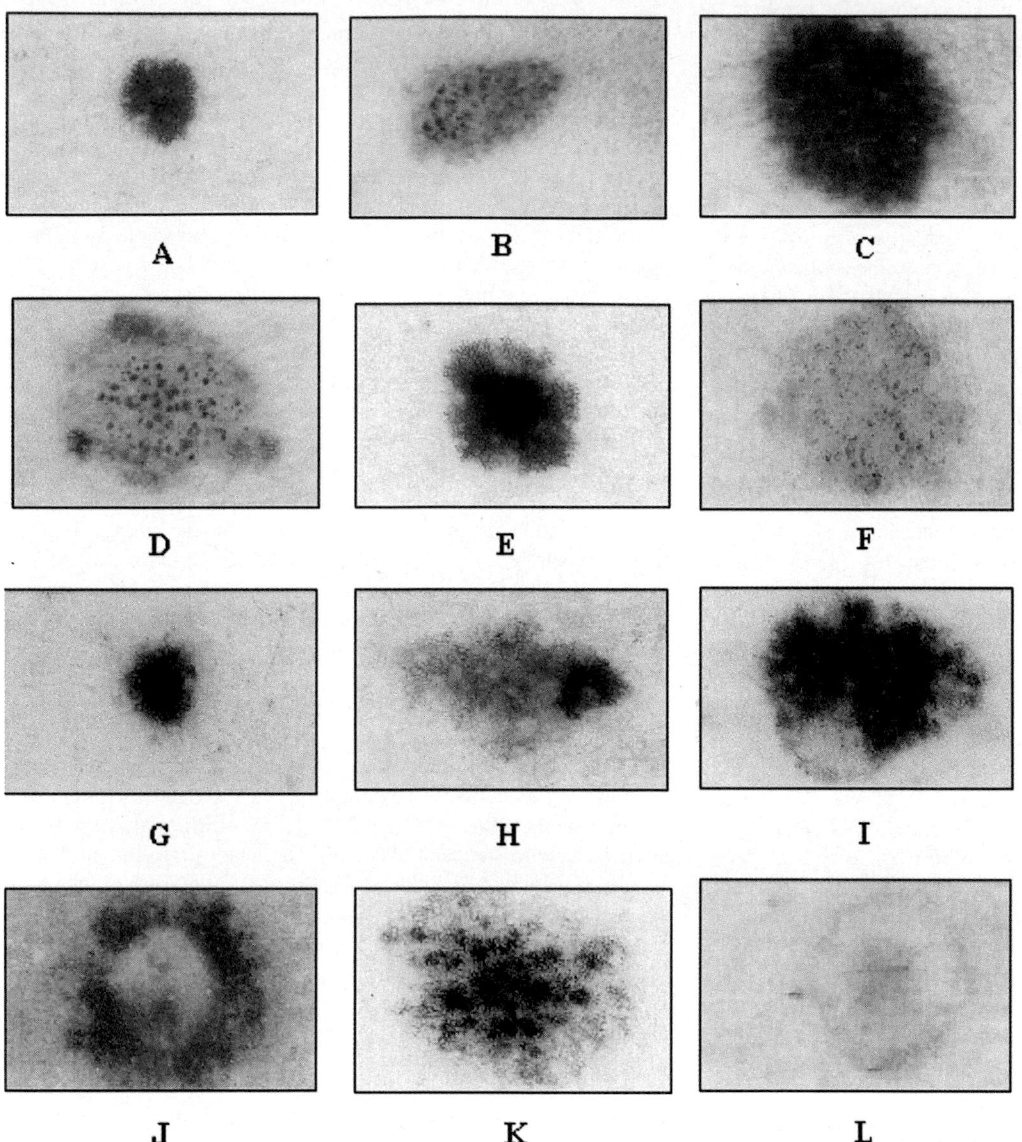

Dermoscopic patterns of atypical melanocytic nevi. The (*A*) reticular pattern with pigment network; (*B*) globular pattern showing numerous globules or dots; (*C*) homogeneous pattern with homogeneous brown pigmentation; (*D*) reticular-globular pattern with ≥3 meshes of pigment network with ≥3 globules or dots; (*E*) reticular-homogeneous pattern with ≥3 meshes of pigment network with homogeneous brown pigmentation in at least one quarter of the lesion; (*F*) globular-homogeneous pattern with ≥3 globules or dots with homogeneous brown pigmentation in at least one quarter of the lesion (*L*) unclassified pattern. Dermoscopic classification of AMN showing (*G*) central hyperpigmentation; (*H*) eccentric peripheral hyperpigmentation; (*J*) central hypopigmentation; (*I*) eccentric peripheral hypopigmentation; (*K*) multifocal hyperpigmentation and hypopigmentation. (*Courtesy of R. Hofmann-Wellenhof, MD.*)

neovascularization (blood vessel proliferation); (3) a proliferation of ellipsoidal and irregularly nested melanocytes disposed at the epidermal basal unit, frequently bridging epidermal rete ridges; (4) nevus cells in the dermis, often associated with impairment of maturation and synthesis of pigment; and (5) extension of intraepidermal melanocytic hyperplasia beyond the shoulders of the dermal nevus component (if a dermal nevus is present).

These criteria[69] have been adopted and modified slightly into two major and four minor criteria recently outlined in a paper by pathologists convened by the World Health Organization (WHO) Melanoma Program to test concordance of interpretation of melanocytic lesions.[70] Diagnosis of AMN by this scheme requires both major criteria and two of the four minor criteria. The major criteria are (1) basilar proliferation of atypical nevomelanocytes, extending three rete ridges beyond a dermal melanocytic component (if a dermal component is present), and (2) a pattern of intraepidermal melanocytic proliferation as one of two types, namely, lentiginous or epithelioid cell. The minor criteria are (1) concentric eosinophilic fibrosis or lamellar fibroplasia, (2) neovascularization, (3) dermal inflammatory response, and (4) fusion of rete ridges. In the WHO Melanoma Program, these predetermined criteria for diagnosis permitted a mean percent concordance of diagnosis for benign acquired nevi, AMN, and radial growth phase melanoma to be 95, 88, and 95 percent, respectively.[70]

The degree of cellular atypia in AMN is often difficult to reproducibly measure. On the one hand, AMN with clear architectural disorder may harbor scant or no melanocyte nuclear atypia. On the other hand, the melanocytic atypia may be so severe that distinction from melanoma is nearly impossible. Cellular atypia of melanocytes is characterized by nuclear enlargement and usually expansion of cell cytoplasm, and expanded retraction artifact (for spindle cells), nuclear

FIGURE 92-5

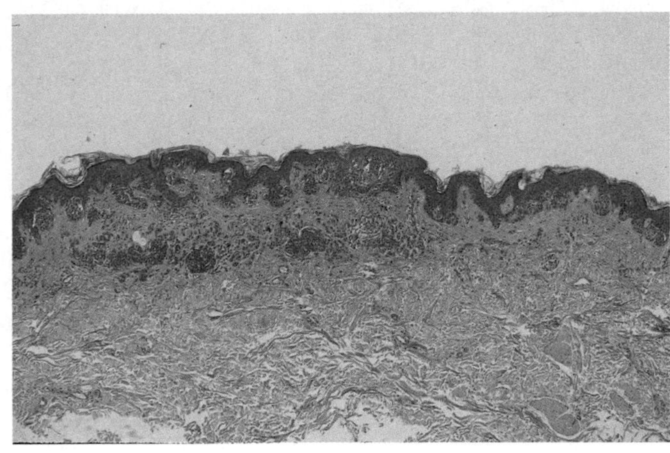

A.

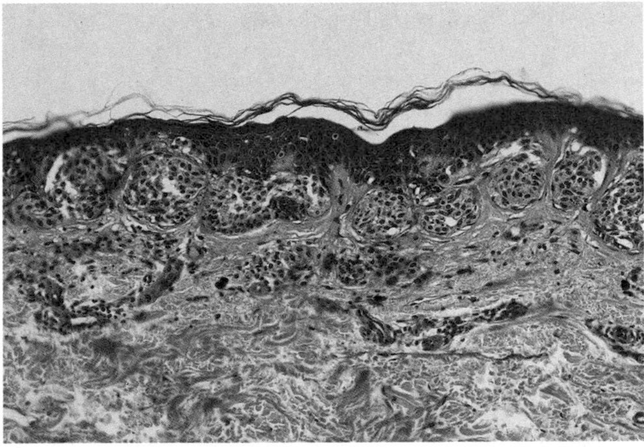

B.

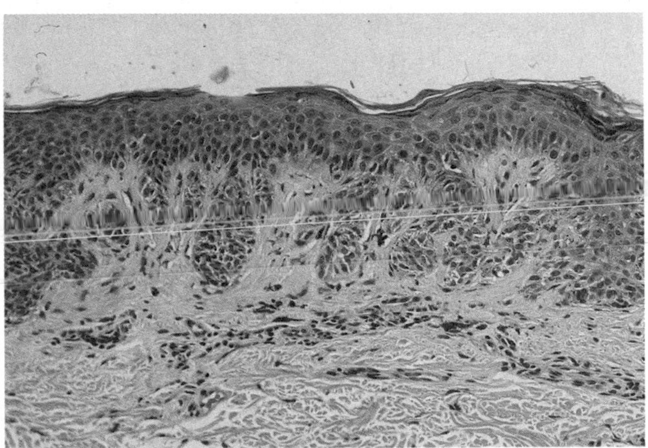

C.

Histopathologic features of a compound dysplastic nevus. *A.* The lesion is asymmetric with centrifugal proliferation of junctional nests which extend well beyond the dermal component ("shoulder phenomenon"). This shoulder results clinically in the irregular macular flare at the border of an atypical mole. *B.* Closer examination reveals an abnormal nesting pattern of melanocytes with moderate epithelioid atypia, concentric eosinophilic fibroplasia, and focal lymphocytic host response. *C.* The presence of cytologic atypia, which is a hallmark of dysplastic nevi, can be appreciated with cells exhibiting marked nuclear pleomorphism and hyperchromasia. (*Photographs courtesy of Artur Zembowicz, MD, PhD.*)

hyperchromasia and pleomorphism, often a prominent nucleolus, and expansion of eosinophilic cytoplasm in spindle cells or finely pink and granular cytoplasm in epithelioid cells.[71] Most nevi that exhibit cellular atypia also possess concomitant architectural changes associated with AMN, including atypical localization of melanocytes in the epidermis, irregular distribution of melanocytes in the junctional zone, and atypical nests of melanocytes.[72] In a multivariate analysis, other histologic features of AMN that were significantly associated with melanocytic nuclear atypia included basal melanocytic hyperplasia, junctional nest disarray, prominent vascularity, and large melanin granules.[73] In another study, dustlike melanin in the cytoplasm of melanocytes, irregular nevoid nests, markedly increased junctional activity, and enlarged melanocytic nuclei were found in half of the AMN and in none of the common typical nevi.[74]

CLINICAL-PATHOLOGIC CORRELATION Suspecting melanocytic dysplasia in a given melanocytic tumor requires a high index of suspicion and experience correlating gross appearance with microscopic patterns of architecture and cellular morphology of melanocytes. With individual lesions clinically, some investigators have found that ill-defined border, macular component, pink color, and especially size (in mm) and irregular border correlate most closely with AMN histology,[75] while others have reported ill-defined border and irregularly distributed pigmentation to be most predictive.[76] However, if histologic criteria of AMN were strictly applied to nevus pathology specimens, a high percentage of benign nevi also exhibit characteristics of AMN. Klein and Barr found that 88 percent of small, clinically benign junctional and compound nevi manifest at least one histologic feature of AMN,[77] while Piepkorn et al. estimated the prevalence of histologic dysplasia in nevi to range from 7 to 32 percent, depending on the observer.[78] As yet, there is no uniform, reproducible consensus to the grading of atypia in AMN.

DIFFERENTIAL DIAGNOSIS AMN must be differentiated from a common nevomelanocytic nevus; intraepidermal (in situ) melanoma; pigmented spindle cell and/or epithelioid cell nevus; blue nevus; combined melanocytic nevus-blue nevus; darkly pigmented solar lentigo; darkly pigmented varieties of lentiginous nevomelanocytic nevi without significant cellular atypia; seborrheic keratosis; pigmented actinic keratosis; pigmented basal cell carcinoma; pigmented varieties of Bowen's disease; traumatic hematoma; pyogenic granuloma; sclerosing hemangioma; and dermatofibroma.

The gross and microscopic features of AMN may not be sufficiently evolved to clearly establish the diagnosis before puberty. However, AMN can develop before puberty, particularly in the familial melanoma setting.[55] It may also be difficult to diagnose nonpigmented varieties of AMN in persons who are relatively deficient in their ability to make melanin.

ATYPICAL MELANOCYTIC NEVI AND MELANOMA RISK Familial, population, and pathologic studies all document an increased risk of cutaneous melanoma among individuals with AMN. Historically, Kraemer initially devised a classification of these families in order to estimate melanoma risk.[12] Persons with sporadic AMN have the lowest risk of developing melanoma, although the risk is still 27 times greater than that for the general population. On the other hand, individuals with familial AMN and a strong family history of cutaneous melanoma have a cumulative risk of melanoma approaching 100 percent by age 75 years;[79] this was approximately 148 times that of the general white population[63] in 1986.

Over the past 20 years, many population- and clinic-based case-controlled studies have reproducibly established an elevated melanoma risk among individuals with atypical nevi.[17,18,60–62,80,81] Because these studies were performed in different parts of the world, the overall impact is unlikely to be biased by specific populations. Patients with a few atypical nevi (<3 to 5 lesions) have an adjusted relative risk of approximately 4 or less. However, individuals with a moderate-to-large number of atypical moles (>5 to 10 lesions) harbor up to a tenfold risk for developing melanoma. More recently, Tucker et al. reported that the presence of even a single AMN conferred a 2.3-fold increase in the risk for melanoma.[18] Prospective cohort studies also consistently show an increased observed-to-expected ratio for developing melanomas among cohorts of patients with atypical nevi.[82–85]

The presence of AMN remnants in histologically confirmed cutaneous melanomas has also been promulgated as evidence for the histiogenic evolution from AMN to malignancy. A contiguous association between melanoma and melanocytic dysplasia has been reported in 6.6 to 70.3 percent of cutaneous melanomas in different case series.[20,63,86–93] Variations in the percentages of precursor AMN reported in the literature most likely reflect differences in the definition of dysplastic nevi and differences in the thoroughness of the histopathologic search (e.g., availability of serial sections). Furthermore, because benign fragments of nevi have also been observed in many studies, the relative rates of transformation to melanoma for AMN and other types of melanocytic hyperplasias are currently unknown.

MANAGEMENT The proper management of people who have AMN, with or without a personal or family history of melanoma, has not been universally established. In general, pathologic confirmation of the clinical diagnosis provides a more solid basis for making additional management recommendations. However, histopathologic examination is not necessary to define an individual at high risk if there are obviously atypical nevi (but none suspicious enough to warrant removal) or prominent nevi (see Table 92-1). It is prudent to offer periodic follow-up to persons who have slightly irregular AMN and/or a prominent nevus pattern, whether or not histopathologic confirmation of the diagnosis of AMN is available. For individuals who have AMN and/or prominent nevi, the goal over time is to excise lesions raising clinical suspicion of melanoma—either new nevi with suspicious features or preexisting nevi that have changed.

Recently, it was suggested that monitoring with digital dermoscopy might be offered to patients with multiple AMN. The potential benefit of this technique is that identification of structural modifications over time enables early detection of melanoma, while decreasing the need for excision of suspicious benign lesions. In a recent study by Kittler et al., 1862 melanocytic skin lesions drawn from 202 patients with multiple AMN were monitored with digital dermoscopy.[94] During follow-up 75 (4%) lesions showed substantial modifications over time and were referred to excision. Eight of the 75 excised lesions were histologically diagnosed as early melanomas. These melanomas initially had not displayed clinical or dermoscopic features of melanoma and the decision to excise relied solely on evidence of morphologic change. Although the value of short-term monitoring with digital dermoscopy is still a matter of ongoing research, it may become a useful procedure for selected patients with multiple AMN, where wholesale removal of all AMN is neither necessary, desirable, nor feasible.

For people who have only one or two lesions suspicious for being AMN, complete excision is reasonable, but periodic examination by a health care provider should be offered for a lifetime. Affected people may be expected to develop new lesions over time. In melanoma-prone families, AMN are usually evident by age 20 years for people destined to have them.[63] Prophylactic removal of every AMN is unnecessary for people who have numerous AMN because most will be benign, few will change over time, and the risk of melanoma cannot be eliminated with such an approach. Lesions that are difficult to monitor (i.e., hairy scalp, perianal area) should be considered for prophylactic excision. Other scenarios requiring consideration for surgical excision include AMN that are extremely atypical in gross appearance, nevi that are documented to be changing or new, and AMN in patients for whom medical follow-up is deemed likely to be inadequate. Despite these approaches, one study reported that in patients with nonfamilial melanoma, only 18 percent of the clinically most atypical nevi show histologic evidence of AMN.[95] Adjunctive measures, such as total-body photography, dermoscopy, patient self-examination, and digital dermoscopy (see above) may improve our ability to identify lesions for surgery.

Although persons who have AMN and a personal and/or family history of melanoma appear to have a greater risk for developing melanoma than do those persons with AMN who do not have a personal or family history of melanoma, the overall management is similar. Those who have AMN should practice self-examination at least once every 1 to 2 months, using full-length mirrors and hand-held mirrors for difficult-to-examine sites. Relatives or spouses should be enlisted to assist in these examinations, particularly the posterior torso and hairy scalp. Affected individuals should be made aware of the signs of early melanoma. Patients who have AMN should be examined by a physician every 3 to 12 months, depending on the history of malignancy and number of AMN, and digital dermoscopy, where available, should be performed. Particular attention should be given to those affected patients during periods of puberty and pregnancy, because nevi may develop or change during these times. For patients who have AMN or melanoma, with or without a family history of melanoma or AMN, it is prudent to recommend examination of first-degree bloodline relatives for AMN and melanoma starting before or around puberty. Early development of melanoma has also been described in the setting of FAMMM.[96–98] In a study of melanoma patients from 23 pedigrees, Goldstein et al. found a mean age of diagnosis to be 36 years[97] as compared to 55 years for the general melanoma population.[99]

Although visual surveillance is universally accepted as part of an ongoing melanoma prevention strategy, there are little data to document its effectiveness. In a Connecticut-based population analysis, skin self-examination, although practiced by only 15 percent of 1159 subjects, was associated with a lower rate of advanced melanoma.[100] Moreover, cutaneous melanomas detected by physicians are thinner, and presumably less life-threatening, than those detected by the patient.[101] Together, these preliminary findings suggest that surveillance of individuals with AMN, either by self-examination or by physician-directed examination, may be beneficial.

In patients with numerous AMN, it should be presumed that excessive UVR exposure, to either artificial or natural sources, may promote cellular alterations that permit the formation of new AMN, de novo melanoma, or cause progression of preexisting AMN to melanoma. Persons who have AMN should avoid sunbathing or getting red in the sun. Cover-up with tightly woven clothing and maximum sunscreen protection to body sites that cannot be covered easily should be used daily for exposed sites during any sun exposure.

Eye care given to people who have AMN is controversial. Although there are case reports and small case series reporting associations between ocular nevi and/or ocular melanoma with AMN and/or cutaneous melanoma,[102–106] formal ophthalmologic recommendations do not currently exist for patients with AMN. Until there is more conclusive information, however, people who have AMN, whether or not there is a personal or family history of cutaneous melanoma, should receive the same level of eye care as that recommended for the general population.

There has also been some recent evidence that individuals from FAMMM kindreds, particularly families with germline *CDKN2A* mutations, have an increased risk of developing pancreatic cancer.[107–109] Moreover, in a population-based analysis, Schenk et al. calculated a twofold risk in pancreatic cancer among patients who developed cutaneous melanoma prior to age 50 years.[110] These findings are still considered preliminary and currently there are no formal recommendations for pancreatic cancer screening among individuals with either familial or sporadic AMN.

Surgical excision is currently the recommended method of removing AMN. Lateral excision margins of 2 to 3 mm should be taken to ensure complete removal of AMN. Because melanoma can arise within lesions, complete histologic examination is essential to rule out melanoma. For lesions with a poorly demarcated outline, dermoscopy or a Wood's lamp (long-wave ultraviolet light) may be useful in defining borders. Incompletely excised AMN may recur and possibly become histologically more atypical over time. Therefore, incompletely excised AMN should be considered for re-excision or close periodic examination for recurrence, depending on degree and quantity of cellular atypia. The deep excision margin of AMN should extend to below the deepest component of the lesion, which for most acquired AMN is the papillary or upper reticular dermis. Destructive modes of therapy for any melanocytic tumor will obfuscate histopathologic confirmation of a benign, intermediate, or malignant lesion.

REFERENCES

1. Elder DE et al: Acquired melanocytic nevi and melanoma, in *Pathology of Malignant Melanoma*, edited by AB Ackerman. New York, Masson, 1981, p 185
2. NIH Consensus conference: Diagnosis and treatment of early melanoma. *JAMA* **268**:1314, 1992
3. Clark WH Jr et al: Origin of familial malignant melanomas from heritable melanocytic lesions: The B-K mole syndrome. *Arch Dermatol* **114**:723, 1978
4. Lynch HT et al: Familial atypical multiple mole-melanoma (FAMMM) syndrome: Segregation analysis. *J Med Genet* **20**:342, 1983
5. Elder DE et al: Dysplastic nevus syndrome: A phenotypic association of sporadic cutaneous melanoma. *Cancer* **46**:1787, 1980
6. Reimer RR et al: Precursor lesions in familial melanoma: A genetic preneoplastic syndrome. *JAMA* **239**:744, 1978
7. Norris W: Case of fungoid disease. *Edinburgh Med Surg J* **16**:562, 1820
8. Munro DD: Multiple active junctional naevi with family history of malignant melanoma. *Proc R Soc Med* **67**:594, 1974
9. Allen AC et al: Histogenesis and clinicopathologic correlation of nevi and malignant melanomas. *Arch Dermatol Syphilol* **69**:150, 1954
10. Frichot BC 3rd et al: New cutaneous phenotype in familial malignant melanoma. *Lancet* **1**:864, 1977
11. Lynch HT et al: Familial atypical multiple mole-melanoma syndrome. *J Med Genet* **15**:352, 1978
12. Kraemer KH et al: Dysplastic naevi and cutaneous melanoma risk. *Lancet* **2**:1076, 1983
13. Nordlund JJ et al: Demographic study of clinically atypical (dysplastic) nevi in patients with melanoma and comparison subjects. *Cancer Res* **45**:1855, 1985
14. Cooke KR et al: Dysplastic naevi in a population-based survey. *Cancer* **63**:1240, 1989
15. Sander C et al: Epidemiology of dysplastic nevus [in German]. *Hautarzt* **40**:758, 1989
16. Augustsson A et al: Prevalence of common and dysplastic naevi in a Swedish population. *Br J Dermatol* **124**:152, 1991
17. Holly EA et al: Number of melanocytic nevi as a major risk factor for malignant melanoma. *J Am Acad Dermatol* **17**:459, 1987
18. Tucker MA et al: Clinically recognized dysplastic nevi. A central risk factor for cutaneous melanoma. *JAMA* **277**:1439, 1997
19. Grob JJ et al: Count of benign melanocytic nevi as a major indicator of risk for nonfamilial nodular and superficial spreading melanoma. *Cancer* **66**:387, 1990
20. Clark WH Jr et al: A study of tumor progression: the precursor lesions of superficial spreading and nodular melanoma. *Hum Pathol* **15**:1147, 1984
21. Salopek TG et al: Dysplastic melanocytic nevi contain high levels of pheomelanin: Quantitative comparison of pheomelanin/eumelanin levels between normal skin, common nevi, and dysplastic nevi. *Pigment Cell Res* **4**:172, 1991
22. Takahashi H et al: Fine structural characterization of melanosomes in dysplastic nevi. *Cancer* **56**:111, 1985
23. Rhodes AR et al: Melanosomal alterations in dysplastic melanocytic nevi. A quantitative, ultrastructural investigation. *Cancer* **61**:358, 1988

24. Greene MH et al: Familial cutaneous malignant melanoma: Autosomal dominant trait possibly linked to the Rh locus. *Proc Natl Acad Sci U S A* **80**:6071, 1983
25. Bale SJ et al: Mapping the gene for hereditary cutaneous malignant melanoma–dysplastic nevus syndrome to chromosome 1p. *N Engl J Med* **320**:1367, 1989
26. Nancarrow DJ et al: Exclusion of the familial melanoma locus (MLM) from the PND/D1S47 and MYCL1 regions of chromosome arm 1p in 7 Australian pedigrees. *Genomics* **12**:18, 1992
27. Cannon-Albright LA et al: Evidence against the reported linkage of the cutaneous melanoma–dysplastic nevus syndrome locus to chromosome 1p36. *Am J Hum Genet* **46**:912, 1990
28. Gruis NA et al: Locus for susceptibility to melanoma on chromosome 1p. *N Engl J Med* **322**:853, 1990
29. Cannon-Albright LA et al: Assignment of a locus for familial melanoma, MLM, to chromosome 9p13-p22. *Science* **258**:1148, 1992
30. Kamb A et al: A cell cycle regulator potentially involved in genesis of many tumor types. *Science* **264**:436, 1994
31. Nobori T et al: Deletions of the cyclin-dependent kinase-4 inhibitor gene in multiple human cancers. *Nature* **368**:753, 1994
32. Hussussian CJ et al: Germline p16 mutations in familial melanoma. *Nat Genet* **8**:15, 1994
33. Lee JY et al: Genetic alterations of p16INK4a and p53 genes in sporadic dysplastic nevus. *Biochem Biophys Res Commun* **237**:667, 1997
34. Park WS et al: Allelic deletion at chromosome 9p21(p16) and 17p13(p53) in microdissected sporadic dysplastic nevus. *Hum Pathol* **29**:127, 1998
35. Boni R et al: Loss of heterozygosity detected on 1p and 9q in microdissected atypical nevi. *Arch Dermatol* **134**:882, 1998
36. Goldstein AM et al: Two-locus linkage analysis of cutaneous malignant melanoma/dysplastic nevi. *Am J Hum Genet* **58**:1050, 1996
37. Goldstein AM et al: Linkage of cutaneous malignant melanoma/dysplastic nevi to chromosome 9p, and evidence for genetic heterogeneity. *Am J Hum Genet* **54**:489, 1994
38. Tsao H et al: Ultraviolet radiation and malignant melanoma. *Clin Dermatol* **16**:67, 1998
39. Nicholls EM: Development and elimination of pigmented moles, and the anatomical distribution of primary malignant melanoma. *Cancer* **32**:191, 1973
40. Augustsson A et al: Regional distribution of melanocytic naevi in relation to sun exposure, and site-specific counts predicting total number of naevi. *Acta Derm Venereol* **72**:123, 1992
41. Gallagher RP et al: Anatomic distribution of acquired melanocytic nevi in white children. A comparison with melanoma: The Vancouver Mole Study. *Arch Dermatol* **126**:466, 1990
42. Harrison SL et al: Body-site distribution of melanocytic nevi in young Australian children. *Arch Dermatol* **135**:47, 1999
43. Rampen FH et al: Prevalence of common "acquired" nevocytic nevi and dysplastic nevi is not related to ultraviolet exposure. *J Am Acad Dermatol* **18**:679, 1988
44. Stierner U et al: Regional distribution of common and dysplastic naevi in relation to melanoma site and sun exposure. A case-control study. *Melanoma Res* **1**:367, 1992
45. Stierner U et al: UVB-induced melanocyte proliferation and 5-S-cysteinyldopa excretion in dysplastic nevus syndrome. *Photodermatol* **5**:218, 1988
46. Noz KC et al: Comet assay demonstrates a higher ultraviolet B sensitivity to DNA damage in dysplastic nevus cells than in common melanocytic nevus cells and foreskin melanocytes. *J Invest Dermatol* **106**:1198, 1996
47. Noz KC et al: UV induction of cyclobutane thymine dimers in the DNA of cultured melanocytes from foreskin, common melanocytic nevi and dysplastic nevi. *Photochem Photobiol* **59**:534, 1994
48. Roth M et al: Thymine dimer repair in fibroblasts of patients with dysplastic naevus syndrome (DNS). *Experientia* **44**:169, 1988
49. Sanford KK et al: Hypersensitivity to G2 chromatid radiation damage in familial dysplastic naevus syndrome. *Lancet* **2**:1111, 1987
50. Caporaso N et al: Cytogenetics in hereditary malignant melanoma and dysplastic nevus syndrome: Is dysplastic nevus syndrome a chromosome instability disorder? *Cancer Genet Cytogenet* **24**:299, 1987
51. Clark WH Jr et al: The developmental biology of induced malignant melanoma in guinea pigs and a comparison with other neoplastic systems. *Cancer Res* **36**:4079, 1976
52. Gomez S et al: Melanocytic carcinogenesis in albino guinea pigs. *Pigment Cell Res* **1**:390, 1988
53. Maiweg C et al: The usefulness of single and combined clinical characteristics for the diagnosis of dysplastic naevi. *Melanoma Res* **1**:377, 1992

54. Roush GC et al: Correlation of clinical pigmentary characteristics with histopathologically-confirmed dysplastic nevi in nonfamilial melanoma patients. Studies of melanocytic nevi IX. *Br J Cancer* **64**:943, 1991
55. Tucker MA et al: Dysplastic nevi on the scalp of prepubertal children from melanoma-prone families. *J Pediatr* **103**:65, 1983
56. Sterry W et al: Quadrant distribution of dysplastic nevus syndrome. *Arch Dermatol* **124**:926, 1988
57. Misago N et al: Unilateral dysplastic nevi associated with malignant melanoma. *J Dermatol* **18**:649, 1991
58. Barnhill RL et al: Interclinician agreement on the recognition of selected gross morphologic features of pigmented lesions. Studies of melanocytic nevi V. *J Am Acad Dermatol* **26**:185, 1992
59. Meyer LJ et al: Interobserver concordance in discriminating clinical atypia of melanocytic nevi, and correlations with histologic atypia. *J Am Acad Dermatol* **34**:618, 1996
60. Marghoob AA et al: Risk of developing multiple primary cutaneous melanomas in patients with the classic atypical-mole syndrome: A case-control study. *Br J Dermatol* **135**:704, 1996
61. Kang S et al: Melanoma risk in individuals with clinically atypical nevi. *Arch Dermatol* **130**:999, 1994
62. Garbe C et al: Markers and relative risk in a German population for developing malignant melanoma. *Int J Dermatol* **28**:517, 1989
63. Greene MH et al: High risk of malignant melanoma in melanoma-prone families with dysplastic nevi. *Ann Intern Med* **102**:458, 1985
64. Halpern AC et al: Natural history of dysplastic nevi. *J Am Acad Dermatol* **29**:51, 1993
65. Pehamberger H et al: In vivo epiluminescence microscopy of pigmented skin lesions. I. Pattern analysis of pigmented skin lesions and early detection of malignant melanoma. *J Am Acad Dermatol* **17**:584, 1987
66. Hofmann-Wellenhof R et al: Dermoscopic classification of atypical melanocytic nevi (Clark nevi). *Arch Dermatol* **137**:1575, 2001
67. Kopf AW et al: Atypical mole syndrome. *J Am Acad Dermatol* **22**:117, 1990
68. Newton-Bishop JA et al: Family studies in melanoma: Identification of the atypical mole syndrome (AMS) phenotype. *Melanoma Res* **4**:199, 1994
69. Elder DE et al: The dysplastic nevus syndrome: Our definition. *Am J Dermatopathol* **4**:455, 1982
70. Clemente C et al: Histopathologic diagnosis of dysplastic nevi: Concordance among pathologists convened by the World Health Organization Melanoma Programme. *Hum Pathol* **22**:313, 1991
71. Rhodes AR et al: Dysplastic melanocytic nevi: A reproducible histologic definition emphasizing cellular morphology. *Mod Pathol* **2**:306, 1989
72. Balkau D et al: Architectural features in melanocytic lesions with cellular atypia. *Dermatologica* **177**:129, 1988
73. Barnhill RL et al: Correlation of histologic architectural and cytoplasmic features with nuclear atypia in atypical (dysplastic) nevomelanocytic nevi. *Hum Pathol* **21**:51, 1990
74. Steijlen PM et al: The efficacy of histopathological criteria required for diagnosing dysplastic naevi. *Histopathology* **12**:289, 1988
75. Barnhill RL et al: Correlation of clinical and histopathologic features in clinically atypical melanocytic nevi. *Cancer* **67**:3157, 1991
76. Kelly JW et al: Clinical diagnosis of dysplastic melanocytic nevi. A clinicopathologic correlation. *J Am Acad Dermatol* **14**:1044, 1986
77. Klein LJ et al: Histologic atypia in clinically benign nevi. A prospective study. *J Am Acad Dermatol* **22**:275, 1990
78. Piepkorn MW et al: A multiobserver, population-based analysis of histologic dysplasia in melanocytic nevi. *J Am Acad Dermatol* **30**:707, 1994
79. Kraemer KH et al: Risk of cutaneous melanoma in dysplastic nevus syndrome types A and B. *N Engl J Med* **315**:1615, 1986
80. Rhodes AR et al: Risk factors for cutaneous melanoma. A practical method of recognizing predisposed individuals. *JAMA* **258**:3146, 1987
81. Augustsson A et al: Common and dysplastic naevi as risk factors for cutaneous malignant melanoma in a Swedish population. *Acta Derm Venereol* **71**:518, 1991
82. Halpern AC et al: A cohort study of melanoma in patients with dysplastic nevi. *J Invest Dermatol* **100**:346S, 1993
83. Rigel DS et al: Dysplastic nevi. Markers for increased risk for melanoma. *Cancer* **63**:386, 1989
84. Tiersten AD et al: Prospective follow-up for malignant melanoma in patients with atypical-mole (dysplastic-nevus) syndrome. *J Dermatol Surg Oncol* **17**:44, 1991
85. Schneider JS et al: Risk factors for melanoma incidence in prospective follow-up. The importance of atypical (dysplastic) nevi. *Arch Dermatol* **130**:1002, 1994
86. Rhodes AR et al: Dysplastic melanocytic nevi in histologic association with 234 primary cutaneous melanomas. *J Am Acad Dermatol* **9**:563, 1983
87. Cook MG et al: Melanocytic dysplasia and melanoma. *Histopathology* **9**:647, 1985
88. McGovern VJ et al: Histogenesis of malignant melanoma with an adjacent component of the superficial spreading type. *Pathology* **17**:251, 1985
89. Black WC: Residual dysplastic and other nevi in superficial spreading melanoma. Clinical correlations and association with sun damage. *Cancer* **62**:163, 1988
90. Duray PH et al: Dysplastic nevus in histologic contiguity with acquired nonfamilial melanoma. Clinicopathologic experience in a 100-bed hospital. *Arch Dermatol* **123**:80, 1987
91. Gruber SB et al: Nevomelanocytic proliferations in association with cutaneous malignant melanoma: A multivariate analysis. *J Am Acad Dermatol* **21**:773, 1989
92. Marks R et al: Do all melanomas come from "moles"? A study of the histological association between melanocytic naevi and melanoma. *Aust J Dermatol* **31**:77, 1990
93. Hastrup N et al: The presence of dysplastic nevus remnants in malignant melanomas. A population-based study of 551 malignant melanomas. *Am J Dermatopathol* **13**:378, 1991
94. Kittler H et al: Follow-up of melanocytic skin lesions with digital epiluminescence microscopy: Patterns of modifications observed in early melanoma, atypical nevi, and common nevi. *J Am Acad Dermatol* **43**:467, 2000
95. Grob JJ et al: Dysplastic naevus in non-familial melanoma. A clinicopathological study of 101 cases. *Br J Dermatol* **118**:745, 1988
96. Kopf AW et al: Familial malignant melanoma. *JAMA* **256**:1915, 1986
97. Goldstein AM et al: Age at diagnosis and transmission of invasive melanoma in 23 families with cutaneous malignant melanoma/dysplastic nevi. *J Natl Cancer Inst* **86**:1385, 1994
98. Lucchina LC et al: Familial cutaneous melanoma. *Melanoma Res* **5**:413, 1995
99. Chang AE et al: The national cancer database report on cutaneous and noncutaneous melanoma. *Cancer* **83**:1664, 1998
100. Berwick M et al: Screening for cutaneous melanoma by skin self-examination. *J Natl Cancer Inst* **88**:17, 1996
101. Epstein, DS et al: Is physician detection associated with thinner melanomas? *JAMA* **281**:640, 1999
102. Rodriguez-Sains RS: Coexistent primary ocular and cutaneous melanoma. *Arch Dermatol* **130**:660, 1994
103. Bataille V et al: Five cases of coexistent primary ocular and cutaneous melanoma. *Arch Dermatol* **129**:198, 1993
104. McCarthy JM et al: Conjunctival and uveal melanoma in the dysplastic nevus syndrome. *Surv Ophthalmol* **37**:377, 1993
105. Rodriguez-Sains RS: Ocular findings in patients with dysplastic nevus syndrome. An update. *Dermatol Clin* **9**:723, 1991
106. Vink J et al: Ocular melanoma in families with dysplastic nevus syndrome. *J Am Acad Dermatol* **23**:858, 1990
107. Goldstein AM et al: Increased risk of pancreatic cancer in melanoma-prone kindreds with $p16^{INK4}$ mutations. *N Engl J Med* **333**:970, 1995
108. Vasen HF et al: Risk of developing pancreatic cancer in families with familial atypical multiple mole melanoma associated with a specific 19 deletion of p16 (p16-Leiden). *Int J Cancer* **87**:809, 2000
109. Hille ETM et al: Excess cancer mortality in six Dutch pedigrees with the familial atypical multiple mole-melanoma syndrome from 1830 to 1994. *J Invest Dermatol* **110**:788, 1998
110. Schenk M et al: The risk of subsequent primary carcinoma of the pancreas in patients with cutaneous malignant melanoma. *Cancer* **82**:1672, 1998

CHAPTER 93

Richard G.B. Langley
Raymond L. Barnhill
Martin C. Mihm, Jr.
Thomas B. Fitzpatrick
Arthur J. Sober

Neoplasms: Cutaneous Melanoma

Cutaneous melanoma is an increasingly common, enigmatic, and potentially lethal malignancy of melanocytes. The salient challenge for clinicians is to detect and excise melanoma in its earliest stage, as tumor thickness remains the most important prognostic indicator for primary cutaneous melanoma.[1–3] Early diagnosis and surgical excision of in situ or early invasive melanomas are curative in most patients. Despite advances in chemotherapy and immunotherapy, the success in the treatment of advanced melanoma remains limited, and the prognosis of metastatic disease is guarded.

DEFINITION

Melanoma results from the malignant transformation of melanocytes. Melanocytes are derived from the neural crest and produce melanin (see Chap. 11). During embryonic life, precursor cells, known as melanoblasts, migrate to the basal-cell layer of the epidermis and, less frequently, to the dermis and sebaceous glands. Melanoma can arise from melanocytes located in these sites and from altered melanocytes called nevus cells in certain precursor lesions.

EPIDEMIOLOGY AND RISK FACTORS

Incidence and Mortality Rates (Table 93-1)

The incidence of melanoma has been steadily increasing in the past several decades. This increased frequency of newly diagnosed melanomas has been seen worldwide and is in the order of 3 to 8 percent per year. This increase in incidence of melanoma has been sustained over time: in the United States, the lifetime risk of invasive melanoma developing was only 1 in 1500 in 1935; in 1960, 1 in 600; in 1992, 1 in 105; in 1996, 1 in 88; and 1 in 75 in 2000 and could reach 1 in 50 by the year 2010.[4] The American Cancer Society estimates that in 2002 alone melanoma will have developed in 87,800 Americans: 53,500 of these tumors will have been invasive and 34,300 will have been in situ.[5] Cutaneous melanoma currently represents 5 percent of all types of newly diagnosed cancer in men, and skin is the fifth most frequent site for cancer to occur overall. Cutaneous melanoma is the leading fatal illness arising in the skin; it is estimated that it will have been the cause of 7400 deaths in the year 2002.[5]

Mortality rates have also been rising over much of this century, but more slowly than incidence rates. The Surveillance, Epidemiology, and End Results Program (SEER) has documented a 32.7 percent increase in mortality rates over the period 1973 to 1995.[6] On the other hand, the overall survival rate has been improving for melanoma in the past 5 decades as a consequence of early detection. In 1940, the 5-year overall survival rate for melanoma was 40 percent. By 1975, the 5-year rate was 67 percent and data from the SEER program indicates this has increased to 88.2 percent for the period 1989 to 1994.[6]

Risk Factors

SUN EXPOSURE There is convincing evidence from epidemiologic studies that exposure to solar radiation is the major cause of cutaneous melanoma in light-pigmented populations and plays a role in the increasing incidence of this malignancy. There are at least four basic lines of evidence that support this relationship, including anatomic differences by sex, migration studies, differences by latitude of residence, and racial differences.[7]

Plotting melanoma cases on anatomic models (Fig. 93-1) illustrates the concentration of melanoma on sites of sun exposure with virtual sparing of consistently covered areas. The pattern of sun exposure appears important because the distribution of melanoma by body site is not consistently related to the areas of maximal ultraviolet radiation exposure in whites, but appears to involve areas intermittently exposed. In men, the trunk, particularly the upper back, is the most common site for melanoma, whereas in women, the most frequent sites are the lower legs and the upper back (Fig. 93-1). Involvement of the head and

TABLE 93-1

Cutaneous Melanoma: Data and Facts

- Melanoma represents 5% of all cancers by incidence in males and 4% in females.
- Estimated number of new cases in the United States for 2002: invasive melanoma: 53,600; melanoma in situ: 34,300
- US lifetime risk of developing invasive melanoma: 1935:1/500; 1961:1/600; 1980:1/150; 1992:1/105; 1996:1/88; 2000:1/75; 2010:1/50. Estimated new melanoma deaths in US, 2002: 7400
- Most frequent sites in whites, male: back, upper extremities
- Most frequent sites in whites, female: back, lower legs
- Most frequent sites in blacks and Asians: soles, mucous membranes, palms, nail beds
- Frequency of melanoma by type of tumor: superficial spreading melanoma: 70%; nodular melanoma: 15%; lentigo maligna melanoma: 5%; acral and unclassified melanoma: 10%
- Important features in recognition: A = asymmetry; B = irregularity of borders, presence of notching;
  C = variegation in color and pigmentation pattern (mixtures of colors in addition to brown and tan);
  D = diameter >6 mm

FIGURE 93-1

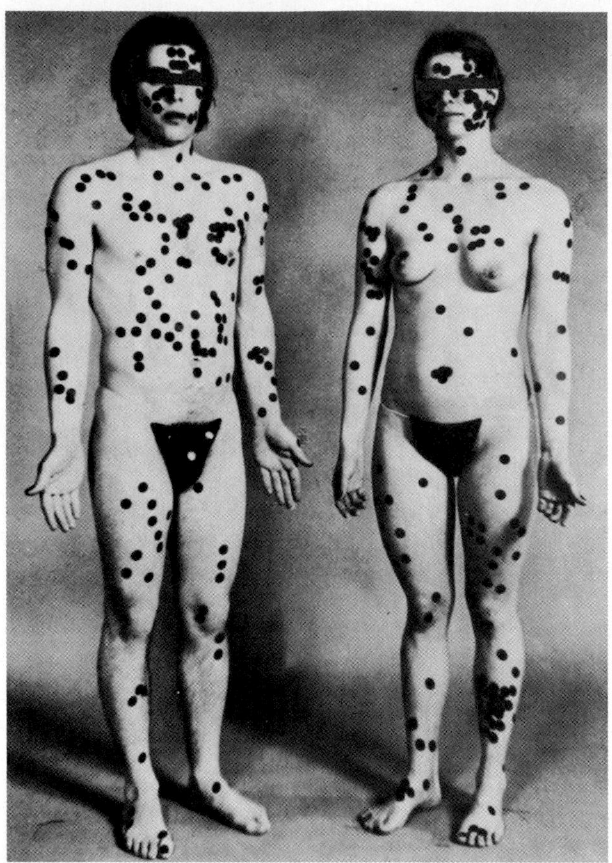

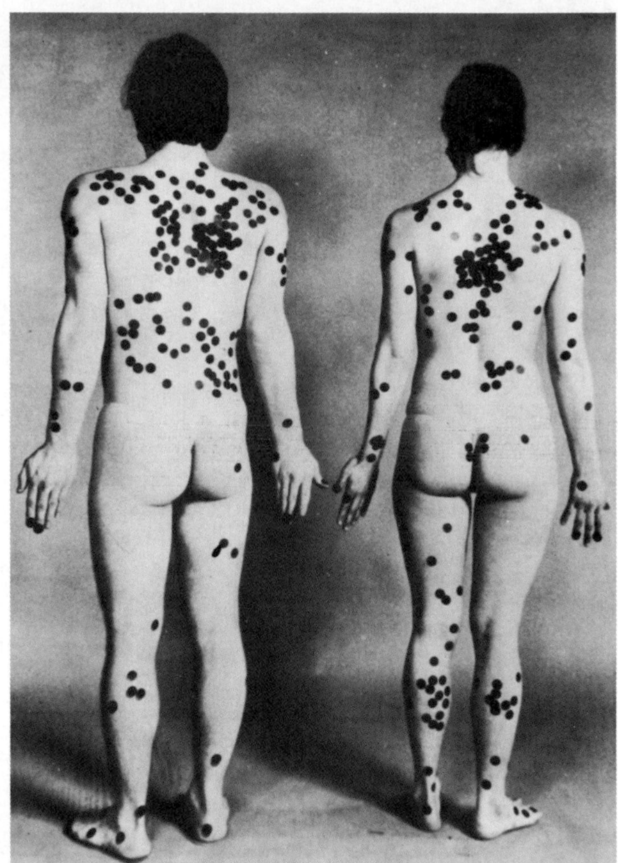

A. *B.*

Anatomic site distribution of melanoma by sex in 731 males and females. (*Courtesy of the Melanoma Cooperative Group*).

neck is less frequent for all subtypes of melanoma apart from lentigo maligna melanoma, for which the link between long-term sun exposure and its development has been more widely accepted. Preferential involvement of sites of intermittent sun exposure has, in part, led to the supposition that for melanoma, intermittent exposure to sunlight is more carcinogenic than continuous exposure. In a critical review of the world's literature, Elwood identified 39 case-control studies involving more than 10,000 melanoma patients investigating the role of melanoma and sun exposure: 20 of these studies examined the role of intermittent exposure to sunlight, with 14 finding a significant positive association; 5 studies failed to show a major association, and 1 study identified a protective effect.[7]

Studies of immigrants to areas with higher levels of ambient solar radiation demonstrate increased rates of melanoma in the immigrants to such areas when compared with similar individuals in their native lands.[8,9] Younger migrants to sunny climates have an increased risk for melanoma as compared with adult migrants. Holman and Armstrong noted that immigrants who migrated to western Australia prior to age 10 years have a fourfold increase in the risk of melanoma as compared with those arriving after the age of 15 years.[10] A study by Holly et al. of women with cutaneous melanoma from the western United States confirmed the importance of intense sun exposure at an early age, but also extended the risk to older ages.[11] Children who sustained frequent severe sunburns before age 12 years had a 3.6 elevated risk of developing melanoma, but sunburns even within the 10 years preceding the diagnosis of melanoma also resulted in a twofold elevation of risk.[11]

Melanoma incidence and mortality among whites correlate inversely with latitude of residence and dose of ultraviolet radiation. This effect has been termed the "latitude gradient," and increased rates of melanoma have been documented when comparing regions of different proximity to the equator in essentially similar populations such as Australia and New Zealand, the United States, and Norway. In these diverse geographic areas, the incidence of melanoma has ranged from being three- to tenfold greater in regions closer to the equator. In one Australian study higher rates were reported in the southwest as compared with the north.[9] This apparent paradoxical relationship to latitude can be resolved after controlling for racial and phenotypic features of the population.

The final line of evidence in support of a role of solar radiation as a cause of melanoma arises from the differences seen between racial groups. Cutaneous melanoma is a greater problem in light-skinned whites,[8] with the incidence of melanoma in blacks living within a similar geographic region roughly one-tenth to one-twentieth that of whites. Among whites, higher rates of melanoma occur among those who are less pigmented. Two reasons cited for the decreased rate of melanoma in darker-pigmented races are the protective effect of melanin against solar radiation and the fewer numbers of nevi that may serve as precursor lesions for melanoma.

Exposure to psoralen and ultraviolet A radiation (PUVA) increases the risk of developing melanoma. The PUVA Follow-up Study is a multicenter, prospective study that evaluated a cohort of 1380 patients who first received PUVA in 1975 to 1976. In the initial report, Stern et. al.[12] documented 11 melanomas in 9 patients who had received PUVA. The relative risk increased over time: it was 1.1 in the study group from 1975 to 1990, but increased to 5.4 for the period 1991 to 1996. An update was recently published,[13] indicating that 23 patients

TABLE 93-2

Risk Factors for Cutaneous Melanoma

Risk factor
Pigmentary characteristics
Blue eyes
Blond, fair, or red hair
Light complexion
Response to sun exposure
Freckling tendency
Inability to tan
Tendency to sunburn
Upper socioeconomic status
Family history of melanoma
p16 mutation; *BRAF* mutation
Nevi
Melanocytic nevi
Dysplastic nevi
Changing mole
Congenital nevus
History of prior melanoma
Immunosuppression

have developed 26 invasive or in situ cutaneous melanomas since 1975. The risk increases in patients exposed to high doses of PUVA.[13]

Taken together, there is compelling epidemiologic evidence that solar radiation is causally related to a significant proportion of cutaneous melanoma. Although the exact quantitative and qualitative nature of this exposure is not clear, it is probable that intermittent exposures and intense exposures with consequent sunburns in a high-risk phenotype are important. While the exact nature of the relationship remains to be precisely defined, it is certain that preventive measures regarding exposure to the sun should be recommended. Exposures to ultraviolet (UV) radiation from early in life should be reduced.

PHENOTYPE Case-control studies have identified certain phenotypic features that are associated with an elevated risk for melanoma[10] (Table 93-2). Such phenotypic features include light skin pigmentation, ease of sun burning, blond or red hair color, pale or light skin, prominent freckling tendency, and blue or green eyes.

REACTION OF SKIN TO SUNLIGHT The manner of reaction of the skin to sun exposure (or skin phototype) is an important indicator of melanoma risk. Increased melanoma risk is associated with erythema or a tendency to sunburn on acute exposure and little or no tendency to tan with long-term exposure[10] (see Chap. 88).

OCCUPATION AND SOCIAL STATUS Multiple case-control studies have documented a relationship between higher socioeconomic status and risk for melanoma.[7] This association may be confounded by factors such as race, degree of pigmentation, greater leisure time, and tendency to take vacations in sunny locations. Elwood[7] reviewed the evidence for an increased relative risk for occupational exposure, noting conflicting results in the 18 studies reported up to 1996. In these studies, a significant increase in the risk of melanoma developing was seen in 4 of 18 cases, with a significant reduction in risk seen in 4 of 18, and no significant difference in the remainder.

FAMILIAL MELANOMA Patients with familial melanoma are estimated to account for 10 to 15 percent of all patients with melanoma. It is important to inquire about family history for relatives with melanoma, as recognition of such cases constitutes an identifiable high-risk group. Patients with at least two first-degree relatives with melanoma are at particular elevated risk. Patients with familial melanoma typically have disease onset at an earlier age, and have an increased frequency of multiple primary melanomas and of dysplastic nevi as compared with nonfamilial melanoma. Dysplastic nevi are markers for individuals at an increased risk for melanoma both in the sporadic and familial settings (see Chap. 92). Patients with familial melanoma appear to have a more favorable prognosis because of higher awareness, as they may have thinner tumors on average at the time of diagnosis. More intensive follow-up may also contribute to earlier melanoma diagnoses in familial cases.

A family history of melanoma should increase the suspicion that melanoma will develop in other relatives, and reported skin examinations should be recommended for all first-degree relatives to facilitate early diagnosis. It is important to inform high-risk persons of the clinical features of early melanoma so that they will be able to recognize suspicious pigmented lesions in themselves and in family members. Genetic linkage studies have identified a familial melanoma gene on chromosome 9p21. A cyclin-dependent kinase inhibitor, $p16^{INK4a}$, has been implicated as candidate tumor-suppressor gene, and has been documented in approximately 40 percent of familial melanoma patients (see below). Future studies to determine the melanoma gene precisely may enable identification of susceptible individuals, and may identify family members who lack the gene, with different counseling, preventive, and follow-up regimens implied.

MELANOCYTIC NEVI Congenital and acquired melanocytic nevi are potential, although infrequent, precursors of cutaneous melanoma. Approximately one-third of melanomas are associated with a nevus remnant. Multiple case-control studies have documented an increased risk developing melanoma, and it is evident that there is both a quantitative and qualitative risk associated with nevi. Quantitative measures of nevi correlate directly with magnitude of melanoma risk.[14] There is also evidence that qualitative abnormalities of nevi are linked to elevated melanoma risk.[14,15] It has been shown that the presence of clinically atypical nevi (dysplastic nevi) in individuals with familial melanoma indicates substantial risk (lifetime relative risk of 148) for melanoma (see Chap. 92). At present, the relative importance of these quantitative versus qualitative factors has not been resolved.

A multicenter prospective case-control study of 716 patients with newly diagnosed melanoma and 1014 controls examined the risk of melanoma according to the number and type of nevi[15] (Table 93-2). An increased risk of melanoma was determined according to the number of nondysplastic and dysplastic nevi. In this study, the presence of a solitary dysplastic nevus doubled the risk of melanoma developing, while having 10 or more dysplastic nevi was associated with a 12-fold elevation of risk. The number of small and large nondysplastic nevi was also associated with an increased risk of melanoma, with the presence of 50 to 99 small nevi or more than 10 large nevi conferring a doubling of risk for the development of melanoma.[15]

GENDER AND HORMONAL FACTORS The possible influence of both endogenous and exogenous hormones on the clinical course of melanoma has been a topic of long-standing interest. Much of this interest stems from several clinical observations unique to melanoma. First, melanoma is rare before puberty, suggesting that development of greater melanoma risk correlates with onset of hormonal changes. Even after adjustment for site and thickness, women still manifest a better prognosis than do men for primary cutaneous melanoma [American Joint Committee on Cancer (AJCC) stages I and II].[16]

The biologic basis of potential hormonal effects on melanoma include the well-known hyperpigmentation associated with pregnancy; elevation of many endogenous hormones during pregnancy [e.g., estrogens, androgens, melanocyte-stimulating hormone (MSH), follicle-stimulating hormone (FSH), and luteinizing hormone (LH)]; induction of melasma by oral contraceptives; and stimulation of melanoma growth in animals after administration of estrogens. There is conflicting evidence on the presence of estrogen receptors on melanoma, as studies employing specific monoclonal antibodies have either failed to verify the presence of estrogen receptors in melanoma or have detected estrogen receptors only to 30 percent of specimens. Because of the influence of sex and other hormonal factors on the course of melanoma, there has been concern about the effects of oral contraceptives on melanoma risk. Review of the studies published so far indicates that there is little, if any, evidence to indicate significant risk for the vast majority of women who have been diagnosed with melanoma and who continue to use oral contraceptives.[17]

TUMORIGENESIS AND CAUSATION

Tumor Progression

Cancer may be viewed as an inherently genetic disease with multiple stages resulting from progressive changes in DNA. These genetic alterations may result from activating mutations of proto-oncogenes, mutations or deletions in tumor-suppressor genes, gross structural changes of chromosomes, and often from all three mechanisms.[18] Aberrations of DNA may contribute not only to tumor progression, but also to alterations in expression and differentiation. Thus, in the evolutionary process from benign cells to fully malignant cells, there are likely to be many causative factors, both endogenous and exogenous, that interact and influence tumorigenesis in a cumulative fashion.

Five stages of tumor progression in the melanocytic system have been suggested based on clinical, histopathologic, immunopathologic, cytogenetic, and in vitro properties:[19] (1) benign melanocytic nevi; (2) dysplastic nevi; (3) primary malignant melanoma, radial growth phase; (4) primary malignant melanoma, vertical growth phase; and (5) metastatic malignant melanoma. It is believed that with each successive step of tumorigenesis, a new clone of cells emerges with growth advantages over the surrounding tissue, resulting in "clonal expansion." Clark and associates postulated that a critical step in tumor progression of melanoma may be the transition from radial to vertical growth phases.[19] The radial growth phase consists of invasion of the papillary dermis by small numbers of melanoma cells that have gained a growth advantage. These cells are thought to have the capacity for autonomous proliferation in this location, but not for aggregative growth. The vertical growth phase is signaled by this property of aggregative growth, resulting in the formation of expansile nests or nodules of cells. It must be emphasized that because the metastatic cascade comprises a complex range of biochemical events, the vertical growth phase is likely to be an oversimplified correlate for the metastatic phenotype.

A discussion of tumorigenesis of melanoma must take into account several important clinical observations: (1) the association between nevi and melanoma in at least 30 percent of cases (an apparent absence of nevi in 70 percent of melanoma); (2) the role of sunlight in the pathogenesis of melanoma; (3) pigmentary phenotype of patients in whom melanoma develops; and (4) family history of melanoma and other genetic factors. In addition, the latter observations are closely related or have complex interactions. When the above observations are considered in light of the multistep process of tumor progression of melanoma, at least two major pathways of tumorigenesis can be envisaged.[20] In the first pathway, melanomas, particularly superficial spreading melanomas (SSMs), develop in association with melanocytic nevi. According to this model, nevi may represent the first stage of tumor progression of melanoma or an initiated clonal proliferation. The most likely initiating agent would be sunlight exposure, perhaps at an early age. There is epidemiologic evidence that sun exposure in the second decade may result in larger numbers of nevi. The number of precursor nevi may be important as greater numbers of initiated cells would increase the target population for another mutational event. Because UV is believed to be a complete carcinogen, sunlight exposure, perhaps of intermittent nature, could lead to this second promotional event of tumor progression.[20]

Another pathway of melanoma development is that of lentigo maligna melanoma (LMM). According to this model, this form of melanoma results from cumulative sun exposure and a corresponding cumulative insult to the DNA of melanocytes of sun-exposed skin. Lentigo maligna (LM) shows the least common association with nevi (3 percent of cases) and the most direct relationship with sun exposure among the different types of melanoma. The age-incidence rates show a steady increase with age, consistent with continuous exposure (initiation) to a carcinogenic agent such as sunlight.

GENETICS Based on the first comprehensive analysis of 22 kindreds of familial melanoma in 1967, Anderson et al. concluded that melanoma appeared to be inherited by an autosomal mechanism, possibly dominant, based on the observed frequent transmission from parent to child, irrespective of sex.[21] However, because of the variation in this mode of transmission, they also observed that inheritance was probably more complex and could involve more than one gene. A formal segregation analysis was conducted by Greene on 401 members of 14 melanoma-prone families and the results were interpreted as consistent with an autosomal dominant mechanism.[22] These studies identified a melanoma susceptibility gene on the short arm of chromosome 1 that was linked to the rhesus blood group locus. By using linkage analysis, Bale et al. later implicated the *1p36* gene on the short arm of chromosome 1p in the pathogenesis of cutaneous melanoma.[23] Subsequently, other researchers worldwide have failed to reproduce linkage to chromosome 1p, leading to controversy regarding the linkage to chromosome 1p.

A tumor-suppression gene, *p16*, has been localized on chromosome 9p[24,25] and was identified as the possible candidate for melanoma susceptibility. This promising information was initiated by cytogenetic studies detecting homozygous and heterozygous deletions of the 9p21-p22 region in melanoma cell lines,[26] and in a patient with multiple primary melanomas and multiple atypical nevi in which cytogenetic rearrangements involving chromosome 5p and 9p were determined.[27] Linkage studies in 11 kindreds with multiple cases of primary melanoma were able initially to link genetic markers to chromosome 9p13-p22.[28] This linkage study identifying markers to the melanoma susceptibility locus to chromosome 9p was subsequently confirmed by investigators studying kindreds from Australia, Holland, Britain, and the United States. These studies were able to identify the locus to within a 2- to 3-Mb region on chromosome 9p21. Nobori et al.[25] and Kamb et al.[24] discovered by positional cloning studies that the gene *p16* is likely the tumor-suppressor gene locus on chromosome 9p21. The current nomenclature for the gene is *CDKN2A (cyclin-dependent kinase inhibitor 2A)*, and the protein is referred to as $p16^{INK4a}$ or INK4a (inhibitor of kinase 4a), although both the gene and protein are often referred to as p16.[29] The p16 locus encodes two gene products: *p16* and an *alternative reading frame (ARF)*. The cyclin-dependent kinase inhibitors bind and inhibit cyclin-dependent kinases, CDK4 and CDK6, which are involved in entry into the cell cycle. p16 thus functions in cell-cycle regulation, because it can bind to CDK4 or CDK6, inhibiting progression of cells through the G1 phase of the cell cycle. Mutations in p16 could allow cells to progress into S phase and result in abnormal proliferation, and ultimately neoplasia.

Germ-line mutations in the p16 gene have been identified in approximately 40 percent of melanoma-prone families.[29] Penetrance studies estimate that 53 percent of individuals with a mutant allele will develop melanoma by the age of 80.[30] Other candidate melanoma susceptibility loci include 3p, 6q, 10q, 11q, and 17p.[29] Deletions in chromosome 10q are believed to be important in melanoma progression with up to 48 percent of metastatic melanomas exhibiting such deletions.

Davies et al. have reported a mutation in the signaling pathway gene *BRAF,* in 66 percent of malignant melanomas.[31] This somatic missense mutation identified a new oncogene likely to play a critical role in our understanding of malignant melanoma. The high frequency of *BRAF* mutations in malignant melanoma may be related to crucial regulations of melanocytes; alpha-melanocyte–stimulating hormone and proopiomelanocortin-derived peptides. These peptides bind to melanocortin receptor I and upregulate CAMP, leading to increased proliferation and melanogenesis in response to UVB radiation.[32] This signaling cascade activates *BRAF,* thus linking a principal melanocyte signaling pathway controlling proliferation and differentiation that operates through activation of *BRAF*. The product of the mutated *BRAF* gene has elevated kinase activity and is transformed in NIH3T3 cells. Inhibiting the kinase may be an important new strategy in the treatment of metastatic melanoma.[31]

PRECURSOR LESIONS

Cutaneous melanoma may arise in a preexisting melanocytic lesion or de novo, in previously normal skin. A preexisting lesion is considered a precursor, implying a temporal and spatial relationship.[33] Such a lesion may occur prior to and at the site of a malignancy. Dysplastic nevi may be precursors and markers of increased risk for cutaneous melanoma (see Chap. 92). Recognition of precursors can facilitate surveillance of a high-risk population for early diagnosis of curable melanomas.

TYPES OF PRIMARY MELANOMA OF THE SKIN

Melanoma can be classified into four main growth patterns, which are defined by their gross and microscopic characteristics and correlated with their life history (Table 93-3). The four major growth patterns of melanoma are termed *lentigo maligna, superficial spreading, nodular,* and *acral lentiginous melanoma.*

Lentigo Maligna

CLINICAL CHARACTERISTICS LM is a type of melanoma in situ with a prolonged radial growth phase that may eventuate into invasive melanoma. Once invasive, LM can be lethal. LM is a macular, freckle-like lesion of irregular shape, with differing shades throughout that occurs on sun-exposed surfaces, most often in elderly patients with sun-damaged atrophic skin (Fig. 93-2*A*). Irregular mottling or flecking may appear as the lesion enlarges. LM grows by spreading radially, increasing in size, and assuming a variety of irregular shapes (Fig 93-2*B*). The exact percentage of LM that progress to LMM is unknown.[34] The lifetime risk of LMM developing from LM is estimated to be 4.7 percent at 45 years of age and 2.2 percent for a person 65 years old.[35]

HISTOPATHOLOGY The histopathology of LM is characterized by an atrophic epidermis with thinning and loss of rete ridges, containing increased numbers of atypical basilar melanocytes (Fig. 93-3). These melanocytes vary in appearance, size, and shape, and have nuclei of different sizes that are variably hyperchromatic. The cytoplasm of these cells, which is usually retracted about the nucleus leaving a space between the cell borders and adjacent melanocytes, is pink to purple to red-brown and irregularly granular. These cells may extend down hair follicles and skin appendages, making the lesion difficult to eradicate by superficial therapies. A mononuclear cell infiltrate is characteristically present in the superficial lesions below the proliferated melanocytes. The dermis shows elastotic changes of the connective tissue from long-term sun damage. Diagnosis can usually be established by biopsy of the darkest portion. Occasionally, the histopathology will not be diagnostic, and either rebiopsy or repeat biopsy over time with close observation will be necessary.

TABLE 93-3

Comparisons of Clinical Features of Cutaneous Melanoma

Type of Melanoma	Frequency (%)	Duration Before Diagnosis Year (Yrs.)	Mean Age at Diagnosis Year (Yrs.)	Site	Clinical Features
Types with radial growth phases					
Superficial spreading melanoma	70	1–7	40–50	Any site; lower legs in females, back in both sexes	Raised border on palpation or inspection; pinks, whites, grays, and blues in brown lesion
Acral lentiginous melanoma (including subungual melanoma)	10	1–10	60	Sole, palms, mucous membranes, subungual	Flat, irregular border; predominantly dark brown with areas of regression
Lentigo maligna melanoma	5	5–20	70	Nose, cheeks, temples	Brown-tan macular lesion with variation in pigment pattern; may be amelanotic
Type with no radial growth phase					
Nodular melanoma	15	Months	40–50	Any site	Nodule arises in apparently normal skin or in a nevus; brown to brown-black; may have bluish hues; may be amelanotic

SOURCE: Modified from Sober AJ et al: Melanoma and other cancers. *Harrison's Principles of Internal Medicine,* 15th ed., edited by E Braunwald et al. New York, McGraw-Hill, 2001, p555

FIGURE 93-2

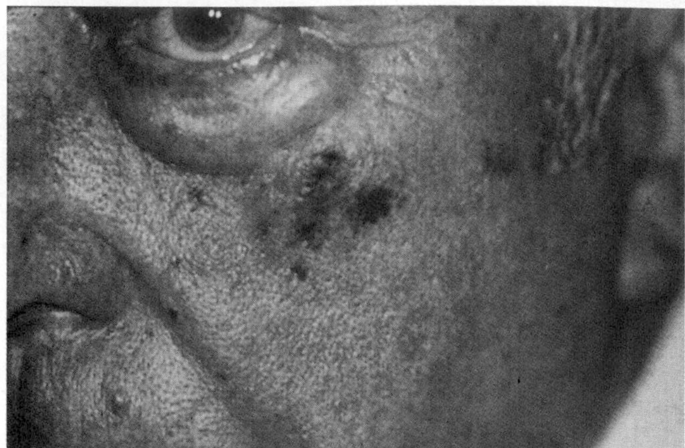

A.

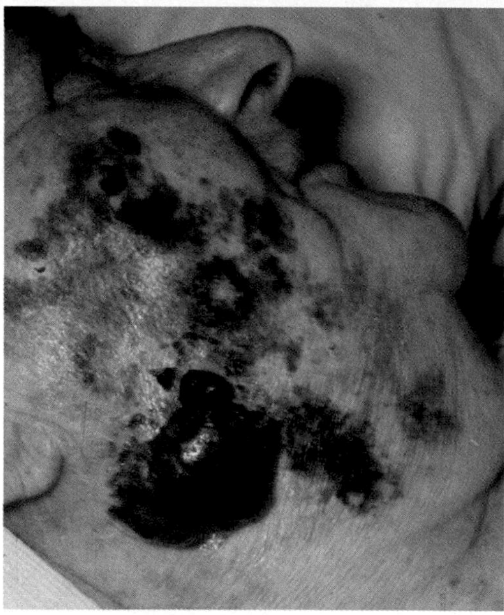

B.

Lentigo maligna and lentigo maligna melanoma. *A.* Lentigo maligna displays prominent asymmetry with irregular borders and variegation of pigmentation. *B.* Extensive lentigo maligna melanoma with large nodules (vertical growth phase) on the face of a patient.

Lentigo Maligna Melanoma

CLINICAL CHARACTERISTICS (Table 93-3) LMM is the least-common type of melanoma (usually 4 to 15 percent of all melanoma patients), although a rising incidence has been reported.[34] LMM is almost exclusively located on sun-exposed skin of the head and neck, with the nose and cheeks the most common sites. Occasionally, LMM may be found on the dorsal aspect of the hands, the lower legs, or, rarely, at other sites. LMM occurs in an older age group, with a median age at diagnosis of approximately 65 years old; it is uncommon before the age of 40 years (Fig. 93-4).[36] Frequently the lesion is quite large (3 to 6 cm or larger), although its nodular portion may vary from only a few millimeters to 1 to 2 centimeters in width (Fig 93-2*B*). The colors in flat areas include tan, brown, black, and, at times, opalescent blue-gray and white. Brown areas may exhibit dark flecks in a black reticular pattern. Regression may be present in blue-gray or white areas (Fig 93-2*B*). Rarely, LM and LMM can be amelanotic. LMM can have extremely convoluted borders with prominent notching. LMM is usually flat, especially in early lesions, and palpability usually indicates invasive melanoma, although clinical examination may be unreliable in early invasive LMM (<1 mm) (Fig. 93-2*A*).

FIGURE 93-3

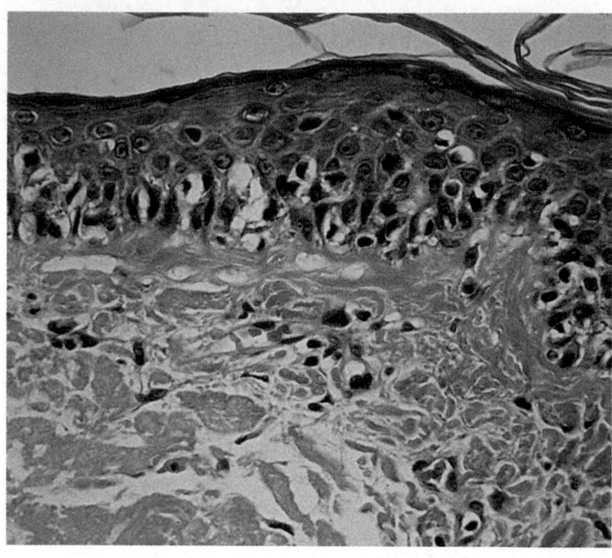

Lentigo maligna. This is a proliferation of pleomorphic melanocytes in the basal cell layer of an atrophic epidermis in sun-damaged skin.

HISTOPATHOLOGY LMM is characterized histologically by extensive variation in the morphologic features of the intraepidermal melanocytes in the tan, brown, and flat black portions of the lesion. Tan areas demonstrate an increased number of melanocytes, some normal, others larger than normal, and others frankly atypical and bizarre, all distributed along the basal layer (Fig. 93-5). In the flat black areas, numerous melanocytes, with variable morphologic character, apparently replace the basal layer and form a sheet along the dermal–epidermal interface, with keratinocytes above it and the papillary layer of the dermis below it. Marked hyperpigmentation and some atrophy of the

FIGURE 93-4

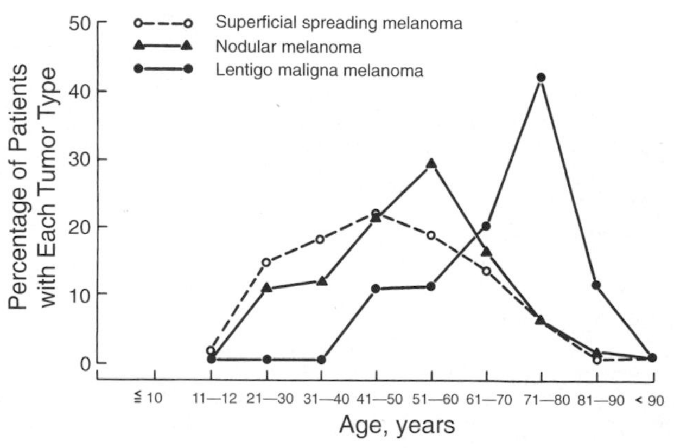

Age distribution by type of melanoma. Superficial spreading (SSM), nodular (NM), and lentigo maligna (LMM) melanomas. (*Melanoma Clinical Cooperative Group data, 1978.*)

FIGURE 93-5

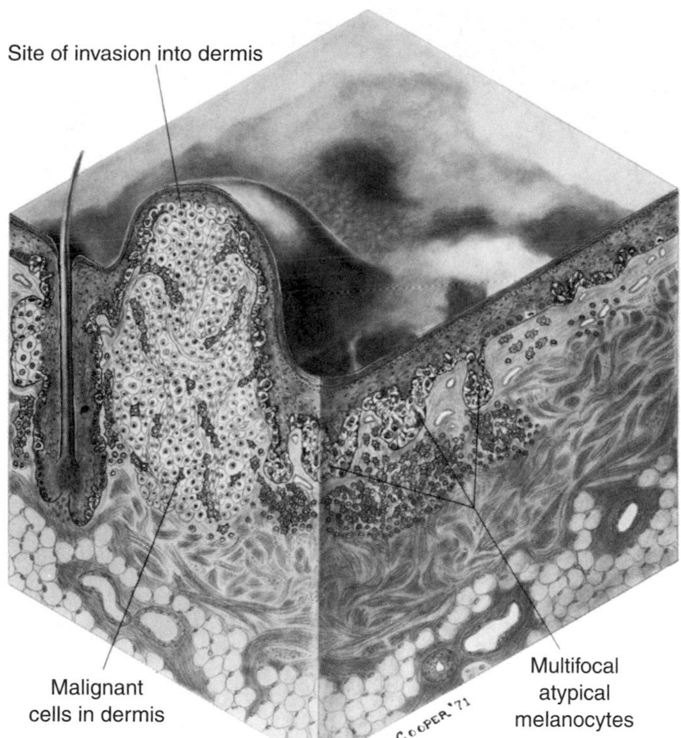

Lentigo maligna melanoma. Illustrated is a large, variegated, freckle-like macule (not elevated above the plane of the skin) with irregular borders; the tan areas show increased numbers of melanocytes, usually atypical and bizarre, and distributed single file along the basal layer; at certain places in the dermis, malignant melanocytes have invaded and formed prominent nests. At the left is a large nodule that is composed of epithelioid cells in this illustration; the nodules of all four types of melanoma are indistinguishable from each other.

keratinocytic epidermis accompany the extensive hyperplasia of atypical melanocytes along the dermal–epidermal interface. The papillary dermis usually contains a dense infiltrate of lymphocytes and macrophages laden with melanin. At certain places in the dermis, invading malignant melanocytes are present and form large nests; these nests correspond to clinically detectable nodules (Fig. 93-6).

Superficial Spreading Melanoma

CLINICAL CHARACTERISTICS (Table 93-3) SSM represents approximately 70 percent of all melanomas and is the most common type of cutaneous melanoma. SSM most commonly occurs on the legs of women and the upper backs of men, although it can occur at any site. SSM is diagnosed most commonly in the fourth and fifth decades. Various clinical presentations of SSM are shown in Figs. 93-7, 93-8, and 93-9. SSM may present as a deeply pigmented macule or barely raised plaque, and initially the fine skin markings may remain intact. The earliest change in a SSM may be a discrete, focal area of darkening within a preexisting nevus. Pigment variegation of SSM involves a mixture of colors, ranging from a dark brown to black to dark blue-gray to a pink or gray-white color (Figs. 93-7 and 93-8). The placement of the different colors is haphazard. The absence of pigmentation within a SSM may represent regression and can be more readily identified with a Wood lamp (long-wave ultraviolet) as a hypopigmented area. As the lesion grows, the surface may appear glossy. The borders of SSM may be irregular with angular indentations (notches) or scalloping (Figs.

FIGURE 93-6

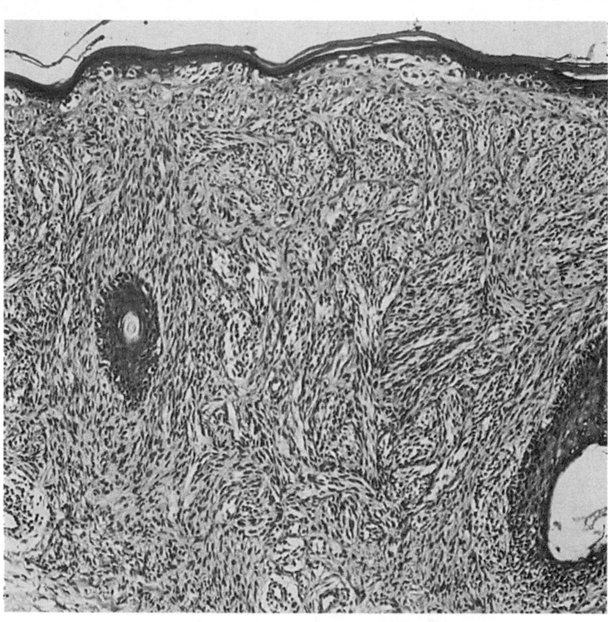

Lentigo maligna melanoma. Extending from the epidermis into the dermis are numerous elongated melanocytes. In LMM these cells are frequently spindle-shaped.

93-7 and 93-8), particularly with enlargement of the SSM. The lesion throughout varies from slightly to definitely elevated (Figs. 93-7, 93-8, and 93-9).

HISTOPATHOLOGY SSM is characterized by a population of melanocytes appearing uniformly atypical; the striking melanocytic pleomorphism so characteristic of LMM is not usually seen. Biopsy of a slightly raised, hyperpigmented portion of SSM reveals a "pagetoid" distribution of large melanocytes throughout the epidermis (Figs. 93-10 and 93-11). The large cells may occur singly or in nests and have a monomorphous appearance. On microscopic examination, biopsies of markedly nodular areas of SSM reveal dense accumulations of malignant cells in the dermis. In areas of invasion, large melanocytes are observed. These large cells have an abundance of cytoplasm containing regularly dispersed, fine particles of melanin; the dusty appearance of the cells, when viewed with the microscope, is the result of these numerous granules.

Nodular Melanoma

CLINICAL CHARACTERISTICS (Table 93-3) The second most common subtype of melanoma is nodular melanoma, with a frequency of 15 to 30 percent of all types. The trunk, head, and neck are the most frequent anatomic sites for nodular melanoma (NM). NM is remarkable for its rapid evolution, often arising over several weeks or months. NM lacks an apparent radial growth phase. It is more common for NM to begin de novo in uninvolved skin than to arise in a preexisting nevus.

NM typically appears as a uniform dark blue-black, bluish-red, or amelanotic papule or nodule, but can present as a polypoid lesion with a stalk.[36] NM may appear as a blueberry-shaped nodule with a thundercloud-gray appearance (Fig. 93-12*A*). Early recognition of NMs can be difficult because they lack many of the conventional clinical features of melanoma. In certain cases, it may be difficult to discriminate between NM and hemangioma, pyogenic granulomas, blue nevus,

FIGURE 93-7

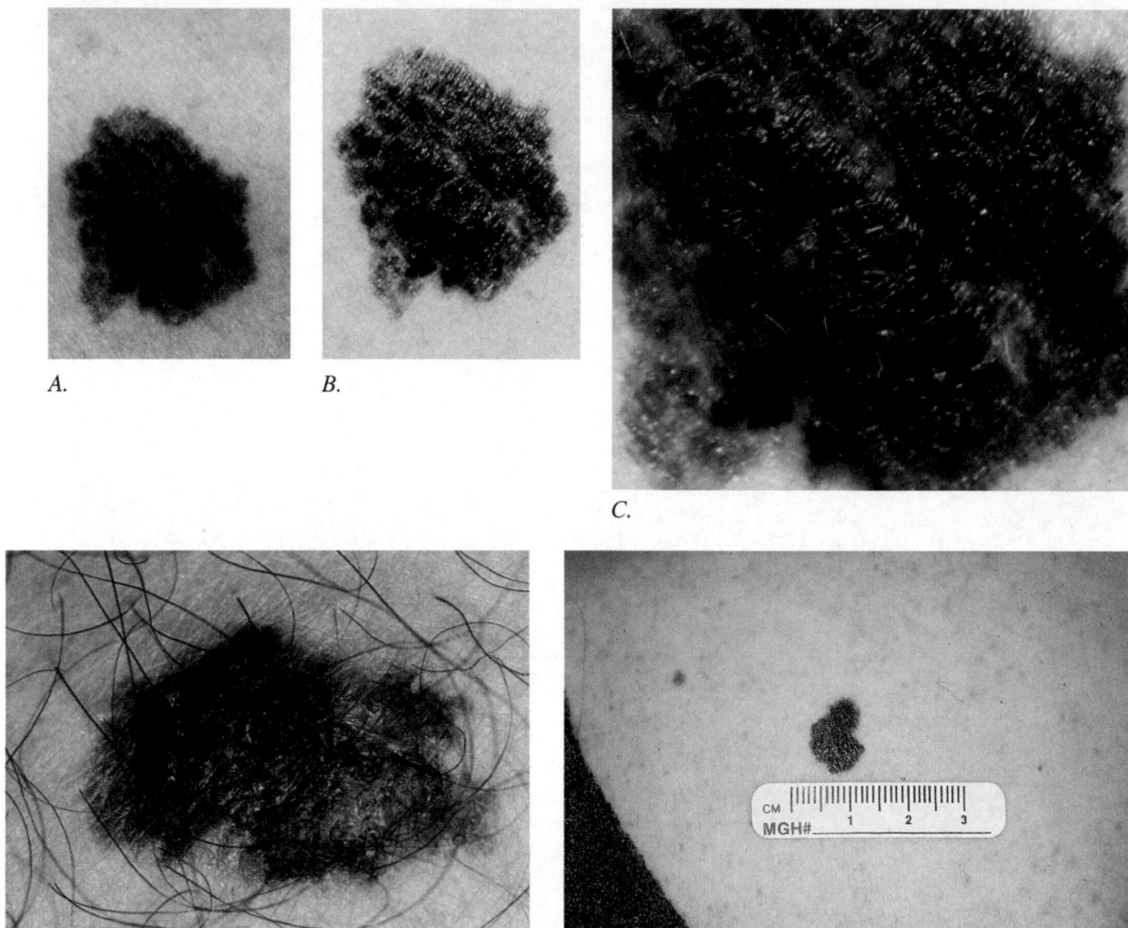

Superficial spreading melanoma. Photographs illustrate the importance of close examination of cutaneous lesions. *A.* One sees the lesion as it would appear to an examiner standing far enough from the patient to include a substantial portion of the body in his or her visual field. Note the notch at 6:30 o'clock. *B.* Close-up view, still with the naked eye, in which pigmentation becomes more obvious. *C.* Under a handheld lens (× 7), bluish coloration and irregular surface typical of melanoma becomes obvious. (*From Hospital Practice, January 1982, with permission.*) *D.* De novo SSM on the back of the thigh, level III (0.49 mm). A classic presentation: There is a pigmented plaque in which all the borders of the lesion are elevated with a central thicker portion. The lesion has the five cardinal features of a superficial spreading melanoma: asymmetry, irregular and scalloped border, mottled color, large diameter, and elevation with surface distortion. *E.* The upper tan portion of the lesion is a dysplastic nevus, and on the lower portion is a blue-black plaque, which is the superficial spreading melanoma.

eccrine poroma, and pigmented basal cell carcinoma on clinical examination (see Figs. 93-12*B* and *C*).

HISTOPATHOLOGY NM demonstrates little tendency for intraepidermal growth. The epidermis lateral to the areas of invasion do not contain atypical melanocytes. Consequently, invasion of the dermis conjointly with any area of intraepidermal invasion is inherent in the concept of NM (Fig. 93-13). This tumor may show large epithelioid cells, spindle cells, small cells, or mixtures of the different cells (Fig. 93-14).

Acral Lentiginous Melanoma

CLINICAL CHARACTERISTICS (Table 93-3) Distinct differences in the frequency of acral lentiginous melanoma (ALM) are seen between racial groups. ALM is relatively infrequent in light-skinned whites (only 2 to 8 percent of melanomas) but represents the most common form in darker-complected individuals (constitutes 60 to 72 percent in blacks, and 29 to 46 percent in Asians[36]). Although darker-pigmented patients have a greater proportion of ALM than other types of melanoma, the incidence of ALM is similar between different ethnic groups. ALM occurs on the palms, soles, or beneath the nail plate, with the sole being the most common site. Not all plantar or palmar melanomas are ALMs; a minority are SSMs or NMs. This subtype is usually diagnosed in older age groups, with a median age at onset of 65 years.

ALM is characterized by a tan, brown to black flat lesion with variegations in color and with irregular borders (Figs. 93-15 and 93-16). Papules or nodules are often present. ALMs that have a flesh-colored appearance can be misdiagnosed as a benign lesion such as a clavus, verruca, or pyogenic granuloma (Fig. 93-16*B*). ALM is considered more aggressive with an associated poorer prognosis; however, this may be a result of late diagnosis of more advanced disease rather than a true difference in biologic nature of the tumor. Early biopsy of suspected lesions is recommended to avoid such delays in the diagnosis.

Subungual melanoma is an uncommon type of cutaneous melanoma and is often considered a variant of the acral lentiginous subtype. The majority of subungual melanomas involve the great toe or the thumb (Fig. 93-16). An early subungual melanoma may be recognized as a

FIGURE 93-8

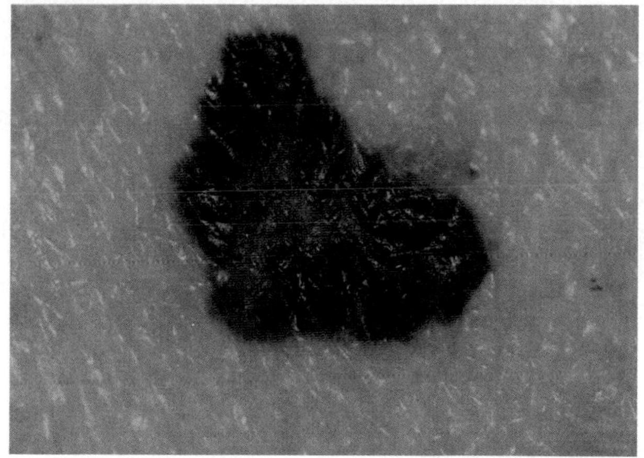

A.

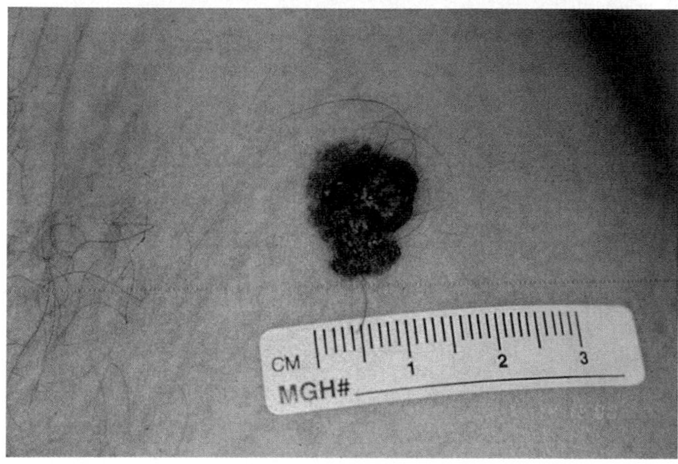

B.

"ABCD's" of melanoma. The two lesions (*A* and *B*) shown here are SSMs: *A, asymmetry:* the melanoma is not symmetrical. Also note the irregular border. *B, border:* note the highly irregular, uneven, and notched border. *C,* color: the color is variegated with different shades of brown, black, tan. *D, diameter:* the diameter is usually >6 mm in melanomas. This does not mean that a melanoma cannot be smaller but, except for atypical (dysplastic) nevi, acquired nevi are usually not >5 mm in diameter.

brown to black discoloration in the nail bed, usually at a proximal location. Hutchinson's sign is the finding of pigmentation of the posterior nail fold and has been considered an ominous finding associated with advanced subungual melanoma (Fig. 93-16*A*). Benign lesions that can mimic subungual melanoma include longitudinal melanonychia, subungual hematoma, onychomycosis, paronychia, ingrown toenail, nevus, or pyogenic granuloma. Subungual hematomas may appear as sharply localized, black, maroon, or multicolored lesions, often within the nail bed or matrix. These lesions are often acutely painful, and a history of trauma at the site can usually be obtained. If the diagnosis is uncertain and the lesion is of recent onset, a diagnostic and therapeutic procedure involves piercing the nail with a large-bore needle to release the blood.

HISTOPATHOLOGY The macular areas exhibit basilar proliferation of large melanocytes with large nuclei showing atypical chromatin patterns. The cytoplasm is filled with melanin granules, and there are elongated dendrites that may extend to the granular cell layer (Fig. 93-17). In the papular or nodular areas, malignant melanocytes are frequently spindle-shaped and extend into the dermis. As discussed

below, desmoplastic–neurotropic patterns of the invasive component are frequently associated with ALM.

Other Melanoma Variants

MELANOMA OF THE MUCOSA Melanoma infrequently can arise from mucosal surfaces. The most common sites are the mucosal surfaces of the head and neck (typically involving the nasal and oral cavity) and vulva or anorectal mucosa. Patients may present with bleeding at these sites or with a mass lesion but most often with a deeply pigmented, irregular mucosa. Melanoma of the mucosa may occur with or without a radial growth phase. The intraepithelial growth phases of malignant melanomas of the vulva and of the conjunctiva can be divided into three subtypes: a pagetoid pattern, which shows the typical characteristics of SSM of the skin; a lentiginous pattern, which shares some features with LM and ALM; and a mixed pattern, in which a profusion of nests of malignant, often ovoid, cells is admixed with a lentiginous proliferation.

LM of the eyelid can involve the conjunctiva and is similar to lentiginous melanocytic hyperplasia of the conjunctiva, without LM, occurring on the palpebral or cutaneous surface. The two lesions, therefore, cannot be distinguished histologically.

DESMOPLASTIC–NEUROTROPIC MELANOMA Desmoplastic melanoma is a rare subtype of melanoma that is locally aggressive with high rates of local recurrence. Desmoplastic melanoma most commonly develops in sun-exposed skin of the head and neck region of elderly individuals, usually in the sixth or seventh decade. Desmoplastic melanomas are variants of invasive melanoma that may arise in association with LM, ALM, and mucosal lentiginous melanoma, as well as de novo. Thus, on clinical examination, one may observe a pigmented macule with or without a nodular component, or a flesh-colored nodule without any surrounding pigmentation. Typically, the latter lesions have a firm, sclerotic or indurated quality.

Histologically, desmoplastic melanoma appears as a nodule of fibrous tissue containing hyperchromatic cells that either are scattered singly, lie in fascicles, or aggregate in nests. Variable degrees of mucin deposition may also be present. Interspersed throughout a dense collagenous tissue are fascicles of hyperchromatic melanoma cells, most often spindle-shaped. Many resemble irregularly shaped fibroblasts. Macrophages filled with melanin may be scattered throughout the dense collagenous tissue.

In general, desmoplastic melanomas have a propensity to infiltrate the perineurium and endoneurium of the cutaneous nerves. The large nerves may have thickened perineurium populated by hyperchromatic cells. Endoneurial involvement usually consists of hypercellularity, with an increase in the size and pleomorphism of the cells. The term *neurotropic melanoma* applies to a subset of desmoplastic melanomas in which the constituent cells, in addition to showing prominent infiltration of nerves, form patterns that resemble nerves or neuroidal structures.[36] The result is a florid proliferation of cells, often with wavy configurations, running parallel to one another, associated with a fibrous response.

The differential diagnosis includes morpheaform (desmoplastic) basal cell carcinoma, desmoplastic nevus, sclerosing variants of blue nevus, scar, fibrous histiocytoma, fibromatosis, atypical fibroxanthoma, malignant fibrous histiocytoma, neurothekeoma, and malignant peripheral nerve sheath tumors (see Chaps. 102 and 107). Helpful features in recognizing desmoplastic malignant melanoma are the usual clinical setting: sun-exposed skin of the head and neck of an elderly individual, an intraepidermal lentiginous melanocytic proliferation, and the presence of cytologic atypia of dermal spindle cells with mitoses. Immunohistochemistry (see below) is usually quite helpful as the tumors

FIGURE 93-9

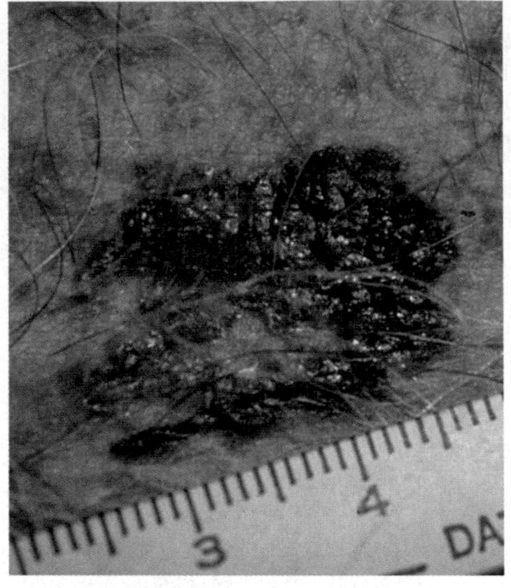

A.

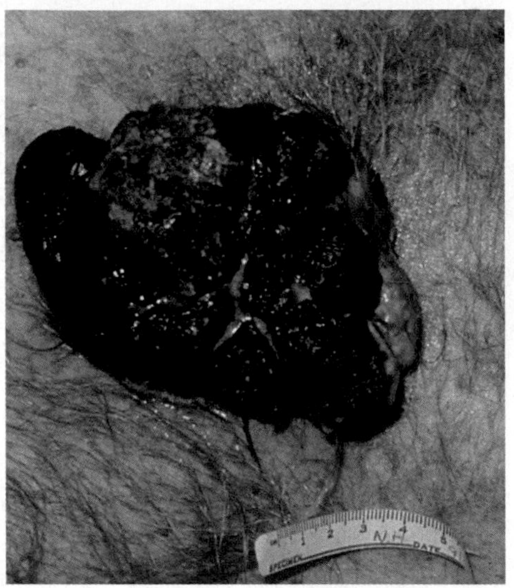

B.

Superficial spreading melanoma. *A.* Lesion had been documented 4 years earlier with biopsy; patient refused treatment. *B.* Three years later, shortly before patient died of metastatic melanoma.(*Courtesy of HC Maguire, Jr, MD.*)

are almost always immunoreactive with S-100 protein and vimentin. However, many tumors are negative for HMB-45. Electron microscopy may not be useful because the spindle cells frequently do not contain melanosomes and may have characteristics of fibroblasts or peripheral-nerve sheath cells.

Most desmoplastic melanomas are deeply invasive at the time of diagnosis. The natural history of these tumors is that of a propensity to local recurrence, frequently multiple, followed by regional metastasis in a smaller subset of cases. The lesions may also exhibit deep local invasion and, when located on the head, even into the skull, result in death.

FIGURE 93-10

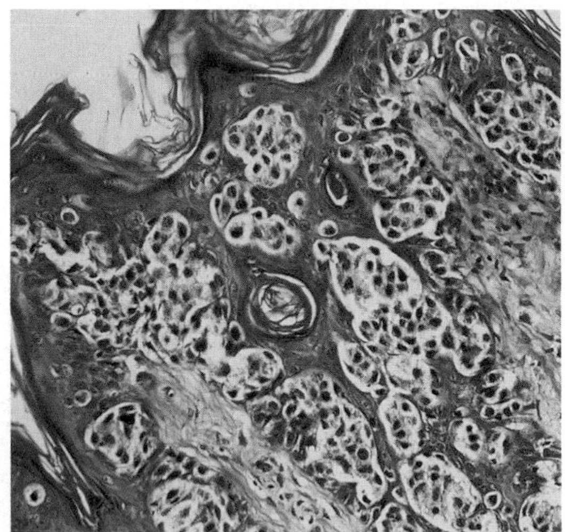

Superficial spreading melanoma. This tumor shows intraepidermal growth. In this photomicrograph, the pagetoid distribution is evident in the epidermis. The cells are relatively uniform and have an abundance of dusty, fine pigment. These relatively large melanoma cells are frequently referred to as epithelioid cell type.

MELANOMA ARISING IN CONGENITAL NEVI

Congenital nevi are recognized potential precursors of melanoma, although the degree of risk is contentious depending on the size of the lesion (see Chap. 91). Specifically, there is convincing evidence that large congenital melanocytic nevi (LCMN) have a significant risk of malignant transformation. Many series arbitrarily define large congenital nevi as greater than 20 cm; however, they have also been defined by area or by ease of surgical excision (inability to close the surgical defect primarily and requiring a skin graft).

Exact quantification of the risk of melanoma developing within a congenital nevus is problematic in that there are a number of methodologic shortcomings of many of the studies reported thus far. Current estimates are in the order of 5 to

FIGURE 93-11

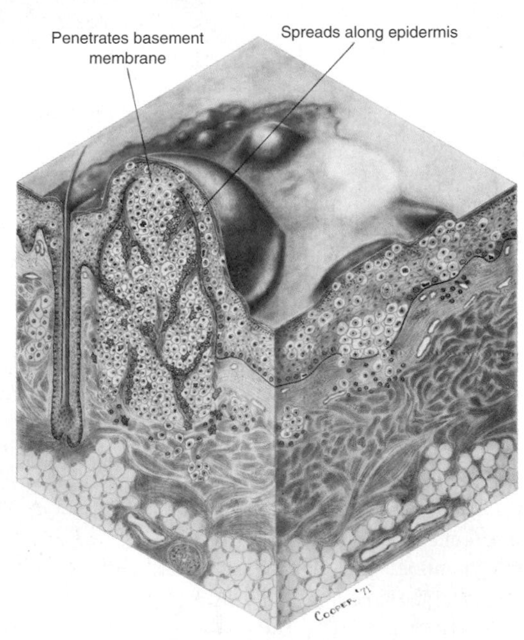

Superficial spreading melanoma. The border is irregular and the lesion is elevated throughout its entirety; biopsy of the area surrounding the large nodule shows a "pagetoid" distribution of large melanocytes and are occurring singly or in nests, and uniformly atypical. On the left is a large nodule, and scattered throughout the surrounding portion of the nodule are smaller papular and nodular areas. The nodule on the left shows malignant melanocytes that are very large, have an abundance of cytoplasm, and often have regularly dispersed fine particles of melanin. The nodules may also show spindle cells or small malignant melanocytes as in lentigo maligna melanoma and nodular melanoma.

42 percent; however, a figure of 6 percent is widely quoted based on a study that estimated the risk from a questionnaire follow-up of patients from the Danish Registry of patients with congenital nevi.[37] A prospective study examining patients from the New York University Registry of LCMN,[38,39] including a review of the world's literature, identified 34 patients with primary cutaneous melanoma in 289 cases of LCMN.[38] Primary cutaneous melanoma developed in 50 percent (17 of 34) of patients before 5 years of age, and 62 percent (21 of 34) died from the disease at a median age of 7.1 years. In general, about half of melanomas developing in giant nevi reportedly do so in the first 3 to 5 years of life compared to malignant transformation after puberty for smaller nevi. In addition to the 34 patients in whom melanoma developed within LCMN, 21 patients had primary melanoma in the central nervous system, and 10 had primary cutaneous melanoma outside the LCMN. In an update of the New York University series, 160 patients were followed prospectively for an average of 5.5 years, with 3 melanomas developing in extracutaneous sites (2 in the central nervous system and 1 retroperitoneally).[39] The cumulative 5-year life table risk for developing melanoma was 2.3 percent, and the relative risk was 101. No melanomas were reported within a LCMN. Four patients developed neurocutaneous melanosis, two of whom had central nervous system melanoma.

FIGURE 93-12

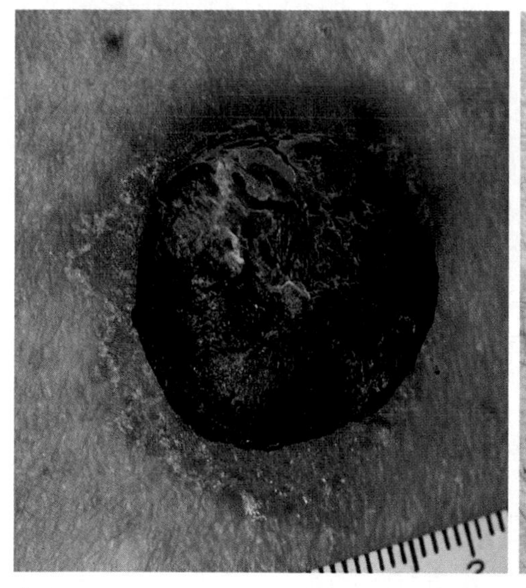

A.

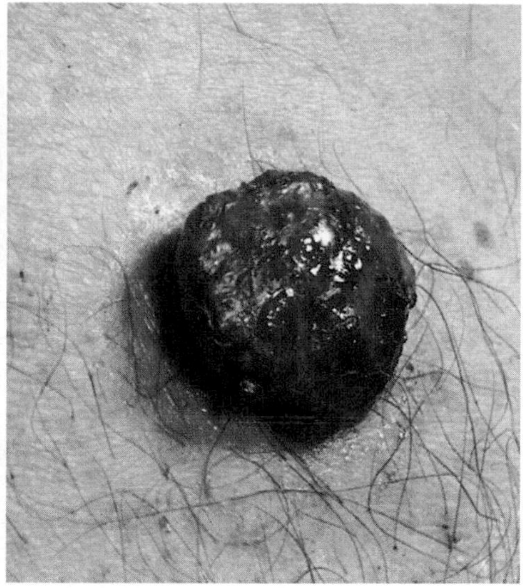

B.

C.

Nodular melanoma. *A.* The lesion consists of a blue-black nodule with scale crust on the surface. *B.* This is a mushroom-shaped 1.5-cm, partially red, otherwise brown, firm tumor, round and sharply demarcated. *C.* This 69-year-old patient presented with an asymptomatic red papule on her right pretibial area. This lesion is an amelanotic nodular melanoma, 2.9 mm in depth, invasive to anatomic level IV. (*From Langley RGB et al.,*[36] *with permission.*)

MELANOMA AND PREGNANCY

The impact of pregnancy on the clinical course of melanoma, whether melanoma is diagnosed concomitantly with, after, or prior to a pregnancy, is uncertain and a source of controversy in the literature. Initial case reports documented a precipitation of melanoma during pregnancy and an overall deleterious effect on the tumor and a fulminant course. Other reports have documented a favorable or protective influence of previous or multiple pregnancies on melanoma. These studies have a number of methodologic shortcomings: many of the previous studies were small; included heterogeneous assortments of patients (e.g., women pregnant before, in some instances many years before, during, or after melanoma); had failed to control for thickness and anatomic site; or were uncontrolled altogether. Critical reviews of the literature on this subject have examined those studies in which the data fulfill more stringent criteria.[40] Driscol et al.[40] noted that of five controlled studies examining this issue none demonstrated a deleterious effect on survival. Two of the studies, however, identified a shorter disease-free survival in pregnant patients. The effect of prior pregnancies on the prognosis of melanoma has also been examined, and there appears to be no adverse effect on prognosis of patients in whom melanoma developed after the woman completed a pregnancy. In fact, one study found an improved survival rate of women with five or more pregnancies after controlling for major prognostic factors. A limited number of controlled studies also suggest that a melanoma developing prior to a pregnancy does not effect the prognosis of a women subsequently diagnosed with melanoma in comparison with controls.[40]

Thus, accumulating data suggest that pregnancy does not affect outcome from melanoma. Based on the evidence to date, women considering pregnancy after melanoma develops should be counseled on prognosis based on standardized microstaging of melanoma (i.e., with tumor thickness and ulceration as the predominant determinant of prognosis for primary cutaneous melanoma). Many authors advise that women delay pregnancy for at least 2 years in order to avoid the period of greatest risk for recurrence. Such advice, however, should be tailored

FIGURE 93-13

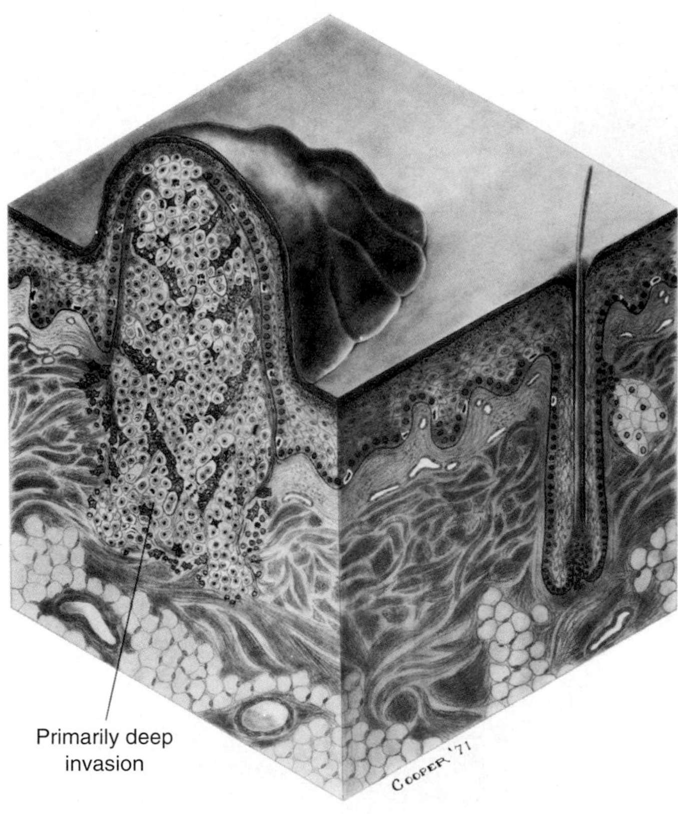

Nodular melanoma. This tumor arises at the dermal–epidermal junction and extends vertically into the dermis; intraepidermal growth is present only in a small group of tumor cells that conjointly are also invading the underlying dermis. The epidermis lateral to the areas of this invasion does not demonstrate atypical melanocytes. As in lentigo maligna melanoma and superficial spreading melanoma, the tumor may show large epithelioid cells, spindle cells, small malignant melanocytes, or mixtures of all three.

FIGURE 93-14

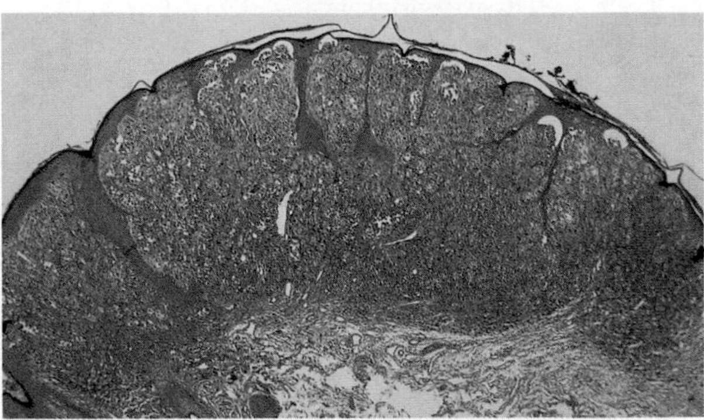

A.

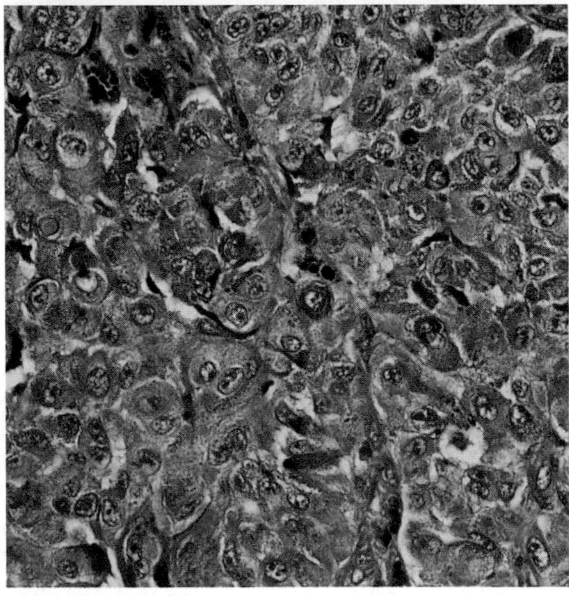

B.

Nodular melanoma. *A.* Low-power photomicrograph demonstrating a dome-shaped expansile tumor located in the upper dermis. *B.* High-power photomicrograph reveals nests of anaplastic epithelioid cells in the tumor.

to the risk of recurrence and is most appropriate for women with higher risk primary (thick or ulcerated) lesions, or those with more advanced disease. We do not routinely recommend avoiding pregnancy for any period in women with thin primary melanomas.

MELANOMA IN CHILDHOOD AND ADOLESCENCE

Melanoma in childhood and adolescence is rare, accounting for approximately 1 to 4 percent of all newly diagnosed melanomas in patients younger than 20 years of age, and 0.3 to 0.4 percent in prepubertal children.[41] Melanoma can develop in a congenital setting due to transplacental spread, or melanomas may arise de novo or in association with a large congenital nevus. A rare but grave presentation of congenital melanoma is that of neurocutaneous melanosis, which is characterized by multiple nevi with meningeal melanosis and melanoma. Particular risk factors for melanoma in childhood include the presence of congenital nevi (Chap. 91), dysplastic nevi (Chap. 92), xeroderma pigmentosum (frequency of melanoma in children is 2000 times greater than it is in children without xeroderma pigmentosum; see Chap. 155), hereditary melanoma, and neurocutaneous melanosis. Immunosuppression may also be relevant in elevating the risk for melanoma.

METASTATIC AND RECURRENT MELANOMA

Approximately 15 to 36 percent of patients with stages I and II melanoma have some form of recurrence or metastasis during their clinical course. Melanoma typically recurs or metastasizes in a stepwise manner. These steps consist of local recurrences, regional metastases, and, finally, distant metastases.

Local Recurrences

A local recurrence is currently defined as any recurrence in close proximity to the surgical scar for primary cutaneous melanoma. A lack of uniformity of a definition exists in the literature: some authors define local recurrence as occurring within the scar, while others include recurrence within 2 cm of the site of the definitive surgical excision scar, recurrences up to 5 cm, and even regional metastatic disease.

FIGURE 93-15

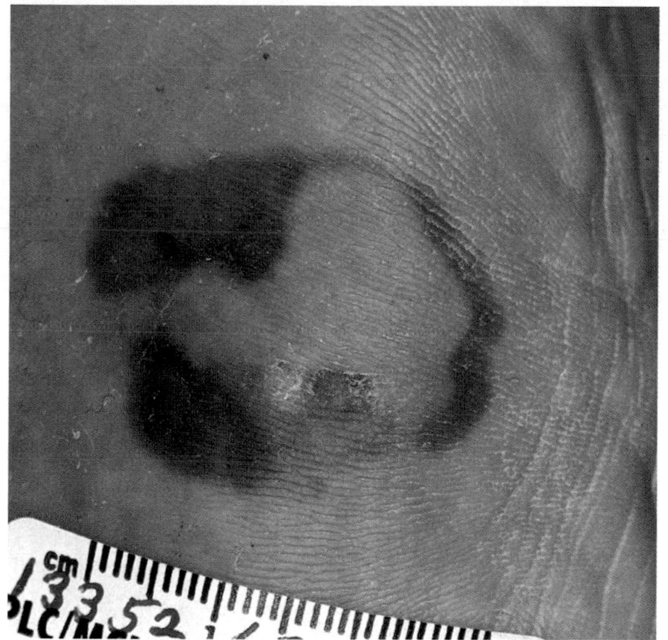

Acral lentiginous melanoma. The lesion is almost entirely macular and exhibits marked irregularity of color. A large confluent central area has a bluish-gray appearance, indicating regression.

Restricting the definition to the distance from the surgical scar is based on the understanding that there is a biologic difference between a local recurrence, which is believed to develop as a result of a failure of the initial local treatment to remove tumor, from that of local metastasis with intralymphatic spread. Based on such understandings of the pathophysiology of recurrent melanoma, a case can be made to restrict the definition to recurrences within the scar. It is difficult to estimate the incidence and prognosis in local recurrences from the literature because of the lack of a consistent definition in the past. The reported frequency of local recurrence is approximately 3 percent, and is related to tumor thickness, with increased rates in patients with thicker primary lesions. Karakousis et al. reported in a multi-institutional randomized surgical trial a local recurrence rate of 2.3 percent for melanomas between 1.0 and 2.0 mm thickness, and 11.7 percent ($p = .001$) in tumors 3.01 to 4.0 mm in thickness.[42] Lesions without ulceration had a local recurrence rate of 1.5 percent, whereas higher local recurrence rates were seen with the presence of ulceration in 10.6 percent ($p = .001$). Local recurrence has historically been associated with a poorer prognosis, and has been considered an indicator of disseminated disease. Karakousis et al. reported that 82 percent of patients with local recurrence died from their disease.[42] A population-based study from Sweden that used strict diagnostic criteria for local recurrence, including only those cases with recurrence in the scar, identified a lower frequency of recurrences: only 1.3 percent (48 of 3706) of patients followed over a period of approximately 20 years.[43] The 5-year disease-free survival rate in patients with local recurrence in this study was 69 percent and the melanoma-specific survival rate was 83 percent, which is favorable in comparison with those reported in the literature.[43] The relatively favorable prognosis reported in this study is likely a result of the strict definition of local recurrence, including only those cases with recurrence in the surgical scar and discriminating such cases from in-transit metastases, which biologically represent intralymphatic spread and potentially more widespread disease.

FIGURE 93-16

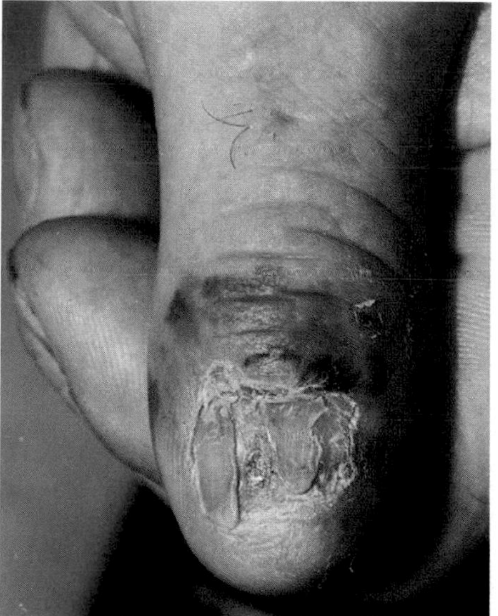

A.

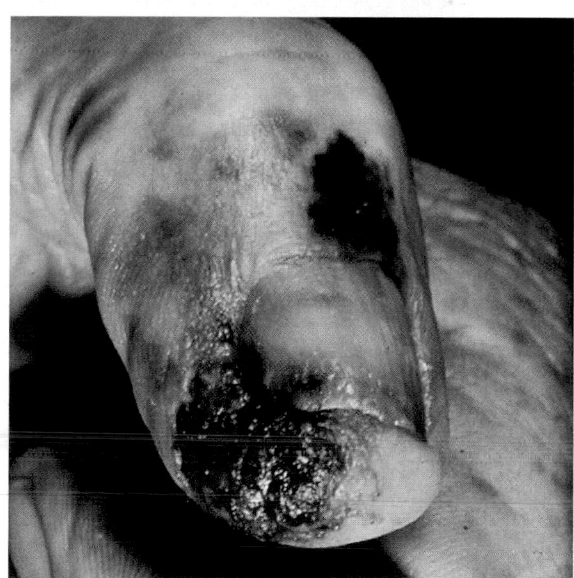

B.

ALM on the thumb. *A.* Extensive involvement of periungual skin (Hutchinson's sign). There is dystrophy and loss of the nail plate secondary to the tumor. *B.* Subungual melanoma. The initial radial growth phase is evident in the periungual skin with blotchy, cloudy macules of various shades of light to dark brown, some ill-, some sharply defined and with irregular borders. There is white, blue, and black close to the ulcerated, nonpigmented subungual tumor (vertical growth phase).

In-Transit and Satellite Metastases

In-transit metastases are currently defined as small tumor emboli within the dermal and subdermal lymphatics between the primary tumor and the regional lymph node basin. In the revised AJCC staging system (see below) in-transit and satellite metastases have been grouped in the same subclassification (N2c).[44] Patients with intralymphatic metastases but no nodal metastases are recognized as having a similar prognosis, and

FIGURE 93-17

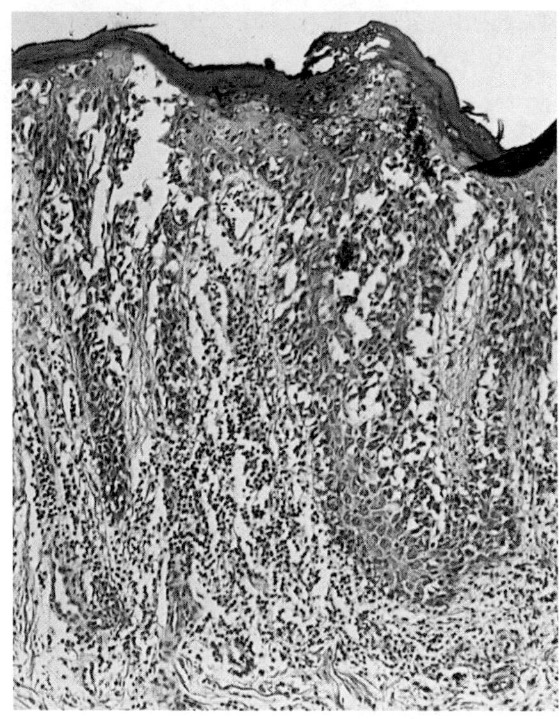

A.

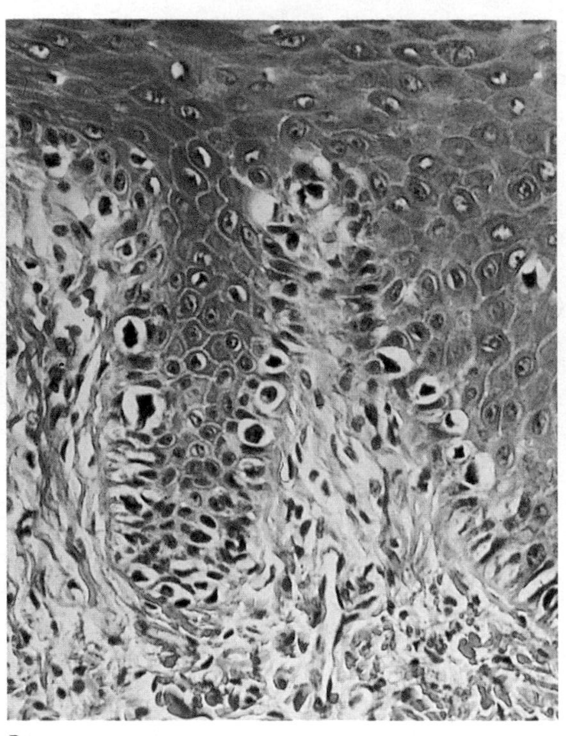

B.

Acral lentiginous melanoma. *A.* Photomicrograph showing hyperkeratosis associated with plantar location of this melanoma. Fibrosis and patchy host response are noted in the dermis. *B.* High-power photomicrograph showing lentiginous proliferation of abnormal melanocytes along the dermal–epidermal junction.

are thus grouped together. Clinically, the lesions are generally multiple, relatively small dermal or subcutaneous nodules, bluish in color or amelanotic. Large lesions are frequently ulcerated.

Regional Lymph Node Metastases

The presence of regional nodal disease is highly predictive of visceral metastases. The risk of regional node metastasis varies by primary tumor thickness (see below): patients with melanomas that are <0.76 mm, 0.76 to 1.49 mm, 1.5 to 4.0 mm, and >4.0 mm have nodal metastases at 3 years in 2 to 3 percent, 25 percent, 57 percent and 62 percent, respectively.

Distant Metastases

Melanoma is well known for its propensity to metastasize to virtually any organ and also for its highly variable clinical course. Nevertheless, melanoma does have certain patterns of metastasis that enable the clinician to manage the disease with some degree of confidence. Melanoma spreads most frequently to nonvisceral sites: skin, subcutaneous tissue, and distant lymph nodes in about 42 to 57 percent of cases. Visceral metastases to the lungs (18 to 36 percent), liver (14 to 20 percent), brain (12 to 20 percent), bone (11 to 17 percent), and intestines (1 to 7 percent) are the next most common sites.[46]

Late Recurrences

The incidence of late recurrence (10 or more years after initial diagnosis and treatment) among melanoma patients is approximately 0.93 to 6.7 percent. The largest series to date involved 7104 patients with melanoma, including 168 patients with late recurrences.[47] This study reported that most of the primary tumors were in the intermediate thickness category (mean thickness, 1.6 mm; range, 0.34 to 6.3 mm) with very few lesions <0.70 mm or >3.0 mm. The mean time to recurrence was 14.3 years for patients having recurrences after 10 years. Another retrospective review of 2766 melanoma patients identified 20 patients with "ultra late" recurrence, defined as recurrences after at least 15 years of disease-free survival.[48] Virtually all tumors were between 0.8 and 2.3 mm in thickness and Clark levels III to IV, and recurred an average of 19 years after initial diagnosis and treatment.

METASTATIC MELANOMA WITH UNKNOWN PRIMARIES

Metastatic melanoma with no known primary site is defined by the presence of histologically confirmed regional lymph node or distant metastases in an individual without a history or evidence of a primary cutaneous, mucosal, or ocular melanoma. This situation occurs in approximately 2 to 6 percent of all melanoma cases. Such metastases involve the lymph nodes in approximately two-thirds of cases, and one-third spread to distant sites, typically the subcutaneous tissue, lung, or brain. In one large series, such patients comprised 4.8 percent of all cases of melanoma, and patients presented with regional lymph node metastases (64 percent) versus distant spread to visceral (21 percent) or nonvisceral (e.g., subcutaneous) sites (15 percent). Most regional lymph node metastases involved the axillae followed by the inguinal nodes. The most frequent sites of visceral metastasis were the lung (54 percent), brain (20 percent), and gastrointestinal tract (13 percent).[49]

The evaluation of such a patient must involve a complete history and a physical examination that includes a thorough Wood lamp examination of the entire skin surface for hypopigmented areas that might suggest a regressed primary lesion, particularly in the areas of regional lymph node drainage. In patients presenting with regional node involvement, particular attention should be focused on areas that drain to that node basin. Any suspicious lesion should be excised to look for residual melanoma or histologic regression (see below). The patient should also have an eye, ear, nose, throat, rectal, and proctoscopic examination; women should also have a gynecologic examination. Staging investigations should also be performed, depending on the clinical presentation. In general, all previously removed melanocytic and other skin lesions should be reviewed histologically to exclude melanoma.

Historically, there has been considerable confusion in the literature about the prognosis of patients with unknown primaries. Early reports indicated that patients had reduced survival compared to a similar group of patients with known primary sites. When controlled for stage of disease, however, subsequent authors have found similar or even improved survival in patients with occult primary melanomas. In the largest study to date, Chang and Knapper observed survival rates of 46 and 41 percent at 5 and 10 years, respectively, in patients with unknown primary and stage III (lymph node) disease.[50] A German study reported that the prognosis of patients with melanoma of unknown primary origin is similar to that of patients with metastasis from a known primary origin if clinical stages of disease are compared.[51] In a review of 3258 melanomas diagnosed over approximately 20 years, 75 cases of melanoma with unknown primary origin were detected. Patients with cutaneous or subcutaneous metastases had a 5-year survival rate of 83 percent, which was significantly better than patients with primary cutaneous melanoma with in-transit metastases in which the 5-year survival rate was 50 percent ($p = .02$).[51] The 5-year survival rate for patients with an unknown primary and lymph node metastases was 50 percent, which compared favorably with patients with a known primary and subsequent lymph node metastasis of 36 percent ($p = 0.14$). The number of nodes involved was not documented in this study, however, which is a significant prognostic indicator, and a key staging criterion in the revised AJCC classification (see below). Finally, the median survival was similar in patients with visceral metastasis with unknown primary or known primary origin of 6 versus 5 months, respectively.[51]

CLINICAL DETECTION OF MELANOMA

Because cutaneous melanoma arises on a readily accessible site, the health professional and patient have a unique and challenging opportunity to diagnose this malignancy at an early, curable time. This is an important challenge given that tumor thickness remains the most critical prognostic indicator in primary cutaneous melanoma.[1–3] Despite the importance of early diagnosis of melanoma, however, there are several reasons why this objective has not yet been fulfilled. Patients with suspicious lesions may delay medical assessment due to lack of knowledge, fear, or denial.[52] In addition, the physician's diagnostic accuracy of melanoma is not perfect, with the sensitivity of diagnosis on the order of 47 to 97 percent.[52]

It must be emphasized that no single clinical feature ensures or excludes a diagnosis of melanoma. Even among expert clinicians, the clinical diagnosis of melanoma can be made in only about 80 to 90 percent of cases, with the remainder being diagnosed only by histologic examination. The clinical diagnosis of melanoma relies on a history of sustained change and assessing a constellation of gross morphologic features, but in essence, is related to the overall degree of order or symmetry of a lesion. In general, the gross morphologic features used in assessing melanocytic lesions include size, coloration, border characteristics, surface topography on tangential or side lighting, and symmetry. For practical purposes the *ABCD rule* can be applied for diagnosis of all types of melanoma, except for NM: *A*, asymmetry of the lesion; *B*, border characteristics (notched, scalloped, irregular); *C*, color (mottled, haphazard display of all shades of brown, black, gray, pink, white, blue); *D*, diameter >6 mm (greater than a pencil eraser) (see Figs. 93-7, 93-8, 93-9A for examples).

Malignant melanomas have an initial pattern of growth in the skin and mucosa, the radial growth phase, common to all types of melanoma with the exception of NM. This stage of proliferation is characterized by a relatively flat or slightly papular surface and horizontally extending growth. In general, irregularity of borders (B) with notching, variation and complexity of color pattern, and asymmetry are present at this stage (see Fig. 93-8). When diagnosed, melanomas are usually >10 mm in largest diameter. Less frequently, they are diagnosed when >6 mm in size (D). There may be obliteration or loss of skin cleavage lines when the lesion is observed with tangential lighting. Pattern of coloration is perhaps the single most important attribute for detection of melanoma (C). Although varying shades of brown typify most melanocytic lesions, striking aspects of black, blue, gray, white, pink, and red coloration may be found in melanoma (Figs. 93-7*C*, *D*; 93-8 and 93-9A). In fact, the presence of blue-black, red, and white hues is particularly suggestive of the diagnosis. Focal black areas, particularly if newly developed, are suspicious for melanoma. Changes of regression usually correspond to foci of white, gray, and pink.

The most suspicious sign suggesting melanoma is a persistently changing pigmented lesion, which should prompt immediate attention. The most frequent signs suggesting early melanoma are changes in size (D) and color (C). Not only darkening, particularly focally, but also lightening (regression) may occur. Loss of pigmentation may involve the lesion in question and take the form of a halo or occur in distant locations, resulting in a process known as melanoma-associated leukoderma. Other findings, such as elevation, ulceration, and bleeding, generally signify more-advanced primary melanoma. These changes typically occur over the course of weeks to months. An alteration of a pigmented lesion within days can usually be attributed to external insult, as from trauma, or an inflamed hair follicle within the lesion.[36]

The development of a new pigmented lesion, particularly in an individual beyond the age of 30 to 40 years and on an anatomic site of the body without similar lesions, is also worthy of close inspection. Also, the development of multiple halo nevi in mid- to late-adult life should lead to a careful inspection of the patient for melanoma (see Chap. 91). The hypopigmented halos in such patients appear around benign pigmented lesions, the melanoma being surrounded by skin of normal color (see below).

Practical Aspects

The skin examination should encompass the entire skin surface, including the scalp and genitalia. The examination should be conducted under optimal lighting, ideally daylight, and with access to a source of side lighting. A magnifying lens, usually handheld, also facilitates the examination. A Wood lamp is useful for accentuation of epidermal hyper- or hypopigmentation, such as in mapping the extent of LM or the detection of a regressed primary melanoma.

Noninvasive Clinical Techniques

The importance of making an early diagnosis of primary melanoma to increase the detection of curable melanomas and the need for improvement in the clinical diagnostic accuracy of melanoma has stimulated interest in the development of noninvasive clinical techniques in the assessment of pigmented skin lesions such as dermoscopy and computerized image analysis.

DERMOSCOPY Dermoscopy [epiluminescence microscopy (ELM)] is a noninvasive in vivo clinical examination technique in which immersion oil is applied to the pigmented lesion and examined with a lens or a handheld device (dermatoscope). More sophisticated stereo microscopes or computerized digital imaging systems can be used. Morphologic structures are observed using this technique that are otherwise not visible to the unaided eye. A new terminology and set of criteria have subsequently been developed based on this subsurface morphology for application in the assessment of pigmented lesions. Dermoscopy improves the clinical diagnosis of melanoma and facilitates the differentiation of other benign and malignant pigmented skin lesions in experienced hands.[53–59] Soyer et al. have thoroughly reviewed the subject.[56]

The pigment network is one of the most recognizable and important structures to identify, to facilitate accurate diagnosis when examining a pigmented skin lesion with dermoscopy (Fig. 93-18, Table 93-4). A pigment network appears on dermoscopy as a series of pigmented lines, because of pigmentation along the rete ridges, and clear holes, which represent the apex of the dermal papillae.[56] Identification of the pigment network invariably indicates that the pigmented lesion is melanocytic, and its absence usually indicates a nonmelanocytic lesion. The pigmented network should be examined closely to determine whether a benign or malignant pattern exists. A benign pigment network pattern, as seen in dermal nevi, has regular, delicate lines with gradual thinning at the margin, whereas melanomas may have a malignant pattern with an irregular, variable, and widened pigment network that ends abruptly at the periphery.[53–55] Lists of many of the important dermoscopy features with clinical pathologic correlations and significance have been published in several studies. Figure 93-18 shows the salient features and Table 93-4 summarizes them.

Different approaches have been developed to facilitate the interpretation of dermoscopy findings, including the pattern analysis method proposed by Pehamberger et al.,[53] the ABCD method,[57] and various others that have been tested and compared to each other in a large multicenter trial.[56] The pattern analysis method has been the most extensively tested method to date, including examination and analysis of over 7000 pigmented lesions.[53–55] In the pattern analysis method, an algorithm is applied in which the dermoscopic features are classified into specific patterns characteristic of different pigmented skin lesions. By using this method, significant improvements were documented in overall diagnostic accuracy: from 60 percent with clinical examination alone to 85 percent with dermoscopy.[54,56]

Although dermoscopy can enhance the diagnostic accuracy of those experienced in using this technique, there is some evidence that dermatologists who are not formally trained in this technique may not benefit by using this technique and that the sensitivity of diagnosis may be lower.[59] Such studies emphasize the need for specific instruction in application of the technique and the need for extensive experience in using the technique if the potential gains in diagnostic accuracy are to be reached. It should be emphasized that the technique is not absolute, and that the presence or absence of dermoscopic features has not been reliably shown to be 100 percent sensitive or specific for the diagnosis of melanoma. Dermoscopy is an aid in the clinical diagnosis of melanoma, however, and dermoscopic examination provides important additional information and affords the opportunity to study and analyze lesional features not visible to the naked eye, particularly in lesions that are small and have not yet developed the full complement of features diagnostic for melanoma. Dermoscopy facilitates a rigorous examination of pigmented lesion morphology and is an important advance in the scientific approach to clinical assessment of pigmented skin lesions.[60]

FIGURE 93-18

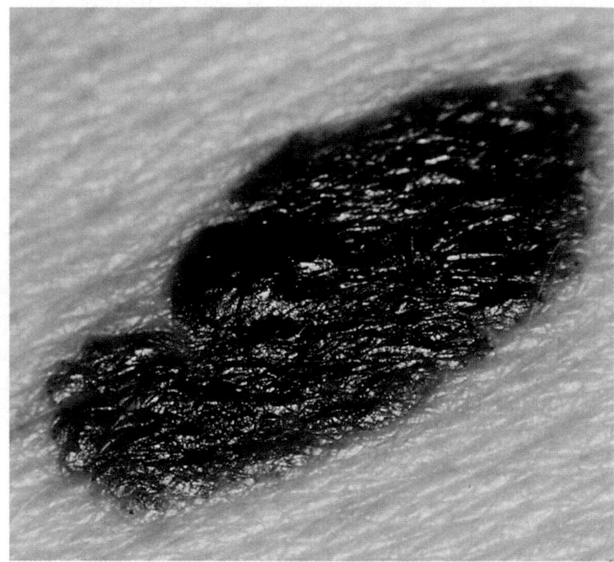

A.

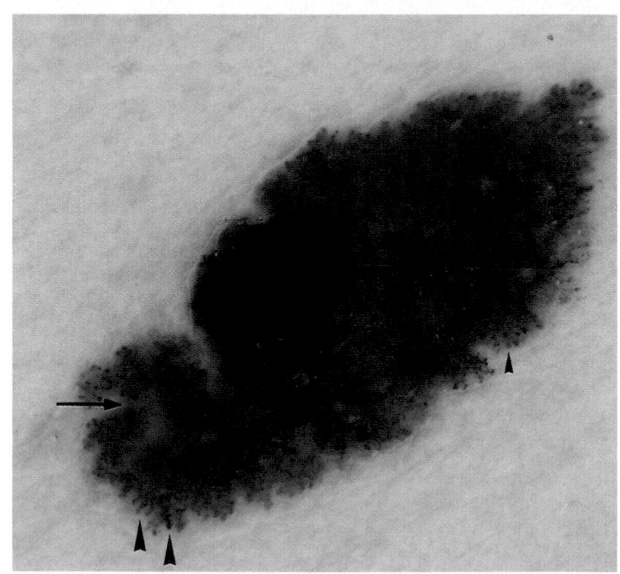

B.

A superficial spreading melanoma as viewed by close inspection with a handheld lens (*A*) and by ELM (i.e., with immersion oil) (*B*). Here new features become apparent, such as the pigment network, brown globules (*small arrowhead*), pseudopods (*large arrowheads*), and depigmentation, extending irregularly to the periphery of the lesion (*arrow*). (*Courtesy of Michael Binder, MD.*)

IMAGE ANALYSIS Computerized digital imaging is another noninvasive in vivo technique currently being investigated for the assessment, diagnosis, and monitoring of pigmented skin lesions. Such images can be retrieved and examined at a later date to permit comparisons, qualitatively or quantitatively, to detect changes over time. Digital dermoscopy [digital epiluminescent microscopy (DELM)] is a significant advance in this field because it enables an enhanced discrimination of melanoma from other pigmented skin lesions. DELM uses computer image analysis programs, which provide objective measurement of changes in pigmented lesions over time (Fig. 93-19), storage and rapid retrieval at low operating cost, transmission of images to experts for further

TABLE 93-4

Dermascopic Features of Pigmented Lesions

Surface Dermoscopy Criteria	Histologic Features	Diagnostic Significance
Pigment network	Pigmented rete ridges	Melanocytic lesion
Regular	Regular distributed rete	Benign melanocytic lesion
Irregular	Irregular distributed rete	Dysplastic nevi or melanoma
Broadened pigment network	Broad rete ridges with increased number of atypical melanocytes	Early melanoma
Black dots	Collections and clumps of pigmented cells in the cornified layer	Melanoma
Pseudopods	Junctional nests at the periphery	Melanoma
Radial streaming	Junctional nests arranged radially	Melanoma, pigmented spindle-cell nevus
Brown globules	Pigmented nests in the papillary dermis and dermal–epidermal junction	Nevomelanocytic nevus (if regular) Melanoma (if irregular)
Maple-leaf–like areas	Pigmented aggregates of basaloid cells	Basal cell carcinoma
Comedo-like openings	Horn pseudocysts	Seborrehic keratosis Papillary dermal nevus
Blue-gray veil	Melanoma with areas of regression	Fibrosis, widened papillary dermis, melanophages
Depigmentation	Areas lacking melanin in the epidermis and dermis. May be fibroplasia or regression of melanoma	Regular and central—benign Irregular and peripheral—malignant

discussion, and extraction of morphologic features for numeric analysis.[60] Such systems even allow the employment of artificial neural networks and can assist screening for melanomas for those untrained in the complexities of dermoscopy or in general dermatology.[60] A recent four-center validation study that used an automated multispectral digital dermatoscope was promising in this regard.[61]

Future Developments

The continued advances in optical imaging technology should translate into improvements in the discrimination of benign pigmented lesions from malignant ones. Ultrasonography, including 20-MHz ultrasound and, more recently, higher frequency (40 to 60 MHz) ultrasound, and magnetic resonance imaging have also been used as noninvasive techniques; however, their value remains to be determined.

The first clinical studies in pigmented lesions using a confocal scanning laser microscope have been reported.[62] The confocal scanning laser microscope (CSLM) allows in vivo visualization of cellular level structures within the epidermis and papillary dermis, including circulating erythrocytes and leukocytes in the superficial plexus. Preliminary analysis of this technique has provided high-resolution in vivo images of pigmented skin lesions.[62] With the technique, melanocytic nevi have cohesive nests of uniformly monomorphic circular cells and increased microvascular blood flow. Melanomas have a polymorphous cytologic structure, containing atypical, pleomorphic cells in disarray and irregular dendritic cells. In this pilot project, CSLM enabled identification of distinct patterns and cytologic features of benign and malignant pigmented skin lesions in vivo.

Continued development of technology for noninvasive imaging of the skin could lead to enhanced diagnostic accuracy of pigmented skin lesions. Improved recognition of benign lesions may result in avoiding unnecessary biopsies while facilitating the diagnosis of early curable melanomas.

ESTABLISHING A HISTOLOGIC DIAGNOSIS

Excision

Patients with lesions clinically suspect for melanoma should, whenever possible, undergo prompt excisional biopsy with narrow margins.

Incisional Biopsy

An incisional biopsy is acceptable, although less desirable, if it is not possible to perform an excisional biopsy because of large size. An incisional or punch biopsy may be obtained through what is considered to be the thickest (most elevated) portion of the clinical lesions. In the case of flat lesions, the darkest (e.g., black) area should be sampled. It must be emphasized that shave biopsies are to be avoided because they usually yield inadequate specimens, frequently disrupt the tumor, and preclude conventional microstaging. There is no evidence that biopsy or incision of a melanoma leads to "seeding" of tissue and adversely affects survival.

Histopathologic Criteria for the Diagnosis of Melanoma

The histologic diagnosis of melanoma is based on the assessment of a constellation of findings with no single feature, particularly architectural, being diagnostic.

Fully evolved cytologic atypia is considered necessary for a diagnosis of melanoma. Although precise definitions are lacking, this degree of atypia generally refers to pronounced cellular enlargement, nuclear enlargement, variations in nuclear size and shape (anisokaryosis), hyperchromasia of nuclei with irregular clumping and distribution of chromatin, and enlarged nucleoli. In melanoma, large epithelioid cells are usually characterized by abundant granular, eosinophilic, or "dusty" cytoplasm; spindle cells have less cytoplasm, which is frequently basophilic or amphophilic, with high nucleus-to-cytoplasm ratios. Architectural features suggestive of melanoma include large size (>5 to 6 mm), asymmetry, and pagetoid spread or intraepidermal upward migration of melanocytes. Also, there is loss of a nevic growth pattern; that is, loss of elongated epidermal rete with variation in the junctional nesting pattern and confluence of nests with dyshesion of cells in nests. Substantial zones of regression and expansile nodule formation in the dermal component are commonly present. Pagetoid spread is usually considered diagnostic of melanoma. However, this finding should be assessed cautiously because of the frequent occurrence of upward migration of cells in acral nevi of children, pigmented spindle-cell nevi, Spitz nevi, and epithelioid cell dysplasia (see Chap 91). In the benign lesions, the upwardly migratory cells have benign cytologic features. The histologic differential diagnosis

icality in the proper clinical context before rendering a diagnosis of melanoma.

FIGURE 93-19

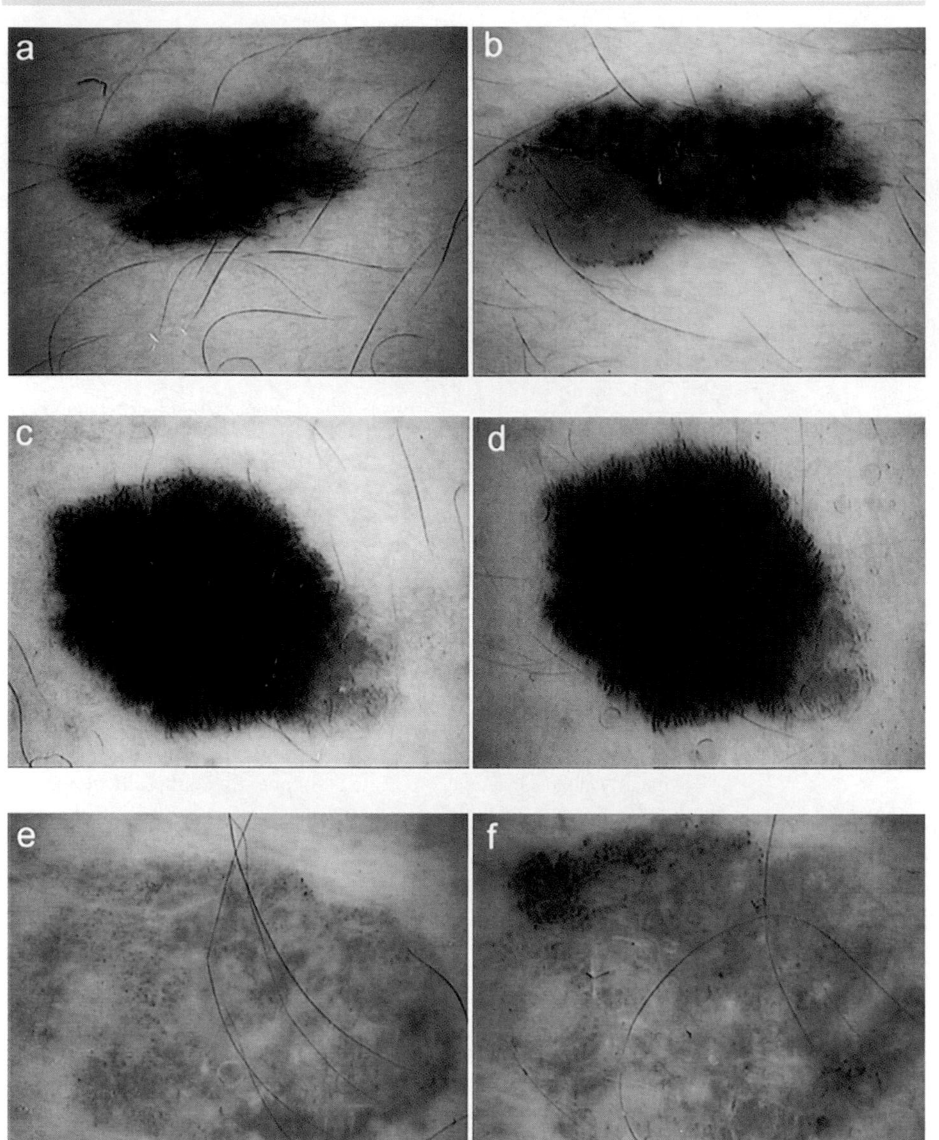

Monitoring of dysplastic nevi (DN) by digital epiluminescence microscopy. All lesions are from patients with the multiple atypical (dysplastic) nevus syndrome. *A*. Image of DN at time of presentation. The lesion shows features of a DN and because the patient has multiple such lesions, clinical monitoring at 6-month intervals was scheduled. *B*. Follow-up of the same lesion after 8 months. The lesion has changed. There is an asymmetrical increase in size and the appearance of a new hypopigmented structure in the periphery on the left. The lesion was excised and histology revealed DN in the right portion of the lesion and SSM <0.75 mm on the left. *C*. This DN is more difficult to evaluate. Typical DN at baseline (*C*.) but after 6 months, (*D*) subtle changes have occurred. There is an increase in size, albeit symmetrical, of the lesion, but the pigment network at the upper and lower margin has transformed into a fringe of fine pseudopods suggesting SSM. Histology confirmed SSM <0.75 mm. *E*. Another DN at baseline. *F*. Follow-up image of the same lesion at 6 months. The most prominent changes are asymmetrical increase in size, appearance of a new irregular pigment network, dots, and globules at the upper left margin of the lesion. Histology revealed SSM <0.75 mm. (*Courtesy of Harald Kittler, MD.*)

of melanoma commonly includes Spitz tumor, pigmented spindle-cell nevus, dysplastic nevus, halo nevus, combined nevus, recurrent nevus (see Chaps. 91 and 92), and cellular blue nevus. Emphasis should be placed on having sufficient architectural and cytologic atyp-

IMMUNOHISTOCHEMISTRY IN THE DIAGNOSIS OF MELANOMA

Immunohistochemistry is used for the diagnosis of melanoma in these situations: primary or metastatic, poorly differentiated malignant neoplasms containing little or no pigment; spindle-cell tumors; tumors with pagetoid epidermal patterns that are not obvious melanoma (e.g., sebaceous carcinoma); and small cell malignant tumors suggesting melanoma, lymphoma, or neuroendocrine carcinoma. The antisera used most often for the routine evaluation of paraffin-embedded specimens include S-100 protein and HMB-45. S-100 protein is expressed by virtually all malignant melanomas and melanocytic nevi, as well as by a variety of other tumors, including peripheral-nerve sheath tumors, cartilaginous tumors, osteosarcomas, eccrine and visceral carcinomas, and Langerhans cell tumors. HMB-45 is a monoclonal antibody with high specificity for malignant melanoma: in general, it is not immunoreactive with carcinomas, lymphomas, or sarcomas. HMB-45 is frequently negative in spindle-cell and desmoplastic melanomas; however, these tumors commonly exhibit vimentin and S-100 protein positivity. In general, these two reagents should be used in concert with a panel of antibodies against other tumor markers, such as cytokeratins, vimentin, and leukocyte common antigen, depending on the clinical and histologic features.

STAGING OF MELANOMA

Accurate documentation of the extent of melanoma is essential for determining the optimal treatment of patients and for assessing prognosis. In addition, melanoma clinical trial design must account for such prognostic factors and stratify patients accordingly to permit comparison of results across institutions and to establish a treatment effect.

The AJCC and the International Union Against Cancer (UICC) tumor node metastasis (TNM) committees have approved a new melanoma staging system, which was implemented in 2002.[44] The changes incorporate information in prognostic variables that have enabled clinicians and pathologists to more accurately stage patients. Specific advances in melanoma staging involve more accurate analysis of primary melanoma tumors (ulceration), regional nodes (sentinel node biopsy), and metastases [site and serum lactic dehydrogenase (LDH)] for determining prognosis of patients. The previous (1997) version of the AJCC staging system did not incorporate this information, prompting the revision of the staging system by a panel of melanoma experts and approval of the current system by the AJCC and UICC TNM committees. Table 93-5 presents the TNM categories and Table 93-6 lists the stage groupings.

In general, approximately 85 percent of patients have localized disease (stages I and II) on presentation, and prognosis and treatment are related to the assessment of the characteristics of the primary tumor, so-called microstaging, as discussed below. Approximately 15 percent of patients have regional nodal disease (stage III), and prognosis is related to evaluating extent of this nodal disease and the presence of ulceration in the primary tumor. Only approximately 2 percent of patients have distant metastases (stage IV) at initial presentation.

the factors examined in the multivariate analysis of the primary tumor. In the analysis of distant metastases, the site of the metastases and the clinical and pathologic features used for the other stages were included.[1] The results are presented in Figs. 93-20, 93-21, 93-22, and 93-23, and are discussed below.

PROGNOSTIC FACTORS INCLUDED IN AJCC STAGING

Tumor thickness Melanoma thickness as measured from the granular layer of the epidermis to the greatest depth of tumor invasion by using an ocular micrometer, as originally described by Breslow (Fig. 93-24), has proved to be the single most important predictor of survival in primary cutaneous melanoma. Survival diminishes with increasing tumor thickness and, in general, there appears to be a linear

CLINICAL AND HISTOPATHOLOGIC PARAMETERS OF POSSIBLE PROGNOSTIC SIGNIFICANCE IN MELANOMA (Table 93-7)

More than 50 multivariate studies have been conducted in an effort to identify clinical and histologic parameters of prognostic significance in melanoma. The factors generally assessed in most studies include age, sex, tumor site, tumor thickness in millimeters (Breslow, see below), anatomic level (Clark, see below), tumor subtype, ulceration, regression, mitotic rate, host response, microscopic satellites, and vascular invasion (Table 93-7). Almost all of these studies have overwhelmingly confirmed the fundamental importance of tumor thickness as predicting the outcome in stages I and II melanoma.

Prognostic Factors for Stages I and II Melanoma

A multicenter AJCC melanoma database was created to validate the new AJCC staging system, and the largest prognostic factor analyses performed to date was conducted.[1] Staging and survival data from 30,450 melanoma patients were contributed from thirteen institutions and cooperative groups. Complete data was available for 17,600 melanomas and a multivariate prognostic factor analysis was performed to validate the new AJCC staging system that included age, sex, site, thickness, Clark's level of invasion, and ulceration. In the examination of the nodal metastases, the prognostic factors examined included the number of metastatic nodes, tumor burden, and

TABLE 93-5

Melanoma TNM Classification*

T Classification	Thickness (mm)	Ulceration Status
T1	≤1.0	a: without ulceration and level II/III b: with ulceration or level IV/V T2
T2	1.01–2.0	a: without ulceration b: with ulceration
T3	2.01–4.0	a: without ulceration b: with ulceration
T4	>4.0	a: without ulceration b: with ulceration

N Classification	No. of Metastatic Nodes	Nodal Metastatic Mass
N1	1	a: micrometastasis† b: macrometastasis‡
N2	2–3	a: micrometastasis† b: macrometastasis‡ c: in-transit met(s)/satellite(s) without metastatic nodes
N3	4 or more metastatic nodes, or matted nodes, or in-transit met(s)/satellite(s) with metastatic node(s)	

M Classification	Site	Serum Lactate Dehydrogenase
M1a	Distant skin, subcutaneous, or nodal metastases	Normal
M1b	Lung metastases	Normal
M1c	All other visceral metastases	Normal
	Any distant metastasis	Elevated

*Six major changes are included in the 2002 version of the AJCC melanoma staging system:

1. Anatomic level is used only in the staging of thin tumors. Thickness and ulceration are primarily used in the T category. The anatomic level of invasion (Clark's levels) is currently understood to be an independent prognostic feature only for thin melanomas. As a result, Clark's levels are incorporated only into staging of thin melanomas (<1.0 mm or category T1).
2. Ulceration of the tumor has been added to the staging system. Ulceration is a independent risk factor and portends a higher risk of developing advanced disease. The presence of ulceration "upstages" all patients with stages I to III disease. In a given T grouping, the new system subclassifies patients as "a" for tumors without ulceration, and "b" for tumors with ulceration.
3. The number of metastatic nodes, rather than the size of nodes, is used as the primary criterion in the N staging.
4. The system incorporates a new convention for categorizing patients both clinically and pathologically. This system incorporates data from lympathic mapping and sentinel node biopsy.
5. In-transit and satellite metastases have been grouped in the same subclassification (N2c). Patients with intralymphatic metastases but no nodal metastases are recongnized as having a similar prognosis, and are thus grouped together.
6. Distant metastatic melanoma is classified by site(s) of metastases and levels of lactic dehydrogenase (LDH) detected in serum.

†Micrometastases are diagnosed after sentinel or elective lymphadenectomy.

‡Macrometastases are defined as clinically detectable nodal metastases confirmed by therapeutic lymphadenectomy or when nodal metastasis exhibits gross extracapsular extension.

SOURCE: From Balch et al.,[44] with permission.

relationship between tumor thickness and survival. In the new staging system, tumor thickness is classified by thresholds that correlate with clinical management (see later) and prognosis of melanoma patients. Tumors are classified by thickness of ≤1.0 mm (T1), 1.01 to 2.0 mm (T2), 2.01 to 4.0 mm (T3), and >4.0 mm (T4).[63,64] In the AJCC melanoma validation study, tumor thickness was the most powerful independent prognostic factor for patients with primary cutaneous melanoma. No natural breakpoints were noted for tumor thickness in the analyses.

Ulceration Ulceration was the second most powerful factor in the AJCC validation study and was highly correlated with survival; consequently, ulceration of the tumor was added to the new staging system. Ulceration is an independent risk factor and portends a higher risk of developing advanced disease. The presence of ulceration "upstages" all patients with stages I to III disease. In a given T grouping, the new system subclassifies patients as "a" for tumors without ulceration and "b" for tumors with ulceration.[44]

Level of invasion Anatomic level of invasion originally described by Clark[2] refers to progressive penetration of certain anatomic barriers in the skin by melanoma[46] (see Fig. 93-24). Level I indicates melanoma is confined to the epidermis. Level II indicates breaching the epidermal–dermal basement membrane by tumor cells extending into the papillary dermis. Level III signifies a further accumulation of tumor cells in the papillary dermis such that the papillary dermis is expanded or distended by a cohesive nodule or plaque of cells or nests of cells. With level IV there is clear-cut extension of tumor cells into the reticular dermis. Finally, level V indicates invasion of the subcutaneous fat. Recognition of these levels provided one of the first objective correlates of survival in stages I and II melanoma.[2] After the description of Breslow's method of measuring tumor thickness,[3] anatomic levels have assumed a less-significant place in the microstaging of melanoma. Much of this has to do with the ease, reproducibility, and objectivity of measuring tumor depth. Assessing anatomic levels can also be cumbersome at certain sites, such as acral skin, and can lack reproducibility in certain instances, for example, level III versus early level IV.

In the AJCC validation study, the level of invasion had a significant impact on survival only within thin melanomas (<1.0 mm). As a result, Clark's levels are incorporated into the revised AJCC staging of thin melanomas only (<1.0 mm or category T1).[44]

TABLE 93-6

Proposed Stage Groupings for Cutaneous Melanoma

	Clinical Staging*			Pathologic Staging†		
	T	N	M	T	N	M
0	Tis	N0	M0	Tis	N0	M0
IA	T1a	N0	M0	T1a	N0	M0
IB	T1b	N0	M0	T1b	N0	M0
	T2a	N0	M0	T2a	N0	M0
IIA	T2b	N0	M0	T2b	N0	M0
	T3a	N0	M0	T3a	N0	M0
IIB	T3b	N0	M0	T3b	N0	M0
	T4a	N0	M0	T4a	N0	M0
IIC	T4b	N0	M0	T4b	N0	M0
III‡	Any T	N1	M0			
		N2				
		N3				
IIIA				T1-4a	N1a	M0
				T1-4a	N2a	M0
IIIB				T1-4b	N1a	M0
				T1-4b	N2a	M0
				T1-4a	N1b	M0
				T1-4a	N2b	M0
				T1-4a/b	N2c	M0
IIIC				T1-4b	N1b	M0
				T1-4b	N2b	M0
				Any T	N3	M0
IV	Any T	Any N	Any M1	Any T	Any N	Any M1

*Clinical staging includes microstaging of the primary melanoma and clinical/radiologic evaluation for metastases. By convention, it should be used after complete excision of the primary melanoma with clinical assessment for regional and distant metastases.
†Pathologic staging includes microstaging of the primary melanoma and pathologic information about the regional lymph nodes after partial or complete lymphadenectomy. Pathologic stage 0 or stage 1A patients are the exception; they do not require pathologic evaluation of their lymph nodes.
‡There are no stage III subgroups for clinical staging.
SOURCE: From Balch et al.,[44] with permission.

TABLE 93-7

Prognostic Factors for Clinical Stage I Melanoma

Factors	Effect on Prognosis
Clinical variables	
Age	Worse prognosis with increasing age
Sex*	Women have better prognosis than men
Anatomic site*	Extremity lesion have more favorable prognosis versus head and neck areas, palms, and soles
Pathologic stage of regional lymph nodes	Histologically negative nodes have better prognosis versus positive nodes
Histologic variables of primary tumor	
Tumor thickness (mm)*	Worse prognosis with increasing thickness
Levels of invasion	Worse prognosis with deeper levels
Radial versus vertical growth phase	Greater likelihood of metastasis with verticle growth phase
Mitotic rate*	Worse prognosis with increasing mitotic rate
Ulceration*	Worse prognosis with presence of ulceration
Lymphoid response (tumor-infiltrating lymphocytes)*	Worse prognosis with diminished lymphoid infiltrates
Regression*	Increased risk for metastasis in tumors <1.0 mm with marked regression
Microscopic satellites	Worse prognosis and increased risk for local, regional, and distant recurrences when present
Vascular invasion	Worse prognosis when present

*Independent predictive value in some multivariate analyses.

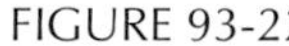

FIGURE 93-20

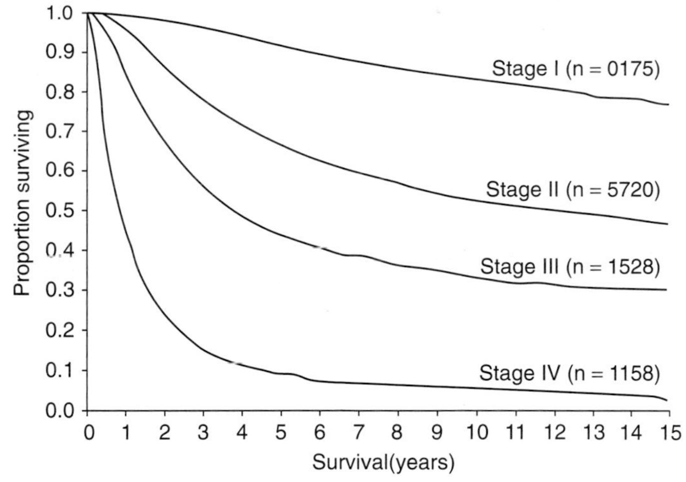

Fifteen-year survival curves comparing localized melanoma (stages II and I), regional metastases (stage III), and distant metastases (stage IV). The numbers in parentheses are patients from the AJCC melanoma staging database used to calculate the survival rates. The differences between the curves are significant ($p < .0001$). (*From Balch CM et al: Final version of the American Joint Committee on Cancer Staging System for Cutaneous Melanoma. J Clin Oncol 1p: 3635, 2001*)

PROGNOSTIC FACTORS NOT INCLUDED IN AJCC STAGING

Although the following prognostic factors also significantly correlate with survival, they have been determined to be less-powerful prognostic factors in multivariate regression models and are not included in the revised 2002 AJCC staging classifications.

Sex A large number of studies have reported women with melanoma as having improved survival rates when compared to men, even after adjustment for tumor thickness and anatomic site (Table 93-7).

Tumor site Multivariate analyses confirm site as an independent predictor of survival.[16] In general, extremity lesions (other than hands and feet) are associated with a better prognosis than tumors located on the trunk, head and neck, and palmar/plantar/subungual sites.[16] In addition, extremity melanomas are associated with a higher proportion of local and regional (in-transit and nodal) recurrences (85.6 percent versus systemic metastases) than are melanomas located on the trunk (77.3 percent local/regional recurrences), and head and neck (62.5 percent local/regional recurrences). Because local and regional recurrences are associated with greater survival than are systemic metastases, the improved survival of patients with extremity lesions appears related to pattern of recurrence. Nonetheless, site has not been confirmed as an independent prognostic factor in many studies. Melanomas of intermediate thickness (0.69 to 1.69 mm) that are localized to the so-called BANS area (back, posterior arm, posterior neck, scalp) have been reported to have a worse prognosis than non-BANS melanomas.[65] However, these findings have not been confirmed in other data bases[16] with the exception of scalp melanomas.

FIGURE 93-21

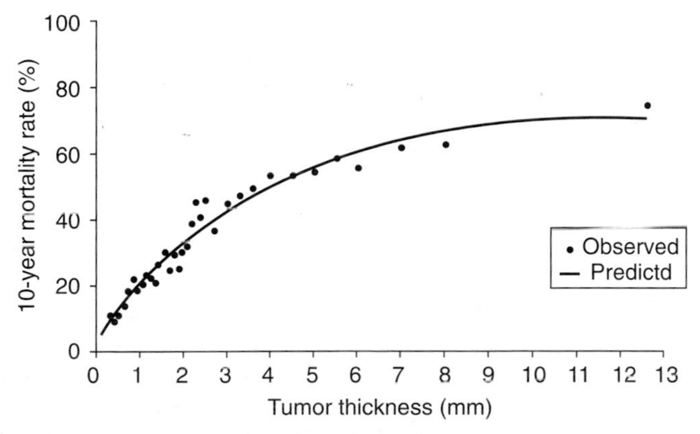

Observed and predicted 10-year mortality rate of 15,320 patients with clinically localized melanoma based on a mathematical model $f(t) = 1 - 0.988e^{(-211t\ +\ 0.0091^2)}$ derived from the AJCC melanoma database. T is the measured tumor thickness (mm) and f(t) is 10-year melanoma-specific mortality rates. $p < .0001$. (*From Balch et al*[1])

FIGURE 93-22

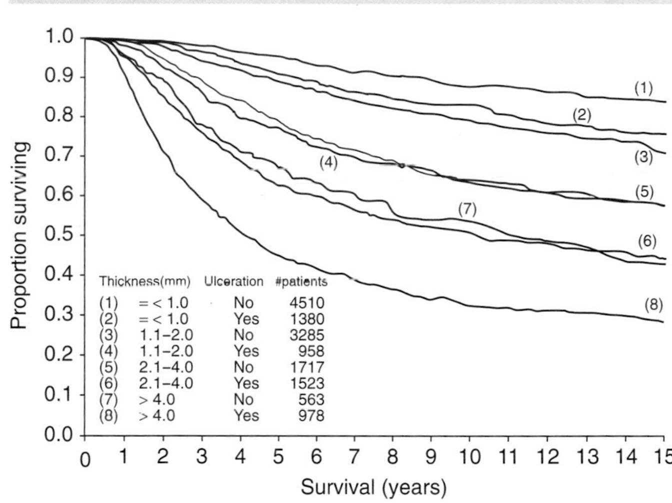

Survival curves of 14,914 patients with localized melanoma stratified by melanoma thickness and presence or absence of ulceration. The correlation of the sub-groups used for defining melanoma TNM staging with melanoma-specific survival is significant ($p < .0001$). (*From Balch et al*[1])

FIGURE 93-23

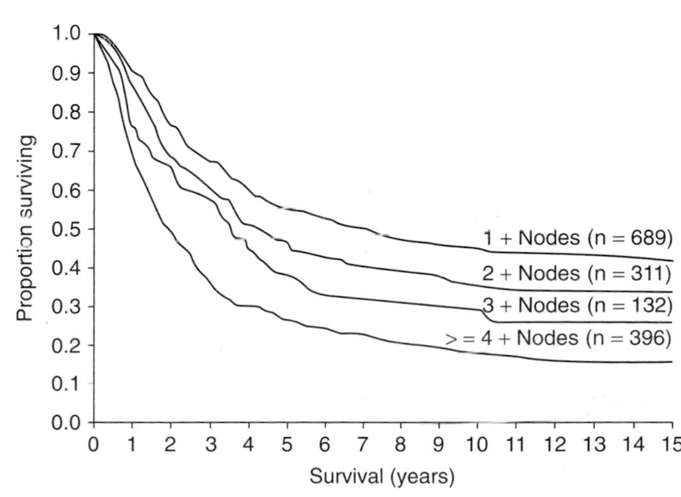

Survival curves of 1528 melanoma patients with lymph node metastases subgrouped by the actual number of metastatic nodes. The correlation is significant ($p < .0001$). (*From Balch et al*[1])

FIGURE 93-24

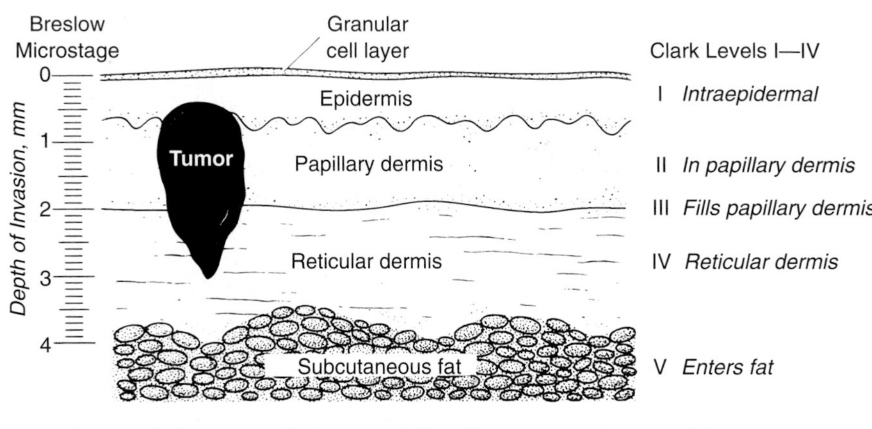

Breslow thickness and anatomic levels of invasion. When using the method described by Breslow, the greatest thickness of melanoma is measured in the vertical dimension from the granular layer (or top of an ulcerated surface) to the point of deepest tumor invasion. The anatomic level of invasion (Clark) refers to the extent of melanoma incursion into the papillary dermis, reticular dermis, and subcutaneous fat.

Age Single-factor and multivariate analysis indicate that advanced age portends a poorer prognosis for patients diagnosed with primary cutaneous melanoma.[16]

Phase of tumor progression The radial and vertical growth phases correlate with thickness and level of invasion. Clark and his colleagues suggested that the vertical growth phase, defined as the presence of an expansile nodule in the papillary dermis, may indicate competence for metastasis, whereas the radial growth phase is associated with no metastatic potential (in the absence of regression).[16] According to these investigators, the generally excellent prognosis of tumors <1.0 mm thick and anatomic level II (almost 100 percent survival at 8 years) is primarily related more to the growth phase than to thickness itself (see below). Other studies, however, have not confirmed the validity of growth phase as an independent prognostic factor.[63]

Histogenetic type For some time after the delineation of histogenetic subtypes of melanoma by Clark, it was reported that LMM had a better prognosis than SSM, and that SSM had a better prognosis than NM. Differences in prognosis among histogenetic subtypes do not remain after controlling for thickness.

Regression There are conflicting reports on the significance of regression on the prognosis of melanoma. Some of the problems in evaluating the contribution of regression can be attributed to lack of standardized definitions of regression and thresholds for recording this phenomenon.

Host response (Table 93-7) There is some evidence that the presence of a lymphoid infiltrate at the base of a melanoma is a favorable prognostic factor indicating a host response to the melanoma.[16] Lymphocytic infiltrates at the tumor base may diminish with increasing tumor thickness. Thus, lymphoid response may be inversely correlated with tumor thickness and have no independent predictive value. The presence of tumor-infiltrating lymphocytes (TILs) is a significant prognostic factor, even after adjustment for other variables, including thickness. TILs were defined as "brisk" if lymphocytes permeated the vertical growth phase nodule and infiltrated the entire base of the vertical growth phase. The presence of "brisk" TILs was one of the most significant prognostic parameters in Clark's model.

Mitotic Rate There is a significant relationship between mitotic activity, usually measured in mitoses/mm^2, and prognosis, particularly in tumors of intermediate thickness.[16] Nonetheless, some investigators have demonstrated an independent effect after adjustment for thickness. One significant problem related to recording mitoses is sampling error. Because of heterogeneity of mitotic activity in most tumors, hot spots or areas with the highest mitotic activity must be assessed for recording purposes.

The prognostic index (PI), defined as *mitoses/mm*^{2} × *thickness*, has been suggested as a better prognostic indicator than thickness alone. Kopf and associates demonstrated that patients with tumors 1.5 to 3.99 mm thick and a PI > 19 had a worse survival rate than patients with comparable tumors and a PI < 19.[64] The effect of PI as an independent variable has not been corroborated in other studies.

Tumor cell type Recognition of melanoma cell type other than spindle- versus non–spindle-cell type has not proved a useful prognostic indicator.[16] In general, the limiting factors in evaluating cell type are the lack of standardized definitions and heterogeneity of tumors.

Vascular invasion This parameter, which is closely related to microscopic satellites, is a strong predictor of nodal metastasis. The usefulness of the finding is limited because of frequent false-positive results (a consequence of tissue-shrinkage artifacts) and the rarity of true positive results.

Prognostic Factors for Stage III Melanoma

The presence of regional lymph node metastasis portends a poorer prognosis for patients with an overall 5-year survival rate of approximately 37 percent and 10-year survival rate of 32 percent.[65] The number of positive lymph nodes is the most important prognostic factor in patients with nodal metastasis. Patients with nodal micrometastases (clinical stages I and II, pathologic stage III) have considerably better survival than clinical stage III (palpable nodes).

In the AJCC melanoma validation study, 1528 melanoma patients with lymph node metastases were analyzed, and the number of metastatic nodes was the most powerful predictor of survival ($P < 0.00001$). Increasing numbers of lymph nodes involved portends a poorer prognosis (Fig. 93-23).[1] The second most significant predictor of outcome was the tumor burden as determined by whether microscopic/clinically occult or macroscopic/clinically apparent disease was present. The only feature of the primary tumor that was a significant predictor of outcome once lymph node involvement was present was tumor ulceration.

Prognostic Factors for Stage IV Melanoma

Once metastases to distant sites have developed, median survival is approximately 6 months. The only variables of prognostic significance are number of metastatic sites, surgical resectability, duration of remission, and location of metastases (Table 93-8). Survival is longer for one metastatic site versus two, and two sites are more favorable than three or more. Solitary resectable metastases in sites such as the lungs, brain, or bowel may be associated with significantly prolonged survival.[46] Patients also have improved survival with nonvisceral sites (skin, subcutaneous tissue, distant lymph nodes) versus visceral (lung, liver, bone, brain).

Site of metastases was the most important prognostic factor in the AJCC melanoma validation study with patients with visceral metastases having a relatively poorer prognosis than nonvisceral (skin, subcutaneous, and distant lymph nodes) sites.

TABLE 93-8

Prognostic Factors for Clinical Stage IV Melanoma

PROGNOSTIC VARIABLE	EFFECT ON PROGNOSIS
Number of metastatic sites	Worse prognosis with increasing number of sites
Location of metastases	Worse prognosis for visceral sites (lung, liver, brain, bone) versus nonvisceral sites (skin, subcutaneous tissue, distant lymph nodes)
Presence of "resectable" metastases	Better prognosis for solitary resectable metastases
Sex*	Worse outcome for males
Duration of remission	Shorter duration of remission associated with worse prognosis

*Not confirmed in all studies.

Melanoma and Hypopigmentation

Both primary and metastatic melanoma may be associated with vitiligo-like hypopigmentation. For details, see Chap. 90.

METASTATIC MELANOMA AND DIFFUSE HYPERMELANOSIS

Advanced metastatic melanoma may be associated with diffuse hypermelanosis and melanogenuria. For details, see Chap. 90.

EVALUATION FOR SUSPECTED OR NEWLY DIAGNOSED MELANOMA

History

A patient with suspected or newly diagnosed melanoma should have an appropriate history taken including risk factor assessment as outlined earlier. (Dr. T.B. Fitzpatrick has proposed an acronym that summarizes the important risk factors for melanoma and is remembered as MM-RISK: M = Moles: atypical; M = Moles: common; R = Red hair and freckling; I = Inability to tan: skin phototypes I and II; S = Sunburn: severe sunburn before age 14 years; K = Kindred: family history of melanoma) (see also Chap. 88). The history should also include the details concerning the lesion in question: how long has the lesion been present; has the lesion changed and how has it changed (e.g., enlargement in area or elevation, change in color, change in borders, ulceration, bleeding, tenderness, itching); duration of changes; how changes were detected or reason for seeking medical attention; occupational exposures; history of other medical conditions; medications; and history of nevi previously removed.

Physical Examination

The patient should have a complete physical examination, including comprehensive examination of the skin. The characteristics of the lesion in question and other relevant pigmented lesions should be assessed with optimal illumination, a source of side-lighting, a hand lens, a Wood lamp, and dermoscopy, as needed. Other gross morphologic parameters such as overall symmetry, regularity of coloration, number of colors, and topography (macular, papular, accentuation or obliteration of skin cleavage lines, ulceration, crusting) should be noted. In general, numbers of nevi and clinically atypical nevi should be recorded because they are markers of increased risk for melanoma. The primary site should be palpated, and the patient examined for evidence of lymphadenopathy and hepatosplenomegaly.

Laboratory Evaluation and Staging

Further evaluation of the patient is aimed at determining the extent of the disease process so that prognosis and therapy are appropriate. In general, additional investigations are directed by symptoms and signs. For example, headache or development of seizures would prompt imaging of the head. Performance of such studies without any clear clinical indication has proved to be of little practical value. As a general rule, individuals with primary cutaneous melanoma may need only a baseline chest x-ray examination as part of an initial evaluation. Patients with melanomas >1.0 mm in thickness may be considered for sentinel lymph node studies (see below).

The presence of lymphadenopathy (clinical stage III disease) generally requires intervention to verify the presence of tumor. Such intervention usually takes the form of a complete lymph node dissection, but lymph node biopsy or fine-needle aspiration may be employed as the first diagnostic maneuver. Additional evaluation of the patient for distant metastases includes liver enzymes, LDH, and CT scans of the chest and abdomen.

MANAGEMENT

This malignancy attracts the interest and requires the expertise of several disciplines. Although there have been significant advances in the management of melanoma, currently the only standard treatment for cutaneous melanoma is early recognition and surgical excision of the primary tumor. The advances in management and evolving treatments are reviewed below.

Therapy for Primary Melanoma (Table 93-9)

The only standard treatment in primary cutaneous melanoma is the complete surgical excision of the primary lesion. The principal debate in the management of primary cutaneous melanoma involves the surgical margin that should be taken. Traditionally, a wide local excision involving a margin of 5 cm was considered the standard of care. The recommendation of a 5-cm margin has been attributed to W. Sampson Handley who, in the 1907 Hunterian lectures, based this recommendation on a single autopsy examination of a 34-year-old patient who had "centrifugal lymphatic spread" of the melanoma cells at a site of cutaneous metastasis. On the basis of this anatomic study, Handley

TABLE 93-9

Guidelines for Surgical Management of Patients with Clinical Stage I and II Melanoma*

TUMOR THICKNESS (MM)	MARGINS OF SURGICAL RESECTION (CM)	CLOSURE	SENTINEL NODE MAPPING
In situ	0.5	Primary	No
≤1.0	1	Primary	No†
1.0–2.0	1–2	Primary	+
2.0–4.0	2	Primary, graft or flap	+
>4.0	2–3	Primary, graft or flap	+

*The treatment of each patient is individualized. It may not be possible to achieve the recommended margins of excision in certain anatomic sites, such as on the face or distal extremities. Also, skin grafts or flaps may be necessary for surgical defects in the latter locations.
†Standard node mapping may be considered for melanoma <1.0 mm if ulcerated, Clark's level IV/V.

recommended a 2.5-cm surgical margin extending to the subcutaneous fat and to 5 cm of the fascial layer.[66] The surgical practice of performing a wide local excision was challenged in 1977, when Breslow and Macht presented a series of 35 patients safely treated with narrower surgical margins.[67] Subsequently, a large number of retrospective and nonrandomized trials have also supported a narrower surgical margin.

Two prospective, randomized surgical trials have provided solid evidence for the safety of narrower excision margins in the surgical management of primary cutaneous melanoma. The World Health Organization (WHO) randomized 612 patients, with melanomas <2 mm thick, to undergo excision with 1- or 3-cm margins.[68] At a mean follow-up of 55 months, there was no significant difference in disease-free survival and survival rates between the groups. An update of this trial was published with a mean follow-up of 90 months, and reported that the 8-year actuarial survival and disease-free survival were similar.[69] The WHO study concluded that margins of 1.0 cm were safe for melanomas 1.0 mm and less in thickness. Based on the trend to local recurrences in the 1.1- to 2.0-mm group, these authors recommended that longer follow-up is needed in this group before issuing a final recommendation.

The Intergroup Melanoma Surgery Trial conducted by Balch et al. prospectively enrolled 486 patients to undergo 2-cm versus 4-cm margins for intermediate-thickness melanomas (between 1 and 4 mm thick).[70] At a median follow-up of 72 months, no statistically significant difference was noted in local recurrence or survival between the study groups. An update has been reported with a median follow-up of 91 months, which update confirmed the effectiveness and safety of a 2-cm margin for intermediate-thickness melanomas.[42] In addition, the local recurrence rate was not significantly different ($p = .72$) groups. The conclusion of these investigators was that a 2-cm margin is satisfactory for eliminating residual disease at the site of primary intermediate-thickness melanomas, and that local recurrences and survival would not be significantly affected by a further 2-cm margin.

Taken together, these well-designed high-quality surgical trials provide strong evidence that 1-cm margins are safe and efficacious for invasive melanomas less than 1 mm in thickness. For melanomas >1 mm in thickness, there remains controversy regarding optimal excision margins. Based on the trend to local recurrences in the 1.1- to 2.0-mm group from the WHO study, and the lack of benefit to any wider excision as determined in the Intergroup study, some centers recommend 2.0-cm margins for intermediate-thickness melanomas, where feasible. The current American Academy of Dermatology (AAD) guidelines of care for cutaneous melanoma recommend a 1.0-cm margin for invasive melanomas <2 mm thick, and 2-cm margins for melanomas >2 mm thick.[71] The lack of a difference in survival or local recurrence with wider margins has led some authors to recommend 1-cm margins for all invasive melanomas,[72] but there are no prospective randomized, controlled surgical trials that support this recommendation.

Prospective randomized studies have not yet evaluated the optimal excision margin for in situ or thick melanomas (>4 mm). A National Institutes of Health consensus conference recommended 0.5-cm margins for melanomas in situ.[73] Despite a lack of good evidence, many surgeons prefer to take margins >3 cm for thick primaries (>4 mm).

It is important to note that strict guidelines should not be routinely recommended in the surgical management of cutaneous primary melanoma, and that each case should be evaluated individually. Primary melanomas near a vital structure may require a reduction in the margin, whereas poor histologic prognostic factors may suggest a biologically more aggressive melanoma and support a wider margin. Melanoma excision at special sites, such as the fingers, toes, sole of the foot, and ear, also require separate surgical and functional considerations. Table 93-9 summarizes current recommendations for surgical margins, based on an evidenced-based approach, and current guidelines.

Elective Lymph Node Dissection

The removal of regional lymph nodes draining the site of a primary cutaneous melanoma in the absence of any clinical evidence of metastasis to those nodes is termed *elective lymph node dissection* (ELND). The decision to perform ELND is a very controversial aspect in the surgical management of melanoma. The debate focuses primarily on the role of ELND in intermediate-thickness melanomas, because thin melanomas (<0.75 mm) have an excellent 5-year survival rate, in the order of 96 to 99 percent with excision of the primary alone, and thick primaries (>4.0 mm) have an elevated risk of systemic metastases, thus reducing any potential survival benefit of prophylactic lymphadenectomy.

The principal rationale for ELND is based on the biologic presumption that melanoma metastasizes in a predictable manner to a regional nodal basin first before spreading to distant organs. Proponents of ELND maintain that by removing regional nodes, draining a primary melanoma, it is possible to eradicate subclinical micrometastases in a timely and potentially curative manner. In further support of early surgical intervention is the recognition that the prognosis is worse with increasing nodal tumor burden. Additional cited benefits of ELND include the accurate staging for prompt initiation of adjuvant therapy and the avoidance of future palliative node dissection.

Opponents of ELND counter that the presumption of regional metastasis may not be valid in melanoma as nodal involvement can be a reflection of systemic metastasis, and that melanoma can metastasize hematogenously, bypassing regional nodes. In addition, it is suggested that removal of regional nodes also reduces the immune response to micrometastasis. Furthermore, in patients with intermediate-thickness melanomas, only approximately 30 percent are expected to have nodal micrometastases, thus subjecting the remaining group to the morbidity of this procedure without any benefit. Additional arguments against prophylactic lymphadenectomy include the morbidity of the procedure, including lymphedema, nerve damage, surgical wound infection, and hematoma, and the chance (although low) of mortality associated with the procedure.

The evidence cited by these groups to support or refute the respective arguments involves the interpretation of both retrospective and prospective studies. Proponents of ELND cite retrospective studies that demonstrate improved prognosis for patients, particularly those with intermediate-thickness lesions. Critics of ELND point to two prospective, randomized trials from WHO and the Mayo Clinic that failed to demonstrate a statistically significant difference in survival from ELND.[74–76] These prospective studies, however, have been criticized on methodologic grounds. Two further randomized, prospective trials that address some of the methodologic shortcomings were subsequently initiated. The Intergroup Melanoma study has been reported with a median follow-up of 7.4 years.[77] This study involved a prospective randomized surgical trial of 740 AJCC stages I and II patients with intermediate-thickness melanomas (1 to 4 mm) of the trunk or extremity. Patients were randomly selected to receive excision of the primary melanoma (with a 2-cm or 4-cm margin) and to receive ELND or observation. This trial failed to show a statistically significant overall 5-year survival benefit from ELND (86 percent) as compared with the observation group (82 percent). A subset analysis did identify a survival benefit in patients who were younger than 60 years of age who had ELND, and in those subgroups having ELND that had nonulcerated lesions, and in melanomas between 1 and 2 mm thick. This trial has been criticized for analyzing subpopulations in this manner, as the trial was not designed to answer this question, and raises the potential of false-positive results. Cascinelli et al. reported for the WHO Melanoma Program that ELND did not significantly improve 5-year survival in patients with trunk melanomas 1.5 mm or greater in thickness.[78] This prospective randomized study in 252 patients determined 5-year survival rates with ELND of 61.7 percent when compared to the rate for delayed node dissection of 51.3 percent ($p = 0.09$). Patients who had occult regional node metastases at the time of ELND had an improved survival rate of 48.2 percent as compared to a rate of 28.6 percent ($p = 0.04$) for those whose nodal dissection was delayed until the appearance of regional node metastases.

Recently, a systematic review and meta-analysis of randomized controlled trials comparing elective lymph node dissection with delayed lymphadenectomy at the time of clinical recurrence was conducted.[79] Three randomized controlled trials comprising 1533 participants met the inclusion criteria. The pooled odds ratio for overall mortality for the 3 trials was 0.86 (95 percent confidence interval, 0.68 to 1.09), and the results were statistically nonsignificant. No significant overall survival benefit for patients undergoing elective lymph node dissection was determined; however, the trials were recognized to contain significant bias. These investigators advised that further research would be required to exclude the possibility that some subgroups may benefit from elective lymph node dissection.

Sentinel Lymph Node Biopsy

Traditionally, staging of regional nodal basins has relied on clinical examination or ELND. A more rational approach to staging nodal basins in patients with melanoma is lymphatic mapping and sentinel lymph node biopsy.[80] This technique is minimally invasive and has decreased morbidity when compared to ELND, particularly in view of the lack of survival benefit from large prospective randomized surgical trials with ELND as outlined in the previous section. This technique is based on the anatomic understanding that the first node draining a lymphatic basin,[80] named the *sentinel node,* would be expected to predict the presence or absence of melanoma in that basin. Preoperative lymphoscintigraphy is typically used to assist operative planning to precisely "map" or locate the nodal basin draining the primary melanoma. Either isosulfan blue or patent blue V is injected around the lesion to permit intraoperative localization of the sentinel node, to which the primary melanoma drains. This allows subsequent histopathologic examination to determine the presence or absence of tumor in the blue sentinel node. Frozen section analysis of sentinel lymph nodes has been reported to have a low sensitivity, and it is recommended that conventional permanent sections be performed. Using sentinel lymph node biopsy, it is possible to identify patients who have subclinical micrometastases to the sentinel node in a minimally invasive way and target them for therapeutic lymph node dissection, without subjecting those patients who lack metastases to the morbidity of ELND. In the original studies, Morton et al.[80] were able to identify a sentinel node in 82 percent of the lymphatic basins, and metastases were detected in 21 percent of lymphadenectomy specimens. The accuracy of the procedure was confirmed as complete lymphadenectomy was performed in all cases, and metastases were present exclusively in 2 of 3079 nonsentinel nodes (1 percent false-negative rate). A single sentinel node was found in 72 percent of the basins, two sentinel nodes were found in 20 percent of the basins, and three or more sentinel nodes were found in 8 percent of the basins.

To facilitate intraoperative identification of the sentinel node, radioactive colloidal tracer may be used for intraoperative mapping. One difficulty of the blue-dye technique is that surgically locating the blue-labeled sentinel node may require considerable surgical dissection, with a success rate in the order of 80 percent.[81] A refinement of the blue-dye technique involves the injection of a radioactive tracer, Technetium (Tc)-99 sulfur colloid, at the site of the primary with intraoperative localization with a handheld gamma probe to help identify the sentinel node.[81] A "hot spot" is identified with the gamma probe, and an incision in the skin over the site of peak transcutaneous counts is made. The sentinel lymph node (SLN) is identified by the radioactivity and the blue staining of the lymphatic channel and the node, with ex vivo correlation. Krag et al. were able to identify 98 percent (118/121) of sentinel nodes with this technique, and with less tissue dissection than with the conventional blue-dye method.[81]

Further refinements of the sentinel node procedure have involved attempts to improve the detection of micrometastases in the sentinel node after it is removed for examination. Conventional pathologic evaluation of lymph nodes, involving sectioning and hematoxylin and eosin staining, underestimates melanoma present in nodes with false negatives occurring. Investigators at the M.D. Anderson Cancer Center examined a consecutive cohort of patients that underwent lymphatic mapping and sentinel node biopsy to determine the patterns of recurrence and causes for failure. It was determined that 11 percent of patients with a histologically negative SLN (AJCC stages I and II) developed recurrence at a median follow-up of 35 months. Serial sectioning and immunohistochemistry, of the 10 patients who developed nodal recurrence in a previously mapped basin, identified occult metastases in 80 percent of these cases.[82] Currently, the assessment of the sentinel node involves careful evaluation of multiple sections of the node with H&E and immunohistochemistry focused on tumor-associated markers (S-100, HMB-45, and Melan-A/MART-1). Attempts to compare PET-FDG (positron emission tomography with [^{18}F]-labeled fluorodeoxyglucose) scanning with SLN biopsy indicate that PET scans are not reliable for detecting micrometastatic melanoma, and that SLN biopsy is superior in identifying metastases in regional basins.

Serial sectioning with standard histopathologic and immunohistologic examination may still fail to detect submicroscopic melanoma metastases in lymph nodes. Reverse transcriptase-polymerase chain reaction (RT-PCR) for tyrosinase is being studied as an adjunct to conventional histopathology and immunohistochemistry to reduce sampling error and to increase sensitivity. Several studies have used RT-PCR to determine that histologically negative SLNs have occult metastases.[83] Nevus cells can be present in lymph nodes and result in false-positive results with this technique. Correlation with conventional histology can reduce this source of error. The significance of micrometastatic melanoma detected by RT-PCR has yet to be definitively determined. One objective of the Sunbelt Melanoma Trial is to determine the survival of patients that have occult metastases in sentinel nodes that are RT-PCR positive, but negative by conventional histopathology. The survival of RT-PCR–positive patients that are observed will be compared to those who undergo node dissection alone, or who undergo node dissection and adjuvant therapy with interferon.

Although the sentinel lymph node procedure provides an elegant method of sampling lymph nodes to determine the presence of subclinical micrometastases, a rigorous, prospective, randomized surgical trial has not yet reported a survival benefit for this procedure. Proponents of this procedure have also advocated this procedure to stage patients for adjuvant interferon therapy. This rationale for performing this procedure is now in question in light of the most recent studies on the use of adjuvant therapy with interferon (see below). As a result, widespread acceptance of this procedure as a standard of care is lacking[83] despite many leading centers and the WHO designation of this procedure as such.[84] The most recent AAD guidelines of care for melanoma note that the value of sentinel node biopsy is "undetermined," and it is neither included nor addressed in the management of primary cutaneous melanoma.[71] The Multicenter Selective Lymphadenectomy Trial (MSLT) is a prospective randomized trial that will examine the impact of SLN on survival. This trial has accrued 1800 patients, and is now closed to enrollment with long-term follow-up results pending. Until the MSLT results are available, current evidence supports the use of the sentinel node biopsy procedure as a staging procedure only, and is generally considered for patients with a melanoma more than 1 mm thick (see Table 93-9 for special consideration).

Therapy for Regional Metastases (Table 93-10)

SURGERY Regional metastases include regional lymph node and in-transit metastases. Treatment for patients with regional node involvement consists of therapeutic lymph node dissection and consideration of adjuvant therapy. The management of in-transit metastases is related to the number of lesions, location, and possible presence of distant metastases. In general, isolated or small numbers of lesions may be surgically excised.

ISOLATED LIMB PERFUSION The technique of isolated limb perfusion (ILP) is principally used to treat locoregional disease of the extremity (in-transit metastases and satellitosis) and for palliation with significant regional disease. The procedure is frequently used in conjunction with surgical excision of in-transit metastases and regional lymph node dissection. The method involves perfusing an isolated extremity with oxygenated blood from an extracorporeal source. Chemotherapeutic agents, especially melphalan (L-phenylalanine mustard), are perfused in high doses to the limb surgically isolated from systemic circulation under hyperthermic conditions [usually 40°C to 41°C (104°F to 105.8°F)] in order to achieve greater tumor destruction. TNF in combination with melphalan compared to melphalan alone is currently the focus of ongoing clinical trial research.

This technique has also been used as adjuvant therapy for high-risk (>1.5 mm) melanomas of the extremities, including acral lentiginous and subungual melanomas. Retrospective series and a recent major prospective multicenter randomized trial failed to demonstrate a benefit of prophylactic ILP, and current evidence does not support this technique as adjuvant therapy in high-risk extremity lesions. Under the auspices of the WHO, North American Perfusion Group, and the European Organization for Research and Treatment of Cancer (EORTC), 832 patients with melanoma greater than 1.5 mm in thickness were randomized to have wide local excision or wide local excision plus ILP with melphalan and hyperthermia.[85] No survival benefit was determined at a median follow-up of 6.4 years. A marginal benefit was noted in patients with melanoma of 1.5- to 2.99-mm thickness, as in-transit metastasis was reduced from 6.6 to 3.3 percent and regional lymph node metastasis was reduced from 16.7 to 12.6 percent.[85]

TABLE 93-10

General Guidelines for Treatment Sequences in Metastatic Melanoma*

METASTATIC SITE	FIRST OPTION	SECOND OPTION	THIRD OPTION
Skin subcutaneous (trunk, head, neck)			
Isolated	Surgery	Radiation	Systemic
Multiple	Radiation, surgery, intralesional	Systemic	
Skin, subcutaneous (extremity)			
Isolated	Surgery	Limb perfusion	Radiation or systemic
Multiple	Limb perfusion (± surgery)	Radiation or systemic	Systemic
Lung			
Isolated	Surgery		
Multiple	Systemic		
Liver	Systemic		
Bone	Radiation (± surgery)	Systemic	
Brain			
Isolated	Surgery + radiation	Radiation	
Multiple	Radiation		
Gastrointestinal tract			
Isolated	Surgery		
Multiple	Systemic		

*Systemic, chemotherapy, or immunotherapy.
SOURCE: Reprinted with permission from Meyers ML et al.,[46] Table 22-9, p 343, with permission.

ADJUVANT THERAPY Adjuvant therapy involves the treatment of a patient after all visible tumor is removed, but the patient is considered at high risk for relapse. The current AJCC staging system helps to define patients at high risk of recurrence (AJCC stages IIb and III) who could be considered for adjuvant therapy. There have been numerous adjuvant trials in patients with melanoma that involved the use of radiotherapy, chemotherapy, regional limb perfusion, and biologic response modifiers and that failed to establish a standard regimen for melanoma in an adjuvant setting. Three randomized trials[86–88] comparing levamisole with placebo in patients with Clark levels II to V or positive nodes, failed to demonstrate a significant difference in survival. One trial conducted by the National Cancer Institute of Canada did show a significant difference in the 5-year survival rates (74 percent in levamisole versus 62 percent in the placebo group, $p = .027$).[89] This improvement in survival, however, was not significant after the multivariate analysis was adjusted for known prognostic factors (sex, age, stage of disease).

The first study to fulfill stringent methodologic criteria and to demonstrate a statistically significant difference in survival in the adjuvant treatment of melanoma was reported by Kirkwood et al. of the Eastern Cooperative Oncology Group (ECOG) 1684 study[90] using interferon alpha-2b (IFN-α2b) conducted under the auspices of the National Cancer Institute. This trial randomized 287 patients who were to receive 52 weeks of IFN-α2b [high-dose interferon (HDI)] or observation. An induction phase for 4 weeks (20 million units/m^2, intravenous, five times weekly) was followed by 48 weeks of maintenance therapy (10 million units/m^2 subcutaneously, three times weekly). Patients selected were at high risk of recurrence, with either thick primaries (>4 mm; AJCC stage IIb, T4N0M0) or presented initially with nodal involvement (AJCC stage III) at ELND or clinically. Patients were also enrolled that had recurrent lymph node metastases after treatment for a primary melanoma. All patients underwent elective lymph node dissection, and those with extracapsular invasion of the lymph nodes were excluded. With a median follow-up of 6.9 years, this trial demonstrated a statistically significant increase in the 5-year survival rate of 11 percent (37 percent for the treatment group as compared with 26 percent for the observation group, $p = .005$), and an increase in the median overall survival by approximately 1 year (3.82 years for the treatment group as compared with 2.78 years for the observation group, $p = .047$). This study led to the FDA approval of IFN-α2b for adjuvant therapy of melanoma in patients with deep primary melanomas (T4), and node-positive patients.

Other randomized trials using interferon in an adjuvant setting in the treatment of melanoma have failed to report a statistically significant benefit. These studies differ from the ECOG study by including patients with extracapsular node involvement, mode of administration (intramuscular/subcutaneous versus intravenous in the induction and subcutaneous in the maintenance phases), dose (lower and shorter course versus high dose), and type of interferon (γ versus α).

The regimen used in the HDI-ECOG-1684 study was associated with significant toxicity, the most frequent being flulike symptoms in almost all patients (fatigue, fever, myalgias, anorexia, headache). Severe (grade 3) and life-threatening (grade 4) reactions were less frequent, but they still occurred in 43 percent (59 of 137) and 14 percent (20 of 143), respectively. While 60 percent of patients were able to complete >80 percent of dosing, adverse effects required discontinuation of interferon in 24 percent of patients. There were two treatment-related deaths caused by hepatotoxicity that occurred early in the trial and prior to close monitoring of liver enzymes. A subsequent study performed a quality-of-life-adjusted survival analysis to compare the interferon treatment group with the observation group after accounting for the decreased quality of life associated with treatment toxicity and that associated with relapse of melanoma.[91] This study determined that the interferon-treated group had more quality-of-life-adjusted time than the observation group even after adjusting for toxicity. This difference was statistically significant, however, only for certain patients who were willing to undergo toxicity in exchange for the increased survival and decreased chance of relapse.

The HDI regimen was reevaluated in the intergroup E1690/S9111/C9190 study, as well as a lower dose of IFN-α2b [low-dose interferon (LDI)] in an effort to administer therapy over a longer period but with less toxicity.[92] Six hundred forty-two patients were treated with wide local excision and randomized to HDI (1684 regimen), LDI (3 million units three times weekly subcutaneously for 2 years), or observation. At a median follow-up of 52 months, no significant benefit in overall survival was reported with HDI, LDI, or observation. HDI did improve disease-free survival (44 percent versus 35 percent; $p = 0.05$) when compared to observation, although LDI did not (40 percent versus 35 percent). Proponents of adjuvant IFN-α2b therapy maintain that the lack of significance of HDI on overall survival in this trial may be a result of confounding factors. In comparing E1684 and E1690, the median survival for the observation arm in 1684 was significantly worse than the observation arm in 1690 (2.8 years versus 6 years in 1690; $p = 0.001$). It was noted that 31 percent of the patients in the observation arm of the 1690 trial who relapsed received "salvage therapy" with interferon. In a post hoc analysis, patients receiving salvage therapy with interferon had an improved overall survival (2.2 years versus 0.8 years; $p = 0.0024$). Still, such post hoc analyses have methodologic flaws, with the possibility of selection bias in a nonrandomized, unblinded setting.

A recent intergroup phase III study (E1694/S9512/C509801) with HDI or GMK vaccine provided evidence in support of a biologic effect of HDI.[93] In this trial, 880 patients were randomized to HDI or GMK vaccine. An interim analysis revealed the HDI arm had significantly improved disease-free survival (62 percent versus 49 percent) and 2-year overall survival (78 percent versus 73 percent). This trial had prespecified early stopping rules; consequently, it was closed by the external safety monitoring committee because of the improved disease-free survival in the interferon-treated arm.

Several studies have also been conducted in LDI, particularly for node-negative patients at high risk of recurrence due to thick, high-risk primary lesions. Pehamberger et al. reported for the Austrian Malignant Melanoma Cooperative Group[94] that adjuvant IFN-α2a treatment diminishes the occurrence of metastases and thus prolongs disease-free survival in patients with resected primary stage II cutaneous melanoma. The prospective randomized study included 311 patients with melanoma who had a Breslow thickness of >1.5 mm who were assigned either to adjuvant IFN-α2a treatment (or observation) after excision of the primary tumor. IFN-α2a was given in a low-dose regimen (3 million international units) subcutaneously. Prolonged disease-free

survival was observed in patients treated with IFN-α2a versus those who underwent surgery alone. The difference was significant ($p = .02$) for all patients enrolled in the study (intention-to-treat analysis) at a mean observation time of 41 months.

A French multicenter randomized trial of LDI was also conducted in patients with >1.5-mm thick primary melanomas. Four hundred eighty-nine patients received excision alone with clinical staging of the nodal basins only (no ELND or sentinel node biopsy), and were randomized to LDI (3 million units subcutaneously three times a week for 18 months) or observation. At a median follow-up of 5 years, a significant improvement was reported in disease-free survival ($p = 0.035$) but not overall survival ($p = 0.059$).[95]

Lens and Dawes recently performed a systematic review of randomized controlled trials that compared regimens with or without IFN-α adjuvant therapy in melanoma patients.[96] Eight trials comprising 3178 patients were analyzed to assess the effect of IFN-α therapy on overall survival, disease-free survival, melanoma recurrences, and toxicity. The authors concluded that no clear benefit of IFN-α therapy on overall survival in patients could be demonstrated. It was proposed that a large randomized controlled trial would be required to answer whether a full regimen of IFN-α therapy is effective and to identify the subgroups of patients who might benefit from IFN-α treatment.[96]

Therapy for Distant Metastases (Stage IV Melanoma)

(Table 93-10)

The treatment of the patient with distant metastatic melanoma must take into account several important factors: average survival for such patients is only 6 months and chemotherapy, immunotherapy, and chemoimmunotherapy have complete responses in a minority of patients that is usually short-lived, although randomized controlled trials are currently evaluating new agents. The aims of therapy in stage IV melanoma must be clearly defined and generally include one or more of the following: (1) to relieve symptoms of a life-threatening problem, (2) to increase length of survival, or (3) to evaluate new therapies.

Therapy should be individualized and should consider the age, underlying medical condition of the patient, number and site(s) of metastasis, previous treatments, and the wishes of the patient and family. Conservative treatment with observation and no active treatment is reasonable in certain patients (asymptomatic, elderly, poor underlying medical condition), particularly given the low probability of cure and potential toxicity associated with certain regimens.

SURGERY Surgical excision (metastasectomy) of isolated metastases in certain sites such as the skin and subcutis, lymph nodes, lung, brain, and gastrointestinal tract can prolong survival.[46] The number of metastatic lesions has prognostic importance, with patients having a solitary lesion performing relatively better than those with two or more sites. Excision of metastatic lesions can achieve significant palliation. For example, resection of a gastrointestinal tract metastasis may relieve life-threatening obstruction or hemorrhage.

RADIATION THERAPY Radiation therapy is indicated in certain patients with stage IV disease with palliative intent. Specific indications include brain metastases, pain associated with bone metastases, and skin and subcutaneous metastases that are superficially located.[46] Spinal cord compression and localized unresectable visceral deposits are special situations in which radiation therapy is also indicated.

CHEMOTHERAPY Chemotherapy is primarily indicated for stage IV, nonresectable metastatic melanoma. A variety of chemotherapy agents have shown activity against melanoma, and have been used as single agents, combination chemotherapy, and chemoimmunotherapy (biochemotherapy) regimens.

Single-agent chemotherapy Dacarbazine (DTIC) has shown the greatest effectiveness as a single agent in most series. The overall response rate in 1936 patients treated with DTIC was 20 percent (382 of 1936).[97] Complete responses occur in approximately 5 percent of patients and are not sustained in the majority of patients.

Other agents used as single therapy that have shown activity against melanoma include nitrosoureas [carmustine (BCNU) and lomustine (CCNU)] and vinca alkaloids (cisplatin and carboplatin), which have had response rates of 10 to 20 percent. Fotemustine is a new class of nitrosourea with a reported response rate in up to 20 percent of patients with metastatic melanoma to the central nervous system (CNS). Temozolomide is a new oral agent with CNS penetration that has also had promising preliminary results in cases of brain metastasis.[98] Other investigational drugs include taxanes and betulinic acid. The use of high-dose chemotherapy with or without autologous bone marrow transplantation (experimental) has also yielded higher response rates, but has not prolonged survival; however, current trials are evaluating this option.

Crosby et al. performed a recent Cochrane Review involving a systematic analyses of all prospective randomized trials using systemic therapy in metastatic cutaneous melanoma.[99] These authors could not find any randomized controlled trials comparing systemic therapy with placebo in metastatic melanoma. No support was found for a "gold standard" therapy in the treatment of metastatic melanoma. The authors noted that DTIC has been used as a control arm in more than 20 prospective randomized clinical trials, and the response rate is in the order of 9.1 to 29 percent. Given the lack of evidence from randomized clinical trials for any systemic therapy versus supportive care, it was proposed that systemic treatments (simple or combination) be compared to single-agent DTIC.

Combination chemotherapy A number of combination chemotherapy regimens have been used in patients with stage IV disease. Most regimens have included agents that have shown efficacy as single therapy and have included various combinations of DTIC, nitrosoureas (BCNU), vinca alkaloids, cisplatin, dactinomycin, hormonal therapy (tamoxifen), and, more recently, fotemustine. One of the more promising regimens is a chemohormonal combination therapy, known as the "Dartmouth regimen" or DBDT. This regimen includes the combination of DTIC, BCNU, cisplatin (DDP), and tamoxifen (TAM). This regimen has been tested predominantly in phase II single-institution studies. A review of all reported clinical experience with this regimen included 384 patients with an overall response in 44 percent, a complete response in 14 percent, and a partial response in 30 percent.[100] The first prospective, randomized placebo-controlled trial conducted under the auspices of the National Cancer Institute of Canada has been reported; it failed to demonstrate a statistically significant difference between groups in response or survival.[101] Such results demonstrate the difficulty in analyzing small uncontrolled studies and support the continued comparison of new agents to single-agent DTIC, which remains the standard chemotherapy agent for stage IV disease.

CHEMOIMMUNOTHERAPY The disappointing results of most chemotherapy regimens in metastatic melanoma have led to clinical investigation using combinations of chemotherapy and immunotherapy (see below), which are believed to have different mechanisms of action, in hopes of a synergistic effect. A number of studies have examined the use of IFN-α in combination with chemotherapy. A review of five phase III randomized trials comparing DTIC/IFN to DTIC $\pm$ TAM indicates that IFN may increase response duration, but in view of added toxicity and absence of improved survival to date, the combination should be restricted to clinical trial investigation.[102] The use of interleukin 2 (IL-2) and IFN-α with the Dartmouth regimen was studied in 42 patients and reported to have an overall response rate of 57 percent, with 24 percent complete responses and 33 percent partial responses. Significant toxicity accompanies such protocols, however, and the duration of response was short-lived. There is some evidence that cisplatin-based biochemotherapy regimens may have improved response rates with some durable remissions.

BIOLOGIC THERAPY The role of the immune system in inducing spontaneous regression of melanoma has stimulated considerable interest in the use of biologic therapy in melanoma. Various strategies for modulating or stimulating the immune response against melanoma have been devised over the years. Principal treatments that have been investigated include interferons, IL-2, adoptive immunotherapy techniques that use IL-2 in combination with lymphokine-activated killer cells (LAKs) or TILs, monoclonal antibodies, and tumor vaccines.

Interferon Interferon is believed to have activity against melanoma based on its antiproliferative effect and the ability to cause upregulation of human leukocyte antigen (HLA) and tumor antigen expression as well as other immunomodulatory effects. Interferon as adjunct treatment was discussed earlier. For advanced disease, IFN-α has been used as a single agent or in combination with chemotherapy. The response rate is on the order of 10 to 20 percent, with a minority of these complete responses. Response duration is typically less than 6 months, and nonvisceral sites have the best response.

Interleukin IL-2 has been used as a single agent in a variety of doses and regimens in metastatic melanoma. Rosenberg et al. published follow-up data for 134 patients treated with high-dose IL-2 from the NCI Surgery branch.[103,104] An overall response was seen in 17 percent, a complete response was seen in 7 percent, and a partial response was seen in 10 percent. Of interest, the complete responses were durable, with patients remaining disease-free for as long as 8 years after initiating therapy. High-dose IL-2 therapy is associated with significant toxicity, including deaths caused by myocardial infarction, arrhythmia, capillary leak syndromes, nephrotoxicity, respiratory distress, and sepsis. Early studies involving IL-2 plus LAK cells suggested increased activity compared to IL-2 alone. Follow-up data, however, fail to demonstrate any significant benefit over IL-2 alone.[105] Another category of IL-2 therapy consists of harvesting TILs, expanding these cells in vitro, and readministering the TILs plus IL-2 to the patient. Summary results of the NCI Surgery branch experience involving 86 patients treated with bolus IL-2 and TIL therapy, determine an overall response rate of 34 percent with 5 complete responses and 24 partial responses.[106] Combinations of IL-2 with IFN results in increased toxicity without significant benefit.[106]

Monoclonal antibodies Murine and human monoclonal antibodies (MAbs) are experimental therapies of potential use in melanoma. MAbs recognize melanoma-associated antigens, such as peptidoglycans, transferrin receptor-related antigens, glycoproteins, high-molecular-weight melanoma-associated antigens, sialoglycoproteins, and gangliosides.[106] MAbs are being developed as direct therapeutic agents to elicit a host immune response, as well as conjugating MAbs to a radioactive isotope for diagnostic imaging of metastases, or to a cytotoxic or other agent for therapeutic effect. Clinical trials using unconjugated murine MAbs have demonstrated clinical responses, particularly using monoclonal antibodies against GD2 and GD3 gangliosides.[106]

Melanoma vaccines Melanoma vaccines have been developed in an attempt to stimulate a specific immune response against melanoma-associated antigens.[107,108] Initial strategies in vaccine therapy included the use of tumor-cell vaccines either using autologous tumor cells or allogeneic melanoma cell lines. Several thousand patients have been treated with such tumor-cell vaccines with an overall response rate of 10 to 20 percent. Attempts to increase immunogenicity of tumor vaccines include treating melanoma cells with viruses (e.g., Newcastle, vaccina), using mechanical lysates, and as using nonspecific immunologic

TABLE 93-11

Advantages and Disadvantages of Melanoma Vaccine Preparations

Type of Vaccine	Advantages	Disadvantages	Examples
Polyvalent			
Whole melanoma cells			
Autologous	HLA specific Invokes broad range of protective responses More immunogenic Less vulnerable to antigenic modulation	Availability of autologous cells May contain immunosuppressive factors Difficult to characterize and reproduce	Autologous vaccines + haptens (DNP, BCG) or cytokines (IL-2, GM-CSF)
Allogeneic	Invokes broad range of protective responses May circumvent TAA heterogeneity More immunogenic Less vulnerable to antigenic modulation Easier to produce, characterize, and reproduce	Irrelevant cellular material Theoretically more toxic May contain immunosuppressive factors Might also induce tolerance or prevent recognition of potentially immunogenic subdominant epitopes	Polyvalent melanoma cell vaccine: PMCV/Cancer-Vex Melacine
Cell lysate	Same as above	Same as above	Vaccinia melanoma cell lysate (VMCL)
Partially purified antigens	Less irrelevant material	Difficult to characterize and reproduce	Shed-antigen vaccine and mechanicial cell lysates
Univalent			
Purified antigens	Minimal irrelevant material	Less immunogenic	GM2-KLH/QS-21
Peptide antigens	Theoretically less toxic Easier to characterize and reproduce	Very vulnerable to antigenic modulation Necessary to match TAA and/or HLA type	Tyrosinase, gp-100

SOURCE: From Curiel-Lewandrowski C, Demierre M: Advances in specific immunotherapy of malignant melanoma. *J Am Acad Dermol* 43:167, 2000 with permission.

adjuvants such as BCG or DETOX.[108] Evolving strategies include the use of vaccines using defined melanoma antigens known to be immunogenic (gangliosides such as GM2), the development of melanoma-derived peptide antigen vaccines (e.g., MART-1, gp-100), and the development of gene therapy to transfect and genetically alter melanoma cells to secrete cytokines of interest or increase immunogenicity by enhanced antigen expression.

The latter approach is based on studies demonstrating that vaccination of mice with cytokine-secreting melanoma cells can protect them from an otherwise lethal challenge with wild-type cancer cells, and can lead to the regression of melanoma cell deposits. Studies have been conducted to test safety, tolerability and, immunostimulatory potency of such cancer vaccines in patients with advanced melanoma.[109] More recently, knowledge of the potent antitumor activity of dendritic cells led to development of dendritic cell vaccines. These vaccines are produced by pulsing autologous dendritic cells with melanoma tumor epitopes to stimulate host antitumor activity.[110] Such novel but exciting therapies remain investigational and are currently the subject of ongoing and future clinical trial research. Table 93-11 reviews the major types of melanoma vaccines and the advantages and disadvantages of each.

FOLLOW-UP EVALUATION

Periodic examination of patients with melanoma is aimed both at detecting recurrence of melanoma and at the development of a second primary. Standardized follow-up schedules have been generated based on the frequency of recurrence for various melanoma thickness categories (Table 93-12). Based on data for 3171 patients with stage I melanoma followed for a mean of almost 10 years, McCarthy and his associates observed that thicker melanomas (>3.0 mm) recurred about eight times more frequently and much more rapidly (50 percent of recurrences within 1 to 1.5 years) than did thin tumors (>0.7 mm).[111] Thus, patients with thick tumors, particularly >1.5 mm, require close surveillance in the first 2 years of follow-up. Thin tumors (<0.76 mm) may be followed less frequently as the risk of recurrence is only approximately 1 percent per year. In general, after 5 years all patients should be followed on a yearly schedule unless they have dysplastic nevi, in which case visits should be every 6 months. The risk of a second primary is significantly increased in patients with dysplastic nevi and a family history of melanoma. Annual examination should continue for a minimum of 10 years and probably for life, as late recurrences develop in about 3 percent of patients. Continued follow-up is also advised for patients with dysplastic nevi.

The history and physical examination are fundamental for the detection of recurrent melanoma. The history should emphasize new or persistently changing lesions and pertinent review of symptoms such as development of cough, headache, or bone pain. The physical examination should include a comprehensive skin examination with attention to the previous primary excision site for local recurrence, regional

TABLE 93-12

Guidelines for Follow-up of Patients with Clinical Stages I and II Melanoma

<1.0 mm	Every 3 months × 1 year, then every 6 to 12 months
>1.0 mm	Every 3 months × 2 years, then every 6 months × 3 years, then every 12 months*

*If a patient has clinically atypical moles or dysplastic nevi, the interval may continue at every 6 months.

lymphatic drainage route, and lymph nodes, liver, and spleen. Patients with dysplastic nevi must be carefully evaluated for changing lesions or nevi sufficiently atypical to require histologic evaluation. Photography is useful for following clinically atypical nevi.

REFERENCES

1. Balch CM et al: Prognostic factors analysis of 17,600 melanoma patients: Validation of the American Joint Committee on Cancer melanoma staging system. *J Clin Oncol* **19**:3622, 2001
2. Clark WH Jr et al: The histogenesis and biologic behavior of primary human malignant melanomas of the skin. *Cancer Res* **29**:705, 1969
3. Breslow A: Thickness, cross-sectional areas and depth of invasion in the prognosis of cutaneous melanoma. *Ann Surg* **172**:902, 1970
4. Rigel DS: Melanoma update: 2001. *Skin Cancer Found J* **19**:13, 2001
5. Ahmedin J et al: Cancer statistics, 2002. *CA Cancer J Clin* **52**:23, 2002
6. Cosary CL et al: SEER Cancer Statistics Review, 1973–1992. Bethesda, MD, National Cancer Institute, NRH Pub. No. 96-2789, 1995
7. Elwood JM: Melanoma and sun exposure. *Semin Oncol* **23**:650, 1996
8. Langley RGB, Sober AJ: A clinical review of the evidence for the role of ultraviolet radiation in the etiology of cutaneous melanoma. *Cancer Invest* **15**:561, 1997
9. Holman CD et al: Epidemiology of pre-invasive and invasive malignant melanoma in western Australia. *Int J Cancer* **25**:317, 1980
10. Holman CD, Armstrong BK: Cutaneous malignant melanoma and indicators of total accumulated exposure to the sun: An analysis separating histogenetic types. *J Natl Cancer Inst* **73**:75, 1984
11. Holly EA et al: Cutaneous melanoma in women: I. Exposure to sunlight, ability to tan, and other risk factors related to ultraviolet light. *Am J Epidemiol* **141**:923, 1995
12. Stern RS et al: Malignant melanoma in patients treated for psoriasis with methoxsalen (psoralen) and ultraviolet A radiation (PUVA). *N Engl J Med* **336**:1041, 1997
13. Stern RS: The risk of melanoma in association with long-term exposure to PUVA. *J Am Acad Dermatol* **44**:755, 2001
14. Holly EA et al: Number of melanocytic nevi as a major risk factor for malignant melanoma. *J Am Acad Dermatol* **17**:459, 1987
15. Tucker MA et al: Clinically recognized dysplastic nevi: A central risk factor for cutaneous melanoma. *JAMA* **277**:1439, 1997
16. Clark WH Jr et al: Model predicting survival in stage I melanoma based on tumor progression. *J Natl Cancer Inst* **81**:1893, 1989
17. Mackie RM: Pregnancy and exogenous female sex hormones in melanoma patients, in *Cutaneous Melanoma,* 3d ed, edited by CM Balch, AN Houghton, AJ Sober, SJ Soong. St Louis, Quality Medical Publishing, 1998, p 187
18. Herlyn M et al: Biology of tumor progression in human melanocytes. *Lab Invest* **56**:461, 1987
19. Clark WH Jr et al: A study of tumor progression: The precursor lesions of superficial spreading and nodular melanoma. *Hum Pathol* **15**:1147, 1984
20. Holman CDJ et al: A theory of the etiology and pathogenesis of human cutaneous malignant melanoma. *J Natl Cancer Inst* **71**:651, 1983
21. Anderson DE et al: Hereditary aspects of malignant melanoma. *JAMA* **200**:741, 1967
22. Greene MH: Familial cutaneous malignant melanoma: Autosomal dominant trait possibly linked to the Rh locus. *Proc Natl Acad Sci U S A* **80**:6071, 1983
23. Bale SJ et al: Mapping the gene for hereditary cutaneous melanoma-dysplastic nevus to chromosome 1p. *N Engl J Med* **320**:1367, 1989
24. Kamb A et al: A cell cycle regulator potentially involved in genesis of many tumor types. *Science* **264**:436, 1994
25. Nobori T et al: Deletions of the cyclin-dependent kinase-4 inhibitor gene in multiple human cancers. *Nature* **368**:753, 1994
26. Fountain JW et al: Homozygous deletions within human chromosome band 9p21 in melanoma. *Proc Natl Acad Sci U S A* **89**:10557, 1992
27. Petty EM et al: Molecular definition of a chromosome 9p21 germ-line deletion in a woman with multiple melanomas and a plexiform neurofibroma: Implications for 9p tumor suppressor gene(s). *Am J Hum Genet* **53**:96, 1993
28. Cannon-Albright LA et al: Assignment of a locus for familial melanoma, MLM, to chromosome 9p13-p22. *Science* **258**:1148, 1992
29. Piepkorn M: Melanoma genetics: An update with focus on the CDKN2A (p16)/ARF tumor suppressors. *J Am Acad Dermatol* **42**:705, 2000
30. Cannon-Albright LA et al: Penetrance and expressivity of the chromosome 9p melanoma susceptibility locus (MLM). *Cancer Res* **54**:6041, 1994
31. Davies et al: Mutations in the BRAF gene in human cancer. *Nature* **9**:1, 2002
32. Halaban R: The regulation of normal melanocyte proliferation. *Pigment Cell Res* **13**:4, 2000
33. Tsao H et al: Precursor lesions and markers of increased risk for melanoma, in *Cutaneous Melanoma,* 3d ed, edited by CM Balch, AN Houghton, AJ Sober, SJ Soon. St. Louis, Quality Medical Publishing, 1998
34. Cohen LM: Lentigo maligna and lentigo maligna melanoma. *J Am Acad Dermatol* **33**:923, 1995
35. Weinstock MA, Sober AJ: The risk of progression of lentigo maligna to lentigo maligna melanoma. *Br J Dermatol* **116**:303, 1987
36. Langley RGB et al: Clinical characteristics, in *Cutaneous Melanoma,* 3d ed, edited by CM Balch, AN Houghton, AJ Sober, SJ Soong. St Louis, Quality Medical Publishing, 1998, p 81
37. Rhodes AR et al: Nonepidermal origin of malignant melanoma associated with a giant congenital nevocellular nevus. *Plast Reconstr Surg* **67**:782, 1981
38. DeDavid M et al: A study of large congenital melanocytic nevi and associated malignant melanomas: Review of cases in the New York University Registry and the world literature. *J Am Acad Dermatol* **36**:409, 1997
39. Bittencourt FV et al: Large congenital melanocytic nevi and the risk for development of malignant melanoma and neurocutaneous melanocytosis. *Pediatrics* **106**:736, 2000
40. Driscol MS et al: Does pregnancy influence the prognosis of malignant melanoma? *J Am Acad Dermatol* **29**:619, 1993
41. Ceballus PI et al: Melanoma in children. *N Engl J Med* **332**:656, 1995
42. Karakousis CP et al: Local recurrence in malignant melanoma: Long-term results of the multi-institutional randomized surgical trial. *Ann Surg Oncol* **3**:446, 1996
43. Cohn-Cedermark G et al: Outcomes of patients with local recurrence of cutaneous malignant melanoma. *Cancer* **80**:1418, 1997
44. Balch CM et al: Final version of the American Joint Committee on Cancer staging system for cutaneous melanoma. *J Clin Oncol* **19**:3635, 2001
45. Balch CM: Surgical management of regional lymph node metastases in cutaneous melanoma. *J Am Acad Dermatol* **3**:511, 1980
46. Meyers ML et al: Diagnosis and treatment of metastatic melanoma, in *Cutaneous Melanoma,* 3d ed, edited by CM Balch, AN Houghton, AJ Sober, SJ Soong. St Louis, Quality Medical Publishing, 1998, p 325
47. Crowley NJ, Seigler HF: Late recurrence of malignant melanoma. *Ann Surg* **212**:173, 1990
48. Tsao H et al: Ultra-late recurrence (15 years or longer) of cutaneous melanoma. *Cancer* **79**:2361, 1997
49. Reintgen DS et al: Metastatic malignant melanoma with an unknown primary. *Surg Gynecol Obstet* **156**:335, 1983
50. Chang P, Knapper WH: Metastatic melanoma of unknown primary. *Cancer* **49**:1106, 1982
51. Schlagenhauff B et al: Metastatic melanoma of unknown primary origin shows prognostic similarities to regional metastatic melanoma: Recommendations for initial staging examinations. *Cancer* **80**:60, 1997
52. Langley RGB, Sober AJ: Causes for the delay in the diagnosis of melanoma, in *Epidemiology, Causes and Prevention of Skin Diseases,* edited by JJ Grob, RS Stern, RM MacKie, WA Weinstock. Cambridge, UK, Blackwell, 1997, p 177
53. Pehamberger H et al: In vivo epiluminescence microscopy of pigmented skin lesions: I. Pattern analysis of pigmented skin lesions. *J Am Acad Dermatol* **17**:571, 1987
54. Steiner A et al: In vivo epiluminescence microscopy of pigmented skin lesions: II. Diagnosis of small pigmented skin lesions and early detection of malignant melanoma. *J Am Acad Dermatol* **17**:584, 1987
55. Pehamberger H et al: In vivo epiluminescence microscopy: Improvement of early diagnosis of melanoma. *J Invest Dermatol* **100**:356S, 1993
56. Soyer HP et al: *Dermoscopy of Pigmented Skin Lesions.* Milan, EDRA Med Publishing and New Media, 2001
57. Nachbar F et al: The ABCD rule of dermatoscopy: High prospective value in the diagnosis of doubtful melanocytic skin lesions. *J Am Acad Dermatol* **30**:551, 1994
58. Langley RGB, Sober AJ: *New Techniques in the Early Diagnosis of Melanoma: Melanogenesis and Malignant Melanoma: Biochemistry, Cell Biology, Molecular Biology, Pathophysiology, Diagnosis, and Treatment.* (International Congress Series 1096.) Excerpta Medica, St Louis, MO 1996, p 233
59. Binder M et al: Epiluminescence microscopy: A useful tool for the diagnosis of pigmented skin lesions for formally trained dermatologists. *Arch Dermatol* 131:286, 1995

60. Wolff K: Why is epiluminescence microscopy important?, in *Cancers of the Skin,* edited by R Dumer, FO Nestle, G Burg. Berlin, Springer, 2002, p 125
61. Elbaum M et al: Automatic differentiation of melanoma from melanocytic nevi with multispectral digital dermoscopy: A feasibility study. *J Am Acad Dermatol* **44**:207, 2001
62. Langley RG et al: Confocal scanning laser microscopy of benign and malignant skin lesions in vivo. *J Am Acad Dermatol* **45**:365, 2001
63. Barnhill RL et al: Predicting five-year outcome for patients with cutaneous melanoma in a population-based study. *Cancer* **79**:423, 1997
64. Kopf AW et al: Prognostic index for malignant melanoma. *Cancer* **59**:1236, 1987
65. Day CL et al: Prognostic factors for melanoma patients with lesions 0.76 mm–1.69 mm in thickness: An appraisal of "thin" level IV lesions. *Ann Surg* **195**:30, 1982
66. Buzzell RA et al: Favorable prognostic factors in recurrent and metastatic melanoma. *J Am Acad Dermatol* **34**:798, 1996
67. Breslow A, Macht SD: Optimal size of resection margin for thin cutaneous melanoma. *Surg Gynecol Obstet* **145**:691, 1977
68. Veronesi U et al: Thin stage I primary cutaneous malignant melanoma. *N Engl J Med* **318**:1159, 1988
69. Veronesi U, Cascinelli N: Narrow excision (1 cm margin). *Arch Surg* **126**:438, 1991
70. Balch CM et al: Efficacy of 2 cm surgical margins for intermediate-thickness melanomas (1 to 4 mm). *Ann Surg* **218**:262, 1993
71. Sober AJ et al: Guidelines of care for primary cutaneous melanoma. *J Am Acad Dermatol* **45**:579, 2001
72. Piepkorn M, Barnhill RL: A factual, not arbitrary, basis for choice of resection margins in melanoma. *Arch Dermatol* **132**:811, 1996
73. NIH Consensus Conference: Diagnosis and treatment of early melanoma. *JAMA* **268**:1314, 1992
74. Veronesi U et al: Inefficacy of immediate node dissection in stage I melanoma of the limbs. *N Engl J Med* **297**:627, 1977
75. Veronesi U et al: Delayed regional node dissection: Delayed regional lymph node dissection in stage I melanoma of the skin of the lower extremities. *Cancer* **49**:2420, 1982
76. Sim FH et al: Lymphadenectomy in the management of stage I malignant melanoma: A prospective randomized study. *Mayo Clin Proc* **61**:697, 1986
77. Balch CM et al: Efficacy of an elective regional lymph node dissection of 1 to 4 mm thick melanomas for patients 60 years of age and younger. *Ann Surg* **224**:255, 1996
78. Cascinelli N et al: Immediate or delayed dissection of regional nodes in patients with melanoma of the trunk: A randomized trial (WHO melanoma programme). *Lancet* **351**:793, 1998
79. Lens MB et al: Elective lymph node dissection in patients with melanoma: Systematic review and meta-analysis of randomized controlled trials. *Arch Surg* **137**:458, 2002
80. Morton DL et al: Technical details of intraoperative lymphatic mapping for early stage melanoma. *Arch Surg* **127**:392, 1992
81. Krag DN et al: Minimal-access surgery for staging of malignant melanoma. *Arch Surg* **130**:654, 1995
82. Gershenwald JE et al: Patterns of recurrence following a negative sentinel lymph node biopsy in 243 patients with stage I or II melanoma. *J Clin Oncol* **16**:2253, 1998
83. Thomas JM, Patocskai EJ: The argument against sentinel node biopsy for malignant melanoma. *BMJ* **321**:3, 2000
84. McMasters et al: Sentinel lymph node biopsy for melanoma: Controversy despite widespread agreement. *J Clin Oncol* **19**:2851, 2001
85. Koops HS et al: Prophylactic isolated limb perfusion for localized, high-risk limb melanoma: Results of a multicenter randomized phase III trial. European Organization for Research and Treatment of Cancer Malignant Melanoma Cooperative Group Protocol 18832, the World Health Organization Melanoma Program Trial 15, and the North American Perfusion Group Southwest Oncology Group-8593. *J Clin Oncol* **16**:2906, 1998
86. Lejeune FJ et al: An assessment of DTIC versus levamisole or placebo in the treatment of high risk stage I patients after surgical removal of a primary melanoma of the skin: A phase III adjuvant study (EORTC protocol 18761). *Eur J Cancer* **24**(suppl 2):81, 1988
87. Loutfi A et al: Double blind randomized prospective trial of levamisole/placebo in stage I cutaneous malignant melanoma. *Clin Invest Med* **10**:325, 1987
88. Spitler LE: A randomized trial of levamisole versus placebo as adjuvant therapy in malignant melanoma. *J Clin Oncol* **9**:736, 1991
89. Quirt IC et al: Improved survival in patients with poor prognosis malignant melanoma treated with adjuvant levamisole: A phase III study by the National Cancer III Trial by the National Cancer Institute of Canada clinical trials group. *J Clin Oncol* **9**:729, 1991
90. Kirkwood JM et al: Interferon alfa-2b adjuvant therapy of high-risk resected cutaneous melanoma: The Eastern Cooperative Oncology Group Trial EST 1684. *J Clin Oncol* **14**:7, 1996
91. Cole BF et al: Quality-of-life-adjusted survival analysis of interferon alfa-2b adjuvant therapy of high-risk resected cutaneous melanoma: The Eastern Cooperative Oncology Group Trial EST 1684. *J Clin Oncol* **14**:2666, 1996
92. Kirkwood JM et al: High- and low-dose interferon alfa-2b in high-risk melanoma: First analysis of intergroup trial E1690/S9111/C9190. *J Clin Oncol* **18**:2444, 2000
93. Kirkwood JM et al: High-dose interferon alfa-2b significantly prolongs relapse-free and overall survival compared with the GM2-KLH/QS-21 vaccine in patients with resected stage IIB-III melanoma: Results of intergroup trial E1694/S9512/C509801. *J Clin Oncol* **19**:2370, 2001
94. Pehamberger H et al: Adjuvant interferon alpha-2a treatment in resected primary stage II cutaneous melanoma. *J Clin Oncol* **16**:1425, 1998
95. Grob JJ et al: Randomized trial of interferon alpha-2a as adjuvant therapy in resected primary melanoma thicker than 1.5mm without clinically detectable node metastases. *Lancet* **351**:1905, 1998
96. Lens MB, Dawes M: Interferon alfa therapy for malignant melanoma: A systematic review of randomized controlled trials. *J Clin Oncol* **20**:1818, 2002
97. Balch CM et al: Cutaneous melanoma, in *Cancer Principles and Practice of Oncology,* 5th ed, edited by VT Devita, S Hellman, SA Rosenberg. Philadelphia, Lippincott Raven, 1997, p 1947
98. Biasco G et al: Treatment of brain metastases of malignant melanoma with temozolomide. *N Engl J Med* **345**:621, 2001
99. Crosby T et al: Systemic treatments for metastatic cutaneous melanoma (Cochrane Review). The Cochrane Library 1, 2002. Oxford: Update Software.
100. McClay MC, McClay MT: Systemic chemotherapy for the treatment of metastatic melanoma. *Semin Oncol* **23**:744, 1996
101. Rusthoven J et al: Randomized, double-blind, placebo-controlled trials comparing the response rates of carmustine, dacarbazine, and cisplatinum with and without tamoxifen in patients with metastatic melanoma. *J Clin Oncol* **14**:2083, 1996
102. Buzaid AC et al: Systemic chemotherapy and biochemotherapy, in *Cutaneous Melanoma,* 3d ed, edited by CM Balch, AN Houghton, AJ Sober, SJ Soong. St Louis, Quality Medical Publishing, 1998, p 405
103. Rosenberg SA et al: Treatment of 283 consecutive patients with metastatic melanoma or renal cell cancer using high dose bolus interleukin-2. *JAMA* **271**:907, 1994
104. Rosenberg SA et al: A progress report on the treatment of 157 patients with advanced cancer using lymphokine-activated killer cells and interleukin-2 or high-dose interleukin-2 alone. *N Engl J Med* **316**:889, 1987
105. Chapman PB et al: Biologic therapy, in *Cutaneous Melanoma,* 3d ed, edited by CM Balch, AN Houghton, AJ Sober, SJ Soong. St Louis, Quality Medical Publishing, 1998, p 419
106. Leong SP: Immunotherapy of malignant melanoma. *Surg Clin North Am* **76**:1355, 1996
107. Fearon ER et al: Interleukin-2 production by tumor cells bypasses T helper function in the generation of an antitumor response. *Cell* **60**:397, 1990
108. Livingston P, Sznol M: Vaccine therapy, in *Cutaneous Melanoma,* 3d ed, edited by CM Balch, AN Houghton, AJ Sober, SJ Soong. St Louis, Quality Medical Publishing, 1998, p 437
109. Schreiber S et al: Immunotherapy of metastatic malignant melanoma by a vaccine consisting of autologous IL-2 transfected cancer cells-outcome of a phase I study. *Proc Nat Acad Sci, USA* **10**:983, 1999
110. Nestle FO et al: Vaccination of melanoma patients with peptide- or tumor lysate-pulsed dendritic cells. *Nat Med* **4**:328, 1998
111. McCarthy WH et al: Time and frequency of recurrence of cutaneous stage I malignant melanoma with guidelines for follow-up study. *Surg Gynecol Obstet* **166**:497, 1988

SECTION 13

INFLAMMATORY AND NEOPLASTIC DISORDERS OF THE DERMIS

CHAPTER 94

Herbert Hönigsmann
Philip R. Cohen
Klaus Wolff

Acute Febrile Neutrophilic Dermatosis (Sweet's Syndrome)

In 1964, Robert Douglas Sweet[1] described eight women who had a distinct, previously unrecognized condition that he termed *acute febrile neutrophilic dermatosis.* This dramatic skin disease is characterized by recurrent painful plaque-forming inflammatory papules or nodules, fever, peripheral leukocytosis, a diffuse dermal neutrophilic infiltrate, and prompt resolution of symptoms and lesions with glucocorticoid therapy. Since Sweet's original paper, several hundred cases of Sweet's syndrome have been reported.[2,3]

INCIDENCE

Sweet's syndrome has a worldwide distribution and no racial predilection.[2,3] The disease presents in three clinical settings (Table 94-1): (1) classic or idiopathic Sweet's syndrome, which may be associated with infection (upper respiratory tract or gastrointestinal tract), inflammatory bowel disease, or pregnancy, (2) malignancy-associated or paraneoplastic Sweet's syndrome, in which the onset and/or recurrence of the dermatosis is temporally associated with the presence of cancer, and (3) drug-induced Sweet's syndrome, which occurs most frequently in patients who are receiving granulocyte colony-stimulating factor (G-CSF) but also may develop during treatment with antibiotics, antiepileptic drugs, antihypertensive agents, oral contraceptives, or retinoids.[4,5]

Idiopathic and drug-induced Sweet's syndrome predominantly affects women. Patients typically range between 30 and 50 years of age, but younger adults and children may be affected.[6,7] The youngest patient recognized was a 7-week-old infant.[6] Malignancy-associated Sweet's syndrome does not have a female predominance (see Table 94-1). In this setting, the dermatosis is usually associated with a hematologic malignancy—most commonly acute myelogenous leukemia.[8] Carcinomas of the genitourinary organs, breast, and gastrointestinal tract are the most frequently occurring cancers in Sweet's syndrome patients with solid tumors.[9] Medications that have been implicated in causing drug-induced Sweet's syndrome are listed in Table 94-2.[5,10]

ETIOLOGY

There is no known cause of Sweet's syndrome. Fever and peripheral leukocytosis suggest a septic process, but antibiotics usually do not influence the course of disease. Although there is no conclusive evidence that a bacterial infection has a causative role, most patients have a febrile upper respiratory tract infection, tonsillitis, or influenza-like illness that precedes their skin lesions by 1 to 3 weeks. Sweet's syndrome reportedly improved with systemic antibiotics in patients who had culture- and serology-confirmed intestinal infection with *Yersinia enterolitica.*[11,12] A case of exclusively photoinduced Sweet's syndrome has been reported; in this patient, an eruption recurred 1 or 2 days after prolonged exposure to the sun every summer for 8 years.[13]

The clinical appearance, course, and histopathology indicate that Sweet's syndrome may represent a form of hypersensitivity reaction to a bacterial, viral, or perhaps tumor antigen.[14] Several characteristics of the skin lesions (clinical appearance, course, and histopathology) support this hypothesis. Also consistent with this concept is the favorable response of the symptoms and lesions to systemic glucocorticoids.

Massive tissue leukocytosis strongly implies a pathogenic role for leukotactic mechanisms.[14] However, contradictory findings have been reported on leukocyte function and their response to chemotactic stimuli.[3,4,15,16] Complement does not appear to be essential to the disease process. Some investigators postulate that dermal dendrocytes may have a prominent role in the pathogenesis of Sweet's syndrome.[17]

A possible role for circulating autoantibodies,[4,18] immune complexes,[8] or cytokines[19,20] has been postulated. Although an increased frequency of HLA-BW54 has been described in Japanese patients with Sweet's syndrome, a subsequent study was unable to demonstrate a significant association between Sweet's syndrome and certain HLA-ABC antigens in Caucasians.[21,22] Antibodies to neutrophilic cytoplasmic antigens (ANCAs) have been observed in some patients,[23] but they likely represent an epiphenomenon.[2,3]

Cytokines that possibly may cause the symptoms and lesions of this disease include G-CSF, granulocyte-macrophage colony-stimulating factor (GM-CSF), interferon-γ (IFN-γ), interleukin 1 (IL-1), IL-3, IL-6, IL-8.[5,19,24–26] GM-CSF was detected in the intraarticular synovial and fluid of an 8-month-old boy with Sweet's syndrome–associated

TABLE 94-1

Clinical Features in Patients with Sweet's Syndrome

	Clinical Form			
Characteristic	Idiopathic[a]	Hematologic Malignancy[a]	Solid Tumor[a]	Drug-Induced[b]
Epidemiology				
Women	80	50	59	71
Prior upper respiratory tract infection	75–90	16	20	21
Recurrence[c]	30	69	41	67
Clinical symptoms				
Fever[d]	80–90	88	79	100
Musculoskeletal involvement	12–56	26	34	21
Ocular involvement	17–72	7	15	21
Lesion location				
Upper extremities	80	89	97	71
Head and neck	50	63	52	43
Trunk and back	30	42	33	50
Lower extremities	Infrequent	49	48	36
Oral mucous membranes	2	12	3	7
Laboratory findings				
Neutrophilia[e]	80	47	60	38
Elevated erythrocyte sedimentation rate[f]	90	100	95	100
Anemia[g]	Infrequent	82	83	100
Abnormal platelet count[h]	Infrequent	68	50	50
Abnormal renal function[i]	11–50	15	7	0

[a] Percentages for idiopathic, hematologic malignancy, and solid tumor–associated Sweet's syndrome.
SOURCE: Adapted from Cohen and Kurzrock[4] with permission.
[b] Percentages for drug-induced Sweet's syndrome.
SOURCE: Adapted from Walker and Cohen[5] with permission.
[c] Recurrence after oral rechallenge testing in patients with drug-induced Sweet's syndrome.
[d] Temperature greater than 38°C.
[e] Neutrophil count greater than 6000 cells/μL.
[f] Erythrocyte sedimentation rate greater than 20 mm/h.
[g] Hemoglobin less than 13 g/dL in men and less than 12 g/dL in women.
[h] Platelet count less than 150,000/μL or greater than 500,000/μL.
[i] Includes hematuria, proteinuria, and renal insufficiency.

acute arthritis.[27] In a patient with myelodysplastic syndrome–associated, non-G-CSF-induced Sweet's syndrome, the levels of G-CSF and IL-6 were elevated.[26]

In a recent study, the patients' serum levels of IL-1α, IL-1β, IL-2, and IFN-γ were significantly elevated, whereas the IL-4 level was within the normal range. It was suggested therefore that the pathogenesis of Sweet's syndrome may be mediated through helper T cell type 1 cytokines (IL-2, IFN-γ) rather than helper T cell type 2 cytokines (IL-4).[28]

TABLE 94-2

Medications Associated with Drug-Induced Sweet's Syndrome*

- Antibiotics
  - Minocycline
  - Nitrofurantoin
  - Trimethoprim-sulfamethoxazole
- Antiepileptics
  - Carbamazepine
- Antihypertensives
  - Hydralazine
- Cytokines
  - Granulocyte colony-stimulating factor
- Oral contraceptives
  - Levonorgestrel-ethinyestradiol
- Retinoids
  - All-*trans*-retinoic acid

*For references, see Cohen and Kurzrock.[10]

CLINICAL FEATURES

The typical skin lesions are red or bluish red papules or nodules that show a strong tendency to coalesce and to form irregular, sharply bordered plaques (Fig. 94-1*A*). Such lesions have been compared with a "relief of a mountain range"[12] (see Fig. 94-1*B*). The pronounced inflammatory edema is often responsible for a transparent vesicular appearance of the lesions, although they are solid on palpation[14] (Fig. 94-2). This phenomenon has been described as an "illusion of vesiculation."[1] In later stages, the tops of the papules occasionally may become studded with tiny pustules, and central clearing may lead to annular or arcuate patterns. The lesions are tender and often painful, tend to enlarge over a period of days or weeks, and resolve eventually without scarring after weeks or months. The eruption may present with a single lesion or multiple lesions, characteristically in an asymmetric distribution (Fig. 94-3). Most commonly, the upper extremities, face, and neck are involved, but lesions also develop on the trunk and lower limbs (see Table 94-1); leg lesions can mimic a panniculitis such as erythema nodosum. Widespread or even generalized forms have been reported (see Fig. 94-2), particularly in the malignancy-associated form, which generally exhibits more severe symptoms of the disease. Involvement of the oral mucosa is uncommon in the idiopathic form; however, it does occur—particularly in patients with hematologic disorders[8] (see Table 94-1). Skin hypersensitivity (cutaneous pathergy) may be present; lesions have occurred at the sites of stimuli such as biopsies, cat scratches, insect bites, intravenous catheter placement sites, and venipuncture sites.[2,3,8] About half of patients experience recurrences, often at previously involved sites.

FIGURE 94-1

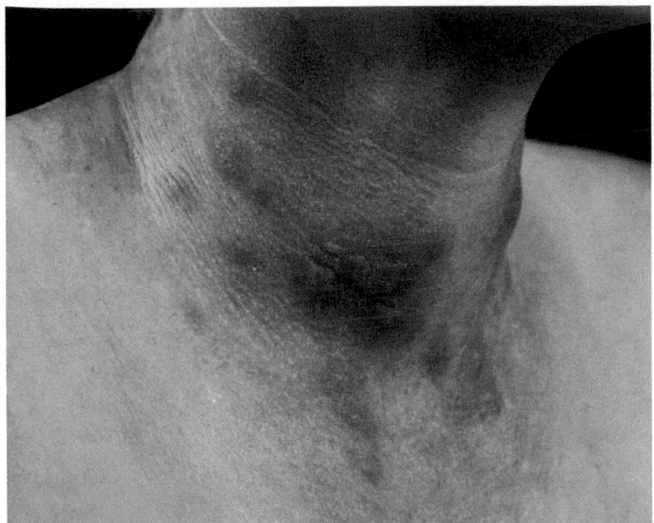

A.

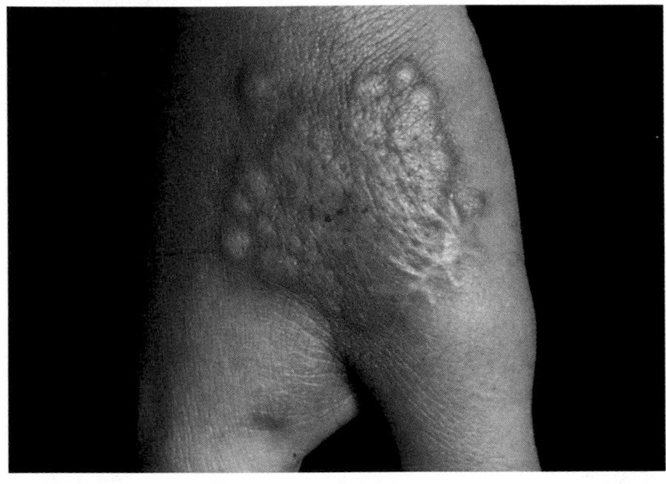

B.

Acute febrile neutrophilic dermatosis. Typical lesions consisting of coalescing, plaque-forming papules. *A.* Bright-red lesions on the neck. *B.* Lesion on the dorsum of the right hand exhibiting the "relief of a mountain range" feature. (*From Hönigsmann and Wolff*[14] *with permission.*)

The systemic symptoms that accompany the skin eruption are fever and leukocytosis, and patients often appear dramatically ill. However, not all patients with Sweet's syndrome express the whole spectrum of symptoms,[4] and fever, neutrophilia, or both may be absent[4,14] (see Table 94-1). A period of fever may precede the skin disease by several days or weeks and may be present throughout the entire course. Additional symptoms that may occur to varying degrees are headache, arthralgia, myalgia, and general malaise. Ocular manifestations such as conjunctivitis and episcleritis may be present; less commonly, conjunctival hemorrhage, glaucoma, iritis, limbal nodules, and ocular congestion have been observed.[2,3,8,29,30]

Extracutaneous manifestations may affect the bone, central nervous system, gastrointestinal tract, kidney, liver, and lung. Dermatosis-related sterile osteomyelitis has been described in children.[2] Neurologic involvement has presented with aseptic meningitis, neurologic and psychiatric symptoms, and neutrophils in the cerebrospinal fluid.[6,31,32] Renal involvement manifests most commonly as proteinuria, less often as hematuria and mesangiocapillary glomerulonephritis.[8,33] Hepatic involvement was shown by liver biopsy, which revealed infiltration of the portal triad and tracts[8,33]; hepatic enzyme abnormalities have been observed in other patients.[2,3] Pulmonary features of Sweet's syndrome were glucocorticoid-responsive, culture-negative infiltrates on chest x-rays and/or neutrophilic infiltrates on open lung biopsies.[3,34]

FIGURE 94-2

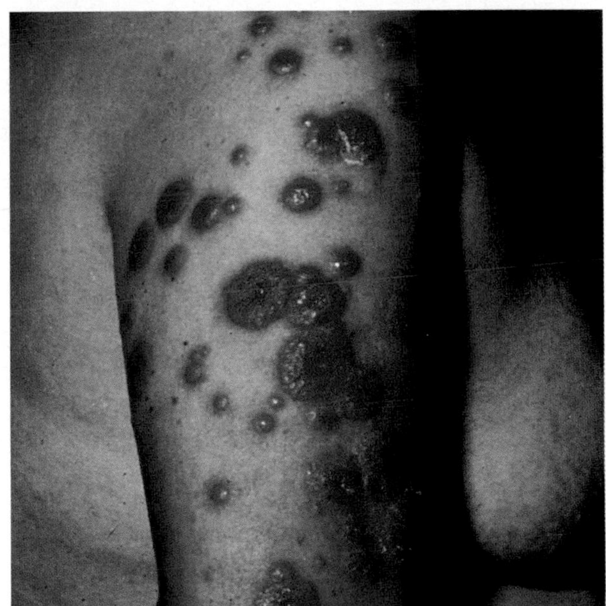

Multiple confluent papules and plaques that at first sight give the illusion of vesiculation but are solid on palpation. (*From Hönigsmann et al: Akute febrile neutrophile Dermatose. Wien Klin Wochenschr 91:842, 1979, with permission.*)

FIGURE 94-3

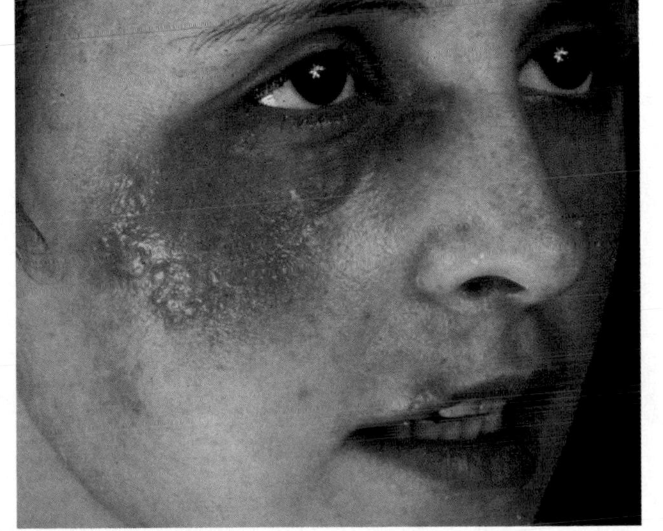

Unilateral lesions around the eye and upper lip consisting of plaques and pseudovesicular papules suggesting herpes simplex.

LABORATORY FINDINGS

An elevated erythrocyte sedimentation rate and peripheral leukocytosis with neutrophilia are the most consistent laboratory findings (see Table 94-1). White blood cell counts range from 10,000 to 20,000/mm^3. However, not all patients with biopsy-confirmed Sweet's syndrome exhibit leukocytosis.[8] In patients with malignancy-associated Sweet's syndrome, anemia, a normal or low neutrophil count, and an abnormal platelet count may be present.[4] Proteinuria occurs in patients with renal involvement.

PATHOLOGY

The most prominent histopathologic features are edema of the dermal papillae and a dense infiltrate of mature leukocytes in the dermis (Fig. 94-4). In some patients with hematologic malignancy–associated Sweet's syndrome, concurrent leukemia cutis has been demonstrated in the lesion.[35] The infiltrate is usually diffuse, with occasional eosinophils and lymphocytes. Fragmented neutrophil nuclei (leukocytoclasia or karyorrhexis) are quite common and, at low magnification, may suggest vasculitis (Fig. 94-5). In some lesions of Sweet's syndrome, secondary vasculitis (occurring as an epiphenomenon in which the affected vessel is most frequently an "innocent bystander" within moderate to extensive, diffuse or bandlike dermal inflammation) has been observed.[36,37] Usually, the epidermis is normal. Spongiosis and exocytosis have been reported, and rarely there may be a subcorneal pustule. In deep-seated nodular lesions, the neutrophilic infiltrates may be confined to the subcutaneous tissue (in the lobules, the septa, or both) or localized within both the dermis and the subcutaneous fat.[14,35,37]

FIGURE 94-4

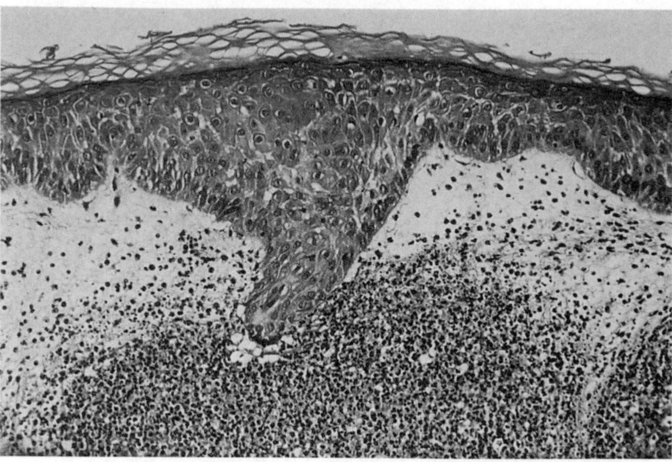

Histopathologic presentation of massive edema of the papillary dermis and a dense diffuse infiltrate of mature neutrophils throughout the upper dermis (hematoxylin and eosin stain). (*From Cohen et al.*[9] *with permission.*)

Electron microscopy does not reveal endothelial cell damage but rather signs of metabolic activation, as indicated by the abundance of endoplasmic reticulum, mitochondria, and multiple Golgi areas in the endothelial cells.[14] The vessels are separated from the cellular infiltrate by a relatively broad electron-lucent zone occupied by multiple concentrically arranged basal laminae and a finely fibrillar and vesicular material consisting of plasma constituents and cell debris, which also may be found in the vascular lumen. Such findings are consistent with endothelial repair and regeneration after endothelial damage.

FIGURE 94-5

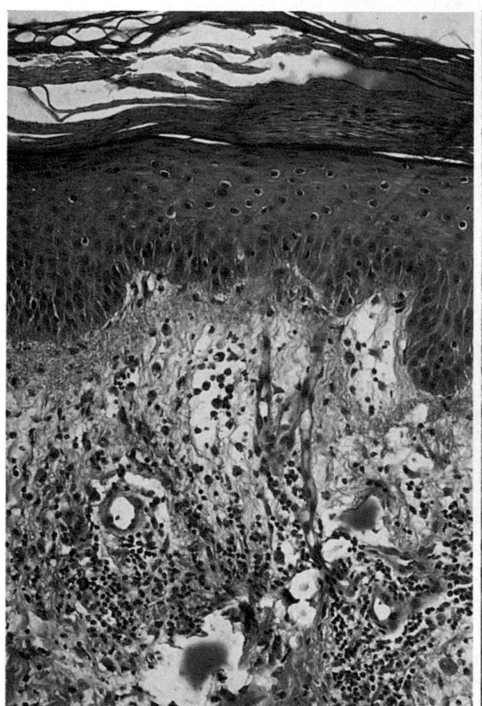

A.

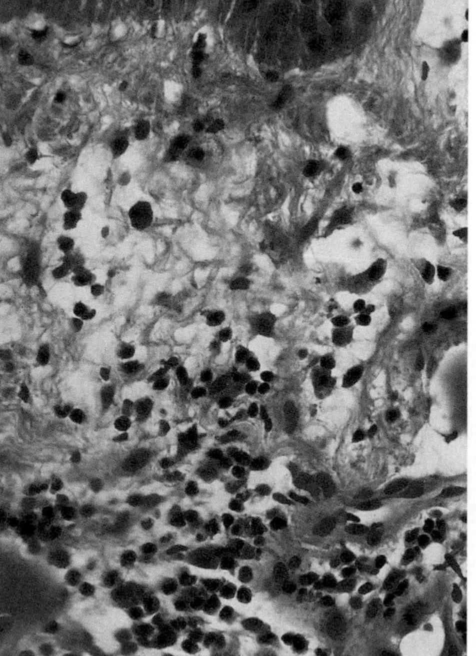

B.

Characteristic histopathologic features of Sweet's syndrome are observed at low (*A*) and high (*B*) magnification: papillary dermal edema, swollen endothelial cells, and a diffuse infiltrate of predominantly neutrophils with leukocytoclasia, yet no evidence of vasculitis (hematoxylin and eosin stain). (*From Cohen et al.*[24] *with permission.*)

IMMUNOFLUORESCENCE

Direct immunofluorescence of lesional skin is noncontributory. Deposits of IgG, IgM, C3, and fibrin are diffusely distributed in a perivascular arrangement, but this distribution may represent only a nonspecific inflammatory exudate.[28,36]

ASSOCIATED DISEASES

Various other conditions have been observed in patients with Sweet's syndrome (Table 94-3). Some of them appear to have a possible etiologic role in the pathogenesis of Sweet's syndrome,[2–5,12,38,39] but others are likely to be coincidental.[10]

TABLE 94-3

Sweet's Syndrome and Associated Conditions

Probably bona fide associated conditions
- Cancer: hematologic malignancies (most commonly acute myelogenous leukemia) and solid tumors (most commonly carcinomas of the genitourinary organs, breast, and gastrointestinal tract)
- Infections: most commonly of the upper respiratory tract (streptococcosis) and the gastrointestinal tract (yersiniosis)
- Inflammatory bowel disease: Crohn's disease and ulcerative colitis
- Medications: most commonly granulocyte colony-stimulating factor
- Pregnancy

Possibly bona fide associated conditions
- Behçet's disease
- Erythema nodosum
- Rheumatoid arthritis
- Sarcoidosis
- Thyroid disease: Grave's disease and Hashimoto's thyroiditis

Validity of associated conditions remains to be established
- Autoimmune disorders: dermatomyositis, lupus erythematosus, relapsing polychondritis, Sjögren's syndrome
- Bronchiolitis obliterans and organizing pneumonia
- Chronic granulomatous disease
- Cirrhosis (cryptogenic)
- Common bile duct and intrahepatic duct stones
- Complement deficiency
- Congenital dyserythropoietic anemia
- Cutis laxa
- Dressler's syndrome (postmyocardial infarction syndrome)
- Fanconi's anemia
- Immunizing agent: BCG vaccination
- Infections: atypical mycobacteria, bartholinitis, chlamydia, cholecystitis, cytomegalovirus, hepatitis (chronic active), histoplasmosis, human immunodeficiency virus, leprosy, lymphadenitis (subacute necrotizing), otitis media, pancreatitis, pyelonephritis, salmonellosis, tonsillitis, toxoplasmosis, tuberculosis, ureaplasmosis, urinary tract, vulvovaginitis
- POEMS syndrome: polyneuropathy, organomegaly, endocrinopathy, M protein, and skin changes
- Psoriasis vulgaris
- Ureter obstruction
- Urticaria pigmentosa

TABLE 94-5

Clinical Differential Diagnosis of Sweet's Syndrome

Cutaneous conditions	Neoplastic conditions
Acral erythema	Chloroma
Drug eruptions	Leukemia cutis
Granuloma faciale	Lymphoma
Halogenoderma	Metastatic tumor
Infectious and inflammatory disorders	Reactive erythemas
Bacterial sepsis	Erythema multiforme
Cellulitis	Erythema nodosum
Erysipelas	Urticaria
Leprosy	Systemic diseases
Lymphangiitis	Behçet's disease
Panniculitis	Bowel bypass syndrome
Pyoderma gangrenosum	Dermatomyositis
Syphilis	Familial Mediterranean fever
Systemic mycosis	Lupus erythematosus
Thrombophlebitis	Vasculitis
Tuberculosis	Erythema elevatum diutinum
Viral exanthem	Leukocytoclastic vasculitis
	Periarteritis nodosa

SOURCE: From Cohen and Kurzrock[4] with permission.

More than 85 percent of patients with malignancies have a hematologic disorder, most commonly acute myeloid leukemia.[4,8,9] In most cases, the skin lesions either precede the diagnosis of leukemia (by up to several months or even years) or appear concurrently with the discovery of malignancy. Because recurrent episodes often herald cancer recurrence, periodic hematologic follow-up of patients with Sweet's syndrome is recommended.[4]

DIAGNOSIS AND DIFFERENTIAL DIAGNOSIS

Diagnostic criteria for classic (idiopathic and malignancy-associated) and drug-induced Sweet's syndrome are summarized in Table 94-4.[2,5] The clinical differential diagnosis of Sweet's syndrome is listed in Table 94-5.[2,8,9] Conditions characterized microscopically by neutrophilic dermatosis are in the histologic differential diagnosis of Sweet's syndrome (Table 94-6).[37,39,40]

TABLE 94-4

Diagnostic Criteria for Classic Sweet's Syndrome versus Drug-Induced Sweet's Syndrome

Classic*	Drug-Induced†
1. Abrupt onset of painful erythematous plaques or nodules	A. Abrupt onset of painful erythematous plaques or nodules
2. Histopathologic evidence of a dense neutrophilic infiltrate without evidence of leukocytoclastic vasculitis	B. Histopathologic evidence of a dense neutrophilic infiltrate without evidence of leukocytoclastic vasculitis
3. Pyrexia >38°C (100.4°F)	C. Pyrexia >38°C (100.4°F)
4. Association with an underlying hematologic or visceral malignancy, inflammatory disease, or pregnancy, *or* preceded by an upper respiratory or gastrointestinal infection or vaccination	D. Temporal relationship between drug ingestion and clinical presentation, *or* temporally related recurrence after oral challenge
5. Excellent response to treatment with systemic glucocorticoids or potassium iodide	E. Temporally-related resolution of lesions after drug withdrawal
6. Abnormal laboratory values at presentation (three of four): erythrocyte sedimentation rate >20 mm/h; positive C-reactive protein; >8,000 leukocytes; >70% neutrophils	

*The presence of both major criteria (1 and 2) and two of the four minor criteria (3, 4, 5, and 6) is required to establish the diagnosis of classic Sweet's syndrome.
†All five criteria (A, B, C, D, and E) are required for the diagnosis of drug-induced Sweet's syndrome.
SOURCE: Adapted from Walker and Cohen[5] with permission.

TABLE 94-6

Histologic Differential Diagnosis of Sweet's Syndrome

DIAGNOSIS	COMMENT
Abscess/cellulitis	Positive culture for infectious agent
Bowel (intestinal) bypass syndrome	History of jejunal-ileal bypass surgery for morbid obesity
Erythema elevatum diutinum	Erythematous asymptomatic plaques often located on the dorsal hands and elbows; younger lesions have microscopic features of leukocytoclastic vasculitis, whereas older lesions have dermal fibrosis and mucin
Granuloma faciale	Yellow to red to brown indurated asymptomatic facial plaques; there is a grenz zone of normal papillary dermis beneath which there is a dense diffuse inflammatory infiltrate of predominantly neutrophils (with microscopic features of leukocytoclastic vasculitis) and numerous eosinophils
Halogenoderma	Neutrophilic dermal infiltrate with necrosis and pseudoepitheliomatous hyperplasia with intraepidermal abscesses; history of ingestion of bromides (leg lesions), iodides (facial lesions), or topical fluoride gel to teeth during tumor radiation therapy to face
Leukemia cutis	Dermal infiltrate consists of immature neutrophils
Leukocytoclastic vasculitis	Vessel wall destruction: extravasated erythrocytes, fibrinoid necrosis of vessel walls, karyorrhexis, and neutrophils in the vessel wall
Neutrophilic eccrine hidradenitis	Neutrophils around eccrine glands, often in patients with acute myelogenous leukemia receiving induction chemotherapy
Pyoderma gangrenosum	Ulcer with overhanging, undermined violaceous edges
Rheumatoid neutrophilic dermatitis	History of rheumatoid arthritis, nodules, and plaques
Sweet's syndrome	Acute onset, fever, neutrophilia, and painful plaques

SOURCE: Adapted from Cohen[40] with permission.

Early Sweet's syndrome clinically may resemble erythema multiforme, but the asymmetric distribution pattern, the usual absence of oral and genital mucosal involvement, the pronounced tenderness of the lesions, the absence of target-like lesions, and the typical histopathology permit the correct diagnosis.

The differential diagnosis of deep-seated lesions also includes erythema nodosum, which can present either concurrently or sequentially in patients with Sweet's syndrome.[24] Solitary lesions of Sweet's syndrome clinically may mimic herpes simplex because of their peculiar transparent, pseudovesicular appearance, but palpation will reveal their solid consistency. Although pyoderma gangrenosum should not give rise to confusion because of its characteristic ulceration, the lesions may be difficult to differentiate clinically in patients with Sweet's syndrome with hematologic malignancies.

TREATMENT

Although the symptoms, fever, and leukocytosis suggest a septic process, the dermatosis usually persists after treatment with antibiotics. Systemic therapy directed toward *Staphylococcus aureus* may result in slight improvement of skin lesions that have become impetiginized secondarily. There are isolated reports of Sweet's syndrome that resolved after treatment with metronidazole in patients with Crohn's disease[41] and after treatment with doxycycline,[11,42] minocycline,[12] or tetracycline[43] in patients with or without an associated *Yersinia* infection.

Prompt relief of cutaneous and systemic symptoms is obtained with systemic prednisone in doses of 30 to 60 mg daily; the dose is tapered to 10 mg within 4 to 6 weeks. In some patients, prolonged treatment with lower doses (10–30 mg on alternate days) for 2 or 3 months may be necessary to suppress recurrences. Localized lesions also respond to either high-potency topical glucocorticoids (0.05% clobetasol propionate) or intralesional glucocorticoids (starting at a dose of approximately 3.0 mg/mL of triamcinolone acetonide).[3,9,44]

A dramatic response to oral potassium iodide (900 mg daily for 2 weeks) was reported in 1980[45] and was confirmed subsequently.[9,46] If potassium iodide tablets are unavailable, an oral saturated solution of potassium iodide (SSKI or Lugol's solution) can be used with either increasing doses [3 drops (in juice) three times each day and increased by 1 drop per day up to a final dose of 10 drops three times each day[14]] or a high dose initially (20 or 30 drops three times each day[39]). Potential drug-induced side effects of potassium iodide include vasculitis and hypothyroidism.[2,47]

Oral colchicine (1.5 mg daily for 7 days with gradual reduction to 0.5 mg daily over 3 weeks) also has been shown to induce rapid regression of Sweet's syndrome.[15,48] However, a common drug-limiting side effect is diarrhea.[39] Other agents,[49] used alone or in combination with glucocorticoids, have been reported (predominantly in case reports) to be effective in the treatment of Sweet's syndrome, including chlorambucil,[50] clofazimine,[2] cyclophosphamide,[51] cyclosporine,[2,52,53] dapsone,[3,16] indomethacin,[54] interferon-α,[44] naproxen,[55] and sulfapyridine.[3]

COURSE AND PROGNOSIS

Acute febrile neutrophilic dermatosis is a benign condition, but it may be the sign of malignancy, especially a hematologic disorder. Without treatment, the eruption may persist for weeks or even months and then involute without leaving scars. Recurrences occur at various intervals after therapy-induced or spontaneous remission in approximately 30 percent of patients and somewhat more frequently in patients with cancer. In the latter group, a recurrence may be the presenting manifestation of recurrent malignancy.

REFERENCES

1. Sweet RD: An acute febrile neutrophilic dermatosis. *Br J Dermatol* **76**:349, 1964
2. von den Driesch: Sweet's syndrome (acute febrile neutrophilic dermatosis). *J Am Acad Dermatol* **31**:535, 1994
3. Fett DL et al: Sweet's syndrome: Systemic signs and symptoms and associated disorders. *Mayo Clin Proc* **70**:234, 1995
4. Cohen PR, Kurzrock R: Sweet's syndrome and cancer. *Clin Dermatol* **11**:149, 1993

5. Walker DC, Cohen PR: Trimethoprim-sulfamethoxazole–associated acute febrile neutrophilic dermatosis: Case report and review of drug-induced Sweet's syndrome. *J Am Acad Dermatol* **34**:918, 1996
6. Dunn TR et al: Sweet's syndrome in a neonate with aseptic meningitis. *Pediatr Dermatol* **9**:288, 1992
7. Boatman BW et al: Sweet's syndrome in children. *South Med J* **87**:193, 1994
8. Cohen PR et al: Malignancy-associated Sweet's syndrome: Review of the world literature. *J Clin Oncol* **6**:1887, 1988
9. Cohen PR et al: Sweet syndrome in patients with solid tumors. *Cancer* **72**:2723, 1993
10. Cohen PR, Kurzrock R: Sweet syndrome: A neutrophilic dermatosis classically associated with acute onset and fever. *Clin Dermatol* **18**:265, 2000
11. Escallier F et al: Sweet's syndrome and *Yersinia enterocolitica* infection. *Ann Dermatol Venereol* **117**:858, 1990
12. Neau D et al: Sweet syndrome and *Yersinia enterocolitica* infection. 2 cases. *Rev Med Interne* **16**:919, 1995
13. Bessis D et al: Photoinduced Sweet syndrome. *Arch Dermatol* **137**:1106, 2001
14. Hönigsmann H, Wolff K: Acute febrile neutrophilic dermatosis (Sweet's syndrome), in *Major Problems in Dermatology*, vol 10, *Vasculitis*, edited by K Wolff, RK Winkelmann, consulting editor A Rook. London, Lloyd-Luke, 1980, p 307
15. Suehisa S et al: Colchicine in the treatment of acute febrile neutrophilic dermatosis (Sweet's syndrome). *Br J Dermatol* **180**:99, 1983
16. Aram H: Acute febrile neutrophilic dermatosis (Sweet's syndrome): Response to dapsone. *Arch Dermatol* **120**:245, 1984
17. Misery L et al: Are neutrophilic dermatoses during granulocytopenia really neutrophilic? (letter). *Arch Dermatol* **132**:832, 1996
18. von den Driesch P, Weber MFA: Are antibodies to neutrophilic cytoplasmic antigens (ANCA) a serologic marker for Sweet's syndrome? (letter). *J Am Acad Dermatol* **29**:666, 1993
19. Cohen PR, Kurzrock R: The pathogenesis of Sweet's syndrome (letter). *J Am Acad Dermatol* **25**:734, 1991
20. Eghrari-Sabet JS, Hartley AH: Sweet's syndrome: An immunologically mediated skin disease? *Ann Allergy* **72**:125, 1994
21. von den Driesch P et al: Analysis of HLA antigens in Caucasian patients with febrile neutrophilic dermatosis (Sweet's syndrome). *J Am Acad Dermatol* **37**:276, 1997
22. Mizoguchi M et al: Human leukocyte antigen in Sweet's syndrome and its relationship to Behçet's syndrome. *Arch Dermatol* **124**:1069, 1988
23. Kemmett D et al: Antibodies to neutrophil cytoplasmic antigens: A serologic marker for Sweet's syndrome. *J Am Acad Dermatol* **24**:967, 1991
24. Cohen PR et al: Concurrent Sweet's syndrome and erythema nodosum: A report, world literature review and mechanism of pathogenesis. *J Rheumatol* **19**:814, 1992
25. Reuss-Borst MA et al: The possible role of G-CSF in the pathogenesis of Sweet's syndrome. *Leukemia Lymphoma* **15**:261, 1994
26. Reuss-Borst MA et al: Sweet's syndrome associated with myelodysplasia: Possible role of cytokines in the pathogenesis of the disease. *Br J Haematol* **84**:356, 1993
27. Tuerlinckx D et al: Sweet's syndrome with arthritis in an 8-month-old boy. *J Rheumatol* **26**:440, 1999
28. Giasuddin AS et al: Sweet's syndrome: Is the pathogenesis mediated by helper T cell type 1 cytokines? *J Am Acad Dermatol* **39**:940, 1998
29. Davies R: Limbal nodules in Sweet's syndrome. *Aust NZ J Ophthalmol* **20**:263, 1992
30. Cohen PR: Sweet's syndrome presenting as conjunctivitis. *Arch Ophthalmol* **111**:587, 1993
31. Furukawa F et al: Neutrophils in cerebrospinal fluid of a patient with acute febrile neutrophilic dermatosis (Sweet's syndrome) (letter). *Int J Dermatol* **31**:670, 1992
32. Chiba S: Sweet's syndrome with neurologic signs and psychiatric symptoms (letter). *Arch Neurol* **40**:829, 1983
33. Matta M, Kurban AK: Sweet's syndrome: Systemic association. *Cutis* **12**:561, 1973
34. Cohen PR, Kurzrock R: Extracutaneous manifestations of Sweet's syndrome: Steroid-responsive culture-negative pulmonary lesions (letter). *Am Rev Respir Dis* **146**:269, 1992
35. Cohen PR: Skin lesions of Sweet's syndrome and its dorsal hand variant contain vasculitis: An oxymoron or an epiphenomenon? (editorial). *Arch Dermatol* **138**:400, 2002
36. Cohen PR: Subcutaneous Sweet's syndrome: A variant of acute neutrophilic dermatosis that is included in the histopathologic differential diagnosis of neutrophilic lobular panniculitis (letter). *J Am Acad Dermatol* (in press)
37. Jordaan HF: Acute febrile neutrophilic dermatosis: A histopathological study of 37 patients and a review of the literature. *Am J Dermatopathol* **11**:99, 1989
38. Cohen PR: Pregnancy-associated Sweet's syndrome: World literature review. *Obstet Gynecol Surv* **48**:584, 1993
39. Su WPD et al: Sweet syndrome: Acute febrile neutrophilic dermatosis. *Semin Dermatol* **14**:173, 1995
40. Cohen PR: Paraneoplastic dermatopathology: Cutaneous paraneoplastic syndromes. *Adv Dermatol* **11**:215, 1995
41. Rappaport A et al: Sweet's syndrome in association with Crohn's disease: Report of a case and review of the literature. *Dis Colon Rectum* **44**:1526, 2001
42. Joshi RK et al: Successful treatment of Sweet's syndrome with doxycycline. *Br J Dermatol* **128**:584, 1993
43. Purdy MJ, Fairbrother GE: Case reports: Acute febrile neutrophilic dermatosis of Sweet. *Australas J Dermatol* **12**:172, 1971
44. Brodkin RH, Schwartz RA: Sweet's syndrome with myelofibrosis and leukemia: Partial response to interferon. *Dermatology* **190**:160, 1995
45. Horio T et al: Treatment of acute febrile neutrophilic dermatosis (Sweet's syndrome) with potassium iodide. *Dermatologica* **160**:341, 1980
46. Myatt AE et al: Sweet's syndrome: A report on the use of potassium iodide. *Clin Exp Dermatol* **12**:345, 1987
47. Cohen PR, Kurzrock R: Treatment of Sweet's syndrome (letter). *Am J Med* **89**:396, 1990
48. Maillard H et al: Colchicine for Sweet's syndrome: A study of 20 cases (letter). *Br J Dermatol* **140**:565, 1999
49. Cohen PR, Kurzrock R: Sweet's syndrome: A review of current treatment options. *Am J Clin Dermatol* **3**:117, 2002
50. Case JD et al: The use of pulse methylprednisolone and chlorambucil in the treatment of Sweet's syndrome. *Cutis* **44**:125, 1989
51. Feliu E et al: Neutrophilic pustulosis associated with chronic myeloid leukemia: A special form of Sweet's syndrome. Report of two cases. *Acta Haematol* **88**:154, 1992
52. Sharpe GR, Leggat HM: A case of Sweet's syndrome and myelodysplasia: Response to cyclosporin. *Br J Dermatol* **127**:538, 1992
53. von den Driesch P et al: Sweet's syndrome: Therapy with cyclosporin. *Clin Exp Dermatol* **19**:274, 1994
54. Jeanfils S et al: Indomethacin treatment of eighteen patients with Sweet's syndrome. *J Am Acad Dermatol* **36**:436, 1997
55. Bello Lopez JL et al: Sweet's syndrome during the chronic phase of chronic myeloid leukemia. *Acta Haematol* **84**:207, 1990

CHAPTER 95

Stephen I. Katz

Erythema Elevatum Diutinum

Erythema elevatum diutinum is a rare, chronic skin disease that is characterized by red, purple, and yellowish papules, plaques, and nodules that are usually distributed acrally and symmetrically over extensor surfaces. It is characterized histologically by a leukocytoclastic vasculitis.

HISTORICAL ASPECTS

In 1894, Radcliffe-Crocker and Williams[1] described a 6-year-old patient with persistent pink and purple nodules over the hands, elbows, knees, and buttocks and reviewed the small number of clinically similar cases reported by Hutchinson[2] and Bury.[3] Inasmuch as the patients could be collectively characterized as having red, raised lesions with a strong tendency toward persistence of lesions rather than toward involution, they suggested the descriptive term *erythema elevatum diutinum.* In that report, Radcliffe-Crocker and Williams distinguished the Bury type of erythema elevatum diutinum, occurring in young females with a family history of gout or "rheumatism," from the Hutchinson type, occurring in elderly males with gout. Radcliffe-Crocker and Williams felt that the two types of erythema elevatum diutinum might be phases of one disease; however, any distinction between these two types has long been abandoned. Although for many years cases of erythema elevatum diutinum were confused with what was later described by Radcliffe-Crocker to be granuloma annulare,[4] these diseases can be clearly differentiated. In the 1930s, extracellular cholesterosis[5] was introduced as a new entity, but it cannot be distinguished from erythema elevatum diutinum[6] and should not be separated nosologically.

ETIOLOGY AND PATHOPHYSIOLOGY

Although the cause of erythema elevatum diutinum is unknown, the finding of C1q binding activity in the sera of some patients, the exacerbation of disease with spontaneous streptococcal infections or with streptokinase-streptodornase skin tests, the Arthus-like histology of all spontaneous and streptokinase-streptodornase-induced lesions, and the positive 4-h streptokinase-streptodornase skin test reactivity in many patients suggest an immune complex etiology.[7] It may be, as Jensen and Esquenazi[8] have proposed from animal studies, that chemoattraction occurs as a direct result of an immune reaction taking place between the chemotactic stimulus and the surface of the responding cell. In the case of erythema elevatum diutinum, the neutrophil surface would have to be coated with a substance that binds bacterial cell products (streptokinase-streptodornase or perhaps others), and the resultant immune complex reaction results in the movement of these neutrophils to the site of antigenic deposition. Others have reported an enhanced response in vitro of neutrophils from patients with erythema elevatum diutinum to interleukin (IL)-8 and increased random migration of neutrophils as well as marked integrin expression in the lesions themselves.[9]

CLINICAL FEATURES AND COURSE

Erythema elevatum diutinum most frequently appears in adults, but may occur at any age.[7] The lesions are multiple and often progress from papules to plaques or nodules. Coalescence of lesions may result in gyrate or irregular forms. The early lesions are often pink or yellowish and may later become red or purple. Early lesions are soft and may be tender, whereas older lesions may become doughy or hard.

The distribution of lesions is highly characteristic. They are usually distributed symmetrically on the extensor surfaces and have a striking predilection for the skin overlying joints, especially on the hands and knees (Figs. 95-1, 95-2, and 95-3). However, lesions may cover large areas of skin (Fig. 95-4). They also have a predilection for the buttocks (Fig. 95-4) and for the skin overlying the Achilles tendon. The face and ears may be affected, but the trunk is generally spared, as are the mucous membranes. Lesions may be round or oval, and their surface is usually smooth with the occasional presence of scale. They are usually freely movable from the underlying tissues. Petechiae or purpura

FIGURE 95-1

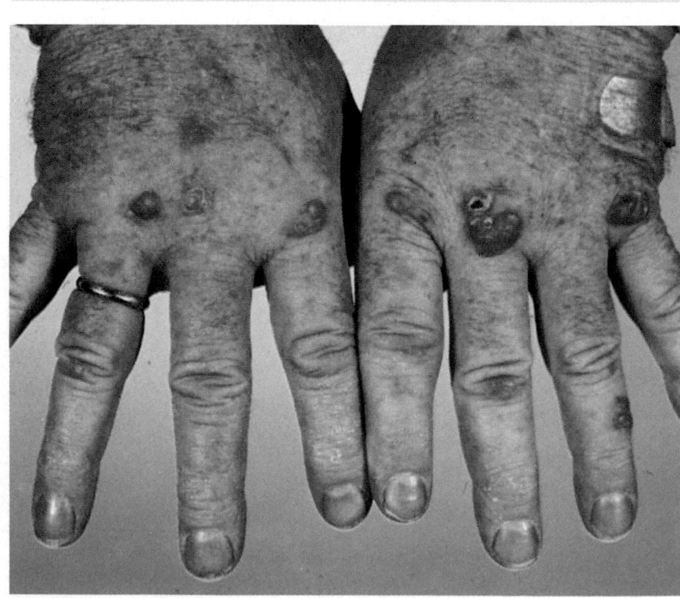

Erythema elevatum diutinum. Nodular lesions on dorsa of hands and on wrists. Each lesion had been present for several years.

FIGURE 95-2

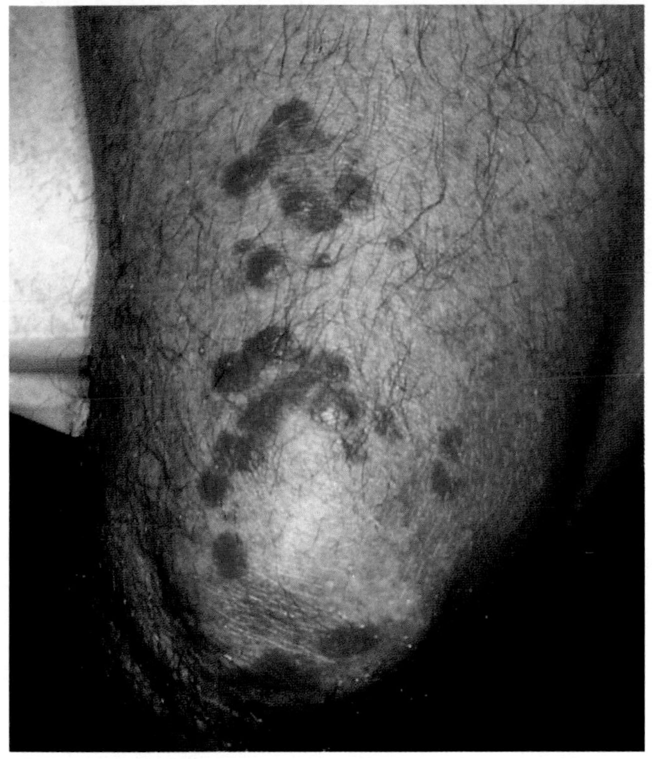

Erythema elevatum diutinum. Papular and nodular lesions on knee.

are sometimes seen in early lesions (especially after discontinuation of dapsone therapy). Bulla formation or hemorrhagic crusting with ulceration may also occur, especially in very edematous lesions. Some old nodules or plaques may become fibrotic and may resemble xanthomas. Occasionally, lesions involute spontaneously and often leave atrophic, wrinkled hyper- or hypopigmented areas with loss of underlying collagen.

FIGURE 95-3

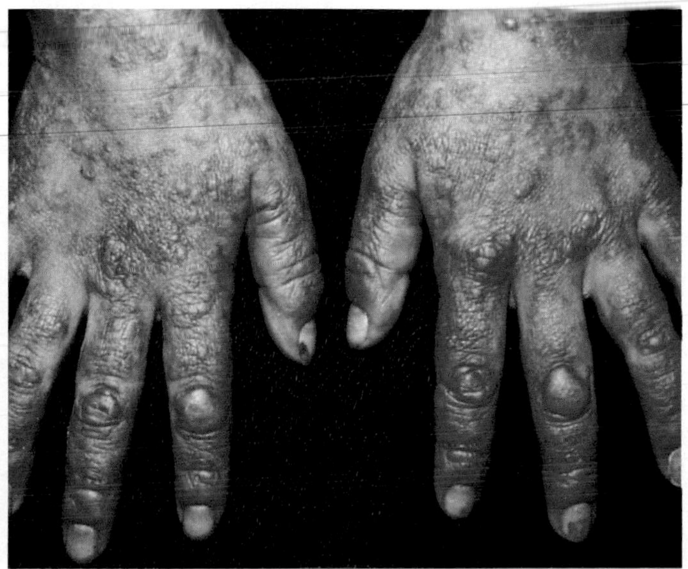

Erythema elevatum diutinum. Papules, nodules, and plaques on dorsa of hands.

FIGURE 95-4

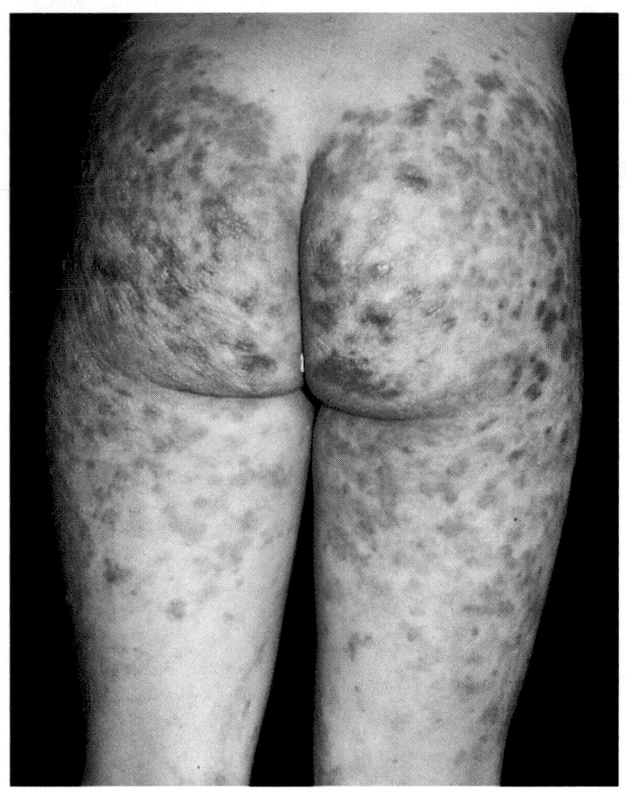

Erythema elevatum diutinum. Papules and nodules on buttocks and thighs.

Symptoms vary; lesions are totally asymptomatic in some and very painful in others. The lesions are sometimes characterized as aching or burning. Often there is an associated systemic abnormality, the most common of which is arthralgia of varying severity.[7] Some patients have had associated rheumatoid arthritis,[10] while others have had ulcerative keratitis.[11] Patients with a long history of recurrent pharyngeal and sinopulmonary infections, most commonly streptococcal, have been described.[7] Several patients have been reported as having associated inflammatory bowel disease with exacerbations in the skin disease at the time of flares in Crohn's disease.[12]

During the past several years, patients infected with HIV have been reported to have erythema elevatum diutinum or a close facsimile to it.[13] Whether lesions occur as a direct result of the virus or as a result of associated bacterial infections is unknown.

The course of the disease is highly variable; there are few well-documented instances of spontaneous long-term resolution. A follow-up study of five patients who were reported in 1977[7] revealed that four of them had disease that had persisted from 24 to 39 years. The fifth patient was lost to follow-up. One of these patients developed an IgA myeloma and another died because of lupus pericarditis. There are periods of waxing and waning; some patients have only one or two lesions or crops of new lesions every 2 to 3 weeks, and others have new lesions once every month or two. Streptococcal infections have been reported to exacerbate the disease.[7] Changes in temperature, and especially cold weather, have also been said to aggravate lesions or to be associated with the eruption of new lesions.

HISTOPATHOLOGY

Erythema elevatum diutinum was one of the first skin diseases designated to be a form of necrotizing vasculitis. Weidman and Besancon[14] felt that the vasculitis with prominent neutrophils along with the marked hyalinization of vessel walls were the outstanding features of this disease, which they clearly differentiated from granuloma annulare. Histologically, the lesions are highly characteristic and are easily differentiated from the other clinical considerations, but they may be difficult to differentiate from other types of leukocytoclastic vasculitis.[7,15] Most small, upper, and mid-dermal blood vessels show endothelial swelling as well as a significant number of neutrophils and their fragments in and around their walls (Fig. 95-5). Fibrinoid degeneration, referred to as toxic hyalin of the vessel walls, is usually present (see Fig. 95-5). An admixture of lymphocytes and a smaller number of eosinophils may be seen perivascularly. Neutrophils and their fragments are also commonly strewn throughout the upper and mid-dermis and may appear in large numbers between collagen bundles. There may be an unaffected zone of collagen just beneath the epidermis as in granuloma faciale. However, the epidermis may be affected as a result of the dermal infiltrate and edema and may show varying degrees of injury from slight acanthosis to frank necrosis. Older lesions may show a fibrotic replacement of the dermis accompanied by capillary proliferation. Even when the dermis appears to be totally replaced by these changes, there can be small foci of the leukocytoclastic vasculitis. In the older lesions, there may be varying amounts of extracellular cholesterol deposits, especially in lesions that have a yellowish xanthomatous appearance clinically. This particular histologic variant of erythema elevatum diutinum, formerly called *extracellular cholesterosis,*[5] is unassociated with disturbances of lipid metabolism. It probably occurs as a result of the heavily damaged tissue with extracellular and intracellular deposits consisting of cholesterol esters. Ultrastructural studies demonstrate that the lipid deposits are mainly intracellular.[16] None of the histologic findings cited is pathognomonic for erythema elevatum diutinum, although the constellation of histologic findings in both recently erupted and older lesions of erythema elevatum diutinum may serve to distinguish this entity from other forms of leukocytoclastic vasculitis. There are occasional solitary cutaneous lesions with histologic features resembling erythema elevatum diutinum in patients who have no other features of the disease.[17]

FIGURE 95-5

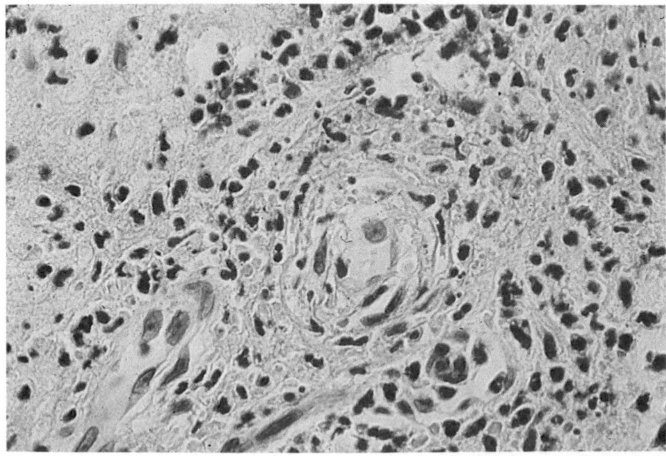

Erythema elevatum diutinum. High-power view showing endothelial swelling, fibrinoid necrosis of the vessel wall ("toxic hyalin"), and neutrophilic fragments in the vessel wall.

LABORATORY FINDINGS

Most patients have elevated erythrocyte sedimentation rates. In addition, in most patients tested, there are markedly positive 4- and 24-h skin test reactions to intradermally injected streptokinase-streptodornase, extracellularly elaborated products of Lancefield group C strains of streptococci.[7,18] Biopsy specimens obtained 4 or 6 h after the skin test show most of the histologic features of leukocytoclastic vasculitis. In addition to the markedly positive skin test reactions, many patients develop satellite lesions peripheral to the skin reactions. These lesions also show the histopathologic features of erythema elevatum diutinum.

Many patients who have IgA (mainly) or IgG or IgM monoclonal gammopathies, or even myeloma, have been reported.[7,19] Elevated levels of IgA in other patients with erythema elevatum diutinum,[7,19–22] and the rarity of both erythema elevatum diutinum and IgA monoclonal gammopathy would suggest that this association may be more than chance. In addition, C1q binding activity (indicative of IgG- or IgM-containing circulating immune complexes) has been identified in the sera of three of five patients.[7] Altered neutrophil chemotaxis has been detected in several patients.[7,9] IgA antineutrophilic antibodies have also been detected in a few patients.[23]

Direct immunofluorescence or immunoperoxidase studies of lesional skin of patients with erythema elevatum diutinum occasionally reveal immunoglobulin and complement deposition in and around blood vessels.[16,24]

DIFFERENTIAL DIAGNOSIS

Although for many years there was confusion between erythema elevatum diutinum and granuloma annulare, there is now little difficulty in differentiating the two clinically and histologically. Recurrent febrile neutrophilic dermatosis of Sweet, characterized by painful red plaques accompanied by fever and neutrophilic leukocytosis, can usually be distinguished from erythema elevatum diutinum by the distribution and character of lesions. Also, although Sweet's syndrome is characterized histologically by the presence of a dense neutrophilic infiltrate, which may be diffuse or, at times, perivascular, there is no leukocytoclastic vasculitis. Xanthomas can easily be distinguished histologically, as can multicentric reticulohistiocytosis. There is occasional difficulty in differentiating erythema elevatum diutinum from granuloma faciale histologically (not clinically); however, the latter lesion usually shows far less vascular involvement, more eosinophilia, and regular sparing of the overlying epidermis. Extracellular cholesterosis of Urbach[5] should be regarded as a variant of erythema elevatum diutinum. Other forms of leukocytoclastic vasculitis may be very difficult to distinguish from erythema elevatum diutinum, especially histologically; the distribution, character, and chronicity of individual lesions is highly suggestive of erythema elevatum diutinum.

TREATMENT

Case reports[18,20,22,25,26] and a study of a series of patients[7] indicate the regularity with which a dramatic response is obtained when patients with erythema elevatum diutinum are treated with dapsone or sulfapyridine. The prompt recurrence of skin lesions and systemic symptoms after sulfone withdrawal is evidence of the suppressive but not curative effect of sulfones in this disease. It seems that the disease exacerbations are more severe with each subsequent withdrawal of medication. A few prior case reports stated that dapsone was ineffective in treating erythema elevatum diutinum, perhaps because of extensive fibrosis in some patients. Dosage, however, varies considerably and is probably crucial. In addition to its beneficial effect in erythema elevatum diutinum, dapsone therapy is occasionally beneficial in other forms of leukocytoclastic vasculitis. Reportedly, niacinamide suppresses erythema elevatum diutinum effectively.[27] Systemic glucocorticoids are generally not effective. However, intralesional and topical high-potency glucocorticoids may be very effective in decreasing the size of lesions, and these glucocorticoids are the preferred treatment for patients with very limited disease.

REFERENCES

1. Radcliffe-Crocker H, Williams C: Erythema elevatum diutinum. *Br J Dermatol* **6**:1, 1894
2. Hutchinson J: On two remarkable cases of symmetrical purple congestion of the skin in patches, with induration. *Br J Dermatol* **1**:10, 1888
3. Bury JS: A case of erythema with remarkable nodular thickening and induration of the skin associated with intermittent albuminuria. *Illus Med News* **3**:145, 1889
4. Radcliffe-Crocker H: Granuloma annulare. *Br J Dermatol* **14**:1, 1902
5. Urbach E et al: Extrazellulare cholesterinose. *Arch Dermatol Syphilol (Berlin)* **166**:243, 1932
6. Herzberg JJ: Die extracellulare Cholesterinose (Kerl-Urbach), eine Variante des Erythema elevatum diutinum. *Arch Klin Exp Dermatol* **205**:477, 1958
7. Katz SI et al: Erythema elevatum diutinum—Skin and systemic manifestations, immunologic studies, and successful treatment with dapsone. *Medicine (Baltimore)* **56**:443, 1977
8. Jensen JA, Esquenazi V: Chemotactic stimulation by cell surface immune reactions. *Nature* **256**:213, 1975
9. Grabbe J et al: Erythema elevatum diutinum-evidence for disease-dependent leucocyte alterations and response to dapsone. *Br J Dermatol* **143**:415, 2000
10. Nakajima H et al: Erythema elevatum diutinum complicated by rheumatoid arthritis. *J Dermatol* **26**:452, 1999

11. Takiwaki H et al: Peripheral ulcerative keratitis associated with erythema elevatum diutinum and a positive rheumatoid factor: A report of three cases. *Br J Dermatol* **138**:893, 1998
12. Elsner J et al: Erythema elevatum and diutinum in Crohn disease. *Hautartz* **47**:701, 1996
13. Muratori S et al. Erythema elevatum diutinum and HIV infection: A report of five cases. *Brit J Dermatol* **141**:335, 1999
14. Weidman FD, Besancon JH: Erythema elevatum diutinum: Role of streptococci, and relationship to other rheumatic dermatoses. *Arch Dermatol Syphilol* **20**:593, 1929
15. Sangueza OP et al: Erythema elevatum diutinum: A clinicopathological study of eight cases. *Am J Dermatopathol* **19**:214, 1997
16. Kanitakis J et al: Ultrastructural study of chronic lesions of erythema elevatum diutinum: "Extracellular cholesterosis" is a misnomer. *J Am Acad Dermatol* **29**:363, 1993
17. Carlson JA, LeBoit PE: Localized chronic fibrosing vasculitis of the skin: An inflammatory reaction that occurs in settings other than erythema elevatum diutinum and granuloma faciale. *Am J Surg Pathol* **21**:698, 1997
18. Cream JJ et al: Erythema elevatum diutinum: An unusual reaction to streptococcal antigen and response to dapsone. *Br J Dermatol* **84**:393, 1971
19. Yiannias JA et al: Erythema elevatum diutinum: A clinical and histopathologic study of 13 patients. *J Am Acad Dermatol* **26**:38, 1992
20. Abdel-Aziz AHM, Robertson DEH: Erythema elevatum diutinum: Immunoglobulin, bacterial skin tests and response to dapsone. *Cutis* **12**:549, 1973
21. Chowdhury MMU et al: Erythema elevatum diutinum and IgA paraproteinaemia: 'A preclinical iceberg'. *Int J Dermatol* **41**:368, 2002
22. Vollum DI: Erythema elevatum diutinum: Vesicular lesions and sulfone response. *Br J Dermatol* **80**:178, 1968
23. Rovel-Guitera P et al: IgA antineutrophilic antibodies in cutaneous vasculitis. *Br J Dermatol* **143**:99, 2000
24. Wolff HH et al: Erythema elevatum diutinum. *Arch Dermatol Res* **261**:17, 1978
25. Fort S, Rodman OG: Erythema elevatum diutinum: A review and report of a case. *Arch Dermatol* **113**:819, 1977
26. Kalkoff KW: Zur Behandlung des Erythema elevatum diutinum mit 3-Sulfanilamido-methox-pyridazin (Lederkyn). *Dermatol Wochenschr* **142**:788, 1960
27. Kohler IK, Lorincz AL: Erythema elevatum diutinum treated with niacinamide and tetracycline. *Arch Dermatol* **116**:693, 1980

CHAPTER 96

Kristin M. Leiferman
Margot S. Peters
Gerald J. Gleich

Eosinophils in Cutaneous Diseases

The eosinophil is a conspicuous cell in cutaneous lesions because of its intense avidity for eosin. Eosinophils are prominent in many skin diseases and often constitute part of the diagnostic histologic patterns (Table 96-1).[1,2] In addition, eosinophils, even when not identifiable in tissue, may participate in the pathogenesis of the disease through the deposition of potently bioactive granule proteins (Table 96-2).

STRUCTURE AND FUNCTION OF EOSINOPHILS

In 1879, Ehrlich named this cell the eosinophil because of the intense staining of its cytoplasmic granules with the acidic dye eosin.[28]

TABLE 96-1

Eosinophils and Cutaneous Diseases

Diseases with peripheral and/or tissue eosinophilia
- Atopic diseases
- Parasitic diseases
- Bullous diseases
- Drug reactions
- Hypereosinophilic syndrome
- Eosinophilia myalgia syndrome
- Toxic oil syndrome
- Eosinophilic fasciitis
- Urticaria and angioedema
- Mastocytosis
- Cutaneous T cell lymphoma
- Eosinophilic panniculitis
- Reactions to arthropod bites and stings

Diseases histologically characterized by tissue eosinophilia
- Kimura's disease and angiolymphoid hyperplasia with eosinophilia
- Wells' syndrome (eosinophilic cellulitis)
- Eosinophilic pustulosis (Ofugi's disease and erythema toxicum neonatorum)
- Granuloma faciale
- Eosinophilic ulcer of the tongue

SOURCE: Adapted from Peters.[2]

By electron microscopy, these distinctive specific granules show an electron-dense core and a less-dense matrix. Because the crystalloid-containing granules are characteristic of eosinophils, their contents have been investigated as a means of understanding eosinophil functions.[29,30] Four cationic proteins comprise the bulk of the granule: major basic protein (MBP), eosinophil peroxidase (EPO), eosinophil-derived neurotoxin (EDN), and eosinophil cationic protein (ECP). MBP constitutes the core of the eosinophil granule; EPO, EDN, and ECP are present in the granule matrix. All the eosinophil granule proteins are cytotoxins, partly because of their basicity.

TABLE 96-2

Deposition of Eosinophil Granule Proteins in Cutaneous Disease

Urticarial and edematous lesions
- Chronic urticaria[3]
- Solar urticaria[4]
- Delayed pressure urticaria[5]
- IgE-mediated late-phase reaction[6]
- Episodic angioedema with eosinophilia[7,8]
- Facial edema with eosinophilia[9]
- GM-CSF reactions[10]
- IL-2 capillary leak syndrome[11]
- Eosinophilic cellulitis[12,13]

Eczematoid dermatitis
- Atopic dermatitis[14–16]
- Onchocercal dermatitis[17]
- Pachydermatous eosinophilic dermatitis[18]
- Prurigo nodularis[19,20]

Blistering disorders
- Herpes (pemphigoid) gestationis[21]
- Bullous pemphigoid[22]
- Bullous morphea[23]
- Incontinentia pigmenti[24]

Vasculitis
- Recurrent cutaneous necrotizing eosinophilic vasculitis[25]
- Eosinophilic vasculitis in connective tissue disease[26]
- Churg-Strauss syndrome[27]

Granule Proteins

MAJOR BASIC PROTEIN MBP has been localized to the eosinophil granule core by biochemical analyses and by immunoelectron microscopy. MBP is a single polypeptide chain of 117 amino acids, 17 of which are arginines, and it has a calculated isoelectric point (pI) of 10.9. It is a potent toxin against helminths, protozoa, bacteria, tumor cells, and many mammalian cells. The cDNA indicates that MBP is translated as a larger preproprotein with an acidic propiece. Because MBP is a potent toxin, its translation as proMBP with an anionic propiece may serve as a mechanism to neutralize the molecule and to protect the cell while MBP is transferred to its sequestered site in the granule core. Of interest is the finding that proMBP is markedly elevated during pregnancy, is produced by the placenta, and serves as an inhibitor for the enzyme, pregnancy-associated plasma protein A (PAPP-A); PAPP-A degrades insulin-like growth factor binding protein 4 and releases insulin-like growth factor activity. The cationic charge of MBP causes it to bind avidly to the anionic surface of target cells; the apolar residues may then insert into and disrupt the lipid milieu, causing nonspecific cell membrane damage and death of target cells. In a noncytotoxic manner, MBP also induces histamine release from human basophils and rat mast cells, activates neutrophils, and is a strong and unique platelet agonist. After instillation into the lungs of primates, MBP increases both respiratory resistance and sensitivity to methacholine. A related protein, MBP homologue, has been identified in eosinophil granules. Its isoelectric point is almost three magnitudes of order less than MBP, but it also has cytotoxic activity.[31] The genes for both MBP and the homologue are localized to chromosome 11q12.[31]

EOSINOPHIL CATIONIC PROTEIN ECP is located in the eosinophil granule matrix and is a strongly basic single polypeptide chain of 133 amino acids, 19 of which are arginines.[29,30] ECP is an enzymatically active member of the ribonuclease supergene family. It also has cytotoxic activity, most likely as a function of its cationic charge. In contrast to MBP, which may increase the permeability of target membranes without formation of transmembrane channels, ECP forms channels across membranes similar to those formed during membrane-complement interactions. ECP is a potent toxin against helminths, protozoa, bacteria, and mammalian cells; it also has neurotoxic activity and antiviral activity.[30]

EOSINOPHIL-DERIVED NEUROTOXIN EDN, contained in the matrix of the eosinophil granule, is a powerful neurotoxin with the ability to damage myelinated neurons.[29,30] The amino acid sequence of EDN has approximately 70 percent identity with that of ECP; the nucleotide sequences of these proteins have an 89 percent similarity index. Like ECP, EDN possesses ribonuclease activity, although it is approximately 100 times more potent, and it has antiviral activity. It is also a member of the ribonuclease supergene family, which includes angiogenin and ribonuclease itself. Both EDN and ECP genes have been localized to the q24-q31 region of human chromosome 14.[29,30]

EOSINOPHIL PEROXIDASE EPO is localized to the matrix of eosinophil granules, and is strongly basic. It consists of two subunits, a heavy chain of 53.0 kDa and a light chain of 12.7 kDa.[29,30] The amino acid sequence of EPO has a high content of arginine, leucine, and aspartic acid. In combination with hydrogen peroxide and a halide, EPO kills bacteria, helminths, and tumor cells. EPO binds to mast cells, and the EPO–mast cell complex catalyzes iodination of proteins in killing microorganisms. At low concentrations, EPO in combination with hydrogen peroxide and halide also causes mast cell degranulation and histamine release in a noncytotoxic reaction. With hydrogen peroxide and halide, EPO inactivates leukotrienes (LT) C_4, D_4, and E_4. Bromide is preferred over chloride in the eosinophil peroxidase reaction, whereas chloride is preferred in the myeloperoxidase reaction. Bromide is present in biologic fluids at concentrations that EPO can use; EPO, hydrogen peroxide, and bromide generate hypobromous acid and the corresponding ion OBr^-, both of which are potent oxidants.

Membrane Proteins

Eosinophils express various membrane receptors that enable communication with the extracellular environment.[29,30] Membrane proteins expressed by eosinophils include receptors for adhesion molecules, chemokines, the Fc portion of immunoglobulins, complement fragments, and soluble substances such as cytokines and lipid mediators.[29,30,32] The presence of IgG and complement receptors is linked to effector functions of the eosinophil toward parasitic and cellular targets. In addition, hypodense eosinophils may possess low-affinity IgE receptors that participate in mediating damage to parasites. Secretory IgA appears to be particularly effective in causing eosinophil degranulation, suggesting that eosinophils possess IgA receptors and participate in mucosal immunity. Based on the activity of the corresponding cytokines, eosinophils possess receptors for interleukin (IL)-3, IL-5, interferon (IFN)-α, IFN-γ, tumor necrosis factor (TNF)-α, and granulocyte-macrophage colony-stimulating factor (GM-CSF). In addition, membrane receptors for leukotriene B_4 (LTB_4) and platelet-activating factor (PAF) are present.[29,30,32]

Oxidative Products

Although eosinophils can ingest and kill microorganisms, their primary role in host defense may be against targets such as helminths and tumor cells. The phagocytic activity of eosinophils is less than that of neutrophils, but the respiratory burst to most stimuli is greater than that of neutrophils. Stimulation of eosinophils results in degranulation with a respiratory burst that forms superoxide anions, hydrogen peroxide, and the hydroxyl radical. Oxygen does not appear to be required for phagocytosis by eosinophils but is used for the generation of toxic oxygen metabolites. In addition, EPO in combination with hydrogen peroxide and a halide generates toxic hypohalous acid.[29,30,32]

Eosinophil Infiltration of Tissues

The factors determining eosinophil infiltration of tissues involve at least three interrelated signals: chemoattractants; adhesion molecules; and activating cytokines such as GM-CSF, IL-3, and IL-5.[33] Several members of the C-C chemokine gene superfamily are chemotactic for eosinophils.[34] These chemoattractants include eotaxin and RANTES (regulated on activation normal T cell-expressed and secreted). Eotaxin is specifically chemotactic for eosinophils, and its activity in inflammation is being delineated. RANTES is potently chemotactic for eosinophils and is also chemotactic for monocytes, T lymphocytes, natural killer (NK) cells, and basophils, but not for neutrophils. In addition to their chemotactic properties, RANTES and eotaxin induce production of reactive oxygen species by eosinophils, indicating that they have both chemotactic and functional activation effects. As an eosinophil chemoattractant, eotaxin is similar in potency to RANTES, but is stronger in inducing reactive oxygen species by eosinophils. Both RANTES and eotaxin are produced by dermal fibroblasts; RANTES is also produced by keratinocytes.

For eosinophils to migrate from the peripheral blood into tissues, the cells must cross blood vessel barriers. Three gene superfamilies contribute to the signaling needed for transmigration. Selectins are involved in the early, high-sheer-force stage of leukocyte adhesion to endothelium, and integrins are cell-surface proteins that recognize counterreceptor members of the immunoglobulin gene superfamily. Together, the integrin-immunoglobulin family interactions promote flattening and migration of cells onto and through the endothelium.[35] After eosinophils migrate through vessels into the extracellular matrix, integrins on the cell surface interact with counterligands such as the fibrous proteins fibronectin, laminin, and collagen, and the glycosaminoglycans hyaluronic acid and chondroitin sulfate. Ongoing studies suggest that integrin expression is critical for the effector functions of eosinophils, including degranulation.[29]

Several lines of investigation indicate that eosinophils are recruited to and activated in tissues by cytokines from a subset of T cells, the T_H2 cells, which produce IL-4, IL-5, IL-10, and IL-13, in addition to some cytokines common to T_H1 cells. Mast cell cytokines may also contribute to eosinophil activation.[36] In addition, human NK cells, which respond to some of the same C-C chemokines as eosinophils, also produce IL-5.[37] Eosinophils themselves elaborate important inflammatory and regulatory cytokines; these include IL-1α, transforming growth factor-α and β_1, GM-CSF, IL-3, IL-5, IL-6, IL-8, TNF-α, and macrophage inhibitory protein-1α.[38] Through expression of major histocompatibility complex (MHC) class II molecules and IL-1α production, eosinophils may act as specialized antigen-presenting cells. The functional diversity of the eosinophils, therefore, may have multiple ramifications in tissues.

Effects of IL-3, IL-5, and GM-CSF

A current model for eosinophil differentiation suggests that totipotent hematopoietic stem cells give rise to pluripotent cells that, in turn, give rise to the cells committed to one or two lines of differentiation.[39] Studies of purified eosinophils from patients with eosinophilia show that eosinophils exist as populations of varying densities, which may reflect their levels of activation. Hypodense eosinophils appear to be activated and generate significantly more superoxide and discharge more granule products than normodense cells. At least three factors are thought to influence eosinophil differentiation in the bone marrow and activation in tissues: GM-CSF, IL-3, and IL-5. Both GM-CSF and IL-3 act by inducing more eosinophil precursors, whereas IL-5 acts later in eosinophil differentiation and regulates cell maturation. IL-5 is also chemotactic for eosinophils. GM-CSF, IL-3, and IL-5 all enhance eosinophil survival. Along with IFN-γ and TNF-α, GM-CSF, IL-3, and IL-5 are cytoprotective and also activate eosinophils, as judged by surface receptor expression and enhancement of the respiratory burst, production of inflammatory mediators, cytotoxicity, and degranulation stimulated by secretory IgA. In vitro exposure to IL-3, IL-5, or GM-CSF alone, or to GM-CSF in association with fibroblasts or endothelial cells can convert normodense eosinophils into hypodense cells.

CUTANEOUS DISEASES ASSOCIATED WITH INCREASED EOSINOPHILS AND/OR EOSINOPHIL DEGRANULATION

Syndromes Associated with Edema

Several cutaneous syndromes show an association between edema and local eosinophilia. Although the etiologic mechanisms are incompletely understood, the ability of eosinophils to elaborate LTC_4 and PAF, to induce histamine release from mediator-containing cells, and to elicit a cutaneous wheal-and-flare reaction in human skin, along with the presence of cationic granule proteins in lesions, support a role for the eosinophil as a primary participant in the inflammation and edema associated with certain cutaneous diseases.

IgE-MEDIATED LATE-PHASE REACTION The mast cell-mediated wheal-and-flare cutaneous reaction is characteristic of IgE-mediated hypersensitivity. In sensitive patients, an intradermal challenge with a particular concentration of allergen elicits a wheal-and-flare followed by a late inflammatory reaction that becomes apparent at 3 to 4 h, peaks at 6 to 12 h, and resolves by 24 to 72 h. At its height, the late-phase reaction is characterized by erythema, warmth, edema, pruritus, and tenderness. Histologic examination of the cutaneous late-phase reaction shows edema; dermal infiltration with mononuclear cells, neutrophils, basophils, and eosinophils; and mast-cell degranulation. The extracellular deposition of neutrophil elastase and MBP indicates that both eosinophil and neutrophil degranulation occur in the late-phase reaction beginning 1 to 3 h after challenge.[6] Electron microscopy confirms that eosinophils degranulate in the tissue and lose their morphologic integrity in the late-phase response. This sequence is considered pertinent to some clinical urticarial diseases, as discussed below.

URTICARIAL REACTIONS Eosinophils are commonly present in urticarial skin lesions, but the histologic patterns are nonspecific. Between 43 and 60 percent of urticarial skin lesions demonstrate prominent extracellular deposition of eosinophil granule proteins.[35] Extracellular granule protein deposition occurs around small blood vessel walls, with granules dispersed in the dermis, and on connective tissue fibers. Autologous serum skin-testing sites in patients with chronic urticaria may also show extracellular MBP deposition.[40] Based on the activities of eosinophil granule proteins, eosinophil degranulation in lesions of chronic urticaria could be of pathogenetic importance.

Sequential biopsy specimens of wheals elicited by either a solar simulator or a dermographometer in patients with solar and delayed pressure urticaria demonstrate a pattern of eosinophil and neutrophil degranulation similar to that seen in the IgE-mediated late-phase reaction with both neutrophil elastase and MBP deposition.

EDEMATOUS SYNDROMES Episodic angioedema associated with eosinophilia was first described in 1984; it is characterized by recurrent angioedema, urticaria, fever, and elevated IgM levels.[7] During attacks, leukocyte counts increase to levels as high as 100,000/mm^3 with up to 90 percent eosinophils, and patients gain up to 31 percent of their body weight in edema fluid (Fig. 96-1). The disease activity waxes and wanes in concert with the number of peripheral eosinophils. Staining of skin biopsy specimens with hematoxylin and eosin shows few eosinophils; but by immunofluorescence, extracellular deposition of MBP can be seen around collagen bundles and blood vessels. Electron microscopy shows alteration of cytoplasmic granules in peripheral blood eosinophils and a spectrum of changes in dermal eosinophils, ranging from abnormal cytoplasmic granules in intact cells to complete cellular disruption, with loss of organelles, including granules, into the spaces among collagen bundles. Analyses of peripheral helper T cells and infiltrating dermal T cells in lesions of episodic angioedema and eosinophilia showed increased activated, HLA-DR+ helper T cells. IL-5 levels are elevated in the serum of patients with this syndrome.[8] The disease responds favorably to prednisone therapy and INF-α therapy (unpublished observations), which may be steroid-sparing in patients with this disease. A variant of episodic angioedema includes recurrent facial edema associated with eosinophilia. Peripheral blood eosinophilia is seen during attacks of localized facial edema; levels of both MBP and Charcot-Leyden crystal protein are elevated in peripheral blood during attacks, and extracellular deposition of MBP is seen in the skin.[9]

An association between T cell activation, eosinophilia, and angioedema has been observed in patients with advanced malignancies undergoing treatment with recombinant IL-2 who experience a capillary leak syndrome with weight gain and peripheral blood eosinophilia. MBP is strikingly elevated in serum and urine, and immunofluorescence analyses of skin specimens show extracellular MBP deposition.[11] IL-5 is elevated in patients undergoing IL-2 therapy.[8,11] Eosinophil degranulation may also be found in skin lesions that develop during GM-CSF therapy.[10]

WELLS' SYNDROME OR EOSINOPHILIC CELLULITIS This entity is characterized by recurrent cutaneous swelling. After prodromal burning or itching, lesions begin with redness and swelling, then evolve in a few days into large areas of edema with violaceous borders; bullae may develop over the surface. Individual lesions persist for days to weeks, and gradually change from bright red to brown-red and, finally, to blue-gray, resembling morphea (Fig. 96-2). The lesions may be single or multiple, may occur in any cutaneous location, and may recur. Familial cases have been reported, and the disease occurs in childhood.[13] The edematous and infiltrative plaques of Wells' syndrome are characterized histologically by dermal foci of amorphous eosinophilic material called *flame figures*. When examined for MBP by immunofluorescence, the flame figures show bright extracellular staining, suggesting that extensive eosinophil degranulation has occurred.[12] Further support for the participation of eosinophils in the formation of flame figures is provided by electron microscopic observations of free eosinophil granules coating collagen fibers in flame figures.

FIGURE 96-1

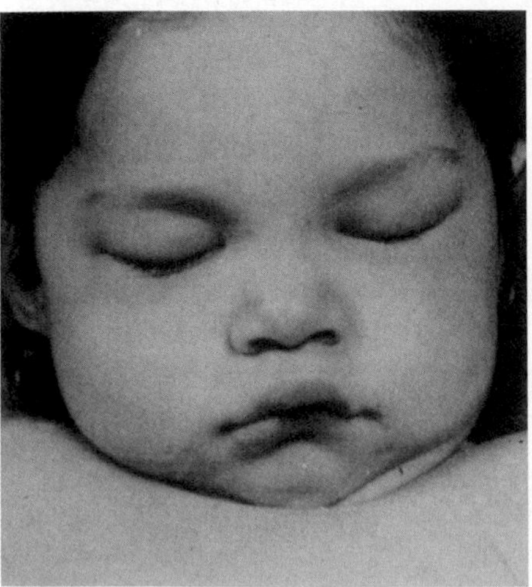
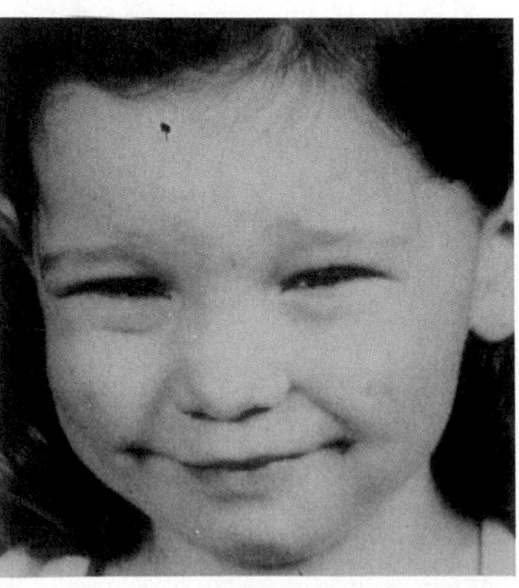

Episodic angioedema with eosinophilia. Facial appearance during an attack, showing marked edema (*left*) and normal appearance (*right*) between episodes. (*From Katzen et al. Hypereosinophilia and recurrent angioneurotic edema in a 2½-year-old girl. Am J Dis Child 140:62, 1986 with permission.*)

Onchocercal Dermatitis, Atopic Dermatitis, and Prurigo Nodularis

An association between peripheral blood eosinophilia and helminth infection was established before 1900, and considerable evidence suggests that eosinophils are important in defense against parasitic diseases.[29] Infection with *Onchocerca volvulus* causes a dermatitis associated with pruritus and lichenification. Slight cutaneous eosinophilia

FIGURE 96-2

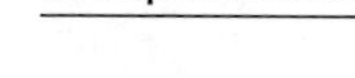

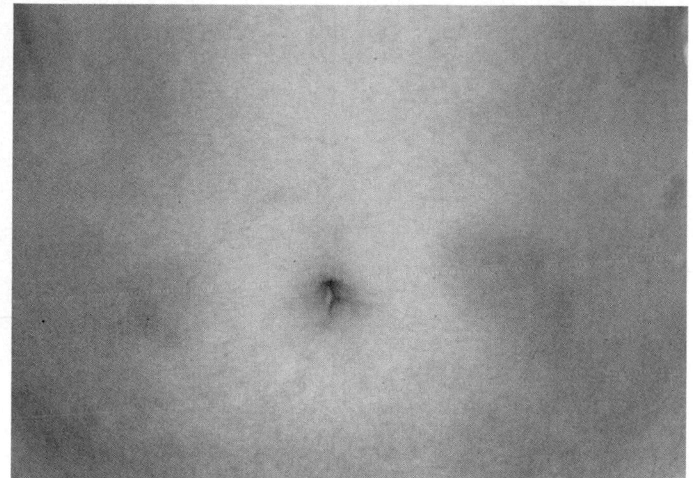

Wells' syndrome. Late lesion resembling morphea.

FIGURE 96-3

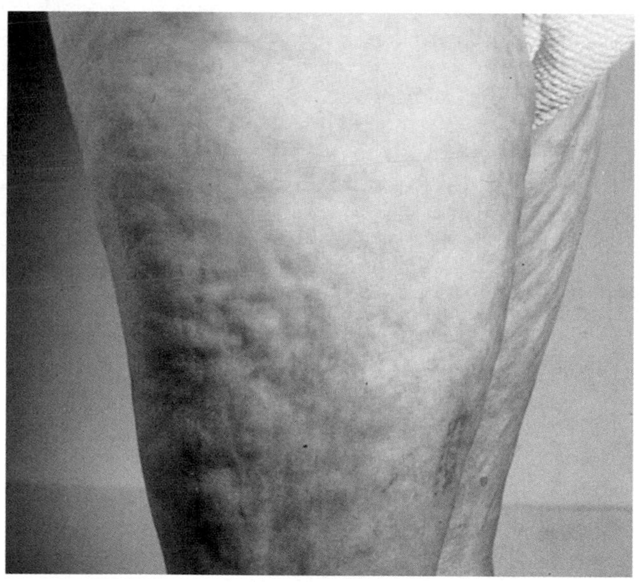

Eosinophilic fasciitis. Puckered skin changes involving the thighs.

and extensive deposition of eosinophil granule proteins throughout the dermis are found in untreated lesions. After treatment, the extracellular deposition of eosinophil granule proteins is located to the areas around degenerating microfilaria in the dermis.[17]

Although eosinophils are rarely a prominent histologic feature of atopic dermatitis, extensive dermal deposition of eosinophil granule proteins, including MBP, EDN, and ECP, is seen in lesions, but not in unaffected skin.[1,14–16] In contrast, neutrophil elastase is absent or minimally present in atopic dermatitis. These observations suggest that composite inflammatory factors differ for atopic dermatitis and urticaria, even though eosinophil involvement is common to both.

A pattern of dermal extracellular eosinophil granule protein deposition similar to that in atopic dermatitis and onchocercal dermatitis is found in prurigo nodularis.[19] Eosinophil granule proteins are deposited in the presence of increased numbers of mast cells but in the absence of neutrophil granule elastase. Comparable extracellular eosinophil granule protein deposition is present in pachydermatous eosinophilic dermatitis.[18] Similar to asthma,[41] eosinophil granule proteins are deposited around cutaneous nerves in both atopic dermatitis (unpublished observations) and prurigo nodularis.[20] The localization of eosinophil granule proteins in these diseases suggests that the eosinophil has deposited its toxic molecules in the tissue, contributing to the cutaneous pathophysiology.

Eosinophils and Blistering

Deposition of eosinophil granule proteins is prominently associated with blister formation in bullous pemphigoid,[22] herpes gestationis,[21] bullous morphea,[23] incontinentia pigmenti,[24] and in blisters developing in Churg-Strauss syndrome.[27] Additionally, eosinophil-active cytokines are found in blister fluid from bullous pemphigoid[22] and Churg-Strauss lesions.[27] These findings imply a connection between eosinophil activation and the pathologic process of blister formation.

Eosinophilic Diseases Associated with Fibrosis

Eosinophils are found in association with fibrotic reactions in a number of diseases, including parasitic infections, pulmonary and hepatic drug-sensitivity reactions, and the hypereosinophilic syndrome. Eosinophils elaborate collagenase that degrades type I and type III collagen; eosinophil extracts stimulate dermal fibroblast DNA synthesis and matrix production. EDN is mitogenic for fibroblasts, and ECP inhibits proteoglycan degradation in fibroblasts. Eosinophil degranulation is prominent in retroperitoneal fibrosis and in the fibrotic areas of orbital pseudotumor.[42] Therefore, eosinophils may be important in the pathogenesis of fibrosis.

EOSINOPHILIC FASCIITIS Eosinophilic fasciitis may be preceded by an episode of marked exertion. The disease commonly presents with pain, erythema, swelling, and induration of the extremities. Lesions are typically confined to the extremities, although truncal and generalized involvement may occur. Peripheral blood eosinophilia, an elevated erythrocyte sedimentation rate, and hypergammaglobulinemia also accompany the disease.[43] Contractures may occur early because of fascial involvement. In addition, fascial involvement may cause separation of muscle groups by a line of demarcation (groove sign), and the veins may appear depressed (sunken veins). Rippling of the skin may develop (Fig. 96-3) as the disease progresses. Histologic findings include thickening of the deep fascia with infiltration of lymphocytes, plasma cells, mast cells, and eosinophils. Later in the course of the disease, the fascia becomes fibrotic. Several features overlap with progressive systemic sclerosis, and the ultimate histologic changes are indistinguishable from those of scleroderma. Eosinophilic fasciitis often responds promptly to systemic glucocorticoids, especially if therapy is initiated early. Cimetidine and methotrexate reportedly are beneficial in treating the process. The pathophysiology of the sclerosing diseases, including eosinophilic fasciitis, is not understood.

EOSINOPHILIA-MYALGIA SYNDROME The eosinophilia-myalgia syndrome (EMS) is characterized by marked peripheral eosinophilia with a spectrum of signs and symptoms, including disabling generalized myalgias, pneumonitis, myocarditis, neuropathy, encephalopathy, and fibrosis.[43] The name derives from the two consistent features of the disease, peripheral blood eosinophilia and myalgias. The clinical picture may progress to one indistinguishable from that of eosinophilic fasciitis. The disease has been related to the ingestion of certain lots of L-tryptophan; epidemiologic studies indicate that the L-tryptophan ingested by the patients was traced to a single manufacturer. The etiology and pathogenesis are unknown, but the implicated lots of L-tryptophan contained a contaminant that was identified as 1,1′-ethylidene *bis* [L-tryptophan]. This contaminant may be the cause of the disease or a marker for another active substance in the preparation that provokes the syndrome.

Cutaneous symptoms associated with EMS include edema, pruritus, a faint erythematous rash, hair loss, and changes suggestive of fasciitis with peau d'orange and morphea-like skin lesions. Several other organ systems have been involved in the disease, including the lungs, heart, and nervous system. Histologic studies of deep-muscle biopsies show a prominent inflammatory cell infiltrate in the perimysium and fascia. Inflammatory cells are scattered diffusely or form sheets or clusters surrounding and often infiltrating the walls of small blood vessels. Some affected vessels have narrow lumina and appear to be occluded, but fibrinoid necrosis of vessel walls is absent; fibrin or platelet thrombi are absent. Perimysial tissue is thickened, and, in some areas, perimysial connective tissue is separated by edema. Striking evidence of eosinophil granule protein deposition is found in areas of skin and around muscle bundles.

Most patients improve with prednisone; however, many of the symptoms, especially painful myalgias and those related to eosinophilic fasciitis, persist. Multiple forms of therapy have been tried, including plasma exchange, methotrexate, and hydroxychloroquine, but a consistently beneficial intervention for refractory signs and symptoms has not been achieved.

TOXIC OIL SYNDROME A condition similar to EMS was described in Spain, in May 1981, and has been termed *toxic oil syndrome* (TOS).[44] Patients presented with acute respiratory symptoms followed by intense myalgias, thromboembolism, weight loss, sicca syndrome, and, lastly, a chronic phase characterized by eosinophilic fasciitis-like lesions, peripheral neuropathy, muscle atrophy, and pulmonary hypertension. The epidemic of TOS was linked to the consumption of adulterated rapeseed oil distributed in the industrial belt around Madrid. The initial clinical manifestation of TOS was pneumonitis along with a nonspecific pruritic, erythematous rash that persisted up to 4 weeks. During the next 2 months, patients developed subcutaneous edema, predominantly in legs, ankles, forearms, face, and hands. The edema was accompanied by myalgias, arthralgias, contractures, and peripheral blood eosinophilia. Histopathologic studies of the skin showed mainly a lymphocytic inflammatory infiltrate in the dermis, fascia, and small vessels of the dermis. The edema was eventually replaced by shiny, indurated skin that adhered to the deep tissues. Years after the onset of the disease, the patients had thin, atrophied, hyperpigmented skin with indurated plaques persisting in pretibial areas and occasionally on the forearms and abdomen.[44] Histologic examination revealed fibrosis and atrophy of sweat glands and hair follicles with extension of the fibrosis into subcutaneous fat. In some tissues, marked hyperplasia of the vessel intima was noted, and the lumina of blood vessels were partially obliterated. Subsequent studies showed eosinophil infiltration and degranulation in tissues, especially during the acute phase of TOS, and serum MBP levels were elevated during all phases, implicating a role for eosinophils in the disease.

TOS was most severe during its first 10 months. Joint contractures were among the most disabling and persistent features; several factors may have contributed to their development, including edema, neuropathy, myositis, and fibrosis of soft tissues. Renal involvement and malabsorption have been reported in only a few patients with TOS. Long-term follow-up studies of TOS patient cohorts at 8 and 12 years showed variable clinical manifestations. The disease had generally improved; however, the most prominent persisting features were muscle cramps, musculoskeletal pain, soft tissue tenderness, Raynaud's phenomenon, carpal tunnel syndrome, chronic lung disease, fatigue, and subjective cognitive impairment. Identification of the triggering agent(s) in TOS and EMS will likely increase understanding of both these multisystem scleroderma-like diseases as well as the effects of eosinophils in tissues.

Hypereosinophilic Syndrome

The hypereosinophilic syndrome is a multisystem disease characterized by peripheral blood eosinophilia and infiltration of eosinophils into many organs, including the skin.[45] Cutaneous involvement occurs in more than 50 percent of patients as either pruritic macular, papular, and nodular lesions over the trunk and extremities or as urticaria and angioedema. Dermographism is reported in over 75 percent of patients. While the hypereosinophilic syndrome is associated with a significant mortality rate, a variant of the disease characterized by mucosal ulcers (Fig. 96-4) carries an unusually grave prognosis—five of seven patients with this subset of hypereosinophilic syndrome died within 2 years of diagnosis. The mucosal ulcers frequently precede or appear concurrently with peripheral blood eosinophilia and are resistant to therapy.

FIGURE 96-4

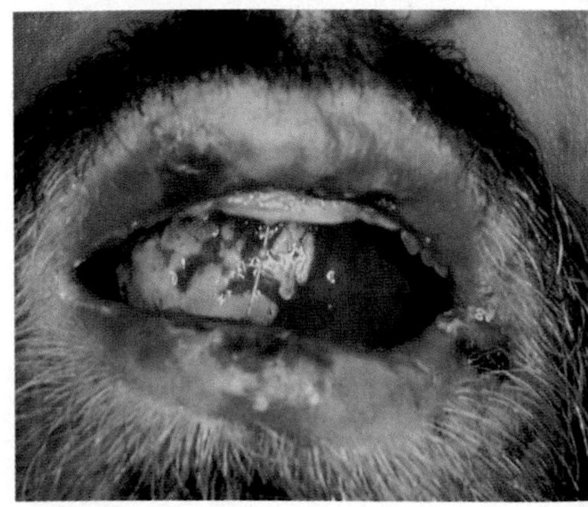

A.

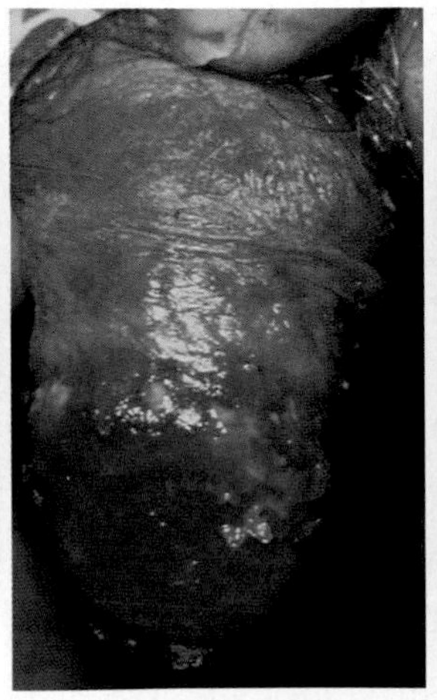

B.

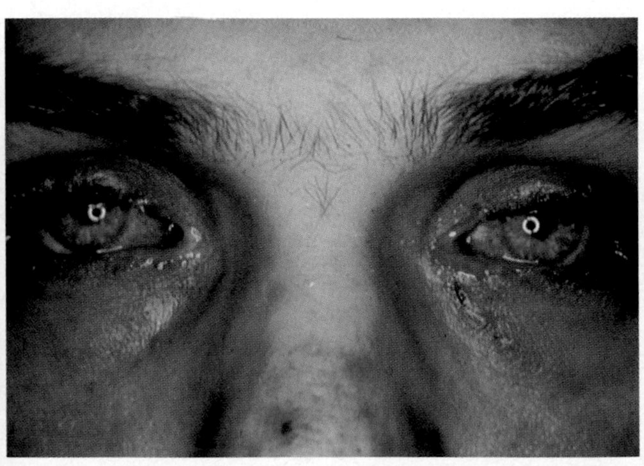

C.

Hypereosinophilic syndrome. Mucosal erosions and ulcers of mouth (*A*) and glans penis (*B*), with conjunctival irritation (*C*).

Criteria for the diagnosis of hypereosinophilic syndrome include persistent peripheral blood eosinophil counts greater than 1500/mm^3 for more than 6 months; failure to diagnose parasitic, allergic, or other known causes of eosinophilia; and presumptive signs and symptoms of organ involvement. Patients satisfying the criteria likely have a constellation of diseases. Recently, a subset of patients with the hypereosinophilic syndrome were found to have unusual T cell clones, CD3– and CD4+, that express T_H2 cytokines, particularly IL-5.[46]

Other organs that may be involved include the bone marrow, sometimes associated with eosinophilic leukemia; the heart, leading to subendocardial fibrosis and restrictive cardiomyopathy; the liver and spleen, with organomegaly; the lung with infiltrates; and the nervous system. The histopathology of skin lesions is nonspecific but frequently shows a heavy dermal infiltrate of eosinophils. Serum MBP levels are usually elevated in patients with the hypereosinophilic syndrome, and eosinophil degranulation is noted in tissues such as the endocardium and the myocardium. Eosinophils from patients with the hypereosinophilic syndrome are hypodense, implying a more activated state.

Glucocorticoids have been used as initial and maintenance therapy for the hypereosinophilic syndrome and are continued until the eosinophilia is under control. In patients unresponsive to prednisone, hydroxyurea is added. Improvement in peripheral eosinophilia correlates with improved cardiac status. Vincristine also has been tried as a therapeutic agent. INF-α therapy has been successfully used to control the disease, including the variant with mucosal ulcerations.[47] Recently, imatinib mesylate (Gleevec), a tyrosine kinase inhibitor useful for treatment of chronic myelogenous leukemia, was found to be remarkably effective for certain patients with hypereosinophilic syndrome, namely those without elevation of IL-5.[48]

The hypereosinophilic syndrome predominantly affects men, and the 5-year survival rates are reported at 80 percent or better. Treatment limits organ involvement and extends survival. The cause of death in patients with the hypereosinophilic syndrome is frequently related to cardiovascular disease, most commonly congestive heart failure.

Angiolymphoid Hyperplasia with Hypereosinophilia and Kimura's Disease

Angiolymphoid hyperplasia with eosinophilia and Kimura's disease are characterized by persistent, recurrent dermal and/or subcutaneous nodules, primarily in the head and neck area. Lesions of both diseases are infiltrated with masses of eosinophils, and peripheral blood eosinophilia is common. Controversy exists as to whether angiolymphoid hyperplasia with eosinophilia and Kimura's disease represent separate disease entities or are part of a single disease spectrum.[49] The features of the two diseases are compared in Table 96-3. Because of the associated tissue and peripheral blood eosinophilia, both syndromes are thought to be hypersensitivity responses; serum IgE is elevated in many cases of Kimura's disease. The pathogenic stimulus for the hypersensitivity response is unknown. Angiolymphoid hyperplasia with eosinophilia has been described in the Occident, and Kimura's disease has been described mainly in the Orient. Compared with Kimura's disease, angiolymphoid hyperplasia with eosinophilia is more varied in its clinical and immunohistologic findings.[50]

Eosinophilic Pustular Folliculitis and Other Pustular Dermatoses

Eosinophilic pustular folliculitis, first described by Ofugi, is characterized by recurrent crops of pruritic follicular papules and pustules that occur mainly on the face, trunk, and extremities. Histologically, the most striking feature is the infiltration of eosinophils, mixed with mononuclear cells, into the epidermis and dermis. Chemotactic factors for neutrophils and eosinophils have been found in stratum corneum extracts from eosinophilic pustular folliculitis lesions. Other studies revealed an epidermal antibody directed against the intercellular substance in the lower epidermis. There are high titers of circulating IgG and IgM directed against the cytoplasm of the epidermal basal cells in the outer sheath of hair follicles. The pathogenesis of eosinophilic pustular folliculitis is unknown, but the disease occurs in conjunction with immunologic disorders including the acquired immunodeficiency syndrome. When bacterial or fungal organisms are cultured, a response to antimicrobial therapy has been demonstrated. Nonsteroidal anti-inflammatory drugs, diaminodiphenylsulfone (dapsone), and topical glucocorticoids may be beneficial. Indomethacin has been suggested as first-line therapy, and improvement is associated with decreases in peripheral blood eosinophils.[51] Other studies suggest that IFN-γ therapy may effectively control the disease.[52]

Granuloma Faciale

Granuloma faciale is characterized by single or multiple brown-red, asymptomatic, indurated facial nodules with prominent follicular orifices and occasional telangiectasias. The lesions never ulcerate and tend to be progressive. Peripheral blood eosinophilia may accompany the disease. Intranasal and laryngeal lesions with similar histopathologic features have been reported. Histologically, granuloma faciale is distinctive: a dense dermal accumulation of neutrophils, eosinophils, monocytes, lymphocytes, plasma cells, and histiocytes is separated from the epidermis by a narrow band of uninvolved dermis. Lesions may contain increased numbers of mast cells. The degree of eosinophil infiltration is variable, from lesions dominated by eosinophils to those

TABLE 96-3

Comparison of Angiolymphoid Hyperplasia with Eosinophilia and Kimura's Disease

Feature	Angiolymphoid Hyperplasia with Eosinophilia	Kimura's Disease
Gender	More often females	Almost exclusively males
Lesion size and location	Small and superficial	Large, deep in subcutis, may involve salivary or parotid glands and regional lymph nodes
Lymphoid follicles	Rarely present in older lesions	Prominent
Mast cell numbers	Commonly increased	Rarely increased
Vascularity	Abundant angiomatoid proliferation with uncanalized masses of endothelial cells	Capillary proliferation, large thickened vessels, swollen canalized endothelial cells
Fibrosis	Absent or present only at lesional edges	Prominent

SOURCE: From Kung et al.,[49] with permission.

with only a few identifiable cells. Evidence for eosinophil degranulation includes extracellular MBP deposition.[53] A vasculitis characterized by vessel wall damage and nuclear dust may be seen. Direct immunofluorescence has shown IgG, IgM, and IgA along the basement membrane zone and striking perivascular fibrin deposition. The disease is resistant to most treatments; surgical excision may be curative, but lesions recur. Diaminodiphenylsulfone (dapsone) therapy has been reported to be helpful.[54]

REFERENCES

1. Leiferman KM: Eosinophils, interleukin-5, and cutaneous disease, in *Interleukin-5: From Molecule to Drug Target For Asthma. Lung Biology in Health and Disease*, vol 125, edited by CJ Sanderson. New York, Marcel Dekker, 1999, pp 95–118
2. Peters MS: The eosinophil, in *Advances in Dermatology*, vol 2, edited by JP Callen et al. Chicago, Year Book, 1987, p 192
3. Peters MS et al: Localization of eosinophil granule major basic protein in chronic urticaria. *J Invest Dermatol* **81**:39, 1983
4. Leiferman KM et al: Evidence for eosinophil degranulation with deposition of granule major basic protein in solar urticaria. *J Am Acad Dermatol* **21**:75, 1989
5. McEvoy MT et al: Immunohistological comparison of granulated cell proteins in induced immediate dermographism and delayed pressure urticaria. *Br J Dermatol* **133**:853, 1995
6. Leiferman KM et al: Extracellular deposition of eosinophil and neutrophil granule proteins in the IgE-mediated cutaneous late phase reaction. *Lab Invest* **62**:579, 1990
7. Gleich GJ et al: Episodic angioedema associated with eosinophilia. *N Engl J Med* **310**:1621, 1984
8. Butterfield JH et al: Elevated serum levels of interleukin-5 in patients with the syndrome of episodic angioedema and eosinophilia. *Blood* **79**:688, 1992
9. Songsiridej V et al: Facial edema and eosinophilia: Evidence for eosinophil degranulation. *Ann Intern Med* **103**:503, 1985
10. Mehregan DR et al: Cutaneous reactions to granulocyte monocyte colony stimulating factor. *Arch Dermatol* **128**:1055, 1992
11. van Haelst-Pisani CM et al: Administration of IL-2 results in increased plasma concentrations of IL-5 and eosinophilia in patients with cancer. *Blood* **78**:1538, 1991
12. Peters MS et al: Immunofluorescence identification of eosinophil granule major basic protein in the flame figures of Wells' syndrome. *Br J Dermatol* **109**:141, 1983
13. Davis MDP et al: Familial eosinophilic cellulitis, dysmorphic habitus and mental retardation. *J Am Acad Dermatol* **38**:919, 1998
14. Leiferman KM et al: Dermal deposition of eosinophil-granule major basic protein in atopic dermatitis: Comparison with onchocerciasis. *N Engl J Med* **313**:282, 1985
15. Leiferman KM: A role for eosinophils in atopic dermatitis. Proceedings of the International Consensus Conference on Atopic Dermatitis. *J Am Acad Dermatol* **45**:S21, 2001
16. Leiferman KM, Plager DA, Gleich GJ. Eosinophils and atopic dermatitis, in *Atopic Dermatitis*, edited by T Bieber, DYM Leung. New York, Marcel Dekker, 2002, p 327
17. Ackerman SJ et al: Eosinophil degranulation: An immunologic determinant in the pathogenesis of the Mazzotti reaction in human onchocerciasis. *J Immunol* **144**:3961, 1990
18. Jacyk WK et al: Pachydermatous eosinophilic dermatitis. *Br J Dermatol* **134**:469, 1996
19. Perez GL et al: Mast cells, neutrophils and eosinophils in prurigo nodularis. *Arch Dermatol* **129**:861, 1993
20. Johansson O, et al: Eosinophil cationic protein- and eosinophil-derived neurotoxin/eosinophil protein X-immunoreactive eosinophils in prurigo nodularis. *Arch Dermatol Res* **292**:371, 2000
21. Scheman AJ et al: Evidence for eosinophil degranulation in the pathogenesis of herpes gestationis. *Arch Dermatol* **125**:1079, 1989
22. Borrego L et al: Deposition of eosinophil granule proteins precedes blister formation in bullous pemphigoid: Comparison with neutrophil and mast cell granule proteins. *Am J Pathol* **148**:897, 1996
23. Daoud MS et al: Bullous morphea: Clinical, pathologic and immunopathologic evaluation of thirteen cases. *J Am Acad Dermatol* **30**:937, 1994
24. Thyresson NH et al: Localization of eosinophil granule major basic protein in incontinentia pigmenti. *Pediatr Dermatol* **8**:102, 1991
25. Chen K-R et al: Recurrent cutaneous necrotizing eosinophilic vasculitis: A novel eosinophil mediated syndrome. *Arch Dermatol* **130**:1159, 1994
26. Chen K-R et al: Eosinophilic vasculitis in connective tissue disease. *J Am Acad Dermatol* **35**:173, 1996
27. Drage LA et al: Evidence for pathogenic involvement of eosinophils and neutrophils in Churg-Strauss Syndrome. *J Am Acad Dermatol* **47**:209, 2002
28. Hirsch JG, Hirsch BI: Paul Ehrlich and the discovery of the eosinophil, in *The Eosinophil in Health and Disease*, edited by AAF Mahmoud, KF Austen. New York, Grune & Stratton, 1980, p 3
29. Kita H: Biology of eosinophils, in *Allergy: Principles & Practice,* Middleton E Jr, Reed CE, Ellis EF, Adkinson NF Jr, Yunginger JW, Busse WW (eds). St. Louis, Mosby, 5th ed, Vol. 1, Ch. 19, 1998, pp 242–260
30. Gleich GJ: Mechanisms of eosinophil-associated inflammation. *J Allergy Clin Immunol* **105**:651, 2000
31. Plager DA et al: A novel human homolog of eosinophil major basic protein. *Immunol Rev* **179**:192, 2001
32. Weller PF: Human eosinophils. *J Allergy Clin Immunol* **100**:283, 1997
33. Broide D, Sriramarao P: Eosinophil trafficking to sites of allergic inflammation. *Immunol Rev* **179**:163, 2001
34. Elsner J, Kapp A. The chemokine network in eosinophil activation. *Allergy Asthma Proc* **22**:139, 2001
35. Bochner BS, Schleimer RP: Mast cells, basophils, and eosinophils: Distinct but overlapping pathways for recruitment. *Immunol Rev* **179**:5, 2001
36. Bradding P et al: Interleukin-4, -5, and -6 and tumor necrosis factor-alpha in normal and asthmatic airways: Evidence for the human mast cell as a source of these cytokines. *Am J Respir Cell Mol Biol* **10**:471, 1994
37. Warren HS et al: Production of IL-5 by human NK cells and regulation of IL-5 secretion by IL-4, IL-10, and IL-12. *J Immunol* **154**:5144, 1995
38. Lacy P, Moqbel R: Eosinophil cytokines. *Chem Immunol* **76**:134, 2000
39. Sehmi R, Denburg JA: Differentiation of human eosinophils. *Chem Immunol* **76**:29, 2000
40. Gratten CEH et al: Eosinophil major basic protein in autologous serum and saline skin tests in chronic idiopathic urticaria [letter]. *Br J Dermatol* **136**:141, 1997
41. Jacoby DB, Costello RM: Eosinophil recruitment to the airway nerves. *J Allergy Clin Immunol* **107**:211, 2001
42. Noguchi H et al: Tissue eosinophilia and eosinophil degranulation in syndromes associated with fibrosis. *Am J Pathol* **140**:521, 1992
43. Varga J, Kahari VM: Eosinophilia-myalgia syndrome, eosinophilic fasciitis, and related fibrosing disorders. *Curr Opin Rheumatol* **9**:562, 1997
44. Diggle GE: The toxic oil syndrome: 20 years on. Int J Clin Prac 55:371, 2001.
45. Leiferman KM: Hypereosinophilic syndrome, in *Cutaneous Medicine and Surgery*, edited by KA Arndt, PE Leboit, JK Robinson, BU Wintroub. Philadelphia, Saunders, 1996, p 352
46. Simon HU et al:: Abnormal clones of T cells producing interleukin-5 in idiopathic eosinophilia. *N Engl J Med* **341**:1112, 1999
47. Butterfield JH, Gleich GJ: Interferon-alpha treatment of six patients with the idiopathic hypereosinophilic syndrome. *Ann Intern Med* **121**:648, 1994
48. Gleich GJ et al: Treatment of the hypereosinophilic syndrome with imatinib mesylate. *Lancet* **359**:1577, 2002
49. Kung ITM et al: Kimura's disease: A clinicopathological study of 21 cases and its distinction from angiolymphoid hyperplasia with eosinophilia. *Pathology* **16**:39, 1984
50. Helander SD et al: Kimura's disease and angiolymphoid hyperplasia with eosinophilia: New observations from immunohistochemical studies of lymphocyte markers, endothelial antigens and granulocyte proteins. *J Cutan Pathol* **22**:319, 1995
51. Ota T et al: Eosinophilic pustular folliculitis (Ofugi's disease): Indomethacin as a first choice of treatment. *Clin Exp Dermatol* **26**:179, 2001
52. Fushimi M et al: Eosinophilic pustular folliculitis effectively treated with recombinant interferon-gamma: Suppression of mRNA expression of interleukin 5 in peripheral blood mononuclear cells. *Br J Dermatol* **134**:766, 1996
53. Dinneen AM et al: Granuloma faciale: Immunohistopathologic study and evidence for eosinophil degranulation [abstract]. *J Invest Dermatol* **96**:568, 1991
54. van de Kerkhof PC: On the efficacy of dapsone in granuloma faciale. *Acta Derm Venereol* **74**:61, 1994

CHAPTER 97

Walter H.C. Burgdorf

Granuloma Faciale

Granuloma faciale is an uncommon disease of unknown origin characterized by single or multiple cutaneous nodules, usually occurring on the face.

HISTORICAL ASPECTS

Although a variety of skin lesions have been called eosinophilic granuloma, the case that Wigley described as eosinophilic granuloma may be the first example of what is now known as granuloma faciale.[1] This rare disease had been lost among the common infectious granulomas and became better recognized only as the latter decreased in number with increasing antibiotic use. Cobane and colleagues used the phrase *facial granuloma with eosinophilia* and separated this entity from other eosinophilic infiltrates of skin and other tissues;[2] Pinkus suggested the name of granuloma faciale.[3]

ETIOLOGY AND PATHOGENESIS

The etiology of granuloma faciale remains a mystery. The literature does not even include any attractive speculations.

CLINICAL MANIFESTATIONS

Granuloma faciale occurs as cutaneous nodules or plaques that are usually solitary.[4] Occasionally, patients have multiple or disseminated lesions. Most often, lesions occur on the face, but they may appear anywhere.[5] Because the disease favors light-exposed areas and sunlight makes some lesions worse, actinic exposure may play a role in the pathogenesis. The disease may appear at any age, but becomes evident primarily in middle life. It seems to be more common in males. Although most have occurred in Caucasians, Lesions have been identified in blacks and Japanese.

The lesions are soft, elevated, well-circumscribed nodules, ranging in size from a few millimeters to several centimeters (Fig. 97-1). Due to sinking of their centers, some lesions become annular. Their color varies; they are seldom bright red, but rather are shades of dull red, brown, blue, and purple. After sun exposure, they may darken. The surface is smooth, but the follicular orifices are accentuated. Lesions are never ulcerated but may be covered by telangiectases (Fig. 97-2). They are usually asymptomatic and chronic or slowly progressive; occasionally, they involute.

FIGURE 97-1

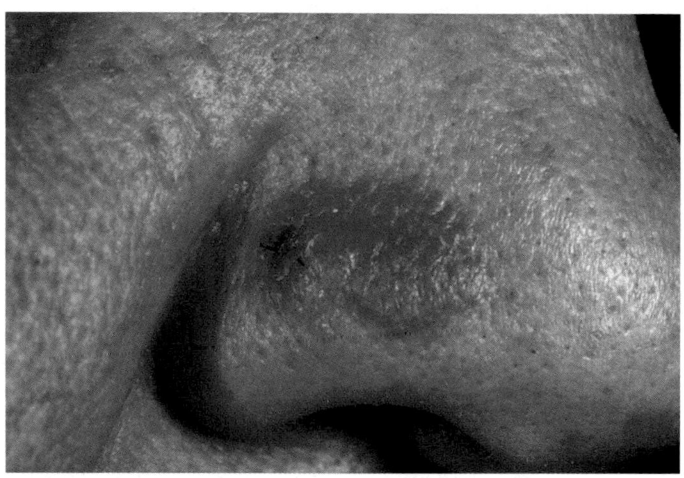

Granuloma faciale. Large reddish brown nodule on the nose.

Extracutaneous involvement is most rare. There have been isolated reports of granuloma faciale–like lesions of the oral mucosa and upper airway, known as eosinophilic angiocentric fibrosis.[6] In one case, the patient had cutaneous granuloma faciale and a histologically similar process in her nasal mucosa, which was causing obstruction.[7] One patient with myelodysplastic syndrome had granuloma faciale, Sweet syndrome, and pyoderma gangrenosum.[8] Even in patients with widespread cutaneous disease, no other internal involvement has been reported.

FIGURE 97-2

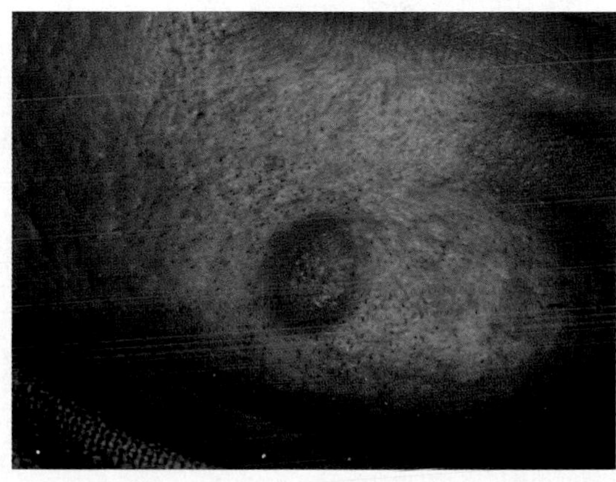

Granuloma faciale. Close-up view of the chin, showing reddish brown nodule with prominent pores and telangiectases.

LABORATORY EXAMINATION

The findings of the laboratory evaluation are normal except for occasional mild blood eosinophilia.

PATHOLOGY

Biopsy of the skin is the most important method of diagnosis, because the histologic changes associated with granuloma faciale are usually distinctive. The epidermis is unaffected except where it is thinned and flattened by the underlying infiltrate. There is usually a narrow Grenz zone of uninvolved dermis between the epidermis and the dense dermal accumulation of inflammatory cells (Fig. 97-3), including neutrophils, eosinophils, monocytes, and lymphocytes. Some cases show a considerable number of mast cells as well. Extravasated red blood cells, hemosiderin, and melanin probably all contribute to the brown color seen clinically. The number of eosinophils varies widely. In some cases, they constitute the largest part of the infiltrate; in others, only a few are seen.

The infiltrate is usually distributed diffusely throughout the involved dermis. At its depth and periphery, it is predominantly perivascular. At times, true vasculitis occurs, causing vessel wall damage and nuclear dust. In other cases, there is fibrinoid or hyaline material within and about the affected blood vessels. In older lesions, considerable fibrosis may occur. Immunofluorescence studies and electron microscopic studies support the vascular involvement and presence of eosinophils. The benign appearance of the cells, as well as the mixed composition, serves to differentiate granuloma faciale from malignant processes.

DIAGNOSIS AND DIFFERENTIAL DIAGNOSIS

Clinically, the reddish brown nodules of granuloma faciale must be differentiated from those associated with a wide variety of other diseases. Many cutaneous infiltrates are similar in appearance, including that of lupus erythematosus, polymorphic light eruption, fixed drug eruption, leukemic infiltrate, and the whole spectrum of benign and malignant lymphoid proliferations. Granulomatous processes ranging from sarcoidosis, granuloma annulare, and foreign body reactions to infections such as tinea faciale, leprosy, and tuberculosis also enter the differential. In children, juvenile xanthogranuloma, mastocytoma, and Spitz nevus are additional possibilities, although one must remember that granuloma faciale is extremely rare in children. The clinical appearance and history usually help to eliminate most of the choices, but histologic findings determine the final diagnosis.

Granuloma faciale and erythema elevatum diutinum appear to be related. Erythema elevatum diutinum is characterized by persistent plaques on the extremities. Histologically, it has more epidermal and vascular involvement with fewer eosinophils.

Several other benign and malignant skin lesions have significant numbers of eosinophils in their infiltrates. Angiolymphoid hyperplasia with eosinophilia also presents as a reddish facial nodule rich in eosinophils, but the prominent endothelial cells and lymphoid proliferation, usually including germinal center formation, allow ready identification on biopsy. Also similar are arthropod bites with both lymphoid and pseudoepitheliomatous hyperplasia and nodular scabies, which usually has less epidermal change. When histiocytosis X involving the skin is rich in eosinophils, differentiation is still possible because its atypical histiocytes exhibit epidermotropism and contain Langerhans granules, which may be identified by immunohistochemical staining or electron microscopy.

FIGURE 97-3

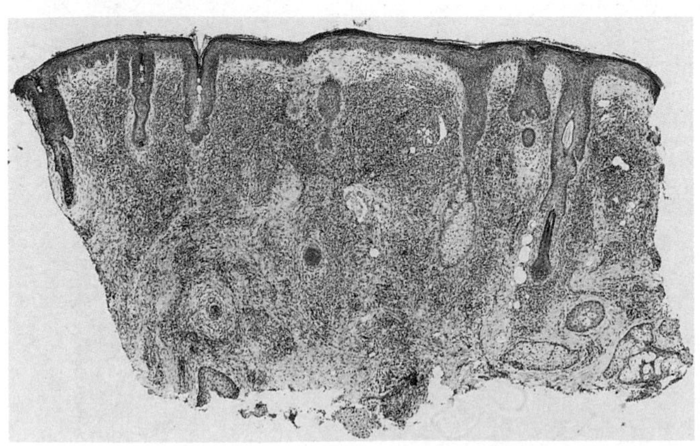

Granuloma faciale. There is a normal epidermis separated from a perivascular infiltrate of lymphocytes and eosinophils by a Grenz zone.

TREATMENT

Facial granulomas are notorious for their stubborn resistance to treatment. Surgical excision may be curative, but both the recurrence of old lesions and the appearance of new lesions are common. Destruction with the 585-nm pulsed dye laser seems promising.[9] Other lasers, electrosurgery, cryosurgery, and dermabrasion have also produced acceptable results.[10] It seems that any destructive treatment may ablate a lesion, but ablation requires treatment deep enough to risk scarring.

Thus, nonscarring intervention is attractive. Local injection of triamcinolone suspension in concentrations of 2.5 to 5 mg/mL with either a fine-gauge needle or pressure injector may be helpful. This approach has been effectively combined with cryotherapy.[11] Several orally administered medications are potentially beneficial. Dapsone in doses of 50 to 150 mg daily has been effective.[12] Although many other therapies havc been the topic of case reports, none has proven consistently successful.

Because of its poor response to therapy and apparent harmlessness, granuloma faciale may be left untreated. However, its facial location and unsightly appearance cause most physicians or patients to at least try some of these remedies.

REFERENCES

1. Wigley JEM: Sarcoid of Boeck? Eosinophilic granuloma. *Br J Dermatol* **57**:68, 1945
2. Cobane JH et al: Facial granulomas with eosinophilia: Their relation to other eosinophilic granulomas of the skin and to reticulogranuloma. *Arch Dermatol Syphilol* **61**:442, 1950
3. Pinkus H: Granuloma faciale. *Dermatologica* **105**:85, 1952
4. Pedace FJ, Perry HO: Granuloma faciale. *Arch Dermatol* **94**:387, 1966
5. Roustan G et al: Granuloma faciale with extrafacial lesions. *Dermatology* **198**:79, 1999
6. Thompson LD, Heffner DK: Sinonasal tract eosinophilic angiocentric fibrosis: A report of three cases. *Am J Clin Pathol* **115**:243, 2001

7. Roberts PF, McCann BG: Eosinophilic angiocentric fibrosis of the upper respiratory tract: A mucosal variant of granuloma faciale? A report of three cases. *Histopathology* **9**:1217, 1985
8. Vazquez Garcia J et al: Multiple neutrophilic dermatoses in myelodysplastic syndrome. *Clin Exp Dermatol* **26**:398, 2001
9. Ammirati CT, Hruza GJ: Treatment of granuloma faciale with the 585-nm pulsed dye laser. *Arch Dermatol* **135**:903, 1999
10. Dinehart SM et al: Granuloma faciale: Comparison of different treatment modalities. *Arch Otolaryngol Head Neck Surg* **116**:849, 1990

11. Dowlati B et al: Granuloma faciale: Successful treatment of nine cases with a combination of cryotherapy and intralesional corticosteroid injection. *Int J Dermatol* **36**:548, 1997
12. van de Kerkhof PC: On the efficacy of dapsone in granuloma faciale. *Acta Derm Venereol* **74**:61, 1994

CHAPTER 98

Klaus Wolff
Georg Stingl

Pyoderma Gangrenosum

Pyoderma gangrenosum is a rare, destructive inflammatory skin disease in which a painful nodule or pustule breaks down to form a progressively enlarging ulcer. Lesions may occur either in the absence of any apparent underlying disorder or in association with systemic disease, such as ulcerative colitis, Crohn's disease, polyarthritis, gammopathy, and other conditions. Pyoderma gangrenosum belongs to the group of neutrophilic dermatoses in which the common cellular denominator is the neutrophil.

ETIOLOGY AND PATHOGENESIS

When Brunsting, Goeckerman, and O'Leary described pyoderma gangrenosum in 1930,[1] they implicated streptococci and staphylococci as causative agents because of the inflammatory and purulent nature of the condition. Seventy years later, the etiology of pyoderma gangrenosum is still unknown, but in all likelihood bacteria do not directly cause the disease, nor is it infectious in nature.

Pyoderma gangrenosum, cystic acne, and pyogenic, aseptic arthritis (PAPA syndrome) have been reported in a three-generation kindred with autosomal dominant transmission and mapped to the long arm of chromosome 15.[2]

A key to the etiologic and pathogenic background of pyoderma gangrenosum may be found in its frequent association with systemic disease, but, because pyoderma gangrenosum exists both as a disease sui generis and in association with a systemic disorder, the cause-effect relationship of such associations is not clear. The phenomenon of pathergy, which describes the development of new lesions or the aggravation of existing ones after trivial trauma and is frequently present in pyoderma gangrenosum, suggests altered, exaggerated, and uncontrolled inflammatory responses to nonspecific stimuli.

The preeminent cell in pyoderma gangrenosum pathology is the neutrophil. Indeed, the condition responds to sulfa drugs, which have an antineutrophilic action (see Chap. 254). Pyoderma gangrenosum has occurred as a side effect of treatment with granulocyte-macrophage colony-stimulating factor (GM-CSF),[3] following treatment with interferon-α2b,[4] and in cases in which IL-8 is overexpressed in the tissue.[5] By contrast, GM-CSF has been successfully used in the treatment of pyoderma gangrenosum.[6] There have been reports of abnormalities of neutrophil function, but no consistent patterns have emerged. Some in vitro studies showed impaired neutrophil chemotaxis,[7] but neutrophil accumulation at a Rebuck skin window was normal[8]; moreover, neutrophils do accumulate at sites of pyoderma gangrenosum. Human skin engrafted to mice with severe combined immunodeficiency and then injected with recombinant adenovirus expressing DNA that encoded human IL-8, which induces a 200-fold increase in IL-8 expression of infected human fibroblasts in vitro, developed massive neutrophilic inflammation and ulceration clinically and histologically resembling pyoderma gangrenosum.[5] A streaking leukocyte factor that enhances migration of leukocytes without altering their chemotactic activity, aberrant neutrophil trafficking, and metabolic oscillations of leukocytes have been observed.[9,10] Impairment of microbicidal activation of leukocytes and impaired neutrophil functions associated with hyperimmunoglobulinemia E have been isolated findings.[11] IgA of multiple myeloma can impair neutrophil chemotaxis in vitro, and IgA gammopathies are not infrequent in pyoderma gangrenosum. Circulating immunoglobulins can affect neutrophil functions, and monoclonal or polyclonal hyperglobulinemia frequently occurs in pyoderma gangrenosum.

The evidence implicating a disturbance of cellular immune functions in pyoderma gangrenosum is insufficient to explain the pathogenesis of the disease. Certainly, the strongest piece of evidence indicating a disturbed immune response is the fact that pyoderma gangrenosum responds to cyclosporine, but no consistent pattern of a disturbed cellular immune response has emerged. Findings include anergy to recall antigens,[12] impairment of both antigen-specific and mitogen-induced lymphocyte proliferation,[13] inhibition of allogeneic and autologous mixed lymphocyte proliferation,[14] and defective monocyte phagocytosis linked to an IgG paraprotein that inhibits Fc-dependent phagocytosis of normal monocytes.[15] All these findings have appeared in some individual patients, but not in others. Thus, although evidence suggests that disturbances of immunoregulation and immunologic effector functions occur in some patients with pyoderma gangrenosum, these disruptions are not detectable in others; it is unclear whether they are epiphenomena.

CLINICAL MANIFESTATIONS

The salient feature of pyoderma gangrenosum is an ulcer with a raised inflammatory border and a boggy, necrotic base. It starts as a deep-seated, painful nodule or as a superficial hemorrhagic pustule (Fig. 98-1*A*), either de novo or after minimal trauma. The lesions break down and ulcerate, discharging a purulent and hemorrhagic exudate (Fig. 98-1*B*). The irregular, crenated border is elevated and is dusky red or purplish; it is undermined, soggy, and often perforated so that pressure releases pus (Fig. 98-1*C* and *D*).

A halo of bright erythema surrounds the margin of an advancing ulceration (Figs. 98-1*B*,98-1*C*, and 98-2*B*), which may expand rapidly in one direction and more slowly in another so that a serpiginous configuration results (Fig. 98-2*B*). The base of such an ulcer is partially covered with necrotic material (Fig. 98-3*A*) and studded with small abscesses (see Figs. 98-1*C* and 98-3*A*). Ulcers may be confined to the dermis, but they often extend into the fat and even down to the fascia (see Figs. 98-1*D*, 98-2*B*, and 98-3).

Lesions are usually solitary, but may arise in clusters that then coalesce to form multicentric, irregular ulcerations. Multiple lesions may arise simultaneously or consecutively in different parts of the body (see Fig. 98-2*A*). Any area of the body may be involved. Mucous membranes are usually spared, but aphthous lesions are sometimes seen in the oral mucosa. Massive ulcerative involvement of the oral cavity, larynx and pharynx, vulva, cervix, and eyes occasionally occurs.

Pyoderma gangrenosum may occur at any age. Its clinical course may follow one of two patterns: (1) an explosive onset with rapid spread of lesions or (2) a slow, indolent progression. Pain, signs of a toxic reaction and fever, hemorrhagic blisters and suppuration, extensive necrosis, and soggy ulcer margins with a highly inflammatory halo characterize the first type of pyoderma gangrenosum (see Figs. 98-1, 98-2, and 98-3). The slow, indolent form clinically exhibits massive granulation within the ulcer from the onset, crusting, and even hyperkeratosis at the margins; it spreads gradually, grazing over large areas of the body for months. Spontaneous regression and healing in one area and progression in another are characteristic of the slow form (Fig. 98-4*A* and *B*). In both forms, healing occurs spontaneously at some time in the disease process, resulting in thin, atrophic, usually cribriform scars.

Rarely, pyoderma gangrenosum may start in the subcutaneous fat, presenting as an extremely painful, suppurative panniculitis

FIGURE 98-1

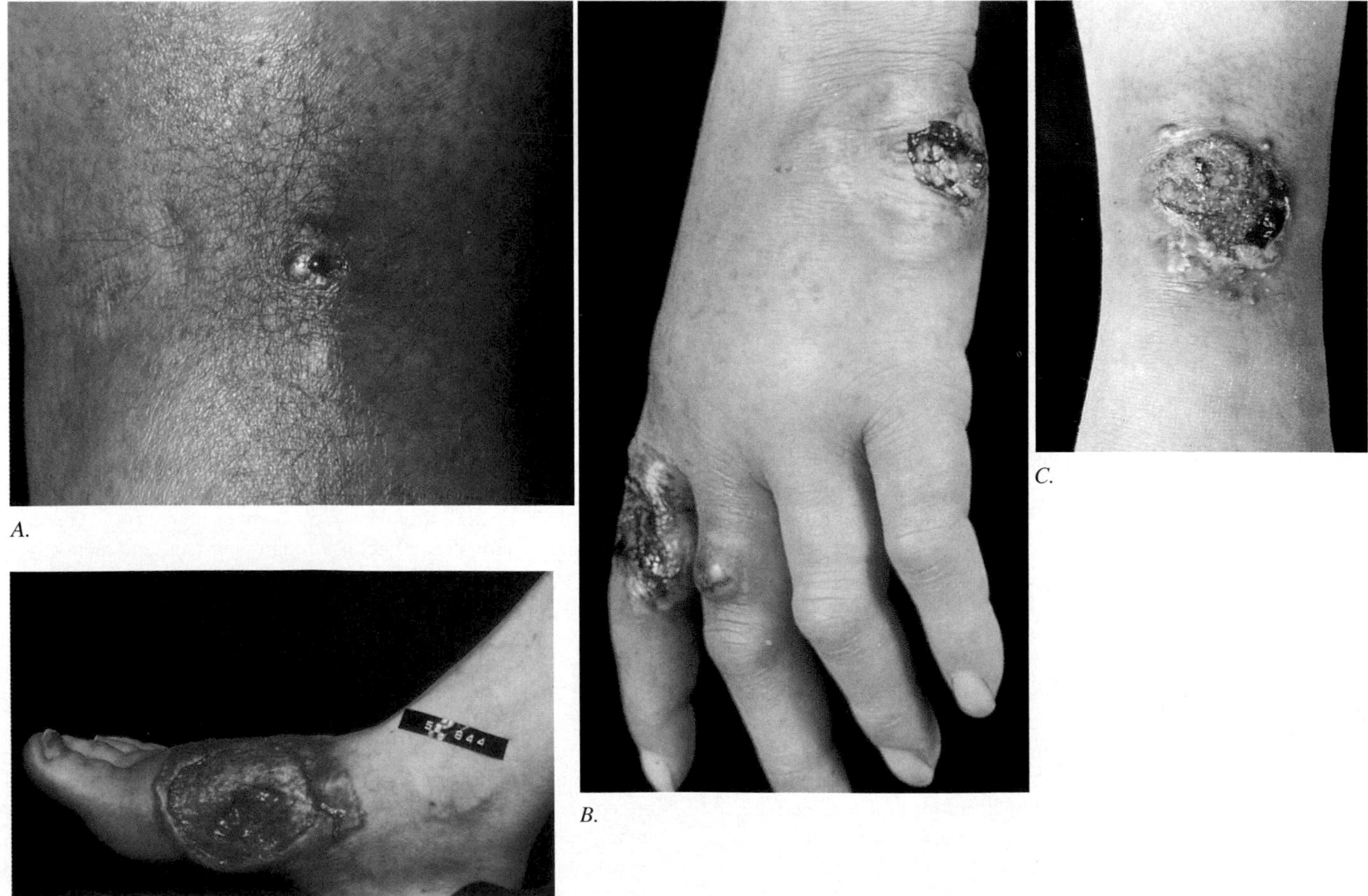

Lesions of pyoderma gangrenosum in various stages of development. *A*. A small, hemorrhagic pustule with an extremely painful red base. *B*. Three rapidly spreading hemorrhagic, bullous lesions that have broken down in the center, revealing a necrotic and purulent base. *C*. A rapidly progressive ulcerative lesion with a soggy, pustular, and partially undermined margin; a granulating necrotic base; and a red inflammatory halo. *D*. A larger ulcerating lesion with undermined bullous margins; a necrotic, purulent base; and a deep ulcer in the center.

FIGURE 98-2

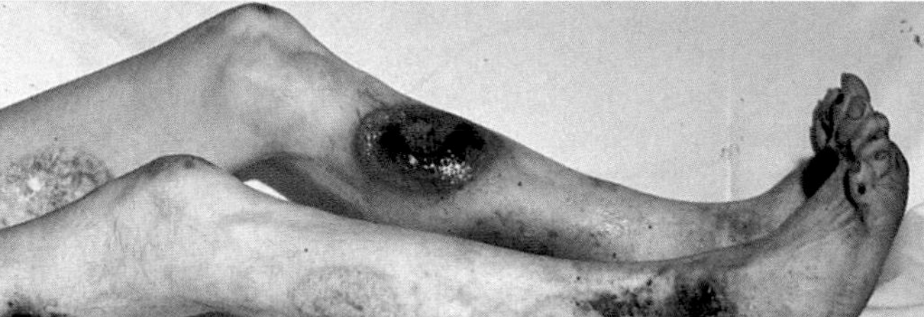

A.

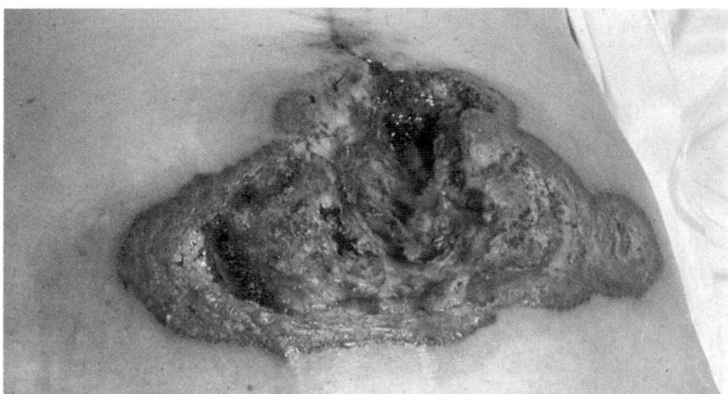

B.

A. Multiple lesions of pyoderma gangrenosum in a patient who later died of Wegener's granulomatosis. Note multiple, atrophic scars that have resulted from previous flareups of pyoderma gangrenosum. *B.* Rapidly enlarging pyoderma gangrenosum triggered by laparotomy. The lesion spread to involve the entire lower abdomen within 5 days.

FIGURE 98-3

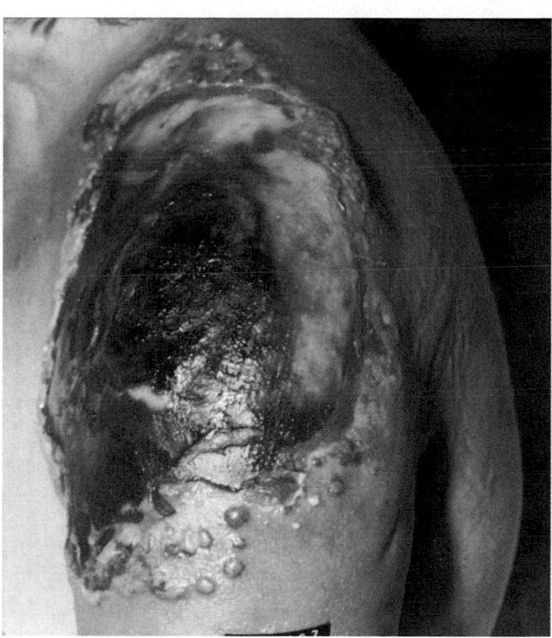

A.

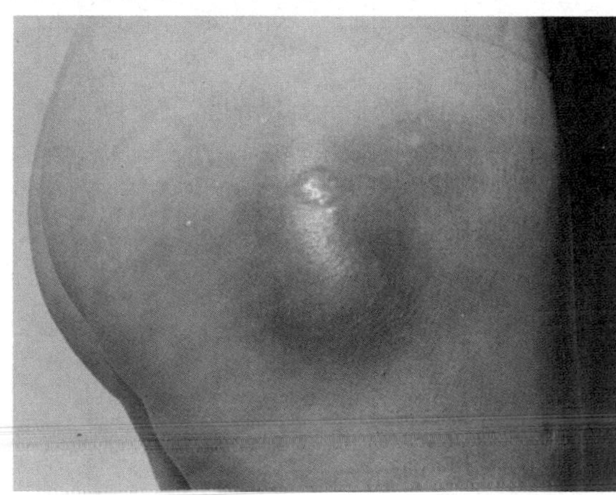

B.

Lesions of pyoderma gangrenosum. *A.* An acute, necrotic ulcer with an elevated purulent border studded with pustules. *B.* Lesion that started in the subcutaneous fat and thus presented as acute, purulent panniculitis. Bullous lesions have developed on the surface. When this lesion broke down, an ulcer similar to that shown in Fig. 98-1 *D* developed, extending all the way down to the fascia.

(Fig. 98-3*B*). Breakdown of the lesion and the centrifugal spread of the resulting ulcer eventually reveal the true nature of the process.

CLINICAL VARIANTS

A localized, vegetative form of pyoderma gangrenosum with verrucous and ulcerative lesions and a more granulomatous histology has been identified and designated superficial granulomatous pyoderma.[16] Most authors consider this condition, originally described as malignant pyoderma,[17] to be a variant of pyoderma gangrenosum,[18] although some of these cases may have actually been a form of Wegener's granulomatosis.[19] Pyostomatitis vegetans, a pustular, vegetative process of the oral mucous membranes often associated with ulcerative and vegetating skin lesions and inflammatory bowel disease, is now also considered a variant of pyoderma gangrenosum.

An atypical, bullous form of pyoderma gangrenosum appears to herald preleukemic or leukemic states.[20,21] It has an acute onset, is more superficial than the typical pyoderma gangrenosum, and is characterized by steadily enlarging, soft purple papules and blue-gray, hemorrhagic bullous lesions. This condition is similar to the bullous form of acute febrile neutrophilic dermatosis (Sweet's syndrome; see Chap. 94).[22,23]

EXACERBATING FACTORS

Intradermal skin testing or injections (including even the injection of saline), pricks, insect bites, biopsies, and operations may induce new lesions of pyoderma gangrenosum. This phenomenon is called pathergy. The lesions shown in Figure 98-2*B* arose after laparotomy for a gynecologic problem. However, pathergy occurs in only 20 percent of patients,[24] and, because some individuals with the disease tolerate even major surgery well, the significance of pathergy is difficult to assess. Pathergy may also be the reason for the rejection of autologous skin grafts and the development of new lesions in donor sites, but again, patients with pyoderma gangrenosum do not always reject skin grafts. Potassium iodide can induce an exacerbation of pyoderma gangrenosum,[1] as can GM-CSF and interferon,[3,4] but, as is true for pathergy after trauma, this exacerbation does not always occur.

FIGURE 98-4

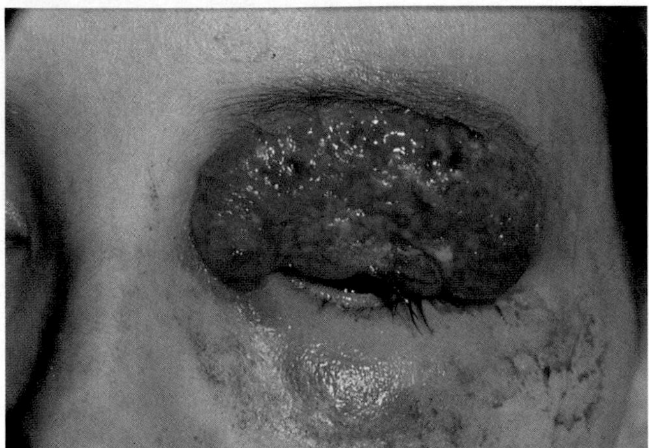

A.

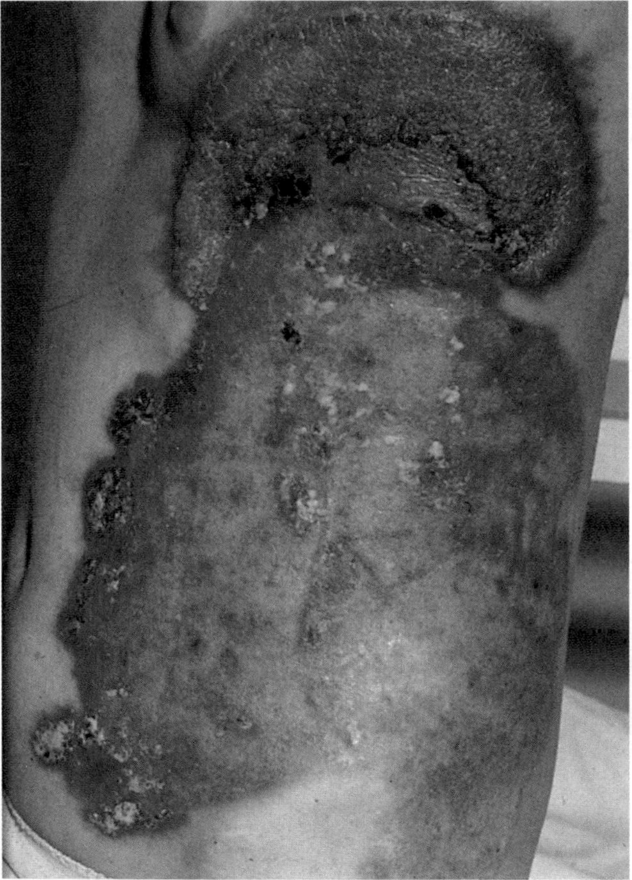

B.

A. Chronic form of pyoderma gangrenosum involving the upper eyelid. The ulcer has an elevated granulating base with multiple small abscesses. *B.* Lesion of chronic pyoderma gangrenosum that slowly spread over months to involve almost the entire trunk. The lesion is less inflammatory than the one shown in *A*; it is progressive at the margins on the abdomen and the lateral chest, while it has spontaneously healed in the center, the hip, and the back.

LABORATORY FINDINGS

No laboratory findings are specific and thus diagnostic of pyoderma gangrenosum. A high erythrocyte sedimentation rate and leukocytosis are invariably present. The level of C-reactive protein may be raised; there may be anemia and a low level of serum iron. Both hyper- and hypoglobulinemia occur. Specific autoantibodies are not known; the complement system is not altered, and circulating immune complexes have not been detected regularly.[7,13,25] HLA typing has not revealed a consistent pattern.[7]

PATHOLOGY

The histopathologic features of pyoderma gangrenosum are not diagnostic. They include edema, massive neutrophilic inflammation, engorgement and thrombosis of small- and medium-sized vessels, necrosis, and hemorrhage. The extremely dense infiltrate of polymorphonuclear leukocytes leads to abscess formation and liquefaction necrosis of the tissue with secondary thrombosis of venules. Lesions further evolve to suppurative granulomatous dermatitis and regress with prominent fibroplasia.[26]

The occurrence of necrotizing vasculitis in lesions of pyoderma gangrenosum was controversial in the past, but a number of authors have now described fibrinoid necrosis, leukocytoclasia,[27,28] and intramural deposition of C3 in vessels of pyoderma gangrenosum lesions[29,30] that are indistinguishable from those associated with immune complex vasculitis. There also exist reports on the concomitant occurrence of pyoderma gangrenosum and necrotizing vasculitis,[28,31–33] and patients with pyoderma gangrenosum have been reported to develop Wegener's granulomatosis.[34] However, the ultimate proof for a pathogenic role of immune complex vasculitis has yet to be provided. When pyoderma gangrenosum is associated with Crohn's disease, lesions may contain granulomatous foci with giant cells.[35] When localized in the fat, it presents as subcutaneous abscess.[36]

ASSOCIATION WITH SYSTEMIC DISEASE

Pyoderma gangrenosum may occur as a disease confined to the skin in 40 to 50 percent of cases (idiopathic pyoderma gangrenosum),[37,38] but it may sometimes manifest itself in extracutaneous sites. Peripheral ulcerative keratitis is an inflammatory keratitis characterized by cellular infiltration, corneal thinning, and ulceration.[39] Cavitating pulmonary infiltrates may also occur in pyoderma gangrenosum.[40,41] Among the systemic diseases sometimes associated with pyoderma gangrenosum are inflammatory large- and small-bowel disease, arthritis, paraproteinemia and myeloma, myeloproliferative disease, and Behçet's syndrome. The heterogeneity of these conditions makes pinpointing a common denominator difficult. Common and less common disease associations are listed in Table 98-1.

Ulcerative Colitis and Crohn's Disease

In its original description, pyoderma gangrenosum was associated with ulcerative colitis in four of five cases,[1] and subsequent series have found a frequency ranging from 30 to 60 percent.[42] These figures are probably too high, for other studies have found a frequency of up to only 15 percent.[43] Also, pyoderma gangrenosum occurs only rarely in ulcerative colitis, with a reported prevalence ranging from 0.6 to

5 percent.[44] Nonetheless, together with erythema nodosum, pyoderma gangrenosum represents the most common dermatologic disorder accompanying ulcerative colitis. In most patients, symptoms of ulcerative colitis precede pyoderma gangrenosum, and exacerbations of the bowel disease frequently correlate with a worsening of the skin lesions. However, pyoderma gangrenosum may persist for long periods while the bowel disease is quiescent.

Pyoderma gangrenosum is also associated with Crohn's disease. In one series, 16.3 percent of patients with pyoderma gangrenosum had Crohn's disease,[45] but the overall prevalence is low (1.2 percent).[46] In inflammatory bowel disease, the most frequent localization of pyoderma gangrenosum is on the lower legs and around a stoma[47] (see Chap. 129).

TABLE 98-1

Systemic Disease Associations with Pyoderma Gangrenosum

	Common	Less Common/Rare
Gastrointestinal	Chronic ulcerative colitis Crohn's disease	Chronic active hepatitis Diverticulitis Primary biliary cirrhosis Gastric and duodenal ulcers
Arthritis	Seronegative with IBD Seropositive without IBD Rheumatoid arthritis	Spondylitis Osteoarthritis
Gammopathy	Monoclonal IgA gammopathy	IgG and IgM gammopathy Congenital IgA deficiency
Hematologic disease	Myeloid leukemia	Myeloma Smoldering leukemia Agnogenic myelodysplasia Myelofibrosis Hairy cell leukemia Polycythemia vera Thrombocytopenic purpura
Collagen-vascular disease	Takayasu's disease (in Japan)	Systemic lupus erythematosus Antiphospholipid antibody/ lupus anticoagulant syndrome Wegener's granulomatosis Necrotizing vasculitis Rheumatoid uveitis and scleritis
Other	None	Behçet's disease Pneumonitis, lung abscess Paroxysmal hemoglobinuria Diabetes Solid tumors

NOTE: IBD, inflammatory bowel disease.

Arthritis

Arthritis is frequently associated with pyoderma gangrenosum and usually precedes it. In one review,[24] arthritis was found in 30 percent of patients with pyoderma gangrenosum. In a study of 86 patients from the Mayo Clinic, arthritis was the most frequently associated disorder.[45] Some patients have classic seropositive rheumatoid arthritis[48]; others have the arthritis associated with inflammatory bowel disease, which is seronegative, acute, oligoarticular, and nondestructive; others have a seronegative rheumatoid-like arthritic syndrome; still others have spondylitis. An association of pyoderma gangrenosum with the synovitis, acne, pustulosis, hyperostosis, and osteitis (SAPHO) syndrome[49,50] and with psoriatic arthritis (see Chap. 43) has been described. In addition, pyoderma gangrenosum is a clinical manifestation of the autosomal dominant PAPA syndrome characterized by pyogenic arthritis, pyoderma gangrenosum, and cystic acne.[2,51]

Monoclonal Gammopathy

Pyoderma gangrenosum is often associated with paraproteinemia, mostly of the IgA type, but also of the IgG and IgM types. In one series,[52] monoclonal gammopathy was found in 5 of 21 patients, and in 4 of the 5 it was of the IgA type. In another series, a monoclonal gammopathy was present in 10 percent of those studied.[45] Although patients with a monoclonal gammopathy do not show progression to malignancy over the short term, some patients with pyoderma gangrenosum have myeloma at presentation or develop it subsequently.[7,24]

Myeloproliferative Disorders

Pyoderma gangrenosum occurs in myelodysplasia,[53] as well as in acute myeloblastic, myelomonocytic, and chronic myeloid leukemia.[42,54,55] A few cases have been associated with smoldering leukemia, hairy cell leukemia, polycythemia vera, erythroid hypoplasia, autoimmune hemolytic anemia, myelofibrosis, and Hodgkin's disease. The features of "atypical bullous" pyoderma gangrenosum overlap with those of Sweet's syndrome presenting as an association with acute leukemia (see Chap. 94).

Other Conditions

Several studies have documented patients with pyoderma gangrenosum and Behçet's syndrome.[56–58] The two diseases share certain features, such as arthritis, pustulation, aphthous lesions of the mucous membranes, and the phenomenon of pathergy. Pyoderma gangrenosum has occurred in association with other purulent diseases, such as acne conglobata and fulminans[59,60] (see Chap. 73), the PAPA syndrome,[2,51] vasculitis,[32,33] erythema elevatum diutinum[61] (see Chap. 95), and Wegener's granulomatosis.[34,62] Figure 98-2*A* shows multiple lesions of pyoderma gangrenosum in a patient who, during the course of the disease, developed necrotizing vasculitis and eventually died of Wegener's granulomatosis. There is an increased frequency (up to 30 percent) of pyoderma gangrenosum in patients with Takayasu's disease in Japan,[63] but not in Europe where such associations are rare.[64] Additional, probably fortuitous, associations are listed in Table 98-1.

Relationship to Other Neutrophilic Dermatoses

The predominant cell in lesions of pyoderma gangrenosum is the neutrophil. This, together with the absence of any sign of infection and the response of pyoderma gangrenosum to sulfa drugs, places pyoderma gangrenosum into the group of etiologically ill-understood neutrophilic dermatoses, such as Sweet's syndrome (see Chap. 94), subcorneal pustular dermatosis (see Chap. 69), Behçet's syndrome (see Chap. 192), neutrophilic eccrine hidradenitis, and rheumatoid neutrophilic dermatitis (see Chap. 179). In the past, pyoderma gangrenosum has been reported in association with generalized, vesiculopustular eruptions, which in retrospect appear to have been subcorneal pustular dermatosis (Sneddon-Wilkinson disease). Indeed, the syndrome consisting of pyoderma gangrenosum, subcorneal pustular dermatosis, and IgA gammopathy, which was first described in 1971,[65] now appears established by a number of case reports.[66–68] Subcorneal pustular dermatosis can be associated with ulcerative colitis and IgA myeloma, and it responds to sulfa drugs (see Chap. 69). These findings also hold true for pyoderma gangrenosum. Generalized pustular eruptions occur in patients with ulcerative colitis; whereas some of these pustular lesions progress to frank pyoderma gangrenosum in some patients, others do not.

DIFFERENTIAL DIAGNOSIS

Because there is no specific laboratory test for pyoderma gangrenosum and the histopathology is only suggestive, the diagnosis rests entirely on the clinical presentation and course. Differential diagnoses include postoperative gangrene, ecthyma gangrenosum, atypical mycobacterial and clostridial infection, deep mycoses, amebiasis, tropical ulcers, bromoderma, North American blastomycosis, and pemphigus vegetans. Stasis ulcers are easily excluded, but artifacts and brown recluse spider bites may occasionally cause problems in early, developing lesions. Wegener's granulomatosis includes involvement of the upper respiratory tract and histopathologically displays necrotizing and granulomatous vasculitis; as mentioned previously, however, the two diseases may occur together.

TREATMENT

In patients with underlying disease, therapy should focus not only on pyoderma gangrenosum, but also and primarily on the systemic disorder. In milder forms and those not associated with systemic disease, a trial of local or topical treatment may be appropriate. Some authorities have advocated the intralesional injection of glucocorticoids into the active border of the lesions; the use of hyperbaric oxygen; or topical treatment with disodium cromoglycate, cyclosporine, or tacrolimus. With the possible exception of the topical use of tacrolimus,[69,70] topical treatment alone is usually insufficient both in patients with associated systemic disease and in most of those having purely cutaneous pyoderma gangrenosum. Although measures directed at cleaning the ulcer and preventing bacterial overgrowth are important, more invasive surgical debridement is generally unwise as it may trigger new lesions. This caveat applies also to excision and grafting, unless systemic treatment has controlled the pyoderma gangrenosum. There have as yet been no enrolled clinical trials for any of the treatments.

Glucocorticoids

The systemic administration of glucocorticoids is the most effective treatment of pyoderma gangrenosum. They dramatically halt the progression of existing ulcerations and prevent the development of new lesions.[43] A high dosage of prednisone, such as 100 to 200 mg/day, may be necessary initially; the dosage is reduced as the inflammatory component of pyoderma gangrenosum disappears and is tapered slowly to discontinuation after the condition has completely resolved. Pulse therapy with suprapharmacologic doses of methylprednisolone (1 g/day for 5 consecutive days) most effectively halts progressive pyoderma gangrenosum,[59,71,72] and it is still the first-line treatment for severe pyoderma gangrenosum in many institutions. However, it is necessary to continue suppressing the inflammatory process after pulse therapy by administering prednisolone or sulfa drugs.[43] Unfortunately, long-term oral therapy with glucocorticoids produces side effects in up to 50 percent of the patients.

Sulfa Drugs

Dapsone, sulfapyridine, and sulfasalazine (Azulfidine) are beneficial drugs for pyoderma gangrenosum, but not all patients respond equally well to them. Initial daily doses of sulfasalazine range from 4 to 6 g; the dosage is gradually reduced to maintenance levels of 0.5 to 1 g/day. It may be necessary to administer sulfa drugs in combination with glucocorticoids (given systemically), particularly in the initial phases of therapy, but there have been patients who have failed to respond to this regimen as well.

The mechanism of action of the sulfa drugs in pyoderma gangrenosum is unknown, but may be related to a stabilizing effect on lysosomes, to their interference with the myeloperoxidase-halide system of polymorphonuclear leukocytes, or to a decrease of glycosaminoglycan viscosity in this condition (see Chap. 254). Dapsone is effective in a host of cutaneous disorders that are all characterized by the abnormal accumulation of polymorphonuclear leukocytes, such as erythema elevatum diutinum, dermatitis herpetiformis, Sneddon-Wilkinson disease, Sweet's syndrome, and pyoderma gangrenosum.

Cyclosporine

The oral administration of cyclosporine[73–77] and tacrolimus[9,78] is very effective in the treatment of pyoderma gangrenosum. In severe cases, cyclosporine given intravenously has been successful.[77] Significant improvement occurs within weeks of the start of oral therapy with cyclosporine in doses that range from 6 to 10 mg/kg per day, and healing is likely to take place within 1 to 3 months. Some patients require low-dose maintenance therapy, but others can tolerate complete withdrawal of the drug. Also, patients may require concomitant medium- to low-dose glucocorticoid therapy. As with other immunosuppressive treatments, patients who use cyclosporine require careful monitoring for side effects.

Other Immunosuppressive Agents

Although not universally successful, 6-mercaptopurine, azathioprine, and methotrexate have been beneficial for some patients. Cyclophosphamide has induced dramatic remissions in some patients,[79,80] and chlorambucil has demonstrated a glucocorticoid-sparing effect.[81,82] Mycophenolate mofetil, either alone or in combination with cyclosporine, has also been useful.[83–85]

Clofazimine

Reports have stressed the efficacy of clofazimine (Lamprene) in pyoderma gangrenosum.[86,87] Dosages of 200 to 300 mg/day supposedly stop progression of lesions within 1 to 2 weeks and lead to complete or partial healing within 2 to 5 months. However, clofazimine may have adverse effects, and some patients do not respond to this drug at all.

Anti–Tumor Necrosis Factor-α

There is no laboratory evidence that tumor necrosis factor-α (TNF-α) plays a pathogenic role in pyoderma gangrenosum. However, monoclonal antibodies to TNF-α are beneficial in Crohn's disease and ulcerative colitis, and such antibodies (infliximab) have also been used in the treatment of pyoderma gangrenosum, apparently with success.[88,89]

Miscellaneous Treatments

Pyoderma gangrenosum has been reported to respond to minocycline, colchicine, and heparin, as well as to the intravenous administration of vancomycin and mezlocillin; although, as indicated by worldwide experience, it is usually unresponsive to any kind of antibiotic. It has been reported to improve with a combination of sulfasalazine and isotretinoin and to respond to interferon-α.[90,91] However, it has also been reported that interferon triggers pyoderma gangrenosum.[4] Plasmapheresis has been successfully used in the treatment of patients with pyoderma gangrenosum.[92,93] Immunoglobulin[94] (given intravenously) and thalidomide are of benefit to patients with pyoderma gangrenosum, both with and without an association with Behçet's disease.[56,57,95]

COURSE AND PROGNOSIS

Pyoderma gangrenosum behaves in an unpredictable way. It may have a dramatic onset with pustular and bullous lesions rapidly breaking down to form ulcers, which progressively enlarge (see Figs. 98-1, 98-2, and 98-3) until arrested by treatment; in these cases, there may be signs of toxicity, fever, and considerable pain. More chronic forms of the disease show ulcers that extend slowly in a creeping fashion (see Fig. 98-4), expanding in one direction and healing spontaneously in another or in the center. In both forms, spontaneous healing can occur, but as old lesions resolve, new lesions may arise. The disease may come to a spontaneous halt for no apparent reason; remain quiescent for months and even years; and exacerbate again after minimal trauma, surgery, or no apparent triggering cause. When associated with ulcerative colitis, the disease activity of pyoderma gangrenosum may parallel that of the bowel disease, but not always. The same is true for patients with associated hematologic disease, in which the underlying condition determines the final prognosis. The overall prognosis of pyoderma gangrenosum per se is good, particularly in those patients who readily respond to treatment, but considerable scarring and disfigurement may occur.

REFERENCES

1. Brunsting LA et al: Pyoderma (ecthyma) gangrenosum: Clinical and experimental observations in five cases occurring in adults. *Arch Dermatol* **22**:655, 1930
2. Yeon HB et al: Pyogenic arthritis, pyoderma gangrenosum, and acne syndrome maps to chromosome 15q. *Am J Hum Genet* **66**:1443, 2000
3. Johnson ML, Grimwood RE: Leukocyte colony-stimulating factors: A review of associated neutrophilic dermatoses and vasculitides. *Arch Dermatol* **130**:77, 1994
4. Montoto S et al: Pyoderma gangrenosum triggered by alpha2b-interferon in a patient with chronic granulocytic leukemia. *Leuk Lymphoma* **30**:199, 1998
5. Oka M et al: Interleukin-8 overexpression is present in pyoderma gangrenosum ulcers and leads to ulcer formation in human skin xenografts. *Lab Invest* **80**:595, 2000
6. Shapiro D et al: Pyoderma gangrenosum successfully treated with perilesional granulocyte-macrophage colony stimulating factor. *Br J Dermatol* **138**:368, 1998
7. Holt PJA et al: Pyoderma gangrenosum: Clinical and laboratory findings in 15 patients with special reference to polyarthritis. *Medicine (Baltimore)* **59**:114, 1980
8. Shore RN: Pyoderma gangrenosum, defective neutrophil chemotaxis, and leukemia. *Arch Dermatol* **112**:792, 1976
9. Abu-Elmagd K et al: Resolution of pyoderma gangrenosum in a patient with streaking leukocyte factor disease after treatment with tacrolimus (FK 506). *Ann Intern Med* **119**:595, 1993
10. Adachi Y et al: Aberrant neutrophil trafficking and metabolic oscillations in severe pyoderma gangrenosum. *J Invest Dermatol* **111**:259, 1998
11. Berbis P et al: Hyperimmunoglobulin E and impaired neutrophil functions in a case of pyoderma gangrenosum: Effect of clofazimine. *Am Acad Dermatol* **18**:574, 1988

12. Lazarus GS et al: Pyoderma gangrenosum, altered delayed hypersensitivity, and polyarthritis. *Arch Dermatol* **105**:46, 1972
13. Breathnach SM et al: Idiopathic pyoderma gangrenosum and impaired lymphocyte functions: Failure of azathioprine and corticosteroid therapy. *Br J Dermatol* **104**:567, 1981
14. Greenberg SJ et al: Pyoderma gangrenosum: Occurrence with altered cellular immunity and circulating serum factor. *Arch Dermatol* **188**:498, 1982
15. Jones RR et al: Defective monocyte function in pyoderma gangrenosum with IgG kappa paraproteinaemia. *Clin Exp Immunol* **82**:685, 1983
16. Wilson Jones E, Winkelmann RK: Superficial granulomatous pyoderma: A localized vegetative form of pyoderma gangrenosum. *Am Acad Dermatol* **18**:511, 1988
17. Perry HO et al: Malignant pyoderma. *Arch Dermatol* **98**:561, 1968
18. Callen JP: Pyoderma gangrenosum and related disorders. *Adv Dermatol* **4**:51, 1989
19. Gibson LE et al: Malignant pyodermas revisited. *Mayo Clin Proc* **72**:734, 1997
20. Perry HO, Winkelmann RK: Bullous pyoderma gangrenosum and leukemia. *Arch Dermatol* **196**:901, 1972
21. Lewis JE et al: Atypical pyoderma gangrenosum with leukemia. *JAMA* **239**:935, 1980
22. Burton JL: Sweet's syndrome, pyoderma gangrenosum, and acute leukemia. *Br J Dermatol* **102**:239, 1980
23. Caughman W et al: Neutrophilic dermatosis of myeloproliferative disorders: Atypical forms of pyoderma gangrenosum and Sweet's syndrome associated with myeloproliferative disorders. *Am Acad Dermatol* **9**:751, 1983
24. Van der Sluis I: Two cases of pyoderma (ecthyma) gangrenosum associated with the presence of an abnormal serum protein (beta2A-paraprotein): With a review of the literature. *Dermatologica* **132**:409, 1966
25. Fernandez Bussy R et al: Evaluation of circulating immune complexes in cutaneous diseases associated with immune disorders. *Allergol Immunopathol (Madr)* **18**:47, 1990
26. Hurwitz RM, Haseman JH: The evolution of pyoderma gangrenosum: A clinicopathologic correlation. *Am Dermatopathol* **15**:28, 1993
27. Benci M et al: Pyoderma gangrenosum, an unusual aspect of cutaneous vasculitis. *Clin Dermatol* **17**:581, 1999
28. Calabrese LH: Cutaneous vasculitis, hypersensitivity vasculitis, erythema nodosum and pyoderma gangrenosum. *Curr Probl Rheumatol* **2**:66, 1990
29. Su WP et al: Histopathologic and immunopathologic study of pyoderma gangrenosum. *J Cutan Pathol* **13**:323, 1986
30. Powell FC et al: Direct immunofluorescence in pyoderma gangrenosum. *Br J Dermatol* **108**:287, 1983
31. English JSC et al: Pyoderma gangrenosum and leukocytoclastic vasculitis in association with rheumatoid arthritis: A report of two cases. *Clin Exp Dermatol* **9**:270, 1984
32. Wong E, Greaves MW: Pyoderma gangrenosum and leukocytoclastic vasculitis. *Clin Exp Dermatol* **10**:72, 1985
33. Callen JP: Cutaneous vasculitis and other neutrophilic dermatoses. *Curr Opin Rheumatol* **5**:33, 1993
34. Thomas RHM et al: Wegener's granulomatosis presenting as pyoderma gangrenosum. *Clin Exp Dermatol* **7**:523, 1982
35. Sanders S et al: Giant cells in pyoderma gangrenosum. *J Cutan Pathol* **28**:97, 2001
36. Hara H et al: Subcutaneous abscesses in a patient with ulcerative colitis. *J Am Acad Dermatol* **42**:363, 2000
37. Hickman JG, Lazarus GS: Pyoderma gangrenosum: A reappraisal of associated systemic diseases. *Br J Dermatol* **110**:235, 1980
38. Powell FC et al: Pyoderma gangrenosum: Classification and management. *J Am Acad Dermatol* **34**:395, 1996
39. Wilson DM et al: Peripheral ulcerative keratitis—An extracutaneous neutrophilic disorder: Report of a patient with rheumatoid arthritis, pustular vasculitis, pyoderma gangrenosum, and Sweet's syndrome with an excellent response to cyclosporine therapy. *J Am Acad Dermatol* **40**:331, 1999
40. Brown TS et al: Cavitating pulmonary infiltrate in an adolescent with pyoderma gangrenosum: A rarely recognized extracutaneous manifestation of a neutrophilic dermatosis. *J Am Acad Dermatol* **43**:108, 2000
41. Kruger S et al: Multiple aseptic pulmonary nodules with central necrosis in association with pyoderma gangrenosum. *Chest* **119**:977, 2001
42. Perry HO: Pyoderma gangrenosum. *South Med J* **62**:899, 1969
43. Hickman JG, Lazarus GS: Pyoderma gangrenosum: New concepts in etiology and treatment, in *Dermatology Update: Review for Physicians*, edited by SL Moschella. New York, Elsevier, 1979, p 325

44. Greenstein AJ et al: The extraintestinal complications of Crohn's disease and ulcerative colitis: A study of 700 patients. *Medicine (Baltimore)* **55**:401, 1976
45. Powell FC et al: Pyoderma gangrenosum: A review of 86 patients. *Am J Med* **55**:173, 1985
46. Bernstein CN et al: The prevalence of extraintestinal diseases in inflammatory bowel disease: A population-based study. *Am J Gastroenterol* **96**:1116, 2001
47. Lyon CC et al: Parastoma pyoderma gangrenosum: Clinical features and management. *J Am Acad Dermatol* **42**:992, 2000
48. Ko CB et al: Pyoderma gangrenosum: Associations revisited. *Int J Dermatol* **31**:574, 1992
49. Claudepierre P et al: SAPHO syndrome and pyoderma gangrenosum: Is it fortuitous? *J Rheumatol* **23**:400, 1996
50. Beretta-Piccoli BC et al: Synovitis, acne, pustulosis, hyperostosis, osteitis (SAPHO) syndrome in childhood: A report of ten cases and review of the literature. *Eur J Pediatr* **159**:594, 2000
51. Lindor NM et al: A new autosomal dominant disorder of pyogenic sterile arthritis, pyoderma gangrenosum, and acne PAPA syndrome. *Mayo Clin Proc* **72**:611, 1997
52. Prystowsky J et al: Present status of pyoderma gangrenosum. *Arch Dermatol* **125**:57, 1989
53. Avivi I et al: Myelodysplastic syndrome and associated skin lesions: A review of the literature. Leuk Res **23**:323, 1999
54. Asai M et al: Pyoderma gangrenosum associated with biphenotypic acute leukemia. *J Am Acad Dermatol* **44**:530, 2001
55. Beele H et al: Pyoderma gangrenosum as an early relevator of acute leukemia. *Dermatology* **200**:176, 2000
56. Munro CS, Cox NH: Pyoderma gangrenosum associated with Behçet's syndrome: Response to thalidomide. *Clin Exp Dermatol* **13**:408, 1988
57. Rustin MHA et al.: Pyoderma gangrenosum associated with Behçet's disease: Treatment with thalidomide. *J Am Acad Dermatol* **23**:941, 1990
58. Lee LA: Behçet disease. *Semin Cutan Med Surg* **20**:53, 2001
59. Velez A et al: Pyoderma gangrenosum associated with acne conglobata. *Clin Exp Dermatol* **20**:496, 1995
60. Kurokawa S et al: Acne fulminans with pyoderma gangrenosum–like eruptions and posterior scleritis. *Dermatol* **23**:37, 1996
61. Wayte JA et al: Pyoderma gangrenosum, erythema elevatum diutinum and IgA monoclonal gammopathy. *Australas J Dermatol* **36**:21, 1995
62. Handfield JS et al: Wegener's granulomatosis presenting as pyoderma gangrenosum. *Clin Exp Dermatol* **117**:197, 1992
63. Kobayashi K et al: A case of pyoderma gangrenosum with Takayasu's arteritis. *J Transpl Med* **42**:181, 1988
64. Frances C et al: Cutaneous manifestations of Takayasu arteritis: A retrospective study of 80 cases. *Dermatologica* **181**:266, 1990
65. Wolff K: Subkorneale pustulöse Dermatose (Sneddon-Wilkinson): Pyoderma gangraenosum mit IgA-Paraproteinämie. *Dermatol Monatsschr* **157**:842, 1971
66. Fraire Murgueytio P et al: Gangrenous pyoderma associated with subcorneal pustular dermatosis (Sneddon-Wilkinson disease). *Med Cutan Iber Lat Am* **17**:105, 1989
67. Marsen JR, Millard LG: Pyoderma gangrenosum, subcorneal pustular dermatosis, and IgA paraproteinemia. *Br J Dermatol* **114**:125, 1986
68. Stone MS, Lyckholm LJ: Pyoderma gangrenosum and subcorneal pustular dermatosis: Clues to underlying immunoglobulin A myeloma. *Am J Med* **100**:663, 1996
69. Reich K et al: Topical tacrolimus for pyoderma gangrenosum. *Br J Dermatol* **139**:755, 1998
70. Petering H et al: Pyoderma gangrenosum—Erfolgreiche toische Therapie mit Tacrolimus (FK 506). *Hautarzt* **52**:47, 2001
71. Johnson RB, Lazarus GS: Pulse therapy, therapeutic efficacy in the treatment of pyoderma gangrenosum. *Arch Dermatol* 118:**76**, 1982
72. Chow RK, Ho VC: Treatment of pyoderma gangrenosum. *J Am Acad Dermatol* **34**:1047, 1996
73. Curley RK et al: Pyoderma gangrenosum treated with cyclosporin A. *Br J Dermatol* **113**:601, 1985
74. Gupta AK et al: Oral cyclosporine in the treatment of inflammatory and noninflammatory dermatoses. *Arch Dermatol* **126**:339, 1990
75. Capella GL et al: The simultaneous treatment of inflammatory bowel disease and associated pyoderma gangrenosum with oral cyclosporin A. *Scand J Gastroenterol* **34**:220, 1999
76. Ho VC et al: Cyclosporine in the treatment of dermatologic disease: An update. *Mayo Clin Proc* **71**:1182, 1996
77. Friedman S et al: Intravenous cyclosporine in refractory pyoderma gangrenosum complicating inflammatory bowel disease. *Inflamm Bowel Dis* **7**:1, 2001
78. Jolles S et al: Combination oral and topical tacrolimus in therapy-resistant pyoderma gangrenosum. *Br J Dermatol* **140**:564, 1999
79. Zonana-Nacach A et al: Intravenous cyclophosphamide pulses in the treatment of pyoderma gangrenosum associated with rheumatoid arthritis. *J Rheumatol* **21**:1352, 1994
80. Reynoso-von Drateln C et al: Intravenous cyclophosphamide pulses in pyoderma gangrenosum: an open trial. *J Rheumatol* **24**:689, 1997
81. Burns JB et al: Chlorambucil is an effective corticosteroid-sparing agent for recalcitrant pyoderma gangrenosum. *J Am Acad Dermatol* **35**:720, 1996
82. Resnik BI et al: Successful treatment of aggressive pyoderma gangrenosum with pulse steroids and chlorambucil. *J Am Acad Dermatol* **27**:635, 1992
83. Hohenleutner U et al: Mycophenolate mofetil and cyclosporin treatment for recalcitrant pyoderma gangrenosum. *Lancet* **350**:1748, 1997
84. Nousari HC et al: The effectiveness of mycophenolate mofetil in refractory pyoderma gangrenosum. *Arch Dermatol* **134**:1509, 1998
85. Gilmour E, Stewart DG: Severe recalcitrant pyoderma gangrenosum responding to a combination of mycophenolate mofetil with cyclosporin complicated by a mononeuritis. *Br J Dermatol* **144**:397, 2001
86. Mensing H: Clofazimine in dermatitis ulcerosa (pyoderma gangrenosum): Open clinical trial. *Dermatologica* **177**:232, 1988
87. Arbeiser JL, Moschella SL: Clofazimine: A review of its medical uses and mechanisms of action. *J Am Acad Dermatol* **32**:241, 1995
88. Tan MH et al: Improvement of pyoderma gangrenosum and psoriasis associated with Crohn disease with anti-tumor necrosis factor alpha monoclonal antibody. *Arch Dermatol* **137**:930, 2001
89. Arnott ID et al: Clinical use of Infliximab in Crohn's disease: The Edinburgh experience. *Aliment Pharmacol Ther* **15**:1639, 2001
90. Smith JB et al: Pyoderma gangrenosum in a patient with cryoglobulinemia and hepatitis C successfully treated with interferon alfa. *J Am Acad Dermatol* **34**:901, 1996
91. Sanchez-Roman J et al: The treatment of cyclosporine A-resistant pyoderma gangrenosum with recombinant interferon alfa-2 [Letter]. *Med Clin (Barc)* **104**:517, 1995
92. Gerard JA et al: Pyoderma gangrenosum: Traitement par exchanges plasmatiques (4 cas). *Ann Med Interne (Paris)* **139** (suppl 1):29, 1988
93. Baumbauer R et al: Drug resistant pyoderma gangrenosum successfully treated with therapeutic plasma exchange. *Transfus Sci* **10**:349, 1989
94. Dirschka T et al: Successful treatment of pyoderma gangrenosum with intravenous human immunoglobulin. *J Am Acad Dermatol* **39**:789, 1998
95. Federman GL, Federman DG: Recalcitrant pyoderma gangrenosum treated with thalidomide. *Mayo Clin Proc* **75**:842, 2000

CHAPTER 99

Walter H. C. Burgdorf

Erythema Annulare Centrifugum and Other Figurate Erythemas

The figurate erythemas include a variety of eruptions characterized by annular and polycyclic lesions; some are fixed, but most are migratory. Many of these conditions appear related to hypersensitivity, be it to drugs, neoplasms, infections, arthropod bites, or self. Classification of the figurate erythemas has always been controversial; the literature about them abounds with contradictions, uncertainties, and a bewildering array of synonyms. The figurate erythemas and other disorders to be considered in their differential diagnosis are listed in Table 99-1.

ERYTHEMA ANNULARE CENTRIFUGUM

Erythema annulare centrifugum (EAC) denotes an eruption with slowly migrating annular and configurate erythematous lesions.

Historical Aspects

Darier first used the term *erythema annulare centrifugum* in 1916,[1] although similar lesions had been described previously under other names.

Etiology and Pathogenesis

Both the annularity and the peripheral spread of EAC have attracted speculation as to a possible mechanism. Most hypotheses have centered about interactions among inflammatory cells, their mediators, and ground substance as foreign antigens diffuse through the skin.[2] The cause of most cases of EAC is unknown. In one series, the conditions of 24 patients were closely evaluated, and in none of the cases was any clear evidence of causality found.[3] There are occasional reports of EAC associated with malignant neoplasms, with the eruption disappearing after treatment of the tumor and often recurring as the tumor recurs.[4,5] Many different infections, inhalants, and medications have been identified as causes of EAC in case reports. Bacterial or candidal infections are most often suspected as triggers.[6,7] Sometimes a true infection can spread peripherally to create an annular pattern; in an immunosuppressed host, there may be no signs of systemic toxicity.[8]

Clinical Manifestations

Erythema annulare centrifugum presents as one or more lesions that begin as erythematous macules or urticarial papules and enlarge by peripheral extension to form ringed, arcuate, or polycyclic figures. They spread gradually to form large rings with central clearing, the edges of the

TABLE 99-1

Figurate Erythemas

DISORDER	KEY FEATURES	SEE CHAPTER
Erythema annulare centrifigum (EAC)	Slowly migrating lesions, often idiopathic	99
Erythema gyratum repens	Rapidly moving; usually cancer marker	184
Erythema migrans	Annular lesions originating from tick bite; skin sign of Lyme disease	203
Annular urticaria	Giant urticaria is annular and overlaps with EAC; should have regular hives elsewhere; more pruritic than EAC	116
Bullous pemphigoid	Bullous pemphigoid often presents with urticarial lesions; sometimes they may be annular	61
Erythema multiforme	Patients have target lesions, oral involvement, acral dominance; some trunk lesions are annular	58
Dermatophyte and tinea versicolor infections	Many fungal rashes are annular and resemble superficial EAC; have peripheral scale that contains hyphae on KOH examination	205 & 206
Annular psoriasis	Pustular psoriasis may present with annular lesions	42
Annular lupus erythematosus (LE)	Most common in neonatal LE; may be seen in adults; usually associated with antibodies against Ro/La (SS-A, SS-B)	171
Erythema marginatum (erythema circinatum)	Specific for rheumatic fever; rapidly spreading, complicated ringed eruption; on occasion, precedes joint involvement	179
Necrolytic migratory erythema	Associated with glucagonoma; usually acral and orificial, but may be annular and scaly on trunk	184
Carriers of chronic granulomatous disease (CGD)	Mothers of boys with CGD may have annular LE-like rash	115
Familial annular erythema	Extremely rare; autosomal dominant	99
Annular erythema of infancy	Probably several diseases; must rule out neonatal LE	99

FIGURE 99-1

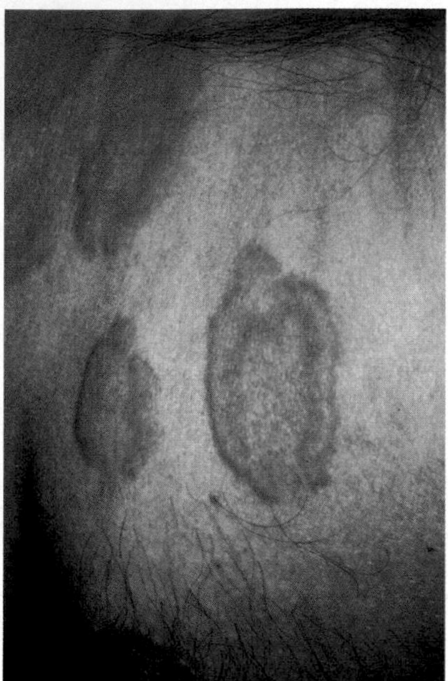

Deep figurate erythema. Annular lesions very similar to urticaria are seen without any scale.

FIGURE 99-2

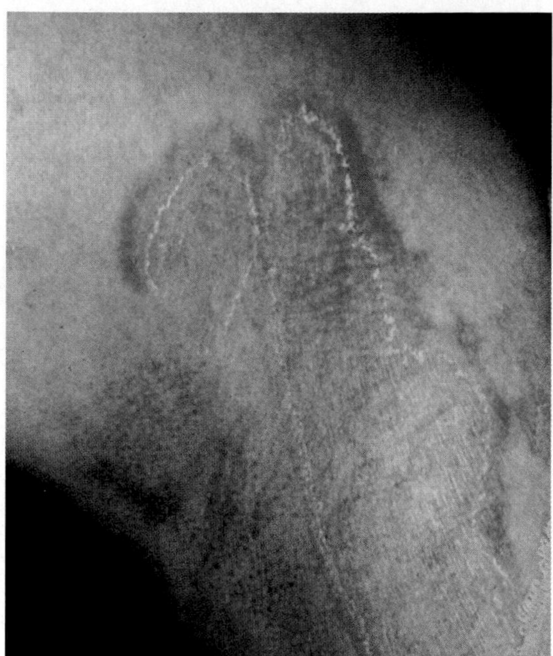

Superficial figurate erythema. A large annular patch has trailing scale behind the advancing erythematous edge.

lesions often advancing several millimeters a day. After a variable period of time, the lesions disappear, often to be replaced by new ones. Erythema annulare centrifugum appears to have no predilection for either sex or any age group.

Bressler and Jones have suggested dropping the term *erythema annulare centrifugum* and instead referring either to (1) deep gyrate erythema that has a firm yet indurated border, lacks scale, and is rarely pruritic (Fig. 99-1) or to (2) superficial gyrate erythema that has an indistinct border, has trailing scale, and is more often pruritic (Fig. 99-2).[9] Although this subdivision is reasonable, it does not help in identifying possible etiologic agents.

Pathology

The typical deep figurate erythemas lack epidermal damage and have intense lymphohistiocytic cuffing about both the superficial and deep vessels. There is minimal papillary dermal edema and no spongiosis (Fig. 99-3). On the other hand, the more superficial figurate erythemas may demonstrate epidermal changes of parakeratosis and spongiosis, with a superficial perivascular infiltrate.

Occasionally, both peripheral blood and tissue eosinophilia occur in EAC. In such cases, EAC may represent an early manifestation of the hypereosinophilic syndrome. The pathologic evaluation may produce other surprises, requiring a new diagnosis. Sometimes a leukocytoclastic vasculitis may be found. A metastatic tumor may occasionally be identified; in this case, the annular lesions usually expand slowly and are permanent.[10]

Diagnosis and Differential Diagnosis

The main differential diagnostic points are summarized in Table 99-1. It is most helpful to observe patients with figurate erythema over a period of weeks to see how they progress and how their rashes evolve. Cases of annular or figurate erythemas may not fit easily into any classification.

Patients may be approached with the following schema:

1. Are there signs or symptoms suggesting a systemic disorder such as a malignancy, infection, or other problems? Many authors feel that there is no distinction between EAC and erythema gyratum repens; since erythema gyratum repens is more often a marker for malignant disease, separation appears valid. Erythema gyratum repens tends to be scalier and move more rapidly than EAC. In addition, erythema gyratum repens often mimics the grain of wood, whereas EAC appears more annular and urticarial.
2. Is there a history of tick bite, or are other manifestations of Lyme disease present? Usually, erythema migrans appears before the rheumatologic or cardiologic problems. In Lyme disease, there are generally one or two annular lesions centered about tick bites. Erythema migrans often evolves into a plaque, which is uncommon for EAC. In EAC, multiple lesions are more common.
3. Are there urticarial or angioedematous lesions elsewhere? Urticaria is more pruritic than EAC and more short-lived.
4. Are bullous lesions present elsewhere? If so, it is wise to consider the annular urticarial phase of bullous pemphigoid or linear IgA disease. An immunofluorescence study of perilesional skin may be helpful.
5. Are the lesions predominantly oral or acral? Are blisters present? An acral distribution is uncommon in EAC and should raise the question of erythema multiforme if it occurs.
6. Is the KOH examination positive?
7. Is the rash psoriasiform? If so, both psoriasis and subacute lupus erythematosus warrant consideration. The clinician should search for psoriasis elsewhere; pustular psoriasis is more likely to present with annular lesions. In Asians and, rarely, in Caucasians, Sjögren's syndrome may present with annular lesions that probably reflect an overlap with subacute lupus erythematosus.[11] Thus, it is helpful to measure antibodies against Ro/La (SS-A, SS-B).
8. Are there other stigmata of rheumatic fever or other rheumatic diseases? Erythema marginatum is more transient than any other figurate erythema.

FIGURE 99-3

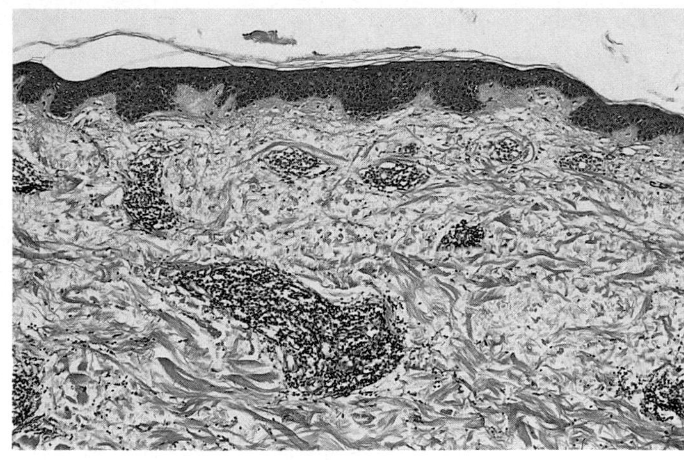

Figurate erythema. Normal epidermis overlies a dermis in which there is tight lymphocytic perivascular cuffing.

9. Are the lesions accompanied by desquamative oral and intertriginous changes or biochemical evidence of excessive glucagon production? These findings suggest necrolytic migratory erythema.
10. Is there a family history of similar lesions or of chronic granulomatous disease? Is phagocytic function normal? In one form of chronic granulomatous disease, the carrier females may have an annular eruption.
11. Is the patient an infant? The approach to figurate erythemas in this age group is slightly different from that used for older age groups. First of all, neonatal lupus erythematosus is usually annular and often occurs in conjunction with congenital heart block. Despite its rarity, it should be excluded first. Second, while there are many discussions of familial annular erythema in the literature, it is extremely rare and not often the correct diagnosis. Third, while dermatophytes and tinea versicolor are most uncommon in infants, it is necessary to exclude such infections. Finally, there are patients meeting none of these criteria who have self-limited annular erythemas, sometimes with atrophy.[12]

Treatment

Although an assiduous search for the underlying cause is the primary goal of treatment, only symptomatic help is truly available. The systemic administration of glucocorticoids usually suppresses EAC, but recurrence is common when these drugs are stopped. Systemic therapy with antipruritics may help, but topical therapy has little effect. Empirical use of antibiotic, antifungal, or anticandidal agents has sometimes been useful. In general, most of the therapeutic approaches employed for chronic urticaria can also be tried for EAC.

FAMILIAL ANNULAR ERYTHEMA

Sometimes associated with other developmental anomalies, familial annular erythema has its onset at an early age.

Historical Aspects

Colcott Fox originally described familial annular erythema in 1881 as erythema gyratum repens.[13] A small number of similar cases have since been described. Beare and colleagues provided a detailed description with color photographs.[14] The disease appears to be inherited in an autosomal dominant fashion and is extremely rare. As EAC can be familial, the diagnosis of familial annular erythema probably can be dropped.

Clinical Manifestations

The eruption appears early, perhaps only a few days after birth. The lesions are similar to those of EAC, but they are more transitory (although the patient is rarely free of them). The eruption persists for many years; the grandfather in one pedigree seems to have outlived his disease.

REFERENCES

1. Darier J: De l'érythème annulaire centrifuge. *Ann Dermatol Syphiligr* **6**:57, 1916
2. Lobitz WC et al: The anergy of annularity. *J Dermatol (Tokyo)* **11**:425, 1984
3. Mahood JM: Erythema annulare centrifugum: A review of 24 cases with special reference to its association with underlying disease. *Clin Exp Dermatol* **8**:383, 1983
4. Yaniv R et al: Erythema annulare centrifugum as the presenting sign of Hodgkin's disease. *Int J Dermatol* **32**:59, 1993
5. Ural AU et al: Erythema annulare centrifugum as the presenting sign of CD 30 positive anaplastic large cell lymphoma—Association with disease activity. *Haematologia (Budap)* **31**:81, 2001
6. Borbujo J et al: Erythema annulare centrifugum and *Escherichia coli* urinary infection. *Lancet* **347**:897, 1996
7. Schmid MH et al: Erythema annulare centrifugum and intestinal *Candida albicans* infection—Coincidence or connection? *Acta Derm Venereol* **77**:93, 1997
8. Czechowicz RT et al: *Pseudomonas aeruginosa* infection mimicking erythema annulare centrifugum. *Australas J Dermatol* **42**:57, 2001
9. Bressler GS, Jones RE Jr: Erythema annulare centrifugum. *J Am Acad Dermatol* **4**:597, 1981
10. Reichel M, Wheeland RG: Inflammatory carcinoma masquerading as erythema annulare centrifugum. *Acta Derm Venereol* **73**:138, 1993
11. Haimowitz JE et al: Annular erythema of Sjögren's syndrome in a white woman. *J Am Acad Dermatol* **42**:1069, 2000
12. Herbert AA, Esterly NB: Annular erythema of infancy. *J Am Acad Dermatol* **14**:339, 1986
13. Colcott Fox T: Erythema gyratum repens. *Trans Clin Soc Lond* **14**:67, 1881
14. Beare JM et al: Familial annulare erythema. *Br J Dermatol* **78**:59, 1966

CHAPTER 100

Mark V. Dahl

Granuloma Annulare

Granuloma annulare is a benign, usually self-limited dermatosis of unknown cause, characterized by necrobiotic dermal papules that often assume an annular configuration. Colcott Fox first described this dermatosis under the name of ringed eruption of the fingers.[1] Radcliffe-Crocker gave it its present title.[2]

EPIDEMIOLOGY

Although it can start at any age, granuloma annulare is predominantly a disease of children and young adults. In a series of 208 patients, the onset was prior to age 30 in more than two-thirds.[3] The disorder affected females twice as often as males. However, most patients with HIV-associated granuloma annulare have been men.

ETIOLOGY AND PATHOGENESIS

Granuloma annulare usually appears for no known reason. It has been reported to follow insect bites; sun exposure; tuberculin skin tests; ingestion of allopurinol; trauma; and viral infections, including Epstein-Barr, HIV, hepatitis C, and herpes zoster. An adenovirus was isolated from a patient with AIDS and granuloma annulare, but the presence of this virus could represent a secondary, unrelated infection in an immunocompromised host.[4] None of 34 consecutive HIV-positive patients with granuloma annulare had the Epstein-Barr virus.[5] Granuloma annulare has occurred in identical twins and siblings and in more than one generation, suggesting hereditary predisposition.[6] Whatever the cause, granuloma annulare evokes a peculiar sort of inflammatory reaction. Most experts believe the reaction is an immunologically mediated one in which inflammation surrounds blood vessels and alters collagen and elastic tissues.[7]

Necrotizing changes suggesting vasculitis are present in dermal blood vessels, although obvious acute leukocytoclastic vasculitis is uncommon.[8] Clinical purpura is rare, but extravasated red blood cells appear in biopsy specimens of about one-third of patients. Immunoglobulins, complement, and fibrinogen are occasionally found in dermal blood vessels in or near the necrobiotic zone.[8,9] The nature of the antigen eliciting the vasculitis is unknown, and the type of immune reaction is debatable. Possible antigens include viruses, altered collagen, altered elastic fibers, or antigens in saliva or infectious agents introduced by arthropod vectors. Vasculitis might result from the deposition of circulating immune complexes, as these complexes have been found in patients with granuloma annulare.[10] The vasculitis also might arise from cytotoxic mediators secreted by cells linked with cell-mediated immunity. Endothelial cells in the dermal capillaries of patients with generalized granuloma annulare contain mysterious rod-shaped bodies resembling Birbeck granules, but their role, if any, in vessel injury is unknown.[11]

The evidence linking cell-mediated immune reactions to granuloma annulare is scantier. The leukocytes of patients with granuloma annulare have produced macrophage inhibitory factor.[12] Activated lymphocytes or lymphoblasts have been noted in the inflammatory infiltrate, but they are widely scattered and not usually prevalent or even evident in 1-mm thick sections. Helper-inducer lymphocytes are common (as they are in most inflammatory skin diseases),[13,14] and fibrin is present within the area of necrobiosis (as it is in many inflammatory disorders).[8,9] Most lymphocytes in the infiltrate are activated and express class II HLA antigens and receptors for interleukin 2 (IL-2).[15] Lesions with histology similar to that of granuloma annulare have occurred in delayed hypersensitivity reactions to intradermally injected bovine collagen.[16] If cell-mediated immunity is important, the granuloma annulare–like lesions that occur in patients with AIDS and sarcoidosis, who have deficiencies of cell-mediated immunity, are difficult to explain.

Vascular damage could also result from non-immune mechanisms. Factor VIII–related antigen circulates in the blood of patients with widespread granuloma annulare.[17] Excessive binding of factor VIII antigen to blood vessels could lead to blood vessel thickening and damage, with secondary deposition of immunoreactants in the vessel walls and a surrounding inflammatory infiltrate.

Blood monocyte function is normal,[18] but tissue monocytes may act abnormally. Release of lysosomal enzymes from macrophages may lead to necrobiosis. Macrophages in lesions of granuloma annulare contain abundant lysozyme,[19] acid phosphatase, and nonspecific esterase, and they abundantly express metaloelastase mRNA in lesional skin.[20] Their epithelioid appearance suggests an active secretory role. Perhaps cytokines from monocytes could activate fibroblasts; this would explain the four- to fivefold increase in Pro alpha 1(I) collagen mRNA,[21] the high activity of prolyl hydroxylase, and the deposition of type III procollagen and fibronectin in the granulomas.[22]

Trauma sometimes resolves the problem of granuloma annulare. Probably every dermatologist has seen the adjacent sides of an annular lesion disappear after biopsy. Just how this happens is speculative, but this phenomenon likely provides an important clue to pathogenesis. Perhaps trauma restores normality to an otherwise disordered inflammatory cascade.

The tendency to develop granuloma annulare may be inherited. In addition to at least 15 reports of familial granuloma annulare, generalized granuloma annulare has been found more frequently among persons who are HLA phenotypes BW35 and A29.[23]

CLINICAL MANIFESTATIONS

Types of Granuloma Annulare

Clinically, granuloma annulare can be divided into a number of more or less distinct types.

FIGURE 100-1

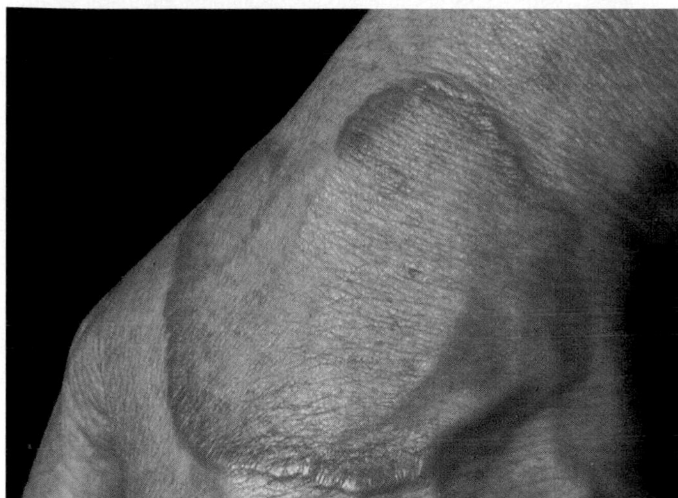

Typical lesion of granuloma annulare demonstrating the elevated rolled border without epidermal change, as well as the frequent violaceous color of the central patch and associated atrophy.

LOCALIZED LESIONS The most common type of granuloma annulare occurs primarily in children and young adults. An annular plaque may be skin-colored, erythematous, or violaceous. Sometimes, dome-shaped papules are arranged in a complete or half circle (Fig. 100-1). Lesions are usually asymptomatic. The epidermal surface is most often undisturbed, but occasionally telangiectatic vessels may appear over individual papules, or epidermal markings may be lost. Centrally, the surface may be slightly hyperpigmented and subtly depressed below the level of surrounding skin. Solitary papules or nodules may also be present. Sometimes these are umbilicated, especially on the fingers.

Localized granuloma annulare most commonly appears on the dorsa of the hands and feet, but it may appear on the forearms, arms, legs, and thighs. It only rarely affects the face and scalp. In about half of the patients, only one ring is present.

GENERALIZED LESIONS About 15 percent of all patients with granuloma annulare have more than 10 lesions. These patients are usually either younger than 10 years old or older than 40. Hundreds or even thousands of individual, 1- to 2-mm, usually skin-colored papules arise anywhere on the cutaneous surface and may form small annular plaques (Fig. 100-2*A*). In contrast to other forms, generalized granuloma annulare usually involves the trunk, and lesions are especially common on the neck, forearms, legs, and extensor surfaces of the elbows. Typically, the rings are less than 5 cm in diameter. They may enlarge centrifugally over the course of weeks or months. Uneven development, skin biopsy, or spontaneous resolution of one side of a lesion may convert annular into arcuate forms (see Fig. 100-2*A*). Sometimes, all the lesions are annular, while at other times, most or all lesions are small papules (Fig. 100-2*B*). They may be slightly violaceous in color, but they are occasionally waxlike and pink, tan, yellow, or dusky gray. Violaceous patches with raised edges, but without epidermal change, are less common. Symmetry is a usual feature. Lesions on the face, palms, soles, and mucous membranes are rare.

SUBCUTANEOUS LESIONS Subcutaneous granuloma annulare consists of large, painless, skin-colored, deep dermal or subcutaneous nodules.[8] Lesions usually occur in children or young adults.[24] About 75 percent of patients develop lesions on the leg or foot, but lesions may also appear on the palms, buttocks, fingers, toes, eyelids, or scalp. They may be solitary or multiple. Occasionally, the skin over the nodules may ulcerate (Fig 100-3). When near the joints, they may be confused with rheumatoid nodules or nodules of rheumatic fever. However, nodules are not associated with arthritis, and rheumatoid factor is not present in serum. Some patients with these "pseudorheumatoid nodules" subsequently develop more ordinary granuloma annulare lesions elsewhere. Diabetes and abnormal glucose tolerance may be more common among patients with this nodular variant.

FIGURE 100-2

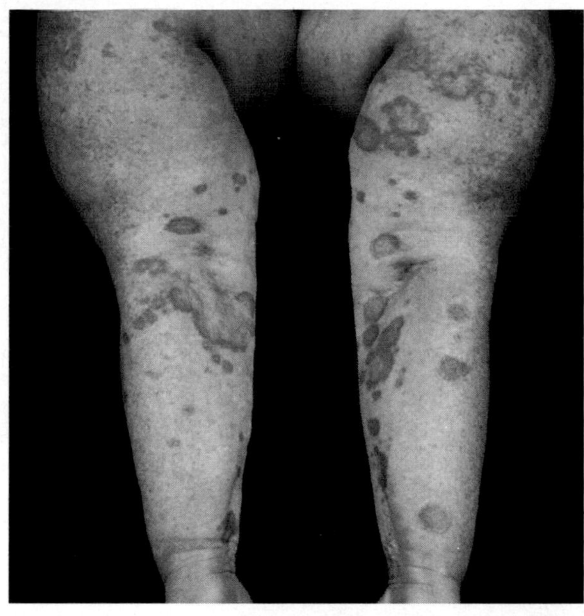

A.

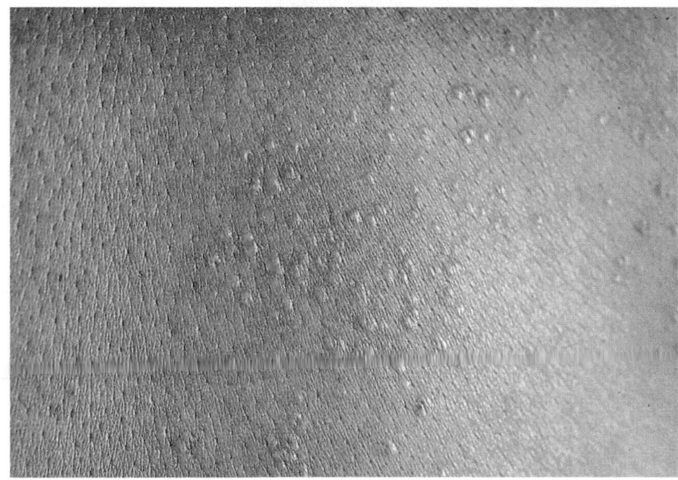

B.

Generalized granuloma annulare. *A.* Numerous annular pink plaques scattered over the arms. *B.* Small papular lesions of generalized granuloma annulare. These lesions are too small to exhibit an annular configuration.

PERFORATING LESIONS Superficial, small papules may develop central umbilication, plugs, or crusts.[25] This occurs most frequently in lesions on the hands and fingers. Frank ulceration with discharge of creamy fluid is rare. In one series, 30 percent of patients with this form had diabetes.[26]

FIGURE 100-3

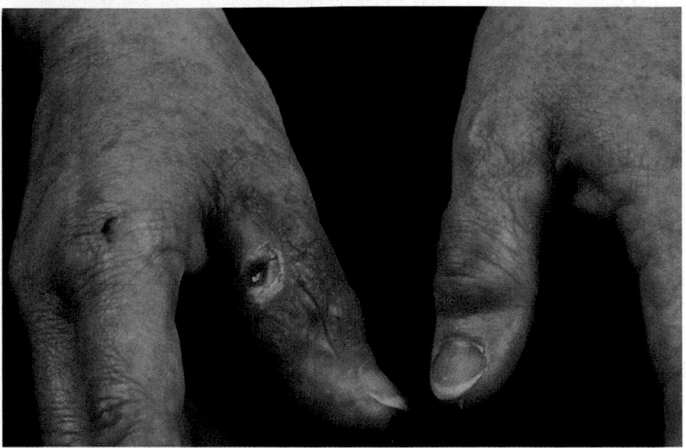

Nodular (subcutaneous) granuloma annulare, with perforation. The necrobiotic granulomas here are large and extend into the subcutaneous fat.

PATCH LESIONS Some patients with granuloma annulare develop subtly pink patches without induration or scale. Most of these patients are women, and most of these lesions occur on the proximal extremities. Both localized and generalized forms are recorded.[27]

ARCUATE DERMAL ERYTHEMA Annular or circinate erythematous lesions that resemble erythema multiforme, erythema migrans, or erythema annulare centrifugum may occur. In such patients, the papular quality is less obvious than the erythema. As in other forms of granuloma annulare, rings may spread centrifugally, and central hyperpigmentation may be present. This form of granuloma annulare, which is uncommon, usually occurs on the trunk. Biopsy rather than clinical inspection generally confirms the diagnosis.

ACTINIC GRANULOMA Sometimes, one or more large annular plaques develop on the face or other actinically damaged skin area.[28] These lesions can become quite large and/or very elevated.

Relationship to Internal Disease

In general, patients with granuloma annulare are in good health. A relationship of granuloma annulare to diabetes mellitus,[26] necrobiosis lipoidica diabeticorum, and rheumatoid nodules has been widely discussed, but not firmly established. Necrobiosis lipoidica coexists with granuloma annulare quite commonly, despite the small number of reported cases. Similarly, some patients with rheumatoid arthritis have developed granuloma annulare. Occasionally, patients with granuloma annulare have arthritis that may worsen when new lesions of granuloma annulare appear. Some of these patients have rheumatoid nodules rather than granuloma annulare. Such patients will nearly always have detectable rheumatoid factor in their sera.

Granuloma annulare may rarely involve fascia and tendons, causing sclerosis, carpal tunnel syndrome, lymphedema, and deformities.[29] Ankylosis of a joint may occur. In one instance, a man with insulin-dependent diabetes, Addison's disease, myxedema, and ulcerative colitis developed small nodules of granuloma annulare in the skin, bowel, mesentery, and peritoneum.[30]

Active vasculopathy or extravascular neutrophilic infiltrates in a skin biopsy specimen showing granuloma annulare is more likely to be associated with underlying systemic disease, particularly in patients with granuloma annulare atypical in location and appearance.

Patients with AIDS have developed granuloma annulare. Painful lesions in atypical locations have been associated with malignant lymphomas.[32]

LABORATORY AND SPECIAL EXAMINATION

The results of laboratory tests are usually normal, although there have been reports of glucose tolerance abnormalities, particularly in patients with the nodular granuloma annulare and in patients with the widespread, disseminated type.[33] Rarely, circulating antithyroid and antinuclear antibodies have been found in the serum of some patients. Levels of complement are normal, but levels of heparin-precipitable cryofibrinogen,[34] fibronectin,[35] serum lysozyme,[36] and benzylamine monoamine oxidase[37] may be elevated, especially in patients with active generalized disease. Serum angiotensin-converting enzyme levels are usually normal.

PATHOLOGY

The chief aid in the diagnosis of granuloma annulare is biopsy.[38,39] The diagnosis is best made at low magnifications (Fig. 100-4). At the

FIGURE 100-4

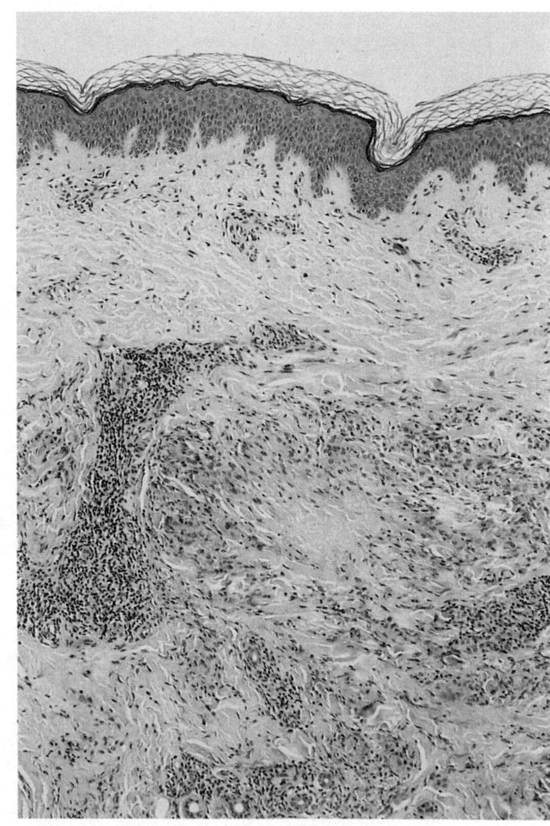

Granuloma annulare. Disease affects the connective tissue of the reticular dermis, characterized by a central area of altered collagen (so-called necrobiosis of collagen) that is surrounded by an inflammatory zone separating altered from normal collagen.

level of the subpapillary plexus of blood vessels, or occasionally somewhat deeper, are single or multiple foci of granulomatous inflammation. These foci have a central core of incomplete and mostly reversible change (necrobiosis) of the connective tissue, surrounded by a wall of palisaded histiocytes. The necrobiotic centers are usually oval in outline, slightly basophilic, devoid of nuclei, and marked by a loss of outline of collagenous and elastic tissue fibers. Characteristically, the necrobiotic foci are not so large or deeply situated as those of rheumatoid nodules or as broad and diffuse as those of necrobiosis lipoidica (diabeticorum). Histochemically, they demonstrate varying amounts of mucinous, PAS-positive, diastase-resistant material and small amounts of lipids. The zone around the necrobiotic focus is composed of palisades of histiocytes intermingled with a few acute inflammatory cells, including neutrophils and eosinophils. Sometimes, histiocytes are large enough to resemble epithelioid cells. Multinucleated giant cells may be present. In some lesions, lines of histiocytes may transverse the necrobiotic focus (the so-called interstitial type). Normal areas of collagen may be found between areas of necrobiosis.

In early lesions, or at the edge of the granuloma, only histiocytic cells may be evident. In these cases, the character of the cellular reaction leads the experienced dermatopathologist to consider the diagnosis of granuloma annulare.

Within the palisading granuloma, inflammation often appears to center around blood vessels, with endothelial swelling and thickening of vessel walls.[12] Vessels may contain PAS-positive, diastase-resistant material. Changes associated with acute leukocytoclastic vasculitis are usually not present, but at times microscopic purpura or a small amount of nuclear dust may be present around one or more blood vessels.[40]

Immunofluorescence examination of biopsied tissue from some lesions of granuloma annulare often reveals C3, IgM, and fibrinogen in some dermal blood vessels and at the dermal-epidermal junction.[8,9,40] Deposits usually occur in only a few vessels, suggesting that complexes may be detectable only at one stage of the indolent pathologic process that causes granuloma annulare. Although deposits of immunoreactants in blood vessels are uncommon, massive deposits of fibrinogen regularly appear throughout the area of necrobiosis. This finding rapidly identifies the areas of necrobiosis, but is not specific.

In subcutaneous forms of granuloma annulare, the foci of necrobiosis are larger and lie in the deep dermis or even the panniculus adiposus. Microscopic differentiation from the more common rheumatoid nodules may be impossible, although mucin deposits are more regularly associated with granuloma annulare. Central ulceration and communication between the area of necrobiosis and the surface characterize perforating granuloma annulare, but serial sections may be necessary to demonstrate the necrobiotic plug.

DIFFERENTIAL DIAGNOSIS

The annular configuration of granuloma annulare often leads to the incorrect diagnosis of tinea corporis, but the lack of epidermal surface change and the failure to detect fungi in scrapings and cultures in tissues taken from patients with granuloma annulare serve to readily distinguish these disorders. Erythema migrans of Lyme disease mimics granuloma annulare, especially the arcuate dermal erythema form. Biopsy helps to distinguish these conditions. Other annular granulomatous eruptions, such as sarcoidosis, cat-scratch disease, or late secondary or tertiary syphilis, may cause some confusion. The clinical differential diagnosis also includes annular lichen planus, tuberculous granulomas, insect bites, xanthomas, lipoid proteinosis, erythema multiforme, erythema annulare centrifugum, subacute cutaneous lupus erythematosus, granuloma multiforme, amyloidosis, creeping eruption, drug reaction (e.g., from angiotensin-converting enzyme inhibitors), and erythema elevatum diutinum.

Annular elastolytic giant-cell granuloma can be confused both clinically and histologically, although the central hypopigmentation, zonal infiltrate, asteroid bodies, giant cells, and absence of true necrobiosis are usually distinctive. Elastic tissue is destroyed in granuloma annulare, and sometimes the result may be secondary anetoderma.[41] Occasionally, as noted earlier, subcutaneous granuloma annulare may simulate rheumatoid nodules both clinically and histologically. Epithelioid sarcoma has necrobiotic features. At times, microscopic and clinical differentiation of granuloma annulare from necrobiosis lipoidica may also be difficult. Lysozyme is abundant in histiocytes of granuloma annulare, but absent or sparse in necrobiosis lipoidica.[19] Interstitial granulomatous drug reactions can cause histologic confusion as well.[42]

Familial granulomatous arthritis, iritis, and skin granulomas (Blau syndrome) comprise an autosomal dominantly inherited syndrome that overlaps both sarcoidosis and granuloma annulare.[43]

TREATMENT

Granuloma annulare is a cosmetic disease in that it is rarely symptomatic and usually has no medical consequence. The cosmetic disfigurement may be severe or mild. Although the disease is usually self-limited, clinicians have used a wide array of treatment methods to hasten resolution. These include the topical application of vitamin E and x-ray therapy, cryotherapy, laser destruction, or intralesional injection of triamcinolone acetonide. Of these, the last seems the most effective. Potent topical glucocorticoids suppress the disease. Glucocorticoids applied topically under occlusion or incorporated into tape may also be beneficial, but side effects such as atrophy may occur. Intralesional injections of recombinant human interferon-γ induced remission in three patients within 3 weeks.[44]

Psoralen plus ultraviolet A (PUVA) therapy may improve the eruption and apparently even cure it.[45] This approach is probably the treatment of choice for patients with widespread disease, because it is quite effective and relatively safe—at least over a short term of treatment. Topical applications of psoralens followed by ultraviolet A radiation can also be effective.[46]

Retinoids given systemically either alone or during PUVA treatments may be effective.[47] Systemic treatment with pentoxifylline, nicotinamide, niacinamide, isotretinoin, salicylates, chlorpropamide, potassium iodide, thyroxine, aspirin, dipyridamole, dapsone, or antimalarials has been advocated and sometimes seems efficacious, but spontaneous resolution makes the evaluation of such treatments difficult. The systemic use of glucocorticoids improves appearance, but risks almost always outweigh benefits. Treatment with low doses of chlorambucil is probably effective, but only very rarely justified because of the severe side effects, including the induction of leukemia and bone marrow depression.

COURSE AND PROGNOSIS

The lesions of granuloma annulare tend to resolve spontaneously. In more than half of 208 cases, cutaneous lesions had disappeared in 2 years.[3] In 40 percent of these, there was recurrence, usually at the original site. Recurrent lesions often disappeared more rapidly than the original ones, and 80 percent of them resolved within 2 years. Although a retrospective study indicates that the prognosis for patients with generalized disease is no worse than the prognosis for those with localized disease,[3] most dermatologists believe that resolution is less likely in middle-aged patients with widespread, generalized granuloma annulare.

REFERENCES

1. Colcott Fox T: Ringed eruption of the fingers. *Br J Dermatol* **7**:91, 1895
2. Radcliffe-Crocker H: Granuloma annulare. *Br J Dermatol* **14**:1, 1902
3. Wells RS, Smith MA: The natural history of granuloma annulare. *Br J Dermatol* **75**:199, 1963
4. Coldiron BM et al: Isolation of adenovirus from a granuloma annulare–like lesion in the acquired immunodeficiency syndrome–related complex. *Arch Dermatol* **124**:654, 1988
5. Toro JR et al: Granuloma annulare and human immunodeficiency virus infection. *Arch Dermatol* **135**:1404, 1999
6. Rubin M, Lynch FW: Subcutaneous granuloma annulare: Comment on familial granuloma annulare. *Arch Dermatol* **93**:416, 1966
7. Dahl MV: Speculations on the pathogenesis of granuloma annulare. *Australas J Derm* **26**:49, 1985
8. Dahl MV et al: Vasculitis in granuloma annulare: Histopathology and direct immunofluorescence. *Arch Dermatol* **113**:463, 1976
9. Thyresson HN et al: Granuloma annulare: Histopathologic and direct immunofluorescent study. *Acta Derm Venereol (Stockh)* **60**:261, 1980
10. Dahl MV et al: Circulating immune complexes in granuloma annulare [Abstract]. *Clin Res* **27**:712A, 1979
11. Kohn S, Friedman-Birnbaum R: Rod-shaped bodies resembling Birbeck granule-like structures in endothelial cells of dermal capillaries in generalized granuloma annulare. *J Dermatol* **28**:5, 2001
12. Baba T et al: Monocyte-modulating activities in the sera of patients with granuloma annulare. *J Dermatol* **15**:248, 1988
13. Buechner SA et al: Identification of T-cell subpopulations in granuloma annulare. *Arch Dermatol* **119**:125, 1983
14. Modlin RL et al: Granuloma annulare: Identification of cells in the cutaneous infiltrate by immunoperoxidase techniques. *Arch Pathol Lab Med* **108**:379, 1984
15. Modlin RL et al: Immunopathologic demonstration of T lymphocyte subpopulations and interleukin 2 in granuloma annulare. *Pediatr Dermatol* **2**:26, 1984
16. Rapaport MJ: Granuloma annulare caused by injectable collagen. *Arch Dermatol* **120**:837, 1984
17. Majewski BBJ et al: Increased factor VIII–related antigen in necrobiosis lipoidica and widespread granuloma annulare without associated diabetes. *Br J Dermatol* **107**:641, 1982
18. Cherney KJ et al: Leukocyte function in granuloma annulare. *Br J Dermatol* **101**:23, 1979
19. Padilla RS et al: Differential staining pattern of lysozyme in palisading granulomas: An immunoperoxidase study. *J Am Acad Dermatol* 121:624, 1985
20. Vaalamo M et al: Enhanced expression of human metalloelastase (MMP-12) in cutaneous granulomas and macrophage migration. *J Invest Dermatol* **112**:499, 1999
21. Tasanen K et al: Quantitation of Pro alpha 1(I) collagen mRNA in skin biopsy specimens: Levels of transcription in normal skin and granuloma annulare. *J Invest Dermatol* **107**:314, 1996
22. Oikarinen A et al: Biochemical and immunohistochemical comparison of collagen in granuloma annulare and skin sarcoidosis. *Acta Derm Venereol (Stockh)* **69**:277, 1989
23. Friedman-Birnbaum R et al: A study of HLA antigen associated in localized and generalized granuloma annulare. *Br J Dermatol* **115**:329, 1986
24. Grogg KL, Nascimento AG: Subcutaneous granuloma annulare in childhood: Clinicopathologic features in 34 cases. *Pediatrics* **107**:E42, 2001
25. Samlaska CP et al: Generalized perforating granuloma annulare. *J Am Acad Dermatol* **27**:319, 1992
26. Castro A et al: Glucose, insulin HGH, and cortisol plasma levels in granuloma annulare patients during glucose tolerance and cortisone glucose tolerance test. *Clin Biochem* **7**:150, 1974
27. Mutasim DF, Bridges AG: Patch granuloma annulare: Clinicopathologic study of 6 patients. *J Am Acad Dermatol* **2**:417, 2000
28. Boneschi V et al: Annular elastolytic giant cell granuloma. *Am J Dermatopathol* **10**:224, 1988
29. Kossad S, Winkelmann RK: Response of generalized granuloma annulare to alkylating agents. *Arch Dermatol* **114**:216, 1978
30. Thomas DJ et al: Visceral and skin granuloma annulare, diabetes, and polyendocrine disease. *Br Med J* **293**:977, 1986
31. Magro CM et al: Granuloma annulare and necrobiosis lipoidica tissue reactions as a manifestation of systemic disease. *Hum Pathol* **27**:50, 1996
32. Barksdale SK et al: Granuloma annulare in patients with malignant lymphoma: Clinicopathologic study of thirteen new cases. *J Am Acad Dermatol* **31**:42, 1994
33. Haim S et al: Carbohydrate tolerance in patients with granuloma annulare. *Br J Dermatol* **88**:447, 1973
34. Dahl MV et al: Elevated heparin precipitable fraction of plasma in granuloma annulare. *Arch Dermatol* **115**:1059, 1979
35. Koh MS et al: Increased plasma fibronectin in diabetes mellitus, necrobiosis lipoidica and widespread granuloma annulare. *Clin Exp Dermatol* **9**:293, 1984
36. Padilla RS et al: Serum lysozyme in patients with localized and generalized granuloma annulare. *Arch Dermatol* **121**:624, 1985
37. Yuen CT et al: Increased activity of serum amine oxidases in granuloma annulare necrobiosis lipoidica and diabetes. *Br J Dermatol* **116**:643, 1987
38. Friedman-Birnbaum R et al: A comparative histopathologic study of generalized and localized granuloma annulare. *Am J Dermatopathol* **11**:144, 1989
39. Dabski K, Winkelmann RK: Generalized granuloma annulare: Histopathology and immunopathology. Systematic review of 100 cases and comparison with localized granuloma annulare. *J Am Acad Dermatol* **20**:28, 1989
40. Bergman R et al: Localized granuloma annulare: Histopathological and direct immunofluorescence study of early lesions, and the adjacent normal-looking skin of actively spreading lesions. *Am J Dermatopathol* **15**:544, 1993
41. Ozkan S et al: Anetoderma secondary to generalized granuloma annulare. *J Am Acad Dermatol* 42:335, 2000
42. Perrin C et al: Interstitial granulomatous drug reaction with a histologic pattern of interstitial granulomatous dermatitis. *Am J Dermatopathol* **23**:295, 2001
43. Blau EB: Familial granulomatous arthritis, iritis, and rash. *J Pediatr* **107**:689, 1985
44. Weiss JM et al: Treatment of granuloma annulare by local injections with low-dose recombinant human interferon gamma. *J Am Acad Dermatol* **39**:117, 1998
45. Hindson TC et al: PUVA therapy of diffuse granuloma annulare. *Clin Exp Dermatol* **13**:26, 1988
46. Grundmann-Kollmann M et al: Cream psoralen plus ultraviolet A therapy for granuloma annulare. *Br J Dermatol* 144:996, 2001
47. Harth W, Richard G: Retinoids in therapy of granuloma annulare disseminatum. *Hautarzt* **44**:693, 1993

CHAPTER 101

Louis Dubertret

Malignant Atrophic Papulosis (Degos' Disease)

Köhlmeier first described malignant atrophic papulosis (Degos' disease) in 1941,[1] and Degos recognized it as a specific entity in 1942.[2] This rare disorder, of which fewer than 200 cases have been reported to date, is a multisystem lymphocytic vasculitis characterized by widespread thrombosis of small vessels not only in the skin, but also, with decreasing frequency, in the gastrointestinal tract and in the ocular and central nervous systems. Local ischemia may also involve the lungs, heart, kidneys, liver, bladder, and prostate gland. Of the patients with documented disease, one-half have died, primarily from intestinal perforations or central nervous system infarcts.

PATHOGENESIS

The pathogenesis of malignant atrophic papulosis is unknown. The occlusion of blood vessels seems to be the consequence of endothelial cell swelling and lymphocytic vasculitis, leading to thrombosis.[3] Besides these constant histologic observations, other physiopathologic phenomena occur, although they have not been uniformly verified in all patients. From time to time, fibrinolytic activity seems to decline within the lesion,[4,5] and a decrease in blood fibrinolytic activity seems to be present in most of the studied patients.[6,7] Some cases have suggested that anticardiolipin antibodies and the lupus anticoagulant play a role in this condition,[8] but a study of 15 patients did not confirm such an association.[9]

By electron microscopy, so-called confronting cylindrical cisternae have been observed in endothelial cells;[10–12] these are now considered products of a cellular reaction to viral infection. An increased content of von Willebrand factor in Weibel-Palade granules has been observed by immunoelectron microscopy, suggesting a secretion defect.[7]

An extract of brain tissue obtained from a surgeon who died of malignant atrophic papulosis produced an extensive subacute spongiform encephalopathy in a chimpanzee and a squirrel monkey.[13] The symptoms of the induced disease were similar to those of Creutzfeldt-Jakob disease. This observation suggests that malignant atrophic papulosis could result from a transmissible agent; however, injections of tissue from other patients' skin lesions into nonhuman primates have not induced the disease.[14]

Four familial cases of malignant atrophic papulosis have been described: (1) a mother and her daughter,[14] (2) a son and his mother,[15] (3) a mother and her five children,[16] and (4) members of three generations in a single family.[17] This emphasizes the possibility of genetic contributing factors in this disease or of slow virus infection and transmission. Findings of an association with AIDS[18] and an exacerbation during immunosuppression[19] also suggest the possible role of an infectious agent.

CLINICAL FEATURES

Malignant atrophic papulosis has been described mainly in Europe and the United States. It nearly always occurs in Caucasians, but two cases have been observed in African American patients and three cases have been reported in Japan. Sixty-one percent of patients are male. Although the disease has occurred in patients of many ages, it is rare in young children.[20,21] Typically, it occurs in young adults.

Cutaneous Manifestations[22,23]

The cutaneous lesions of malignant atrophic papulosis, which pass through progressive stages, are pathognomonic. They can be few in number, but are usually multiple—up to 600 lesions on the same patient. Lesions predominate on the trunk and upper limbs. The disease does not affect the scalp and usually spares the palms, soles, and face.

The evolution of the lesion is characteristic. In the early phase, a small, firm papule from 2 to 5 mm in diameter appears. Its color may be pink, gray, or yellow, and a normal epidermis covers it. Dermal edema may be evident. Within a few days, the papule becomes umbilicated, and a typical central white, porcelain-like zone of atrophy appears (Fig. 101-1). A scale may cover this central zone, and an erythematous border, generally 1 to 2 mm in width and sometimes slightly raised, may encircle it. This border may be pink or violaceous and is covered by telangiectasia. With time, the border disappears, leading to a varicelliform scar.

FIGURE 101-1

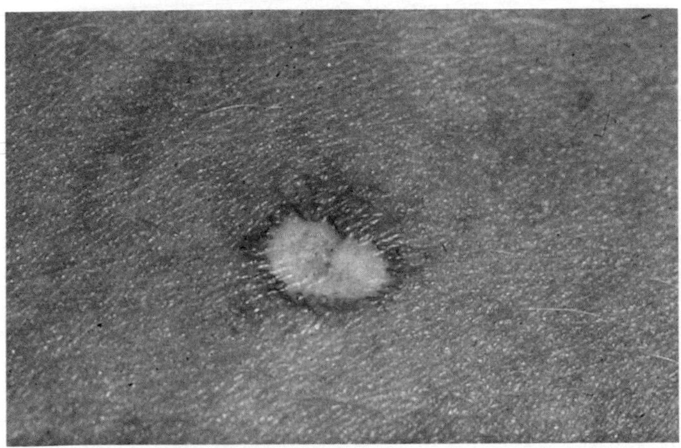

Malignant atrophic papulosis. Characteristic evolution of papules into typical porcelain-white atrophic lesions.

Crops of new elements occur from time to time, and lesions of different ages can be evident in the same patient. Skin lesions are asymptomatic or slightly pruritic. Usually, the lesions are separated from each other, but they may coalesce, leading to polycyclic atrophic areas or to skin ulcerations.

Gastrointestinal Manifestations [22,23]

In general, gastrointestinal lesions occur a few months after the onset of skin lesions, but they may not occur until many years later. Thus, it is difficult to determine the percentage of patients with gastrointestinal manifestations. According to the published cases without long-term follow-up, 61 percent of patients with malignant atrophic papulosis suffer from gastrointestinal lesions. Gastrointestinal tract involvement may remain unsymptomatic and may be discovered only at autopsy of patients who died of encephalitis.[24] Sometimes, patients suffer only from dyspepsia, but there is usually an abdominal emergency such as vomiting, acute abdominal pain, hematemesis, or melena that reveals the intestinal involvement. Symptomatic gastrointestinal involvement signifies a poor prognosis, even though the results of a radiologic examination of the intestine remain normal.

Laparoscopy or laparotomy reveals white, avascular patches scattered on the surface of the small intestine, colon, or stomach, sometimes with perforation leading to peritonitis. The rectum can also be involved.

Among mucosal lesions, ocular involvement is predominant. It is present in one-third of patients,[25,26] occurring mainly on the conjunctiva but also on the sclera, episclera, retina, choroid, and the optic nerves. Lesions appear as avascular patches on the conjunctiva (Fig. 101-2) or on chorioretinal sites, sometimes with depigmentation. Telangiectasia with microaneurysms has also been observed. Involvement of the buccal mucosa and of the genitalia is rare.

In most cases, cutaneous manifestations precede visceral symptoms. When gastrointestinal or neurologic manifestations precede those of the skin, the diagnosis is hardly possible clinically and requires the histologic examination of specimens obtained by abdominal surgery or at autopsy.

Neurologic Manifestations[27,28]

Twenty percent of patients experience neurologic manifestations of malignant atrophic papulosis. These symptoms are polymorphic and include hemiparesis, aphasia, multiple cranial nerve involvement, monoplegia, sensory disturbances, and seizures. The cerebrospinal fluid is usually abnormal, with pleocytosis and increased protein content. Neuropathologic findings are multiple infarcts, with or without hemorrhage, in the brain, cerebellum, and spinal cord. The meningeal vessels can also be occluded.

Neurologic manifestations usually occur in the course of the acute form of malignant atrophic papulosis, where the prognosis is dependent mainly on the intestinal involvement. However, progressive neurologic involvement sometimes leads to death. This has been the case in some rare cases of malignant atrophic papulosis occurring in children.[29]

Other Visceral Manifestations

Postmortem examination reveals infarcts in many organs (heart, kidneys, bladder, lungs, pleura, liver, pancreas). These lesions are rarely symptomatic during life. However, pleuritis and pericarditis have been observed, and death has occasionally resulted from respiratory insufficiency (five patients). In one infant, death resulted from disseminated myocardial infarcts.[20]

Other Disease Associations

Malignant atrophic papulosis–like lesions have been described in collagen vascular disease,[30] and lesions have been reported in one patient who also had AIDS.[18]

HISTOPATHOLOGY

The histologic lesions of malignant atrophic papulosis are characteristic.[2] Classically, there is a definite area of dermal necrosis situated just below an atrophic epidermis, with or without hyperkeratosis (Fig. 101-3). The first histologic description of typical lesions emphasized the absence of adnexae, vessels, and inflammatory cells in the necrobiotic zone. Just beneath the necrobiotic zone, there is considerable vascular pathology with endothelial cell swelling, proliferation, and thrombosis. The vessel walls are thickened, and fibrinoid necrosis is often present (Fig. 101-4). Vascular damage occurs predominantly in the arterioles, but it may also occur in the small, deep venules.

FIGURE 101-2

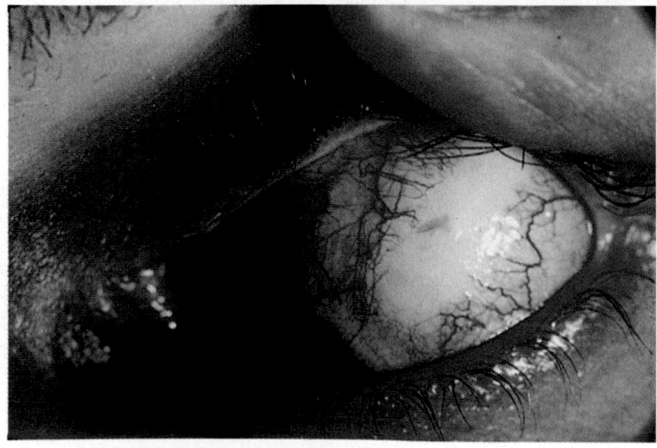

Ocular involvement in malignant atrophic papulosis: a typical avascular patch on the conjunctiva surrounded by injected collateral vessels.

FIGURE 101-3

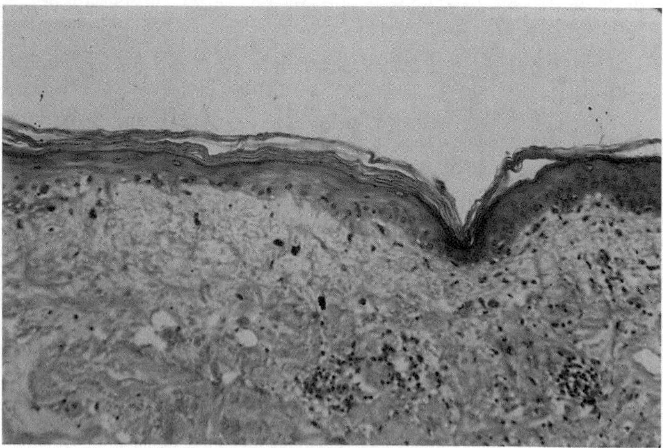

Early lesion of malignant atrophic papulosis with the beginning of ischemic necrolysis of the epidermis and dermis on the left and sparse superficial lymphocytic infiltrates on the right. (*Courtesy of Olivier Verola, MD*)

FIGURE 101-4

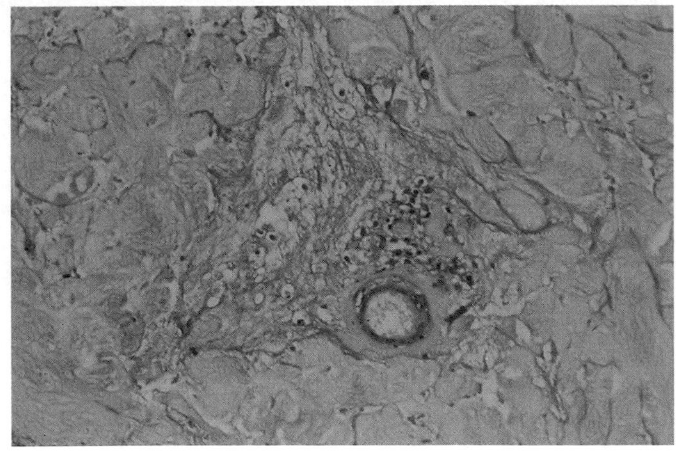

Early lesion of malignant atrophic papulosis showing fibrinoid necrosis of an arteriole, a sparse inflammatory infiltrate, and mucin deposition. *(Courtesy of Bernard Cribier, MD)*

The classical abscence of inflammatory cells[2] is a questionable criterion for diagnosis as it is characteristic only for old lesions. Most of the early lesions show features of lymphocytic vasculitis associated with the alterations of endothelial cells of arterioles and venules (see Fig. 101-4).[3,31] Demyelination and degenerative alterations of small nerves may occur. Fibrin deposits are frequently evident within and around the skin vessels. Mucin deposits are common in the dermis.[32]

Immunofluorescence studies have not detected immunoglobulin or complement deposits in the lesions. Circulating immune complexes have not been found.[33]

Electron microscopy indicates that the essential features of malignant atrophic papulosis are focal endothelial cell degeneration and hypertrophy with fibrin deposits. Paramyxovirus-like inclusions have appeared in the endothelial cells and fibroblasts of some patients.[11,12] These structures are now called confronting cylindrical cysternae and are considered products of a cellular reaction to an unknown, possibly infectious agent; they are a not uncommon sequela of certain viral infections and/or virus-induced neoplasms in different species.[34] These structures, which can be induced in vitro by interferon,[34,35] are commonly found in association with Kaposi's sarcoma.[36]

LABORATORY FINDINGS

Patients with malignant atrophic papulosis have a normal CBC and a normal erythrocyte sedimentation rate; hypergammaglobulinemia can be observed in a few patients. Some abnormalities in blood coagulation have been reported: an increase in plasma fibrinogen level,[37–43] increased platelet aggregation,[7,9,38,40] and a decrease of local[4] and systemic fibrinolytic activity.[6,7] Thus, the possibility of consumption coagulopathy has been entertained.[40] Antiarterial antibodies have been observed in a few patients.[41–43] The results of skin tests to common recall antigens are normal.

DIFFERENTIAL DIAGNOSIS

The clinical and histologic patterns of the skin lesions are diagnostic of malignant atrophic papulosis. As noted earlier, however, when visceral lesions precede the skin lesions, diagnosis may be impossible. Similar skin lesions have appeared in patients with systemic lupus erythematosus.[44] Individual lesions of atrophie blanche can mimic the disease, but the topography of the lesions and the absence of papules excludes the diagnosis.[45] A skin biopsy can exclude allergic necrotizing vasculitis, acute parapsoriasis, or lymphomatoid papulosis, when necessary.

TREATMENT

Proposed therapies for malignant atrophic papulosis are unfortunately not based on controlled studies because of the rarity of the disease and its unpredictable and variable evolution. Glucocorticoids not only seem to be inefficient, but also may increase the risk of intestinal perforation.

Anticoagulants, mainly heparin, have been used without demonstrable effect.[46] Therapy with dipyridamole (50 mg three times a day) and aspirin (325 mg daily) has been beneficial in some patients who demonstrate increased platelet aggregation.[38,39] Fibrinolytic therapy with phenformin and ethylestrenol has been useful in some cases,[47] but ineffective in others.[48] Ethylestrenol has been used as an anabolic steroid; like danazol, it has fibrinolytic activity, but danazol has not been tested in malignant atrophic papulosis. Pentoxifyllin plus aspirin has been reported beneficial in one case.[49] Dextran perfusion has not proved useful. Surgery of intestinal lesions is usually ineffective.

PROGNOSIS

Classically, the prognosis is poor, and death usually occurs after a few years as the consequence of intestinal lesions or neurologic involvement. However, some patients have survived for 15 years with only skin lesions.[50] Thus, as more observations are made, the spectrum of the disease seems more and more polymorphic with both acute and chronic forms, with lesions either limited to the skin or associated with visceral involvement, and with or without the presence of detectable coagulation abnormalities. When platelet aggregation is increased, treatment to inhibit the aggregation seems logical and useful.

REFERENCES

1. Köhlmeier W: Multiple Hautnekrosen bei Thrombangiitis obliterans. *Arch Dermatol Syphilol* **181**:783, 1941
2. Degos R et al: Dermatite papulo-squameuse atrophiante. *Bull Soc Fr Dermatol Syphiligr* **49**:148, 281, 1942
3. Soter NA et al: Lymphocytes and necrosis of the cutaneous microvasculature in malignant atrophic papulosis: A refined light microscope study. *J Am Acad Dermatol* **7**:620, 1982
4. Black MM et al: The role of dermal blood vessels in the pathogenesis of malignant atrophic papulosis (Degos' disease): A study of two cases using enzyme histochemical, fibrinolytic, electron-microscopical and immunological techniques. *Br J Dermatol* **83**:213, 1973
5. Muller SA, Landry M: Malignant atrophic papulosis (Degos disease): A report of two cases with clinical and histological studies. *Arch Dermatol* **112**:357, 1976
6. Daniel F et al: Papulose atrophiante maligne avec insuffisance de la fibrinolyse sanguine. *Ann Dermatol Venereol* **109**:763, 1982
7. Caux F et al: Anomalies de la fibrinolyse dans la maladie de Degos. *Ann Dermatol Venereol* **121**:537, 1994
8. Englert HJ et al: Degos' disease: Association with anticardiolipin antibodies and the lupus anticoagulant. *Br Med J* **289**:576, 1984

9. Assier H et al: Absence of antiphospholipid and anti-endothelial cell antibodies in malignant atrophic papulosis: A study of 15 cases. *J Am Acad Dermatol* **33**:831, 1995
10. Olmos L, Laugier P: Ultrastructure de la maladie de Degos (Apport d'un nouveau cas et revue de la littérature). *Ann Dermatol Venereol* **104**:280, 1977
11. Olmos L et al: Microcylinders of endoplasmic reticulum in histiocytes in patients suffering from Degos' syndrome and dermatomyositis. *Br J Dermatol* **100**:137, 1979
12. Bioulac P et al: La papulose atrophiante maligne de Degos: Étude ultrastructurale d'un nouveau cas. *Ann Anat Pathol (Paris)* **25**:111, 1980
13. Gajdusek DC et al: Transmission of subacute spongiform encephalopathy to the chimpanzee and squirrel monkey from a patient with papulosis atrophicans maligna of Köhlmeier-Degos. *Proceedings of the Tenth International Congress of Neurology*, Series 319, edited by A Subirana, JM Espadaler, EH Burrows. Amsterdam, Excerpta Medica, 1973–1974, p 390
14. Moulin G et al: Papulose atrophiante de Degos familiale (mère-fille). *Ann Dermatol Venereol* **111**:149, 1984
15. Hall-Smith R: Malignant atrophic papulosis (Degos' disease): Two cases occurring in the same family. *Br J Dermatol* **81**:817, 1969
16. Kisch LS, Bruynzeel DP: Six cases of malignant atrophic papulosis (Degos' disease) occurring in one family. *Br J Dermatol* **111**:469, 1984
17. Katz SK et al: Malignant atrophic papulosis (Degos' disease) involving three generations of a family. *J Am Acad Dermatol* **37**:480, 1997
18. Requena L et al: Degos disease in a patient with acquired immunodeficiency syndrome. *J Am Acad Dermatol* **38**:852, 1998
19. Powell J et al: Benign familial Degos disease worsening during immunosuppression. *Br J Dermatol* **141**:524, 1999
20. Cabré J et al: Papulose atrophiante maligne de Degos chez un nourrisson. *Bull Soc Fr Dermatol Syphiligr* **81**:652, 1974
21. Enjolras O et al: Un cas juvenile de maladie de Degos. *Bull Soc Fr Dermatol Syphiligr* **81**:205, 1974
22. Degos R: Malignant atrophic papulosis. *Br J Dermatol* **100**:21, 1979
23. Barrière H: Papulose atrophiante maligne (maladie de Degos). *Ann Dermatol Venereol* **105**:733, 1978
24. Huriez CL et al: Forme à prédominance cérébrale d'une maladie de Degos. *Bull Soc Fr Dermatol Syphiligr* **82**:276, 1975
25. Henkind P, Clark WE: Ocular pathology in malignant atrophic papulosis Degos' disease. *Am J .Ophthalmol* **65**:164, 1968
26. Sibillat M et al: Papulose atrophiante maligne (maladie de Degos): Revue clinique. *J Fr Ophthalmol* **9**:299, 1986
27. Petit WA Jr et al: Degos' disease: Neurologic complications and cerebral angiography. *Neurology* **32**:1305, 1982
28. Label LS et al: Myelomalacia and hypoglycorrhachia in malignant atrophic papulosis. *Neurology* **33**:936, 1983
29. Rosemberg S et al: Childhood Degos' disease with prominent neurological symptoms: Report of a clinicopathological case. *J Child Neurol* **3**:42, 1988
30. Tsao H et al: Lesions resembling malignant atrophic papulosis in a patient with dermatomyositis. *J Am Acad Dermatol* **36**:317, 1997
31. Thiers H et al: Papulose atrophiante de Degos: Particularités histologiques. *Bull Soc Fr Dermatol Syphiligr* **75**:657, 1968
32. Feuerman EJ et al: Malignant atrophic papulosis with mucin in dermis: A clinical and pathological study including autopsy. *Arch Pathol* **90**:310, 1970
33. Tribble K et al: Malignant atrophic papulosis: Absence of circulating immune complexes or vasculitis. *J Am Acad Dermatol* **15**:365, 1986
34. Luu J et al: Tubular structures and cylindrical confronting cisternae: A review. *Hum Pathol* **20**:617, 1989
35. Orenstein JM et al: The relationship of serum alpha-interferon and ultrastructural markers in HIV-seropositive individuals. *Ultrastruct Pathol* **11**:673, 1987
36. Rappersberger K et al: Endemic Kaposi's sarcoma in human immunodeficiency virus type-1 seronegative persons: Demonstration of retrovirus-like particles in cutaneous lesions. *J Invest Dermatol* **95**:371, 1990
37. Roenigk HH, Farmer RG: Degos' disease (malignant papulosis): Report of three cases with clues to etiology. *JAMA* **206**:1508, 1968
38. Stahl D et al: Malignant atrophic papulosis: Treatment with aspirin and dipyridamole. *Arch Dermatol* **114**:1687, 1978
39. Drucker CR: Malignant atrophic papulosis: Response to antiplatelet therapy. *Dermatologica* **180**:90, 1990
40. Dastur DK et al: CNS involvement in malignant atrophic papulosis (Köhlmeier-Degos disease): Vasculopathy and coagulopathy. *J Neurol Neurosurg Psychiatry* **44**:156, 1981
41. Degos R et al: Papulose atrophiante maligne avec présence d'anticorps anti-artère. *Bull Soc Fr Dermatol Syphiligr* **74**:715, 1967
42. Basset A et al: Papulose atrophiante maligne de Degos avec atteinte du système nerveux central et présence d'anticorps anti-artères. *Bull Soc Fr Dermatol Syphiligr* **76**:333, 1969
43. Repay VI: Über das Krankheitsbild "Papulose atrophiante maligne Degos." *Dermatol Wochenschr* **155**:325, 1969
44. Dubin HV, Stawiski MA: Systemic lupus erythematosus resembling malignant atrophic papulosis. *Arch Intern Med* **134**:321, 1974
45. Black MM, Hudson PM: Atrophie blanche closely resembling malignant atrophie papulosis (Degos' disease) in systemic lupus erythematosus. *Br J Dermatol* **95**:649, 1976
46. Rivoire J: Papulose atrophiante maligne de Degos. Evolution après 28 mois de traitement aux anticoagulants. *Bull Soc Fr Dermatol Syphiligr* **78**:18, 1971
47. Delaney TJ, Black MM: Effect of fibrinolytic treatment in malignant atrophic papulosis. *Br Med J* **3**:415, 1975
48. Howsden SM et al: Malignant atrophic papulosis of Degos: Report of a patient who failed to respond to fibrinolytic therapy. *Arch Dermatol* **112**:1582, 1976
49. Victor C, Schulz-Ehrenburg U: Malignant atrophic papulosis (Uëhlweier-Degos): Diagnosis, therapy and course. *Hautarzt* **52**:734, 2001
50. Su WPD et al: Clinical and histologic findings in Degos' syndrome (malignant atrophic papulosis). *Cutis* **35**:131, 1985

CHAPTER 102

Christopher R. Shea
Victor G. Prieto

Fibrous Lesions of Dermis and Soft Tissue

Lesions characterized by (1) proliferations of fibroblasts or myofibroblasts and/or (2) increased or altered extracellular deposits of collagen or elastic tissue are discussed in this chapter. Classification into traditional nosologic categories is problematic. Fibrous lesions often are composed predominantly of stroma, and only in certain high-grade sarcomas is the neoplastic nature of the lesion obvious. The presence of defined chromosomal abnormalities suggests a neoplastic status for some fibrous lesions traditionally considered to be reactive.

THE FIBROMATOSES

Fibromatoses are proliferations composed of fibrous tissue with varying degrees of cellularity, often exhibiting myofibroblastic differentiation. Lesions in childhood often remit spontaneously, whereas in adults fibromatoses tend to be locally aggressive but nonmetastatic. Fibromatoses of most interest to the dermatologist may arise in fascia (e.g., palmoplantar fibromatosis) or musculoaponeuroses (e.g., fibromatosis colli); a few are dermal (e.g., infantile digital fibromatosis). While most fibromatoses are considered nonmalignant, lesions affecting vital viscera (e.g., abdominal desmoid tumors) can be fatal through local complications. The nosologic status of fibromatoses is disputed. Clonal chromosome aberrations (e.g., trisomies 8 and 20 and loss of 5q material) occur in 46 percent of desmoid tumors and in 10 percent of superficial types.[1]

CHILDHOOD FIBROMATOSES

Solitary Lesions

FIBROMATOSIS COLLI (STERNOMASTOID TUMOR OF INFANCY) This benign proliferation of fibrous tissue infiltrating the lower third of the sternocleidomastoid or shoulder region is the most common cause of neonatal torticollis. Possibly a consequence of birth trauma, it usually is present at birth and remits spontaneously. Fine-needle aspiration reveals clusters of spindled fibroblasts with plump, ovoid nuclei.[2]

INFANTILE DIGITAL FIBROMATOSIS (INCLUSION BODY FIBROMATOSIS, REYE TUMOR) This lesion usually occurs as a small, asymptomatic, nodular, dermal fibrous proliferation at the extensor or lateral surface of a finger or toe (Fig. 102-1) but occasionally is seen at other sites, such as breast or tongue. Typically, onset is in the first year of life, and the lesion may involute spontaneously without scarring after several years. Recurrence after local excision is common; thus management by observation is usually the best approach. Histologically, myofibroblasts in poorly circumscribed, interlacing bundles contain pathognomonic, eosinophilic, paranuclear inclusion bodies that stain red with Masson's trichrome stain and purple with phosphotungstic acid–hematoxylin.[3]

FIGURE 102-1

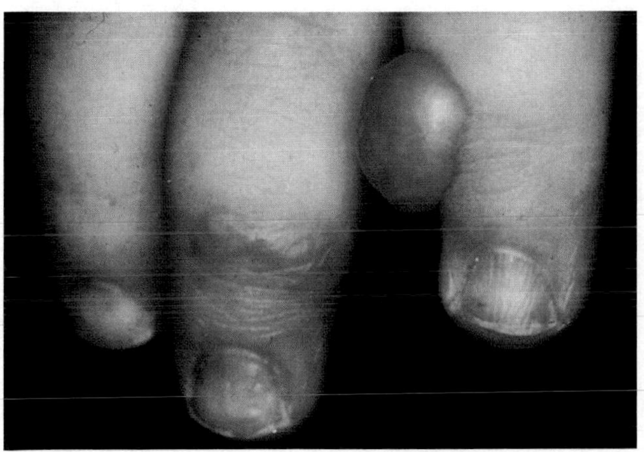

Infantile digital fibromatosis (Reye's tumor) in a 2-year-old child.

CALCIFYING APONEUROTIC FIBROMA This lesion usually presents as a painless, solitary, deep fibrous nodule, often adherent to tendon, fascia, or periosteum, on the hands and feet.[4] Histologically, fascicles of spindled fibroblasts and scattered epithelioid cells border chondroid areas with or without calcification. This lesion is best managed by conservative local excision.

Multifocal Lesions

AGGRESSIVE INFANTILE FIBROMATOSIS This lesion is characterized by rapidly growing nodules on the trunk that infiltrate skeletal muscle and only rarely regress spontaneously.[5] The pathologic appearance varies from immature mesenchymal cells to collagenous and desmoid patterns. Treatment is by complete local excision, but this often cannot be accomplished because of muscular involvement. Distant metastases, e.g., to lungs, can occur.

INFANTILE MYOFIBROMATOSIS This lesion is usually solitary (solitary infantile myofibroma), but patients with multicentric presentation (congenital generalized fibromatosis) often also have visceral involvement, and in these there may be a 75 percent mortality rate. Occasionally, familial cases are reported. Most lesions present at or soon after birth as rubbery masses in skin or muscle in the head and neck, upper extremity, or trunk; they may simulate hemangiomas clinically. Similar lesions occur rarely in adults.[6] This biphasic tumor is composed of (1) interlacing fascicles or whorled nodules of eosinophilic spindle cells in a collagenous or myxoid stroma and (2) centrally, vascular proliferation resembling hemangiopericytoma admixed with primitive-appearing round to spindle cells. Mitotic figures, vascular invasion, and tumor necrosis may be seen and are not evidence of malignancy. The cells express vimentin and muscle actin. Because solitary lesions of skin and bone usually regress spontaneously, surgical excision is limited to lesions interfering with function.

JUVENILE HYALINE FIBROMATOSIS This very rare, possibly autosomal recessive disease occurs from early childhood to adulthood. It presents as slow-growing, pearly white or skin-colored dermal or subcutaneous papules or nodules on the face, scalp, and back that may be confused clinically with neurofibromatosis. The course generally progresses to ulceration, joint contractures, deformities, and lytic bone lesions. Associated clinical features include gingival hyperplasia, growth retardation, and papillomatous perianal lesions. Histologically, cords of spindled myofibroblasts, often with cytoplasmic vacuoles, occur in a hyalinized or chondroid stroma. Infantile systemic hyalinosis shows similar features affecting viscera.[7]

FIBROMATOSES MAINLY OF ADULT ONSET

Dupuytren's Contracture (Palmar Fibromatosis)

This bilateral, progressive fibrosis of the palmar fascia usually presents as nodules over the fourth or fifth metacarpal head and progresses to flexion deformity of the fingers. While most lesions are asymptomatic, about one-fifth of patients have tingling, edema, changes in temperature sensation, sweating, or pain. Dupuytren's disease predominantly affects males of northern European descent. Some patients have associated plantar fibrosis (Ledderhose's disease), usually over the medial side of the sole and rarely associated with contractures.[8] These two processes share the same histologic and ultrastructural features.[9] Knuckle pads are also associated (see below).

Chronic trauma appears an unlikely etiology. Decreases in conduction velocity of the ulnar nerve occur in some patients, as do abnormal cervical vertebrae. The disease has a hereditary component, and there is an association with alcoholic liver disease, epilepsy, diabetes mellitus, and smoking.[10] Histologically, the palmar aponeurosis and adipose tissue exhibit nodules of fibroblasts in a dense reticulin network. In older lesions, thick, acellular collagen bundles predominate.[11] Early lesions contain fibroblasts and collagen type III, intermediate lesions have myofibroblasts, and late lesions contain fibrocytes and collagen type I.[12] Basic fibroblast growth factor and transforming growth factor alpha are overexpressed,[13] as is epidermal growth factor receptor, suggesting a possible autocrine stimulatory loop.[14]

The early, nodular lesions may respond to intralesional steroids or colchicine.[15] Older lesions usually require partial fasciectomy. Recurrence is more common in highly cellular lesions in which mitotic figures can be seen, as opposed to the more mature, hypocellular lesions.[16]

Peyronie's Disease (Induratio Penis Plastica)

This fibrosing condition involves the dorsum of the penis and, in particular, the fibrous septa between the corpus spongiosum and corpora cavernosa. It is occasionally associated with Dupuytren's contracture. The etiology is unknown. Propranolol has been suspected as an inciting agent,[17] but the condition existed long before propanolol was used as a drug. Over several years, most patients have spontaneous regression.[18] The histology is very similar to that of Dupuytren's fibromatosis.

Knuckle Pads

These are circumscribed, keratotic, fibrous growths over the dorsa of the interphalangeal joints.[19] Many patients have coexisting fibromatosis of the palmar, plantar, or penile aponeurosis or fascia.[20] Pathologically, there is intradermal fibroblastic and myofibroblastic proliferation without atypia or inflammation, eventuating in fibrosis. *False knuckle pads* are caused by repetitive mechanical trauma or factitious injury such as chewing or gagging in bulemics.

Pachydermodactyly

This superficial dermal fibromatosis presents as poorly circumscribed symmetric, infiltrative, asymptomatic soft-tissue hypertrophy of the proximal fingers, typically sparing the thumbs and fifth fingers and rarely extending proximally to the wrists or occurring distally.[21] Most cases occur in young men. It may be associated with tuberous sclerosis, atrophia maculosa varioliformis cutis, and carpal tunnel syndrome. Histologically, it exhibits a thickened, fibrotic dermis entrapping eccrine glands.

Progressive Nodular Fibrosis of the Skin

This lesion presents with progressive dermal nodules of fibroblasts in a collagenous stroma. In vitro, increased synthesis of procollagen and decreased synthesis of collagenase suggest expansion of a clone of fibroblasts having these reciprocal abnormalities.[22]

DESMOID TUMOR

This rare mesenchymal tumor may develop anywhere on the body, most often on the anterior abdominal wall and shoulder girdle (Fig. 102-2). More frequent in women, desmoids may develop following childbirth or in abdominal scars. Injury precedes a minority of cases.[23] The desmoids slowly, relentlessly invade surrounding structures, sometimes causing fatality. Retroperitoneal desmoids occur in Gardner's syndrome, especially after intraabdominal operations. Rarely, desmoid tumors transform into classic fibrosarcomas.[24] Desmoid tumors have chromosomal abnormalities, such as trisomies 20 and 8. The latter may behave less aggressively.[25]

Histologically, a poorly circumscribed growth of mature fibrous tissue arises from a musculoaponeurosis. Regarding differential diagnosis, in contrast with fibrosarcomas, desmoids tend to be less cellular and more monomorphous. In contrast with nodular fasciitis, desmoids lack significant myxoid background or mitotic figures.

Due to diffuse infiltration, surgical excision is very difficult. When feasible, aggressive wide resection is the treatment of choice because the lesions recur often (see Fig. 102-2), and death may result from local infiltration. Metastases do not occur. Radiotherapy can be used to control recurrent disease and may be the primary therapy to avoid a mutilating resection, particularly of extraabdominal desmoids. Antiestrogens can be used when surgery is not possible or in recurrent disease.[26] Chemotherapy with doxorubicin, dacarbazine, and carboplatin can be

FIGURE 102-2

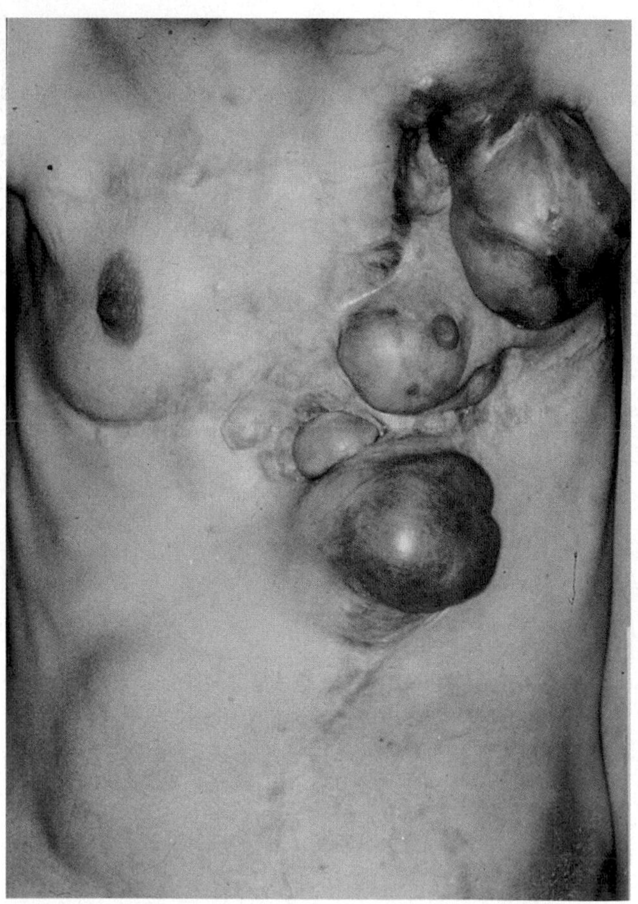

Desmoid tumors involving upper chest and epigastric region. These represent recurrences after multiple surgical interventions. This patient also had intraabdominal desmoid tumors.

used for recurrent extraabdominal desmoid tumors where surgery is contraindicated.[27]

REACTIVE AND DEGENERATIVE FIBROUS LESIONS

Hypertrophic Scars and Keloids

Both are abnormal growths of fibrous tissue following cutaneous injury. A hypertrophic scar remains confined to the site of original injury, whereas a keloid grows beyond it. Keloids and hypertrophic scars are most common around the shoulders (Fig. 102-3), upper back, and chest (Fig. 102-4), where the skin is thick and under tension, and on the earlobe following piercing. Hypertrophic scars are usually linear following surgical trauma and papular or nodular following inflammatory and ulcerating lesions, as in cystic acne or burns (see Fig. 102-3). Both hypertrophic scars and keloids are disfiguring and can produce contractures. A keloid appears as a firm, mildly tender, irregular nodule or plaque (see Fig. 102-4). The overlying epidermis is thin, and there may be focal ulceration. The borders are well demarcated but irregular. The color is pink to purple and may be accompanied by hyperpigmentation. Both lesions may be pruritic; in addition, keloids are often painful and hyperesthetic.

Hypertrophic scars occur at any age. Keloids usually present in the third decade. Although both sexes are affected, more females seek help for keloids, especially when the lesions appear in the face, such as after ear piercing. Dark-skinned and blood group A individuals are more susceptible to keloid formation. Growth of a keloid may be stimulated by pregnancy. Surgical resection of a keloid may be followed by recurrence of a larger growth; if a skin graft has been used, a keloid may occur in the donor site as well.

Early scars show a proliferation of fibroblasts running parallel to the epidermis in an edematous, myxoid stroma. Blood vessels are prominent. After a few weeks to months, cellularity and edema are replaced by mature collagen. In a hypertrophic scar, areas of eosinophilic collagen are admixed haphazardly with areas of myxoid stroma. In addition to the immature stroma, a keloid has thick, eosinophilic, acellular bands of collagen (Fig. 102-5). Mast cells and plasma cells are seen in increased numbers[28]; mast cells are degranulated and closely apposed to myofibroblasts, suggesting a pathogenic role.[28] However, the differences in mast cell numbers are not significant between the scarred area and the surrounding dermis.[29] Elastin is usually absent, in contrast to a normal mature scar, which does contain elastin. Electron microscopy confirms the presence of fibroblasts and myofibroblasts.[30] The collagen bundles are dense and homogeneous. The intercellular ground substance is increased, with a fibrillar appearance instead of the normal globular deposits.

Hypertrophic scars are associated with HLA-DRβ16,[31] perhaps explaining the predisposition to keloid formation in certain individuals. In most studies, keloids and scars show the same biochemical and pathologic abnormalities. In contrast, some studies have identified

FIGURE 102-3

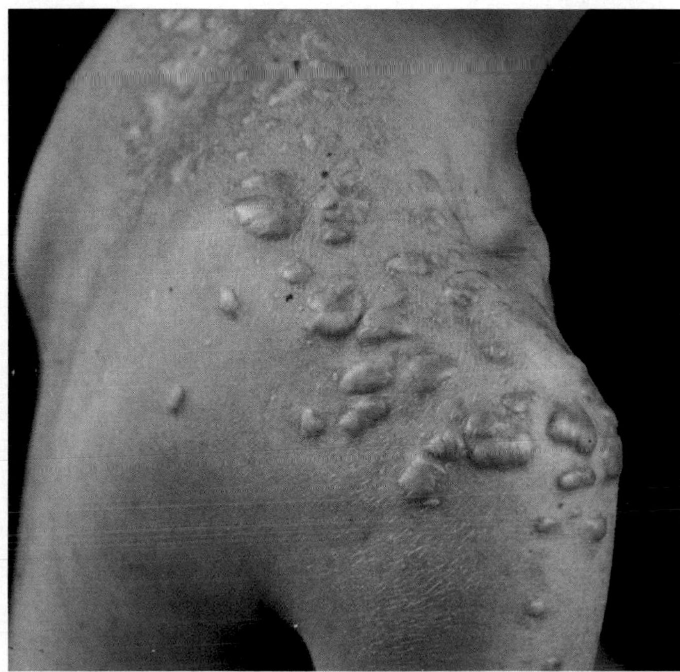

Hypertrophic keloidal scars following cystic acne.

FIGURE 102-4

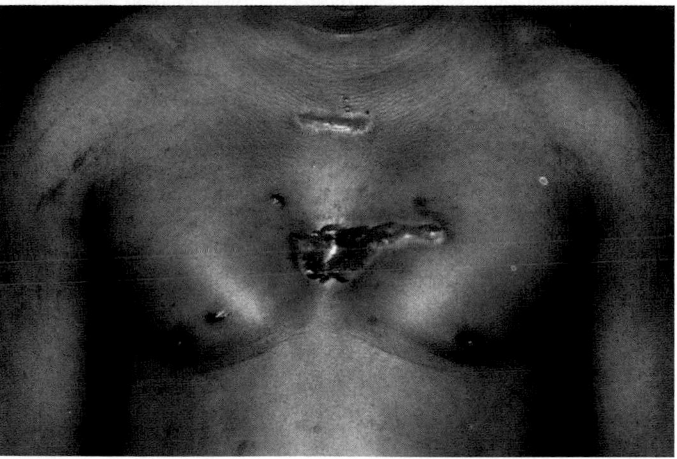

Two keloids in the presternal region, a typical location.

FIGURE 102-5

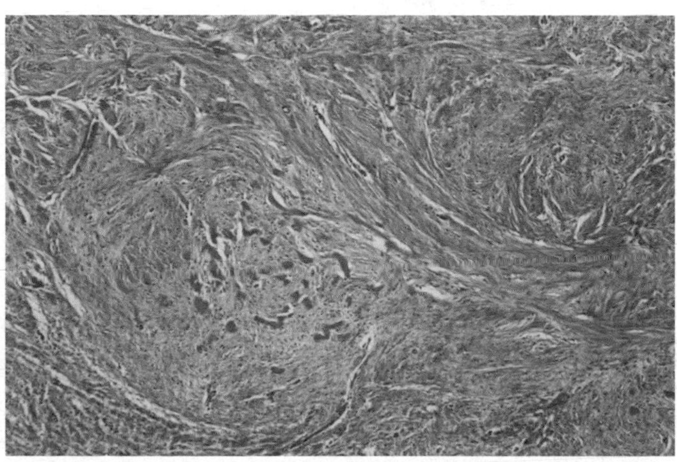

Photomicrograph showing whorls of collagen characteristic of hypertrophic scar. The thick eosinophilic bundles of collagen on the left are typical of keloid.

antinuclear antibodies in keloids but not in scars. Keloids express increased levels of the gli-1 protein, an oncogene product also present in neoplasms such as basal cell carcinoma.[32] Collagen synthesis and collagenase activity are increased in both keloids and hypertrophic scars. $Alpha_1$ globulin (a collagenase inhibitor usually not present in normal scars) may contribute to increased collagen deposits. Hypertrophic scars have increased levels of the profibrotic agent tumor necrosis factor.[31] Keloids contain tenascin C, a protein associated with inflammation and wound healing.[33] Fibroblasts from keloid-prone patients have altered cytokine patterns[34] and increased sensitivity to transforming growth factor $\beta 1$ (TGF-$\beta 1$),[35] TGF-$\beta 2$,[36] and epidermal growth factor.[37] Along these lines, CO_2 laser treatment reduces TGF-$\beta 1$ levels in keloids.[38] At least part of the fibroblast stimulation may be secondary to infiltration of the scar by activated T cells.[39] Also, there seem to be decreased levels of apoptosis (as shown by TUNEL technique) and increased bcl-2 and p53 expression in keloid-associated fibroblasts.[40] Electron-microscopic studies show partially or totally occluded blood vessels in granulation tissue, hypertrophic scars, and keloids. Blood vessel occlusion may be due primarily to endothelial cell proliferation, resulting in anoxia and stimulation of growth of fibroblasts.[41] However, this theory is difficult to accept because constant pressure on a hypertrophic scar flattens the lesion, presumably due to anoxia. Hypertrophic scars and, even more so, keloids appear to be proliferative lesions based on quantitation of silver-stained nucleolar organizer regions (AgNORs).

Intralesional steroids (e.g., triamcinolone acetonide, 10–40 mg/mL) given every few weeks will stop growth of the keloid or hypertrophic scar, and continued use leads to significant flattening in most instances. Cryotherapy immediately before injection softens the tumor thus allowing easier instillation of the steroid. Leakage of steroid into tissues surrounding the keloid/hypertrophic scar likely will cause atrophy; therefore, steroids should be injected into the center of the lesion. Too superficial an injection leads to visible collections of chalky material, which can be removed surgically. Other side effects of steroid injections include hypopigmentation and occasional sloughing of the keloid. Adrenal suppression is very rare.

Larger keloids are best treated by excision combined with steroid infiltration at the edges of the lesion, immediate skin grafting, and pressure bandaging. After such treatment, there is a reduction in pro-$alpha_1$ type I collagen gene expression.[42] Pressure should be applied to both the resected area and the donor site. Pressure (around 24 mmHg) alone often will prevent hypertrophic scars in burn patients and, if used in early hypertrophic scars, may induce regression.

Radiation therapy may prevent keloid formation and decrease recurrence when used in the early postoperative period (24–48 h).[43] However, it is sometimes difficult to find a radiotherapist willing to use this modality for a benign indication. Laser therapy results have been mixed, but one study did show a decrease in collagen production after therapy, as well as clinical improvement.[44] The 585-nm flashlamp and pulsed-dye lasers are effective in the treatment of keloids and hypertrophic scars. In contrast, the recurrence rate is fairly high when CO_2 lasers are used.

Retinoids decrease fibroblast proliferation and collagen synthesis. Topical retinoid creams have been partially effective in treating keloids.[45] Intralesional interferon alpha 2b also has decreased both collagen production and glycosaminoglycans in keloidal fibroblasts, both in vivo and in vitro.[46] Intralesional interferon alpha 2b does not improve mature keloids[47] but reduces recurrence after treatment with carbon dioxide laser ablation.[48] Silicone oil has been used as a silicone cream or silicone gel sheet in the treatment of both keloids and hypertrophic scars.[49,50] The mechanism of action is still unclear; however, hydration and occlusion rather than the silicone itself are felt to play an important role. Since it is painless and noninvasive, this silicone solution appears especially useful in the treatment of children. In summary, a combined surgical and medical therapeutic approach may be the best approach to treatment and prevention of keloid recurrence.

Nodular Fasciitis

Nodular fasciitis typically occurs after trauma and is probably a reactive proliferation rather than a neoplasm. It usually presents as a very rapidly growing, firm, variably painful mass in the subcutis, fascia, or muscle of the forearm, upper arm, or thigh, with onset in the third and fourth decade. Involvement of the head and neck (*cranial fasciitis*) is most common in children. The dermal analogue of this lesion has been designated *postoperative/posttraumatic spindle cell nodule of the skin*. Despite its somewhat alarming clinical presentation (and histology; see below), nodular fasciitis is self-limiting and rarely recurs (1–2 percent); any recurrent lesion warrants careful scrutiny because it might represent a misdiagnosed sarcoma. Local excision is the treatment of choice, although some cases have been reported to regress spontaneously.

Histologically, there is a poorly circumscribed nodule in the subcutis, fascia, or occasionally dermis composed of spindled fibroblasts and myofibroblasts in a loose, myxoid, highly vascular stroma resembling granulation tissue, often with associated hemorrhage and infiltrates of lymphocytes, plasma cells, and mast cells. The cellularity and stromal quality (myxoid, fibrotic) vary from area to area. The cells have a feathery "tissue culture fibroblast" appearance and vesicular nuclei. Mitotic figures are often prominent, but atypical forms or nuclear pleomorphism are not present. Besides these classic features, the spectrum includes granulation tissue–like areas, solid and whorled myofibroblastic proliferations with multinucleated cells, mucoid cysts, and "ancient" forms with dense, refractile strands of keloidal collagen.[51] Occasionally, giant cells resemble osteoclasts. Related lesions include *proliferative fasciitis*,[52] distinguished by the presence of ganglion-like giant cells; *proliferative myositis*, of intramuscular location; *ischemic fasciitis*, on pressure points, often in bedridden patients; and *intravascular fasciitis*, involving veins. These variants tend to occur in older patients than classic nodular fasciitis. Immunohistochemically, nodular fasciitis expresses smooth muscle and muscle-specific actins, vimentin, and CD68, consistent with dual myofibroblastic and "histiocytic" differentiation. The lesions are negative for cytokeratin, S-100 protein, and desmin.[51]

Elastofibroma Dorsi

The lesion may be a reparative phenomenon or perhaps a degenerative end-stage response to chronic trauma. A subcutaneous, tender nodule, up to several centimeters in diameter, typically occurs in women in the sixth to the eighth decade. It is often attached to ribs and fascia on the back and tends to protrude from beneath the tip of the scapula. Occasionally, it arises around other articular bursae. Radiology shows a poorly circumscribed soft-tissue mass; signal intensity on MRI is similar to that of muscle interlaced with linear areas of fat.[53] Histologically, fibrous tissue and fat are admixed with thick globules and strands of dense eosinophilic elastic tissue. Ultrastructural and immunohistochemical studies suggest abnormal elastogenesis.[54]

Degenerative Collagenous Plaques of the Hands (Synonyms: Keratoelastoidosis Marginalis, Digital Papular Calcific Elastosis)

Progressive, firm, glistening, linear plaques are located symmetrically on the medial and lateral aspects of the fingers and thumbs.[55] They are probably due to actinic damage, possibly in concert with repetitive mechanical trauma. Histologically, the epidermis is hyperkeratotic, and the reticular dermis has a bandlike deposition of dense collagen. Solar elastosis is prominent, and calcification is characteristic.

Pachydermoperiostosis (Primary Hypertrophic Osteoarthropathy)

Digits are enlarged from pachydermia, periostosis, and clubbing related to altered proteoglycan synthesis.[56] The lesion is commonly associated with arthralgia and other cutaneous signs, including cutis verticis gyrata and seborrhea, and is familial.

Acrokeratoelastoidosis of Costa

This familial condition is characterized by multiple keratotic papules on the dorsum of hands and feet, palms, and soles. Electron microscopy shows rarified, abnormal elastic tissue; fibroblasts contain dense granules at the periphery of their cytoplasm without elastic extracellular fibers, suggesting abnormal secretion of elastic material.[57]

Fibroepithelial Polyp (Synonyms: Acrochordon, Skin Tag, Soft Fibroma)

These flesh-colored, pedunculated papules or nodules have an irregular or smooth surface (Fig. 102-6). They occur mostly on eyelids, neck, and axillae. Usually asymptomatic, they may undergo infarction if the pedicle twists. The larger lesions that occur on the groin and thighs sometimes are associated with diabetes. The clinical differential diagnosis includes wart, nevus, neurofibroma, and seborrheic keratosis.

These exophytic or pedunculated lesions may have a flattened, acanthotic-hyperpigmented, or folded and frondlike epidermis. The stroma has loose connective tissue with dilated blood vessels resembling the papillary dermis.[58] Nerves are reduced or absent, and no appendages are present. Pseudosarcomatous fibroepithelial polyps show scattered, bizarre stromal cells similar to those seen in degenerating angiofibroma and vaginal pseudosarcomatous polyp.[59] Lesions containing adipose tissue in addition to the loose fibrous stroma are called *lipofibromas* or *dermatolipomas* and may be associated with diabetes mellitus (N. S. McNutt, personal communication). Similar lesions occurring in a dermatomal or other patterned distribution are seen in nevus lipomatosus superficialis.

If requested, simple snipping with curved scissors, cryotherapy, and electrodesiccation are all appropriate treatments. Simple excision may be needed in the larger lesions.

HAMARTOMAS AND RELATED SYNDROMES

Fibrous Hamartoma of Infancy

This rapidly growing, painless, ill-defined subcutaneous or intradermal nodule is generally solitary and less than 5 cm in size[60]; rarely, multiple lesions occur synchronously. Onset is almost always within the first or second year of life and is congenital in 20 percent of cases. Boys are affected twice as often as girls. The axilla, upper arm, shoulder, groin, and external genitalia are involved most often. Histopathologically, a triphasic pattern comprises (1) orderly interlacing fascicles of fibroblasts and myofibroblasts embedded in a densely collagenous stroma, (2) primitive mesenchymal cells in organoid nests, concentric whorls, and bands, often in a myxoid stroma, and (3) mature adipose tissue intimately admixed with the other components; some cases include disorganized, immature-appearing adipocytes.[61] The treatment of choice is local excision, but recurrence may follow partial excision.

Connective Tissue Nevus

These may be present at birth or appear within the first few years. They are elevated, soft to firm, vary from 0.5 to several centimeters in diameter, and may be grouped, linear, or irregularly distributed. The overlying epithelium is usually smooth. Lesions often are centered on hair follicles and form irregular aggregates ("cobblestones"). They may be flesh-colored, brown, or hypopigmented; a yellow color usually reflects high elastic tissue content. *Familial cutaneous collagenoma* is an autosomally inherited symmetric eruption of nodules and plaques (Fig. 102-7) occurring predominantly over the upper back in adolescents. The autosomal dominant *Buschke-Ollendorf syndrome* (dermatofibrosis lenticularis disseminata) is asymmetric, occurs on the lower trunk and extremities, is composed of papules of elastin tissue, and is associated with osteopoikilosis, i.e., multiple round or oval densities of long bones, pelvis, hands, and feet.[62,63] Connective tissue nevi also may occur in focal dermal hypoplasia (Goltz syndrome), macrodactyly, and hemihypertrophy, as well as the shagreen patches of tuberous sclerosis. Histologically, the dermis may contain abnormally compact collagen, adipose tissue, or increased or decreased elastic fibers.[64] However, because the cellularity is normal, routine histology may be unremarkable.

FIGURE 102-6

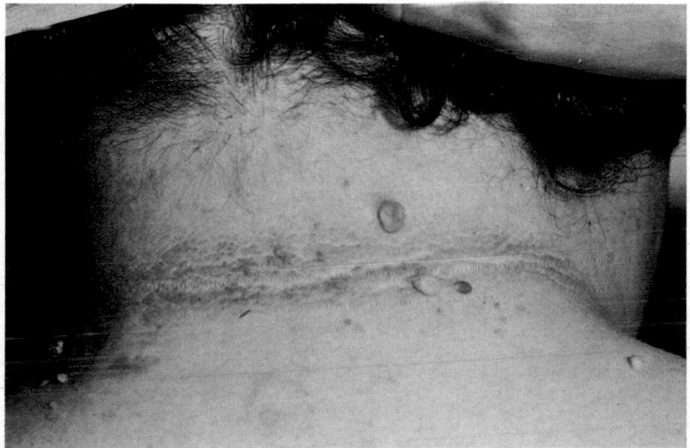

Soft fibromas or skin tags on the neck of a female patient who also had (endocrine) acanthosis nigricans.

FIGURE 102-7

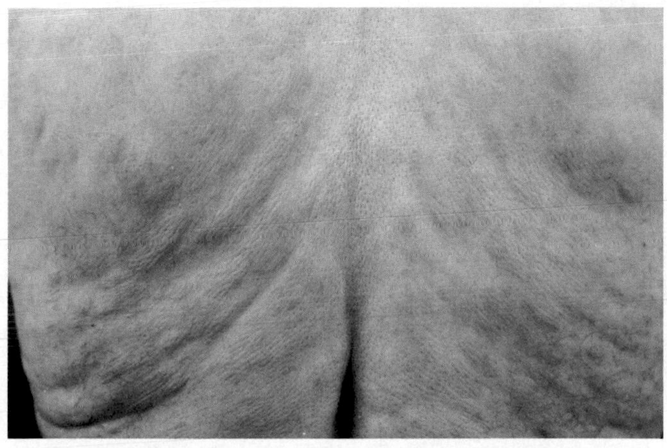

Cutaneous collagenoma, a connective tissue nevus involving almost the entire back.

BENIGN NEOPLASMS

Angiofibroma (See also Chap. 189)

These lesions are small, reddish brown or even flesh-colored, smooth, shiny, 0.1- to 0.3-cm papules present over the sides of the nose and the medial portions of the cheeks (Fig. 102-8). They are usually associated with the tuberous sclerosis complex and are dealt with in detail in Chap. 189. However, solitary lesions are quite common and clinically resemble small basal cell carcinomas. In the penile coronal sulcus, similar lesions are called *pearly penile papules.* Histopathologically, there is a proliferation of dense collagen surrounding appendages and ectatic blood vessels (Fig. 102-9).

Fibrofolliculoma (See also Chap. 85)

Fibrofolliculomas are 2 to 4 mm in diameter, dome-shaped, yellowish or skin-colored papules usually located on the head, neck, and upper trunk. Multiple lesions usually are inherited in an autosomal dominant pattern. The association with trichodiscomas and skin tags constitutes the Birt-Hogg-Dubé syndome.[65]

Sclerotic Fibroma (Circumscribed Storiform Collagenoma, Plywood Fibroma)

This uncommon benign neoplasm occurs as an isolated lesion in healthy individuals.[66] Multiple lesions are a cutaneous marker for the multiple hamartoma (Cowden's) syndrome (see Chap. 184). This autosomal dominant syndrome involves the *PTEN/MMAC1* gene (chromosome 10q)[67] and leads to multiple organ involvement, including trichilemmoma, oral papillomatosis, gastrointestinal polyps and carcinoma, thyroid goiter and carcinoma, fibrocystic disease/gynecomastia, leukemia, lymphoma, and Lhermitte-Duclos disease (dysplastic cerebellar gangliocytoma).

Histologically, sclerotic fibromas reveal dermal hypocellularity and stromal sclerosis with eosinophilic, hyalinized collagen bundles in a parallel or whorled ("plywood") arrangement. Occasional patients express CD34, raising the possibility of misdiagnosis with hypocellular areas of dermatofibrosarcoma protuberans. There is a striking microscopic similarity between sclerotic fibroma and perineurinoma. The latter can express CD34, but in contrast to sclerotic fibroma, it also expresses epithelial membrane antigen (EMA).

FIGURE 102-8

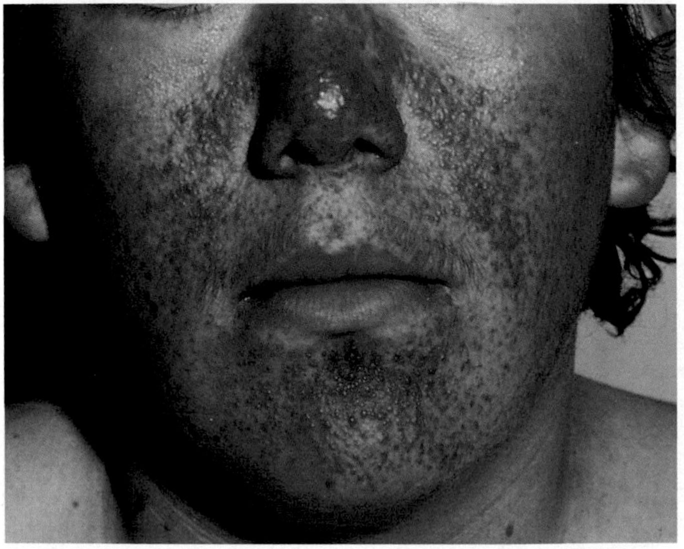

Multiple angiofibromas in a patient with tuberous sclerosis complex.

FIGURE 102-9

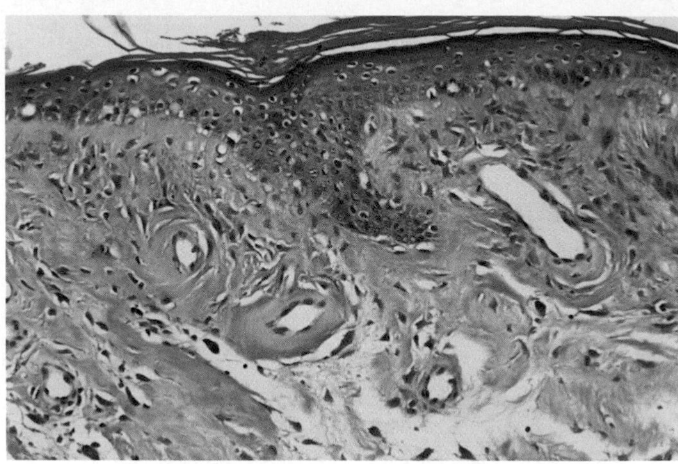

Solitary angiofibroma of the face. The upper dermis shows fibrosis and an increased number of stellate and dendritic cells. Telangiectatic vessels are also present, and so are melanophages in the superficial portion of the dermis.

Giant Cell Collagenoma

This rare, solitary, slowly growing, symmetric, well-circumscribed, dome-shaped nodule occurs on the trunk, upper extremities, and face of young and middle-aged individuals. Histologically, it has hyalinized collagen bundles in a whorled, storiform pattern that is indistinguishable from sclerotic fibroma; however, it also contains a population of plump, bizarre, multinucleated giant cells expressing vimentin.[68]

Pleomorphic Fibroma

This presents as a polypoid to dome-shaped dermal fibrous lesion on the torso, extremities, or face of adults.[69] Histologically, it is sparsely cellular but has striking nuclear atypia and rare mitotic figures. Immunohistochemical staining for vimentin and actin supports fibroblastic differentiation. The lesion is biologically benign, and the atypia may be a degenerative phenomenon akin to that seen in an "ancient" schwannoma. Lesions otherwise resembling sclerotic fibromas but with a similar high degree of atypia also have been described.[70] It has been proposed that there is a spectrum between sclerotic fibroma and pleomorphic fibroma based on the occurrence of cases showing transition between these poles.[71]

Desmoplastic Fibroblastoma (Collagenous Fibroma)

A painless, slowly growing mass, often of long duration, typically involves the arm, shoulder girdle, posterior neck, upper back, feet, ankles, leg, hand, abdominal wall, or hip in middle-aged men.[72] It is a relatively well-circumscribed lesion that predominantly involves subcutaneous tissue but may involve fascia or skeletal muscle. Microscopically, it is composed of bland, stellate or spindled myofibroblasts in a hypovascular fibrous or fibromyxoid stroma; mitotic figures are minimal. Simple conservative excision suffices.

Solitary Fibrous Tumor

This lesion most often involves the pleura but also may occur in the skin (among other organs).[73] It is a well-circumscribed, nonencapsulated tumor composed of uniform spindle cells expressing CD34.[74] Histologically, it exhibits alternating hypercellular and hypocellular areas, often with prominent hemangiopericytoma-like (stag-horn vessels) regions.

Dermatofibroma (Cutaneous Benign Fibrous Histiocytoma)

The concept of fibrohistiocytic lesions is attended by long-standing controversy. Originally, the notion was based on apparent features of both fibroblastic and histiocytic morphology of neoplastic cells when cultured in vitro. However, it is now recognized that the cytologic features of these differentiation pathways are not specific. Even the term *histiocyte* is controversial, and some authors[75] have proposed to rename those cells by more specific terms, e.g., interdigitating dendritic cells in lymph nodes or dermal dendrocytes (dendritic cells) in the skin. However, most authors still use the term *histiocyte,* putatively of monocyte-macrophage lineage, to describe cells with prominent evidence of phagocytosis. Such cells usually have abundant eosinophilic cytoplasm and vesicular, irregular nuclei. The specificity of histiocytic markers is also challenged. For example, the CD68 antigen seems to be present in lysosomes and therefore could be detected in any lesion formed by cells with significant numbers of lysosomes, including granular cell tumors,[76] neural neoplasms,[77] and even melanomas.[78] For all these reasons, the concept of fibrous histiocytoma has been criticized (and especially in regard to the malignant fibrous histiocytoma; see below). However, most clinicians are familiar with this term, and it is still used in the World Health Organization (WHO) classification of mesenchymal neoplasms. Accordingly, this terminology is retained here for convenience.

Some authors distinguish between a fibrous form (*dermatofibroma*) with spindled cells in a collagenous stroma and a *fibrous histiocytoma* form rich in histiocytes. However, many lesions show different areas with varying degrees of these two basic patterns, so they are best considered to represent poles of one entity that exhibits both myofibroblastic and histiocytic differentiation.[79]

Dermatofibroma is perhaps the most common mesenchymal growth of the skin. It has a predilection for the lower legs of women in their early twenties. The surface may be shiny or keratotic, and the color is usually brown, sometimes with a play of colors (Fig. 102-10). Characteristically, a dermatofibroma is firm and mobile and measures from 0.5 mm to 1 cm in diameter. Lateral compression produces a dimple-like depression in the overlying skin. Generalized lesions have been described, as have occasional unusual tumors confined to the palms and soles. Usually asymptomatic, they occasionally are pruritic and may ulcerate following trauma. Some tumors grow very rapidly, whereas others remain static for many years. Regression may leave hypopigmentation. Dermatofibromas arising on the face are uncommon but require special mention. They are more often of cellular type, extend into the subcutaneous fat or muscle, and frequently recur; therefore, a wider initial excision is recommended.[80]

Trauma, such as insect bites, has been thought to induce some lesions. For this reason, some authors classify these as reactive/reparative lesions rather than as neoplasms. However, the recent demonstration of chromosome abnormalities in at least some cases of dermatofibroma supports a neoplastic nature.[81] Of note, the karyotypic changes identified are different from those in dermatofibrosarcoma. A viral etiology also has been considered.

Histologically, the epidermis is usually hyperplastic and hyperpigmented ("dirty fingernail" sign). There is sometimes a curious induction phenomenon, whereby the basilar epidermis proliferates to form basaloid aggregates. While these may simulate superficial basal cell carcinoma, they more often resemble an early stage in fetal development of a hair follicle and lack the myxoid stroma and retraction effect usually seen in basal cell carcinoma. Regardless, rarely basal cell carcinoma has been reported to arise in a dermatofibroma, but this diagnosis should be reserved for unequivocal cases showing deep nodular growth or necrosis. The dermis has haphazardly arranged fascicles of plump spindle cells that lack atypia in most cases. The edges of the lesion are poorly defined, with individual cells infiltrating between collagen bundles that are often thickened and hyalinized ("keloidal"). Mitotic figures may be present, but atypical forms are not a feature.

A cellular variant characterized by increased cellularity, storiform arrangement, larger size, and location in the deep dermis, often with extension into the superficial subcutaneous tissue, may be difficult to differentiate from dermatofibrosarcoma protuberans. In such circumstances, immunohistochemical expression of factor XIIIa rather than CD34 is often helpful. Because about 20 percent of cellular dermatofibromas recur after simple biopsy, a conservative complete excision

FIGURE 102-10

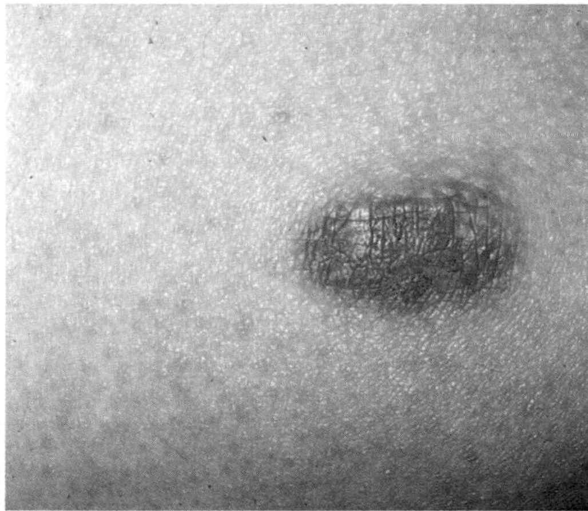

A.

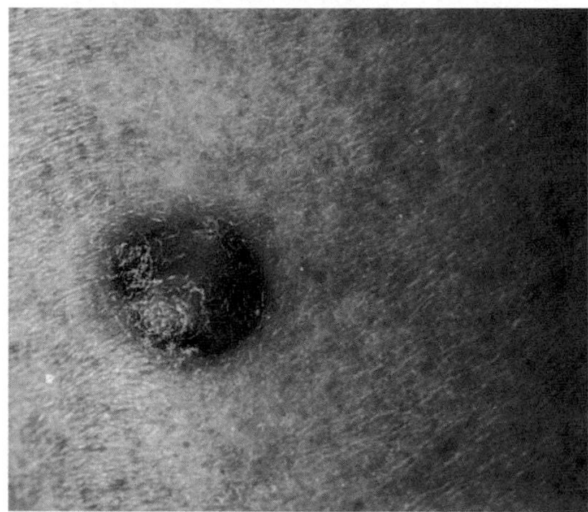

B.

Dermatofibroma. *A.* This is a firm, flat nodule with a variegated yellowish to brown color. Lateral compression will produce a dimple-like depression in the center of the overlying skin. *B.* This dermatofibroma is also variegated in color, with a red center and a brownish to black periphery. In contrast to melanoma, it is hard and shows the dimple-like depression on lateral compression.

may be indicated. There is a report of two cellular dermatofibromas that underwent metastasis to lymph nodes and lungs.[82] Notably, both original lesions were two cm in diameter, an unusually large size for dermatofibroma, and had recurred locally prior to metastasis.

Several other histologic variants exist, more than one of which may be present in a single lesion, so-called combined dermatofibroma.[83] A vascular variant, rich in endothelial-lined spaces and hemosiderin pigment, formerly was termed *sclerosing hemangioma.* The epithelioid histiocytoma[84] is characterized by large, angulated cells and presents clinically as a solitary raised vascular nodule resembling pyogenic granuloma. A granular cell variant of dermatofibroma is described.[85] Dermatofibroma with monster cells is an interesting lesion in which many of the cells have notable nuclear enlargement and prominent nucleoli.[86,87] This morphologic change generally is considered a degenerative phenomenon of little clinical import.

There is a rare group of atypical fibrous histiocytomas[88] characterized by pleomorphic, plump, spindle, or polyhedral cells with large, hyperchromatic, irregular, or bizarre nuclei set in a background of classic features of fibrous histiocytoma, including a storiform pattern and keloidal collagen. Some lesions attained a diameter of more than 2 cm, invaded the superficial subcutis, or exhibited geographic necrosis. Atypical mitotic figures have been noted, as have local recurrence and distant metastases. Thus lesions with such atypical features must be excised completely and the patients followed up carefully.

A different lesion is the indeterminate histiocytic lesion of skin,[89] which has several features intermediate between dermatofibroma and dermatofibrosarcoma protuberans. These include overlying acanthosis and densely cellular fascicles with focal storiform areas. Prominent cytologic atypia has been observed. All lesions have keloidal dermal collagen, infiltrate the subcutis in a honeycomb pattern, and have low mitotic counts without atypical forms. All are diffusely immunoreactive for factor XIIIa as well as CD34. However, double immunolabeling shows no significant coexpression of these two antigens by individual cells. A single recurrence was documented. These indeterminate fibrohistiocytic lesions of skin suggest a possible spectrum between dermatofibroma and dermatofibrosarcoma protuberans. Their potential for local recurrence suggests that performing a complete conservative excision may be prudent.

Immunolabeling for factor XIIIa is usually positive in dermatofibroma[90] but not in dermatofibrosarcoma protuberans.[91] In addition, the more cellular forms of dermatofibroma tend to express alpha-smooth-muscle actin, whereas the lesions with more epithelioid cells and giant cells tend to express histiocytic markers.[92]

Dermatomyofibroma

This benign lesion[93] occurs typically on the shoulder area of young women, presenting as a firm, asymptomatic, intradermal 1- to 2-cm plaque. Histologically, it forms a well-circumscribed platelike lesion in the middermis that is arranged parallel to the epidermal surface and composed of elongated fascicles of spindle cells lacking atypia or mitotic figures. The neoplastic cells express vimentin and muscle-specific actin; initially, expression of alpha-smooth-muscle actin was reportedly negative, but in our experience, it is usually positive. By electron microscopy, the cells have typical features of myofibroblasts, including prominent rough endoplasmic reticulum, pinocytotic vesicles, and subplasmalemmal linear densities.

Superficial Acral Fibromyxoma

This recently described lesion[94] presents as a solitary dermal or subcutaneous mass of the toe, finger, or palm, and it often involves the nail region. Histologically, it is composed of spindled and stellate-shaped cells with random, loose storiform or fascicular growth patterns embedded in a myxoid/collagenous stroma. There is generally only slight nuclear atypia, and mitotic figures are infrequent. There is expression of CD34, epithelial membrane antigen, and CD99.

INTERMEDIATE-GRADE NEOPLASMS (OF LOW METASTATIC POTENTIAL)

Dermatofibrosarcoma Protuberans

Dermatofibrosarcoma protuberans (DFSP) is a locally aggressive dermal and subcutaneous mesenchymal neoplasm that typically occurs during the third and fourth decades of life on the trunk and proximal extremities of patients. It often grows to several centimeters in diameter and may form large tumors (Fig. 102-11). The clinical morphology is variable. The most common presentation is as an indurated plaque with firm, bosselated, flesh-colored to red-brown nodules (see Fig. 102-11). It also can present as a nonprotuberant, atrophic, violaceous lesion (Fig. 102-12) simulating sclerosing basal cell carcinoma, anetoderma, or scar. Large nodular tumors occur (Fig. 102-13). The epidermis is often atrophic and may ulcerate focally. Local recurrences even following wide excision are common; metastases are extremely rare,[95] being hematogenous in two-thirds of cases and nodal in one-third of cases.

DFSP is a poorly circumscribed dermal proliferation of monomorphous, slender or slightly plump spindle cells with little pleomorphism arranged in a storiform pattern (Fig. 102-14). The proliferation commonly infiltrates the subcutaneous fat, isolating adipocytes to form lucencies ("honeycomb" or "Swiss cheese" pattern). In contrast to dermatofibroma, the tumor is much more cellular and usually does not have mature collagen interspersed between fascicles of spindle cells.

Variable histologic patterns described include myxoid, neuroid, fibrosarcomatous, myoid,[96] and granular cell types. The tumor may be relatively monomorphous or show combinations of various patterns within the original tumor or in the recurrences. As discussed below, some lesions show overlap between giant cell fibroblastoma

FIGURE 102-11

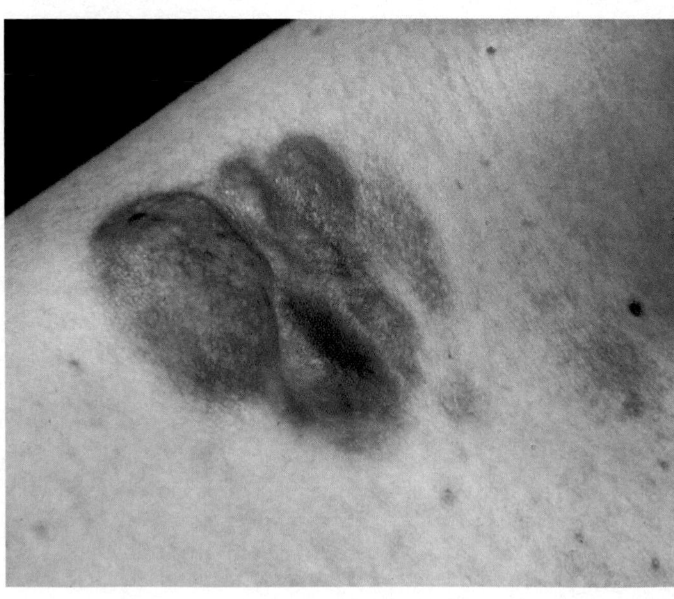

Dermatofibrosarcoma protuberans presenting as reddish brown confluent flat nodules.

FIGURE 102-12

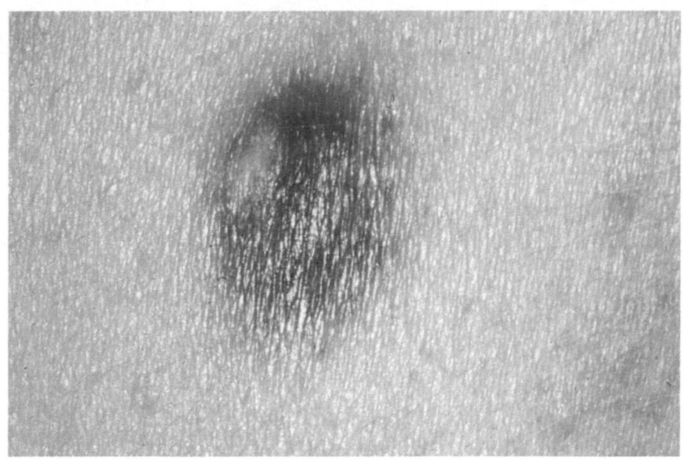

Atrophic variant of dermatofibrosarcoma protuberans.

and DFSP.[97] The fibrosarcomatous variant has basic features of DFSP but focal areas in which the cells exhibit a high grade of atypia and are arranged in long fascicles in a herringbone (fibrosarcoma-like) pattern. Several series indicate an increased biologic aggressiveness of this type compared with ordinary DFSP; thus in a series from Memorial Sloan Kettering Cancer Center, patients with the fibrosarcomatous variant versus classic DFSP had a 5-year recurrence-free survival rate of 81 and 28 percent, respectively.[98] On the other hand, in a series from the Cleveland Clinic, patients with sarcomas arising in DFSP did not have an increased risk of distant metastasis within a 5-year follow-up period, provided they were treated by wide local excision with negative margins.[99]

The histogenesis of DFSP is uncertain; fibrohistiocytic, purely fibroblastic, and neural-related differentiation have all been hypothesized. A very sensitive, although nonspecific, marker for DFSP is CD34. A distinctive cell population within normal nerves has been shown to express CD34, consistent with a neural-related histogenesis of DFSP. CD34 can help distinguish between DFSP and scar tissue in reexcision specimens because scars are CD34-negative.[79] However, myxoid or fibrosarcomatous areas may be negative[100]; therefore, a focally negative CD34 immunostain does not rule out DFSP. Another interesting marker is low-affinity nerve growth receptor (p75), reported to be positive in DFSP but negative in dermatofibroma.[101] This antigen is

FIGURE 102-13

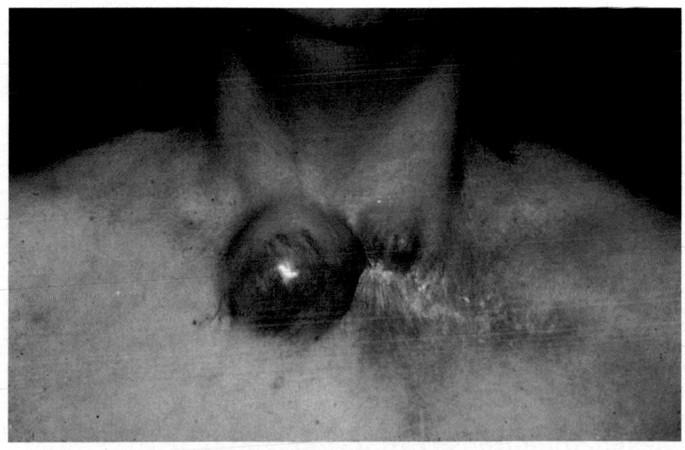

Large nodular dermatofibrosarcoma protuberans. This is a recurrence after the primary tumor had been excised.

FIGURE 102-14

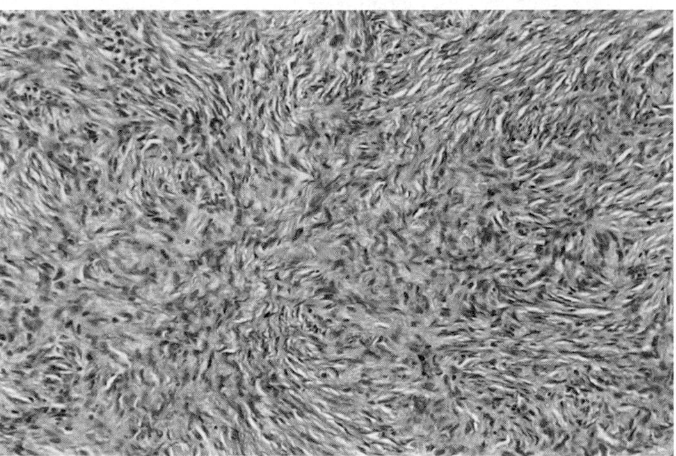

Dermatofibrosarcoma protuberans showing fibroblastic spindle cells that are arranged in interlacing fascicles. These intersect and bend at acute angles producing a starburst (storiform) pattern.

also consistently expressed in many neural neoplasms and in embryonal and alveolar rhabdomyosarcoma, synovial sarcoma, and spindle cell hemangioendothelioma, as well as in a variable number of cases of fibrosarcoma variants, solitary fibrous tumor, hemangiopericytoma, spindle cell lipoma, Ewing's sarcoma, mesenchymal chondrosarcoma, and malignant melanoma.

At the molecular level, DFSP exhibits the reciprocal translocation t(17;22)(q22;q13), producing a fusion of the collagen type I alpha 1 gene (*COL1A1*) and the platelet-derived growth factor B-chain gene (*PDGFB*). Current techniques permit sensitive and specific detection of these fusion transcripts in paraffin-embedded DFSP tumor specimens by reverse transcription polymerase chain reaction (PCR).[102] Both fibrosarcomatous transformation of DFSP and some cases of superficial fibrosarcoma have been shown to harbor these fusion transcripts, suggesting a close affinity between DFSP and fibrosarcoma.[103]

DFSP is a low-grade malignant tumor, often infiltrating diffusely through the dermis and into the subcutaneous fat but seldom metastasizing. Increased age, high mitotic index, and increased cellularity are predictors of poor clinical outcome.[98] About 30 to 50 percent of DFSPs recur locally after simple excision, so it is generally recommended that a wide excision with at least 2-cm free margins be performed (see Fig. 102-13). Pathologic examination of margins during surgery is helpful in delineating the extent of the tumor. Mohs surgery has shown good results in some practitioners' hands.[104] Adjuvant radiation therapy may help decrease the local recurrence rate.[105]

Giant Cell Fibroblastoma

This rare tumor, commonly considered a juvenile variant of DFSP, occurs occasionally in adults.[106] It usually presents as a dermal or subcutaneous mass on the back, inguinal, or thigh areas. Tumors with a DFSP component have been described, suggesting that giant cell fibroblastoma is a variant of DFSP.[107] Recurrences are common (50 percent); metastases have not been reported. Treatment is adequate surgical excision.

Spindle cells with moderate nuclear atypia are seen in a loose fibrous or mucinous stroma infiltrating the dermis and subcutis. Angiectoid spaces lined by multinucleated tumor giant cells are prominent in the deeper portions of the tumor. Immunohistochemically, the cells are positive for CD34 and occasionally $alpha_1$ antichymotrypsin and negative for factor VIII and S-100. Ultrastructural studies are compatible with fibrohistiocytic differentiation.

Atypical Fibroxanthoma (AFX)

This relatively common rapidly growing but low-grade neoplasm occurs mainly on sun-exposed skin (face, neck, and hands) of elderly individuals (Fig. 102-15). The anatomic distribution and the presence of cyclobutane pyrimidine dimers support a pathogenic role for ultraviolet radiation.[108] Some tumors occur 10 to 15 years after local ionizing irradiation. The lesion usually presents as a solitary nodule, often ulcerated, and usually less than 3 cm in diameter. Metastases are rare[109]; vascular invasion, necrosis, and deep subcutaneous invasion may be associated with greater metastatic potential. Recurrences are common, predominantly those involving the subcutaneous tissue. Mohs' micrographic surgery may lead to a better outcome than conventional wide local excision.[110] AFX is now considered a subtype of malignant fibrous histiocytoma (MFH) that, because of its small size and superficial location, behaves in a much less aggressive fashion. Additionally, it has been suggested that unlike deep MFH, AFX may lack some mutations in *ras* oncogenes, possibly also contributing to its more favorable biologic course.[111]

Specimens often are partially exophytic tumors with ulceration of the overlying epidermis. A Grenz zone may be present, but usually the tumor abuts onto the dermal-epidermal junction. However, evidence for true origin from the epidermis is lacking. A poorly circumscribed hypercellular tumor often extends deeply into the reticular dermis or subcutis. It consists of spindle cells in a collagenous or occasionally myxoid stroma admixed with multinucleated giant cells and epithelioid cells (Fig. 102-16). The neoplastic cells display pronounced atypia, with bizarre, large, round or ovoid hyperchromatic nuclei with numerous mitotic figures (some of them atypical); large, prominent eosinophilic nucleoli; and abundant, occasionally vacuolated cytoplasm. Some cells may contain fine droplets of lipid, demonstrable by oil red O stains on frozen tissue. The spindle cell subtype of AFX occurs in the same clinical setting as an ulcerated tumor and is characterized by a monomorphous proliferation of spindle cells with very little pleomorphism. Immunohistochemically, AFX has variable profiles, but cells usually express vimentin and histiocytic markers such as $alpha_1$-antitrypsin, $alpha_1$-antichymotrypsin, HAM-56 antigen, and CD68. A few express factor XIIIa. Recently, expression of CD99 has been proposed to be a relatively sensitive (73 percent of cases) and, in context, specific marker for these tumors.[112] Expression of S-100A6 also appears to be a sensitive marker for AFX.[113]

FIGURE 102-15

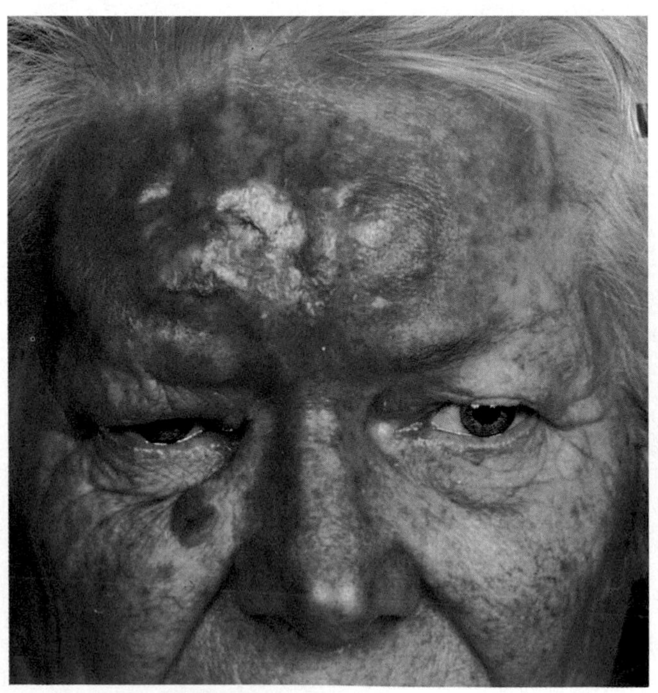

Atypical fibroxanthoma presenting as a flat, bosselated tumor on the forehead of an elderly woman. Note the yellowish to reddish color.

FIGURE 102-16

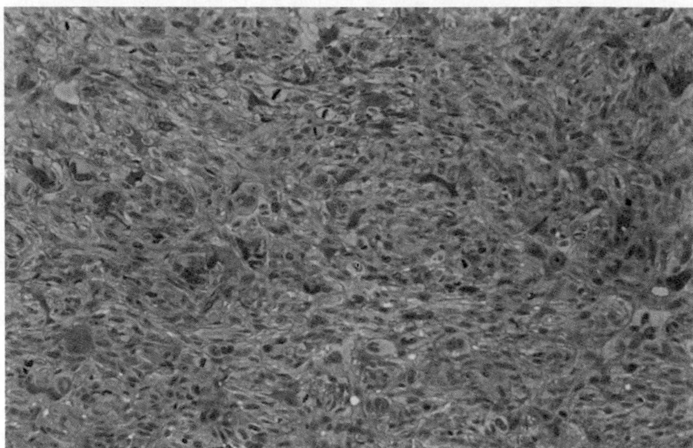

Atypical fibroxanthoma showing atypical plump spindle cells and multinucleated giant cells.

By electron microscopy, the tumor cells differentiate along histiocytic (multiple phagolysosomes), fibroblastic (abundant rough endoplasmic reticulum), or myofibroblastic (subplasmalemmal condensations of intermediate filaments, pinocytosis) lines. Tumor cells lack features of epithelial (desmosomes or tonofilaments) or melanocytic (melanosomes) differentiation.

The histologic differential diagnosis includes squamous cell carcinoma and malignant melanoma and some types of sarcoma. Some pathologists argue that all AFX cases are actually dedifferentiated (sarcomatoid) squamous cell carcinomas, but we prefer to designate as squamous cell carcinoma only those lesions having expression of epithelial markers such as cytokeratin, showing histologic evidence of keratinization, or arising in the setting of squamous cell carcinoma in situ. Most melanomas exhibit at least focal areas of melanoma in situ and express S-100 protein, gp100 (with HMB-45), and MART-1 (see Chap. 93). In AFX, in contrast, the neoplastic cells are S-100–negative, although scattered S-100–positive dendritic cells may infiltrate the tumor. Diagnosis of specific histogenic types of sarcoma requires immunohistochemical or ultrastructural evidence for a particular pathway of differentiation.

MALIGNANT NEOPLASMS

Malignant Fibrous Histiocytoma (MFH)

This tumor is presently considered to be the most common malignant soft tissue tumor, having replaced fibrosarcoma in that position some years ago. However, the future of this entity is in doubt. Some authorities deride the concept of MFH, considering it to be a diagnostic wastebasket. According to this view, MFH is merely a morphologic pattern rather than a defined pathologic entity.[114] Moreover, this school argues that, in most cases, careful immunohistochemical and ultrastructural examination permits probable or definite classification into defined histogenetic subtypes of sarcoma; the remaining minority might be better designated as pleomorphic sarcoma not otherwise classified rather than using an ambiguous and potentially misleading term such as MFH. It has been questioned whether an exhaustive attempt to subclassify pleomorphic sarcomas into defined histogenetic categories is clinically significant or worthwhile. However, MFH tumors reclassified as myogenic sarcoma had a worse prognosis and a shorter interval before metastasis compared with nonmyogenic tumors of the same stage.[115] Accordingly, there is much merit in the attacks on MFH as a term and entity. However, most pathologists and clinicians are familiar with this term and use it to describe mesenchymal proliferations of markedly atypical cells that lack any more definitive differentiation. Accordingly, we shall continue to use this terminology, but without implying a defined fibrohistiocytic differentiation of such lesions.

MFH occurs mainly in the deep soft tissue (skeletal muscle) of the limbs or retroperitoneum, but virtually any anatomic site, including the heart, gall bladder, and other viscera, can be affected. It rarely occurs in children except for the dermal/subcutaneous angiomatoid variant. Recurrences occur in half of patients, and at least one-third of deep tumors metastasize within 2 years, primarily to lung, lymph nodes, liver, and bone. As with several other soft tissue tumors (leiomyosarcoma, liposarcoma), MFH originating in the dermis or subcutis (atypical fibroxanthoma) is associated with a better prognosis than when the deep soft tissue is involved.

The predominant pattern may be storiform, myxoid, giant cell, or inflammatory. Large size, histologic grade, and positive surgical margins are all significantly negative prognostic factors for survival.[115] The most common appearance is of spindle cells in a storiform pattern. The stroma may be finely fibrillary, myxoid, or densely collagenous. Bizarre epithelioid and giant cells may be present and may contain small amounts of lipid. Many mitotic figures, bizarre giant cells, and necrosis are common. Ultrastructurally, the neoplastic cells have features consistent with fibroblastic, myofibroblastic, and histiocytic differentiation. Immunohistochemistry using a broad antibody panel is required to rule out metastatic carcinoma, lymphoma, leiomyosarcoma, melanoma, and similar lesions.

Complete surgical resection at presentation offers the best chance for survival. Radiation therapy plays an important role in combination with surgery for better local control, particularly in high-grade lesions and in patients with positive surgical margins after wide complete gross excision. Adjuvant chemotherapy is investigational.[116]

Epithelioid Sarcoma

This aggressive sarcoma[117] occurs most often on the hands and fingers of young males (mean age 27 years). Proximally located tumors (e.g., groin, thigh, vulva, and axilla) have a much worse prognosis.[118] Because the classic location on distal extremities often discourages early deep biopsy, and because epithelioid sarcoma may closely mimic various nonneoplastic lesions histologically such as granuloma annulare, it often evades diagnosis at an early, localized stage. The etiology is obscure; possibly trauma plays some a role. Epithelioid sarcoma usually presents as a firm dermal or subcutaneous nodule, sometimes with ulceration or sinus formation (Fig. 102-17). Linear subcutaneous nodules due to progressive multifocal spread along tendons, nerves, and fascia may give a sporotrichoid appearance. The tumor has recurrence rates of 50 to 77 percent and nodal or hematogenous metastasis in 40 to 50 percent of patients. The lung and pleura are the most common sites of metastatic disease; local recurrence (size of 5 cm or larger) and re-

FIGURE 102-17

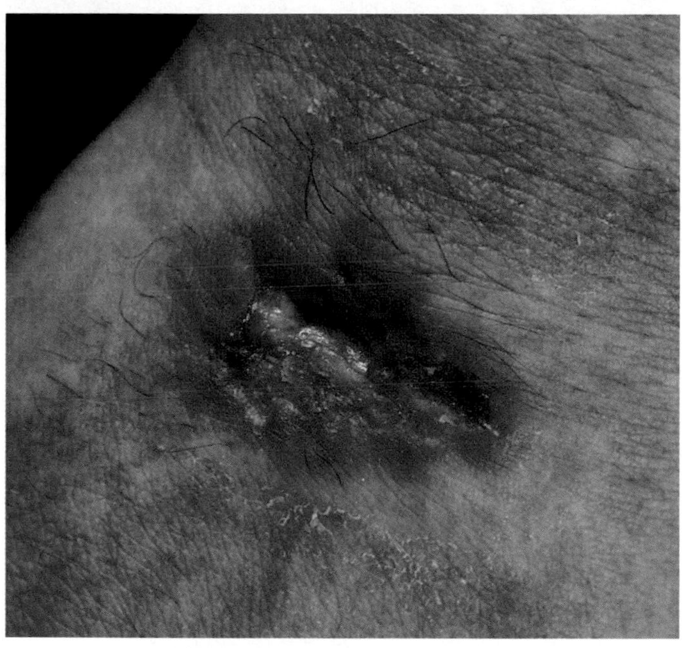

Epithelioid sarcoma typically occurring over the wrist. Note ulceration and granuloma-like border.

gional metastasis events are predictive of worse distant-metastasis-free survival.[119]

Radical excision traditionally has been the treatment of choice, but recurrences occur even with amputation. Recently, conservative (limb-sparing) surgery combined with pre- or postoperative radiation therapy has been tried, with results comparable with those reported with radical amputation.[120] Chemotherapeutic regimens have not been successful. Surgical excision of a solitary metastasis is occasionally helpful.

Most lesions occur in fascia, tendon, or subcutaneous septa; approximately 25 percent arise in the dermis. The tumor usually presents as a multinodular mass composed of epithelioid cells with abundant eosinophilic, often vacuolated, cytoplasm admixed with spindle cells in a collagenous and myxoid stroma. Characteristically, there is central necrosis with a surrounding palisade of tumor cells. A high mitotic rate, large areas of necrosis, vascular invasion, and size greater than 5 cm are associated with worse prognosis. Proximal tumors often have a rhabdoid appearance.[118] Other histologic variants include spindle cell (fibroma-like)[121] and angiomatoid types.

The cell of origin is uncertain. Tumor cells express vimentin and epithelial markers. In a large series, epithelial membrane antigen was present in 96 percent of patients, and muscle-specific actin and CD34 were noted in 41 and 52 percent of the patients, respectively. The angiomatoid, fibroma-like, and large cell–rhabdoid variants had immunohistochemical profiles similar to the classic cases. S-100 protein is usually absent. Ultrastructural findings suggest myofibroblastic differentiation, but others conclude that the tumor is composed of immature mesenchymal tissue.

The pathologic differential diagnosis includes necrobiosis lipoidica, granuloma annulare, rheumatoid nodule, and necrotizing infectious granuloma. In addition, other malignant neoplasms include epithelioid forms of angiosarcoma, malignant peripheral nerve sheath tumor (malignant schwannoma), malignant melanoma, synovial sarcoma, and fibrosarcoma. Deep biopsy, immunohistochemical workup, and review of all previous material may be necessary before the correct diagnosis is reached.

REFERENCES

1. De Wever I et al: Cytogenetic, clinical, and morphologic correlations in 78 cases of fibromatosis: A report from the CHAMP study group. Chromosomes and morphology. *Mod Pathol* **13**:1080, 2000
2. Kurtycz DF et al: Diagnosis of fibromatosis colli by fine-needle aspiration. *Diagn Cytopathol* **23**:338, 2000
3. Fringes B et al: Identification of actin microfilaments in the intracytoplasmic inclusions present in recurring infantile digital fibromatosis (Reye tumor). *Pediatr Pathol* **6**:311, 1986
4. Fetsch JF, Miettinen M: Calcifying aponeurotic fibroma: A clinicopathologic study of 22 cases arising in uncommon sites. *Hum Pathol* **29**:1504, 1998
5. Hoffman CD et al: Aggressive infantile fibromatosis: Report of a case undergoing spontaneous regression. *J Oral Maxillofac Surg* **51**:1043, 1993
6. Guitart J et al: Solitary cutaneous myofibromas in adults: Report of six cases and discussion of differential diagnosis. *J Cutan Pathol* **23**:437, 1996
7. Landing BH, Nadorra R: Infantile systemic hyalinosis: Report of four cases of a disease, fatal in infancy, apparently different from juvenile systemic hyalinosis. *Pediatr Pathol* **6**:55, 1986
8. Classen DA, Hurst LN: Plantar fibromatosis and bilateral flexion contractures: A review of the literature. *Ann Plast Surg* **28**:475, 1992
9. de Palma L et al: Plantar fibromatosis: An immunohistochemical and ultrastructual study. *Foot Ankle Int* **20**: 253, 1999
10. Frey M: Risks and prevention of Dupuytren's contracture. *Lancet* **350**:1568, 1997
11. Ushijima M et al: Dupuytren-type fibromatoses: A clinicopathologic study of 62 cases. *Acta Pathol Jpn* **34**:991, 1984
12. Meister P et al: Palmar fibromatosis, "Dupuytren's contracture": A comparison of light electron and immunofluorescence microscopic findings. *Pathol Res Pract* **164**:402, 1979
13. Berndt A et al: TGF beta and bFGF synthesis and localization in Dupuytren's disease (nodular palmar fibromatosis) relative to cellular activity, myofibroblast phenotype and oncofetal variants of fibronectin. *Histochem* **27**:1014, 1995
14. Margo G et al: Myofibroblasts of palmar fibromatosis coexpress transforming growth factor-alpha and epidermal growth factor receptor. *J Pathol* **181**:213, 1997
15. Dominguez-Malagon HR et al: Clinical and cellular effects of colchicine in fibromatosis. *Cancer* **69**:2478, 1992
16. Rombouts JJ et al: Prediction of recurrence in the treatment of Dupuytren's disease: Evaluation of a histologic classification. *J Hand Surg* **14A**:644, 1989
17. Coupland WW: Fibrosing conditions and propranolol. *Med J Aust* **2**:137, 1977
18. Williams G, Green NA: The non-surgical treatment of Peyronie's disease. *Br J Urol* **52**: 392, 1980
19. Guberman D et al: Knuckle pads—a forgotten skin condition: Report of a case and review of the literature. *Cutis* **57**:241, 1996
20. Caroli A et al: Epidemiological and structural findings supporting the fibromatosis origin of dorsal knuckle pads. *J Hand Surg* **168**:258, 1991
21. Tompkins SD et al: Distal pachydermodactyly. *J Am Acad Dermatol* **38**:359, 1998
22. Bauer EA et al: Progressive nodular fibrosis of the skin: Altered procollagen and collagenase expression by cultured fibroblasts. *J Invest Dermatol* **87**:210, 1986
23. Ben-Izhak O et al: Fibromatosis (desmoid tumor) following radiation therapy for Hodgkin's disease. *Arch Pathol Lab Med* **118**:815, 1994
24. Lowy M et al: Desmoid tumor: Transformation into fibrosarcoma (author's translation). *Dermatologica* **163**:125,1981
25. Fletcher JA et al: Chromosome aberrations in desmoid tumors: Trisomy 8 may be a predictor of recurrence. *Cancer Genet Cytogenet* **79**:139, 1995
26. Wilcken N, Tattersall MH: Endocrine therapy for desmoid tumors. *Cancer* **68**:1384, 1991
27. Hamilton L et al: Chemotherapy for desmoid tumours in association with familial adenomatous polyposis: A report of three cases. *Can J Surg* **39**:247, 1996
28. Lee YS, Vijayasingam S: Mast cells and myofibroblasts in keloid: A light microscopic, immunohistochemical and ultrastructural study. *Ann Acad Med Singapore* **24**:902, 1995
29. Beer TW et al: Mast cells in pathological and surgical scars. *Br J Ophthalmol* **82**:691, 1998
30. Kischer CW: Contributions of electron microscopy to the study of the hypertrophic scar and related lesions. *Scanning Microsc* **7**:921, 1993
31. Castagnoli C et al: TNF production and hypertrophic scarring. *Cell Immunol* **147**:51, 1993
32. Kim A et al: Are keloids really "gli-loids"? High-level expression of *gli-1* oncogene in keloids. *J Am Acad Dermatol* **45**:707, 2001
33. Dalkowski A et al: Increased expression of tenascin C by keloids in vivo and in vitro. *Br J Dermatol* **141**:50, 1999
34. McCauley RL et al: Altered cytokine production in black patients with keloids. *J Clin Immunol* **12**:300, 1992
35. Younai S et al: Modulation of collagen synthesis by transforming growth factor-beta in keloid and hypertrophic scar fibroblasts. *Ann Plast Surg* **33**:148, 1994
36. Smith P et al: TGF-beta2 activates proliferative scar fibroblasts. *J Surg Res* **82**:319, 1999
37. Kikuchi K et al: Effects of various growth factors and histamine on cultured keloid fibroblasts. *Dermatology* **190**:4, 1995
38. Nowak KC et al: The effect of superpulsed carbon dioxide laser energy on keloid and normal dermal fibroblast secretion of growth factors: A serum-free study. *Plast Reconstr Surg* **105**:2039, 2000
39. Castagnoli C et al: Characterization of T-cell subsets infiltrating post-burn hypertrophic scar tissues. *Burns* **23**:565, 1997
40. Ladin DA et al: p53 and apoptosis alterations on keloids and keloid fibroblasts. *Wound Repair Regen* **6**:28, 1998
41. Kischer CW et al: Perivascular myofibroblasts and microvascular occlusion in hypertrophic scars and keloids. *Hum Pathol* **13**:819, 1982
42. Kauh YC et al: Major suppression of pro-alpha1(I) type I collagen gene expression in the dermis after keloid excision and immediate intrawound injection of triamcinolone acetonide. *J Am Acad Dermatol* **37**:586, 1997
43. Sallstrom KO et al: Treatment of keloids with surgical excision and postoperative x-ray radiation. *Scand J Plast Reconstr Surg Hand Surg* **23**:211, 1989
44. Sherman R, Rosenfeld H: Experience with the Nd:YAG laser in the treatment of keloid scars. *Ann Plast Surg* **21**:231, 1988
45. Daly TJ, Weston WL: Retinoid effects on fibroblast proliferation and collagen synthesis in vitro and on fibrotic disease in vivo. *J Am Acad Dermatol* **15**:900, 1986
46. Berman B, Duncan MR: Short-term keloid treatment in vivo with human interferon alpha-2b results in a selective and persistent normalization of keloidal fibroblast collagen, glycosaminoglycan, and collagenase production in vitro. *J Am Acad Dermatol* **21**:694, 1989
47. Wong TW et al: Intralesional interferon alpha-2b has no effect in the treatment of keloids. *Br J Dermatol* **130**:683, 1994
48. Conejo-Mir JS et al: Carbon dioxide laser ablation associated with interferon alpha-2b injections reduces the recurrence of keloids. *J Am Acad Dermatol* **39**:1039, 1998
49. Tilkorn H et al: The protruding scars: Keloids and hypertrophic diagnosis and treatment with silicon-gel sheeting. *Polim Med* **24**:31, 1994
50. Fulton JE Jr: Silicone gel sheeting for the prevention and management of evolving hypertrophic and keloid scars. *Dermatol Surg* **21**:947, 1995
51. Montgomery EA, Meis JM: Nodular fasciitis. Its morphologic spectrum and immunohistochemical profile. *Am J Surg Pathol* **15**:942, 1991
52. Kiryu H et al: Proliferative fasciitis. Report of a case with histopathologic and immunohistochemical studies. *Am J Dermatopathol* **19**:396, 1997
53. Naylor MF et al: Elastofibroma dorsi: Radiologic findings in 12 patients. *AJR* **167**:683, 1996
54. Fukuda Y et al: Histogenesis of unique elastinophilic fibers of elastofibroma: Ultrastructural and immunohistochemical studies. *Hum Pathol* **18**:424, 1987
55. Jordaan HF, Rossouw DJ: Digital papular calcific elastosis: A histopathological, histochemical and ultrastructural study of 20 patients. *J Cutan Pathol* **17**:358, 1990
56. Wegrowski Y et al: Alteration of matrix macromolecule synthesis by fibroblasts from a patient with pachydermoperiostosis. *J Invest Dermatol* **106**:70, 1996
57. Masse R et al: Costa's acrokerato-elastoidosis: Ultrastructural study (author's translation). *Ann Dermatol Venereol* **104**:441, 1977
58. Brodell RT, Pokorney DR: Fibroepithelial polyps and pathologic evaluation. *Arch Dermatol* **133**:915, 1997
59. Williams BT et al: Cutaneous pseudosarcomatous polyp: A histological and immunohistochemical study. *J Cutan Pathol* **23**:189, 1996.
60. Dickey GE, Sotelo-Avila C: Fibrous hamartoma of infancy: Current review. *Pediatr Dev Pathol* **2**:236, 1999
61. Groisman G, Lichtig C: Fibrous hamartoma of infancy: An immunohistochemical and ultrastructural study. *Hum Pathol* **22**:914, 1991

62. Schirren H et al: Papular elastorrhexis: A variant of dermatofibrosis lenticularis disseminata (Buschke-Ollendorff syndrome)? *Dermatology* **189**:368, 1994
63. Assmann A et al: Buschke-Ollendorff syndrome—differential diagnosis of disseminated connective tissue lesions. *Eur J Dermatol* **11**:576, 2001
64. DePadova-Elder S et al: Multiple connective tissue nevi. *Cutis* **42**:222, 1988
65. Lindor NM et al: Birt-Hogg-Dubé syndrome: An autosomal dominant disorder with predisposition to cancers of the kidney, fibrofolliculomas, and focal cutaneous mucinosis. *Int J Dermatol* **40**:653, 2001
66. Donati P et al: Sclerotic (hypocellular) fibromas of the skin. *Br J Dermatol* **124**:395, 1991
67. Steck PA et al: Identification of a candidate tumour suppressor gene, *MMAC1,* at chromosome 10q23.3 that is mutated in multiple advanced cancers. *Nature Genet* **15**:356, 1997
68. Brito H et al: Giant cell collagenoma: Case report and review of the literature. *J Cutan Pathol* **29**:48, 2002
69. Kamino H et al: Pleomorphic fibroma of the skin: A benign neoplasm with cytologic atypia. A clinicopathologic study of eight cases. *Am J Surg Pathol* **13**:107, 1989
70. Garcia-Doval I et al: Pleomorphic fibroma of the skin, a form of sclerotic fibroma: An immunohistochemical study. *Clin Exp Dermatol* **23**:22, 1998
71. Chen TM et al: Pleomorphic sclerotic fibroma: A case report and literature review. *Am J Dermatopathol* **24**:54, 2002
72. Miettinen M, Fetsch JF: Collagenous fibroma (desmoplastic fibroblastoma): A clinicopathologic analysis of 63 cases of a distinctive soft tissue lesion with stellate-shaped fibroblasts. *Hum Pathol* **29**:676, 1998
73. Okamura JM et al: Solitary fibrous tumor of the skin. *Am J Dermatopathol* **19**:515, 1997
74. Westra WH et al: Solitary fibrous tumor: Consistent CD34 immunoreactivity and occurrence in the orbit. *Am J Surg Pathol* **18**:992, 1994
75. Headington JT: The histiocyte: In memoriam. *Arch Dermatol* **122**:532, 1986
76. Tsang WY, Chan JK: KP1 (CD68) staining of granular cell neoplasms: Is KP1 a marker for lysosomes rather than the histiocytic lineage? *Histopathology* **21**:84, 1992
77. Tos AP et al: KP1 (CD68) expression in benign neural tumours: Further evidence of its low specificity as histiocytic/myeloid marker. *Histopathology* **23**:185, 1993
78. Banerjee SS, Harris M: Morphological and immunophenotypic variations in malignant melanoma. *Histopathology* **36**:387, 2000
79. Prieto VG et al: CD34 immunoreactivity distinguishes between scar tissue and residual tumor in re-excisional specimens of dermatofibrosarcoma protuberans. *J Cutan Pathol* **21**:324, 1994
80. Mentzel T et al: Benign fibrous histiocytoma (dermatofibroma) of the face: Clinicopathologic and immunohistochemical study of 34 cases associated with an aggressive clinical course. *Am J Dermatopathol* **23**:419, 2001
81. Vanni R et al: Cytogenetic evidence of clonality in cutaneous benign fibrous histiocytomas: A report of the CHAMP study group. *Histopathology* **37**:212, 2000
82. Colome-Grimmer MI, Evans HL: Metastasizing cellular dermatofibroma. Report of two cases. *Am J Surg Pathol* **20**:1361, 1996
83. Zelger BG et al: Combined dermatofibroma: Co-existence of two or more variant patterns in a single lesion. *Histopathology* **36**:529, 2000
84. Jones EW et al: Epithelioid cell histiocytoma: A new entity. *Br J Dermatol* **120**:185, 1989
85. Soyer HP et al: Granular cell dermatofibroma. *Am J Dermatopathol* **19**:168, 1997
86. Rudolph P et al: Differential expression of CD34 and Ki-M1p in pleomorphic fibroma and dermatofibroma with monster cells. *Am J Dermatopathol* **21**:414, 1999
87. Goodman WT et al: Giant dermatofibroma with monster cells. *Am J Dermatopathol* **24**:36, 2002
88. Kaddu S et al: Atypical fibrous histiocytoma of the skin: Clinicopathologic analysis of 59 cases with evidence of infrequent metastasis. *Am J Surg Pathol* **26**:35, 2002
89. Horenstein MG et al: Indeterminate fibrohistiocytic lesions of the skin: Is there a spectrum between dermatofibroma and dermatofibrosarcoma protuberans? *Am J Surg Pathol* **24**:996, 2000
90. Cerio R et al: Identification of factor XIIIa in cutaneous tissue. *Histopathology* **13**:362, 1988
91. Kutzner H: Expression of the human progenitor cell antigen CD34 (HPCA-1) distinguishes dermatofibrosarcoma protuberans from fibrous histiocytoma in formalin-fixed, paraffin-embedded tissue. *J Am Acad Dermatol* **28**:613, 1993
92. Prieto VG et al: Immunohistochemistry of dermatofibromas and benign fibrous histiocytomas. *J Cutan Pathol* **22**:336, 1995
93. Kamino H et al: Dermatomyofibroma: A benign cutaneous, plaque-like proliferation of fibroblasts and myofibroblasts in young adults. *J Cutan Pathol* **19**:85, 1992
94. Fetsch JF et al: Superficial acral fibromyxoma: A clinicopathologic and immunohistochemical analysis of 37 cases of a distinctive soft tissue tumor with a predilection for the fingers and toes. *Hum Pathol* **32**:704, 2001
95. Lal P et al: Dermatofibrosarcoma protuberans metastasizing to lymph nodes: A case report and review of literature. *J Surg Oncol* **72**:178, 1999
96. Calonje E, Fletcher CD: Myoid differentiation in dermatofibrosarcoma protuberans and its fibrosarcomatous variant: Clinicopathologic analysis of 5 cases. *J Cutan Pathol* **23**:30, 1996
97. Sigel JE et al: A morphologic study of dermatofibrosarcoma protuberans: Expansion of a histologic profile. *J Cutan Pathol* **27**:159, 2000
98. Bowne WB et al: Dermatofibrosarcoma protuberans: A clinicopathologic analysis of patients treated and followed at a single institution. *Cancer* **88**:2711, 2000
99. Goldblum JR et al: Sarcomas arising in dermatofibrosarcoma protuberans: A reappraisal of biologic behavior in eighteen cases treated by wide local excision with extended clinical follow up. *Am J Surg Pathol* **24**:1125, 2000
100. Orlandi A et al: Myxoid dermatofibrosarcoma protuberans: Morphological, ultrastructural and immunohistochemical features. *J Cutan Pathol* **25**:386, 1998
101. Fanburg-Smith JC, Miettinen M: Low-affinity nerve growth factor receptor (p75) in dermatofibrosarcoma protuberans and other nonneural tumors: A study of 1150 tumors and fetal and adult normal tissues. *Hum Pathol* **32**:976, 2001
102. Wang J et al: Detection of *COL1A1-PDGFB* fusion transcripts in dermatofibrosarcoma protuberans by reverse transcription-polymerase chain reaction using archival formalin-fixed, paraffin-embedded tissues. *Diagn Mol Pathol* **8**:113, 1999
103. Wang J et al: *COL1A1-PDGFB* fusion transcripts in fibrosarcomatous areas of six dermatofibrosarcomas protuberans. *J Mol Diagn* **2**:47, 2000
104. Huether MJ et al: Mohs' micrographic surgery for the treatment of spindle cell tumors of the skin. *J Am Acad Dermatol* **44**:656, 2001
105. Sun LM et al: Dermatofibrosarcoma protuberans: Treatment results of 35 cases. *Radiother Oncol* **57**:175, 2000
106. Shmookler BM et al: Giant cell fibroblastoma: A juvenile form of dermatofibrosarcoma protuberans. *Cancer* **64**:2154, 1989
107. Galinier P et al: Giant-cell fibroblastoma and dermatofibrosarcoma protuberans: The same tumoral spectrum? Report of two cases of association in children. *Eur J Pediatr Surg* **10**:390, 2000
108. Sakamoto A et al: Immunoexpression of ultraviolet photoproducts and *p53*mutation analysis in atypical fibroxanthoma and superficial malignant fibrous histiocytoma. *Mod Pathol* **14**:581, 2001
109. Sankar NM et al: Metastasis from atypical fibroxanthoma of skin. *Med J Aust* **168**:418, 1998
110. Davis JL et al: A comparison of Mohs' micrographic surgery and wide excision for the treatment of atypical fibroxanthoma. *Dermatol Surg* **23**:105, 1997
111. Sakamoto A et al: *H-, K-,* and *N-ras* gene mutation in atypical fibroxanthoma and malignant fibrous histiocytoma. *Hum Pathol* **32**:1225, 2001
112. Monteagudo C et al: CD99 immunoreactivity in atypical fibroxanthoma: A common feature of diagnostic value. *Am J Clin Pathol* **117**:126, 2002
113. Fullen DR et al: S100A6 expression in fibrohistiocytic lesions. *J Cutan Pathol* **28**:229, 2001
114. Hollowood K, Fletcher CD: Malignant fibrous histiocytoma: Morphologic pattern or pathologic entity? *Semin Diagn Pathol* **12**:210, 1995
115. Fletcher CD et al: Clinicopathologic reevaluation of 100 malignant fibrous histiocytomas: Prognostic relevance of subclassification. *J Clin Oncol* **19**:3045, 2001
116. Belal A et al: Malignant fibrous histiocytoma: A retrospective study of 109 cases. *Am J Clin Oncol* **25**:16, 2002
117. Chase DR, Enzinger FM: Epithelioid sarcoma: Diagnosis, prognostic indicators, and treatment. *Am J Surg Pathol* **9**:241, 1985
118. Hasegawa T et al: Proximal-type epithelioid sarcoma: A clinicopathologic study of 20 cases. *Mod Pathol* **14**:655, 2001
119. Spillane AJ et al: Epithelioid sarcoma: The clinicopathological complexities of this rare soft tissue sarcoma. *Ann Surg Oncol* **7**:218, 2001
120. Callister MD et al: Epithelioid sarcoma: Results of conservative surgery and radiotherapy. *Int J Radiat Oncol Biol Phys* **51**:384, 2001
121. Tan SH, Ong BH: Spindle cell variant of epithelioid sarcoma: An easily misdiagnosed tumor. *Australas J Dermatol* **42**:139, 2001

CHAPTER 103

Suzanne Virnelli Grevelink
John Butler Mulliken

Vascular Anomalies and Tumors of Skin and Subcutaneous Tissues

Proper diagnosis of vascular anomalies has been hampered by contradictory and confusing descriptive nomenclature. The old terminology derives from the appearance of the anomaly and/or the concept of maternal impressions, as expressed in such terms as *strawberry hemangioma, cherry angioma, port-wine stain,* and *Salmon patch.* The first histopathologic classification by Virchow categorized vascular anomalies into three main types: *angioma simplex, angioma cavernosum,* and *angioma racemosum.* Variations on this confusing terminology persist in modern textbooks and are still used. Thus the generic term *hemangioma* is applied to lesions that predictably grow and involute and also to acquired vascular lesions in adults that do not regress and often progress. The nineteenth-century descriptive term *port-wine stain* applies to a permanent vascular abnormality that unfortunately is often called *capillary hemangioma.* Virchow's term, *cavernous hemangioma,* has been used mistakenly to describe deep cutaneous vascular anomalies and vascular anomalies of bone, muscle, and viscera that never regress. These categorizations of cutaneous anomalies based on descriptive terms or histopathologic terms, without clinical correlations, are confusing and lead to incorrect diagnosis and therapy and misdirected research efforts.[1]

A BIOLOGIC CLASSIFICATION

In 1982, Mulliken and Glowacki proposed a classification system for vascular birthmarks that correlated natural history and physical examination with cellular features.[2] This schema divided vascular lesions of infancy and childhood into two major types: *hemangiomas,* which exhibit endothelial hyperplasia, and *malformations,* which have normal endothelial turnover (Table 103-1). The terminological key is the Greek suffix *oma* that originally meant "swelling or tumor." Today, this suffix should be appended to terms describing lesions that grow by cellular proliferation, such as the common hemangioma. Most hemangiomas of infancy are not present at birth but appear postnatally. They grow rapidly during the first year (*proliferating phase*), undergo slow, spontaneous regression during childhood (*involuting phase*), and remain stable thereafter (*involuted phase*). Histologically, the proliferating phase is characterized by increased mitotic activity, whereas the involuting phase is characterized by apoptosis, gradual fibrosis, and variable fatty infiltration.

Vascular malformations are errors of morphogenesis that are presumed to occur between the fourth and tenth weeks of intrauterine life. Most vascular malformations are present at birth, although they may not be apparent; others do not appear until years later. Once manifest, they grow proportionately with the patient; however, rapid enlargement can occur as a result of trauma, hormonal changes (puberty, pregnancy, oral contraceptive), thrombosis, infection, or surgical intervention. Histologically, vascular malformations are characterized by dilated channels with abnormal walls lined by normal, quiescent endothelium.

This binary biologic classification has gained wide acceptance and has required only minor modifications to incorporate new information. Rather than specify all vascular birthmarks as either *hemangioma* or *malformation,* it is more appropriate to use the categorical terms *vascular tumors* and *vascular malformations* (Table 103-2). Vascular malformations are subclassified according to the basic structural components into capillary, venous, lymphatic, arterial, and combined forms. In addition, it is clinically useful to separate rheologically vascular anomalies into *slow-flow* (capillary, lymphatic, venous, combined) and *fast-flow* (arterial, combined) types. Abbreviated designations are formed by the first letter of the major anomalous channel(s).

TRANSLATION OF TERMINOLOGY

The old descriptive nomenclature can be translated into the current biologic classification. For example, *strawberry, cherry, and capillary* hemangiomas are all forms of superficial hemangioma of infancy. The

TABLE 103-1

Distinguishing Features of Vascular Tumors (Hemangiomas) and Vascular Malformations

	Tumors	Malformations
Present at birth	Usually postnatal, 30 percent nascent, rarely fully grown	100 percent (presumably), not always obvious
Male:female ratio	1:3–1:5	1:1
Incidence	1–2.6 percent at birth; 10–12 percent at 1 year	0.3–0.5 percent "port-wine" stain
Natural history	Phases: Proliferating, involuting, and involuted	Proportionate growth, can expand
Cellular	Endothelial hyperplasia	Normal endothelial turnover
Skeletal changes	Occasional mass effect on adjacent bone; rare hypertrophy	Slow flow: distortion, hypertrophy, or hypoplasia Fast flow: destruction, distortion, or hypertrophy

SOURCE: Modified from Mulliken and Young.[1]

TABLE 103-2

Classification of Vascular Anomalies

- Congenital*
  - Hemangioma
  - Kaposiform hemangioendothelioma
  - Tufted angioma
  - Hemangiopericytoma
- Acquired*
  - Pyogenic granuloma
  - Acquired tufted angioma
  - Targetoid hemosiderotic hemangioma
  - Unilateral nevoid telangiectasia
  - Angiolymphoid hyperplasia with eosinophilia
  - Intravascular papillary endothelial hyperplasia
  - Spindle cell hemangioendothelioma
  - Kaposi's sarcoma
  - Endovascular papillary angioendothelioma
  - Epithelioid hemangioendothelioma
  - Retiform hemangioendothelioma
  - Angiosarcoma
  - Macular stain†
  - Cutis marmorata†
- Capillary malformation (CM)
  - Port-wine stain
  - Phakomatosis pigmentovascularis
  - Telangiectasias
  - Spider angioma
  - Cutis marmorata telangiectasia congenita
- Lymphatic malformation (LM)
  - Localized, diffuse, macro- or microcystic
- Venous malformation (VM)
  - Venous lake
  - Blue rubber bleb nevus
  - Glomangioma
- Arterial
  - Arterial malformation (AM)
  - Arteriovenous fistula (AVF)
  - Arteriovenous malformation (AVM)
- Combined
  - Slow-flow: capillary-lymphaticovenous malformation (CLVM)
  - Fast-flow: capillary-arteriovenous malformation (CAVM)

*"Congenital" by definition means present at birth. "Acquired" is used variably; it usually refers to cutaneous lesions that manifest after 1 year of age. However, the nidus of any vascular birthmark may be present at birth, but not clinically evident.

†These common lesions tend to fade completely over time. There is little evidence they are dermatopathologic lesions.

term *cavernous hemangioma* should be abandoned; it has been used to refer both to a deep hemangioma and to a venous malformation. *Nevus flammeus*, stork bite, and salmon patch should not be used interchangeably for a capillary malformation because they are minor dermal capillary ectasias that usually fade. In contrast, capillary malformation (port-wine stain) is a permanent vascular anomaly. All of the rare vascular anomalies, such as unilateral nevoid telangiectasia and "acquired" lymphangioma circumscriptum, fit comfortably into this biologic schema. This classification also accommodates various eponymous malformation syndromes, such as Sturge-Weber and Klippel-Trenaunay, Parkes Weber, and Maffucci syndromes by delineation of the various slow-flow or fast-flow channel types.

TUMORS

Hemangioma of Infancy

EPIDEMIOLOGY Hemangioma is the most common tumor of infancy. The incidence in the newborn nursery is between 1.0 and 2.6 percent[3,4] in white, black[3] and Japanese infants.[5] An incidence of 10 to 12 percent has been reported in white children by 1 year of age.[6] Hemangiomas develop in premature infants weighing between 1500 and 2500g at a frequency equal to that in full-term babies, whereas 23 percent of premature infants weighing less than 1000 g manifest a hemangioma.[7] Females are affected more commonly than males in a 3:1 ratio.[8] Approximately 30 percent of hemangiomas are nascent at birth; two-thirds become apparent during the first to fourth weeks of life. A family history of hemangioma can be elicited in 10 percent of children, but this may be more related to the frequency in whites rather than to an inheritable predisposition.[9]

The hemangioma's initial proliferative phase of rapid postnatal growth lasts for 3 to 9 months; rarely beyond 18 months (Figs. 103-1 and 103-2). Proliferative-phase hemangiomas express high levels of angiogenic molecules, specifically basic fibroblast growth factor (bFGF) and vascular endothelial growth factor/vascular permeability factor (VEGF/VPF). Enzymes involved in remodeling of extracellular matrix, e.g., type IV collagenase, urokinase, proteases, and metalloproteinases, are also present in the proliferative phase. There is also evidence for diminished levels of an endogenous inhibitor of angiogenesis, interferon-β (IFN-β).[10] Hemangiomas represent clonal expansions of endothelial cells that may result from somatic mutations in one or more genes regulating endothelial cell proliferation.[11]

The phase of involution occurs gradually over 2 to 6 years and is complete by the age of 7 to 10 years[1,12] (Figs. 103-2 and 103-3). The rate of involution varies greatly between children and does not correlate with the size, location, or appearance of the lesion. An increase in cellular apoptosis during the second year of life is associated with the initiation of the involuting phase.[13] During regression, levels of IFN-β return to normal. Mast cells are prominent in the involuting phase, along with upregulation of tissue inhibitor of metalloproteinase (TIMP), clusterin, and mitochondrial cytochrome.[14] About 50 percent of children have normal skin after involution, whereas the remainder have variable telangiectasias, atrophy, fibrofatty residuum, or scarring (particularly if there was ulceration during infancy).

DESCRIPTION The initial signs of a nascent hemangioma can be a hypopigmented blanched macule with or without telangiectasia (similar in appearance to a *nevus anemicus*) or an erythematous to ecchymotic patch that is superficial,[5] often with an irregular surface and borders. Several large draining veins typically radiate from the tumor. Most hemangiomas grow to between 0.5 and 5.0 cm in diameter, whereas some involve large areas of the face, trunk, or extremities (see Figs. 103-1 and 103-3). Eighty percent of affected infants have a single lesion, most commonly located on the head and neck (60 percent), followed by the trunk (25 percent), and the extremities (15 percent).[8] Multiple hemangiomas occur in 20 percent of affected infants. Often these cutaneous tumors are tiny, dome-shaped lesions associated with hemangiomas in visceral organs such as the liver.

ATYPICAL PRESENTATIONS There are several unusual presentations, including deep (subcutaneous) hemangioma, telangiectatic hemangioma, arteriovenous malformation (AVM)–like hemangioma, multiple cutaneous hemangiomas, and congenital hemangioma.

Deep hemangioma Deep hemangiomas (old term, *cavernous hemangioma*) proliferate in the lower dermis and subcutaneous tissue without penetration of the papillary dermis. They present as a localized, firm, rubbery subcutaneous mass that can be slightly raised with a bluish color or with telangiectasias involving the overlying skin, or they may be deep enough that the overlying skin is completely flat and of normal hue (Fig. 103-4). Hemangiomas that involve the papillary

FIGURE 103-1

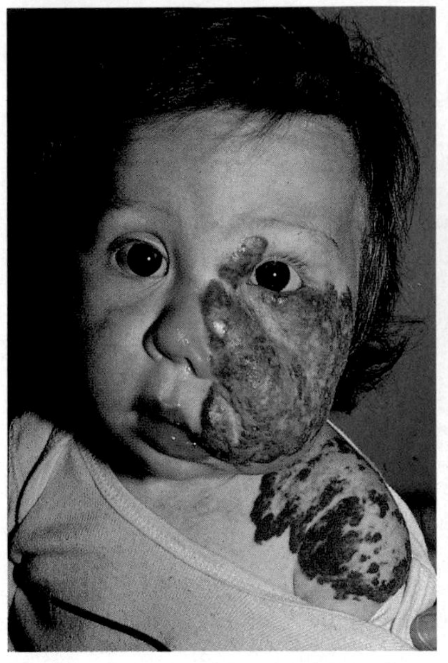

A.

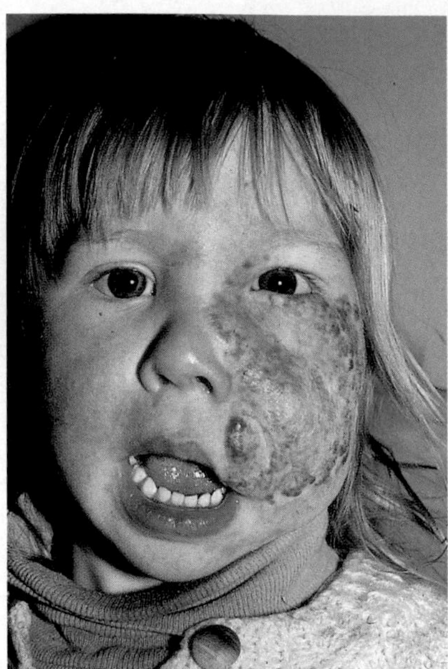

B.

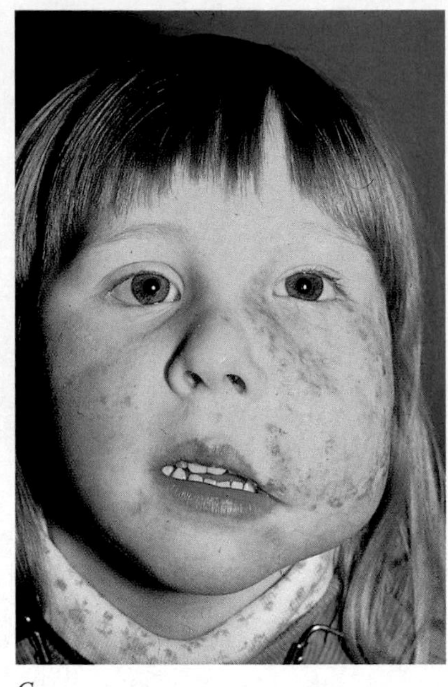

C.

Natural history of hemangioma. *A*. Age 11 months, at peak of proliferating phase. *B*. Age 2 years, involuting phase, apoptosis is maximal. *C*. Age 4 years, some further involution expected.

dermis, and deeper tissues have the typical bright-red surface as well as a subcutaneous component and can be called *superficial* and *deep hemangiomas*.

Telangiectatic hemangioma Telangiectatic hemangiomas are flat or slightly elevated and deep red with an array of superficial dilated capillaries radiating over the surface (Fig. 103-5). This tumor resembles a port-wine stain but involutes spontaneously with the usual time course of all postnatal hemangiomas, leaving telangiectasias and occasionally a minor fibrofatty residuum. Extensive telangiectatic hemangiomas can be associated with fast flow, congestive heart failure, and ulcerations.

AVM-like hemangioma There can be a localized hemangioma with shunting, sometimes referred to as *AVM-like hemangioma*. Reported complications include episodic bleeding, venous thrombosis, and increased cardiac output and failure.[15] Involution is slow, often these tumors can be resected. Histologic examination reveals endothelial proliferation within arteries and venous walls indicative of persistent fast flow.

Multiple infantile hemangiomas Hemangiomas also can present as multiple small (1 to 20 mm) lesions involving the skin alone (called *benign cutaneous hemangiomatosis*) or involving both the skin and

FIGURE 103-2

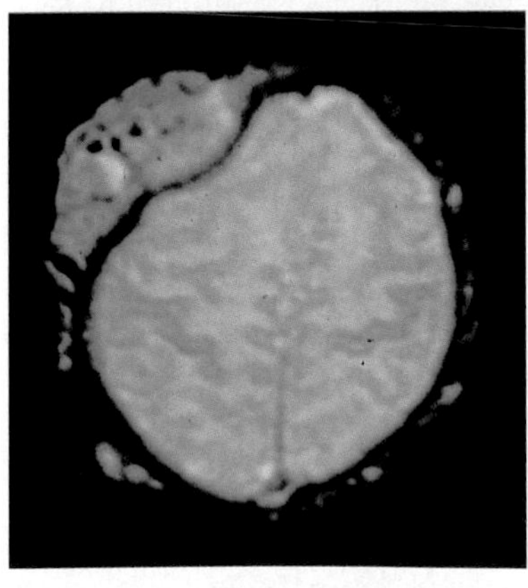

A.

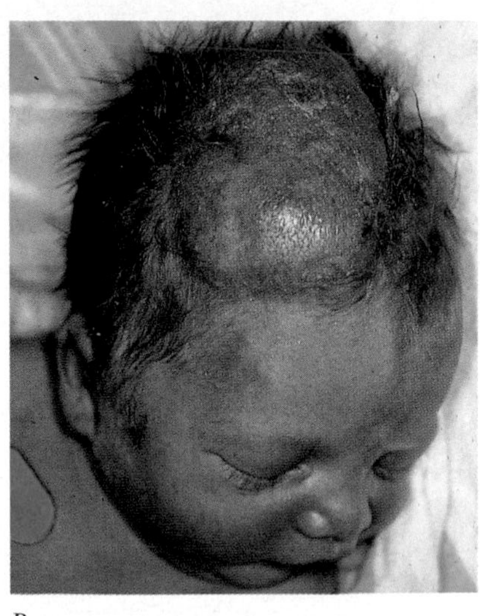

B.

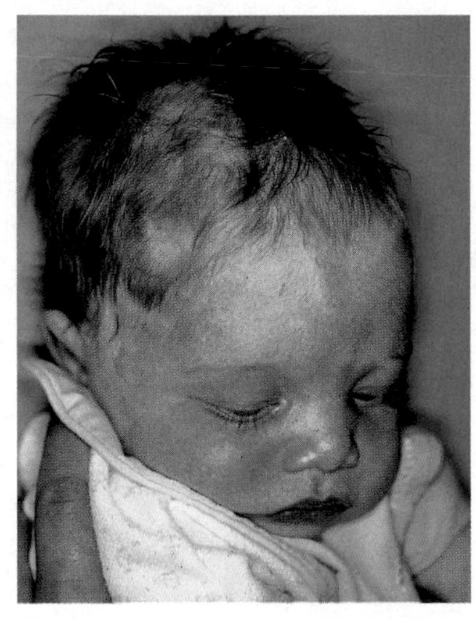

C.

Congenital hemangioma. *A*. Fetal ultrasonography reveals tumor on right parietal scalp with fast-flow vessels and cranial deformation. *B*. Fully grown tumor as seen at birth. *C*. Rapid involution at age 1 month; color faded before 1 year.

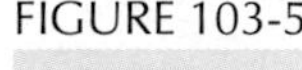

FIGURE 103-3

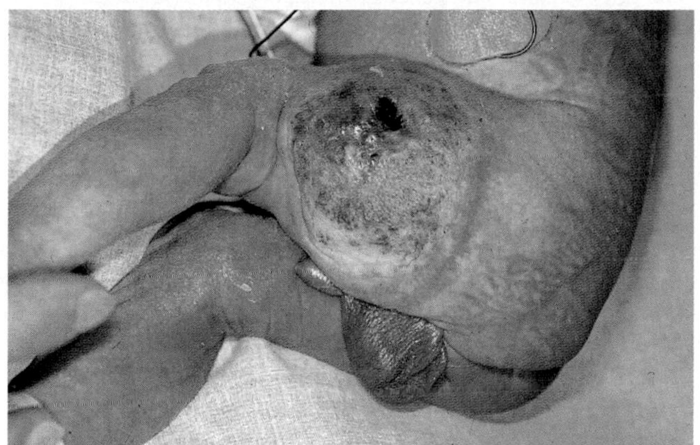

A.

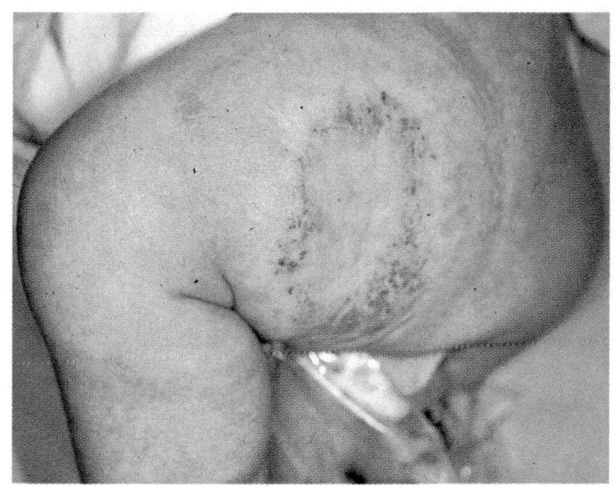

B.

Congenital hemangioma on left thigh. *A.* Note central ulceration, violaceous color, and pale periphery. Fast-flow vessels detected on Doppler examination. *B.* Rapid regression at age 2 months.

viscera (called *diffuse neonatal hemangiomatosis*) (Fig. 103-6). It is unknown whether *hemangiomatosis* represents multifocal involvement or metastatic spread. Visceral hemangiomas have been reported in the lymph nodes, liver, spleen, brain and meninges, iris, retina, salivary glands, heart, thymus, gastrointestinal tract, lung, urinary bladder, kidney, gallbladder, pancreas, and adrenal gland.[16] Hepatic hemangiomas can be solitary or multiple and can be associated with a mortality as high as 30 to 40 percent because of high-output cardiac failure. Involution of

FIGURE 103-4

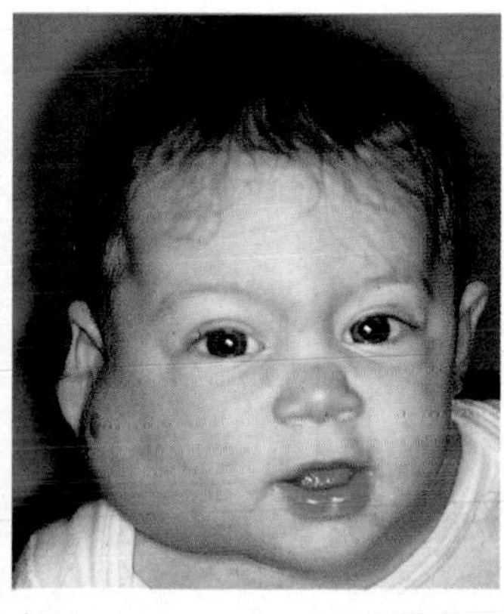

A.

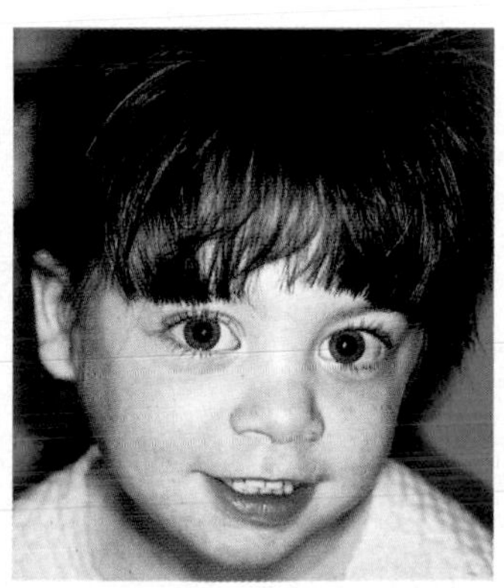

B.

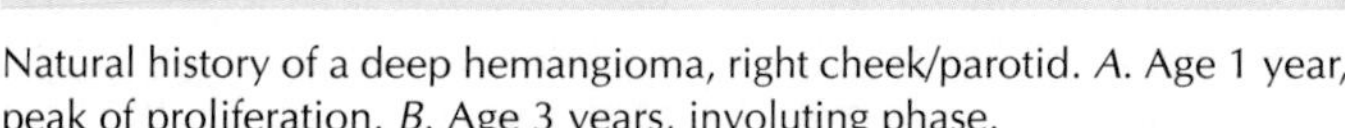

Natural history of a deep hemangioma, right cheek/parotid. *A.* Age 1 year, peak of proliferation. *B.* Age 3 years, involuting phase.

FIGURE 103-5

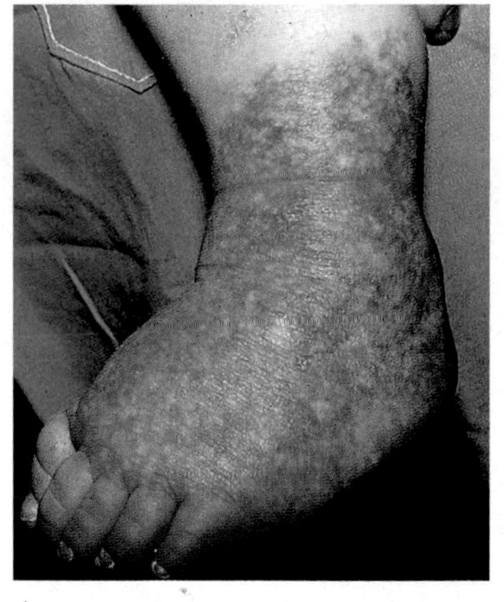

A.

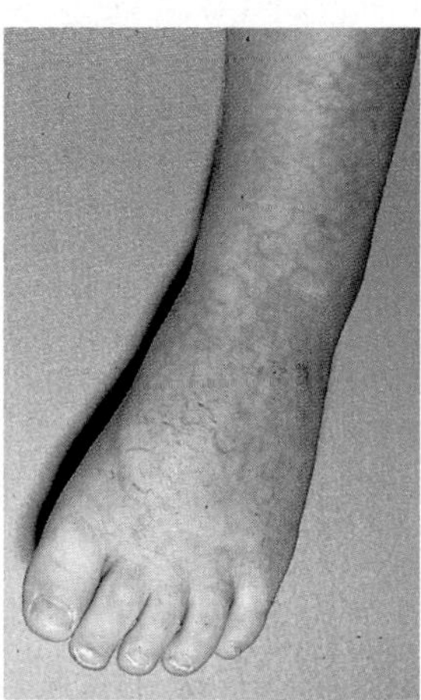

B.

Telangiectatic hemangioma, left foot. This lesion could be confused with a port-wine stain. *A.* Reticulated stain and minor soft-tissue hypertrophy. *B.* Only fine telangiectasias remain at age 11 years (involuted phase).

FIGURE 103-6

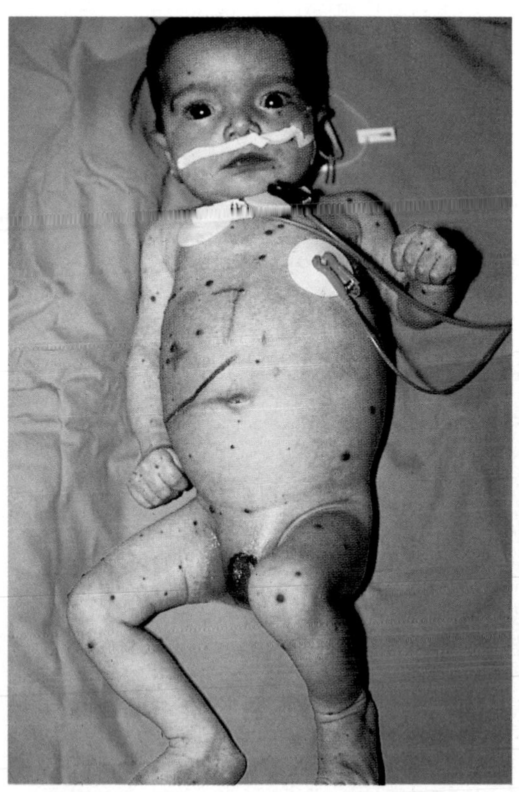

Infant with multiple dome-shaped cutaneous hemangiomas, hepatic hemangiomas, and high-output congestive heart failure. Tumors and cardiac failure responded to systemic glucocorticoid therapy.

multiple cutaneous hemangiomas often begins after just 3 to 6 months and is complete within 1 to 2 years—much sooner than with the more common solitary lesions.[16]

Congenital hemangioma Hemangiomas can develop in fetal life, proliferate in utero and present as fully formed tumors at birth. This is the definition of a congenital hemangioma. Congenital hemangiomas can be subdivided according to natural history into rapidly involuting congenital hemangiomas (RICH) and noninvoluting congenital hemangiomas (NICH). It is not clear whether or not these two subtypes are really the same vascular tumor that behaves differently because of prenatal and postnatal influences. The important observation is that there is no rapid proliferation in the neonate. Curiously, neither RICH nor NICH have the marked female preponderance of common infantile hemangiomas.

Rapidly Involuting Congenital Hemangiomas RICH present as violaceous hemispheric nodules with overlying telangiectasia, pale dusky borders, and large veins at the periphery (see Fig. 103-2). Alternatively, they may appear as firm, erythematous to violaceous plaques infiltrating the dermis or subcutaneous tissue. Regression becomes obvious in early infancy, resulting in disappearance of these lesions more rapidly than common hemangiomas that regress postnatally (by 14 months versus 5 to 9 years). Approximately 50 percent of RICHs involute prior to 7 months of age.[12]

Noninvoluting Congenital Hemangiomas NICH are uncommon vascular lesions that grow proportionately with the child and do not regress. NICH have many similar features to RICH in appearance, size, and location. Characteristic features of NICH include coarse overlying telangiectasia, pale halos at the rims, and intermingled areas of pallor (Fig. 103–7). Lesions have an average diameter of 5 cm and are located (in order of frequency) on the head/neck, extremities, and trunk. Radiologic studies, specifically Doppler and arteriography, demonstrate fast flow. Histologically, NICH differ from common involuting hemangiomas in several ways, including larger and more irregular intralobular vessels, higher cellularity, and multiple microscopic arteriovenous fistulas. Excision is generally the treatment of choice.[17]

FIGURE 103-7

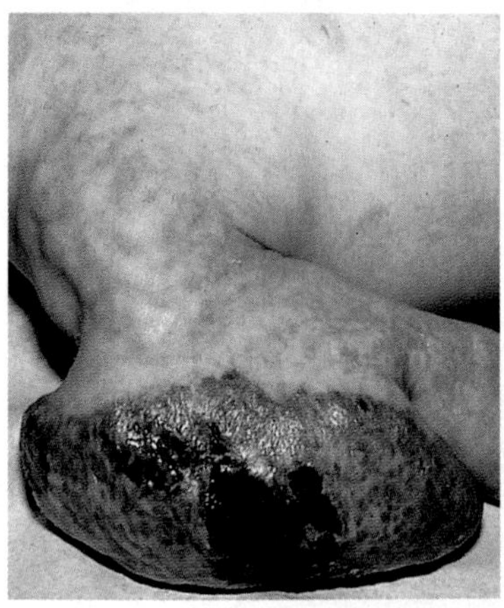

A.

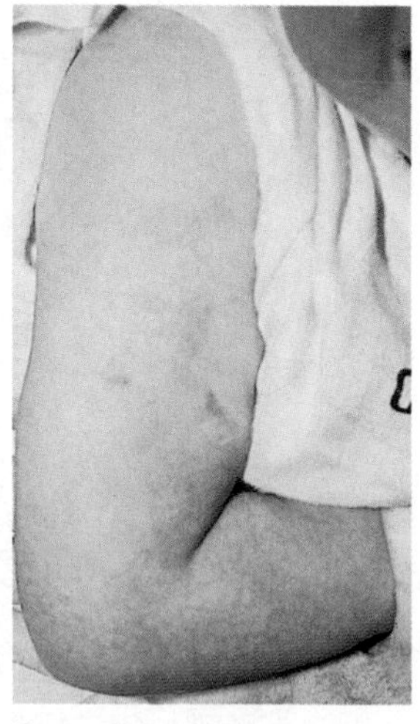

B.

Noninvoluting congenital hemangioma (NICH). Hemangioma with persistent fast flow. *A.* Girl at 1 year of age with pedunculated tumor right upper limb with rapid flow, ulceration, and bleeding. *B.* Two years after resection, large draining veins have regressed.

ASSOCIATED STRUCTURAL ANOMALIES Hemangiomas are rarely associated with underlying anomalies, and in these unusual cases, a marked female preponderance has been documented. Large cervicofacial hemangiomas may present with (1) ocular abnormalities such as microphthalmia, congenital cataract, and optic nerve hypoplasia, (2) sternal nonunion and supraumbilical raphe, (3) arterial abnormalities such as persistent embryonic intra- and extracranial embryonic arteries, absence of ipsilateral carotid/vertebral vessels, and coarctation of a right-sided aortic arch, and (4) posterior fossa malformations, including the Dandy-Walker malformation. The acronym *PHACE* has been proposed as an mnemonic for these associations: posterior fossa malformations, hemangioma (especially a segmental lesion), arterial abnormalities, coarctation of the aorta, and eye abnormalities.[18] However, this term does not include other structural anomalies that can be associated with hemangiomas. For example, lumbosacral hemangiomas may signal the presence of spinal dysraphism and should be evaluated by magnetic resonance imaging (MRI). These hemangiomas are often clinically distinctive, being telangiectatic, macular, or diffuse, sometimes with an acrochordon. Pelvic and perineal hemangiomas may be associated with urogenital and anorectal anomalies (e.g., anterior or vestibular anus, hemiclitoris, atrophy or absence of the labia minora, and hypospadias).

DIAGNOSIS Hemangiomas almost always can be diagnosed accurately by clinical presentation and history alone. The hemangioma is nonblanching and is firm to rubbery on palpation. In some infants with ambiguous, atypical, or deep lesions, observation of change over time or radiologic investigation is necessary to confirm the diagnosis. Biopsy of any vascular lesion is indicated whenever there is the slightest suspicion of malignancy.

Ultrasonography with color flow imaging is, in experienced hands, a useful and cost-effective method,[19] but it does not portray the extent of the lesion or its relation to adjacent structures. MRI provides the most useful information, including exact localization, extent of involvement, and with midline lesions the presence of associated cranial or spinal dysraphism. MRI is also useful for differential diagnosis of an atypical lesion, since hemangiomas have an appearance on MRI distinct from vascular malformations, dermoid cysts, meningoceles, and other benign and malignant infantile tumors. Computed tomography (CT) is less informative than MRI because it cannot distinguish between fast-flow and slow-flow lesions, although it does display skeletal abnormalities. These noninvasive imaging techniques have essentially replaced arteriography.

High endothelial immunoreactivity for the erythrocyte-type glucose transporter protein GLUT1 is observed in hemangiomas of infancy in all phases as well as in other microvessels of blood-tissue barrier function, including brain and placenta. Vascular malformations do not exhibit any GLUT1 immunoreactivity.[20] GLUT1 may provide a diagnostic tool to differentiate hemangioma from vascular malformation. RICH and NICH do not stain with antibodies to GLUT1, however.

COMPLICATIONS Potential problems in the proliferative phase include ulceration; bleeding; infection; distortion of the cornea; obstruction of the visual axis, nasal passages, larynx, or auditory canals; congestive heart failure; skeletal distortion; and rarely, skeletal overgrowth. Spontaneous ulceration, bleeding, and secondary infection occur in approximately 5 percent of superficial lesions and are seen most often in hemangiomas involving the lips and genital areas, where abrasion is common. Rarely, ulceration and subsequent infection can result in extensive necrosis and destruction of facial soft tissues and the cartilaginous framework of the nose or ear.

Hemangiomas in the upper eyelid can obstruct the visual axis, resulting in deprivation amblyopia and failure to develop binocular vision (Fig. 103-8). Obstruction need be present for only 1 to 2 weeks to cause blindness. More important, even a small hemangioma in the upper

FIGURE 103-8

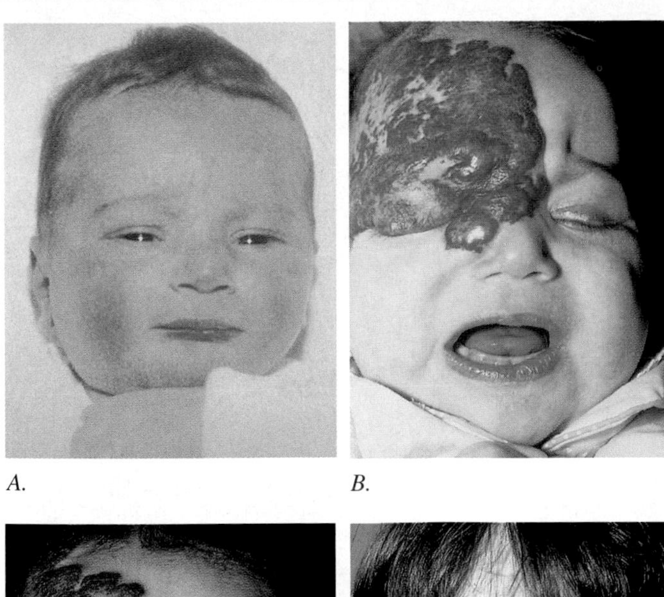

A. B.

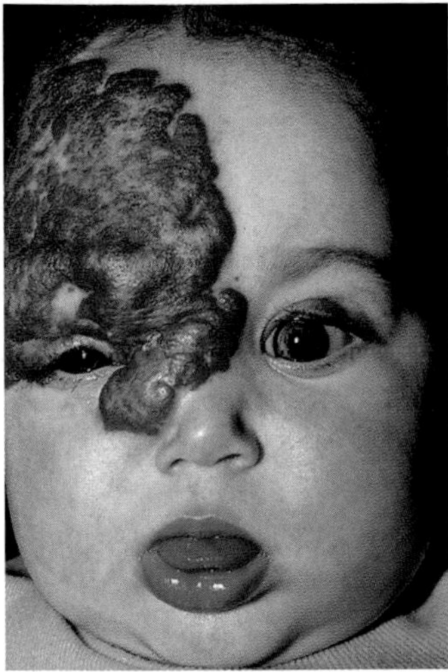

C.

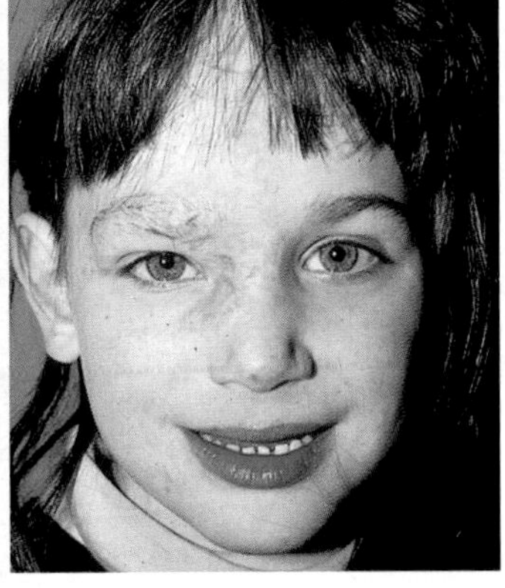

D.

Vision-endangering hemangioma treated with systemic glucocorticoids. *A.* No premonitory signs of tumor seen on infant's photograph. *B.* By age 3 months, extensive hemangioma has infiltrated upper lid and surrounding tissue, causing blocked vision. *C.* Eyelid opened within 2 weeks of glucocorticoid therapy. *D.* Involuted tumor, age 6 years.

eyelid or supraorbital region can distort the cornea, leading to refractive errors, both astigmatic and myopic. Periorbital hemangiomas require prompt consultation with a pediatric ophthalmologist. Another ocular complication is strabismus, an abnormal alignment of the eyes due to amblyopia or to infiltration of the extraocular muscles by the hemangioma.

Blockage of the nasal passages typically develops so gradually that the infant adapts by breathing through the mouth. However, subglottic obstruction can be life-threatening. It develops insidiously, manifesting as biphasic stridor with or without respiratory distress. A child with a subglottic hemangioma often presents with a mistaken diagnosis of laryngotracheitis or multiple episodes of croup. Half of infants with subglottic hemangiomas have an associated cutaneous tumor in the cervicofacial skin.[1] Furthermore, infants with a cutaneous hemangioma in a beard distribution (preauricular areas, chin, anterior neck, and lower lip) are at increased risk for upper airway or subglottic involvement.[21]

High-output failure is another potentially life-threatening complication. It is usually associated with multiple hepatic hemangiomas; however, it also can occur with a single large cutaneous hemangioma. The proliferation of a hemangioma within the vascular hepatic parenchyma produces the hemodynamic changes characteristic of a large left-to-right shunt. Hepatic hemangiomas can be single or multiple; the latter are often associated with multiple small (2 to 15 mm in diameter) hemispherical cutaneous hemangiomas. Liver hemangiomas can also occur in the absence of cutaneous lesions. Infants with multiple hepatic tumors present within the first 16 weeks of life with a clinical triad of hepatomegaly, congestive heart failure, and anemia.[22] The rare infant with a hepatic arteriovenous malformation or a single large hepatic hemangioma typically presents at birth with the same triad.

TREATMENT The decision to treat a hemangioma is based on many factors, including size and location of the lesion, psychosocial implications, and risks and benefits of the proposed therapy. For the majority of small hemangiomas, active nonintervention is the most appropriate approach. This does not mean doing nothing. The parents need a thorough explanation of the natural history of their child's hemangioma, including photographs of the likely outcome for a similar lesion. The infant should be seen frequently, and the parents must be reassured constantly. Over the past decade, there has been an increase in parental pressure for intervention. Treatment is probably indicated in about 25 percent of hemangiomas—the 5 percent that ulcerate; the 20 percent that compress, distort, or obstruct vital structures such as the eyes, nose, ears, or larynx; and the less than 1 percent of truly life-threatening tumors.

Ulceration is managed with gentle cleansing and application of topical antibiotics and barrier creams. Biocclusive dressings may be helpful, especially in the anogenital area, where the tumor is frequently contaminated. Systemic antibiotics are used for infection. Other modalities for treatment of ulcerated hemangioma include intralesional and systemic corticosteroids, excision, and interferon-α. Pain may be controlled with topical lidocaine ointment and oral acetominophen with or without codeine. Ulcerations generally heal within 2 to 3 weeks with topical care, leaving a scar. Treatment with the pulsed-dye laser may reduce healing time and pain; one study reported that 50 percent of ulcerated hemangiomas treated with pulsed-dye laser showed a definite improvement, but 18 percent showed no change, and one hemangioma showed definite worsening.[23]

Pharmacologic therapy Intralesional glucocorticoids can be used for small hemangiomas (1 to 2 cm) localized to critical sites such as the lip, nasal tip, cheek, or ear. Triamcinolone is injected slowly and at low pressure at a dose of 3 to 5 mg/kg every 4 to 6 weeks for 1 to 5 total injections. Injection into an upper eyelid hemangioma carries a slight risk of retrobulbar hematoma, and there are two case reports of microvascular embolism causing blindness due to occlusion of the central retinal artery.[24,25] Glucocorticoid injections also can be effective in the treatment of minor ulceration. The response rate for intralesional steroid injections is the same as for systemic steroid therapy.[26] The high-potency topical steroid clobetasol propionate may be used to treat small superficial lesions.[27]

Systemic glucocorticoids are the first-line pharmacologic treatment for deforming, endangering, or life-threatening hemangiomas. Prednisone or prednisolone is given at a dose of 2 to 3 mg/kg per day for 4 to 6 weeks, after which time the dosage is tapered gradually for several months. If the drug dosage is lowered or stopped before the age of 8 to 10 months, rebound growth often occurs.

The response to oral glucocorticoids is excellent, with approximately 84 percent showing accelerated involution or cessation of growth (response rate) with a mean prednisone equivalent daily dose of 2.9 mg/kg given over 1.8 months[28] (see Fig. 103-8). The optimal dosage is controversial. Response is 75 percent with a dosage of prednisone between 2 and 3 mg/kg per day, whereas a dosage higher than 3 mg/kg results in a response as high as 94 percent but greater adverse effects. Dosages lower than 2 mg/kg per day result in a 69 percent response rate, but the rebound rate (enlargement after tapering after response occurred) is 70 percent. If there is no response after 2 to 3 weeks of therapy, the tumor is unlikely to respond to a higher dose, and the glucocorticoids should be discontinued. Short-term complications of glucocorticoid therapy include cushingoid facies (71 percent), personality changes (29 percent), gastric irritation (21 percent), fungal infection (oral or perineal, 6 percent), and diminished gain of height (35 percent) and weight (42 percent) during treatment. Over 90 percent of children with diminished gain of height return to their pretreatment growth curve for height by 24 months of age.[29]

Interferon-α2a and -2b are indicated in the treatment of endangering and life-threatening hemangiomas, specifically for tumors unresponsive to glucocorticoids. The drug is given subcutaneously at a dose of 3 million U/m^2 daily for 6 to 12 months.[30,31] Side effects include transient fever, neutropenia, and minor elevations in liver enzymes. Spastic diplegia develops in approximately 5 to 10 percent of infants treated with interferon.[32] The neurologic signs are reversible after stopping the drug. Obviously, periodic neurologic examination is indicated during treatment.

Laser therapy Treatment of hemangiomas with the flash-lamp pulsed-dye laser has been a subject of considerable controversy over the past decade. This laser uses a wavelength of 585 nm, specific for the absorption of oxyhemoglobin, the treatment target. In addition, the pulse duration is extremely short (400 ms), allowing for effective coagulation of vessels without extensive thermal diffusion to surrounding tissue that could result in scarring. Histologically, the flash-lamp pulsed-dye laser produces selective intravascular and perivascular coagulation necrosis, seen clinically as purpura. On resolution of the purpura, histologic examination shows an absence of dermal ectatic vessels and an otherwise normal unaltered epidermis and dermis. With darker skin types, laser treatment can cause damage to melanocytes in the basal cell layer, resulting in hypopigmentation.

It is generally accepted that the pulsed-dye laser is the treatment of choice for residual telangiectasias during or after involution. More controversial is the treatment of a proliferating hemangioma or a precursor lesion in an effort to prevent or diminish growth. Laser treatment of the superficial dermal component of the tumor has no effect on proliferation of the deeper component.[33] Thus laser treatment is ineffective in reducing the bulk of deep hemangiomas.[34] Some authors think that laser treatment can accelerate involution and diminish the growth phase if therapy is begun early enough; however, this has not been substantiated by controlled trials. Laser treatment is most effective in telangiectatic-type hemangiomas, and it typically results in complete clearing of the lesion after a mean of two laser sessions.[34] However, it is important to remember that telangiectatic hemangiomas are generally macular or slightly elevated—the very tumors that tend to regress spontaneously leaving minimal to no residua.[35] Potential side effects of pulsed-dye laser treatment include ulceration with scarring and hypopigmentation that becomes evident only after regression.

The pulsed-dye laser should be considered in the treatment of ulcerated hemangiomas. One small pilot study showed that 6 of 10 ulcerations healed after a single laser treatment, and pain was subjectively decreased in all patients within 2 to 3 days after one treatment.[36] Controlled trials are needed to confirm these findings.

Surgical therapy Surgical resection may be indicated at any time during the life cycle of a hemangioma. Excision is often necessary for fibrofatty tissue and abnormal skin after involution (when the child is 8 to 12 years old). Surgical intervention in early childhood should be considered for special situations. For example, a localized pedunculated hemangioma on the upper eyelid unresponsive to pharmacologic therapy sometimes can be totally excised, thereby quickly correcting astigmatism. An ulcerated hemangioma that bleeds frequently and is largely necrotic can take as long as 4 to 8 weeks to heal and is often associated with significant pain. Such tumors may be excised, leaving a scar that is likely to be more cosmetically acceptable than the scar resulting from natural regression.[35]

Surgical excision should be considered during the preschool age, before the child begins to manifest a facial or body image. A spheroidal hemangioma in the nasal tip usually causes cutaneous expansion and splayed alar cartilages. For psychosocial reasons, subtotal excision to improve nasal contour should be considered during early childhood. Hemangiomas of the vermilion border, glabella, eyebrow, and eyelid (Fig. 103-9) often are excised prior to the child's entry into school. In some instances, it is best to wait until regression is nearly complete before resecting the fibrofatty residuum or atrophic skin. In summary, excision in early childhood is indicated (1) if it is obvious that resection is inevitable (because of postulcerative scarring unalterably expanded skin, or likely fibrofatty residuum), (2) if the scar would be the same length or appearance if excision were postponed, and (3) if the scar can be easily concealed.[35]

FIGURE 103-9

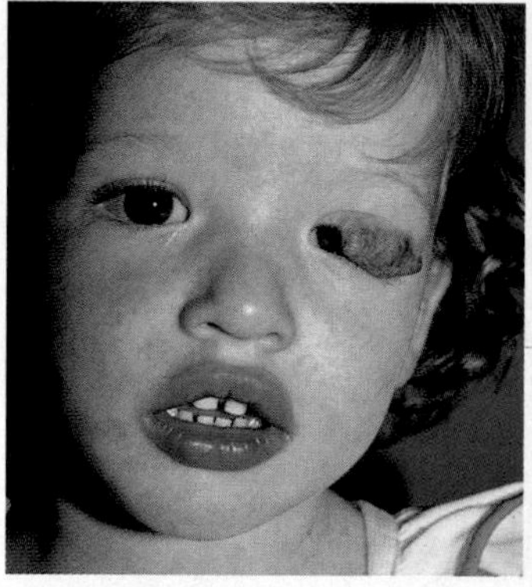

A.

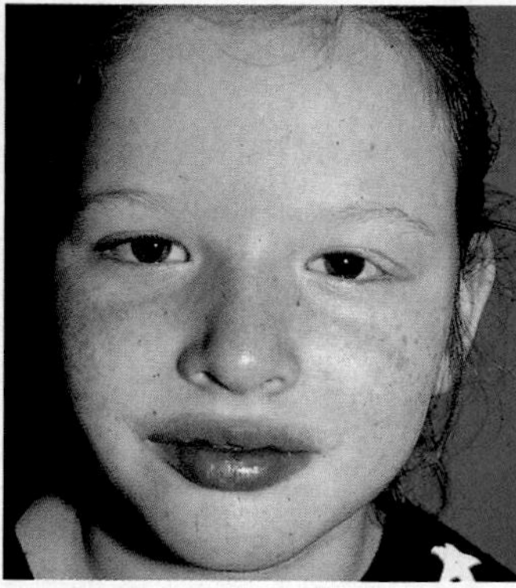

B.

Surgical correction of involuting-phase hemangioma. *A.* Three-year-old girl with protuberant tumor on upper eyelid. *B.* Age 9 years, after staged surgical resection, including vertical shortening of eyelid, repair of blepharoptosis, and formation of tarsal crease.

Other Vascular Tumors of Infancy

KASABACH-MERRITT PHENOMENON/KAPOSIFORM HEMANGIOENDOTHELIOMA The association of a giant capillary hemangioma with thrombocytopenia was first reported in 1940 by Kasabach and Merritt. In addition to thrombocytopenia, there is a superimposed disseminated intravascular coagulation manifested by anemia, prolongation of the prothrombin and partial thromboplastin times, low fibrinogen level, and elevated levels of D-dimers and fibrin split products. This disorder is not a true syndrome; it is best termed *Kasabach-Merritt phenomenon* because it is pathogenically heterogeneous.

Clinical manifestations Hemangiomas of infancy are not associated with Kasabach-Merritt coagulopathy. Usually the tumor is a kaposiform hemangioendothelioma (KHE), a more aggressive vascular lesion that is distinctive histologically, clinically, and radiographically.[37,38] Approximately 50 percent of KHEs are congenital; the remainder appear during the first year of life. The tumor grows rapidly to a large size (5 cm) and is characterized by a deep-red to violaceous color, induration, and a centrifugally advancing rim of ecchymosis (Fig. 103-10). The anatomic distribution of KHE is retroperitoneum (52 percent), proximal lower limb (19 percent), upper limb (19 percent), and the cervicofacial region (10 percent).[38]

FIGURE 103-10

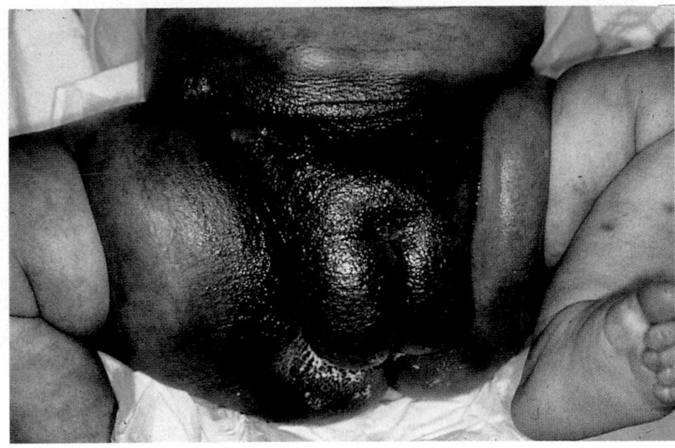

A.

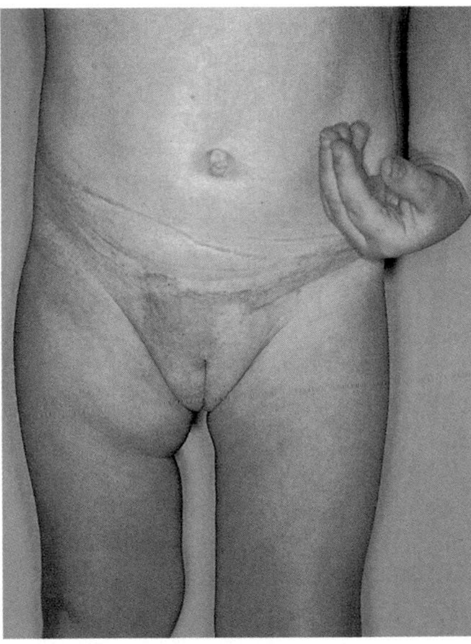

B.

Kasabach-Merritt phenomenon (KMP) secondary to KHE. *A.* Indurated, purpuric tumor appeared at age 3 months, seen here at age 8 months. KHE confirmed by MRI and biopsy. Platelet count less than 5000/mm^3. *B.* Age 2 years, after successful treatment with interferon alfa-2a for 6 months and a 3-day course of cyclophosphamide.

Pathology The histopathology of this vascular neoplasm shows remarkable similarity to Kaposi sarcoma with infiltrating interconnecting sheets of slender endothelial cells lining slitlike vessels interspersed with nests of epithelioid endothelial cells with a prominent eosinophilic cytoplasm.

Diagnosis and treatment MRI shows distinctive findings, i.e., diffuse enhancement with poorly defined margins, cutaneous thickening, edema, and stranding of subcutaneous fat. The mortality is high (30 to 40 percent) despite a variety of treatments, e.g., blood products, antifibrinolytic agents, compression, embolization, glucocorticoids, and chemotherapy. In one review, interferon-α2a accelerated tumor regression and corrected coagulopathy in 6 of 14 infants; the mortality rate was 19 percent (4 of 21).[38] Vincristine is also effective and is currently the first-line drug if there is no response to corticosteroids. Spontaneous regression can occur from 1 to 5 years of age; however, residual dormant KHE is common after the resolution of thrombocytopenia and coagulopathy.[39] There are some rare examples of recrudescence of thrombocytopenia in late childhood and adolescence.

FIGURE 103-11

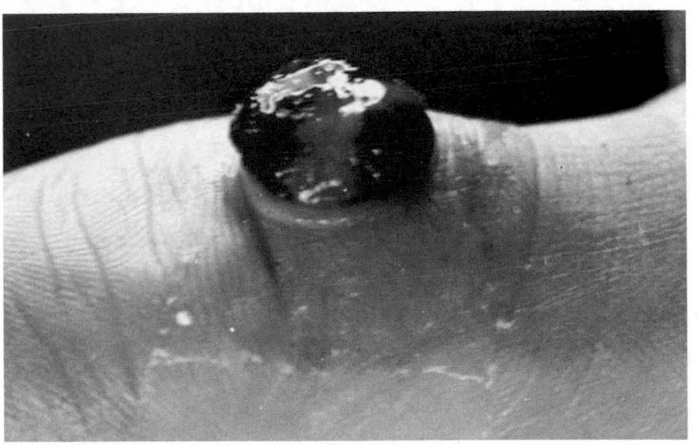

Pyogenic granuloma. An early lesion. An ulcerated, glistening, reddish papule is surrounded by a collarette.

PYOGENIC GRANULOMA

Clinical manifestations Pyogenic granuloma is a rapidly developing vascular lesion that often arises at sites of minor trauma; it may represent a reactive phenomenon. Pyogenic granuloma is common. Lesions are solitary, small (average size 6.5 mm), eroded papules or nodules that bleed spontaneously or after trauma (Fig 103-11). Common locations include the face, fingers, toes, and trunk. Pyogenic granuloma rarely appears prior to 6 months of age; mean age at presentation in children is 6.7 years.[40] Pyogenic granuloma frequently presents in adults. The lesions can appear within an existing capillary malformation (port-wine stain), but most commonly there is no history of a preexisting dermatologic condition.

Pathology Histopathology reveals well-circumscribed lobular aggregates of proliferating capillaries within an edematous stroma infiltrated by numerous neutrophils. The epidermis is often eroded.

Treatment Treatment is by surgical excision or curettage with electrodesiccation of the base. Smaller lesions (< 5mm) in cosmetically important areas can be treated with the pulsed-dye laser. Other rare vascular proliferations[41–47] are summarized in Table 103-3.

VASCULAR MALFORMATIONS

There are two common vascular phenomena in infants that are characterized by transient, macular, blotchy, erythematous staining. Because they typically fade and disappear, these are not true vascular malformations but rather a transitory phenomenon related to vasodilatation.

Cutis Marmorata

Cutis marmorata is a marbled, bluish discoloration of the skin that occurs in a netlike pattern on the trunk and extremities of an infant. It occurs as a physiologic response to cooling and resolves on rewarming of the child. This typically resolves during the first year of life, and treatment is usually unnecessary. Cutis marmorata may persist in patients with the De Lange syndrome, Down syndrome, and trisomy.[22]

TABLE 103-3

Other Vascular Tumors

Name	Clinical Manifestations	Histopathology	Biologic Behavior
Tufted angioma [41,42] (Fig. 103-12)	Deep to dusky red telangiectatic plaque on upper back, shoulder, or neck; present at birth or during Ist year; growth phase for 0.5 to 10 years, followed by stabilization; only occasional remission	Round tufts of capillaries (cannon balls) in middle to lower dermis (histologic features overlap with KHE)	Benign
Hemangiopericytoma[43,44]	Painless subcutaneous nodule on lower extremities, retroperitoneum, and nonuterine pelvis, upper extremities, trunk, and paraspinal area	Capillary lumina lined by single layer of endothelium surrounded by pericytes; branching vessels have "antler-like configuration"	Classified as benign, bordeline malignant or malignant based on degree of anaplasia, mitoses, etc: prognosis correlates with size of tumor and cellular maturity
Targetoid hemosiderotic hemangioma[45,46]	Violaceous papule surrounded by pale rim and peripheral ecchymotic halo on trunk and extremities; halo can fade with time	Dilated vascular channels with intraluminal papillary projections dissecting into collagen bundles in subcutis; extravasated erythrocytes and hemosiderin	Benign
Unilateral nevoid telangiectasia[47]	Multiple telangiectasias located unilaterally in the C3–T1 dermatomes; congenital or acquired (associated with pregnancy, puberty, hormonal therapy, cirrhosis)	Dilated capillaries in superficial dermis	Benign
Angiolymphoid hyperplasia with eosinophilia (see Chap. 159)	Papules or nodules on head (ears, forehead, scalp) > trunk, extremities; young adults	Irregular vessels lined by plump endothelial hobnail cells protruding into lumen; endothelial walls may be 2–3 cells thick with smooth muscle coat; extensive infiltrate of lymphocytes, histiocytes, and eosinophils	Inflammatory (reactive) process
Intravascular papillary endothelial hyperplasia (Masson's pseudoangiosarcoma)	Extremities, especially fingers	Papillated vascular structures extending from wall within vascular lumina occluded by thrombus	Reactive hyperplasia after intravascular thrombosis
Spindle-cell hemangioendothelioma (Fig. 103–13)	Mean age 34 (range, 8–78); reddish brown nodules (3 mm–3 cm); extremities; solitary or multiple; may be associated with Maffucci syndrome*	Thin-walled dilated vessels, juxtaposed to cellular spindled zones; > 50 percent entirely or partially intravascular	Benign, reactive vascular proliferation within preexisting vascular malformation
Kaposi's sarcoma (see Chap. 104)	Four variants: (1) classic— elderly, violaceous nodules on legs, (2) African-endemic—nodular (like classic), lymphadenopathic (children, lesion in lymph nodes, skin), (3) immunosuppressive-drug associated (like classic), (4) AIDS-associated—violaceous macules, papules, nodules on face, oral mucosa, trunk, extremities	No fundamental differences in the four clinical groups; early lesions: jagged, vascular spaces lined by thin endothelium; scattered necrotic cells; vessels are distributed around adnexal structures and blood vessels, later lesions: increased spindle cells lining slitlike vascular spaces; nuclear atypia, pleomorphism, mitotic figures; intra- and extra-cellular hyaline globules	Biologic behavior based on clinical type; (1) classic—mortality 10–20 percent in 10 years; (2) African-endemic—lymphadenopathic-fulminant, usually fatal within 2–3 years; (3) immunosuppressive-drug associated—regresses after discontinuation of drug; (4) AIDS-associated—overall 41 percent mortality in short period
Endovascular papillary angioendothelioma (Dabska's tumor)	Age range, 4 months to 54 years; dermal nodule or diffuse swelling on head, neck, extremities	Narrow to wide vascular channels lined by atypical endothelial cells; papillary plugs of atypical endothelium $\pm$ central hyalinized core projecting into lumina in "glomeruloid" pattern	Low-grade angiosarcoma
Epithelioid hemangioendothelioma	Rare in childhood; extremities; tender nodule in skin or soft tissue; usually solitary, may be multiple	Plump epithelioid cells in fibromyxoid or sclerotic stroma; intracytoplasmic vacuoles; slight cellular pleomorphism	Low-grade angiosarcoma; <50 percent of patients with metastases die of disease

(continued)

TABLE 103-3 (*Continued*)

Name	Clinical Manifestations	Histopathology	Biologic Behavior
Retiform hemangioendothelioma	Age range, 9–78; plaques and nodules on extremities > scalp, trunk, other; multiple lesions	Arborizing dermal blood vessels in "retiform" pattern (similar to rete testis), lined by hobnail endothelial cells with minimal atypia	Low-grade angiosarcoma; frequent recurrence but low metastatic rate and no tumor-related deaths
Angiosarcoma (Fig. 103-14)	M > F, elderly; scalp and upper forehead, also in areas of localized lymphedema (Stewart-Treves syndrome); purpuric macule, plaque, or nodule ± edema, ulceration; multifocal	Irregularly dilated vascular channels lined by hyperchromatic, pleomorphic endothelial cells with prominent mitoses	High-grade malignancy; 12 percent 5-year survival

*Spindle-cell hemangioendothelioma may be seen in association with Maffucci syndrome (5 percent), comprised of asymmetric superficial and deep venous malformations, enchondromas, and possible development of chondrosarcoma and angiosarcoma.

Fading Macular Stain

Fading macular stain (old terms, *stork bite, salmon patch, angel's kiss, nevus flammeus neonatorum*) consists of a faint pink, blanchable patch with irregular borders. Studies document an incidence of 42 percent in white neonates, 31 percent in blacks,[3] and 23.4 percent in Chinese and Malaysian infants.[48] These stains are located most commonly on the nape of the neck (81 percent), the eyelids (45 percent), and the glabella (33 percent).[4] The macular stain becomes more obvious during crying or when the infant is febrile. They typically fade slowly and usually disappear completely after 1 year of age. Nuchal lesions fade more slowly and less completely than facial lesions; if they persist in this location, the term *nevus of Unna* has been applied. A fading macular stain is often listed as a dermatologic finding in various syndromes, including Beckwith-Wiedemann and Rubenstein-Taybi syndromes. However, the high incidence of these macular stains argues against any true association with such syndromes.

True vascular malformations are subdivided according to the rate of flow and predominant vessel type. *Slow-flow* anomalies include capillary malformation (CM), lymphatic malformation (LM), and venous malformation (VM), whereas *fast-flow* anomalies include arterial malformation (AM), arteriovenous fistula (AVF), and arteriovenous malformation (AVM).

FIGURE 103-12

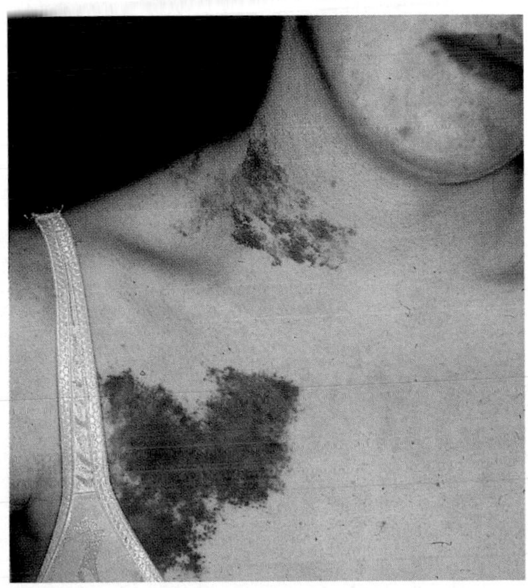

Tufted angioma, acquired tumor in an adolescent girl. The tumor failed to respond to pulsed-dye laser therapy.

Capillary Malformation

CLINICAL MANIFESTATIONS *Port-wine stain* is the nineteenth-century term for the most common type of CM. It is a light-pink to deep-red macule occurring in 0.3 percent of neonates.[4] The lesion can be small or can cover extensive areas of the body in a geographic pattern or a dermatomal distribution (Fig. 103-15). The color deepens gradually with time, becoming dark red during adolescence and violaceous during middle age. In addition, with age, the surface thickens, slowly becoming raised and nodular. CM is usually considered sporadic, but there are well-documented pedigrees showing autosomal dominant inheritance. A CM can be associated with combined vascular anomalies (see Table 103-4).

PATHOLOGY Microscopy reveals dilated ectatic vessels in the papillary and upper reticular dermis lined by normal-appearing, flat endothelial cells. Stains for factor VIII, fibronectin, and basement membrane proteins fail to show any difference between a CM and normal dermal vessels. However, a paucity of nerves was documented by S100 staining; decreased perivascular neural elements could account for altered modulation of vascular tone and subsequent gradual ectasia.[49]

TREATMENT Many therapeutic methods have been used for CM, including scarification, electrocautery, cosmetic tattooing, dermabrasion,

FIGURE 103-13

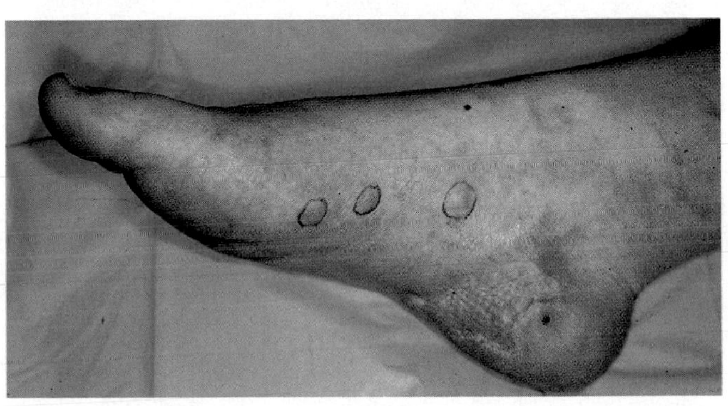

Spindle-cell hemangioendotheliomas on the foot of a young woman with Maffucci syndrome.

FIGURE 103-14

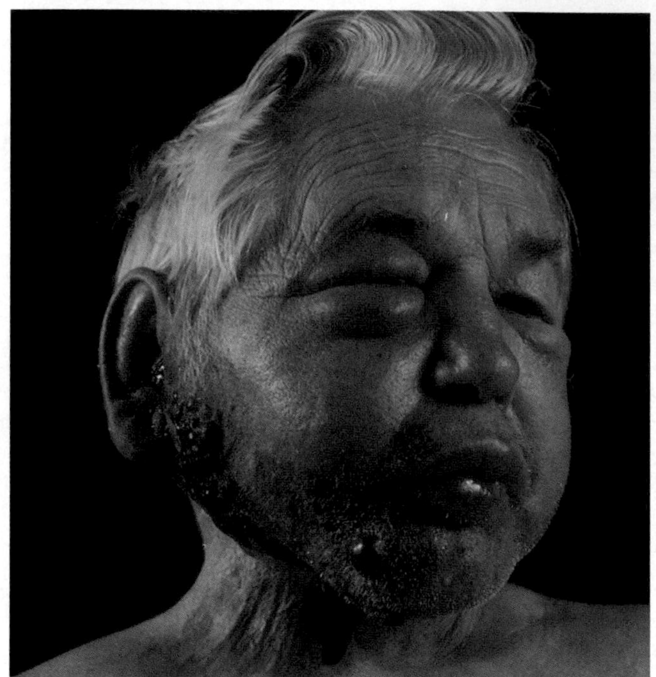

A.

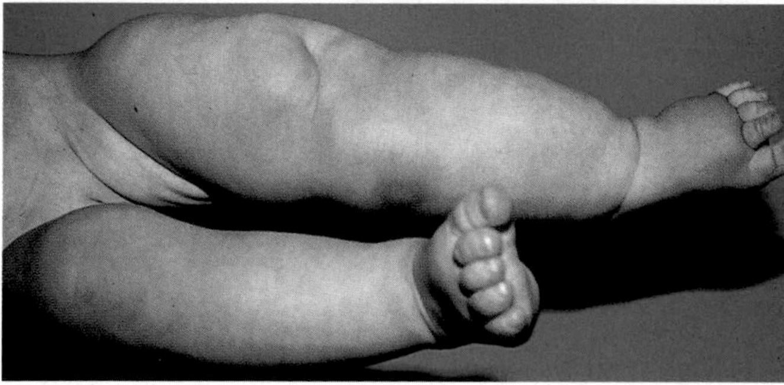

B.

A. An advanced lesion of angiosarcoma. The tumor has infiltrated the jaw, maxillary bone and sinus, and neck. Note pronounced accompanying edema. *B.* Six-month-old girl with congenital lymphedema, left lower extremity. Ecchymotic, firm area appeared below the medial knee and biopsy confirmed angiosarcoma. Congenital lymphedema as well as acquired lymphedema can presage angiosarcoma (Stewart-Treves syndrome).

cryosurgery, and cosmetic makeup. These methods are no longer used because of ineffectiveness and scarring; however, camouflage using either Dermablend or Covermark remains an option for some patients. Laser therapy is the treatment of choice for most patients with facial CM.

The flash-lamp, pumped, pulsed-dye laser was introduced in the late 1970s for treatment of CM.[50] This system differs from the argon laser in that it uses a wavelength of 585 nm, specific for the absorption of oxyhemoglobin. In addition, as discussed earlier, the pulse duration is extremely short (400 ms), allowing for effective coagulation of vessels without extensive thermal diffusion to surrounding tissue (i.e., selective photothermolysis).[51] The pulsed-dye laser (PDL) offers effective treatment for infants and children with a very low risk of hypopigmentation (1.4 percent) or scarring (atrophic, 4.3 percent; hypertrophic,

FIGURE 103-15

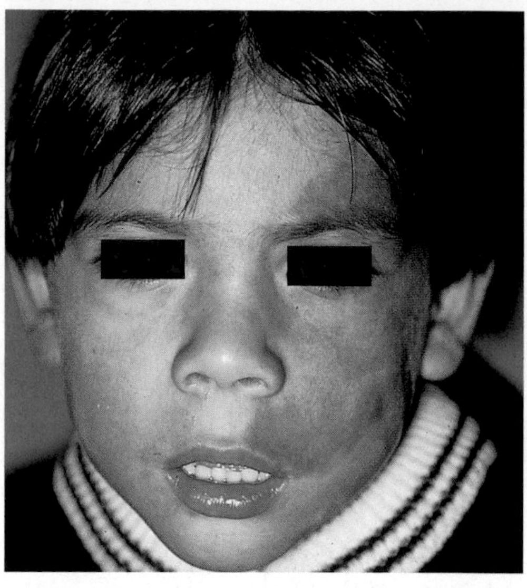

Capillary malformation (port-wine stain) involving V_1–V_2 dermatomes, left face; patients with CM in the V_2 distribution are at risk for the Sturge-Weber syndrome.

0.7 percent).[52] Approximately 65 percent of patients treated with PDL will achieve between 50 and 90 percent lightening, and 15 percent will have more than 90 percent lightening of their lesion.[53] Multiple treatment sessions (6 to 12) are often needed to obtain optimal lightening of lesions, and lesions may recur several years after treatment.[53] General anesthesia is safe and significantly less traumatic for infants and small children,[54] but precautions must be taken to avoid flash fires resulting from ignition of oxygen from the endotracheal tube. Refinements of PDL include the use of longer pulses and longer wavelengths that penetrate more deeply, thereby producing greater lightening. In addition, the use of a dynamic cooling device to cool the epidermis allows the use of higher fluences, effectively producing greater lightening and reducing the number of treatments needed.[55]

Phakomatosis Pigmentovascularis

Phakomatosis pigmentovascularis refers to the coexistence of a CM (port-wine stain) with various melanocytic lesions, including dermal melanocytosis (Mongolian spots), nevus spilus, and nevus of Ota. Fewer than 100 cases have been reported since the original description in 1947[56]; most reports are in the Japanese literature. Phakomatosis pigmentovascularis is categorized into four types, each of which is further subclassified according to the presence or absence of associated systemic findings (Table 103-5). Developmental abnormalities of neural crest–derived vasomotor nerves and melanocytes are thought to be involved in the pathogenesis. Aberrant neural regulation of blood vessels coupled with abnormal migration of melanocytes could explain the coexistence of CM and melanocytic lesions.

Telangiectases

These lesions are composed of dilated capillaries that manifest clinically as tiny erythematous to violaceous cutaneous vessels. These may blanch but do not tend to fade with time. They may be sporadic or associated with several syndromes (Table 103-6).

Familial telangiectasia (Osler-Rendu-Weber disease) This process, a vascular anomaly transmitted as a simple dominant trait, affects the skin, the mucous membranes, the gastrointestinal and genitourinary tracts, and occasionally the nervous system (see Chap. 188). The basic lesion is probably a defect in the vessel wall. The lesions range from

TABLE 103-4

Vascular Syndromes

Syndrome Name	Flow Type	Location of Vascular Malformation	Associated Findings
Klippel-Trenaunay (Fig. 103-23)	Slow	Limbs, trunk, perineum	CVM, CLVM, skeletal hypertrophy (rare hypotrophy), lymphatic hypoplasia, lymphedema
Maffucci (Fig. 103-24)	Slow	Distal extremities	VM, LVM, enchondromas, short stature, chrondrosarcoma (15–20 percent)
Proteus	Slow	Any cutaneous site	CM, LM, CVM, CLM, lipoma, epidermal nevus, palmar/plantar hyperplasia, macrodactyly, scoliosis macrocephaly, asymmetric bony and soft tissue hypertrophy, cataracts
Cobb	Slow ± fast	Over spine	VM or AVM of spinal cord ± cord compression
Solomon	Slow ± fast	CM, VM (any cutaneous site), AVM (intracranial)	Epidermal nevi, skeletal hypertrophy
Sturge-Weber (Fig. 103-15)	Slow ± fast	Face in V1-V2 dermatome	CM, VM or AVM in ipsilateral choroid and meninges, gyriform calcifications "tram-tracks," facial soft-tissue/skeletal hypertrophy, choroidal vascular anomaly, glaucoma
Parkes-Weber (Fig. 103-25)	Fast	Limbs	CAVM, CAVF, soft-tissue/skeletal hypertrophy
Bonnet-Dechaume-Blanc (Wyburn-Mason)	Fast	Unilateral vascular stain	Ipsilateral AVM of optic tract

the size of a pinhead to 3 mm or more, are of bright-red or violaceous color, and blanch under pressure (see Fig. 166-6). Some of them form small vascular papules 2 to 3 mm in diameter. Located sparsely in the skin of any part of the body, they first appear during childhood, enlarge during adolescence, and may assume spidery forms, resembling, in late adult life, the cutaneous telangiectases of cirrhosis. The lesions cause trouble only because of their tendency to hemorrhage. During adult years, they may give rise to severe and repeated epistaxis or gastric, intestinal, or urinary tract hemorrhages. Chronic blood loss may result in an iron-deficiency anemia.

Lesions may form in either the spinal cord or brain and produce apoplectic syndromes, or an intermittently progressive cerebral syndrome may result from a succession of small hemorrhages. Diagnosis of an unexplained gastrointestinal, genitourinary, intracranial, or intraspinal hemorrhage warrants a search for these small cutaneous lesions, which are easily overlooked. Pulmonary fistulas constitute another important feature of the generalized vascular dysplasia. Such patients are subject to brain abscesses, like the patient with congenital heart disease (see Chap. 166). Although cautery eradicates a bleeding lesion, satellites tend to re-form. Prophylaxis has proved to be unsatisfactory. The pulmonary arteriovenous malformation can be excised, if not too large, and the common hepatic vascular malformation as well.

TABLE 103-5

Classification of Phakomatosis Pigmentovascularis*

Type	CM	Dermal Melanocytosis	Nevus Anemicus	Nevus Spilus	Other
I a,b	+	−	−	−	Nevus pigmentosus et verrucosus
II a,b	+	+	±	−	
III a,b	+	−	±	+	
IV a,b	+	+	±	+	

*a = cutaneous involvement only; b = cutaneous and systemic involvement. Systemic involvement includes: + = present; − = not present; ± = may or may not be present; nevus anemicus = localized pale macule with irregular borders that usually presents at birth and is most often located on the upper trunk. The lesion is a pharmacologic anomaly rather than a structural one; the involved vessels exhibit increased reactivity to catecholamines resulting in persistent vasoconstriction.

SPIDER ANGIOMA Spider angioma is a localized network of dilated capillaries radiating from a central feeding arteriole. Lesions appear most often on the face, forearms, and hands and occur in approximately 40 percent of children. They can fade spontaneously, but more commonly they persist. Pulsed-dye laser treatment usually can eradicate these lesions completely (Fig. 103-16).

Cutis Marmorata Telangiectasia Congenita (CMTC)

Old terms for CMTC include *congenital generalized phlebectasia, nevus vascularis reticularis, congenital livedo reticularis,* and *van Lohuizen syndrome*.

CLINICAL MANIFESTATIONS CMTC, first described in 1922 by van Lohuizen, is characterized by a distinct, deeply erythematous to violaceous, reticulate vascular network that can be localized or generalized. Lesions are often segmental and unilateral and are present, in order of decreasing frequency, on the extremities (Fig. 103-17), trunk, face, and scalp.[56] CMTC is present at birth. Approximately 75 percent of children will show improvement of the marbled vascular pattern over time, with the most significant change occurring during the first 2 years of life. The skin within the reticulated network can be normal in color or erythematous to violaceous. The reticulated pattern is always present and is enhanced by crying, exercise, or cold temperatures. With time, the dilated veins become more prominent as the overlying skin becomes increasingly atrophic.

Associated findings have been reported in approximately 27 percent of patients; however, it is unknown whether these findings occur more frequently in CMTC patients compared with the normal population.[57] The most frequent findings include ulceration, cutaneous atrophy, and hypertrophy or atrophy of the affected limb. Other findings in association with CMTC include (1) craniofacial abnormalities such as cleft palate, high arched palate, micrognathia, dytrophic teeth, congenital glaucoma, macrocephaly, dolichocephaly, optic nerve atrophy, facial asymmetry, and frontal bossing; (2) neurologic abnormalities such as mental retardation, delayed motor development, and hypotonia; (3) vascular anomalies such as CM; (4) cutaneous abnormalities such as hyperelastic skin and aplasia cutis; (5) syndactyly of the toes; and (6) hypospadias.[58]

TABLE 103-6

Syndromes with Telangiectasia

DISORDER	COMMON LOCATION OF TELANGIECTASIA	ASSOCIATED FINDINGS
Generalized essential telangiectasia	Lower extremities	None
Hereditary hemorrhagic telangiectasia	Face, tongue, lips, nasal and oral mucous membranes, conjunctiva, palmar fingers, nail beds, internal mucous membranes	Epistaxis, hematemesis, hematuria, melena, AVM in brain, spinal cord, liver, and lungs
Ataxia-telangiectasia (see Chap. 191)	Nasal and temporal bulbar conjunctiva, face, neck, upper chest, flexor forearms	Cerebellar ataxia, progressive neuromotor degeneration, endocrine dysfunction, chromosomal instability, growth retardation, sinopulmonary infection, lymphoreticular malignancy

CMTC is considered to be a sporadic disorder; however, two sisters with CMTC have been reported.[56]

PATHOLOGY Histopathologic examination reveals dilated capillaries and veins, as well as vascular fibrosis. Hyperkeratosis, dilated lymphatics, and venous thrombosis also can be seen. In some biopsies, there are few to no histologic changes. Diagnosis is generally made by the characteristic clinical features.

TREATMENT Management begins with careful evaluation of the child for possible associated abnormalities. Ulcerations may require topical or systemic antibiotics. PDL treatment potentially could help to lighten areas of CMTC.

Lymphatic Malformation

Old terms for LM include *lymphangioma circumscriptum, lymphangioma,* and *cystic hygroma*.

CLINICAL MANIFESTATIONS LM are composed of micro-to macroscopic vesicles and channels filled with clear or serosanguinous fluid or soft, subcutaneous nodules or large masses composed of dilated ectatic lymphatic channels (Fig. 103-18). Lesions typically present at birth or prior to 2 years of age. Occasionally, LMs may not manifest until childhood or adulthood. LMs very rarely involute spontaneously; they usually expand or contract according to changes in the flow of lymphatic fluid and the presence of inflammation or intralesional bleeding. They are subcategorized as microcystic (*lymphangioma*), macrocystic (*cystic hygroma*), or combined.

LM is often associated with bony hypertrophy, especially in the face or extremity. Difficulty in differentiating LM from VM is due to spontaneous intralesional bleeding or blood flow within LM and the fact that many lesions at their onset are a combined lymphaticovenous malformation (LVM). Lymphedema is caused by LM in an extremity.

TREATMENT Intralesional bleeding causes pain and is managed with rest and analgesics. Bacterial infection should be treated promptly with antibiotics; often prolonged administration is necessary. Long-term management involves sclerotherapy and resection for appearance and functional problems.

FIGURE 103-16

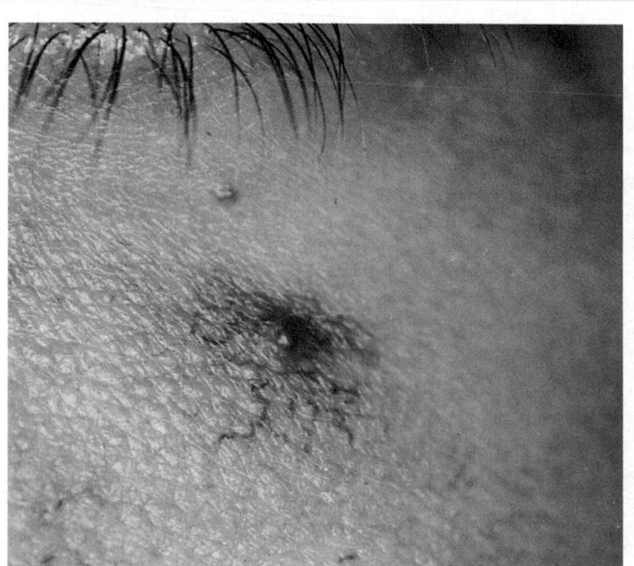

Spider hemangioma. A red lesion with a central papular punctum at the site of the feeding arterial vessel, with macular, radiating, telangiectatic vessels. On diascopy, the central arterial vessels can be seen to pulsate.

FIGURE 103-17

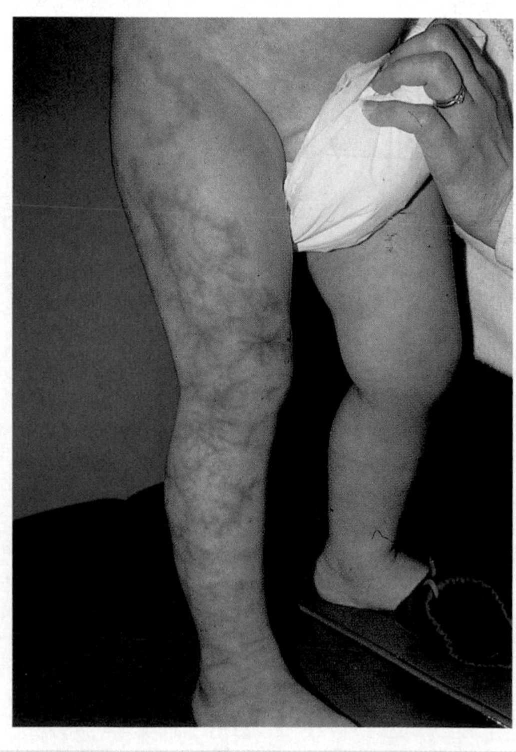

Cutis marmorata telangiectasia congenita, right lower limb in a young boy.

FIGURE 103-18

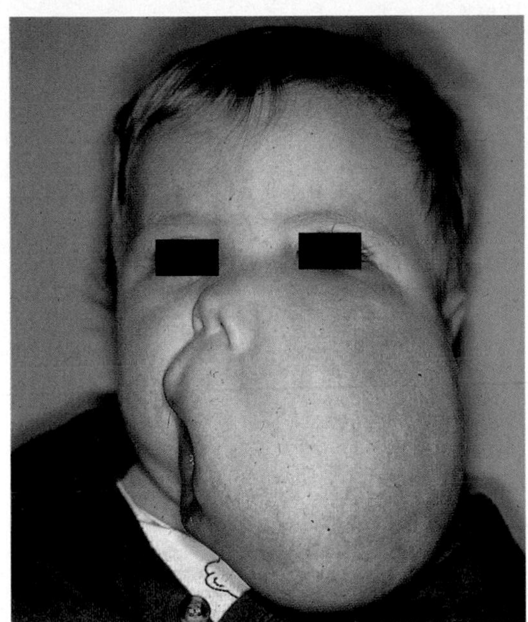

Macro-/microcystic lymphatic malformation involving soft tissues on the left face. This patient has had multiple bouts of cellulitis.

Capillary-Lymphatic Malformation (CLM)

Old terms for CLM include *hypertrophic nevus flammeus*, *verrucous hemangioma, hemangiolymphangioma,* and *angiokeratoma circumscriptum*.

CLINICAL MANIFESTATIONS CLM is a well-demarcated, pink to bluish red, raised lesion consisting of dilated protuberant vascular and lymphatic channels (Fig. 103-19A). These lesions are commonly located on the lower extremities, but CLM may be found also on the chest, abdomen, and arms. If the surface is rough, hyperkeratotic, and wartlike, lesions are called angiokeratomas (see Fig. 103-19*B*).

All the angiokeratomas can be considered as variations of CLM, including angiokeratoma of Mibelli, angiokeratoma of Fordyce, angiokeratoma circumscriptum, angiokeratoma corporis diffusum universale (Fabry disease, see Chap. 151), and fucosidosis (Table 103-7).

PATHOLOGY CLMs are composed of dilated vessels with deficient elastic fibers in the dermis and subcutaneous tissues. The caliber of vessels ranges from capillary to large venule. Larger ectatic lymphatic vessels also can be present, containing proteinaceous material. There may be reactive epidermal hyperkeratosis and parakeratosis.

FIGURE 103-19

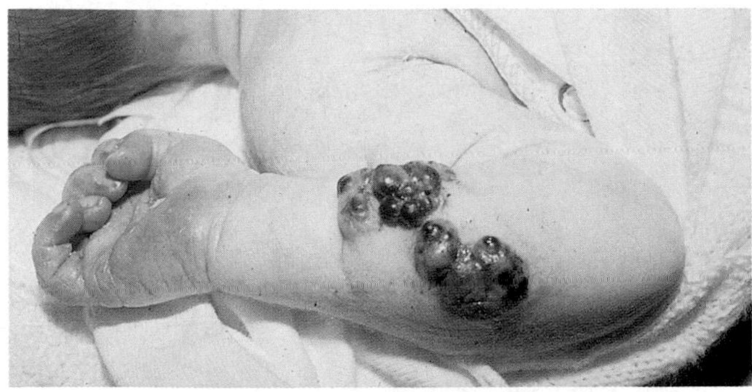

A.

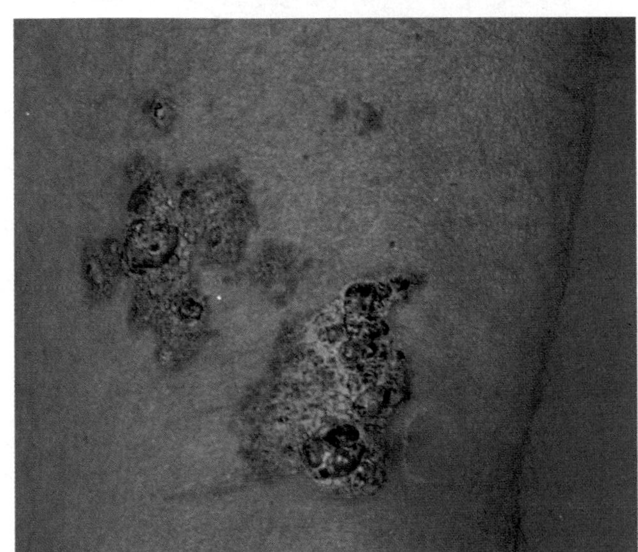

B.

A. Capillary-lymphatic malformation, right forearm; treated by resection *B.* Angiokeratoma circumscriptum. Keratotic violaceous plaques whose edges are jagged.

TABLE 103-7

The "Angiokeratomas"

NAME OF ANGIOKERATOMA	AGE AT ONSET	LOCATION OF LESIONS	ASSOCIATED FINDINGS
Mibelli	10–15 years	Dorsal and volar hands and feet > ankles, knees, palms, elbows	Acrocyanosis, chilblain, frostbite
Fordyce	>60 years	Genitalia, abdomen, or thigh	None
Solitary papular	10–40 years	Legs, can be anywhere	None
Circumscriptum	Birth	Lower leg or foot > thigh, buttock, elsewhere	
Fabry disease (angiokeratoma corporis diffusum) (see Chap. 151)	Prior to puberty	"Bathing trunk" area: thighs, groin, buttocks, lower abdomen	Painful episodes, dry hypohidrotic skin, HTN, CVA, CAD, renal disease
Fucosidosis	Between 6 months and 8 years	Trunk and thighs: similar distribution to Fabry's disease	MR, spasticity, seizures, sinus and pulmonary infections

HTN, hypertension; CVA, cerebrovascular accident; CAD, coronary artery disease; and MR, mental retardation.

FIGURE 103-20

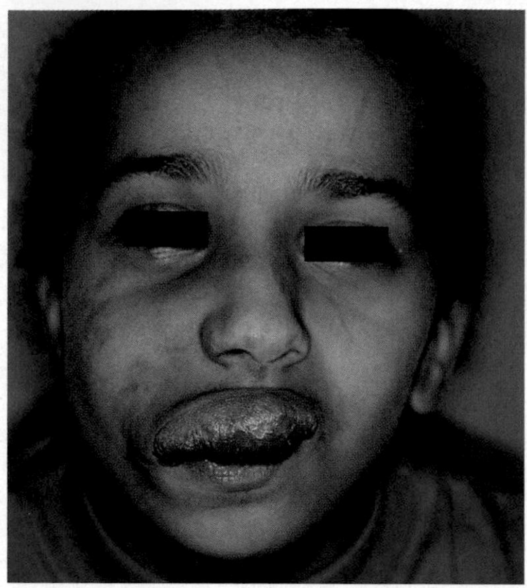

Nine-year-old girl with extensive cutaneous-intramuscular VM of upper lip and cheek.

Venous Malformation

CLINICAL MANIFESTATIONS VM is present at birth but may not be evident clinically until childhood or adulthood. Typical lesions are violaceous to blue in color and consist of patches or soft, compressible papules, plaques, or nodules. They may be localized or more extensive, involving an entire anatomic region. VMs are located most frequently on the face (Fig. 103-20), trunk, or extremities but may be present in the oronasopharynx and any of the viscera, as well as in bone. Typically, VMs are solitary; however, multiple cutaneous and visceral lesions may occur. Multifocal VM suggests an inheritable disorder or syndrome (see Table 103-4).

VMs are easily compressible and swell when the affected part is dependent. Patients often complain of intermittent pain in the VM, particularly on wakening in the morning. Presumably this is due to stasis and possibly thrombosis within this slow-flow vascular anomaly. Phleboliths, noted by either palpation or radiographically, are the hallmark of VMs.

Skeletal alterations can occur with VMs. Craniofacial VMs typically cause facial asymmetry and gradual progressive distortion of facial features. Intraorbital VMs are associated with expansion of the orbital cavity, and oral VMs cause dental malalignment. An extremity VM may induce bony hypertrophy, resulting in length discrepancy, although undergrowth due to disuse may also occur.

DIAGNOSIS Ultrasonography is the easiest way to confirm the diagnosis of a deep VM and to differentiate the lesion from a deep hemangioma versus lymphatic malformation. However, MRI is considered the gold standard for diagnosis of VMs and for documentation of their extent and involvement of surrounding tissues. Patients with an extensive VM should be evaluated for the possibility of localized intravascular coagulopathy caused by stasis within the interstices of the VM; this is a different bleeding disorder than that seen in Kasabach-Merritt phenomenon. A coagulation profile may reveal a slightly low platelet count (100,000 to 150,000/mm^3 range), low fibrinogen (150 to 200 mg/dL), and increased D-dimers, with normal prothrombin and partial thromboplastin times.

TREATMENT Indications for treatment of VM include appearance, pain, and functional impairment. Conservative management involves the use of custom-made elastic support, especially for extremity VMs. Episodes of painful thrombosis may be minimized with low-dose aspirin (80 mg qd to qod). Small cutaneous VMs at any site may be injected with a sclerosant such as 1% sodium tetradecyl sulfate. Patients with a large VM, either cutaneous or intramuscular, also may be sclerosed, but they require general anesthesia with real-time fluoroscopic monitoring. The most commonly used sclerosant in the United States is absolute ethanol (100%), whereas Ethibloc (a corn protein, ethanol, and contrast medium) is used commonly in Europe. Possible complications include blistering, hemoglobinuria, deep ulceration, nerve damage, renal toxicity, and cardiac arrest.[59] Multiple therapeutic sessions may be necessary because VM has a tendency for recanalization and reexpansion. Surgical excision is best done after sclerotherapy to decrease tissue bulk or to improve function.

Blue Rubber Bleb Nevus Syndrome

Blue rubber bleb nevus syndrome (BRBNS) is composed of the constellation of multiple cutaneous and gastrointestinal venous malformations. The first description of this entity was in 1860 by Gascoyen, and in 1958, Bean reported two cases and coined the term *blue rubber bleb nevus syndrome*.[56] Cutaneous lesions may be present at birth or appear during early childhood and, once present, remain unchanged. The lesions are soft, compressible, 0.1- to 5.0-cm blue nodules commonly located on the trunk and extremities, but they can be located anywhere on the skin and mucosa. Lesions are usually asymptomatic but can be tender, and occasionally, patients have pain in the lesions (likely secondary to thromboses). Most cases are sporadic, but there are several reports suggesting autosomal dominant inheritance.

BRBNS lesions are the most common type of intestinal venous anomaly. Gastrointestinal lesions occur most commonly in the small intestine; however, any portion of the gastrointestinal tract can be involved, including the oral and anal mucosa. In contrast to cutaneous lesions, the gastrointestinal lesions are friable and often bleed, causing iron-deficiency anemia. Acute gastrointestinal hemorrhage, intussusception, volvulus, bowel infarction, and rectal prolapse have been described. The VMs that constitute blue rubber bleb nevus syndrome also can involve other organ systems, including the eye, nasopharynx, brain, meninges, heart, lung, liver, spleen, gallbladder, kidney, adrenal gland, uterus, muscle and joints.[56]

PATHOLOGY Histopathologic examination reveals ectatic vessels of various sizes in the deep dermis and subcutaneous fat.

TREATMENT Treatment options for cutaneous lesions include excision, sclerotherapy, and laser (pulsed-dye or CO_2) for the smaller new lesions. Treatment of these patients should include periodic stool guaiac examinations, complete blood count, and endoscopic cauterization or sclerosis or bowel resection, if necessary.

Glomuvenous Malformations (GVMs)

Old term *glomangiomas.*

CLINICAL MANIFESTATIONS GVM arise from the arterial segment of the cutaneous glomus, the Suquet-Hoyer canal. Glomus cells are of smooth muscle origin and are polyhedral in shape, in contrast

FIGURE 103-21

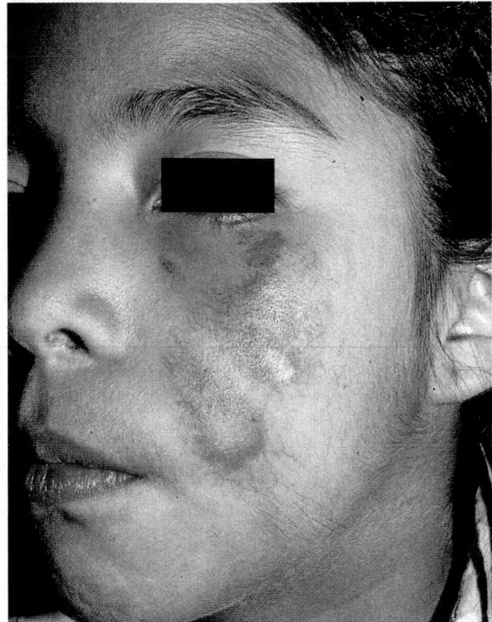

Stage I arteriovenous malformation on the left face. Cheek is warm; only tiny dermal blush seen on MRI.

to the usual elongated form. These cells comprise specialized vascular structures, called *glomus formations,* that are present in abundance in the distal pads and nail beds of the fingers and to a lesser degree on the volar aspect of the hands and feet, in the skin of the ears, and on the central face. Glomus formations are special arteriovenous shunts that appear to play a role in thermoregulation.

GVM are distinct from the more common glomus tumors, which present as solitary, painful papules that are a few millimeters in diameter on the extremities, especially in the nail bed. GVM is a type of slow-flow vascular malformation consisting of multiple, nontender vascular lesions that may reach a size of several centimeters. They are usually scattered over the body but may be localized to one area such as the face.[60] GVMs are generally asymptomatic, although paroxysmal attacks of pain have been described, occasionally related to menstruation or pregnancy. GVMs arise during childhood or during the second decade of life. Men are more commonly affected than women. In many cases of GVM, a strong family history has been reported, with incomplete

FIGURE 103-22

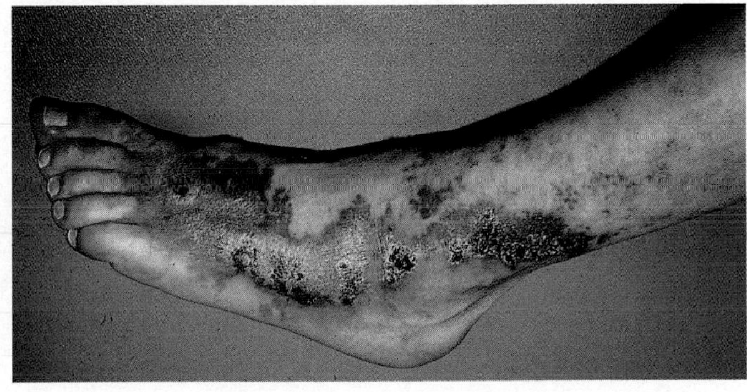

Teenage girl with stage III AVM in her left foot, with pseudo-Kaposi cutaneous changes.

FIGURE 103-23

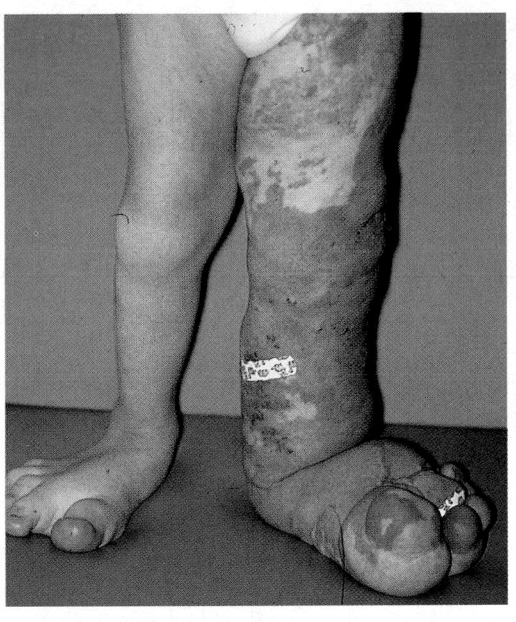

Capillary-lymphaticovenous malformation (CLVM) (old term, *Klippel-Trenauney syndrome*), lower limb.

to complete penetrance.[61] Gastrointestinal involvement, so common in the blue rubber bleb nevus syndrome, has not been described.

TREATMENT Treatment options include excision, electrosurgery, sclerotherapy, electron-beam irradiation, and laser therapy with the CO_2, argon, and pulsed ruby lasers.

Arteriovenous Malformation and Fistula

CLINICAL MANIFESTATIONS *Arterial malformation* (AM) is a general term for embryonic vascular anomalies, such as aneurysm, coarctation, hypoplasia, and stenosis. AVM is the most common fast-flow anomaly in children. AVMs are present at birth but may not be evident clinically until later. The most common location for an AVM is intracranial, followed by extremities, trunk, and viscera. The initial presentation may be a faint or ill-defined area of macular erythema resembling a port-wine stain (Fig. 103-21). Expansion of an AVM often occurs in puberty or following trauma or infection and results in an altered clinical appearance: a deeply erythematous to violaceous color, an underlying subcutaneous mass (possibly pulsatile), warmth, a thrill, and a bruit. End-stage lesions are characterized by ulceration, intractable pain, bleeding and multiple violaceous papules and nodules—pseudo Kaposi sarcomatous changes (Fig. 103-22).

DIAGNOSIS Diagnosis of AVM is primarily clinical and is confirmed by ultrasonography and color Doppler examination. MRI is superior for evaluation of the extent of an AVM. Diagnostic angiography is usually done at the same time as embolization or sclerotherapy. The Schobinger staging system has been proposed to facilitate clinical research and outcome studies[62]: stage I (quiescence): stain and warmth; stage II (expansion): enlargement, tortuous, tense veins, pulsations,

FIGURE 103-24

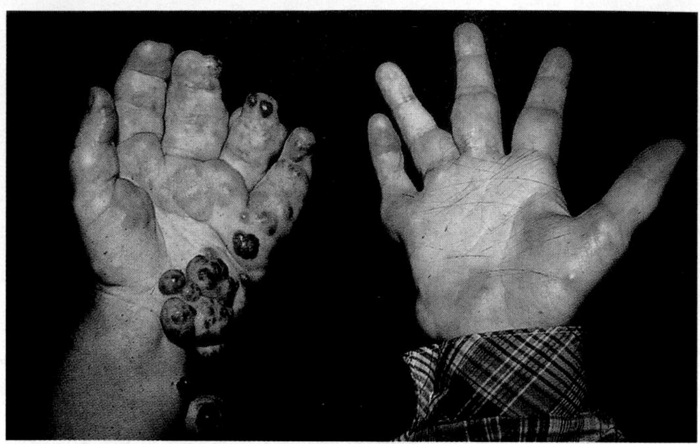

Lymphaticovenous anomalies (LVM) of hands; radiographs show enchondromas (Maffucci syndrome).

thrill, and bruit; stage III (destruction): dystrophic changes, ulceration, bleeding, and persistent pain; and stage IV (decompensation): cardiac failure.

FIGURE 103-25

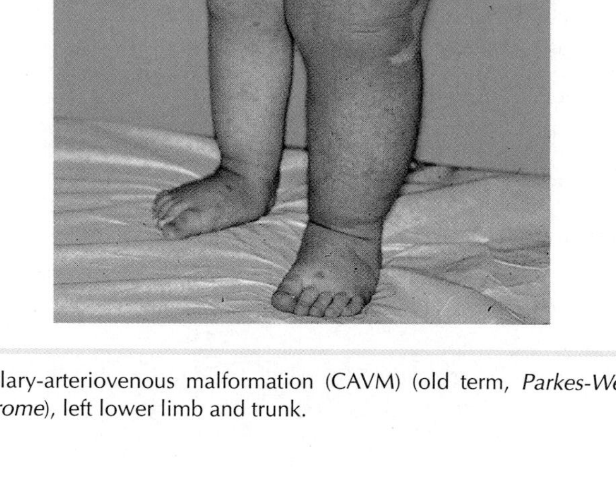

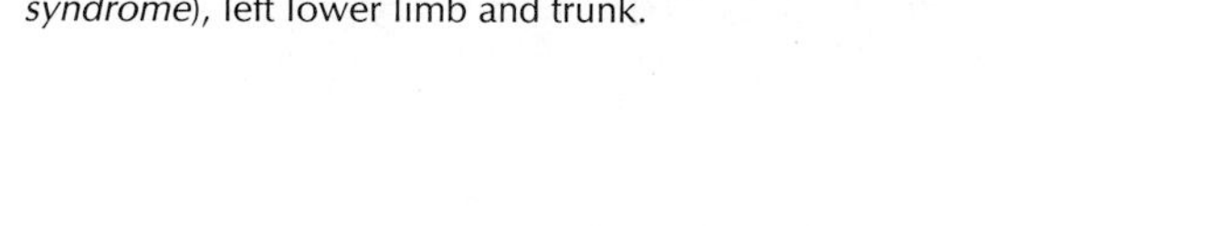

Capillary-arteriovenous malformation (CAVM) (old term, *Parkes-Weber syndrome*), left lower limb and trunk.

TREATMENT Intervention for AVM is considered whenever endangering signs or symptoms develop—Schobinger stage III or IV. Early intervention for a quiet AVM (stages I to II) is debatable but should be considered if resection is achieved easily without disfigurement. Palliative embolization can be done but almost never will cure an AVM, in contrast to closure of an AVF by embolization. The concept for cure is to obliterate and resect the nidus or epicenter of the AVM. This requires embolization or sclerotherapy followed by resection (whenever possible). Following combined embolization-resection, the patient must be followed for years by clinical examination, ultrasonography, and/or MRI. There are extensive AVMs for which only palliative embolization is possible. Pharmacologic treatment of such AVMs is evolving.

TABLE 103-8

Genetic Information for Selected Vascular Anomalies

Disorder	Genetic Information*
Fabry Disease (see Chap. 151)	Alpha-galactosidase A gene, Xq
Fucosidosis[63]	Alpha-fucosidase gene (*FUCA 1*), 1p36.1-p.34.1
Hereditary hemorrhagic telangiectasia[64]	*HHT1*: endoglin gene, 9q33-34 *HHT2* activin-like receptor tyrosine kinase, 12q11-14
Ataxia= telangiectasia[65] (see Chap. 191)	*ATM*: (ataxia telangiectasia mutated) gene, 11q22-23
Familial cutaneomucosal VM[66]	*TIE2* mutation, 9p21-22
Venous malformation with glomus cells[67]	*VMGLOM* locus, 1p21-p22
Cerebral capillary-venous malformation[68]	*CCM1* gene, 7q21-22 encoding KRIT 1 protein; two other loci: 3q25-27 and 7p13-15
Lymphedema (autosomal dominant): Milroy syndrome, Meige syndrome (lymphedema praecox, lymphedema distichiasis syndrome, yellow-nail syndrome) (see also Chap.167)[69]	Milroy: *VEGFR3* gene, 5q35 All AD lymphedema syndromes: forkhead transcription factor, FOXC2, 16
Bannayan-Riley Ruvalcava syndrome[70]	*PTEN* tumor suppressor
Proteus-like syndrome[71]	*PTEN* tumor suppressor

*The genetic information tabulated above is not in any way comprehensive. It is possible that genes on other chromosomes may also be responsible for the anomalies.

Combined Malformations

Combined vascular malformations (CVMs) include, CLM, CLVM, and CLAVM and are also subdivided as either slow flow or fast flow (Figs. 103-23, 103-24, and 103-25). There is often associated soft tissue and skeletal hypertrophy. Many of the combined malformations are known by well-worn eponyms (see Table 103-4).

Genetics of Vascular Malformations

Advances in molecular genetics have led to the discovery of the genes and/or chromosomal locations for many inheritable vascular anomalies. Genetic information regarding several well-known vascular disorders is listed in Table 103-8 and in references 64, 65, 66, 67, 68, 69, 70 and 71.

REFERENCES

1. Mulliken JB, Young AE: *Vascular Birthmarks: Hemangiomas and Malformations*. Philadelphia, Saunders 1988
2. Mulliken JB, Glowacki J: Hemangiomas and vascular malformations in infants and children: A classification based on endothelial characteristics. *Plast Reconstr Surg* **69**:412, 1982
3. Pratt AG: Birthmarks in infants. *Arch Dermatol* **67**:302, 1953
4. Jacobs AH, Walton RG: The incidence of birthmarks in the neonate. *Pediatrics* **58**:218, 1976
5. Hidano A, Nakajima S: Earliest features of the strawberry mark in the newborn. *Br J Dermatol* **87**:138, 1972
6. Holmadahl K: Cutaneous hemangiomas in premature and mature infants. *Acta Paediatr* **44**:370, 1955
7. Amir J et al: Strawberry hemangioma in preterm infants. *Pediatr Dermatol* **3**:331, 1986
8. Finn MC et al: Congenital vascular lesions: Clinical application of a new classification. *J Pediatr Surg* **18**:894, 1983
9. Cheung DS et al: Hemangioma in twins. *Ann Plast Surg* **38**:269, 1997
10. Bielenberg DR et al: Progressive growth of infantile cutaneous hemangiomas is directly correlated with hyperplasia and angiogenesis of adjacent epidermis and inversely correlated with expression of the endogenous angiogenesis inhibitor, IFN-beta. *Int J Oncol* **14**:401, 1999
11. Boye E et al: Clonality and altered behavior of endothelial cells in hemangiomas. *J Clin Invest* **107**:665, 2001
12. Enjolras O, Mulliken JB: The current management of vascular birthmarks. *Pediatr Dermatol* **10**:311, 1993
13. Razon MJ et al: Increased apoptosis coincides with onset of involution in infantile hemangioma. *Microcirculation* **5**:189, 1998
14. Hasan Q et al: Altered mitochondrial cytochrome *b* gene expression during the regression of hemangioma. *Plast Reconstr Surg* **108**:1471, 2001
15. Martinez-Perez D et al: Not all hemangiomas look like strawberries: Uncommon presentations of the most common tumor of infancy. *Pediatr Dermatol* **12**:1, 1995
16. Esterly NB et al: The management of disseminated eruptive hemangiomata in infants. *Pediatr Dermatol* **1**:312, 1984
17. Enjolras O et al: Noninvoluting congenital hemangioma: A rare cutaneous vascular anomaly. *Plast Reconstr Surg* **107**:1647, 2001
18. Frieden IJ et al: PHACE syndrome: The association of posterior fossa brain malformations, hemangiomas, arterial anomalies, coarctation of the aorta and cardiac defects, and eye abnormalities. *Arch Dermatol* **132**:307, 1996
19. Paltiel HJ et al: Soft-tissue vascular anomalies: Utility of US for diagnosis. *Radiology* **214**:747, 2000
20. North PE et al: GLUT1: A newly discovered immunohistochemical marker for juvenile hemangiomas. *Hum Pathol* **31**:11, 2000
21. Orlow SJ et al: Increased risk of symptomatic hemangiomas of the airway in association with cutaneous hemangiomas in a "beard" distribution. *J Pediatr* **131**:643, 1997
22. Boon LM et al: Hepatic vascular anomalies in infancy: A twenty-seven year experience. *J Pediatr* **129**:346, 1996
23. Kim HJ et al: Ulcerated hemangiomas: Clinical characteristics and response to therapy. *J Am Acad Dermatol* **44**:962, 2001
24. Ellis PO: Occlusion of the central retinal artery after retrobulbar corticosteroid injection. *Am J Ophthalmol* **85**:352, 1978
25. Deans RM et al: Surgical dissection of capillary hemangiomas: An alternative to intralesional corticosteroids. *Arch Ophthalmol* **110**:1743, 1992
26. Sloan GM et al: Intralesional corticosteroid therapy for infantile hemangiomas. *Plast Reconstr Surg* **83**:459, 1989
27. Elsas FJ, Lewis AR: Topical treatment of periocular capillary hemangioma. *J Pediatr Ophthalmol Strabismus* **31**:153, 1994
28. Bennett ML et al: Oral corticosteroid use is effective for cutaneous hemangiomas: An evidence-based evaluation. *Arch Dermatol* **137**:1208, 2001
29. Boon LM et al: Complications of systemic corticosteroid therapy for problematic hemangioma. *Plast Reconstr Surg* **104**:1616, 1999
30. Ezekowitz RA et al: Interferon-α2a therapy for life-threratening hemangiomas of infancy. *New Engl J Med* **326**:1456, 1992
31. Tamayo L et al: Therapeutic efficacy of interferon-α2b in infants with life-threatening giant hemangiomas. *Arch Dermatol* **133**:1567, 1997
32. Barlow CF et al: Spastic diplegia as a complication of interferon-α2a treatment of hemangiomas of infancy. *J Pediatr* **132**:527, 1998
33. Ashinoff R, Geronemus RG: Failure of the flashlamp-pumped pused-dye laser to prevent progression to a deep hemangioma. *Pediatr Dermatol* **10**:77, 1993
34. Scheepers JH, Quaba AA: Does the pulsed tunable dye laser have a role in the management of infantile hemangiomas: Observations based on 3 years' experience. *Plast Reconstr Surg* **95**:305, 1995
35. Mulliken JB: Management of hemangiomas. *Pediatr Dermatol* **14**:60, 1997
36. Morelli JG et al: Treatment of ulcerated hemangiomas with the pulsed tunable dye laser. *Am J Dis Child* **145**:1062, 1991
37. Enjolras O et al: Infants with Kasabach-Merritt syndrome do not have "true" hemangiomas. *J Pediatr* **130**:631, 1997
38. Sarkar M et al: Thrombocytopenic coagulopathy (Kasabach-Merritt phenomenon) is associated with kaposiform hemangioendothelioma and not with common infantile hemangioma. *Plast Reconstr Surg* **100**:1377, 1997
39. Enjolras O et al: Residual lesions after Kasabach-Merritt phenomenon in 41 patients. *J Am Acad Dermatol* **42**:225, 2000
40. Patrice SJ et al: Pyogenic granuloma (lobular capillary hemangioma): A clinicopathologic study of 178 cases. *Pediatr Dermatol* **8**:267, 1991
41. Jones EW, Orkin M: Tufted angioma (angioblastoma): A benign progressive angioma, not to be confused with Kaposi's sarcoma or low-grade angiosarcoma. *J Am Acad Dermatol* **20**:214, 1989
42. Suarez SM et al: Response of deep tufted angioma to interferon-α. *J Am Acad Dermatol* **33**:124, 1995
43. Pitluk HC, Conn JJ: Hemangiopericytoma: Literature review and clinical presentations. *Am J Surg* **137**:413, 1979
44. Enzinger FM, Smith BH: Hemangiopericytoma: An analysis of 106 cases. *Hum Pathol* **7**:61, 1976
45. Santa Cruz DJ, Aronberg J: Targetoid hemosiderotic hemangioma. *J Am Acad Dermatol* **19**:550, 1988
46. Vion B, Frenk E: Targetoid hemosiderotic hemangioma. *Dermatology* **184**:300, 1992
47. Hynes LR, Shenefelt PD: Unilateral nevoid telangiectasia: Occurrence in two patients with hepatitis C. *J Am Acad Dermatol* **36**:819, 1997
48. Tan KL: Nevus flammeus of the nape, glabella, and eyelids: A clinical study of frequency, racial distribution, and association with congenital anomalies. *Clin Pediatr* **11**:112, 1972
49. Smoller BR, Rosen S: Port-wine stains: A disease of altered neural modulation of blood vessels? *Arch Dermatol* **122**:177, 1986
50. Anderson RR, Parrish JA: Microvasculature can be selectively damaged using dye lasers: A basic theory and experimental evidence in human skin. *Lasers Surg Med* **1**:263, 1981
51. Anderson RR, Parrish JA: Selective photothermolysis: Precise microsurgery by selective absorption of pulsed radiation. *Science* **220**:524, 1983
52. Seukeran DC et al: Adverse reactions following pulsed tunable dye laser treatment of port-wine stains in 701 patients. *Br J Dermatol* **36**:725, 1997
53. Orten SS et al: Port-wine stains: An assessment of 5 years of treatment. *Arch Otolaryngol Head Neck Surg* **122**:1174, 1996
54. Grevelink JM et al: Pulsed laser treatment in children and the use of anesthesia. *J Am Acad Dermatol* **37**:75, 1997
55. Waldorf HA et al: Effect of dynamic cooling on 585-nm pulsed dye laser treatment of port-wine stain birthmarks. *Dermatol Surg* **23**:657, 1997
56. Requena L, Sangueza OP: Cutaneous vascular anomalies: Hamartomas, malformations, and dilatation of preexisting vessels. *J Am Acad Dermatol* **37**:523, 1997
57. Picascia DD, Esterly NB: Cutis marmorata telangiectasia congenita: Report of 22 cases. *J Am Acad Dermatol* **20**:1098, 1989
58. Ben-Amitai D et al: Cutis marmorata telangiectatica congenita and hypospadias: Report of 4 cases. *Am Acad Dermatol* **45**:131, 2001
59. Berenguer B et al: Sclerotherapy of craniofacial venous malformations: Complications and results. *Plast Reconstr Surg* **104**:1, 1999
60. Mounayer C et al: Facial "glomangiomas": Large facial venous malformations wit glomus cells. *J Am Acad Dermatol* **45**:239, 2001
61. Rudolph B: Familial multiple glomangiomas. *Ann Plast Surg* **30**:183, 1993
62. Kohout MP et al: Arteriovenous malformations of the head and neck: Natural history and management. *Plast Reconstr Surg* **102**:643, 1998
63. Cragg H et al: Fucosidosis: Genetic and biochemical analysis of eight cases. *J Med Genet* **34**:105, 1997
64. Guttmacher AE et al: Hereditary hemorrhagic telangiectasia. *New Engl J Med* **333**:918, 1995
65. Savitsky K et al: A single ataxia-telangiectasia gene with a product similar to PI-3 kinase. *Science* **268**:1749, 1995
66. Vikkula M et al: Vascular dysmorphogenesis caused by an activating mutation in the receptor tyrosine kinase TIE2. *Cell* **87**:1181, 1996
67. Boon LM et al: A gene for inherited cutaneous venous anomalies ("glomangiomas") localizes to chromosome 1p21–22. *Am J Hum Genet* **65**:125, 1999
68. Eerola I et al: KRIT1 is mutated in hyperkeratotic cutaneous capillary-venous malformation associated with cerebral capillary malformation. *Hum Mol Genet* **22**:1351, 2000
69. Finegold DN et al: Truncating mutations in *FOXC2* cause multiple lymphedema syndromes. *Human Molecular Genetics* **10**:1185, 2001
70. Vikkula M et al: Molecular genetics of vascular malformations. *Matrix Biology* **20**:327, 2001
71. Zhou X et al: Germline and germline mosaic PTEN mutation associated with a Proteus-like syndrome of hemohypertrophy, lower limb asymmetry, arteriovenous malformations, and lipomatosis. *Hum Mol Genet* **9**:765, 2000

CHAPTER 104

Klemens Rappersberger
Georg Stingl
Klaus Wolff

Kaposi's Sarcoma

GENERAL CONSIDERATIONS

In 1872, the Austro-Hungarian dermatologist Moriz Kaposi described five patients with multicentric cutaneous and extracutaneous neoplasms that primarily affected older individuals. This disease, originally described as "idiopathic, multiple, pigment sarcoma" was later eponymously designated *Kaposi's sarcoma* (KS) and is now called *classic KS* (CKS). In the 1950s, endemic KS was described in certain areas of central Africa (endemic African KS) and subsequently in iatrogenically immunosuppressed patients (immunosuppression KS). This disease, however, raised little interest in the general medical community until its epidemic spread among young male homosexuals was recognized as a hallmark of the new disease AIDS (AIDS-associated KS). While these different clinical and epidemiologic variants run rather distinct clinical courses, the phenotypic features of the proliferating vascular elements are quite uniform. The discovery of the presence of a new human herpesvirus [human herpesvirus (HHV)-8, alternatively designated Kaposi's sarcoma-associated herpesvirus (KSHV)] in all KS-variants and the identification of a humoral immune response against this putative infectious agent, has shed new light onto the postulated infectious etiology of the disease. Subsequently, various molecular mechanisms were identified as to how HHV-8 initiates and sustains KS cell growth and proliferation. However, it remains to be seen whether HHV-8 is the sole etiologic agent and how genetic, social, immunologic, and endocrine factors influence the pathogenesis and course of this disease.

EPIDEMIOLOGY AND CLINICAL MANIFESTATIONS

Classic KS

The annual incidence of CKS in the United States is estimated to be 0.02 to 0.06 percent of all malignant tumors. Among those afflicted, there is a distinct preponderance of people of either Jewish or Mediterranean descent.[1] Recent epidemiologic studies in Sweden and Denmark, countries with very small nonclustered Jewish populations, indicate a twofold increase in the incidence of classic KS in the late 1960s (Sweden), and incidence rates of 0.40 and 0.22 per 1,000,000 population among men and women, respectively.[2–5] Although the clustered occurrence of CKS in the Mediterranean (Sardinia, Peloponnesos) and the preponderance of KS in several Jewish populations suggest a critical role for genetic factors, no disease-defining human leukocyte antigen (HLA) marker has yet been identified.[6] Although previously reported to have a very high male:female ratio, current studies indicate that there is a slight preponderance for males with a male:female ratio of approximately 3:1, the mean age of onset is 65 years.

CKS usually starts as single or multiple pea-sized bluish-red macules on the distal portions of the lower extremities (Fig. 104-1). In most instances, the lesions progress very slowly and may coalesce to form large plaques and, subsequently, nodules and tumors. Unilateral involvement, seen at the onset of the disease, changes to a bilateral and later to a more disseminated, multicentric pattern spreading in a centripetal fashion (Fig. 104-2). As the lesions age, they become brownish in color and may display a verrucous and hyperkeratotic surface. KS may show eczematous changes, and the lesions can erode and even ulcerate. In severe cases, there are large, partly eroded and ulcerated plaques or tumors involving the feet, hands, and even an entire extremity. Early, angiomatous lesions are soft and spongy to the touch, but older tumors are firm. An initially pitting edema of the surrounding tissue is often present, particularly on the lower extremities, where it may evolve into a fibrotic swelling of the limb that causes considerable discomfort.

CKS may develop on various mucous membranes, especially in the oral cavity and within the gastrointestinal tract.[5] Gastrointestinal lesions mostly evolve without any clinical symptoms and are often found only at autopsy. Upon thorough examination (e.g., gastroscopy, x-ray, and tests for occult blood), one may detect gastrointestinal involvement in up to 90 percent of patients. CKS usually develops very slowly and therefore runs a rather benign course (mean duration, 3 to 8 years), however, rapid courses with involvement of the lungs, spleen, heart, and gastrointestinal tract may occur.[7]

FIGURE 104-1

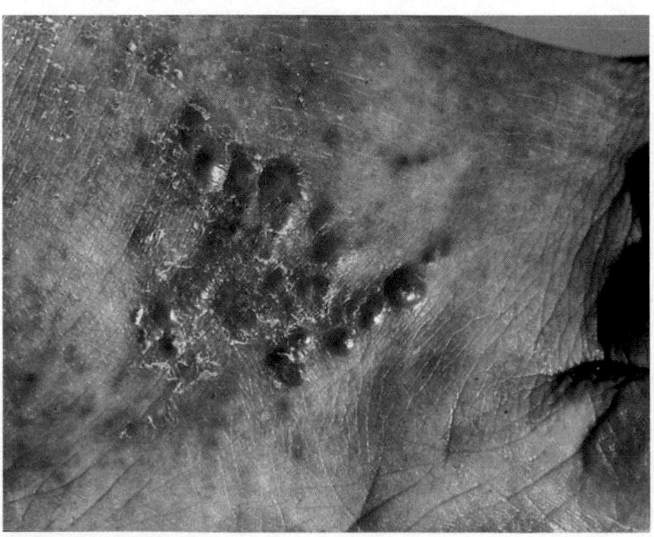

Classic variant. Multiple papules and nodules are localized on the dorsum of the foot, a site of predilection of classic KS.

FIGURE 104-2

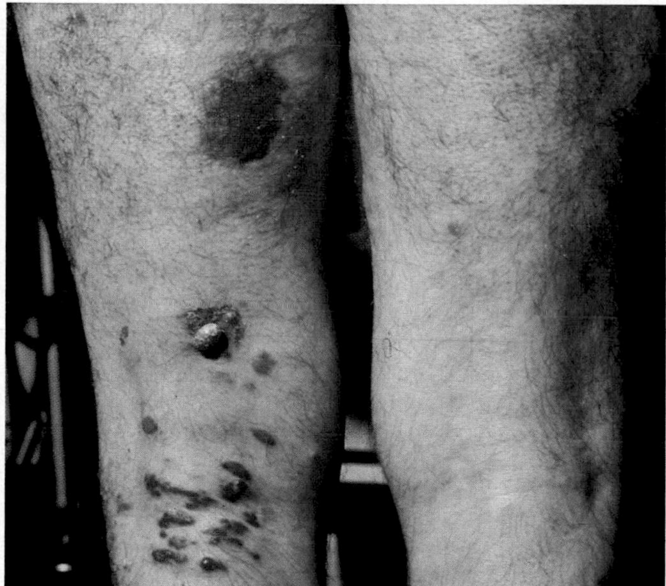

Mediterranean variant. Involvement of extremities by KS lesions at different stages of development. As is usually seen in non-AIDS cases, the disease started on both feet and evolved in a centripetal fashion.

African Endemic KS

KS is a common tumor in black Africans and accounts for up to 9 percent of all malignancies in central Africa.[8] Its endemic occurrence was first noted in the 1950s, thus antedating the outbreak of the AIDS pandemic by several decades. Epidemiologic studies indicate a clear-cut prevalence of male patients, with ratios ranging from 3 to 1 in children and up to 18 to 1 in adults. The mean age at onset is 36 years for females and 48 years for males. The disease runs a faster course with earlier generalization in females as compared to males. In children, fulminant courses with rapid dissemination to the visceral organs are seen.

According to clinicopathologic features African endemic KS (AKS) is classified into four subvariants: nodular-, florid-, infiltrative-, and lymphadenopathic-type (for review, see Ref. 8). Nodular KS runs a rather benign course, with a mean duration of 5 to 8 years, and resembles CKS. The florid/vegetating and infiltrative variants are characterized by a more aggressive biologic behavior and may extend deeply into the dermis, subcutis, muscle, and bone. Lymphadenopathic AKS predominantly affects children and young adults; skin and mucosa are affected to a lesser degree. Ninety percent of AKS patients develop asymptomatic gastrointestinal involvement that is found at autopsy only.

KS in Iatrogenically Immunocompromised Patients

With the development of immunosuppressive therapy, KS has been described with increasing frequency in organ-transplant recipients.[9] It has also been reported in individuals who had undergone chronic immunosuppressive therapy for autoimmune diseases and, sporadically, in cancer patients having received cytotoxic chemotherapy. The risk of developing KS in association with cyclosporin A immunosuppression is four times higher than with conventional immunosuppressive therapy (e.g., glucocorticoids and azathioprine) and the onset of the disease is much earlier.[9] Males are more frequently affected than females (ratios range from 3:1 to 7:1). A particularly high KS frequency has been documented in a transplantation center in Tel Aviv, where it was found in 2.5 percent of all kidney transplant recipients. This observation further strengthens the hypothesis of a genetic predisposition in KS. KS in immunocompromised patients is strikingly dependent on the dose of the immunosuppressive drug employed. Complete regression of KS lesions can be achieved by reduction/withdrawal of the immunosuppression and, vice versa, rapid tumor progression may occur after increase of the dosage.[10]

Epidemic HIV-Associated KS

In the late 1970s, clusters of KS cases were observed in the New York and San Francisco areas among young homosexual men with signs of a profound immunosuppression.[11,12] Subsequently, it became clear that KS occurred almost exclusively in homo- or bisexual men and, to a lesser degree, in female partners of the latter, and in women from certain regions of Africa and the Caribbean, who had heterosexually acquired HIV infection.[13] In contrast, in other AIDS risk groups (i.e., intravenous drug users of both sexes, hemophiliacs, blood transfusion recipients, and children born to HIV-positive mothers) the occurrence of KS is rare. Recent epidemiologic studies clearly have shown that homosexual men with KS tend to be sexually more active, frequently report histories of sexually transmitted diseases and are more likely to have partners from areas with a high frequency of AIDS-associate KS. Moreover, this population practices sexual contacts such as "rimming" (oral-anal contacts) and "fisting" (insertion of the hand into the partner's rectum). The hypothesis that AIDS-KS is caused by a sexually transmissible infectious agent that is cotransmitted with HIV was subsequently supported by a steady decline in its incidence, paralleled by a decrease in the incidence of HIV-1 seroconversion in male homosexuals. This trend has been attributed to an increased use of condoms and avoidance of a high-risk sexual behavior of the male homosexual population.[13]

In pediatric AIDS patients in the United States, KS is a rare event: among 4954 children it was found in 8 patients, much less frequently than other AIDS-defining tumors such as lymphomas that accounted for 102 cases.[14] However, in Africa, KS is the most frequent tumor among children suffering from AIDS, and even occurs more frequently than Burkitt's lymphoma. Among 318 children with AIDS, KS was diagnosed in 36 patients and Burkitt's lymphoma was diagnosed in 33 cases.[15]

Early AIDS-KS lesions appear either as small round or oval pink to reddish macules, mimicking insect bites or as dermatofibroma-like small, tense, brownish papules. In contrast to other variants of KS, the initial lesions in AIDS patients frequently develop on the face, especially on the nose, eyelids, and ears, and on the trunk, where the lesions follow the lines of cleavage (Fig. 104-3). In prolonged courses, KS lesions may be disseminated over the entire face, head, and trunk, often coalescing to form large plaques. Involvement of the deep subcutaneous tissue, skeletal muscle, or bone is usually absent. A pronounced lymphedema is observed when tumors arise on the eyelids or in acral areas.

The oral mucosa, primarily the palate, is the initial site of localization in 10 to 15 percent of all HIV-KS patients (Fig. 104-4) and severe involvement of the epipharynx and larynx are not uncommon. These localizations may cause considerable discomfort, interfere with eating and speech, may lead to respiratory distress and carry the risk of life-threatening bleeding.

Extracutaneous KS is most frequently encountered in the lymph nodes, gastrointestinal tract, and lungs. Gastrointestinal KS is found in up to 80 percent of AIDS patients, especially when extensive cutaneous lesions are present; however, patients with exclusively gastrointestinal involvement have been described.[16] Although KS can be found throughout the gastrointestinal tract, the stomach and duodenum

FIGURE 104-3

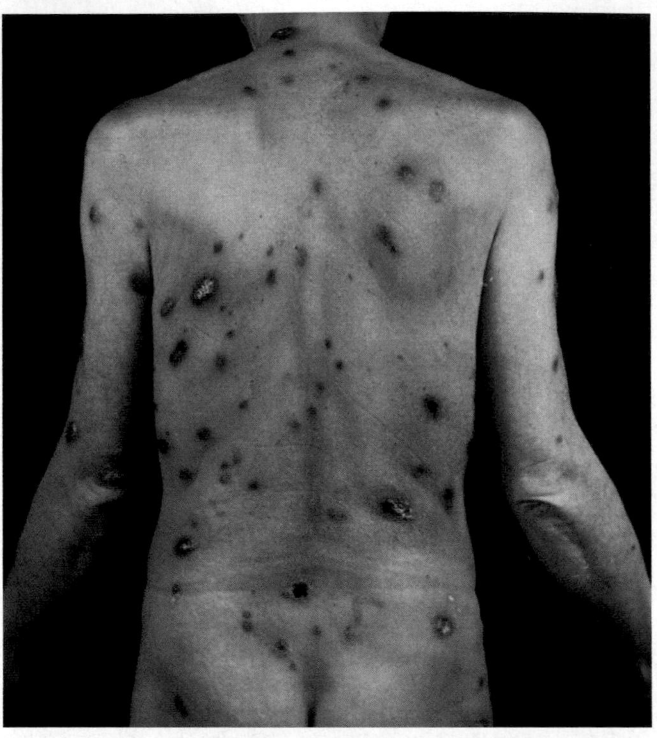

Epidemic variant. Multiple lesions at all stages of development (macules, papules, nodules) are located on the trunk. Note that the lesions follow the lines of cleavage.

FIGURE 104-4

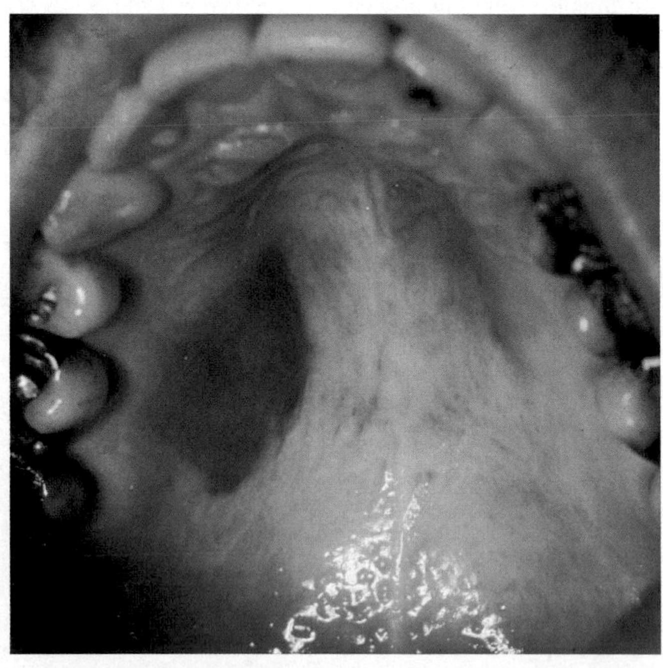

Epidemic variant. The localization of KS macules on the hard palate is a typical finding in AIDS patients.

represent predilection sites. The lesions frequently cause clinical symptoms (e.g., nausea, ulceration, bleeding, perforation, and ileus). Visible by gastroscopy, such lesions are underdiagnosed histologically because they are located in the submucosa and may escape the biopsy forceps. Pulmonary KS can cause such diverse symptoms as bronchospasm, intractable coughing, and progressive respiratory insufficiency. These symptoms are very similar to those described in *Pneumocystis carinii* pneumonia. Although chest x-ray generally reveals diffuse interstitial infiltrates in both diseases, pulmonary nodules and pleural effusions are more common in KS. Bronchoscopy with bronchoalveolar lavage is the most appropriate diagnostic tool to explore pulmonary KS. The prognosis of pulmonary KS is poor and justifies aggressive systemic chemotherapy.

PATHOLOGY

Like other skin neoplasms, KS evolves through stages of macules, papules/plaques, and nodules/tumors. Early patchlike lesions exhibit rather discrete histopathologic changes, which consist of a proliferation of oval or spindle-shaped cells within the interstitium around the superficial vascular plexus.[17] These neoplastic cells outline irregular, tiny, bizarre slits and clefts that may display features of lymphangioma. KS papules and plaques show multiple dilated and angulated vascular spaces outlined by an attenuated endothelium. These structures dissect the collagen bundles of the entire dermis, leaving a spongy network of collagen tissue. A characteristic sign of KS papules is the presence of solid cords and fascicles of spindle cells arranged between the jagged vascular channels (Fig. 104-5). This biphasic angiomatous and solid tumor morphology changes to a clear-cut sarcomatous morphology with progression of the disease. Tumorous lesions almost exclusively consist of spindle cells arranged in bundles and interlacing fascicles. Advanced lesions may display pronounced pleomorphism, nuclear atypia, and mitotic figures. At the periphery of solid tumors, (lymph) angiomatous-like portions of KS with bizarre vascular lumina and intravascular and extravasated erythrocytes, as well as siderophages, may be preserved. Erythrocytes, which appear as eosinophilic globules, are trapped within the slits and clefts formed by the spindle cells and occasionally erythrophagocytosis is observed. A moderate inflammatory infiltrate of lymphocytes, histiocytes, plasma cells, and, sporadically, neutrophils is always present in all stages of KS.

FIGURE 104-5

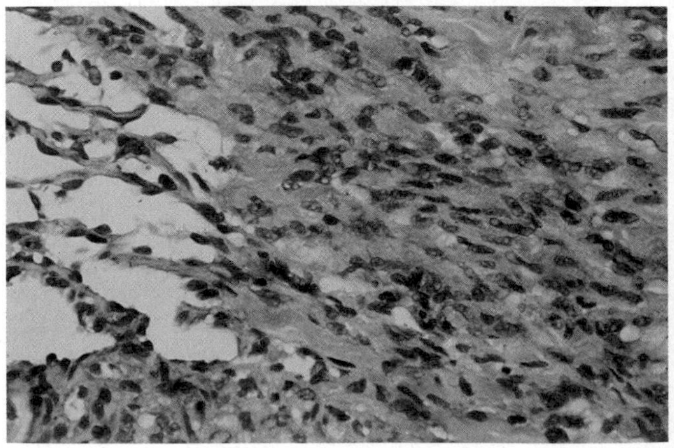

Histopathology of KS (biopsy taken from a KS papule). The neoplastic process follows a biphasic growth pattern: angiomatous portions, reminiscent of a lymphangioma, as well as solid, sarcomatous fascicles are present.

Considerable controversy still exists whether KS is a reversible proliferative disorder or a true malignant neoplasia. Assessing the methylation pattern of the human androgen receptor gene (*HUMARA*), several investigators showed that KS can be both, a clonal and polyclonal proliferation, respectively. Moreover, multiple lesions that arise in an individual patient may develop independently from distinct transformed cells and later acquire clonal characteristics.[18] Studies of HHV-8 terminal repeat sequences in KS-lesions support these findings and indicate that KS starts as a polyclonal disease with subsequent evolution to a monoclonal process.[19]

HISTOGENESIS

The histogenetic derivation of the KS cells, the cell lining the irregular vascular-like spaces of angiomatous lesions and composing the bundles and interlacing fascicles of solid tumors, has been the subject of considerable controversy: the histopathologic features of KS lesions and the immunophenotype of the proliferating cell (e.g., CD31+, CD34+, vimentin+, collagen type 4+/–, laminin+/–, vWF+/–) strongly favored the concept of an endothelial origin. However, because KS cells do not react with PAL-E, a specific marker for blood endothelial cells, but express markers for smooth muscle cells, macrophages, and dendritic cells, other authors suggest that KS cells may derive from a pluripotent mesenchymal precursor or represent a heterogeneous cell population.[20,21] Recent immunomorphologic and ultrastructural studies show that KS cells express vascular endothelial growth factor (VEGF) receptor-3 and podoplanin, proteins that are specific for lymphatic endothelial cells.[22,23] Moreover, there are significant morphologic similarities between KS cells and the endothelium of dermal lymphatic capillaries. Thus, KS cells are considered to be most closely related to or are even derived from the lymphatic endothelial cell lineage.[24] However, because cultured spindle cells, derived from peripheral blood mononuclear cells (PBMCs) of patients with or at risk for KS, displayed both, common endothelial cell antigens and macrophage markers, the mere possibility remains that the KS is derived from a circulating progenitor/endothelial stem cell/angioblast.[25,26]

ETIOLOGY

Human Herpesvirus-8/Kaposi's Sarcoma-Associated Herpesvirus

In 1994, Chang and colleagues identified DNA sequences in AIDS-KS coding for amino acids that shared a striking homology (30 to 50 percent) with two lymphotropic, oncogenic gamma-herpesviruses: Epstein-Barr virus and herpesvirus saimiri.[27] These findings were confirmed and extended by several molecular studies of all clinical variants of KS, suggesting that a new human herpesvirus, designated HHV-8, might be causally related to KS.[28,29] The subsequent observation that KSHV can be also detected in PBMCs in more than 50 percent of AIDS-KS patients, and, moreover, that the detection may precede the onset of KS lesions by months, further corroborated the hypothesis that HHV-8 represents the causative agent of KS.[30,31]

Currently, four HHV-8 subtypes—A, B, C, and D— are known, and each has a close association with the geographic and ethnic backgrounds of the infected individuals.[8] Subtype A is present in western Europe and North America, B is found almost exclusively in Africans, and subtype C in Middle East and Mediterranean Europe. Subtype D has been described in individuals from the Pacific islands. Another subtype (E) has been described in PBMC and saliva of Amerindians in Brazil in whom KS was not reported.[32] Molecular studies have localized the HHV-8-DNA to the nuclei of KS tumor cells but not to regular endothelial cells in KS lesions.[33] These findings were corroborated by immunomorphologic studies that used monoclonal antibodies against the major viral latency-associated nuclear antigen (LANA-1/LNA-1), that is expressed in virtually all HHV-8 infected cells.[34] During the development of KS lesions there is a steady increase of spindle cells positive for LANA-1: in early patchlike lesions HHV-8 is present only in approximately 10 percent of spindle cells, whereas in nodular lesions, more than 90 percent of spindle cells are positive.[34] Evidence that HHV-8 may induce productive/lytic infection was provided by Renne, who established HHV-8+ cell lines from body cavity-based lymphomas (BCBLs).[35] Stimulation of HHV-8–harboring cells with the phorbol ester 12-*O*-tetradecanoyl phorbol-13-acetate induced a dramatic inhibition of cell growth accompanied by widespread transcription of the viral genome, including the gene for the viral capsid protein that is expressed only late in the viral life cycle. Electron microscopic studies revealed the presence of lytic cells that displayed mature herpesvirus-like particles within their nuclei and cytoplasm, and also within the cell-free supernatant of the cultures. Further evidence for production and transmission of mature (infectious) viral particles came from coculture experiments using a BCBL cell line and the CD19+ cell fraction of umbilical cord blood mononuclear cells.[36] The assumption that a lymphoid cell may serve as the original site of HHV-8 replication was also supported by the observation that KS tissue harbors intact HHV-8, but in a latent, circular-episomal form, whereas the linear form of HHV-8/DNA indicative of replication occurs in PBMCs.[37] Moreover, the observation of virus replication in vivo, confined to CD34+ cells localized within the lumen of KS slits and in CD34+ circulating PBMCs, also points to a lymphoid (precursor) cell as the target for original HHV-8 infection/replication.[38,39] This is further supported by the occurrence of HHV-8 in Castleman's disease and pleural effusion lymphoma.[34] One would thus expect that KSHV may undergo a continuous infectious life cycle also in vivo, as it has already been shown in vitro by the production of DNAse-resistant filterable viruses transmitted into and released from kidney embryonic epithelial cells.[40]

Infections with human herpesviruses are ubiquitous, usually occur during infancy and childhood, and result in the persistence of the viral genome throughout life.

Several seroepidemiologic studies support the hypothesis that HHV-8 is the causative agent of KS and suggest various routes of virus transmission: HHV-8 DNA is present in all types of KS lesions and all patients with KS, independent of their HIV-status, have HHV-8 antibodies.[41] Seroconversion seems to reflect a primary infection with HHV-8, because viremia is detectable close to the point of seroconversion.[42] The persistence of HHV-8 antibodies indicates that continuous antigen presentation is taking place. This suggests that the virus remains present in a latent or lytic form of replication somewhere in the body.[42] As best exemplified in HIV-positive individuals, the time from seroconversion to overt KS may last up to 15 years (median 63.5 months), with a higher incidence of KS when HIV-infection was acquired before HHV-8 seroconversion.[43] This phenomenon may be due to inadequate immune responses to HHV-8 in HIV-infected individuals, with subsequent higher HHV-8 virus loads.[44,45] Moreover, there is now clear epidemiologic evidence of a prevalence of HHV-8 seropositivity in people who have acquired HIV more likely via sexual contacts than via clotting-factor concentrates or other blood products. These observations support previous epidemiologic data suggesting an association of KS with promiscuity and risky sexual behavior,[13] and are also true for HIV-seropositive and high-risk HIV-seronegative women, especially those who are engaged in commercial sex and have a history of sexually transmitted disease (syphilis, gonorrhea).[46] Nevertheless, the prevalence of HHV-8 seropositivity in females is much lower than in males.

A direct correlation apparently exists between human herpesvirus-8 seroprevalence and the incidence of the Mediterranean- and Jewish-variant of classic KS.[47,48] Seroprevalence for HHV-8 is also increased among family members. The most important risk factors for adult individuals to test positive for HHV-8 were place of birth and seropositivity of spouses; in children, maternal seropositivity was the discriminating factor.[48] These observations also confirm what several HHV-8 seroepidemiologic studies in Africa indicate: the familial aggregation of HHV-8 seroprevalence in the population of endemic KS areas in Africa indicates early infection in childhood and adolescence, mostly from mother to child or between siblings.[49] Thus, nonsexual routes of infection, that is, "casual/household infections," are obviously of major importance in endemic areas.

It is interesting in this context that HHV-8 DNA is frequently detectable in saliva/nasal secretions, but only rarely in genitourinary secretions (i.e., semen, prostate secretion, and cervicovaginal fluids) of KS-patients and individuals at risk for the development of KS.[50–52] Recent investigations in homosexual men identified the oral mucosa as the major site of HHV-8 shedding. Thus, one can assume that oral exposure to infectious saliva (oro-penile contact, deep kissing) is a potential risk factor for the acquisition of HHV-8 and one can easily imagine that casual, nonsexual transmission of the virus via infectious saliva also occurs in close familial contacts, among siblings, spouses and between mother and child.[53]

Because circulating CD34+ cells may serve as HHV-8 carriers, there exists a certain risk to transmit HHV-8 through blood. Several studies have shown an increased risk among needle-sharing IV drug users.[45] Vertical transmission from a mother to her newborn can occur, albeit as an exceedingly rare event.[54] However, the risk of acquiring HHV-8 by transfusion of white blood cell (WBC)-depleted blood components seems to be negligible.[55] In contrast, HHV-8 seroconversions in organ transplant recipients are frequently observed and occur more often in liver, than in renal, transplant recipients. Renal transplant recipients have a higher risk of developing KS, whereby reactivation of a preexisting HHV-8 infection seems to play a greater role than incident infection. Therefore, there is a need to perform routine screening for HHV-8 antibodies in organ transplant donors and recipients.[56,57]

PATHOGENESIS (see Fig. 104-6)

Several in vivo and in vitro studies indicate that KS results from a mutual, cytokine-driven, autocrine and paracrine stimulation of KS cells and passenger leucocytes (for review, see Refs. 8, 58, and 59). KS cells express a wide array of various proinflammatory cytokines, such as intercellular adhesion molecule (ICAM)-I, platelet-activating factor, monocyte chemotactic protein 1/2, IL-6, and IL-8, that may attract and activate leucocytes. Attracted inflammatory cells then exert growth stimulatory effects through the secretion of, for example, oncostatin-M, IL-1, tumor necrosis factor (TNF)-α, interferon (IFN)-γ, and granulocyte macrophage colony-stimulating factor. In addition, KS cells express receptors for potent endothelial cell mitogens such as platelet-derived growth factor (PDGF)-β, IL-1, and VEGF (e.g., VEGF-KDR and -flt-1). VEGF production is upregulated by PDGF and IL-1. The observation that VEGF-stimulated microvascular endothelial cells injected into mice induced KS-like angiogenic lesions, led to the speculation that these cytokines regulate angiogenesis in KS in vivo.

Because AIDS-KS displays a much more aggressive biology, several investigators have speculated that HIV-gene products could account for this phenomenon. This was first exemplified by the demonstration that male, HIV-tat transgenic mice develop KS-like angiomatous skin lesions.[60] Interestingly, tat-expression in these animals was essentially confined to the epidermis. Because epidermal Langerhans cells in humans are the major cutaneous target of HIV-1[61] it is conceivable that tat production in these cells and subsequent release into the dermis may provide the appropriate mitogenic stimulus required for cutaneous endothelial cells to progress to KS-like angiomatous tumors.[8,58,59] Alternatively, growth-stimulating mechanisms might be initiated by HIV-expressing leucocytes (monocytes/macrophages, dendritic cells) present in KS lesions in situ that produce high levels of HIV-tat and cytokines mentioned above, thereby stimulating the proliferation of a certain responder cell, most likely the KS-precursor, that then becomes autonomous. These inflammatory cytokines induce normal endothelial cells to acquire characteristics as KS cells, stimulate the constitutive synthesis and release of bioactive β-fibroblast growth factor (FGF), and enhance their ability to form angiogenic KS-like lesions in athymic nude mice. Moreover, after exposure to cytokine-rich supernatants of T cell cultures from AIDS patients, normal endothelial cells express the receptors for tat, $\alpha_v\beta_1$- and $\alpha_v\beta_3$-integrins and become responsive to the mitogenic effects of tat protein. Subsequently, they start proliferation and migration and even

FIGURE 104-6

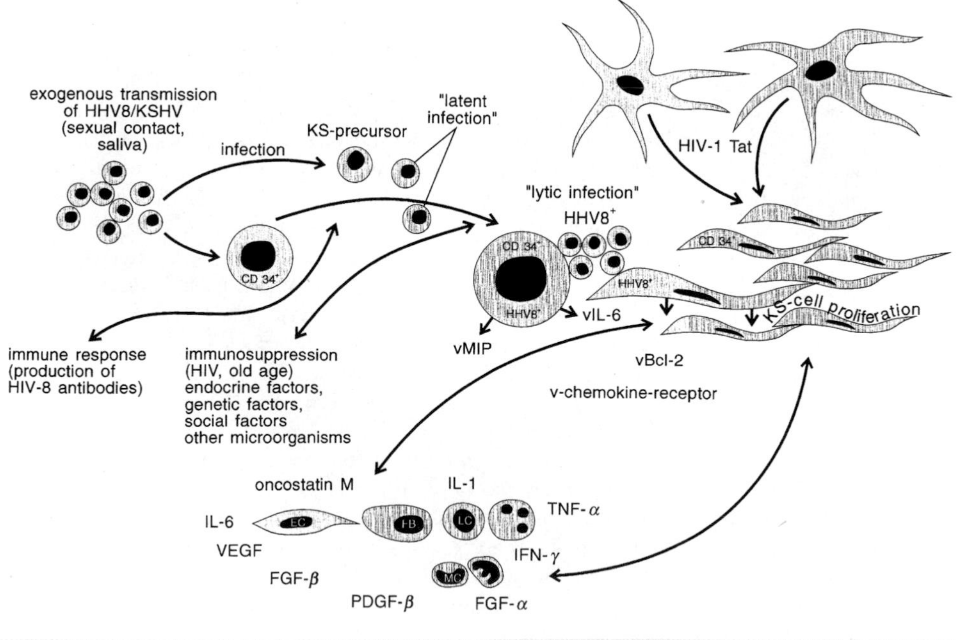

The etiopathogenesis of KS: a hypothesis. EC, endothelial cell; FB, fibroblast; LC, lymphocyte; MC, monocyte.

degrade basement membrane collagen type IV, indicative of the acquisition of an invasive potential.

Together, these studies indicate that chronic immune stimulation via the release of inflammatory cytokines may contribute to the pathogenesis of KS, an effect that is dramatically increased by tat protein in AIDS-KS.

What is the connection, if any, between these events and HHV-8 infection? There is now clear evidence that HHV-8 encodes for various genes that may directly contribute to the pathogenesis of KS.[58,59] Several factors have been identified that promote KS-cell growth, for example, vIL-6, viral interferon regulatory factor (vIRF) and v-cyclin; others inhibit KS cell apoptosis, such as vFLIP, LANA, vBcl-2, K15/LAMP, and vIRF. Additional factors, such as K1, vGPCR, Kaposin, and vIRF, may guarantee a limitless replicative potential of KS cells. Moreover, HHV-8 possibly encodes for paracrine factors that promote leucocytes attraction, for example, vIL-6, MIP-1, -2, and -3. The genes for some of these factors can be upregulated by the addition of phorbol esters, indicating their expression during virus replication in the lytic phase.[62]

In summary, current data suggest that HHV-8, exogenously acquired (e.g., from saliva, sexual contact, organ transplant), initially most likely infects a B lymphoid precursor, or, alternatively, the KS precursor cell, integrates and subsequently enters a latent phase of infection. Upon activation of the virus through immunosuppression (AIDS, iatrogenic) or various other endocrine, metabolic, microbiologic, and social stimuli (sexual practices), as well as a genetic predisposition (Jews and Mediterranean People), HHV-8 genes are activated and transcribed. Robust activation allows HHV-8 to enter a productive/lytic life cycle. Full transcriptive activity is achieved and cytokine homologues, proteins that stimulate inflammation and cell proliferation or inhibit apoptosis, are produced. Concomitantly, inflammatory cells attracted by HHV-8 gene products provide additional proliferative stimuli to maintain and support the proliferation of KS-cells, which then increases the release of appropriate tumor-promoting mediators. Most likely, these circumstances also result in the replication and release of mature, infectious HHV-8, which subsequently may infect other host cells. However, if this mutual stimulation is perturbed, for example, by reconstitution of immune competence [highly active antiretroviral therapy (HAART)], the cascade of pathobiologic events would be adversely influenced resulting in delayed tumor growth or even tumor regression (see Fig. 104-6).

TREATMENT

The choice of treatment of KS depends on the extent and the localization of lesions as well as on the clinical type of the disease. Solitary lesions of all KS variants may be excised or subjected to laser irradiation. Superficial and flat lesions can be successfully treated with liquid nitrogen and photodynamic therapy.[63,64]

Ionizing Radiation

Radiation therapy plays a major role in the management of solitary and disseminated mucocutaneous KS.[65] Types of radiation, dosage and application-form depend on the extent and size of lesions. Flat lesions are usually irradiated with superficial x-ray; high-energy beams, including cobalt therapy, are commonly used in the treatment of large tumors. Other possibilities are (un)fractionated half-body irradiation with electron beams and/or photon beams. High-dose microelectron brachytherapy has fewer adverse effects than external beam radiotherapy.[66]

(Poly)chemotherapy

Patients with rapidly progressive disease require (poly)chemotherapy with cytotoxic drugs. Good efficacy has been reported for liposomal-doxorubicin, and liposomal-daunorubicin.[67] Paclitaxel has been used as a single agent with moderate success, and the vinca alkaloids are currently preferred in combination with adriamycin and bleomycine.[68]

Interferon and Antiretroviral Drugs

INF-α has been widely used in the treatment of KS and it has yielded quite contradictory results. However, there seem to be some beneficial effects, especially when the immunosurveillance is, at least partially, intact.[69] It is now well established that the treatment of HIV-infected individuals with antiretroviral agents may prolong survival and improve the quality of life. Most important was the introduction of HAART into the management of HIV infection, which has dramatically decreased the incidence of AIDS-KS. These observations have been explained by supportive effects of HAART on the immune system. However, recent investigations clearly demonstrate direct antiangiogenic properties of HIV protease inhibitors in vitro and in vivo.[70–72]

Experimental Therapy

The establishment of long-term KS spindle cell cultures and of KS mouse models has enabled us to test new therapeutic concepts. Some of these concepts were assessed for safety, tolerability, and efficacy in experimental trials in KS patients. Such studies were performed with substances that interact with neoangiogenesis, matrix metalloproteinase inhibitors, as well as topical retinoic acid and "immunomodulators." Treatment with the β chain of human chorionic gonadotropin did not keep its early promise.[73] Large clinical trials are needed to ultimately determine the efficacy and, thus, the future applicability of these experimental treatment modalities.

REFERENCES

1. Safai B: Kaposi's sarcoma: An overview of classical and epidemic forms, in *AIDS, Modern Concepts and Therapeutic Challenges,* edited by S Broder. New York, Marcel Dekker, 1987, p 205
2. Fenig E et al: Classic Kaposi's sarcoma: Experience at Rabin Medical Center in Israel. *Am J Clin Oncol* **21**:498, 1998
3. Bendsöe N: Increased incidence of Kaposi's sarcoma in Sweden before the AIDS epidemic. *Eur J Cancer* **26**:699, 1990
4. Hjalgrim H et al: Epidemiology of classic Kaposi's sarcoma in Denmark between 1970 and 1992. *Cancer* **77**:1373, 1996
5. Rappersberger K et al: Endemic Kaposi's sarcoma in human immunodeficiency virus type 1-seronegative persons: Demonstration of retrovirus-like particles in cutaneous lesions. *J Invest Dermatol* **95**:371, 1990
6. Brunson M et al: HLA and Kaposi's sarcoma in solid organ transplantation. *Hum Immunol* **29**:56, 1990
7. Iscovich J et al: Classic Kaposi's sarcoma: Epidemiology and risk factors. *Cancer* **88**:500, 2000
8. Boshoff C, Weiss RA: Epidemiology and pathogenesis of Kaposi's sarcoma-associated herpesvirus. *Phil Trans R Soc Lond B* **356**:517, 2001
9. Penn I: The changing pattern of posttransplant malignancies. *Transplant Proc* **23**:1101, 1991
10. Wijnveen AC et al: Disseminated Kaposi's sarcoma—Full regression after withdrawal of immunosuppressive therapy: Report of a case. *Transplant Proc* **19**:3735, 1987
11. Centers for Disease Control: Kaposi's sarcoma and *Pneumocystis carinii* pneumonia among homosexual men—New York City and California. *MMWR Morb Mortal Wkly Rep* **25**:305, 1981
12. Centers for Disease Control: Special report: Epidemiologic aspects of the current outbreak of Kaposi's sarcoma and opportunistic infections. *N Engl J Med* **306**:258, 1982
13. Beral V et al: Is risk of Kaposi's sarcoma in AIDS patients in Britain increased if sexual partners come from the United States or Africa? *BMJ* **324**:624, 1991
14. Biggar RJ et al: Risk of cancer in children with AIDS. AIDS-cancer Match registry study group. *JAMA* **284**:205, 2000

15. Newton R et al: A case-control study of human immunodeficiency virus infection and cancer in adults and children residing in Kampala, Uganda. *Int J Cancer* **92**:622, 2001
16. Ioachim HL et al: Kaposi's sarcoma of internal organs: A multiparameter study of 86 cases. *Cancer* **75**:1376, 1995
17. Ackerman AB: Subtle clues to diagnosis by conventional microscopy: The patch stage of Kaposi's sarcoma. *Am J Dermatopathol* **1**:165, 1979
18. Gil PS et al: Evidence for multiclonality in multicentric Kaposi's sarcoma. *Proc Natl Acad Sci USA* **95**:8257, 1998
19. Judde JG et al: Monoclonality or oligoclonality of human herpesvirus 8 terminal repeat sequences in Kaposi's sarcoma and other diseases. *J Natl Cancer Inst* **92**:729, 2000
20. Regezi JA et al: Human immunodeficiency virus-associated oral Kaposi's sarcoma: A heterogeneous cell population dominated by spindle-shaped endothelial cells. *Am J Pathol* **143**:240, 1993
21. Uccini S et al: Kaposi's sarcoma cells express the macrophage-associated antigen mannose receptor and develop in peripheral blood cultures of Kaposi's sarcoma patients. *Am J Pathol* **150**:929, 1997
22. Weninger W et al: Expression of vascular endothelial growth factor receptor-3 and podoplanin suggests a lymphatic endothelial cell origin of Kaposi's sarcoma tumor cells. *Lab Invest* **79**:243, 1999
23. Kriehuber E et al: Isolation and characterization of dermal lymphatic and blood endothelial cells reveal stable and functionally specialized cell lineages. *J Exp Med* **194**:797, 2001
24. Sauter B et al: Immunoelectronmicroscopic characterization of human dermal lymphatic microvascular endothelial cells. Differential expression of CD31, CD34 and type IV-collagen with lymphatic endothelial cells versus blood capillary endothelial cells in normal human skin, lymphangioma and hemangioma, in situ. *J Histochem Cytochem* **46**:165, 1998
25. Browning PF et al: Identification and culture of Kaposi's sarcoma-like spindle cells from the peripheral blood of human immunodeficiency virus-1–infected individuals and normal controls. *Blood* **84**:2711, 1994
26. Sirianni MC et al: Circulating spindle cells: Correlation with human herpesvirus-8 (HHV-8) infection and Kaposi's sarcoma. *Lancet* **349**:255, 1997
27. Chang Y et al: Identification of herpesvirus-like DNA sequences in AIDS-associated Kaposi's sarcoma. *Science* **266**:1865, 1994
28. Moore PS, Chang Y: Detection of herpesvirus-like DNA sequences in Kaposi's sarcoma in patients with and those without HIV infection. *N Engl J Med* **332**:1181, 1995
29. Huang YQ, Li JJ, Kaplan MH et al: Human herpesvirus-like nucleic acid in various forms of Kaposi's sarcoma. *Lancet* **345**:759, 1995
30. Whitby D et al: Detection of KS associated herpesvirus in peripheral blood of HIV-infected individuals and progression to Kaposi's sarcoma. *Lancet* **346**:799, 1995
31. Parry JP, Moore PS: Corrected prevalence of Kaposi's sarcoma (KS)-associated herpesvirus infection prior to onset of KS. *AIDS* **11**:127, 1997
32. Biggar R et al: Human herpesvirus 8 in Brazilian Amerindians: A hyper-endemic population with a new subtype. *J Infect Dis* **181**:1562, 2000
33. Boshoff C et al: Kaposi's sarcoma associated herpesvirus infects endothelial cells and spindle cells. *Nat Med* **1**:1274, 1995
34. Dupin N et al: Distribution of human herpesvirus-8 latently infected cells in Kaposi's sarcoma, multicentric Castleman's disease and primary effusion lymphoma. *Proc Natl Acad Sci USA* **96**:4546, 1999
35. Renne R et al: Lytic growth of Kaposi's sarcoma-associated herpesvirus (human herpesvirus 8) in culture. *Nat Med* **2**:342, 1996
36. Mesri EA et al: Human herpesvirus-8/Kaposi's sarcoma associated herpesvirus is a new transmissible virus that infects B cells. *J Exp Med* **183**:2385, 1996
37. Decker LL et al: The Kaposi's sarcoma associated herpesvirus (KSHV) is present as an intact latent genome in KS tissue but replicates in the peripheral blood mononuclear cells of KS patients. *J Exp Med* **184**:283, 1995
38. Orenstein JM et al: Visualization of human herpesvirus type 8 in Kaposi's sarcoma by light and transmission electron microscopy. *AIDS* **11**:F35, 1997
39. Henry M et al.: Infection of circulating CD34+ cells by HHV-8 in patients with Kaposi's sarcoma. *J Invest Dermatol* **113**:613, 1999
40. Foreman KE et al: Propagation of a human herpesvirus from AIDS associated Kaposi's sarcoma. *N Engl J Med* **336**:163, 1997
41. Katano H et al: Identification of antigenic proteins encoded by human herpesvirus 8 and seroprevalence in the general population and among patients with and without Kaposi's sarcoma. *J Virol* **74**:3478, 2000
42. Goudsmit J et al: Human herpesvirus 8 infections in the Amsterdam Cohort Studies (1984–1997): Analysis of seroconversion to ORF65 and ORF73. *Proc Natl Acad Sci USA* **97**:4383, 2000
43. O'Brien TR et al: Evidence for concurrent epidemics of human herpesvirus 8 and human immunodeficiency virus type 1 in US homosexual men: rates, risk factors, and relationship to Kaposi's sarcoma. *J Infect Dis* **180**:1010, 1999
44. Renwick N et al.: Seroconversion for human herpesvirus 8 during HIV infection is highly predictive of Kaposi's sarcoma. *AIDS* **12**:2481, 1998
45. Cannon MJ et al: Blood-borne and sexual transmission of human herpesvirus 8 in women with a risk for human immunodeficiency virus infection. *N Engl J Med* **344**:637, 2001
46. Greenblatt RM et al.: Human herpesvirus 8 infection and Kaposi's sarcoma among human immunodeficiency virus-infected and uninfected women. *J Infect Dis* **183**:1130, 2001
47. Santarelli R et al: Direct correlation between human herpesvirus-8 seroprevalence and classic Kaposi's sarcoma incidence in northern Sardinia. *J Med Virol* **65**:368, 2001
48. Davidovici B et al: Seroepidemiology and molecular epidemiology of Kaposi's sarcoma associated herpesvirus among Jewish population groups in Israel. *J Natl Cancer Inst* **93**:194, 2001
49. Plancoulaine Sabel L et al: Human herpesvirus-8 transmission from mother to child and between siblings in an endemic population. *Lancet* **356**:1062, 2000
50. Gessain A et al: Human herpesvirus 8 primary infection occurs during childhood in Cameroon, Central Africa. *Int J Cancer* **81**:189, 1999
51. Koelle DM et al: Frequent detection of Kaposi's sarcoma-associated herpesvirus in saliva of human immunodeficiency virus-infected men: Clinical and immunological correlates. *J Infect Dis* **176**:94, 1997
52. Calabro ML et al: Detection of human herpesvirus 8 in cervicovaginal secretions and seroprevalence in human immunodeficiency virus type 1-seropositive and seronegative women. *J Infect Dis* **179**:1534, 1999
53. Pauk K et al: Mucosal shedding of human herpesvirus 8 in men. *N Engl J Med* **343**:1369, 2000
54. Mantina H et al: Vertical transmission of Kaposi's sarcoma associated herpesvirus. *Int J Cancer* **94**:749, 2001
55. Challine D et al: Seroprevalence of human herpes virus 8 antibody in populations at high or low risk of transfusion, graft, or sexual transmission of virus. *Transfusion* **41**:1120, 2001
56. Milliancourt C et al: Human herpesvirus-8 seroconversion after renal transplantation. *Transplantation* **72**:1319, 2001
57. Andreoni M et al.: Prevalence, Incidence and correlates of HHV-8/KSHV infection and Kaposi's sarcoma in renal and liver transplant recipients. *J Infect* 43:195, 2001
58. Stürzl, M et al: Human herpesvirus-8 and Kaposi's sarcoma: Relationship with the multistep concept of tumorigenesis. *Adv Cancer Res* **81**:125, 2001
59. Moore PS, Chang Y: Molecular virology of Kaposi's sarcoma-associated herpesvirus. *Philos Trans R Soc Lond B Biol Sci* **356**:499, 2001
60. Vogel J et al: The HIV tat gene induces dermal lesions resembling Kaposi's sarcoma in transgenic mice. *Nature* **335**:606, 1988
61. Rappersberger K et al: Langerhans cells are an actual site of HIV-1 replication. *Intervirology* **29**:185, 1988
62. Montaner S et al: The Kaposi's sarcoma-associated herpesvirus G protein coupled receptor promotes endothelial cell survival through the activation of Akt/protein kinase B. *Cancer Res* **61**:2641, 2001
63. Lenz P et al: Treatment of HIV-Kaposi's sarcoma. *Derm Therapy* **12**:77, 1999
64. Mitsuyasu RT: Update no the pathogenesis and treatment of Kaposi sarcoma. *Curr Opin Oncol* **12**:174, 2000
65. Kirova YM et al: Radiotherapy in the management of epidemic Kaposi's sarcoma: A retrospective study of 643 cases. *Radiother Oncol* **46**:19, 1998
66. Syndikus I et al: High dose rate microselectron radiation for Kaposi's sarcoma of the palate. *Radiother Oncol* **42**:167, 1997
67. Nunez M et al: Response to liposomal doxorubicin and clinical outcome of HIV-1–infected patients with Kaposi's sarcoma receiving highly active antiretroviral therapy. *HIV Clin Trials* **2**:429, 2001
68. von Roenn J et al: Management of AIDS associated Kaposi's sarcoma: A multidisciplinary perspective. *Oncology* **12**(suppl 3):1, 1998
69. Krown SE: Interferon-alpha: Evolving therapy for AIDS-associated Kaposi's sarcoma. *J Interferon Cytokine Res* **18**:1112, 1998
70. Holkova B et al: Effect of highly active antiretroviral therapy on survival in patients with AIDS-associated pulmonary Kaposi's sarcoma treated with chemotherapy. *J Clin Oncol* **19**:3848, 2001
71. Jones JL et al: Incidence and trends in Kaposi's sarcoma in the era of effective antiretroviral therapy. *J Acquir Immune Defic Syndr* **24**:270, 2000
72. Sgadari C et al: HIV protease inhibitors are potent anti-angiogenic molecules and promote regression of Kaposi sarcoma. *Nat Med* **8**:225, 2002
73. Gill PS et al: The effects of preparations of human chorionic gonadotropin on AIDS-related Kaposi's sarcoma. *N Engl J Med* **335**:1261, 1996

CHAPTER 105

Walter H.C. Burgdorf

Anetoderma and Other Atrophic Disorders of the Skin

Anetoderma is a localized laxity of the skin with herniation or outpouching resulting from abnormal dermal elastic tissue. Because atrophy is not an essential component of this process, the term *anetoderma* (Greek *anetos,* relaxed; *derma,* skin) more accurately describes the phenomenon than does the alternative name, macular atrophy.

HISTORICAL ASPECTS

Far too many proper names have been associated with anetoderma. The idiopathic version without preceding lesions is named after Schweninger and Buzzi, while the postinflammatory form is attributed to Jadassohn, Pellizari, and others.

ETIOLOGY AND PATHOGENESIS

The key defect is damage to the dermal elastic fibers. However, the exact mechanisms of damage remain a mystery. Both cell-mediated and humoral damage have been postulated, but specific antielastin reactivity has not been shown. The occurrence of anetoderma with acrodermatitis chronica atrophicans, a proven borreliosis (see Chap. 203), suggests that anetoderma may have an infectious cause in some cases. Anetoderma may occur as an early finding in HIV infections, sometimes without clinically apparent inflammation[1] but more often secondary to well-characterized eruptions.[2] In addition, a variety of autoimmune phenomena have been reported in patients with anetoderma; most common appears to be the presence of antiphospholipid antibodies,[3] sometimes associated with systemic lupus erythematosus[4] or HIV infection. Rare familial cases have been described.

The mechanism of elastin destruction remains unclear, but there are multiple ways in which the structures can be altered. Electron microscopy may show fragmented and irregular elastic fibers, occasionally engulfed by macrophages.[5] Many different inflammatory and enzymatic pathways have been studied, but no unifying concept has emerged. When anetoderma is secondary to an obvious dermatosis or tumor, the whole spectrum of inflammatory processes as well as simple pressure combine to produce diminished elastic fibers. In adults, the capacity for repair of elastin is limited. Attempts to unequivocally separate anetoderma from other forms of scarring are futile, as ordinary scars from any cause may also be atrophic and lack elastin.

CLINICAL MANIFESTATIONS

All forms of anetoderma are characterized by a circumscribed loss of normal skin elasticity. As a result, a soft bladder-like pouch is created. The examining finger can press this pouch into the dermis and sometimes seems to fall through into the subcutaneous layer without meeting resistance. The sensation is similar to palpating an inguinal hernia. When the finger is removed, the skin pushes outward again. The epidermis is wrinkled, thinned, and often depigmented with telangiectases apparent. Despite the thinness, ulceration is uncommon (Figs. 105-1 and 105-2).

Attempts to distinguish between Schweninger-Buzzi and Jadassohn-Pellizari types of anetoderma are artificial. Clearly all anetoderma must have a precursor phase with inflammation and elastic fiber damage; whether one can recognize this feature or not is an individual variable, not a disease-defining feature. Patients often have several types of lesions simultaneously, some inflammatory, some noninflammatory, some spontaneous, and some secondary to minor trauma.[6] The best established causes of primary anetoderma are the antiphospholipid syndrome and HIV/AIDS.

Many dermatoses produce a true secondary anetoderma in which the pouched lesions develop at the sites of inflammation; the most common causes today are probably acne and varicella. Anetoderma following secondary syphilis was formerly common. Persistent irritation and inflammation, such as with prurigo nodularis, may also evolve into anetoderma.[7] Anetoderma can also appear with acrodermatitis chronica atrophicans, especially at the periphery of such lesions. In some forms of granulomatous inflammation, dermal elastolysis and anetoderma may be seen. Anetoderma may also follow the resolution of cutaneous tumors such as juvenile xanthogranulomas,[8] pilomatricomas,[9] or lymphomas.[10,11] Finally, in Sicily, leech application appears to be a common cause; here there is no mystery as to the origin of the trauma.[12]

FIGURE 105-1

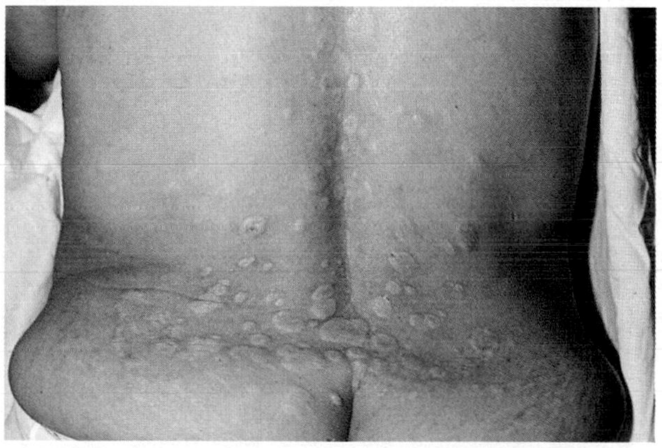

Anetoderma. Patulous herniations are seen on the lower back.

FIGURE 105-2

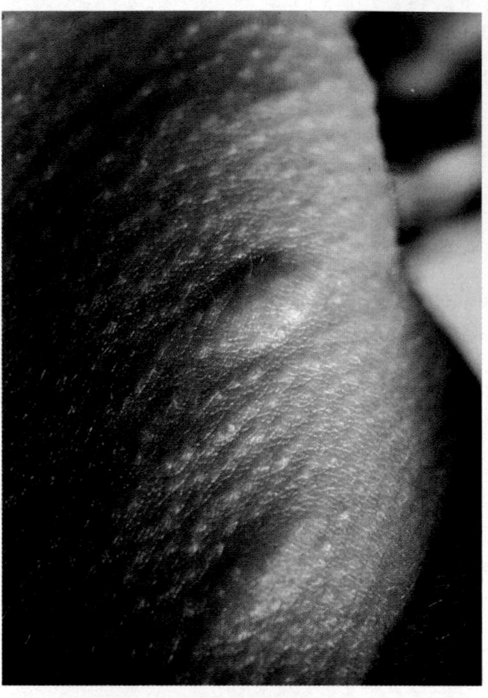

Anetoderma. A closer view.

Children may be affected with anetoderma; they are similar in every way to adult cases.[13] In contrast, in premature infants a distinct type of anetoderma may be seen, clearly suspected to be caused by electrocardiographic electrodes or adhesives.[14,15]

PATHOLOGY

The predominant defect resides in the elastic fibers, which are fragmented, shortened, and, in some lesions, have almost completely disappeared (Fig. 105-3). In a study of 45 biopsies from 17 patients with anetoderma, the elastin was generally absent, but the fine microfibrils were still present.[16] Presumably the weakening of the elastic network leads to flaccidity and herniation. The collagen fibers appear normal. Mononuclear inflammatory cells have been found in all types of anetoderma, regardless of whether the lesions were thought to be clinically inflamed.

RELATED DISORDERS

A number of other defects of elastin that have been described are similar to anetoderma. For example, endocrine disorders may produce changes in dermal connective tissue resulting in localized loss of elasticity. Perhaps related to anetoderma are the common striae of pregnancy, puberty, Cushing disease, and long-term glucocorticoid therapy. Transverse striae of the back[17] also have many similarities.

The ophthalmologic literature contains a number of reports of eyelid laxity following chronic and recurrent lid dermatitis, as well as that

FIGURE 105-3

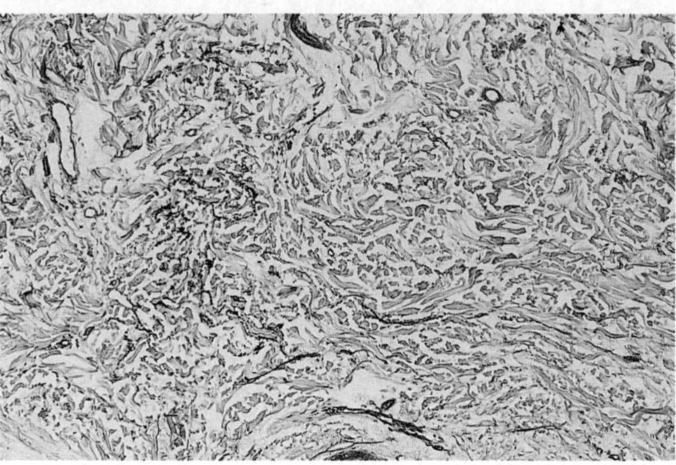

Anetoderma. The section of skin is stained with an elastin stain and viewed at high power. There are far more elastin fibers visible as black strands on the left, or normal, side than on the right, or anetodermic, side.

developing spontaneously. Idiopathic lid laxity can exist alone or associated with redundancy of the upper lip (Ascher's syndrome) or with cutis laxa. Lid laxity is also part of the aging process.

Penicillamine is the only drug that produces anetoderma. It is plausible that penicillamine produces this process by interfering with lysyl oxidase, a copper-dependent enzyme essential to normal manufacture of elastin fibers. There is no other evidence of abnormal copper metabolism in patients with the disease.

Diffuse damage to elastic tissue, whether congenital or acquired, is designated cutis laxa (see Chap. 154), but overlaps between anetoderma and cutis laxa exist. Postinflammatory elastosis and cutis laxa has been described primarily in African children who experience apparent insect bites that heal with atrophic scars resembling anetoderma. At the same time, the children develop more diffuse atrophy without a clear preceding event. A similar case has been reported in a North American child.[18]

While changes in elastin are a well-known part of both aging and actinic damage, occasionally such changes occur in localized areas in relatively young patients. Some young women develop focal loss of mid-dermal elastin, leading to wrinkling and protrusion of tiny papules of nonfollicular skin known as mid-dermal elastolysis.[19] The same process is also associated with systemic lupus erythematosus.[20] A similar clinical and histologic appearance has been described in a patient with pancreatic carcinoma. Presumably, elastases from the tumor caused the dermal damage.[21]

Sometimes the elastin changes are localized about hair follicles, producing perifollicular elastolysis. A similar process may produce the common papular acne scars, which also lack elastin.[22] Elastolysis in aging skin may produce both pseudoxanthoma elasticum–like changes and white fibrous papules of the neck, which seem to combine fibrosis and elastolysis.[23]

DIAGNOSIS AND DIFFERENTIAL DIAGNOSIS

Lesions of anetoderma must be distinguished from other forms of localized loss of substance or circumscribed protrusion of the skin. Atrophic conditions include scars, discoid lupus erythematosus, lichen sclerosus et atrophicus, and more esoteric cutaneous atrophies. The following conditions are included in this list:

1. Atrophoderma of Pasini and Pierini is a major source of confusion both etymologically and clinically. Patients have larger lesions with a sharp peripheral border dropping into a depression with no outpouching. It may be a nonsclerotic variant of morphea, more common in adolescent females. On biopsy, elastin is normal, while collagen may be thickened, but this finding is difficult to quantify. Patients have been identified who clinically best fit atrophoderma but have clear-cut elastolysis; the term *atrophoderma elastolytica discreta* has been proposed for this variant.[24]
2. Patients with atrophia maculosa varioliformis cutis are typically young with subtle, slightly depressed lesions on the temples and cheeks.[25] While the clinical impression is that of pits and scars, perhaps following varicella, no supporting history is obtained. Familial cases have been described. Histologic studies are limited, but in some cases elastic fibers have been damaged.
3. Glucocorticoid-induced atrophy occurs typically over the triceps or buttocks. The lesions resemble atrophoderma, but patients have a history of injection of glucocorticoids. Polarization may show the steroid crystals in the dermis; at other times only dermal atrophy and inflammation are seen.[26] One should be most reluctant to diagnose idiopathic atrophoderma at sites where injections are usually given.
4. Perifollicular atrophoderma is most prominent on the backs of the hands and is often associated with multiple basal cell carcinomas and hair abnormalities in the Bazex syndrome. It is also a feature of the Conradi-Hünermann syndrome, better designated as X-linked dominant ichthyosis or X-linked dominant chondrodysplasia punctata. Perifollicular atrophy has also been described in extreme forms of keratosis pilaris, in which large keratin plugs may produce a dilated patulous follicle. This condition, usually found on the cheeks of young children, has been given a variety of long names. Both of these lesions mimic perifollicular anetoderma but lack elastin changes.

Other protuberant lesions are neurofibromas, connective tissue nevi, lipomatous nevus of Hoffman and Zurhelle, and the adipose herniations in focal dermal hypoplasia. In the last condition, thinning or absence of the dermis, rather than changes in elastin fibers, accounts for the proximity of the subcutis to the epidermis.

TREATMENT

Cosmetically objectionable areas of anetoderma may be excised. No other therapy is of value. Appropriate treatment of inflammatory conditions might forestall later development of atrophy.

REFERENCES

1. Ruiz-Rodriguez R et al: Anetoderma and human immunodeficiency virus infection. *Arch Dermatol* **128**:661, 1992
2. Lindstrom J et al: Increased anticardiolipin antibodies associated with the development of anetoderma in HIV-1 disease. *Int J Dermatol* **34**:408, 1995
3. Stephansson EA, Niemi KM: Antiphospholipid antibodies and anetoderma: Are they associated? *Dermatology* **191**:204, 1995
4. Montilla C, Alarcon-Segovia D: Anetoderma in systemic lupus erythematosus: Relationship to antiphospholipid antibodies. *Lupus* **9**:545, 2000
5. Zaki I et al: Primary anetoderma: Phagocytosis of elastic fibres by macrophages. *Clin Exp Dermatol* **19**:388, 1994
6. Venencie PY et al: Anetoderma: Clinical findings, associations, and long-term follow-up. *Arch Dermatol* **120**:1032, 1984
7. Hirschel-Scholz S et al: Anetodermic prurigo nodularis (with Pautrier's neuroma) responsive to arotinoid acid. *J Am Acad Dermatol* **25**:437, 1991
8. Ang P, Tay TK: Anetoderma in a patient with juvenile xanthogranuloma. *Br J Dermatol* **140**:541, 1999
9. Shames BS et al: Secondary anetoderma involving a pilomatricoma. *Am J Dermatopathol* **16**:557, 1994
10. Child FJ et al: Multiple cutaneous immunocytoma with secondary anetoderma: A report of two cases. *Br J Dermatol* **143**:165, 2000
11. Kasper RC et al: Anetoderma arising in cutaneous B-cell lymphoproliferative disease. *Am J Dermatopathol* **23**:124, 2001
12. Siragusa M et al: Anetoderma secondary to the application of leeches. *Int J Dermatol* **35**:227, 1996
13. Karrer S et al: Primary anetoderma in children: Report of two cases and literature review. *Pediatr Dermatol* **13**:382, 1996
14. Prizant TL et al: Spontaneous atrophic patches in extremely premature infants. Anetoderma of prematurity. *Arch Dermatol* **132**:671, 1996
15. Colditz PB et al: Anetoderma of prematurity in association with electrocardiographic electrodes. *J Am Acad Dermatol* **41**:479, 1999
16. Venencie PY, Winkelmann RK: Histopathologic findings in anetoderma. *Arch Dermatol* **120**:1040, 1984
17. Burket JM et al: Linear focal elastosis (elastotic striae). *J Am Acad Dermatol* **20**:633, 1989
18. Lewis PG et al: Postinflammatory elastolysis and cutis laxa. A case report. *J Am Acad Dermatol* **22**:40, 1990
19. Kim JM, Su WP: Mid-dermal elastolysis with wrinkling. Report of two cases and review of the literature. *J Am Acad Dermatol* **26**:169, 1992
20. Boyd AS, King LE Jr: Mid-dermal elastolysis in two patients with lupus erythematosus. *Am J Dermatopathol* **23**:136, 2001
21. Slater DN, Messenger A: Eruptive elastolysis: A new manifestation of pancreatic carcinoma. *J R Soc Med* **79**:237, 1986
22. Wilson BB et al: Papular acne scars. *Arch Dermatol* **126**:797, 1990
23. Rongioletti F, Rebora A: Fibroelastolytic patterns of intrinsic skin aging: Pseudoxanthoma elasticum-like papillary dermal elastolysis and white fibrous papulosis of the neck. *Dermatology* **191**:19, 1995
24. Carrington PR et al: Atrophoderma elastolytica discreta. *Am J Dermatopathol* **18**:212, 1996
25. Dall'Oglio F et al. Familial atrophia maculosa varioliformis cutis: An ultrastructural study. *Pediatr Dermatol* **18**:230, 2001
26. Schetman D et al: Cutaneous changes following local injection of triamcinolone. *Arch Dermatol* **88**:820, 1963

CHAPTER 106

Walter H.C. Burgdorf

Ainhum and Pseudoainhum

AINHUM

The name *ainhum* is derived from a word in the Nagos language of East Africa meaning "to saw." It aptly describes the development of constricting bands about digits that then undergo autoamputation. In the United States, more attention has been focused on the other constricting bands that may mimic ainhum and have been designated *pseudoainhum*.

Epidemiology

Ainhum is traditionally a disease of middle-aged African males accustomed to going barefoot,[1] although it occurs throughout the world in both sexes and all races. In one series it was present in 2 percent of all patients admitted to University Hospital in Ibadan, Nigeria.[2] Occasional isolated cases are reported in North America.[3] Ainhum has been reported in children, but these cases most likely represent a postinfectious or posttraumatic process.

Etiology and Pathogenesis

Chronic trauma, infection, hyperkeratosis, decreased vascular supply, and impaired sensation may alone or in combination produce excessive fibroplasia in a susceptible host. As they tend to form keloids, some blacks appear to respond to relatively minor damage with an excessive fibroblastic reaction. But keloids are not a problem in the scarred digital stumps of ainhum. Impaired blood supply to the little toe has been identified in four patients with ainhum.[4] All had attenuation of the posterior tibial artery and absence of the plantar arterial arch; perhaps poor perfusion predisposed the toe to mechanical trauma.

Clinical Manifestations

Ainhum usually affects the fifth toe (Fig. 106-1); it may be unilateral, but 75 percent of the cases are bilateral. In the beginning, a groove or sulcus appears at the plantar junction of the toe with the sole. The formation of the sulcus has been blamed on rotational stress applied to the bare, mechanically unstable foot, perhaps comparable to the way a piece of plastic is damaged by repeated flexing. As this sulcus deepens, edema develops distally and roentgenographic examination shows resorption of the underlying bone. Slowly and often painfully, the process of autoamputation proceeds, until the digit is dangling by a twisted piece of soft tissue. Eventually, this tenuous connection necroses and amputation is complete. Accompanying problems other than infection and gangrene are uncommon. The entire process is usually slowly progressive, and the disease may require many years to run its full course.

Pathology

The constricting bands consist of fibrous tissue density resembling scar tissue. The band usually extends deep into the subcutaneous layers and may impinge upon underlying skeletal and vascular structures. In addition, there may be moderate inflammation and the overlying epidermis may be hyperplastic or verrucous.[5]

Treatment

Surgery is the mainstay of therapy, for in most cases of ainhum, prompt amputation may allow the patient to escape pain and infection. Early cases may respond to conservative plastic repair with a Z-plasty or similar relaxing closure.

PSEUDOAINHUM

Pseudoainhum or constricting bands are far more common than ainhum outside of Africa and constitute the only differential diagnostic consideration. There are three main categories of pseudoainhum: (1) congenital constricting bands; (2) constricting bands secondary to

FIGURE 106-1

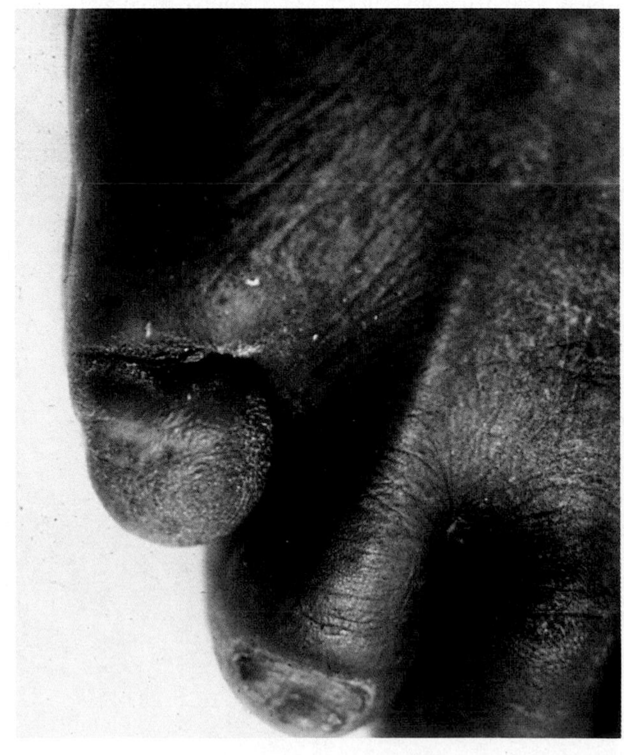

Ainhum in an African male. (*Courtesy of Wayne M. Meyers, MD.*)

FIGURE 106-2

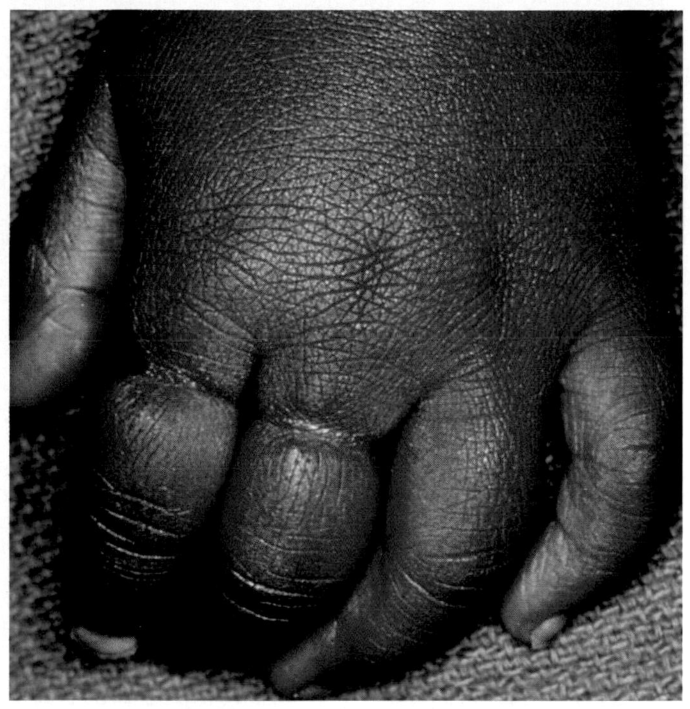

Congenital constricting bands about two digits. No etiology was identified.

hyperkeratosis, trauma, chronic infections, and a variety of other conditions; and (3) constriction by external forces, such as hairs or threads.

Clinical Manifestations

Congenital constricting bands are usually caused by the umbilical cord. They usually involve more than one part of the body and frequently encircle large structures such as limbs or even the trunk. They persist throughout life and interfere with normal growth of the involved segment unless surgically treated[6] (Fig. 106-2).

Acquired constricting bands are seen in a variety of conditions. When associated with chronic trauma and infection of the extremities, they blend with ainhum. In general, pseudoainhum is more likely to involve any of the toes or even the hands, rather than being confined to the little toes. In children, chronic dermatophyte infection can be identified and appropriately treated, with apparent complete reversal of the constriction. Pseudoainhum has been seen in a number of seemingly unrelated diseases with vascular abnormalities (Raynaud's disease, diabetes mellitus, linear scleroderma), systemic sclerosis, sensory changes (leprosy, tertiary syphilis, syringomyelia), or scar formation (burns, frostbite, trauma).

Hyperkeratosis is also associated with constricting bands and subsequent loss of digits. This sequence is common in the verrucous hyperkeratotic plantar lesions of yaws. Rarer hereditary forms include Vohwinkel's syndrome or keratoderma hereditaria mutilans, in which palmar and plantar hyperkeratoses as well as starfish-like and linear keratoses on the extremities are seen with the constricting bands. Genetic studies have provided surprising insight into the etiology of Vohwinkel's syndrome. Two different genes are involved. Mutations in the gene for loricrin (1q21), a major component of the epidermal differentiation complex forming the cornified cell envelope lead to Vohwinkel's syndrome with ichthyosis[7,8] or progressive symmetric erythrokeratoderma.[9] On the other hand, mutations in connexin 26 (GJB2) (13q11-q13) lead to Vohwinkel's syndrome with neurosensory deafness. Connexin 26 is a crucial protein in the formation of gap junctions and docking with adjacent cells.[10,11] Other less-distinctive palmar and plantar keratodermas have also been reported to be accompanied by constricting bands (see Chap. 52).

Even a disease as common as psoriasis may present with pseudoainhum. For example, a 68-year-old black woman presented with constricting casts about her fingers and an acute pustular hand dermatitis but shortly thereafter she developed typical psoriasis elsewhere.[12] Pseudoainhum was also described in a Caucasian woman with erythropoietic protoporphyria, which generally is not considered a cause of acral scarring.[13]

Artifactitious pseudoainhum may prove to be a most challenging diagnosis. Strands of hair, fibers, or threads may be wrapped around digits or other body parts. This phenomenon is encountered in children or mentally deranged adults. Because of soft-tissue swelling, the ligating band may not be visible and the true cause of the condition not immediately recognized.[14]

Pathology

The constricting bands in all these conditions tend to be more superficial than in ainhum but are otherwise similar. There may be histologic clues to the associated disorder, such as dermatophytosis, foreign bodies, or distinct patterns of keratinization.

Treatment

Constricting bands can be treated with a Z-plasty or similar relaxing closure. Early surgery may avoid further disease progression and damage to underlying structures.[14]

Impending amputation in Vohwinkel's syndrome can sometimes be aborted by therapy with oral etretinate. When chronic fungal or bacterial infections are diagnosed in the early phase of band formation, treatment may reverse the threat to the digit. Other predisposing causes of underlying diseases should be treated aggressively in the hope of preventing loss of a digit.

REFERENCES

1. Browne SG: True ainhum: Its distinctive and differentiating features. *J Bone Joint Surg Br* **47**:52, 1965
2. Cole GJ: Ainhum: An account of fifty-four patients with special reference to etiology and treatment. *J Bone Joint Surg Br* **47**:43, 1965
3. Greene JT, Fincher RM: Case report: Ainhum (spontaneous dactylolysis) in a 65-year-old American black man. *Am J Med Sci* **303**:118, 1992
4. Dent DM et al: Ainhum and angiodysplasia. *Lancet* **2**:396, 1981
5. Kerhisnik W: The surgical pathology of ainhum (dactylolysis spontanea). *J Foot Surg* **25**:95, 1986
6. Ray M et al: Amniotic band syndrome. *Int J Dermatol* **27**:312, 1988
7. Camisa C, Rossana C: Variant of keratoderma hereditaria mutilans (Vohwinkel's syndrome): Treatment with orally administered isotretinoin. *Arch Dermatol* **120**:1323, 1984
8. Maestrini E et al: A molecular defect in loricrin, the major component of the cornified cell envelope, underlies Vohwinkel's syndrome. *Nat Genet* **13**:70, 1996
9. Ishida-Yamamoto A et al: The molecular pathology of progressive symmetric erythrokeratoderma: A frameshift mutation in the loricrin gene and perturbations in the cornified cell envelope. *Am J Hum Genet* **61**:581, 1997
10. Solis RR et al: Vohwinkel's syndrome in three generations. *J Am Acad Dermatol* **44**:376, 2001
11. Maestrini E et al: A missense mutation in connexin 26, D66H, causes mutilating keratoderma with sensorineural deafness (Vohwinkel's syndrome) in three unrelated families. *Hum Mol Genet* **8**:1237, 1999
12. McLaurin CI: Psoriasis presenting with pseudoainhum. *J Am Acad Dermatol* **7**:132, 1982
13. Christopher AP et al: Pseudoainhum and erythropoietic protoporphyria. *Br J Dermatol* **118**:113, 1988
14. Pickus EJ et al: Digital constriction bands in pseudoainhum: Morphological, radiographic, and histological analysis. *Ann Plast Surg* **47**:194, 2001

CHAPTER 107

Steffen Albrecht

Neoplasias and Hyperplasias of Neural and Muscular Origin

TUMORS OF SKELETAL MUSCLE

This group of lesions includes the nonneoplastic neuromuscular and rhabdomyomatous mesenchymal hamartomas, as well as neoplasms with striated muscle differentiation, that is, benign rhabdomyomas and malignant rhabdomyosarcomas. Contrary to most other classes of mesenchymal tumors where benign neoplasms are more frequent than malignant ones, rhabdomyosarcomas far outnumber rhabdomyomas. Interestingly, both types of neoplasms have been described in patients with Gorlin's nevoid basal cell carcinoma syndrome.[1]

Neuromuscular Hamartoma

This is a very rare entity of which less than 20 cases have been reported in the English language literature;[2] it is also known as *neuromuscular choristoma* or *benign triton tumor*. Most reported cases involved large nerves; dermal location is unusual. Histologically, the lesion is composed of bundles of nerves and fascicles of mature skeletal muscle fibers, all of which are intimately intermingled to the point where some muscle fibers actually grow within the nerve fascicles. This very unusual growth pattern along with the lack of other mesenchymal elements distinguish the neuromuscular hamartoma from the rhabdomyomatous mesenchymal hamartoma described below.

Rhabdomyomatous Mesenchymal Hamartoma

Rhabdomyomatous mesenchymal hamartoma (RMH) is a rare entity; only about two dozen cases have been described.[3] It is also known as *striated muscle hamartoma, hamartoma of cutaneous adnexa and mesenchyma,* or *congenital midline hamartoma*. It presents as a pedunculated nodule ("skin tag"), usually on the face around the eyes, nose, or mouth. Most are solitary; rare patients with multiple lesions have been described. Although most are congenital, a few have been noted only in adults. Histologically, the dermis contains randomly oriented, mature, striated muscle fibers with admixed mesenchymal elements (adipose tissue, vessels, collagen) and prominent nerves. Skin appendages are also prominent. Excision is curative. Patients with RMH of the ocular adnexa invariably have ocular malformations[3] and some patients with nonocular RMH have other malformations, including cerebral ones. In fact, as reviewed elsewhere,[3] some patients with RMH and multiple associated malformations fulfill the criteria for Delleman's oculocerebrocutaneous syndrome or Goldenhar's oculoauriculovertebral syndrome, which may be related. A diagnosis of RMH in a patient thus should prompt further investigations, especially to rule out brain malformations.

Rhabdomyoma

Cardiac rhabdomyomas occur in about 30 to 50 percent of patients with tuberous sclerosis (TS) and, conversely, a similar proportion of patients with cardiac rhabdomyoma have TS.[4] Sporadic examples are usually solitary, whereas TS-associated cases are often multiple. A minority becomes symptomatic by obstructing cardiac flow or by causing dysrhythmias. Because it is now well established that many cardiac rhabdomyomas regress spontaneously with age, surgical removal is reserved for patients with severe hemodynamic compromise or refractory dysrhythmias.[4]

Extracardiac rhabdomyomas are not associated with TS.[5] They are subdivided into three types: adult, fetal, and genital.[5] The designation as "adult" or "fetal" refers to the tumor's resemblance to adult or fetal skeletal muscle, not to the age of the patient. While the adult type is indeed seen mostly in adults, many fetal rhabdomyomas also occur in older children and adults.[5] Both types occur predominantly in male patients and usually arise in the soft tissues or mucosal surfaces of the head and neck region. As such, they are unlikely to come to the attention of a dermatologist. The fetal type, however, has been repeatedly associated with Gorlin's syndrome.[5] Genital rhabdomyomas usually occur as small polypoid vaginal or vulvar lesions in middle-aged women.[5]

Rhabdomyosarcoma

Rhabdomyosarcomas are aggressive sarcomas occurring most commonly in children. There are four histologic types: embryonal, alveolar (ARMS—alveolar rhabdomyosarcoma), pleomorphic, and undifferentiated. ARMS is characterized at the molecular level by novel fusion genes combining the forkhead (*FKHR*) gene with either the *PAX3* or the *PAX7* gene, producing a t(2;13) or t(1;13), respectively.[6] Rhabdomyosarcoma is the most frequent soft tissue sarcoma of childhood and involves predominantly the head and neck region, the genitourinary tract, and the extremities.[7] Only about 0.7 percent occur as primary skin lesions;[7] nevertheless, in one series, rhabdomyosarcoma was the most frequent primary malignant pediatric skin tumor, making up about one-third of such cases[8] and very rare cases of primary cutaneous rhabdomyosarcoma have been reported in adults.[9] Some of these cases arose in giant congenital nevi either pure or as part of a mixed malignant neoplasm.[10] A deep soft tissue rhabdomyosarcoma can also extend into the overlying skin and present as a cutaneous nodule. Metastases to the skin also occur.[7] In fact, in children, rhabdomyosarcoma is the most common nonhematological cutaneous metastatic tumor.[11]

About a dozen cases of congenital ARMS have been reported.[6,7,12] Roughly half of these patients presented as a "blueberry muffin baby" with multiple cutaneous and subcutaneous metastases. Prognosis has been dismal, with all patients dying in spite of aggressive therapy, usually within a few weeks to months after diagnosis. Interestingly, none of four cases examined for the typical ARMS-associated fusion genes was positive,[6,12] leading one group to postulate that congenital ARMS is a clinically and genetically distinct entity with very poor prognosis.[6] Rhabdomyosarcoma has been reported in association with Gorlin's syndrome[1] and an embryonal rhabdomyosarcoma has been described in a patient with cardiofaciocutaneous syndrome.[13] There is also definitely an increased incidence of rhabdomyosarcoma in type 1 neurofibromatosis (NF1).[14]

TUMORS OF SMOOTH MUSCLE

The dermis contains smooth muscle fibers in the arrectores pilorum muscles, in the walls of dermal blood vessels, and in the dartos muscle of the scrotum, vulva, nipple, and areola. As with striated muscle tumors, there are three types of cutaneous smooth muscle lesions: hamartomas, leiomyomas, and leiomyosarcomas. Whether neoplastic or not, smooth muscle cells are recognized histologically by their spindle cell shape, their eosinophilic, fibrillary cytoplasm, and their blunt ended, oval ("cigar-shaped") nuclei. By immunohistochemistry, they express smooth muscle actin (also called α-actin) and the muscle-specific intermediate filament desmin, but are negative for S-100 protein and epithelial membrane antigen (EMA).

Congenital Smooth Muscle Hamartoma

First described by Stokes in 1923,[15] congenital smooth muscle hamartoma (CSMH) has been increasingly recognized during the last two decades. Most cases are congenital; a prevalence of up to 0.2 percent in children has been reported.[16] Notwithstanding the name, some cases appear to be acquired.[16,17] CSMH usually arises on the trunk or an extremity and may take one of several forms: a solitary patch or plaque with or without a follicular pattern, multiple lesions (rarely with a linear distribution), and diffuse skin involvement producing a "Michelin-tire baby."[18,19] Vellus hairs may be prominent. Clinically, most lesions cause concern because of their congenital nature or for cosmetic reasons. Some can produce worm-like movements ("vermiculation") and stroking may induce transient induration with piloerection (pseudo-Darier's sign).

Histologically, there is a marked increase of smooth muscle fibers in the dermis, especially in its deeper portions. The fibers are grouped in sharply circumscribed bundles that are arranged haphazardly and are not necessarily attached to hair follicles. There may be basal hyperpigmentation, as well as acanthosis and papillomatosis of the overlying epidermis. The grouping of the smooth muscle fibers into discrete bundles and the fact that these bundles do not intermingle with the dermal collagen fibers distinguish smooth muscle hamartomas from pilar leiomyomas. Smooth muscle hamartoma shares some clinical and histologic features with Becker's nevus; some authors consider these lesions as part of a spectrum,[16] while others prefer to keep them separate.[17,20] No specific treatment is indicated. Although the localized form is usually not associated with other malformations,[16] some of the children with the generalized form did have multiple associated congenital malformations[21] and growth, as well as psychomotor retardation.[21,22]

Leiomyoma

Leiomyomas of the skin are generally divided into three categories: (1) solitary or multiple pilar leiomyomas arising from the arrectores pilorum muscles; (2) angioleiomyomas, which are thought to arise from vascular smooth muscle; and (3) dartoic leiomyomas originating in the dartos muscles of the genitalia, areola, and nipple. Most are acquired.

Pilar leiomyomas range in size from several millimeters to a centimeter and are fixed to the skin but freely moveable with it over underlying structures. The skin often has a reddish brown color (Fig. 107-1). The tumors can coalesce to form plaques. The extensor surfaces of limbs, trunk, and sides of face and neck are most commonly involved. The lesions are often sensitive to touch or cold and may be spontaneously painful. Angioleiomyomas are mostly seen on the legs in women and can reach a size of several centimeters. Dartoic leiomyomas are usually solitary, deep, and occasionally pedunculated. Leiomyomas involving the nipple are surprisingly rare.[23] Smooth muscle proliferations resembling pilar leiomyomas have been reported in some cases of nevus sebaceous.[24]

FIGURE 107-1

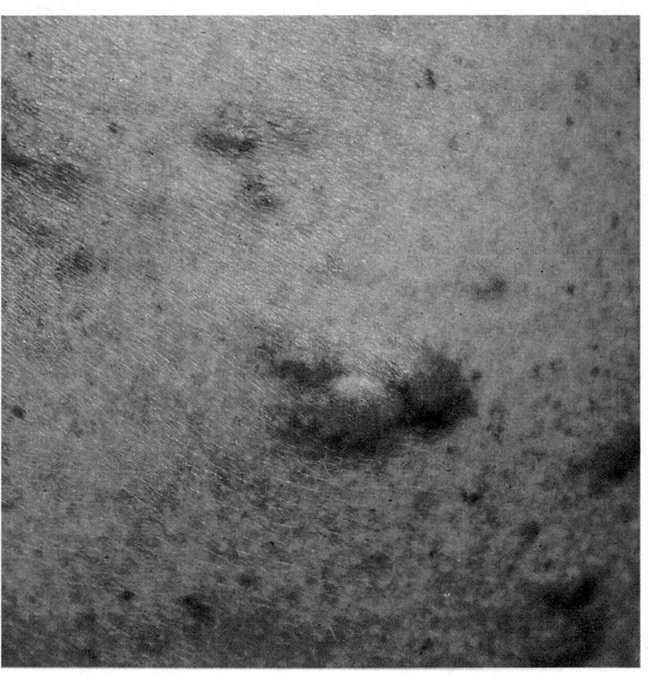

Clinical photograph showing multiple leiomyomas involving the back.

Histologically, pilar leiomyomas are made up of a poorly circumscribed proliferation of haphazardly arranged smooth muscle fibers located in the dermis that appear to infiltrate the surrounding tissue and may extend into the subcutis (Fig. 107-2). They are usually separated from the epidermis by a thin grenz zone. On the other hand, angioleiomyomas are well circumscribed, richly vascularized dermal or subcutaneous nodules composed of well-differentiated smooth muscle fibers (Fig. 107-3). Occasionally, the vessel of origin can be identified. Dartoic leiomyomas resemble pilar leiomyomas which are distinctive lesions, not easily confused with other tumors. Angioleiomyoma should be distinguished from schwannoma; this is discussed in the latter section. Excision is the treatment of choice for solitary leiomyomas if pain is a problem or because of cosmetic concern.

Special mention should be made of patients with multiple pilar leiomyomas. Starting in early adulthood, these patients develop increasing numbers of tumors and can have hundreds to thousands of them; transmission appears to be autosomal dominant with variable penetrance.[25] One patient with multiple leiomyomas was also mentally retarded and had craniofacial dysmorphism (and a similarly affected sister); the patient's karyotype showed anomalies of chromosomes 9 and 18.[26] However, other workers found normal karyotypes in three patients with multiple leiomyomas without other lesions.[27] Women affected by the condition may also have uterine smooth muscle tumors, an entity named *familial leiomyomatosis cutis et uteri* or *Reed's syndrome*.[25] Pain may be a major problem in these patients and excision of all lesions is obviously not feasible. The pain may respond to treatment with nitroglycerin, phenoxybenzamine, or nifedipine.[25,28] Trials assessing the effect of a given medication on cold-induced pain may be helpful

FIGURE 107-2

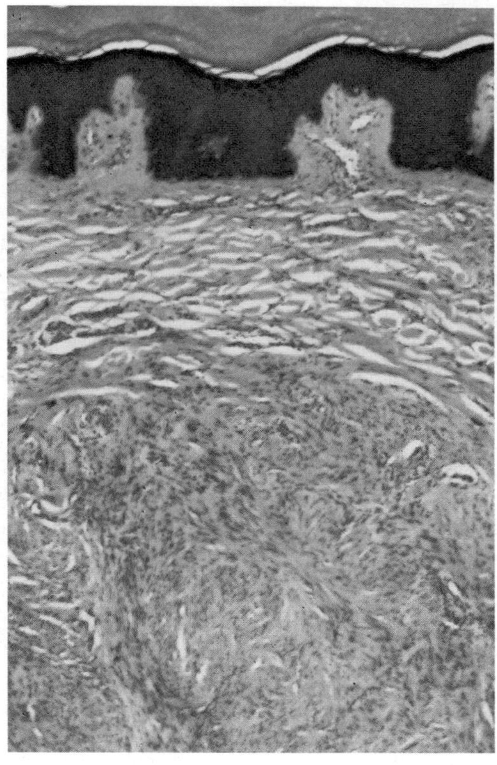

Histologic appearance of a pilar leiomyoma. The tumor has an irregular outline. It is composed of fascicles of smooth muscle fibers with intermingled dermal collagen and is separated from the epidermis by a grenz zone of uninvolved dermis. (H&E, ×40.)

FIGURE 107-3

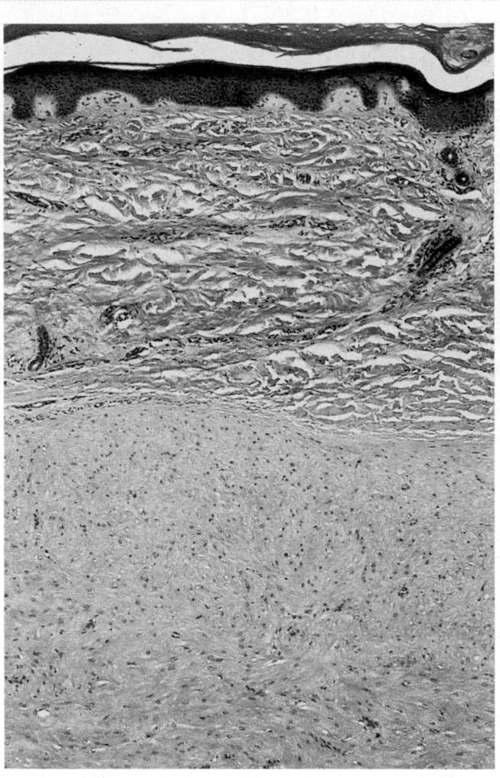

Histologic appearance of an angioleiomyoma. Compared to the pilar leiomyoma, this tumor is more sharply circumscribed (but not encapsulated). Furthermore, the smooth muscle fibers form a solid nodule with little, if any, intervening collagen. (H&E, ×40.)

in selecting an agent effective for a particular patient. Occasionally, the tumors are associated with polycythemia and erythropoietin-like activity has been demonstrated in tumor extracts.[29] Recently, an association between familial cutaneous leiomyomas and a peculiar histological variant of renal cell carcinoma with linkage to chromosome arm 1q has been reported.[30]

Leiomyosarcoma

Leiomyosarcomas are malignant mesenchymal tumors usually found in the uterus, the retroperitoneum, gastrointestinal tract, or deep soft tissue. They do, however, rarely occur as primary skin tumors. The legs are the favored site. Some cases arise in fields of prior radiotherapy or at sites of previous trauma.[31] They may be painful or tender. Some patients have multiple lesions; four of seven such patients in one series had a previous retroperitoneal leiomyosarcoma,[32] raising the possibility that the cutaneous lesions could be metastases. Cutaneous (or "superficial") leiomyosarcomas are divided into either a dermal or subcutaneous type, based on their origin.[31] Dermal lesions usually present as small (<2 cm) nodules that are fixed to the epidermis and can be ulcerated. Subcutaneous tumors tend to be larger and are usually not associated with epidermal changes.

Histologically, the tumor cells are still identifiable as having smooth muscle differentiation. However, their malignant character is evidenced by nuclear hyperchromasia, prominent nucleoli, mitotic activity, and possibly necrosis. The cells are arranged in irregular, intersecting bundles and fascicles. The tumors may be more or less circumscribed or frankly infiltrative. *Granular cell, epithelioid cell, myxoid,* and *sclerosing* (or *desmoplastic*) variants have been described.[33] Leiomyosarcomas have to be distinguished from other malignant spindle cell tumors of the skin, such as spindle cell melanoma, spindle cell squamous cell carcinoma, or atypical fibroxanthoma. Immunohistochemistry and electron microscopy can be very useful in this regard.

As reviewed elsewhere,[31] the most important prognostic factor is the origin of the tumor: although both dermal and subcutaneous lesions may recur locally in up to one-third to one-half of cases, the risk of metastasis is about 5 to 10 percent for the former versus up to 50 to 60 percent for the latter.[31] Standard therapy for either type consists of wide local excision and reexcision for recurrent lesions.[31] Especially in acral locations, complete excision may require amputation.[31] Alternative treatment modalities that may be applicable to selected patients include the Mohs technique, cryosurgery, and isolated limb perfusion with chemotherapeutic agents.[31,34]

BENIGN PROLIFERATIONS OF NERVES—NEUROMAS

Quite literally, neuromas are tumors composed of a proliferation of nerves; that is, they contain both Schwann cells and axons. This is not to say, however, that they constitute true neoplasms; on the contrary, these lesions appear to represent nonneoplastic overgrowths of preexisting neural structures. The first three lesions in this section are mentioned mostly for sake of completeness because they are usually not seen by dermatologists.

Morton's Neuroma

This lesion is not a neuroma in the strict sense, but rather a chronic compressive neuropathy typically involving the third digital plantar nerve along its course through its intermetatarsal space.[35] Repeated microtrauma to the nerve causes epi- and perineurial fibrosis, leading to nerve enlargement, which makes the nerve still more susceptible to trauma. Middle-aged women are predominantly affected; "nonsensible" footwear (i.e., pointed high-heeled shoes) may be partly to blame. Conservative measures include a metatarsal pad or steroid injections; surgical removal is curative.[35]

Hyperplastic/Hypertrophic Pacinian Corpuscle ("Pacinian Neuroma")

Pacinian corpuscles are the largest sensory corpuscles in the body,[36] normally measuring 1 to 2 mm on average. They are mechanoreceptors involved in deep touch and vibrational sense. More than 30 cases of hyperplasia and/or hypertrophy of pacinian corpuscles ("pacinian neuroma") have been reported.[36,37] This presents clinically as an extremely painful and exquisitely tender nodule or swelling of the digital pulp. (Their painfulness is somewhat surprising, given that normal pacinian corpuscles are not thought to be involved in pain perception.) A history of preceding local trauma is present in about half the patients. Treatment is by excision. These lesions should not be confused with rare cases of true nerve sheath neoplasms such as neurofibromas and schwannomas that can occasionally have structures resembling pacinian or meissnerian corpuscles.

Traumatic (Amputation) Neuroma

When a nerve is partially or completely severed, the axons distal to the point of transection undergo Wallerian degeneration, whereas the axons and Schwann cells of the proximal stump proliferate. If the two nerve segments are reapproximated, and if the Schwann cells and the endoneurium of the distal segment remain intact, it can be reinnervated. However, if there is interposition of tissue between the two segments (e.g., because of scarring) or if the distal segment is lost (e.g., by amputation), axons and Schwann cells will still grow out of the proximal stump but will fail to reach their target and form instead a disorganized tangle of nerve twiglets extending into the surrounding soft tissue, thus forming a traumatic neuroma. The pain associated with traumatic neuromas may be caused by contraction of the scar tissue leading to nerve compression or ischemia.[38] The nerve proliferation typical of accessory digits may also represent an example of traumatic neuroma. Treatment can be conservative or surgical; the latter aims either at preventing axonal growth or at isolating the nerve from injury.[38]

Palisaded Encapsulated Neuroma

This lesion was initially described by Reed et al. in 1972,[39] and although by no means uncommon, it received relatively little attention until the last decade or so.[40–45] Palisaded encapsulated neuroma (PEN) presents in adults, mostly in their third to fifth decade, as an asymptomatic papule, usually less than 6 mm in diameter, located on the face in approximately 80 percent of cases.[42–44] The sex distribution is roughly equal. Although it makes up approximately a quarter of benign cutaneous neural lesions,[44] PEN is almost never diagnosed clinically; the most common misdiagnoses are nevus, basal cell carcinoma, and adnexal tumor.

Histologically, there is a well-demarcated dermal nodule composed of fascicles of Schwann cells (Fig. 107-4). Contrary to what the name implies, the capsule is rarely complete and the palisading typical of schwannomas is often indistinct at best. This has led one author to propose rechristening these tumors *circumscribed solitary neuromas of skin*.[41] Special stains demonstrate variable numbers of axons within the lesion. A dermal nerve twig is often seen in continuity with the neuroma and its perineurium merges with the tumor capsule. Immunohistochemical data[40,41,43] also support a perineurial phenotype of the tumor capsule as opposed to the Schwannian phenotype of the cells making up the lesion proper. In fact, some PENs may actually be small dermal schwannomas that contain a few residual entrapped axons.[45]

FIGURE 107-4

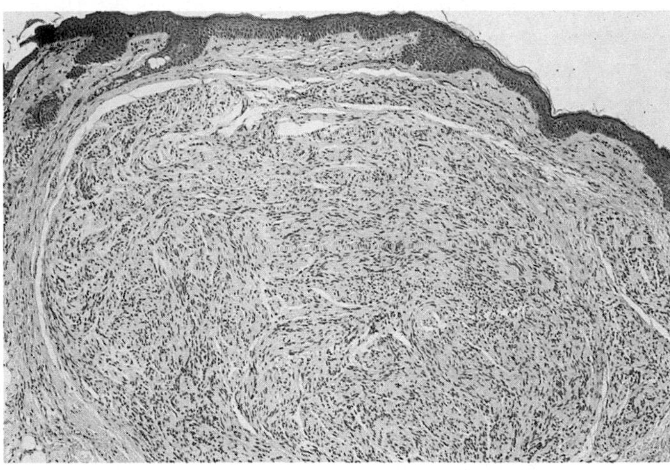

Histologic appearance of a typical palisaded encapsulated neuroma. The tumor is composed of fascicles of Schwann cells and surrounded by a delicate capsule best seen on the left. There is a suggestion of nuclear palisading but this is not as pronounced as that seen in a schwannoma. (The axons that are normally also present cannot be seen on this stain.) (H&E, ×40.)

Excision is the treatment of choice. There is no evidence of an association between PEN and neurofibromatosis, and although the individual lesions may be histologically quite similar, there is also no evidence linking PEN to the multiple endocrine neoplasia syndrome type 2B (multiple mucosal neuroma syndrome).

Multiple Endocrine Neoplasia Syndrome Type 2B (Multiple Mucosal Neuromas)

Multiple endocrine neoplasia syndrome type 2 (MEN2) is an autosomal dominant disease associated with hyperplasia and/or tumors of the calcitonin-producing cells of the thyroid gland (C cells), the adrenal medulla, the parathyroids, and the enteric autonomic nervous system. MEN2A is characterized by the triad of medullary carcinoma of the thyroid gland, pheochromocytoma, and parathyroid hyperplasia. The neoplastic spectrum of MEN2B is similar, but in addition, these patients have malformations (marfanoid habitus, facial dysmorphism) and overgrowth of mucosal nerves giving rise the so-called mucosal neuromas. MEN2A and 2B are caused by different germ-line mutations of the *RET* proto-oncogene located on chromosome 10q11.2.[46]

The neuromas appear by 2 years of age and thus serve as an important clinical marker for identifying affected individuals in MEN2B families.[46] They involve all mucosal surfaces; those accessible to clinical examination (oral mucosa, lips, tongue, conjunctivae), appear as pink, pedunculated nodules. The lips become enlarged and bulging, and the eyelids may be everted. Histologically, there is hypertrophy of the mucosal nerves; some lesions may resemble palisaded encapsulated neuromas. Other cutaneous lesions include café-au-lait spots, facial lentigines and hyperpigmentation of the hands and feet.

The main threat to these patients is the development of tumors. Virtually all will have a medullary carcinoma of the thyroid by early adulthood and about half will develop pheochromocytomas. The thyroid carcinoma is highly aggressive. Early detection and prophylactic thyroidectomy by 5 years of age are essential.[46]

BENIGN NERVE SHEATH NEOPLASMS

Cells that make up the nerve sheath include the Schwann cells and the endo- and perineurial fibroblasts. Benign nerve sheath tumors used to be simply divided into neurofibromas and schwannomas. In recent years, however, several new subtypes as well as two "new" lesions have been added. Unfortunately, the nomenclature is at times quite confusing with identical lesions receiving different names and identical names referring to different lesions.

Schwannoma

Schwannomas are also called *neurinomas, neurolem(m)omas,* or *neurilem(m)omas*. They usually arise in cranial nerves, especially the vestibular nerve (the so-called acoustic neuromas are actually schwannomas of the vestibular division of the eighth cranial nerve); they also occur in other peripheral nerves and spinal roots. Therefore, most schwannomas are either intracranial, intraspinal, or deep soft-tissue lesions; dermal location is uncommon. Schwannomas occur sporadically or in association with NF2, which is discussed in greater detail in Chap. 190. Briefly, the hallmark of NF2 is the presence of bilateral vestibular schwannomas. Patients with NF2 also frequently develop meningiomas, schwannomas of the spinal roots, and gliomas. The NF2 gene is located on the long arm of chromosome 22 (22q12). It codes for a protein that is variously called merlin or schwannomin and which has tumor-suppressor activity.[47]

In the skin, schwannomas present as rather nondescript, asymptomatic papules or nodules. Because a schwannoma is a neoplastic proliferation composed only of Schwann cells and devoid of axons, it grows as an eccentric nodule, displacing its nerve of origin. This growth pattern and its cellular composition distinguish schwannoma from neurofibroma (Fig. 107-5). Histologically, schwannomas are well encapsulated; in fact, the capsule is derived from the epineurium of the schwannoma's nerve of origin. The tumor cells are typically slender, spindled, elongated, and "wavy" in appearance. Areas of high cellularity (Antoni A) alternate with areas of hypocellularity (Antoni B), which can have a myxoid quality. In the cellular A areas, adjacent cells have a tendency to align, creating stacks of nuclei known as palisades. These palisades are separated by an anuclear area made up of stacked cytoplasmic extensions; these stacks of nuclei and cell processes form the so-called Verocay bodies (Fig. 107-6). Tumor blood vessels are characteristically thick and hyalinized. By immunohistochemistry, schwannomas are strongly positive for S-100 protein and negative for EMA and smooth muscle markers (desmin, α-actin), which distinguishes them from perineuriomas (S-100 negative, EMA positive, desmin and α-actin negative) and leiomyomas (S-100 and EMA negative, desmin and α-actin positive).

Several histological variants of schwannoma are recognized. Some tumors have extensive degeneration with cyst formation, old hemorrhage, and marked hyalinization (*ancient schwannoma*). This may be accompanied by bizarre nuclear morphology that does not imply malignancy. Other schwannomas are quite cellular and poor in hypocellular areas with few palisades or Verocay bodies. These tumors have been called *cellular schwannomas;*[48] they may have significant mitotic activity but behave in a benign fashion. This type only rarely involves subcutaneous tissue. Some schwannomas are melanotic. A rare and unusual variant is melanotic and also contains concentrically lamellated microcalcifications called psammoma bodies.[49] Although this *psammomatous melanotic schwannoma* only rarely involves the skin, it is noteworthy that roughly half the affected patients have Carney's syndrome and that about 10 percent of cases metastasize.[49]

In recent years, attention has been drawn to the *plexiform* variant of schwannoma. As the name implies, this tumor grows within a nerve, forming an agglomeration of small nodules and interconnected cords. Contrary to ordinary schwannomas, plexiform schwannomas have a distinct predilection for the dermis and subcutaneous tissue. The relationship between plexiform schwannoma and neurofibromatosis is

FIGURE 107-5

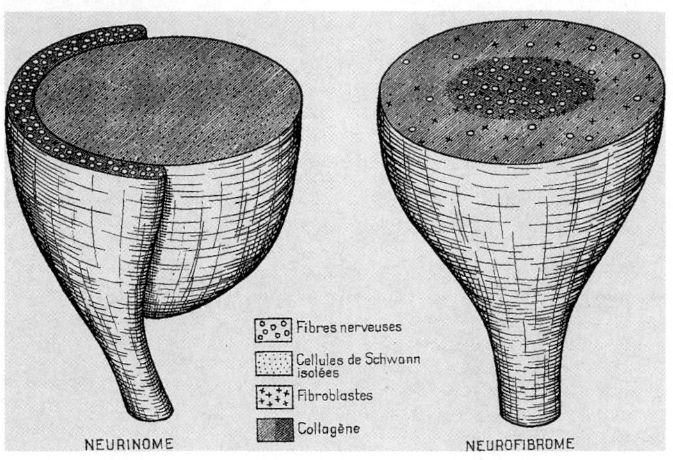

Diagram illustrating the difference between a schwannoma and a neurofibroma. A schwannoma (*left*) is a circumscribed tumor composed only of Schwann cells which arises eccentrically from a nerve. A neurofibroma (*right*), on the other hand, is a segmental hyperplasia of all the nerve's constituent elements. This also illustrates why a schwannoma can often be resected without sacrificing its nerve of origin whereas resection of a neurofibroma always requires transection of that nerve. (*Reproduced from Escourolle R, Poirier J: Manuel élémentaire de neuropathologie, 2nd ed. Paris, Masson Publishing, 1977, p 36, with permission.*)

FIGURE 107-6

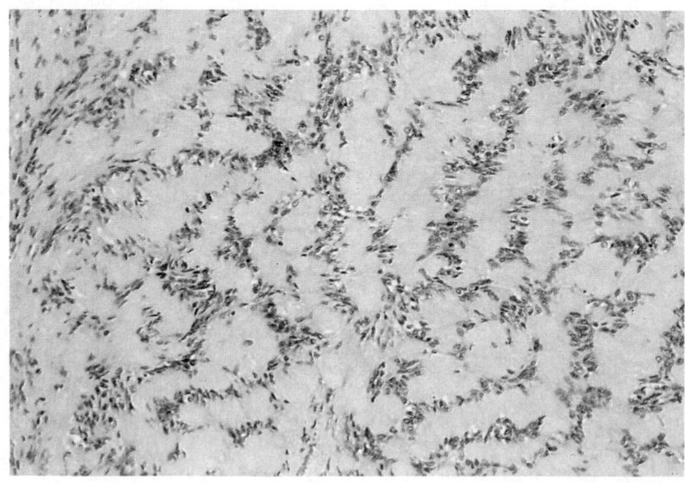

Photomicrograph of a schwannoma showing orderly arrangement of tumor cells into palisades and Verocay bodies. (H&E, ×100.)

somewhat ill defined, because of confusing nomenclature and because some authors do not distinguish between NF1 and NF2. Judging from the literature, most plexiform schwannomas are not associated with either type of NF,[50–53] especially if they are solitary. Some solitary, and especially multiple, plexiform schwannomas, however, are definitely associated with NF2.[52,53]

Finally, there is an entity called *neurolemmomatosis* or *schwannomatosis* in which patients present with multiple cutaneous, soft tissue, or spinal schwannomas, but without vestibular schwannomas or other central nervous system (CNS) tumors typical of NF2 (such as meningiomas or ependymomas); this entity is usually sporadic but can rarely be familial. Based on the literature, it may well represent more than one entity. Some of these patients probably have unrecognized NF2, either because they have had insufficient cranial imaging to exclude small vestibular schwannomas or because they are still too young to exclude the eventual growth of such tumors.[54] Among those in whom vestibular schwannomas have been definitively excluded, a minority do nevertheless carry germ-line mutations of the NF2 gene.[54,55] Some patients are in fact somatic mosaics, which could explain the limited extent of their disease.[56,57] However, the majority of schwannomatosis patients (including those with the familial form) do not have germ-line mutations of NF2, even though their schwannomas do harbor the typical somatic mutations seen in NF2-associated schwannomas.[56] This intriguing finding led the authors of the study to surmise that this type of schwannomatosis is due to an inheritable predisposition to somatic NF2 mutations.[56] Finally, a last group of patients has neither germline nor somatic NF2 mutations;[56] in these individuals, an as yet unknown gene may be involved.

Excision is the treatment of choice for schwannoma. Plexiform schwannomas may recur, but this probably reflects incomplete excision due to their multifocal nature rather than true recurrence.

Neurofibroma

Neurofibroma can be seen as a sporadic lesion or in the context of NF1 which is covered in detail in Chap. 190. At this point, suffice it to say that patients with NF1 have multiple cutaneous and noncutaneous neurofibromas as well as café-au-lait spots, axillary and/or inguinal freckling, iris hamartomas (Lisch nodules), and certain bony malformations. They may also develop other tumors, especially pilocytic astrocytomas of the optic pathways, malignant nerve sheath neoplasms, rhabdomyosarcoma, and pheochromocytoma as well as myeloid leukemia.[14] The gene for NF1 is located on the long arm of chromosome 17 (17q11.2). At least one of the functions of the NF1 protein, which is called *neurofibromin,* appears to be regulation of the *ras* oncogene.[14]

Neurofibromas arise in nerves, and, consequently, are found wherever nerves are found. Those likely come to the attention of the dermatologist are the ones located in the dermis and subcutaneous tissue. Cutaneous neurofibromas present as protuberant to pedunculated, flesh-colored papules or nodules that are typically quite soft on palpation, contrary to what the term "fibroma" might imply. They can be very pruritic. Subcutaneous neurofibromas are usually larger than dermal ones and consist of a fusiform swelling involving a larger nerve. In patients with NF1, the tumors start appearing in early childhood and may be quite variable in size. NF1 has a highly variable expressivity, even among patients from the same kindred who have identical germline mutations.[58] Patients may therefore have from a few to thousands of lesions with corresponding degrees of disfigurement and functional impairment. A special type of neurofibroma is the *plexiform* variant, which involves an entire large nerve and its branches (Fig. 107-7), forming a mass of tangled, ropelike structures that feel like a "bag of worms" on palpation and that can reach an enormous size and be associated with massive soft tissue overgrowth leading to significant functional impairment. A plexiform neurofibroma is considered to be pathognomonic of NF1.

FIGURE 107-7

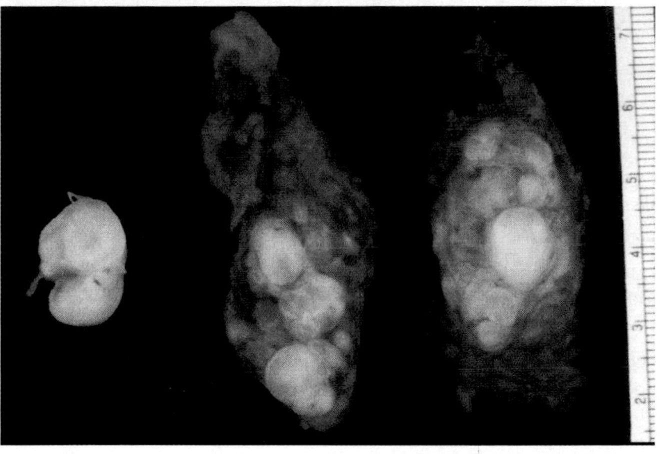

Cross-sections of a plexiform neurofibroma of the facial nerve in a child with NF1. The main nerve is on the left. Note its massive enlargement and involvement of its branches.

Neurofibromas are polyclonal proliferations[59] and can be regarded as hyperplasias of all the nerve's elements (see Fig. 107-5). Histologically, a neurofibroma is composed of Schwann cells, fibroblasts, endothelial cells, perineurial fibroblasts, mast cells, and axons, all arranged haphazardly in a matrix that contains collagen and myxoid ground substance in various proportions (Fig. 107-8). Dermal neurofibromas are circumscribed but unencapsulated nodules. A rare subtype of neurofibroma is the *diffuse* variant that involves the skin and subcutaneous tissue in a plaquelike fashion, surrounding rather than displacing preexisting structures such as skin appendages. Plexiform neurofibromas have the same histologic appearance as ordinary neurofibromas but instead of involving merely a segment of a nerve, they involve an entire nerve and its branches; they also infiltrate the surrounding soft tissue. Rarely, neurofibromas can contain structures resembling meissnerian or pacinian corpuscles. A variant with a very unusual histologic appearance was recently described as *dendritic cell neurofibroma with pseudorosettes*.[60] Finally, some neurofibromas are melanotic.

FIGURE 107-8

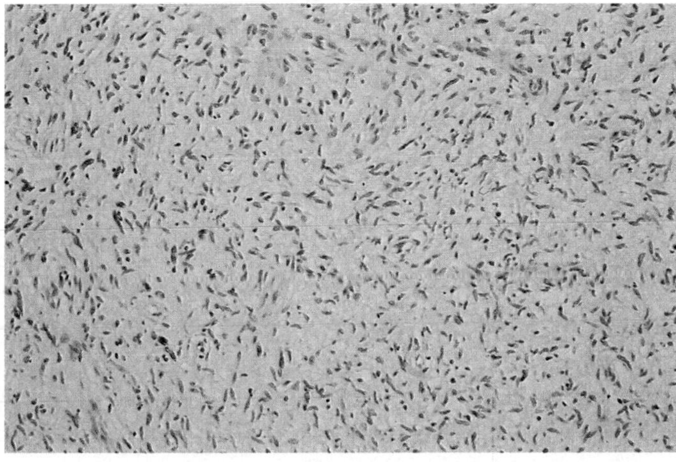

Histology of a neurofibroma. Neurofibromas lack the orderly arrangement of cells that is typical of schwannomas. (H&E, ×100.)

Solitary dermal neurofibromas can be simply excised. Resection of a neurofibroma involving an identifiable nerve by definition implies sacrificing the nerve. Management of patients with NF1 is discussed in Chap. 190.

Neurothekeoma

As is often the case with rare lesions, this one goes under a disturbing variety of names, including *nerve sheath myxoma* (the most frequently used alternate name), *benign myxoid tumor of nerve sheath, perineurial myxoma, bizarre cutaneous neurofibroma,* and *pacinian neurofibroma,* the last two being real misnomers. Two large series established it as an entity;[61,62] most of the literature concerning this lesion has been reviewed recently.[63]

Three-fourths of these tumors arise in the dermis of the head, neck, shoulder, or arm where they present as nondescript, asymptomatic papules. The "classical" neurothekeoma is hypocellular, very myxoid, with a distinctly lobulated growth pattern, and immunohistochemical evidence of nerve-sheath derivation.[63] The tumor expands the dermis, leaving a grenz zone. Variants of neurothekeoma that are more cellular and lack the myxoid matrix have been reported as *cellular neurothekeoma,* but these tumors often lack evidence of nerve sheath differentiation and may be more closely related to fibrohistiocytic tumors.[63,64] Neurothekeomas are clinically benign and there is no recurrence after complete excision. There is no evidence at this point that they are associated with NF1, NF2, or other types of phakomatosis.

Perineurioma

There are two forms of perineurioma. One is *intraneural* and presents as a fusiform swelling of a major nerve, often with signs of mononeuropathy. Histologically, the tumor is confined to the nerve and composed of very delicate, elongated spindle cells that grow around axons, forming whorls composed of multiple concentric layers.[65] These whorls are similar to the "onion bulbs" seen in certain types of hypertrophic neuropathy and especially in the older literature, intraneural perineurioma is often called *localized hypertrophic neuropathy*. However, the cells in perineurioma clearly differentiate along perineurial lines, as shown by ultrastructure and immunohistochemistry,[65] whereas the "onion bulbs" of hypertrophic neuropathy are composed of Schwann cells. Furthermore, cytogenetic evidence indicates that intraneural perineurioma is a true neoplasm.[65] The other form of perineurioma is *extraneural*. It usually arises in soft tissue, but recently, cutaneous examples are increasingly being reported, possibly due to more routine use of immunohistochemistry for the diagnosis of cutaneous spindle cells tumors. This clearly identifies tumors with perineurial differentiation (EMA positive; S-100 protein, α-actin, and desmin negative) and has already led to the description of several histological variants.[66–70] Excision is curative. Neither intra- nor extraneural perineuriomas appear to be associated with NF1 or NF2, but chromosome 22 deletions have been described in one intraneural and two cutaneous perineuriomas.[65,66,71] Analysis of these tumors for somatic NF2 mutations would clearly be of interest.

MALIGNANT TUMORS OF NERVE

Malignant Peripheral Nerve Sheath Tumor

Malignant peripheral nerve sheath tumor (MPNST) is also known as *neurofibrosarcoma, neurogenic sarcoma,* and *malignant schwannoma,* but because its histogenesis is uncertain, the noncommittal term MPNST is preferred. These neoplasms arise mostly in the deep soft tissues; primary cutaneous MPNSTs are rare but are being increasingly recognized.[72,73] MPNSTs often have a relatively nonspecific "spindle-cell sarcoma" histology; the classical features of Schwannian differentiation are only seldom seen. Often, the major reason for calling such a tumor MPNST is that it shows some (often very focal) immunoreactivity for S-100 protein and arises within a nerve or a neurofibroma; origin from either of these can be demonstrated in many cases.[74] Plexiform neurofibromas and neurofibromas involving medium-sized to large nerves are the ones most likely to undergo malignant degeneration, which does not occur in cutaneous neurofibromas.[74] Benign schwannomas on the other hand almost never undergo malignant transformation; one recent compilation presents only nine well-documented cases reported in the last six decades.[75] MPNSTs can contain (malignant) heterologous components such as bone, cartilage, glandular or squamous epithelium, and skeletal muscle; an MPNST with a rhabdomyosarcomatous component is called a *malignant triton tumor*. In some MPNSTs, the tumor cells have an epithelioid appearance and this variant must be distinguished from (metastatic) melanoma.[76] Recently, perineurial rather than Schwannian differentiation has been described in a minority (<5 percent) of MPNTs.[77]

Depending on the series, about 20 to 70 percent of MPNSTs occur in patients with NF1.[10] These are aggressive tumors with a tendency to recur and metastasize. Outcome is guarded with reported 5-year survival rates of no more than 50 percent in spite of aggressive therapy;[10] however, primary cutaneous MPNSTs may have a better prognosis.[72,73] A low-grade plexiform MPNST of infancy and childhood has been proposed as a distinct clinicopathologic entity,[78] but its malignant nature has been disputed.[79]

Primitive Neuroectodermal Tumor

Several types of peripheral primitive neuroectodermal tumors (PNETs) seen mostly in children, such as neuroblastoma and Ewing's sarcoma, can metastasize to the skin.[11] Especially with neuroblastoma, cutaneous metastases can be very numerous and involve multiple sites. In about half the patients with such metastases, they were the initial clinical presentation.[11] Somewhat paradoxically, neuroblastoma patients with multiple skin, liver, and bone marrow lesions (without any other involved organs) actually have a good prognosis with their tumors often undergoing spontaneous regression; this stage is called IV-S (for "special"). Extremely rare cases of peripheral PNETs arising as primary cutaneous or subcutaneous tumors have also been reported.[80]

MISCELLANEOUS TUMORS

Granular Cell Tumor

Granular cell tumors (GCTs) are neoplasms of uncertain histogenesis, but with a typical histological appearance, that have been reported in (almost) every anatomic site but are most often seen in the tongue and skin.[81] Multiple GCTs are seen in approximately 10 to 25 percent of patients.[81] Most cutaneous GCTs are asymptomatic papules or nodules less than 3 cm in diameter; they can be verrucous.

The classical histologic picture is that of an ill-defined, dermal, nonencapsulated nodule composed of large, polyhedral cells, that grow in a sheetlike fashion, with distinct cell borders; small, round, central nuclei; and abundant, granular cytoplasm. The cytoplasmic granules stain strongly with the PAS stain and retain this characteristic after diastase digestion. By immunohistochemistry, the granular cells are strongly positive for S-100 protein (Fig. 107-9). Ultrastructurally, the granules consist of phagolysosomes containing granular and membranous debris.[81] An unusual plexiform variant has been described.[82]

FIGURE 107-9

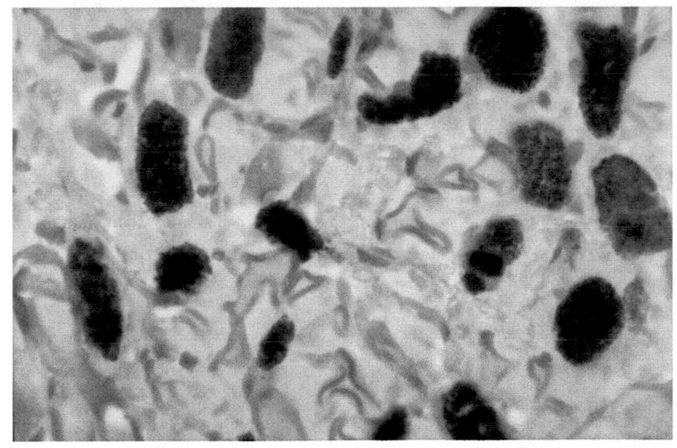

Granular cell tumor stained immunohistochemically with an antibody against S-100 protein. Note strong positivity of the granular cells. (Hematoxylin counterstain, ×400.)

Cutaneous and mucosal lesions typically have pseudoepitheliomatous hyperplasia of the overlying epithelium. Few tumors have created as much controversy about their "cell of origin" as granular cell tumors and this debate has created a body of literature far out of proportion to the importance of the problem. Suffice it to say that current opinion favors neural crest origin.[81]

Excision is the treatment of choice. The major threat to the patient lies in overdiagnosing the pseudoepitheliomatous hyperplasia as carcinoma, a possibility especially with superficial biopsies or excisions that contain only epidermis and miss the underlying dermal tumor.

Only 1 to 2 percent of granular cell tumors are malignant.[81] Clinical findings that should raise concern are a size greater than 4 to 5 cm, location in deep soft tissue (as opposed to dermis), and recurrence.[81] Histological warning signs are the presence of increased cellularity, cytological atypia, and especially mitotic figures and necrosis.[81] However, some clinically malignant GCTs were small and/or histologically innocuous.[81] Therefore, the only definite proof of malignancy is metastasis. Other malignant cutaneous tumors that can contain a subpopulation of cells with granular cytoplasm, such as leiomyosarcoma, melanoma, or angiosarcoma, have to be excluded pathologically.

Cutaneous Lesions with Meningothelial Cells

Meningiomas are neoplasms that arise from meningothelial (arachnoid) cells and usually grow on the inner surface of the cranial or spinal dura. Multiple intracranial and/or intraspinal meningiomas are seen in patients with NF2. Cutaneous lesions containing meningothelial cells also exist. In adults, these usually represent the cutaneous or subcutaneous extension of an aggressive intracranial meningioma that invades through the skull into the pericranial soft tissues and scalp. The meningioma itself may cause surprisingly few neurologic symptoms and patients may actually present because of a growing "lump" on their scalp. In children, skin nodules composed of fibrous tissue and islands of meningothelial cells occur mostly in the scalp over the midline or more rarely along the spine. They are variously called *rudimentary* or *acoelic meningocele, meningeal hamartoma,* or *cutaneous heterotopic meningeal nodules*. These are most likely developmental defects related to meningoceles, which would explain their locations and their invariably congenital nature, along with the fact that some contain a central lumen and may be connected to the dura by a fibrous band running through a skull or vertebral defect.[83] This possibility should be kept in mind at the time of surgical excision and preoperative imaging is indicated to exclude it. Rare familial cases have been reported.[84,85] Exceptionally, a skull or facial bone fracture may cause a tear in the dura with entrapment of meningeal cells in the overlying skin and subsequent development of a posttraumatic cutaneous meningioma.[86]

Myxopapillary Ependymoma

Myxopapillary ependymoma (MPE) is a peculiar variant of ependymoma that typically arises intradurally from the filum terminale of the spinal cord. However, histologically identical lesions also rarely occur as primary extradural tumors of the sacrococcygeal soft tissue, where they present as subcutaneous masses. They are thought to arise from subcutaneous ependymal rests, which are quite common in this region.[87]

These tumors generally present in young patients as a sacrococcygeal or more rarely gluteal mass that is asymptomatic in most cases and can reach a size of several centimeters. Histologically, they are composed of papillae covered by ependymal cells. The cores of the papillae contain abundant myxoid ground substance, hence the name. While intradural MPEs are usually benign, the subcutaneous type is more aggressive with a significant risk of local recurrence and even metastasis.[87]

Cutaneous Ganglioneuroma and Ganglion Cell Tumor

Ganglioneuromas are neoplasms composed of large mature neurons (ganglion cells) growing in a Schwann cell stroma. Pure ganglion cell tumors (or gangliocytomas) do not contain the Schwann cell component. Although they are usually seen as tumors of the autonomic nervous system, some very rare examples have been encountered in the skin or subcutis where they presented as small papules or nodules. Of the half dozen or so reported cases,[88,89] only one was congenital.[88] These lesions have to be distinguished from cutaneous metastases from a neuroblastoma, which can mature into ganglioneuroma. Furthermore, some plexiform neurofibromas in patients with neurofibromatosis arise in autonomic ganglia and can therefore contain residual, entrapped ganglion cells.[90]

Cerebral Heterotopia

Cutaneous cerebral heterotopias arise from CNS tissue that is entrapped in dural diverticula. This can occur during craniofacial development and sometimes fail to regress.[91] In other words, these lesions are now considered as malformations related to encephaloceles,[92] and not as neoplasms as the older designation, "nasal glioma," implied. They occur most often in or on the nose but are also seen on the face, scalp, lip, tongue, as well as in the oro- and nasopharynx, and orbit.[92] Histologically, there are various admixtures of neurons, astrocytes, oligodendrocytes, ependyma, and choroid plexus. There may be significant fibrosis, which can obscure the neuroglial component.[92] Treatment is by excision. Preoperative CT and/or MRI of the head is imperative to determine whether the lesion is connected to the CNS, because this will determine the surgical approach.[91]

REFERENCES

1. Gorlin RJ: Nevoid basal-cell carcinoma syndrome. *Medicine (Baltimore)* **66**:98, 1987
2. Tiffee JC, Barnes EL: Neuromuscular hamartomas of the head and neck. *Arch Otolaryngol Head Neck Surg* **124**:212, 1998

3. Read RW et al: Rhabdomyomatous mesenchymal hamartoma of the eyelid. Report of a case and literature review. *Ophthalmology* **108**:798, 2001
4. Freedom RM et al: Selected aspects of cardiac tumors in infancy and childhood. *Pediatr Cardiol* **21**:299, 2000
5. Weiss SW, Goldblum JR: *Enzinger and Weiss's Soft Tissue Tumors*. St. Louis, Mosby, 2001, p 769
6. Grundy R et al: Congenital alveolar rhabdomyosarcoma. Clinical and molecular distinction from alveolar rhabdomyosarcoma in older children. *Cancer* **91**:606, 2001
7. Schmidt D et al: Rhabdomyosarcomas with primary presentation in the skin. *Pathol Res Pract* **189**:422, 1993
8. Orozco-Covarrubias M et al: Malignant cutaneous tumors in children. Twenty years of experience at a large pediatric hospital. *J Am Acad Dermatol* **30**:243, 1994
9. Colleoni M et al: Primary cutaneous rhabdomyosarcoma in adults—description of an uncommon aggressive disease. *Acta Oncol* **35**:494, 1996
10. Wong T-Y, Suster S: Primary cutaneous sarcomas showing rhabdomyoblastic differentiation. *Histopathology* **26**:25, 1995
11. Wesche A et al: Non-hematopoietic cutaneous metastases in children and adolescents: Thirty years experience at St. Jude Children's Research Hospital. *J Cutan Pathol* **27**:485, 2000
12. Godambe SV, Rawal J: Blueberry muffin rash as a presentation of alveolar cell rhabdomyosarcoma in a neonate. *Acta Paediatr* **89**:115, 2000
13. Bisogno G et al: Rhabdomyosarcoma in a patient with cardio-facio-cutaneous syndrome. *J Pediatr Hematol Oncol* **21**:424, 1999
14. Korf BR: Malignancy in neurofibromatosis type 1. *Oncologist* **5**:477, 2000
15. Stokes JH: Nevus pilaris with hyperplasia of nonstriated muscle. *Arch Dermatol Syphil* **7**:479, 1923
16. De la Espriella J et al: Hamartome musculaire lisse: Caractères anatomo-cliniques et limites nosologiques. *Ann Dermatol Venereol* **120**:879, 1993
17. Darling TN et al: Acquired cutaneous smooth muscle hamartoma. *J Am Acad Dermatol* **28**:844, 1993
18. Gerdsen R et al: Congenital smooth muscle hamartoma of the skin: Clinical classification. *Acta Derm Venereol* **79**:408, 1999
19. Jang HS et al: Linear congenital smooth muscle hamartoma with follicular spotted appearance. *Br J Dermatol* **142**:138, 2000
20. Gagné EJ, Su WPD: Congenital smooth muscle hamartoma of the skin. *Pediatr Dermatol* **10**:142, 1993
21. Schnur RE et al: Variability in the Michelin tire syndrome. A child with multiple anomalies, smooth muscle hamartoma, and familial paracentric inversion of chromosome 7q. *J Am Acad Dermatol* **28**:364, 1993
22. Oku T et al: Folded skin with an underlying cutaneous smooth muscle hamartoma. *Br J Dermatol* **129**:606, 1993
23. Tsujioka K et al: Cutaneous leiomyoma of the male nipple. *Dermatologica* **170**:98, 1985
24. Burden PA et al: Piloleiomyoma arising in an organoid nevus: A case report and review of the literature. *J Dermatol Surg Oncol* **13**:1213, 1987
25. Fernández-Pugnaire MA, Delgado-Florencio V: Familial multiple cutaneous leiomyomas. *Dermatology* **191**:295, 1995
26. Fryns JP et al: 9p trisomy/18p distal monosomy and multiple cutaneous leiomyomata. Another specific chromosomal site (18pter) in dominantly inherited multiple tumors? *Hum Genet* **70**:284, 1985
27. Turleau C et al: Etude cytogénétique de trois cas de léiomyomatose cutanée multiple [letter]. *Ann Dermatol Venereol* **115**:483, 1988
28. Tiffee JC, Budnick SD: Multiple cutaneous leiomyomas. Report of a case. *Oral Surg Oral Med Oral Pathol* **76**:716, 1993
29. Venencie PY et al: Multiple cutaneous leiomyomata and erythrocytosis with demonstration of erythropoietic activity in the cutaneous leiomyomata. *Br J Dermatol* **107**:483, 1982
30. Kiuru M et al: Familial cutaneous leiomyomatosis is a two-hit condition associated with renal cell cancer of characteristic histopathology. *Am J Pathol* **159**:825, 2001
31. Auroy S et al: Léiomyosarcomes cutanés primitifs: 32 cas. *Ann Dermatol Venereol* **126**:235, 1999
32. Dahl I, Angervall L: Cutaneous and subcutaneous leiomyosarcoma. A clinicopathologic study of 47 patients. *Pathol Europ* **9**:307, 1974
33. Diaz-Cascajo C et al: Desmoplastic leiomyosarcoma of the skin. *Am J Dermatopathol* **22**:251, 2000
34. Häffner AC et al: Complete remission of advanced cutaneous leiomyosarcoma following isolated limb perfusion with high-dose tumor necrosis factor-α and melphalan. *Br J Dermatol* **141**:935, 1999
35. Wu KK: Morton neuroma and metatarsalgia. *Curr Opin Rheumatol* **12**:131, 2000
36. Reznik M et al: Painful hyperplasia and hypertrophy of Pacinian corpuscles in the hand. Report of two cases with immunohistochemical and ultrastructural studies, and a review of the literature. *Am J Dermatopathol* **20**:203, 1998
37. Rinaldi P et al: Iperplasia paciniana digitale. Descrizione di un caso con associata reazione da corpo estraneo. *Pathologica* **92**:36, 2000
38. Whipple RR, Unsell RS: Treatment of painful neuromas. *Orthop Clin North Am* **19**:175, 1988
39. Reed RJ et al: Palisaded, encapsulated neuromas of the skin. *Arch Dermatol* **106**:865, 1972
40. Albrecht S et al: Palisaded encapsulated neuroma: an immunohistochemical study. *Mod Pathol* **2**:403, 1989
41. Fletcher CDM: Solitary circumscribed neuroma of the skin (so-called palisaded, encapsulated neuroma). A clinicopathologic and immunohistochemical study. *Am J Surg Pathol* **13**:574, 1989
42. Kutzner H et al: Das solitäre, umkapselte Neurom. *Hautarzt* **41**:620, 1990
43. Eckert F et al: Das umkapselte Neurom der Haut. Eine klinische, histologische und immunohistologische Studie. *Hautarzt* **41**:378, 1990
44. Dakin MC et al: The palisaded, encapsulated neuroma (solitary circumscribed neuroma). *Histopathology* **20**:405, 1992
45. Kossard S et al: Neural spectrum: Palisaded encapsulated neuroma and Verocay body poor dermal schwannoma. *J Cutan Pathol* **26**:31, 1999
46. Stratakis CA: Clinical genetics of multiple endocrine neoplasias, Carney complex and related syndromes. *J Endocrinol Invest* **24**:370, 2001
47. Pollack IF, Mulvihill JJ: Neurofibromatosis 1 and 2. *Brain Pathol* **7**:823, 1997
48. Casadei GP et al: Cellular schwannoma. A clinicopathologic, DNA flow cytometric, and proliferation marker study of 70 patients. *Cancer* **75**:1109, 1995
49. Carney JA: Carney complex: The complex of myxomas, spotty pigmentation, endocrine overactivity, and schwannomas. *Semin Dermatol* **14**:90, 1995
50. Fletcher CDM, Davies SE: Benign plexiform (multinodular) schwannoma: A rare tumour unassociated with neurofibromatosis. *Histopathology* **10**:971, 1986
51. Kao GF et al: Solitary cutaneous plexiform neurilemmoma (schwannoma): A clinicopathologic, immunohistochemical, and ultrastructural study of 11 cases. *Mod Pathol* **2**:20, 1989
52. Reith JD, Goldblum JR: Multiple cutaneous plexiform schwannomas. Report of a case and review of the literature with particular reference to the association with types 1 and 2 neurofibromatosis and schwannomatosis. *Arch Pathol Lab Med* **120**:399, 1996
53. Val-Bernal JF et al: Cutaneous plexiform schwannoma associated with neurofibromatosis type 2. *Cancer* **76**:1181, 1995
54. Pulst SM et al: Spinal scwannomatosis. *Neurology* **48**:787, 1997
55. Honda M et al: Neurofibromatosis 2 and neurilemmomatosis gene are identical. *J Invest Dermatol* **104**:74, 1995
56. Jacoby LB et al: Molecular analysis of the NF2 tumor-suppressor gene in schwannomatosis. *Am J Hum Genet* **61**:1293, 1997
57. MacCollin M et al: Schwannomatosis resulting from somatic mosaicism of the NF2 gene. *Ann Neurol* **42**:513, 1997
58. Zwarthoff EC: Neurofibromatosis and associated tumour suppressor genes. *Pathol Res Pract* **192**:647, 1996
59. Fialkow PJ et al: Multiple cell origin of hereditary neurofibromas. *N Engl J Med* **284**:298, 1972
60. Michal M et al: Dendritic cell neurofibroma with pseudorosettes. A report of 18 cases of a distinct and hitherto unrecognized neurofibroma variant. *Am J Surg Pathol* **25**:587, 2001
61. Gallager RL, Helwig EB: Neurothekeoma—a benign cutaneous tumor of neural origin. *Am J Clin Pathol* **74**:759, 1980
62. Pulitzer DR, Reed RJ: Nerve-sheath myxoma (perineurial myxoma). *Am J Dermatopathol* **7**:409, 1985
63. Laskin WB et al: The "neurothekeoma": Immunohistochemical analysis distinguishes the true nerve sheath myxoma from its mimics. *Hum Pathol* **31**:1230, 2000
64. Zelger BG et al: Cellular "neurothekeoma": An epithelioid variant of dermatofibroma? *Histopathology* **32**:414, 1998
65. Emory TS et al: Intraneural perineurioma. A clonal neoplasm associated with abnormalities of chromosome 22. *Am J Clin Pathol* **103**:696, 1995
66. Burgues O et al: Cutaneous sclerosing Pacinian-like perineurioma. *Histopathology* **39**:498, 2001
67. Fetsch JF, Miettinen M: Sclerosing perineurioma. A clinicopathologic study of 19 cases of a distinctive soft tissue lesion with a predilection for the fingers and palms of young adults. *Am J Surg Pathol* **21**:1433, 1997
68. Graadt van Roggen JF et al: Reticular perineurioma. A distinctive variant of soft tissue perineurioma. *Am J Surg Pathol* **25**:485, 2001
69. Michal M: Extraneural retiform perineuriomas. A report of four cases. *Pathol Res Pract* **195**:759, 1999
70. Robson AM, Calonje E: Cutaneous perineurioma: A poorly recognized tumour often misdiagnosed as epithelioid histiocytoma. *Histopathology* **37**:332, 2000

71. Sciot R et al: Cutaneous sclerosing perineurioma with a cryptic *NF2* gene deletion. *Am J Surg Pathol* **23**:849, 1999
72. Coady MSE et al: Cutaneous malignant peripheral nerve sheath tumour (MPNST) of the hand: A review of the current literature. *J Hand Surg* **18B**:478, 1993
73. Misago N et al: Malignant peripheral nerve sheath tumor of the skin: A superficial form of this tumor. *J Cutan Pathol* **23**:182, 1996
74. Woodruff JM: Pathology of tumors of the peripheral nerve sheath in type 1 neurofibromatosis. *Am J Med Genet* **89**:23, 1999
75. Woodruff JM et al: Schwannoma (neurilemoma) with malignant transformation. A rare, distinctive peripheral nerve tumor. *Am J Surg Pathol* **18**:882, 1994
76. King R et al: Metastatic malignant melanoma resembling malignant peripheral nerve sheath tumor: Report of 16 cases. *Am J Surg Pathol* **23**:1499, 1999
77. Hirose T et al: Perineurial malignant nerve sheath tumor (MPNST). A clinicopathologic, immunohistochemical, and ultrastructural study of seven cases. *Am J Surg Pathol* **22**:1368, 1998
78. Meis-Kindblom JM, Enzinger FM: Plexiform malignant peripheral nerve sheath tumor of infancy and childhood. *Am J Surg Pathol* **18**:479, 1994
79. Woodruff JM, Scheithauer BW: Nerve sheath tumors [letter]. *Am J Surg Pathol* **19**:608, 1995
80. Taylor GB, Chan YF: Subcutaneous primitive neuroectodermal tumour in the abdominal wall of a child: Long-term survival after local excision. *Pathology* **32**:294, 2000
81. Ordóñez NG: Granular cell tumor: A review and update. *Adv Anat Pathol* **6**:186, 1999
82. Lee J et al: Plexiform granular cell tumor. A report of two cases. *Am J Dermatopathol* **16**:537, 1994
83. El Shabrawi-Caelen L et al: Rudimentary meningocele: Remnant of a neural tube defect? *Arch Dermatol* **137**:45, 2001
84. Miyamoto T et al: Primary cutaneous meningioma on the scalp: Report of two siblings. *J Dermatol* **22**:611, 1995
85. Tron V et al: Familial cutaneous heterotopic meningeal nodules. *J Am Acad Dermatol* **28**:1015, 1993
86. Walters GA et al: Posttraumatic cutaneous meningioma of the face. *Am J Neuroradiol* **15**:393, 1994
87. Kline MJ et al: Extradural myxopapillary ependymoma: Report of two cases and review of the literature. *Pediatr Pathol Lab Med* **16**:813, 1996
88. Gambini C, Rongioletti F: Primary congenital cutaneous ganglioneuroma. *J Am Acad Dermatol* **35**:353, 1996
89. Hammond RR, Walton JC: Cutaneous ganglioneuromas: A case report and review of the literature. *Hum Pathol* **27**:735, 1996
90. Rios JJ et al: Cutaneous ganglion cell choristoma. *J Cutan Pathol* **18**:469, 1991
91. Pensler JM et al: Craniofacial gliomas. *Plast Reconstr Surg* **98**:27, 1996
92. Argenyi ZB: Cutaneous neural heterotopias and related tumors relevant for the dermatopathologist. *Semin Diagn Pathol* **13**:60, 1996

CHAPTER 108

Mark Lebwohl

Acquired Perforating Disorders

DEFINITION AND HISTORICAL ASPECTS

The acquired perforating disorders consist of a group of conditions characterized by transepithelial elimination of dermal material. Umbilicated papules with central white, keratotic crusts are the clinical hallmarks of the perforating disorders. Historically, reactive perforating collagenosis, Kyrle's disease, and perforating folliculitis have been differentiated from one another histologically. In 1982, reactive perforating collagenosis was described as associated with diabetes and renal disease.[1] In retrospect, cases of Kyrle's disease and perforating folliculitis had also been associated with diabetes and renal failure[2,3] and reexamination of histologic sections in some of those cases revealed transepidermal elimination of collagen consistent with reactive perforating collagenosis. Because of the common association with diabetes and renal failure, one group of authors suggested that the diseases be called reactive perforating collagenosis of diabetes and renal failure.[4] More recently, another group of authors suggested the term acquired perforating dermatosis,[5] and similar terminology has been used by several authors over the past decade.

Elastosis perforans serpiginosa is a unique perforating disorder characterized by transepidermal elimination of elastic fibers and distinctive clinical lesions, which are serpiginous in distribution and can be associated with specific diseases. Consequently, the latter condition is dealt with separately.

In 1916, Kyrle described[6] hyperkeratosis follicularis et parafollicularis in cutem penetrans, the disorder reported in patients with liver disease, diabetes, or renal disease. Many authors now include it under the general term of acquired perforating dermatosis, although others still distinguish Kyrle's disease as a unique entity. Of interest, the original patient reported by Kyrle did not have diabetes, but developed it 8 years later.[7]

Perforating folliculitis was first described by Mehregan and Coskey in 1968.[8] As with Kyrle's disease, some now include this with the acquired perforating dermatoses but others maintain the term perforating folliculitis as a unique entity. Mehregan also described reactive perforating collagenosis in 1967,[9] and this condition has also been included by some in the acquired perforating disorders.

ETIOLOGY AND PATHOGENESIS

Although there are several theories that seek to explain the etiology of the perforating disorders, none have been proven. Several features in the pathogenesis of the disorder have been suggested, however.

Components of the dermal extracellular matrix are extruded from the dermis through the epidermis to form the central keratotic crusts that are apparent in these skin lesions. It is clear that many patients exhibit the Koebner phenomenon and lesions can be produced experimentally by traumatizing the skin.[10] Noting a microvasculopathy in the dermis of affected patients, one study hypothesizes that perforating disorders are triggered by trauma to the skin that results in an abnormal cutaneous response due to the dermal vasculopathy.[11] Yet another group of investigators has shown increased serum or extracellular matrix fibronectin, suggesting that fibronectin may result in increased epithelial migration that ultimately results in perforation.[12] Other theories have attributed perforating disorders to elevated plasma silicon in patients on dialysis[13]or to vitamin A deficiency.[14,15]One patient with perforating folliculitis, however, was found to have elevated serum levels of vitamin A.[16] While none of these theories concerning the etiology of the perforating disorders has been proven, all agree that affected patients have an abnormal cutaneous response to trauma.

Another study examined the evolution of skin lesions through light and electron microscopic examination of biopsies. Excoriations developed in a chronic mass containing collagen bundles that were contiguous with the reticular dermis. As lesions evolved, new epidermis regenerated between the necrotic mass and the reticular dermis with bundles of collagen connecting the necrotic mass with the reticular dermis through epithelial tunnels. The authors suggest that the regenerated epidermis forms a thick horny layer that lifts up the necrotic mass and its collagen bundles from the dermis through these epidermal channels.[17] Yet another author has demonstrated that at least some of the collagen being eliminated in reactive perforating collagenosis stains with antibodies against type IV collagen, suggesting that the collagen eliminated in this disorder may originate in the basement membrane.[18]

CLINICAL MANIFESTATIONS

The acquired perforating disorders are characterized by umbilicated papules with central white, keratotic crusts (Fig. 108-1). Lesions most often develop on the arms and legs, but any site on the cutaneous surface can be affected including trunk and scalp. Lesions have even been described on the conjunctiva and buccal mucosa of a patient with Kyrle's disease.[19] Virtually all patients complain of pruritus, and scratching can lead to a Koebner phenomenon, with linear umbilicated papules arising in excoriated skin.

In the original description of reactive perforating collagenosis, renal failure and diabetes were not noted.[9] Nevertheless, most acquired perforating disorders are seen in association with kidney failure, diabetes, or both. Associations with hyperparathyroidism, hypothyroidism, and liver disorders,[20] as well as HIV infection[21] and primary sclerosing cholangitis,[22] have also been reported, but these may be coincidental.

FIGURE 108-1

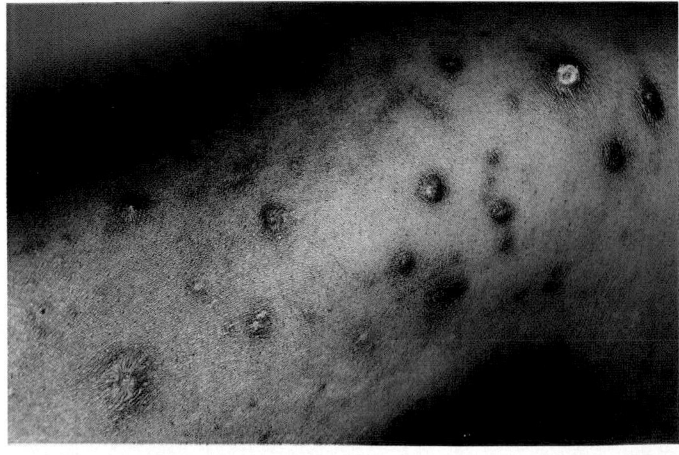

Acquired perforating dermatosis. Umbilicated, keratotic papules on the arm of a patient with diabetes and renal failure.

HISTOPATHOLOGY

Histologically, the acquired perforating disorders are characterized by invagination of the epidermis with extrusion of dermal material through the cup-shaped epidermal depression into the necrotic basophilic tissue within the invaginated epidermis. In the classic description of reactive perforating collagenosis, collagen bundles were observed crossing from the reticular dermis through the epidermis (Fig. 108-2). More recently, one group of investigators found that elastic fibers accompanied the collagen in a small group of patients.[5]

In Kyrle's disease, an amorphous extracellular dermal material was extruded through the epidermis. Descriptions of Kyrle's disease report an invagination of the epidermis that is filled with a keratotic plug containing a parakeratotic column. Within the epidermal invagination, there is a focus of vacuolated dyskeratotic cells, which extends to the basal cell layer and eventually penetrates into the dermis, leaving fragments of parakeratotic keratin in the dermis with a surrounding inflammatory and granulomatous reaction. Subsequent studies using Masson trichrome stains have found bundles of collagen perforating through the epidermis into the base of the invagination.

Perforating folliculitis is characterized histologically by follicular perforation. There is a focal inflammatory infiltrate adjacent to areas of perforation of the follicular epithelium. Degenerating collagen and extracellular matrix tissues mixed with inflammatory cells and orthokeratotic and parakeratotic material fill the dilated hair follicle. Occasionally, a hair is seen. One author suggested that lesions begin as follicular pustules and develop into perforating folliculitis and, ultimately, into prurigo nodularis.[23]

FIGURE 108-2

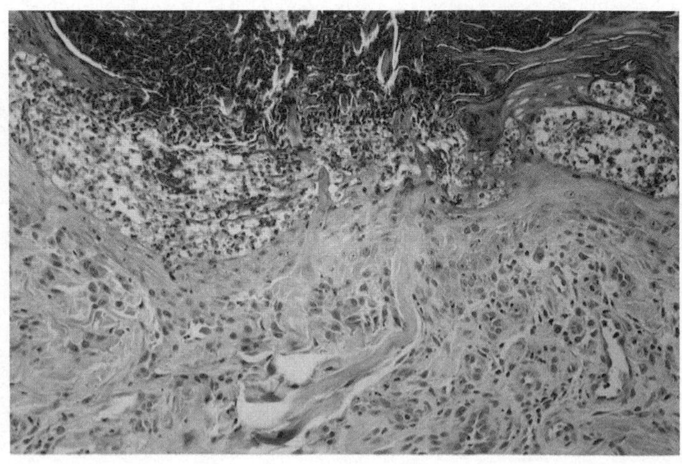

Reactive perforating collagenosis. Collagen bundles can be seen crossing from the reticular dermis through the epidermis into an epidermal depression containing necrotic debris (Hematoxylin and eosin stain).

ELASTOSIS PERFORANS SERPIGINOSA

Definition and History

After several clinical descriptions of the entity we now call elastosis perforans serpiginosa, Miescher described the histopathology of this condition in 1955,[24] and in 1958, the term *elastosis perforans serpiginosa* (EPS) was coined.[25] EPS is characterized by keratotic papules that are often, but not always distributed in a serpiginous pattern (Fig. 108-3). It is associated with Down's syndrome,[26] as well as with a number of inherited disorders of connective tissue (see below). It also occurs as a result of treatment with oral penicillamine. Histologically, lesions are characterized by transepidermal elimination of elastic fibers.

Etiology and Pathogenesis

Alterations of elastic fibers have been described in patients with penicillamine-induced EPS and this condition has usually occurred after long-term therapy of Wilson's disease[27] or cystinuria, and has also been reported in a child treated with D-penicillamine for juvenile rheumatoid arthritis.[28] Abnormal elastic fibers have been found in the lungs as well as the skin of penicillamine-treated patients,[29] and abnormalities of collagen have also been described in patients with EPS.[30,31] The precise mechanism by which penicillamine induces EPS is not entirely known, but the drug chelates copper, the cofactor for lysyl oxidase, which is the enzyme that cross-links elastin. The abnormal elastin is eliminated through the epidermis.

Familial cases of EPS have been reported with different modes of inheritance. In at least one family, autosomal dominant inheritance with variable expression of EPS was suggested.[32] Several inherited disorders of connective tissue have also been associated with EPS, suggesting that various pathways can lead to the abnormal elastin that results in this condition.

FIGURE 108-3

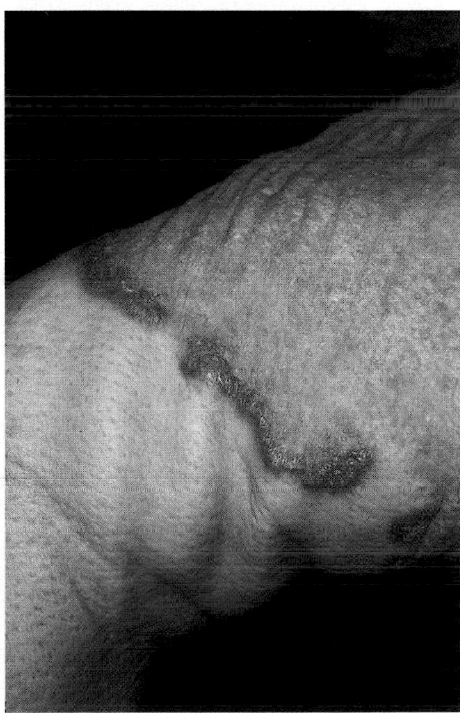

Elastosis perforans serpiginosa. Erythematous, hyperkeratotic papules in a serpiginous distribution on the arm.

Clinical Manifestations

Skin lesions consist of hyperkeratotic papules raging from 2 mm to 1 cm in diameter in a serpiginous distribution. Skin within these serpiginous arcs is often atrophic. The most common site of involvement is the neck, but lesions can also occur on the extremities and, more rarely, on the trunk. In rare instances systemic involvement occurs with involvement of elastic tissue in the endocardium, bronchiolar walls, and arteries. Rupture of the aorta has been reported.[33]

Elastosis perforans serpiginosa is associated with numerous inherited disorders including osteogenesis imperfecta,[34] cutis laxa,[35] acrogeria,[36] Ehlers-Danlos syndrome, Marfan's syndrome, Rothmund-Thompson syndrome,[37] and Down's syndrome.[26] It is also associated with pseudoxanthoma elasticum,[38,39] but at least one author has questioned that association,[40] believing that most reported cases of EPS in patients with pseudoxanthoma elasticum represent perforating pseudoxanthoma elasticum.

Histopathology

On pathologic examination of skin biopsy specimens, typical changes can be identified and consist of an inflammatory response around abnormal elastic tissue in the papillary dermis. The elastic tissue penetrates through channels in the acanthotic epidermis. The channels may be straight or tortuous, and there may be multinucleated giant cells in the surrounding inflammatory infiltrate. In addition to elastic tissue, the channels contain necrobiotic material with degenerated epithelial cells and parakeratotic nuclei of inflammatory cells. The top of the epidermal channels is also filled with keratotic material.

Therapy

While some have reported spontaneous disappearance of perforating disorders with stabilization of renal disease,[41] most of the perforating diseases continue for years unless treated. With renal transplantation, lesions can resolve.[42]

Both reactive perforating collagenosis[43,44] and Kyrle's disease[45] are reported to respond to topical retinoids, but these are not always effective. In patients refractory to topical therapy, phototherapy with UVB[46] and PUVA[47] are reported to clear the disease.

In recent years, oral retinoids, including isotretinoin[48] and acitretin,[49] have been used effectively for Kyrle's disease, and phototherapy has also been used effectively for perforating folliculitis.[23] Because some authors attribute perforating disorders to low serum levels of vitamin A, it should not be surprising that oral retinoids are effective. In fact, there is one report of perforating folliculitis improving dramatically upon treatment with oral vitamin A.[15] Other treatments that have been used for perforating disorders include surgical removal,[50] transcutaneous electrical nerve stimulation,[51] oral antibiotics, and topical corticosteroids.[23] Most recently, there have been several reports of success in treating perforating disorders with oral allopurinol.[52–54]

Many of the treatments that have been applied to the other perforating disorders have also been used for EPS. In recent years, isotretinoin has been used to treat this disorder.[55] Destructive modalities such as cryotherapy have been effective,[56] and, most recently, lasers have been used for EPS.[57,58]

Differential Diagnosis

Other perforating dermatoses can simulate the acquired perforating disorders. EPS is easily distinguished when characteristic serpiginous lesions are present and by the finding of elastic fibers in the perforating tissue on histology. In contrast to the other perforating dermatoses, which are usually associated with diabetes or renal failure, EPS has an entirely different group of disease associations as mentioned above.

Individual lesions of perforating pseudoxanthoma elasticum can simulate those of the acquired perforating dermatoses, but patients with pseudoxanthoma elasticum have characteristic yellow papules and plaques on the neck, axillae, and other flexural sites. Moreover, on skin biopsy, von Kossa stains show calcification of elastic fibers and Verhoeff van Gieson stains show fragmentation and clumping of elastic tissue. The lesions of perforating granuloma annulare can also simulate acquired perforating disorders, but on biopsy, palisading granulomas are seen. Flegel disease is characterized by keratotic papules, but these are smaller and usually involve the palms and soles. Histologically, this is not a perforating condition, but occasionally it has been confused with perforating disorders.[59]

EPS is easily distinguished from the acquired perforating disorders in that the latter conditions are often associated with diabetes and renal disease. There is a single case report of EPS in a patient with renal disease.[60] Histologically, however, the perforating elastic fibers of EPS usually allow differentiation although fragments of elastic fibers may be found in the necrobiotic plug of other perforating disorders. At least one study reports the transepidermal elimination of elastic fibers in follicular occlusion disease, distinguishing that disorder from EPS.[61] The differentiation of EPS from perforating pseudoxanthoma elasticum is easily accomplished because the eliminated elastic fibers in EPS are not calcified in contrast to the von Kossa–staining fibers of pseudoxanthoma elasticum.

REFERENCES

1. Poliak SC et al: Reactive perforating collagenosis associated with diabetes mellitus. *N Engl J Med* **306**:81, 1982
2. Harman M et al: Kyrle's disease in diabetes mellitus and chronic renal failure. *J Eur Acad Dermatol Venereol* **11**:87, 1998
3. Hurwitz RM et al: Perforating folliculitis in association with hemodialysis. *Am J Dermatopathol* **4**:101, 1982
4. Cochran RJ et al: Reactive perforating collagenosis of diabetes mellitus and renal failure. *Cutis* **31**:55, 1983
5. Rapini RP et al: Acquired perforating dermatosis. Evidence for combined transepidermal elimination of both collagen and elastic fibers. *Arch Dermatol* **125**:1074, 1989
6. Kyrle J: Über einen ungewöhnlichen fall von universeller folliculärer und parafollikulärer hyperkeratose (hyperkeratosis follicularis et parafollicularis in cutem penetrans). *Arch Dermatol Syph (Berlin)* **123**:466, 1916
7. Kren O: Keratosis follicularis in cutem penetrans (Kyrle). *Dermatology* **78**:57, 1924
8. Mehregan AH, Coskey RJ: Perforating folliculitis. *Arch Dermatol* **97**:394, 1968
9. Mehregan AH et al: Reactive perforating collagenosis. *Arch Dermatol* **96**:277, 1967
10. Bovenmyer DA: Reactive perforating collagenosis. Experimental production of the lesion. *Arch Derm* **102**:31, 1970
11. Kawakami T, Saito R: Acquired reactive perforating collagenosis associated with diabetes mellitus: Eight cases that meet Faver's criteria. *Br J Dermatol* **140**:521, 1999
12. Morgan MB et al: Fibronectin and the extracellular matrix in the perforating disorders of the skin. *Am J Dermatopathol* **20**:147, 1998
13. Saldanha LF et al: Silicon-related syndrome in dialysis patients. *Nephron* **77**:48, 1997
14. Neill SM et al: Phrynoderma and perforating folliculitis due to vitamin A deficiency in a diabetic. *J R Soc Med* **81**:171, 1988
15. Barr DJ et al: Bypass phrynoderma. Vitamin A deficiency associated with bowel-bypass surgery. *Arch Dermatol* **120**:919, 1984
16. Bardach HG: Generalized perforating folliculitis in chronic kidney insufficiency [in German]. *Hautarzt* **33**:584, 1982
17. Yanagihara M et al: The pathogenesis of the transepithelial elimination of the collagen bundles in acquired reactive perforating collagenosis. A light and electron microscopical study. *J Cutan Pathol* **23**:398, 1996
18. Herzinger T et al: Reactive perforating collagenosis—Transepidermal elimination of type IV collagen. *Clin Exp Dermatol* **21**:279, 1996
19. Alyahya GA et al: Ocular changes in a case of Kyrle's disease. 20-year follow-up. *Acta Ophthalmol Scand* **78**:585, 2000
20. Faver IR et al: Acquired reactive perforating collagenosis. Report of six cases and review of the literature. *J Am Acad Dermatol* **30**:575, 1994
21. Rubio FA et al: Perforating folliculitis: Report of a case in an HIV-infected man. *J Am Acad Dermatol* **40**:300, 1999
22. Kahana M et al: Perforating folliculitis in association with primary sclerosing cholangitis. *Am J Dermatopathol* **7**:271, 1985
23. Hurwitz RM: The evolution of perforating folliculitis in patients with chronic renal failure. *Am J Dermatopathol* **7**:231, 1985
24. Miescher G: Elastoma intrapapillare perforans verruciform. *Dermatologica* **110**:254, 1955
25. Dammet K, Putkonen T: Keratosis follicularis serpiginosa Lutz. *Dermatologica* **116**:143, 1958
26. Siragusa M et al: Localized elastosis perforans serpiginosa in a boy with Down syndrome. *Pediatr Dermatol* **14**:244, 1997
27. Hill VA et al: Penicillamine-induced elastosis perforans serpiginosa and cutis laxa in Wilson's disease. *Br J Dermatol* **142**:560, 2000
28. Sahn EE et al: D-Penicillamine–induced elastosis perforans serpiginosa in a child with juvenile rheumatoid arthritis. Report of a case and review of the literature. *J Am Acad Dermatol* **20**:979, 1989
29. Bardach H et al: "Lumpy-bumpy" elastic fibers in the skin and lungs of a patient with a penicillamine-induced elastosis perforans serpiginosa. *J Cutan Pathol* **6**:243, 1979
30. Ludatscher RM et al: Structural alterations of collagen fibrils in the reactive type of elastosis perforans serpiginosa. *Arch Dermatol Res* **280**:319, 1988
31. Holbrook KA, Byers PH: Structural abnormalities in the dermal collagen and elastic matrix of patients with inherited connective tissue disorders. *J Invest Dermatol* **79**:7s, 1982
32. Langeveld-Wildschut EG et al: Familial elastosis perforans serpiginosa. *Arch Dermatol* **129**:205, 1993
33. Eide J: Elastosis perforans serpiginosa with widespread arterial lesions: A case report. *Acta Derm Venereol* **57**:533, 1977
34. Relias A et al: Lutz-Miescher elastosis perforans serpiginosa and osteogenesis imperfecta. *Ann Dermatol Syph (Paris)* **95**:491, 1968
35. Korting GW: Elastosis perforans serpiginosa as an ectodermal border symptom in cutis laxa. *Arch Klin Exp Dermatol* **224**:437, 1966
36. Tafelkruyer J, Mees R: Acrogeria and elastosis perforans serpiginosa [proceedings] *Dermatologica* **156**:309, 1978
37. Mehregan AH: Elastosis perforans serpiginosa: A review of the literature and report of 11 cases. *Arch Dermatol* **97**:381, 1968
38. Katagiri K et al: Heterogeneity of clinical features of pseudoxanthoma elasticum: Analysis of thirteen cases in Oita Prefecture from a population of 1,240,000. *J Dermatol* **18**:211, 1991
39. Caro I et al: Pseudoxanthoma elasticum and elastosis perforans serpiginosa. Report of two cases. *Dermatologica* **150**:36, 1975
40. Lund HZ, Gilbert CF: Perforating pseudoxanthoma elasticum. Its distinction from elastosis perforans serpiginosa. *Arch Pathol Lab Med* **100**:544, 1976.
41. Chang P, Fernandez V: Acquired perforating disease: Report of nine cases. *Int J Dermatol* **32**:874, 1993
42. White CR Jr et al: Perforating folliculitis of hemodialysis. *Am J Dermatopathol* **4**:109, 1982
43. Cullen SI: Successful treatment of reactive perforating collagenosis with tretinoin. *Cutis* **23**:187, 1979
44. Berger RS: Reactive perforating collagenosis of renal failure/diabetes responsive to topical retinoic acid. *Cutis* **43**:540, 1989
45. Petrozzi JW, Warthan TL: Kyrle disease. Treatment with topically applied tretinoin. *Arch Dermatol* **110**:762, 1974
46. Vion B, Frenk E: Acquired reactive collagen disease in the adult: Successful treatment with UV-B light [in German]. *Hautarzt* **40**:448, 1989
47. Serrano G et al: Reactive perforating collagenosis responsive to PUVA. *Int J Dermatol* **27**:118, 1988
48. Saleh HA et al: Kyrle's disease. Effectively treated with Isotretinoin. *J Fla Med Assoc* **80**:395, 1993
49. Baumer FE et al: The Kyrle disease entity and its therapeutic modification by acitretin (etretin) [in German]. *Z Hautkr* **64**:286, 289, 1989.
50. Ford TC et al: Kyrle's disease. A rare case report and surgical treatment. *J Am Podiatr Med Assoc* **80**:151, 1990
51. Chan LY et al: Treatment of pruritus of reactive perforating collagenosis using transcutaneous electrical nerve stimulation. *Eur J Dermatol* **10**:59, 2000
52. Querings K et al: Treatment of acquired reactive perforating collagenosis with allopurinol. *Br J Dermatol* **145**:174, 2001

53. Munch M et al: Treatment of perforating collagenosis of diabetes and renal failure with allopurinol. *Clin Exp Dermatol* **25**:615, 2000
54. Kruger K et al: Acquired reactive perforating dermatosis. Successful treatment with allopurinol in 2 cases [in German]. *Hautarzt* **50**:115, 1999
55. Ratnavel RC, Norris PG: Penicillamine-induced elastosis perforans serpiginosa treated successfully with isotretinoin. *Dermatology* **189**:81, 1994
56. Tuyp EJ, McLeod WA: Elastosis perforans serpiginosa: treatment with liquid nitrogen. *Int J Dermatol* **29**:655, 1990
57. Kaufman AJ: Treatment of elastosis perforans serpiginosa with the flashlamp pulsed dye laser. *Dermatol Surg* **26**:1060, 2000
58. Abdullah A et al: Localized idiopathic elastosis perforans serpiginosa effectively treated by the Coherent Ultrapulse 5000C aesthetic laser. *Int J Dermatol* **39**:719, 2000
59. Price ML et al: Flegel's disease, not Kyrle's disease. *J Am Acad Dermatol* **18**:1366, 1988
60. Schamroth JM et al: Elastosis perforans serpiginosa in a patient with renal disease. *Arch Dermatol* **122**:82, 1986
61. Hyland CH, Kheir SM: Follicular occlusion disease with elimination of abnormal elastic tissue. *Arch Dermatol* **116**:925, 1980

SECTION 14
DISORDERS OF SUBCUTANEOUS TISSUE

CHAPTER 109

Michael J. Camilleri
W. P. Daniel Su

Panniculitis

The subcutaneous fat or panniculus adiposus is the cushioning tissue that lies between the dermis and the fascia. The subcutaneous fat has two important functions: a protective function from thermal and mechanical injuries and a metabolic function, acting as a depot of energy in the form of stored fat. The subcutaneous fat is composed of adipocytes and fibrocytes, which are embryologically derived from primitive mesenchymal cells. Mature adipocytes are characterized by polygonal-shaped cells that have a small dark eccentric nucleus and a large cytoplasmic lipid vacuole. Small cohesive collections of adipocytes form the primary microlobules, which aggregate into secondary lobules that are separated from each other by discernible fibrous septa or trabeculae. The pannicular fibrous septa contain blood vessels (arteries and veins), lymphatics, and nerves. Arteriolar branches from the septal arteries, which traverse between the pannicular lobules, give off a capillary network that surrounds each adipocyte[1,2] (see Chap. 6).

The panniculitides are a diverse group of cutaneous disorders that are characterized by an inflammatory process that predominantly affects the subcutaneous fat. A wide range of etiological factors may result in panniculitis[3] (Table 109-1). Weber-Christian disease (synonyms: idiopathic nodular panniculitis, nodular panniculitis, and relapsing febrile nonsuppurative nodular panniculitis) was formerly described as an idiopathic type of lobular panniculitis with mixed inflammation characterized by erythematous subcutaneous nodules, often accompanied by systemic involvement. Most authorities now agree that this type of panniculitis should no longer be considered as a distinctive entity, because an alternative specific cause of the lobular panniculitis is detected in most cases.[4,5] Lipoatrophy is characterized by atrophy of subcutaneous fat and may represent either an end-stage result of various inflammatory panniculitides or may be a primary process not associated with inflammation, also known as lipodystrophy.[5]

PANNICULITIS IN CONNECTIVE TISSUE DISORDERS

Lupus Panniculitis (See Chap. 171)

Lupus panniculitis (LP), also known as lupus profundus or Kaposi-Irgang disease, is an uncommon form of chronic cutaneous lupus erythematosus that is characterized by chronic, recurrent pannicular inflammation.[6]

HISTORICAL ASPECTS LP was first described by Kaposi in 1883, and the term lupus erythematosus profundus was coined by Irgang in 1940.[6]

EPIDEMIOLOGY LP is seen in 1 to 5 percent of patients with lupus erythematosus, with a mean age incidence of 40 years (age range: 30 to 60 years). Females are more commonly affected, with a 4:1 female-to-male ratio.[7]

CLINICAL MANIFESTATIONS The cutaneous lesions of LP are characterized by multiple, deep, symmetric, painful subcutaneous nodules or plaques that characteristically heal with persistent, large areas of depression or delling secondary to lipoatrophy (Fig. 109-1*A*). LP may be associated with an overlying chronic discoid lupus erythematosus (CDLE) lesion and may ulcerate. LP commonly affects the proximal upper and lower extremities, trunk, and head, but may also involve unusual sites, including the breast, orbital, and periparotid tissue.[3,6,7] Aggravating factors for LP include trauma (scars and injections) and ultraviolet radiation. LP may rarely present as morphea-like lesions, in a linear arrangement, or in association with neonatal lupus erythematosus (LE).[5]

LP may precede, occur simultaneous with, or follow discoid LE in 33 percent of LP.[7] In 10 percent of cases, LP may be associated with systemic LE.[7] The LE tends to be less severe and includes arthralgias, Raynaud's phenomenon, lymphadenopathy, pleurisy, and livedo reticularis.[6] Other autoimmune disorders associated with LP include Hashimoto's thyroiditis, chronic ulcerative colitis, and autoimmune hepatitis.[7]

LABORATORY FINDINGS Patients with LP may have a positive low-titer antinuclear antibody (65 percent), anti–double-stranded DNA antibody (15 percent), rheumatoid factor (12 percent) and anti-RNP (ribonucleoprotein) (14 percent). Leukopenia, an elevated sedimentation rate, a low total hemolytic complement activity (CH50), and a low C2 and C4 level have also been reported.[7]

PATHOLOGY The main histopathologic characteristic of LP is a predominantly lobular panniculitis without any vasculitis. In the early stages of LP, there is marked lobular (usually periseptal) inflammation composed of lymphocytic aggregates that are often arranged as lymphoid follicles with central germinal centers (Fig. 109-1*B*). The inflammatory infiltrate may also extend into the pannicular septa.

TABLE 109-1

Etiologic Classification of the Panniculitides[1,3]

Causes of Panniculitis	
Connective Tissue Disorders	***Noninfectious Granulomatous Panniculitides***
Lupus panniculitis	Erythema nodosum
Deep morphea and its variants	Subcutaneous sarcoidosis (Darier-Roussy sarcoid) (see Chap. 183)
Other connective tissue disorder-related panniculitides	Palisading granulomatous disorders
Vascular Disorders	Subcutaneous granuloma annulare (see Chap. 100)
Vasculitis	Necrobiosis lipoidica (see Chap. 168)
Polyarteritis nodosa (see Chap. 174)	Rheumatoid nodule (see Chap. 179)
Superficial thrombophlebitis (see Chap. 167)	Necrobiotic xanthogranuloma (see Chap. 161)
Nodular vasculitis	Metastatic Crohn's disease (see Chap. 164)
Leukocytoclastic vasculitis (see Chap. 175)	***Infectious Panniculitides*** (see also Chaps. 194, 196, 197, 200, 201, and 207)
Leprosy reactions—Erythema nodosum leprosum and Lucio's phenomenon (see Chap. 202)	***Physical Panniculitis***
Vascular Calcification	Traumatic panniculitis
Calciphylaxis	Cold panniculitis
Oxalosis	***Chemical/Foreign Body Panniculitis***
Sclerosing Panniculitis	***Childhood Panniculitides***
Other Systemic Disorders	Sclerema neonatorum
Pancreatic Panniculitis	Subcutaneous fat necrosis of the newborn
α_1-Antitrypsin deficiency-associated panniculitis	Poststeroid panniculitis
Gouty panniculitis (see Chap. 179)	
Cytophagic Histiocytic Panniculitis	***Lipodystrophy*** (see Chap. 110)

Lymphocytic vasculitis, lymphocytic nuclear dust, and eosinophils are also frequently noted. In more advanced stages of LP, there is hyaline fibrosis of the pannicular lobules and septa (Fig. 109-1*C*) with calcification, increased mucin deposition and a decrease in the degree of inflammation. Associated overlying epidermal and dermal changes of discoid lupus may also be observed.[5,6] Direct immunofluorescence demonstrates granular deposition of IgM, IgG, and C3 at the dermoepidermal junction (lupus band) in 70 percent of cases.[6]

TREATMENT AND PROGNOSIS The treatment of LP includes bed rest, avoidance of trauma, photoprotection, and the use of immunosuppressive agents.[6,7] Potent topical corticosteroids under occlusion,[8] intralesional and systemic corticosteroids,[7] antimalarials,[7] dapsone,[9] thalidomide,[10] cyclophosphamide,[7] and cyclosporine[11] have all been used with success. LP follows a chronic, recurrent course. Evidence exists supporting the possibility that some cases of LP may exhibit phenotypic and genomic abnormalities suggesting a subcuticular T cell lymphoid dyscrasia in which subcutaneous T cell lymphoma forms part of the spectrum.[12]

Deep Morphea (See Chap. 173)

Deep morphea (DM), also known as scleroderma panniculitis, is a fibrosing inflammatory process primarily involving the subcutaneous fat, with variable involvement of the deep dermis, fascia, and muscle. Various types of DM are described,[13] including:

- Subcutaneous morphea characterized by predominant involvement of the panniculus.
- Morphea profunda characterized by predominant involvement of both the panniculus and fascia.
- Eosinophilic fasciitis characterized by predominant involvement of the fascia with extension into the panniculus and muscle (see Chap. 173).
- Pansclerotic morphea of childhood, characterized by involvement of the deep dermis, panniculus, fascia, muscle and bone (see Chap. 173).

ETIOLOGY AND PATHOGENESIS Most cases of DM are idiopathic, although a number of specific factors have been observed in some variants of DM. In eosinophilic fasciitis, prior physical exertion has been observed in 50 percent of cases.[13] Toxins such as L-tryptophan in eosinophilia-myalgia syndrome, and ingestion of adulterated rapeseed oil in toxic-oil syndrome, are also implicated. Other etiologic agents for DM variants include infections (acute brucellosis[14] and Lyme disease), malignancies (lymphoproliferative malignancies, breast and prostate carcinoma) in cancer-associated fasciitis panniculitis,[15] radiation (postirradiation pseudosclerodermatous panniculitis[16]), and the late stage of graft-versus-host disease.

CLINICAL MANIFESTATIONS The cutaneous manifestations of DM include stable or progressively enlarging, bound down, indurated plaques or nodules, which heal with atrophy and hyperpigmentation. The sites of involvement vary with the clinical subtype, predominantly involving the proximal upper extremities and trunk in subcutaneous morphea and morphea profunda (Fig. 109-2*A*), bilateral forearms and legs in eosinophilic fasciitis, and generalized in pansclerotic morphea of childhood.[13]

PATHOLOGY The main histopathologic manifestations of DM include a predominantly septal panniculitis without vasculitis. The histologic hallmark of the disease is marked fibrous thickening of the pannicular septa with lymphoplasmacytic inflammatory aggregates at the septal–lobular junction (Fig. 109-2*B*). The homogenous, eosinophilic, thickened collagen bundles replace the fat surrounding adnexal structures, which also become atrophic. Calcification may also be seen.[13]

TREATMENT AND PROGNOSIS Therapeutic modalities for the treatment of DM include intralesional corticosteroids, systemic corticosteroids, antimalarials, penicillamine, and methotrexate. Usually, DM's response to treatment is poor with progressive sclerosis and atrophy of the affected areas.[13]

FIGURE 109–1

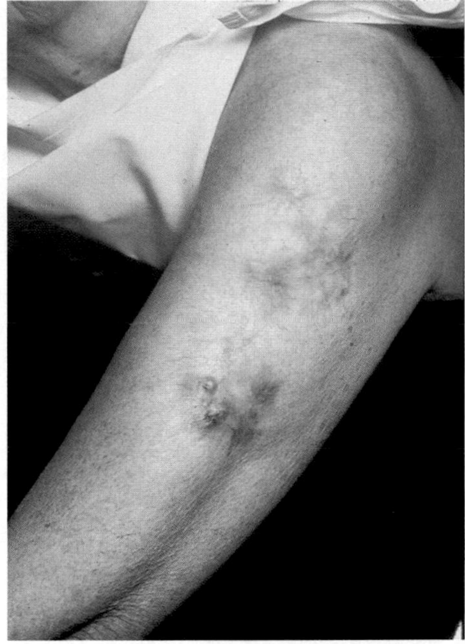

A.

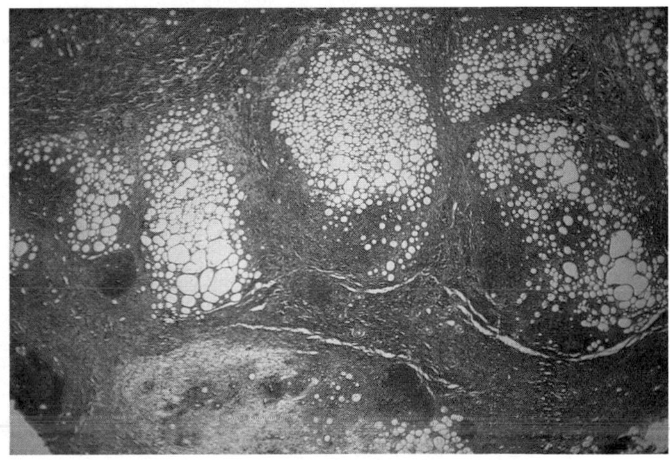

B.

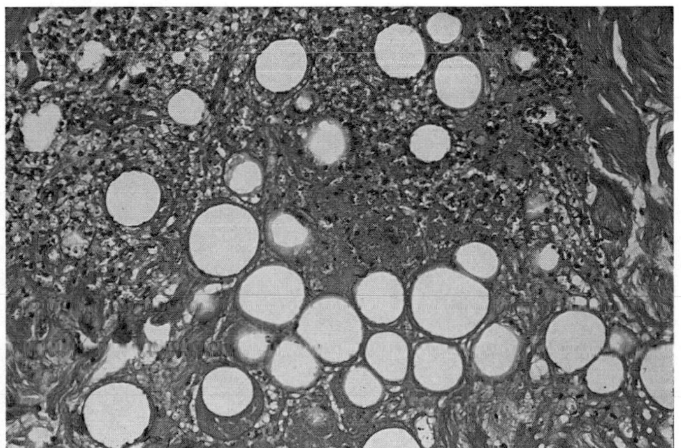

C.

Lupus panniculitis. *A.* Erythematous nodules with central delling (lipoatrophy) involving the lateral arm. Histopathologic features of (*B*) early lupus panniculitis with lobular lymphocytic pannicular inflammation and lymphoid follicle formation and (*C*) more advanced lupus panniculitis with the characteristic hyaline fibrosis of pannicular lobules.

Other Connective Tissue Disease–Associated Panniculitides

Dermatomyositis is rarely associated with either a lobular lipophagic panniculitis secondary to subcutaneous calcification or a lymphoplasmacytic lobular panniculitis with hyaline sclerosis, similar to LP.[17]

Sjögren's syndrome is rarely associated with a lobular panniculitis, characterized by a granulomatous, lymphocytic or plasma cell–rich inflammatory infiltrate.[18]

Mixed connective tissue disease is also associated with a lobular lipophagic panniculitis secondary to subcutaneous calcification.[19]

VASCULAR DISORDERS

Nodular Vasculitis

Nodular vasculitis (NV), is a reactive inflammatory lobular panniculitis associated with vasculitis.

HISTORICAL ASPECTS Erythema induratum was first described in 1861 by Bazin, and in 1900, French dermatologists linked this condition to tuberculosis, including it with the tuberculids. In 1905, Whitfield described cases of erythema induratum without any associated tuberculosis and in 1945, Montgomery, O'Leary, and Barker proposed the term *nodular vasculitis* for these cases of erythema induratum. A consensus has been reached considering erythema induratum of Bazin, erythema induratum of Whitfield, and nodular vasculitis as the same entity.[5]

EPIDEMIOLOGY NV is an uncommon condition that mainly affects obese middle-aged females,[3] who also have venous insufficiency. The incidence of NV has risen with the reemergence of tuberculosis due to the HIV pandemic.[20]

ETIOLOGY AND PATHOGENESIS NV is a reactive, probably immune complex-mediated vasculitis, which results in ischemic injury of fat with secondary pannicular necrosis and inflammation. The most common cause of NV is tuberculosis, but cases without any evidence of a tuberculous focus have also been described (see Chap. 200). Most nontuberculous cases are idiopathic, but case reports of NV associated with underlying hepatitis C infection[21] and propylthiouracil[22] have been described. Rheumatoid arthritis rarely has been associated with a lobular panniculitis with vasculitis similar to NV (neutrophilic lobular panniculitis or pustular panniculitis associated with rheumatoid arthritis).[23]

CLINICAL MANIFESTATIONS The main cutaneous manifestations of NV include recurrent, bilateral, painful, erythematous subcutaneous nodules and plaques that commonly affect the posterior legs, but which also may affect the thighs, as well as other sites of the body. The lesions characteristically become bluish-red in color and break down into slowly healing ulcers with violaceous margins, eventually resulting in atrophic scars (Fig. 109-3*A*). The condition tends to occur in cold, winter months and has a prolonged recurrent course, with new crops of lesions occurring at irregular intervals, and it may last for many years. Associated erythrocyanosis, cutis marmorata, perifollicular erythema, features of venous insufficiency, and swollen, column-like calves may be observed. Individuals with NV tend to have no systemic involvement.[3,5]

LABORATORY FINDINGS Patients with NV should be evaluated for tuberculosis with a chest x-ray and a tuberculin test.

FIGURE 109-2

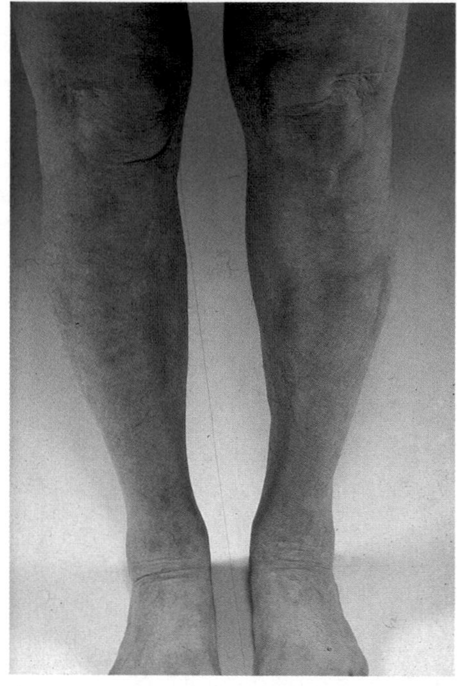

A.

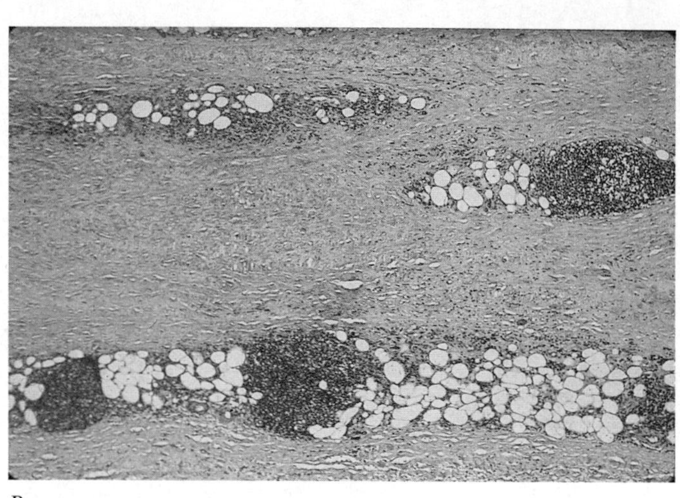

B.

Deep morphea. *A.* Bilateral, bound down, indurated plaques with atrophy and hyperpigmentation involving the legs. Histopathologic features of deep morphea with fibrous thickening of the pannicular septa and lymphoplasmacytic aggregates at the septal–lobular junction.

FIGURE 109-3

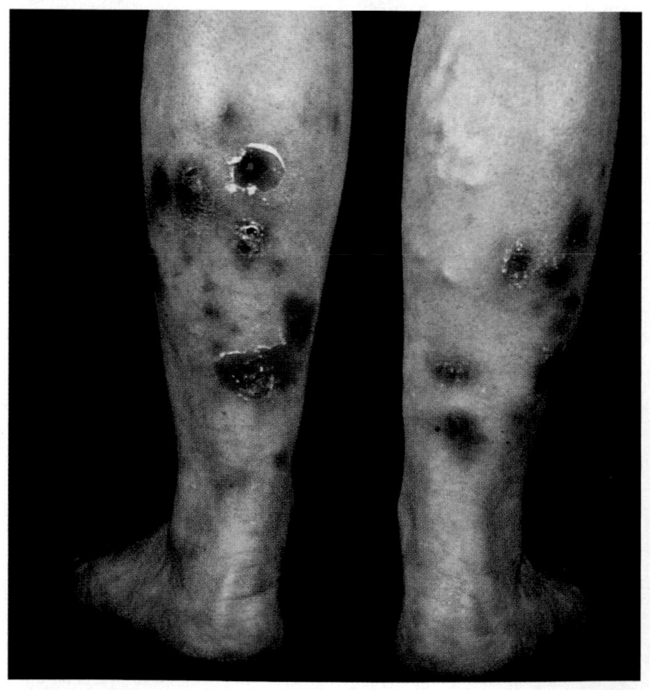

A.

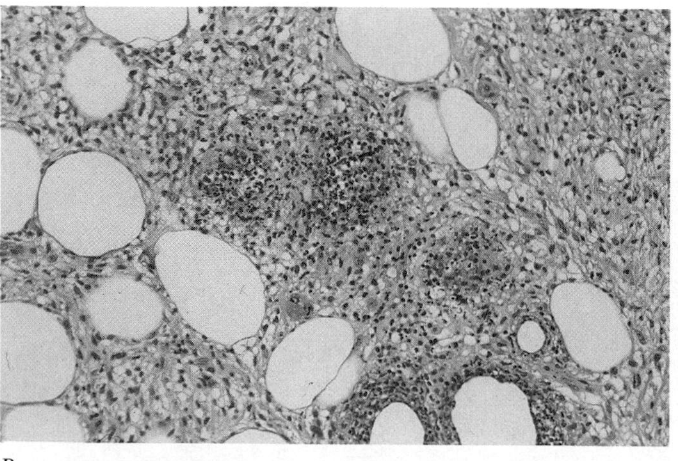

B.

Nodular vasculitis. *A.* Note overall configuration of the legs, deep-seated erythematous and bluish nodules, ulceration, and scarring. *B.* Histopathologic features of nodular vasculitis with a mixed lobular panniculitis and neutrophilic vasculitis.

PATHOLOGY NV is characterized histopathologically by a predominantly lobular panniculitis with vasculitis. There is an intense neutrophilic vasculitis of blood vessels (both arteriolar and venular) of different sizes in both the septa and lobules (Fig. 109-3*B*). In early lesions, there is a neutrophil-rich inflammatory infiltrate with extensive fat necrosis. In later lesions, there is a granulomatous inflammatory infiltrate composed of foamy histiocytes, epithelioid histiocytes and multinucleated giant cells in association with caseation necrosis, The inflammatory infiltrate may extend to the dermis and results in epidermal ulceration. In advanced cases, the inflammatory infiltrate is replaced by fibrosis.[5] In those cases associated with tuberculosis, *Mycobacterium tuberculosis* complex DNA may be demonstrated by polymerase chain reaction (PCR) within the cutaneous biopsy specimen.[24]

TREATMENT AND PROGNOSIS All cases of NV require bed rest and nonsteroidal anti-inflammatory agents for pain. Further treatment of NV depends on the underlying cause. Triple-agent antituberculous therapy is indicated in NV associated with evidence of a tuberculous infection. NV not associated with tuberculosis may be treated with systemic steroids, tetracycline, or potassium iodide.[25]

Calciphylaxis

Calciphylaxis, also known as calcifying panniculitis and vascular calcification-cutaneous necrosis syndrome, is a necrotic and ulcerative form of panniculitis resulting from ischemia secondary to calcification of the cutaneous vessel walls.

HISTORICAL ASPECTS In 1962, Selye[26] described the pathogenic factors leading to calciphylaxis in an animal experimental model. He observed that two requirements were needed: a critical period of sensitization by a variety of factors (parathyroid hormone, vitamin D, and a high calcium and phosphorus diet, all potentiated by nephrotoxic agents) followed by exposure to a challenging agent (trauma, metal salts, glucocorticoids, albumin, and mast cell degranulators).

EPIDEMIOLOGY Calciphylaxis occurs in about 4 percent of patients on hemodialysis. The mean age affected is 50 years and there is a predilection in females and whites.[27]

ETIOLOGY AND PATHOGENESIS Ischemic necrosis and ulceration of the skin in calciphylaxis occurs as a result of medial calcification, intimal hyperplasia and occlusion of the small cutaneous arterioles.[27] The most common cause of calciphylaxis is end-stage chronic renal failure (ESRF), with associated secondary hyperparathyroidism and raised calcium-phosphorus product. Precipitating factors for calciphylaxis in ESRF include arterial hypertension, obesity, diabetes mellitus, trauma, corticosteroids, immunosuppression, posthemodialysis metabolic alkalosis, and hypercoagulable defects, especially protein C and S deficiency.[27] Calciphylaxis may occur in patients with ESRF and normal calcium and phosphorus levels. Calciphylaxis may rarely occur in individuals with normal renal function, including patients with primary hyperparathyroidism,[28] malignancies (metastatic breast carcinoma,[29] cholangiocarcinoma,[30] and multiple myeloma[31]) and end-stage liver disease.[32]

CLINICAL MANIFESTATIONS The early lesions of calciphylaxis include symmetric, violaceous, mottled to reticulated patches and plaques (livedo reticularis-like) with occasional bullae. The lesions most commonly involve the lower extremities (especially the thighs), but other less-common sites of involvement include the upper extremities, trunk, and penis. As the lesions evolve, they become indurated, necrotic plaques that break down into very painful, large, deep, nonhealing ulcers covered with black eschar[33] (Fig. 109-4*A*). Associated ischemic digital pain and gangrene has also been described. Calciphylaxis may rarely affect extracutaneous sites, particularly the eyes and the tracheal mucosa (tracheopathia chondro-osteoplastica).[5,27]

FIGURE 109-4

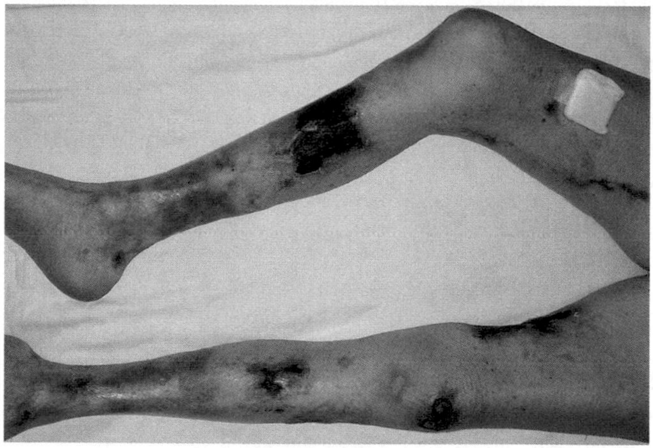

A.

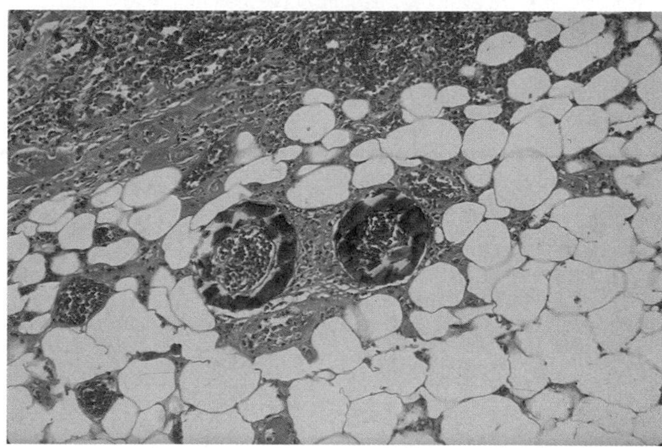

B.

Calciphylaxis. *A.* Bilateral necrotic, ulcerating plaques with black eschar. *B.* Histopathologic features of calciphylaxis with lobular inflammation and medial vascular wall calcification.

LABORATORY FINDINGS Patients with calciphylaxis often have end-stage renal failure with elevated creatinine, BUN, and parathyroid hormone, as well as elevated calcium and phosphorus levels. Radiographs of affected areas may demonstrate vascular calcification.

PATHOLOGY Calciphylaxis is characterized by a predominantly lobular panniculitis without any vasculitis. Vascular wall calcification, capillary congestion, prominent fat necrosis, and lobular calcification accompany a sparse lobular inflammatory infiltrate composed of lymphocytes, neutrophils and foamy histiocytes. The vascular wall calcification (Fig. 109-4*B*) is the histopathologic hallmark of calciphylaxis and usually consists of segmental or circumferential calcium depositions in the media of small- to medium-sized arteries/arterioles in the reticular dermis and pannicular septa. Associated overlying dermal and epidermal necrosis is usually seen. Pseudoxanthoma elasticum-like elastic fiber calcification in the lower dermis and pannicular septa has also been observed in some cases of calciphylaxis.[5]

TREATMENT AND PROGNOSIS Calciphylaxis has a poor prognosis with a mortality rate of up to 60 to 70 percent, this being mainly caused by sepsis that results from secondary infection of the necrotic ulcers. Proximal extremity and truncal involvement are poor prognostic factors as compared to distal extremity involvement. Supportive therapy is of utmost importance in the treatment of calciphylaxis and includes wound care, control of the ESRF and the prevention and treatment of secondary hyperparathyroidism.[27] Parathyroidectomy[34,35] and hyperbaric oxygen therapy[36,37] reportedly are effective in the treatment of calciphylaxis. Studies are underway to assess the therapeutic efficacy of hyperbaric oxygen therapy with subcutaneous fractionated heparin.[27]

Oxalosis

Oxalosis is a rare crystal deposition disorder characterized by the accumulation and deposition of calcium oxalate crystals, which may result in histopathologic features similar to calciphylaxis: a lobular panniculitis with both vascular and extravascular calcification. There are two main types of oxalosis: primary and secondary oxalosis. Primary oxalosis, which presents with miliary, palmar deposits, is an autosomal recessive genetic disorder. Secondary oxalosis, which presents with livedo reticularis and digital gangrene, occurs in association with chronic renal failure, intestinal disease, excessive oxalate/glycolic acid ingestion, methoxyflurane anesthesia, and ethylene glycol poisoning. Both forms of oxalosis may result in a crystal deposition arthropathy and renal failure.[5]

Sclerosing Panniculitis

Sclerosing panniculitis (SP), also known as hypodermatitis sclerodermiformis, lipodermatosclerosis, lipomembranous change in chronic panniculitis, venous stasis panniculitis, and sclerous atrophic cellulitis, is a chronic form of lower extremity panniculitis associated with venous insufficiency[38] (see Chap. 167).

EPIDEMIOLOGY SP is a common cause of panniculitis most commonly affecting obese middle-aged to elderly females.[39]

ETIOLOGY AND PATHOGENESIS SP results from venous insufficiency of the lower extremity, this leading to decreased venous return with sludging of the blood in the lobular capillaries, thus resulting in pannicular ischemia, fat necrosis, and fibrosis. Venous insufficiency commonly results from varicose veins or deep venous thrombosis.

CLINICAL MANIFESTATIONS The cutaneous manifestations of SP are characterized by a clinical spectrum with an acute inflammatory phase at one end and a chronic fibrotic stage at the other end.[40] Progressive, symmetric, erythematous, woodlike, indurated plaques that involve the lower extremities in a stocking distribution characterize the acute phase. Associated features of lower extremity stasis including edema, telangiectasia, hyperpigmentation, dermatitis, and ulceration commonly accompany the acute phase of SP. As the disease advances there is extensive sclerosis and atrophy of the subcutaneous tissue resulting in an inverted champagne bottle deformity[5,38] (see Chap. 167).

LABORATORY FINDINGS Venous Doppler ultrasound studies will reveal incompetence of the lower extremity veins.

PATHOLOGY The main histopathologic finding of SP is a predominantly lobular panniculitis without any vasculitis. There is septal thickening and sclerosis with atrophy of the fat lobules surrounded by a lipophagic granulomatous inflammatory infiltrate composed of lymphocytes, plasma cells and foamy histiocytes. The atrophic fat lobules are characterized by fatty microcysts lined by an amorphous, PAS-positive, eosinophilic corrugated membrane, known as lipomembranous or membranocystic change.[5,39] Although the latter finding is characteristic for SP, it is not diagnostic because it is seen as a late feature in other panniculitides.[39] Overlying dermal angioplasia and fibrosis are also observed.

TREATMENT AND PROGNOSIS The management of SP includes treating venous insufficiency with leg elevation, elastic compression stockings (20 to 40 mmHg); in some difficult cases, the condition may be improved with the additional use of the fibrinolytic agent, stanozol.[5,38]

OTHER PANNICULITIDES ASSOCIATED WITH SYSTEMIC DISORDER

Pancreatic Panniculitis

Pancreatic panniculitis (PP) is a panniculitis that results from the saponification of fat as a result of the release of pancreatic enzymes in pancreatic disease.

EPIDEMIOLOGY PP is rare, occurring in 2 to 3 percent of all patients with pancreatic disorders.[41] The average age incidence of PP is 60 years and males are affected more commonly than females, especially in cases associated with pancreatic carcinoma (5:1), but also, to a lesser extent, in cases associated with pancreatitis (3:1).[42]

ETIOLOGY AND PATHOGENESIS The most common pancreatic disorders associated with PP are acute or chronic pancreatitis (especially alcohol-related) and pancreatic carcinoma (usually the acinar cell type and less frequently the islet cell type). Rarely, other pancreatic disorders may be associated with PP, including pancreatic pseudocysts, pancreas divisum (unfused ducts of Wirsung and Santorini), and vascular-pancreatic fistulas.[5,42] The released pancreatic enzymes (particularly lipases) are thought to result in pannicular fat necrosis by saponification and secondary pannicular inflammation.

CLINICAL MANIFESTATIONS The cutaneous lesions of PP include multiple, variably painful, erythematous, fluctuant subcutaneous nodules that tend to ulcerate and exude a brown oily material (Fig. 109-5*A*). The most common sites of involvement of PP are the distal extremities (knees and ankles), although the proximal lower extremities, abdomen, and arms may also be affected. PP associated with a pancreatic carcinoma tends to be more extensive, more persistent, more recurrent, and more ulcerative than cases associated with pancreatitis.[5,42] Systemic manifestations of PP include periarticular fat necrosis with secondary acute arthritis, especially of the ankles (60 percent) polyserositis (pleuritis, peritonitis, and pericarditis), fat necrosis of the bone marrow, and mesenteric thrombosis.[42]

LABORATORY FINDINGS Diagnostic findings that demonstrate pancreatic disease include elevated serum pancreatic enzymes (amylase and lipase) and pancreatic imaging (ultrasonography or computed tomographic scan). A leukemoid reaction and eosinophilia are common findings in association with PP.[42]

PATHOLOGY The main histopathologic feature of PP is a predominantly lobular panniculitis without any vasculitis. A predominantly neutrophilic lobular inflammatory infiltrate is seen surrounding a characteristic type of fat necrosis—saponification of fat (Fig. 109-5*B*). This pancreatic fat necrosis is characterized by a collection of ghost adipocytes, which are anucleate and contain intracytoplasmic fine,

FIGURE 109-5

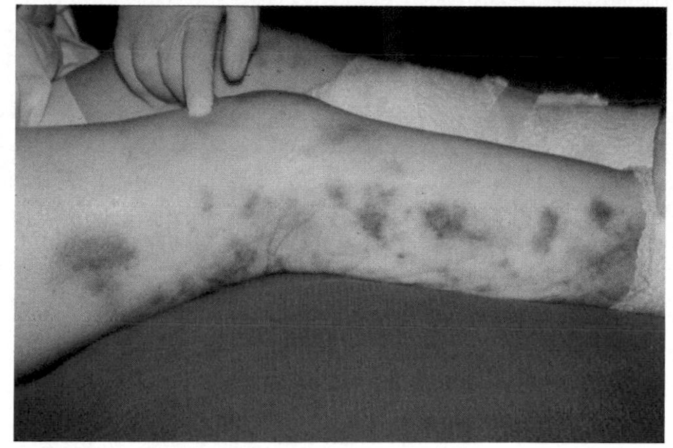

A.

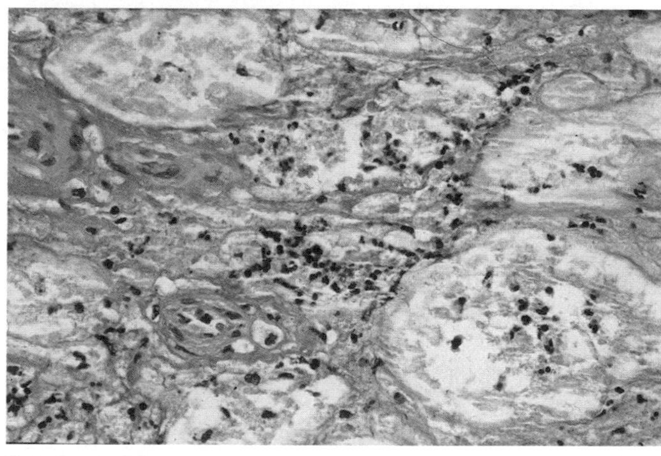

B.

Pancreatic panniculitis. *A.* Erythematous, ulcerating nodules in lower extremity. *B.* Histopathologic features of pancreatic panniculitis with saponification necrosis and neutrophilic pannicular inflammation.

basophilic granular material (calcification) from saponification of the fat secondary to the action of the pancreatic enzymes. In more advanced lesions, the infiltrate is more granulomatous (foamy histiocytes and multinucleated giant cells) and fewer ghost cells are observed.[5,42]

TREATMENT AND PROGNOSIS The mainstay of treatment of PP is treatment of the underlying pancreatic disorder, which may include surgery.[43] The prognosis is worse for cases of PP associated with pancreatic carcinoma.

α_1-Antitrypsin Deficiency–Associated Panniculitis

α_1-Antitrypsin deficiency–associated panniculitis (α_1-ATDP) is a rare form of panniculitis that results from the uncontrolled activity of proteases on the subcutaneous tissue as a result of a deficiency in the serine proteinase inhibitor, α_1-antitrypsin (α_1-AT).

EPIDEMIOLOGY α_1-ATDP is a rare type of panniculitis that is usually seen in adults. It has no sexual predilection.

ETIOLOGY AND PATHOGENESIS α_1-ATDP results from a deficiency of the serine proteinase inhibitor α_1-AT (α_1 proteinase inhibitor). This hepatic-derived enzyme normally inhibits the activity of a number of serine proteases including trypsin, chymotrypsin, plasmin, thrombin, neutrophilic elastase, pancreatic elastase, collagenase, factor VII, and kallikrein. It is thought that the unchecked overactivity of these enzymes, particularly elastases and collagenase, will result in damage to the skin, as well as activation of lymphocytes and phagocytes, thus resulting in severe inflammation and necrosis. Trauma is a common precipitant of α_1-ATDP.[44]

GENETICS α_1-AT deficiency is inherited in an autosomal codominant fashion. There are 33 different alleles for the gene for α_1-AT, the commonest being the M, S, and Z alleles. Individuals with the phenotype, PiMM have normal levels of α_1-AT, whereas those individuals with the PiZZ phenotype have a severe deficiency.[44] The PiMS and PiMZ heterozygote phenotypes are associated with a moderate deficiency of α_1-AT. α_1-ATDP usually occurs in individuals with the homozygous phenotype PiZZ, although reports of α_1-ATDP occurring in association with other phenotypes (PiMZ, PiSS,[45] PiSZ[46]) have also been described.

CLINICAL MANIFESTATIONS The cutaneous lesions of α_1-ATDP are characterized by ill-defined, subcutaneous, erythematous nodules or plaques (similar to cellulitis) commonly seen on the lower extremities, arms, trunk, and face. The lesions commonly ulcerate, exuding an oily material (derived from necrotic adipocytes),[44,45,47] and heal with atrophic scars. They are commonly seen in sites of trauma (Fig. 109-6*A*). Other cutaneous manifestations of α_1-ATDP include vasculitis, acquired angioedema, severe psoriasis, and Marshall's syndrome (Sweet's syndrome and acquired cutis laxa).[5] Systemic manifestations of α_1-AT deficiency include emphysema, hepatitis (commonly neonatal) and cirrhosis.[5]

LABORATORY FINDINGS Low levels of α_1-AT and an abnormal phenotype are the key tests for the diagnosis of this form of panniculitis.

PATHOLOGY α_1-ATDP is characterized histopathologically by a predominantly lobular panniculitis without vasculitis. Early lesions consist of focal areas of severe fat necrosis associated with a predominantly neutrophilic lobular inflammatory infiltrate (Fig. 109-6*B*), surrounded by large areas of normal adipose tissue. Within the overlying reticular dermis of early lesions, there is splaying of the collagen bundles by an interstitial neutrophilic inflammatory infiltrate (Fig. 109-6*C*).[5,44,48] Late lesions are characterized by replacement of fat lobules by an infiltrate of lymphocytes and foamy histiocytes and fibrosis.

PROGNOSIS AND TREATMENT Effective therapies that have been used for α_1-ATDP include dapsone,[49] systemic corticosteroids,[44] doxycycline,[46] minocycline,[50] intravenous infusions of exogenous α_1-protease inhibitor concentrate[44,45,51] (60 mg/kg per week), and liver transplantation.[52] Trauma or surgical débridement should be avoided, as well as smoking and exposure to potential hepatotoxins. The prognosis of α_1-ATDP is poor when there is associated pulmonary and hepatic involvement.

CYTOPHAGIC HISTIOCYTIC PANNICULITIS

Cytophagic histiocytic panniculitis (CHP) is a biologically aggressive, autonomous cellular proliferation affecting the panniculus and is characterized by a cytokine-driven histiocytic cytophagocytosis.[53]

HISTORICAL ASPECTS Winkelmann and Bowie first described CHP in 1980.[54]

EPIDEMIOLOGY CHP is a rare form of panniculitis that is most commonly seen in middle-aged to elderly individuals.[55]

FIGURE 109-6

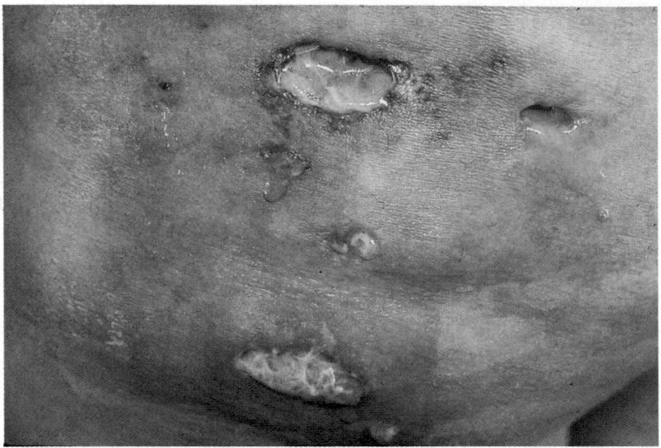

A.

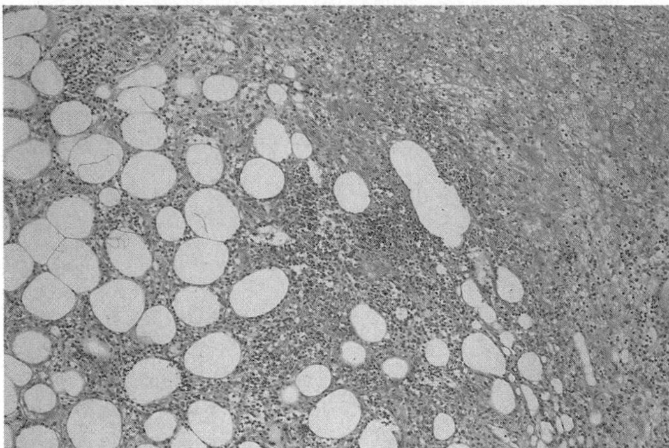

B.

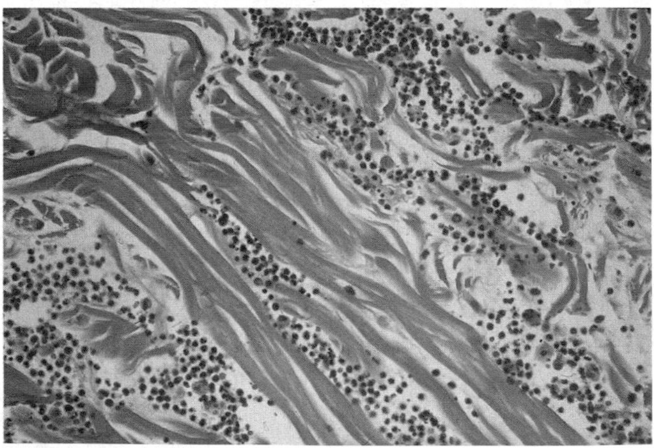

C.

α_1-Antitrypsin deficiency–associated panniculitis. *A.* Subcutaneous, erythematous, ulcerating nodules exuding an oily material. Histopathologic features include neutrophilic lobular pannicular inflammation (*B*) and splaying of collagen in the pannicular septa (*C*).

ETIOLOGY AND PATHOGENESIS The current concept of CHP is that it represents a spectrum of lymphoproliferative disorders that characteristically induce secondary histiocytic cytophagocytosis. Histiocytes are stimulated to undertake cytophagocytosis by a number of cytokines, especially interferon-γ and macrophage inflammatory protein-1α (MIP-1α). Nonneoplastic and neoplastic lymphocytes, endothelial cells, and macrophages themselves elaborate these cytokines.

Studies suggest that CHP represents an early stage of a lymphoproliferative disorder, where the underlying lymphoid clone is difficult to detect, but in which there is a natural progression to develop into a lymphoma.[20,56] In most cases, this non-Hodgkin's lymphoma is a subcutaneous panniculitic T cell lymphoma (SPTL), with either the α/β or the γ/δ cytophenotypes. Rarely, natural killer cell lymphoma (NKL) or some B cell lymphomas have also been described. Epstein-Barr virus infection is associated with CHP, especially those cases associated with SPTL or NKL.[53] Exogenous interferon therapy and the altered immunologic milieu in bone marrow transplantation are associated with CHP[53] (see Chap. 158).

CLINICAL MANIFESTATIONS The main cutaneous manifestations of CHP are multiple, large erythematous, subcutaneous plaques and nodules, which commonly have associated overlying ecchymoses and spontaneous ulcerations. The main sites of involvement include the upper and lower extremities (Fig. 109-7*A*) and, to a lesser extent, the trunk and face. Associated features of the hemophagocytic syndrome (HPS) include pyrexia, weight loss, lymphadenopathy, hepatosplenomegaly, pancytopenia, and a consumptive coagulopathy.[3,5,20,55,57]

LABORATORY FINDINGS CHP is characterized by the laboratory findings of HPS—characterized by pancytopenia, elevated liver enzymes, and a consumptive coagulopathy.

PATHOLOGY The main histopathologic manifestation of CHP is a predominantly lobular panniculitis without vasculitis. The inflammatory infiltrate is composed of lymphocytes and histiocytes, the latter exhibiting the pathognomonic finding of cytophagocytosis that is characterized by intrahistiocytic intact and fragmented erythrocytes, leukocytes, and lymphocytes—"bean-bag" cells (Fig. 109-7*B*). The lymphocytes have a benign morphology in CHP, while they are atypical in SPTL, usually forming a ring around the necrotic adipocytes.[3,5,55]

TREATMENT AND PROGNOSIS The prognosis and treatment of CHP depends on two main poor prognostic factors: (1) the presence of HPS and (2) the presence of an underlying lymphoma. In cases of CHP not associated with these poor prognostic factors, prednisone, potassium iodide, and cyclosporine have been used with success. Multiagent chemotherapy with CHOP (cyclophosphamide, doxorubicin, vincristine, and prednisone) combined with cyclosporine is used in cases of CHP associated with HPS or an underlying lymphoma.[57]

NONINFECTIOUS GRANULOMATOUS PANNICULITIDES

Erythema Nodosum

Erythema nodosum (EN) is a reactive dermatosis that occurs in response to a myriad of conditions, characterized by tender, erythematous subcutaneous nodules primarily affecting the lower extremities.

HISTORICAL ASPECTS Willan, in 1798, with further contributions by Wilson in 1842 and Hebra in 1866, first described EN. Several variants of EN were described: erythema nodosum migrans by Bafverstedt

FIGURE 109-7

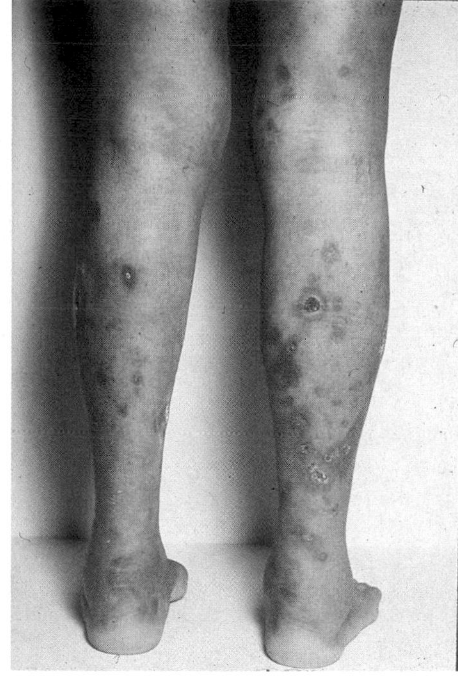

A.

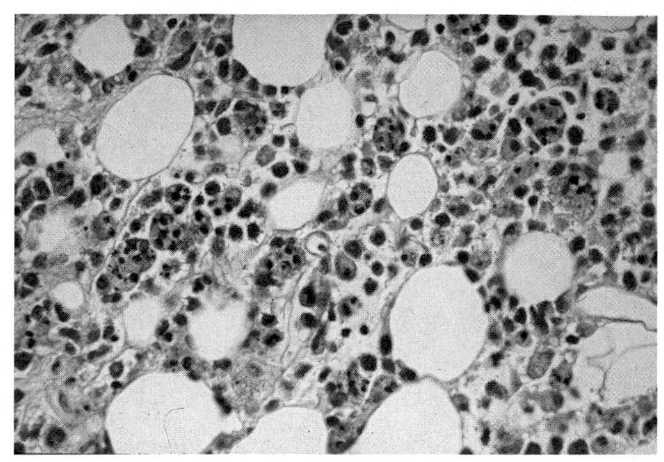

B.

Cytophagic histiocytic panniculitis. *A.* Multiple, ulcerating erythematous nodules and plaques involving the lower extremities. *B.* Histopathologic features with mixed lobular pannicular inflammation and the pathognomonic feature of cytophagocytosis—"bean-bag" cells.

in 1954, and acute nodular migratory panniculitis by Vilanova and Pinol in 1956, and by Perry and Winkelmann in 1964. The term *chronic erythema nodosum* was coined by Fine and Meltzer, in 1969, to encompass both erythema nodosum migrans and acute nodular migratory panniculitis.[1]

EPIDEMIOLOGY EN is the most common type of panniculitis, with a peak age incidence of 20 to 30 years. Females are three to six times more commonly affected than males. However, any age may be affected, and in children, there is less of a female predominance.[1,3]

ETIOLOGY AND PATHOGENESIS EN is a reactive hypersensitivity reaction that may occur in response to a number of antigenic stimuli. Table 109-2 presents an extensive list of the various reported causes of EN.[1] Streptococcal infections are the leading cause of EN in children, while in adults, the most common causes of EN include drugs, sarcoidosis, and inflammatory bowel disease. The underlying cause of EN may also be idiopathic.[1]

CLINICAL MANIFESTATIONS EN is characterized by the sudden onset of symmetric, painful, erythematous, warm, nonulcerating nodules and plaques commonly affecting the knees, shins, and ankles (Fig. 109-8*A*), but they may also be seen on the thighs, arms, face, and neck. As the lesions of EN advance, they become flat and undergo color changes similar to a bruise, becoming purple after a few days and then acquiring a greenish-yellow hue. EN lesions finally resolve without any scarring or atrophy. Associated systemic manifestations include pyrexia, malaise, headache, cough, arthralgias, conjunctivitis, and gastrointestinal upset. Recurrent episodes of EN frequently occur.[1,3]

A variant of EN is chronic erythema nodosum (synonyms: erythema nodosum migrans and subacute nodular migratory panniculitis) that is characterized by unilateral subcutaneous nodules or plaques, which are fewer, less tender, and more persistent than those in classic EN. The

TABLE 109-2

Causes of Erythema Nodosum[1,3]

Infections	Other
Bacterial	***Drugs***
Streptococcal infections	Sulfonamides
Tuberculosis	Bromides and iodides
Yersiniosis	Oral contraceptives
Other: Salmonella, campylobacter, shigella, brucellosis, psittacosis, and mycoplasma	Other: Minocycline, gold salts, penicillin, and salicylates
Fungal	***Malignancies***
Coccidioidomycosis, blastomycosis, histoplasmosis, sporotrichosis, and dermatophytosis	Hodgkin's and non-Hodgkin's lymphoma, leukemia, renal cell carcinoma
Viral	***Other***
Infectious mononucleosis, hepatitis B, orf, and herpes simplex	Sarcoidosis
	Inflammatory bowel disease: ulcerative colitis and Crohn's disease
Other	Behçet's disease
Amebiasis, giardiasis, and ascariasis	

FIGURE 109-8

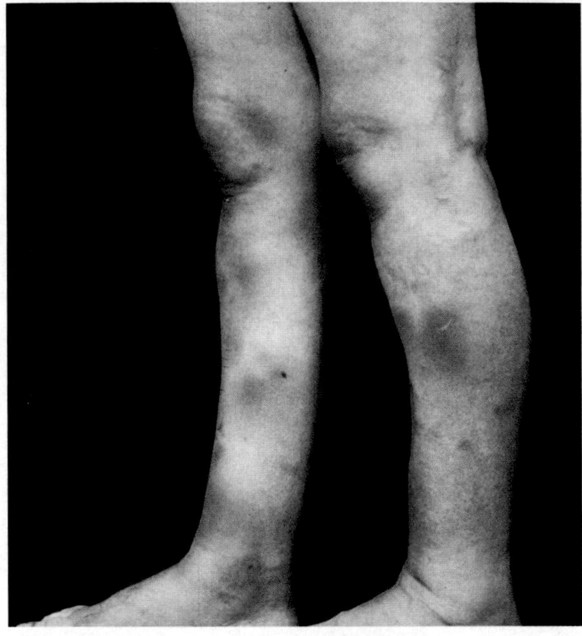

A.

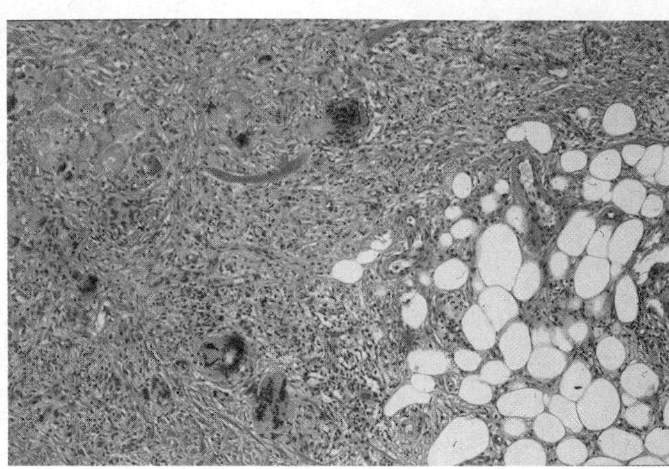

B.

Erythema nodosum. *A.* Bilateral erythematous nodules in lower extremities. *B.* Histopathologic features of erythema nodosum with a granulomatous septal panniculitis.

individual lesions of chronic EN tend to extend peripherally with central clearing.[58]

LABORATORY FINDINGS An elevated sedimentation rate and a leukocytosis commonly accompany an acute episode of EN. Diagnostic tests to search for an underlying cause of EN depend on the geographic location, age, and clinical presentation of the patient. All patients should have a chest roentgenogram and complete blood count.

PATHOLOGY EN is characterized histopathologically by a predominantly septal panniculitis without any vasculitis. The histopathologic features vary with the stage of the disease, but are characterized throughout all the stages of the lesion by pannicular septal thickening containing Miescher's radial granulomas, which are small aggregates of histiocytes, surrounding a stellate-shaped cleft. The septal widening in the early stages is due to edema, hemorrhage, and predominantly neutrophilic inflammatory infiltrate surrounding the Miescher's radial granulomas, while in late-stage lesions, there is septal fibrosis and a predominantly granulomatous inflammatory infiltrate with multinucleated giant cells and lymphocytes (Fig. 109-8*B*). As the lesions advance, there is a sparser inflammatory infiltrate with granulation tissue at the dermal–pannicular interface. The septal pannicular inflammation is associated with some peripheral lobular inflammation and a superficial and deep dermal lymphocytic inflammatory infiltrate.[1,3]

TREATMENT AND PROGNOSIS The treatment of EN depends upon identifying and treating any underlying associated condition. In most cases, EN resolves spontaneously within a few weeks, and bed rest and a nonsteroidal anti-inflammatory agent (aspirin, indomethacin, or naproxen)[59] for analgesia are all that is required. In more chronic or recurrent cases of EN, potassium iodide[25] (400 to 900 mg daily) or oral prednisone[20] may be used.

TABLE 109-3

Microorganisms that May Cause an Infectious Panniculitis[60–63]

BACTERIA	FUNGI	OTHER
Gram-Positive Bacteria	Chromomycosis	*Amoeba histolytica*
Streptococcus pyogenes	*Sporothrix schenckii*	*Acanthamoeba*
Staphylococcus aureus	*Cryptococcus neoformans*	Helminthic infestations
Trophermyma whippleii (causing Whipple's disease)	*Histoplasma capsulatum*	
Gram-Negative Bacteria	*Aspergillus* spp.	
Pseudomonas aeruginosa	*Fusarium* spp.	
Klebsiella spp.	*Candida* spp.	
Other		
Nocardia spp., *Actinomyces israelii* *mycobacteria* (*M. tuberculosis,* atypical mycobacteria, and *M. leprae*)		
Treponema pallidum (gummatous syphilis)		

INFECTIOUS PANNICULITIS

ETIOLOGY AND PATHOGENESIS

The process occurs commonly in immunosuppressed patients[3,5] and a large variety of microorganisms may cause the subcutaneous infections[60–63] (Table 109-3). The source of infection may be local or hematogenous. Local infection may result from direct inoculation (e.g., most subcutaneous mycoses), or at sites of an occlusive dressing (e.g., aspergillosis), or from direct extension from lymph nodes or viscera (e.g., actinomycosis, amebiasis, and tuberculosis). Hematogenous spread of infection usually, but not always, occurs in immunosuppressed individuals (e.g., candidiasis, opportunistic fungal infections, pseudomonas infections, and atypical mycobacterial infections).

CLINICAL MANIFESTATIONS The cutaneous lesions of an infectious panniculitis are characterized by erythematous subcutaneous nodules and plaques, some of which ulcerate and discharge a necrotic and/or pustular material. The site of involvement varies with the type of infection.[3,5]

PATHOLOGY The characteristic histopathologic features of an infectious panniculitis may be a predominantly lobular or predominantly septal, or a mixed lobular and septal panniculitis, usually being accompanied by dermal involvement. Fat necrosis and vascular thrombosis usually accompanies a variably mixed inflammatory infiltrate of neutrophils, plasma cells, histiocytes, and multinucleated giant cells. Microorganism may be seen within the inflammatory infiltrate or necrotic debris.[3,5] Special stains (Gram's, Fite, PAS with and without diastase, and Gomori methenamine stains) may be needed to identify the microorganisms. In subcutaneous Whipple's disease, a predominantly septal panniculitis with foamy histiocytes containing pathognomonic PAS-positive, diastase-resistant intracytoplasmic granular material is seen.[63] Anti-BCG immunostaining may be used as a highly sensitive screen for bacterial or fungal microorganisms.[64] PCR techniques for specific organisms may also be used to identify the specific DNA of the causative microorganism.

TREATMENT AND PROGNOSIS The therapy of an infectious panniculitis involves antimicrobials dictated by the causative microorganism. The prognosis depends mainly on other sites of involvement and the immune status of the patient.[5]

PHYSICAL PANNICULITIDES

Traumatic Panniculitis

ETIOLOGY AND PATHOGENESIS Traumatic panniculitis (TP) usually results from blunt trauma to the subcutaneous fat resulting in fat necrosis and inflammation. A number of situations may result in physical trauma to the subcutaneous fat and may be accidental, factitial, or secondary to a procedure.

CLINICAL MANIFESTATIONS TP is clinically characterized by subcutaneous nodules or plaques, which may or may not be erythematous. TP may involve any site of the body. The most common sites of involvement of accidental TP are the lower extremities (shins; anterolateral thighs in females who repeatedly knock them against a desk at work—lipoatrophia semicircularis), elbows, and breasts (especially in obese 20- to 60-year-old females with large breasts—traumatic fat necrosis of the breast). Factitial TP is commonly seen following self-inflicted blunt trauma to the distal extremities—l'oedeme bleu. TP has also been seen following cupping or acupuncture. Mobile encapsulated lipoma (synonyms: nodular-cystic fat necrosis and encapsulated fat necrosis) is an end stage of TP, characterized by a persistent, well-demarcated, mobile nodule at sites of injury.[3,5]

PATHOLOGY TP is characterized histopathologically by a predominantly lobular panniculitis without vasculitis. Variably sized and variably shaped cystic spaces of fat necrosis are surrounded by various degrees of fibrosis, hemorrhage, and a lipophagic inflammatory infiltrate. In later stages, there may be lipomembranous change, extracellular and intracellular hemosiderin, and encapsulation of lipocytes (both normal and necrotic) by a fibrous capsule—mobile encapsulated lipoma.[3,5,65]

TREATMENT AND PROGNOSIS TP is usually self-limited often resulting in a residual subcutaneous nodule (mobile encapsulated lipoma), which may be surgically excised.

Cold Panniculitis

Cold panniculitis (CP) is a form of traumatic panniculitis that results from cold injury to the subcutaneous fat.

HISTORICAL ASPECTS In 1966, Duncan et al. reproduced a lymphohistiocytic lobular panniculitis 49 to 72 hours after application of ice cubes on the skin.[5]

EPIDEMIOLOGY This is an uncommon cause of panniculitis that is commonly seen in infants and, to a lesser extent, adult females.

ETIOLOGY AND PATHOGENESIS The main risk factor for cold injury to the subcutaneous fat is age, where it is seen most commonly in infants, who have a higher content of saturated fat that solidifies more rapidly at low temperatures. CP is seen in the cheeks of infants following sucking of ice cubes, ice packs, or ice popsicles—popsicle panniculitis. CP may also occur in adults following activities that involve prolonged exposure to cold temperature—sledding, motorcycling, and horseback riding (equestrian panniculitis).[3,5] Contributing risk factors for CP in adults are the female sex, tight fitting or noninsulating clothing, a chilblain type of circulation, paralysis and cold agglutinin disease.[66] Adult CP especially occurs in the buttocks and lateral thighs of females. CP involving the scrotum may also be seen in prepubertal males.

CLINICAL MANIFESTATIONS The cutaneous manifestations of CP are indurated, erythematous plaques with ill-defined margins that occur on the face and extremities in winter. The plaques slowly soften and resolve after a few days with temporary hyperpigmentation but no scarring.[3,5]

PATHOLOGY Cold panniculitis is characterized by a predominantly lobular panniculitis without vasculitis. Fat necrosis usually accompanies a lymphohistiocytic pannicular inflammatory infiltrate. Papillary dermal edema and a superficial and deep perivascular dermal lymphocytic infiltrate are also seen.[3,5]

TREATMENT Cold panniculitis usually resolves with avoidance of cold exposure. In equestrian panniculitis, looser-fitting trousers are helpful.

CHEMICAL/FOREIGN BODY PANNICULITIS

Panniculitis may result from the introduction of a variable number of different chemicals within the subcutaneous fat—chemical/foreign body panniculitis (CFBP).

ETIOLOGY AND PATHOGENESIS In CFBP, the introduction of a variety of chemicals in the subcutaneous fat may be either for factitial or therapeutic/cosmetic reasons[67–70] (Table 109-4).

TABLE 109-4

Causes of Chemical/Foreign Body Panniculitis[67–70]

Factitial	Therapenutic/Cosmetic
Acids/alkalis	Meperidine
Mustard	Vitamin K_1
Oils	Povidone
Urine/feces	Paraffin
Microbiologically contaminated material	Silicone
	PMMA-microspheres (Artecoll)
	Polymethylsiloxane (Bioplastique)

CLINICAL MANIFESTATIONS The main cutaneous manifestations of CFBP are subcutaneous nodules or plaques, which may or may not be erythematous or ulcerated.

PATHOLOGY The main histopathologic feature of CFBP is usually a predominantly lobular panniculitis without vasculitis. The inflammatory infiltrate is predominantly neutrophilic in early lesions, becoming predominantly granulomatous in more advanced lesions. The inciting foreign material (commonly polarizable) may be identified and, sometimes, specific features that help identify the injected material may also be observed (Table 109-5). Spectroscopic analysis also helps to identify the injected material.[3,5]

TREATMENT AND PROGNOSIS Treatment of CFBP depends on the underlying cause. In cases that are factitial, psychiatric advice should be sought and any associated underlying secondary infection should be appropriately treated. In cases associated with material injected for cosmetic purposes such as silicone, the material should be removed.

CHILDHOOD PANNICULITIS (See also Chap. 143)

Sclerema Neonatorum

EPIDEMIOLOGY Sclerema neonatorum (SN) is a rare form of panniculitis, mainly affecting seriously ill, low birth weight and/or premature neonates, usually in their first days of life.

ETIOLOGY AND PATHOGENESIS The high ratio of saturated to unsaturated fatty acids in the adipose tissue of low birth weight or premature neonates predisposes them to the changes in the adipose tissue that result in SN.

CLINICAL MANIFESTATIONS The characteristic cutaneous manifestations of SN are diffuse yellow-white, woody, indurated plaques that start on the buttocks and thighs and rapidly expand to involve large areas of the body with immobility of the extremities. SN occurs in association with a serious underlying systemic illness such as an infection or congenital heart disease or any other major developmental anomaly.[5]

PATHOLOGY The main histopathologic characteristics of SN include a predominantly lobular panniculitis with a sparse to absent lymphohistiocytic inflammatory infiltrate with a few multinucleated giant cells. The characteristic histopathologic findings are radial needle-shaped clefts within the adipocytes and the few multinucleated giant cells. Fat necrosis is not present in SN and the pannicular septa are thickened and bandlike.[5]

TREATMENT AND PROGNOSIS The management of SN is usually treatment of the underlying systemic illness. Exchange transfusions may help to decrease mortality, while corticosteroids are ineffective in this disorder.[5] The prognosis if SN is very poor, with infants dying within a few days of the onset of disease.[71] Survivors of this disorder usually have normal skin without any long-term complications or calcification.

TABLE 109-5

Pathognomonic Histopathologic Findings of Injectable Materials in Chemical/Foreign Body Panniculitis[5,67–70]

Material Injected	Characteristic Features on Histopathology
Povidone	Blue, foamy intrahistiocytic deposits that are positive for Congo red, chlorazol-fast, and PAS stains
Pentazocine	Lipophagic granulomas and fat necrosis with associated marked dermal and pannicular septal sclerosis and vascular thrombosis
Vitamin K_1	Septal panniculitis with lymphoplasmacytic inflammation and septal fibrosis (similar to morphea profunda)
Paraffinoma	Sclerosing lipogranuloma: Granulomatous inflammation and fibrosis surrounding multiple variably sized spaces (Swiss cheese–like) that replace the fat lobules
Silicone	Granulomatous inflammation surrounds polygonal translucent angulated foreign bodies
PMMA-microspheres (Artecoll)	Granulomatous inflammation and sclerosis surround regularly sized and shaped spaces containing sharply circumscribed, round, translucent, nonbirefringent foreign bodies
Polymethylsiloxane (Bioplastique)	Granulomatous inflammation surrounding irregularly sized and shaped spaces containing jagged, translucent nonbirefringent foreign bodies

Subcutaneous Fat Necrosis of the Newborn

EPIDEMIOLOGY Subcutaneous fat necrosis of the newborn (SFNN) is a rare form of neonatal panniculitis that is mainly seen in the first days of the neonatal period, but rarely are lesions present at birth.[72]

ETIOLOGY AND PATHOGENESIS Various etiologic factors are associated with SFNN, including hypercalcemia, obstetric trauma, induced hyperthermia for cardiac surgery, prostaglandin E administration, brown fat deficiency, serum lipid/lipoprotein abnormalities, use of cocaine by the mother during pregnancy, and intrapartum administration of calcium-channel blockers, and in association with thrombocytopenia. It is felt that the large surface-area-to-weight ratio and the greater ratio of saturated

TABLE 109-6

Clinical Clues to the Diagnosis of the Etiology of Panniculitis

Disease	Age	Sex	Site	Surface Changes	Systemic Involvement
Lupus Panniculitis	30–60 years	F > M	Proximal UE & LE and face	Overlying features of DLE; heal with lipoatrophic scars	Features of SLE
Morphea Profunda	20–60 years	M = F	Proximal UE & trunk	Heal with hyperpigmentation and atrophy	None
Polyarteritis Nodosa	50–60 years	M > F	LE	Ulcerations & livedo vascularis	Pyrexia, arthralgias, myalgias, malaise, & fatigue. Renal involvement, peripheral neuropathy, intestinal involvement in the systemic variant
Superficial Thrombophlebitis	Middle age to elderly	M = F	LE, migratory	None	Associated malignancy or hypercoagulable state
Nodular Vasculitis	Middle age	F > M	Posterior LE	Slowly healing ulcerations; heal with lipoatrophic scars	None, except for any associated tuberculosis
Calciphylaxis	50–60 years	F > M	LE, UE, and trunk	Violaceous necrotic ulcers with black eschar	Associated renal failure
Sclerosing Panniculitis	Elderly	F > M	Distal LE	Stasis changes, heal with atrophy & sclerosis	None
Pancreatic Panniculitis	Middle age to elderly	M > F	Distal LE & abdomen	Ulcerations and oily discharge	Features of pancreatic disease and arthritis
α_1-Antitrypsin Deficiency–Associated Panniculitis	Adults	M = F	LE, UE, and trunk	Ulceration and oily discharge; heal with lipoatrophy	Emphysema, hepatitis and cirrhosis, vasculitis, angioedema, & severe psoriasis
Cytophagic Histiocytic Panniculitis	Middle age to elderly	M = F	UE & LE	Ulceration and ecchymoses	Features of HPS—pyrexia, hepatosplenomegaly, lymphadenopathy, pancytopenia, and coagulopathy
Erythema Nodosum	20–30 years	F > M (3-6:1)	LE, UE, & face	None	Pyrexia, arthritis, malaise
Subcutaneous Sarcoidosis	40–60 years	F > M	LE	None	Precedes systemic sarcoidosis
Subcutaneous Granuloma Annulare	Children & young adults	M = F	Head, hands, & LE	None	None
Necrobiosis Lipoidica	Young to middle age	F > M (3:1)	Legs	Ulceration	Associated diabetes mellitus
Rheumatoid Nodule	↑ with age	F > M (3:1)	Elbows & fingers	None	Associated features of rheumatoid disease
Necrobiotic Xanthogranuloma	Middle age	M = F	Periorbital region	Central atrophy, telangiectasia, & ulceration	Hepatosplenomegaly, associated paraproteinemia (IgG κ type)
Infectious Panniculitis	Variable	F = M	Variable	Ulceration and purulent discharge; heal with lipoatrophic scars	Underlying immunosuppression
Traumatic Panniculitis	Variable	M = F	LE & breasts	Ulceration	None
Cold Panniculitis	Infants	M = F	Cheeks	None	None
Chemical/Foreign Body Panniculitis	Adults	M = F	Variable	Ulceration	Psychiatric disease in factitial disease
Sclerema Neonatorum	Neonates	M = F	Buttocks & thighs	None	Associated serious illness
Subcutaneous Fat Necrosis of the Newborn	Neonates	M = F	Proximal extremity	None	Hypercalcemia
Poststeroid Panniculitis	Infants	M = F	Cheeks, arms, & trunk	None	Weight gain from steroid use

ABBREVIATIONS: DLE, discoid lupus erythematosus; F, female; HPS, hemophagocytic syndrome; LE, lower extremities; M, male, SLE, systemic lupus erythematosus; UE, upper extremities

TABLE 109-7

Diagnostic Tests for the Etiology of Panniculitis

CUTANEOUS BIOPSY	
Hematoxylin and eosin	See Tables 109–8 and 109–9
Special tests for microorganisms	Anti-BCG immunostaining screens for bacteria and fungi Special stains (Gomori methenamine stain, PAS stain, Gram's stain, Fite stain) Tissue culture for bacteria, fungi, and mycobacteria PCR tests for specific micoorganisms (e.g., *Mycobacterium tuberculosis*)
Special tests for lymphoma/leukemia	Immunohistochemistry stains (CD43, CD3, CD4, CD8, CD20, CD56, lysozyme, myeloperoxidase, TIA, and granzyme B) Genetic studies for T and B cell gene rearrangement by PCR and Southern blot techniques
Special tests for foreign bodies	Polarizing microscopy Spectroscopic analysis
BLOOD TESTS	
Pancreatic enzymes (lipase and amylase)	*Antistreptolysin O antibody and other microbiological serologic tests (e.g., fungal serologies)*
α_1-Antitrypsin levels and phenotype	*Angiotensin-converting enzyme level*
Antinuclear antibodies	*Fasting serum glucose/glycosylated hemoglobin*
Extractable nuclear antigen antibodies	*Serum protein electrophoresis*
Anti–double-stranded DNA	*Serum calcium, phosphorus, and PTH*
Rheumatoid factor	*Serum uric acid*
Anti-neutrophilic cytoplasmic antibody	
DIAGNOSTIC IMAGING	
Chest radiography	*Lower extremity venous Doppler ultrasound studies*
CT scan of thorax, abdomen, and pelvis	
OTHER	
Tuberculin skin test	*Colonoscopy*
Lepromin skin test	

to unsaturated fatty acids in the neonate favor release of hydrolases, induced by minor trauma, resulting in the breakdown of unsaturated fatty acids.[5,72]

CLINICAL MANIFESTATIONS The cutaneous manifestations of SFNN consist of indurated, erythematous subcutaneous nodules or plaques mainly affecting the buttocks, thighs, shoulders, and cheeks. Although many underlying conditions are associated with SFNN, this form of panniculitis is usually seen in healthier individuals.[5,72]

LABORATORY FINDINGS Hypercalcemia is a common associated laboratory finding in SFNN.[5,72]

PATHOLOGY The histopathologic characteristics of SFNN are a lobular panniculitis without any vasculitis. Fat necrosis occurs in association with a dense inflammatory infiltrate, composed of lymphocytes, histiocytes, foamy histiocytes, multi-nucleated giant cells and eosinophils. Characteristic of SFNN are needle-shaped clefts (triglyceride crystals) that are present within both lipocytes and histiocytes. Advanced lesions will have septal fibrosis and calcification.[5,72]

TREATMENT AND PROGNOSIS SFNN has an excellent prognosis, regressing within a few days without any sequelae.

Poststeroid Panniculitis

Poststeroid panniculitis (PSP) is a rare type of childhood panniculitis that occurs in children who are withdrawn from high doses of systemic steroids.

EPIDEMIOLOGY PSP is very rare and has only been seen in children.

ETIOLOGY AND PATHOGENESIS PSP is most commonly seen 1 to 10 days following rapid withdrawal of high doses of systemic corticosteroids used in infants for several conditions, including rheumatic fever, leukemia, nephrotic syndrome, and cerebral edema.[73,74] The exact pathogenesis of this type of panniculitis is unclear, although it may result from lipocyte injury secondary to the accelerated removal of the excess fat gained during corticosteroid use.

CLINICAL MANIFESTATIONS The characteristic cutaneous lesions of PSP are erythematous, 1 to 4 cm, occasionally pruritic subcutaneous nodules that develop up to 2 weeks following cessation of high-dose corticosteroids. The most common sites of involvement are the cheeks, arms, and trunk. Although no extracutaneous manifestations are usually seen with poststeroid panniculitis, a fatal case of intestinal fat necrosis has been reported.[5,73,74]

PATHOLOGY The main histopathologic feature of PSP includes a lobular panniculitis without vasculitis. The inflammatory infiltrate is composed of lymphocytes and foamy histiocytes that contain intracytoplasmic needle-shaped clefts similar to subcutaneous fat necrosis of the newborn.[5]

TREATMENT AND PROGNOSIS Mild cases of poststeroid panniculitis do not usually require any treatment, because there is gradual resolution over a period of a few weeks. In more severe cases, where ulceration and scarring of the cheeks may occur, readministration of high-dose systemic corticosteroids followed by a gradual tapering of the dose is indicated.[5]

DIAGNOSTIC APPROACH TO PANNICULITIS

The diagnosis of the etiology of panniculitis can be made in most cases after careful clinical assessment (Table 109-6) and appropriate diagnostic testing (Table 109-7). The diagnosis of the cause of a panniculitis is usually established on assessment of a number of dermatopathologic parameters, which include the location of the inflammatory infiltrate (septal or lobular), the presence or absence of vasculitis, and the nature of the inflammatory infiltrate[75] (Tables 109-8 and 109-9).

TABLE 109-8

Histopathologic Differential Diagnosis of Predominantly Septal Panniculitides

WITH VASCULITIS

- *Small vessel involvement* → *Leukocytoclastic vasculitis*
- *Large vessel involvement*
  - → *Veins* → *Superficial thrombophlebitis*
  - → *Arteries* → *Polyarteritis nodosa*

WITHOUT VASCULITIS

- *Predominant lymphoplasmacytic inflammation* → *Morphea profunda*
- *Predominant granulomatous inflammation*
  - → *Miescher's granuloma* → *Erythema nodosum*
  - → *Palisading granuloma*
    - → *Central necrobiosis and mucin* → *Subcutaneous granuloma annulare*
    - → *Central necrobiosis and fibrin* → *Rheumatoid nodule*
    - → *Alternating zones of necrobiosis and inflammation* → *Necrobiosis lipoidica*
    - → *Broad zones of necrobiosis and cholesterol clefts* → *Necrobiotic xanthogranuloma*

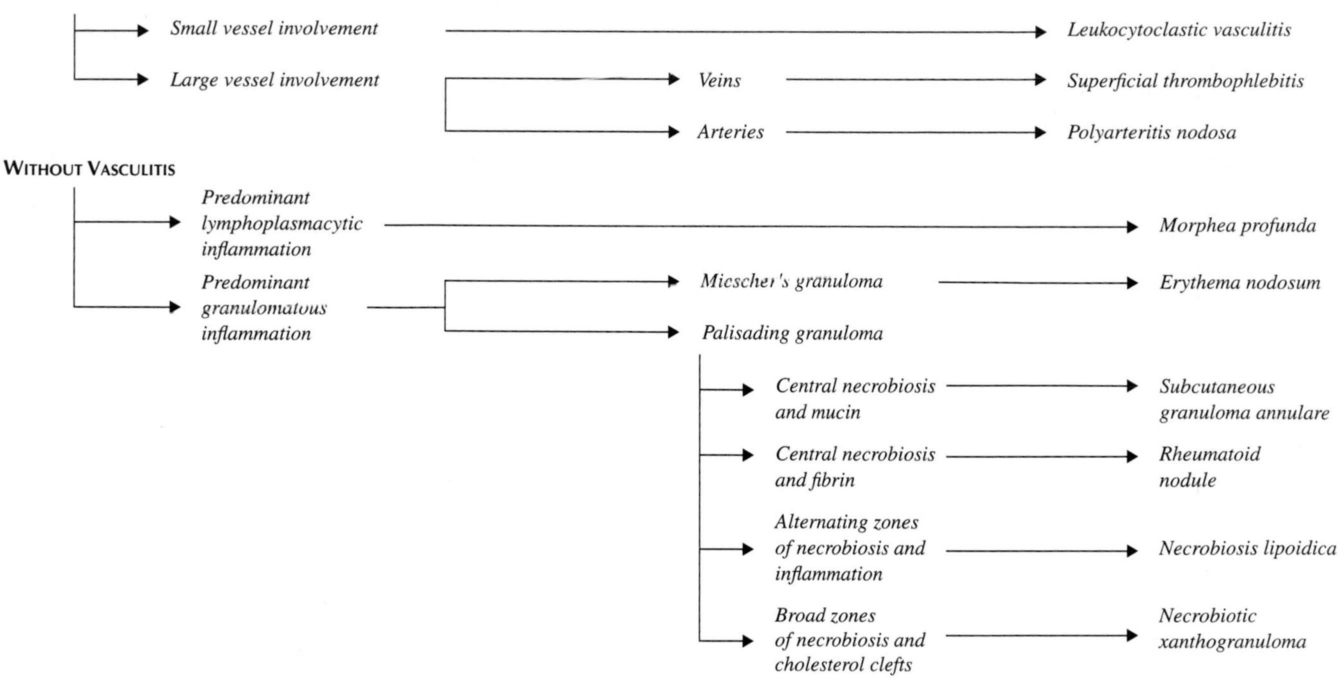

TABLE 109-9

Histopathologic Differential Diagnosis of Predominantly Lobular Panniculitides

WITH VASCULITIS

- *Small vessel involvement* → *Leprosy reactions*
  - *a. Erythema nodosum leprosum*
  - *b. Lucio's phenomenon*
- *Small, medium, and large vessel involvement* → *Nodular vasculitis*

WITHOUT VASCULITIS

- *Minimal inflammation*
  - → *Needle-shaped clefts in lipocytes* → *Sclerema neonatorum*
  - → *Vascular calcification* → *Calciphylaxis; oxalosis*
  - → *Lipomembranous and stasis change* → *Sclerosing panniculitis*
- *Predominant lymphocytic inflammation*
  - → *Lymphoid follicles, hyaline sclerosis, and features of LE* → *Lupus panniculitis*
  - → *Superficial and deep dermal lymphocytic inflammation* → *Cold panniculitis*
- *Predominant neutrophilic inflammation*
  - → *Extensive saponification* → *Pancreatic panniculitis*
  - → *Dermal interstitial neutrophilia* → *α_1-Antitrypsin deficiency*
  - → *Microorganisms* → *Infectious panniculitis*
- *Predominant granulomatous inflammation*
  - → *Cytophagocytosis* → *Cytophagic histiocytic panniculitis*
  - → *Needle-shaped clefts* → *Subcutaneous fat necrosis of newborn; poststeroid panniculitis*
  - → *Microorganisms* → *Infectious panniculitis*
  - → *Foreign bodies* → *Foreign body panniculitis*
  - → *Naked granulomas* → *Subcutaneous sarcoidosis*

REFERENCES

1. Raquena L, Sanchez Yus E: Panniculitis. Part I. Mostly septal panniculitis. *J Am Acad Dermatol* **45**:163, 2001
2. Ackermann AB et al: *Histologic Diagnosis of Inflammatory Skin Disease: An Algorithmic Method Based on Pattern Analysis,* 2nd ed. Baltimore, Williams and Wilkins, 1997, p 31
3. Peters MS, Su WPD: Panniculitis. *Dermatol Clin* **10**:37, 1992
4. White JW, Winkelmann RK: Weber-Christian panniculitis: A review of 30 cases with this diagnosis. *J Am Acad Dermatol* **39**:56, 1998
5. Requena L, Sanchez Yus E: Panniculitis. Part II. Mostly lobular panniculitis. *J Am Acad Dermatol* **45**:325, 2001
6. Peters MS, Su WPD: Lupus erythematosus panniculitis. *Med Clin North Am* **73**:1113, 1989
7. Martens PM et al: Lupus panniculitis: Clinical perspectives from a case series. *J Rheumatol* **26**:68, 1999
8. Yell JA, Burge SM: Lupus erythematosus profundus treated with clobetasol propionate under hydrocolloid dressing. *Br J Dermatol* **128**:103, 1993
9. Yamada Y et al: Lupus erythematosus profundus: Report of a case treated with dapsone. *J Dermatol* **16**:379, 1989
10. Burrows NP et al: Lupus erythematosus profundus with partial C4 deficiency responding to thalidomide. *Br J Dermatol* **125**:62, 1991
11. Saeki Y et al: Maintaining remission of lupus erythematosus profundus (LEP) with cyclosporin A. *Lupus* **9**:390, 2000
12. Magro CM et al: Lupus profundus, indeterminate lymphocytic lobular panniculitis and subcutaneous T-cell lymphoma: A spectrum of subcuticular T-cell lymphoid dyscrasia. *J Cutan Pathol* **28**:235, 2001
13. Peterson LS et al: Classification of morphea (localized scleroderma). *Mayo Clin Proc* **70**:1068, 1995
14. Zuckerman E et al: Fasciitis-panniculitis in acute brucellosis. *Int J Dermatol* **33**:57, 1994
15. Naschitz JE et al: Cancer-associated fasciitis panniculitis. *Cancer* **73**:231, 1994
16. Winkelmann RK et al: Pseudosclerodermatous panniculitis after irradiation: An unusual complication of megavoltage treatment of breast carcinoma. *Mayo Clin Proc* **68**:122, 1993
17. Chao YY, Yang LJ: Dermatomyositis presenting as panniculitis. *Int J Dermatol* **39**:140, 2000
18. Tait PT et al: Sjögren's syndrome and granulomatous panniculitis. *Aust J Dermatol* **41**:187, 2000
19. Itoh O et al: Mixed connective tissue disease with severe pulmonary hypertension and extensive subcutaneous calcification. *Intern Med* **37**:421, 1998
20. Phelps RG, Shoji T: Update on panniculitis. *Mt Sinai J Med* **68**:262, 2001
21. Cardinali C et al: Hepatitis C virus: A common triggering factor for both nodular vasculitis and Sjögren's syndrome? *Br J Dermatol* **142**:187, 2000
22. Wolf D et al: Nodular vasculitis associated with propylthiouracil therapy. *Cutis* **49**:253, 1992
23. Tran TA et al: Neutrophilic lobular (pustular) panniculitis associated with rheumatoid arthritis: A case report and review of the literature. *Am J Dermatopathol* **21**(3):247, 1999
24. Yen A et al: Detection of *Mycobacteria tuberculosis* in erythema induratum of Bazin using polymerase chain reaction. *Arch Dermatol* **133**:532, 1997
25. Hori T et al: Potassium iodide in the treatment of erythema nodosum and nodular vasculitis. *Arch Dermatol* **117**:29, 1981.
26. Selye H: *Calciphylaxis*. Chicago, IL, University of Chicago Press, 1962, pp 1–100
27. Mathur RV et al: Calciphylaxis. *Postgrad Med J* **77**:557, 2001
28. Mirza I et al: An unusual presentation of calciphylaxis due to primary hyperparathyroidism. *Arch Pathol Lab Med* **125**:1351, 2001
29. Mastruserio DN et al: Calciphylaxis associated with metastatic breast carcinoma. *J Am Acad Dermatol* **41**:295, 1999
30. Riegert-Johnson DL et al: Calciphylaxis associated with cholangiocarcinoma treated with low-molecular-weight heparin and vitamin K. *Mayo Clin Proc* **76**:749, 2001
31. Raper RD, Ibels LS: Osteosclerotic myeloma complicated by diffuse arteritis, vascular calcification and extensive cutaneous necrosis. *Nephron* **39**:389, 1985
32. Fader DJ, Kang S: Calciphylaxis without renal failure. *Arch Dermatol* **132**:837, 1996
33. Dahl PR et al: The vascular calcification: cutaneous necrosis syndrome. *J Am Acad Dermatol* **33**:53, 1995
34. Hafner J et al: Uremic small-artery disease with medial calcification and intimal hyperplasia (so-called calciphylaxis): A complication of chronic renal failure and benefit from parathyroidectomy. *J Am Acad Dermatol* **33**:954, 1995
35. Girotto JA et al: Parathyroidectomy promotes wound healing and prolonged survival in patients with calciphylaxis from secondary hyperparathyroidism. *Surgery* **130**:645, 2001
36. Vassa N et al: Hyperbaric oxygen therapy in calciphylaxis-induced skin necrosis in a peritoneal dialysis patient. *Am J Kidney Dis* **23**:878, 1994
37. Podymow T et al: Hyperbaric oxygen in the treatment of calciphylaxis: A case series. *Nephrol Dial Transplant* **16**:2176, 2001
38. Jorizzo JL et al: Sclerosing panniculitis: A clinicopathological assessment. *Arch Dermatol* **127**:554, 1991
39. Snow JL, Su WPD: Lipomembranous (membranocystic) fat necrosis: Clinicopathological correlation of 38 cases. *Am J Dermatopathol* **18**:151, 1996
40. Kirsner RS et al: The clinical spectrum of lipodermatosclerosis. *J Am Acad Dermatol* **28**:623, 1993
41. Sibrack LA, Goutermann IH: Cutaneous manifestations of pancreatic diseases. *Cutis* **21**:763, 1978
42. Dahl PR et al: Pancreatic panniculitis. *J Am Acad Dermatol* **33**:413, 1995
43. Lambiase P et al: Resolution of panniculitis after placement of pancreatic duct stent in chronic pancreatitis. *Am J Gastroenterol* **91**:1835, 1996
44. Su WPD et al: α_1-Antitrypsin deficiency panniculitis: A histopathological and immunopathological study of 4 cases. *Am J Dermatopathol* **9**:483, 1987
45. Pittelkow MR et al: Alpha$_1$-antitrypsin deficiency and panniculitis: Perspectives on disease relationship and replacement therapy. *Am J Med* **84**:80, 1988
46. Ching WJ, Henderson CA: Suppurative panniculitis associated with alpha$_1$-antitrypsin deficiency (PiSZ phenotype) treated with doxycycline. *Br J Dermatol* **144**:1261, 2001
47. Smith KC et al: Clinical and pathologic correlations in 96 patients with panniculitis, including 15 patients with deficient levels of α_1-antitrypsin. *J Am Acad Dermatol* **21**:1192, 1989
48. Geller JD, Su WPD: A subtle clue to the histopathological diagnosis of early α_1-antitrypsin deficiency panniculitis. *J Am Acad Dermatol* **31**:241, 1994
49. Smith KC et al: Panniculitis associated with severe α_1-antitrypsin deficiency: Treatment and review of the literature. *Arch Dermatol* **123**:1655, 1987
50. Ginarte M et al: Treatment of alpha$_1$-antitrypsin-deficiency panniculitis with minocycline. *Cutis* **68**(2):86, 2001
51. Furey NL et al: Treatment of alpha$_1$-antitrypsin deficiency, massive edema and panniculitis with alpha$_1$protease inhibitor. *Ann Intern Med* **125**:699, 1996
52. O'Riordan K et al: Alpha$_1$-antitrypsin deficiency-associated panniculitis: Resolution with intravenous alpha$_1$-antitrypsin administration and liver transplantation. *Transplantation* **63**:480, 1997
53. Wick MR, Patterson JW: Cytophagic histiocytic panniculitis—A critical reappraisal. *Arch Dermatol* **136**:922, 2000
54. Winkelmann RK, Bowie EJ: Hemorrhagic diathesis associated with benign histiocytic cytophagic panniculitis and systemic histiocytosis. *Arch Intern Med* **140**:1460, 1980
55. Chin-Yao EW, Su WPD: Subcutaneous panniculitic T-cell lymphoma. *Int J Dermatol* **35**:1, 1996
56. Marzano AV et al: Cytophagic histiocytic panniculitis and subcutaneous panniculitis-like T-cell lymphoma. Report of 7 cases. *Arch Dermatol* **136**:889, 2000
57. Weenig RH et al: Subcutaneous panniculitis-like T-cell lymphoma. An elusive case presenting as lipomembranous panniculitis and a review of 72 cases in the literature. *Am J Dermatopathol* **23**:206, 2001
58. De Almeida Prestes C et al: Septal granulomatous panniculitis: Comparison of the pathology of erythema nodosum migrans (migratory panniculitis) and chronic erythema nodosum. *J Am Acad Dermatol* **22**:477, 1990
59. Ubogy Z, Persellin RM: Suppression of erythema nodosum by indomethacin. *Acta Derm Venereol (Stockh)* **107**:209, 1982
60. Patterson JW et al: Infection-induced panniculitis. *J Cutan Pathol* **16**:183, 1989
61. Bartralot R et al: Cutaneous infections due to non-tuberculous mycobacteria: Histopathological review of 28 cases. Comparative study between lesions observed in immunosuppressed patients and normal hosts. *J Cutan Pathol* **27**:124, 2000
62. Rosenberg AS, Morgan MB: Disseminated acanthamoebiasis presenting as lobular panniculitis with necrotizing vasculitis in a patient with AIDS. *J Cutan Pathol* **28**:307, 2001
63. Tarroch X et al: Subcutaneous nodules in Whipple's disease. *J Cutan Pathol* **28**:368, 2001
64. Byrd J et al: Utility of anti-bacillus Calmette-Guerin antibodies as a screen for organisms in sporotrichoid infections. *J Am Acad Dermatol* **44**:261, 2001

65. Kiryu H et al: Encapsulated fat necrosis: a clinicopathological study of 8 cases and a literature review. *J Cutan Pathol* **27**:19, 2000
66. De Silva BD et al: Equestrian perniosis associated with cold agglutinins: A novel finding. *Clin Exp Dermatol* **25**:285, 2000
67. Kossard S et al: Povidone panniculitis. Polyvinylpyrrolidone panniculitis. *Arch Dermatol* **116**:704, 1980
68. Palestine RF et al: Skin manifestations of pentazocine abuse. *J Am Acad Dermatol* **2**:47, 1980
69. Delage C et al: Mammary silicone granuloma. *Arch Dermatol* **108**:104, 1973.
70. Rudolph CM et al: Foreign body granulomas due to injectable aesthetic microimplants. *Am J Surg Pathol* **23**:113, 1999

71. Warwick W et al: Sclerema neonatorum: A sign not a disease. *JAMA* **184**:680, 1963
72. Burden AD, Krafchik BR: Subcutaneous fat necrosis of the newborn: A review of 11 cases. *Pediatr Dermatol* **16**:384, 1999
73. Silverman RA et al: Poststeroid panniculitis. *Pediatr Dermatol* **5**:92, 1988
74. Saxena AK, Nigam PK: Panniculitis following steroid therapy. *Cutis* **42**:341, 1988
75. Cascajo CD et al: Panniculitis: Definition of terms and diagnostic strategy. *Am J Dermatopathol* **22**:530, 2000

CHAPTER 110

Lipodystrophy

Ervin H. Epstein, Jr.

The syndromes of partial lipodystrophy (PL) and generalized lipodystrophy (GL) are a heterogeneous group of diseases characterized by the absence of subcutaneous fat over part or all of the body surface.[1]

CLASSICAL PARTIAL LIPODYSTROPHY

Etiology

The causes of most instances of PL, the more common of the syndromes, are unknown. There are conflicting data regarding a possible genetic predisposition to the usual cephalothoracic type. For example, in two instances one identical twin had PL with glomerulonephritis, decreased C3, and the presence of C3 nephritic factor, but her twin sister had none of these abnormalities.[2] By contrast, one family was reported in which an affected mother had two normal and two affected children.

Clinical Features

Over several years, patients with "classical" acquired (Barraquer-Simons) PL gradually lose their subcutaneous fat in clearly demarcated, generally symmetric areas of the body. The wasting usually begins on the face, spreads downward, and may stop at any level, most often above or at the middle of the thighs. Occasionally, the lower portion of the body may be affected while the upper portion remains uninvolved. The unaffected part of the body often appears obese, partly because of the contrast with the gaunt appearance of the thin portion. Excess fat deposition over the hips and thighs frequently occurs in postpubertal women with PL. Eighty percent of patients are female, and the disease develops in most patients before the age of 15 years. A clinically apparent inflammatory phase does not precede the fat loss, but patients often correlate the onset with some acute febrile illness.

The face appears cachectic. Buccal fat pads disappear, leaving a relative prominence of the chin and zygomas (Fig. 110-1). With loss of retroorbital and periorbital tissue, the eyes may sink deeply into the sockets. Smiling produces many wrinkles and a prematurely aged expression. Unshielded by the usual blanket of fat, the veins and muscles of the trunk and upper extremities appear hypertrophied. The overlying skin itself is of normal color, texture, and elasticity. Visceral fat stores underlying the thin areas also are absent.

Patients with the clinically quite separate syndrome of localized lipodystrophy, or lipoatrophy, have one or more scattered areas of loss of subcutaneous fat. There may be myositis underlying these areas, and the loss may represent the end stage of lymphocytic panniculitis (see Chap. 109). Lipoatrophia semicircularis is a bandlike depression of the skin mainly on the lower extremities and caused by pressure and trauma.[3]

Histopathology

Subcutaneous fat cells may be detected microscopically but in markedly decreased number.[4]

Laboratory Findings and Associated Internal Disease

The most common laboratory abnormality in patients with PL is decreased serum complement: C3 was diminished in 70 percent of unselected PL patients, and this may be due both to decreased synthesis and to increased catabolism. Associated with this is the presence of C3 nephritic factor, an immunoglobulin that binds to factor H (an inhibitor of C3) and hence allows uncontrolled activation of C3. Many PL patients have glomerulonephritis. These serologic abnormalities may be found in patients with glomerulonephritis without PL, and currently the weight of evidence, albeit it mostly circumstantial, favors the hypothesis that the nephritic factor predisposes to glomerulonephritis via direct toxicity and/or via hypocomplementemia.[5,6] Furthermore, there is experimental evidence that serum that contains nephritic factor is toxic to adipocytes in vitro, leading to the suggestion that this factor contributes directly to the loss of fat.[7] Patients with these complement abnormalities may have histologically detectable glomerulonephritis before renal disease is apparent clinically.[8] The percentage of patients

FIGURE 110-1

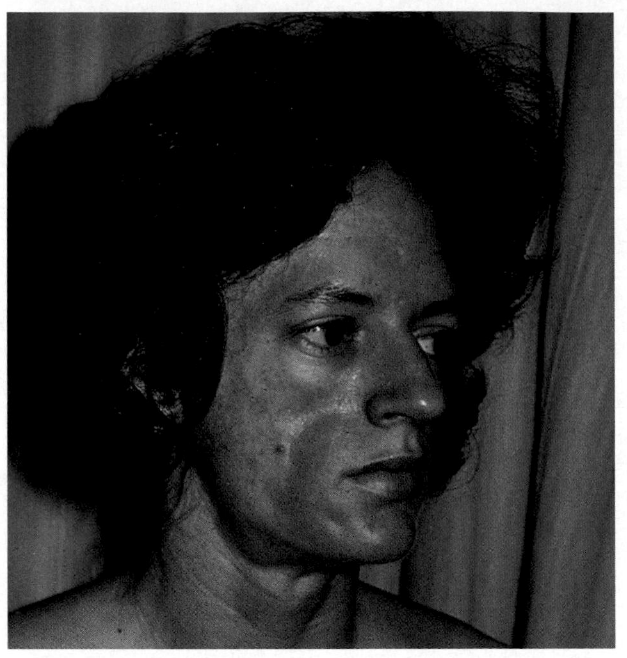

Partial lipodystrophy. Emaciated facies results from a loss of buccal fat pads. (*Courtesy of John Reeves, MD.*)

who eventually develop significant renal disease is not known. In some patients with PL, resistance to infection is decreased, possibly because of the C3 deficiency.[9] Some of the patients have had pancreatitis with eosinophilia.[10] Women with PL may be at increased risk for third-trimester intrauterine death.[11] Development of diabetes is common.

Treatment

Effective therapy for the underlying defect is not available. Because fat may be resorbed rapidly, implantation of fat from unaffected areas is of inconsistent benefit, but one patient had good cosmetic results more than a year following subcutaneous implantation of muscle harvested from the abdomen.[12] Subcutaneous lipectomy and liposuction may improve the appearance of lower extremities in which excessive subcutaneous fat is deforming.[13] Patients with uremia have had successful renal transplants.

DUNNIGAN TYPE OF LIPODYSTROPHY

Etiology and Pathogenesis

More rarely, patients lose subcutaneous fat only from the limbs with maintenance of fat on the trunk and face or they lose fat from both the limbs and trunk and maintain fat on the face. In some families, this syndrome is inherited as an autosomal dominant trait, the Dunnigan-Kobberling syndrome (D-PL; MIM #151660).[14–17] Mutations in *LMNA*, the gene that encodes lamins A and C, underlie D-PL.[18–20] Other mutations in the same gene can cause autosomal forms of muscular dystrophy, dilated cardiomyopathy, Charcot-Marie-Tooth neuropathy, and mandibuloacral dysplasia, in which affected individuals have not only lipodystrophy but also several other abnormalities including mottled hyperpigmentation and alopecia.[21] The nuclear lamins belong to the family of intermediate filament proteins and are attached to the inner surface of the nuclear envelope. This localization contrasts with that of other intermediate filament proteins such as the keratins, which are cytoplasmic and are attached to the inner surface of the plasma membrane. One report suggested association of lamin A/C gene polymorphisms and obesity in non-PL individuals.[22] In a unique mother and son with insulin-resistance, hypocalcemia, and PL, similar clinically to that of the Dunnigan type, there was a missense mutation in a calcium-sensing receptor at the cell surface.[23]

Clinical Features, Laboratory Findings, and Associated Internal Disease

In patients with D-PL, the fat loss of the extremities and trunk begins at puberty and is accompanied by fat deposition on the face and upper back as well as by maintenance of fat within the truncal cavities and bone marrow.[24] Despite maintenance of some fat, the acanthosis nigricans (see Chap. 185) and metabolic problems of insulin resistant diabetes of these patients resemble more those of patients with GL, rather than PL. These metabolic abnormalities are more common in women than in men with D-PL.[25]

Treatment

Thus far, the recent insights into the genetic basis of this disease have yet to produce new therapeutic options.

HIV-ASSOCIATED LIPODYSTROPHY[26,27]

(see also Chap. 225)

Etiology and Pathogenesis

Soon after the introduction in the mid-1990s of highly active antiretroviral therapy (HAART) for the treatment of patients with HIV disease, redistribution of body fat—analogous to PL—in treated patients was reported. The incidence of this complication increases with duration of therapy and may affect one-third to two-thirds of patients treated for 2 years or longer. Although the incidence of PL clearly increased markedly after the introduction of protease inhibitors (PI), several reports document the development of PL in patients who had not received PI. Evidence for several disparate mechanisms of action of HAART components in causing PL has been reported,[28,29] but a unifying hypothesis is lacking. For now, it appears that different classes of anti-HIV drugs may contribute and that within each class different drugs may be more or less associated with PL. Although some of the changes may be long-term effects of HIV infection, unmasked by HAART prolongation of life, patients treated early after HIV infection also may develop PL, suggesting more direct drug effects.

Clinical Features

Starting as soon as several months after institution of HAART, patients notice loss of subcutaneous fat from their limbs (both upper and lower) (Fig. 110-2) and from their face. Fat increases at the posterior neck/upper back (a "buffalo hump" similar to that in patients with Cushing's disease), in the abdomen (with increased waist:hip ratio, and with feelings of bloating and distention), and on the breasts (sometimes with marked pain).

Histopathology

Subcutaneous fat is atrophic and adipocyte apoptosis is present.[30]

FIGURE 110-2

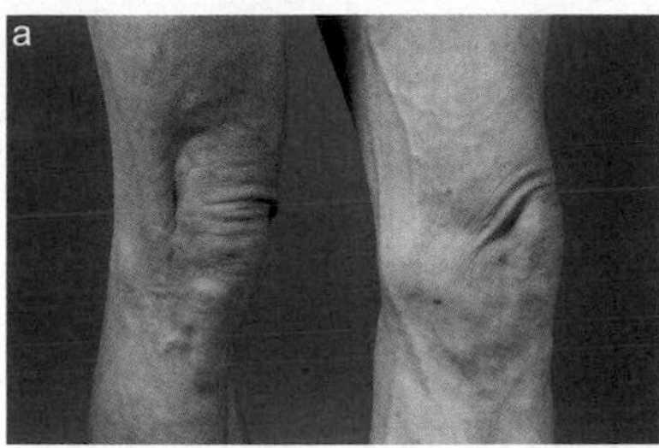

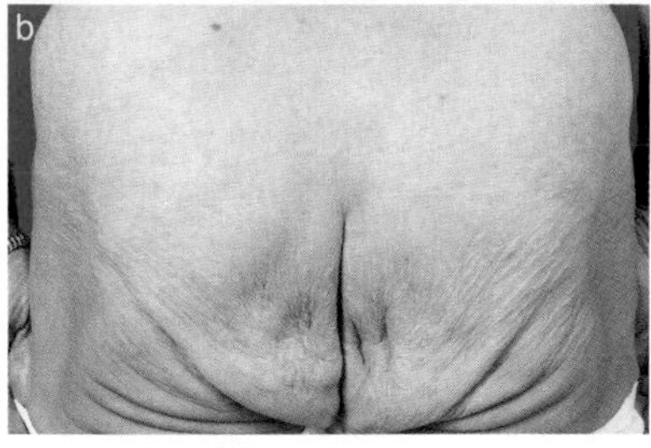

Partial lipodystrophy associated with HIV and HAART. Note protruding veins and excessive skin folds over knees and loss of fat of the buttocks in this 35-year-old patient. Also note increased fat on the hips. *(Courtesy of Armin Rieger MD.)*

Laboratory Findings and Associated Internal Disease

Patients generally have insulin resistance and hyperglycemia, progressing in some cases to frank non-insulin-dependent diabetes mellitus, hypertriglyceridemia, and hypercholesterolemia. This constellation of metabolic abnormalities clearly is associated in the non-HIV population with accelerated atherosclerosis, and these patients, too, may be at increased risk for cardiovascular disease.[31] The development of HIV-PL may be more common in those with a better therapeutic response to HAART, as measured by recovery of peripheral blood CD4+ lymphocytes.[32]

Treatment

Some patients find the cosmetic and symptomatic changes of HIV-PL to be so debilitating as to require changes in their HIV treatment. Changes between or within a class of drugs may ameliorate the disease as may treatment with recombinant human growth hormone (rhGH), metformin, dehydroepiandrosterone plus nonsteroidal anti-inflammatory drugs, or PPAR-γ agonists.[33,34] However, although they may be associated with improvement in both the metabolic abnormalities and in the intraabdominal fat deposition, these therapies have not led to cosmetically-significant reaccumulation of facial or limb subcutaneous fat. Statins may be helpful in reducing the hyperlipidemia and, hopefully, in reducing the risk of accelerated atherosclerosis. Liposuction of the upper back may reduce the cosmetic disfigurement of the "buffalo hump."[35]

GENERALIZED LIPODYSTROPHY

Etiology and Pathogenesis

Patients with congenital GL (MIM #269700) cluster in consanguineous families, most of whom have linkage evidence of abnormalities at the BSCL 1 locus on chromosome 9q34,[36] or the BSCL 2 locus on chromosome 11q13. The mutated gene at the latter site is the G-protein seipin.[37] Patients with later onset GL appear not to have seipin mutations. Seipin's strong expression in normal brain and absent expression in normal adipose tissue are consistent with the earlier hypotheses of a primary hypothalamic dysfunction with secondary adipose and other tissue effects.[38] Transgenic mice engineered to have specific loss of white adipose tissue have metabolic abnormalities that are reversed by transplantation of normal fat, indicating the likelihood of a causal effect of the fat loss.[39,40] Therefore, the most likely pathogenesis is that hypothalamic abnormalities cause loss of adipose tissue, which, in turn, causes the metabolic abnormalities.

Clinical Features

Patients with GL lack both subcutaneous fat and extracutaneous adipose tissue. This condition may be congenital (Berardinelli-Seip syndrome) or acquired later in life (Seip-Lawrence syndrome), in which patients' loss of fat may be extremely rapid.[41] Acanthosis nigricans (see Chap. 185), hypertrichosis, generalized hyperpigmentation, and unusually thick, curly scalp hair (*cf.* the development of curly hair coincident with the onset of HIV-associated PL[42]) often are present. During infancy and childhood linear growth is accelerated, and adult height may be greater than that predicted by the height of the parents. Daily energy consumption is increased noticeably; patients eat voraciously, perspire excessively, and may be heat-intolerant despite normal thyroid function; and the basal metabolic rate is elevated. In infants, hepatosplenomegaly causes abdominal protuberance. This may resolve in later childhood. Because of generalized absence of fat, the muscles appear hypertrophic; however, usually the age at which the child sits and walks is normal, and muscle strength is not increased.[43] The external genitalia often are enlarged, with the large clitoris or penis and rippling muscles suggesting precocious puberty. Moderate mental retardation is frequent but not uniform.[44]

Laboratory Findings and Associated Internal Disease

The characteristic laboratory abnormality is decreased glucose tolerance, and the syndrome is often termed *lipoatrophic diabetes*. Diabetes may become apparent clinically only in the second or third decade, but insulin resistance can be detected earlier. Hyperglycemia (reportedly due mostly to increased glucose production), glycosuria, and insulin resistance are often marked, but life-threatening ketoacidosis does not develop. Nonetheless, renal, retinal, and neuropathic diabetic changes may occur. Patients' endogenous insulin is normal biologically, immunologically, and in its proportion of proinsulin.[45] Conflicting findings of decreased or normal binding of insulin to cell receptors have been reported in patients with congenital GL. Fasting reduces the serum insulin and increases cell surface binding of insulin by peripheral blood leukocytes, and it is uncertain whether the putative decreased binding in vivo is a primary cause of insulin resistance or is a result of the high circulating insulin. Some believe the insulin resistance to be the result of a postreceptor defect.[46] A separate group of patients without lipodystrophy but with insulin resistance, acanthosis nigricans, hirsutism, and accelerated early growth have a definitely decreased number of insulin receptors, but insulin binding does not increase with fasting.[47,48] Also, patients with various other syndromes with associated insulin resistance and acanthosis nigricans have been reported, some of whom have insulin-receptor gene mutations.[49]

Nearly all patients with GL have hepatomegaly, resulting initially from increased fat; the liver may shrink with fasting. As with fatty liver resulting from other causes, cirrhosis may develop and the patient may die of hepatic failure.[50]

Significant kidney disease (without hypocomplementemia), mental retardation, and crippling schizophrenia have occurred in patients with GL. In one patient with diabetic nephropathy, a transplanted kidney was damaged acutely by massive lipid deposition.[51] Several women with GL have had frank virilization with polycystic ovarian disease,[52,53] but several affected patients have had normal children.[54]

Reduced fat around the viscera and increased fat in the liver can be detected by abdominal computed tomography (CT) scan and ultrasonography.[55] Enlarged cerebral ventricles have been reported, but cerebral CT scans are usually normal.[56] Radiographic changes of bony sclerosis and cystic changes have been described frequently.[55] Hyperlipoproteinemia occurs with a rapid turnover of plasma free fatty acids, presumably derived from peripheral lipolysis of triglycerides[57] and with overproduction of very-low-density lipoproteins.[58,59] Eruptive xanthomas may occur (see Chap. 150). Patients with GL, thickened dermis, frank scleroderma, and Hodgkin's disease have been reported.[60]

Treatment

There is no treatment confirmed to restore the storage of fat or to forestall the sequelae of long-term diabetes. Although the hyperglycemia persists despite therapy with very large doses of insulin, hyperglycemia and hyperinsulinemia both fall following treatment with insulin-like growth factor 1 (IGF-1).[61,62] Whether this will be helpful or harmful[44] for the patients is unknown. Reduction of food intake, for example, by treatment with fenfluramine or simply by caloric restriction alone, may reduce the hypermetabolic state, but the long-term benefits are unproven,[44] and fenfluramine may cause significant morbidity. Etretinate caused clearing of acanthosis nigricans in one patient.[63] One group found improvement in the metabolic abnormalities and some regain of subcutaneous fat in patients with various forms of lipodystrophy treated with the PPAR-γ agonist troglitazone. This drug has been removed from the US market because of hepatotoxicity but has been succeeded by pioglitazone and rosiglitazone, which are expected to be similarly beneficial.[64] Leptin infusion can reverse metabolic abnormalities in murine transgenic lipoatrophic mice but the sensitivity to this agent depends on the model used.[65,66] Combination therapy of lipoatrophic mice with leptin plus adiponectin may be more effective.[67] Nine women treated with leptin for 4 months had significant amelioration of their metabolic and endocrine abnormalities and reduction in liver hypertrophy and abnormal transaminases.[68,69]

REFERENCES

1. Garg A: Lipodystrophies. *Am J Med* **108**:143, 2000
2. Bier DM et al: Cephalothoracic lipodystrophy with hypocomplementemic renal disease: Discordance in identical twin sisters. *J Clin Endocrinol Metab* **46**:800, 1978
3. Nagore E et al: Lipoatrophia semicircularis—A traumatic panniculitis: Report of seven cases and review of the literature. *J Am Acad Dermatol* **39**:879, 1998
4. Bernstein RS et al: Adipose cell morphology and control of lipolysis in a patient with partial lipodystrophy. *Metabolism* **28**:519, 1979
5. Mathieson PW, Peters K: Are nephritic factors nephritogenic? *Am J Kidney Dis* **24**:964, 1994
6. Williams DG: C3 nephritic factor and mesangiocapillary glomerulonephritis. *Pediatr Nephrol* **11**:96, 1997
7. Mathieson PW et al: Complement-mediated adipocyte lysis by nephritic factor sera. *J Exp Med* **177**:1827, 1993
8. Bennett WM et al: Mesangiocapillary glomerulonephritis type II (dense-deposit disease): Clinical features of progressive disease. *Am J Kidney Dis* **13**:469, 1989
9. Alper CA et al: Increased susceptibility to infection in a patient with type II essential hypercatabolism of C3. *N Eng J Med* **288**:601, 1973
10. Smith PM et al: Lipodystrophy, pancreatitis, and eosinophilia. *Gut* **16**:230, 1975
11. Fitch N, Tulandi T: Progressive partial lipodystrophy and third-trimester intrauterine fetal death. *Am J Obstet Gynecol* **156**:1195, 1987
12. Coessens BC, Van Geertruyden JP: Simultaneous bilateral facial reconstruction of a Barraquer-Simons lipodystrophy with free TRAM flaps. *Plast Reconstr Surg* **95**:911, 1995
13. Ketterings C: Lipodystrophy and its treatment. *Ann Plast Surg* **21**:536, 1988
14. Kobberling J, Dunnigan MG: Familial partial lipodystrophy: Two types of an X linked dominant syndrome, lethal in the hemizygous state. *J Med Genet* **23**:120, 1986
15. Lloyd J et al: Subtotal lipodystrophy with autosomal dominant inheritance. *J R Soc Med* **86**:477, 1993
16. Johansen K et al: An unusual type of familial lipodystrophy. *J Clin Endocrinol Metab* **80**:3442, 1995
17. Jackson SN et al: Dunnigan-Kobberling syndrome: An autosomal dominant form of partial lipodystrophy. *QJM* **90**:27, 1997
18. Cao H, Hegele RA: Nuclear lamin A/C R482Q mutation in Canadian kindreds with Dunnigan-type familial partial lipodystrophy. *Hum Mol Genet* **9**:109, 2000
19. Shackleton S et al: LMNA, encoding lamin A/C, is mutated in partial lipodystrophy. *Nat Genet* **24**:153, 2000
20. Speckman RA et al: Mutational and haplotype analyses of families with familial partial lipodystrophy (Dunnigan variety) reveal recurrent missense mutations in the globular C-terminal domain of lamin A/C. *Am J Hum Genet* **66**:1192, 2000
21. Novelli G et al: Mandibuloacral dysplasia is caused by a mutation in LMNA-encoding lamin A/C. *Am J Hum Genet* **71**:426, 2002
22. Hegele RA et al: Genetic variation in LMNA modulates plasma leptin and indices of obesity in aboriginal Canadians. *Physiol Genomics* **3**:39, 2000
23. Vigouroux C et al: A new missense mutation in the calcium-sensing receptor in familial benign hypercalcaemia associated with partial lipoatrophy and insulin resistant diabetes. *Clin Endocrinol* **53**:393, 2000
24. Garg A et al: Adipose tissue distribution pattern in patients with familial partial lipodystrophy (Dunnigan variety). *J Clin Endocrinol Metab* **84**:170, 1999
25. Garg A: Gender differences in the prevalence of metabolic complications in familial partial lipodystrophy (Dunnigan variety). *J Clin Endocrinol Metab* **85**:1776, 2000
26. John M et al: Antiretroviral therapy and the lipodystrophy syndrome. *Antivir Ther* **6**:9, 2001
27. Strawford A, Hellerstein MK: Metabolic Complications of HIV and AIDS. *Curr Infect Dis Rep* **3**:183, 2001
28. Murata H et al: The mechanism of insulin resistance caused by HIV protease inhibitor therapy. *J Biol Chem* **275**:20251, 2000
29. Caron M et al: The HIV protease inhibitor indinavir impairs sterol regulatory element-binding protein-1 intranuclear localization, inhibits preadipocyte differentiation, and induces insulin resistance. *Diabetes* **50**:1378, 2001
30. Domingo P et al: Subcutaneous adipocyte apoptosis in HIV-1 protease inhibitor-associated lipodystrophy. *AIDS* **13**:2261, 1999
31. Hadigan C et al: Metabolic abnormalities and cardiovascular disease risk factors in adults with human immunodeficiency virus infection and lipodystrophy. *Clin Infect Dis* **32**:130, 2001
32. Wurtz R, Ceaser S: The possible benefits of the improved CD4 response outweigh the metabolic and cosmetic problems associated with lipodystrophy is not known. *Clin Infect Dis* **31**:1497, 2000
33. Hadigan C et al: Metformin in the treatment of HIV lipodystrophy syndrome. *JAMA* **284**:472, 2000
34. Smith KJ, Skelton HG: Peroxisomal proliferator-activated ligand therapy for HIV lipodystrophy. *Clin Exp Dermatol* **26**:155, 2000
35. Chastain MA et al: HIV lipodystrophy: Review of the syndrome and report of a case treated with liposuction. *Dermatol Surg* **27**:497, 2001
36. Garg A et al: A gene for congenital generalized lipodystrophy maps to human chromosome 9q34. *J Clin Endocrinol Metab* **84**:3390, 1999
37. Magre J et al: Identification of the gene altered in Berardinelli-Seip congenital lipodystrophy on chromosome 11q13. *Nat Genet* **28**:365, 2001
38. Corbin A et al: Diencephalic involvement in generalized lipodystrophy: Rational and treatment with the neuroleptic agent, pimozide. *Acta Endocrinol (Copenh)* **77**:209, 1974
39. Shimomura I et al: Insulin resistance and diabetes mellitus in transgenic mice expressing nuclear SREBP-1c in adipose tissue: Model for congenital generalized lipodystrophy. *Genes Dev* **12**:3182, 1998
40. Gavrilova O et al: Surgical implantation of adipose tissue reverses diabetes in lipoatrophic mice. *J Clin Invest* **105**:271, 2000
41. Andreelli F et al: Normal reproductive function in leptin-deficient patients with lipoatrophic diabetes. *J Clin Endocrinol Metab* **85**:715, 2000

42. Colebunders R et al: Curly hair and lipodystrophy as a result of highly active antiretroviral treatment? *Arch Dermatol* **136**:1064, 2000
43. Garg A et al: Skeletal muscle morphology and exercise response in congenital generalized lipodystrophy. *Diabetes Care* **23**:1545, 2000
44. Seip M, Trygstad O: Generalized lipodystrophy, congenital and acquired (lipoatrophy). *Acta Pediatr Suppl* **413**:2, 1996
45. Sovik O, Oseid S: Studies in congenital generalized lipodystrophy. VI. Suppressible and non-suppressible insulin-like activities of plasma. *Acta Endocrinol (Copenh)* **79**:720, 1975
46. Sovik O et al: Studies of insulin resistance in congenital generalized lipodystrophy. *Acta Pediatr Suppl* **413**:29, 1996
47. Kahn CR et al: The syndromes of insulin resistance and acanthosis nigricans: Insulin-receptor disorders in man. *N Engl J Med* **294**:739, 1976
48. Podskalny JM, Kahn CR: Cell culture studies on patients with extreme insulin resistance: 1. Receptor defects on cultured fibroblasts. *J Clin Endocrinol Metab* **54**:261, 1982
49. Moller DE et al: Prevalence of mutations in the insulin receptor gene in subjects with features of the type A syndrome of insulin resistance. *Diabetes* **43**:247, 1994
50. Case records of the Massachusetts General Hospital: Case 1-1975. *N Engl J Med* **292**:35, 1975
51. Casali RE et al: Renal Transplantation in a patient with lipoatrophic diabetes. *Transplantation* **26**:174, 1978
52. Huseman CA et al: Congenital lipodystrophy. II. Association with polycystic ovarian disease. *J Pediatr* **95**:72, 1979
53. Penney LL et al: Congenital lipodystrophy and polycystic ovarian disease. *J Reprod Med* **26**:145, 1981
54. Catalano PM et al: Successful pregnancy outcome in association with lipoatrophic diabetes mellitus. *Obstet Gynecol* **76**:978, 1990
55. Westvik J: Radiological features in generalized lipodystrophy. *Acta Pediatr Suppl* **413**:44, 1996
56. Wilson TA et al: Cerebral computed tomography in lipodystrophy. *Arch Neurol* **39**:733, 1982
57. Boucher BJ et al: Plasma free fatty acid turnover in total lipodystrophy. *Clin Endocrinol (Oxf)* **4**:83, 1975

58. Chait A et al: Lipodystrophy with hyperlipidaemia: The role of insulin in very low density lipoprotein over-synthesis. *Clin Endocrinol (Oxf)* **10**:173, 1979
59. Rossini AA et al: Metabolic and endocrine studies in a case of lipoatrophic diabetes. *Metabolism* **26**:637, 1977
60. Hall SW et al: Generalized lipodystrophy, scleroderma, and Hodgkin's disease. *Arch Intern Med* **138**:1303, 1978
61. Kuzuya H et al: Trial of insulin-like growth factor I therapy for patients with extreme insulin resistance syndromes. *Diabetes* **42**:696, 1993
62. Moses AC et al: Insulin-like growth factor I (rhIGF-I) as a therapeutic agent for hyperinsulinemic insulin-resistant diabetes mellitus. *Diabetes Res Clin Pract* **28**(Suppl):S185, 1995
63. Mork NJ et al: Treatment of acanthosis nigricans with etretinate (Tegison) in a patient with Lawrence-Seip syndrome (generalized lipodystrophy). *Acta Derm Venereol (Stockh)* **66**:173, 1986
64. Arioglu E et al: Efficacy and safety of troglitazone in the treatment of lipodystrophy syndromes. *Ann Intern Med* **133**:263, 2000
65. Shimomura I et al: Leptin reverses insulin resistance and diabetes mellitus in mice with congenital lipodystrophy. *Nature* **401**:73, 1999
66. Ebihara K et al: Transgenic overexpression of leptin rescues insulin resistance and diabetes in a mouse model of lipoatrophic diabetes. *Diabetes* **50**:1440, 2001
67. Yamauchi T et al: The fat-derived hormone adiponectin reverses insulin resistance associated with both lipoatrophy and obesity. *Nat Med* **7**:941, 2001
68. Oral EA et al: Leptin-replacement therapy for lipodystrophy. *N Engl J Med* **346**:570, 2002
69. Oral EA et al: Effect of leptin replacement on pituitary hormone regulation in patients with severe lipodystrophy. *J Clin Endocrinol Metab* **87**:3110, 2002

CHAPTER 111

Karl H. Anders

Neoplasms of the Subcutaneous Fat

Benign lipomatous tumors of the subcutaneous fat are very common, whereas cutaneous liposarcomas are exceptionally rare. The recently described variants of lipomas are encountered infrequently,[1–4] but recognition of their characteristics is important so as to avoid erroneous diagnoses and excessive surgery.

In general, lipomas and all their variations are grossly and microscopically symmetric, well circumscribed, and smooth bordered. In contrast, malignant neoplasms of adipocytes (lipocytes) and of lipoblasts, the embryonic precursors of lipocytes (i.e., liposarcomas), are asymmetric and infiltrative. Usually lipomas do not persist at the local site once they have been completely excised. This is equally true for most liposarcomas, although their poor circumscription often precludes complete resection.

Benign and malignant lipomatous tumors often demonstrate repeatable karyotypic abnormalities, thereby offering a potential, albeit usually impractical, diagnostic tool for their elucidation. A discussion of these chromosomal aberrations is beyond the scope of this chapter, and the interested reader is referred elsewhere.[1,2,5]

LIPOMA

Clinical Features

Lipomas are the most common mesenchymal neoplasms.[1] They may be found at any subcutaneous site but are especially frequent on the neck and trunk. Although lipomas usually are solitary, they may be multiple. Most lipomas are small, mobile, slowly growing, and asymptomatic, but some may be large (>15 cm). Lipomas may occur at any age but usually become evident in middle age. Characteristically, they are disk-shaped, round or ovoid, lobulated, yellow masses, usually within the

FIGURE 111-1

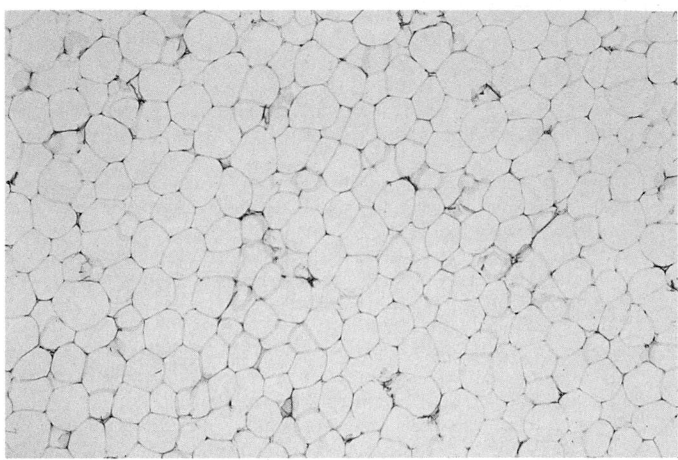

Lipoma.

subcutaneous tissue, with a doughy consistency. Lipomas are easily "shelled out" surgically because they are well demarcated. Recurrences are uncommon. Lipomas practically never eventuate in liposarcoma.

Histopathologic Findings

Subcutaneous lipomas tend to be well-circumscribed neoplasms surrounded by a thin, fibrous capsule. They are composed of sheets of mature, uniform adipocytes (i.e., large clear cells), spherical to polygonal, characterized by a single, large, lipid vacuole that compresses and displaces the nucleus to the periphery of the cell (Fig. 111-1). Adipocytes in a lipoma are indistinguishable from those in the adjacent subcutaneous fat and, like them, are encircled by capillaries. Thin strands of fibrous tissue intersect the sheets of adipocytes, but they are not arranged in the fenestrated pattern characteristic of fibrous septa in the normal subcutaneous fat.

Lipomas may extend into or arise within skeletal muscle (*intramuscular lipomas*), a phenomenon usually seen on the trunk[6] (Fig. 111-2).

FIGURE 111-2

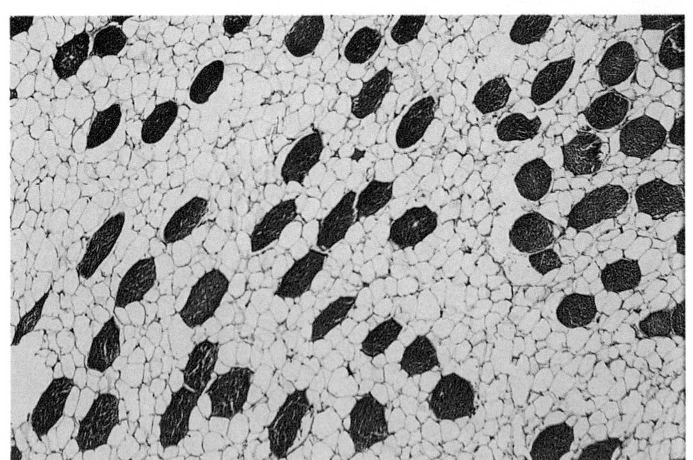

Intramuscular lipoma.

FIGURE 111-3

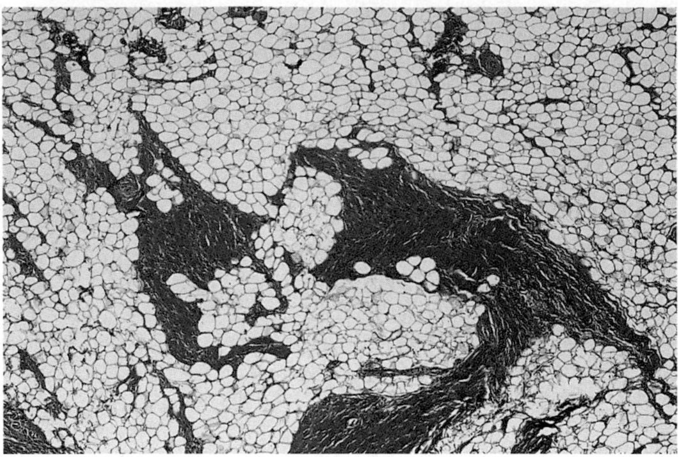

Fibrolipoma.

Intramuscular lipomas are often poorly delineated and thus more prone to recur because their excision often is incomplete. *Adenolipomas* are characterized by the presence of eccrine glands and ducts within a lipoma.[7]

Some lipomas contain mesenchymal elements other than fat. For example, *fibrolipomas* exhibit many thick bundles of collagen (Fig. 111-3). *Sclerotic lipomas* demonstrate primarily thickened collagen bundles, with few persisting adipocytes, and mimic sclerotic fibromas.[4,8] *Myxolipomas* show extensive stromal deposits of mucopolysaccharides (Fig. 111-4) and may mimic myxoma. *Myelolipomas* manifest ectopic hematopoietic bone marrow elements; *osteolipomas* display metaplastic bone.

Trauma and ischemia can cause necrosis en masse of adipocytes. *Infarcted lipomas* demonstrate necrotic fat surrounded by multinucleate histiocytic giant cells, lipophages, lymphocytes, and extravasated erythrocytes (Fig. 111-5). Pseudocysts may form consequent to absorption of necrotic adipocytes, and fibrosis and dystrophic calcification are late sequelae.

FIGURE 111-4

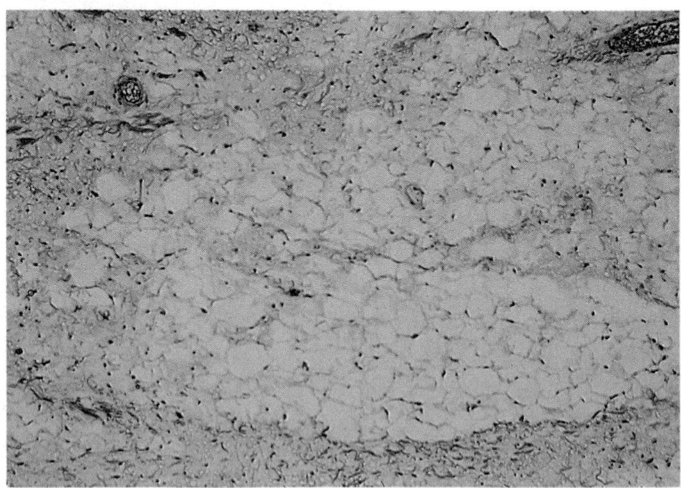

Myxolipoma.

FIGURE 111-5

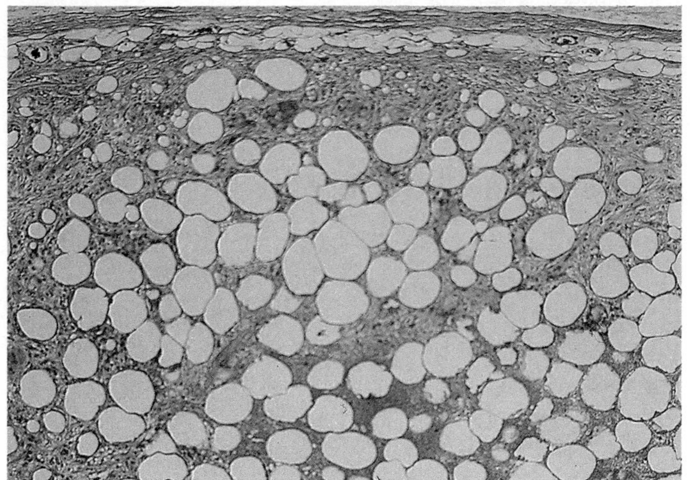

Infarcted lipoma.

MULTIPLE LIPOMA SYNDROMES

Some patients bear numerous subcutaneous lipomas.[1] These neoplasms are microscopically indistinguishable from the solitary lipomas just described but are of clinical interest.

Familial multiple lipomas are transmitted in autosomal dominant fashion, with incomplete penetrance, and usually have become apparent by the third decade of life.[9] Patients may have hundreds of discrete, slowly growing, asymptomatic, subcutaneous lipomas of various sizes and in widespread distribution (Fig. 111-6). The lesions are often more pronounced on the extremities, especially the forearms.

FIGURE 111-6

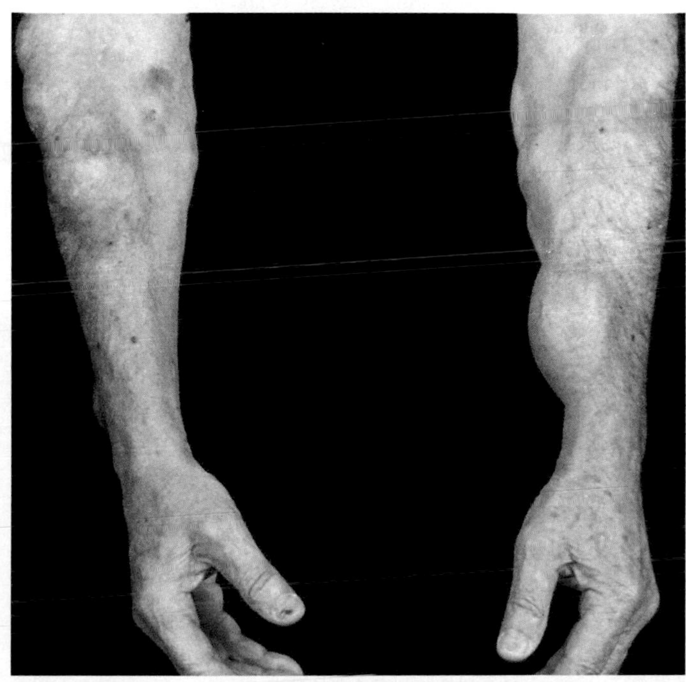

Multiple, symmetric lipomas of variable size on the forearms of a middle-aged man.

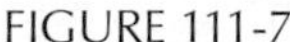

FIGURE 111-7

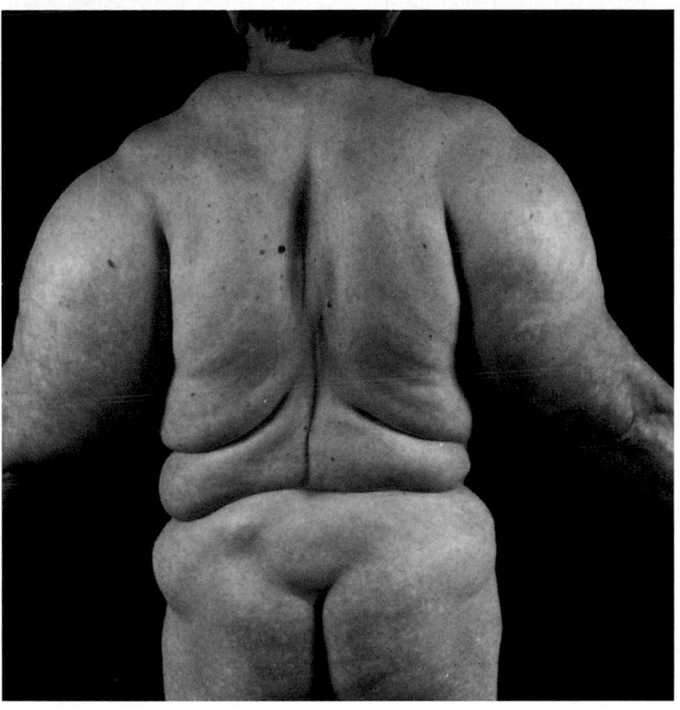

Symmetric lipomatosis.

Diffuse lipomatosis is characterized by widespread, noncircumscribed overgrowth of mature adipocytes.[1] The lesions usually are situated on the trunk or proximal extremity. They may be huge and cosmetically disfiguring. Persistence at the local site is common because resection of these lesions is often incomplete; they may be treated with suction lipectomy.

Symmetric lipomatosis (Madelung's disease) is an uncommon disorder characterized by numerous, symmetrically distributed, nontender, poorly demarcated fatty tumors in the subcutaneous and deeper tissues. These masses are situated mostly in the neck, suboccipital region, proximal (but not distal) extremities, and upper part of the trunk[10] (Fig. 111-7). Confluence of these lesions results in a disfiguring "horse collar" appearance that, when severe, may interfere with mobility of the neck and with respiration. This idiopathic condition is not hereditary and usually afflicts middle-aged alcoholic men.

Adiposis dolorosa (Dercum's disease) is a rare idiopathic disorder that favors middle-aged, obese, menopausal women.[11] In this condition, many slowly growing, exquisitely tender lipomas are present, especially on the arms, trunk, and periarticular soft tissues. Pain is episodic and may be debilitating. Sustained therapy with analgesics may be required for symptomatic relief of painful paroxysms. Weight loss is reputed to be beneficial, and surgical excision may eliminate pain at a local site.

Congenital lipomatosis is usually diagnosed during the first few months of life, presenting as large, irregular, subcutaneous masses of adipose tissue.[12] These masses are found mostly on the chest, where they permeate skeletal muscle (i.e., *infiltrating lipomas*). Since their resection is often incomplete, the lesions frequently persist at the local site.

Congenital lipomatosis may also be a manifestation of the *Proteus syndrome*[13,14] (see Chap. 188), in which, in addition to lipomas, there are partial gigantism of the hands or feet, hemihypertrophy, exostoses, scoliosis, melanocytic nevi, and other cutaneous neoplasms (i.e., hemangiomas, lymphangiomas, mesenchymomas). The disorder may be sporadic or inherited in autosomal recessive fashion. It is now thought that the "Elephant Man" was afflicted with the Proteus syndrome.

The *Bannayan-Zonana syndrome,* an autosomal dominant disorder manifest in children, consists of multiple lipomas, hemangiomas, lymphangiomas, and macrocephaly without ventricular enlargement.[14] Patients with the Bannayan-Zonana syndrome often demonstrate delayed motor and speech development and motor dysfunction.

ANGIOLIPOMA

Clinical Features

Angiolipomas resemble lipomas clinically but tend to develop in young adults and are less prevalent (representing about 5 percent of fatty tumors). They are usually numerous, frequently painful or tender on palpation, and sometimes surprisingly mobile.[1] The forearms and trunk are favored sites. Angiolipomas tend to be small (<5 cm), firm, well-circumscribed, yellow to red subcutaneous tumors. Rarely, these neoplasms present as large, ill-defined masses with jagged extensions into skeletal muscle (i.e., *infiltrating angiolipomas*). Familial angiolipomatosis is uncommon but does occur.[15]

Histopathologic Findings

Angiolipomas are usually sharply circumscribed neoplasms composed of a mixture of adipocytes and small blood vessels (Fig. 111-8). Blood vessel proliferation is most pronounced at the periphery of the neoplasm, and the vascular component comprises at least 10 percent of the tumor's volume. Some angiolipomas, however, contain very few vessels, in contrast to others that are richly vascular in a lobular pattern that mimics a hemangioma. Intraluminal spaces are often filled with erythrocytes or fibrin thrombi. Oval-shaped pericytes, mast cells, and fibrous tissue also may be present.

Angiolipomas that exhibit a prominent vascular pattern and little fat are often highly cellular (i.e., *cellular angiolipoma*), and when they are poorly circumscribed or removed in fragmented fashion, they have been confused with Kaposi's sarcoma and hemangioendothelioma.[16] Endothelial cells in angiolipomas are small and monomorphous; no mitotic figures are detectable.

SPINDLE CELL LIPOMA

Clinical Features

Spindle cell lipomas comprise about 1.5 percent of neoplasms of adipocytes. They usually are small (< 5 cm), firm, subcutaneous masses that become apparent in middle-aged men.[1,17] Generally only one spindle cell lipoma is present, but patients with multiple tumors—including familial clusters—have been reported.[18] The lesions are slowly growing, painless nodules situated principally on the upper part of the back, shoulders, or lower posterior neck, although they may present at almost any site. On gross inspection, they are yellow to gray-white.

Histopathologic Findings

Spindle cell lipomas consist of mature adipocytes, oval to spindle-shaped cells, and a stroma replete with collagen and mucin within which mast cells are scattered (Fig. 111-9). The relative proportion of these elements varies markedly, even within a particular lesion. Most tumors are subcutaneous and well circumscribed, but some are intradermal and poorly delineated.[3,19] Spindle cell lipomas rarely are dominated by mucinous stroma and may be diagnosed incorrectly as a myxoma or myxoid liposarcoma. An entity described as *dendritic fibromyxolipoma* appears to be a variant of spindle cell lipoma that is replete with mucinous stroma and stellate mesenchymal cells.[4,19]

The "spindle" cells characteristic of spindle cell lipoma usually have small, oval, monomorphous nuclei and pale cytoplasm. In some foci, there are only a few oval cells among numerous adipocytes; in others, there are sheets of oval cells that may obscure the fundamental adipose character of the neoplasm. Rarely, the oval cells exhibit pleomorphism and multinucleation, analogous to changes seen in "ancient schwannomas." Mitotic figures are hardly ever seen. Some spindle cell lipomas demonstrate large, irregular clefts and slitlike spaces that resemble blood vessels, described as the *pseudoangiomatous variant* of spindle cell lipoma.[4,21]

Although the origin of the oval cells has yet to be elucidated, electron microscopy reveals them to display features consistent with fibroblasts

FIGURE 111-8

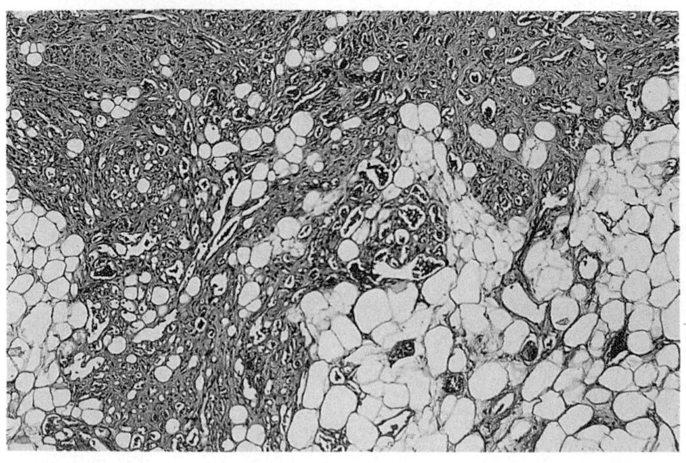

Angiolipoma.

FIGURE 111-9

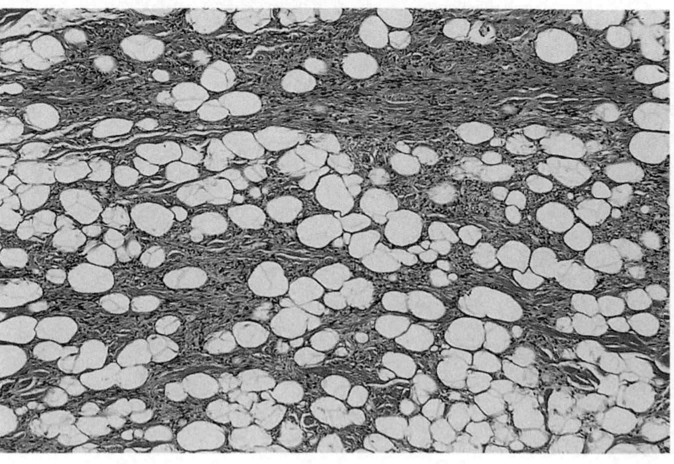

Spindle cell lipoma.

or prelipoblastic mesenchymal cells.[17,20,22] Unlike myolipomas, no evidence of smooth muscle differentiation is found within the oval cells of spindle cell lipoma, which are desmin- and actin-negative but strongly positive for CD34.[1]

Spindle cell lipoma may be confused with dermatofibrosarcoma protuberans, fibrosarcoma, and liposarcoma but can be differentiated from those malignant neoplasms by its sharply circumscribed border, monomorphous nuclei, and absence of mitotic figures and of lipoblasts.[17]

PLEOMORPHIC LIPOMA

Clinical Features

Pleomorphic lipomas are uncommon neoplasms that cannot be distinguished clinically from spindle cell lipomas.[1,23] Because of their similarity clinically and ultrastructurally,[23] and because of identical chromosomal alterations,[5] these tumors are now generally accepted as pleomorphic variants of spindle cell lipomas.

Histopathologic Findings

In the overall setting of a spindle cell lipoma, there are bizarre, multinucleate giant cells, termed *floret cells* (Fig. 111-10). These cells, which also may be seen in pleomorphic fibroma and fibroepithelial papillomas, have abundant eosinophilic cytoplasm and many crowded, overlapping dark nuclei that resemble, vaguely, the petals of a flower. Floret cells in a particular pleomorphic lipoma may be few or many, localized or diffuse. The precise nature of floret cells has yet to be established, but they are probably prelipoblastic mesenchymal cells.[22] Occasional lipoblast-like cells may be scattered throughout a pleomorphic lipoma, and the adipocytes may show nuclear hyperchromasia.

Although pleomorphic lipomas are benign, they may be misinterpreted histopathologically as a sarcoma, especially liposarcoma, because of the presence of the peculiar floret cells. Pleomorphic lipomas can be differentiated from liposarcomas by their circumscription, infrequent (nonatypical) mitotic figures, only rare lipoblasts, absence of necrosis, and distinct cytogenetic alterations.[5]

FIGURE 111-10

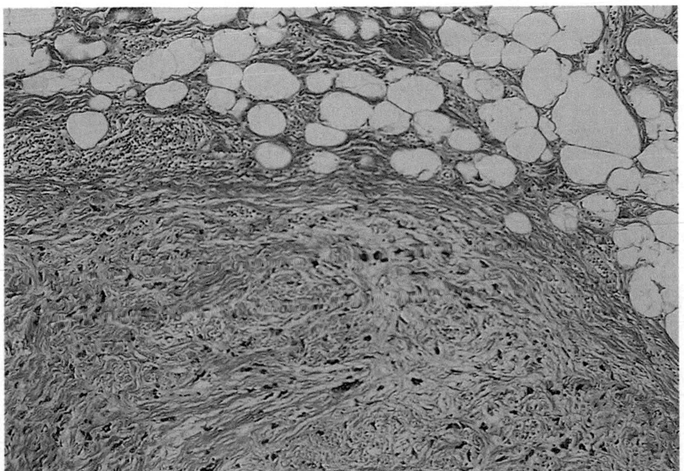

Pleomorphic lipoma.

CHONDROID LIPOMA

Clinical Features

This neoplasm is extremely uncommon and found mostly in women.[14,24,25] It usually appears in the subcutaneous fat or in muscles of the hips and extremities. Chondroid lipomas are small (<5 cm) lesions with a rubbery, yellow, cut surface.

Histopathologic Findings

The neoplasm is sharply circumscribed and composed of lobules of eosinophilic, vacuolated cells that resemble chondroblasts or lipoblasts admixed with a variable number of mature adipocytes.[24–26] The vacuolated cells are often arranged in sheets, nests, or cords and are situated in a collagenous and mucinous stroma that resembles cartilage. The vacuolated cells contain hyperchromatic nuclei that sometimes have scalloped borders and are replete with cytoplasmic fat, as demonstrated by oil-red O stains[25,26]; they are S-100 protein positive. In some foci, the tumor appears mostly chondroid; in other regions, adipocytes predominate, and it is there that the lipomatous nature of the neoplasm is apparent. Blood vessels are prominent, and hemorrhage and hemosiderin are common. Ultrastructurally, most chondroid lipomas show features consistent with origin from white fat.[26]

While clinically benign, chondroid lipoma may be misinterpreted histopathologically as extraskeletal myxoid chondrosarcoma or myxoid liposarcoma, but it is distinguished from these malignant neoplasms by its sharp circumscription and absence of nuclear atypia and mitotic figures.

MYOLIPOMA

Clinical Features

Sometimes known as *lipoleiomyomas,* these rare neoplasms clinically resemble large lipomas.[1,4,27] They usually arise in subcutaneous or deeper abdominal tissues of adults. Grossly, they are generally large (>15 cm) and well demarcated, with a soft to slimy yellow-white cut surface.

Histopathologic Findings

Myolipomas are biphasic neoplasms that consist of a mixture of mature adipocytes and smooth muscle cells, the latter demonstrating immunoreactivity with actin and desmin but not CD34, features that are useful in differentiating these tumors from spindle cell lipomas.[27] In some fields the smooth muscle cells may predominate, and the lesions may mimic leiomyomas, but thorough study always reveals many adipocytes. The prominent vascular component so characteristic of angiomyolipoma is not seen. There is no nuclear atypia or mitotic activity, a feature useful in distinguishing myolipoma from dedifferentiated liposarcoma.

ANGIOMYOLIPOMA

Clinical Features

Angiomyolipomas (*angiolipoleiomyomas*) occur mostly in the kidneys, generally in patients with tuberous sclerosis. Rarely, these neoplasms appear in the dermis or subcutis, usually in acral skin or in skin near the elbows and ears. Cutaneous angiomyolipomas usually arise in adult men and are not associated with tuberous sclerosis or with renal angiomyolipomas.[28,29] They are slowly growing, usually asymptomatic, circumscribed neoplasms. Clinically, they are often confused with cysts, conventional lipomas, and giant cell tumors of tendon sheath.

Histopathologic Features

Like their more common renal counterparts, cutaneous angiomyolipomas contain a variable admixture of thick-walled blood vessels, smooth muscle bundles, and mature adipocytes. The smooth muscle cells are desmin- and actin-positive and may show atypia that is of no prognostic significance. Unlike renal angiomyolipomas, smooth muscle cells in cutaneous angiomyolipomas do not stain with HMB-45. Stromal mucin may be present and is accompanied by mast cells.

FIBROHISTIOCYTIC LIPOMA

Clinical Features

Fibrohistiocytic lipomas are uncommon benign neoplasms that arise in the subcutaneous tissues of young men, especially on the anterior torso.[4,30] These tumors are small (<5 cm), solitary, and well circumscribed; complete excision is curative.

Histopathologic Findings

Fibrohistiocytic lipomas are smooth bordered and are characterized by an admixture of mature adipocytes and spindle cells that resemble those seen in fibrous histiocytoma. Fibrohistiocytic lipomas lack atypia, mitotic activity, xanthoma cells, and inflammation; their spindle cells are CD34- and calponin-positive.

The differential diagnosis of fibrohistiocytic lipoma includes spindle cell lipoma, fibrous histiocytoma, and dermatofibrosarcoma protuberans. Spindle cell lipoma has a different clinical presentation and demonstrates no calponin staining but very strong CD34 positivity. Unlike fibrohistiocytic lipoma, fibrous histiocytoma demonstrates no adipocytes, no calponin positivity, and the presence of inflammatory cells. Dermatofibrosarcoma protuberans has a distinctive infiltrative growth pattern and lacks calponin immunoreactivity.

HEMOSIDEROTIC FIBROHISTIOCYTIC LIPOMATOUS LESION

Clinical Features

Hemosiderotic fibrohistiocytic lipomatous lesions are extremely rare, usually occurring around the ankle or feet of middle-aged women.[31] There is often a history of prior trauma at the site, suggesting that they are reactive or reparative proliferations. Hemosiderotic fibrohistiocytic lipomatous lesions are subcutaneous, well circumscribed, and yellow-brown.

Histopathologic Findings

The morphology of hemosiderotic fibrohistiocytic lipomatous lesions overlaps with that of fibrohistiocytic lipoma, in that both contain mature adipocytes and a proliferation of spindle cells. Hemosiderotic fibrohistiocytic lipomatous lesions also demonstrate numerous plump fibroblastic cells, some with atypia and multinucleation, abundant hemosiderin pigment, and the presence of mixed inflammatory cell infiltrates.

HIBERNOMA

Clinical Features

Hibernomas are uncommon benign neoplasms that clinically resemble common lipomas.[1,32] They are solitary and reside in the subcutaneous tissues of the interscapular, lower cervical, or axillary region of young adults. Hibernomas tend to be small, mobile, and tan to reddish brown.

Histopathologic Findings

Hibernomas are distinguished by their similarity to embryonic brown fat. The neoplasms are formed by lobules of plump, round or oval vacuolated cells that resemble mulberries (Fig. 111-11). "Mulberry cells" have large, round central nuclei, often with prominent nucleoli, and abundant granular eosinophilic cytoplasm. Small intracytoplasmic lipid vacuoles are numerous in mulberry cells. Larger univacuolar adipocytes, i.e., white fat cells, are often present in these lesions, especially at the periphery. In some neoplasms, there are features of both conventional lipomas and hibernomas. Electron microscopy reveals numerous large mitochondria that account for the granular cytoplasm of the cells and the brown gross appearance of these neoplasms.[32]

LIPOBLASTOMA/LIPOBLASTOMATOSIS

Clinical Features

Lipoblastomas are uncommon neoplasms that appear only in infants and children, usually in the first 5 years of life.[1,33,34] They are solitary subcutaneous masses, usually situated on the trunk or limbs, that may be present at birth. Growth of the neoplasm is slow, but in time it may become large, i.e., >12 cm.

Two variants of lipoblastoma are recognized, i.e., the benign and the diffuse, terms that are confusing because they are not contrasting.

FIGURE 111-11

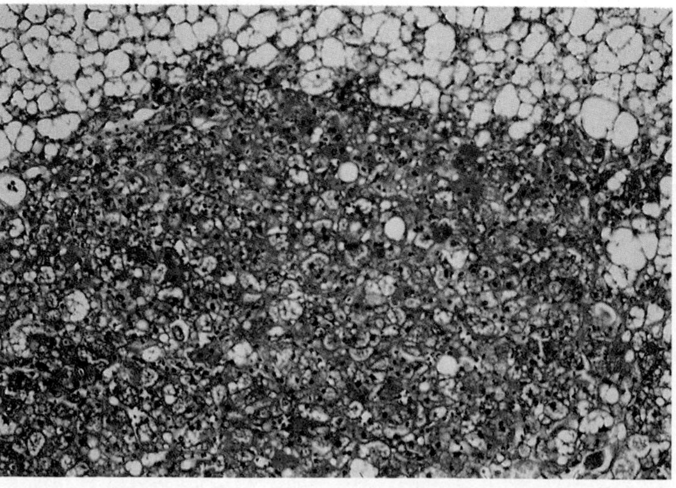

Hibernoma.

FIGURE 111-12

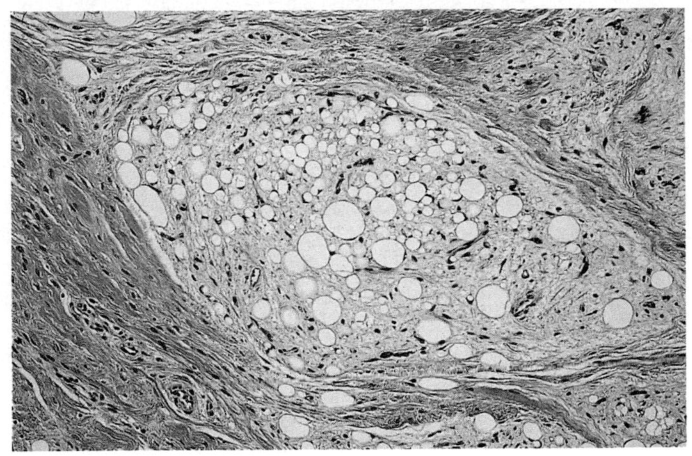

Lipoblastoma.

Benign lipoblastomas are subcutaneous, discrete, and suggestive clinically of lipoma. *Diffuse lipoblastomas (lipoblastomatosis)* are seated more deeply and infiltrate skeletal muscle and other soft tissues. Diffuse lipoblastomas are more likely to persist because their resection tends to be incomplete. The cut surface of lipoblastomas reveals pale-yellow lobulated tissue, often with mucinous stroma.

Histopathologic Findings

Lipoblastomas consist of a variable admixture of mature adipocytes, lipoblasts, and primitive stellate mesenchymal cells situated in a myxoid stroma (Fig. 111-12). The lipoblasts are separated into small lobules by fibrovascular septa. Most lipoblasts demonstrate a single cytoplasmic fat vacuole that causes the nucleus to be compressed to the periphery of the cell, resulting in a "signet ring" appearance. Some lipoblasts have numerous cytoplasmic vacuoles and scalloped nuclear contours. Scattered mature adipocytes are present in variable numbers and sometimes predominate; rarely, hibernoma-like brown fat cells are noted.

Histopathologically, lipoblastomas are easily confused with myxoid liposarcomas. Lipoblastomas occur only in children, in contrast to liposarcomas, which practically never affect children. There are few mitotic figures, no bizarre lipoblasts, and no giant cells in lipoblastomas. At times, however, the histopathologic distinction between lipoblastoma and myxoid liposarcoma may be nearly impossible. Cytogenetic studies can be a useful diagnostic aid, if they have been submitted, because they show characteristic genetic abnormalities that allow these entities to be distinguished.[1,5]

Biologically, lipoblastomas are benign. With the passage of time, the lipoblasts of a lipoblastoma mature to become adipocytes, and the microscopic appearance then becomes that of a conventional lipoma.

LIPOSARCOMAS

Clinical Features

Liposarcomas are among the most common soft tissue malignancies. They are discovered mostly in middle-aged and elderly adults, practically never in children and young adults. Almost always, liposarcomas arise de novo rather than in a preexisting lipoma.[35–38] Most liposarcomas present in the deep soft tissues, but they may involve the skin.

Liposarcomas that arise primarily in the dermis or subcutaneous tissues are very rare but well-documented and have a predilection for the scalp.[3,36–38] Their superficial location generally allows them to be detected and treated when they are relatively small. Primary cutaneous liposarcomas may recur at the local site, but metastases are uncommon, even if the tumor is of high histologic grade.[3,38] As with other cutaneous sarcomas, e.g., leiomyosarcoma, atypical fibroxanthoma, and dermatofibrosarcoma protuberans, their superficial location seems to impart a favorable prognosis.

Usually when liposarcoma involves the skin it is by secondary extension—or metastatic spread—from a deep-seated primary site. These tumors present themselves as nonmobile, often rapidly enlarging masses that cause pain by compression or infiltration of nerves. The skin above such liposarcomas may be stretched, inflamed, ulcerated, or infiltrated by tumor. Successful management requires wide and deep complete resection, in conjunction with local radiation and/or chemotherapy for higher-grade lesions.

Histopathologic Findings

Several types of liposarcomas are recognized on the basis of their characteristic biology, cytogenetic, and histopathologic changes. Common to all are abnormal lipoblasts. The various types of liposarcoma are as follows:

1. *Well-differentiated liposarcomas* have highly variable histopathologic patterns, all of which imply a favorable prognosis. *Lipoma-like liposarcomas* closely resemble, and are often misdiagnosed as, lipomas, especially at scanning magnification (Fig. 111-13). There is greater variation, however, in the size of adipocytes, some of which have enlarged, hyperchromatic nuclei. Abnormal primitive mesenchymal cells are present in thickened fibrous septa. Lipoblasts are also seen occasionally. These neoplasms are sometimes incorrectly classified as *atypical lipomas*[2,35] but, unlike lipomas, frequently recur following surgical resection and may dedifferentiate into higher-grade sarcomas capable of metastasis. *Sclerosing liposarcoma* is typified by abundant dense and fibrillary collagen that contains bizarre, hyperchromatic (sometimes multinculeate) mesenchymal cells and only rare lipoblasts. When a dense infiltrate of lymphocytes and plasma cells is present in the setting of a well-differentiated liposarcoma, a diagnosis of *inflammatory liposarcoma* can be rendered. *Spindle cell liposarcoma* is a recently recognized variant of well-differentiated liposarcoma found in the

FIGURE 111-13

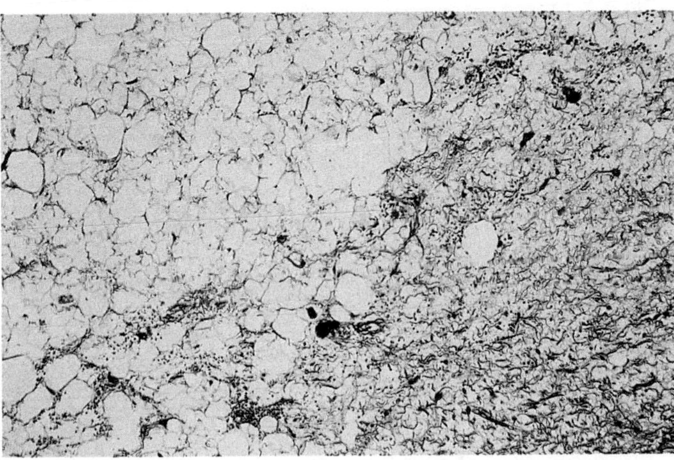

Well-differentiated lipoma-like liposarcoma.

FIGURE 111-14

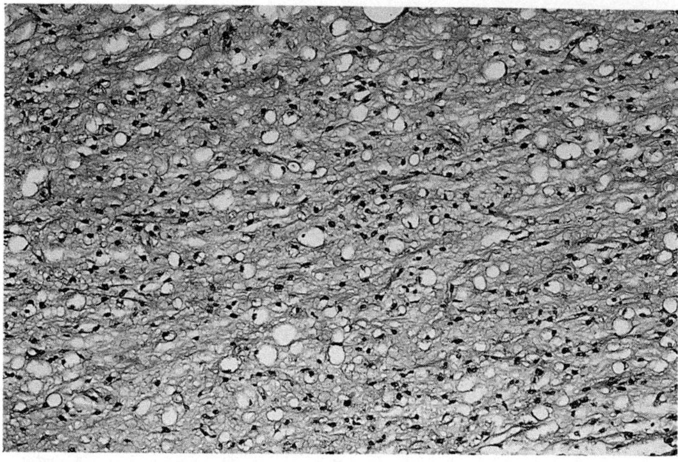

Myxoid liposarcoma.

subcutaneous tissues, generally on the shoulder and upper limbs of middle-aged adults. It is characterized by a slightly atypical spindle cell proliferation demonstrating mitotic activity and associated with adipocytes and lipoblasts. Like other low-grade liposarcomas, spindle cell liposarcoma will recur if excised incompletely and may dedifferentiate.[4,39] With the passage of time and repeated local recurrences, well-differentiated liposarcomas may evolve to become *dedifferentiated liposarcoma,*[35,40] a higher-grade tumor of variable histologic pattern that is capable of metastasis and of causing death.

2. *Myxoid and round cell liposarcomas* have in common a reciprocal translocation between chromosomes 12 and 16. *Myxoid liposarcomas* are the most common variant of liposarcoma (Fig. 111-14), resembling fetal fat, with abundant mucinous stroma, a complex capillary network, and variable numbers of abnormal lipoblasts and stellate cells. Like well-differentiated liposarcomas, myxoid liposarcomas have a favorable prognosis; they often recur following incomplete resection but only rarely metastasize. *Round cell liposarcomas* (Fig. 111-15) are now generally considered to be the most malignant of myxoid liposarcomas, consisting of sheets of primitive, round or oval neoplastic cells that often house a single cytoplasmic lipid vacuole ("signet ring" lipoblasts) and scattered multivacuolated lipoblasts. Stroma is scant but mucinous. It is not uncommon to see evolution focally of an otherwise low-grade myxoid liposarcoma into a round cell liposarcoma.

FIGURE 111-15

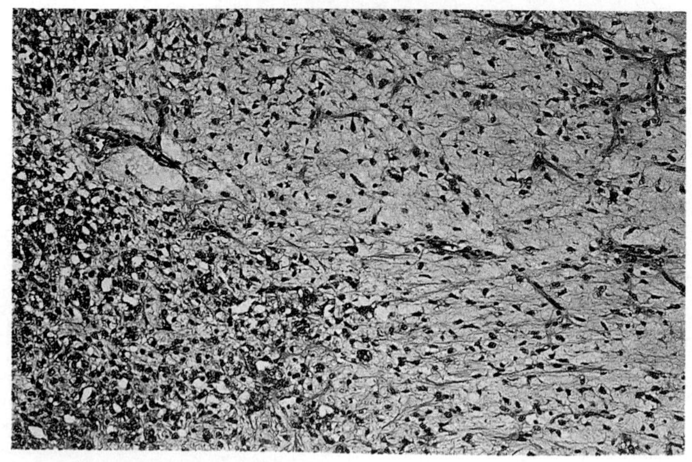

Round cell liposarcoma.

3. *Poorly differentiated (pleomorphic) liposarcomas* exhibit bizarre, markedly abnormal lipoblasts intermingled with smaller pleomorphic cells. The cellularity of the tumor is high, with plentiful mitosis (often atypical) and extensive necrosis. Stroma is usually scant. The neoplasm may be difficult to diagnose as liposarcoma by conventional microscopy alone; electron microscopy may be necesary. Like round cell liposarcoma, these tumors are highly malignant and capable of widespread metastases.

REFERENCES

1. Weiss SW, Goldblum JR: Benign lipomatous tumors, in *Soft Tissue Tumors,* 4th ed. St Louis, Mosby, 2001, p 571
2. Mentzel T, Fletcher CDM: Lipomatous tumors of soft tissues: An update. *Virchows Arch* **427**:353, 1995
3. Mentzel T: Cutaneous lipomatous neoplasms. *Semin Diagn Pathol* **18**:250, 2001
4. Guillou L, Coindre JM: Newly described adipocytic lesions. *Semin Diagn Pathol* **18**:238, 2001
5. Fletcher CDM et al: Correlation between clinicopathological features and karyotype in lipomatous tumors: A report of 178 cases from the chromosomes and morphology (CHAMP) collaborative study group. *Am J Pathol* **148**:623, 1996
6. Fletcher CDM, Bates EM: Intramuscular and intermuscular lipoma: Neglected diagnoses. *Histopathology* **12**:275, 1988
7. Hitchcock MG et al: Adenolipoma of the skin: A report of nine cases. *J Am Acad Dermatol* **29**:82, 1993
8. Zelger BH et al: Sclerotic lipoma: Lipomas simulating sclerotic fibroma. *Histopathology* **31**:174, 1997
9. Leffell DJ, Braverman IM: Familial multiple lipomatosis: Report of a case and a review of the literature. *J Am Acad Dermatol* **15**:275, 1986
10. Uhlin SR: Benign symmetric lipomatosis. *Arch Dermatol* **115**:94, 1979
11. Held JL et al: Surgical amelioration of Dercum's disease: A report and review. *J Dermatol Surg Oncol* **15**:1294, 1989
12. Nixon HH, Scobie WG: Congenital lipomatosis: A report of four cases. *J Pediatr Surg* **6**:742, 1971
13. Viljoen DL et al: Cutaneous manifestations of the Proteus syndrome. *Pediatr Dermatol* **5**:14, 1988
14. Bialer MG et al: Proteus syndrome versus Bannayan-Zonana syndrome: A problem in differential diagnosis. *Eur J Pediatr* **148**:122, 1988
15. Kumar R et al: Autosomal dominant inheritance in familial angiolipomatosis. *Clin Genet* **35**:202, 1989
16. Hunt SJ et al: Cellular angiolipoma. *Am J Surg Pathol* **14**:75, 1990
17. Fletcher CDM, Martin-Bates E: Spindle-cell lipoma: A clinicopathological study with some original observations. *Histopathology* **11**:803, 1987
18. Fanburg-Smith JC et al: Multiple spindle cell lipomas: A report of 7 familial and 11 nonfamilial cases. *Am J Surg Pathol* **22**:40, 1998
19. French CA et al: Intradermal spindle cell/pleomorphic lipoma: A distinct subset. *Am J Dermatopathol* **22**:496, 2000
20. Suster S et al. Dendritic fibromyxolipoma: Clinicopathologic study of a distinctive benign soft tissue lesion that may be mistaken for a sarcoma. *Ann Diagn Pathol* **2**:111, 1998
21. Hawley IC et al: Spindle cell lipoma: A pseudoangiomatous variant. *Histopathology* **24**:565, 1994
22. Pitt MA et al: Spindle cell and pleomorphic lipoma: An ultrastructural study. *Histopathology* **19**:475, 1995
23. Shmookler BM, Enzinger FM: Pleomorphic lipoma: A benign tumor simulating liposarcoma. A clinicopathologic analysis of 48 cases. *Cancer* **47**:126, 1981
24. Meis JM, Enzinger FM: Chondroid lipoma: A unique tumor simulating liposarcoma and myxoid chondrosarcoma. *Am J Surg Pathol* **17**:1103, 1993
25. Thomson TA et al: Cytogenetic and cytologic features of chondroid lipoma of soft tissue. *Mod Pathol* **12**:88, 1999
26. Kindblom LG, Meis-Kindblom JM: Chondroid lipoma: An ultrastructural and immunohistochemical analysis with further observations regarding its differentiation. *Hum Pathol* **26**:706, 1995
27. Meis JM, Enzinger FM: Myolipoma of soft tissue. *Am J Surg Pathol* **17**:121, 1991

28. Fitzpatrick JE et al: Cutaneous angiolipoleiomyoma. *J Am Acad Dermatol* **23**:1093, 1990
29. Argenyi ZB et al: Cutaneous angiomyolipoma: A light-microscopic, immunohistochemical, and electron-microscopic study. *Am J Dermatopathol* **13**:497, 1991
30. Marshall-Taylor C, Fanburg-Smith JC: Fibrohistiocytic lipoma: Twelve cases of a previously undescribed benign fatty tumor. *Ann Diagn Pathol* **4**:354, 2000
31. Marshall-Taylor C, Fanburg-Smith JC: Hemosiderotic fibrohistiocytic lipomatous lesion: Ten cases of a previously undescribed fatty lesion of the foot/ankle. *Mod Pathol* **13**:1192, 2000
32. Fleishman JS, Schwartz RA: Hibernoma: Ultrastructural observations. *J Surg Oncol* **23**:285, 1983
33. Mentzel T et al: Lipoblastoma and lipoblastomatosis: A clinicopathological study of 14 cases. *Histopathology* **23**:527, 1993
34. Collins MH, Chatten J: Lipoblastoma/lipoblastomatosis: A clinicopathologic study of 25 tumors. *Am J Surg Pathol* **21**:1131, 1997
35. Weiss SW, Goldblum JR: Liposarcoma, in *Soft Tissue Tumors,* 4th ed. St Louis, Mosby, 2001, p 641
36. Weitzner S, Kornblum S: Subcutaneous liposarcoma of forearm. *Am Surg* **38**:176, 1972
37. McKee PH et al: Subcuteaneous liposarcoma. *Clin Exp Dermatol* **8**:593, 1983
38. Dei Tos AP et al: Primary liposarcoma of the skin: A rare neoplasm with unusual high grade features. *Am J Dermatopathol* **20**:332, 1998
39. Dei Tos AP et al: Spindle cell liposarcoma, a hitherto unrecognized variant of liposarcoma: Analysis of six cases. *Am J Surg Pathol* **18**:913, 1994
40. McCormick D et al: Dedifferentiated liposarcoma: Clinicopathologic analysis of 32 cases suggesting a better prognostic subgroup among pleomorphic sarcomas. *Am J Surg Pathol* **18**:1213, 1994

SECTION 15
DISORDERS OF THE MUCOCUTANEOUS INTEGUMENT

CHAPTER 112

Jonathan A. Ship
Joan Phelan
A. Ross Kerr

Biology and Pathology of the Oral Mucosa

The mucosal tissues that extend from the vermilion border of the lips to the posterior border of the oral pharynx play a critical role in the protection and maintenance of oral and systemic health. The oral mucosa is a unique tissue that is designed to protect the host; to provide oral-facial sensory feedback to the brain; to facilitate mastication, deglutition, and chemosensory function; and to assist in phonation. Impaired oral mucosal health may lead to numerous oral and systemic complications, including pain, malnutrition, infection, compromised immune function, and exacerbation of medical disorders. Many systemic conditions appear initially in the oral cavity, and prompt diagnosis and management can help minimize disease progression and organ destruction. Further, the oral and systemic implications of oral mucosal diseases can have deleterious consequences for a person's health and quality of life.[1–4] The diagnosis, management, and prevention of oral mucosal diseases are a joint responsibility of dental and medical health care professionals.

BIOLOGY OF THE ORAL MUCOSA

Anatomy and Histology of the Oral Mucosa

The two major functional roles of the oral mucosa are (1) to cover and protect the tissues beneath it and (2) to convey sensory information from the surface. As a covering layer, it provides resistance to insult and protects against infection and toxic substances. In its specialized sensory role, the oral mucosa provides taste sensation and transmits pain, touch, and temperature information. The oral mucosa is classified into three functional types: lining mucosa, masticatory mucosa, and specialized mucosa.

Orthokeratinized stratified squamous epithelium covers the vermilion of the lips. An abrupt interface with the labial oral mucosa occurs just inside the oral cavity. Lining mucosa includes the labial and buccal mucosa, the mucosa covering the ventral surface of the tongue and floor of the mouth, and the mucosa covering the soft palate and the alveolar processes that extend to the gingiva (Fig. 112-1). The lining epithelium is moderately thicker than that of skin and is usually nonkeratinized, but it may be orthokeratinized in areas subject to persistent friction, such as the buccal mucosal tissues adjacent to the occlusal plane (i.e., the interface between the maxillary and the mandibular teeth). The trenchlike configurations that form where the buccal and labial mucosae attach to the maxilla and mandible are called maxillary and mandibular, buccal and labial vestibules.

The second type of oral mucosa, the masticatory mucosa, includes the mucosa covering the hard palate and gingiva. The surface of these areas is orthokeratinized stratified squamous epithelium. The free gingiva occurs where the oral mucosa meets the surface of a tooth and is just a few millimeters in thickness. The mucosa covering the alveolar bone of the maxilla and mandible is called the attached gingiva, and the lining mucosa that extends from the attached gingiva to the buccal and labial mucosa is called the alveolar mucosa. When teeth have been extracted, the resulting area is called the alveolar ridge.

The third type of oral mucosa is the specialized mucosa. This type of mucosa consists primarily of two types of papillae (filiform and fungiform) that cover the dorsal surface of the tongue (Fig. 112-2). The filiform papillae are located on the anterior portion of the tongue and consist of fronds of keratinized epithelium covering thin connective tissue cores. Fungiform papillae are scattered among the filiform papillae. Dark pink in color, they consist of thin nonkeratinized squamous epithelium covering well-vascularized fibrous connective tissue

FIGURE 112-1

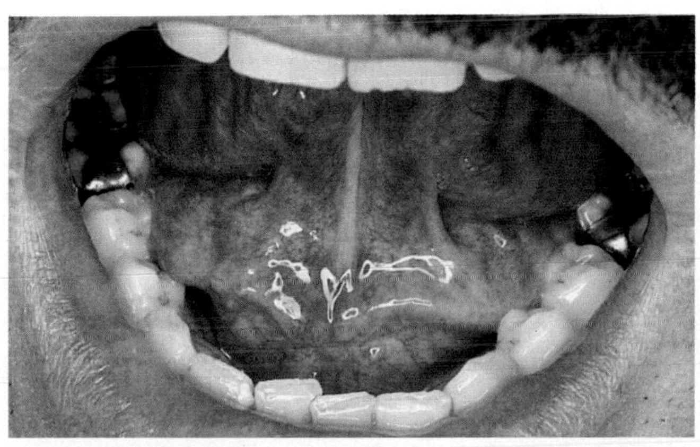

Normal teeth and anterior floor of the mouth. The patient is raising the tongue toward the upper incisor teeth. Visible are the lingual frenum, dark-colored veins on the ventrum of the tongue, and the ridges corresponding to the submandibular (Wharton's) duct.

FIGURE 112-2

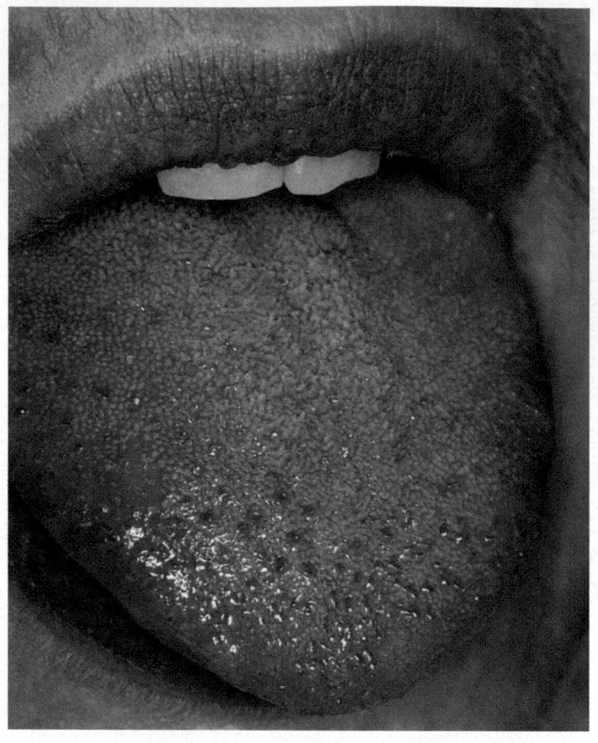

Normal tongue. Note the rough surface, with filiform papillae, and the red, punctate, fungiform papillae scattered, especially in the anterior and lateral regions.

cores. The specialized mucosa of the tongue also includes circumvallate papillae and rudimentary foliate papillae. Circumvallate papillae are located on the posterior dorsal surface of the tongue and are arranged in a V-shaped pattern with the apex of the V at the foramen cecum (Fig. 112-3). These appear as round (4 mm in diameter), erythematous, and slightly exophytic structures. Foliate papillae appear as vertical ridges or folds of tissue on the posterior lateral borders of the tongue.

Several different specialized structures lie in the oral cavity. The most numerous of these are the minor salivary glands. The majority

FIGURE 112-3

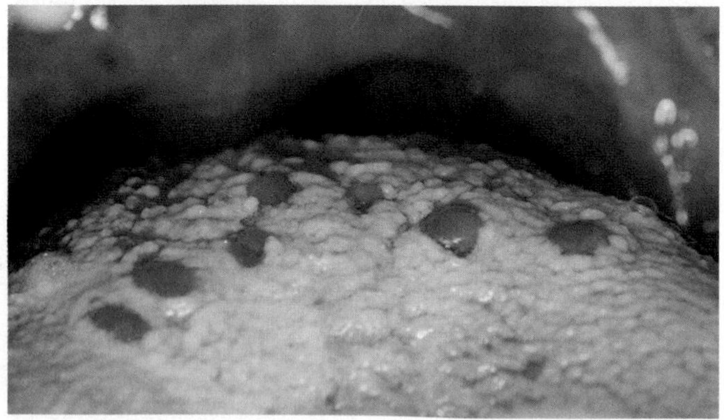

Normal dorsal tongue, with circumvallate papillae. A white coating makes the papillae stand out in sharp relief.

occur in the mucosa of the lower lip and junction of the hard and soft palate, but these glands also appear in many other locations, including the upper lip, the buccal mucosa, and the tongue. The vast majority are mucus-secreting glands. Serous minor salivary glands are found on the tip of the tongue and bilaterally on the posterior lateral aspect of the tongue.

Taste buds are in the mucosa of the tongue, the soft palate, and the pharynx. Three types of lingual papillae contain taste buds: fungiform (anterior two-thirds of the tongue), foliate (lateral borders of the tongue), and circumvallate (posterior border of the tongue). Also commonly found in the oral mucosa, sebaceous glands appear as yellowish-white, slightly raised, granule-appearing structures located on labial and buccal mucosal surfaces. They are referred to as Fordyce's granules and are true sebaceous glands, but have no identified function in the oral cavity.

Three major pairs of salivary glands secrete saliva into the oral cavity: parotid, submandibular, and sublingual glands. The orifice of the excretory duct of the parotid glands (Stenson's duct) is visible on a raised papilla on the buccal mucosa opposite the maxillary molars. The submandibular gland saliva enters the oral cavity through ducts with orifices that open into the floor of the mouth (Wharton's duct; see Fig. 112-1). The sublingual gland is composed of collections of mucous glands; the majority share the same excretory duct as the submandibular gland, while others excrete saliva directly into the floor of the mouth through individual ducts.

Finally, there are dendritic and lymphoid cells located in the oral mucosal tissues. The dendritic Langerhans cells and melanocytes are present in multiple layers of the oral mucosal epithelium. Aggregates of lymphoid tissue, referred to collectively as Waldeyer's ring, are located in the posterior oral pharynx. This tissue forms the lingual (soft, yellowish-red, nodular tissue on the posterior lateral aspect of the tongue), palatine, and pharyngeal tonsils.

Oral Physiology

The oral cavity serves three essential functions in human physiology: (1) the production of speech and communication, (2) the initiation of alimentation, and (3) the protection of the host from pathogens and trauma. Many specialized oral-facial tissues have evolved to carry out these vital functions. The teeth, the periodontium (Fig. 112-4), and the muscles of mastication prepare food for deglutition. The tongue, besides

FIGURE 112-4

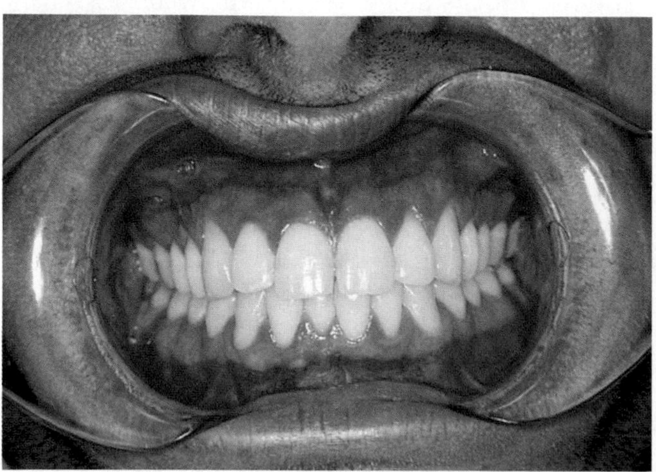

Normal teeth, gingival tissues, and periodontium. The mucogingival line, between the pink attached gingiva and red vestibular mucosa, is well demonstrated.

occupying a central role in communication, is a key participant in food bolus preparation and translocation. Salivary glands provide a secretion with multiple functions. In addition to lubricating all oral mucosal tissues to keep them intact and pliable, saliva moistens the developing food bolus, permitting it to be fashioned into a swallow-acceptable form. All these activities are finely coordinated, and a disturbance in any one function can significantly compromise speech and/or alimentation and diminish the quality of a person's life.

Because of its exposure to the external world, the oral cavity is potentially vulnerable to a limitless number of environmental insults. Extensive mechanisms have evolved to protect the mouth and permit normal oral function. The oral cavity is richly endowed with sensory systems that not only contribute to the enjoyment of food, but also alert an individual to potential problems. These systems include mechanisms for taste (and its inextricable relationship with smell); thermal, textural, and tactile sensations; and pain discrimination. Also, saliva plays an important protective role through its broad spectrum of antimicrobial proteins that modulate oral microbial colonization. Other proteins maintain the functional integrity of the teeth by keeping saliva supersaturated with calcium and phosphate salts and, in effect, repairing incipient caries (tooth decay) by a remineralization process.

Many of these functions and tissues can remain remarkably intact throughout the aging process in healthy persons. Conversely, numerous systemic diseases and their treatment (e.g., medications, surgery, head and neck radiation) can cause significant impairments to oral health, particularly in older adults. These problems can subsequently lead to impaired communication, malnutrition, and diminished host immunity.

PATHOLOGY OF THE ORAL MUCOSA

Leukoplakic Lesions

Leukoplakic, or white, lesions are among the most prevalent oral mucosal conditions found in people of all ages. They range from benign to malignant, and all require appropriate diagnosis.

LEUKOPLAKIA A white plaque that cannot be wiped off and cannot be diagnosed as any other distinct lesion is called leukoplakia.[5] The histologic appearance of leukoplakia varies, ranging from hyperkeratosis and epithelial hyperplasia to epithelial dysplasia and squamous cell carcinoma. When the diagnosis of a white lesion is definitive, the term *leukoplakia* is no longer appropriate. The histologic diagnosis of the lesion determines the appropriate treatment of clinical leukoplakia.

LEUKOEDEMA A variant of normal, leukoedema appears as a grayish-white opalescence of the buccal mucosa, more frequently observed in blacks. The mucosa attains a normal pink color if stretched. Histologically, the epithelium of leukoedema exhibits acanthosis, and the cells of the spinous layer appear larger and more transparent than those of normal epithelium. Because leukoedema is a variant of normal, no treatment is required.

FRICTIONAL KERATOSIS Chronic friction against another surface may result in a white lesion called frictional keratosis. There is a marked thickening of the keratin on the epithelial surface that may be accompanied by acanthosis. Identification and elimination of the cause of the friction (e.g., sharp tooth, rough or overextended denture border) should resolve the lesion. If not, biopsy and histologic examination are warranted.

CHRONIC LIP, TONGUE, AND CHEEK CHEWING Individuals who chronically chew their lip, tongue, and cheek may develop a white lesion that is a form of frictional keratosis. The surface appears rough, and a clinician can easily remove keratin scales from the surface. When this occurs on the buccal mucosa, a wedge-shaped configuration is observed that is broader at the anterior aspect and narrower at the posterior aspect.

LINEA ALBA Forming most commonly on the buccal mucosa at the edge of the teeth (occlusal plane), linea alba is a white, raised line. The line follows the pattern of the teeth at the occlusal plane and may extend onto the labial mucosa as well. In some patients with a teeth-clenching habit, linea alba becomes prominent. Histologically, the white raised line is due to epithelial hyperplasia with overlying hyperkeratosis. No treatment is indicated.

NICOTINE STOMATITIS In response to pipe, cigar, and cigarette smoking, nicotine stomatitis may develop.[6] With this condition, the keratin surface of the hard palate thickens. Because the increase in the surface keratin obstructs the minor salivary gland ducts on the palatal surface, the ducts become inflamed.. They appear as raised, erythemic dots, 2 to 5 mm in diameter, representing the opening of the minor salivary glands on the posterior hard palate and the soft palate. The white appearance will resolve with cessation of smoking; however, it may take several weeks for a change in the lesion to become noticeable. Diagnosis is based upon signs and symptoms, and it is not considered to be a premalignant lesion. Except for cessation of smoking, there is no successful treatment.

TOBACCO CHEWER'S WHITE LESION Individuals who chew tobacco may develop a white lesion in the area where they habitually place tobacco.[7] The mucosa appears granular or wrinkled, and lesions are most commonly located in the mucobuccal fold. Long-standing lesions have a more opaque and corrugated appearance than newer lesions do. Histologically, these white lesions show epithelial hyperplasia and hyperkeratosis. Long-term exposure to smokeless tobacco has been associated with an increased risk of intraoral squamous cell carcinoma. Lesions usually resolve when the individual no longer places tobacco in the area. If resolution does not occur, biopsy and histologic examination are warranted.

HAIRY TONGUE A condition characterized by elongation of the filiform papillae on the dorsal surface of the tongue, hairy tongue may be white, black, or brown; in fact, it can be stained almost any color by candies or lozenges dissolved in the mouth (Fig. 112-5). The color of black hairy tongue is attributed to chromogenic bacteria, whereas the color of brown hairy tongue is associated with tobacco smoking. The etiology is unknown, although chemical mouth rinses (e.g., hydrogen peroxide), radiation-induced xerostomia, and systemic antibiotic and glucocorticoids have all been proposed. Gentle brushing of the tongue may be helpful in decreasing the length of the papillae.

ASPIRIN/CHEMICAL BURN An aspirin burn of the oral mucosa occurs when a patient with a toothache places an aspirin tablet directly on the painful tooth instead of swallowing the tablet. As a result, the nearby mucosal tissues become necrotic. The necrotic tissue in this white and painful lesion is loosely adherent to the underlying connective tissue and easily sloughs off.

Phenol is a component of some nonprescription products advertised for the relief of oral pain. When these products contact oral mucosa, they destroy tissue in a way that appears identical to aspirin burns. Diagnosis is usually established from patient history, signs, and symptoms.

FIGURE 112-5

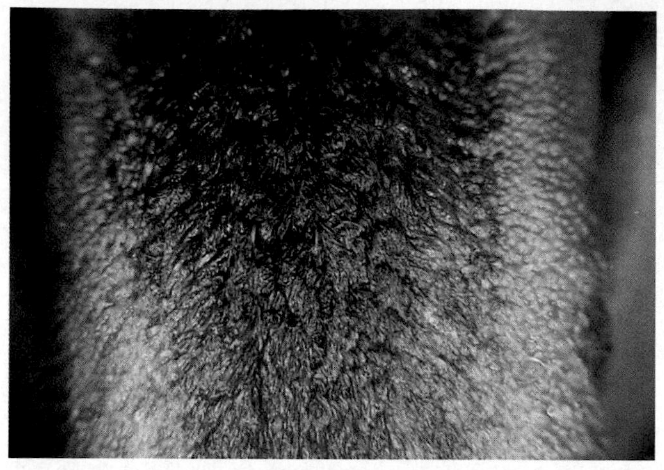

Hairy tongue. There is hyperplasia of the filiform papillae of the dorsum of the tongue. The pigmentation results from overgrowth of pigment-producing strains of microbial flora as a result of antibiotic therapy.

OTHER WHITE LESIONS Keratoacanthoma and squamous acanthoma have occurred in the oral cavity. Submucous fibrosis, a potentially premalignant condition, has a generalized white appearance of the oral mucosa that has been attributed to betel nut chewing, seen in India and Southeast Asia.[8] White sponge nevus, a white lesion of the oral mucosa that follows an autosomal dominant inheritance pattern, is usually diagnosed from family history (Fig. 112-6). Lichen planus and candidiasis (described below) may also appear as white lesions.

Leukoplakic and/or Erythemic Lesions

DYSPLASIA AND SQUAMOUS CELL CARCINOMA Lesions with erythroplakic components appear red because of inflammation, hemorrhage, increased angiogenesis, epithelial atrophy, acantholysis, or ulceration. Among the most significant erythroplakic conditions of the oral cavity are dysplasia and squamous cell carcinoma.[9,10] In their early stages, the lesions are generally unilateral and asymptomatic, appearing as white (leukoplakic), red/white (erythroleukoplakic), or red (erythroplakic) lesions. Suspicious lesions have erythroplakic components with poorly defined borders, nonhomogenous coloration, and ulcerations (Fig. 112-7).[11]

FIGURE 112-6

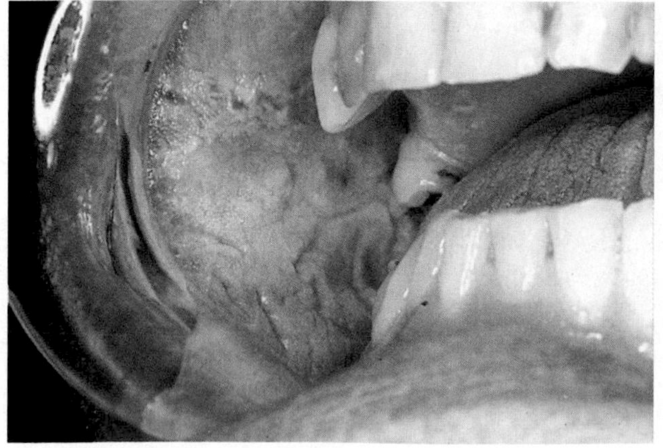

White sponge nevus. These lesions appeared in a nonsmoking young adult with a family history of white sponge nevus.

FIGURE 112-7

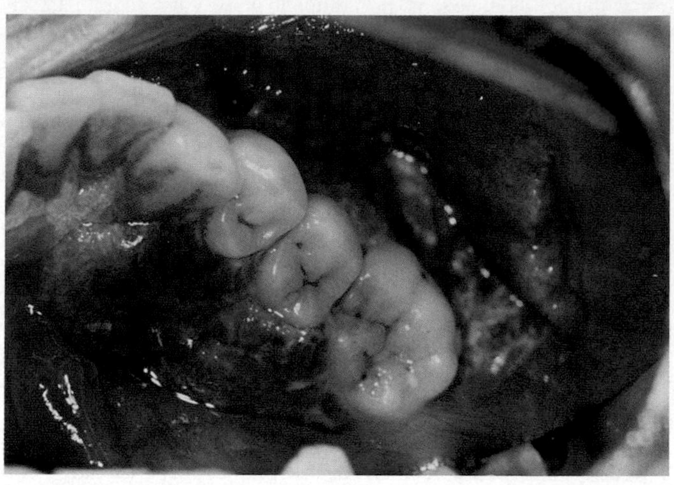

A squamous cell carcinoma involving the alveolar ridge, gingiva, floor of the mouth, and buccal mucosal tissues.

High-risk sites for developing oral cancer are the lower lip, lateral border of the tongue, oropharynx, and floor of the mouth (Fig. 112-8). High-risk factors are age greater than 50 years, and excessive tobacco and/or alcohol use. It is important not to rely on clinical appearance alone, and all lesions that persist for longer than 3 weeks without a definitive diagnosis should undergo biopsy with either scalpel[12] or transepithelial brush,[13] followed by histopathologic examination. Toluidine blue staining is helpful for facilitating biopsy site selection.[14]

Treatment of dysplastic lesions involves complete excision (i.e., by scalpel or CO_2 laser), risk reduction, and close follow-up for recurrences. Recurrent lesions may respond to antioxidant micronutrients.[15] Treatment of squamous cell carcinoma begins with tumor staging.[16] Surgery is the treatment of choice for accessible localized disease, while tumors with lymph node involvement usually require surgery followed by external beam head and neck radiotherapy.

FIGURE 112-8

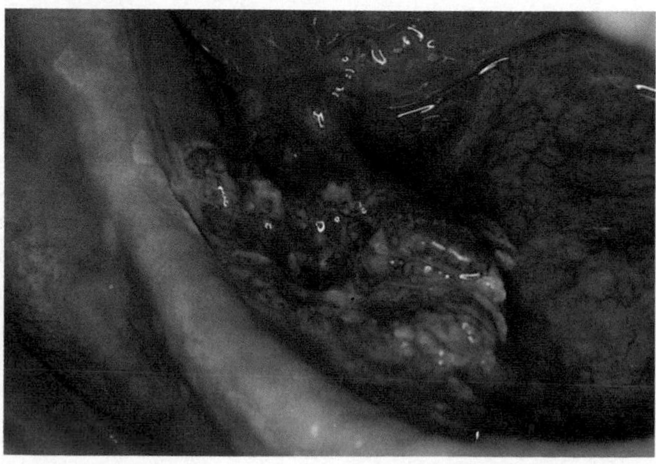

Invasive oral squamous cell carcinoma on the floor of the mouth of an edentulous patient.

FIGURE 112-9

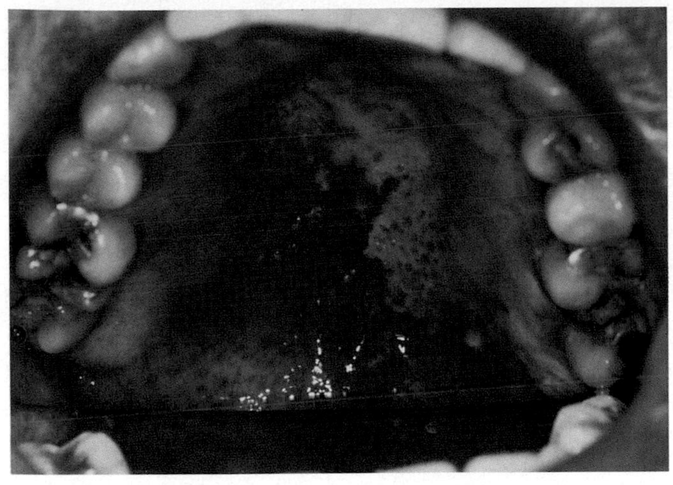

Pseudomembraneous candidiasis, the most common intraoral manifestation of *Candida albicans,* on the hard palate.

ORAL CANDIDIASIS The commensal fungus *Candida albicans* is the primary cause of candidiasis (see Chap. 206). The condition develops as a result of compromised oral and systemic immune function (e.g., salivary hypofunction, HIV infection, diabetes), and immunosuppressant drugs or broad-spectrum antibiotics.[17,18] Oral fungal infections are common beneath removable prostheses, especially in the presence of poor oral and denture hygiene. There are four clinical manifestations showing a range of white, red/white, or red appearances:

1. *Pseudomembraneous candidiasis* (thrush) is asymptomatic and has a diagnostically characteristic appearance of curdlike white patches that can easily be wiped off to reveal an underlying erythema (Figs. 112-9 and 112-10).
2. *Erythematous candidiasis* may manifest as (a) a generalized oral erythema (Fig. 112-11) with symptoms of burning (e.g., atrophic candidiasis secondary to antibiotic therapy), (b) a sharply defined erythematous area under dentures (denture stomatitis), and (c) a midline dorsal tongue atrophy and erythema (median rhomboid glossitis).

FIGURE 112-10

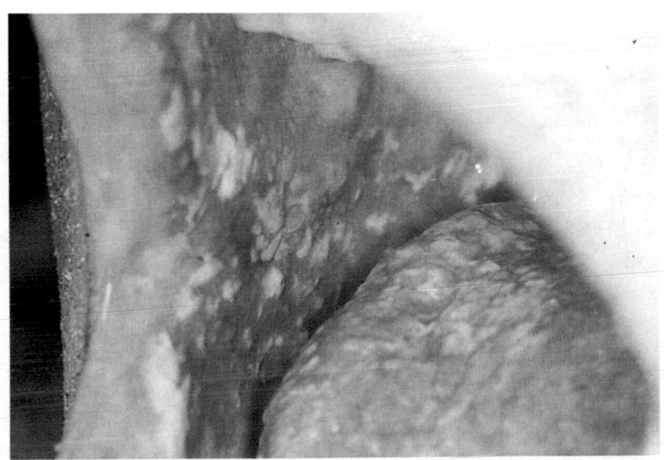

Pseudomembraneous oral candidiasis of the buccal mucosa and tongue dorsum.

FIGURE 112-11

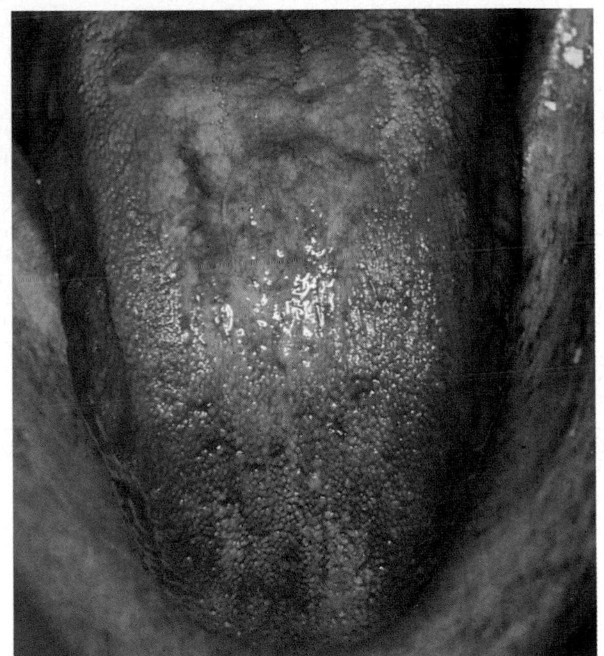

A.

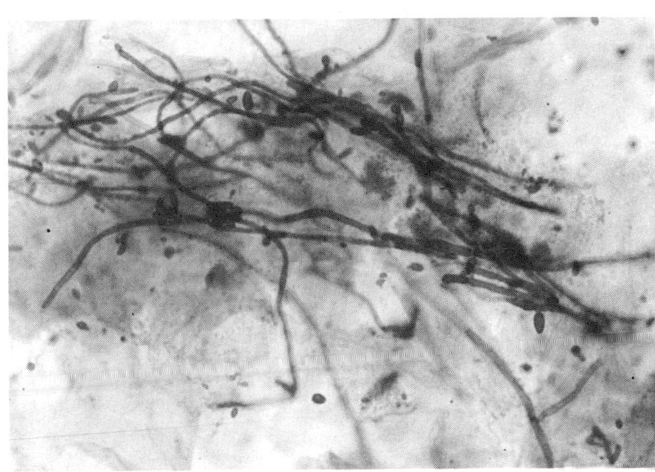

B.

Erythematous candidiasis. *A.* Papillary atrophy on the dorsum of the tongue of a patient with AIDS. *B.* Cytologic smear showing yeast cells and pseudomycelia of *Candida* (periodic acid–Schiff stain).

3. *Angular cheilitis,* not exclusively attributed to candidiasis, manifests as erythema with cracking and crusting of the labial commissures. It is commonly seen concomitant with other forms of candidiasis (Fig. 112-12).
4. *Hyperplastic candidiasis,* a relatively uncommon form, is a thickened and firm nonremovable white lesion. It affects smokers and sites of friction, such as the anterior buccal mucosa.

Diagnosis of candidiasis is initially based on the clinical presentation, positive findings on a KOH examination, and a favorable response to antifungal therapy. When the clinical signs are less obvious, smears or biopsies stained with periodic acid–Schiff (PAS) or cultures to identify candidal species are required (see Fig. 112-11*B*). The clinical

FIGURE 112-12

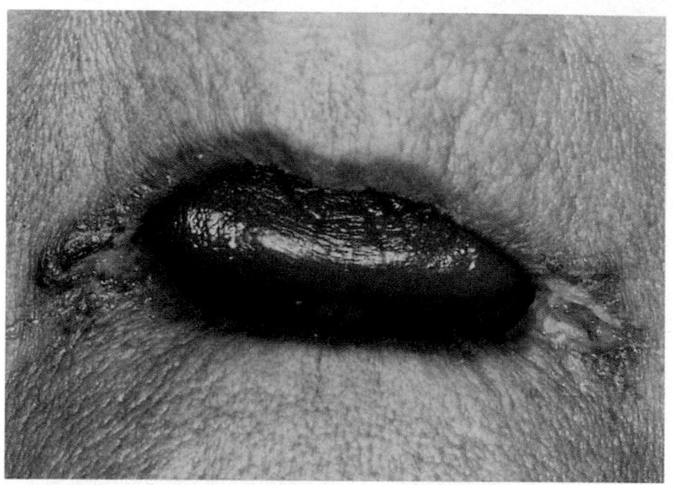

Angular cheilitis resulting from *Candida albicans* infection of the bilateral labial commissures.

circumstances dictate the choice of antifungal therapy (Table 112-1).[19] Topical antifungals are the first line of treatment, delivered as troches, rinses, or creams. Systemic antifungals are indicated for refractory and more extensive lesions, but their use increases the risk for drug interactions and adverse effects.

GEOGRAPHIC TONGUE Also known as benign migratory glossitis, geographic tongue is a very common oral inflammatory condition affecting approximately 2 percent of the population. Lesions manifest as mixed red/white annular areas of dorsal tongue depapillation, sharply demarcated by a whitish rim (Fig. 112-13). Geographic tongue intermittently recurs and is associated with fissured tongue. Lesions migrate around the tongue dorsum, revealing an ever-changing maplike or "geographic" appearance. Lesions may occasionally occur on sites other than the tongue in a condition known as areata migrans. Treatment with topical steroid ointments is reserved for symptomatic patients.

RADIOTHERAPY- AND CHEMOTHERAPY-INDUCED MUCOSITIS Oral and pharyngeal mucositis is one of the most common short-term complications of head and neck radiotherapy and some chemotherapeutic regimens.[20] Causes are direct tissue damage by radiotherapy and chemotherapy, resulting in mucosal ulceration, pain, and epithelial cell death. Radiation mucositis begins after 1 to 2 weeks of radiotherapy with mucosal erythema. Ulcerations develop with pseudomembranes that can hemorrhage readily, with associated stomatodynia and dysphagia. Ulcers form readily in areas where trauma is unavoidable (e.g., buccal/labial mucosa, tongue dorsum). Healing begins after completion of radiotherapy.

Chemotherapy-induced mucositis has a similar clinical appearance. Radiotherapy- and chemotherapy-induced salivary hypofunction frequently accompanies the mucositis, which increases pain and mucosal friability (Fig. 112-14). Desiccated lips and oral mucosal surfaces, dental caries, oral fungal infections, and poorly fitting dentures are common signs of salivary hypofunction.

Palliative therapies include avoidance of mucosal irritation by careful oral care and application of water-based lubricants, oral rinsing with saline or bicarbonate solutions, oral cooling with ice chips, topical coating agents (e.g., kaolin-pectin, aluminum or magnesium hydroxide, sucralfate), topical anesthetic agents, and analgesics.[21] Dietary counseling can help avoid dehydration and nutritional disorders.

ORAL LICHEN PLANUS A common epithelial immune-mediated condition, oral lichen planus affects 1 to 2 percent of adults.[22] It has many forms (leukoplakic, erosive, atrophic) that reflect the degree of epithelial damage and the host's capacity for repair. Lesions affect the buccal mucosa most frequently, although the tongue, palate, gingiva, or lips are also involved (Fig. 112-15). The reticular form of oral lichen planus has a predominant network of lace-like white striae and, on occasion, plaques or papules (Fig. 112-16). Atrophy, erosion, ulceration, and rarely, the formation of bullae mark the epithelial destruction, as seen in the erosive form. Typically, erosive oral lichen planus is painful, particularly following the ingestion of acidic or spicy foods. Tissue biopsy establishes the diagnosis.

Oral lichenoid drug reactions, contact sensitivities, and oral graft-versus-host disease all have an almost identical clinical and histologic presentation. All patients, particularly those with erosive disease, need long-term follow-up care to identify early signs of dysplastic change.[23] Treatment begins with the removal of local traumatic factors (e.g., sharp teeth) and rigorous oral hygiene. Topical treatment and/or intralesional injections with immunosuppressants are reserved for patients with symptomatic disease, and systemic treatment with immunosuppressants should be used in patients with significant oral and/or cutaneous lesions[24,25] (Table 112-2).

LUPUS ERYTHEMATOSUS Both discoid and systemic lupus erythematosus may produce oral lesions similar in appearance to those of oral lichen planus or lichenoid drug reactions (Fig. 112-17). The course of oral lesions frequently parallels that of systemic manifestations. A biopsy may be required for accurate diagnosis.

TABLE 112-1

Treatment of Oral Fungal Infections

Infections of Lips and Oral Mucosal Tissues

- Nystatin oral suspension 100,000 units/mL. Disp: 60 mL. Sig: Swish and swallow 5 mL qid for 5 min. Contains sugar.
- Nystatin ointment. Disp: 15-g tube. Sig: Apply thin coat to affected areas after each meal and qhs.
- Nystatin pastilles 200,000 units. Disp: 70 pastilles. Sig: Let 1 pastille dissolve in mouth 5 times/day.
- Clotrimazole troches 10 mg. Disp: 70 troches. Sig: Let 1 troche dissolve in mouth 5 times/day.

Infections of Removable Prostheses

- Improve oral hygiene of appliance, keep denture out of mouth for extended periods and while sleeping.
- Soak for 30 min in solutions containing benzoic acid, 0.12% chlorhexidine, or 1% sodium hypochlorite and thoroughly rinse.
- Apply a few drops of nystatin oral suspension or a thin film of nystatin ointment to inner surface of denture after each meal.

Refractory Candidiasis

- Ketoconazole 200 mg (20 tabs, 1 tab daily for 2–4 weeks)
- Fluconazole 100 mg (20 tabs; 2 tabs stat, then 1 tab daily for 2–4 weeks)
- Itraconazole 100 mg (20 tabs, 1 tab bid for 2–4 weeks)
- In the patient with salivary gland dysfunction at risk for dental caries, avoid the sugar content of nystatin and clotrimazole troches by substituting with vaginal nystatin tablets.

FIGURE 112-13

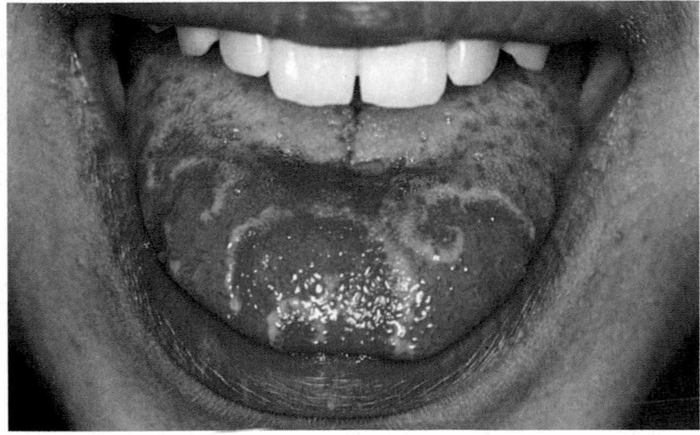

Geographic tongue. Irregular linear white lesions enclose areas of erythema and mucosal atrophy.

Pigmented and Vascular Lesions

MELANOCYTIC LESIONS

Melanin pigmentation In general, melanin pigmentation is a variant of normal seen in patients with more deeply pigmented skin.[26] Any areas of the oral mucosal tissues can appear brown and pigmented. Edentulous patients may present with melanin pigmentation on the alveolar ridge. Histologically, melanin pigment is visible in the basal layer of the epithelium and in the subjacent connective tissue. Focal areas of melanin pigmentation may follow inflammation, and increased melanin pigmentation of the anterior attached gingiva may be associated with smoking (referred to as smoker's melanosis or smoking-associated melanosis).

Oral melanotic macule Flat, small (<1 cm in diameter), well-circumscribed, brown lesions, oral melanotic macules are of unknown etiology. The lesions exhibit a focal increase in melanin deposition in the basal layer of the epithelium, as well as in the subjacent connective tissue and normal stratified squamous epithelium.[27] A labial melanotic macule is a similar lesion occurring on the vermilion of the lips. The labial melanotic macule darkens with exposure to sunlight. Lesions may require biopsy and histologic examination to confirm the diagnosis. No treatment is necessary once the diagnosis has been established.

FIGURE 112-14

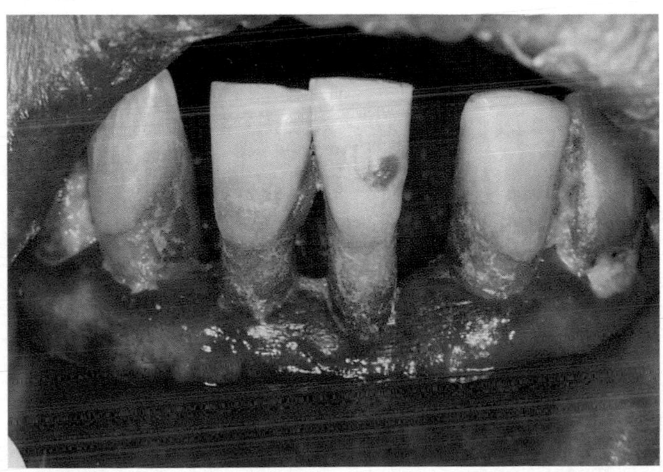

Salivary hypofunction and xerostomia, which frequently occur after external beam radiotherapy (for head and neck cancers), chemotherapy, and multiple prescription and nonprescription medications.

FIGURE 112-15

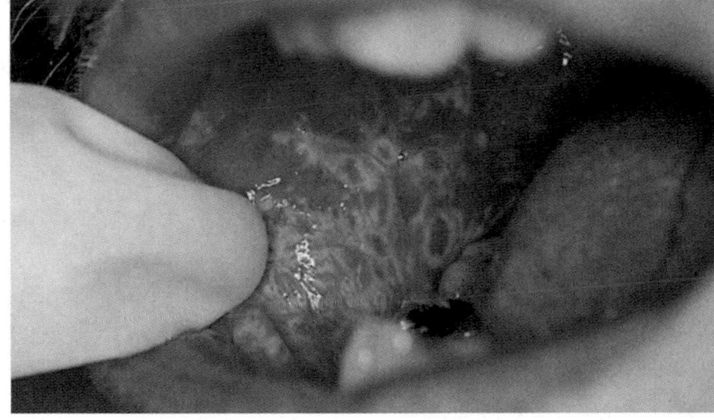

Irregular white striae of classic oral lichen planus on the buccal mucosa, right side.

Melanocytic nevi Intraoral melanocytic nevi are uncommon, yet junctional, compound, intramucosal, and blue nevi have all been reported to occur in the oral cavity.[28] Most melanocytic nevi arise on the palate or gingiva, although they may appear on any oral mucosal site. Biopsy and histologic examination are required, as early oral malignant melanoma can mimic a melanocytic nevus.

Malignant melanoma A rare oral disease, malignant melanoma affects adults in the sixth to seventh decade of life. Most oral melanomas occur on the hard palate or maxillary gingiva. Early oral melanomas appear as brown to black macules with irregular borders. The macules thicken, enlarge, and ulcerate. Diagnosis requires biopsy, and treatment involves complete surgical removal. The prognosis for oral melanoma is extremely poor.

Peutz-Jeghers syndrome Freckle-like lesions of the skin are a characteristic of Peutz-Jeghers syndrome. They frequently involve the perioral area and occasionally the intraoral mucosa. These melanocytic lesions do not darken with exposure to sunlight. The syndrome is inherited (autosomal dominant), but new mutations also occur. Components

FIGURE 112-16

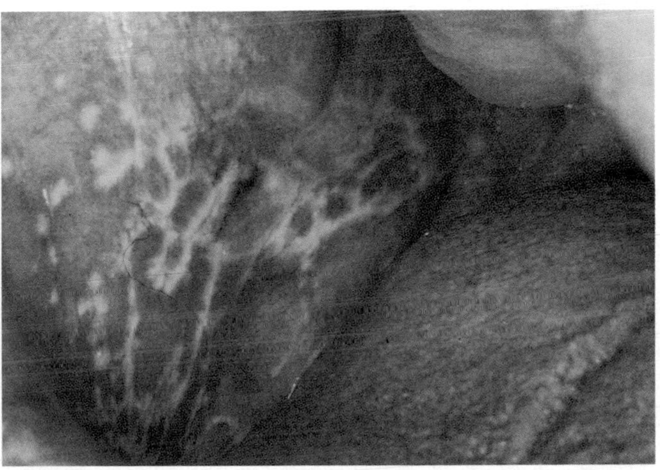

Erosive lichen planus and reticular lichen planus of the posterior buccal mucosa. The leukoplakic striations are referred to as "Wickham's striae."

TABLE 112-2

Treatment of Common Oral Vesiculobullous and Erosive Diseases

MEDICATION	REGIMEN
Topical Treatments[1–3]	
Fluocinonide gel 0.05%	Apply to affected regions tid and qhs
Triamcinolone acetonide in gel base 0.1%	
Clobetasol propionate gel 0.05%	
Oral Rinse Rinses[2–4]	
Dexamethasone elixir 0.5 mg/5 mL	Rinse and spit 10 mL qid for 5 min
Diphenhydramine elixir 12.5 mg/5 mL	
Systemic Medications[2,5]	
Prednisone 5 mg	12 tabs qod × days, decreasing by 2 tabs every other day
Azathioprine 50 mg	1 tab bid

[1] If extensive gingival lesions are present, use with a custom-fabricated tray.
[2] Oral candidiasis may result, and concomitant antifungal therapy may be necessary.
[3] Taper as indicated by clinical response.
[4] Treatment can be combined in a 1:1 mixture with sucralfate, Kaopectate, or Maalox.
[5] Dose and duration depend on severity of disease and concomitant systemic diseases. Azathioprine in combination with prednisone permits use of lower doses of prednisone.

of the syndrome include hamartomatous intestinal polyposis and tumors of the pancreas, breast, and ovaries; there also is an increased risk of gastrointestinal carcinoma.

EXOGENOUS PIGMENTED LESIONS The deposition of amalgam particles causes the amalgam tattoo, a flat, bluish-gray lesion. The introduction of amalgam particles into the mucosa can occur during the placement or removal of an amalgam restoration or during a tooth extraction if a piece of amalgam fractures and remains in the extraction site tissue. The metal particles disperse in the connective tissue and produce a permanent pigmentation. Amalgam tattoos most commonly occur on the gingiva or on an edentulous alveolar ridge, with occasional lesions in the mandibular vestibule, floor of the mouth, and buccal mucosa. The identification of the metal particles in the tissue on a dental radiograph often can confirm the diagnosis. Biopsy and histologic examination are occasionally required for diagnosis. No treatment is necessary.

A blue-gray line along the free gingival margin has been reported to occur with lead and bismuth toxicity.

FIGURE 112-17

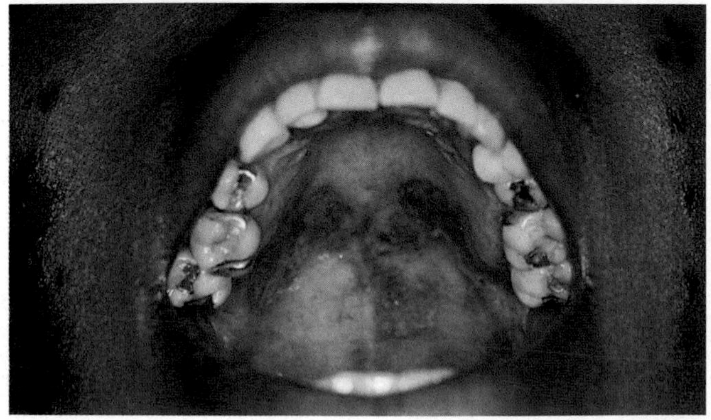

Discoid lupus erythematosus. Painful ulcers with inflammation are evident on the palate.

VASCULAR LESIONS

Varicosities/varices Oral varicosities are multiple, asymptomatic, bluish-purple elevated nodules that are most commonly found on the ventral and lateral aspects of the tongue and lips in individuals more than 45 years of age. Oral mucosal varices are not associated with systemic disease, and generally, no treatment is indicated. Biopsy and histologic examination are required to confirm the diagnosis if thrombi and phleboliths are associated with oral varices.

Hemangioma Oral mucosal hemangiomas are benign proliferations of blood vessels that appear as raised, bluish-red nodular lesions. They may be either capillary or cavernous. Capillary hemangiomas contain a proliferation of capillary-sized blood vessels, whereas cavernous hemangiomas exhibit larger dilated blood vessels. Thromboses and phleboliths may form in hemangiomas. Oral hemangiomas are primarily tumors of childhood, although they may also occur in adults. When they occur in infants and children, they tend to regress with time. Treatment for adults includes surgical removal, laser therapy, and injection with sclerosing agents.

Kaposi's sarcoma Oral Kaposi's sarcoma is rare except in association with HIV infection.[29] Histologically, Kaposi's sarcoma consists of a proliferation of spindle-shaped cells mixed with slitlike vascular spaces. Lesions are usually bluish-red and vary from single to multiple and from flat to nodular.[30] The most common locations are the gingiva and the hard palate. A viral etiology has been proposed for Kaposi's sarcoma, in particular human herpesvirus type 8. The use of highly active antiretroviral therapy (HAART) has reduced the prevalence of HIV-associated Kaposi's sarcoma. Because treatment is not curative, its purpose is to reduce the size of lesions via surgical debulking, radiation therapy, and chemotherapy.

BLEEDING DIATHESES

Oral mucosal petechiae, ecchymoses, hematomas, and spontaneous gingival bleeding Oral mucosal lesions such as petechiae, ecchymoses, hematomas, and spontaneous gingival bleeding may occur in patients with blood dyscrasias, including severe thrombocytopenia and coagulation defects.[31] The etiology includes a variety of medical disorders (e.g., hemolytic anemia, von Willebrand's disease) and medications (e.g., chemotherapy, anticoagulants). Thrombocytopenia-associated oral lesions do not usually become evident until the platelet level falls below 100,000/mm^3, and they resolve when platelet levels increase.

Polycythemia The oral mucosa in individuals with primary or secondary polycythemia appears deeper red in color than normal and may resemble the mucosa seen in erythematous candidiasis. A history of polycythemia or a serologic bleeding profile confirms the diagnosis.

Hereditary hemorrhagic telangiectasia (Rendu-Osler-Weber syndrome) An autosomal dominant syndrome, hereditary hemorrhagic telangiectasia involves multiple telangiectasias of the mucosa and skin. Oral mucosal telangiectasias are most frequently found on the vermilion of the lips, tongue, and buccal mucosa. Frequent episodes of epistaxis because of telangiectasias of the nasal mucosa often lead to the initial diagnosis. However, the oral mucosal telangiectasias may be the most easily recognized component of the syndrome.

FIGURE 112-18

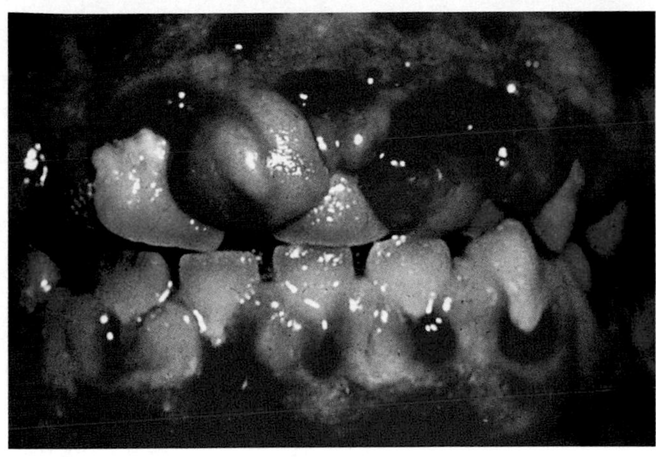

Gingival hyperplasia caused by phenytoin.

GINGIVAL AND PERIODONTAL DISEASES

Drug-induced gingival enlargement Characterized by an increase in free and attached gingiva, particularly involving the interdental papillae (gingival tissue between teeth),[32] gingival enlargement results from the use of certain medications: phenytoin, calcium channel blockers (nifedipine, diltiazem, felodipine, nitrendipine, verapamil), other dihydropyridines, and cyclosporine (Fig. 112-18).[33] When the patient has used two drugs known to cause gingival enlargement concurrently, the enlargement may be more severe. Signs and symptoms establish the diagnosis. Management includes meticulous oral hygiene, and moderate to severe cases require surgical removal of the enlarged tissue (gingivectomy). Recurrences are frequent, especially if the patient continues to use the causative drug.

HIV/AIDS-associated gingival and periodontal disease When associated with HIV infection and AIDS, gingival disease appears as a distinct linear gingival erythema (Fig. 112-19).[30] The etiology is unknown, and the prevalence remains unclear. Necrotizing, ulcerative gingivitis and more extensive periodontitis with bone involvement may also occur in conjunction with HIV infection and AIDS. Bacterial species commonly associated with inflammatory periodontal diseases are generally responsible. The signs and symptoms establish the diagnosis. Treatment involves debridement of the necrotic tissue, the administration of antibiotics (e.g., metronidazole, tetracycline), and meticulous oral hygiene.

FIGURE 112-19

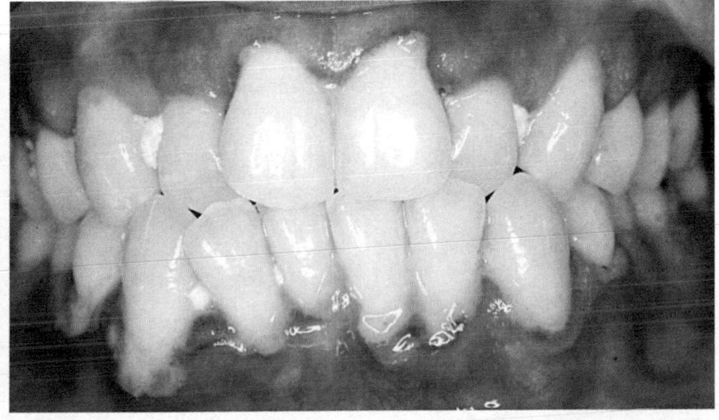

AIDS-related periodontitis, with painful erosions of the marginal gingiva and exudate from the gingival sulcus.

Cyclic neutropenia A cyclic decrease in the number of circulating neutrophils characterizes cyclic neutropenia, an autosomal dominant disease. Cycles are usually at intervals of 21 to 27 days and persist for 2 to 3 days. Oral manifestations of cyclic neutropenia include ulcerative gingivitis and oral mucosal ulcers. With repeated cycles of neutropenia, gingivitis progresses into periodontal disease and bone loss. Oral lesions usually improve when the neutrophil count returns to normal. Antibiotic therapy is occasionally used to prevent the development of alveolar bone loss.

Langerhans cell disease Formerly called histocytosis X, Langerhans cell disease is characterized by the proliferation of Langerhans cells accompanied by eosinophils. The etiopathogenesis is unclear. Ulcerating or proliferating gingival lesions with bone destruction may be evident in chronic disseminated disease (Hand-Schuller-Christian disease) and in solitary eosinophilic granuloma. Diagnosis requires tissue biopsy, and treatment involves curettage of the affected tissue and/or low doses of external beam radiation.

Papillary and Verrucous Lesions

REACTIVE PAPILLARY HYPERPLASIA Mechanical trauma from dentures and/or *Candida albicans* colonization may cause reactive papillary hyperplasia. An erythemic and papillary hyperplastic condition, the disease typically affects the palate beneath an ill-fitting removable prosthesis. Symptoms range from none to soreness and burning. The palatal mucosa covered by the prosthesis is bright red, with short papillary projections that may appear either packed together or scattered. The clinical appearance and fungal culture indicate the diagnosis. If initial therapy is ineffective, definitive diagnosis requires tissue biopsy. Therapy begins with antifungal treatment of both prosthesis and palatal mucosa (see Table 112-1). Ill-fitting dentures require relining with temporary and permanent materials and, possibly, reconstruction.

ORAL HAIRY LEUKOPLAKIA Epstein-Barr virus infection of mucosal keratinocytes is associated with oral hairy leukoplakia, a proliferative epithelial lesion. Originally, reports of the disorder involved almost exclusively homosexual men infected with HIV-1, but now the disorder also affects immunodeficient and HIV-negative adults, typically after organ transplant therapy or chemotherapy. Oral hairy leukoplakia appears as an accentuation of the normal vertical folds at the lateral border of the tongue, with elongation of the papillae (Fig. 112-20). It is homogenously leukoplakic, and as the lesion progresses, it coalesces and thus takes on a shaggy appearance.

The condition is asymptomatic unless infected with *Candida albicans,* which may cause pain and burning. The clinical appearance is the basis for the diagnosis of oral hairy leukoplakia. If certain risk factors are present (e.g., HIV-1 infection, immunodeficiency, smoking, alcohol use), then tissue biopsy can help rule out dysplastic or neoplastic conditions. Frictional keratosis, another benign mucosal proliferative condition, shares many of the clinical attributes of oral hairy leukoplakia, but it has no HIV-1/immunodeficiency association.

Oral hairy leukoplakia rarely requires treatment, unless the clinical appearance is bothersome to the patient. Surgical removal is helpful in the short term, but the lesion will recur. If oral hairy leukoplakia is associated with candidiasis, then appropriate antifungal therapy must be initiated (see Table 112-1). A few symptomatic patients have benefited from the application of podophyllum resin solution.

VERRUCOUS CARCINOMA Also referred to as verrucous hyperplasia and proliferative verrucous leukoplakia, verrucous carcinoma is

FIGURE 112-20

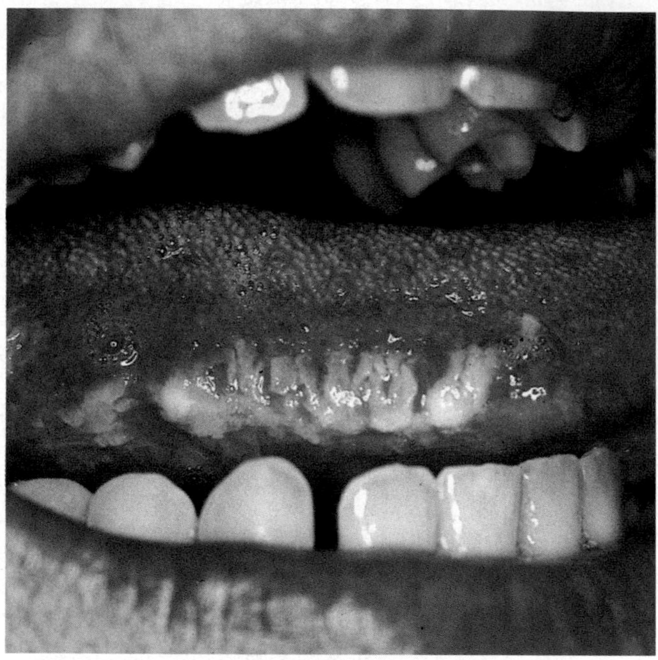

Oral hairy leukoplakia. White corrugated folds occur on the lateral aspects of the tongue. Rubbing with gauze cannot remove the lesion.

a mucosal proliferation condition commonly affecting older adults, particularly those who use tobacco. Lesions present as thickened, rough, white areas; diagnosis is a challenge, because the lesions have clinical and microscopic features intermediate between those of frictional or reactive keratosis and squamous cell carcinoma (Fig. 112-21). The buccal mucosa is a common location, but the disorder may involve any oral site. Early lesions may be relatively inconspicuous, but become more prominently thick, rough, and leukoplakic over time. Tissue biopsy confirms the diagnosis, although the fact that many specimens show intermediate features of hyperplasia and neoplasia complicates the diagnostic process.

Treatment consists of eliminating tobacco and alcohol use, and removing irrevocably altered mucosa by surgery, laser, cautery, or cryotherapy. Patients require frequent reevaluation and episodic treatment in order to identify and eliminate potentially preneoplastic tissue.

SQUAMOUS PAPILLOMA Although squamous papilloma is a small, exophytic, papillary mucosal growth that can occur on any oral mucosal surface, it occurs most frequently on the palate, tongue, lips, and gingiva. Most papillomas are small (less than 1 cm in diameter), asymptomatic pedunculated growths, with a similar color to that of the surrounding mucosa (Fig. 112-22). The etiology of these lesions is unknown, although there is a strong association with human papillomavirus. Tissue biopsy establishes the diagnosis, and treatment requires complete excision (preferably, by scalpel), including the base of the lesion. Failure to remove the entire lesion may result in recurrence.

VERRUCA VULGARIS The lesions of verruca vulgaris are small, sessile, finely papillated, and exophytic epithelial proliferations that are etiologically associated with human papillomavirus (particularly types 2 and 4). They can occur singly or in small clusters, which is suggestive of autoinoculation. Lesions more commonly occur on the masticatory mucosa, the lips, and the perioral skin. Tissue biopsy establishes the diagnosis, and treatment requires complete excision. Recurrence is possible if there are lesions elsewhere that can serve as sources for reinoculation of the virus.

FIGURE 112-21

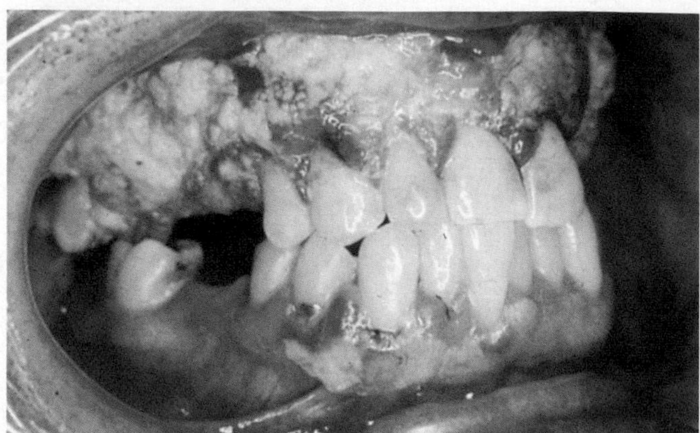

Verrucous squamous cell carcinoma.

CONDYLOMA ACUMINATUM Another papillary epithelial hyperplasia with a human papillomavirus as a contributing factor (most commonly type 6 or 11) is condyloma acuminatum. These lesions frequently affect the anogenital mucosa, but can also occur in the oral cavity, primarily as a result of sexual activity. The clinical appearance is nearly identical to that of verruca vulgaris or squamous papilloma, and lesions can occur on any oral mucosal tissue. Tissue biopsy is necessary for diagnosis, yet recurrence or growth of new lesions at different oral sites occurs, possibly because of reinoculation or different latency periods in lesions that were initiated at the same time.

VERRUCIFORM XANTHOMA A small (less than 2 cm), asymptomatic, sessile, rough-surfaced growth, verruciform xanthoma appears white or yellow in color. It affects any oral mucosal site, most commonly in older adults. The etiology is uncertain, but it is hypothesized that the cause may be low-grade epithelial damage resulting from irritation or minor trauma, with the accumulation of lipid from the damaged cells. Diagnosis is made by tissue biopsy. This is an innocuous lesion that seldom recurs after conservative excision; it is necessary to distinguish the lesions from dysplastic epithelial proliferations, which require more aggressive treatment.

FIGURE 112-22

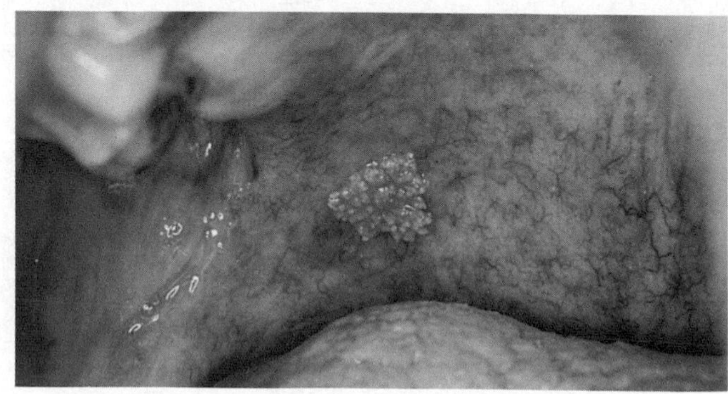

Papilloma on the soft palate.

UNCOMMON PAPILLARY AND VERRUCOUS ORAL LESIONS

Among the uncommon papillary and veruccous lesions that occur in the oral cavity are warty dyskeratoma (focal acantholytic dyskeratosis), focal epithelial hyperplasia (Heck's disease), acanthosis nigricans, and focal dermal hypoplasia (Gorlin-Goltz syndrome).

Submucosal Nodules

SOLITARY NODULES

Parulis Found at the distal opening of an intraoral sinus tract, a parulis is a mass of inflamed granulation tissue related to an abscess associated with the root of a tooth. The parulis is asymptomatic, as the abscess has already drained. Diagnosis involves dental radiographs and identification of the tooth involved. Treatment involves endodontic therapy, dental-alveolar surgery, or extraction of the tooth.

Irritation fibroma A tumor-like lesion, an irritation fibroma contains dense fibrous connective tissue with a surface of intact stratified squamous epithelium. Most fibromas are sessile lesions, but pedunculated fibromas also occur. Chronic irritation of the fibroma may result in a thicker keratin surface, and acute trauma may result in surface ulceration. This type of fibroma is not a true tumor, but rather a reactive lesion resulting from local irritation or trauma. Diagnosis requires tissue biopsy. Treatment involves conservative surgical excision, and irritation fibromas generally do not recur.

Giant cell fibroma Another fibrous lesion, the giant cell fibroma, can occur on any oral mucosal surface with distinct histopathologic features: well-vascularized fibrous connective tissue covered by stratified squamous epithelium. In the superficial connective tissue, there are numerous large, stellate-shaped, and multinucleated fibroblasts. The giant cell fibroma may be sessile or pedunculated, and the surface may appear nodular; it is asymptomatic. There is no known etiology. Diagnosis requires tissue biopsy, treatment involves conservative surgical excision, and lesions generally do not recur.

Pyogenic granuloma Characteristic of this commonly occurring lesion is a proliferation of granulation tissue infiltrated by neutrophils, lymphocytes, and plasma cells. There is no known cause. The lesion appears as an ulcerated and pedunculated mass, most often on the gingiva. It is more common in children and young adults than in older adults. Diagnosis requires tissue biopsy, and treatment involves conservative surgical excision. If not treated, fibrosis may occur, resulting in an oral mucosal fibroma.

The term *pyogenic granuloma* is a misnomer, because the lesion is neither pyogenic nor a granuloma. Pyogenic granulomas that develop on the gingiva in pregnant women are often called *pregnancy tumors*. These may resolve, decrease in size, or undergo fibrosis after pregnancy.

Peripheral giant cell lesion (granuloma) Occurring only on the gingiva or edentulous alveolar ridge, the peripheral giant cell lesion (peripheral giant cell granuloma) contains multinucleated giant cells, extravasated red blood cells, hemosiderin, and inflammatory cells, with osteoid and bone formation. The peripheral giant cell lesion is thought to be a reactive lesion, not a true tumor. Diagnosis requires tissue biopsy, and treatment involves conservative surgical excision. Recurrence of these lesions has been reported.

A lesion exhibiting the same histologic appearance also occurs within the bone of the maxilla and mandible. In this location, it is called a central giant cell lesion or central giant cell granuloma. In addition, the "brown tumor" of hyperparathyroidism is histologically indistinguishable from the central giant cell lesion.

Peripheral ossifying fibroma Only the gingiva is affected by a peripheral ossifying fibroma. It is composed of a cellular, fibrous proliferation with formation of calcified material that consists of osteoid and bone trabeculae, rounded cementoid calcifications, or dystrophic calcifications. The peripheral ossifying fibroma is a reactive lesion, most commonly occurring in teenagers and young adults, that presents as an ulcerated, sessile or pedunculated gingival mass. Diagnosis requires tissue biopsy, treatment involves conservative surgical excision, and the condition may recur.

Lipoma A benign tumor of fat, a lipoma occasionally develops in the oral cavity. A well-circumscribed mass of mature fat cells, sometimes in a lobular arrangement, makes up the lipoma. Microscopic variants of oral lipomas include fibrolipoma, angiolipoma, myxoid lipoma, spindle cell lipoma, and pleomorphic lipoma. Oral lipomas present as soft, yellowish-pink nodules that can occur on any oral mucosal surface. Diagnosis requires tissue biopsy, treatment involves conservative surgical excision, and recurrences are rare.

Neurogenic lesions Benign neurogenic lesions occur in the oral cavity, although all are uncommon (see Chap. 107). Oral neurogenic lesions require tissue biopsy for diagnosis, and treatment involves conservative surgical excision. There are several types:

- A traumatic neuroma is a reactive proliferation of nerve tissue that develops when the proximal portion of a peripheral nerve attempts to regenerate after it has been damaged. Such neuromas appear as nonulcerated nodules, most commonly in the mental foramen area, that are occasionally painful.
- The neurofibroma is an asymptomatic mass, most commonly located on the tongue or buccal mucosa, that exhibits a well-delineated diffuse proliferation of spindle-shaped Schwann cells. Malignant transformation of a solitary neurofibroma has been reported.
- The neurilemoma (Schwannoma) is another benign tumor of Schwann cell origin that presents as a slow-growing, occasionally painful mass.
- The granular cell tumor is a benign mesenchymal tumor also of Schwann cell origin, that infiltrates regional striated muscle. It presents as an asymptomatic, sessile mass most commonly located on the dorsal tongue.

MULTIPLE NODULES Several different oral mucosal conditions can produce multiple submucosal nodules. For example, multiple neurofibromas or neurolemomas are evident in neurofibromatosis. Multiple mucosal neuromas are a common component of multiple endocrine neoplasia, type III. Multiple oral mucosal fibroepithelial nodules occur in multiple hamartoma syndrome (Cowden's disease). Finally, primary and secondary amyloidosis may present as multiple oral mucosal nodules.

Salivary Gland Diseases

BENIGN SALIVARY GLAND DISEASES Common problems affecting salivary glandular tissue result from the obstruction of salivary secretions from either fluid-producing acinar cells or ductal cells. The most common lesion is a mucocele, occurring on the lower lip or floor of the mouth (Fig. 112-23). It is a smooth-surfaced, exophytic, fluid-containing recurrent lesion, which is caused by a traumatic rupture of the minor salivary gland duct. Long-term fibrosis can develop if chronic draining and refilling occurs.

Lesions affecting the main excretory duct of the submandibular or sublingual gland are called ranulas. Usually larger than mucoceles, ranulas produce a fluctuant mass covered by translucent mucosa, causing an elevation of the tongue. Diagnosis and treatment of a minor gland mucocele requires complete excision. Complete excision is also necessary in the treatment of a ranula, and the required excision may also involve the submandibular or sublingual gland.

Glandular obstructions can also result from the formation of mucous plugs or sialoliths (salivary gland stones). The cause is a reduced salivary output (see Fig. 112-14), which may be due to numerous medications (e.g., antihypertensives, antipsychotics, anticholinergics),

FIGURE 112-23

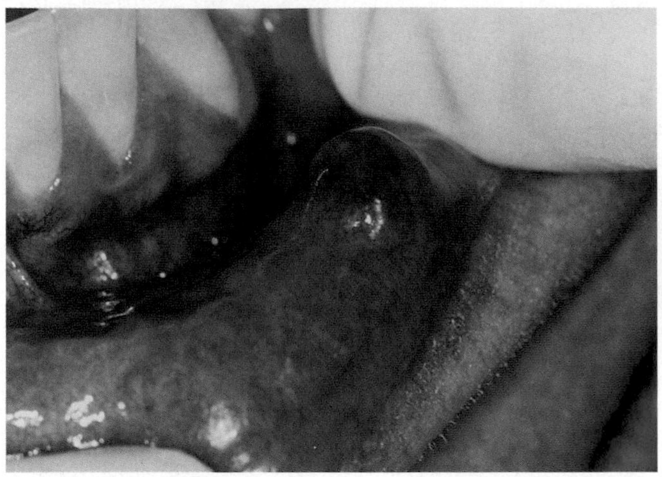

Mucocele: a smooth-surfaced, exophytic, fluid-containing, recurrent lesion caused by a traumatic rupture of the minor salivary gland duct.

dehydration, head and neck radiotherapy, or certain medical disorders (e.g., Sjögren's syndrome, diabetes). Signs and symptoms include painful swellings of the major salivary gland regions, and palpation of the glands produces either viscous or no salivary secretions. Excision of swellings may be necessary to restore salivary gland function if stimulation is not successful and to exclude the possibility of a glandular neoplasm.

SALIVARY GLAND NEOPLASMS Fewer than 10 percent of all oral malignancies are salivary gland neoplasms, but they can affect all major and minor glands located in the palate, labial and buccal mucosa, retromolar areas, floor of the mouth, and the base of the tongue.[16,34] Common findings are a swelling, with or without pain, with surface morphology ranging from smooth to ulcerated. Pleomorphic adenomas, adenoid cystic carcinomas, and polymorphous low-grade adenocarcinomas affect minor as well as major glands, whereas acinic cell carcinomas and mucoepidermoid carcinomas affect major glands. Pleomorphic adenomas are the most common benign salivary gland neoplasm; they grow slowly and respond well to conservative excision. Mucoepidermoid carcinomas are the most common malignant tumors of salivary glands and frequently require aggressive therapies, including excision of tumors and surrounding lymph nodes and postoperative external beam radiotherapy. Adenoid cystic carcinomas are aggressive tumors that invade the perineural areas.

Diagnosis of all salivary gland tumors requires tissue biopsy. If a neoplasm is suspected, then incisional/excisional biopsy with a margin of uninvolved tissue is the preferred diagnostic procedure. However, highly suspicious tumors warrant referral to an oncologic surgeon who will eventually participate in the definitive care of the patient.

Ulcerative, Vesicular, and Bullous Oral Lesions

Ulcerative and vesiculobullous lesions of the oral mucosa can be subdivided into four groups: (1) traumatic, (2) immune-mediated, (3) infectious, and (4) neoplastic. In general, treatment starts with removal of any possible source of trauma (e.g., sharp teeth or restorations), particularly in a patient with diminished salivary flow or with an oral movement disorder, and/or pharmacologic therapy based on the clinical appearance of the lesion. If no resolution occurs within 2 to 3 weeks, then reevaluation with consideration of tissue biopsy for histopathologic diagnosis is necessary.

FIGURE 112-24

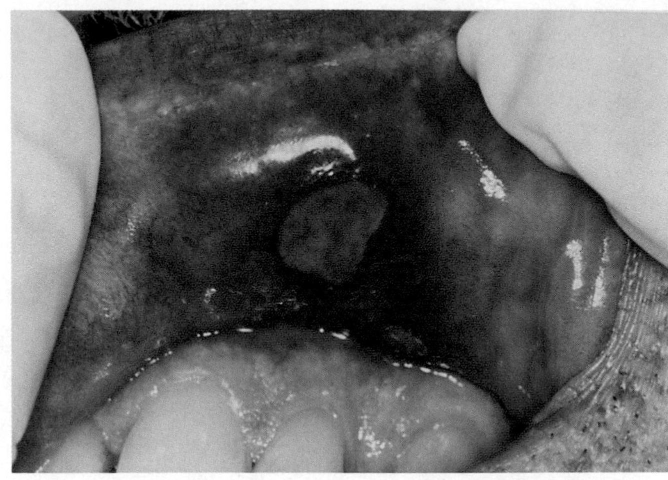

A minor recurrent aphthous stomatitis lesion on the inner aspect of the lower lip. This well-circumscribed lesion has a characteristic erythematous halo with a gray pseudomembranous and necrotic center.

RECURRENT APHTHOUS STOMATITIS The most common immune-mediated oral ulcerative condition is recurrent aphthous stomatitis (RAS). There are three types of RAS (minor, major, and herpetiform) that all produce acute, painful, and recurring ulcers, usually involving nonkeratinized oral mucosa.[35,36] Minor RAS (canker sores) have a high prevalence in healthy adults (5 to 25 percent) and manifest as one or more small shallow ulcers (5 to 10 mm in diameter) with a necrotic gray center and an erythematous halo (Figs. 112-24 and 112-25). The ulcer lasts 7 to 10 days, with recurrences averaging two to three times a year. Not only are major RAS ulcers less common, but also they are larger (>10 mm in diameter), penetrate deeper, can last up to 6 weeks, and often scar after healing (Fig. 112-26). Herpetiform RAS ulcers (unrelated to herpes infection) are the least common, characterized by multiple small painful ulcers (1 to 3 mm in diameter) on nonkeratinized oral mucosa; they coalesce to produce large irregular ulcers.

The etiology of RAS includes heredity, allergy to certain foods or drugs, hematologic and immunologic disorders, emotional stress, and tissue trauma. In addition, RAS is an oral manifestation of several systemic diseases, such as HIV infection; Behçet's syndrome; Reiter's syndrome; Crohn's disease; cyclic neutropenia; nutritional and hematinic deficiencies; gluten-sensitive enteropathy; and periodic fever, aphthous stomatitis, pharyngitis, and adenitis (FAPA). History and clinical

FIGURE 112-25

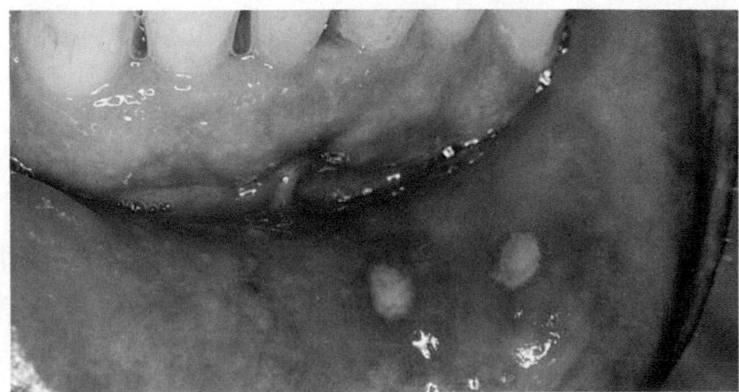

Minor aphthous stomatitis ulcers of the labial mucosa and vestibule. A pair of aphthae, each exhibiting a well-circumscribed, flat, erythematous border, surround an ulcer with a fibrin-covered base.

FIGURE 112-26

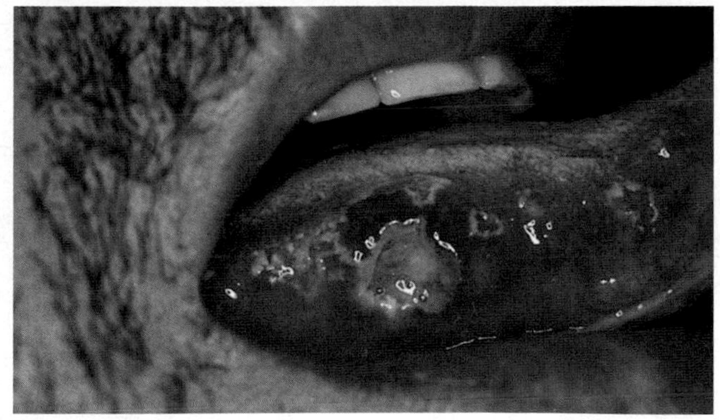

Major aphthous stomatitis ulcer of the lateral border of the tongue.

appearance form the basis for diagnosis. In patients with frequently occurring outbreaks, systemic diseases should be ruled out.

Treatment is supportive for minor RAS, and the topical or intralesional administration of glucocorticoids is beneficial for major RAS, as well as for frequently recurring and painful minor RAS[37] (see Table 112-2). Ulcers refractory to topical medications may require the use of systemic glucocorticoids and immunosuppressants. Second-line systemic therapy includes dapsone, thalidomide (particularly in HIV-associated aphthous), colchicine, and pentoxyfylline.

ERYTHEMA MULTIFORME An acute immune-mediated ulcerative mucocutaneous disease, erythema multiforme commonly affects healthy young adults (see Chap. 58). The cause is often unestablished, although there is an association with emotional stress, infections (herpes simplex and *Mycoplasma*), and medications (especially antibiotics and antiepileptics). Erythema multiforme may involve only lip and oral mucosal sites, or it may affect multiple sites on the skin and other mucous membranes (i.e., Stevens-Johnson syndrome). The oral presentation depends on the severity of the disorder; it may range from lip swelling and erythematous, target-like erosions to widespread ulcerations with bleeding and crusting. Lesions are usually painful, causing difficulty with chewing and swallowing. They will resolve within 14 days. Chronic erythema multiforme is rare, but recurrence is possible. The most severe forms of erythema multiforme (i.e., Stevens-Johnson syndrome and toxic epidermal necrolysis) can be fatal.

Treatment is palliative with topical anesthetics and analgesics, yet may require hospitalization in severely dehydrated and nutritionally depleted patients. Severe forms of erythema multiforme require the systemic administration of glucocorticoids and other immunosuppressants.

CICATRICIAL PEMPHIGOID Another chronic immune-mediated ulcerative condition is cicatricial pemphigoid (see Chap. 62). This disorder has a predilection for females in the sixth decade and results in the deposition of autoimmune complexes, leading to subepithelial separation, bulla formation, desquamation of the epithelium, and significant discomfort.[38] Oral lesions involve gingival tissues (referred to as desquamative gingivitis), and the tongue, palate, buccal mucosa, and oropharynx (Fig. 112-27). Ocular involvement warrants an ophthalmologic evaluation, because mucosal scarring can lead to blindness. Diagnosis is predicated on tissue biopsy for histopathologic study (characteristic appearance of subepithelial separation) and examination by direct immunofluorescence (IgG and C3 deposition at the basement membrane).

Treatment of cicatricial pemphigoid depends on the severity and location of the involvement. Improved oral hygiene and the use of high-potency topical glucocorticoids are indicated for mild disease

FIGURE 112-27

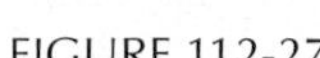

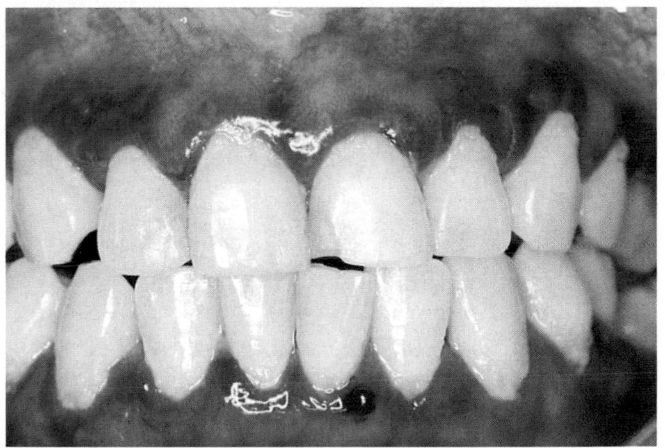

Cicatricial pemphigoid lesions on the maxillary and mandibular attached gingival. The erythemic and fragile mucosa on the gingival tissues (desquamative gingivitis) was tender and bled easily.

(see Table 112-2), while the systemic administration of glucocorticoids, with or without steroid-sparing drugs (e.g., azathioprine and cyclophosphamide), dapsone, sulfonamides, and tetracyclines, have been shown to be effective for more extensive disease.

PEMPHIGUS VULGARIS The presentation of pemphigus vulgaris is similar to that of cicatricial pemphigoid (see Chap. 59).[39] It affects male and female adults in the fifth to seventh decades, particularly Ashkenazi Jews. The oral mucosa, where it appears as shallow irregular ulcerations of gingival and buccal mucosal tissues (Fig. 112-28), is the first site of involvement in the majority of cases. Disease progression leads to involvement of skin and other mucosal sites. Untreated, pemphigus vulgaris can lead to high rates of morbidity and mortality. The basis for diagnosis is tissue biopsy for histopathologic study (finding of acantholysis) and direct immunofluorescence examination (finding of intraepithelial spider-web deposition of IgG and C3).

Topical glucocorticoids are helpful for limited oral lesions. Disseminated pemphigus vulgaris requires the systemic administration of glucocorticoids, often in conjunction with steroid-sparing drugs

FIGURE 112-28

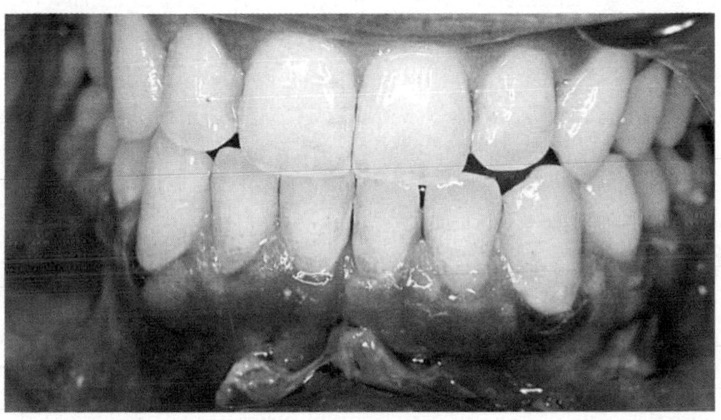

Pemphigus vulgaris lesions on the maxillary and mandibular gingival and labial vestibular tissues. Multiple eroded areas are visible on both masticatory and lining mucosa.

FIGURE 112-29

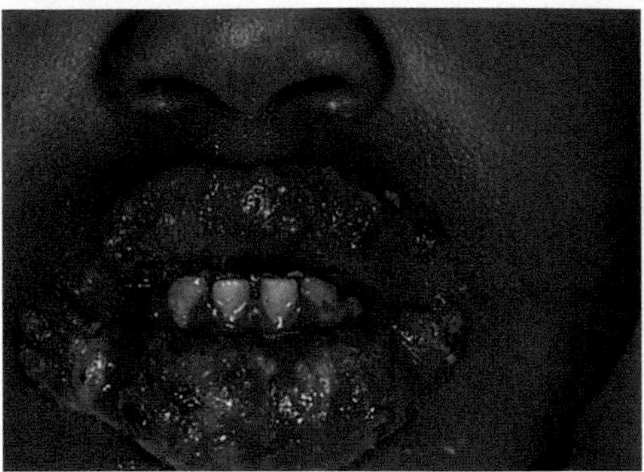

Primary herpetic gingivostomatitis.

(e.g., azathioprine, cyclophosphamide), and other immunosuppressants (e.g., mycophenolate mofetil).

HERPES SIMPLEX VIRUS INFECTIONS The most common viral infection producing oral ulcerations is the herpes simplex viral (HSV) infection (see Chap. 214).[40] Primary HSV infection occurs frequently as a subclinical infection during childhood, resulting in a lifelong latent condition. However, some patients develop acute primary herpetic gingivostomatitis, with fever, malaise, lymphadenopathy, and generalized painful ulcers of gingival and oral mucosal tissues (Fig. 112-29). The signs and symptoms establish the diagnosis.

Reactivation of the HSV occurs in patients of all ages and follows triggering events (e.g., stress, tissue trauma, sunlight) and/or immunosuppression. The most common recurrence manifests as herpes labialis (known as a cold sore): several painful vesicles form on the lip, coalesce, and then produce a crusted scab in 5 to 7 days (Fig. 112-30). Intraoral recurrent HSV infection produces a painful focal eruption of vesicles on keratinized tissues (e.g., hard palate, gingivae) that coalesce into a poorly defined ulceration.

In the immunocompetent patient, treatment is palliative. The topical use of antiviral medications (e.g., penciclovir, acyclovir) produces limited relief, and the systemic administration of antivirals (e.g., acyclovir, valacyclovir) provides prophylactic benefit to patients who experience frequent recurrences. In immunocompromised patients, HSV infections can produce extensive and long-lasting oral ulcerations that lead to significant morbidity.[30] Diagnosis is by viral culture, and treatment requires high doses of antiviral drugs.

VARICELLA ZOSTER VIRUS INFECTIONS The primary infection of varicella zoster virus is chicken pox, which causes oral ulcers in children (see Chap. 215). The secondary infection, herpes zoster (shingles), represents a reactivation of the varicella zoster virus and frequently involves the trigeminal nerve in adults. Involvement of the maxillary branch of the trigeminal nerve manifests intraorally as unilateral palatal ulcerations. The signs and symptoms indicate the diagnosis, and a smear or viral culture confirms it. Early treatment with the systemic administration of high-dose antivirals (e.g., famciclovir, valacyclovir) minimizes the risk for developing postherpetic neuralgia.[41] Other viral infections that can cause oral ulcerations include cytomegalovirus, measles, and coxsackievirus (causing herpangina and hand, foot, and mouth disease).

FIGURE 112-30

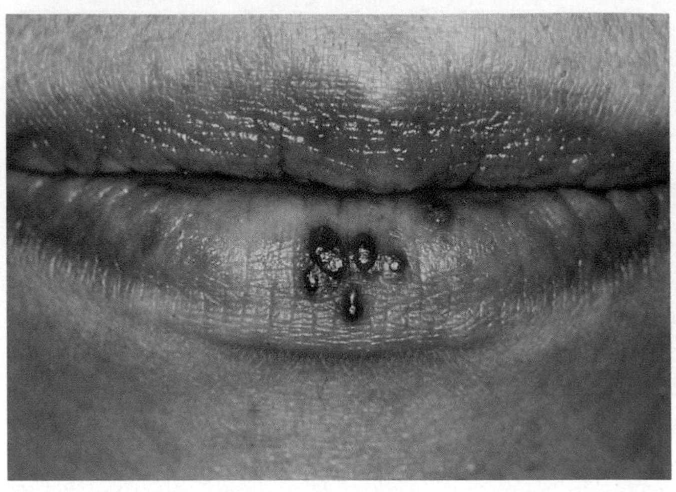

Recurrent herpes labialis of the lower lip. Small fluid-filled vesicles are early characteristics of the condition; they will coalesce and form a scab within 7 days.

BACTERIAL AND DEEP FUNGAL INFECTIONS Rarely do the bacterial and deep fungal infections that cause oral ulceration occur in the immunocompetent patient, with the exception of the sexually transmitted bacterial diseases.[42] Syphilis produces oral mucosal ulcers as the primary chancre, but most often as the secondary mucous patch (Fig. 112-31) or the tertiary gumma. Gonorrhea has a greater predilection for the nasopharynx than for the oral cavity. Tuberculosis has also been reported to occur in the mouth. Deep fungal infections (e.g., histoplasmosis, cryptococcosis) are seen almost exclusively in the immunocompromised patient.[43]

OTHERS Neoplastic diseases, such as oral squamous cell carcinoma (see above), and oral lymphomas can present as ulcers in the oral cavity.

FIGURE 112-31

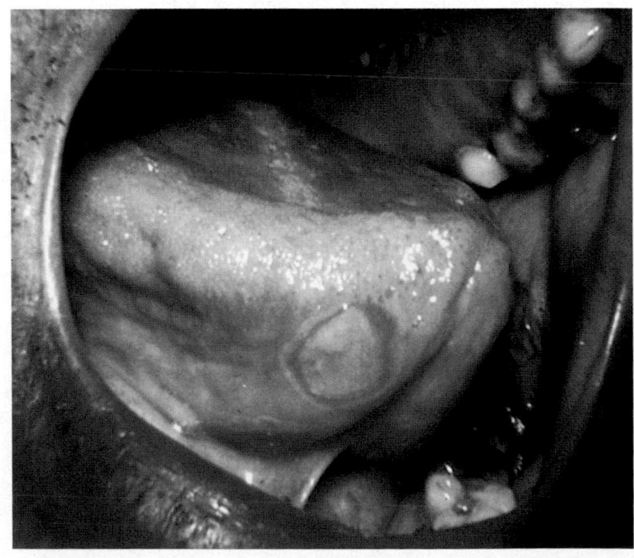

Mucous patch of the anterior-lateral border of the tongue. It may be the only sign of secondary syphilis. This patch is a large painless erosion simulating an aphthous lesion.

REFERENCES

1. Greenberg M, Glick M: *Burket's Oral Medicine: Diagnosis and Treatment*, 10th ed. Hamilton, Ontario, Canada; BC Decker, 2003
2. Neville BW et al: *Oral and Maxillofacial Pathology*. Philadelphia, WB Saunders, 1995
3. Regezi JA, Sciubba JJ: *Oral Pathology: Clinical Pathological Correlations*. Philadelphia, WB Saunders, 1999
4. Silverman S Jr et al: *Essentials of Oral Medicine*, 1st ed. Hamilton, Ontario, Canada, BC Decker, 2001
5. Scully C, Porter S: ABC of oral health: Swellings and red, white, and pigmented lesions. *BM J* **321**:225, 2000
6. Hoffmann D, Djordjevic MV: Chemical composition and carcinogenicity of smokeless tobacco. *Adv Dent Res* **11**:322, 1997
7. Johnson GK et al: Development of smokeless tobacco-induced oral mucosal lesions. *J Oral Pathol Med* **27**:388, 1998
8. Zain RB et al: Oral mucosal lesions associated with betel quid, areca nut and tobacco chewing habits: Consensus from a workshop held in Kuala Lumpur, Malaysia, November 25–27, 1996. *J Oral Pathol Med* **28**:1, 1999
9. Silverman SJ: *Oral Cancer*, 4th ed. Hamilton, Ontario, Canada, The American Cancer Society, 1998
10. Ship JA et al: Evaluation and management of oral cancer. *Home Health Care Consult* **6**:2, 1999
11. Axell T et al: Oral white lesions with special reference to precancerous and tobacco-related lesions: Conclusions of an international symposium held in Uppsala, Sweden, May 18–21, 1994. International Collaborative Group on Oral White Lesions. *J Oral Pathol Med* **25**:49, 1996
12. Golden DP, Hooley JR: Oral mucosal biopsy procedures: Excisional and incisional. *Dent Clin North Am* **38**:279, 1994
13. Sciubba JJ: Improving detection of precancerous and cancerous oral lesions: Computer-assisted analysis of the oral brush biopsy. U.S. Collaborative Oral CDx Study Group. *J Am Dent Assoc* **130**:1445, 1999
14. Epstein JB et al: The utility of toluidine blue application as a diagnostic aid in patients previously treated for upper oropharyngeal carcinoma. *Oral Surg Oral Med Oral Pathol Oral Radiol Endod* **83**:537, 1997
15. Anderson WF et al: Secondary chemoprevention of upper aerodigestive tract tumors. *Semin Oncol* **28**:106, 2001
16. Million RR, Cassisi NJ: *Management of Head and Neck Cancer*, 2nd ed. Philadelphia, JB Lippincott, 1994
17. Reichart PA et al: Pathology and clinical correlates in oral candidiasis and its variants: A review. *Oral Diseases* **6**:85, 2000
18. Farah CS et al: Oral candidosis. *Clin Dermatol* **18**:553, 2000
19. Meis JF, Verweij PE: Current management of fungal infections. *Drugs* **61**(suppl 1):13, 2001
20. Scully C, Epstein JB. Oral health care for the cancer patient. *Oral Oncol* **32B**:281, 1996
21. Plevova P: Prevention and treatment of chemotherapy- and radiotherapy-induced oral mucositis: A review. *Oral Oncol* **35**:453, 1999
22. Sugerman PB et al: Oral lichen planus. *Clin Dermatol* **18**:533, 2000
23. Silverman S Jr: Oral lichen planus: A potentially premalignant lesion. *J Oral Maxillofac Surg* **58**:1286, 2000
24. Eisen D: The therapy of oral lichen planus. *Crit Rev Oral Biol Med* **4**:141, 1993
25. McCreary CE, McCartan BE: Clinical management of oral lichen planus. *Br J Oral Maxillofac Surg* **37**:338, 1999
26. Batsakis J et al: The pathology of head and neck tumors: Mucosal melanomas. *Head Neck Surg* **4**:404, 1982
27. Buchner A, Hansen L: Melanotic macule of the oral mucosa: A clinical pathologic study of 105 cases. *Oral Surg Oral Med Oral Pathol* **48**:244, 1979
28. Buchner A, Hansen L; Pigmented nevi of the oral mucosa: A clinical pathologic study of 36 new cases and review of 155 cases from the literature. Part II: Analysis of 191 cases. *Oral Surg Oral Med Oral Pathol* **63**:676, 1987
29. Ficarra G et al: Kaposi's sarcoma of the oral cavity: A study of 134 patients and a review of the pathogenesis, epidemiology, clinical aspects, and treatment. *Oral Surg Oral Med Oral Pathol* **66**:543, 1988
30. Patton LL, van der Horst C: Oral infections and other manifestations of HIV disease. *Infect Dis Clin North Am* **13**:879, 1999
31. Patton LL, Ship JA: Treatment of patients with bleeding disorders. *Dent Clin North Ar* **38**:465, 1994
32. Meraw SJ, Sheridan PJ: Medically induced gingival hyperplasia. *Mayo Clin Proc* **73**:1196, 1998
33. Ship JA, Crow HC: Diseases of periodontal tissues in the elderly: Description, epidemiology, aetiology, and drug therapy. *Drugs Aging* **5**:346, 1994
34. Lopes MA et al: A clinicopathologic study of 196 intraoral minor salivary gland tumours. *J Oral Pathol Med* **28**:264, 1999
35. Porter SR et al: Recurrent aphthous stomatitis. *Clin Dermatol* **18**:569, 2000
36. Ship JA et al: Recurrent aphthous stomatitis. *Quintessence Int* **31**:95, 2000
37. Ship JA, Mohammad AR: *Clinician's Guide to Oral Health in Geriatric Patients*, 1st ed. Baltimore, American Academy of Oral Medicine, 1999
38. Scully C et al: Update on mucous membrane pemphigoid: A heterogeneous immune-mediated subepithelial blistering entity. *Oral Surg Oral Med Oral Pathol Oral Radiol Endod* **88**:56, 1999
39. Sirois D et al: Oral pemphigus vulgaris preceding cutaneous lesions: Recognition and diagnosis. *J Am Dent Assoc* **131**:1156, 2000
40. Birek C. Herpesvirus-induced diseases: Oral manifestations and current treatment options. *J Calif Dent Assoc* **28**:911, 2000
41. Johnson R. Herpes zoster—Predicting and minimizing the impact of post-herpetic neuralgia. *J Antimicrob Chemother* **47**(suppl T1):1, 2001
42. Siegel MA. Syphilis and gonorrhea. *Dent Clin North Am* **40**:369, 1996
43. Scully C et al: The deep mycoses in HIV infection. *Oral Diseases* **3**(suppl 1): S200, 1997

CHAPTER 113

Richard Allen Johnson

Diseases and Disorders of the Male Genitalia

The male genital skin is markedly varied in its anatomy, microecology, and physiology. Anatomically, the glans penis and inner surface of the prepuce (i.e., the preputial sac) are covered with nonkeratinized epithelium. This sac is continually moist and may accumulate smegma, the product of mucosal turnover and adnexal gland secretion, unless daily hygiene is performed. Smegma provides an excellent growth substrate for various infectious agents that are capable of causing balanoposthitis. Amputation of the prepuce, i.e., circumcision, eliminates the preputial sac and thus prevents many types of acute and chronic balanoposthitis and reduces the risk for many sexually transmitted infections (STDs),[1] as well as penile squamous cell carcinoma (SCC).[2]

DISEASES AND DISORDERS OF THE PENIS AND SCROTUM RELATING TO ITS SPECIALIZED ANATOMY AND FUNCTION

BALANITIS AND BALANOPOSTHITIS Balanitis is an inflammatory condition of the glans penis; posthitis is an inflammation of the foreskin; and balanoposthitis is an inflammation of the contiguous and opposing mucosa of the glans penis and prepuce. Balanoposthitis does not occur in an adequately circumcised male. In young males, the incidence of balanoposthitis is highest in those 2 to 5 years of age, in whom the foreskin is either partly or completely nonretractable; characteristic findings include erythema, swelling, discharge, dysuria, bleeding, and ulceration of the glans. In most cases, no single infectious agent is the cause; bacterial cultures of the exudate in the space commonly produce a mixed growth, but, at times, *Staphylococcus aureus* and group A (GAS) or group B β-hemolytic *Streptococcus* (GBS) can be recovered alone. At times, perianal streptococcal cellulitis, cause by GAS, can be accompanied by acute balanoposthitis.

In adult uncircumcised males, balanoposthitis most commonly occurs as an intertrigo, with no specific etiologic agent identifiable. Diabetes mellitus with glucosuria is a common predisposing disease. Sexually transmissible agents that can cause balanoposthitis include *Candida albicans,* GBS, gonococcus, *Gardnerella vaginalis,* and *Trichomonas vaginalis*. Clinical findings include "rash," itching, burning sensation, erythema, erosion/ulceration, pseudomembrane, and/or subpreputial exudate. Invasive infection can complicate balanoposthitis (penile cellulitis), especially in the immune-compromised host. The differential diagnosis of balanoposthitis includes trauma, allergic or irritant contact dermatitis, psoriasis (inverse pattern), plasma cell balanitis, balanitis circinata (Reiter's syndrome), fixed drug eruption, squamous cell carcinoma in situ, and extramammary Paget's disease.

Management of acute balanoposthitis is based on elimination of any predisposing factors in the pathogenesis, identification of a specific etiologic agent, and retraction of the foreskin, if possible, to eliminate the preputial sac, allowing the opposing epithelial surfaces to dry out. Castellani's paint applied daily is effective in acute symptomatic cases. In some cases of recurrent balanoposthitis, the sexual partner also must be treated to prevent recolonization of the specific infectious agent; circumcision is indicated in some cases, especially if phimosis exists.

BALANITIS XEROTICA OBLITERANS (BXO) This is the end stage of some cases of chronic balanoposthitis.[3] The most common disorder associated with BXO is lichen sclerosus (LS); however, BXO also occurs in males with chronic nonspecific balanoposthitis. The onset and evolution of BXO is insidious, evolving over many years. Patients usually seek medical consultation because of a reduced urinary stream or an acute, painful exacerbation of balanoposthitis with resulting phimosis or paraphimosis. Clinically, the prepuce is thickened, contracted, fissured, and fixed over the glans and cannot be retracted even with moderate tension, i.e., phimosis (Fig. 113-1). Patients with LS may have associated urethral narrowing and stricture. BXO may respond to potent topical corticosteroids.[4] Circumcision is curative in patients with phimosis secondary to chronic balanoposthitis. Invasive SCC has been reported to arise in LS with long-standing BXO.

PEARLY PENILE PAPULES (PPPs) These are common, normal anatomic structures located on the proximal glans penis. The papules are asymptomatic but often arouse some anxiety when first noticed by patient or physician. Clinically, PPPs appear as skin-colored 1- to 2-mm, discrete, domed papules evenly distributed circumferentially around the corona and extending proximally on each side of the frenulum (Fig. 113-2). Histologically, the lesions are angiofibromas with dense connective tissue and a rich vascular complex. No treatment other than reassurance is indicated.

FIGURE 113-1

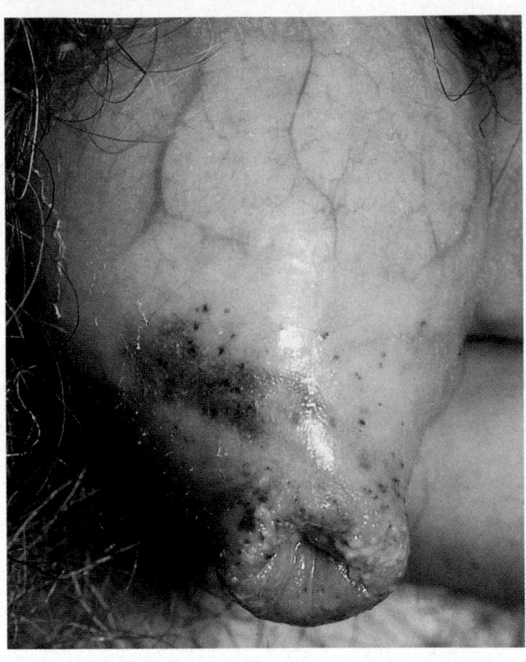

Balanitis xerotica obliterans with phimosis. The prepuce is fixed, covering the glans, and cannot be retracted.

PLASMA CELL BALANITIS (BALANITIS CIRCUMSCRIPTA PLASMACELLULARIS OR ZOON'S BALANITIS This presents as a solitary, persistent plaque on the glans of uncircumcised, middle-aged to older men. The etiology and pathogenesis are unknown. The duration of the lesion prior to presentation ranges from several months to a decade or more. The clinical presentation is usually an erythematous, shiny,

FIGURE 113-2

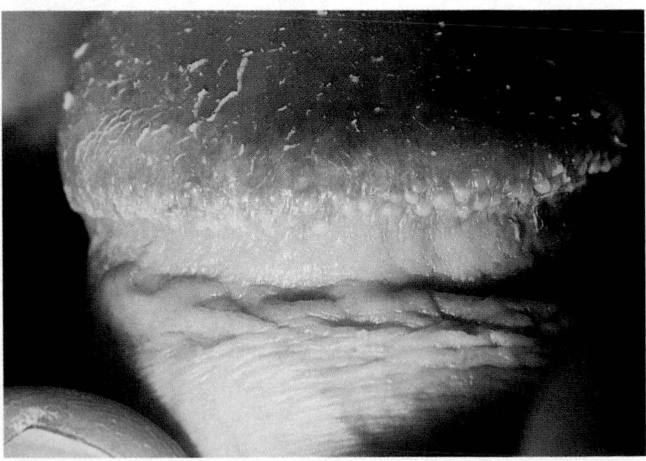

Pearly penile papules. Pink (skin-colored), 1- to 2-mm papules are seen regularly spaced along the corona of the glans penis. These structures, which are part of the normal anatomy of the glans, are commonly mistaken for condylomata or molluscum contagiosum.

FIGURE 113-3

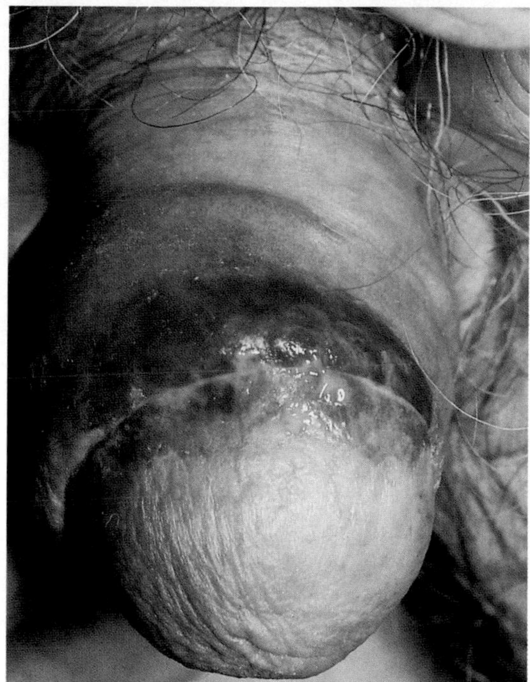

Plasma cell (Zoon's) balanitis. A single red, glistening plaque is seen on the glans penis, extending onto the adjacent prepuce.

moist, and glistening macular to slightly raised plaque(s) (Fig. 113-3) on the glans penis. At times, the coronal sulcus and the inner surface of the prepuce may be involved. The color of the lesion is usually bright red, but it may be the color of cayenne pepper due to microhemorrhage and hemosiderin deposition. Solitary lesions are more common, but multiple lesions may occur in some patients. Clinical variants including erosive and vegetative types have been reported. The differential diagnosis includes psoriasis, eczema, lichen simplex chronicus, lichen planus, lichen sclerosus, SCC, balanitis circinata, fixed drug eruption, HPV infections (external genital warts, SCC in situ or invasive), and extramammary Paget's disease. Histologic features include a thinned epidermis showing "lozenge" keratinocytes (i.e., diamond-shaped acanthocytes), an occasional dyskeratotic keratinocyte, and mild spongiosis. Dermal findings include a dense bandlike or lichenoid mixed infiltrate with a predominance of plasma cells and vascular proliferation. There is poor response to all local modalities of therapy[5]; circumcision is curative.

LICHEN SCLEROSUS (LS) This is a chronic idiopathic dermatosis characterized by white papules or plaques occurring most commonly on the anogenital skin. Penile LS is diagnosed most commonly in middle age. Penile LS is often asymptomatic; some men are aware of subtle visual changes occurring over months to years. Symptomatic individuals report itching, burning with urination, painful erections, diminished sensation of the glans, or diminution in the caliber and force of the urinary stream. In uncircumcised males, a sclerotic, constricting band forms 1 to 2 cm from the distal end of the prepuce; in time, phimosis may occur. Obstruction of urinary flow may occur if the urethral orifice is involved or if phimosis becomes severe. BXO occurs if the sclerotic process progresses untreated.

Clinically, ivory- or porcelain-white macules and plaques (Fig. 113-4) are noted in all patients; the anemic color is caused by a loss of dermal vasculature with or without depigmentation. The surface of lesions is usually smooth but in some patients may be hyperkeratotic and may be elevated above or in the same plane as normal skin. Hemorrhage may occur beneath the surface of macules and plaques,

FIGURE 113-4

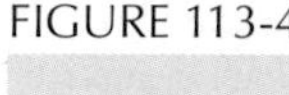

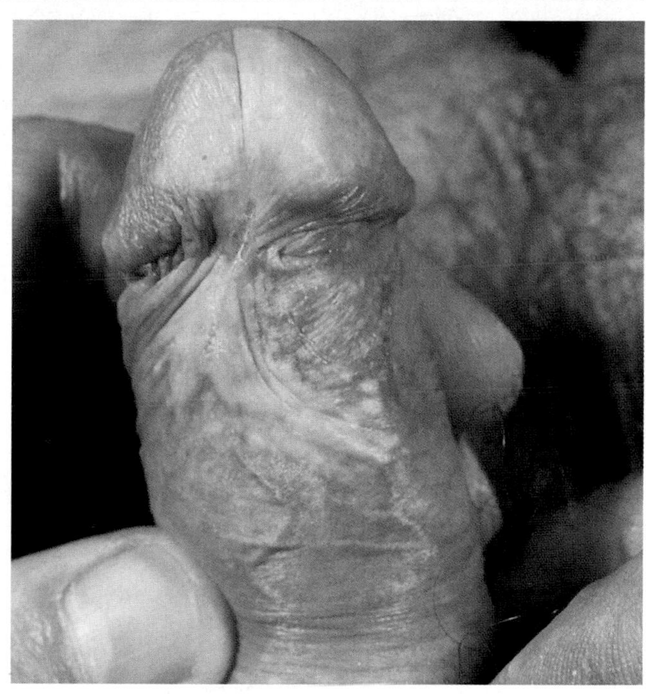

Lichen sclerosus, chronic. A white sclerotic plaque is seen on the glans and prepuce.

resulting in ecchymotic sites or hemorrhagic bullae within the lesions. The epidermis of atrophic lesions may sheer off, resulting in eroded or ulcerated loci within the lesions. LS occurs most commonly on the glans and inner aspect of the prepuce; in some individuals, it may occur circumferentially around the urethral meatus, resulting in varying degrees of stricture and obstruction of urinary flow. BXO is usually associated with phimosis and paraphimosis (once retracted, the prepuce cannot be replaced over the glans). A rare complication of LS and/or BXO is the development of SCC of the penis arising in involved sites.[6] The differential diagnosis of LS includes vitiligo, postinflammatory hypopigmentation, and posttraumatic or surgical scar. Clobetasol ointment has proven very effective for treatment of early disease.[7] Circumcision is helpful in LS-induced phimosis.[8] Patients should be monitored on a regular basis; focal persistent hyperkeratotic or ulcerated sites within the involved sites should be biopsied to rule out evolution to SCC.

PSEUDOEPITHELIOMATOUS, KERATOTIC, AND MICACEOUS BALANITIS (PEKMB) This is a rare, idiopathic, papulosquamous dermatosis occurring on the glans penis that may represent a premalignancy or low-grade SCC. PEKMB is usually asymptomatic but may be associated with pain during intercourse. Clinically, a solitary, well-demarcated, laminated (micaceous) hyperkeratotic plaque is seen on the circumcised glans penis; the surface is thick, often resembling a sheet of mica from which thin folia can be peeled. Invasive SCC should be considered in nodular lesions arising within the plaque, whether hyperkeratotic or erosive.

PEYRONIE'S DISEASE (PENILE FIBROMATOSIS) This is an idiopathic disorder of the penis that leads to distortion or angulation of the erect penis. Onset is usually in middle age. Dupuytren's contracture of the hand and plantar fibromatosis may present concurrently. Symptomatically, erection may be associated with pain, especially in the early stages of the disease, caused by fibrosis of the tunica albuginea, the covering sheaths of the corpora cavernosa. The inflammatory plaque begins in the dorsal midline connective tissue near the base and extends to the adjacent tissue. Reduction in the normal erectile property of the dorsal penis results in an upward painful curvature when the penis is erect. Progressive fibrosis and curvature preclude coitus. Intralesional injection of corticosteroid into the fibrotic plaque may be helpful in some patients. Anti-inflammatory agents have been used, and surgical procedures have been developed.

CUTANEOUS DISORDERS INVOLVING THE MALE GENITALIA

PSORIASIS VULGARIS (see Chap. 42) This is the most common noninfectious dermatosis occurring on the penis. In circumcised males, penile psoriasis presents most commonly as a well-demarcated erythematous plaque(s) with varying degrees of scale (Fig. 113-5), similar to psoriasis at other nonoccluded sites. In uncircumcised individuals, psoriatic plaques occur on both the glans and the inner aspect of the foreskin and lack any scale (inverse psoriasis) (Fig. 113-6). Genital psoriasis is frequently accompanied by asymptomatic, unrecognized intertriginous psoriasis, perianally and in the intergluteal cleft, which appears as an elongated, well-demarcated, erythematous plaque(s). The diagnosis usually can be made on the local clinical findings, assisted by findings of psoriasis at other sites such as the scalp or intergluteal cleft and of nail changes. In that the differential diagnosis includes human papilloma virus (HPV) infections [genital warts, squamous intraepithelial lesion (SIL), and invasive SCC], the diagnosis may be confirmed by lesional biopsy in older uncircumcised males with preputial lesions. The course of anogenital psoriasis tends to wax and wane for years and is usually minimally symptomatic. Topical corticosteroids are effective, but their use should be minimized to avoid atrophy. Newer topical agents such as vitamin D preparations (calcipotriol), tacrolimus, and pimecrolimus may be effective and appear to be safe for long-term use.

FIGURE 113-5

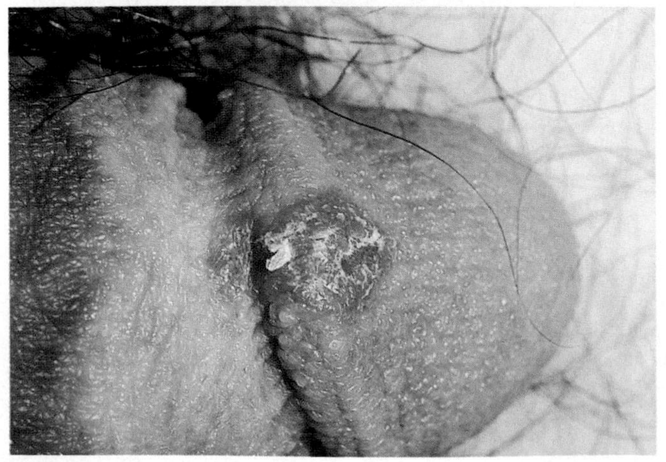

Psoriasis vulgaris. A scaling plaque is seen on the glans penis of this circumcised male.

FIGURE 113-6

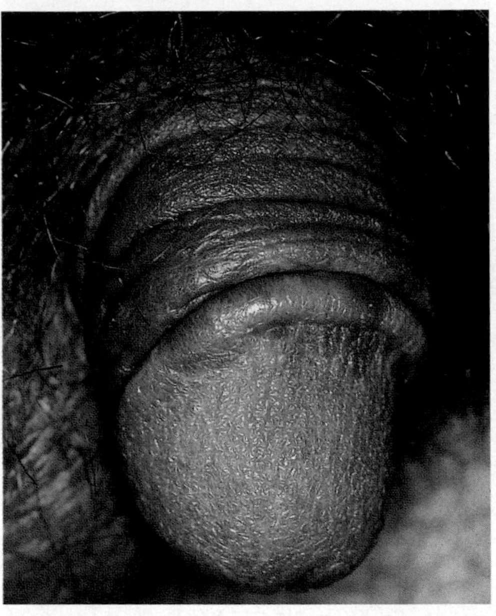

Psoriasis vulgaris, "inverse pattern." A well-demarcated nonscaling plaque is seen under the prepuce and on the proximal glans of this uncircumcised male.

Epithelial Precancerous and Cancerous Lesions of the Penis and Scrotum (see Chap. 79)

SQUAMOUS CELL CARCINOMA IN SITU (SCCIS) Several presentations of penile SCCIS occur. One is a solitary lesion arising on the epithelium of the glans/inner surface of the prepuce known as *erythroplasia of Queyrat* (EQ). EQ occurs in those not circumcised in infancy and with poor hygiene, i.e., associated chronic low-grade balanoposthitis. Another presentation is HPV-associated high-grade squamous intraepithelial lesions (HSIL), which usually occur as multiple lesions on the penis and may be associated with lesions at other anogenital sites.[9] In addition, SCCIS occurs in chronic inflammatory dermatoses such as lichen sclerosus, lichen planus, BXO, etc. HPV-B has been detected recently in EQ and may be a factor in oncogenesis.[10,11] Non-EQ penile SCCIS is associated with HPV-16 and -18. Additional etiologic factors include immunocompromised patients (HIV disease, solid-organ transplantation) and PUVA therapy. Clinically, EQ presents as a well-defined, irregularly bordered, red patch with a glazed to velvety surface (Fig. 113-7); a nodule or ulcer within EQ usually represents invasive SCC arising within the SCCIS. Histologically, approximately 10 percent of EQ lesions show invasion. Effective modalities of therapy for EQ include electrosurgery, cryosurgery, laser surgery, photodynamic therapy, and topical application of 5-fluorouracil.[12,13]

INVASIVE SCC OF THE PENIS (see Chap. 80) This is an uncommon cancer in the United States, accounting for 2 percent of all male genital cancers, having a mean age at diagnosis of 59 years. Geographically, penile SCC is 10 times greater in certain regions of Africa than in industrialized countries. Invasive penile SCC usually arises within SCCIS, i.e., EQ, HPV-induced SIL, or inflammatory dermatoses. The tumor usually presents as a warty, exophytic papule or nodule, erythematous compared with the normal color of the penis, and it usually feels indurated, often arising in an area of SCCIS (Figs. 113-8 and 113-9). Less commonly, lesions may be flat and ulcerative. The tumor arises most commonly on the glans, prepuce, or coronal sulcus. Inguinal lymphadenopathy is indicative of secondary bacterial infection of the tumor or metastatic disease.

FIGURE 113-7

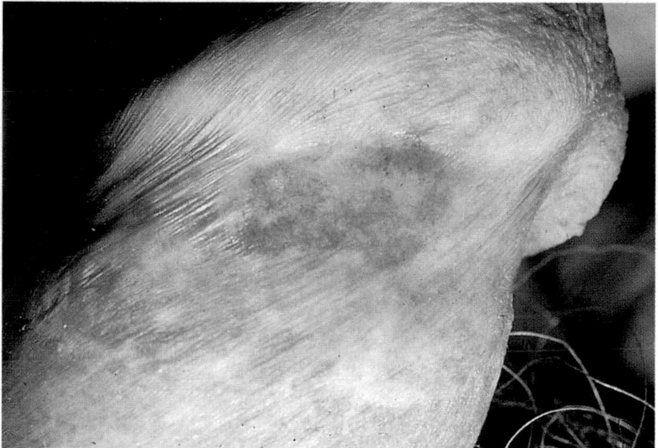

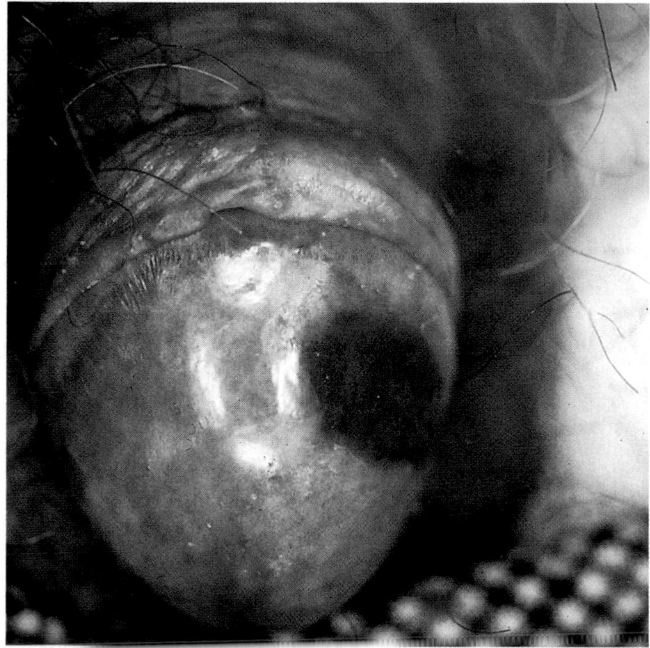

B.

A. Squamous intraepithelial lesion (SIL) of the prepuce. Pink plaque on the prepuce. A circumcision had been performed recently because of "chronic balanitis." Histology of the excised specimen showed high-grade SIL. The lesion cleared following topical 5-fluorouracil therapy. *B.* Squamous cell carcinoma in situ of the glans penis (erythroplasia of Queyrat). A solitary red plaque on the glans of this uncircumcised male must be differentiated from plasma cell balanitis and psoriasis. (*Courtesy of Alfred Eichmann, MD.*)

SCC OF THE SCROTUM (see Chap. 80) This is much less common than SCC of the penis. Industrial carcinogens such as tar have long been implicated in the pathogenesis ("soot warts," chimney sweeps' disease); other agents include inorganic arsenic and HPV. Clinically, early scrotal SCC presents as a slowly growing, painless nodule; older, more advanced lesions tend to be indurated, ulcerated, and/or painful, in some cases with unilateral inguinal adenopathy.

GENITAL VERRUCOUS CARCINOMA (GVC) (see Chap. 80) This is a slowly growing SCC, accounting for up to 25 percent of penile cancers. Etiologic factors include HPV infection. GVC arises most frequently on the glans penis and prepuce and less often on the scrotum and perianal regions; it often presents as a large, chronic fungating tumor mass. With continuing growth, the tumor erodes exophytically through the prepuce; however, at times, it may erode inwardly into the urethra and corpora cavernosa with subsequent compression and destruction. Areas of more aggressive SCC may exist within a GVC. Because of the low-grade aggressive nature of GVC, the prognosis is usually excellent.[14,15] However, in long-standing tumors, more aggressive behavior can develop and regional and distant lymphatic metastasis occur.

FIGURE 113-8

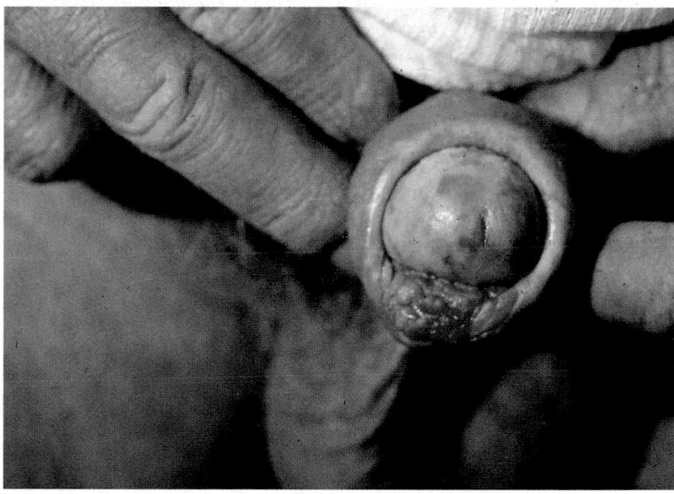

Invasive squamous cell carcinoma of the penis arising in chronic lichen sclerosus. A large eroded tumor is seen arising on the prepuce.

FIGURE 113-9

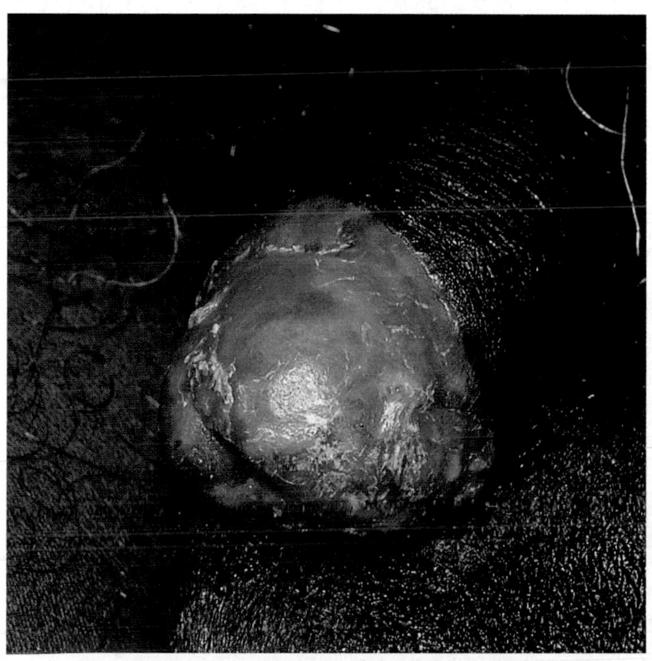

Invasive squamous cell carcinoma of the penis arising in pseudoepitheliomatous keratotic and micaceous balanitis of Civatte. The superior aspect of the glans shows micaceous balanitis with a large nodule inferolaterally.

BASAL CELL CARCINOMA (BCC) OF THE PENIS AND SCROTUM (see Chap. 81) BCC, the most common malignancy in geographic regions populated by fair-skinned individuals, rarely arises in the penis or scrotum.[16] Ultraviolet radiation exposure, which is a major etiologic factor in BCC at other sites, is an uncommon factor in the pathogenesis of anogenital lesions. As with other skin cancers, BCC of the genital skin is much more common in fair-skinned than heavily melanized males. Clinically, the most common presentation of penile and scrotal BCCs is a pearly papule with surface telangiectases, but ulcerative, cicatricial, and superficial multicentric variants also occur.

EXTRAMAMMARY PAGET'S DISEASE (EMPD) This is a rare neoplasia that arises most commonly within apocrine glands present in the anogenital, anorectal, and axillary regions.[17] Rarely, it is associated with rectal or urothelium carcinoma. EMPD of the glans penis associated with a urethral or bladder carcinoma may present up to 7 years after treatment of the primary malignancy. Clinically, EMPD appears as a macular to slightly raised plaque with well-demarcated borders (Fig. 113-10) that is pink, red, to tan or brown; the surface may appear glistening red or scaly. Secondary changes of excoriations and lichen simplex chronicus from scratching may be a prominent part of the clinical appearance. A nodular area within a plaque of EMPD may represent a site of deeper invasion into the dermis. In males, the most common sites for EMPD are the perianal, scrotal, penile, and axillary regions. Perianal EMPD may extend up to the anal canal. Scrotal lesions tend to extend to the thigh or onto the shaft of the penis. A shiny red patch of EMPD occurring periurethrally on the glans penis may herald carcinoma of the urethra, periurethral gland, or bladder. Metastasis to regional inguinal or femoral lymph nodes or to distant lymph nodes may occur late in the course of the disease. The most common underlying primary carcinomas found in association with male anogenital EMPD are adenocarcinoma of the sweat glands and rectal carcinoma.

FIGURE 113-10

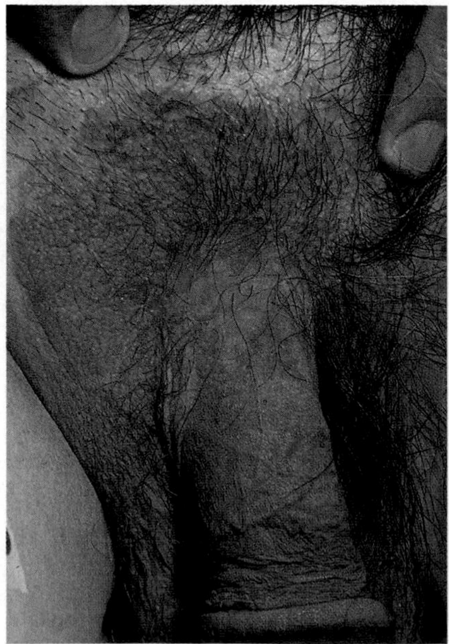

Extramammary Paget's disease. A large brown-pink plaque at the base of the penis and the pubic region.

Benign Epithelial and Appendegeal Tumors

The most common benign nonviral tumor of the anogenital regions is seborrheic keratosis. These lesions usually can be distinguished from external genital warts on clinical findings.

VERRUCIFORM XANTHOMA This occurs on the male genitalia as well as in the mouth.[18] Clinically, the presentation is of hyperkeratotic plaques occurring at the coronal sulcus which, if large, can cause phimosis. The pathogenesis is unknown but is thought to represent an initial epidermal irritation or degeneration followed by a dermal histiocytic response. SCC may arise within the lesion.

SCROTAL CYSTS These are a relatively common occurrence, whereas those arising on the penis are infrequent. Epidermal inclusion cysts may arise in a circumcision or other scars. Medical raphe cysts lined with epithelium of combined epidermal and urothelial origin occur on the shaft. *Sebaceous glands* occur normally on the shaft of the penis in association with hair follicles. *Syringomas,* benign tumors of the eccrine sweat duct, occur on the penis, presenting as discrete, skin-colored, dome-shaped papules 1 to 3 mm in diameter located on the dorsal and lateral aspects of the shaft. The differential diagnosis of appendageal tumors includes normal sebaceous glands, lichen nitidus, condylomata acuminata, and mollusca contagiosa.

Disorders of Melanocytes: Disorders of Pigmentation (see Chap. 90)

HYPERPIGMENTATION Postinflammatory hyperpigmentation commonly occurs following various inflammatory disorders of the genitalia, more frequently in individuals with darker skin types. Following a fixed drug eruption, a violaceous-brown macule persists for many months after the acute lesion has resolved. Recurrences of the eruption at the same site leave the skin progressively darker. A similar pigmentation occurs during the course of lichen planus, associated with pigment incontinence. Epidermal hyperpigmentation occurs following many genital infections such as genital herpes.

LEUKODERMA Penile postinflammatory hypopigmentation occurs commonly following recurrent episodes of genital herpes, especially in individuals with darker skin types. LS often presents with macular white areas on the glans and shaft that are caused by decreased dermal vasculature rather than decreased melanin pigmentation. Depigmentation is seen most commonly with vitiligo but also as a chemical or occupational leukoderma or following exposure to rubber-containing devices such as condoms and pessaries. The isomorphic phenomenon occurs in vitiligo, i.e., depigmentation at sites of injury; as such, an individual with vitiligo may develop depigmentation on the genital skin following infections such as genital herpes or gonorrhea or inflammatory disorders. Vitiligo, either idiopathic or chemically induced, appears as sharply demarcated, macular white lesions. The entire cutaneous surface should be examined, looking for other depigmented areas, using a Wood's lamp; hypopigmented areas show little accentuation of pigmentary differences.

Disorders of Melanocytes: Benign Neoplasias, Hyperplasias, and Dysplasias of Melanocytes

(see Chaps. 92 and 93)

PENILE MELANOSIS This condition is characterized clinically by large size, irregular borders, multifocality, and variegated pigmentation and histologically by basalar hyperpigmentation without melanocytic hyperplasia.[19] The condition is usually idiopathic but has been associated with ultraviolet A irradiation with or without psoralens. The macules may be solitary or multiple, tan to brown in color, with variation in

FIGURE 113-11

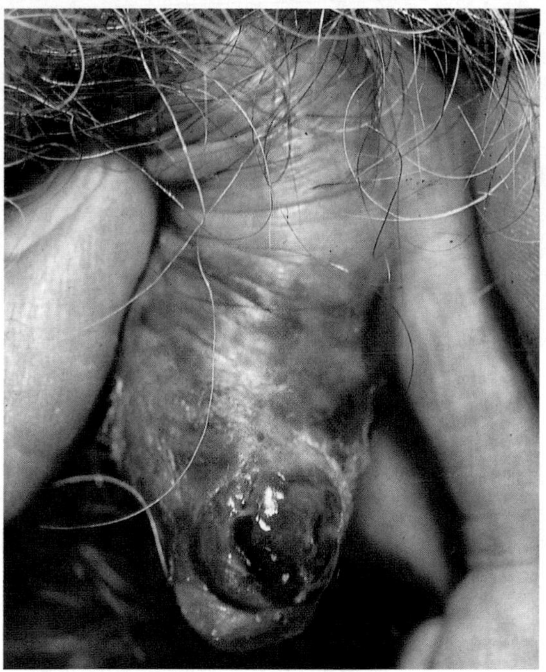

Malignant melanoma arising on the penis. A large, highly variegated plaque on the penis with an eroded invasive nodule.

the pigmentation from macule to macule. Borders are regular with round or oval shapes. However, melanosis on the glans penis may show some variegation of color and/or irregularity of the borders. Genital lentigines may be part of systemic disorders such as the LAMB syndrome (vulvar and other mucocutaneous lentigines, atrial myoxoma, and blue nevi) and multiple lentigines syndrome (lentigines and hypertrophic cardiomyopathy). Penile melanosis must be differentiated from in situ malignant melanoma, Peutz-Jeghers syndrome, and Ruvalcaba-Myhre-Smith syndrome (pigmented penile macules, macrocephaly, hamartomatous intestinal polys, and a unique lipid storage myopathy).

MALIGNANT MELANOMA This tumor arising on the male genitalia is rare, accounting for 0.1 to 0.2 percent of all nonocular melanomas and 1 percent of all penile carcinomas; the most common histologic type is acrolentiginous melanoma. As with melanoma at other sites, that occurring on genital skin can arise either from a preexisting pigmented lesion or de novo from epidermal melanocytes. Penile melanomas appear as macules or papules with variegation of brown-black color, irregular borders, and often with an area of ulceration averaging 1 cm in diameter at time of diagnosis (Fig. 113-11). The most common sites are the glans, prepuce, urethral meatus, penile shaft, and coronal sulcus. The prognosis of penile melanoma is poor because of late presentation, delay in treatment, early metastases via lymphatic vessels, and anatomic constraints regarding surgical excision; the majority of patients die within 1 to 3 years.[20–22]

Epidermal-Dermal Inflammatory Conditions of Unknown Etiology

LICHEN PLANUS (LP) (see Chap. 49) LP of the penis may be the sole manifestation of the condition, but it is more often part of a more widespread eruption. Clinically, violaceous flat-topped papules with a lacy white surface pattern are seen, most commonly on the glans (Fig. 113-12). Older lesions may have a grayish hue associated with melanin incontinence into the dermis. Annular lesions occur on the glans and penile shaft. In some individuals, the epithelium may slough,

FIGURE 113-12

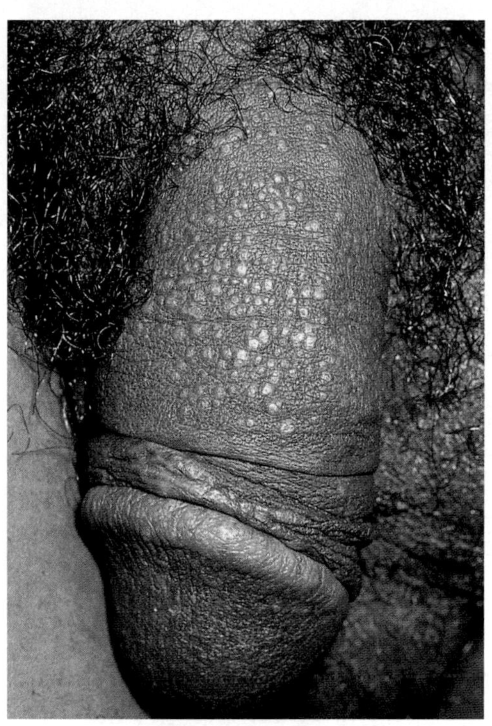

Lichen planus. Small papules with a follicular pattern resemble lichen nitidus; however, the lesions are larger than those seen in lichen nitidus, and typical findings of lichen planus were present at other sites. Flattopped violaceous papules are also seen on the glans.

resulting in eroded portions of lesions (erosive LP). SCC is a rare complication of chronic LP.[23] In the majority of cases, penile LP undergoes spontaneous remission after several years with residual postinflammatory hyperpigmentation in darker-skinned individuals. Erosive penile LP, as with the oral involvement, may persist for decades. Papular lesions can be treated with mild topical corticosteroid ointment; erosive lesions respond to intralesional triamcinolone injection. Topical tacrolimus or pimecrolimus may be effective without the risk of cutaneous atrophy.

LICHEN NITIDUS (see Chap. 50) This is an uncommon, asymptomatic cutaneous disorder characterized by the appearance of small, discrete, skin-colored papules occurring most commonly on the penis, abdomen, and arms. Clinically, shiny, 1- to 2-mm, well-demarcated, domed, skin-colored papules are seen on the shaft of the penis. The lesions remain discrete and usually are not grouped or confluent; however, a linear arrangement may be seen with the isomorphic or Koebner phenomenon. The course of penile lichen nitidus is chronic, extending over years.

Neoplasms, Pseudoneoplasms, Hyperplasias, and Mucinoses of Supporting Tissue Origin

SCROTAL CALCINOSIS This is characterized by variable numbers of subcutaneous, hard, marble-like, scrotal nodules (Fig. 113-13) that probably arise from epidermoid cysts.[24] The nodules are of varying diameters and are attached neither to the underlying structures nor to the overlying epidermis. Soft tissue radiologic examination shows calcified nodules. Histologically, accretions of homogeneous material that stains for calcium are seen scattered throughout the dermal connective tissue,

FIGURE 113-13

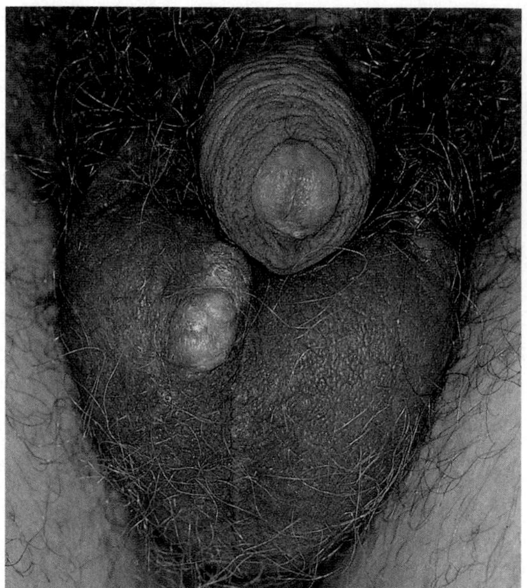

A.

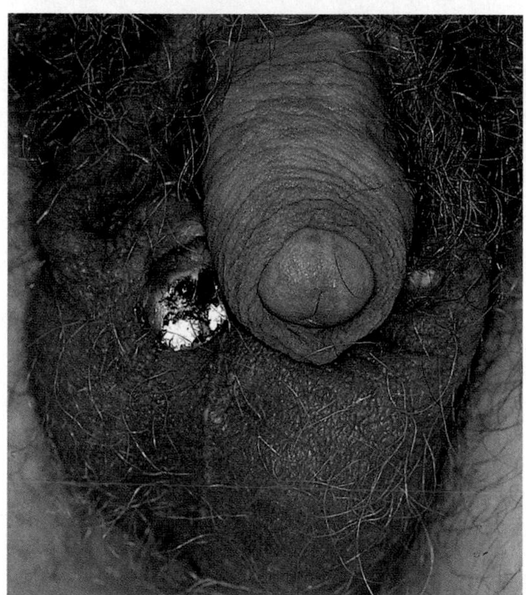

B.

Idiopathic calcification of the scrotum. *A.* White nodule on the scrotum. *B.* The contents of one cyst, a white chalky material, seen after incision and expression.

with an inflammatory infiltrate composed of lymphocytes, histiocytes, and giant cells; cyst walls can be seen in some cases. Scrotal calcinosis slowly progresses throughout life; the lesions remain discrete and do not become confluent. Symptomatic single or groups of nodules can be excised surgically.

Vascular Neoplasms, Pseudoneoplasms, and Hyperplasias (see Chap. 103)

ANGIOKERATOMAS Angiokeratomas of the scrotum and penis are common genital lesions characterized by ectasia of superficial der-

FIGURE 113-14

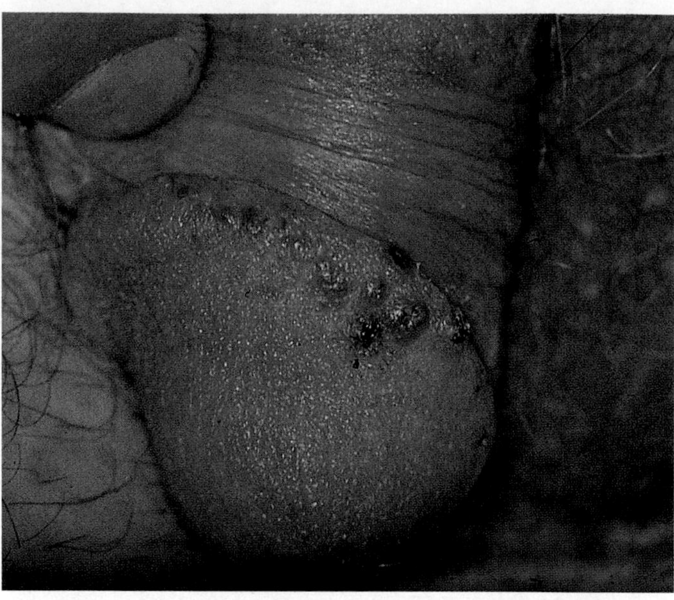

Angiokeratomas of Fordyce. Multiple violaceous and red papules on the glans.

mal blood vessels and hyperkeratosis. Lesions occur on the scrotum or periurethral glans, may be solitary or multiple, and increase in number with age. Penile angiokeratomas are thin-walled and occasionally bleed spontaneously with trauma. Clinically, the lesions are soft and compressible, purple, 1- to 5-mm papules. Angiokeratomas are occasionally solitary but are more commonly multiple with up to 50 to 100 caviar-like scrotal papules (Fig. 113-14). The differential diagnosis includes angiokeratoma corporis diffusum of Fabry's disease, which appears as multiple, 1- to 4-mm lesions concentrated in the bathing-trunk area but also on the gentalia. Symptomatic lesions can be eradicated by electrodesiccation or laser surgery.

DARTOIC LEIOMYOMA This is a smooth muscle tumor arising in the dartoic muscle within the scrotal sac; its occurrence is rare, accounting for only 0.1 percent of scrotal tumors. Like other types of leiomyomas, this solitary, pink, firm dermal nodule may be painful and may contract following touch or cold stimulus. Multiple lesions can occur.

APHTHOUS ULCERS (AUs) (see Chap. 112) These arise on the scrotum and penis, less commonly than vulvovaginal involvement in females. Genital ulcers, indistinguishable from AUs, occur during the course of the acute retroviral syndrome (HIV disease), resolving within a few weeks. When chronic AUs occur, the diagnosis of Behçet's syndrome always should be considered; genital aphthae are a major diagnostic criterion for the syndrome and occur in 60 to 90 percent of cases. Lesions are usually painful and solitary, with a gray, necrotic, fibrin-filled base surrounded by a halo of erythema (Fig. 113-15). Unlike AUs of the mouth, the diagnosis of AUs of the genitalia must be made by ruling out other causes of genital ulcer disease. Intralesional triamcinolone is quite effective in treatment.

Eczematous Dermatitis

ALLERGIC CONTACT DERMATITIS (ACD) (see Chap. 121) This occurs on the penis and scrotum and often is more florid and symptomatic than on other sites. In nonsensitized individuals, a minimum of 5 to 7 days elapses from the time of contact to onset of symptoms. In a previously sensitized individual, however, the time varies with the

FIGURE 113-15

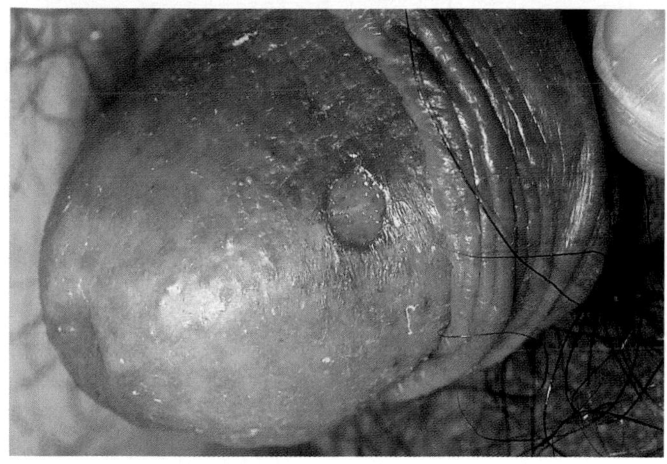

Aphthous ulcer. A sharply marginated ulcer with a red rim is seen on the glans; the diagnosis is made by ruling out other causes of genital ulcer disease. Identical lesions occur in Behçet's syndrome.

quantity of allergen and the individual reactivity but can be as short as 4 to 6 h. The extreme reactivity and tremendous vascularity of the penis maximize the intensity of the ACD. Sensitizing haptens make contact with the penis in three ways: hand-to-penis contact occurs in phytodermatitis (poison ivy or oak); during sexual intercourse, a sensitizing agent may be applied directly to the penis or from a sexual partner; and as involvement in a generalized contact dermatitis. Symptomatically, acute ACD is heralded by intense pruritus and a burning sensation at times prior to any visible changes.

Clinically, gential ACD presents with erythema and marked edema and, in time, with microvesiculation and exudation (Fig. 113-16). Older lesions may become crusted. Intense pruritus often causes the patient to

FIGURE 113-16

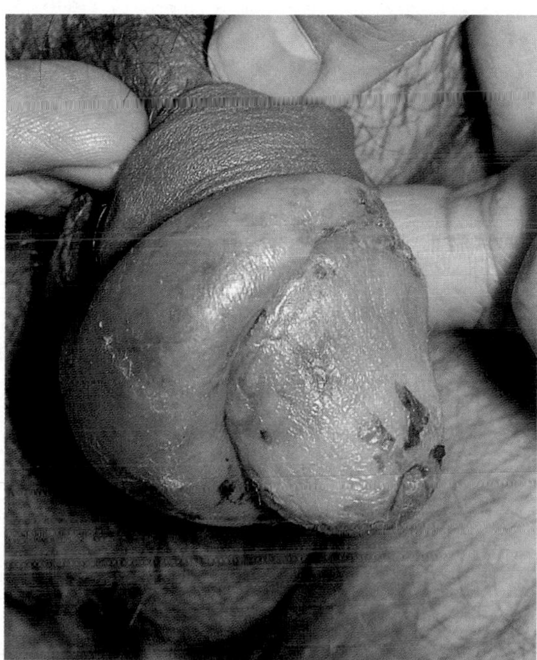

Allergic contact dermatitis; neomycin. Striking skin-colored edema of the distal penile shaft was attributed to neomycin application. (The red color on the glans is Castellani's paint.)

scratch, resulting in excoriations and larger erosions. Finding eczematous dermatitis on the inguinal area, thighs, perianal area, axillae, hands, or face is helpful in making a diagnosis of an ACD. The differential diagnosis includes atopic dermatitis, seborrheic dermatitis, genital herpes, cellulitis, inguinal dermatophyte infection, balanoposthitis, intertrigo, psoriasis, lichen planus, and balanitis circinata. Untreated and with no further exposure to the contactant, ACD of the penis usually resolves in 2 weeks or less. Reexposure to the hapten can result in repeated flares of the dermatitis even months or years later. Most cases of acute dermatitis respond to short courses of potent topical corticosteroids. Prednisone (70 mg initially tapered by 10 mg per day) is indicated for severe symptomatic involvement.

ATOPIC DERMATITIS (see Chap. 122) Individuals with atopic dermatitis frequently have involvement of the penis or scrotum as part of either flexural or generalized dermatitis. Atopic patients can have the dermatitis confined to a single area of lichen simplex chronicus on the scrotum (Fig. 113-17) for years or decades. Lichen simplex chronicus is best treated with intralesional triamcinolone (3–5 mg/mL), combined with the application of a corticosteroid ointment for a limited time. Topical macrolides (tacrolimus or pimecrolimus) may be useful.

SEBORRHEIC DERMATITIS (see Chap. 124) This occurs in the pubic area or scrotum, usually associated with involvement of the scalp, retroauricular area, face (eyebrows and nasolabial fold), presternal chest, and axillae. Genital involvement can occur in isolation, characterized by mild erythema, mild scaling, and at times, follicular involvement only. Individuals with psoriasis may have more erythema and scaling, i.e., seborrhiasis of the pubic and scrotal skin; inverse pattern psoriasis also may be present. Symptomatic patients can be treated with a mild topical corticosteroid or a topical macrolide (tacrolimus or pimecrolimus).

Photomedicine

EFFECT OF PUVA THERAPY ON THE MALE GENITALIA (see Chap. 265) Neither natural sunlight nor artificial ultraviolet B

FIGURE 113-17

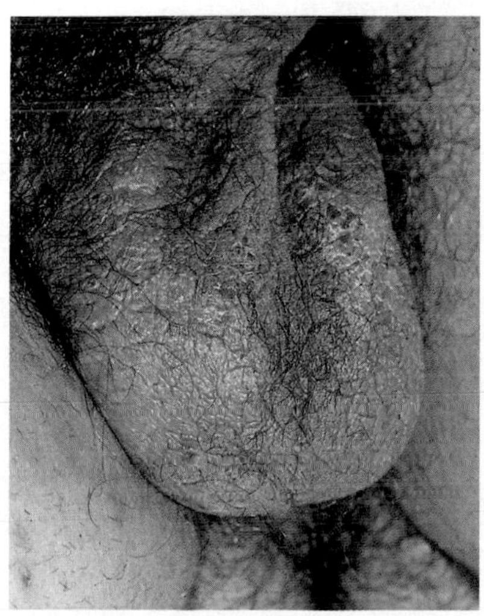

Lichen simplex chronicus. Lichenification, erythema, and hypopigmentation on the scrotum have been present for 20 years. The pruritus and lichen simplex chronicus resolved following intralesional triamcinolone injection.

exposure on the male genital skin appears to be an etiologic factor in photodamage or precancerous or cancer lesions at this site. Photochemotherapy (oral psoralen plus ultraviolet A; PUVA) has been used to treat extensive refractory psoriasis for two decades and has been implicated occasionally in the etiology of genital malignancies in males.[25,26] PUVA-induced ultraviolet damage can be avoided easily by covering the penis and scrotum with clothing during therapy.

ADVERSE CUTANEOUS DRUG REACTIONS (ACDRs)

ACDRs such as urticarial and exanthematous types are systemic reactions. Genital involvement is usually minor and part of the generalized cutaneous reaction.

FIXED DRUG ERUPTIONS (FDEs) These follow ingestion of a sensitizing drug, occurring most commonly in males on the penis, with or without lesions at other mucocutaneous sites. Patients often give a history of having identical lesions occurring at the same site. Because of the recurrent nature of an FDE, many patients are misdiagnosed as having genital herpes. Common drugs causing fixed eruptions include phenazones, tetracyclines, sulfonamides, dapsone, barbiturates, griseofulvin, and carbamazepine. Clinically, FDEs occur initially as inflammatory plaque(s) 2 to 3 cm in diameter that become bullous in some cases (Fig. 113-18). The most common site is on the glans and distal shaft. The lesion may be solitary or associated with similar lesions at other cutaneous or oral sites. Patients with previous FDEs often have macular violaceous to brown hyperpigmentation at the site that persists for many months after the previous outbreak. Phosphonoformate, used in the treatment of cytomegalovirus and acyclovir-resistant HVS infections, causes erosive and ulcerative penile lesions (Fig. 113-19), an irritant effect from high concentration of the drug in urine, which should be differentiated from FDE.

FIGURE 113-18

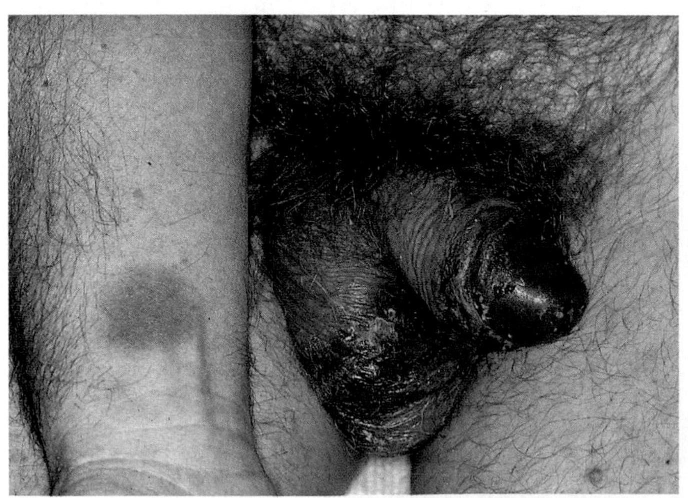

Adverse cutaneous drug reaction. Fixed drug eruption: phenolphthalein. Bright-red erosions on the glans and scrotum and a red plaque on the wrist were associated with extensive oral erosions following self-administration of phenolphthalein in a laxative. The patient had a history of three identical reactions following ingestion of the drug.

FIGURE 113-19

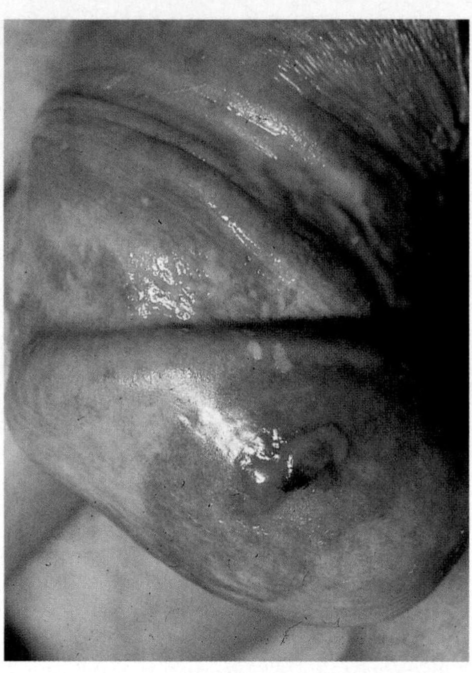

Adverse cutaneous drug reaction: erosions secondary to foscarnet. Erosion and ulceration are seen on the glans associated with foscarnet therapy of cytomegalovirus retinitis in an individual with advanced HIV disease.

GLUCOCORTICOID-INDUCED ATROPHY Prolonged used of moderate to potent glucocorticoids may result in epithelial and dermal atrophy. Clinically, chronic corticosteroid application to the penis is characterized by an atrophic appearance to the skin, prominent blood vessels, spontaneous ecchymoses, and striae on the glans and shaft. Corticosteroid-induced atrophy occurs more commonly in the inguinal region than the genitalia (Fig. 113-20).

TOPICAL 5-FLUOROURACIL This has been used in the treatment of HPV-induced lesions (external genital warts, squamous intraepithelial lesion). An irritant dermatitis occurs most commonly on the intertriginous skin between the anterior scrotum and the underside of the penis. Clinically, the dermatitis can begin within 3 to 5 days after onset of application and may present as mild dermatitis to extensive erosive lesions.

INTRAVENOUS DRUG USE Intravenous injections into penile veins or soft tissue result in venous thrombosis, thrombophlebitis, cellulitis, lymphangitis, and abscess formation. Localized gangrene of the scrotum and penis can follow injection of heroin into the femoral artery. Injection of particulate matter into the microcirculation of the genitalia results in arterial thrombosis, ischemia, and subsequent gangrene.

ORAL RETINOIDS Isotretinoin can cause erythema and stickiness of the epithelium, including the glans penis and urethral meatus. At times, the opposing surfaces of the distal urethral mucosa may adhere together, resulting in a diverted stream of urine flow.

SYSTEMIC DISEASES INVOLVING THE MALE GENITALIA

LEUKEMIA CUTIS This can present on the scrotum, heralding the relapse of acute myelogenous or chronic lymphocytic leukemia.[27]

FIGURE 113-20

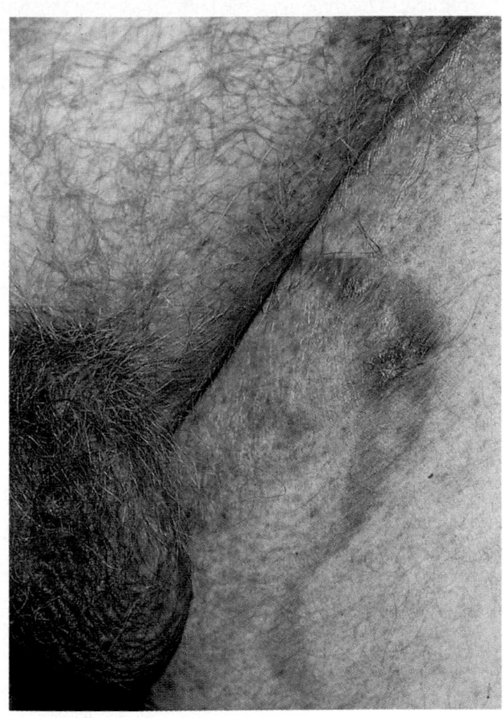

Adverse cutaneous drug reaction: topical glucocorticoid-induced atrophy and striae. The scrotum and inguinal area show erythema, telangiectasias, and striae formation follow chronic application of a class III glucocorticoid cream.

Chronic herpetic ulcers occur commonly in individuals with hematologic malignancies. Priapism also has been reported to occur with both acute and chronic types of leukemia. Multiple myeloma, when associated with hyperglobulinemia and hyperviscosity, also has been reported to cause priapism. An exophytic, ulcerative penile lesion may occur as the initial presentation of Langerhans' cell histiocytosis. A yellow or red-brown papular eruption in the diaper and inguinal areas, at times with nodules within the eruption, may be the only manifestation of Langerhans' cell histiocytosis in male infants.

CUTANEOUS CHANGES IN PERIPHERAL VASCULAR DISEASE

Severe Raynaud's phenomenon associated with progressive systemic sclerosis can reduce penile arterial blood flow and cause impotence. In diabetics, occulsion of arterioles commonly results in neuropathy and erectile dysfunction and, rarely, infarction/gangrene of the penis. Penile gangrene can be associated with penile calciphylaxis, occurring in diabetes mellitus with renal failure. Phlebothrombosis and thrombosis of the penile veins are rare and, when present, are attributed to trauma, infection, internal malignancy, or injecting drug use. Clinically, they present as a subcutaneous cord that is usually nontender and lacks any signs of inflammation. Lymphangitis and thrombophlebitis cannot be distinguished on clinical grounds.

LYMPHATIC DISORDERS Sclerosing lymphangitis of the penis (nonvenereal sclerosing lymphangitis) represents a thrombosed or sclerosed lymphatic vessel. The etiology is unknown but often follows vigorous sexual activity. Clinically, a painless, firm, at times nodular, translucent cord appears suddenly, usually parallel to the corona or on the glans. The lesion resolves spontaneously in a period of weeks to months.

SCROTAL AND/OR PENILE EDEMA This is characteristically painless, nontender, and nonerythematous and may be acute or chronic

and occur as a result of local or distant disorders of lymphatic vessel inflammation, fibrosis, or obstruction. Because of the loose connective support and the abundant vasculature of the genitalia, lymphedema is often confined to the penis and scrotum and does not involve the abdominal wall. The most common etiologies of acute edema are allergic contact dermatitis, angioedema, parenteral fluid overload, and peritonitis. Penile venereal edema is associated with gonorrhea ("bull-headed clap"), *Chlamydia trachomatis, Ureaplasma urealyticum, Mycoplasma genitalium,* and HSV infections. Reversible, iatrogenic genital edema occurs in patients with parenteral fluid overload and in 10 percent of patients with renal failure treated with peritoneal dialysis. Chronic lymphedema may be idiopathic or secondary to inflammation, postoperative state, neoplasms, radiation, hypoproteinemia, injection of foreign material such as silicone or paraffin, and other medical conditions. In countries where endemic filariasis is common, genital lymphedema is much more common and may be associated with massive lymphedema, i.e., elephantiasis.

SYSTEMIC VASCULITIS (see Chap. 174) Henoch-Schönlein purpura (HSP) can present with tender edema and hemorrhage of the penis and/or scrotum in boys and may herald the onset of other, more typical cutaneous and systemic signs and symptoms. Scrotal swelling occurs in 15 percent of young male patients with HSP, at times associated with pain that mimics testicular torsion; scrotal swelling and pain may be the presenting symptom of HSP.[28] Polyarteritis nodosa (PAN) also can present with scrotal swelling that is painful. Vasculitis of the testicle or epididymis may be the sole manifestation of the PAN early in its course and often results in ischemic damage to the skin with subsequent infarction and ulceration, Testicular biopsy showing large-vessel vasculitis is often helpful in making the diagnosis of PAN. Wegner's granulomatosisis is a systemic vasculitis that has been associated with penile necrosis secondary to large-vessel vasculitis.

REITER'S SYNDROME (see Chap. 182) This is characterized by an episode of peripheral arthritis and urethritis and frequently is accompanied by circinate balanitis (CB) (25 percent), conjunctivitis, stomatitis, and keratoderma blenorrhagica. In noncircumcised males with CB, superficially erosive plaques with ragged margins occur around the corona, with smaller satellite lesions on the glans and prepuce. In circumcised males, balanitis circinata sicca is seen, the lesions resembling those seen in psoriasis. A mucoid urethral discharge with periurethral erythema is frequently present.

SARCOIDOSIS (see Chap. 183) Rarely, this can be limited to the penis and scrotum.[29] Penile involvement is reportedly characterized by tender, erythematous induration of the distal shaft and yellow-tan plaques on the dorsum of the glans. There may be associated urethral obstruction.

GLUCAGONOMA SYNDROME Glucagonoma syndrome with superficial migratory necrolytic erythema (MNE) presents with inflammatory plaques that occur in the anogenital region.[30] The lesions enlarge with central clearing, resulting in confluence and a geographic pattern; borders may show vesiculation to bulla formation, crusting, and scaling. In addition to the anogenital region, axillae, umbilicus, perioral skin, and fingertip lesions, glossitis, angular cheilitis, and blepharitis are also seen.

METASTATIC CANCER TO THE PENIS/SCROTUM Despite the rich vascularization of the penis, metastasis of distant carcinomas to the region is rare; metastatic scrotal tumors are even rarer.[31] Sites of origin of penile or scrotal metastases include adenocarcinoma of the prostate

FIGURE 113-21

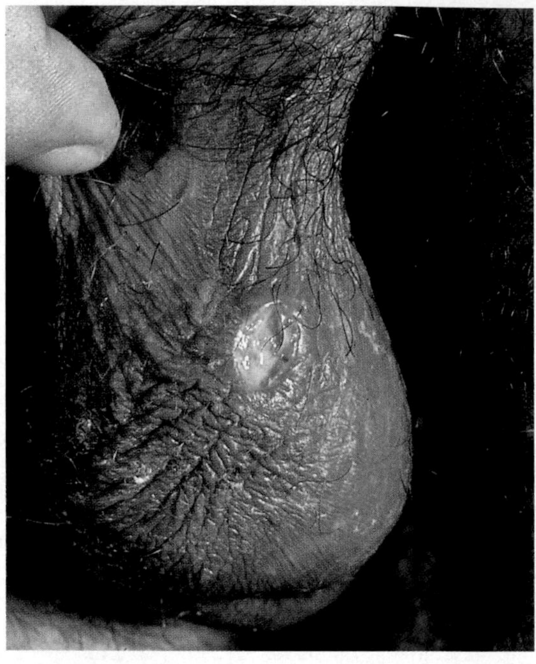

Behçet's syndrome with aphthous ulcer of scrotum. A chronic scrotal ulcer was associated with oral aphthous ulcers and central nervous system symptoms.

(30 percent), transitional cell carcinoma of the bladder (30 percent), rectosigmoid tumors (16 percent), and renal cell carcinoma (11 percent). The presentation is either as dermal or subcutaneous nodule(s), gangrene, carcinoma erysipelatodes, penile pain, or priapism.

BEHÇET'S SYNDROME (see Chap. 192) In Turkish males with Behcet's syndrome, 89 percent had experienced scrotal ulceration, 6 percent epididymitis, and 3 percent sterile urethritis. In a report from Korea, 99 percent had oral ulcers, 83 percent genital ulcers, and 84 percent skin lesions.[32] Large, painful, deep aphthous-type ulcerations occur commonly on the scrotum and penis (Fig. 113-21). MAGIC syndrome (mouth and genital ulcers with inflamed cartilage) is an overlap syndrome of Behçet's syndrome with relapsing polychondritis.

INFECTIOUS DISEASES OF MALE GENITALIA

Bacterial Diseases (See Chap. 194)

STAPHYLOCOCCUS AUREUS This organism causes primary infections in the anogenital region (folliculitis, impetigo, bullous impetigo, furuncles, carbuncles), secondary infection of dermatoses (atopic dermatitis, lichen simplex chronicus, and at times, psoriasis), or superinfection (genital herpes, chancres, or *Candida* intertrigo). Group A (GAS) and group B β-hemolytic *Streptococcus pyogenes* (GBS) colonize the anogenital region and may cause a superficial erosive intertrigo, e.g., perianal streptococcal "cellulitis." *Erythrasma* presents as a uniformly colored, pink to tan, well-demarcated plaque on the medial thigh, most commonly with symmetric bilateral involvement; the adjacent scrotum and penis are usually uninvolved. *Trichomycosis pubis* presents on the pubic area, with hair appearing to be thicker than the normal and with a yellow, red, or black layer coating.

CELLULITIS OF THE SCROTUM AND PENIS This is an uncommon condition probably because of the rich vasculature of the tissue. In the immunocompetent host, aggressive pathogens such as groups GAS, GBS, or *S. aureus* can enter a break in the epithelium, i.e., normal skin, underlying dermatosis such as psoriasis or at the site of a superficial infection such as a balanoposthitis with resulting cellulitis. GBS is the most common bacterial pathogen in the neonatal period and can cause cellulitis following circumcision. In the immune compromised host, pathogens such as *Pseudomonas aeruginosa,* especially in the setting of neutropenia, can cause soft tissue infections such as ecthyma gangrenosum. Symptomatically, early infection is associated with local pain and fever. Clinically, the genital skin is red, hot, and tender and may be associated with an obvious portal of entry.

FOURNIER'S GANGRENE This process is a necrotizing soft tissue infection of the genital and anorectal regions characterized by tissue necrosis (cellulitis, fasciitis, and myositis), rapid progression, lack of frank suppuration, severe systemic toxicity.[33] Major etiologic factors included diabetes mellitus, periurethritis with urinary extravasation, indwelling catheter placement, after instrumentation, after genitourinary surgery, after traumatic injury, injecting drug use into the dorsal vein of the penis, and infiltration of the urethra from a bladder tumor. In the majority of cases the infection was polymicrobial; *S. aureus,* GAS, or *Escherchia coli* may be the sole isolate in some cases. The onset can be insidious, with a discrete area of necrosis on the scrotum that progresses to advanced skin necrosis rapidly over 1 to 2 days. The infection tends to be superficial, limited to skin and subcutaneous tissue, and extending to the base of the scrotum; the testes, glans penis, and spermatic cord usually are spared in that they have a separate blood supply. The infection may extend to the perineum and the anterior abdominal wall through fascial planes. Symptomatically, patients with urogenital necrotizing infection show marked systemic toxicity, urinary retention, abdominal discomfort, and peroneal pain out of proportion to the physical findings. Clinically, local findings of Fournier's gangrene involving the scrotum and penis universally include edema, erythema, skin necrosis, crepitus, and bulla formation. Fever and leukocytosis are seen in nearly all patients.

TUBERCULOSIS OF THE PENIS This is a rare problem even in developing countries, where the prevalence of tuberculosis remains relatively high. Tuberculosis of the penis may be a primary infection acquired through sexual contact with genital or oral tuberculosis or may be associated with coexisting infection at some other site. Penile tuberculosis presents as subacute or chronic, painful, usually multiple ulcers; there may be associated inguinal lymphadenopathy.

ACUTE LYME BORRELIOSIS (see Chap. 203) This disease can present with either erythema migrans, which occurs at the site of the tick bite, often the groin or pubic area, and lymphocytoma cutis, which also occurs at the bite site, often on the scrotum. Lymphocytoma cutis is characterized by an inflammatory nodule, usually solitary but occasionally multiple, occurring on the scrotum; it is part of the clinical spectrum of European Lyme borreliosis but very uncommon in North American Lyme borreliosis. Young males are most commonly infected, the lesion occurring at the site of the tick bite. There may be coexisting systemic symptoms.

Fungal Diseases

DERMATOPHYTOSIS (see Chap. 205) This commonly involves the inguinal area, i.e., tinea cruris, but rarely causes superficial infection of the scrotum or penis. Tinea cruris is always associated with tinea pedis, the dermatophyte being transferred by the hand from the feet to the crural area. Clinically, tinea cruris presents as an erythematous to tan plaque with well-demarcated, scalloped borders advancing inferiorly down the anterior thigh. Chronic scratching may induce an eczematous dermatitis or lichen simplex chronicus on the scrotum or, less commonly, on the penis. Chronic application of topical corticosteroids can mask the clinical presentation (tinea incognito).

CANDIDIASIS (see Chap. 206) *C. albicans* is often a resident flora of the bowel and can be cultured from the intertriginous skin of the preputial sac, the inguinal folds, and the perineal area. Etiologic factors for intertriginous candidiasis include uncontrolled diabetes mellitus, impaired immunity during the course of a disease or immunosuppressive therapy, and severe debilitating illness. Candidal intertrigo in males usually represents overgrowth of endogenous *C. albicans*. With recurrent balanoposthitis, the source is exogenous from the sexual partner. Clinically, the primary lesions of candidal intertrigo are small papules and pustules that quickly increase in number, merging to form erosive patches and plaques. The central eroded area has ragged edges and is surrounded by satellite pustules. The most common sites are the preputial sac (balanoposthitis) and the inguinal regions. Bacterial superinfection with *S. aureus* or *Streptococcus* is associated with more pain and exudation than with candidal infection alone.

PITYRIASIS (TINEA) VERSICOLOR This occurs uncommonly as an asymptomatic scaling hypo- or hyperpigmented macular eruption on the shaft of the penis. This superficial fungal infection may occur only on the penis but is usually present on the upper trunk as well.

Viral Diseases

HERPES SIMPLEX VIRUS (HSV) (see Chap. 214) Genital herpes is a recurrent infection caused by herpes HSV-2 more commonly than HSV-1. Primary genital HSV infection is most commonly asymptomatic. Symptomatic males note fragile grouped vesicles on a red base that soon rupture and leave superficial erosions. Unilateral tender lymphadenitis often accompanies symptomatic primary infection but not recurrences. Headache associated with aseptic meningitis occurs in some patients with primary HSV infection and less often with each recurrence. Recurrent genital herpes is often heralded by a tingling, burning, or sensitivity 24 h prior to the appearance of vesicles. Groups of vesicles (Fig. 113-22) appear and are quickly eroded; the size of recurrent lesions is usually much less than that of primary infection. Genital herpes occurs more commonly on the prepuce, glans penis, and shaft and least commonly on the scrotum. Uncommonly, herpetic urethritis associated with a scant discharge and dysuria may occur with few lesions on the external penile epithelium. Primary and recurrent HSV proctitis or lesions in the anal canal or perianal area may follow receptive anal intercourse. Chronic herpetic ulcers (CHUs) occur in immunocompromised individuals. HIV disease is the most common underlying disorder associated with CHUs; other underlying disorders include cancer chemotherapy, hematologic malignancies, and bone marrow and solid-organ transplantation. CHUs appear as painful erosions or ulcerations that may have rolled borders and are located most commonly on the penis, scrotum, and inguinal areas (Fig. 113-23). Older ulcers may become crusted or hyperkeratotic. Giant ulcers may occur in patients with acyclovir-resistant strains of HSV.

FIGURE 113-22

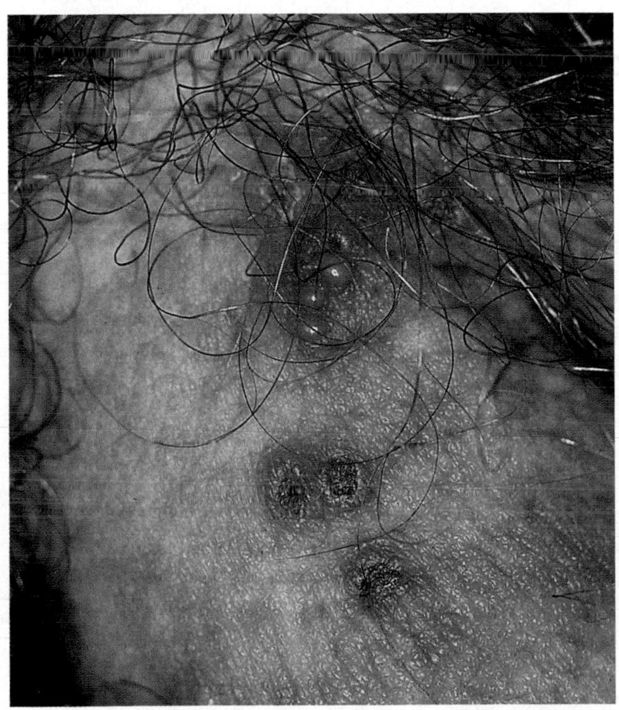

Herpes simplex virus infection: recurrent. Clusters of small vesicles on the penile shaft.

FIGURE 113-23

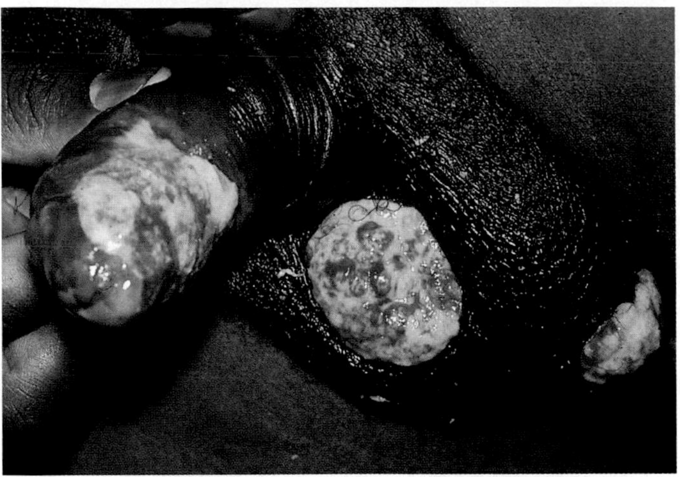

Herpes simplex virus infection: chronic. Larger ulcers on the penis and scrotum caused by an acyclovir-resistant HSV strain resolved with intravenous cidofovir.

HERPES ZOSTER (see Chap. 215) Herpes zoster infection of the third or fourth sacral sensory nerves involves the penis, scrotum, and perianal skin. Symptomatically, zoster is often associated with varying degrees of neuritic pain. Pain prior to the appearance of any cutaneous findings can be confused with an acute surgical problem. Clinically, zoster is characterized by grouped vesicles in a dermatomal distribution.

MOLLUSCUM CONTAGIOSUM (MC) (see Chap. 221) This is a poxvirus skin infection characterized by clustered 1- to 5-mm domed papules with central umbilication. The clusters evolve at sites of primary inoculation following autoinoculation. The anogenital area is a common site in children. In adult men, the penis is a common site for sexually transmitted MC. Commonly, MC varies from this classic description following trauma or spontaneous involution, becoming hyperkeratotic and/or inflamed, such that the skin-colored, centrally umbilicated dome becomes a red scaling papule. As such, MC becomes clinically indistinguishable from condylomata acuminata.

HUMAN PAPILLOMAVIRUS (HPV) (see Chap. 223) HPV infects the moist epithelium of the anogenital region and gives rise to a spectrum of lesions in males ranging from genital warts, squamous intraepithelial

FIGURE 113-24

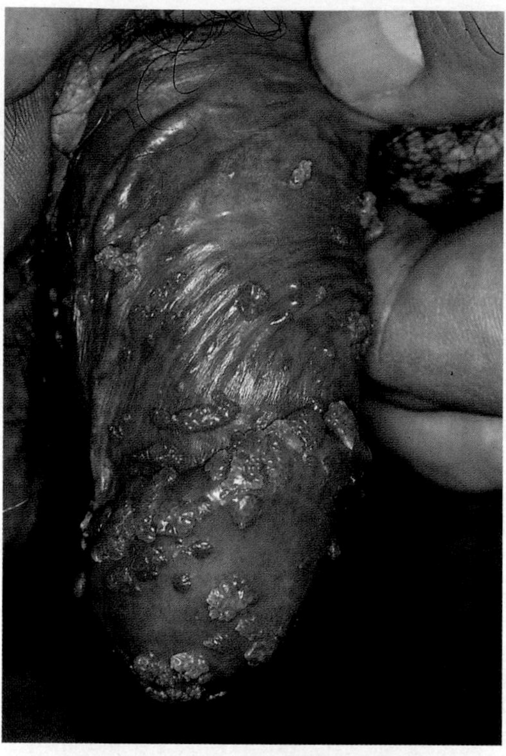

Human papillomavirus infection: condylomata acuminata. Multiple skin-colored papules on the shaft and glans penis.

lesions (SIL), and invasive SCC. More than 60 HPV types have been detected; however, types 6 and 11 most commonly infect anogenital epithelium, as well as types 16, 18, 31, and 33. Types 16, 18, 31, and 33 are linked etiologically to intraepithelial neoplasia and invasive SCC. Anogenital HPV infections/genital warts are the most common sexually transmitted diseases, infecting 30 to 40 million individuals in the United States. The majority of cases of genital HPV infection are subclinical; i.e., no clinical lesions can be detected on routine examination.

External genital warts (EGWs) The majority of anogenital HPV infections are subclinical. When clinically detectable, EGWs appear as papules, condyloma acuminatum (cauliflower floret–like papules), flat-topped plaques, and hyperkeratotic papules/nodules (Fig. 113-24). The color is that of the normal genital skin but may be pink or hyperpigmented. Lesions much darker in color than the normal genital skin may be SIL. The most common sites for genital warts to occur in males are the frenulum corona, glans, prepuce, shaft, scrotum, urethral meatus, and urethra. Perineal, perianal, and anal canal genital warts are associated with receptive anal intercourse. EGWs cannot be distinguished on clinical findings from SIL; lesional biopsy is indicated in immunocompromised individuals. EGWs recur after appropriate therapy in a high percentage of patients due to persistence of latent HPV in normal-appearing perilesional skin. The major significance of HPV infection is the oncogenic potential. HPV types 16, 18, 31, and 33 are the major etiologic factors for SIL and invasive SCC of the cervix, anus, and external genitalia. Subclinical genital infection persists for months to years. The current approach is to treat visible lesions with a variety of destructive modalities, the most commonly used of which is cryosurgery with liquid nitrogen. Topical imiquimod 5% cream is an immunomodulatory molecule that upregulates T_H1 cytokine response, causing specific immune response to HPV.

FIGURE 113-25

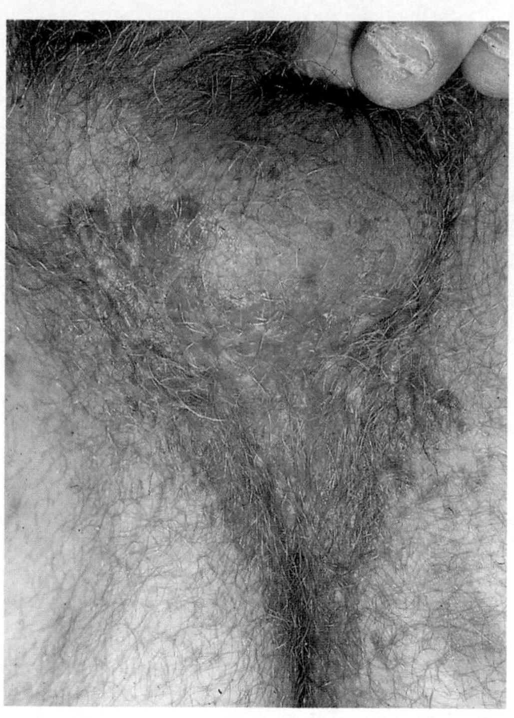

Human papillomavirus infection: squamous cell carcinoma in situ. A huge cobblestoned plaque composed of confluent brown and pink papules on the penis, scrotum, inguinal folds, and perineum in an individual with advanced HIV disease.

Squamous intraepithelial lesions (SIL) SIL of the anogenital skin are characterized by multifocal maculopapular lesions occurring on the cervix, anus, and external anogenitalia. Intraepithelial neoplasia is caused by HPV type 16 most commonly but also by types 18, 31, and 33. Commonly, patients have a prior history of EGWs or female sexual partners with cervical or anal SIL. Immunosuppression associated with HIV disease,[34] iatrogenically induced immunosuppression in solid-organ transplantation,[35] and prolonged immunosuppressive therapy have been linked with an increased incidence. Clinically, SIL appears as erythematous macules and lichenoid (flat-topped) or pigmented papules (several millimeters) occurring as solitary lesions, scattered lesions, or confluent larger plaques (Fig. 113-25). The surfaces of lesions are usually smooth or velvety; the color is tan, brown, pink, red, violaceous, or white. Patients with SIL should be followed frequently, and new lesions should be treated to minimize the risk of progression to invasive SCC. HAART does not appear to have reduced the incidence of SIL.[36] Long-term survivors with immune compromise continue to be at risk for invasive SCC.

HUMAN IMMUNODEFICIENCY VIRUS DISEASE
(see Chap. 225)

Sexually Transmitted Diseases

SYPHILIS (see Chap. 228) Syphilis is manifested by anogenital lesions during the primary, secondary, tertiary, and congenital stages of the infection. A syphilitic chancre develops at the site of entry of the treponeme, beginning as a button-like papule/nodule that often erodes and ulcerates centrally. The lesion, which is usually not painful or tender on palpation, feels like a firm dermal lozenge, varying in size from 1 or 2 cm. Chancres are most often solitary but may occur as "kissing" lesions. The most common sites of anogenital chancres are on the inner prepuce, coronal sulcus of the glans, penile shaft and base, anus, and rectum. In secondary syphilis, condylomata lata appear as soft, flat-topped, moist, red to pale papules, nodules, or plaques that may become confluent, occurring in the anogenital region. Uncommonly, lesions of secondary syphilis and a chancre of primary syphilis may coexist. Annular polycyclic lesions may occur, especially in dark-skinned individuals.

CHANCROID (see Chap. 230) Chancroid is characterized clinically by a painful ulcer at the site of inoculation, often associated with painful inguinal lymphadenitis. The initial lesion, a papule, occurs at the site of inoculation 4 to 7 days after exposure, evolving into an ulcer with sharp, often undermined borders and a friable base of granulation tissue, often covered with a gray to yellow exudate. The most common sites of ulceration are the prepuce, frenulum, coronal sulcus, glans, and shaft. Edema of the prepuce and penis is common. Multiple lesions may occur due to autoinoculation. Inguinal lymphadenitis (usually unilateral), occurring in approximately half of patients within 1 to 2 weeks after the appearance of the primary lesion, is common in untreated patients. Abscess formation may occur within the infected lymph nodes with bubo formation; these have erythema of the overlying epidermis and may drain spontaneously with formation of a sinus tract.

LYMPHOGRANULOMA VENEREUM (LGV) (see Chap. 231) LGV is manifested by an infrequent primary genital lesion, secondary lymphadenitis with bubo formation and/or proctitis, and late infrequent sequelae of fibrosis, edema, and fistula formation. Clinically, primary infection is characterized by a papule, shallow erosion, ulcer, grouped small erosions, or ulcers (herpetiform) on the coronal sulcus, frenulum, prepuce, penile shaft, urethra, glans, or scrotum at the portal of entry. Lymphatic infection is manifested by a cordlike lymphangitis of the dorsal penis or lymphangial nodule (bubonulus); complications of lymphatic involvement include rupture, formation of sinuses and fistulas of the urethra, and deforming scars of the penis. When the inoculation site occurs intraurethrally, the presentation is of a nonspecific urethritis with a thin, mucopurulent discharge. Subacute or chronic LGV is manifested by the inguinal syndrome, anogenitorectal syndrome, and genital edema. In the inguinal syndrome, bubo formation occurs in the inguinal lymph nodes, more commonly unilaterally, with edema, erythema of the overlying skin, and rupture in one-third of cases. The inflammatory mass of femoral and inguinal nodes separated by a depression or groove made by Poupart's ligament is called the *groove sign*. In the anogenitorectal syndrome, proctocolitis, as well as hyperplasia of intestinal and perirectal lymphatic tissue, occurs with formation of perirectal abscesses, ischiorectal and rectovaginal fistulas, anal fistulas, or rectal stricture. Overgrowth of lymphatic tissue results in lymphorrhoids (resembling hemorrhoids) or perianal condylomata. Genital edema can occur years after the primary infection.

DONOVANOSIS (GRANULOMA INGUINALE) (see Chap. 232) Granuloma inguinale is characterized by ulceration and epitheliomatous hyperplasia. This STD is endemic in some developing geographic areas (Papua New Guinea, India, and South America) and is infrequently diagnosed in the industrialized nations of North America or Europe. The primary lesion is a relatively painless, button-like papule or subcutaneous nodule that ulcerates within a few days of appearance, occurring on the prepuce, glans, penile shaft, or scrotum. Ulcers have a beefy-red granulation tissue base with sharply defined edges. Ulcerations may enlarge by direct extension or autoinoculation to the inguinal and perineal regions. Fibrosis occurs concurrently with extension of the ulcer. Long-standing, untreated infection is associated with chronic lymphedema, which, if severe, may result in elephantiasis of the penis and scrotum. Variants of chronic donovanosis include ulcerovegetative with large, spreading exuberant ulcers, nodular with soft, red nodules that eventually ulcerate with bright red granulating bases, hypertrophic with formation of large vegetating masses, and cicatricial with spreading scar tissue formation associated with spread of infection. Regional lymph node enlargement is uncommon: however, a large subcutaneous nodule may mimic an enlarged lymph node, i.e., pseudobubo.

GONORRHEA (see Chap. 233) This is most commonly manifested as an acute urethritis in males associated with a purulent urethral discharge usually within 5 days after exposure. Clinically, the most common presentation of gonorrhea in males is a urethral discharge, which may be scanty or copious, clear or purulent. Uncircumcised individuals are more likely to experience meatal edema, balanoposthitis, erosion or ulceration of the glans, or penile edema. Untreated patients may experience a deeper infection of the urothelium with infection of the sebaceous glands of Tyson, periurethral glands, Littré's glands, lacunae of Morgagni, subepithelial and periurethral tissue of the urethra, median raphe, and Cowper's ducts and glands. Uncommonly, abscess of a periurethral gland may point and drain on the glans penis with formation of a small fistula. Rarely, gonococcal periprosthetic infection of a penile implant has been reported. The differential diagnosis of gonococcal urethritis is that of urethritis. A serious complication of gonococcal infection is disseminated gonococcal infection (DGI), which occurs more commonly in homosexual men with asymptomatic rectal or pharyngeal gonorrhea.

Infestations (See Chap. 236)

LYMPHATIC FILARIASIS (TROPICAL ELEPHANTIASIS) This is caused by the filarial worms *Wuchereria bancrofti, Brugia malayi,* and *B. timori,* which are estimated to infect approximately one-quarter of a billion individuals in tropical climes. In some geographic areas, up to 25 percent of the adult male population have lymphatic filariasis with thickened scrotal skin and hydrocele. The adult worms lodge in lymphatic vessels, resulting in a chronic inflammation, lymphatic obstruction, and chronic lymphedema. Clinically, early signs of infection include swelling, erythema, and tenderness of the scrotum. Long-standing disease may result in orchitis, hydrocele, thickening of the scrotal skin, scrotal elephantiasis, secondary bacterial cellulitis or lymphangitis, and a verrucous epidermal hypertrophy.

CUTANEOUS LARVA MIGRANS (CREEPING ERUPTION) This is caused by nematodes, which do not normally infest humans, and is characterized by serpiginous tracks on the skin overlying the path of migrating parasites. Larvae tunnel within the subcutaneous tissue. An inflammatory response is mounted with a resulting pruritic urticarial lesion over the larvae; as the parasites wander, a serpiginous track is created about the sites of penetration, i.e., the groin or buttocks.

SCHISTOSOMIASIS (BILHARZIASIS) Shistosomiasis with paragenital granulomas and fistulous tracts occurs in highly endemic areas and is caused by a variety of schistosomal blood flukes. The presence of adult flukes within the vasculature results in granulomatous inflammatory masses, which form condylomata, sinuses, and fistulas on the genitalia, perineum, groin, and buttocks.

AMEBIASIS Caused by *Entamoeba histolytica,* this is a common infestation is South America and Southeast Asia. Genital and perianal ulcers occur either at the site of penetration of the ameba, most commonly on the penis of homosexual males, or as a consequence of enteric amebiasis. Ulcers associated with enteric amebiasis begin about the anus or buttocks and enlarge to form large, deep, very painful ulcerations with serpiginous borders.

Bites and Stings (See Chap. 237)

Scabies presents with pruritus associated with small serpiginous tunnels on the penis and/or scabetic nodules on the scrotum and penis; eczematous dermatitis occurs secondary to scratching. Hyperkeratotic scabies occurs in immune-compromised individuals, presenting with hyperkeratotic and crusted lesions of the penis, extremities, and other sites. *Pediculosis pubis* (crabs, crab lice, pubic lice) is most commonly manifested in the pubic hair. Clinical findings include adult lice, appearing as 1- to 2-mm brownish gray specks in the pubic, scrotal, and inguinal hairy sites, eggs (nits) attached to the hair, papular urticaria (small erythematous papules at bite sites), secondary changes of lichenification, excoriations, impetiginized excoriations, and maculae caeruleae (tache bleues), slate-gray or bluish gray macules 0.5 to 1.0 cm in diameter on the lower abdominal wall, buttocks, and upper thighs.

DISEASES AND DISORDERS OF THE PERINEUM AND ANUS

PRURITUS ANI This is a common symptom, defined as an unpleasant cutaneous sensation that induces the desire to scratch the skin around the anal orifice, occurring in the absence of any identifiable dermatologic disorder, more common in males than in females (4:1 ratio). The onset occurs throughout life but is more common in the fifth and sixth decades. The pathogenesis is multifactorial in the majority of patients: fecal contamination and irritation [aggravated by poor hygiene, anorectal disease (fissures, hemorrhoids, chronic diarrhea, fistulas, impaction, or partial obstruction), diet (excessive liquids, spicy foods), drugs (mineral oil, colchicine, quinidine)] and anal sphincter dysfunction. The normal pH of the perianal skin and feces is acidic; factors that make it more alkaline may cause pruritus. Secondary infection (*S. aureus,* GAS, GBS, erythrasma, dermatophytosis, candidiasis, and HSV) may be a factor in some cases.

Symptomatically, pruritus ani is characterized by local itching. Clinically, the perianal skin may show erosions, excoriations, and lichenification. Erythema is more pronounced with secondary infection. Treatment should be directed at identifying and correcting local factors such as infection and anorectal anatomic disorders and eliminating irritant foods or drugs. All mechanical traumas should be minimized. Zinc oxide ointment is helpful in protecting the perianal skin from irritants. Castellani's paint is effective in reducing exudation from inflamed skin acutely. Topical macrolides (tacrolimus, pimecrolimus) may be effective and appear to be safe with long-term use. Fluorinated corticosteroid preparations should be avoided because of the possibility of atrophy with prolonged usage. Intralesional injection of triamcinolone is helpful in patients with lichen simplex chronicus. Oral antihistamines are helpful at controlling nocturnal rubbing and scratching.

PSORIASIS VULGARIS (see Chap. 42) This commonly occurs in the intergluteal cleft and perianal regions. In these sites, psoriasis is often asymptomatic, although some persons (atopics) may experience pruritus. Clinically, perianal psoriasis presents as very well demarcated linear erythema in the intergluteal cleft that may extend perianally. It is often helpful to examine the intergluteal cleft for, psoriasis to confirm the diagnosis in those with minimal disease.

HIDRADENITIS SUPPURATIVA (see Chap. 77) This may present with involvement in the perianal region and buttocks with inflammatory nodules, abscesses, fistulas, and sinus tracts, often accompanied by involvement of the axillae and inguinocrural region. In the absence of hidradenitis suppurativa at other sites, diagnosis of the disorder with involvement of the perineum and buttocks is often missed. The differential diagnosis includes acne, *S. aureus* folliculitis, furuncles, pilonidal infection, and inflammatory bowel disease with fistulas.

PILONIDAL CYSTS AND SINUSES These present as midline inflammatory nodules overlying the sacrum or coccyx. Secondary infection may occur, resulting in deeper infection and cellulitis. Rarely, a chronically inflamed pilonidal cyst may give rise to SCC.

PERIANAL STREPTOCOCCAL CELLULITIS (PSC) This is a superficial infection (intertrigo) caused by GAS and characterized symptomatically by perianal pruritus and mild pain and clinically by a ring of perianal erythema and edema. It is most common in prepubertal children but also occurs in adults. Several members of one family may be infected simultaneously, some with streptococcal pharyngitis and others with perianal cellulitis.[37] In some patients, a coexisting GABHS proctocolitis and vulvovaginitis may occur. Subjective findings include pruritus, painful defecation, fecal hoarding behavior, and blood staining the underpants in these children. A well-demarcated erythematous plaque is seen perianally.

REFERENCES

1. Auvert B et al: Male circumcision and HIV infection in four cities in sub-Saharan Africa. *AIDS* **15** (suppl 4):S31, 2001
2. Mallon E et al: Circumcision and genital dermatoses. *Arch Dermatol* **136**:350, 2000
3. Das S, and Tunuguntla HS: Balanitis xerotica obliterans: A review. *World J Urol* **18**:382, 2000
4. Kiss A et al: The response of balanitis xerotica obliterans to local steroid application compared with placebo in children. *J Urol* **165**:219, 2001
5. Tang A et al: Plasma cell balanitis of Zoon: Response to Trimovate cream. *Int J STD AIDS* **12**:75, 2001
6. Dillner J et al: Etiology of squamous cell carcinoma of the penis. *Scand J Urol Nephrol Suppl* **205**:189, 2000
7. Riddell L et al: Clinical features of lichen sclerosus in men attending a department of genitourinary medicine. *Sex Transm Infect* **76**:311, 2000
8. Aynaud O et al: Incidence of preputial lichen sclerosus in adults: Histologic study of circumcision specimens. *J Am Acad Dermatol* **41**:923, 1999
9. von Krogh G, Horenblas S: Diagnosis and clinical presentation of premalignant lesions of the penis. *Scand J Urol Nephrol Suppl* **205**:201, 2000
10. Wieland U et al: Erythroplasia of Queyrat: Coinfection with cutaneous carcinogenic human papillomavirus type 8 and genital papillomaviruses in a carcinoma in situ. *J Invest Dermatol* **115**:396, 2000
11. Rubin MA et al: Detection and typing of human papillomavirus DNA in penile carcinoma: Evidence for multiple independent pathways of penile carcinogenesis. *Am J Pathol* **159**:1211, 2001
12. van Bezooijen BP et al: Laser therapy for carcinoma in situ of the penis. *J Urol* **166**:1670, 2001
13. Stables GI et al: Erythroplasia of Queyrat treated by topical aminolaevulinic acid photodynamic therapy. *Br J Dermatol* **140**:514, 1999
14. Cubilla AL et al: Warty (condylomatous) squamous cell carcinoma of the penis: A report of 11 cases and proposed classification of "verruciform" penile tumors. *Am J Surg Pathol* **24**:505, 2000
15. Bezerra AL et al: Clinicopathologic features and human papillomavirus dna prevalence of warty and squamous cell carcinoma of the penis. *Am J Surg Pathol* **25**:673, 2001
16. Gibson GE, Ahmed I: Perianal and genital basal cell carcinoma: A clinicopathologic review of 51 cases. *J Am Acad Dermatol* **45**:68, 2001
17. Park S et al: Extramammary Paget's disease of the penis and scrotum: Excision, reconstruction and evaluation of occult malignancy. *J Urol* **166**:2112, 2001
18. Mohsin SR et al: Cutaneous verruciform xanthoma: A report of five cases investigating the etiology and nature of xanthomatous cells. *Am J Surg Pathol* **22**:479, 1998
19. Barnhill RL et al: Genital lentiginosis: A clinical and histopathologic study. *J Am Acad Dermatol* **22**:453, 1990
20. Oldbring J, Mikulowski P: Malignant melanoma of the penis and male urethra: Report of nine cases and review of the literature. *Cancer* **59**:581, 1987

21. Larsson KB et al: Primary mucosal and glans penis melanomas: The Sydney Melanoma Unit experience. *Aust NZ J Surg* **69**:121, 1999
22. Honda S et al: Six cases of metastatic malignant melanoma with apparently occult primary lesions. *J Dermatol* **28**:265, 2001
23. Leal-Khouri S, Hruza GJ: Squamous cell carcinoma developing within lichen planus of the penis: Treatment with Mohs micrographic surgery. *J Dermatol Surg Oncol* **20**:272, 1994
24. Dini M, Colafranceschi M: Should scrotal calcinosis still be termed idiopathic? *Am J Dermatopathol* **20**:399, 1998
25. Stern RS: Genital tumors among men with psoriasis exposed to psoralens and ultraviolet A radiation (PUVA) and ultraviolet B radiation: The Photochemotherapy Follow-up Study. *N Engl J Med* **322**:1093, 1990
26. Aubin F et al: Genital squamous cell carcinoma in men treated by photochemotherapy: A cancer registry-based study from 1978 to 1998. *Br J Dermatol* **144**:1204, 2001
27. Gatto-Weis C et al: Ulcerative balanoposthitis of the foreskin as a manifestation of chronic lymphocytic leukemia: Case report and review of the literature. *Urology* **56**:669, 2000
28. Ben-Sira L, Laor T: Severe scrotal pain in boys with Henoch-Schonlein purpura: Incidence and sonography. *Pediatr Radiol* **30**:125, 2000
29. Wei H et al: Multiple indurated papules on penis and scrotum *J Cutan Med Surg* **4**:202, 2000
30. Alkemade JA et al: Delayed diagnosis of glucagonoma syndrome. *Clin Exp Dermatol* **24**:455, 1999
31. Fujimoto N et al: Metastasis to the penis in a patient with squamous cell carcinoma of the lung with a review of reported cases. *Lung Cancer* **34**:149, 2001
32. Bang D et al: Epidemiologic and clinical survey of Behcet's disease in Korea: The first multicenter study. *J Korean Med Sci* **16**: 615, 2001
33. Basoglu M et al: Fournier's gangrene: Review of fifteen cases. *Am Surg* **63**:1019, 1997
34. Aboulafia DM, Gibbons R: Penile cancer and human papilloma virus (HPV) in a human immunodeficiency virus (HIV)–infected patient. *Cancer Invest* **19**:266, 2001
35. Penn I: Cancers of the anogenital region in renal transplant recipients: Analysis of 65 cases *Cancer* **58**:611, 1986
36. Palefsky JM et al: Effect of highly active antiretroviral therapy on the natural history of anal squamous intraepithelial lesions and anal human papillomavirus infection. *J AIDS* **28**:422, 2001
37. Barzilai A, Choen HA: Isolation of group A streptococci from children with perianal cellulitis and from their siblings. *Pediatr Infect Dis J* **17**:358, 1998

CHAPTER 114

Libby Edwards

Diseases and Disorders of the Anogenitalia of Females

The diagnosis of vulvar skin disease and the management of women with such conditions require modification of some dermatologic principles, evaluation for and correction of vaginitis, and careful patient education regarding expectations and therapy. In general, women with vulvovaginal symptoms assume that their problems are produced by a curable infectious disease, particularly a yeast infection. Patients require reassurance and an explanation that dermatoses generally are controllable, although not curable. These women cannot be evaluated and treated in a 10-minute office visit; rather, they require adequate time for reassurance and education.

Vulvar skin disease, even more than skin disease in other areas of the body, is often multifactorial with subtle clinical abnormalities sometimes causing significant symptoms. Vulvar skin disease is often accompanied and driven by a secondary yeast infection or bacterial colonization, even in the absence of obvious clincal findings. The infection can be purely cutaneous, purely vaginal, or both. Thus vaginal secretions should be examined microscopically or cultured. Irritant contact dermatitis from multiple applied topical agents often exacerbates the symptoms.

Extremely severe itching and pain of the vulva are sometimes associated with unimpressive physical findings. Lichenification manifested only by a slight texture change can be associated with excruciating pruritus deserving of and responsive to aggressive therapy. Many clinicians make the mistake of overlooking or dismissing subtle physical findings.

The warm, moist environment of the vulva produces an altered morphology of some diseases. For example, scaling dermatoses may lack clinically obvious scale, and diseases that usually exhibit well-demarcated plaques may be less well formed. In addition, diseases that normally do not produce scarring of keratinized skin or oral mucosa can induce agglutination (resorption) of the labia minora, narrowing of the introitus, and scarring of the clitoral hood. Thus vulvar scarring can occur from any inflammatory condition, including lichen sclerosus, lichen planus, pemphigus vulgaris, and even a single episode of a blistering form of erythema multiforme.

THE VAGINA

Vulvar symptoms cannot be divorced from vaginal abnormalities. Irritating or infected vaginal secretions are a common cause of vestibulular (introital) symptoms. Vaginal cultures sometimes yield surprises such as a nonalbicans *Candida* infection, a pathogen that can be responsible for significant symptoms but is difficult to see on microscopic smears. However, a microscopic evaluation of vaginal smears can be extremely helpful and generally is more important than an examination of the vaginal mucosa. In addition to an inspection for *Candida albicans, Trichomonas,* and bacterial vaginosis, a microscopic examination for other abnormalities such as an increased number of white blood cells or the presence of immature epithelial cells is important. These abnormalities may be markers for inflammatory skin diseases such as lichen planus or other causes of desquamative inflammatory vaginitis, for estrogen deficiency, for a foreign body, or for a pyogenic bacterial infection.

Normal women of childbearing age and postmenopausal women on adequate estrogen-replacement therapy exhibit moist, pink mucous membranes with prominent vaginal rugae. Normal vaginal secretions show mature, differentiated epithelial cells that are large, flattened, and cuboidal with small nuclei. Immature epithelial cells are rounded basaloid cells that are shed from erosions or from thin, fragile, poorly estrogenized epithelium. Immature epithelial cells serve as a sign of erosions, extreme inflammatory disease, or estrogen deficiency. Epithelial cells that are stippled with surface bacteria and have borders obscured by these bacteria (clue cells) are markers for bacterial vaginosis.

Scattered white blood cells are usual, in a ratio of one or fewer leukocytes to one epithelial cell. Significantly more white blood cells suggest bacterial vaginitis, *Trichomonas,* or noninfectious inflammation. Abundant lactobacilli in the form of long rods are normally present and produce an acidic vaginal pH. Lactobacilli are often absent when vaginal inflammation is intense, and lactobacilli are always lacking when estrogen levels are low.

Group B *Streptococcus* (*Streptococcus agalactiae*) is often cultured from the asymptomatic vagina and generally is regarded as colonizing bacteria. More recently, there is evidence that this organism is sometimes associated with vulvovaginal inflammation.[1]

COMMON NORMAL VARIANTS

Erythema of varying degrees is present in most asymptomatic premenopausal women, but this redness is rarely noticed before the onset of discomfort. Several normal structures can resemble genital warts. Vulvar papillae, a common normal variant, are monomorphous, soft, tubular papillae with rounded tips seen in up to half of premenopausal women. These differ from warts by their monomorphous, symmetric distribution. Some patients demonstrate a variant of vulvar papillae characterized by diffuse plaques of short, dome-shaped, discrete but closely set papules that form a monotonous, cobblestoned texture.

Some physicians presume that whitening of the epithelium after the application of 5% acetic acid (white vinegar) to the vulva (*acetowhitening*) is diagnostic of genital warts or epithelial dysplasia. However, this is a nonspecific sign that occurs with any inflamed, acanthotic, or hyperkeratotic skin, as well as in the normal skin of many women. Acetowhite skin should be biopsied before making a diagnosis of wart, although some pathologists overcall human papillomavirus infection because of the presence of pseudokoilocytes.

Fordyce spots are prominent sebaceous glands that occasionally are confused with genital warts. These occur as normal findings on the modified mucous membranes of most premenopausal women. Although Fordyce spots were once believed to produce itching, they are now known to be common, normal findings.

The labia minora exhibit a wide range of asymmetry and size, which is usually obvious to the examiner. However, normal but very small labia minora may be difficult to differentiate from agglutination produced by inflammatory skin disease.

Although a wide range in color, consistency, and volume of vaginal secretions is normal, any changes are likely to be interpreted by the patient as infection, particularly yeast. The quantity of vaginal secretions varies among women both by time of the menstrual recycle and as a result of other poorly understood factors unrelated to infection or disease. Some women experience copious secretions that are otherwise normal. Vaginal secretions that have an acid pH of less than 5.0, mature epithelial cells, normal numbers of leukocytes, no yeast forms, no *Trichomonas,* no clue cells, multiple lactobacilli, and a negative culture indicate an absence of pathology. This diagnosis of a physiologic discharge is unpopular with patients, and some of these patients can be irritated by the ever-present moisture. However, careful patient education can end an ongoing search for diagnosis. Sometimes excess wetness from a "vaginal discharge" is actually perspiration from the groin area, and the problem can be controlled by an antiperspirant.

Some patients also complain of unpleasant odor. Although bacterial vaginosis is the classic cause, some patients are unaware that vulvovaginal odor is normally present in varying degrees. Sometimes perceived vaginal odor is actually skin odor, and this can be controlled by the application of a deodorant.

INFLAMMATORY DERMATOSES

Clinically subtle inflammation of the vulva sometimes produces remarkable symptoms. Therefore, a very careful examination with a high index of suspicion for a dermatosis is required.

Eczema/Lichen Simplex Chronicus

The most common inflammatory but noninfectious dermatosis is eczema (atopic dermatitis, lichen simplex chronicus). The morphologic manifestations of this disease when it occurs on the vulva vary from remarkable lichenification, edema, and even elephantiasis nostra verrucosum to minimal hyperpigmentation and dullness of texture of the modified mucous membranes (Figs. 114-1 and 114-2). Erythema can be subtle on the labia majora because hair obscures the skin, and the modified mucous membranes are normally pink. Sometimes, hydrated, thickened eczema appears white, mimicking lichen sclerosus or premalignant leukoplakia of intraepithelial neoplasia (Fig. 114-3).

FIGURE 114-1

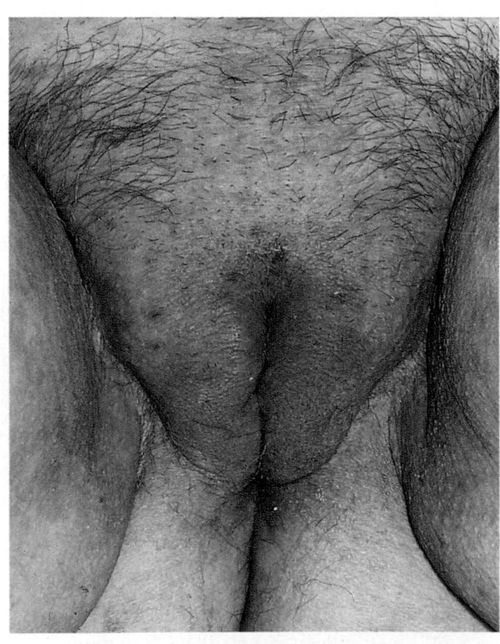

Dusky erythema, lichenification, excoriations, and loss of hair from rubbing are classic findings of skin eczema. Staphylococcal folliculitis as seen in this patient demonstrates the frequent occurrence of a secondary infection that often drives pruritus.

FIGURE 114-2

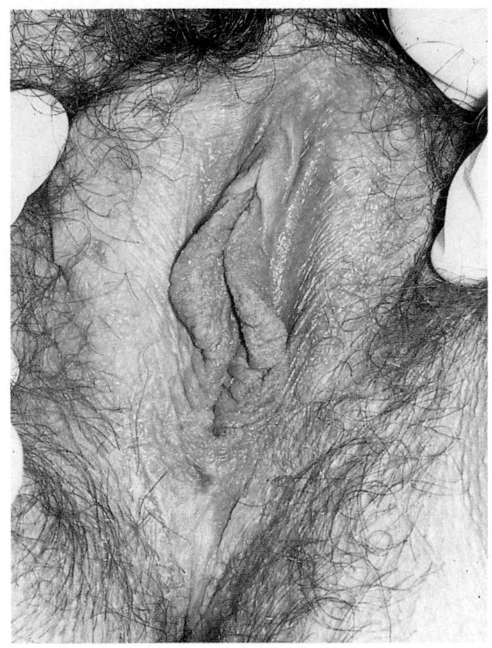

Often clinical findings in patients with very symptomatic eczema are minimal, with lichenification of the inner right labium majus most notable when the texture of the left modified mucous membrane is compared to that of the right.

Excoriations and fissures within skin folds are common but heal quickly and may not be seen in the office.

Although the histology, differential diagnosis, and therapy are the same for vulvar eczema as for eczema on other parts of the body, there are several notable modifications in the management of vulvar eczema.

FIGURE 114-3

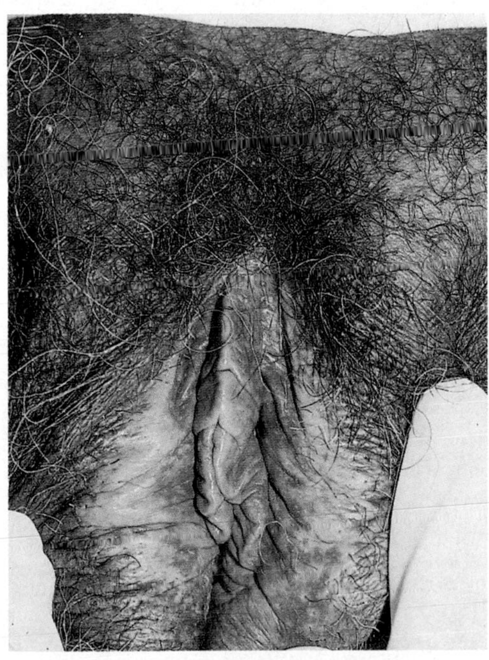

When occurring in moist areas such as the vulva, the acanthosis of eczema frequently appears white, mimicking the clinical findings of lichen sclerosus or lichen planus.

Subtle skin and vaginal infections are extremely common and often drive eczema. Therefore, a vaginal culture should be performed on any patient who does not improve as expected or who requires ongoing middle- or high-potency topical glucocorticoid therapy for control. A negative microscopic examination of a vaginal smear is an inadequate evaluation. As with eczema in other areas, nighttime sedation is crucial to interrupt the itch-scratch cycle. However, moisturization is not needed because of the occluded, naturally moist nature of the skin. In fact, the occlusive property of lubricants sometimes can increase pruritus.

Topical glucocorticoid therapy is a mainstay in the treatment of eczema, but prompt alleviation of symptoms often requires a higher-potency preparation than is standard for intertriginous skin. Although a low-potency glucocorticoid usually is recommended for genital skin, most patients with vulvar eczema are much better served with a high-potency glucocorticoid initially. Those with significant lichenification do well with an ultrapotent preparation such as clobetasol propionate for the first few weeks. However, these patients should be reevaluated monthly and warned about side effects in the surrounding areas where atrophy is especially likely to occur, such as the inguinal crease, proximal medial thighs, and perianal skin. The potency or frequency can be decreased as the patient improves.

Although tacrolimus or pimecrolimus can be used on vulvar skin, there is little experience with these medications. Stinging can occur with initial application, although this is generally well tolerated.

Patients with eczema that is not intensely inflamed or excoriated generally prefer medications in a cream base because an ointment can be too occlusive. However, inflamed or eroded vulvar skin often stings when treated with a cream or a gel.

Irritant Contact Dermatitis

Irritant contact dermatitis is a common complicating factor in vulvar symptoms. A patient with vulvar symptoms will have tried multiple local therapies by the time she sees a dermatologist. Topical medications, washing, soaps, and home remedies are the most common causes of a chronic irritant contact dermatitis. Because soap and water, douches, disinfectants, and very hot or cold water often are not considered relevant, the use of these home remedies frequently is not volunteered by patients, and very careful questioning is warranted.

The resulting chronic irritant contact dermatitis is characterized by poorly demarcated erythema or hyperpigmentation that can be difficult to appreciate because the vulva normally is pink or dusky. Lichenification, scale, and pruritus are suggestive of either this diagnosis, chronic allergic contact dermatitis, or eczema. Often the skin appears nearly normal.

Acute irritant dermatitis occurs most often in response to caustic therapies such as fluorouracil or podophyllum resin for genital warts. In addition, some topical antifungal creams can produce an immediate and brisk reaction, as can topical gentian violet therapy, a medication used by some gynecologists for unusually recalcitrant vulvovaginal yeast infections. An acute irritant contact dermatitis is essentially a chemical burn, so the diagnosis is relatively easy because the patient experiences immediate burning on contact with the offending substance. Deeper erythema is common; vesiculation can occur on keratinized skin, whereas erosion is usual on modified mucous membranes.

An irritant contact dermatitis also can obscure underlying disease, and women with chronic symptoms often are well served by discontinuing all topical therapies. Cleansing can be a accomplished by gentle flushing of the area once a day with clear water (or mild soap and water) and patting the area dry. Triamcinolone ointment 0.1% applied twice daily can hasten improvement. Reevaluation 1 or 2 weeks later may reveal the underlying process.

Allergic Contact Dermatitis

Vulvar dermatoses can be complicated by allergic contact dermatitis. This is true in part because of exposure to multiple allergens in the form of medications and cleansers applied to alleviate symptoms and in part because the vulvar skin is thin, damp, and permeable. Although the British have found allergic contact dermatitis to be a common finding on the vulva, American physicians report few relevant positive patch tests on patients with eczematous vulvar skin.[2,3] However, women with refractory vulvar symptoms should be evaluated clinically and historically for allergic contact dermatitis.

Allergic contact dermatitis of the genital area often presents somewhat differently than allergic contact dermatitis of dry, keratinized skin. The classic confluent vesicles that normally result from acute allergic contact dermatitis often erode as quickly as they form on the vulva, producing exudative, painful plaques. Chronic allergic contact dermatitis is manifested more often by erythema, which is often mild, and edema, which can be subtle in this area with loose connective tissue. Scale is frequently inapparent. More severe chronic disease can produce lichenification and secondary changes due to itching and scratching, causing the physician to make a diagnosis of eczema and to overlook an underlying allergic contact dermatitis.

Common allergens include topical medications such as diphenhydramine, neomycin, polymyxin, sulfonamides, some anesthetics, some antifungal creams, spermacides, glucocorticoids, some antiseptics, and preservatives and fragrances. As can occur with eyelid dermatitis, allergens can be carried inadvertently from fingertips to the vulva during the course of scratching or wiping. In addition, the habits of sexual partners can be important. For example, a woman allergic to latex can experience symptoms caused by a rubber condom (*consort dermatitis*).

The therapy for vulvar allergic contact dermatitis is the same as for this disease occurring in other areas.

Psoriasis (See Chap. 42)

Although vulvar psoriasis generally is accompanied by psoriasis in other typical locations, the vulva is a common site of initial involvement. Vulvar psoriasis usually affects only fully keratinized skin, sparing the modified mucous membrane of the inner labia majora and the labia minora. Vulvar psoriasis typically exhibits dusky red, well-demarcated, scaling plaques. Most often the scale is not typical psoriasiform scale but is more likely to exhibit the moistness of inverse psoriasis or a glazed, shiny surface texture. Extension of erythema into the gluteal cleft is characteristic of psoriasis.

Therapy for genital psoriasis is difficult. First-line therapy consists of a topical glucocorticoid. A middle- or high-potency glucocorticoid generally is required for significant clinical or symptomatic improvement. Glucocorticoid atrophy is surprisingly uncommon on the modified mucous membranes of the vulva, but the proximal medial thighs, the crural crease, and the perianal skin become atrophic quite easily. Calcipotriene ointment can be tried as well, but some patients find this too irritating. Some clinicians suggest topical tar as a useful therapy, but this medication should be used carefully because of irritation in skin folds of some patients. Tar can be used in a bath or as a 5% liquor carbonis detergens mixed with topical glucocorticoid cream applied twice daily. Most often vulvar psoriasis is controlled adequately by a topical glucocorticoid, but otherwise, systemic medications such as methotrexate, oral retinoids, and cyclosporine are required.

Of paramount importance to the comfort of women with psoriasis is control of local factors. The thickened epithelium, scale, warmth, and moisture promote infection and maceration. Yeast infections are especially common, particularly when patients are treated with topical glucocorticoids. The identification of infection on red, scaling, and often exudative skin can be difficult and should be pursued actively in patients with recalcitrant symptoms. Patients with recurrent documented yeast infections can be maintained free of *Candida albicans* with fluconazole 150 mg by mouth each week.

Candida Vulvovaginitis

Although most *Candida* infections produce mild or no erythema of the vulva, this infection is occasionally accompanied by deeply erythematous plaques with scale and peripheral erosions, pustules, or collarettes. Because warm, damp skin folds are a good environment for yeast, skin fold fissures are especially common. Vulvar candidiasis is often prominent in women who have treated their *Candida* vaginitis with an intravaginal topical antifungal medication, neglecting the vulva.

Candida vulvitis can be treated effectively in any of several ways. Topical azole creams applied two to four times a day are the most commonly prescribed therapies. However, cream vehicles sometimes produce unacceptable stinging on very inflamed vulvar skin. Nystatin is available in a soothing ointment base. The vagina generally also requires treatment when topical medications are used. Oral fluconazole is effective for the vulva and vagina in a single 150-mg dose.

Lichen Sclerosus (et Atrophicus)

Lichen sclerosus et atrophicus, its name now shortened to *lichen sclerosus* by the International Society for the Study of Vulvovaginal Disease, is a skin disease that occurs most often on vulvar skin. Other names include *kraurosis vulvae* and *hypoplastic dystrophy*. The disease usually occurs on the vulva, although occasionally it can be found on the glans penis and on other keratinized skin surfaces. Previously, lichen sclerosus was believed to occur most often in postmenopausal women, but it is now known that this disease occurs in all ages but tends to be most symptomatic in a setting of the estrogen deficiency of early or late life.

A likely but unproven etiology is that of an autoimmune mechanism.[4] Lichen sclerosus clusters with other autoimmune diseases, and histologic similarities exist between lichen sclerosus and several other immunologically mediated skin diseases, including lichen planus, graft-versus-host diseases, and lupus erythematosus. Other theories include abnormalities of keratin synthesis and defects in androgen metabolism or receptor function.[5] Abnormal keratins, decreased collagenase, increased collagen inhibitors, and an increase in elastase activity all have been reported as well.[6] Although an association of both lichen sclerosus and morphea with serologic evidence of past *Borrelia bergdorferi* infection, has been documented in some areas, women in the United States with vulvar lichen sclerosus have not exhibited increased seropositivity to this organism.[7] Finally, there is a known but small hereditary predisposition for this disease.

Lichen sclerosus begins asymptomatically in most patients. Many women, by the time they are seen with the classic symptoms of itching or pain, exhibit late signs of lichen sclerosus, including remarkable textural changes and scarring. Often women tolerate their disease comfortably until they develop a superimposed complicating event, such as candidiasis or atrophic vaginitis, that produces itching followed by scratching, and the process becomes self-perpetuating.

The most common symptom is that of pruritus. Itching can be mild or severe. Because vulvar skin affected by lichen sclerosus is fragile, scratching often produces painful erosions. With late scarring and narrowing of the introitus, pain with, and even an inability to tolerate, intercourse may occur.

Lichen sclerosus begins with white papules or plaques that often occur first on the anterior vulva and periclitorally. Although these papules

FIGURE 114-4

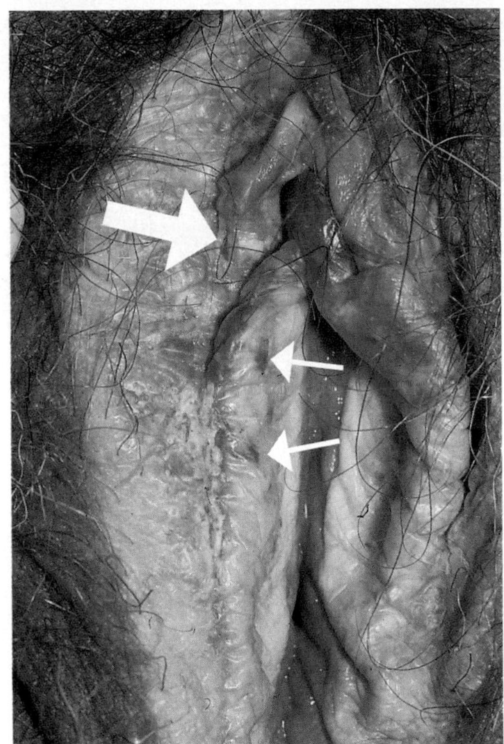

In addition to the well-demarcated, white vulvar plaque that is classic for lichen sclerosus, the waxy or crinkled texture, purpura (*small arrows*), and erosions (*large arrow*) are diagnostic.

FIGURE 114-5

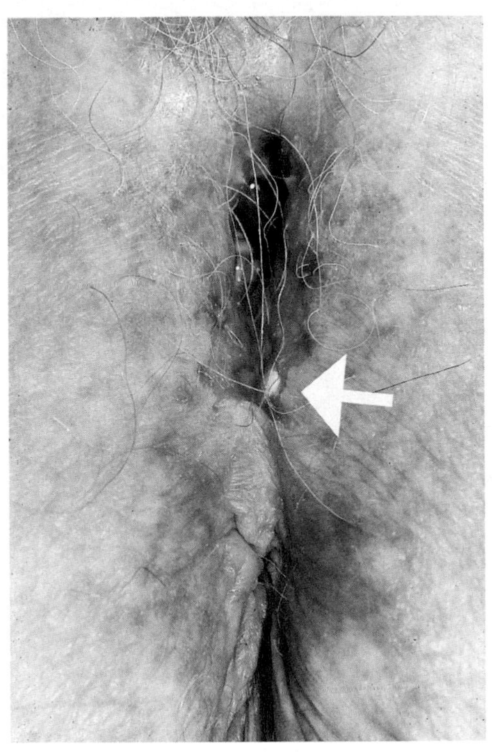

Late lichen sclerosus results in resorption of the labia minora and clitoral hood and narrowing of the introitus. A thickened, white hyperkeratotic squamous cell carcinoma at the posterior fourchette (*arrow*) required a conservative vulvectomy in this elderly woman with recalcitrant disease.

and plaques are sometimes smooth and somewhat waxy, especially when occurring on moist skin, the classic presentation is one of a hypopigmented, well-demarcated plaque with a crinkled or cellophane paper–like texture (Fig. 114-4). Although other diseases such as lichen planus can produce hypopigmentation and scarring, this characteristic crinkled texture occurs only in lichen sclerosus. Generally, the skin is quite fragile and thin, with erosions and purpura being common manifestations. Some women, particularly those who are excruciatingly itchy, exhibit thickened, hyperkeratotic skin and accompanying changes of eczema.

Many patients with lichen sclerosus experience progressive scarring. Resorption of the labia minora and scarring of the clitoral hood, which buries the clitoris, are common in long-standing disease (Fig. 114-5). Although this end result is classic for lichen sclerosus, it is a nonspecific scarring caused also by lichen planus, cicatricial pemphigoid, and other chronic, inflammatory dermatoses that affect the modified mucous membranes of the vulva.

Unfortunately, lichen sclerosus is sometimes subtle or a mimic of other diseases. Superimposed changes of eczema and hyperkeratosis can obscure underlying pathognomonic texture changes. Because an ultrapotent glucocorticoid dramatically improves both eczema and lichen sclerosus, diagnostic changes of lichen sclerosus may not be obvious clinically. Occasionally, lichen sclerosus lacks the characteristic white color or texture. These patients deserve a skin biopsy, although in this circumstance initial biopsies are sometimes nondiagnostic.

Lichen sclerosus never affects the vagina. Published reports of oral lesions of lichen sclerosus exist but are extremely uncommon.[8] However, some clinicians report caring for a number of patients with oral lesions clinically and histologically typical for lichen sclerosus. Oral lesions morphologically and microscopically characteristic of lichen planus also have been described in women with lichen sclerosus, and the coexistence of vulvar lichen sclerosus and vulvar lichen planus is reported. Extragenital lichen sclerosus of keratinized skin occurs in a minority of women with vulvar lichen sclerosus, and lesions most often are located on the upper trunk and arms. Usually, extragenital lesions are asymptomatic.

Although an association of lichen sclerosus with circulating autoantibodies has been reported, there are no associations with autoimmune diseases sufficient to prompt laboratory testing. Well-developed lichen sclerosus has an easily recognized histologic picture, although very early or late disease may be quite subtle. Thinning and effacement of the epidermis with hyperkeratosis is usual, although acanthosis is present occasionally. A chronic inflammatory infiltrate is present in early lesions in the upper dermis, abutting the epidermis. Vacuolar degeneration of the basal cell layer occurs, and a characteristic homogenization of the upper dermis is characteristic and pathognomonic. With later lesions, this zone of edematous and homogenized dermis displaces the inflammatory response from the upper dermis into the middermis.

Fully developed lichen sclerosus with hypopigmentation and distinctive shiny or crinkled texture changes is easily recognized. However, lichen sclerosus often is obscured by and mistaken for secondary lichen simplex chronicus. Also, disease with more subtle texture changes can be mistaken for vitiligo. Lichen planus occasionally exhibits uniform white papules or plaques and scarring that resembles lichen sclerosus, although vulvar lichen planus usually is accompanied by oral or vaginal disease. Also, lichen planus and lichen sclerosus occur together more often than predicted by chance. Scarring identical to that produced by lichen sclerosus also occurs with immunobullous disease and by any intensely inflammatory process. When doubt of the diagnosis exists, a biopsy is indicated because the course and long-term management of lichen sclerosus differ from those of these other diseases.

FIGURE 114-6

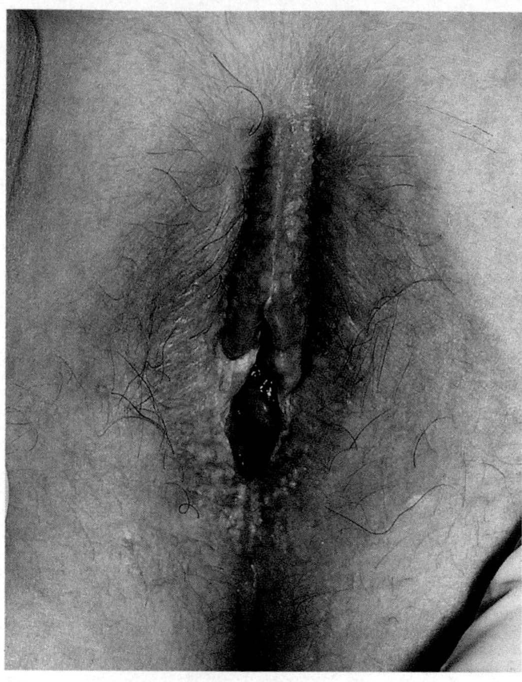

Prepubertal girls can develop lichen sclerosus, and this 11-year-old child has secondarily lichenified the area from rubbing despite the use of a midpotency topical glucocorticoid.

FIGURE 114-7

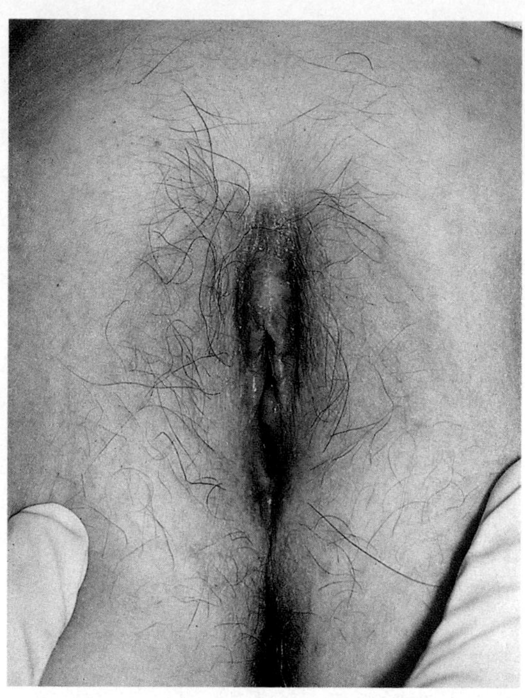

After 4 months of daily application of the ultrapotent glucocorticoid clobetasol propionate, the skin appears nearly normal. Although symptoms resolved within 1 week, prolonged therapy is required for adequate control.

The management of patients with lichen sclerosus has become far easier in the past few years since the effectiveness of ultrapotent topical glucocorticoids such as clobetasol propionate has been realized.[9] Although midpotency topical glucocorticoids reduce symptoms, they do not normalize the skin texture or prevent scarring. The application of an ultrapotent topical preparation such as clobetasol propionate once or twice a day alleviates symptoms within a few days, but several months of therapy are required for reversion of the clinical texture and color changes to normal (Figs. 114-6 and 114-7). Patients should be followed monthly to monitor the skin for steroid side effects and for improvement so that the frequency of application can be decreased.

Most patients require 3 to 5 months of once- or twice-daily application reach maximal improvement. Chronic maintenance therapy is required, but there is no proven optimal schedule.[10] Most patients do well with the chronic application of an ultrapotent glucocorticoid thrice weekly on an ongoing basis. Although this therapy eliminates itching and pain, restores a normal texture and resiliency to the skin, and usually eliminates hypopigmentation, any preexisting scarring of vulvar structures remains unchanged.

Most women very quickly experience dramatic relief from itching or pain with a superpotent glucocorticoid. However, women with especially severe itching or pain, patients with significant secondary eczematous changes or hyperkeratosis, and estrogen-deficient females, such as prepubertal children and postmenopausal women, often improve more quickly with additional therapy for the first 2 weeks to control scratching and secondary infection. Nighttime therapy with sedating doses of an antihistamine or a tricyclic antidepressant helps to control scratching and hasten healing. Women with hyperkeratosis, lichenification, and excoriation are likely to experience secondary bacterial infection with the addition of a topical glucocorticoid. This risk is also increased for patients whose skin is further thinned by low estrogen levels. Patients who appear to have secondary infection or who may be at high risk for this are best treated for the first 2 weeks with an oral antistaphylococcal antibiotic such as cephalexin, dicloxacillin, or erythromycin. Because the combination of antibiotics and glucocorticoids is particularly likely to allow for the development of a yeast infection, the clinician should seriously consider the addition of 150 mg of oral fluconazole weekly to prevent this occurrence during antibiotic therapy. Estrogen deficiency in postmenopausal women should be corrected with topical therapy, achieved by insertion of an estrogen cream or estradiol vaginal tablet three nights a week.

No other treatments for lichen sclerosus produce the striking and prompt benefit of ultrapotent glucocorticoid, and other therapies generally have shown benefit only in open-label series. Oral retinoids have been reported to be useful for some.[11] Beneficial effects have been reported with topical progesterone and topical estrogen, but the benefit is minimal and equivalent to that of lubrication alone. Topical tretinoin 0.025% sometimes produces improvement, but its usefulness is limited by its remarkable irritant properties.[12] An unduplicated report of benefit with oral potassium aminobenzoate also has been published. One case report describes a good outcome following treatment with the 585-nm flashlamp-pumped dye laser. The Chinese literature abounds with reports of benefit with traditional Chinese herbs and acupuncture for lichen sclerosus.

Although topical testosterone is a time-honored therapy for lichen sclerosus, its effectiveness has been substantiated almost exclusively by open trials rather than by placebo-controlled, double-blind studies.[13] Recent controlled trials have shown that topical testosterone and placebo are equally effective, producing a significant improvement in 66.6 and 75 percent of women, respectively.[14] Also, another study compared testosterone, its vehicle, and the ultrapotent glucocorticoid clobetasol propionate.[15] This trial showed that topical testosterone and vehicle produced similar improvement in patients but that clobetasol propionate exerted a far superior effect when compared with either. In addition, topical testosterone does not control lichen sclerosus after clearing by an ultrapotent corticosteroid, but the addition of this hormone tends to increase irritation.[16] At this time, there is no place for topical testosterone in the treatment of any vulvar dermatosis.

In the past, surgical therapy, including cryotherapy, vulvectomy, and carbon dioxide laser vaporization, had been advocated for lichen sclerosus. Ablation of lichen sclerosus is regularly followed by recurrence. However, surgical intervention is required for patients who develop a secondary squamous cell carcinoma and for those whose lichen sclerosus is well controlled but who experience scarring that results in dysfunction. Surgery for scarring should never be performed before the skin disease has been controlled with glucocorticoid therapy. Surgery is also advocated by some physicians for the rare patient whose lichen sclerosus is not adequately treated medically. Although recurrence is expected, recurrent disease is sometimes better controlled with the early reinstitution of medical therapy.

Sometimes patients with lichen sclerosus who are treated with an ultrapotent glucocorticoid either fail to improve or experience a relapse following initial improvement. These women should be reexamined to evaluate them specifically for several events: (1) the possibility of an intercurrent bacterial or yeast infection, (2) the occurrence of contact dermatitis to the topical medication, cleansers, topical anesthetics, etc., (3) the presence of a secondary squamous cell carcinoma, and (4) the possibility of a different or additional diagnosis; e.g., erosive lichen planus can produce white plaques and scarring but often does not respond well to therapy.

Lichen sclerosus is not eliminated permanently by therapy, and disease recurs gradually when medication is discontinued. However, the disease generally can be controlled chronically with the twice- or thrice-weekly application of ultrapotent glucocorticoid, although this conclusion is supported only by anecdotal experience. Despite earlier reports that childhood vulvar lichen sclerosus generally remits spontaneously, more recent series show that most patients continue to exhibit signs but not necessarily symptoms of lichen sclerosus.[17]

Reports published before the advent of topical glucocorticoid therapy show that about 5 percent of patients develop a local squamous cell carcinoma in the natural course of lichen sclerosus.[18] Squamous cell carcinomas occur primarily in patients with chronic hyperkeratosis or erosions. Although the likelihood of intercurrent squamous cell carcinoma theoretically will decline as more patients receive topical glucocorticoid therapy, this is not yet supported by data, and patients should continue to be followed carefully.

Vulvar Fissures

Small, linear fissures on the vulva are common causes of dyspareunia, itching, and stinging. Sometimes these fissures present clinically as painful, erythematous lines in skin folds and at other times as obvious linear erosions.

Most well recognized are fissures at the posterior fourchette that split during intercourse (Fig. 114-8). These produce tearing pain initially, followed by burning and stinging when alkaline semen touches the area. The skin heals quickly, but splits recur with intercourse. The cause is unknown, although some patients exhibit tight, inelastic skin at the posterior fourchette, and others simply may have fragility of the area. The condition usually occurs suddenly, after years of comfortable coitus. Adequate lubrication and the woman positioned on top can minimize tearing. Otherwise, surgical excision is required, with the vertical fissure excised and the skin closed front to back with advancement of the vaginal mucosa to cover the area.

Recurrent fissuring within skin folds of the vulva rather than the posterior fourchette is a much less well recognized but common cause of stinging and irritation of the vulva. Women typically complain of a sensation of "paper cuts." Intercourse and tight clothing often are precipitating events. Clinically, subtle fissures or linear erythema occur within skin folds, especially in the interlabial sulci. Skin fold fissures

FIGURE 114-8

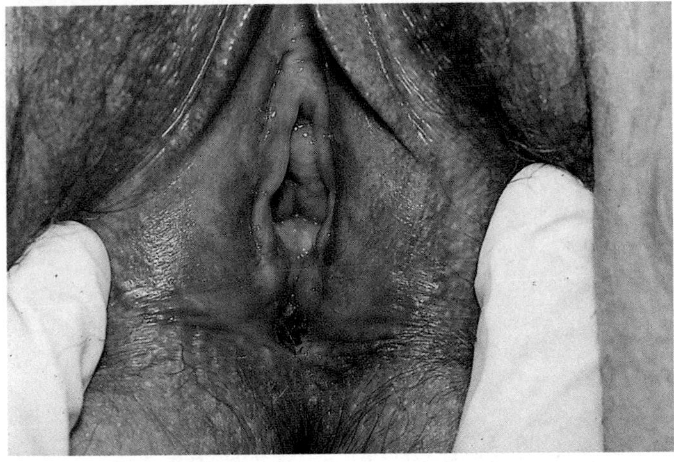

A posterior fourchette fissure is a painful, recurring split that occurs with intercourse.

result from any inflammatory dermatosis, including eczema, psoriasis, seborrhea, and lichen sclerosus. Isolated fissuring is associated most often with bacterial (especially group B *Streptococcus*) or *Candida* colonization or infection. When one of these factors is identified, treatment obviously is directed toward correction of infection or skin disease. When no specific underlying cause is found, a topical glucocorticoid ointment combined with an oral antibiotic and anticandidal medication usually eliminates this fissuring. However, almost immediate recurrence is common, and prolonged therapy may be required to break this cycle.

BULLOUS AND EROSIVE DISEASES

Lichen Planus (See Chap. 49)

Symptomatic vulvovaginal lichen planus is generally of the erosive form. Although formerly believed to be rare, an increased awareness of this disease has shown that it is actually very common, although exact numbers are not known.[19] Lichen planus is believed to be a disease of cell-mediated autoimmunity.

Vulvovaginal lichen planus presents with symptoms of itching, burning, rawness, and dyspareunia. Occurring most often in postmenopausal women, this disease has a very wide variety of clinical manifestations. Although vulvar lichen planus usually is associated with oral and/or vaginal disease, accompanying lesions on keratinized skin are unusual. White, lacy, reticulate striae resembling papular oral lichen planus sometimes occur on the modified mucous membranes the vulva (Fig. 114-9). Less easily recognized are solid, uniformly hypopigmented, flat white plaques that mimic lichen sclerosus except for the absence of crinkled cellophane paper–like texture. Finally, erosive lichen planus sometimes is manifested by red, painful erosions that are either nonspecific or surrounded by typical white epithelial changes (Fig. 114-10).

Lichen planus, especially when erosive, produces remarkable scarring. Resorption of the labia minora and obliteration of the clitoris under an agglutinated clitoral hood are very common. Narrowing of the introitus occurs more often and more severely than with lichen sclerosus, and vaginal adhesions can close the vagina, preventing intercourse and

FIGURE 114-9

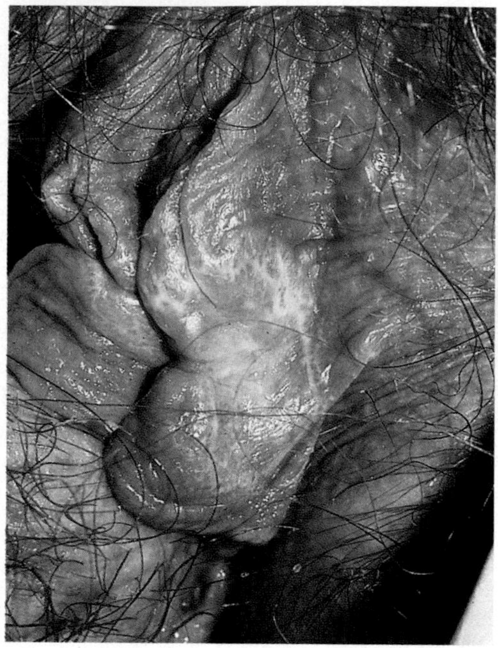

Lichen planus of the modified mucous membranes of the vulva sometimes appears identical to lichen planus of the buccal mucosa, exhibiting white, lacy striae.

FIGURE 114-10

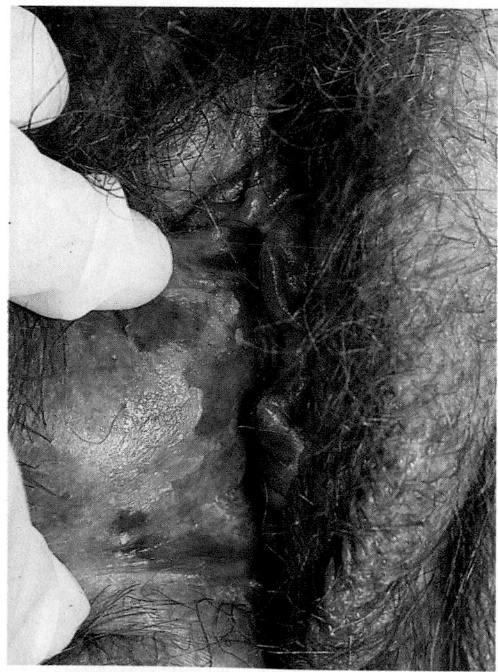

Lichen planus of the vulva also can show white, solid plaques that resemble lichen sclerosus, although the texture does not show the crinkled or waxy changes of lichen sclerosus. Erosive lichen planus is often manifested by nonspecific erosions, but a biopsy of any white surrounding epithelium, when present, is diagnostic.

FIGURE 114-11

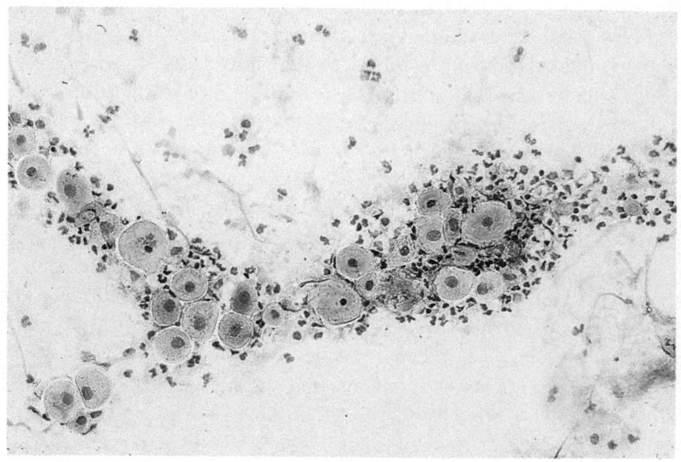

Although the vaginal erosions of lichen planus can be difficult to visualize, a microscopic examination of vaginal secretions can detect disease. An abundance of neutrophils and immature, rounded squamous epithelial cells shed from the base of erosions, rather than the usual large, flat, cuboidal mature surface cells, is characteristic.

introduction of the speculum. Rectal and perianal diseases are common and often produce pain.

Although nonerosive lichen planus of the vulva may appear bland, significant and symptomatic accompanying erosive vaginal disease is often present. Irritating inflammatory vaginal secretions can produce symptoms of introital burning and stinging due to an irritant contact dermatitis. Vaginal erosions are often obvious, appearing as bright-red patches, but sometimes equally painful disease can be more subtle and show only mild erythema on a speculum examination. However, an examination of vaginal smears is a sensitive test for the presence of a vaginal inflammation. Large, flat, cuboidal mature desquamated vaginal epithelial cells are replaced by smaller, rounded basal cells shed from erosions and rapidly proliferative inflamed vaginal epithelium (Fig. 114-11). Often vaginal secretions exhibit sheets of leukocytes as well.

Vulvovaginal lichen planus is usually accompanied by erosive oral disease. In addition to the more common buccal mucosa disease, erosive gingival lichen planus is likely to occur.

A biopsy normally shows irregular acanthosis, hyperkeratosis, hypergranulosis, and a lichenoid infiltrate with basal cell degeneration. Cytoid bodies are usual. On mucous membrane and modified mucous membrane skin, epidermal thinning and effacement are common, and parakeratosis rather than hypergranulosis may be seen.

The diagnosis of lichen planus is made either by the identification of classic lacy lesions in association with other typical mucous membrane lesions or by biopsy. Lichen planus is confused most often with lichen sclerosus because both produce hypopigmentation and scarring. However, lichen planus does not exhibit the characteristic texture changes of lichen sclerosus, and purpura is absent. In addition, lichen sclerosus essentially never affects the vagina or the mouth.

Mucosal immunobullous diseases can be indistinguishable from erosive lichen planus, as can blistering erythema multiforme and fixed drug eruptions. These diseases are differentiated by biopsy and onset.

Pruritic, noneroded, papular vulvar lichen planus is usually quite well managed simply by the application of a potent topical glucocorticoid. Unfortunately, severe erosive vulvovaginal lichen planus can be an extraordinarily difficult therapeutic problem.

The treatment of vaginal lichen planus is crucial for patient comfort. Standard therapy includes the use of an antibiotic for its anti-inflammatory effects. A common choice is oral clindamycin or doxycycline or topical clindamycin vaginal cream. Hydrocortisone acetate

25-mg rectal suppositories can be inserted nightly into the vagina as well. Any vulvar patient receiving both an antibiotic and a glucocorticoid should receive prophylactic anticandidal therapy such as oral fluconazole 150 mg each week.

Although topical cyclosporine has been found effective for oral lichen planus, its usefulness in vulvovaginal lichen planus is limited by its cost, its tendency to burn with application, and its minimal effectiveness. Other medications that have been reported primarily in open trials as useful for erosive mucous membrane lichen planus include hydroxychloroquine, oral retinoids, azathioprine, and cyclophosphamde.[20,21] Although topical tacrolimus has been reported to be useful for vulvar lichen planus, this medication is irritating and, when inserted into the vagina, produces significant blood levels of medication.[22] Case reports suggest that some patients may improve with oral thalidomide, although some clinicians describe disappointing results in their patients.[23]

Meticulous local care with early treatment of infection, minimization of external irritants, and attention to superimposed atrophy of estrogen deficiency are important measures that enhance patient comfort. Emotional support and careful patient education regarding the nature disease, its prognosis, and its therapy are vital.

There is little tendency for erosive vulvovaginal lichen planus to remit. The severity tends to wax and wane, sometimes as a result of secondary infections, irritants, or stress but more often for no identifiable cause. Bursts of oral prednisone can be helpful for flares.

Finally, squamous cell carcinoma has been well described in patients with erosive genital lichen planus. The magnitude of this risk is not known, but patients should be evaluated for this regularly.

Stevens-Johnson Syndrome, Toxic Epidermal Necrolysis (Bullous Erythema Multiforme)

(See Chap. 58)

Blistering erythema multiforme nearly always affects mucous membranes, with the vulva and vagina frequently involved. Although the diagnosis is often obvious, many physicians do not specifically examine for or address complications of bullous erythema multiforme that are unique to the vulva and vagina.

Sometimes manifestations of blistering erythema multiforme are limited to oral and vulvovaginal erosions. In these patients, vulvar erosions generally are smaller than 1 cm, well demarcated, and sparing of surrounding hair-bearing skin. Frequently, surrounding inflammation is minimally apparent. With more severe disease, vulvovaginal blistering and erosions are often extensive. Secondary vulvovaginal infection is common, and permanent scarring including vaginal adhesions sometimes occurs. One retrospective survey of 40 women with toxic epidermal necrolysis revealed 28 with vulvovaginal involvement, of whom 5 experienced permanent scarring.[24] These patients were unable to engage in intercourse, even after corrective surgery.

Unfortunately, patients with severe disease at risk for significant sequelae are women who are extremely ill and little attention is given to their genitalia. However, as with eye involvement, local care during the serious phase of this illness can prevent long-term dysfunction arising from scarring. Prompt treatment of secondary bacterial or candidal infection may be important. In addition, daily insertion of a vaginal dilator or syringe cover can ensure patency.

Cicatricial Pemphigoid (see Chap. 62)

Cicatricial pemphigoid regularly produces multiple erosions, often without accompanying blisters on keratinized skin. Surrounding epithelium is sometimes white from hydrated hyperkeratotic skin. The nonspecific, painful erosions of the vulva and surrounding epithelium can be clinically indistinguishable from lichen planus and lichen sclerosus. Vulvar erosions generally are accompanied by nonspecific vaginal

erosions that can, like lichen planus, eventuate in significant vaginal scarring. Like lichen planus, desquamative gingivitis and other oral mucosal erosions are usual. Eye involvement is much more common in cicatricial pemphigoid than in erosive lichen planus. A high index of suspicion and characteristic biopsies are required for this diagnosis in patients without blistering of keratinized skin.

Management consists of both local glucocorticoid therapy and traditional systemic treatments. Recently, intravenous immunoglobulin therapy has shown promise in the therapy of this disease.[25] Again, local care, the use of vaginal dilators, and secondary infection control are important factors in management.

Pemphigus Vulgaris (See Chap. 59)

Because pemphigus vulgaris often presents with mucosal erosions before the appearance of blisters or erosions on keratinized skin, this disease sometimes can be confused with erosive lichen planus, erythema multiforme, or cicatricial pemphigoid. The fragility of vulvovaginal epithelium results in deepening erosions that mimic those of cicatricial pemphigoid. In addition, although pemphigus vulgaris usually is considered to be a nonscarring disease, vulvovaginal involvement can eventuate in scarring, with obliteration of vulvar architecture and vaginal adhesions. As for cicatricial pemphigoid, a high index of suspicion and confirmatory biopsies are important in the correct diagnosis.

The mainstay of therapy is oral glucocorticoids, with antimetabolites conferring possible steroid-sparing effects. More recently, pulse intravenous cyclophosphamide therapy and oral mycophenolate have been reported beneficial.[26,27]

Fixed Drug Eruption

Erosions due to fixed drug eruption sometimes occur on the vulva. Common offenders include acetaminophen, allopurinol, barbiturates, nonsteroidal anti-inflammatory medications, tetracyclines, penicillin, sulfa drugs, oral contraceptives, and furosemide.[28] These are most often located in the vestibule or on the modified mucous membranes of labia minora or medial labia majora. Unlike the classic, round, edematous plaques or blisters seen on keratinized skin, the erosions of a fixed drug eruption on the vulva are often irregular, sometimes with a slightly shaggy border (Fig. 114-12). Often there are one or a few typical lesions on keratinized skin, or there are oral erosions. The deepening hyperpigmentation seen on keratinized skin affected by recurrent fixed drug eruptions is usually absent on the modified mucous membranes of the vulva. This condition generally can be differentiated from other erosive diseases by the history of ingestion of a potentially causitive medication, the sudden onset, and the pattern of involvement.

ULCERS

Aphthae (See Chap. 112)

The most common noninfectious ulcers of the vulva are aphthae. These usually occur in women who have a history of oral aphthae, although oral and genital ulcers may not be present concomitantly. These recurrent ulcerations occur most often on the modified mucous membrane of the vulva but are larger, more irregular, and deeper than oral aphthae (Fig. 114-13). Often, as with oral aphthae, the base of a vulvar lesion is covered with white fibin debris. Unlike oral aphthae, significant scarring may occur on the vulva. Some women experience only one episode of genital ulceration, whereas others develop frequently recurrent or chronic crops of ulcerations.

FIGURE 114-12

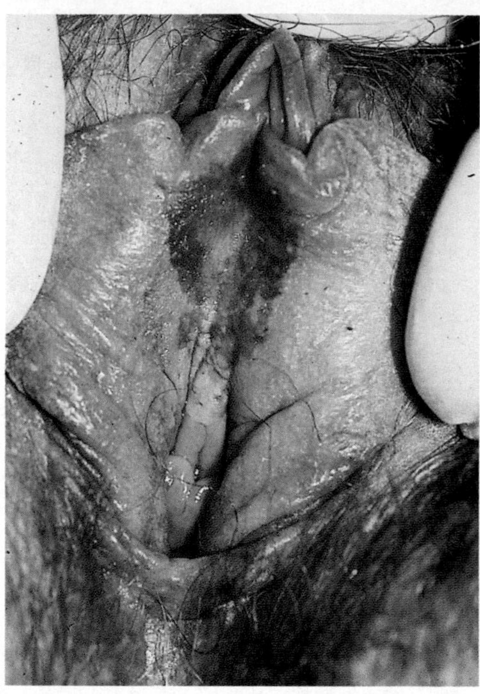

A fixed drug eruption of the vulva occurs most often on the modified mucous membranes and may be round in shape, as seen here, or more irregular.

The diagnosis is made after ruling out infectious causes of ulceration as well as sterile inflammatory diseases such as Crohn's disease and hidradenitis suppurativa. Women without a typical history of recurrent aphthae or with atypical lesions should undergo biopsy. The treatment of vulvar aphthae is the same as when these ulcers occur in the mouth. A burst of oral prednisone is indicated when outbreaks are occasional. Topical potent glucocorticoid ointments can hasten healing of mild aphthae. Daily dapsone alone or with colchicine often suppresses or

FIGURE 114-13

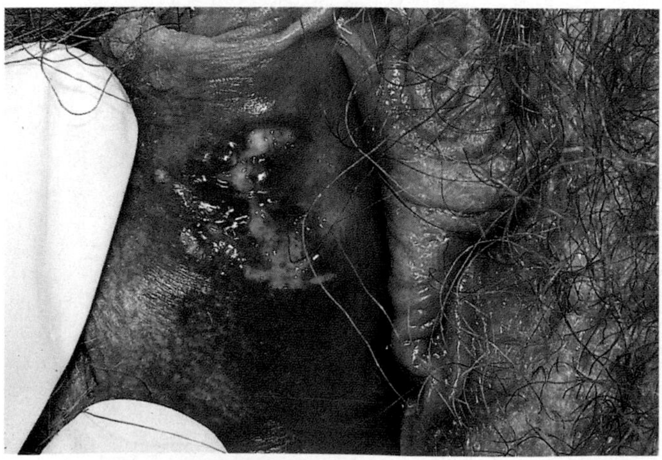

Aphthae of the vulva usually are larger and more irregular than those on the oral mucosa, and the base may show either the classic white fibrin or red granulation tissue.

decreases the frequency and severity of aphthae, and thalidomide is very beneficial but toxic.[29,30]

Crohn's Disease

Although this sterile disease of granulomatous inflammation primarily involves the bowel, vulvar and perianal skin sometimes are affected. Draining sinus tracts and fistulas from the bowel to the overlying skin are classic manifestations. However, cutaneous ulcers that do not extend to the bowel occur at times. These ulcers characteristically are linear, resemble lacerations, and lie in skin folds. Nonspecific painless, firm edema and erythema also can represent Crohn's disease. The diagnosis is made on the basis of a characteristic granulomatous biopsy and identification of the bowel disease. The primary disease to be differentiated from anogenital Crohn's disease is hidradenitis suppurativa (see below), and treatment consists of systemic therapy for underlying intestinal Crohn's disease. In addition to systemic glucocorticoids, infliximab and oral tacrolimus have been shown to be effective in some patients with Crohn's disease.[31,32] Topical and intralesional glucocorticoids and local care can help to induce healing of ulcerations.

Hidradenitis Suppurativa (See Chap. 77)

Hidradenitis suppurativa, sometimes called *apocrine acne* or *inverse acne,* generally is manifested by red papules and nodules that suppurate and drain, sometimes causing ulcerations. Not only is the clinical presentation similar to that Crohn's disease, but these two conditions reportedly coexist more often than predicted by chance.

One manifestation of hidradenitis suppurativa is that of chronic ulceration as inflamed cysts break down. This can occur on keratinized, hair-bearing areas of the vulva but also can occur on the modified mucous membranes. Ulcerations are especially likely to occur in the setting of chronic edema.

The diagnosis is made by the setting and by the elimination of infectious causes. Ulcerations usually heal with long-term suppressive antibiotic therapy for the underlying disease. Although oral retinoids are useful in the short term, long-term results are poor.[33] Surgical excision is a treatment of choice, and removal of individual lesions is often practical and beneficial.[34,35] More recently, cyclosporine and finasteride have been reported beneficial for some.[36,37]

VULVODYNIA (VULVAR DYSESTHESIA)

Vulvodynia is the symptom of chronic vulvar burning, soreness, stinging, or rawness in the absence of objective physical signs. By definition, whenever a specific etiology is defined, the name of the causitive disease is substituted for the term *vulvodynia*. For example, pain produced by vaginal lichen planus is not referred to as *vulvodynia* but rather as *vaginal lichen planus*. Vulvodynia previously was held to be a rare occurrence, but this symptom now is known to be quite common. In the past, vulvodynia was believed to be a psychosomatic disease. By the 1980s, candidiasis (or hypersensitivity to colonizing yeast) was believed to cause vulvodynia, but the poor response of patients to antifungal therapy and recent evidence have shown yeast to be a minor factor in most patients.[38] Subclinical human papillomavirus infection is believed by some to produce vulvodynia, but this concept also has been shown to be unlikely in other studies.[39,40] When all other causes of pain are ruled out, the cause of vulvodynia is believed to be neuropathic pain, especially complex regional pain syndrome.[41] Associated with and complicating neuropathy as a cause of vulvodynia is pelvic floor muscle dysfunction.[42]

Patients with vulvodynia describe burning, irritation, rawness, or soreness, often associated with self-perceived redness and swelling.

Many of these women present with a presumed diagnosis of chronic yeast infections. Although an occasional patient with vulvodynia describes itching, this is a minor aspect of the symptomatology. She denies both scratching and pleasure with scratching. Usually, women report dyspareunia and pain with constrictive clothing. Women with vulvodynia are uniformly depressed, often anxious, and usually have experienced significant disruption in their lives and relationships.

There are no characteristic laboratory findings, and biopsies reveal only nonspecific chronic perivascular inflammation, sometimes with mild squamous hyperplasia. However, patients are likely to report an increased frequency of headaches, interstitial cystitis, irritable bowel syndrome, chronic fatigue syndrome, fibromyalgia, poor sleeping, and low energy levels.

Patients with vulvodynia should be examined carefully for any underlying skin disease or infection. Very subtle findings sometimes can produce very significant symptoms. Irritant contact dermatitis, vulvar fissures (see above), and lichen planus are the most common skin diseases to be mistaken for vulvodynia. A significant proportion of women with symptoms of vulvar dysesthesia are found to have a sterile, inflammatory vaginitis manifested by grossly and microscopically purulent vaginal secretions and immature epithelial cells similar to those seen with lichen planus. Biopsies are nonspecific, and a relationship of this inflammation to symptoms is sometimes tenuous.

Nonalbicans *Candida* infections such as *C. glabrata, C. krusei,* and *Saccharomyces cerevisiae* and vaginal group B streptococcal infection or colonization are the most common infections that can account for chronic vulvovaginal pain. These infections are easily missed without a culture and can be resistant to therapy. Often, when these infections are cleared, symptoms remit. However, these infections not infrequently are coincidental rather than causitive.

Women with vulvar dysesthesia fall into two major groups: those who experience provoked pain only at the introitus (pain only when touched and only in this localized area) and those who experienced unprovoked, spontaneous symptoms in any area, not necessarily worsened by touch.[43] Pain limited to touch in the introitus is referred to as *vulvar vestibulitis,* whereas more generalized or migratory pain that is not necessarily provoked by touch is called *dysesthetic vulvodynia.*[44,45] The primary importance of a distinction between these two groups is the management option of surgical excision in those women with introital, well-localized, provoked pain.

The management of women with vulvar dysesthesias first includes attention to depression and sexual dysfunction. Most patients benefit from referral for counseling to help these women cope with such debilitating symptoms. Local care and topical anesthetics improve day-to-day quality of life. The elimination of irritants, including overwashing and topical medications, can improve symptoms significantly. Topical lidocaine jelly 2% is useful for many patients.

Tricyclic antidepressants such as amitriptyline or desipramine, beginning at very low doses and increasing up to 150 mg or until the patient is comfortable, is a first-line treatment for neuropathic pain.[45] For women who do not tolerate tricyclic antidepressants or who experience suboptimal improvement, gabapentin has been used.[46]

Most women with vulvar pain syndrome exhibit abnormal pelvic floor muscle function that can contribute to their symptoms. These patients are more likely than symptom-free women to show abnormally high resting pelvic floor tension, fasiculations, but poor contractile strength on surface electromyography. These women benefit remarkably from pelvic floor rehabilitation and subsequently are able to engage in comfortable sexual activity.[47,48] However, improvement is slow, and trial-and-error therapy with support by the physician is required frequently. Other anecdotal therapies include a low-oxalate diet with calcium citrate supplementation, topical estrogen, topical capsaicin, and chronic suppressive antifungal therapy. Acupuncture has been useful in a small open study as well.[50]

PRURITUS VULVAE

Like the burning of vulvar pain or irritation, itching can occur with minimal physical findings. The most common cause of acute itching is an infection, usually caused by *C. albicans*. Otherwise, even in the absence of significant physical findings, itching is often caused by eczema and responds well to empirical therapy with a topical corticosteroid, nighttime sedation, and control of infection.

A small proportion of women have itching and no clinical findings and do not respond to treatment for eczema. Additionally, these patients generally do not respond to topical doxepin, anesthetics, or tacrolimus. Some of these patients may have pruritus on the basis of neuropathy and respond to therapy directed toward this. In other women, depression and anxiety play a major role, and this must be addressed.

REFERENCES

1. Honig E et al: Can group B streptococcus cause symptomatic vaginitis? *Infect Dis Obstet Gynecol* **7**:206, 1999
2. Marren P et al: Allergic contact dermatitis and of vulvar dermatoses. *Br J Dermatol* **126**:52, 1992
3. Bauer A et al: Allergic contact dermatitis and patients with anogenital complaints. *J Reprod Med* **45**:649, 2000
4. Gross T et al: Identification of TIA+ and granzyme B+ cytotoxic T cells in lichen sclerosus et atrophicus. *Dermatology* **202**:198, 2001
5. Neill SM et al: The cytokeratin profile of normal vulval epithelium and vulval lichen sclerosus. *Br J Dermatol* **123** (suppl 37):62, 1990
6. Ridley CM: Lichen sclerosus. *Dermatol Clin* **10**:309, 1992
7. Fugiwara H et al: Detection of *Borrelia burgorferi* DNA (*B. garinii* or *B. afzelii*) in morphea and lichen sclerosus et atrophicus tissues of German and Japanese but not of U.S. patients. *Arch Dermatol* **41**:1133, 1997
8. de Araujo VC et al: Lichen sclerosus at atrophicus. *Oral Surg Oral Med Oral Pathol* **60**:655, 1985
9. Dalziel KL et al: The treatment of vulval lichen sclerosus with a very potent topical steroid (clobetasol propionate 0.05%) cream. *Br J Dermatol* **124**:461, 1991
10. Dalziel KL, Wojnarowski F: Long-term control of vulva lichen sclerosus after treatment with a topical steroid cream. *J Reprod Med* **38**:25, 1993
11. Bousema MT et al: Acetretin in the treatment of severe lichen sclerosus at atrophicus of the vulva: A double-blind, placebo-controlled study. *J Am Acad Dermatol* **30**:225, 1994
12. Virgili A et al: Open study of topical 0.025% tretinoin in the treatment of lichen sclerosus: One year of therapy. *J Reprod Med* **40**:614, 1995
13. Joura EA et al: Short-term effects of topical testosterone in vulvar lichen sclerosus. *Obstet Gynecol* **89**:297, 1997
14. Sideri M et al: Topical testosterone in the treatment of vulvar lichen sclerosus. *Int J Gynaecol Obstet* **46**:53, 1994
15. Bornstein J et al: Clobetasol dipropionate 0.05% versus testosterone propionate 2% topical application for severe vulvar lichen sclerosus. *Am J Obstet Gynecol* **178**:80, 1998
16. Cattaneo A et al: Testosterone maintenance therapy: Effects on vulvar lichen sclerosus treated with clobetasol propionate. *J Reprod Med* **41**:99, 1996
17. Ridley CM: Genital lichen sclerosus (lichen sclerosus at atrophicus) in childhood and adolescents. *J R Soc Med* **86**:68, 1998
18. Scurry JP, Vanin K: Vulvar squamous cell carcinoma and lichen sclerosus. *Australas J Dermatol* **38**(suppl 1):S20, 1997
19. Eisen D: The vulvovaginal gingival syndrome: The clinical characteristics of two patients. *Arch Dermatol* **130**:1379, 1994
20. Eisen D: Hydroxychloroquine sulfate (Plaquenil) improves oral lichen planus: An open trial. *J Am Acad Dermatol* **28**:609, 1993
21. Lear JT, English JS: Erosive and generalized lichen planus responsive to azathioprine. *Clin Exp Dermatol* **21**:56, 1996
22. Lener EV et al: Successful treatment of erosive lichen planus with topical tacrolimus. *Arch Dermatol* **137**:411, 2001
23. Camisa C, Popovski JL: Effective treatment of oral erosive lichen planus with thalidomide. *Arch Dermatol* **136**:1442, 2000
24. Meneux L et al: Vulvovaginal sequelae in toxic epidermal necrolysis. *J Reprod Med* **42**:153, 1997

25. Urcelay ML et al: Cicatricial pemphigoid treated with intravenous immunoglobulin. *Br J Dermatol* **137**:467, 1997
26. Fleischli ME et al: Pulse intravenous cyclophosphamde therapy in pemphigus. *Arch Dermatol* **135**:57, 1999
27. Enk AH et al: Mycophenolate is effective in the treatment of pemphigus vulgaris. *Arch Dermatol* **135**:54, 1999
28. Litt J: Drugs responsible for 100 common reaction patterns, in *Drug Eruption Reference Manual 2001,* edited by J Litt. New York, Parthenon Publishing Group, 2001, p 373
29. Rosen T, Brown TJ: Genital ulcers: Evaluation and treatment. *Dermatol Clin* **16**:673, 1998
30. Moraes M, Russo G: Thalidomide and its dermatologic uses. *Am J Med Sci* **34**:159, 1995
31. Panaccione R: Canadian Consensus Group on the use of infliximab in Crohn's disease. *Can J Gastroenterol* **15**:371, 2001
32. Ierardi E et al: Oral tacrolimus (FK 506) in Crohn's disease complicated by fistulae of the perineum. *J Clin Gastroenterol* **30**:200, 2000
33. Boer J, van Gemert MJ: Long-term results of isotretinoin in the treatment of 68 patients with hidradenitis suppurativa. *J Am Acad Dermatol* **41**:73, 1999
34. Endo Y et al: Perianal hidradenitis suppurativa: Early surgical treatment gets good results in chronic or recurrent cases. *Br J Dermatol* **139**:906, 1998
35. Golcman R: Subcutaneous fistulectomy in bridging hidradenitis suppurativa. *Dermatol Surg* **25**:795, 1999
36. Buckley DA, Rogers S: Cyclosporin-responsive hidradenitis suppurativa. *J Soc Med* **88**:289P, 1998
37. Farrell AM et al: Finasteride as a therapy for hidradenitis suppurativa. *Br J Dermatol* **141**:1138, 1999
38. Bornstein J et al: Pure versus complicated vulvar vestibulitis: A randomized trial of fluconazole treatment. *Gynaecol Obstet Invest* **50**:194, 2000
39. Bornstein J et al: A repetitive DNA sequence that characterizes human papillomavirus integration site into the human genome is present in vulvar vestibulitis. *Eur J Obstet Gynecol Reprod Biol* **89**:173, 2000
40. Orgoni M at al: Human papillomavirus with coexisting vulvar vestibulitis syndrome and vestibule or papillomatosis. *Int J Gynaecol Obstet* **64**:259, 1999
41. Cox JT: Deconstructing vulval pain. *Lancet* **345**:53, 1995
42. Glazer HI et al: Electromyographic comparisons of the pelvic floor in women with dysesthetic vulvodynia and asymptomatic women. *J Reprod Med* **43**:959, 1998
43. McKay M: Vulvodynia: Diagnostic patterns. *Dermatol Clin* **10**:423, 1992
44. Marinoff S, Turner MLC: Vulvar vestibulitis syndrome: An overview. *Am J Obstet Gynecol* **165**:1228, 1991
45. McKay M: Dysesthetic ("essential") vulvodynia: Treatment with amitriptyline. *J Reprod Med* **38**:9, 1993
46. Ben-David B, Friedman M: Gabapentin therapy for vulvodynia. *Anesth Analg* **89**:1459, 1999
47. Bergeron S: A randomized comparison of group-behavioral therapy, surface electromyographic biofeedback, and vestibulodynia in the treatment of dyspareunia resulting from vulvar vestibulitis. *Pain* **91**:297, 2001
48. Glazer HI: Dysesthetic vulvodynia: Long-term follow-up after treatment with surface electromyography-assisted pelvic floor muscle rehabilitation. *J Reprod Med* **45**:798, 2000
49. McCormick WM, Spence MR: Evaluation of the surgical treatment of vulvar vestibulitis. *Eur J Obstet Gynecol Reprod Biol* **86**:135, 1999
50. Powell J, Wojnarowska F: Acupuncture for vulvodynia. *J R Soc Med* **92**:579, 1999

SECTION 16

CUTANEOUS CHANGES IN DISORDERS OF ALTERED REACTIVITY

CHAPTER 115

Amy S. Paller

Genetic Immunodeficiency Diseases

Immunodeficiency disorders may be associated with a variety of cutaneous abnormalities, and recognition of these clinical features may allow an early diagnosis of primary immunodeficiency. Cutaneous abnormalities may include cutaneous infections, atopic- or seborrheic-like dermatitis, macular erythemas, alopecia, poor wound healing, purpura, petechiae, telangiectasias, pigmentary dilution, cutaneous granulomas, angioedema, and lupus-like changes (Table 115-1). Other clinical consequences of impaired immunocompetence often include failure to thrive, visceral infection, autoimmune disorders, allergic reactions, and neoplasia.

The classification of genetic immunodeficiency disorders includes (1) disorders of lymphocytes, including antibody-deficiency disorders, severe combined immunodeficiency, partial combined immunodeficiency, and predominantly T cell defects; (2) disorders of phagocytic cells; and (3) disorders of complement proteins. The characteristic clinical signs of each group suggest proper classification, and laboratory tests may be employed to confirm the diagnosis. In the past decade, great advances have been made in the prenatal diagnosis of immunodeficiency, the elucidation of the underlying molecular basis of several immunodeficiencies, and early gene therapy.

SIGNS OF IMMUNODEFICIENCY

In general, immunodeficiency should be suspected when patients have recurrent infections of increased duration and severity, particularly with unusual organisms. Incomplete clearing of infections or poor response to antibiotics may be associated. Affected infants often grow poorly (failure to thrive). The most common noncutaneous abnormalities are infections, diarrhea, vomiting, hepatosplenomegaly, arthritis, adenopathy or lack of nodes where they would be expected, and hematologic abnormalities. The clinical characteristics of each group of immunodeficiency disorders are outlined in Table 115-2.

ANTIBODY-DEFICIENCY DISORDERS

X-Linked Hypogammaglobulinemia

X-linked hypogammaglobulinemia (XLH, Bruton's disease) is characterized by recurrent pyogenic infections that often begin approximately 9 months after birth with the disappearance of maternal immunoglobulins.[1,2] Recurrent otitis, sinusitis, bronchitis, and staphylococcal pneumonitis are the earliest infectious manifestations and usually are caused by pneumococci, staphylococci, or *Haemophilus*. Untreated pulmonary infections may lead to chronic progressive bronchiectasis. Other common bacterial infections include conjunctivitis, osteomyelitis, septic arthritis, and meningitis. Protracted diarrhea may be due to infection, particularly with *Giardia, Salmonella, Campylobacter,* or *Cryptosporidium* spp.

Skin infections, especially furunculosis and impetigo, occur in 28 percent of patients and often surround body orifices. An atopic-like eczematous eruption that fails to improve with immunoglobulin therapy has been described in many affected children. Pyoderma gangrenosum and cutaneous granulomas have been reported. Childhood exanthematous disorders are handled appropriately, but the infections may recur owing to a failure to develop specific antibodies. Three virus groups cause problems: enterovirus, hepatitis B virus, and rotavirus. Patients have developed paralysis after administration of polio vaccine. A rheumatoid-like arthritis, characterized by chronic inflammation and swelling of the large joints, may develop in as many as one-third to one-half of boys with XLH and is often due to mycoplasmal infection (*Ureaplasma urealyticum*). Disseminated echovirus infection has caused meningoencephalitis and a dermatomyositis-like disorder with brawny edema, induration of the muscles with accompanying weakness, muscle contractures, and poikiloderma.

The underlying defect in XLH is a failure of maturation of the pre-B cell to a differentiating B cell; B cell precursors are found in the bone marrow in normal numbers. Serum concentrations of IgG, IgA, and IgM

TABLE 115-1

Cutaneous Manifestations of Immunodeficiency Disorders

Atopic-like dermatitis	Cutaneous granulomas
X-linked hypogammaglobulinemia	Chronic granulomatous disease
IgA deficiency	Ataxia-telangiectasia
IgM deficiency	X-linked hypogammaglobulinemia
Elevated IgM with hypogammaglobulinemia	Common variable immunodeficiency
Common variable immunodeficiency	Severe combined immunodeficiency
Wiskott-Aldrich syndrome	Pyoderma gangrenosum–like ulcerations
Hyperimmunoglobulinemia E syndrome	X-linked hypogammaglobulinemia
Chronic granulomatous disease	IgA deficiency
Seborrheic-like dermatitis	Leukocyte adhesion deficiency
Severe combined immunodeficiency	Chronic granulomatous disease
Ataxia-telangiectasia	Hyperimmunoglobulinemia E syndrome
Leiner's disease	Chédiak-Higashi syndrome
Cutaneous abscesses	Cutaneous candidal infections
Hyperimmunoglobulinemia E syndrome	Severe combined immunodeficiency
Chronic granulomatous disease	Di George syndrome
Leukocyte adhesion deficiency	Nezelof syndrome
Petechiae and/or purpura	Chronic mucocutaneous candidiasis
Wiskott-Aldrich syndrome	Angioedema
Chédiak-Higashi syndrome	Hereditary angioedema
Griscelli syndrome	Lupus-like cutaneous changes
Mucocutaneous telangiectases	IgA deficiency
Ataxia-telangiectasia	Elevated IgM with hypogammaglobulinemia
Pigmentary dilution	Carriers of chronic granulomatous disease
Chédiak-Higashi syndrome	Deficiency of early complement components
Griscelli syndrome	
Graft-versus-host disease	
Severe combined immunodeficiency	
Di George syndrome	
Nezelof syndrome	

TABLE 115-2

Classification of Genetic Immunodeficiency Disorders by Clinical Characteristics

Features of antibody deficiency disorders
- Recurrent infections with pathogenic extracellular encapsulated bacteria
- Chronic sinopulmonary infections
- Normal handling of fungal and viral infections, except enterovirus infections
- Minimal growth retardation
- Paucity of palpable lymphoid tissue (XLH)
- Compatible with survival for many years except if persistent enteroviral infections, malignancy, or autoimmune disease

Features of cellular (T lymphocyte) immunodeficiency
- Recurrent infections with low-grade or opportunistic infections, particularly with fungi, *Pneumocystis carinii*, and viruses
- Growth retardation, wasting, diarrhea
- Susceptible to graft-versus-host disease, fatal infections from live vaccines
- High incidence of malignancy
- Shortened life span

Features of neutrophil disorders
- Recurrent skin and pulmonary infections
- Lymphadenopathy, hepatosplenomegaly
- Ulcerative stomatitis

Features of complement deficiency disorders (see Chaps. 33 and 117)
- Autoimmune disorders (early components)
- Bacterial infections, especially neisserial (alternative, late components)
- Angioedema (C1 esterase inhibitor deficiency)

are far below the 95 percent confidence limits for appropriate controls (usually less than 100 mg/dL total immunoglobulin). Cell-mediated immunity is normal. Early intravenous immunoglobulin replacement markedly reduces the risk of infections, although it may not be helpful in diminishing the risk and morbidity of chronic enterovirus infection or of lymphoreticular malignancy (as high as 6 percent).

The gene for XLH encodes Btk (Bruton's or B cell tyrosine kinase).[3,4] The *btk* gene is expressed early in B cell development but not in T cells or plasma cells; it is likely to be required for B cell maturation. Several mutations in all parts of the *btk* gene have been identified. Carrier detection is possible by analyzing the patterns of X-chromosome inactivation, with selective inactivation of the abnormal X chromosome in B lymphocytes from female carriers.

Common Variable Immunodeficiency

Common variable immunodeficiency (CVID) commonly presents in young adults, but 45 percent of cases are diagnosed before the age of 21 years.[5] Patients have infections similar to those in patients with XLH, particularly sinopulmonary infections, but are less susceptible to enteroviral infections and more susceptible to *Giardia* infections. Many patients with CVID have malabsorption syndromes; and noncaseating granulomas of skin (Fig. 115-1), lungs, liver, and spleen have been reported. Lymphoid tissues often are enlarged, and splenomegaly with hypersplenism is found in 25 percent of patients. Autoimmune disorders are especially frequent (22 percent), particularly autoimmune thrombocytopenia, autoimmune hemolytic anemia, rheumatoid arthritis, sicca syndrome, and pernicious anemia. Alopecia areata and lupus also have been described. In 11 percent of patients, other family members also are immunodeficient (hypogammaglobulinemia, IgA deficiency). The incidences of lymphoreticular malignancy and gastric carcinoma are markedly increased, particularly in the fifth and sixth decades of life.[6]

Immunoglobulin levels may be as low as or lower than those in X-linked hypogammaglobulinemia probably because of intrinsic abnormalities in B cells. The numbers of circulating T and B lymphocytes are usually normal. Approximately one-half of patients have T cell dysfunction as well (Fig. 115-2), with the incidence increasing with advancing age. Molecular genetic studies have suggested that both CVID and IgA deficiency are linked to the same susceptibility gene, the complement 4A (C4A) locus on chromosome 6 in the class III major histocompatibility complex (MHC) region.[7]

Selective Immunoglobulin Disorders

IgA deficiency occurs in approximately 1 in 600 persons, and most of those affected are healthy. However, affected individuals tend to have an increased incidence of upper respiratory tract infections (especially viral), allergies and atopic dermatitis, chronic gastroenteritis, and autoimmune disorders with circulating autoimmune antibodies.[8] Approximately one-third of patients with IgA deficiency have IgE

FIGURE 115-1

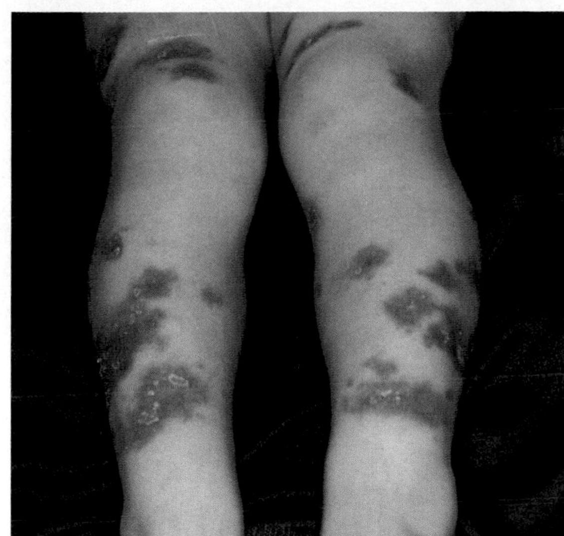

Noncaseating granulomas on the legs of a child with common variable immunodeficiency. Cultures and special stains showed no organisms.

anti-IgA antibody and risk transfusion reactions if immunoglobulin is given. Selective IgM deficiency is associated with an increased risk of pneumococcal and neisserial infections, warts, and eczema.

Patients with hypogammaglobulinemia associated with elevated IgM levels have recurrent respiratory tract infections, eczematous dermatitis, an increased incidence and severity of warts, and oral ulcerations, sometimes in association with neutropenia.[9,10] The disorder usually occurs in males, with X-linked inheritance in approximately 70 percent of affected individuals. In addition to pyogenic and opportunistic infections, including *Pneumocystis carinii,* patients tend to develop autoimmune disorders of the hematopoietic system. Uncontrolled proliferation of IgM-producing plasma cells often occurs during the second decade of life, at times resulting in potentially fatal, massive infiltration of the gastrointestinal tract, liver, and gallbladder. Patients with hyper-IgM syndrome also have an increased risk of abdominal

FIGURE 115-2

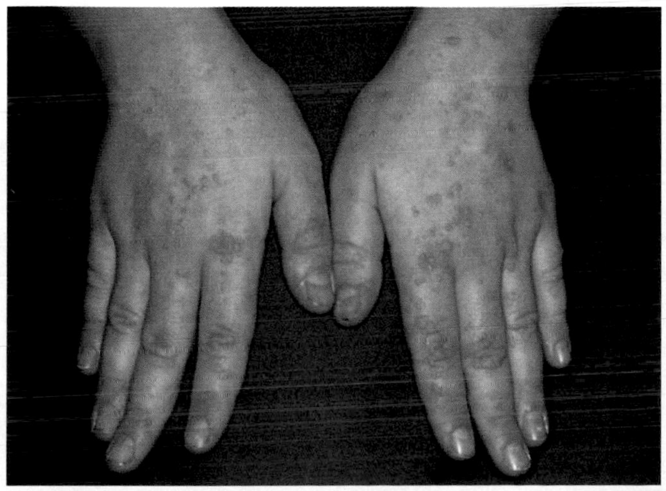

Flat warts on the hands of a girl with CVID. The warts were widespread, including face, trunk, and extremities, and did not respond to therapy during a 3-year treatment period.

cancer. The sera of patients with hyper-IgM syndrome have very low amounts of IgG, IgA, and IgE but normal or high concentrations of IgM and IgD. The condition is treated prophylactically with intravenous gamma globulin; the autoimmune neutropenia also may respond well to granulocyte-macrophage colony-stimulating factor. Allogencic bone marrow transplantation may correct the disorder.

Hyper-IgM syndrome is caused by a defect of B cell differentiation.[11] Normally, the humoral immune response begins with production of IgM and IgD antibodies. Subsequently, IgG, then IgA, and finally IgE antibodies are produced. The sequential production of different classes of immunoglobulins is called *class switching.* This mechanism enables the immune system to produce antibodies with different effector functions while retaining variable region specificity. In hyper-IgM syndrome, B cells are unable to switch from IgM/IgD secretion to the production of other immunoglobulin isotypes.

Normally, isotype switching in B cells requires a contact-dependent signal from T cells. B cells have on their surface CD40, a glycoprotein. This molecule interacts with CD40 ligand on activated T cells. The hyper-IgM syndrome is caused by a defect in the gene that encodes for the CD40 ligand. T cells from patients with the syndrome cannot synthesize CD40 ligand, or in some cases a nonfunctional ligand is produced. B cells respond to antigen and produce specific antibodies; however, they are restricted to the IgM isotype, and there is no memory response. In contrast to the case in X-linked hypogammaglobulinemia, female carriers of the hyper-IgM syndrome have random inactivation of the X chromosome in T lymphocytes because the CD40 ligand is not required for the normal development of T lymphocytes.

X-Linked Lymphoproliferative Disease (Duncan's Disease)

X-linked lymphoproliferative (XLP) disease, or Duncan's disease, is characterized by an abnormal immune response to Epstein-Barr virus (EBV) infection.[12] Before EBV infection, patients with XLP have normal immunologic responses. With EBV infection, however, patients respond abnormally to the antigen and fail to develop EBV-specific serologic responses. Clinical features include fever, maculopapular rash, pharyngitis, lymphadenopathy, hepatosplenomegaly with jaundice, and purpura. Most patients die early because of severe hepatitis, liver necrosis, and hepatic failure. Patients who survive the acute EBV infection (25 percent) tend to develop acquired dysgammaglobulinemia and chronic infectious mononucleosis, progressing to malignant lymphoma and marked T lymphocyte depletion of lymph nodes, thymus, and spleen. Overall, 70 percent of affected boys die by 10 years of age. XLP disease results from mutations in the gene encoding SH2D1A, which affects intracellular signaling.[13]

COMBINED ANTIBODY AND T CELL DEFICIENCY

Wiskott-Aldrich Syndrome

The Wiskott-Aldrich syndrome (WAS) is an X-linked recessive disorder characterized by hemorrhage due to thrombocytopenia and platelet dysfunction, recurrent pyogenic infections, and recalcitrant dermatitis, although this classic triad appears in only 27 percent of patients.[14,15] WAS usually manifests initially during the first weeks or months of life with bleeding, especially with bloody diarrhea. Epistaxis, hematemesis, hematuria, mucocutaneous petechiae, and intracranial

FIGURE 115-3

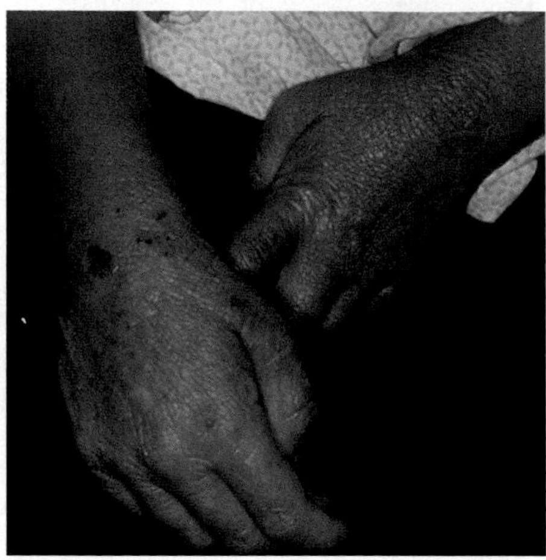

Severe atopic dermatitis in a patient with Wiskott-Aldrich syndrome. Note the serosanguineous crust.

FIGURE 115-4

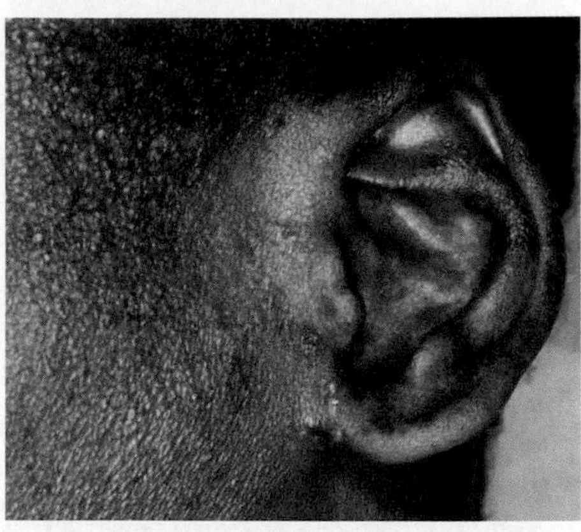

Herpetic infection with pustules on the ear of a patient with Wiskott-Aldrich syndrome. The patient was blind in his left eye owing to previous ocular involvement with herpes simplex. Following the pictured infection, the patient was administered prophylactic oral acyclovir and had no subsequent herpetic infections during 5 years of follow-up. (*From Paller AS: Hereditary immunodeficiency disorders, in* Genetic Disorders of the Skin, *edited by JC Alper. Chicago, Mosby–Year Book, 1991, pp 105–123.*)

hemorrhage also may occur. Recurrent bacterial infections begin in infancy as levels of placentally transmitted maternal antibodies diminish. These infections include furunculosis, conjunctivitis, otitis media and externa, pansinusitis, pneumonia, meningitis, and septicemia. Infections with encapsulated bacteria such as pneumococcus, *H. influenzae,* and *Neisseria meningitidis* predominate. With advancing age, T cell function deteriorates progressively, and patients become increasingly susceptible to infections due to herpes and other viruses and to *P. carinii.*

The atopic dermatitis associated with WAS, which occurs in approximately 80 percent of patients, usually develops during the first few months of life and may be quite severe. The face, scalp, and flexural areas are the most severely involved, although patients commonly have widespread involvement with progressive lichenification. The rash is often more exfoliative than that of atopic dermatitis in individuals without WAS, and excoriated areas frequently have serosanguineous crusts (Fig. 115-3). Secondary bacterial infection of eczematous lesions is common, as are eczema herpeticum (Fig. 115-4) and molluscum.

Hepatosplenomegaly is common, and lymphadenopathy, transient arthritis with joint effusions, nephropathy, and nodular vasculitis with arteritis are present occasionally. IgE-mediated allergic problems such as urticaria, food allergies, and asthma are seen in addition to the atopic dermatitis.

The thrombocytopenia of WAS is persistent, and platelet counts may range from 1000 to 80,000 platelets per microliter. The platelets are small, and platelet aggregation is defective. Patients also may have Coombs-positive hemolytic anemia, leukopenia, lymphopenia, and eosinophilia. Levels of IgM and sometimes IgG are low, and isohemagglutinins are absent. IgA, IgE, and IgD levels usually are elevated. Delayed hypersensitivity skin test reactivity is diminished, and patients fail to respond to polysaccharide antigens. The number of T lymphocytes and the response in vitro to mitogens may be normal in early life but often decrease with advancing age.

Many patients with WAS die during infancy, usually as a result of severe infections, especially of the respiratory and central nervous systems, or as a result of severe hemorrhage, especially intracranial. Twenty percent of patients with WAS develop lymphoreticular malignancies, especially non-Hodgkin's lymphoma, with a predominance of extranodal and brain involvement. Ten percent of patients die from these malignancies, usually as adolescents or young adults.

Appropriate antibiotics and transfusions of platelets and plasma decrease the risk of fatal infections and hemorrhage. Intravenous infusions of gamma globulin are useful in some patients. Splenectomy has been advocated to ameliorate the bleeding abnormality in patients with recurrent severe hemorrhage, but this procedure increases the risk of infection from encapsulated bacterial organisms in these patients who cannot mount a response to vaccination. Bone marrow transplantation is the treatment of choice for patients with recurrent problems. Full engraftment results in normal platelet numbers and functions, normal immunologic status, and clearance of the dermatitis (T lymphocyte engraftment). Topical glucocorticoid preparations and systemic gamma globulin may improve the dermatitis, and chronic administration of oral acyclovir is appropriate for patients with recurrent eczema herpeticum.

Lymphocytes from patients with WAS lack microvilli formed by actin bundles. Additionally, sialoglycoproteins (e.g., CD43 and others) are not stably expressed by WAS lymphocytes and platelets. The defective gene is *WAS,* which encodes WASP, a 53-kDa protein that functions in signaling and cytoskeletal organization.[16]

Female carriers of *WAS* mutations may be detected by the selective inactivation of the abnormal X chromosome in T and B cells and in platelets. Studies of maternal X-chromosome inactivation also have been used to diagnose boys with atypical WAS. Prenatal diagnosis has been achieved in the first trimester with DNA markers.[17]

Ataxia-Telangiectasia

Ataxia-telangiectasia (AT) is an autosomal recessive disorder characterized by ataxia, oculocutaneous telangiectases, sinopulmonary infections, immunodeficiency, and the development of lymphoreticular malignancies.[18] The gene for AT (*ATM*) encodes a protein that resembles phosphoinositol-3 kinases and is involved in DNA repair and cell-cycle control.[19] Ataxia-telangiectasia is covered in detail in Chap. 191.

SEVERE COMBINED IMMUNODEFICIENCY

Severe combined immunodeficiency (SCID) includes a group of heterogeneous disorders characterized by similar clinical manifestations and immunologic deficiencies of both humoral and cell-mediated immunity.[20–22] Most patients with SCID are boys (95 percent) with an X-linked recessive inheritance pattern (50–60 percent), but autosomal recessive and sporadic modes have been described. The overall incidence of SCID is from 1 in 100,000 to 500,000 live births.

Infants with SCID usually fail to gain weight by 3 to 6 months of age, following the onset of recurrent infections. Persistent mucocutaneous candidiasis is often present at the time of diagnosis, and systemic candidal infections occur occasionally. Patients with SCID also may have chronic diarrhea and malabsorption caused by viral infections. *P. carinii* pneumonia is often a presenting feature. Although bacterial infections usually respond to systemic antibiotics, viral infections tend to be fatal. Infants with SCID lack palpable lymphoid tissue despite recurrent infections.

In addition to cutaneous bacterial and candidal infections, the most common cutaneous eruptions are morbilliform or resemble seborrheic dermatitis. In some infants with SCID, biopsy sections show graft-versus-host disease (GVHD). GVHD may result from the in utero exposure to maternal lymphocytes or from transfusion with nonirradiated blood products, or it may follow bone marrow transplantation.

All patients with SCID share most clinical features and have abnormalities of both cell-mediated and humoral immunity, although the extent of deficiency is variable. However, the underlying bases of SCID are quite heterogeneous. The genetic defect in X-linked SCID is a mutation in γ_c chain of the interleukin 2 (IL-2) receptor, which is shared with several other interleukin receptors, thus explaining the severity of the immunodeficiency. Several of these receptors are required for the early development of T cells, so female carriers with the mutation have nonrandom inactivation of T cells, which do not survive if the mutated allele is activated.

The most common forms of autosomal recessive SCID result from mutations in the genes for the purine-degradation enzymes adenosine deaminase and purine nucleoside phosphorylase and account for 20 percent of cases of SCID. SCID also may result from deficiency of MHC class I or MHC class II molecules (HLA-DP, -DQ, -DR).[23] MHC class I deficiency is due to mutations in TAP1 or TAP2, proteins that transport peptides to assemble the class I molecule. Affected children have a deficiency of CD8 and natural killer (NK) cells. The pathogenesis of MHC class II deficiency is complex and relates to defects in transactivating factors (e.g., class II transactivator, RFX5, RFXAP, or RFX-B). Patients with MHC class II deficiency have insufficiency of CD4 and not CD8 cells, and their T cells do not react to specific antigens. Affected children have hypogammaglobulinemia, although the B cell number is normal. Patients with SCID also may have defects in lymphocyte activation, including defects in the CD3 T cell receptor, in cytokine production (especially IL-2 production), and in signal transduction (e.g., ZAP-70 deficiency).

SCID must be differentiated from acquired immunodeficiency syndrome (HIV infection). In addition to the lack of HIV antigen and anti-HIV antibodies in patients with SCID, other features help to differentiate the disorders. Despite the lymphopenia of SCID, the inverted CD4/CD8 ratio of HIV infection is not found. Most patients with SCID have low levels of immunoglobulins, in contrast to the hypergammaglobulinemia of infants with HIV infection. The subtype of SCID is determined generally by DNA analysis, although detection of cells by fluorescence-activated cell sorting (e.g., T, B, and NK cells) and by analysis for the presence of surface markers is confirmatory.

In families with a previously affected sibling of a known phenotype, prenatal detection of SCID is possible by DNA analysis if the specific gene defect is known, by fluorescence-activated cell sorting of fetal blood with monoclonal antibodies, or by analysis of enzyme levels in cultured amniocytes. Carrier mothers of boys with X-linked SCID may be detected by the selective inactivation of the abnormal X chromosome in T and B cells.

The definitive treatment of choice for SCID is bone marrow transplantation.[24] Affected children with most forms of SCID rarely survive beyond 2 years without transplantation. Removal of postthymic cells from parental marrow may diminish the risk of GVHD in patients with SCID without an HLA-identical donor. In utero transfer of haploidentical CD34 cells[25] and gene therapy[26] have been successful for patients with γ_c- and adenosine deaminase (ADA)–deficient forms of SCID. Patients with IL-2 deficiency have been treated with IL-2 injections. Enzyme replacement therapy with polyethylene glycol modified bovine ADA administered subcutaneously once weekly has resulted in clinical and immunologic improvement in patients with ADA deficiency.

SELECTIVE T LYMPHOCYTE DISORDERS

Chronic Mucocutaneous Candidiasis

Patients with chronic mucocutaneous candidiasis (CMC) have recurrent, progressive infections of the skin, nails, and mucous membranes most commonly due to *Candida albicans* and in some cases due to dermatophytes as well.[27] The clinical features of CMC may be seen in a variety of immunologic disorders, all characterized by ineffective defense mechanisms against *Candida*. In general, the patients with greater severity and an earlier onset of cutaneous candidal infections have more severe immunologic alterations.

The clinical presentation ranges from recurrent, recalcitrant thrush (Fig. 115-5) to mild erythematous scaling plaques with a few dystrophic nails to severe generalized, crusted granulomatous plaques (Fig. 115-6). The cutaneous plaques occur most commonly in intertriginous and on periorificial sites and the scalp, but they may be more generalized. The nails are thickened, brittle, and discolored, and the paronychial areas are often erythematous, swollen, and tender. Scalp infections may lead to scarring and alopecia. Although the oral mucosa is the most frequent site of mucosal alteration, esophageal, genital, and laryngeal mucosae may be affected. Patients with CMC rarely develop systemic candidiasis but may develop recurrent or severe infections other than candidal, including bacterial septicemia, particularly if other immune defects are present. Concomitant dermatophyte infections are not uncommon.

Many patients with CMC have *a*utoimmune *p*oly*e*ndocrinopathy-*c*andidiasis-*e*ctodermal *d*ysplasia (APECED) syndrome,[28] owing to

FIGURE 115-5

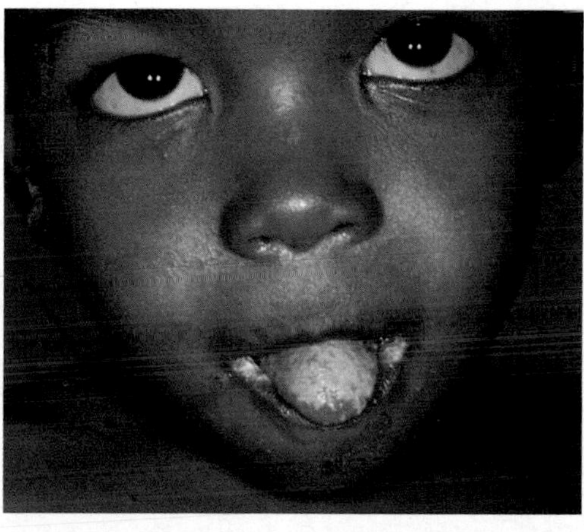

Recurrent thrush and candidal cheilitis in a patient with chronic mucocutaneous candidiasis.

FIGURE 115-6

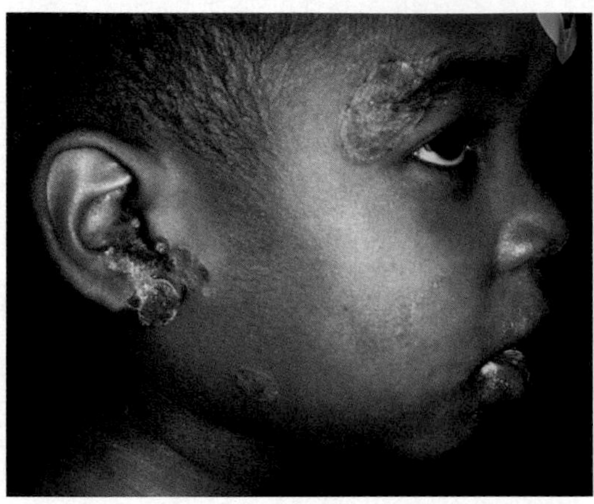

Cutaneous candidal infections with a hyperkeratotic candidal granuloma. The child responded to oral ketoconazole but not to topical agents.

FIGURE 115-7

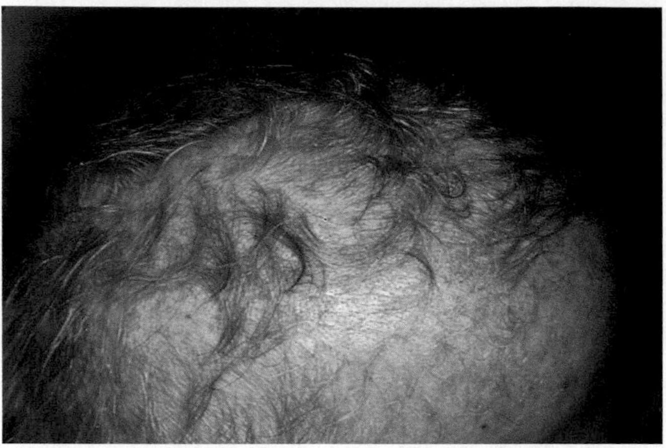

Sparse hypopigmented hair in a patient with the cartilage-hair hypoplasia syndrome. (*From Brennan and Pearson*[34] *with permission.*)

mutations in the *a*uto*i*mmune *re*gulator (*AIRE*) gene. The candidal infections tend to begin by 5 years of age, although the endocrinologic dysfunction may not be apparent until 12 to 13 years of age. Associated endocrinopathies have been described. Most common are hypoparathyroidism (88 percent) and hypoadrenocorticism (60 percent). One-third of patients have candidiasis, hypoparathyroidism, and defective adrenal function. Other associated endocrinopathies or autoimmune disorders include gonadal insufficiency (45 percent), alopecia areata (20 percent), pernicious anemia (16 percent), thyroid abnormalities (12 percent), chronic active hepatitis or juvenile cirrhosis (9 percent), vitiligo, diabetes mellitus, and hypopituitarism. Chronic diarrhea and malabsorption have been reported in 25 percent of patients and usually are associated with hypoparathyroidism. Some affected patients also have pulmonary fibrosis, dental enamel hypoplasia, and keratoconjunctivitis. Patients with APECED often have autoimmune antibodies, including antithyroglobulin, antimicrosomal antibodies, antiadrenal and antimelanocyte antibodies, and rheumatoid factor. Autoantibodies also have been found in patients with CMC who do not have clinical endocrinologic disease.

Scrapings and cultures from cutaneous or mucosal lesions demonstrate candidal organisms. Most patients with CMC have defective cell-mediated immunity, although no uniform alteration is found.[29,30] Some 25 to 35 percent of patients with CMC have no demonstrable immunologic defects.

Candidal lesions in patients with CMC generally respond to systemically administered azole antifungal agents (itraconazole, fluconazole).[31] Ketoconazole is no longer used becaused of the risk of hepatitis. Cutaneous granulomas often are less responsive despite clearance of infection. Recurrences are common, and the antifungal agents must be used intermittently. The drugs have no effect on the abnormal cell-mediated immunity. Patients who are resistant usually respond to amphotericin B with or without flucytosine.

Di George Syndrome

Di George syndrome (congenital thymic aplasia) is a member of a group of disorders that result from deletion of chromosome 22q11 (catch 22/Di George/velocardiofacial syndrome).[32] The disorder results from developmental defects of the third and fourth pharyngeal pouches due to haploinsuffienciency of Tbx1, a member of the t-box transcription factor.[33] Although most patients have T cell defects, some have only mild T cell abnormalities, whereas others have SCID with B cell immunodeficiency as well, presumably due to the effect of T cells on B cell function. The thymic shadow is absent or reduced at birth. Infants often have neonatal tetany with hypocalcemia due to the aplastic parathyroid glands. The cardiac anomalies are most commonly truncus arteriosus, septal defects, and abnormal aortic arch vessels. Characteristic facial features of Di George syndrome include a short philtrum, low-set malformed ears, and hypertelorism.

Many patients have recurrent mucocutaneous candidal infections as neonates, as well as increased susceptibility to viral infections, *P. carinii,* and other fungal infections. GVHD may develop in infants given nonirradiated blood products.

Cartilage-Hair Hypoplasia Syndrome

Cartilage-hair hypoplasia syndrome is an autosomal recessive disorder that is most common in Amish and Finnish individuals.[34] Patients have fine, sparse, hypopigmented hair (Fig. 115-7) and metaphyseal dysostosis that results in short-limbed dwarfism. Patients may have soft, doughy skin with degenerated elastic tissue. Associated pleiotropic features include Hirschsprung's disease, deficient erythrogenesis, and an increased risk of malignancies,[35] particularly non-Hodgkin's lymphoma and basal cell carcinomas. The disorder results from mutations in the RNA component of a ribonucleoprotein endoribonuclease,[36] RNase MRP, that in mitochondria cleaves RNA primers responsible for DNA replication and in the nucleolus processes pre-rRNA. Most patients have defective cell-mediated immunity, and patients may be particularly susceptible to severe disseminated varicella.[37] A subset of patients who have additional defective humoral immunity has been described.

Nezelof Syndrome

Most patients with Nezelof syndrome present later in infancy or childhood with infections similar to those of patients with SCID. Gram-negative sepsis and pneumonia are common, as are candidal infections of the mouth, perianal area, skin (Fig. 115-8), esophagus, and gastrointestinal tract that do not respond to topical therapy. Severe viral and *P. carinii* infections also may occur. Patients characteristically have lymphopenia, but other leukocyte counts are normal. T cells are deficient, but immunoglobulin levels are normal or near normal. Despite the presence of immunoglobulin, antibody production is suboptimal or absent. A subgroup of patients with Nezelof syndrome has purine

FIGURE 115-8

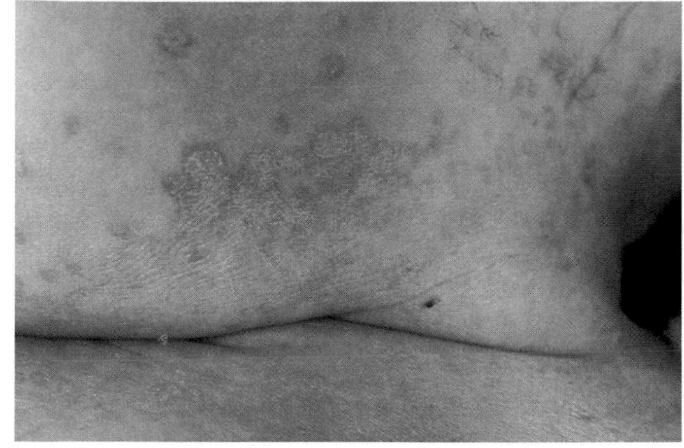

Cutaneous candidal infection in an infant with Nezelof syndrome.

nucleoside phosphorylase (PNP) deficiency, an autosomal recessive disorder that is due to absence of an enzyme of the purine salvage pathway (see discussion of SCID earlier). Between 10 and 15 percent of children with ADA deficiency have a less severe form of Nezelof syndrome with the onset of T cell immunodeficiency after 6 months of age and normal immunoglobulin levels.

DISORDERS OF PHAGOCYTIC CELLS

Chronic Granulomatous Disease

Chronic granulomatous disease (CGD) is a heterogeneous group of X-linked and autosomal recessive disorders characterized by severe recurrent infections due to an inability of phagocytic leukocytes to kill intracellular organisms by generation of oxidative metabolites.[38,39] Ninety percent of patients with the disorder are male, and the overall incidence is 1 in 250,000 to 500,000 persons. The recurrent infections of patients with CGD usually begin during the first year of life. Pyodermas with associated regional lymphadenopathy and dermatitis, especially periorificial, may occur during infancy. Staphylococcal abscesses are common, particularly of the perianal area. Cutaneous granulomas occur less frequently than cutaneous infections and are nodular and often necrotic. The granulomas can occlude vital structures, especially of the gastrointestinal and genitourinary systems. Intraoral ulcerations resembling aphthous stomatitis, chronic gingivitis, perioral ulcers, scalp folliculitis, and seborrheic dermatitis have been described in many patients.

The lymph nodes, lungs, liver, spleen, and gastrointestinal tract are the most frequent areas of noncutaneous involvement. Suppurative lymphadenitis with abscess and fistula formation usually affects cervical nodes. Pneumonia occurs in almost all affected children and may lead to abscess formation, cavitation, and empyema. Hepatosplenomegaly has been reported in 80 to 90 percent of patients; more than 30 percent of patients develop hepatic abscesses, and hepatic granuloma formation is common.

Normal bactericidal activity after phagocytosis requires the nicotinamide adenine dinucleotide (NADPH) oxidase system, which consists of NADPH, an unusual phagocyte cytochrome b, and several cytosolic proteins. Patients with CGD have deficient killing because this membrane-associated NADPH oxidase system fails to produce superoxide and other toxic oxygen metabolites. In X-linked kindreds (60–76 percent of patients), the gene encoding the gp91^{phox} (*ph*agocyte *ox*idase) subunit of cytochrome b_{558} is mutated. Patients with autosomal recessive CGD (40 percent) are deficient in NADPH oxidase cytosolic factors (p47^{phox} or p67^{phox}); occasionally the p22^{phox}(γ subunit of cytochrome b_{558}) is deficient. It is thought that cytochrome b_{558} is the membrane attachment site for these cytosolic factors that translocate from the cytosol to the plasma membrane, assembling oxidase components to allow activation of the oxidase.

The types of microbial organisms that cause infections in patients with CGD are usually catalase-positive and require intracellular killing; such organisms include *Staphylococcus aureus, Klebsiella, Pseudomonas, Escherichia coli, Serratia,* and *Aspergillus.* The intensive humoral and granulomatous responses can be explained as compensatory reactions. The screening test for CGD is the nitroblue tetrazolium (NBT) reduction assay. Quantitative NBT tests and chemiluminescence assays also may be performed. Immunoblot analysis confirms the absence of the phagocyte oxidase component; because deficiency of one component of cytochrome b_{558} leads to absence of the other, sequencing of the *gp91^{phox}* or *p22^{phox}* genes is necessary if absence is noted by immunoblot analysis. Patients frequently have leukocytosis, anemia, elevated sedimentation rate, and hypergammaglobulinemia, but immune function is otherwise normal. Heterozygous carriers for X-linked CGD do not have the increased risk of infections but may have discoid or systemic lupus erythematosus, severe aphthous stomatitis, or granulomatous cheilitis.

Therapy of CGD includes antimicrobial agents for infections and debridement and drainage of abscesses. Long-term prophylactic trimethoprim-sulfamethoxazole therapy decreases the incidence of bacterial infection without increasing the incidence of fungal infection, whereas itraconazole therapy effectively lowers the risk of *Aspergillus* infection.[40,41] Leukocyte transfusions have been used for rapidly progressive, life-threatening infections. Bone marrow transplantation has been performed in some patients with CGD. Interferon-γ induces the mRNA that codes for the defective cytochrome b, and it has been shown to increase the functional cytochrome b, superoxide generation, and bactericidal activity.[42] Patients with both X-linked CGD and autosomal recessive CGD showed clinical improvement after receiving interferon-γ. Systemic glucocorticoids have been helpful for patients with obstructive visceral granulomas. Stem cell gene therapy has been used for patients with the p47^{phox}-deficient form.[43] Prenatal diagnosis has been performed by the NBT slide test and now can be based on molecular analysis.

Hyperimmunoglobulinemia E Syndrome

The hyperimmunoglobulinemia E (HIE) syndrome is characterized by (1) markedly increased levels of IgE, (2) recurrent cutaneous and systemic pyogenic infections, (3) atopic-like dermatitis, (4) peripheral eosinophilia, and (5) defective neutrophil chemotaxis. Buckley's syndrome and Job's syndrome are subsets of the HIE syndrome. The disorder is thought to be autosomal dominant with variable expressivity; many patients show a partial phenotype.[44,45] The gene has been mapped to chromosome 4q, although it has not yet been identified.[46]

The dermatitis of HIE syndrome begins in infancy and resembles atopic dermatitis, often with extensive lichenification (Fig. 115-9). Many patients have other manifestations of atopy. Early skin manifestions may include vesicular lesions and cutaneous candidal infections. *Candida* also may affect mucosal sites and nails. Patients develop progressive coarsening of facial features (Fig. 115-10). Staphylococcal skin infections include impetigo, furunculosis, paronychia, cellulitis, and characteristic abscesses ("cold" abscesses; see Fig. 115-10) that do not demonstrate the anticipated degree of erythema, warmth, and

FIGURE 115-9

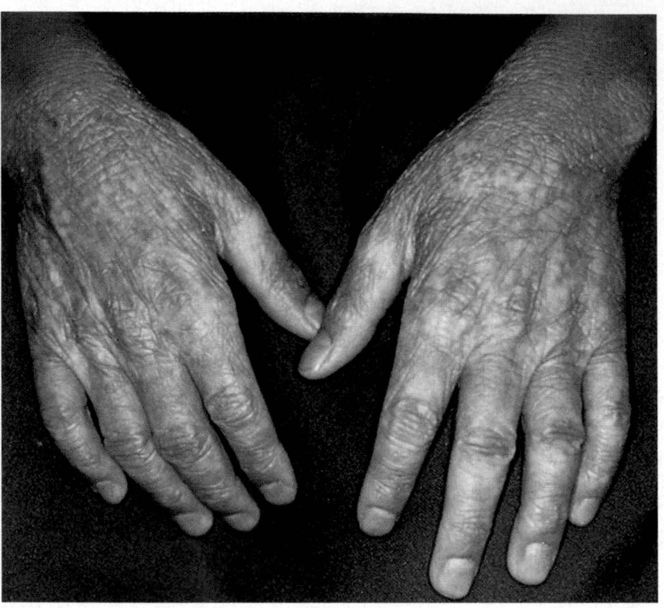

Extensive lichenification in a patient with hyperimmunoglobulinemia E syndrome and severe atopic dermatitis.

purulence. The abscesses occur most commonly on the head and neck and in intertriginous areas. Pulmonary bacterial pneumonia, abscesses, and empyema are the most frequent systemic infections and may result in pneumatoceles that become the nidus for further bacterial and fungal infections. The most common infecting organisms are *S. aureus* and *H. influenza.* Osteopenia is common, and 57 percent of patients have had at least three fractures, especially of the long bones, ribs, and pelvis. Scoliosis occurs in 76 percent of adult patients and hyperextensibility of joints in 68 percent of patients. Dental anomalies include retention of primary teeth and lack of eruption of secondary teeth.

Elevated serum IgE levels (>2000 IU; may be considerably lower in infancy but still markedly elevated from standard levels) are characteristic and may be related to defective T suppressor cell function. Cell-mediated immunity is often abnormal. The most common functional defect in host resistance is defective neutrophil chemotaxis, particularly during severe infections. Mononuclear cells from patients with HIE syndrome fail to exhibit the normal stimulation of IgE production by IL-4[47] and cannot produce normal levels of interferon-γ even after cells are stimulated by IL-12.[48]

Antistaphylococcal antibiotics are effective for most cutaneous infections in patients with HIE. Ascorbic acid and cimetidine have decreased the number of infections and the chemotactic defect in some patients. Isotretinoin has been reported to eliminate the recurrent staphylococcal abscesses in an isolated patient without any change in immunologic status. Gamma globulin and interferon-γ also have been used successfully; the former may decrease IgE levels without altering IgG or IgM levels, whereas the latter improves the chemotactic response. The cutaneous and pulmonary abscesses often require incision and drainage and may require partial lung resections.

Leukocyte Adhesion Deficiency

Leukocyte adhesion deficiency (LAD) is a rare autosomal recessive disorder that affects the adherence of neutrophils, lymphocytes, and monocytes.[49] Patients have frequent skin infections, mucositis, and otitis. The skin infections often present as necrotic abscesses that resemble pyoderma gangrenosum (Fig. 115-11),[50] but the inflammatory response and production of purulent material are impaired. Patients may have delayed separation of the umbilical cord. Cellulitis of the face and perirectal area is common. Gingivitis with periodontitis results in loss of teeth. Life-threatening severe bacterial or fungal infections may occur. Poor wound healing leads to paper-thin or dysplastic cutaneous scars.

Adherence of leukocytes relates in part to a group of cell surface glycoproteins (β_2 integrins) that share a common 95-kDa β_2 subunit (CD18) encoded on the distal portion of the long arm of chromosome 21. This β_2 subunit may be linked to three distinct α chains to form three different surface glycoproteins. These glycoproteins—the iC3b receptor (CR3), LFA-1, and p150,95 (CR4)—are absent or deficient in affected patients with LAD1. As a result, neutrophil and monocyte chemotaxis and phagocytosis are impaired. The severity of clinical involvement is proportional to the degree of glycoprotein deficiency. Death usually occurs by 2 years of age unless successful bone marrow transplantation is performed. The normal CD18 subunit gene has been introduced into hematopoietic stem cells and may provide the

FIGURE 115-10

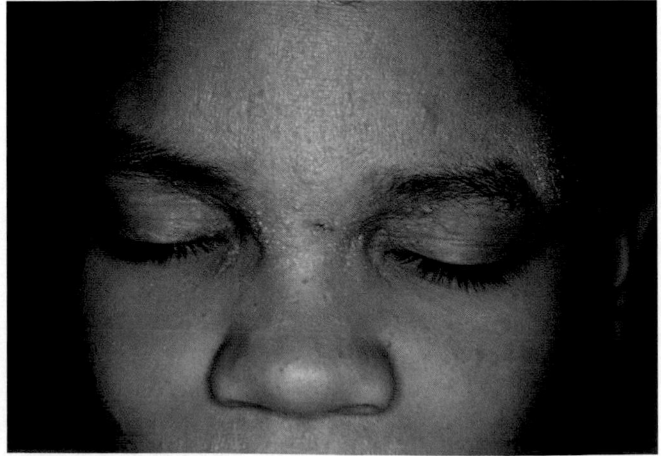

Coarse facial features and "cold" abscess and furuncle in a patient with hyperimmunoglobulinemia E syndrome.

FIGURE 115-11

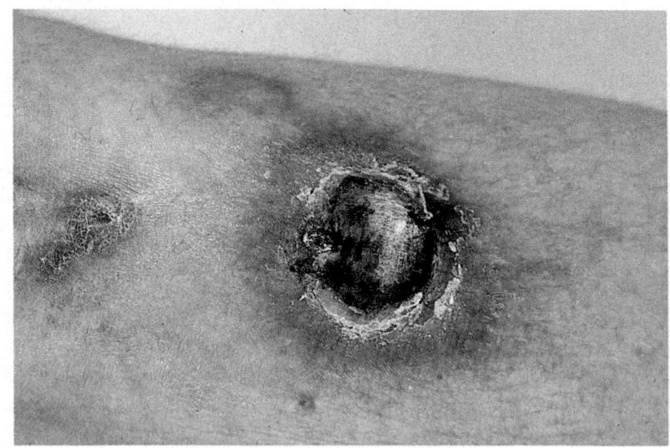

A necrotic ulcer on the leg of a boy with leukocyte adhesion deficiency type 1. Note the presence of heaped-up edges of the ulcer and extensive crusting. Biopsies showed essentially no neutrophils invading.

basis for gene therapy.[51] Another adhesion molecule deficiency (LAD2) that results from absence of the neutrophil sialyl-Lewis X ligand of E-selectin on vascular endothelium has been described. Clinical features and markedly decreased neutrophil motility resemble that of LAD1.[52] Oral fucose administration has been helpful in some patients.[53]

Chédiak-Higashi Syndrome

This rare autosomal recessive disorder is characterized by incomplete oculocutaneous albinism and severe recurrent infections.[54,55] Parental consanguinity is often reported. Pigmentary dilution is present in 75 percent of patients. Ocular hypopigmentation may cause photophobia, and strabismus and nystagmus are common. The skin is typically fair, but slate-colored areas of pigmentation may be present. The hair frequently has a silvery sheen (Fig. 115-12*A*). Infections most commonly involve the skin, lungs, and respiratory tract and usually are due to *S. aureus, Streptococcus pyogenes,* and *Pneumococcus.* Deep ulcerations resembling pyoderma gangrenosum have been described. Seizures and progressive neurologic deterioration, with muscle weakness and cranial and peripheral neuropathy, occur in some patients in early childhood.

An accelerated phase that resembles lymphoma occurs by late childhood and is characterized by widespread visceral infiltration by atypical lymphoid and histiocytic cells. This lymphoma-like stage is precipitated by viruses, particularly by EBV infection. Hepatosplenomegaly, lymphadenopathy, pancytopenia, jaundice, a leukemia-like gingivitis, and pseudomembraneous sloughing of the buccal mucosa are associated. The thrombocytopenia and depletion of coagulation factors lead to petechiae, bruising, and gingival bleeding. The mean age of death for patients with Chédiak-Higashi syndrome is 6 years, usually from overwhelming infection or hemorrhage during the lymphoma-like accelerated phase.

Giant granules typically are found in circulating neutrophils, melanocytes, renal tubular cells, and neurons. Hair shafts have finely clumped pigment granules (see Fig. 115-12*B*), in contrast to the larger pigmentary clumping of Griscelli syndrome (see Fig. 115-12*C*). The granules are thought to result from markedly delayed discharge of lysosomal and peroxidative enzymes from cells, perhaps because of a defective protein involved in membrane fusion. Diminished chemotaxis of neutrophils and decreased antibody-dependent cellular cytotoxicity and NK cell function are often associated.

The gene that is mutated in the Chédiak-Higashi syndrome is the lysosomal trafficking regulator (*LYST*).[56] The protein appears to regulate the secretion of intracellular lysosomal vesicles and melanosomes. Cytotoxic T lymphocyte–associated antigen is trapped in abnormally large vesicles rather than on the cell surface and thus may be unable to regulate T cell activation, increasing the risk of lymphoproliferative disease.[57]

Prenatal diagnosis has been achieved by examination of hair from fetal scalp biopsies and of leukocytes from fetal blood samples. The treatment of choice for patients with Chédiak-Higashi syndrome is bone marrow transplantation, which corrects the immunologic status but does not affect pigment dilution. Acyclovir, high-dose intravenous gamma globulin, vincristine, cyclosporine, and prednisone have been used to control the accelerated phase. Ascorbic acid corrects the microtubular defects in vitro but has no clinical ameliorative effect. Interferon has been demonstrated by some authors to partially restore NK cell function.

Griscelli Syndrome

As in Chédiak-Higashi syndrome, patients with Griscelli syndrome have pigmentary dilution with silver-gray hair, recurrent systemic and cutaneous pyogenic infections, and cutaneous abscesses.[58] Early hepatosplenomegaly, progressive neurologic deterioration, lymphohistiocytosis, and neutropenia and thrombocytopenia may occur. Large

clumps of pigment are present in the hair shaft (see Fig. 115-12*C*), and melanosomes accumulate in melanocytes. Patients with Griscelli syndrome also have hypogammaglobulinemia and defective cell-mediated immunity. Polymorphonuclear leukocytes do not show giant granules.

FIGURE 115-12

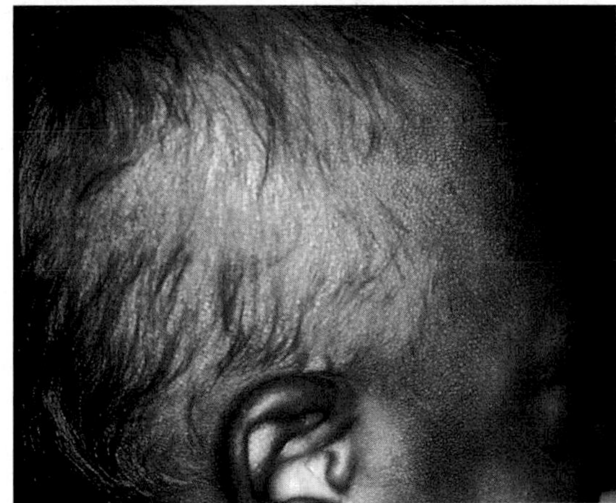

A.

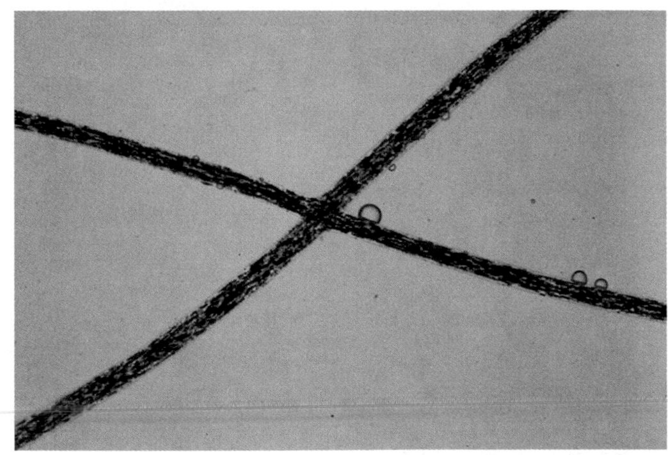

B.

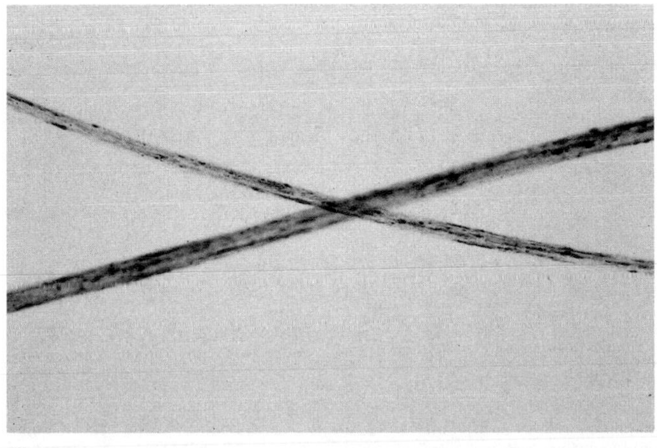

C.

Chédiak-Higashi syndrome. *A.* Silvery sheen to hair in a black infant; patient had darkly pigmented eyes and skin. *B.* Clumped pigment granules in hairs. *C.* Larger aggregates of clumped pigmentation in hairs of a patient with Griscelli syndrome.

Mutations that lead to Griscelli syndrome occur in either *myosin Va*[59] or *RAB27a*.[60] Griscelli syndrome has been uniformly fatal but now can be reversed by successful bone marrow transplantation. Prenatal diagnosis has been achieved by examination of hair from fetal scalp biopsies and of leukocytes from fetal blood samples.

COMPLEMENT-DEFICIENCY DISORDERS

(See also Chaps. 33 and 117)

Leiner's Disease

Leiner's disease is characterized by severe seborrheic dermatitis, diarrhea, failure to thrive, and recurrent gram-negative and candidal infections during infancy. Although originally reported as a disorder due to defective yeast opsonization from dysfunctional C5, it is now clear that so-called Leiner's syndrome describes a constellation of clinical findings that may be manifestations of a variety of immunodeficiency disorders, including defective yeast opsonization, C3 deficiency, severe combined immunodeficiency, hypogammaglobulinemia, and hyperimmunoglobulinemia E.[61]

REFERENCES

1. Rosen FS et al: The primary immunodeficiencies. *N Engl J Med* **333**:431, 1995
2. Minegishi Y et al: Recent progress in the diagnosis and treatment of patients with defects in early B-cell development. *Curr Opin Pediatr* **11**:528, 1999
3. Vetrie D et al: The gene involved in X-linked agammaglobulinaemia is a member of the *src* family of protein-tyrosine kinases. *Nature* **361**:226, 1993
4. Tsukada S et al: Deficient expression of a B cell cytoplasmic tyrosine kinase in human X-linked agammaglobulinemia. *Cell* **72**:279, 1993
5. Cunningham-Rundles C, Bodian C: Common variable immunodeficiency: Clinical and immunological features of 248 patients. *Clin Immunol* **92**:34, 1999
6. Cunningham-Rundles C et al: Incidence of cancer in 98 patients with common varied immunodeficiency. *J Clin Immunol* **7**:294, 1987
7. Schaffer FM et al: Individuals with IgA deficiency and common variable immunodeficiency share complex polymorphisms of major histocompatibility complex class III genes. *Proc Natl Acad Sci USA* **86**:8015, 1989
8. Sennhauser FH et al: Anti-IgA antibodies in IgA-deficient children. *J Clin Immunol* **8**:356, 1988
9. Schneider LC: X-linked hyper IgM syndrome. *Clin Rev Allergy Immunol* **19**:205, 2000
10. Chang MW et al: Mucocutaneous manifestations of the hyper-IgM immunodeficiency syndrome. *J Am Acad Dermatol* **38**:191, 1998.
11. DiSanto JP et al: CD40 ligand mutations in X-linked immunodeficiency with hyper-IgM. *Nature* **361**:541, 1993
12. Seemayer TA et al: X-linked lymphoproliferative disease: Twenty-five years after the discovery. *Pediatr Res* **38**:471, 1995
13. Sylla B et al: The X-linked lymphoproliferative syndrome gene product SH2D1A is associated with p62^{dok} (Dok1) and activates NF-κB. *Proc Natl Acad Sci USA* **97**:7470, 2000
14. Ochs HD: The Wiskott-Aldrich syndrome. *Semin Hematol* **35**:332, 1998
15. Thrasher AJ, Kinnon C: The Wiskott-Aldrich syndrome. *Clin Exp Immunol* **120**:2, 2000
16. Snapper SB, Rosen FS: The Wiskott-Aldrich syndrome protein (WASP): Roles in signaling and cytoskeletal organization. *Annu Rev Immunol* **17**:905, 1999.
17. Giliani S et al: Prenatal molecular diagnosis of Wiskott-Aldrich syndrome by direct mutation analysis. *Prenat Diagn* **19**:36, 1999
18. Gatti RA: Ataxia-telangiectasia. *Dermatol Clin* **13**:1, 1995
19. Savitsky K et al: A single ataxia telangiectasia gene with a product similar to PI-3 kinase. *Science* **268**:1749, 1995
20. Fischer A: Severe combined immunodeficiencies (SCID). *Clin Exp Immunol* **122**:143, 2000
21. Gaspar HB et al: Severe combined immunodeficiency: Molecular pathogenesis and diagnosis. *Arch Dis Child* **84**:169, 2001
22. Gennery AR, Cant AJ: Diagnosis of severe combined immunodeficiency. *J Clin Pathol* **54**:191, 2001
23. DeSandro A et al: The bare lymphocyte syndrome: Molecular clues to the transcriptional regulation of major histocompatibility complex class genes. *Am J Hum Genet* **65**:279, 1999
24. Haddad E et al: Long-term immune reconstitution and outcome after HLA-nonidentical T-cell depleted bone marrow reconstitution for SCI: A European retrospective study of 116 patients. *Blood* **91**:3636, 1998
25. Buckley RH et al: Hematopoeietic stem cell transplantation for the treatment of severe combined immunodeficiency. *N Engl J Med* **340**:508, 1999
26. Cavazzana-Calvo M et al: Gene therapy of human severe sombined immundeficiency (SCID)-X1 disease. *Science* **288**:669, 2000
27. Kirkpatrick CH: Chronic mucocutaneous candidiasis. *Pediatr Infect Dis J* **20**:197, 2001
28. Ahonen P et al: Clinical variation of autoimmune polyendocrinopathy-candidiasis-ectodermal dystrophy (APECED) in a series of 68 patients. *N Engl J Med* **322**:1829, 1990
29. Lilic D, Gravenor I: Immunology of chronic mucocutaneous candidiasis. *J Clin Pathol* **54**:81, 2001
30. de Moraes-Vasconcelos D et al: Characterization of the cellular immune function of patients with chronic mucocutaneous candidiasis. *Clin Exp Immunol* **123**:247, 2001
31. Tosti A et al: Itraconazole in the treatment of two young brothers with chronic mucocutaneous candidiasis. *Pediatr Dermatol* **14**:146, 1997
32. Hong R: The Di George anomaly. (catch 22, Di George/velocardiofacial syndrome). *Semin Hematol* **35**:282, 1998
33. Merscher S et al: TBX1 is responsible for cardiovascular defects in velo-cardiofacial/Di George syndrome. *Cell* **104**:619, 2001
34. Brennan T, Pearson R: Abnormal elastic tissue in cartilage-hair hypoplasia. *Arch Dermatol* **124**:1411, 1988
35. Makitie O et al: Increased incidence of cancer in patients with cartilage-hair hypoplasia. *J Pediatr* **134**:315, 1999
36. Ridanpaa M et al: Mutations in the RNA component of RNase MRP cause a pleiotropic human disease, cartilage-hair hypoplasia. *Cell* **104**:195, 2001
37. Makitie O et al: Deficiency of humoral immunity in cartilage-hair hypoplasia. *J Pediatr* **137**:487, 2000
38. Winkelstein JA et al: Chronic granulomatous disease: Report on a national registry of 368 patients. *Medicine* **79**:155, 2000
39. Segal BH et al: Genetic, biochemical, and clinical features of the chronic granulomatous disease. *Medicine* **79**:170, 2000
40. Margolis DM et al: Trimethoprim-sulfamethoxazole prophylaxis in the management of chronic granulomatous disease. *J Infect Dis* **162**:723, 1990
41. International Chronic Granulomatous Disease Cooperative Study Group: A controlled trial of interferon gamma to prevent infection in chronic granulomatous disease. *N Engl J Med* **324**:509, 1991
42. Mouy R et al: Long-term itraconazole prophylaxis against *Aspergillus* infections in thirty-two patients with chronic granulomatous disease. *J Pediatr* **125**:998, 1994
43. Malech HL: Progress in gene therapy for chronic granulomatous disease. *J Infect Dis* **2**:S318, 1999
44. Grimbacher B et al: Hyper-IgE syndrome with recurrent infections: An autosomal dominant multisystem disorder. *N Engl J Med* **340**:692, 1999
45. Borges WG et al: The face of Job. *J Pediatr* **133**:303, 1998
46. Grimbacher B et al: Genetic linkage of hyper-IgE syndrome to chromosome 4. *Am J Hum Genet* **65**:735, 1999
47. Garraud O et al: Regulation of immunoglobulin production in hyper-IgE (Job's) syndrome. *J Allerg Clin Immunol* **103**:333, 1999
48. Borges WG et al: Defective interleukin-12/interferon-γ pathway in patients with hyperimmunoglobulinemia E syndrome. *J Pediatr* **136**:176, 2000
49. Arnaout MA: Leukocyte adhesion molecule deficiency: Its structural basis, pathophysiology and implications for modulating the inflammatory response. *Immunol Rev* **114**:145, 1990
50. Paller AS et al: Leukocyte adhesion deficiency: Recurrent childhood skin infections. *J Am Acad Dermatol* **31**:316, 1994
51. Hibbs M et al: Transfection of cells from patients with leukocyte adhesion deficiency with an integrin beta subunit (CD18) restores lymphocyte function associated antigen-1 expression and function. *J Clin Invest* **85**:674, 1990
52. Marquardt T et al: Leukocyte adhesion deficiency II syndrome, a generalized defect in fucose metabolism. *J Pediatr* **134**:681, 1999
53. Marquardt T et al: Correction of leukocyte adhesion deficiency type II with oral fucose. *Blood* **94**:3976, 1999
54. Blume RS, Wolff SM: The Chédiak-Higashi syndrome: Studies in four patients and review of the literature. *Medicine* **51**:247, 1972

55. Anderson LL et al: Chédiak-Higashi syndrome in a black child. *Pediatr Dermatol* **9**:31, 1992
56. Introne W et al: Clinical, molecular, and cell biological aspects of Chédiak-Higashi syndrome. *Mol Genet Metab* **68**:283, 1999
57. Barrat FJ et al: Defective CTLA-4 cycling pathway in Chédiak-Higashi syndrome: A possible mechanism for deregulation of T lymphocyte activation. *Proc Natl Acad Sci USA* **96**:8645, 1999
58. Mancini A et al: Partial albinism with immunodeficiency: Griscelli syndrome. Report of a case and review of the literature. *J Am Acad Dermatol* **38**:295, 1998

59. Pastural E et al: Griscelli disease maps to chromosome 15q21 and is associated with mutations in the *myosin-Va* gene. *Nature Genet* **16**:289, 1997
60. Menasche G et al: Mutations in RAB27A cause Griscelli syndrome associated with haemophagocytic syndrome. *Nature Genet* **25**:173, 2000
61. Glover M et al: Syndrome of erythroderma, failure to thrive and diarrhea in infancy: A manifestation of immunodeficiency. *Pediatrics* **81**:66, 1988

CHAPTER 116

Nicholas A. Soter
Allen P. Kaplan

Urticaria and Angioedema

Urticaria and angioedema occur as clinical manifestations of immunologic and inflammatory mechanisms, or they may be idiopathic. They may develop after IgE- or IgE receptor–dependent reactions, in association with abnormalities of the complement system and other plasma effector systems, after direct mast cell degranulation, and in relation to activation of cellular arachidonic acid metabolic pathways (Table 116-1). In addition to the skin and mucous membranes, the respiratory and gastrointestinal tracts as well as the cardiovascular system may be involved in any combination.

HISTORICAL ASPECTS

In China, cutaneous lesions thought to be urticaria have been recognized since about 1000 B.C. Hippocrates (460–377 B.C.) described pruritic lesions caused by nettles and mosquitoes that he termed *knidosis*, which is derived from the Greek word for nettle (*knide*). Plinius (A.D. 32–79) used the term *uredo* (burning), Zedler in 1740 used the word *urticatio*, and William Cullen in 1769 introduced the word *urticaria*. Some physical urticarias initially were recognized in the eighteenth century. Angioedema was described by Donato in 1586, and hereditary angioedema was reported by Osler in 1888.

EPIDEMIOLOGY

Urticaria and angioedema are common. Age, race, sex, occupation, geographic location, and season of the year may be implicated in urticaria and angioedema only insofar as they may contribute to exposure to an eliciting agent. Of a group of college students, 15 to 20 percent reported having experienced urticaria, and 1 to 3 percent of the patients referred to hospital dermatology clinics in the United Kingdom noted urticaria and angioedema. In the National Ambulatory Medical Care Survey data from 1990 to 1997 in the United States, women accounted for 69 percent of patient visits. There was a bimodal age distribution in patients aged birth to 9 years and 30 to 40 years.[1]

Urticaria/angioedema is considered to be acute if it lasts less than 6 weeks. Most acute episodes are due to adverse reactions to foods in children or to viral illnesses. Episodes of urticaria/angioedema persisting beyond 6 weeks are considered chronic and most likely represent

TABLE 116-1

Classification of Urticaria/Angioedema

Immunologic IgE- and IgE receptor–dependent urticaria/angioedema
- Atopic diathesis
- Specific antigen sensitivity (foods, drugs, therapeutic agents, aeroallergens, animal danders, Hymenoptera venom, helminths)
- Physical urticaria/angioedema
- Contact urticaria
- Autoimmune urticaria

Urticaria/angioedema mediated by the complement system and other plasma effector systems
- Hereditary angioedema
- Acquired angioedema with $\overline{C1}$INH deficiency and malignant disorders or autoantibody
- Urticarial venulitis
- Serum sickness
- Reactions to blood products
- Infections
- Angiotensin-converting enzyme inhibitors

Urticaria/angioedema after direct mast cell degranulation
- Opiate analgesics
- Polymyxin B
- Curare, D-tubocurarine
- Radiocontrast media

Urticaria/angioedema relating to abnormalities of arachidonic acid metabolism
- Aspirin and nonsteroidal anti-inflammatory agents
- Azo dyes and benzoates

Idiopathic urticaria/angioedema
- Cyclic episodic angioedema

idiopathic urticaria or urticaria that is autoimmune. Physically induced urticaria/angioedema is not included in the definition. Various types of physical urticaria/angioedema may last for years, but the individual lesions last fewer than 2 h and are intermittent. Whereas 85 percent of children experience only urticaria, approximately 50 percent of adult patients with urticaria also experience angioedema.

About 50 percent of patients with urticaria alone are free of lesions within 1 year, 65 percent within 3 years, and 85 percent within 5 years; fewer than 5 percent have lesions that last for more than 10 years. Angioedema alters the natural history, and only 25 percent of patients experience resolution of lesions within 1 year.

PATHOGENESIS

The mast cell (see Chap. 32) is the major effector cell in most forms of urticaria and angioedema, although other cell types may be involved. Cutaneous mast cells adhere to fibronectin and laminin through the very late activation (VLA) β_1 integrins VLA-3, VLA-4, and VLA-5 and to vitronectin through the $\alpha v\beta_3$ integrin. Cutaneous mast cells, but not those from other sites, release histamine in response to compound 48/80, C5a, morphine, and codeine. The neuropeptides substance P (SP), vasoactive intestinal peptide (VIP), and somatostatin, but not neurotensin, neurokinins A and B, bradykinin, and calcitonin gene–related peptide (CGRP), activate mast cells for histamine secretion. Dermal microdialysis studies of the application of SP on skin indicate that it induces histamine release only at 10^{-6} M, which suggests that after physiologic nociceptor activation, SP does not release histamine.[2] Not all potential biologic products are produced when cutaneous mast cells are stimulated. For example, SP releases histamine from cutaneous mast cells but does not generate prostaglandin D_2 (PGD_2). Vascular permeability in skin is produced predominantly by H_1 histamine receptors, although H_2 histamine receptors sometimes may participate.

The participation of the mast cell in vivo in urticaria and angioedema has been studied by analysis of morphologic alterations of mast cells and by identification and quantitation of mast cell products in tissues or biologic fluids. Aspirates of experimental suction blisters generated over lesional and control skin have provided biologic fluid for analysis. The skin chamber model has been useful particularly because the presentation of antigen into the chamber is controlled, and the mast cell products appearing in the fluid can be assessed quantitatively and serially. Scanning laser Doppler imaging has been used to study dermal blood perfusion, and dermal microdialysis has been used to detect the presence of biochemical mediators and the consequences of their actions. A current hypothesis suggests that the release of mast cell products leads to alterations in vasopermeability with the appearance of adhesion molecules on endothelial cells and the subsequent rolling and attachment of blood leukocytes that enter the cutaneous microenvironment.

Various forms of physical urticaria/angioedema have provided experimental models to study urticaria/angioedema by allowing the observation of the elicited clinical response, examination of lesional and normal skin biopsy specimens, assay of chemical mediators released into the blood or tissues, and characterization of peripheral leukocyte responses. The intracutaneous injection of specific antigen in sensitized individuals has provided an experimental model for analysis of the role of IgE and its interaction with the mast cell. In some subjects, the challenged cutaneous sites demonstrate a biphasic response, with a transient, pruritic, erythematous wheal-and-flare reaction followed by a tender, deep, erythematous, poorly demarcated area of swelling that persists for up to 24 h.

In a study of the histamine-induced wheal-and-erythema reaction with dermal microdialysis and scanning laser Doppler imaging, the wheal began to develop at 1 to 2 min and reached a maximum at 10 min. The flare reached a steady state between 7 and 10 min. Although the rate of development of the flare was independent of the histamine concentration, the steady-state flare area at 10 min was concentration-dependent. The fact that histamine was detected in the wheal but not in the flare implies that the flare is a neurogenic reflex.[3]

The possibility that chronic idiopathic urticaria may be an autoimmune disorder arose from data that suggested an association of chronic idiopathic urticaria with autoimmune thyroiditis and, more specifically, with the presence of IgG autoantibodies to thyroglobulin and peroxidase.[4] In the original studies, the incidence of such antibodies was 12 to 14 percent in patients with chronic idiopathic urticaria; more recently, the incidence of antibodies to either antigen or to both of them is 24 percent.

It was demonstrated subsequently that approximately 10 percent of patients with chronic idiopathic urticaria had circulating IgG anti-IgE antibodies. Then IgG antibodies to the α subunit of the high-affinity IgE receptor FcεRIα were detected in about 30 percent of patients with chronic idiopathic urticaria. Autologous serum injected into their skin induced a wheal-and-flare reaction.

The autoantibodies to FcεRIα and IgE are associated with IgG_1 and IgG_3.[5,6] Consistent with the latter subclass distribution are data that demonstrate a role for complement in the degranulation of basophils or cutaneous mast cells. IgG alone is effective at plasma concentrations, but the reaction is augmented in the presence of C5a in serum.[7] Blocking antibody to the C5a receptor inhibits the ability of serum to augment basophil histamine release caused by the patient's IgG autoantibodies; therefore, the complement agonist is C5a.[8] The circulating basophils of patients with chronic idiopathic urticaria behave as if they are nonspecifically desensitized, with reduced histamine release in response to challenge with anti-IgE; there is a peripheral basopenia.

Immunoblot analysis initially was thought to be a method to screen patients for the FcεRIα autoantibody and to seek evidence of serum IgG binding to a cloned α subunit after sodium dodecylsulfate (SDS) gel electrophoresis. However, there are both false-positive and false-negative reactions when this assay is used,[7] and a functional assay is required to demonstrate the presence of the autoantibody. Although the autologous serum skin test can be used as a screening method that identifies some patients, serum is injected and clotting leads not only to bradykinin formation but also to enzymatic cleavage of C5 to release C5a, which may result in false-positive reactions.

The autoantibody to FcεRIα has been detected in 35 to 40 percent of patients with chronic idiopathic urticaria and in some individuals with dermatomyositis, systemic lupus erythematosus, pemphigus vulgaris, and bullous pemphigoid; it has not been detected in patients with atopic dermatitis or psoriasis. Sera obtained from patients with chronic idiopathic urticaria but not from those with other autoimmune diseases released histamine from peripheral blood basophils and cutaneous mast cells.[5,6] The explanation for the observation that the autoantibodies to either IgE or FcεRIα can be present but not functional is unclear. Considerations are antibody affinity, subclass distribution, and differences in epitope recognition. In addition to patients with chronic idiopathic urticaria, autoantibodies to IgE that are not functional also may be found in 5 to 10 percent of sera from patients with atopic dermatitis and from normal control subjects.

Some patients with chronic urticaria and thyroid autoimmunity have IgG autoantibodies to thyroglobulin and peroxidase.[4] In a study of 116 patients with chronic idiopathic urticaria, 19.8 percent exhibited IgG autoantibodies to peroxidase, and 88 percent of these individuals also exhibited IgE autoantibodies to peroxidase.[9] These IgE autoantibodies were functional and released β-hexosaminidase from mouse mast cells. This finding has not been corroborated, however.[10]

Partially characterized histamine-releasing factors obtained from sera of patients with chronic idiopathic urticaria and from mononuclear cells, neutrophils, and platelets suggest that cytokines or chemokines may provide alternative mechanisms.

HLA-DRB1*04, HLA-DQB1*0302, HLA-DRB1*15, and HLA-DQB1*06 are present with increased frequency in patients with chronic idiopathic urticaria as compared with a control population.[11] In patients with FcεRIα autoantibody, HLA-DRB1*04, HLA-DQB1*0301/4, and HLA-DQB1*0302 are present with increased frequency.

FIGURE 116-1

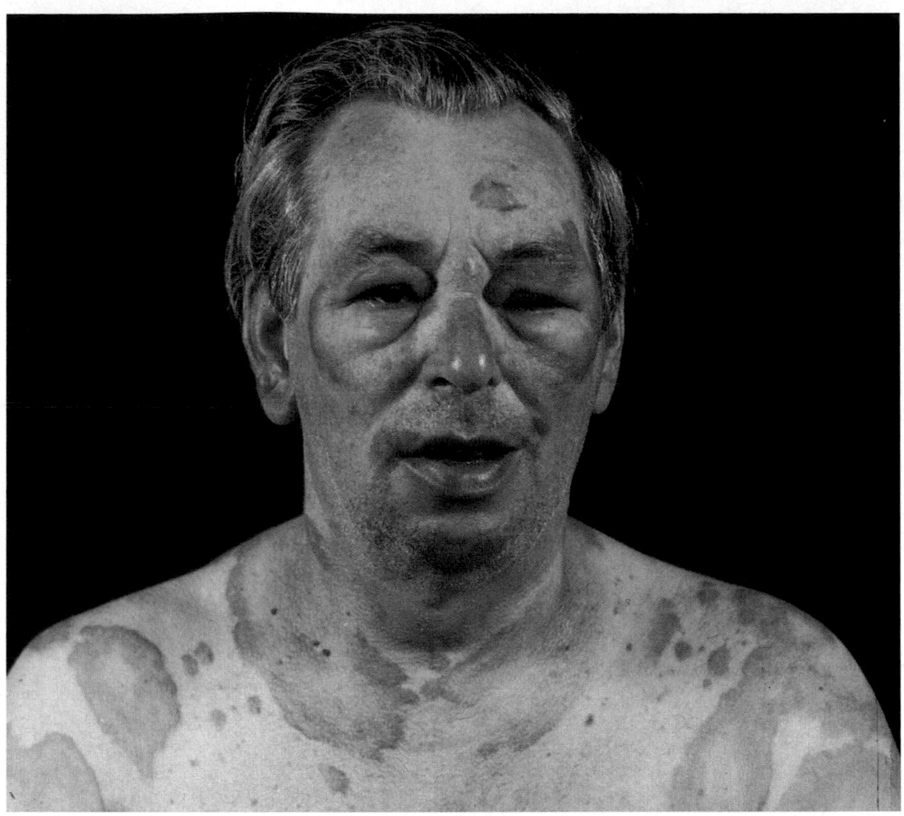

Urticaria. This patient has urticaria occurring on the face, neck, and upper trunk with angioedema about the eyes.

CLINICAL MANIFESTATIONS

Circumscribed, raised, erythematous, usually pruritic, evanescent areas of edema that involve the superficial portion of the dermis are known as *urticaria* (Fig. 116-1); when the edematous process extends into the deep dermis and/or subcutaneous and submucosal layers, it is known as *angioedema* (Fig. 116-2). Urticaria and angioedema may occur in any location together or individually. Angioedema commonly affects the face or a portion of an extremity, may be painful but not pruritic, and may last several days. Involvement of the lips, cheeks, and periorbital areas is common, but angioedema also may affect the tongue and pharynx. The individual lesions of urticaria arise suddenly, rarely persist longer than 24 to 48 h, and may continue to recur for indefinite periods.

Immunologic IgE- and IgE Receptor–Dependent Urticaria/Angioedema

ATOPIC DIATHESIS Episodes of acute urticaria/angioedema that occur in individuals with a personal or family history of asthma, rhinitis, or eczema are presumed to be IgE-dependent. In clinical practice, however, urticaria/angioedema infrequently accompanies an exacerbation of asthma, rhinitis, or eczema. The prevalence of chronic urticaria/angioedema is not increased in atopic individuals.

SPECIFIC ANTIGEN SENSITIVITY Common examples of specific antigens that provoke urticaria/angioedema include foods, such as shellfish, nuts, and chocolate; drugs and therapeutic agents, notably penicillin; aeroallergens; and Hymenoptera venom. Urticaria in patients with helminthic infestations has been attributed to IgE-dependent processes; however, proof of this relationship is often lacking. Specific allergens and nonspecific stimuli may activate local reactions, termed *recall urticaria*, at sites previously injected with allergen immunotherapy.

PHYSICAL URTICARIA/ANGIOEDEMA[12,13] (Table 116-2)

Dermographism Dermographism is the most common form of physical urticaria. It appears as a linear wheal with a flare at a site in which the skin is briskly stroked with a firm object. A transient wheal appears rapidly and usually fades within 30 min; however, normal skin is typically pruritic so that an itch-scratch sequence may appear. The prevalence of dermographism in the general population was 1.5 and 4.2 percent, respectively, in two studies, and its prevalence in patients with chronic idiopathic urticaria is 22 percent. It is not associated with atopy. The peak prevalence occurs in the second and third decades. In one study, the duration of dermographism was greater than 5 years in 22 percent of individuals and greater than 10 years in 10 percent.

Elevations in blood histamine levels have been documented in some patients after experimental scratching, and increased levels of histamine, tryptase, SP, and VIP, but not CGRP, have been detected in experimental suction-blister aspirates. The dermographic response has been passively transferred to the skin of normal subjects with serum or IgE.

Delayed dermographism Delayed dermographism develops 3 to 6 h after stimulation, either with or without an immediate reaction, and lasts 24 to 48 h. The eruption is composed of linear red nodules. This condition may be associated with delayed pressure urticaria. Cold-dependent dermographism is a condition that occurs only after cold exposure. Cholinergic dermographism is a rare form that develops as punctate wheals in patients with cholinergic urticaria.

Pressure urticaria Delayed pressure urticaria appears as erythematous, deep, local swellings, often painful, that arise from 0.5 to 6 h after sustained pressure has been applied to the skin. Spontaneous episodes are elicited after sitting on a hard chair, under shoulder straps and belts, on the feet after running, and on the hands after manual labor. The peak prevalence occurs in the third decade. Delayed pressure urticaria may be associated with fever, chills, arthralgias, and myalgias, as well as with an elevated erythrocyte sedimentation rate and leukocytosis. In one study, it occurred in 37 percent of patients with chronic

FIGURE 116-2

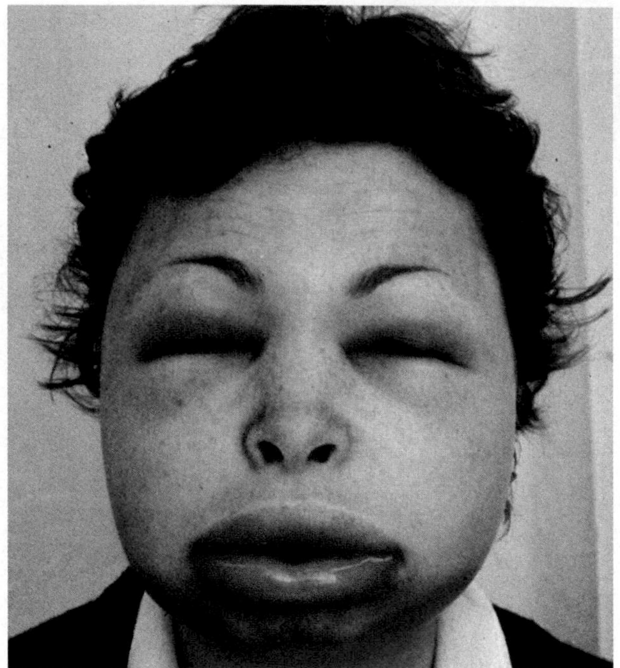

A.

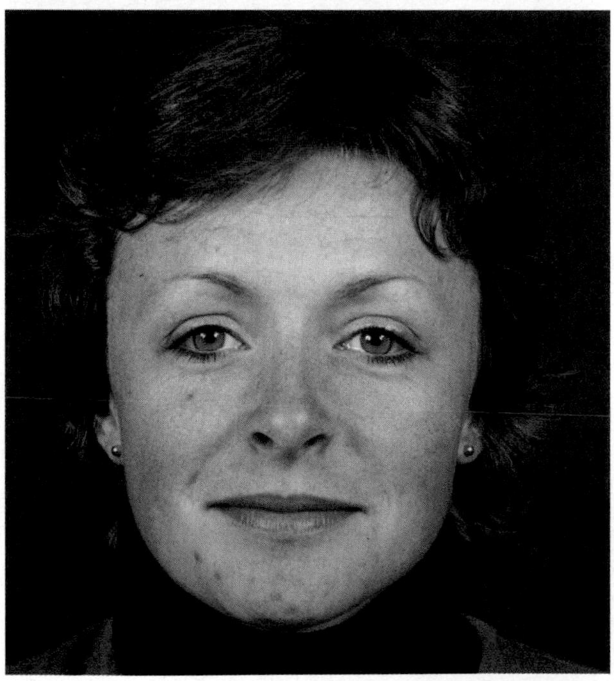

B.

Hereditary angioedema. Extensive involvement (*A*) is to be contrasted with this patient's normal facies (*B*).

idiopathic urticaria plus dermographism. An IgE-mediated mechanism has not been demonstrated; however, histamine and interleukin 6 (IL-6) have been detected in lesional experimental suction-blister aspirates and in fluid from skin chambers, respectively; leukotriene B_4 (LTB_4), 12- and 15-hydroxyeicosatetraenoic acids, and IL-1 were absent.

Immediate pressure urticaria is a rare idiopathic disorder. It has been described in patients with the hypereosinophilic syndrome.

Vibratory angioedema Vibratory angioedema may occur as an acquired idiopathic disorder, in association with cholinergic urticaria, or after several years of occupational exposure to vibration. It has been described in a family with an autosomal dominant pattern of inheritance. The heritable form often is accompanied by facial flushing. An increase in the level of plasma histamine was detected during an experimental attack in patients with the hereditary form and in patients with acquired disease.

Cold urticaria There are both acquired and inherited forms of cold urticaria/angioedema. The acquired forms are more common. Idiopathic or primary acquired cold urticaria may be associated with headache, hypotension, syncope, wheezing, shortness of breath, palpitations, nausea, vomiting, and diarrhea. Attacks occur within minutes after exposures that include changes in ambient temperature and direct contact with cold objects. The elicitation of a wheal after the application of ice has been called a *diagnostic cold contact test.* If the entire body is cooled, as in swimming, hypotension and syncope, which are potentially lethal events, may occur. In rare instances, acquired cold urticaria has been associated with underlying cryoglobulins, cryofibrinogens, cold agglutinins, and cold hemolysins, especially in children with infectious mononucleosis.

Passive transfer of cold urticaria with serum or IgE to the skin of a normal recipient has been documented. Histamine, chemotactic factors for eosinophils and neutrophils, PGD_2, cysteinyl leukotrienes, platelet-activating factor, and tumor necrosis factor α (TNF-α) have been released into the circulation after experimental challenge. Histamine, SP, and VIP, but not CGRP, have been detected in experimental suction-blister aspirates. Histamine has been released in vitro from chilled skin biopsy specimens that have been rewarmed. Neutrophils harvested from the blood of an experimentally cold-challenged arm manifested an impaired chemotactic response. Whereas complement has no role in primary acquired cold urticaria, the challenge of patients with cold urticaria who have circulating immune complexes, such as cryoglobulins, can provoke a cutaneous necrotizing venulitis with complement activation.

Rare forms of acquired cold urticaria that have been described mainly in case reports include systemic cold urticaria, localized cold urticaria, cold-induced cholinergic urticaria, cold-dependent dermographism, and localized cold reflex urticaria. Two forms of dominantly inherited cold urticaria have been described. *Familial cold urticaria,* which also has been termed *familial cold autoinflammatory syndrome* and is considered a type of periodic fever,[14] is an autosomal dominant disorder with a genetic linkage to chromosome 1q44. The responsible gene has been identified as *CIAS1,* which codes for a protein involved in regulation of inflammation and apoptosis.[15] The eruption occurs as erythematous macules and infrequent wheals and is associated with burning or pruritus. Fever, headaches, conjunctivitis, arthralgias, and a neutrophilic leukocytosis are features of attacks. The delay between cold exposure and onset of symptoms is 2.5 h, and the average duration of an episode is 12 h. Renal disease with amyloidosis occurs infrequently. Skin biopsy specimens show mast cell degranulation and an infiltrate of neutrophils. The cold contact test and passive transfer with serum have been negative. Serum levels of IL-6 and granulocyte colony-stimulating factor (G-CSF) were elevated in one patient. *Delayed cold urticaria* occurs as erythematous, edematous, deep swellings that appear 9 to18 h after cold challenge. Lesional biopsy specimens show edema with minimal numbers of mononuclear cells; mast cells are not degranulated; and complement proteins, immunoglobulins, and fibrin are not detected. Cold immersion does not release histamine, and the condition cannot be passively transferred.

Cholinergic urticaria Cholinergic urticaria develops after an increase in core body temperature, such as during a warm bath or shower, exercise, or episodes of fever. The highest prevalence is observed in

TABLE 116-2

Physical Urticaria/Angioedema

Stimulus and Type of Response	Clinical Presentation
Mechanical	
Acute brisk trauma	
Dermographism	Erythema, wheal, pruritus
Delayed dermographism	Erythema, wheal, nodules, pruritus
Pressure	
Immediate pressure urticaria	Erythema, angioedema
Delayed pressure urticaria	Erythema, angioedema, tenderness or pain, fever, chills, arthralgia, myalgia, leukocytosis
Vibration	Erythema, angioedema, flushing (may be familial)
Temperature	
Cold	
Primary acquired	Erythema, wheal, angioedema, pruritus, headache, hypotension, syncope, wheezing, shortness of breath, palpitations, nausea, vomiting, diarrhea
Familial	Erythema, macules, wheals, burning, fever, headache, conjunctivitis, arthralgia, leukocytosis (dominantly inherited
Delayed	Erythema, deep local swelling (dominantly inherited)
Heat	
Cholinergic	Erythema, small wheals, pruritus, dizziness, headache, syncope, flushing, wheezing, shortness of breath, nausea, vomiting, diarrhea (may be familial)
Local	Erythema, wheal, pruritus (may be familial)
Light	
Solar	Erythema, wheal, angioedema, pruritus, headache, syncope, dizziness, wheezing, nausea
Exercise	
Exercise-induced anaphylaxis	Erythema, wheal, angioedema, hoarseness, difficulty swallowing, syncope
Stress	
Adrenergic	Erythema, wheal with halo, pruritus
Water	
Aquagenic	Erythema, small wheals, pruritus (may be familial)

individuals aged 23 to 28 years. The eruption appears as distinctive, pruritic, small, 1- to 2-mm wheals that are surrounded by large areas of erythema (Fig. 116-3); occasionally, the lesions may become confluent, or angioedema may develop. Systemic features include dizziness, headache, syncope, flushing, wheezing, shortness of breath, nausea, vomiting, and diarrhea. An increased prevalence of atopy has been reported. The intracutaneous injection of cholinergic agents, such as methacholine chloride, produces a wheal locally in approximately one-third of patients. Alterations in pulmonary function have been documented during experimental exercise challenge or after the inhalation of acetylcholine.

Familial cases have been reported only in men in four families. This observation suggests an autosomal dominant pattern of inheritance. One of these individuals had coexisting dermographism and aquagenic urticaria.

After exercise challenge, histamine and factors chemotactic for eosinophils and neutrophils have been released into the circulation. Tryptase has been detected in lesional suction-blister aspirates. The urticarial response has been passively transferred on one occasion; however, most other attempts to do so have been unsuccessful.

Local heat urticaria Local heat urticaria is a rare form of urticaria in which wheals develop within minutes after exposure to locally applied heat. An increased incidence of atopy has been reported. Passive transfer has been negative. Histamine, neutrophil chemotactic activity, and PGD_2 have been detected in the circulation after experimental challenge. In two individuals, there were alterations in factor B levels, which suggested activation of the alternative complement pathway. A familial delayed form of local heat urticaria in which the urticaria occurred 1 to 2 h after challenge and lasted up to 10 h has been described.

Solar urticaria Solar urticaria occurs as pruritus, erythema, wheals, and occasionally angioedema that develop within minutes after exposure to sun or artificial light sources. Headache, syncope, dizziness, wheezing, and nausea are systemic features. Most commonly, solar urticaria appears during the third decade.[16] In one study, 48 percent of patients had a history of atopy. Although solar urticaria may be associated with systemic lupus erythematosus and polymorphous light eruption, it is usually idiopathic. The development of skin lesions under experimental conditions in response to specific wavelengths has allowed classification into six subtypes; however, individuals may respond to more than one portion of the light spectrum. In type I, elicited by wavelengths of 285 to 320 nm, and in type II, elicited by wavelengths of 400 to 500 nm, the responses have been passively transferred with serum. In type I, the wavelengths are blocked by window glass. Type VI, which occurs in erythropoietic protoporphyria and is due to ferrochelatase deficiency, has been reported in a single patient.

Histamine and chemotactic factors for eosinophils and neutrophils have been identified in blood after exposure of the individuals to

FIGURE 116-3

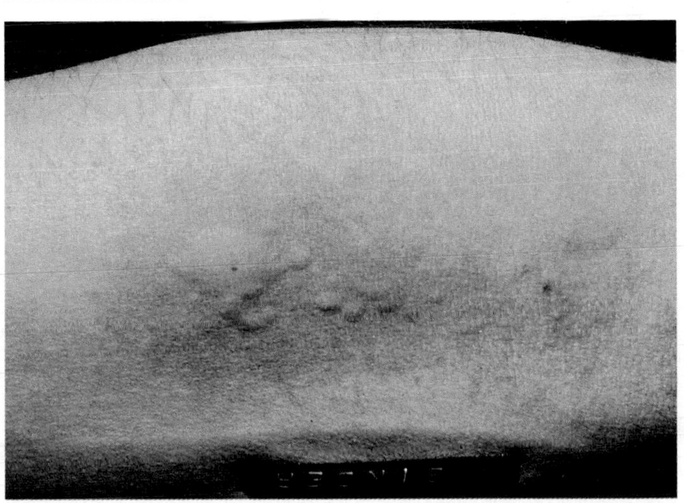

Cholinergic urticaria showing small wheals with surrounding erythema.

ultraviolet A (UVA), UVB, and visible light. In some individuals, uncharacterized serum factors with molecular weights ranging from 25 to 1000 kDa, which elicit cutaneous wheal-and-erythema reactions after intracutaneous injection, have been implicated in the development of lesions.

Exercise-induced anaphylaxis Exercise-induced anaphylaxis is a clinical symptom complex consisting of pruritus, urticaria, angioedema (cutaneous, laryngeal, and intestinal), and syncope that is distinct from cholinergic urticaria. In most patients, the wheals are not punctate but are normal in size. There is a high prevalence of an atopic diathesis. Various types of this syndrome have been described, including exercise-induced anaphylaxis requiring exercise alone as a stimulus, food-dependent exercise-induced anaphylaxis requiring both exercise and food as stimuli, and a variant form in which punctate wheals appear after exercise. The administration of aspirin before the ingestion of food allergens induced urticaria in some patients with food-dependent exercise-induced anaphylaxis.[17] Analysis of a questionnaire study of individuals with exercise-induced anaphylaxis for more than a decade[18] disclosed that the frequency of attacks had decreased in 47 percent and had stabilized in 46 percent. Forty-one percent had been free of attacks for one year. Rare familial forms have been described. In exercise-induced anaphylaxis, pulmonary function tests are normal, biopsy specimens show mast cell degranulation, and histamine and tryptase are released into the circulation.

Adrenergic urticaria Adrenergic urticaria occurs as wheals surrounded by a white halo that develop during emotional stress. The lesions can be elicited by the intracutaneous injection of norepinephrine.

Aquagenic urticaria and aquagenic pruritus Contact of the skin with water of any temperature may result in pruritus alone or, more rarely, urticaria. The eruption consists of small wheals that are reminiscent of cholinergic urticaria. Aquagenic urticaria has been reported in more than one member in five families.[19] Aquagenic pruritus without urticaria is usually idiopathic but also occurs in elderly persons with dry skin and in patients with polycythemia vera, Hodgkin's disease, the myelodysplastic syndrome, and the hypereosinophilic syndrome. Patients with aquagenic pruritus should be evaluated for the emergence of a hematologic disorder. After experimental challenge, blood histamine levels were elevated in subjects with aquagenic pruritus and with aquagenic urticaria. Mast cell degranulation was present in lesional tissues. Passive transfer was negative.

CONTACT URTICARIA Urticaria may occur after direct contact with a variety of substances. It may be IgE-mediated or nonimmunologic. The transient eruption appears within minutes, and when it is IgE mediated, it may be associated with systemic manifestations. Passive transfer has been documented in some instances. Proteins from latex products are a prominent cause of IgE-mediated contact urticaria. Latex proteins also may become airborne allergens, as demonstrated by allergen-loaded airborne glove powder used in inhalation challenge tests (see Chap. 137). These patients may manifest cross-reactivity to fruits, such as bananas, avocado, and kiwi. Associated manifestations include rhinitis, conjunctivitis, dyspnea, and shock. The risk group is dominated by biomedical workers and individuals with frequent contact with latex, such as children with spina bifida. Agents such as stinging nettles, arthropod hairs, and chemicals may release histamine directly from mast cells.

Papular urticaria occurs as episodic, symmetrically distributed, pruritic, 3- to 10-mm urticarial papules that result from a hypersensitivity reaction to insect bites, such as mosquitoes, fleas, and bedbugs. This condition appears mainly in children. The lesions tend to appear in groups on exposed areas, such as the extensor aspects of the extremities.

AUTOIMMUNE URTICARIA Circulating autoantibodies have been recognized in the sera of some patients with chronic idiopathic urticaria, leading to the term *autoimmune urticaria.* These antibodies are estimated to be present in at least 35 to 40 percent of patients with chronic idiopathic urticaria and are discussed under "Pathogenesis" above. A positive autologous serum skin test is defined as a red wheal with a diameter that is 1.5 mm greater than the saline-induced response at 30 min.[20] Patients with autoantibodies have a greater number of wheals with a wider distribution, more severe pruritus, and systemic features of nausea, abdominal pain, diarrhea, and flushing.[21]

Urticaria/Angioedema Mediated by the Complement System and Other Plasma Effector Systems

HEREDITARY AND ACQUIRED ANGIOEDEMA Hereditary angioedema is a dominantly inherited disorder that is characterized by recurrent attacks of angioedema that involve the skin and mucous membranes of the respiratory and gastrointestinal tracts (see Chap. 117). Urticaria is not a manifestation. There is a functional deficiency of the inhibitor of the activated first component of the complement system (C$\bar{1}$INH). Acquired angioedema with depletion of C$\bar{1}$INH has two forms. One is associated with malignant disorders, notably B cell lymphomas and autoantibody to paraproteins. The other form is associated with an autoantibody directed against the C$\bar{1}$INH molecule.

A clinical symptom complex that resembles hereditary angioedema and has an X-linked pattern of inheritance was described in women with angioedema without urticaria and with laryngeal edema and abdominal pain. C4 and C$\bar{1}$INH levels and function are normal.[22]

An estrogen-dependent form of angioedema that resembles hereditary angioedema has been reported in a single family with seven affected individuals in three generations, suggesting an autosomal dominant pattern of inheritance.[23] Clinical features include angioedema without urticaria, laryngeal edema, and abdominal pain with vomiting. Attacks occur during pregnancy and with the administration of exogenous estrogens. Although the molecular mechanism is unknown, C$\bar{1}$INH levels and function are normal, and the 5' flanking region of the gene encoding factor XII, which contains an estrogen response element, is normal.

URTICARIAL VENULITIS Chronic urticaria and angioedema may be manifestations of cutaneous necrotizing venulitis, which is known as *urticarial venulitis.*[24] Associated features include fever, malaise, arthralgia, abdominal pain, and less commonly, conjunctivitis, uveitis, diffuse glomerulonephritis, obstructive and restrictive pulmonary disease, and benign intracranial hypertension (see Chap. 175). Serum complement abnormalities have been reported in some patients with this disorder. The term *hypocomplemententemic urticarial vasculitis syndrome* is used in patients with more severe clinical manifestations of urticarial venulitis with hypocomplementemia and a low-molecular-weight 7S C1q-precipitin that has been identified as an IgG autoantibody directed against the collagen-like region of C1q. Urticarial venulitis also may occur in individuals with serum sickness, connective tissue disorders, hematologic malignant conditions, an IgM$_K$M component, and infections and as an idiopathic disorder.

SERUM SICKNESS Serum sickness, which was defined originally as an adverse reaction that resulted from the administration of heterologous serum to humans, may occur after the administration of drugs. Serum sickness occurs 7 to 21 days after the administration of the offending agent and is manifested by fever, urticaria, lymphadenopathy, myalgia, arthralgia, and arthritis. Symptoms are usually self-limited and last 4 to 5 days. More than 70 percent of patients with serum sickness experience urticaria, which may be pruritic or painful. The initial manifestation of urticaria may appear at the site of injection. It is not clear whether the urticaria is due to IgE antibodies to the offending allergen or to immune complexes that activate the complement system leading to C5a or both.

REACTIONS TO THE ADMINISTRATION OF BLOOD PRODUCTS Urticaria/angioedema may develop after the administration of blood products. It usually is the result of immune complex formation and complement activation that leads to direct vascular and smooth muscle alterations and indirectly, via anaphylatoxins, to mast cell mediator release. This mechanism has been delineated clearly in the case of urticarial or anaphylactic reactions to blood, plasma, or immunoglobulin in patients with antibodies to IgA, which may arise after transfusion or by placental transfer. These antibodies form complexes with donor IgA and may activate the complement system.

Urticarial or anaphylactic reactions to the administration of immunoglobulin do not, however, always depend on antibody to IgA. Aggregates of IgG may activate mast cells by binding to FcγRIII or by activating complement. The intradermal administration of aggregated IgG to humans leads within 10 min to swelling and erythema that becomes tender and persists up to 24 to 48 h. Biopsy specimens of these reactions show neutrophilic infiltrates at 6 and 24 h, with a mononuclear infiltrate appearing at 24 h. The implication that aggregated IgG is responsible for most human reactions is strengthened by the fact that the administration of IgG from which aggregates have been removed is not associated with urticaria or anaphylaxis.

An uncommon mechanism for the development of urticaria after the administration of blood products is the transfusion of IgE of donor origin directed toward an antigen to which the recipient is subsequently exposed. Another mechanism may be the transfusion of a soluble antigen present in the donor preparation into a previously sensitized recipient.

INFECTIONS Episodes of acute urticaria can be associated with upper respiratory tract viral infections, most commonly in children. The acute urticaria resolves within 3 weeks. Hepatitis B virus infection has been associated with episodes of urticaria lasting up to 1 week that are associated with fever and arthralgias as part of the prodrome.

ANGIOTENSIN-CONVERTING ENZYME INHIBITORS Angioedema has been associated with the administration of angiotensin-converting enzyme (ACE) inhibitors.[25] The frequency of angioedema occurring after ACE inhibitor therapy is 0.1 to 0.7 percent. Angioedema develops during the first week of therapy in up to 72 percent of affected individuals and usually involves the head and neck, including the mouth, tongue, pharynx, and larynx. Urticaria occurs only rarely. Cough and angioedema of the gastrointestinal tract are associated features. It has been suggested that therapy with ACE inhibitors is contraindicated in patients with a prior history of idiopathic angioedema, hereditary angioedema, and acquired C1INH deficiency.[25]

The mechanism is believed not to be immunologic because the angioedema may occur within hours of the first dose and may develop after the administration of ACE inhibitors of various structures. The pathobiologic mechanism is believed to be related to the kallikrein-kinin plasma effector system. One hypothesis is that bradykinin, which is normally degraded in part by ACE, accumulates in tissues when an ACE inhibitor is given.

Urticaria/Angioedema after Direct Mast Cell Degranulation

Various therapeutic and diagnostic agents have been associated with urticaria/angioedema. Up to 8 percent of patients receiving radiographic contrast media experience such reactions, which occur most commonly after intravenous administration. Opiate analgesics, polymyxin B, curare, and D-tubocurarine release histamine from mast cells and basophils. Decreased serum alternative pathway complement protein lev-

els and increased serum histamine levels have been detected in patients receiving radiocontrast media. A greater risk for urticaria/angioedema and anaphylactic-like reactions in women is suggested by one study in which 70 percent of those experiencing such a reaction were women.

Urticaria/Angioedema Relating to Abnormalities of Arachidonic Acid Metabolism

Intolerance to aspirin manifested as urticaria/angioedema occurs in otherwise normal individuals or in patients with allergic rhinitis and/or bronchial asthma. Urticaria/angioedema in response to aspirin and nonsteroidal anti-inflammatory drugs (NSAIDs) occurred in approximately 10 to 20 percent of individuals referred to a hospital dermatology clinic in the United Kingdom. Patients intolerant of aspirin also may react to indomethacin and to other NSAIDs.

Reactions to aspirin are shared with other NSAIDs because they reflect inhibition of prostaglandin endoperoxide synthase 1 (PGHS-1, cyclooxygenase 1) rather than inhibition of the inducible PGHS-2 (cyclooxygenase 2). Sodium salicylate and choline salicylate generally are well tolerated because of their weak activity against PGHS-1. In a single-blind, placebo-controlled oral provocation study with PGHS-2 inhibitors in 82 patients with urticaria and angioedema who were intolerant to NSAIDs, 74.5 percent were cross-reactors.[26] The reaction rates were 33.3 percent for celecoxib, 21.3 percent for nimesulide, 17.3 percent for meloxicam, and 3.0 percent for rofecoxib. Reactions to NSAIDs increase the levels of cysteinyl leukotrienes,[27] which may relate to the appearance of urticaria, although their role in NSAID-induced asthma is better characterized. Prick skin tests are of no diagnostic value, passive transfer reactions are negative, and neither IgG nor IgE antibodies have been associated with clinical disease. The clinical manifestations elicited by aspirin challenge of aspirin-intolerant patients are blocked when such patients are protected with a cysteinyl leukotriene receptor blocker or biosynthetic inhibitor; this finding confirms a pathobiologic role for the cysteinyl leukotrienes rather than acetylation of PGHS-2 by aspirin. However, in two patients with aspirin-induced urticaria, the administration of a cysteinyl leukotriene receptor 1 antagonist provoked urticaria.[28]

Idiopathic Urticaria/Angioedema

In at least 70 percent of individuals with chronic idiopathic urticaria/angioedema, the cause is unknown. Because this clinical entity is common, has a capricious course, and is recognized easily, it is frequently associated with concomitant events. Such attributions must be interpreted with caution. Although infections, metabolic and hormonal abnormalities, malignant conditions, and emotional factors have been claimed as causes, proof of their etiologic relationship often is lacking. In a meta-analysis of chronic idiopathic urticaria and *Helicobacter pylori* infection,[29] resolution of the urticaria was four times more likely when the *H. pylori* infection was eradicated successfully by antibiotic therapy than when it was not. However, only one-third of patients with chronic urticaria will undergo remission with successful eradication of infection. The hypothesis that urticaria is associated with internal malignant disease has been based primarily on anecdotal reports. There is no convincing evidence to support a causal relationship.

Although idiopathic urticaria/angioedema is the most prevalent form, the diagnosis remains one of exclusion. Cyclic episodic angioedema with urticaria/angioedema has been associated with fever, weight gain, absence of internal organ damage, a benign course, and peripheral blood eosinophilia.[30] Biopsy specimens of tissues show eosinophils, eosinophil granule proteins, and CD4 lymphocytes exhibiting HLA-DR. Blood levels of IL-1, soluble IL-2 receptor, and IL-5 are elevated.

LABORATORY FINDINGS

The evaluation of patients (Table 116-3) with urticaria/angioedema begins with a comprehensive history, with particular emphasis on the recognized causes, and a physical examination. Some varieties of urticaria may be identified by their characteristic appearance, such as the small wheals with a large erythematous flare of cholinergic urticaria, the linear wheals in dermographism, and the localization of lesions to exposed areas in light- or cold-induced urticaria. If suggested by the history, the physical examination in all patients with urticaria should include tests for physical urticaria, such as a brisk stroke to elicit dermographism, the use of a weight to elicit delayed pressure urticaria, and application of a cold or warm stimulus for cold-induced urticaria and localized heat urticaria, respectively. Exercise, such as running in place, may elicit cholinergic urticaria and, in some instances, exercise-induced anaphylaxis. Phototests to elicit solar urticaria usually are performed in referral centers, as are challenges for exercise-induced anaphylaxis.

In most patients with chronic urticaria/angioedema, no underlying disorders or causes can be discerned. Diagnostic studies should be based on findings elicited by the history and physical examination. There is no recommended diagnostic laboratory evaluation for chronic urticaria/angioedema, and routine screening laboratory tests are of no value.[31] Serum hypocomplementemia is not present in chronic idiopathic urticaria, and mean levels of serum IgE are normal.

Cryoproteins should be sought in patients with acquired cold urticaria. An antinuclear antibody test should be obtained in patients with solar urticaria. Autoantibodies to thyroglobulin and peroxidase may be present in individuals with autoimmune thyroid disease and urticaria/angioedema; routine screening in patients with chronic urticaria for thyroid autoimmunity is suggested by some investigators but not by others. Assessment of serum complement proteins may be helpful in identifying patients with urticarial venulitis, as well as those with hereditary and acquired forms of $C\bar{1}$INH deficiency.

Skin biopsy of chronic urticarial lesions should be undertaken only to identify urticarial venulitis.

TABLE 116-3

Investigation of Chronic Idiopathic Urticaria/Angioedema

In all patients
- History and physical examination
- Provocative tests for physical urticarias

In selected patients
- Complete blood count with differential analysis
- Erythrocyte sedimentation rate
- Urinalysis
- Blood chemistry profile
- Stool examination for ova and parasites
- Hepatitis B virus surface antigen and hepatitis B and C antibodies
- Thyroid microsomal and peroxidase antibodies
- Antinuclear factor
- Cryoproteins
- Skin tests for IgE-mediated reactions
- Radioallergosorbent test (RAST) for specific IgE
- Skin biopsy

There is little role for routine prick skin testing or the radioallergosorbent test (RAST) in the diagnosis of specific IgE-mediated antigen sensitivity in chronic urticaria/angioedema. Inhalant materials are uncommon causes of urticaria/angioedema, and food skin tests may be difficult to interpret. The tests for drugs are limited to penicillin but cannot be performed in patients with dermographism. The RAST should be reserved for those in whom skin testing is contraindicated, unavailable, or unrevealing despite a highly suspected history. Use of the autologous serum skin test to seek autoantibodies to FcεRIα or IgE remains a research technique.

The release of histamine from peripheral basophilic leukocytes has supported the diagnosis of anaphylactic sensitivity to a variety of antigens, which include pollens and insect venom, and may suggest the presence of a FcεRIα autoantibody, but this assay also remains a research technique.

PATHOLOGY

Edema involving the superficial portion of the dermis is characteristic of urticaria, whereas angioedema involves the deeper dermis and subcutaneous tissue. Both disorders are associated with dilation of the venules. Mast cell numbers are comparable in lesional and nonlesional skin of patients with chronic idiopathic urticaria and are not different from the numbers in control skin of unaffected individuals, although in a few studies mast cell numbers were observed to be increased in the lesional skin of patients with chronic idiopathic urticaria.

In chronic idiopathic urticaria, the dermal infiltrating inflammatory cells may be sparse or dense in amount and include more CD4 than CD8 T lymphocytes, neutrophils, eosinophils, and basophils[32,33] without B lymphocytes or natural killer (NK) cells. In some specimens, neutrophils are the predominant cell type. Increased expression of TNF-α and IL-3 on endothelial cells and perivascular cells was detected in the upper dermis of patients with acute urticaria, chronic idiopathic urticaria, and delayed-pressure urticaria and in one patient with cold urticaria.[34] TNF-α also was detected on epidermal keratinocytes in lesional and nonlesional biopsy specimens. In chronic idiopathic urticaria, CD11b and CD18 cells were detected about the blood vessels in the superficial and deep dermis. Direct immunofluorescence tests for immunoglobulins and complement proteins were negative.

Major basic protein and eosinophil cationic protein (ECP), which are derived from the eosinophil granule, are present around blood vessels and are dispersed in the dermis in lesions of acute urticaria, chronic idiopathic urticaria, delayed-pressure urticaria, cholinergic urticaria, and solar urticaria. In chronic idiopathic urticaria, free eosinophil granules in the dermis were increased in wheals of greater than 24 h duration as compared with wheals lasting fewer than 24 h. The secreted form of ECP and eosinophil-derived neurotoxin were detected on cells in greater amounts in biopsy specimens from patients with chronic idiopathic urticaria without autoantibodies as compared with those with autoantibodies. P-selectin, E-selectin, intercellular adhesion molecule 1 (ICAM-1), and VCAM-1 have been demonstrated on the vascular endothelium of patients with chronic idiopathic urticaria and dermographism. Major histocompatability complex (MHC) class II antigen also is upregulated on the endothelial cells of patients with chronic idiopathic urticaria, and the peripheral blood lymphocytes have increased CD40 ligand expression and higher Bcl-2 expression; these observations suggest an augmentation of autoimmune phenomena.[35]

In papular urticaria, the epidermis is thick, with intercellular edema and lymphocytes. In the dermis, there is edema with an infiltrate containing T lymphocytes, macrophages, eosinophils, and neutrophils without B lymphocytes or the deposition of immunoglobulins, fibrin, and C3.

DIAGNOSIS AND DIFFERENTIAL DIAGNOSIS

Urticaria and angioedema are easily recognizable disorders. Urticarial eruptions are episodic and evanescent, with multiple lesions occurring in various stages of evolution and resolution. Seldom do individual urticarial lesions persist for more than 48 h except in patients with urticarial venulitis. Angioedema may persist for several days. Several disorders are included in the differential diagnosis. Edematous, papulovesicular, or bullous eruptions with mucosal involvement and typical iris, or target, lesions characterize erythema multiforme. One or more annular, edematous plaques that may expand in diameter (erythema migrans) occur in Lyme borreliosis. Edematous and erythematous plaques that are indolent with or without bullae are features of bullous pemphigoid. Urticaria pigmentosa is a generalized, red-brown, macular, papular, or nodular mast cell infiltration in which the skin lesions become edematous when rubbed. The syndrome of perceptive deafness, fever with urticaria, and renal insufficiency consequent to amyloidosis is readily excluded.

Cellulitis, congestive heart failure, renal insufficiency, myxedema, thrombophlebitis, the superior vena cava syndrome, and the Melkersson-Rosenthal syndrome should be considered as causes for edematous processes resembling angioedema.

TREATMENT (Table 116-4)

The pathobiologic areas at which the treatment of urticaria and angioedema are directed include the initiating stimulus, effector cells and their inflammatory mediators, and receptor sites on target tissues. Therapy directed at mast cells involves blocking the release or generation of mediators or the effects of released mediators. Release can be blocked by stabilizing the membrane and by modulating cyclic nucleotide levels or calcium flux. Therapy also can be directed at other effector cells, such as lymphocytes. In one study, allergists and dermatologists were demonstrated to have more expertise in caring for patients with urticaria/angioedema than other specialists. Allergists were the least likely to use a systemic glucocorticoid (6 percent of visits), whereas internists were the most likely (29 percent of visits).[1]

The ideal treatment for urticaria/angioedema is identification and removal of its cause. Many patients with acute urticaria and angioedema probably are not treated by physicians because the cause is identified by the individual or the course is limited. Treatment of chronic idiopathic urticaria focuses on measures that provide symptomatic relief. The physician should provide not only medications but also support and reassurance. In a questionnaire study, patients with chronic idiopathic urticaria considered the worst aspects to be pruritus and the unpredictable nature of the attacks.[36] Affected individuals reported sleep disturbances, diminished energy, social isolation, and altered emotional reactions as well as difficulties in relation to work, home activities, social life, and sex life. Another study showed a correlation between the severity of chronic idiopathic urticaria and depression. In a questionnaire study, individuals with delayed-pressure urticaria and cholinergic urticaria had the most quality-of-life impairment.[37] Those with cholinergic urticaria suffered in relation to their sporting activities and sexual relationships. Although urticaria/angioedema may be a source of frustration to both physicians and patients, most individuals can achieve acceptable symptomatic control of their disease without identification of the cause. In some individuals it is important to avoid aspirin and other NSAIDs. Antipruritic lotions, cool compresses, and ice packs may provide temporary relief.

H_1-type antihistaminic drugs are the mainstays in the management of urticaria/angioedema (see Chap. 258). The older H_1-type antihistamines are known as classic, traditional, or first-generation H_1-type antihistamines. Newer, low-sedating, or second- and third-generation H_1-type antihistamines with reduced sedative and anticholinergic side effects have become the initial therapeutic agents of choice. Antihistaminic agents should be administered initially at a low dose and increased to tolerance. The drug should be taken on a regular basis and not as needed. If the initial drug chosen is ineffective, an agent from a different pharmacologic class should be used. If the initial drug chosen is partially beneficial, an agent from a different pharmacologic class can be added. Thus combinations of agents from different classes may be used. The combination of H_1- and H_2 antihistamines may benefit a few patients with chronic idiopathic urticaria. The tricyclic antidepressant doxepin, which has activity against both H_1 and H_2 histamine receptors, may be useful. Terbutaline, a β-adrenergic agonist, in combination with an H_1-type antihistamine, has been reported to benefit a few patients with chronic idiopathic urticaria. Although clinical trials have been carried out with many of the H_1-type antihistamines, in many instances the therapeutic approaches are based on clinical experience.

For patients with refractory, chronic idiopathic urticaria who have failed to benefit from conventional therapy, novel and anecdotal therapeutic measures may be considered. Nifedipine has been shown in a double-blind crossover study to be useful as an adjunctive therapeutic agent with H_1 antihistamines. In open trials, zafirlukast and montelukast had beneficial responses,[38] and zileuton was used successfully in some patients. In a double-blind, placebo-controlled trial, the combination of montelukast and cetirizine was of benefit to patients with intolerance to food additives or acetylsalicylic acid.[39] In a study of 18 patients with chronic idiopathic urticaria, the addition of zafirlukast or montelukast to an H_1 antihistamine was beneficial.[40] In a single female who experienced urticaria after treatment with piroxicam, zafirlukast prevented a flare of urticaria on subsequent use of piroxicam.[41] Stanozolol and sulfasalazine[42] have been of benefit in some patients with chronic idiopathic urticaria. One report suggested that colchicine in combination with an H_1 antihistamine was of value to 5 of 7 patients with chronic idiopathic urticaria, in which the dermal infiltrate is rich in neutrophils and eosinophils. Cyclosporine was effective in chronic idiopathic urticaria in a randomized, double-blind study[43]; however, the appropriate dose has not yet been determined.[44] Methotrexate was used in 3 patients with benefit. Plasmapheresis was of value in patients with circulating autoantibodies, but relapse occurred as the antibody formed again. Intravenous immunoglobulin was of limited benefit in a few patients.[45] In one study, the use of narrow-band UVB phototherapy achieved improvement in 71 percent and resolution in 28 percent of patients

TABLE 116-4

An Approach to the Management of Chronic Urticaria/Angioedema

- Identification and removal of precipitating cause when possible
- Administration of H_1 antihistamines with empirical trials of each pharmacologic subclass
- Various combination of H_1 antihistamines
- Administration of H_1 and H_2 antihistamines
- Addition of a β-adrenergic agonist to an H_1 antihistamine
- Avoidance of epinephrine except in instances of respiratory tract compromise or cardiovascular collapse
- Alternate-day systemic glucocorticoids and trials of novel and anecdotal therapeutic agents in refractory disease

with chronic idiopathic urticaria.[46] The subcutaneous administration of interferon α in two controlled trials was of no benefit. In one study of 7 euthyroid patients with thyroid autoantibodies and chronic idiopathic urticaria, all experienced resolution within 4 weeks after the administration of thyroxine. In 5 of the 7 patients, the urticaria recurred after the treatment was discontinued. In a few individuals, hypnosis may be useful. Acupuncture has been reported to be of benefit in the treatment of urticaria in Asia.

The use of prednisone in the management of acute urticaria has been advocated in emergency rooms, but this form of therapy should not be routine. Epinephrine is used widely, particularly in hospital emergency departments, but its use is indicated only in cases of laryngeal edema or cardiovascular collapse. Systemic glucocorticoids have no place in the regular therapy of chronic idiopathic urticaria. When glucocorticoids are used, alternate-day administration is recommended. Prednisone is used at a dose of 15 to 20 mg every other day and is tapered gradually by 2.5 to 5.0 mg every 3 weeks, depending on the patient's response. At that rate, it often can be discontinued in a 4- to 5-month period. The alternate-day dose rarely exceeds 20 mg of prednisone or its equivalent. Side effects are minimized with dietary discretion and exercise. Patients requiring alternate-day glucocorticoids beyond this period should be examined annually by an ophthalmologist for cataracts or glaucoma, and a bone density scan is obtained to seek osteoporosis.

In the treatment of the physical urticarias, patient education and avoidance of the inciting stimulus are important. Most forms of physical urticaria are treated with antihistamines. Induction of refractoriness has been achieved in some patients with primary acquired cold urticaria, solar urticaria, and local heat urticaria. In cholinergic urticaria, hydroxyzine and cetirizine are the initial agents of choice. In anecdotal reports and in small numbers of patients in open trials, delayed-pressure urticaria may respond to NSAIDs, dapsone, cetirizine, sulfasalazine, and systemic glucocorticoids but not to colchicine and uncommonly to H_1 antihistamines. During hypothermic cardiopulmonary bypass, cold urticaria was managed successfully with the administration of H_1 and H_2 antihistamines. Plasmapheresis has been used successfully in patients with solar urticaria with a circulating photoallergen. Propranolol hydrochloride may prevent attacks of adrenergic urticaria. A few patients with some forms of physical urticaria have responded to treatment with broadband UVB phototherapy and PUVA photochemotherapy. In exercise-induced anaphylaxis, there are no controlled therapeutic trials. Although treatment for acute exercise-induced anaphylaxis is the same as that for anaphylaxis of any cause, an important aspect of therapy is modification of exercise programs and food intake.

In hereditary angioedema, therapy is directed toward treatment of the acute attack, to preoperative and dental prophylaxis, and to chronic prophylactic suppression of attacks (see Chap. 117).

The role of dietary manipulation in urticaria/angioedema is difficult to assess. Information gained from the routine trial of elimination diets may be confusing due to the placebo effect and the variability of the course of urticaria. It is generally thought that if a food is truly responsible for exacerbation of urticaria, its ingestion should be followed routinely by lesions within 2 h. In addition to foods, ingested preservatives, food colorings, and natural salicylates in foods may be responsible for the genesis or aggravation of chronic idiopathic urticaria, although these associations may be spurious.

REFERENCES

1. Henderson RL Jr et al: Allergists and dermatologists have far more expertise in caring for patients with urticaria than other specialists. *J Am Acad Dermatol* **43**:1084, 2000
2. Weidner C et al: Acute effects of substance P and calcitonin gene-related peptide in human skin: A microdialysis study. *J Invest Dermatol* **115**:1015, 2000
3. Petersen LJ et al: Histamine is released in the wheal but not the flare following challenge of human skin in vivo: A microdialysis study. *Clin Exp Allergy* **27**:284, 1997
4. Turktas I et al: The association of chronic urticaria and angioedema with autoimmune thyroiditis. *Int J Dermatol* **36**:187, 1997
5. Ferrer M et al: Comparative studies of functional and binding assays for IgG anti-FcεRIα (α-subunit) in chronic urticaria. *J Allergy Clin Immunol* **101**:672, 1998
6. Fiebiger E et al: Anti-FcεRIα autoantibodies in autoimmune-mediated disorders: Identification of a structure-function relationship. *J Clin Invest* **101**:243, 1998
7. Kikuchi Y, Kaplan AP: Mechanisms of autoimmune activation of basophils in chronic urticaria. *J Allergy Clin Immunol* **107**:1056, 2001
8. Kikuchi Y, Kaplan AP: A role for C5a in augmenting IgG-dependent histamine release from basophils in chronic urticaria. *J Allergy Clin Immunol* **109**:114, 2002
9. Hanau A et al: Functional thyroid peroxidase autoantibodies of IgE class in patients with chronic urticaria. *J Invest Dermatol* **117**:776, 2001
10. Tedeschi A et al: Anti-thyroid peroxidase IgE in patients with chronic urticaria. *J Allergy Clin Immunol* **108**:467, 2001
11. O'Donnell BF et al: Human leukocyte antigen class II associations in chronic idiopathic urticaria. *Br J Dermatol* **140**:853, 1999
12. Gorevic PD, Kaplan AP: The physical urticarias. *Int J Dermatol* **19**:417, 1980
13. Soter NA: Physical urticaria/angioedema. *Semin Dermatol* **6**:302, 1987
14. Hoffman HM et al: Familial cold autoinflammatory syndrome: Phenotype and genotype of an autosomal dominant periodic fever. *J Allergy Clin Immunol* **108**:615, 2001
15. Hoffman HM et al: Mutation of a new gene encoding a putative pyrin-like protein causes familial cold autoinflammatory syndrome and Muckle-Wells syndrome. *Nature Genet* **29**:301, 2001
16. Uetsu N et al: The clinical and photobiological characteristics of solar urticaria in 40 patients. *Br J Dermatol* **142**:32, 2000
17. Harada S et al: Aspirin enhances the induction of type I allergic symptoms when combined with food and exercise in patients with food-dependent exercise-induced anaphylaxis. *Br J Dermatol* **145**:336, 2001
18. Shadick NA et al: The natural history of exercise-induced anaphylaxis: Survey results from a 10-year follow-up study. *J Allergy Clin Immunol* **104**:123, 1999
19. Luong KV, Mguyen LT: Aquagenic urticaria: Report of a case and review of the literature. *Ann Allergy Asthma Immunol* **80**:483, 1998
20. Sabroe RA et al: The autologous serum skin test: A screening test for autoantibodies in chronic idiopathic urticaria. *Br J Dermatol* **140**:446, 1999
21. Sabroe RA et al: Chronic idiopathic urticaria: Comparison of the clinical features of patients with and without anti-FcεRI or anti-IgE autoantibodies. *J Am Acad Dermatol* **40**:443, 1999
22. Bork K et al: Hereditary angioedema with normal C1-inhibitor activity in women. *Lancet* **356**:213, 2000
23. Binkley KE, Davis A III: Clinical, biochemical, and genetic characterization of a novel estrogen-dependent inherited form of angioedema. *J Allergy Clin Immunol* **106**:546, 2000
24. Soter NA: Urticarial venulitis. *Derm Ther* **13**:400,2000
25. Sabroe RA, Kobza Black A: Angiotensin-converting enzyme (ACE) inhibitors and angio-oedema. *Br J Dermatol* **136**:153, 1997
26. Sanchez Borges M et al: Tolerability to new COX-2 inhibitors in NSAID-sensitive patients with cutaneous reactions. *Ann Allergy Asthma Immunol* **87**:201, 2001
27. Israel E et al: The pivotal role of 5-lipoxygenase products in the reaction of aspirin-sensitive asthmatics to aspirin. *Am Rev Respir Dis* **148**:1447, 1993
28. Ohnishi-Inoue Y et al: Aspirin-sensitive urticaria: Provocation with a leukotriene receptor antagonist. *Br J Dermatol* **138**:483, 1998
29. Federman DG et al: The effect of antibiotic therapy for *H. pylori*–infected patients with chronic urticaria. *J Am Acad Dermatol* (in press)
30. Gleich GJ et al: Episodic angioedema associated with eosinophilia. *New Engl J Med* **310**:1621, 1984
31. Kozel MMA et al: The effectiveness of a history-based diagnostic approach in chronic urticaria and angioedema. *Arch Dermatol* **134**:1575, 1998
32. Hoskin SL et al: Basophil infiltration of wheals in chronic idiopathic urticaria. *J Allergy Clin Immunol* **109**:587, 2002
33. Ying S et al: T_h1/T_h2 cytokines and cell infiltration in skin from chronic idiopathic urticaria: Comparison with allergen-induced skin late-phase reactions and normal controls. *J Allergy Clin Immunol* **109**:S88, 2002

34. Hermes B et al: Upregulation of tumor necrosis factor α and interleukin-3 expression in lesional and uninvolved skin in different types of urticaria. *J Allergy Clin Immunol* **103**:307, 1999
35. Toubi E et al: Immune aberrations in B and T lymphocytes derived from chronic urticaria patients. *J Clin Immunol* **20**:371, 2000
36. O'Donnell BF et al: The impact of chronic urticaria on the quality of life. *Br J Dermatol* **136**:197, 1997
37. Poon E et al: The extent and nature of disability in different urticarial conditions. *Br J Dermatol* **140**:667, 1999
38. Nettis E et al: Comparison of montelukast and fexofenadine for chronic idiopathic urticaria. *Arch Dermatol* **137**:99, 2001
39. Pacor ML et al: Efficacy of leukotriene receptor antagonist in chronic urticaria: A double-blind, placebo-controlled comparison of treatment with montelukast and cetirizine in patients with chronic urticaria with intolerance to food additive and/or acetylsalicylic acid. *Clin Exp Allergy* **31**:1607, 2001
40. Bensch G, Borish L: Leukotriene modifiers in chronic urticaria. *Ann Allergy Asthma Immunol* **83**:348, 1999

41. Asero R: Leukotriene receptor antagonists may prevent NSAID-induced exacerbations in patients with chronic urticaria. *Ann Allergy Asthma Immunol* **85**:156, 2000
42. Jaffer AM et al: Sulfasalazine in the treatment of chronic urticaria (CU). *J Allergy Clin Immunol* **109**:S127, 2002
43. Grattan CEH et al: Randomized double-blind study of cyclosporine in chronic "idiopathic" urticaria. *Br J Dermatol* **143**:365, 2000
44. Toubi E et al: Low-dose cyclosporin A in the treatment of severe chronic idiopathic urticaria. *Allergy* **52**:312, 1997
45. O'Donnell BF et al: Intravenous immunoglobulin in autoimmune chronic urticaria. *Br J Dermatol* **138**:101, 1998
46. Clark C et al: TI-01 phototherapy for chronic idiopathic urticaria: 14 years' experience. *Br J Dermatol* **145**(suppl.59):136, 2001

CHAPTER 117

Irma Gigli
Fred S. Rosen

Angioedema Associated with Complement Abnormalities

Angioedema is a reaction characterized by swellings of the subcutaneous tissue that occurs in the skin and the mucosae, including those of the respiratory and gastrointestinal tracts. In certain patients, angioedema and urticaria may present with abnormalities of the serum complement system. This presentation is seen most often with an underlying cutaneous necrotizing venulitis or systemic lupus erythematosus, after the injection of blood products or the administration of diagnostic agents, or in the presence of a number of autoantibodies. Angioedema/urticaria without complement abnormalities may occur in association with antigen-initiated IgE-dependent reactions, anti-IgE, or anti-Fc_{ε} receptor 1 autoantibodies; with reactions to non-steroidal anti-inflammatory agents; or with contact and physical stimuli. It also may occur without apparent cause.[1] Less frequently, angioedema is caused by a genetic or acquired defect in the inhibitor of the activated first component of the complement system (C1INH). The genetic deficiency of C1INH results in the disease termed *hereditary angioedema* (HAE). A nonhereditary form of C1INH deficiency designated *acquired C1INH deficiency* (or acquired angioedema, AAE) may be due to a monoclonal B cell disease or to autoantibodies to C1INH.[2] Urticaria does not accompany the angioedema in patients with the genetic or acquired deficiency of C1INH.

CLASSIFICATION AND CLINICAL MANIFESTATIONS (Table 117-1)

Hereditary Angioedema (Genetic C1INH Deficiency)

HAE is a rare form of angioedema with life-threatening consequences. It was described initially by Robert Graves in 1843. In 1882, Quincke reported circumscribed swellings occurring in members of two consecutive generations of the same family. Osler pointed out that angioedema, in certain instances, seems to adhere to a clear pattern of inheritance; he named this entity *hereditary angioneurotic edema*. Landerman et al.[3] reported a biochemical abnormality in HAE, observing that individuals with this disease were unusually reactive to the intracutaneous injection of a kallikrein. Simultaneously, Donaldson and

TABLE 117-1

Classification of Angioedema

- Normal or elevated serum complement levels
  - IgE mediated (atopic, specific antigen, exercise)
  - Induced by physical agents (cold pressure)
  - Induced by aspirin and nonsteroidal anti-inflammatory agents
  - Dyes, contrast media
  - Opiates
  - Polyanionic antibiotics
- Low serum complement levels
  - Low C1INH (protein, function, or both)
    - Genetic (HAE)
      - C1INH deficiency type I (no protein)
      - C1INH deficiency type II (dysfunctional protein)
    - Acquired (AAE)
      - Lymphoproliferative disorders (type I, low protein)
      - Anti-C1INH antibodies (type II, dysfunctional protein)
  - Normal C1INH
    - Serum sickness
    - Blood products reactions
    - Necrotizing vasculitis
    - Idiosyncratic
    - Dyes, contrast media

Evans[4] demonstrated that the sera of such patients lacked the protein C1INH. It was established subsequently that this inhibitor also was active against kallikrein.[5] Although HAE is believed to account for only a small fraction of all cases of angioedema, it is the most common disorder caused by the deficiency of a complement protein.

Clinically, HAE is characterized by recurrent, circumscribed, nonpruritic, nonpitting, subepithelial edema (see Fig 116-2). Cutaneous angioedema may develop over several hours at any given site and may be preceded by a faint macular or serpiginous erythema. Patients frequently are aware of a peculiar tingling or twitching sensation in the affected area. The skin swells progressively within hours, returning to normal in 24 to 72 hours. The lesions may involve an area a few centimeters in diameter or may evolve to include an entire extremity. Swelling of the face and lips may progress to involve the upper airways. The patients do not have urticaria associated with the angioedema.[6]

All patients with cutaneous manifestations report varying degrees of intestinal symptoms. Recurrent abdominal pain in multiple family members has been reported as the sole manifestation of HAE.[7] Angioedema of the small bowel frequently is associated with colicky, severe abdominal pain without fever or leukocytosis. When the large intestine is involved, copious watery diarrhea may ensue. Hemoconcentration is evidenced by an increased hematocrit and prerenal azotemia. During these abdominal crises, undiagnosed patients frequently are subjected to unnecessary exploratory laparotomies. Other associated symptoms frequently observed are urinary retention and central nervous system involvement, including severe headaches, transient aphasia, and hemiplegia.

The onset of HAE is extremely variable. Most patients date the initial appearance of their symptoms to early childhood and become dramatically worse at pubescence. However, symptoms can begin in the second decade of life and even later. Most commonly, the attacks decrease in frequency and severity after age 50 and may even disappear.[2] The precipitating factors are not clear. Patients state that attacks of angioedema follow minor trauma to any body part, and some recognize an association with extreme heat or cold, vigorous exercise, and infections. Some female patients note an increase in the frequency of attacks during menses and while they are taking birth control pills. In contrast, most women report a marked decrease in the frequency of attacks during the last two trimesters of pregnancy. Most menopausal females do not improve. The term *hereditary angioneurotic edema* was used because affected individuals are known to respond to stress with an episode of angioedema. Evaluation of a large number of these patients reveals no increase in psychiatric disorders. Systemic lupus erythematosus, lupus-like disorders, and Sjögron's syndrome have been diagnosed in members of families with HAE.[1,8–10]

GENETICS OF C1INH DEFICIENCY HAE is inherited as an autosomal dominant trait. Each patient is heterozygous for the defect; thus every affected individual has an affected and a normal parent. There is no linkage with the human leukocyte antigen system, and there is no sex preference. About 10 percent of patients have new mutations and two normal parents, but these mutations are transmitted to their offspring in a Mendelian dominant fashion.[11]

There are two genetic variants of HAE.[12,13] In the more common form (type I), between 5 and 30 percent of the normal antigenic and functional C1INH protein is present in the blood, whereas in the less common form (type II), a normal or increased amount of an abnormal, dysfunctional C1INH protein is found together with low levels of the normal protein. Of patients with HAE, 85 percent have type I and 15 percent have type II.[13] Patients with type I HAE have one normally expressed C1INH gene and one deleted or non-expressed abnormal gene. Patients with type II HAE have one normal gene and one expressed abnormal gene with missense mutations that result in the synthesis of a dysfunctional protein. One family has been identified in which the disease is transmitted as an autosomal recessive trait due to a mutation in the promoter region of the gene.[14]

The gene encoding the C1INH maps to the long arm of chromosome 11.2-q13.[15,16] It encodes a single-chain protein composed of 478 amino acid residues. The secreted protein is cleaved by various serum proteases at an arginine-threonine bond between residues 444 and 445.[16] The carboxyl-terminal 33 amino acids are set free, and this peptide has no known biologic function. Mutations are found throughout the 12 exons of the *C1INH* gene. In type II HAE, the mutations are almost exclusively at or around the bait site Arg^{444}–Thr^{445}.[17] Arginine is usually substituted by a histidine[18] or a cysteine[19] and renders the inhibitor nonfunctional. Other mutations have been found in the hydrophobic amino acid residues just amino-terminal to the arginine at position 444.[20] These mutations apparently distort the tertiary structure of the C1INH in a hydrophobic region that is critical for maintaining the binding site exposed and determining the substrate specificity. A mutant protein with a substitution at position 443 (Ala^{443}–Val) has diminished inhibitory activity toward C1r and C1s but normal activity toward contact system proteases.[21] One other mutation is due to deletion of a lysine codon at residue 251. The lysine deletion creates a glycosylation signal that appears to distort the conformation of the molecule.[22] In type I HAE there are nonsense mutations resulting in premature stop codons. Twenty percent of patients have unequal crossovers between Alu sequences in the introns.[23,24] Deletions and duplications in the gene occur in other cases of HAE.[25]

The sequence of the C1INH, as determined by the combination of protein and DNA sequence analysis, shows that it belongs to the superfamily of protease inhibitors called *serpins.*[15,16] It has 40 to 50 percent amino acid sequence homology with antithrombin III and α_1-antitrypsin, but it differs from the other serpins in that it is heavily glycosylated. The functional role of this carbohydrate-rich domain is unknown.

C1INH is synthesized mainly in hepatocytes, but it also can be synthesized in blood monocytes, skin fibroblasts, and umbilical endothelial cells. The expression of C1INH in vivo is enhanced by androgens, and in vitro synthesis can be upregulated greatly by interferon-γ and interleukin 6 (IL-6).[26] As a result of the presence of a single functional gene,[22] the rate of synthesis of C1INH in cells of patients with HAE is only 30 to 40 percent of normal.[27] When the turnover of radiolabeled C1INH is measured in patients with HAE, the fractional catabolic rate is found to be almost twice normal.[28] Thus the decreased synthesis of C1INH is inadequate to maintain the equilibrium in the spontaneous activation of the complement system as well as other proteolytic enzymes. The activation of these enzymes results in increased C1INH consumption. For these reasons, patients with HAE have far less than the anticipated 50 percent of normal C1INH in their sera. Functionally, C1INH inhibits the activation of the first component of complement (C1) and the esteratic activity of two of its subcomponents, C1r and C1s. Although C1INH is the only serum inhibitor of these complement proteins, it also inhibits factors XIa, XIIa, and XIIf, kallikrein, and plasmin.[5,29]

MECHANISM OF INCREASED VASCULAR PERMEABILITY IN HAE A number of studies have implicated the activation of the classical pathway of the complement system as the mechanism of angioedema.[2] During attacks, activated C1s can be detected in fluids from the involved area, and the natural substrates of C1, complement proteins C4 and C2, are cleaved, thus resulting in markedly reduced blood levels of these proteins.[30] Because this activation occurs in the body fluids rather than on antigen-antibody aggregates, the concentrations of C3 and the late-acting complement components (C5 to C9) usually are normal. The reason for the episodic activation of C1 during attacks remains unclear. C1 may be activated by enzymes such as factor XIIa and plasmin.[31] The capacity of C1INH to inhibit these enzymes

FIGURE 117-1

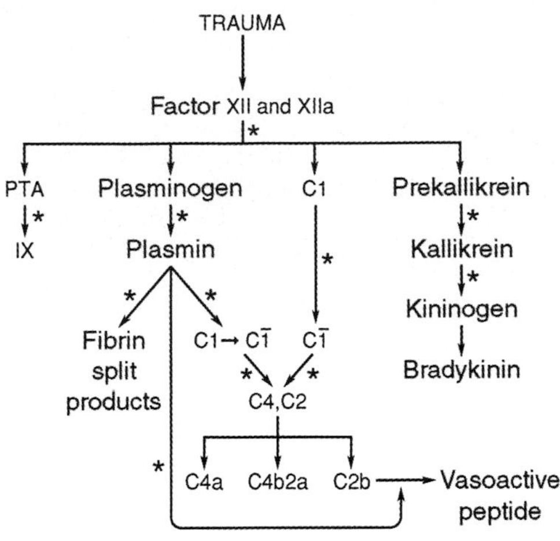

Sites of action of C1INH in the contact phase of coagulation, fibrinolysis, kinin generation, and complement activation. PTA, plasma thromboplastin antecedent; C1̄, activated C1. Deficiency of C1INH leads to the generation of bradykinin and a complement-derived vasoactive peptide.

suggests that the activation of factor XII in traumatized tissues may be responsible for the further activation of C1 (Fig. 117-1).

Multiple clinical studies support the view that uninhibited C1 can elicit angioedema. The intradermal injection of C1s into normal persons induces local edema that is not painful and does not itch.[32] The active site of C1s is required for this activity. Individuals deficient in C2 fail to respond, whereas one C3-deficient patient responded normally. Plasma obtained from patients with HAE during asymptomatic intervals spontaneously generates smooth muscle contracting activity during incubation; this activity is associated with a heat-stable kinin-like polypeptide.[33] The generation of this peptide is inhibited by addition to the plasma of purified C1INH, heparin, or antibodies to C4 and C2 but not by antibodies to C3. The polypeptide enhances vascular permeability when injected intradermally and causes histamine release from mast cells in vitro.[34] However, neither antihistamines nor histamine-depleting substances such as 48/80 inhibit the angioedema induced by the local injection of activated C1s or the polypeptide. Furthermore, a kinin-like peptide has been generated from mixtures of purified C1s, C4, C2, and plasmin; the requirement for C4 was abrogated by a large input of C2. Other studies have shown that plasmin releases several small peptides from C2 cleaved by C1s (C2b) with kinin activity and the ability to increase vascular permeability.[34] Moreover, a 38-amino-acid fragment released from the carboxyl terminal portion of C2b can cause angioedema. This peptide differs from bradykinin in size, electrophoretic mobility, isoelectric point, and susceptibility to trypsin.

Other studies suggest that the source of the kinin-like activity in HAE plasma is bradykinin rather than C2. This hypothesis is based on the following observations: The levels of bradykinin and cleaved high-molecular-weight kininogen are elevated in the plasma of patients with angioedema, and plasma levels of factor XIIa are significantly increased during attacks.[35–37] The intracutaneous injection of small amounts of factor XIIa (Hageman factor) induces a localized increase in vascular permeability. Blister fluid obtained from suction blisters induced in the skin of patients with HAE contain large amounts of kallikrein.[35] Moreover, members of a family with a mutant C1INH (Ala^{443}–Val) that inhibits the proteases of the kinin-forming system but is a poor inhibitor of C1r and C1s have not developed angioedema.[20]

Further evidence for the role of bradykinin in HAE has been obtained from studies with mice genetically deficient in the *C1INH* gene or in both the *C1INH* gene and the bradykinin 2 receptor (*Bk2R*) gene.[38] The C1INH deficiency results in increased vascular permeability that could be reversed with the infusion of C1INH, whereas the animals deficient in the *C1INH* and *Bk2R* genes did not display increased vascular permeability. Because bradykinin is the only known ligand for the bradykinin 2 receptor, these data strongly suggest that the symptoms of angioedema are mediated, at least in part, by bradykinin via the bradykinin 2 receptor. Although a receptor for C2 kinin has not yet been identified, it is possible that mediator(s) generated during activation of complement also may play a role.

PATHOLOGY OF HAE Pathologic alterations in HAE have been described on the basis of studies of cutaneous and jejunal biopsies obtained at autopsies or laparotomies of affected individuals during attacks. Skin changes consisted primarily of subcutaneous edema. Laryngeal edema was characterized by spongiosis of the mucosal epithelial cells with cytoplasmic vacuole formation and submucosal edema with masking of fibrous structures. When edema and hemorrhage of the lungs were present, they were attributed to asphyxiation. Jejunal tissue showed edema of the lamina propria, particularly of the superficial portion of the villi, giving rise to a club-shaped appearance. No submucosal edema was present, nor were there any cellular infiltrates.

The increased vascular permeability is due to the creation of gaps between the endothelial cells in the postcapillary venules. Under electron microscopy, the contraction of the endothelial cells is denoted by wrinkling and indentation of the nuclei. Degranulation of adjacent mast cells is also seen. However, the lesion is not mediated by histamine, and it cannot be aborted by antihistamines or by depleting the skin of its histamine content with compound 48/80 or polysorbate.[39]

Acquired C1INH Deficiency

An acquired form of C1INH deficiency with angioedema (AAE) has been observed in patients in the fifth and sixth decades of life without a family history of the disorder. The clinical manifestations of this form of angioedema resemble those of the hereditary type of C1INH deficiency, i.e., non-pruritic subcutaneous edema without urticaria and with upper respiratory and gastrointestinal tract involvement. There are two forms of AAE, type I and type II.[40] AAE type I was described initially as a clinical entity in association with lymphoproliferative disorders. Most, but not all, of these patients have monoclonal B cell disease such as myeloma, Waldenström's macroglobulinemia, B cell lymphoma, or chronic lymphocytic leukemia and, less commonly, other types of malignancies. In some patients, the immunochemical abnormalities and episodes of angioedema appear several years before the underlying malignancy of the lymphocytes (Table 117-2). When these patients are relieved of their tumor burden, the acquired C1INH deficiency improves. The immunoglobulin isotypes expressed in the abnormal B cells include gamma, mu, and alpha heavy chains, as well as both kappa and lambda light chains. Neither epsilon nor delta heavy-chain disease has been associated with acquired C1INH deficiency. It became apparent that these patients have anti-idiotypic antibodies to their monoclonal immunoglobulins.[41] A markedly decreased serum level of C1 distinguishes acquired C1INH deficiency from the hereditary form, in which the level of C1 is within the normal range. It is possible that the idiotype–anti-idiotype interaction fixes C1 and preferentially consumes C1INH. In AAE type II, autoantibodies to the C1INH are present in the sera of patients.[42] The antibodies to the C1INH usually are of the IgG_1 class and bind to the reactive center of the inhibitor at residues 448–459, with lower affinity to residues 438–449. The C1INH in the complex has lost its proteinase regulatory capacity. In some of these patients the anti-C1INH antibodies may

TABLE 117-2

Disease Association in Acquired C1INH Deficiency

Pathologic Diagnosis	Presenting Symptom
IgA myeloma	Cutaneous angioedema, gastrointestinal symptoms
Chronic lymphatic leukemia	Cutaneous angioedema, laryngeal edema
Non-Hodgkin's B cell lymphoma	Cutaneous angioedema
Histiocytic lymphoma	Laryngeal edema
Chronic lymphatic leukemia	Cutaneous angioedema
Lymphosarcoma	Cutaneous angioedema
Lymphocytic lymphomas	Cutaneous angioedema
Undefined neoplastic lymphoproliferative disorder	Cutaneous angioedema
Waldenström's macroglobulinemia	Cutaneous angioedema
Essential cryoglobulinemia	Cutaneous angioedema
Monoclonal gammopathy	Cutaneous angioedema
Adenocarcinoma	Cutaneous angioedema
Myelofibrosis	Cutaneous angioedema
Autoimmunity	Cutaneous angioedema
Anti-C1INH autoantibodies	Cutaneous angioedema

be part of the serologic abnormalities associated with systemic lupus erythematosus, rheumatoid arthritis, and Sjögren's syndrome. Although C1INH synthesis is normal or increased in both types of AAE, in type I the levels of the inhibitor in blood are reduced, whereas in type II the inhibitor remains in the circulation as an inactive protein.

LABORATORY FINDINGS

The diagnosis of HAE is not straightforward. On immunochemical measurement of C1INH, 85 percent of patients with HAE are identified by decreased serum levels (type I), but 15 percent (type II) are missed because they have normal levels or increased levels of abnormal C1INH protein. C4 levels usually are measured at the same time because almost all patients with HAE have decreased serum levels of C4 (Table 117-3). However, some affected individuals, especially young children, may not exhibit this decrease; therefore, it may be necessary in some cases to assay C1INH functionally to be certain of the diagnosis.[2]

The acquired form of C1INH deficiency can be diagnosed readily because the serum level of C1 is markedly decreased in contrast to the normal level of C1 in sera from patients with HAE. C4 levels are not helpful because they are decreased in both the genetic and acquired forms of C1INH deficiency. The underlying cause for acquired C1INH deficiency must be investigated carefully. Patients with AAE are clinically and biochemically heterogeneous, and they have different responses to treatment.[2]

TABLE 117-3

Complement Abnormalities in Hereditary and Acquired Angioedema

	C1INH						
	Antigenic	Functional	CH_{50}	C1	C4	C2*	C3
HAE type 1	↓↓	↓↓	N or ↓	N	↓↓	↓	N
HAE type 2	N	↓↓	N or ↓	N	↓↓	↓	N
AAE type 1	↓↓	↓↓					
AAE type 2	N†	↓↓	↓↓	↓↓	↓↓	↓↓	N

NOTE: ↓, depressed; ↓↓, markedly depressed; N, normal.
*↓ during attacks of hereditary angioedema.
†Normal or depressed.

DIFFERENTIAL DIAGNOSIS

Complement-mediated angioedema, by definition, excludes clinically similar syndromes mediated by other pathways, such as those involving IgE or abnormalities in arachidonic acid metabolism uncovered by the administration of nonsteroidal anti-inflammatory agents. Acute IgE-mediated reactions in humans are characterized by respiratory symptoms, hypotension or vascular collapse, and angioedema/urticaria. These clinical manifestations begin within minutes of antigen exposure, and the diagnosis can be confirmed by the demonstration of specific IgE by in vitro techniques. The adverse reactions that occur after the ingestion of aspirin include angioedema/urticaria, rhinitis (with associated nasal polyps), and bronchial asthma. In each of these clinical settings, localized angioedema may occur without any other symptoms or signs.

Although angioedema usually is recognized easily because of its episodic and evanescent nature, several other disorders should be included in the differential diagnosis. Contact dermatitis may occur as recurrent episodes of swelling at sites of contact with the responsible antigen. Historical information, additional cutaneous changes, and patch tests are useful in establishing the diagnosis. Cellulitis or erysipelas may, at times, resemble angioedema. Lymphedema may occur after cutaneous pyoderma. Surgery, congestive heart failure, and obstruction of the superior vena cava may produce recurrent swelling.

TREATMENT

Acute attacks of HAE are potentially life-threatening; thus patients should be advised about prevention. Care should be taken to avoid trauma. Before dental or surgical procedures, appropriate prophylactic therapy should be given.

Airway obstruction is the most threatening event during an attack. It is a medical emergency, and a patent airway must be established. Epinephrine is of little value, as are antihistamines and glucocorticoids. Freshly reconstituted freeze-dried plasma has been used for acute attacks.[43] However, besides replacing the C1INH, the plasma provides the substrates of C1, C4, and C2. The intravenous injection of purified C1INH or recombinant C1INH is the most effective modality of treatment; however, neither has been approved for use in the United States.[44] Demerol compounds are effective in controlling the excruciating pain associated with abdominal attacks.

In 1960, testosterone was found to be effective in preventing attacks of angioedema. Subsequently, attenuated androgens with reduced virilizing effects but retained anabolic activity also were found to be prophylactic agents.[45] Stanozolol (0.5–2 mg daily) and danazol (50–400 mg daily) are now used widely to prevent attacks of angioedema. The optimal daily dose must be determined for each patient.[46] Because the latent period to achieve an effect is approximately 5 days, these agents are of little value in treating acute attacks. When surgical procedures or dental work is contemplated, it is prudent to give two to three times the doses stated earlier for 5 days before the anticipated trauma. Androgens are contraindicated in children except for short courses before surgery or dental work. This therapeutic approach may not be justified in patients with limited manifestations of the disease, and some patients prefer to live with their symptoms rather than take prophylactic androgens. The most common side effects of androgen treatment include irregular menstruation but rarely amenorrhea and hirsutism and less frequently hepatic dysfunction.

The two types of acquired C1INH deficiency require distinct therapeutic approaches. Whereas patients with lymphoproliferative disorders (AAE type I) respond to attenuated androgens, those with anti-C1INH autoantibodies (AAE type II) respond to glucocorticoids.[40]

REFERENCES

1. Zuraw BL: Urticaria, angioedema, and autoimmunity. *Clin Lab Med* **17**:559, 1997
2. Cicardi M et al: Pathogenetic and clinical aspects of C1 inhibitor deficiency. *Immunobiology* **199**:366, 1998
3. Landerman NS et al: Hereditary angioneurotic edema: II. Deficiency of inhibitor for serum globulin permeability factor and/or plasma kallikrein. *J Allergy* **33**:330, 1962
4. Donaldson VH, Evans RR: A biochemical abnormality in hereditary angioneurotic edema: Absence of serum inhibitor of C′1-esterase. *Am J Med* **35**:37, 1963
5. Gigli I et al: Interaction of plasma kallikrein with the C1 inhibitor. *J Immunol* **104**:574, 1970
6. Winnewisser J et al: Type I hereditary angio-oedema: Variability of clinical presentation and course within two large kindreds. *J Int Med* **241**:39, 1997
7. Weinstock LB et al: Recurrent abdominal pain as the whole manifestation of hereditary angioedema. *Gastroenterology* **93**:1116, 1987
8. Kohler PF et al: Hereditary angioedema and "familial" lupus erythematosus in identical twin boys. *Am J Med* **56**:406, 1974
9. Donaldson VH et al: Lupus-erythematosus-like disease in three unrelated women with hereditary angioedema. *Ann Intern Med* **86**:312, 1977
10. Suzuki Y et al: Association of Sjögren's syndrome with hereditary angioneurotic edema: Report of a case. *Clin Immunol Immunopathol* **84**:95, 1997
11. Ariga T et al: A de novo deletion in the C1 inhibitor gene in a case of sporadic hereditary angioneurotic edema. *Clin Immunol Immunopathol* **69**:103, 1993
12. Oltvai ZN et al: C1 inhibitor deficiency: Molecular and immunologic basis of hereditary and acquired angioedema. *Lab Invest* **65**:381, 1991
13. Rosen FS et al: Genetically determined heterogeneity of the C1 esterase inhibitor in patients with hereditary angioneurotic edema. *J Clin Invest* **50**:2143, 1971
14. Verpy E et al: Exhaustive mutation scanning by fluorescence-assisted mismatch analysis discloses new genotype-phenotype correlations in angioedema. *Am J Hum Genet* **59**:289, 1996
15. Davis AE et al: Human inhibitor of the first component of complement, C1: Characterization of cDNA clones and localization of the gene to chromosome 11. *Proc Natl Acad Sci USA* **83**:3161, 1986
16. Bock SC et al: Human C1 inhibitor: Primary structure, cDNA cloning and chromosomal localization. *Biochemistry* **25**:4292, 1986
17. Davis AE et al: C1 inhibitor hinge region mutations may convert the inhibitor to a substrate or may result in diminished ability to interact with target proteases. *Nature Genet* **1**:354, 1992
18. Aulak KS et al: Dysfunctional C1 inhibitor (At), isolated from a type II hereditary angioedema plasma, contains a P1 "reactive center" (Arg[444]–His) mutation. *Biochem J* **253**:615, 1988
19. Skriver K et al: CpG mutations in the reactive site of human C1 inhibitor. *J Biol Chem* **264**:3066, 1989
20. Zahedi R et al: C1 inhibitor: Analysis of the role of amino acid residues within the reactive center loop in target protease recognition. *J Immunol* **167**:1500, 2001
21. Zahedi R et al: Role of the P2 residue of complement 1 inhibitor (Ala[443]) in determination of target protease specificity: Inhibition of complement and contact system proteases. *J Immunol* **159**:983, 1997
22. Parad RB et al: Dysfunctional C1 inhibitor Ta: Deletion of Lys-251 results in acquisition of an *N*-glycosylation site. *Proc Natl Acad Sci USA* **87**:6786, 1990
23. Stoppa-Lyonet D et al: Clusters of intragenic Alu repeats predispose the human C1 inhibitor locus to deleterious rearrangements. *Proc Natl Acad Sci USA* **87**:1551, 1990
24. Ariga T et al: Recombination between Alu repeat sequences that result in partial deletions within the C1 inhibitor gene. *Genomics* **8**:607, 1990
25. Bissler JJ et al: A cluster of mutations within a short triplet repeat in the C1 inhibitor gene. *Proc Natl Acad Sci USA* **91**:9622, 1994
26. Prada AE et al: Regulation of C1 inhibitor synthesis. *Immunobiology* **199**:377, 1998
27. Kramer J et al: Synthesis of C1 inhibitor in fibroblasts from patients with type I and type II hereditary angioneurotic edema. *J Clin Invest* **87**:1614, 1991
28. Quastel M et al: Behavior in vivo of normal and dysfunctional C1 inhibitor in normal subjects and patients with hereditary angioneurotic edema. *J Clin Invest* **7**:1041, 1983
29. Kaplan AP et al: The intrinsic coagulation/kinin-forming cascade: Assembly in plasma and cell surfaces in inflammation. *Adv Immunol* **66**:225, 1997
30. Donaldson VH et al: Action of complement in hereditary angioneurotic edema: Role of C1-esterase. *J Clin Invest* **43**:2204, 1964
31. Ratnoff OD et al: The conversion of C′1s to C′1 esterase by plasmin and trypsin. *J Exp Med* **125**:337, 1967
32. Klemperer MR et al: Effect of C′1 esterase on vascular permeability in man: Studies in normal and complement deficient individuals and in patients with hereditary angioneurotic edema. *J Clin Invest* **47**:604, 1968
33. Donaldson VH et al: Permeability-increasing activity in hereditary angioneurotic edema plasma: II. Mechanism of formation and partial characterization. *J Clin Invest* **48**:642, 1969
34. Strang CJ et al: Angioedema induced by a peptide derived from complement component C2. *J Exp Med* **168**:1685, 1988
35. Curd JG et al: Detection of active kallikrein in induced blister fluids of hereditary angioedema patients. *J Exp Med* **152**:742, 1980
36. Cugno M et al: Activation of factor XII and cleavage of high molecular weight kininogen during acute attacks in hereditary and acquired C1-inhibitor deficiencies. *Immunopharmacology* **33**:361, 1996
37. Cugno M et al: Activation of the coagulation cascade in C1-inhibitor deficiencies. *Blood* **89**:3213, 1997
38. Han ED et al: Enhanced vascular permeability in C1 inhibitor–deficient mice is mediated via the bradykinin type 2 receptor. *J Clin Invest* **109**:1007, 2002
39. Granerus G et al: Studies on the histamine metabolism and the complement system in hereditary angioneurotic edema. *Acta Med Scand* **182**:11, 1967
40. Markovic SN et al: Acquired C1 esterase inhibitor deficiency. *Ann Intern Med* **132**:144, 2000
41. Geha RS et al: Acquired C1-inhibitor deficiency associated with antiidiotypic antibody to monoclonal immunoglobulins. *N Engl J Med* **312**:534, 1985
42. Alsenz J et al: Autoantibody-mediated acquired deficiency of C1 inhibitor. *N Engl J Med* **316**:1360, 1987
43. Jaffe CJ et al: Hereditary angioedema: The use of fresh frozen plasma for prophylaxis in patients undergoing oral surgery. *J Allergy Clin Immunol* **155**:386, 1975
44. Waytes AT et al: Treatment of hereditary angioedema with a vapor-heated C1 inhibitor concentrate. *N Engl J Med* **334**:1630, 1996
45. Gelfand JA et al: Treatment of hereditary angioedema with danazol: Reversal of clinical and biochemical abnormalities. *N Engl J Med* **295**:1444, 1976
46. Cicardi M et al: Long-term treatment of hereditary angioedema with attenuated androgens: A survey of a 13-year experience. *J Allergy Clin Immunol* **87**:768, 1991

CHAPTER 118

Thomas D. Horn

Graft-versus-Host Disease

Dermatologists play an important role in the evaluation and management of patients at risk for or diagnosed with graft-versus-host disease (GVHD). Of all organ dysfunction associated with GVHD, the skin serves as the earliest and most frequent target. To evaluate patients, optimally, the dermatologist must know the type of marrow transplant, any manipulation of marrow before infusion, the preparative regimen used, the date of marrow infusion, the peripheral white blood cell count, medications administered, and the course of hospitalization.

The field of marrow transplantation has evolved greatly over the past several decades. Early observations of GVHD were made among patients who received their marrow transplants with little or no prophylaxis. The flagrant disease that ensued then no longer occurs, and dermatologists must evaluate patients in the setting of significant prophylactic immunosuppression that blunts the clinical and histologic expression of GVHD. Viewed most simply, a marrow transplant is merely a form of dose intensification. With the recognition that the development of GVHD partially protects against tumor relapse, interest in immunologic manipulations that allow or even induce GVHD (in the autologous setting) arose. The frontiers of marrow transplantation expand constantly, as evidenced by a xenograft between a human recipient of baboon marrow.[1] Recently, transplantation of actual marrow has diminished in favor of the use of peripheral blood stem cells for both allogeneic and autologous transplants.

The clinical manifestations, histopathology, treatment, and pathogenesis of GVHD with emphasis on the skin are considered in this chapter, and its organization follows the types of marrow transplants to highlight the fact that skin disease after marrow ablation varies with subsequent therapy. Table 118-1 provides definitions for several common terms used.

TABLE 118-1

Terms and Definitions

TERM	DEFINITION
Allogeneic	Between two individuals
Autologous	From the same person
Syngeneic	Between two individuals with identical genetic material
Xenograft	Transplanted tissue from another species
Graft-versus-host disease (GVHD)	The totality of organ dysfunction attributable to immunocompetent lymphocytes targeting recipient tissues
Graft-versus-host reaction (GVHR)	The expression of GVHD in a specific organ, e.g., cutaneous GVHR
Stage	A term referring to clinical findings
Grade	A term referring to histopathologic findings

ERUPTIONS OF LYMPHOCYTE RECOVERY

The concept of cutaneous eruptions developing at the time of peripheral recovery of lymphocytes after marrow ablative therapy unifies all diagnoses considered in this chapter.[2] As defined initially, the eruption of lymphocyte recovery occurred with the earliest return of lymphocytes to the peripheral circulation of patients with acute leukemia who did not receive a marrow transplant.[3] The eruptions consisted of erythematous coalescing macules, predominantly on the trunk and proximal extremities. Skin biopsy specimens revealed nonspecific changes, with an upper dermal perivascular infiltrate of lymphocytes and variable epidermal spongiosis but no significant epidermal cell necrosis. An acute elevation in temperature accompanied the cutaneous eruptions. Resolution of the eruption occurred with multiline hematologic recovery.

This concept of lymphocyte recovery eruption has application to the field of marrow transplantation because graft-versus-host reactions (GVHRs) develop at the time of peripheral lymphocyte recovery and represent this phenomenon with immunologic differences between donor and recipient or in the setting of some immunologic manipulation. Indeed, some histologically nonspecific cutaneous eruptions among patients at risk for GVHD may represent the eruption of lymphocyte recovery rather than a true GVHR, in the sense that the acute cutaneous GVHR requires the epidermis to be targeted for cytotoxic damage by an effector lymphocyte population.

CUTANEOUS GRAFT-VERSUS-HOST REACTIONS AFTER ALLOGENEIC MARROW TRANSPLANTATION

Acute Cutaneous GVHR

CLINICAL DESCRIPTION Marrow ablative regimens vary. Combinations of cyclophosphamide, busulfan, total-body ionizing radiation, methotrexate, and thio-TEPA are employed. The acute cutaneous GVHR develops in 20 to 80 percent of patients, usually 10 to 30 days after marrow infusion. Factors that predispose to the occurrence of GVHD include mismatch in the major histocompatibility complex (MHC), transplantation between unrelated individuals (Table 118-2), older age, and prophylactic regimen, among others. Patients receive cyclosporine in high dose at the time of marrow infusion to promote engraftment and prevent maximal expression of GVHD. Other modalities used to diminish the severity of GVHD include counterflow centrifugal elutriation, a mechanism of sorting lymphocytes by size to remove smaller,

TABLE 118-2

Overview of Acute GVHD by Type of Transplant

Marrow Transplant	Incidence and Severity of GVHD	Cutaneous Manifestations	Treatment	Histopathology
Allogeneic, matched	++	Erythematous macules and papules, variable distribution, bullae rare	Prednisone FK-506 Anti-thymocyte globulin Monoclonal antibodies	Dermal infiltrate of lymphocytes, > 4 necrotic epidermal cells per linear millimeter, subepidermal bulla
Allogeneic, mismatched	+++	Generally greater distribution and intensity than allogeneic, matched	Same	Same
Allogeneic, unmatched	++++	Generally greater distribution and intensity than allogeneic, matched	Same	Same
Allogeneic, unmatched, unrelated	++++	Generally greater distribution and intensity than allogeneic, matched	Same	Same
Syngeneic	+	Generally less widely distributed than allogeneic, matched	Usually none	Fewer lymphocytes, fewer necrotic keratinocytes than allogeneic, matched
Autologous	+	Generally less widely distributed than allogeneic, matched	Usually none	Changes resemble eruption of lymphocyte recovery
Autologous with cyclosporine	++	Generally less widely distributed than allogeneic, matched	Usually none	Fewer lymphocytes, fewer necrotic keratinocytes than allogeneic, matched
Autologous with cyclosporine and interferon-γ	++	Eruption more widespread, erythroderma more common than autologous with/or without cyclosporine	Prednisone rarely for erythroderma	Spongiosis often a prominent feature with fewer necrotic epidermal cells than allogeneic, matched

mature effector cells, and application of various antibodies to the graft to remove putative effector cell populations.

The eruption generally begins with faint erythematous macules on any skin surface but often the palms, soles, and pinnae (stage 1) (Fig. 118-1). The specificity of palmoplantar erythema in the diagnosis of a cutaneous GVHR is questionable because chemotherapy alone, in the absence of marrow support, may cause acral erythema.[4] Edema and tenderness often accompany the erythema regardless of cause. Pruritus is an uncommon complaint. As a GVHR evolves, the distribution of erythematous macules increases, becoming confluent over broad surfaces, commonly the upper back (stages 2 to 3). On the trunk, the erythematous macules may be observed in a perifollicular array at a very early stage (Fig. 118-2). At later stages, erythroderma may ensue (Fig. 118-3). Development of bullae (stage 4) portends a poor prognosis. These bullae are subepidermal with a necrotic roof, greatly resembling toxic epidermal necrolysis. The staging scheme is detailed in Table 118-3. This progression of the acute cutaneous GVHR generally occurs over several weeks. An explosive variant is described in which erythroderma evolves rapidly, with subsequent quick evolution to a lichen planus–like eruption resembling chronic disease.[5] Factors predisposing to this form of the acute cutaneous GVHR are not known.

While the skin is the earliest and most commonly involved organ in GVHD, liver and gastrointestinal disease are frequent; the presence of elevated total bilirubin levels and diarrhea often aids in establishing the diagnosis when skin findings are not specific. Isolated liver or gastrointestinal involvement is uncommon. Retrospective analysis of a large series of patients revealed that the extent of the cutaneous eruption, total bilirubin value, and stool output per day provided significant prognostic information when considered separately or in aggregate.[6] Ocular and oral involvement in the acute phase may occur but are less common than in chronic GVHD.

With successful treatment, the eruption resolves with desquamation in the same general progression as its appearance. A brown-gray discoloration of the skin may evolve as a postinflammatory change with very slow or, in some cases, no resolution. Significant blister formation results in widespread denudation with exposed dermis, placing the patient at greater risk of sepsis as well as fluid and electrolyte imbalance.

An acute cutaneous GVHR may arise after maternal-fetal transfer of lymphocytes,[7] as well as after blood transfusion[8] and solid organ transplant, most commonly a liver containing numerous immunocompetent lymphocytes.[9]

The clinical differential diagnosis of the acute cutaneous GVHR includes drug hypersensitivity eruption, viral exanthem, transient acantholytic dermatosis, and in the presence of bullae, toxic epidermal necrolysis. As discussed below, findings in a skin biopsy specimen help to differentiate a GVHR from a drug eruption or a viral exanthem. Transient acantholytic dermatosis is an incidental finding in febrile patients receiving antineoplastic chemotherapy, with or without marrow support.[10,11] Sampling more palpable lesions predisposes to obtaining this spurious diagnosis. Confident differentiation between a stage 4 acute cutaneous GVHR and toxic epidermal necrolysis generally is not possible, although dermatologists are often asked to try. Affected patients have received numerous medications known to cause toxic

FIGURE 118-1

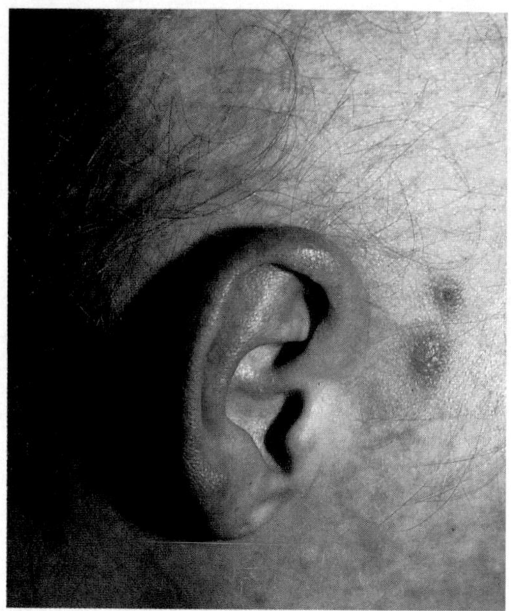

A.

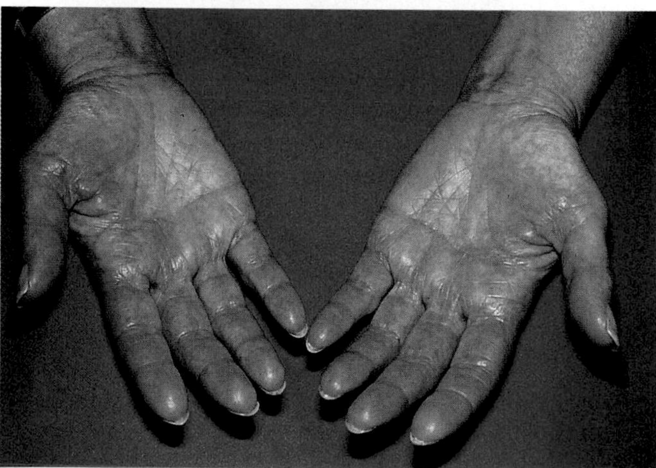

B.

Acute cutaneous GVHR. Erythematous macules involving the pinna (*A*), palms (*B*), and soles are typical in early stages of the cutaneous GVHR after allogeneic and autologous marrow transplantation.

epidermal necrolysis, but rational criteria to exclude a GVHR in this setting do not exist.

HISTOPATHOLOGY The changes of an interface dermatitis appear in all phases of a cutaneous GVHR, including chronic sclerodermoid disease. The grading scheme for the histopathology of an acute cutaneous GVHR is given in Table 118-4. Minimal criteria for the diagnosis include an infiltrate of lymphocytes in the dermis, basal vacuolar alteration, and necrosis of epidermal cells at a frequency of at least four per linear millimeter of epidermis (grade 2).[12] Extension of lymphocytes into the epidermis is common (Fig. 118-4). The direct apposition of a lymphocyte to a necrotic keratinocyte is known as *satellite cell necrosis* and may occur in many types of interface dermatitis in which cell death is mediated by lymphocytes. Some quantitation of necrotic

FIGURE 118-2

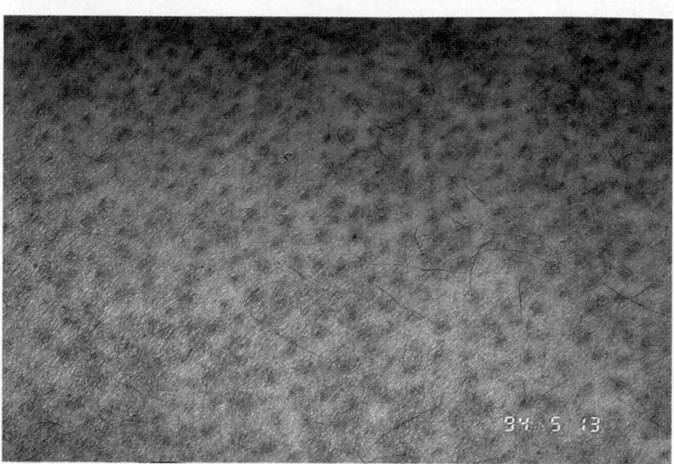

Follicular GVHR. In some patients, the earliest manifestation of the acute cutaneous GVHR is perifollicular erythema, as seen in this photograph at day 15 after marrow transplantation.

epidermal cells is advised because changes referable to the preparative regimen clearly include this finding, but in lower numbers than in a GVHR.[6,12,13] Other histologic findings attributable to marrow ablative measures include loss of polarity of keratinocytes, large and bizarrely shaped keratinocytes with unusual mitotic figures, and irregular nuclear forms.[14] This "dysmaturation" should be avoided when seeking to establish the diagnosis of a GVHR inasmuch as it may prevent adequate assessment of the specimen. Significant infiltration by lymphocytes typically does not accompany changes due to the preparative regimen, provided there is no erosion or ulceration.

In accordance with the clinical observation that the acute cutaneous GVHR begins around the hair follicle, early histopathologic changes

FIGURE 118-3

Acute cutaneous GVHR. Diffuse erythema may evolve in the acute cutaneous GVHR and is often faint.

TABLE 118-3

Clinical Staging Scheme for the Acute Cutaneous GVHR

Stage	Description
1	Cutaneous eruption involving less than 25% of surface area
2	Cutaneous eruption involving 25–50% of surface area
3	Erythroderma
4	Vesicles and bullae

SOURCE: Adapted from Glucksberg H et al: Clinical manifestations of graft-versus-host disease in human recipients of marrow from HLA-matched sibling donors. *Transplantation* **18**:295, 1974.

also begin in a perifollicular array. At the follicular epithelium, evidence of interface changes is observed with necrosis of follicular keratinocytes and extension of lymphocytes into follicular epithelium. The pattern of inflammation seems to be along the entire follicular infundibulum, but evidence to suggest targeting of the bulge region, specifically the pleuripotent stem cells harbored there, does exist.[15]

Grade 1 changes are not specific and may represent a GVHR in evolution, drug eruption, viral exanthem, or the eruption of lymphocyte recovery. Clinicians monitor patients at risk for GVHD closely and sample cutaneous eruptions very early in evolution. It is not surprising, then, that the histopathology is not fully manifest. Resampling is recommended as clinically indicated when diagnostic changes are absent.

Evaluations of the immunologic changes in the skin during acute cutaneous GVHD document upregulation of keratinocyte expression of MHC class II and intercellular adhesion molecule 1. Inflammatory infiltrates contain a mixture of CD4+ (helper/inducer), CD8+ (cytotoxic/suppressor), and CD56+ natural killer (NK) cell lymphocytes with extension of all subsets into the epidermis.[16] CD8+ cells accumulate preferentially.[17] After the preparatory regimen, the number of Langerhans cells gradually diminishes over 1 to 4 weeks to undetectable levels.[18] Repopulating cells are derived from the donor. In a murine model, Langerhans cell number and function decreased more in animals developing GVHD than in those undergoing the preparative regimen alone.[19]

Evidence of endothelial damage exists in GVHD, based on extravasation of anticoagulation factor VIII. Other findings correlating with the presence of GVHD include nuclear debris in the perivascular dermis and expression of endothelial LN3, an epitope on MHC class II.[20,21]

PATHOGENESIS The precise pathophysiology of GVHD is not known. A distillation of many lines of evidence implicates allostimulation of donor lymphocytes by major and/or minor transplantation antigens, with subsequent targeting of host tissues, mostly epithelial, for cytotoxic damage. It is unclear whether direct lymphocyte-mediated damage occurs via molecules such as granzyme and perforin, whether cytokines are the main mediators of cell death, or whether both mechanisms are operative.[22] Epithelial cell death ensues by apoptosis, with

TABLE 118-4

Histologic Grading Scheme for the Acute Cutaneous GVHR

Grade	Description
0	Normal skin or changes not referable to GVHD
1	Basal vacuolization of the dermal-epidermal junction
2	Basal vacuolization, necrotic epidermal cells, lymphocytes in the dermis and/or epidermis
3	Subepidermal cleft formation plus grade 2 changes
4	Separation of epidermis from dermis plus grade 2 changes

SOURCE: Adapted from Lerner KG et al: Histopathology of graft-versus-host reaction (GVHR) in human recipients of marrow from HLA-matched sibling donors. *Transplantation* **18**:367, 1974.

FIGURE 118-4

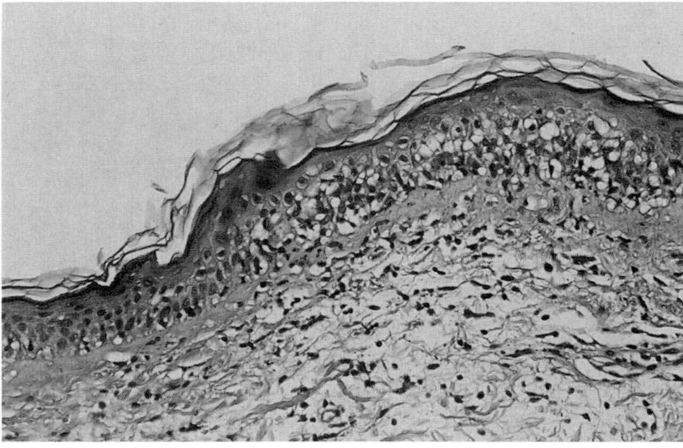

Histopathology of the acute cutaneous GVHR, grade 2. Inflammation of the upper dermis is evident with extension of lymphocytes into the epidermis and interface change.

evidence indicating T cell–mediated mechanisms as well as noncellular triggers.[23–25]

It is unlikely that a specific lymphocyte subset consistently mediates GVHD. Many epitopes on major and minor histocompatibility antigens are likely to promote allostimulation, resulting in numerous populations of effector lymphocytes in target organs. Indeed, several cytotoxic T cell clones have been isolated and identified from the skin of a single patient.[26] CD4+ and CD8+ cell lines are capable of mediating epidermal damage. In a murine model of GVHD, the effector population mediating the cutaneous GVHR varied with the strains used in the transplant,[27] suggesting that among humans each donor-recipient pair is nearly unique, with the potential to employ different lymphocyte subsets in subsequent GVHD. Evidence exists to implicate CD4+ T cells as major mediators of human disease.[28] These considerations are likely to explain the variability of disease expression, irrespective of MHC match or mismatch.

Other cell types are likely involved in mediating GVHD. The presence of numerous NK cells in the dermal and epidermal infiltrates of cutaneous GVHRs suggests that these cells are recruited once the antigen-specific recognition phase of the immunologic reaction has occurred in a target tissue.[29] NK cells lack a hypermutable molecule such as the T cell receptor and are nonspecific mediators of epidermal damage. Mast cells and dermal dendrocytes increase in number in the superficial dermis during acute phases of the disease.[30,31]

Why cutaneous involvement in GVHD is so frequent and early compared with liver and gastrointestinal disease is unknown. Expression of the cutaneous lymphocyte antigen by lymphocytes returning to the peripheral circulation after marrow engraftment would explain homing to the skin.

DIAGNOSIS AND DIFFERENTIAL DIAGNOSIS The diagnosis of the acute cutaneous GVHR rests on the combination of clinical findings, including the onset of variably distributed erythematous macules and papules at the time of peripheral lymphocyte recovery (generally more than 10 to 14 days after transplantation), and a minimum of grade 2 histopathologic changes. Since stage 1 disease generally is not treated, eruptions with limited distribution may not warrant sampling. If eruptions persist or progress despite initial nonspecific histopathologic changes, resampling is very helpful because diagnostic changes evolve as the rash evolves. Emphasis on very early sampling of eruptions, while logical, promotes this dilemma.

Despite some distinguishing clinical features, the acute allogeneic cutaneous GVHR lacks absolutely specific findings. Other considerations include a drug hypersensitivity reaction and a viral exanthem. Differentiation of a stage 4 cutaneous GVHR from toxic epidermal necrolysis was discussed earlier. In addition, in some patients a poorly characterized cutaneous eruption seems to occur at the time of marrow engraftment but before the appearance of peripheral lymphocytes. This eruption develops prior to day 14 after transplantation and consists of variably distributed erythematous macules. It should not be confused with a GVHR because this "engraftment" or "cytokine-release" eruption clearly occurs very early and without a discernible rise in peripheral leukocytes.

What is the role of the biopsy specimen? There is more ability to establish the diagnosis of a GVHR than to exclude drug eruption and viral exanthem from consideration. The causes that may underlie grade 1 changes generally defy identification. It is sufficient to relate "not GVHD" rather than to speculate about the cause where objective criteria are lacking. Holding to the standard of an infiltrate of lymphocytes, basal vacuolization, and at least four necrotic epidermal cells per millimeter of epidermis helps to diminish the effects of the preparative regimen and heighten the specificity, and thus the significance, of the histologic changes. This standard should be employed in diagnostic dermatopathlogy as well as in prospective and retrospective investigations of the specificity of the histologic changes of the acute cutaneous GVHR. Although not documented in the literature, rare patients display early clinical and histologic features of a drug hypersensitivity reaction, including eosinophils in the tissue, only to have typical grade 2 GVHR histopathology 7 to 10 days later, after engraftment. Once allogeneic lymphocytes predominate and infiltrate the site of prior inflammation, effector function changes, allowing expression of GVHR.

TREATMENT Patients receiving allogeneic transplants are placed on cyclosporine, methotrexate, or both before marrow infusion. With the diagnosis of a cutaneous GVHR, usually greater than stage 1, typical therapy is systemic administration of glucocorticoids. In the face of worsening disease, additional immunosuppressive therapy may include FK-506, anti-thymocyte globulin,[32] or administration of monoclonal antibodies directed against effector cell populations or cytokines.[33,34] Dosages and specific regimens vary among transplantation centers. As indicated earlier, manipulation of the marrow graft before transplantation reduces the incidence and severity of GVHD. Cutaneous and systemic disease both persist at some level, however. These maneuvers may lessen the incidence of GVHD but also may prevent prompt engraftment and the protection against tumor relapse afforded by GVHD (see below).

Therapy directed specifically at the skin includes topical glucocorticoids and ultraviolet (UV) radiation. Psoralen plus UVA (PUVA) produces improvement in clinical features of the cutaneous GVHR, but whether this treatment improves survival is unknown.[35] UV radiation must be administered cautiously to avoid increasing the erythema of the GVHR and thereby inciting more inflammation. Extracorporeal photopheresis has reported benefit in acute disease, including steroid-refractory GVHD, possibly by promoting a shift from a T_H1 to T_H2 lymphocyte distribution.[36,37] Pretreatment of the graft with UVA prevents disease in a murine model of transfusion GVHD.[38]

Chronic Cutaneous GVHR

CLINICAL DESCRIPTION Traditionally, chronic GVHD is divided into lichenoid and sclerodermoid forms. The lichenoid phase generally develops earlier than the sclerodermoid phase, and both usually occur more than 60 days after transplantation. Some patients experience both forms of the disease sequentially or concurrently. The greatest predictor for the development of a chronic GVHR is prior acute GVHD.[39] The incidence of a chronic cutaneous GVHR is roughly 25 percent. Rare reports of a chronic GVHR after autologous transplantations exist.[40]

FIGURE 118-5

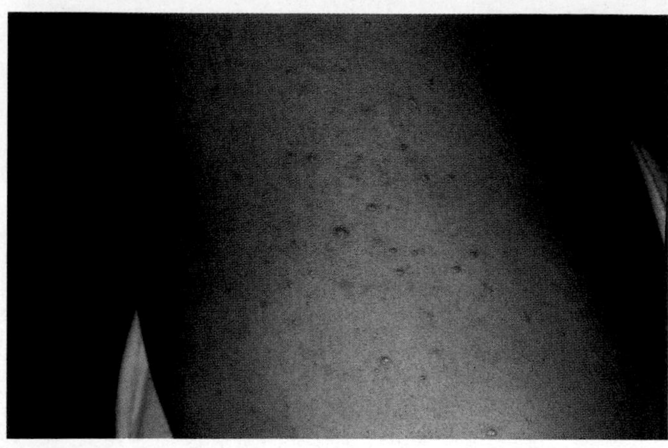

Lichenoid GVHR. These violaceous lichenoid papules developed approximately 100 days after allogeneic bone marrow transplantation.

The lichenoid form greatly resembles lichen planus, with erythematous to violaceous polygonal papules (Fig. 118-5) arising on flexor surfaces; subsequent greater distribution occurs in some patients. A keratotic variant with individual lesions resembling warts has been described.[41] Oral involvement is typical, with white lacy patches on the buccal mucosa. Rare patients display oral changes only. The lichenoid phase resolves with postinflammatory hyperpigmentation.

The sclerodermoid phase greatly resembles scleroderma in that variably distributed plaques of thickened skin arise with a shiny, somewhat atrophic appearance and varied hyper- and hypopigmentation (Fig. 118-6*A*). The plaques display erythema and progressive loss of the pilosebaceous apparatus. Some patients develop very few sclerodermoid plaques and do not require therapy. Other patients develop widespread disease associated with joint contractures, chronic cutaneous ischemia with erosion (see Fig. 118-6*B*), alopecia, and a syndrome of general wasting. In certain patients, the main anatomic site of collagen alteration is fascial. This fasciitis is similarly debilitating and is suggested in patients in whom the skin seems supple but the deeper soft tissue is hard. Joint contracture is quite common in this group of patients. Bacterial skin infections recur, consonant with the general immunodeficiency that characterizes chronic GVHD. This immunocompromise promotes sepsis, a common cause of death in these patients. Sicca symptoms resembling Sjögren's syndrome often accompany the sclerodermoid phase due to diminished lacrimal and salivary output.

The sharp separation of lichenoid and sclerodermoid phases of chronic GVHD is artificial. The two forms of disease clearly overlap in many patients. Furthermore, lichen planus–like forms of GVHD occur soon after transplantation.[42] Since immunomodulation and variability in histocompatibility are likely to result in differing clinical expression of all forms of the cutaneous GVHR, rigid adherence to the concept of time as an accurate discriminant of the phases of GVHD may not be appropriate.

HISTOPATHOLOGY Fully evolved histologic features of lichen planus may occur in the lichenoid chronic GVHR. In general, the degree of inflammation is less in the GVHR, but acanthosis, orthohyperkeratosis, wedge-shaped hypergranulosis, sharply pointed rete ridges, basal

FIGURE 118-6

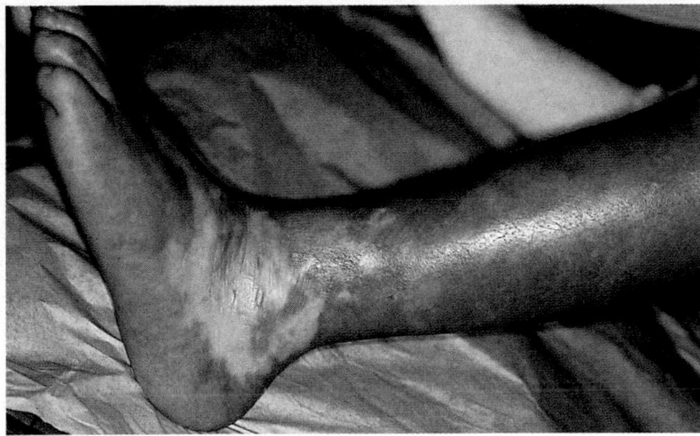

A.

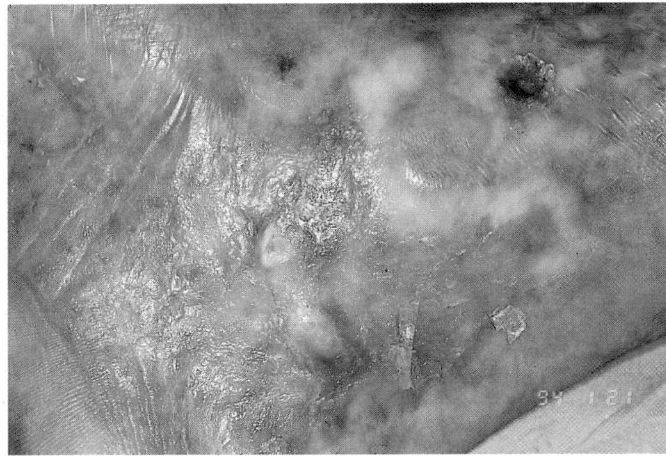

B.

Sclerodermoid GVHR. A. Shiny bound-down skin with variable pigmentation is evident. B. The inflammation and collagen alteration combine to cause erosion and some crust formation, as seen in this photograph of a patient with overlap features of lichenoid and sclerodermoid disease.

vacuolization, necrotic epidermal cells, and melanophages in the upper dermis characterize the fully evolved lesion (Fig. 118-7). The only distinction between a lichenoid chronic GVHR and the acute GVHR lies in recognition of the lichen planus–like epidermal changes, since both entities are considered to represent interface dermatitides.

The sclerodermatous chronic GVHR displays thickened bundles of collagen with loss of interstices, entrapment of eccrine coils, and progressive loss of pilosebaceous units (Fig. 118-8). The dermal-epidermal junction is ill-defined with basal vacuolization and melanophages. Necrotic epidermal cells are rare. Unlike scleroderma, the progression of collagen alteration in the sclerodermatous GVHR is reportedly from the papillary dermis downward.[43] Panniculitis is an uncommon finding.

Specimens of oral mucosa and minor salivary glands may aid in the diagnosis of chronic GVHD.[44] Interface changes along the epithelium may occur but generally without associated acanthosis and other epidermal features of the lichenoid chronic GVHR in the skin. Similar to the changes in Sjögren's syndrome, lymphocytes infiltrate glandular elements of the salivary glands, with progressive destruction and loss of acini. Lacrimal glands are sampled less often but show similar changes.

FIGURE 118-7

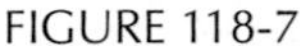

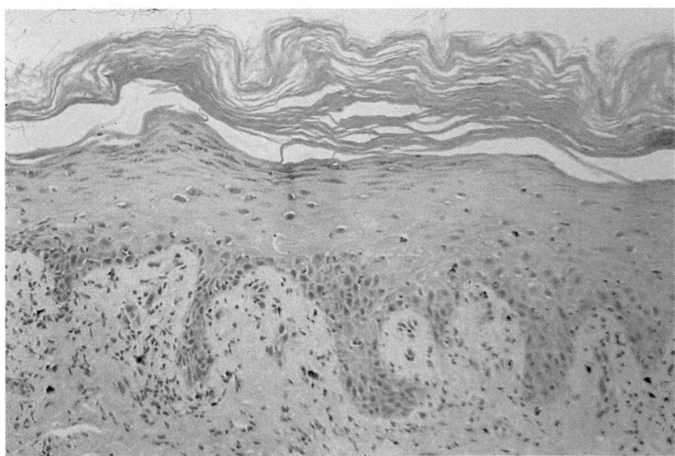

Histopathology of the lichenoid GVHR. Epidermal features of lichen planus are present with acanthosis, hypergranulosis, hyperkeratosis, and pointed rete ridges. The inflammatory infiltrate in the upper dermis is less intense than the typical case of idiopathic lichen planus.

PATHOGENESIS Chronic GVHD in the skin bears great similarity to various diseases presumed to be autoimmune in origin. Empirical observation suggests the connection between lichen planus, scleroderma, and Sjögren's syndrome with phases of cutaneous GVHRs. Improper regulation of autoreactive elements of the immune system is proposed as an explanation for the development of these findings.[45] Strong evidence links transforming growth factor β (TGF-β) to the development of skin and visceral changes in sclerodermoid GVHD with neutralizing antibodies capable of reversing the fibrosis in a mouse model.[46]

FIGURE 118-8

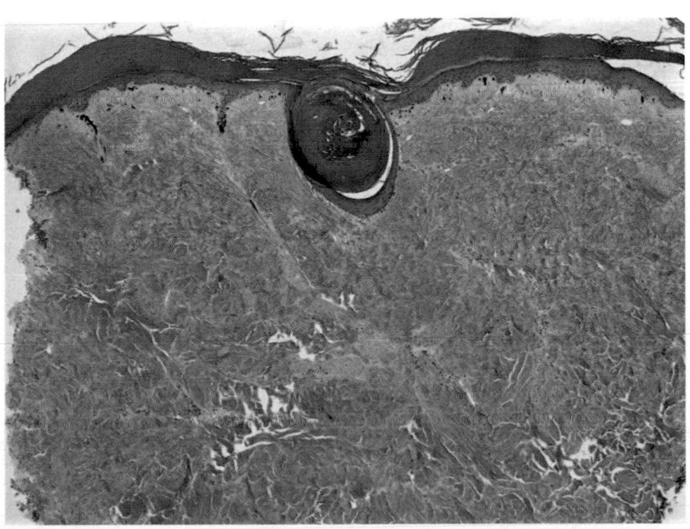

Histopathology of sclerodermoid GVHR. The epidermis shows mild, compact hyperkeratosis and keratotic plugging. There is hyalinization of the collagen throughout the dermis with loss of the appendageal structures.

In women with scleroderma, persistent chimerism of male fetal tissue is identified. A fetal antimaternal immunologic reaction is proposed as the graft-versus-host–like (GVH-like) mechanism mediating the disease.[47] Cutaneous fibroblasts in sclerodermatous skin express MHC class II and make abnormally large amounts of type I collagen.

As the use of peripheral blood stem cell transplantation increases, it is important to note a possible higher associated incidence of chronic GHVD.[48]

DIAGNOSIS The diagnosis of a sclerodermatous GVHR is generally apparent on the basis of the clinical and histologic findings detailed earlier. If superficial biopsy specimens fail to show changes consistent with sclerodermatous disease, then consideration should be given to fascial involvement, which requires incisional sampling. The distinction between the acute cutaneous GVHR and some cases of lichenoid chronic GVHR is more challenging. Rigid adherence to time after transplantation as a reliable discriminant between the two phases results in confusion.[42] Clinical and histologic features resembling lichen planus should lead to the diagnosis of "lichen planus–like GVHR," with less emphasis placed on whether the disease is necessarily acute or chronic.

PROGNOSIS A graft-versus-tumor effect is recognized in patients who develop GVHD.[49] The incidence of tumor relapse is reduced, resulting in a dichotomous view of the disease. GVHD is the most common cause of morbidity and mortality after allogeneic marrow transplantation, yet mild disease modulated by immunosuppression increases the chance of cure. Systemic infection is the most common cause of death in patients with chronic GVHD. Patients with sclerodermatous disease demonstrate better survival than patients with lichenoid disease because they have overcome the earlier phases of acute and chronic GVHD and have lived longer, on average. Patients with skin biopsy specimens showing fully evolved features of lichenoid disease have a 5.6-fold increased risk for death due to GVHD.[42] No other histologic finding is known to correlate with outcome, specifically not in the early phases of GVHD.

TREATMENT Although most chronic GVHD is manifested only in the skin, oral immunosuppressive therapy is used because the disease is considered to be systemic. Thus glucocorticoids, cyclosporine, and azathioprine are given in various combinations. Thalidomide has received renewed interest as an immunomodulating agent due to its ability to ameliorate chronic GVHD.[50]

The dermatologist is involved in treating chronic cutaneous infections, manifestations of lichenoid disease, and sclerodermatous disease. Intermittent cultures for bacteria and fungi should be taken as necessary. Chronic administration of antibiotics becomes necessary in cases of recurrent pyoderma. The incidence of cutaneous and oral mucosal squamous cell carcinoma is increased in long-term survivors with risk factors that include older age, treatment with cyclosporine, and prior administration of ionizing radiation.[51–53]

For the lichenoid manifestations, PUVA treatment generally controls widespread disease effectively.[54] Tapering PUVA is recommended after several months of clearance. Therapies claiming efficacy in the sclerodermatous GVHR are difficult to evaluate because the disease is relatively rare and remits spontaneously in some cases. It is unclear whether PUVA is able to reverse the cutaneous changes in sclerodermatous disease. Photopheresis has been reported as beneficial.[55] Etretinate has received attention as a treatment of the sclerotic GVHR.[56] Halofuginone, an inhibitor of collagen type I synthesis, has a reported beneficial effect.[57]

ACUTE CUTANEOUS GVHR AFTER AUTOLOGOUS AND SYNGENEIC MARROW TRANSPLANTATION AND PERIPHERAL STEM CELL TRANSPLANTATION

Protocols employing autologous marrow support are becoming increasingly popular as a means of dose intensification. Immunologic manipulations designed to enhance autoimmunity and hopefully to promote GVH-like phenomena are being investigated for potential graft-versus-tumor effect and improved survival.

Cutaneous eruptions simulating acute allogeneic GVHRs occur after autologous and syngeneic transplants in up to 10 percent of patients.[58] Prospective evaluation of eruptions in patients receiving peripheral stem cell transplants has not been undertaken, but mild eruptions do occur at the time of peripheral lymphocyte recovery. Peripheral stem cells are harvested by selecting and concentrating CD34+ cells (hematopoietic progenitor antigen) with reinfusion after marrow ablative therapy.[59,60]

The administration of chronic low-dose cyclosporine in the setting of autologous marrow transplants promotes a GVH-like eruption in roughly 60 percent of patients. Theoretically, cyclosporine, given in low dose, promotes escape from thymic and peripheral mechanisms regulating expression of self-targeted mechanisms, thus allowing expression of autoimmunity.[43] This autoimmunity resembles a mild acute cutaneous allogeneic GVHR. Again with the goal of enhancing graft-versus-tumor effect, protocols exist that add interferon-γ (IFN-γ) and interleukin 2 (IL-2) to cyclosporine regimens. These cytokines support general immunologic reactions and expand T cell populations, and it is hoped they will prime any graft-versus-tumor effect that may accrue with autologous transplants. Eruptions in this setting are more common and more severe, leading to erythroderma (stage 3 disease), an otherwise uncommon finding after autologous transplants.[61]

Whether these eruptions are truly GVHRs as seen after allogeneic transplants is uncertain. Because autologous marrow and peripheral stem cell transplant programs increasingly are performed outside university centers, dermatologists will encounter these eruptions more frequently. To assess clinical trial outcomes adequately, dermatologists and pathologists in academic centers must assess the occurrence of GVH-like reactions accurately.

CLINICAL DESCRIPTION Erythematous macules and papules appear in variable locations and distributions at the time of peripheral lymphocyte recovery and are self-limited. Resolution with desquamation occurs without therapy. Stage 1 and stage 2 disease is most common after the administration of cyclosporine, whereas stage 3 disease is common after the addition of IFN-γ and is accompanied by significant pruritus. Stage 4 disease, manifestations of chronic GVHD, and extracutaneous involvement are exceedingly rare.

HISTOPATHOLOGY Unmodified autologous transplants result in eruptions that are histologically indistinguishable from that of lymphocyte recovery.[62] The administration of cyclosporine results in some cutaneous eruptions that histopathologically resemble grade 2 acute cutaneous GVHR after allogeneic transplantation, but the findings are usually mild without evolution to grade 3 or grade 4. Transplants modified by the administration of cyclosporine and IFN-γ result in eruptions that combine the histologic features of a GVHR and eczematous dermatitis, as evidenced by more marked exocytosis and intercellular edema.[61]

PATHOGENESIS In rodents and humans, evidence exists that autoimmunity is directed against an epitope(s) on the MHC class II molecule.[63] Since IFN-γ upregulates MHC class II expression (ideally on tumor cells), and since cyclosporine promotes MHC class II–reactive T lymphocytes, this therapy combined with the dose intensification of autologous marrow transplants leads to enhanced GVH-like cutaneous reactions and possibly the beneficial graft-versus-tumor effect.

DIAGNOSIS Separation of autologous GVHRs from the eruption of lymphocyte recovery may be difficult. Applying the same histologic criteria as for the acute allogeneic GVHR is recommended.

TREATMENT No significant morbidity is associated with autologous GVHD, and the cutaneous eruptions resolve without therapy. Patients with erythroderma after autologous marrow transplants modified by cyclosporine and IFN-γ may require systemic glucocorticoids to control the intense itching that accompanies the eczematous changes seen histologically.

REFERENCES

1. Fricker J: Baboon xenotransplant fails but patient improves. *Lancet* **347**:457, 1996
2. Horn TD: Acute cutaneous eruptions after marrow ablation: Roses by other names? *J Cutan Pathol* **21**:385, 1994
3. Horn TD et al: Cutaneous eruptions of lymphocyte recovery. *Arch Dermatol* **105**:1512, 1989
4. Blaack BR, Burgdorf WHC: Chemotherapy-induced acral erythema. *J Am Acad Dermatol* **24**:457, 1991
5. Vogelsang GB et al: Explosive graft-versus-host disease. *Blood* **82**:422a, 1993
6. Darmstadt GL et al: Clinical, laboratory, and histopathologic indicators of the development of progressive acute graft-versus-host disease. *J Invest Dermatol* **99**:397, 1992
7. Grogan TM et al: Graft-versus-host reaction (GVHR): A case report suggesting GVHR occurred as a result of maternofetal cell transfer. *Arch Pathol* **99**:330, 1975
8. Tanei R et al: Transfusion-associated graft-versus-host disease: An in situ hybridization analysis of the infiltrating donor-derived cells in the cutaneous lesion. *Dermatology* **199**:20,1999
9. Schmuth M et al: Cutaneous lesions and the presenting sign of acute graft-versus-host disease following liver transplantation. *Br J Dermatol* **141**:901,1999
10. Horn TD, Groleau GE: Transient acantholytic dermatosis in immunocompromised febrile patients with cancer. *Arch Dermatol* **123**:238, 1987
11. Harvell JD et al: Grover's-like disease in the setting of bone marrow transplantation and autologous peripheral blood stem cell infusion. *Am J Dermatopathol* **20**:179, 1998
12. Horn TD et al: Reappraisal of histologic features of the acute cutaneous graft-versus-host reaction based upon an allogeneic rodent model. *J Invest Dermatol* **100**:546a, 1993
13. LeBoit PE: Subacute radiation dermatitis: A histologic imitator of acute cutaneous graft-versus-host disease. *J Am Acad Dermatol* **20**:236, 1989
14. Horn TD: Antineoplastic chemotherapy, sweat and the skin. *Arch Dermatol* **133**:905, 1997
15. Murphy GF et al: Cytotoxic folliculitis in GvHD: Evidence of follicular stem cell injury and recovery. *J Cutan Pathol* **18**:309, 1991
16. Horn TD, Haskell J: The lymphocyte infiltrate in acute cutaneous allogeneic graft-versus-host reactions lacks evidence for phenotypic restriction in donor-derived cells. *J Cutan Pathol* **25**:210, 1998
17. Paller AS et al: T-lymphocyte subsets in the lesional skin of allogeneic and autologous bone marrow transplant patients. *Arch Dermatol* **124**:1795, 1988
18. Murphy GF et al: Depletion and repopulations of epidermal dendritic cells after allogeneic bone marrow transplantation in humans. *J Invest Dermatol* **84**:210, 1985
19. Breathnach SM et al: Immunologic aspects of acute cutaneous graft-versus-host-disease: Decreased density and antigen-presenting function of Ia+ Langerhans cells and absent antigen-presenting capacity of Ia+ keratinocytes. *J Invest Dermatol* **86**:226, 1986
20. Sviland L et al: Endothelial changes in cutaneous graft-versus-host disease: A comparison between HLA matched and mismatched recipients of bone marrow transplantation. *Transplantation* **7**:35, 1991
21. Synovec MS et al: LN-3: A diagnostic adjunct in cutaneous graft-versus-host disease. *Mod Pathol* **3**:643, 1990

22. Graubert TA et al: Perforin/granzyme-dependent and independent mechanisms are both important for the development of graft-versus-host disease after murine BMT. *J Clin Invest* **100**:904, 1997
23. Gilliam AC et al: Apoptosis is the predominant form of epithelial target cell injury in acute experimental graft-versus-host disease. *J Invest Dermatol* **107**:377, 1996
24. Yoo YH et al: Experimental induction and ultrastructural characterization of apoptosis in murine acute cutaneous graft-versus-host disease. *Arch Dermatol Res* **289**:389, 1997
25. Jerome KR et al: Keratinocyte apoptosis following bone marrow transplantation: Evidence for CTL-dependent and -independent pathways. *Bone Marrow Transplant* **22**:359, 1998
26. Gaschet J et al: Acute graft-versus-host disease due to T lymphocytes recognizing a single HLA-DPB1*0501 mismatch. *J Clin Invest* **98**:100, 1996
27. Murphy GF et al: Characterization of target injury of murine acute graft-versus-host disease directed to multiple minor histocompatibility antigens elicited by either CD4+ or CD8+ effector cells. *Am J Pathol* **183**:983, 1991
28. Nikaein A et al: Characterization of skin-infiltrating cells during acute graft-versus-host disease following bone marrow transplantation using unrelated marrow donors. *Hum Immunol* **40**:68, 1994.
29. Acevedo A et al: Identification of natural killer (NK) cells in lesions of human cutaneous graft-versus-host disease: Expression of a novel NK-associated surface antigen (Kp43) in mononuclear infiltrates. *J Invest Dermatol* **97**:659, 1991
30. Stuart SP et al: Kinetics of mast cell, fibroblast, and epidermal cell proliferation during acute graft-versus-host disease in the neonatal rat. *J Invest Dermatol* **88**:369, 1987
31. Yoo YH et al: Dermal dendrocytes participate in the cellular pathology of experimental actue graft-versus-host disease. *J Cutan Pathol* **25**:426, 1998
32. Durrant S et al: Combination therapy with tacrolimus and anti-thymocyte globulin for the treatment of steroid-resistant acute graft-versus-host disease developing during cyclosporine prophylaxis. *Br J Haematol* **113**:217, 2001
33. Hiscott A, McLellan DS: Graft-versus-host disease in allogeneic bone marrow transplantation: The role of monoclonal antibodies in prevention and treatment. *Br J Biomed Sci* **57**:163, 2000.
34. Herve P et al: Phase I–II trial of a monoclonal anti-tumor necrosis factor alpha antibody for the treatment of refractory severe acute graft-versus-host disease. *Blood* **79**:3362, 1992
35. Wiesmann A et al: Treatment of acute graft-versus-host disease with PUVA (psoralen and ultraviolet irradiation): Results of a pilot study. *Bone Marrow Transplant* **23**:151, 1999
36. Klosner G et al: Treatment of peripheral blood mononuclear cells with 8-methoxypsoralen plus ultraviolet A radiation induces a shift in cytokine expression from a Th1 to a Th2 response. *J Invest Dermatol* **116**:459, 2001
37. Greinix HT et al: Extracorporeal photochemotherapy in the treatment of severe steroid-refractory acute graft-versus-host disease: A pilot study. *Blood* **96**:2426, 2000
38. Grass JA et al: Prevention of transfusion associated graft versus-host disease by photochemical treatment. *Blood* **93**:3140, 1999
39. Loughran TP et al: Value of day 100 screening studies for predicting the development of chronic graft-versus-host disease after allogeneic bone marrow transplantation. *Blood* **76**:228, 1990
40. Pimpinelli N: Localized scleroderma-like lesions in autologous bone marrow transplantation. *Eur J Dermatol* **2**:12, 1992
41. Kossard S, Ma DD: Acral keratotic graft-versus-host disease simulating warts. *Australas J Dermatol* **40**:161, 1999
42. Horn TD et al: Lichen planus–like histopathologic characteristics in the cutaneous graft-versus-host reaction. *Arch Dermatol* **133**:961, 1997
43. Bos GMJ et al: Chronic cyclosporine-induced autoimmune disease in the rat: A new experimental model for scleroderma. *J Invest Dermatol* **93**:610, 1989
44. Horn TD et al: The significance of oral mucosal and salivary gland pathology after allogeneic bone marrow transplantation. *Arch Dermatol* **131**:964, 1995
45. Hess AD et al: Effector mechanisms in cyclosporin-induced syngeneic graft-versus-host disease. *J Immunol* **145**:526, 1990
46. McCormick LL et al: Anti-TGF-beta treatment prevents skin and lung fibrosis in murine sclerodermatous graft-versus-host disease: A model for human scleroderma. *J Immunol* **163**:5693, 1999

47. Artlett CM et al: Identification of fetal DNA and cells in skin lesions from women with systemic sclerosis. *N Engl J Med* **338**:1186, 1998
48. Storek J et al: Allogeneic peripheral blood stem cell transplantation may be associated with a high risk of chronic graft-versus-host disease. *Blood* **90**:4705, 1997
49. Weiden PL et al: Anti-leukemic effect of chronic graft-versus-host disease: Contribution to improved survival after allogeneic bone marrow transplantation. *N Engl J Med* **304**:1529, 1981
50. Vogelsang GB et al: Thalidomide therapy of chronic graft-versus-host disease. *N Engl J Med* **326**:1055, 1992
51. Kolb HJ et al: Malignant neoplasms in long-term survivors of bone marrow transplantation. *Ann Intern Med* **131**:738, 1999
52. Bhatia S et al. Solid cancers after bone marrow transplantation. *J Clin Oncol* **19**:464, 2001
53. Gmeinhart B et al. Anaplastic squamous cell carcinoma (SCC) in a patient with chronic cutaneous graft-versus-host disease (GVHD). *Bone Marrow Transplant* **23**:1197, 1999
54. Vogelsang GB et al: Treatment of chronic graft-versus-host disease with ultraviolet radiation and psoralen (PUVA). *Bone Marrow Transplant* **17**:1061, 1996
55. Dippel E et al: Long-term extracorporeal photoimmunotherapy for treatment of chronic cutaneous graft-versus-host disease: Observations in four patients. *Dermatology* **198**:370, 1999.
56. Marcellus DC et al: Etretinate therapy for refractory sclerodermatous chronic graft-versus-host disease. *Blood* **93**:66, 1999
57. Nagler A, Pines M: Topical treatment of cutaneous chronic graft-versus-host disease with halofuginone: A novel inhibitor of collagen type I synthesis. *Transplantation* **68**:1806, 1999
58. Hood AF et al: Acute graft-versus-host disease: Development following autologous and syngeneic bone marrow transplantation. *Arch Dermatol* **123**:745, 1987
59. Kessinger A: Autologous transplantation with peripheral blood stem cells: A review of clinical results. *J Clin Apheresis* **5**:97, 1990
60. Watanabe T et al: Peripheral blood stem cell transplantation: An update. *J Med Invest* **44**:25, 1997
61. Horn TD et al: Erythroderma after autologous bone marrow transplantation modified by administration of cyclosporine and interferon gamma for breast cancer. *J Am Acad Dermatol* **34**:413, 1996
62. Bauer DJ et al: Histologic comparison of autologous graft-versus-host reaction and cutaneous eruption of lymphocyte recovery. *Arch Dermatol* **129**:855, 1993
63. Geller RB et al: Successful in vitro graft-versus-tumor effect against an Ia-bearing tumor using cyclosporine-induced syngeneic graft-versus-host disease in the rat. *Blood* **74**:1165, 1989

CHAPTER 119

Andrew Blauvelt

Mucocutaneous Manifestations of the Non-HIV-Infected Immunosuppressed Host

This chapter is focused on dermatologic manifestations of patients with acquired immunodeficiency when the cause is not HIV infection. The changes associated with HIV infection are described in Chap. 225. Most individuals included in this group have cancer, have received an organ transplant, and/or are receiving immunosuppressive therapy. Some have diabetes mellitus or are transiently immunosuppressed following surgery. Since relatively few skin diseases manifest exclusively in an immunosuppressed host, many conditions discussed in this chapter also can occur in immunocompetent individuals. However, salient clinical features particularly associated with immunosuppression are emphasized here.

Like those infected with HIV, other immunosuppressed patients commonly present with skin disease characterized by unusual presentations of common dermatoses, as well as by infections with atypical or opportunistic pathogens. These features make both diagnosis and treatment of cutaneous disease difficult in this population. Prompt clinical evaluation, judicious use of skin biopsy and culture, and aggressive treatment often are necessary to alleviate significant morbidity and mortality.

Individuals with cancer often have immune system defects prior to aggressive cytotoxic, radiation, or surgical therapy.[1] Environmental exposures and systemic defects in tumor immune surveillance that induce the primary cancer can make individuals more vulnerable to opportunistic pathogens as well. In addition, tumors from patients with established malignancy often secrete immunosuppressive factors, e.g., transforming growth factor β (TGF-β), that help evade normal immune responses and lead to further systemic immunosuppression. Ravaging side effects of cancer therapies debilitate cancer patients further. Primary cutaneous infections and systemic infections with secondary skin involvement are common complications in this setting.[2]

Solid-organ transplantation is a therapeutic option for many human diseases. Unfortunately, however, individuals who have received grafts often require lifelong immunosuppressive drugs to maintain function of the transplanted organ. Cyclosporine, tacrolimus, prednisone, and azathioprine are the drugs used most commonly to prevent graft-versus-host disease, predominately by impairing cell-mediated immunity, i.e., T cell function.[3] Humoral immunity, i.e., B cell function, remains relatively intact in these patients. Thus opportunistic diseases are dominated by viral and fungal infections, intracellular bacterial infections, and viral-associated malignancies,[4,5] conditions that are controlled predominantly by cell-mediated immune mechanisms in immunocompetent hosts. As with cancer patients, the skin is a commonly affected organ in posttransplant patients.

Graft-versus-host disease, the cutaneous manifestations of HIV disease, skin signs associated with primary immunodeficiency disorders, and side effects of cancer chemotherapeutic agents and cytokines are covered in other chapters (see Chaps. 118, 140, 225, and 256). Idiopathic CD4+ lymphocytopenia, which occurs in the absence of HIV infection, is a recently described rare condition that immunologically and clinically resembles AIDS. The cutaneous manifestations of these patients are very similar to those experienced by AIDS patients[6] (see Chap. 225) and will not be further discussed in this chapter.

INFECTIONS

The diversity of cutaneous infections that occurs in immunosuppressed patients can pose a significant diagnostic challenge. To aid in the evaluation of these patients, it is helpful to know and understand the underlying immune defects that are associated with the medical condition(s) of the patient (Table 119-1). This helps to focus the history and physical examination toward skin manifestations of specific pathogens. In particular, the skin can be critical in the evaluation of immunosuppressed patients who are ill because the initial diagnosis of systemic infection often can be established by careful examination and biopsy of cutaneous lesions.

Fungal Infections

CANDIDIASIS (See Chap. 206) Candidiasis is the most common fungal infection in immunosuppressed patients.[2,4,5] Medical conditions that cause defects in cell-mediated immunity or neutropenia, chronic immunosuppressive drug or broad-spectrum antibiotic therapy, hyperglycemia, intravenous catheterization, and prolonged hospitalization all can predispose to candidal infection[7] (see Table 119-1). Neutropenic patients and those with indwelling catheters are particular susceptible. Importantly, disseminated candidiasis should be suspected when evaluating acutely ill patients with one of these predisposing conditions. The classic triad of fever, myalgias, and erythematous skin lesions in a septic patient not responding to antibiotic therapy is highly suggestive of disseminated candidiasis. Fungus may seed numerous organs, causing myositis, meningitis, endocarditis, pneumonitis, cerebritis, esophagitis, bursitis, osteomyelitis, arthritis, and endophthalmitis. Accordingly, prognosis is poor, and mortality rates range as high as 75 percent.

Cutaneous lesions are present in only 5 to 10 percent of persons with disseminated candidiasis.[8] Lesions are characteristically nonpainful, nonblanching, discrete, erythematous macules, papules, or nodules (Fig. 119-1) that may become purpuric, pustular, or necrotic within the centers of the lesions. They are usually generalized, but occasionally patients may present with a few lesions limited to the proximal extremities. The major clinical differential diagnosis includes infections caused by other opportunistic pathogens and drug eruptions. Histologically, periodic acid–Schiff-positive yeast forms are seen in the dermis, usually associated with vascular damage and mild inflammation.

Candida can be grown from skin lesions in approximately 50 percent of patients, and success correlates with the ability to isolate organisms from blood. *C. albicans* is isolated in over 50 percent of patients; other pathogenic species include *C. tropicalis* (25 percent), *Torulopsis glabrata* (8 percent), *C. parapsilosis* (7 percent), and *C. kruzei* (4 percent).[9] *C. tropicalis* is more likely than the other strains to cause skin lesions (up to 25 percent of patients). In general, less common strains are less virulent than *C. albicans*, although they are more likely to demonstrate fluconazole resistance. The treatment of choice for disseminated candidiasis is intravenous amphotericin B, with or without oral flucytosine; oral or intravenous fluconazole may be used as alternative treatment.

TABLE 119-1

Opportunistic Infections That Are Commonly Associated with Specific Underlying Immune Defects

IMMUNE DEFECT	USUAL CONDITIONS	COMMON BACTERIAL PATHOGENS	COMMON VIRAL PATHOGENS	COMMON FUNGAL PATHOGENS
Cell-mediated immunity	Organ transplantation, metastatic cancer, Hodgkin's disease, glucocorticoid or cyclosporine therapy	*Listeria, Salmonella, Nocardia, M. avium-intracellulare, M. tuberculosis, Legionella*	Cytomegalovirus, herpes simplex virus, varicella-zoster virus	*Candida, Cryptococcus, Histoplasma, Coccidioides*
Humoral immunity	Multiple myeloma, chronic lymphocytic leukemia	*Streptococcus pneumoniae, H. influenzae, N. meningitidis*	Enteroviruses	—
Neutropenia	Cancer chemotherapy, acute leukemia, adverse drug reaction	Aerobic gram-negative bacteria. *Staphylococcus, aureus, Streptococcus viridans, Staphylococcus epidermidis*	Herpes simplex virus	*Candida, Aspergillus*
Neutrophil function	Chronic granulomatous disease, myeloperoxidase deficiency	Catalase-positive bacteria: *Staphylococcus, aureus E. coli*	—	*Candida*
Chemotaxis	Diabetes, alcoholism, renal failure, systemic lupus, trauma	*Staphylococcus aureus, Streptococcus*	—	*Candida*
Hyposplenism	Splenectomy, hemolytic anemia	*Streptococcus pneumoniae, H. influenzae*	—	—
Complement components	Congenital or acquired deficiencies	*Streptococcus pneumoniae* (C2, 3, 5 alternate), *H. influenzae* (C2, 3, alternate), *S. aureus* (C5), Enterobacteriaceae (C5), *Salmonella* (alternate), *N. meningitidis* (C6–8)	—	—
Skin barrier disruption	Intravascular catheters, decubitus ulcers, burns	*Staphylococcus, M. fortuitum,* gram-negative bacteria, anaerobes	—	*Candida, Aspergillus, Mucor*

FIGURE 119-1

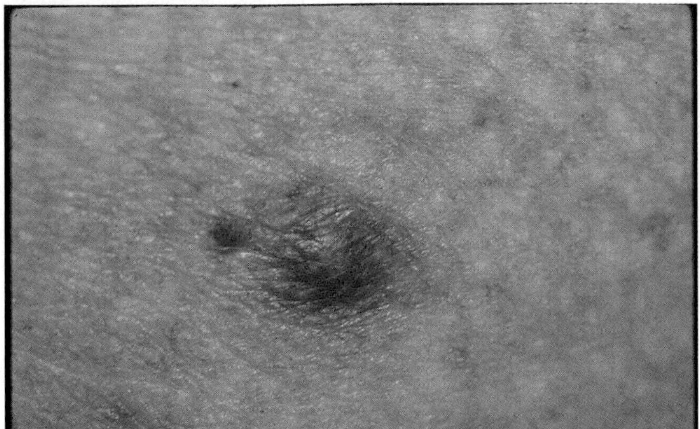

Early cutaneous lesion of disseminated candidiasis in a neutropenic patient following chemotherapy for non-Hodgkin's lymphoma.

Although less serious than disseminated candidiasis, candidiasis confined to mucosal and skin surfaces is also a very common complication observed in immunosuppressed hosts.[10] The conditions that predispose to mucocutaneous disease are the same that predispose to systemic infection. Approximately 10 percent of organ transplant patients exhibit oral candidiasis.[11] In patients receiving immunosuppressive therapy or broad-spectrum antibiotics, oral and/or vaginal candidiasis can develop within 1 month of initiating therapy. Patients with chronic mucocutaneous candidiasis have specific underlying immune deficits in fighting candidal infections and usually have chronic widespread disease (without systemic involvement).

Patients with oral mucosal candidiasis most commonly present with pseudomembranous, white, friable plaques that are removed easily by scraping (see Chaps. 112 and 206). Less common oral lesions include erythematous or atrophic plaques, as well as angular cheilitis. Esophageal involvement should be suspected in any patient with oral candidiasis complaining of pain or difficulty in swallowing. Women with vaginitis secondary to *Candida* present with pruritus, irritation, and a thick, white discharge. Cutaneous candidiasis commonly occurs in moist intertriginous areas as tender erythematous papules and satellite pustules. Onychomycosis and paronychia also may be caused by *Candida* and are common in patients with chronic mucocutaneous candidiasis. For mucocutaneous disease, topical therapy with nystatin or clotrimazole and oral fluconazole are the treatments of choice. Prophylactic treatment with fluconazole is often recommended in patients at high risk for infection, such as patients who have recently undergone organ transplant surgery.

ASPERGILLOSIS (See Chap. 207) Aspergillosis is caused by ubiquitous saprophytes found in soil and water. *Aspergillus fumigatus* is the most common cause of disseminated infections, whereas *A. flavus* is associated most commonly with primary cutaneous disease.[12] After candidiasis, aspergillosis is the second most common opportunistic fungal infection in immunosuppressed patients[2,4,5]; disease is rare in immunocompetent hosts. In organ transplant recipients, aspergillosis accounts for 20 percent of all opportunistic fungal infections. Normal functioning of both neutrophils and macrophages is required to prevent infection. Thus neutropenic patients (e.g., individuals with leukemia or those receiving chemotherapy) and patients receiving high-dose glucocorticoids (which impair macrophage function) are at high risk for aspergillosis. Environmental factors also contribute to the development of disease, including hospital construction (which increases spore counts in ventilation systems), indwelling catheters (which provide portals of entry for organisms), and contaminated tape and arm boards used to secure catheters.

FIGURE 119-2

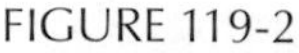

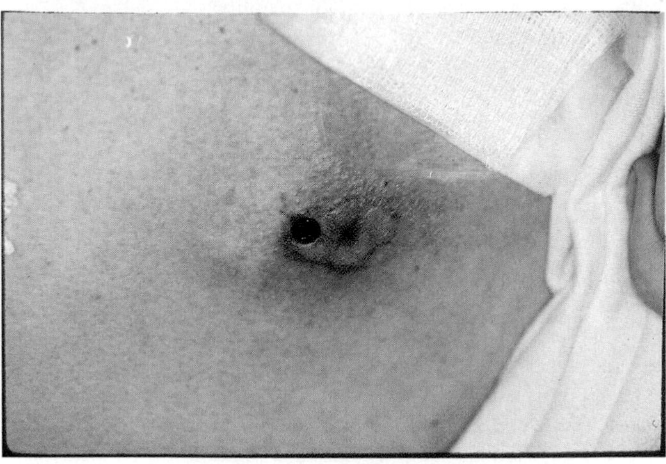

Primary cutaneous aspergillosis at an intravenous catheter site in a child with leukemia. (*Courtesy of Alexa Boer-Kimball, M.D., Stanford University.*)

Primary infection usually occurs by inhalation of spores. Patients with disseminated aspergillosis often present with unremitting fever despite antibiotic use, necrotizing pneumonia, and sinusitis. The central nervous system, heart, kidneys, and gastrointestinal tract also may be involved. Cutaneous manifestations of disseminated aspergillosis are uncommon, occurring in 5 to 10 percent of patients.[12] Lesions begin as single or multiple, painful, erythematous papules, nodules, or plaques. They rapidly expand and develop central hemorrhagic vesicles or bullae, which in turn rapidly progress to central ulcers with black eschars (Fig. 119-2). Lesions of primary cutaneous aspergillosis that develop at indwelling catheter sites appear initially as cellulitis and progress quickly to necrotic ulcers with black eschars. In patients with *Aspergillus* sinusitis, necrotic ulcers with black eschars can occur in the anterior nares, nasal septum, palate, and skin overlying the nasal bridge. Cutaneous necrosis caused by *Aspergillus* is secondary to invasion of fungi within deep blood vessels.

Primary pulmonary, cutaneous, or sinus infection commonly leads to disseminated disease, and the prognosis is very poor (usually greater than 90 percent mortality). In tissue sections, diagnosis can be made by demonstration of nonpigmented septated hyphae that branch at acute angles. Blood cultures often are not positive or reliable because *Aspergillus* is found commonly as a laboratory contaminant. The treatment of choice is high-dose intravenous amphotericin B; oral itraconazole is used as alternative treatment. Surgical removal of isolated lesions of primary cutaneous aspergillosis can be attempted, although this may not necessarily prevent secondary disseminated infection in patients with persistent neutropenia. Laminar flow rooms, low-dose amphotericin B, and aerosolized amphotericin B nasal spray have been used in attempts to prevent infection.

MUCORMYCOSIS (See Chap. 207) Mucormycosis is the third most common opportunistic fungal infection in immunosuppressed hosts, accounting for 5 to 15 percent of all fungal infections.[2,4,5] The causative agents are "bread molds" of the phylum Zygomycetes, order Mucorales, and include species of *Mucor, Rhizopus, Absidia, Mortierella,* and *Cunninghamella.* Like aspergillosis, mucormycosis is rare in individuals without underlying immunodeficiency or predisposing conditions,

FIGURE 119-3

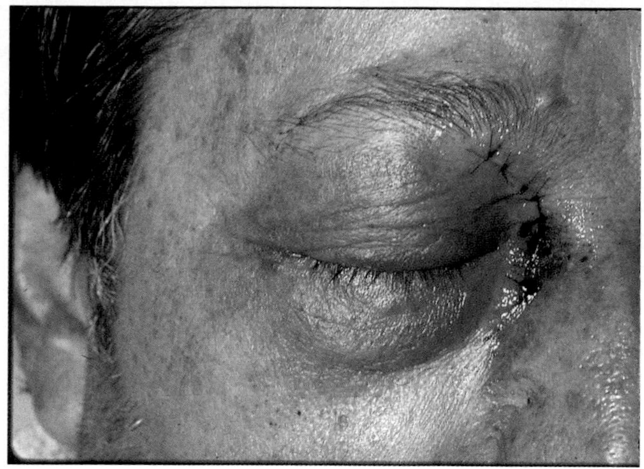

Rapidly progressing mucormycosis in a man with diabetes.

which include neutropenia, organ transplantation, high-dose systemic glucocorticoid or cytotoxic therapy, cancer (especially leukemia), diabetes, intravenous drug use, hepatic or renal disease, anemia, burns, and severe malnutrition. Primary infection in these individuals can occur by inhalation, by direct inoculation into damaged skin, or by ingestion. In particular, diabetes and metabolic acidosis predispose patients to primary rhinocerebral and pulmonary infection, wounds and burn injuries predispose to primary cutaneous infection, and malnutrition and gastrointestinal disease predispose patients to primary gastrointestinal tract infection. Each type of primary infection can lead to hematogenous spread and disseminated infection of numerous organs (especially the brain). In such patients, prognosis is poor.

The clinicopathologic hallmarks of cutaneous mucormycosis are vascular invasion, ischemic infarction, and necrosis, resulting in painful erythematous nodules and plaques that ulcerate rapidly and form central black eschars.[13] Rhinocerebral mucormycosis typically begins with facial edema and erythema (Fig. 119-3), bloody nasal discharge, and ulceration of the palate or nasal septum. Within a few days, necrotic skin lesions, headache, focal neurologic defects, exophthalmos, and altered vision develop and can progress to seizures, stupor, coma, and death. Primary cutaneous mucormycosis, which can develop rapidly in burn wounds, indwelling catheter sites, diabetic ulcers, and surgical wounds, manifests as necrotic ulcers with profuse, malodorous, purulent exudate. Diagnosis of mucormycosis usually is made by demonstration of nonseptated hyphae (with branching at right angles) within infected tissue. The treatment of choice for disseminated disease is intravenous amphotericin B and surgical debridement. If possible, reversal or removal of underlying predisposing conditions always should be attempted.

FUSARIOSIS *Fusarium* is a filamentous mold found in soil and plants. Leukemic patients with prolonged neutropenia are particularly susceptible to infection.[14] Primary infection usually occurs by inhalation of spores, although primary cutaneous infection can occur at indwelling catheter sites. Other than the lungs, disseminated infection commonly involves the sinuses and skin (75 percent of patients have skin lesions). Cutaneous lesions caused by *Fusarium* resemble lesions caused by *Aspergillus* and appear as painful, erythematous nodules and plaques that ulcerate rapidly and form black eschars. Unlike *Aspergillus, Fusarium* can be cultured readily from skin and blood of infected patients. Prognosis is poor because no effective therapy is available.

TRICHOSPORONOSIS *Trichosporon beigelii,* a yeastlike organism that causes white piedra in the tropics, may produce acute systemic infection in immunosuppressed patients, most commonly in the setting of neutropenia.[15] As with disseminated candidiasis, persons with disseminated trichosporonosis are acutely ill. They may have fever, hypotension, pulmonary infiltrates, renal involvement, and hepatosplenomegaly. Skin lesions occur in 30 percent of patients and appear similar to cutaneous lesions of disseminated candidiasis. Definitive diagnosis is made by culture, and the treatment of choice is fluconazole; amphotericin B resistance is not uncommon.

CRYPTOCOCCOSIS (See Chap. 207) *Cryptococcus neoformans* is a yeastlike encapsulated fungus that is ubiquitous and is found commonly in soil enriched with pigeon feces. Primary infection is acquired via the respiratory tract by inhalation of airborne spores and usually is asymptomatic. However, immunosuppressed patients, particularly those receiving high-dose systemic glucocorticoids, are susceptible to hematogenous spread and disseminated infection.[16,17] In fact, 70 percent of individuals with disseminated cryptococcosis have some form of underlying immune defect. The central nervous system is involved most commonly, although infection may occur throughout the body, including the lungs, bone marrow, heart, liver, spleen, kidneys, thyroid, lymph nodes, and adrenal glands.

Cutaneous lesions occur in 10 to 15 percent of patients with disseminated infection and may be protean.[10] In transplant patients, erythematous, edematous, warm, painful plaques (clinically indistinguishable from bacterial cellulitis) have been reported commonly. Umbilicated papules (resembling molluscum contagiosum), nodules, pustules, vesicles, and ulcers also may occur (Fig. 119-4). Oral mucosal cryptococcal nodules and ulcerations also have been described. Lesions may be isolated or multiple and can be quite painful. Although any area of the skin and oral mucosa may be involved, there is a predilection for disseminated disease to involve the head and neck region. Localized cryptococcal cellulitis is most common on the extremities.

Although primary skin disease may occur in the absence of pulmonary infection, diagnosis of cutaneous cryptococcosis always warrants an investigation for systemic infection, especially since disseminated disease may not always be evident clinically. This is usually accomplished by examining cerebrospinal fluid for cryptococcal polysaccharide antigens. For evaluating skin lesions, budding

FIGURE 119-4

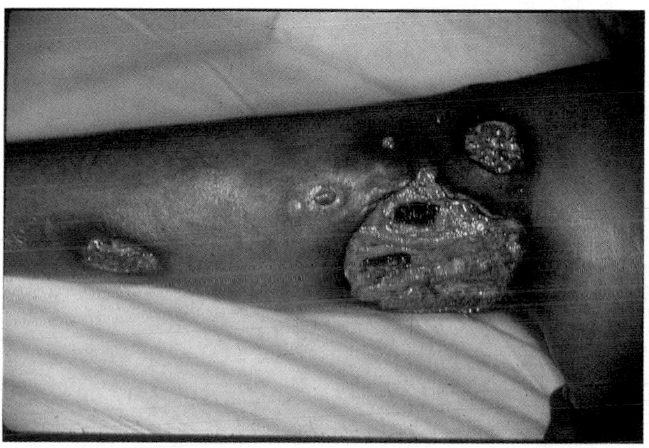

Cryptococcal cellulitis with ulceration in a woman receiving long-term high-dose glucocorticoids for systemic lupus erythematosus.

encapsulated yeasts can be identified readily in tissue biopsies, as well as in purulent material obtained from skin lesions. They stain red with periodic acid–Schiff and mucicarmine stains and black with methenamine silver stain. *Cryptococcus* also can be isolated in culture from cutaneous tissue. The treatment of choice for cryptococcosis is intravenous amphotericin B with or without flucytosine. Fluconazole is used as alternative primary treatment. However, fluconazole is the treatment of choice for prophylaxis in individuals at high risk for primary or recurrent infection.

HISTOPLASMOSIS (See Chap. 207) *Histoplasma capsulatum* is a dimorphic fungus that is found commonly in soil in central and eastern regions of the United States. Endemic foci also exist in South America, Africa, and Asia. As with cryptococcosis, inhalation of airborne spores causes primary pulmonary infection that usually leads to self-limited disease in otherwise healthy individuals. However, disseminated disease may occur, particularly in individuals with deficiencies in cell-mediated immunity.[18] In addition to pneumonia, immunosuppressed hosts may present with fever, renal failure, central nervous system involvement, hepatosplenomegaly, lymphadenopathy, and myelosuppression.

With disseminated infection, skin lesions occur in 5 to 25 percent of patients and may be an initial sign of disease.[10] Mucocutaneous lesions commonly manifest as painful nodules or plaques that progress to ulcers with indurated borders. However, numerous other morphologies have been described, including molluscum-like papules, acneiform papules and pustules, and cellulitis. In addition, as with cryptococcosis, the head and neck region is involved most commonly. In fact, the oropharynx is the most common site for lesions of mucocutaneous histoplasmosis. Because the organism grows very slowly in culture, histoplasmosis is best diagnosed by direct examination of tissue. Numerous small, oval, yeastlike fungi can be seen within the cytoplasm of dermal macrophages. The treatment of choice for disseminated histoplasmosis in an immunosuppressed host is intravenous amphotericin B. For patients who are not acutely ill, oral itraconazole may be used; itraconazole is also recommended for immunosuppressed patients to prevent recurrent disease.

COCCIDIOIDOMYCOSIS (See Chap. 207) *Coccidioides immitis*, the causative agent of coccidioidomycosis, is endemic to soil in the southwestern United States, and primary pulmonary infection is acquired through inhalation of spores.[19] Although progressive primary infection may occur in immunosuppressed patients, reactivation of prior, clinically inapparent infection appears to be more common. The risks of dissemination and fatal infection are greater among pregnant women, non-Caucasians, and immunosuppressed patients with defects in cell-mediated immunity, e.g., transplant patients receiving cyclosporine. Thus disseminated coccidioidomycosis can occur in any immunocompromised patient who lives or has lived previously in an endemic area.

Immunosuppressed patients with disseminated disease may present with fever, pneumonia, bone involvement, and meningitis. Mortality is high. Cutaneous lesions are common and appear as reddish brown papules and nodules, pustules, abscesses, or ulcers. Lesions occur most commonly on the face. Definitive diagnosis of coccidioidomycosis is made by demonstrating characteristic endosporulating spherules in smears or biopsy specimens or by culture of infected tissue. For disseminated infections in immunosuppressed hosts, treatments include intravenous amphotericin B and oral fluconazole.

BLASTOMYCOSIS (See Chap. 207) *Blastomyces dermatiditis* is endemic to the soil of the Ohio and Mississippi river valleys. Infection is acquired through inhalation of spores. Immunosuppressed patients are prone to disseminated disease involving the lungs, bone, genital tract, and skin.[18] The most common lesion appears as a verrucous or crusted plaque with serpiginous borders located on the head, neck, or distal extremities. Subcutaneous nodules and ulcers are also not uncommon. Diagnosis is made on demonstration of broad-based, budding, thick-walled yeasts in pus or skin scrapings from the edges of lesions or by tissue culture. In life-threatening disseminated infection, intravenous amphotericin B is the treatment of choice; however, less severe disease is treated with oral itraconazole.

DERMATOPHYTOSIS (See Chap. 205) Dermatophytes commonly infect normal hosts and typically cause superficial scaly annular plaques and onychomycosis. However, immunosuppressed patients may have widespread, aggressive infection that can be resistant to topical and systemic therapy.[10] The morphology of individual lesions in immunosuppressed patients is usually similar to lesions seen in normal individuals. However, both white superficial onychomycosis and proximal subungual onychomycosis are types of fungal nail infections that are uncommon in immunocompetent hosts. In the former, the surfaces of affected nails have a white chalky appearance (Fig. 119-5), and hyphae are observed readily in superficial nail plate scrapings. These conditions should prompt a search for underlying immune deficiency.

OTHER FUNGAL INFECTIONS *Penicillium marneffei* is a dimorphic fungus that has emerged as an opportunistic pathogen in immunosuppressed patients (most but not all AIDS patients) who live in or who have traveled to Southeast Asia.[20] Initial infection is acquired through inhalation or ingestion of spores. Patients with disseminated disease develop fever, weight loss, anemia, pneumonia, hepatosplenomegaly, lymphadenopathy, and molluscum-like papules on the head and upper body (70–80 percent of patients). The mold *Scedosporium prolificans* can cause asymptomatic colonization, localized infection related to trauma or surgery, and disseminated infection.[21] The latter is particularly common in patients with neutropenia secondary to hematologic malignancies. *Alternaria* is a common saprophytic fungus that can cause opportunistic infection in the setting of hypercorticism (e.g., glucocorticoid treatment, Cushing's disease) and skin fragility.[22] *Paecilomyces lilacinus*, a fairly new opportunistic fungal pathogen, has been reported to contaminate topical preparations and cause deep-seated cutaneous nodules in immunosuppressed patients.[23] A number of dematiaceous fungi cause primary cutaneous phaeohyphomycosis. Immunosuppressed patients are particularly susceptible to infection and

FIGURE 119-5

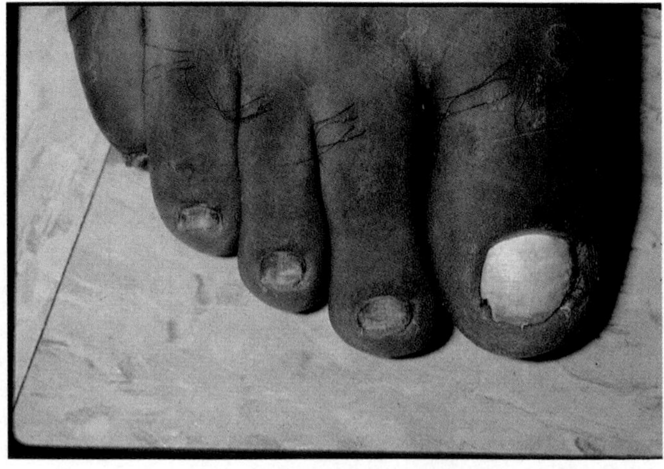

White superficial onychomycosis in a renal transplant patient receiving cyclosporine.

present with subcutaneous abscesses or cysts at sites of inoculation.[24] Chromomycosis, which typically occurs in patients in tropical and subtropical areas, is caused by dematiaceous fungi and can develop in immunosuppressed patients from other geographic areas. Typical lesions occur as scaly verrucous or crusted plaques on the extremities. Immunosuppressed patients may develop disseminated sporotrichosis, although this is not common. Tinea versicolor and folliculitis caused by *Pityrosporum ovale* (also known as *Malassezia furfur*) may be widespread and persistent in immunosuppressed hosts.[25] In addition, *Malassezia* has been reported to cause indwelling catheter–associated fungemia in immunosuppressed hosts.

Viral Infections

HERPESVIRUSES There are eight known human herpesviruses, including herpes simplex viruses (HSV) 1 and 2, varicella-zoster virus (VZV), Epstein-Barr virus (EBV), cytomegalovirus (CMV), human herpesviruses (HHV) 6 and 7, and Kaposi's sarcoma–associated herpesvirus (KSHV). As a family, herpesviruses are large DNA viruses that infect their hosts for life, typically remaining dormant in nuclei of latently infected cells. Clinical manifestations of primary infection, which generally occurs in childhood (except for HSV-2 and KSHV), are discussed in other chapters (see Chaps. 214 and 215). Acquired defects in cell-mediated immunity often lead to herpesvirus reactivation (i.e., a latent to lytic switch) and recurrent or chronic disease. Interestingly, decreasing or stopping immunosuppressive drug therapy can improve or prevent recurrent herpesvirus-associated disease.

Recurrent HSV-1, HSV-2, and VZV infections occur commonly in cancer and posttransplant patients.[26,27] As many as 70 to 80 percent of these persons will experience reactivation with at least one of these three viruses. Eczema herpeticum, which is HSV infection involving previously damaged skin, can occur in patients with less obvious immune dysfunction, including individuals with atopic or other forms of dermatitis, cutaneous T cell lymphoma, or burns. Typical recurrent mucocutaneous lesions are grouped (for HSV) or dermatomal (for VZV) vesicles and crusted erosions, although lesions are commonly atypical in morphology and distribution. For example, recurrent lesions due to HSV or VZV in immunosuppressed hosts may be isolated, nondermatomal, disseminated, necrotic, ulcerative, or verrucous (Figs. 119-6 and 119-7). In the mouth, chronic recurrent HSV infection can form white plaques and can be confused clinically with candidiasis. Severe pain often is associated with both skin and oral lesions, and postherpetic neuralgia (for VZV) occurs commonly. Protracted clinical courses of recurrent HSV or VZV infection are also more common in the setting of immunosuppression. In short, any painful, eroded lesion in an immunocompromised patient, regardless of its distribution or age, should be evaluated for both HSV and VZV by Tzanck preparation, viral antigen detection by immunofluorescence, polymerase chain reaction (PCR), and viral culture. Importantly, systemic infection involving the lungs, central nervous system, liver, heart, and gastrointestinal tract may occur. Treatment with systemic acyclovir or a related newer antiherpesvirus drug is always necessary, whereas prophylactic treatment to prevent recurrent episodes should be considered for individual patients if warranted. Foscarnet is the drug of choice for acyclovir-resistant viruses.

Reactivation and recurrent disease associated with CMV (see also Chap. 216) are major causes of morbidity and mortality in patients with marked immunosuppression, occurring in up to one-third of transplant patients.[28] This is not as common in cancer patients. In patients with transplants, most disease is caused by reactivation of preexisting CMV, although CMV may be transmitted from donor to host via the transplanted organ. Cytomegalovirus retinitis, gastroenteritis, hepatitis, and pneumonitis are the most common clinical disease manifestations. Mucocutaneous lesions caused by CMV are indicative of systemic disease.[28] Oral ulcers caused by CMV are common, particularly on the lateral aspects of the tongue. However, skin involvement

FIGURE 119-6

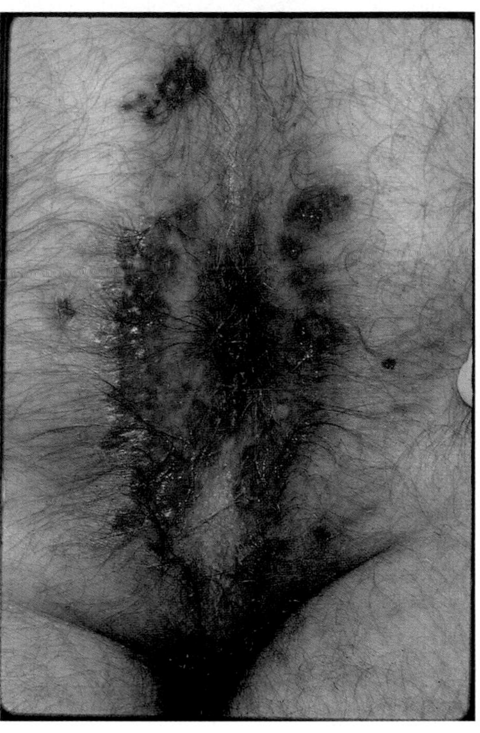

Severe chronic herpes simplex 2 infection in a patient receiving long-term high-dose glucocorticoids for autoimmune disease.

FIGURE 119-7

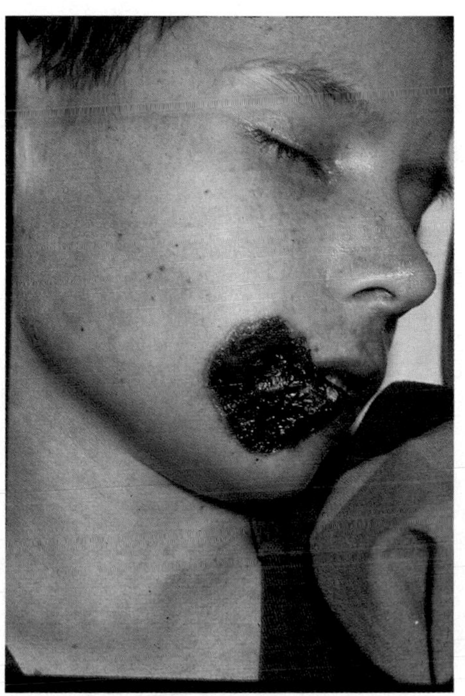

Severe recurrent varicella-zoster virus infection in a child with acute lymphocytic leukemia.

with CMV is unusual, the lesions are nonspecific, and it is difficult to prove that they actually are caused by the virus. Cytomegalovirus skin lesions have been described as ulcers, macules, papules, vesicles, petechiae, and purpura.[28] Painful punched-out perianal ulcers have been reported frequently and are probably the most specific type of skin lesion attributable to CMV infection. Tzanck preparation from the bases of ulcers may show multinucleated giant cells, and CMV-infected dermal endothelial cells may be seen in tissue sections by routine microscopy, appearing as large cells with intranuclear inclusions surrounded by clear halos (owl-eye nuclei). In addition, CMV can be cultured from infected skin. Ulcers containing both CMV and HSV also have been reported. The treatment of choice for systemic CMV disease is intravenous ganciclovir, although intravenous foscarnet, cidofovir, or CMV immunoglobulin also may be effective. Human herpesvirus 6 and HHV-7, herpesviruses most closely related to CMV, also can cause widespread multiorgan infection in immunosuppressed individuals.[29]

Epstein-Barr virus and KSHV (see also Chap. 217) infections are distinguished from the other herpesviruses infections in that they are associated with malignancies in the setting of immunosuppression. Specifically, chronic reactivated EBV infection is associated with non-Hodgkin's lymphoma and other lymphoproliferative disorders,[30] whereas chronic KSHV infection is associated with Kaposi's sarcoma (discussed below), primary effusion lymphoma, and the plasmablastic variant of Castleman's disease.[29] In addition, reactivation of EBV within oral mucosal epithelial cells causes oral hairy leukoplakia in immunosuppressed individuals (see also Chap. 225). Between 10 and 15 percent of transplant patients have this disease.[11] Lesions appear as adherent, white, corrugated plaques on the lateral aspects of the tongue. By contrast, oral candidiasis, which clinically can appear similar to oral hairy leukoplakia, is removed easily by scraping. Histologically, there is hyperkeratosis and vacuolated suprabasal epithelial cells. Oral hairy leukoplakia may respond to topical podophyllin or high-dose acyclovir; however, it is usually asymptomatic and does not require treatment. Although it has been regarded as a poor prognostic indicator in HIV-infected individuals, the clinical significance of oral hairy leukoplakia in transplant patients is not known.

HUMAN PAPILLOMAVIRUSES (See Chap. 223) Warts caused by human papillomavirus (HPV) infection are a common problem in posttransplant patients and in others receiving long-term immunosuppressive drug therapy.[31] Cyclosporine-based regimens are associated with a higher prevalence of warts compared with immunosuppressed patients not taking cyclosporine.[32] In addition, the prevalence of warts increases with a longer duration of immune compromise, with up to 80 percent of individuals affected 5 years following transplant surgery. In this setting, lesions are numerous, persistent, and difficult to eradicate. The morphology of the lesions may be typical or atypical. The atypical lesions appear as scaly macules and plaques, occur more commonly in sun-exposed areas, and are associated with HPV types observed in patients with epidermodysplasia verruciformis, e.g., HPV types 5 and 8. Several recent studies have reported that systemic retinoids, i.e., isotretinoin or acitretin, can prevent or decrease wart formation and prevent a variety of premalignant and malignant cutaneous lesions in posttransplant patients.[33–36] In these patients, the association between HPV infection and cutaneous genital and nongenital squamous cell carcinoma is complex, as discussed below.

OTHER VIRAL INFECTIONS Molluscum contagiosum (see also Chap. 221) infection also can be a problem in individuals with non-HIV-associated immune deficiency.[37] In patients who have received organ transplants, however, molluscum lesions are not nearly as common as warts. Lesions typically manifest as numerous umbilicated papules that are difficult to eradicate in the setting of immunosuppression. Measles (see also Chap. 210), a paramyxovirus, can occur in immunocompromised patients and is associated with a very high mortality rate.[38] Specifically, individuals with defects in cell-mediated immunity, as opposed to those with humoral immune deficits, are particularly susceptible to severe infection. Patients may present without classic maculopapular lesions or with widespread and purpuric lesions. Secondary complications, including otitis media, pneumonia, and encephalitis, are common in this setting. Treatment may include intravenous ribavirin or immunoglobulin, as well as aggressive supportive care to prevent and treat secondary complications.

Bacterial Infections

PSEUDOMONAS (See Chap. 197) Patients with neutropenia, cystic fibrosis, or extensive burns are particularly susceptible to systemic *Pseudomonas aeruginosa* infection.[2] Skin lesions occur in approximately 30 percent of individuals with *Pseudomonas* bacteremia.[8] Ecthyma gangrenosum is the most characteristic lesion, and classically, it appears as a painful erythematous nodule or plaque that rapidly develops a central pustule or hemorrhagic vesicle, followed by a central area of necrosis (Fig. 119-8). The groin, perianal area, and axillae are the most common locations for this condition. There may be one or many lesions. Usually, ecthyma gangrenosum is a manifestation of *Pseudomonas* septicemia, although rarely it can represent a primary focus cutaneous infection. Other organisms are also capable of causing ecthyma gangrenosum–like lesions, including *Staphylococcus aureus, Aeromonas hydrophilia, Serratia marcescens, Aspergillus* spp., and Mucorales. Other cutaneous manifestations of *Pseudomonas* septicemia may present initially as grouped vesicles, cellulitis, subcutaneous nodules, petechiae, purpura, or folliculitis. All these types of lesions can progress to destructive ulcerative lesions more characteristic of ecthyma gangrenosum. Necrosis is secondary to underlying focal vasculitis, which can be observed on skin biopsy. Diagnosis is made by culture of the organism from skin or blood. The treatment of choice is an intravenous antipseudomonal penicillin combined with an aminoglycoside.

NOCARDIOSIS (See Chap. 201) *Nocardia asteroides* is a filamentous rod found in soil that is a fairly common opportunistic pathogen.[39] Transplant recipients are particularly susceptible. The mean onset of infection in these patients is 9 months (although it can occur as early

FIGURE 119-8

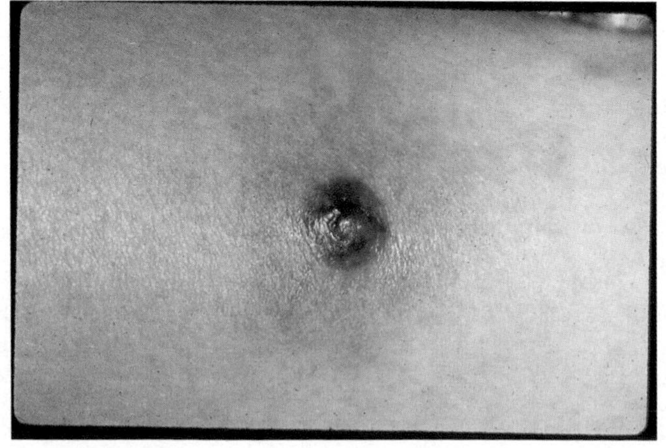

Early lesion of *Pseudomonas aeruginosa* sepsis (ecthyma gangrenosum) in a neutropenic cancer patient following chemotherapy.

FIGURE 119-9

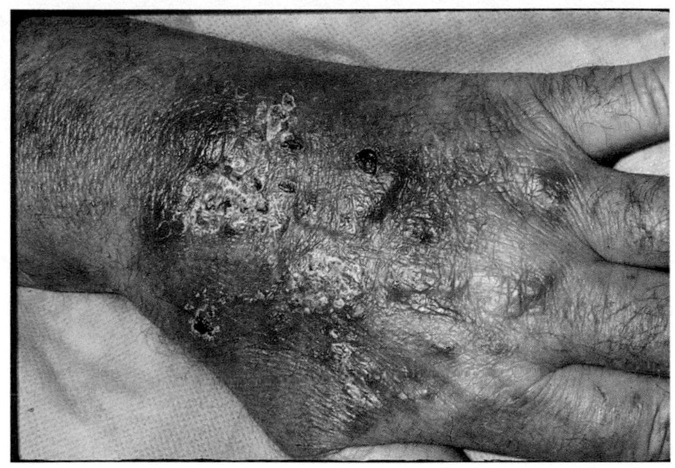

Nocardiosis in a man with glioblastoma.

as 1 month) following transplantation. A history of local trauma or occupational exposure is elicited often in healthy individuals but usually is absent in immunosuppressed patients. The most common sites of infection are the lungs, central nervous system, and skin. Several types of skin lesions have been described, including abscesses with sinus tract formation, subcutaneous nodules with pustules (Fig. 119-9), mycetoma, sporotrichoid nodules, and cellulitis.[40] Cutaneous nocardiosis may represent primary skin infection or foci of infection in 30 percent of patients with disseminated disease. Thus a diagnosis of cutaneous nocardiosis always requires a search for systemic infection. Diagnosis is based on demonstration of gram-positive, partially acid-fast, branching bacilli in tissue or tissue exudate or is based on tissue culture, although it often takes several weeks for organisms to grow. The treatment of choice is trimethoprim-sulfamethoxazole; numerous other antibiotics have been reported to be efficacious as well. Transplant patients may require long-term prophylactic therapy to prevent recurrent disease. In addition, incision and drainage of cutaneous abscesses should be performed.

MYCOBACTERIAL INFECTIONS (See Chap. 200) Atypical mycobacteria are ubiquitous organisms found in soil and water. The most common organisms in this group include *Mycobacterium marinum, M. chelonei, M. fortuitum, M. kansasii, M. haemophilum,* and *M. avium-intracellulare*. Postoperative patients, individuals with neutropenia or defects in cell-mediated immunity, and persons with interleukin-12 receptor or interferon-γ receptor deficiency are prone to infection, particularly with non-*marinum* species.[41] Atypical mycobacterial infections in the skin are characterized by diverse morphologies, including reddish brown nodules and plaques (Fig. 119-10), abscesses (Fig. 119-11), and ulcers.[42] *M. avium-intracellulare* and *M. haemophilum* commonly cause disseminated infection that can involve the lungs, lymph nodes, liver, spleen, bone marrow, and skin. Organisms can be identified with special stains or by culture from affected skin. Specific antimycobacterial antibiotic treatment regimens are complex and depend on the mycobacterial species, sensitivity results, extent and severity of disease, and the presence or absence of underlying immune defects.[43]

M. tuberculosis infection is a common worldwide problem, especially in individuals with impaired immunity. For example, individuals receiving high-dose glucocorticoids are prone to active pulmonary tuberculosis. Cutaneous tuberculosis is usually more common in the setting of immunosuppression. Specifically, scrofuloderma (tuberculous lymphadenitis with extension to overlying skin) and numerous cutaneous lesions of miliary tuberculosis may occur more commonly in patients with underlying immune defects.[44,45]

FIGURE 119-10

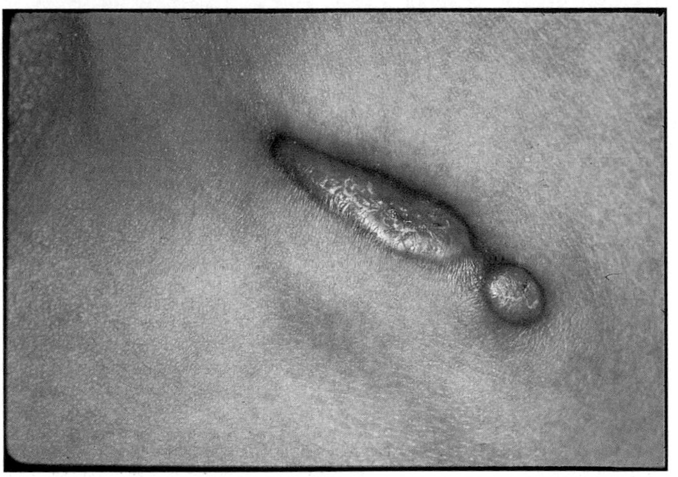

Cutaneous *Mycobacterium avium-intracellulare* infection in a child with an inherited interleukin 12 receptor deficiency.

BACILLARY ANGIOMATOSIS (See Chap. 198) Bacillary angiomatosis is caused by infection with the rickettsia-like organisms *Bartonella henselae* or *B. quintana* and usually occurs in immunocompromised hosts.[46] Cutaneous lesions appear as painful, dome-shaped vascular papules and nodules (resembling pyogenic granulomas). Disseminated infection may occur and involve the liver, spleen, bone marrow, and brain. Patients often have a history of scratches or bites by cats, the natural reservoir for *B. henselae* and *B. quintana*. Diagnosis is made by demonstration of pleomorphic bacilli in tissue specimens with Warthin-Starry or silver stain. Preferred treatments include oral erythromycin or doxycycline.

FIGURE 119-11

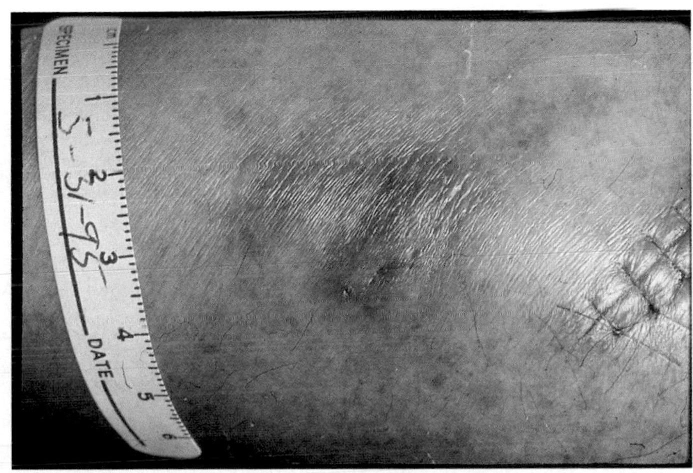

Mycobacterium chelonei in a patient receiving long-term high-dose glucocorticoid treatment.

FIGURE 119-12

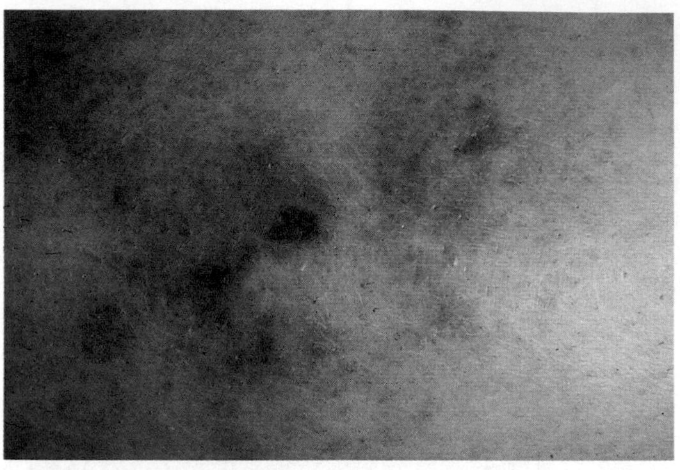

A.

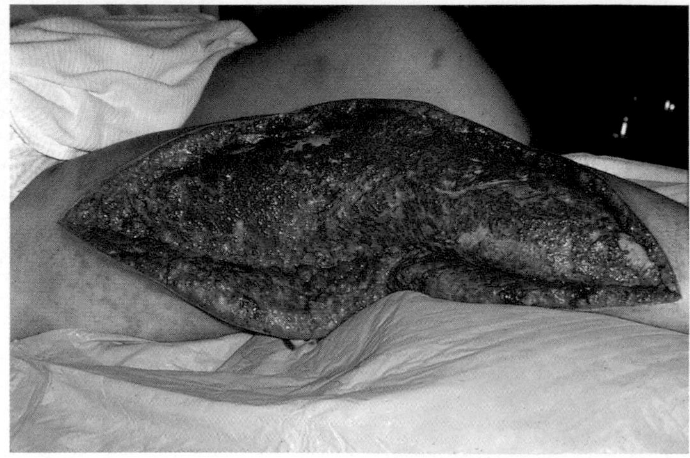

B.

Early (*A*) and late (after surgical debridement, (*B*) lesions of necrotizing fasciitis caused by *Streptococcus pyogenes* in an intravenous drug abuser with underlying Job's syndrome.

STAPHYLOCOCCUS* AND *STREPTOCOCCUS (See Chaps. 194 and 196) Staphylococcal and streptococcal infections in posttransplant patients occur most commonly within 1 month of transplant surgery and are most commonly the result of poor aseptic surgical techniques or inadequate wound care.[47] Other immunocompromised hosts are prone to wound-associated cutaneous infections with common gram-positive organisms as well. Folliculitis, furunculosis, and cellulitis are additional manifestations of local staphylococcal or streptococcal infections. Importantly, cellulitis caused by *Streptococcus pyogenes, S. pneumoniae,* or *Staphylococcus aureus* may progress rapidly and cause necrotizing fasciitis in immunosuppressed patients (Fig. 119-12). Solid-organ recipients also may develop recurrent cellulitis of the elbow, a condition termed *transplant elbow,* that has been attributed to staphylococcal infection. Bone marrow transplant patients and other patients with neutropenia are prone to streptococcal bacteremia and may develop facial flushing, a widespread erythematous maculopapular eruption, and desquamation of the palms and soles. Staphylococcal scalded skin syndrome, which typically occurs in children (see Chap. 195), can occur in immunosuppressed adults.[48]

NECROTIZING SOFT-TISSUE INFECTIONS Patients with neutropenia, diabetes, or peripheral vascular disease, as well as postoperative patients and intravenous drug users, are prone to cellulitis and necrotizing fasciitis.[49] Both aerobic and anaerobic bacteria have been implicated in these infections, most commonly *S. pyogenes, S. aureus, Clostridium perfringens, S. pneumoniae, Peptostreptococcus* spp., *Bacteroides fragilis,* and *Escherichia coli.* Patients present with rapidly evolving cellulitis and require aggressive surgical debridement and intravenous antibiotics to control spread of infection.

OTHER BACTERIAL INFECTIONS (See Chap. 197) Individuals with underlying complement deficiencies (loss of late phase components C5–C9) or alcoholism are susceptible to infection with *Neisseria meningitidis.*[50] Patients present with acute septicemia, meningitis, disseminated intravascular coagulation, and widespread petechiae and purpura (Fig. 119-13). Persons with underlying hepatic disease (commonly alcoholic cirrhosis or hemochromatosis) are prone to infection with *Vibrio vulnificus,* a gram-negative bacillus commonly found in seawater, shellfish, clams, and oysters.[51] Infection occurs by ingestion of contaminated seafood or by direct cutaneous inoculation after contact with contaminated seawater, and patients classically present with rapidly evolving septicemia and painful cellulitis, bullae, or ulcers on the lower extremities (Fig. 119-14). *Capnocytophaga canimorsus* is a commensal bacterium found in the saliva of dogs and cats that is transmitted to humans by bites or scratches.[52] Immunosuppressed hosts (postsplenectomy patients, alcoholics) are particularly susceptible to septicemia and widespread organ involvement. Skin lesions occur commonly and include macules, papules, purpura, and gangrene. In immunosuppressed patients, *Salmonella enteritidis* has been associated with cutaneous abscesses of the head and neck.[53]

FIGURE 119-13

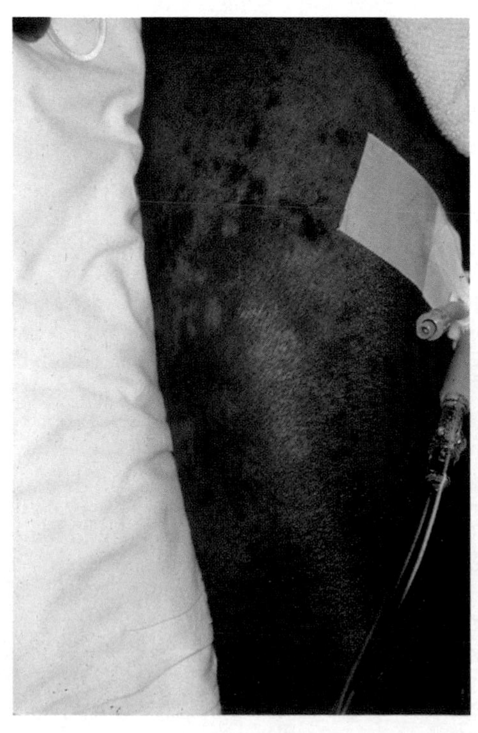

Acute meningococcemia in a man with acquired complement deficiency.

FIGURE 119-14

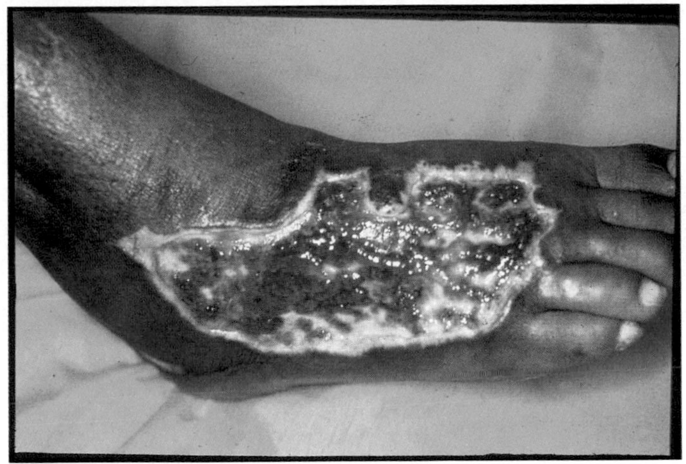

Vibrio vulnificus infection in an alcoholic patient following minor trauma sustained while swimming in the ocean.

Parasitic Infections

NORWEGIAN SCABIES (See Chap. 238) Keratotic (or Norwegian) scabies infection typically occurs in the settings of mental deficiency, malnutrition, or immunosuppression.[54] Clinically, patients present with multiple, widespread, thick, gray or yellowish scaly plaques (Fig. 119-15), with numerous mites present within lesions. Unlike common scabies, pruritus may be minimal. Several courses of treatment with topical lindane or permethrin, as well as keratolytics, may be necessary to cure patients. Oral ivermectin is useful in these patients.

DEMODEX In immunosuppressed hosts, overgrowth of *Demodex* mites as well as abnormal immune responses triggered by *Demodex* mites may lead to rosacea-like disease[55] and eosinophilic folliculitis,[56] respectively. Topical permethrin, sometimes on a chronic basis, is required to treat these patients.

OTHER PARASITIC DISEASES (See Chaps. 235 and 236) Individuals with defects in cell-mediated immunity are more likely to develop parasitic infections.[57] Cutaneous lesions of amebiasis include painful ulcers in the genital or perianal area (due to direct extension for intestinal foci of infection), urticaria, and pruritus.[58] Trypanosomiasis caused by *Trpanosoma cruzi,* or Chagas' disease, can lead to severe heart disease that requires cardiac transplantation. Paradoxically, immunosuppressive therapy required to maintain the transplanted heart may lead to reactivation of Chagas' disease.[59] Cutaneous lesions appear as subcutaneous nodules. In immunocompromised individuals, strongyloidiasis caused by *Strongyloides stercoralis* may be severe and cause pneumonia, severe gastrointestinal symptoms, urticaria, generalized pruritus, and larva currens (rapidly moving larvae under skin of covered areas).[60]

FIGURE 119-15

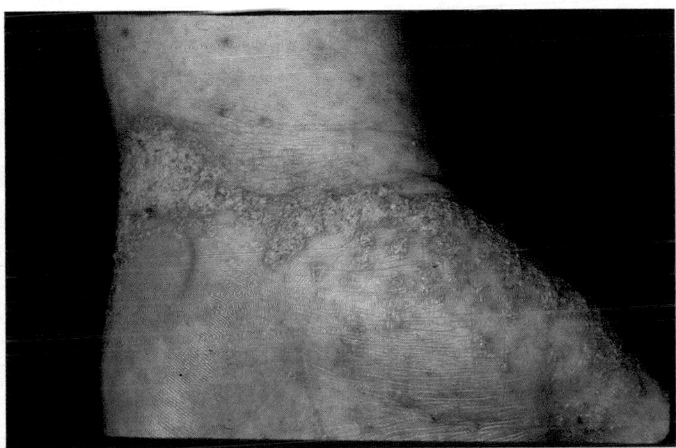

Norwegian scabies in a man with non-Hodgkin's lymphoma.

CANCERS

Nonmelanoma Skin Cancer (See also Chaps. 80 and 81)

Individuals who have received a solid-organ transplant are at high risk for developing nonmelanoma skin cancers.[61,62] The risk for developing skin cancer in other immunosuppressed populations is probably increased as well, but this group of individuals is not nearly as well studied. In posttransplant Caucasian patients, the incidence and prevalence of both squamous cell carcinomas and basal cell carcinomas are staggering, occurring in up to 40 and 70 percent of patients within 5 and 20 years following transplant surgery, respectively[63]; initial cancers usually occur within 2 to 3 years of surgery.[64] At a minimum, these numbers represent a 20-fold increase in nonmelanoma skin carcinoma incidence when compared with immunocompetent Caucasians. In addition, renal transplant patients have a 100-fold increase in anogenital carcinomas compared with the general population.[65] In skin, most studies show that squamous cell carcinomas occur more commonly than basal cell carcinomas (approximately 2:1 ratio). The incidence of other epidermal proliferative diseases is greatly increased as well, including actinic keratoses, keratoacanthomas, porokeratosis, and Bowen's disease.

The pathogenesis of nonmelanoma skin cancers in posttransplant patients is multifactorial and has been studied extensively. Sun exposure is probably the most important factor. Epidemiologically, patients with fair skin types, those living near the equator (e.g., Australians), and those with documented histories of significant sun exposure (e.g., farmers) are at highest risk.[64] In addition, mutations in the tumor suppressor gene *p*53 within nonmelanoma skin cancers from transplant patients suggest gene inactivation by ultraviolet light.[35,66] The next most important factor in skin cancer development in immunosuppressed hosts is HPV infection. Clinically, squamous cell carcinomas have been reported to arise from common warts. Epidermodysplasia verruciformis–associated HPV (types 5, 8, and many others) also is detected commonly in tumors from these patients.[67] Although known oncogenic HPV (types 16, 18, 31, and 33) is not involved in cutaneous cancers in transplant patients, such types do contribute to the development of anogenital carcinomas in this population[65] (see Chap. 223). Genetically, certain HLA types (e.g., HLA-B27 or HLA-DR7) may predispose to development of nonmelanoma skin cancer.[68] Immunosuppressive drugs required for maintenance of solid-organ grafts also probably contribute to cancer development by impairing immune surveillance of tumor cells. In summary, cumulative effects of sunlight, HPV infection, genetics, and systemic immunosuppression contribute to the high incidence of skin cancer in posttransplant patients.

Squamous cell and basal cell carcinomas occur most commonly on sun-exposed areas of the body. Importantly, these cancers (especially squamous cell carcinomas) can be particularly aggressive. Local invasion, recurrence following primary treatment, and distant metastases are not uncommon. Fatalities caused by metastatic squamous cell carcinoma in immunocompromised patients also have been reported. Thus careful and regular examination of skin is required for all Caucasian posttransplant patients, with an emphasis on monitoring all potential premalignant lesions (e.g., actinic keratoses, porokeratosis) for morphologic changes. Recently, the use of topical or oral retinoids has been advocated in the prophylaxis of nonmelanoma skin cancers following transplantation surgery. Regular use of topical tretinoin, oral etretinate, and oral acitretin has been shown to decrease the incidence of both benign and malignant epidermal diseases.[33–36]

Kaposi's Sarcoma (See also Chap. 104)

Kaposi's sarcoma (KS) is a multifocal inflammatory and proliferative disease that (in most cases) is probably not a true malignancy. It typically occurs in distinct populations, including patients receiving immunosuppressive therapy.[69] This form of KS is commonly called *iatrogenic KS*. Interestingly, Chang and Moore first identified KSHV in KS lesions from AIDS patients in 1994,[70] and subsequently, this virus was detected within tumor spindle cells of all clinical forms of KS.[71,72] Although KSHV is now generally believed to be the etiologic agent for KS, exact mechanisms involved in KS pathogenesis remain unclear.[29]

KS accounts for approximately 0.5 percent of new neoplasms in organ transplant patients. Lesions appear soon after transplantation and more commonly in patients with liver transplants compared with those with renal transplants. In addition, individuals on cyclosporine-based immunosuppressive regimens are affected more commonly than individuals not taking cyclosporine. Because cyclosporine potently suppresses T cell function, this finding suggests that T cells are involved in normal immune surveillance and control of KS tumors. Epidemiologically, iatrogenic KS occurs more commonly in individuals of Mediterranean, Arabic, Jewish, and African descent compared with persons of northern European descent.[69] This pattern of clinical disease correlates with the incidence and distribution of KSHV seroprevalence,[29] again providing further evidence for a role of KSHV in the pathogenesis of KS.

Clinically, skin lesions of iatrogenic KS are identical to other forms of KS. Typically, early KS lesions are deep red to violaceous macules or patches. With time, lesions develop into papules, plaques, nodules, or tumors. Surface characteristics vary and may be smooth, crusted, necrotic, verrucous, or scaly. Significant edema may be associated with lower leg lesions. KS lesions are found most commonly on the lower legs and feet, although the groin and oral cavity are also common locations. In general, iatrogenic KS is a more aggressive disease than classic (Mediterranean type) KS but usually not as severe as cases of epidemic (HIV-associated) KS and endemic (African) KS. Systemic KS involvement can occur in up to 40 percent of cases in immunosuppressed individuals. The most common sites for internal disease include the lymph nodes, gastrointestinal tract, and lungs.

The first line of treatment for iatrogenic KS is to remove or decrease immunosuppressive therapy. This can lead to complete clearing of KS in up to 30 percent of patients. However, these patients remain at risk for developing KS at later times if immunosuppressive therapy is reinstituted. The decision to decrease or stop immunosuppressive drugs can be complex and should take into consideration the severity and extent of KS, as well as the importance of the immunosuppressive medications in maintaining overall health, e.g., in maintaining a potentially lifesaving transplanted organ. Otherwise, guidelines for KS therapy are no different from those for other forms of KS. Options include local excision or radiation, intralesional therapy, or systemic chemotherapy.

Other Cancers

The incidence of malignant melanoma and widespread atypical melanocytic nevi may be increased in transplant recipients and in other immunosuppressed patients.[73,74] Most melanomas arise from precursor nevi in these patients. Fatal Merkel cell carcinoma has been reported in a renal transplant patient.[75] Oral mucosal leukoplakia and oral carcinoma also occur more commonly in immunocompromised individuals.[76] Lip lesions are particularly common, suggesting a pathogenic role for sunlight in lesion formation. Finally, cutaneous lesions secondary to non-Hodgkin's lymphoma or other lymphoproliferative processes may occur in the setting of iatrogenic immunosuppression.[30] Disease is nearly always linked with EBV infection and is tightly controlled by the immune system; e.g., lesions may resolve following reductions in immunosuppressive drug therapy.

MISCELLANEOUS CONDITIONS

Acute neutrophilic febrile dermatosis (see Chap. 94), or Sweet's syndrome, has been reported in association with malignancies, especially acute myeloid leukemia[77,78] (see also Chap. 184). Lesions can occur prior to the onset of both initial and recurrent leukemic episodes (Fig. 119-16). There is not a female preponderance with malignancy-associated Sweet's syndrome (as there is with idiopathic Sweet's syndrome). Pyoderma gangrenosum (see Chap. 98) has been associated with a wide variety of diseases, including individuals with underlying leukemia.[77,78] Both Sweet's syndrome and pyoderma gangrenosum may represent manifestations of abnormal neutrophil function.

Multiple dermatofibromas and multiple lesions of porokeratosis can occur in association with immunosuppressive therapy for autoimmune disease or in the posttransplant setting, although the reasons for this are unclear.[79] Pseudo–hairy leukoplakia is described as adherent, white, corrugated plaques on the lateral aspects of the tongue,[76] clinical features that are identical to EBV-associated oral hairy leukoplakia, as described earlier. Histologic features of these two conditions are also identical. However, EBV and other known viruses cannot be detected in these lesions; thus the etiology is unknown. Although this condition has been reported in transplant patients, its clinical significance in these patients is unclear.[76] Trichomegaly of the eyelashes has been reported in AIDS patients, patients taking cyclosporine, and cancer patients[80]

FIGURE 119-16

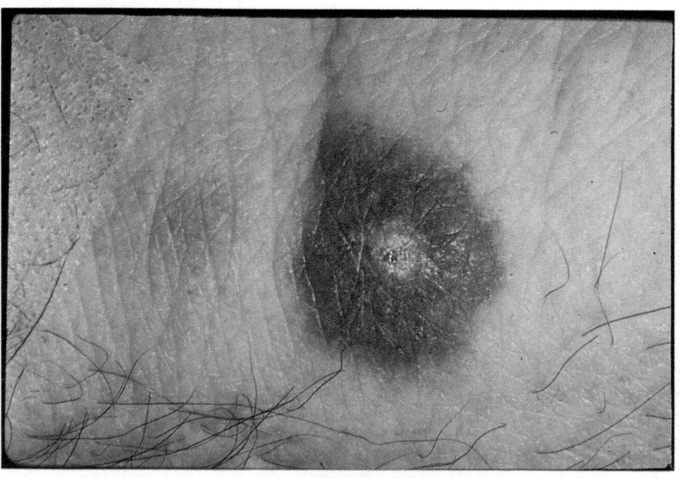

Sweet's syndrome in a man with new-onset acute myeloid leukemia.

FIGURE 119-17

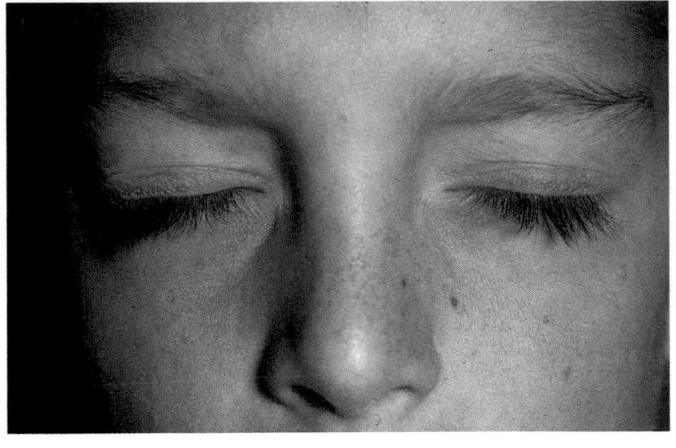

Acquired trichomegaly of the eyelashes in a child with advanced rhabdomyosarcoma.

(Fig. 119-17). The etiology is unclear, but it appears to be a manifestation of severe underlying immunodeficiency.

REFERENCES

1. Kavanaugh DY, Carbone DP: Immunologic dysfunction in cancer. *Hematol Oncol Clin North Am* **10**:927, 1996
2. Emmanouilides C, Glaspy J: Opportunistic infections in oncologic patients. *Hematol Oncol Clin North Am* **10**:841, 1996
3. Yocum DE: Cyclosporine, FK-506, rapamycin, and other immunomodulators. *Rheum Dis Clin North Am* **22**:133, 1996
4. Kontoyiannis DP, Rubin RH: Infection in the organ transplant recipient: an overview. *Infect Dis Clin North Am* **9**:811, 1995
5. Patel R, Paya CV: Infections in solid-organ transplant recipients. *Clin Microbiol Rev* **10**:86, 1997
6. Kurwa HA, Marks R: Protracted cutaneous disorders in association with low CD4+ lymphocyte counts. *Br J Dermatol* **133**:625, 1995
7. Wright WL, Wenzel RP: Nosocomial *Candida:* Epidemiology, transmission, and prevention. *Infect Dis Clin North Am* **11**:411, 1997
8. Bodey GP: Dermatologic manifestations of infections in neutropenic patients. *Infect Dis Clin* **8**:655, 1994
9. Wingard JR: Importance of *Candida* species other than *C. albicans* as pathogens in oncology patients. *Clin Infect Dis* **20**:115, 1995
10. Conant MA: Fungal infections in immunocompromised individuals. *Dermatol Clin* **14**:155, 1996
11. King GN et al: Prevalence and risk factors associated with leukoplakia, hairy leukoplakia, erythematous candidiasis and gingival hyperplasia in renal transplant recipients. *Oral Surg Oral Med Oral Pathol Radiol Endod* **78**:718, 1994
12. Isaac M: Cutaneous aspergillosis. *Dermatol Clin* **14**:137, 1996
13. Adam RD et al: Mucormycosis: Emerging prominence of cutaneous infections. *Clin Infect Dis* **19**:67, 1994
14. Boutati EI, Anaissie EJ: *Fusarium,* a significant emerging pathogen in patients with hematologic malignancy: Ten years' experience at a cancer center and implications for management. *Blood* **90**:999, 1997
15. Hajjeh RA, Blumberg HM: Bloodstream infection due to *Trichosporon beigelii* in a burn patient: Case report and review of therapy. *Clin Infect Dis* **20**:913, 1995
16. White MH, Armstrong D: Cryptococcosis. *Infect Dis Clin* **8**:383, 1994
17. Pema K et al: Disseminated cutaneous cryptococcosis: Comparison of clinical manifestations in the pre-AIDS and AIDS eras. *Arch Intern Med* **154**:1032, 1994
18. Bradsher RW: Histoplasmosis and blastomycosis. *Clin Infect Dis* **22**:S102, 1996
19. Stevens DA: Coccidioidomycosis. *N Engl J Med* **332**:1077, 1995
20. Duong TA: Infection due to *Penicillium marneffei,* an emerging pathogen: Review of 155 reported cases. *Clin Infect Dis* **23**:125, 1996
21. Berenguer J et al: Deep infections caused by *Scedosporium prolificans*: A report on 16 cases in Spain and a review of the literature. *Medicine* **76**:256, 1997
22. Machet L et al: Cutaneous alternariosis: Role of corticosteroid-induced cutaneous fragility. *Dermatology* **193**:342, 1996
23. Itin PH et al: Cutaneous manifestations of *Paecilomyces lilacinus* infection induced by a contaminated skin lotion in patients who are severely immunosuppressed. *J Am Acad Dermatol* **39**:401, 1998
24. Rinaldi MG: Phaeohyphomycosis. *Dermatol Clin* **14**:147, 1996
25. Assaf RR, Weil ML: The superficial mycoses. *Dermatol Clin* **14**:57, 1996
26. Whitley RJ et al: Herpes simplex viruses. *Clin Infect Dis* **26**:541, 1998
27. Cohen JI et al: Recent advances in varicella-zoster virus infection. *Ann Intern Med* **130**:922, 1999
28. Drago F et al: Cytomegalovirus infection in normal and immunocompromised humans: A review. *Dermatology* **200**:189, 2000
29. Blauvelt A: Skin diseases associated with human herpesvirus 6, 7, and 8 infection. *J Investig Dermatol Symp Proc* **6**:197, 2001
30. Nalesnik MA: Posttransplantation lymphoproliferative disorders (PTLD): Current perspectives. *Semin Thorac Cardiovasc Surg* **8**:139, 1996
31. Bouwes JNB, Berkhout RJ: HPV infections and immunosuppression. *Clin Dermatol* **15**:427, 1997
32. Barba A et al: Analysis of risk factors for cutaneous warts in renal transplant recipients. *Nephron* **77**:422, 1997
33. Rook AH et al: Beneficial effect of low-dose systemic retinoid in combination with topical tretinoin for the treatment and prophylaxis of premalignant and malignant skin lesions in renal transplant recipients. *Transplantation* **59**:714, 1995
34. Bavinck JN et al: Prevention of skin cancer and reduction of keratotic skin lesions during acitretin therapy in renal transplant recipients: A double-blind, placebo-controlled study. *J Clin Oncol* **13**:1933, 1995
35. Gibson GE et al: *p*53 tumor suppressor gene protein expression in premalignant and malignant skin lesions of kidney transplant recipients. *J Am Acad Dermatol* **36**:924, 1997
36. Yuan ZF et al: Use of acitretin for the skin complications in renal transplant recipients. *N Z Med J* **108**:255, 1995
37. Birthistle K, Carrington D: Molluscum contagiosum virus. *J Infect* **34**:21, 1997
38. Kaplan LJ et al: Severe measles in immunocompromised patients. *JAMA* **267**:1237, 1992
39. Lerner PI: Nocardiosis. *Clin Infect Dis* **22**:891, 1996
40. Warren NG: Actinomycosis, nocardiosis, and actinomycetoma. *Dermatol Clin* **14**:85, 1996
41. deJong R et al: Severe mycobacterial and *Salmonella* infections in interleukin-12 receptor-deficient patients. *Science* **280**:1435, 1998
42. Weitzul S et al: Nontuberculous mycobacterial infections of the skin. *Dermatol Clin* **18**:359, 2000
43. Tartaglione T: Treatment of nontuberculous mycobacterial infections: Role of clarithromycin and azithromycin. *Clin Ther* **19**:626, 1997
44. Kawabata E et al: Bilateral inguinal scrofuloderma during steroid therapy in a patient with bullous pemphigoid. *J Dermatol* **22**:582, 1995
45. Libraty DH, Byrd TF: Cutaneous miliary tuberculosis in the AIDS era: Case report and review. *Clin Infect Dis* **23**:706, 1996
46. Spach DH, Koehler JE: *Bartonella*-associated infections. *Infect Dis Clin* **12**:137, 1998
47. Donnelly JP: Bacterial complications of transplantation: diagnosis and treatment. *J Antimicrob Chemother* **36**:59, 1995
48. Strauss G et al: Staphylococcal scalded skin syndrome in a liver transplant patient. *Liver Transplant Surg* **3**:435, 1997
49. Stone DR, Gorbach SL: Necrotizing fasciitis: The changing spectrum. *Dermatol Clin* **15**:213, 1997
50. Salzman MB, Rubin LG: Meningococcemia. *Infect Dis Clin* **10**:709, 1996
51. Kumamoto KS, Vukich DJ: Clinical infections of *Vibrio vulnificus*: A case report and review of the literature. *J Emerg Med* **16**:61, 1998
52. Lion C et al: *Capnocytophaga canimorsus* infections in humans: Review of the literature and cases report. *Eur J Epidemiol* **12**:521, 1996
53. Ray J et al: A rare case of *Salmonella* neck abscess. *J Laryngol Otol* **111**:489, 1997
54. Orkin M: Scabies: What's new? *Curr Probl Dermatol* **22**:105, 1995
55. Ivy SP et al: Demodicidosis in childhood acute lymphoblastic leukemia: An opportunistic infection occurring with immunosuppression. *J Pediatr* **127**:751, 1995
56. Evans TRJ et al: Eosinophilic folliculitis occurring after bone marrow autograft in a patient with non-Hodgkin's lymphoma. *Cancer* **73**:2512, 1994
57. Ambroise-Thomas P: Parasitic diseases and immunodeficiencies. *Parasitology* **122**:S65, 2001
58. Marshall MM et al: Waterborne protozoan pathogens. *Clin Microbiol Rev* **10**:67, 1997

59. Tomimori-Yamashita J et al: Cutaneous manifestation of Chagas' disease after heart transplantation: Successful treatment with allopurinol. *Br J Dermatol* **137**:626, 1997
60. Kramer MR et al: Disseminated strongyloidiasis in AIDS and non-AIDS immunocompromised hosts: Diagnosis by sputum and bronchoalveolar lavage. *South Med J* **83**:1226, 1990
61. Veness MJ et al: Aggressive cutaneous malignancies following cardiothoracic transplantation: The Australian experience. *Cancer* **85**:1758, 1999
62. Otley CC, Pittelkow MR: Skin cancer in liver transplant recipients. *Liver Transplant* **6**:253, 2000
63. Bouwes JNB et al: The risk of skin cancer in renal transplant recipients in Queensland, Australia: A follow-up study. *Transplantation* **61**:715, 1996
64. Espana A et al: Skin cancer in heart transplant recipients. *J Am Acad Dermatol* **32**:458, 1995
65. Wright TC, Sun XW: Anogenital papillomavirus infection and neoplasia in immunodeficient women. *Obstet Gynecol Clin North Am* **23**:861, 1996
66. McGregor JM et al: *p*53 mutations implicate sunlight in post-transplant skin cancer irrespective of human papillomavirus status. *Oncogene* **15**:1737, 1997
67. Berkhout RJ et al: Nested PCR approach for detection and typing of epidermodysplasia verruciformis–associated human papillomavirus types in cutaneous cancers from renal transplant recipients. *J Clin Microbiol* **33**:690, 1995
68. Bouwes JNB et al: Relation between HLA antigens and skin cancer in renal transplant recipients in Queensland, Australia. *J Invest Dermatol* **108**:708, 1997
69. Gotti E, Remuzzi G: Post-transplant Kaposi's sarcoma. *J Am Soc Nephrol* **8**:130, 1997
70. Chang Y et al: Identification of herpesvirus-like DNA sequences in AIDS-associated Kaposi's sarcoma. *Science* **266**:1865, 1994
71. Moore PS, Chang Y: Detection of herpesvirus-like DNA sequences in Kaposi's sarcoma in patients with and those without HIV infection. *N Engl J Med* **332**:1181, 1995
72. Boshoff C et al: Kaposi's-sarcoma-associated herpesvirus in HIV-negative Kaposi's sarcoma. *Lancet* **345**:1043, 1995
73. Frezza EE et al: Non-lymphoid cancer after liver transplantation. *Hepatogastroenterology* **44**:1172, 1997
74. Richert S et al: Widespread eruptive dermal and atypical melanocytic nevi in association with chronic myelocytic leukemia: Case report and review of the literature. *J Am Acad Dermatol* **35**:326, 1996
75. Douds AC et al: Fatal Merkel-cell tumour (cutaneous neuroendocrine carcinoma) complicating renal transplantation. *Nephrol Dial Transplant* **10**:2346, 1995
76. Seymour RA et al: Oral lesions in organ transplant patients. *J Oral Pathol Med* **26**:297, 1997
77. Kurzrock R, Cohen PR: Mucocutaneous paraneoplastic manifestations of hematologic malignancies. *Am J Med* **99**:207, 1995
78. Huang W, McNeely MC: Neutrophilic tissue reactions. *Adv Dermatol* **13**:33, 1997
79. Herranz P et al: High incidence of porokeratosis in renal transplant recipients. *Br J Dermatol* **136**:176, 1997
80. Velez A et al: Acquired trichomegaly and hypertrichosis in metastatic adenocarcinoma. *Clin Exp Dermatol* **20**:237, 1995

CHAPTER 120

Donald V. Belsito

Allergic Contact Dermatitis

Allergic contact dermatitis (ACD) is one of the more frequent, vexing, and costly dermatologic problems. When the incidence of all occupationally related illness in the United States was last estimated, ACD accounted for 7 percent, at an annual cost of $250 million in lost productivity, medical care, and disability payments.[1] Given data suggesting that the actual annual incidence rate of ACD may be 10 to 50 times greater than reported in the US Bureau of Labor Statistics data, the total annual cost of occupational ACD alone may reach $1.25 billion.[1] It should be noted that these estimates were based on the assumption that 80 percent of occupational contact dermatitis (OCD) is irritant and 20 percent allergic. However, recent data from the United Kingdom[2] and the United States[3] suggest that the percentage of OCD due to allergy may be much higher, ranging between 50 and 60 percent, thus raising the economic impact of occupational ACD to greater than $3 billion annually. The additional costs of nonoccupational contact dermatitis are difficult to assess. In one study, nonoccupational ACD was found three times more frequently than occupational disease.[3] Furthermore, these estimates do not include the economic impact of retraining workers and "quality of life" issues.

HISTORICAL ASPECTS

Although ACD has probably plagued humans for millennia, the term *allergy* and its clinical recognition by patch testing are barely a century old. With the advent of experimental animal models for ACD in the 1920s, studies concerning its pathophysiology became possible. Despite all the clinical and scientific research since, a thorough understanding of the disease remains elusive.

EPIDEMIOLOGY

Incidence and Prevalence of Disease

The relatively few population-based studies assessing incidence and prevalence rates of ACD have primarily centered on specific allergens. Occupational data provide most of the available estimates. However, as previously noted, these data are subject to considerable underreporting. In one of the few population-based studies available, 86 (15.2 percent) of 567 randomly recruited adults had evidence of at least 1 allergic reaction to the 23 allergens tested.[4] Of note, more women (18.8 percent) were found to have contact allergies than men (11.5 percent) in this study. However, it must be understood that these numbers refer to the prevalence of ACD in the population (i.e., the number of individuals who have the capability to develop ACD when exposed to an allergen), and not to its incidence (i.e., number of individuals who develop ACD over a defined period of time).

Age-Related Effects

Clinically, aged individuals have various defects in the induction and/or elicitation of ACD.[5] In studies on Rhus reactivity, younger (18 to 25 years) individuals had a quicker onset and a quicker resolution of the dermatitis than did older persons.[6] When sensitization rates to standard allergens were evaluated as a function of age, incidence rates dropped significantly in individuals older than 70 years.[6] For potent allergens such as dinitrochlorobenzene (DNCB), the effect of age on the induction of sensitization is more controversial.[7,8] The precise reason for this age-related decline in contact sensitivity is unknown. Experiments in which contact-sensitized aged mice were reconstituted with naïve young T cells so that they subsequently demonstrated normal responses upon antigenic challenge suggest that a failure of T cell amplification signals and/or the generation of sufficient T effector cells may be the primary deficiencies in aged animals.[9]

The competency of T cell–mediated immune reactions in children is controversial.[5] It was believed that children rarely developed ACD because of an immature immune system. However, as suggested by Strauss[10] who was able to sensitize 35 of 48 infants (1 to 4 days old) to *Toxicodendron* oleoresin, the apparent hyporesponsiveness of children may be due to limited exposure and not to deficient immunity. Thus, documented allergic reactions are seen mostly in older pediatric patients and are secondary to topical medications, plants, nickel, fragrances, or shoe-related allergens.[5]

Patterns of Exposure

Allergen exposure, and, hence, the likelihood of sensitization, varies not only with age, but also with social customs, environmental factors, avocation, and occupation. Although most of the gender-related and geographic variations in ACD have been attributed to social and environmental factors,[5] avocation and occupation have more pronounced effects. Allergic reactions to thiurams (and other rubber constituents), topical medicaments (benzocaine and neomycin), and nickel are common among sports enthusiasts, who are frequently exposed to these materials.[11] Health care workers have high rates of sensitization to thiurams in gloves, while dental personnel and endoscopic technicians frequently react to glutaraldehyde, which is a rare allergen in the general population.[12] Finally, one must be constantly vigilant for the arrival of potentially new allergens into the environment. For example, the North American Contact Dermatitis Group recently added a number of amide anesthetics, once considered rare sensitizers, to its screening tray given the recent widespread use of topical anesthetic creams containing these agents.

Concomitant Disease

Impairment of cell-mediated immunity has been reported in certain diseases. In addition to the obvious disorders associated with immunologic deficiency, such as AIDS or severe combined immunodeficiency, diseases as diverse as lymphoma, sarcoidosis, lepromatous leprosy, and atopic dermatitis have been associated with diminished reactivity or anergy. However, while atopic individuals may be less-readily sensitized, the repeated application of topical preparations to their damaged skin can result in a significant incidence of ACD in this population.[13]

PATHOPHYSIOLOGY

The Allergens

Most environmental allergens are haptens, simple chemicals that must link to proteins to form a complete antigen before they can sensitize. These haptens are primarily small ($\leq$ 500 kDa) electrophilic molecules that bind to carrier proteins via covalent bonds (Table 120-1). Although there are more than 3700 known environmental allergens,[15] not all electrophilic, protein-binding substances are haptens. The nature of the antigenic determinants, the type of binding that the hapten undergoes with the carrier, the final three-dimensional configuration of the conjugate, and a variety of unknown factors contribute to the antigenicity of a chemical. However, the importance of the carrier for the hapten cannot be underestimated because potent contact sensitizers, when complexed to nonimmunogenic carriers, can induce tolerance rather than sensitization. HLA-DR or class II antigens on the surface of the antigen-presenting Langerhans cells (LCs) act as the binding site (carrier) for contact allergens. The pathophysiologic basis of ACD, a type IV, cell-mediated, delayed hypersensitivity is reviewed in Chap. 23.

Induction and Elicitation

In order for ACD to develop, a genetically susceptible individual must have biologically significant, and often repeated, contact with the allergen. As delineated by Friedmann[16] in his review of the dose/response induction of ACD to DNCB, "An apparently ineffective sensitizing stimulus is . . . registered immunologically . . . [and results in] enhanced subsequent responses to the same antigen." This progressive subclinical induction of disease is consistent with the multitude of clinical observations that induction of allergy often takes months to years of exposure to low levels of the allergen.[17] Furthermore, a variety of endogenous and exogenous factors can influence both the induction and elicitation of allergic reactions (Table 120-2).

The concentrations for inducing ACD are probably the same as those for eliciting the disease in "real life," as opposed to the higher concentrations of allergen required to induce and elicit disease acutely in the laboratory. The point is reinforced by the data on incidence rates of occupational ACD, for example, to chromium in cement workers chronically exposed to low levels (10 to 50 ppm) of the sensitizing hexavalent form of this metal.[18] Because cement is diluted with water prior to use, chromium concentrations necessary for induction and elicitation of clinical disease in cement workers are significantly lower than the chromium concentrations typically used for inducing or eliciting the allergy by patch testing (2500 to 5000 ppm).

Primary Sensitization

The route of primary sensitization has a profound effect on the subsequent immunologic response. Tolerance induction has been reported after primary systemic injection or oral ingestion of allergens, and after primary epicutaneous application of allergens to areas deficient in HLA-DR–positive LCs. The exact mechanism by which tolerance ensues is controversial and partly depends on the route of exposure. In most instances, either induction of hapten-specific suppressor T cells or clonal deletion of the responding T cells seems responsible. Antibodies

TABLE 120-1

The Twenty-five Most Frequent Allergens in the United States: 1996 to 1998*†

ALLERGEN	NO. OF PATIENTS TESTED	POSITIVE REACTIONS (%)	POSITIVE REACTIONS CONSIDERED RELEVANT (%)
Nickel sulfate	3429	14.2	49.1
Neomycin sulfate	3436	13.1	46.2
Balsam of Peru	3439	11.8	82.9
Fragrance mix‡	4095	11.7	86.9
Thimerosal	4087	10.9	16.8
Sodium gold thiosulfate	4101	9.5	40.6
Formaldehyde	3440	9.3	63.2
Quaternium-15	3436	9.0	88.7
Cobalt	4095	9.0	55.1
Bacitracin	4103	8.7	50.4
MDBGN/PE	4054	7.6	59.1
Carba mix¶	3437	7.3	71.7
EU-MF	4095	7.2	65.9
Thiuram mix§	3435	6.9	79.8
Para-phenylenediamine	3441	6.0	53.1
Propylene glycol	4095	3.8	82.8
Diazolidinyl urea	4095	3.7	91.5
Lanolin	3442	3.3	78.9
Imidazolidinyl urea	4094	3.2	91.7
2-Bromo-2-nitropropane-1,3,diol	4094	3.2	68.5
MCI/MI	4083	2.9	87.2
Potassium dichromate	3440	2.8	54.3
Ethylenediamine dihydrochloride	3439	2.6	23.9
DMDM hydantoin	4093	2.6	93.4
Glutaraldehyde	4094	2.6	48.1

*The population studied consisted of patients with suspected ACD referred for patch testing and is therefore not necessarily representative of the general population. EU/MF, Ethyleneurea/melamine formaldehyde; MCI/MI, Methylchloroisothiazolinone/methylisothiazolinone (Kathon CG), MDBGN/PE, methyldibromo-glutaronitrile/phenoxyethanol (Euxyl K400).

†Although *Toxicodendron* oleoresin in poison ivy/oak and sesquiterpene lactones in Compositae are frequent causes of ACD, they are not listed because they were not tested in this study.

‡Cinnamic alcohol 1%, cinnamic aldehyde 1%, hydroxycitronellal 1%, amylcinnamaldehyde 1%, geraniol 1%, eugenol 1%, isoeugenol 1%, oakmoss absolute 1%.

¶1,3-Diphenylguanidine 1%, zinc diethyldithiocarbamate 1%, zinc dibutyldithiocarbamate 1%.

§Tetramethylthiuram disulfide 0.25%, tetramethylthiuram monosulfide 0.25%, tetraethylthiuram disulfide 0.25%, dipentamethylenethiuram disulfide 0.25%.

SOURCE: Data from Marks et al.[14]

directed against the antigen recognition site of the T cell receptor (anti-idiotypic antibodies) may also play a role in tolerance. After tolerance is induced, it is long-lived and difficult to break. The mechanism(s) of tolerance induction is reviewed elsewhere.[19]

GENETIC FACTORS

Specific Allergens

Although animal studies show strain (presumably genetic) variation in cell-mediated immunity, the evidence for a genetic influence in humans is slight. Studies on the induction of ACD to DNCB and para-nitrosodimethylaniline (PNDA) suggest a genetic association.[20] However, attempts to correlate HLA haplotype with nickel sensitivity or other contact allergies have shown no association. Thus, definitive evidence of class II-related influences on ACD in humans has been meager, probably because of our diverse genetic pool and the limitations of technology.

Racial Differences

Whether African Americans develop significantly fewer reactions than do Caucasians to potent allergens such as DNCB, PNDA, or para-phenylenediamine (PPD) is controversial.[6] However, in the limited studies performed to date, the rate of sensitization to weaker allergens (e.g., nickel and neomycin) seem to be reduced in African Americans when compared to Caucasians.[6] This reduced rate of sensitization most likely relates to the greater compaction and lipid content in the stratum corneum of African American in contrast to white skin. This enhanced barrier function of African American skin, which is also thought to account for reduced rates of irritant contact dermatitis in this population, likely results in the observed differences in ACD, rather than any innate, genetically based, immunologic factors.[6]

Studies regarding ACD in other racial groups are very limited. In human "maximization tests" of cosmetic ingredients, Japanese individuals showed more severe allergic reactions than did Caucasians, although incidence rates for reactivity were the same.[21] Furthermore, Goh found no differences in the incidence of ACD among the indigenous (Malay, Chinese, and Indian) subpopulations in Singapore.[22] Additional studies evaluating racial influences on immunologic and nonimmunologic (e.g., barrier function) factors affecting ACD are needed.

Gender

The genetic effects of gender on ACD remain controversial because few studies have looked at induction of sensitization under similar circumstances in men and women. When the "human repeat insult patch testing" method was used to assess induction rates to 10 common allergens, women were found to be more often sensitized to 7 of the 10 allergens studied.[23] However, in "maximization studies" looking at allergens of different potencies, women reacted more frequently only to the weakest sensitizers.[24] Nonetheless, when challenged with the potent allergen DNCB, women had significantly more severe reactions at lower doses than did men.[25] Thus, female gender seems to correlate with higher rates of sensitization and frequently more severe reactivity, at least for some allergens. Notwithstanding this, most gender differences

TABLE 120-2

Endogenous and Exogenous Factors Affecting Thresholds for Allergic Contact Dermatitis

ENDOGENOUS	EXOGENOUS
Application site	Vehicle
• State of stratum corneum	pH
• Follicular shunting	Exposure time
• Epidermal thickness	Exposure area
Immunologic state of the host	Occlusion
• Medications/disease states	Ambient temperature
• Sunlight exposure	Ambient humidity
• Concomitant exposure	Concomitant exposures

in ACD seem to relate to cultural patterns and/or exposures in the workplace.[5]

PREVENTION

Avoidance of Allergens

In most cases, "prevention" of ACD has been through avoidance of allergen(s) once the individual has become sensitized. However, for some chemicals (such as the metals nickel and chromium), avoidance once sensitization has occurred does not necessarily result in symptomatic improvement. Burrows[18] found that more than 70 percent of chromium-sensitive workers in Northern Ireland had persistence of their skin disease for greater than 10 years. The persistence of ACD to metals, especially nickel and chrome, may partly be related to their trace levels in foods. Investigators have demonstrated that levels of nickel and/or chromium similar to those in foods are capable of eliciting allergic reactions in some sensitized individuals.[26]

Overall, the prognosis for occupationally acquired allergy is poor. In an Australian study of nearly 1000 workers with occupational skin disease, 54.7 percent had persistent problems, including many of the >40 percent who changed jobs.[27] Thus, allergen avoidance once sensitization occurs is inadequate prevention. Furthermore, advising workers with ACD to leave their current positions may not be the best advice, especially if a job change will result in a significantly negative economic impact.

Induction Thresholds

True prevention of ACD lies in the determination of thresholds for induction of disease. Armed with this information, products can be marketed and workplaces designed that contain allergens at levels below these thresholds. Led by Denmark, the European Economic Community (EEC) has restricted nickel content in metals that can contact the skin to $\leq 0.5\ \mu g$ nickel per cm^2 of skin per week. A decreased rate of nickel dermatitis has been noted.[28] Recently, some authors have argued for restrictions on chromium content in consumer products to ≤ 5 ppm to reduce rates of nonoccupational chromate dermatitis.[29] Already, many European countries add ferrous sulfate to cement to lessen the concentration of hexavalent chromium below the 10 to 50 ppm range, and hence reduce the sensitizing capacity of cements. As with nickel restriction, these occupational measures have significantly reduced the development of new cases of contact dermatitis to chromium in those countries where they have been instituted. Recently, European Economic Community (EEC) investigators have begun to focus on threshold induction levels for certain allergenic fragrances, such as isoeugenol.

In the US and EEC, labeling laws give the consumer access to the specific ingredients contained in cosmetics and over-the-counter/ prescription medicaments, but do not guarantee that these have been formulated to minimize sensitization by potential allergens. Although the safety of individual cosmetic ingredients is reviewed by the Cosmetic Ingredient Review's (CIR's) Expert Panel (Washington, DC), and although the panel has set limits on the use of specific ingredients based upon their ability to sensitize [e.g., parabens should not be used in products designed for use on damaged skin and the concentration of methylchloroisothiazolinone/methylisothiazolinone (MCI/MI) should be ≤ 7.5 ppm in "leave on" products], the panel's findings are not binding upon manufacturers unless the US Food and Drug Administration (FDA) chooses to enforce its rulings. However, one might anticipate that manufacturers would not take the legal and/or financial risks of marketing a product that sensitizes a significant proportion of consumers, especially if the sensitizer has been restricted by CIR.

In workplaces in the US, individuals have less assurance regarding exposure to potential allergens. Although material safety data sheets (MSDS) should be available for materials handled occupationally, many times the contents are labeled proprietary. In addition, MSDS sheets do not need to list chemicals present in amounts <1 percent, unless they are carcinogenic. Unfortunately, many common sensitizers, such as biocides, are present at ≤ 1 percent. Even latex, the cause of life-threatening urticarial reactions in some individuals, is labeled on medical, but not nonmedical, products.

Currently, prevention requires postsensitization counseling and allergen avoidance. The success of such efforts after the diagnosis of ACD largely depends upon how rapidly the correct diagnosis is made. The longer the dermatitis persists before adequate treatment, the poorer the prognosis for complete resolution. Furthermore, patient education regarding allergen avoidance is crucial to improving outcome. In a study of 230 workers,[30] only one-third accurately recalled their diagnosis and treatment regimens and, among those workers who could not remember, persistent dermatitis was three times more likely.

CLINICAL MANIFESTATIONS

Physical Findings

The clinical appearance of ACD can vary depending on its location and duration. In most instances, acute eruptions are characterized by macular erythema and papules, vesicles, or bullae, depending on the intensity of the allergic response (Fig. 120-1). However, in acute ACD in certain areas of the body, such as the eyelids, penis, and scrotum, erythema

FIGURE 120-1

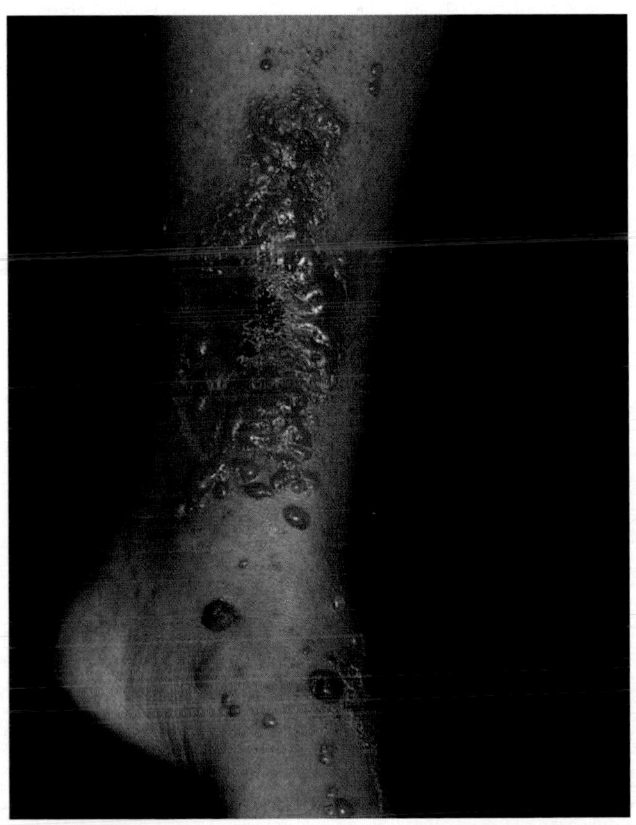

Acute dermatitis due to poison ivy. Note the linear arrangement of the lesions typical of phytodermatitis acquired by inadvertent contact with the plant. The severe vesiculobullous reaction is typical for urushiol, the pentadecylcatechol of *Toxicodendron* spp.

and edema usually predominate rather than vesiculation. In contrast, chronic ACD of nearly all cutaneous sites presents as a lichenified, scaling, occasionally fissured dermatitis, with or without accompanying papulovesiculation (Figs. 120-2 and 120-3).

At its inception, ACD usually involves the cutaneous site of principal exposure. However, as it evolves, it can spread to other more distant sites either by inadvertent contact or, under certain circumstances, by autosensitization (see Chap. 121). Of note, the scalp, palms, and soles are relatively resistant to ACD; these areas may exhibit little pathology despite contact with an allergen that produces significant dermatitis in adjacent areas.

A Geographic Approach

While the failure of an eczematous dermatitis to respond to standard treatments may suggest the possibility of ACD, the shape and location(s) of the eruption provide the most important clues, especially to the causal allergen. ACD due to plants (e.g., poison ivy, poison oak, *Primula obconica,* and English ivy) is often characterized by linear lesions (Fig. 120-1). Aeroallergens, such as the sesquiterpene lactones in Compositae, involve the more exposed areas of skin with relative sparing of clothed areas (Fig. 120-4). In contrast, textile-related allergens (azoaniline dyes or urea formaldehyde resins) produce dermatitis of clothed areas with accentuation about the posterior neck, upper back, lateral thorax, waistband, flexor surfaces, and periaxillary areas with relative sparing of the axillary vault and undergarment areas. This pattern of textile-related ACD points out the importance of such nonimmunologic factors as pressure, friction, heat, and perspiration on the ultimate clinical response.

A careful clinical assessment of the patient is required before any diagnostic tests to correctly identify causal allergens. Krasteva et al.[31] have published on the most frequently encountered causes of ACD in the major anatomic areas of the body. Summarized below is an overview of regional contact dermatitis.

HEAD AND NECK ACD of the head and neck can present particular difficulties in determining the causative allergen(s) because many substances could potentially be responsible. One must consider not only the components of facial cosmetics (vehicles, preservatives, emulsifiers, fragrances), airborne allergens (plant resins, fragrances), or photocontact allergens (see Chap. 136), but also grooming aids such as eyelash curlers (nickel, rubber) or make-up applicators (rubber). In addition, allergy to chemicals applied to the scalp, which has a greater resistance to ACD, may manifest itself on the face, ears, and neck while sparing the scalp (e.g., ACD from para-phenylenediamine in hair dyes). Finally, the hands can be an unwitting source of transmission of allergens to the face, ear, and neck, yet manifest no evidence of dermatitis themselves. Indeed, in women, a frequent cause of patchy ACD over the eyelids, face, and neck, but not the hands, are allergens in nail-care products (see Fig. 120-2).

HANDS Dermatitis of the hands, especially when chronic, is the bane of patients and practitioners alike. A history of atopy is frequently seen in many of these patients. In occupationally induced skin diseases, the hand is involved in one-third or more of cases. Among certain "wet work" occupations (health care, food handlers, cosmetologists, etc.), the number of cases of hand dermatitis is even higher.[1]

The etiology of hand dermatitis is complex because multiple factors, in addition to atopy, contribute to its development. In some patients, an acute allergic or irritant contact dermatitis unmasks an endogenous disease (dyshidrosis, psoriasis, etc.) that otherwise might not have produced clinical symptoms. Not unusually, a secondary ACD of the hands

FIGURE 120-2

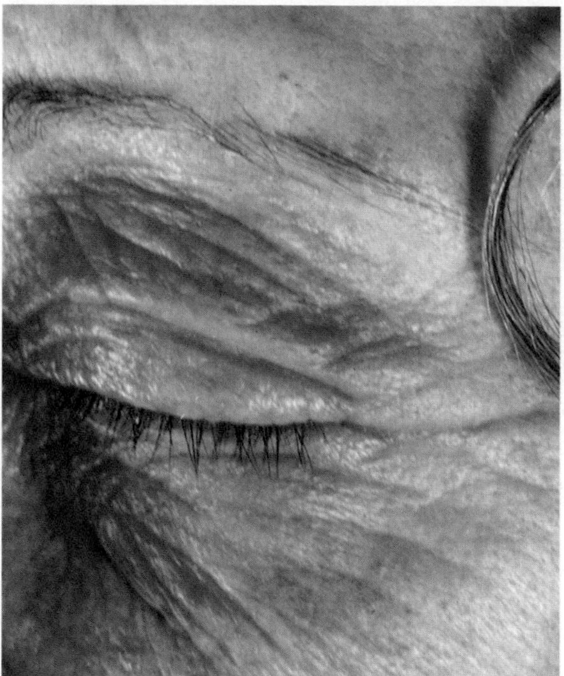

A.

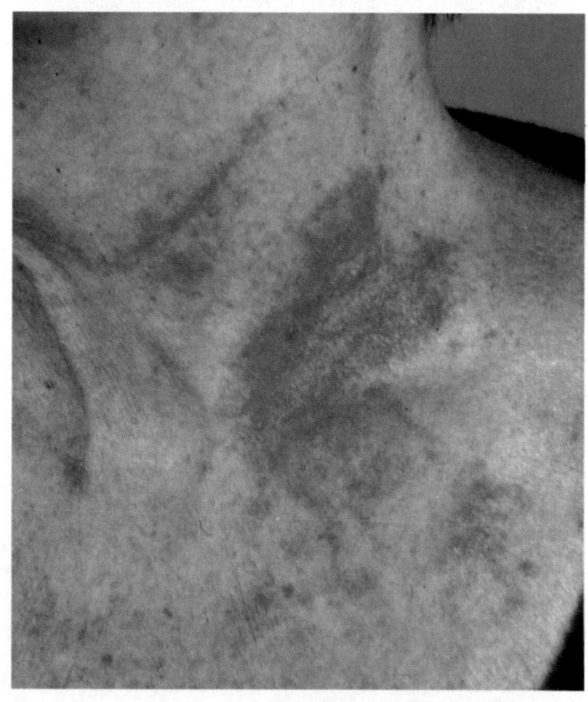

B.

Chronic dermatitis of (*A*) the eyelids and (*B*) the neck, but not the hands, from an allergen in nail-care products. The patient was allergic to tosylamide/formaldehyde resin in her nail polish. Similar reactions caused by tosylamide/epoxy resin in nail polish, or to cyanoacrylate-containing nail glue and other acrylic products used about the nails, can be observed. The absence of an associated dermatitis of the fingers or hands is not unusual.

will develop in a patient with an underlying, nonallergic hand dermatitis who begins using rubber gloves and/or topical creams and who becomes sensitized to a chemical in these products (see Fig. 120-3*A*). Significantly greater involvement of the finger webs and dorsa of the hands, rather than the palms, suggests ACD if the allergen contacts all

FIGURE 120-3

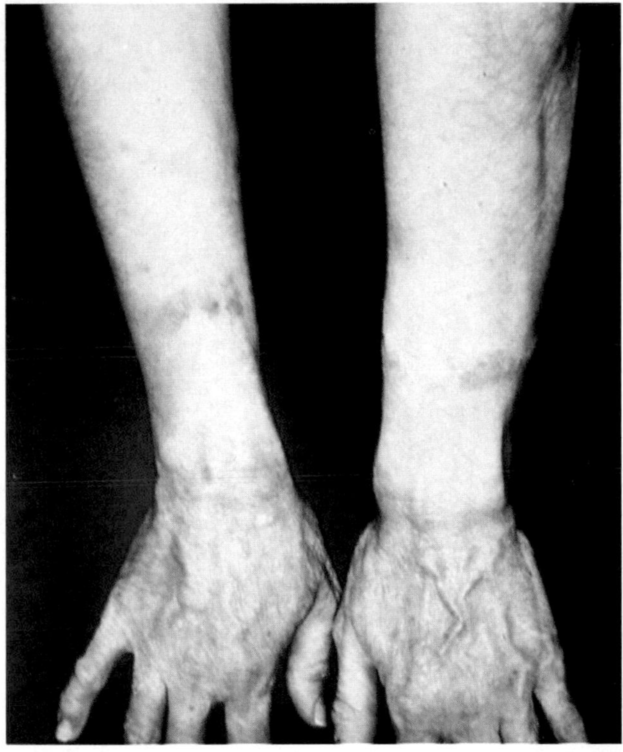

A.

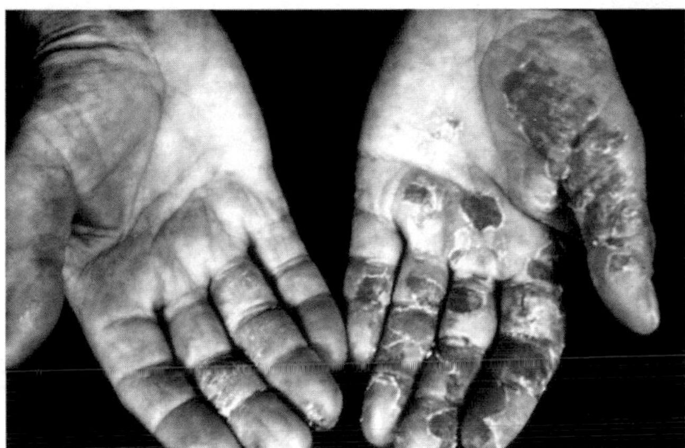

B.

Chronic dermatitis of the hands. *A*. ACD involving the dorsal aspects of the hands and the distal forearms, but with minimal involvement of the palms, due to thiuram present in rubber gloves prescribed for treatment of an irritant hand dermatitis. *B*. ACD involving primarily the palms in a florist allergic to Tuliposide A, the allergen in *Alstroemeria* spp. Note the more prominent involvement of the dominant hand.

FIGURE 120-4

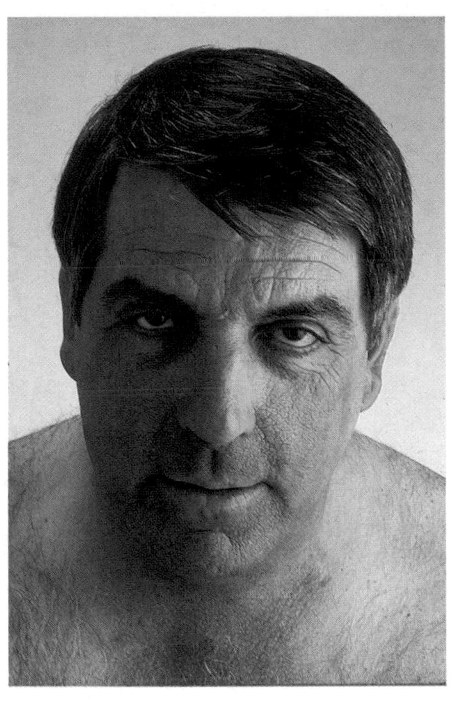

Airborne ACD to sesquiterpene lactones in ragweed (Ambrosia). This outdoorsman had annually developed increasingly more severe outbreaks of dermatitis about the face, neck, upper chest, and forearms beginning in late summer and lasting through the fall. The involvement of the submental area/upper neck and posterior auricular areas helps to differentiate airborne contact from photocontact. Although he reacted strongly to the crushed leaf and stem of native ragweed, he did not react to the commercially available sesquiterpene lactone mix. The failure to react to the commercial mix is not unusual and testing to the plant (as is) should be undertaken, if possible. Although some authors feel that ragweed dermatitis can be photo-accentuated, this was not the case for this patient.

areas of the hand equally (Fig. 120-3*A*). However, the floral worker who snaps the stems and leaves of Peruvian lilies (*Alstroemeria* spp.) with the palmar aspects of the dominant hand and fingers may present with dermatitis restricted primarily to these areas (Fig. 120-3*B*). When seeking an allergic cause for hand dermatitis, one must pay particular attention to those chemicals, listed in standard texts,[32,33] that are encountered in the occupation(s) and hobbies of the patient. In addition, the many household and cosmetic products used must be identified.

FEET ACD of the feet is usually recognizable because, like the palms of the hands, the soles of the feet are relatively resistant to the manifestations of ACD. Thus, the typical picture is a dermatitis over the dorsal feet that is frequently accentuated over the joints of the toes. When the plantar aspects of the feet are involved, ACD typically spares the arch, toe creases, and webs. Nonetheless, despite a clinical picture suggesting allergy, the clinician must consider other diseases (psoriasis, dyshidrosis, juvenile plantar dermatosis, etc.), even when dermatitis is confined only to the feet. When allergic, the principal allergens are rubber accelerators (present in rubber-based liners and/or glues), isocyanates (present in foam rubber), *p*-tert-butylphenol formaldehyde resin (glue), or potassium dichromate (tanned leather) present in shoes.[34] Dyes (in either shoes or socks) are a rare cause of ACD of the feet.

Because the range of potential allergens in shoes frequently goes beyond that in standard testing kits (e.g., dithiodimorphilone and isocyanates),[34] patch testing with materials taken from the shoe can be helpful. When testing with pieces of the shoe, the length of adhesion of the patch to the skin often must be exaggerated beyond 48 hours, perhaps as long 1 week. Before testing, it is important to rule out underlying fungal disease, because at least one investigator has transmitted dermatophyte infection with such patch testing (William P. Jordan, Jr., MD, personal communication). Finally, when evaluating dermatitis of the feet, it is important to note that many cases of secondary ACD develop in individuals applying topical antibiotics (neomycin/bacitracin) and/or topical steroids to an underlying nonallergic dermatitis.[34] As with hand dermatitis, the clinical picture can be confusing.

FIGURE 120-5

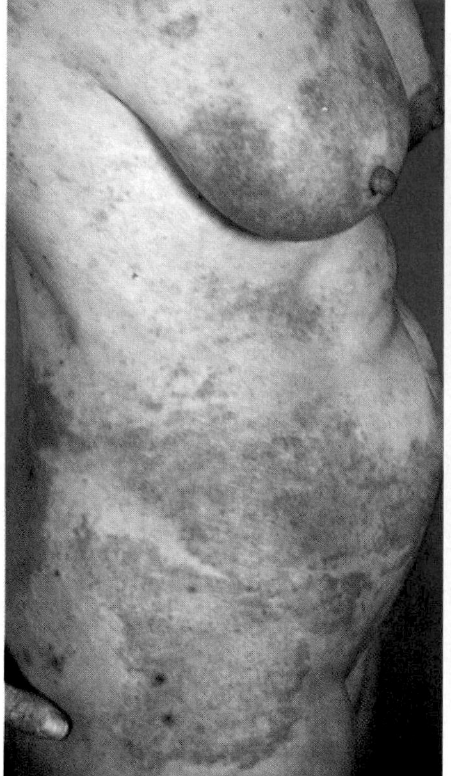

A.

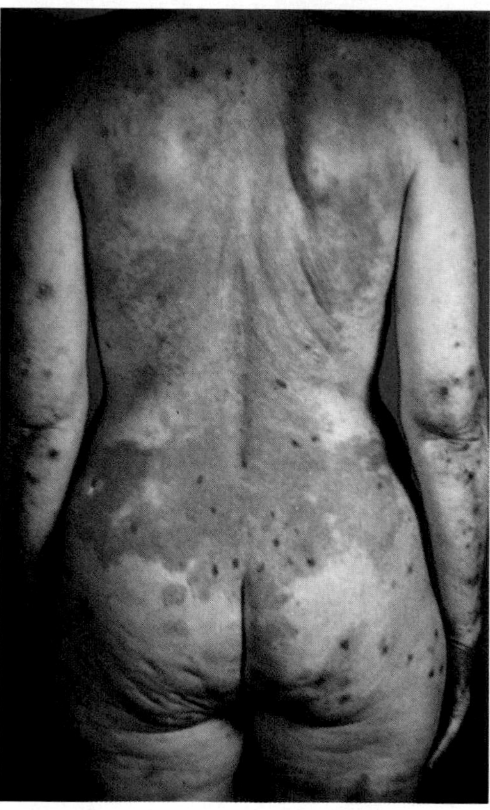

B.

Systemic contact dermatitis due to balsam of Peru. The patient had a history of chronic constipation and used a variety of suppositories. For 7 months she had been bothered by pruritus ani but only recently developed this generalized eruption unresponsive to glucocorticoids and light therapy. The multiple areas of excoriation are indicative of the intense pruritus. The rash was particularly severe about the anus and, for unknown reasons, about the lower torso, buttocks, and genital areas. Her dermatitis cleared when suppositories were discontinued and she was placed on a balsam-free diet. Colonoscopic examination revealed only minimal irritation of the sigmoid colon and rectum compatible with spastic colitis.

IATROGENIC Iatrogenic ACD must always be suspected when the primary dermatitis does not respond to usual therapies. A secondary ACD of the hands can develop in a patient with nonallergic hand dermatitis who uses rubber gloves to protect the hands (Fig. 120-3*A*). Iatrogenic contact dermatitis can also develop from the various topical preparations, including prescriptions, that patients apply. In a recent study, 9 of 70 (12.9 percent) individuals with suspected ACD of the foot had iatrogenic disease secondary to topical steroids (1 of 9), topical antifungals (1 of 9), or topical antibiotics (7 of 9).[34] It can be particularly difficult to identify the allergic nature of iatrogenic ACD because the eczematous quality can be muted by the underlying disease for which the topical preparation was used.

MUCOSAL AND OTHER INTERNAL EXPOSURES ACD of the mucosa is rare.[20,35] Patients allergic to flavorings such as cinnamic aldehyde in toothpastes or mouthwashes frequently present not with intraoral complaints but with a perioral dermatitis extending onto, but not past, the vermilion border of the lips. The unusual individual reacting to nickel, mercury, palladium, or gold in dental amalgams may present with a localized stomatitis and/or systemic contact dermatitis (see below). Given the widespread exposure of the oral mucosa to allergens, the scarcity of reports in the literature makes it obvious that patients only rarely react to allergens intraorally. Thus, one should be wary to ascribe cutaneous symptoms beyond the perioral area to contact with known intraoral allergens (e.g., a patient with scalp dermatitis, nickel allergy and dental amalgams containing nickel most likely has seborrhea or psoriasis and probably will not experience relief of the scalp disease following removal of the amalgams).

The paucity of intraoral ACD has frequently been ascribed to the dilutional effects of saliva. Similarly, tearing of the eyes has been thought to explain why ACD to preservatives, such as thimerosal, in eye drops presents as pronounced erythema and edema of the eyelids with only mild injection of the conjunctiva. Although the dilutional effects of mucosal secretions in modifying ACD cannot be discounted, other unknown factors peculiar to mucosal surfaces are likely to account for the diminished responsiveness. The rectal mucosa, where chemicals are unlikely to be diluted or necessarily promptly swept away, is rarely involved in allergic reactions. ACD from medications and other materials administered per rectum presents as a perianal dermatitis and/or systemic contact dermatitis with little or no rectal pathology (Fig. 120-5).

Although mucosal exposure to allergens infrequently causes symptoms, other internal exposures are even rarer causes of dermatitis. Given the frequency of nickel and cobalt sensitivity in the population, and given the large number of orthopedic implants performed worldwide, the very small number of reports linking dermatitis to intraarticular metals makes it unlikely, although not impossible, that the nickel or cobalt allergic individual with a dermatitis and an artificial joint is reacting to metals in the orthopedic appliance. The literature linking metals in cardiac pacemakers and other implantable devices to dermatitis is even scarcer than that for orthopedic appliances. In a recent controversial article that suggested an increased risk of cardiac stent stenosis in individuals with ACD to nickel and/or molybdenum, none of the 10 patients with metal allergies exhibited evidence of active dermatitis, although one had a history of metal intolerance.[36] Similarly, intramuscular administration of small amounts of an allergen is unlikely to generate a cutaneous reaction. For example, it has been shown that >90 percent of thimerosal-allergic individuals can be safely vaccinated intramuscularly with thimerosal-containing vaccines. The small percentage of reactors develop a dermatitis about the vaccination site, most likely secondary to accidental skin contamination.[37] Although not as well studied, the same is likely true for neomycin-sensitive individuals exposed to neomycin in vaccines.

Systemic Manifestations

Systemic contact dermatitis is an uncommon condition that highlights one of the poorly understood aspects of ACD: the potential for long-lasting immunologic memory in previously sensitized areas of skin. The phenomenon occurs in an individual who has been sensitized topically to an allergen and is subsequently exposed systemically. Although the clinical reaction is typically a dermatitis limited to the site of the original sensitization (recall reaction), a more pronounced eruption ranging from an extensive, bizarre-appearing dermatitis (Fig. 120-5) to erythroderma may rarely occur.

GENERALIZED DERMATITIS Generalized and/or bizarre patterns of dermatitis are not only caused by systemic exposures, but can also follow topical exposure to allergens that are ubiquitous in the environment. Nickel is a frequent offender as it is present not only in jewelry, but also in hair and eyelash curlers, hooks and buttons, eyelets of shoes, dental amalgams, some of our coinage, and a multitude of other products.[38] Indeed, nickel is also found in food and water and is believed by many Scandinavian dermatologists to cause recurrent, vesicular hand dermatitis (pompholyx) in some patients. Fortunately, most patients are aware of contact with metal-based products. This is not true of other common environmental allergens.

Formaldehyde is not only ubiquitous but is frequently present in materials in which it is not suspected. Among these many products are insulating materials, rugs, paper products (including sanitary napkins and toilet tissue), and even smoke.[38] Many preservatives used in cosmetics, pharmaceuticals, and industry can release formaldehyde, such as 2-bromo-2-nitropropane-1,3-diol (Bronopol), quaternium-15 (Dowicil), DMDM hydantoin (Glydant), *tris*-(hydroxymethyl)-nitro-methane (Tris Nitro), imidazolidinyl urea (Germal I), and diazolidinyl urea (Germal II). The urea formaldehyde resins used to impart color-fastness and wrinkle resistance to clothing can also release free formaldehyde. Thus, ACD to formaldehyde can present with a variety of clinical pictures, which can be confusing to the practitioner. Furthermore, although many wash-off products (e.g., shampoos and liquid soaps) are preserved with formaldehyde or its releasers, they are rarely problematic because the material is rapidly diluted and quickly rinsed off. Nonetheless, in areas where the product can be trapped (ear canals, under rings), or in the exquisitely formaldehyde-sensitive patient, such wash-off products can cause ACD.

Balsam of Peru or its cross-reacting allergens can, like formaldehyde, be present but unsuspected in a variety of products. The allergen is itself a mixture of many chemicals derived from wounding the bark of *Myroxolon pereirae*, a tree native to El Salvador. Approximately two-thirds of the native balsam consists of a volatile oil containing cinnamic acid, cinnamyl cinnamate, benzyl benzoate, benzoic acid, and benzyl alcohol, among other ingredients. The remaining one-third, which is thought to harbor the principal allergen, contains esterified polymers of coniferyl alcohol with benzoic acid and cinnamic acid.[38] Peruvian balsam is used as a "tacking" agent in cosmetics, topical medications, suppositories, and dental liquids/cements. Furthermore, as might be expected of a substance containing numerous constituent chemicals, balsam of Peru can cross-react with many other substances including benzoic acid, benzoin, benzyl alcohol, benzyl benzoate, cinnamic acid, cinnamon, clove, eugenol, and isoeugenol, among others. The balsam itself or, more typically, modified fractions are frequently used as fragrance and flavoring additives. In a recent publication,[39] 47 percent of balsam of Peru- and/or fragrance-allergic patients required dietary modification to control their dermatitis, while 18 percent of patients who failed to modify their diet had persistent disease and only 36 percent improved without some form of dietary modification. Thus, the patient allergic to balsam of Peru can present with a spectrum of clinical symptoms ranging from limited dermatitis at the site of application of a cosmetic product to a more generalized dermatitis bordering on erythroderma (see Fig. 120-5).

Both natural and synthetic rubber are also ubiquitous. ACD to rubber products can therefore produce patchy dermatitis in various areas of the body. Among the sites most frequently involved are the face (make-up sponges), ear canals (ear plugs), periocular area (goggles), brassiere and/or waistline areas (elasticized undergarments), genital areas (condoms, diaphragms, pessaries), hands (gloves), feet (shoes), and/or joints (orthopedic braces). The allergens are typically either the accelerants (thiurams, carbamates, guanidines, and/or benzothiazoles) or the antioxidants (para-phenylenediamine derivatives) that are found in both natural and synthetic rubber.[38]

Noneczematous Variants of ACD

ACD need not be eczematous in appearance.[20] Noneczematous variants (Table 120-3) include lichenoid contact, erythema multiforme (EM), the cellulitic-like appearing dermal contact hypersensitivity, contact leukoderma, contact purpura, and erythema dyschromicum perstans, among others. Of these, the lichenoid and EM-like variants are seen most frequently.

Metals are the most likely cause of lichenoid allergic contact reactions, and have been linked to some cases of oral lichen planus. Many drugs can also cause a systemic lichenoid hypersensitivity,[20] the

TABLE 120-3

Etiologic Factors in Noneczematous Allergic Contact Dermatitis

APPEARANCE	ALLERGENS
Lichenoid	Metals/tattoo pigments (mercury, palladium, silver, gold, cobalt, chromium, nickel), para-phenylenediamine derivatives (e.g., black rubber mix), photographic color developers (CD2 and CD3), flavoring agents (menthol and peppermint), aminoglycoside antibiotics, fragrances (especially musk ambrette), plants *(Primula obconica),* Red Sea coral, α-amylase
Erythema multiforme	Exotic woods (rosewood, jacaranda, palissandre, pao ferro, caviuana), plants [poison ivy, primula, mugwort, costus, tea tree oil (melaleuca), and terpene extract], medications (bufexamac, chloramphenicol, econazole, furazolidone, mafenide acetate, mephenesin, neomycin, nifuroxime, nitrogen mustard, penicillin, phenylbutazone, promethazine, scopolamine, sulfonamides, and vitamin E) and miscellaneous topical allergens [balsam of Peru, 9-bromofluorene, cobalt, cutting oils, DNCB, diphenylcyclopropenone, disperse dyes, epoxy resins, ethylenediamine dihydrochloride, formaldehyde, isopropyl-*p*-phenylenediamine (black rubber), latex rubber, methyl parathion, nickel, phenyl sulfone derivatives, para-chlorobenzene sulfonylglycolic acid nitrile, para-phenylenediamine]
Dermal contact (especially in atopics)	Formaldehyde, gold, neomycin, nickel, ragweed oleoresin, vitamin K
Allergic contact leukoderma	Para-phenylenediamine
Allergic contact purpura	*N*-Isopropyl-*N*-phenylenediamine (black rubber), para-phenylenediamine, urea formaldehyde textile resins, balsam of Peru, epoxy resins, fiberglass (irritant, not allergic), oxyquinoline, quinidine

most notorious being the quinine derivatives, hydroxyurea, angiotensin-converting enzyme inhibitors, beta blockers, and antiepileptic agents. EM-like ACD is most frequently seen following contact with exotic woods, common plants, and topical medications. The other noneczematous variants of ACD are rare, most likely because they have many fewer causal agents. Of note, most cases of contact leukoderma are due to either postinflammatory hypopigmentation or direct chemical toxicity (e.g., hydroquinones, catechols, phenols, mercaptoamines).[40]

Allergic Contact Urticaria

As noted above, chemicals in rubber, especially those contained in black rubber mix, can cause a variety of noneczematous ACD, which includes not only those patterns delineated in Table 120-3, but also rarely plantar pustulosis, pitted keratolysis, and pyoderma gangrenosum. However, in addition to contact dermatitis, natural rubber latex (but not synthetic rubber) is responsible for a currently ongoing epidemic of allergic contact urticaria (ACU), an IgE-mediated phenomenon pathophysiologically distinct from the T cell–mediated ACD reactions discussed earlier in this chapter. Since 1979, when Nutter first called attention to ACU induced by latex, thousands of cases have been reported worldwide.

There are few good studies designed to look at the prevalence of immediate hypersensitivity to latex in the US. In 1996, Ownby et al.[41] evaluated 1000 volunteer blood donors in southeastern Michigan. They specifically targeted donors at mobile workplace sites and excluded all health facility sites. These authors found that, overall, 6.4 percent of their population was latex allergic. While this study revealed a remarkably high incidence rate of latex allergy in the general population, it may have underestimated the true rate because health care workers were specifically excluded, as were certain (but unknown) proportions of systemically medicated atopic patients. Both of these excluded populations have high incidence rates of latex urticaria. Among hospital workers most likely to be exposed to natural rubber latex gloves, the rate of latex ACU has been reported to range from a low of 5.5 percent[42] to as high as 38 percent.[43]

Atopic dermatitis predisposes to the development of ACU, as does mucosal exposure to latex. In one study, three of seven patients developed ACU following mucosal exposure.[44] In two of these individuals, anaphylactic reactions developed within minutes of contact. Thus, in addition to hospital personnel, paraplegics (especially patients with spina bifida), sexually active individuals exposed to latex condoms, and others with repeated mucosal exposure to latex must be considered high-risk groups for development of ACU. The failure to detect ACU to latex can have grave consequences in the allergic patient.

The presentation of ACU from latex is varied. For many patients, the symptoms are immediate burning, stinging, or itching with or without localized urticaria upon contact with latex. In some, symptoms include disseminated urticaria, allergic rhinitis, asthma, and/or anaphylaxis. The respiratory symptoms are frequently a result of the latex allergen binding to, and being aerosolized by, glove powder. Patients with latex ACU may also present with an eczematous-appearing dermatitis. This clinical pattern is usually due to concomitant ACD to a rubber additive, which, in many cases, precedes the development of ACU.[44] However, some patients presenting with an eczematous pattern may have protein contact dermatitis, an IgE-mediated reaction to proteins (especially in foods) that clinically has the appearance of ACD.

In contrast to those with ACD from rubber gloves, many patients with ACU from latex gloves present with the palmar aspects of the hands as involved as, or more involved than, the dorsal surfaces. This may relate to the lipid composition of the palmar epidermis, which allows it to be more easily penetrated by the water-soluble protein allergens of latex. Urticarial reactions can occur to any combination of at least 10 different water-soluble proteins within latex (termed Hev b 1 through Hev b 10) rather than to just one, or a few, proteins. This makes the diagnosis very difficult. However, with cloning of these allergens (except Hev b 4) as recombinant proteins, more precise diagnostic tools may soon be available.[45]

Among the commercially available in vitro tests for IgE-mediated latex allergy, the CAP system, a solid-phase immunoassay (Kabi-Pharmacia, Uppsala, Sweden), seems to perform better than Ala STAT, the liquid-phase immunoassay (DPC, Los Angeles, California). For CAP, the sensitivity is 94 percent and the specificity is 82 percent; for Ala STAT, the sensitivity is 74 percent and the specificity is 92 percent.[46] Recently, an in-office serum dipstick method (Allergodip, Allergopharma, Reinbek, Germany) has been tested against the CAP assay and found to have nearly equivalent sensitivity and specificity.[47] However, the Allergodip is not yet FDA-approved. Furthermore, these in vitro tests do miss some individuals with ACU to latex. Therefore, in vivo prick and/or use testing are necessary if the in vitro tests are negative and ACU to latex remains a consideration.

When performing in vivo tests, one would ideally want the purified allergens extracted from natural latex; however, although cloned, these are not yet commercially available. Instead, one can leach out the responsible allergen(s) by soaking the rubber material in water at room temperature for 30 min.[48] In most, but not all, cases, use of such an eluate for prick testing is sufficient for detecting ACU. Whenever in vivo testing for latex is performed, the investigator must be aware of the potential for life-threatening anaphylactic reactions, especially in patients whose symptoms suggest prior systemic reactions to latex products. Such reactions may even follow prick testing.

LABORATORY FINDINGS

In Vivo Tests for ACD: The Patch Test

The only useful and reliable method for the diagnosis of ACD remains the patch test. Only 23 commercially prepared allergens are currently available in the United States (Table 120-4). A comparison of Table 120-1 with Table 120-4 makes it apparent that some, but not all, of the common allergens in the environment are contained on this tray. Therefore, given the fact that there are more than 3700 potential environmental allergens, practitioners interested in fully evaluating patients with ACD must be prepared to perform tests with other materials. For physicians compounding their own allergens, texts detailing appropriate concentrations and vehicles are available.[15]

Relevance

As with any in vivo assay, patch testing is subject to pitfalls. A primary concern is that even when a chemical is found to be allergenic for a given patient, it cannot de facto be assumed to be the cause of ACD. As Table 120-1 shows, the relevance of presumably true-positive reactions to episodes of ACD ranges from as low as 16.8 percent for thimerosal to as high as 93.4 percent for DMDM hydantoin. This lack of relevance does not mean that patients are not allergic to the chemical in question, but rather that the specific allergen is not responsible for the current dermatitis. The temptation to "force" relevance for an irrelevant allergen can frustrate and disappoint the patient. This is particularly true for allergens that historically have low relevance, such as thimerosal. Many patients with positive patch tests to thimerosal have been asymptomatically sensitized by vaccines.[49]

To determine the relevance of a positive patch test requires correlation with the materials encountered by the involved areas of skin.

Furthermore, even in some instances when patients are allergic to chemicals in products they are using, the allergen may be present in only minimal amounts and may not be responsible for the dermatitis. In this regard, "repeat open application testing" (ROAT), in which the patient applies the commercial product to normal skin several times daily for 1 to 2 weeks, can be helpful. With use of such provocative tests, members of the North American Contact Dermatitis Group (NACDG) found that 5 of 10 individuals who tested positive to MCI/MI at 100 ppm in water did not react to a generic skin care lotion preserved with 15 ppm MCI/MI.[50] This is of particular note given the CIR's recommendation that MCI/MI not be used in "leave on" cosmetics above 7.5 ppm.

TABLE 120-4

Allergens Currently Available in the United States*

Allergens	Principal Sources of Contact
Balsam of Peru	Fragrances, flavorings
Black rubber mix	Rubber products
Caine mix	Aminobenzoate (*not* amide) anesthetics
Carba mix	Rubber products, fungicides
Cobalt	Metals, blue pigments (paint, cosmetics, tattoos), vitamin B_{12}
Colophony/rosin	Adhesives, waxes, turpentine, other pine tree extracts
Epoxy resin	Glues, plastics
Ethylenediamine dihydrochloride	Stabilizer in cosmetics and medicaments, hardener in plastics, cutting oils, certain antihistamines
Formaldehyde	Preservative in many materials
Fragrance mix	Fragrances, flavorings
Lanolin (wool) alcohol	Vehicle for cosmetics, cutting oils, polishes
Mercaptobenzothiazole	Rubber products, fungicides, cutting oils
Mercapto mix	Rubber products, fungicides, cutting oils
MCI/MI	Preservative in many materials
Neomycin sulfate	Antibiotics (cross reactions with other aminoglycosides), vaccines
Nickel	Metals (including high-sulfur stainless steel), foods
Paraben mix	Preservative in cosmetics, medicaments, foods
para-Phenylenediamine	Dyes, especially hair
p-tert-Butylphenol formaldehyde resin	Adhesives, shoe glues, plastics
Potassium dichromate	Leather, cement/spackling compounds, green pigments (paint, cosmetics, tattoos), detergents
Quaternium-15	Preservative in cosmetics and cutting oils
Thimerosal	Preservative in medications and vaccines
Thiuram mix	Rubber products, fungicides, animal repellents

*The European Standard Tray is similar; however, it does not contain carba mix, ethylenediamine dihydrochloride, or thimerosal. Instead, the European Tray has two screening agents for plant allergens (sesquiterpene lactone mix and primin), two screening agents for steroid allergens (budesonide and tixocortol pivalate), and clioquinol (Vioform). The Japanese standard is nearly equivalent to the US standard, with the addition of two screening agents for plants (primin and urushiol).

False Positives and Negatives

Physicians performing patch tests must also be concerned with the possibility of false-positive and false-negative reactions. False-positive reactions due either to the use of allergens at irritant concentrations or to the "excited skin syndrome" have received much attention in the literature.[51] In addition, metal allergens can produce irritant pustular reactions and cobalt is notorious for producing a "cayenne pepper" appearance to the skin, which represents deposition of cobalt in the pores and is not an allergic reaction.[35] The "false" nature of these reactions can usually be resolved by repeating the patch tests individually and/or in lower concentrations, or by ROAT. In contrast, false-negative reactions require high levels of suspicion and diligence to uncover.

One common and easily correctable cause of false-negative reactions is the failure to perform a second reading of the test sites after the initial 48-h inspection. This second reading, sometime between 3 and 7 days after application of the patches, is particularly important for elderly patients, who take longer to mount an allergic reaction.[8] A second reading is also important in detecting positive reactions to allergens such as neomycin, more than half of which are not evident until 96 h after application of the patch test.[52] False-negative reactions can also occur when the allergen is used in too low a concentration for patch testing, as can happen when cosmetic products are used as is. Therefore, if clinical suspicion warrants, and despite a negative patch test, additional testing such as ROAT with the suspect product can unmask the cause of ACD. In doing so, one must be aware of the "paraben paradox" and "lanolin paradox":[53] neither chemical seems to be a potent allergen when applied to intact skin; however, when they are applied to dermatitic skin (e.g., stasis dermatitis), ACD may ensue.

With more than 3700 potential allergens,[15] negative reactions may simply indicate that the responsible chemical has not been tested. There is a particular problem in the US, where only 23 allergens have been FDA-approved (Table 120-4). Contrasting this table with Table 120-1 reveals that 40 percent of the 25 most common allergens in the US are not readily available for testing!

Although it has been widely quoted that 70 to 80 percent of patients with ACD can be diagnosed with use of screening trays such as the TRUE Test (Kabi Pharmacia Service A/S, Hillerød, Denmark), these numbers have recently been questioned. In an analysis of the 1994–1996 NACDG data on 3120 patients,[54] it was found that 62 percent had at least one positive reaction to an allergen present on the TRUE Test, of which 45 percent were relevant to the current dermatitis. However, by expanding the panel from 23 to 50 allergens, additional allergens of potential relevance were identified in 31 percent. In their study of 732 patients over 5.5 years, Cohen et al.[55] found that only 23 percent of patients reacted exclusively to allergen(s) on a similar (but not identical) standard series, 37 percent reacted to allergens on both the standard series and other supplementary tests, and 40 percent reacted only to supplementary allergens. Thus, to maximally benefit patients, practitioners must use allergens beyond those present on "standard" trays. In the case of fragrance allergens, Larsen et al.[56] found that the addition of a "natural mix" of 2% jasmine absolute, 2% ylang-ylang oil, 2% narcissus absolute, 2% sandalwood oil, and 2% spearmint oil increased the sensitivity of detecting fragrance allergy to 95 percent from the 81 percent detected by using only the "standard" allergens, fragrance mix and balsam of Peru.

In Vitro Tests for ACD

In vitro and animal tests for the diagnosis of ACD have received much attention in the past decade. Laboratory studies such as lymphocyte transformation or macrophage migration inhibition have been evaluated as measurements of ACD in both humans and animals. A major problem in developing in vitro systems is the lack of knowledge about what constitutes the antigenic moiety of a particular chemical.

Nonetheless, these assays are now being extensively studied and reliably standardized. In a review of 209 chemicals, the accuracy of the local mouse lymph node assay (LLNA, a lymphocyte transformation test) versus all guinea pig tests (GPTs) was 86 percent and versus human data was 72 percent, whereas that of all GPTs versus human tests was 73 percent.[57] In terms of accuracy, sensitivity, specificity, and positive/negative predictability, the performance of the LLNA was similar to that of the GPT. Equally important, the performance of the LLNA and the GPT were similar when each was compared with human data.

In vitro predictive methodologies have been hampered by the lack of LC lines. Recent advances in culturing LC-like dendritic cells from CD34+ precursors under appropriate cytokine conditions and the development of stable LC-like cell lines should enhance the utility of in vitro methodologies. Based upon current data, a chemical that enhances CD86 expression and interleukin (IL)-1β production, downregulates E-cadherin, causes endocytosis of surface major histocompatibility complex (MHC) class II, and induces tyrosine phosphorylation in LC cultures will likely be sensitizing.[57] However, given the variability in these assays among individuals, more work needs to be done in this area. Finally, studies are continuing in order to improve the predictive capabilities of LC/T cell cocultures and skin equivalent/reconstituted epidermal cultures. Thus, although in vivo patch testing, in which the skin can process the allergen for presentation, currently remains the "gold standard," there are exciting prospects for in vitro testing in the future.

Computer Modeling

Quantitative structure–activity relationships (QSAR) represent a chemistry-based predictive approach that uses computer modeling. DEREK ("deductive estimation of risks from existing knowledge") has been tested extensively for its ability to predict allergenicity. Based upon data from animal studies, DEREK uses a set of $\geq$50 rules describing chemical substructures responsible for sensitization. Although the predictive capabilities of DEREK are high ($\geq$80 percent),[58] further refinements in the scope of existing rules and the generation of new rules based on a chemical's biological activity are needed to enhance its validity. Data derived from the LLNA should enhance the capabilities of QSAR.

PATHOLOGY AND DIFFERENTIAL DIAGNOSES

Eczematous Dermatitis

For most episodes of ACD, the end result of the exquisitely orchestrated interplay of cytokines and adhesion molecules is the entrance into the skin of T helper (T_H)-1 cells secreting IL-2 and interferon (IFN)-γ (Chap. 23). IFN-γ acts in a number of ways to amplify the immune response.[59] It activates cytotoxic T cells, natural killer (NK) cells, and macrophages. In addition, the induction of interferon-inducible protein 10 on keratinocytes adds to the recruitment of monocytes/macrophages, as does the IL-1- and tumor necrosis factor (TNF)-α–enhanced production of monocyte chemoattractant-1, monocyte chemotactic and activating factor, and macrophage inflammatory protein-2 by keratinocytes. This collection of monocytes/macrophages and proliferating T cells, along with their chemical mediators, is responsible for the epidermal spongiosis (intercellular edema) and superficial, perivascular, lymphohistiocytic dermal infiltrate that are the histologic hallmarks of ACD (Fig. 120-6). The clinicopathologic differential diagnoses include irritant contact, atopic, nummular, dyshidrotic, and autosensitization dermatitis.

FIGURE 120-6

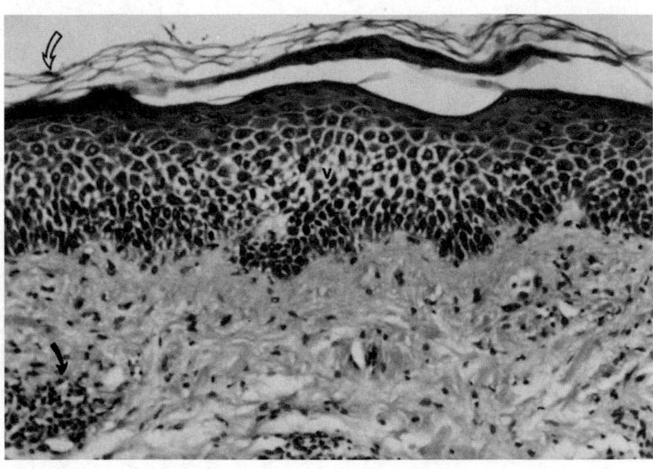

Histopathology of acute allergic contact dermatitis. The biopsy shows epidermal intercellular edema and microvesiculation (*v*), which are characteristic of an allergic response, as well as other eczematous dermatitides. The superficial perivascular infiltrate (*solid arrow*) consists of lymphocytes, macrophages, and, occasionally, eosinophils. The orthokeratotic stratum corneum (*open arrow*) is indicative of the acute nature of this eruption. In subacute to chronic allergic reactions, the stratum corneum is parakeratotic.

Noneczematous Variants

The pathologic findings of the noneczematous variants of ACD are nearly identical to the diseases they simulate. Lichenoid ACD does have some features that help to distinguish it from idiopathic lichen planus (Chap. 49), including a less-intense lichenoid infiltrate with more eosinophils and neutrophils, less epidermal hyperplasia with fewer necrotic keratinocytes, and some degree of epidermal spongiosis.[60] In contrast, EM-like ACD has no epidermal spongiosis and the findings are indistinguishable from other causes of EM (Chap. 58). Dermal contact hypersensitivity also lacks spongiosis, but has the characteristic lymphohistiocytic, perivascular infiltrate that often goes deeper in the dermis (mid-dermal) than eczematous ACD.[61] The histopathology of acute allergic contact leukoderma has not been studied. In the best-documented cases,[62] eczematous patch test reactions to PPD subsequently depigmented, at which time the biopsy was indistinguishable from chemically induced vitiligo (Chap. 90). Allergic contact purpura is pathologically similar to the eczematous variant of ACD, but with a capillaritis that results in extravasated red blood cells.[63] It is difficult to separate from the other pigmented purpuric dermatoses (Chap. 176).

In all of the noneczematous and eczematous variants of ACD, patch testing is the only means for accurate diagnosis. The history, physical examination, and/or pathology are not diagnostic. For example, it has been reported that 46 percent of patients with a clinically apparent nickel-induced dermatitis are, in fact, not allergic to nickel.[64]

TREATMENT

Allergic Contact Dermatitis

ALLERGEN AVOIDANCE The treatment of ACD lies in identifying its cause and thoroughly instructing the patient to avoid the responsible allergen(s). For certain allergens (e.g., vehicles, preservatives, stabilizers, and emulsifiers) found in topical preparations, it is important to impress upon patients the need to read labels. In addition, a recurrently updated, electronic database of ingredients in cosmetics and over-the-counter/prescription topical preparations (CARD: Contact Allergen Database) is available on the Internet (www.contactderm.org) and allows practitioners to generate a unique list of topical preparations appropriate for the individual with specified allergies.

Patients with allergies to preservatives must be aware that these materials can be found in any water-based formulation, such as latex paint. Furthermore, the name given a chemical used in a cosmetic or pharmaceutical product is frequently changed when it is used in a commercial product. For instance, the cosmetic preservative quaternium-15, when used in industry, is referred to as Dowicil 100 or Dowicil 200. Practitioners guiding patients through the synonymic jungle of these chemicals are advised to consult standard texts on the subject.[33,38]

Unfortunately for patients and physicians, the allergenic component of many materials will almost never be labeled. Rubber-, textile-, and metal-related allergens are but a few examples. In counseling patients with reactions to these materials, the physician must provide information about what kinds of products are likely to contain the allergen, as well as appropriate replacements. Such information can be found in standard texts.[33,38,65] Furthermore, some allergens are incompletely labeled. Given the proprietary nature of a fragrance's formulation, the individual fragrances that have been combined in the product are never listed. Patients with an allergic reaction to a fragrance should be advised to use fragrance-free materials, which include not only topical preparations but also a variety of other products such as toilet paper and sanitary napkins.[38,65] It is important to realize that products labeled "unscented" contain masking fragrances, although they are usually present in very low concentrations and do not cause problems.

Because many allergens may share common antigenic moieties, the patient must be instructed not only about the known allergen, but also about possible cross-reacting allergens. For example, the individual allergic to benzocaine must be aware of the many potentially cross-reacting substances, which include agents as diverse as other anesthetics (e.g., procaine), certain medications (e.g., sulfonamides), hair dyes (e.g., para-phenylenediamine), textile dyes (e.g., aniline dyes), some sunscreens (e.g., para-aminobenzoic acid), and other products.[38] Because cross-reactions are not always evident to the nonchemist (e.g., benzoyl peroxide with cocaine), physicians must consult standard texts[38,65] when instructing their patients.

SYMPTOMATIC THERAPY In addition to avoidance of further contact with the allergen and its cross-reactants, treatment of ACD should be directed to amelioration of symptoms. Acute vesicular, weeping eruptions benefit from drying agents such as topical aluminum sulfate/calcium acetate; chronic, lichenified eruptions are best treated with emollients. Pruritus can be controlled with topical antipruritics or oral antihistamines; topical antihistamines or anesthetics are best avoided because of the risk of inducing a secondary allergy in already dermatitic skin. Treatment with physicochemical agents that downregulate responsiveness may also be required. Glucocorticoids, macrolactams, and ultraviolet radiation are most widely used.

A variety of other pharmacologic agents have been reported to interfere with the induction and/or elicitation of ACD in mouse models.[66] These include calcium channel blockers, amiloride, pentoxifylline, pentamidine, clonidine, spiperone, *N*-acetylcysteine, and flavonoids. Of these, only pentoxifylline has been evaluated in humans, where it was found to induce a slight reduction in responsiveness, perhaps by an effect on TNF-α. Whether the other pharmacologic agents exert any effect on the human response remains to be determined. Of note, with the possible exception of azelastine,[66] H_1-antihistamines do not affect the induction or elicitation of ACD. H_2-antihistamines enhance induction, but have no effect on elicitation.[67]

Topical glucocorticoids or macrolactams (pimecrolimus or tacrolimus) usually suffice for treating most patients with ACD. However, individuals with involvement of greater than 25 percent of their body surface area and/or those exposed to certain allergens [such as *Toxicodendron (Rhus)* oleoresin, which may persist locally in the skin

for weeks after exposure] may require treatment with systemic glucocorticoids. In those patients in whom systemic steroid therapy is inappropriate, phototherapy with UVB or PUVA can be beneficial. Individuals with occupational ACD who are economically unable to discontinue working with the offending allergen and who are also unable to work with gloves or effective barrier creams may also benefit from chronic maintenance therapy with UVB or PUVA. The advent of topical macrolactams, which do not cause cutaneous atrophy, are another option for these chronically exposed workers. In the future, inhibitors of cellular metabolic activity, inhibitors of cell adhesion molecules, targeted skin application of regulatory cytokines, and neutralization of proinflammatory cytokines with antisense oligonucleotides, anticytokine antibodies, or soluble cytokine receptors, may also be added to the therapeutic armamentarium.

PHYSICOCHEMICAL BARRIERS While prevention of ACD rests with avoidance of the allergen, for various reasons, principally economic, this is not always possible. Many chemicals, especially organic molecules, can rapidly penetrate vinyl and synthetic or natural latex rubber gloves, and exposed workers may be unable to avoid daily contact with the allergen. These individuals may benefit from a plastic glove made of a proprietary laminate (4H, North Safety Products, Cranston, Rhode Island). In clinical trials, the 4H glove, which is only 0.07 mm thick, was impervious to more than 90 percent of all randomly selected organic chemicals for 4 h at 35°C (95°F).[68] However, this glove is not form-fitting and is thought by many professionals to impede the fine dexterity needed in their work. In the future, barrier creams may be available to help such patients. Now, however, barrier creams are available for only a limited number of allergens (principally poison ivy and poison oak), are effective only if the protected area is washed within several hours of contact with the allergen, and are objectionable to many patients because of their thick tack and greasy consistency.

HYPOSENSITIZATION Although the possibility of hyposensitization for ACD has intrigued dermatologists for decades, it remains a nonviable alternative. Despite early encouraging work, Kligman[69] concluded that "complete desensitization of the highly sensitive subject by oral or intramuscular administration is impossible," a statement later echoed by others. In these studies, months of treatment with *Toxicodendron* oleoresin resulted in a temporary lessening of the intensity, but not ablation, of the allergic response. Of the topical desensitization programs, only that for mechlorethamine hydrochloride (nitrogen mustard) has shown any success in a limited number of patients.[70] However, this success has been contested by others, as has the nature of the reaction (allergic or irritant) to mechlorethamine hydrochloride.[71]

TOLERANCE INDUCTION One theoretical possibility for prevention of occupational ACD is the induction of tolerance to known occupational allergen(s) before employment. When an antigen to which an individual has not yet been sensitized is administered either systemically or topically to areas deficient in functional LCs, long-lived tolerance rather than sensitization often ensues. However, because allergic reactions to otherwise apparently innocuous materials, such as nickel, persist in the human genotype, one must question on a Darwinian basis whether there is selective advantage to the trait. In the absence of information concerning the antigenic moieties of many simple chemicals and how they might relate to antigenically more complex viruses and malignancies, one cannot assume that simple chemical allergens do not cross-react with viral- or tumor-related antigens. At present, it is a matter of debate whether it is ethical to induce tolerance to even the most problematic environmental allergens given the theoretical risk of enhancing susceptibility to potentially more life-threatening diseases.

TABLE 120-5

Latex Alternative and Other Information

OSHA–General
http://www.osha-slc.gov/SLTC/latexallergy/index.html
Spina Bifida Association of America–Home and Hospital
http://www.sbaa.org/html/sbaa_latex.html
Alert, Inc.–Dental Products
http://www.execpc.com/~alert/dentprod.html
Elastic Inc.–Latex-Free Alternatives for the Home
http://www.latex–allergy.org/resources.htm#when

Allergic Contact Urticaria

The treatment of latex allergy, and other contact urticarial reactions, is straightforward: avoid the allergen. However, this can be difficult. Regarding latex, Yunginger et al.[72] have shown a 3000-time variation in allergen levels among gloves produced by different manufacturers. In general, nonsterile, examination gloves had significantly more latex than sterile surgical gloves. Powered gloves also had much higher latex levels because the glove powder tends to concentrate the allergen and because nonpowdered gloves are typically treated with chlorine (which reduces protein levels) during their manufacture. Among "hypoallergenic gloves," 11 of 24 brands had significant levels of latex allergen;[72] this is because "hypoallergenic" refers to the absence of delayed-type hypersensitivity without concern for IgE-mediated urticaria.

Various methods exist to decrease the allergenicity of latex by removing residual protein. Those which have been shown to be most beneficial include: distilled water washing with or without agitation at 60°C (140°F), chlorination, 0.59 M ammonia , 0.28 M trichloroacetic acid, and steam autoclaving.[73] In contrast, methods such as wet-gel leaching, surface swabbing, autoclaving in dry air, and variations in vulcanization have produced clinically insignificant decreases in protein levels.[73] The use of powder-free gloves also results in lower allergen levels, as described above. In countries such as Finland, where there has been a shift to low-protein natural latex products, there appears to be a decline in the incidence of new cases of ACU.

Given that there is no movement to label nonmedical latex, avoidance can be quite frustrating to the consumer. Fortunately, there is a significant amount of information on allergen alternatives available through the Internet. Table 120-5 lists some of the more valuable Internet sites for alternative materials and other information related to latex allergy. In addition to avoiding latex, it is important that latex-allergic individuals wear a medical alert tag and, depending upon their symptomatology, carry oral antihistamines and/or injectable epinephrine. If these individuals suffer respiratory symptoms, a search must be performed for potential airborne exposures. Finally, these patients need to be aware of the potential for cross-reactivity with the various foods that have been reported to be problematic for individuals with latex allergy (Table 120-6).

TABLE 120-6

Problematic Foods for Patients with Allergy to Latex

Fruits	Banana,* kiwi,* avocado,* peach, mango, plum, cherry, papaya, fig, melon, apple, and pear
Vegetables	Tomato, celery, and potato
Nuts	Chestnuts, hazelnuts, and other tree nuts

*Most frequently reported cross-reacting food allergens.

REFERENCES

1. Burnett CA et al: Occupational dermatitis causing days away from work in US private industry, 1993. *Am J Ind Med* **34**:568, 1998
2. Meyer J et al: Occupational contact dermatitis in the UK: A surveillance report from EPIDERM and OPRA. *Occup Med* **50**:265, 2000
3. Kucenic MJ, Belsito DV: Occupational allergic contact dermatitis is more prevalent than irritant contact dermatitis: A five-year study. *J Am Acad Dermatol* **46**:695, 2002
4. Nielsen NH, Menne T: Allergic contact sensitization in an unselected Danish population. The Glostrup Allergy Study, Denmark. *Acta Derm Venereol* **72**:456, 1992
5. Kwangsukstith C, Maibach HI: Effect of age and sex on the induction and elicitation of allergic contact dermatitis. *Contact Dermatitis* **33**:289, 1995
6. Robinson MK: Population differences in skin structure and physiology and the susceptibility to irritant and allergic contact dermatitis: Implications for skin safety testing and risk assessment. *Contact Dermatitis* **41**:65, 1999
7. Schwartz M: Eczematous sensitization in various age groups. *J Allergy* **24**:143, 1952
8. Przybilla B et al: Evaluation of the immune status in vivo by the 2,4-dinitro-1-chlorobenzene contact allergy time (DNCB-CAT). *Dermatologica* **167**:1, 1983
9. Belsito DV, Possick LE: Age-related changes in allergic contact hypersensitivity: Functional T cell deficiencies are primarily responsible. *J Invest Dermatol* **90**:546, 1988
10. Strauss HW: Artificial sensitization of infants to poison ivy. *J Allergy* **2**:137, 1931
11. Ventura MT et al: Contact dermatitis in students practicing sports: Incidence of rubber sensitization. *Br J Sports Med* **35**:100, 2001
12. Shaffer MP, Belsito DV: Allergic contact dermatitis to glutaraldehyde in health-care workers. *Contact Dermatitis* **43**:150, 2000
13. Whitmore SE: Should atopic individuals be patch tested? *Dermatol Clin* **12**:491, 1994
14. Marks JG et al: North American Contact Dermatitis Group Patch Test Results, 1996–1998. *Arch Dermatol* **136**:272, 2000
15. de Groot AC: *Patch Testing: Test Concentrations and Vehicles for 3700 Allergens,* 2nd ed. Amsterdam, Elsevier, 1994
16. Friedman PS: The immunology of allergic contact dermatitis: The DNCB story. *Adv Dermatol* **5**:175, 1990
17. Wilkinson JD, Shaw S: Contact dermatitis: Allergic, in *Rook/Wilkinson/Ebling Textbook of Dermatology,* 6th ed, edited by RH Champion, JL Burton, DA Burns, and S.M. Breathnach. London, Blackwell Science, 1998, p 769
18. Burrows D: Adverse chromate reactions on the skin, in *Chromium: Metabolism and Toxicity,* edited by D. Burrows. Boca Raton, FL, CRC Press, 1983, p 137
19. Sosroseno W: A review of the mechanisms of oral tolerance and immunotherapy. *J R Soc Med* **88**:14, 1995
20. Belsito DV: The diagnostic evaluation, treatment, and prevention of allergic contact dermatitis in the new millennium. *J Allergy Clin Immunol* **105**:409, 2000
21. Rapaport MJ: Patch testing in Japanese subjects. *Contact Dermatitis* **11**:93, 1984
22. Goh CL: Prevalence of contact allergy by sex, race and age. *Contact Dermatitis* **14**:237, 1986
23. Jordan WP Jr, King SE: Delayed hypersensitivity in females. The development of allergic contact dermatitis in females during the comparison of two predictive patch tests. *Contact Dermatitis* **3**:19, 1977
24. Leyden JJ, Kligman AM: Allergic contact dermatitis: Sex differences. *Contact Dermatitis* **3**:333, 1977
25. Rees JL et al: Sex differences in susceptibility to development of contact hypersensitivity to dinitrochlorobenzene (DNCB). *Br J Dermatol* **120**:371, 1989
26. Sertoli A et al: Effetto della somministrazione orale de apteni in soggetti sensibilizzati affetti de eczema allergico de contatto. *Giorn It Derm Vener* **120**:212, 1985
27. Wall LM, Gebauer KA: A follow-up study of occupational skin disease in western Australia. *Contact Dermatitis* **24**:241, 1991
28. Liden C: Legislative and preventive measures related to contact dermatitis. *Contact Dermatitis* **44**:65, 2001
29. Basketter D et al: Investigation of the threshold for allergic reactivity to chromium. *Contact Dermatitis* **44**:70, 2001
30. Holness DL, Nethercott JR: Is a worker's understanding of their diagnosis an important determinant of outcome in occupational contact dermatitis? *Contact Dermatitis* **25**:296, 1991
31. Krasteva M, Nicolas JF: Eczéma de contact: Perspectives thérapeutiques. *Objectif Peau* **4**:442, 1996
32. Adams RM ed: *Occupational Skin Disease,* 3rd ed. Philadelphia, WB Saunders, 1999
33. Kanerva L et al: *Handbook of Occupational Dermatology.* Berlin, Springer-Verlag, 2000

34. Shackelford KE, Belsito DV: The etiology of foot dermatitis: A five-year retrospective study. *J Am Acad Dermatol* **47**:715, 2002
35. Storrs FJ: All the things I knew were true about contact dermatitis that aren't. *Cutis* **52**:301, 1993
36. Köster R et al: Nickel and molybdenum contact allergies in patients with coronary in-stent restenosis. *Lancet* **356**:1895, 2000
37. Audicana M et al: Allergic contact dermatitis from mercury antiseptics and derivatives. Study protocol of tolerance to intramuscular injections of thimerosal. *Am J Contact Dermatitis* **13**:3, 2002
38. Rietschel RL, Fowler JF Jr: *Fisher's Contact Dermatitis,* 5th ed. Philadelphia, Lippincott, Williams & Wilkins, 2001
39. Salam TN, Fowler JF Jr: Balsam-related systemic contact dermatitis. *J Am Acad Dermatol* **45**:377, 2001
40. Fisher AA: The differential diagnosis of contact chemical leukoderma. *Am J Contact Dermatitis* **8**:52, 1997
41. Ownby DR et al: The prevalence of anti-latex IgE antibodies in 1000 volunteer blood donors. *J Allergy Clin Immunol* **97**:1188, 1996
42. Kaczmarek RG et al: Prevalence of latex-specific IgE antibodies in hospital personnel. *Ann Allergy Asthma Immunol* **76**:51, 1996
43. Yassin MS et al: Latex allergy in hospital employees. *Ann Allergy* **72**:245, 1994
44. Belsito DV: Contact urticaria caused by rubber: An analysis of seven cases. *Dermatol Clin* **8**:61, 1990
45. Yip L et al: Skin prick test reactivity to recombinant latex allergens. *Int Arch Allergy Immunol* **121**:292, 2000
46. Grüber C et al: Is there a role for immunoblots in the diagnosis of latex allergy? Intermethod comparison of in vitro and in vivo IgE assays in spina bifida patients. *Allergy* **55**:476, 2000
47. Niggemann B, Wahn U: A new dipstick test (Allergodip) for in vitro diagnosis of latex allergy—Validation in patients with spina bifida. *Pediatr Allergy Immunol* **11**:56, 2000
48. Turjanmaa K et al: Comparison of diagnostic methods in latex surgical glove contact urticaria. *Contact Dermatitis* **19**:241, 1988
49. Suneja T, Belsito DV: Thimerosal in the detection of clinically relevant allergic contact reactions. *J Am Acad Dermatol* **45**:23, 2001
50. Marks JG Jr et al: Methylchloroisothiazolinone/methylisothiazolinone (Kathon CG) Biocide—United States multicenter study of human skin sensitization. *Am J Contact Dermatitis* **1**:157, 1990
51. Mitchell JC: Multiple concomitant positive patch test reactions. *Contact Dermatitis* **3**:315, 1975
52. Belsito DV et al: Reproducibility of patch tests: A US multicenter study. *Am J Contact Dermatitis* **3**:193, 1992
53. Wolf R: The lanolin paradox. *Dermatology* **192**:198, 1996
54. Marks JG Jr et al: North American Contact Dermatitis Group patch test results for the detection of delayed-type hypersensitivity to topical allergens. *J Am Acad Dermatol* **38**:911, 1998
55. Cohen DE et al: Utility of a standard allergen series alone in the evaluation of allergic contact dermatitis: A retrospective study of 732 patients. *J Am Acad Dermatol* **36**:914, 1997
56. Larsen W et al: A study of new fragrance mixtures. *Am J Contact Dermatitis* **9**:202, 1998
57. Ryan CA et al: Approaches for the development of cell-based in vitro methods for contact sensitization. *Toxicol In Vitro* **15**:43, 2001
58. Barratt MD, Langowski JJ: Validation and subsequent development of the DEREK skin sensitization rule base by analysis of the BgVV list of contact allergens. *J Chem Inf Comput Sci* **39**:294, 1999
59. Tau G, Rothman P: Biologic functions of the IFN-γ receptors. *Allergy* **54**:1233, 1999
60. West AJ et al: A comparative histopathologic study of photodistributed and non-photodistributed lichenoid drug eruptions. *J Am Acad Dermatol* **23**:689, 1990
61. Hogan KP, Wyre HW: Dermal contact dermatitis to a disposable electrode plate. *Cutis* **27**:157, 1981
62. Taylor JS et al: Contact leukoderma associated with the use of hair colors. *Cutis* **52**:273, 1993
63. Calnan CD, Peachey RDG: Allergic contact purpura. *Clin Allergy* **1**:287, 1971
64. Kieffer M: Nickel sensitivity: Relationship between history and patch test reaction. *Contact Dermatitis* **5**:398, 1979
65. Guin JD: *Practical Contact Dermatitis*. New York, McGraw-Hill, 1995
66. Belsito DV: Patch-testing: After 100 years, still the gold standard in diagnosing cutaneous delayed-type hypersensitivity, in *Regulatory Control and Standardization of Allergenic Extracts: The Eighth International Paul-Ehrlich-Seminar,* edited by R Kurth YL Devries, and U Wagner. Stuttgart, Germany, Gustav Fischer, 1997, pp 195–202
67. Belsito DV et al: Cimetidine-induced augmentation of allergic contact hypersensitivity reactions in mice. *J Invest Dermatol* **94**:441, 1990
68. Henriksen HR et al: *Beskyttelsesklaeder mod Kemikalier, Oplosningsparametre og Taethed*. Lyngby, Denmark, Instituttet for Kemiindustri, 1986
69. Kligman AM: Hyposensitization against *Rhus* dermatitis. *Arch Dermatol* **78**:47, 1958
70. Waldorf DS et al: Cutaneous hypersensitivity and desensitization to mechlorethamine in patients with mycosis fungoides lymphoma. *Ann Intern Med* **67**:282, 1967
71. Leshaw S et al: Failure to induce tolerance to mechlorethamine hydrochloride. *Arch Dermatol* **113**:1406, 1977
72. Yunginger JW et al: Extractable latex allergens and proteins in disposable medical gloves and other rubber products. *J Allergy Clin Immunol* **93**:836, 1994
73. Dalrymple SJ, Audley BG: Allergenic proteins in dipped products: Factors influencing extractable protein levels. *Rubber Develop* **45**:51, 1992

CHAPTER 121

Donald V. Belsito

Autosensitization Dermatitis

CLINICAL MANIFESTATIONS

Autosensitization dermatitis refers to a phenomenon in which an acute dermatitis develops at cutaneous sites distant from an inflammatory focus and where the secondary acute dermatitis is not explained by the inciting cause of the primary inflammation. The term was coined in 1921 by Whitfield to describe reaction patterns ranging from a generalized, erythematous, morbilliform, and urticarial eruption following blunt trauma to a generalized, petechial, papulovesicular dermatitis after the acute irritation of chronic stasis dermatitis.[1] Over the next several decades, the cutaneous, vesicular "id" reactions associated with

may change in a manner consistent with the chronicity (i.e., vesicles to scale).

FIGURE 121-1

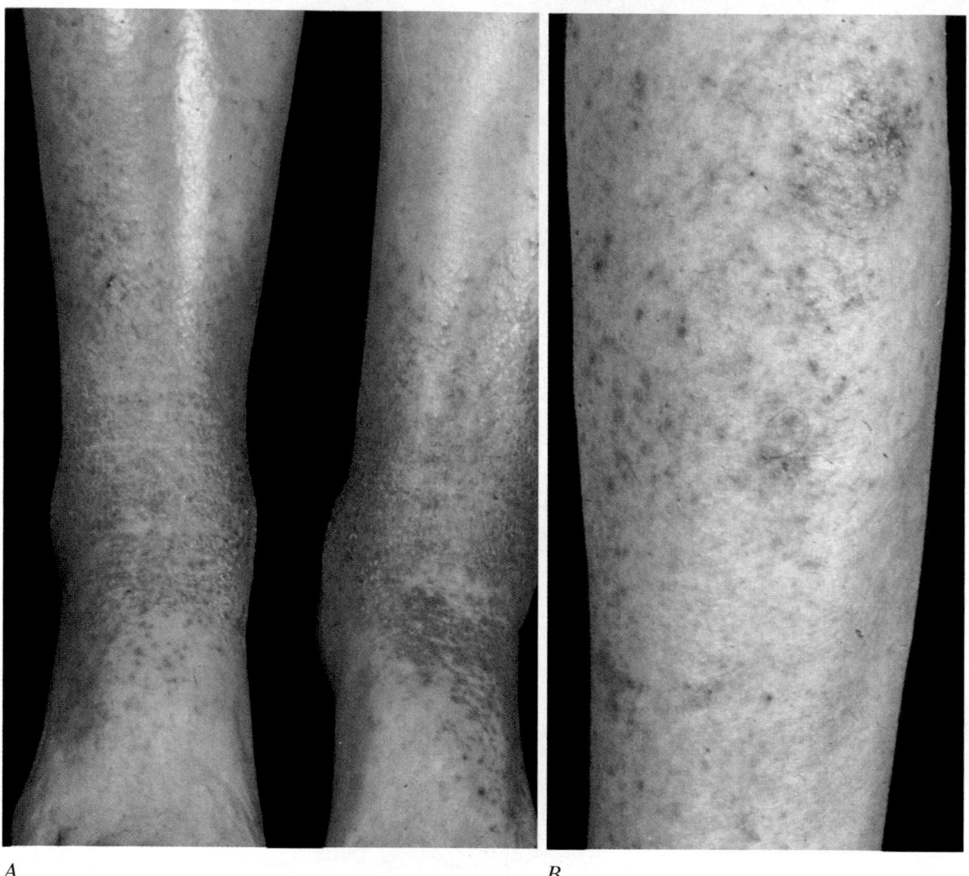

Stasis dermatitis with autosensitization. An elderly woman with a long-standing history of stasis dermatitis presented with gradual worsening of the edema; pruritus; and multiple, punctate, superficial, excoriated ulcers overlying the medial malleoli (*A*). Nine days after the ulcers appeared, she developed an acute, extremely pruritic, erythematous, papulovesicular eruption over the forearms (*B*), which progressively involved the upper arms, upper torso, and hands. The acute papulovesicular dermatitis also involved the lower extremities and can be noted overlying the chronic stasis dermatitis (*A*).

infections caused by tuberculosis,[2] dermatophytes,[3] and bacteria[4] were considered to be pathophysiologically equivalent phenomena.[5–7] During this time, the concept that the process involves an urticarial component was dismissed, and the term was limited to a secondary papulovesicular eruption.[5–7] In the more recent past, the precipitating factors for this phenomenon have been broadened to include the application of irritant or sensitizing chemicals[8] and ionizing radiation.[9] The "excited skin syndrome,"[10] an entity well described by Mitchell,[11] could also be included under this rubric.

The classic presentation of autosensitization is that seen in patients with venous stasis disease[12] where, in the past, as many as 37 percent of patients have been reported to develop autosensitization.[13] Although still observed (Fig. 121-1), the incidence of autosensitization in stasis dermatitis is probably much lower today, given the dearth of reports in the current literature. Typically, 1 to 2 weeks after an acute inflammation of the lower leg, an extremely pruritic, symmetric, scattered, erythematous, eruption with macules, papules, and vesicles develops. The eruption involves the forearms, thighs, legs, trunk, face, hands, neck, and feet in descending order of frequency.[7,13] The rash often persists and spreads until the underlying causative primary site of inflammation is treated. During the evolution of the dermatitis, its morphology

ETIOLOGY

Although the disease was originally thought to be due to autosensitization to epidermal antigens,[1] this concept has not been experimentally verified. In murine studies designed to determine whether keratinocyte-derived proteins can serve as antigenic carriers for hapten, Fehr et al.[14] derived major histocompatibility complex (MHC)-restricted, T cell receptor (TCR) α/β, CD4+ T cell clones that proliferated in response to keratinocyte extracts unconjugated to hapten. In these studies, such autoreactive T cell clones could not be derived following treatment with irritants. These authors speculated that T cells autoreactive to keratinocyte antigens may be generated during the course of contact hypersensitivity and lead to the development of an "id" reaction. However, they could not exclude the possibility that the derived T cell clones were reacting to an inherently antigenic substance or a tumor antigen present on the keratinocytes (PAM 212, a line derived from a murine squamous cell carcinoma) used to sensitize the mice. Furthermore, they did not inject the mice with the putative autoreactive clones to determine whether a dermatitis similar to autosensitization could be induced. Finally, this model would not explain the development of id reactions following irritant contact dermatitis.

In the most extensive study to date,[12] only 4 of 81 patients with autosensitization dermatitis had serum antibodies cytotoxic to autologous or homologous skin. However, the role of such autoantibodies in mediating the disorder, even in these four patients, must be interpreted cautiously, given the high frequency of epidermal autoantibodies in the normal adult population.[15] Unfortunately, this study was performed before the technology to evaluate autoreactive T cells was widely available.

One problem in defining the etiology of autosensitization is the lack of an accepted experimental model. In an experiment in which guinea pigs were injected with autologous skin, Wilhelmj et al.[16] reported cutaneous disease characterized by hair loss in 3 of 11 and dermatitis in 2 of 11 guinea pigs, but it was not clear whether these reactions were immunologic and, if so, what the causal allergen(s) was. Indeed, other investigators using similar techniques have been unable to induce cutaneous disease in animals by means of epidermal extracts.[17] These results in animals are in contrast to those in humans, where intradermal challenge with water-soluble extracts of autologous epidermal scale precipitated some form of reaction in 19 of 24 patients with active autosensitization.[18]

The term autosensitization may be a misnomer, and the disease could be due not to an allergy to one's own skin but to a conditioned hyperirritability of the skin induced by either immunologic or nonimmunologic stimuli. Thus, animal studies, in which acute skin irritation lowered the irritancy threshold to the same irritant chemical at remote sites, may be relevant.[19] In 2 percent of chronically irritated animals, antibodies to epidermis could be found;[20] this proportion is comparable to that reported for patients experiencing autosensitization[12] and enhances the validity of the model. Furthermore, states akin to autosensitization can be triggered in animals, as in humans, not only by irritant chemicals, but also by acute allergic dermatitis or chronic ulceration of the skin.[19] Although cytotoxic antibody to skin does not appear to be responsible, the factor(s) involved remains elusive.

In 1933, Turck proposed that hematogenous dissemination of "cytosts" released from inflamed tissues could induce damage in distant organs.[21] In 1939, Brown proposed that these "cytosts" might be responsible for autosensitization.[5] Currently, "cytosts" are more properly termed *cytokines*. Indeed, factors such as irritation, sensitization, infection, and wounding, which are known to precipitate autosensitization, have been reported to release a variety of epidermal cytokines.[22,23] Once hematogenously disseminated in sufficient amounts, these cytokines could heighten the sensitivity of skin to a variety of nonspecific, but otherwise innocuous, stimuli, producing a pattern of "spillover" reactions[24] that have been classically termed *autosensitization*. Such an hypothesis would account for (1) the results in humans of delayed-type hypersensitivity testing with autologous epidermal scale,[18] (2) the histopathologic findings noted in the disease (see below), and (3) the activated T lymphocytes observed in the blood of one patient with autosensitization.[25] The characteristic distribution of the disease might perhaps be explained if the skin overlying the arms and legs was found to contain increased numbers of, or more avid receptors for, various cytokines than the skin of the face or hands. Such a geographic variation in the distribution of bullous pemphigoid antigen has been observed and hypothesized to account for the clinical patterns of this truly autoimmune disease.[26] Application of modern biotechnological tools should provide insight into the mysteries of autosensitization.

HISTOPATHOLOGY

The lesions of autosensitization are characterized by spongiotic epidermal vesicles associated with a superficial, perivascular lymphohistiocytic infiltrate, which may contain scattered eosinophils.[27] Immunophenotypic studies of skin from experimental models have revealed that most of the lymphohistiocytic cells are CD3+, that is, T lymphocytes.[24] Those T cells present in the epidermal vesicles are primarily CD8+ (cytotoxic/suppressor cells), whereas those in the dermal infiltrate are primarily CD4+ (helper cells). Consistent with earlier reports that cytotoxic antibodies could not be found in the majority of individuals with autosensitization,[12] deposition of antibody or complement in affected skin was not detected. Thus, the histopathologic findings in autosensitization are not pathognomonic, but can be seen in other conditions including allergic or irritant contact dermatitis, nummular dermatitis, and dyshidrosis.[27] In addition, vesicular dermatophytic infections can have a similar appearance, although the presence of hyphae in the stratum corneum helps to distinguish this entity.[27]

DIAGNOSIS AND TREATMENT

The diagnosis of autosensitization remains one of exclusion. As clinically indicated, patients with an underlying focus of inflammation who present with the acute onset of disseminated papulovesicular disease should be tested to exclude secondary allergic contact dermatitis and/or secondary bacterial, fungal, viral, or parasitic disease. After other potential underlying causes for the widespread dermatitis have been eliminated, treatment is best directed toward the inciting disease. Concomitantly, the frequently weeping, vesicular eruption of autosensitization benefits from drying agents such as aluminum sulfate and calcium acetate. Given the likely involvement of cytokines and inflammatory mediators sensitive to glucocorticoids[28] or macrolactams,[29,30] systemic and/or topical treatment with glucocorticoids or macrolactams (cyclosporin A, tacrolimus, pimecrolimus) may be helpful. To prevent the secondary effects of excoriation, pruritus must be controlled with topical antipruritic agents or oral antihistamines. As in the case of treatment for allergic contact dermatitis (Chap. 120), one must remain alert to the possibility of inducing an allergy in existing dermatitic skin from such topical medicaments.

REFERENCES

1. Whitfield A: Lumelian lectures on some points in the aetiology of skin disease. *Lancet* **2**:122, 1921
2. Darier J: Des tuberculides cutanées. *Ann Dermatol Venereol* **7**:1431, 1896
3. Guth A: Uber lichenoide (Kleinpapulose, spinulost) Trichophytie. *Arch Dermatol Syphilis* **118**:856, 1914
4. Andrews GC et al: Recalcitrant pustular eruption of palms and soles. *Arch Dermatol* **29**:548, 1934
5. Brown WH: Some clinical manifestations of endogenous sensitization eruptions following local infection or injury. *Br J Dermatol* **51**:197, 1939
6. Hopkins HH, Burky EL: Cutaneous autosensitization: Role of staphylococci in chronic eczema of the hands. *Arch Dermatol* **49**:124, 1944
7. Smith SW: Eczema autolytica. *Br Med J* **1**:628, 1945
8. Bendl BS: Nummular eczema of stasis origin: The backbone of a morphologic pattern of diverse etiology. *Int J Dermatol* **18**:129, 1979
9. Roa WH et al: Generalized autosensitization to a localized eczematoid dermatitis induced by ionizing radiation. *J Am Acad Dermatol* **30**:489, 1994
10. Maibach HI: The E.S.S.—Excited skin syndrome (alias the "angry back"), in *New Trends in Allergy*, edited by J Ring, G Burg. New York, Springer, 1981, p 208
11. Mitchell JC: Multiple concomitant positive patch test reactions. *Contact Dermatitis* **3**:315, 1975
12. Parish WE et al: A study of auto-allergy in generalized eczema. *Br J Dermatol* **77**:479, 1965
13. Haxthausen H: Generalized "ids" ("autosensitization") in varicose eczema. *Acta Derm Venereol (Stockh)* **35**:271, 1955
14. Fehr BS et al: T cells reactive to keratinocyte antigens are generated during induction of contact hypersensitivity in mice. A model for autoeczematization in humans? *Am J Contact Dermat* **11**:145, 2000
15. Ackermann-Schopf C et al: Natural and acquired epidermal autoantibodies in man. *J Immunol* **112**:2063, 1974
16. Wilhelmj CM Jr et al: Production of hypersensitivity to skin of animals. *Arch Dermatol* **86**:161, 1962
17. Rosenthal SA et al: Failure to sensitize to autologous skin. *Proc Soc Exp Biol Med* **97**:279, 1958
18. Esplin BM, Cormia FE: Further studies in autoeczematization. *Arch Dermatol* **64**:31, 1951
19. Roper SS, Jones HE: An animal model for altering the irritability threshold of normal skin. *Contact Dermatitis* **13**:91, 1985
20. Parish WE: Autosensitization to skin, in *Progress in Biological Sciences in Relation to Dermatology*, edited by A Rook. Cambridge, England, Cambridge University Press, 1960, p 259
21. Turck FB: *The Action of the Living Cell*. London, Macmillan, 1933
22. Williams IR, Kupper TS: Immunity at the surface: Homeostatic mechanisms of the skin immune system. *Life Sci* **58**:1485, 1996
23. Uchi H et al: Cytokines and chemokines in the epidermis. *J Dermatol Sci* **24**(suppl 1):S29, 2000
24. Bruynzeel DP et al: Allergic reactions, "spillover" reactions, and T cell subsets. *Arch Dermatol Res* **275**:80, 1983

25. Cunningham MJ et al: Circulating activated (DR-positive) T lymphocytes in a patient with autoeczematization. *J Am Acad Dermatol* **14**:1039, 1986
26. Goldberg DJ et al: Bullous pemphigoid antibodies: Human skin as a substrate for indirect immunofluorescence assay. *Arch Dermatol* **121**:1137, 1985
27. Ackerman AB: *Histologic Diagnosis of Inflammatory Skin Disease: An Algorithmic Method Based on Pattern Analysis,* 2nd ed. Baltimore, MD, Williams & Wilkins, 1997
28. Almawi WY et al: Regulation of cytokine and cytokine receptor expression by glucocorticoids. *J Leukoc Biol* **60**:563, 1996
29. Paul C et al: Ascomycins: Promising agents for the treatment of inflammatory skin diseases. *Expert Opin Investig Drugs* **9**:69, 2000
30. Dumont FJ: FK506, an immunosuppressant targeting calcineurin function. *Curr Med Chem* **7**:731, 2000

CHAPTER 122

Donald Y.M. Leung
Lawrence F. Eichenfield
Mark Boguniewicz

Atopic Dermatitis (Atopic Eczema)

Atopic dermatitis (AD) is a chronically relapsing skin disease that occurs most commonly during early infancy and childhood. It is frequently associated with elevated serum IgE levels and a personal or family history of AD, allergic rhinitis, and/or asthma. There is no single distinguishing feature of AD or a diagnostic laboratory test. Thus, the diagnosis is based on the constellation of clinical findings listed in Table 122-1.

HISTORICAL ASPECTS

This disorder was probably first reported by Robert Willan,[1] in 1808, as a *prurigo*-like condition. The term *disseminated neurodermatitis* was proposed by Brocq and Jacquet, in 1891, to emphasize that the disorder was emotionally based. In 1892, Besnier delineated the prurigo group of diseases and described the association of hay fever and asthma with AD. He suggested that these disorders tended to be familial and occurred in the constitutionally predisposed. Besnier also believed that pruritus played a primary role in the pathogenesis of AD and called the disorder *prurigo diathesique,* a term that was soon changed to Besnier's prurigo.

In 1923, Coca and associates[2] introduced the term *atopy* for [no(a)-place(top)-ness(y)] to describe some of the clinical manifestations of human hypersensitivity that characterized asthma and hay fever. Coca and Cooke later included patients with "the pruritic rash" in this group. In the 1930s, Sulzberger and associates[3] suggested the term *atopic dermatitis* to be used in place of disseminated neurodermatitis. The term AD has the advantage of connoting a close relationship among skin manifestations, asthma, and allergic rhinitis in patients with an atopic diathesis.

EPIDEMIOLOGY

Because there are no precise clinical definitions of AD, epidemiologic studies must be carefully interpreted as they can be plagued by problems of bias ascertainment. Despite these limitations, several well-designed studies suggest that there has been at least a two- to threefold increase in the prevalence of AD during the past three decades (reviewed in Ref. 4). Indeed, the most recent estimates indicate that AD is a major public health problem worldwide, with a prevalence in children of 10 to 20 percent in the United States, northern and western Europe, urban Africa, Japan, Australia, and other industrialized countries.[5] The prevalence of AD in adults is approximately 1 to 3 percent. Interestingly, the prevalence of AD is much lower in agricultural countries such as China and in eastern Europe, rural Africa, and Central Asia. There is also a female preponderance for AD, with an overall female/male ratio of 1.3:1.

The basis for this increased prevalence of AD is not well understood. However, wide variations in prevalence have been observed within countries inhabited by similar ethnic groups, suggesting that

TABLE 122-1

Clinical Features of Atopic Dermatitis

Major features
- Pruritus
- Facial and extensor eczema in infants and children
- Flexural eczema in adults
- Chronic or relapsing dermatitis
- Personal or family history of atopic disease

Associated features
- Xerosis
- Cutaneous infections
- Nonspecific dermatitis of the hands or feet
- Ichthyosis, palmar hyperlinearity, keratosis pilaris
- Pityriasis alba
- Nipple eczema
- White dermatographism and delayed blanch response
- Anterior subcapsular cataracts, keratoconus
- Elevated serum IgE levels
- Positive immediate-type allergy skin tests
- Early age of onset
- Dennie-Morgan infraorbital folds, orbital darkening
- Facial erythema or pallor
- Perifollicular accentuation
- Course influenced by environmental and/or emotional factors

environmental factors are critical in determining disease expression. Some of the potential risk factors that have received attention as being associated with the rise in atopic disease include small family size, increased income and education both in whites and blacks, migration from rural to urban environments, and increased use of antibiotics, that is, the so-called Western lifestyle.[6] This has resulted in the "hygiene hypothesis," first proposed by Strachan, that allergic diseases might be prevented by "infection in early childhood transmitted by unhygienic contact with older siblings."[7] This hypothesis is supported by recent studies demonstrating that allergic responses are driven by T helper type (T_H) 2 immune responses whereas infections are induced by T_H1 immune responses.[8] T_H1 responses antagonize the development of T_H2 cells. Therefore, a decreased number of infections during early childhood could predispose to enhanced T_H2 allergic responses.

ETIOLOGY AND PATHOGENESIS

Complex interactions among genetic, environmental, skin barrier, pharmacologic, and immunologic factors contribute to the pathogenesis of AD. The development of new techniques for the study of naturally occurring and experimentally induced skin lesions have provided valuable new insights into the pathogenesis of AD. The concept that AD has an immunologic basis is supported by the observation that patients with primary T cell immunodeficiency disorders frequently have elevated serum IgE levels and eczematoid skin lesions indistinguishable from AD. In patients with Wiskott-Aldrich syndrome, clearing of the skin rash occurs following correction of their immunologic defect by successful bone marrow transplantation.[9] These data suggest that AD is not caused by a constitutive skin defect but is mediated by a bone marrow–derived cell(s).

The Systemic Response (Table 122-2)

Most patients with AD have peripheral blood eosinophilia and increased serum IgE levels (reviewed in Ref. 10). Nearly 80 percent of children with AD develop allergic rhinitis or asthma, suggesting that respiratory allergy and AD have a common systemic link. Because serum IgE levels are strongly associated with the prevalence of asthma, it suggests that allergen sensitization through the skin predisposes to respiratory disease due to its effects on the systemic allergic response (reviewed in Ref. 11). Indeed, when mice are sensitized epicutaneously with protein antigen, it induces allergic dermatitis, elevated serum IgE, airway eosinophilia, and hyperresponsiveness to methacholine, suggesting that epicutaneous exposure to allergen in AD may enhance the development of allergic asthma.[12]

TABLE 122-2

Systemic Immune Abnormalities in Atopic Dermatitis

- Increased synthesis of IgE
- Increased specific IgE to multiple allergens, including foods, aeroallergens, microorganisms, bacterial toxins, autoallergens
- Increased expression of CD23 (low affinity IgE receptor) on B cells and monocytes
- Increased basophil histamine release
- Impaired delayed-type hypersensitivity response
- Eosinophilia
- Increased secretion of IL-4, IL-5, and IL-13 by T_H2 cells
- Decreased secretion of IFN-γ by T_H1 cells
- Increased soluble IL-2 receptor levels
- Elevated levels of monocyte CAMP-phosphodiesterase with increased IL-10 and prostaglandin-E_2

Peripheral blood mononuclear cells (PBMC) from AD patients have a decreased capacity to produce interferon-gamma (IFN-γ). IFN-γ generation ex vivo is inversely correlated with serum IgE concentrations in AD. There are also a number of studies demonstrating an increased frequency of allergen-specific T cells producing increased interleukin (IL)-4, IL-5, and IL-13, but little IFN-γ, in the peripheral blood of patients with AD.[10] These immunologic alterations are important because IL-4 and IL-13 are the only cytokines that induce germ-line transcription at the Cε exon, thereby promoting isotype switching to IgE. IL-4 and IL-13 also induce the expression of vascular adhesion molecules such as vascular cell adhesion molecule (VCAM)-1 involved in eosinophil infiltration and downregulate T_H1 cell function. In contrast, IFN-γ inhibits IgE synthesis as well as the proliferation of T_H2 cells and expression of the IL-4 receptor on T cells. Peripheral blood monocytes from AD patients are also activated, have an abnormally low incidence of spontaneous apoptosis, and are unresponsive to IL-4 induced apoptosis following stimulation. The likely cause of this inhibition of apoptosis is increased production of GM-CSF by circulating monocytes of AD patients.[13]

Immunologic Triggers

FOODS Well-controlled studies demonstrate that food allergens induce skin rashes in children with AD (reviewed in Ref. 14). Based on double-blind, placebo-controlled food challenges, approximately 40 percent of infants and young children with moderate to severe AD have food allergy. Although the dermatology literature has frequently not supported a role for foods in AD, a study by Eigenmann et al.[15] reported that 37 percent of unselected children with moderate to severe AD followed at a university dermatology clinic had food allergy. Food allergies in AD patients may induce eczematous dermatitis in some patients, while in others urticarial reactions, contact urticaria, or other noncutaneous symptoms are elicited. In a study of 250 children with AD, Guillet and Guillet[16] found that increased severity of AD symptoms and younger age of patients was correlated directly with the presence of food allergy. Removal of food allergens from the patient's diet can lead to significant clinical improvement but requires a great deal of education because most of the common allergens (e.g., egg, milk, wheat, soy, and peanut) contaminate many foods and are therefore difficult to avoid.[17]

Laboratory studies support a role for food allergy in AD. Infants and young children with moderate to severe AD generally have positive immediate skin tests or serum IgE directed to various foods (even in the face of normal total serum IgE levels). Positive food challenges are accompanied by significant increases in plasma histamine levels and eosinophil activation. Children with AD who are chronically ingesting foods to which they are allergic have increased spontaneous basophil histamine release compared with children without food allergy. In mouse models of AD, oral sensitization with foods results in the elicitation of eczematous skin lesions on repeat oral food challenges.[18] In patients, however, immediate skin tests to specific allergens do not always indicate clinical sensitivity. Therefore, clinically relevant food allergy must be verified by controlled food challenges or carefully investigating the effects of a food elimination diet that is being done in the absence of other exacerbating factors.

Importantly, food allergen-specific T cells have been cloned from the skin lesions of patients with AD.[19] In support of a role for food allergen-specific T cells in AD, patients with food-induced AD have been studied to analyze the relationship between tissue specificity of a clinical reaction to an allergen and expression of the skin homing receptor cutaneous lymphoid antigen (CLA) on T cells activated in vitro by the relevant allergen.[20] Casein-reactive T cells from patients with milk-induced eczema were found to have significantly higher levels of CLA than *Candida albicans*-reactive T cells from the same patients, casein- or

C. albicans-reactive T cells from nonatopic controls, or noneczematous controls with milk-induced gastroenteropathy. Overall, these studies provide strong scientific evidence that foods can play a role in the pathogenesis of AD in young children. Most food allergic children, however, outgrow their food hypersensitivity in the first few years of life, so food allergy is not a common trigger factor in older patients with AD.

AEROALLERGENS Walker reported, in 1918, that several of his patients had exacerbation of AD following exposure to horse dander, timothy grass, or ragweed pollen.[21] In the 1950s, Tuft and co-workers reported that in patients with AD, pruritus and eczematoid skin lesions developed after intranasal inhalation challenge with either Alternaria or ragweed pollen, but not placebo. More recently, double-blind, placebo-controlled challenges have demonstrated that inhalation of house dust mites by bronchial challenge can result in new AD skin lesions and exacerbation of a previous skin rash.[22] Epicutaneous application of aeroallergens by patch test techniques on uninvolved atopic skin elicits eczematoid reactions in 30 to 50 percent of patients with AD (reviewed in Ref. 23). Positive reactions have been observed to various aeroallergens, including dust mite, weeds, animal danders, and molds. In contrast, patients with respiratory allergy and healthy volunteers rarely have positive allergen patch tests.

Several studies have examined whether avoidance of aeroallergens results in clinical improvement of AD. Most of these reports have involved uncontrolled trials in which patients were placed in mite-free environments, such as hospital rooms, through the use of acaricides or impermeable mattresses covers. Such methods have invariably led to improvement in AD. One double-blind, placebo-controlled study using a combination of effective mite-reduction measures, as compared to no treatment, in the home showed that a reduction in house dust mites is associated with significant improvement in AD.[24]

Laboratory data supporting a role for inhalants include the finding of IgE antibody to specific inhalant allergens in most patients with AD. Indeed, a recent study found that 95 percent of sera from AD patients continued IgE to house dust mites as compared to 42 percent of asthmatic subjects.[25] The degree of sensitization to aeroallergens is directly associated with the severity of AD.[26] The isolation from AD skin lesions and allergen patch test sites of T cells that selectively respond to *Dermatophagoides pteronyssinus* and other aeroallergens provides further evidence that the immune response in AD skin can be elicited by aeroallergens.[23]

MICROBIAL PRODUCTS Patients with AD have an increased tendency to develop bacterial, viral, and fungal skin infections. Immune responses to the products of *Staphylococcus aureus* have provided insights into mechanisms underlying skin inflammation in AD. *S. aureus* is found in more than 90 percent of AD skin lesions.[10] In contrast, only 5 percent of normal subjects harbor this organism. The density of *S. aureus* on inflamed AD lesions without clinical superinfection can reach up to 10^7 colony-forming units per cm^2 on lesional skin. The importance of *S. aureus* is supported by the observation that even AD patients without overt infection show a greater reduction in severity of skin disease when treated with a combination of antistaphylococcal antibiotics and topical corticosteroids as compared to topical corticosteroids alone.[27]

One strategy by which *S. aureus* exacerbates or maintains skin inflammation in AD is by secreting a group of toxins known to act as superantigens that stimulate marked activation of T cells and macrophages. The skin lesions of over half of AD patients contain *S. aureus* that secrete superantigens such as enterotoxins A and B, and toxic shock syndrome toxin-1.[28,29] An analysis of the peripheral blood skin homing CLA+ T cells from these patients, as well as T cells in their skin lesions, reveals that they have undergone a T cell receptor (TCR) Vβ expansion consistent with superantigenic stimulation.[30,31] Most AD patients make specific IgE antibodies directed against the staphylococcal superantigens found on their skin.[28,29] Basophils from patients with IgE antibodies directed to superantigens release histamine on exposure to the relevant superantigen, but not in response to superantigens to which they have no specific IgE.[28] This raises the interesting possibility that superantigens induce specific IgE in AD patients and mast cell degranulation in vivo when the superantigens penetrate the disrupted epidermal barrier. This promotes the itch-scratch cycle critical to the evolution of skin rashes in AD.

A correlation has also been found between the presence of IgE anti-superantigens and severity of AD.[29] Using a humanized murine model of skin inflammation, the combination of *S. aureus* superantigen plus allergen has been shown to have an additive effect in inducing skin inflammation.[32] Superantigens also augment allergen-specific IgE synthesis and induce corticosteroid resistance suggesting that several mechanisms exist by which superantigens could aggravate the severity of AD.[33,34] Fulfilling Koch's postulates, application of the superantigen SEB to the skin can induce skin changes of erythema and induration accompanied by the infiltration of T cells that are selectively expanded in response to SEB.[35,36] Furthermore, in a prospective study of patients recovering from toxic shock syndrome, it was found that 14 of 68 patients developed chronic eczematoid dermatitis, whereas no patients recovering from gram-negative sepsis developed eczema.[37] These investigators concluded that superantigens may induce an atopic process in the skin. It is therefore of interest that superantigens have been demonstrated to induce T cell expression of the skin homing receptor via stimulation of IL-12 production.[38]

Aside from superantigens, staphylococci can produce other toxins that likely contribute to skin inflammation.[39] AD *S. aureus* isolates that do not secrete superantigenic toxins produce alpha-toxin. All staphylococcal strains also express staphylococcal protein A. There are significant differences in the action of these toxins on keratinocytes. Superantigenic toxins as well as protein A do not induce significant cytotoxic damage on keratinocytes but cause the delayed release of tumor necrosis factor (TNF)-α. In contrast, alpha-toxin induces profound keratinocyte cytotoxicity and immediate release of TNF-α. Keratinocyte cytotoxicity induced by alpha-toxin demonstrates the morphologic and functional characteristics of necrosis, but not apoptosis.

Increased binding of *S. aureus* to AD skin is likely related to underlying atopic skin inflammation. This concept is supported by several lines of investigation. First, it has been found that treatment with topical corticosteroids or tacrolimus will reduce *S. aureus* counts on atopic skin although they have no antibiotic actions.[40,41] Second, acute inflammatory lesions have more *S. aureus* than chronic AD skin lesions or normal-looking atopic skin. Scratching likely enhances *S. aureus* binding by disturbing the skin barrier and exposing extracellular matrix molecules known to act as adhesins for *S. aureus,* for example, fibronectin and collagens. Finally, in studies of *S. aureus* binding to skin lesions of mice undergoing T_H1 versus T_H2 inflammatory responses, bacterial binding was significantly greater at skin sites with T_H2-mediated inflammation.[42] Importantly, this increased bacterial binding did not occur in IL-4 gene knockout mice, indicating that IL-4 plays a crucial role in the enhancement of *S. aureus* binding to skin. IL-4 appears to enhance *S. aureus* binding to the skin by inducing the synthesis of fibronectin, an important *S. aureus* adhesin. Interestingly in studies of human AD, a role for fibrinogen in the binding of *S. aureus* to atopic skin has been found.[43] Because acute exudative lesions likely have increased plasma-derived fibrinogen, this may provide a mechanism for further binding of *S. aureus* to acute AD lesions.

AUTOALLERGENS In the 1920s, several investigators reported that human skin dander could trigger immediate hypersensitivity reactions in the skin of patients with severe AD suggesting that they made IgE against autoantigens in the skin.[44] The potential molecular basis for these observations was recently demonstrated by Valenta et al. (reviewed in Ref. 45) who reported that the majority of sera from patients with severe AD contain IgE antibodies directed against human proteins. One of these IgE-reactive autoantigens has been cloned from a human epithelial cDNA expression library and designated *Hom s 1,* which is a 55-kDa cytoplasmic protein in skin keratinocytes.[46] Such antibodies were not detected in patients with chronic urticaria, systemic lupus erythematosus (SLE), graft versus host disease (GVHD), or healthy controls. Although the autoallergens characterized to date have mainly been intracellular proteins, they have been detected in IgE immune complexes of AD sera, suggesting that release of these autoallergens from damaged tissues could trigger IgE- or T cell–mediated responses. These data suggest that while IgE immune responses are initiated by environmental allergens, allergic inflammation can be maintained by human endogenous antigens, particularly in severe AD.

Immune Response in AD Skin

ROLE OF CYTOKINES T_H2- and T_H1-type cytokines contribute to the pathogenesis of skin inflammation in AD. As compared with the skin of normal controls, unaffected skin of AD patients have an increased number of cells expressing IL-4 and IL-13, but not IL-5, IL-12, or IFN-γ, mRNA.[47,48] Acute and chronic skin lesions, when compared to normal skin or uninvolved skin of AD patients, have significantly greater numbers of cells that are positive for IL-4, IL-5, and IL-13 mRNA. However, acute AD does not contain significant numbers of IFN-γ or IL-12 mRNA expressing cells.

Chronic AD skin lesions have significantly fewer IL-4 and IL-13 mRNA-expressing cells, but increased numbers of IL-5, granulocyte-macrophage colony-stimulating factor (GM-CSF), IL-12, and IFN-γ mRNA-expressing cells than does acute AD. Thus, acute T cell infiltration in AD is associated with a predominance of IL-4 and IL-13 expression, whereas maintenance of chronic inflammation is associated with increased IL-5, GM-CSF, IL-12, and IFN-γ expression, and is accompanied by the infiltration of eosinophils and macrophages. The increased expression of IL-12 in chronic AD skin lesions is of interest as that cytokine plays a key role in T_H1 cell development and its expression in eosinophils and/or macrophages may initiate the switch to T_H1 or T_H0 cell development in chronic AD.

This biphasic pattern of T cell activation has also been demonstrated after epicutaneous application of aeroallergens using patch test techniques (reviewed in Ref. 49). Twenty-four hours after allergen application to the skin, increased expression of IL-4 mRNA and protein is observed, after which IL-4 expression declines to baseline levels. In contrast, IFN-γ mRNA expression is not detected in 24-h patch-test lesions, but is strongly expressed at the 48- to 72-h time points. Furthermore, T cell clones obtained from early time points of evolving allergen patch test sites secrete T_H2-type cytokines, whereas the majority of allergen-specific T cell clones derived from later patch-test sites (>48 h) exhibit a T_H1- or T_H0-type cytokine profile. Interestingly, the increased expression of IFN-γ mRNA in atopic patch test lesions is preceded by a peak of IL-12 expression coinciding with the infiltration of macrophages and eosinophils.

Activated T cells infiltrating the skin of AD patients have also been found to induce keratinocyte apoptosis contributing to the spongiotic process found in AD skin lesions.[50] This process is mediated by IFN-γ released from activated T cells that upregulates Fas on keratinocytes. The lethal hit is delivered to keratinocytes by Fas-ligand expressed on the surface of T cells that invade the epidermis and soluble Fas-ligand released from T cells.

CHEMOATTRACTANT FACTORS IL-16, a chemoattractant for CD4+ T cells, is more highly expressed in acute than chronic AD skin lesions.[51] The C-C chemokines, RANTES (regulated on activa-

tion, normal T cell expressed and secreted), monocyte chemotactic protein-4, and eotaxin are also increased in AD skin lesions and likely contribute to the chemotaxis of eosinophils and T_H2 lymphocytes into the skin.[52,53] Recent studies suggest a role for cutaneous T cell attractant chemokine (CTACK/CCL27) in the preferential attraction of CLA+ T cells to the skin.[54] The chemokine receptor CCR3, which is found on eosinophils and T_H2 lymphocytes and can mediate the action of eotaxin, RANTES, and MCP-4, has been reported to be increased in nonlesional and lesional skin of patients with AD.[53] Selective recruitment of CCR4 expressing T_H2 cells into AD skin may also be mediated by the chemokines MDC and TARC, which are increased in AD.[55]

PERSISTENT SKIN INFLAMMATION Chronic AD is linked to the prolonged survival of eosinophils and monocyte-macrophages in atopic skin. IL-5 expression during chronic AD likely plays a role in prolonging eosinophil survival and enhancement of their function. In chronic AD, the increased GM-CSF expression plays an important role in maintaining the survival and function of monocytes, Langerhans' cells and eosinophils.[13] Epidermal keratinocytes from AD patients express significantly higher levels of RANTES following stimulation with TNF-α and IFN-γ than keratinocytes from psoriasis patients.[56] This may serve as one mechanism by which the TNF-α and IFN-γ production during chronic AD enhances the chronicity and severity of eczema. Mechanical trauma can also induce the release of TNF-α and many other proinflammatory cytokines from epidermal keratinocytes. Thus, chronic scratching plays a role in the perpetuation and elicitation of skin inflammation in AD.

Factors Controlling T_H2 Cell Development

A number of determinants support T_H2 cell development early in the atopic skin process and provide opportunities for therapeutic intervention. These include the cytokine milieu in which T cell development is taking placing, the host's genetic propensity to produce T_H2-type cytokines, pharmacologic factors, the costimulatory signals used during T cell activation, the antigen-presenting cell, and skin barrier function (reviewed in Ref. 10).

ROLE OF CYTOKINES IL-4 promotes T_H2 cell development, whereas IL-12, produced by macrophages, dendritic cells, or eosinophils, induces T_H1 cells. The IL-12 receptor (IL-12R) β_2 subunit, which is the binding and signal transducing component of the IL-12R, is expressed on T_H1 but not T_H2 clones. Interestingly, IL-4 inhibits the expression of IL-12Rβ_2 on T cells. In contrast, IL-12, IFN-α and IFN-γ induce expression of the IL-12Rβ_2 chain, thereby providing a basis by which these cytokines induce differentiation of T_H1 cells. IL-4 has also been demonstrated to inhibit IFN-γ production and to downregulate the differentiation of T_H1 cells. Furthermore, mast cells and basophils also provide a source of T_H2-type cytokines that can be released upon cross-linking of their high affinity IgE receptor. Consequently, the increased systemic and local skin expression of IL-4 by T cells and mast cells/basophils in AD might promote T_H2 cell development.

PHARMACOLOGIC FACTORS Mononuclear cells from patients with AD have increased cyclic adenosine monophosphate (CAMP)-phosphodiesterase (PDE) enzyme activity.[57] This cellular abnormality contributes to the increased IgE synthesis by B cells and IL-4 production by T cells in AD as IgE and IL-4 production can be decreased in vitro by PDE inhibitors. The elevated CAMP PDE in atopic monocytes also contributes to the secretion of increased IL-10 and prostaglandin E_2. Both monocyte-derived IL-10 and PGE_2 inhibit IFN-γ production by T cells and might contribute to the decreased IFN-γ production by cultured AD PBMC. PDE inhibitors have also been found to reduce superantigen-induced, IL-12–dependent expression of the CLA skin homing receptor on T cells from patients with AD.[58]

COSTIMULATORY SIGNALS Complete activation of resting T cells requires costimulatory signals independent of the engagement of T cell receptors with the MHC plus peptide complex on antigen-presenting cells (APC). In mice, the generation of T_H2 cells depends on the interaction of CD28 with B7.2 (CD86).[59] The expression of B7.2 on B cells of AD patients is significantly higher than in normals or in patients with psoriasis.[60] In contrast, there was no significant difference in B7.1 (CD80) expression among the three subject groups. Importantly, total serum IgE from AD patients and normal subjects correlated significantly with B7.2 expression on B cells suggesting a role for B7.2+ B cells in IgE synthesis. Antihuman B7.2, but not B7.1, monoclonal antibody (MAb) significantly decreased IgE production by PBMC stimulated with IL-4 and anti-CD40 MAb. These data support the concept that B7.2 expression in AD promotes IgE synthesis. IL-4 and IL-13 also induce B7.2 expression on B cells, thereby providing an amplification loop for IgE synthesis in AD.

Langerhans cells (LC) in the lesional skin of AD predominantly express B7.2 as compared to B7.1.[61] Furthermore, antibodies to B7.2 completely inhibited T cell proliferation stimulated with *D. pteronyssinus* (house dust mite antigen) in the presence of LC. These data suggest that CD86 expression on LC plays an important role as a costimulatory molecule for T cell activation and may account for the increased T_H2 responses that occur after repeated antigen presentation by LC.

ANTIGEN-PRESENTING CELLS AD skin contains an increased number of IgE-bearing LC that appear to play an important role in cutaneous allergen presentation to T_H2 cells (reviewed in Ref. 62). In this regard, IgE bearing LC from AD skin lesions, but not LC which lack surface IgE, are capable of presenting house dust mite allergen to T cells. These results suggest that cell-bound IgE on LC facilitates capture and internalization of allergens into LC prior to their processing and antigen presentation to T cells. IgE-bearing LC that have captured allergen likely activate memory T_H2 cells in atopic skin but they may also migrate to the lymph nodes to stimulate naïve T cells there to further expand the pool of systemic T_H2 cells.

Binding of IgE to LC occurs primarily via high affinity IgE receptors. The clinical importance of these IgE receptors on LC is supported by the observation that the presence of FcεRI-expressing, LC-bearing IgE molecules is required to provoke eczematous skin lesions by application of aeroallergens on the skin of atopic patients. In contrast to mast cells and basophils, where the FcεRI is a tetrameric structure constitutively expressed at high levels, this receptor on LC lacks the classical β chain and its expression varies depending on the donor. Normal individuals and patients with respiratory allergy have low-level surface expression of FcεRI on their LC, whereas FcεRI is expressed at high levels in the inflammatory environment of AD. High-level FcεRI expression not only enhances binding and uptake of allergens but the activation of LC upon receptor ligation. Surface expression of FcεRI has been found to correlate with IgE serum levels. Furthermore, IL-4 strongly induces the cytoplasmic expression of the α chain of FcεRI in dendritic cells and upregulates the expression of the skin homing structures, E-cadherin and CLA. In contrast, IFN-γ inhibits FcεRIα and E-cadherin expression.

DECREASED SKIN BARRIER FUNCTION AD skin has a marked decrease in barrier function associated with reduced ceramide levels and enhanced transepidermal water loss.[63] These epidermal changes likely contribute to increased antigen absorption into the skin. Because epicutaneous, as compared to systemic or airway, sensitization to allergen results in higher level T_H2 responses, decreased skin barrier function could lead to more vigorous systemic T_H2 responses, thereby acting as a sensitization site for allergic responses.[12,64]

GENETICS

AD is familially transmitted with a strong maternal influence. Although many genes are likely to be involved in the development of allergic diseases, there has been particular interest in the potential role of chromosome 5q31-33 because it contains a clustered family of cytokine genes—IL-3, IL-4, IL-5, IL-13, and GM-CSF—which are expressed by T_H2 cells.[65] A case-control comparison has suggested a genotypic association between the T allele of the –590C/T polymorphism of the IL-4 gene promoter region with AD. Because the T allele is associated with increased IL-4 gene promoter activity when compared to the C allele, this suggests that genetic differences in transcriptional activity of the IL-4 gene influence AD predisposition. In addition, an association of AD with a gain-of-function mutation in the α subunit of the IL-4 receptor has been reported. These data support the concept that IL-4 gene expression plays a critical role in the expression of AD. A functional mutation in the promoter region of the C-C chemokine RANTES and an IL-13 coding region variant may also be involved in the pathogenesis of AD. These candidate gene approaches have identified genes that suggest that AD has a common genetic basis with other atopic diseases.

A significant association between a specific polymorphism in the mast cell chymase gene and AD has been identified. It has no association with asthma or allergic rhinitis. This finding suggests that a genetic variant of mast cell chymase, which is a serine protease secreted by skin mast cells, may have organ-specific effects and contribute to the genetic susceptibility for AD. Two recent genome-wide linkage studies have also been performed to identify susceptibility loci for AD. A study by Lee et al.[66] suggested linkage for AD on chromosome 3q21, a region that encodes the costimulatory molecules CD80 and CD86. In contrast, Cookson et al.[67] reported linkage of AD to chromosome 1q21 and 17q25, identifying loci which closely coincide with regions linked to psoriasis. This suggests that AD is influenced by genes that modulate skin responses independent of allergic mechanisms.

CLINICAL MANIFESTATIONS

The diagnosis of AD is based on the constellation of clinical features summarized in Table 122-1. AD typically begins during infancy. Approximately 50 percent of patients develop this illness by the first year of life and an additional 30 percent between the ages of 1 and 5 years. Nearly 80 percent of patients with AD eventually develop allergic rhinitis or asthma later in childhood. Many of these patients outgrow their AD as they are developing respiratory allergy.

Skin Reaction Patterns

Intense pruritus and cutaneous reactivity are cardinal features of AD. Pruritus may be intermittent throughout the day but is usually worse in the early evening and night. Its consequences are scratching, prurigo papules (Fig. 122-1), lichenification (Fig. 122-2), and eczematous skin lesions. The pathogenesis of cutaneous pruritus is not well understood but is thought to be induced by various products of inflammatory effector cells including neuropeptides, histamine, leukotrienes, and

FIGURE 122-1

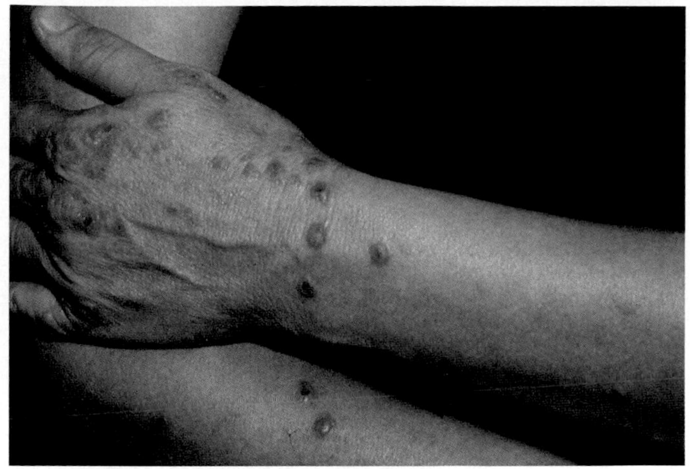

Prurigo papules in a patient with AD.

proteolytic enzymes. Patients with AD also have a reduced threshold for pruritus. Clinically, this is supported by the observation that allergens, reduced humidity, excessive sweating, and low concentrations of irritants (e.g., wool, acrylic, soaps, and detergents) can exacerbate pruritus and scratching.

Several skin reaction patterns are commonly seen in AD. Acute skin lesions are characterized by intensely pruritic, erythematous papules associated with excoriation, vesicles over erythematous skin, and serous exudate (Fig. 122-3). Subacute dermatitis is characterized by erythematous, excoriated, scaling papules (Fig. 122-4). Chronic AD is characterized by thickened plaques of skin, accentuated skin markings (lichenification), and fibrotic papules (prurigo nodularis) (Fig. 122-5). In chronic AD, all three stages of skin reactions frequently coexist in the same individual. At all stages of AD, patients usually have dry, lackluster skin (Fig. 122-6).

The distribution and skin reaction pattern varies according to the patient's age and disease activity. During infancy, the AD is generally more acute and primarily involves the face, scalp, and the extensor surfaces of the extremities (Fig. 122-7). The diaper area is usually spared. In older children, and in those who have long-standing skin disease, the patient develops the chronic form of AD with lichenification and localization of the rash to the flexural folds of the extremities (Fig. 122-8). AD often subsides as the patient grows older, leaving an adult with skin that is prone to itching and inflammation when exposed to exogenous irritants. Chronic hand eczema may be the primary manifestation of many adults with AD (Fig. 122-9). Other associated features of AD are listed in Table 122-1.

FIGURE 122-2

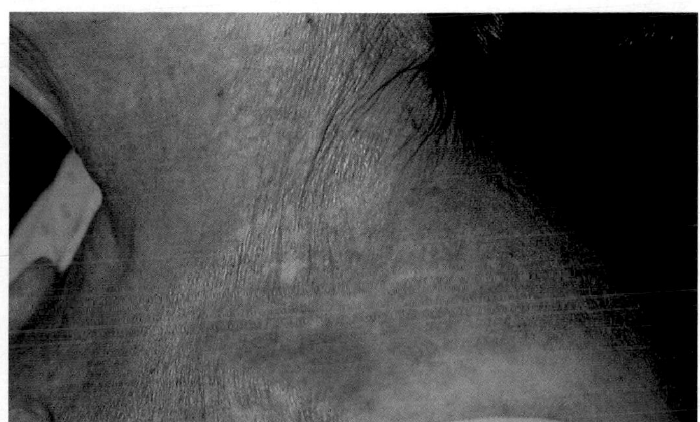

Lichenification of the neck and shoulders in an adult with AD.

FIGURE 122-3

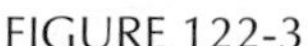

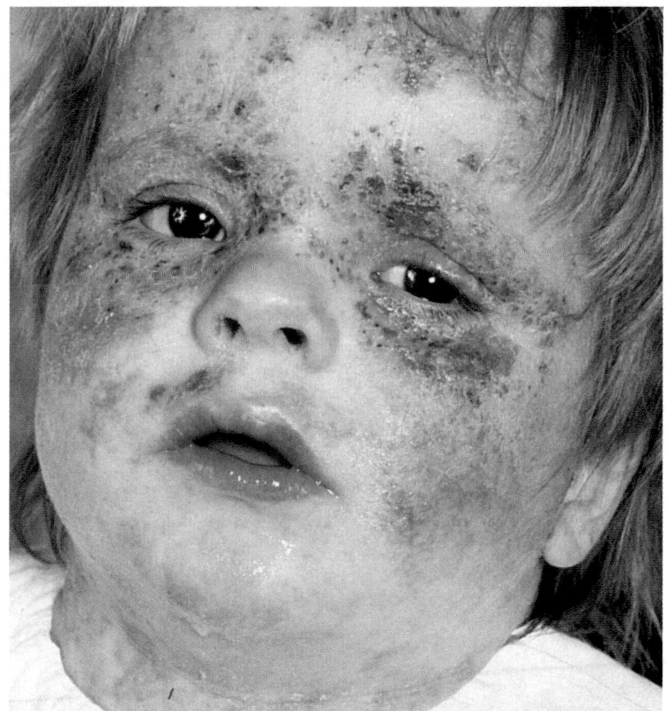

A.

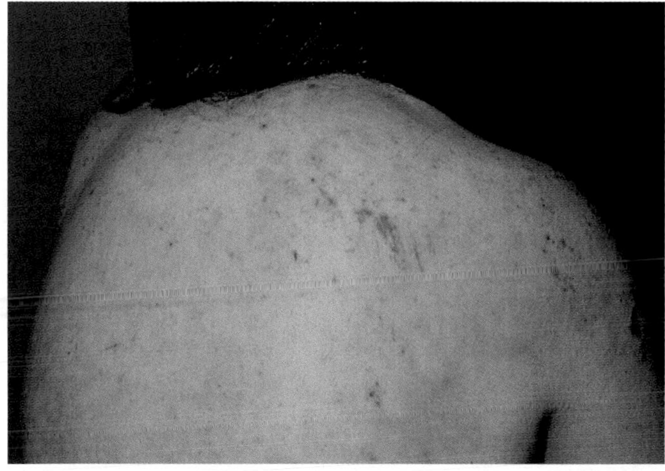

B.

A. Pronounced weeping and crusting of eczematous lesions in childhood AD. *B.* Excoriated papules and crusting in an acute flare of AD.

Complications

OCULAR PROBLEMS Eye complications associated with severe AD can lead to significant morbidity. Eyelid dermatitis and chronic blepharitis are commonly associated with AD and may result in visual impairment from corneal scarring. Atopic keratoconjunctivitis is usually

FIGURE 122-4

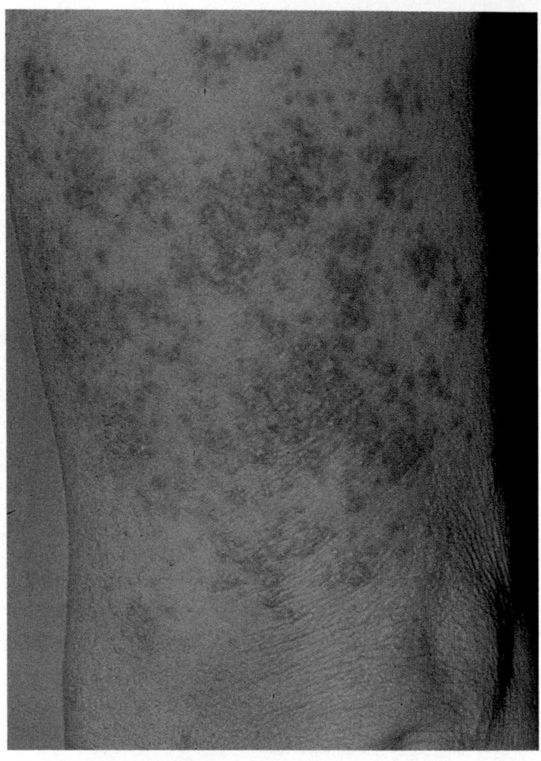

Erythematous papules in a patient with subacute AD.

FIGURE 122-5

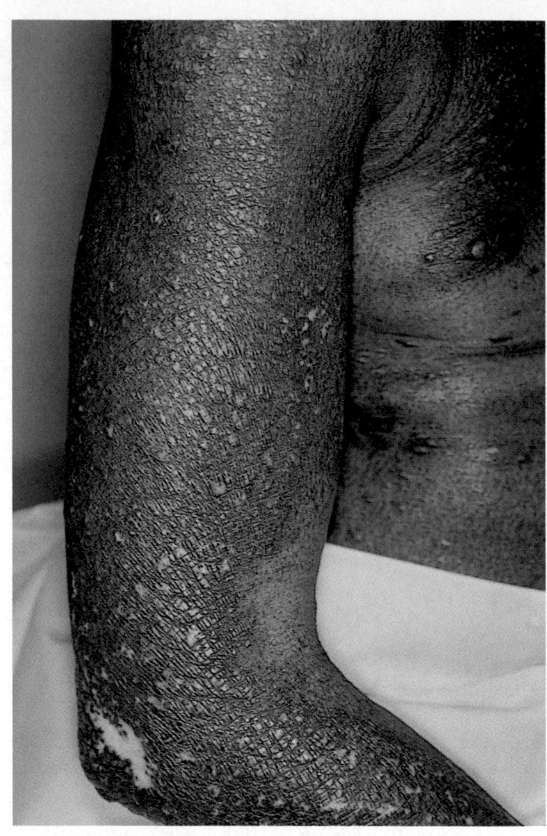

Severe lichenification and hyperpigmented prurigo papules seen in a patient with chronic AD.

bilateral and can have disabling symptoms that include itching, burning, tearing, and copious mucoid discharge. Vernal conjunctivitis is a severe bilateral recurrent chronic inflammatory process associated with papillary hypertrophy, or cobblestoning of the upper eyelid conjunctiva. It usually occurs in younger patients and has a marked seasonal incidence, often in the spring. The associated intense pruritus is exacerbated by exposure to irritants, light, or sweating. Keratoconus is a conical deformity of the cornea believed to result from chronic rubbing of the eyes in patients with AD and allergic rhinitis. Cataracts were reported in the early literature to occur in up to 21 percent of patients with severe AD. However, it is unclear whether this was a primary manifestation of AD or the result of the extensive use of systemic and topical glucocorticoids, particularly around the eyes. Indeed, more recent studies suggest that routine screening for cataracts in patients with AD may not be productive unless there is concern about potential side effects from steroid therapy.

INFECTIONS AD can be complicated by recurrent viral skin infections that may reflect local defects in T cell function. The most serious viral infection is herpes simplex, which can affect patients of all ages, resulting in Kaposi's varicelliform eruption or eczema herpeticum. After an incubation period of 5 to 12 days, multiple, itchy, vesiculopustular lesions erupt in a disseminated pattern; vesicular lesions are umbilicated, tend to crop, and often become hemorrhagic and crusted (Fig. 122-10). Punched out and extremely painful erosions result. These lesions may coalesce to large, denuded and bleeding areas that can extend over the entire body.

Although smallpox infections have been eradicated worldwide since the late 1970s, threats of bioterrorism (with smallpox and other infectious agents) have made nations reconsider their policies toward

FIGURE 122-6

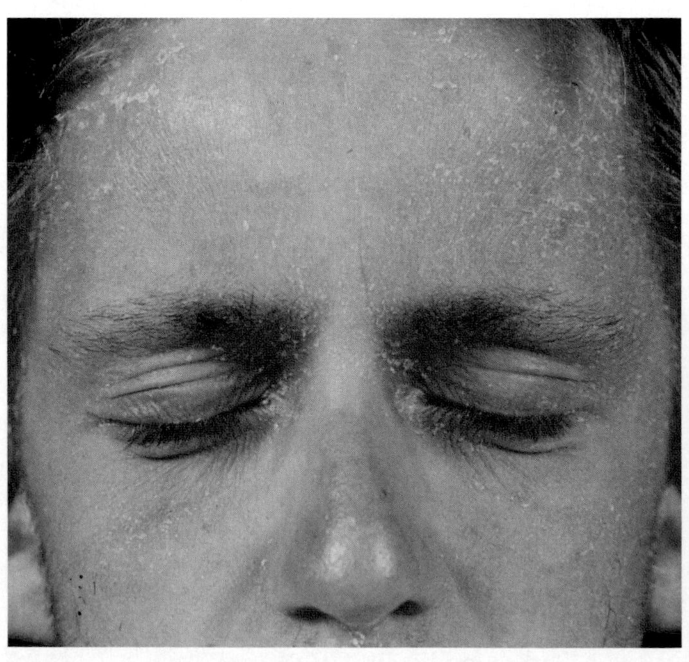

Infiltrated, erythematous facial skin with scaliness in an adolescent with AD. Note lateral thinning of eyebrows and infraocular (Morgan's) fold.

FIGURE 122-7

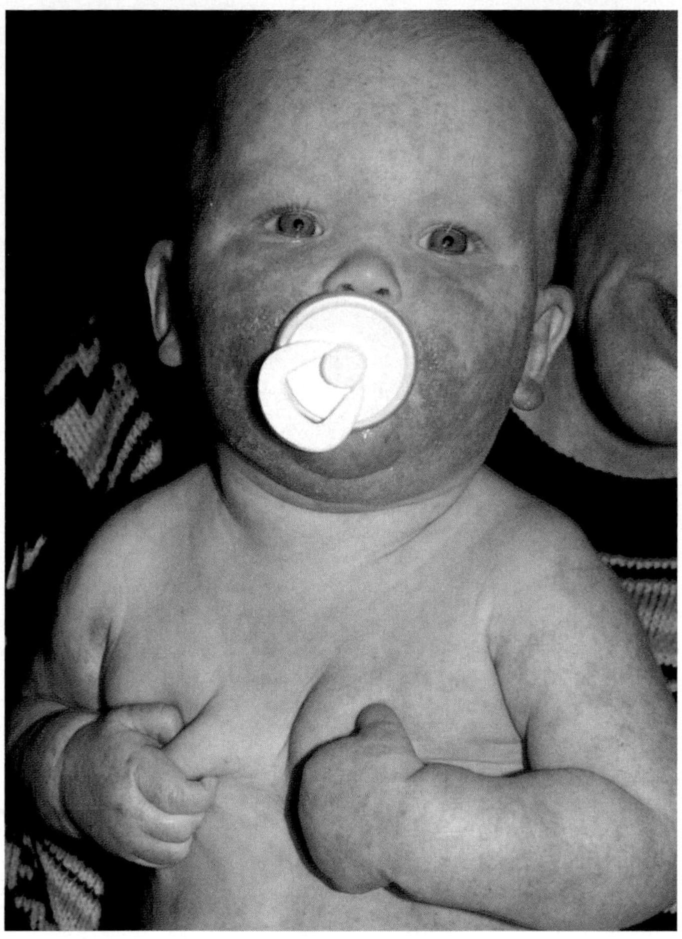

Itching infant with AD. (*Courtesy of Oholm Larsen, MD.*)

FIGURE 122-8

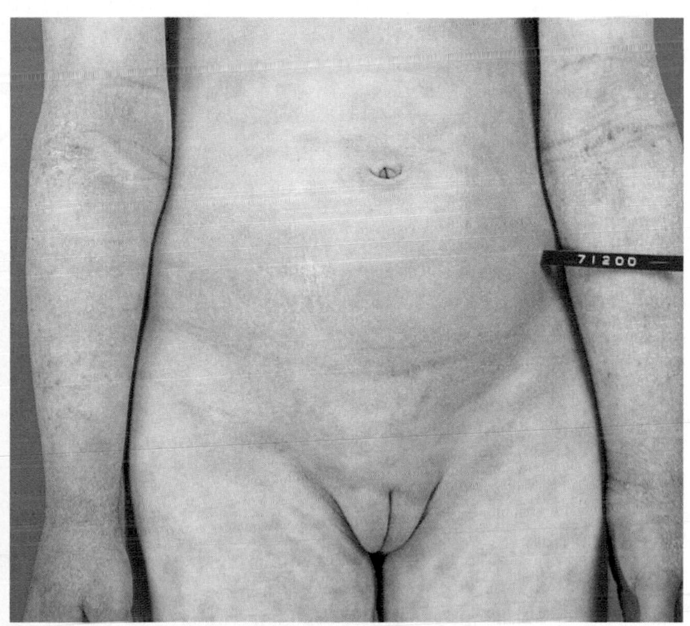

Childhood AD with lichenification of antecubital fossae and generalized severely pruritic eczematous plaques.

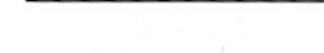

FIGURE 122-9

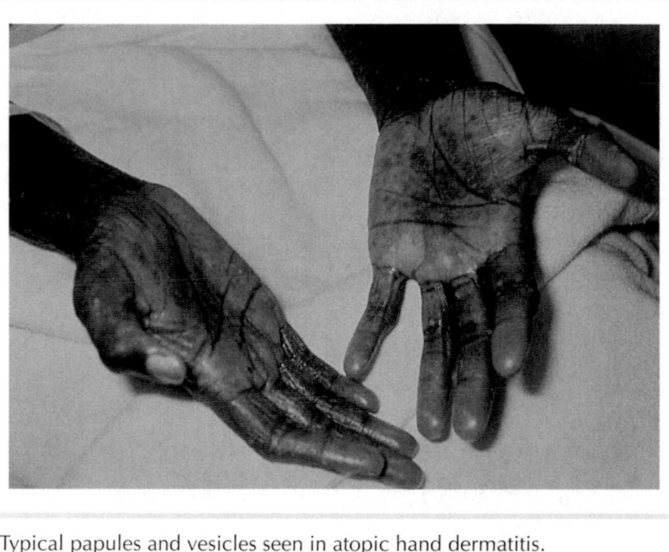

Typical papules and vesicles seen in atopic hand dermatitis.

initiating vaccination programs. In AD patients, smallpox vaccination (or even exposure to vaccinated individuals) may cause a severe widespread eruption (called eczema vaccinatum) that appears very similar to eczema herpeticum. Thus, in patients with AD, vaccination is contraindicated unless there is a clear risk of smallpox. In addition, decisions regarding vaccination of family members should take into consideration the potential of eczema vaccinatum in household contacts.

Superficial fungal infections are also more common in atopic individuals and may contribute to the exacerbation of AD. Patients with AD have an increased prevalence of *Trichophyton rubrum* infections compared to nonatopic controls. There has been particular interest in the role of *Malassezia furfur* (*Pityrosporum ovale* or *P. orbiculare*) in AD. *M. furfur* is a lipophilic yeast commonly present in the seborrheic areas of the skin. IgE antibodies against *M. furfur* are commonly found in AD patients and most frequently in patients with head and neck dermatitis. In contrast, IgE sensitization to *M. furfur* is rarely observed in normal controls or asthmatics. Positive allergen patch test reactions to this yeast have also been demonstrated. The potential importance of *M. furfur* as well as other dermatophyte infections is further supported by the reduction of AD skin severity in such patients following treatment with antifungal agents.

As discussed earlier, *S. aureus* is found in more than 90 percent of AD skin lesions. Honey-colored crusting, folliculitis, and pyoderma are indicators of secondary bacterial skin infection, usually due to *S. aureus* that requires antibiotic therapy. Regional lymphadenopathy is common in such patients. The importance of *S. aureus* in AD is supported by the observation that patients with severe AD, even those without overt infection, can show clinical response to combined treatment with antistaphylococcal antibiotics and topical glucocorticoids. Although recurrent staphylococcal pustulosis can be a significant problem in AD, deep seated *S. aureus* infections occur rarely and should raise the possibility of an immunodeficiency syndrome such as hyper-IgE syndrome.

HAND DERMATITIS Patients with AD often develop a nonspecific, irritant hand dermatitis. It is frequently aggravated by repeated wetting and by washing of the hands with harsh soaps, detergents, and disinfectants. Atopic individuals with occupations involving wet work are prone to develop an intractable hand dermatitis in the occupational setting. This is a common cause of occupational disability.

FIGURE 122-10

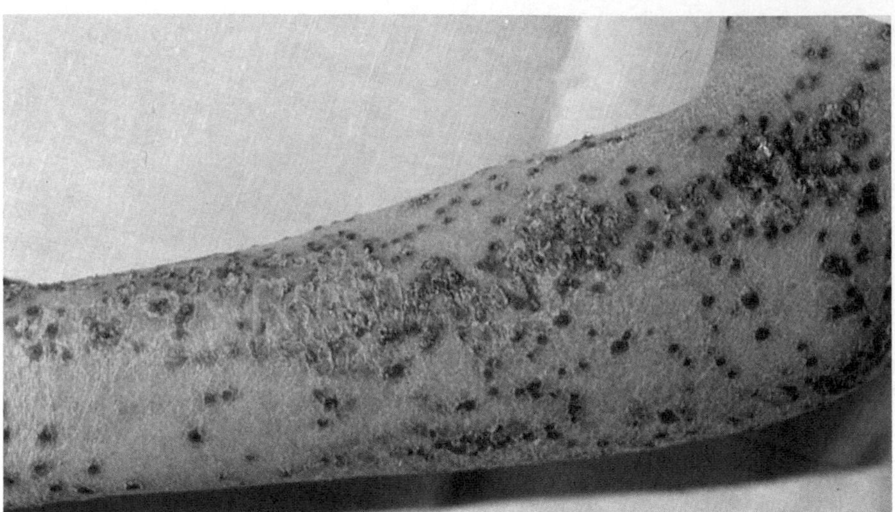

Eczema herpeticum. Typical vesicles and crusting in a patient with disseminated disease.

EXFOLIATIVE DERMATITIS Patients with extensive skin involvement may develop exfoliative dermatitis. This is associated with generalized redness, scaling, weeping, crusting, systemic toxicity, lymphadenopathy, and fever (see Chap. 44). Although this complication is rare, it is potentially life-threatening. It is usually due to superinfection, for example, with toxin-producing *S. aureus* or herpes simplex infection, continued irritation of the skin, or inappropriate therapy. In some cases, the withdrawal of systemic glucocorticoids used to control severe AD may be a precipitating factor for exfoliative erythroderma.

LABORATORY FINDINGS

Serum IgE levels are elevated in the majority of patients with AD. Approximately 85 percent of patients have positive immediate skin tests or serum IgE antibody directed to a variety of food, inhalant, and microbial allergens. The majority of patients with AD also have peripheral blood eosinophilia. Unlike eosinophils from normal donors, peripheral blood eosinophils from AD patients are primed for chemotaxis and transendothelial transmigration.[11] Furthermore, serum levels of eosinophil cationic protein and urinary eosinophil protein X are elevated in AD and levels of these markers of eosinophil activation correlate with the severity of skin disease. Patients with AD also have increased spontaneous histamine release from basophils. These findings likely reflect a systemic T_H2 immune response in AD. Importantly, the peripheral blood skin homing CLA+ T cells in AD expressing either CD4 or CD8 spontaneously secrete IL-5 and IL-13, which functionally prolong eosinophil survival and induce IgE synthesis.

PATHOLOGY

Clinically unaffected skin of AD patients is not normal but reveals mild epidermal hyperplasia and a sparse perivascular T cell infiltrate.[47] Acute eczematous skin lesions are characterized by marked intercellular edema (spongiosis) of the epidermis. Dendritic APC (e.g., LC, macrophages) in lesional and, to a lesser extent, in nonlesional skin of AD exhibit surface-bound IgE molecules. A sparse epidermal infiltrate consisting primarily of T lymphocytes is also frequently observed. In the dermis of the acute lesion, there is a marked perivenular T cell infiltrate with occasional monocyte-macrophages. The lymphocytic infiltrate consists predominantly of activated memory T cells bearing CD3, CD4, and CD45 RO (suggesting previous encounter with antigen). Eosinophils, basophils, and neutrophils are rarely present in acute AD. Mast cells are found in normal numbers in different stages of degranulation.

Chronic lichenified lesions are characterized by a hyperplastic epidermis with elongation of the rete ridges, prominent hyperkeratosis, and minimal spongiosis. There is an increased number of IgE-bearing LC in the epidermis, and macrophages dominate the dermal mononuclear cell infiltrate. Mast cells are increased in number but are generally fully granulated. Increased numbers of eosinophils are observed in chronic AD skin lesions. These eosinophils undergo cytolysis with release of granule protein contents into the upper dermis of lesional skin. Eosinophil-derived extracellular major basic protein can be detected in a fibrillar pattern associated with the distribution of elastic fibers throughout the upper dermis. Eosinophils are thought to contribute to allergic inflammation by the secretion of cytokines and mediators that augment allergic inflammation and induce tissue injury in AD through the production of reactive oxygen intermediates and release of toxic granule proteins.

DIAGNOSIS AND DIFFERENTIAL DIAGNOSIS

Table 122-1 lists the clinical features of AD. Of the major features, pruritus and chronic or remitting eczematous dermatitis with typical morphology and distribution are essential for diagnosis. Other features, including exogenous allergy or elevated IgE are variable, and some of the "associated features" in the table may not be useful discriminators of individuals with AD from the unaffected general population. Various diagnostic criteria have been proposed to assist with clinical diagnosis, definition of patients for clinical studies, and epidemiologic population studies.[68] A refined list of diagnostic criteria suitable for epidemiologic studies has been derived and validated by workers in the United Kingdom.[69] The sensitivity and specificity of these criteria have varied greatly in studies to date.

Table 122-3 lists a number of inflammatory skin diseases, immunodeficiencies, skin malignancies, genetic disorders, infectious diseases, and infestations that share symptoms and signs with AD. These should be considered and ruled out before a diagnosis of AD is made. Infants presenting in the first year of life with failure to thrive, diarrhea, a generalized scaling erythematous rash, and recurrent cutaneous and/or systemic infections should be evaluated for severe combined immunodeficiency syndrome. Wiskott-Aldrich syndrome is an X-linked recessive disorder characterized by cutaneous findings almost indistinguishable from AD. It is associated with thrombocytopenia, variable abnormalities in humoral and cellular immunity, and recurrent severe bacterial infections. The hyperimmunoglobulin-E syndrome is characterized by markedly elevated serum IgE levels, defective T cell function, recurrent deep-seated bacterial infections, including cutaneous abscesses due to *S. aureus* and/or pruritic skin disease due to *S. aureus* pustulosis, or by recalcitrant dermatophytosis. Although *S. aureus* is an important pathogen in this disorder, infection with other bacteria, viruses, and fungi may occur, particularly when patients are on chronic antistaphylococcal antibiotic prophylaxis. The pruritic dermatitis in this rare syndrome may be difficult to distinguish from AD.

It is important to recognize that an adult who presents with an eczematous dermatitis with no history of childhood eczema, respiratory allergy, or atopic family history may have allergic contact dermatitis (see Chap. 120). A contact allergen should be considered in any patient whose AD does not respond to appropriate therapy. Of note, topical glucocorticoid contact allergy has been reported increasingly in patients with chronic dermatitis on topical corticosteroid therapy. In addition, cutaneous T cell lymphoma must be ruled out in any adult presenting with chronic dermatitis poorly responsive to topical glucocorticoid therapy. Ideally, biopsies should be obtained from three separate sites, because the histology may show spongiosis and cellular infiltrate similar to AD. Eczematous dermatitis has been also reported with HIV as well as with a variety of infestations such as scabies. Other conditions that can be confused with AD include psoriasis, ichthyoses, and seborrheic dermatitis.

TABLE 122-3

Differential Diagnosis of Atopic Dermatitis

Congenital disorders
- Netherton's syndrome
- Familial keratosis pilaris

Chronic dermatoses
- Seborrheic dermatitis
- Contact dermatitis (allergic or irritant)
- Nummular eczema
- Lichen simplex chronicus deficiency
- Psoriasis
- Ichthyoses

Infections and Infestations
- Scabies
- HIV-associated dermatitis
- Dermatophytosis

Malignancies
- Cutaneous T cell lymphoma (Mycosis fungoides/ Sézary syndrome)
- Letterer-Siwe disease

Immunologic disorders
- Dermatitis herpetiformis
- Pemphigus foliaceus
- Graft versus host disease
- Dermatomyositis

Metabolic disorders
- Zinc deficiency
- Pyridoxine (vitamin B_6) and niacin
- Multiple carboxylase deficiency
- Phenylketonuria

Immunodeficiencies
- Wiskott-Aldrich syndrome
- Severe combined immunodeficiency
- Hyper-IgE syndrome

TREATMENT AND PROGNOSIS

Successful treatment of AD requires a systematic, multipronged approach that incorporates skin hydration, pharmacologic therapy, and the identification and elimination of flare factors such as irritants, allergens, infectious agents, and emotional stressors.[70] Many factors lead to the symptom complex characterizing AD. Thus, treatment plans should be individualized to address each patient's skin disease reaction pattern, including the acuity of the rash, and the trigger factors that are unique to the particular patient. In patients refractory to conventional forms of therapy, alternative anti-inflammatory and immunomodulatory agents may be necessary.

Topical Therapy

CUTANEOUS HYDRATION Patients with AD have reduced skin barrier function and dry skin (xerosis) contributing to disease morbidity by the development of microfissures and cracks in the skin, which serve as portals of entry for skin pathogens, irritants, and allergens. This problem can become aggravated during the dry winter months and in certain work environments. Lukewarm soaking baths for at least 20 min followed by the application of an occlusive emollient to retain moisture can give such patients excellent symptomatic relief. Use of an effective emollient combined with hydration therapy will help to restore and preserve the stratum corneum barrier, and may decrease the need for topical glucocorticoids. Moisturizers are available in the form of lotions, creams, or ointments. Lotions and creams may be irritating due to added preservatives, solubilizers, and fragrances. Lotions containing water may be drying due to an evaporative effect. Hydrophilic ointments can be obtained in varying degrees of viscosity according to the patient's preference. Occlusive ointments are sometimes not well tolerated because of interference with the function of the eccrine sweat ducts and the induction of folliculitis. In these patients, less occlusive agents should be used.

Hydration, by baths or wet dressings, promotes transepidermal penetration of topical glucocorticoids. Dressings may also serve as an effective barrier against persistent scratching, allowing more rapid healing of excoriated lesions. Wet dressings are recommended for use on severely affected or chronically involved areas of dermatitis refractory to therapy. However, overuse of wet dressings may result in maceration of the skin complicated by secondary infection. Wet dressings or baths also have the potential to promote drying and fissuring of the skin if not followed by topical emollient use. Thus, wet dressing therapy is reserved for poorly controlled AD and should be closely monitored by a physician.

TOPICAL GLUCOCORTICOID TREATMENT Topical glucocorticoids are the cornerstone of treatment for anti-inflammatory eczematous skin lesions. Because of potential side effects, most physicians use topical glucocorticoids only to control of acute exacerbations of AD. However, recent studies suggest that once control of AD is achieved with a daily regimen of topical glucocorticoid, long-term control can be maintained with twice weekly applications of topical fluticasone to areas that have healed but are prone to developing eczema.[71]

Patients should be carefully instructed in the use of topical glucocorticoids in order to avoid potential side effects. The potent fluorinated glucocorticoids should be avoided on the face, the genitalia, and the intertriginous areas. A low-potency glucocorticoid preparation is generally recommended for these areas. Patients should be instructed to apply topical glucocorticoids to their skin lesions and to use emollients over uninvolved skin. Failure of a patient to respond to topical glucocorticoids is sometimes due in part to an inadequate supply. It is important to remember that it takes approximately 30 g of cream or ointment to cover the entire skin surface of an adult once. To treat the entire body twice daily for 2 weeks requires approximately 840 g (2 lb) of topical glucocorticoids.

There are seven classes of topical glucocorticoids, ranked according to their potency based on vasoconstrictor assays (see Chap. 243). Because of their potential side effects, the ultrahigh-potency glucocorticoids should be used only for very short periods of time and in areas that are lichenified but not on the face or intertriginous areas. The goal is to use emollients to enhance skin hydration and low-potency glucocorticoids for maintenance therapy. Midpotency glucocorticoids can be used for longer periods of time to treat chronic AD involving the trunk and extremities. Glucocorticoids in gels are usually in a propylene glycol base and are irritating to the skin in addition to promoting dryness, thus limiting their use to the scalp and beard areas.

Side effects from topical glucocorticoids are directly related to the potency ranking of the compound and the length of use, so it is incumbent on the clinician to balance the need for a more potent steroid with the potential for side effects. In addition, ointments have a greater potential to occlude the epidermis, resulting in enhanced systemic absorption when compared to creams. Side effects from topical glucocorticoids can be divided into local side effects and systemic side effects resulting from suppression of the hypothalamic-pituitary-adrenal axis. Local side effects include the development of striae and skin atrophy. Systemic side effects are related to the potency of the topical glucocorticoid, the site of application, the occlusiveness of the preparation, the percentage of the body surface area covered, and the length of use. The potential for potent topical glucocorticoid to cause adrenal suppression is greatest in infants and young children.

TOPICAL IMMUNOMODULATORS

Tacrolimus Topically applied FK-506 or tacrolimus, a calcineurin inhibitor that acts by binding to FK binding protein, has been successfully used in the treatment of AD (see Chap. 250). Tacrolimus inhibits the activation of a number of key cells involved in AD including T cells, Langerhans cells, mast cells, and keratinocytes. Atopic Dermatitis patients receiving this form of therapy can have markedly diminished pruritus within 3 days of initiating therapy. Skin biopsy results after treatment demonstrate markedly diminished T cell and eosinophilic infiltrates as well as decreased FcεRI expression on both Langerhans cells and inflammatory dendritic epidermal cells. Multicenter, blinded, vehicle-controlled phase 3 trials with tacrolimus ointment, 0.03% and 0.1%, in both adults and children with AD have shown tacrolimus to be both safe and effective.[72,73] A local burning sensation has been the only common adverse event. In adults, but not children, a dose-response effect was seen between 0.03% and 0.1% tacrolimus, particularly for patients with severe skin disease. Long-term open-label studies with tacrolimus ointment applied on up to 100 percent of body surface area have been performed for up to 12 months in adults and children with demonstrated sustained efficacy and no significant side effects; for example, no increased skin infections have been observed. Indeed, *S. aureus* colonization decreases during long-term therapy with tacrolimus ointment.[41] In addition, unlike topical corticosteroids, tacrolimus ointment does not cause cutaneous atrophy and has been used safely for facial and eyelid eczema. Tacrolimus ointment (Protopic) 0.03% is approved by the FDA for short-term and intermittent long-term use in moderate to severe AD for children 2 to 15 years of age; and 0.03%, as well as 0.1%, has been approved for adults.

Pimecrolimus Ascomycin compounds, which act by binding to macrophilin 12 to interfere with calcineurin action, have been developed in topical and oral forms that appear to have preferential drug distribution to the skin (see Chap. 250). Like tacrolimus, they inhibit T_H1 and T_H2 cytokine production and also inhibit mediator release from mast cells and basophils. Topical pimecrolimus (Elidel) 1% cream applied twice daily in a randomized, double-blind, placebo-controlled, right-and-left comparison trial in adult patients with moderate AD was significantly more effective than either a vehicle cream or once daily treatment over a 21-day period.[74] No significant drug-related adverse effects were noted.[75] In a vehicle- and betamethasone-17-valerate 0.1% cream-controlled dose-finding study of 260 adults with AD, pimecrolimus 1.0% cream was found to be the most effective concentration. Of note, the 0.1% betamethasone-17-valerate was more effective than the pimecrolimus creams tested in this study. However, the authors suggested that the efficacy plateau was not reached with the pimecrolimus creams during the 3 weeks of treatment. Further therapeutic trials are in progress with this new drug.

Identification and Elimination of Triggering Factors

GENERAL CONSIDERATIONS Patients with AD are more susceptible to irritants than are normal individuals. Thus, it is important to identify and eliminate aggravating factors that trigger the itch-scratch cycle. These include soaps or detergents, contact with chemicals, smoke, abrasive clothing, and exposure to extremes of temperature and humidity. Alcohol and astringents found in toiletries are drying. When soaps are used, they should have minimal defatting activity and a neutral pH. New clothing should be laundered prior to wearing to decrease levels of formaldehyde and other added chemicals. Residual laundry detergent in clothing may be irritating. Using a liquid rather than powder detergent and adding a second rinse cycle will facilitate removal of the detergent.

Recommendations regarding environmental living conditions should include temperature and humidity control to avoid problems related to heat, humidity, and perspiration. Every attempt should be made to allow children to be as normally active as possible. Certain sports such as swimming may be better tolerated than other sports involving intense perspiration, physical contact, or heavy clothing and equipment, but chlorine should be rinsed off immediately after swimming and the skin lubricated. While ultraviolet light may be beneficial to some patients with AD, sunscreens should be used to avoid sunburn. However, because sunscreens can be irritants, care should be used to identify a nonirritating product.

SPECIFIC ALLERGENS Foods and aeroallergens such as dust mites, animal danders, molds, and pollens have been demonstrated to exacerbate AD. Potential allergens can be identified by taking a careful history and carrying out selective skin prick tests. Negative skin tests or serum tests for allergen-specific IgE have a high predictive value for ruling out suspected allergens. A normal total serum IgE level, however, does not rule out the possibility of allergen-specific IgE being present. Positive skin or in vitro tests, particularly to foods, often do not correlate with clinical symptoms and should be confirmed with controlled food challenges and elimination diets. Avoidance of foods implicated in controlled challenges results in clinical improvement.[14,17] Extensive elimination diets, which in some cases can be nutritionally deficient, are rarely, if ever, required, because even with multiple positive skin tests, the majority of patients will react to three or fewer foods on controlled challenge. In dust mite–allergic patients with AD, prolonged avoidance of dust mites has been found to result in improvement of their skin disease. Avoidance measures include use of dust mite proof encasings on pillows, mattresses, and box springs; washing bedding in hot water weekly; removal of bedroom carpeting; and decreasing indoor humidity levels with air conditioning. Because there are many triggers contributing to the flares of AD, attention should be focused on identifying and controlling the flare factors that are important to the individual patient. Infants and young children are more likely to have food allergies, whereas older children and adults are more likely to be sensitive to environmental aeroallergens.

EMOTIONAL STRESSORS Although emotional stress does not cause AD, it often exacerbates the illness. AD patients often respond to frustration, embarrassment, or other stressful events with increased pruritus and scratching. In some instances, scratching is simply habitual and less commonly associated with significant secondary gain. Psychological evaluation or counseling should be considered in patients who have difficulty with emotional triggers or psychological problems, contributing to difficulty in managing their disease. It may be especially useful in adolescents and young adults who consider their skin disease disfiguring. Relaxation, behavioral modification, or biofeedback may be helpful in patients with habitual scratching.

INFECTIOUS AGENTS Antistaphylococcal antibiotics are very helpful in the treatment of patients who are heavily colonized or infected with *S. aureus*. Erythromycin and the newer macrolide antibiotics (azithromycin and clarithromycin) are usually beneficial for patients who are not colonized with a resistant *S. aureus* strain. However, for macrolide-resistant *S. aureus,* a penicillinase-resistant penicillin (dicloxacillin, oxacillin, or cloxacillin) may be preferred. First-generation cephalosporins also offer effective coverage for both staphylococci and streptococci. Topical mupirocin offers some utility in the treatment of impetiginized lesions; however, in patients with extensive superinfection, a course of systemic antibiotics is most practical.

Herpes simplex can provoke recurrent dermatitis and may be misdiagnosed as *S. aureus* infection. The presence of punched-out erosions, vesicles, and/or infected skin lesions that fail to respond to oral antibiotics should initiate a search for herpes simplex. This can be diagnosed by a Giemsa-stained Tzanck smear of cells scraped from the vesicle base or by viral culture. For infection suspected to be caused by herpes simplex, topical glucocorticoids are best discontinued, at least temporarily. Antiviral treatment for cutaneous herpes simplex infections is of critical importance in the patient with widespread AD because life-threatening dissemination has been reported. Acyclovir, 400 mg three times daily for 10 days or 200 mg four times daily for 10 days by oral administration (or an equivalent dosage of one of the newer antiherpetic medications), is useful in adults with herpes simplex confined to the skin. Intravenous treatment may be necessary for severe disseminated eczema herpeticum. The dosage should be adjusted according to weight in children.

Dermatophyte infections can complicate AD and may contribute to exacerbation of disease activity. Patients with dermatophyte infection or IgE antibodies to *P. ovale* may benefit from a trial of topical or systemic antifungal therapy.

Pruritus

The treatment of pruritus in AD should be directed primarily at the underlying causes. Reduction of skin inflammation and dryness with topical glucocorticoids and skin hydration, respectively, will often symptomatically reduce pruritus. Inhaled and ingested allergens should be eliminated if documented to cause skin rash in controlled challenges. Systemic antihistamines act primarily by blocking the H_1 receptors in the dermis, thereby ameliorating histamine-induced pruritus. However, histamine is only one of many mediators that can induce pruritus of the skin. Therefore, certain patients may derive minimal benefit from antihistaminic therapy. Some antihistamines are also mild anxiolytics and may offer symptomatic relief through tranquilizing and sedative effects. Studies of newer nonsedating antihistamines show variable results in the effectiveness of controlling pruritus in AD, although they may be useful in the small subset of AD patients with concomitant urticaria.

Because pruritus is usually worse at night, the sedating antihistamines, for example, hydroxyzine or diphenhydramine, may offer an advantage with their soporific side effects when used at bedtime. Doxepin hydrochloride has both tricyclic antidepressant and H_1- and H_2-histamine receptor-blocking effects. It can be used in doses of 10 to 75 mg orally at night or up to 75 mg bid in adult patients. If nocturnal pruritus remains severe, short-term use of a sedative to allow adequate rest may be appropriate. Treatment of AD with topical antihistamines is generally not recommended because of potential cutaneous sensitization. However, short-term (1 week) application of topical 5% doxepin cream has been reported to reduce pruritus without sensitization. Of note, sedation is a side effect of widespread application of doxepin cream.

Tar Preparations

Coal tar preparations may have antipruritic and anti-inflammatory effects on the skin. The anti-inflammatory properties of tars, however, are not well characterized and are usually not as pronounced as those of topical glucocorticoids. Tar preparations may be useful in reducing the potency of topical glucocorticoids required in chronic maintenance therapy of AD. Newer coal tar products have been developed that are more acceptable with respect to odor and staining of clothes than some older products. Tar shampoos can be beneficial for scalp dermatitis and are often helpful in reducing the concentration and frequency of topical glucocorticoid applications. Tar preparations should not be used on acutely inflamed skin, because this often results in skin irritation. Side effects associated with tars include folliculitis and photosensitivity. There is a theoretical risk of tar being a carcinogen based on observational studies of workers using tar components in their occupations.

Phototherapy

Natural sunlight is frequently beneficial to patients with AD. However, if the sunlight occurs in the setting of high heat or humidity, thereby triggering sweating and pruritus, it may be deleterious to patients. Broad-band ultraviolet B, broad-band ultraviolet A, narrow-band ultraviolet B (311 nm), UVA-1 (340 to 400 nm), and combined UVAB phototherapy can be useful adjuncts in the treatment of AD. Investigation of the photoimmunologic mechanisms responsible for therapeutic effectiveness indicates that epidermal Langerhans cells and eosinophils may be targets of ultraviolet A phototherapy with and without psoralen, while UVB exerts immunosuppressive effects via blocking of function of antigen-presenting Langerhans cells and altered keratinocyte cytokine production. Photochemotherapy with PUVA may be indicated in patients with severe, widespread AD, although studies comparing it with other modes of phototherapy are limited. Short-term adverse effects with phototherapy may include erythema, skin pain, pruritus, and pigmentation. Long-term adverse effects include premature skin aging and cutaneous malignancies (see Chaps. 265 and 266 for detailed discussion of phototherapy and photochemotherapy).

Hospitalization

AD patients who appear erythrodermic or who have widespread severe skin disease resistant to outpatient therapy should be hospitalized before considering systemic alternative therapies (see below). In many cases, removing the patient from environmental allergens or emotional stresses, intense patient education, and assurance of compliance with therapy result in a sustained improvement in their AD. Clearing of the patient's skin during hospitalization also allows the patient to undergo allergen skin testing and appropriately controlled provocative challenges to correctly identify potential allergens.

Phosphodiesterase Inhibitors

Leukocytes from patients with AD have increased CAMP-PDE enzyme activity. This abnormality is most pronounced in atopic monocytes, which have a unique, highly active PDE isoenzyme. Monocytes from AD patients produce elevated levels of PGE_2 and IL-10, which both inhibit IFN-γ production by T cells. Clinical studies using topical application of high-potency PDE inhibitors have demonstrated clinical benefit in AD.[57]

Systemic Therapy

SYSTEMIC GLUCOCORTICOIDS The use of systemic glucocorticoids, such as oral prednisone, is rarely indicated in the treatment of chronic AD. Some patients and physicians prefer the use of systemic glucocorticoids to avoid the time-consuming skin care involving hydration and topical therapy. However, the dramatic clinical improvement that may occur with systemic glucocorticoids is frequently associated with a severe rebound flare of AD following the discontinuation of systemic glucocorticoids. Short courses of oral glucocorticoids may be appropriate for an acute exacerbation of AD while other treatment measures are being instituted. If a short course of oral glucocorticoids is given, it is important to taper the dosage and to begin intensified skin care, particularly with topical glucocorticoids and frequent bathing followed by application of emollients, in order to prevent rebound flaring of AD.

ALLERGEN IMMUNOTHERAPY Unlike allergic rhinitis and extrinsic asthma, immunotherapy with aeroallergens is not proven to be efficacious in the treatment of AD. There are anecdotal reports of both disease exacerbation and improvement. Well-controlled studies are still required to determine the role for immunotherapy with this disease, and this form of treatment for AD should be reserved for individuals who have a clear-cut demonstrable history of aeroallergen-induced AD such as seasonal exacerbations to pollen.

INTERFERONS IFN-γ is known to suppress IgE responses and downregulate T_H2 cell proliferation and function. Several studies of patients with AD, including a multicenter, double-blind, placebo-controlled trial, have demonstrated that treatment with recombinant IFN-γ results in clinical improvement. Reduction in clinical severity of AD correlated with the ability of IFN-γ to decrease total circulating eosinophil counts. Influenza-like symptoms arc commonly observed side effects early in the treatment course.

Recombinant IFN-α has also been used to treat patients with AD in several small, uncontrolled trials. Although a few reports suggest some clinical benefit using this immunomodulator, other studies have not confirmed this finding; however, a significant decrease in circulating eosinophils was noted. A single study of two patients with AD suggests improvement in their AD when recombinant IFN-γ and IFN-α were used sequentially. Further controlled studies are required before any firm conclusion can be made regarding the role of interferon therapy in AD.

CYCLOSPORINE Cyclosporine is a potent immunosuppressive drug that acts primarily on T cells by suppressing cytokine transcription. The drug binds to cyclophilin, an intracellular protein, and this complex, in turn, inhibits calcineurin, a molecule required for initiation of cytokine gene transcription. Multiple studies demonstrate that both children and adults with severe AD, refractory to conventional treatment, can benefit from short-term cyclosporine treatment. Various oral-dosing regimens have been recommended: 5 mg/kg has generally been used with success in short-term and long-term (1 year) use, while some authorities advocate body-weight–independent daily dosing of adults with 150 mg (low dose) or 300 mg (high dose) daily of cyclosporine microemulsion. Treatment with cyclosporine is associated with reduced skin disease and an improved quality of life (see Chap. 262 for further discussion). However, discontinuation of treatment generally results in rapid relapse of skin disease. Elevated serum creatinine or more significant renal impairment and hypertension are specific side effects of concern with cyclosporine use.

ANTIMETABOLITES Mycophenolate mofetil (MMF) is a purine biosynthesis inhibitor used as an immunosuppressant in organ transplantation, that has been used for treatment of refractory inflammatory skin disorders (see Chap. 262). Open-label studies report that short-term oral MMF 2 g daily as monotherapy results in clearing of skin lesions in adults with AD resistant to other treatment including topical and oral steroids and PUVA. The drug has generally been well tolerated with the exception of one patient developing herpes retinitis that may have been secondary to this immunosuppressive agent. Dose-related bone marrow suppression has also been observed. Similar results were previously reported in another open study of 10 patients with a mean reduction in the SCORAD index of 68 percent in all 10 patients. Of note, not all patients benefit from treatment. Therefore the medication should be discontinued if patients do not respond within 4 to 8 weeks. Dose finding and well-controlled studies are needed for this drug.

Methotrexate is an antimetabolite with potent inhibitory effects on inflammatory cytokine synthesis and cell chemotaxis. Methotrexate has been used for AD patients with recalcitrant disease, although controlled trials are lacking. Dosing is more frequent than the weekly dosing used for psoriasis. Azathioprine is a purine analogue with anti-inflammatory and antiproliferative effects; azathioprine has been used for severe AD, although no controlled trials have been reported. Myelosuppression is a significant adverse effect, and thiopurinemethyl transferase levels may predict individuals at risk.

EXTRACORPOREAL PHOTOPHERESIS This treatment consists of the passage of psoralen-treated leukocytes through an extracorporeal UVA light system. Clinical improvement in skin lesions associated with reduced IgE levels has been reported in a few patients with severe, resistant AD who were treated with extracorporeal photopheresis and topical glucocorticoids.

Other Therapies

Disturbances in the metabolism of essential fatty acids (EFA), involved in the generation of inflammatory mediators, has been suggested in patients with AD. Consequently, clinical trials have been conducted with either fish oil as a source of Ω-3 series EFA, or oil extracted from the seeds of *Oenothera biennis,* evening primrose, as a source of Ω-6 series EFA. Conflicting results were reported in earlier studies; however, recent better-controlled studies failed to demonstrate clinical benefit with either primrose oil or fish oil.

Several placebo-controlled clinical trials have suggested that patients with severe AD benefit from treatment with traditional Chinese herbal therapy. They had significantly reduced skin disease and decreased pruritus. The beneficial response of Chinese herbal therapy, however, is often temporary, and effectiveness may wear off despite continued treatment. The possibility of hepatic toxicity, cardiac side effects, or idiosyncratic reactions remains a concern. The specific ingredients of the herbs also remain to be elucidated and some preparations have been found to be contaminated with corticosteroids. At present, Chinese herbal therapy for AD is considered investigational.

There are many different alternative therapies that could be efficacious in AD, but it is not possible to review them all. However, it is clear that AD is an illness associated with a multitude of immunoregulatory abnormalities. Future directions in therapy are likely to focus on a number of different immunologic targets in this illness.

Prognosis

The natural history of AD is not completely known because studies have been flawed in terms of inadequate sample size, an unclear definition of remission, inadequate length of follow-up, selection bias in the initial cohort, and excessive loss of patients to follow-up. Nevertheless, although the outcome of AD may be difficult to predict in any given individual, the disease generally tends to be more severe and persistent in young children. Periods of remission appear more frequently as the patient grows older. Spontaneous resolution of AD has been reported to occur after age 5 years in 40 to 60 percent of patients affected during infancy, particularly if their disease is mild. While earlier studies suggested that approximately 84 percent of children outgrow their AD by adolescence, more recent studies have reported that AD disappears in approximately 20 percent of children followed from infancy until adolescence, but becomes less severe in 65 percent. In addition, more than half of adolescents treated for mild dermatitis may experience a relapse of disease as adults.

Importantly for occupational counseling, adults whose childhood AD has been in remission for a number of years may present with hand dermatitis, especially if daily activities require repeated hand wetting. The following predictive factors correlate with a poor prognosis for AD: widespread AD in childhood; associated allergic rhinitis and asthma; family history of AD in parents or siblings; early age at onset of AD; being an only child; and very high serum IgE levels (Table 122-2).

REFERENCES

1. Willan R: *On Cutaneous Diseases,* Johnson, London, 1808
2. Coca AF et al: On the classification of the phenomena of hypersensitiveness. *J Immunol* **8**:163, 1923
3. Hill LW et al: Evolution of atopic dermatitis. *Arch Dermatol* **32**:451, 1935
4. Schultz-Larsen F, Hanifin JM: Epidemiology of atopic dermatitis. *Immunol Allergy Clin North Am* **22**:1, 2002
5. Williams H et al: Worldwide variations in the prevalence of symptoms of atopic eczema in the International Study of Asthma and Allergies in Childhood. *J Allergy Clin Immunol* **103**:125, 1999
6. von Mutius E: The environmental predictors of allergic disease. *J Allergy Clin Immunol* **105**:9, 2000
7. Strachan DP: Hay fever, hygiene, and household size. *BMJ* **299**:1259, 1989
8. Romagnani S: The role of lymphocytes in allergic disease. *J Allergy Clin Immunol* **105**:399, 2000
9. Saurat JH: Eczema in primary immune-deficiencies. Clues to the pathogenesis of atopic dermatitis with special reference to the Wiskott-Aldrich syndrome. *Acta Derm Venereol Suppl* **114**:125, 1985
10. Leung DYM: Atopic dermatitis: New insights and opportunities for therapeutic intervention. *J Allergy Clin Immunol* **105**:860, 2000
11. Beck LA, Leung DYM: Allergen sensitization through the skin induces systemic allergic responses. *J Allergy Clin Immunol* **106**:S258, 2000
12. Spergel JM et al: Epicutaneous sensitization with protein antigen induces localized allergic dermatitis and hyperresponsiveness to methacholine after single exposure to aerosolized antigen in mice. *J Clin Invest* **101**:1614, 1998
13. Bratton DL et al: Granulocyte macrophage colony-stimulating factor contributes to enhanced monocyte survival in chronic atopic dermatitis. *J Clin Invest* **95**:211, 1995
14. Sampson HA: Food allergy. Part 1: Immunopathogenesis and clinical disorders. *J Allergy Clin Immunol* **103**:717, 1999
15. Eigenmann PA et al: Prevalence of IgE-mediated food allergy among children with atopic dermatitis. *Pediatrics* **101**:E8, 1998
16. Guillet G, Guillet MH: Natural history of sensitizations in atopic dermatitis. A 3-year follow-up in 250 children: Food allergy and high risk of respiratory symptoms. *Arch Dermatol* **128**:187, 1992
17. Lever R et al: Randomised controlled trial of advice on an egg exclusion diet in young children with atopic eczema and sensitivity to eggs. *Pediatr Allergy Immunol* **9**:13, 1998
18. Li XM et al: Murine model of atopic dermatitis associated with food hypersensitivity. *J Allergy Clin Immunol* **107**:693, 2001
19. van Reijsen FC et al: T-cell reactivity for a peanut-derived epitope in the skin of a young infant with atopic dermatitis. *J Allergy Clin Immunol* **101**:207, 1998
20. Abernathy-Carver KJ et al: Milk-induced eczema is associated with the expansion of T cells expressing cutaneous lymphocyte antigen. *J Clin Invest* **95**:913, 1995
21. Walker IC: Causation of eczema, urticaria, and angioneurotic edema by proteins other than those derived from foods. *JAMA* **70**:897, 1918
22. Tupker RA et al: Induction of atopic dermatitis by inhalation of house dust mite. *J Allergy Clin Immunol* **97**:1064, 1996
23. Wheatley LM, Platts-Mills TAE: Role of inhalant allergens in atopic dermatitis, in *Allergic Skin Disease: A Multidisciplinary Approach,* edited by DYM Leung, MW Greaves. New York, Marcel Dekker, 2000, p 423
24. Tan BB et al: Double-blind controlled trial of effect of house dust-mite allergen avoidance on atopic dermatitis. *Lancet* **347**:15, 1996
25. Scalabrin DM et al: Use of specific IgE in assessing the relevance of fungal and dust mite allergens to atopic dermatitis: A comparison with asthmatic and nonasthmatic control subjects. *J Allergy Clin Immunol* **104**:1273, 1999
26. Schafer T et al: Association between severity of atopic eczema and degree of sensitization to aeroallergens in schoolchildren. *J Allergy Clin Immunol* **104**:1280, 1999
27. Leyden JJ, Kligman AM: The case for steroid–antibiotic combinations. *Br J Dermatol* **96**:179, 1977
28. Leung DYM et al: Presence of IgE antibodies to staphylococcal exotoxins on the skin of patients with atopic dermatitis. Evidence for a new group of allergens. *J Clin Invest* **92**:1374, 1993
29. Breuer K et al: Severe atopic dermatitis is associated with sensitization to staphylococcal enterotoxin B (SEB). *Allergy* **55**:551, 2000
30. Bunikowski R et al: Evidence for a disease-promoting effect of *Staphylococcus aureus*-derived exotoxins in atopic dermatitis. *J Allergy Clin Immunol* **105**:814, 2000
31. Strickland I et al: Evidence for superantigen involvement in skin homing of T cells in atopic dermatitis. *J Invest Dermatol* **112**:249, 1999
32. Herz U et al: A human-SCID mouse model for allergic immune response bacterial superantigen enhances skin inflammation and suppresses IgE production. *J Invest Dermatol* **110**:224, 1998
33. Hofer MF et al: Staphylococcal toxins augment specific IgE responses by atopic patients exposed to allergen. *J Invest Dermatol* **112**:171, 1999
34. Hauk PJ et al: Induction of corticosteroid insensitivity in human PBMCs by microbial super antigens. *J Allergy Clin Immunol* **105**:782, 2000
35. Strange P et al: Staphylococcal enterotoxin B applied on intact normal and intact atopic skin induces dermatitis. *Arch Dermatol* **132**:27, 1996
36. Skov L et al: Application of staphylococcal enterotoxin B on normal and atopic skin induces up-regulation of T cells by a superantigen-mediated mechanism. *J Allergy Clin Immunol* **105**:820, 2000
37. Michie CA, Davis T: Atopic dermatitis and staphylococcal superantigens. *Lancet* **347**:324, 1996
38. Leung DYM et al: Bacterial superantigens induce T cell expression of the skin-selective homing receptor, the cutaneous lymphocyte-associated antigen, via stimulation of interleukin 12 production. *J Exp Med* **181**:747, 1995
39. Ezepchuk YV et al: Staphylococcal toxins and protein A differentially induce cytotoxicity and release of tumor necrosis factor-alpha from human keratinocytes. *J Invest Dermatol* **107**:603, 1996
40. Nilsson EJ et al: Topical corticosteroids and *Staphylococcus aureus* in atopic dermatitis. *J Am Acad Dermatol* **27**:29, 1992
41. Remitz A et al: Tacrolimus ointment reduces staphylococcal colonization of atopic dermatitis lesions. *J Allergy Clin Immunol* **107**:196, 2001
42. Cho SH et al: Preferential binding of *Staphylococcus aureus* to skin sites of T_H2-mediated inflammation in a murine model. *J Invest Dermatol* **116**:658, 2001
43. Cho SH et al: Fibronectin and fibrinogen contribute to the enhanced binding of *Staphylococcus aureus* to atopic skin. *J Allergy Clin Immunol* **108**:269, 2001
44. Keller P: Beitrag zu den beziehungen von asthma und ekzem. *Arch Derm Syph Berl* **148**:82, 1924
45. Valenta R et al: Autoallergy: A pathogenetic factor in atopic dermatitis? *J Allergy Clin Immunol* **105**:432, 2000
46. Valenta R et al: Molecular characterization of an autoallergen, *Hom s* 1, identified by serum IgE from atopic dermatitis patients. *J Invest Dermatol* **111**:1178, 1998
47. Hamid Q et al: Differential in situ cytokine gene expression in acute versus chronic atopic dermatitis. *J Clin Invest* **94**:870, 1994
48. Hamid Q et al: In vivo expression of IL-12 and IL-13 in atopic dermatitis. *J Allergy Clin Immunol* **98**:225, 1996
49. Grewe M et al: A role for T_H1 and T_H2 cells in the immunopathogenesis of atopic dermatitis. *Immunol Today* **19**:359, 1998

50. Trautmann A et al: T cell-mediated Fas-induced keratinocyte apoptosis plays a key pathogenetic role in eczematous dermatitis. *J Clin Invest* **106**:25, 2000
51. Laberge S et al: Association of increased CD4+ T-cell infiltration with increased IL-16 gene expression in atopic dermatitis. *J Allergy Clin Immunol* **102**:645, 1998
52. Taha RA et al: Evidence for increased expression of eotaxin and monocyte chemotactic protein-4 in atopic dermatitis. *J Allergy Clin Immunol* **105**:1002, 2000
53. Yawalkar N et al: Enhanced expression of eotaxin and CCR3 in atopic dermatitis. *J Invest Dermatol* **113**:43, 1999
54. Morales J et al: CTACK, a skin-associated chemokine that preferentially attracts skin-homing memory T cells. *Proc Natl Acad Sci U S A* **96**:14470, 1999
55. Galli G et al: Macrophage-derived chemokine production by activated human T cells in vitro and in vivo: Preferential association with the production of type 2 cytokines. *Eur J Immunol* **30**:204, 2000
56. Giustizieri ML et al: Keratinocytes from patients with atopic dermatitis and psoriasis show a distinct chemokine production profile in response to T cell-derived cytokines. *J Allergy Clin Immunol* **107**:871, 2001
57. Hanifin JM et al: Type 4 phosphodiesterase inhibitors have clinical and in vitro anti-inflammatory effects in atopic dermatitis. *J Invest Dermatol* **107**:51, 1996
58. Santamaria LF et al: Rolipram inhibits staphylococcal enterotoxin B-mediated induction of the human skin-homing receptor on T lymphocytes. *J Invest Dermatol* **113**:82, 1999
59. Kuchroo VK et al: B7-1 and B7-2 costimulatory molecules activate differentially the T_H1/T_H2 developmental pathways: Application to autoimmune disease therapy. *Cell* **80**:707, 1995
60. Jirapongsananuruk O et al: Enhanced expression of B7.2 (CD86) in patients with atopic dermatitis: A potential role in the modulation of IgE synthesis. *J Immunol* **160**:4622, 1998
61. Ohki O et al: Functional CD86 (B7-2/B70) is predominantly expressed on Langerhans cells in atopic dermatitis. *Br J Dermatol* **136**:838, 1997
62. Von Bubnoff D et al: Antigen-presenting cells in allergy. *J Allergy Clin Immunol* **108**:329–339, 2001
63. Imokawa G: Lipid abnormalities in atopic dermatitis. *J Am Acad Dermatol* **45**:S29, 2001
64. Herrick CA et al: T_H2 responses induced by epicutaneous or inhalational protein exposure are differentially dependent on IL-4. *J Clin Invest* **105**:765, 2000
65. Forrest S et al: Identifying genes predisposing to atopic eczema. *J Allergy Clin Immunol* **104**:1066, 1999
66. Lee YA et al: A major susceptibility locus for atopic dermatitis maps to chromosome 3q21. *Nat Genet* **26**:470, 2000
67. Cookson WO et al: Genetic linkage of childhood atopic dermatitis to psoriasis susceptibility loci. *Nat Genet* **27**:372, 2001
68. Williams HC: Diagnostic criteria for atopic dermatitis: Where do we go from here? *Arch Dermatol* **135**:583, 1999
69. Williams HC et al: The U.K. Working Party's Diagnostic Criteria for Atopic Dermatitis. I. Derivation of a minimum set of discriminators for atopic dermatitis. *Br J Dermatol* **131**:383, 1994
70. Hoare C et al: Systematic review of treatments for atopic dermatitis. *Health Technol Assess* **4**:1, 2000
71. Van Der Meer JB et al: The management of moderate to severe atopic dermatitis in adults with topical fluticasone propionate. The Netherlands Adult Atopic Dermatitis Study Group. *Br J Dermatol* **140**:1114, 1999
72. Hanifin JM et al: Tacrolimus ointment for the treatment of atopic dermatitis in adult patients: part I, efficacy. *J Am Acad Dermatol* **44**:S28, 2001
73. Paller A et al: A 12-week study of tacrolimus ointment for the treatment of atopic dermatitis in pediatric patients. *J Am Acad Dermatol* **44**:S47, 2001
74. Van Leent EJ et al: Effectiveness of the ascomycin macrolactam SDZ ASM 981 in the topical treatment of atopic dermatitis. *Arch Dermatol* **134**:805, 1998
75. Luger T et al: SDZ ASM 981: An emerging safe and effective treatment for atopic dermatitis. *Br J Dermatol* **144**:788, 2001

CHAPTER 123

Nicholas A. Soter

Nummular Eczema and Lichen Simplex Chronicus/Prurigo Nodularis

NUMMULAR ECZEMA

Nummular eczema, which is also known as *discoid eczema,* is defined by its clinical appearance as coin-shaped, circular, or oval lesions with a definite border.

Historical Aspects

In 1845, Rayer described a condition with patches of vesicles and an illustration that resembled nummular eczema. Nummular eczema as a term was introduced by Devergie in 1857.

Epidemiology

Nummular eczema in adults occurs more frequently in men than in women. The peak age of onset in both sexes is between 55 and 65 years; in women, another peak is observed at 15 to 25 years. Nummular eczema is uncommon in children, rarely appears before one year of age, and its frequency tends to increase with age.[1]

Etiology and Pathogenesis

Although the cause is unknown, many factors, acting alone or in combination, have been proposed as etiologic agents. Staphylococci and micrococci have been incriminated both as a direct cause and through the mechanism of hypersensitivity; however, their pathogenic role remains unresolved.[2] Immediate skin test reactions have been elicited by intradermal injections of antigens prepared from *Staphylococcus aureus* and micrococci. Subjects aged 60 to 85 years showed more delayed-type contact sensitivity reactions as assessed by patch tests to *Candida albicans, Dermatophagoides farinae,* and house dust than did age-matched control subjects.[3] In other individuals, positive patch tests to rubber chemicals, formaldehyde, neomycin, chrome, and nickel have been thought to have clinical relevance.[4] Nummular eczema in adults is unrelated to the atopic disorders. In children, however, nummular lesions occur in atopic dermatitis.

There is a frequent association with dry skin, and the incidence of nummular eczema reaches a peak during the winter months. Patients with nummular eczema showed a low hydration state of the stratum corneum as assessed by high-frequency electrical conductors.[3] Of patients whose condition became worse in the summer months, men predominated with exacerbations after exertion in hot, humid situations.[5] Substances implicated with exacerbations include wool, soaps, water during frequent bathing, and topically applied medicaments. An association with emotional stress and with the ingestion of alcoholic beverages has been suggested.

Systemically administered drugs, notably gold, methyldopa, streptomycin, aminosalicylic acid, isoniazid, and isotretinoin,[6] as well as mercury in dental amalgam,[7] have been implicated in nummular eczema, but a direct association often is difficult to prove.

In cutaneous sensory nerves, increased amounts of substance P (SP), vasoactive intestinal polypeptide (VIP), and calcitonin gene–related peptide (CGRP) are present in the dermal fibers. Increased amounts of SP and CGRP are present in epidermal fibers.[8] These observations implicate neuropeptides as a potential mechanism for mast cell degranulation.

Clinical Manifestations

The acute eruption appears as vesicles and papules that may enlarge by becoming confluent or by peripheral extension to form the characteristic, discrete, erythematous, coin-shaped areas (Fig. 123-1). Lesions that are more than 10 cm in diameter are seldom seen. Subsequently, there may be central clearing, which leads to morphologic configurations that resemble superficial fungal infections. Edema and exudation with crusts occur in acute lesions, whereas scale and lichenification are present in chronic lesions. Excoriations may be a prominent feature. Pruritus and occasionally burning occur in the lesional sites. The eruption occurs on the legs, the upper extremities including the dorsal surfaces of the hands, and the trunk; the lower extremities are the most commonly affected areas. The eruption may begin as a single lesion or several lesions that appear in episodes; individual lesions may persist for prolonged periods and commonly recur at previously affected sites.

Laboratory Findings

If the history does not suggest an underlying cause for pruritus, no laboratory tests should be obtained. Scale may be examined for fungi. Patch tests at times may be of value. Serum IgE levels are normal.[9]

FIGURE 123-1

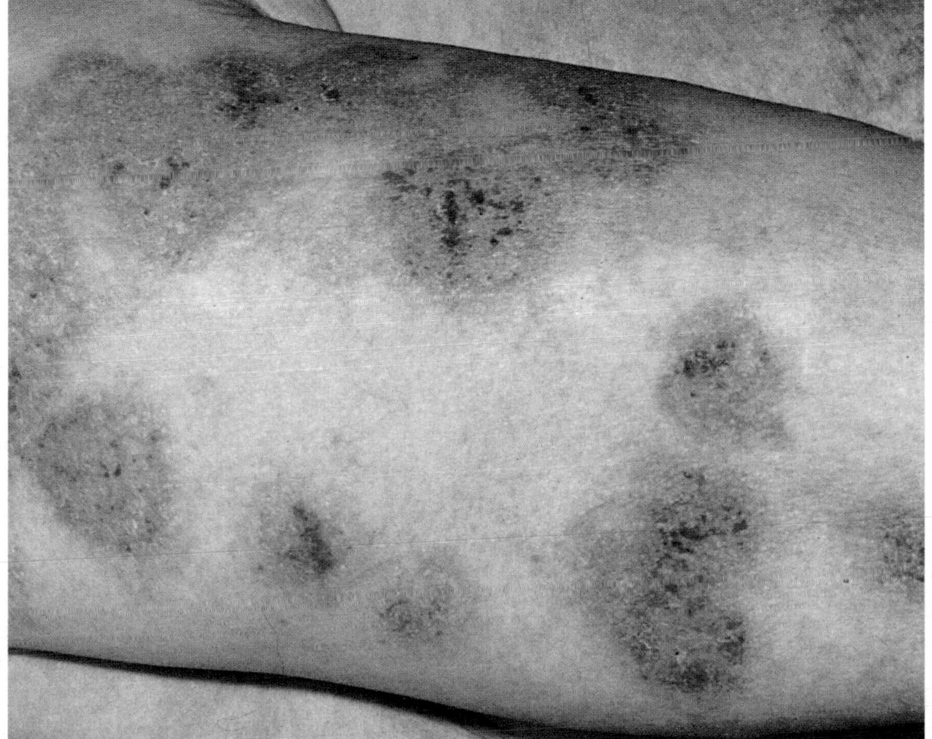

Nummular eczema. Coin-shaped plaques composed of papules and vesicles on an erythematous base with some excoriations also present.

Pathology

The histopathologic alterations (Fig. 123-2) reflect the stage of evolution of the clinical lesion at the time of biopsy. In acute lesions, epidermal intercellular edema with vesicles of various sizes is associated with a dermal, perivenular infiltrate of lymphocytes and macrophages. In chronic lesions, hyperplasia of the epidermis with retention of the rete ridge pattern, hyperkeratosis, and an increase in the granular-cell layer are present. Minimal amounts of epidermal intercellular edema (spongiosis) may occur. Fibrosis of the papillary dermis may be present with lymphocytes and macrophages disposed about venules. The majority of the lymphocytes in the epidermis are CD8+ T lymphocytes. In the dermis, the lymphocytes are CD4+ T lymphocytes and exhibit CDw29.

In the dermis, most of the mast cells are the MC_{TC} type, which contain tryptase and chymase. Some of the mast cells are the MC_T type, which contain only tryptase. This latter type of mast cell has increased contacts with the dermal–epidermal basement membrane zone.[10] Some of the mast cells contain interleukin-4 immunoreactivity.[11]

Diagnosis and Differential Diagnosis

Nummular eczema must be differentiated from the erythematous, annular areas with scale and erosions that may appear in dry skin. At times, nummular eczema may resemble dermatophyte infections or

FIGURE 123-2

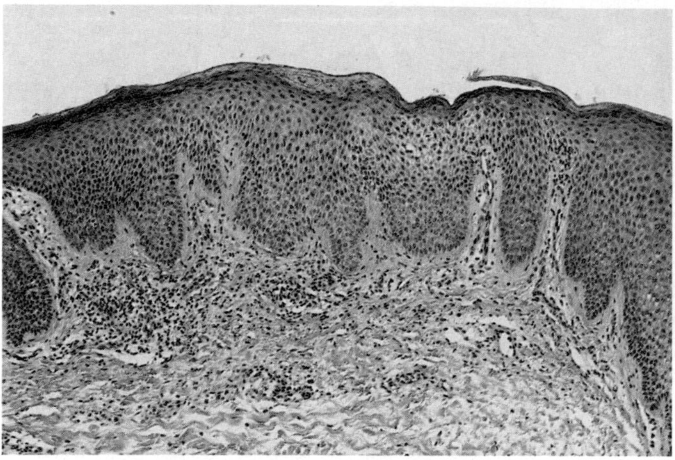

Parakeratosis containing plasma and neutrophils (scale crust) and psoriasiform epidermal hyperplasia with intercellular edema (spongiosis) are present with a superficial, dermal, perivascular infiltrate of lymphocytes, macrophages, and eosinophils. H&E 50×.

impetigo. Allergic contact dermatitis and atopic dermatitis should be considered.

Treatment and Prognosis

The skin should be hydrated by baths containing oil additives and the application of emollients. Topical anti-inflammatory agents include tar preparations, glucocorticoids, tacrolimus or pimecrolimus. Systemic antibiotics should be administered if a cutaneous infection is present. The humidity of the room should be regulated to avoid drying of the skin. If wool garments are to be worn, they should be lined with nonirritating material. The pruritus may be treated with the administration of H_1 antihistamines. Both broad-band and narrow-band ultraviolet B phototherapy may be effective. The systemic administration of glucocorticoids should be reserved for severe, refractory cases and should be administered in short courses.

In one series of patients followed for various intervals up to 2 years, 22 percent were without disease, 25 percent had periods without lesions ranging from weeks to years, and 53 percent were never free of lesions except when using local therapy.[5] Furthermore, it was evident that the eruption would clear within 1 year after onset if it cleared at all; after that time, it tended to persist and recur for many years.

LICHEN SIMPLEX CHRONICUS/PRURIGO NODULARIS

Lichen simplex chronicus, which is also known as *circumscribed neurodermatitis,* and prurigo nodularis are alterations in the skin that result from repetitive rubbing, scratching, and picking of the skin, owing to a variety of pruritogenic stimuli.

Historical Aspects

The term *lichen simplex chronicus* initially was used by Vidal, and this condition was further characterized by Brocq in 1891. In 1880, Hardaway described a skin disease characterized by multiple tumors associated with pruritus. In 1909, this entity was named prurigo nodularis by Hyde.

Epidemiology

Lichen simplex chronicus is uncommon in childhood. The peak incidence occurs between 30 and 50 years of age. Women are affected more frequently than are men. Individuals with prurigo nodularis can be divided into an atopic and a nonatopic group.[12] Prurigo nodularis patients in the group associated with atopic dermatitis have a younger mean age of onset of 19 ± 5 years and a high incidence of reactivity to multiple environmental allergens. In contrast, those patients with prurigo nodularis without atopic dermatitis have an older mean age of onset of 48 ± 14 years without hypersensitivity to environmental allergens.

Etiology and Pathogenesis

The underlying stimulus for the development of lichen simplex chronicus and prurigo nodularis is pruritus. Hypotheses regarding the pruritus focus on underlying medical disorders, associated dermatologic disorders, proliferation of nerves, and psychological aspects with emotional tension. The underlying medical disorders include chronic renal failure, obstructive biliary disease, Hodgkin's lymphoma, polycythemia rubra vera, hyperthyroidism, gluten-sensitive enteropathy, and human immunodeficiency infection. The important pruritic dermatoses are atopic dermatitis, allergic contact dermatitis, insect bites, and stasis dermatitis.

In prurigo nodularis, eosinophils, which contain eosinophil cationic protein and eosinophil-derived neurotoxin/eosinophil protein X, are increased in the dermis.[13] The basic proteins possess the ability to degranulate mast cells. HLA-DR and S-100 Langerhans cells are more numerous in the dermis.

The number of nerves containing immunoreactive CGRP and SP are increased in the dermis in prurigo nodularis but not lichen simplex chronicus.[14] Depletion of SP as demonstrated by confocal laser scanning microscopy associated with clinical improvement of prurigo nodularis lends support for the role of neuropeptides.[15] The number of nerves showing immunoreactive somatostatin, VIP, peptide histidine-isoleucine, galanin, and neuropeptide Y were the same in lichen simplex chronicus, prurigo nodularis, and normal skin. It has been suggested that the nerve proliferation results from mechanical trauma, such as scratching. SP and CGRP may release histamine from mast cells, which further enhances the pruritus. Schwann cell membranes and perineurium cells show increased expression of p75 nerve growth factor, which perhaps results in neural hyperplasia.[16] In the dermal papillae and upper dermis, alpha-melanocyte–stimulating hormone (α-MSH)-like immunoreactivity was visualized in the endothelial cells of the capillaries.[17] Although the role of α-MSH in prurigo nodularis is unknown, it may function in immunosuppression to counter cutaneous inflammation.

Clinical Manifestations

Lichen simplex chronicus appears as circumscribed, erythematous plaques with lichenification and excoriations. Often there is a single lesion (Fig. 123-3*A*). Commonly involved sites include the posterior and lateral aspects of the neck, extensor aspects of the forearms, lower legs, vulva, scrotum, and perianal area. Localized variants are known lichen nuchae, pruritus vulvae, pruritus scroti, and pruritus ani.

Prurigo nodularis is a nodule that develops at a local site in which persistent picking and scratching occur. The lesions appear as dome-shaped nodules, which often have an eroded surface with scale and crusts (Fig. 123-3*B*). They range in size from several millimeters to 2 cm. Multiple lesions may be distributed on the extremities. The intervening skin may be normal or show changes such as erythema, scales, excoriations, lichenification, postinflammatory pigmentary changes, and scars.

FIGURE 123-3

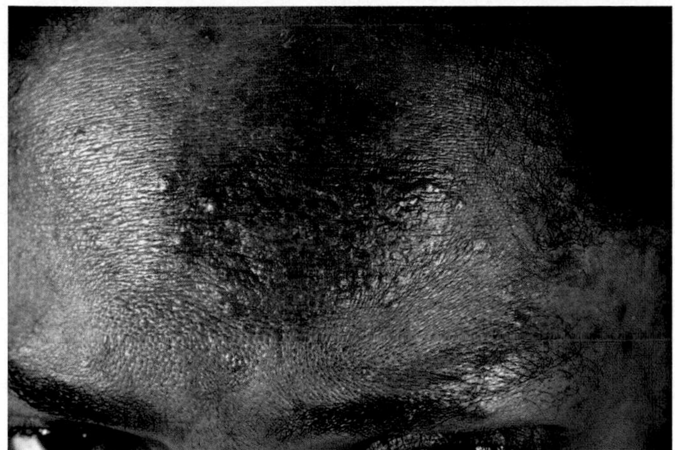

A.

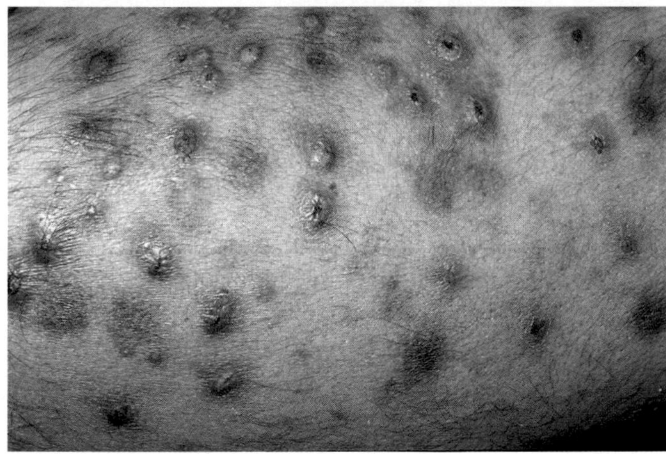

B.

A. Lichen simplex chronicus. Lichenified plaque with erythema and excoriations. *B.* Prurigo nodularis. Several dome-shaped nodules, some with a depressed center.

Laboratory Findings

If an underlying systemic disease is suspected, a complete blood count with differential analysis, a blood chemistry profile that includes liver and renal function tests, thyroid function tests, and a chest radiograph may be obtained. Further laboratory studies depend on the history and on the results of the initial laboratory tests. Serum IgE levels may be elevated in atopic prurigo nodularis but are normal in those with nonatopic prurigo nodularis.[12]

Pathology

The histopathologic findings in lichen simplex chronicus include orthokeratosis, hypergranulosis, and epidermal hyperplasia with regular elongation of the rete ridges. A perivascular infiltrate of lymphocytes, macrophages, and fibroblasts may be present. The histopathologic features of prurigo nodularis are similar to those of lichen simplex chronicus; additional findings are a dome-shaped configuration, proliferation of Schwann cells, and neural hyperplasia.

Diagnosis and Differential Diagnosis

The diagnosis of lichen simplex chronicus or prurigo nodularis requires the elimination of primary dermatologic causes of pruritus and

the search for underlying medical disorders. Lichen simplex chronicus must be differentiated from psoriasis, mycosis fungoides, dermatophyte infections, lichen planus, and lichen amyloidosis. Prurigo nodularis must be differentiated from keratoacanthomas, hypertrophic lichen planus, and perforating disorders.

Treatment and Prognosis

Lichen simplex chronicus and prurigo nodularis require similar therapeutic approaches. The traumatic perpetuation of the lesions should be explained to the patient. Treatment includes potent topical glucocorticoids, glucocorticoids under plastic-film occlusion, and intralesional injection of glucocorticoids. Doxepin cream can be used. Capsaicin cream has been used with clinical benefit in an open trial of 33 patients.[15] Oral H_1 antihistamines may be administered. Broad-band and narrow-band ultraviolet B phototherapy and psoralen plus ultraviolet A (PUVA) photochemotherapy may be of benefit. In some patients with prurigo nodularis, thalidomide, cyclosporine, azathioprine, and liquid nitrogen cryotherapy have been used. One patient with prurigo nodularis was successfully treated with a 585-nm pulsed dye laser.

The prognosis for lichen simplex chronicus and prurigo nodularis is variable, owing to the variety of causes of pruritus and the psychological status of the patient. When an underlying medical condition is present, improvement in pruritus may be achieved by treating the associated disorder.

REFERENCES

1. Goh CL, Akarapanth R: Epidemiology of skin disease among children in a referral skin clinic in Singapore. *Pediatr Dermatol* **11**:125, 1994
2. Krogh H-K: Nummular eczema: Its relationship to internal foci of infection. A survey of 84 case records. *Acta Derm Venereol Suppl (Stockh)* **40**:114, 1960
3. Aoyama H et al: Nummular eczema: An addition of senile xerosis and unique cutaneous reactivities to environmental aeroallergens. *Dermatology* **199**:135, 1999
4. Fleming C et al: Patch testing in discoid eczema. *Contact Dermatitis* **36**:261, 1997
5. Cowan MA: "Nummular eczema": A review, follow-up and analysis of a series of 325 cases. *Acta Derm Venereol Suppl (Stockh)* **41**:453, 1961
6. Bettoli V et al: Nummular eczema during isotretinoin treatment. *Arch Dermatol* **16**:617, 1987
7. Adachi A et al: Mercury-induced nummular dermatitis. *J Am Acad Dermatol* **43**:383, 2000
8. Järvikallio A et al: Neuropeptides SP, VIP and CGRP are increased in lesions of atopic dermatitis and nummular eczema. *J Invest Dermatol* **106**:891, 1996
9. O'Loughlin S et al: Serum IgE in dermatitis and dermatosis: An analysis of 497 cases. *Arch Dermatol* **113**:309, 1977
10. Järvikallio A et al: Quantitative analysis of tryptase- and chymase-containing mast cells in atopic dermatitis and nummular eczema. *Br J Dermatol* **136**:871, 1997
11. Horsmanheimo L et al: Mast cells are one major source of interleukin-4 in atopic dermatitis. *Br J Dermatol* **131**:348, 1994
12. Tanaka M et al: Prurigo nodularis consists of two distinct forms: Early onset atopic and late-onset non-atopic. *Dermatology* **190**:269, 1995
13. Johansson O et al: Eosinophil cationic protein- and eosinophil-derived neurotoxin/eosinophil protein X immunoreactive eosinophils in prurigo nodularis. *Arch Dermatol Res* **292**:371, 2000
14. Vaalasti A et al: Calcitonin gene-related peptide immunoreactivity in prurigo nodularis: A comparative study with neurodermatitis circumscripta. *Br J Dermatol* **120**:619, 1989
15. Ständer S et al: Treatment of prurigo nodularis with topical capsaicin. *J Am Acad Dermatol* **44**:471, 2001
16. Liang Y et al: Light and electron microscopic immunohistochemical observations of p75 nerve growth factor receptor-immunoreactive dermal nerves in prurigo nodularis. *Arch Dermatol Res* **291**:14, 2000
17. Liang Y et al: Endothelial cells express an α-melanocytic-stimulatory-hormone-like immunoreactivity in prurigo nodularis. *Br J Dermatol* **144**:1262, 2001

CHAPTER 124

Gerd Plewig
Thomas Jansen

Seborrheic Dermatitis

Seborrheic dermatitis is a common chronic papulosquamous dermatosis that is usually easily recognized. It affects infants and adults and is often associated with increased sebum production (seborrhea) of the scalp and the sebaceous follicle-rich areas of the face and trunk. The affected skin is pink, edematous, and covered with yellow-brown scales and crusts. The disease varies from mild to severe, including psoriasiform or pityriasiform patterns and erythroderma.[1] Seborrheic dermatitis is one of the most common skin manifestations in patients with human immunodeficiency virus (HIV) infection.[2] Consequently, it is included in the spectrum of premonitory lesions and should be carefully evaluated in high-risk patients.

INCIDENCE

Seborrheic dermatitis has two age peaks, one in infancy within the first 3 months of life and the second around the fourth to the seventh decades of life. No data are available on the exact incidence of seborrheic dermatitis in infants, but the disorder is common. The disease in adults is believed to be more common than psoriasis, for example, affecting at least 3 to 5 percent of the population in the United States.[3] Men are affected more often than women in all age groups. There does not appear to be any racial predilection. Seborrheic dermatitis is found in up to 85 percent of patients with HIV infection.[2]

ETIOLOGY AND PATHOGENESIS

Although many theories abound, the cause of seborrheic dermatitis remains unknown.

Seborrhea

The disease is associated with oily-looking skin (seborrhea oleosa), although an increased sebum production cannot always be detected in these patients.[4] Even if seborrhea does provide a predisposition, seborrheic dermatitis is not a disease of the sebaceous glands. The high incidence of seborrheic dermatitis in newborns parallels the size and activity of the sebaceous glands at this age. It has been shown that newborns have large sebaceous glands with high sebum secretion rates similar to adults.[5] In childhood, sebum production and seborrheic dermatitis are closely connected. In adulthood, however, they are not, as the sebaceous gland activity peaks in early puberty and decades later seborrheic dermatitis may occur.

The sites of predilection—face, ears, scalp, and upper part of the trunk—are particularly rich in sebaceous follicles. Two diseases are prevalent in these regions: seborrheic dermatitis and acne. In patients with seborrheic dermatitis, the sebaceous glands are often particularly large on cross-sectional histologic specimens. In one study, skin surface lipids were not elevated but the lipid composition was characterized by an increased proportion of cholesterol, triglycerides, and paraffin, and a decrease in squalene, free fatty acids, and wax esters.[6] However, mild abnormalities in the skin surface lipids could well result from the ineffective keratinization, which is often demonstrable histopathologically. Seborrheic dermatitis seems to be more frequent in patients with parkinsonism, in whom sebum secretion is increased. Similarly, after reduction of sebum production induced by levodopa and by promestriene,seborrheic dermatitis may improve.

The synonym *eczéma flannelaire* stems from the idea that a retention of skin surface lipids by clothing and rubbing of the rough textiles on the skin—cotton (flannel), wool, or synthetic underwear in particular—promotes or aggravates seborrheic dermatitis.

Microbial Effects

Unna and Sabouraud, who were among the first to describe the disease, favored an etiology involving bacteria, yeasts, or both. This hypothesis has remained unsupported, although bacteria and yeast can be isolated in great quantities from affected skin sites.

In infancy, *Candida albicans* is often found in dermatitic skin lesions and in stool specimens. Although intracutaneous tests with candidin, positive agglutinating antibodies in serum, and positive lymphocyte-transformation tests in affected infants revealed sensitization to *C. albicans,* these observations cannot be convincingly linked to the pathogenesis.

Aerobic bacteria were recovered from the scalp of patients with seborrheic dermatitis (140,000 bacteria/cm^2 versus 280,000 in normal individuals and 250,000 in persons with dandruff). In contrast, *Staphylococcus aureus* was rarely seen in normal persons or those with dandruff. *Staphylococcus* was recovered in about 20 percent of patients with seborrheic dermatitis, accounting for an average of about 32 percent of the total skin flora.[7]

Propionibacterium acnes counts were low in patients with seborrheic dermatitis (7550 bacteria/cm^2 in those without dandruff). The small quantities of *P. acnes* in patients with seborrheic dermatitis may explain the low yield of free fatty acids from their skin surfaces.

The lipophilic yeast *Pityrosporum* is abundant in normal skin (504,000 organisms/cm^2 versus 922,000 in individuals with dandruff and 665,000 in patients with seborrheic dermatitis).[7] This organism has received particular attention in recent years. Some authors claim strong evidence in favor of a pathogenic role for these microbes, whereas others do not share this view. Their argument is that *Pityrosporum ovale* is not the causative organism, but is merely present in large numbers. In patients with pityriasis versicolor[8] and *Pityrosporum* folliculitis,[9] seborrheic dermatitis has been found in a higher percentage than expected. Clearing of seborrheic dermatitis by selenium sulfide and continued suppression of *P. ovale* with topical amphotericin B caused a relapse of the disease on inflamed scalp skin.[10] In seborrheic dermatitis, both normal and high levels of serum antibodies against *P. ovale* have been demonstrated. A cell-mediated immune response to *P. ovale* has been found in normal individuals using *Pityrosporum* extracts in lymphocyte-transformation studies.[11] Overgrowth of *P. ovale* may lead to inflammation, either through introduction of yeast-derived metabolic products into the epidermis or as a result of the presence of yeast cells on the skin surface. The mechanism of production of inflammation would likely then be through Langerhans cell and T lymphocyte activation by *Pityrosporum* or its by-products. When *P. ovale* comes into contact with serum, it can activate complement via the direct and alternative pathways and this may play some part in the introduction of inflammation.[12] A possible role for this yeast in the pathogenesis of seborrheic dermatitis is supported by the fact that seborrheic dermatitis–like lesions have been shown to be reproducible in animal models by inoculation of *P. ovale*.[13]

Miscellaneous

DRUGS Several drugs have been reported to produce seborrheic dermatitis–like lesions, including arsenic, gold, methyldopa, cimetidine, and neuroleptics.

NEUROTRANSMITTER ABNORMALITIES Seborrheic dermatitis is often associated with a variety of neurologic abnormalities, pointing to a possible influence of the nervous system. These neurologic conditions include postencephalitic parkinsonism, epilepsy, supraorbital injury, facial paralysis, unilateral injury to the ganglion of Gasser, poliomyelitis, syringomyelia, and quadriplegia. Emotional stress seems to aggravate the disease; a high rate of seborrhea is reported among combat troops in times of war.

PHYSICAL FACTORS It has been suggested that cutaneous blood flow and skin temperature may be responsible for the distribution of seborrheic dermatitis.[14] Seasonal variations in temperature and humidity are related to the course of the disease. Low fall and winter temperatures and low humidity in centrally heated rooms are known to worsen the condition. Seborrheic dermatitis of the face was observed in 8 percent of 347 patients receiving PUVA therapy for psoriasis and occurred within a few days to 2 weeks after the beginning of treatment;[15] the patients had no previous history of facial psoriasis or seborrheic dermatitis. Lesions were avoided by masking the face during irradiation.

ABERRANT EPIDERMAL PROLIFERATION Epidermal proliferation is increased in seborrheic dermatitis, like psoriasis, explaining why cytostatic therapeutic modalities may improve the condition.[16]

NUTRITIONAL DISORDERS Zinc deficiency in patients with acrodermatitis enteropathica and acrodermatitis enteropathica–like conditions may be accompanied by dermatitis mimicking seborrheic dermatitis of the face. Seborrheic dermatitis is, however, not associated with zinc deficiency nor does it respond to supplementary zinc therapy.

Seborrheic dermatitis in infancy may have a different pathogenesis. Biotin deficiency, whether secondary to a holocarboxylase deficiency or a biotinidase deficiency, and abnormal metabolism of essential fatty acids have been proposed as possible mechanisms.[17]

IMMUNODEFICIENCY AND SEBORRHEIC DERMATITIS

The development of seborrheic dermatitis either de novo or as a flare of preexisting disease also may serve as a clue to the presence of HIV infection. The first report of this association in 1984 was followed by

FIGURE 124-1

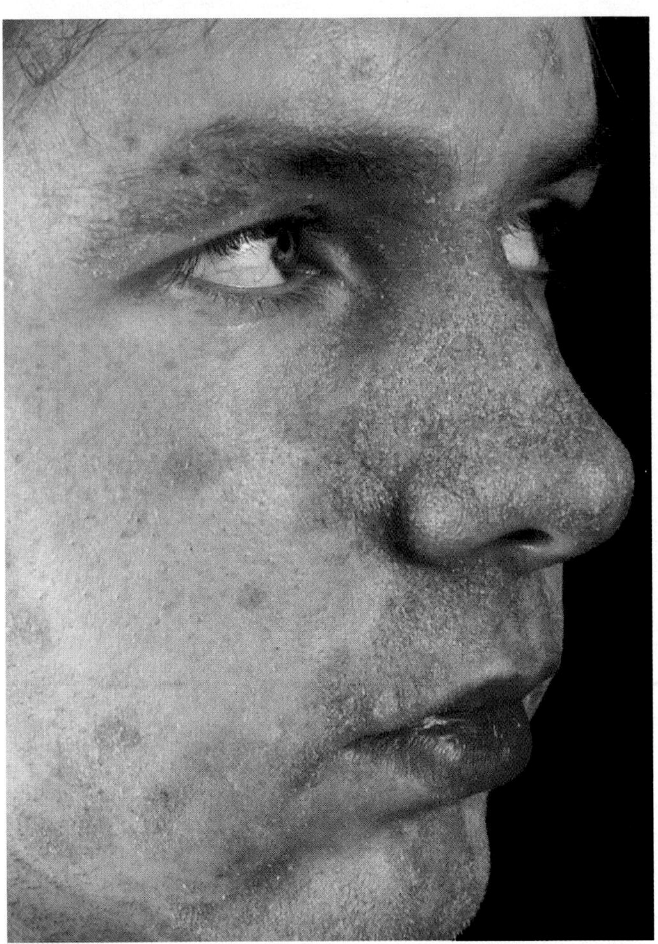

Seborrheic dermatitis with involvement of nasolabial folds, cheeks, eyebrows, and nose.

observations from all parts of the world.[2] The expression of the disease differs in several aspects from its classical form seen in HIV seronegative individuals (Figs. 124-1 to 124-4): the distribution is extensive, severity is marked, and treatment often difficult (Fig. 124-5). Even the histopathologic changes differ somewhat from those seen in commonly encountered seborrheic dermatitis (Table 124-1).

The increased incidence and severity of seborrheic dermatitis in HIV seropositive individuals has led to speculation that unchecked growth of *Pityrosporum* in immunosuppressed patients is responsible. However, a study that compared quantitative *Pityrosporum* cultures in AIDS patients with and without seborrheic dermatitis failed to demonstrate increased yeast colonization in patients with seborrheic dermatitis.[18]

PSORIASIS AND SEBORRHEIC DERMATITIS

In patients with a psoriatic diathesis, particularly adults, seborrheic dermatitis is said to evolve into psoriasis. The term *sebopsoriasis* is sometimes used for these overlapping conditions. It should be used with caution because psoriasis, especially of the scalp, is clinically and histopathologically almost indistinguishable from seborrheic dermatitis.

FIGURE 124-2

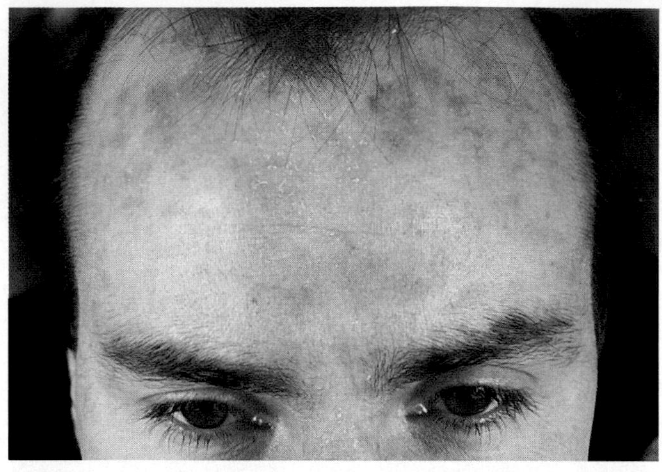

Seborrheic dermatitis of forehead and scalp.

FIGURE 124-4

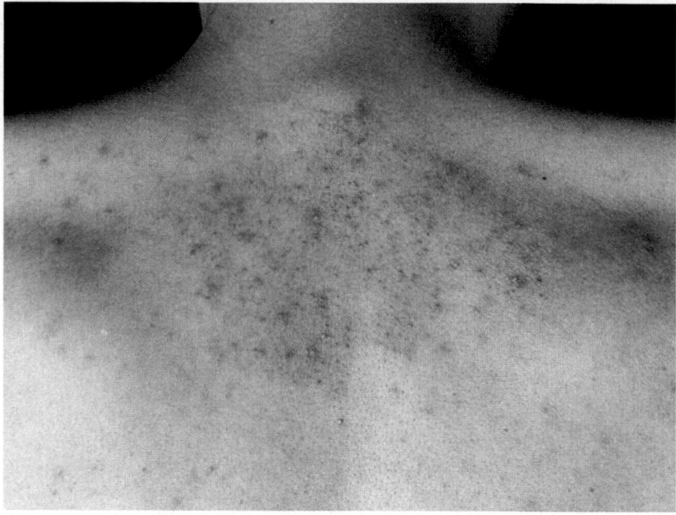

Seborrheic dermatitis of the upper back.

PITYRIASIS AMIANTACEA

Pityriasis amiantacea (synonyms: tinea amiantacea, porrigo amiantacea, tinea asbestina, fausse teigne amiantacée, keratosis follicularis amiantacea) is the name given to a disease of the scalp in which heavy scales extend onto the hairs and separate and bind together their proximal portions.

Pityriasis amiantacea is a reaction of the scalp, often without evident cause, that may occur at any age. It may be observed as a complication or sequel of streptococcal infection, seborrheic dermatitis, atopic dermatitis, lichen simplex, and it also occurs in psoriasis, of which it may be the first clinical manifestation.[19]

The process may be circumscribed or diffuse. It is only slightly inflammatory with dry, micaceous scales, or markedly inflammatory with admixture of a crust (Fig. 124-6). Removal of the scales reveals normal or erythematous, edematous epidermis. The process is not followed by atrophy, scarring, or alopecia. If scarring alopecia occurs, it may be related to secondary infection. A common form complicates chronic or recurrent fissuring behind one or both ears mostly in young girls. The sticky scales extend several centimeters into the neighboring scalp. Another form extends from patches of lichen simplex and is seen mainly in middle-aged women.

FIGURE 124-3

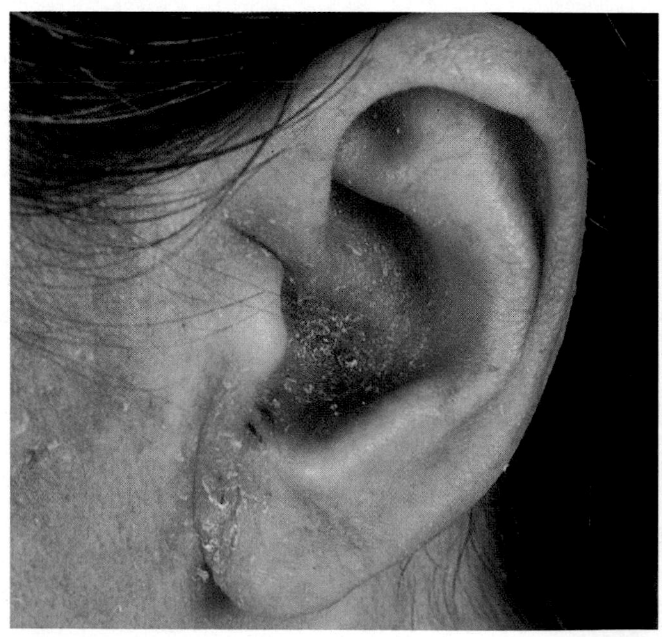

Seborrheic dermatitis of the ear lobe. The ear canal is also affected.

HISTOPATHOLOGY

The histopathologic picture varies according to the stage of the disease: acute, subacute, or chronic.[20,21] In acute and subacute seborrheic dermatitis, there is a sparse superficial perivascular infiltrate of lymphocytes and histiocytes, slight to moderate spongiosis, slight psoriasiform hyperplasia, follicular plugging by orthokeratosis and parakeratosis, and scale-crusts containing neutrophils at the tips of the follicular ostia (see Table 124-1). In chronic seborrheic dermatitis, there are markedly dilated capillaries and venules in the superficial plexus, in addition to the above-mentioned features.

Clinically and histopathologically the lesions of chronic seborrheic dermatitis are psoriasiform and often difficult to distinguish from those of psoriasis.[20] Abortive forms of psoriasis share many features with seborrheic dermatitis. There are lesions that resemble psoriasis and may persist over many years before they finally turn into overt psoriasis. The most important diagnostic signs of seborrheic dermatitis are mounds of scale-crust containing neutrophils at the tips of the dilated horn-filled follicular infundibula. Acrosyringia and acroinfundibula may be plugged by corneocyte casts.

The most consistent findings in pityriasis amiantacea are spongiosis, parakeratosis, migration of lymphocytes into the epidermis, and a variable degree of acanthosis.[22] The essential features responsible for

FIGURE 124-5

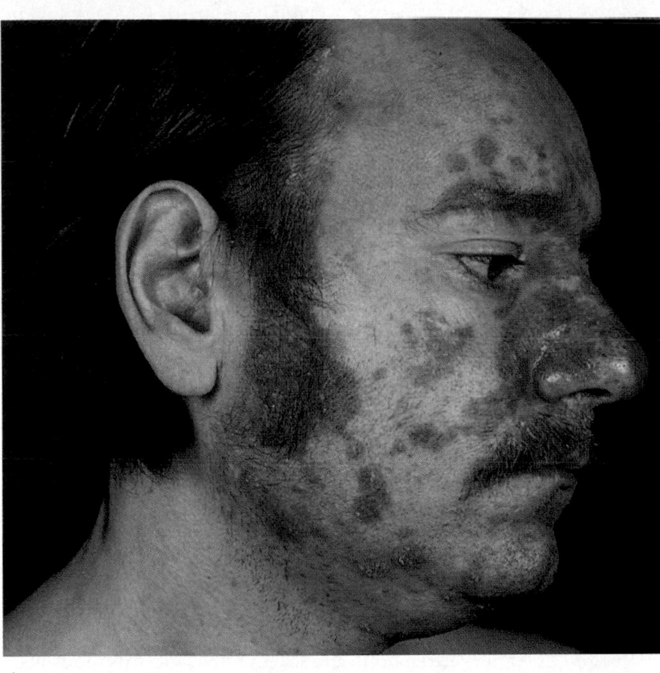

A.

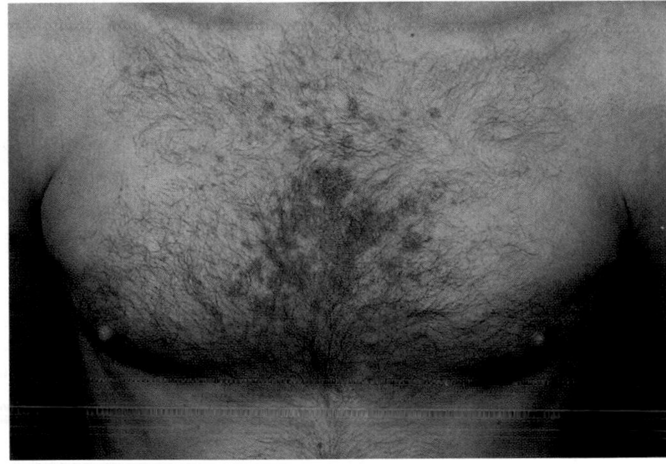

B.

Widespread unusual distribution pattern of seborrheic dermatitis in a patient with AIDS. *A.* Moist patches on the centrofacial region and hairy scalp. *B.* Moist lesions on the chest. In patients with AIDS, the disease responds poorly to conventional therapy.

the asbestosis-like scaling are diffuse hyperkeratosis and parakeratosis together with follicular keratosis in which each hair is surrounded by a sheath of corneocytes and debris.

EXFOLIATIVE CYTOLOGY

Cytologic abnormalities of superficial horny cells (corneocytes) including ortho- and parakeratotic (nucleated) cells, horny cells in different stages of nuclear decomposition (halo cells), and masses of leukocytes can be evaluated by exfoliative cytology. Seborrheic dermatitis and psoriasis, however, present similar findings compared with other conditions of the dermatitis-eczema group.[23]

TABLE 124-1

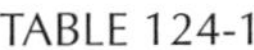

Histopathologic Differences Between AIDS-Associated Seborrheic Dermatitis and Classical Seborrheic Dermatitis

AIDS-Associated Seborrheic Dermatitis	Classical Seborrheic Dermatitis
Epidermis	
Widespread parakeratosis	Limited parakeratosis
Many necrotic keratinocytes	Rare necrotic keratinocytes
Focal interface obliteration with clusters of lymphocytes	No interface obliteration
Sparse spongiosis	Prominent spongiosis
Dermis	
Many thick-walled vessels	Thin-walled vessels
Increased plasma cells	Rare plasma cells
Focal leukocytoclasis	No leukocytoclasis

SOURCE: From Soeprono FF et al: Seborrheic-like dermatitis of acquired immunodeficiency syndrome: A clinicopathologic study. *J Am Acad Dermatol* **14**:242, 1986

CLINICAL FINDINGS

In all patients with seborrheic dermatitis there is a so-called seborrheic stage, which is often combined with a gray-white or yellow-red skin discoloration, prominent follicular openings, and mild to severe pityriasiform scales. Several forms can be distinguished (Table 124-2).

Seborrheic Dermatitis in Infants

The disease occurs in infants predominantly within the first months of life as an inflammatory disease mainly affecting the hairy scalp and intertriginous folds with greasy-looking scales and crusts. Other regions such as the center of the face, chest, and neck may also be affected. Scalp involvement is fairly characteristic. The frontal and parietal scalp regions are covered with an oily-looking, thick, often fissured crust (*crusta lactea, milk crust* or *cradle cap*). Hair loss does not occur and inflammation is sparse. In the course of the disease, the redness

FIGURE 124-6

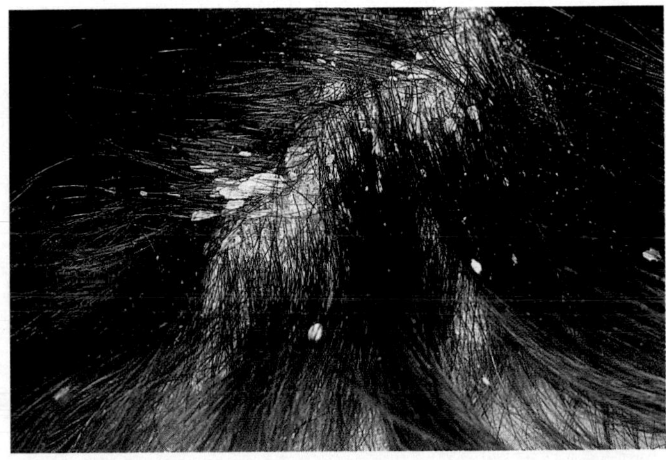

Pityriasis amiantacea. Masses of sticky silvery scales adhere to the scalp and are attached in layers to the shafts of the hairs that they surround.

TABLE 124-2

Clinical Patterns of Seborrheic Dermatitis

Infantile
- Scalp (cradle cap)
- Trunk (including flexures and napkin area)
- Leiner's disease
  - Nonfamilial
  - Familial C5 dysfunction

Adult
- Scalp
- Face (may include blepharitis)
- Trunk
  - Petaloid
  - Pityriasiform
  - Flexural
  - Eczematous plaques
  - Follicular
- Generalized (may be erythroderma)

increases and the scaled areas form clearly outlined erythematous patches topped by a greasy scale. Extension beyond the frontal hairline occurs. The retroauricular folds, the pinna of the ear, and the neck may also be involved. Otitis externa is often a complicating factor. Semiocclusive clothing and diapers favor moisture, maceration, and intertriginous dermatitis, particularly in the folds of the neck, axillae, anogenital area, and groins. Opportunistic infection with *C. albicans, S. aureus,* and other bacteria occurs. The clinical aspect reminds one of psoriasis vulgaris, hence the expressions *psoriasoid* or *napkin psoriasis.*

COURSE The disease is usually protracted over weeks to months. Exacerbation and, rarely, generalized erythroderma desquamativum may occur. The prognosis is good. There is no indication that infants with seborrheic dermatitis are more likely to suffer from the adult form of the disease.

DIFFERENTIAL DIAGNOSIS The differential diagnosis in seborrheic dermatitis of infancy includes atopic dermatitis (which usually starts after the third month of life); psoriasis in newborns, a rare disease; scabies; and Langerhans cell histiocytosis. The most useful distinguishing feature between atopic dermatitis and seborrheic dermatitis is the increased number of lesions on the forearms and shins in the former and in the axillae in the latter. The development of skin lesions solely in the diaper area favors a diagnosis of infantile seborrheic dermatitis. RAST (radioallergosorbent assay test) screening to egg white and milk antibodies or other geographically or ethnically relevant allergens (e.g., soybean), and, to a lesser extent, total IgE levels, may be useful in diagnosing atopic dermatitis at an early stage and distinguishing it from infantile seborrheic dermatitis. Absent to mild pruritus is considered a significant feature of infantile seborrheic dermatitis. Some authors believe that infantile seborrheic dermatitis is a clinical variant of atopic dermatitis rather than a separate entity.[24]

Erythroderma Desquamativum (Leiner's Disease)

This complication of seborrheic dermatitis in infants (dermatitis seborrhoides infantum) was described in 1908 by Leiner.[25] There is usually a sudden confluence of lesions, leading to a universal scaling redness of the skin (erythroderma). The young patients are severely ill with anemia, diarrhea, and vomiting. Secondary bacterial infection is common. The prognosis is very good unless proper intensive care and skin care are provided. The disease is both a familial and a nonfamilial form. The former is noted for having a functional deficiency of C5 complement, resulting in defective opsonization. These patients respond to antibiotics and infusions of fresh-frozen plasma or whole blood. The true nature of this disease remains obscure.

Seborrheic Dermatitis in Adults

The clinical picture and course of this disease differ in adults and infants.

Seborrheic eczematid is the mildest form of the disease (eczematid = eczema-like, dermatitis-like). It is associated with seborrhea, scaling, mild redness, and often pruritus of the scalp, eyebrows, nasolabial folds, and retroauricular area, as well as over the sternum and the shoulder blades (see Figs. 124-1 to 124-4). Asymptomatic fluffy, white dandruff of the scalp represents the mild end of the spectrum of seborrheic dermatitis and has been referred to as *pityriasis sicca. Erythema paranasale,* more common in young women than men, may be part of this disease spectrum.

Patchy seborrheic dermatitis is the classical, well-known disease with chronic recurrent lesions. Lesions have a predilection for scalp, temples, retroauricular folds (see Fig. 124-3), external ear canals (see Fig. 124-3), inner parts of the eyebrows and glabella with nasolabial folds (see Fig. 124-2), and V-shaped areas of the chest and back (*eczema mediothoracicum*). Less frequently, intertriginous areas such as the side of the neck, axillae, submammary region, umbilicus, and genitocrural folds are involved.

Skin lesions are characterized by a yellow color, mild to severe erythema, mild inflammatory infiltrate, and oily, thick scales and crusts. This has occasionally been referred as *pityriasis steatoides.* Patients report pruritus, particularly on the scalp and in the ear canal. The lesions start with follicular and perifollicular redness and mounds; they spread until they form clearly outlined, round to circinate (petaloid) patches (Greek *petalon,* a thin plate or leaf). The pityriasiform type of seborrheic dermatitis is seen on the trunk and mimics the lesions of pityriasis rosea, producing oval scaly lesions whose long axes tend to parallel the ribs. In some individuals, only one or two sites are involved. Chronic otitis externa may be the sole manifestation of seborrheic dermatitis often mistaken for mycotic infections. Another possible manifestation is blepharitis with honey-colored crusts along the rim of the eyelid and casts of horny cell debris around the eyelashes. In men, a more follicular type of seborrheic dermatitis may extend over large parts of the back, flanks, and abdomen.

COURSE Usually the disease lasts for years to decades with periods of improvement in warmer seasons and periods of exacerbation in the colder months. Widespread lesions may occur as a result of improper topical treatment or sun exposure. The extreme variant of the disease is a generalized exfoliative erythroderma (seborrheic erythroderma).

DIFFERENTIAL DIAGNOSIS The differential diagnosis varies from site to site: *scalp:* dandruff, psoriasis, atopic dermatitis, impetigo; *ear canal:* psoriasis or contact dermatitis, irritant or allergic; *face:* rosacea, contact dermatitis, psoriasis, impetigo; *chest and back:* pityriasis versicolor, pityriasis rosea; *eyelids:* atopic dermatitis, psoriasis, *Demodex folliculorum* infestation (demodicosis, demodicidosis); *intertriginous areas:* psoriasis, candidiasis.

THERAPY

In general, therapy is directed toward loosening and removal of scales and crusts, inhibition of yeast colonization, control of secondary infection, and reduction of erythema and itching. Adult patients should be informed about the chronic nature of the disease and understand that therapy works by controlling the disease rather than by curing it. The prognosis of infantile seborrheic dermatitis is excellent because the condition is benign and self-limited.

Infants

SCALP Treatment consists of the following measures: removal of crusts with 3 to 5% salicylic acid in olive oil or a water-soluble base; warm olive oil compresses; application of low-potency glucocorticosteroids (e.g., 1% hydrocortisone) in a cream or lotion for a few days; topical antifungal agents such as imidazoles (in a shampoo); mild baby shampoos; proper skin care with emollients, creams, and soft pasts.

INTERTRIGINOUS AREAS Treatment measures include drying lotions, such as 0.2 to 0.5% clioquinol in zinc lotion or zinc oil. In cases of candidiasis, nystatin or amphotericin B lotion or cream can be applied followed by soft and stiff pastes. In cases of oozing dermatitis, application of 0.1 to 0.25% gentian violet where still available in combination with cotton or muslin diapers is often helpful. Imidazole preparations (e.g., 2% ketoconazole in soft pastes, creams, or lotions) may also be effective.

DIET Milk-free and high-protein, low-fat diets have not been shown to be of value nor has the efficacy of oral or intramuscular biotin, vitamin B complex, or essential fatty acids been established.

Adults

Because the disease runs an unpredictably long course, careful and mild treatment regimens are recommended. Anti-inflammatory agents and, when indicated, antimicrobial or antifungal agents have to be used.

SCALP Frequent shampooing with shampoos containing 1 to 2.5% selenium sulfide, imidazoles (e.g., 2% ketoconazole), zinc pyrithione, benzoyl peroxide, salicylic acid, coal or juniper tar where still available, or detergents is recommended. Crusts or scales can be removed by overnight application of glucocorticosteroids or salicylic acid in water-soluble bases or, when necessary, under occlusive dressings. Tinctures, alcoholic solutions, hair tonics, and similar products usually aggravate the inflammatory state and should be avoided.

In pityriasis amiantacea, scales should be removed by the use of Oil of Cade ointment or a topical tar/salicylic ointment. Either preparation should be washed out of the scalp after 4 to 6 h with a suitable shampoo (e.g., tar or imidazole shampoo). Potent topical corticosteroid scalp creams or liquids may be beneficial in some cases, preferably under plastic occlusion in the initial phase. If topical treatment fails, systemic glucocorticosteroids (e.g., 0.5 mg prednisolone/kg body weight per day for approximately 1 week) in combination with topical treatment (steroid under occlusion, followed by open application) is worthwhile. Concomitant antimicrobial treatment (e.g., macrolides, sulfonamides) is reserved for stubborn cases, especially if bacterial coinfection of the scalp is proven or suspected. Of course, the underlying condition must be treated. Treatment remains difficult, and relapses occur frequently.

FACE AND TRUNK Patients should avoid greasy ointments and reduce or omit the use of soaps. Alcoholic solutions or pre- or aftershave lotions should not be recommended. Low-potency glucocorticosteroids (1% hydrocortisone is usually sufficient) are helpful early in the course of the disease. Uncontrolled long-term applications will lead to side effects such as steroid dermatitis, steroid rebound phenomenon, steroid rosacea, and perioral dermatitis.

SEBORRHEIC OTITIS EXTERNA Seborrheic otitis externa can be best treated with a low-potency glucocorticoid cream or ointment. Many otic preparations (solutions) that contain neomycin and other antibiotics, often in combination, are strong sensitizers and should be avoided. Once dermatitis is under control, the glucocorticoid should be discontinued and a solution containing aluminum acetate should be applied once or twice daily to maintain control. This acts as a drying agent and reduces the microbial flora. Basic ointments or plain petroleum jelly, gently applied into the ear canal (without cotton tips), are often helpful to maintain satisfaction of the patient.

SEBORRHEIC BLEPHARITIS Special consideration is given to the treatment of seborrheic blepharitis. The use of hot compresses with gentle débridement with a cotton-tipped applicator and baby shampoo one or more times daily is recommended. Stubborn cases may require the use of a topical antibiotic such as sodium sulfacetamide ophthalmic ointment. The use of ocular preparations containing glucocorticosteroids should be deferred to an ophthalmologist. If *D. folliculorum* mites occur in large numbers, they should be treated with antiparasitic drugs such as lindane (γ-hexachlorocyclohexane), crotamiton, permethrin, or benzyl benzoate.

Antifungals

Good results are achieved with topical application of antifungal agents, especially imidazoles. Clinical studies have reported response rates ranging from 63 percent[26] up to 90 percent[27] after 4 weeks. In these trials, imidazoles such as itraconazole, miconazole, fluconazole, econazole, bifonazole, and ciclopiroxolamine were studied. The imidazole compound that has been mostly used is ketoconazole. In several clinical studies, 2% ketoconazole cream has been found as effective as glucocorticosteroid creams, and this often results in more prolonged remissions.[26,28] Comparative studies of topical antifungal agents, however, are lacking. Personal experience, though based on open uncontrolled studies only, favors 2% ketoconazole cream. Other antifungal agents may also be effective. In a limited trial, 1% butenafine cream, a benzylamine derivative, demonstrated efficacy in the topical treatment of seborrheic dermatitis.

Oral antifungal agents such as ketoconazole and terbinafine are also effective, but because of potential side effects and pharmacoeconomic considerations, should probably be limited to severe or refractory cases. Antifungal agents have a wide spectrum of effects, including anti-inflammatory properties and inhibition of cell wall lipid synthesis. This efficacy is not proof of a causal relationship between *P. ovale* and seborrheic dermatitis.

Metronidazole

Topical metronidazole is a worthwhile alternative in the treatment repertoire of seborrheic dermatitis. It has been used successfully in patients with rosacea. Extemporaneous formulations (1 to 2% in a cream base) or commercial products (0.75% gel, cream, or lotion, 1% cream) are used once or twice daily. Recently, a significant benefit of using 1% metronidazole gel over placebo in the treatment of seborrheic dermatitis was demonstrated.[29]

Lithium Succinate

Another topical agent that is effective in the treatment of seborrheic dermatitis is lithium succinate, which possesses antifungal properties.[30]

Vitamin D_3 Analogues

Vitamin D_3 analogues (calcipotriol cream or lotion, calcitriol ointment, or tacalcitol ointment) are also recommended and useful in selected patients.[31] Their anti-inflammatory properties may be responsible for their efficacy in seborrheic dermatitis.

Isotretinoin

Oral isotretinoin (13-*cis*-retinoic acid) is a useful, although not officially approved, drug for this indication. Low to very-low doses (0.05 to 0.1 mg/kg body weight daily) given for several months clear stubborn seborrheic dermatitis in many cases. The lowest available dose (10 mg) is given daily with a fat-rich food for better absorption. The frequency can be reduced to 3 to 5 days per week. In women of child-bearing age, all precautions against pregnancy must be met.

Phototherapy

Narrow-band UVB phototherapy appears to be an effective and safe treatment option for patients with severe and refractory seborrheic dermatitis.[32] PUVA therapy has been used successfully in the erythrodermic form of the disease.[33]

REFERENCES

1. Fox BJ, Odom RB: Papulosquamous diseases: A review. *J Am Acad Dermatol* **12**:597, 1985
2. Soeprono FF et al: Seborrheic-like dermatitis of acquired immunodeficiency syndrome: A clinicopathologic study. *J Am Acad Dermatol* **14**:242, 1986
3. Johnson M, Roberts J: *Prevalence of dermatological diseases among persons 1–74 years of age.* Publication No. (PHS) 79-1660. Washington, DC, US Department of Health and Human Services, 1977
4. Burton JL, Pye PJ: Seborrhoea is not a feature of seborrhoeic dermatitis. *Br Med J* **286**:1169, 1983
5. Agache P et al: Sebum levels during the first year of life. *Br J Dermatol* **103**:643, 1980
6. Gloor M et al: Über Menge und Zusammensetzung der Hautoberflächenlipide beim sogenannten seborrhoischen Ekzem. *Dermatol Monatsschr* **158**:759, 1972
7. McGinley K et al: Quantitative microbiology of the scalp in non-dandruff, dandruff, and seborrheic dermatitis. *J Invest Dermatol* **64**:401, 1975
8. Faergemann J, Fredriksson T: Tinea versicolor with reference to seborrhoeic dermatitis. *Arch Dermatol* **115**:966, 1979
9. Bäck O et al: *Pityrosporum* folliculitis: A common disease of the young and middle-aged. *J Am Acad Dermatol* **12**:56, 1985
10. Leyden JJ et al: Role of microorganisms in dandruff. *Arch Dermatol* **112**:333, 1976
11. Sohnle PG, Collins-Lech C: Relative antigenicity of *P. orbiculare* and *C. albicans*. *J Invest Dermatol* **75**:279, 1980
12. Sohnle PG, Collins-Lech C: Activation of complement by *Pityrosporum orbiculare*. *J Invest Dermatol* **80**:93, 1983
13. Faergemann J, Fredriksson T: Experimental infections in rabbits and humans with *Pityrosporum orbiculare* and *P. ovale*. *J Invest Dermatol* **77**:314, 1981
14. Hale EK, Bystryn JC: Relation between skin temperature and location of facial lesions in seborrheic dermatitis. *Arch Dermatol* **136**:559, 2000
15. Tegner E: Seborrhoeic dermatitis of the face induced by PUVA treatment. *Acta Derm Venereol Suppl (Stockh)* **63**:335, 1983
16. Shuster S: The aetiology of dandruff and the mode of action of therapeutic agents. *Br J Dermatol* **111**:235, 1984
17. Tollesson A et al: Essential fatty acids in infantile seborrheic dermatitis. *J Am Acad Dermatol* **28**:957, 1993
18. Wikler JR et al: Quantitative skin cultures of *Pityrosporum* yeasts in patients seropositive for the human immunodeficiency virus with and without seborrheic dermatitis. *J Am Acad Dermatol* **27**:37, 1992
19. Ring DS, Kaplan DL: Pityriasis amiantacea: A report of 10 cases. *Arch Dermatol* **129**:913, 1993
20. Braun-Falco O et al: Histologische Differentialdiagnose von Psoriasis vulgaris und seborrhoischem Ekzem des Kapillitium. *Hautarzt* **30**:478, 1979
21. Metz J, Metz G: Zur Ultrastruktur der Epidermis bei seborrhoischem Ekzem. *Arch Dermatol Forsch* **252**:285, 1975
22. Knight AG: Pityriasis amiantacea: A clinical and histopathological investigation. *Clin Exp Dermatol* **2**:137, 1977
23. Goldschmidt H, Thew MA: Exfoliative cytology of psoriasis and other common dermatoses: Quantitative analysis of parakeratotic horny cells in 266 patients. *Arch Dermatol* **106**:476, 1972
24. Podmore P et al: Seborrheic eczema—A disease entity or a clinical variant of atopic eczema? *Br J Dermatol* **115**:341, 1986
25. Leiner C: Über Erythrodermia desquamativa, eine eigenartige universelle Dermatose der Brustkinder. *Arch Dermatol Syphilol (Berlin)* **89**:65, 1908
26. Pari T et al: Randomised double blind controlled trial of 2% ketoconazole cream versus 0.05% clobetasol 17-butyrate cream in seborrheic dermatitis. *J Eur Acad Dermatol Venereol* **10**:89, 1998
27. Green CA et al: Treatment of seborrhoeic dermatitis with ketoconazole: II. Response of seborrheic dermatitis of the face, scalp and trunk to topical ketoconazole. *Br J Dermatol* **116**:217, 1987
28. Katsambas A et al: A double-blind trial of treatment of seborrheic dermatitis with 2% ketoconazole cream compared with 1% hydrocortisone cream. *Br J Dermatol* **121**:353, 1989
29. Parsad D et al: Topical metronidazole in seborrheic dermatitis—A double-blind study. *Dermatology* **201**:35, 2001
30. Cuelenaere C et al: Use of topical lithium succinate in the treatment of seborrheic dermatitis. *Dermatology* **184**:194, 1992
31. Nakayama J: Four cases of sebopsoriasis or seborrheic dermatitis of the face and scalp successfully treated with 1α-24 (R)-dihydroxycholecalciferol (tacalcitol) cream. *Eur J Dermatol* **10**:528, 2000
32. Pirkhammer D et al: Narrow-band ultraviolet B (ATL-01) phototherapy is an effective and safe treatment option for patients with severe seborrheic dermatitis. *Br J Dermatol* **143**:964, 2000
33. Dahl KB, Reymann F: Photochemotherapy in erythrodermic seborrheic dermatitis. *Arch Dermatol* **113**:1295, 1977

CHAPTER 125

Alexa Boer Kimball

Vesicular Palmoplantar Eczema

Vesicular palmoplantar eczema is an endogenous dermatitis of the hands and feet characterized clinically by small to large blisters and histologically by spongiotic vesicles. It can be present as an acute and/or as a chronic problem.

The nomenclature and the clinical presentations of the variants of hand dermatitis, including vesicular palmoplantar eczema, often overlap, rendering the diagnostic categories imprecise. Moreover, some variants are frequently caused or exacerbated by more that one factor. For example, patients with pompholyx, the most acute form of vesicular palmoplantar eczema, have been noted to have a higher incidence of both atopy and contact dermatitis than controls.

With the above caveat in mind, vesicular palmoplantar dermatitis can be divided into four categories: pompholyx, chronic vesiculobullous hand dermatitis (often mistermed *dyshidrotic hand dermatitis*), hyperkeratotic hand dermatitis, and id reactions. Some authors have grouped these conditions in the category of endogenous hand dermatitis, to distinguish them from dermatitis clearly caused by exogenous factors such as contact allergy or irritation.[1]

Pompholyx is a term best reserved for acute explosive outbreaks of small to large vesicles and bullae on the palms and soles. It tends to occur more often in the spring and fall and may be associated with stress. Other etiologic factors are less well established. Cheiropompholyx and podopompholyx are terms occasionally used to describe cases affecting the palms or soles, respectively.

Chronic vesiculobullous hand dermatitis, also known as *dyshidrotic hand eczema* or *dyshidrotic hand dermatitis,* is usually characterized by small vesicles on the inner aspects of the fingers. "Dyshidrosis," a dysfunction of the sweat gland, is disproved as a cause, but the term, unfortunately, persists.

A third category is *chronic hyperkeratotic hand dermatitis,* an entity that generally occurs on the central palms. Although vesicles do not dominate the clinical presentation, spongiosis observed histologically is indistinguishable from the other forms.

An *id reaction* is a vesiculobullous process, generally appearing on the lateral aspects of the fingers, elicited by an infection elsewhere in the body. The most common cause is a fungal infection. Treatment of the underlying cause usually leads to resolution.

Endogenous hand dermatitis can, of course, be exacerbated by exogenous factors, most notably irritant dermatitis and allergic contact dermatitis. In addition, atopy may, in some cases, predispose to the development of vesicular palmoplantar eczema.

HISTORICAL ASPECTS

The clinical presentation of an acute blistering disorder confined to the palms and the soles was first described by Fox in 1873.[1] He attributed the blisters to a disorder of the sweat gland, giving rise to the term "dyshidrosis." Not long thereafter, Hutchison[2] described acute explosive blisters on the hands, which he termed "pompholyx" from the Greek word meaning bubble.

EPIDEMIOLOGY

Differences in classification and definition have made it difficult to assess the true incidence of endogenous hand disorders and most studies have focused on the prevalence of allergic contact and irritant contact dermatitis in occupational settings.

Pompholyx is the least-common presentation of hand dermatitis; in one Swedish series, pompholyx accounted for 6 percent (51 of 827) of the cases of hand eczema.[3]

ETIOLOGY AND PATHOGENESIS

With the exception of the id reaction, a direct cause of vesicular palmoplantar hand dermatitis is rarely identified. Although previous theories about "dyshidrosis," a dysfunction of the acrosyringium, have been debunked, hyperhidrosis may be an exacerbating factor.[4] An increased number of Langerhans cells has been observed, similar to that seen in other forms of dermatitis affecting the hands.[5,6] Stress has been cited to be an exacerbating factor, and hot weather during the summer months worsens the condition.[7] Pompholyx has been reported after intravenous immunoglobulin therapy,[8,9] ingestion of piroxicam,[10] and after ingestion of certain metals in predisposed or sensitized patients.[11] There has been one case report of pompholyx occurring after implantation of a nickel-containing pacemaker in a nickel-allergic patient.[12]

EXACERBATING FACTORS

Contact allergy is common in patients affected with vesicular palmoplantar eczema, especially the chronic type, but the causal relationship is not always clear.[13] There are cases where contact allergy has exacerbated preexisting dermatitis and reports that ingestion of certain metals, including nickel, cobalt, and chromium, have caused flares. However, in other cases, the causal relationship may be the reverse[4] so that the skin's impaired barrier function in vesiculobullous hand dermatitis might, in some cases, lead to sensitization and a higher prevalence of contact dermatitis.

Investigations into the role of atopy have yielded mixed results. Some studies show levels of personal or familial atopy as high as

50 percent in affected subjects, as compared to 11.5 percent of controls,[7] but other studies demonstrate no difference in the prevalence in people with vesiculobullous hand dermatitis versus controls.[13]

GENETICS

Genetics does not appear to play a major role in hand dermatitis, with the possible exception of the genetic tendency to atopy.

PREVENTION

Prevention is a critical part of therapy in most cases, especially when known exacerbating factors are present. Avoidance of commonly encountered allergens, such as foods and plants, and irritants such as soaps, detergents, solvents, acids, and alkalis can be helpful. Modification of environmental exposure to exacerbating factors, such as friction and cold air, may also help with persistent or refractory disease.

CLINICAL MANIFESTATIONS

Vesiculobullous attacks can range from the inconvenient to the severe; rarely, it can lead to hospitalization. In true acute pompholyx, there is an explosive outbreak of deep-seated vesicles on the palms, the lateral aspects of the fingers and sometimes the soles, usually in a symmetric pattern. (Figs. 125-1 and 125-2). Discomfort and itching usually precede the development of the blisters, which have been described as having a "tapioca" appearance (Figure 125-3). Blisters may coalesce, then desiccate and resolve without rupture. Large blisters can be drained but should not be unroofed.

This phase is generally followed by desquamation of the affected areas. Individual outbreaks are usually self-limited over 2 to 3 weeks, although they may recur. Secondary bacterial infection may occur and should be treated as it may evolve into cellulitis or lymphangitis. Attacks are most common among adolescents and young adults and seem to be more common in the spring and summer months.

FIGURE 125-1

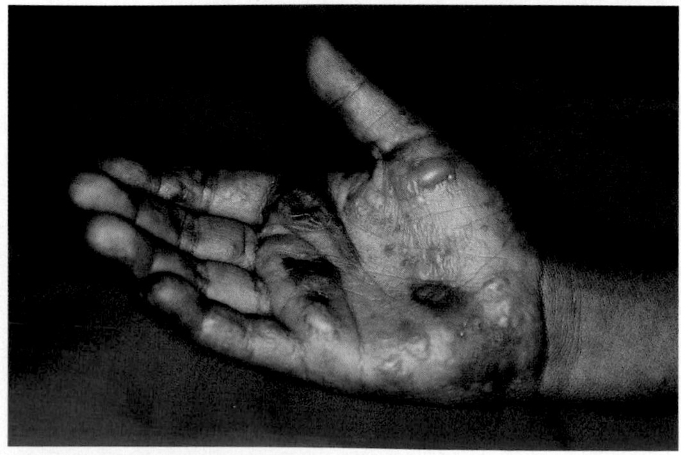

Acute pompholyx (cheiropompholyx).

FIGURE 125-2

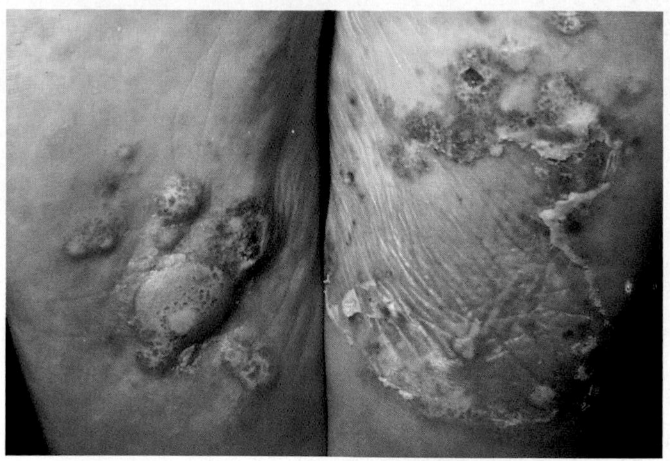

Podopompholyx.

Chronic vesiculobullous hand dermatitis is more common than true pompholyx and more difficult to manage because of its relapsing course. The clinical presentation includes small, 1- to 2-mm vesicles filled with clear fluid, on the lateral aspects of the fingers, palms, and soles (see Fig. 125-3). As the condition becomes more chronic, the clinical appearance may evolve and subsequently appear more fissured and hyperkeratotic. A clear history of vesicles or exacerbations characterized by blistering may help to narrow the classification of a given presentation of hand dermatitis.

Patients with hyperkeratotic hand dermatitis are usually male and generally present with a chronic keratotic pruritic plaques, sometimes with fissures on the central palm (Fig 125-4). This condition may be the end result of allergy, excoriation, and irritation, but generally the cause is not identifiable and contact allergy does not seem to play an important role. This type of eczema commonly occurs in middle-aged to elderly men and is normally very refractory to treatment.[14] Frictional factors or lichen simplex chronicus (neurodermatitis) may be an important factor in some cases. Plantar involvement is present in a minority of cases. In an ID reaction, erythematous vesicles usually are noted on the

FIGURE 125-3

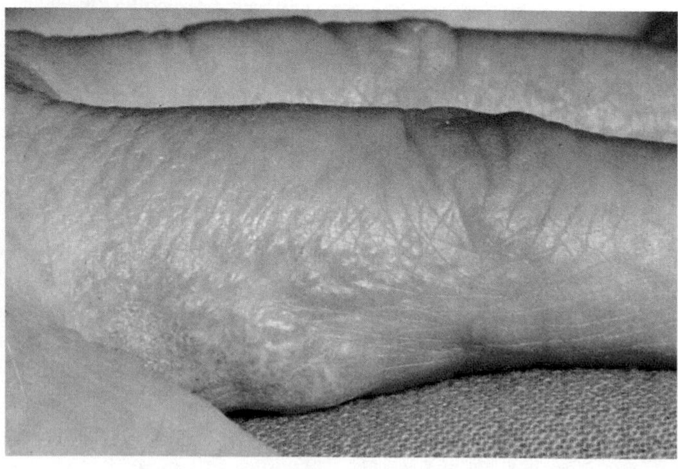

Vesiculobullous eczematous dermatitis on the lateral fingers. Note the tapioca-like, deep-seated vesicles on the sides of the fingers.

FIGURE 125-4

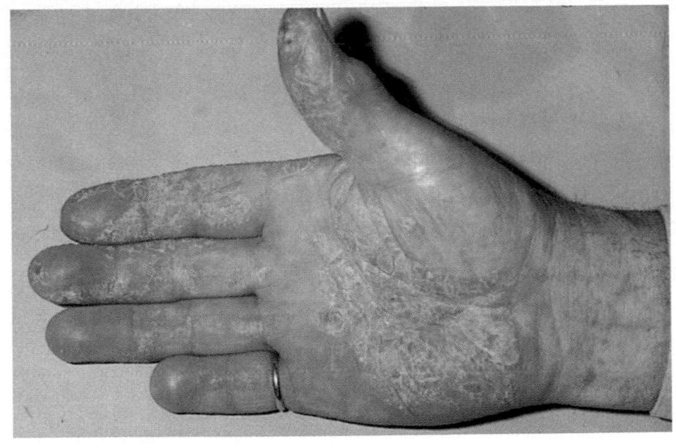

Hyperkeratotic hand eczema.

lateral aspects of the fingers and the palms in the setting of a distant inflammatory reaction (Figs 125-5). The vesicles are usually pruritic and resolve with treatment of the underlying condition.

LABORATORY FINDINGS

There are no distinctive laboratory findings characteristic of vesicular palmoplantar eczema, although IgE levels may be elevated in atopic patients.

PATHOLOGY

The histology of these entities depends on the chronicity of the disease. The primary vesicle appears as an intraepidermal spongiotic vesicle that does not involve the acrosyringia[15] on both conventional and electron microscopy. Lymphocytic infiltration is common in the epidermis with a mixed infiltrate observed in the dermis. In more chronic cases, the epidermis may show hyperproliferation, hyperkeratosis, or even psoriasiform epidermal hyperplasia. PAS (periodic acid–Schiff) staining can be helpful in excluding fungal elements.

FIGURE 125-5

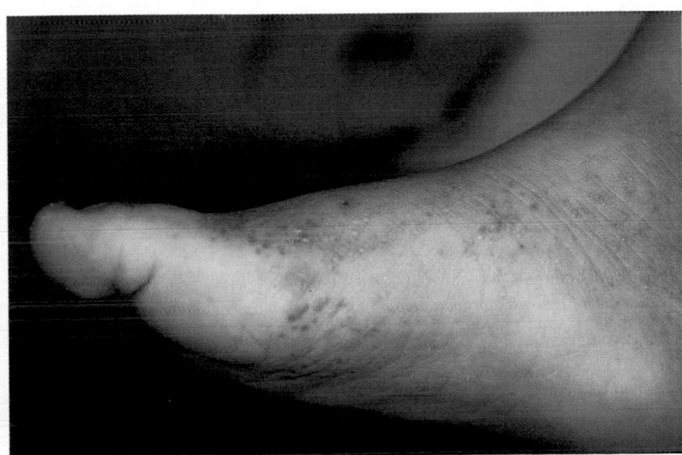

Id reaction to tinea infection.

DIAGNOSIS AND DIFFERENTIAL DIAGNOSIS

The diagnosis of vesiculobullous hand dermatitis is usually made on the basis of clinical presentation, history, and, sometimes, histology. Patch testing may be useful in helping to distinguish this entity from other palmoplantar disorders or in eliminating other exacerbating factors such as irritant exposure and contact allergy.

There are many other skin conditions of the hands and feet that can be difficult to distinguish from vesiculobullous hand dermatitis. Several of these diagnoses may coexist.

Differential Diagnoses

Allergic contact dermatitis may be clinically indistinguishable from constitutional forms of hand eczema, and patch testing should always be performed in those with recurrent, atypical, or persistent forms of the disease. Common allergens include nickel, potassium dichromate, rubber, fragrances, formaldehyde, and lanolin.

Irritant contact dermatitis is by far the most common hand dermatitis and is often exacerbated by occupational exposures. It is usually symmetric, chronic, and affects the dorsal fingertips and web spaces.

Atopic hand dermatitis is associated with a number of factors: hand dermatitis before age 15 years, persistent eczema on the body, dry or itchy skin in adult life, and widespread atopic dermatitis in childhood. The backs of the hands, particularly the fingers are affected with erythema, vesiculation, crusting, excoriation, and scale.

Infections, most commonly from tinea,[16] can mimic endogenous hand dermatitis. In cases of asymmetric or atypical cases, or in cases of small vesicles confined to the feet, a potassium hydroxide exam may be useful in ruling out primary tinea infection.

In chronic cases of hand dermatitis, fungal and bacterial infections may be superimposed and treatment may result in improvement in clinical symptoms.

Herpes simplex may, in unusual cases, present as blisters on the hands.[17]

Bazex's acrokeratosis paraneoplastica is a rare, acute, erythematous, scaling vesiculobullous hand dermatitis with nail dystrophy associated with neoplasia, usually squamous carcinomas of the upper digestive and respiratory tracts, although there have been some reports of similar findings in patients with colon cancer and genitourinary tumors.

Psoriasis and *psoriasiform hand dermatitis* are most prominent over pressure points. Psoriasis can normally be distinguished by its sharply marginated, nummular, or circinate scaly plaques; the silvery scales; and the presence of psoriasis elsewhere. Psoriasiform hand dermatitis can occur without a family or personal history of psoriasis. It is a diagnosis made primarily on clinical and histologic presentation. At times, however, it appears as though eczematous, hyperkeratotic, and psoriatic diatheses coexist. Repeated pressure or friction may cause hyperkeratosis in some individuals.

Pustular hand dermatitis is generally easy to distinguish because, unlike the presentation of uninfected vesiculobullous hand dermatitis, pustules are the primary lesion. For example, in pustular psoriasis, the vesicles are cloudy and painful.

Keratolysis exfoliativa (recurrent focal palmar peeling), is a chronic asymptomatic noninflammatory peeling of the palms and soles, most commonly during the summer months. It is thought to occur more frequently in people with hyperhidrosis in these areas. Scaling usually starts from one to two fine points and expands outward to larger circular areas. The asymptomatic condition is usually self-limited, requiring only emollients.

Other blistering diseases, such as pemphigoid, pemphigus, or epidermolysis bullosa, may affect the hands and feet, but usually do so in the setting of blisters elsewhere on the body.[18]

TREATMENT AND PROGNOSIS

Treatment of vesiculobullous hand dermatitis should be based on the acuity of the condition, the severity of the disease, the prominence of blisters versus chronic changes, and any relevant history that reveals possible cofactors. There are few published, randomized, controlled therapeutic studies of hand dermatitis; thus, most therapy is empiric.

Topical Therapy

Topical glucocorticoids, usually of high potency, remain the mainstay of treatment. They are often more effective if used under occlusion, although this approach may increase the chance of infection. Topical drying agents such as Domeboro soaks, Burrow's solution (aluminum subacetate), or dilute potassium permanganate solution (1:8000) may be useful in acute forms with a predominance of vesicles. Newer therapies include topical tacrolimus and pimecrolimus.

For maintenance, frequent ointment applications and avoidance of irritants are generally helpful. Vinyl gloves, rather than latex, are recommended because of the risk of either having an underlying allergy or of developing one in the setting of impaired barrier function. Tap-water iontophoresis with pulsed direct current showed no benefit in time to improvement for subjects with hand dermatitis over controls, but those who were treated had much longer remissions by a factor of months.[19,20] Hyperkeratotic palmar eczema is notoriously difficult to manage. In addition to potent topical glucocorticoids, intralesional glucocorticoids may prove to be of some benefit. Retinoids, keratolytics in high concentrations, and tar preparations are also used.

Systemic Therapy

For pompholyx, oral steroids may be required and are often effective. However, because of their side effects, they are inappropriate for long-term management. Large blisters may need to be drained and bacterial superinfection may require treatment with systemic antibiotics.

Other treatments for severe cases have included UVB, systemic, topical and bathwater PUVA, and UVA1.[21–23] For severe cases, systemic immunosuppressives have been tried, including low-dose methotrexate,[24] mycophenolate mofetil,[25] and cyclosporine[26] in doses ranging from 2.5 to 5.0 mg/kg. Superficial radiotherapy (Grenz ray) is still used at a few centers. This condition may be one of the last indications for this treatment modality, although there is controversy as to its efficacy in double-blind studies.[27,28]

Disulfiram (200 mg per day for 8 weeks) was used in an open-label study to treat a small group of women with nickel allergy as chelation therapy and resulted in improvement in 10 women.[29] The role of ingested allergens in provoking vesicular hand eczema remains controversial. Patients with troublesome and persistent vesicular palmar eczema who are found to be allergic to substances that may be ingested may benefit from elimination diets.

For the hyperkeratotic variant of hand dermatitis, treatment can be exceedingly challenging. If topical glucocorticoid options fail, acitretin may be of benefit, and success with cyclosporine has been reported.

Two severity indices, the dyshidrosis area and severity index (DASI)[30] and the total sign and symptoms score (TSS), have been validated and may prove useful in clinical trials to better assess the effectiveness of some of these approaches.

For id reactions, treating the underlying condition is the most useful intervention, and should result in the resolution of the lesions. The same treatments described above may also be helpful.

Pompholyx tends to occur as intermittent explosive outbreaks, which fortunately, become less frequent with middle age. The more chronic forms of vesicular palmoplantar eczema, however, are much more persistent and frustrating to manage and often require multiple therapeutic approaches over time.

REFERENCES

1. Epstein E: Hand dermatitis: Practical management and current concepts. *J Am Acad Dermatol* **10**:395, 1984
2. Hutchinson J: Cheiropompholyx. *Lancet* **1**:630, 1876
3. Agrup GG: Hand eczema and hand dermatoses in south Sweden. *Acta Derm Venereol* **49**(suppl 61):1, 1969
4. Yokozeki H et al: The role of metal allergy and local hyperhidrosis in the pathogenesis of pompholyx. *J Dermatol* **19**:964, 1992
5. Rosen K: Pustulosis palmoplantaris and chronic eczematous hand dermatitis. Treatment, epidermal Langerhans cells and association with thyroid disease. *Acta Derm Venereol Suppl (Stockh)* **137**:1, 1988
6. Rosen K et al: Epidermal Langerhans' cells in chronic eczematous dermatitis of the palms treated with PUVA and UVB. *Acta Derm Venereol* **69**:200, 1989
7. Lodi A et al: Epidemiological, clinical and allergological observations on pompholyx. *Contact Dermatitis* **26**:17, 1992
8. Iannaccone S et al: Pompholyx (vesicular eczema) after i.v. immunoglobulin therapy for neurologic disease. *Neurology* **53**:1154, 1999
9. Ikeda K et al: Pompholyx after IV immunoglobulin therapy for neurologic disease. *Neurology* **54**:1879, 2000
10. Youn JI et al: Piroxicam photosensitivity associated with vesicular hand dermatitis. *Clin Exp Dermatol* **18**:52, 1993
11. Fisher AA: Hand dermatitis resembling pompholyx in nickel sensitive patients. *Cutis* **47**:157, 1991
12. Landwehr HA, Vanketel KG: Pompholyx after implantation of a nickel-containing pacemaker in a nickel-allergic patient. *Contact Dermatitis* **9**:147, 1983
13. Lehucher-Michel MP et al: Dyshidrotic eczema and occupation: A descriptive study. *Contact Dermatitis* **43**:200, 2000
14. Hersle K, Mobacken H: Hyperkeratotic dermatitis of the palms. *Br J Dermatol* **107**:195, 1982
15. Kutzner H et al: Are acrosyringia involved in the pathogenesis of "dyshidrosis"? *Am J Dermatopathol* **8**:109–116, 1986
16. Nakagawa T et al: Trichosporon cutaneum (*Trichosporon asahii*) infection mimicking hand eczema in a patient with leukemia. *J Am Acad Dermatol* **42**:929, 2000
17. Parker RK, Guin JD: Hand eczema herpeticum. *Cutis* **52**:227–228, 1993
18. Barth JH et al: Palmo-plantar involvement in auto-immune blistering disorders—Pemphigoid, linear IgA disease and herpes gestationis. *Clin Exp Dermatol* **13**:85, 1988
19. Wollina U et al: Therapy of hyperhidrosis with tap water iontophoresis. Positive effect on healing time and lack of recurrence in hand–foot eczema. *Hautarzt* **49**:109, 1998
20. Odia S et al: Successful treatment of dyshidrotic hand eczema using tap water iontophoresis with pulsed direct current. *Acta Derm Venereol* **76**:472, 1996
21. Behrens S et al: PUVA-bath photochemotherapy (PUVA-soak therapy) of recalcitrant dermatoses of the palms and soles. *Photodermatol Photoimmunol Photomed* **15**:47, 1999
22. Schmidt T et al: UVA1 irradiation is effective in treatment of chronic vesicular dyshidrotic hand eczema. *Acta Derm Venereol* **78**:318, 1998
23. Davis MD et al: Topical psoralen-ultraviolet A therapy for palmoplantar dermatoses: Experience with 35 consecutive patients. *Mayo Clin Proc* **73**:407, 1998
24. Egan CA et al: Low-dose oral methotrexate treatment for recalcitrant palmoplantar pompholyx. *J Am Acad Dermatol* **40**:612, 1999

25. Pickenacker A et al: Dyshidrotic eczema treated with mycophenolate mofetil. *Arch Dermatol* **134**:378, 1998
26. Granlund H et al: Comparison of cyclosporine and topical betamethasone-17,21-dipropionate in the treatment of severe chronic hand eczema. *Acta Derm Venereol* **76**:371, 1996
27. Lindelof B et al: A double-blind study of Grenz ray in chronic eczema of the hands. *Br J Drematol* **117**:77, 1987
28. Cartwright PH, Nowell NR: Comparison of Grenz rays versus placebo in the treatment of chronic hand eczema. *Br J Dermatol* **117**:73, 1987
29. Kaaber K et al: Antabuse treatment of nickel dermatitis. Chelation—A new principle in the treatment of nickel dermatitis. *Contact Dermatitis* **5**:221, 1979
30. Vocks E et al: The Dyshidrotic Eczema Area and Severity Index—A score developed for the assessment of dyshidrotic eczema. *Dermatology* **198**:265, 1999

SECTION 17

SKIN CHANGES DUE TO MECHANICAL AND PHYSICAL FACTORS

CHAPTER 126

Gérald Piérard
Isabelle Fumal
Claudine Piérard-Franchimont

Cold Injuries

The human capacity for physiologic adaptation to cold is minimal. This may cause problems because seasonal changes in the outdoor environment are quite prominent even in the temperate zone of the world. In this context, skin is important in preserving homeostasis between the body and its environment. One of its main roles is thermoregulation, where cutaneous blood flow and the resulting skin temperature may vary widely in order to help preserve the core body temperature.[1,2] There are physiologic, behavioral, and environmental factors that predispose to skin alterations following cold exposure.

PHYSIOLOGIC RESPONSE TO COLD

Core body temperature is maintained within a narrow range by thermoregulatory mechanisms that rely largely on control of the cutaneous blood flow. Arteriovenous anastomoses are abundant in acral areas, and they regulate the blood volume that passes through the skin. When the skin is cooled, there is usually an immediate acute shutdown in the amount of blood that flows to the surface. These events result in changes in skin temperature, heat loss, and color. Skin reactivity and the anatomic pattern of blood supply differ in the skin of newborns, adults, and older people. For instance, a reticulate appearance of cooled skin is a common finding in young infants (Fig. 126-1).

The parallel arrangement of large arteries and veins in the limbs allows countercurrent exchange of heat. Vasoconstriction due to cold results in shunting of blood from the superficial to the deep venous system, and heat is transferred from arteries to veins. Thus the blood going to the acral part of the limbs is precooled, and less heat is lost to the environment. With such thermoregulation, the body can maintain a constant core temperature of approximately 37°C over a range of external temperatures between 15 and 54°C.

Normally, the skin is to some extent adapted to a cooler environment than the 37°C of internal organs. With the presence of many cold-adapted enzymes, the skin may even function more effectively when slightly cooled. In the case of adipose tissue, mild chronic exposure to cooling may lead to a progressive better insulation. Chronically cold-exposed skin also develops a more efficient system for shunting blood away from the surface. These adaptive mechanisms are most flexible during the first years of life. Tissues in the aged are less able to develop new shunts.

The body fluid balance is affected by prolonged cold exposure, leading to hemoconcentration, extracellular fluid expansion, and diuresis. Increased sympathetic nerve activity and release of histamine can be observed. A reduction in plasma volume is, in part, due to venoconstriction and raised intracapillary pressure, which lead to enhanced filtration of intravascular fluid into the interstitium. In cold water, this is counteracted to some extent by hydrostatic forces. An interesting feature of winter swimmers is rapid rewarming of the interscapular region, providing circumstantial evidence that winter swimming may improve cold tolerance through nonshivering thermogenesis. The effect of cold water swimming following the extreme heating of the sauna[3] is somewhat comparable to the threat of accidental cold water immersion. Well-being in both groups and survival in the latter group largely depend on the degree of subcutaneous insulation. Overweight persons, as well as those who are well clothed, survive prolonged accidental cold water exposure.[4]

Viscosity of fluids increases as temperature decreases. However, blood is a nonnewtonian fluid exhibiting thixotropy, by which it

FIGURE 126-1

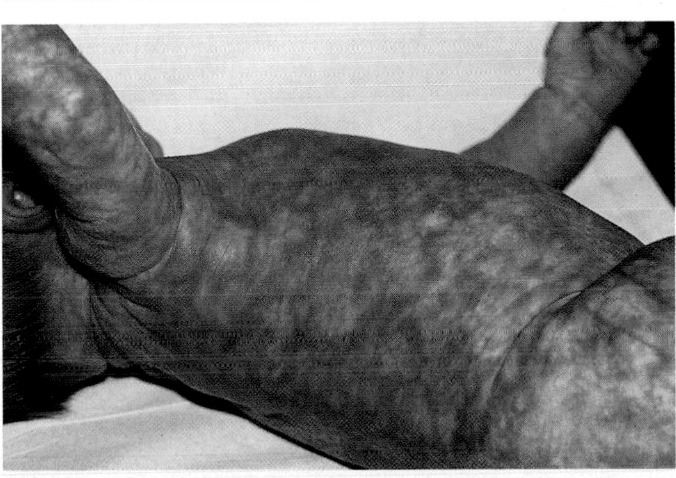

Reticulate appearance of cooled skin in the newborn due to the anatomic pattern of the blood supply and factors influencing flow, such as arteriolar vasoconstriction and the increased viscosity of cooled blood.

becomes less viscous with increasing flow velocity independent of temperature. This effect is strongly influenced by hematocrit and by packing of erythrocytes. Normally, rouleau formation maintains some flexibility of the erythrocyte columns, but defects in erythrocyte flexibility, such as are present in sickle cell anemia, can lead to severe disturbances of flow, especially in slow-flow conditions. Disordered erythrocyte flexibility can present as a decrease in the sedimentation rate. In persons who suffer from inflammatory diseases and a blood sedimentation rate lower than 2 mm/h, erythrocyte flexibility disorders should be considered. Such a situation is not uncommon in patients suffering from cold disorders. Macrophages also can block capillaries when developing pseudopods as a result of reduced flow. The combination of slow flow and leukocyte conformational changes is, in part, a physiologic process enabling these cells to migrate through the endothelial lining.[5] Other factors affecting blood viscosity include increased platelet adhesiveness, changes in concentrations of proteins, and the presence of abnormal proteins. Fibrinogen level is particularly important.

To some extent the skin becomes stiffer when cooled. The deformability and elasticity of the epidermis and dermis, and especially the capacity of the adipose tissue to dissipate the distorting forces of compression, are altered. These physical changes may influence the clinical signs of skin cold injuries. The interplay of these factors with a global depression of metabolism determines the normal skin response to cold and influences the related pathologic manifestations.

THERMOREGULATION AND HUNTING REACTION

Local and systemic thermoregulation is complex. A group of neurons of the hypothalamus responds directly to temperature. When the temperature decreases, the rate of discharges decreases. From this brain temperature-sensitive area, signals radiate to various other portions of the hypothalamus to control either heat production or heat loss. Stimuli that influence the autonomic nervous system, such as painful stimulation, mental stress, arousal stimuli, and deep breaths, can all produce cutaneous vasoconstriction in warm subjects but vasodilation in cold subjects.[6] The extent and direction of cutaneous vasomotor reflex responses depend therefore on skin temperature. Furthermore, the responses in the hands may differ from simultaneous responses in the feet, suggesting that there is spatial organization of vasomotor control. The response of the skin to cooling in atopic dermatitis and in disorders of sympathetic control often differ from normal.[7] Indeed, neuromediators synthesized and released by cutaneous cells play a prominent role in these regulations.

Cold exposure produces an initial massive cutaneous vasoconstriction, resulting in a fall in skin temperature. This change serves to maintain core temperature, but at the expense of the skin. Conversely, cold-induced vasodilation represents a protective mechanism against skin necrosis. This physiologic reflex, known as the *hunting reaction of Lewis,* involves transient cyclic vasodilation caused by the opening of arteriovenous anastomoses.[8] For instance, when a finger is immersed in water at 0°C, an initial drop in skin temperature to 2 to 4°C is followed by a rise of 7 to 13°C. With continued cold exposure, the temperature drops again, and the cycle is repeated over and over, especially in people acclimatized to cold, who have rapid cycling times and higher final skin temperatures. When core temperature is threatened, the hunting phenomenon ceases, and vasoconstriction persists.[7]

COLD, WIND, AND HUMIDITY

A cold environment can be a threat to the skin, with a subsequent fall in core body temperature. Many physiologic, behavioral, and environmental factors predispose to the global effects of cold injuries. Marked increases in convective, conductive, or radiant heat loss are responsible for the immediate effects of cold exposure. For instance, touching of metal objects considerably increases conductive cooling. Other predisposing factors increasing heat loss and/or decreasing heat production and clothing insulation make people especially susceptible to cold.[9]

There is ample evidence that the effect of low temperature on skin biology is, in part, a function of environmental humidity, wind speed, and altitude. In these respects, the wind chill index is indicative of the convective heat loss. Its value affects the gradients of temperature and water content across the stratum corneum, resulting in an imbalance in condition between outer and deeper epidermal layers.[10] High altitude, which reduces the oxygen supply to tissues, also contributes to increasing the skin damage induced by cold.

Environmental absolute humidity is a key factor for cold injuries. This parameter indicates the mass of water vapor present in a unit volume of the atmosphere, unlike relative humidity (RH), which is the ratio of the quantity of water vapor present in the atmosphere to the quantity that would saturate it at the actual temperature. An accurate representation of the amount of moisture in the air as a function of temperature is given by the calculation of the dew point,[11] which is defined as the temperature of the air at which the gaseous moisture begins to condense, i.e., when RH reaches 100 percent.

Poor clothing insulation is a common reason for cold injuries. The insulation can be insufficient when clothing is too light, wet, tight, permeable to wind, or inadequate to cover the cold sensitive body parts. Individual factors predisposing to cold injuries are physical injuries, leanness, inadequate behavior, low physical fitness, fatique, dehydration, previous cold injuries, sickness, trauma, poor peripheral circulation, tight constrictive clothing, and old age.[9] Newborns, the elderly, and individuals with impaired mental faculties remain the most vulnerable. Severity of damage is often increased by alcohol, smoking, and psychotropic drug intake.

Severe cold injuries have always represented a dramatic threat to human history. In particular, they have affected the outcome of battles and wars.[12,13] American troops at Valley Forge during the winter of 1777 were endangered more by the cold than by the British army. During the Napoleonic wars, the Grand Army of France lost more than four-fifths of its troops in the Russian campaign primarily due to cold injuries. During World War I, the British recorded about 115,000 cases of frostbite and trench foot. The number of casualties declined after the winter of 1916 with the enforcement of disciplinary measures including a second pair of dry socks, mandatory arrangements for drying socks, and time provided for sock changes. During World War II, American cold casualties were greater than 90,000 in the European theater alone, and only 15 percent of these soldiers returned to combat. Approximately one-third of these casualties had trench foot, and one-third had frostbite. In the Korean War, about 9000 cold casualties occurred, most of which were frostbite. Peacetime military operations also may be responsible for similar threats.[14]

Today, cold injuries are becoming more prevalent among the general population.[15] Many cases are associated with alcohol consumption, homelessness in urban centres, and car breakdown. Frostbite also prevails in winter sport enthusiasts, such as cross-country skiers and backpackers who get lost or trapped in a snowstorm.[2,16–18]

Adaptation to cold protects one from responding inappropriately, and a moderate degree of exposure to cooling might be health-promoting by stimulating a responsive and protective vasculature. In contrast, individuals who have experienced severe cold injury may have a profoundly delayed or abolished hunting reaction in the affected limbs.[19] They are rendered more susceptible to recurrent cold injury with pain, hyperesthesia, or paresthesia.[20] Some of these subjects also have coldness of the skin, which is very persistent and probably related to a functional imbalance in the sympathetic nervous system resulting from increased α-adrenergic receptor density or affinity for norepinephrine.[21] In addition, changes of vascular structure may cause reduced vasocompliance subsequent to cold exposure. In addition, there may be impairment of normal vascular reflexes to a series of stimuli including deep inspiration, venous occlusion, neck cooling, and ipsilateral skin cooling.[21]

BIOMETROLOGY APPLIED TO COLD EXPOSURE

Objective and quantitative assessments of the skin following cold exposure are possible using a series of biometrologic methods. Standardization of measuring conditions and procedures is required for skin temperature and blood flow assessments.

Thermography is the measurement and recording of the temperature at the skin surface. Contact and noncontact devices are available. The most popular methods are based on thermal conductance and infrared or microwave thermography. They suffer from relatively poor sensitivity.

The most widely used method to assess skin blood flow relies on laser-Doppler flowmetry. This method is designed to provide a continuous noninvasive measurement of microvascular perfusion in terms of relative changes in blood volume and velocity. The method is based on the effect of the light on moving erythrocytes and static components of a limited volume of tissue. Laser-Doppler imaging was designed to overcome contact measurements and spatial variability. These devices are based on the laser-Doppler principle, and data are collected without touching the skin. They generate a color-coded image of tissue perfusion. Photoplethysmography, using red or infrared emitting diodes, is well correlated with laser-Doppler velocimetry. It consists of a continuous recording of light intensity scattered by the skin. The signal is generated by the amount of blood present in a given skin area. The higher the hemoglobin content, the higher is the amount of light that is absorbed. Hence the method is sensitive to blood volume. The velocity of erythrocytes also may influence the readings through changes in the optical transmittance due to changes in their orientation relative to their speed.

CLASSIFICATION OF SKIN COLD INJURIES

Freezing and nonfreezing injuries basically can be distinguished according to the severity and duration of chilling. However, the nature of damage caused depends on many variables other than the actual temperature. Skin conditions caused by cold temperature are not uncommon. Recognition is generally easy at a clinical level, but awareness of the much less common underlying disorders is important. Treatment, both physical and pharmacologic, is aimed at keeping the body warm and maintaining vasodilation.

Frostbite is the consequence of extreme and prolonged freezing conditions. In addition, the whole body may cool down so much that life-threatening hypothermia may ensue. This condition can occur in many regions of the world. It is an especially important concern among people who enjoy cold weather sports, particularly in mountains and circumpolar regions. Prompt recognition and treatment are of paramount

FIGURE 126-2

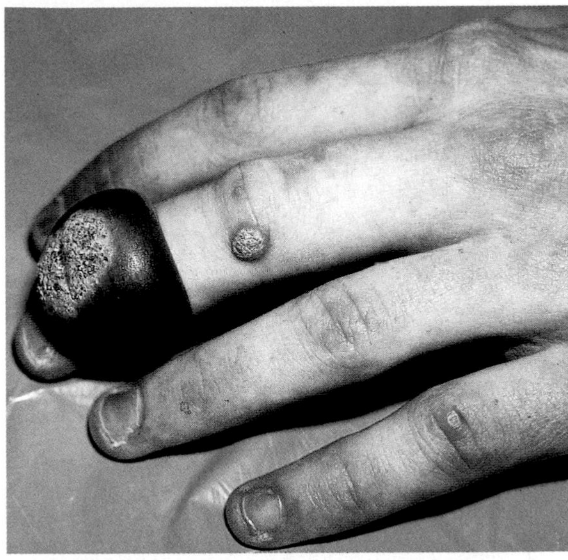

Necrosis of the skin induced by freezing a wart with liquid nitrogen.

importance because many hypothermia victims can recover from very low body temperatures. Treatment in an adequate medical facility can make the difference between full recovery and lifelong problems. Even if someone appears to be dead from exposure to cold, resuscitative efforts should be started and continued until the proper core body temperature is reached.[15]

Extreme and often conductive heat loss at a given body site freezes the tissues and results in localized blistering and necrosis (Fig. 126-2). Several cutaneous disorders also occur when the tissue temperature is maintained just above freezing for long periods. These conditions include chilblains, cold urticaria, cold panniculitis, erythrocyanosis, and acrocyanosis, among others. This may be a consequence of impaired blood flow, reduced sensory perception, or a change in the physical properties of components of the tissues, such as may occur in adipose tissue.

Minor but chronic cold exposure combined with environmental desiccation may have profound effects on the biology of the epidermis. As a result, winter xerosis develops.[22,23] Persistent erythema of the face and the hands is not a rare finding (Fig. 126-3).

FROSTBITE

Frostbite occurs when tissue freezes after exposure to extreme cold air, liquids, or metals. The clinical effects of accidental injury that leads to death of tissues are similar to those caused by cryosurgery.[24] The components of tissue that may lead to damage when frozen are water, with formation of ice crystals at 0°C, and lipids such as fat globules or cell membrane constituents.

The rate of freezing determines the focus of freezing injury.[25] The extracellular formation of ice occurs most commonly with slow freezing, whereas fast freezing tends to produce intracellular ice. The formation of ice crystals in the extracellular space alters the osmotic properties of the tissues and disturbs the flow of water and electrolytes across the

FIGURE 126-3

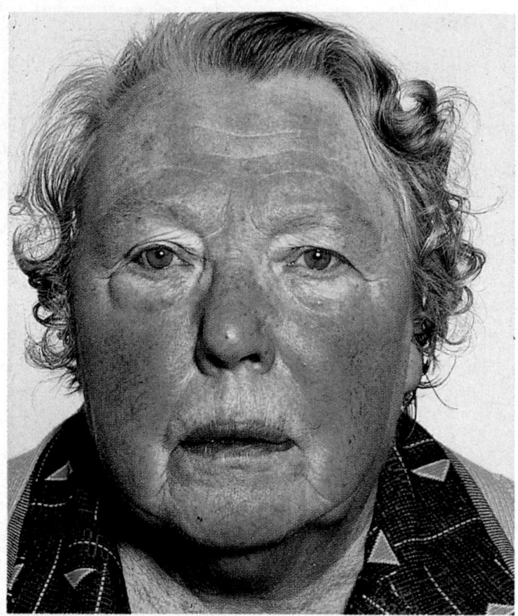

Facial redness in a person exposed to temperate climate with cold winters.

cell membranes. Thawing may be as damaging as the freezing itself, and repeated freeze and thaw cycles, as may occur in accidental injury, compound the injury, making available more water, which rapidly provides intracellular flooding. The rewarming rate is also important. In slow rewarming, ice crystals become larger and more destructive. Cells are also exposed to a high concentration of electrolytes for a longer period than with rapid rewarming.

As the body cools, there is a reflex constriction of the arteries and veins in the extremities. This results in increased venous pressure, decreased capillary perfusion, and sludging. Cooling also creates a left shift in the oxygen dissociation curve, and hemoglobin gives up its oxygen less readily. These two conditions result in hypoxia and damage to the capillaries and surrounding tissue. Oxygen tension is further decreased by thrombus formation in the microvasculature resulting in arteriovenous shunting. Arterial and arteriolar constriction, mediated by sympathetic outflow, initiates and probably maintains circulatory impairment. In addition, segmental vascular necrosis occurs in areas of erythrostasis, suggesting that ultimate damage may depend more on insufficient clearance of toxic substances than on initial vasoconstriction.

Cell types vary in their susceptibility to cold injury. Melanocytes are very sensitive to cold, and damage may occur at −4 to −7°C. This sensitivity explains the hypopigmentation that follows cryotherapy. In addition, it appears that black persons are more susceptible to frostbite than whites. Nerve axons are also easily damaged by cold, and nerve injury may occur with axonal degeneration of large myelinated fibers. Autonomic fibers are also affected, and this may account for the abnormal sweating and cold sensitivity that follow nonfreezing cold injury.[26,27] Nerve sheaths are quite resistant to cold, as are bone and cartilage.[19] Desolidification of lipids in adipose tissue and disruption of endothelial cells lining blood vessels and lymphatics, with secondary disturbances of permeability and blood flow, are other consequences of severe cold. In the overall assessment, there are marked similarities in the pathologic processes to those seen in thermal burns and in ischemia-perfusion injuries.

TABLE 126-1

Consequences of Cold Injuries

1. Arterial and arteriolar vasoconstriction
2. Excessive venular and capillary vasodilation
3. Increased endothelial leakage
4. Erythrostasis
5. Arteriovenous shunting
6. Segmental vascular necrosis
7. Massive thrombosis

Three stages of cooling are recognized. The first is massive vasoconstriction, which causes a rapid fall in skin temperature. In a second step, the hunting reaction follows with a cyclic rise and fall in skin temperature. If cold exposure continues, the third stage of freezing occurs as the skin temperature falls to approach ambient temperature. The events that ensue in freezing and nonfreezing cold injuries are similar.[12,28] They are listed in Table 126-1.

Frosbite usually affects a finger, toe, ear, nose, or cheek. The clinical presentation of frostbite falls into three categories corresponding to mild frostbite or frostnip, superficial frostbite, and deep frostbite with tissue loss.

Frostnip involves only the skin and causes no irreversible damage. There is sensation of severe cold progressing to numbness followed by pain. Erythema is usually present on the cheeks, ears, nose, and extremities (Fig. 126-4). There is no edema or bleb formation. Frostnip is the only form of frostbite that can be treated safely in the field with first aid measures.

Superficial frostbite involves the skin and immediate subcutaneous tissues. It includes the previously described signs but with progression of pain subsiding to feelings of warmth. This is a sign of severe involvement. The skin has a waxy appearance, but deeper tissues remain soft and resilient. Clear blebs form, accompanied by edema and erythema, within 24 to 36 h after thawing. Lesions may become eroded (Fig. 126-5).

Deep frostbite extends to the deep subcutaneous tissue. The injured skin becomes white or bluish white with a variable degree of anesthesia. Most often the affected skin becomes deceptively pain-free, and the discomfort of feeling cold vanishes. The tissue is totally numb, indurated with immobility of joints and extremities. Muscles may be paralyzed. Nerves, large blood vessels, and even bone may be damaged. Large

FIGURE 126-4

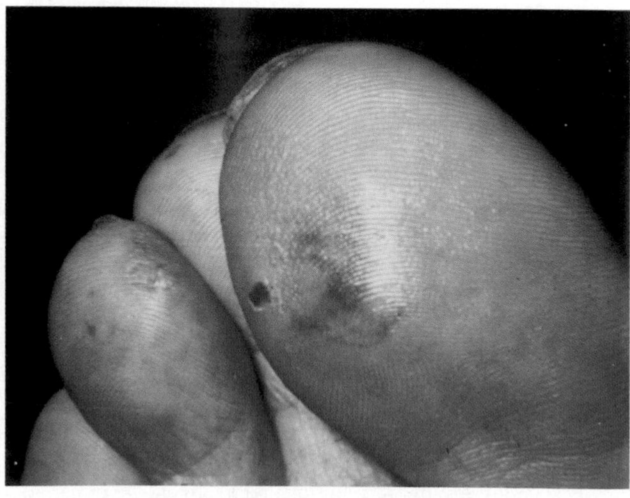

Frostnip.

FIGURE 126-5

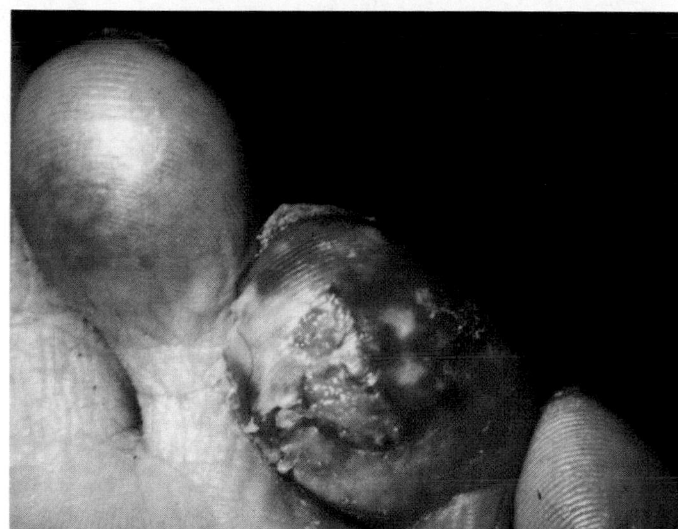

Superficial frostbite.

blisters form 1 to 2 days after rewarming, and they can be classified according to depth, as in heat-induced burns. Frostbite blister fluid contains high amounts of prostaglandins, including prostaglandin F_{2a} and thromboxane A_2. These mediators may contribute to increased vasoconstriction, platelet aggregation, leukocyte adhesiveness, and ultimately progressive tissue injury. The blister fluid begins to be resorbed within 5 to 10 days, leading to formation of hard, black gangrene. Weeks later, a line of demarcation occurs, and the tissues distal to the line undergo autoamputation.

Preparation is the key to protecting individuals from the effects of cold weather; and frostbite, frostnip, and hypothermia always should be taken seriously.[25,29] Prognostic factors are listed in Table 126-2. Nonmedicated ointments are traditionally used for protection against facial frostbite without evidence of their benefit. The thermal insulation they provide is indeed minimal. Protective emollients seem to cause a false sensation of safety, leading to an increased risk of frostbite, probably through neglect of efficient protective measures.[30,31] However, in less extreme conditions, some specific topical formulations bring beneficial effects.[32]

TABLE 126-2

Prognostic Signs of Frostbite

Good prognostic signs	Large, clear blebs extending to the tips of the digits
	Rapid return of sensation
	Rapid return of normal (warm) temperature to the injured area
	Rapid capillary filling time after pressure blanching
	Pink skin after rewarming
Poor prognostic signs	Hard, white, cold, insensitive skin
	Cold and cyanotic skin without blebs after rewarming
	Dark hemorrhagic blebs
	Early evidence of mummification
	Constitutional signs of tissue necrosis, such as fever and tachycardia
	Cyanotic or dark red skin persisting after pressure
	Freeze-thaw-refreeze injury

SOURCE: From ref. 12 with permission.

The first consideration in frostbite treatment is to be aware that the victim may be suffering from hypothermia.[33] Because of the difficulty in assessing the depth of frostbite injury, conservative waiting after the frostbite episode is often encouraged to try to delineate the extent of tissue loss. Barring this, the main principles are to avoid trauma, friction, pressure, massaging with snow, and refreezing. Slow rewarming increases tissue damage, and therefore, rapid rewarming is the keystone of treatment.[14] It should be performed in a water bath no warmer than 40 to 42°C until the most distal part is flushed. Large amounts of analgesics may be required. The damaged part should be elevated, and blisters should be left intact. Surgical debridement is often delayed by 1 to 3 months after demarcation. However, triple-phase bone scans, magnetic resonnace imaging, and magnetic resonance angiography can be used to predict ultimate tissue loss and to assess the possibility of earlier surgical intervention.[28,34,35]

There is no uniformly accepted protocol for other measures allegedly beneficial in the treatment of frostbite injury. Intraarterial reserpine and sympathectomy have been used to reverse vasospasm, which may contribute to tissue loss. Their role is controversial, although some patients have benefited from the therapy. To counteract vasoconstriction caused by local release of inflammatory mediators, topical aloe vera, which inhibits thromboxane synthetase, and systemic ibuprofen, which inhibits cyclooxygenase, have been advocated. In addition, several adjunctive therapies, including vasodilators, thrombolysis, and hyperbaric oxygen, are sometimes useful. Tetanus toxoid should be given in case of open wounds.

Sequelae of frostbite include hypersensitivity to cold and hyperhidrosis.[26] Squamous cell carcinoma is a rare outcome, usually on the heel 20 to 30 years later. Epiphyseal plate damage or premature fusion may occur in children. Premature fusion can result in shortened digits, joint deviation, and dystrophic nails. In addition, frostbite arthritis, resembling osteoarthritis, may occur weeks to years later.

NONFREEZING COLD INJURY AND DAMPNESS

Nonfreezing cold injury occurs when tissues are cooled to temperatures between about 15°C and their freezing point for prolonged periods. This type of injury, which is exacerbated by dampness, has claimed numerous casualties in warfare.[12,13] Nonfreezing cold injury may be followed by cold sensitivity and hyperhidrosis, which may persist for years.

During World War I, trench foot was identified as a separate entity. Wet conditions at temperatures above freezing and limb dependency due to immobility and constrictive footwear were important pathogenic factors. Three stages were described. Stage I consisted of initial erythema, edema, and tenderness. Stage II followed within 24 h with paresthesia, marked edema, numbness, and sometimes blisters. Stage III corresponded with progression to a usually superficial gangrene. Immersion foot was described in shipwreck survivors during World War II. It was similar to trench foot clinically and followed four phases corresponding to exposure, prehyperemia, hyperemia, and posthyperemia.

Tropical immersion foot was described during the Pacific campaign in World War II. Occurring after exposure to the warm, wet conditions of jungle warfare, this condition differed from classic trench foot and immersion foot by causing less tissue destruction, numbness, and anesthesia and by yielding quicker complete recovery. The role of temperature

FIGURE 126-6

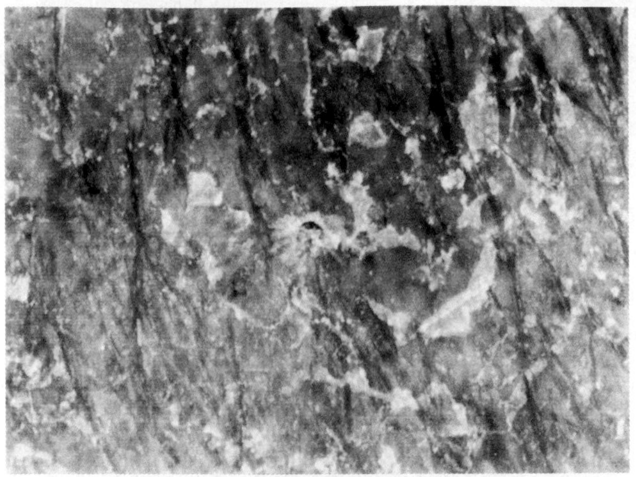

Winter xerosis observed under ultraviolet light.

in tropical immersion foot is unclear and may not be important.[36] As with trench foot and immersion foot, prevention is most important.

Another specific condition known as "pulling-boat hands" was described as erythematous macules and plaques present on the dorsum of the hands and fingers of sailors aboard rowboats.[37] Small vesicles developed later, accompanied by itching, burning, and tenderness. These individuals were exposed to long periods of high humidity, cool air, and wind, an ideal setting for the development of nonfreezing cold injury. In addition, hours of vigorous rowing daily provided repetitive hand trauma.

WINTER XEROSIS

Many subjects present with dryness of the skin, particularly on the lower extremities, during wintertime. The hands, forearms, cheeks, lips, and trunk also may be affected. Itch, a dry appearance, chapping, and cracking of the stratum corneum are more or less prominent (Fig. 126-6). The condition is markedly influenced by cold environments, especially in combination with low humidity.[21,22] Predisposing factors include atopic dermatitis, ichthyosis, and increasing age. Excessive washing exacerbates winter xerosis. Indeed, irritant dermatitis of the hands worsens in a cold and dry environment.[38] Emollients and improvement in the environmental temperature and humidity are helpful in controlling this skin condition.

ACROCYANOSIS

Acrocyanosis is a bilateral dusky, mottled discoloration of the entire hands, feet, and sometimes the face. It is persistent and accentuated by cold exposure. When the temperature is very low, the skin may be bright red. Trophic changes and pain do not occur, and pulses are present. This condition must be distinguished from Raynaud's phenomenon, which is clearly episodic and often segmental, as well as from obstructive arterial disease.

Acrocyanosis is genetically determined and usually starts in adolescence. Chronic vasospasm of small cutaneous arterioles or venules with a secondary dilatation of the capillaries and subpapillary venous plexus has been postulated. Stasis in the papillary loops with aneurysmal dilatation at the tips redistributes blood flow to the subpapillary venous plexus. The blood flow may be compromised by altered erythrocyte flexibility, increased platelet adhesiveness, and other plasma viscosity factors.

FIGURE 126-7

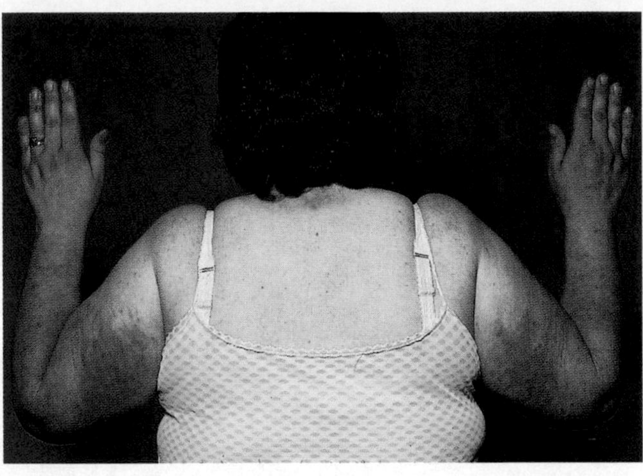

Erythrocyanosis of plump upper arms of a woman.

Acrocyanotic tissues are less sclerotic than in Raynaud's phenomenon. They contain twisted collagen fibrils and large pericytes. In cases developing for the first time late in life, a search for an underlying myeloproliferative disorder should be performed. Remittent necrotizing acrocyanosis is associated with enhanced susceptibility to cooling and pain, as well as ulceration and gangrene of the fingers. Arteriolar occlusion may occur by thrombi or intima proliferation.

There is no curative treatment for acrocyanosis. Supportive measures to keep the skin warm are helpful.

ERYTHROCYANOSIS

Erythrocyanosis is a dusky cyanotic discoloration, worse in winter, that occurs over areas with a thick layer of subcutaneous fat (Fig. 126-7). The condition is seen most often on the lower legs and thighs of adolescent girls and middle-aged women. Nodular lesions similar to chilblains may occur and have been described in women with severe erythrocyanosis and paraplegia. Keratosis pilaris, angiokeratomas, and telangiectases are commonly associated (Fig. 126-8). Spontaneous improvement often occurs after a few years. However, the disease may persist with longstanding edema and fibrosis.

Warm clothes and weight reduction are important to decease the insulating effect of the subcutaneous fat, which is responsible for a chronically lower skin temperature. The outcome remains unpredictable.

CHILBLAINS

Chilblains, also called *pernio* or *perniosis* (Fig. 126-9*A*), are localized inflammatory lesions caused by continued exposure to cold above the freezing point.[39] Dampness and wind that increase cold conductivity and convection play a part. Absolute temperature is less important than cooling of nonadapted tissue. The condition shows a genetic predisposition. It has been described most often in temperate regions, where

FIGURE 126-8

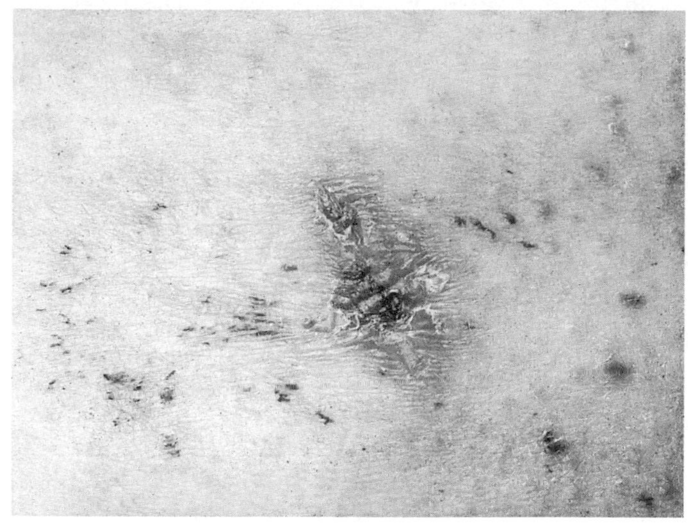

Angiokeratomas occurring on the upper arm of erythrocyanotic skin of the patient shown in Fig. 126-7.

winters are occasionally cold and damp. Chilblains are seen less often in very cold climates, where well-heated houses and warm clothing are essential. Both acrocyanosis and chilblains appear to be more common in children, women, and persons with low body mass. As such, anorexia nervosa is a predisposing factor. Spontaneous healing is common when spring arrives, and relapse is frequent on the following winters. However, chilblains do not always occur at the time of maximum cold.

Chilblains develop acutely as single or multiple, burning, erythematous, or purplish swellings. Patients may complain of itching, burning, or pain. In severe cases, blisters (see Fig. 126-9*B*), pustules, and ulceration may occur. Characteristic locations include the proximal phalanges of the fingers and toes and the plantar surfaces of the toes, heels, nose, and ears. Lesions usually resolve in 1 to 3 weeks but may become chronic in elderly people with venous stasis. Tight garments such as gloves, stockings, and shoes are especially to be avoided where there is also peripheral vascular disease. A papular form of chilblains resembles erythema multiforme and occurs at all times of the year, usually as crops on the sides of the fingers,[40] often superimposed on a background of acrocyanosis.

A peculiar clinical presention may occur in young women riding horses for several hours daily during winter.[41,42] Indurated red to violet tender plaques develop on the lateral calves and thighs (see Fig. 126-9*C*). The condition is quite similar to the nodular perniotic lesions described in adolescent girls with erythrocyanosis. With respect to prophylaxis, experienced riders usually wear baggy breeches that give insulation and are not tight enough to compromise the circulation.

Perniotic lesions have been described in association with myeloproliferative disorders,[43] probably as a consequence of blood flow changes, presence of cold agglutinins, and altered inflammatory response on cooling.

Idiopathic perniosis is characterized histologically by edema of the papillary dermis and by superficial and deep perivascular lymphocytic infiltrates. Necrotic keratinocytes and lymphocytic vasculitis also have been reported. Thickening of blood vessel walls with intimal proliferation may lead to obliteration of the vascular lumen.[44]

Chilblain lupus is a distinct disease similar to discoid lupus erythematosus.[45] Lupus pernio is a variant of sarcoidosis.

Unfamiliarity of physicians with chilblains sometimes gives rise to unnecessary hospital admissions with expensive laboratory and radiologic evaluations and, at times, hazardous therapy. The most important point in management is prophylaxis with adequate, loose, insulating clothing and appropriate warm housing and workplace. Maintaining the blood circulation by avoiding immobility is also helpful. A short course of ultraviolet light at the beginning of winter was a tradition that has been challenged.[46] Once chilblains occur, treatment is symptomatic with rest, warmth, and topical antipruritics. Calcium channel inhibiting drugs may be effective in the treatment of severe recurrent perniosis.[47] However, headache and flushing are troubling to some patients. In cases of crippling severity, thyrocalcitonin and hemodilution may be helpful.

COLD URTICARIA AND POLYMORPHOUS COLD ERUPTION

Cold urticaria (Fig. 126-10) occurs at sites of localized cooling, usually when the area is rewarmed. It may be idiopathic or associated with some serologic abnormality.[48] It accounts for about 2 percent of cases of urticaria.

Most cases fall into the group of essential cold urticaria. They can be subdivided into a rare familial type and an acquired form. IgE and, more rarely, IgM have been implicated in the pathogenesis. The antigen is likely a normal metabolite produced on exposure to cold. Histamine is one of the most important mediators, but leukotrienes, platelet-activating factor, and others have been incriminated. In this disease, exposure to cold causes prolonged edematous swellings, often with headache, fever, arthralgia, and leukocytosis. Swelling of the oral mucosa and esophagus may occur on ingestion of cold liquids. A rather distinctive combination of cold urticaria with dermographism or with cholinergic urticaria is not uncommon. Alarming signs resembling histamine shock are responsible for loss of consciousness. Death may occur while swimming in cold water.

Familial cold urticaria is a rare autosomal dominant condition with onset at an early age. Urticaria develops when the patient is exposed to generalized cooling, particularly chilling wind, rather than local cold application. The delayed type of familial cold urticaria is characterized by localized angioedema developing 9 to 18 h after cold exposure.

Cold urticaria may occur in 3 to 4 percent of patients with cryoglobulinemia, and it also may be associated with cold agglutinins, cryofibrinogens, and cold hemolysins. Cold urticaria has been reported in cases of infectious mononucleosis in association with either cryoglobulins or cold agglutinins, but such occurrences are rare. *Helicobacter pylori* could be involved as a causative agent in some cases of acquired cold urticaria.[49]

Diagnosis of cold urticaria is confirmed by placing an ice cube wrapped in a plastic bag on the skin of the forearm for periods varying from 30 s to 10 min. Weals form on rewarming. Sometimes water at 7°C is more effective because it presumably causes less severe vasoconstriction.

Cold erythema seems to be a related disorder with erythema and pain but without urticaria. Familial polymorphous cold eruption is a rare autosomal dominant disease characterized by childhood-onset, nonpruritic, erythematous eruptions often accompanied by influenza-like symptoms after generalized exposure to cold, a negative ice-cube test, and leukocytosis. The pathogenesis remains unknown. The disease frequently has been referred to as familial cold urticaria, although the skin lesions are not urticarial.[50]

Avoiding cold wind exposure and swimming in cold water are important preventive measures. Antihistamines lower the clinical signs. Desensitization to cold is possible by immersing one arm on a daily basis into water at 15°C for 5 min.

FIGURE 126-9

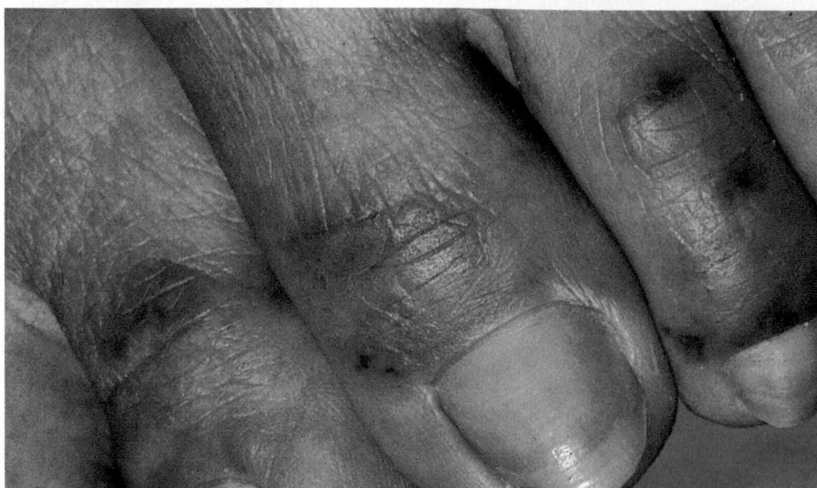

A.

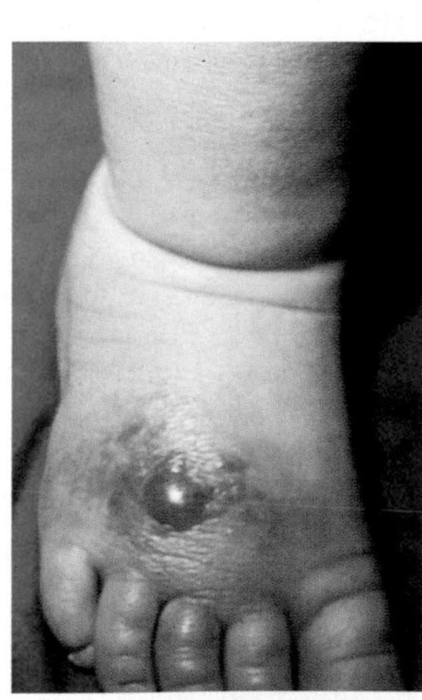

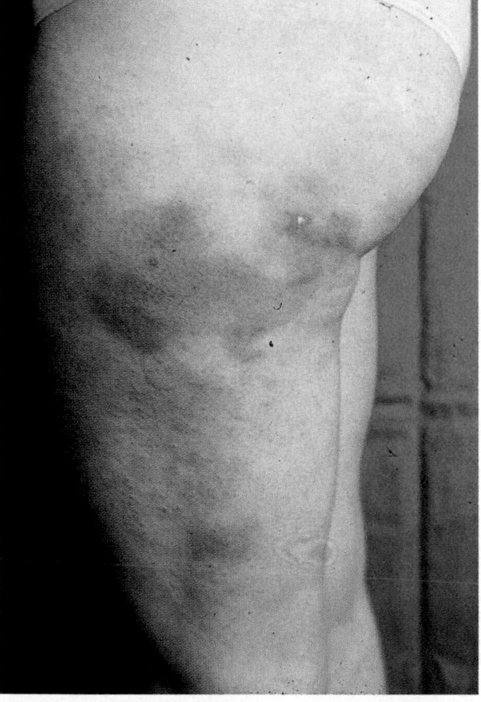

B. C.

Chilblains are common at such sites as the hands and feet when they are exposed to both cooling and tight garments. *A.* Chilblains on the toes. *B.* Chilblains on the dorsum of the foot. Children and the elderly are most commonly affected, perhaps because they take less care to protect themselves from cooling. *C.* Equestrian chilblains from horse riding on a cold morning with inadequate clothing.

COLD PANNICULITIS AND RELATED ENTITIES

Cold injuries may affect the subcutaneous tissue in different ways. The freezing injury in deep frostbite results in tissue gangrene. Nonfreezing injuries also can alter the hypodermis. Among them, cold panniculitis is more common in children than in adults. It affects the cheeks and legs most commonly. Tender erythematous subcutaneous nodules appear 1 to 3 days after exposure and subside spontaneously within 2 to 3 weeks. Ice-cube challenge to the child's skin for 10 min results in the development of an erythematous plaque 12 to 18 h later.

A perivascular mixed infiltrate with neutrophils, lymphocytes, and histiocytes is present at the dermal subcutaneous junction after 24 h, followed by a well-developed panniculitis at 48 to 72 h. Some lipocytes are necrotic. They rupture to form cystic spaces, and the reaction subsides completely by 2 weeks. Infants have a higher content of saturated fatty acids in adipose tissue than do adults, and this may result in solidification at lower temperatures.[51] Cold panniculitis should be distinguished from other related disorders, including erythrocyanosis with nodules, sclerema neonatorum, and subcutaneous fat necrosis of the newborn.

SCLEREMA NEONATORUM AND SUBCUTANEOUS FAT NECROSIS OF THE NEWBORN

Sclerema neonatorum and subcutaneous fat necrosis of the newborn are distinct disorders involving the subcutaneous fat of the newborn. Infant fat differs from adult fat by having a higher saturated to unsaturated fatty acid ratio, resulting in solidification at a higher temperature. Prematurity and immature enzyme systems may result in a relative inability to desaturate fatty acids, altering the ratio further. Sepsis, dehydration, chilling, infection, and other stresses also may inhibit the enzyme system. Thus infants in general and premature or otherwise compromised newborns in particular are susceptible to such disorders.

Sclerema neonatorum is a rare disorder characterized by diffuse, rapidly spreading hardening of the skin and subcutaneous tissue of infants. It starts on the buttocks and trunk, usually in the first week of life. Palms, soles, and scrotum are spared. Fifty percent of affected infants are premature. They have difficulty feeding, are lethargic, and many are otherwise debilitated. Septicemia is frequent, and the prognosis is poor. Cold exposure does not seem to be important in the etiology of sclerema neonatorum; however, similar clinical findings have been seen in cases of primary cold injury. It seems likely that sclerema neonatorum results from the effect of severe illness and prematurity on the desaturating enzyme system in neonatal fat, resulting in an exaggeration of the usual saturated to unsaturated fatty acid ratio in infants. The subcutaneous layer is greatly thickened by enlarged fat cells and wide, fibrous bands. There is no fat necrosis, and many of the fat cells contain fine needle-like clefts.[52]

Treatment of sclerema neonatorum involves correcting dehydration and electrolyte imbalance and treating possible septicemia. The value of systemic glucocorticoids is controversial. Successful treatment with exchange transfusions has been reported.[53]

Subcutaneous fat necrosis of the newborn is characterized by discrete red to violaceous mobile plaques and nodules that usually appear within a few days of birth. The back, thighs, and cheeks are affected most commonly. Fat necrosis and crystallization are the hallmarks of the

FIGURE 126-10

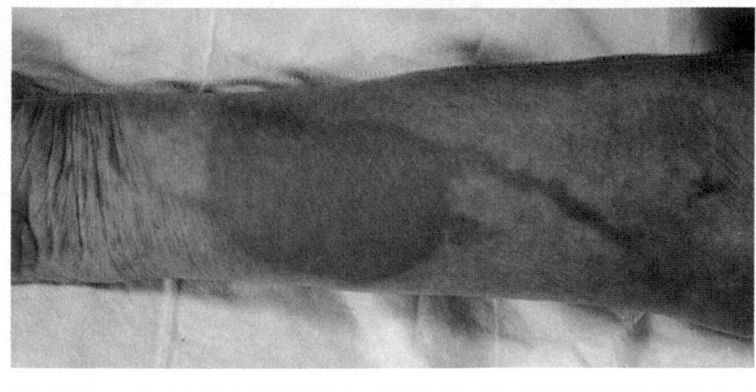

Cold urticaria induced by the application of ice to the skin.

disease. There may be a granulomatous inflammatory response with foci of calcification. In most cases, the condition is benign and self-limited, although it has been associated with hypercalcemia and death.[54]

As in sclerema neonatorum, there is no clear etiologic relationship to cold, and the etiology is likely multifactorial. It has been postulated that an underlying defect in fat composition, poor nutrition, and various physical stresses such as hypothermia may be important.

ERYTHROMELALGIA

Erythromelalgia is a rare chronic cutaneous disorder characterized by erythema, burning discomfort, and warmth of the extremities. Its pathogenesis and histopathologic characteristics have not yet been clearly identified.[55–58] Vasoconstriction apparently precedes reactive hyperaemia, similar to that seen in Raynaud's phenomenon. An early-onset type and an adult-onset type have been recognized. When the extremity is lowered or heat is applied, the pain is intensified. The application of cold or elevation of the extremity has the opposite effect of decreasing the pain. Idiopathic erythromelalgia may be due to increased thermoregulatory arteriovenous shunt flow.[56] Secondary erythromelalgia is associated commonly with myeloproliferative syndrome–related thrombocythemia and is mostly evident in the adult-onset condition.

Treatment for adults with erythromelalgia includes a single daily dose of acetylsalicylic acid, but children who have no associated underlying disorder find little to no relief with the drug.

RAYNAUD'S PHENOMENON (See Chap. 173)

CRYOGLOBULINEMIA (See Chap. 177)

LIVEDO RETICULARIS (See Chap. 167)

REFERENCES

1. Page EH, Shear NH: Temperature-dependent skin disorders. *J Am Acad Dermatol* **18**:1003, 1988
2. Claes G et al: La peau, le froid et les sports d'hiver. *Rev Med Liege* **56**:257, 2001
3. Kauppinen K: Sauna and winter swimming. *Arct Med Res* **47**:71, 1989
4. Keatinge WR et al: Exceptional case of survival in cold water. *BMJ* **292**:171, 1986
5. Schmid Schoenlein GW: Activated leukocytes and endothelium in chronic venous insufficiency. *Phlebology* **10**(suppl 1):90, 1995
6. Oberle J et al: Temperature-dependent interaction between vasoconstrictor and vasodilator mechanisms in human skin. *Acta Physiol Scand* **132**:149, 1988
7. Hornstein OP, Heyer G: Responses of skin temperature to different thermic stimuli. *Acta Derm Venereol (Stockh)* **144**(suppl):149, 1989
8. Dana AS Jr et al: The hunting reaction. *Arch Dermatol* **99**:441, 1969
9. Rintamaki H: Predisposing factors and prevention of frostbite. *Int J Cicumpolar Health* **59**:114, 2000
10. Piérard-Franchimont C et al: Skin surface patterns of xerotic legs: The flexural and accretive types. *Int J Cosmet Sci* **23**:121, 2001
11. Paquet F et al: Sensitive skin at menopause: Dew point and electrometric properties of the stratum corneum. *Maturitas* **28**:221, 1998
12. Corbett DW: Cold injuries. *J Assoc Milit Dermatol* **8**:34, 1982
13. Francis TJR: Nonfreezing cold injury: A historical review. *J R Nav Med Serv* **70**:134, 1984
14. Taylor MS: Cold weather injuries during peacetime military training. *Mil Med* **157**:602, 1992
15. Murphy JV et al: Frostbite: Pathogenesis and treatment. *J Trauma Injury Infect Crit Care* **48**:171, 2000
16. Miller BJ, Chasmar LR: Frostbite in Saskatoon: A review of 10 winters. *Can J Surg* **23**:423, 1980
17. Fritz RL, Perrin DH: Cold exposure injuries: Prevention and treatment. *Clin Sports Med* **8**:111, 1989
18. Foray J: Mountain frosbite: Current trends in prognosis and treatment (from results concerning 1261 cases). *Int J Sports Med* **13**(suppl 1):193, 1992
19. Burge S et al: Effect of freezing the helix and rim or edge of the human and pig ear. *J Dermatol Surg Oncol* **10**:816, 1984
20. Cooke E et al: Reflex sympathetic dystrophy and repetitive strain injury: Temperature and microcirculatory changes following mild cold stress. *J R Soc Med* **86**:69, 1993
21. Arvesen A et al: Skin microcirculation in patients with sequelae from local cold injuries. *Int J Microcirc Exp* **14**:335, 1994
22. Middleton JB, Allen BM: The influence of temperature and humidity on stratum corneum and its relation to skin chapping. *J Soc Cosmet Chem* **24**:239, 1974
23. Piérard-Franchimont C, Piérard GE: Beyond a glimpse at seasonal dry skin: A review. *Exog Dermatol* **1**:3, 2002
24. Dawber RPR: Cold kills. *Clin Exp Dermatol* **13**:138, 1993
25. Gage AA: What temperature is lethal for cells? *J Dermatol Surg Oncol* **5**:459, 1979
26. Irwin MS et al: Neuropathy in non-freezing cold injury (trench foot). *J R Soc Med* **90**:433, 1997
27. Ervasti O et al: Sequelae of moderate finger frostbite as assessed by subjective sensations, clinical signs, and thermophysiological responses. *Int J Circumpolar Health* **59**:137, 2000
28. Kibbi AG, Tannous Z: Skin diseases caused by heat and cold. *Clin Dermatol* **16**:91, 1998
29. Hamlet MP: Prevention and treatment of cold injury. *Int J Circumpolar Health* **59**:108, 2000
30. Lehmuskallio E: Emollients in the prevention of frostbite. *Int J Circumpolar Health* **59**:122, 2000
31. Lehmuskallio E et al: Thermal effects of emollients on facial skin in the cold. *Acta Derm Venereol (stockh)* **80**:203, 2000
32. Claes G, Piérard GE: Biometrological assessment of skin protectors against moderate cold threat. *Exog Dermatol* **1**:92, 2002
33. Hirvonen J: Some aspects on death in the cold and concomitant frostbites. *Int J Circumpolar Health* **59**:131, 2000
34. Mehta RC, Wilson MA: Frostbite injury: Prediction of tissue viability with triple-phase bone scanning. *Radiology* **170**:511, 1989
35. Barker JR et al: Magnetic resonance imaging of severe frostbite injuries. *Ann Plast Surg* **38**:275, 1997
36. Taplin D et al: The role of temperature in tropical immersion foot syndrome. *JAMA* **202**:210, 1967
37. Toback AC et al: Pulling boat hands: A unique dermatosis from coastal New England. *J Am Acad Dermatol* **12**:649, 1985

38. Uter W et al: An epidemiological study of the influence of season (cold and dry air) on the occurrence of irritant skin changes of the hands. *Br J Dermatol* **138**:266, 1998
39. Goette DK: Chilbain (perniosis). *J Am Acad Dermatol* **23**:257, 1990
40. Wesagowit P et al: Papular perniosis mimicking erythema multiforme: The first case report in Thailand. *Int J Dermatol* **39**:527, 2000
41. Dowd PM et al: Nifedipine in the treatment of chilblains. *BMJ* **293**:923, 1986
42. Beacham BE et al: Equestrian cold panniculitis in women. *Arch Dermatol* **116**:1025, 1980
43. Kelly JW, Dowling JP: Pernio: A possible association with chronic myelomonocytic leukemia. *Arch Dermatol* **121**:1048, 1985
44. Wall LM, Smith NP: Perniosis: A histopathological review. *Clin Exp Dermatol* **6**:263, 1981
45. Doutre MS et al: Chilblain lupus erythematosus: Report of 15 cases. *Dermatology* **184**:26, 1992
46. Langtry JAA, Diffey BL: A double-blind study of ultraviolet phototherapy in the prophylaxis of chilblains. *Acta Derm Venereol (stockh)* **69**:320, 1989
47. De Silva BD et al: Equestrian perniosis associated with cold agglutinins: A novel finding. *Clin Exp Dermatol* **25**:285, 2000
48. Wanderer AA: Cold urticaria syndromes: Historical background, diagnostic classification, clinical and laboratory characteristics, pathogenesis, and management. *J Allergy Clin Immunol* **85**:965, 1990
49. Kranke B et al: *Helicobacter pylori* in acquired cold urticaria. *Contact Dermatitis* **44**:57, 2001
50. Urano Y et al: An unusual reaction to cold: A sporadic case of familial polymorphous cold eruption? *Br J Dermatol* **139**:504, 1998
51. Lowe LB Jr: Cold panniculitis in children. *Am J Dis Child* **115**:709, 1968
52. Kellum RE et al: Sclerema neonatorum. *Arch Dermatol* **97**:372, 1968
53. Fretzin DF, Arias AM: Sclerema neonatorum and subcutaneous fat necrosis of the newborn. *Pediatr Dermatol* **4**:112, 1987
54. Thomsen RJ: Subcutaneous fat necrosis of the newborn and idiopathic hypercalcemia. *Arch Dermatol* **116**:1155, 1980
55. Cohen JS. Erythromelalgia: New theories and new therapies. *J Am Acad Dermatol* **43**:841, 2000
56. Mork C et al: Microvascular arteriovenous shunting is a probable pathogenic mechanism in erythromelalgia. *J Invest Dermatol* **114**:643, 2000
57. Mork C, Kvernebo K: Erythromelalgia: A mysterious condition? *Arch Dermatol* **136**:406, 2000
58. Davis MD et al: Natural history of erythromelalgia: Presentation and outcome in 168 patients. *Arch Dermatol* **136**:330, 2000

CHAPTER 127

Robert Sheridan

Evaluation and Management of the Thermally Injured Patient

Despite increased awareness and focused prevention measures, burn injury remains a significant source of mortality and a major source of morbidity in the general population. The prognosis of those who do suffer serious burn injury has improved dramatically over the past 20 years, largely because of a recognition of the importance of early wound excision and biologic closure.[1,2] The epidemiology of the injuries remains age specific in that the very young and the very old are at higher risk. Hot liquid is the injury agent in approximately 70 percent of pediatric burns, whereas a similar proportion of adults are injured by flame in the home or in the workplace. Although smoke alarms, tap water temperature limits, and other prevention strategies have had significant impact, the basic epidemiology has not changed over many years. This chapter provides a general overview of the management of the burned patient, with attention to our growing understanding of the pathophysiology of the injury.

NATURAL HISTORY AND PATHOPHYSIOLOGY

The development of an envelope of skin was a crucial component of the adaptation of aquatic sea animals to the land environment. The vapor and fluid barrier created by the epidermal layer facilitates the maintenance of fluid and electrolyte homeostasis within very narrow limits. The dermis provides strength and flexibility, and the reactive dermal vasculature facilitates control of internal body temperature within very narrow limits. The appendages provide lubrication and prevent desiccation. All of these critical functions are lost when substantial areas of the skin are burned.

There is both a local and a systemic response to the burn wound. The local response consists of coagulation of tissue with progressive thrombosis of surrounding vessels in the zone of stasis over the first 12 to 48 postinjury hours. An ability to truncate this secondary microvascular injury and its associated tissue loss is a major area of ongoing investigation. In larger burns, a systemic response develops that is driven initially by release of mediators from the injured tissue, with a secondary diffuse loss of capillary integrity and accelerated transeschar fluid losses. This systemic response is subsequently fueled by byproducts of bacterial overgrowth within the devitalized eschar.

Burn wounds are initially clean but are rapidly colonized by endogenous and exogenous bacteria. As bacteria multiply within the eschar over the days following injury, proteases result in eschar liquefaction and separation. This leaves a bed of granulation tissue or healing burn, depending on the depth of the original injury. In patients with large wounds involving 40 percent or more of the body surface, the local infectious challenge generally cannot be localized by the immune system with resulting systemic infection. This explains the rare survival of patients managed in an expectant fashion with burns of this size.

The systemic response to injury is characterized clinically by fever, a hyperdynamic circulatory state, increased metabolic rate, and muscle catabolism. This stereotypical response to injury has been retained by all mammalian species. It is effected by a complex cascade of mediators, including changes in hypothalamic function resulting in increases in glucagon, cortisol, and catecholamine secretions; deficient gastrointestinal barrier function with translocation of bacteria and their byproducts into the systemic circulation; bacterial contamination of the burn wound with systemic release of bacteria and bacterial byproducts; and some element of enhanced heat loss via transeschar evaporation.[3] It is likely that this response has significant survival value, but control of some of the adverse aspects of this response, particularly muscle catabolism, is an active area of ongoing investigation.

INITIAL EVALUATION OF THE BURNED PATIENT

The tendency to allow the burn wound to distract one from the performance of an organized and complete evaluation should be vigorously avoided, as many burn patients have sustained concurrent injuries. Ideally, the evaluation is done in a warm environment, as such patients are highly likely to become hypothermic. The most important component of the initial evaluation involves assessment and maintenance of airway patency. Airway resistance increases as the fourth power of the radius, and, particularly in small children, airway edema sufficient to cause obstruction can occur rapidly after the inhalation of noxious chemicals and superheated air. In equivocal cases, flexible bronchoscopy will allow for accurate assessment of the need for endotracheal intubation. Secure venous access, via the central or the peripheral approach, will allow for administration of adequate resuscitative fluids and reliable medication delivery. In children suffering from profound hypovolemia secondary to burn shock, intravenous access can be difficult, and temporary intraosseous access will allow for administration of initial resuscitative fluids. A functioning nasogastric tube will prevent acute gastric dilation, which can lead to emesis and aspiration. Placement of a bladder catheter permits accurate assessment of the adequacy of urine output, an important guide to fluid resuscitation. The core temperature should be monitored frequently.

An organized and complete burn-specific secondary survey should follow the initial evaluation, again not allowing the wound to distract the examiner from a complete examination. This survey should include a complete history, vital signs, a detailed physical examination, and selected laboratory and radiographic studies. Often, an accurate history can be obtained in the emergency department only from the rescuing emergency medical personnel, highlighting the importance of attention to this detail during the initial evaluation. Important details of history include the mechanism of injury, past medical and surgical history, time of the last meal, status of tetanus immunization, medications, and allergies. Vital signs should be interpreted in an age-appropriate fashion.

Neurologic status should be carefully evaluated at first presentation. Patients with serious burns often become obtunded over the succeeding hours and days because of fluid shifts and the need for analgesics and sedatives. If the injury mechanism is consistent with a possible head injury, central nervous system imaging should be performed. The head and neck should be carefully inspected for other injuries. The corneal epithelium should be examined prior to the development of adnexal edema, which will make the examination more difficult. Topical fluorescein staining will facilitate an accurate evaluation of the corneal epithelium. Upper airway edema should be suspected if there are perioral or intraoral burns, carbonaceous sputum, or a hoarse voice. A clinical judgment must be made regarding the need for endotracheal intubation to guard the airway. Often, flexible bronchoscopy will facilitate this decision making.

The torso should be examined for the adequacy and symmetry of breath sounds and the presence of abdominal distention or tenderness. The abdomen should be imaged if the mechanism of injury is such that an intraabdominal injury is a possibility. Gastric distention is very common, particularly in smaller children, and nasogastric decompression should be performed at this time. Nasogastric tube position and functioning should be regularly verified during the subsequent hours. Gastric ulcer prophylaxis should be instituted at this time.

The status of peripheral perfusion should be verified at initial presentation and throughout the subsequent 48 h. Blood flow may be compromised by intracompartmental edema in patients with very deep thermal burns or electrical injuries, but more commonly it is compromised by overlying circumferential eschar that will not stretch as underlying soft tissue swells. Ideally, compromised perfusion is detected by monitoring the flow in low-pressure distal vasculature, such as the palmar arch or digital vessels, rather than by monitoring the presence of radial or pedal pulses. This is because the tissue pressure is lower than the mean arterial pressure in these large vessels, and it is possible to have flow detectable by Doppler in these higher pressure vessels with ischemic soft tissues distally. If peripheral perfusion is compromised by overlying eschar, escharotomies should be performed (Figure 127-1). It can be very difficult to detect the presence of intracompartmental pressure elevations in obtunded burn patients. When compartments become firm on serial examination, decompression should be done in the operating room. Selected patients may be followed with serial compartment pressure measurements, acknowledging the risk of seeding compartments by performing such measurements through burn. Most can be adequately evaluated with careful serial clinical examination.

The wound is evaluated after higher priority evaluations are complete. The wound should be assessed for depth, size, and circumferential components. It is difficult to estimate burn depth accurately on initial examination, as most injuries will become deeper in the 24 h following injury because of progressive microvascular thrombosis at the margins

FIGURE 127-1

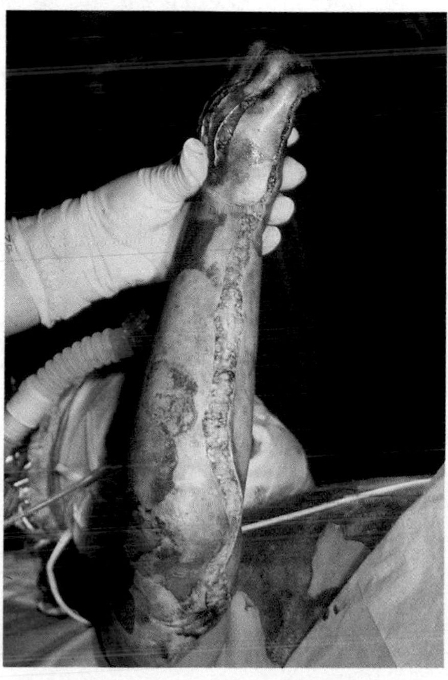

If peripheral perfusion is compromised by overlying eschar, escharotomies should be performed.

FIGURE 127-2

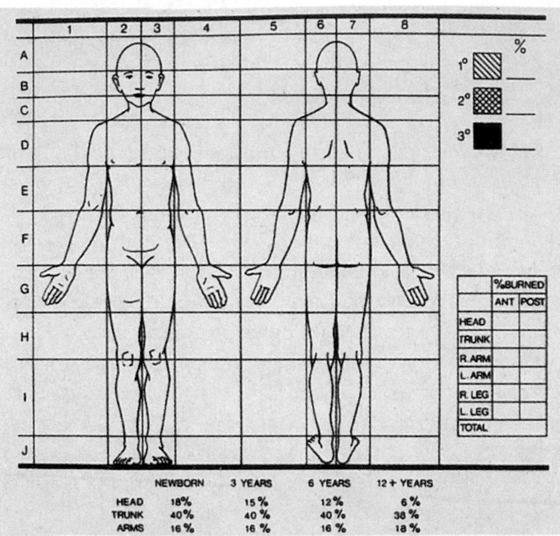

An age-specific burn diagram should be used to determine total burn size.

of the zone of coagulation. However, an exact determination of the burn depth is irrelevant to the initial resuscitation. Burn size in children is best estimated with an age-specific chart (Fig. 127-2) because body proportions change with growth. In adolescents and adults, the rule of nines facilitates accurate evaluation. Irregular burns can be estimated by remembering that the surface of the palm of the hand (excluding the digits) represents approximately 0.5 percent of the body surface area in all age groups. Patients with large burns, greater than 15 percent of the body surface area, are often best served by care in a specialized facility (Fig. 127-3).

Selected laboratory and radiographic studies that are of value during the initial evaluation include a blood gas analysis with carboxyhemoglobin determination in those exposed to noxious fumes; routine hematology, chemistry, and coagulation studies; and urinalysis. Chest radiographs facilitate the documentation of proper position of resuscitative cannulae.

FIGURE 127-3

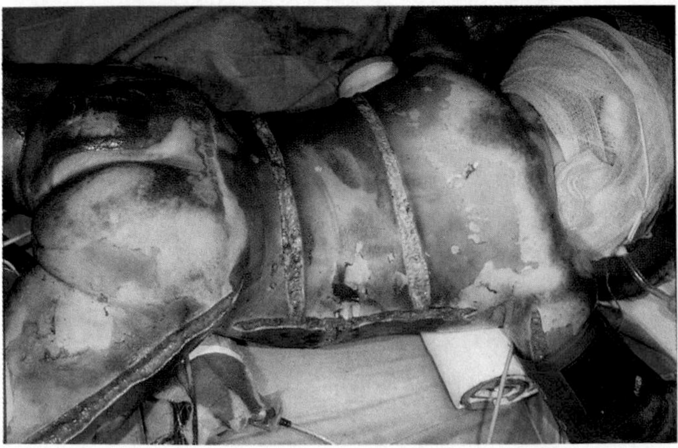

Patients with large burns, greater than 15 percent of the body surface area, are often best served by care in a specialized facility.

INITIAL EVALUATION OF SPECIAL SITUATIONS

There are certain patients who are referred to burn units routinely for care of specialized burns, nonburn injuries, and other conditions.[4] Such injuries include electrical, chemical, tar, or abuse-related burns that require unique evaluations. Nontraumatic conditions commonly referred to burn units include purpura fulminans, toxic epidermal necrolysis, staphylococcal scalded skin syndrome, and major soft tissue injuries. Such patients benefit from the unique combination of surgical, wound care, and critical care resources available in burn units. Unique aspects of the evaluation of these patients will be presented here.

Patients with electrical injuries can be conveniently divided into three exposure types: low voltage or household current, intermediate voltages between household and 1000 volts (V), and high voltage, which is defined as greater than 1000 V. Intermediate range and even low-voltage exposures, combined with a good quality electrical contact, can result in locally destructive injuries. A patient with high-voltage exposure often has multiple injuries and should be approached as a polytrauma patient. It is important to determine the presence of pigment in the urine promptly so that this can be appropriately treated with volume loading and judicious use of loop and osmotic diuretics. Involved extremities must be monitored carefully for subtle signs of evolving intracompartmental edema so that timely decompression can be performed in the operating room. Patients with serious tissue destruction should undergo all needed decompression operations within the first hours after injury and subsequently should be taken to the operating room within 72 h with a goal of definitive débridement and wound closure. Such is often facilitated by the use of local and distant flaps in addition to split-thickness autograft.

Patients sustaining chemical injury should undergo prompt irrigation at the scene, including dusting off dry chemicals and removing all clothing. Acidic wounds are generally well irrigated after 30 min of high-volume tap water irrigation. Alkaline injuries may require a longer time for adequate irrigation. The adequacy of irrigation of alkaline wounds can be evaluated by determining that the soapy feel on the fingers of a gloved hand has resolved or by checking the skin with litmus paper. Hydrofluoric acid exposures can be complicated by life-threatening hypocalcemia.[5] This should be suspected and treated appropriately with intravenous calcium supplementation and subeschar 10% calcium gluconate. It is important to contact poison control services to facilitate the proper management of patients exposed to one of the thousands of chemical agents in common industrial and home use.

Tar injuries should be cooled with tap water irrigation, and the tar removed later with appropriate lipophilic solvents. Underlying burns are generally very deep as these thermoplastic road materials are liquefied in the region of 300°C to 700°C (572°F to 1292°F).

Patients with purpura fulminans are often referred to burn units for definitive management. This is a condition, usually seen in a setting of meningococcal sepsis, that is thought to be induced by a transient protein C deficiency with diffuse microvascular thrombosis and soft tissue necrosis. These patients commonly develop organ failure secondary to the initial meningococcal sepsis and from infection of their deep wounds. Treatment requires management of organ failures and excision and grafting of the wounds, which are usually quite deep and have a characteristic "cookie cutter" appearance.

Toxic epidermal necrolysis is a variant of erythema multiforme major with a diffuse slough of the epidermis at the dermal–epidermal junction. Prominent mucous membrane and conjunctival involvement is common, and when particularly notable, the disease process is often called Stevens-Johnson syndrome (see Chap. 58). A differentiation from staphylococcal scalded skin syndrome is generally made on clinical grounds, but skin biopsy is diagnostic. Treatment involves

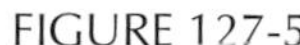

FIGURE 127-4

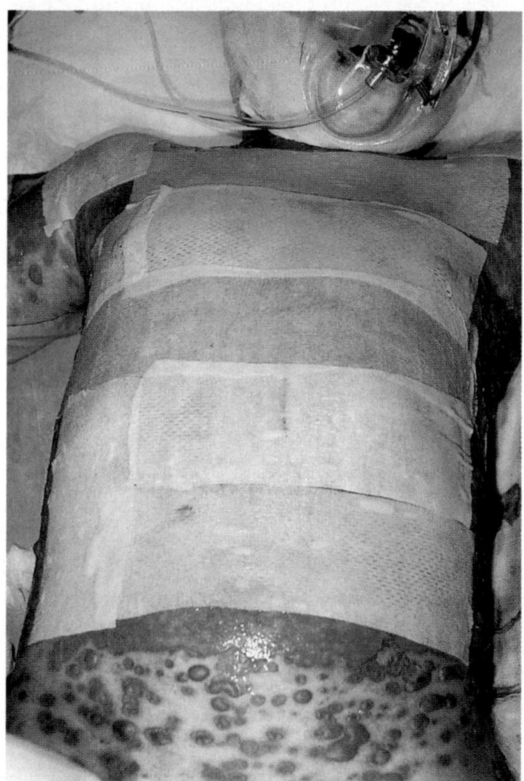

Large areas of open confluent wound in patients with toxic epidermal necrolysis should be dressed with a biologic membrane such as porcine xenograft.

management of any sepsis-associated organ failures, prevention of wound desiccation and superinfection, topical antimicrobial use (generally 0.5% silver nitrate solution), and xenografting of large areas of confluent wound (Fig. 127-4). Ophthalmic evaluation is important as long-term sequelae often occur. Intense oropharyngeal involvement may make handling of secretions difficult, mandating intubation for airway protection and enteral feedings.

Staphylococcal scalded skin syndrome is a staphylococcal exotoxin-induced separation of the epidermis at the granular layer (see Chap. 195). Mucous membrane and conjunctival involvement are not seen. These patients often have simply an area of colonization without an infection, but a careful search for focus of the staphylococcal infection is warranted while empiric antistaphylococcal antibiotics are initiated.

Epidermolysis bullosa consists of a group of diseases that result in epidermal loss over varying areas (see Chap. 65). If extensive, this may be complicated by sepsis. On occasion, children with particularly severe diffuse lesions are referred to burn units, particularly when these are complicated by sepsis. Management strategy requires prevention of desiccation and superinfection of wounds and support of failing organs system during septic episodes.

Finally, it is important to be sensitive to abuse as a possible etiologic agent. The index of suspicion should be raised when there is delay in the presentation for reasonable medical care or when there are conflicting histories of the event given by caregivers. Suspicious burn patterns include those demonstrating sharply demarcated margins or uniform depth; scald injuries without splash marks; flexor sparing (particularly in the antecubital or popliteal fossae); or sparing of areas in forced contact with the tub or sink. Also suspicious are localized, very deep contact or dorsal contact injuries. All suspicious cases should be reported to appropriate state authorities, and all such children should be admitted to the hospital regardless of the severity of their injuries. Imaging of the head and long bones should be considered (Fig. 127-5).

FIGURE 127-5

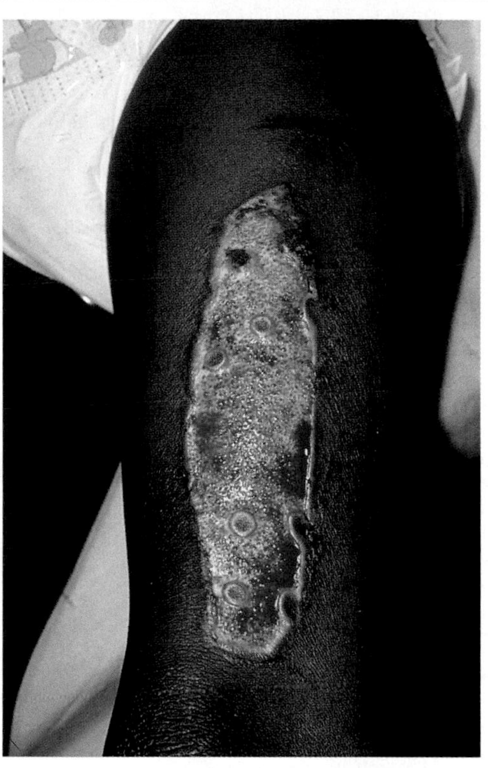

If the history or burn pattern is suggestive, children suffering injuries of abuse should be hospitalized, and their cases filed with state authorities for further investigation and intervention.

MANAGEMENT

The management of an acutely burned adult or child is a challenging task requiring the exercise of skills in critical care, surgery, physical and occupational therapy, nursing, and psychology. The following discussion outlines the management of such injuries by describing fluid resuscitation, initial wound excision and biologic closure, definitive wound closure, selected critical care issues, and reconstruction and reintegration.

Fluid Resuscitation

Patients with large burns will require fluid resuscitation. There are many fluid resuscitation formulas in common use. The variability in their prediction of an individual burn patient's needs is a tribute to the inherent inaccuracy in any formula that attempts to predict individual needs in this group. A fluid resuscitation formula cannot therefore replace the bedside presence of a knowledgeable physician constantly reevaluating the physiologic effects of the fluid therapy and adjusting it appropriately. A commonly used consensus formula is the modified Brooke formula (Table 127-1). However, all such predictions are inherently inaccurate, and failure to adjust infusions based on the patient's physiology is fraught with hazard.

TABLE 127-1

The Modified Brooke Formula

First 24 h
Adults and children weighing > 10 kg
  Ringer's lactate: 2–4 mL/kg per % burn (half in first 8 h)
  Colloid: none
Children weighing between 10 and 30 kg
  Ringer's lactate: 2–3 mL/kg per % burn (half in first 8 h)
  Ringer's lactate with 5% dextrose: calculated maintenance rate
  Colloid: none

Second 24 h
All patients
  Crystalloid: to maintain urine output. If silver nitrate is used, sodium leaching will mandate continued isotonic crystalloid. If other topicals are used, free water requirement is significant. Serum sodium should be monitored closely. Nutritional support should begin, ideally by the enteral route.
  Colloid (5% albumin in Ringer's lactate graded with burn size):
    0–30% burn: none
    30–50% burn: 0.3 mL/kg per % burn
    50–70% burn: 0.4 mL/kg per % burn
    > 70% burn: 0.5 mL/kg per % burn

The physiology behind the various resuscitation formulas is still very poorly understood, although it is thought that vasoactive mediators are released from injured tissue and result in a diffuse systemic capillary leak that is graded with burn size. This results in extravasation of both crystalloid and colloid for the first 18 to 24 h after injury. This physiologic reaction explains the enormous crystalloid requirements calculated by resuscitation formulas and the fact that most withhold colloid until 12 to 24 h has elapsed. To a certain extent, fluid requirements during this period are an artifact of the resuscitation end points chosen. Children are commonly thought to require fluid in excess of that predicted by various formulas, but this may be in part an artifact of setting 2 mL/kg of body weight per hour of urine output as a resuscitation end point. In infants and very young children, whose renal concentrating abilities are not completely mature, this is required. However, in older children, renal concentrating abilities are more fully developed and targeting urine flow of 0.5 to 1 mL/kg per hour results in overall resuscitative fluid requirements much closer to that of the adult patient. Patients who have suffered inhalation injury commonly require substantially more fluid than predicted for adequate resuscitation, and this may be secondary to the release of vasoactive mediators from injured pulmonary tissue.

During the first 24 h, Ringer's lactate is the primary resuscitative fluid. Young children can develop hypoglycemia if glucose is not administered, therefore Ringer's lactate or half-normal saline with 5% dextrose is infused at a maintenance rate. However, the primary resuscitation fluid should be Ringer's lactate without dextrose, because if dextrose-containing fluids are used as the primary resuscitation fluid, hyperglycemia and osmotic diuresis will occur. It is ideal to reevaluate the patient every 30 to 60 min during resuscitation and gradually increase or decrease infusions based on age-specific resuscitation end points.

If the resuscitation is not going as predicted, one should consider the early use of low-dose dopamine to facilitate renal perfusion, the early institution of colloid, and/or the insertion of a pulmonary artery catheter to facilitate monitoring and accurate fluid administration. Patients with obvious pigment in the urine, secondary to deep thermal or electrical burns, must be identified early, and the pigment cleared with additional intravenous crystalloid. Alkalinization of the urine is appropriate in selected patients. Occasionally, a forced diuresis with mannitol is beneficial.

During the second 24 h, colloid administration is appropriate as the capillary leak that characterizes the early postinjury period has abated. During this period, crystalloid requirements markedly diminish, and transeschar free water loss dominates the electrolyte situation except when an aqueous topical antimicrobial agent such as 0.5% silver nitrate is used. There is significant morbidity to rapid changes in serum sodium concentration, so diligent electrolyte monitoring during this period, with appropriate correction, is critical. Enteral nutritional support should start during this period as well.

Initial Wound Excision and Biologic Closure

Although most is written about patients with large, deep burns, the majority of patients have small, superficial burns, which can be very well managed, often in the outpatient setting, with a number of topical agents (Fig. 127-6). All topical care plans for such patients share the common goals of general cleanliness, prevention of wound desiccation, reduction of wound colonization, monitoring for infection, and minimizing mechanical trauma and pain. A wide variety of topical agents can be employed effectively to this end.

An essential element of modern care for patients with larger injuries is the prompt identification and removal of necrotic tissue with immediate biologic closure. This surgical maneuver modifies the natural history of burn injury by eliminating the process of wound colonization, infection, liquefaction, and separation. Such expectant management of large burn wounds results in predictable sepsis of the host, with a resulting maximum survivable burn size of 40 to 50 percent of the body surface area. The policy of early burn wound excision and closure is now widely practiced in North America and is typically carried out as a series of staged excisions of all deep partial- and full-thickness components of the wound (except for the face, palms, soles, and genitals) over the first postinjury week.[6] This approach results in enhanced survival in patients with large injuries, truncated hospital stays,[7] decreased costs, and fewer painful dressing changes.

This policy of prompt definitive wound excision presupposes an ability to estimate burn depth accurately, which is still best judged by the eye of an experienced examiner. There is a rich history of efforts to

FIGURE 127-6

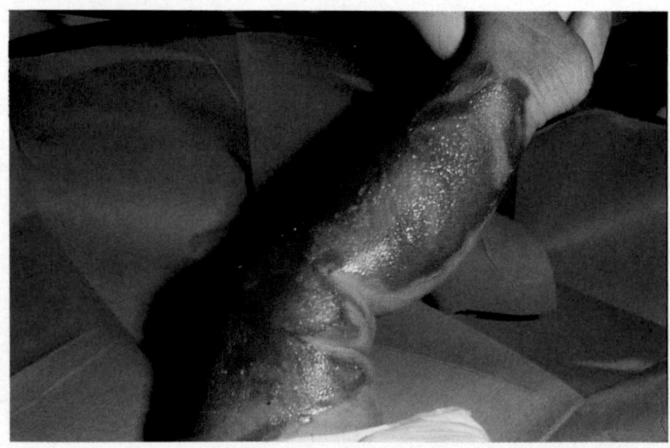

Patient with superficial burns that can be managed in an out-patient setting.

quantify burn depth objectively by using devices such as laser Doppler flow meters, burn wound biopsy, intravenous fluorescence, thermography, light reflectance, and fluorescence of intravenous dyes.[8] However, nothing has yet surpassed the eye of an experienced examiner in accuracy, reliability, or practicality. If the patient presents with an overall wound size that is not large and there is a significant area of indeterminate depth, it is reasonable to treat this wound with topical antimicrobials for 3 to 5 days, at which time the full-thickness component becomes clear.

The topical wound care agents in general use have specific advantages and disadvantages that determine their use on the variety of wounds seen in clinical practice. The three most commonly used are silver sulfadiazine, mafenide acetate, and silver nitrate, the latter as an aqueous 0.5% solution. Silver sulfadiazine is painless on application, has relatively poor eschar penetration, has no metabolic side effects, and a broad antibacterial spectrum. Mafenide acetate is painful on application, penetrates eschar extremely well, is a carbonic anhydrase inhibitor, and has a broad antibacterial spectrum. Aqueous silver nitrate is painless on application, penetrates eschar poorly, and leaches electrolytes, yet it has a very broad spectrum of action, including against fungal organisms, which renders it quite useful.

The techniques of burn excision have evolved greatly since the initial reports, in the early 1970s,[9,10] of conserving techniques of layered excision. These procedures should be done in a well-planned fashion in an operating room adequately heated and humidified to minimize evaporative heat loss. Keeping the patient euthermic during the procedure will greatly facilitate the effectiveness of innate clotting mechanisms.

Once necrotic eschar is excised to a bed of viable tissue, immediate biologic closure is essential. In most patients, immediate autografting is performed. However, when donor sites are insufficient for this purpose, temporary biologic closure is necessary. Such coverage will ideally prevent desiccation and superinfection and provide a vapor and bacterial barrier over the excised wound. Ideal to this purpose is cryopreserved human allograft, placed in a meshed, unexpanded fashion. There are a number of other temporary closure options available, and this is an area of ongoing investigation. A large, excised wound that is left open will become further desiccated and be a source of bacterial invasion and ongoing fluid and vapor loss.

Among the exciting new alternative biologic closure resources is a synthetic bilayered membrane that has an inner layer of homogenized bovine collagen, created so that the pore size forms an inviting lattice for fibrovascular ingrowth. Upon this layer is poured liquid silicone, which congeals into an outer membrane that bonds with the collagen. This bilaminar structure is laid upon freshly excised wounds, and fibrovascular ingrowth occurs. After 2 to 3 weeks, the outer membrane is removed and replaced with a very thin autograft. Initial experience with this procedure is encouraging.[11,12]

Definitive Wound Closure

After the first postburn week, under ideal conditions, the patient has undergone near-complete wound excision, and permanent or temporary biologic cover has been achieved. Subsequently, it is predictable that the patient's physiology will normalize and the need for critical care will decrease. It is at this point that the definitive wound closure phase can be said to begin. It is during this phase of management that temporary covers are removed and replaced with autograft and areas of small physiologic surface area but high complexity, such as the face, hands, and genitals, are addressed surgically. In patients with extraordinarily extensive burns and very limited donor sites, there are a number of emerging technologies that will make a contribution to definitive wound closure. However, for the large majority of patients, split-thickness autografts continue to provide the most durable and reliable of covers.

Because of the thickness and well-developed skin appendages of the central face, relatively deep burns in this area will frequently heal with a good result. Therefore, unless burns in the central face are of extraordinary depth, they are treated with topical antimicrobial agents for 2 weeks. At that time, unhealed wounds are excised and autografted. Ideally, the face should be resurfaced in cosmetic units[13] by using sheet autografts of maximal thickness and of optimally matched pigmentation.

Burns of the ocular adnexa are quite common. The paramount concern during the acute phase of management is protection of the globe. During the initial few days after injury, adnexal edema generally results in complete coverage of the globe with excellent lubrication. As wound contracture occurs, exposure and desiccation can ensue and result in keratitis and corneal ulceration. If this is unresponsive to ocular lubrication, acute lid release should be performed. Tarsorrhaphy is an ineffective alternative, as wound contraction forces will disrupt the sutures and damage the lids. When the lid substance is destroyed but the globe is intact, a difficult wound problem ensues. However, in general, this can be successfully managed by mobilizing the remnant palpebral conjunctiva from the inferior and superior lids and closing them over the globe, placing split-thickness skin graft over this. Subsequently, the resulting membrane can be opened, creating an eyelid-like structure that, with difficulty, can provide a reasonable functional alternative.

Burns of the external ear are treated with topical mafenide acetate, as it will reliably penetrate the cartilage of the ear and prevent auricular chondritis. It is important to avoid pressure on the burned auricle. Deep burns of the external ear with full-thickness skin loss are resurfaced, carefully preserving underlying viable cartilage.

Management of hand burns is critical to a good outcome, and it is important to address this issue from the very beginning of the hospital stay, no matter what the burn size. Critical components include a complete examination ruling out other injuries and ongoing attention to perfusion of the digits throughout the resuscitative period. As the mean arterial pressure in named vessels is much higher than tissue pressure, it is not enough to ensure that there is detectable flow in the ulnar or radial arteries. If the burned hand is cool and firm with decreased flow in the digital pulp, decompression should be performed to ensure adequate perfusion. In patients with very deep thermal burns or with high-voltage electrical injury, the need for urgent fasciotomy is predicted by progressive firmness of the compartments of the hands and forearm. The evaluation for the need for fasciotomy can be facilitated by documenting a compartment pressure of 30 mmHg; however, in most cases serial, physical examination is enough to make this determination. Even in the most obtunded patient, the burned hand should be taken through a complete range of passive motion twice a day and splinted in a functional position with the metacarpophalangeal joints at 70 to 90 degrees and the interphalangeal joints in extension. The only interruption in this program should be the time required to obtain sheet autograft closure of the wounds. Therapy is then advanced to an active and strength-enhancing program. Fourth-degree hand burns, with involvement of the underlying extensor mechanism, joint capsule, or bone, are significantly more difficult management problems. However, outcomes consistent with performing independent activities of daily living are the expectation in the large majority of these patients.[14]

Burn Critical Care

During the period of progressive wound closure, the burn patient often requires sophisticated life support to maintain homeostasis. Advanced techniques in burn critical care have played an important role in

TABLE 127-2

Complications after Burn Injury

Neurologic

1. *Transient delirium* occurs in up to 30% of patients and generally resolves with supportive therapy when the possibilities of anoxia, metabolic disturbance, and structural lesions are eliminated by appropriate studies.
2. *Seizures* most commonly result from hyponatremia or abrupt benzodiazepine withdrawal.
3. *Peripheral nerve injuries* occur from direct thermal injury, compression from compartment syndrome or overlying nonelastic eschar, major metabolic disturbances, or improper splinting techniques.
4. *Delayed peripheral nerve and spinal cord deficits* develop weeks or months after or months after high-voltage injury secondary to small vessel injury and demyelinization

Renal

1. *Early acute renal failure* follows inadequate perfusion during resuscitation or myoglobinuria.
2. *Late renal failure* complicates sepsis and multiorgan failure or the use of nephrotoxic agents.

Adrenal

1. *Acute adrenal insufficiency* secondary to hemorrhage into the gland presents with hypotension, fever, hyponatremia, and hyperkalemia.

Cardiovascular

1. *Endocarditis and suppurative thrombophebitis* are intravascular infections that typically present with fever and bacteremia without signs of local infection.
2. *Hypertension* occurs in up to 20% of children and is best managed with β-adrenergic blockers.
3. *Venous thromboembolic complications* are so infrequent in patients with large burns that routine prophylaxis is not currently routine.
4. *Iatrogic catheter insertion complications* are minimized by meticulous technique.

Pulmonary

1. *Carbon monoxide intoxication,* which is best managed acutely with effective ventilation with pure oxygen, can be associated with delayed neurologic sequelae.
2. *Pneumonia* may occur with or without antecedent inhalation injury and is treated with pulmonary toilet and antibiotics.
3. *Respiratory failure* may occur early postinjury secondary to inhalation of noxious chemicals or later in the course secondary to sepsis or pneumonia.

Hematologic

1. *Neutropenia and thrombocytopenia* as well as *disseminated intravascular coagulation* are common indicators of impending sepsis and should prompt appropriate investigations.
2. *Global immunologic deficits* associated with burn injury contribute to a high rate of infectious complications.

Otologic

1. *Auricular chondritis* secondary to bacterial invasion of cartilage results in rapid loss of viable tissue and is prevented by the routine use of topical mafenide acetate on all burned ears.
2. *Sinusitis and otitis media* can be caused by transnasal instrumentation and are treated by relocation of tubes, antibiotics, and judicious surgical drainage.
3. *Complications of endotrachael intubation* include nasal alar and septal necrosis, vocal cord erosions and ulcerations, tracheal stenosis, and tracheoesophageal and tracheoinominate artery fistulae. The occurrence of such complications is minimized by compulsive attention to tube position, avoidance of oversized tubes, and attention to cuff pressures.

Enteric

1. *Hepatic dysfunction,* secondary to transient hepatic blood flow deficits and manifested as transaminase elevations, is extremely common during resuscitation from large burns and resolves with volume restitution. Late hepatic failure, beginning with elevations of cholestatic chemistries and progressing through coagulopathy and frank failure, complicates sepsis and multiorgan failure.
2. *Pancreatitis,* beginning with amylase and lipase elevations and ileus and progressing through hemorrhagic pancreatitis, is generally coincident with splanchnic flow deficits early and sepsis-induced organ failures later in the hospital course.
3. *Acalculous cholecystitis* can present as sepsis without localized symptoms or signs accompanied by rising cholestatic chemistries. A standard radiographic evaluation can be followed by bedside percutaneous cholecystostomy in unstable patients.
4. *Gastroduodenal ulceration,* secondary to splanchnic flow deficits that degrade mucosal defenses, is extremely common and often life-threatening if routine histamine receptor blockers and antacids are not administered.
5. *Intestinal ischemia,* which can progress to infarction, is secondary to inadequate resuscitation and splanchnic flow deficits.

Ophthalmic

1. *Ectropia,* from progressive contraction of burned occular adnexae, results in exposure of the globe. This requires acute eyelid release. Tarsorrhaphy is rarely helpful, more often resulting in injury to the tarsal plate as contraction forces pull out tarsorrhapy sutures.
2. *Corneal ulceration,* which develops after initial epithelial injury or later exposure secondary to ectropion, can progress to full-thickness corneal destruction if secondary infection occurs. This is prevented by careful globe lubrication with topical antibiotics in the former case and acute lid release in the latter.
3. *Symblepharon,* or scarring of the lid to the denuded conjunctiva following chemical burns or corneal epithelial defects complicating toxic epidermal necrolysis, is prevented by daily examination and adhesion disruption with a fine glass rod.

Genitourinary

1. *Urinary tract infections* are minimized by maintaining bladder catheters only when absolutely required and are treated with appropriate antibiotics. Neither catheterization nor colonic diversion is required for management of perineal and genital burns.
2. *Candida cystitis* occurs in those patients treated with bladder catheters and broad-spectrum antibiotics. Catheter change and amphotericin irrigation for 5 days is generally successful. If infections are recurrent, the upper genitourinary tract should be screened ultrasonographically.

Musculoskeletal

1. *Burned exposed bone* is generally débrided with a dental drill until viable cortical bone is reached, which is then allowed to granulate and is autografted. Patients whose overall condition and wounds are appropriate are managed with local or distant flaps.
2. *Fractured and burned extremities* are best immobilized with external fixators while overlying burns are grafted. Burn patients with coincident fractures in unburned extremities benefit from prompt internal fixation.

Continued

TABLE 127-2

Complications after Burn Injury (*Continued*)

3. *Heterotopic ossification* develops weeks after injury, is seen most commonly around deeply burned major joints such as the triceps tendon and presents with pain and decreased range of motion. Most patients respond to physical therapy, but some require excision of heterotopic bone to achieve full function.

Soft tissue

1. *Hypertrophic scar formation* is a major cause of long-term functional and cosmetic deformities seen in burn patients. This poorly understood process is heralded by a secondary increase in neovascularity between 9 to 13 weeks after epithelialization. Management options include grafting of deep dermal and full-thickness wounds, compression garments, judicious steroid injections, topical silicone products, and scar release and resurfacing procedures.

salvage of those patients with large injuries. The core components of this contribution are management of failing organ systems, support of the predictable hypermetabolic response to injury, nutritional support, and early detection and treatment of infectious foci.

The most common organ failure addressed in the burn unit is acute respiratory failure. This has multiple etiologies, including inhalation injury, pneumonia or other pulmonary infections, systemic sepsis, and as a component of multiorgan failure. The pathophysiology of inhalation injury is complex, but there are three major clinical components. The first is early upper airway obstruction secondary to edema. This is most likely to occur in smaller children with their decreased airway diameter, is generally a problem early during the course of injury, and is managed with endotracheal intubation for airway protection. Endotracheal tubes are removed when airway swelling has decreased, as manifested by decreased facial edema and an air leak around an appropriately sized endotracheal tube at a moderate pressure. The second problem is impaired gas exchange, which commonly becomes an increasing problem 3 to 5 days after injury. The degree of gas exchange dysfunction varies with the aerosolized toxins that the individual patient has inhaled and is difficult to predict, even when flexible bronchoscopy is used. Management of impaired gas exchange requires mechanical ventilation designed to minimize ventilator-induced lung injury.[15] The third problem, which is generally seen toward the end of the first postburn week, is pulmonary infection. This takes the form of either pneumonia or tracheobronchitis. Both present with fevers, impaired gas exchange, and purulent sputum. The management of pulmonary infection is with specific antibiotics and aggressive pulmonary toilet, often facilitated by toilet bronchoscopy.

Patients injured in structural fires may have been exposed to a hypoxic environment, high levels of carbon monoxide, and high levels of cyanide. These factors, combined with hemodynamic instability, may contribute to neurologic compromise. Such patients should be ventilated with 100% oxygen from the time of extrication. Selected patients with severe carbon monoxide exposures who are stable enough from a hemodynamic and pulmonary perspective to be managed safely in a monoplane hyperbaric chamber are appropriate candidates for hyperbaric oxygen treatment to facilitate more rapid clearance of carbon monoxide from hemoglobin and cellular enzyme systems.[16]

Nutritional support is a critically important component of burn critical care. The hypermetabolic response to injury is intense and lasts well beyond the time of complete wound closure, and this physiologic state must be supported if optimal outcomes are to be achieved. This response consists clinically of fever, a hyperdynamic circulatory state with high cardiac output and low afterload, increased gluconeogenesis and protein catabolism not suppressed with glucose infusion, decreased albumin synthesis, and increased acute-phase protein production. Accurate nutritional support is essential, because overfeeding is associated with hepatic steatosis and hepatic dysfunction as well as increased CO_2 production, which will exacerbate respiratory failure, while underfeeding results in poor wound healing. Patients with significant burns should be given a caloric load approximately 1.5 times their calculated basal metabolic rate and approximately 2.5 g/kg per day of protein. The accuracy of this program should be continually reassessed, ideally by indirect calorimetry and protein balance studies.

Throughout the intensive care course of the seriously burned patient, a vigilant search for the legion of predictable complications is an essential aspect of management, as prompt treatment markedly reduces morbidity and mortality associated with these problems (Table 127-2).

Rehabilitation, Reconstruction, Reintegration

With the increasing frequency with which patients suffering large burns survive, the importance of specific attention to the critical aspects of rehabilitation, reconstruction, and reintegration is increasing. It is clearly the duty of the burn unit team to place great importance on these aspects of care and to address these issues from the time of the initial burn management. Burn rehabilitation begins during burn resuscitation. This may initially be limited to splinting, antideformity positioning, and passive range of motion twice a day. As wound closure becomes complete, these activities expand to fill the bulk of the patient's day with active motion, ranging, strengthening, and work-hardening programs. These important activities are carefully planned to continue after discharge from the acute care hospital. It is ideal if the burn unit team can direct these activities after the patient has left inpatient status.

Psychosocial adaptation after severe burns can be very difficult. This is particularly true in patients with serious injury to the hands or face. The coordinated involvement of psychiatric, psychological, and social work staff will facilitate achieving the optimal emotional outcome. It is important to plan for funding for these activities.

Hypertrophic scar formation is a major source of long-term morbidity after burns (Fig. 127-7*A*). All healed and grafted burns will become hypervascular shortly after successful epithelization, but this neovascularity should involute between 9 and 13 weeks after the injury.[17] Additional collagen forms, and contraction occurs over the next 4 to 6 months in those wounds that go on to become hypertrophic. Typically, the hypervascular and erythematous nature of the wounds will become more prominent over the next months, peaking at 6 to 8 months after injury. Subsequently, this will involute, leaving a mature scar. The physiology of this reaction is very poorly understood. Wounds that are most commonly associated with scar hypertrophy are deep dermal burns that heal on their own over more than 3 weeks and full-thickness burns that heal by epithelial migration from the edges. Wounds across highly elastic surfaces, such as flexor surfaces and the anterior neck and submental area, are also highly prone to hypertrophic scar formation.

Our ability to influence the development of hypertrophic scars favorably is limited. Current methods include compression garments, topical silicone, wound massage, intradermal steroid injections, and surgery. The mechanism of action for these techniques has not been

FIGURE 127-7

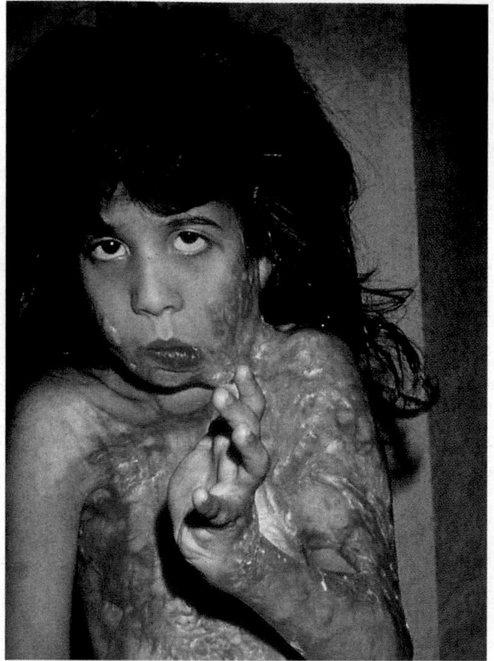

A.

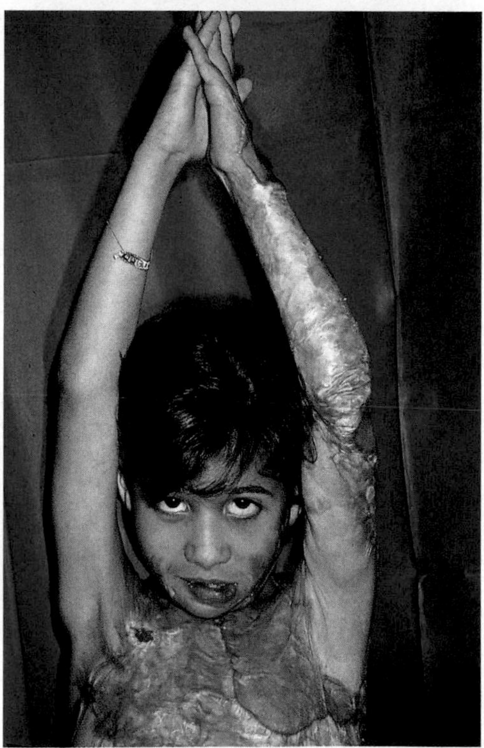

B.

A. Hypertrophic scarring is a major source of morbidity in burn patients. *B.* Release and autografting of these injuries is an important component of ongoing care.

fully elucidated, and none is of enormous benefit; however, when used in appropriate combination they can be helpful. Carefully planned reconstructive surgery plays a critical role in these patients (Fig. 127-7*B*). Cosmetic or functionally limiting areas of hypertrophic scar are incised or excised, and the resulting wounds are replaced with sheet autograft. Tissue expanders are of great value in selected locations. Traditionally, it is considered ideal to wait for a fully mature scar prior to considering reconstructive surgery, but earlier surgery is indicated when function is threatened.

ON THE HORIZON

On the horizon are exciting potential adjuncts to current burn care; however, none will ever replace the sound practice of clinical burn care. These adjuncts include permanent skin substitutes, critical care technologies, modifiers of the injury response, growth factors, and new modes of wound management and evaluation. Definitive wound closure that uses materials other than autograft remains the "holy grail" of burn care. It is an area of enormous interest and ongoing research. Multiple substitutes currently in early clinical trials include epidermal and dermal analogues and composite substitutes of either a temporary or permanent nature. Of the plethora of materials in trial, the most commonly described are cultured autologous epithelium, cryopreserved allograft dermis, and the synthetic bilaminar artificial skin of Yannas and Burke previously described. Cultured epidermal autografts can be of value in patients with massive burns in whom there are insufficient donor sites available for wound closure. However, the low initial engraftment rates, relatively poor quality of the resulting wound closure, and significant expense make this an imperfect solution to this difficult problem. Cryopreserved allograft dermis with overlying thin autograft is in initial clinical trials, and preliminary results are encouraging. However, this technology is also associated with significant additional expense. This area of research offers a major potential benefit to our patients.

Critical care technologies under development include newer modes of ventilation that allow for the complete avoidance of ventilator-induced lung injury, partial liquid ventilation, inhaled nitric oxide, and extracorporeal support. As these technologies are incorporated into burn care, our patients will gain the same benefits as other critically ill populations who suffer respiratory failure.

Better targeted nutritional support, provision of conditionally essential nutrients, and modifiers of the hypermetabolic response all offer potential advantages by improving the support of the response to injury. However, the complex cellular and subcellular biology involved should temper our blind enthusiasm for administration of powerful biologic substances without clear understanding of their effects.

Innovations in wound evaluation and management include the possible wider application of technologies that will allow us a better determination of burn depth, such as laser Doppler flow meters or fluorescence of intravenously administered dyes. The potential use of scanning CO_2 lasers and debriding enzymes for bloodless burn débridement are exciting technologies that may further improve burn care.

Epidermal growth factor and human growth hormone have been in clinical trials for some time and may be associated with shortened donor-site healing time in burn patients. Ongoing animal and clinical work with transforming growth factors, fibroblast growth factors, platelet-derived growth factor, and colony-stimulating factors may further enhance our understanding of the biology of wound healing and may ultimately lead to improvements in clinical care. However, caution must be exercised when giving large doses of these potent substances to our patients without a clear understanding of their complex biology.

Over the past 20 years, the field of burn care has changed dramatically. Regionalization of care, early surgery modifying the natural history of the disease process, and more focused attention on long-term outcomes has resulted in a much improved outlook for our patients. However, the disease process remains a very difficult one and requires an aggressive and multidisciplinary approach to achieve consistently favorable outcomes.

REFERENCES

1. Sheridan RL et al: Long-term outcomes of children surviving massive burns. *JAMA* **283**:69, 2000
2. Sheridan RL et al. Current expectations for survival in pediatric burns. *Arch Pediatrs Adolesc Med* **154**:245, 2000
3. Youn YK et al: The role of mediators in the response to thermal injury. *World J Surg* **16**:30, 1992
4. Sheridan RL et al: The burn unit as a resource for the management of acute nonburn conditions in children. *J Burn Care Rehabil* **16**:62, 1995
5. Sheridan RL et al: Emergency management of major hydrofluoric acid exposures. *Burns* **21**:62, 1995
6. Sheridan RL et al: Management of burn wounds with prompt excision and immediate closure. *J Intensive Care Med* **9**:6, 1994
7. Herndon DN et al: A comparison of conservative versus early excision. Therapies in severely burned patients. *Ann Surg* **209**:547, 1989

8. Heimbach D et al: Burn depth: A review. *World J Surg* 16:10, 1992
9. Janzekovic Z: A new concept in the early excision and immediate grafting of burns. *J Trauma* **10**:1103, 1970
10. Tompkins RG et al: Prompt eschar excision: A treatment system contributing to reduced burn mortality. A statistical evaluation of burn care at the Massachusetts General Hospital (1974–1984). *Ann Surg* **204**:272, 1986
11. Heimbach D et al: Artificial dermis for major burns. A multi-center randomized clinical trial. *Ann Surg* **208**:313, 1988
12. Sheridan RL: Skin substitutes in burns. *Burns* **25**:97, 1999
13. Gonzalez-Ulloa M: Restoration of the face covering by means of selected skin in regional aesthetic units. *Br J Plast Surg* **9**:212, 1956
14. Sheridan RL et al: The acutely burned hand: Management and outcome based on a ten-year experience with 1047 acute hand burns. *J Trauma* **38**:406, 1995
15. Sheridan RL et al: Permissive hypercapnia as a ventilatory strategy in burned children: Effect on barotrauma, pneumonia, and mortality. *J Trauma* **39**:854, 1995
16. Sheridan RL, Shank ES: Hyperbaric oxygen: A brief overview of a controversial topic. *J Trauma* **47**:426, 1999
17. Kischer CW: The microvessels in hypertrophic scars, keloids and related lesions. *J Submicrosc Cytol Pathol* **24**:281, 1992

CHAPTER 128

Frederick D. Malkinson
Renato G. Panizzon

Radiobiology and Radiotherapy of Skin Diseases

RADIOBIOLOGY OF THE SKIN

Radiobiologic events in the skin are best interpreted from a knowledge of the general responses of cells and tissues to ionizing radiation. These responses to electromagnetic radiation (x-rays, gamma-rays) and to particulate radiation (electrons, neutrons, protons, alpha particles, etc.) may be studied in the whole organism or at the tissue, cellular, or molecular levels.

Clinical and microscopic changes in skin and its appendages were among the first reactions seen after accidental or therapeutic exposure to x-rays. In the late 1890s, Becquerel and Pierre Curie both noted erythema and ulceration in their own radiation-exposed skin sites after accidental and deliberate exposure respectively. Our current knowledge of radiation responses in skin derives from clinical observations and animal studies. The latter sources are important, because certain data for humans can only be provided by accidental radiation exposure.

Mechanisms of Radiation Injury

Electromagnetic radiation with energies above 125eV (x-rays, ^{60}Co gamma rays) produce indirect ionization by ejecting orbital electrons from atoms in tissues or cells. These fast electrons ionize other atoms and break chemical bonds. The resultant free radicals (atoms or molecules carrying an unpaired electron in the outer orbital shell) have half-lives of 10^{-5} seconds, are largely formed from tissue water molecules and oxygen, and react with cell or tissue organic molecules, altering their structure and function. The activated cellular response pathways mediating cytoprotective and cytotoxic responses of cell survival or death[1] and the roles of cytokines in normal tissue radiation reactions have been reviewed.[2,3] Resulting biological, biochemical, and/or metabolic changes appear within minutes, hours, days, weeks, or longer.

Cellular Radiation Effects

Although functional cell loss in nonproliferating cell systems may only follow large radiation doses (100 Gy; 1 Gy = 100 rad), reproductive integrity is usually lost after exposure to only 3 to 4 Gy. Cell death may occur within hours but usually occurs after one to five postradiation division cycles. Normal and malignant cells have similar radiation sensitivities. Chromosomal DNA is the main target for cell killing via chromosome and chromatid alterations. Cellular necrosis, reproductive failure, and apoptosis are the principal mechanisms of post-radiation cell death. Recent studies also suggest that microvascular endothelial cells may be a primary radiation target, contributing to consequent tissue or cell death.[4]

DNA and Chromosome Damage

Differences in numbers of chromosome sets (ploidy) affect radiation sensitivity.[5] Ionizing radiation impairs the synthesis of DNA, thymidine kinase, and DNA polymerase. Genetic damage from irradiation may occur in the gene at the molecular level or in the chromosome at the cellular level. Chromosome breaks may follow exposure to only 1 cGy (1 rad). Single strand breaks are common and readily repaired, but erroneous repair may induce mutation(s). Double-strand breaks, however, may be irreparable. Increased genome-wide instability in future cell generations may also occur. Chromosomal translocations or inversions may result in oncogene activation and malignancy.

Cell Cycle Effects

Cells in the division cycle are usually more radiosensitive than nondividing cells. In vitro and in vivo data reveal that radiosensitivity varies significantly in different phases of the cell cycle.[6] For most cell lines G_2- and M-phase cells are the most radiosensitive. Late S-phase and early G_1-phase cells are relatively radioresistant. Changes in DNA replication states and sulfhydryl compound content (radioprotectors) may affect cell cycle phase radiosensitivity. Overall, radiosensitivity varies by a factor of 2.5 to 3.0 among the various cell cycle phases.

Division Delay

Ionizing radiation produces cell division delay of 1 hour per Gy in a 2 to 10 Gy range. The delay is greatest for cells in G_2 phase. Molecular checkpoint genes arrest cells in G_2 phase to allow chromosomes to be checked for integrity and to be repaired before mitosis occurs. Cells lacking normal checkpoint genes will likely be more sensitive to radiation killing and malignant change. Shorter division delays occur in S cells and are least for G_1 cells.

Radiation Modifiers

There are two principal groups of radiation modifiers, radiosensitizers and radioprotectors,[7] both of which have been widely studied in skin and hair. For these agents, toxic effects, technological limitations, and, often, a lack of differential effects on tumors versus normal tissues, limit their usefulness. Only a few of these modifiers are discussed here.

OXYGEN AS A RADIOSENSITIZER The addition of oxygen to low prevailing pressures of 0 to 30 mmHg increases the effectiveness of sparsely ionizing radiation (x-rays, gamma-rays) up to threefold for a dose greater than 2 Gy. To produce this effect, mediated by free radical and H_2O_2 formation, oxygen must be present during the irradiation time. No further sensitization occurs after oxygen concentrations of 2 percent are reached. Oxygen enhancement ratios are least for densely ionizing radiations (neutrons, alpha particles). Hypoxic areas in tumors are best overcome by fractionation treatment schedules and use of densely ionizing radiation where feasible. Hyperbaric oxygen therapy is markedly compromised by sharp falls in oxygen levels during tissue and tumor diffusion.

ELECTRON-AFFINIC AGENTS AS RADIOSENSITIZERS Electron-affinic agents interact with radiation-damaged DNA, blocking repair of injury produced by free radicals. The agents are cytotoxic to hypoxic cells and bind to intracellular radioprotectors (glutathione), further enhancing radiosensitivity effects. Unlike oxygen, these agents diffuse over greater distances and are more slowly metabolized. The principal compounds used are nitroimidazoles, including metronidazole (Flagyl) and misonidazole. Cytotoxic effects (neuropathies) have limited their usefulness, but newer, less-lipophilic agents, have shorter tissue half-lives and display significantly enhanced sensitization potentials. Some of these agents also potentiate chemotherapeutic drug effects. Certain compounds have been evaluated in clinical trials.[8]

HYPERTHERMIA-INDUCED RADIOSENSITIZATION Heating skin before, during, or after irradiation enhances cutaneous reactions in mouse or human skin. At temperatures over 41.5°C (106.7°F) structural, chromosomal and/or repair proteins are damaged, and RNA, DNA, and protein synthesis are impaired. Above 43°C (109.4°F) cell survival curves are similar to those for ionizing radiation. Hyperthermia also induces apoptosis in some cell lines. Overall, normal and malignant cells have similar heat sensitivities. In the clinical and experimental use of hyperthermia with radiation, heat at temperatures of 43°C (109.4°F) or higher is usually administered within 4 hours before radiation. Thermal enhancement ratios range from 2 to 4 for single doses, but are lower for fractionated therapy. Combination treatment produces more partial and complete tumor responses than radiation alone, but the sole use of hyperthermia has little effect. Cooling reduces tissue oxygen tension through vasoconstriction, decreasing radiosensitivity.

RADIOPROTECTORS With sparsely ionizing radiation, dose reduction factors of 2 to 2.5 have been found with thiol and disulfide compounds (cysteine, glutathione) which scavenge free radicals. The most effective of these is WR-2721 (amifostine),[9] but toxicity (hypotension) may limit its effectiveness. Leukotrienes and, especially, prostaglandins are effective radioprotectors in microgram amounts, yielding dose reduction factors up to 6 for misoprostol, although their protective mechanism is not fully elucidated. Given before radiation, their efficacy depends on the presence of receptors for the individual agent.[10] Prostaglandins are radioprotective after local or systemic administration, greatly reducing, for example, experimental radiation-induced alopecia.[11] They also protect against chemotherapeutic agent toxicity as well, especially for doxorubicin and cyclophosphamide.[11,12] Misoprostol holds clinical promise for the protection of normal tissues (hair, mucous membranes) lying in the path of a radiation beam, while experimentally it fails to protect tumors against radiation effects.[13,14]

Radiobiology of the Skin and Hair

Within 2 to 3 weeks after exposure of human skin to high doses of fractionated radiation, acute erythema, moist desquamation, erosions, and epilation occur, followed by healing. The intensity of radiation erythema depends on age, gender, anatomic site, dose, and dose rate. These early changes reflect injury, apoptosis, and reproductive failure in germinative epidermal and hair matrix cells, reduced division rates in surviving cells, and vascular damage.[15] Epidermal cell replacement occurs from the third to the fifth week after radiation. Later chronic postradiation changes result largely from injury to dermal structures, particularly the vasculature, and fibrosis, which is actually an early (within 1 week) but progressive postradiation event that is cytokine mediated.[15–17]

The character and magnitude of cutaneous responses to radiation depend on total dose and dose fractionation, radiation quality and ionization density, area or volume of tissue irradiated, anatomic site, and vascular supply. The responses of irradiated skin and the effects on postradiation skin changes of radioprotectors, radiosensitizers, and hyperthermia have been reviewed.[15,18] The subjects of increased radiosensitivity and carcinogenesis in genetic disorders characterized by defective cellular and DNA repair processes have been summarized.[19]

Postradiation changes in the highly proliferative anagen hair matrix cells induce hair dysplasia and reduced hair lengths and growth rates. In humans, 3 Gy produces complete, reversible anagen alopecia; permanent alopecia begins to occur at 5 Gy. In mice, G_0 telogen matrix cells are 2.5 times more radioresistant than anagen cells. Differences in cell proliferation states and vascular supply between anagen and telogen hairs probably explain these differences. Altered matrix cell uptake of isotopically labeled amino acids, incidence of hair dysplasia, measurements of reduced hair shaft diameters, and quantitative assessments of surviving hairs or later regrown hairs have all been used as biologic end points to study general cellular radiation effects, as well as radioprotective or radiosensitizing actions of numerous pharmacologic or physical agents.[15,20]

Radiobiologic Effects on Melanocytes and Pigment Formation

Low-dose radiation induces cutaneous hyperpigmentation after minimal inflammation. Pigmentation is directly related to dose rate and total dose, and is characterized by increased numbers of melanocytes with increased tyrosinase activity, and by enhanced melanin transfer to epidermal cells. Higher radiation doses destroy melanocytes with resultant depigmentation. Similar radiation effects occur in mid-anagen hair follicles. At higher dose rates, hair melanocytes are far more susceptible to radiation destruction than epidermal melanocytes. In mice, telogen melanocytes are much more radiosensitive than anagen melanocytes. Melanocyte survival in hair follicle squashes and depigmentation of hair in laboratory animals have both been used to quantitate combined drug-radiation effects.

Radiobiologic Effects on Langerhans Cells

Although Langerhans cells (LC) are relatively radioresistant,[21] in one study, single doses of 20 Gy in mice reduced LC numbers to 18 percent within 10 days; repopulation was complete 30 days later. Whole-body irradiation to the bone marrow delayed repopulation another 3 weeks. In mice, the effects of such radiation early in life markedly increased skin LC loss in aged animals, perhaps reflecting dermal fibrosis and reduced blood flow.[21] Loss of LCs and their immunologic functions may contribute to increased postradiation tumorigenesis and to reduced susceptibility to contact hypersensitivity in affected sites.

RADIOTHERAPY OF SKIN DISEASES

Soon after the discovery of x-rays by Röntgen in 1895, the therapeutic potential of radiation was recognized. The first patient treated for a squamous cell carcinoma of the nose was treated in 1900. Soon thereafter, radiation therapy was used empirically for a host of conditions, both benign and malignant. In many situations, in which no effective therapeutic alternatives existed, radiation therapy may have been one of the few treatment options available. This was true until the 1950s. Thereafter, radiation treatment declined for two major reasons: One reason was awareness of the deleterious late effects of radiation, including the potential for the induction of malignancy. In addition, advances in surgical techniques and the development of effective medical therapies such as corticosteroids and antibiotics provided effective alternatives to the use of ionizing radiation. Nonetheless, dermatologists should retain primary expertise in the indication and treatment with x-rays for skin diseases either benign or malignant.[22] There are situations in which ionizing radiation remains an accepted therapeutic alternative or even the treatment of choice for certain skin diseases. Dermatologists, often in collaboration with radiation oncologists, can assist the patient and referring physician in selecting the treatment regimen with the highest therapeutic ratio for a particular individual (Table 128-1). In many cases, the morbidity of radiation is low when compared to the morbidity or even mortality associated with alternative therapies, or with the complications associated with progressive or recurrent disease.

Benign Skin Diseases

The use of ionizing radiation for benign skin diseases has decreased considerably as new and better systemic and local treatments have become available. In some diseases, radiation treatment is a useful therapeutic alternative, for example, for keloids. In certain dermatoses, for example eczema, radiotherapy should be applied only after other therapeutic methods have failed. Improved x-ray technology, accurate dosimetry, and strict adherence to safety rules have reduced cutaneous and noncutaneous side effects to a minimum.[23] The use of x-rays for benign diseases in all medical specialties has been evaluated by the National Academy of Sciences and these recommendations are now endorsed by the Food and Drug Administration (FDA).[24] In addition, the following rules for the irradiation of benign skin diseases are emphasized by dermatologists and radiooncologists:[23]

- The diagnosis must be clearly established, if possible by biopsy.
- Radiotherapy should start at the earliest possible time, e.g., in keloids.
- There should be a reasonable expectation that radiotherapy will lead to an improvement.
- All patients should be questioned about previous irradiations ("passport").

TABLE 128-1

Radiation Qualities

Type	kV	FSD (cm)	HVL (mm)	$D_{1/2}$ (mm)
Grenz rays (ultrasoft, supersoft, Bucky therapy)	10–20	10–30	0.03 Al	0.2–1.0
Soft x-ray	20–100	10–30	0.1–2.0 Al	1–20
Contact therapy (chaoul therapy)	50–60	1.5–3.0	2.0–4.0 Al	4–30
Superficial x-ray (low voltage)	60–150	15–30	0.7–2.0 Al	7–10
Orthovoltage therapy (deep x-ray therapy, conventional x-ray therapy)	150–400	50–80	2–4 Cu	50–80
Supervoltage therapy	400–800	50–80	5–10 Pb	80–110
Megavoltage therapy (betatron, particle accelerators)	>1000	80	>10 Pb	10–200

FSD, focus-skin distance; HVL, half-value layer; $D_{1/2}$, half-value depth.

- No area of the skin should be subjected to more than 12 Gy of soft or superficial x-rays (20 to 150 kV) or 50 Gy of grenz rays per lifetime and radiation field.
- No local treatment should be applied prior to radiotherapy in order to avoid irritating effects (e.g., 5-fluorouracil) or a reduction of the x-ray effect (e.g., zinc preparations).

For very superficial skin conditions, especially epidermal processes, grenz-ray treatment (5 to 19 kV) is preferred. Lindelöf and colleagues conducted a large-scale investigation of grenz-ray therapy and concluded that even doses up to 100 Gy are not associated with any significant side effects.[25]

Most inflammatory dermatoses have their pathology in the first millimeter of the skin and the rest in the first 3 mm. Grenz-ray therapy may be expected to be beneficial because 50 percent of grenz radiation administered is absorbed by the first 0.5 mm of the skin. This form of radiation is extremely suitable if one considers the sparing effect on hair roots, sebaceous and sweat glands, as well as eyes and gonads. Grenz-ray therapy may be indicated for these dermatoses:[26]

- Psoriasis
- Lichen simplex chronicus
- Pruritus ani et vulvae
- Seborrheic dermatitis
- Nummular eczema or persistent eczematous conditions
- Lichen planus
- Hailey-Hailey disease

The possible side effects of grenz-ray therapy are qualitatively identical to those of conventional x-rays, the principal adverse effects being erythema and pigmentation. Grenz-ray erythema is relatively asymptomatic, and its latent period is shorter than that of conventional x-ray erythema. It is ordinarily not followed by sequelae other than pigmentation. For this reason, close shielding should be avoided in order to not produce a sharp line at the edge of the treated area. Pigmentation so induced varies with race, age, and body region, but is seldom permanent.

In the following paragraphs the specific indications for the x-ray treatment of benign skin diseases with grenz rays or superficial x-rays are reviewed.

Psoriasis

Once a widely used treatment modality, x-ray therapy is used as a last resort in recalcitrant localized legions, especially where other treatment modalities are not very effective, for example psoriasis of the scalp and psoriasis of the nails. If properly used, radiation therapy is not associated with any major side effects. In general, there is no difference between conventional superficial x-ray therapy and grenz-ray therapy in more than 70 percent of the patients. Some authors found that the effect of superficial x rays were longer lasting than grenz rays.[26] Although grenz rays may be tried in psoriatic nails of normal thickness, it has been shown that they are less effective in thickened, diseased nails.[23] In accordance with other reports in the literature, we recommend the dose schedule described in Table 128-2.

Eczema/Dermatitis

If superficial x-rays are used, the least-penetrating quality should be preferred; in most cases, grenz rays (5 to 19 kV) are suitable.[23] However, in some chronic, long-standing eczematous conditions, especially of the palms and soles, more penetrating radiation qualities, that is, soft x-rays (20 to 150 kV) are more effective. There were different studies performed, all with favorable response rates, for hyperkeratotic eczemas or chronic lichenified eczemas. The weekly doses range from 0.5 to 1 Gy. It has also been shown that under certain indications, especially hyperkeratotic eczemas, a total dose of 3 Gy of conventional superficial x-ray was superior to 9 Gy of grenz rays. In atopic dermatitis, ionizing radiation is rarely advisable because of its high tendency to recur, whereas lichen simplex chronicus responds quickly to radiation therapy, because the antipruritic effect of radiation in this dermatosis is striking. Recent surveys indicate that the group of eczematous disorders constitute the most frequent indication for radiotherapy of benign lesions, especially in older patients with contraindications to systemic steroids or to the continued use of topical steroids. Table 128-2 lists our dose recommendations.

Keloids

For unknown reasons, certain individuals have a predisposition to keloid formation after surgery or other skin injury.[27] Lesions appear to occur frequently among those of African or Asian ancestry. In addition to cosmetic problems, keloids can become painful, pruritic, or fibrotic, and can produce significant morbidity. A variety of treatment options have been described. The use of pressure postoperatively is important as an additional treatment as are injections of corticosteroids. Radiation therapy has been employed successfully in the treatment of keloids. In most series, external kilovoltage or electron beam radiation is directed at the surgical bed within 24 to 72 hours after surgery.[23,28]

It has been shown that recurrence rates after keloid irradiation are much lower if radiation is administered following excision (25 to 36 percent) than the recurrence rate without prior excision (63 to 74 percent).[23] Typical dose-fractionation schemes range from 9 to 16 Gy in 3 to 4 Gy fractions. There does not appear to be a significant dose–response relationship in this dose range. The technique for the treatment of keloids is relatively straightforward: the reexcision scar, plus a 1- to 2-cm margin is treated. All suture sites should be included. Superficial x-rays can be used. The overall profile of morbidity and efficacy compares favorably with that of other treatments for keloids. Table 128-2 lists dose recommendations.

TABLE 128-2

Recommended Doses: Dermatoses

Diagnosis	kV	Fractionation (Gy)	Total Dose (Gy)	Time Interval (Days)
Eczema, chronic	12	6–12 × 1	6–12	4–7
	20	6–12 × 0,5	3–6	4–7
Eczema, seborrheic	12	6–12 × 1	6–12	
Psoriasis	12	4–12 × 2	8–24	4–7
	20	4–12 × 1	4–12	4–7
Erythrodermas	50/Teleroentgen	6–12 × 0,5	3–6	4–7
Lichen planus	20–50	6–12 × 0,5	3–6	4–7
Lichen planus, verrucous	20–50	4–12 × 1	4–12	4–7
Venous ulcer, painful	20–50	5–10 × 0,2	1–2	daily
Pruritus ani or vulvae	12	4–8 × 1	4–8	4–7

Lymphocytoma Cutis (Lymphocytoma Cutis Benigna, Lymphoid Hyperplasia)

This entity represents a pseudolymphoma and occurs as a localized or disseminated type. Because there are different etiologic agents, a therapeutic trial with antibiotics may not induce quick resolution of the lesion. The localized and circumscribed type responds well to small doses of x-rays.[23,29] Early lesions are more radiosensitive than older lesions. Cases of cutaneous lymphoid hyperplasia have also been reported in conjunction with the acquired immunodeficiency syndrome (AIDS), and progression to malignant lymphoma occurs in some cases. It is also possible to treat lymphomatoid papulosis with x-rays.[30] In general, the dose recommendations are similar to those for lymphomas (see below).

Other Indications

There are other rare indications for radiotherapy such as severely pruritic and refractory cases of the *verrucous type of lichen planus,* particularly on the legs.[23]

We earlier mentioned the possible indication of treating *Hailey-Hailey disease,* especially with grenz rays. These represent an excellent alternative to other treatment modalities and have a long-lasting effect. In rare cases, the treatment has to be repeated.[23] The dose schedule is the same as for eczema.

Another possible indication is *Peyronie's disease* (Induratio penis plastica), characterized by the development of penile plaques, arising from fibrosis of the corpus cavernosum. This disorder is characterized by a penile curvature during erection, and the presence of penile plaques or induration, often leading to pain during erection or intercourse. The disease may be self-limited in many cases. Indications and rationale for radiotherapy include the following:[31]

- There is a high rate of success when compared with other treatments: palliation of pain in approximately 80 percent of patients; decreased size of plaque in approximately 61 percent of patients; improvement of curvature in approximately 57 percent of patients.
- Treatment is painless, localized to the penis, without systemic side effects, and completed in 1 to 2 weeks.
- Failure of other therapies does not preclude a response to radiotherapy, and failure of radiotherapy does not preclude the use of other modalities.

Pain is the most reliable palliated symptom, with lesser rates of palliation achievable for induration and curvature.

Vasculitic painful leg ulcers are another potential indication for very-low-dose x-rays, that is, 0.2 Gy.[23,32] The doses are applied daily and the pain relief is quite striking after a few sessions. Table 128-2 shows the treatment schedule.

Erythroderma[33] or *generalized senile pruritus* may also be treated with x-rays.[23]

There is no longer an indication for the treatment of acne, hemangiomas or verrucae with radiation therapy.

RADIATION THERAPY OF MALIGNANT SKIN DISEASES/TUMORS Carcinomas of the skin are the most accessible cancers, the diagnosis is readily made and the limits of the lesion are usually easy to define. No single treatment method is best for all cancers of the skin. If the sole criterion of success is eradication of the lesion, surgery and radiotherapy yield similar results. Most cutaneous cancers are sufficiently sensitive to radiation to be eradicated by doses that are well tolerated by the surrounding normal tissue. If appropriate principles are followed and precautions are taken, x-irradiation is a safe and effective method of therapy.[22] Our discussion is deliberately limited to radiotherapy of cutaneous cancers of moderate size that can be effectively treated with grenz rays, superficial x-rays, or contact therapy units (see Table 128-1). Larger and more complicated skin cancers should be referred to Mohs surgeons and/or radiation oncologists for treatment with higher kilovoltage, megavoltage, or electron-beam techniques, or for implants with radioactive isotopes.

When treating skin cancer, the *advantages* of soft- or superficial x-ray therapy include:

- Performable on an outpatient basis
- Painless
- Usable for physically or psychologically handicapped patients (also patients over 90 years old[34])
- Usable for anticoagulated patients
- Usable in patients in whom there exists a contraindication for a surgical intervention
- Healthy tissue or certain organs can be protected
- Usually a wide margin of normal-appearing skin (wider than in surgical excisions)
- Atraumatic intervention

However, there also are *disadvantages* to radiation therapy about which the patient should be informed:

- The treatment cannot be done in one single session
- If the patient has already received full tumor doses in a radiation field, this particular field cannot be irradiated a second time
- Radiation treatment is followed by alopecia (except if treated by grenz rays)
- Chronic radiation dermatitis tends to be accentuated with time

What is the ideal indication for radiotherapy? Radiotherapy is particularly valuable for medium-sized tumors of 1 to 4 cm in diameter on the face of elderly people, because smaller tumors are mostly treated by surgery and larger lesions are mostly treated either by Mohs surgery or by a combination of surgery and megavoltage treatment.

What are the best areas to be treated by radiation therapy? The real superiority of irradiation over excision lies in its greater preservation of uninvolved tissue. In certain anatomic regions this may pose a problem for the surgeon but not for the radiotherapist who can easily adjust the size of the field to the required area of treatment. Therefore, radiation is often the treatment of choice in areas where tissue cannot be readily sacrificed for cosmetic and/or functional reasons. There is general agreement that ionizing radiation is often preferable to other methods of treatment for cutaneous tumors of the following areas:[22]

- Eyelids
- Medial or lateral canthi of the eyes
- Nose
- Ears
- Lips
- Nasolabial folds
- Preauricular areas
- Larger tumors of the cheek

On the other hand the skin of the trunk and extremities has a greater tendency to develop radiation sequelae, particularly telangiectasias and changes in pigmentation.[35]

Before radiation therapy of a lesion is begun, the diagnosis must be confirmed by biopsy.

Why biopsy? The histologic examination determines

- the type of the tumor.
- the radiosensitivity of the tumor.
- the exact extension of the tumor.
- the depth of the tumor.
- the exclusion of an error.

Concerning the radiosensitivity of skin tumors, *four categories* are distinguishable (Table 128-3): (1) *Highly indicated* and unique advantage:

TABLE 128-3

Indications/Radiosensitivity of Different Skin Tumors

INDICATION	TUMOR
Highly indicated	Cutaneous T cell lymphomas (CTCL) Some B cell lymphomas Kaposi's sarcoma
Good indication	Basal cell carcinoma (BCC) Squamous cell carcinoma (SCC) Keratoacanthoma Bowens'disease Queyrat's erythroplasia Merkel cell tumor
Sometimes indicated	Angiosarcoma melanoma (LMM)
Rarely indicated	Carcinoma of the scrotum, or palms/soles fibrosarcoma

Kaposi's sarcoma, mycosis fungoides, and other lymphomas of the skin. (2) *Good indication:* basal cell and squamous cell carcinomas, keratoacanthoma, Bowen's disease, Queyrat's erythroplasia, Merkel cell carcinoma. (3) *Sometimes indicated:* angiosarcoma, melanoma. (4) *Rarely indicated:* fibrosarcoma, carcinomas of the scrotum, soles, and palms.

We also distinguish between *curative* radiotherapy in tumors such as basal cell carcinomas; squamous cell carcinomas; keratoacanthomas; precancerous lesions and melanomas of the lentigo maligna type; and *palliative* radiation therapy in tumors such as Merkel cell carcinoma, Kaposi's sarcoma, and most lymphomas.

The contraindications for radiotherapy with soft x-rays include:

- Tumors penetrating into cartilage or bone
- Intraoral tumors
- Tumors penetrating into the nostrils
- Tumors in scars of osteomyelitis, burns, chronic ulcers, or in chronic radiodermatitis
- No retreatment of previously irradiated skin carcinomas
- Genodermatoses that are prone to neoplasms such as basal cell nevus syndrome or xeroderma pigmentosum

Which radiation quality? Since the work done in England, Germany, and United States, and with the introduction of the beryllium-windowed x-ray units, as a rule of thumb, radiation qualities with a half-value depth (HVD $= D_{1/2}$) corresponding to the depth of the tumor have been proposed. Most of the radiation will then be absorbed in the pathologic tissue and the possibility of undesirable radiation effects to underlying uninvolved tissue will be markedly reduced. The depth of the tumor can either be reasonably estimated by inspection and palpation or by an exact histopathologic description of the tumor depth, preferably by an experienced dermatopathologist. Several studies show that 50 percent of all basal cell and squamous cell cancers infiltrate to a depth of only 2 mm or less, and 75 percent of such tumors infiltrate to a depth of 5 mm or less.[22]

With grenz and superficial x-ray machines, the kilovoltage is in a fixed combination with filters in order to avoid filter mistakes and thus application of faulty dosages. These x-ray machines have a kilovoltage between 10 and 50 kV, sometimes up to 100 or even 150 kV. With filter combinations, a HVD ($= D_{1/2}$) from 1 mm to 20 mm can be reached. For dermatologic purposes, it is rarely necessary to irradiate tumors thicker than 20 mm.

Why fractionated doses? Fractionation of radiation dosage is based on the assumptions that tissues recover at different rates from the effects of radiation and that tumor tissue recovers more slowly than normal tissue. When a given dose of radiation is divided into several increments and delivered over a period of several days, the biological effect is usually less pronounced than that of the same radiation administered in a single dose. This lesser damage with fractionation appears to be related to cell recovery between increments and to the capabilities of recovering cells to adapt to radiation-induced alterations of the surrounding tissues. Small tumors and radiation fields support higher single doses than do large tumors with large irradiation fields that have to be irradiated with smaller single doses. In addition, in large irradiation fields, we have to consider an additional backscatter factor.

Much work has been done in an attempt to define optimum time-dose-volume relationships for carcinomas of the skin. There is no consensus as to the total dose needed to eradicate a cutaneous cancer and when to terminate radiotherapy. Different authors have recommended different dosages.[22] The tendency is to use standardized schedules (Table 128-4).

TABLE 128-4

Recommended Doses: Malignant Tumors

DIAGNOSIS	kV	FIELD (cm)	FRACTIONATION (Gy)	TOTAL DOSE (Gy)	TIME INTERVAL (DAYS)
Lentigo maligna	12	<2 >2	5–6 × 20 or 10–12 × 10	100–120 100–120	4–7 3–4
Bowen's disease or Queyrat's erythroplasia	20	<2 >2	3–4 × 8 8 × 10 × 4	24–32 32–40	4–7 3–4
Keratosis, senile	12 20	<2	5–7 × 8 2–3 × 8 5–7 × 4	40–56 16–24 20–28	4–7 4–7 3–4
Basal cell carcinoma/squamous cell carcinoma	20–50	<2 2–5 >5	5–6 × 8 10–12 × 4 26–28 × 2	40–48 40–48 52–56	4–7 3–4 daily
Mycosis fungoides/other malignant lymphomas/leukemic infiltrates	20–50 Teleroentgen		3–7 × 2 4–10 × 1	6–14 4–10	3–4 3–7
Lentigo maligna melanoma/melanoma metastases	20–50		7–9 × 6	42–54	4–7
Kaposi's sarcoma	20–50	<2 >2	3–5 × 8 5–10 × 4	24–40 20–40	4–7 3–4

It is still worthwhile to observe the patient's reaction during radiation therapy and to look for an exudative or erosive reaction in the irradiated margin. When larger individual doses are administered, the recommended total dose is usually smaller than in cases where smaller individual doses were used.

FIGURE 128-1

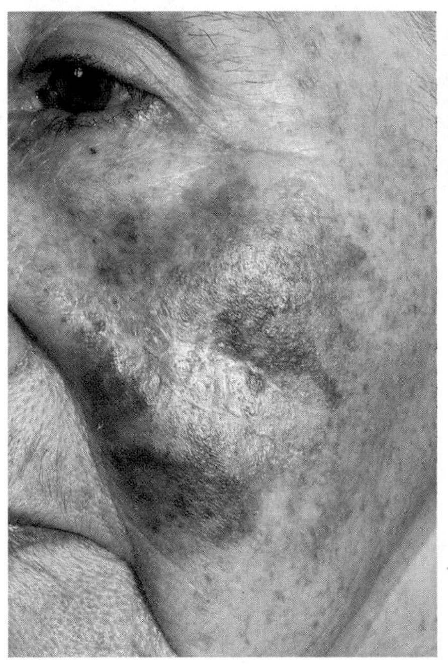

A.

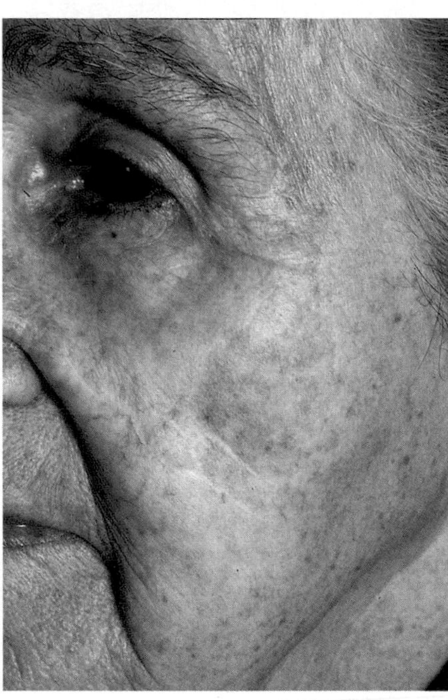

B.

A. Extensive lentigo maligna on the left cheek of a 76-year-old female patient before and (*B*) 2 years after grenz ray treatment [10 times 10 Gy (100 Gy), twice per week].

Disseminated Actinic Keratoses

Usually, there is agreement that small actinic keratoses are best treated by surgical excision or other equivalent methods. The problem arises in extensive and disseminated actinic keratoses as, for example, on the scalp. Here, again, there are possibilities with topical treatments such as 5-fluorouracil or imiquimod cream, but usually recurrence rates are higher or appear sooner than after treatment with radiotherapy. Because these lesions are intraepidermal and often in an atrophic epidermis, the ideal treatment is with grenz rays. The treatment consists of six sessions of 6 Gy twice weekly applied on one or several divided fields.[36] At the end of the treatment, an erythema or an exudative reaction will occur. If there is marked pruritus, topical glucocorticoid creams may be of help to the patient. One month after the end of treatment, the erythema has mostly gone. The patient has to be told to continue sun protection with a hat and application of a sunscreen. Rarely, it is necessary to perform a second treatment years later.

Table 128-4 shows the dose schedule.

Bowen's Disease/Queyrat's Erythroplasia

This carcinoma in situ is treated in a similar fashion to actinic keratosis, but histopathologically, these lesions are thicker. Even in elderly patients, it is possible to apply grenz rays with a $D_{1/2}$ of 1 mm. If the lesions are more infiltrated, soft x-rays with quality of 20 kV or more are necessary. The dose schedule can be adapted (see Table 128-4). Again fractions of single doses of 6 Gy up to total dose around 40 Gy may be used. Single doses with soft x-rays would be 4 Gy. Exudative reactions have to be expected a little earlier in the genitoanal area. Treatment results are excellent.[36]

Table 128-4 shows the dose schedule.

Lentigo Maligna

This is another precancerous lesion that is an excellent indication for radiation treatment. This treatment modality is not well known because it is always thought that it is not curative. Recent reports show that treatment results are at least as good as surgical procedures.[37–39] As mentioned earlier, the inclusion of a wide enough margin is not a problem for the radiation therapist; consequently, large lentigo malignas are an excellent indication for radiotherapy. The classical treatment schedule is named after Miescher who proposed 5 to 6 doses of 20 Gy grenz rays for medium-sized lesions (around 2.5 cm in diameter). For larger lesions we prefer 10 to 12 doses of 10 Gy grenz rays (see Table 128-4). The epidermis in the elderly is atrophic, and with a HVD of 1 mm we reach even atypical melanocytes in the hair follicles. Figure 128-1 shows a grenz-ray treatment result.

Basal Cell Carcinoma, Squamous Cell Carcinoma, Keratoacanthoma

These tumors represent the classical indications for radiotherapy with soft x-rays or superficial x-rays, because most of these tumors are well circumscribed and rarely larger than 2.5 cm. In addition, 75 percent of these tumors are less than 5 mm thick. Some treatment centers use the same treatment schedules for basal cell carcinomas (BCCs) and squamous cell carcinomas (SCCs), although one could imagine that SCC should be treated with a higher total dose, because it represents a more aggressive tumor.[22] Elderly patients prefer not to come every day for the treatment sessions. Therefore, medium-sized lesions can be treated with, for example, a 4-Gy single dose in three fractions per week. There is even the possibility of applying a higher single dose, for example 6 to 8 Gy per fraction twice a week, to small lesions that cannot be excised. We agree that large lesions, (larger than 4 cm) are best treated with daily fractions of 2 or 3 Gy (see Table 128-4). Figure 128-2 shows the results of treating a BCC as described here.

We want to stress the importance of knowing the histopathology of BCC and SCC for the outcome of the treatment. A large study has shown that if the histopathology shows a sclerosing type rather than a nodular type of BCC or SCC, the recurrence rate rises immediately.[36] Consequently, the sclerosing histologic type is not well suited for treatment with soft x-rays. There are two possibilities: (1) if the patient is operable, Mohs surgery is the preferred method, or (2) if surgery is contraindicated, megavoltage therapy should be chosen.

For keratoacanthomas the same dose schedule is used as for SCCs.[40] Carcinomas of the skin appendages and carcinomas penetrating into cartilage or bone, localized in the mucous membranes, or arising in chronic scars, are not an indication for soft x-ray therapy.

FIGURE 128-2

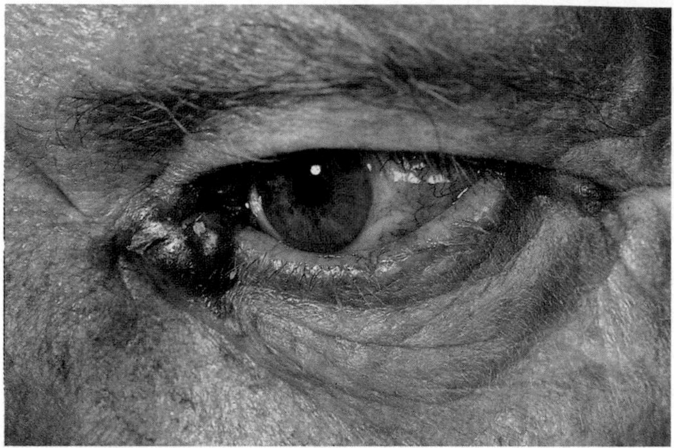

A.

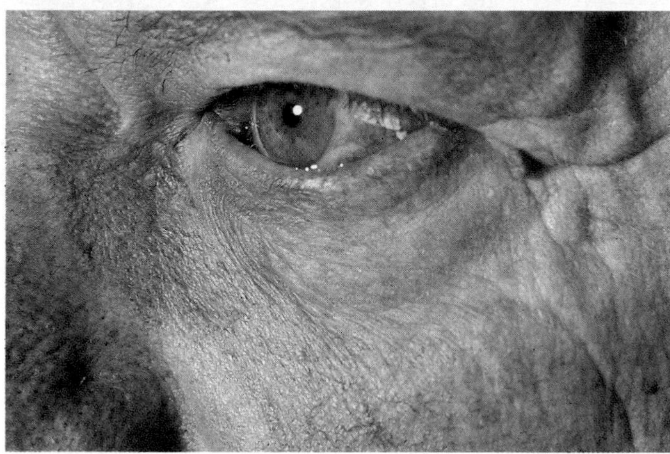

B.

A. Basal cell carcinoma on the left inner canthus of a 64-year-old man before and (*B*) 6 months after soft x-ray treatment (40 kV) [12 times 4 Gy (48 Gy), twice per week].

Radiation treatment is possible for BCCs, SCCs, or keratoacanthomas that were not completely excised or were incompletely treated by electrodesiccation or cryotherapy. The techniques are the same as for primary tumors. The functional and the cosmetic results after irradiation of such treated tumors are usually satisfactory.[22]

Melanoma of the Lentigo Maligna Type

Since the time of Miescher, it has been well known that not only lentigo malignas (LMs), but also lentigo maligna melanomas (LMMs) respond well to radiation treatment.[37–39] In contrast to lentigo malignas, LMMs penetrate into the dermal tissues. As a result, grenz-ray treatment is not recommended; instead, soft or superficial x-rays, that is, radiation qualities of at least 20 kV or more, are recommended. We want to stress that LM and LMM are not to be considered radioresistant; instead, they may be tumors with a *reduced radiosensitivity* for the following reasons:[41]

- High percentage of nonproliferating cells
- High percentage of hypoxic cells
- High probability of potentially lethal repair
- Subpopulations of cells with different radiosensitivity in the "shoulder" region of the survival curve
- Synthesis of the prostaglandins (radioprotectors) in the tumor cells
- Melanin is a scavenger of "radicals"

Therefore, higher doses per fractions are recommended, mostly situated around 6 Gy per fraction. Table 128-4 shows the proposed dose schedule.

Our results from treatment of 64 patients show a similar outcome for radiation treatment as for surgical treatment, with a cure rate of approximately 90 percent.[38] This rate is for both LM and LMM, especially for large lesions on the face of elderly patients, which lets these patients avoid major surgical procedures and scarring. From the cosmetic and functional point of view, the outcome is excellent.

Paget's Disease

Paget's disease of the nipple shows mostly an underlying carcinoma. In extramammary Paget's disease, seldom is an underlying carcinoma found. In these situations, we are dealing with a superficial lesion and thus grenz rays can be used. The dose schedule is similar to that used for Bowen's disease.

Merkel Cell Tumor

Merkel cell tumor is a rare primary skin tumor and occurs most frequently in the seventh and eighth decades. Tumors occur with greatest frequency in the head and neck region (50 percent). Tumors are characterized by a high rate of local recurrence after surgical excision (25 to 60 percent) and by frequent involvement of regional lymph nodes (45 to 79 percent); distant metastatic failure is common (22 to 48 percent).[42] Several series have shown promising results when radiation therapy is added to the initial surgical management of Merkel cell carcinoma. At the M.D. Anderson Cancer Center, 83 percent of patients showed disease control when they were treated with surgery and radiation therapy for palpable neck disease. Doses of 50 Gy at conventional fractionation appear adequate for the treatment of subclinical disease, but when microscopic or gross residual disease exists, boosting the doses to 60 to 70 Gy is indicated.[43]

Cutaneous Lymphomas

In general, the lesions of cutaneous lymphomas, that is, T cell or B cell lymphomas, are very radiosensitive.[44,45] With the exception of certain circumscribed B cell lymphomas or localized CD30+ lymphomas where radiotherapy is curative, the radiation treatment for lymphomas is palliative. Total doses in the range of 20 to 30 Gy are commonly used and offer excellent palliation. Doses in this range may result in a relapse rate of up to 30 percent. Single doses of 2 Gy, either daily or three times per week, seem to offer the best local control. See also Table 128-4.

Because of the possible need for the subsequent treatment in adjacent areas, it is important to document the treated areas with photographs, accurate drawings, and, if feasible, tattooing of the corners of the fields with India ink. In most patients, the lesions will not clear during or at the completion of irradiation and it may take up to 6 to 8 weeks for complete response (Fig. 128-3). For individual skin lesions, energies may range from orthovoltage to electron beam. The depth of infiltration defines the energy of the beam required. Larger, bulkier lesions, such as deep ulcers or lymph nodes, may be treated by either Cobalt or 4 to 6 MeV photons. (see Table 128-1)

FIGURE 128-3

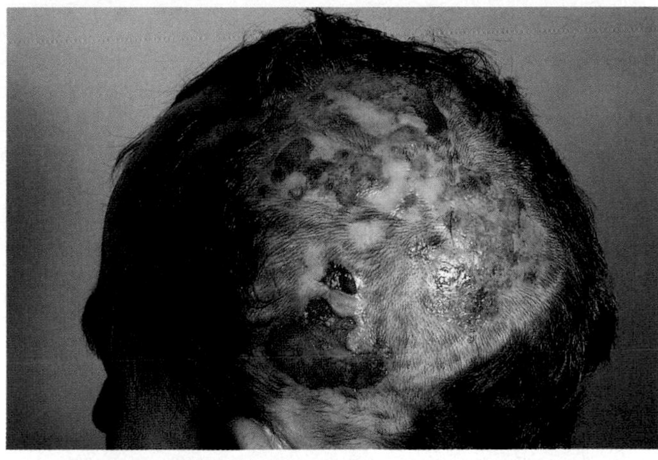

A.

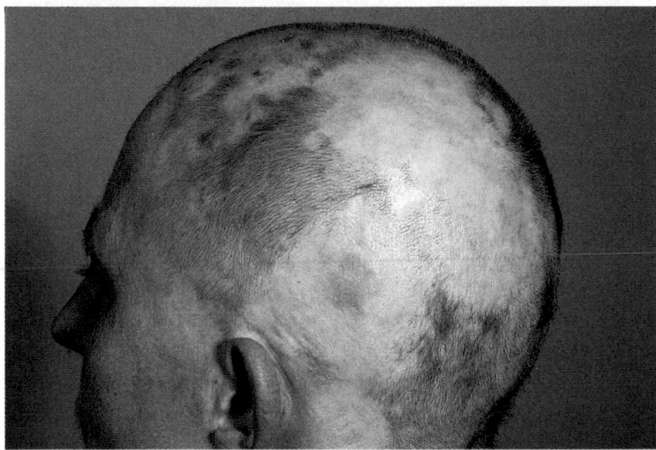

B.

A. Mycosis fungoides in a 42-year-old woman before and (*B*) 1 month after soft x-ray treatment (40 kV) [6 times 2Gy (12 Gy), 3 times per week].

Kaposi's Sarcoma

NON–AIDS-ASSOCIATED KAPOSI'S SARCOMA Local irradiation of Kaposi's sarcoma (KS) includes the lesion plus a normal tissue border of approximately 1 to 2 cm. Thin, cutaneous lesions can be effectively treated either by superficial x-ray therapy (e.g., 20 to 150 kV) or relatively low-energy electron beams (e.g., 4 to 6 MeV). Thick nodules are best treated by electron beams that encompass the entire lesion homogeneously but spare underlying normal tissues. Lesions on the eyelids are treated most easily by superficial x-rays with protective shields over the optic lens.[36,46]

Based on the available evidence, both local therapy and elective regional therapy are effective techniques for the treatment of classical KS. The literature supports the use of a wide range of doses and fractionation patterns. As long as a sufficient dose is delivered (e.g., 20 to 30 Gy in 10 fractions or, for small lesions, 8 Gy in 1 fraction), a salutary outcome is likely.[47] Table 128-4 shows a treatment schedule.

AIDS-ASSOCIATED KAPOSI'S SARCOMA Usually, the same dose schedules are used and no difference is evident, although it may take 3 to 4 months for the tumors to resolve. Radiation-induced edema of the feet or face, as well as symptomatic mucositis, are more severe in patients with AIDS than in other patients.[47]

Radiation therapy may be reserved for specific indications such as pain, ulceration, bleeding, functional impairment (e.g., on the legs), or improvement of the appearance of cosmetically disfiguring lesions (e.g., the eyelids). In the case of palliative radiation therapy for AIDS-associated Kaposi's sarcoma:

- Sufficient dose should be delivered to accomplish the desired goal and maintain that state for as long as possible.
- The treatment should be delivered as rapidly as possible.
- Distressing side effects should not be induced by the treatment.

Other Skin Tumors

Other possible indications for radiation therapy include:[26]

- Angiosarcoma
- Leukemic infiltrates of the skin (e.g., infiltrations of chronic myelogenous leukemia, or chronic lymphatic leukemia)
- Metastatic nodules of melanoma
- Metastatic nodules of breast carcinoma

REFERENCES

1. Schmidt-Ullrich RK et al: Signal transduction and cellular radiation responses. *Radiat Res* **153**:245, 2000
2. Herskind C et al: The role of cytokines in the development of normal-tissue reactions after radiotherapy. *Strahlenther Onkol* **174**(suppl 3):12, 1998
3. Rosen EM et al: The molecular and cellular basis of radiosensitivity: Implications for understanding how normal tissues and tumors respond to therapeutic radiation. *Cancer Invest* **17**:56, 1999
4. Davis ST et al: Prevention of chemotherapy-induced alopecia in rats by CDK inhibitors. *Science* **291**:134, 2001
5. Schwartz JL et al: The contribution of DNA ploidy to radiation sensitivity in human tumor cell lines. *Br J Cancer* **79**:744, 1999
6. Sinclair WK, Morton RA: X-ray sensitivity during cell generation cycle of cultured Chinese hamster cells. *Radiat Res* **29**:450, 1966
7. Maisin JR: Bacq and Alexander Award lecture—Chemical radioprotectors: Past, present, and future prospects. *Int J Radiat Biol* **73**:443, 1998
8. Lorimore SA et al: Oral (PO) dosing with RS 1069 or RB 6145 maintains their potency as hypoxic cell sensitizers and cytotoxics but reduces systemic toxicity compared with parenteral (IP) administration in mice. *Int J Radiat Oncol Biol Phys* **21**:387, 1991
9. Wasserman T: Radioprotective effects of amifostine. *Semin Oncol* **26**(2 suppl 7):89, 1999
10. Hanson WR et al: Prostaglandin-induced protection from radiation or doxorubicin is tissue specific in mice. *J Invest Dermatol* **104**:606, 1995
11. Geng L et al: Topical or systemic 16,16-dimethyl prostaglandin E_2 or WR-2721 (WR-1065) protects mice from alopecia after fractionated irradiation. *Int J Radiat Biol* **61**:533, 1992
12. Malkinson FD et al: Prostaglandins protect against murine hair injury produced by ionizing radiation or doxorubicin. *J Invest Dermatol* **101**(suppl):135, 1993
13. Hanson WR et al: The prostaglandin E_2 analog, misoprostol, a normal tissue protector, does not protect four murine tumors in vivo from radiation injury. *Radiat Res* **142**:281, 1995
14. Khan AM et al: A prospective randomized placebo-controlled double-blinded pilot study of misoprostol rectal suppositories in the prevention of acute and chronic radiation proctitis symptoms in prostate cancer patients. *Am J Gastroenterol* **95**:1961, 2000
15. Malkinson FD, Hanson WR: Radiobiology of the skin, in *Physiology, Biochemistry, and Molecular Biology of the Skin,* vol II, 2nd ed, edited by LA Goldsmith. Oxford, Oxford University Press, 1991, p 976
16. Panizzon RG et al: Ionizing radiation induces early, sustained increases in collagen biosynthesis: A 48-week study in mouse skin and fibroblast cultures. *Radiat Res* **116**:145, 1988
17. Randall K, Coggle JE: Expression of transforming growth factor-β_1 in mouse skin during the acute phase of radiation damage. *Int J Radiat Biol* **68**:301, 1995

18. Archombeau JO et al: Pathophysiology of irradiated skin and breast. *Int J Radiat Oncol Biol Phys* **31**:1171, 1995
19. Malkinson FD: Radiobiology of the skin, in *Dermatology in General Medicine,* vol I, 5th ed, edited by IM Freedberg, AZ Eisen, K Wolff, KF Austen, LA Goldsmith, SI Katz, TB Fitzpatrick. New York, McGraw-Hill, 1999, p 1514
20. Kyoizumi S et al: Radiation sensitivity of human hair follicles in SCID-hu mice. *Radiat Res***149**:11, 1998
21. Cole S et al: Langerhans cells: Quantitative indicators of x-ray damage in mouse skin? *Br J Cancer* **53**(suppl VII):75, 1986
22. Goldschmidt H: Treatment planning, in *Modern Dermatologic Radiation Therapy,* edited by H Goldschmidt, RG Panizzon. New York, Springer, 1991, pp 49–63
23. Goldschmidt H: Chronic radiation effects and radiation protection, in *Modern Dermatologic Radiation Therapy,* edited by H Goldschmidt, RG Panizzon. New York, Springer, 1991, pp 37–48
24. Goldschmidt H: FDA recommendations on radiotherapy of benign diseases. *J Dermatol Surg Oncol* **4**:619, 1978
25. Lindelöf B, Eklund G: Incidence of malignant skin tumors in 14,140 patients after grenz ray treatment for benign skin disorders. *Arch Dermatol* **122**:1391, 1986
26. Lindelöf B: Grenz ray therapy, in *Modern Dermatologic Radiation Therapy,* edited by H Goldschmidt, RG Panizzon. New York, Springer, 1991, pp 155–159
27. Luo S et al: Abnormal balance between proliferation and apoptotic cell death in fibroblasts derived keloid lesions. *Plast Reconstr Surg* **107**:87, 2001
28. Wagner W et al: Results of prophylactic irradiation in patients with resected keloids, a retrospective analysis. *Acta Oncol* **39**:217, 2000
29. Gillian AC, Wood GS: Cutaneous lymphoid hyperplasias. *Semin Cutan Med Surg* **19**:133, 2000
30. Kaufmann T et al: Lymphomatoid papulosis: Case report of a patient managed with radiation therapy an of the literature. *Am J Clin Oncol* **15**:412, 1992
31. Mira JG et al: The value of radiotherapy for Peyronie's disease: Presentation of 56 new case studies and review of the literature. *Int J Radiat Oncol Biol Phys* **6**:161, 1980
32. Trott KR: Therapeutic effects of low radiation doses. *Strahlenther Onkol* **170**:1, 1994
33. Holloway KB et al: Therapeutic alternatives in cutaneous T-cell lymphoma. *J Am Acad Dermatol* **27**:367, 1992
34. Mitsuhashi N et al: Cancer in patients aged 90 years or older: Radiation therapy. *Radiology* **211**:829, 1999
35. Panizzon RG, Goldschmidt H: Radiation reactions and sequels, in *Modern Dermatologic Radiation Therapy,* edited by H Goldschmidt, RG Panizzon. New York, Springer, 1991, pp 25–36
36. Panizzon RG: Radiotherapie des précancéroses et tumeurs malignes de la peau. *Med Hyg* **56**:461, 1998
37. Gaspar ZS, Dawber RP: Treatment of lentigo maligna. *Australas J Dermatol* **38**:1, 1997
38. Panizzon RG: Radiotherapy of lentigo maligna and lentigo maligna melanoma. *Skin Cancer* **14**:203, 1999
39. Schmid-Wndtner MH et al: Fractionated radiotherapy of lentigo maligna and lentigo maligna melanoma in 64 patients. *J Am Acad Dermatol* **43**:477, 2000
40. Caccialanza M, Sopelama N: Radiation therapy of keratoacanthomas: Results in 55 patients. *Int J Radiat Oncol Biol Phys* **16**:475, 1988
41. Panizzon RG. Radiation therapy of melanomas, in *Modern Dermatologic Radiation Therapy,* edited by H Goldschmidt, RG Panizzon. New York, Springer, 1991, pp 133–137
42. Pilotti S et al: Clinicopathologic correlations of cutaneous neuroendocrine Merkel cell carcinoma. *J Clin Oncol* **6**:1863, 1988
43. Wegmuller EA Jr et al: Merkel cell carcinoma of the ear. *Head Neck* **13**:68, 1991
44. Bekkenk MW et al: Treatment of multifocal primary cutaneous B-cell lymphoma: A clinical follow-up study of 29 patients. *J Clin Oncol* **17**:2471, 1999
45. Micaily B, Vonderheid EC: Cutaneous T-cell lymphoma in *Principles and Practice of Radiation Oncology,* edited by CA Perez, LW Brady. Philadelphia, Lippincott-Raven, 1997, p 763
46. Goldschmidt H Radiation therapy of other cutaneous tumors, in *Modern Dermatologic Radiation Therapy,* edited by H Goldschmidt, RG Panizzon. New York, Springer, 1991, pp 123–131
47. Cooper JS: Classic and acquired immunodeficiency syndrome (AIDS)-related Kaposi's sarcoma, in *Principles and Practice of Radiation Oncology,* edited by CA Perez, LW Brady. Philadelphia, Lippincott-Raven, 1997, p 745

CHAPTER 129

Calum C. Lyon
Michael H. Beck

Skin Problems in Amputees and Ostomates

PROBLEMS IN AMPUTEES*

The skin of an amputation stump is not designed to withstand the physical insults it encounters within a prosthetic limb. While some adaptation will occur, for example to friction or pressure, some skin problems are inevitable. If these dermatoses cannot be prevented or rapidly resolved by prosthesis adjustment or medical intervention, they can incapacitate the patient, particularly those who have a lower-limb prosthesis. As a result, the patient may suffer social isolation, emotional distress, or even financial deprivation if the patient is unable to work.

Although modern limb prostheses allow many of today's amputees to lead an active life with good mobility,[1] as many as one-third of amputees will experience a skin problem that interferes with the normal use of their artificial limb.[2]

In most centers, artificial limbs are made by using a modular construction technique. The stump is placed in a thermoplastic socket that is then fitted into the main body of the limb. The bulk of the prosthesis comprises a metal frame with articulations and an outer casing of acrylic resin or carbon composite material. Before fitting the limb many patients place their stump in a liner designed to reduce friction on the

*We wish to acknowledge S. William Levy, MD, the previous author of this chapter for his enormous contribution to the field of dermatoses in amputees and for stimulating our interest in the subject.

FIGURE 129-1

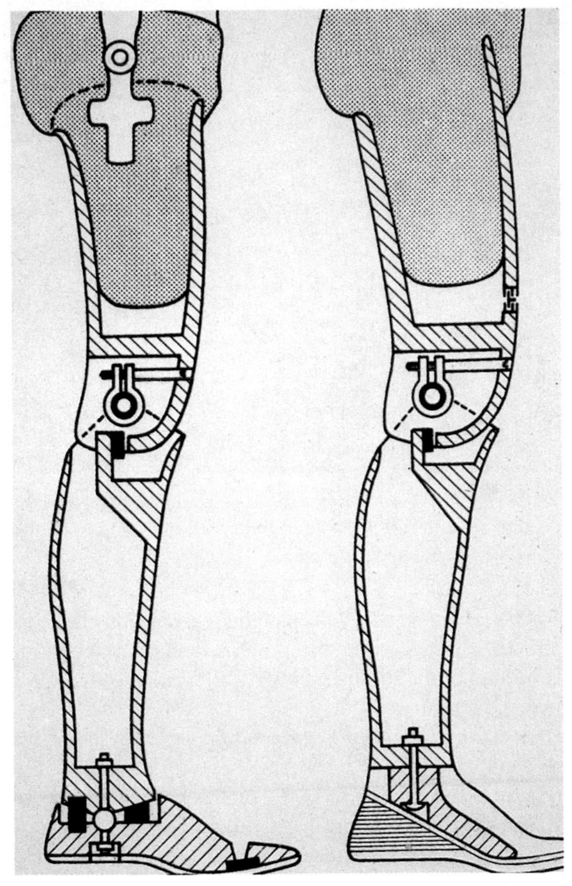

Above-knee prosthesis. Suction-socket prosthesis.

FIGURE 129-2

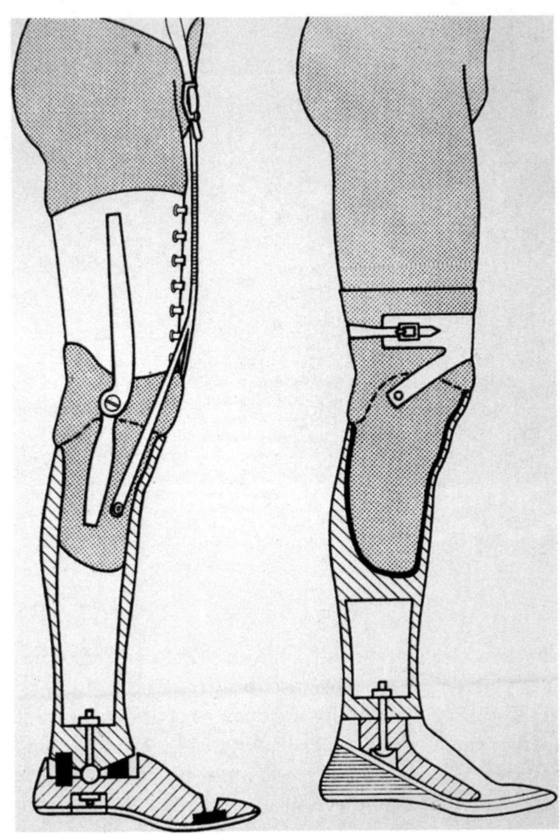

Below-knee prosthesis. Patellar–tendon-bearing cuff suspension.

skin. This may be an expanded plastic cup, a silicon/mineral oil sleeve, or a cotton sock. The prosthetic limb, once fitted, is held in position by one of a range of suspension elements. In above-knee (Fig. 129-1) or proximal arm amputations, this is usually a fabric belt arrangement worn around the waist or shoulders, respectively. Below-knee amputees require a different system using either a butyl rubber sleeve or corset to hold the appliance firmly onto the thigh (Fig. 129-2). Many patients with above-knee amputations now use a suction socket device that provides sufficient suspension, holding the prosthesis in place by negative pressure without the need for additional belts (Fig. 129-1).

Skin problems may occur because of allergy or chemical irritation to materials in contact with the skin, as well as from trauma and occlusion. Examples of physical stresses on the skin include shearing and friction from elements in the socket and pressure on load-bearing areas, especially on the tibial tuberosity in below-knee amputations and the ischial tuberosity, adductor region, or groin in above-knee amputations. In all cases, the occlusion results in increased humidity from trapped perspiration increasing the likelihood of irritation, allergy, and infection.

The great majority of artificial limb wearers are amputees, although a small proportion are people with congenital limb malformations. Lower-limb amputees are the most numerous and are also the group at greatest risk of skin problems. The reasons for this are clear when one considers the environmental stresses to which the stump skin is subjected. These stresses include heat, humidity, friction, shearing stress, and pressure, both positive and negative. In lower-limb prostheses, the greater load bearing and need for more secure attachment means that all these effects are amplified.

The common skin disorders in amputation stumps can be classified into diseases related to the reasons for the amputation, physical effects of a prosthesis, infection, contact dermatitis and other cutaneous disorders.

Dermatoses Related to the Reasons for Amputation

Several disorders resulting in the need for amputation can have a significant impact on skin integrity. In general, younger patients require artificial limbs because of traumatic amputations, congenital abnormalities, or malignancy, whereas in the older age group, arterial disease and vascular complications of diabetes mellitus predominate. Amputations following trauma or severe vasculitis may be associated with scarring that makes for a suboptimal prosthesis fit (Fig. 129-3). However, it is diabetes mellitus that is particularly associated with protracted skin problems as a result of impaired wound healing, susceptibility to infection, abnormal sensory nerve function, and disruption of normal tissue fluid balance.[3] Diabetic amputees as a group require more frequent clinical review in order to prevent complications. Treatment of the diabetic amputee not only requires good control of the blood glucose level but possibly a change of the stump environment through adjustment or redesign of the artificial limb. The diabetic amputee highlights the need for close links with a prosthetics department, which allow rapid referral of patients for assessment.

Physical Dermatoses

The physical effects of wearing a prosthesis are the commonest causes of skin problems.[2,4] These can be divided into those resulting from repeated direct trauma and those secondary to disturbance of tissue fluid dynamics.

FIGURE 129-3

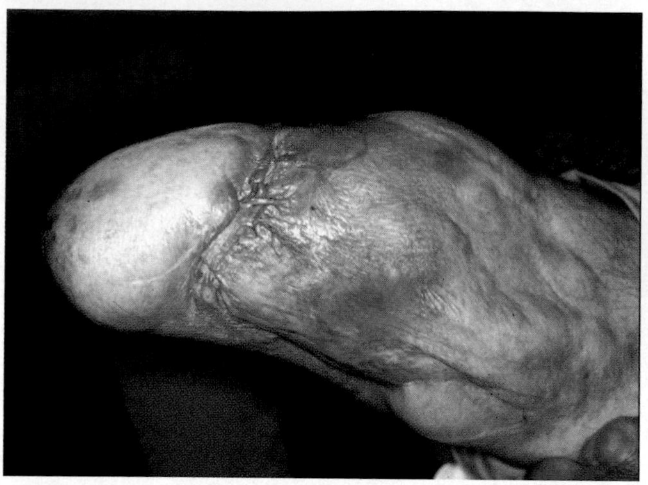

Scarring of the stump following amputation for severe postinfective vasculitis.

DIRECT PHYSICAL TRAUMA

Ulceration Ulceration and callus formation are seen where there is chronic pressure or repeated frictional forces on stump skin. Ulceration may also be caused by infection or poor cutaneous nutrition particularly secondary to diabetes mellitus (Fig. 129-4). Stump ulcers should be treated early as malignancy may develop in long-standing ulceration. With repeated infection and ulceration, an amputation scar on the distal stump skin can erode further. In some cases, the skin may become completely adherent to bone and develop thick, callus-like hyperkeratosis (Fig. 129-5), which may necessitate revision of the distal bony surface. In every instance, the cause of the ulceration must be determined in order to resolve a chronic process that can become totally disabling.

FIGURE 129-4

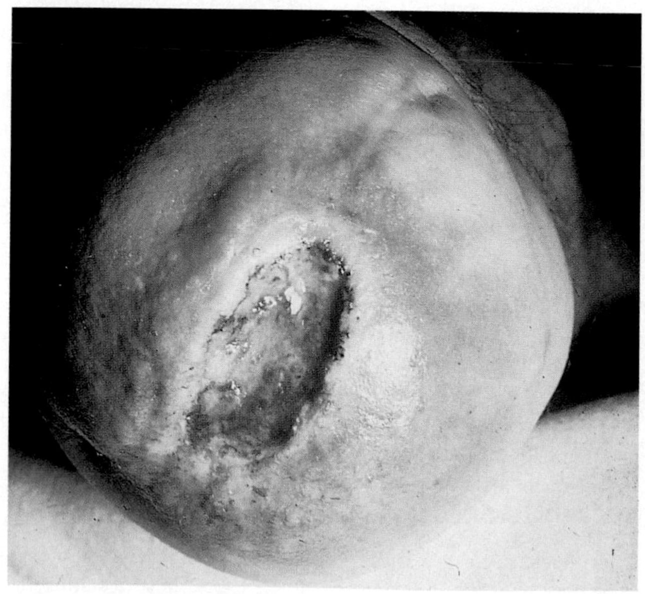

Chronic ulcer of stump skin.

FIGURE 129-5

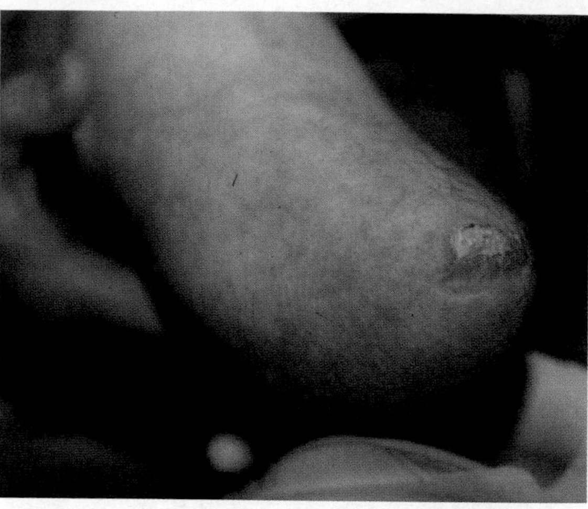

Chronic ulceration resulting in thick hyperkeratosis and scab formation adherent to the underlying bone.

Physical dermatitis In some patients, eczema may be caused by a poorly fitted or misaligned prosthesis or by edema and congestion of the terminal portion of the stump; only with alleviation of these problems does the condition clear.

Epidermoid cysts and follicular keratoses These are two ends of a spectrum of the same disorder. They are a consequence of repeated pressure and friction from the prosthesis that appears to cause invagination of keratin around hair follicles, which then result in a foreign-body reaction. Follicular keratoses are therefore the earliest changes.[5] These are very common, often multiple, and distributed at sites of weight bearing such as the anterior tibial area, popliteal fossa, and the adductor or inguinal areas of the thigh (Fig. 129-6*A*). Fortunately, they cause little trouble in many cases, but they can become inflamed and painful, particularly if the patient picks at them to extract the keratin plug or if they become infected. Inflamed follicular keratoses can have an acneiform appearance leading some to suggest that they represent a form of acne mechanica.[6] When the continued pressure and friction causes the keratin to extend deeper into the dermis, larger cystic lesions, 1 to 3 cm in diameter, form; these are commonly termed *posttraumatic epidermoid cysts*. Deeper cysts can be very tender when compressed by the prosthesis. Some cysts have an obvious punctum and patients may express keratinous material from them. Large cysts can be so painful that the patient can no longer wear a weight-bearing prosthesis each day (Fig. 129-6*B*). Distention of the overlying epidermis can occur, followed by spontaneous rupture. A serous or purulent fluid, often mixed with blood, is then discharged. The resulting sinus is difficult to occlude and the discharge continues as long as the prosthesis is worn. Intercommunicating sinuses can appear and spontaneous ruptures may occur. In far-advanced cases, a granulomatous reaction occurs around the cyst, with considerable capillary dilation, vascularization, and a heavy inflammatory infiltrate progressing to abscess formation (see Fig. 129-6*B*).

Management of this condition can be difficult. Clearly, prevention is the ideal but is not always possible despite regular prosthetic assessments. The fit of the prosthesis is the single most important method of preventing cyst formation. The problem can sometimes be improved or successfully eliminated by proper fitting and aligning of the prosthesis and continued adjustment by the prosthetist. Rough surfaces in areas of increased contact pressure in the socket, particularly the suction socket, tend to catch the skin, increasing the shearing forces. For this reason, the lining of the socket should be kept smooth. With the idea of inserting a buffer between the skin and the socket, protective devices such as

FIGURE 129-6

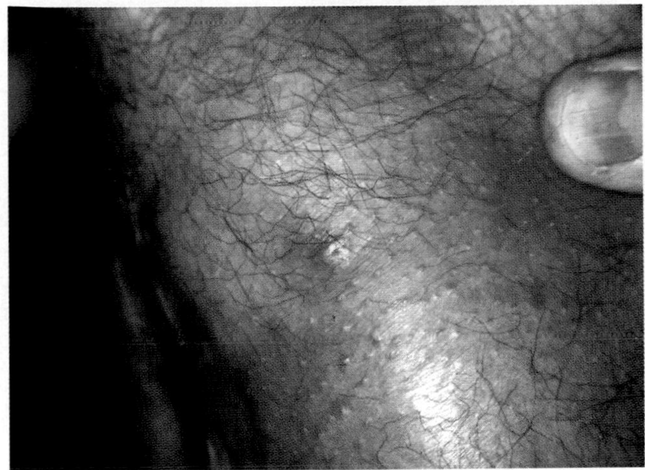

A.

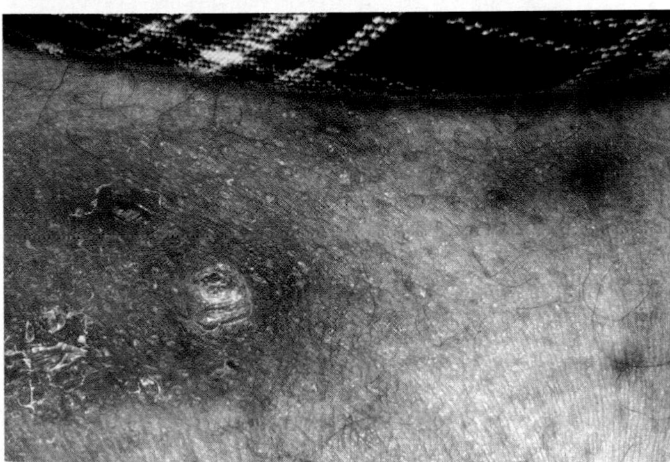

B.

Epidermoid cysts in different stages. *A*. Early follicular keratoses in the popliteal fossa of a man with below-knee amputation. *B*. Hemorrhagic and inflamed large epidermoid abscess in a man with an above-knee prosthesis. Note the follicular hyperkeratosis.

liners and stump socks are used. Various synthetic films and adhesives, such as Teflon, have been found satisfactory as liners. They allow for a smooth, gliding action of the prosthetic socket wall or brim against the skin. Applying a vapor-permeable adhesive membrane to the skin before fitting the appliance can also help to reduce frictional trauma. Topical glucocorticoids can be used at night to reduce inflammation and provide symptomatic relief. Intralesional injection of glucocorticoids into the cysts and their channels has also resulted in temporary improvement.

Surgical intervention is useful in cases with a few lesions that are not infected. Lesions can be surgically incised and drained. In other instances, removal of the prosthesis is sufficient to cause the lesion to involute, provided that the cyst has not become too large. However, spontaneous rupture, incision and drainage, and even spontaneous resorption of the lesion are of only temporary benefit. When the prosthesis is worn again, these cysts can recur so that surgical excision is not always the treatment of choice, especially in continually rubbed areas.

In selected cases, systemic retinoid therapy may be appropriate to minimize hyperkeratosis. One author found oral isotretinoin to be effective in a patient described as having acne mechanica.[6]

DISTURBANCES OF TISSUE FLUID DYNAMICS

Edema Amputation of a lower extremity greatly disturbs the normal pattern of blood and lymph channels, as well as the relationship of pressure both inside the vessels and in the surrounding tissues of the stump. An important feature of care during convalescence after amputation is the reduction of edema and stabilization of new circulatory patterns in the stump. Swelling can be partially prevented by gradual compression of the stump tissues with an elastic bandage or "shrinker" sock before fitting the prosthesis and socket.

When an amputee begins to wear a suction-socket prosthesis, the skin must adapt to an entirely new environment. The patient can expect edema, reactive hyperemia for days or weeks, a reddish-brown pigmentation resulting from capillary hemorrhage, and, occasionally, serous exudation and crusting of the skin of the distal portion of the stump. These changes are the almost inevitable result of the altered conditions forced on the skin and the subcutaneous tissues. They are relatively innocuous, usually short-lived, and do not usually require therapy.

The extent to which edema may persist or recur in the healed stump depends on many factors.[7] Edematous portions of the skin of the distal part of the stump may become pinched and strangulated within the socket. Such areas may ulcerate if they catch in the spring-valve opening and become gangrenous as a result of the impaired blood supply. Therapy includes eliminating all mechanical factors contributing to the edema, such as choking by the socket and poor fitting and misalignment. Excessive negative pressure in a suction-socket prosthesis also contributes to circulatory congestion and edema. Treatment should be directed toward better support of the distal soft tissues. Occasional use of an oral diuretic sometimes allows the edema to resolve.

Verrucous hyperplasia This term refers to a reactive hyperplastic condition, characterized morphologically by numerous, coalescent warty papules (Fig. 129-7). It occurs when the chronic pressure effects of a poor prosthetic fit disrupt vascular and lymphatic channels resulting in chronic tissue edema. The same appearance is seen around long-standing leg ulcers where there is an element of lymphoedema (see Chap. 167). Histologic examination can show evidence of pseudoepitheliomatous hyperplasia, although the condition itself is benign and potentially reversible. However, in neglected cases, malignant change can occasionally occur (see Fig. 129-7). Bacterial infection may play a role in the development of pseudoverrucous hyperplasia, as secondary mixed flora infections are common because of the poor superficial blood flow and the convoluted surface. External compression is the best method of treatment, in combination with topical control of bacterial infection. In below-knee amputees, the distal part of the stump is edematous; the stump dangles freely in the socket or has no distal support or partial end-bearing. When the stump end is supported in the socket by a temporary cushion or platform, compression gradually reduces and slowly clears the verrucous condition. The greater the compression on the distal stump, the more immediate and lasting is the improvement. The use of compression bandaging, shrinker socks and other pads, and partial end-bearing all have a definite place in therapy and can be skillfully applied by the prosthetist. Short courses of oral diuretics may be indicated to reduce edema of the stump. The medication can be gradually decreased when the stump and its skin return to normal.

Acroangiodermatitis This disorder occurs when the chronic pressure changes result in vessel proliferation in the upper and mid-dermis. There is also extravasation of red blood cells and these features combine to give a purplish hue to the papules and plaques that appear on a background of edematous skin. Some authors suggest that acroangiodermatitis occurs in above-knee amputees who use a suction socket prosthesis that exerts negative pressure.[8] However, there are reports of acroangiodermatitis in below-knee amputees,[9] and the same condition is seen in chronic venous insufficiency and in those patients with

FIGURE 129-7

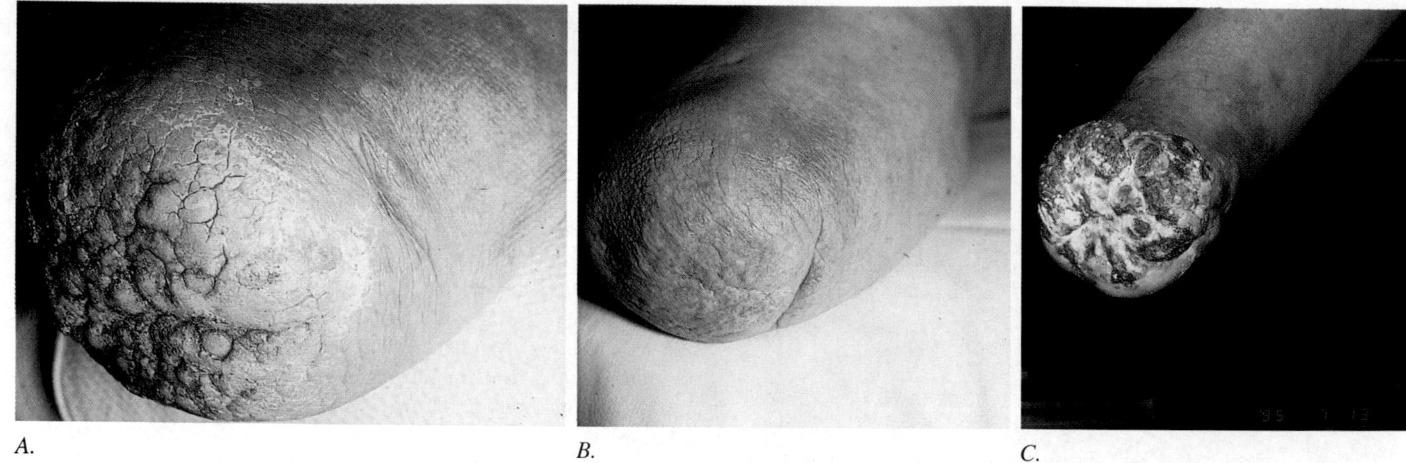

A. B. C.

Verrucous hyperplasia of the distal stump skin. *A*. Before compression therapy. *B*. Total resolution after compression therapy. *C*. Malignant degeneration into squamous cell carcinoma.

arteriovenous shunts (acroangiodermatitis of Mali). Management of this condition is the same as for stump edema and verrucous hyperplasia (above).

Bacterial and Fungal Infections

The bacterial flora of amputation stumps have been examined in small groups of patients,[10,11] the commonest species encountered being *Staphylococcus epidermidis*, *S. aureus,* and *Streptococcus* species. The moist, occluded environment under a prosthesis is ideal for fungal and bacterial growth so that minor skin infections occur fairly frequently. In a study by the authors, *S. aureus* folliculitis or *Trichophyton rubrum* infection were identified in 3 percent of the study population.[2] Infections are more common during hot weather and in those amputees who pay insufficient attention to stump hygiene, partly because in these situations the skin becomes macerated more readily and follicular infections become more likely. Although folliculitis (Fig. 129-8) and furuncles are more common, superficial infections of the skin itself may also occur. Superficial dermatophyte and candidal infection are also common, and may be difficult to eradicate because of the ideal environment for fungal growth within a prosthesis.

The diagnosis of infection is usually obvious when the rash extends onto skin not covered by the prosthesis. Underneath the prosthesis any superficial infection may present as a nonspecific scaling erythema indistinguishable from that caused, for example, by chronic irritation. All stump rashes should be swabbed for bacterial and fungal culture.

Superficial fungal infections respond to appropriate topical imidazole or terbinafine preparations. Infection can, however, be hard to completely eradicate because of the favorable conditions for fungal growth and because a widespread tinea corporis can occur. In this situation, systemic antifungal therapy is useful.

In the management of bacterial infections, oral antibacterial therapy should be directed by bacterial culture and sensitivity. Topical antiseptics or antibacterials can be used but some antiseptic preparations can cause irritation and there is also the potential for sensitization.

FIGURE 129-8

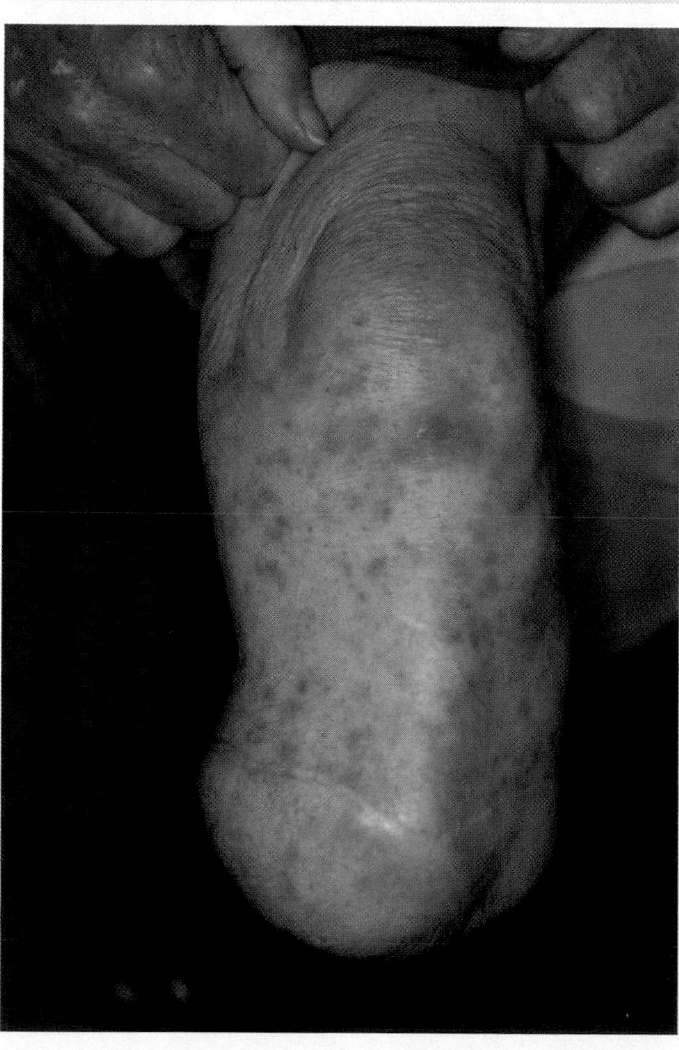

Folliculitis of stump skin showing the typical distribution in the occluded area.

Contact Dermatitis (See also Chap. 120)

The clinical presentations of irritant and allergic contact dermatitis affecting amputation stumps are indistinguishable (Fig. 129-9), ranging

FIGURE 129-9

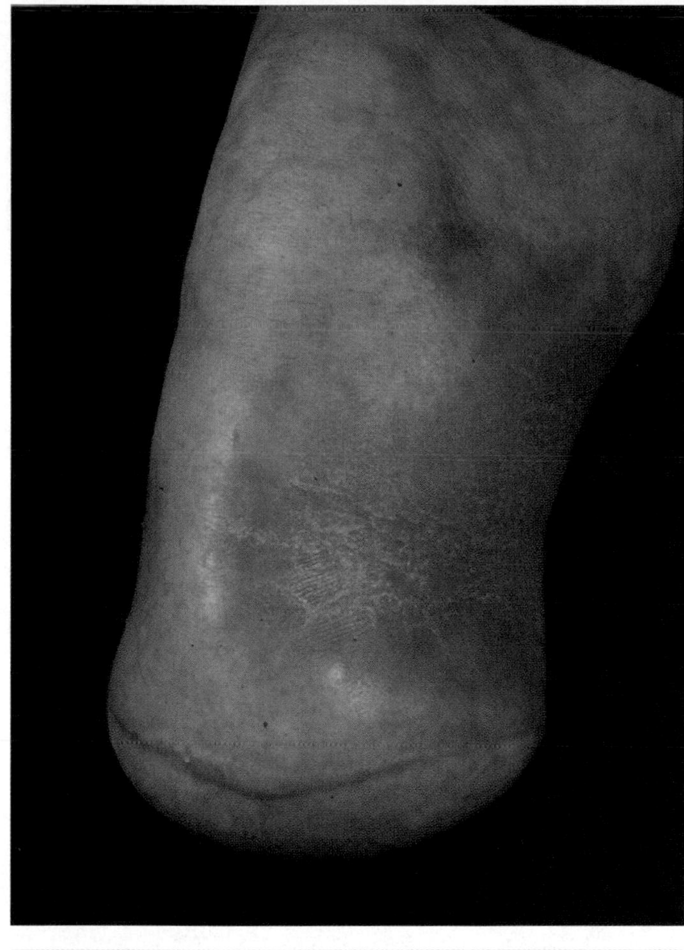

Allergic contact dermatitis to formaldehyde-releasing biocides in a lubricating "baby oil." Note the nonspecific dry eczematous appearance.

from dry, scaling erythema to weeping eczema.[2] Indeed, the morphologic features may be the same as nonspecific eczematization where no irritant, allergic, or infectious cause is found, and where there is no history of eczema or atopy. Consequently, a careful history and examination is essential if one is to identify irritant or allergic causes. This includes accurate timing of the onset of dermatitis in relation to changes in the patient's appliance routine or the composition of the prosthesis. The distribution of rash typically matches the site of the contactant. To identify a primary irritant or allergen, it is particularly important for the dermatologist to observe the patient removing and refitting their limb, making note of the construction and any medicaments or other agents such as talcs and creams that the patient uses. Knowledge of the materials used in prosthesis manufacture and the patient's use of any topical agents is necessary when considering potential sensitizers and irritants. This is best achieved by liaison with one's local prosthetist, as different construction techniques may be used in different areas. In general, modern modular prostheses are fabricated with sockets, liners, and casings that may contain acrylic resins, carbon composites, and thermoplastics. Epoxy and, occasionally, polyester resins are still used by some manufacturers. Acrylate-based thread sealants are commonly used in socket bolts and metalwork. Butyl or black rubber material may be used to conceal access points to the metal frame. Rubber materials can also be found in some suction socket valves. Suspension elements often include leather in straps and sometimes have metal fastenings, rivets, or screws containing nickel. Glues containing *para*-tertiary butylphenol (PTBP) formaldehyde resins are often used.

Repairs or adjustments to prostheses can introduce new irritants and allergens. For example, sockets sometimes have additional leather linings cemented to points of friction or pressure. Volatile solvents in these cements can be irritating and the resins potentially allergenic. Leather itself will often contain allergenic dichromates.

A proportion of patients regularly use an emollient cream or oil either as part of a skin care regimen or to lubricate the stump when fitting a socket. Talc may also be used to dry the skin or to ease the fitting of a socket. These products may contain allergens such as fragrances or preservatives and patients should be advised to avoid such products. Colored stump socks may contain potentially allergenic nylon dyes.

Irritant dermatitis can be due to contact with volatile solvents in glues or resins, uncured monomers in a variety of resins, or from fragrances, preservatives, and emulsifiers in topical medicaments or lubricants. Soaps and other washing materials used to clean appliances can cause irritation if they are not removed by proper washing.

Contact allergy should always be considered as a cause of inflammatory and dermatitic disorders affecting the stump especially if there is secondary spread. In addition to standard series patch testing, we recommend an extra series of allergens to include components of plastics including acrylic, epoxy, and polyester resin systems, as well as an azo dyes series. It is important to test with pieces of the prostheses and all materials applied to the stump skin, including emollients, cleansers, powders, medicaments, and cosmetics. In our experience, the most common relevant allergens are nickel, acrylates, rubber, chromate (in leather), PTBP formaldehyde resin and components of topical applications.[2]

Other Cutaneous Disorders

Common skin diseases, for example, eczema and psoriasis, may affect amputation stumps by virtue of their typical distribution on limbs. Those diseases that exhibit the Koebner phenomenon, especially psoriasis or lichen planus, have been reported on amputation stumps with little involvement of other areas of skin.

Constitutional eczematous processes can also become localized to stump skin, as can acne vulgaris. In these cases, it is important to diagnose and treat the generalized skin condition. Atopic dermatitis with eczematization of the stump skin is often seen as a persistent, weeping or dry and scaly, itching area of dermatitis over the distal portion of the stump, as well as over the stump in general.

Temporary symptomatic topical therapy with glucocorticoid preparations can be effective, but the condition frequently recurs unless its cause can be eliminated. A short course of oral glucocorticoids may help control the process.

Benign keratoses, warts, nevi, and a variety of cutaneous papillomas may occur on stump skin and occasionally cause discomfort when a prosthesis is worn. Malignancies have also been described and squamous cell carcinoma may develop in nonhealing chronic stump ulcers or verrucous hyperplasia (Fig 129-7*C*). Patients who have amputations for lymphangiomas may develop the Stewart-Treves syndrome and metastatic lymphangiosarcoma.

Treatment of these benign and malignant tumors is the same as when they occur elsewhere on the skin. Healing after tumor excision may take weeks during which time the artificial limb may not be worn.

General Management Considerations

Many of the commoner skin problems can be prevented or controlled by adherence to an appropriate hygiene and skin-care regimen in conjunction with regular prosthetics reviews, which ensure that the prosthesis remains appropriate and correctly adjusted. To this end, it is important that good contacts exist between the dermatologist and prosthetist, which will allow rapid referrals of patients before skin disorders become established.

As a general routine, the stump skin should be washed at night rather than in the morning, because newly washed skin is hydrated and swollen, thereby increasing the likelihood of friction and shearing trauma. Nonperfumed soap should be used to minimize contact with potential sensitizers and fully removed with tepid water and gentle rubbing with a nonabrasive towel.

Soaps or washes containing hexachlorophene, triclocarban, or triclosan have a bacteriostatic effect in addition to their cleansing action and can reduce the possibility of infection. However, these antiseptic preparations can cause irritation or allergy in a small number of cases and patients should be warned about this.

If a stump sock is worn, it should be changed daily and washed and rinsed fully as soon as it is taken off, before perspiration is allowed to dry within it.

FIGURE 129-10

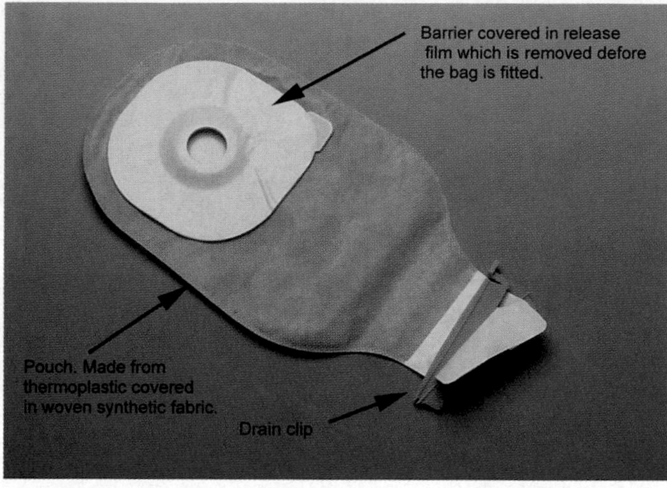

A typical drainable stoma bag.

SKIN PROBLEMS IN PATIENTS WITH ABDOMINAL STOMAS (OSTOMATES)

A stoma is a surgically created opening onto the skin of an abdominal viscus. Stomas may be intended to be temporary or permanent. The most frequently performed stomas are ileostomies, colostomies, and ileal conduits (urostomies). The most common reasons for ileostomy and colostomy surgery are inflammatory bowel disease and malignancy. Urostomies are most frequently performed because of renal tract malignancy or for neurologic problems. A patient with a stoma is usually termed an "ostomist" or "ostomate." There are more than one million ostomates in the United States and 100,000 in the United Kingdom. There have been considerable advances in the design of collecting devices for stoma effluent allowing for a high degree of comfort and convenience. Essentially, the device is a pouch or bag held in place over the stoma by an adhesive skin barrier made solely or partly from hydrocolloid (Fig. 129-10). Many ileostomists and urostomists use two-piece appliances where the barrier remains on the skin for 2 to 4 days and is detachable; disposable bags are changed as necessary. Appliances with convexity on the surface next to the skin are available for patients with short or buried stomas.

At least two-thirds of ostomates experience skin problems that interfere with the normal use of their stoma appliance.[12] The majority of these problems are irritant reactions, usually dermatitis secondary to leaks from the stoma, however there are also a number of other well-defined irritant reactions. Common coincidental dermatoses, particularly psoriasis and constitutional eczema, account for around 15 percent of the diseases seen.

Irritant Reactions

DERMATITIS This most frequently results from the chronic leakage of effluent onto the skin because the patient is using an inappropriately shaped appliance or one with too large a hole for their stoma. The most common cause is the remodeling of the stoma and abdominal wall that occurs in the months after surgery, whereby a stoma usually becomes a little shorter and thinner, resulting in leaks unless a correctly fitting appliance is selected (Fig. 129-11). Leaks will also occur when patients gain a lot of weight after surgery and the effective length of their stoma diminishes because it becomes buried by subcutaneous fat. Irregular scarring after surgery or retraction of the stoma, may also be associated with chronic leakage. Chronically irritated skin can become markedly hyperkeratotic and acanthotic. These problems can be prevented and resolved by careful postsurgical follow-up by the enterostomal therapist (ET; stoma nurse specialist) to ensure that the correct appliance is being used. Severe, acute irritant dermatitis can be effectively treated with a short course of topical corticosteroid while longer-term appliance modifications are being undertaken.

In ileostomy patients with short bowel, the output may be very high and corrosive due to the enzyme content. In this situation, some leaks are inevitable, despite the use of proprietary barrier preparations or soothing lotions. Where the irritation has resulted in an eroded dermatitis, sucralfate powder applied at every stoma bag change can be

FIGURE 129-11

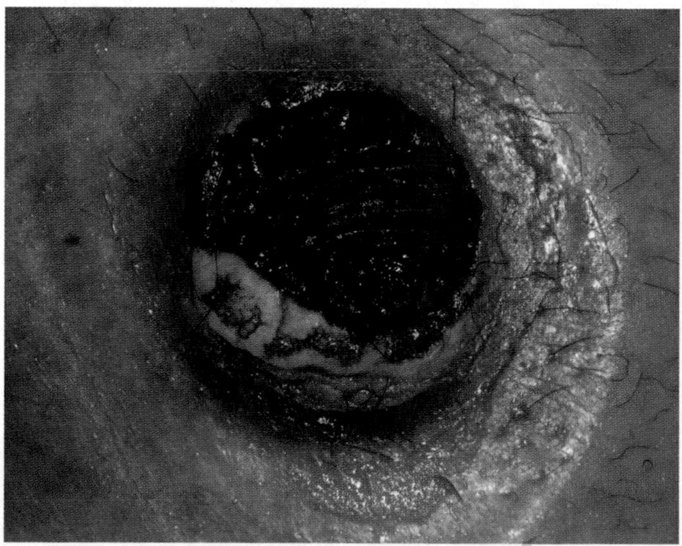

Peristomal dermatitis due to fecal irritation. The skin beneath the stoma was chronically exposed to feces because a bag with too large an aperture was used.

very effective. In addition to forming a sticky barrier, the preparation is thought to promote healing.[13]

Approximately 15 percent of ostomates with skin problems suffer from a chronic dermatitis for which no irritant, allergic, or infective cause can be found, and where primary skin disease is ruled out.[12] In the absence of a primary treatable cause, the authors have used topical corticosteroid lotions. Most patients require only occasional short courses for a maximum of 4 weeks duration. A small number of patients require intermittent applications longer term. Provided that the frequency of application is no more than once every 10 days, steroid atrophy of the skin appears to be unusual.

Excessively frequent bag changing may cause an irritant dermatitis. This can be the result of patient anxiety concerning leaks. Whatever the cause of skin inflammation, a vicious cycle can develop when the damaged skin prevents proper bag adhesion necessitating more frequent bag changes. Careful counseling is usually necessary in order to reassure the patient regarding leaks.

CHRONIC PAPILLOMATOUS DERMATITIS This term refers to clinical appearance of warty excrescences around urostomies resulting from leaks and pooling of urine on the peristomal skin. Recurrent urinary tract infections appear to increase the likelihood of chronic papillomatous dermatitis (CPD) probably due to the presence of ammonia from urea-splitting bacteria. Histologically, there is massive hyperkeratosis and acanthosis. Pseudoepitheliomatous hyperplasia may also be a feature but is not universal. In severe cases, the lesions can encroach on the stoma and cause stenosis (Fig. 129-12). When the leaking of urine is caused by a receding stoma, CPD will resolve rapidly if a convex-backed appliance is used to increase the effective length of the urostomy and thereby stop leaks. Acetic acid soaks (10% domestic vinegar in water[14]) at each bag change are effective in some cases. Larger excrescences may be shaved off under local anesthetic to allow a bag with a smaller aperture to be used. In severe cases, surgical revision of the stoma may be required.

GRANULOMAS The term *granuloma* is commonly used for a range of papular lesions, which are probably all secondary to irritation. The authors have only seen the condition affecting ileostomies or colostomies and not urostomies. They may affect the stoma itself (inflammatory colonic or ileal polyps) or the mucocutaneous junction, or may be found more widely, extending onto the peristomal skin (Fig. 129-13). The latter is more frequent in patients with colostomies, and in this situation, the papules may become very extensive. This occurs when the patient enlarges the stoma bag aperture to accommodate a papule, thereby exposing normal skin to fecal irritation. The irritation precipitates further lesions and prompts the patient to enlarge the aperture still further. In this way, progressively, areas several centimeters in diameter can become covered with these polyps. Histologically, the lesions contain a chronic inflammatory infiltrate, granulation tissue, and metaplastic bowel mucosa where the metaplasia is probably a response to fecal irritation.

FIGURE 129-12

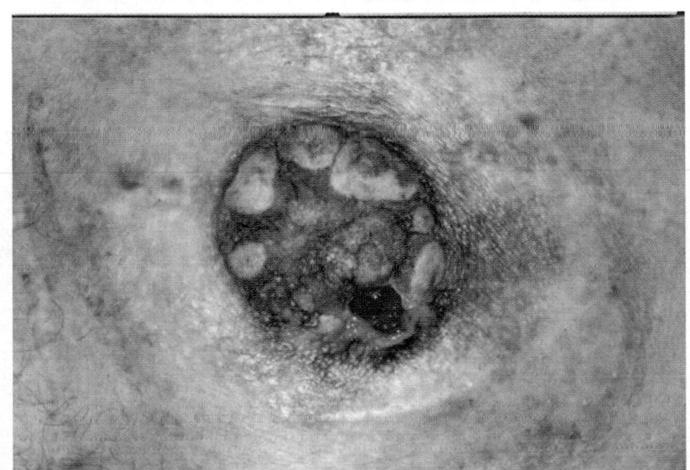

Chronic papillomatous dermatitis affecting a urostomy in a patient who is using a bag with too large an aperture. The red area is stoma and is becoming stenosed by the warty papules. The brown pigmentation is a typical finding in long-standing urostomies in all races. (Courtesy of Anita Eriksson, Karolinska Institute, Stockholm, Sweden)

FIGURE 129-13

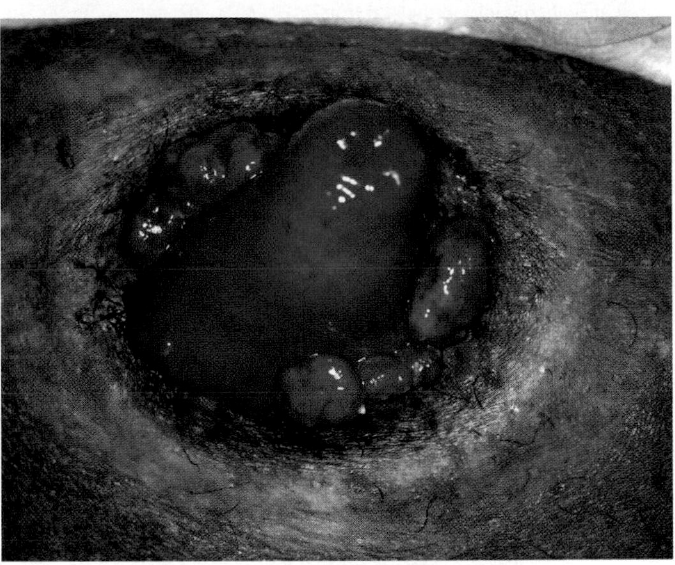

"Granulomas" around a colostomy. The patient has cut the bag aperture larger to accommodate the original lesion and the area thus exposed is seen as a ring of postinflammatory hyperpigmentation in which new lesions developed.

Asymptomatic, solitary lesions can be left, although they may be painful and bleed easily, leading to poor stoma bag adhesion. In these cases, they can be destroyed by cautery (thermal or silver nitrate) or by cryotherapy, using a liquid nitrogen spray. Larger and proliferating lesions around colostomies are best removed by shave and cautery under local anesthetic and an appliance with a correctly sized aperture fitted in order to prevent massive proliferation.

PSORIASIS Psoriasis is a common cause of peristomal skin disease because it may appear in irritated and traumatized skin (Koebner's phenomenon). Peristomal psoriasis presents as a glazed erythema similar to flexural psoriasis and can be treated in the same way with topical corticosteroids although at the peristomal site, a nongreasy base should be selected. Resolution of psoriasis under hydrocolloid occlusion has been described,[15] which is of relevance to stoma patients because 50 percent of cases of peristomal psoriasis will resolve if a bag is selected with a thicker, hydrocolloid-only barrier. Where the patient can tolerate the stoma being temporarily unprotected from leaks, UV phototherapy is effective as for psoriasis elsewhere. The mucous membranes of the stoma should be protected from UV light. Although irritating topical psoriasis treatments are not usually tolerated, some patients have had success with creams containing hydrocortisone 1% and coal tar 3%, the application being left on the skin for 1 h each day before wiping off and applying a stoma bag. While the cream is in place, a nonadhesive bag can be worn, held in place with a waist belt, provided that the patient is sedentary during this time. Superficial x-ray (grenz-ray) therapy has been used in recalcitrant cases.

INFECTIONS The most frequent peristomal skin infection is staphylococcal folliculitis, usually, but not exclusively, in those individuals with hairy abdomens who shave regularly to help the bags to stick. It responds to oral antibiotics and to a reduction in shaving frequency to no more than once per week. Although antiseptic washes can be a useful additional therapeutic measure, they can cause irritant reactions if the skin is not correctly rinsed before being occluded by the stoma bag. Localized skin infections, usually staphylococcal or streptococcal, can produce a rash indistinguishable from irritant dermatitis or primary skin disease such as psoriasis or eczema. Furthermore, preexisting psoriasis or eczema can become secondarily infected under occlusion. Therefore, all peristomal rashes should be swabbed for microbiological investigation and appropriate antibiotics prescribed based on microbiological sensitivities. In tropical climates, cutaneous fungal infections are common, whereas in more temperate regions, *Candida albicans* is an occasional problem and dermatophyte infection is rare.

PYODERMA GANGRENOSUM This rare, inflammatory, ulcerative neutrophilic dermatosis (see Chap. 98) is more common in peristomal skin than would be expected from its frequency in the general population.[16] Clearly, this is partly due to its strong association with inflammatory bowel disease. There is some evidence, however, that the increased use of convex-backed appliances may contribute to the incidence via the pathergic effect of increased pressure on the skin. Although some cases of pyoderma gangrenosum (PG) are associated with active inflammatory bowel disease, the association is not universal; indeed, peristomal PG occurs in ostomates who have no history of inflammatory bowel disease.

Small, superficial, and solitary ulcers respond to topical steroids. Because of the problems with greasy preparations causing lifting of stoma bags, alternative vehicles are usually necessary. These include triamcinolone in carmellose sodium paste, gauze soaked in aqueous prednisone, and scalp gels or lotions that do not contain oils or propylene glycol. Adhesive tapes impregnated with corticosteroids are useful in this and many of the other conditions. Larger ulcers, and those not responding to topical therapy, require topical tacrolimus or systemic treatment as for PG elsewhere (see Chap. 98).

Contact Allergy

Most patients and many health professionals regard contact hypersensitivity as an important cause of peristomal rashes. The authors have patch tested more than 100 ostomates with unexplained dermatitis and relevant positive allergic reactions were found in only two cases. Stoma bags are made largely from food-grade materials with a low potential for sensitization. Nonetheless, there are many case reports of sensitivities to individual ingredients including Gantrez resins, epoxy resins, and acrylate adhesives. Furthermore, there is a potential for contact allergy from deodorizers and topically applied preparations. Patch testing is indicated in patients with persisting problems where infection, irritation, and constitutional skin disease has been ruled out.[17]

General Management

The necessity for good adhesion between the skin and appliance presents problems for topical treatment of peristomal dermatoses. While some patients can apply therapies in a cream base, most patients find that any greasy preparation will make the bag lift and cause leaks; consequently, they will not use them. Dressings under the bag to cover a greasy topical agent can be used in selected cases, but are not universally practical. Alternative vehicles are usually required and a number of alternatives can be tried. Adhesive tapes and lotions are a useful compromise, particularly for corticosteroids, and lotions are available as scalp applications formulated in 40% isopropyl alcohol. The alcohol can cause stinging on broken skin. In such cases, the lotion can be applied to the barrier and allowed to evaporate for 20 min before fitting to the skin.

REFERENCES

1. Marks LJ, Michael JW: Artificial limbs. *BMJ* **323**:732, 2001
2. Lyon CC et al: Skin disorders in amputees. *J Am Acad Dermatol* **42**:501, 2000
3. Feingold KE et al: Endocrine skin interactions: Diabetes mellitus. *J Am Acad Dermatol* **17**:921, 1987
4. Levy SW: Skin problems of the leg amputee. *Prosthet Orthot Int* **4**:37, 1980
5. Ibbotson SH et al: Follicular keratoses at amputation sites. *Br J Dermatol* **130**:770, 1994
6. Strauss RM, Harrington CI: Stump acne: A new variant of acne mechanica and a cause of immobility. *Br J Dermatol* **144**:647, 2001
7. Barnes GH et al: *Problems of the Amputee; Stump Edema. Illustrated Pamphlet*. University of California, Biomechanics Laboratory, 1964.
8. Suarez EC et al: Circulatory disorders in amputation stumps. *J Am Acad Dermatol* **44**:723, 2001
9. Gucluer H, et al: Kaposi-like acroangio-dermatitis in an amputee. *Br J Dermatol* **141**:380, 1999
10. Allende MF et al: The bacterial flora of the skin of amputation stumps. *J Invest Dermatol* **36**:165, 1961
11. Kohler P et al: Bacteria on stumps of amputees and the effect of antiseptics. *Prosthet Orthot Int* **13**:149, 1989
12. Lyon CC et al: The spectrum of skin disorders in abdominal stoma patients. *Br J Dermatol* **143**:1248, 2000
13. Lyon CC et al: Topical sucralfate in the management of peristomal skin disease. An open study. *Clin Exp Dermatol* **25**:584, 2000
14. Jeter KF. Hyperplasia or what? *J Enterostomal Ther* **10**:181, 1983
15. Griffiths CE et al: Prolonged occlusion in the treatment of psoriasis: A clinical and immunohistological study. *J Am Acad Dermatol* **35**:283, 1996
16. Lyon CC et al: Parastomal pyoderma gangrenosum: Clinical features and management. *J Am Acad Dermatol* **42**:992, 2000
17. Lyon CC, Beck MH, Smith A (eds): *Abdominal Stomas and Their Skin Disorders*. London, Martin Dunitz, 2001, pp 43–47

CHAPTER 130

Thomas M. DeLauro

Corns and Calluses

Every human being is vulnerable to the development of corns and calluses because our skin is subjected to regular mechanical stress. The prevalence of corns and calluses can be readily appreciated by the number of nonprescription products aimed at reducing or preventing them—a billion dollar annual market!

HISTORICAL ASPECTS

The earliest known discussion of these lesions can be found in the writings of Cleopatra, who authored a textbook on cosmetics.[1] Corns and calluses have plagued humankind since antiquity, affecting all socioeconomic levels.

EPIDEMIOLOGY

All human beings, with the exception of non–weight-bearing infants, are subject to the development of corns and calluses. As discussed below, certain foot types and regions are prone to mechanically induced skin thickening, regardless of race, gender, or age.

ETIOLOGY AND PATHOGENESIS

Corns (clavus or heloma, clavi or helomata) and calluses (tyloma, tylomata) are, respectively, keratotic papules and plaques that occur in response to chronic, excessive, mechanical shear or friction forces. In theory, these forces induce hyperkeratinization, leading to a thickening of the stratum corneum, although the precise mechanism by which this occurs remains unknown. If the abnormal forces are distributed over a broad area (i.e., more than one square centimeter), a callus occurs. In contrast, a corn will form if the same forces are applied to a focused location, wherein the lamellae of the stratum corneum become impacted to form a hard central core known as the radix or nucleus.

GENETICS

Mechanical keratoses are not determined genetically. Heredity does play a role, however, in configuring our skeletal architecture. A family history of bony abnormality or ligamentous laxity predisposes one to sites of increased cutaneous friction or shear.

PREVENTION

These lesions can only be prevented by reducing or eliminating the mechanical forces that created them. Usually, this is a daunting, if not impossible, task. Repetitive occupational motions are often unavoidable, patients are commonly reluctant to alter shoe styles, and osseous architecture is predetermined through heredity.

CLINICAL MANIFESTATIONS

Corns and calluses produce painful symptoms often described as burning in character, especially when weight-bearing and/or in shoe gear. This discomfort is thought to result from microtearing of the thickened, inflexible skin. The lesions occur in predictable pedal locations, corresponding to a structural deformity or biomechanical fault. Crookedness of the lesser toes leads to prominence of the proximal and/or distal interphalangeal joints. Keratoses can therefore form either dorsal to those joints, between the toes (Fig. 130-1), at the distal end of the toe, or on the lateral aspect of the fifth toe and/or toenail (the lateral toenail corn, aka Durlacher's corn, Fig. 130-2). Interdigital corns (those between toes) can be hard when adjacent to the interphalangeal joint(s), or soft when deep within the fourth interdigital space. The softness of this last corn results from trapped perspiration, leading to maceration of the keratotic tissue.

FIGURE 130-1

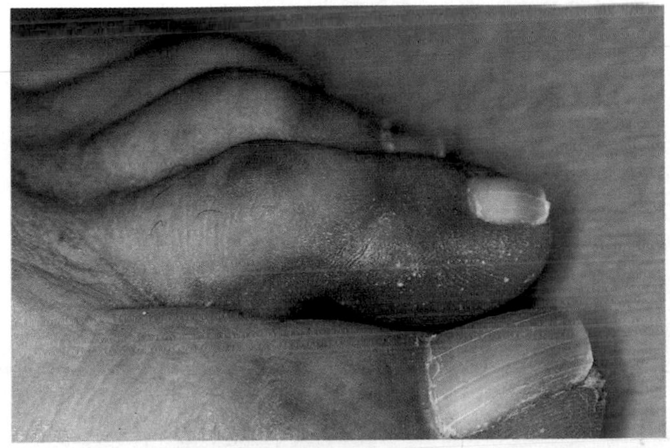

An interdigital corn at the medial aspect of the second distal interphalangeal joint.

FIGURE 130-2

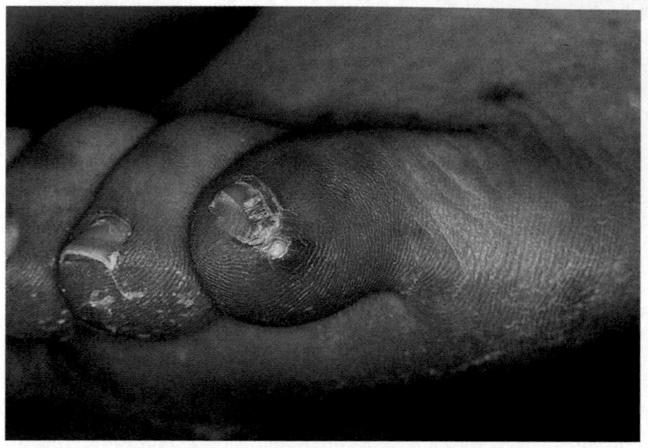

A Durlacher's corn at the lateral nail groove of the fifth toe.

In patients with bunions (hallux valgus), a callus usually forms at the medioplantar aspect of the hallux. During gait, one rolls off that portion of the great toe due to its incorrect position. The skin is subsequently pinched to form a "pinch callus" (Fig. 130-3). In addition, the first metatarsal often does not bear its fair share of the weight-bearing load. Weight is therefore transferred laterally to the second metatarsal head, usually leading to an additional corn or callus beneath that bone.

Other favored locations for lesser metatarsal head keratosis include:

1. Beneath the first and fifth metatarsal heads in cavus foot types;
2. Beneath the fifth metatarsal head alone in cases with tailor's bunions (bunionette);

FIGURE 130-3

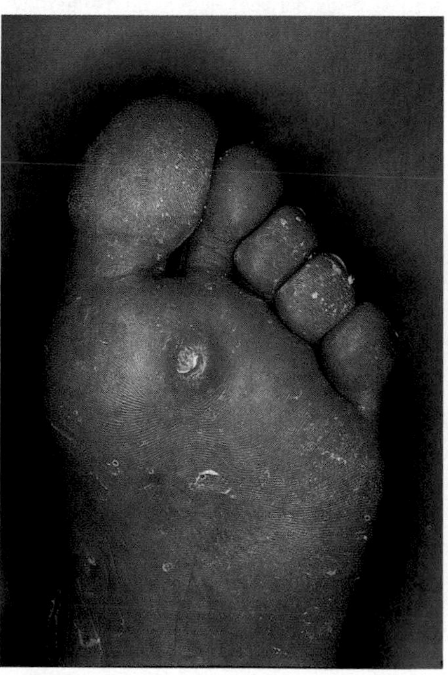

A patient exhibiting both an exquisitely painful, intractable plantar keratosis (IPK) (beneath the second metatarsal head) and a "pinch" callus (at the medioplantar hallux).

3. Beneath the second through fourth metatarsal heads when multiple hammertoes or an equinus deformity coexist; and
4. Erratic locations (e.g., subthird and fifth metatarsal heads, isolated third or fourth metatarsal head lesions, second and fourth metatarsal heads) in structural abnormalities such as brachymetatarsia or dislocated metatarsophalangeal joints as in rheumatoid arthritis or neuroarthropathy.

Another variant of corn is that referred to as heloma miliare, or seed corn. This title is derived from their clinical appearance: multiple guttate keratoses that are easily pared. When seamed nylon hosiery was fashionable, the garment was considered the etiologic factor. However, patients still present with seed corns even though they have never worn seamed stockings.

LABORATORY FINDINGS

Because corns and calluses are the result of mechanical friction and shear alone, there are no associated laboratory abnormalities.

PATHOLOGY

In contrast to nonmechanically induced keratoses, corns and calluses exhibit changes within the epidermis, dermis, and adipose layer. Corns demonstrate a parakeratotic plug within the stratum corneum, with a pressure-related loss of the stratum granulosum, as well as atrophy of the stratum malpighii. The dermis will display significant fibrosis, dilated eccrine ducts and blood vessels, hypertrophied nerves, and scar tissue replacement of subcutaneous fat. Overall, the histologic changes in calluses are less pronounced, and include a thickened stratum corneum but intact stratum granulosum. The ratio of stratum corneum to stratum malpighii is commonly 1:1.[2]

DIAGNOSIS AND DIFFERENTIAL DIAGNOSIS

Corns and calluses are easily recognized by the finding of a thickened stratum corneum adjacent to a bony prominence. Patients who have undergone transmetatarsal amputation can develop corns and calluses at the stump's distal aspect when an Achilles tendon lengthening is not performed simultaneously. Charcot neuroarthropathy affecting the midfoot can lead to collapse and reversal of the longitudinal arch ("rocker bottom foot"), with corns or calluses forming midsole. In patients with flatfeet or who pronate excessively, it is common to find a diffuse keratotic ridge at the medioplantar aspect of the heel.

On occasion, one encounters patients with excruciatingly painful corns (Fig. 130-3). The central nucleus is deeper and wider, and mediolateral compression of the lesion elicits discomfort. A variety of terms have been used to describe such lesions, albeit interchangeably: neurofibrous or neurovascular corn, intractable plantar keratosis (IPK), or porokeratosis plantaris discretum. Treatment is the same as for other pressure-induced keratoses, which are described below.

Unlike verrucae, corns and calluses do not exhibit pinpoint hemorrhage, a papilliform surface, or interrupted skin lines when pared.

Corns and calluses *not* overlying a bony prominence should prompt a search for another etiology (e.g., genokeratosis, cutaneous neoplasm).

RELEVANCE TO THE DIABETIC FOOT

Lower extremity amputation is a dominant fear in most diabetic patients. These amputations are most often preceded by a history of foot ulceration. Although a number of comorbidities contribute to the development of ulceration (e.g., peripheral vascular disease, neuropathy, limited joint mobility), minor trauma via repetitive pressure is the pivotal precipitating event. As markers of repetitive friction and shear, corns and calluses in the diabetic foot are of special significance. Simple débridement of these hyperkeratotic lesions decreases peak plantar pressures by as much as 26 percent.[3] In a recent retrospective review of more than 200 diabetic foot ulcerations, patients who had their corns and calluses pared frequently experienced a statistically significant decrease in the incidence of foot ulceration, hospitalization, and surgical intervention.[4] Hemorrhage within a corn or callus is an especially ominous sign, indicating subcutaneous breakdown with a strong potential for ulceration.

TREATMENT AND PROGNOSIS

If left untreated, corns and calluses result in painful ambulation, and also in subhelomal bursitis and blistering that can rupture to the surface. Given the close proximity of some corns to joints and bone, septic arthritis and/or osteomyelitis can ensue. The mechanical forces that cause corns and calluses can also rupture portions of the subcutaneous vascular plexus, leading to hemorrhage within keratotic tissue. In healthy patients, these observations are of minor significance, but in other cases (e.g., in diabetics and patients with connective tissue disease), they may herald extensive skin ulceration or vasculitis.

Paring is the simplest treatment for corns and calluses. In the case of corns, the central radix or nucleus must also be débrided for pain to be relieved. Felt dispersion padding should be applied when paring is completed; the padding protects the tender underlying skin. Keratolytics may be employed by either the health care provider or patient, but must be used cautiously. Unmonitored usage is contraindicated in patients with comorbid peripheral neuropathy or arterial disease.

Soft corns and IPKs may also respond to biweekly infiltrations of a sclerosing solution of 4% alcohol mixed with local anesthetic. Typically, up to seven injections may be required with darkening and thrombosis of the lesion heralding a cure.[5,6] Lastly, osseous surgical procedures designed to redistribute weightbearing pressures may be employed to eliminate corns and calluses. However, not all lesions can be cleared using this method.

REFERENCES

1. Block BH: *Foot Talk.* New York, Arbor House, 1984
2. Lemont H: Histologic differentiation of mechanical and non-mechanical keratoses of the sole. *Clin Dermatol* **1**:44, 1983
3. Young MJ, Cavanagh PR, Thomas G, et al: The effect of callus removal on dynamic plantar foot pressures in diabetic patients. *Diabet Med* **9**:55, 1992
4. Sage RA, Webster JK, Fisher SG: Outpatient care and morbidity reduction in diabetic foot ulcers associated with chronic pressure callus. *J Am Podiatr Med Assoc* **91**:275, 2001
5. Costello MJ, Gibbs RC: *The Palms and Soles in Medicine.* Springfield, IL, Charles C. Thomas, 1967
6. Dockery GL, Nilson RZ: Intralesional injections. *Clin Podiatr Med Surg* **3**:473, 1986

CHAPTER 131

Dirk M. Elston

Sports Dermatology

SPORTS AND THE DERMATOLOGIST

Skin problems are extremely common among athletes. During an 8-week survey of university athletic teams, 40 percent reported skin problems.[1] In a recent study of mountain biking injuries, skin lesions accounted for 75 percent of all injuries.[2] Skin lesions account for 35 percent of all in-line skating injuries.[3] Minor skin injuries frequently become infected, and close physical contact during sports increases the risk of skin infection. As a result, skin infections are more prevalent in top athletes than in the general population.[4] The training environment is frequently the source of infection.

Skin-related complaints are especially common in warm, humid climates. During the 1993 Central American and Caribbean Games, held in Puerto Rico, 1 of every 100 athletes had a skin-related complaint severe enough to require medical care.[5] Similarly, sports that involve repeated immersion in water are associated with an increased incidence of skin injury and infection.[6]

Skin injuries frequently result in lost training time, and after months of dedication and training, an athlete may be disqualified from competition because of an infectious skin lesion. Thus, a knowledgeable dermatologist can be a great asset in the prevention and therapy of sports-related skin disease.

The views expressed are those of the author and are not to be construed as official or as representing those of the Army Medical Department or the Department of Defense. This work is in the public domain. The work is original and has not been published or presented elsewhere. The author has no conflicts of interest to disclose.

TABLE 131-1

Unique Sports-Associated Skin Conditions

Bikini bottom: bacterial folliculitis on the buttocks of swimmers
Jazz ballet bottom: buttock cleft abscess
Jogger's nipples: painful, swollen, eroded, or hyperkeratotic nipples
Karate cicatrices: linear scars on the dorsal aspects of the hands
Mogul skier's palm: traumatic hypothenar ecchymosis
Painful piezogenic pedal papules: transdermal fat herniations
Ping pong patches: traumatic ecchymotic patches
Pool palms: smooth, shiny, tender palms secondary to rough pool surfaces
Pulling boat hands: friction and damp cold produce a pernio-like condition
Rower's rump: lichenification
Runner's nails: multiple Beau's lines or periodic shedding of a nail plate (Fig. 131-1)
Runner's rump: ecchymoses of the superior gluteal cleft
Stingray hickey: bite ecchymosis
Stretcher's scrotum: scrotal hematoma
Swimmer's shine: facial oiliness seen in swimmers
Swimmer's shoulder: abrasion of shoulder by beard during crawl stroke
Talon noir (black heal): intradermal hemorrhage.
Tennis toe: subungual hematoma with or without subungual hyperkeratosis or nail dystrophy (jogger's toe, hiker's toe, and skier's toe are similar)
Turf toe: metatarsophalangeal joint sprains

FIGURE 131–1

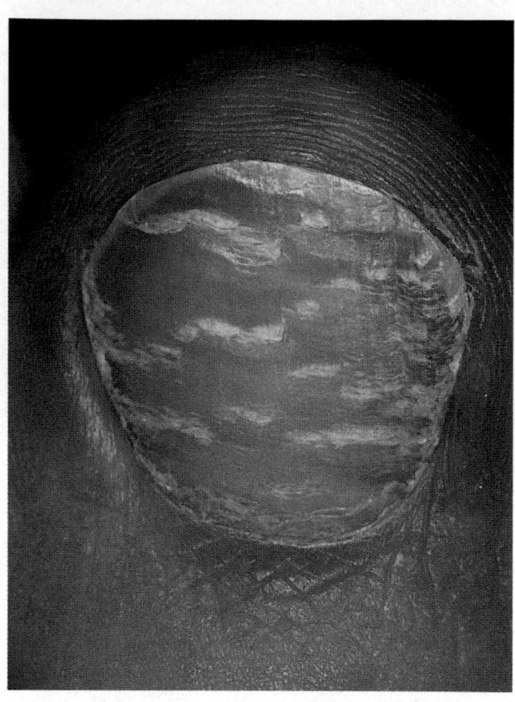

Runner's nail; in this case, multiple Beau's lines with onychoschizia.

New treatments, including hydroactive wound dressings, have advanced the treatment of superficial wounds. Application of a hydroactive dressing can provide a protective barrier that allows the athlete to return to competition. Long used for deeper soft tissue injuries, nonsteroidal anti-inflammatory drugs may play a role in the treatment of skin and superficial soft tissue injuries, providing symptomatic relief to allow continued participation in competition.

Sports dermatology has produced some of the most vivid and alliterative diagnostic terms to be found in medicine. Table 131-1 lists some of the more memorable of these unique conditions.

Pyogenic Skin Infections

Outbreaks of furuncles may spread rapidly within an athletic team. Attack rates of approximately 25 percent have been described in high school athletic teams. Epidemiologic data implicate direct contact with infected individuals, rather than fomites, as the major route of transmission,[7] although fomites may play some role. Factors associated with the spread of furunculosis include the lack of readily available shower facilities, sharing of athletic pads, and sharing of towels.[8]

Group A streptococcal infections may also spread rapidly among team members.[9] Epidemic pyoderma with a nephritogenic streptococcus caused an epidemic of scrum kidney (glomerulonephritis) in a rugby team.[10] In addition to impetigo, streptococci may produce erysipelas and lymphangitis.

Pseudomonas infections are commonly associated with water. Type O:11 *Pseudomonas* is implicated most commonly. Other serotypes, including O:1, O:3, O:8, O:10, and O:16, have been reported.[11] Hot tub, whirlpool, and swimming pool folliculitis present with intensely pruritic papules and pustules involving intertriginous and "bathing suit" areas. Outbreaks are associated with both chlorine- and bromine-treated water.[12] Contamination of well water or bathroom components may result in *Pseudomonas* folliculitis related to bathing or showering.[13] Biopsy of a pruritic papule demonstrates suppurative folliculitis. Generally, organisms are not seen with special stains, but can be cultured from the lesions and from the source of infection. Loofah sponges enhance the growth of gram-negative organisms, and have been implicated as reservoirs of *Pseudomonas* organisms.[14] Most cases of *Pseudomonas* folliculitis resolve spontaneously; in cases requiring antibiotics, fluoroquinolones offer effective therapy.[15]

Diving suit dermatitis is an unusual manifestation of *Pseudomonas* folliculitis that presents as widespread crusted papules and pustules on the trunk and extremities. The lesions may be painful rather than pruritic, and are restricted to areas covered by the wetsuit. Diving suit dermatitis has been reported with both fresh and salt water diving.[16,17]

Green nails are caused by *Pseudomonas* colonization in persons habitually exposed to water. Frequently, patients have preexisting hand eczema or psoriasis with distal onycholysis. *Candida* colonization can perpetuate and worsen the onycholysis, creating a deep, moist nidus for *Pseudomonas* growth. Effective treatment may require applications of an anticandidal agent, as well as topical antibiotic or acidic (acetic acid, aluminum acetate) measures against *Pseudomonas*. Chronic hand dermatitis and psoriasis often initiate the onycholysis and *Pseudomonas* colonization. Recurrences are common unless the underlying cause of onycholysis is addressed.

Pseudomonas is also a common cause of webspace infection and otitis externa in swimmers.[18] Webspace infection is commonly associated with occlusive footwear and preexisting interdigital tinea pedis. If not treated appropriately, prolonged disability may result. Topical aluminum acetate or dilute acetic acid may be helpful in this setting. Webspaces should be thoroughly dried with a fan or cool blow-dryer after each soak. Topical gentamicin or an oral fluoroquinolone may be required.

Severe contact dermatitis may occur as a result of treatment of otitis externa with a topical suspension containing neomycin, polymyxin B, and hydrocortisone. The offending agent is usually neomycin or thimerosal (a preservative present in the otic suspension but not the solution). Otic aluminum acetate solutions can be an effective alternative. Treatment of the contact dermatitis may require potent topical or oral steroids. Invasive *Pseudomonas* infections (malignant otitis externa) may be associated with sepsis and require parenteral antibiotics.

Pseudomonas keratitis may occur as a result of exposure to contaminated whirlpools.[19] This infection can have devastating consequences, and prompt consultation with an ophthalmologist is essential. *Pseudomonas* osteomyelitis has been associated with nail puncture wounds through tennis shoes.[20]

Prevention of Contagious Skin Infections

Herpes simplex virus (HSV) can be transmitted by skin to skin contact during any contact sport. Herpes gladiatorum (Fig. 131-2) is recognized as a major problem among wrestlers. Attack rates as high as 34 percent have been reported.[21] Ocular involvement is a serious complication. Wrestlers with active infections should be barred from participation. Because abrasive shirts may contribute to the spread of HSV infections among wrestlers,[22] they should be avoided. Oral antiviral drugs, such as acyclovir, valacyclovir, and famciclovir, can be used to shorten the course of an outbreak. It is likely that all three of these drugs will be shown to be useful in preventing outbreaks of herpes gladiatorum by means of long-term or periodic prophylaxis, as they are used for prophylaxis against genital herpes outbreaks.

Other infectious diseases, including pyogenic infections and tinea corporis can be spread by means of contact sports. Tinea pedis may be spread on floors around swimming pools.[23] Tinea infection is particularly common among wrestlers.[24] Prevalence among runners increases with age, and asymptomatic carriers are common.[25] Prompt identification and treatment of infected individuals, as well as use of protective clothing and footwear, reduces the incidence of infection. Periodic treatment of carriers with topical agents to prevent clinical disease may be possible. Intermittent doses of oral antifungal agents, such as itraconazole 200 mg bid for 1 day every 2 weeks, may be effective for prophylaxis against dermatophytosis in contact sports such as wrestling.[26]

There is growing concern about possible transmission of bloodborne pathogens during contact sports. Minor cuts and abrasions are both a source of contamination and a portal of entry for HIV and hep-

FIGURE 131-2

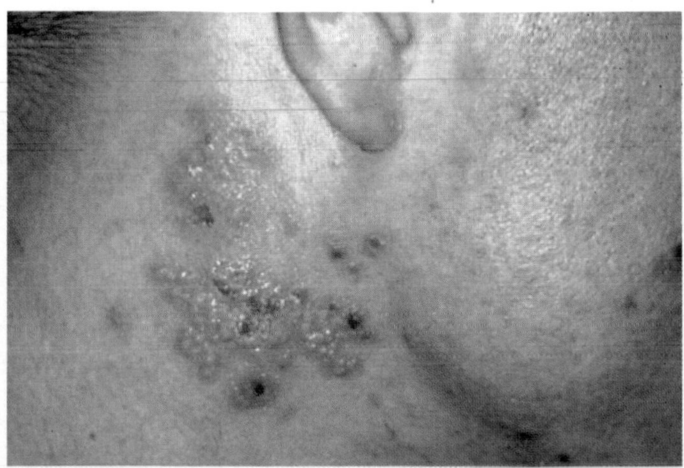

Herpes gladiatorum. (*Courtesy of Rita George, MD, Wilford Hall Air Force Medical Center.*)

atitis viruses. Lacerations should be covered with self-adherent biosynthetic dressings to prevent blood transmission from minor wounds during contact sports.[27]

Heat and Cold Injury (See also Chap. 126)

Heat injury is a common cause of morbidity during sports. The skin serves as the major organ of thermal regulation. Regular exercise modifies the responsiveness of cutaneous vessels, increasing cutaneous perfusion during periods of activity.[28] The duration of exercise can be safely increased in hot environments if a volume of fluid at least equal to that lost in sweat is ingested within 60 min prior to and during exercise.[29] Adequate skin surface must be exposed during exercise in order to reduce the risk of heat stress injury. Evaporative cooling from forearm skin is more efficient than that from the upper trunk.[30] Short sleeve shirts are advisable when competing in a hot environment. Clothing should be lightweight and have high water permeability in order to facilitate evaporative cooling.[31] At high humidity, evaporative cooling from skin is inefficient and the risk of heat stress increases. Spraying of water on the skin during exercise can reduce skin temperature, but this results in vasoconstriction and does not reduce core body temperature.[32]

Younger athletes have a greater skin surface area, which places them at greater risk for hypothermia in cold environments.[33] Skin injury, such as frostbite and perniosis are seen in sports enthusiasts who engage in cold weather sports. The decreased oxygen tension at high altitudes contributes to peripheral vasoconstriction, and decreased peripheral blood flow increases the risk of frostbite.[34] Frostbite is also a problem among joggers, and may occur on the face, hands, feet, and penis. Clothing must remain dry in order to retain its insulating properties. Frequent changes of socks and periodic breaks in a warm environment are important safeguards. If frostbite occurs, rapid rewarming should be accomplished as soon as the individual is in a safe environment with no risk of refreezing. Rarely, frostbite may be related to the use of ice packs in a training environment.[35]

Friction Blisters

Friction blisters occur as a result of mid-epidermal necrosis and are a major cause of disability in athletes (Fig. 131-3). Proper fitting of footwear and the use of gloves and chalk can reduce the incidence of blistering. Heat, sweating, and maceration increase the risk of blistering. Antiperspirants have been used in an attempt to reduce the incidence of blistering, but results have been mixed and they may cause irritant dermatitis. Attempts to reduce the incidence of irritant dermatitis with the addition of emollients reduces the efficacy of the antiperspirant.[36] In a study of cross-country hikers, a 20% solution of aluminum chloride hexahydrate in anhydrous alcohol reduced the rate of blister formation from 48 percent to 21 percent, but the incidence of irritant dermatitis was high and noncompliance with the treatment regimen was common.[37] Closed-cell neoprene insoles, acrylic socks or thin polyester socks combined with thick wool, or polypropylene socks that maintain their bulk can reduce the incidence of blisters.[38] Mesh top footwear can decrease the risk of blistering by providing a cooler, dryer environment without the use of antiperspirants.

Small blisters should be left intact to maintain sterility. An adhesive bandage or thin self-adhesive hydrocolloid dressing can be applied over the area, or a "doughnut" of moleskin can be applied around the blister to decrease discomfort. Larger blisters should be drained. The blister roof may be left in place as a biological dressing. A thin self-adhesive hydrocolloid dressing can be applied over the entire lesion. Antibiotics should be used if secondary infection is present.

FIGURE 131-3

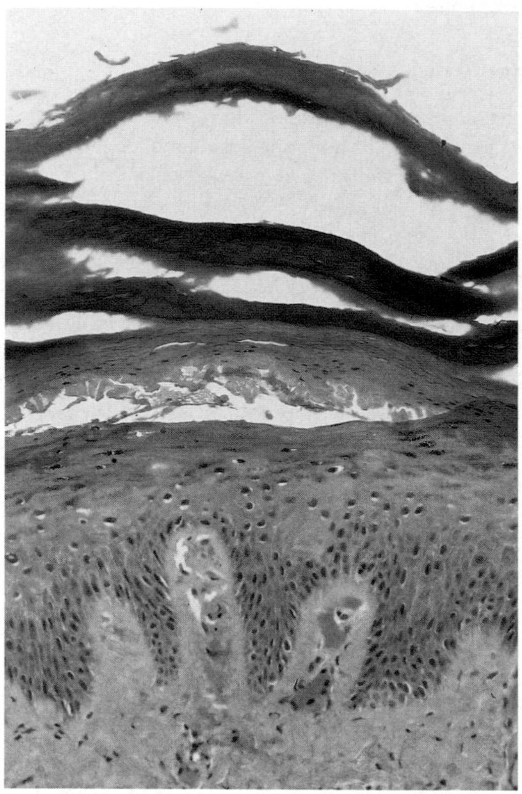

Friction blisters are a manifestation of intraepidermal necrosis.

Lime Burns

The use of calcium oxide (quicklime) or calcium hydroxide (slaked lime) instead of calcium carbonate (chalk) to line sports fields may result in chemical burns, especially in wet weather. In one report, 75 percent of football players developed chemical burns from lime used to mark a playing field. Such burns were predominantly located on the torso, buttocks and proximal lower extremities—areas occluded by football gear. Little reaction occurred on exposed skin. Second- and third-degree burns occurred, and the severity and extent of burns were related to the number of minutes played, and to delays in showering after the game.[39] Lime may also result in severe inhalation and ocular injuries.[40]

Soccer and rugby players may develop similar chemical burns. Calcium oxide (quicklime) converts to calcium hydroxide in wet environments. Calcium oxide is often used in Europe to mark soccer and rugby touchlines. Varying proportions of calcium compounds are often found in marking powders.[41] A lack of international regulations regarding marking materials has contributed to the problem.[42] Uniform regulations should be adopted by all sports federations.

Calluses and Corns (Clavi)

Callus formation is a physiologic protective mechanism. Large calluses can interfere with function, and may require treatment. Corns or clavi are particularly common in golfers, and can be treated with chemical or physical débridement. Liquid nitrogen and lasers can be useful in the treatment of corns. Prevention requires properly fitted footwear. Cushioning pads and metatarsal pads can be helpful.

Athlete's Nodules

Collagenous "surfer's nodules" are a well-described complication of surfboarding.[43] Boxers, marbles players, and football players are also prone to collagenous nodules.[44] These nodules occur at areas of pressure, trauma, and friction. Surgical excision may be required.[45]

Actinic Damage (See also Chaps. 134 and 247)

Actinic irradiation can cause burns and a risk of skin cancer in later life. Even relatively short periods of exposure during sports is associated with an increase risk for basal cell carcinoma.[46] Sweating alters hydration of the stratum corneum and lowers the minimal erythema dose (MED) to ultraviolet B (UVB) by as much as 40.9 percent after just 15 min of jogging.[47] Participation in water sports is an independent risk factor for melanoma.[48] Professional cyclists experience intense ultraviolet exposure with a mean daily average exposure of 8.1 MED of UVB. During mountain segments, cyclists may have exposures of more than 17 MED.[49] Lifeguards have daily exposures from 3.6 to 9.5 MED, mountain guides have exposures from 4.4 to 17.1 MED, and ski instructors from 2.8 to 8.8 MED.[50]

Phototoxic reactions may occur in athletes treated with drugs such as tetracycline and sulfa. Actinic radiation in the UVA range is important in the induction of phototoxic reactions. Unfortunately, most currently available sunscreens do not block UVA well, although sunblocks with Parsol 1789 and "physical" sunblocks, such as titanium dioxide, offer better UVA protection. Application technique has a significant impact on the effectiveness of sunscreens. Sunblock should be applied evenly prior to sun exposure. Reapplication as often as every 2 h may be necessary after perspiration or water exposure.

Sun exposure may reactivate orolabial herpes infections. Although sunscreens are commonly recommended to decrease the risk of recurrence, a controlled trial did not confirm their effectiveness.[51] Oral antiviral drugs can be used effectively to prevent herpes reactivation following sun exposure.[52]

Allergic Contact Dermatitis

Rubber allergens are the most common cause of sports-associated allergic contact dermatitis. Rubber adhesives and rubber chemicals in the box toe and cushioning materials of footwear can cause dermatitis (Fig. 131-4). Contact dermatitis also results from swimming goggles,

FIGURE 131-4

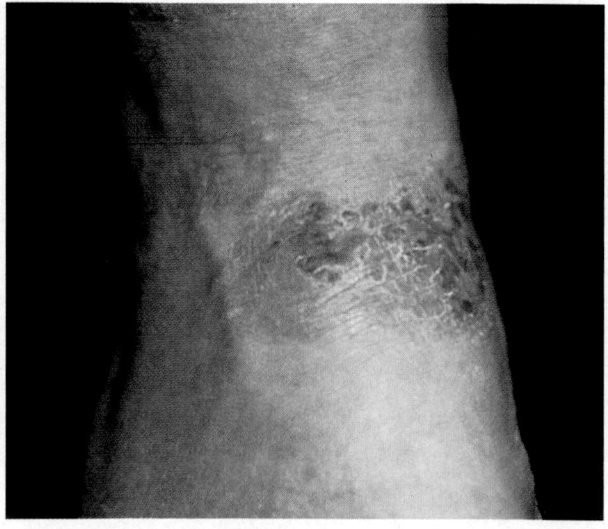

Allergic contact athletic shoe dermatitis.

diving equipment, swimming pool chemicals, bathing caps, nose clips, athletic tape, and topical creams and sprays that contain salicylates. The eruptions will respond to topical and systemic corticosteroids, but will recur unless the offending allergen is identified and eliminated. Patch testing can identify the allergen, and allow substitution of a suitable alternative.

SKIN PROBLEMS RELATED TO WATER SPORTS

Recreational swimming in lake water can result in significant transdermal absorption of water pollutants.[53] Hyperchlorinated rinsing pools may also cause cutaneous injury.

Water serves as a common source of infection, and an increased incidence of skin infections has been noted in swimmers exposed to polluted sea water.[54] Bathers are also at increased risk for gastroenteritis, acute febrile illness, and ear and eye infections. Illness is closely linked to contamination of water with domestic sewage.[55] Microscopic examination of formed stools found in swimming pools has demonstrated a significant rate of infestation with intestinal parasites.[56] Monitoring of water for fecal coliforms has been practiced for years, and has proved to be a better predictor of the risk of skin disease than of gastrointestinal disease.[57] Although many skin eruptions from recreational water probably go unreported, those that are reported account for almost half of all illness from recreational water.[58]

Storm run-off contaminating recreational waters results in a predominance of organisms linked to respiratory and skin infections. Current surveillance, which focuses on fecal contamination, may be inadequate to detect such contamination.[59] It has been suggested that monitoring for staphylococci could result in improved evaluation of the risk of skin disease.

Swimmers are prone to xerosis, especially during winter months. Contributing factors include loss of sebum and chlorine exposure while swimming, as well as long showers after swimming and the irritating liquid soap often supplied by the pool. Prevention and treatment include limiting showers, using mild soap and cooler water, and application of petrolatum before swim practice and a moisturizer after showering.[60]

Exposure to the rough surfaces of diving boards can result in a chronic plantar dermatosis. The fingers can also be affected (Fig. 131-5). Some of these individuals have a history of atopic dermatitis, psoriasis, or juvenile plantar dermatosis. The rough interior of swimming pools can result in "pool palms." The skin appears taught, shiny, and erythematous with loss of dermatoglyphics. Avoidance of rough pool surfaces will result in healing, but divers and swimmers are seldom willing to give up their sport. Topical steroids and tars can occasionally be of some benefit.

FIGURE 131-5

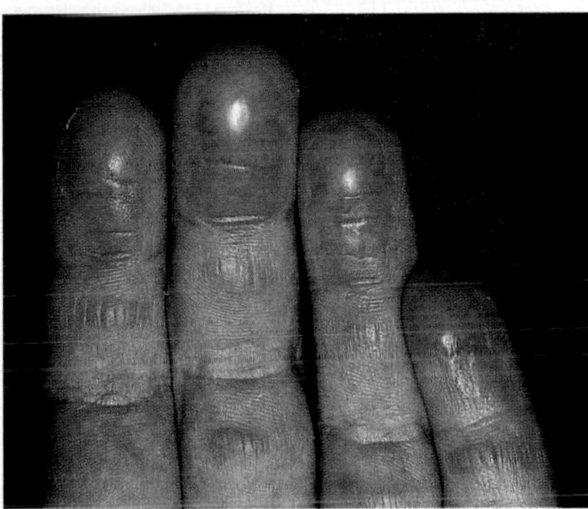

Finger dermatitis in this diver paralleled the intensity of her training. It resolved during breaks from training.

Water slide alopecia has been described as symmetric alopecic patches of the posterolateral aspects of the calves.[61] The patches are associated with repeated frictional trauma to the areas.

Green hair is related to copper in pool water. Copper pipes or algicides may be the source of the high copper levels. Acidic pH, fluoridation of water, and swimming pool chlorination all contribute to the release of copper into pool water.[62] Previous damage to the hair shaft, frequent contact with chlorinated water, or the use of alkaline shampoos may predispose to the development of green hair. Hair damage induces cysteic acid and related sulfonate groups that adsorb copper. Green hair has been treated with hot vegetable oil, hydrogen peroxide, edetic acid (EDTA),[63] and 1-hydroxyethyl diphosphonic acid.[64] Penicillamine shampoo has also been used successfully.

Swimming pool water may be treated with chlorine, bromine, and ozone ionization. All three methods are acceptable, although bromine with ozone may be associated with a slightly lower risk of cutaneous reactions. Skin rashes with onset less than 24 h after swimming is reported by up to 8 percent of swimmers, while eye redness and itching is reported in up to 33 percent.[65] Swim goggles have a protective effect against eye irritation.

Swimmer's Itch (See also Chap. 237)

Swimmer's itch is generally produced by the penetration of avian schistosome cercariae through exposed skin. In endemic areas, a less-severe dermatitis is caused by penetration of the cercariae of human schistosomes. Eutrophication of lakes due to excessive nutrient input favors proliferation of schistosomes. Newly created bodies of water, such as recently abandoned quarries, have a lower incidence of swimmer's itch. Praziquantel, given to ducks inhabiting a lake, can reduce the incidence of swimmer's itch.[66] Chemical control or mechanical removal of snails can also be effective. The rash heals spontaneously in 2 to 3 weeks. Topical steroids and antihistamines may be beneficial.

Seabather's Eruption (Sea Lice) (See also Chap. 237)

Seabather's eruption occurs under the bathing suit area. Some outbreaks are caused by jellyfish larvae;[67] others are caused by sea anemone larvae.[68] The eruption runs its course in about 2 weeks. Topical corticosteroids and antihistamines may provide some relief, but are frequently ineffective. Of interest, topical thiabendazole and systemic thiabendazole have been reported as effective.[69] The mechanism for this reported effect in the treatment of what appears to be tiny coelenterate stings is unclear. During epidemics, children, people with a prior history of seabather's eruption, and surfers are at greatest risk. Length of time spent in the water is not a major risk factor. Showering with one's bathing suit off after seabathing reduces the incidence of the eruption.[70]

Other Skin Problems Related to Sea Water (See also Chap. 237)

Corals, especially fire coral, can produce contact dermatitis in divers. Their stinging cells produce a powerful irritant that can produce severe local reactions, including reactions that resemble full-thickness burns.

Sea urchin spines are brittle, and readily break off in the skin, potentially causing delayed contact sensitivity. Sarcoidal granulomas can occur.

FIGURE 131-6

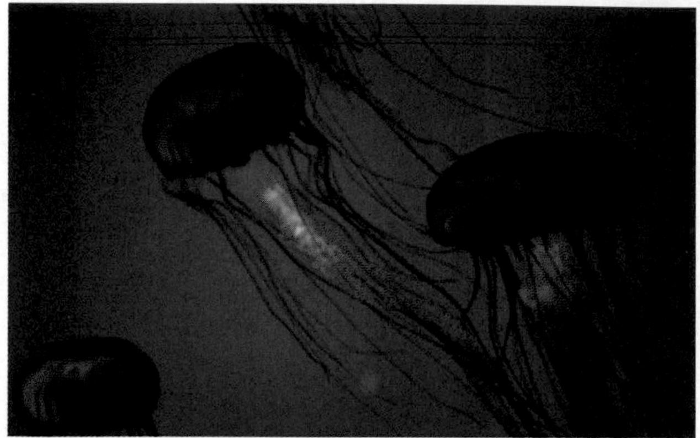

A.

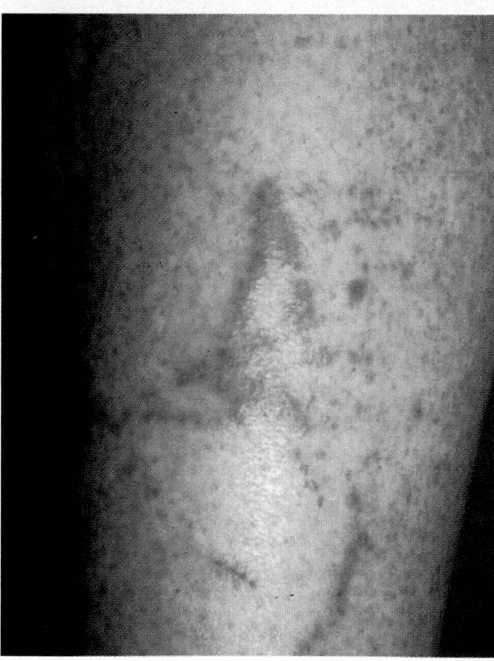

B.

Free-floating jellyfish tentacles (*A*) may cause stings (*B*) identical to those caused by contact with an intact jellyfish. (*Photograph of clinical lesions is from the Wilford Hall Air Force Medical Center Dermatology teaching file.*)

Jellyfish stings cause both immediate pain and delayed allergic reactions (Fig. 131-6). Local reactions may be severe, and can result in gangrene and contractures. Delayed allergic reactions generally consist of local reactivation, but generalized reactions and erythema nodosum can also occur. Portuguese man-of-war (*Physalia physalis*) stings are more severe than those of most other jellyfish. Pacific box jellyfish (*Chironex fleckeri*) venom contains hemolytic, dermonecrotic, and myocardial toxins, and can cause severe cardiorespiratory reactions. Antivenin can neutralize cardiovascular effects of sea wasp envenomation in an animal model. In contrast, verapamil does not neutralize cardiovascular effects and increases mortality in the same animal model.[71] Vinegar is routinely used to inactivate undischarged box jellyfish nematocysts. It may also cause discharge of nematocysts of some other species of jellyfish, including some *Physalia*.[72] Cold packs provide effective analgesia during the acute painful stage of jellyfish stings.

Contact with seaweed has been implicated in vesiculobullous reactions. Algal organisms in seaweed can cause "stinging seaweed dermatitis" and pustular folliculitis.

Mycobacterium marinum (see Chap. 200) can cause epidemics of "swimming pool granuloma". Mycobacterial infections are also commonly acquired in brackish coastal waters. Lesions can present as a smoldering tenosynovitis. Accurate diagnosis is essential because intralesional steroid injections for an "inflammatory joint" can cause severe sequelae.

Marine vibrio infections occur in brackish coastal waters. Many cases are related to ingestion of oysters, but skin and soft tissue injury in brackish water may also result in infection. Sepsis may occur, especially in those with preexisting liver disease (most commonly cirrhosis). Culture of wounds contaminated with sea water have a greater yield if thiosulfate-citrate-bile-sucrose agar is used, and the cultures are performed both at room temperature and 30°C (86°F).[73]

Stingrays lash with their toxin-containing barbed tails when stepped on. Cutaneous and neurologic injury may result. Embedded barbs are associated with bacterial and deep fungal infection.

Decompression injury may affect the skin of divers, commonly causing livido reticularis. In a porcine model of decompression injury, vascular congestion and vasculitis were common skin biopsy findings.[74]

HISTAMINE-MEDIATED REACTIONS

Exercise-associated urticarial reactions include cholinergic urticaria, solar urticaria, symptomatic dermatographism, pressure-induced urticaria, cold urticaria, aquagenic urticaria, latex-induced contact urticaria, and exercise-induced anaphylaxis, which is the most severe of these reactions. In many cases, the reaction requires "priming" by an ingested allergen prior to exercise. These entities are discussed in more detail in Chap. 116.

ACNEIFORM LESIONS

Acne mechanica is common among athletes. It is caused by physical factors including pressure, occlusion, friction, and heat. It commonly occurs under chin straps, helmets, and shoulder pads. The lesions may respond better to keratolytics than to antibacterial agents.[75] They remit with the season's end.

Severe acne may be a sign of anabolic steroid use, which is widespread among athletes of all ages. Anabolic steroids cause enlargement of sebaceous glands, alter skin lipids and promote the growth of *Propionibacterium acnes*. Hirsutism and androgenic alopecia may also be present. Clinicians should be alert for skin signs of possible anabolic steroid use, as these drugs may have serious consequences, including peliosis hepatis.

OTHER SPECIAL DERMATOLOGIC PROBLEMS OF ATHLETES

Athletes with atopic eczema present special problems with exercise. Overheating may lead to bouts of pruritus. Individuals with atopic dermatitis demonstrate abnormal sweating and vasoconstriction patterns. However, there is evidence that the sweating[76] and vascular response improve with athletic training, and that athletics may not interfere with treatment of atopic dermatitis.[77] Application of an emollient after showering and short periods of rest can inhibit sweat-induced itching in atopic athletes, and regular moderate exercise does not cause deterioration in the condition of their skin.[78]

The athlete treated with oral retinoids also faces special problems. Arthralgia, staphylococcal colonization, photosensitization, and fatigue may result in lost training time or lost seasons. Retinoids cause disruption of epidermal integrity and skin fragility. The stratum corneum becomes loose and loses its barrier function. Greater trochanter enthesopathy (pain at the site of tendon insertion) may be a complication of short-term oral retinoid therapy in athletes.[79] For these reasons, when possible, retinoid treatment should be planned between seasons.

REFERENCES

1. Strauss RH et al: Illness and absence among wrestlers, swimmers, and gymnasts at a large university. *Am J Sports Med* **16**:653, 1988
2. Gaulrapp H et al: Injuries in mountain biking. *Knee Surg Sports Traumatol Arthrosc* **9**:48, 2001
3. Heitkamp HC et al: In-line skating: Injuries and prevention. *J Sports Med Phys Fitness* **40**:247, 2000
4. Brenner IK et al: Infection in athletes. *Sports Med* **17**:86, 1944
5. Perz-Perdomo R et al: Description of morbidity notified in the epidemiologic surveillance system of the XVII Central American and Caribbean Sport Games, Puerto Rico, 1993. *Puerto Rico Health Sci J* **13**:267, 1993
6. Shephard RJ: Science and medicine of canoeing and kayaking. *Sports Med* **4**:19, 1987
7. Sosin DM et al: An outbreak of furunculosis among high school athletes. *Am J Sports Med* **17**:828, 1989
8. Bartlett PC et al: Furunculosis in a high school football team. *Am J Sports Med* **10**:371, 1982
9. Falck G: Group A streptococcal infections after indoor association football tournament. *Lancet* **347**:840, 1996
10. Ludlam H et al: Scrum kidney: Epidemic pyoderma caused by a nephritogenic *Streptococcus pyogenes* in a rugby team. *Lancet* **2**:331, 1986
11. Maniatis AN et al: Pseudomonas aeruginosa folliculitis due to non-O:11 serotypes: Acquisition through the use of contaminated synthetic sponges. *Clin Infect Dis* **21**:437, 1995
12. Penn C et al: *Pseudomonas* folliculitis: and outbreak associated with bromine-based disinfectants. *Can Dis Wkly Rep* **16**:31, 1990
13. Zichichi L et al: *Pseudomonas aeruginosa* folliculitis after shower/bath exposure. *Int J Dermatol* **39**:270, 2000
14. Bottone EJ et al: Loofah sponges are reservoirs and vehicles in the transmission of potentially pathogenic bacterial species to human skin. *J Clin Microbiol* **32**:469, 1994
15. Rolston KV et al: *Pseudomonas aeruginosa* infection in cancer patients. *Cancer Invest* **10**:43, 1992
16. Lacour JP et al: Diving suit dermatitis caused by *Pseudomonas aeruginosa*: Tow cases. *J Am Acad Dermatol* **31**:1055, 1994
17. Saltzer KR et al: Diving suit dermatitis: A manifestation of *Pseudomonas* folliculitis. *Cutis* **59**:245, 1997
18. Agger WA: *Pseudomonas aeruginosa* infections of intact skin. *Clin Infect Dis* **20**:302, 1995
19. Insler MS et al: *Pseudomonas* keratitis and folliculitis from whirlpool exposure. *Am J Ophthalmol* **101**:41, 1986
20. Molina DN et al: Unusual presentation of *Pseudomonas aeruginosa* infections: A review. *Bol Asoc Med P R* **83**:160, 1991
21. Belogna EA et al: An outbreak of herpes gladiatorum at a high school wrestling camp. *N Engl J Med* **325**:906, 1991
22. Strauss RH et al: Abrasive shirts may contribute to herpes gladiatorum among wrestlers. *N Engl J Med* **320**:598, 1989
23. Bolanos B: Dermatophyte feet infection among students enrolled in swimming pool courses at a university pool. *Bol Asoc Med P R* **83**:181, 1991
24. Adams B: Tinea corporis gladiatorum: A cross-sectional study. *J Am Acad Dermatol* **43**:1039, 2000
25. Auger P et al: Epidemiology of tinea pedis in marathon runners: Prevalence of occult athlete's foot. *Mycoses* **36**:35, 1993
26. Hazen et al: Itraconazole in the prevention and management of dermatophytosis in competitive wrestlers. *J Am Acad Dermatol* **36**:481, 1997
27. Hazen PG et al: Management of lacerations in sports: The use of a biosynthetic dressing during competitive wrestling. *Cutis* **56**:301, 1995
28. Kvernmo HD et al: Enhanced endothelium-dependent vasodilatation in human skin vasculature induced by physical conditioning. *Eur J Applied Physiol Occup Physiol* **79**:30, 1998
29. Lindinger MI: Exercise in the heat: Thermoregulatory limitations to performance in humans and horses. *Can J Appl Physiol* **24**:152, 1999
30. Kato M et al: Thermophysiological effects of two different types of clothing under warm temperatures. *Appl Hum Sci* **14**:119, 1995
31. Gonzalez RR: Biophysiological integration of proper clothing for exercise. *Exerc Sport Sci Rev* **15**:261, 1987
32. Bassett DR, et al: Thermoregulatory responses to skin wetting during prolonged treadmill running. *Med Sci Sports Exerc* **19**:28, 1987
33. Squire DL: Heat illness. Fluid and electrolyte issues for pediatric and adolescent athletes. *Pediatr Clin North Am* **37**:1085, 1990
34. Fisher AA: Sports-related cutaneous reactions: Part 1. Dermatoses due to physical agents. *Cutis* **63**:134, 1999
35. O'Toole G, Rayatt S: Frostbite at the gym: A case report of an ice pack burn. *Br J Sports Med* **33**:278, 1999
36. Knapik JJ et al: Friction blisters. Pathophysiology, prevention, and treatment. *Sports Med* **20**:136, 1995
37. Knapik JJ et al: Influence of an antiperspirant on foot blister incidence during cross-country hiking. *J Am Acad Dermatol* **39**:202, 1998
38. Kawabata A et al: Effects of two kinds of sport shoes with different structure on thermoregulatory responses. *Ann Physiol Anthropol* **12**:165, 1993
39. Baker JG: Lime disease? *Arch Dermatol* **136**:1277, 2000
40. Potts A: Toxic responses of the eye, in, *Toxicology,* edited by M Amdur. New York, McGraw-Hill, 1993, p 524
41. Gelmetti C et al: Caustic ulcers caused by calcium hydroxide in 2 adolescent football players. *Contact Derm* **27**:265, 1992
42. Fisher AA: Sports-related cutaneous reactions: Part III. Sports identification marks. *Cutis* **63**:256, 1999
43. Erickson JG et al: Surfer's nodules and other complications of surfboarding. *JAMA* **201**:134, 1967
44. Cohen PR et al: Athlete's nodules: Sports-related connective tissue nevi of the collagen type (collagenomas). *Cutis* **50**:131, 1992
45. Cohen PR et al: Athlete's nodules. Treatment by surgical excision. *Sports Med* **10**:198, 1990
46. Rosso S et al: The multicenter south European study "Helios" II: Different sun exposure patterns in the aetiology of basal cell and squamous cell carcinomas of the skin. *Br J Cancer* **73**:1447, 1996
47. Moehrle M et al: Reduction of minimal erythema dose by sweating. *Photodermatol Photoimmunol Photomed* **16**:260, 2000
48. Herzfeld PM et al: A case-control study of malignant melanoma of the trunk among white males in upstate New York. *Cancer Detect Prev* **17**:601, 1993
49. Moehrle M et al: Extreme UV exposure of professional cyclists. *Dermatology* **201**:44, 2000
50. Moehrle M et al: *Bacillus subtilis* spore film dosimeters in personal dosimetry for occupational solar ultraviolet exposure. *Int Arch Occup Environ Health* **73**:575, 2000
51. Mills J et al: Recurrent herpes labialis in skiers. Clinical observations and effect of sunscreen. *Am J Sports Med* **15**:76, 1987
52. Spruance SL et al: Acyclovir prevents reactivation of herpes simplex labialis is skiers. *JAMA* **260**:1597, 1988
53. Moody RP et al: Dermal exposure to environmental contaminants in the Great Lakes. *Environ Health Perspect* **103**:103, 1995
54. von Schirnding YE et al: Morbidity among bathers exposed to polluted seawater. A prospective epidemiologic study. *S Afr Med J* **81**:543, 1992
55. Fleisher JM et al: Estimates of the severity of illnesses associated with bathing in marine recreational waters contaminated with domestic sewage. *Int J Epidemiol* **27**:722, 1998
56. Prevalence of parasites in fecal material from chlorinated swimming pools—United States. 1999. *MMWR Morb Mortal Wkly Rep* **50**:410, 2001
57. Zmirou D et al: Evaluation des indicateurs microbiens du risque sanitaire lie aux baignades en riviere. *Rev Epidemiol Sante Publique* **38**:101, 1990
58. Kramer MH et al: Surveillance for waterborne-disease outbreaks—United States, 1993–1994. *MMWR CDC Surveill Sum* **45**:1, 1996
59. O'Shea ML et al: Detection and disinfection of pathogens in storm-generated flows. *Can J Microbiol* **38**:267, 1992
60. Basler RS et al: Special skin symptoms seen in swimmers. *J Am Acad Dermatol* **43**:299, 2000
61. Adams B: Water-slide alopecia. *Cutis* **67**:399, 2001
62. Fisher AA: Green hair: Causes and management. *Cutis* **63**:317, 1999
63. Mascaro JM et al: Green hair. *Cutis* **56**:37, 1995
64. Melnik BC et al: Green hair: Guidelines for diagnosis and therapy. *J Am Acad Dermatol* **15**:1065, 1986
65. Kelsall HL, Sim MR: Skin irritation in users of brominated pools. *Int J Environ Health Res* **11**:29, 2001
66. Reimink RL et al: Efficacy of praziquantel in natural populations of mallards infected with avian schistosomes. *J Parasitol* **81**:1027, 1995

67. Wong DE et al: Seabather's eruption. Clinical, histologic, and immunologic features. *J Am Acad Dermatol* **30**:399, 1994
68. Freudenthal AR et al: Seabather's eruption. *N Engl J Med* **329**:542, 1993
69. Burnett JW: Seabather's eruption. *Cutis* **50**:98, 1992
70. Kumar S et al: Risk factors for seabather's eruption: a prospective study. *Public Health Rep* **112**:59, 1997
71. Tibballs J et al: The effects of antivenom and verapamil on the haemodynamic actions of *Chironex fleckeri* (box jellyfish) venom. *Anaesth Intensive Care* **26**:40, 1998
72. Fenner PJ et al: First aid treatment of jellyfish stings in Australia. Response to a newly differentiated species. *Med J Aust* **158**:498, 1993
73. Reed KC et al: Skin and soft-tissue infections after injury in the ocean: Culture methods and antibiotic therapy for marine bacteria. *Mil Med* **164**:198, 1999
74. Buttolph TB et al: Cutaneous lesions in swine after decompression: Histopathology and ultrastructure. *Undersea Hyperb Med* **25**:115, 1998
75. Basler R: Acne mechanica in athletes. *Cutis* **50**:125, 1992
76. Parkkinen MU et al: Sweating response to moderate thermal stress in atopic dermatitis. *Br J Dermatol* **126**:346, 1992
77. Salzer B et al: Gruppensport als adjuvante Therapie fur Patienten mit atopischem Ekzem. *Hautarzt* **45**:751, 1994
78. Heyer GR, Hornstein OP: Recent studies of cutaneous nociception in atopic and non-atopic subjects. *J Dermatol* **26**:77, 1999
79. Stitik TP et al: Greater trochanter enthesopathy: An example of "short course retinoid enthesopathy": A case report. *Am J Phys Med Rehab* **78**:571, 1999

CHAPTER 132

Joel M. Gelfand
David J. Margolis

Decubitus (Pressure) Ulcers and Venous Ulcers

Chronic wounds are a common medical problem that result in dramatic alterations in quality of life due to the associated pain, disability, and social isolation. Chronic wounds also result in excessive medical costs, health care provider visits, hospitalizations, and death. They disproportionately affect the elderly and, therefore, are increasing in incidence and prevalence as this segment of the population expands. Two of the most common types of chronic wounds are decubitus (pressure) ulcers and venous leg ulcers. Dermatologists are frequently involved in the care of patients with these problems.

Decubitus ulcers, preferably called pressure ulcers but also known as pressure sores and bedsores, are wounds that occur in areas of bony prominence as localized areas of necrosis of the skin and deeper soft tissues. These wounds tend to occur in individuals who are immobile. The pathophysiology involves unrelieved pressure, shearing, and frictional forces exerted on skin and subcutaneous tissues by bedding or seating surfaces. Pressure ulcers are initially evident as areas of blanchable or nonblanchable erythema, without a break in the continuity of the epidermis. They can progress to involve muscle, tendon, and bone. Treatment centers on relieving pressure.

Venous leg ulcers are wounds that occur on the lower extremity, most commonly in the gaiter area, which is located approximately between the lower half of the calf and 1 inch below the malleolus. The pathophysiology involves venous abnormalities of the lower extremity that result in ambulatory venous hypertension of the superficial venous system. The clinical diagnosis of venous leg ulcer is often made in any individual with a chronic wound in the gaiter area, with other signs of venous abnormalities (such as varicose veins, venous blush, lipodermatosclerosis), and an adequately functioning lower limb arterial system (e.g., an ankle brachial index of > 0.80, presence of a palpable distal limb pulse).[1] Venous leg ulcers frequently extend to the deep dermis and are often exudative wounds caused by the underlying abnormalities in venous circulation. Treatment centers on improving venous hemodynamics.

HISTORICAL ASPECTS

Management of chronic wounds dates back to one of the oldest known medical manuscripts, circa 2200 B.C. in which the need to wash the wound and bandage it are described. Pressure ulcers have been identified on a mummy of an elderly priestess of Amen.[2] Amboise Paré of the sixteenth century was one of the first to describe the significance of immobility and pressure in the cause of decubiti. He wrote of the importance of using a soft bed and local wound care; he also shunned the use of boiling oil to treat wounds, which was the routine at the time. Brown-Séquard believed that skin moisture was an important factor, while Charcot described the "neurotropic theory" of decubiti. Sir James Paget wrote about the importance of prevention of decubiti, particularly in those who are immobilized.

Writings on venous leg ulcers also date to antiquity.[3] Hippocrates wrote about the treatment of lower extremity varicosities. In the fourteenth century, Guy de Chauliac described the mechanical treatment of venous leg ulcers using lead plates. P.G. Unna developed the zinc paste bandage for treatment of venous leg ulcers in 1885. With the development of antiseptic techniques by Sir Joseph Lister, the use of surgical approaches increased with pioneering efforts by Friedrich Trendelenburg, Max Schede, Theodor Kocher, and William Babcock.

EPIDEMIOLOGY

Pressure Ulcers

Incidence and prevalence rates of pressure ulcers (Table 132-1) have varied with definition of incidence or prevalence used, study

TABLE 132-1

Incidence and Prevalence of Pressure Ulcers by Population

Population	Incidence	Prevalence
General	Unknown	0.5%
Acute care	0.4–38%	10–17%
Long-term care	2.2–23.9%	2.3–28%
Home care	0–17%	0–29%
Spinal cord injury patients	20–31%	10.2–30%
Elderly	0.18 to 3.36 per 100-person years	0.31–10%
Hip fracture patients	19.1–55%	Unknown

methodology, population studied, and imprecision due to small sample size. Pressure ulcers affect approximately 0.5 to 2.2 percent of the total population and in the United States, the cost is an estimated $1.335 billion dollars annually.[4,5] The age distribution includes one peak in younger, mostly neurologically impaired (e.g., spinal cord injuries) individuals, and another peak in older, geriatric patients, with the elderly accounting for 70 percent of all pressure ulcers.[6] The incidence and prevalence is highly dependent on clinical setting (e.g., intensive care unit, nursing home, community settings) and patient factors, such as age, and related infirmities, such as hip fractures, spinal cord injuries, and other immobilizing conditions.

The prevalence of pressure ulcers in the acute care setting in the late 1990s was estimated to be 10 to 17 percent, with 48 to 53 percent of these ulcers being acquired while in the hospital.[6] The majority of pressure ulcers in the acute care setting are stage I or II and are located on the sacrum and coccyx, followed by the heel. The incidence of pressure ulcers in the long-term care setting in the 1990s varied from 2.2 to 23.9 percent[6] and the prevalence ranged from 2.3 to 28 percent.[7] In the home care setting, incidence was 0 to 17 percent and prevalence was 0 to 29 percent.[6,7]

Certain patient factors affect incidence and prevalence of pressure ulcers. The incidence and prevalence of pressure ulcers in patients with spinal cord injuries in the 1990s was 20 to 31 percent, and 10.2 to 30 percent, respectively.[6,8] The overall prevalence rate in the elderly is estimated to be 5 to 10 percent.[6] Studies in elderly outpatients however, have found an annual prevalence between 0.31 and 0.70 percent with an incidence of 0.18 to 3.36 per 100-person years.[9] The incidence of pressure ulcers in patients with hip fractures varies from 19.1 to 55 percent.[6]

Venous Leg Ulcers

The epidemiology of venous leg ulcers has been investigated in several community-based population studies that are limited by the lack of a "gold standard" diagnostic for a large population sample. Therefore, data on venous leg ulcers are often extrapolated from studies of chronic ulcerations of the lower extremity. It is estimated that 40 to 70 percent of chronic lower extremity wounds are venous leg ulcers.[10] The prevalence of leg ulcers increases with age and disproportionately affects women with an observed female to male ratio of 1.6:1.[11] Chronic ulcerations of the leg occur in 0.8 percent of the general population, 1 percent of the adult population, and 3.6 percent of those older than 65 years of age, based on a mail survey of a Scottish community.[12] The prevalence of active ulcerations of the lower extremity is estimated to be 1.48/1000[13] and the incidence of venous leg ulcers is estimated to be 18 per 100,000 person years. Chronic wounds of the lower extremity typically have a prolonged course with greater than 50 percent being present for more than a year.[14] Therefore, the prolonged course of venous leg ulcers results in a high prevalence of the disease relative to its incidence. Once healed, venous ulcers frequently recur with an annual recurrence rate of 33 to 42 percent.[15,16] It is estimated that the annual cost of caring for a venous leg ulcer is $7460 with annual U.S. costs in excess of $1.9 billion.[11]

ETIOLOGY AND PATHOGENESIS

Pressure Ulcers

Central to the pathophysiology of the development of pressure ulcers is the interface of pressure between the skin and subcutaneous tissue, and the bedding or seating surface. Studies consistently find that pressures in excess of 32 mmHg are required to initiate skin breakdown.[17] Skin and subcutaneous tissue overlying bony prominences such as the occiput, sternum, scapulae, sacrum, coccyx, iliac crests, trochanters, patellae, malleoli, heel, and lateral edge of the foot, are particularly apt to develop high pressures. Certain subcutaneous tissues, such as muscle, are more sensitive to hypoxia than the overlying epidermis, and may undergo substantial injury prior to clinical signs of epidermal injury.[17]

Elevated cutaneous pressure results in tissue hypoxia, as a result of impairment in capillary flow. Pressure forces also lead to impairment in removal of toxic metabolites, such as free radicals, because of obstruction of venules. Initial tissue injury is physiologically responded to by vasodilation and resultant hyperemia (clinically seen as blanchable erythema), which may paradoxically lead to further tissue damage through further generation of free radicals. Elevated pressures result in hemorrhage into the tissues, clinically observed as nonblanchable erythema. An inverse relationship between amount of pressure and duration of pressure exists in terms of the force necessary to yield tissue necrosis. Low pressure over a long duration of time, however, results in greater tissue injury than does high pressure exerted over a short time period.[17]

Pressure alone is not the only cause of pressure ulcers. In humans, pressure ulcers occur when soft tissues are exposed to less pressure and time gradients than those required to create tissue necrosis in experimental models. Additional forces involved are shear and friction. Forces that are parallel to an area are called shearing forces and can reduce, especially in deep tissues and blood vessels, the amount of pressure required to create necrosis by half.[18,19] Frictional forces result in damage to the stratum corneum and epidermis resulting in an impairment of barrier function and a greater susceptibility to tissue necrosis.[17] Excessive moisture results in increased adhesiveness of the skin to bed linens, generating greater frictional and shearing forces.[17]

Venous Leg Ulcers

Chronic ambulatory venous hypertension is central to the pathophysiology of venous leg ulcers.[20] Venous return from the lower extremity involves the superficial veins, the communicating or perforator veins, and the deep veins. The superficial veins consist of the long and short saphenous veins and their tributaries. The superficial veins can enter directly into the deep veins or connect to the deep veins by small communicating or perforator veins. The deep veins are classified as either intramuscular or intermuscular. The deep venous system involves three sets of paired tibial veins, which merge to become the popliteal vein, which becomes the superficial femoral vein. The superficial femoral vein merges with the deep femoral vein in the femoral triangle to become the common femoral vein. Superficial, communicating, and deep veins have one-way bicuspid valves that allow flow only in the cephalad direction. Blood is returned to the heart primarily through the pumping action of leg muscles.[11,21]

During ambulation, in an individual with a properly functioning venous system, the pressures in the superficial system fall toward zero. In an individual with venous disease, superficial venous pressure is elevated during ambulation to as high as 40 to 100 mmHg.[20] Venous hypertension may occur through four mechanisms: (1) dysfunction of valves in the superficial and/or communicating veins because of congenital or acquired (e.g., phlebitis, trauma) incompetence; (2) dysfunction in the valves of the deep system from congenital absence, inherent weakness, or thrombotic damage; (3) deep venous outflow obstruction from a mass or obesity; and (4) from muscle pump failure secondary to inflammatory conditions of the joints or muscles, fibrosis, or neuropathies.[11]

Why patients with ambulatory venous hypertension develop venous-associated wounds is not clear. The most popular theories concern the deposition of pericapillary fibrin in the small venules surrounding the ulcers,[20] the trapping of inflammatory cells within the venules surrounding the ulcers resulting in the liberation of proteolytic enzymes, and the trapping of essential growth factors by macroglobulins within the venules and dermis surrounding the ulcers.[22] None of these theories have been fully validated by experimental evidence. Central to all of these theories is an alteration in venous hemodynamics of the lower limb resulting in abnormally elevated ambulatory venous pressure. The importance of ambulatory venous hypertension in the pathophysiology of venous leg ulcers is validated by the centrality of lower-limb compression therapy in the treatment of these wounds.

Genetics

The role of genetics in the development of pressure ulcers and venous leg ulcers has not been clearly delineated. Factor V Leiden mutations resulting in resistance to activated protein C occur with increased prevalence in patients with postthrombotic venous leg ulcers relative to control subjects.[23,24] Venous leg ulcers have also been reported in men with sex chromosome abnormalities, such as Klinefelter's syndrome.

PREVENTION

Pressure Ulcers

Prevention of pressure ulcers involves a multidisciplinary approach. Aggressive programs to prevent pressure ulcers may lower their incidence by 25 to 30 percent.[25,26] The first step is the identification of individuals at risk for pressure ulcer development. Several scoring systems, including the Norton Scale,[27] the Waterlow Scale,[28] and the Braden Scale,[29] have been developed to identify such patients. These instruments evaluate variables such as mobility, moisture exposure, nutrition, and patient factors (e.g., health status, age, body weight). They have variable sensitivity and specificity, and are limited by poor predictive value because the incidence of pressure ulcers is relatively low in most settings, thus limiting the scale's clinical application.[4]

Relief of pressure is believed to be important in the prevention of pressure ulcers. Efforts to turn the patient, use of proper positioning, and improvement of passive activity, while important empirically, have not been validated by published data. Bioengineering advances have led to the development of alternating air mattresses and low-air-loss beds, which minimize the amount of pressure exerted on the skin. These specially designed pressure-reducing mattresses reduce the risk of pressure ulcers by 70 percent when compared to standard mattresses.[4] No dramatic advantage of type of pressure-reducing mattress (e.g., alternating air versus low-air-loss) has been demonstrated in clinical trials.[4] Therefore, the choice of pressure-reducing device in the prevention of pressure ulcers is based on cost, local availability, and patient factors.

The nutritional status of the patient is also believed to be important in the development of pressure ulcers. Patients who develop pressure ulcers frequently have low serum albumin, which is a marker of poor nutritional status. However, studies evaluating the use of oral and enteral feeding supplements have not demonstrated efficacy in the prevention of pressure ulcers.[4]

Venous Leg Ulcers

Efforts aimed at prevention of venous leg ulcers have centered on reversing ambulatory venous hypertension. Compression therapy is believed to prevent venous leg ulcers in patients with ambulatory venous hypertension, and to prevent recurrence of leg ulcers.[30,31] Controlled data on the primary prevention of venous leg ulcers in those with venous stasis, however are limited. Furthermore, the use of compression therapy in the prevention of the recurrence of venous leg ulcers has been evaluated by the Cochrane group, which found no controlled studies that demonstrate the efficacy of compression in this setting.[32] Preliminary data suggests that surgical correction of isolated superficial venous reflux may reduce the long-term recurrence rate of venous leg ulcers.[33] These data await confirmation by a controlled trial.

CLINICAL MANIFESTATIONS

Pressure Ulcers

The clinical appearance of a pressure ulcer depends on its stage of evolution (Table 132-2). The earliest sign of pressure ulcer is blanchable erythema. Stage I ulcers appear as nonblanchable erythema without breakdown of the epidermis (Fig. 132-1) and can be difficult to detect in patients with darkly pigmented skin. Stage II ulcers have partial-thickness skin loss involving the epidermis or the epidermis and dermis. Stage III ulcers demonstrate full-thickness skin loss that may extend to, but not include, the fascia. Stage IV ulcers show extensive necrosis with tissue destruction down to muscle, bone, or supporting structures (Fig. 132-2).[5] An overhanging border of epidermis may be seen in advanced pressure ulcers, masking the true extent of the tissue destruction. Pressure ulcers occur predominantly over areas of bony prominence such as the occiput, scapulae, elbows, sternum, sacrum, ischial tuberosities, iliac crest, trochanters, heels, and knees. They may also occur on the nose, ears, or lips. Pressure ulcers are often painful and can be particularly distressful to patients and families.

Venous Leg Ulcers

The early signs of venous hypertension include varicosities of the superficial veins, red brown hyperpigmentation of the leg resulting from red cell extravasation, and an eczematous dermatitis manifested as erythema, scaling, and, in some instances, a serosanguineous exudate.

TABLE 132-2

Staging of Pressure Ulcers

Stage	Definition
I	Nonblanchable erythema of intact skin
II	Partial-thickness skin loss involving epidermis, dermis, or both
III	Full-thickness skin loss involving damage or necrosis of subcutaneous tissue that may extend down to, but not through, underlying fascia
IV	Full-thickness skin loss with extensive necrosis, or damage to muscle, bone, or supporting structures

FIGURE 132-1

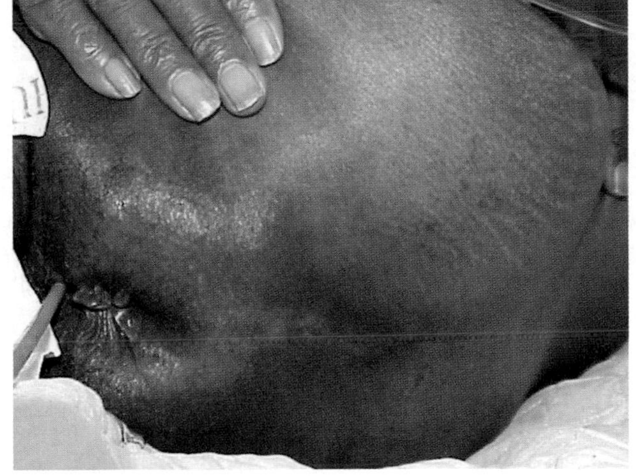

Extensive stage I pressure ulcer of the sacral area.

Lipodermatosclerosis, a sclerosing panniculitis, is seen in some patients with venous disease and is manifested by epidermal atrophy, yielding a shiny texture to the skin with a woody or indurated texture. The process often results in the lower leg resembling an inverted champagne bottle. An additional finding in some patients is atrophie blanche, which is manifested as porcelain-white atrophic lesions with telangiectasia that can be exquisitely painful.

Venous ulcers typically have a beefy red base with an edematous bluish border, termed *venous blush* (Fig. 132-3). Frank necrosis or eschar is rarely seen. The ulcers typically involve the middle to deep dermis, and rarely involve deeper tissue such as fascia, muscle, or bone. They can be large, exceeding 550 cm^2 in size, circumferential, commonly located between the lower half of the calf and 1 inch below the malleolus (gaiter area). The medial aspect of the leg is more commonly involved; however, venous ulcers can affect the lateral aspect. The calf has been reported to be involved in 5 percent of cases and the foot in 8 percent.[34] Pain is frequent and common features include burning, throbbing, cramping, and aching pain. Pain is often relieved with

FIGURE 132-2

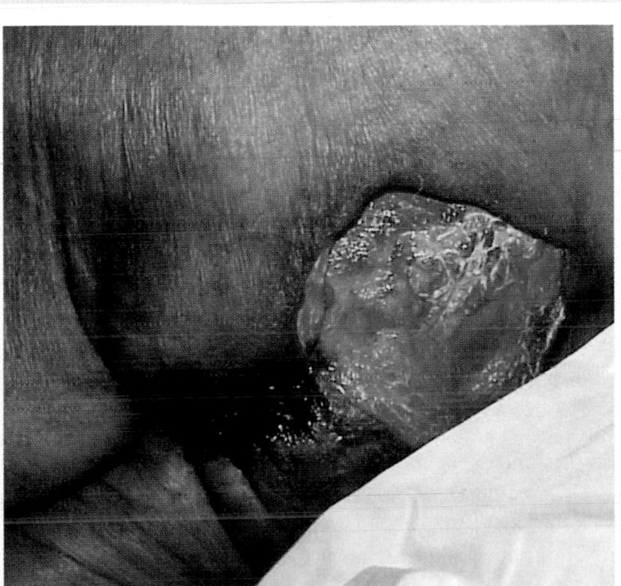

Extensive stage IV pressure ulcer of the sacral area.

FIGURE 132-3

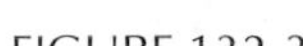

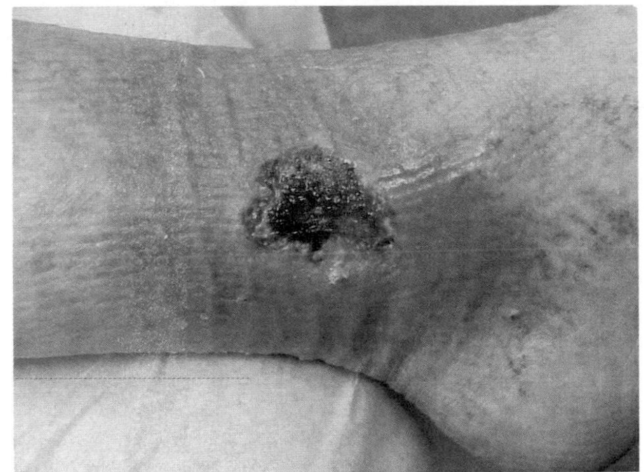

Venous stasis ulcer of the medial leg. Note the characteristic features of beefy red base, venous blush of wound edges, and varicosities.

leg elevation or ambulation. Foul smell may be present and socially isolating.

Venous leg ulcers are often preceded by phlebitis and deep venous thrombosis (DVT) (e.g., postphlebitic syndrome) in some individuals.[21] Diagnosis and treatment of these conditions is important to help improve venous hemodynamics, as well as to prevent potential fatal sequelae of DVT such as pulmonary embolus. Venous leg ulcers are also associated with infection and contact dermatitis (particularly to topical steroids). Chronic wounds, such as pressure ulcers and venous leg ulcers, may also be complicated by the development of squamous cell carcinoma (Fig. 132-4).

FIGURE 132-4

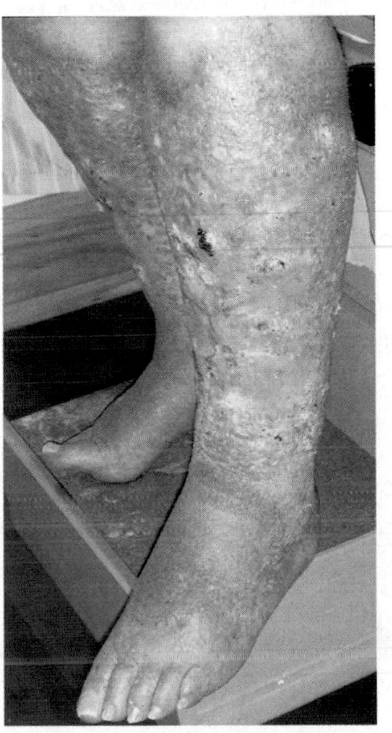

Development of multiple squamous cell carcinomas in a patient with a history of venous leg ulcers and stasis dermatitis.

LABORATORY FINDINGS

There are no specific laboratory findings in patients with pressure ulcers or venous leg ulcers. As with any patient with a chronic wound, laboratory tests to evaluate nutritional status (e.g., serum albumin, total lymphocyte count), and infection (white blood count with differential) should be considered. In individuals with evidence of hypercoagulability (e.g., recurrent deep vein thrombosis) an appropriate hematologic workup should be considered.

For patients with suspected venous leg ulcers, function of the lower extremity superficial and deep venous system can be studied with venography, plethysmography, or ultrasound (duplex and continuous wave). These diagnostic tests confirm the diagnosis of venous leg ulcers (which is often made on a clinical basis), provide prognostic information (e.g., venous leg ulcers associated with deep venous reflux respond poorly to treatment), and help to localize the anatomic site of reflux for potential surgical correction. In addition, the clinician can perform the Trendelenburg test at the bedside to determine if the origin of the reflux is from the superficial or deep system.[35] To perform this maneuver, the patient's leg is elevated until the veins collapse. A tourniquet is then placed above the level of suspected reflux (typically just below the saphenofemoral junction at the groin). The patient then stands with the tourniquet in place. If the distal varicosity fills quickly, then the point of reflux has not been correctly identified or the deep veins or communicating veins are incompetent. If the veins fill very slowly, but then fill rapidly with removal of the tourniquet, the reflux originates from the superficial system (and therefore may be more amenable to treatment or surgical correction).

For ulcers on the lower extremity, arterial vascular disease should be assessed, particularly in patients that are treated with compression therapy. Options include physical examination (e.g. examination of pulses), determination of peak velocity ratio (PVR) by Doppler ultrasound, arteriography, or measuring the ankle-brachial index (ABI). The ABI is determined with the patient in the supine position. The systolic pressure is measured in both upper extremities by using Doppler measurement of the pulse and in the lower extremity with the pressure cuff around the calf. The dorsal pedal or posterior tibial pulse is determined with Doppler. A ratio (systolic ankle pressure divided by the higher of the two systolic brachial pressures) of >1 is normal, and a ratio of < 0.8 suggests lower extremity arterial disease.

PATHOLOGY

Pressure Ulcers

The pathologic findings in pressure ulcers depend on the stage of evolution. Witkowski and Parish studied the pathological changes of pressure ulcers in 59 patients.[36] In blanchable erythema the histologic changes are primarily in the papillary dermis, where a mild perivascular lymphocytic infiltrate is seen. Occasionally, degenerative changes of adnexal structures and fibrin thrombi of deep dermal vessels are present. In stage I ulcers vessels are engorged with red blood cells and there is prominent hemorrhage. Degeneration of adnexal structures and subcutaneous fat is occasionally noted. In early ulceration, the epidermis is not present; however, the dermal papillae are seen. In addition to a perivascular lymphocytic infiltrate, neutrophils are seen. The necrotic changes in the appendages and fat are more pronounced. In ulcers with eschar the tissue appears basophilic with loss of the cellular details in the dermis. An inflammatory infiltrate is often not seen with this level of tissue destruction.

Venous Leg Ulcers

The histopathology of venous leg ulcer typically reveals absence of the epidermis with stigmata of venous stasis. The surrounding epidermis may show acanthosis, parakeratosis, and variable spongiosis. Hemosiderin deposition is notable. A superficial infiltrate of lymphocytes and, occasionally, both histiocytes and plasma cells surrounding thickened capillaries and venules with fibrin deposits are often seen, as well as dermal fibrosis. In some instances the vascular proliferation may resemble Kaposi's sarcoma. In lipodermatosclerosis, pathologic changes extend to the adipose tissue. In early lesions, there is a sparse lymphocytic infiltrate between the collagen bundles of the septae and necrosis of adipocytes in the center of the lobules. In later lesions, there is fibrosis and thickening of the septae with atrophy of the fat and a variable infiltrate of foamy macrophages, lymphocytes, plasma cells, and lipophagic granulomas.

DIAGNOSIS AND DIFFERENTIAL DIAGNOSIS

A pressure ulcer is any lesion caused by unrelieved pressure resulting in damage to the underlying tissue. The diagnosis is readily made in the proper clinical setting. The clinical diagnosis of venous leg ulcer is made in any individual with a chronic wound in the gaiter area, with other signs of venous abnormalities (such as varicose veins, venous blush, lipodermatosclerosis), and an adequately functioning lower-limb arterial system (e.g., an ankle brachial index of > 0.80, presence of a palpable distal limb pulse).[1] Venous ulcers have also been described on the upper leg and the foot.[34] The definitions of pressure ulcer and venous leg ulcer are broad and may actually represent syndromes of distinct disease entities that have not been delineated.

The differential diagnosis of a chronic wound is broad (Table 132-3). Common alternative etiologies to venous or pressure wounds of the lower extremity include arterial ulcers and diabetic foot (neuropathic) ulcers, which must be excluded by further diagnostic testing (e.g., Doppler ultrasound of arterial flow, ankle-brachial indexes, neurologic testing) because these disorders require different treatment. Furthermore, ulcers with an arterial component may be exacerbated by therapies for venous leg ulcers, such as compression. The reader is referred to Table 132-3 for a comprehensive differential diagnosis of chronic wounds. Biopsies and tissue culture of chronic wounds thought to be venous leg ulcers or pressure ulcers should be considered if they are not responding appropriately to treatment or if clinical signs indicate the potential for an alternative etiology.

TREATMENT AND PROGNOSIS

Pressure Ulcers

PROGNOSIS Pressure ulcers often have a prolonged course. About 80 percent will heal without surgery; however, 61 percent of patients will have ulcers for at least 6 months.[37] Pressure ulcers are frequently complicated by infections that play an important role in morbidity and mortality. The incidence of bacteremia from pressure ulcers is estimated to be 1.7 per 10,000 hospital discharges and osteomyelitis was found to occur in 38 percent of patients with infected ulcers.[4,37,38] Pressure ulcers are also associated with excess risk of mortality. Patients who developed a pressure ulcer in the acute care setting had a 67 percent risk of dying in a year as compared to a 15 percent mortality rate of patients who were at risk for development of a pressure ulcer but did not develop one.[4] In the long-term care setting, patients who developed a pressure ulcer within 3 months of admission had a 92 percent mortality rate as compared to a 4 percent mortality rate in patients who did not develop a pressure ulcer.[40] It appears, however, that pressure ulcers may be a marker of other comorbidities and not necessarily causally associated with death. Correction for comorbidities eliminates the association of pressure sores with death,[41] and the severity of pressure ulcer has not been linked to risk of death.

TREATMENT The majority of the treatment recommendations for pressure ulcers are based on clinical experience and have not been validated by rigorously controlled trials. Treatment of pressure ulcers involves assessment of the patient, management of tissue loads, local wound care, management of bacterial colonization and infection, surgical intervention when indicated, and proper pain management (see Table 132-4).[5] Assessment of the patient should include proper evaluation of the ulcer, a thorough history and physical examination, identification and treatment of comorbid conditions, a nutritional assessment, an evaluation of pain, a psychosocial evaluation, and an evaluation of the individual's risk for developing additional pressure ulcers.

Assessment of the pressure ulcer itself includes identifying stage, location, undermining, tunneling, exudate, necrotic tissue, and the presence or absence of granulation tissue and reepithelization. Proper assessment of the ulcer is important because pressure ulcers may appear shallow on initial inspection despite deep involvement. The ulcer should be reevaluated weekly for complications or more often if dictated by a change in patient status. It should be anticipated that assessing response to treatment may take several weeks to months of observation.

Peripheral vascular disease, diabetes mellitus, immune deficiencies, collagen vascular diseases, malignancies, mental health disorders, immobility, and incontinence should be evaluated and treated because they may impede wound healing. Possible complications of pressure ulcers, such as maggot infestation, sinus tract or abscess formation, osteomyelitis, cellulitis, bacteremia, sepsis, septic arthritis, meningitis, and endocarditis, should be treated. Additional complications of chronic pressure ulcers include amyloidosis, heterotopic bone formation, perineal-urethral fistula, pseudoaneurysm, and development of squamous cell carcinoma in the wound.[5] Side effects of treatment including contact dermatitis and systemic effects of local treatment (e.g., iodine toxicity) should also be monitored.

Nutritional assessment is also essential to the care of patients with pressure ulcers. The stage of ulcer may correlate with degree of malnutrition, particularly protein deficiency and hypoalbuminemia.[42] Markers of malnutrition include albumin less than 3.5 mg/dL, total lymphocyte count less than 1800/mm^3, and patient body weight less than 80 percent of ideal.[43] Inability to take food by mouth and a history of involuntary weight loss are important risk factors for malnutrition.

TABLE 132-3

Differential Diagnosis of Chronic Wounds

- Predilection for lower extremity
  - Arterial, neuropathic (diabetic), Buerger's disease, pernio, necrobiosis lipoidica diabeticorum, lymphedema
- Site independent
  - Pyoderma gangrenosum
  - Calciphylaxis
  - Infectious
    - Bacterial, fungal, mycobacterial
  - Vasculitis
    - Leukocytoclastic vasculitis, polyarteritis nodosa, Wegener's granulomatosis, rheumatoid vasculitis
  - Vasoocclusive
    - Cryoglobulinemia, cryofibrinogenemia, antiphospholipid syndrome, cholesterol emboli (often lower extremity), oxalosis, sickle cell disease
  - Malignancy
    - Basal cell carcinoma, squamous cell carcinoma, lymphoma, metastatic disease
  - Ulcerating panniculitis
    - α_1-Antitrypsin deficiency, pancreatic panniculitis, nodular vasculitis (often lower extremity)
  - Factitial

TABLE 132-4

Wound Care

- Evaluation
  - Extent of wound
  - Identify and treat underlying infection
  - Identify and treat comorbidities that impair wound healing (diabetes, arterial disease, malnutrition, collagen vascular disease)
  - Address precipitants (e.g., unrelieved pressure, venous hypertension)
  - Biopsy (to rule out alternative diagnosis, to evaluate for development of squamous cell carcinoma, to identify bacterial pathogen)
- Cleansing
  - Use cleanser, such as normal saline, that is physiologic and nontoxic to epithelial cells and fibroblasts. A 35-mL syringe with 19-gauge angiocatheter is necessary to provide adequate pressure (e.g., 4 to 15 psi) to remove bacteria and necrotic debris without harming healthy tissue
- Dressing
  - Use nonadherent dressing that promotes moisture of wound bed without macerating surrounding normal skin
- Debridement
  - Remove fibrinous debris, devitalized tissue, eschar
    - Sharp debridement
      - Often indicated when there is extensive devitalized tissue or infection
    - Mechanical debridement (wet-to-dry dressings, hydrotherapy, wound irrigation)
    - Enzymatic debridement
    - Autolytic debridement (avoid in infected wounds)
- Antibiotics
  - Use systemic antibiotics for infectious complications of wounds (e.g., cellulitis, osteomyelitis, sepsis)
  - Topical antibiotics for wounds not responding to treatment or for foul-smelling wounds
- Pain management
  - For chronic pain associated with a chronic wound
  - For acute pain associated with infection, debridement, dressing changes, transferring

Nutrition should be reassessed every 3 months in patients at risk while treating a patient with a pressure ulcer. Vitamins and minerals important to wound healing, such as vitamin C and zinc, should be supplemented in individual patients with deficiencies. However, supplementation with vitamin C or zinc in patients without deficiency has not been shown to be helpful in clinical trials, and zinc may be harmful to wound healing when given at high doses.[44,45] Alimentation of 30 to 35 calories/kg/day and 1.25 to 1.50 g of protein/kg/day is recommended to maintain a positive nitrogen balance in order to improve healing.[46] Enteral tube feeding to supplement protein and calories in an effort to improve wound healing has not been effective in all studies, however.

Management of tissue loads is a critical component of treating pressure ulcers. The distribution of pressure on the tissues, as well as the frictional and shear forces, must be managed. Positioning and repositioning techniques are necessary to offload pressure forces away from bony prominences (e.g., trochanters) and pressure ulcers. Pillows and foam wedges may be useful positioning devices. Donut-type devices are to be avoided as they result in venous congestion and may be deleterious.[47] To minimize shearing forces on the sacral area, the head of the bed should be maintained at the lowest degree of elevation tolerable by the patient's medical condition.

A variety of support devices are available for patients with pressure ulcers. They can be rated based on cost and performance characteristics. These characteristics include level of support, low moisture retention, reduced heat accumulation, shear reduction, pressure reduction, and dynamic changes in forces exerted. Examples include (in order from highest cost and best performance characteristics to lowest cost and performance): air-fluidized, low-air loss, alternating air, static flotation (air or water), foam, and standard mattresses.

There is no compelling evidence that one support surface consistently performs better than all others in all circumstances.[4,5] Static support surfaces are recommended for patients who can assume multiple positions without bearing weight on a pressure ulcer and without bottoming out (e.g., fully compressing the static support surface by having less than 1 inch of support material underneath areas of pressure).[48] Dynamic support surfaces, such as air-fluidized, low-air-loss, or alternating air, are recommended for patients who cannot assume a variety of positions without bearing weight on an ulcer. They should also be used if the patient bottoms out, or if the ulcer does not show evidence of healing.[5]

For patients with large stage III or IV pressure ulcers on multiple turning surfaces, a low–air-loss or air-fluidized bed may be indicated. Air-fluidized beds may benefit patients in the acute care setting with large ulcers; however, these beds are limited by their cumbersome size and weight, the difficulties they cause for nurses in transferring patients, and their excessive cost. Low-air-loss beds are generally cheaper than air-fluidized beds and are better equipped for transferring patients. A review of four randomized controlled trials totaling 259 patients showed improvement in wound healing rates for low-air-loss beds from 64 to 80 percent as compared to 47 to 68 percent of controls.[5] The comparative efficacy of air-fluidized and low–air-loss beds has not been studied in head-to-head trials; air-fluidized beds, however, have the theoretical advantage of improved shear reduction. Air-fluidized and low-air-loss beds may also be indicated for patients in whom moisture is leading to maceration and skin breakdown.

For patients who are able to sit in a chair, techniques are necessary to prevent pressure ulcer development and to minimize exacerbation of existing ulcers. Individuals who are able should reposition themselves every 15 min.[5] If the patient cannot self-reposition then they should be repositioned at least every hour or be returned to bed.

Proper care and dressing of the wound is an important aspect of treating pressure ulcers. Proper care includes debriding, cleansing, and dressing. Ulcers with devitalized, necrotic tissue should be debrided by using sharp, mechanical, enzymatic, or autolytic methods. An exception to this recommendation is heel ulcers that do not exhibit edema, erythema, fluctuance, or drainage.[5] The sharp method involves use of a scalpel or other sharp instruments and may require use of an operating room for larger ulcers. When stage IV ulcers are debrided in the operating room, a bone biopsy for culture should be considered to evaluate the presence of osteomyelitis. Sharp debridement is generally indicated when there is frank evidence of infection, sepsis in which the wound is the source, or cellulitis.

Mechanical debridement involves techniques such as wet-to-dry dressings, hydrotherapy (e.g., whirlpool), or wound irrigation. Wet-to-dry dressings should be changed every 4 to 6 h and additional pain control may be necessary during dressing changes. The main disadvantage of wet-to-dry dressings is that they are nonselective and may remove healthy granulation tissue. Wound irrigation can remove dead tissue and bacteria when using a 35-mL syringe and 19-gauge angiocatheter to provide adequate force (e.g., 4 to 15 psi).[49]

Enzymatic debridement can be accomplished using topical debriding agents such as collagenase, papain/urea, or papain/urea-chlorophyll. Enzymatic treatments poorly penetrate thick eschars, however, and the benefit of enzymatic debridement on wound healing rate is unclear. Autolytic debridement can be performed by the use of occlusive dressings that allow the wound's own exudate to break down devitalized tissue. The autolytic method should be avoided in infected wounds.

Wound cleansing should occur with dressing changes. Cleansing should be performed gently to minimize trauma to healing tissues. Skin cleansers and antiseptics such as povidone-iodine, iodophor, sodium hypochlorite solution, hydrogen peroxide, acetic acid should be avoided because they are toxic to wound tissue.[50] Normal saline is preferred as it is most physiologic and will not harm healing tissue.

Wound dressings should maintain moisture of the wound bed at all times to maximize wound healing[51] (see Chap. 272). It has been demonstrated experimentally that dressings that promote moisture of the wound bed heal 40 percent faster then air-exposed wounds.[52] Occlusive dressings, such as polymer films, polymer foams, hydrogels, hydrocolloids, alginates, and biomembranes, are appropriate. The type of dressing that promotes moisture is not clearly significant as long as wound bed moisture is maintained. Choice should be based on the individual wound with the goal of promoting a moist wound environment without causing maceration of the wound edges.

Management of bacterial colonization and wound infection is important in the healing process. It has been demonstrated experimentally that pressure ulcers are more susceptible to bacterial colonization than wounds not subjected to pressure.[52] Healing is impaired when bacterial counts exceed 10^5 per gram of tissue. Proper wound debridement, cleansing, and bandaging help to minimize bacterial colonization and risk of infection. Because bacterial colonization (particularly *Pseudomonas aeruginosa* and *Providencia* species) is associated with delayed wound healing, a trial of topical antibiotic active against gram-positive, gram-negative, and anaerobic bacteria (silver sulfadiazine, triple antibiotic) should be considered for nonhealing or exudative wounds.[4,5] Clinical trials of topical antibiotics in decubiti have demonstrated improvement in the appearance of these wounds and therefore may be helpful in wound healing.[4] Topical metronidazole may be helpful for wounds colonized by anaerobic bacteria, clinically recognized as foul-smelling wounds.

Systemic antibiotics should be reserved for clinical infections such as cellulitis, bacteremia, sepsis, and osteomyelitis. *Staphylococcus aureus*, gram-negative rods, and *Bacteroides fragilis* are frequent causes of sepsis in these patients. Because it should be anticipated that all chronic wounds will be colonized by bacteria, swab cultures of wound beds should not be used to diagnose infection.[53] Only samples obtained by tissue biopsy are reliable for determining the pathogen of a clinically infected wound. It should be emphasized that quantitative tissue cultures alone are insufficient to determine infection in a chronic wound, and therefore clinical signs such as pain, erythema, fever, and exudate are necessary to diagnose infection.

Beyond medical therapies, a variety of surgical techniques are also available to repair pressure ulcers. These techniques include direct closure, skin grafts, skin flaps, and myocutaneous flaps. Patients must be carefully selected for surgical intervention and the patient's therapeutic goals and ability to tolerate surgery should be considered. Surgical repairs of pressure ulcers are limited by high cost and high postoperative recurrence rate.[4] Thus, the efficacy of surgical repair of pressure ulcers has been questioned even in young patients.

Venous Leg Ulcers

PROGNOSIS Venous leg ulcers take a prolonged time period to heal and many patients will never achieve complete wound healing. Within 24 weeks of therapy the best success rates vary from 30 to 60 percent, and within a year the best success rates vary from 70 to 85 percent.[54,55] Several risk factors are associated with failure of venous leg ulcers to heal, including wound area; wound duration; history of venous ligation or stripping; history of hip or knee replacement surgery; ankle brachial index of less then 0.80; deep vein involvement on noninvasive testing; fixed limb joints; and general immobility.[55,56] Venous leg ulcers are also frequently complicated by contact dermatitis, particularly to topical steroids, and can be a frequent source of infection, such as cellulitis.[57]

TREATMENT Treatments for venous leg ulcer are aimed at reducing ambulatory venous hypertension. Elevation of the legs above heart level for 30 min, three to four times per day, allows for improvement in leg swelling. Leg elevation at night can be accomplished by raising the foot end of the bed by 15 to 20 cm. Walking and exercise further improve venous circulation through calf muscle pump action.[9,11]

The standard of care for venous leg ulcers centers on the use of compression therapy.[58,59] Since 1966, MEDLINE has listed more than 1200 studies concerning the treatment of venous leg ulcers. These papers describe alleviating venous hypertension; removing lower limb edema; wound debridement; wound cleansing; wound bandaging and dressing; the use of systemic and topical compounds to augment healing; the use of mechanical devices to augment healing; and the use of surgery to improve venous hemodynamics. Unfortunately, none of these studies have been able to demonstrate a consistent and reproducible advantage over lower-limb compression;[60] consequently, compression therapy remains the cornerstone of treatment. Compression therapy increases transcutaneous oxygen pressure,[61] improves lymph transport, enhances fibrinolysis, improves reflux in the deep venous system,[62] improves deep venous valve function, and reduces the release of macromolecules into the extravascular space.[63]

The most popular compression bandage for venous leg ulcers was introduced by P.G. Unna in 1885, and has not been substantially improved upon since.[59] This form of lower-limb compression is gauze impregnated with zinc and fitted to the patient's leg. Although not appreciated by Unna, the essential component of this technique is the compression of the lower limb afforded by this bandage and not the zinc.[64] The consensus is that 35 to 40 mmHg at the ankle is required for therapeutic efficacy.[11]

Compression therapy can be applied via a rigid inelastic dressing, such as the Unna boot, or by elastic or multilayered bandages.[65] Rigid dressings provide high pressure with muscle contraction but little pressure at rest, and do not accommodate for changes in volume of the leg associated with changes in edema. Rigid dressings may be particularly useful for reducing edema in the acute management of venous leg ulcers. Rigid dressings cannot absorb exudate from wounds efficiently and therefore can create irritant dermatitis, as well as foul odors. Less-rigid alternatives to the Unna boot dressing include short-stretch dressing such as Unna-Flex and Comprilan.

Long-stretch elastic compression bandages may allow for more frequent dressing changes, which may be appropriate for exudative wounds. Long-stretch bandages provide higher resting pressures and therefore may be more useful after the initial edema has been resolved with rigid dressings. Elastic compression bandages need to be applied with 50 percent overlap as they progress up the leg in order to produce sustained pressure and require skill in their application.[66] Multilayered bandages such as three-layered systems (Dynaflex) and four-layered systems (Profore) may provide for faster healing rates when compared to rigid Unna boot dressings.[67] Multilayered dressings can be used for legs of various sizes and can provide sustained pressures of 40 to 45 mmHg at the ankle; however, their use is limited by their cost.

After a leg ulcer is healed, compression therapy should be continued empirically to prevent recurrence. This recommendation is based on clinical experience and has not been rigorously validated by clinical trials.[32] Elastic compression stockings are suitable for this indication. Compression class I (20 to 30 mmHg), class II (30 to 40 mmHg), class III (40 to 50 mmHg), and class IV (> 60 mmHg) are available. Elastic compression stockings should be replaced every 6 months to maintain adequate function. Custom fitting may be indicated for some individuals. Aids have been developed to assist patients in the donning and removal of compression stockings and are available at medical supply stores.

Dressing of the wound is important in providing pain relief, improving wound healing by promoting a moist wound environment, and for absorption of wound exudate. Hydrogels, alginates, hydrocolloids, foams, and films do not necessarily improve healing relative to simple nonadherent dressings, but may have relative advantages for individual patients and practitioners.[68] As with pressure ulcers, the goal is to maintain moisture of the wound bed while minimizing maceration of the wound edges. Removal of necrotic debris and or fibrinous exudates can be accomplished with sharp debridement, enzymatic debridement (such as collagenase), or by mechanical debridement (e.g., wet-to-dry dressing, whirlpool therapy).

Few systemic treatments for venous leg ulcers have been rigorously investigated. Pentoxifylline has shown mixed results in a number of randomized controlled trials. A grouped analysis of these studies demonstrated the benefit of pentoxifylline as an adjuvant to compression therapy.[69] Recent studies suggest that higher doses of pentoxifylline (800 mg po tid) may be necessary for efficacy.[70] Surgical treatment of venous leg ulcers is generally reserved for patients who are not responding to treatment or for patients with large ulcers. Split-thickness skin grafts have been reported as beneficial, but their success rate is variable.[71] Possible risk factors for failure to heal with a split-thickness skin graft include comorbidities, living alone, stasis dermatitis, and prolonged duration of wound. Superficial vein ligation or sclerosis may decrease recurrence of venous leg ulcers if the deep veins are competent.[72] Tissue-engineered skin equivalents such as Apligraf were approved for use by the Food and Drug Administration and have demonstrated clinical efficacy in one randomized controlled trial.[73]

Other Therapies for Chronic Wounds

Numerous therapies for chronic wounds have been and continue to be investigated. Laser, ultrasound, ultraviolet, infrared, electrotherapy, electromagnetic therapy, hyperbaric oxygen, topical application of growth factors, and topical application of phenytoin have shown promise in some reports, however, all await more rigorous investigation to validate their efficacy.[5,74–76] Studies of therapies for chronic wounds often report wound healing rate and clinical appearance of the wound as outcomes, however, complete wound healing is the gold standard outcome for assessing efficacy of a wound healing agent.

Pain Control

Adequate assessment and treatment of pain is a critical component in caring for patients with chronic wounds. Both venous leg ulcers and pressure ulcers may be associated with severe pain. Appropriate treatment of chronic pain with additional medication for breakthrough episodes (e.g., dressing changes or debridement during turning or transferring) is indicated. Systemic analgesics including acetaminophen, nonsteroidal anti-inflammatories, and opiates may be necessary.

REFERENCES

1. Stromber K et al: Regulatory concerns in the development of topical recombinant ophthalmic and cutaneous wound healing biologics. *Wound Repair Regen* **2**:155, 1994
2. Rowling JT: Pathological changes in mummies. *Proc R Soc Med* **54**:409, 1961
3. Scholz A: Historical aspects, in *Leg Ulcers: Diagnosis and Treatment,* edited by W Westerhof. Elsevier, Elsevier Science Publishers, 1993
4. Thomas DR: Issues and dilemmas in the prevention and treatment of pressure ulcers: A review. *J Gerontol* **56A**:M328, 2001
5. Bergstrom N et al: *Treatment of Pressure Ulcers. Clinical Practice Guideline, No. 15.* Rockville, MD, US Department of Health and Human Services, 1994
6. Cuddigan J et al: *Pressure Ulcer in America: Prevalence, Incidence, and Implications for the Future.* Reston, VA, National Pressure Ulcer Advisory Panel, 2001
7. Berquist S et al: Pressure ulcers in community-based older adults receiving home health care. Prevalence, incidence, and associated risk factors. *Adv Wound Care* **12**:339, 1999
8. Garber SL et al: Pressure ulcer risk in spinal chord injury: Predictors of ulcer status over three years. *Arch Phys Med Rehab* **81**:465, 2000
9. Margolis et al: The incidence and prevalence of pressure ulcers among elderly patients in general medical practice. *Ann Epidemiol* **12**:321, 2002
10. Lee TA et al: Prevalence of lower limb ulceration in an urban health district. *Br J Surg* **79**:1032, 1992
11. Valencia IC et al: Chronic venous insufficiency and venous leg ulceration. *J Am Acad Dermatol* **44**:401, 2001
12. Dale JJ et al: Chronic ulcers of the leg: A prevalence study in a Scottish Community. *Health Bull* **41**:310, 1983
13. Callam MJ et al: Chronic ulceration of the leg: Extent of the problem and provision of care. *Br Med J* **290**:1855, 1985
14. Cornwall JV et al: Leg ulcers: Epidemiology and aetiology. *Br J Surg* **73**:893, 1986
15. Nelzén O et al: Long-term prognosis for patients with chronic leg ulcers: A prospective cohort study. *Eur J Vasc Endovasc Surg* **13**:500, 1997
16. Heit JA et al: Trends in the incidence of venous stasis syndrome and venous ulcer: A 25-year population-based study. *J Vasc Surg* **33**:1022, 2001
17. Maklebust J et al: Pressure ulcers: Guidelines for prevention and nursing management. Springhouse, PA, Springhouse, 1996
18. Bennett L et al: Shear vs. pressure as causative factors in skin blood flow occlusion. *Arch Phys Med Rehabil* **60**:309, 1979
19. Dinsdale SM: Decubitus ulcers: Role of pressure and friction in causation. *Arch Phys Med Rehabil* **55**:147, 1974
20. Baker SR et al: Aetiology of chronic leg ulcers. *Eur J Vasc Surg* **6**:245,1992
21. Alguire PC et al: Chronic venous insufficiency and venous ulceration. *J Gen Intern Med* **12**:374, 1997
22. Falanga V et al: The trap hypothesis of venous ulceration. *Nature* **341**:1006, 1993
23. Gaber Y et al: Resistance to activated protein C due to factor V Leiden mutation: High prevalence in patients with post-thrombotic leg ulcers. *Br J Dermatol* **144**:546, 2001
24. Hafner J et al: Factor V Leiden mutation in postthrombotic and non-postthrombotic venous ulcer. *Arch Dermatol* **137**:599, 2001
25. Berlowitz DR et al: Are we improving the quality of nursing home care: The case of pressure ulcers. *J Am Geriatr Soc* **48**:59, 2000
26. Hopkins B et al: Reducing nosocomial pressure ulcers in an acute care facility. *J Nurs Care Qual* **14**:28, 2000
27. Norton D et al: *An Investigation of Geriatric Nursing Problems in Hospitals.* Edinburgh, Churchill-Livingstone, 1975
28. Waterlow J: Pressure scores: A risk assessment card. *Nurse Times* **8**:49, 1985
29. Bergstrom N et al: The Braden scale for predicting pressure sore risk. *Nurse Res* **36**:205, 1987
30. Franks PJ et al: Factors associated with healing leg ulceration with high compression. *Age Aging* **24**:407, 1995
31. Margolis DJ. The treatment of lower extremity venous ulceration. *Hosp Pract* **27**:32, 1992
32. Nelson EA et al: Compression for preventing recurrence of venous ulcers. *Cochrane Database Syst Rev* **4**:CD002303, 2000
33. Barwell JR et al: Surgical correction of isolated superficial venous reflux reduces long-term recurrence rate in chronic venous leg ulcers. *Eur J Vasc Endovasc Surg* **4**:363, 2000
34. London NJM et al: ABC of arterial and venous disease. Ulcerated lower limb. *BMJ* **320**:1589, 2000
35. Feied C. Venous insufficiency, in *Emedicine Dermatology Online Textbook,* edited by James, WD and Elston, DM. Available at www.emedicine.com
36. Witkowski JA et al: Histopathology of the decubitus ulcer. *J Am Acad Dermatol* **6**:1014, 1982
37. Petersen NC et al: The epidemiology of pressure ulcers. *Scand J Plast Reconstr Surg* **5**:62, 1971
38. Bryan CS et al: Bacteremia associated with decubitus ulcers. *Arch Intern Med* **143**:2093, 1983
39. Sugarman B et al: Osteomyelitis beneath pressure sores. *Arch Intern Med* **143**:683, 1983.
40. Bergstrom N et al: A prospective study of pressure sore risk among institutionalized elderly. *J Am Geriatr Soc* **40**:747, 1992
41. Thomas DR et al: Pressure ulcers and risk of death. *J Am Geriatr Soc.* **44**:1435, 1996
42. Pinchcofsky-Devin GD et al: Correlation of pressure sores and nutritional status. *J Am Geriatr Soc* **34**:435, 1986
43. Greer et al: Nutrition Screening Manual for Professionals Caring for Older Americans: Nutrition Screening Initiative. Washington, DC, The Nutrition Screening Initiative, 1991
44. Ter Riet G et al: Randomized controlled trial of ascorbic acid in the treatment of pressure ulcers. *J Clin Epidemiol* **48**:1453, 1995
45. Thomas DR. The role of nutrition in prevention and healing of pressure ulcers. *Clin Geriatr Med* **13**:497, 1997
46. Breslow RA et al: The importance of dietary protein in healing pressure ulcers. *J Am Geriatr Soc* **41**:357, 1993
47. Crewe RA. Problems of rubber ring nursing cushions and a clinical survey of alternative cushions for ill patients. *Care Sci Pract* **5**:9, 1987
48. Ferrell BA et al: A randomized trial of low air loss beds for treatment of pressure ulcers. *JAMA* **269**:494, 1993
49. Stevenson TR et al: Cleansing the traumatic wound by high pressure syringe irrigation. *JACEP* **5**:17, 1976
50. Johnson AR et al: Comparison of common topical agents for wound treatment: Cytotoxicity for human fibroblasts in culture. *Wounds* **1**:186, 1989
51. Gorse GJ et al: Improved pressure sore healing with hydrocolloid dressings. *Arch Dermatol* **123**:766, 1987
52. Krizek T et al: Biology of surgical infection. *Surg Clin North Am* **55**:1261, 1975
53. Garner JS et al: CDC guidelines for the prevention and control of nosocomial infections. *Am J Infect Control* **16**:177, 1988
54. Marston WA et al: Healing rates and cost efficacy of outpatient compression treatment for leg ulcers associated with venous insufficiency. *J Vasc Surg* **30**:491, 1999
55. Margolis DJ et al: Risk factors associated with the failure of a venous leg ulcer to heal. *Arch Dermatol* **135**:920, 1999
56. Franks PJ et al: Factors associated with healing leg ulceration with high compression. *Age Aging* **24**:407, 1995
57. Wilkinson SM. Hypersensitivity to topical corticosteroids. *Clin Exp Dermatol* **19**:1, 1994
58. Abu-Own A et al: Effect of leg elevation on the skin microcirculation in chronic venous insufficiency. *J Vasc Surg* **20**:705, 1994
59. Margolis DJ. Management of chronic venous ulcers: a literature guided approach. *Clin Dermatol* **12**:19, 1994
60. Fletcher A et al: A systematic review of compression treatment for venous leg ulcers. *BMJ* **315**:576, 1997
61. Kolari PJ et al: Effects of intermittent compression treatment on skin perfusion and oxygenation in lower legs with venous ulcers. *Vasa* **16**:312, 1987
62. Christopoulos D et al: Venous reflux: Quantification and correlation with the clinical severity of chronic venous disease. *Br J Surg* **75**:352, 1988
63. Van de Scheur M et al: Pericapillary fibrin cuffs in venous disease. *J Dermatol Surg Oncol* **23**:955, 1997
64. Agren MS. Studies on zinc in wound healing. *Acta Derm Venereol Suppl (Stockh)* **154**:1, 1990

65. Partsch H. Compression therapy of the legs: A review. *J Dermatol Surg Oncol* **17**:575, 1991
66. Simon DA et al: Approaches to venous leg ulcer within the community: Compression, pinch skin grafts, and simple venous surgery. *Ostomy Wound Manag* **42**:34, 1996
67. Phillips TJ et al: Successful methods of treating leg ulcers: The tried and the true, plus the novel and new. *Postgrad Med* **105**:159, 1999
68. Freak L et al: Comparative study of three primary dressings in the healing of chronic venous ulcers. *Br J Surg* **79**:1235, 1992
69. Jull AB et al: Oral pentoxifylline for the treatment of venous leg ulcers. *Cochrane Database Syst Rev.* **2**:CD00173, 2000
70. Falanga F et al: Systemic treatment of venous leg ulcer with high doses of pentoxifylline: Efficacy in a randomized, placebo-controlled trial. *Wound Repair Regen* **7**:208, 1999
71. Kirsner RS et al: Split-thickness skin grafting of leg ulcers. *J Dermatol Surg* **21**:701, 1995
72. Barwell et al: Surgical correction of isolated superficial venous reflux reduces long-term recurrence rate in chronic venous ulcer. *Eur J Vasc Endovasc Surg* **4**:363, 2000
73. Falanga V et al: Rapid healing of venous leg ulcers and lack of clinical rejection with an allogeneic cultured human skin equivalent. *Arch Dermatol* **134**:293, 1998
74. Cullum N et al: Systematic reviews of wound care management: (5) beds; (6) compression; (7) laser therapy, therapeutic ultrasound, electrotherapy and electromagnetic therapy. *Health Technol Assesss (Rockv)* **5**:1, 2001
75. Payne WG et al: Long-term outcome study of growth factor-treated pressure ulcers. *Am J Surg* **181**:81, 2001
76. Rhodes RS et al: Topical phenytoin treatment of stage II decubitus ulcers in the elderly. *Ann Pharmacother* **35**:675, 2001

SECTION 18
PHOTOMEDICINE

CHAPTER 133

Irene E. Kochevar
Charles R. Taylor

Photophysics, Photochemistry, and Photobiology

Why should a clinical dermatologist be interested in reading a chapter on photophysics, photochemistry, and photobiology? Simply put, knowledge of the interaction of sunlight with the skin is fundamental to understanding the pathogenesis, diagnosis, and treatment of more than 100 cutaneous disorders. The material in this chapter provides the foundation for all photodermatology: phototesting, photopatch testing, photosensitivity, the porphyrias, photodermatoses, phototherapy, photochemotherapy, photodynamic therapy, photopheresis, photoprotection, laser surgery and photocarcinogenesis. Whenever ultraviolet (UV) radiation is used to treat a skin condition, important principles of photophysics involving absorption and emission of light underlie the success of the therapy. When a patient suffers from increased sun sensitivity, critical photochemistry has occurred. Sunscreen recommendations rely on an understanding of solar UV radiation and the ways in which the causative wavelengths can be minimized. Skin cancer is an epidemic clinical problem, and its pathophysiology necessitates comprehension of the photophysical, photochemical, and photobiological events described in this chapter.

Almost every ancient civilization worshipped a god of the sun whose healing powers were believed to be broad reaching. Even today, sun exposure is widely felt to induce a sense of well being. In addition, sunlight is important for the synthesis of vitamin D_3 and the setting of internal clocks. On the negative side, sunlight causes deleterious acute and chronic effects such as sunburn, skin cancer, and photoaging, and can elicit adverse reactions to certain drugs (Fig. 133-1). Abnormal responses to sunlight occur in polymorphic light eruption, solar urticaria, certain porphyrias, and many other conditions (Chaps. 135, 136, 149). While the sun is a major source of UV and visible radiation that interacts with human skin, UV and/or visible radiation are also emitted from common sources such as fluorescent lights, incandescent bulbs, photocopy machines, and phototherapy lamps. Tanning salons are another familiar example. Dentists use UV for hardening of acrylates, as do nail salon estheticians. Thus, UV and visible radiation are a constant part of the human environment and play a role in health, disease, and therapy. Photomedicine is the study of this interaction between human tissue and UV or visible radiation, usually from the sun, but from artificial sources as well. To understand the responses of skin to UV and visible radiation, it is essential to be acquainted with the properties of electromagnetic (EM) radiation and with the principles governing the interaction of EM radiation with biomolecules.

FIGURE 133-1

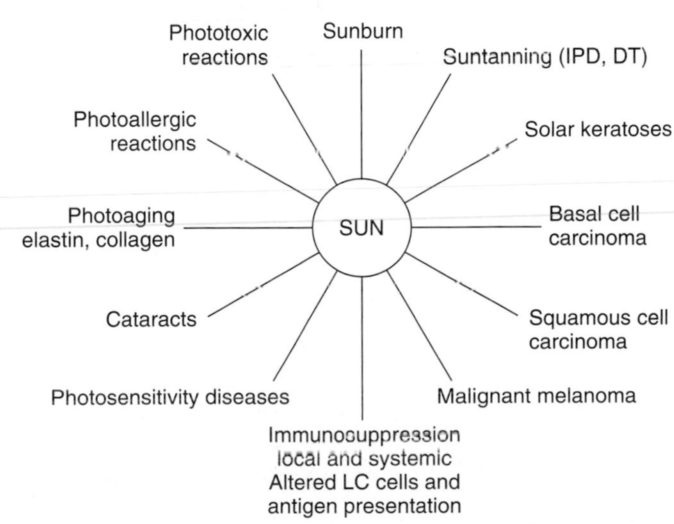

Deleterious effects of UV and visible radiation in human skin and eye. DT, delayed tanning; IPD, immediate pigment darkening; LC, Langerhans cells.

ELECTROMAGNETIC RADIATION

Electromagnetic radiation is a form of energy. UV and visible radiation are part of the continuous EM spectrum. The wavelengths of EM radiation vary from fractions of nanometers to thousands of meters along a continuous spectrum. Specific wavelengths are classified into wave bands and given the names shown in Table 133-1 and Fig. 133-2.

Short wavelengths and high energy are properties of x-rays and gamma rays. Such wavelengths are useful for destroying tumors because they generally ionize molecules (remove electrons) indiscriminately. Consequently, they are known as ionizing radiations, the subject of radiobiology (Chap. 128). Longer wavelengths and lower energy are associated with infrared radiation. Infrared wavelengths may be felt as

TABLE 133-1

Electromagnetic Radiation According to Wavelength

WAVEBAND	WAVELENGTH RANGE (NM)
X-ray	0.1–10
Vacuum UV	10–200
Ultraviolet C (UVC)	200–290
Ultraviolet B (UVB)	290–320
Ultraviolet A (UVA)	320–400
UVAI	340–400
UVAII	320–340
Visible	400–760
Violet	400
Blue	470
Green	530
Yellow	600
Red	700
Near infrared	760–1000
Far infrared	1000–100,000
Microwaves and radiowaves	$> 10^6$

heat, and they can trigger a variety of disorders such as cholinergic urticaria.

The UV and visible radiation region lies between the x-ray/gamma ray portion and infrared radiation. This part of the EM spectrum is of special interest because dozens of skin disorders are aggravated by wavelengths in these regions. Moreover, many popular therapies, such as UVB phototherapy, photochemotherapy (PUVA), blue-light aminolevulinic acid (ALA)-photodynamic therapy, and several routine lasers (e.g., pulsed dye laser, Q-switched ruby) all function using wavelengths in this region.

For medical photobiology, the UV range is broken into certain convenient subdivisions (Table 133-1; Fig. 133-2). A division was made at 290 nm because wavelengths from the sun shorter than 290 nm do not reach the earth's surface at sea level. The energy is absorbed by the ozone layer in the stratosphere. Such wavelengths in the range of 200 to 290 nm are referred to as UVC. When produced by artificial sources, these wavelengths are absorbed by DNA, RNA, and proteins of cells, as well as by the stratum corneum, and they can be lethal to viable cells of the epidermis. Because germicidal lamps emit 254-nm radiation within this waveband, the UVC region of the spectrum is often called *germicidal radiation*.

FIGURE 133-2

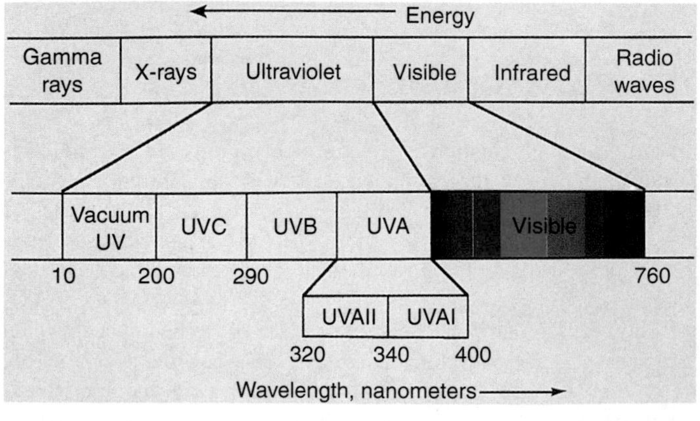

Electromagnetic spectrum divided into major wavelength regions. The lower band emphasizes the UV and visible bands that are important for photobiological responses in human skin.

Another division is made at 320 nm, the upper limit of the most erythemogenic wavelengths reaching the earth's surface. Also, ordinary window glass filters out wavelengths shorter than about 320 nm. The range 290 to 320 nm is known as UVB and is often referred to as *mid-UV* or *sunburn spectrum*. Most sunscreens work very efficiently at minimizing the effects of this waveband. In fact, the sun protection factor (SPF) is actually based on testing against this waveband. Properly used, a sunscreen with a SPF rating of 15 effectively means that 15 times more incident UVB is needed to give the same degree of erythema.

Long-wave UV or UVA (320 to 400 nm) is sometimes referred to as *black light* because it is not visible to the human eye and causes certain substances to emit visible fluorescence. Recently, UVA has been divided into UVA-I (340 to 400 nm) and UVA-II (320 to 340 nm) because the latter band is more damaging to unsensitized skin than the longer wavelengths. It is important to remember that there may be great variation in the biologic effects of different wavelengths within these subdivisions. For example, 297-nm radiation is nearly 100 times more erythemogenic than 313-nm radiation, although both are in the UVB region.

Certain principles are better illustrated by conceptualizing EM radiation as a *wave,* whereas others are better understood by thinking of it as packets of energy called *photons*. These two descriptions are entirely complementary. The concepts of "*light as waves*" and "*light as photons*" are discussed below.

EM Radiation Considered as Waves

Waves consist of periodic motion or oscillations that travel through a medium or space. When the motion is perpendicular to the direction of propagation, such as waves traveling down a length of rope, the waves are called *transverse waves*. EM radiation travels as a transverse wave. EM radiation consists of oscillating electric and magnetic fields at right angles to each other and to the direction of propagation.

EM radiation may be described either by its frequency (number of oscillations per second) or by its wavelength (distance traveled per oscillation). Since all EM radiation propagates at the same velocity through space, frequency and wavelength have an inverse relationship, which is expressed as:

$$\nu = \frac{c}{\lambda}$$

where ν = frequency of oscillations per second, c = velocity of radiation (the speed of light, 3×10^8 m/s), and λ = wavelength in meters. When light is considered as a wave, specific colors of UV and visible radiation are associated with specific wavelengths of the EM spectrum. For example, red wavelengths occur around 700 nm, while blue ones occur around 470 nm (Table 133-1).

EM Radiation Considered as a Particle

In addition to its wave character, EM radiation may be described as a stream of discrete packets of energy known as *quanta* or *photons*. Photons have no mass; when the energy of a photon is absorbed by a molecule the photon ceases to exist. The amount of energy in a photon (quantum) is directly proportional to the frequency of the radiation and inversely proportional to the wavelength of radiation, as expressed by Planck's theory:

$$E = h\nu = \frac{hc}{\lambda}$$

where E = the energy of the photon in joules (J), h = Planck's constant (6.626×10^{-34} J × s), ν = frequency of oscillations per second, c = velocity of radiation (3×10^8 m/s), and λ = wavelength in meters.

This relationship shows that the energy (E) of the photon increases when the wavelength is shorter and decreases when the wavelength is longer. Consequently, radiation of shorter wavelength has greater energy per photon. For example, a 300-nm photon has twice the energy of a 600-nm photon. Because of their lower energies, wavelengths longer than about 800 nm usually do not cause photochemical reactions. Primarily UV radiation is implicated in many normal and abnormal reactions in human skin. Skin responses to visible light usually require a higher than normal concentration of an endogenous chromophore (e.g., protoporphyrin) or the presence of an exogenous dye or drug to absorb the light.

FROM EM RADIATION TO DERMATOLOGY

Skin is affected by UV and visible radiation that is absorbed by molecules in skin. The pathway from light absorption to biological response can be broken into several steps (Fig. 133-3). In the first step, molecules in skin such as pyrimidine nucleotides, DNA (e.g., thymidine, cytosine), and urocanic acid absorb radiation. A light-absorbing molecule is referred to as a *chromophore*. In some cases, the chromophore is an exogenous agent such as an ingested photosensitizing drug, for example, tetracycline or 8-methoxypsoralen. After absorbing the energy of the radiation, the chromophore is in an *excited state*. Although this highly energetic species exists for only a fraction of a second, a chemical change may occur during this time to transform the molecule into a *photoproduct* such as an oxidized membrane lipid,[1,2] pyrimidine dimer,[3] or psoralen-DNA adduct.[4] The presence of photoproducts in cells provokes biochemical responses, beginning with signal transduction processes that often involve adding and removing

FIGURE 133-3

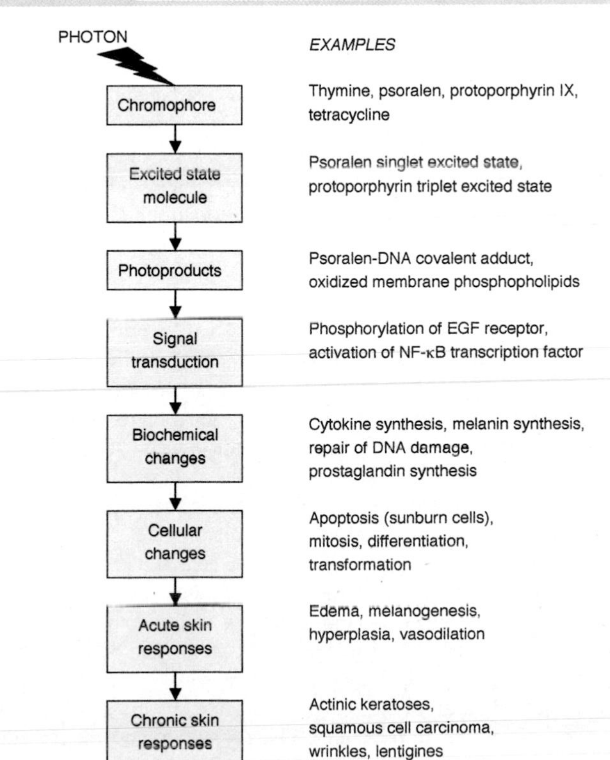

Generalized steps in the response of skin to UV or visible radiation.

phosphate groups from proteins such as the growth factor receptors in the plasma membrane.[5,6] These changes may activate transcription factors such as AP-1[7,8] and NF-kB[9,10] and thereby initiate cellular synthesis of new proteins, for example, melanin,[11,12] cytokines,[13–15] cyclooxygenase,[16,17] and matrix metalloproteinase-1.[18,19] Other important processes, such as repair of UV-induced DNA damage, also occur in response to photoproducts.[20,21] These biochemical responses culminate in cellular effects, such as proliferation, secretion of cytokines, and apoptosis that are observed as acute skin responses. For example, in the case of the patient who has taken tetracycline and overdone sun exposure, one might see exaggerated sunburn as a classic example of a phototoxic reaction. A similar series of steps is also responsible for responses to chronic exposure to UV radiation such as actinic keratoses and wrinkles (photoaging).

Absorption of EM Radiation

Skin is composed mainly of water, organic molecules (proteins, lipids, nucleic acids), and inorganic ions such as sodium and chloride. The organic molecules may absorb in the UVA, UVB, and visible spectral regions. The specific wavelengths of UV or visible radiation absorbed by these molecules (called their absorption spectra) are determined by the electronic structure of the molecules. It is important to understand that only absorbed radiation can initiate biologic responses. In fact, the first law of photochemistry set forth by Grotthus and Draper, in 1818, is precisely the principle that only absorbed light can cause a photochemical change.

The absorption spectrum of a compound is a plot of the probability of absorption (y-axis) against wavelength (x-axis). The wavelengths that have the highest probability of absorption are called absorption maxima, λ_{max}, and are often used as identifying characteristics of a compound (e.g., DNA, λ_{max} = 260 nm; porphyrin, λ_{max} = 400 to 420 nm). Absorption maxima are important in the design of various therapies. Consider the recently introduced ALA-photodynamic therapy for the treatment of actinic keratoses.[22] Topically applied ALA is metabolized to protoporphyrin IX. Because the λ_{max} of the porphyrins lies in the range of 400 to 420 nm, a blue light source is chosen for the irradiation.[22]

Compounds that have absorption maxima in the UV spectrum include aromatic amino acids in proteins (280 to 300 nm), the purine and pyrimidine bases in DNA and RNA (~260 nm), urocanic acid (280 nm), NADH (340 nm), and 7-dehydrocholesterol (7-DHC) (~285 nm). Most photosensitizing drugs absorb some radiation in the UVA range although their absorption maxima are at shorter wavelengths. For example, the absorption maxima for psoralens are in the UVB, but for PUVA they are activated by UVA. Some photosensitizing drugs, such as sulfa antibiotics and the thiazide diuretics, also absorb in the UVB spectrum because of structural differences that allow for photon absorption in that range. Many endogenous cutaneous biomolecules absorb longer wavelengths of light (visible) because their structures include double bonds, heteroatoms (oxygen, nitrogen, sulfur) and charged groups. Examples include hemoglobin (410 nm), bilirubin (~450 nm), and beta-carotene (460 nm). Melanin absorbs throughout the UV and visible spectrum without a distinct absorption maximum wavelength.

Excited States of Molecules

For each molecule, a series of *electronic states* exists, each of which corresponds to a certain distribution of electrons in space around the nuclei. A specified energy is also associated with each electronic state. According to quantum mechanics, only certain energies are allowed; thus fixed energy gaps exist between electronic states. At room temperature almost all molecules are in the electronic state with the lowest energy, the so-called *ground state*. Molecules in states with higher energy are in *excited electronic states*. Energy absorbed by a molecule in the ground state promotes it to an excited electronic state.

The nuclei in molecules are in relatively fixed positions and are surrounded by negatively charged electrons in defined volumes known as orbitals. Each orbital holds a maximum of two electrons. In addition to their electronic charge, electrons have property called *spin*, an angular momentum that makes electrons act like tiny bar magnets. According to the Pauli exclusion principle, electrons in the same orbital must have opposite spins. Most ground-state molecules have two electrons in each orbital, and their spins are in opposite directions; these are called *singlet states*. Absorption of a photon does not change the electron spins. Some excited states have two electrons in different orbitals with the same spin and these are called *triplet states*. The chemical reactions that an excited-state molecule undergoes are modulated by the spin state (singlet or triplet) of the molecule. An excited-state molecule can discharge its energy by chemical reaction to form photoproducts, by emission of light, by decay to heat (internal conversion), by transfer of the energy to another molecule, and by changing from singlet to triplet or from triplet to ground state (intersystem crossing). Formation of photoproducts by reactions of the chromophore are of greatest interest to dermatologists and photobiologists since photoproducts initiate photobiologic responses. Excited singlet states usually exist for less than 100 ns (10^{-7} s) and triplets less than 10 μs (10^{-5} s) in tissue.

Emission of light is called *fluorescence* when it originates from a singlet excited state of a molecule and *phosphorescence* when it is from a triplet excited state of the molecule. A common example of fluorescence occurs every time a Wood's light is used. UVA emitted from this lamp causes autofluorescence of dermal collagen fibers. To the examining physician, this fluorescence is viewed through the overlying epidermis. Thus, any epidermal lesions such as lentigines tend to have their borders accentuated by contrast because the fluorescence is observed most brightly around the lesion.

The internal conversion pathway for loss of electronic excitation energy proceeds by conversion of the electronic energy into vibrational energy within the molecule. This energy is quickly transferred to neighboring molecules, especially water, in the tissue; if enough is transferred, heating may be detectable. The thermal destruction of tissue by visible laser irradiation is possible because many photons are absorbed in a small volume of tissue and the excited-state molecules decay by heat-producing internal conversion.

Formation of Photoproducts

During a photochemical reaction, the chromophore is transformed into a new molecule, the photoproduct. Often, the photoproduct is the result of bonding between the chromophore and a cell molecule. An important example is the formation of covalent adducts between psoralen, the chromophore, and DNA (Chap. 266). In other cases, the chromophore is not chemically changed; instead, it causes a chemical change in another molecule. The chromophore is then called a *photosensitizer* and the reaction is called a *photosensitized reaction*. Protoporphyrin IX, the porphyrin that accumulates to abnormally high levels in red blood cells of patients with erythropoietic protoporphyria (EPP, Chap. 149) is a photosensitizer that absorbs blue light (400 to 420 nm). The initially formed excited singlet state converts to an excited triplet state which then transfers that energy to oxygen molecules to form a highly reactive excited state of oxygen called singlet oxygen.[23] Singlet oxygen subsequently reacts with lipids, proteins, and DNA to form stable photoproducts. The term *photosensitizer* is often used also when the chromophore bonds to a cellular molecule. For example, psoralens are called photosensitizers because they alter DNA by binding to it.

The efficiency for photochemical reactions vary. Not all of the chromophore molecules that absorb a photon undergo a photochemical reaction because, as noted above, several pathways are available to molecules in excited states. In addition to forming photoproducts, the excited state molecule may emit fluorescence and phosphorescence, transfer energy to oxygen, and return to the ground state. The term *quantum yield* is used to define the likelihood that one of these processes occurs. For example, the quantum yield for forming a certain photoproduct is:

$$\text{Quantum yield} = \frac{\text{Number of photoproduct molecules formed}}{\text{Number of photons absorbed}}$$

From Photoproducts to Skin Responses

Progress is being made in establishing how the photoproducts formed in skin lead to specific responses (see Fig. 133-3). Often the response involves multiple photoproducts and multiple responses may result from a single type of photoproduct. An example of beneficial photoproduct formation is production of previtamin D_3 in skin. 7-Dehydrocholesterol absorbs a photon of UVB radiation and is converted by a bond rearrangement into previtamin D_3. The previtamin D_3 thermally isomerizes to vitamin D_3 which binds to vitamin D-binding protein in the capillaries and is carried from the skin to the liver and then to the kidney. In skin, vitamin D_3 enhances keratinocyte differentiation and inhibits proliferation, which are believed to underlie the effectiveness of vitamin D_3 analogues in psoriasis therapy.[24,25] The signal transduction and biochemical steps for these responses have been studied extensively for development of related therapeutic agents.[26]

Absorption of blue light by the high concentrations of protoporphyrin IX in the skin of patients with EPP results in the formation of singlet oxygen, a highly reactive oxidizing species, by energy transfer from excited state protoporphyrin molecules. The photoproducts are oxidized lipids and proteins, especially in the cell membranes where the majority of protoporphyrin molecules localize in cells. How these photoproducts lead to the erythema, wheals, and pain that EPP patients experience in sunlight is still being investigated. One possibility is that the membranes of mast cells are altered when the lipid and protein components in the membranes are oxidized by singlet oxygen. Release of histamine and synthesis of prostaglandin D_2 (PDG_2) by these stimulated mast cells would lead to the vasodilation and increased vasopermeability responsible for the erythema and wheal formation.

The photoproducts initiating a skin response may also be derived from exogenously administered (systemically or topically) photosensitizers (Chaps. 135, 136). These responses are referred to as phototoxicity and photoallergy and the agent usually is a drug or plant material. Many phototoxic drugs and phytochemicals absorb in the UVA range and form singlet oxygen in the same manner as described above for protoporphyrin IX. This reactive form of oxygen then oxidizes nearby molecules in the cell. The differences in light-induced skin responses between those caused by phototoxic agents and that produced by protoporphyrin IX may be due to different tissue locations of the photosensitizer (e.g., epidermis, dermis, or vasculature). These photosensitizers may also be in different locations in the cells (i.e., nucleus, mitochondria, or cell membranes) which would influence the photoproducts formed. In some individuals, sunscreens (e.g., oxybenzone), may not induce an allergic rash until sun exposure occurs. The photoproducts that are possibly produced after oxybenzone absorbs UV radiation may be the cause.[27] Phototherapy of diseases such as psoriasis makes use of the phototoxicity of compounds such as 8-methoxypsoralen and its covalent photoaddition reaction with DNA (Chap. 266). In this case, light-induced cellular changes in DNA are apparently beneficial to the total organism.

Action Spectrum

The *action spectrum* for a photobiologic response indicates which wavelengths produce the response most effectively. Knowing the action spectrum of a patient's photosensitivity is helpful in determining the treatment plan. On the other hand, phototherapy will be most efficient when the emission of the lamp most closely matches the action spectrum for the beneficial response.

In an ideal case, the action spectrum corresponds to the absorption spectrum for the chromophore. Determination of an action spectrum is, therefore, a powerful tool for identification of the putative chromophore for a given photobiologic reaction. Peaks in the action spectrum correspond to the most effective wavelengths. An action spectrum is most accurately plotted as the reciprocal of the number of incident photons required to produce a given effect (y-axis) against wavelength (x-axis). Conventionally in dermatology, the reciprocal of the minimum fluence (dose) is plotted versus wavelength. Such a graph is shown in Fig. 133-4 for wheal formation in a patient with erythropoietic protoporphyria.[28] The maximum of the action spectrum at 400 nm is close to the maximum in the absorption spectrum for protoporphyrin supporting biochemical evidence for protoporphyrin as the chromophore for the photosensitivity.

Lack of correspondence between an experimentally determined action spectrum and the absorption spectrum of the actual chromophore may occur due to tissue optics. Light that impinges on a tissue is usually absorbed by other chromophores in the tissue; it is also reflected and scattered (Fig. 133-5). These effects decrease the amount of light transmitted to a specific depth in tissue and vary with wavelength. One familiar example is that of psoralen, which has absorption maxima around 295 and 330 nm with slight absorption extending into the longer UVA waveband in vitro (Chap. 266). However, determinations of the psoralen photosensitization action spectrum in vivo show that maximum responses occur with wavelengths >320 nm, possibly due to skin optical properties.[29,30] Whenever possible, decisions about which wavelengths to use for a treatment should be based on action spectra rather than on the in vitro absorption spectrum of the photochemotherapeutic drug.

FIGURE 133-4

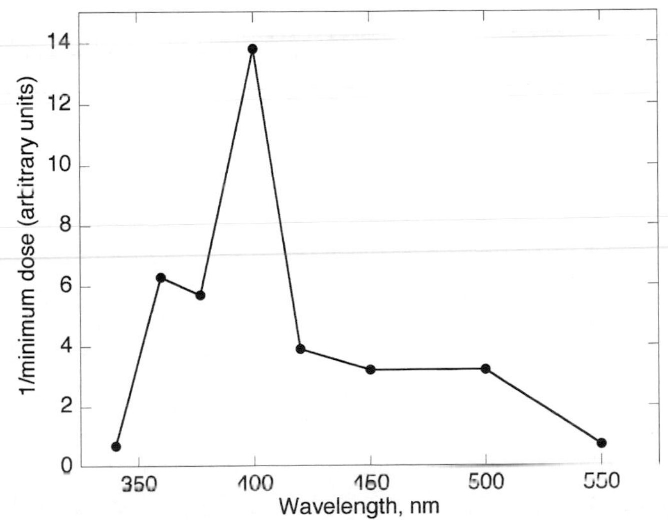

Action spectrum for wheal formation in erythropoietic protoporphyria patient. The *y*-axis is the reciprocal of the minimal dose required to produce a wheal. This dose of radiation (exposure time × irradiance) is expressed in arbitrary units. A monochromator with a quartz-xenon lamp was used to deliver selected narrow wavebands. (*From Magnus IA et al.,*[28] *with permission.*)

FIGURE 133-5

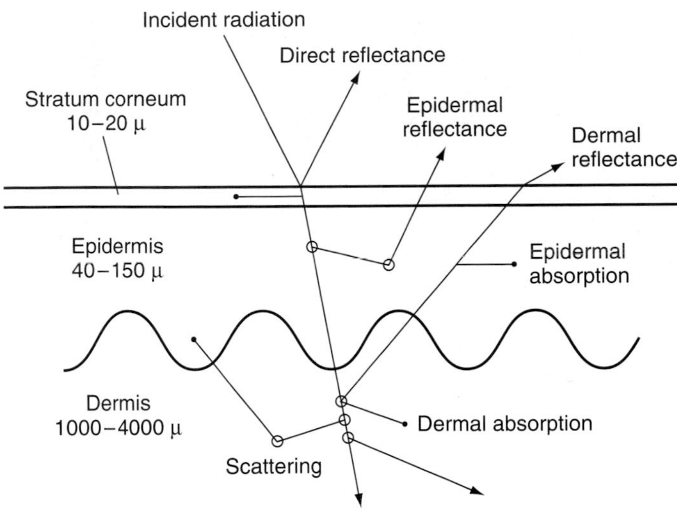

The interaction of UV and visible radiation with skin. The incident radiation is reflected from the surface, scattered (*circles*), and absorbed (*black dots*) as it travels through the skin.

OPTICAL PROPERTIES OF SKIN

When radiation strikes the skin, part is remitted (reflected and scattered), part is absorbed in various layers, and part is transmitted inward to successive layers of cells, until the energy of the incident beam has been dissipated[31,32] (see Fig. 133-5). A very small fraction of the absorbed radiation is reemitted at longer wavelengths as fluorescence. The amounts of absorption and scattering of UV and visible radiation vary with wavelength.

UV wavelengths less than 320 nm are mostly absorbed by proteins and other components of epidermal cells, which, along with scattering, accounts for the low penetration of these wavelengths into skin (Fig. 133-6). For example, approximately 90 percent of 300 nm radiation is dissipated by about 14 nm into the epidermis, and only 10 percent of 350 nm radiation reaches the dermal–epidermal junction (~140 nm). Between 5 and 10 percent of incident light is reflected by the outer surface of the stratum corneum. This surface or so-called specular reflectance is relatively constant for all visible wavelengths and accounts for the surface appearance of skin, which is especially glossy if the surface is smooth, wet, or oily. It is by this surface component of the total skin reflectance that we have learned to judge roughness of the skin. Moisturizers applied to the skin reduce this rough appearance by smoothing out the many air-surface interface irregularities, thus reducing specular reflectance and making the skin look shinier.

In addition to the surface reflectance, white skin remits about 50 percent of the incident visible light by backward scattering from within the dermis. *Scattering* includes any process that deflects the path of optical radiation. For example, skin with scales, as in psoriasis, scatters more light than does normal skin. During phototherapy, application of emollients to the psoriatic plaques helps reduce the scattering of UVR and allows more of the effective wavelengths to penetrate into the viable tissue. In fair white skin, the bulk of the visible remittance is light that has penetrated the epidermis and has been scattered from various depths within the dermis back through the epidermis and skin surface.

FIGURE 133-6

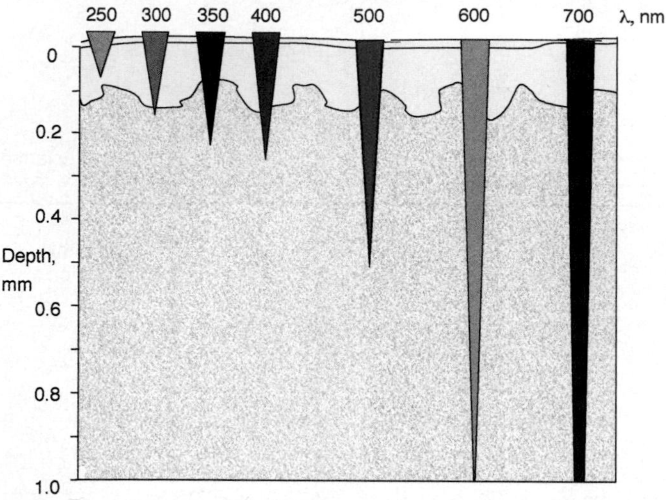

Representation of the variation in penetration of UV and visible radiation into skin.

Melanin, which absorbs relatively uniformly over the visible wavelengths and is normally present only in the epidermis, acts largely as a density (gray) filter to diminish dermal remittance. Melanosomes in darker-skinned individuals are larger and singly dispersed as compared to those of fairer-skinned individuals. By being larger, they absorb more. By being singly dispersed, they also create a darker color for the skin. Consider, for example, how the octopus changes color by shifting all its pigment. When widely dispersed, the octopus looks dark; when the pigment is gathered together in tight clusters it looks lighter.

Blood within the dermis absorbs the shorter (blue) visible wavelengths, diminishing these spectral regions of the dermal remittance component, and giving a reddish hue to our perception of the total remittance. Abnormal location and quantity of these or other pigments account for the appearance of the skin in pathologic conditions (e.g., melasma with extra pigment in the epidermis and/or dermis; vitiligo with an absence of epidermal melanin).

SOURCES OF EM RADIATION

Solar Radiation

The shortest wavelength of the solar spectrum reaching the earth's surface at sea level is approximately 290 nm; at higher altitudes, shorter wavelengths (up to 285) nm have been detected.[33] Although the sun emits shorter UV wavelengths, they are filtered out by the ozone layer and molecular oxygen of the stratosphere. Depending on the geographic location and the season, it has been estimated that sunlight produces between 2 and 6 mW/cm^2 of UV radiation between 290 and 400 nm. Filtering of wavelengths less than 290 nm by ozone is a very important process because the shorter UV wavelengths are highly damaging to animals and plants. Ozone is present in the stratosphere and is constantly being generated and degraded. Halocarbons from industrial and domestic uses rise to the stratosphere where photochemical reactions cause them to release the chlorine and bromine atoms that catalyze ozone destruction. Because the transmission of solar UVB through the atmosphere varies exponentially with ozone concentration, small changes in the ozone layer may result in hazardous increases in UV irradiance at the earth's surface. Calculations of the effects of ozone depletion on skin cancer incidence predict a doubling by 2100 even if the Montreal Protocol restrictions on ozone-depleting substances are followed.[34] Similarly, a decrease in the ozone layer was predicted to lead to greater UVB suppression of cellular immunity based on experimental studies.[35]

The recently introduced UV Index represents an attempt to quantify the risks attendant with solar radiation at a given time and place. Among other factors, the effects of altitude and clouds are considered. The scale goes up to 15 and any UV Index >10 is considered a high-risk day for possible overexposure on that day and in that locale.

FIGURE 133-7

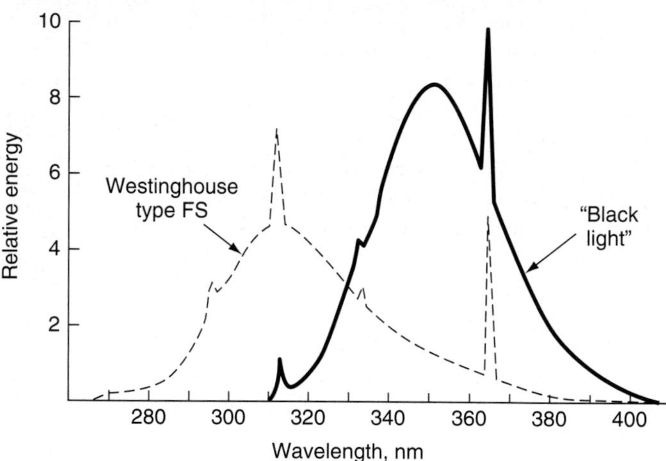

A.

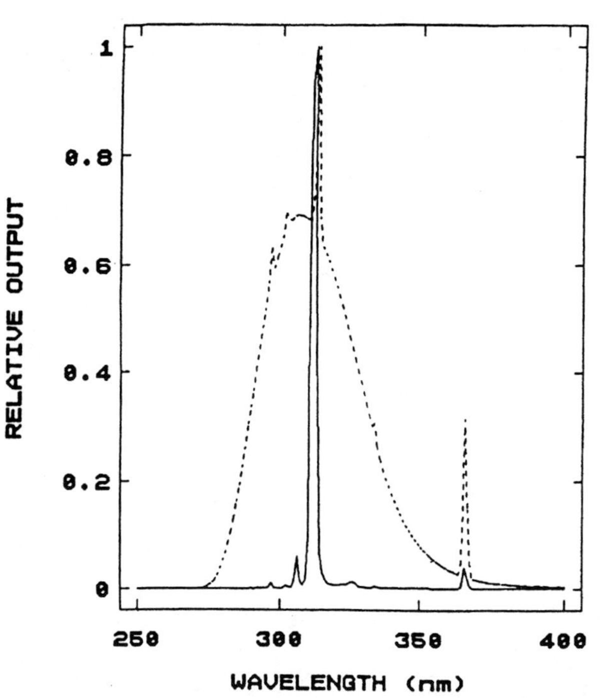

B.

Emission spectra of some of the fluorescent lamps used in phototherapy. *A.* The broadband type FS fluorescent lamps and black light lamps are often referred to as UVB and UVA lamps, respectively. *B.* The TL01 lamp (*full line*) has its main emission at 311 nm and the TL12 (*dotted line*) is a broadband UVB lamp. (*From reference El-Ghorr AA, Norval M,*[38] *with permission.*)

Artificial Sources of Radiation

INCANDESCENT SOURCES The electric light bulb is an incandescent source. An electric current passed through a metal filament increases the filament temperature to that of incandescence. Most of the radiation emitted is in the visible and infrared spectrum. Only the occasional patient with solar urticaria, chronic actinic dermatitis or some porphyrias is bothered by the output of ordinary incandescent sources. Wavelengths shorter than 360 nm are usually not emitted because the hot filaments are encased in glass envelopes which transmit only UVA and visible radiation. Tungsten-halogen incandescent lamps, often used as floodlamps, emit UVA and visible radiation. Some quartz iodide incandescent lamps may produce significant UVA and some UVB emission.

ARC SOURCES In arc lamps, electrons are driven at high velocity by a potential difference between two electrodes. Gaseous molecules between the electrodes are ionized and electronically excited and subsequently release radiant energy. The spectral power distribution depends on the gas used, the arc temperature, the pressure within the lamp, the electrical input to the lamp, and the lamp wall material. Most of the radiation is emitted at wavelengths corresponding to the transition energies, between orbitals particular to the gas in the lamp. In addition to these spectral emission lines, a continuum of wavelengths is emitted by high-temperature arc lamps.

Xenon arc Xenon gas under 20 to 40 atm of pressure is heated to a high temperature in a rigid quartz envelope to produce intense visible and UV radiation. At these pressures the xenon spectrum becomes a continuum; that is, all wavelengths are emitted rather than just specific wavelengths. Xenon arc lamps are now the most common sources used in solar simulators. Photoprovocation testing for polymorphic eruption is often done with such sources. Filters are used to limit the wavelengths for phototesting with solar simulators. Xenon arcs are also used in some phototherapy and photobiologic research applications.

Mercury arc At low pressure, mercury vapor lamps emit 85 percent of the radiant energy at 254 nm and 5 percent at 185 nm. When the material used for the lamp envelope is quartz, nearly all the 254-nm radiation is transmitted. UVC is lethal to microorganisms and these are, therefore, called *germicidal lamps*. Because the operating temperature is low, they are also known as *cold quartz lamps*. With increasing pressure (1 atm), the primary 254-nm emission is absorbed by other mercury atoms within the lamp and reemitted at longer wavelengths (297, 302, 313, 334, and 365 nm, and visible wavelengths). With further pressure increases (2 to 100 atm), these spectral lines broaden and decrease relative to the intensity of the continuous spectral background. In medical practice, medium- and high-pressure mercury lamps (*hot quartz*) are used mainly as sources of UVB, although their spectral power distribution is mainly in the UVA and visible range.

FLUORESCENT LAMPS A fluorescent lamp is a glass tube containing low-pressure mercury with electrodes at both ends. Electric current passing through the tube ionizes the mercury atoms, which subsequently emit at 254 nm (germicidal radiation). When the inner surface of the glass envelope is coated with phosphor, the 254-nm radiation is absorbed and then reemitted at longer wavelengths. The composition of the phosphor determines which wavelengths are reemitted. In general, fluorescent lamps have a relatively wide, bell-shaped emission spectra, with spectral emission lines of mercury superimposed, and are referred to as *broadband light sources*.

UVB lamps Fluorescent sunlamps (type FS) emit mainly in the UVB range (Fig. 133-7). They are often referred to as UVB lamps, even though they emit a portion of UVA radiation, because the therapeutically significant radiation is in the UVB range (Table 133-2). A fluorescent lamp with a major emission peak at 311 nm (Philips TL01) was developed for use in phototherapy (Fig. 133-7).[36–38] This lamp is an efficient source for psoriasis phototherapy since, compared to a conventional UVB lamp, the energy emitted almost entirely overlaps with the action spectrum for clearance of psoriasis.[39] Ironically, this lamp has been successfully employed for the treatment of vitiligo, atopic dermatitis, and polymorphic light eruption, all of whose action spectra are unknown and may well vary from that for psoriasis.

UVA lamps High-intensity, UVA-emitting fluorescent lamps are most often used in PUVA therapy of psoriasis, vitiligo, and other skin diseases. The most efficient UVA source for PUVA therapy would maximize the emission of 320- to 360-nm radiation for photoactivation of psoralen molecules, while minimizing the UVB emission. Table 133-2 shows the percentage of total emission that is in the 320- to 360-nm range from several UVA-emitting light sources that are used in phototherapy units.

Wood's lamps Current versions of Wood's lamps are small, low-pressure, UVA-emitting fluorescent lamps with a UVA-transmitting, visible-absorbing glass envelope. Wood's lamps are invaluable in clinical practice because the fluorescent emission from normal and abnormal components of skin, hair, and urine may be diagnostic (e.g., in porphyria, vitiligo, and fungal infection).

HALIDE LAMPS The metal halide lamp usually consists of a high-pressure mercury lamp with metal halides as additives. The continuous range of wavelengths emitted from halide lamps makes them preferable to medium-pressure mercury arc lamps that emit in narrow wavelength ranges. Approximately 20 percent of the power consumption can be UVA radiation. Because of the high-intensity continuum emission in the UVB and especially the UVA range, this lamp, with appropriate filters, is used increasingly as a UVB, as well as a UVA, source for phototherapy and photochemotherapy.

LASERS Laser is an acronym for Light Amplification by Stimulated Emission of Radiation. Lasers produce intense beams of monochromatic optical radiation. The laser operates by exciting molecules to a

TABLE 133-2

***Approximate* Spectral Power Distribution of UVB and UVA Radiation Expressed as Percentage of Total Emission in the UV Waveband in Common Phototherapy Sources**

	% UVB	% UVA
Broadband UVB (Westinghouse Sunlamp)	60	40
Narrow-band UVB* (Phillips Fluorescent UVB, TL01, 311 nm)	80	20
Broadband UVA (Houva Lite; Black Light by Sylvania, Westinghouse and General Electric; Sylvania Puva Lite Line; Dermalight Metal)	2	98
UVA-1† (Dermalight UltrA1, Dr. K. Hönle Medizintechnik GmbH)	0	100
Wood's light‡ (RA Fisher; Spectronics)	0	100
Halide lamps§ (Dermalight Systems; Dr. K. Hönle Medizintechnik GmbH)	0	100

*Most (~95% of the UVB emission of the typical narrow-band UVB source is centered around 311 nm.)
†This UVA emission is above 340 nm.
‡The filter used (so-called Wood's filter) is glass with nickel oxide phosphor. Consequently, UVB is screened. A moderate amount of visible light is produced.
§The actual amount depends on the model purchased and the filters used (glass versus quartz). Some models allow the operator to change the filters readily and thus increase the amount of UVB to >50% of the irradiance.

metastable excited state from which photon emission is stimulated by a subsequent photon incident upon the excited molecule. The emitted photon and the stimulating photon are then each capable of stimulating emission of yet other excited molecules, eventually producing an avalanche of photons of the same wavelength, phase, and direction of propagation. Lasers emit UV, visible, or infrared wavelengths and may operate as either continuous or pulsed sources. Applications of lasers in dermatology utilize their capacity to concentrate large amounts of energy in a small volume of tissue (Chap. 267).

ULTRAVIOLET RADIATION DOSIMETRY

The basic unit of energy is the joule (J). Power is the rate of energy flow or dissipation, given in watts (W), or joules per second (W = J/s). The rate at which radiant energy is delivered to a surface such as skin is expressed as the power delivered per unit area of surface [W/cm^2 = (J/s) per cm^2]. This quantity is called *irradiance*. The total radiant energy delivered per unit area of skin surface, the *exposure dose*, or fluence, is the product of irradiance and time: Irradiance (W/cm^2) $\times$ time(s) $=$ exposure dose (J/cm^2)

For most photobiologic phenomena, it is the exposure dose at a particular wavelength that determines the magnitude of the response. The rate of energy delivery generally does not affect the response (Bunsen-Roscoe law of reciprocity). A common office example demonstrating the law of reciprocity occurs with PUVA boxes. A PUVA box with half as many bulbs in it would take twice as long to deliver a given dose as would one with twice as many bulbs of the same age, make and individual output.

The irradiance delivered by a source as a function of wavelength is called the *spectral irradiance*, expressed as units of irradiance per nanometer [(W/cm^2) per nm]. The purpose of a *spectroradiometer* is to measure the spectral irradiance of a light source at the position of the skin. If one is interested only in measuring the irradiance provided by a source over a given spectral region, a detector might be used that measures only those wavelengths of interest (broadband radiometric measurements). For example, a broadband radiometric measurement of wavelengths less than 315 nm provides a rough indication of the erythemally effective wavelengths emitted by a source of UV radiation.

There is, however, no substitute for knowing the full spectral irradiance delivered by a source, as determined by a spectroradiometer. If spectral irradiance, exposure field size, angles of incidence, exposure duration, and environmental conditions such as humidity and temperature are recorded, the important conditions of the exposure are described with precision and may be repeated with some accuracy. These considerations are of practical importance in phototesting, phototherapy, and photochemotherapy. For example, in phototesting, only the wavelengths of interest should be employed. To assess endogenous UVA sensitivity, the UVB portion of a source's emission, if present, must be filtered out so that the more erythemogenic UVB wavelengths do not lead to a falsely lowered erythema threshold in the UVA range. The spectroradiometer is critical in defining the full spectral output.

REFERENCES

1. Girotti AW: Lipid hydroperoxide generation, turnover, and effector action in biological systems. *J Lipid Res* **39**:1529, 1998
2. Geiger PG et al: Lipid peroxidation in photodynamically stressed mammalian cells: use of cholesterol hydroperoxides as mechanistic reporters. *Free Radic Biol Med* **23**:57, 1997
3. Cadet J et al: Effects of UV and visible radiations on cellular DNA. *Curr Probl Dermatol* **29**:62, 2001
4. Moor AC, Gasparro FP: Biochemical aspects of psoralen photochemotherapy. *Clin Dermatol* **14**:353, 1996
5. Katiyar SK: A single physiologic dose of ultraviolet light exposure to human skin in vivo induces phosphorylation of epidermal growth factor receptor. *Int J Oncol* **19**:459, 2001
6. Wan YS et al: Ultraviolet irradiation activates PI 3-kinase/AKT survival pathway via EGF receptors in human skin in vivo. *Int J Oncol* **18**:461, 2001
7. Djavaheri-Mergny M, Dubertret L: UV-A-induced AP-1 activation requires the Raf/ERK pathway in human NCTC 2544 keratinocytes. *Exp Dermatol* **10**:204, 2001
8. Fisher GJ, Voorhees JJ: Molecular mechanisms of photoaging and its prevention by retinoic acid: Ultraviolet irradiation induces MAP kinase signal transduction cascades that induce AP-1–regulated matrix metalloproteinases that degrade human skin in vivo. *J Invest Dermatol Symp Proc* **3**:61, 1998
9. Abeyama K et al: A role for NF-kappaB–dependent gene transactivation in sunburn. *J Clin Invest* **105**:1751, 2000
10. Legrand-Poels S et al: NF-kappa B: An important transcription factor in photobiology. *J Photochem Photobiol B* **45**:1, 1998
11. Gilchrest BA, Eller MS: DNA photodamage stimulates melanogenesis and other photoprotective responses. *J Invest Dermatol Symp Proc* **4**:35, 1999
12. Sturm RA: Human pigmentation genes and their response to solar UV radiation. *Mutat Res* **422**:69, 1998
13. Beissert S, Schwarz T: Mechanisms involved in ultraviolet light-induced immunosuppression. *J Invest Dermatol Symp Proc* **4**:61, 1999
14. Scholzen TE et al: Effect of ultraviolet light on the release of neuropeptides and neuroendocrine hormones in the skin: Mediators of photodermatitis and cutaneous inflammation. *J Invest Dermatol Symp Proc* **4**:55, 1999
15. Duthie MS, Kimber I and Norval M: The effects of ultraviolet radiation on the human immune system. *Br J Dermatol* **140**:995, 1999
16. Tang Q et al: Role of cyclic AMP responsive element in the UVB induction of cyclooxygenase-2 transcription in human keratinocytes. *Oncogene* **20**:5164, 2001
17. Isoherranen K et al: Ultraviolet irradiation induces cyclooxygenase-2 expression in keratinocytes. *Br J Dermatol* **140**:1017, 1999
18. Brenneisen P et al: Ultraviolet-B induction of interstitial collagenase and stromelyin-1 occurs in human dermal fibroblasts via an autocrine interleukin-6-dependent loop. *FEBS Lett* **449**:36, 1999
19. Fisher GJ et al: Pathophysiology of premature skin aging induced by ultraviolet light. *N Engl J Med* **337**:1419, 1997
20. Cleaver JE: Common pathways for ultraviolet skin carcinogenesis in the repair and replication defective groups of xeroderma pigmentosum. *J Dermatol Sci* **23**:1, 2000
21. McGregor WG: DNA repair, DNA replication, and UV mutagenesis. *J Invest Dermatol Symp Proc* **4**:1, 1999
22. Jeffes EW et al: Photodynamic therapy of actinic keratoses with topical aminolevulinic acid hydrochloride and fluorescent blue light. *J Am Acad Dermatol* **45**:96, 2001
23. Klotz LO et al: UVA and singlet oxygen as inducers of cutaneous signaling events. *Curr Probl Dermatol* **29**:95, 2001
24. Johansen C et al: 1Alpha, 25-dihydroxyvitamin D_3-induced differentiation of cultured human keratinocytes is accompanied by a PKC-independent regulation of AP-1 DNA binding activity. *J Invest Dermatol* **114**:1174, 2000
25. Griner RD et al: 1,25-Dihydroxyvitamin D_3 induces phospholipase D-1 expression in primary mouse epidermal keratinocytes. *J Biol Chem* **274**:4663, 1999
26. Kowalzick L: Clinical experience with topical calcitriol (1,25-dihydroxyvitamin D_3) in psoriasis. *Br J Dermatol* **144**:21, 2001
27. Tokura Y: Immune responses to photohaptens: Implications for the mechanisms of photosensitivity to exogenous agents. *J Dermatol Sci* **23**:S6, 2000
28. Magnus IA et al: Erythropoietic protoporphyria. A new porphyria syndrome with solar urticaria due to protoporphyrinemia. *Lancet* **ii**:448, 1961
29. Pathak MA: Mechanism of psoralen photosenstization and in vivo biological action spectrum of 8-methoxypsoralen. *J Invest Dermatol* **37**:397, 1961
30. Buck HW et al: The action spectrum of 8-methoxypsoralen for erythema in human skin. *Br J Dermatol* **72**:249, 1960
31. Anderson RR: Optics of the skin, in *Clinical Photomedicine*, edited by HW Lin, NA Soter. New York, Marcel Dekker, 1993, p 19

32. Anderson RR: Tissue optics and photoimmunology, in *Photoimmunology*, edited by JA Parrish, W Morison, M Kripke. New York, Plenum Medical, 1983, p 73
33. Cadle RD, Allen ER: Atmospheric photochemistry. *Science* **167**:243, 1970
34. Slaper H et al: Estimates of ozone depletion and skin cancer incidence to examine the Vienna Convention achievements. *Nature* **384**:256, 1996
35. Garssen J et al: Estimation of the effect of increasing UVB exposure on the human immune system and related resistance to infectious diseases and tumours. *J Photochem Photobiol B* **42**:167, 1998
36. Green C et al: 311 nm UVB phototherapy—An effective treatment for psoriasis. *Br J Dermatol* **119**:691, 1988

37. van Weelden H et al: A new development in UVB phototherapy of psoriasis. *Br J Dermatol* **119**:11, 1988
38. El-Ghorr AA, Norval M: Biological effects of narrow-band (311 nm TL01) UVB irradiation: A review. *J Photochem Photobiol B* **38**:99, 1997
39. Parrish JA, Jaenicke KF: Action spectrum for phototherapy of psoriasis. *J Invest Dermatol* **76**:359, 1981

CHAPTER 134

Susan L. Walker
John L.M. Hawk
Antony R. Young

Acute and Chronic Effects of Ultraviolet Radiation on the Skin

ULTRAVIOLET RADIATION

Extraterrestrial sunlight is electromagnetic radiation energy comprising mainly the ultraviolet (UV), visible, and infrared spectra, although both shorter (ionizing) and longer (microwave and radiofrequency) wavelengths are also present. They are modified significantly by their passage through the atmosphere, so that only about two-thirds of this energy reaches ground level.

UV radiation (UVR) comprises approximately 5 percent of terrestrial solar radiation and is defined as those wavelengths between 100 and 400 nm. By the official designation of the Commission Internationale de l'Eclairage (CIE), it is subdivided into UVA (315 to 400 nm), UVB (280 to 315 nm), and UVC (100 to 280 nm), but by popular convention the ranges are 320 to 400, 290 to 320, and 100 to 290 nm, respectively. Recently, UVA was divided into UVAI (340 to 400 nm) and UVAII (320 to 340 nm) because the biological effects of UVAII are mechanistically similar to those of UVB. Solar UVR at the earth's surface is approximately 95 to 98 percent UVA and 2 to 5 percent UVB, all the UVC having been completely absorbed by stratospheric ozone. The precise amount and composition of solar UVR depend on a number of factors, particularly the solar zenith angle, which varies with the time of day, season, and latitude; the stratospheric ozone concentration; and pollution, cloud cover, and altitude.

INTRODUCTION TO MOLECULAR AND CLINICAL EFFECTS OF UVR

The most obvious acute clinical effects of UVR on normal skin are sunburn inflammation (erythema) and tanning (melanogenesis). However, as will be discussed, UVR has a wide range of other acute effects, such as DNA photodamage, immunosuppression, and vitamin D synthesis. Chronic exposure to sunlight leads to photoaging and skin cancer (see Chap. 38). The acute effects of solar UVR are amenable to controlled laboratory investigation but logistics and ethics prevent the study of such effects over the decades necessary for the appearance of chronic effects. The determination of long-term effects requires an epidemiologic or clinicopathologic approach. By definition, chronic effects are the consequence of a series of acute effects or, less probably, the delayed outcome of a single acute event. In the understanding of long-term effects there is, therefore, a need to look at the interrelation between acute and long-term effects, as well as the mechanisms of acute effects. It has been useful to clinically assign sun-sensitivity according to skin phototype, as shown in Table 134-1, a classification that also shows a relationship between acute and chronic effects (see Chap. 88).

It is widely assumed that sensitivity to UVR is directly and solely related to pigmentation or tanning ability, an assumption primarily based on epidemiologic evidence showing skin cancers are much less common in people who tan well (e.g., skin phototypes III and IV) or who have high levels of constitutive pigmentation (e.g., skin phototypes V and VI). Furthermore, studies comparing dark-skinned people with related albinos show the latter to have a higher incidence of photodamage and nonmelanoma skin cancer. However, comparisons based on pigmentation alone may fail to take into account other factors important in UVR sensitivity, such as DNA repair capacity and sensitivity to UVR-induced immunosuppression (see Chap. 39), now also widely believed to be important in human skin cancer.

MEASUREMENT OF HUMAN EXPOSURE TO UVR

In photobiology, radiant exposure (fluence, dose) is denoted precisely in physical units of J/cm^2. However, a biological dose unit, the minimal

TABLE 134-1

Classification of Human Skin Types with Respect to Relative Response to Acute and Long-term Solar Exposure

Skin Type	Susceptibility to Sunburn	Constitutive Skin Color	Facultative Tanning Ability	Susceptibility to Skin Cancer
I	High	White	Very poor	High
II	High	White	Poor	High
III	Moderate	White	Good	Moderate
IV	Low	Olive	Very good	Low
V	Very low	Brown	Very good	Very low
VI	Very low	Black	Very good	Very low

erythemal dose (MED), is more commonly used. An MED is the lowest UVR dose required to produce either a just perceptible erythema (MED_{JP}) on exposed skin of a given individual after 24 h or an erythema with sharp margins after 24 h. Clearly these end points refer to different physical doses, and it is therefore essential to define the measure on each occasion. In one study, the interobserver error in determining the MED_{JP} was significantly less than that for sharp margins,[1] and this definition thus appears preferable. In general, individuals with higher skin types have higher MEDs. However, as shown in Fig. 134-1, there is considerable overlap of MED_{JP} within skin types I to IV exposed to solar-simulated radiation (SSR). It was recently proposed that a new term, the standard erythema dose (SED), be used as a standardized measure of erythemogenic UVR.[2] The SED is equivalent to an erythemally weighted dose of 100 J/m^2, and about 1.5 SED is equivalent to an MED in a skin type I person.

FIGURE 134-1

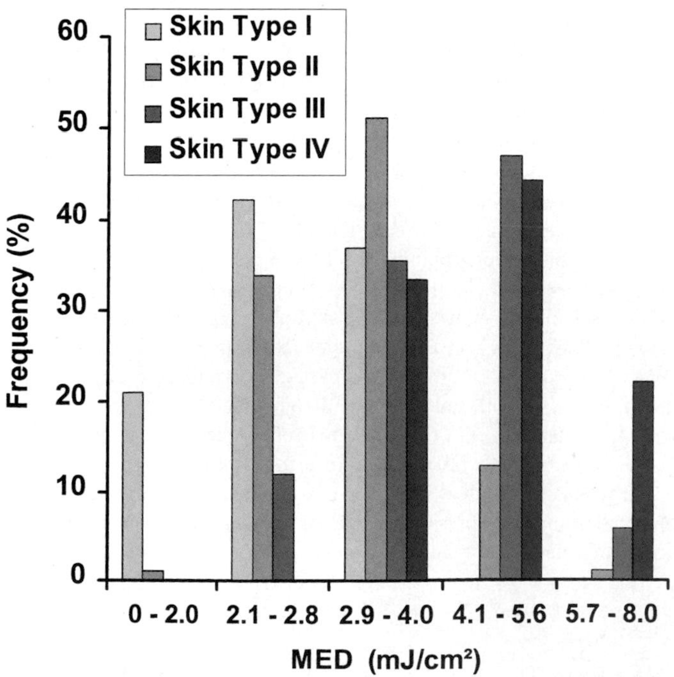

There is considerable overlap for SSR (just perceptible MED on previously unexposed buttock skin) in different white skin types. Mean MED for skins types I, II, III, and IV are 2.9 (SD ± 0.7), 3.5 (SD ± 1.0), 4.5 (SD ± 1.2), and 5.3 (SD ± 1.2) J/cm^2, respectively.

Most human UVR exposure is to sunlight, although other sources include medical phototherapy lamps, sun beds, arc-welding apparatus, and unshielded fluorescent and tungsten-halogen lamps. Individual skin exposure to solar UVR depends on the ambient levels of UVR, fraction of ambient exposure received on different body sites, exposure behavior and time spent outdoors, as well as clothing, hat, and sunscreen use. Studies on indoor workers in Northern Europe have shown an annual exposure of about 200 SED, mainly from weekend and vacation activities, which represents about 5 percent of the total ambient available.[3] A study of children in the UK and Australia shows the importance of behavior. The median daily dose in Australia was 1.7 SED as compared to 0.9 SED in England, each being about 5 percent of the ambient UVR. However, on any given day 17 percent of the English children received more UVR than the Australian median exposure, and 26 percent of the Australian children had lower doses than the English median dose.[4]

ACUTE EFFECTS OF UVR

DNA Photodamage and Mutation

The photophysical and photochemical basis of photobiology is discussed in Chap. 133. The epidermis and the dermis contain UVR-absorbing chromophores including urocanic acid, aromatic amino acids (proteins), and melanin precursors.[5] However, there is increasing evidence that epidermal DNA is the most important chromophore for many of the acute and long-term effects of solar exposure. The absorption of UVR by DNA results in the formation of characteristic dipyrimidine lesions such as cyclobutane pyrimidine dimers (CPD) and pyrimidine (6-4) pyrimidone photoproducts in human epidermis (keratinocytes and melanocytes) in situ after suberythemal or erythemal exposures of SSR, UVB, and UVA.[6–8] Figure 134-2 shows the action spectrum (the relative efficacies of different wavelengths) for the induction of thymine dimers (T=T), a specific type of CPD, in different epidermal layers, in human skin types I and II. It is clear that solar range UVB causes considerable DNA damage in the basal layer, but UVA can also induce epidermal CPD, albeit with much higher doses. Unless repaired, the molecular rearrangement of adjacent pyrimidine bases (cytosine or thymine) may give rise to highly characteristic UVR, so-called signature, mutations, namely C $\rightarrow$T or CC $\rightarrow$TT at dipyrimidine sites.[9]

Human studies have shown that, after a single exposure of SSR, global (i.e., whole genome) (6-4) photoproduct repair in situ is relatively rapid, while global CPD repair is much slower, many lesions persisting for at least 24 h.[6,10] Such slow repair means that lesions may accumulate if skin is again exposed to UVR the following day, as is often the case in normal life. There is also evidence that cytosine-containing lesions (C=C, C=T) are repaired more rapidly than those with thymine only (T=T),[10] perhaps because photodamage to thymine is of less importance than to cytosine because of the "A rule," which dictates that adenine (the correct base match for thymine) be used in DNA repair in cases of uncertainty. There is also some evidence that epidermal DNA repair may be inducible by repeated SSR exposure in skin types that tan well (IV) but not in skin types that tan poorly (II).[11]

FIGURE 134-2

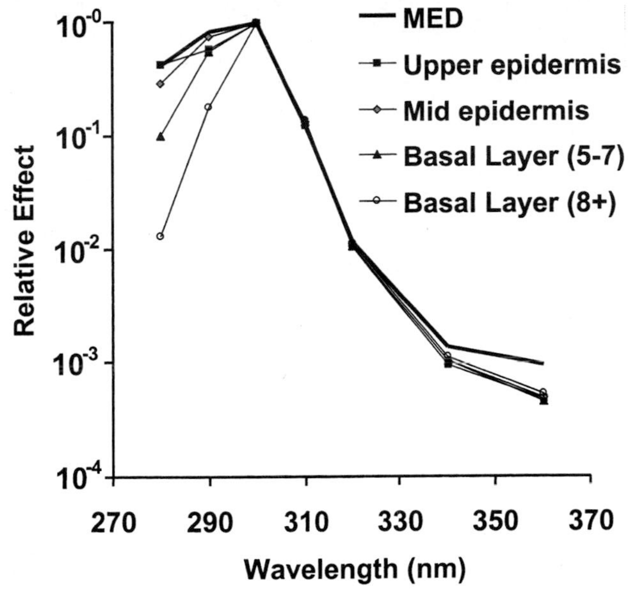

Comparison of action spectra for erythema and epidermal DNA photodamage (thymine dimers) in the same group of 40 skin-type I/II volunteers. From Young et al.[7]

The tumor suppressor p53 protein is not detectable in normal human epidermis but is readily induced by a single exposure to UVR, as shown in Fig. 134-3*A*. This protein, which acts as a transcription factor, induces cell cycle (G1) arrest to allow time for the repair of DNA photolesions, thus minimizing the transfer of potentially carcinogenic mutations to daughter cells.[12]

Sunburn Inflammation

Sunburn inflammation (erythema) is the most conspicuous and well-recognized acute cutaneous response to UVR, particularly in fair-skinned individuals, and is associated with the classic signs of inflammation, namely, redness, warmth, pain, and swelling. Generally, the degree of such erythema is determined by the total UVR energy administered, doubling of the irradiance and halving of the irradiation time thus leading to the same degree of sunburn, a relationship known as reciprocity. Such a relationship holds true over a very wide range of times and irradiances, except with very high irradiances and short times (e.g., with lasers), which often result in thermal rather than photochemical events, and very low irradiances and long times, which may enable repair processes to keep pace with damage or inflammatory mediators to diffuse away as they are formed.[13]

Erythema is UVR dose-dependent, solar range UVB (300 nm and 313 nm) and UVA (365 nm) erythemas having similar slopes, although the slopes for UVC (254 nm) and nonsolar UVB (280 nm) are much less steep.[14] Studies with 2 MED SSR in skin types I/II show the onset of erythema at about 6 h, a peak response at 18 to 24 h with marked erythema persisting for at least 1 week.[6] Repeated daily suberythemal SSR exposures result instead in a marked erythema after a few days, especially in sun-sensitive skin types.[11,15]

Erythemal Effectiveness of Different UVR Wavelengths

Figure 134-2 shows one assessment of the action spectrum for erythema in skin types I and II. Erythemal effectiveness declines rapidly with increasing wavelength, with for example 360 nm (UVA) radiation requiring 1280 times more energy than 300 nm (UVB) radiation to produce the same effect. Therefore, the relatively small UVB component of solar UVR accounts for the majority of its erythemal effect, as shown in Fig. 134-4, which also shows the reference CIE action spectrum[16] for erythema, widely used for UVR hazard assessment. Fig. 134-2 also shows the action spectra for thymine dimers and for erythema in the same pool of volunteers are very similar, thereby providing strong indirect evidence that DNA is a major chromophore for erythema. Another erythema action spectrum determined with truly monochromatic irradiation from lasers shows results that are essentially similar to those of Figs. 134-2 and 134-4, but with a secondary peak at 362 nm,[17] strongly suggestive of a chromophore other than DNA in the UVA region,

FIGURE 134-3

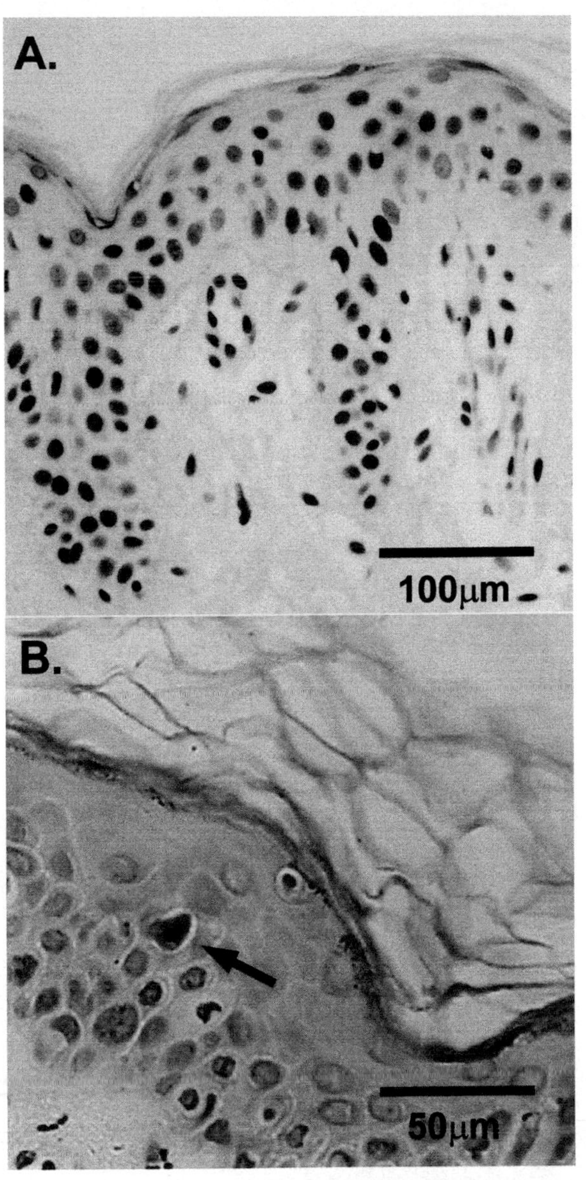

Epidermal responses in patients with skin type II at 24 h after 2 MED_{JP} with solar-simulated radiation. *A*. Wild-type p53 (immunostained brown with DO-7 antibody) is expressed maximally. *B*. Sunburn cell counts are maximal. Note shrunken eosinophilic cytoplasm and condensed pyknotic nucleus after staining with hematoxylin and eosin. (*Photomicrographs courtesy of John Sheehan.*)

FIGURE 134-4

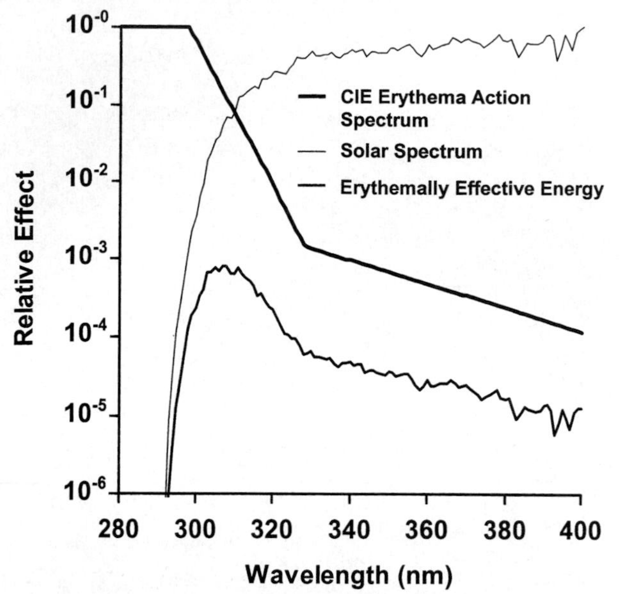

Standardized CIE erythema action spectrum,[16] noontime summer spectral irradiance in London, UK (51°N 29′), and resultant erythemal effectiveness spectrum. These data show that the 4.9 percent of the UVB (< 320 nm) in the solar spectrum contributes 80 percent of the erythemal effectiveness of the solar UVR spectrum.

presumably acting through photosensitization reactions that are characteristically oxygen dependent. This observation supports earlier clinical studies showing that UVA-induced, but not UVB-induced, erythema is oxygen dependent.[18]

Pharmacologic Mediators

UVR exposure induces the synthesis and release of an extensive array of mediators including histamine, by-products of arachidonic metabolism, proinflammatory and immunosuppressive cytokines, chemokines, adhesion molecules, growth factors, neurohormones and neurotransmitters, all of which may profoundly influence the biological function of the skin.

Epidermal keratinocytes are often reported to be the prime target for UVB-induced damage, in that in vitro models suggest that little UVB penetrates into the dermis. However, in situ studies in human skin demonstrate that 2 MED of UVB (300 nm) induces specific DNA lesions in both dermal cells and hair follicle keratinocytes,[7] suggesting that UVB does have a direct effect on most resident skin cells.

Mast cells present in the upper dermis are important in the development of the early phase of erythema as they contain preformed mediators, particularly histamine, serotonin, and tumor necrosis factor (TNF), which stimulate vasodilation and the synthesis of prostaglandins and leukotrienes in neighboring cells.[19–21] Mast cell products can be detected within an hour of UVR exposure. The synthesis of prostaglandins and leukotrienes can also be initiated by UVR-induced oxidative damage to cell membranes by lipid peroxidation and their release parallels the development of erythema in humans in vivo.[22] The primary cytokine interleukin (IL)-1α is also stored preformed in keratinocytes and may be released as well at an early stage after UVR damage.

For the most part, however, mediators are not stored as preformed molecules but are synthesized following the activation of a variety of transcription factors. This leads to the upregulation of many genes central to the initiation of inflammation and recruitment of inflammatory cells to UVR-exposed skin.[23,24] As a result, proinflammatory cytokines,[25,26] chemokines,[26] complement components,[27] and adhesion molecules[26] are all readily detectable in human skin after in vivo UVR exposure.

An inflammatory infiltrate consisting largely of neutrophils and T lymphocytes appears in the upper dermis from as early as 3 h after UVB exposure and increases rapidly until 48 h. At 48 to 72 h, neutrophils and macrophages are also present in the epidermis.[28,29] These infiltrating cells contribute to the inflammatory process through the release of cytokines, superoxide, chemotactic factors, and proteases that alter the microenvironment and guide the recruitment of further immune effector cells.[30] Macrophages peak at 72 h after exposure and these may play an important role in the resolution of erythema, having been reported as the major producers of the immunosuppressive cytokine IL-10,[31] shown to downregulate a broad spectrum of proinflammatory cytokines.[32] Keratinocytes and macrophages also release transforming growth factor (TGF)-β, which may also play a role in the resolution of inflammation.[33,34]

Neuropeptides

Afferent sensory nerves innervating the epidermis and dermis are also capable of releasing a variety of neuropeptides after UVR exposure.[35] These products, such as substance P and calcitonin gene-related peptide (CGRP), may act as mediators for pain and itch as well as for inflammation and immune modulation. In addition, a range of skin cells, including melanocytes, keratinocytes, and endothelial cells, upregulate the production of neurotrophins and hormones such as proopiomelanocortin (POMC) peptides and their receptors. These mediators can then stimulate vasodilation, mast cell degranulation, the augmentation of UVR-induced cytokine production, chemokine production, and cellular adhesion molecule expression, all required for the activation and trafficking of inflammatory cells into the skin. There is also evidence that the mediators α-melanocyte stimulating hormone (α-MSH) and CGRP play an important role in the resolution of UVR inflammation.

Immunosuppression (See also Chap. 39)

It is well established that UVR exposure suppresses cutaneous cell-mediated immunity in humans. The depletion of Langerhans cells, the principal antigen-presenting cells in the epidermis, recruitment of macrophages into the dermis and epidermis, and release of inflammatory mediators such as TNF-α, IL-10, TGF-β, α-MSH, and CGRP, are all important events in the initiation of immunosuppression.[31,33–36] These changes result in an alteration to the antigen presentation process leading to the generation of regulatory T cells that inhibit cell-mediated immune responses to newly encountered antigens. Such UVR-induced immunosuppression plays an important role in the emergence and growth of nonmelanoma skin cancers in mice and a similar role is suspected in humans, because transplant patients maintained on immunosuppressive therapy have an elevated risk of both nonmelanoma and melanoma skin cancer, especially if they also have a history of high sun exposure.[37] Exposure to UVR also increases the incidence and severity of infectious diseases in animal models and suppresses the elicitation of immunity to some infectious agents in humans, therefore having theoretical implications for susceptibility to infectious diseases and vaccine effectiveness in humans.

Susceptibility to UVR-induced immunosuppression appears to be skin-type dependent. Thus, patients of skin phototypes I/II, who are at greater risk of skin cancer, are also more readily immunosuppressed

FIGURE 134-5

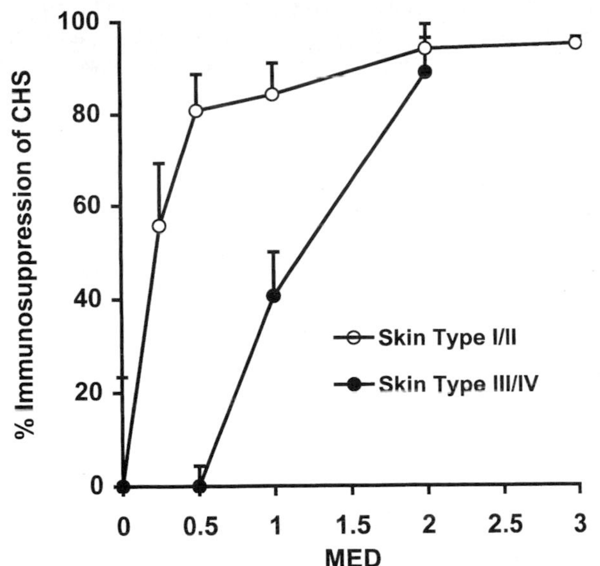

Erythema is a poor indicator of suppression of the induction phase of the contact hypersensitivity response. Patients with skin types I/II are suppressed with suberythemal exposure to solar simulated radiation, whereas erythemal exposures are necessary to suppress the CHS response in skin types III/IV. From Kelly et al.[38]

than patients of skin phototypes III/IV. Figure 134-5 shows that a single suberythemal exposure of SSR, of either 0.25 MED or 0.5 MED, can suppress cutaneous cell-mediated immune responses by 50 and 80 percent, respectively, in normal volunteers of skin types I/II, whereas a full MED may only induce 40 percent suppression in those of skin type III/IV.[38] Such data suggest that skin-type–dependent sensitivity to immunosuppression may be a risk factor for skin cancer.

DNA seems to be an important chromophore for UVR-induced immunosuppression because the enhanced repair of CPD inhibits immunosuppression in animal models and the release of immunoregulatory cytokines such as TNF and IL-10 in vitro.[39] The photoisomerization of *trans*-urocanic acid (UCA), a component of stratum corneum, has also been implicated in such immunosuppression, perhaps by triggering the degranulation of mast cells.[36]

Adaptive Responses of the Skin After UVR Exposure

TANNING (See also Chap. 88) It is important to distinguish between true melanogenesis, also known as delayed tanning, and immediate pigment darkening (IPD). Thus, the latter is an immediate but transitory grayish color induced by UVA and visible radiation and is believed to result from the photo-oxidation of existing melanins and the redistribution of melanocytic melanosomes from a perinuclear position into the peripheral dendrites, to which cellular microfilament and microtubular activity may contribute. Persistent pigment darkening (PPD) may then be regarded as that portion of the IPD response that remains stable for up to 2 h post exposure. There is no evidence that IPD and PPD are photoprotective.

Delayed tanning following UVR exposure is the result of increased epidermal melanin formation, the pigment becoming visible within days after UVB exposure. With exposure to the longer UVA wavelengths, tanning occurs earlier, sometimes blending with the IPD/PPD. Thus, with UVA, no apparent latency may be observed, while the tanning may also persist for prolonged periods. The action spectrum for tanning is broadly similar to that for erythema. However, for the UVB wavelengths, UVR effectiveness is greater for erythema than tanning in fair-skinned individuals,[40] while for UVA in darker-skinned subjects, it is greater for pigmentation. From these data, it is therefore likely that the mechanisms of melanin synthesis following UVB and UVA exposure are distinct.

UVB delayed tanning is associated with an increase in the activity and numbers of melanocytes. In general, single exposures increase only activity, while repeated doses are required to increase numbers. Melanocyte tyrosinase activity also increases, melanocyte dendrites elongate and branch, and melanosomes increase in number and size. This may sometimes result in small freckles, particularly in fair-skinned individuals, while large single exposures, such as might occur in severe sunburn, may lead instead to large freckles or even to solar lentigines.

UVA tanning has distinct effects that are wavelength dependent. Thus UVAI produces an increased melanin density localized to the basal cell layer, whereas UVAII increases the synthesis and transfer of melanized melanosomes to the epidermis, similar to the changes seen with UVB.

MECHANISMS OF UVR-INDUCED SKIN PIGMENTATION (See also Chap. 11) The rate-limiting enzyme in melanogenesis is tyrosinase, a copper-binding transmembrane glycoprotein localized to the melanosome. Thus, tyrosinase activity correlates closely with the melanin content of cultured pigment cells and increases during tanning. The mechanisms of melanogenesis have been reviewed by Gilchrest et al.,[41] who advocated an important role for DNA photodamage and its repair. This is supported by the known enhancement of melanogenesis in vitro and in animal skin in vivo after the administration of a synthetic thymidine dinucleotide (pTpT) that mimics bases excised during the repair of UVR-induced DNA damage. Such damage may also upregulate cell surface receptors for a variety of keratinocyte-derived melanogenic factors, in particular MSH. In addition, there may be an increase in the production and release of factors such as basic fibroblast growth factor (bFGF), nerve growth factor (NGF), endothelin-1, and POMC-derived products such as MSH, adrenocorticotrophic hormone (ACTH), β-lipotropic hormone (LPH), and β-endorphin, all of which regulate the molecular and cellular aspects of melanogenesis. Gilchrest et al.[41] also proposed that melanogenesis is a so-called mammalian SOS (i.e., survival) response to UVR exposure, which would suggest a relationship between skin type and the effectiveness of DNA repair. In accordance with this hypothesis, Sheehan et al.[11] provided the first evidence for better epidermal DNA repair after repeated SSR exposure in patients with skin type IV, which tans well, as compared with skin type II, which tans poorly.

PHOTOPROTECTION FROM UVR-INDUCED TANNING Several in vivo and in vitro human studies suggest that the acute photoprotection afforded by constitutive (racial) and facultative (induced) pigmentation against DNA photodamage in keratinocytes and melanocytes and against sunburn is equivalent to the wearing of a sunscreen with a sun protection factor (SPF) of 2 to 4[42] (see Chap. 247). Such comparable results for both DNA photodamage and erythema provide additional evidence that DNA is an important chromophore for erythema. Protection factors of 2 to 3 should clearly result in a 50 to 60 percent reduction of biologically effective dose and such a reduction, if maintained over long periods, would theoretically be significant in terms of long-term risk of skin cancer. However, the maintenance of a facultative tan requires repeated exposures to UVR from the sun or artificial sources and it seems highly likely that this would be associated instead with the accumulation of epidermal DNA photodamage[11] sufficient to negate the benefits of the protection. There are, however, conflicting data about the role of a tan in affording protection against the development of malignant melanoma in women, with Weinstock et al.[43] suggesting that a tan may afford some protection and Holly et al.[44] reporting no benefit.

HYPERPLASIA Hyperplasia of the dermis, epidermis, and stratum corneum also follow UVR exposure, a period of initial growth and cellular arrest for 24 to 48 h followed by increased activity for days thereafter. For example, 2 weeks of daily suberythemal SSR results in a 20 to 40 percent increase in the number of cell layers in the stratum corneum in patients of skin types I, II, III, and IV.[45] A number of studies suggest that such UVR-induced hyperplasia, particularly of the stratum corneum, plays a major role in photoprotection particularly in the fair-skinned, whereas other studies suggest a much more limited effect.[15]

ANTIOXIDANT DEFENSES Various enzymatic and nonenzymatic antioxidants protect against oxidative damage in UVR-exposed skin, and are dramatically depleted after UVR exposure. Thus enzymes of this type that repair oxidative injury include superoxide dismutase, catalase, and thioredoxin reductase, while natural antioxidants such as vitamins A, C, and E, as well as glutathione, also act directly to prevent oxygen radical damage. Antioxidants inhibit the human sunburn response,[46] immunosuppression, and photocarcinogenesis in mice.[47,48] Genetic variation at the glutathione S-transferase locus is also linked to variable susceptibility to sunburn[49] and to nonmelanoma and melanoma skin cancer risk in humans.[50,51]

Photosynthesis of Vitamin D

The apparent single beneficial effect of UVR on skin is the photochemistry that leads to the production of vitamin D_3 (cholecalciferol).[52] For most people, this vitamin derives mostly from the action of solar UVB on the skin, with dietary sources providing only a minor component of the daily requirement. During exposure to sunlight, UVB is absorbed by 7-DHC (previtamin D_3) situated in the plasma membrane of epidermal and dermal cells, and the resulting photoproduct, known as previtamin D_3, is converted over a day or so into vitamin D_3 through a thermally dependent rearrangement of its double bonds. Once this product is synthesized, it enters the circulation, bound with high specificity to vitamin D_3-binding protein, and travels to the liver to be hydroxylated to 25-hydroxyvitamin D [25(OH)D]. This is the major circulating form of vitamin D_3, which is, in turn, hydroxylated in the kidney to its active form, 1,25-dihydroxyvitamin D_3[1,25$(OH)_2$D]. 1,25$(OH)_2$D then interacts with vitamin D_3 receptors (VDRs) in the small intestine to increase the efficacy of intestinal calcium and phosphorus absorption, as well as with VDRs on osteoblasts to promote the mineralization of bone. VDRs are also present on keratinocytes as targets mediating calcitriol-associated induction of keratinocyte differentiation and inhibition of cell proliferation. As a result of these properties, topical vitamin D derivatives are now being used with therapeutic success in psoriasis. Skin immune cells also express VDRs, and studies suggest a constitutive immunosuppressive role for 1,25-$(OH)_2$D.[53]

Vitamin D intoxication cannot result from excessive sunlight exposure because both previtamin D_3 and vitamin D_3 are photolabile and are converted to other biologically inactive photoproducts. Furthermore, during repeated UVB exposure, photoprotection from tanning and hyperplasia decrease cutaneous vitamin D synthesis, as does constitutive pigmentation, white individuals producing the highest levels, followed by Orientals and Asians, while production is extremely attenuated in black skin. Elderly individuals have lower serum 25(OH)D levels, when compared with their younger counterparts, as a result of the progressive decrease in epidermal 7-DHC, such that acute UVB exposure in aged subjects also results in reduced serum vitamin D responses.

CHRONIC EFFECTS OF UVR

Skin Cancer: From DNA Photodamage to Tumors

(See also Chap. 38)

Basal cell carcinoma (BCC), squamous cell carcinoma (SCC), and malignant melanoma are reviewed in Chaps. 81, 80, and 93, respectively. A relationship between solar exposure and all types of skin cancer has long been established by extensive epidemiologic studies, and animal studies show that UVR, especially UVB, is a causal factor. Molecular epidemiology has also provided a direct link between nonmelanoma skin cancer and UVR-induced damage to epidermal DNA. At least 50 percent of BCC contain UVR signature mutations (C $\rightarrow$T or CC $\rightarrow$TT) at p53 sites that appear to be UVR mutation hotspots.[12] Chronic sun exposure leads to actinic keratoses (AK), which may spontaneously regress, but in some circumstances may progress instead to SCC. Brash et al.[12] investigated the cutaneous p53 mutations induced by UVR and noted that those present in more than 90 percent of SCC were also found in AK. UVR signature mutations have also been found in the PTCH gene in BCC[9] and in p53 in malignant melanoma,[54] all of which supports the epidemiologic data suggesting a causal role for solar UVR in cutaneous carcinogenesis.

UVB irradiation induces early epidermal apoptosis in the form of highly characteristic sunburn cells (SBC) that are apparent within 30 min of exposure and maximal at 24 h. Histologically, when stained with hematoxylin and eosin, SBCs have pyknotic nuclei and shrunken glassy, eosinophilic cytoplasm, as shown in Fig. 134-3*B*. SBC formation is thought to be a way of eliminating keratinocytes with carcinogenic potential, namely cells that have failed to adequately repair DNA. Inactivating p53 in mouse skin reduces the appearance of SBC, leading Brash et al.[12] to propose a relationship between sunburn and p53 in the onset of skin cancer. Thus, these authors suggest that UVR-induced p53 mutations result in a reduced SBC apoptotic response, which gives rise to a sunburn-based selection for clonal expansion of a p53-mutated cell into an actinic keratosis with possible further progression to an SCC. UVR thus may have a role as both tumor initiator and promoter.

The frequent appearance of clonal patches of p53-mutated keratinocytes in normal human skin (especially in chronically exposed sites)[55] supports the hypothesis that these mutations arise from aberrant stem cell proliferation rather than as random mutation events. This stem cell theory is further supported by the observation that these abnormal colonies are often arranged as conical clones, arguably arising from putative stem cells. Thus, protection from apoptosis results in a sunlight-induced selection pressure for clones of p53-mutated cells that are resistant to apoptosis and so able to accumulate further UVR-induced mutations that may lead to skin cancer. p53 clonal expansion is, however, a function of continuing UVR exposure rather than time, because these patches regress in mouse skin in the absence of continuing exposure.[56] p53-mutated keratinocyte clones are more frequent and larger in sun exposed skin. However, this does not necessarily mean all will become cancerous; rather, it means that larger colonies provide bigger targets with a greater chance for secondary mutations that can lead to cancer. Jonason et al.[55] suggested that p53 clonal expansion occurs by quantized colonization by the nonaggressive expansion of clones into compartments left empty by adjacent cells that have undergone UVR-induced apoptosis.

Our current understanding of nonmelanoma skin cancer is that DNA photodamage is the immediate acute effect that initiates a chain of molecular, mutational, cellular, and immunologic events that may lead to a skin tumor.

Photoaging (See also Chap. 144)

Photoaging is distinct from normal chronological aging. Clinically, photoaged skin is dry, deeply wrinkled, inelastic, leathery and telangiectatic, often with irregular pigmentation, freckling and lentigo formation (dermatoheliosis, Fig. 134-6). Histologically, such skin shows marked quantitative and qualitative abnormalities, particularly of the dermal connective tissue, including the accumulation of abnormal elastotic material, namely, elastosis, and proteoglycans. Furthermore, the degradation and disorganization of collagen fibrils, responsible for the strength and resilience of skin, have been observed.

There are no comprehensive epidemiologic data on photoaging but sunlight is firmly implicated through comparison of adjacent sun-exposed and sun-protected skin, and animal studies provide conclusive evidence for a significant role for UVR, especially UVB. Recently, it was hypothesized that UVR-induced tissue-degrading matrix metalloproteinases (MMPs) may be involved in photoaging.[57] MMPs belong to a family of zinc-dependent endopeptidases that degrade structural proteins such as collagens and elastin in connective tissue. Their proteolytic activity is regulated by endogenous tissue inhibitors of metalloproteinases (TIMPs) that inhibit the active MMPs by the formation of tight noncovalent 1:1 complexes. Single exposures of UVB and environmentally relevant doses of SSR induce MMPs and TIMPs gene expression in human skin within 24 h,[57,58] but the induction of MMP-1 is much greater than TIMP-1 at the mRNA level. MMP induction occurs through the activation of the AP-1 transcription factor. A current model of photoaging proposes that UVR-induced MMPs degrade the dermal matrix, which is followed by imperfect matrix repair. With repeated MMP induction over time, the faulty repair gives rise to a "solar scar" that manifests as skin wrinkling.[57] The chromophores for photoaging have not been investigated; these may well be molecules within cell surface receptors,[57] as well as DNA.[59]

FIGURE 134-6

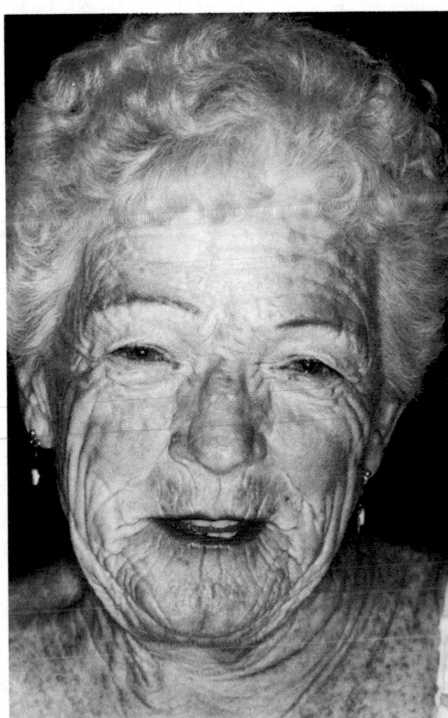

Dermatoheliosis. Severe fine and deep wrinkling. The skin appears waxy with a yellowish hue due to actinic elastosis.

REFERENCES

1. Quinn AG: Definition of minimal erythemal dose used for diagnostic phototesting. *Br J Dermatol* **131**:56, 1994
2. Diffey BL et al: The standard erythema dose: A new photobiological concept. *Photodermatol Photoimmunol Photomed* **13**:64, 1997
3. Diffey BL: Ultraviolet radiation and human health. *Clin Dermatol* **16**:83, 1998
4. Diffey BL, Gies HP: The confounding influence of sun exposure in melanoma. *Lancet* **351**:1101, 1998
5. Young AR: Chromophores in human skin. *Phys Med Biol* **42**:789, 1997
6. Young AR et al: The in situ repair kinetics of epidermal thymine dimers and 6-4 photoproducts in human skin types I and II. *J Invest Dermatol* **106**:1307, 1996
7. Young AR et al: The similarity of action spectra for thymine dimers in human epidermis and erythema suggests that DNA is the chromophore for erythema. *J Invest Dermatol* **111**:982, 1998
8. Young AR et al: Human melanocytes and keratinocytes exposed to UVB or UVA in vivo show comparable levels of thymine dimers. *J Invest Dermatol* **111**:936, 1998
9. Wikonkal NM, Brash DE: Ultraviolet radiation induced signature mutations in photocarcinogenesis. *J Invest Dermatol Symp Proc* **4**:6, 1999
10. Xu G et al: Effect of age on the formation and repair of UV photoproducts in human skin in situ. *Mutat Res* **459**:195, 2000
11. Sheehan JM et al: Repeated ultraviolet exposure affords the same protection against DNA photodamage and erythema in human skin types II and IV but is associated with faster DNA repair in skin type IV. *J Invest Dermatol* **118**:825, 2002
12. Brash DE et al: Sunlight and sunburn in human skin cancer: p53, apoptosis, and tumor promotion. *J Invest Dermatol Symp Proc* **1**:136, 1996
13. Anderson RR et al: A survey of the acute effects of UV lasers on human and animal skin, in *Lasers in Photomedicine and Photobiology,* edited by R Pratesi, A Sacchi. Berlin, Springer-Verlag, 1980, p 109
14. Diffey BL, Farr PM: Quantitative aspects of ultraviolet erythema. *Clin Phys Physiol Meas* **12**:311, 1991
15. Sheehan JM et al: Tanning in human skin types II and III offers modest photoprotection against erythema. *Photochem Photobiol* **68**:588, 1998
16. McKinlay AF, Diffey BL: A reference action spectrum for ultraviolet induced erythema in human skin. *CIE J* **6**:17, 1987
17. Anders A et al: Action spectrum for erythema in humans investigated with dye lasers. *Photochem Photobiol* **61**:200, 1995
18. Auletta M et al: Effect of cutaneous hypoxia upon erythema and pigment responses to UVA, UVB and PUVA (8-MOP + UVA) in human skin. *J Invest Dermatol* **86**:649, 1986
19. Gilchrest BA et al: The human sunburn reaction: Histologic and biochemical studies. *J Am Acad Dermatol* **5**:411, 1981
20. Pentland AP et al: Enhanced prostaglandin synthesis after ultraviolet injury is mediated by endogenous histamine stimulation. A mechanism for irradiation erythema. *J Clin Invest* **86**:566, 1990
21. Walsh LJ: Ultraviolet B irradiation of skin induces mast cell degranulation and release of tumour necrosis factor-α. *Immunol Cell Biol* **73**:226, 1995
22. Black AK et al: Time course changes in levels of arachidonic acid and prostaglandins D_2, E_2, F_2 alpha in human skin following ultraviolet B irradiation *Br J Clin Pharmacol* **10**:453, 1980
23. Bender K et al: UV-induced signal transduction. *J Photochem Photobiol B: Biol* **37**:1, 1997
24. Abeyama K et al: A role for NF-kappaB–dependent gene transactivation in sunburn. *J Clin Invest* **105**:1751, 2000
25. Barr RM et al: Suppressed alloantigen presentation, increased TNF-α, IL-1, IL-1Ra, IL-10 and modulation of TNF-R in UV-irradiated human skin. *J Invest Dermatol* **112**:692, 1999
26. Strickland I et al: TNF-α and IL-8 are upregulated in the epidermis of normal human skin after UVB exposure: Correlation with neutrophil

accumulation and E-selectin expression. *J Invest Dermatol* **108**:763, 1997
27. Rauterberg A et al: Complement deposits in epidermal cells after ultraviolet B exposure. *Photodermatol Photoimmunol Photomed* **9**:135, 1993
28. Tadashi T et al: Occurrence of neutrophils and activated T_H1 cells in UVB-induced erythema. *Acta Derm Venereol* **81**:8, 2001
29. Meunier L et al: In human dermis, ultraviolet radiation induces expansion of a CD36+ CD11b+ CD1− macrophage subset by infiltration and proliferation; CD1+ Langerhans-like dendritic antigen-presenting cells are concomitantly depleted. *J Invest Dermatol* **105:**782, 1995
30. Savage JE et al: Activation of neutrophil membrane-associated oxidative metabolism by ultraviolet radiation. *J Invest Dermatol* **101:**532, 1993
31. Kang K et al: CD11b+ macrophages that infiltrate human epidermis after in vivo ultraviolet exposure potently produce IL-10 and represent the major secretory source of epidermal IL-10 protein. *J Immunol* **153**:5256, 1994
32. Moore KW et al: Interleukin-10 and the interleukin-10 receptor. *Ann Rev Immunol* **19**:683, 2001
33. Lee H-ST et al: Modulation of TGF-β1 production from human keratinocytes by UVB. *Exp Dermatol* **6**:105, 1997
34. Stevens SR et al: Suppressor T cell-activating macrophages in ultraviolet-irradiated human skin induce a novel, TGF-β–dependent form of T cell activation characterized by deficient IL-2rα expression. *J Immunol* **155**:5601, 1995
35. Scholzen TE et al: Effect of ultraviolet light on the release of neuropeptides and neuroendocrine hormones in the skin: mediators of photodermatitis and cutaneous inflammation. *J Invest Dermatol Symp Proc* **4**:55, 1999
36. Hart PH et al: Mast cells in UVB-induced immunosuppression. *J Photochem Photobiol B: Biol* **55**:81, 2000
37. Euvrard S et al: Skin cancers in organ transplant recipients. *Ann Transplant* **2**:28, 1997
38. Kelly DA et al: Sensitivity to sunburn is associated with susceptibility to UVR-induced suppression of cutaneous cell-mediated immunity. *J Exp Med* **191**:561, 2000
39. Vink AA, Rosa L: Biological consequences of cyclobutane pyrimidine dimers. *J Photochem Photobiol B: Biol* **65**:101, 2001
40. Parrish JA et al: Erythema and melanogenesis action spectra of normal human skin. *Photochem Photobiol* **36**:187, 1982
41. Gilchrest BA et al: Mechanisms of ultraviolet light-induced pigmentation. *Photochem Photobiol* **63**:1, 1996
42. Young AR, Sheehan JM: UV-induced pigmentation in human skin, in *Sun Protection in Man,* edited by PU Giacomoni. Elsevier Science BV, St Louis, MO, 2001, p 357
43. Weinstock MA et al: Melanoma and the sun: The effect of swimsuits and a "healthy" tan on the risk of nonfamilial malignant melanoma in women. *Am J Epidemiol* **134**:462, 1991
44. Holly EA et al: Cutaneous melanoma in women. I. Exposure to sunlight, ability to tan, and other risk factors related to ultraviolet light. *Am J Epidemiol* **141**:923, 1995
45. Young AR et al: Photoprotection and 5-MOP photochemoprotection from UVR-induced DNA damage in humans: The role of skin type. *J Invest Dermatol* **97**:942, 1991
46. Montenegro L et al: Protective effect evaluation of free radical scavengers on UVB-induced human cutaneous erythema by skin reflectance spectrophotometry. *Int J Cosmet Sci* **17**:91, 1995
47. Steenvoorden DP, Beijersbergen van Henegouwen G: Protection against UV-induced systemic immunosuppression in mice by a single topical application of the antioxidant vitamins C and E. *Int J Radiat Biol* **75**:747, 1999
48. Black, H: The defensive role of antioxidants in skin carcinogenesis, in *Oxidative Stress in Dermatology,* edited by J Fuchs, L Packer. New York, Marcel Dekker, 1993, p 243
49. Kerb R et al: Deficiency of glutathione S-transferases T1 and M1 as heritable factors of increased cutaneous UV sensitivity. *J Invest Dermatol* **108**:229, 1997
50. Heagerty AH et al: Glutathione S-transferase GSTM1 phenotypes and protection against cutaneous tumours. *Lancet* **343**:266, 1994
51. Lafuente A et al: Phenotype of glutathione S-transferase Mu (GSTM1) and susceptibility to malignant melanoma. Multidisciplinary Malignant Melanoma Group. *Br J Cancer* **72**:324, 1995
52. Holick MF: Environmental factors that influence the cutaneous production of vitamin D. *Am J Clin Nutr* **61**(suppl):638s, 1995
53. Muller K, Bendtzen K: 1,25-Dihydroxyvitamin D_3 as a natural regulator of human immune functions. *J Invest Dermatol Symp Proc* **1**:68, 1996
54. Zerp SF et al: p53 mutations in human cutaneous melanoma correlate with sun exposure but are not always involved in melanoma genesis. *Br J Cancer* **79**:921, 1999
55. Jonason AS et al: Frequent clones of p53-mutated keratinocytes in normal human skin. *Proc Natl Acad Sci U S A* **93**:14025, 1996
56. Berg RJ et al: Early p53 alterations in mouse skin carcinogenesis by UVB radiation: Immunohistochemical detection of mutant p53 protein in clusters of preneoplastic epidermal cells. *Proc Natl Acad Sci U S A* **93**:274, 1996
57. Fisher GJ, Voorhees JJ: Molecular mechanisms of photoaging and its prevention by retinoic acid: Ultraviolet irradiation induces MAP kinase signal transduction cascades that induce AP-1 regulated matrix metalloproteinases that degrade human skin in vivo. *J Invest Dermatol Symp Proc* **3**:61, 1998
58. Lahmann C et al: Induction of mRNA for matrix metalloproteinase-1 and tissue inhibitor of metalloproteinases-1 in human skin in vivo by solar simulated radiation. *Photochem Photobiol* **73**:657, 2001
59. Hawk J: Skin photoaging and the health benefits of cutaneous photoprotection, in *Photobiology for the 21st Century,* edited by TP Coohill, DP Valenzeno. Valdenmar Publishing, Overland Park, Kansas, 2001, p 31

CHAPTER 135

John L.M. Hawk
Paul G. Norris
Herbert Hönigsmann

Abnormal Responses to Ultraviolet Radiation: Idiopathic, Probably Immunologic, and Photoexacerbated

Abnormal responses to ultraviolet radiation (UVR) exposure can be broadly categorized into four groups (Table 135-1): acquired idiopathic, probably immunologic photodermatoses; DNA repair-defective photodermatoses; photosensitization by exogenous drugs or chemicals; and dermatoses exacerbated by UVR. The first group, the idiopathic, probably immunologic photodermatoses, and the last, the photoexacerbated dermatoses, as well as the approach to assessing a photosensitive patient, are all discussed in this chapter; the other groups are covered in Chaps. 136, 149, and 155.

POLYMORPHIC (POLYMORPHOUS) LIGHT ERUPTION

Polymorphic (or polymorphous) light eruption (PMLE) is a common acquired disorder characterized clinically by the abnormal occurrence, within hours to a day or so of UVR exposure, of itchy, nonscarring, erythematous papules, vesicles, or plaques of some or, less commonly, all light-exposed skin. The lesions are generally symmetric, and they resolve completely over days to a week or two. Histologically, there is a dense, dermal, predominantly perivascular, lymphocytic cellular infiltrate.

Epidemiology

PMLE is the most common photodermatosis: approximately 20 percent of Scandinavians[1] and 10 to 15 percent of those living in the northern United States[2] and the United Kingdom[3] appear to suffer from the condition. Conversely, only 5 percent of Australians[3] and virtually no equatorial Singaporeans[4] have the disease. The prevalence of the condition thus increases steadily with increasing distance from the equator.

The disorder[1,2,5] usually has onset in the first three decades of life and affects females two to three times more often than males. It may occur in all skin types and racial groups but appears more commonly to affect relatively fair-skinned individuals. A positive family history is present in about a sixth of the patients.[1]

Etiology and Pathogenesis

A delayed-type hypersensitivity response to a sunlight-induced, cutaneous neoantigen, first proposed in 1942 by Stephen Epstein because of the hours usually taken for the eruption to develop, and the lesional histologic appearances, has proved almost certainly to be the cause of PMLE, although the now fairly substantial evidence for this remains circumstantial. The underlying reason for the occurrence of the disorder in any given patient appears likely to be genetic, perhaps 70 percent of all subjects having a tendency to the condition, but its actual expression depends on the degree of gene penetrance.[6] Furthermore, the inherited defect may be a diminished capacity in patients for normal UV-induced cutaneous immunosuppression.

INDUCTION OF PMLE Difficulty in the reliable laboratory induction of clinical lesions has long frustrated investigations into the

TABLE 135-1

Abnormal Reactions of Ultraviolet Irradiation

Acquired idiopathic, probably immunologic, photodermatoses	Polymorphic light eruption (PMLE) Actinic prurigo Hereditary PMLE of Native Americans Hydroa vacciniforme Solar urticaria Chronic actinic dermatitis
DNA repair-defective disorders	Xeroderma pigmentosum Cockayne's syndrome Trichothiodystrophy Bloom's syndrome Rothmund-Thomson syndrome (probable)
Photosensitization by exogenous drugs or exogenous or endogenous chemicals	Porphyrias Acute inflammatory reactions (phototoxicity) Eczematous reactions (photoallergy)
Dermatoses exacerbated by ultraviolet irradiation	

pathogenesis of PMLE. This frequent lack of response, often to adequate doses of artificially produced UVR, by patients who react readily to just suberythemogenic doses of natural sunlight, appears to relate to a number of variables. These include in particular the size of the UV irradiation site and its location and the irradiation of small, normally unaffected areas perhaps not eliciting sufficient immunologic stimulus to activate the response. It also may relate to the UV irradiation spectrum, irradiation dose, irradiation dose rate, and degree of cutaneous immunologic tolerance, which may be increased by any recent prior exposure.[7]

The complex interrelationships between factors such as these have contributed significantly to the conflicting nature of reports concerning the most effective wavelengths for PMLE induction. In most series, UVA (315 to 400 nm) has been more reliably effective than UVB (280 to 315 nm).[7,8] Thus, in one of these studies,[8] following exposures of buttock skin to UVA or UVB daily for 4 to 8 days, the action spectrum was in the UVA range in 56 percent, UVB in 17 percent, and both in 27 percent. However, Miyamoto[9] later confirmed earlier reports that induction with UVB can also be successful in a high proportion (57 percent) of selected patients. This apparent diversity in action spectrum for the induction of PMLE may very possibly be the result of different UV-evoked inducing antigens, as also appears likely in solar urticaria,[10] and perhaps also of different cutaneous levels for these antigens.

Contradictory results regarding the action spectrum for PMLE induction could also conceivably be accounted for by the presence of inhibitory wavelengths in some patients. Pryzbilla et al.[11] reported patients in whom the condition could not be induced by broad-spectrum UVA; however, lesions developed at sites deprived of the shorter UVA wavelengths by filters, suggesting an inhibiting effect by this waveband. This phenomenon has not been confirmed by other investigators, however, and remains speculative, but theoretically could be due to interference with photoallergen induction or with subsequent reactions, as are also suggested to occur on occasion in solar urticaria.[12]

Although chromophores for PMLE have not been identified, one study suggested that a form of heat shock protein may be responsible.[13] In addition, the induction of lesions by a UVA sunbed in the nontanning sacral pressure area[14] further suggests that the UV-chromophore interaction in some patients may be oxygen-independent.

Variation in the proportions of UVA and UVB present in terrestrial sunlight may also explain certain clinical characteristics of PMLE. Thus, the greater proportion of UVA to UVB in temperate climates and during the spring and fall months might be expected to contribute to a higher incidence of PMLE in temperate rather than tropical regions,[3] with greater susceptibility to the condition in spring and occasionally fall, rather than summer, in most patients. Moreover, the higher proportion of UVB to UVA in summer sunlight probably inhibits PMLE development through a predominantly UVB-induced cutaneous immunosuppressive mechanism. Paradoxically, the use of sunscreens, which often predominantly remove UVB but are also generally advised for PMLE patients and are required for normal sun protection, might also have the same UVA- and PMLE-enhancing effect.

IMMUNOLOGIC ASPECTS Early immunohistochemical characterization of the inflammatory infiltrate in naturally occurring PMLE lesions of uncertain and varying age gave inconsistent results. However, a later study[15] of timed biopsies from such lesions induced by low-dose, solar-simulated radiation demonstrated the consistent appearance of a T cell-dominated perivascular infiltrate within 5 h, peaking by 72 h. CD4+ T cells were most numerous in the early lesions, whereas after 72 h CD8+ T cells were predominant, perhaps helping to limit the previous immunologically mediated tissue damage. Increased numbers of dermal and epidermal Langerhans cells and dermal macrophages were also present. These findings are similar to those in allergic contact dermatitis and the tuberculin reaction, both known delayed-type hypersensitivity reactions, thus supporting a similar mechanism for PMLE.

Intercellular adhesion molecule-1 (ICAM-1), which assists lymphocyte tissue trafficking, is absent from resting keratinocytes but strongly induced on them by interferon-γ. Such expression has previously been demonstrated in the tuberculin reaction[16] and allergic contact dermatitis,[17] but not irritant contact dermatitis or following irradiation with two minimal erythema doses (MEDs) of UVB on normal skin.[16] ICAM-1 may therefore be a marker for immunologically specific responses, and its presence on keratinocytes overlying the perivascular infiltrate in PMLE[18] is probably secondary to interferon-γ release by immunologically activated lymphocytes in the underlying dermis, further supporting an immunologic basis for PMLE. Finally, in a study of PMLE patients, high-dose UVB and UVA irradiation increased the stimulatory capability of epidermal cells in unidirectional culture with autologous peripheral blood mononuclear cells,[19] again consistent with immune sensitization against autologous UV-modified antigens.

Beyond this, unpublished results by one of us (JH) indicate that patients with PMLE cutaneously immunosuppress significantly less easily than do normal subjects following solar simulated irradiation, such that they are more easily sensitized to dinitrochlorobenzene (DNCB) after UVR exposure than are normal subjects. This is very likely the genetically determined factor mentioned previously,[6] which leads to the putative immune recognition of photoinduced cutaneous antigen in PMLE but not normal subjects, although the antigen is presumably expressed in all individuals.

VARIATIONS IN ARACHIDONIC ACID METABOLISM In 13 of 23 patients with PMLE, the topical application of indomethacin for 2 h after irradiation inhibited UVB but not UVA erythema, as in normal subjects, whereas in the remaining 10 patients, it caused an abnormal augmentation of both UVB and UVA responses.[20] The 10 patients in the latter group had clinically more severe disease and more persistent lesions, and in general, they demonstrated abnormal erythemal responses to monochromatic UVA and sometimes to UVB irradiation. Such findings probably result from variations in disease severity rather than pathogenesis. However, polyunsaturated fatty acids compete with arachidonic acid as a substrate for prostaglandin A_2 resulting in the formation of less active prostanoids, and dietary supplementation with fish oil rich in omega-3 polyunsaturated fatty acids is reported to reduce both basal and UVB-generated prostaglandin levels in skin and to increase PMLE UVA-induced provocation thresholds,[21] leading to trials of their use in treatment.

Clinical Features

The eruption of PMLE[5] (Fig. 135-1) typically begins each spring, on sunny vacations, or after recreational sunbed use, often moderating with continuing exposure. Rarely, it occurs in winter after exposure to UVR reflected from snow; it may also occur only through window glass. Individual susceptibility varies considerably, the period of sun exposure needed to trigger the eruption usually being from 30 min to several hours, occasionally more or less, but often up to several days on vacations. Following exposure, new lesions appear after a latent interval of hours to days, but not less than about 30 min, although itching may develop sooner. In the absence of further exposure, all the lesions gradually subside completely without scarring over 1 to 7 days, occasionally 2 weeks, or, very rarely, longer in severe cases. In a given patient, the eruption tends always to affect the same skin sites, although its distribution may gradually spread or recede overall. Lesions also generally occur symmetrically and affect only some exposed sites, often those normally covered in winter such as the upper chest and arms.

FIGURE 135-1

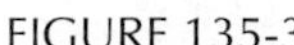

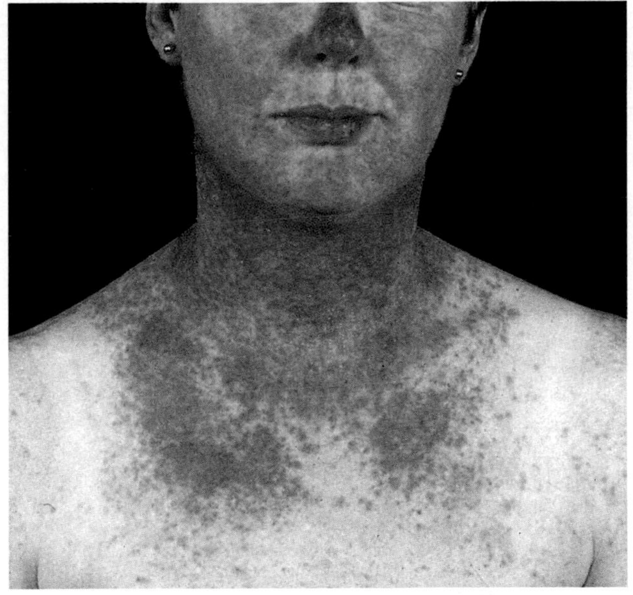

Polymorphous light eruption. Lesions are on habitually exposed sites, which is unusual because they most often occur on areas normally covered in winter.

Associated systemic symptoms are rare, but chills, headache, fever, nausea, and a variety of other sensations are possible. Over 7 years, 64 of 114 patients (57 percent) reported steadily diminishing sun sensitivity, including 12 (11 percent) who totally cleared.[22] There is a higher chance than normal of prior PMLE in patients with lupus, but very few patients with PMLE ever develop that condition.[23]

PMLE has many morphologic variants, while any combination of these is also possible. Thus, papular, papulovesicular (Fig. 135-2), plaque (Fig. 135-3), vesiculobullous, eczematous, insect bite-like, and erythema multiforme-like variants have been described, relating mostly to the clinical severity of the disorder and its site. Rarely, only pruritus may occur.[24] Such subdivisions do not apparently relate to differences in disease pathogenesis. The papular form, of either large or small separate or confluent lesions (generally tending to be in clusters), is the most common, followed by the papulovesicular and plaque variants; the others are rare. The eczematous form probably does not exist, representing instead chronic actinic dermatitis (see below), although PMLE may on occasion become secondarily lichenified or eczematized during resolution. Differing morphologies may also occur at different skin sites in the same patient; thus, diffuse facial erythema and swelling, for example, may accompany typical papular lesions at other sites. Complete sparing of small or large areas of exposed skin is an important characteristic distinguishing the disorder from other photodermatoses. Juvenile spring eruption,[25] which affects mainly boys, apparently represents an extreme example of this phenomenon. This condition is a self-limited eruption of pruritic grouped papules and vesicles confined to the light-exposed helices of the ears and characterized by a dense perivascular lymphocytic infiltration, although typical PMLE may sometimes coexist in the same patient. A final morphologic variant, a small papular form generally sparing the face and occurring after several days' exposure, has been designated as benign summer light eruption in continental Europe.

FIGURE 135-2

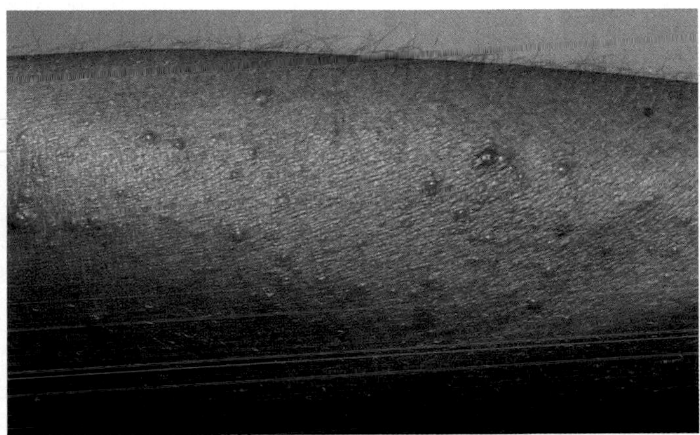

Polymorphous light eruption. Rash composed of papulovesicular lesions on an arm.

FIGURE 135-3

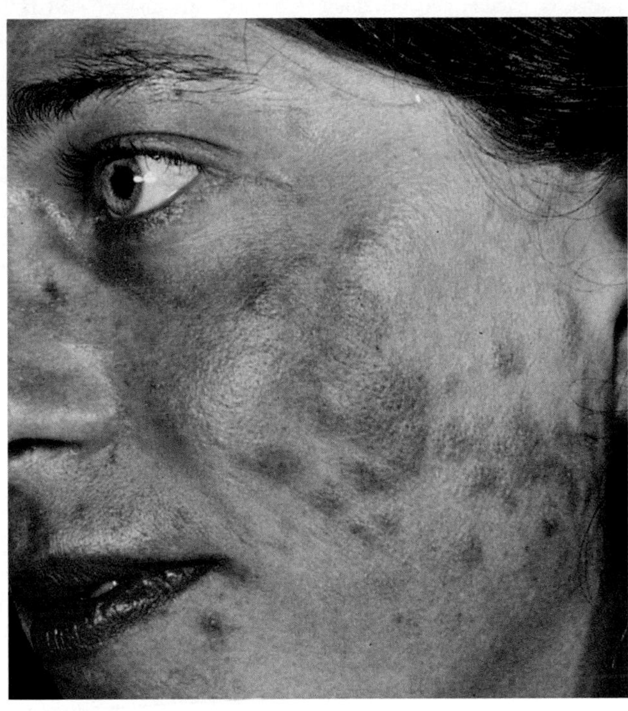

Polymorphous light eruption. Variably sized plaques on cheek, simulating lupus erythematosus. However, they disappear in a few days.

Histology

The histologic features[26] of PMLE are characteristic but not pathognomonic and vary with the different clinical presentations. There is a moderate to intense, tight, perivascular infiltrate in the upper dermis and mid-dermis in all clinical types, the infiltrate consisting predominantly of T cells. Neutrophils are also present, while eosinophils are infrequent. Other common features are upper dermal and perivascular edema and endothelial cell swelling, and while epidermal changes may be absent or variable in severity, spongiosis, occasional dyskeratosis, exocytosis, and basal cell vacuolization are common.

Diagnosis

Diagnosis is made largely on clinical grounds, particularly based on the time course for lesion evolution and the morphology of the eruption, particularly because the responses to routine phototesting are often normal except in very photosensitive patients. Subacute cutaneous lupus erythematosus, not generally itchy as in PMLE, must be excluded by measurement of the circulating antinuclear, anti-SSA and anti-SSB antibody titers. Persistent plaque-type PMLE must also be differentiated from Jessner's lymphocytic infiltrate of the skin, while the photoexacerbation of dermatoses, such as atopic and seborrheic eczema, may occur in susceptible subjects with the same time course as for PMLE, but with differing and characteristic morphologies. Erythropoietic protoporphyria must also be distinguished from the pruritic variant of PMLE without eruption, as must any exaggerated sunburn of patients with xeroderma pigmentosum or very fair skin. Finally, solar urticaria may be readily differentiated on history, its lesions being wheals and typically appearing within just 5 to 10 min and resolving within only 1 to 2 h.

Treatment

The mild disease of many patients is satisfactorily controlled by the moderation of sun exposure at times of high UVR intensity and the regular application of broad-spectrum sunscreens with high protection factors, particularly against UVA. However, as stated earlier, sunscreens protecting against mostly UVB may be ineffective, perhaps delaying the onset of protective cutaneous immunosuppression while permitting longer UVA exposure before sunburning. More severely affected subjects suffering frequent attacks of their disease throughout the summer, may instead require courses of prophylactic low-dose photo(chemo)therapy (see Chap. 266). Thus, in a controlled trial in which UVR exposure was monitored by means of polysulfone film lapel badges, PUVA was more effective than UVB, satisfactorily controlling symptoms in 91 percent, as compared with 62 percent, of cases.[27] Furthermore, in another study[8] of 122 patients treated with PUVA, total protection was achieved in 64 percent and partial protection in 26 percent; only 10 percent did not respond. The use of narrow-band 312 nm UVB phototherapy is now also becoming popular, being simpler to administer, as safe as or safer than, and apparently of comparable efficacy to PUVA (see Chap. 265).[28] Prophylactic PUVA or UVB may sometimes trigger the eruption, particularly in severely affected subjects, necessitating concurrent systemic corticosteroid therapy on occasion; this approach is usually effective.[29]

Patients who only develop their disorder during infrequent vacations also generally respond well to oral corticosteroids prescribed for them in advance.[29] If their eruption should develop, the medication is taken at the first sign of pruritus and then each morning till clear, usually after at most several days. Rare adverse effects of nausea or depression only occasionally necessitate stopping the drug. The treatment, if suitable and effective, may then be repeated every few months if required. Patients who are unsuitable for this approach or remain uncontrolled, however, may need phototherapy.

If none of the above therapies is effective or suitable, other potential therapies may be tried, but none are of certain efficacy. Such remedies include hydroxychloroquine,[30] which is occasionally helpful although not as much as tradition has long suggested; thalidomide,[31] which is helpful for some persistent forms; beta-carotene,[32] which is rarely useful; nicotinamide, which is probably not at all effective; and omega-3 polyunsaturated fatty acids, which are, perhaps, of moderate assistance in some patients.[21]

There then remains a small proportion of patients who are unsuitable for, unable to tolerate, or not helped by any of the above therapeutic measures. UVR avoidance may then be the only reasonable option. However, very few patients are so sensitive that they are continuously affected in spite of all reasonable UVR avoidance measures and, for them, intermittent immunosuppressive therapy with azathioprine or cyclosporine may be considered appropriate, their use having led to marked clinical improvement in a few patients.[33,34]

ACTINIC PRURIGO

Actinic prurigo (AP) is a not infrequent, persistent, pruritic, excoriated, papular or nodular eruption of the sun-exposed and, to a lesser extent, non-exposed skin. It is worse in summer and frequently fails to clear completely in winter, while also usually arising in childhood and sometimes remitting at puberty. The condition appears likely to be a persistent variant of the sometimes coexistent PMLE but is clinically different. A similar condition is hereditary or familial PMLE, which predominantly affects North, Central, or South Americans of native or mixed race; this form of the disease is normally more severe and persists into adulthood.

Pathogenesis

UVR exposure appears to be the inducer of AP in that the disorder is more severe in spring and summer, and that abnormal skin responses to monochromatic irradiation are present in up to two-thirds of patients, more commonly with UVA than with UVB.[5] In addition, solar-simulated radiation may occasionally evoke a response resembling that of PMLE, while a dermal, perivascular mononuclear cell infiltrate, also similar to that of PMLE, may sometimes be seen in early lesions. This has not yet been investigated immunohistochemically. Finally, the reported augmentation of UVA erythema[35] by the topical application of indomethacin, as in some patients with PMLE, again suggests that AP may be immunologically mediated.

AP on balance may thus be a slowly evolving, excoriated form of PMLE, and thus also a delayed type hypersensitivity reaction. This is supported by the fact that more AP patients than expected have close relatives with PMLE;[6] that human leukocyte antigen (HLA) DR4, occurring in some 30 percent of normal subjects, is present in around 80 to 90 percent of those with AP; and that the DR4 subtype DRB1*0407, occurring in some 6 percent of normal subjects and not infrequently also in Native Americans, is present in approximately 60 percent of those with AP.[36,37] This feature may be the genetic component responsible for converting PMLE into AP. In addition, some patients with the genetic characteristics of AP demonstrate clinical PMLE but have persistent lesions, while some with clinical AP may change to clinical PMLE and vice versa,[37] further suggesting a relationship between the two conditions. Inducing chromophores have not been studied, but may be the same as for PMLE.

Clinical Features

AP is more common in females and usually begins by the age of 10 years;[5] it then tends to improve and resolve by adolescence, but may on occasion persist into adult life. A positive family history occurs in some 15 to 50 percent of patients,[5] while atopy occurs in approximately 10 percent.[30] The AP eruption is often present throughout the year, but is generally worse in summer; very occasionally it occurs in winter instead, or else in both spring and fall, tolerance in these instances apparently developing during the summer. Furthermore, lesional exacerbations tend to occur in sunny weather rather than clearly following episodes of sun exposure, although PMLE-like outbreaks are possible. Lesions are typically pruritic, often excoriated, papules or nodules

FIGURE 135-4

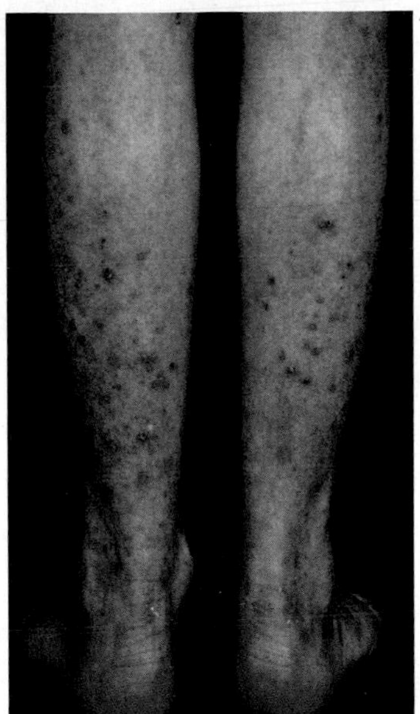

Actinic prurigo. Papules and nodules on legs of 15-year-old female.

(Fig. 135-4), associated with eczematization, lichenification, or crusting, at least on some sites. All exposed areas are usually involved, the condition being most severe on consistently uncovered sites but fading gradually toward normally covered skin. The latter is often also mildly affected, particularly over the sacral area and buttocks. Cheilitis, particularly of the lower lip, is also possible, while facial lesions may sometimes heal with small, pitted or shallow, linear scars.

Some patients clearly have PMLE or AP or both, but others may have a sufficiently mixed clinical picture to make precise diagnosis difficult. Thus, while AP almost always begins before age 10 years, PMLE may also begin in childhood. Furthermore, although individual AP lesions are generally more persistent than those of PMLE, lasting for weeks to months, those of PMLE may also be present on occasion for at least days to weeks. In addition, while AP is usually present all year round, patients with severe PMLE may also rarely be affected by winter sunshine. Finally, AP may be associated with a tendency to eczematization, but this might occasionally occur in PMLE, especially during its resolution phase. However, the often marked excoriation, the occasional mild scarring, and the usual fading of lesions toward and into covered skin sites in AP are very rare indeed in PMLE and their presence or absence tends usually to clarify the diagnosis.

Histology

Early papular lesions show changes similar to those of PMLE, namely mild acanthosis, exocytosis, and spongiosis in the epidermis and moderate lymphohistiocytic, dermal perivascular infiltration. In persistent, excoriated lesions, however, the epidermal features include also orthokeratosis, acanthosis, and sometimes hypergranulosis.

Diagnosis

Diagnosis is suspected on clinical grounds in the first instance, but there may be abnormal photosensitivity to monochromatic irradiation in up to two-thirds of patients,[5] which may involve the UVB, UVB and UVA, or, rarely, just UVA, wavelengths. In addition, lupus should be excluded by assessment of the circulating antinuclear factor and anti-SSA and anti-SSB antibody titers. Hepatic porphyria may occasionally need to be excluded by appropriate screening. Biopsy rarely aids diagnosis.

Treatment

The restriction of sun exposure and use of broad-spectrum, high-protection sunscreens may occasionally help milder cases, but these usually provide inadequate control. However, intermittent courses of low-dose thalidomide (50 to 200 mg at night) are very effective within a few weeks in the majority of patients,[38] although immediate, generally mild, side effects may include drowsiness, headache, constipation, and weight gain (see Chap. 264). To avoid peripheral neuropathy, the careful monitoring of nerve conduction every few months is also essential, while pregnancy must also be avoided because of the high risk of teratogenicity. If thalidomide is unavailable or unsuitable, PUVA therapy may occasionally be helpful. Thus, Farr and Diffey[39] successfully treated 5 patients twice weekly over 15 weeks, the skin shielded during treatment continuing to show abnormal UV sensitivity, however, suggesting a local mechanism of action. Nevertheless, this therapy seems to work more reliably as a prophylactic measure if the skin lesions are cleared first by thalidomide or by oral steroids. Chloroquine is not useful.

HEREDITARY POLYMORPHIC LIGHT ERUPTION OF NATIVE AMERICANS

This condition, which may affect North, Central, or South American patients of Native American or mixed race, appears indistinguishable from white AP except that it persists much more frequently into adulthood,[40] is clinically more severe, and regularly affects the lips and conjunctivae of patients. In addition, many patients have a positive family history and demonstrate the same HLA-DR4 and DRB1*0407 subtype positivity as their white counterparts.[41,42] Onset is in childhood and affected females outnumber males by 2 to 1, while the clinical features are similar to those of white AP, namely a pruritic, excoriated, papular, eczematized eruption of the sun-exposed areas of the face and limbs with minimal scarring. As stated earlier, there is also a marked associated tendency to cheilitis and conjunctivitis.

HYDROA VACCINIFORME

Hydroa vacciniforme (HV) is a very rare photodermatosis of unknown etiology that principally starts in childhood. It is characterized by recurrent crops of papulovesicles or vesicles most commonly on the face and the dorsa of the hands but other sun-exposed areas of the skin may also be involved. The vesicles resolve with pocklike scarring. The disease was first described by Bazin in 1862, and it is possible that before the clear definition of erythropoietic protoporphyria by Magnus and associates (see Chap. 149), some of the cases that were classified as hydroa may have been protoporphyria.

Pathogenesis

The pathogenesis of hydroa vacciniforme is unknown. No chromophores have been identified as yet. The UVB MED reaction is normal in the majority of patients but reduced UVA MED values have been found in some patients.[43] Blood, urine, and stool porphyrins are negative and all other laboratory parameters, including immunologic tests, are within normal limits. The course, distribution of lesions and histopathology, with a perivascular lymphocytic infiltrate, are somewhat reminiscent of polymorphic light eruption. However, the clinical features are quite different. The action spectrum lies in the UVA region and repetitive irradiation with broad spectrum UVA has been shown to elicit typical skin lesions that are clinically and histologically identical to those produced by natural sunlight.[44,45] Recent reports of an association with Epstein-Barr virus infection and lymphoma are interesting, but some of these cases are atypical, and may not represent the usual form of HV.[46–49]

Incidence

Although HV occurs in early childhood and may resolve spontaneously at puberty, some patients may suffer from life-long photosensitivity. There is a male predominance for the severe manifestations, whereas milder forms are more common in females.[43,45] Familial incidence is exceptional. In a recent study, the estimated prevalence of HV was about 0.34 cases per 100,000 with an approximately equal sex ratio. Males had a later onset and longer duration of disease than did females.[45]

Clinical Features

Erythema with a burning or itching sensation, and sometimes with associated swelling, begins within hours of sufficient sun exposure in light-exposed skin areas, particularly on the face and the hands. This is followed by the appearance of symmetrically scattered tender papules within 24 h. These generally later become vesicular, umbilicated, and, on occasion, confluent and hemorrhagic (Fig. 135-5). Within a few weeks, crusting followed by detachment of the lesions leaves permanent, depressed, hypopigmented scars. Vesicles and bullae, as well as the scars, resemble the lesions of vaccinia. Occasional systemic features include headache, malaise, and fever. HV usually occurs only during the summer months, and sometimes, but not always, improves or resolves in adolescence.[43,45]

FIGURE 135-5

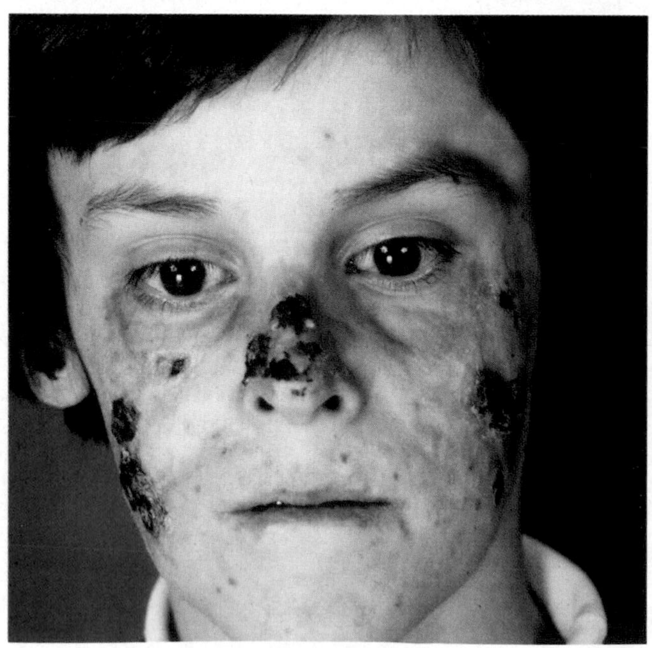

Hydroa vacciniforme. Vesicular, bullous, and crusted lesions on the face that will result in vacciniform scars.

Histology

Distinctive histologic changes include initial intraepidermal vesicle formation with later focal epidermal keratinocyte necrosis and spongiosis in association with dermal perivascular neutrophile and lymphocyte infiltration. Vasculitic features have also been reported.[43] Immunofluorescence findings are nonspecific.

Diagnosis

The differential diagnosis includes several photosensitivity states. However, the typical history and the clinical features are characteristic. Of particular importance, however, is the exclusion of erythropoietic protoporphyria which may rarely have similar morphology. An evaluation of erythrocyte protoporphyrin levels, red cell photohemolysis, and stool analysis will exclude protoporphyria.

Treatment

The treatment of HV consists of restriction of sun exposure and use of broad-spectrum sunscreens. Occasionally, antimalarials have been helpful, but their true value remains to be established. Similar observations have been made with beta-carotene, which in our hands, was ineffective in three cases. As in polymorphic light eruption, prophylactic phototherapy with narrowband UVB or PUVA may be helpful, particularly the latter, although it should be administered with care to avoid exacerbations.[43–45]

SOLAR URTICARIA

Solar urticaria (SU) is a rare but severely disabling, rarely even life-threatening, photosensitive disease in which UVR or visible irradiation leads to whealing of some or all exposed skin.

Pathogenesis

SU is due to an immediate type I hypersensitivity response to a cutaneous or circulating photoallergen generated from a precursor after the absorption of light energy. Both a circulating photoallergen and reaginic antibodies have been demonstrated.

Two types of SU have been proposed. Type I is an IgE-mediated hypersensitivity to specific photoallergens generated only in SU patients. Type II is an IgE-mediated hypersensitivity to a nonspecific photoallergen that is generated in both SU patients and others.[50] Therefore, in type I SU, passive transfer tests may be positive or negative, while, in type II, passive transfer tests are always positive. The diversity of the action spectra reported in the literature can be attributed to differences in photoallergens. Patients with type I appear to have a photoallergen of molecular mass 25 to 34 kDa and an action spectrum in the visible region, while those with type II may have a photoallergen of molecular mass 25 to 1000 kDa and a variable action spectrum.[50]

Urticaria develops on exposure to specific, characteristic, and usually broad-spectrum UVB, UVA, visible light, or a combination of these.[51] Susceptibility to the condition can occasionally disappear spontaneously, while the range of eliciting wavelengths can also narrow or broaden over months to years. However, the determination of action spectra has not led to the identification of chromophores.

Exposure to longwave visible or UVA radiation before, during, or after the urticaria-inducing irradiation inhibits whealing in some patients, possibly by inactivation of the initial active photoproduct or the inhibition of subsequent reactions. Conversely, Horio and Fujigaki[52] reported a patient with SU induced by 320 to 420 nm light in whom preirradiation with 450 to 500 nm visible light augmented the whealing. Postirradiation with the same spectrum failed to increase the response, suggesting that the energy in those wavelengths was absorbed by a precursor of the photosensitizer, altering it to a state more readily reactive to the urticaria-eliciting radiation (for references see Ref. 51).

Although mast cell degranulation and histamine release are implicated in SU, antihistamine therapy is only sometimes effective. This suggests the possible importance of other mediators, such as neutrophil and eosinophil chemotactic factors that accompany histamine in the venous blood draining irradiated skin. The initial mast cell degeneration is followed by the recruitment of circulating neutrophils and eosinophils, along with the tissue distribution of eosinophil major basic protein, which may, in turn, amplify the whealing response.[51]

True SU must not be confused with rare reactions due to photosensization by topical chemicals (e.g., tar, pitch, or dyes), protoporphyrin in erythropoietic protoporphyria, or some drugs (e.g., benoxaprofen) as these reactions are clinically different (see Chap. 136); only one patient with erythropoietic protoporphyria associated with SU has been reported. SU is not associated with an atopic background.

Clinical Features

SU is slightly more common in females, usually beginning between 10 and 50 years of age and persisting indefinitely, occasionally slowly worsening or gradually improving. Within 5 to 10 min of sun exposure, patients experience itching, erythema, and patchy or confluent whealing (Fig. 135-6), which resolves generally with sun avoidance within 1 to 2 h; very rarely, however, the onset of symptoms has been reported to be delayed by several hours.[53] SU may affect only normally covered skin, sparing the face and hands, because of a hardening phenomenon or usually all exposed sites, while sharp demarcation at lines of clothing is often seen in more severe cases; bruised skin appears particularly susceptible.[54] Attacks may be accompanied by headache, nausea, bronchospasm, faintness, and syncope, especially if extensive areas of the skin are affected.

FIGURE 135-6

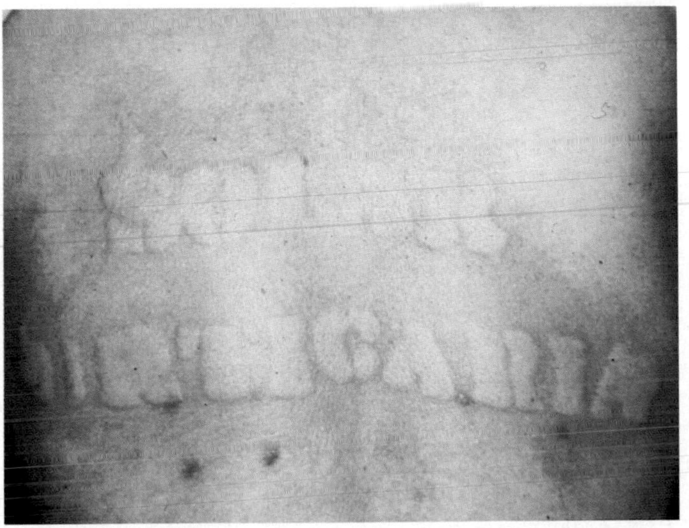

Solar urticaria. These lesions appeared within 15 min of sun exposure, with wheals and marked pruritus. They were produced by irradiating the back of this patient through a template.

Differential Diagnosis

The primary diagnostic criteria are itching, burning, erythema, and whealing, which only appear after sun exposure and usually disappear within 1 to 2 h. The timing criterion is a guideline for the differential diagnosis from PMLE, which has the same localization, but PMLE lesions usually appear between hours to days after sun exposure and generally take 2 to 6 days to disappear after its avoidance. In addition, the lesions are not limited to wheals. Confirmation of the diagnosis of SU is given by phototesting, with transient itching or burning erythema and whealing occurring at the immediate reading. Primary SU should be differentiated by history from drug- or chemical-induced phototoxicity, which can also cause a burning sensation within minutes of sun exposure.

Histology

There is dermal vasodilation and edema, while light-microscopic study of timed biopsies of induced lesions of SU has demonstrated a dose-dependent increase, predominantly perivascular, in upper dermal neutrophil and eosinophil numbers at 5 min and 2 h but not at 24 h. Endothelial cell swelling is also observed in early lesions, while late infiltration by mononuclear cells is seen only following high doses of radiation. In addition, staining by indirect immunofluorescence for eosinophil granule major basic protein shows extensive extracellular deposition in the dermis at 2 and 24 h, suggesting eosinophil degranulation.[55]

Diagnosis

Phototesting with an irradiation monochromator or broad-spectrum irradiation source generally allows confirmation of the diagnosis and definition of the action spectrum of SU. Several lamps can be used for phototesting, such as inexpensive fluorescent tubes or a more sophisticated solar simulator, while the most detailed phototesting procedure involves a xenon lamp combined with a monochromator; the urticarial reaction usually disappears in a few minutes. It is very important to realize that a negative phototest from a single light source does not exclude a diagnosis of solar urticaria, it being necessary to continue provocative testing with other light sources, such as polychromatic light sources, a slide projector, or even directly with sunlight.

Treatment

High-protection-factor sunscreens and appropriate clothing cover may be useful in UVB-sensitive subjects, but are much less effective in those sensitive to UVA and particularly visible light. However, nonsedating H_1 antihistamines may help significantly, increasing the minimum whealing dose tenfold or more. The addition of H_2 blockers rarely may offer a slight further advantage. In many patients chronically exposed skin, such as on the face and the hands, becomes tolerant. Based on this observation, therefore, patients with SU can be treated with repeated artificial UV exposures; this can be done with narrowband UVB, broadband UVB, UVA alone, a combination of UVB and UVA, and even visible light. The major disadvantage of phototherapy is that the tolerance obtained usually lasts only a few days, although a more lasting effect is obtained with PUVA, the protection provided lasting several weeks. Such regimens do not alter tissue histamine content or mast cell numbers, however, and they may act via nonspecific photoinduced stabilization of the mast cell activation mechanism or possibly through the persistent occupation of IgE-binding sites with photoallergen.[55] Multiple exposures with increasing doses within a day ("rush hardening") also appear to be quite successful.[56] In addition, in patients with a detectable serum factor, removal of this by plasmapheresis has resulted in clinical remissions persisting several months.[57,58]

CHRONIC ACTINIC DERMATITIS

Chronic actinic dermatitis is a persistent, generally eczematous, sometimes pseudolymphomatous eruption, worse in summer, with corresponding histologic features. It is induced and maintained by exposure to often very small amounts of UVB, often UVA, and sometimes also visible radiation; rarely, UVA alone appears responsible. It most commonly affects elderly men with outdoor interests, although many other subjects are also susceptible. The syndromes of persistent light reactivity, actinic reticuloid, photosensitive eczema, and photosensitivity dermatitis (Table 135-2), each independently named more than 30 or more years ago, are now all considered variants of the same condition. The disorder appears in all respects to have the features of allergic contact dermatitis, and thus may be an acquired, delayed-type hypersensitivity reaction to endogenous, photoinduced, epidermal antigen(s).

Historical Aspects (See Table 135-2)

The possibility of persistent light reactivity appears to have been first mentioned in 1933 by Haxthausen, who described continuing photosensitivity in a patient intravenously injected with trypaflavine, following which Wilkinson, in 1961, reported an epidemic in older males of a prolonged photoallergy to tetrachlorosalicylanilide, an antibacterial agent present in soaps and hair toiletries. Jillson and Baughman then named this condition persistent light reaction.[60] Thus, following continuing cutaneous contact with photoallergens such as the halogenated salicylanilides, musk ambrette, or quinoxaline dioxide, occasional patients developed a photoallergic contact dermatitis to these substances, and a very few progressed to a persisting abnormal photosensitivity of not just exposed skin but often also covered sites, despite an apparent complete avoidance of exposure to the offending chemicals. Further, whereas the action spectrum for the initiating photocontact reaction generally encompassed just the UVA wavelengths, that of the persistent disorder generally included the UVB, and occasionally visible light.

In 1969, Ive et al.[61] introduced the term actinic reticuloid to describe a similar, but apparently more severe, dermatosis; in this case, however, there was no apparent prior photoallergen. Nevertheless, the condition again affected mostly elderly males, and it was characterized by infiltrated, erythematous plaques, on an eczematous background, predominantly affecting exposed sites. The histopathologic features tended to resemble cutaneous T cell lymphoma, and there were abnormal cutaneous photobiologic responses to UVB, UVA, and, occasionally, visible radiation. Furthermore, although the authors noted a resemblance to persistent light reactivity, photopatch tests to all common photoallergens were negative in their patients. Similar, but purely eczematous variants of the condition, also without overt preceding photoallergy, were also described, with action spectra limited to the UVB (photosensitive eczema)[62] or UVB ± UVA (photosensitivity dermatitis).[63]

In 1979, Hawk and Magnus[64] proposed that actinic reticuloid, photosensitive eczema, and photosensitivity dermatitis be incorporated into the one syndrome of chronic actinic dermatitis (CAD), the validity of which was supported by reports of the transition of actinic reticuloid to photosensitive eczema,[65] and the occasional association of the clinicopathologic features of actinic reticuloid with just UVB photosensitivity, a variant with no specific name. Furthermore, in view of the close clinical, histological, and photobiological resemblances between persistent light reactivity and CAD, the end-stage persistent light reactivity syndrome and CAD also appear to be the same. Patients who do not demonstrate increased sensitivity to UVB irradiation on covered skin in the absence of an external photoallergen are excluded, however, thereby differentiating the persistent photosensitivity of CAD from the transient light reactivity of photoallergic contact dermatitis, which may nevertheless rarely eventually progress to CAD (see also Chap. 136).

Etiology and Pathology

The mechanism underlying the transition from photoallergy to CAD, in cases in which this disorder is in fact a precursor, remains unclear. Any explanation needs to account for the increased UVB, rather than just UVA, sensitivity of skin that has had no direct contact with any relevant chemical. However, it seems very possible[66] that during the initial localized photoallergic reaction, a normal skin constituent is altered to become antigenic, the induction of the local response apparently beginning with UVA-dependent covalent photochemical binding of hapten to endogenous protein, followed by an eczematous delayed-type hypersensitivity response. In the localized reaction, hapten must be present, but with the progression to CAD, UVB ± UVA irradiation alone may trigger the immune response at any site, very possibly by the continuing formation of antigenic photoproduct from the ubiquitous endogenous carrier protein alone. This outcome now also appears possible, and, in fact, usual, without any prior photoallergy. Kochevar and Harber,[67] using an in vitro model with the photosensitizer tetrachlorosalicylanilide, provided theoretical support for such a mechanism, demonstrating that the phototoxic oxidation of histidine with the modification of carrier protein into weak antigen was indeed possible. Although the chromophores for such putative antigen formation have not been

TABLE 135-2

Original Published Criteria for Eczematous Photosensitivity Disorders

Persistent light reactivity (Wilkinson, 1961)[59]	Eczematous eruption predominantly affecting light-exposed skin associated with photosensitivity to UVB ± UVA with preceding acute photoallergic contact dermatitis.
Actinic reticuloid (Ive et al., 1969)[61]	Infiltrated papules and plaques on light-exposed skin associated with lymphoma-like histologic appearances in some cases, photosensitivity to UVB + UVA, sometimes also visible light, and negative photopatch tests.
Photosensitive eczema (Ramsay and Kobza-Black, 1973)[62]	Morphologic and histologic changes of eczema predominantly affecting light-exposed skin, with photosensitivity confined to UVB, and negative photopatch tests.
Photosensitivity dermatitis (Frain-Bell et al., 1974)[63]	Morphologic and histologic changes of eczema predominantly affecting light-exposed skin, with photosensitivity to UVB ± UVA, and positive (photo) patch tests in proportion of cases.
Chronic actinic dermatitis (Hawk and Magnus, 1979)[64]	A syndrome including photosensitive eczema, photosensitivity dermatitis, and actinic reticuloid; persistent light reactivity is now also included.

identified, the action spectrum for CAD induction resembles that for sunburn inflammation,[68] at least in many instances, for which DNA is already considered the most likely main target. Thus, perhaps DNA, or a similar or related molecule, may also act as an antigen in CAD.

The histologic and immunohistochemical features of CAD, including adhesion molecule expression, are essentially the same as those of persistent allergic contact dermatitis,[69,70] or, in more severe cases, cutaneous T cell lymphoma (CTCL). In particular, the dermal infiltrate consists predominantly of T lymphocytes with a significant trend toward lower CD4+/CD8+ ratios in patients with more florid histology,[69] features that may also all occur in persistent, pseudolymphomatous forms of allergic contact dermatitis. Thus, the occurrence of the actinic reticuloid variant of CAD may, in fact, reflect prolonged and marked endogenous antigenic stimulation.

Allergic contact dermatitis commonly coexists with CAD, often preceding the onset of any photosensitivity,[71] reactivity to one or more allergens occurring in 75 percent of patients.[72] Sesquiterpene lactone extracts from Compositae plants are implicated most commonly, but other allergens may include fragrance, colophony, rubber, and sunscreens. Such substances do not cause positive photopatch test reactions, although they may cause phototoxic reactions in vitro,[73,74] including the ability to oxidize histidine, and might contribute additionally to altering endogenous protein to antigenic forms leading to CAD. As also proposed for persistent light reactivity, the avoidance of such substances may conceivably result in gradual resolution of the condition.[75] In addition, chronic cutaneous immunostimulation from constant patient exposure to airborne allergens during simultaneous ultraviolet exposure, as in gardening, may enhance cutaneous immune recognition of the putative, presumed weak, endogenous photoallergen.

Although photoallergy may progress to CAD and then to the actinic reticuloid variant[76] in a proportion of patients, there is often no evidence of preceding photoallergy. CAD is thus likely to represent an end state that may arise from a number of predisposing conditions, namely photoallergic contact dermatitis, allergic contact dermatitis to substances with possible phototoxic potential, endogenous eczema,[77] perhaps photosensitivity from oral medication, possibly polymorphic light eruption, and human immunodeficiency virus infection.[78] Finally, CAD also appears not uncommonly to arise de novo in normal subjects.

Significant exposure to sunlight, both photoaging the skin and activating putative endogenous photosensitizer, may lead to CAD in men such as gardeners, who are also regularly exposed to important airborne antigens such as Compositae oleoresins. Aged skin may also be more susceptible as a result of reduced barrier function and allergen removal. Finally, because only small doses of UVR are needed to evoke the eruption, the increased melanin of black skin does not apparently protect against the condition.

Clinical Features

Chronic actinic dermatitis usually affects the middle-aged or elderly throughout many areas of the world,[74,78,79] approximately 90 percent of patients being male. Occurrence under 50 years of age is unusual, unless patients have coexistent atopic eczema.[77] The eruption is usually worse in summer and after sun exposure, although patients may often fail to recognize this, particularly if affected year-round. Patchy or confluent eczematous changes are present on the exposed skin of the backs of the hands, face (Figs. 135-7 and 135-8), scalp, and upper chest, often with some degree of sparing of the skin of the finger webs, of the upper cyelids, behind the ears, and in the depths of skin creases. Severely affected patients also characteristically demonstrate shiny, erythematous, infiltrated papules or confluent plaques on exposed sites, sometimes abruptly adjacent to patches of normal exposed skin. Irregular hyper- and hypopigmentation, sometimes marked, may also

FIGURE 135-7

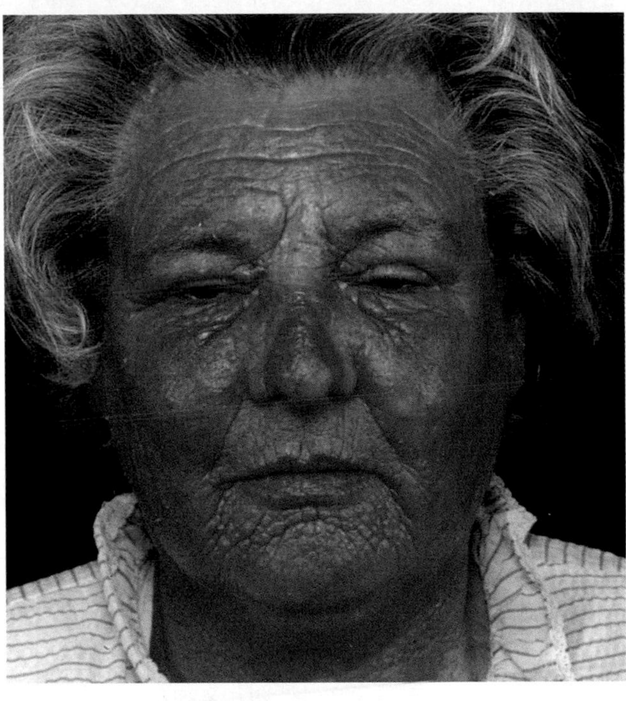

Chronic actinic dermatitis. Infiltrated eczematous eruption on face.

occur. In addition, there is the occasional progression to erythroderma, often, but not always, accentuated on exposed sites. Large numbers (up to 20 percent) of circulating CD8+ Sézary cells may be found in such patients without any suggestion of malignancy.[80] An association with lymphoma has, however, been reported but such reports are rare and any association may be coincidental, particularly because T cell receptor and immunoglobulin gene rearrangement studies fail to demonstrate any evidence of clonal lymphoid proliferation.[81]

Histology

Histologic features[26] include epidermal spongiosis, acanthosis, and, sometimes, hyperplasia, along with a predominantly perivascular lymphocytic cellular infiltrate confined to the upper dermis, milder cases having the appearance of chronic eczema. Severe CAD, however, may mimic CTCL histologically, with epidermal Pautrier-like microabscesses and a deep, dense epidermotropic mononuclear cell infiltrate, sometimes with hyperchromatic convoluted nuclei and giant cells, but no marked increase in mitoses.

Diagnosis

Phototesting of the skin is essential to confirm the diagnosis of CAD, and is characterized by abnormally low erythemal thresholds with eczematous or pseudolymphomatous responses characteristic of the disorder itself following irradiation with UVB, and, in the majority of patients, also UVA. A minority of patients react also to the visible wavelengths, while a very small number may be sensitive to UVA alone, although drug or chemical photosensitivity must be carefully excluded in such instances. Such testing must be performed on uninvolved skin not exposed to systemic or topical corticosteroid administration over the preceding 3 to 4 days to avoid false-negative results. Broad-spectrum

FIGURE 135-8

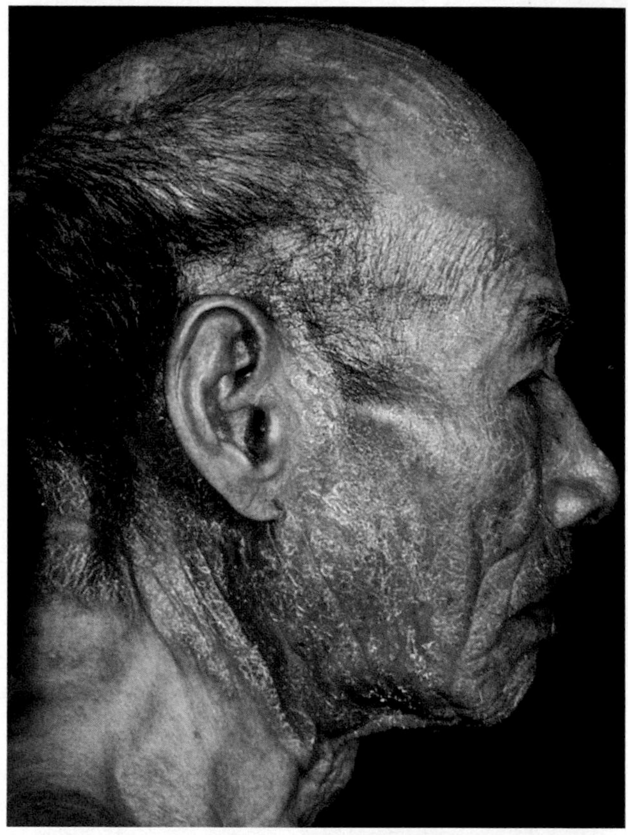

A.

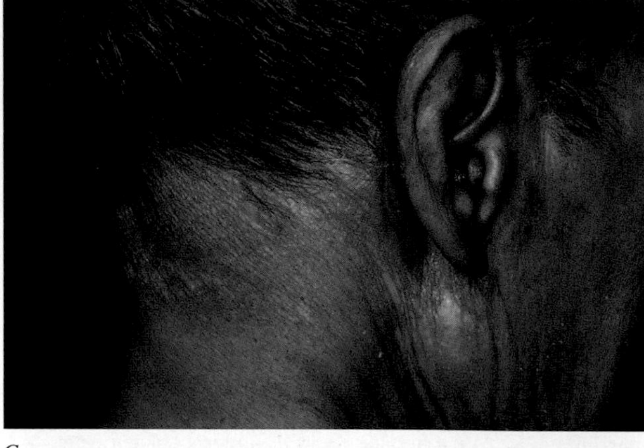

C.

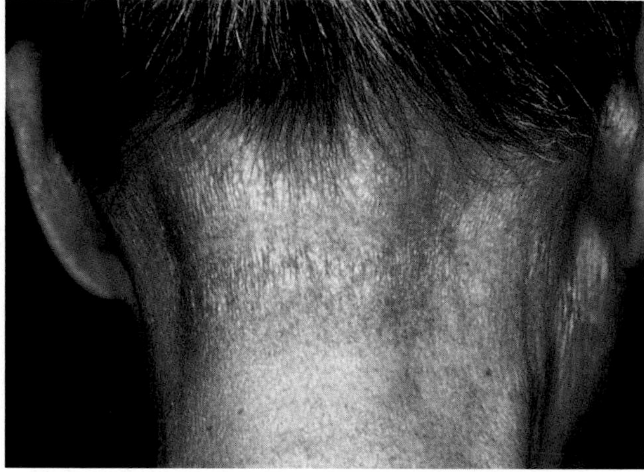

D.

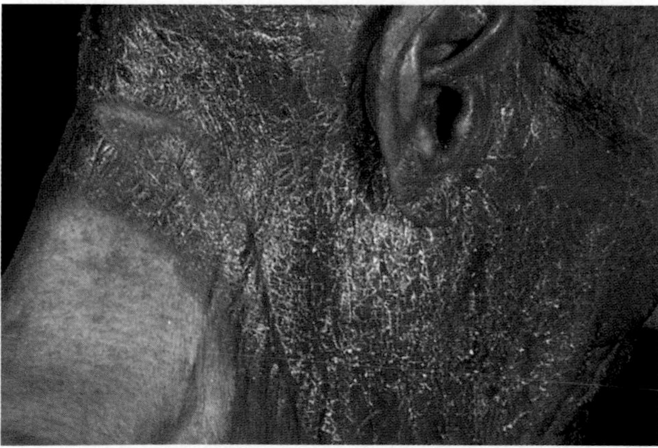

B.

Chronic actinic dermatitis. *A, B.* Severe involvement of face and neck with marked eczematous dermatitis. *C, D.* In this instance, the disease resolved with a course of oral PUVA photochemotherapy over several weeks. Oral corticosteroids were necessary initially, however, to control the exacerbation induced by irradiation.

or monochromatic sources may both be effective at inducing abnormal responses, although the latter determine the action spectrum for the disease more precisely. Light-exacerbated endogenous eczemas must be distinguished by their differing clinical features and usually normal light tests, while CTCL may also rarely be photosensitive, more commonly to UVA than UVB. Such photosensitivity, however, is usually clinically mild.

Patch and photopatch tests are also essential in suspected CAD. Contact sensitivity to airborne or other ubiquitous allergens such as Compositae oleoresins, perfume, or colophony are able to mimic or coexist with CAD. In addition, secondary contact or photocontact sensitivity to sunscreens or topical applications may also occur. Finally, photopatch testing may also detect primary photoallergic contact dermatitis such as to the fragrance, musk ambrette.

Treatment

The treatment of CAD is usually difficult and often only partially effective. In the first instance, the rigorous avoidance of UVR and exacerbating allergen exposure and regular application of broad-spectrum topical sunscreens of low irritancy and allergenic potential (e.g., containing microfine titanium dioxide) are essential but rarely adequate as sole measures. Topical steroids and emollients and occasionally topical tacrolimus or pimecrolimus may help, but, in approximately two-thirds of resistant patients, azathioprine, 50 mg twice or three times daily, achieves remission within several months,[82] following which the drug dose may be reduced. However, recurrent therapeutic courses, generally each summer, are usually necessary. Cyclosporine too has been used and may give excellent results,[83] while mycophenolate mofetil can also be helpful. Finally, low-dose PUVA, and perhaps narrow-band UVB therapy, may be effective (see Chap. 266), although potent oral and topical steroid cover is generally necessary to avoid disease flares early on. As a result of these interventions, most CAD patients can now lead a reasonable life, until, in due course, many gradually recover from their disorder.[75]

PHOTOEXACERBATED DERMATOSES

Photoexacerbated (or photoaggravated) dermatoses represent a heterogeneous group of conditions that share one common feature: they can be precipitated or exacerbated by exposure to sunlight or to therapeutic or cosmetic UVR in at least a proportion of cases (Table 135-3). It is however important to recognize that these diseases are not true photodermatoses because they commonly develop without exposure to radiation. The precise underlying mechanisms of their exacerbations are generally undetermined, but UV irradiation apparently contributes specifically to pathogenesis in some disorders, such as lupus erythematosus, while in others, it may be just a nonspecific factor able to worsen the condition. Some of the disorders most frequently and importantly affected in this way are discussed below.

Acne (See also Chap. 73)

Acne aestivalis, as first described by Hjorth et al.,[84] was characterized by pruritic, 1- to 3-mm, pink or pale, dome-shaped papules occurring after sun exposure, usually on the face, neck, or trunk. Nieboer[85] then further reported two patients, describing the disorder as actinic superficial folliculitis with a predominantly follicular, pustular, nonpruritic rash occurring several hours after sun exposure, on the upper trunk and arms. Verbov[86] finally described patients with overlapping features of both acne aestivalis and actinic superficial folliculitis, suggesting the unifying term actinic folliculitis. The condition appears to be a form of UVR-exacerbated acne, for which high-protection-factor sunscreens, standard acne treatments, including topical retinoic acid,

TABLE 135-3

Diseases Exacerbated by Ultraviolet Irradiation

Acne
Atopic eczema
Carcinoid syndrome
Cutaneous T cell lymphoma
Dermatomyositis
Disseminated superficial actinic porokeratosis
Erythema multiforme
Familial benign chronic pemphigus (Hailey-Hailey disease)
Granuloma annulare
Keratosis follicularis (Darier's disease)
Lichen planus
Lupus erythematosus
Pellagra
Pemphigus foliaceus (erythematosus)
Pityriasis rubra pilaris
Psoriasis
Reticulate erythematous mucinosis syndrome
Rosacea
Seborrheic eczema
Transient acantholytic dermatosis (Grover's disease)
Viral infections

and topical and systemic antibiotics have not generally been helpful. Oral isotretinoin was however prophylactic and highly effective in two cases.[87]

Darier's Disease (See also Chap. 54)

There are not many reports of photosensitivity in Darier's disease. However, controlled tests with mainly UVB radiation have shown that lesions can be induced that exhibit the clinical and histopathologic criteria of the disease. The exacerbation of Darier' s disease after sun exposure is also well-documented, and one of the authors found exacerbation in two patients experimentally treated with psoralen photochemotherapy (PUVA).

Disseminated Superficial Actinic Porokeratosis (See also Chap. 56)

Disseminated superficial actinic porokeratosis (DSAP) may be induced or exacerbated by sun exposure, or by immunosuppression,[88] which suggests that the exacerbation by sunlight in part reflects the UVR-induced impairment of local cutaneous immunity.

Several authors have also reported the induction of new lesions or exacerbation of preexisting ones following exposure to artificial UVR radiation sources, in particular, during the long-term treatment of psoriasis,[89,90] and the disorder has also been aggravated by suntan parlor exposure. Furthermore, in a study of potentially provocative wavelengths, UVB plus UVA was more effective in inducing new or exacerbating preexisting lesions than either wavelength alone.[91]

Herpes Simplex (See also Chap. 214)

It is common knowledge that many patients experience herpes simplex eruptions after sun exposure, particularly while sunbathing, mountain hiking, or skiing at higher altitudes. The mechanisms for viral activation by UVR are unknown but may be related to localized UVR immune suppression. However, several other nonspecific stimuli, such as fever, hormonal changes (menses), or heat, can trigger herpes lesions. Reports on sunlight-induced erythema multiforme may actually reflect the fact that herpes may precipitate erythema multiforme. Finally, relapsing gluteal herpes simplex is not uncommon in patients treated with UVB or PUVA (see Chap. 266).

Lichen Planus Actinicus (See also Chap. 49)

In addition to being able to trigger lichen planus as a Koebner reaction to sunburn injury, UV irradiation in suberythemogenic doses can also induce a lichenoid reaction known as lichen planus actinicus.[92] The condition most commonly affects dark-skinned subjects, particularly from the Middle East, but patients have also been reported from India, Europe, and the United States. Several clinical patterns have been described. The most common consists of annular, hyperpigmented plaques predominantly on the face and dorsa of the hands. Others include pigmented melasma-like patches on the face and neck, or skin-colored, closely aggregated, pinhead papules particularly on the face and dorsa of the hands.[92,93] The peak age of onset is the third decade, and the lesions are generally only mildly pruritic, developing mainly on exposed sites during spring and summer and improving or remitting in winter. Experimental reproduction of lesions was successful in one patient with UVB but not with UVA.[94] Histopathology is identical to classic lichen planus.

Eczema (See also Chaps. 122 and 124)

Patients with atopic or seborrheic eczema occasionally report mild to moderate, nonspecific exacerbation of their condition following sun exposure. Normal responses are generally demonstrated on phototesting, thus allowing distinction from chronic actinic dermatitis. However, the majority of patients with atopic dermatitis actually benefit from both sunlight and artificial UV irradiation.

Lupus Erythematosus (See also Chap. 171)

Photosensitivity has been reported for several so-called collagen vascular diseases such as lupus erythematosus or dermatomyositis. However, only in lupus erythematosus (LE) is the correlation between sunlight exposure and the development of skin lesions well established. Therefore, photosensitivity that results in a specific skin rash has been added to the American Rheumatological Association (ARA) list of criteria to diagnose systemic lupus. The estimated prevalence of photosensitivity in this disease ranges from 30 to 70 percent in the white population. It is important to recognize that different subsets of lupus erythematosus show different degrees of photosensitivity. Chronic cutaneous LE with typical discoid lesions is usually not photoaggravated. However, discoid lesions occur primarily on sun-exposed areas such as the face, scalp, and ears, and some patients with discoid LE will progress to systemic LE. Whether such progression occurs in photosensitive patients only is unclear. In systemic LE, the typical butterfly rash may appear suddenly after sun exposure. Also widespread lesions may develop in other exposed skin areas associated with systemic exacerbation. The subset that exhibits photosensitivity most strikingly is subacute cutaneous LE. About 50 percent of these patients fulfill the ARA criteria for systemic LE but systemic manifestations tend to be milder than in patients with classical systemic LE.[95,96] Patients with subacute cutaneous LE tend to have anti-Ro (SSA) antibodies that represent predictors of photosensitivity. Thus, several studies have supported the hypothesis that UVB irradiation may induce Ro antigens in the disease to translocate to the keratinocyte membrane by a glycosylation and microfilament-dependent process. At the membrane, they are bound by Ro autoantibodies, which leads to immunologic cell lysis, probably by antibody-dependent cellular cytotoxicity.[97–99]

The action spectrum for the induction of LE skin lesions includes both UVB and UVA and there are reports about exacerbation during photochemotherapy for psoriasis. Lehmann et al.[100] investigated the reproduction of LE lesions with artificial UVR in 128 patients. They found the development of lesions on exposure to UVA and UVB in 53 percent, on exposure to UVA alone in 14 percent, and on exposure to UVB in 33 percent. Interestingly, lesions were induced in 64 percent of patients with subacute cutaneous LE, in 42 percent of patients with chronic discoid LE, and in only 25 percent of patients with systemic LE.[100] This strongly supports the idea that discoid LE is photoaggravatable. In view of this study and several previous investigations, photosensitivity to broadband UVR in LE is a well-documented phenomenon.[101] Because exacerbations can be provoked by UVA and UVB, appropriate broad-spectrum sun protection should be recommended for all forms of LE.[95]

Pellagra (See also Chap. 145)

Pellagra is characterized clinically by skin abnormalities, gastroenteritis, and encephalopathy, the cutaneous features often being sunlight-induced, appearing in the spring and summer and improving in winter. Pruritus and erythema occur initially on exposed areas, followed by vesicles, bullae, and essentially symmetric, chronic, scaly, hyperpigmented, thickened sclerotic papules and plaques. Dusky erythema and powdery scaling of the nose, a scaling collarette around the neck with sternal extension (Casal's necklace), glossitis, and mucous membrane ulcerations are also typical. The inducing wavelengths are unknown, as no lesions or other abnormalities have been demonstrated following artificial irradiation. It seems likely that decreased availability of NADP and NADPH resulting from niacin deficiency may prevent the oxidation/reduction reactions necessary for the normal repair of UVR-induced epidermal damage.

Pemphigus (See also Chap. 59)

Pemphigus vulgaris is not clinically associated with photosensitivity, although artificial UVR induction of lesions with typical acantholysis has been noted. Pemphigus foliaceus and erythematosus may however be aggravated or induced by sun exposure, characteristic lesions having also been produced in both variants with experimental UVR.[102,103]

Bullous Pemphigoid (See also Chap. 61)

A few patients have been described who developed bullous pemphigoid lesions after UVB exposure. However, more cases have been reported in which photochemotherapy (PUVA), given for unrelated diseases, was the triggering mechanism.[104]

Psoriasis (See also Chap. 42)

Some patients with psoriasis report exacerbation of their disease after sunbathing, particularly, after sunburn. Several groups have also attempted to estimate the prevalence of photosensitivity in psoriasis from surveys and questionnaires. Ros et al. sent questionnaires to 2000 patients with psoriasis in Stockholm, and after telephone interviews, considered the prevalence of photosensitivity to be 5.5 percent. In this study, in addition, the light-sensitive patients with psoriasis had a history of PMLE with a secondary exacerbation of their psoriasis in 43 percent of cases, and were more likely to have skin phototype I, psoriasis affecting their hands, a family history of psoriasis, and an advanced age.[105] Interestingly, despite photosensitivity, such patients can be successfully treated with PUVA. It is thus very likely that the phenomenon of photosensitive psoriasis represents a Koebner type of reaction to either PMLE or sunburn in fair-skinned subjects.

APPROACH TO THE PATIENT WITH PHOTOSENSITIVITY

Clinical Features

History taking is frequently the most important element in diagnosis of the photodermatoses, particularly of the intermittent conditions in which the eruption is often not present at the time of consultation. The following features of the eruption are of particular importance.

Exposure:
Latent interval between exposure and eruption
Seasonal variation
Minimum exposure duration to elicit eruption
Response to irradiation through window glass or clothing
Eruption:
Duration
Distribution
Morphology
Accompanying or premonitory symptoms (such as pruritus, dizziness, burning sensation, swelling)

Patient:
Age at onset
Sex
Occupation (outdoor or indoor, such as sailor, farmer, welder, roofer, gardener, phototherapist)
Topical applications or contacts (such as cosmetics, sunscreen, plants, chemicals, perfumes, sprays, aftershaves)
History of skin response to sun exposure (rash or susceptibility to sunburn)
History of effectiveness of sunscreens in prophylaxis
Systemic medications
Leisure activities such as gardening, outdoor pursuits
Family history

To establish the relationship between an eruption and UVR exposure, it is important in most patients to determine whether the exposed sites are affected predominantly, whether the condition is worse in summer, and whether the lesions develop only in association with UVR exposure. If photosensitivity is present, the eruption tends to occur on the forehead; bridge of nose; upper cheeks; chin; rims of ears; back and sides of the neck; upper chest; dorsa of the hands and feet; and extensor surfaces of the arms and lower legs. On the other hand, sparing characteristically occurs below the eyebrows; under the hair fringe; on the upper eyelids; below the nose, lower lip, and chin; behind the earlobes; in the webspaces of the fingers; and at the bottom of skin folds or creases. Involvement of the latter sites can sometimes occur, however, if allergic contact dermatitis to airborne allergens or extreme photosensitivity is present.

Central to the diagnosis of the acute intermittent photodermatoses is the time course of the eruption following sun exposure. Thus, onset within 5 to 10 min with resolution in an hour or so is typical of solar urticaria and photosensitivity due to certain drugs such as benoxaprofen (which has been withdrawn from the market) or amiodarone. A delay of 20 min to several hours with lesions lasting for several days is characteristic of PMLE, HV, erythropoietic protoporphyria, subacute cutaneous LE and other light-exacerbated dermatoses, and xeroderma pigmentosum, as well as drug photosensitivity to, for example, thiazide diuretics.

A description of the morphology of the eruption is also of great diagnostic importance. Patients with SU describe raised pruritic wheals, sometimes confluent, whereas those with erythropoietic protoporphyria or drug photosensitivity to amiodarone or previously benoxaprofen complain of an often severe, painful, burning sensation with initially no visible signs. Later they may develop diffuse swelling and erythema of the exposed sites with prolonged exposure. HV is differentiated from PMLE by its characteristic blistering response always leading to varioliform scarring. Helpful in distinguishing PMLE from subacute cutaneous LE are the usual lack of pruritus and the presence of discrete scaling plaques in the latter, although an eruption indistinguishable from PMLE has also been described in some subacute cutaneous LE patients.

Photoexacerbated dermatoses must be distinguished by their morphologies and distribution. Xeroderma pigmentosum and most drug-induced photosensitivity, on the other hand, can lead to an exaggerated sunburn-like response, which, in the case of xeroderma pigmentosum, may not reach its peak until 48 to 72 h after exposure.

In patients who report a more persistent, apparently photosensitive eruption, the morphology of lesions should be carefully considered. Persistent pruritic papules, occurring mostly on exposed sites but also involving the upper limbs and sometimes buttocks, are suggestive of AP. An eczematous eruption accentuated on or limited to the exposed sites suggests CAD, particularly if there is a history of exposure to potential airborne contact allergens such as the Compositae oleoresins or colophony, but this must be differentiated from light-aggravated endogenous eczema and perhaps eczematous drug-induced photosensitivity (e.g., thiazide-induced) (see Chap. 136), although the latter seems rare. Fragility and blistering with scarring of the exposed skin, worse in the summer, suggests a hepatic porphyria or pseudoporphyria, particularly if drug or excessive alcohol ingestion, or frequent sunbed exposure, has occurred (see Chap. 149).

Other important general points in the history, often helpful in diagnosis, include the age at onset—young girls most often suffer from AP, children from HV, young women from PMLE, and elderly men from CAD. A family history of photosensitivity is sometimes present in AP, PMLE, and the porphyrias. Finally, a reaction to sun exposure through window glass may assist in diagnosis and treatment by suggesting the action spectrum of the eruption, as UVB radiation is absorbed by glass. Certain occupations or leisure activities may permit exposure to allergens or photocontact allergens, such as in outdoor workers or enthusiasts, in whom CAD is possible. Deterioration in the condition despite regular sunscreen application should suggest the possibility of allergic contact dermatitis to one of the sunscreen constituents.

Laboratory Studies

Unless the diagnosis is otherwise certain, important investigations in all cases of photosensitivity include measurement of the circulating antinuclear factor, anti-SSA (Ro) and anti-SSB (La) antibody titers, and of blood, urine, and stool porphyrin concentrations. Lesional skin histology, particularly in PMLE, HV, and CAD, may also be helpful, but rarely diagnostic. Direct immunofluorescence, however, can assist in the diagnosis of LE. On the other hand, phototesting of unaffected skin, usually of the back with narrow-waveband or monochromatic irradiation, may induce the eruption and thus define the action spectrum in certain disorders. This type of testing is however only moderately reliable overall, while solar simulating and broad-waveband irradiation are more effective eruption inducers but give less idea of the action spectrum. In eczematous photosensitivity, patch and photopatch testing are also important to identify any inducing or exacerbating allergens. Finally, special techniques, such as the measurement of DNA excision repair or the rate of recovery of RNA synthesis in cultured fibroblasts following UV irradiation, are also required to make the diagnosis in certain genophotodermatoses.

Phototesting

Phototesting of the unaffected skin, usually on the back, may assist in the diagnosis of photosensitivity and help to identify the responsible wavelengths by demonstrating reduced erythemal thresholds or reproducing the typical lesions. Table 135-4 lists the disorders in which such testing is likely to be helpful. Several suitable protocols have been described, either relatively simply with broad-spectrum light sources and filters if necessary, or, preferably, for precise definition of the action spectrum, with an irradiation monochromator. Sunlight with filters may also be used in some parts of the world but is generally too unpredictable for regular and reliable use (for references see Refs. 106 and 107).

Solar simulators produce imitation sunlight from xenon arc lamps; excitation of the highly compressed gas produces a continuous emission spectrum approximating fairly closely that of terrestrial sunlight after the unwanted wavelengths shorter than 285 nm and longer than 700 nm have been removed by appropriate filters. Such sources most reliably induce the typical eruption of the photodermatoses, enabling confirmation of the diagnosis, while further filters can also be used to enable some degree of action spectrum determination.

An irradiation monochromator (normally incorporating a xenon arc source, input slit, collimating mirror, and output slit) is required to establish precise action spectra, but the experience necessary for its

TABLE 135-4

Phototest Responses in Photosensitivity Disorders

	ACTION SPECTRUM	FREQUENCY OF ABNORMAL FINDINGS
Actinic prurigo	UVA > UVB	Sometimes
Chronic actinic dermatitis	UVB ± UVA ± visible light	Always
Drug-induced photosensitivity	UVA > UVB	Frequent
Hydroa vacciniforme	UVA	Sometimes
Photoallergic contact dermatitis	UVA	Frequent (if allergen present)
Polymorphic light eruption	UVA > UVB	Sometimes
Solar urticaria	UVB, UVA, visible or combination	Frequent

correct use and the appropriate interpretation of results is such that this sophisticated and expensive equipment is not generally available. The apparatus emits any chosen narrow waveband with reliable purity, although usually relatively low irradiance, which may be accurately quantified with an appropriate radiometer such as a thermopile.

A number of other less expensive, more versatile, and more robust radiation sources have also been used to investigate patients with photosensitivity. For example, mercury vapor arc lamps emit throughout most of the solar spectrum but with superimposed isolated lines of relatively high output, rather than the smoothly continuous spectrum produced by the xenon arc. Thus, the Kromayer lamp has been a widely available, convenient, mobile, medium-pressure source emitting mostly in the UVB and UVC regions, but the difficulty in precise determination of the wavelengths and doses of light emitted have made it useful mainly for rapid nonquantitative studies or occasionally treatment. Fluorescent lamps on the other hand are low-pressure mercury arc glass tubes coated on their inner surfaces with fluorescent phosphors made of alkaline earth salts, which then convert the internally emitted 254-nm mercury line into a variety of external broadband outputs, for example, UVA or UVB. Such lamps can be used for phototesting in relatively inexpensive and easily constructed systems, if necessary with filters. However, they are even more useful for phototherapy and, in the case of UVA lamps, also for photopatch testing.

Phototesting is usually performed on the unaffected skin of the back, although the attempted induction, for example of PMLE, is best undertaken on previously involved skin. Systemic glucocorticoids in high doses should not have been administered nor test sites treated with topical glucocorticoids in the preceding few days in order to avoid false-negative results. Furthermore, both patient and investigator must wear protective goggles.

Photopatch Testing (See also Chap. 136)

Photopatch testing is a well-established method to use for identifying phototoxic or photoallergic substances. It should be performed whenever a phototoxic reaction or photoallergic contact dermatitis is suspected. Diseases of the CAD spectrum are also indications for testing. In the latter, contact sensitivity may also be noted to airborne allergens such as plant oleoresins, which may have an inducing or exacerbating role in CAD. Other photodermatoses, such as PMLE, HV, SU (see above), or porphyrias, are diagnosed according to specific criteria of these entities and do not represent an indication for the photopatch test.

For patients who present with unclear photoreactions that cannot be associated with a genuine photodermatosis, photopatch testing should also be performed. This holds true in particular for patients with eczema in a photodistribution, or those with exacerbated sunburn reactions. Such lesions are suspicious for photoallergic or phototoxic reactions, respectively, and a careful history should evaluate all drugs and topical preparations. Among those, the photosensitizer should be identified in the photopatch test. Following such stringent criteria for photopatch testing, unnecessary test procedures are avoided and the positive test reactions obtained are likely to be highly relevant for the patients.

Test materials are applied to the back in a duplicate set, one for irradiation, the other as a control. Patches to be irradiated are left on the skin for 24 h; control patches are applied for either 24 or 48 h. Nonirradiated patches are used as controls to exclude nonphotoinduced plain contact sensitivity. Test sites are evaluated before and immediately after irradiation as well as 24, 48, and 72 h later. Control sites are read shortly after removal of the patches as well as 24 and 48 h later.

Until the early 1980s, the photopatch test procedure was not standardized. Differences between the recommended test procedures included variations in the range of test substances, the irradiation doses, the precise irradiating wavelengths, the timing of the irradiation, the irradiance used, and the delay before reading the responses. The first attempt to devise a standard method was initiated by the Scandinavian Photodermatitis Research Group (SPRG).[108] Following this example, the German photopatch test working group was founded in 1984 in Germany, Austria, and Switzerland. This group also established a standardized protocol for photopatch testing.[109]

REFERENCES

1. Ros A, Wennersten G: Current aspects of polymorphous light eruption in Sweden. *Photodermatology* **3**:298, 1986
2. Morison WL, Stern RS: Polymorphous light eruption: A common reaction uncommonly recognized. *Acta Derm Venereol (Stockh)* **62**:237, 1982
3. Pao C et al: Polymorphic light eruption: Prevalence in Australia and England. *Br J Dermatol* **130**:62, 1994
4. Khoo SW et al: Photodermatoses in a Singapore skin referral center. *Clin Exp Dermatol* **21**:263, 1996
5. Norris PG, Hawk JLM: The idiopathic photodermatoses: polymorphic light eruption, actinic prurigo and hydroa vacciniforme, in *Photodermatology*, edited by JLM Hawk. London, Arnold, 1999, pp 178–190
6. McGregor JM et al: Genetic modeling of abnormal photosensitivity in families with polymorphic light eruption and actinic prurigo. *J Invest Dermatol* **115**:471, 2000
7. Hölzle E et al: Polymorphous light eruption: Experimental reproduction of skin lesions. *J Am Acad Dermatol* **7**:111, 1982
8. Ortel B et al: Polymorphous light eruption: Action spectrum and photoprotection. *J Am Acad Dermatol* **14**:748, 1986
9. Miyamoto C: Polymorphous light eruption: Successful reproduction of skin lesions, including papulovesicular light eruption, with ultraviolet B. *Photodermatology* **6**:69, 1989
10. Leenutaphong V et al: Pathogenesis and classification of solar urticaria: A new concept. *J Am Acad Dermatol* **21**:237, 1989
11. Pryzbilla B et al: Polymorphous light eruption: Eliciting and inhibiting wavelengths. *Acta Derm Venereol* **68**:173, 1988
12. Leenutaphong V et al: Solar urticaria induced by visible light and inhibited by UVA. *Photodermatology* **5**:170, 1988
13. McFadden JP et al: Heat shock protein 65 immunoreactivity in experimentally induced polymorphic light eruption. *Acta Derm Venereol (Stockh)* **74**:283, 1994.
14. Tegner E, Bradin AM: Polymorphous light eruption in hypopigmented pressure areas with a UVA sunbed. *Acta Derm Venereol (Stockh)* **66**:446, 1986
15. Norris PG et al: Polymorphic light eruption: An immunopathological study of evolving lesions. *Br J Dermatol* **120**:173, 1989
16. Norris PG et al: The expression of endothelial leukocyte adhesion molecule (ELAM-1), intercellular adhesion molecule-1 (ICAM-1), and vascular cell adhesion molecule-1 (VCAM-1) in experimental cutaneous

inflammation: A comparison of ultraviolet B erythema and delayed hypersensitivity. *J Invest Dermatol* **96**:763, 1991
17. Vejlsgaard GL et al: Kinetics and characterization of intercellular adhesion molecule-1 (ICAM-1) expression on keratinocytes in various inflammatory skin lesions and malignant cutaneous lymphomas. *J Am Acad Dermatol* **20**:782, 1989
18. Norris PG et al: Adhesion molecule expression in polymorphic light eruption. *J Invest Dermatol* **99**:104, 1992
19. Gonzales-Amaro R et al: Immune sensitization against epidermal antigen in polymorphous light eruption. *J Am Acad Dermatol* **24**:70, 1991
20. Farr PM, Diffey BL: Effects of indomethacin on UVB- and UVA-induced erythema in polymorphic light eruption. *J Am Acad Dermatol* **21**:230, 1989
21. Rhodes L et al: Dietary fish oil reduces basal and ultraviolet B-generated PGE_2 levels in skin. *J Invest Dermatol* **105**:532, 1995
22. Jansen CT, Darvonen J: Polymorphous light eruption. A seven-year follow-up evaluation of 114 patients. *Arch Dermatol* **120**:862, 1984
23. Murphy GM, Hawk JLM: The prevalence of antinuclear antibodies in patients with apparent polymorphic light eruption. *Br J Dermatol* **125**:448, 1991
24. Dover JS, Hawk JLM: Polymorphic light eruption sine eruptione. *Br J Dermatol* **118**:73, 1988
25. Hawk J: Juvenile spring eruption is a variant of polymorphic light eruption. *N Z Med J* **109**:389, 1996
26. Hawk JLM et al: The photosensitivity disorders, in *Lever's Histopathology of the Skin* edited by DE Elder, R Elenitsas, C Jaworsky, B Johnson Jr. Philadelphia, Lippincott-Raven, 1997, pp 305–310
27. Murphy GM et al: Prophylactic PUVA and UVB therapy in polymorphic light eruption—a controlled trial. *Br J Dermatol* **116**:531, 1987
28. Bilsland D et al: A comparison of narrow band phototherapy (TL-01) and photochemotherapy (PUVA) in the management of polymorphic light eruption. *Br J Dermatol* **129**:708, 1993
29. Patel DC et al: Efficacy of short-course oral prednisolone in polymorphic light eruption: A randomized controlled trial. *Br J Dermatol* **143**:828, 2000
30. Murphy GM et al: Hydroxychloroquine in polymorphic light eruption: A controlled trial with drug and visual sensitivity monitoring. *Br J Dermatol* **116**:379, 1987
31. Saul A et al: Polymorphous light eruption: Treatment with thalidomide. *Australas J Dermatol* **17**:17, 1976
32. Corbett MF et al: Controlled therapeutic trials in polymorphous light eruption. *Br J Dermatol* **107**:571, 1982
33. Norris PG, Hawk JLM: Successful treatment of severe polymorphic light eruption with azathioprine. *Arch Dermatol* **125**:1377, 1989
34. Shipley DR, Hewitt JB: Polymorphic light eruption treated with cyclosporin. *Br J Dermatol* **144**:446, 2001
35. Farr PM, Diffey BL: Augmentation of ultraviolet erythema by indomethacin in actinic prurigo: Evidence of mechanism of photosensitivity. *Photochem Photobiol* **47**:413, 1988
36. Menagé H et al: HLA-DR4 may determine expression of actinic prurigo in British patients. *J Invest Dermatol* **106**:362, 1996
37. Grabczynska SA et al: Actinic prurigo and polymorphic light eruption: Common pathogenesis and the importance of HLA-DR4/DRB1*0407. *Br J Dermatol* **140**:232, 1999
38. Lovell CR et al: Thalidomide in actinic prurigo. *Br J Dermatol* **108**:467, 1983
39. Farr PM, Diffey BL: Treatment of actinic prurigo with PUVA: Mechanism of action. *Br J Dermatol* **120**:411, 1989
40. Birt AR, Davis RA: Hereditary polymorphous light eruption of American Indians. *Int J Dermatol* **14**:105, 1975
41. Bernal JE et al: Actinic prurigo among the Chimila Indians in Colombia: HLA studies. *J Am Acad Dermatol* **22**:1049, 1990
42. Sheridan DP et al: HLA typing in actinic prurigo. *J Am Acad Dermatol* **22**:1019, 1990
43. Sonnex TS, Hawk JLM: Hydroa vacciniforme: A review of ten cases. *Br J Dermatol* **118**:101, 1988
44. Jaschke E, Hönigsmann H: Hydroa vacciniforme—Aktionsspektrum, UV-Toleranz nach Photochemotherapie. *Hautarzt* **32**:350, 1981
45. Gupta G, Man I, Kemmett D: Hydroa vacciniforme: A clinical and follow-up study of 17 cases. *J Am Acad Dermatol* **42**:208, 2000
46. Murphy GM. Diseases associated with photosensitivity. *J Photochem Photobiol: B Biol* **64**:93, 2001
47. Steger GG et al: Permanent cure of hydroa vacciniforme after treatment of Hodgkin's disease with C-MOPP/AS VD regimen. *Br J Dermatol* **119**:684, 1988
48. Ohtsuka T et al: Hydroa vacciniforme with latent Epstein-Barr virus infection. *Br J Dermatol* **145**:509, 2001
49. Cho KH et al: Epstein-Barr virus associated peripheral T-cell lymphoma in adults with hydroa vacciniforme-like lesions. *Clin Exp Dermatol* **26**:242, 2001
50. Leenutaphong V et al: Pathogenesis and classification of solar urticaria: A new concept. *J Am Acad Dermatol* **21**:237, 1989
51. Uetsu N et al: The clinical and photobiological characteristics of solar urticaria in 40 patients. *Br J Dermatol* **142**:32, 2000
52. Horio T, Fujigaki K: Augmentation spectrum in solar urticaria. *J Am Acad Dermatol* **18**:1189, 1988
53. Monfrecola G et al: Solar urticaria: A report on 57 cases. *Am J Contact Dermatol* **11**:89, 2000
54. Norris PG, Hawk JLM: Bruising and susceptibility to solar urticaria. *Br J Dermatol* **124**:393, 1991
55. Roelandts R, Ryckaert S: Solar urticaria: The annoying photodermatosis. *Int J Dermatol* **38**:411, 1999
56. Beissert S, Ständer H, Schwarz T: UVA rush hardening for the treatment of solar urticaria. *J Am Acad Dermatol* **42**:1030, 2000
57. Duschet P et al: Solar urticaria—Effective treatment by plasmapheresis. *Clin Exp Dermatol* **12**:185, 1987
58. Bissonnette R et al: Treatment of refractory solar urticaria with plasma exchange. *J Cutan Med Surg* **3**:236, 1999
59. Wilkinson DS: Photodermatitis due to tetrachlorosalicylanilide. *Br J Dermatol* **73**:213, 1961
60. Jillson OF, Baughman RD: Contact photodermatitis from bithionol. *Arch Dermatol* **88**:409, 1963
61. Ive FA et al: "Actinic reticuloid": A chronic dermatosis associated with severe photosensitivity and the histological resemblance to lymphoma. *Br J Dermatol* **81**:469, 1969
62. Ramsay CA, Kobza-Black A: Photosensitive eczema. *Trans St John's Hosp Dermatol Soc* **59**:152, 1973
63. Frain-Bell W et al: The syndrome of chronic photosensitivity dermatitis and actinic reticuloid. *Br J Dermatol* **91**:617, 1974
64. Hawk JLM, Magnus IA: Chronic actinic dermatitis—An idiopathic photosensitivity syndrome including actinic reticuloid and photosensitive eczema. *Br J Dermatol* **101**(suppl 17):24, 1979
65. Hawk JLM, Magnus IA: Resolution of actinic reticuloid with transition to photosensitive eczema. *J R Soc Med* **71**:608, 1978
66. Norris PG, Hawk JLM: Chronic actinic dermatitis-a unifying concept. *Arch Dermatol* **126**:376, 1990
67. Kochevar IE, Harber LC: Photoreactions of 3,3′,4′,5-tetrachlorosalicylanilide with proteins. *J Invest Dermatol* **68**:151, 1977
68. Menagé H et al: The action spectrum for induction of chronic actinic dermatitis is similar to that for sunburn inflammation. *Photochem Photobiol* **62**:976, 1995
69. Norris PG et al: Chronic actinic dermatitis: An immunohistological and photobiological study. *J Am Acad Dermatol* **21**:966, 1989
70. Menagé H et al: A study of the kinetics and pattern of adhesion molecule expression in induced lesions of chronic actinic dermatitis. *Br J Dermatol* **134**:262, 1996
71. Murphy G et al: Allergic airborne dermatitis to Compositae with photosensitivity—Chronic actinic dermatitis in evolution. *Photodermatol Photoimmunol Photomed* **7**:38, 1990
72. Menagé H et al: Contact and photocontact sensitization in chronic actinic dermatitis: Sesquiterpene lactone mix is an important allergen. *Br J Dermatol* **132**:543, 1995
73. Addo HA et al: A study of Compositae plant reactions in photosensitivity dermatitis. *Photodermatology* **2**:68, 1995
74. Menagé HduP, Hawk JLM: The idiopathic photodermatoses: Chronic actinic dermatitis (photosensitivity dermatitis/actinic reticuloid syndrome), in *Photodermatology*, edited by JLM Hawk. London, Arnold, 1999, pp 127–142
75. Dawe RS et al: The natural history of chronic actinic dermatitis. *Arch Dermatol* **136**:1215, 2000
76. Wolf C, Hönigsmann H: Persistent light reaction-actinic reticuloid. *Hautarzt* **39**:635, 1988
77. Creamer D et al: Chronic actinic dermatitis occurring in young patients with atopic dermatitis. *Br J Dermatol* **139**:1112, 1998
78. Lim H et al: Chronic actinic dermatitis: An analysis of 51 patients evaluated in the United States and Japan. *Arch Dermatol Res* **130**:1284, 1994
79. Healy E, Rogers S: Photosensitivity dermatitis/actinic reticuloid syndrome in an Irish population: A review and some unusual features. *Acta Derm Venereol* **75**:72, 1995
80. Chu AC et al: Immunologic differentiation of the Sézary syndrome due to cutaneous T-cell lymphoma and chronic actinic dermatitis. *J Invest Dermatol* **86**:134, 1986

81. Menagé H et al: Analysis of T-cell receptor genes in chronic actinic dermatitis: No evidence of clonality. *J Invest Dermatol* **98**:546, 1992
82. Murphy GM et al: A double-blind controlled trial of azathioprine in chronic actinic dermatitis. *Br J Dermatol* **117**:16, 1987
83. Norris PG et al: Actinic reticuloid: Response to cyclosporin A. *J Am Acad Dermatol* **21**:307, 1989
84. Hjorth N et al: Acne aestivalis—Mallorca acne. *Acta Derm Venereol* **52**:61, 1972
85. Nieboer C: Actinic superficial folliculitis: A new entity? *Br J Dermatol* **112**:603, 1985
86. Verbov J: Actinic folliculitis. *Br J Dermatol* **112**:630, 1985
87. Norris PG, Hawk JLM: Actinic folliculitis—Response to isotretinoin. *Clin Exp Dermatol* **14**:69, 1989
88. Lederman JS et al: Immunosuppression: A cause of porokeratosis? *J Am Acad Dermatol* **13**:75, 1985
89. Hazen PG et al: Disseminated superficial actinic porokeratosis: Appearance associated with photochemotherapy for psoriasis. *J Am Acad Dermatol* **12**:1077, 1985
90. Allen AL, Glaser DA: Disseminated superficial actinic porokeratosis associated with topical PUVA. *J Am Acad Dermatol* **43**:720, 2000
91. Neumann RA et al: Disseminated superficial actinic porokeratosis: Experimental induction and exacerbation of skin lesions. *J Am Acad Dermatol* **21**:1182, 1989
92. Bedi TR: Summertime actinic lichenoid eruption. *Dermatologica* **157**:115, 1978
93. Verhagen AR, Koten JW: Lichenoid melanodermatitis. *Br J Dermatol* **101**:651, 1979
94. van der Schroeff JG et al: Induction of actinic lichen planus with artificial UV sources. *Arch Dermatol* **119**:498, 1983
95. Millard TP et al: Photosensitivity in lupus. *Lupus* **9**:3, 2000
96. Catherine H et al: The pathophysiology of photosensitivity in lupus erythematosus. *Photodermatol Photoimmunol Photomed* **17**:95, 2001
97. Furukawa F et al: Binding of antibodies to ENA SS-A/Ro and SS-B/La is induced in the surface of human keratinocytes by UVL: Implications for the pathogenesis of cutaneous lupus. *J Invest Dermatol* **94**:77, 1990
98. Furukawa F et al: Susceptibility to UVB light in cultured keratinocytes of cutaneous lupus erythematosus. *Dermatology* **189**:18, 1994
99. Wang B et al: SSA/Ro antigen expressed on membrane of UVB-induced apoptotic keratinocytes is pathogenic but not detectable in supernatant of cell culture.*Chin Med J (Engl)* **112**:512, 1999
100. Lehmann P et al: Experimental reproduction of skin lesions in lupus erythematosus by UVA and UVB radiation. *J Am Acad Dermatol* **22**:181, 1990
101. Kuhn A et al: Phototesting in lupus erythematosus: A 15–year experience. *J Am Acad Dermatol* **45**:86, 2001
102. Cram DL, Winkelmann RK: Ultraviolet-induced acantholysis in pemphigus. *Arch Dermatol* **92**:7, 1965
103. Dechamps P et al: Photoinduction of lesions in a patient with pemphigus erythematosus. *Photodermatology* **1**:38, 1984
104. Perl S et al: Bullous pemphigoid induced by PUVA therapy. *Dermatology* **193**:245, 1996
105. Ros AM: Photosensitive psoriasis. *Semin Dermatol* **11**:267, 1992
106. Roelandts R: The diagnosis of photosensitivity. *Arch Dermatol* **136**:1152, 2000
107. Neumann NJ, Lehmann P: Photodiagnostic modalities, in *Dermatological Phototherapy and Photodiagnostic Methods*, edited by J Krutmann, H Hönigsmann, CA Elmets, PR Bergstresser. Berlin, Springer, 2001, pp 329–337
108. Thune P, et al: The Scandinavian Multicenter Photopatch Test Study 1980–1985: Final report. *Photodermatology* **5**:261, 1988
109. Neumann NJ et al: Photopatch testing: The 12-year experience of the German, Austrian, and Swiss Photopatch Test Group. *J Am Acad Dermatol* **42**:183, 2000

CHAPTER 136

Henry W. Lim

Abnormal Responses to Ultraviolet Radiation: Photosensitivity Induced by Exogenous Agents

Photosensitivity induced by chemicals can be caused by exogenous or endogenous agents. Exogenous photosensitizers can be categorized into those administered systemically and agents applied topically. Well-characterized examples of photosensitivity induced by endogenous photosensitizers are the porphyrias, which are associated with enzymatic defects in heme biosynthetic pathways, resulting in elevated levels of porphyrins, known phototoxic agents (Chap. 149).

Photosensitivity induced by exogenous agents can be divided into phototoxicity and photoallergy. Phototoxicity is the result of a direct tissue injury caused by the phototoxic agent and radiation; it can occur in all individuals exposed to adequate doses of the agent and the appropriate radiation (Table 136-1). In contrast, photoallergy is a type IV delayed hypersensitivity response; it has a sensitization phase, occurs only in sensitized individuals, and requires only a minimal concentration of the photoallergen (see Table 136-1).

INCIDENCE

There are more than 300 medications in the United States that have been reported to cause photosensitivity, however, only a small number of them induce frequent reactions or have been well-studied.[1,2] The estimated incidence of photosensitivity induced by exogenous agents ranges from 16 to 25 percent for chlorpromazine, 3 percent for doxycycline, and 0.025 to 15 percent for fluoroquinolones.[3,4] The percentage of photopatch-tested patients who have clinically relevant reactions leading to a diagnosis of photoallergic contact dermatitis ranges from 4 to 20 percent.[5,6]

TABLE 136-1

Characteristics of Phototoxicity and Photoallergy

	PHOTOTOXICITY	PHOTOALLERGY
Clinical presentation	Sunburn reaction: erythema, edema, vesicles and bullae; frequently resolves with hyperpigmentation	Eczematous lesions, usually pruritic
Histology	Necrotic keratinocytes, epidermal degeneration; sparse dermal infiltrate of lymphocytes, macrophages, and neutrophils	Spongiotic dermatitis, dermal lymphohistiocytic infiltrate
Pathophysiology	Direct tissue injury	Type IV delayed hypersensitivity response
Occurrence after first exposure	Yes	No
Onset of eruption after exposure	Minutes to hours	24 to 48 h
Dose of agent needed for eruption	Large	Small
Cross reactivity with other agents	Rare	Common
Diagnosis: Topical agent	Clinical	Photopatch tests
Systemic agent	Clinical + phototests	Clinical + phototests; possibly photopatch tests

HISTORICAL ASPECTS

The earliest documented clinical application of a photosensitizing agent was in 1400 B.C., when psoralens-containing seeds of the plant *Psoralia corylifolia* plus sunlight were used in India to treat vitiligo.[7] Around the twelfth century A.D., the Egyptians obtained psoralens from flowers of another plant, *Ammi majus;* the flowers were ground and rubbed on the leukodermic skin before sun exposure.

In 1913, Meyer-Betz reported one of the earliest experiments that conclusively demonstrated the photosensitizing effect of a systemically administered agent, hematoporphyrin. In 1916, Freund described mild erythema resolving with marked hyperpigmentation in patients using perfume containing 5-methoxypsoralen. Because the perfume was often applied to the chest, the ensuing dermatitis was referred to as *berloque* (French for pendant) or necklace dermatitis. In the 1920s and 1930s, the synergistic effect of crude coal tar and light in the treatment of psoriasis was reported by Goeckermann at the Mayo Clinic.

The current understanding of phototoxicity and photoallergy was pioneered by the studies of Stephen Epstein. In 1939, he reported data obtained from volunteers injected intradermally with sulfanilamide and subsequently irradiated with a hot quartz mercury vapor lamp. He observed and defined the *phototoxic* response, which occurred in all individuals within 24 h, and the *photoallergic* response, which occurred in only a small number of individuals 10 days later.

Since 1974, 8-methoxypsoralen has been widely used in psoralen plus ultraviolet A (PUVA) photochemotherapy and, more recently in extracorporeal photopheresis (see Chap. 266). Porphyrin derivatives and other photosensitizers are currently used in the photodynamic therapy of tumors of the skin and internal organs.[8]

PHOTOTOXICITY

Clinical Manifestations

ACUTE PHOTOTOXICITY This occurs usually within hours of exposure to the phototoxic agent and light. The patient complains of a burning and stinging sensation on light-exposed areas, such as forehead, nose, V-area of the neck and dorsum of hands. These subjective complaints are especially pronounced after exposure to tar and pitch, and are referred to as "tar smarts." Erythema and edema appear within hours of light exposure; in severe cases, vesicles and bullae may develop. Light-protected areas, such as nasolabial folds, postauricular and submental areas, and areas covered by clothing, are spared (Fig. 136-1). A notable exception to the above-described kinetics is psoralen induced phototoxicity, where the acute response appears in 24 h, and peaks at

FIGURE 136-1

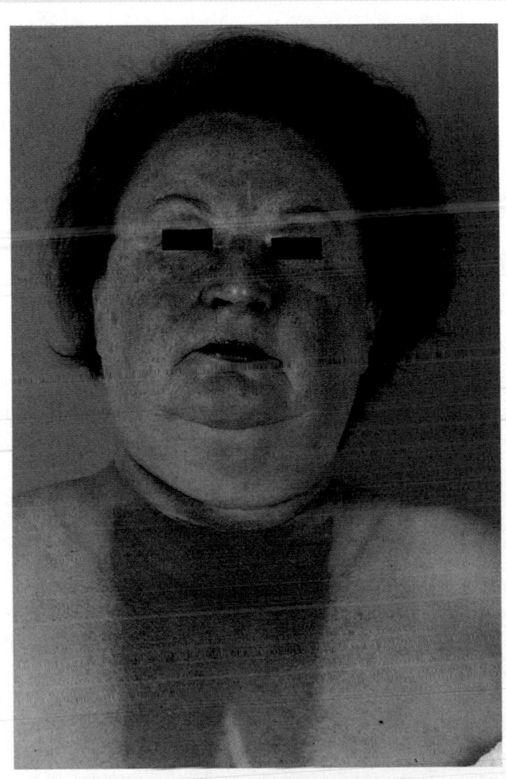

Phototoxicity associated with a heterocyclic antidepressant. Note erythema and edema on sun-exposed areas and sparing of sun-protected chest and shaded upper lip and neck. *(Courtesy of Dr. Adrian Tanew)*

FIGURE 136-2

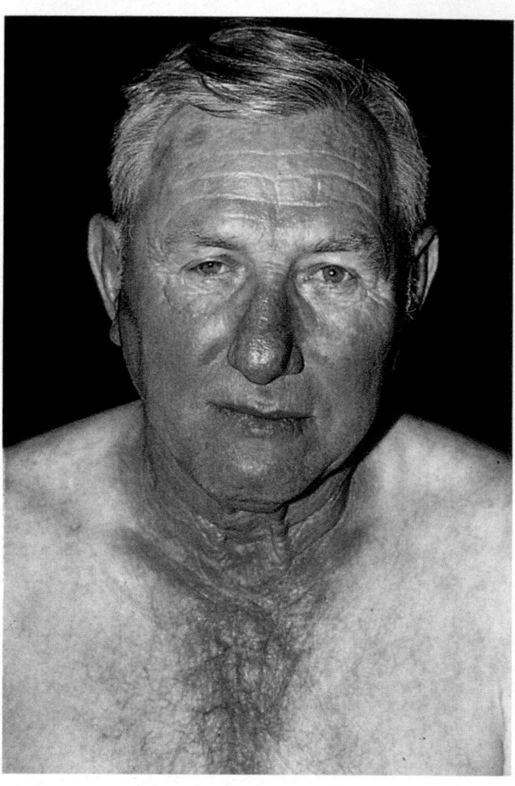

Amiodarone-induced phototoxicity. Note the erythema and slate-gray pigmentation (nose, forehead) on the sun-exposed area.

FIGURE 136-3

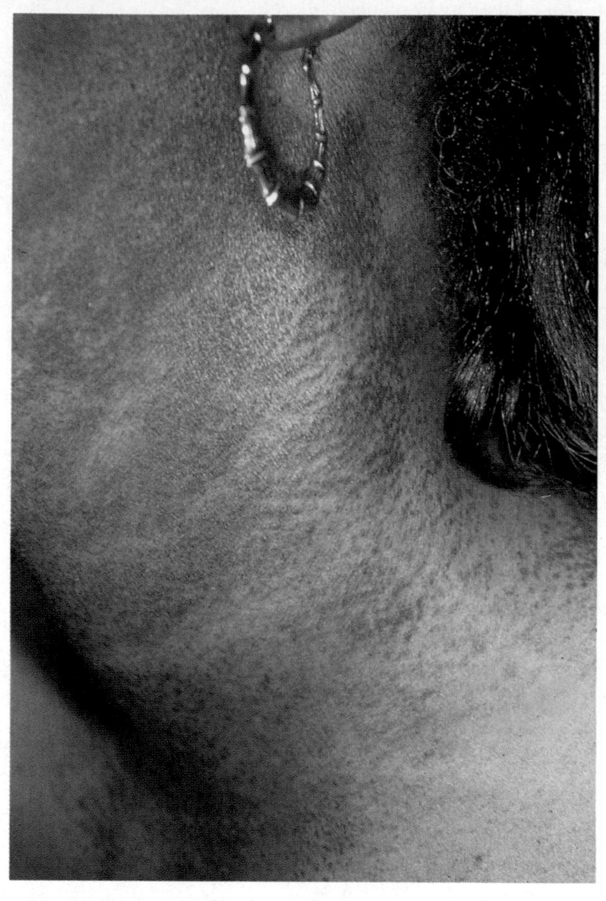

Slate-gray, reticulated patches on sun-exposed areas in a patient taking diltiazem. Note the sparing of the postauricular area and skin folds on the neck.

48 to 72 h. This is the rationale of administering PUVA photochemotherapy doses 48 h apart. The phototoxic response usually resolves with a varying degree of hyperpigmentation, which may last for months.

PHOTO-ONYCHOLYSIS Separation of the distal nail from the nail bed is a manifestation of acute phototoxicity. It has been reported with *doxycycline* and other *tetracyclines, fluoroquinolones, psoralens, benoxaprofen, chlorazepate dipotassium,* and *quinine.*[9,10]

SLATE-GRAY PIGMENTATION (see also Chap. 90) Blue-gray pigmentation on sun exposed areas has been associated with exposure to several agents.[11,12] One to 10 percent of patients taking *amiodarone* develop this side-effect (Fig. 136-2). *Chlorpromazine* can induce a similar change. The tricyclic antidepressants *imipramine* and, less commonly, *desipramine* have also been reported to cause slate-gray pigmentation; a drug metabolite-melanin complex has been postulated to be the cause of this alteration. Chronic exposure to *diltiazem,* a benzothiazepine calcium channel blocker, has resulted in photodistributed, reticulated, slate-gray pigmentation (Fig. 136-3); pigmentary incontinence and melanosome complexes are the prominent histologic and electron microscopic findings. Slate-gray pigmentation seen in *argyria* involves lunulae of nails, mucous membranes, and sclerae. A photochemical reaction involving silver granules deposited in the dermis results in these pigmentary alterations.

LICHENOID ERUPTION This has been reported following exposure to *fenofibrate, quinine, quinidine, hydrochlorothiazide, demeclocycline, enalapril, pyrazinamide, chloroquine,* and *hydroxychloroquine.*[9,13] Patients present with lichen planus-like lesions on sun-exposed areas; some consider this a variant of photoallergy.

PSEUDOPORPHYRIA The development of porphyria cutanea tarda-like cutaneous changes of skin fragility, vesicles, and subepidermal blisters is associated with several phototoxic agents (see Chap. 149). While histologic and immunofluorescence findings are similar to porphyria cutanea tarda, the porphyrin profile is normal in these patients.[14] *Naproxen* is the most commonly reported agent. Other drugs incriminated include *nabumetone, oxaprozin, ketoprofen, mefenamic acid, tiaprofenic acid, diflunisal, celecoxib, tetracyclines, nalidixic acid, amiodarone, furosemide,* and *etretinate.*[14,15]

PHOTODISTRIBUTED TELANGIECTASIA Telangiectasia on sun-exposed areas has been reported with calcium channel blockers including *nifedipine* and *amlodipine,* and with the antibiotic *cefotaxime.* Provocation with UVA resulted in the development of telangiectasia.[16]

PERSISTENCE OF PHOTOSENSITIVITY AND EVOLUTION TO CHRONIC ACTINIC DERMATITIS While phototoxicity usually resolves following discontinuation of the exposure to the causative agent, there are reports of persistence of photosensitivity many years after the cessation of exposure, resulting in the development of chronic actinic dermatitis (see photoallergy below). This has been reported with *thiazides, quinidine,* and *quinine.*[17]

FIGURE 136-4

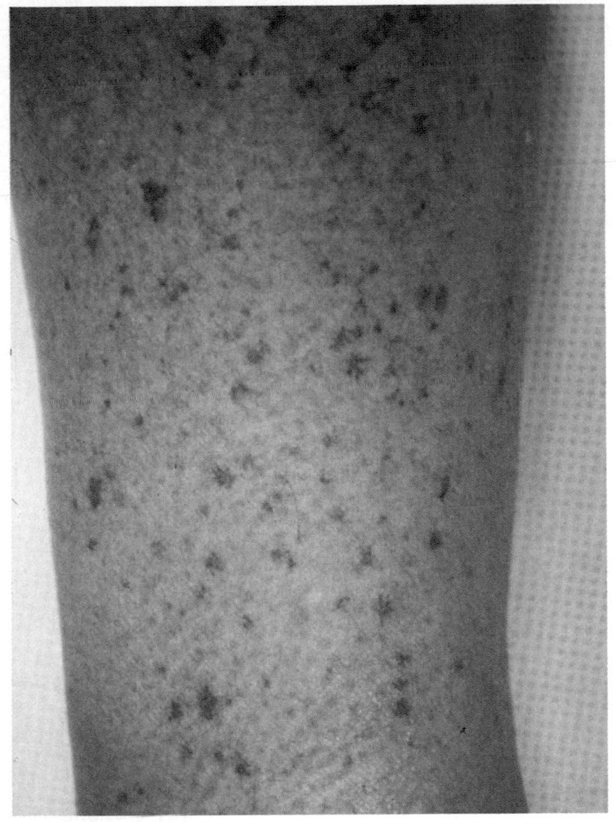

Lentigines on the forearm of a patient who had received high cumulative PUVA exposure.

CHRONIC EFFECTS Cutaneous effects of chronic, repeated phototoxic tissue injury are best exemplified by patients who had received long-term PUVA photochemotherapy. These include premature aging of the skin, lentigines (Fig. 136-4), squamous cell and basal cell carcinomas, and melanoma.[18] These are discussed in greater detail in Chap. 266.

Phototoxic Agents

TOPICAL AGENTS Table 136-2 lists the major topical phototoxic agents; therapeutic or occupational exposures to these agents are the common route of contact. The action spectrum is in the UVA range for most of them.

Furocoumarins Topical exposures to *furocoumarins* may occur in certain occupations (bartenders, salad chefs, gardeners), and in patients receiving topical photochemotherapy with *psoralens.* Such exposure could also occur among users of tanning preparations or perfumes containing *5-methoxypsoralen (bergapten),* although these preparations are not longer available in most countries.[19]

Tar Crude coal tar used in dermatologic therapy is the product of the destructive distillation of coal; it is a complex mixture of over 10,000 compounds including many phototoxic polyaromatic hydrocarbons. It may produce "tar smarts" upon exposure to UVA. In addition to phototoxicity, occupational exposure to tar is associated with increased risk of nonmelanoma skin cancers; however, the carcinogenicity of coal tar used in dermatologic therapy remains controversial.[20]

TABLE 136-2

Topical Phototoxic Agents

AGENT	EXPOSURE
Rose bengal	Ophthalmologic examination
Furocoumarins	Occur naturally in plants (especially Compositae species), fruits and vegetables (lime, lemon, celery, fig, parsley and parsnip); used in perfumes and cosmetics; used for topical photochemotherapy
Tar	Topical therapeutic agent; roofing materials

SYSTEMIC AGENTS Table 136-3 lists the major systemic phototoxic agents; most are therapeutic or diagnostic agents.[1,2] They produce an exaggerated sunburn reaction. However, some may also induce an eczematous photoallergic response, especially following topical exposure; phenothiazines, sulfonamides, quinine, and ketoprofen are examples of such agents.[21–25] As a rule, the action spectra are in the UVA range; exceptions include sulfonamides and vinblastine, whose action spectra are in the UVB range,[9] and the porphyrins, fluorescein, and other dyes, whose action spectra are in the visible range.[8]

The more commonly encountered systemic phototoxic agents are described below, following the sequence given in Table 136-3.

Antianxiety drugs Phototoxicity has been reported following systemic administration of *alprazolam* and *chlordiazepoxide.*[21]

Anticancer drugs *Dacarbazine, fluorouracil,* and *vinblastine* are well-documented phototoxic agents.[9] *Methotrexate* is known to be able to reactivate UVB-induced and PUVA-induced erythema.[26]

Antidepressants Phototoxicity induced by the tricyclics *amitriptyline* and *imipramine* is mediated by oxygen free radicals.[27] *Imipramine* and *desipramine* have been reported to induce slate-gray pigmentation in sun-exposed distribution, which is due to deposition of drug metabolite-melanin complexes.[11]

Antifungal *Griseofulvin* is a known phototoxic agent; it may also induce photoallergic reactions.[28]

Antimalarials The property of *chloroquine* as a phototoxic agent is unclear. Clinically, it is implicated as causing photosensitivity; however, a study involving 25 patients showed that chloroquine or hydroxychloroquine did not affect the response to UVA and UVB radiation.[29] *Quinine* is a phototoxic agent; in addition, it can induce a positive photopatch test,[24] lichenoid eruption,[23] and chronic actinic dermatitis.[30]

Antimicrobials All *quinolones* tested have been shown to be phototoxic, mediated by reactive oxygen species, and, in some, by photoproducts.[31,32] Some of these are also photoallergens.[33] *Clinafloxacin, fleroxacin, lomefloxacin,* and *sparfloxacin,* all molecules with a halogen atom at position 8, have the highest potential for phototoxicity. *Ciprofloxacin, gemifloxacin, moxifloxacin, norfloxacin,* and *ofloxacin* produce only mild phototoxic reactions. *Enoxacin, lomefloxacin,* and *nalidixic acid* also elicit photoallergic responses. The quinolones were shown to have potential photocarcinogenic properties in an animal model, and are capable of inducing DNA breaks in vitro.[32] The *sulfonamides* are both phototoxic and photoallergic.[22] Among the *tetracyclines, demeclocycline* (used to treat diabetes insipidus) and *doxycycline* are the most potent phototoxic agents; the respective incidence is 1 to 2 percent, and 3 percent.[4,34]

Antipsychotics The *phenothiazines* are phototoxic agents that can also induce photoallergic reactions, usually after an inadvertent topical exposure in a patient care environment.[23,35] *Chlorpromazine* can also induce blue-gray pigmentation on light-exposed skin.

Cardiac medications *Amiodarone* induces an acute phototoxic response, occurring in up to 50 percent of patients;[36] it also results in a slate-gray pigmentation in sun-exposed areas (Fig. 136-2). *Quinidine*

TABLE 136-3

Systemic Phototoxic Agents

Property	Generic Name (*US Trade Name*)	Property	Generic Name (*US Trade Name*)
Antianxiety drugs	Alprazolam (*Xanax*)		Hydrochlorothiazide (*Accuretic; Aldactazide; Aldoril; Atacand; Avalide; Capozide; Diovan; Dyazide; HydroDIURIl*)*
	Chlordiazepoxide (*Librax; Librium; Limbitrol*)	Dye	Fluorescein (*AK-Fluor; Fluor-I-Strip; Fluorescite*)
Anticancer drugs	Dacarbazine (*DTIC-Dome*)		Methylene blue (*Urised*)
	Fluorouracil (*Adrucil*)	Furocoumarins	Psoralens:
	Methotrexate (*Rheumatrex*)		5-Methoxypsoralen*
	Vinblastine (*Velban*)		8-Methoxypsoralen (*Oxsoralen-Ultra*)*
Antidepressants	Tricyclics:		4,5′,8-Trimethylpsoralen*
	Amitriptyline (*Elavil; Limbitrol; Triavil*)	Hypoglycemics	Sulfonylureas:
	Desipramine (*Norpramin*)		Acetohexamide
	Imipramine (*Tofranil*)		Chlorpropamide (*Diabinase*)
Antifungal	Griseofulvin (*Fulvicin; Grifulvin V; Gris-PEG*)		Glipizide (*Glucotrol*)
Antimalarials	Chloroquine (*Aralen*)		Glyburide (*DiaBeta; Glucovance; Glynase Pres Tab; Micronase*)
	Quinine		Tolazamide (*Tolinase*)
Antimicrobials	Quinolones:		Tolbutamide (*Orinase*)*
	Ciprofloxacin (*Cipro*)	NSAIDs	Acetic acid derivative:
	Enoxacin (*Penetrex*)		Diclofenac (*Arthrotec; Cataflam; Voltaren*)
	Gemifloxacin		Anthranilic acid derivative:
	Lomefloxacin (*Maxaquin*)*		Mefenamic acid (*Ponstel*)
	Moxifloxacin (*Avelox*)		Enolic acid derivative:
	Nalidixic acid (*NegGram*)*		Piroxicam (*Feldene*)*
	Norfloxacin (*Chibroxin; Noroxin*)		Propionic acid derivatives:
	Ofloxacin (*Floxin; Ocuflox*)		Ibuprofen (*Advil; Motrin; Nuprin; Vicoprofen*)
	Sparfloxacin (*Zagam*)*		Ketoprofen (*Orudis; Oruvail*)
	Sulfonamides		Naproxen (*Aleve; Naprelan; Naprosyn*)*
	Tetracyclines		Oxaprozin (*Daypro*)
	Demeclocycline (*Declomycin*)*		Tiaprofenic acid
	Doxycycline (*Monodox; Periostat; Vibramycin*)*		Salicyclic acid derivative:
	Minocycline (*Dynacin; Minocin*)		Diflunisal (*Dolobid*)
	Tetracycline (*Helidac; Sumycin*)		Others:
	Trimethoprim (*Bactrim; Polytrim; Primsal; Septra*)		Celecoxib (*Celebrex*)
Antipsychotic drugs	Phenothiazines:		Nabumetone (*Relafen*)*
	Chlorpromazine (*Thorazine*)*	Photodynamic Therapy Agents	Porfimer (*Photofrin*)*
	Perphenazine (*Triavil; Trilafon*)		Verteporfin (*Visudyne*)*
	Prochlorperazine (*Compazine*)*	Retinoids	Acitretin (*Soriatane*)
	Thioridazine (*Mellaril*)		Isotretinoin (*Accutane*)
	Trifluoperazine (*Stelazine*)		Etretinate
Cardiac Medications	Amiodarone (*Cordarone; Pacerone*)*	Other	Flutamide (*Eulexin*)
	Quinidine (*Quinaglute; Quinidex*)		Hypericin
Diuretics	Furosemide (*Lasix*)*		Pyridoxine (vitamin B6)
	Thiazides:		Ranitidine (*Zantac*)
	Bendroflumethiazide (*Corzide*)		
	Chlorothiazide (*Aldoclor; Diuril*)*		

*Commonly reported

induces lichenoid photodermatitis[23] and an evolution to chronic actinic dermatitis;[17] although it has been considered to be a phototoxic agent, most studies now show that it is a systemic and topical photoallergen.[37]

Diuretics The *thiazides* are well known phototoxic agents (Fig. 136-1);[23] they can induce persistence of photosensitivity for many years.[17] *Furosemide* reportedly induces pseudoporphyria.[14]

Dyes *Fluorescein* and *methylene blue* reportedly induce phototoxicity.[38,39]

Furocoumarins These are formed by the fusion of a furan with a coumarin. They occur naturally in many fruits, vegetables, and plants, including lime, lemon, fig, celery, parsley, and parsnip. The phototoxic properties of *5-methoxypsoralen, 8-methoxypsoralen,* and *4,5,8-trimethylpsoralen* are used therapeutically in the treatment of psoriasis, vitiligo, cutaneous T cell lymphoma, and other conditions (see Chap. 266).

Hypoglycemics Photosensitivity has been reported with the *sulfonylureas*; the mechanism involves reactive oxygen species.[40]

Nonsteroidal anti-inflammatory drugs (NSAIDs) *Piroxicam,* an enolic acid derivative, generates a metabolite that is phototoxic in mice and in tissue culture. Clinically, piroxicam-induced photosensitivity is associated with eczematous skin lesions and positive photopatch tests to piroxicam and its photoproducts, strongly indicating that this is a photoallergic response.[41]

Generation of a photoproduct is responsible for the phototoxicity associated with *diclofenac*. *Ibuprofen,* a propionic acid derivative introduced in 1963, reportedly causes phototoxicity with a lowered minimal erythema dose (MED) to UVA;[9] however, ibuprofen-induced photosensitivity is a rare event. The phototoxicity of the other *propionic acid-derived NSAIDs* have been demonstrated in vitro, in an animal model, and in human volunteers; reactive oxygen species are partially responsible for the process.[25] Similar to the phenothiazines, topical exposure to this group of NSAIDs can result in photoallergic contact dermatitis.[25,42] Pseudoporphyria has been reported with many NSAIDs, including *naproxen* (the most common precipitating agent), *nabumetone* (whose chemical structure is very similar to naproxen), and the cyclooxygenase-2 inhibitor *celecoxib.*[15] *Benoxaprofen,* a highly phototoxic NSAID, was withdrawn from the market in 1982 because of its cholestatic hepatitis side effect.

Photodynamic therapy agents The phototoxic properties of these agents are used therapeutically in photodynamic therapy[8] (see Chap. 266).

Retinoids Phototest results were normal in patients taking isotretinoin and suppressed in two of nine patients taking etretinate, with an action spectrum at 300 to 365 nm.[43] The decreased stratum corneum thickness may play a major role in this retinoid "photosensitivity."

Others Phototoxicity has also been reported to be induced by *flutamide,* a nonsteroidal antiandrogen, and *ranitidine,* an H_2 histamine receptor antagonist.[44,45] *Hypericin,* an extract of St. John's wort, has antiretroviral activity in vitro but not in vivo, and is used in the management of depression. Up to 48 percent of patients developed phototoxicity at high doses, but not at the doses used for depression.[46] It is being investigated as an agent for photodynamic therapy.[47] Phototoxicity due to *pyridoxine (vitamin B_6)* is rare; it is caused by the generation of toxic photoproducts.[48]

Histopathology

Acute phototoxicity is characterized by necrotic keratinocytes, and in severe cases, epidermal necrosis. There may be epidermal spongiosis, dermal edema, and mild infiltrates consisting of neutrophils, lymphocytes, and macrophages. *Slate-gray pigmentation* is associated with increased dermal melanin, and dermal deposits of the drug or its metabolite.[11,12] Histologic features of *lichenoid eruptions* are similar to those of idiopathic lichen planus; however, there may be a greater degree of spongiosis and dermal eosinophilic and plasma cell infiltrates, and a larger number of necrotic keratinocytes and cytoid bodies. Similar to porphyria cutanea tarda, there is dermal–epidermal separation at the lamina lucida in *pseudoporphyria,* and deposits of immunoglobulins at the dermal–epidermal junction and blood vessel walls.[14]

Pathophysiology

PHOTODYNAMIC PROCESSES Upon absorption of light energy by the photosensitizer (P) at its ground state, formation of an excited (usually triplet) state (^{3}P) molecule occurs. The excited state molecule may then participate in oxygen-dependent processes (i.e., photodynamic processes) in two major pathways: type I or type II reactions that both result in cytotoxic injury.[8]

The *type I reaction* involves transfer of an electron or a hydrogen atom to the excited state photosensitizer (^{3}P), resulting in the formation of free radicals (Eq. 1). These may then participate in an oxidation-reduction reaction that results in peroxide formation and subsequent cell damage (*Eqs. 2* and *3*).

$$^3P + RH \rightarrow PH\cdot + R\cdot \qquad (1)$$

$$PH\cdot + PH\cdot \rightarrow P + PH_2 \qquad (2)$$

$$PH_2 + O_2 \rightarrow P + \underset{\text{hydrogen peroxide}}{H_2O_2} \qquad (3)$$

Interaction of ^{3}P with ground state oxygen could result in the formation of superoxide anion ($O_2^{\cdot-}$), which, in turn, can be converted into highly reactive and cytotoxic hydroxyl radicals (OH·).

The *type II reaction* is also known as an energy transfer process. Transfer of energy to ground state oxygen results in the formation of singlet oxygen ($^1O_2$), which is highly reactive and has a lifetime of 50 nsec (*Eq. 4*).

$$^3P + O_2 \rightarrow P + {}^1O_2 \qquad (4)$$

Cytotoxic injury occurs upon singlet oxygen-induced oxidation of amino acids and unsaturated fatty acids; interaction with the latter results in the formation of hydroperoxides, which initiate lipid and protein oxidation.

Phototoxicity induced by porphyrins,[8] quinolones,[32] and nonsteroidal anti-inflammatory agents[25,49] are examples of photodynamic phototoxic reactions.

GENERATION OF PHOTOPRODUCTS With some photosensitizers, exposure to radiation may result in the generation of stable photoproducts, which are responsible for tissue injury. Phototoxic products have been demonstrated upon irradiation of chlorpromazine, tetracyclines, quinolones, and nonsteroidal anti-inflammatory agents.[32,49]

BINDING TO SUBSTRATE Another mechanism of phototoxicity is radiation-mediated binding of the photosensitizer to its biologic substrate. A photoaddition reaction occurs when the excited state molecule covalently binds to a ground state molecule. An example is the covalent binding of 8-methoxypsoralen to pyrimidine bases of the DNA molecules, resulting in the formation of a cross-link of the DNA chains.

INFLAMMATORY MEDIATORS Mediators of inflammation and inflammatory cells participate in phototoxic tissue injury. Biologically active products of complement activation, mast cell-derived mediators, eicosanoids, proteases, and polymorphonuclear leukocytes contribute to the development of phototoxicity induced by porphyrins, demeclocycline, and chlorpromazine.[50,51]

Management

Identification and avoidance of the causative phototoxic agent is the most important step in the management. Sun avoidance is central. Because the action spectrum for most agents is in the UVA spectrum, broad-spectrum sunscreens should be used. Acute phototoxicity could be managed with topical corticosteroids and compresses; systemic corticosteroids should be reserved only for the most severely affected patients. Management of patients with slate-gray pigmentation, a lichenoid eruption, pseudoporphyria, and photodistributed telangiectasia is symptomatic only, because it will take months after the discontinuation of the offending agent before the resolution of the eruption. Patients with NSAID-induced pseudoporphyria who require NSAIDs should be switched to a different class of agents, or to those that are less photosensitizing, such as indomethacin or sulindac.[14] Management of chronic actinic dermatitis evolving from exposure to exogenous agents is identical to that of chronic actinic dermatitis in general.

PHOTOALLERGY

Clinical Manifestations

The presence of photoallergen and the appropriate radiation is necessary for the clinical manifestation of photoallergy. In sensitized individuals, exposure to the photoallergen and sunlight results in the development of a pruritic, eczematous eruption within 24 to 48 hours after exposure (see Table 136-1, Fig. 136-5). This eruption is clinically indistinguishable from allergic contact dermatitis, is initially confined to light exposed areas, but, in contrast to phototoxic reactions, may spread beyond the exposed site. Lesions usually resolve with erythema; postinflammatory hyperpigmentation does not occur as commonly as in phototoxicity. The action spectrum is mostly in the UVA range.

The incidence of photoallergy in the United States peaked in the 1960s due to the widespread use of halogenated salicylanilide containing soaps and cleansers;[52] these have been now removed from personal care products in the United States. In the late 1970s and 1980s, fragrances in cosmetics and sunscreens, especially musk ambrette and 6-methylcoumarin, were common photoallergens. The removal of these agents has lessened their frequency. In the 1990s, sunscreen agents were the most common cause of photoallergy in the United States, United Kingdom, and France, which is a reflection of the current widespread use of sunscreens.[5,53,54] In Germany, Austria, and Switzerland, NSAIDs, antibacterials, and phenothiazines are the most common photoallergens.[6]

FIGURE 136-5

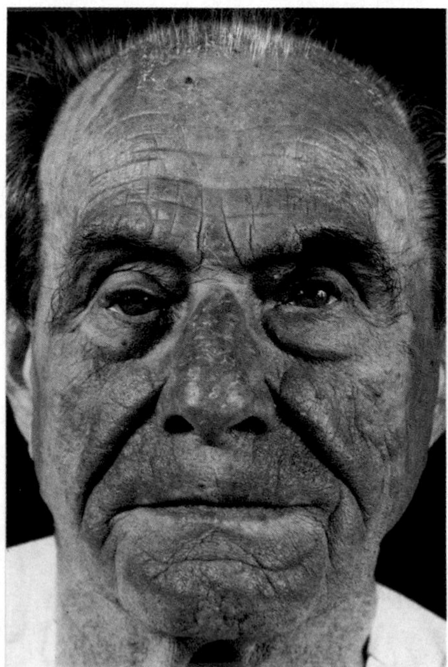

Photoallergic dermatitis. This eruption is clinically indistinguishable from allergic contact dermatitis, except it is distributed predominantly in sun-exposed areas.

PERSISTENCE OF PHOTOSENSITIVITY AND EVOLUTION TO CHRONIC ACTINIC DERMATITIS (See also Chap. 135) Similar to phototoxicity, persistence of photosensitivity and evolution to chronic actinic dermatitis have been reported following exposure to photoallergens, including halogenated salicylanilides, musk ambrette, ketoprofen, dioxopromethazine, and quinidine.[17,55,56] The mechanism is not completely understood. One possible explanation is that UV radiation induces alteration of the carrier protein that originally binds the photoallergen; this results in the formation of a neoantigen that chronically stimulates the immune system. This is supported by the observation that the histidine moiety in albumin can undergo oxidation in the presence of salicylanilide that binds to albumin.

Photoallergens

Topical exposure to photosensitizers is the most common route of sensitization to photoallergens. Table 136-4 lists the common groups of photoallergens, which are discussed below.

SUNSCREENS Photoallergy has been reported with practically all organic chemical sunscreen agents. Currently, the most commonly reported photoallergen is *benzophenone-3,* followed by *dibenzoylmethane.*[5,52,53,57,58] It should be noted that while sunscreen agents are a common cause of photoallergic contact dermatitis, the true prevalence of photosensitivity reaction to sunscreens is very low. Therefore, the potential for photoallergy should not deter one from using sunscreens.

Para-aminobenzoic acid (PABA) and its esters, *octyl dimethyl PABA* and *amyl dimethyl PABA,* can cause photoallergy. Amyl dimethyl PABA is no longer used in the United States or the European Union, although it is approved for use in Japan and Australia.[58] Individuals with a positive patch or photopatch test result to PABA or its esters may cross-react with other related chemicals such as *p-phenylenediamine* (hair dye), *procaine* and *benzocaine* (anesthetics), *procainamide* (antiarrhythmic agent), *sulfonamides* (antimicrobials) and *sulfonylureas* (hypoglycemic agents).[57]

FRAGRANCES Fragrances are the second most common cause of photoallergic reactions after sunscreens in the United States.[5,53] *6-Methylcoumarin* is a known photoallergen that was used as a fragrance in suntanning lotions in the 1970s; it has been removed from the market.[57] *Musk ambrette* was commonly used in the 1970s in after-shave colognes; it was a common photosensitizer. It is much less commonly used now following the recommendation of the International Fragrance Association (IFA), in 1982, that it not be used in products intended for skin application; however, there are still products that contain this agent. *Sandalwood oil* infrequently causes photoallergic reactions.

ANTIBACTERIALS This is another group of common photosensitizers.[6,59] *Halogenated salicylanilides* are well-characterized photoallergens. In the United States, they are no longer used in soaps and personal cleansers; however, they are used as surface disinfectants and mold inhibitors. They may also be present in personal care products sold in other countries. *Chlorhexidine, dimethylol-dimethyl hydantoin,* and *hexachlorophene* are used as skin cleansers. *Bithionol* is a potent photoallergen. It is no longer used in personal care products in the United States and Japan; however, it is used in industrial cleaners and in agricultural and veterinary products. It cross-reacts with hexachlorophene and halogenated salicylanilides. *Dichlorophene* and *triclosan* are present in personal care products; both have a low level of photoallergenicity. Triclosan is the most commonly used halogenated phenolic antibacterial agent worldwide.

TABLE 136-4

Topical Photoallergens

GROUP	INCI NAME/CHEMICAL NAME/TRADE NAME*
Sunscreens	*UVB absorbers:*
	para-Aminobenzoic acids (PABA):
	Amyl dimethyl PABA (*Padimate A; Escalol 506*)†
	PABA (*Pabanol*)†
	Ethylhexyl dimethyl PABA (octyl dimethyl PABA; *Padimate O; Escalol 507*)†
	Cinnamates:
	Cinoxate (2-ethoxyethyl-*p*-methoxycinnamate; *Phiasol*)
	Ethylhexyl methoxycinnamate (octyl methoxycinnamate; *Parsol MCX; Escalol 557*)
	Salicylate:
	Homosalate (metahomomenthyl salicylate; *Eusolex HMS*)
	UVA absorbers:
	Anthranilate:
	Menthyl anthranilate (cyclohexanol; *Trivent MA*)
	Benzophenones:
	Benzophenone-3 (oxybenzone; *Escalol 567*)†
	Benzophenone-4 (sulisobenzone; *Escalol 577*)†
	Dibenzoylmethane:
	Butyl methoxydibenzoylmethane (avobenzone; *Parsol 1789*)†
Fragrances	6-Methylcoumarin†
	Musk ambrette†
	Sandalwood oil
Antibacterials	Dibromosalicylanilide (dibromsalan; DBS)†
	Tetrochlorosalicylanilide (TCSA; *Impregon; Irgasan BS200*)†
	Tribromosalicylanilide (tribromsalan; TBS)*
	Chlorhexidene (*Hibiclens*)
	Dimethylol-dimethyl hydantoin
	Hexachlorophene (*pHisoHex*)
	Bithionol (thiobisdichlorophenol; bisphenol; *Actamar*)†
	Dichlorophene (G4)
	Triclosan (*Irgasan DP300*)
Antifungals	Fentichlor (thiobischlorophenol)*
	Jadit (butylchlorosalicylamide; buclosamide)
	Multifungin (bromochlorosalicylanilide; BCSA)
Others	Chlorpromazine (*Thorazine*)*
	Clioquinol
	Ketoprofen (*Orudis*)
	Olaquindox
	Promethazine (*Phenergan*)*
	Quinidine (*Cardioquin; Quinidex*)
	Thiourea (thiocarbamide)

* INCI: International Nomenclature of Cosmetic Ingredients.
†Commonly reported photoallergens.

ANTIFUNGALS *Fenticlor* (thiobisdichlorophenol) is an antifungal agent used in personal care products particularly in Canada, the United Kingdom, and Australia.[59] *Jadit* (butylchlorosalicylamide) and *multifungin* (bromochlorosalicylanilide) are antifungals used primarily in Australia and Europe; both are structurally related to halogenated salicylanilides.

OTHERS Exposure to the phenothiazines (*chlorpromazine* and *promethazine*) usually occurs in individuals handling medications. *Promethazine* is used as a topical antipruritic agent in some countries.[56] *Clioquinol* and *olaquindox* are antibiotics that are added to cattle feed; pig breeders are the most commonly exposed group.[60,61] *Ketoprofen* is a NSAID used topically and systemically; it produces phototoxic and photoallergic reactions. It cross-reacts with fenofibrate (a triglyceride-lowering agent), tiaprofenic acid (a NSAID), and benzophenones (sunscreen agents).[25,42,55,62] *Quinidine,* an antiarrhythmic agent, is a topical and systemic photoallergen.[37] *Thiourea (thiocarbamide)* is used in photocopy paper, photography, and rubber products.[57]

SYSTEMATIC PHOTOALLERGENS Photoallergy caused by systemic agents is much less frequent compared to that induced by topical agents. Table 136-5 lists the major photoallergens. All are also phototoxic agents and have been previously discussed in this chapter. *Pyridoxine*-induced photoallergy is rare but has been reported.[63,64]

Histopathology

The histology of photoallergy is similar to that of allergic contact dermatitis. There is epidermal spongiosis associated with infiltrate of mononuclear cells in the dermis (see Table 136-1).

Pathophysiology

Photoallergy is a type IV delayed hypersensitivity response in which the concomitant presence of photoallergen and the appropriate radiation is necessary.[9] Following the absorption of light energy, a photoallergen may be converted to an excited state molecule, which subsequently reverts to ground state by releasing the energy. In this process, the molecule may conjugate with a carrier protein to form a complete antigen. This is thought to be the mechanism of photoallergy induced by halogenated salicylanilides, chlorpromazine, and *p*-aminobenzoic acid. Alternately, a photoallergen may form a stable photoproduct upon exposure to radiation, which, in turn, may conjugate with a carrier protein to form a complete antigen. Sulfanilamide and chlorpromazine have both been shown to participate in this reaction.

Once the complete antigen is formed, the mechanism of photoallergy is identical to that of contact allergy. The antigen is taken up and processed by epidermal Langerhans cells, which then migrate to regional lymph nodes to present the antigen to T lymphocytes. Cutaneous lesions develop when the activated T lymphocytes circulate to the exposed site to initiate an inflammatory response.

Management

This is identical to that of phototoxicity; namely, identification and avoidance of photoallergen, sun protective measures, and symptomatic therapy.

TABLE 136-5

Systemic Photoallergens

PROPERTY	GENERIC NAME (US TRADE NAME)
Antifungal	Griseofulvin (*Fulvicin-U/F*)
Antimalarial	Quinine
Antimicrobials	Quinolone:
	Enoxacin (*Penetrex*)
	Sulfonamides
Cardiac medication	Quinidine (*Quinaglute, Quinidex*)
Nonsteroidal	Ketoprofen (*Orudis, Oruvail*)
	Piroxicam (*Feldene*)
Vitamin	Pyridoxine hydrochloride (vitamin B_6)

TABLE 136-6

Interpretation of Photopatch Tests

Reaction at Nonirradiated Site	Reaction at Irradiated Site	Interpretation
Negative	Positive	Photoallergic contact dermatitis
Positive	Positive (equal intensity)	Allergic contact dermatitis
Positive	Positive (more intense)	Allergic and photoallergic contact dermatitis

EVALUATION OF PATIENTS WITH PHOTOTOXICITY AND PHOTOALLERGY

The evaluation is similar to that of patients with other photosensitivity disorders and is described in greater detail in Chap. 135. Specifically, exposure to known photosensitizers needs to be obtained from the history. Development of lesions after the first exposure would suggest phototoxicity, while eruptions following a sensitization phase would suggest photoallergy. Furthermore, it is helpful to ascertain whether window glass-filtered sunlight can induce the cutaneous eruption, because UVB is filtered out by window glass. Distribution of the cutaneous eruption is a helpful clue to the type of photosensitizer responsible. Widespread eruption would suggest systemic photosensitizers while topical photosensitizers would produce lesions only in areas that have been exposed to both sensitizers and radiation. Vesicular and bullous eruptions are most commonly associated with phototoxicity, while eczematous eruptions would suggest photoallergy; the former is associated with a burning sensation, the latter with pruritus. Skin biopsy may also be helpful in differentiating these two conditions: necrotic keratinocytes are commonly seen in phototoxicity, whereas spongiotic dermatitis is associated with photoallergy (see Table 136-1).

An integral part of the evaluation of photosensitivity are phototests and photopatch tests. Approximately 4 to 20 percent of patients who undergo photopatch tests have clinically relevant positive photopatch test results, eventuating in the diagnosis of photoallergic contact dermatitis.[5,6]

The procedures for phototests and photopatch tests are as follows, although there are variations in testing methods.[65] On day 1, exposure to UVB, UVA, and visible light for MED determination is performed and duplicate sets of photoallergens are applied symmetrically to the back and covered by opaque tape. On day 2, the MEDs are quantitated. One set of patches is removed and exposed to 10 J/cm^2 of UVA, or 50 percent of the MED to UVA, whichever is lower. After irradiation, the test sites are covered again with opaque tape. On day 3, both irradiated and nonirradiated test sites are uncovered and the reactions are graded. On day 5 or day 8, the irradiated and nonirradiated sites are evaluated for delayed reactions. Table 136-6 outlines the interpretation of photopatch test reactions. Well-defined erythema that resolves promptly indicates an irritant dermatitis.

OTHER EXOGENOUS AGENT-INDUCED PHOTODERMATOSIS AND PHOTOEXACERBATED DERMATOSES

PORPHYRIA CUTANEA TARDA Ingestion of wheat treated with *hexachlorobenzene* as a preservative resulted in an outbreak of a porphyria cutanea tarda-like syndrome in Turkey in the 1950s.[66] Inhibition of the enzyme uroporphyrinogen decarboxylase by hexachlorobenzene was responsible for the clinical manifestations (see Chap. 149).

LUPUS ERYTHEMATOSUS Although a long list of medications are associated with drug-induced lupus erythematosus, it has been reported most frequently with *procainamide* and *hydralazine*.[67] Arthralgia and systemic symptoms are common; photosensitivity is a rare manifestation. Most patients have antibodies to histones. Individuals whose hepatic *N*-acetyltransferase system expresses a "slow acetylator" phenotype are most susceptible to develop this syndrome (see Chap. 171).

PELLAGRA (See Chap. 145) Skin changes of pellagra (from the Italian *pelle agra,* "rough skin") are associated with isoniazid, 6-mercaptopurine, 5-fluorouracil, chloramphenicol, sulfapyridine, anticonvulsants, and antidepressants.[68] The pathogenesis of drug-induced pellagra probably is related to the inhibition of conversion of niacin to NAD and NADP by the drug.

REFERENCES

1. Litt, JZ: *Drug Eruption Reference Manual 2001*. New York, Parthenon, 2001, pp 400–401
2. Drugs that cause photosensitivity. *Med Lett* **37**:35, 1995
3. González E, González S: Drug photosensitivity, idiopathic photodermatoses, and sunscreen. *J Am Acad Dermatol* **35**:871, 1996
4. Layton AM, Cunliffe WJ: Phototoxic eruptions due to doxycycline—A dose-related phenomenon. *Clin Exp Dermatol* **18**:425, 1993
5. Fotiades J et al: Results of evaluation of 203 patients for photosensitivity in a 7.3-year period. *J Am Acad Dermatol* **33**:597, 1995
6. Neumann NJ et al: Photopatch testing: The 12-year experience of the German, Austrian, and Swiss photopatch test group. *J Am Acad Dermatol* **42**:183, 2000
7. Harber LC, Bickers DR: *Photosensitivity Diseases. Principles of diagnosis and treatment,* 2nd ed. Toronto, BC Decker, 1989
8. Kalka K et al: Photodynamic therapy in dermatology. *J Am Acad Dermatol* **42**:389, 2000
9. Gould JW et al: Cutaneous photosensitivity diseases induced by exogenous agents. *J Am Acad Dermatol* **33**:551; 1995
10. Yong CK et al: An unusual presentation of doxycycline-induced photosensitivity. *Pediatrics* **106**:E13, 2000
11. Ming ME et al: Imipramine-induced hyperpigmentation: Four cases and a review of the literature. *J Am Acad Dermatol* **40**:159, 1999
12. Scherschun L et al: Diltiazem-associated photodistributed hyperpigmentation: A review of 4 cases. *Arch Dermatol* **137**:179, 2001
13. Choonhakarn C, Janma J: Pyrazinamide-induced lichenoid photodermatitis. *J Am Acad Dermatol* **40**:645, 1999
14. Green JJ, Manders SM: Pseudoporphyria. *J Am Acad Dermatol* **44**:100, 2001
15. Cummins R et al: Pseudoporphyria induced by celecoxib in a patient with juvenile rheumatoid arthritis. *J Rheumatol* **27**:2938, 2000
16. Borgia R et al: Photodistributed telangiectasia following use of cefotaxime. *Br J Dermatol* **143**:674, 2000
17. Lim HW et al: Chronic actinic dermatitis: Study of the spectrum of chronic photosensitivity in twelve patients. *Arch Dermatol* **126**:317, 1990
18. Morison WL et al: Consensus workshop on the toxic effects of long-term PUVA therapy. *Arch Dermatol* **134**:595, 1998
19. Moysan A et al: Evaluation of phototoxic and photogenotoxic risk associated with the use of photosensitizers in suntan preparations: Application to tanning preparations containing bergamot oil. *Skin Pharmacol* **6**:282, 1993
20. Pion IA et al: Is dermatologic usage of coal tar carcinogenic? A review of the literature. *J Dermatol Surg Oncol* **21**:227, 1995
21. Harth Y, Rapoport M: Photosensitivity associated with antipsychotics, antidepressants and anxiolytics. *Drug Saf* **14**:252, 1996

22. Epstein S: Photoallergy and primary photosensitivity to sulfanilamide. *J Invest Dermatol* **2**:43, 1939
23. Johnson BE, Ferguson J: Drug and chemical photosensitivity. *Semin Dermatol* **9**:39, 1990
24. Ljunggren B et al: Systemic quinine photosensitivity with photoepicutaneous cross-reactivity to quinidine. *Contact Dermatitis* **26**:1, 1992
25. Bagheri H et al: Photosensitivity to ketoprofen: Mechanisms and pharmacoepidemiological data. *Drug Saf* **22**:339, 2000
26. Okamoto H et al: Reactivation of phototoxicity test for psoralen plus ultraviolet A by low-dose methotrexate. *Photodermatol Photoimmunol Photomed* **10**:134, 1994
27. Viola G et al: In vitro studies of the phototoxic potential of the antidepressant drugs amitriptyline and imipramine. *Farmaco* **55**:211, 2000
28. Matsuo I et al: Possible involvement of oxidation of lipids in inducing griseofulvin photosensitivity. *Photodermatol Photoimmunol Photomed* **7**:213, 1990
29. Seidman P, Ros AM: Sensitivity to UV light during treatment with chloroquine in rheumatoid arthritis. *Scand J Rheumatol* **21**:245, 1992
30. Guzzo C, Kaidbey K: Persistent light reactivity from systemic quinine. *Photodermatol Photoimmunol Photomed* **7**:166, 1990
31. Stahlmann R, Lode H: Toxicity of quinolones. *Drugs* **58**(suppl 2):37, 1999
32. Man I et al: Recent development in fluoroquinolone phototoxicity. *Photodermatol Photoimmunol Photomed* **15**:32, 1999
33. Ohshima A et al: Formation of antigenic quinolone photoadducts on Langerhans cells initiates photoallergy to systemically administered quinolone in mice. *J Invest Dermatol* **114**:569, 2000
34. Kapusnik-Uner JE et al: Antimicrobial agents, in *Goodman & Gilman's The Pharmacological Basis of Therapeutics,* 9th edi, edited by JG Hardman, LE Limbird, PB Molinoff, RW Ruddon, A Goodman Gilman. New York, McGraw-Hill, 1996, p 1129
35. Eberlein-Konig B et al: Phototoxic properties of neuroleptic drugs. *Dermatology* **194**:131, 1997
36. Charlmers RTC et al: High incidence of amiodarone-induced photosensitivity in North-West England. *Br Med J* **285**:341, 1982
37. Schurer NY et al: Photosensitivity induced by quinidine sulfate: Experimental reproduction of skin lesions. *Photodermatol Photoimmunol Photomed* **9**:78, 1992
38. Danis RP et al: Phototoxicity from systemic sodium fluorescein. *Retina* **20**:370, 2000
39. Porat R et al: Methylene blue-induced phototoxicity: an unrecognized complication. *Pediatrics* **97**:717, 1996.
40. Vargas F et al: Studies on the in vitro phototoxicity of the antidiabetes drug glipizide. *In Vitr Mol Toxicol* **13**:17, 2000
41. Serrano G et al: Oxicam-induced photosensitivity. Patch and photopatch testing studies with tenoxicam and piroxicam photoproducts in normal subjects and in piroxicam-droxicam photosensitive patients. *J Am Acad Dermatol* **26**:545, 1992
42. Matsushita T, Kamide R: Five cases of photocontact dermatitis due to topical ketoprofen: Photopatch testing and cross-reaction study. *Photodermatol Photoimmunol Photomed* **17**:26, 2001
43. Ferguson J, Johnson BE: Photosensitivity due to retinoids: Clinical and laboratory studies. *Br J Dermatol* **115**:275, 1986
44. Yokote R et al: Photosensitive drug eruption induced by flutamide. *Eur J Dermatol* **8**:427, 1998
45. Todd P et al: Ranitidine-induced photosensitivity. *Clin Exp Dermatol* **20**:146, 1995
46. Schempp CM et al: Single-dose and steady-state administration of *Hypericum perforatum* extract (St. John's wort) does not influence skin sensitivity to UV radiation, visible light, and solar-simulated radiation. *Arch Dermatol* **137**:512, 2001
47. Vantieghem A et al: Different pathways mediate cytochrome *c* release after photodynamic therapy with hypericin. *Photochem Photobiol* **74**:133, 2001
48. Maeda T et al: Vitamin B_6 phototoxicity induced by UVA radiation. *Arch Dermatol Res* **292**:562, 2000
49. Encinas S et al: Phototoxicity associated with diclofenac: A photophysical, photochemical, and photobiological study on the drug and its photoproducts. *Chem Res Toxicol* **11**:946, 1998
50. Lim HW et al: Role of complement and polymorphonuclear cells in demethylchlortetracycline-induced phototoxicity. *J Clin Invest* **71**:1326, 1983
51. Torinuki W, Tagami H: Role of complement in chlorpromazine-induced phototoxicity. *J Invest Dermatol* **86**:142, 1986
52. Nehal KS, Lim HW: Phototoxicity and photoallergy. *Dermatol Nurs* **7**:227, 1995
53. DeLeo VA et al: Photoallergic contact dermatitis: Results of photopatch testing in New York, 1985 to 1990. *Arch Dermatol* **128**:1513, 1992
54. Darvey A et al: Photoallergic dermatitis is uncommon. *Br. J. Dermatol* **145**:597, 2001
55. Albes B et al: Prolonged photosensitivity following contact photoallergy to ketoprofen. *Dermatology* **201**:171, 2000
56. Schauder S: Dioxopromethazine-induced photoallergic contact dermatitis followed by persistent light reaction. *Am J Contact Dermat* **9**:182, 1998
57. Rietschel RL, Fowler JF Jr: *Fisher's Contact Dermatitis,* 5th ed. Philadelphia, Lippincott Williams & Wilkins, 2001
58. *IARC Handbook of Cancer Prevention. Vol. 5: Sunscreen*. Lyon, France, International Agency for Research on Cancer, 2001
59. Marks JG Jr, DeLeo VA: Photoallergens, in *Contact and Occupational Dermatology,* 2nd ed. St. Louis, Mosby, 1997, p 200
60. Rivara G et al: Photosensitivity in a patient with contact allergic dermatitis from clioquinol. *Photodermatol Photoimmunol Photomed* **8**:225, 1991
61. Schauder S et al: Olaquindox-induced airborne photoallergic contact dermatitis followed by transient or persistent light reaction in 15 pig breeders. *Contact Dermatitis* **35**:344, 1996
62. Le Coz CJ et al: Photocontact dermatitis from ketoprofen and tiaprofenic acid: Cross-reactivity study in 12 consecutive patients. *Contact Dermatitis* **38**:245, 1998
63. Tanaka M et al: Photoallergic drug eruption due to pyridoxine hydrochloride. *J Dermatol* **23**:708, 1996
64. Murata Y et al: Photosensitive dermatitis caused by pyridoxine hydrochloride. *J Am Acad Dermatol* **39**:314, 1998
65. Kim JJ, Lim HW: Evaluation of the photosensitive patient. *Semin Cutan Med Surg* **18**:253, 1999
66. Herrero C et al: Urinary porphyrin excretion in a human population highly exposed to hexachlorobenzene. *Arch Dermatol* **135**:400, 1999
67. Hahn BH: Systemic lupus erythematosus, in *Harrison's Principles of Internal Medicine,* 15th ed., edited by E Braunwald, AS Fauci, DL Kasper, S Hauser, DL Longo, JL Jameson. New York, McGraw-Hill, 2001, p 1922
68. Hendricks WM: Pellagra and pellagra-like dermatoses: Etiology, differential diagnosis, dermatopathology, and treatment. *Semin Dermatol* **10**:282, 1991

SECTION 19

DISORDERS DUE TO DRUGS AND CHEMICAL AGENTS

CHAPTER 137

James S. Taylor
Apra Sood

Occupational Skin Disease

Occupational dermatoses are any abnormal conditions of the skin caused or aggravated by substances or processes associated with the work environment. Disorders range from erythema, urticaria, and eczematous reactions to acneiform, pigmentary, ulcerative, granulomatous, and neoplastic conditions. Often overlooked is the importance of the skin as a major portal of entry for chemical exposure to systemic toxins.

HISTORICAL ASPECTS AND RESOURCES

Paracelsus (1498–1541), in his *Morbis Metallicus,* was the first to write about occupational diseases, including changes in the skin caused by salt compounds. At about the same time, Agricola described deep skin ulcers in his book about metal workers. And in 1700, Ramazzini, the father of modern occupational medicine, made many observations about occupational skin diseases in his classical work *De Morbis Artificium Diatriba*. Beginning in 1775, when Percival Pott described carcinoma of the scrotum among chimney sweeps, a number of other European authors described and studied occupational skin diseases and contact dermatitis. Earlier twentieth century texts include Prosser White's *The Dermatergoses or Occupational Afflictions of the Skin,* in 1915, and Schwartz, Tulipan, and Birmingham's *Occupational Diseases of the Skin* in 1957. Selected current resources for more in depth information include Taylor JS (ed), *Dermatologic Clinics* (6:1–129, 1988 and 12:461–600, 1994); Marks and DeLeo's *Contact and Occupational Dermatology* (1997); Adams' *Occupational Skin Disease* (1999); Kanerva et al.'s *Handbook of Occupational Dermatology* (2000); *Fisher's Contact Dermatitis* (2001); and Rycroft et al.'s *Textbook of Contact Dermatitis* (2001).

EPIDEMIOLOGY

The US Department of Labor publishes annual incidence statistics on the safety and health of employees in private industry (www.osha.gov). In 2000, 5.7 million nonfatal job-related injuries and illnesses were reported, a rate of 6.1 per 100 equivalent full-time workers. This is the lowest rate ever recorded. Illnesses accounted for 362,500 cases, the majority of which were repeated trauma disorders, such as carpal tunnel syndrome, followed by skin diseases or disorders, accounting for 41,800 cases. The number of skin disease cases has declined significantly since data collection began in the 1970s, and the drop has been more precipitous in the past 4 years. Reasons for this decline are not clear but include better prevention and a change in the ease with which workers' compensation cases are accepted, or a change in reporting patterns of employees or employers, or other factors.[1] Earlier studies showed significant underreporting of all classes of work-related disorders. Some cases are never reported but instead are filed with the employer's private health insurance. This decline in OSHA-reported occupational skin diseases has been widespread across industry sectors. Manufacturing and service industries account for about three-fourths of all skin disease cases, and contact dermatitis is the most frequent diagnosis (1994 data). One-third of workers with occupational skin disease missed more than 5 days of work [14.5 percent missed 6 to 10 days, 8.3 percent (11 to 20 days), 3.3 percent (21 to 30 days), and 5.8 percent (more than 31 days)]; two-thirds missed 1 to 5 days (1994 data). [2] Data from Germany and Denmark indicate that the incidence rate for skin disease among hairdressers and cooks is more than 10 to 20 times the average of all cases.[3] For years, skin disorders were considered an invariable accompaniment of work, but ideally, all occupational skin disease can and should be prevented.

IRRITANT CONTACT DERMATITIS

Irritant contact dermatitis (ICD), the most common occupational skin disease, is a nonimmunologic inflammatory reaction following exposure of the skin to an external chemical or physical agent. Irritation accounts for up to 80 percent of occupational skin disease cases and affects the most often exposed areas of skin, such as the hands and forearms. The clinical spectrum of irritation is very broad and in addition to the more common acute and chronic eczematous reactions also includes ulceration, folliculitis, acneiform eruptions, miliaria, pigmentary alterations, alopecia, contact urticaria and granulomatous reactions (Table 137-1).[4]

TABLE 137-1

Clinical Features That May Suggest the Etiology of Irritant Dermatitis*

Eczema (acute and cumulative irritant exposure)
- Industrial cleaners
- Water, soaps, and detergents
- Weak acids and alkalies
- Oils and organic solvents
- Oxidizing agents (H_2O_2, benzoyl peroxide)

Ulcerations/burns
- Strong acids, especially chromic, hydrofluoric, nitric, hydrochloric, sulfuric
- Strong alkalis, especially calcium oxide, sodium hydroxide, potassium hydroxide, ammonium hydroxide, calcium hydroxide, sodium metasilicate, sodium silicate, potassium cyanide, trisodium phosphate
- Salts, especially arsenic trioxide, dichromates
- Solvents, especially acrylonitrile, carbon bisulfide
- Gases, especially ethylene oxide, acrylonitrile

Folliculitis and acneiform eruptions
- Arsenic trioxide
- Glass fibers
- Oils and greases
- Tar
- Asphalt
- Chlorinated naphthalenes
- Polyhalogenated biphenyls

Miliaria
- Occlusive clothing
- Adhesive tape
- Ultraviolet and infrared radiation
- Aluminum chloride

Pigmentary changes

Hyperpigmentation
- Any irritant or allergen, especially phototoxic agents such as psoralens, tar, asphalt, phototoxic plants, others
- Metals,* such as inorganic arsenic (systemically), silver, gold, bismuth, mercury
- Radiation: ultraviolet, infrared, microwave, ionizing

Hypopigmentation*
- *p-tert*-Amylphenol and butylphenol
- Hydroquinone
- Monobenzyl and monomethyl ether of hydroquinone
- *p-tert*-Catechol
- *p*-Cresol
- 3-Hydroxyanisole
- Butylated hydroxyanisole
- 1-*tert*-Butyl-3,4-catechol
- 1-Isopropyl-3,4-catechol
- 4-Hydroxypropriophenone

Alopecia
- Borax
- Chloroprene dimers

Urticaria
- Numerous chemicals, cosmetics, animal products, foods, plants, textiles, woods

Granulomas*
- Keratin
- Silica
- Beryllium
- Talc
- Cotton fibers
- Bacteria
- Fungi
- Parasites and parasite parts

*Some are allergens.
SOURCE: Lammintausta K et al.[4]

Major Categories

The two major types of irritant contact dermatitis are acute ICD, including chemical burns, and cumulative ICD.

ACUTE ICD, INCLUDING CHEMICAL BURNS Acute eczematous dermatitis after exposure to a potent irritant, often to a single chemical acid or alkali solution, may overlap with chemical burns. Highly irritating chemicals induce a reaction in any person's skin if the concentration and duration of action are sufficient; the intrinsic nature of the chemical is also important. Strong alkalis and acids, such as sodium and potassium hydroxides and hydrochloric and sulfuric acids are common irritants, among others. In national statistics for work-related injuries, acute ICD reactions are often classified as chemical burns (Fig. 137-1).

CUMULATIVE ICD Cumulative ICD, the most common type of ICD, develops slowly after cumulative but additive subthreshold exposures to mild irritants (soap, water, detergents, industrial cleansers, solvents, etc.) under a variety of conditions. Dermatitis is usually localized to the finger webspaces, but later spreads to the sides and dorsal surface of the hands, and finally to the palmar surface. The volar aspect of the wrist is usually spared in contrast to allergic hand eczema. The hallmark is the absence of vesicles and the predominance of dryness and chapping. However, the diagnosis is complicated by hybrids, where there is a combination of ICD and allergic contact dermatitis, or of ICD and atopy, or even of all three.[5] High-risk occupations for cumulative ICD include bakers, canners, caterers, cleaners, cooks, health care workers such as dental assistants and technicians and nurses, hairdressers, mechanics, printers, and butchers.[6]

FIGURE 137-1

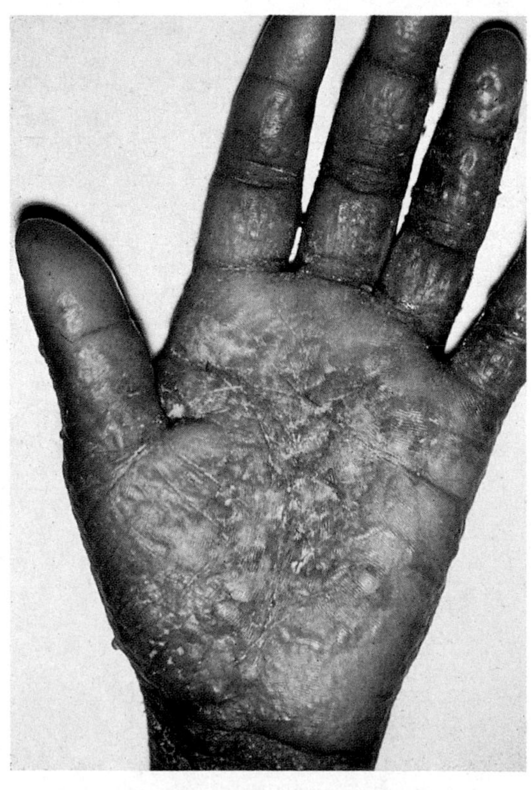

Vesiculobullous hand eruption in a 42-year-old man from prolonged wearing of solvent-soaked gloves.

Other Categories

To more accurately define irritant dermatitis, other types have been described; some represent subcategories or overlap forms:

ACUTE DELAYED ICD Reaction is not seen until 8 to 24 h after exposure and may be misdiagnosed as allergic contact dermatitis. Examples include anthralin, bromine,[7] hexanediol diacrylate, podophyllin, ethylene oxide, and propylene glycol.

IRRITANT REACTION Irritant reaction is an early, almost subclinical dermatitis, or sentinel event, often seen on the hands of individuals exposed to wet work, such as hair dressers or metal workers, in their first several months of training.[5,8] The eruption is monomorphous and is characterized by one or more of the following signs: dryness, erythema, vesicles, pustules, and erosions.

TRAUMATIC ICD See posttraumatic eczema in the section "Physical Causes."

NONERYTHEMATOUS ICD Another subclinical type characterized by changes in the stratum corneum barrier function without a clinical correlate.

SUBJECTIVE ICD Also called sensory ICD, this condition is characterized by lack of clinical signs but is accompanied by burning and stinging after contact with certain chemicals, such as lactic acid.

PREDISPOSING FACTORS IN ICD

Specific factors Occupational ICD, especially of the chronic, cumulative type, is a prime example of the concept of multifactorial causation of disease. Not only are the *properties of the irritating substance* important (pH, solubility, and detergent action), but also its *physical state* (gaseous, liquid, or solid). Important *host factors* include the presence or absence of occlusion, sweating, pigmentation, dryness, and sebaceous activity, and the simultaneous presence of another skin disease, especially one that is reactivated by contact with irritant(s). Important *environmental factors* include temperature, humidity, friction, pressure, occlusion, and coexisting lacerations. A *worker's age, gender, skin type,* and *genetic background* may also be important.

Other factors Atopy is one of the most important contributing factors to ICD. Individuals with a personal or past history of atopic eczema (see Chap. 122) have an increased susceptibility to skin irritation and account for a large percentage of workers compensation dermatitis claims.

Low relative humidity in the workplace, especially in atopics is also an important factor in developing dermatitis, especially with the presence of other irritants. With relative humidity below 35 to 40 percent, the stratum corneum becomes drier and more brittle, with increasing permeability to marginal irritants. *Low humidity dermatitis* has been reported in closed, windowless offices, in manufacturing of soft contact lenses, and in the clean rooms of silicon-chip manufacturing plants. Symptoms, such as pruritus and burning may be the only complaints and are more distressing than physical signs, which may involve exposed or covered areas. Differential diagnosis includes airborne irritation, other dermatoses, and psychogenic causes. Treatment includes liberal use of emollients and increasing the indoor relative humidity to about 50 percent, if possible.

Airborne Irritant Dermatitis

Airborne irritants are an important cause of contact dermatitis. The pattern is fairly characteristic with distribution on the face, neck, anterior chest and arms. The most frequent causes are irritating dusts and volatile chemicals, such as solvents, ammonia, formaldehyde, epoxy resins and their hardeners, cement dust, fibrous glass, and sawdust-especially from irritating woods.

Diagnosis of Irritant Dermatitis

There are no reliable confirmatory tests for the diagnosis of ICD. Diagnosis is primarily based on a history of exposure to a known potential irritant that is consistent with the observed clinical appearance and anatomic distribution. Because of their close resemblance to allergic contact dermatitis, subacute and chronic irritant dermatitis are almost always diagnoses of exclusion and it is necessary to patch test most affected patients. Rietschel[9] has proposed criteria for the clinical diagnosis of ICD (Table 137-2).

Common Occupational Irritants

Examples of common occupational irritants are described in the following sections.

SOAPS AND DETERGENTS Most toilet soaps do not irritate normal skin in normal usage. If the skin is already even slightly damaged from contact with other irritants, the use of industrial skin cleansers, designed to remove heavy industrial soil from the skin, can be very irritating, especially to atopic skin. Industrial skin cleansers are available commercially as cakes, liquids, powders, or creams. The choice of cleanser varies with the job for which it is intended. Machinists and auto-mechanics need a cleanser with a high detergent and abrasive action. Borax has been used for years for this purpose, and has the advantage of dissolving as it cleans. Somewhat more irritating are abrasives of vegetable origin. Sand and pumice have been used in some hand cleansers but are highly irritating and should generally be avoided or used sparingly, mainly on the palms and only for removal of the most tenacious soils.

TABLE 137-2

Diagnostic Criteria of Irritant Contact Dermatitis

Major	Minor
Subjective	
1. Onset of symptoms within minutes to hours of exposure	1. Onset of dermatitis within 2 weeks of exposure
2. Pain, burning, stinging, or discomfort exceeding itching early in the clinical course	2. Many people in the environment affected similarly
Objective	
1. Macular erythema, hyperkeratosis, or fissuring predominating over vesiculation	1. Sharp circumspection of the dermatitis
2. Glazed, parched, or scalded appearance of the epidermis	2. Evidence of gravitational influence, such as a dripping effect
3. Healing process begins promptly on withdrawal of exposure to the offending agent	3. Lack of tendency of the dermatitis to spread
4. Patch testing is negative	4. Morphologic changes suggesting small concentration differences or contact time produce large differences in skin damage

SOURCE: Rietschel et al.[9]

TABLE 137-3

Selected Burns That Require Unique Therapies

CHEMICAL	TREATMENT
Burning metal fragments of sodium, potassium, and lithium	Extinguish with sand, cover with mineral oil, and irrigate with water before mechanically extracting particles
Hydrofluoric acid	Running water; then calcium gluconate: gel (2.5%) followed by intralesional injection, if needed
Phosphorus	Remove particles mechanically; soap and water, then copper (II) sulfate in water for several minutes; remove black copper phosphide and wash with water
Phenolic compounds	Initial soap and water washing followed by polyethylene glycol 300 or 400 or ethanol (10%) in water
Bromine or iodine	Wash frequently with soap and water followed by treatment with 5% sodium thiosulfate

SOURCE: Bruze M et al.[11]

WATERLESS HAND CLEANSERS Waterless hand cleansers are formulated to remove difficult oil and grease stains and are widely used at worksites where there is no convenient source of water. These products should not be used for skin cleaning when ordinary hand soaps would suffice, and they may provoke dermatitis from unnecessary overuse. They should be used sparingly during the workday, because they contain a higher percentage of petroleum-derived solvent. Rags are often used to remove these cleansers, and by the end of a shift they can be saturated with a variety of irritants. After use, the potentially irritating residual film should be washed off with mild soap and water. Disposable towels or presaturated wipes from dispensers are better choices and are useful in many situations, especially in the clean rooms of the semiconductor industry. They usually contain antibacterial agents as preservatives, which also may be contact allergens. Instant hand sanitizers, often containing high concentrations of alcohol, are now available. Some of these can be drying to skin.

Many chemicals are capable of causing skin damage, making chemical burns an important cause of occupational injury.[10] Copious washing is the primary measure required in treating all chemical burns. However, certain types of burns require specific antidotes and therapies (Table 137-3).[11]

Acids and Alkalis, Including Chemical Burns

Inorganic acids are used in enormous quantities in industry, especially sulfuric, hydrochloric, chromic, hydrofluoric, nitric, and phosphoric acids. *Sulfuric acid* is one of the largest chemical commodities produced in the United States and is widely used in the manufacture of fertilizers, inorganic pigments, textile fibers, explosives, pulp and paper. *Hydrochloric acid* is used in the production of fertilizers, dyes, paints, and soaps. Sodium and potassium hydroxide, ammonium hydroxide, sodium and potassium carbonate and calcium oxide are widely used in the manufacture of bleaches, dyes, vitamins, plastics, pulp and paper, soaps and detergents.[12] Many of these acids and alkalis are common causes of chemical burns. Strong acids cause erythema, blistering and necrosis, and may discolor the skin. Strong alkalis saponify surface lipids and penetrate easily, leading to more severe and extensive tissue destruction, including deep ulcerations that heal very slowly.

Organic acids, such as acetic, acrylic, formic, glycolic, benzoic and salicylic acids, tend to be less irritating than inorganic acids, but especially after prolonged exposure, even in weak concentrations, they can cause chronic irritant dermatitis. *Formic acid* is used in the textile industry in dyeing and finishing, as a delimer and neutralizer in leather manufacture, and as a coagulant in the production of natural latex, among other uses. It has greater corrosive potential than most other organic acids. *Acrylic acid,* used chiefly as a monomer for acrylic plastics, is irritating and corrosive to the skin. Fatty acids, such as palmitic, oleic, and stearic acids tend to be less irritating.[12]

HYDROFLUORIC ACID Hydrofluoric acid (HF) is a strong acid with many uses including etching and frosting of glass, rust removal, and "spot cleaning" in dry cleaning. HF is extremely irritating to skin, even in concentrations of 15 to 20 percent. Fluoride ions penetrate deep into the tissues and bind to the calcium and magnesium ions, causing severe tissue damage including bone destruction, especially of the terminal digits of the hand.[11] Following exposure to lower concentrations of HF, the onset of symptoms may be delayed until release of fluoride ions occurs in deep tissues. Exposure to HF is a medical emergency requiring topical or subcutaneous calcium gluconate after lavage to bind the fluoride ions (Table 137-3).

CEMENT Exposure to wet cement may cause severe alkaline and thermal burns due to the exothermic reaction of calcium oxide with water forming calcium hydroxide.[13] Kneeling in wet cement for prolonged periods leads to deep burns of the knees (cement knees) and shins; [14] lesions may become deep enough to require excision and grafting. Burns may also result from the trapping of wet cement in gloves and boots.

CHROMIC ACID Chromic acid is highly irritating to the skin, causing ulcerations of the skin ("chrome holes") and perforation of the nasal septum. Exposures occur in chrome plating, copper stripping, and aluminum anodizing operations. Chromic acid may be absorbed and lead to renal failure.[15]

PHOSPHORUS Phosphorus is used in the manufacture of insecticides and fertilizers, and can cause deep, destructive burns. It ignites spontaneously on exposure to air so that the affected area should be kept moist until the chemical is completely removed. Severe metabolic derangements have been reported following phosphorus burns and patients should be closely monitored for multiorgan failure.[16]

ETHYLENE OXIDE Ethylene oxide is used commercially and in hospital central supply units for sterilization of surgical and medical instruments and devices as well as textiles and plastic material. Burns may result from contact with porous materials and devices that have been sterilized with ethylene oxide but not properly aerated.[17]

PHENOL Phenol is rapidly absorbed through intact skin and can cause local necrosis and nerve damage.

METAL SALTS Arsenic compounds such as arsenic trioxide, the dust of which can be contacted during the smelting of copper, gold, lead, and other metals, can cause a persistent folliculitis in addition to systemic poisoning. In the semiconductor industry, exposure to arsenic can occur during maintenance activities and especially during the handling of raw materials. Allergic contact dermatitis has been reported from sodium arsenate. *Beryllium compounds* are employed in the aerospace and other industries for the production of hard, corrosion-resistant alloys, among other uses. They may cause an irritant dermatitis, but especially characteristic are ulcerating granulomas from implantation of beryllium salts.[12] Allergic contact dermatitis and allergic granulomas are also reported. *Calcium oxide* (quicklime), used as a refractory, as a flux in the manufacture of steel (among many other uses) is a strong skin irritant that releases heat on contact with water, causing painful skin ulcerations. *Copper salts* are skin irritants and occasionally contact allergens. Inorganic arsenic may contaminate coppers ores. Metal fume fever, a flulike illness of brief duration, may result from inhalation of the fine particle of oxides of copper, as well as from magnesium and zinc. Today, it is usually associated with welding operations performed with inadequate ventilation.[18] *Cobalt salts,* used in alloys, ceramics, electroplating, electronics, magnets, paints and varnishes, cosmetics, and the like, may be irritants and also cause allergic contact dermatitis. When used in hard metal alloys, the dust may also cause pulmonary sensitization.[19] Inorganic mercury exposure sometimes causes a bluish linear pigmentation on the gums and tongue, which should be considered a marker for systemic poisoning. *Compounds of mercury* have been widely used as bactericides, dental amalgams, catalysts, and the like. Alkyl mercury compounds cause severe burns and corrosion of the skin. Exposure to *selenium compounds* can cause a conjunctivitis termed *rose eye,* as well as a reddish discoloration of the skin and hair. Selenium dioxide and selenium oxychloride are strong skin vesicants.

SOLVENTS Millions of workers are exposed to solvents daily. Until recently, most solvents were used to dissolve other substances or as diluents for adhesives or surface coatings. Today the chief uses are in the manufacture of other chemicals; as carriers for chemical reactions; as pressure transmitters for hydraulic systems; and in coatings, industrial cleaners, printing inks, and pharmaceuticals. After water, the most common solvents are aliphatic and aromatic hydrocarbons, esters, ethers, ketones, amines, and nitrated and chlorinated hydrocarbons (Table 137-4).[20] Volatile solvents, especially, act by dissolving the intercellular lipid of the epidermis, causing "whitening" of the skin and a feeling of dryness. By dissolving the skin's lipid barrier layer, percutaneous absorption of the solvent, and any chemical it contains is increased. The more lipophilic the solvent, the greater the absorption. Prolonged skin contact with solvent-soaked clothing can result in systemic symptoms, as well as severe burns, and sometimes even death. There is an inverse correlation between the boiling point of a solvent and its primary irritant effect.[21]

TABLE 137-4

Selected Industrial Solvents That Are Skin Irritants

Solvent Class/Solvent	Comments
Coal tar solvents: Benzene, toluene, xylene, ethyl, benzene, cumene	Industrial use reduced by environmental regulation; benzene associated with aplastic anemia/leukemia
Petroleum solvents: Gasoline, kerosene, Stoddard solvent, hexane	Stoddard solvent widely used; gasoline vapors may induce narcosis; *N*-hexane may cause sensory/motor neuropathy
Chlorinated hydrocarbon solvents: Carbon tetrachloride, trichloroethane, tetrachloroethane, trichloroethylene (TCE), methylene chloride, ethylene dichloride	Many are degreasers with systemic (especially liver, renal, and CNS) toxicity; alcohol ingestion after TCE exposure causes degreaser's flush
Alcohol solvents: Methyl-, ethyl-, and isopropyl alcohols	Methyl alcohol ingestion and inhalation causes blindness
Ethylene glycol ether solvents: Glycidyl ethers; ethyl-amyl-, and butyl acetates	Solvents for paints and dyes; lower molecular weight glycidyl ethers are contact allergens
Others: Turpentine, ethyl ether, acetone, methyl ethyl ketone, carbon disulfide, DMSO, dioxane, styrene	Acetone widely used; turpentine is a contact allergen

SOURCE: Wahlberg JE et al.[20]

Workers are rarely exposed to a single solvent. More often they are exposed to mixtures of several solvents, but clinically, it is often difficult to demonstrate the relative importance of an individual ingredient of a mixture. Mineral spirits, kerosene, gasoline, and various thinners are widely used as mixtures.

FIBROUS GLASS Glass fibers, also called man-made vitreous fibers (MMVF), causes a characteristic highly pruritic contact dermatitis, that may resemble scabies. Fibers larger than 3.5 μm are generally responsible, causing pruritus and furious scratching and excoriations. Symptoms usually subside in a week or two and workers can usually return to the same work without recurrence. Patients with atopic eczema or dermographism may have to change jobs. Pathogenesis is via direct, indirect (through clothing), or airborne irritant dermatitis. Symptoms may occur through simple mechanical irritation by sting, penetration of fibers into the skin and a secondary allergic contact dermatitis from the associated finishing resins, for example, epoxy.

FABRICS Wool and rough synthetic clothing are well known to cause itching dermatitis, especially in atopic individuals. Fire-retardant fabrics, "NCR" paper, and paper face masks, as used in the semiconductor and other industries, also frequently induce irritation in such persons.

PLANTS Irritant dermatitis is the most frequent type of plant-related dermatitis and can appear as erythema, hyperkeratosis of the hands and fingers, papules, vesicles, necrosis, abrasions, or granulomas. Plant families most commonly associated with irritation are the *Euphorbiaceae* (various spurges, crotons, poinsettias, manchineel tree); *Ranunculaceae* (buttercup) and *Cruciferae,* also termed *Brassicaceae* (black mustard); *Urticaceae* (nettles); *Solanaceae* (pepper, capsaicin); and *Opuntia vulgaris* (prickly pear).[22] Many plants cause only simple irritation, as from spines, thorns, sharp-edged weeds, and trichromes and barbs (glochids) of certain cacti.[23] Sabra dermatitis, for example, is a term used for dermatitis caused by contact with tiny glochids on the surface of the Indian fig (*Opuntia ficus-indica*), which penetrate the skin and cause a dermatitis resembling scabies. Sometimes foreign-body granulomas are formed.

The chemicals present in various sections of plants are responsible for much of the irritation from plants. These include oxalic, formic and acetic acids; various glycosides; proteolytic enzymes; phorbol esters; isothiocyanates; and crystals of calcium oxalate.[24] Phototoxic eruptions from plants (phytophotodermatitis) are fairly common among farm workers, nursery personnel, florists, and gardeners, and occur more frequently than photoallergic reactions. Plants containing furocoumarins, such as 5-methoxypsoralen (bergapten, 5-MOP), are the most common causes of phototoxic reactions, which result from contact with the plant followed by exposure to ultraviolet light (UVA) at wavelengths of 320 to 400 nm in sunlight. Large bullae appear on exposed skin, which are almost always nonpruritic. After resolving in a week or so, characteristic linear, hyperpigmented streaks remain, which may last for months. Outdoor workers exposed to moist plants, either from fog or irrigation, and sunlight may develop these characteristic lesions, which usually appear a few hours after exposure but sometimes not until 36 to 48 h later. Plant families responsible for most of these eruptions are the *Umbelliferae* (parsley, celery, parsnip, giant hogweed, and others), *Rutaceae* (rue, burning bush or gas plant, bergamot), and *Moraceae* (fig tree).

A widespread phytophotodermatitis may result from contact with weeds, such as cow parsley (*Anthrisis sylvestris*) and hogweed (*Heracleum sphondylium*). The term *strimmer dermatitis* (or "weed-whacker dermatitis") is applied to a photodermatitis caused by contact with newly mowed, moist plant fragments on sunny days. The eczematous eruption is often bullous, leaving characteristic hyperpigmented streaks.

Celery harvesters and grocery clerks handling celery may develop a phytophotodermatitis, as well as bartenders squeezing limes, especially out-of-doors on sunny days. By testing celery pickers with serial dilutions of 8-methoxypsoralen, 5-methoxypsoralen, and trimethylpsoralen, Ljunggren was able to differentiate allergy from phototoxicity.[25]

ALLERGIC CONTACT DERMATITIS (See also Chap. 120)

Allergic contact dermatitis (ACD) in the working environment is reported less frequently to workers' compensation authorities than irritant dermatitis, in part because most workers with contact dermatitis are never patch tested to determine the presence of contact allergy; thus many cases are not diagnosed and reported. In a recent multicenter study from the North American Contact Dermatitis Group, of 839 occupational dermatitis cases (29 percent of 2889 patients referred for evaluation of contact dermatitis), 54 percent were primarily allergic, 32 percent irritant, and 14 percent were diagnoses other than contact dermatitis, aggravated by work.[26] In this series, nursing was the occupation most commonly found to have allergic contact dermatitis. Other occupations were assemblers, nurse's aides and orderlies, machinists, students, machine operators, auto mechanics, compressing and compacting jobs, and cooks. Allergens strongly associated with occupational exposure were rubber (thiuram and carbamate accelerators), epoxy resin, and ethylenediamine. The hands are the most commonly affected site in occupational allergic contact dermatitis. The dorsal hands are typically involved along with the finger webspaces and the forearms. Nail dystrophy may occur if there is involvement of the periungual areas.

Table 137-5[27] lists the principal occupational contact allergens and Table 137-6[28] lists blind spots in the diagnosis of allergic contact dermatitis. Also see "Patch Testing" later in this chapter.

The mechanism of ACD is discussed in Chap. 120. It is important to remember, however, that the induction of allergic sensitization to a specific allergen in a nonsensitive individual requires 4 or 5 days or more. Following subsequent contact with the allergens, the sensitive person will develop a clearly defined reaction, appearing as early as 24 to 48 h later. This information is important in determining when and where sensitization took place. If ACD develops in a worker after only 2 or 3 days following initial contact with an allergen, the induction of sensitivity must have occurred previously, perhaps during an earlier occupation.

TABLE 137-5

Major Occupational Contact Allergens

Biocides: isothiazolinones, formaldehyde releasers
Chromate
Cobalt
Colophony
Dyes
Epoxy resin systems (may need to test with worker's own resin)
Formaldehyde
Formaldehyde resins
Fragrances and essences
Nickel—primarily, usually nonoccupational
Plants and woods
Rubber processing chemicals

SOURCE: Rycroft RJG.[27]

TABLE 137-6

Blind Spots in the Diagnosis of Allergic Contact Dermatitis (ACD)

BLIND SPOT	EXAMPLE
ACD may be identical to another disease	Seborrheic dermatitis–like ACD caused by hair tonic
	Tinea pedis misdiagnosed as occupational ACD; positive KOH prep made the diagnosis
	Factitial dermatitis of the hand diagnosed as occupational ACD; cured with Unna boot occlusive dressing
	ACD caused by sunscreen ingredient benzophenone 3 in a utility lineman; misdiagnosed as sunburn
Failure to make a second diagnosis	ACD from neomycin; misdiagnosed as flare of atopic eczema
	Chronic actinic dermatitis of the face with ACD from topical corticosteroids in a roofer
Occult exposure to an allergen	Keys in pants pocket caused ACD of the lateral thigh in a nickel plater allergic to nickel
	ACD caused by preservative imidazolidinyl urea in a sunscreen with a label that listed only active ingredients
	Chronic hand eczema and contact allergic to thiourea mix in a rubber worker caused by neoprene beverage holder
Inadequate or deceptive history—patient does not recall exposure to specific allergens	Patient with chronic hand eczema worsened by doxepin cream and identified only from a pharmacy prescription list
	Patient allergic to neomycin with persistent periorbital eczema caused by tobramycin-containing ointment, not recognized as a cross-reacting allergen
Failure of patch testing	Occupational contact dermatitis of the hands attributed to a false-positive irritant patch test reaction to a cleanser
	Occupational contact dermatitis of the hands with a false-negative patch test reaction to latex surgical gloves; further patch testing indicated an allergy to thiurams, present as accelerators in the gloves

SOURCE: Shelly WB et al.[28]

CONTACT URTICARIA AND IMMEDIATE CONTACT REACTIONS

There are three varieties of contact urticaria (CU): (1) nonimmunologic (NICU); (2) Immunologic (ICU), a type I IgE-mediated reaction; and (3) CU of uncertain mechanism (see also Chap. 116).

NICU

In NICU, nearly all exposed individuals will develop reactions without previous sensitization, depending on the nature of the substance, its concentration, the area of skin exposed, and mode of exposure. The reaction usually remains localized, and systemic symptoms of wheezing, rhinorrhea and syncope usually do not occur. Among the most potent ubiquitous urticants causing this type of CU are benzoic acid, sorbic acid, cinnamic acid, cinnamic aldehyde, and nicotinic acid esters.[29] Gardeners (nettles, various plants, caterpillar hairs, moths, and other insects), cooks (fish, mustard, cayenne pepper, and thyme), and medical and related personnel (alcohol, balsam of Peru, benzocaine, methyl salicylate, tar extracts, tincture of benzoin, witch hazel, and DMSO) are some of the occupational groups that may be affected.

ICU

ICU, an IgE-mediated, immediate allergic reaction, occurs in persons previously sensitized to a specific agent. Individuals with a history of atopy, especially atopic dermatitis, are more susceptible. The paradigm for occupational ICU is natural rubber latex (NRL) allergy, which results from a reaction to one or more of the 240 proteins present in NRL. The highest prevalence of NRL allergy is in spina bifida patients. Also affected are health care workers, kitchen workers, cleaners, rubber band, surgical glove, and latex doll manufacturing workers, and others who wear NRL gloves. Greatest risk is from exposure to dipped NRL devices (gloves, especially if powdered; balloons; condoms; catheters; and dental dams) in contrast to dry-molded rubber products (syringes, plungers, vial stoppers, etc.), which contain lower residual or extractable protein levels.[30] See Chap. 120 and the section "Prevention" in this chapter for more information on NRL allergy. Besides latex, the next most common cause of ICU is foodstuffs, occurring in cooks, grocery workers, and handlers of meat, fish, and other foodstuffs. Raw potato, meat (especially liver), and raw fish are common causes, as are antibiotics and other medications, preservatives, disinfectants, fragrances, epoxy resin hardeners, several woods, birch pollen, formaldehyde in clothing, and many others.

Uncertain Mechanism

Of uncertain mechanism are reactions to ammonium persulfate, used as a "booster" in bleaching hair to obtain a platinum blonde effect. The dermatitis, occurring mostly in clients, is sudden in onset and characterized by erythema, edema, severe itching, urticaria, and, occasionally, syncope, with wheezing and dyspnea. Hairdressers should be made aware of the seriousness of this problem.

Clinical Features/Other Terms

The term *contact urticaria* typically refers to a wheal-and-flare reaction elicited, usually at the site of contact, within 20 to 30 min of exposure; delayed onset CU (up to 4 to 6 h) has been described, as has delayed onset (24 h) and prolonged (1 week) CU. The concept of CU has been expanded and the precise usage of related terms varies considerably in the literature and includes (1) immediate contact reaction, the broadest concept, referring to both immunologic and nonimmunologic urticarial or nonurticarial reactions, but says nothing about the appearance of the reaction; (2) protein contact dermatitis with allergic or nonallergic eczematous immediate reactions, often dyshidrosis caused by proteins—initially described in food handlers; (3) contact urticaria syndrome with local reactions in the skin, and systemic reactions (angioedema, asthma, and anaphylaxis) in other organs; usually immunologic; (4) atopic contact dermatitis, a historical term referring to an immediate urticarial or eczematous IgE-mediated contact reaction in an atopic person; and (5) immediate-type irritancy with nonallergic urticarial or nonurticarial reactions.

Other than for NRL, there is little statistical data on CU. Data from Finland lists farmers with the most cases and bakers as having the highest rate.[31] Cow dander was the number one cause of CU and was also the most frequent cause of occupational rhinitis and asthma in Finland. This is in contrast to other reports of respiratory and food allergy that have only occasionally been associated with contact urticaria. This association is assumed to be uncommon, because it is thought that the responsible large protein molecules do not ordinarily penetrate intact skin, but require inflamed skin. The Finnish data also identified several low molecular weight chemicals as a cause of contact urticaria: methyltetrahydrophthalic anhydrides, diglycidyl ether of bisphenol, an epoxy resin, polyfunctional aziridines nickel, and reactive dyes. Diagnosis of ICU typically involves skin testing with the suspected substance and serologic assays for specific IgE. Where a chemical hapten is suspect, it is necessary to centrifuge it with a protein, usually human serum albumin, a nonstandard procedure.

Contact urticaria occurs from direct contact with skin (most examples) or mucosa (latex and chlorhexidine; the latter may be associated with systemic toxicity), or by airborne contact (cinchona, mulberry, xylene). Exposure may be accidental or due to equipment failure (xylene). Ingredients (Tinofix) or trace contaminants or impurities (an anhydride present in sorbitan sesquioleate) may be responsible. Contact urticaria may be associated with other urticaria, such as delayed pressure urticaria.[32] Occasionally, only erythema, burning, and itching occur, but at least some people should develop urticaria at the application site to be regarded as contact urticaria. Combined CU and delayed allergic eczematous reactions may occur.[32]

BIOLOGICAL CAUSES

Potential exposure to infectious agents is significant in many occupations. Service workers in the health, food, cleaning, and personal service jobs develop most of the cases, but many are never reported, especially those among agricultural workers.

Establishing a definite relationship between the work and a specific infection is not always simple. Laboratory isolation of the infective organism and a supporting medical history and examination are helpful, but often the evidence is based on conjecture. However, the circumstantial evidence is sometimes so strong that a definite connection can be made, as, for example, herpes simplex on the ungloved finger of a dental assistant or tinea pedis in a sewage worker with frequently wet feet.

Bacterial Infections

STAPHYLOCOCCAL AND STREPTOCOCCAL INFECTIONS (See also Chap. 194) Secondary bacterial skin infections due to *Staphylococcus* and *Streptococcus* are common complications of abrasions, lacerations, burns and puncture wounds. Butchers and meat handlers are likely to develop infected cuts and scratches; paronychia, abscesses, and lymphangitis. Folliculitis and boils are common in farm workers and construction workers. Workers in hot, humid, and dirty environments (Fig. 137-2) or those working in close contact with infected persons, such as nurses, hairdressers and manicurists are at risk. Staphylococcal colonization of individuals with active atopic dermatitis limits their work in food service and health care jobs. The increase in multidrug-resistant bacterial strains and widespread cross-resistance to antibiotics may present a therapeutic challenge in some cases.[33]

FIGURE 137-2

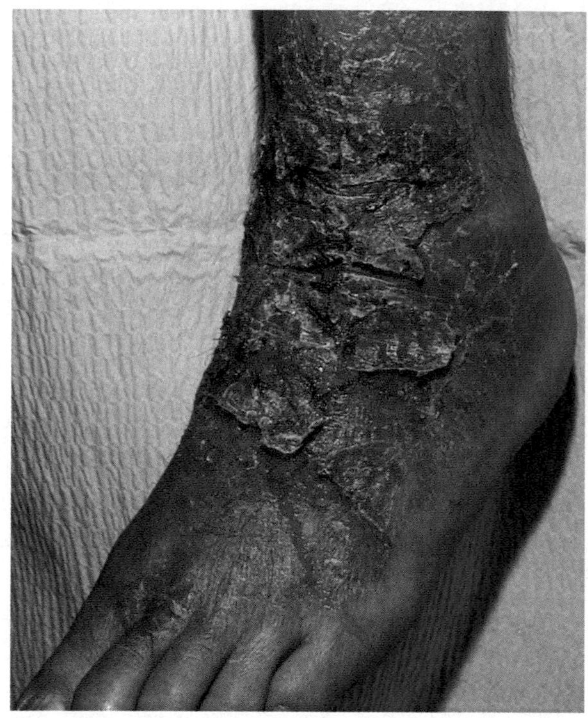

Infectious eczematoid dermatitis frequently follows contact dermatitis that is untreated and in an area where there is constant rubbing. In this case, the patient was a logger working in an area with poor access to medical attention.

FIGURE 137-3

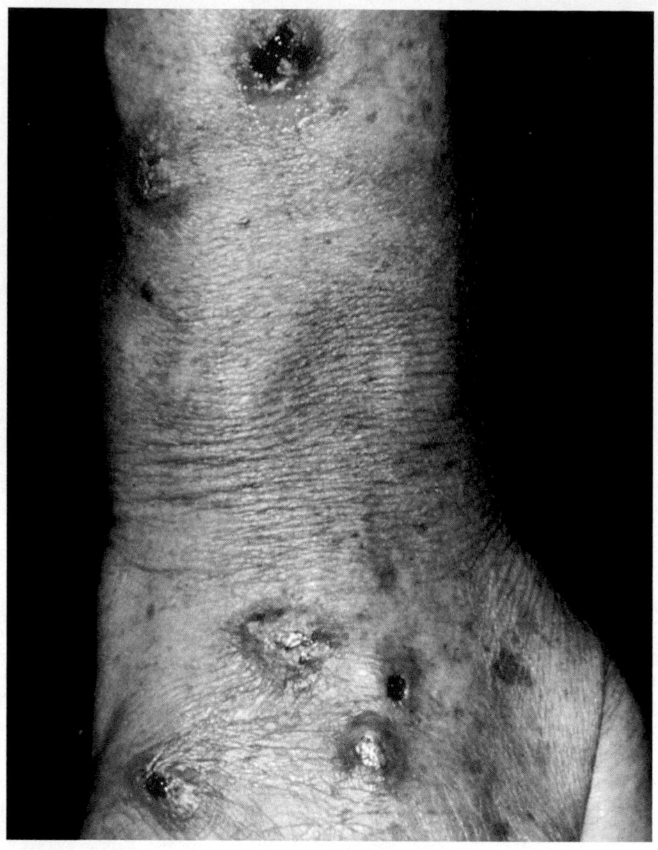

Sporotrichoid atypical mycobacterial infection with *M. marinum* in a woman who worked in a shop selling tropical fish.

ANTHRAX (See also Chap. 199) Anthrax, caused by *Bacillus anthracis,* is primarily an animal disease seen in cattle, sheep, horses, goats, and wild herbivores. Agricultural workers, stockbreeders, butchers, and meat-processors can become infected by contact with diseased animals. Contaminated hides, goat hair, wool, and bones can infect longshoremen, freight handlers, warehouse workers, and employees of processing plants where these products are treated for use. Tanners, carpet makers, and upholsterers are also at risk. The cutaneous form is more common and begins as a papule at the site of inoculation. This progresses to a characteristic, usually painless necrotic eschar surrounded by brawny edema. Regional lymphadenopathy is common, and constitutional symptoms and a generalized maculopapular eruption may be seen. A vaccine is available for those in high-risk occupations.

Anthrax spores are highly infectious, making it a desirable agent of germ warfare, especially for the development of the often-fatal pulmonary anthrax. However, of the 22 cases of anthrax recently reported in the United States as a result of bioterrorism, 12 were the cutaneous form. Immunohistochemistry (IHC) was crucial to the diagnosis. All demonstrated *Bacillus anthracis* cell wall antigen by IHC, including the New York City index case, which had a negative culture and Gram's stain. A cutaneous anthrax management algorithm has been published and is available online at www.aad.org.

CUTANEOUS TUBERCULOSIS

Typical mycobacterial infections (See also Chap. 200) The classic example of work-acquired tuberculosis of the skin is tuberculosis cutis verrucosa, a slow-growing warty growth acquired by the inoculation of *Mycobacterium tuberculosis hominis* or *M. bovis*. It is usually seen in pathologists and morgue attendants (prosectors or necrogenic wart). Surgeons, veterinarians, farmers, and butchers are also at risk.

Atypical mycobacterial infections *Mycobacterium marinum* causes swimming pool or fish-tank granuloma, a solitary or disseminated granulomatous infection in fishermen, fish-tank cleaners (Fig 137-3), and workers cleaning contaminated swimming pools; surgeons are also at risk. *M. ulcerans, M. fortuitum, M. avium, M. intracellulare, M. kansasii,* or *M. chelonae* may also cause infection, especially in persons with suppressed immunity.[12]

BRUCELLOSIS (See also Chap. 199) Brucellosis is a zoonosis transmitted to humans from contact with infected animals or ingestion of untreated milk or milk products. The organism is a nonmotile, gram-negative rod, with any of the four species capable of causing infection: *Brucella melitensis* from goats, sheep and camels; *B. abortus* from cattle; *B. suis* from pigs; and *B. canis* from dogs. Skin manifestations are nonspecific and include maculopapular eruptions, purpura and petechiae, chronic ulcerations, abscesses, discharging sinuses, and superficial thrombophlebitis. Farmers, livestock-breeders, meatpackers, veterinarians, and laboratory workers are at risk. An epidemic caused by sniffing bacterial cultures has been reported.[34] When cases go undiagnosed and unreported, they constitute a major health hazard. As a result, chronic forms occur, which may present as endocarditis, meningitis, and other organ infections. Although the disease is rarely fatal, it is a potential agent of bioterrorism.

TULAREMIA (See also Chap. 199) Tularemia is caused by *Francisella tularensis,* a gram-negative, pleomorphic, non–spore-forming bacillus, transmitted by ticks, fleas, and deer flies. Animal reservoirs include wild rabbits, squirrels, birds, sheep, beavers, muskrats, and domestic dogs, and cats. In nature, the most common form is ulceroglandular tularemia, presenting as an ulcerative lesion with eschar formation at the site of inoculation, with regional lymphadenopathy and lymphadenitis. A generalized maculopapular eruption and constitutional symptoms resembling typhoid may be seen in other forms of the disease, which may also be weaponized in germ warfare. Tularemia is ordinarily seen in hunters, trappers, game wardens, butchers, fur handlers, and laboratory workers. This highly infectious organism readily penetrates unbroken skin, and great care should be exercised in handling infected tissues and excreta.

ERYSIPELOID (See also Chap. 199) Erysipeloid is almost always an occupational disease caused by *Erysipelothrix rhusiopathiae,* a slender, gram-negative rod that infests freshwater and saltwater fish, ducks, emus, turkeys, chicken, and other farmed animals such as sheep.[35] Butchers, fishermen, and retailers of fish and poultry are commonly affected. Infection usually follows puncture wounds and lacerations and presents as a painful, purplish-red, nonvesicular papule or plaque with burning or itching, which gradually disappears in 3 to 4 weeks.

Viral Infections

HERPES SIMPLEX (See also Chap. 214) The most common viral infection of occupational origin is herpes simplex virus (HSV) type 1. HSV type 1, or, occasionally, HSV type 2, are seen in occupations where there is exposure to infected secretions from the mouth or the respiratory tract. Dentists, dental assistants, nurses, and respiratory technicians are particularly vulnerable. When localized to the fingers, it is termed herpetic whitlow and is characterized by erythema and edema resembling a bacterial infection. Herpes gladiatorum refers to HSV infection on the body surfaces of wrestlers and rugby players, and is temporarily disqualifying for infected athletes. The rapid appearance of grouped vesicles usually clarifies the diagnosis, which is confirmed by culture of the vesicle fluid. The use of protective gloves, safety glasses, and masks is the best preventive measure, and has greatly reduced the incidence of the infection.

VIRAL WARTS (See also Chap. 223) Handlers of meat, poultry, and fish have a high prevalence of viral warts. Minor cuts and abrasions acquired during work by butchers and slaughterhouse workers are predisposing factors. Human papilloma virus-7 has been isolated more frequently in this group of patients.[36]

MOLLUSCUM CONTAGIOSUM (See also Chap. 221) This infection may be seen in professional wrestlers and boxers, as well as in runners and swimmers.

ORF (ECTHYMA CONTAGIOSUM) (See also Chap. 220) Orf, caused by a parapox virus, is endemic in sheep and goats, and is easily transmitted to humans through direct contact. Veterinarians, farmers, and shepherds are at risk. Usually one or two rather large (1 to 2 cm) painful nodules appear on the hands and may be accompanied by fever, lymphangitis, and regional lymphadenopathy. Lesions are self-healing in 3 to 6 weeks, occasionally with secondary infection, and second attacks are common.

MILKER'S NODULES (See also Chap. 222) The paravaccinia virus, infecting the udders of cows and producing ulcers in the mouths of calves, can be transmitted to dairy farmers and veterinarians causing milker's nodules (or pseudocowpox). The lesions are commonly seen on the hands as relatively painless erythematous nodules (Fig. 137-4). There is regional lymphadenopathy, but the disease is benign, disappearing after 4 to 6 weeks and confers permanent immunity.

FIGURE 137-4

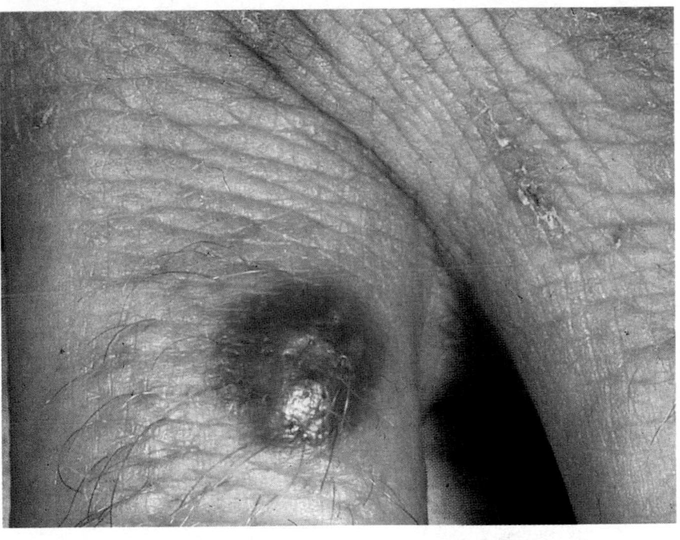

Milker's nodule is a self-limited condition on the fingers.

Occupational Aspects of Bioterrorism

Twelve agents are of highest concern for germ warfare: anthrax, plague, small pox, botulism, tularemia, two filoviruses (Ebola and Marburg), and five arenaviruses (Lassa and four South American viruses: Guanarito, Junin, Machupo, and Sabia). All have cutaneous manifestations with the exception of botulism and Lassa fever.[37] Risk of human-to-human transmission is high for pneumonic plague, for small pox, and for the viral hemorrhagic fevers, putting health care workers at risk. In Uganda, a number of hospital employees have succumbed to Ebola hemorrhagic fever despite strict isolation measures.[38] Anthrax, tularemia, and botulism are not contagious. Personal protection, decontamination, vaccination, and/or quarantine are important measures for preventing occupational spread of these diseases.[37]

Fungal Infections (See also Chap. 205)

DERMATOPHYTE SKIN INFECTIONS Dermatophyte skin infections are frequent in certain occupations, especially in farmers and those tending cattle who may develop infections with *Trichophyton verrucosum,* a zoophilic dermatophyte. Infections with *T. rubrum* and *T. mentagrophytes,* which are seen in the general population, may occur in work situations involving increased perspiration and occlusion. *Microsporum gypseum* and *T. mentagrophytes* are geophilic fungi, which cause infection in agricultural and other outdoor workers (Fig. 137-5). *M. canis* infects small animals as well as veterinarians and laboratory workers.

CANDIDIASIS (See also Chap. 206) Infection with *Candida albicans* is common in occupations that expose the skin to moisture and occlusion, such as wearing gloves for long periods of time. Food handlers, nurses, dental assistants, dishwashers, and laundry workers are at risk.

SPOROTRICHOSIS (See also Chap. 207) Sporotrichosis, caused by the saprophytic fungus *Sporothrix schenckii,* is acquired by inoculation through puncture wounds with thorns, sticks, or splinters. It is seen in farmers, nursery and forestry workers, and in other outdoor occupations.

FIGURE 137-5

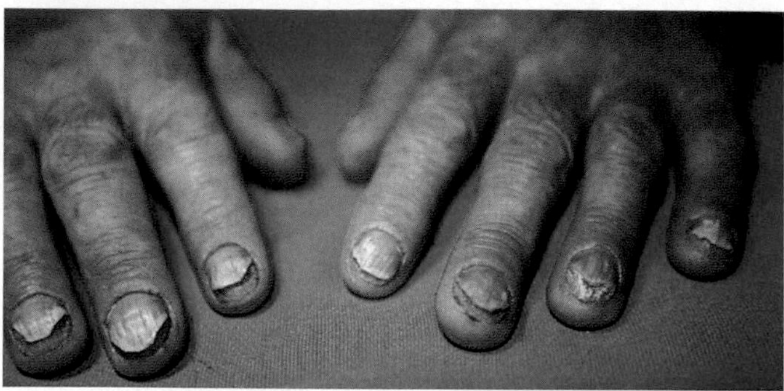

Fungal infection of the fingernails in a greengrocer. Trauma from repeatedly opening boxes of produce, in addition to the almost constant wetness, contributed to its development.

Gardeners working with sphagnum moss used for packing plant roots may also be at risk.

MYCETOMA (MADURA FOOT) (See also Chap. 207) Mycetoma, caused by various species of fungi and actinomycetes, is seen mainly in farmers and outdoor workers, who walk barefoot in tropical and subtropical countries. The organisms become implanted after trauma and lesions present as chronic, localized granulomatous infections of the feet or hands, with multiple draining sinuses.

CHROMOBLASTOMYCOSIS (See also Chap. 207) Chromoblastomycosis, a deep mycosis, often follows a puncture wound or other trauma, during which soil inhabiting fungi of *Phialophora, Hormodendrum,* and *Fonsecaea* species are injected deep into the tissues. Agricultural and other outdoor workers are at risk.

BLASTOMYCOSIS (See also Chap. 207) Blastomycosis, caused by a dimorphic fungus, *Blastomyces dermatitidis,* is found in the southeastern United States and northern Mexico. It is primarily an infection of the lungs, but dissemination occurs frequently with skin involvement. Those at risk include agricultural, forest, and construction workers, farmers, and persons working with heavy earth-moving equipment.

COCCIDIOIDOMYCOSIS (See also Chap. 207) Coccidioidomycosis is seen in the southwestern United States and Central and South America. Infection is acquired by inhalation of dust containing the spores of *Coccidioides immitis*. The clinical picture is usually of a self-limiting upper respiratory tract infection, often followed by the development of erythema nodosum, and, in rare instances, dissemination. Occasionally, a primary cutaneous infection follows a traumatic puncture wound. Farmers, construction workers, bulldozer and heavy equipment operators, professional baseball players and laboratory workers are susceptible.

Parasitic Diseases (See also Chap. 235)

Leishmaniasis, caused by *Leishmania tropica* (oriental sore) and by *L. brasiliensis* (American leishmaniasis) is endemic in the Middle East and Central and South America, respectively. Cutaneous ulcers and mucocutaneous lesions are common and workers in rural areas are infected, the vector is a tiny sandfly.

The larvae of *Ancylostoma braziliense* and *Necator americanus* cause creeping eruption (larva migrans) in agricultural workers, fishermen, sewer workers, and lifeguards. Feces of dogs, cats, and cattle contain the larvae, and humans are the final host. Skin divers, lifeguards, dockworkers, and caretakers who maintain lakes and ponds are prone to develop swimmer's itch caused by the cercariae of a schistosome. The cercariae penetrate human skin inadvertently, causing itching within minutes of leaving the water; uncovered areas of skin are involved. A secondary stage follows in 10 to 15 h with an intensely pruritic, urticarial, and occasionally vesicular eruption. In contrast, sea-bather's eruption, caused by different larvae or other marine toxins, occurs on covered body areas. Dogger bank itch is an allergic eczematous eruption of fishermen and dockworkers in the North Sea, who are exposed to the marine bryozoan, *Alcyonidium gelatinosum*.

FIGURE 137-6

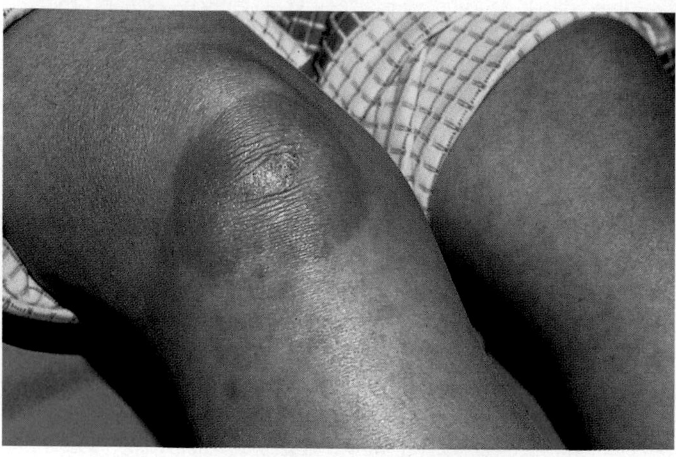

Erythema surrounding a tick bite that is several weeks old. Erythema chronicum migrans is common following such bites and may last for months. Lyme disease, transmitted by ticks of the genus *Ixodes,* frequently follows such reactions.

Arthropods (See also Chap. 239)

The bites of bees, wasps, hornets, ants, ticks, mites, centipedes, and millipedes frequently cause work-related skin disease. Outdoor workers, food handlers, chicken farmers (chicken mites), workers in food processing plants, restaurant workers, and dockworkers may be affected. Epidemics of *scabies* have occurred in nursing homes, hospitals, and other residential facilities for the aged. An infected employee is often the source.

Lyme disease (Fig. 137-6) (see also Chap. 203) is transmitted through a tick bite and can affect outdoor workers, loggers, ranchers and construction workers in wilderness areas.

PHYSICAL CAUSES

Mechanical Trauma

Mechanical trauma, an accompaniment of many different occupations, is a primary factor in many cases of occupational skin disease, and accounts for a number of skin manifestations. The skin may be subjected to friction, pressure, cuts, lacerations, and abrasions. Repeated mechanical trauma such as low-intensity pressure or friction, the most common mechanical trauma, leads to hyperpigmentation and lichenification, whereas heavier and persistent friction leads to hyperkeratosis and callus formation (Fig. 137-7). Sudden shearing forces may lead to the formation of friction blisters, erosions, or ulcers.[39] Prolonged

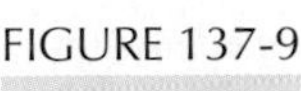

FIGURE 137-7

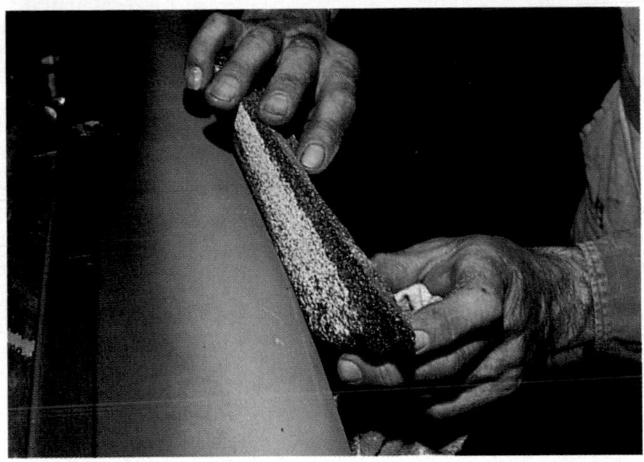

In spite of growing automation of many jobs, the hands are still useful tools. Here a bodyshop worker is sanding a fender in preparation for painting.

and excessive pressure may produce erythema, vesicobullae, and later necrosis, but usually only hyperpigmentation and thickening, which are so characteristic as the stigmata of various occupations[40] (Fig. 137-8). In athletes, repetitive trauma from running may lead to black heel or "talon noir," which represents punctate petechiae on the heels as a result of ruptured dermal papillary capillaries. Corns may also develop due to extreme pressure associated with bony deformities, poor foot mechanics, or improper footwear.[41]

Underlying skin conditions such as psoriasis and lichen planus are aggravated by the occupational trauma as a result of the isomorphic response of Koebner. Patients with psoriasis may develop lesions at the sites of repeated friction or pressure and should be advised to avoid occupations that may subject them to mechanical injury.

Workers, often of middle age, engaged in manual work and nearing retirement, may present with a chronic hyperkeratotic, scaly, fissured dermatitis involving the palms (Fig. 137-9). Chronic callus formation after years of repeated trauma may result in permanent disability, contributing to early retirement. This is termed *hyperkeratotic hand eczema* and is a relatively severe and recalcitrant condition. Repeated friction and pressure is thought to play a role. Although it may be a manifestation of psoriasis, a review concluded that it was an independent entity, unrelated to psoriasis and mechanical irritation.[42]

FIGURE 137-8

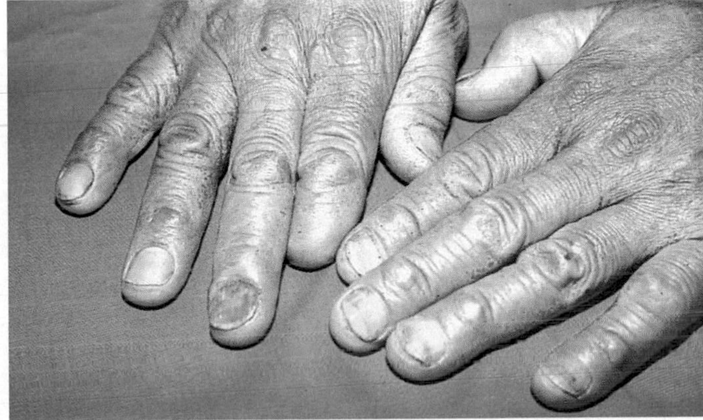

Nail dystrophy in a slaughterhouse worker. Holding a knife in his right hand to cut off the hide, he pulled and tugged on the hide with his left. Note the calluses over the distal interphalangeal joints on the left.

FIGURE 137-9

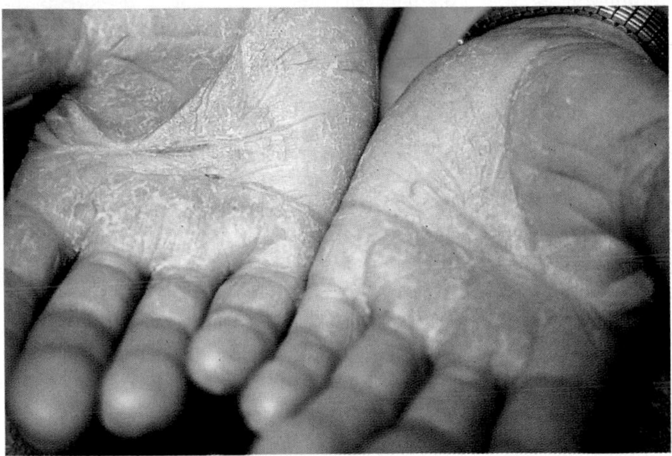

Chronic hypertrophic dermatosis of the palms in a 59-year-old machinist. He was transferred to work in a storeroom, where he continually handled tools, and was forced to retire because of persistence of the dermatosis with its fissuring and bleeding.

A dry, scaly, fissuring, painful dermatitis may be seen on the fingertips, especially in women engaged in domestic work. This is a form of frictional dermatitis known as *pulpitis.* It may sometimes affect only the thumb and first two fingers of the dominant hand, indicating an occupational basis, such as that seen in persons handling newspapers repeatedly.[43] Kanerva et al. have reported a similar condition, in which paresthesia on the fingertips are prominent symptoms, in dental personnel allergic to acrylates.[44]

Before the onset of automation of industry, the location and nature of calluses were considered representative of a person's occupation.[40] Besides calluses and corns, occupational marks include discolorations, telangiectases, tattoos, odors, deformities, and other changes caused by specific work activities. Occupational marks are less common today because of greater automation and better protective clothing, especially a wider selection of gloves.

Mathias reported a series of patients with *posttraumatic eczema,* which is defined as the occurrence of dermatitis at the site of cutaneous trauma. The trauma is insufficient to cause obvious tissue damage accompanied by inflammation or tissue regeneration. The eczema usually develops within a few weeks of the acute injury and may persist or recur for long periods of time.[45] The damaged, functionally altered skin is thought to play a role in precipitating the eczema. It has to be distinguished from posttraumatic psoriasis and secondary allergic contact dermatitis from topical medicaments applied to the injured skin. Table 137-7 lists the types of posttraumatic eczema.[45]

TABLE 137-7

Clinical Classification of Posttraumatic Eczema

Idiopathic reaction (endogenous eczema absent)
Isomorphic reaction
Primary (precedes endogenous eczema)
Secondary (follows endogenous eczema)

SOURCE: From Mathias CGT.[45]

Occupational skin granulomas may form due to the penetration of the skin by foreign material. Substances such as beryllium, zirconium, chromium, and tattoo pigments may induce an allergic reaction in the skin, leading to the formation of immunogenic granulomas.[46] Granulomas formed as a reaction to oils, starch, suture material, silk, wool, liquid paraffin, thorns, cactus spikes, and wood splinters are nonallergic or foreign-body granulomas. The penetration of human hair into the interdigital spaces of barbers, and of cow and sheep hair into the hands of animal tenders, can also produce foreign-body granulomas.

Preexisting dermatitis caused by friction and pressure may predispose to the development of allergic sensitization. It is well known that allergic contact dermatitis and contact urticaria to natural rubber latex gloves develops when these are worn over dermatitic skin. Hard metal workers are predisposed to develop cobalt allergy due to the trauma sustained during work. The microtrauma facilitates the entry of allergens and irritants into the skin and contributes to irritant and allergic contact dermatitis. Even minor lacerations and abrasions, which may not be serious, can increase the likelihood of contact sensitization to allergens present in the immediate environment.

HEAT

Thermal Burns

Workers are at risk for thermal burns as a result of scalding, contact with liquid metal, hot equipment and tar, and flame burns following explosions. Kitchen workers and adolescents working in fast food restaurants may develop scalds from hot grease.[47] Roofers frequently experience hot tar burns, whereas explosives and use of flammable liquids cause most industrial burns. Persons working in foundries and smelting plants are at risk for molten metal burns.

In evaluating impairment (see section "Impairment and Disability Evaluation") of patients scarred or otherwise disfigured from burns, the degree of scarring, pigmentary changes and cosmetic disfigurement are the chief considerations. Superficial partial thickness burns heal without scarring but may become hyperpigmented, especially in those with darker skin types. Deeper burns are associated with scarring, and some persons heal with hypertrophic scars, limiting movement. Leukoderma may also occur with deep burns; when there is total pigment loss, actinic damage and skin malignancy can result, especially in outdoor workers. Pigmentary changes alone may be cosmetically disfiguring. While hyperpigmentation often disappears in a year or two, in some cases permanent pigmentary changes may be severe enough to limit occupational possibilities.

Electrical Burns

In industrial settings electrical burns are usually high voltage injuries, which may result in serious tissue destruction, as well as potentially fatal cardiac arrhythmias. Extensive muscle injury carries a risk of renal failure. Low voltage injuries appear mild, but deceptively extend away from the edges of the visible wound, penetrating deep into tissue along nerves and blood vessels. Lightening burns, an ever present hazard of outdoor workers, may show characteristic bizarre feather- and/or fern-like patterns.

Erythema ab Igne

Erythema ab igne is a reticular, telangiectatic, and pigmented dermatosis resulting from prolonged or repeated exposure to infrared radiation (heat) insufficient to produce a burn. Persons working over a heat source, including stokers, blacksmiths, glassblowers, and bakers, may develop this condition, which may progress to skin cancer after a number of years.

Miliaria (See also Chap. 76)

Miliaria is a common work-related condition, caused by sweat retention resulting from pore closure. The clinical picture, depending upon the degree and duration of heat exposure, ranges from mild erythema (miliaria crystallina), patches of erythema studded with tiny vesicles (miliaria rubra), and deep-seated vesicles and papules (miliaria profunda) associated with symptoms of heat exhaustion if left untreated. Miliaria rubra, or prickly heat, is commonly misdiagnosed as contact dermatitis.

Intertrigo

Intertrigo is a macerated, superficial erythematous eruption seen in the body folds, caused by excessive sweating and sweat retention, especially in obese persons. It is commonly seen in the interdigital spaces of workers whose hands are continuously wet, such as from wearing rubber gloves for prolonged periods. Secondary infection with *Candida albicans* is common.

Other Conditions

Acne vulgaris and *rosacea* may be aggravated by the heat of open furnaces, heat torches, ovens, and stoves. *Herpes simplex* may also be triggered by heat exposure. *Heat-induced urticaria* may result from excessive physical exercise.

COLD (See also Chap. 126)

Frostbite, Chilblains, Immersion Foot

Frostbite, chilblains, immersion foot, and *cold urticaria* are common in workers employed in cold environments. Military personnel stationed in cold climates are most commonly affected with these conditions, but firefighters, icemakers, liquefied-gas makers, refrigeration workers, persons engaged in winter sports, and others who work outdoors in the cold may be affected. Cold urticaria is described in Chap. 116.

FROSTBITE Frostbite is due to the freezing of the skin and subcutaneous tissue resulting in formation of ice crystals, causing tissue injury. The extent of skin damage is dependent on temperature, duration of insult, and rate of cooling. If the rate of rewarming is slow then tissue damage is greater.

CHILBLAINS Chilblains (perniosis) represent the mildest form of cold injury, with reddish blue, swollen and boggy lesions with bullae and ulceration. Gangrene and loss of tissue rarely occur. Exposed fingers, toes, nose, ears, and lower legs are especially affected. Treatment is symptomatic and calcium channel blockers such as nifedipine have been recommended.

IMMERSION FOOT Immersion foot results from exposure to temperatures a few degrees above freezing for several days, in the presence of moisture and constrictive clothing, such as ill-fitting boots. It is not as severe as frostbite, and gangrene does not occur. However, there may be prolonged vasomotor instability, hyperhidrosis, and persistent sensitivity to cold. Treatment is the same as for frostbite.

VIBRATION SYNDROME

The vibration of handheld tools may induce a type of vascular spasm in the fingers and hands, known as " white fingers," "dead fingers," and "vibration-induced white finger disease."[48] This syndrome is one of a growing list of cumulative trauma disorders that primarily affect the musculo-tendinous-osseous-nervous system. Operators of vibrating impact and power tools such as jackhammers, pounding machines, riveting hammers, chain saws, and hand grinders may develop this condition, especially in cold climates. The vasospastic symptoms may be associated with neuromuscular and arthritic symptoms, and even with bone degeneration.[49] Symptoms commonly appear after a few years, but may be seen as early as 3 months. Earlier symptoms are mild and consist of numbness and tingling, followed by blanching and stiffness of one or more fingers. Initial symptoms are often ignored by the worker; when they progress and workers develop paresthesias and weakening of grip, the condition can become disabling, sometimes causing workers to lose their jobs. Vibration frequencies between 30 and 300 Hz are most strongly associated with vibration syndrome; smoking is also considered a risk factor. Improvement in the design of chain saws and other vibrating tools has resulted in a decrease in the prevalence of vibration-induced symptoms.

OCCUPATIONAL CONNECTIVE TISSUE DISORDERS

The occurrence of Raynaud's phenomenon and scleroderma-like skin lesions with osteolytic changes in the bones of the fingers is well described in vinyl chloride workers.[50] The syndrome has been called occupational acro-osteolysis; systemic abnormalities such as thrombocytopenia, portal and hepatic fibrosis, and hepatic angiosarcoma were associated. Only 3 percent of workers cleaning the reactor tanks containing the vinyl chloride monomers were affected. Today, the condition is rare because of better engineering controls.[50] Exposures to other organic solvents have also been reported to cause scleroderma-like disease.[50]

There are now a number of reports of systemic sclerosis and sclerodermatous skin changes associated with silica exposure and pulmonary silicosis, especially in underground miners (coal, gold, uranium, lead) or stone masons and related occupations.[50] The simultaneous operation of vibration tools during mining, a common activity in mining, contributes to the development of the disease.[50]

OCCUPATIONAL AND ENVIRONMENTAL ACNE

Oil Acne

Oil acne is a folliculitis consisting of follicular papules and pustules occurring on skin that contacts oils, especially heavy industrial oils or straight cutting oils in machinists. The skin areas where there is the greatest exposure to oil-soaked clothing, such as the arms and thighs, are most frequently involved. Topical and systemic treatment is the same as for acne vulgaris. With better engineering controls and greater emphasis on personal cleanliness, and protective clothing, its frequency has greatly diminished in the past several decades.

Coal Tar and Pitch Acne

Coal tar oils, creosote, and pitch can produce a comedonal type of acne, which often shows a predilection for exposed areas, particularly the malar regions.[51] Coal tar plant workers, roofers, road maintenance workers, and construction workers are among those at risk. Coal tar acne may be complicated by phototoxic reactions affecting both the skin and the eyes and resulting in hyperpigmentation known as coal tar melanosis. Late complications include the development of pitch and tar papillomas, keratoses, and acanthomas.[52]

Chloracne (See also Chap. 73)

Chloracne is one of the most sensitive biological indicators of occupational or environmental exposure to certain highly toxic halogenated aromatic hydrocarbons, which often occur as trace contaminants during synthesis of industrial chemicals. Chloracne appears regardless of whether chemical exposure has occurred via skin contact, the usual route, or by inhalation or ingestion. One of the most potent inducers of chloracne is 2,3,7,8- tetrachlorodibenzo-*p*-dioxin (TCDD). Table 137-8 lists other chloracnegenic chemicals that reportedly cause chloracne.[53] Chloronaphthalenes and polychlorinated biphenyls (PCBs) caused chloracne in the pre-World War II era. Since then, trace contaminants formed during the manufacture of PCBs and other polyhalogenated compounds, especially herbicides, have been the major causes. These include polyhalogenated dibenzofurans, polychlorinated dibenzo-*p*-dioxins, especially TCDD and chlorinated azo- (TCAOB) and azoxy- (TCAB) benzene compounds.

Most outbreaks have been occupationally related with more recent reports from the United States, Britain, and Mexico (chlorobenzenes), and China (dioxins and furans during pentachlorophenol production). Nonoccupational, environmental chloracne has resulted from some of the largest outbreaks, affecting hundreds of persons. These episodes have resulted from industrial accidents affecting the surrounding population (TCDD in Italy in 1976), contaminated industrial waste (Missouri horse arenas in the 1970s) and poisoned food products [PBBs in Michigan in the 1970's, PCBs in Japan (1968) and Taiwan (1979), and dioxins and furans in Spain in 1982].[53,54]

Clinical features of chloracne include multiple closed comedones and straw-colored cysts distributed primarily over the malar crescents and retroauricular folds, typically sparing the nose. This pattern of distribution is of significant diagnostic importance. As toxicity increases, the posterior neck, trunk, and extremities, buttocks, scrotum, and penis

TABLE 137-8

Chloracne-Producing Chemicals

Polyhalogenated biphenyls
Polychlorinated biphenyls (PCBs)
Polybrominated biphenyls (PBBs)
Polychlorodibenzofurans
Contaminants of polychlorophenol compounds, especially herbicides
2,4,5-tetra and pentachlorophenol, and herbicide intermediates,
2,4,5-trichlorophenol and 2,3,7,8-tetrachlorodibenzo-*p*-dioxin (TCDD)
Hexachlorodibenzo-*p*-dioxin
Tetrachlorodibenzofuran
Contaminants of 3,4-dichloroaniline and related herbicides (e.g., Propanil, Methazole)
3,4,3′,4′-Tetrachlorozooxybenzene
3,4,3′,4′-Tetrachloroazobenzene
Others
1,2,3,4-Tetrachlorobenzene (experimental)
Dichlobenil (Cararon) herbicide
DDT (crude tichlorobenzene)

SOURCE: From Taylor.[53]

TABLE 137-9

Clinical Features of Acne Vulgaris as Compared to Chloracne

Clinical Features	Acne Vulgaris	Chloracne
Usual age	Teenage	Any
Comedones	Present	Many (if absent, not chloracne); pathognomonic
Straw-colored cysts	Rare	
Temporal comedones	Rare	Diagnostic
Inflammatory papules and cysts	Common	Uncommon
Retroauricular involvement	Uncommon	Common
Nose involvement	Often spared	Often spared
Associated systemic findings	Rare	Common

may become involved. Dermatologic findings associated with specific exposures include hyperpigmentation (PCBs, TCDD); mucous membrane and nail hyperpigmentation (PCBs); follicular hyperkeratosis (PCBs, TCDD); conjunctivitis and meibomian gland changes (PCBs); facial erythema and edema (trichlorophenol); hypertrichosis (TCDD); hyperhidrosis of palms and soles (TCDD, PCBs); and actinic elastosis (TCDD). PCBs and dibenzofurans are transplacental dermatotoxins producing dystrophic finger and toe nails and hyperpigmented toe nails in exposed children whose mothers had accidentally ingested PCBs; dental abnormalities, growth deficit, and developmental delay also occur.

Diagnosis of chloracne requires documentation of exposure to known chloracnegen chemicals, compatible clinical findings, and absence of other causes of acneiform eruptions. Following initial chemical exposure there is a delay of 2 weeks to a month or more before the appearance of chloracne lesions. Based on clinical findings alone it may be difficult to differentiate chloracne from early acne vulgaris (Table 137-9) and senile (solar) comedones of the Favre-Racouchot syndrome. Dowling-Degos' disease also can be considered in the clinical differential diagnosis. Table 137-10 differentiates chloracne from other types of environmental acne such as oil folliculitis, pitch acne, and tropical acne.[54]

Threshold concentrations of dibenzodioxins and dibenzofurans in blood lipids associated with chloracne were determined in workers from a pentachlorophenol production facility in China. The blood levels were converted to toxicity equivalents and indicate that in addition to tetra isomers, the hepta and hexa congeners may cause chloracne.[55]

The mechanism for chloracne development is still unclear. TCDD is known to have an effect on in vitro keratinocyte differentiation, which may include changes of the epithelium of the pilosebaceous unit. Contrary to data from animal experiments, changes in epidermal retinol have not been observed in epidermal tissue from humans with chloracne.[55]

Systemic findings of liver disease, porphyria cutanea tarda, peripheral neuropathy, hyperlipidemia, plus involvement of other systems have been reported with chloracne, usually depending on the level of chemical exposure. Long-term follow-up of dioxin-exposed populations suggests an increased risk for soft tissue sarcoma, and non-Hodgkin's lymphoma.[54] Treatment, which is often unsatisfactory, consists in use of acne medications, including topical tretinoin, oral isotretinoin, and antibiotics. Acne surgery, light cautery, and dermabrasion have also been used.[55] Olestra, a nondigestible and nonabsorbable dietary fat substitute was recently reported to increase fecal excretion of TCDD in amounts sufficient to reduce the elimination half-life of TCDD from about 7 years to 1 to 2 years.[56]

TABLE 137-10

Differential Diagnosis of Various Forms of Occupational and Environmental Acne

Disease	Etiology	Location	Lesions
Chloracne	Halogenated aromatics	Malar; retroauricular; mandibular	Comedones; straw-colored cysts (0.1 to 1.0 cm)
Oil folliculitis	Oil	Arms; thighs; buttocks	Erythematous papules, pustules
Coal tar/pitch acne	Tar/pitch	Exposed facial areas, especially malar	Open comedones
Tropical acne	Heat/humidity	Back; neck; buttocks; proximal extremities	Nodules; cysts

SOURCE: McDonnell K et al.[54]

OCCUPATIONAL SKIN CANCER

Nonmelanoma skin cancer (NMSC) is the most common cancer in whites. Approximately 1.2 million cases of nonmelanoma skin cancers occur each year in the United States, with approximately 300,000 being squamous cell carcinomas and 900,000 being basal cell carcinomas. How many of these cases are induced by the work environment is disputed; some studies suggest that in as many as 70 to 80 percent the work environment contributed to their development,[57] but other studies indicate a much lower percentage.[58] Although cancer registries are operative in most countries, an accurate count of skin cancer, even malignant melanoma, is impossible because many, if not most, skin cancers are entirely treated in physicians' offices and not reported. Furthermore, physicians treating these cancers rarely consider the role of the patient's occupation in its etiology. The proposition that sunlight exposure is the most important causative stimulus is supported by the observation that the majority of NMSCs occur on exposed areas of skin, such as the head and neck.

The skin is an ideal organ for the study of cancer. Indeed, it was the skin that occasioned the first report of an occupational cancer by the English physician Percival Pott in 1775; he described scrotal cancer in chimney sweeps, stating, "it seems to derive its origin from a lodgment of soot in the rugae of the scrotum. . . ." Pott's astute and remarkably accurate observation initiated a study of chemical carcinogenesis that has continued unabated to the present. Even today, scrotal cancer is almost always considered occupational. Other malignancies found to have a definite occupational etiology are angiosarcoma of the liver in workers exposed to polyvinyl chloride, bladder cancer in workers exposed to certain dyes, and lung cancer in asbestos workers (with the added factor of cigarette smoking).

In the occupational environment, the most common causes of skin cancer are ultraviolet (UV) light, polycyclic aromatic hydrocarbons, arsenic trauma, and ionizing radiation.

ULTRAVIOLET LIGHT (See also Chap. 38)

Ultraviolet (UV) radiation from the sun is a carcinogen to which we all are exposed. UV light within the spectrum of UVB (290 to 320 nm) is a primary cause of skin cancer in humans. UVA (320 to 400 nm) augments UVB carcinogenesis and in large amounts can also induce skin cancers. UVC (100 to 290 nm) does not reach the earth but exposure to shorter wavelength rays can occur in industrial settings such as emissions from germicidal lamps and welding arcs.

Sunlight acts as a tumor initiator by inducing specific mutations in the p53 tumor suppressor gene (TP53).[59] In one study, these mutations were detected in more than 90 percent of squamous cell carcinomas and in more than 50 percent of basal cell carcinomas.[60] They are also found in actinic keratosis, implying an early role for potential conversion to squamous cell carcinoma. UV radiation also favors the clonal expansion of these mutated p53 cells, thus acting as a tumor promoter in addition to initiating the process of carcinogenesis.[59] The measurement of this unique pattern of mutations may be useful as a molecular marker of UV exposure and as a possible predictor of risk for skin cancer. It may also prove to be useful in cancer risk assessment in occupationally predisposed individuals.

The relationship between sunlight-induced skin cancer and outdoor exposure has been studied extensively.[61–63] Most studies report a significant association between work-related sun exposure and skin cancer,[61] as well as the appearance of precancerous actinic keratoses[64] (Fig. 137-10). However, other studies have found no definite association between skin cancer and outdoor work,[63] or have found a very slight increase in the risk of such an association.[62] These latter findings may be a result of self-selection for indoor jobs in those with fair and medium skin types and a tendency to burn, as compared to those with less-susceptible skin types.[63]

UV exposure plays a critical role in the pathogenesis of malignant melanoma.[65] Prolonged occupational exposure to sunlight has been implicated in the development of melanomas of the head, face, and neck. However, some studies fail to show an increased risk of developing melanoma in outdoor workers as compared to indoor workers.[66] Occupational exposure to nonsolar radiation such as welding torches and fluorescent light is reportedly associated with an increased risk of melanoma.

FIGURE 137-10

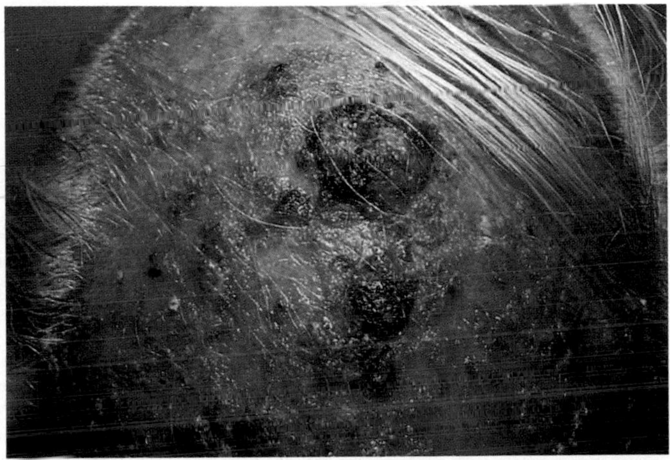

Severe actinic damage with actinic keratoses and squamous cell carcinomas in an elderly man who had worked outdoors as a fruit picker for most of his life.

Whereas exposure to intermittent high-dose UV exposure is implicated in the pathogenesis of malignant melanoma, chronic, repeated low-dose exposure is thought to be the likely cause of nonmelanoma skin cancers.[65] These findings may be the reason for a better correlation between nonmelanoma skin cancers and occupational UV exposure.[67] The association of squamous cell carcinoma with cumulative UV exposure is stronger, making outdoor occupations a significant risk factor. However, other occupational exposures, such as to chemical carcinogens, may also play a critical role,[68] and a cumulative effect cannot be excluded. A similar association between cumulative UV exposure and basal cell carcinoma is less clear,[69] although the occurrence of basal cell carcinoma on exposed areas has been shown to be related to UV exposure. In one case-control study artificial tanning devices were associated with an increase in the risk for basal and squamous cell skin cancers.[70]

Solitary keratoacanthomas may result from occupational exposures. The combination of sunlight, prolonged contact with tar and oil, mechanical trauma, and burns contribute to their development. These tumors grow rapidly, with a central keratin core surrounded by squamous cell growth.

Physicians are frequently asked to determine the role the workplace played in the development of actinic skin damage, including skin cancer. This information is important for medicolegal reasons, specifically for workers' compensation determination of permanent disability. Physicians who evaluate these patients must obtain a detailed occupational history, with job descriptions beginning with the first job after leaving school. Activities, especially sports, as a child and teenager are also important. Nonoccupational activities, hobbies and sports, and other recreational pursuits are important. After this information has been collected and evaluated, it should be possible to decide the significance of work-related actinic exposure on the current skin condition and even to assign a percentage of the work activity responsible for the actinic damage and resulting malignancy and/or premalignant lesions.

POLYCYCLIC AROMATIC HYDROCARBONS

Among the chemical carcinogens found at the work place, polycyclic aromatic hydrocarbons (PAHs) account for most of the reported occupational skin tumors.[71] PAHs are hydrophobic, nonpolar compounds that act both as initiators of carcinogenesis as well as complete carcinogens due to their ability to form DNA adducts.[72] Coal tar and petroleum products such as tar, pitch, coke, carbon black (soot), creosote, anthracene, crude paraffin, asphalt fuel and diesel oils, lubrication and coolant oils, untreated mineral oils, as well as oils, waxes, and tars from the distillation products of shale oil and lignite, contain PAHs and can play an important role in occupation related carcinogenesis.[73] High occupational exposure to PAHs occurs in several industries and occupations such as aluminum production, coal gasification, coke production, iron and steel foundries, tar distillation, shale oil extraction, and wood impregnation. Workers can be exposed to PAHs through inhalation or skin contact. High dermal exposure is a risk factor for skin cancer.

Clear epidemiologic evidence demonstrates that early formulations of mineral oil in metal machining and in cotton and jute spinning were carcinogenic to the skin. Mineral oils are a complex mixture of aliphatic hydrocarbons, naphthenics, and aromatics. The end products may contain PAHs (particularly benz[a]pyrene), nitrosamines, chlorinated paraffins, and long-chain aliphatics, the relative distribution of which depends on the source of the oil and the method of refinement. However, current formulations of mineral oils have lower concentrations of PAHs and nitrosamines. The potential presence of multiple carcinogens in the mixtures makes epidemiologic studies difficult and complicated. Although the risk for melanoma and internal cancers has been reported to be increased in oil refinery workers, it is unlikely that chemical carcinogens are a major cause of melanoma.[76]

Shale oil products have been found to be especially carcinogenic. In 1993, Cruickshank and Squire[77] noted the association with scrotal cancers and the use of cutting oils, probably related to the addition of shale oil. Coal tar pitch appears to be more carcinogenic than petroleum-derived tars. An additive action exists between polycyclic aromatic hydrocarbons and UVB, which has been used for years in the so-called Goeckerman regimen for the treatment of recalcitrant psoriasis. A parallel may be seen in the development of skin cancer in outdoor workers such as roofers, cable layers, timber treaters, and others who contact polycyclic aromatic hydrocarbons in their work. Creosote used in wood treatment has been suggested as a cause of skin and lip cancer when associated with sunlight exposure.[78] Roofers and road pavers are also at increased risk for skin cancers and internal cancers due to the potential carcinogenicity of bitumen, and PAHs from coal tar products.[79] Tar refinery workers are at increased risk of developing nonmelanoma skin cancers, mainly on the facial areas, forearms, and hands.[80] UV exposure is known to be a factor in the development of tar-induced skin cancers, although some authors believe that its role is now less important. Callahan et al. note that molecular epidemiology is a way to study cancer risk. They hypothesize that there are different p53 mutations for tar in contrast to UV-induced skin cancers.[76]

The clinical sequence of events leading to cancer includes repeated episodes of photosensitization dermatitis on exposed skin, accompanied by burning and pigment formation. After several years and many repeated episodes of burning, poikilodermatous changes appear, especially on the face, neck, and exposed parts of the arms and hands. Keratotic papillomas (tar warts) appear, sometimes as long as 20 years after onset of the first signs. Squamous cell carcinomas develop from many, but not necessarily all, of these verrucous keratoses. Basal cell carcinoma and keratoacanthomas also develop in the sun-damaged areas. Older skin appears to be more susceptible to these changes, with the appearance of malignancy after a shorter period of time. Heredity plays a very important role in skin carcinogenesis; persons of Celtic heritage are far more susceptible. The protective effect of melanin in the skin is considerable; deeply pigmented blacks rarely develop actinic skin cancers regardless of the amount of UV radiation they receive throughout their lives. The hereditary disease complex known as xeroderma pigmentosum, with several defective enzymes responsible for incomplete DNA repair following exposure to UV radiation, is marked by the presence, beginning even in young adulthood, of highly aggressive skin cancers, which often lead to premature death (see Chaps. 35 and 38). Following organ transplantation and the use of drugs causing immunosuppression, an increase of cutaneous malignancy, mainly squamous cell carcinoma, has been reported.[81] Occupational sunlight exposure is also an important factor in the development of these lesions.

ARSENIC

Arsenic is widely distributed in nature in the form of metalloids or chemical compounds. Arsenic-containing drinking water is clearly associated with various skin and internal organ malignancies.[82] However, arsenic does not easily induce cancer in animal models. Recent advances in the knowledge of arsenic carcinogenesis indicate that the methylated, trivalent form of arsenic is more toxic than the pentavalent form.[83] Arsenic has been shown to induce chromosomal abnormalities both in experimental systems and in human tissues. It has been implicated in causing the expression of heme oxygenase; the oxidative stress protein and altering growth factors leading to cell proliferation.[83] Another mechanism may be indirect DNA damage by inhibiting DNA repair.[84] Further studies are required to understand the exact mechanism of arsenic genotoxicity and carcinogenicity.

Commercially, arsenic is used in industrial processes associated with glass production; copper, zinc, and lead smelters, and the manufacture of semiconductors.[82] Farmers exposed to arsenic pesticides are reported to be at risk for development of nonmelanoma skin cancers.[85] Although the commercial use and production of substances containing arsenic has decreased, it is still an important occupational hazard.[76]

Exposure to arsenic in the workplace may occur through ingestion of food or water, and to a lesser extent from inhalation of air-borne arsenic. Chronic arsenic exposure may lead to arsenical keratosis, squamous cell and basal cell carcinomas, and Bowen's disease. Merkel cell carcinoma has also been reported in a person with chronic arsenicalism.[86]

Arsenical keratoses are the characteristic feature of chronic arsenic exposure. These consist of multiple, yellow, punctate keratoses distributed symmetrically on the palms and soles. Mild erythema and hyperhidrosis may precede their appearance. From some of these keratoses, aggressive squamous cell carcinomas develop. More commonly associated with arsenicalism are Bowen's intraepidermal squamous cell carcinomas, which only rarely become aggressive. Callen[87] has reported that patients with Bowen's disease have an approximately 10 percent chance of developing internal malignancy, thus it is appropriate to recommend that patients with Bowen's disease have a regular physical examination with appropriate laboratory testing for their age group, but without extensive searches for internal malignancy, unless clearly indicated.

TRAUMA

Although trauma as a cause of skin cancer has been a controversial subject since Virchow first proposed a relationship in 1863, the concept has not gained universal acceptance. Proving that mechanical injury has lead to the development of a cutaneous neoplasm may be difficult. Not infrequently patients themselves report that a single injury preceded the appearance of a skin cancer. Workers' compensation courts will often accept a relationship between trauma and cancer if testimony indicates a greater than 50 percent probability that a given cancer was caused by trauma. Ewing's original criteria for establishing a relationship between a single trauma and malignancy,[88] modified by Stoll and Crissey,[89] still probably hold true for medicolegal purposes:

1. The skin must previously have been normal.
2. Adequate and authenticated trauma must have occurred, preferably confirmed by a medical person.
3. A positive diagnosis of nonmetastatic carcinoma must be made, and the tumor must be histologically consistent with the tissues of that site.
4. The carcinoma must originate from the exact point of injury.
5. A reasonable time interval between the trauma and the first appearance of the carcinoma must be present.
6. There must be continuity of physical signs from the traumatic event to the appearance of carcinoma.

The fact that mechanical injuries may predispose to epidermal neoplasms has been demonstrated in mouse skin, using dimethylbenzanthracene as the initiator. The epidermal regeneration that follows abrasions results in epidermal hyperplasia that may function as a tumor promoter. However, surgically induced ulceration has not been shown to initiate carcinogenesis.[90] These experiments support the assertion that from a scientific viewpoint trauma most likely acts as a cocarcinogen or final trigger, rather than as a true carcinogen.

Marjolin ulcer is a term synonymous with malignant transformation of chronic ulcers, sinus tracts, and burn scars. The Kangri cancer of Kashmir[91] and the Kairo cancer of Japan are well recognized examples of burn scar neoplasms. It is easier to explain the appearance of malignancy in these settings of chronic irritation and scarring than those following single incidents of trauma.

Most malignancies are epithelial, although melanoma[92] and sarcoma[93] arising in burn scars have been described. Squamous cell carcinomas are more frequent than basal cell carcinomas by a ratio of 3:1. The growth usually arises from the margin and is solitary. The latent period may be long, posing difficulties for occupational physicians, insurance companies, and compensation boards.[94]

IONIZING RADIATION

Ionizing radiation as a cause of occupational skin cancer has been known since the early 1900s, only a few years after Roentgen's discovery of x-rays in 1895. Following high acute or cumulative exposures to ionizing radiation, in addition to radiodermatitis, several types of cancers may result, in skin, thyroid, liver, bone, and blood-forming tissues. Yamada et al.,[95] in reporting a follow-up of atomic bomb survivors, found that the occurrence of basal cell and squamous cell carcinomas increased with the estimated ionizing radiation dose. In 1991, the International Commission on Radiological Protection indicated the probability of skin cancer following exposure to ionizing radiation to be 2×10^{-4}/Sv.[96] High-dose radiation exposure has also been found to shorten life, to contribute to premature aging, and to result in teratogenic and reproductive abnormalities. Even with relatively small doses of radiation, such as 500 to 1000 mGy (50 to 100 rad) received irregularly over many years, progressive dryness of the skin, loss or scantiness of hair, irregular areas of hyperpigmentation, and signs of premature aging develop. Squamous cell carcinomas of x-ray origin tend to be more invasive than those of actinic origin, with metastases occurring in 20 to 26 percent of patients, as opposed to only 3 percent of sunlight-induced squamous cell cancers[97] (Fig 137-11). Radiation carcinomas constitute approximately 1 percent of all occupational skin cancers.[94]

FIGURE 137-11

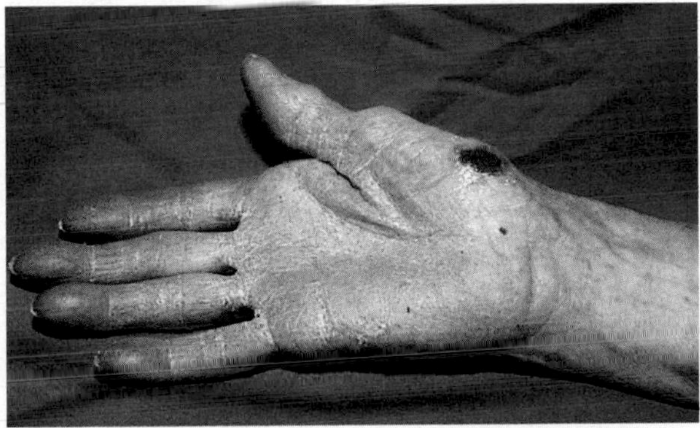

Radiodermatitis and squamous cell carcinoma in a woman who had worked as an x-ray technician for years, holding young patients still, but without protection, during x-ray examinations, including fluoroscopy.

DIAGNOSIS OF OCCUPATIONAL SKIN DISEASE

Medical determinations in putative occupational skin disorders and in workers compensation cases involve several dilemmas for the physician: (1) Patient assertions and demands concerning work relatedness of disease, job changes, and job modifications. (2) Social gate keeping concerning time off and date of return to work. (3) Lack of adequate workplace information: job description, list of work chemicals, and exposures including material safety data sheets. (4) Clinical judgment versus technology (determining whether hand eczema and negative patch tests in a machinist is work related). (5) Causation in the legal arena usually only requires probability (within reasonable certainty or greater than 50 percent medical certainty), rather than absolute certainty such as fulfilling Koch's postulates.[98]

Thus essentials in evaluating occupational skin disorders include:

1. *Accurate diagnosis,* which includes a detailed medical and occupational history, complete cutaneous examination and ancillary diagnostic tests as indicated. Information obtained should include the appearance of the lesions, site of the eruption, course of the disease and predisposing or contributing factors. Diagnostic tests may include patch testing and other allergy tests, KOH exams and fungal, bacterial and viral smears and cultures, and skin biopsies. Sufficient time is necessary to make a detailed diagnosis and determine the role of the work environment, which may be difficult or impossible initially. Because the initial diagnosis becomes the basis for future evaluations, and is often the one accepted by insurance companies, legal and rehabilitation personnel, and even other physicians, it becomes difficult to change a diagnosis that has been previously made.
2. *Causation.* Mathias[99] has proposed that a "yes" answer to four of the following seven questions would generally be adequate to establish occupational causation and aggravation in contact dermatitis cases and establish probable cause:
   a. Is the clinical appearance compatible with contact dermatitis?
   b. Are there workplace exposures to potential irritants or allergens?
   c. Is the anatomic distribution of the eruption compatible with job exposure?
   d. Is the temporal relationship between exposure and onset consistent with contact dermatitis?
   e. Have nonoccupational exposures been excluded as causes?
   f. Does the dermatitis improve away from work exposure to the suspected irritant or allergen?
   g. Do patch or provocation tests identify a probable cause?
3. *Recommendations* for treatment, prevention, disability (if any), job placement, rehabilitation, and use of other resources (industrial hygiene consultation and other medical specialists, such as allergy, pulmonary, or occupational medicine consultations).

DIAGNOSTIC TESTING FOR ALLERGY

Patch Testing

Because of the importance of allergic contact dermatitis in the etiology of occupational skin disease, patch testing should be performed in almost all cases of contact dermatitis, even in those patients who initially are thought to have only irritant dermatitis. Testing should be done with commercially prepared allergens. Further testing is sometimes indicated with the worker's environmental substances, including topical medications, protective equipment such as gloves, sensitizing ingredients in cleansers or other products, and, occasionally, the products themselves (cutting oils, etc.). Testing with irritants, such as most solvents, soaps, cement, and the like, should not be done, and patch testing with other environmental chemicals should only be performed by individuals knowledgeable in the procedure, in order to avoid false-positive irritant reactions. Standard texts can be consulted for patch test concentrations.

Tests for Immediate Hypersensitivity

The diagnosis of immediate contact reactions is often overlooked. If the dermatosis is thought to be due to type I immediate hypersensitivity (contact urticaria) then testing suspected agents in nonirritating concentrations can be carried out in the following manner and sequence:

- Application to normal skin
- If negative, application to previously affected, yet normal appearing, skin.
- If negative, test on eczematous skin on an area showing only slight erythema, so that an urticarial response can be observed.
- If all of the above tests are negative then perform occluded patch tests on normal or previously affected skin and read at 10 and 45 min.
- If still negative, perform prick testing. Intradermal tests are more likely to be associated with anaphylaxis and are rarely reported to document contact urticaria.
- If available, a commercial radioallergosorbent assay test (RAST) can be performed for diagnosis of specific causes of contact urticaria such as latex. The RAST is generally considered to be less sensitive than a prick test.[100]

Other Tests

Photopatch testing is important in the evaluation of patients with photosensitivity (see Chap. 136). Other procedures include the repeat open application use test, in which a small amount of the suspected allergen is rubbed into the skin twice daily, usually near the antecubital fossae. If dermatitis appears within 1 week, the test is considered positive. Chemical analysis may be helpful in situations where it is difficult to determine whether the patient has actually been exposed to the suspected substance. The dimethylgloxime test for nickel is readily available. More complicated tests are available for other chemicals such as formaldehyde and chromate.[101]

TREATMENT

Initial therapy of occupational skin disease depends upon the etiology and is essentially the same as diseases of nonoccupational origin. However it is important that patients are told the specific cause(s) of their disease and methods to avoid recurrences, and given information on appropriate use of skin cleansers, topical therapy, and protective clothing along with other preventive measures.

Fitness for Work and Workplace Accommodation

The Americans with Disabilities Act of 1990 brought to the fore issues of job placement and accommodation. Few instances of skin disease exclude a person from performing a given job, although a specific skin disorder may be considered a basis for exclusion in certain circumstances. Table 137-11 discusses fitness to work with skin disease and lists selected conditions, which may disqualify an individual for work.[101] Most individuals with chronic skin conditions can perform normal work activities, but in some instances require accommodation in the workplace. Table 137-12 lists some work-aggravated skin disorders that may require accommodation by employers.[101]

Prognosis and Persistence

The prognosis for acute irritant and allergic contact dermatitis is quite good in most cases, especially in a well-motivated worker with a cooperative plant management. Recurrence is likely with repeated, chronic exposures to low levels of irritants and allergens. Certain diagnoses, such as chromium sensitivity, have a poor prognosis and are notoriously long lasting. Negative influences in prognosis also include atopic eczema, especially in occupations where there is heavy contact with water, soaps, and detergents, food products, and the like. A number of studies confirm the guarded prognosis of chronic occupational contact dermatitis. Factors determining return to work for dermatologic disorders include severity of the condition, site and extent of involvement, effect of therapy and comorbid conditions, frequency of recurrences, age, effect of job availability and of alternative work, and recommendations of health care providers, including results of diagnostic tests.[98,102]

Of the several causes of persistence of occupational skin disease, the most important is an incomplete or incorrect diagnosis. Other factors include failure to eliminate the cause(s), improper job placement, improper therapy, the presence of secondary diagnoses (e.g.,

TABLE 137-11

Selected Dermatologic Conditions That, Under Some Circumstances, May Exclude an Individual from Work

Disorder	Excluded Job
1. Herpes simplex virus whitlow of a finger recurrent and not controllable	Health care worker with direct patient contact
2. Dermatophyte infection of the palms recurrent and not controllable	Massage therapy
3. Recurrent impetigo in chronic pyogenic staphylococcus aureus infection	Health care workers
4. Dermatoses of the feet	Police and fire work
5. Thermoregulatory skin disorders: anhidrotic ectodermal dysplasia	Extreme hot with potential for prolonged heat stress
6. Thermoregulatory skin disorders: patients with chronic erythroderma	Extremely cold indoor or outdoor jobs
7. Physical agent intolerance: lupus erythematosus	Extensive outdoor work
8. Physical agent intolerance: Raynaud's disease	Prolonged cold exposure
9. Physical agent intolerance: cold urticaria	Prolonged cold exposure; ocean or lake lifeguard
10. Hand dermatitis	May limit grip strength

SOURCE: Veien NK.[101]

TABLE 137-12

Selected Dermatologic Conditions That May Require Accommodation

DISORDER	ACCOMMODATION
1. Dermatophyte infection of the palms	Gloves because a large innoculum is required to transmit the infection
2. Psoriasis and lichen planus	Frequent trauma that induces Koebner phenomenon, e.g., welder
3. Vitiligo	Disfiguring cosmetically, but does not impair work unless in strong sunlight
4. Endogenous eczema or atopic dermatitis	Avoid wet work as much as possible; inhalant allergens and heavy physical work may aggravate the condition
5. Contact dermatitis	Avoidance, allergen substitution, protective equipment
6. Hyperhidrosis	Certain tasks such as handling paper documents and work with cement and other chemicals
7. Stasis ulcers recurrent in a setting of post-phlebitic syndrome	Prolonged standing may aggravate the condition
8. Type 1 fair complexion (patient always sunburns and never tans)	Prolonged outdoor work in sunlight may be a hazard even with sunscreens and clothes
9. Hereditary or acquired bullous disorders	Physical work involving friction and pressure

SOURCE: Veien NK.[101]

allergy to topical medications or multiple contact allergies), exposure to cross-reacting substances in home or vocational activities, and improper cleansing of the skin. Prolonged rubbing and scratching may lead to lichen simplex chronicus, which is often self-perpetuating. Rarely, self-inflicted lesions are used surreptitiously to maintain disease activity and an attractive compensation status.[98]

Impairment and Disability Evaluation

Detailed evaluation of patients with disabling skin disorders is discussed in more detail in other sources. However, dermatologists should be familiar with the existence of the *Guides to the Evaluation of Permanent Impairment,* published by the American Medical Association. The *Guides'* chapter on skin disease has been used for more than 30 years to evaluate patients with permanently impairing skin disorders (diseases that have reached maximum medical improvement—often after 6 to 12 months duration) of occupational and nonoccupational origin. The *Guides* are used by a number of state workers' compensation authorities and provide examples of five classes of impairment ranging from 0 percent to 95 percent.

Prevention

Most occupational skin disorders are preventable and multidimensional control measures are required, involving environmental, personal, and medical methods.[103]

ENVIRONMENTAL METHODS Environmental methods are the preferred, but most expensive, control measures and use industrial hygiene and environmental engineering interventions such as (1) hazard identification; (2) substitution of less irritating and allergenic chemicals, such as rubber gloves without thiurams and carbamates, an alternative resin (phenolic or polyester) for epoxy resins, and an alternative metal working fluid without a sensitizing additive; (3) isolation and enclosure of the process; (4) local exhaust ventilation and chemical dispensers; and (5) good housekeeping.

WORKPLACE VISITS Workplace visits are an important, but often overlooked part of the evaluation of workers with occupational skin disease. Hazard identification and assessment of methods of exposure can be evaluated by direct observation and may be requisite for problem solving, especially when more than one worker is affected.

PERSONAL METHODS

Barrier creams Barrier creams have been called invisible gloves, but in fact they are rarely an adequate substitute for protective clothing. Nevertheless, they are often used in situations in which glove, sleeves, and face masks cannot be conveniently or safely used. Because they are washed out before coffee breaks and at mealtimes, they encourage cleanliness and at the same time remove industrial dirt from the skin. Several types are available: ordinary emollient creams, water repellant creams, oil- and solvent-resistant creams, and miscellaneous products for use against poison ivy and oak. Over the years, their effectiveness has been greatly overrated. The most effective products are sunscreens and blocks, which ideally should be worn by all outdoor workers.

Problems associated with the use of barrier creams are a false sense of security, improper selection and use, allergy to an ingredient (often a preservative or fragrance), potential for increased absorption of occupational chemicals, and inadequate or infrequent application.

SKIN CLEANSERS (See "Common Occupational Irritants" earlier in this chapter.)

PROTECTIVE CLOTHING Many types of protective clothing are available ranging from gloves, aprons, hoods, boots, and work shoes to full body clothing. Fabrics that resist heat, cold, acids, alkalis, solvents, and UV radiation are available. Certain types are mildew and fire resistant. Federal Occupational and Safety Administration (OSHA) requirements for personal protective equipment (PPE), as amended in 1994, are described in the US Government Code of Federal Regulations (29 CFR Part 1910). Other privately promulgated national and international standards also exist. Manufacturers of PPE provide catalogues with guidelines for selection of clothing for various exposures. A handy reference guide is also very useful: Forsberg K, Mansdorf SZ. *Quick Selection Guide to Chemical Protective Clothing,* 3rd ed. New York, Wiley, 1997. Table 137-13 lists major glove materials and general guidance for their suitability for use with certain chemicals. Several important factors to consider in glove selection are that (1) completely impermeable PPE does not exist, and no single item of clothing can provide a barrier to all chemicals; (2) chemicals ultimately penetrate gloves and can do so without evidence of damage to the glove; (3) gloves should not be worn if torn or damaged; and (4) frequent donning and doffing of gloves may allow contamination of their interior surfaces with work chemicals.

MEDICAL METHODS Physicians often overlook certain medical aspects of prevention. Basic considerations include the following:

TABLE 137-13

General Recommendations for Use of Glove Materials with Certain Chemicals*

Glove Material	Protects Against	Comments
Natural rubber	Soaps and detergents (heavy weight), water-soluble irritants, dilute acids and alkalis	Avoid with organic solvents, strong acids and alkalis, many other organic compounds
Butyl rubber (isobutene, isoprene)	Aldehydes, some amines; amides; ketones; formaldehyde resins; epoxy resins; glycol ethers; most acrylates; isocyanates; hydroxyl compounds (e.g., ethanol)	Avoid with aliphatic and aromatic halogen and hydrocarbon compounds (e.g., vinyl chloride, chlorobenzenes, kerosene, cumene)
Chloroprene (neoprene)	Soaps; detergents; dilute acids and alkalis; certain amines and esters; most alcohols; vegetable oils	Avoid with most aliphatic and aromatic halogen and hydrocarbon compounds (e.g., vinyl chloride, chlorobenzenes, heptane, cumene)
Nitrile rubber	Organic acids; certain alcohols, amines, ethers, peroxdes, inorganic alkalis, vegetable oils	Some protection against some organophosphorus compounds
Viton (copolymer of hexafluoropropylene and vinylidene fluoride)	Organic solvents, particularly halogenated and aromatic hydrocarbons	Avoid with acrylics and ethers; cost 30 to 40 times more than natural rubber
Polyvinyl alcohol	Several organic solvents, esters	Not resistant to water or aqueous solutions
Polyvinyl chloride (vinyl)	Soaps and detergents, oils, metalworking fluids, dilute acids and alkalis, vegetable oils	Not good for most organic solvents
4H and Silvershield (polyethylene/ethylene vinyl alcohol copolymer)	Epoxy resins; acrylic resins; glyceryl thioglycolate; many other chemicals	Can be worn under other gloves as they are bulky to wear
Polyethylene	Used by food handlers	Not good for most chemicals

*Consult with manufacturer for specific glove recommendations.
SOURCE: Modified from Refs.[20,27,104,105]

(1) Initial and subsequent employment physical examinations should include appraisals of the skin and evaluation of fitness for work (Table 137-11). (2) Workers with skin disease may require accommodation in the workplace (see Table 137-12). (3) Avoid potentially sensitizing topical preparations (neomycin, bacitracin, Furacin, benzocaine, etc.) when treating occupational dermatoses. (4) Medical and vocational rehabilitation of well-motivated workers with occupational skin disease is important and is often covered by many workers compensation plans. It is important that the personnel of rehabilitation agencies understand the nature of skin disease and especially the chemicals found in specific jobs.

Health Risk Assessment

The current scientific approach to risk reduction in occupational health is based upon risk assessment, which is separated into four basic elements:[1,106]

1. *Hazard identification* involves determining whether exposure to an agent can cause disease or injury. Material Safety Data Sheets (MSDSs) are often used as the basis for this determination. All employers are required to provide MSDSs to their employees. The sheets provide basic chemical and health and safety information only about substances that are considered hazardous; those present in concentrations under 1 percent are not routinely required to be listed. Accordingly, many chemicals are not listed, but this information can be obtained by telephone from a number present on the first page of the MSDS. A physician can then decide whether any ingredient is a known allergen and patch test accordingly.
2. *Dermal exposure assessment* is the term used to describe the nature and size of various populations exposed to a chemical agent via the skin, as well as the magnitude and duration of the exposure. Dermal toxicity depends upon a number of factors including the degree, duration and route of exposure, the bioavailability of the chemical and the presence of dermatitis. Published data for workplace exposures (Threshold Limit Values or TLV's) to a number of chemicals by the American Conference of Governmental Industrial Hygienists is based upon measurement of airborne exposures. Skin notations for a number of substances indicate only the potential significant contribution to overall exposure by the cutaneous route and convey no quantitative information. Some of the best data exists for pesticides, where percutaneous absorption can result in significant systemic toxicity. Practical considerations for exposure include the method of exposure: spills, contaminated tools or rags, aerosols or sprays, or permeation of protective clothing. Thus, work activity (task duration and frequency; amount of chemical used), work substance (molecular weight, particle size, solubility, volatility, etc.), and worker (surface area exposed, personal hygiene, presence of dermatitis) are three major considerations. Methods for measuring dermal exposure to chemicals include wipe samples, hand or skin rinses, dermal dosimeter patches and fluorescent tracers; there is no gold standard. Studies on bioavailability of nickel show that plasma is more effective than heat or water in dissolving nickel from earrings, which is also dependent on the metallurgy and composition of various nickel-containing alloys.
3. *Dose response assessment* describes the quantitative relationship between the dose at the target and the toxicologic effect. Studies in allergic contact dermatitis have shown a wide range in the maximum and minimum concentrations of nickel and other chemicals, which will elicit contact allergy. Thus very small quantities of some allergens may provoke a reaction in some sensitized individuals. Persons with atopic dermatitis have increased transepidermal water loss and enhanced reactivity to irritants.
4. *Risk characterization* involves the integration of the data from the other three steps to determine safe exposure by comparing exposure levels with no observed adverse effect levels (NOAEL), while allowing for a safe margin of error. With the possible exception of nickel and chrome, few skin exposures have been characterized in this way and it may be difficult to do so. Additionally in determining risk assessment for cutaneous exposure to chemicals, at least as much attention needs to be given to percutaneous absorption as to dermal exposure.

REFERENCES

1. Emmett EA: Occupational contact dermatitis II. Risk assessment and prognosis. *Am J Contact Dermat*. In press.
2. Burnett CA et al: Occupational dermatitis causing days away from work in U.S. private industry, 1993. *Am J Ind Med* **34**:568, 1998
3. Coenraads JP et al: Epidemiology, in *Textbook of Contact Dermatitis* 3rd ed, edited by RJG Rycroft, T Menne, P Frosch, JP Lepoittevin. Berlin, Springer, 2001, p 200
4. Lammintausta K, Maibach HI: Contact dermatitis due to irritation, in *Occupational Skin Disease,* 2nd ed, edited by RM Adams. Philadelphia, Saunders, 1990, p 11
5. Frosch PJ: Clinical aspects of irritant contact dermatitis, in *Textbook of Contact Dermatitis* 3rd ed, edited by RJG Rycroft, T Menne, P Frosch, JP Lepoittevin. Berlin, Springer, 2001, p 313
6. Bruze H, Emmett EM: Occupational exposure to irritants, in *Irritant Contact Dermatitis,* edited by EM Jackson, R Goldner. New York, Marcel Dekker, 1990, p 81
7. Kim IH, Seo SH: Occupational chemical burns caused by bromine. *Contact Dermatitis* **41**:43, 1999
8. Schwanitz HJ, Uter W: Interdigital dermatitis: sentinel skin damage in hairdressers. *Br J Dermatol* **142**:1011, 2000
9. Rieschel RL: Diagnosing irritant contact dermatitis, in *Irritant Contact Dermatitis,* edited by EM Jackson, R Goldner. New York, Marcel Dekker, 1990, p 167
10. Singer A et al: Chemical burns: Our 10-year experience. *Burns* **18**:250, 1992
11. Bruze M, Fregert S: Chemical skin burns, in *Handbook of Occupational Dermatology,* edited by L Kanerva, P Elsner, JE Wahlberg, HI Maibach. Springer, Berlin, 2000, p 325
12. Adams RM: Occupational skin disease, in *Dermatology in General Medicine,* 5th ed, edited by IM Freedberg, AZ Eisen, K Wolff, KE Austen, LA Goldsmith, SI Katz, TB Fitzpatrick, New York, McGraw-Hill, 1999, p 1609
13. Spoo J, Elsner P: Cement burns: A review 1960–2000. *Contact Dermatitis* **45**:68, 2001
14. Fisher AA: Cement injuries: Part II. Cement burns resulting in necrotic ulcers due to kneeling on wet cement. *Cutis* **61**:121, 1998
15. Terrill PJ, Gowar JP: Chromic acid burns; beware, be aggressive, be watchful. *Br J Plast Surg* **43**:699, 1990
16. Eldad A et al: Phosphorus burns: Evaluation of various modalities for primary treatment. *J Burn Care Rehabil* **16**:49, 1995
17. Karacalar A, Karacalar SA: Chemical burns due to blood pressure cuff sterilized with ethylene oxide. *Burns* **26**:760, 2000
18. Lewis R: Metals, in *Occupational Medicine,* edited by J LaDou. Stamford, CT, Appleton & Lange, 1997, p 434
19. Schwartz I et al: Allergic dermatitis due to metallic cobalt. *J Allergy* **16**:51, 1945
20. Wahlberg JE, Adams RM: Solvents, in *Occupational Skin Disease,* 3rd ed, edited by RM Adams. Philadelphia, Saunders, 1999, p 484
21. Klauder JV, Brill FA: Correlation of boiling ranges of some petroleum solvents with irritant action on skin. *Arch Dermatol* **56**:197, 1947
22. Zug K, Marks JG Jr: Plants and woods, in *Occupational Skin Disease,* 3rd ed, edited by RM Adams. Philadelphia, Saunders, 1999, p 567
23. Lovell CR: *Plants and the Skin*. Oxford, Blackwell Scientific, 1993
24. Epstein WL: House and garden plants, in *Irritant Contact Dermatitis,* edited by EM Jackson, R Goldner. New York, Marcel Decker, 1990, p 127
25. Ljunggren B: Psoralen photoallergy caused by plant contact. *Contact Dermatitis* **3**:85, 1977
26. Rietschel RL et al: A preliminary report of the occupation of patients evaluated in patch test clinics. *Am J Contact Dermat* **12**:72, 2001
27. Rycroft RJG: Occupational contact dermatitis, in *Textbook of Contact Dermatitis,* 3rd ed, edited by RJG Rycroft, T Menne, P Frosch, JP Lepoittevin. Berlin, Springer, 2001, p 555
28. Shelley WB, Shelley ED: *Contact Dermatitis, Advanced Dermatologic Diagnosis*. Philadelphia, WB Saunders, 1992
29. Lahti A: Immediate contact reactions, in *Textbook of Contact Dermatitis,* edited by RJG Rycroft, T Menne, PJ Frosch, JP Lepoittevin. Berlin, Springer-Verlag, 1995, p 69
30. Taylor JS et al: Latex allergy, in *1999 Yearbook of Dermatology and Dermatological Surgery,* edited by Thiers BH, Lang PG. St. Louis, Mosby, 1999, p 1
31. Kanerva L et al: Statistical data on occupational contact urticaria. *Contact Dermatitis* **35**:229, 1996
32. Taylor JS et al: Contact urticaria, in *Occupational Skin Disease* 3rd ed, edited by RM Adams. Philadelphia, Saunders, 1999, p 111
33. Nichols RL: Optimal treatment of complicated skin and skin structure infections. *J Antimicrob Chemother* **44**:19, 1999
34. Grammont-Cupillard M et al: Brucellosis from sniffing bacteriological cultures. *Lancet* **348**:1733, 1996
35. Brooke CJ, Riley TV: Erysipelothrix rhusiopathiae: Bacteriology, epidemiology and clinical manifestations of an occupational pathogen. *J Med Microbiol* **48**:789, 1999
36. Keefe M et al: Cutaneous warts in butchers. *Br J Dermatol* **132**:166, 1995
37. McGovern T: Can derm warfare fight germ warfare? *Medscape Dermatol* 2001. Available at: http://www.medscape.com/medscape/Dermatology/journal/2001/vo2.no6/md1115.01.mcgov. Accessed November 15, 2001
38. Ebola hemorrhagic fever (Uganda). *MMWR Morb Mortal Wkly Rep* **50**:73, 2001
39. Freeman S, Rosen RH: Irritant contact dermatitis resulting from repeated low-grade frictional trauma, in *The Irritant Contact Dermatitis Syndrome,* edited by P van der Valk, HI Maibach. Boca Raton, FL, CRC Press, 1996 p 205
40. Ronchese F: *Occupational Marks and Other Physical Signs. A Guide to Personal Identification.* New York, Grune & Stratton, 1948
41. Rogachefsky AS, Taylor JS: Professional sports: Skin disorders in athletes, in *Handbook of Occupational Dermatology,* edited by L Kanerva, P Elsner, JE Wahlberg, HI Maibach. Berlin, Springer, 2000, p 1072
42. Menne T: Hyperkeratotic dermatitis of the palms, in *Hand Eczema,* edited by T Menne, HI Maibach. Boca Raton, FL, CRC Press, 1994, p 95
43. Wilkinson DS: Introduction, definition and classification, in *Hand Eczema,* edited by T Menne, HI Maibach. Boca Raton, FL, CRC Press, 1994, p 1
44. Kanerva L et al: Allergic contact dermatitis from dental composite resins due to aromatic epoxy acrylates and aliphatic acrylates. *Contact Dermatitis* **20**:201, 1989
45. Mathias CGT: Post-traumatic eczema. *Dermatol Clin* **6**:35, 1988
46. Rietschel RL, Fowler JF: Noneczematous contact dermatitis, in *Fisher's Contact Dermatitis,* 5th ed, edited by RL Rietschel, JF Fowler. Philadelphia, Lippincot Williams & Wilkins, 2001, p 71
47. Riina LH et al: Burn injury in kitchen workers: A cause for prevention. *J Burn Care Rehabil* **21**:563, 2000
48. Taylor JS: Vibration syndrome in industry: Dermatological viewpoint. *Am J Ind Med* **8**:415, 1985
49. Kanerva L: Physical causes and radiation effects, in *Occupational Skin Disease,* 3rd ed, edited by RM Adams. Philadelphia, Saunders, 1999, p 35
50. Haustein UF, Haupt B: Occupational connective tissue disorders, in *Handbook of Occupational Dermatology,* edited by L Kanerva, P Elsner, JE Wahlberg, HI Maibach. Berlin, Springer, 2000, p 295
51. Adams BB et al: Periorbital comedones and their relationship to pitch tar: A cross-sectional analysis and a review of the literature. *J Am Acad Dermatol* **42**:624, 2000
52. Taylor JS: The pilosebaceous unit, in *Occupational and Industrial Dermatology,* 2nd ed, edited by HI Maibach. Chicago, Year Book Medical, 1987, p 105
53. Taylor JS: Environmental chloracne: Update and overview. *Ann N Y Acad Sci* **320**:295, 1979
54. McDonnell K, Taylor JS: Occupational and environmental acne, in *Handbook of Occupational Dermatology,* edited by L Kanerva, P Elsner, JE Wahlberg, HI Maibach. Berlin, Springer, 2000, p 225
55. Coenraads PJ et al: Blood lipid concentrations of dioxins and dibenzofurans causing chloracne. *Br J Dermatol* **141**:694, 1999
56. Geusau A et al: Olestra increases faecal excretion of 2,3,7,8-tetrachlorodibenzo-*p*-dioxin. *Lancet* **354**:1266, 1999
57. Schottenfield P, Haas F: Carcinogens in the workplace. *CA Cancer J Clin* **29**:144, 1979
58. Doll R: Relevance of epidemiology to policies for the prevention of cancer. *J Occup Med* **23**:601, 1981
59. Wikonkal NM, Brash DE: Ultraviolet radiation induced signature mutations in photocarcinogenesis. *J Investig Dermatol Symp Proc* **4**:6, 1999
60. Brash DE et al: Sunlight and sunburn in human skin cancer: p53, apoptosis, and tumor promotion. *J Investig Dermatol Symp Proc* **1**:136, 1996
61. Lear JT et al: A comparison of risk factors for malignant melanoma, squamous cell carcinoma and basal cell carcinoma in the UK. *Int J Clin Pract* **52**:145, 1998
62. Freedman DM et al: Residential and occupational exposure to sunlight and mortality from non-Hodgkin's lymphoma: Composite (threefold) case-control study. *BMJ* **314**:1451, 1997
63. Green A et al: Skin cancer in a subtropical Australian population: Incidence and lack of association with occupation. The Nambour Study Group. *Am J Epidemiol* **144**:1034, 1996
64. Suzuki T et al: Incidence of actinic keratosis of Japanese in Kasai City, Hyogo. *J Dermatol Sci* **16**:74, 1997

65. Gilchrest BA et al: The pathogenesis of melanoma induced by ultraviolet radiation. *N Engl J Med* **340**:1341, 1999
66. Pion IA et al: Occupation and the risk of malignant melanoma. *Cancer* **75**:637, 1995
67. Gallagher RP et al: Sunlight exposure, pigmentation factors, and risk of nonmelanocytic skin cancer. II. Squamous cell carcinoma. *Arch Dermatol* **131**:164, 1995
68. Gallagher RP et al: Chemical exposures, medical history, and risk of squamous and basal cell carcinoma of the skin. *Cancer Epidemiol Biomarkers Prev* **5**:419, 1996
69. Gallagher RP et al: Sunlight exposure, pigmentary factors, and risk of nonmelanocytic skin cancer. I. Basal cell carcinoma. *Arch Dermatol* **131**:157, 1995
70. Kavages MR et al: Use of tanning devices and risk of basal cell and squamous cell cancers. *J Natl Cancer Inst* **94**:224, 2002
71. Emmett EA: Occupational skin cancer—A review. *J Occup Med* **17**:44, 1975
72. Ingram AJ et al: DNA adducts produced by oils, oil fractions and polycyclic aromatic hydrocarbons in relation to repair processes and skin carcinogenesis. *J Appl Toxicol* **20**:165, 2000
73. Porru S et al: [The toxicology and prevention of the risks of occupational exposure to aromatic polycyclic hydrocarbons. III. The effects: epidemiological evidence, early effects. Individual hypersusceptibility. Health surveillance]. *G Ital Med Lav Ergon* **19**:152, 1997
74. Boffetta P et al: Cancer risk from occupational and environmental exposure to polycyclic aromatic hydrocarbons. *Cancer Causes Control* **8**:444, 1997
75. Tolbert PE: Oils and cancer. *Cancer Causes Control* **8**:386, 1997
76. Callahan CP, Merk HF: Occupational skin cancer and tumors, in *Handbook of Occupational Dermatology,* edited by L Kanerva, P Elsner, JE Wahlberg, HI Maibach. Berlin Springer, 2000, p 248
77. Cruickshank CN, Squire JR: Skin cancer in the engineering industry from the use of mineral oil. 1949. *Br J Indust Med* **50**:289, 1993
78. Karlehagen S et al: Cancer incidence among creosote-exposed workers. *Scand J Work Environ Health* **18**:26, 1992
79. Partanen T, Boffetta P: Cancer risk in asphalt workers and roofers: Review and meta-analysis of epidemiologic studies. *Am J Ind Med* **26**:721, 1994
80. Letzel S, Drexler H: Occupationally related tumors in tar refinery workers. *J Am Acad Dermatol* **39**:712, 1998
81. Ramsay HM et al: Clinical risk factors associated with nonmelanoma skin cancer in renal transplant recipients. *Am J Kidney Dis* **36**:167, 2000
82. Basu A et al: Genetic toxicology of a paradoxical human carcinogen, arsenic: A review. *Mutat Res* **488**:171, 2001
83. Kitchin KT: Recent advances in arsenic carcinogenesis: modes of action, animal model systems, and methylated arsenic metabolites. *Toxicol Appl Pharmacol* **172**:249, 2001
84. Hartwig A et al: Interaction of arsenic (III) with nucleotide excision repair in UV-irradiated human fibroblasts. *Carcinogenesis* **18**:399, 1997
85. Spiewak R: Pesticides as a cause of occupational skin diseases in farmers. *Ann Agric Environ Med* **8**:1, 2001
86. Tsuruta D et al: Merkel cell carcinoma, Bowen's disease and chronic occupational arsenic poisoning. *Br J Dermatology* **139**:291, 1998
87. Callen JP: Bowen's disease and internal malignant disease. *Arch Dermatol* **124**:675, 1988
88. Ewing J: Relation of trauma to malignant tumors. *Am J Surg* **40**:30, 1926
89. Stoll HI, Crissey JT: Epithelioma from single trauma, in *Cancer Dermatology,* edited by F Helm. Philadelphia, Lea & Febiger, 1979, p 25
90. Hasegawa R et al: Evaluation of epidermal cell kinetics following freezing or wounding of mouse skin and their potential as initiators of carcinogenesis. *J Invest Dermatol* **88**:652, 1987
91. Aziz SA et al: Profile of Kangri cancer: A prospective study. *Burns* **24**:763, 1998
92. Jerbi G et al: Melanoma arising in burn scars: Report of 3 observations and a literature review. *Arch Dermatol* **135**:1551, 1999
93. Can Z et al: Sarcoma developing in a burn scar: Case report and review of the literature. *Burns* **24**:68, 1998
94. Epstein JH et al: Occupational skin cancer, in *Occupational Skin Disease,* 3rd ed, edited by RM Adams. Philadelphia, Saunders, 1998, p 142
95. Yamada M et al: Prevalence of skin neoplasms among the atomic bomb survivors. *Radiat Res* **146**:223, 1996
96. ICRP (International Commission on Radiological Protection): *Recommendations of the ICRP. Annals of the ICRP 21:(1–3). ICRP Publication 60.* Oxford, Pergamon Press, 1991
97. Schwartz RA, Stoll HL Jr: Squamous cell carcinoma, in *Dermatology in General Medicine,* 5th ed, edited by IM Freedberg, AZ Eisen, K Wolff, KE Austen, LA Goldsmith, SI Katz, TB Fitzpatrick. New York, McGraw-Hill, 1999, p 840
98. Taylor JS: Dermatology, in *Disability Evaluation,* edited by SL Demeter, GBJ Andersson, GM Smith. St. Louis, Mosby, 1996, p 415
99. Mathais CGT: Contact dermatitis and workers' compensation: Criteria for establishing occupational causation and aggravation. *J Am Acad Dermatol* **20**:842, 1989
100. Warner MR et al: Agents causing contact urticaria. *Clin Dermatol* **15**:623, 1997
101. Veien NK: Diagnostic procedures for eczema patients: Exogenous dermatoses, in *Environmental Dermatitis,* edited by T Menne, MI Maibach, Boca Raton, FL, CRC Press, 1991
102. Nethercott JR: Fitness to work with skin disease and the Americans with Disability Act of 1990. *Occup Med* **9**:11, 1994
103. Taylor JS: The skin and occupational dermatoses, in *Fundamentals of Industrial Hygiene,* edited by B Plog, PJ Quinlan. Itasca, IL, National Safety Council, 2002
104. Estlander T, Jolanki R: How to protect the hands. *Dermatol Clin* **6**:105, 1988
105. Berardinelli SP: Prevention of occupational skin disease through use of chemical protective glove. *Dermatol Clin* **6**:115, 1988
106. Paustenbach D et al: Health risk assessment, in *Occupational Skin Disease,* 3rd ed, edited by RM Adams. Philadelphia, Saunders, 1998, p 291

CHAPTER 138

Neil H. Shear
Sandra R. Knowles
John R. Sullivan
Lori Shapiro

Cutaneous Reactions to Drugs

Complications from drug therapy are a major cause of patient morbidity and account for a significant number of patient deaths.[1] Approximately 14 percent of adverse drug reactions in hospital patients are cutaneous or allergic in nature.[2] Drug eruptions range from common nuisance eruptions to rare or life-threatening drug-induced diseases. Drug reactions can be solely limited to the skin, or they may be part of a systemic reaction, such as the drug hypersensitivity syndrome or toxic epidermal necrolysis (TEN).

Drug eruptions are distinct disease entities and must be approached as any other cutaneous disease. A precise diagnosis of the reaction pattern can help narrow possible causes, as different drugs are more commonly associated with different types of reactions.

PATHOGENESIS OF DRUG ERUPTIONS

Constitutional factors influencing the risk of cutaneous eruption include pharmacogenetic variation in drug-metabolizing enzymes and human leukocyte antigen (HLA) associations. Acetylator phenotype alters the risk of developing drug-induced lupus due to hydralazine, procainamide, and isoniazid. Acetylator phenotype is also important in many other drug eruptions. Fast acetylator status appears to partially protect against the risk of developing TEN and the drug hypersensitivity syndrome due to sulfonamide antibiotics.[3] HLA-DR4 is significantly more common in individuals with hydralazine-related drug-induced lupus than in those with idiopathic systemic lupus erythematosus.[4] HLA factors may also influence the risk of bullous drug reactions.[5]

Many drugs associated with severe idiosyncratic drug reactions are metabolized by the body to form reactive, or toxic, drug products.[6] These reactive products comprise only a small proportion of a drug's metabolites and are usually rapidly detoxified. However, patients with the drug hypersensitivity syndrome, TEN, and Stevens-Johnson syndrome (SJS), resulting from treatment with sulfonamide antibiotics and the aromatic anticonvulsants (e.g., carbamazepine, phenytoin, and phenobarbital), show increased sensitivity in in vitro assessments to the oxidative, reactive drug metabolites of these drugs as compared to control subjects.[7,8]

Acquired factors also alter an individual's risk of drug eruption. Active viral infection and concurrent medications have been shown to alter frequency of drug-associated eruptions. Drug–drug interactions may also alter risk of cutaneous eruption. Valproic acid increases the risk of severe cutaneous adverse reactions to lamotrigine, another anticonvulsant.[9] The basis of these interactions and reactions is unknown but may represent a mixture of factors including alteration in drug metabolism, drug detoxification, antioxidant defenses, and immune reactivity.

The course and outcome of drug-induced disease are also influenced by host factors. Older age may delay the onset of drug eruptions and has been associated with a higher mortality rate in some severe reactions; a higher mortality rate is also observed in patients with severe reactions with underlying malignancy.[10] Reactivation of latent viral infection with human herpesvirus (HHV)-6 also appears common in the drug hypersensitivity syndrome and may be partially responsible for some of the clinical features and/or course of the disease.[11]

The pathogenesis of most drug eruptions is not understood, although the clinical features of most drug eruptions are consistent with immune-mediated disease. The immune system may target the native drug, its metabolic products, altered self, or a combination of these factors.

MORPHOLOGIC APPROACH TO DRUG ERUPTIONS

Exanthematous Eruptions

Exanthematous eruptions, known also as morbilliform or maculopapular, are the most common form of drug eruptions, accounting for approximately 95 percent of skin reactions.[12] Simple exanthems are erythematous changes in the skin without evidence of blistering or pustulation. The eruption typically starts on the trunk and spreads peripherally in a symmetric fashion. Pruritus is almost always present. These eruptions usually occur within 1 week of starting therapy and resolve within 7 to 14 days. Resolution occurs with a change in color from bright red to a brownish-red, which may be followed by scaling or desquamation. The differential diagnosis in these patients includes a viral

exanthem, collagen vascular disease, and bacterial and rickettsial infections.

Exanthematous eruptions can be caused by many drugs including the penicillins, sulfonamides, nonnucleoside reverse transcriptase inhibitors (e.g., nevirapine), and antiepileptic medications.[12] Clinical experience and laboratory data have indicated that T cells are involved in these reactions because they are able to recognize the drug directly, without covalent hapten modification of proteins or peptides.[13] In patients who have concomitant infectious mononucleosis, the risk of developing an exanthematous eruption while being treated with an aminopenicillin (e.g., ampicillin) increases to 60 to 100 percent.[14] Patients are able to tolerate all beta-lactam antibiotics, including the aminopenicillins, after the infectious process has resolved. A similar drug–viral interaction has been observed in 50 percent of HIV-infected patients who are exposed to sulfonamide antibiotics.[15]

An exanthematous eruption in conjunction with fever and internal organ involvement (e.g., liver, kidney, central nervous system) signifies a more serious reaction, known as the *hypersensitivity syndrome reaction* (HSR). HSR occurs most frequently on first exposure to the drug, with initial symptoms starting 1 to 6 weeks after exposure. Fever and malaise are often the presenting symptoms. Atypical lymphocytosis with a subsequent eosinophilia may occur during the initial phases of the reaction in some patients. Even though most patients present with an exanthematous eruption, more serious cutaneous manifestations may be evident (Fig. 138-1). Internal organ involvement can be asymptomatic. Some patients may become hypothyroid approximately 2 months after the first symptoms appear.[16]

The formation of toxic metabolites by the aromatic anticonvulsants, namely phenytoin, carbamazepine, and phenobarbital, may play a pivotal role in the development of the HSR.[7] Approximately 70 to 75 percent of patients who develop anticonvulsant HSR in response to one aromatic anticonvulsant show cross-reactivity to the other aromatic anticonvulsants. In addition, in vitro testing shows that there is a familial occurrence of HSR due to anticonvulsants.[7] Thus, counseling of family members and disclosure of risk is essential.

Sulfonamide antibiotics are also metabolized to toxic metabolites, namely hydroxylamines and nitroso compounds. Because siblings and other first-degree relatives are at an increased risk (perhaps as high as 1 in 4) of developing a similar adverse reaction, counseling of family members is essential.

FIGURE 138-1

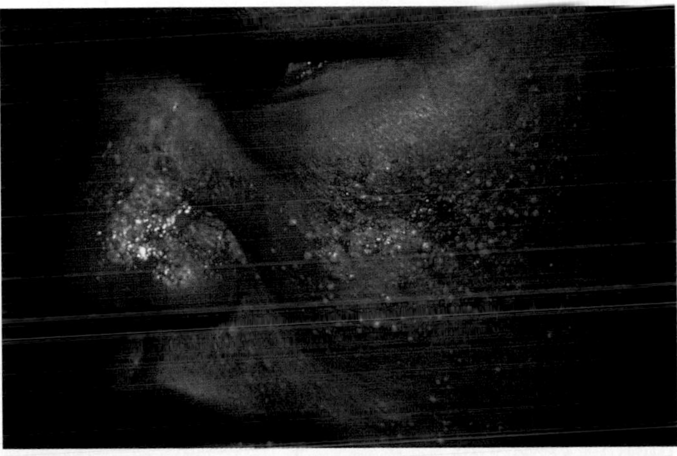

Hypersensitivity syndrome reaction, characterized by fever, a pustular eruption, and hepatitis, in a 23-year-old man after 18 days of treatment with minocycline.

Urticarial Eruptions

Urticaria is characterized by pruritic red wheals of various sizes. Individual lesions generally last for less than 24 h, although new lesions can continually develop. When deep dermal and subcutaneous tissues are also swollen, the reaction is known as *angioedema*. Angioedema is frequently unilateral and nonpruritic and lasts for 1 to 2 h, although it may persist for 2 to 5 days.

Urticaria and angioedema, when associated with drug use, are usually indicative of an IgE-mediated immediate hypersensitivity reaction; this mechanism is typified by immediate reactions to penicillin and other antibiotics. Nonimmunologic activation of inflammatory mediators may also result in urticarial reactions. For example, narcotic analgesics may directly cause release of histamine from mast cells independent of IgE[17] (see Chap. 116).

Angiotensin-converting enzyme (ACE) inhibitors are frequent causes of angioedema.[18] The onset is usually within hours of starting ACE-inhibitor therapy but can occur as late as 1 week to several months into therapy. Angioedema usually resolves within 48 h with treatment. Angioedema has also been reported to occur with angiotensin II antagonists; in many of these patients, a prior history of angioedema related to an ACE-inhibitor was documented.[19]

Serum sickness-like reactions are defined by the presence of fever, rash (usually urticarial), and arthralgias 1 to 3 weeks after initiation of drug. Lymphadenopathy and eosinophilia may also be present; however, in contrast to true serum sickness, immune complexes, hypocomplementemia, vasculitis, and renal lesions are absent.

Cefaclor is associated with an increased relative risk of serum sickness-like reactions. In genetically susceptible hosts, a reactive metabolite is generated during the metabolism of cefaclor that may bind with tissue proteins and elicit an inflammatory response manifesting as a serum sickness–like reaction.[20]

Pustular Eruptions

Acneiform eruptions are associated with iodides, bromides, adrenocorticotropic hormone (ACTH), glucocorticoids, isoniazid, androgens, lithium, actinomycin D, and phenytoin. Drug-induced acne may appear in atypical areas, such as on the arms and legs, and is most often monomorphous. Comedones are usually absent. The fact that acneiform eruptions do not affect prepubertal children indicates that previous hormonal priming is a necessary prerequisite. In cases where the offending agent cannot be discontinued, topical tretinoin may be useful.[21]

Acute generalized exanthematous pustulosis (AGEP) is an acute febrile eruption that is often associated with leukocytosis[22] (Fig. 138-2). After drug administration, it may take 1 to 3 weeks before skin lesions appear; however, in previously sensitized patients, the skin symptoms may occur within 2 to 3 days. The lesions often start on the face or main skin creases. Generalized desquamation occurs approximately 2 weeks later. The estimated incidence rate of AGEP is approximately 1 to 5 cases per million per year.[23] Differential diagnosis includes pustular psoriasis, the hypersensitivity syndrome reaction with pustulation, subcorneal pustular dermatosis (Sneddon-Wilkinson disease), pustular vasculitis, or TEN, especially in severe cases of AGEP. The typical histopathologic analysis of AGEP lesions shows spongiform subcorneal and/or intraepidermal pustules, an often marked edema of the papillary dermis, and perivascular infiltrates with neutrophils and exocytosis of some eosinophils.[23]

Bullous Eruptions

Pseudoporphyria is a cutaneous phototoxic disorder that can resemble either porphyria cutanea tarda (PCT) in adults or erythropoietic protoporphyria (EPP) in children (see Chap. 149). Pseudoporphyria of the PCT variety is characterized by skin fragility, blister formation, and scarring in photodistribution; it occurs in the presence of normal porphyrin levels. The other clinical pattern mimics EPP and manifests as cutaneous burning, erythema, vesiculation, angular chicken pox-like scars, and waxy thickening of the skin. The eruption may begin within 1 day of initiation of therapy or may be delayed for as long as 1 year. The course is prolonged in some patients, but most reports describe symptoms that disappear several weeks to several months after the offending agent is withdrawn. Because of the risk of permanent facial scarring, the implicated drug should be discontinued if skin fragility, blistering, or scarring occurs.[24] In addition, broad-spectrum sunscreen and protective clothing should be recommended.

FIGURE 138-2

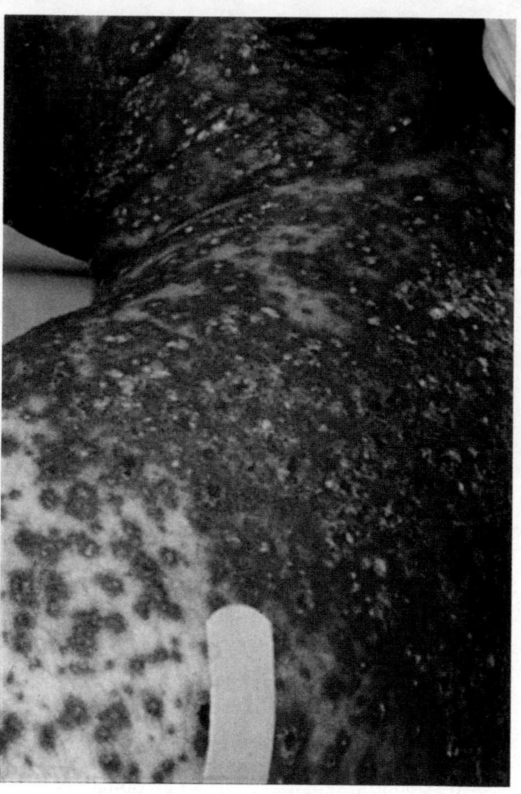

Acute generalized exanthematous pustulosis (AGEP) in a 48-year-old man who developed nonfollicular pustules and fever after 7 days of treatment with diltiazem.

Both idiopathic and *drug-induced linear IgA* disease are heterogeneous in clinical presentation. Cases of the drug-induced type have morphologies resembling erythema multiforme, bullous pemphigoid, and dermatitis herpetiformis. The drug-induced disease may differ from the idiopathic entity in that mucosal or conjunctival lesions are less common, spontaneous remission occurs once the offending agent is withdrawn, and immune deposits disappear from the skin once the lesions resolves.

Biopsy specimens are necessary for diagnosis. Histologically, the two entities are similar. A study suggests that, as in the idiopathic variety, the target antigen is not unique in the drug-induced disease. While 13 to 30 percent of patients with sporadic linear IgA have circulating basement membrane zone antibodies, these antibodies have not been reported in drug-induced cases.[25] In patients with linear IgA bullous disease proven by direct immunofluorescence, the index of suspicion of drug induction should be higher in cases with only IgA and no IgG in the basement membrane zone.

Pemphigus may be considered as drug-induced or drug-triggered (i.e., a latent disease that is unmasked by the drug exposure). Drug-induced pemphigus caused by penicillamine and other thiol drugs tends to remit spontaneously in 35 to 50 percent of cases, presents as pemphigus foliaceus, has an average interval to onset of 1 year, and is associated with the presence of antinuclear antibodies in 25 percent of patients.

Most patients with nonthiol drug-induced pemphigus manifest clinical, histologic, immunologic, and evolutionary aspects similar to those of idiopathic pemphigus vulgaris with mucosal involvement with a 15 percent rate of spontaneous recovery after drug withdrawal. Treatment of drug-induced pemphigus begins with drug withdrawal. Systemic glucocorticoids are often required until all symptoms of active disease disappear. Vigilant follow-up is required after remission to monitor the patient and the serum for autoantibodies to detect an early relapse.[26]

Drug-induced bullous pemphigoid (see Chap. 61) can encompass a wide variety of presentations, ranging from the classic features of large, tense bullae arising from an erythematous, urticarial base, with moderate involvement of the oral cavity, through mild forms with few bullous lesions, or scarring plaques and nodules with bullae.[26] In contrast to the idiopathic form, patients with drug-induced bullous pemphigoid are generally younger; as well, the histopathologic findings are of a perivascular infiltration of lymphocytes with few eosinophils and neutrophils, intraepidermal vesicles with foci of necrotic keratinocytes, thrombi in dermal vessels, and a possible lack of tissue-bound and circulating antibasal membrane zone IgG.

In the acute, self-limited condition, resolution occurs after the withdrawal of the culprit agent, with or without glucocorticoid therapy. However, in some patients, the drug may actually trigger the idiopathic form of the disease.

Erythema multiforme-major (EM-major), SJS, and *TEN* (see Chap. 58), which may represent variants of the same disease process, encompass a spectrum of serious dermatologic eruptions (Fig. 138-3). The more severe the reaction, the more likely it is that it has been drug-induced. A large percentage of cases of EM/SJS are not drug related and may develop after a variety of other predisposing factors including infections (e.g., herpes simplex, *Mycoplasma pneumoniae*), neoplasia, and autoimmune diseases. The risk of TEN has been estimated to be 1 per million per year and 1 to 6 per million per year for SJS.[27]

The pathogenesis of severe cutaneous adverse drug reactions is unknown, although a metabolic basis has been hypothesized.[7]

Treatment of EM, SJS, and TEN includes discontinuation of the suspected drug and supportive measures, such as careful wound care, hydration, and nutritional support. The use of glucocorticoids to treat SJS and TEN is controversial.[28,29] Intravenous immunoglobulin (IVIG, 0.2 to 0.75 g/kg for 4 consecutive days) has rapidly reversed disease progression within 48 hours.[30] A limited number of patients have been treated with cyclophosphamide[31] and cyclosporine.[32] Patients who have developed a severe cutaneous adverse reaction (i.e., EM/SJS/TEN) should not be rechallenged with the drug or undergo desensitization with the medication.

FIGURE 138-3

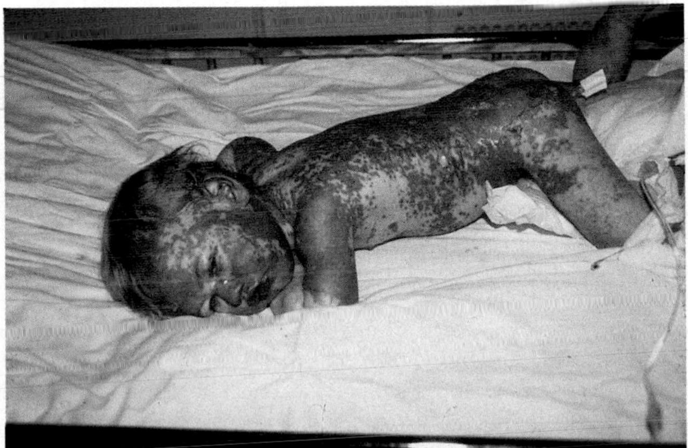

Toxic epidermal necrolysis in a child after 18 days of treatment with phenobarbital for febrile seizures.

Fixed Drug Eruptions

Fixed drug eruptions (FDE) usually appear as solitary, erythematous, bright red or dusky red macules that may evolve into an edematous plaque; bullous-type lesions may be present. FDE are most commonly found on the genitalia and in the perianal area, although they can occur anywhere on the skin surface. Some patients may complain of burning or stinging, and others may have fever, malaise, and abdominal symptoms. FDE can develop 30 min to 8 to 16 h after ingestion of the medication. After the initial acute phase lasting days to weeks, residual grayish or slate-colored hyperpigmentation develops. Upon rechallenge, not only do the lesions recur in the same location, but also new lesions often appear.

More than 100 drugs have been implicated in FDE, including ibuprofen, sulfonamides, and tetracyclines. A haplotype linkage in the setting of trimethoprim-sulfamethoxazole–induced FDE was recently documented.[33]

Histologically, FDE resembles erythema multiforme, with an interface dermatitis with lymphocytes at the dermal–epidermal junction and degenerative changes of epithelium with dyskeratosis. However, there is also evidence of chronic injury in FDE, which is manifested by acanthosis, hyperkeratosis, and hypergranulosis. Eosinophils and neutrophils are also present. The numbers of helper and suppressor T lymphocytes are increased in lesional skin. The T cells may persist in lesional skin and are believed to contribute to immunologic "memory."[34]

A challenge or provocation test with the suspected drug may be useful in establishing the diagnosis. Patch testing at the site of a previous lesion yields a positive response in up to 43 percent of patients. In some patients, prick and intradermal skin tests may be positive in 24 and 67 percent of patients, respectively.[35]

Coumarin-Induced Skin Necrosis

Coumarin-induced skin necrosis (Fig. 138-4) begins 3 to 5 days after initiation of treatment. Early, red, painful plaques develop in adipose-rich sites such as breasts, buttocks, and hips. These plaques may blister, ulcerate, or develop into necrotic areas. It is estimated that 1 in

FIGURE 138-4

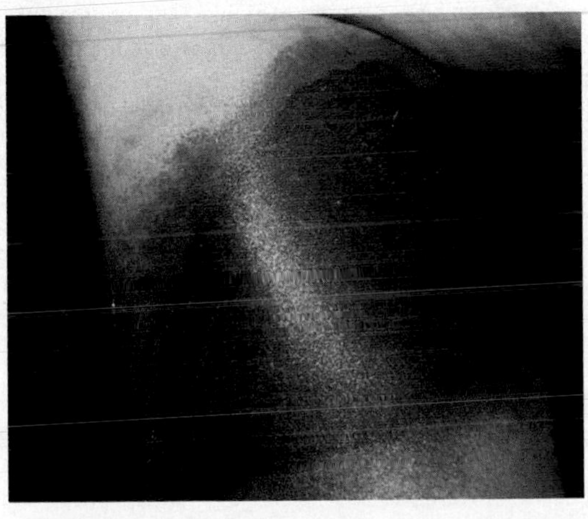

Skin necrosis in a patient after 4 days of warfarin therapy.

10,000 persons who receive the drug is at risk of this adverse event.[36] The incidence is four times higher in women, especially in obese women, with a peak incidence in the sixth and seventh decades of life. Afflicted patients often have been given a large initial loading dose of coumarin in the absence of concomitant heparin therapy. An accompanying infection such as pneumonia, viral infection, or erysipelas may be seen in up to 25 percent of patients. An association with protein C and protein S deficiencies exists, but pretreatment screening is not warranted. An association with a heterozygote for the factor V Leiden mutation has been reported recently.[37]

Treatment involves the discontinuation of coumarin, administration of vitamin K, and infusion of heparin at therapeutic doses. Fresh-frozen plasma and purified protein C concentrates have been used.[38] Supportive measures for the skin are a mainstay of therapy. The morbidity rate is high; 60 percent of affected individuals require plastic surgery for remediation of full thickness skin necrosis by skin grafting. These patients may be treated with coumarin in the future, but small doses (2 to 5 mg daily) are recommended with initial treatment under heparin coverage.

The pathogenesis of this adverse event is the paradoxical development of occlusive thrombi in cutaneous and subcutaneous venules due to a transient hypercoagulable state. This results from the suppression of the natural anticoagulant protein C at a greater rate than the suppression of natural procoagulant factors.

Drug-Induced Lichenoid Eruptions

Drug-induced lichen planus produces lesions that are clinically and histologically indistinguishable from idiopathic lichen planus; however, lichenoid drug eruptions often appear initially as eczematous with a purple hue and involve large areas of the trunk. Usually the mucous membranes and nails are not involved. Histologically, focal parakeratosis, focal interruption of the granular layer, cytoid bodies in the cornified and granular layers, the presence of eosinophils and plasma cells in the inflammatory infiltrate, and an infiltrate around the deep vessels favor a lichenoid drug eruption.[39] Many drugs, including beta blockers, penicillamine, and ACE-inhibitors, especially captopril, reportedly produce this reaction. The mean latent period is between 2 months and 3 years for penicillamine, approximately 1 year for β-adrenergic blocking agents, and 3 to 6 months for ACE inhibitors. The latent period may be shortened if the patient has been previously exposed to the drug.[39] Resolution usually occurs with 2 to 4 months. Rechallenge with the culprit drug has been attempted in a few patients, with reactivation of symptoms within 4 to 15 days.[40]

Drug-Induced Cutaneous Pseudolymphoma

Pseudolymphoma is a process that simulates lymphoma but has a benign behavior and does not meet the criteria for malignant lymphoma. Drugs are a well-known cause of cutaneous pseudolymphomas, but the condition may also be provided by foreign agents such as insect bites, infections (e.g., HIV), and idiopathic causes.[41]

Anticonvulsant-induced pseudolymphoma generally occurs after 1 week to 2 years of exposure to the drug. Within 7 to 14 days of drug discontinuation, the symptoms generally resolve. The eruption often manifests as single lesions but can also be widespread erythematous papules, plaques, or nodules. Most patients also have fever, marked lymphadenopathy and hepatosplenomegaly, and eosinophilia.[42] Mycosis fungoides-like lesions are also associated with these drugs.[43]

Drug-Induced Vasculitis

Drug-induced vasculitis represents approximately 10 percent of the acute cutaneous vasculitides and usually involves small vessels.[44] Drugs that are associated with vasculitis include allopurinol, penicillins, and thiazide diuretics. The average interval from initiation of drug therapy to onset of drug-induced vasculitis is 7 to 21 days.[45]

The clinical hallmark of cutaneous vasculitis is palpable purpura, classically found on the lower extremities. Urticaria can be a manifestation of small vessel vasculitis, with individual lesions remaining fixed in the same location for more than 1 day. Other features include hemorrhagic bullae, urticaria, ulcers, nodules, Raynaud's disease, and digital necrosis.[46] The same vasculitic process may also affect internal organs such as the liver, kidney, gut, and central nervous system and can be potentially life-threatening.

Drug-induced vasculitis can be difficult to diagnose and is often a diagnosis of exclusion. In some cases, serology has revealed the presence of perinuclear-staining antineutrophil cytoplasmic autoantibodies (p-ANCA) against myeloperoxidase.[47] Alternative etiologies for cutaneous vasculitis such as infection or autoimmune disease must be eliminated. Treatment consists of drug withdrawal. Systemic glucocorticoids may be of benefit.

Drug-Induced Lupus (See Chap. 171)

Drug-induced lupus is characterized by frequent musculoskeletal complaints, fever, weight loss, pleuropulmonary involvement in more than half of patients, and, rarely, renal, neurologic, or vasculitic involvement.[48] Most patients have no cutaneous findings of lupus erythematosus. The most common serologic abnormalities are positivity for antinuclear antibodies with a homogeneous pattern, as well as the presence of antihistone antibody. The recent identification of minocycline as a cause of drug-induced lupus makes it important for dermatologists to recognize this syndrome. Minocycline-induced lupus typically occurs after 2 years of therapy. The patient presents with a symmetric polyarthritis. Hepatitis is often detected on laboratory evaluation.[49] Cutaneous findings include livedo reticularis, painful nodules on the legs, and nondescript eruptions. Antihistone antibody is seldom present. A study of HLA class II alleles revealed the presence of HLA-DR-4 or HLA-DR-2 in many of the patients.[50]

In contrast, *drug-induced subacute cutaneous lupus erythematosus* (SCLE) is characterized by a papulosquamous or annular cutaneous lesion, which is often photosensitive, and absent or mild systemic involvement; circulating anti-Ro (SSA) antibodies have also been identified in many patients. The most commonly reported causative agents are thiazide diuretics, calcium channel blockers, and ACE inhibitors. The number of patients who develop SCLE during treatment with these medications is very small, and these drugs are thought to have low risk for causing or exacerbating cutaneous lupus.[51]

DIAGNOSIS AND MANAGEMENT

These iatrogenic disorders are distinct disease entities, although they may closely mimic many infective or idiopathic diseases. A drug cause should be considered in the differential diagnosis of a wide spectrum of dermatologic diseases, particularly when the presentation or course is atypical.

The diagnosis of a cutaneous drug eruption involves the precise characterization of reaction type (Tables 138-1 and 138-2). A wide variety of cutaneous drug-associated eruptions may also warn of associated internal toxicity (Table 138-3). Even the most minor cutaneous eruption should trigger a clinical review of systems, as the severity of systemic involvement does not necessarily mirror that of the skin.[52] Hepatic, renal, joint, respiratory, hematologic, and neurologic changes should be sought, and any systemic symptoms or signs investigated. Fever, malaise, pharyngitis, and other systemic symptoms or signs should be investigated. A usual screen would include a full blood count, liver and renal function tests, and a urine analysis.

TABLE 138-1

Drug Eruptions

Clinical Presentation	Pattern and Distribution of Skin Lesions	Mucous Membrane Involvement	Implicated Drugs	Treatment
Erythema multiforme	Target lesions, limbs	Absent	Anticonvulsants (including lamotrigine), sulfonamide antibiotics, allopurinol, nonsteroidal anti-inflammatory drugs (e.g., piroxicam), dapsone	Supportive*
Stevens-Johnson syndrome	Atypical targets, widespread	Present	As above	IVIG, cyclosporine
Toxic epidermal necrolysis	Epidermal necrosis with skin detachment	Present	As above	
Pseudoporphyria	Skin fragility, blister formation in photodistribution	Absent	Tetracycline, furosemide, naproxen	Supportive
Linear IgA disease	Bullous dermatosis	Present/absent	Vancomycin, lithium, diclofenac, piroxicam, amiodarone	Supportive
Pemphigus	Flaccid bullae, chest	Present/absent	Penicillamine, captopril, piroxicam, penicillin, rifampin	Supportive
Bullous pemphigoid	Tense bullae, widespread	Present/absent	Furosemide, penicillamine, penicillins, sulfasalazine, captopril	Supportive

*Supportive: systemic glucocorticoids are often required until all symptoms of active disease disappear.

Skin biopsy should be considered for all patients with potentially severe reactions, such as those with systemic symptoms, erythroderma, blistering, skin tenderness, purpura, and pustulation, or in those cases where diagnosis is uncertain. Some cutaneous reactions, such as FDE, are virtually always due to drug therapy, and nearly 90 percent of TEN cases are also drug related.[27] Other more common eruptions, including exanthematous or urticarial eruptions, have many nondrug causes.

There is no gold standard investigation for confirmation of a drug cause. Instead, diagnosis and assessment of cause involve analysis of a constellation of features such as timing of drug exposure and reaction onset, course of reaction with drug withdrawal or continuation, timing and nature of a recurrent eruption on rechallenge, a history of a similar reaction to a cross-reacting medication, and previous reports of similar reactions to the same medication. Investigations to exclude nondrug causes are similarly helpful.

Several in vitro investigations can help to confirm causation in individual cases, but their exact sensitivity and specificity remain unclear. Investigations include the lymphocyte toxicity and lymphocyte transformation assays.[7,9] Penicillin skin testing with major and minor determinants is useful for confirmation of an IgE-mediated immediate

TABLE 138-2

Clinical Features of Cutaneous Reactions to Drugs

Clinical Presentation	Drug Eruption	Fever	Internal Organ Involvement	Arthralgia	Lymphadenopathy	Implicated Drugs
Hypersensitivity syndrome reaction	Exanthem Exfoliative dermatitis Pustular eruptions Erythema multiforme-major Stevens-Johnson syndrome Toxic epidermal necrolysis	Present	Present	Absent	Present	Aromatic anticonvulsants (e.g., phenytoin, phenobarbital, carbamazepine), sulfonamide antibiotics, dapsone, minocycline, allopurinol
Serum sickness-like reaction	Urticaria Exanthem	Present	Absent	Present	Present	Cefaclor, cefprozil, bupropion, minocycline
Drug-induced lupus	Usually absent	Present	Present/absent	Present	Absent	Procainamide, hydralazine, isoniazid, minocycline, acebutolol
Drug-induced subacute cutaneous lupus erythematosus	Papulosquamous or annular cutaneous lesion (often photosensitive)	Absent	Absent	Absent	Absent	Thiazide diuretics, calcium channel blockers, ACE inhibitors
AGEP	Nonfollicular pustules on an edematous erythematous base	Present	Absent	Absent	Absent	Beta-blockers, macrolide antibiotics, calcium channel blockers

TABLE 138-3

Clinical Features That Warn of a Potentially Severe Drug Reaction

Systemic

- Fever and/or other symptoms of internal organ involvement such as pharyngitis, malaise, arthralgia, cough, and meningism
- Lymphadenopathy

Cutaneous

- Evolution to erythroderma
- Prominent facial involvement +/− edema or swelling
- Mucous membrane involvement (particularly if erosive or involving conjunctiva)
- Skin tenderness, blistering, or shedding
- Purpura

hypersensitivity reaction to penicillin.[53] Patch testing has been used in patients with ampicillin-induced exanthematous eruptions[54] and in the ancillary diagnosis of fixed drug eruptions. Patch testing has greater sensitivity if performed over a previously involved area of skin.[55]

Cutaneous drug eruptions do not usually vary in severity with dose. Less-severe reactions may abate with continued drug therapy (e.g., transient exanthematous eruptions associated with commencement of a new HIV antiretroviral regimen). However, a reaction suggestive of a potentially life-threatening situation should prompt immediate discontinuation of the drug, along with discontinuation of any interacting drugs that may slow the elimination of the suspected causative agent(s). Resolution of the reaction over a reasonable time frame after the drug is discontinued is consistent with drug cause but also occurs for many infective and other causes of transient cutaneous eruptions. Patients should not be rechallenged if they have suffered a potentially serious reaction.

PREVENTION

Cutaneous reactions to drugs are largely idiosyncratic and unexpected; serious reactions are rare. Once a reaction has occurred, however, it is important to prevent future similar reactions in the patient with the same drug or a cross-reacting medication. For patients with hypersensitivity and severe reactions, wearing a bracelet (e.g., MedicAlert) detailing the nature of the allergy is advisable, and patient records should be appropriately labeled.

Host factors appear important in many reactions. Some of these can be inherited, placing first-degree relatives at increased risk over the general population of a similar reaction to the same or a metabolically cross-reacting drug. This finding appears to be important in SJS, TEN, and drug hypersensitivity syndrome.[7,56]

Reporting reactions to the manufacturer or regulatory authorities is important. Postmarketing voluntary reports of rare, severe, or unusual reactions remain crucial to enhance the safe use of pharmaceutical agents.

REFERENCES

1. Lazarou J et al: Incidence of adverse drug reactions in hospitalized patients: A meta-analysis of prospective studies. *JAMA* **279**:1200, 1998
2. Leape LL et al: The nature of adverse events in hospitalized patients. Results of the Harvard Medical Practice Study II. *N Engl J Med* **324**:377, 1991
3. Wolkenstein P et al: A slow acetylator genotype is a risk factor for sulphonamide-induced toxic epidermal necrolysis and Stevens-Johnson syndrome. *Pharmacogenetics* **5**:255, 1995
4. Batchelor JR et al: Hydralazine-induced systemic lupus erythematosus: Influence of HLA-DR and sex on susceptibility. *Lancet* **1**:1107, 1980
5. Roujeau JC et al: HLA phenotypes and bullous cutaneous reactions to drugs. *Tissue Antigens* **28**:251, 1986
6. Uetrecht J: Is it possible to more accurately predict which drug candidates will cause idiosyncratic drug reactions? *Curr Drug Metab* **1**:133, 2000
7. Shear N, Spielberg S: Anticonvulsant hypersensitivity syndrome, in vitro assessment of risk. *J Clin Invest* **82**:1826, 1988
8. Shear N et al: Differences in metabolism of sulfonamides predisposing to idiosyncratic toxicity. *Ann Intern Med* **105**:179, 1986
9. Sullivan JR, Shear NH: What are some of the lessons learnt from in vitro studies of severe unpredictable drug reactions? *Br J Dermatol* **142**:205, 2000
10. Bastuji-Garin S et al: SCORTEN: A severity-of-illness score for toxic epidermal necrolysis. *J Invest Dermatol* **115**:149, 2000
11. Hashimoto K, Tohyama M: HHV-6–associated drug eruptions. *Allergologie* **24**:219, 2001
12. Bigby M et al: Drug-induced cutaneous reactions: A report from the Boston Collaborative Drug Surveillance Program on 15,438 consecutive inpatients, 1975 to 1982. *JAMA* **256**:3358, 1986
13. Pichler W, Yawalkar N: Allergic reactions to drugs: Involvement of T cells. *Thorax* **55**(suppl 2):S61, 2000
14. Kerns D et al: Ampicillin rash in children. *Am J Dis Child* **125**:187, 1973
15. Coopman S et al: Cutaneous disease and drug reactions in HIV infection. *N Engl J Med* **328**:1670, 1993
16. Gupta A et al: Drug-induced hypothyroidism: The thyroid as a target organ in hypersensitivity reactions to anticonvulsants and sulfonamides. *Clin Pharmacol Ther* **51**:56, 1992
17. Fisher M et al: Anaphylactoid reactions to narcotic analgesics. *Clin Rev Allergy* **9**:309, 1991
18. Pracy J et al: Angioedema secondary to angiotensin-converting enzyme inhibitors. *J Laryngol Otol* **108**:696, 1994
19. Warner K et al: Angiotensin II receptor blockers in patients with ACE inhibitor-induced angioedema. *Ann Pharmacother* **34**:526, 2000
20. Kearns G et al: Serum sickness-like reactions to cefaclor: role of hepatic metabolism and individual susceptibility. *J Pediatr* **125**:805, 1994
21. Remmer H, Falk W: Successful treatment of lithium-induced acne. *J Clin Psychiatry* **47**:48, 1986
22. Beylot C et al: Acute generalized exanthematous pustulosis. *Semin Cutan Med Surg* **15**:244, 1996
23. Sidoroff A et al: Acute generalized exanthematous pustulosis (AGEP): A clinical reaction pattern. *J Cutan Pathol* **28**:113, 2001
24. Lang B, Finlayson L: Naproxen-induced pseudoporphyria in patients with juvenile rheumatoid arthritis. *J Pediatr* **124**:639, 1994
25. Primka E et al: Amiodarone-induced linear IgA disease. *J Am Acad Dermatol* **31**:809, 1994
26. Ruocco V, Sacerdoti G: Pemphigus and bullous pemphigoid due to drugs. *Int J Dermatol* **30**:307, 1991
27. Roujeau J et al: Medication use and the risk of Stevens-Johnson syndrome or toxic epidermal necrolysis. *N Engl J Med* **333**:1600, 1995
28. Patterson R et al: Effectiveness of early therapy with corticosteroids in Stevens-Johnson syndrome: Experience with 41 cases and a hypothesis regarding pathogenesis. *Ann Allergy* **73**:27, 1994
29. Barone C et al: Treatment of toxic epidermal necrolysis and Stevens-Johnson syndrome in children. *J Oral Maxillofac Surg* **51**:264, 1993
30. Viard I et al: Inhibition of toxic epidermal necrolysis by blockade of CD95 with human intravenous immunoglobulin. *Science* **282**:490, 1998
31. Heng M, Allen S: Efficacy of cyclophosphamide in toxic epidermal necrolysis. *J Am Acad Dermatol* **25**:778, 1991
32. Sullivan J, Watson A: Lamotrigine-induced toxic epidermal necrolysis treated with intravenous cyclosporin: A discussion of pathogenesis and immunosuppressive management. *Australas J Dermatol* **37**:208, 1996
33. Ozkaya-Bayazit E, Akar U: Fixed drug eruption induced by trimethoprim-sulfamethoxazole: Evidence for a link to HLA-A30 B13 Cw6 haplotype. *J Am Acad Dermatol* **45**:712, 2001
34. Crowson A, Magro C: Recent advances in the pathology of cutaneous drug eruptions. *Dermatol Clin* **17**:537, 1999
35. Barbaud A et al: The use of skin testing in the investigation of cutaneous adverse drug reactions. *Br J Dermatol* **49**:139, 1998
36. Bauer K: Coumarin-induced skin necrosis. *Arch Dermatol* **129**:766, 1993
37. Freeman B et al: Factor V Leiden mutation in a patient with warfarin-associated skin necrosis. *Surgery* **127**:595, 2000

38. Schramm W et al: Treatment of coumarin-induced skin necrosis with a monoclonal antibody purified protein C concentrate. *Arch Dermatol* **19**:753, 1993
39. Halevy S, Shai A: Lichenoid drug eruptions. *J Am Acad Dermatol* **29**:249, 1993
40. Thompson D, Skaehill P: Drug-induced lichen planus. *Pharmacotherapy* **14**:561, 1994
41. Rijlaarsdam J, Willemze R: Cutaneous pseudolymphoma: Classification and differential diagnosis. *Semin Dermatol* **13**:187, 1994
42. Souteyrand P, d'Incan M: Drug-induced mycosis-fungoides-like lesions. *Curr Probl Dermatol* **19**:176, 1990
43. Rijlaarsdam J et al: Cutaneous pseudo-T-cell lymphomas. *Cancer* **69**:717, 1992
44. Sanchez N et al: Clinical and histopathologic spectrum of necrotizing vasculitis: Reports of findings in 101 cases. *Arch Dermatol* **121**:220, 1985
45. Dubost J et al: Drug-induced vasculitides. *Ballieres Clin Rheumatol* **5**:119, 1991
46. Roujeau JC, Stern R: Severe adverse cutaneous reactions to drugs. *N Engl J Med* **331**:1272, 1994
47. Colakovski H, DL: Propylthiouracil-induced perinuclear-staining antineutrophil cytoplasmic autoantibody-positive vasculitis in conjunction with pericarditis. *Endocr Pract* **7**:37, 2001

48. Price E, Venables P: Drug-induced lupus. *Drug Saf* **12**:283, 1995
49. Gough A et al: Minocycline-induced autoimmune hepatitis and systemic lupus erythematosus-like syndrome. *BMJ* **312**:169, 1996
50. Dunphy J et al: Antineutrophil cytoplasmic antibodies and HLA class II alleles in minocycline-induced lupus-like syndrome. *Br J Dermatol* **142**:461, 2000
51. Callen J: Drug-induced cutaneous lupus erythematosus, a distinct syndrome that is frequently unrecognized. *J Am Acad Dermatol* **45**:315, 2001
52. Sullivan JR, Shear NH: The drug hypersensitivity syndrome: What is the pathogenesis? *Arch Dermatol* **137**:357, 2001
53. Sogn D et al: Results of the National Institute of Allergy and Infectious Diseases Collaborative Clinical Trial to test the predictive value of skin testing with major and minor penicillin derivatives in hospitalized adults. *Arch Intern Med* **152**:1025, 1992
54. Romano A et al: Aminopenicillin allergy. *Arch Dis Child* **76**:513, 1997
55. Philips K et al: The importance of patch testing on previously affected skin in the diagnosis of type IV drug allergy. *Allergologie* **24**:224, 2001
56. Shear NH, Bhimji S: Pharmacogenetics and cutaneous drug reactions. *Semin Dermatol* **8**:219, 1989

CHAPTER 139

James E. Fitzpatrick

Mucocutaneous Complications of Antineoplastic Therapy

The last decade has seen an explosion of new treatment modalities for neoplastic diseases. Prolonged survival and even cures of many cancers can now be attributed to advances in chemotherapy, radiation therapy, surgery, and, more recently, drugs that augment the immune response or target specific receptors or antigenic targets on tumor cells. Some chemotherapeutic agents have also found a role in the treatment of immunologically mediated systemic and skin disease, making it even more important that dermatologists are cognizant of the side effects that may be encountered from these drugs.

More than 70 drugs now are classified as antineoplastic agents, and several excellent reviews have been published summarizing the clinical[1,2] and histopathologic[3,4] findings associated with them. Because there is an unavoidable delay from the time that new drugs are introduced until many of the cutaneous reactions are described in the literature, dermatologists are frequently faced with evaluating patients who are taking new chemotherapeutic agents for which all of the side effects are not yet known. This chapter is organized by clinical presentation rather than by a discussion of specific drugs and their side effects because the clinical presentation is more relevant for patient evaluation. Because related chemotherapeutic agents often have similar side effects, it is also useful to understand the mechanism of action of drugs and how they are related. Table 139-1 lists the drugs by class with a brief discussion of the mechanisms of action.

This chapter focuses on mucocutaneous reactions that are unique to (e.g., acral erythema), specific for (e.g., bleomycin-induced flagellate hyperpigmentation), or commonly associated with (e.g., asparaginase-induced urticaria) chemotherapeutic agents. It does not discuss drug reactions that can be associated with any drug class (e.g., erythema multiforme, spongiotic drug eruptions, fixed drug eruptions, pruritus).

PHARMACOLOGY

Alkylating Agents

Alkylating agents can be subdivided into mustard gas derivatives (e.g., chlorambucil, cyclophosphamide, mechlorethamine hydrochloride) and heavy metal alkylating agents (e.g., cisplatin). The nonplatinum alkylating drugs work by producing intrastrand and interstrand crosslinks of DNA strands, which, in turn, block the synthesis of DNA, RNA, and, ultimately, protein. The heavy metal alkylating agents primarily work by producing interstrand DNA crosslinks. The effect for all drugs in this class is cell-cycle phase-nonspecific. Some authorities prefer to place carboplatin and cisplatin in a separate category because they are heavy metal complex alkylating agents with a platinum atom surrounded by two ammonia molecules. Chlorambucil is the slowest-acting and least toxic of the drugs in this class.

Antibiotics

Most of the cytotoxic antibiotics work by intercalating with the DNA molecule and inhibiting DNA synthesis. This action blocks DNA-dependent RNA synthesis and, ultimately, protein synthesis. Mitomycin, although classified as an antibiotic, works like an alkylating

TABLE 139-1

Classification of Antineoplastic Agents

GENERIC	TRADE NAME(S)	GENERIC	TRADE NAME(S)
Alkylating Agents		Antiestrogens	
• Busulfan	Myleran	• Anastrozole	Arimidex
• Carboplatin	Paraplatin	• Estramustine	Emcyt
• Carmustine (BCNU)	BiCNU, Gliadel	• Letrozole	Femara
• Chlorambucil	Leukeran	• Tamoxifen	Nolvadex, Tamofen
• Cisplatin (cis-platinum)	Platinol	• Toremifene	Fareston
• Cyclophosphamide	Cytoxan	Estrogens	
• Dacarbazine (DTIC)	DTIC-Dome	• Estrogen	Estratab, Menest, Premarin
• Ifosfamide	Ifex	• Ethinyl estradiol	Estinyl
• Lomustine (CCNU)	CeeNU	Gonadotropin-releasing hormone analogues	
• Mechlorethamine (nitrogen mustard)	Mustargen	• Goserelin	Zoladex
• Melphalan	Akeran	• Leuprolide	Lupron
• Thiotepa	Thioplex	Progestins	
Antibiotic Agents		• Megestrol	Megace
• Bleomycin	Blenoxane	*Mitotic Inhibitors*	
• Dactinomycin (actinomycin D)	Cosmegen	Epipodophyllotoxins	
• Daunorubicin	Cerubidine, DaunoXome	• Etoposide	Etopophos, Topoxar, VePesid
• Doxorubicin hydrochloride	Adriamycin, Doxil, Rubex	• Teniposide	Vumon
• Idarubicin	Idamycin	Taxanes	
• Mitomycin	Mutamycin	• Docetaxel	Taxotere
• Mitoxantrone	Novantrone	• Paclitaxel	Taxol
• Plicamycin	Mithracin	Vinca alkaloids	
Antimetabolite Agents		• Vinblastine	Velban, Velbe
Folic acid analogues		• Vincristine	Oncovin, Vincasar
• Methotrexate	Folex, Mexate, Rheumatrex	• Vinorelbine	Navelbine
• Trimetrexate	Neutrexin	*Miscellaneous Agents*	
Nucleotide analogues, NOS		Anthracyclines	
• Fludarabine	Fludara	• Epirubicin	Ellence
• Gemcitabine	Gemzar	Fusion proteins	
Pyrimidine analogues		• Denileukin diftitox	Ontak
• Capecitabine	Xeloda	Hydrazine derivatives	
• Cytarabine (ara-C, cytosine arabinoside)	Cytosar-U	• Procarbazine	Matulane, Natulan
• Floxuridine	FUDR	Naphylureas	
• Fluorouracil (5-FU)	Adrucil, Efudex, Fluoroplex	• Suramin	
Purine analogues		Topoisomerase I inhibitors	
• Cladribine	Leustatin	• Irinotecan	Camptosar
• Mercaptopurine (6-MP)	Purinethol	• Topotecan	Hycamtin
• Thioguanine		Triazine derivatives	
Urea analogue		• Altretamine	Hexalen
• Hydroxyurea	Hydrea	*Immune Modulators*	
Antineoplastic Enzymes		• Levamisole	Ergamisol
• Asparaginase	Colaspase, Elspar	• Interferon-α2b	Intron
Hormonal Agonists/Antagonists		• Interferon-α2a	Roferon-A
Adrenocortical suppressant agents		• Interleukin-2 (aldesleukin)	Proleukin
• Aminoglutethimide	Cytadren	• Rituximab	Rituxan
• Mitotane	Lysodren	• Trastuzumab	Herceptin
Androgens		• Filgrastim (granulocyte colony-stimulating factor)	Neupogen
• Methyltestosterone	Android, Testrid	• Sargramostim (granulocyte-macrophase colony-stimulating factor)	Leukine
• Testolactone	Teslac		
• Testosterone	Numerous trade names		
Antiandrogens			
• Bicalutamide	Casodex		
• Flutamide	Eulexin		
• Nilutamide	Nilandron		

agent; it exerts its cytotoxic activity by forming cross-links between strands of DNA and inhibiting DNA, RNA, and protein synthesis. All of the antibiotics are cell-cycle phase-nonspecific. Bleomycin is inactivated by a hydrolase enzyme that is found in all tissues except lung and skin. This fact may account for the high incidence of bleomycin-related side effects in these tissues.

Antimetabolites

The antimetabolites constitute a diverse group of antineoplastic agents. The folic acid analogues (i.e., methotrexate, trimetrexate) block folic acid participation in nucleic acid synthesis by binding competitively and irreversibly to dihydrofolate reductase with a stronger affinity than folic acid. The pyrimidine analogues (capecitabine, floxuridine, and fluorouracil) compete for thymidine synthetase, the enzyme required for synthesis of thymidine and ultimately DNA. These drug are cell-cycle phase-specific and affect the S phase. Cytarabine is a pyrimidine analogue that is believed to interfere with DNA synthesis by blocking conversion of cytidine to deoxycytidine. It may also be incorporated into the RNA molecule. It is specific for the S phase during DNA synthesis, but under some conditions it may also prevent cells from going from G_1 to S phase. The purine analogues (mercaptopurine, thioguanine) compete with hypoxanthine and guanine for hypoxanthine guanine phosphoribosyltransferase and ultimately interfere with purine synthesis by multiple mechanisms. Hydroxyurea is a synthetic analogue of urea that blocks the incorporation of thymidine into DNA and may also damage DNA directly.

Enzymes

Asparaginase is a polypeptide enzyme that catalyzes the hydrolysis of asparagine to aspartic acid and ammonia, which depletes the extracellular asparagine necessary for synthesis of DNA. Because normal cells are able to synthesize asparagine and some malignant cells cannot, asparaginase is selectively cytotoxic for these malignant cells. The drug is cell-cycle phase-nonspecific and is primarily used in the treatment of acute leukemias.

Hormonal Agonists/Antagonists

A discussion of the mechanisms of the hormonal agonists and antagonists is beyond the scope of this chapter. In general, glucocorticoids are used for their lympholytic effects and ability to suppress lymphocyte mitotic activity. Thus, they are often included in many lymphocytic leukemia and lymphoma regimens. Another category of hormonal antagonist includes adrenocortical suppressant drugs (e.g., aminoglutethimide, mitotane) that are used primarily to treat adrenal carcinomas. Androgens (e.g., testolactone) and estrogens are used for their effect in breast carcinoma but have been largely supplanted by the antiestrogens (e.g., tamoxifen). Progestins are second-line hormonal drugs useful in the treatment of breast and endometrial carcinomas that have hormonal receptors on tumor cells. Gonadotropin-releasing analogues (i.e., goserelin, leuprolide) are used to treat prostatic carcinoma and breast cancer because they inhibit the secretion of luteinizing hormone (LH) and follicle stimulating hormone (FSH) and ultimately produce profound depression in the levels of testosterone and estrogen. Bicalutamide and flutamide are nonsteroidal antiandrogens that uniquely work by inhibiting the translocation of the androgen receptor from the nucleus to the cytoplasm in the prostate and hypothalamus. Because they inhibit the binding of androgen to its intracellular receptor, these drugs are useful to treat prostatic carcinoma.

Mitotic Inhibitors

The mitotic inhibitors include the vinca alkaloids, epipodophyllotoxins, and taxanes. The vinca alkaloids are cell-cycle phase-specific drugs that bind to tubulin and block the assembly into microtubules, thus arresting cells in metaphase. The taxanes bind directly to the microtubules that are needed for the interphase phase of cell mitosis. This action stabilizes the microtubule network and results in inhibition of cells that are mitotically active. The epipodophyllotoxins, although semisynthetic derivatives of podophyllotoxin, do not arrest cells in mitosis; instead, they work by complexing with topoisomerase II and producing single and double-stranded DNA breaks. These drugs remain attached to the free end of the DNA and also inhibit resealing of the break by topoisomerase II. Cells in S and G_2 phases are susceptible to these drugs.

Miscellaneous Cytotoxic Agents

Procarbazine is a hydrazine derivative that is cell-cycle phase-specific for cells in S phase. Its precise mechanism is unknown. It is metabolized to multiple cytotoxic metabolites that methylate DNA and ultimately suppress mitotically active cells in interphase and also produce chromatid breaks and translocations. Irinotecan and topotecan are inhibitors of topoisomerase I, an enzyme required for the relaxation of supercoiled double-stranded DNA. By binding to this enzyme, these agents allow uncoiling but prevent recoiling, thereby causing a break between the two strands. Altretamine is a synthetic cytotoxic thiazine derivative that structurally resembles some alkylating agents but does not appear to work as an alkylating agent. It binds to DNA, but it is not known whether this action is relevant; the precise mechanism of action is unknown.

MUCOCUTANEOUS COMPLICATIONS

Hair Follicle Complications

ALOPECIA Chemotherapy-induced alopecia is the most common mucocutaneous side effect associated with cancer treatment, and it is often the most distressing to the patient's self-image. Chemotherapy-induced alopecia is primarily an anagen effluvium due to toxic effects on the rapidly dividing hair matrix cells. This effect is dependent on the chemotherapeutic agent, dose, schedule, and route of administration. Even at the same dose, intravenous infusion produces more severe alopecia than oral administration. Although numerous drugs produce alopecia (Table 139-2), doxorubicin, cyclophosphamide, and vincristine have the highest potential to do so.[5] Chemotherapy-induced alopecia typically occurs 7 to 10 days after induction of therapy and continues to progress over 1 to 2 months. In severe cases, more than 90 percent of the hair is lost; the remaining hairs are spared because they were in telogen at the time of therapy, but with prolonged treatment, even these will be shed. Although loss of scalp (Fig. 139-1) and eyebrow hair is clinically most noticeable, patients also shed eyelashes and body hair. To a lesser degree, telogen effluvium also participates in chemotherapy-induced alopecia secondary to weight loss, fevers, and other medications, and secondary to the effects of the cancer itself. The alopecia typically resolves after therapy is stopped, although hair may regrow with a different color or texture. Permanent alopecia was documented in 6 of 22 patients who received busulfan and cyclophosphamide.[6] Different methods have been used to prevent chemotherapy-induced alopecia, and a scalp cooling system has proved the most effective. The diagnosis is usually easily made clinically, but in those rare cases in which biopsies are performed for diagnosis, the hair follicles demonstrate a cell-poor alopecia with numerous necrotic follicular keratinocytes.[3]

FOLLICULITIS (ACNEIFORM ERUPTION) Folliculitis is most commonly associated with dactinomycin (actinomycin D)[7] and less commonly with methotrexate and cisplatin. Patients initially develop erythema of the face, followed over a 2- to 3-day period by the appearance of papules and pustules on the face and upper trunk. As the follicular erythema and pustules resolve over 10 days, comedones may persist. Biopsies of fully developed lesions are not specific and demonstrate an acute folliculitis with replacement of the pilosebaceous unit by neutrophils. Acne vulgaris may also be aggravated by androgens used as chemotherapeutic agents.

TABLE 139-2

Adverse Mucocutaneous Reactions to Antineoplastic Agents

Complication	Agent(s)
Follicular Reactions	
Alopecia	Altretamine, bleomycin, busulfan, carboplatin, carmustine, chlorambucil, cyclophosphamide, cytarabine, dacarbazine, dactinomycin, daunorubicin, docetaxel, doxorubicin, epirubicin, etoposide, fluorouracil, gemcitabine, GM-CSF, hydroxyurea, idarubicin, ifosfamide, interferon-α, irinotecan, levamisole, mechlorethamine, megestrol, melphalan, methotrexate, mitomycin, mitoxanthrone, paclitaxel, procarbazine, tamoxifen, teniposide, thiotepa, topotecan, vinblastine, vincristine, vinorelbine
Eyelash growth	Interferon-α
Flag hair	Methotrexate
Folliculitis	Cisplatin, dactinomycin, methotrexate
Nail Reactions	
Beau's lines	Bleomycin, cisplatin, cyclophosphamide, dactinomycin, docetaxel, doxorubicin, etoposide, melphalan, vincristine
Onycholysis/ onychomadesis	Bleomycin, capecitabine, cyclophosphamide, docetaxel, doxorubicin, etoposide, fluorouracil, hydroxyurea, methotrexate, trastuzumab
Mee's lines	Daunorubicin
Photo-onycholysis	Docetaxel, mercaptopurine
Hyperpigmentation	Bleomycin, busulfan, cisplatin, cyclophosphamide, dacarbazine, daunorubicin, docetaxel, doxorubicin, docetaxel, etoposide, fluorouracil, hydroxyurea, idarubicin, ifosfamide, melphalan, methotrexate, mitomycin, mitoxantrone, paclitaxel
Hypopigmentation (leukonychia)	Cisplatin, cytarabine, daunorubicin, melphalan, vincristine
Sweat gland effects	
Eccrine syringosquamous metaplasia	Bleomycin, cisplatin, cyclophosphamide cytarabine, daunorubicin, doxorubicin, etoposide, fluorouracil, mitoxantrone, suramin
Increased sweating	Nilutamide, toremifene
Neutrophilic hidradenitis	Bleomycin, chlorambucil, cytarabine, daunorubicin, doxorubicin, G-CSF, mitoxantrone, vincristine
Epidermal effects	
Acral erythema	Cisplatin, cyclophosphamide, cytarabine, daunorubicin, docetaxel, doxorubicin, etoposide, fluorouracil, floxuridine, hydroxyurea, idarubicin, lomustine, melphalan, mercaptopurine, methotrexate, mitomycin, paclitaxel, suramin, vinblastine, vincristine
Exfoliative dermatitis	Chlorambucil/busulfan, cisplatin, irinotecan, methotrexate
Fixed drug eruptions	Dacarbazine, procarbazine
Hyperpigmentation	
Acral	Cyclophosphamide, fluorouracil, ifosfamide
Diffuse (Addison-like)	Busulfan, dactinomycin, doxorubicin, hydroxyurea, procarbazine
Flagellate	Bleomycin
Occluded areas	Etoposide, ifosfamide, thiotepa
Patchy	Bleomycin, paclitaxel, plicamycin, vinblastine, vincristine, vinorelbine
Pressure areas	Cisplatin
Polycyclic	Daunorubicin
Serpentine	Fluorouracil, vinorelbine
Sun-exposed	Daunorubicin, fluorouracil, methotrexate
NOS	Mercaptopurine
Inflammation of keratoses	
Actinic keratoses	Cisplatin, dacarbazine, doxorubicin, fluorouracil
Seborrheic keratoses	Cytarabine
Phototoxic reactions	Dacarbazine, dactinomycin, doxorubicin, fluorouracil, hydroxyurea, methotrexate, mitomycin, procarbazine, thioguanine, vinblastine
Photoallergic reactions	Fluorouracil, flutamide
Pseudodermatomyositis	Hydroxyurea
Radiation enhancement	Bleomycin, chlorambucil, cisplatin, dactinomycin, doxorubicin, fluorouracil, hydroxyurea, mercaptopurine, methotrexate
Recall reactions	
Heat recall	Bleomycin
Radiation recall	Bleomycin, cyclophosphamide, cytarabine, dactinomycin, daunorubicin, doxorubicin, docetaxel, etoposide, fluorouracil, gemcitabine, hydroxyurea, idarubicin, lomustine, melphalan, methotrexate, mitomycin, paclitaxel, tamoxifen, trimetrexate, vinblastine
Sunburn recall	Methotrexate, suramin
Toxic erythema	Busulfan, cytarabine, etoposide, methotrexate
Vesiculobullous reactions	
Dermatitic (spongiotic)	Interleukin-1, mitomycin
Pemphigus	Rituximab
TEN	Rituximab

(*continued*)

TABLE 139-2 (*Continued*)

COMPLICATION	AGENT(S)
Dermal effects	
Immediate hypersensitivity reactions	
Angioedema	Asparaginase, bleomycin, interferon-α2b, methotrexate
Urticaria	Asparaginase, carboplatin, cisplatin, interferon-α2b, interferon-α2a, levamisole, mitoxanthrone, rituximab, thiotepa
Local injury	
Chemical cellulitis/necrotic reactions	Bleomycin, carboplatin, carmustine, cisplatin, dacarbazine, dactinomycin, daunorubicin, doxorubicin, epirubicin, etoposide, fluorouracil, idarubicin, melphalan, mechlorethamine, mitomycin, mitoxantrone, paclitaxel, plicamycin, vinblastine, vincristine, vinorelbine
Phlebitis	Cyclophosphamide, dacarbazine, dactinomycin, daunorubicin, docetaxel, doxorubicin, epirubicin, etoposide, fluorouracil, idarubicin, ifosfamide, mechlorethamine, mitomycin, mitoxantrone, paclitaxel, plicamycin, thiotepa, vinblastine, vincristine, vinorelbine
Morbilliform eruptions	Aminoglutethimide, azathioprine, fluorouracil, GM-CSF, gemcitabine, suramin
Pruritus	Altretamine, aminoglutethimide, bleomycin, carboplatin, cladribine, cisplatin, dacarbazine, estramustine, gemcitabine, GM-CSF, interferon-α, interleukin-2, levamisole, megestrol, paclitaxel
Raynaud's phenomenon	Bleomycin (increased risk if combined with vinblastine), cisplatin + gemcitabine
Sclerotic reactions	Bleomycin, docetaxel
Sweet's syndrome	G-CSF
Mucosal Reactions	
Conjunctivitis	Carmustine, cisplatin, cytarabine
Hyperpigmentation	Busulfan, cisplatin, cyclophosphamide, doxorubicin, fluorouracil, hydroxyurea, floxuridine
Stomatitis	Bleomycin, capecitabine, carboplatin, cyclophosphamide, cytarabine, dactinomycin, daunorubicin, docetaxel, doxorubicin, epirubicin, floxuridine, fludarabine, fluorouracil, hydroxyurea, idarubicin, interleukin-2, mercaptopurine, mechlorethamine, methotrexate, mitomycin, paclitaxel, plicamycin, procarbazine, teniposide, thioguanine, topotecan, vinblastine, vincristine, vinorelbine

G-CSF, granulocyte colony-stimulating factor; GM-CSF, granulocyte-macrophage colony-stimulating factor.

Nail Complications

BEAU'S LINES/ONYCHOLYSIS/ONYCHOMADESIS Nail toxicity is frequently associated with chemotherapeutic agents. Some antineoplastic agents (e.g., paclitaxel) produce nail changes in up to 40 percent of patients. Anthracyclines (e.g., daunorubicin, doxorubicin, idarubicin) and taxanes (e.g., paclitaxel, docetaxel) are the groups of drugs that most commonly produce severe nail toxicity. Mild toxic reactions produce Beau's lines, while severe toxic reactions produce onycholysis and even onychomadesis (Fig. 139-2). The first toe is the most common digit affected and may be the only digit affected in milder cases. In severe cases, all of the nails of the hands and feet may be involved. Less common findings include severe nail pain, nail thickening, nail thinning, splinter hemorrhages, and subungual hemorrhage. Nail toxicity is dose dependent and is more common with high dosage

FIGURE 139-1

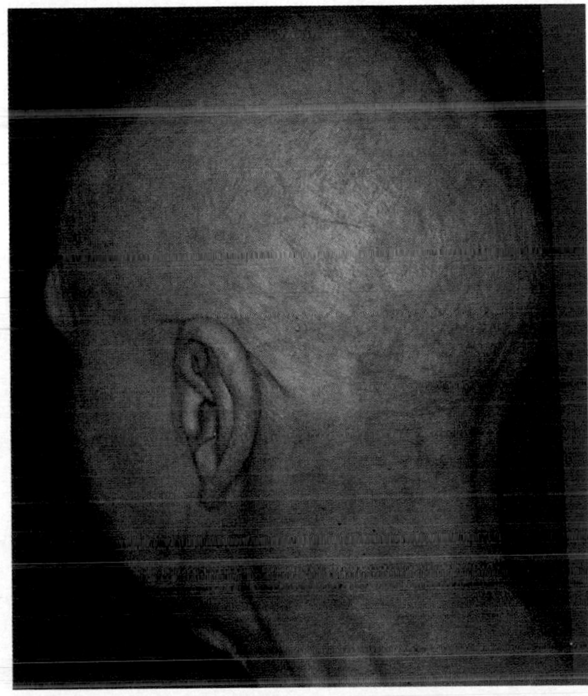

Alopecia after the administration of combined chemotherapy (cyclophosphamide, doxorubicin, vincristine).

FIGURE 139-2

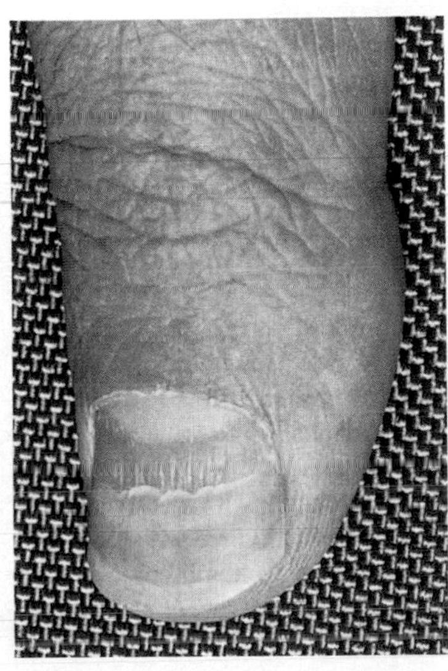

Presence of a proximal indented Beau's line and distal band of leukonychia due to cyclophosphamide 3 months after bone marrow transplantation.

regimens and prolonged therapy. These reactions are not life-threatening and rarely warrant changes in chemotherapy. The mechanism is probably due to direct toxicity to the nail plate, although inhibition of nail bed angiogenesis has been proposed. Clinical evidence suggests that for the taxanes sunlight exposure may either aggravate or actually be necessary for the development of onycholysis.[8]

NAIL PIGMENT ABNORMALITIES Drugs from many different classes produce either hypopigmentation (leukonychia or transverse white banding) or hyperpigmentation of the nail. The mechanisms for the development of the various patterns of leukonychia are unknown but are presumed to be cytotoxic in nature (Fig. 139-2). Hyperpigmentation may appear as longitudinal hyperpigmentation, horizontal hyperpigmentation, pigmentation confined to the lunula, and diffuse hyperpigmentation. Chemotherapy-induced nail hyperpigmentation appears to be more common in black patients, presumably due to the increased numbers of melanocytes in the nail matrix.[9] Nail hyperpigmentation most commonly develops 10 days to 6 months after chemotherapy except for treatment with hydroxyurea when it develops after chronic therapy (1 to 3 years).[10] Chemotherapy-induced nail hyperpigmentation has not been critically studied by biopsies; but in those rare cases where it has been examined, there has been increased melanin in the ventral nail plate. The mechanism is not understood, but it has been hypothesized to be due to increased activity of the melanocytes. In the cases of daunorubicin and doxorubicin, it has been hypothesized that the increased melanocytic activity may be due to increased melanocyte-stimulating hormone (MSH) or corticotropin release, or secondary to a conjugate of the chemotherapeutic agent and MSH.[9]

Sweat Gland Complications

NEUTROPHILIC HIDRADENITIS Neutrophilic hidradenitis may occur in patients undergoing therapy with several different antineoplastic agents, most commonly cytarabine. Less commonly implicated antineoplastic agents include bleomycin and granulocyte colony-stimulating factor.[11,12] This reaction is manifested as tender, erythematous macules, papules, and plaques of the trunk, neck, and extremities that develop days to months after induction. The lesions resolve spontaneously over a period of several days. Histologic changes are distinctive and include a neutrophilic infiltrate involving and surrounding the sweat gland coils. The eccrine coils are most commonly affected, but apocrine involvement may also occur.[13] The mechanism is most likely secondary to high concentrations of the cytotoxic drug being secreted in the sweat gland coils. This hypothesis is supported by the demonstration that bleomycin injected into normal human skin produces changes that resemble those seen with systemic administration of the drug. Because similar histologic findings have been reported in patients receiving drugs that are not chemotherapeutic agents (e.g., acetaminophen) and in other diseases (e.g., idiopathic palmoplantar eccrine hidradenitis of childhood), other pathogenic mechanisms can also produce this histologic pattern.

SYRINGOSQUAMOUS METAPLASIA (ECCRINE SQUAMOUS METAPLASIA) Chemotherapy-induced syringosquamous metaplasia is a clinicopathologic reaction that is closely related to neutrophilic hidradenitis. It has occurred with multiple different chemotherapeutic regimens.[14,15] Like neutrophilic hidradenitis, it is thought to be secondary to direct toxic injury of sweat ducts by the antineoplastic agents. Clinically, these reactions have most commonly presented as erythematous papular eruptions that resemble miliaria. The papules resolve over a period of weeks after therapy is discontinued. The histologic findings are distinct and consist of marked squamous metaplasia of the upper sweat duct associated with necrotic ductal epithelial cells. There is usually a minimal host response, although scattered neutrophils and lymphocytes are often present.[4]

Epidermal Complications

CHEMOTHERAPY-INDUCED TOXIC ERYTHEMA Chemotherapy-induced toxic erythema is one of the most common adverse reactions to high-dose or multiple-drug regimens. In multiple-drug regimens, a single drug cannot usually be implicated because these regimens almost always include two or more drugs that are cytotoxic to the skin. Single drugs that commonly produce this reaction when administered in high-dose regimens are busulfan,[16] cytarabine, etoposide,[17] and methotrexate. The reaction typically begins with a prodrome of pain or tingling of the skin. Increasingly tender erythema and edema of the skin resembling toxic epidermal necrolysis rapidly follow the initial symptoms. The distribution varies with the drug regimen and may range from generalized to accentuated in acral areas, areas of pressure, intertriginous folds, or under tape. In some cases, the reaction may be localized to areas where the drug is infused in higher concentrations. Examples include intraarterial infusions of limbs, where the toxic reaction is confined to that limb, or intrathecal infusions, where the reaction is confined to the skin overlying the spine. In milder reactions, this is followed by desquamation, while in severe reactions, it is followed by bullae. Long-term hydroxyurea therapy produces a unique form of toxic erythema that clinically resembles dermatomyositis (drug-induced pseudodermatomyositis). In the largest study, 7 of 21 patients developed dermatomyositis-like changes on the hands, often in association with leg ulcers.[18]

Biopsies of early chemotherapy-induced lesions of toxic erythema demonstrate a cell-poor, interface tissue reaction manifesting as vacuolar alteration and necrotic keratinocytes.[3,4] Older lesions may demonstrate varying degrees of epidermal dysmaturation with larger-than-normal keratinocytes and edematous-abundant eosinophilic cytoplasm. If the patients continue to receive chemotherapy, the epidermis may eventually become attenuated because it cannot be replenished with new cells. Etoposide and busulfan produce distinct histologic findings. Etoposide produces "starburst cells," which are enlarged, pale-staining keratinocytes in mitotic arrest manifesting absence of the nuclear membrane associated with fragments of chromosomes haphazardly arranged in the cytoplasm.[17] Busulfan produces "busulfan cells," which are abnormal keratinocytes with strikingly large nuclei (up to 22 μm in diameter) that have irregular contours and prominent nucleoli. Similar cells are seen in other epithelial-lined surfaces such as lung, gastrointestinal tract, and bladder.[16]

CHEMOTHERAPY-INDUCED ACRAL ERYTHEMA Since its description in 1982,[19] there have been numerous case reports and series documenting that many chemotherapeutic agents can produce a distinctive toxic reaction manifesting a painful acral erythema. The exact mechanism is unknown, but the concentration of drug in eccrine structures of the palms and soles has been postulated to play a role. This hypothesis is supported by the presence of syringosquamous metaplasia in conjunction with acral erythema.[20] Although numerous drugs have been implicated (see Table 139-2), this reaction is most common with high-dose cytarabine, with a reported incidence of 20 percent,[21] and doxorubicin, with an incidence of 29 percent. The reaction typically develops 4 to 23 days after chemotherapy is begun and manifests as painful, sharply demarcated erythema of the palmar and plantar surfaces (Fig. 139-3). In severe cases, the toxic reaction may progress to large bullae, may extend over the dorsum of the hands and feet, or may involve other cutaneous sites. The pain is sometimes so intense that patients cannot walk and they keep their hands immobile in a partially flexed position. Histologic changes can be difficult to distinguish from graft-versus-host reactions and demonstrate an interface tissue reaction with

FIGURE 139-3

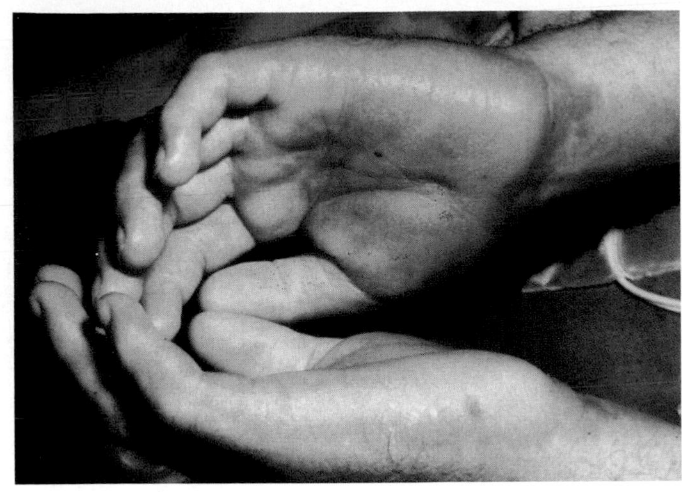

Cytarabine-induced painful acral erythema with marked edema.

vacuolar alteration of the basal cell layer, necrotic keratinocytes, variable dysmaturation, and a minimal superficial perivascular lymphocytic infiltrate. The lesions resolve spontaneously with desquamation over a period of 2 to 3 weeks. Therapy is limited to analgesics and emollients.

INFLAMMATION OF KERATOSES A number of different chemotherapeutic agents and chemotherapeutic combination protocols produce inflammation of actinic keratoses and seborrheic keratoses. Fluorouracil is the most common cause of toxic reactions in actinic keratoses, and this selective reaction is the basis for the use of this drug in the topical treatment of actinic keratoses.[22] The reaction usually develops within 1 week of initiating chemotherapy. The actinic keratoses may resolve or remain after therapy is discontinued. A similar reaction in seborrheic keratoses has been reported to occur with cytarabine.

HYPERPIGMENTATION Bleomycin commonly produces a unique form of flagellate (linear) hyperpigmentation with an incidence that has varied from 8 to 66 percent depending on the treatment protocol.[23] Typically this reaction starts within days after bleomycin therapy is initiated and manifests as severely pruritic, erythematous linear lesions that are slowly replaced by brown linear lesions (Fig. 139-4). The eruption resolves without treatment over a period of weeks to months. In one patient who developed flagellate hyperpigmentation, the subsequent use of a heating pad reproduced these areas of hyperpigmentation confined to the area of treatment.[24] The pathogenesis is unknown. Some authors have noted the development of these streaks in areas of excoriation. One group of investigators induced lesions in a patient by rubbing the skin during bleomycin administration. Other investigators have not been able to reproduce these lesions with trauma. The incidence of skin reactions secondary to bleomycin may be due to the absence of hydrolase, the enzyme that inactivates bleomycin, in the skin. The clinical findings of bleomycin-induced flagellate hyperpigmentation are so characteristic that biopsies are usually not required. Biopsies of early lesions demonstrate vacuolar alteration and necrotic keratinocytes with minimal inflammation, whereas biopsies of later lesions demonstrate hyperpigmentation of the basilar keratinocytes and melanin incontinence.[4] Bleomycin may also produce patchy pigmentation in areas of pressure, palmar creases, and striae distensae.[1]

Several chemotherapeutic agents, including fluorouracil[25] and vinorelbine,[26] also produce a unique form of hyperpigmentation manifesting as serpentine supravenous areas of hyperpigmentation. This reaction may follow the intravenous administration of fluorouracil and also occurs with several multiple-drug chemotherapeutic regimens. The reaction resolves spontaneously with time. Daunorubicin also produces a unique form of pigmentation manifesting as polycyclic bands of pigmentation of the scalp.[9]

Numerous antineoplastic drugs produce other patterns of hyperpigmentation including patchy, acral, photoaccentuated, polycyclic, occlusion (e.g., tape) accentuated (Fig. 139-5), pressure accentuated, or generalized hyperpigmentation that may resemble Addison's disease (see Table 139-2). The causes of these patterns of chemotherapy-induced hyperpigmentation are unknown. Postulated mechanisms include a direct toxic effect on melanocytes, increased drug deposition due to increased blood flow, increased toxicity secondary to secretion in the sweat, endocrinologic abnormalities (e.g., increased MSH), and drug-induced depletion of tyrosinase inhibitors.[1]

PHOTOSENSITIVITY Most cases of chemotherapy-induced photosensitivity are phototoxic in terms of pathogenesis, although photoallergic reactions may also occur (see Table 139-2). Phototoxic reactions mimic sunburns and present as burning and erythema; vesiculobullous

FIGURE 139-4

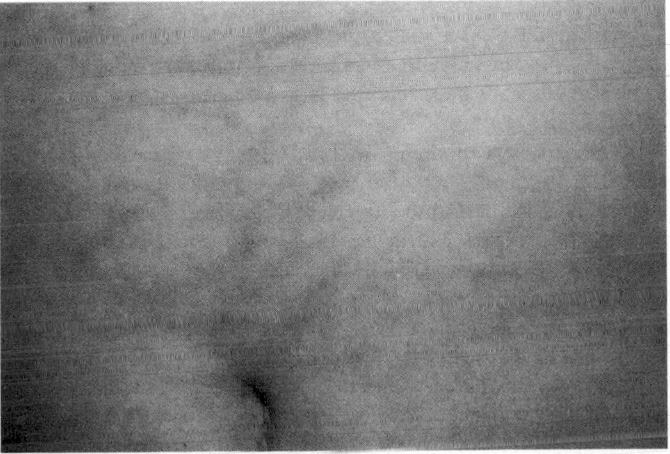

Flagellate hyperpigmentation 2 weeks after administration of bleomycin.

FIGURE 139-5

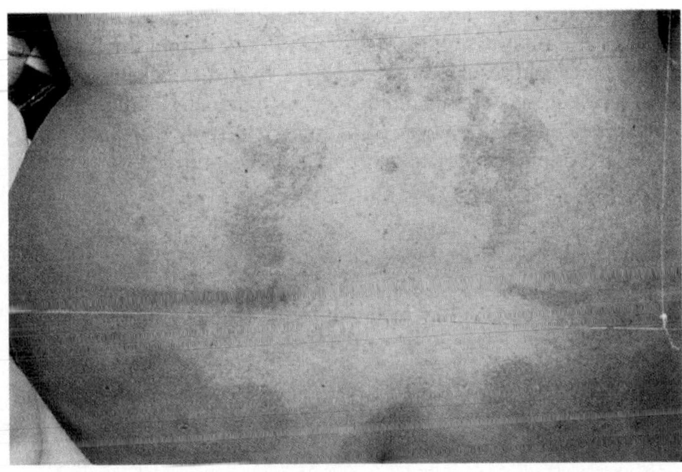

Hyperpigmentation at sites occluded during infusion of thiotepa.

FIGURE 139-6

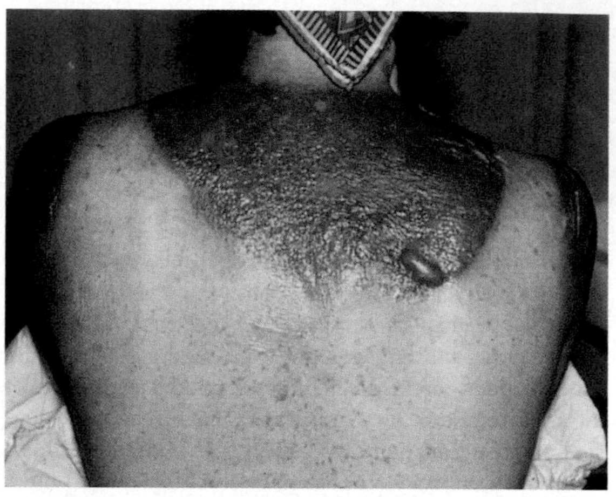

Reactivation of solar erythema 2 days after high-dose methotrexate administration to a young woman with choriocarcinoma. (*From Bronner and Hood: Cutaneous complications of chemotherapeutic agents. J Am Acad Dermatol 9:645,1983 with permission.*)

lesions appear in severe cases. As the erythema fades, varying degrees of desquamation develop. Biopsies demonstrate a cell-poor interface tissue reaction with necrotic keratinocytes.[27] Photoallergic reactions present as dermatitis reactions that often have a papulovesicular appearance. In contrast to phototoxic reactions, photoallergic reactions may not occur when the drug is started but may develop weeks or months later. Biopsies of photoallergic reactions demonstrate a spongiotic dermatitis that is primarily mediated by lymphocytes.[4]

SUNBURN RECALL REACTIONS Methotrexate produces a unique reactivation of sunburn when it is given 1 to 3 days after sun exposure; at least one case occurred as late as 8 days.[28] These reactions present as erythema confined to the area of previous sunburn with severe cases developing superficial blisters as in second-degree sunburns (Fig. 139-6). This reaction is not prevented by leucovorin rescue. The pathogenesis is not understood, but it has been postulated to be due to the fact that ultraviolet-damaged keratinocytes undergoing enhanced DNA, RNA, protein synthesis are further damaged by the methotrexate.

RADIATION ENHANCEMENT DERMATITIS Radiation enhancement is defined as a synergistic reaction between an antineoplastic drug and radiation. Radiation enhancement is often a desired effect on the tumor but is not desirable when it affects the skin. Radiation-enhanced skin reactions are most commonly associated with orthovoltage or megavoltage radiation, but they also can occur with electron beam therapy.[29] The mechanism for most drugs has not been established, but, for the vinca alkaloids, in vitro studies suggest that treated cells accumulate in G_2/M-phase of the cell cycle and that cells in this state are more susceptible to radiation-induced apoptosis. In most cases, the drug and radiation are administered within 1 week of each other, but in occasional cases, the window for enhancement appears to be longer. Although a number of chemotherapeutic agents produce this reaction, doxorubicin and dactinomycin are most commonly implicated. The reaction presents initially as pain and erythema followed by desquamation and hyperpigmentation. Radiation-induced alopecia also appears to be enhanced by these drugs within the treatment port.

FIGURE 139-7

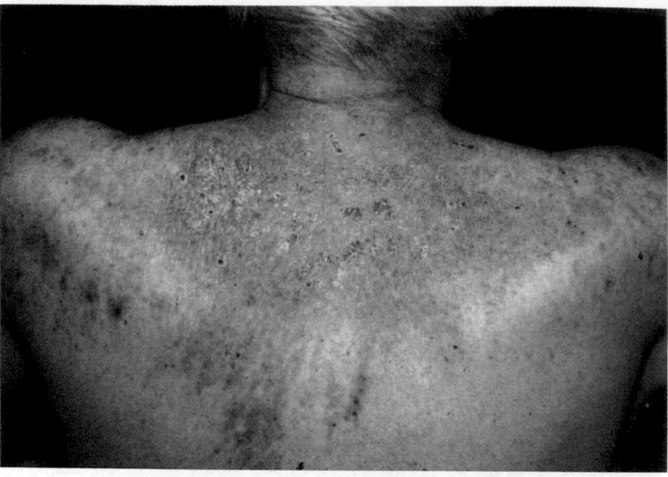

Radiation recall reaction appearing 2 weeks after the administration of methotrexate.

RADIATION RECALL DERMATITIS Radiation recall reactions are defined as cutaneous cytotoxicity that develops in a previously quiescent radiation field with the administration of an antineoplastic agent.[30] The mechanism for this reaction is unknown, but it has been hypothesized that the radiation depletes the cutaneous stem cells from the treatment field and that surviving cells are more susceptible to cytotoxic drugs. Another hypothesis is that the surviving stem cells within the radiation field are damaged by the initial treatment and thus more sensitive to the cytotoxic drugs. Radiation recall reactions may occur from days to as long as 15 years after radiation therapy. Recall usually occurs with induction chemotherapy and is sometimes absent or often milder with rechallenge.[31] Clinically, it resembles acute radiodermatitis with burning and erythema confined to the radiation field followed by desquamation and blisters in severe cases (Fig. 139-7). Treatment consists of discontinuing the offending drug and supportive local care. Although there are anecdotal reports of improvement with topical or systemic glucocorticoids, the value of this treatment is questionable given the pathogenesis and absence of prospective studies.

Dermal Complications

LOCAL INJURY The delivery of chemotherapeutic agents by intravenous or occasionally intraarterial routes (i.e., limb perfusion) is associated with a risk of extravasation estimated to be 0.1 to 6 percent in adults and even higher in children.[1] Those agents having minimal toxicity produce only chemical cellulitis or phlebitis and are classified as being irritants. Those agents having severe toxicity produce tissue necrosis and are classified as vesicants. The degree of injury is related to the drug, rate of delivery, concentration, and amount extravasated. Chemical cellulitis manifests as erythema, induration, and pain at the injection site; sometimes it may follow the course of the vein. Chemical cellulitis is usually of relatively short duration and resolves without treatment. Chemotherapy-related phlebitis manifests as linear cords and may be associated with discomfort.

Chemotherapy-induced tissue necrosis secondary to extravasation can be a devastating complication. Histologic studies of doxorubicin-associated extravasation suggest that the earliest findings are degenerative changes of blood vessels associated with extravasation of red blood cells.[32] This is followed by necrosis of the epidermis and collagen. The absence of significant numbers of inflammatory cells argues against the use of topical or intralesional glucocorticoids. Although a number of

FIGURE 139-8

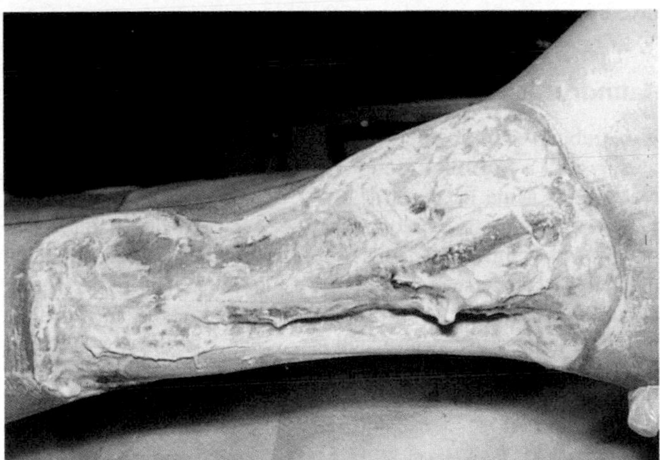

Severe tissue necrosis after extravasation of doxorubicin.

drugs have been implicated, doxorubicin is considered to be the most potent drug causing tissue necrosis.[33] Doxorubicin may produce ulcers that progress from 1 to 3 months and may eventually reach the level of tendons and bone (Fig. 139-8). Extravasation should be treated by immediate discontinuation of perfusion and the application of either hot or cold packs. Cold packs are used for all chemotherapeutic agents except vinca alkaloids to localize the drug and promote localized degradation. Vinca alkaloids are treated with hot packs because the application of cold promotes tissue necrosis.[1] Other treatments advocated but not proven include the application of potent topical glucocorticoids under occlusion, topical dimethylsulfoxide (DMSO), DMSO and α-tocopherol in conjunction, and locally injected hyaluronidase for vinca alkaloid and etoposide injections.[1] Severe ulcerations may require wide excision of the ulcer with grafting.

IMMEDIATE HYPERSENSITIVITY REACTIONS Dermatologists are rarely called on to treat immediate hypersensitivity reactions to chemotherapeutic agents, but these reactions are caused by a number of antineoplastic agents (e.g., cisplatin).[34] The most common causative agent is asparaginase, which produces urticaria, angioedema, or anaphylaxis in up to 65 percent of patients.[1] Because immediate hypersensitivity reactions to this agent are so common, it is recommended that intradermal testing be done before the initial dose is administered and repeated if the drug is used after an interval of 1 week or more.

SCLEROTIC DERMAL REACTIONS Bleomycin[35] and docetaxel[36] produce sclerotic tissue reactions that may be localized, regional, or diffuse. Localized tissue reactions may mimic morphea or progressive systemic sclerosis. Melphalan has been reported to produce a unique form of reticulate scleroderma after limb perfusion.[37] In some cases, these reactions have resolved after withdrawal of the offending drug.[35,36] The mechanism has not been established, but in vitro bleomycin upregulates α_1(I) collagen, fibronectin, and decorin gene expression in both normal and scleroderma skin fibroblasts.[38] Biopsies demonstrate dermal sclerosis that is indistinguishable from morphea or progressive systemic sclerosis.

RAYNAUD'S PHENOMENON Raynaud's phenomenon, with or without digital ulcerations, is most often associated with bleomycin,[39] cisplatin,[40] or cisplatin in combination with gemcitabine. This reaction may occur either with systemic chemotherapy or after intralesional injection to treat verruca vulgaris.[41] The mechanism is unknown; but bleomycin is known to be toxic to endothelial cells, and in addition

FIGURE 139-9

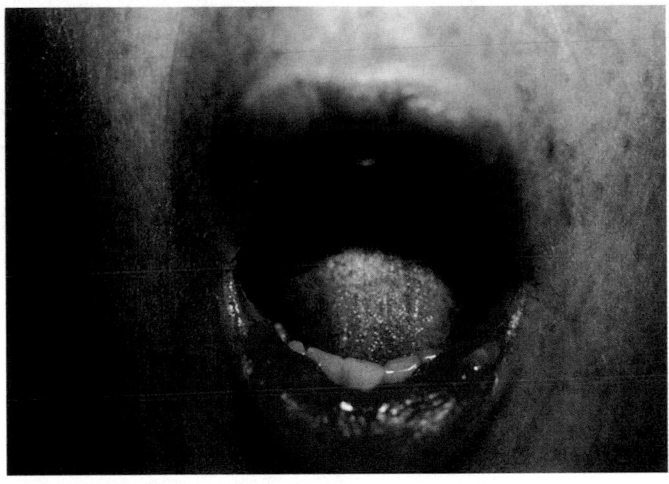

Stomatitis induced by cytarabine, doxorubicin, and methotrexate. *(Courtesy of Allan C. Harrington, MD.)*

to Raynaud's phenomenon, it has produced acral leukocytoclastic vasculitis with acral ulcerations and digital gangrene. In a study of 90 patients receiving bleomycin for testicular cancer, 37 percent developed Raynaud's phenomenon, with 7 percent having transient disease.[39] Risk factors for the development of Raynaud's phenomenon include combination therapy with vinblastine and high cumulative doses of bleomycin.

Mucosal Complications

STOMATITIS Mucosal epithelium, because of its high mitotic activity, is extremely susceptible to several classes of chemotherapeutic agents including those that affect the synthesis of DNA or RNA and those that act as mitotic inhibitors. Oral complications occur in approximately 40 percent of patients receiving chemotherapy. Young patients, because of their higher mitotic index, and patients with preexisting oral disease are more susceptible to severe reactions.[1] Patients typically note burning and increased mucosal erythema within days after administration of the chemotherapy followed by erosions and ulcerations that are characteristically intensely painful (Fig. 139-9). The oral mucosa is most commonly affected, especially the buccal mucosa and tongue, but any mucosal surface, including ocular mucosa, may be involved. Eating and drinking may aggravate the pain; this problem sometimes necessitates altering the dosage regimen.[42] The mucositis is often accompanied by secondary bacterial and fungal infections. Meticulous, but not overly aggressive, oral hygiene may reduce the incidence of secondary infection, but antibiotics and antifungal agents are often needed to augment healing and reduce the incidence of septicemia. Oral hemorrhage secondary to chemotherapy-induced thrombocytopenia is also often present.

MUCOSAL HYPERPIGMENTATION The mucosa may develop various patterns of hyperpigmentation including linear, patchy, and macular. Specific agents may affect certain anatomic areas such as the gingival margin (e.g., cyclophosphamide) or tongue (e.g., fluorouracil). The mechanism is not understood. The hyperpigmentation slowly resolves over a period of weeks to months except for the oral hyperpigmentation produced by cyclophosphamide, which may be permanent.

Reactions to Immune Modifiers

The immune modifiers are discussed separately because they work by modifying or intensifying the host immune response to the tumor. Their side effects are totally different from those of the classic chemotherapeutic agents.

INTERLEUKINS Interleukin-2 (IL-2) is a cytokine produced by antigen-activated T cells. It stimulates T cell proliferation, potentiates the apoptotic cell death of antigen-activated T cells, and stimulates the proliferation and effector functions of natural killer cells and B cells. It is used primarily for the treatment of malignant melanoma, but the mechanism of action in the treatment of tumors is unknown. Clinically, it is associated with a dose-related *capillary leak syndrome,* manifesting as peripheral and central edema.[43] It has also been reported to produce a persistent macular erythema with associated pruritus and burning, usually localized to the head and neck region. The eruptions desquamate and resolve after IL-2 administration is discontinued. Skin biopsies demonstrate papillary edema associated with a superficial mononuclear infiltrate. Other mucocutaneous complications of IL-2 administration include stomatitis, telogen effluvium, punctate superficial cutaneous ulcers, erosions in surgical scars, erythema nodosum, and exacerbation of psoriasis.

Denileukin diftitox is a fusion protein consisting of diphtheria toxin and IL-2. Because some leukemias and lymphomas express the high affinity form of the IL-2 receptor, the fusion protein attaches to the receptor and produces cell death within hours. Cutaneous reactions include hypersensitivity reactions, dermatitis at the site of injection, generalized dermatitis, pruritus, and increased sweating. Premedication with steroids decreases the incidence and severity of skin reactions without compromising the clinical response.[44]

INTERFERONS Interferon-α2a and interferon-α2b are cytokines that have a variety of actions including inhibition of viral replication, increasing the lytic potential of natural killer cells, and stimulation of the development of T_H1 cells. Although flulike symptoms such as fever, chills, fatigue, and myalgias are the most frequent complications, cutaneous reactions are also common and include alopecia, pruritus, nonspecific dermatitis, and transient dermatitis.[45] Local reactions, such as erythema at the site of injection or inflammation of the nasal mucosa, have also been noted. Other cutaneous reactions include radiation enhancement, exacerbation of psoriasis, reactivation of oral herpes simplex, and increased growth of eyelashes. The eyelash growth is reversible.[46] In the largest study of ocular complications, increased eyelash growth occurred in 2 of 36 patients (6 percent). The mechanism for this unique reaction is not known. Paradoxically, alopecia is the most common generalized cutaneous manifestation of interferon-α therapy.

MONOCLONAL ANTIBODIES The development of monoclonal antibodies that target specific binding sites on tumors is one of the most exciting areas in oncology. Recently approved drugs include rituximab and trastuzumab. Rituximab is a genetically engineered chimeric/human monoclonal antibody directed against the CD20 antigen found in normal and malignant B cells. It is indicated for the treatment of low-grade or follicular, CD20-positive B cell lymphomas. Cutaneous reactions include toxic epidermal necrolysis, pemphigus, urticaria, and vasculitis.[47,48] Trastuzumab is a monoclonal antibody that selectively binds to the human epidermal growth factor receptor 2 protein, HER2, which is overexpressed in 25 to 30 percent of breast cancers. Cutaneous reactions include anaphylactoid reactions, dermatitis, and possible activation of herpes zoster.

COLONY-STIMULATING FACTORS The hematopoietic colony-stimulating factors, granulocyte-macrophage colony-stimulating factor (GM-CSF) and granulocyte colony-stimulating factor (G-CSF), have increasingly been used in chemotherapeutic regimens to enhance leukemic cell proliferation before cell-cycle–specific antileukemic therapy or for chemotherapy-induced neutropenia.

This class of drugs has been most commonly associated with macular or papular dermatitis that often demonstrates an accumulation of granulocytes, macrophages, and lymphocytes (GM-CSF)[49] or granulocytes (G-CSF). G-CSF is also associated with Sweet's syndrome. An X inactivation study performed in one case demonstrated clonality in the skin biopsy, suggesting that the Sweet's syndrome was due to induced differentiation of sequestered leukemic cells.[50]

REFERENCES

1. Susser WS et al: Mucocutaneous reactions to chemotherapy. *J Am Acad Dermatol* **40**:367, 1999
2. Koppel RA, Boh EE: Cutaneous reactions to chemotherapeutic agents. *Am J Med Sci* **321**:327, 2001
3. Fitzpatrick JE, Hood AF: Histopathologic reactions to chemotherapeutic agents. *Adv Dermatol* **3**:161, 1988
4. Fitzpatrick JE: The cutaneous histopathology of chemotherapeutic reactions. *J Cutan Pathol* **20**:1, 1993
5. Hussein AM: Chemotherapy-induced alopecia: New developments. *South Med J* **86**:489, 1993
6. Baker B et al: Busulphan/cyclophosphamide conditioning for bone marrow transplantation may lead to failure of hair regrowth. *Bone Marrow Transplant* **7**:43, 1991
7. Epstein EH, Lutzner MH: Folliculitis induced by actinomycin D. *N Engl J Med* **281**:1094, 1969
8. Hussain S et al: Onycholysis as a complication of systemic chemotherapy. Report of five cases associated with prolonged weekly paclitaxel therapy and review of the literature. *Cancer* **88**:2367, 2000
9. Anderson LL et al: Cutaneous pigmentation after daunorubicin chemotherapy. *J Am Acad Dermatol* **26**:255, 1992
10. Don PC, Sadjadi MM: Nail and skin pigmentation associated with hydroxyurea therapy for polycythemia vera. *Int J Dermatol* **32**:731, 1993
11. Fitzpatrick JE et al: Neutrophilic eccrine hidradenitis associated with induction chemotherapy. *J Cutan Pathol* **14**:272, 1987
12. Bachmeyer C et al: Neutrophilic eccrine hidradenitis induced by granulocyte colony-stimulating factor. *Br J Dermatol* **139**:354, 1998
13. Brehler R et al: Neutrophilic hidradenitis induced by chemotherapy involves eccrine and apocrine glands. *Am J Dermatopathol* **19**:73, 1997
14. Bhawan J, Malhotra R: Syringosquamous metaplasia: A distinctive eruption in patients receiving chemotherapy. *Am J Dermatopathol* **12**:1, 1990
15. Hurt MA et al: Eccrine squamous syringometaplasia: A cutaneous sweat gland reaction in the histologic spectrum of "chemotherapy-associated eccrine hidradenitis" and "neutrophilic eccrine hidradenitis." *Arch Dermatol* **126**:73, 1990
16. Hymes SR et al: Cutaneous busulfan effect in patients receiving bone-marrow transplantation. *J Cutan Pathol* **12**:125, 1985
17. Yokel BK et al: Cutaneous pathology following etoposide therapy. *J Cutan Pathol* **14**:326, 1987
18. Vassallo C et al: Muco-cutaneous changes during long-term therapy with hydroxyurea in chronic myeloid leukaemia. *Clin Exp Dermatol* **26**:141, 2001
19. Burgdorf WHC et al: Peculiar acral erythema secondary to high-dose chemotherapy for acute myelogenous leukemia. *Ann Intern Med* **97**:61, 1982
20. Rongioletti F et al: Necrotizing eccrine squamous syringometaplasia presenting as acral erythema. *J Cutan Pathol* **18**:453, 1991
21. Demircay Z et al: Chemotherapy-induced acral erythema in leukemic patients: A report of 15 cases. *Int J Dermatol* **36**:593, 1997
22. Omura EF, Torre D: Inflammation of actinic keratoses due to systemic fluorouracil therapy. *JAMA* **208**:150, 1969
23. Guillet G et al: Cutaneous pigmented stripes and bleomycin treatment. *Arch Dermatol* **122**:381, 1986
24. Kukla LJ, McGuire WP: Heat-induced recall of bleomycin skin changes. *Cancer* **50**:2283, 1982
25. Hrushesky WJ: Serpentine supravenous 5-fluorouracil hyperpigmentation. *Cancer Treat Rep* **60**:639, 1976

26. Cecchi R et al: Supravenous hyperpigmentation induced by vinorelbine. *Dermatology* **188**:244, 1994
27. Yung CW et al: Dacarbazine-induced photosensitivity reaction. *J Am Acad Dermatol* **4**:541, 1981
28. Westwick TJ et al: Delayed reactivation of sunburn by methotrexate: Sparing of chronically sun-exposed skin. *Cutis* **39**:49, 1987
29. Solberg LA Jr et al: Doxorubicin-enhanced skin reaction after whole-body electron-beam irradiation for leukemia cutis. *Mayo Clin Proc* **55**:711, 1980
30. Yeo W, Johnson PJ: Radiation-recall skin disorders associated with the use of antineoplastic drugs. Pathogenesis, prevalence, and management. *Am J Clin Dermatol* **1**:113, 2000
31. Camidge R, Price A: Characterizing the phenomenon of radiation recall dermatitis. *Radiother Oncol* **59**:237, 2001
32. Luedke DW et al: Histopathogenesis of skin and subcutaneous injury induced by Adriamycin. *Plast Reconstr Surg* **61**:86, 1978
33. Tsavaris NB et al: Conservative approach to the treatment of chemotherapy-induced extravasation. *J Dermatol Surg Oncol* **16**:519, 1990
34. Goldberg A et al: Anaphylaxis to cisplatin: Diagnosis and value of pretreatment in prevention of recurrent allergic reactions. *Ann Allergy* **73**:271, 1994
35. Cohen IS et al: Cutaneous toxicity of bleomycin treatment. *Arch Dermatol* **107**:553, 1973
36. Hassett G et al: Scleroderma in association with the use of docetaxel (Taxotere) for breast cancer. *Clin Exp Rheumatol* **19**:197, 2001
37. Landau M et al: Reticulate scleroderma after isolated limb perfusion with melphalan. *J Am Acad Dermatol* **39**:1011, 1998
38. Yamamoto T et al: Bleomycin increases steady-state levels of type I collagen, fibronectin, and decorin mRNAs in human skin fibroblasts. *Arch Dermatol Res* **292**:556, 2000
39. Berger CC et al: Secondary Raynaud's phenomenon and other late vascular complications following chemotherapy for testicular cancer. *Eur J Cancer* **31A**:2229, 1995
40. Lee TC et al: Severe exfoliative dermatitis associated with hand ischemia during cisplatin therapy. *Mayo Clin Proc* **69**:80, 1994
41. Vanhooteghem O et al: Raynaud's phenomenon after treatment of verruca vulgaris of the sole with intralesional injection of bleomycin. *Pediatr Dermatol* **18**:249, 2001
42. Bell KA et al: Mucositis as a treatment-limiting side effect in the use of capecitabine for the treatment of metastatic breast cancer. *J Am Acad Dermatol* **45**:790, 2001
43. Gaspari AA et al: Dermatologic changes associated with interleukin-2 administration. *JAMA* **258**:1624, 1987
44. Foss FM et al: Biologic correlates of acute hypersensitivity events with DAB389IL-2 (denileukin diftitox, ONTAK) in cutaneous T cell lymphoma: Decreased frequency and severity with steroid premedication. *Clin Lymphoma* **1**:298, 2001
45. Berglund EF et al: Hypertrichosis of the eyelashes associated with interferon-alpha therapy for chronic granulocytic leukemia. *South Med J* **83**:363, 1990
46. Stafford-Fox V, Guindon KM: Cutaneous reactions associated with alpha interferon therapy. *Clin J Oncol Nurs* **4**:164, 2000
47. Dillman RO: Infusion reactions associated with the therapeutic use of monoclonal antibodies in the treatment of malignancy. *Cancer Metastasis Rev* **18**:465, 1999
48. Dereure O et al: Rituximab-induced vasculitis. *Dermatology* **203**:83, 2001
49. Horn TD et al: Intravenous administration of recombinant human granulocyte-macrophage colony-stimulating factor causes a cutaneous eruption. *Arch Dermatol* **127**:49, 1991
50. Magro CM et al: Sweet's syndrome in the setting of CD34-positive acute myelogenous leukemia treated with granulocyte colony stimulating factor: Evidence for a clonal neutrophilic dermatoses. *J Cutan Pathol* **28**:90, 2001

CHAPTER 140

Maria L. Chanco Turner

Cutaneous Reactions to Cytokines and Growth Factors

Discoveries and developments in molecular biology and recombinant gene technology have made possible the synthesis of large amounts of pure proteins such as cytokines and growth factors (see Chap. 26). The ready availability of these recombinant proteins has permitted their use in analysis of cellular signaling pathways as well as in therapeutic applications. As a result of the increase in the use of cytokines as therapeutic agents, adverse reactions associated with their use have been recognized. In this chapter we use a classification of cytokines based on their major function.[1] Those with antiviral properties are classified as *interferons;* cytokines produced by leukocytes with major effects on other white blood cells are called *interleukins;* and those that cause proliferation and differentiation of stem cells are classified as *colony-stimulating factors*. Just as the biologic effects of cytokines have a tendency to overlap or to be redundant, the same is true of their adverse effects. This is due to the tendency of cytokines with similar structures to bind to the same receptors and to the limited number of extracellular domains on the five "superfamilies" of cytokine receptors.[2] The discussion below focuses on the adverse cutaneous reactions to cytokines already approved for therapeutic use. Recognition of these reaction patterns facilitates differentiation of these complications from cutaneous reactions to other drugs or disease processes occurring in the complicated settings in which these cytokines are frequently used.

INTERFERONS

When originally discovered, interferons (IFNs) were thought to have only antiviral effects. However, they have since been shown to have potent immunoregulatory and antiproliferative actions as well.[3] Based on their sources, there are three groups of interferons: IFN-α (leukocyte IFN), which is produced by null lymphocytes and macrophages; IFN-β (fibroblast IFN), which is produced by fibroblasts, macrophages, and epithelial cells; and IFN-γ (immune IFN), which is produced by T lymphocytes, natural killer cells, and macrophages. IFN-α and

IFN-β share the same receptor and have some homology, properties that explain the similarity in their biologic and adverse effects.[3]

Interferon-α (IFN-α)

Recombinant IFN-α is approved for use as a single agent or as adjuvant therapy for hairy cell leukemia, AIDS-related Kaposi's sarcoma, melanoma, chronic myelogenous leukemia, genital human papillomavirus infection, and hepatitis B and C virus infections. IFN-α causes multiple adverse cutaneous reactions.

CUTANEOUS NECROSIS AND ULCERATIONS AT INJECTION SITES These are the most dramatic, although extremely rare, adverse cutaneous complications of subcutaneous injections of any of the various forms of IFN-α. These complications have been observed in patients with AIDS who are receiving IFN-α for Kaposi's sarcoma[4,5] and in patients with chronic myelogenous leukemia,[6] multiple sclerosis,[7] and hepatitis C virus (HCV) infection.[8] The lesions start out as painful or pruritic red to purple indurated plaques at injection sites 2 months to 3 years after initiation of treatment. While some plaques clear spontaneously, others break down into necrotic ulcers (Fig. 140-1). Histopathologically, microthromboses of deep dermal and subcutaneous vessels are apparent.[7] Most ulcers heal after discontinuation of treatment; some heal after the dose is decreased; and some heal despite continuation of therapy. Some ulcers require debridement, with or without excision and closure. Ulcers can be prevented by rotating injection sites and avoiding erythematous and/or pruritic areas until they resolve.

DIGITAL NECROSIS This reaction is even more rare than ulcerations at injection sites. This complication is seen most often when IFN-α is given to patients who are also receiving cytotoxic agents for the treatment of malignancies. In two cases, histology revealed small-vessel thromboses without vasculitis.[9] In three patients with HCV infection and cryoglobulinemia-related ischemic disease, systemic manifestations improved with a combination of treatments including IFN-α. In contrast, digital necrosis worsened and required amputation in two patients and resulted in enlargement of the ulcer in another.[10] A localized procoagulant effect of IFN-α may be the reason for this reaction.

FIGURE 140-1

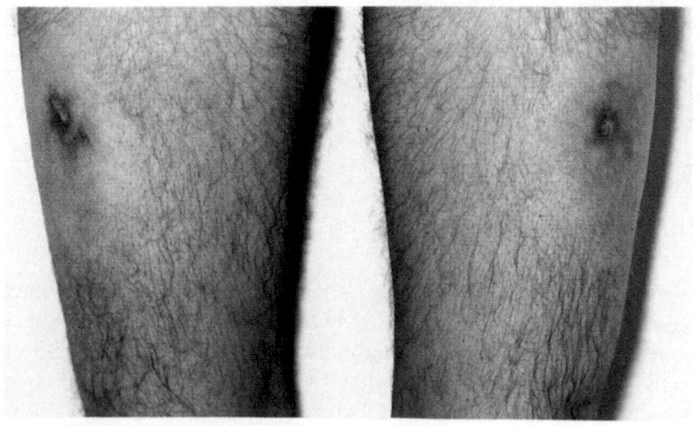

Bilateral punched-out ulcers at IFN-α injection sites. Note absence of hair around perimeter of injection site ulcers.

PSORIASIS Psoriasis appears to be a relatively common complication of IFN-α therapy across the spectrum of patients treated with this cytokine. Wolfer et al.[11] chronicled 20 patients in whom psoriasis was exacerbated or induced by IFN-α therapy. Psoriasis has occurred at injection sites, and it waxes and wanes with IFN-α dosing. Severity appears to be dose-related. IFN-α–induced or –exacerbated psoriasis usually clears on discontinuation of therapy, and it responds to the usual antipsoriatic treatments. Since IFN-α upregulates both inflammatory and immune responses,[3] the pathogenesis of this side effect seems clear whether psoriasis is viewed as an autoimmune disease mediated by activated T cells[12] or as an epidermal hyperproliferative disorder mediated by inflammation.

HAIR ABNORMALITIES Hair loss is a frequent complaint with IFN-α therapy. Tosti et al.[13] described telogen effluvium in 5 of 10 patients who were followed with trichograms and the pull test. The authors did not feel that the onset and severity of hair loss were related to the dose of IFN-α or the duration of therapy.

Ill-defined patches of hair loss around nonindurated injection sites and around an ulcerated injection site have been reported.[14] No "exclamation point" hairs were noted. Histology revealed perifollicular and intrafollicular lymphocytic infiltration. In all cases, hair regrew after injection sites were switched.

LICHEN PLANUS The literature is replete with case reports relating to the induction, aggravation, or improvement of lichen planus due to the use of IFN-α for the treatment of HCV infection. There are also some case reports calling attention to this association in patients with lymphoma and melanoma. In a group of 120 patients with chronic viral hepatitis who were treated with IFN-α, 3.3 percent developed mild lichen planus.[15] All had antinuclear antibodies before initiation of therapy. Because HCV infection itself is thought to be associated with an increased incidence of lichen planus, it is possible that the upregulation of immune function brought on by IFN-α further stimulates a system that is already primed for the development of lichen planus. Lichen planus associated with IFN-α therapy does not require discontinuation of therapy except in cases of recalcitrant erosive mucosal lichen planus.

SARCOIDOSIS There have been case reports of cutaneous and systemic sarcoidosis coincident with IFN-α treatment of HCV infection[16] and of chronic myelogenous leukemia.[17] It has been postulated that the upregulation of T_H1 responses by IFN-α may unmask an innate predilection of patients with these diseases to develop sarcoidosis. This theory is supported by the observation that systemic sarcoidosis tends to remit with dose reduction or discontinuation of IFN-α therapy. Although purely cutaneous lesions can be managed successfully with topical glucocorticoid therapy, systemic involvement often requires the addition of systemic glucocorticoids.

AUTOIMMUNE REACTIONS Cutaneous autoimmune reactions other than psoriasis and lichen planus have been reported in isolated cases. These include leukocytoclastic vasculitis, periarteritis nodosa, autoimmune bullous diseases, and systemic lupus erythematosus with cutaneous manifestations.[18] Vitiligo was noted at sites distant from lesions of metastatic melanoma in three patients who were being treated with IFN-α. The vitiligo was associated with a favorable response to treatment.[19]

MISCELLANEOUS REACTIONS These non-dose-limiting reactions include skin dryness, itching, erythemas, and urticaria. They have been reported in 10 percent of IFN-α recipients.

Interferon-β (IFN-β)

IFN-β is also known as *fibroblast interferon*. Although natural IFN-β is available, the recombinant forms (IFN-β1a and IFN-β1b) are more widely used for the treatment of multiple sclerosis, condylomata acuminata, malignant melanoma, and HCV infection. Cutaneous adverse reactions to the various forms are similar but seem to occur more frequently with IFN-β1b.

INJECTION-SITE REACTIONS These reactions are the most common adverse event in patients receiving subcutaneous IFN-β. Reactions consist of local pain, soreness, erythema, bruising, and rarely, sclerotic plaques. They have been reported in as many as 85 percent of patients. They generally appear within the first month of treatment and diminish over the next 6 months. Discontinuation of therapy is not often required and can be avoided by administering IFN-β by deep intramuscular injections.[20]

Single or multiple, painful, deep, necrotic ulcerations suggesting vascular compromise were found to develop in 5 percent of IFN-β subcutaneous injection sites.[20] They were more likely to appear within the first few months of treatment. Deep biopsies revealed thrombosis of venules in the deep dermis and subcutaneous tissue with a mild superficial perivascular lymphocytic infiltrate.[21] It was hypothesized that thrombosis of the deep dermal vessels is related to a localized clotting abnormality caused by increased platelet aggregation. Necrotic ulcers could be prevented by regularly switching injection sites, by changing to intramuscular injections, by warming the injectable solution to room temperature, and by massaging the injection site to promote dispersion of the drug.[20] Conservative local therapy alone was frequently sufficient to promote healing. Surgical excision of the ulcer speeds the healing process. It also has been possible to continue IFN-β therapy despite the ulcers.[20]

MISCELLANEOUS REACTIONS A flare of pustular psoriasis,[22] the appearance of psoriatic plaques at all injection sites (author's unpublished case) (Fig. 140-2), subacute cutaneous lupus,[23] and contact dermatitis with a positive patch test to the ophthalmic form of natural IFN-β[18] have been observed.

Interferon-γ (IFN-γ)

IFN-γ, also known as *immune interferon,* is produced by activated T cells and natural killer (NK) cells. Recombinant IFN-γ is approved for the treatment of chronic granulomatous disease, renal cancer, and congenital osteopetrosis. Unlike IFN-α and IFN-β, there are only a few reports of cutaneous adverse reactions to IFN-γ. Psoriasis at injection sites[18] and erythema nodosum leprosum (ENL) are two such reactions. ENL was induced in 60 percent of patients with lepromatous leprosy who received recombinant IFN-γ over a period of 6 to 7 months in comparison with a 15 percent incidence in the group not treated with recombinant IFN-γ.[24]

FIGURE 140-2

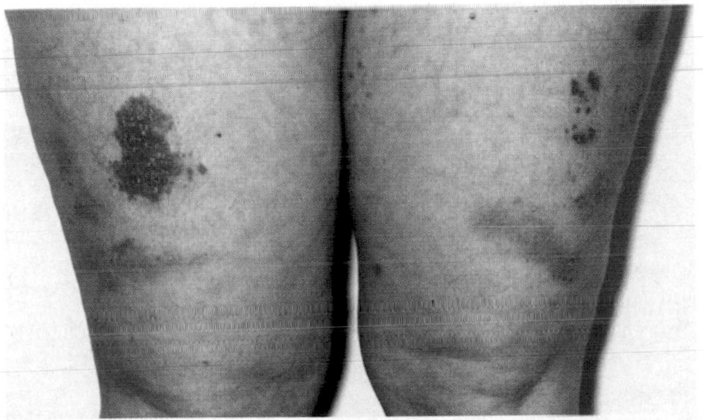

Psoriasis at IFN-β injection sites. Note sharp-angled, erythematous, nonscaly plaques resulting from tape irritation. This eventually became psoriatic as well.

INTERLEUKINS

Interleukins are a heterogeneous group of cytokines produced by T cells, monocytes-macrophages, and at times, somatic cells. These agents have major effects on immune function and inflammation by virtue of their influence on the growth, differentiation, and activation of leukocytes.

Interleukin 2 (IL-2)

IL-2 is produced by activated T cells. By promoting the proliferation, growth, and activity of T, B, and NK cells, Il-2 not only upregulates immunity but also has marked proinflammatory effects.[2] The level of proinflammatory cytokines induced by the administered dose of IL-2 determines its toxicity. Recombinant IL-2 is approved for the treatment of metastatic renal cell carcinoma and metastatic melanoma in high-dose regimens. Low-dose regimens for HIV are currently in clinical trials. In the high-dose intravenous regimen used by Rosenberg et al.,[25] the dose-limiting toxicity was "capillary leak syndrome," characterized by massive weight gain, hypotension, tachycardia, and hypoxemia, symptoms also seen in septic shock syndrome. High fevers and chills were universal. For these reasons, patients are hospitalized for this form of therapy. The clinical and histologic descriptions of the cutaneous side effects that occur with the high-dose regimen are described by Gaspari et al.[26] and Wolkenstein et al.[27]

IL-2 DERMATITIS The markedly pruritic rash consists of various combinations of erythema, edema, blistering, and desquamation. At its worst, the initial presentation is that of an erythrodermic, somewhat edematous patient who has a very severe "sunburn" (Fig. 140-3). The eruption generally starts on the face within 48 to 72 hours of the initiation of infusions. This eruption may be accompanied by petechiae and tense bullae, especially of the lower extremities. The dermatitis clears on termination of therapy and results in scaling that varies from fine desquamation to sheetlike peeling, especially on the palms and soles. These reactions are not clearly dose-related. The findings on histologic examination and immunophenotyping of the infiltrate are consistent with "dermatitis." In the author's experience, antihistamines are only minimally helpful in relieving the pruritus and only when taken to the point of sedation. In these patients, if the use of topical steroids is interdicted by protocol requirements, treatment can be with bland or mentholated lubricating lotions.

MUCOSITIS AND GLOSSITIS Erosions of the tongue and oral mucous membranes occurred simultaneously with the skin changes. Glossitis was seen in 6 of 20 patients[27] and, together with the mucositis, cleared soon after discontinuation of IL-2.

AUTOIMMUNE DERMATOSES Gaspari[28] reviewed the cases of pemphigus, psoriasis, and vitiligo that had been reported in association with IL-2 therapy. The occurrence of vitiligo in patients being

FIGURE 140-3

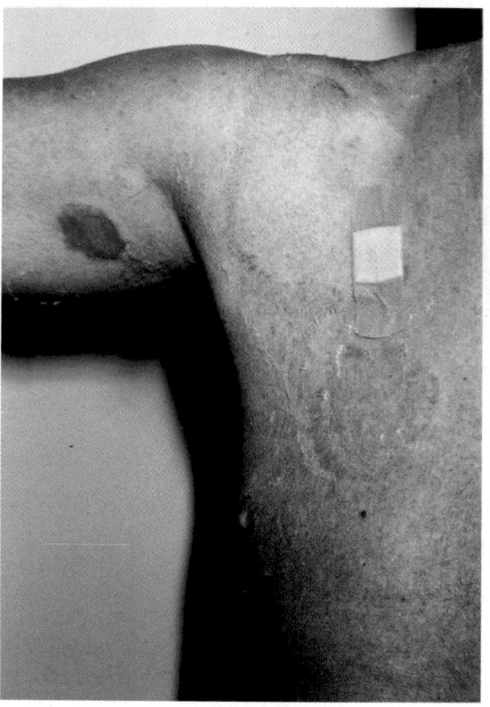

Sunburn-like erythema with desquamation and an erosion in a patient receiving high-dose IL-2 therapy.

treated with IL-2 for metastatic melanoma was seen to be a predictor of a favorable response. High doses of IL-2 result in widespread immune activation. Thus the rarity of these autoimmune reactions suggests that the presence of risk factors such as preexisting mild disease or a family history may be necessary precursors of these side effects.

DRUG REACTIONS Patients who receive IL-2 at least 2 weeks before exposure to iodine-containing contrast media are reported to be 2 to 4 times more likely than those who are not treated with IL-2 to develop a reaction consisting of flushing, flulike symptoms, rash, pruritus, joint pains, wheezing, hypotension, edema, and oliguria.[29] These complications are likely to occur within 1 to 4 h of exposure to contrast media and can be avoided by premedication with systemic steroids. The use of noniodinated contrast media has been suggested to prevent this reaction. Multifocal fixed drug eruption in response to acetaminophen, tropisetron, and ondansetron has been reported.[30] The author has encountered a very similar case with IL-2 treatment.

MISCELLANEOUS ERUPTIONS There are isolated case reports of IL-2–induced grade II to III cutaneous graft-versus-host disease in autologous transplant patients, recall of subcutaneous injection-site reactions after intravenous dosing, telogen effluvium, urticaria, and erythema nodosum.

HEMATOPOIETIC GROWTH FACTORS

Hematopoietic growth factors (HGFs) are cytokines that trigger the proliferation, differentiation, and survival of hematopoietic stem and progenitor cells. The availability of recombinant forms of HGFs has made possible dose intensification of chemotherapeutic regimens. The four approved, commercially available HGFs in the United States are erythropoietin (EPO), oprelvekin (IL-11), granulocyte-macrophage colony-stimulating factor (GM-CSF), and granulocyte colony-stimulating factor (G-CSF).

EPO stimulates the production and differentiation of red cells, whereas oprelvekin has similar effects on platelets. Neither is immunomodulatory, and they do not appear to have adverse cutaneous side effects except for mild injection-site reactions.[31,32]

Granulocyte-Macrophage Colony-Stimulating Factor (GM-CSF)

There are two recombinant forms, one of which, filgrastim, is approved by the Food and Drug Administration (FDA) for the treatment of neutropenic states after chemotherapy and myeloablative treatment. GM-CSF is a panstimulator of all granulocytes and induces the production of inflammatory cytokines, an effect not shared with G-CSF. Vascular leak syndrome leading to massive edema, similar to that which occurs with IL-2, is the major dose-limiting toxic effect of GM-CSF.[33]

Injection-site reactions are common, severe, and exhibit "recall." In a study with 5 mg/g per day given subcutaneously, all patients developed pruritic and burning erythemas that recurred after each injection so that treatment had to be discontinued.[34] In another protocol, generalized cutaneous reactions occurred in 21 of 26 patients who received GM-CSF by subcutaneous injection.[35] The eruption ranged from urticaria to exfoliative dermatitis, causing therapy to be discontinued in 13 patients and continued at a reduced dose in 3. Peripheral and tissue eosinophilia were noted in this cohort.

Granulocyte Colony-Stimulating Factor (G-CSF)

G-CSF stimulates the production, differentiation, and activity of neutrophils. A recombinant form is approved for the treatment of neutropenic states due to chemotherapy and myeloablative therapy. The same action accounts for its cutaneous side effects, which are uncommon and are mild enough not to cause discontinuation of therapy.

Neutrophilic dermatoses, consisting of eruptions such as Sweet's syndrome and bullous pyoderma gangrenosum (Fig. 140-4), are sometimes associated with malignancies, especially myeloproliferative ones. These eruptions have been reported as a complication of G-CSF therapy as single cases or in a small series. Typical is a report that G-CSF exacerbated a tendency of patients with myeloid leukemia to develop

FIGURE 140-4

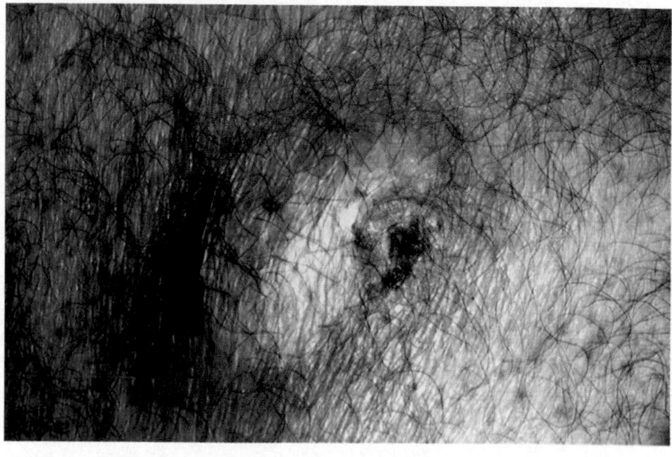

Bullous pyoderma gangrenosum–like lesion in a patient receiving G-CSF after chemotherapy for non-Hodgkin's lymphoma.

Sweet's syndrome.[36] These neutrophilic dermatoses also have been reported in association with nonhematologic malignancies treated with G-CSF.[37]

Leukocytoclastic vasculitis limited to the skin occurred in patients treated with G-CSF for malignant disease as well as for chronic benign neutropenias.[38] This complication was likely to occur when the absolute neutrophil count was above 800/mm^3. Folliculitis involving the face and upper torso, recurring with each dose of G-CSF, has been reported in a patient with myelodysplasia as well as in a normal volunteer.[39] Histology revealed a mixed inflammatory infiltrate around hair follicles and eccrine glands.

The histopathology of a cutaneous reaction to G-CSF demonstrates numerous large, atypical histiocytes with mitotic figures. This is a G-CSF effect and should not be mistaken for a malignancy.[40]

This author has observed all the foregoing reactions to G-CSF in addition to injection-site reactions and exacerbation of preexisting dermatoses such as psoriasis and rosacea, and is of the opinion that allergic reactions to simultaneously administered drugs tend to be more florid and last longer. In general, G-CSF is safe and well-tolerated.

REFERENCES

1. Parkin J, Cohen B: An overview of the immune system. *Lancet* **357**:1777, 2001
2. Oppenheim JJ: Cytokines: Past, present, and future. *Int J Hematol* **74**:3, 2001
3. Pfeffer LLM et al: Biological properties of recombinant α-interferons: 40th anniversary of the discovery of interferons. *Cancer Res* **58**:2489, 1998
4. Orlow SJ, Friedman-Kein AE: Cutaneous ulcerations secondary to interferon-α therapy of Kaposi's sarcoma. *Arch Dermatol* **128**:566, 1992
5. Virgili A et al: Cutaneous lesions due to interferon seem not to be related to dosage. *J Eur Acad Dermatol Venereol* **13**:141, 1999
6. Krainick U et al: Local cutaneous necrotizing lesions associated with interferon injections. *J Interferon Cytokine Res* **18**:823, 1998
7. Sheremata WA et al: More on interferon-induced cutaneous necrosis. *N Engl J Med* **333**:1223, 1995
8. Sickler JB et al: Cutaneous necrosis associated with interferon-α2b. *Am J Gastroenterol* **93**:463, 1998
9. Bachmeyer C et al: Raynaud's phenomenon and digital necrosis induced by interferon-alpha. *Br J Dermatol* **135**:481, 1996
10. Cid MC et al: Interferon-alpha may exacerbate cryoglobulinemia-related ischemic manifestations: An adverse effect potentially related to its antiangiogenic activity. *Arthritis Rheum* **42**:1051, 1999
11. Wolfer LU et al: Interferon-alpha–induced psoriasis vulgaris. *Hautarzt* **47**:124, 1996
12. Griffiths CEM, Voorhees JJ: Psoriasis, T cells and autoimmunity. *J R Soc Med* **89**:315, 1996
13. Tosti A et al: Telogen effluvium due to recombinant interferon-α2b. *Dermatology* **184**:124, 1992
14. Lang A et al: Localized interferon alpha-2b–induced alopecia. *Arch Dermatol* **135**:1126, 1999
15. Dalekos GN et al: A prospective evaluation of dermatological side effects during alpha-interferon therapy for chronic viral hepatitis. *Eur J Gastroenterol Hepatol* **10**:933, 1998
16. Eberlein-Koenig B et al: Cutaneous sarcoid foreign body granulomas developing in sites of previous skin injury after systemic interferon-alpha treatment for chronic hepatitis C. *Br J Dermatol* **140**:358, 1999
17. Pietropaoli A et al: Interferon-α therapy associated with the development of sarcoidosis. *Chest* **116**:569, 1999
18. Vial T, Descotes J: Immune-mediated side effects of cytokines in humans. *Toxicology* **105**:31, 1995
19. LeGal F-A et al: More on cutaneous reactions to recombinant cytokine therapy. *J Am Acad Dermatol* **35**:650, 1996
20. Bayas A, Rieckmann P: Managing the adverse effects of interferon-beta therapy in multiple sclerosis. *Drug Saf* **22**:149, 2000
21. Elgart GW et al: Cutaneous reaction to recombinant human interferon beta-1b: The clinical and histologic spectrum. *J Am Acad Dermatol* **37**:553, 1997
22. Webster GF et al: Cutaneous ulcerations and pustular psoriasis flare caused by recombinant interferon beta injections in patients with multiple sclerosis. *J Am Acad Dermatol* **34**:365, 1996
23. Nousari HC et al: Subacute cutaneous lupus erythematosus associated with interferon beta-1b. *Lancet* **352**:1825, 1998
24. Sampaio EP et al: Prolonged treatment with recombinant interferon gamma induces erythema nodosum leprosum in lepromatous leprosy patients. *J Exp Med* **175**:1729, 1992
25. Rosenberg SA et al: A progress report on the treatment of 157 patients with advanced cancer using lymphokine-activated killer-cells and interleukin-2 or high-dose interleukin-2 alone. *N Engl J Med* **316**:889, 1987
26. Gaspari AA et al: Dermatologic changes associated with interleukin 2 administration. *JAMA* **258**:1624, 1987
27. Wolkenstein P et al: Cutaneous side effects associated with interleukin 2 administration for metastatic melanoma. *J Am Acad Dermatol* **28**:66, 1993
28. Gaspari AA: Autoimmunity as a complication of interleukin 2 immunotherapy: Many unanswered questions. *Arch Dermatol* **130**:894, 1994
29. Choyke P et al: Delayed reactions to contrast media after interleukin-2 immunotherapy. *Radiology* **183**:111, 1992
30. Bernard S et al: Multifocal fixed drug eruption to paracetamol, tropisetron and ondansetron induced by interleukin 2. *Dermatology* **201**:148, 2000
31. Markam A, Bryson HM: Epoietin alpha: A review of its pharmacodynamic and pharmacokinetic properties and therapeutic use in nonrenal applications. *Drugs* **49**:232, 1995
32. Moreland L et al: Results of a phase I–II randomized, masked, placebo-controlled trial of recombinant human interleukin 11 (rhIL-11) in the treatment of subjects with active rheumatoid arthritis. *Arthritis Res* **3**:247, 2001
33. Lieschke GJ, Burgess AW: Granulocyte colony-stimulating factor and granulocyte-macrophage colony-stimulating factor (part 1). *N Engl J Med* **327**:28, 1992
34. Locker GJ et al: Cutaneous side effects in breast cancer patients treated with cytostatic polychemotherapy with rhGM-CSF: Immune phenomena or drug toxicity. *Breast Cancer Res Treat* **34**:213, 1995
35. Mehregan DR et al: Cutaneous reactions to granulocyte-monocyte colony-stimulating factor. *Arch Dermatol* **128**:1055, 1992
36. Paydas S et al: Sweet's syndrome accompanying leukaemia: Seven cases and review of the literataure. *Leuk Res* **24**:83, 2001
37. Johnson ML, Grimwood RE: Leukocyte colony-stimulating factors: A review of associated neutrophilic dermatoses and vasculitides. *Arch Dermatol* **130**:88, 1994
38. Jain KK: Cutaneous vasculitis associated with granulocyte colony-stimulating factor. *J Am Acad Dermatol* **31**:213, 1994
39. Paul C et al: Cutaneous effects of granulocyte colony-stimulating factor in healthy volunteers. *Arch Dermatol* **134**:111, 1998
40. Farina MC et al: Histopathology of cutaneous reaction to granulocyte colony-stimulating factor: Another pseudomalignancy. *J Cutan Pathol* **25**:559, 1998

CHAPTER 141

Miguel Sanchez

Cutaneous Manifestations of Drug Abuse

Drug abuse can be suspected or diagnosed on the basis of skin findings. The parenteral administration of drugs causes skin lesions and eruptions predominantly through local or systemic, toxic or hypersensitivity-induced effects of the drug itself, adulterants, or infectious agents. Intravenous administration can produce a number of recognizable stigmata, which may identify an individual abusing drugs to anyone with experience in illicit drug use.

Behavior associated with drug abuse is an important factor in the spread of HIV infection. In the United States, 25 percent of all reported cases of AIDS in adults and adolescents resulted solely from sharing needles. In addition, 6.5 percent of cases occurred in men who have sex with men and inject drugs. Current or former drug users transmit most of the 11 percent of AIDS cases acquired through heterosexual contact. Parenteral drug users also have high risks for contracting hepatitis B and C and other blood-borne infections. About 60 percent of all new hepatitis C infections in the United States are attributed to syringe and needle sharing with an infected individual. In some user populations, hepatitis C is transmitted so rapidly that within 6 months of beginning drug use, one-third of users are infected, and within 2 years, 90 percent have contracted the infection.[1] Drug addicts also have higher incidences of sexually transmitted diseases, depression, accidental injuries, and trauma due to criminal violence or domestic abuse. Numerous sociologic problems, such as loss of work productivity and increases in crime, prison occupancy, and property damage, result from drug abuse and dependence. In 1992, the National Institute on Drug Abuse and the National Institute on Alcohol Abuse and Alcoholism estimated that the annual economic cost to society from drug abuse exceeded $97.7 billion.

DEFINITIONS

Drug abuse is a maladaptive pattern involving misuse or overuse of prescribed or recreational drugs, which results in related legal problems, social or interpersonal problems, failure to sustain major obligations at work, at school, or at home, or continued use despite potential physical harm.[2] In contrast, *drug dependence* is a pattern of recurrent or excessive drug use that has produced clinically significant physical, emotional, or social impairment or distress (especially with the induction of tolerance). It is characterized by recurrent and excessive use of drugs to avoid withdrawal symptoms associated with abstinence (Table 141-1). *Tolerance* is a physiologic state in which progressive increases in the dose of a drug are needed to achieve intoxication or the desired effects previously experienced at smaller doses. Drug dependence may be physical or psychological or both. Some drugs, particularly opiates, chiefly induce physical dependence, a neurobiologic state of physiologic adaptation to a drug that results in withdrawal symptoms during abstinence. Other drugs, such as marijuana, cocaine, amphetamines, and hallucinogens, cause predominantly *psychological dependence*, a biopsychosocial state characterized by a need to administer a drug repeatedly to produce desired psychological effects and prevent feelings of discontent.

TABLE 141-1

Criteria for Drug Dependence (DSM-IV)

The presence of three (or more) of the following, occurring at any time in the same 12-month period:

- Continued drug use despite awareness of the presence of a persistent or recurrent physical or psychological problem caused or exacerbated by the drug
- Sustained intent or unsuccessful efforts to abate drug use
- Tolerance
- Withdrawal symptoms
- Administration of drug in higher doses and longer duration than initially intended
- Significant time devoted to obtaining the drug or recovering from its effects
- Relinquishment or reduction of social, occupational, or recreational activities because of drug abuse

COMMONLY ABUSED DRUGS

Cannabis (marijuana, Mary Jane, pot, herb, weed, boom) is a mixture of dried shredded leaves and flowers of *Cannabis sativa* that contains the chemical delta-9-tetrahydrocannabinol (THC). Diacetylmorphine (heroin, junk, smack, horse, scag), the fastest-acting and most potent opiate, accounts for 90 percent of the opiate abuse in this country. A "rush" develops within 7 to 8 seconds if the opiate is injected intravenously or within 10 to 15 min if it is snorted or smoked. Persons addicted to opiates may alternate injections of heroin and cocaine (crisscrossing) or inject highly addictive "speedballs" of the two drugs together. Cocaine (coke, blow, toot, flake, and snow) is an alkaloid stimulant and topical anesthetic that is extracted from the leaves of the coca shrub. Crack (base, rock, hubba, gravel, girl), or crystallized, freebase cocaine, is far more addictive than heroin. Crystallized methamphetamine (ice, crystal, glass) may be inhaled or injected intravenously. The powder form may be ingestion or snorted. Because withdrawal symptoms are so intense, methamphetamine addiction is more difficult than any other addiction to treat. 3,4-Methylenedioxymethamphetamine, often abbreviated as MDMA (ecstasy, Adam, XTC, hug, beans, love drug) is a synthetic psychoactive drug with stimulant and mildly hallucinogenic properties. It is widely available at raves, clubs, and all-night parties. Lysergic acid diethylamide (LSD, acid) continues to be a popular hallucinogen.

STATISTICS

In 2000, an estimated 14.0 million persons in the United States (6.3 percent of the population over 12 years of age) used an illicit drug one or more times during the previous month. Of these, approximately 59 percent consumed only marijuana, 17 percent used marijuana and another illicit drug, and the remaining 24 percent used an illicit drug but not marijuana. Pain relievers (3.8 million persons) are the most commonly used illicit drugs, followed by cocaine (1.2 million persons), hallucinogens (1.0 million persons), tranquilizers (1.0 million persons), stimulants (0.8 million persons), sedatives (200,000 persons), and heroin (130,000 persons). The actual number of individuals who use heroin is difficult to determine because in the past decade there has been a growing tendency to sniff, snort (shabbang), or smoke (chase the dragon) rather than to inject heroin intravenously (shoot up) or subcutaneously (skin pop). In contrast to individuals who inject opiates intravenously, those who inhale opiates less often seek help for their addiction and are not detected by the usual cutaneous stigmata associated with injections. Offsetting the slow decline in use of the many addictive drugs has been a spiraling increase in the use of methamphetamine, especially by young people. More than 7 million persons have tried MDMA (ecstasy) at least once in their lifetime. The popularity of other so-called club drugs, such as benzodiazepin, flunitrazepam (Rohypnol, roofies), and the depressant gamma-hydroxybutyrate (GHB) waxes and wanes. However, GHB, known as the date rape drug, is being used increasingly by bodybuilders, who believe that it helps to metabolize fat and build muscle. In 2000, approximately 3.6 percent of male and 0.9 percent of female twelfth graders in the United States had used anabolic steroids. Although the number of adult users has not been determined, it is estimated to be in the hundreds of thousands.

PATHOGENESIS

Studies in concordant twins have shown a strong influence of genetic inheritance on the susceptibility to drug abuse.[3] The processes by which genes regulate physical reactions to addictive drugs have not been elucidated. Repeated exposure to cocaine causes a change at the level of gene expression that leads to altered levels of a specific brain protein called *cyclin-dependent kinase-5*. This protein regulates the action of dopamine, which potentiates the euphoric effects of cocaine and other drugs.[4] In mice, the absence of a gene for one of the receptors of serotonin predisposes to the use of cocaine.[5] However, environmental factors are clearly important.

The mechanisms leading to tolerance and dependence are complex, but drugs appear to cause these effects at least partly by stimulating the release of dopamine through activation of the mesolimbic system, especially the nucleus accumbens, augmenting the hedonic tone. Drugs also inhibit or excite neuronal activity in various areas of the nervous system. To compensate for these alterations, neuroadaptation develops with either formation of new neuroreceptor sites (upregulation) or diminished synthesis and sensitivity of neurotransmitters and neuroreceptor sites. Discontinuation of the drug reverses the neuroadaptation process and results in an exaggerated neural response that produces withdrawal symptoms.

CLINICAL MANIFESTATIONS

Fibrotic Changes and Ulcerations

The most specific sign of drug abuse by injection is the presence of *skin tracks* (Fig. 141-1). Initially, punctures, ecchymoses, and crusted lesions trail along the length of the vein (Fig. 141-2). With repeated injections of irritating drugs and adulterants, the veins become inflamed and scarred.[6] Due to their easy access, the veins of the arms and hands are injected initially by most novice addicts. However, to avoid the presence of incriminating tracks, some addicts prefer injections on the legs and feet. When these areas become scarred, drugs are injected into the vessels of the neck, abdomen, axillae, groin, sublingual area, genitals, hemorrhoids, or any visible or palpable vein or artery. When intact veins cannot be found, the skin may be cut superficially with razor blades or knifes and powdered drugs rubbed into the lacerations. Some young addicts actually prefer this technique. Subcutaneous and intradermal injections cause irregular, round, leukodermic, atrophic depressions known as *skin popping scars* (Fig. 141-3). In some cases, indurated, linear, hypertrophic, or keloidal scars form.

Intradermal injections or accidental extravasation of certain drugs and adulterants can cause tissue injury. Heroin and other powder drugs are frequently "cut" with fillers such as lactose, mannitol, dextrose, baking soda, and flour.[7] Injection of sclerosing adulterants and drugs can produce tender and inflammatory plaques or nodules that ulcerate and heal with epidermal pigmentary changes, woody induration of the dermis and subcutaneous tissue, and retracted cicatrices. Quinine, which is popular because of its bitter taste similar to heroin and its enhancement of the narcotic euphoria, is destructive to lymphatics, and repeated injections can lead to chronic, nonpitting hand or limb edema.[6] Drugs also can cause severe tissue damage. Injected propoxyphene produces thrombophlebitis and skin necrosis.[8,9] Cocaine is a vasoconstrictor and can produce tissue ischemia, especially when extravasated. It does not regularly form tracks, but cutaneous fibrotic scars on the extremities resulting from intracutaneous injection have been reported.[10] Even inhalation of cocaine can cause skin and muscle infarction.[11] Extensive necrosis of the nose and upper lip accompanied by a necrotizing infection of the subcutaneous soft tissue of the cheeks, forehead, and temporal regions has been caused by forced intranasal impaction of crack

FIGURE 141-1

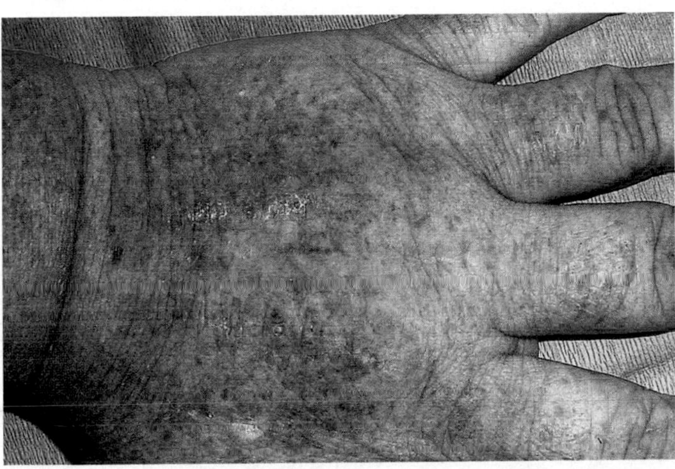

Skin tracks along the veins of the dorsal hand.

FIGURE 141-2

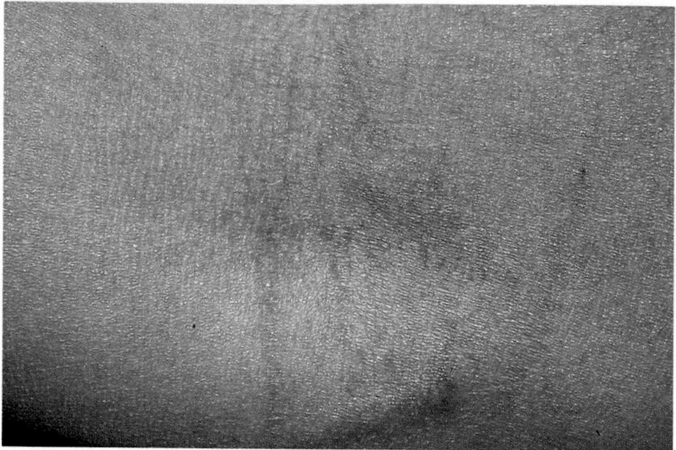

Purpuric puncture marks on several veins, suggesting intravenous drug use.

cocaine.[12] Injection into soft tissue of barbiturates, which are highly alkaline, results in tender, erythematous, indurated plaques that break down into deep ulcers and frequently become infected. Trepalonamine (pyribenzamine), an antihistamine usually injected in combination with pentazocine or another opioid, also induces tissue necrosis and ulceration. Pentazocine injection alone can cause brawny, fibrotic skin and large, irregularly shaped, deeply penetrating ulcers that may extend to muscle.[13]

Granulomas

Pulmonary foreign body granulomas have been found in 30 percent of addicts on whom autopsies have been performed. Although cutaneous granulomas are not common, they can develop months and up to 50 years after the last intravenous or subcutaneous injection because granuloma formation requires conversion of silica to its colloidal form.[14] Most granulomas are caused by the injection of hydrous magnesium silicate (talc) and, less often, starch into the subcutaneous tissue, deep dermis, and walls of veins. The lesions are firm, movable cutaneous nodules (Fig. 141-4). Talc granulomas also may develop in the liver, lymph nodes, spleen, and bone marrow. In addition to being a popular adulterant for powder drugs, talc is the main ingredient in some narcotic tablets that are crushed, diluted in liquid, and injected.[14]

FIGURE 141-3

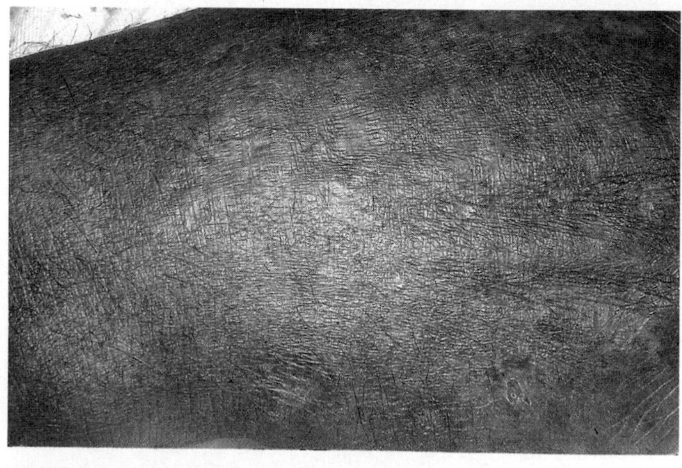

Depressed, circular scars ("pop scars") due to subcutaneous heroin injection.

FIGURE 141-4

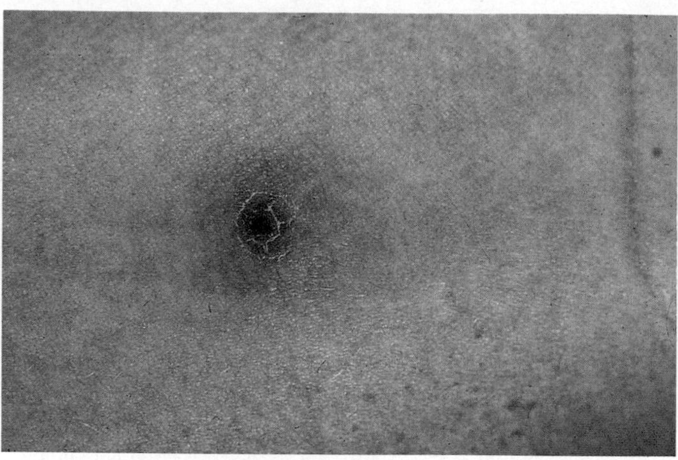

Foreign body granuloma from subcutaneous injection of adulterated heroin.

Burns

Burns from lit matches, cigarettes, paraphernalia, and contact with fire during cooking are common during the altered state of consciousness produced by drug intoxication. Cigarette burns, most commonly on the digits and sternum, occur from lit cigarettes that addicts were smoking before falling asleep. The *necklace sign* is produced by cigarette ashes that fall on the neck when the smoking addict dozes off.[6] Singeing of the eyelashes and eyebrows, resulting in madorosis, may be caused by rising hot vapors during smoking of crack cocaine. Individuals who use crack also may develop linear, circular, or oval blackened, hyperkeratotic lesions caused by the heat of the glass pipe.[15] The areas affected are the thenar eminences of the thumbs (*crack thumbs*) and the palm (*crack hands*) of the dominant hand. More severe thermal burns may be incurred on the hands while lighting a crack-cocaine pipe with a butane lighter directed downward onto the pipe.

Solvent inhalation has been gaining in popularity among adolescents. Minor, superficial burns have been reported as a result of flash fires caused by the ignition of lighter fluid composed of butane and isobutane in enclosed spaces while the fumes were being inhaled. Patients recovered with conservative medical care. However, extensive explosion burns can occur involving the face, neck, arms, and hands, as well as the trunk and/or lower extremities.[16] Severe burns also occur when other solvents, such as paint thinner or petrol, become ignited by a cigarette that the sniffer is simultaneously smoking.

Pigmentary Changes

Postinflammatory pigmentary changes are more common in persons with darkly pigmented skin. Circumferential pigmented bands due to pressure from tourniquets are common in dark-skin intravenous drug users. *Soot tattoos* are black macules produced by inadvertent injection of residual carbon that remains on the needle after flaming. Persons who abuse methamphetamine develop grayish, dry, leathery skin with a strange odor.

Vascular Lesions

The most common vascular lesions in addicts are ecchymosis and hematomas from extravasated blood along injected vessels. Petechiae may form distal to tourniquets. Addicts who inject drugs intraarterially are at risk of developing vascular compromise of the hands with discoloration, edema, and cold temperature. Arterial constriction or emboli can lead to gangrene and loss of digits or a limb.[17] Repeated vascular injury and infection of the digits may cause irreversible contractures (camptodactylia) that resemble Dupuytren's disease. It is important to evaluate any patient with contractures, inflammation, or edema of the hand for soft tissue infection, as well as for underlying musculoskeletal complications, such as fibrous myopathy, joint restriction, muscle contractures, inflexible ankylosis, and suppurative tenosynovitis. Distal thrombosis with extensive infarctive skin lesions and associated hepatitis and glomerulonephritis may follow intravenous injection of cocaine into an arm vein.[18] Painful discoloration with resulting ulceration of the palm also can result from injection of cocaine into the radial artery.

Necrotizing vasculitis from injected drugs usually develops on the neck or extremity as a warm, firm, tender mass that may be misdiagnosed as an abscess. Cocaine may produce superficial or deep venous thrombosis, which is treated with parenterally administered antibiotics, bed rest, elevation of the involved extremity, and anticoagulation, once a mycotic aneurysm, which can bleed, has been excluded.[8,19] Mycotic aneurysms occur in 15 to 25 percent of patients with infective endocarditis, most frequently in the femoral artery, and require immediate surgery. Pseudoaneurysms result from infected injury to arteries during intraarterial injection of drugs ("hitting the pinkie") and are most common in the extremities and groin. The typical lesion is a tender, diffusely indurated, pulsatile mass with an associated bruit (50 to 60 percent of cases) and decreased peripheral pulses (25 percent). Local suppuration, petechiae, and purpura are often present. Half resolve with antibiotics alone, but expanding lesions require proximal ligation of the vessel, resection of the pseudoaneurysm, and appropriate drainage.

An erythematous, tender cord is the hallmark sign of superficial septic thrombophlebitis. However, patients with deep vein thrombophlebitis present with a tender, swollen extremity, with or without erythema, that resembles cellulitis or an abscess. Indeed, infection may be simultaneously present, further complicating the diagnosis.

Cases of Henoch-Schonlein purpura, polyareritis nodosa, and necrotizing angiitis with renal and pulmonary disease have been reported.

Vesiculobullous Lesions

Traumatic vesicles or bullae at the site of injection are observed occasionally. Comatose patients who have overdosed with barbiturates or other sedative drugs often develop pressure erythema, bullae, and ulcers.[7] Unlike bedridden patients, who typically develop pressure-induced lesions on the sacral or ischial areas, elbows or heels, addicts may present with bullae in unusual body areas and configurations, depending on the body position in which they lost consciousness.

Acne

Anabolic steroid abuse can cause acne, cysts, oily hair and skin, male and female pattern alopecia, increased hair growth in women, gynecomastia in men, coarse skin, edema, testicular atrophy, and clitoral enlargement. There have been reports in habitual users of MDMA (ecstasy) of a papulopustular, facial, acneiform eruption that may indicate a higher risk of systemic adverse effects, such as hepatic damage. In some cases, the eruption responded to topical metronidazole.[20] Acne and other skin eruptions are anecdotally worsened by cannabis.

Pruritus

Chronic cocaine use coupled with marijuana inhalation may cause pruritus. Prolonged use of cocaine may lead to the development of formication, tactile hallucinations during which the individual senses that insects are crawling on or under the skin (*coke bugs*). Foraging behavior, involving compulsive searching for pieces of crack cocaine in locations where it was once used, has been reported by some long-term users. Repetitive, stereotypical skin picking leading to excoriations and skin ulcers on the face and extremities has been observed in individuals who abuse methamphetamine. The feeling of euphoria provided by heroin may be accompanied by skin flushing and itching, as well as dry mouth, watery eyes, and runny nose. Heroin addicts often have dry skin that becomes easily irritated and pruritic.

Generalized or focal, especially genital, itching after drug administration has been named *"high" pruritus*. Hypoesthesia is a manifestation of low-dose exposure to phencyclidine (PCP).

Mucous Membrane Lesions

The abuse of drugs via an intranasal route is an increasingly prevalent pattern of behavior. Snorting cocaine causes erythema and erosion of the nasal turbinates, nasopharynx, and soft palate. With continued use, the erosions progress to necrosis, atrophy, and eventual perforation of the nasal septum and even the palate[21] (Fig. 141-5). The pathogenesis is vasoconstriction with resulting ischemia and occasionally infection. Chronic rhinitis, epistaxis, osteolytic sinusitis, gingival retraction, and bruxism are other complications. Halitosis and frequent lip smacking are signs of cocaine abuse. Cuts from chipped glass pipes and thermal burns may be present on the lips of some crack users. Sniffing heroin less often causes these changes. However, invasive fungal rhinosinusitis appears to be a complication unique to intranasal narcotic abuse.[21] A case of pemphigus vegetans, Neumann type, restricted to the intranasal tissue was reported to have been induced by inhalation of heroin. The patient responded to systemic glucocorticoids.[22]

Xerotic cheilitis is observed commonly in methamphetamine and heroin addicts.[7] Methamphetamine users also have red, dry noses. Transient eyelid edema has been described with opiate abuse. The typical red or "bloodshot" eye frequently occurs with marijuana and sometimes with cocaine or PCP use. Scleral hemorrhages in drug addicts are usually traumatic but may be caused by septic emboli due to endocarditis. There are reports of men applying cocaine powder to their glans penis to postpone ejaculation and of women rubbing cocaine on their genitals to enhance pleasure. These practices can lead to priapism, irritant dermatitis, and even ulcerations. Priapism can follow crack inhalation.[23] Penile ulcers have developed after injection of heroin into the shaft veins.

Marked dental decay and gingival disease are common in hard core users of opiates as a result of the effects of opiates and poor hygiene.

FIGURE 141-5

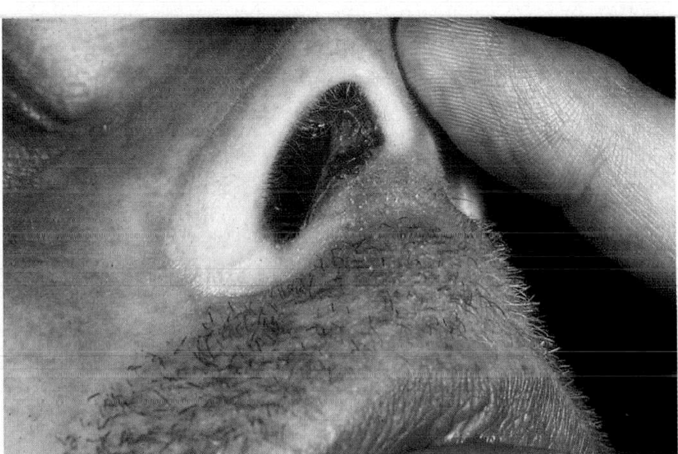

Cocaine-induced granuloma of the nasal septum.

Hallucinogen-induced xerostomia also predisposes to caries. Persons addicted to methamphetamine, especially snorters, have higher tooth wear caused by teeth clenching. Habitual chewing of betel palm seeds, which contain a narcotic stimulant—a practice in some areas of Southeast Asia—stains the teeth. A noted habit of children born to mothers who smoked marijuana during pregnancy is thumb sucking.

Pilosebaceous Effects

Hyperhidrosis is a common adverse effect of amphetamines.[20] Piloerection, paresthesias, and percutaneous flushings are manifestations of the somatic but not the perceptual phase of LSD intoxication. Together with constricted pupils and runny nose, gooseflesh skin is a sign of opiate intoxication.

BACTERIAL INFECTION

Skin and soft tissue infections are the most common disorders for which drug addicts seek health care or are hospitalized.[24–26] In a study of 127 hospitalized intravenous drug users, the diagnoses were cellulitis (40.9 percent), abscess with cellulitis (32.3 percent), abscess alone (16.5 percent), infected skin ulcers (10.2 percent), necrotizing fasciitis (7.1 percent), and septic phlebitis with cellulitis (5.5 percent).[27] Cellulitis usually presents as one or more red, tender, warm, edematous, indurated plaques. However, only tenderness and edema may be apparent initially, and erythema may be difficult to assess in dark-skinned patients. Lymphangitis may accompany skin infection. In any addict with soft tissue infection, the possible presence of osteomyelitis or pyogenic arthritis should be considered. Since upper extremity vessels are used preferentially, cellulitis of the hand, arm, and forearm is very common and should be treated aggressively. In a 5-year review of 103 patients with upper extremity infection who required admission, 92 percent had cellulitis, which in one-third was associated with ulceration at the site of injection. Seven percent presented with gangrene.[17] The inclusion of vancomycin (for methacillin-resistant *Staphylococcus aureus*) and clindamycin (for anaerobes) in the antibiotic regimen has been recommended for hand infections[17] and, arguably, should be considered in any limb or life-threatening infection. About 10 percent of hand infections may require amputation of digits or of the hand, even after appropriate antibiotic and surgical treatment.[17]

In parenteral drug users, *S. aureus* is the most frequently cultured bacteria from soft issue infections, followed by streptococcal species.[27,28] An attempt to obtain a culture is prudent because skin infection by gram-negative bacteria, anaerobes, and unusual organisms is also common.[17] Notably, the flora spectrum of street heroin has no relationship to the bacteria causing infections in intravenous drug users.[17] However, tripelennamine and pentazocine may allow for the selective survival of *Pseudomonas aeruginosa*. The use of quinine to adulterate heroin appears to predispose to *Clostridium* infection. Wound botulism due to *Clostridium botulinum* type A occurs almost exclusively in drug addicts.[29] Several cases have been reported from California and other western states during the past decade.[30] It is associated with parenteral injection, especially skin popping of black tar heroin, a form that derives its color from impurities during its manufacture and from adulterants. This form of heroin is highly hygroscopic and has a high water content that supports the growth of organisms. The spores of *C. botulinum* are not destroyed by heating the contaminated heroin and are inoculated into the subcutaneous tissue, where they germinate and produce toxin. There is pain, tenderness, and swelling, but in the early stages a cellulitis or abscess may not be prominent. In cocaine snorters, the intranasal septum or paranasal sinuses may become infected.[31] Necrotizing cellulitis of the scrotum and penis has been reported in addicts who accidentally injected drugs into the femoral artery instead of the vein.[32]

Due to the popularity of skin popping, the incidence of abscesses has been increasing. Abscesses from such subcutaneous drug injection are often multilobulated and deep and have extensive necrosis that requires exploration and debridement. Superficial abscesses may rupture spontaneously, leaving punched-out ulcers. Abscesses may develop in any skin area of the body in which the addict injected drugs. In more than half of the abscesses, only one pathogen is cultured, but in 33 to 45 percent of abscesses, more than one organism is present.[27] Fever and leukocytosis are not absolutely reliable measures of severity and are absent in about half of cases. Any bacteria may be recovered from an abscess, but the more commonly cultured ones are *S. aureus* (20 to 60 percent), *Streptococcus* species (25 percent), and gram-negative rods (up to 25 percent). Anaerobic bacteria are also common, especially in polymicrobial infections. In one study, anaerobic bacteria were recovered from two-thirds of abscesses, and in one-third of these, they were the only cultured organism.[33] *Eikinella corrodens,* an oral flora bacterium, is cultured from some abscesses caused by injections of methylphenidate. Curiously, some abscesses develop months after a patient has ceased to use drugs.

Abscesses may be contiguous with bone when osteomyelitis of the long bones is present. Cervical abscesses usually occur in the anterior cervical triangle and may cause life-threatening complications such as mediastinitis, pneumomediastinum, airway obstruction, internal jugular vein thrombosis, and extension into the carotid sheath. Abscesses in the groin may present with only tenderness and edema. These abscesses can be deep and extensive, especially if they originate in the femoral triangle. The degree of pain usually exceeds that suspected from clinical findings. Computed tomographic (CT) scanning is needed to determine the extent of involvement of deep abscesses and abscesses in regions such as the neck and groin.

Necrotizing fasciitis with or without myositis often presents with lesions characterized by erythema (77 percent), fluctuance (20 percent), edema (20 percent), or induration (43 percent) that clinically resemble an abscess[34] but which require extensive subfascial debridement. In some cases, only swelling or inconspicuous cellulitis is apparent. However, severe pain, disproportionate to the clinical signs, is present in 94 percent of cases.[35] If the clinician disregards the patient's complaint merely as a request for narcotics, the outcome may be devastating. Fever and leukocytosis are common, but at the time of presentation, the classic cutaneous findings of bullae, tissue crepitance, and skin necrosis are only present in 3, 3, and 10 percent of cases, respectively.[34] For this reason, surgical exploration is mandatory in any addict with cellulitis and unexplainable severe pain. Multiple organisms are cultured in 59 to 85 percent of cases. The presence of gas is not pathognmonic for *Clostridium* infection. In most cases, the infection is polymicrobial, and multiple organisms are recovered. Anaerobes are present in 12 percent of cases. The infection will progress in 75 percent of patients treated with parenteral antibiotics without debridement.[36] A decrease in the mortality rate from 27 to 7 percent was reported with a protocol consisting of early diagnosis, intravenous wide-coverage antimicrobial therapy, supportive care, early subfascial debridement, and repeated wound debridement every 8 to 12 h until no necrotic tissue is formed. Between two and four debridements are needed.[34]

Sporadic cases of toxic shock syndrome related to intravenous heroin abuse have been reported. Nephrotic syndrome from amyloidosis has been reported in skin poppers and intravenous drug users with chronically draining skin lesions.[37]

Bacterial endocarditis is the most common systemic bacterial infection in intravenous drug users and accounts for 5 to 8 percent of hospitalizations. Although in some reports a third of hospitalized addicts with skin and soft tissue infection have positive blood cultures, bacteremia from skin infection is not common.[8] Several cutaneous signs (arterial emboli, conjunctival hemorrhages, splinter hemorrhages, Janeway lesions, Osler nodes) may be present.

FUNGAL INFECTION

Even in the absence of HIV infection, the incidence of dermatophytosis, including onychomycosis, tinea pedis, tinea cruris, and tinea corporis, is higher among intravenous drug addicts.[38] Injections of brown heroin have caused disseminated candidiasis due to yeast overgrowth in the lemon juice used to dissolve the heroin. The initial symptoms are high fever, rigors, headaches, myalgia, and occasionally jaundice, but at this stage, blood and urine cultures rarely grow organisms. After approximately 7 days, 88 percent of the patients develop pustular folliculitis and painful nodules on the scalp and other hairy areas. The folliculitis is often misdiagnosed as bacterial, but potassium hydroxide examination and biopsy demonstrates the presence of yeasts. Other complications include ocular disease (uveitis, endophthalmitis), monarthritis, osteochondritis, and pleuritis.[39] Unlike HIV infection, intravenous drug use is a predisposing factor to zygomycosis. The charcteristic cutaneous lesion is a cellulitic plaque or abscess that becomes necrotic.

DRUG-INDUCED REACTIONS

As expected, hypersensitivity reactions to drugs, especially exanthematous eruptions, urticaria, fixed drug reactions, leukocytoclastic vasculitis, erythema multiforme, and toxic epidermal necrolysis, occur more frequently in users of illicit drugs than in the general population. Dermatographism was found in 26 percent of patients comatose from heroin overdose.[40] Pigmented patches on the skin and mucous membranes may be extensive in addicts with fixed drug eruptions.

Narcotic abuse is a common cause of falsely reactive nontreponemal tests for syphilis (VDRL, RPR). In these cases, treponemal tests (MHATP, FTA-ABS) will be nonreactive. However, in addicts who have had syphilis, not only will both tests be positive but the titers of the treponemal test also may not decrease after treatment.

ASSOCIATED NONINFECTIOUS SKIN DISEASES

Seborrheic dermatitis may be more frequent in chronic cocaine users. Eczemas, especially contact dermatitis, have been reported to occur more frequently. Drug abuse may indirectly cause skin lesions through congenital malformations in the offspring, domestic violence, or systemic disease. Pseudoacanthosis nigricans has been observed in heroin addicts.

REFERENCES

1. Garfein RS et al: Viral infections in short-term injection drug users: The prevalence of the hepatitis C, hepatitis B, human immunodeficiency, and human T-lymphotropic viruses. *Am J Public Health* **86**:655, 1996
2. American Psychiatric Association: *Diagnostic and Statistical Manual of Mental Disorders IV-TR,* 4th ed. Washington, DC, American Psychiatric Press, 2000
3. Tsuang MT et al: The Harvard twin study of substance abuse: What we have learned. *Harvard Rev Psych* **9**:267, 2001
4. Bibb JA et al: Effects of chronic exposure to cocaine are regulated by the neuronal protein Cdk5. *Nature* **410**:376, 2001
5. Castanon N et al: Modulation of the effects of cocaine by 5-HT1B receptors: A comparison of knockouts and antagonists. *Pharmacol Biochem Behav* **67**:559, 2000
6. Young AW: Cutaneous stigmas of heroin addiction. *Arch Dermatol* **104**:80, 1971
7. Burnett JW: Drug abuse. *Cutis* **49**:307, 1992
8. Levine DP: Skin and soft tissue infections in intravenous drug abusers, in *Infections in Intravenous Drug Abusers,* edited by DP Levine, JD Sobel. New York, Oxford University Press, 1991, p 183
9. Tennant FS: Complications of propoxyphene abuse. *Arch Intern Med* **132**:191, 1973
10. Kircik LH et al: Scars on the legs: Cutaneous fibrosis resulting from intracutaneous injection of cocaine. *Arch Dermatol* **128**:1644, 1992
11. Zamora-Quezada JC et al: Muscle and skin infarction after free-basing cocaine (crack). *Ann Intern Med* **108**:564, 1988
12. Tierney BP, Stadelmann WK: Necrotizing infection of the face secondary to intranasal impaction of "crack" cocaine. *Ann Plast Surg* **43**:640, 1999
13. Furner BB: Parenteral pentazocine: Cutaneous complications. *J Am Acad Dermnatol* **22**:694, 1990
14. Posner DI, Guill A: Cutaneous foreign body granulomas associated with intravenous drug abuse. *J Am Acad Dermatol* **13**:869, 1985
15. Feeney CM, Briggs S: Crack hands: A dermatologic effect of smoking crack cocaine. *Cutis* **50**:193, 1992
16. Ho WS et al: Burn injuries during paint thinner sniffing. *Burns* **24**:757, 1998
17. Smith DJ et al: Drug injection injuries of the upper extremity. *Ann Plast Surg* **22**:19, 1989
18. Heng M, Haberfeld G: Thrombotic phenomena associated with intravenous cocaine. *J Am Acad Dermatol* **16**:462, 1987
19. Lisse JR et al: Cocaine abuse and deep venous thrombosis. *Ann Intern Med* **110**:571, 1989
20. Wollina U et al: Ecstasy pimples: A new facial dermatosis. *Dermatology* **197**:171, 1998
21. Yewell J et al: Complications of intranasal prescription narcotic abuse. *Ann Otol Rhinol Laryngol* **111**:174, 2002
22. Downie JB et al: Pemphigus vegetans, Neumann variant associated with intranasal heroin abuse. *J Am Acad Dermatol* **39**:872, 1998
23. Altman AL et al: Cocaine associated priapism. *J Urol* **161**:817, 1999
24. Organ CH: Surgical procedures upon the drug addict. *Surg Gynecol Obstet* **134**:947, 1972
25. Orangio GR et al: Soft tissue infections in parenteral drug abusers. *Ann Surg* **199**:97, 1984
26. White AG: Medical disorders in drug addicts: 200 consecutive admissions. *JAMA* **223**:1469, 1973
27. Hasan SB et al: Infectious complications in IV drug abusers. *Infect Surg* **7**:218, 1988
28. Tuazon CU, Sheagren JN: Staphylococcal endocarditis in parenteral drug abusers: Source of the organism. *Ann Intern Med* **82**:788, 1975
29. MacDonald KL et al: The changing epidemiology of adult botulism in the United States. *Am J Epidemiol* **124**:794, 1986;
30. CDC: Wound botulism—California, 1995. *Morbid Mortal Weekly Rep* **44**:889, 1995
31. Kudrow DB et al: Botulism associated with *Clostridium botulinum* sinusitis after intranasal cocaine abuse. *Ann Intern Med* **109**:984, 1988
32. Alguire PC: Necrotizing cellulitis of the scrotum: A new complication of heroin addiction. *Cutis* **34**:93, 1984
33. Webb D, Thadepalli H: Skin and soft tissue polymicrobial infections from intravenous abuse of drugs. *West J Med* **130**:200, 1979
34. Callahan TE et al: Necrotiizng soft tissue infection masquerading as cutaneous abscess following illicit drug injection *Arch Surg* **133**:813, 1998
35. Sudarsky LA et al: Improved results from a standardized approach in treating patients with necrotizing fasciitis. *Ann Surg* **206**:661, 1987
36. Clark DD: Surgical management of infections and other complications resulting from drug abuse. *Arch Surg* **101**:619, 1970
37. Neugarten J et al: Amyloidosis in subcutaneous heroin abusers ("skin poppers' amyloidosis"). *Am J Med* **81**:635, 1986
38. Gaeta GB et al: Mucocutaneous diseases in drug addicts with or without HIV infection: A case-controlled study. *Infection* **22**:77, 1994
39. Dupont B, Drouhet E: Cutaneous, ocular, and osteoarticular candidiasis in heroin addicts: New clinical and therapeutic aspects in 38 patients. *J Infect Dis* **152**:577, 1985
40. Cotliar RW et al: Dermatographism, erythema and flare: Clinical signs of drug overdose in the comatose patient. *South Med J* **66**:1277, 1973

INDEX

NOTE: Bold number indicates the start of the chapter that contains the main discussion of the topic; numbers followed with "f" and "t" refer to figure and table pages.

Set 0-07-138076-0

FREEDBERG / DIGM6 (SET)

ISBN 0-07-138066-3

FREEDBERG / DIGM6 (VOL. I)

ISBN 0-07-138067-1

FREEDBERG / DIGM6 (VOL. II)